Bailey & Love's
SHORT PRACTICE of SURGERY

26th EDITION

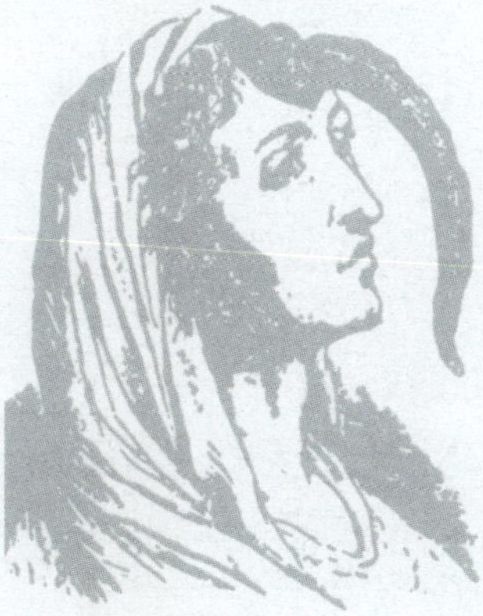

Sebaceous horn
(The owner, the widow Dimanche, sold water-cress in Paris)

A favourite illustration of Hamilton Bailey and McNeill Love, and well known to readers of earlier editions of Short Practice.

Bailey & Love's
SHORT PRACTICE of SURGERY

26th EDITION

Edited by

NORMAN S. WILLIAMS MS FRCS FMed Sci
Professor of Surgery and Director of Surgical Innovation,
Barts and the London School of Medicine and Dentistry,
Queen Mary, University of London and President,
The Royal College of Surgeons of England, London, UK

CHRISTOPHER J.K. BULSTRODE MCh FRCS(T&O)
Emeritus Professor, University of Oxford, Oxford, UK

P. RONAN O'CONNELL, MD FRCSI, FRCPS Glas.,
Head, Surgery and Surgical Specialties,
UCD School of Medicine and Medical Sciences
Consultant Surgeon, St Vincent's University Hospital,
Dublin, Ireland

CRC Press
Taylor & Francis Group
Boca Raton London New York

CRC Press is an imprint of the
Taylor & Francis Group, an **informa** business

First published in Great Britain in 1932
25th edition published in 2008
This 26th edition published in 2013 by
CRC Press
Taylor & Francis Group
6000 Broken Sound Parkway NW, Suite 300
Boca Raton, FL 33487-2742

CRC Press is an imprint of Taylor & Francis Group, an Informa business
No claim to original U.S. Government works
Typeset in 9.5/11 pt Goudy by Phoenix Photosetting, Chatham, Kent
Printed and bound in India by Replika Press Pvt. Ltd.
Version Date: 20120813
International Standard Book Number: 978-1-4441-2127-8
ISBN-13 [ISE] 978-1-4441-2128-5 (International Students' Edition, restricted territorial availability)
1 2 3 4 5 6 7 8 9 10

Contents

Contributors

Derek Alderson MD FRCS
Barling Chair of Surgery and Head of Department, Queen Elizabeth Hospital, Edgbaston, Birmingham, UK

Gina Allen BM DCH MRCGP MRCP FRCR
Oxford Soft Tissue Injury Clinic (Ostic), St Luke's Hospital, Oxford, UK

Jonathan R Anderson MD
Department of Cardiothoracic Surgery, Imperial College Healthcare NHS Trust, Hammersmith Hospital, London, UK

Andrew Barnett FRCS(Orth)
Consultant Orthopaedic Surgeon, Robert Jones and Agnes Hunt Orthopaedic Hospital, Gobowen, Shropshire, UK

Grant Bates BSc BM Bch FRCS (deceased)
Ear, Nose and Throat Surgeon, John Radcliffe Hospital, Oxford and Lecturer, University of Oxford, Oxford, UK

Philip Bejon MD
Bone Infection Unit, Nuffield Orthopaedic Centre, Oxford, UK

Tony Belli MD FRCS(SN)
Reader in Trauma, Neurosurgery, University of Birmingham, Birmingham, UK

Satyajit Bhattacharya MS MPhil FRCS
Consultant Hepato-Pancreato-Biliary Surgeon, The Royal London Hospital, London, UK

Martin Birchall M(Cantab) FRCS FRCS(Oto) FRCS(ORL)
Professor of Laryngology, University College London, Consultant in Otolaryngology, Head and Neck Surgery, The Royal National Throat, Nose and Ear Hospital, UCLH NHS Trust, London, UK

Ken Boffard BSC(Hons) MB BCh FRCS FRCS(Ed) FRCPS(Glas) FACS FCS(SA)
Professor and Head, Department of Surgery, Johannesburg Hospital, University of the Witwatersrand, Johannesburg, South Africa

Gavin Bowden MB BCh FCS(SA)(Orth)
Consultant Spinal Surgeon, St Lukes Hospital, Oxford, UK

J Andrew Bradley MB ChB PhD FRCS Ac Med Sci
Professor of Surgery, University of Cambridge, and Consultant Surgeon, Addenbrooke's Hospital, Cambridge, UK

Karim Brohi FRCS FRCA
Professor of Trauma Sciences, Barts and the London School of Medicine and Dentistry, Queen Mary University of London, London, UK

Harry Bulstrode MA Cantab BMBCh MRCS(Eng)
Academic Clinical Fellow in Neurosurgery, Division of Neurosciences, Southampton General Hospital, Southampton, UK

Gordon Carlson BSc MD FRCS
Consultant Surgeon, Honorary Professor of Surgery, University of Manchester; Honorary Professor of Biomedical Science, University of Salford, Salford, UK

Christopher Chan BSC PhD FRCS FRCS(Gen Surg)
Consultant Colorectal Surgeon, Academic Surgical Unit, Barts Health NHS Trust, London, UK

Ian Chetter MB ChB FRCSMD FRCS(Gen Surg) PG Cert Medical Ultrasound PG Dip Clinical Education
Professor of Surgery, Hull York Medical School, University of Hull; Honorary Consultant Vascular Surgeon, Hull and East Yorkshire NHS Trust, Academic Vascular Surgical Unit, Old Doctors Residence, Hull Royal Infirmary, Hull, UK

Sue Clark MD FRCS(Gen Surg)
Consultant Colorectal Surgeon, St Mark's Hospital, Harrow, UK

Kevin C Conlon MA MCh MBA FRCSI FACS FRCPS(Glas) FTCD
Professor of Surgery, Trinity College Dublin; Consultant Surgeon, St. Vincent's University Hospital and The Adelaide and Meath Hospital, Dublin, Ireland

Paul Cool MD MedSc(Res) FRCS(Ed) FRCS(Orth)
Consultant Orthopaedic and Oncological Surgeon, Robert Jones and Agnes Hunt Orthopaedic Hospital, Gobowen, Shropshire, UK

Ara Darzi PC KBE HonFrEng FmedSci
Professor the Lord Darzi of Denham, Professor of Surgery, Imperial College London, St Mary's Hospital Campus, London, UK

Pradip K Datta MBE MS FRCS(Ed) FRCS FRCSI FRCPS(Glas)
Honorary Consultant Surgeon, Caithness General Hospital, Wick, Caithness, UK

Brian R Davidson MD FRCS
Consultant Surgeon, Royal Free Hospital and Professor of Surgery, Hampstead Campus, University College London, London, UK

Sanjay De Bakshi MB BS MS FRCS FRCS(Ed)
Consultant Surgeon, Unit of Surgical Gastroenterology, Calcutta Medical Research Institute, Kolkata, India

Ian Eardley MA MChir FRCS (Urol) FEBU
Consultant Urologist, Department of Urology, St James University Hospital, Leeds, UK

Michael Earley MB MCh FRCSI FRCS(Plast)
Consultant Plastic Surgeon and Associate Clinical Professor, The Children's University Hospital, Temple Street and Mater Misericordiae University Hospital, Dublin, Ireland

Jonothan Earnshaw DM FRCS
Consultant Vascular Surgeon, Gloucestershire Royal Hospital, Gloucester, UK

Deborah Eastwood FRCS
The Catterall Unit, Royal National Orthopaedic Hospital, Stanmore, Middlesex, UK

Hilary Edgcombe BA BM BCh(Oxon) FRCA(Lon)
Consultant Anaesthetist, Oxford University Hospitals, Oxford, UK

Jonathan Epstein MA MD FRCS
Specialist Registrar in General Surgery, Hope Hospital, Salford, UK

Roger Feakins MB BCh BAO BA MD FRCPI FRCPath
Consultant Histopathologist and NHS Professor of Gastrointestinal Pathology, Department of Histopathology, Barts Health NHS Trust, London, UK

Kenneth Fearon MD FRCPS(Glas) FRCS(Ed) FRCS
Professor of Surgical Oncology and Honorary Consultant Colorectal Surgeon, Clinical Surgery, School of Clinical Science, University of Edinburgh, Royal Infirmary, Edinburgh, UK

Pierre Foex DPhil FRCA FMedSci
Nuffield Division of Anaesthetics, John Radcliffe Hospital, Headley Way, Oxford, UK

Christopher G Fowler BSc MB BS MA MS FRCP FRCS(Urol) FEBU FHEA
Professor, Department of Urology, The Royal London Hospital, London, UK

O James Garden BSc MB ChB FRCPS(Glas) FRCS(Ed) FRCP(Ed) FRCSCan FRACS(Hon)
Regius Professor of Clinical Surgery, School of Clinical Sciences, University of Edinburgh, Royal Infirmary, Edinburgh, UK

Sudip Ghosh MB BS MS FRCS(Plast)
Consultant Plastic Surgeon, Stoke Mandeville Hospital, Aylesbury, UK

Peter Giannoudis MD FRCS
Professor of Trauma and Orthopaedic Surgery, School of Medicine, University of Leeds, Leeds, UK

Tim Goodacre MD FRCS
Senior Clinical Lecturer and Consultant Plastic Surgeon, Oxford Radcliffe Hospitals, Oxford, UK

William Gray MB MD FRCSI FRCS(SN)
Professor of Functional Neurosurgery, Institute of Psychological Medicine and Clinical Neurosciences, Cardiff University, Cardiff, UK

Adam Greenbaum MB BS MBA PhD FRCS(Plast) FEBOPRAS
Consultant Plastic Surgeon, The Aesthetic Body Centre, Hamilton, New Zealand

Jagannath Haldar MB BS MD FRCA
Consultant Anaesthetist and Clinical Lead, Oxford University Hospitals NHS Trust, Honorary Clinical Lecturer, Oxford Brooke's University, Oxford, UK

Freddie Hamdy MD MA FRCS FRCS(Ed)(Urol) FMedSci
Director, Division of Surgery and Oncology, Oxford Radcliffe Hospitals NHS Trust, John Radcliffe Hospital, Oxford, UK

Bob Handley MB ChB FRCS
John Radcliffe Hospital, Oxford, UK

Jim Hill MB ChB ChM FRCS
Consultant General and Colorectal Surgeon, Manchester Royal Infirmary, Manchester, UK

Shervanthi Homer-Vanniasinkam BSc MD FRCS(Ed) FRCS
Consultant Vascular Surgeon, The General Infirmary at Leeds; Clinical Sub-Dean, University of Leeds Medical School Chair, Translational Vascular Medicine, University of Bradford; Director, Northwick Park Institute for Medical Research, London Honorary Professor, Division of Surgical and Interventional Sciences, University College London, London, UK

Ian Hunt MB BS BSc(Hons) FRCS(C-Th)
Consultant Thoracic Surgeon, Department of Cardiothoracic Surgery, St George's Hospital, London, UK

Ian Jackson MB ChB FRCA
Consultant Anaesthetist, Past President British Association of Day Surgery, York Teaching Hospital NHS Foundation Trust, York, UK

Kath Jenkins BM BS FRCA
Consultant Anaesthetist, North Bristol NHS Trust, Bristol, UK

Kevin D. Johnston MBChB (Hons) BDS BSc MFDSRCS FRCA
Specialist Registrar in Anaesthetics, Nuffield Department of Anaesthetics, John Radcliffe Hospital, Oxford, UK

Sanjeev Kanoria FRCS
HPB and Liver Transplant Unit, University Department of Surgery, Royal Free Hospital, London, UK

Frank Keane MD FRCSI FRCS FRCS(Ed) FRCPS(Glas) FRCPI
Associate Professor of Surgery, Trinity College, and Consultant Colorectal Surgeon, Adelaide and Meath Hospital, Dublin, Ireland

Stephen Kennedy
Professor of Reproductive Medicine and Head of Department, Nuffield Department of Obstetrics and Gynaecology, University of Oxford, Oxford University Hospitals NHS Trust, The Women's Centre, Oxford, UK

Irfan Khan MB BS MRCS
Specialty Doctor, Orthopaedics, Gloucestershire Hospitals NHS Trust, Gloucestershire, UK

Jay Kini MB BS DA MD FFARCSI
Consultant Anaesthetist, Nuffield Department of Anaesthetics, John Radcliffe Hospital, Oxford, UK

Charles H Knowles BChir PhD FRCS
Clinical Professor of Surgical Research and Hononary Consultant Colorectal Surgeon, Centre for Digestive Diseases, Blizard Institute, Barts and the London School of Medicine and Dentistry, Queen Mary University, London, UK

Rahul S Koti MD FRCS
Honorary Lecturer in Surgery, Department of Surgery, University College London; Department of Surgery, Royal Free Hospital, London, UK

Zygmunt H Krukowski PhD FRCS FRCP
Surgeon to the Queen in Scotland; Consultant Surgeon, Aberdeen Royal Infirmary; Professor of Clinical Surgery, University of Aberdeen, Aberdeen, UK

Pawanindra Lal MS DNB FIMSA FRCS(Ed) FRCPS(Glas) FRCS FACS
Professor of Surgery, Maulona Azad Medical College & Associated Lok Nayak Hospital, New Delhi, India

Peter Lamont MB ChB MD FRCS FEBVS
Consultant Vascular Surgeon, Department of Vascular Surgery, Bristol Royal Infirmary, Bristol, UK

Anthony Lander Phd FRCS(Paed) DCH
Consultant Paediatric Surgeon, Birmingham Children's Hospital, Birmingham, UK

Richard Langford MD FRCA FFPMRCA
Professor of Anaesthesia and Pain Medicine and Directory, Pain and Anaesthesia Research Centre, St Bartholomew's and Royal London Hospitals, Barts Health NHS Trust, London UK

Chris Lavy OBE MD MCh FRCS
Honorary Professor and Consultant Orthopaedic Surgeon, Nuffield Department of Orthopaedics, Rheumatology and Musculoskeletal Sciences (NDORMS), University of Nuffield, Nuffield Orthopaedic Centre, Oxford, UK

Tom WJ Lennard MD FRCS
Professor of Surgery, Newcastle University, Newcastle upon Tyne, UK

James Lindsay PhD FRCP
Consultant and Senior Lecturer in Gastroenterology, Digestive Diseases Clinical Academic Unit, Barts and the London School of Medicine and Dentistry, Queen Mary University of London, London, UK

Peter Lunniss BSc MS FRCS
Senior Lecturer, Honorary Consultant Coloproctologist, Royal London Hospital Whitechapel, London, UK

Peter McCollum BA MB BCh BAO MCh FRCSI FRCS(Ed)
Professor of Vascular Surgery, Hull York Medical School; Honorary Consultant Vascular Surgeon, Hull & East Yorkshire Hospitals NHS Trust, Hull Royal Infirmary, Hull, UK

John MacFie MB ChB R Nutr MD FRCS FRCP
Professor of Surgery/Consultant Surgeon, PGMI, University of Hull/Scarborough Hospital, Scarborough, UK

Martin McNally MD FRCS(Ed) FRCS(Orth)
Consultant in Limb Reconstruction Surgery, Bone Infection Unit, Nuffield Orthopaedic Centre; Honorary Senior Lecturer in Orthopaedics

Enda McVeigh
Senior Fellow in Reproductive Medicine, Nuffield Department of Obstetrics and Gynaecology, University of Oxford, Oxford University Hospitals NHS Trust, The Women's Centre, Oxford, UK

Douglas McWhinnie MD(Hons) FRCS
Consultant General and Vascular Surgeon, Past President British Association of Day Surgery, Milton Keynes NHS Foundation Trust, Milton Keynes, UK

Matthew Matson MRCP FRCR
Consultant Radiologist, Royal London Hospital, London, UK

Philippa Matthews MSc MRCP FRCPath DPhil
Academic Clinical Lecturer in Infectious Diseases and Microbiology, Oxford University Hospitals NHS Trust, Oxford, UK

Vivek Mehta MD FRCA FFPMRCA
Consultant in Pain Medicine, Deputy Director, Pain and Anaesthesia Research Centre, St Bartholomew's and Royal London Hospitals, Barts Health NHS Trust, London, UK

Alastair J Munro BSc FRCP(E) FRCR
Professor of Radiation Oncology, University of Dundee, Tayside Cancer Centre, Ninewells Hospital and Medical School, Dundee, UK

Dinesh Nathwani MB ChB MSc FRCSI(Tr & Orth)
Consultant and Honorary Senior Clinical Lecturer, Department of Trauma and Orthopaedic Surgery, Imperial College Healthcare, Academic Health Sciences Centre, London, UK

David E Neal FMedSci MS FRCS
University Department of Oncology, Addenbrooke's Hospital, Cambridge, UK

Stephen J Nixon FRCS(Ed) FRCP(Edin)
Consultant Surgeon, Department of Surgery, Royal Infirmary of Edinburgh, Edinburgh, UK

Iain J Nixon MB ChB FRCS(Ed)(ORL-HNS)
Clinical Fellow, Head and Neck Service, Memorial Sloan Kettering Cancer Center, New York, NY, USA

Karen Nugent MA MS FRCS
Professorial Surgical Unit, Southampton General Hospital, Southampton, UK

Colm O'Brien MD FRCS FRCOphth
Professor of Ophthalmology and Consultant Ophthalmic Surgeon, University College Dublin and Mater Misericordiae University Hospital, Dublin, Ireland

P Ronan O'Connell MD FRCSI FRCPS(Glas)
Professor of Surgery, University College Dublin; Consultant Surgeon, St Vincent's University Hospital, Dublin, Ireland

Hemant G Pandit FRCS(Orth) DPhil (Oxford)
Honorary Senior Clinical Lecturer in Orthopaedics, Nuffield Orthopaedic Centre and Nuffield Department of Orthopaedics, Rheumatology and Musculoskeletal Sciences (NDORMS), Oxford, UK

Charles Perkins FDSRCS FFDRCSI FRCS
Consultant Oral and Maxillofacial Surgeon, Department of Oral and Maxillofacial Surgery, Gloucestershire Royal Hospital, Gloucester, UK

Niall Power
Royal London Hospital, London, UK

Ashley Poynton MD FRCSI FRCS(TrandOrth)
Consultant Spinal Surgeon, National Spinal Injuries Unit, Mater Misericordiae University Hospital, Dublin, Ireland

John N Primrose MB ChB(Hons) FRCS MD
Professor, University Surgical Unit, Southampton General Hospital, Southampton, UK

Sanjay Purkayastha BSc MB BS MD FRCS(Gen Surg)
Locum Consultant, General & Bariatric Surgery, St Mary's Hospital, Paddington, Imperial College Healthcare NHS Trust, London, UK

Mridula Rai MB BS MD FRCA
Consultant Anaesthetist, Nuffield Department of Anaesthetics, Modular Building, John Radcliffe Hospital, Oxford, UK

Mamoon Rashid FRCS FCPS(Pak)
Professor of Plastic and Reconstructive Surgery, Shifa College of Medicine; Consultant Plastic Surgeon and Programme Director, Shifa International Hospital, Islamabad, Pakistan

Robert W Ruckley MB ChB FRCS FRCS(Ed)
Consultant Ear Nose and Throat and Head and Neck Surgeon (retired), Darlington Memorial Hospital, Darlington, UK

David A Russell MB ChB MD FRCS(Gen Surg)
Consultant Vascular Surgeon, Leeds Vascular Institute, Leeds General Infirmary, Leeds, UK

Richard Sainsbury MD FRCS
Consultant Breast Surgeon, Southampton University Hospitals NHS Foundation Trust, Southampton, UK

Anand Sardesai MB BS MD FRCA
Consultant Anaesthetist, Addenbrook's Hospital, Cambridge, UK

Robert Sayers
Professor of Vascular Surgery, Leicester Royal Infirmary, Leicester, UK

Rishi Sharma MRCS DOHNS
Specialist Registrar, Ear Nose and Throat Surgery, Guy's and St Thomas' Hospital, London, UK

Bob Sharp BMBCh MA FRCS FRCS(Tr & Orth)
Consultant Orthopaedic Surgeon, Oxford University Hospitals, The Nuffield Orthopaedic Centre, Oxford, UK

Greg L Shaw MD FRCS(Urol)
Clinical Lecturer in Urology, Cambridge University, Cambridge, UK

Mohan de Silva MS FRCS(Ed) FCSSL
Professor of Surgery and Dean, Faculty of Medical Sciences, University of Sri Jayawardenepura Gangodawila, Nugegoda, Colombo, Sri Lanka

Parminder J Singh MB BS MRCS FRCS(Tr & Orth) MS
Consultant Orthopaedic Surgeon, Maroondah Hospital and Honorary Senior Lecturer, Monash and Deakin University, Melbourne, Australia

V Sitaram MS FRCPS(Glas)
Professor of Surgery, Department of Hepatic, Pancreatic & Biliary (HPB) Surgery, Christian Medical College, Vellore, India

William P Smith FDSRCS FRCS(Ed) FRCS
Consultant Maxillofacial Surgeon, Northampton General Hospital NHS Trust, Northampton, UK

Robert JC Steele MB ChB MD FRCS(Ed)
Professor, Head of Academic Surgery, Ninewells Hospital and Medical School, Dundee, UK

Vinay Takwale MB MS FRCS(Tr & Orth)
Consultant Orthopaedic Surgeon, Gloucestershire Hospital, Gloucester, UK

Carol Tan MB ChB FRCS(C-Th)
Consultant Thoracic Surgeon, St George's Hospital, London, UK

William EG Thomas MS FRCS FSACS(Hon)
Consultant Surgeon and Honorary Senior Lecturer in Surgery, Sheffield, UK

Kevin Tremper PhD MD
Robert B Sweet Professor and Chair, Department of Anesthesiology, University of Michigan, Ann Arbor, MI, USA

Bruce Tulloh MB MS(Melb) FRACS FRCS(Ed)
Department of Surgery, Royal Infirmary of Edinburgh, Edinburgh, UK

Michael Tyler FRCS(Plast) MB CHM
Stoke Mandeville Hospital, Aylesbury, UK

Timothy J Underwood BSc(Hons) MB BS PhD FRCS
MRC Clinician Scientist and Honorary Consultant Surgeon, University Surgical Unit, Southampton General Hospital, Southampton, UK

Medha Vanarase MB BS MD FRCA(Cert Ed)
Consultant Anaesthetist, Oxford Radcliffe Hospitals NHS Trust, Oxford, UK

Robert Wheeler MS FRCS FRCPCH LLB(Hons) LLM
Consultant Paediatric Surgeon, Child Health, University Hospitals of Southampton, Southampton, UK

Birgit Whitman PhD
Head of Research Governance, University of Bristol, Bristol, UK

Joseph Windley MB BS BSc(Hons) MRCS
Specialist Registrar, Department of Trauma and Orthopaedic Surgery, Imperial College Healthcare, Academic Health Sciences Centre, London, UK

Mustafa Zakkar PhD
Department of Cardiothoracic Surgery, Imperial College Healthcare NHS Trust, Hammersmith Hospital, London, UK

Preface

In this age of rapid electronic access to scientific papers and erudite surgical opinion one has to ask whether there is still a place for a comprehensive surgical textbook that takes several years to compile and risks losing its immediacy. The success of the 25th edition of *Bailey & Love* together with the numerous positive communications we have received since its publication suggest that the answer is very much in the affirmative. However, it is essential that in producing further editions cognisance is taken of what the "customer" wants. Consequently before preparing the 26th edition of this venerable text we conducted considerable market research as to what had succeeded in the previous edition, what had been omitted and how we could improve content and presentation. Readers from a range of backgrounds from undergraduates to hard bitten and, dare we say, cynical senior consultants were asked for their opinion. Their musings and frank criticisms were all taken very seriously and many of their suggestions were adopted for this edition. A few chapters were removed or consolidated into others; new chapters have been added focusing on the important topics of patient safety, day case surgery and bariatric surgery.

All existing chapters have been radically revised and have been thoroughly brought up to date. We have attempted to ensure more conformity with regard to illustrations; however, we have kept faith with Hamilton Bailey and McNeil Love's original concept of ensuring clinical photographs are liberally used to not only enhance the text but more importantly illuminate a clinical point. Many new photographs have been introduced, some of which have been provided by our readers, which is very much a *Bailey & Love* tradition.

Although we have been ruthless in removing old material we make no excuse for retaining the odd original pen drawing taken from the first few editions. This is not just for nostalgia's sake but because they illustrate a pertinent point not easily captured by a modern photograph. Another tradition beloved of readers has of course been the autobiographical notes. These have all been painstakingly researched and added to by Pradip Datta.

We recognise that despite very careful attention to detail by our authors there may be an occasional error in the text that we and our proof readers have failed to spot. It would not be surprising in a text of this length. We apologise in advance for any errors and thank our eagle-eyed readers whom we know from experience will let us know of any that they find. This is a *Bailey & Love* tradition and we value all contributions that can improve accuracy.

Several editions ago we introduced the concept of learning objectives and summary boxes in order to help examination candidates in their revision. The feedback regarding these innovations was extremely positive and we have attempted to ensure that these are comprehensive, standardised and liberally dispersed through the text.

The authors of the chapters have been carefully chosen not just for their undoubted experience and expertise in their specialty but also their ability to write both accurately and succinctly. Writing is a skill honed by practice; it is a labour of love and takes time and patience to perfect. The best authors are like gifted musicians who, after numerous rehearsals, are able to deliver a perfect recital. It is our belief that our contributors have done just this and we the editors have attempted wherever possible to ensure there is a rhythm and harmony flowing through the pages. However, at the end of the day we appreciate it will be up to the audience to decide how successful we and our authors have been in this endeavour.

It has been a pleasure and privilege to edit this historic textbook beloved of so many students and trainees through the decades. However, we are conscious that previous reputation counts for very little unless the present product meets expectations and is relevant to the present era. This thought has always been in our minds when preparing the content of the 26th edition. We very much hope it fits the bill and fulfils your requirements whether you, the reader, are studying for an exam, checking on an area of practice that you may be unfamiliar with or just refreshing your memory about some forgotten fact or biographical detail.

Norman S. Williams
Christopher J.K. Bulstrode
P. Ronan O'Connell
2012

Acknowledgements

Sometimes a new edition of *Bailey & Love* feels like a swan swimming swiftly but serenely across a lake. From afar it may look effortless (and beautiful we hope), but to those who are closer to the action you can glimpse the webbed feet paddling away furiously beneath the surface driving that swan forward. The three editors are one part of a huge orchestra too large to mention all by name. However, it is a pleasure to acknowledge some of the most notable amongst the players.

Gavin Jamieson initiated the new edition as commissioning editor under the supervision of Jo Koster, who then took over following Gavin's departure. Sarah Penny and Stephen Clausard took on the awesome responsibility of pulling all things 'manuscript-related' together. Susie Bond, Alyson Thomas and Theresa Mackie have done a great job with the copy editing and proof reading, while the index has been compiled ably by Christopher Boot. Mr Pradip Datta FRCS completely revamped the historical footnotes, going back all the way to the first edition to check that we had left no 'jewels' out of the crown. Mr Hemant Pandit FRCS, Dr Medha Vanarese FRCA and Mr Parminder Singh FRCS helped enormously with the commissioning and editing of the orthopaedic, anaesthetic and trauma chapters respectively.

Chapter 4, *Basic surgical skills and anastomoses*, contains some material from '*Basic surgical skills and anastomoses*' by David J. Leaper. The material has been revised and updated by the current author.

Chapter 5, *Surgical infection*, contains some material from '*Surgical infection*' by David J. Leaper. The material has been revised and updated by the current author.

Chapter 8, *Principles of paediatric surgery*, contains some material from 'Principles of paediatric surgery' by Mark Stringer. The material has been revised and updated by the current author.

Chapter 11, *Surgical ethics and law*, contains some material from '*Surgical ethics*' by Len Doyal. The material has been revised and updated by the current author.

Chapter 16, *Preoperative preparation*, contains some material from '*Preoperative preparation*' by Lisa Leonard and Sarah J. Barton. The material has been revised and updated by the current authors.

Chapter 18, *Care in the operating room*, contains some material from '*Care in the operating room*' by Sunny Deo and Vipul Mandalia. The material has been revised and updated by the current authors.

Chapter 19, *Perioperative management of the high-risk surgical patient*, contains some material from '*Perioperative management of the high-risk surgical patient*' by Rupert M. Pearse and Richard M. Langford. The material has been revised and updated by the current authors.

Chapter 20, *Nutrition and fluid therapy*, the author would like to thank Marcel Gatt MD FRCS, who provided some illustrations and helped with proofreading the text.

Chapter 21, *Postoperative care*, contains some material from '*Postoperative care*' by Alistair Pace and Nicholas C.M. Armitage. The material has been revised and updated by the current author.

Chapter 25, *Head injury*, contains some material from '*Head injury*' by Richard Stacey and John Leach. The material has been revised and updated by the current authors.

Chapter 34, *Sports medicine and sports injuries*, contains some material from '*Sports medicine and sports injuries*' by D.L. Back and Jay Smith. The material has been revised and updated by the current author.

Chapter 36, *Upper limb – pathology, assessment and management*, contains some material from '*Upper limb – pathology, assessment and management*' by Srinath Kamineni. The material has been revised and updated by the current authors.

Chapter 37, *Hip and knee*, contains some material from '*Hip and knee*' by Vikas Khanduja and Richard N. Villar. The material has been revised and updated by the current authors.

Chapter 38, *Foot and ankle*, contains some material from '*Foot and ankle*' by Mark Davies, Matthew C. Solan and Vikas Khanduja. The material has been revised and updated by the current author.

Chapter 41, *Paediatric orthopaedics*, contains some material from '*Paediatric orthopaedics*' by the current author and Joanna Hicks, which has been revised and updated for this edition.

Chapter 43, *Elective neurosurgery*, contains some material from '*Elective Neurosurgery*' by John Leach and Richard Kerr. The material has been revised and updated by the current authors.

Chapter 44, *The eye and orbit*, contains some material from '*The eye and orbit*' by Jonathan D. Jagger and Hugo W.A. Henderson. The material has been revised and updated by the current author.

Chapter 48, *The pharynx, larynx and neck*, contains some material from '*The pharynx, larynx and neck*' by Jonathan D. Jagger and Hugo W.A. Henderson. The material has been revised and updated by the current author.

Chapter 52, *The adrenal glands and other abdominal endocrine disorders*, contains some material from '*Adrenal glands and other endocrine disorders*' by Matthias Rothmund. The material has been revised and updated by the current author.

Chapter 54, *Cardiac surgery*, contains some material from '*Cardiac surgery*' by Jonathan Anderson and Ian Hunt. The material has been revised and updated by the current authors.

Chapter 55, *The thorax*, contains some material from '*The thorax*' by Tom Treasure. The material has been revised and updated by the current authors.

Chapter 56, *Arterial disorders*, contains some material from '*Arterial disorders*' by John A. Murie. The material has been revised and updated by the current author.

Chapter 57, *Venous disorders*, contains some material from '*Venous disorders*' by Kevin Burnand. The material has been revised and updated by the current authors.

Chapter 58, *Lymphatic disorders*, contains some material from '*Lymphatic disorders*' by Shervanthi Homer-Vanniasinkam and Andrew Bradbury. The material has been revised and updated by the current authors.

Chapter 59, *History and examination of the abdomen*, contains some material from '*History and examination of the abdomen*' by Simon Paterson-Brown. The material has been revised and updated by the current authors.

Chapter 60, *Abdominal wall, hernia and umbilicus*, contains some material from '*Hernias, umbilicus and abdominal wall*' by Andrew N. Kingsnorth, Giorgi Giorgobiani and David H. Bennett. The material has been revised and updated by the current authors.

Chapter 61, *The peritoneum, omentum, mesentery and retroperitoneal space*, contains some material from '*The peritoneum, omentum, mesentery and retroperitoneal space*' by Jerry Thompson. The material has been revised and updated by the current author.

Chapter 65, *The liver*, contains some material from '*The liver*' by Brian R. Davidson. The material has been revised and updated by the current authors.

Chapter 69, *The small and large intestines*, contains some material from '*The small and large intestines*' by Neil J. McC Mortensen and Shazad Ashraf. The material has been revised and updated by the current authors.

Chapter 70, *Intestinal obstruction*, contains some material from '*Intestinal obstruction*' by Marc Christopher Winslet. The material has been revised and updated by the current author.

Chapter 76, *The urinary bladder*, contains some material from '*The urinary bladder*' by David E. Neal. The material has been revised and updated by the current author.

Chapter 78, *Urethra and penis*, contains some material from '*Urethra and penis*' by Christopher G. Fowler. The material has been revised and updated by the current author.

Chapter 79, *Testis and scrotum*, contains some material from '*Testis and scrotum*' by Christopher G. Fowler. The material has been revised and updated by the current author.

Sayings of the great

Both Hamilton Bailey and McNeill Love, when medical students, served as clerks to Sir Robert Hutchinson, 1871–1960, who was Consulting Physician to the London Hospital and President of the Royal College of Physicians. They never tired of quoting his 'medical litany', which is appropriate for all clinicians and, perhaps especially, for those who are surgically minded.

> From inability to leave well alone;
> From too much zeal for what is new and contempt for what is old;
> From putting knowledge before wisdom, science before art, cleverness before common sense;
> From treating patients as cases; and
> From making the cure of a disease more grievous than its endurance,
> Good Lord, deliver us.

To which may be added:

> The patient is the centre of the medical universe around which all our works revolve and towards which all our efforts trend.
>
> J.B. Murphy, 1857–1916, Professor of Surgery, Northwestern University, Chicago, IL, USA

> To study the phenomenon of disease without books is to sail an uncharted sea, while to study books without patients is not to go to sea at all.
>
> Sir William Osler, 1849–1919, Professor of Medicine, Oxford, UK

> A knowledge of healthy and diseased actions is not less necessary to be understood than the principles of other sciences. By and acquaintance with principles we learn the cause of disease. Without this knowledge a man cannot be a surgeon. … The last part of surgery, namely operations, is a reflection on the healing art; it is a tacit acknowledgement of the insufficiency of surgery. It is like an armed savage who attempts to get that by force which a civilised man would by stratagem.
>
> Hunter, 1728–1793, Surgeon, St George's Hospital, London, UK

Investigating Nature you will do well to bear ever in mind that in every question there is the truth, whatever our notions may be. This seems perhaps a very simple consideration; yet it is strange how often it seems to be disregarded. If we had nothing but pecuniary rewards and worldly honours to look to, our profession would not be one to be desired. But in its practice you will find it to be attended with peculiar privileges; second to none in intense interest and pure pleasures. It is our proud office to tend the fleshy tabernacle of the immortal spirit, and our path, if rightly followed, will be guided by unfettered truth and love unfeigned. In the pursuit of this noble and holy calling I wish you all God-speed.

Promoter's address, Graduation in Medicine, University of Edinburgh, August, 1876, by Lord Lister, the Founder of Modern Surgery

Surgery has undergone many great transformations during the past fifty years, and many are to be thanked for their contributions – yet when we think of how many remain to be made, it should rather stimulate our inventiveness than fuel our vanity.

Sir Percival Pott, 1714–88, Surgeon, St Bartholomew's Hospital, London, UK

If you cannot make a diagnosis at least make a decision!
Sir Harry Platt, 1897–1986,
Professor of Orthopaedics, Manchester, and President of the Royal College of Surgeons England, London, UK

If the surgeon cuts a vessel and knows the name of that vessel, the situation is serious; if the anaesthetist knows the name of that vessel, the situation is irretrievable.

Maldwyn Morgan 1938–
Anaesthetist, Hammersmith Hospital, London, UK

CHAPTER 1

Metabolic response to injury

LEARNING OBJECTIVES

To understand:
- Classical concepts of homeostasis
- Mediators of the metabolic response to injury
- Physiological and biochemical changes that occur during injury and recovery
- Changes in body composition that accompany surgical injury
- Avoidable factors that compound the metabolic response to injury
- Concepts behind optimal perioperative care

BASIC CONCEPTS IN HOMEOSTASIS

In the eighteenth and nineteenth centuries, a series of eminent scientists laid the foundations of our understanding of homeostasis and the response to injury. The classical concepts of homeostasis and the response to injury are:

- 'The stability of the "milieu intérieur" is the primary condition for freedom and independence of existence' (Claude Bernard); i.e. body systems act to maintain internal constancy.
- 'Homeostasis: the co-ordinated physiological process which maintains most of the steady states of the organism' (Walter Cannon); i.e. complex homeostatic responses involving the brain, nerves, heart, lungs, kidneys and spleen work to maintain body constancy.
- 'There is a circumstance attending accidental injury which does not belong to the disease, namely that the injury done, has in all cases a tendency to produce both the deposition and means of cure' (John Hunter); i.e. responses to injury are, in general, beneficial to the host and allow healing/survival.

In essence, the concept evolved that the constancy of the 'milieu intérieur' allowed for the independence of organisms, that complex homeostatic responses sought to maintain this constancy, and that within this range of responses were the elements of healing and repair. These ideas pertained to normal physiology and mild/moderate injury. In the modern era, such concepts do not account for disease evolution following major injury/sepsis or the injured patient who would have died but for artificial organ support. Such patients exemplify less of the classical homeostatic control system (signal detector–processor–effector regulated by a negative feedback loop) and more of the 'open loop' system, whereby only with medical/surgical resolution of the primary abnormality is a return to classical homeostasis possible.

As a consequence of modern understanding of the metabolic response to injury, elective surgical practice seeks to reduce the need for a homeostatic response by minimising the primary insult (minimal access surgery and 'stress-free' perioperative care). In emergency surgery, where the presence of tissue trauma/sepsis/hypovolaemia often compounds the primary problem, there is a requirement to augment artificially homeostatic responses (resuscitation) and to close the 'open' loop by intervening to resolve the primary insult (e.g. surgical treatment of major abdominal sepsis) and provide organ support (critical care) while the patient comes back to a situation in which homeostasis can achieve a return to normality (Summary box 1.1).

Summary box 1.1

Basic concepts

- Homeostasis is the foundation of normal physiology
- 'Stress-free' perioperative care helps to preserve homeostasis following elective surgery
- Resuscitation, surgical intervention and critical care can return the severely injured patient to a situation in which homeostasis becomes possible once again

This chapter aims to review the mediators of the stress response, the physiological and biochemical pathway changes associated with surgical injury and the changes in body composition that occur following surgical injury. Emphasis is laid on why knowledge of these events is important to understand the rationale for modern 'stress-free' perioperative and critical care.

John Hunter, 1728–1793, surgeon, St George's Hospital, London, UK. He is regarded as 'The Father of Scientific Surgery'. To further his knowledge of venereal disease he inoculated himself with syphilis in 1767.

Claude Bernard, 1813–1878, Professor of Physiology, The College de France, Paris, France.
Walter Bradford Cannon, 1871–1945, Professor of Physiology, Harvard University Medical School, Boston, MA, USA.

THE GRADED NATURE OF THE INJURY RESPONSE

It is important to recognise that the response to injury is graded: the more severe the injury, the greater the response (Figure 1.1). This concept not only applies to physiological/metabolic changes but also to immunological changes/sequelae. Thus, following elective surgery of intermediate severity, there may be a transient and modest rise in temperature, heart rate, respiratory rate, energy expenditure and peripheral white cell count. Following major trauma/sepsis, these changes are accentuated, resulting in a systemic inflammatory response syndrome (SIRS), hypermetabolism, marked catabolism, shock and even multiple organ dysfunction (MODS). It is important to recognise that genetic variability plays a key role in determining the intensity of the inflammatory response. Moreover, in certain circumstances, the severity of injury does not lead to a simple dose-dependent metabolic response, but rather leads to quantitatively different responses.

Not only is the metabolic response graded, but it also evolves with time. In particular, the immunological sequelae of major injury evolve from a proinflammatory state driven primarily by the innate immune system (macrophages, neutrophils, dendritic cells) into a compensatory anti-inflammatory response syndrome (CARS) characterised by suppressed immunity and diminished resistance to infection. In patients who develop infective complications, the latter will drive ongoing systemic inflammation, the acute phase response and continued catabolism.

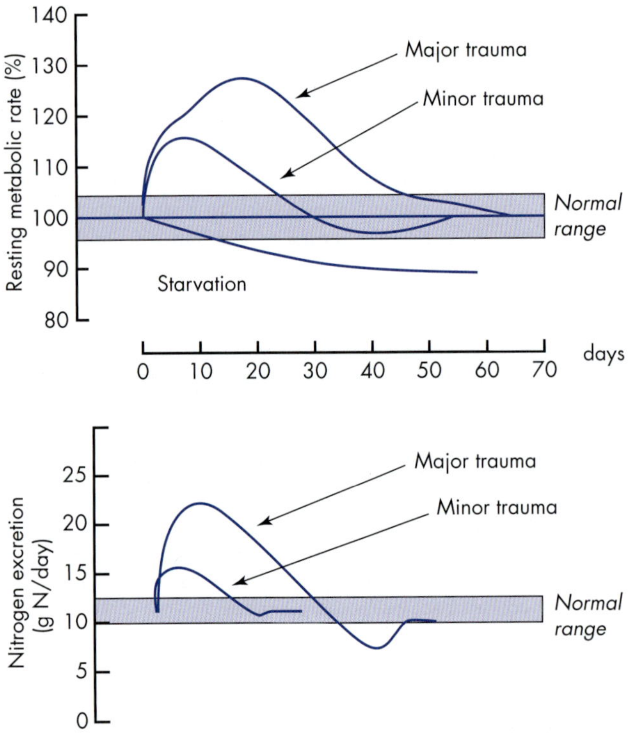

Figure 1.1 Hypermetabolism and increased nitrogen excretion are closely related to the magnitude of the initial injury and show a graded response.

MEDIATORS OF THE METABOLIC RESPONSE TO INJURY

The classical neuroendocrine pathways of the stress response consist of afferent nociceptive neurones, the spinal cord, thalamus, hypothalamus and pituitary (Figure 1.2). Corticotrophin-releasing factor (CRF) released from the hypothalamus increases adrenocorticotrophic hormone (ACTH) release from the anterior pituitary. ACTH then acts on the adrenal to increase the secretion of cortisol. Hypothalamic activation of the sympathetic nervous system causes release of adrenalin and also stimulates release of glucagon. Intravenous infusion of a cocktail of these 'counter-regulatory' hormones (glucagon, glucocorticoids and catecholamines) reproduces many aspects of the metabolic response to injury. There are, however, many other players, including alterations in insulin release and sensitivity, hypersecretion of prolactin and growth hormone (GH) in the presence of low circulatory insulin-like growth factor-1 (IGF-1) and inactivation of peripheral thyroid hormones and gonadal function. Of note, GH has direct lipolytic, insulin-antagonising and proinflammatory properties (Summary box 1.2).

Summary box 1.2

Neuroendocrine response to injury/critical illness

The neuroendocrine response to severe injury/critical illness is biphasic:

- **Acute phase** characterised by an actively secreting pituitary and elevated counter-regulatory hormones (cortisol, glucagon, adrenaline). Changes are thought to be beneficial for short-term survival
- **Chronic phase** associated with hypothalamic suppression and low serum levels of the respective target organ hormones. Changes contribute to chronic wasting

The innate immune system (principally macrophages) interacts in a complex manner with the adaptive immune system (T cells, B cells) in co-generating the metabolic response to injury (Figure 1.2). Proinflammatory cytokines including interleukin-1 (IL-1), tumour necrosis factor alpha (TNFα), IL-6 and IL-8 are produced within the first 24 hours and act directly on the hypothalamus to cause pyrexia. Such cytokines also augment the hypothalamic stress response and act directly on skeletal muscle to induce proteolysis while inducing acute phase protein production in the liver. Proinflammatory cytokines also play a complex role in the development of peripheral insulin resistance. Other important proinflammatory mediators include nitric oxide ((NO) via inducible nitric oxide synthetase (iNOS)) and a variety of prostanoids (via cyclo-oxygenase-2 (Cox-2)). Changes in organ function (e.g. renal hypoperfusion/impairment) may be induced by excessive vasoconstriction via endogenous factors such as endothelin-1.

Within hours of the upregulation of proinflammatory cytokines, endogenous cytokine antagonists enter the circulation (e.g. interleukin-1 receptor antagonist (IL-1Ra) and TNF-soluble receptors (TNF-sR-55 and 75)) and act to control the proinflammatory response. A complex further series of adaptive

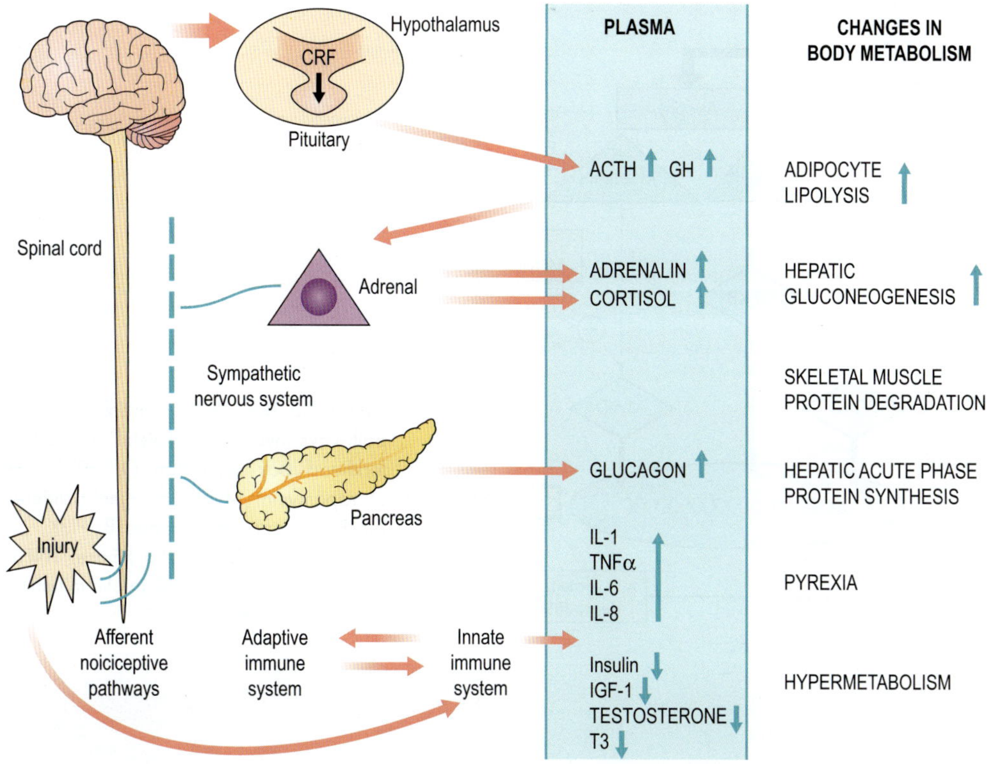

Figure 1.2 The integrated response to surgical injury (first 24–48 hours): there is a complex interplay between the neuroendocrine stress response and the proinflammatory cytokine response of the innate immune system.

changes includes the development of a Th2-type counterinflammatory response (regulated by IL-4, -5, -9 and -13 and transforming growth factor beta (TGFβ)) which, if accentuated and prolonged in critical illness, is characterised as the CARS and results in immunosuppression and an increased susceptibility to opportunistic (nosocomial) infection (Summary box 1.3). Within inflamed tissue the duration and magnitude of acute inflammation as well as the return to homeostasis are influenced by a group of local mediators known as specialised pro-resolving mediators (SPM) that include essential fatty acid-derived lipoxins, resolvins, protectins and maresins. These endogenous resolution agonists orchestrate the uptake and clearance of apoptotic polymorphonuclear neutrophils and microbial particles, reduce proinflammatory cytokines and lipid mediators as well as enhance the removal of cellular debris in the inflammatory milieu. Thus both at the systemic level (endogenous cytokine antagonists – see above) and at the local tissue level, the body attempts to limit/resolve inflammation driven dyshomeostasis.

Summary box 1.3

Systemic inflammatory response syndrome following major injury

- Is driven initially by proinflammatory cytokines (e.g. IL-1, IL-6 and TNFα)
- Is followed rapidly by increased plasma levels of cytokine antagonists and soluble receptors (e.g. IL-1Ra, TNF-sR)
- If prolonged or excessive may evolve into a counterinflammatory response syndrome

There are many complex interactions between the neuroendocrine, cytokine and metabolic axes. For example, although cortisol is immunosuppressive at high levels, it acts synergistically with IL-6 to promote the hepatic acute phase response. ACTH release is enhanced by proinflammatory cytokines and the noradrenergic system. The resulting rise in cortisol levels may form a weak feedback loop attempting to limit the proinflammatory stress response. Finally, hyperglycaemia may aggravate the inflammatory response via substrate overflow in the mitochondria, causing the formation of excess free oxygen radicals and also altering gene expression to enhance cytokine production.

At the molecular level, the changes that accompany systemic inflammation are extremely complex. In a recent study using network-based analysis of changes in mRNA expression in leukocytes following exposure to endotoxin, there were changes in the expression of more than 3700 genes with over half showing decreased expression and the remainder increased expression. The cell surface receptors, signalling mechanisms and transcription factors that initiate these events are also complex, but an early and important player involves the nuclear factor kappa B (NFκB)/*relA* family of transcription factors. A simplified model of current understanding of events within skeletal muscle is shown in Figure 1.3.

THE METABOLIC STRESS RESPONSE TO SURGERY AND TRAUMA: THE 'EBB AND FLOW' MODEL

In the natural world, if an animal is injured, it displays a characteristic response, which includes immobility, anorexia and catabolism (Summary box 1.4).

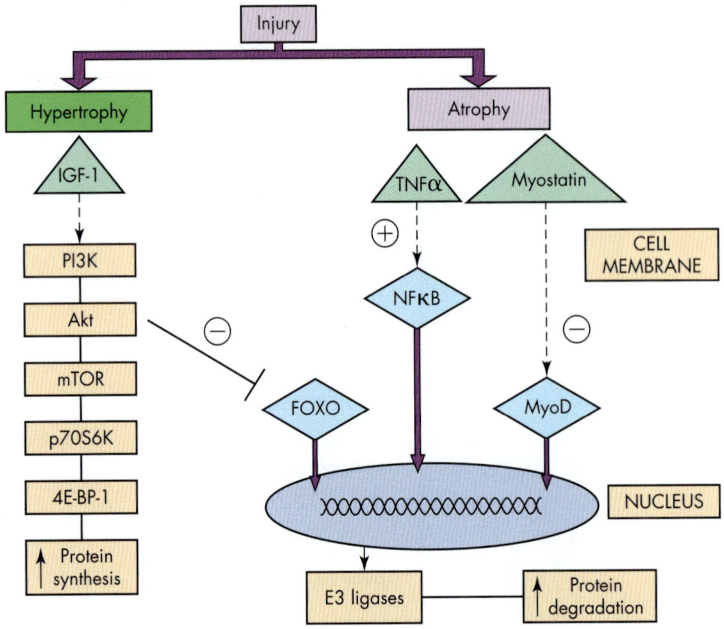

Figure 1.3 The major catabolic and anabolic signalling pathways involved in skeletal muscle homeostasis. FOXO, forkhead box sub-group O; mTOR, mammalian target of rapamycin; MyoD, myogenic differentiation factor D; NFκB, nuclear factor kappa B; PI3K, phosphatidylinositol 3-kinase; p70S6K, p70S6 kinase; TNFα, tumour necrosis factor alpha; 4E-BP-1, eukaryotic initiation translation factor 4E binding protein 1.

Summary box 1.4

Physiological response to injury

The natural response to injury includes:

- Immobility/rest
- Anorexia
- Catabolism

The changes are designed to aid survival of moderate injury in the absence of medical intervention.

In 1930, Sir David Cuthbertson divided the metabolic response to injury in humans into 'ebb' and 'flow' phases (Figure 1.4). The ebb phase begins at the time of injury and lasts for approximately 24–48 hours. It may be attenuated by proper resuscitation, but not completely abolished. The ebb phase is characterised by hypovolaemia, decreased basal metabolic rate, reduced cardiac output, hypothermia and lactic acidosis. The predominant hormones regulating the ebb phase are catecholamines, cortisol and aldosterone (following activation of the renin–angiotensin system). The magnitude of this neuroendocrine response depends on the degree of blood loss and the stimulation of somatic afferent nerves at the site of injury. The main physiological role of the ebb phase is to conserve both circulating volume and energy stores for recovery and repair.

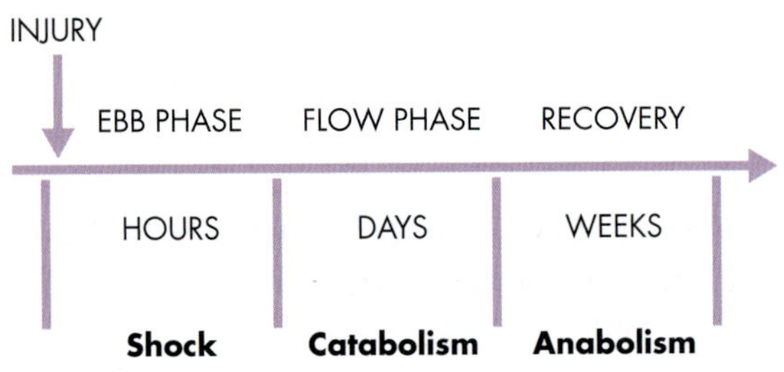

Figure 1.4 Phases of the physiological response to injury (after Cuthbertson 1930).

Following resuscitation, the ebb phase evolves into a hypermetabolic flow phase, which corresponds to SIRS. This phase involves the mobilisation of body energy stores for recovery and repair, and the subsequent replacement of lost or damaged tissue. It is characterised by tissue oedema (from vasodilatation and increased capillary leakage), increased basal metabolic rate (hypermetabolism), increased cardiac output, raised body temperature, leukocytosis, increased oxygen consumption and increased gluconeogenesis. The flow phase may be subdivided into an initial catabolic phase, lasting approximately 3–10 days, followed by an anabolic phase, which may last for weeks if extensive recovery and repair are required following serious injury. During the catabolic phase, the increased production of counter-regulatory hormones (including catecholamines, cortisol, insulin and glucagon) and inflammatory cytokines (e.g. IL-1, IL-6 and TNFα) results in significant fat and protein mobilisation, leading to significant weight loss and increased urinary nitrogen excretion. The increased production of insulin at this time is associated with significant insulin resistance and, therefore, injured patients often exhibit poor glycaemic control. The combination of pronounced or prolonged catabolism in association with insulin resistance places patients within this phase at increased risk of complications, particularly infectious and cardiovascular. Obviously, the development of complications will further aggravate the neuroendocrine and inflammatory stress responses, thus creating a vicious catabolic cycle (Summary box 1.5).

Sir David Paton Cuthbertson, 1900–1989, biochemist, Director of the Rowett Research Institute, Glasgow, UK.

Summary box 1.5

Purpose of neuroendocrine changes following injury

The constellation of neuroendocrine changes following injury acts to:

- Provide essential substrates for survival
- Postpone anabolism
- Optimise host defence

These changes may be helpful in the short term, but may be harmful in the long term, especially to the severely injured patient who would otherwise not have survived without medical intervention.

KEY CATABOLIC ELEMENTS OF THE FLOW PHASE OF THE METABOLIC STRESS RESPONSE

There are several key elements of the flow phase that largely determine the extent of catabolism and thus govern the metabolic and nutritional care of the surgical patient. It must be remembered that, during the response to injury, not all tissues are catabolic. Indeed, the essence of this coordinated response is to allow the body to reprioritise limited resources away from peripheral tissues (muscle, adipose tissue, skin) and towards key viscera (liver, immune system) and the wound (Figure 1.5).

Hypermetabolism

The majority of trauma patients (except possibly those with extensive burns) demonstrate energy expenditures approximately 15–25 per cent above predicted healthy resting values. The predominant cause appears to be a complex interaction between the central control of metabolic rate and peripheral energy utilisation. In particular, central thermodysregulation (caused by the proinflammatory cytokine cascade), increased sympathetic activity, abnormalities in wound circulation (ischaemic areas produce lactate, which must be metabolised by the adenosine triphosphate (ATP)-consuming hepatic Cori cycle; hyperaemic areas cause an increase in cardiac output), increased protein turnover and nutritional support may all increase patient energy expenditure. Theoretically, patient energy expenditure could rise even higher than observed levels following surgery or trauma, but several features of standard intensive care (including bed rest, paralysis, ventilation and external temperature regulation) counteract the hypermetabolic driving forces of the stress response. Furthermore, the skeletal muscle wasting experienced by patients with prolonged catabolism actually limits the volume of metabolically active tissue (Summary box 1.6; see below).

Summary box 1.6

Hypermetabolism

Hypermetabolism following injury:

- Is mainly caused by an acceleration of energy-dependent metabolic cycles
- Is limited in modern practice on account of elements of routine critical care

Alterations in skeletal muscle protein metabolism

Muscle protein is continually synthesised and broken down with a turnover rate in humans of 1–2 per cent per day, and with a greater amplitude of changes in protein synthesis (± two-fold) than breakdown (± 0.25-fold) during the diurnal cycle. Under normal circumstances, synthesis equals breakdown and muscle bulk remains constant. Physiological stimuli that promote net muscle protein accretion include feeding (especially extracellular amino acid concentration) and exercise. Paradoxically, during exercise, skeletal muscle protein synthesis is depressed, but it increases again during rest and feeding.

During the catabolic phase of the stress response, muscle wasting occurs as a result of an increase in muscle protein degradation (via enzymatic pathways), coupled with a decrease in muscle protein synthesis. The major site of protein loss is peripheral skeletal muscle, although nitrogen losses also occur in the respiratory muscles (predisposing the patient to hypoventilation and chest infections) and in the gut (reducing gut motility). Cardiac muscle appears to be mostly spared. Under extreme conditions of catabolism (e.g. major sepsis), urinary nitrogen losses can reach 14–20 g/day; this is equivalent to the loss of 500 g of skeletal muscle per day. It is remarkable that muscle catabolism cannot be inhibited fully by providing artificial nutritional support as long as the stress response continues. Indeed, in critical care, it is now recognised that 'hyperalimentation' represents a metabolic stress in itself, and that nutritional support should be at a modest level to attenuate rather than replace energy and protein losses.

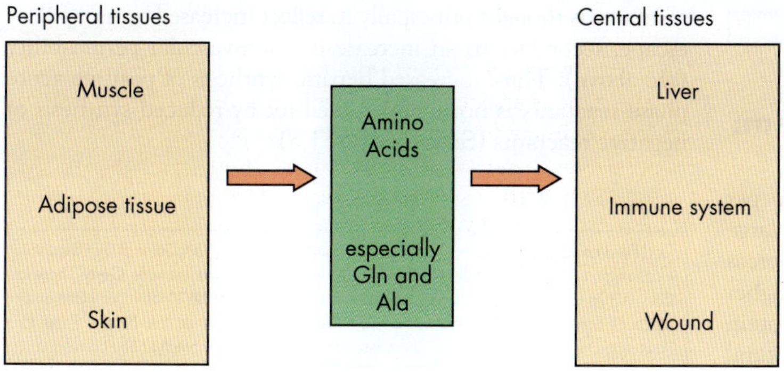

Figure 1.5 During the metabolic response to injury, the body reprioritises protein metabolism away from peripheral tissues and towards key central tissues such as the liver, immune system and wound. One of the main reasons why the reutilisation of amino acids derived from muscle proteolysis leads to net catabolism is that the increased glutamine and alanine efflux from muscle is derived, in part, from the irreversible degradation of branched chain amino acids. Ala, alanine; Gln, glutamine.

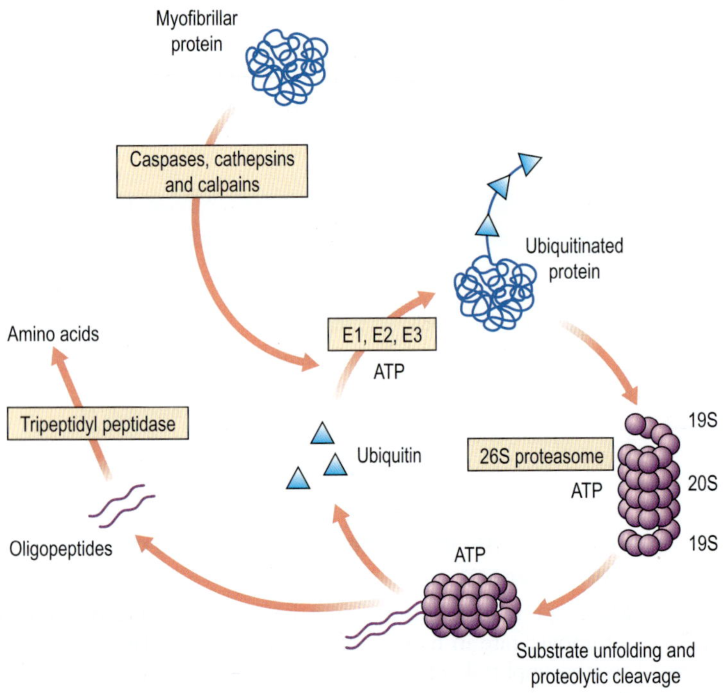

Figure 1.6 The intercellular effector mechanisms involved in degrading myofibrillar protein into free amino acids. The ubiquitin–proteasome pathway is a complex multistep process, which requires adenosine triphosphate and results in the tagging of specific proteins with ubiquitin for degradation of proteasome. E1, ubiquitin-activating enzyme; E2, ubiquitin-conjugating enzyme; E3, ubiquitin ligase.

The predominant mechanism involved in the wasting of skeletal muscle is the ATP-dependent ubiquitin–proteasome pathway (Figure 1.6), although the lysosomal cathepsins and the calcium–calpain pathway play facilitatory and accessory roles.

Clinically, a patient with skeletal muscle wasting will experience asthenia, increased fatigue, reduced functional ability, decreased quality of life and an increased risk of morbidity and mortality. In critically ill patients, muscle weakness may be further worsened by the development of critical illness myopathy, a multifactorial condition that is associated with impaired excitation–contraction coupling at the level of the sarcolemma and the sarcoplasmic reticulum membrane (Summary box 1.7).

Summary box 1.7

Skeletal muscle wasting

- Provides amino acids for the metabolic support of central organs/tissues
- Is mediated at a molecular level mainly by activation of the ubiquitin–proteasome pathway
- Can result in immobility and contribute to hypostatic pneumonia and death if prolonged and excessive

Alterations in hepatic protein metabolism: the acute phase protein response

The liver and skeletal muscle together account for >50 per cent of daily body protein turnover. Skeletal muscle has a large mass but a low turnover rate (1–2 per cent per day), whereas the liver has a relatively small mass (1.5 kg) but a much higher protein turnover rate (10–20 per cent per day). Hepatic protein synthesis is divided roughly 50:50 between renewal of structural proteins and synthesis of export proteins. Albumin is the major export protein produced by the liver and is renewed at the rate of about 10 per cent per day. The transcapillary escape rate (TER) of albumin is about ten times the rate of synthesis, and short-term changes in albumin concentration are most probably due to increased vascular permeability. Albumin TER may be increased three-fold following major injury/sepsis.

In response to inflammatory conditions, including surgery, trauma, sepsis, cancer or autoimmune conditions, circulating peripheral blood mononuclear cells secrete a range of pro-inflammatory cytokines, including IL-1, IL-6 and TNFα. These cytokines, in particular IL-6, promote the hepatic synthesis of positive acute phase proteins, e.g. fibrinogen and C-reactive protein (CRP). The acute phase protein response (APPR) represents a 'double-edged sword' for surgical patients as it provides proteins important for recovery and repair, but only at the expense of valuable lean tissue and energy reserves.

In contrast to the positive acute phase reactants, the plasma concentrations of other liver export proteins (the negative acute phase reactants) fall acutely following injury, e.g. albumin. However, rather than represent a reduced hepatic synthesis rate, the fall in plasma concentration of negative acute phase reactants is thought principally to reflect increased transcapillary escape, secondary to an increase in microvascular permeability (see above). Thus, increased hepatic synthesis of positive acute phase reactants is not compensated for by reduced synthesis of negative reactants (Summary box 1.8).

Carl Ferdinand Cori, 1896–1984, Professor of Pharmacology, and later of Biochemistry, Washington University Medical School, St Louis, MI, USA and his wife Gerty Theresa Cori, 1896–1957, who was also Professor of Biochemistry at the Washington University Medical School. In 1947 the Coris were awarded a share of the Nobel Prize for Physiology or Medicine 'for their discovery of how glycogen is catalytically converted'.

Summary box 1.8

Hepatic acute phase response

The hepatic acute phase response represents a reprioritisation of body protein metabolism towards the liver and is characterised by:

- **Positive** reactants (e.g. CRP): plasma concentration ↑
- **Negative** reactants (e.g. albumin): plasma concentration ↓

Insulin resistance

Following surgery or trauma, postoperative hyperglycaemia develops as a result of increased glucose production combined with decreased glucose uptake in peripheral tissues. Decreased glucose uptake is a result of insulin resistance which is transiently induced within the stressed patient. Suggested mechanisms for this phenomenon include the action of proinflammatory cytokines and the decreased responsiveness of insulin-regulated glucose transporter proteins. The degree of insulin resistance is proportional to the magnitude of the injurious process. Following routine upper abdominal surgery, insulin resistance may persist for approximately 2 weeks.

Postoperative patients with insulin resistance behave in a similar manner to individuals with type II diabetes mellitus. The mainstay of management of insulin resistance is intravenous insulin infusion. Insulin infusions may be used in either an intensive approach (i.e. sliding scales are manipulated to normalise the blood glucose level) or a conservative approach (i.e. insulin is administered when the blood glucose level exceeds a defined limit and discontinued when the level falls). Studies of postoperatively ventilated patients in the intensive care unit (ICU) have suggested that maintenance of normal glucose levels using intensive insulin therapy can significantly reduce both morbidity and mortality. Furthermore, intensive insulin therapy is superior to conservative insulin approaches in reducing morbidity rates. However, the mortality benefit of intensive insulin therapy over a more conservative approach has not been proven conclusively. The observed benefits of insulin therapy are probably simply as a result of maintenance of normoglycaemia, but the glycaemia-independent actions of insulin may also exert minor, organ-specific effects (e.g. promotion of myocardial systolic function).

CHANGES IN BODY COMPOSITION FOLLOWING INJURY

The average 70-kg male can be considered to consist of fat (13 kg) and fat-free mass (or lean body mass: 57 kg). In such an individual, the lean tissue is composed primarily of protein (12 kg), water (42 kg) and minerals (3 kg) (Figure 1.7). The protein mass can be considered as two basic compartments, skeletal muscle (4 kg) and non-skeletal muscle (8 kg), which includes the visceral protein mass. The water mass (42 litres) is divided into intercellular (28 litres) and extracellular (14 litres) spaces. Most of the mineral mass is contained in the bony skeleton.

The main labile energy reserve in the body is fat, and the main labile protein reserve is skeletal muscle. While fat mass can be reduced without major detriment to function, loss of protein mass results not only in skeletal muscle wasting, but also depletion of visceral protein status. Within lean issue, each 1 g of nitrogen is contained within 6.25 g of protein, which is contained in approximately 36 g of wet weight tissue. Thus, the loss of 1 g of nitrogen in urine is equivalent to the breakdown of 36 g of wet weight lean tissue. Protein turnover in the whole body is of the order of 150–200 g per day. A normal human ingests about 70–100 g protein per day, which is metabolised and excreted in urine as ammonia and urea (i.e. approximately 14 g N/day). During total starvation, urinary loss of nitrogen is rapidly attenuated by a series of adaptive changes. Loss of body weight follows a similar course (Figure 1.8), thus accounting for the survival of hunger strikers for a period of 50–60 days. Following major injury, and particularly in the presence of ongoing septic complications, this adaptive change fails to occur, and there is a state of 'autocannibalism', resulting in continuing urinary nitrogen losses of 10–20 g N/day (equivalent to 500 g of wet weight lean tissue per day). As with total starvation, once loss of body protein mass has reached 30–40 per cent of the total, survival is unlikely.

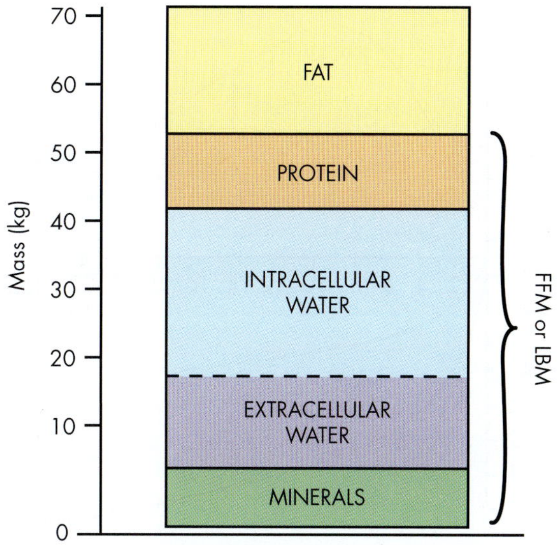

Figure 1.7 The chemical body composition of a normal 70-kg male. FFM, fat-free mass; LBM, lean body mass.

Critically ill patients admitted to the ICU with severe sepsis or major blunt trauma undergo massive changes in body composition (Figure 1.8). Body weight increases immediately on resuscitation with an expansion of extracellular water by 6–10 litres within 24 hours. Thereafter, even with optimal metabolic care and nutritional support, total body protein will diminish by 15 per cent in the next 10 days, and body weight will reach negative balance as the expansion of the extracellular space resolves. In marked contrast, it is now possible to maintain body weight and nitrogen equilibrium following major elective surgery. This can be achieved by blocking the neuroendocrine stress response with epidural analgesia and providing early enteral feeding. Moreover, the early fluid retention phase can be avoided by careful intraoperative management of fluid balance, with avoidance of excessive administration of intravenous saline (Summary box 1.9).

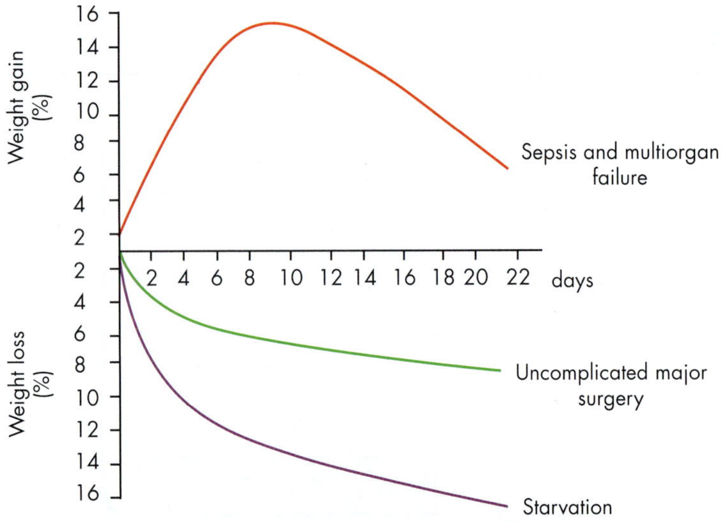

Figure 1.8 Changes in body weight that occur in serious sepsis, after uncomplicated surgery and in total starvation.

Summary box 1.9

Changes in body composition following major surgery/critical illness

- Catabolism leads to a **decrease** in fat mass and skeletal muscle mass
- Body weight may paradoxically **increase** because of expansion of extracellular fluid space

AVOIDABLE FACTORS THAT COMPOUND THE RESPONSE TO INJURY

As noted previously, the main features of the metabolic response are initiated by the immune system, cardiovascular system, sympathetic nervous system, ascending reticular formation and limbic system. However, the metabolic stress response may be further exacerbated by anaesthesia, dehydration, starvation (including preoperative fasting), sepsis, acute medical illness or even severe psychological stress (Figure 1.9). Attempts to limit or control these factors can be beneficial to the patient (Summary box 1.10).

Summary box 1.10

Avoidable factors that compound the response to injury

- Continuing haemorrhage
- Hypothermia
- Tissue oedema
- Tissue underperfusion
- Starvation
- Immobility

Volume loss

During simple haemorrhage, pressor receptors in the carotid artery and aortic arch, and volume receptors in the wall of the left atrium, initiate afferent nerve input to the central nervous system (CNS), resulting in the release of both aldosterone and antidiuretic hormone (ADH). Pain can also stimulate ADH release. ADH acts directly on the kidney to cause fluid retention. Decreased pulse pressure stimulates the juxtaglomerular apparatus in the kidney and directly activates the renin–angiotensin system, which in turn increases aldosterone release.

Aldosterone causes the renal tubule to reabsorb sodium (and consequently also conserve water). ACTH release also augments the aldosterone response. The net effects of ADH and aldosterone result in the natural oliguria observed after surgery and conservation of sodium and water in the extracellular space. The tendency towards water and salt retention is exacerbated by resuscitation with saline-rich fluids. Salt and water retention can result in not only peripheral oedema, but also visceral oedema (e.g. stomach). Such visceral oedema has been associated with reduced gastric emptying, delayed resumption of food intake and prolonged hospital stay. Careful limitation of intraoperative administration of colloids and crystalloids (e.g. Hartmann's solution) so that there is no net weight gain following elective surgery has been proven to reduce postoperative complications and length of stay.

Hypothermia

Hypothermia results in increased elaboration of adrenal steroids and catecholamines. When compared with normothermic controls, even mild hypothermia results in a two- to three-fold increase in postoperative cardiac arrhythmias and increased catabolism. Randomised trials have shown that maintaining normothermia by an upper body forced-air heating cover reduces wound infections, cardiac complications and bleeding and transfusion requirements.

Tissue oedema

During systemic inflammation, fluid, plasma proteins, leukocytes, macrophages and electrolytes leave the vascular space and accumulate in the tissues. This can diminish the alveolar diffusion of oxygen and may lead to reduced renal function. Increased capillary leak is mediated by a wide variety of mediators including cytokines, prostanoids, bradykinin and nitric oxide. Vasodilatation implies that intravascular volume

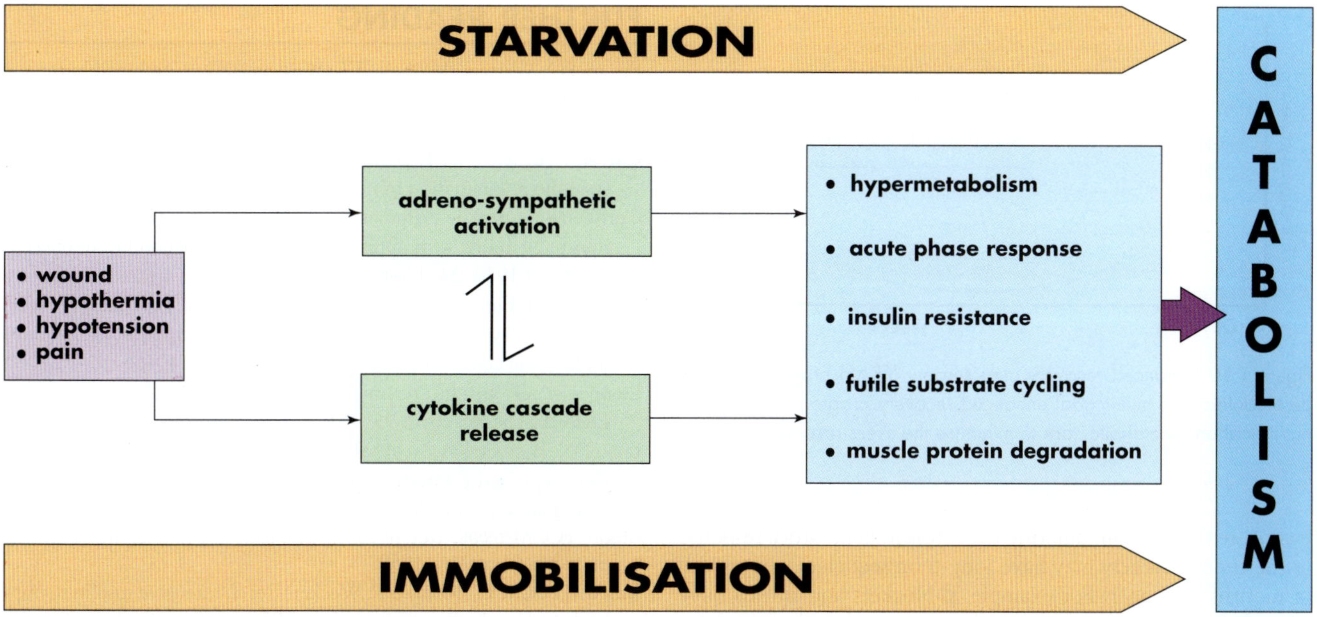

Figure 1.9 Factors that exacerbate the metabolic response to surgical injury include hypothermia, controlled pain, starvation, immobilisation, sepsis and medical complications

decreases, which induces shock if inadequate resuscitation is not undertaken. Meanwhile, intracellular volume decreases, and this provides part of the volume necessary to replenish intravascular and extravascular extracellular volume.

Systemic inflammation and tissue underperfusion

The vascular endothelium controls vasomotor tone and microvascular flow, and regulates trafficking of nutrients and biologically active molecules. When endothelial activation is excessive, compromised microcirculation and subsequent cellular hypoxia contribute to the risk of organ failure. Maintaining normoglycaemia with insulin infusion during critical illness has been proposed to protect the endothelium, probably in part, via inhibition of excessive iNOS-induced NO release, and thereby contribute to the prevention of organ failure and death. Administration of activated protein C to critically ill patients has been shown to reduce organ failure and death and is thought to act, in part, via preservation of the microcirculation in vital organs.

Starvation

During starvation, the body is faced with an obligate need to generate glucose to sustain cerebral energy metabolism (100 g of glucose per day). This is achieved in the first 24 hours by mobilising glycogen stores and thereafter by hepatic gluconeogenesis from amino acids, glycerol and lactate. The energy metabolism of other tissues is sustained by mobilising fat from adipose tissue. Such fat mobilisation is mainly dependent on a fall in circulating insulin levels. Eventually, accelerated loss of lean tissue (the main source of amino acids for hepatic gluconeogenesis) is reduced as a result of the liver converting free fatty acids into ketone bodies, which can serve as a substitute for glucose for cerebral energy metabolism. Provision of 2 litres of intravenous 5 per cent dextrose as intravenous fluids for surgical patients who are fasted provides 100 g of glucose per day and has a significant protein-sparing effect. Avoiding unnecessary fasting in the first instance and early oral/enteral/parenteral nutrition form the platform for avoiding loss of body mass as a result of the varying degrees of starvation observed in surgical patients. Modern guidelines on fasting prior to anaesthesia allow intake of clear fluids up to 2 hours before surgery. Administration of a carbohydrate drink at this time reduces perioperative anxiety and thirst and decreases postoperative insulin resistance.

Immobility

Immobility has long been recognised as a potent stimulus for inducing muscle wasting. Inactivity impairs the normal meal-derived amino acid stimulation of protein synthesis in skeletal muscle. Avoidance of unnecessary bed rest and active early mobilisation are essential measures to avoid muscle wasting as a consequence of immobility.

CONCEPTS BEHIND OPTIMAL PERIOPERATIVE CARE

Current understanding of the metabolic response to surgical injury and the mediators involved has led to a reappraisal of traditional perioperative care. There is now a strong scientific rationale for avoiding unmodulated exposure to stress, prolonged fasting and excessive administration of intravenous (saline) fluids (Figure 1.10). The widespread adoption of minimal access (laparoscopic) surgery is a key change in surgical practice that can reduce the magnitude of surgical injury and enhance the rate of patients' return to homeostasis and recovery. It is also impor-

Alexis Frank Hartmann, 1898–1964, paediatrician, St Louis, MO, USA.

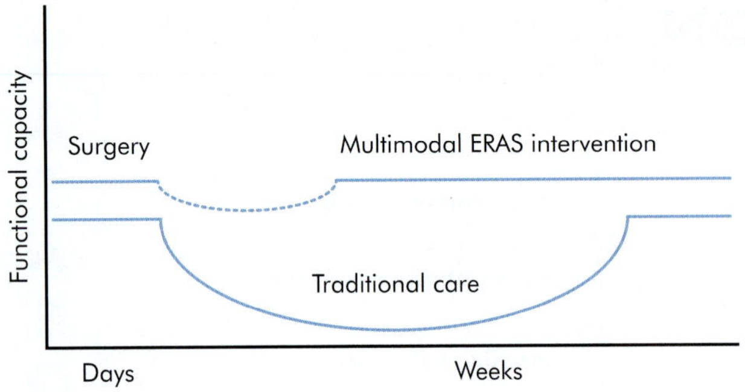

Figure 1.10 Enhanced recovery after surgery (ERAS) programmes can be modulated by multimodal enhanced recovery programmes (optimal nutritional and metabolic care to minimise the stress response).

tant to realise that modulating the stress/inflammatory response at the time of surgery may have long-term sequelae over periods of months or longer. For example, β-blockers and statins have recently been shown to improve long-term survival after major surgery. It has been suggested that these effects may be due to suppression of innate immunity at the time of surgery. Equally, the use of epidural analgesia to reduce pain, block the cortisol stress response and attenuate postoperative insulin resistance may, via effects on the body's protein economy, favourably affect many of the patient-centred outcomes that are important to postoperative recovery but have largely been unmeasured to date, such as functional capacity, vitality and ability to return to work (Summary box 1.11).

Summary box 1.11

A proactive approach to prevent unnecessary aspects of the surgical stress response

- Minimal access techniques
- Blockade of afferent painful stimuli (e.g. epidural analgesia)
- Minimal periods of starvation
- Early mobilisation

FURTHER READING

Bessey PQ, Watters JM, Aoki TT, Wilmore DW. Combined hormonal infusion simulates the metabolic response to injury. *Ann Surg* 1984; **200**: 264–81.

Calvano SE, Xioa W, Richards DR *et al.* A network-based analysis of systemic inflammation in humans. *Nature* 2005; **437**: 1032–7.

Cuthbertson DP. The disturbance of metabolism produced by bone and non-bony injury, with notes on certain abnormal conditions of bone. *Biochem J* 1930; **24**: 1244.

Fearon KCH, Ljungqvist O, von Meyenfeldt M *et al.* Enhanced recovery after surgery: a consensus review of clinical care for patients undergoing colonic resection. *Clin Nutr* 2005; **24**: 466–77.

Ljungqvist O. Insulin resistance and outcomes in surgery. *J Clin Endocrinol Metab* 2010; **95**: 4217–19.

Lobo DN, Bostock KA, Neal KR *et al.* Effect of salt and water balance on recovery of gastrointestinal function after elective colonic resection: a randomised controlled trial. *Lancet* 2002; **359**: 1812–18.

Moore FO. *Metabolic care of the surgical patient.* Philadelphia, PA: WB Saunders Company, 1959.

Van den Berghe G, Wonters P, Weckers F *et al.* Intensive insulin therapy in the critically ill patient. *N Engl J Med* 2001; **345**: 1359–67.

Vanhorebeek O, Langounche L, Van den Berghe G. Endocrine aspects of acute and prolonged critical illness. *Nat Clin Pract Endocrinol Metab* 2006; **2**: 20–31.

Varadhan KK, Neal KR, Dejong CH *et al.* The enhanced recovery after surgery (ERAS) pathway for patients undergoing major elective open colorectal surgery: a meta-analysis of randomised controlled trials. *Clin Nutr* 2010; **29**: 434–40.

Wilmore DW. From Cuthbertson to fast-track surgery: 70 years of progress in reducing stress in surgical patients. *Ann Surg* 2002; **236**: 643–8.

Francis Daniels Moore, 1913–2001, Moseley Professor of Surgery at Peter Bent Brigham Hospital, Boston. 'Franny' to his colleagues, did pioneering work on metabolic response to surgery and published his seminal work in 1959, *Metabolic care of the surgical patient.* At the age of 34 he became the youngest Chairman of Surgery in Harvard's history. His leadership led to the first ever kidney transplantation between identical twins in his department by Joe Murray in 1954. He was often regarded as 'the ultimate communicator'.

CHAPTER 2

Shock and blood transfusion

LEARNING OBJECTIVES

To understand:

- The pathophysiology of shock and ischaemia–reperfusion injury
- The different patterns of shock and the principles and priorities of resuscitation
- Appropriate monitoring and end points of resuscitation
- Use of blood and blood products, the benefits and risks of blood transfusion

INTRODUCTION

Shock is the most common and therefore the most important cause of death of surgical patients. Death may occur rapidly due to a profound state of shock, or be delayed due to the consequences of organ ischaemia and reperfusion injury. It is important therefore that every surgeon understands the pathophysiology, diagnosis and priorities in management of shock and haemorrhage.

SHOCK

Shock is a systemic state of low tissue perfusion which is inadequate for normal cellular respiration. With insufficient delivery of oxygen and glucose, cells switch from aerobic to anaerobic metabolism. If perfusion is not restored in a timely fashion, cell death ensues.

Pathophysiology

Cellular

As perfusion to the tissues is reduced, cells are deprived of oxygen and must switch from aerobic to anaerobic metabolism. The product of anaerobic respiration is not carbon dioxide but lactic acid. When enough tissue is underperfused, the accumulation of lactic acid in the blood produces a systemic metabolic acidosis.

As glucose within cells is exhausted, anaerobic respiration ceases and there is failure of sodium/potassium pumps in the cell membrane and intracellular organelles. Intracellular lysosomes release autodigestive enzymes and cell lysis ensues. Intracellular contents, including potassium are released into the blood stream.

Microvascular

As tissue ischaemia progresses, changes in the local milieu result in activation of the immune and coagulation systems. Hypoxia and acidosis activate complement and prime neutrophils, resulting in the generation of oxygen free radicals and cytokine release. These mechanisms lead to injury of the capillary endothelial cells. These, in turn, further activate the immune and coagulation systems. Damaged endothelium loses its integrity and becomes 'leaky'. Spaces between endothelial cells allow fluid to leak out and tissue oedema ensues, exacerbating cellular hypoxia.

Systemic

Cardiovascular

As preload and afterload decrease, there is a compensatory baroreceptor response resulting in increased sympathetic activity and release of catecholamines into the circulation. This results in tachycardia and systemic vasoconstriction (except in sepsis – see below).

Respiratory

The metabolic acidosis and increased sympathetic response result in an increased respiratory rate and minute ventilation to increase the excretion of carbon dioxide (and so produce a compensatory respiratory alkalosis).

Renal

Decreased perfusion pressure in the kidney leads to reduced filtration at the glomerulus and a decreased urine output. The renin–angiotensin–aldosterone axis is stimulated, resulting in further vasoconstriction and increased sodium and water reabsorption by the kidney.

Endocrine

As well as activation of the adrenal and renin–angiotensin systems, vasopressin (antidiuretic hormone) is released from the hypothalamus in response to decreased preload and results in vasoconstriction and resorption of water in the renal collecting system. Cortisol is also released from the adrenal cortex contributing to the sodium and water resorption and sensitizing the cells to catecholamines.

Table 2.1 Cardiovascular and metabolic characteristics of shock.

	Hypovolaemia	Cardiogenic	Obstructive	Distributive
Cardiac output	Low	Low	Low	High
Vascular resistance	High	High	High	Low
Venous pressure	Low	High	High	Low
Mixed venous saturation	Low	Low	Low	High
Base deficit	High	High	High	High

Ischaemia–reperfusion syndrome

During the period of systemic hypoperfusion, cellular and organ damage progresses due to the direct effects of tissue hypoxia and local activation of inflammation. Further injury occurs once normal circulation is restored to these tissues. The acid and potassium load that has built up can lead to direct myocardial depression, vascular dilatation and further hypotension. The cellular and humoral elements activated by the hypoxia (complement, neutrophils, microvascular thrombi) are flushed back into the circulation where they cause further endothelial injury to organs such as the lungs and the kidneys. This leads to acute lung injury, acute renal injury, multiple organ failure and death. Reperfusion injury can currently only be attenuated by reducing the extent and duration of tissue hypoperfusion.

Classification of shock

There are numerous ways to classify shock, but the most common and most clinically applicable is one based on the initiating mechanism (Summary box 2.1).

All states are characterised by systemic tissue hypoperfusion and different states may coexist within the same patient.

Summary box 2.1

Classification of shock

- Hypovolaemic shock
- Cardiogenic shock
- Obstructive shock
- Distributive shock
- Endocrine shock

Hypovolaemic shock

Hypovolaemic shock is due to a reduced circulating volume. Hypovolaemia may be due to haemorrhagic or non-haemorrhagic causes. Non-haemorrhagic causes include poor fluid intake (dehydration), excessive fluid loss due to vomiting, diarrhoea, urinary loss (eg. diabetes), evaporation, or 'third-spacing' where fluid is lost into the gastrointestinal tract and interstitial spaces, as for example in bowel obstruction or pancreatitis.

Hypovolaemia is probably the most common form of shock, and to some degree is a component of all other forms of shock. Absolute or relative hypovolaemia must be excluded or treated in the management of the shocked state, regardless of cause.

Cardiogenic shock

Cardiogenic shock is due to primary failure of the heart to pump blood to the tissues. Causes of cardiogenic shock include myocardial infarction, cardiac dysrhythmias, valvular heart disease, blunt myocardial injury and cardiomyopathy. Cardiac insufficiency may also be due to myocardial depression due to endogenous factors (e.g. bacterial and humoral agents released in sepsis) or exogenous factors, such as pharmaceutical agents or drug abuse. Evidence of venous hypertension with pulmonary or systemic oedema may coexist with the classical signs of shock.

Obstructive shock

In obstructive shock there is a reduction in preload due to mechanical obstruction of cardiac filling. Common causes of obstructive shock include cardiac tamponade, tension pneumothorax, massive pulmonary embolus or air embolus. In each case, there is reduced filling of the left and/or right sides of the heart leading to reduced preload and a fall in cardiac output.

Distributive shock

Distributive shock describes the pattern of cardiovascular responses characterising a variety of conditions, including septic shock, anaphylaxis and spinal cord injury. Inadequate organ perfusion is accompanied by vascular dilatation with hypotension, low systemic vascular resistance, inadequate afterload and a resulting abnormally high cardiac output.

In anaphylaxis, vasodilatation is due to histamine release, while in high spinal cord injury there is failure of sympathetic outflow and adequate vascular tone (neurogenic shock). The cause in sepsis is less clear but is related to the release of bacterial products (endotoxin) and the activation of cellular and humoral components of the immune system. There is maldistribution of blood flow at a microvascular level with arteriovenous shunting and dysfunction of cellular utilization of oxygen.

In the later phases of septic shock there is hypovolaemia from fluid loss into interstitial spaces and there may be concomitant myocardial depression, complicating the clinical picture (Table 2.1).

Endocrine shock

Endocrine shock may present as a combination of hypovolaemic, cardiogenic or distributive shock. Causes of endocrine shock include hypo- and hyperthyroidism and adrenal insufficiency. Hypothyroidism causes a shock state similar to that of neuro-

Table 2.2 Clinical features of shock.

	Compensated	Mild	Moderate	Severe
Lactic acidosis	+	++	++	+++
Urine output	Normal	Normal	Reduced	Anuric
Conscious level	Normal	Mild anxiety	Drowsy	Comatose
Respiratory rate	Normal	Increased	Increased	Laboured
Pulse rate	Mild increase	Increased	Increased	Increased
Blood pressure	Normal	Normal	Mild hypotension	Severe hypotension

genic shock due to disordered vascular and cardiac responsiveness to circulating catecholamines. Cardiac output falls due to low inotropy and bradycardia. There may also be an associated cardiomyopathy. Thyrotoxicosis may cause a high-output cardiac failure.

Adrenal insufficiency leads to shock due to hypovolaemia and a poor response to circulating and exogenous catecholamines. Adrenal insufficiency may be due to pre-existing Addison's disease or be a relative insufficiency due to a pathological disease state, such as systemic sepsis.

Severity of shock

Compensated shock

As shock progresses, the body's cardiovascular and endocrine compensatory responses reduce flow to non-essential organs to preserve preload and flow to the lungs and brain. In compensated shock, there is adequate compensation to maintain central blood volume and preserve flow to the kidneys, lungs and brain. Apart from a tachycardia and cool peripheries (vasoconstriction, circulating catecholamines), there may be no other clinical signs of hypovolaemia.

However, this cardiovascular state is only maintained by reducing perfusion to the skin, muscle and gastrointestinal tract. There is a systemic metabolic acidosis and activation of humoral and cellular elements within the underperfused organs. Although clinically occult, this state will lead to multiple organ failure and death if prolonged due to the ischaemia–reperfusion effect described above under Ischaemia–reperfusion syndrome. Patients with occult hypoperfusion (metabolic acidosis despite normal urine output and cardiorespiratory vital signs) for more than 12 hours have a significantly higher mortality, infection rate and incidence of multiple organ failure (see below under Multiple organ failure).

Decompensation

Further loss of circulating volume overloads the body's compensatory mechanisms and there is progressive renal, respiratory and cardiovascular decompensation. In general, loss of around 15 per cent of the circulating blood volume is within normal compensatory mechanisms. Blood pressure is usually well maintained and only falls after 30–40 per cent of circulating volume has been lost.

Mild shock

Initially there is tachycardia, tachypnoea, a mild reduction in urine output and the patient may exhibit mild anxiety. Blood pressure is maintained although there is a decrease in pulse pressure. The peripheries are cool and sweaty with prolonged capillary refill times (except in septic distributive shock).

Moderate shock

As shock progresses, renal compensatory mechanisms fail, renal perfusion falls and urine output dips below 0.5 mL/kg per hour. There is further tachycardia, and now the blood pressure starts to fall. Patients become drowsy and mildly confused.

Severe shock

In severe shock, there is profound tachycardia and hypotension. Urine output falls to zero and patients are unconscious with laboured respiration.

Pitfalls

The classic cardiovascular responses described (Table 2.2) are not seen in every patient. It is important to recognise the limitations of the clinical examination and to recognise patients who are in shock despite the absence of classic signs.

Capillary refill

Most patients in hypovolaemic shock will have cool, pale peripheries, with prolonged capillary refill times. However, the actual capillary refill time varies so much in adults that it is not a specific marker of whether a patient is shocked, and patients with short capillary refill times may be in the early stages of shock. In distributive (septic) shock, the peripheries will be warm and capillary refill will be brisk, despite profound shock.

Tachycardia

Tachycardia may not always accompany shock. Patients who are on beta-blockers or who have implanted pacemakers are unable to mount a tachycardia. A pulse rate of 80 in a fit young adult who normally has a pulse rate of 50 is very abnormal. Furthermore, in some young patients with penetrating trauma, where there is haemorrhage but little tissue damage, there may be a paradoxical bradycardia rather than tachycardia accompanying the shocked state.

Blood pressure

It is important to recognise that hypotension is one of the last signs of shock. Children and fit young adults are able to maintain blood pressure until the final stages of shock by dramatic

Thomas Addison, 1799–1860, physician, Guy's Hospital, London, UK, described the effects of disease of the suprarenal capsules in 1849.

increases in stroke volume and peripheral vasoconstriction. These patients can be in profound shock with a normal blood pressure.

Elderly patients who are normally hypertensive may present with a 'normal' blood pressure for the general population but be hypovolaemic and hypotensive relative to their usual blood pressure. Beta-blockers or other medications may prevent a tachycardic response. The diagnosis of shock may be difficult unless one is alert to these pitfalls.

Consequences

Unresuscitatable shock

Patients who are in profound shock for a prolonged period of time become 'unresuscitatable'. Cell death follows from cellular ischaemia and the ability of the body to compensate is lost. There is myocardial depression and loss of responsiveness to fluid or inotropic therapy. Peripherally there is loss of the ability to maintain systemic vascular resistance and further hypotension ensues. The peripheries no longer respond appropriately to vasopressor agents. Death is the inevitable result.

This stage of shock is the combined result of the severity of the insult and delayed, inadequate or inappropriate resuscitation in the earlier stages of shock. Conversely, when patients present in this late stage, and have minimal responses to maximal therapy, it is important that the futility of treatment is recognised and valuable resources are not wasted.

Multiple organ failure

As techniques of resuscitation have improved, more and more patients are surviving shock. Where intervention is timely and the period of shock is limited, patients may make a rapid, uncomplicated recovery. However, the result of prolonged systemic ischaemia and reperfusion injury is end-organ damage and multiple organ failure.

Multiple organ failure is defined as two or more failed organ systems (Summary box 2.2).

Summary box 2.2

Effects of organ failure

- Lung: Acute respiratory distress syndrome
- Kidney: Acute liver insufficiency
- Clotting: Coagulopathy
- Cardiac: Cardiovascular failure

There is no specific treatment for multiple organ failure. Management is supporting of organ systems with ventilation, cardiovascular support and haemofiltration/dialysis until there is recovery of organ function. Multiple organ failure currently carries a mortality of 60 per cent; thus prevention is vital by early aggressive identification and reversal of shock.

RESUSCITATION

Immediate resuscitation manoeuvres for patients presenting in shock are to ensure a patent airway and adequate oxygenation and ventilation. Once 'airway' and 'breathing' are assessed and controlled, attention is directed to cardiovascular resuscitation.

Conduct of resuscitation

Resuscitation should not be delayed in order to definitively diagnose the source of the shocked state. However, the timing and nature of resuscitation will depend on the type of shock and the timing and severity of the insult. Rapid clinical examination will provide adequate clues to make an appropriate first determination, even if a source of bleeding or sepsis is not immediately identifiable. If there is initial doubt about the cause of shock, it is safer to assume the cause is hypovolaemia and begin with fluid resuscitation, and then assess the response.

In patients who are actively bleeding (major trauma, aortic aneurysm rupture, gastrointestinal haemorrhage), it is counterproductive to institute high-volume fluid therapy without controlling the site of haemorrhage. Increasing blood pressure merely increases bleeding from the site while fluid therapy cools the patient and dilutes available coagulation factors. Thus operative haemorrhage control should not be delayed and resuscitation should proceed in parallel with surgery.

Conversely, a patient with bowel obstruction and hypovolaemic shock must be adequately resuscitated before undergoing surgery otherwise the additional surgical injury and hypovolaemia induced during the procedure will exacerbate the inflammatory activation and increase the incidence and severity of end-organ insult.

Fluid therapy

In all cases of shock, regardless of classification, hypovolaemia and inadequate preload must be addressed before other therapy is instituted. Administration of inotropic or chronotropic agents to an empty heart will rapidly and permanently deplete the myocardium of oxygen stores and dramatically reduce diastolic filling and therefore coronary perfusion. Patients will enter the unresuscitatable stage of shock as the myocardium becomes progressively more ischaemic and unresponsive to resuscitative attempts.

First-line therapy, therefore, is intravenous access and administration of intravenous fluids. Access should be through short, wide-bore catheters that allow rapid infusion of fluids as necessary. Long, narrow lines, such as central venous catheters, have too high a resistance to allow rapid infusion and are more appropriate for monitoring than fluid replacement therapy.

Type of fluids

There is continuing debate over which resuscitation fluid is best for the management of shock. There is no ideal resuscitation fluid, and it is more important to understand how and when to administer it. In most studies of shock resuscitation there is no overt difference in response or outcome between crystalloid solutions (normal saline, Hartmann's solution, Ringer's lactate) or colloids (albumin or commercially available products). Furthermore, there is less volume benefit to the administration

Alexis Frank Hartmann, 1898–1964, paediatrician, St Louis, MO, USA, described the solution; should not be confused with the name of Henri Albert Charles Antoine Hartmann, French surgeon, who described the operation that goes by his name.

Sidney Ringer, 1835–1910, Professor of Clinical Medicine, University College Hospital, London, UK.

of colloids than had previously been thought, with only 1.3 times more crystalloid than colloid administered in blinded trials. On balance, there is little evidence to support the administration of colloids, which are more expensive and have worse side-effect profiles.

Most importantly, the oxygen carrying capacity of crystalloids and colloids is zero. If blood is being lost, the ideal replacement fluid is blood, although crystalloid therapy may be required while awaiting blood products.

Hypotonic solutions (dextrose etc.) are poor volume expanders and should not be used in the treatment of shock unless the deficit is free water loss (eg. diabetes insipidus) or patients are sodium overloaded (eg. cirrhosis).

Dynamic fluid response

The shock status can be determined dynamically by the cardiovascular response to the rapid administration of a fluid bolus. In total, 250–500 mL of fluid is rapidly given (over 5–10 minutes) and the cardiovascular responses in terms of heart rate, blood pressure and central venous pressure are observed. Patients can be divided into 'responders', 'transient responders' and 'non-responders'.

Responders have an improvement in their cardiovascular status which is sustained. These patients are not actively losing fluid but require filling to a normal volume status.

Transient responders have an improvement which then reverts to the previous state over the next 10–20 minutes. These patients have moderate ongoing fluid losses (either overt haemorrhage or further fluid shifts reducing intravascular volume).

Non-responders are severely volume depleted and are likely to have major ongoing loss of intravascular volume, usually through persistent uncontrolled haemorrhage.

Vasopressor and inotropic support

Vasopressor or inotropic therapy is not indicated as first-line therapy in hypovolaemia. As discussed above, administration of these agents in the absence of adequate preload rapidly leads to decreased coronary perfusion and depletion of myocardial oxygen reserves.

Vasopressor agents (phenylephrine, noradrenaline) are indicated in distributive shock states (sepsis, neurogenic shock) where there is peripheral vasodilatation, and a low systemic vascular resistance, leading to hypotension despite a high cardiac output. Where the vasodilatation is resistant to catecholamines (e.g. absolute or relative steroid deficiency) vasopressin may be used as an alternative vasopressor.

In cardiogenic shock, or where myocardial depression complicated a shock state (e.g. severe septic shock with low cardiac output), inotropic therapy may be required to increase cardiac output and therefore oxygen delivery. The inodilator dobutamine is the agent of choice.

Monitoring

The **minimum** standard for monitoring of the patient in shock is continuous heart rate and oxygen saturation monitoring, frequent non-invasive blood pressure monitoring and hourly urine output measurements. Most patients will need more aggressive invasive monitoring, including central venous pressure and invasive blood pressure monitoring (Summary box 2.3).

Summary box 2.3

Monitoring for patients in shock

Minimum
- ECG
- Pulse oximetry
- Blood pressure
- Urine output

Additional modalities
- Central venous pressure
- Invasive blood pressure
- Cardiac output
- Base deficit and serum lactate

Cardiovascular

Cardiovascular monitoring at a minimum should include continuous heart rate (ECG), oxygen saturation and pulse waveform and non-invasive blood pressure. Patients whose state of shock is not rapidly corrected with a small amount of fluid should have central venous pressure monitoring and continuous blood pressure monitoring through an arterial line.

Central venous pressure

There is no 'normal' central venous pressure (CVP) for a shocked patient, and reliance cannot be placed on an individual pressure measurement to assess volume status. Some patients may require a CVP of 5 cmH_2O, whereas some may require a CVP of 15 cmH_2O or higher. Further, ventricular compliance can change from minute to minute in the shocked state, and CVP is a poor reflection of end diastolic volume (preload).

CVP measurements should be assessed dynamically as response to a fluid challenge (see above). A fluid bolus (250–500 mL) is infused rapidly over 5–10 minutes.

The normal CVP response is a rise of 2–5 cmH_2O which gradually drifts back to the original level over 10–20 minutes. Patients with no change in their CVP are empty and require further fluid resuscitation. Patients with a large, sustained rise in CVP have high preload and an element of cardiac insufficiency or volume overload.

Cardiac output

Cardiac output monitoring allows not only assessment of the cardiac output but also the systemic vascular resistance and, depending on the technique used, end diastolic volume (preload) and blood volume. Use of invasive cardiac monitoring using pulmonary artery catheters is becoming less frequent as new non-invasive monitoring techniques, such as Doppler ultrasound, pulse waveform analysis and indicator dilution methods, provide similar information without many of the drawbacks of more invasive techniques.

Measurement of cardiac output, systemic vascular resistance and preload can help distinguish the types of shock present (hypovolaemia, distributive, cardiogenic), especially when they coexist. The information provided guides fluid and vasopressor therapy by providing real-time monitoring of the cardiovascular response.

Christian Johann Doppler, 1803–1853, Professor of Experimental Physics, Vienna, Austria, enunciated the Doppler principle in 1842.

Measurement of cardiac output is desirable in patients who do not respond as expected to first-line therapy, or who have evidence of cardiogenic shock or myocardial dysfunction. Early consideration should be given to instituting cardiac output monitoring on patients who require vasopressor or inotropic support.

Systemic and organ perfusion

Ultimately, the goal of treatment is to restore cellular and organ perfusion. Ideally, therefore, monitoring of organ perfusion should guide the management of shock. The best measures of organ perfusion and the best monitor of the adequacy of shock therapy remains the urine output. However, this is an hourly measure and does not give a minute-to-minute view of the shocked state. The level of consciousness is an important marker of cerebral perfusion, but brain perfusion is maintained until the very late stages of shock, and hence is a poor marker of adequacy of resuscitation (Table 2.3).

Currently, the only clinical indicators of perfusion of the gastrointestinal tract and muscular beds are the global measures of lactic acidosis (lactate and base deficit) and the mixed venous oxygen saturation.

Base deficit and lactate

Lactic acid is generated by cells undergoing anaerobic respiration. The degree of lactic acidosis, as measured by serum lactate level and/or the base deficit, is sensitive for both diagnosis of shock and monitoring the response to therapy. Patients with a base deficit over 6 mmol/L have a much higher morbidity and mortality than those with no metabolic acidosis. Furthermore, the duration of time in shock with an increased base deficit is important, even if all other vital signs have returned to normal (see occult hypoperfusion below under End points of resuscitation).

These parameters are measured from arterial blood gas analyses, and therefore the frequency of measurements is limited and they do not provide minute-to-minute data on systemic perfusion or the response to therapy. Nevertheless, the base deficit and/or lactate should be measured routinely in these patients until they have returned to normal levels.

Mixed venous oxygen saturation

The per cent saturation of oxygen returning to the heart from the body is a measure of the oxygen delivery and extraction by the tissues. Accurate measurement is via analysis of blood drawn from a long central line placed in the right atrium. Estimations can be made from blood drawn from lines in the superior vena cava, but these values will be slightly higher than those of a mixed venous sample (as there is relatively more oxygen extraction from the lower half of the body). Normal mixed venous oxygen saturation levels are 50–70 per cent. Levels below 50 per cent indicate inadequate oxygen delivery and increased oxygen extraction by the cells. This is consistent with hypovolaemic or cardiogenic shock.

High mixed venous saturations (>70 per cent) are seen in sepsis and some other forms of distributive shock. In sepsis, there is disordered utilization of oxygen at the cellular level, and arteriovenous shunting of blood at the microvascular level. Thus less oxygen is presented to the cells, and those cells cannot utilise what little oxygen is presented. Thus, venous blood has a higher oxygen concentration than normal.

Patients who are septic should therefore have mixed venous oxygen saturations above 70 per cent; below this level, they are not only in septic shock but also in hypovolaemic or cardiogenic shock. Although the S_vO_2 level is in the 'normal' range, it is low for the septic state, and inadequate oxygen is being supplied to cells that cannot utilize oxygen appropriately. This must be corrected rapidly. Hypovolaemia should be corrected with fluid therapy, and low cardiac output due to myocardial depression or failure should be treated with inotropes (dobutamine), to achieve a mixed venous saturation greater than 70 per cent (normal for the septic state).

New methods for monitoring regional tissue perfusion and oxygenation are becoming available, the most promising of which are muscle tissue oxygen probes, near-infrared spectroscopy and sublingual capnometry. While these techniques provide information regarding perfusion of specific tissue beds, it is as yet unclear whether there are significant advantages over existing measurements of global hypoperfusion (base deficit, lactate).

Table 2.3 Monitors for organ/systemic perfusion.

	Clinical	Investigational
Systemic perfusion		Base deficit
		Lactate
		Mixed venous oxygen saturation
Organ perfusion		
Muscle	–	Near-infrared spectroscopy
		Tissue oxygen electrode
Gut	–	Sublingual capnometry
		Gut mucosal pH
		Laser Doppler flowmetry
Kidney	Urine output	–
Brain	Conscious level	Tissue oxygen electrode
		Near-infrared spectroscopy

End points of resuscitation

It is much easier to know when to start resuscitation than when to stop. Traditionally, patients have been resuscitated until they have a normal pulse, blood pressure and urine output. However, these parameters are monitoring organ systems whose blood flow is preserved until the late stages of shock. A patient therefore may be resuscitated to restore central perfusion to the brain, lungs and kidneys and yet continue to underperfuse the gut and muscle beds. Thus activation of inflammation and coagulation may be ongoing and lead to reperfusion injury when these organs are finally perfused, and ultimately multiple organ failure.

This state of normal vital signs and continued underperfusion is termed 'occult hypoperfusion'. With current monitoring techniques, it is manifested only by a persistent lactic acidosis and low mixed venous oxygen saturation. The duration patients spend in this hypoperfused state has a dramatic effect on outcome. Patients with occult hypoperfusion for more than 12 hours have two to three times the mortality of patients with a limited duration of shock.

Resuscitation algorithms directed at correcting global perfusion end points (base deficit, lactate, mixed venous oxygen saturation) rather than traditional end points have been shown to improve mortality and morbidity in high-risk surgical patients. However, it is clear that despite aggressive regimens, some patients cannot be resuscitated to normal parameters within 12 hours by fluid resuscitation alone. More research is underway to identify the pathophysiology behind this and investigate new therapeutic options.

HAEMORRHAGE

Haemorrhage must be recognised and managed aggressively to reduce the severity and duration of shock and avoid death and/or multiple organ failure. Haemorrhage is treated by arresting the bleeding – not by fluid resuscitation or blood transfusion. Although necessary as supportive measures to maintain organ perfusion, attempting to resuscitate patients who have ongoing haemorrhage will lead to physiological exhaustion (coagulopathy, acidosis and hypothermia) and subsequently death.

Pathophysiology

Haemorrhage leads to a state of hypovolaemic shock. The combination of tissue trauma and hypovolaemic shock leads to the development of an endogenous coagulopathy called acute traumatic coagulopathy (ATC). Up to 25 per cent of trauma patients develop ATC within minutes of injury and it is associated with a four-fold increase in mortality. It is likely that ATC exists whenever there is the combination of shock and tissue trauma (e.g. major surgery). ATC is the component of trauma-induced coagulopathy (TIC) which is ultimately multifactorial (Figure 2.1).

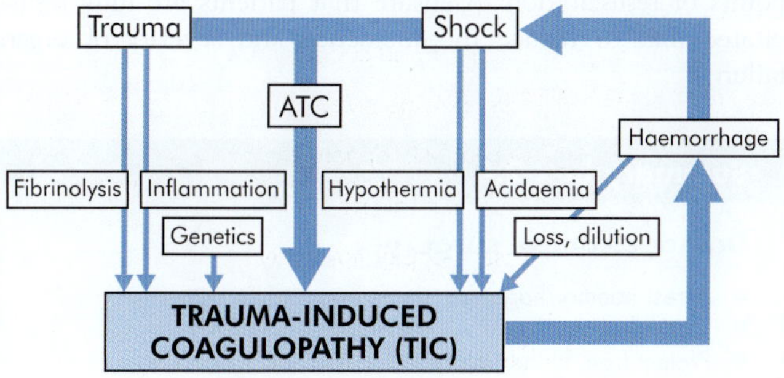

Figure 2.1 Trauma-induced coagulopathy.

Ongoing bleeding with fluid and red blood cell resuscitation leads to a dilution of coagulation factors which worsens the coagulopathy. In addition, the acidosis induced by the hypoperfused state leads to decreased function of the coagulation proteases, resulting in coagulopathy and further haemorrhage. The reduced tissue perfusion includes reduced blood supply to muscle beds. Underperfused muscle is unable to generate heat and hypothermia ensues. Coagulation functions poorly at low temperatures and there is further haemorrhage, further hypoperfusion and worsening acidosis and hypothermia. These three factors result in a downward spiral leading to physiological exhaustion and death (Figure 2.1).

Medical therapy has a tendency to worsen this effect. Intravenous blood and fluids are cold and exacerbate hypothermia. Further heat is lost by opening body cavities during surgery. Surgery usually leads to further bleeding and many crystalloid fluids are themselves acidic (e.g. normal saline has a pH of 6.7). Every effort must therefore be made to rapidly identify and stop haemorrhage, and to avoid (preferably) or limit physiological exhaustion from coagulopathy, acidosis and hypothermia.

Definitions

Revealed and concealed haemorrhage

Haemorrhage may be revealed or concealed. Revealed haemorrhage is obvious external haemorrhage, such as exsanguination from an open arterial wound or from massive haematemesis from a duodenal ulcer.

Concealed haemorrhage is contained within the body cavity and must be suspected, actively investigated and controlled. In trauma, haemorrhage may be concealed within the chest, abdomen, pelvis, retroperitoneum or in the limbs with contained vascular injury or associated with long-bone fractures. Examples of non-traumatic concealed haemorrhage include occult gastrointestinal bleeding or ruptured aortic aneurysm.

Primary, reactionary and secondary haemorrhage

Primary haemorrhage is haemorrhage occurring immediately due to an injury (or surgery). Reactionary haemorrhage is delayed haemorrhage (within 24 hours) and is usually due to dislodgement of clot by resuscitation, normalisation of blood pressure and vasodilatation. Reactionary haemorrhage may also be due to technical failure, such as slippage of a ligature.

Secondary haemorrhage is due to sloughing of the wall of a vessel. It usually occurs 7–14 days after injury and is precipitated by factors such as infection, pressure necrosis (such as from a drain) or malignancy.

Surgical and non-surgical haemorrhage

Surgical haemorrhage is due to a direct injury and is amenable to surgical control (or other techniques such as angioembolisation). Non-surgical haemorrhage is the general ooze from all raw surfaces due to coagulopathy and cannot be stopped by surgical means (except packing). Treatment requires correction of the coagulation abnormalities.

Degree and classification

The adult human has approximately 5 litres of blood (70 mL/kg children and adults, 80 mL/kg neonates). Estimation of the amount of blood that has been lost is difficult, inaccurate and usually underestimates the actual value.

External haemorrhage is obvious, but it may be difficult to estimate the actual volume lost. In the operating room, blood collected in suction apparatus can be measured and swabs soaked in blood weighed.

The haemoglobin level is a poor indicator of the degree of haemorrhage as it represents a concentration and not an absolute amount. In the early stages of rapid haemorrhage, the haemoglobin concentration is unchanged (as whole blood is lost). Later, as fluid shifts from the intracellular and interstitial spaces into the vascular compartment, the haemoglobin and haematocrit levels will fall.

The amount of haemorrhage can be classified into classes 1–4 based on the estimated blood loss required to produce certain physiological compensatory changes (Table 2.4). Although conceptually useful, there is variation across ages (the young compensate well, the old very poorly), variation between individuals (athletes versus the obese) and variation due to confounding factors (e.g. concomitant medications, pain).

Treatment should therefore be based upon the degree of hypovolaemic shock according to vital signs, preload assessment, base deficit and, most importantly, the dynamic response to fluid therapy. Patients who are 'non-responders' or 'transient responders' are still bleeding and must have the site of haemorrhage identified and controlled.

Table 2.4 Traditional classification of haemorrhagic shock.

	Class			
	1	2	3	4
Blood volume lost as percentage of total	<15%	15–30%	30–40%	>40%

Management

Identify haemorrhage

External haemorrhage may be obvious, but the diagnosis of concealed haemorrhage may be more difficult. Any shock should be assumed to be hypovolaemic until proved otherwise, and similarly, hypovolaemia should be assumed to be due to haemorrhage until this has been excluded.

Immediate resuscitative manoeuvres

Direct pressure should be placed over the site of external haemorrhage. Airway and breathing should be assessed and controlled as necessary. Large-bore intravenous access should be instituted and blood drawn for cross-matching (see Cross-matching below). Emergency blood should be requested if the degree of shock and ongoing haemorrhage warrants this.

Identify the site of haemorrhage

Once haemorrhage has been considered, the site of haemorrhage must be rapidly identified. Note this is not to definitively identify the exact location, but rather to define the next step in haemorrhage control (operation, angioembolisation, endoscopic control).

Clues may be in the history (previous episodes, known aneurysm, non-steroidal therapy for gastrointestinal (GI) bleeding) or examination (nature of blood – fresh, melaena; abdominal tenderness, etc.). For shocked trauma patients, the external signs of injury may suggest internal haemorrhage, but haemorrhage into a body cavity (thorax, abdomen) must be excluded with rapid investigations (chest and pelvis x-ray, abdominal ultrasound or diagnostic peritoneal aspiration).

Investigations for blood loss must be appropriate to the patient's physiological condition. Rapid bedside tests are more appropriate for profound shock and exsanguinating haemorrhage than investigations such as computed tomography (CT) which take time. Patients who are not actively bleeding can have a more methodical, definitive work-up.

Haemorrhage control

The bleeding, shocked patient must be moved rapidly to a place of haemorrhage control. This will usually be in the operating room but may be the angiography or endoscopy suites. These patients require surgical and anaesthetic support and full monitoring and equipment must be available.

Haemorrhage control must be achieved rapidly so as to prevent the patient entering the triad of coagulopathy–acidosis–hypothermia and physiological exhaustion. There should be no unnecessary investigations or procedures prior to haemorrhage control to minimize the duration and severity of shock. This includes prolonged attempts to volume resuscitate the patient prior to surgery, which will result in further hypothermia and clotting factor dilution until the bleeding is stopped. Attention should be paid to correction of coagulopathy with blood component therapy to aid surgical haemorrhage control.

Surgical intervention may need to be limited to the minimum necessary to stop bleeding and control sepsis. More definitive repairs can be delayed until the patient is haemodynamically stable and physiologically capable of sustaining the procedure. This concept of tailoring the operation to match the patient's physiology and staged procedures to prevent physiological exhaustion is called 'damage control surgery' – a term borrowed from the military which ensures continued functioning of a damaged ship above conducting complete repairs which would prevent rapid return to battle (Summary box 2.4).

Once haemorrhage is controlled, patients should be aggressively resuscitated, warmed and coagulopathy corrected. Attention should be paid to fluid responsiveness and the end points of resuscitation to ensure that patients are fully resuscitated and to reduce the incidence and severity of organ failure.

Summary box 2.4

Damage control surgery

- Arrest haemorrhage
- Control sepsis
- Protect from further injury
- Nothing else

Damage control resuscitation

These concepts have been combined into a new paradigm for the management of trauma patients with active haemorrhage called damage control resuscitation (DCR). The four central strategies of DCR are:

1. Anticipate and treat acute traumatic coagulopathy
2. Permissive hypotension until haemorrhage control
3. Limit crystalloid and colloid infusion to avoid dilutional coagulopathy
4. Damage control surgery to control haemorrhage and preserve physiology.

Damage control resuscitation strategies have been shown to reduce mortality and morbidity in patients with exsanguinating trauma and may be applicable in other forms of acute haemorrhage.

TRANSFUSION

The transfusion of blood and blood products has become commonplace since the first successful transfusion in 1818. Although the incidence of severe transfusion reactions and infections is now very low, in recent years it has become apparent that there is an immunological price to be paid from the transfusion of heterologous blood, leading to increased morbidity and decreased survival in certain population groups (trauma, malignancy). Supplies are also limited, and therefore the use of blood and blood products must always be judicious and justifiable for clinical need (Table 2.5).

Table 2.5 History of blood transfusion.

1492	Pope Innocent VIII suffers a stroke and receives a blood transfusion from three ten-year-old boys (paid a ducat each). All three boys died, as did the pope later that year
1665	Richard Lower in Oxford conducts the first successful canine transfusions
1667	Jean-Baptiste Denis reports successful sheep–human transfusions
1678	Animal–human transfusions are banned in France because of the poor results
1818	James Blundell performs the first successful documented human transfusion in a woman suffering post-partum haemorrhage. She received blood from her husband and survived
1901	Karl Landsteiner discovers the ABO system
1914	The Belgian physician Albert Hustin performed the first non-direct transfusion, using sodium citrate as an anticoagulant
1926	The British Red Cross instituted the first blood transfusion service in the world
1939	The Rhesus system was identified and recognised as the major cause of transfusion reactions

Blood and blood products

Blood is collected from donors who have been previously screened before donating, to exclude any donor whose blood may have the potential to harm the patient or to prevent possible harm that donating a unit of blood may have on the donor. In the UK, up to 450 mL of blood is drawn, a maximum of three times each year. Each unit is tested for evidence of hepatitis B, hepatitis C, HIV-1, HIV-2 and syphilis. Donations are leukodepleted as a precaution against variant Creutzfeldt–Jakob disease (this may also reduce the immunogenicity of the transfusion). The ABO and rhesus D blood group is determined, as well as the presence of irregular red cell antibodies. The blood is then processed into subcomponents.

Whole blood

Whole blood is now rarely available in civilian practice as it is an inefficient use of the limited resource. However, whole blood transfusion has significant advantages over packed cells as it is coagulation factor rich and, if fresh, more metabolically active than stored blood.

Packed red cells

Packed red blood cells are spun-down and concentrated packs of red blood cells. Each unit is approximately 330 mL and has a haematocrit of 50–70 per cent. Packed cells are stored in a SAG-M solution (saline–adenine–glucose–mannitol) to increase shelf life to 5 weeks at 2–6°C. (Older storage regimens included storage in CPD – citrate–phosphate–dextrose solutions which have a shelf life of 2–3 weeks.)

Fresh-frozen plasma

Fresh-frozen plasma (FFP) is rich in coagulation factors and is removed from fresh blood and stored at −40 to −50°C with a two-year shelf life. It is the first-line therapy in the treatment of coagulopathic haemorrhage (see below under Management of coagulopathy). Rhesus D-positive FFP may be given to a rhesus D-negative woman although it is possible for seroconversion to occur with large volumes due to the presence of red cell fragments, and rhesus D immunization should be considered.

Cryoprecipitate

Cryoprecipitate is a supernatant precipitate of FFP and is rich in factor VIII and fibrinogen. It is stored at −30°C with a two-year shelf life. It is given in low fibrinogen states or factor VIII deficiency.

Platelets

Platelets are supplied as a pooled platelet concentrate and contain about 250 × 10^9/L. Platelets are stored on a special agitator at 20–24°C and have a shelf life of only 5 days. Platelet transfusions are given to patients with thrombocytopenia or with platelet dysfunction who are bleeding or undergoing surgery.

Patients are increasingly presenting on antiplatelet therapy such as aspirin or clopidogrel for reduction of cardiovascular risk. Aspirin therapy rarely poses a problem but control of haemorrhage on the more potent platelet inhibitors can be extremely difficult. Patients on clopidogrel who are actively bleeding and undergoing major surgery may require almost continuous infusion of platelets during the course of the procedure. Arginine vasopressin or its analogues (DDAVP) have also been used in this patient group, although with limited success.

Hans Gerhard Creutzfeldt, 1885–1946, neurologist, Kiel, Germany.
Alfons Maria Jakob, neurologist, Hamburg, Germany.

Prothrombin complex concentrates

Prothrombin complex concentrates (PCC) are highly purified concentrates prepared from pooled plasma. They contain factors II, IX and X. Factor VII may be included or produced separately. It is indicated for the emergency reversal of anticoagulant (warfarin) therapy in uncontrolled haemorrhage.

Autologous blood

It is possible for patients undergoing elective surgery to predonate their own blood up to 3 weeks before surgery for retransfusion during the operation. Similarly, during surgery blood can be collected in a cell-saver which washes and collects red blood cells which can then be returned to the patient.

Indications for blood transfusion

Blood transfusions should be avoided if possible, and many previous uses of blood and blood products are now no longer considered appropriate use. The indications for blood transfusion are as follows:

- acute blood loss, to replace circulating volume and maintain oxygen delivery;
- perioperative anaemia, to ensure adequate oxygen delivery during the perioperative phase;
- symptomatic chronic anaemia, without haemorrhage or impending surgery.

Transfusion trigger

Historically, patients were transfused to achieve a haemoglobin >10 g/dL. This has now been shown to not only be unnecessary but also to be associated with an increased morbidity and mortality compared to lower target values. A haemoglobin level of 6 g/dL is acceptable in patients who are not actively bleeding, not about to undergo major surgery and are not symptomatic. There is some controversy as to the optimal haemoglobin level in some patient groups, such as those with cardiovascular disease, sepsis and traumatic brain injury. Although conceptually a higher haemoglobin improves oxygen delivery, there is little clinical evidence at this stage to support higher levels in these groups (Table 2.6).

Table 2.6 Perioperative red blood cell transfusion criteria.

Haemoglobin level (g/dL)	Indications
<6	Probably will benefit from transfusion
6–8	Transfusion unlikely to be of benefit in the absence of bleeding or impending surgery
>8	No indication for transfusion in the absence of other risk factors.

Blood groups and cross-matching

Human red cells have on their cell surface many different antigens. Two groups of antigens are of major importance in surgical practice – the ABO and rhesus systems.

ABO system

These are strongly antigenic and are associated with naturally occurring antibodies in the serum. The system consists of three allelic genes – A, B and O which control synthesis of enzymes that add carbohydrate residues to cell surface glycoproteins. A and B genes add specific residues while O gene is an amorph and does not transform the glycoprotein. The system allows for six possible genotypes although there are only four phenotypes. Naturally occurring antibodies are found in the serum of those lacking the corresponding antigen (Table 2.7).

Blood group O is the universal donor type as it contains no antigens to provoke a reaction. Conversely, group AB individuals are 'universal recipients' and can receive any ABO blood type as they have no circulating antibodies.

Rhesus system

The rhesus D (Rh(D)) antigen is strongly antigenic and is present in approximately 85 per cent of the population in the UK. Antibodies to the D antigen are not naturally present in the serum of the remaining 15 per cent of individuals, but their formation may be stimulated by the transfusion of Rh-positive red cells, or acquired during delivery of a Rh(D)-positive baby.

Acquired antibodies are capable, during pregnancy, of crossing the placenta and, if present in a Rh(D)-negative mother, may cause severe haemolytic anaemia and even death (hydrops fetalis) in a Rh(D)-positive fetus *in utero*. The other minor blood group antigens may be associated with naturally occurring antibodies, or may stimulate the formation of antibodies on relatively rare occasions.

Transfusion reactions

If antibodies present in the recipient's serum are incompatible with the donor's cells, a transfusion reaction will result. This usually takes the form of an acute haemolytic reaction. Severe immune-related transfusion reactions due to ABO incompatibility result in potentially fatal complement-mediated intravascular haemolysis and multiple organ failure. Transfusion reactions from other antigen systems are usually milder and self-limiting.

Febrile transfusion reactions are non-haemolytic and are usually caused by a graft-versus-host response from leukocytes in transfused components. Such reactions are associated with fever, chills or rigors. The blood transfusion should be stopped immediately. This form of transfusion reaction is rare with leukodepleted blood.

Cross-matching

To prevent transfusion reactions, all transfusions are preceded by ABO and rhesus typing of both donor and recipient blood to ensure compatibility. The recipient's serum is then mixed with the donor's cells to confirm ABO compatibility and to test for rhesus and any other blood group antigen–antibody reaction.

Full cross-matching of blood may take up to 45 minutes in most laboratories. In more urgent situations, 'type specific' blood is provided which is only ABO/rhesus matched and can be issued within 10–15 minutes. Where blood must be given emergently, group O (universal donor) blood is given (O− to females, O+ to males).

Karl Landsteiner, 1868–1943, Professor of Pathological Anatomy, University of Vienna, Austria. In 1909 he classified the human blood groups into A, B, AB and O. For this he was awarded the Nobel Prize for Physiology or Medicine in 1930.

Table 2.7 ABO blood group system.

Phenotype	Genotype	Antigens	Antibodies	Frequency (%)
O	OO	O	Anti-A, anti-B	46
A	AA or AO	A	Anti-B	42
B	BB or BO	B	Anti-A	9
AB	AB	AB	None	3

When blood transfusion is prescribed and blood is administered, it is essential that the correct patient receives the correct transfusion. Two healthcare personnel should check the patient details against the prescription and the label of the donor blood. In addition, the donor blood serial number should also be checked against the issue slip for that patient. Provided these principles are strictly adhered to, the number of severe and fatal ABO incompatibility reactions can be minimized.

Complications of blood transfusion

Complications from blood transfusion can be categorised as those arising from a single transfusion and those related to massive transfusion.

Complications from a single transfusion

Complications from a single transfusion include:

- incompatibility haemolytic transfusion reaction
- febrile transfusion reaction
- allergic reaction
- infection
  - bacterial infection (usually due to faulty storage)
  - hepatitis
  - HIV
  - malaria
- air embolism
- thrombophlebitis
- transfusion-related acute lung injury (usually from FFP).

Complications from massive transfusion

Complications from massive transfusion include:

- coagulopathy
- hypocalcaemia
- hyperkalaemia
- hypokalaemia
- hypothermia.

In addition, patients who receive repeated transfusions over long periods of time (e.g. patients with thalassaemia) may develop iron overload. (Each transfused unit of red blood cells contains approximately 250 mg of elemental iron.)

Management of coagulopathy

Correction of coagulopathy is not necessary if there is no active bleeding or haemorrhage is not anticipated (not due for surgery). However, coagulopathy following or during massive transfusion should be anticipated and managed aggressively. Standard guidelines are as follows:

- FFP if prothrombin time (PT) or partial thromboplastin time (PTT) >1.5 times normal
- cryoprecipitate if fibrinogen <0.8 g/L
- platelets if platelet count <50 × 109/mL.

However, in the presence of non-surgical haemorrhage these tests take time to arrange and may underestimate the degree of coagulopathy. Treatment should then be instituted on the basis of clinical evidence of non-surgical bleeding.

There are pharmacological adjuncts to blood component therapy, although their indications and efficacy are yet to be established. Antifibrinolytics such as tranexamic acid and aprotinin are the most commonly administered. Recombinant factor VIIa is also under investigation for the treatment of non-surgical haemorrhage.

Blood substitutes

Blood substitutes are an attractive alternative to the costly process of donating, checking, storing and administering blood – and due to the immunogenic and potential infectious complications associated with transfusion.

There are several oxygen-carrying blood substitutes under investigation in animal or early clinical trials. Blood substitutes are either biomimetic or abiotic. Biomimetic substitutes mimic the standard oxygen-carrying capacity of the blood and are haemoglobin based. Abiotic substitutes are synthetic oxygen carriers and are currently primarily perfluorocarbon based.

Haemoglobin is seen as the obvious candidate for developing an effective blood substitute. Various engineered molecules are under clinical trials, based on human, bovine or recombinant technologies. Second-generation perfluorocarbon emulsions are also showing potential in clinical trials.

FURTHER READING

Alam HB. An update on fluid resuscitation. *Scand J Surg* 2006; **95**: 136–45.

Duchesne JC, McSwain NE Jr, Cotton BA *et al.* Damage control resuscitation: the new face of damage control. *J Trauma* 2010; **69**: 976–90.

Otero RM, Nguyen HB, Huang DT *et al.* Early goal-directed therapy in severe sepsis and septic shock revisited: concepts, controversies and contemporary findings. *Chest* 2006; **130**: 1579–95.

Roussaint R, Cerny V, Coats TJ *et al.* Key issues in advanced bleeding care in trauma. *Shock* 2006; **26**: 322–31.

Sihler KC, Nathans AB. Management of severe sepsis in the surgical patient. *Surg Clin N Am* 2006; **86**: 1457–81.

CHAPTER 3

Wounds, tissue repair and scars

LEARNING OBJECTIVES

To understand:

- Normal healing and how it can be adversely affected
- How to manage wounds of different types, of different structures and at different sites
- Aspects of disordered healing that lead to chronic wounds
- The variety of scars and their treatment

INTRODUCTION

Wound healing is a mechanism whereby the body attempts to restore the integrity of the injured part. This falls far short of tissue regeneration by pluripotent cells, seen in some amphibians, and is often detrimental, as seen in the problems created by scarring, such as adhesions, keloids, contractures and cirrhosis of the liver. Several factors may influence healing (Summary box 3.1). However, a clean incised wound in a healthy person where there is no skin loss will follow a set pattern as outlined below.

Summary box 3.1

Factors influencing healing of a wound

- Site of the wound
- Structures involved
- Mechanism of wounding
  - Incision
  - Crush
  - Crush avulsion
- Contamination (foreign bodies/bacteria)[a]
- Loss of tissue
- Other local factors
  - Vascular insufficiency (arterial or venous)
  - Previous radiation
  - Pressure
- Systemic factors
  - Malnutrition or vitamin and mineral deficiencies
  - Disease (e.g. diabetes mellitus)
  - Medications (e.g. steroids)
  - Immune deficiencies (e.g. chemotherapy, acquired immunodeficiency syndrome (AIDS))
  - Smoking

[a] In explosions, the contamination may consist of tissue such as bone from another individual.

NORMAL WOUND HEALING

This is variously described as taking place in three or four phases, the most commonly agreed being:

1. the inflammatory phase;
2. the proliferative phase;
3. the remodelling phase (maturing phase).

Occasionally, a haemostatic phase is referred to as occurring before the inflammatory phase, or a destructive phase following inflammation consisting of the cellular cleansing of the wound by macrophages (Figure 3.1).

The inflammatory phase begins immediately after wounding and lasts 2–3 days. Bleeding is followed by vasoconstriction and thrombus formation to limit blood loss. Platelets stick to the damaged endothelial lining of vessels, releasing adenosine diphosphate (ADP), which causes thrombocytic aggregates to fill the wound. When bleeding stops, the platelets then release several cytokines from their alpha granules. These are platelet-derived growth factor (PDGF), platelet factor IV and transforming growth factor beta (TGFβ). These attract inflammatory cells such as polymorphonuclear lymphocytes (PMN) and macrophages. Platelets and the local injured tissue release vasoactive amines, such as histamine, serotonin and prostaglandins, which increase vascular permeability, thereby aiding infiltration of these inflammatory cells. Macrophages remove devitalised tissue and microorganisms while regulating fibroblast activity in the proliferative phase of healing. The initial framework for structural support of cells is provided by fibrin produced by fibrinogen. A more historical (Latin) description of this phase is described in four words: rubor (redness), tumour (swelling), calor (heat) and dolour (pain).

The proliferative phase lasts from the third day to the third week, consisting mainly of fibroblast activity with the production of collagen and ground substance (glycosaminoglycans and proteoglycans), the growth of new blood vessels as capillary loops (angioneogenesis) and the re-epithelialisation of the

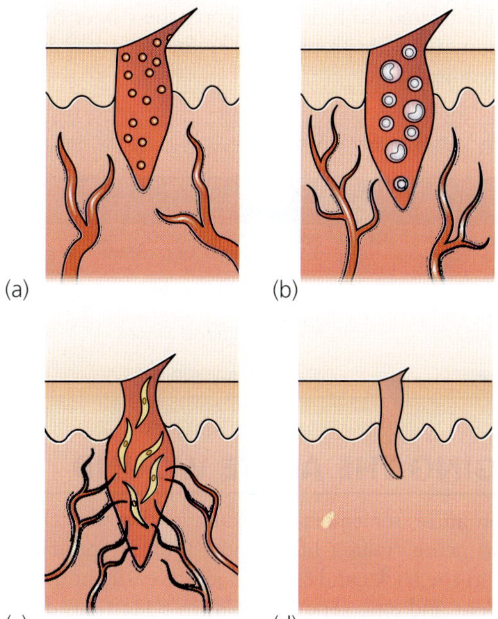

Figure 3.1 The phases of healing. (a) Early inflammatory phase with platelet-enriched blood clot and dilated vessels. (b) Late inflammatory phase with increased vascularity and increase in polymorphonuclear lymphocytes and lymphocytes (round cells). (c) Proliferative phase with capillary buds and fibroblasts. (d) Mature contracted scar.

wound surface. Fibroblasts require vitamin C to produce collagen. The wound tissue formed in the early part of this phase is called granulation tissue. In the latter part of this phase, there is an increase in the tensile strength of the wound due to increased collagen, which is at first deposited in a random fashion and consists of type III collagen.

The remodelling phase is characterised by maturation of collagen (type I replacing type III until a ratio of 4:1 is achieved). There is a realignment of collagen fibres along the lines of tension, decreased wound vascularity and wound contraction due to fibroblast and myofibroblast activity.

NORMAL HEALING IN SPECIFIC TISSUES

Bone

The phases are as above, but periosteal and endosteal proliferation leads to callus formation, which is immature bone consisting of osteoid (mineralised by hydroxyapatite and laid down by osteoblasts). In the remodelling phase, cortical structure and the medullary cavity are restored. If fracture ends are accurately opposed and rigidly fixed, callus formation is minimal and primary healing occurs. If a gap exists, then secondary healing may lead to delayed union, non-union or malunion.

Nerve

Distal to the wound, Wallerian degeneration occurs. Proximally, the nerve suffers traumatic degeneration as far as the last node of Ranvier. The regenerating nerve fibres are attracted to their receptors by neurotropism, which is mediated by growth factors, hormones and other extracellular matrix trophins. Nerve regeneration is characterised by profuse growth of new nerve fibres which sprout from the cut proximal end. Overgrowth of these, coupled with poor approximation, may lead to neuroma formation.

Tendon

While following the normal pattern of wound healing, there are two main mechanisms whereby nutrients, cells and new vessels reach the severed tendon. These are **intrinsic**, which consists of vincular blood flow and synovial diffusion, and **extrinsic**, which depends on the formation of fibrous adhesions between the tendon and the tendon sheath. The random nature of the initial collagen produced means that the tendon lacks tensile strength for the first 3–6 weeks. Active mobilisation prevents adhesions limiting range of motion, but the tendon must be protected by splintage in order to avoid rupture of the repair.

ABNORMAL HEALING

Some of the adverse influences on wound healing are listed in Summary box 3.1. Delayed healing may result in loss of function or poor cosmetic outcome. The aim of treatment is to achieve healing by primary intention and so reduce the inflammatory and proliferative responses (Summary box 3.2).

Healing by primary intention is also known as healing by first intention. This occurs when there is apposition of the wound edges and minimal surrounding tissue trauma that causes least inflammation and leaves the best scar. Delayed primary intention healing occurs when the wound edges are not opposed immediately, which may be necessary in contaminated or untidy wounds. The inflammatory and proliferative phases of healing are well established when delayed closure of the wound is carried out. This is also called healing by tertiary intention in some texts and will result in a less satisfactory scar than would result after healing by primary intention. Secondary healing or healing by secondary intention occurs in wounds that are left open and allowed to heal by granulation, contraction and epithelialisation.

Summary box 3.2

Classification of wound closure and healing

- Primary intention
  - Wound edges opposed
  - Normal healing
  - Minimal scar
- Secondary intention
  - Wound left open
  - Heals by granulation, contraction and epithelialisation
  - Increased inflammation and proliferation
  - Poor scar
- Tertiary intention (also called delayed primary intention)
  - Wound initially left open
  - Edges later opposed when healing conditions favourable

Augustus Volney Waller, 1816–1870, a general practitioner of Kensington, London, UK (1842–1851), who subsequently worked as a physiologist in Bonn, Germany; Paris, France; Birmingham, UK; and Geneva, Switzerland.

Louis Antoine Ranvier, 1835–1922, physician and histologist who was a professor in the College of France, Paris, France, described these nodes in 1878.

TYPES OF WOUNDS – TIDY VERSUS UNTIDY

The site injured, the structures involved in the injury and the mechanism of injury (e.g. incision or explosion) all influence healing and recovery of function. This has led to the management of wounds based upon their classification into tidy and untidy (Table 3.1 and Figure 3.2). The surgeon's aim is to convert untidy to tidy by removing all contaminated and devitalised tissue.

Primary repair of all structures (e.g. bone, tendon, vessel and nerve) may be possible in a tidy wound, but a contaminated wound with dead tissue requires debridement on one or several occasions before definitive repair can be carried out (the concept of 'second look' surgery). This is especially true in injuries caused by explosions, bullets or other missiles, where the external wound itself may appear much smaller than the wider extent of the injured tissues deep to the surface. Multiple debridements are often required after crushing injuries in road traffic accidents or in natural disasters such as earthquakes, where fallen masonry causes widespread muscle damage and compartment syndromes (see Compartment syndromes below). Any explosion where there are multiple victims at the same site or where there has been a suicide-related explosion will carry the risk of tissue and viral contamination. Appropriate tests for hepatitis and HIV viruses are required.

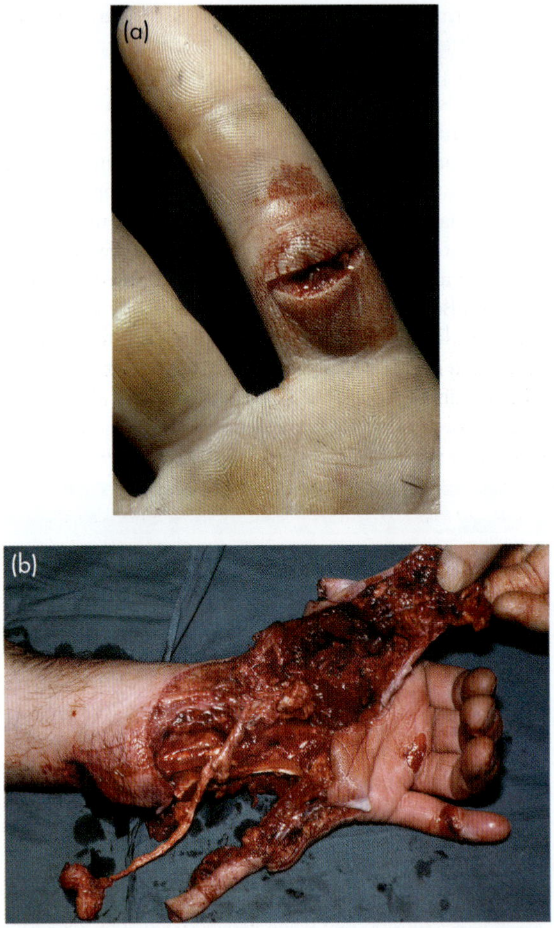

Figure 3.2 (a) Tidy incised wound on the finger. (b) Untidy avulsed wound on the hand.

The term '**debridement**' was introduced by the great French surgeon in Napoleon's army, Dominique Jean Larrey (1766–1842). He used it to describe the removal of bullets, bits of cloth, loose bits of bone and soft tissue.

Table 3.1 Tidy versus untidy wounds.

Tidy	Untidy
Incised	Crushed or avulsed
Clean	Contaminated
Healthy tissues	Devitalised tissues
Seldom tissue loss	Often tissue loss

MANAGING THE ACUTE WOUND

The surgeon must remember to examine the whole patient according to acute trauma life support (ATLS) principles. A stab wound in the back can be missed just as easily in the reality of the accident and emergency room as in a fictitious detective novel. The wound itself should be examined, taking into consideration the site and the possible structures damaged (Figure 3.3). It is essential to assess movement and sensation while watching for pain and listening to the patient. Tetanus cover should be noted and appropriate treatment carried out.

A bleeding wound should be elevated and a pressure pad applied. Clamps should not be put on vessels blindly as nerve damage is likely and vascular anastomosis is rendered impossible.

In order to facilitate examination, adequate analgesia and/or anaesthesia (local, regional or general) are required. General anaesthesia is often needed in children. In limb injuries, particularly those of the hand, a tourniquet should be used in order to facilitate visualisation of all structures. Due care should be taken with tourniquet application, avoiding uneven pressure and noting the duration of tourniquet time.

After assessment, a thorough debridement is essential. Abrasions, 'road rash' (following a fall from a motorbike) and explosions all cause dirt tattooing and require the use of a scrubbing brush or even excision under magnification. A wound should be explored and debrided to the limit of blood staining. Devitalised tissue must be excised until bleeding occurs with the obvious

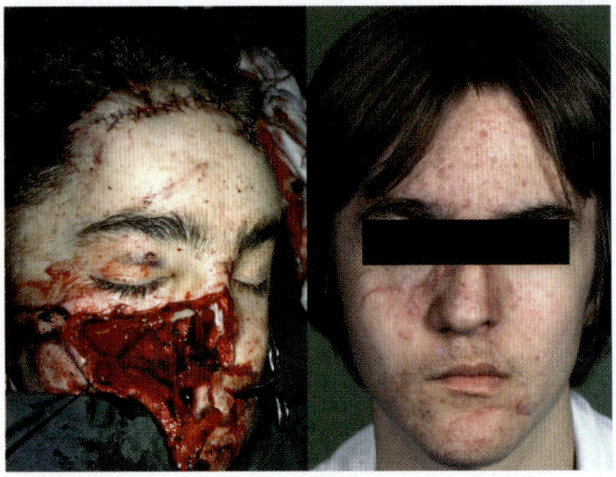

Figure 3.3 Facial trauma – apparent tissue loss but none found after careful matching.

exception of nerves, vessels and tendons. These may survive with adequate revascularisation subsequently or by being covered with viable tissue such as that brought in by skin or muscle flaps.

The use of copious saline irrigation or pulsed jet lavage (where the instrumentation is available) can be less destructive than knife or scissors when debriding. However, it has been suggested that pulsed jet lavage can implant dirt into a deeper plane and care should be taken to avoid this complication. Muscle viability is judged by the colour, bleeding pattern and contractility.

In a tidy wound, repair of all damaged structures may be attempted. Repair of nerves under magnification (loupes or microscope) using 8/0 or 10/0 monofilament nylon is usual. Vessels such as the radial or ulnar artery may be repaired using similar techniques. Tendon repairs, particularly those in the hand, benefit from early active mobilisation as this minimises adhesions between the tendon and the tendon sheath (see above under Tendon for extrinsic tendon healing mechanism).

Skin cover by flap or graft may be required as skin closure should always be without tension and should allow for the oedema typically associated with injury and the inflammatory phase of healing. A flap brings in a new blood supply and can be used to cover tendon, nerve, bone and other structures that would not provide a suitable vascular base for a skin graft. A skin graft has no inherent blood supply and is dependent on the recipient site for nutrition.

SOME SPECIFIC WOUNDS

Bites

Most bites involve either puncture wounds or avulsions. Small animal bites are common in children (Figure 3.4) and require cleansing and treatment according to the principles outlined in Summary box 3.3, usually under general anaesthetic.

Ear, tip of nose and lower lip injuries are most usually seen in victims of human bites. A boxing-type injury of the metacarpophalangeal joint may result from a perforating contact with the teeth of a victim. Anaerobic and aerobic organism prophylaxis is required as bite wounds typically have high virulent bacterial counts.

Puncture wounds

Wounds caused by sharp objects should be explored to the limit of tissue blood staining. Needle-stick injuries should be treated according to the well-published protocols because of hepatitis and human immunodeficiency virus (HIV) risks. X-ray examination should be carried out in order to rule out retained foreign bodies in the depth of the wound.

Summary box 3.3

Managing the acute wound

- Cleansing
- Exploration and diagnosis
- Debridement
- Repair of structures
- Replacement of lost tissues where indicated
- Skin cover if required
- Skin closure without tension
- All of the above with careful tissue handling and meticulous technique

Haematoma

If large, painful or causing neural deficit, a haematoma may require release by incision or aspiration. In the gluteal or thigh region, there may be an associated disruption of fat in the form of a fat fracture, which results in an unsightly groove but intact skin. An untreated haematoma may also calcify and therefore require surgical exploration if symptomatic.

Degloving

Degloving occurs when the skin and subcutaneous fat are stripped by avulsion from its underlying fascia, leaving neurovascular structures, tendon or bone exposed. A degloving injury may be open or closed. An obvious example of an open degloving is a ring avulsion injury with loss of finger skin (Figure 3.5). A closed degloving may be a rollover injury, typically caused by a motor vehicle over a limb. Such an injury will extend far further than expected, and much of the limb skin may be non-viable (Figure 3.6). Examination under anaesthetic is required with a radical excision of all non-bleeding skin, as judged by bleeding dermis. Fluoroscein can be administered intravenously while the patient is anaesthetised. Under ultraviolet light, viable (perfused) skin will show up as a fluorescent yellowish green colour, and the non-viable skin for excision is clearly mapped out. However, the main objection to this method is that of possible anaphylactic shock due to fluoroscein sensitivity. Most surgeons therefore rely upon serial excision until punctate dermal bleeding is obvious.

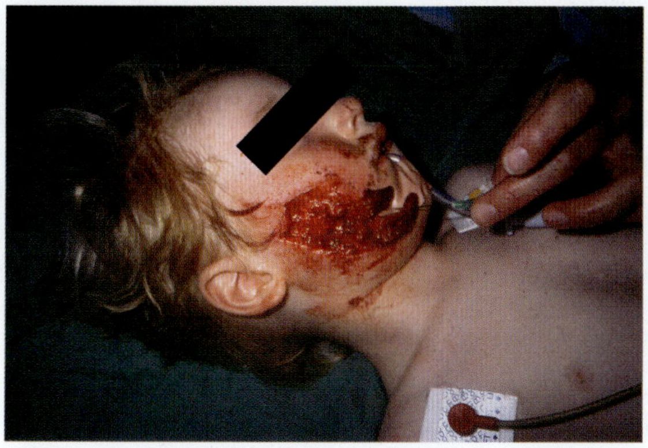

Figure 3.4 Dog bite in a child.

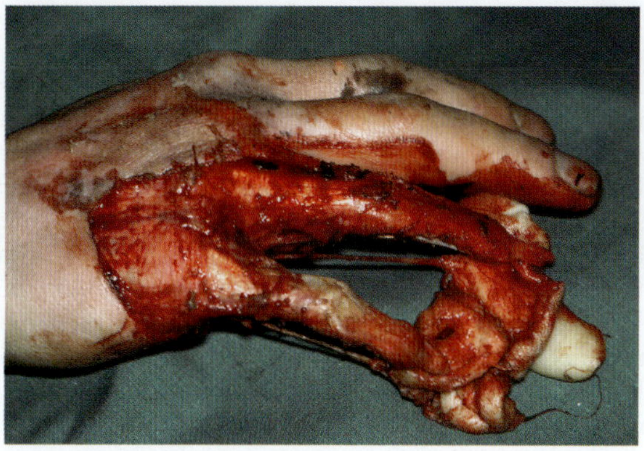

Figure 3.5 Degloving hand injury.

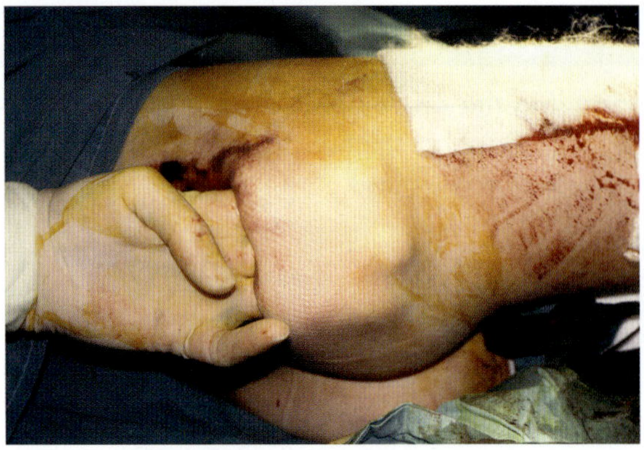

Figure 3.6 Degloving buttock injury.

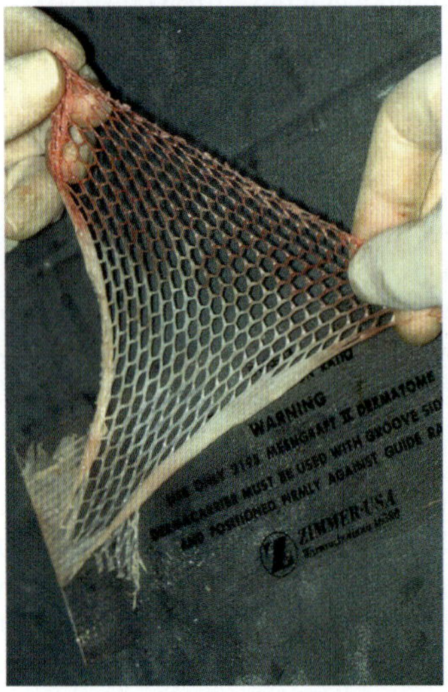

Figure 3.7 Meshed split-skin graft.

Split-skin grafts can be harvested from the degloved non-viable skin and meshed (Figure 3.7) to cover the raw areas resulting from debridement.

Compartment syndromes

Compartment syndromes typically occur in closed lower limb injuries. They are characterised by severe pain, pain on passive movement of the affected compartment muscles, distal sensory disturbance and, finally, by the absence of pulses distally (a late sign). They can occur in an open injury if the wound does not extend into the affected compartment.

Compartment pressures can be measured using a pressure monitor and a catheter placed in the muscle compartment. If pressures are constantly greater than 30 mmHg or if the above clinical signs are present, then fasciotomy should be performed. Fasciotomy involves incising the deep muscle fascia and is best carried out via longitudinal incisions of skin, fat and fascia (Figure 3.8). The muscle will be then seen bulging out through the fasciotomy opening. The lower limb can be decompressed via two incisions, each being lateral to the subcutaneous border of the tibia. This gives access to the two posterior compartments and to the peroneal and anterior compartments of the leg. In crush injuries that present several days after the event, a late fasciotomy can be dangerous as dead muscle produces myoglobin which, if suddenly released into the bloodstream, causes myoglobinuria with glomerular blockage and renal failure. In the late treatment of lower limb injuries, therefore, it may be safer to amputate the limb once viable and non-viable tissues have demarcated.

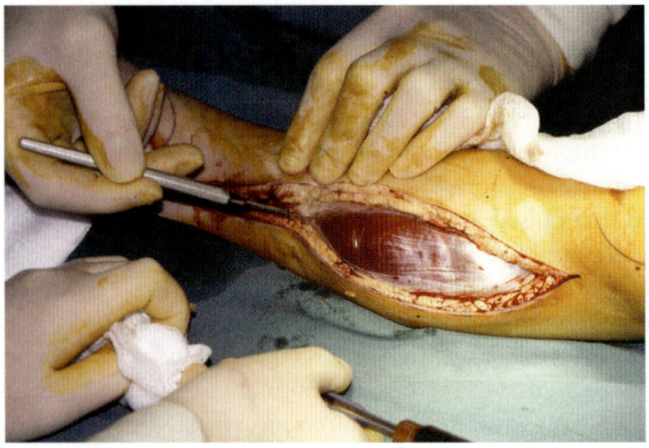

Figure 3.8 Fasciotomy of the lower leg.

High-pressure injection injuries

The use of high-pressure devices in cleaning, degreasing and painting can cause extensive closed injuries through small entry wounds. The liquid injected spreads along fascial planes, a common site being from finger to forearm. The tissue damage is dependent upon the toxicity of the substance and the injection pressure. Treatment is surgical with wide exposure, removal of the toxic substance and thorough debridement. Preoperative x-rays may be helpful where air or lead-based paints can be seen. It should be noted that amputation rates following high-pressure injection injuries are reported as being over 45 per cent. Delayed or conservative treatment is therefore inappropriate.

CHRONIC WOUNDS

Leg ulcers

In developed countries, the most common chronic wounds are leg ulcers. An ulcer can be defined as a break in the epithelial continuity. A prolonged inflammatory phase leads to overgrowth of granulation tissue, and attempts to heal by scarring leave a fibrotic margin. Necrotic tissue, often at the ulcer centre, is called slough. The more common aetiologies are listed in Summary box 3.4.

Summary box 3.4

Aetiology of leg ulcers

- Venous disease leading to local venous hypertension (e.g. varicose veins)
- Arterial disease, either large vessel (atherosclerosis) or small vessel (diabetes)
- Arteritis associated with autoimmune disease (rheumatoid arthritis, lupus, etc.)
- Trauma – could be self-inflicted
- Chronic infection – tuberculosis/syphilis
- Neoplastic – squamous or basal cell carcinoma, sarcoma

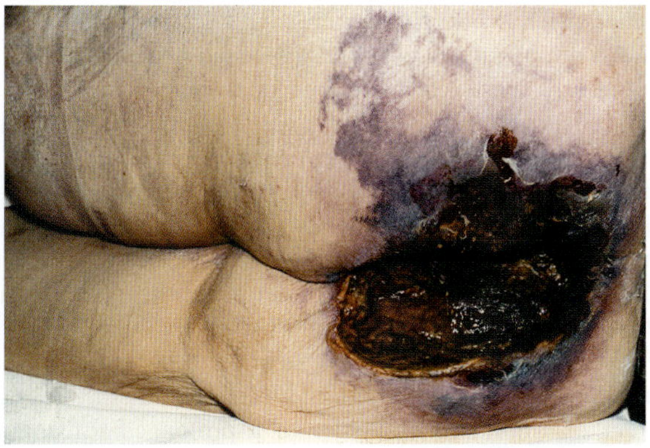

Figure 3.9 Pressure ulcer.

Table 3.2 Staging of pressure sores.

Stage	Description
1	Non-blanchable erythema without a breach in the epidermis
2	Partial-thickness skin loss involving the epidermis and dermis
3	Full-thickness skin loss extending into the subcutaneous tissue but not through underlying fascia
4	Full-thickness skin loss through fascia with extensive tissue destruction, maybe involving muscle, bone, tendon or joint

A chronic ulcer, unresponsive to dressings and simple treatments, should be biopsied to rule out neoplastic change, a squamous cell carcinoma known as a Marjolin's ulcer being the most common. Effective treatment of any leg ulcer depends on treating the underlying cause, and diagnosis is therefore vital. Arterial and venous circulation should be assessed, as should sensation throughout the lower limb. Surgical treatment is only indicated if non-operative treatment has failed or if the patient suffers from intractable pain. Meshed skin grafts (Figure 3.7) are more successful than sheet grafts and have the advantage of allowing mobilisation, as any tissue exudate can escape through the mesh. It should be stressed that the recurrence rate is high in venous ulceration, and patient compliance with a regime of hygiene, elevation and elastic compression is essential.

Pressure sores

These can be defined as tissue necrosis with ulceration due to prolonged pressure. Less preferable terms are bed sores, pressure ulcers and decubitus ulcers. They should be regarded as preventable but occur in approximately 5 per cent of all hospitalised patients (range 3–12 per cent in published literature). There is a higher incidence in paraplegic patients, in the elderly and in the severely ill patient. The most common sites are listed in Summary box 3.5.

> **Summary box 3.5**
>
> **Pressure sore frequency in descending order**
>
> - Ischium
> - Greater trochanter
> - Sacrum
> - Heel
> - Malleolus (lateral then medial)
> - Occiput

A staging system for description of pressure sores devised by the American National Pressure Ulcer Advisory Panel is shown in Table 3.2.

If external pressure exceeds the capillary occlusive pressure (over 30 mmHg), blood flow to the skin ceases leading to tissue anoxia, necrosis and ulceration (Figure 3.9). Prevention is obviously the best treatment with good skin care, special pressure dispersion cushions or foams, the use of low air loss and air-fluidised beds and urinary or faecal diversion in selected cases. Pressure sore awareness is vital, and the bed-bound patient should be turned at least every 2 hours, with the wheelchair-bound patient being taught to lift themselves off their seat for 10 seconds every 10 minutes.

Surgical management of pressure sores follows the same principles involved in acute wound treatment (Summary box 3.4). The patient must be well motivated, clinically stable with good nutrition and adhere to the preventative measures advised postoperatively. Preoperative management of the pressure sore involves adequate debridement, and the use of vacuum-assisted closure (VAC) may help to provide a suitable wound for surgical closure (see below). The aim is to fill the dead space and to provide durable sensate skin. Large skin flaps that include muscle are best and, occasionally, an intact sensory innervated area can be included (e.g. extensor fascia lata flap with lateral cutaneous nerve of the thigh). If possible, use a flap that can be advanced further if there is recurrence and that does not interfere with the planning of neighbouring flaps that may be used in the future.

Vacuum-assisted closure

This is now more correctly known as negative pressure wound closure. Applying intermittent negative pressure of approximately −125 mmHg appears to hasten debridement and the formation of granulation tissue in chronic wounds and ulcers. A foam dressing is cut to size to fit the wound. A perforated wound drain is placed over the foam, and the wound is sealed with a transparent adhesive film. A vacuum is then applied to the drain (Figure 3.10). Negative pressure may act by decreasing oedema, by removing interstitial fluid and by increasing blood flow. As a result, bacterial counts decrease and cell proliferation increases, thereby creating a suitable bed for graft or flap cover.

NECROTISING SOFT-TISSUE INFECTIONS

These are rare but often fatal. They are most commonly polymicrobial infections with Gram-positive aerobes (*Staphylococcus aureus*, *S. pyogenes*), Gram-negative anaerobes (*Escherichia coli*,

Hans Christian Joachim Gram, 1853–1938, Professor of Pharmacology (1891–1900) and of Medicine (1900–1923), Copenhagen, Denmark, described this method of staining bacteria in 1884.

Jean-Nicholas Marjolin, 1780–1850, surgeon, Paris, France, described the development of carcinomatous ulcers in scars in 1828.

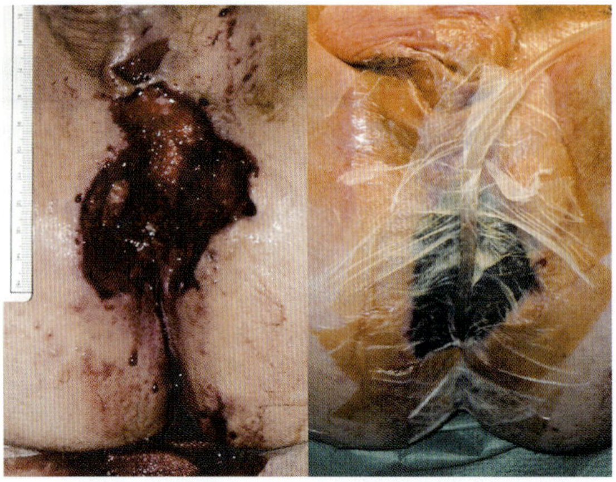

Figure 3.10 Vacuum-assisted closure dressing of a large wound.

Pseudomonas, *Clostridium*, *Bacteroides*) and β-haemolytic *Streptococcus*. There is usually a history of trauma or surgery with wound contamination. Sometimes, the patient's own defence mechanism may be deficient. These infections are characterised by sudden presentation and rapid progression. The fact that deeper tissues are involved often leads to a late or missed diagnosis (Figure 3.11). Clinical signs are shown in Summary box 3.6.

Summary box 3.6

Signs and symptoms of necrotising infections

- Unusual pain
- Oedema beyond area of erythema
- Crepitus
- Skin blistering
- Fever (often absent)
- Greyish drainage ('dishwater pus')
- Pink/orange skin staining
- Focal skin gangrene (late sign)
- Shock, coagulopathy and multiorgan failure

There are two main types of necrotising infections: clostridial (gas gangrene) and non-clostridial (streptococcal gangrene and necrotising fasciitis). The variant of necrotising fasciitis with toxic shock syndrome results from *Streptococcus pyogenes* and is often called the 'flesh-eating bug' in this situation. Treatment is surgical excision with tissue biopsies being sent for culture and diagnosis. Wide raw areas requiring skin grafting often result.

SCARS

The maturation phase of wound healing has been discussed above and represents the formation of what is described as a scar. The immature scar becomes mature over a period lasting a year or more, but it is at first pink, hard, raised and often itchy. The disorganised collagen fibres become aligned along stress lines with their strength being in their weave rather than in their amount (this has been compared with steel wool being slowly woven into a cable). As the collagen matures and becomes denser, the scar becomes almost acellular as the fibroblasts and blood vessels reduce. The external appearance of the scar becomes paler, while the scar becomes softer, flattens and its itchiness diminishes. Most of these changes occur over the first three months but a scar will continue to mature for one to two years. Tensile strength will continue to increase but would not be expected to exceed 60–80 per cent that of normal skin.

Scars are often described as being atrophic, hypertrophic and keloid. An atrophic scar is pale, flat and stretched in appearance, often appearing on the back and areas of tension. It is easily traumatised as the epidermis and dermis are thinned. Excision and resuturing may only rarely improve such a scar.

A hypertrophic scar is defined as excessive scar tissue that does not extend beyond the boundary of the original incision or wound. It results from a prolonged inflammatory phase of wound healing and from unfavourable scar siting (i.e. across the lines of skin tension). In the face, these are known as the lines of facial expression.

A keloid scar is defined as excessive scar tissue that extends beyond the boundaries of the original incision or wound (Figure 3.12). Its aetiology is unknown, but it is associated with elevated levels of growth factor, deeply pigmented skin, an inherited tendency and certain areas of the body (e.g. a triangle whose points are the xiphisternum and each shoulder tip).

The histology of both hypertrophic and keloid scars shows excess collagen with hypervascularity, but this is more marked in keloids where there is more type III collagen.

The treatment of both hypertrophic and keloid scars is difficult and is summarised in Summary box 3.7.

Hypertrophic scars improve spontaneously with time, whereas keloid scars do not.

Summary box 3.7

Treatment of hypertrophic and keloid scars

- Pressure – local moulds or elasticated garments
- Silicone gel sheeting (mechanism unknown)
- Intralesional steroid injection (triamcinolone)
- Excision and steroid injections[a]
- Excision and postoperative radiation (external beam or brachytherapy)[a]
- Intralesional excision (keloids only)
- Laser – to reduce redness (which may resolve in any event)
- Vitamin E or palm oil massage (unproven)

[a]All excisions have high rates of recurrence.

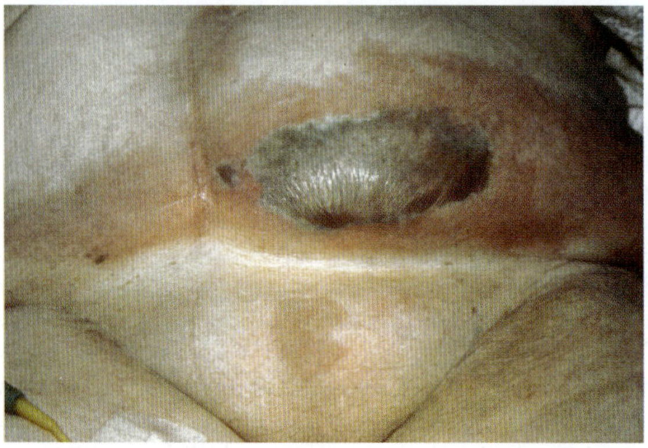

Figure 3.11 Necrotising fasciitis of the anterior abdominal wall.

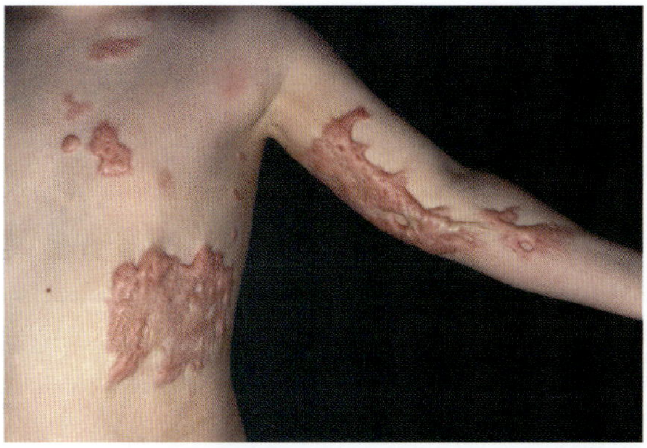

Figure 3.12 Multiple keloid scars.

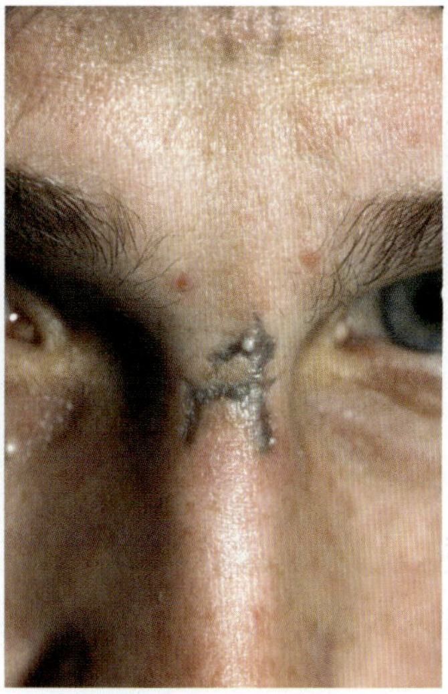

Figure 3.13 Dirt-ingrained scar.

AVOIDABLE SCARRING

If an acute wound has been managed correctly (Summary box 3.4), most of the problems described above should not occur. However, the surgeon should always stress to the patient that there will be a scar of some description after wounding, be it planned or accidental. A dirt-ingrained (tattooed) scar is usually preventable by proper initial scrubbing and cleansing of the wound (Figure 3.13). Late treatment may require excision of the scar or pigment destruction by laser.

Mismatched or misaligned scars result from a failure to recognise normal landmarks, such as the lip vermilion/white roll interface, eyelid and nostril free margins and hair lines such as those relating to eyebrows and moustache. Treatment consists of excision and resuturing.

Poorly contoured scars can be stepped, grooved or pincushioned. Most are caused by poor alignment of deep structures such as muscle or fat, but trapdoor or pincushioned scars are often unavoidable unless the almost circumferential wound can be excised initially. Late treatment consists of scar excision and correct alignment of deeper structures or, as in the case of a trapdoor scar, an excision of the scar margins and repair using W- or Z-plasty techniques.

Suture marks may be minimised by using monofilament sutures that are removed early (3–5 days). Sutures inserted under tension will leave marks. Wounds can be strengthened post-suture removal by the use of sticky strips. Fine sutures (6/0 or smaller) placed close to the wound margins tend to leave less scarring. Subcuticular suturing avoids suture marks either side of the wound or incision.

CONTRACTURES

Where scars cross joints or flexion creases, a tight web may form restricting the range of movement at the joint. This may be referred to as a contracture and can cause hyperextension or hyperflexion deformity (Figure 3.14). In the neck, it may interfere with head extension (Figure 3.15). Treatment may be simple involving multiple Z-plasties (Figure 3.16) or more complex requiring the inset of grafts or flaps. Splintage and intensive physiotherapy are often required postoperatively.

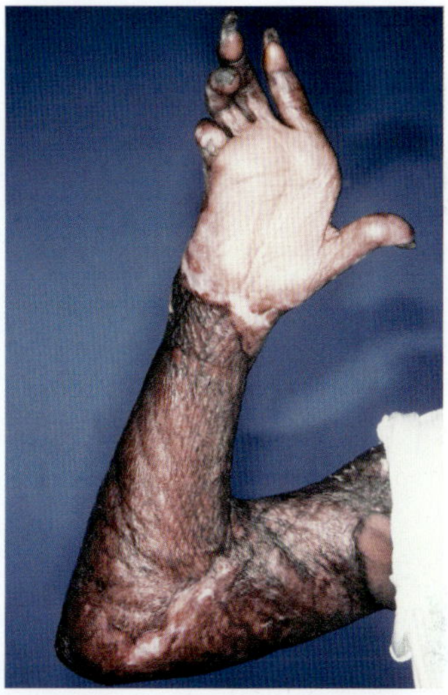

Figure 3.14 Burn contractures showing hyperextended fingers and hyperflexed elbow.

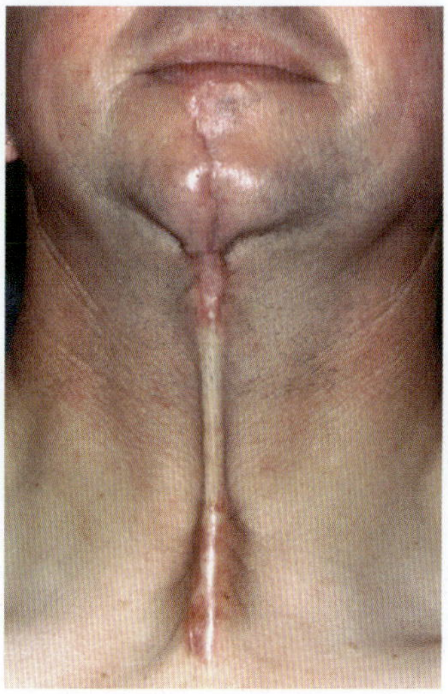

Figure 3.15 Post-traumatic (chainsaw) midline neck contracture.

Laser is an acronym for **L**ight **A**mplification by **S**timulated **E**mission of **R**adiation. A laser is an intense beam of monochromatic light.

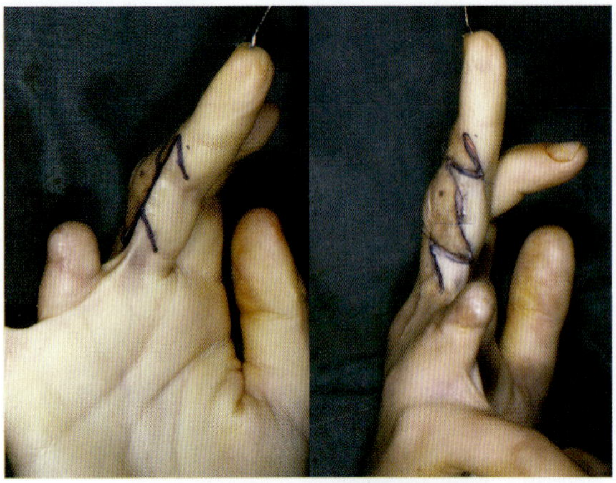

Figure 3.16 Multiple Z-plasty release of finger contracture.

FURTHER READING

Brown DL, Borschel GH. *Michigan manual of plastic surgery*. Baltimore, MD: Lippincott, Williams & Wilkins, 2004.

Georgiade GS, Riefkokl R, Levin LS. *Georgiade plastic, maxillofacial and reconstructive surgery*, 3rd edn. Baltimore, MD: Williams & Wilkins, 1997.

McGregor AD, McGregor, IA. *Fundamental techniques of plastic surgery*, 10th edn. Edinburgh, Churchill Livingstone, 2000.

Richards AM, MacLeod T, Dafydd H. *Key notes on plastic surgery*. Oxford, Wiley-Blackwell, 2012.

Thomas S. An introduction to the use of vacuum assisted closure. *World Wide Wounds* 2005; available from: www.worldwide-wounds.com.

Westaby S. *Wound care*. London: William Heinemann Medical Books Ltd, 1985.

CHAPTER 4

Basic surgical skills and anastomoses

LEARNING OBJECTIVES

To understand:
- The principles of skin and abdominal incisions
- The principles of wound closure

To know the principles in performing:
- Bowel anastomoses
- Vascular anastomoses

To be aware of:
- The principles of drain usage
- The principles of diathermy, ligasure and harmonic scalpel

INCISIONS

Skin incisions

Skin incisions should be made with a scalpel with the blade being pressed firmly down at right angles to the skin and then drawn gently across the skin in the desired direction to create a clean incision, the site and extent of which should have been clearly planned by the surgeon. It is important not to incise the skin obliquely as such a shearing mechanism can lead to necrosis of the undercut edge. The incision is facilitated by tension being applied across the line of the incision by the fingers of the non-dominant hand, but the surgeon must ensure that at no time is the scalpel blade directed at their own fingers as any slip may result in a self-inflicted injury. Blades for skin incisions usually have a curved cutting margin, while those used for an arteriotomy or drain site insertion have a sharp tip (Figure 4.1). Scalpels should at all times be passed in a kidney dish rather than by a direct hand-to-hand process as this can lead to a needle stick-like injury. Diathermy, laser and harmonic scalpels can be used instead of blades when opening deeper tissues, as it is felt that they can reduce blood loss and save operating time, and may reduce postoperative pain.

When planning a skin incision, four factors should be considered:

1. **Skin tension lines** (Langer's lines). These lines represent the orientation of the dermal collagen fibres and any incision placed parallel to these lines result in a better scar (Figure 4.2).
2. **Anatomical structure**. Incisions should avoid bony prominences and crossing skin creases if possible, and take into consideration underlying structures, such as nerves and vessels.
3. **Cosmetic factors**. Any incision should be made bearing in mind the ultimate cosmetic result, especially in exposed parts of the body, as an incision is the only part of the operation the patient sees.
4. **Adequate access for the procedure**. The incision must be functionally effective for the procedure in hand as any compromise purely on cosmetic grounds may render the operation ineffective or even dangerous.

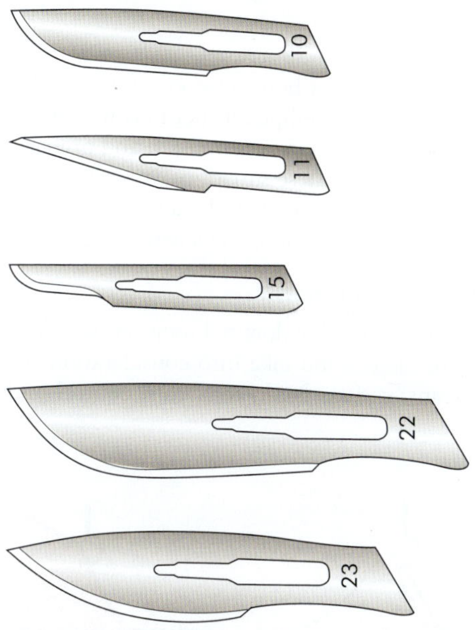

Figure 4.1 Scalpel blade sizes and shapes. The 22-blade is often used for abdominal incisions, the 11-blade for arteriotomy and the 15-blade for minor surgical procedures.

Occasionally, it may be necessary to excise a skin lesion with a circular incision in an area when the direction of Langer's lines are not apparent. However, once the circular incision has been made, it can often be observed that the circular incision is converted to an ellipse thus indicating the lines of tension. This circular incision should then be formally converted into an elliptical incision, remembering the rule of thumb that 'an elliptical incision must be at least three times as long as it is wide'

Karl Ritter Von Langer, Austrian anatomist, 1847–1888.

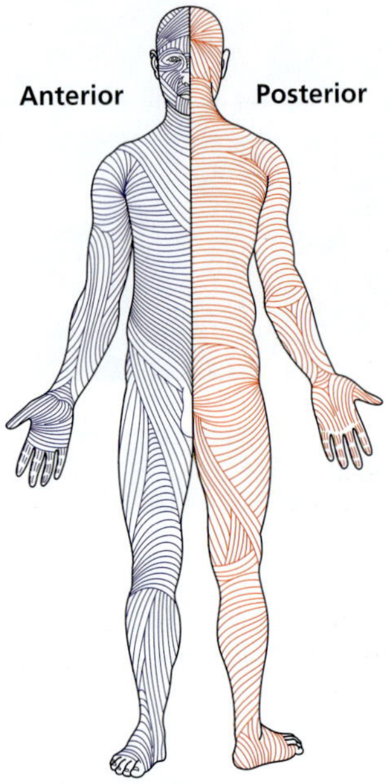

Figure 4.2 Langer's lines. These depict the orientation of the dermal collagen fibres. Reproduced with permission from Thomas WEG, Senninger N (eds). *Short stay surgery*. Berlin: Springer-Verlag, 2008.

for the wound to heal without tension. Occasionally, 'dog ears' remain in the corner of elliptical incisions in spite of adequate care having been taken during formation and primary closure of an elliptical wound. In these situations, it is advisable to pick up the 'dog ear' with a skin hook and excise it as shown in Figure 4.3. This allows for a satisfactory cosmetic outcome.

Abdominal incisions

As for skin incisions, all abdominal incisions should be planned in advance of surgery and take into consideration access to the relevant organs, surface landmarks, pain control and cosmetic outcome, e.g. transverse incisions tend to be associated with fewer respiratory complications and a better cosmetic outcome. In the past, traditionally vertical midline or paramedian incisions were used for the majority of abdominal procedures, but there is a current trend to utilise transverse incisions wherever possible as this minimises postoperative complications. The incision should be carried deeper through the subcutaneous tissues and then, depending on the site of the incision (Figure 4.4), the muscle layers should be divided or split, and the peritoneum displayed. This should be picked up between two clips and gently incised to ensure there is no damage to the underlying organs. This is particularly important in the emergency situation when there may be dilatation of the bowel. Every incision should be made with closure in mind, and the layers appropriately delineated. Mass closure of the abdominal wall is usually advocated using large bites and short steps in the closure technique using either non-absorbable (e.g. nylon or polypropylene) or very slowly absorbable suture material (e.g. polydioxanone suture (PDS)). It has been estimated that for abdominal wall closure, the length of the suture material should be at least four times the length of the wound to be closed to minimise the risk of abdominal dehiscence or later incisional hernia. Similar attention to detail applies to laparoscopic surgery, where access is of equal importance as correct port site placement and closure is crucial to the success of the operative procedure.

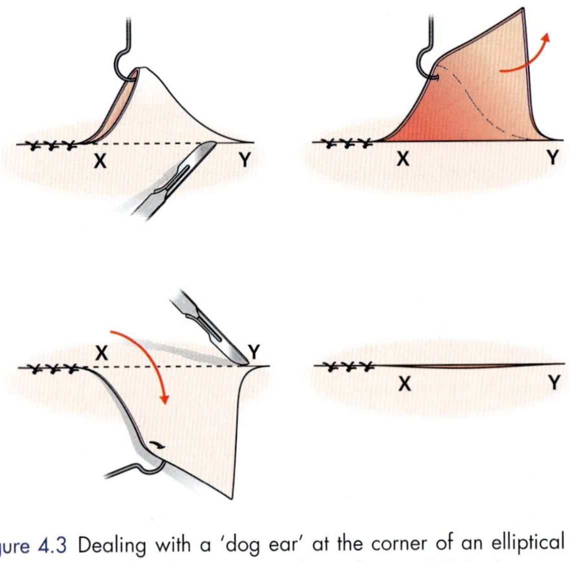

Figure 4.3 Dealing with a 'dog ear' at the corner of an elliptical incision. Reproduced with permission from Thomas WEG, Senninger N (eds). *Short stay surgery*. Berlin: Springer-Verlag, 2008.

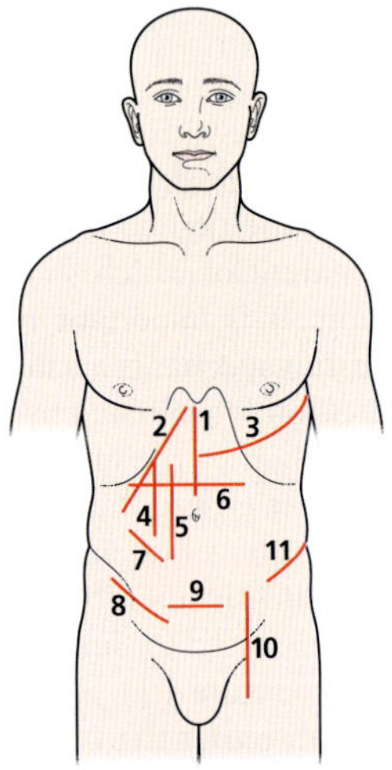

Figure 4.4 Abdominal incisions. Reproduced with permission from Thomas WEG. *Preparation and revision for the MRCS*. London: Churchill Livingstone (Elsevier Limited), 2004. 1, Midline; 2, Kocher's; 3, thoracoabdominal; 4, rectus split; 5, paramedian; 6, transverse; 7, McBurney's gridiron; 8, inguinal; 9, pfannenstiel; 10, McEvedy; 11, Rutherford Morison.

WOUND CLOSURE

The suturing of any incision or wound needs to take into consideration the site and tissues involved and the technique for closure should be chosen accordingly. There is no ideal wound closure technique that would be appropriate for all situations, and the ideal suture has yet to be produced, although many of the desired characteristics are listed in Summary box 4.1. Therefore, the correct choice of suture technique and suture material is vital, but will never compensate for inadequate

> **Summary box 4.1**
>
> **Suture material: desired characteristsics**
>
> - Easy to handle
> - Predictable behaviour in tissues
> - Predictable tensile strength
> - Sterile
> - Glides through tissues easily
> - Secure knotting ability
> - Inexpensive
> - Minimal tissue reaction
> - Non-capillary
> - Non-allergenic
> - Non-carcinogenic
> - Non-electrolytic
> - Non-shrinkage

operative technique, and for any wound to heal well, there must be a good blood supply and no tension on the closure.

Clean uninfected wounds with a good blood supply heal by primary intention and so closure simply requires accurate apposition of the wound edges. However, if a wound is left open, it heals by secondary intention through the formation of granulation tissue, which is tissue composed of capillaries, fibroblasts and inflammatory cells. Wound contraction and epithelialisation assist in ultimate healing, but the process may take several weeks or months. Delayed primary closure or tertiary intention is utilised when there is a high probability of the wound being infected. The wound is left open for a few days and then if any infective process is resolved then the wound is closed to heal by primary intention. Skin grafting is another form of tertiary intention healing (Summary box 4.2).

> **Summary box 4.2**
>
> **Types of wound healing**
>
> - Primary intention
>   - Clean wound
> - Secondary intention
>   - Healthy granulation tissue
>   - Over-exuberant granulation tissue
>   - Infected sloughy wound
>   - Black eschar
> - Tertiary intention
>   - Delayed closure
>   - Skin grafting

When choosing suture materials, there are certain specific requirements depending on the tissues to be sutured, e.g. vascular anastomoses require smooth, non-absorbable, non-elastic material, while biliary anastomoses require an absorbable material that will not promote tissue reaction or stone formation. When using absorbable material, the time in which wound support is required and maintained will vary according to the tissues in which it is inserted. Furthermore, certain tissues require wound support for longer than others, for example muscular aponeuroses compared with subcutaneous tissues. It is therefore crucial for the surgeon to select the suture material and suture technique that will most effectively achieve the desired objective for each wound closure or anastomosis.

Suture materials

History

> Sutures are best made of soft thread, not too hard twisted that it may sit easier on the tissue, nor are too few nor too many of either of them to be put in.
>
> Aurelius Cornelius Celsus, 25BC–AD50

Multiple examples of early surgery abound, with East African tribes ligating blood vessels with tendons strips, and closing wounds with acacia thorns pushed through the wound with strips of vegetable matter wound round these in a figure of eight. A South American method of wound closure involved using large black ants to bite the wound together with their pincers or jaws acting like skin clips, and then the ant's body was twisted off leaving the head in place keeping the wound apposed. By 1000BC, Indian surgeons were using horsehair, cotton and leather sutures while in Roman times, linen and silk and metal clips, called fibulae, were commonly used to close gladiatorial wounds. By the end of the nineteenth century, developments in the textile industry led to major advances, and both silk and catgut became popular as suture materials. Lister believed that catgut soaked in chromic acid (a form of tanning) prevented early dissolution in body fluids and tissues, while Moynihan felt that chromic catgut was ideal as it could be sterilised, was non-irritant to tissues, kept its strength until its work was done and then disappeared. However, catgut is no longer in use as it causes an inflammatory cellular reaction with release of proteases and may also carry the risk of prion transmission if of bovine origin.

Suture characteristics

There are five characteristics of any suture material that need to be considered:

1 **Physical structure**. Suture material may be monofilament or multifilament. Monofilament suture material is smooth and tends to slide through tissues easily without any sawing action, but is more difficult to knot effectively. Such material can be easily damaged by gripping it with needle holder or forceps and this can lead to fracture of the suture material. Multifilament or braided sutures are much easier to knot, but have a surface area of several thousand times that of monofilament sutures and thus have a capillary action and interstices where bacteria may lodge and be responsible for persistent infection or sinuses. In order to overcome some of these problems, certain materials are produced as a braided suture which is coated with silicone in order to make it smooth.

2 **Strength**. The strength of a suture material depends upon its constituent material, its thickness and how it is handled in the tissues. Suture material thickness is classified according to its diameter in tenths of a millimetre (Table 4.1), although

> **Berkley George Andrew Moynihan, (Lord Moynihan of Leeds)**, 1865–1936, Professor of Clinical Surgery, University of Leeds, Leeds, UK. Moynihan felt that English surgeons knew little about the work of their colleagues both at home and abroad. Therefore, in 1909, he established a small travelling club which in 1929 became the Moynihan Chirurgical Club. It still exists today. He took a leading part in founding the British Journal of Surgery in 1913 and became the first chairman of the editorial committee until his death.

Aurelius Cornelius Celsus, Roman physician, 25BC–AD50.
Joseph Lister (Lord Lister), Professor of Surgery in Glasgow, Edinburgh and King's College Hospital, London and Vice President of Royal College of Surgeons of England, 1827–1912.
Alexis Carrel, 1873–1944, a surgeon from Lyons in France who worked at the Rockefeller Institute for Medical Research in New York, NY, USA. He received the Nobel Prize for Physiology or Medicine in 1912 'in recognition for his works on vascular suture and the transplantation of blood vessels and organs'.
Gladiators were so called because they fought with a Roman sword called a '*gladius*'.

Table 4.1 Size of suture material.

Metric (EurPh)	Range of diameter (mm)	USP ('old')
1	0.100–0.149	5–0
1.5	0.150–0.199	4–0
2	0.200–0.249	3–0
3	0.300–0.349	2–0
3.5	0.350–0.399	0
4	0.400–0.499	1
5	0.500–0.599	2

the figure assigned is also dependent upon the nature of the material, e.g. absorbable material and non-absorbable material, such as polypropylene, may differ in their designations. The tensile strength of a suture can be expressed as the force required to break it when pulling the two ends apart, but is only a useful approximation as to its strength in the tissues, as what matters is the material's *in vivo* strength. Absorbable sutures show a decay of this strength with the passage of time and although a material may last in the tissues for the stated period in the manufacturer's product profile, its tensile strength cannot be relied on *in vivo* for this entire period. Materials such as catgut (no longer in use in the UK) has a tensile strength of only about a week while PDS will remain strong in the tissues for several weeks. However, even non-absorbable sutures do not necessarily maintain their strength indefinitely, and may degrade with time. Those non-absorbable materials of synthetic origin, such as polypropylene, probably retain their tensile strength indefinitely and do not change in mass in the tissues, although it is still possible for them to fracture. Non-absorbable materials of biological origin, such as silk, will definitely fragment with time and lose their strength, and such materials should never be used in vascular anastomoses for fear of late fistula formation.

3 **Tensile behaviour**. Suture materials behave differently depending upon their deformability and flexibility. Some may be 'elastic' in which the material will return to its original length once any tension is released, while others may be 'plastic' in which case this phenomenon does not occur. Sutures may be deformable in that a circular cross-section may be converted to an oval shape, or they may be more rigid and have the somewhat irritating capacity to kink and coil. Many synthetic materials demonstrate 'memory' in which they keep curling up in the shape that they adopted within the packaging. A sharp but gentle pull on the suture material helps to diminish this memory, but the more memory a suture material has, the less is the knot security. Therefore, knotting technique also plays a significant role in any suture line's tensile strength and it is important to recognise that sutures lose 50 per cent of their strength at the knot.

4 **Absorbability**. Suture materials may be absorbable (Table 4.2) or non-absorbable (Table 4.3) and this property must be taken into consideration when choosing suture materials for specific wound closures or anastomoses. Sutures for use in the biliary or urinary tract need to be absorbable in order to minimise the risk of stone production. However, a vascular anastomosis requires a non-absorbable material and it is wise to avoid braided material as platelet adherence may predispose to distal embolisation. Non-absorbable materials tend to be preferred where persistent strength is required and, as an artificial graft or prosthesis never heals fully or integrates into a host artery, persistent monofilament suture materials, such as polypropylene, are almost universally used.

5 **Biological behaviour**. The biological behaviour of suture material within the tissues depends upon the constituent raw material. Biological or natural sutures, such as catgut, are proteolysed, but this involves a process that is not entirely predictable and can cause local irritation and such materials are therefore seldom used. Man-made synthetic polymers are hydrolysed and their disappearance in the tissues is more predictable. However, the presence of pus, urine or faeces influences the final result and renders the outcome more unpredictable. There is also some evidence that in the gut, cancer cells may accumulate at sites where sutures persist, possibly giving rise to local recurrence. For this reason, synthetic materials that have a greater predictability and elicit minimal tissue reaction may have an important non-carcinogenic property.

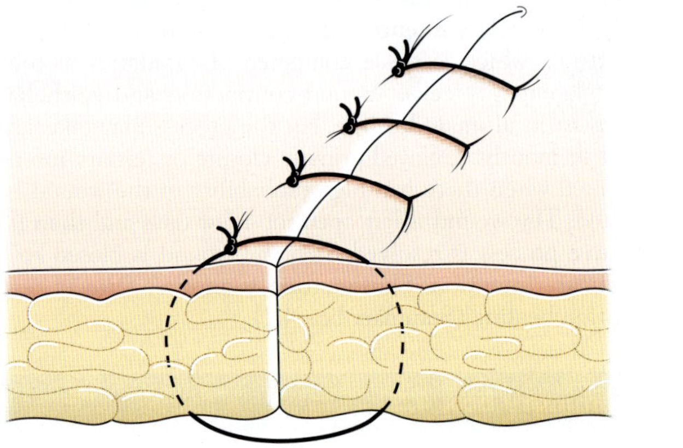

Figure 4.5 Interrupted suture technique. Reproduced with permission from Royal College of Surgeons of England. *The intercollegiate basic surgical skills course participants handbook*, edns 1–4. London: RCS.

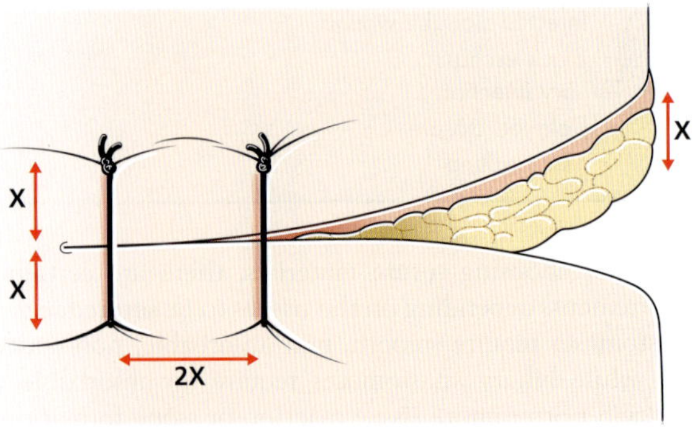

Figure 4.6 The siting of sutures. As a rule of thumb, the distance of insertion from the edge of the wound should correspond to the thickness of the tissue being sutured (x). Each successive suture should be placed at twice this distance apart (2x). Reproduced with permission from Royal College of Surgeons of England. *The intercollegiate basic surgical skills course participants handbook*, edns 1–4. London: RCS.

Table 4.2 Non-absorbable suture materials.

Suture	Types	Raw material	Tensile strength	Absorption rate	Tissue reaction	Contraindications	Frequent uses	How supplied
Silk	Braided or twisted multifilament. Dyed or undyed. Coated (with wax or silicone) or uncoated	Natural protein Raw silk from silkworm	Loses 20% when wet; 80–100% lost by 6 months. Because of tissue reactions and unpredictability, silk is increasingly not recommended	Fibrous encapsulation in body at 2–3 weeks Absorbed slowly over 1–2 years	Moderate to high Not recommended Consider suitable absorbable or non-absorbable	Not for use with vascular prostheses or in tissues requiring prolonged approximation under stress Risk of infection and tissue reaction makes silk unsuitable for routine skin closure	Ligation and suturing when long-term tissue support is necessary For securing drains externally	10/0–2 with needles, 4/0–1 without needles
Linen	Twisted	Long staple flax fibres	Stronger when wet Loses 50% at 6 months; 30% remains at 2 years	Non-absorbable Remains encapsulated in body tissues	Moderate	Not advised for use with vascular prostheses	Ligation and suturing in gastrointestinal surgery. No longer in common use in most centres	3/0–1 with needles, 3/0–1 without needles
Surgical steel	Monofilament or multifilament	An alloy of iron, nickel and chromium	Infinite (>1 year)	Non-absorbable Remains encapsulated in body tissues	Minimal	Should not be used in conjunction with prosthesis of different metal	Closure of sternotomy wounds Previously found favour for tendon and hernia repairs	Monofilament: 5/0–5 with needles; multifilament: 5/0–3/0 with needles
Nylon	Monofilament or braided multifilament Dyed or undyed	Polyamide polymer	Loses 15–20% per year	Degrades at approximately 15–20% per year	Low	None	General surgical use, e.g. skin closure, abdominal wall mass closure, hernia repair, plastic surgery, neurosurgery, microsurgery, ophthalmic surgery	Monofilament: 11/0–2 with needles (including loops in some sizes), 4/0–2 without needles; multifilament: 6/0–2 with needles, 3/0–1 without needles
Polyester	Monofilament or braided multifilament Dyed or undyed Coated (polybutylate or silicone) or uncoated	Polyester (polyethylene terephthalate)	Infinite (> 1 year)	Non-absorbable: remains encapsulated in body tissues	Low	None	Cardiovascular, ophthalmic, plastic and general surgery	Monofilament: (ophthalmic) 11/10; 10/0 with needles; multifilament: 5/0–1 with needles
Polybutester	Monofilament. Dyed or undyed	Polybutylene terephthalate and polytetramethylene ether glycol	Infinite (>1 year)	Non-absorbable: remains encapsulated in body tissues	Low	None	Exhibits a degree of elasticity. Particularly favoured for use in plastic surgery	7/0–1 with needles
Polypropylene	Monofilament. Dyed or undyed	Polymer of propylene	Infinite (>1 year)	Non-absorbable: remains encapsulated in body tissues	Low	None	Cardiovascular surgery, plastic surgery, ophthalmic surgery, general surgical subcuticular skin closure	10/0–1 with needles

Table 4.3 Absorbable suture materials.

Suture	Types	Raw material	Tensile strength retention *in vivo*	Absorption rate	Tissue reaction	Contraindications	Frequent uses	How supplied
Catgut	Plain	Collagen derived from healthy sheep or cattle	Lost within 7–10 days Marked patient variability Unpredictable and not recommended	Phagocytosis and enzymatic degradation within 7–10 days	High	Not for use in tissues which heal slowly and require prolonged support Synthetic absorbables are superior	Ligate superficial vessels, suture subcutaneous tissues Stomas and other tissues that heal rapidly	6/0–1 with needles; 4/0–3 without needles
Catgut	Chromic	Collagen derived from healthy sheep or cattle Tanned with chromium salts to improve handling and to resist degradation in tissue	Lost within 21–28 days Marked patient variability Unpredictable and not recommended	Phagocytosis and enzymatic degradation within 90 days	Moderate	As for plain catgut Synthetic absorbables superior	As for plain catgut	6/0–3 with needles; 5/0–3 without needles
Polyglactin	Braided multifilament	Copolymer of lactide and glycolide in a ratio of 90:10, coated with polyglactin and calcium stearate	Approximately 60% remains at 2 weeks Approximately 30% remains at 3 weeks	Hydrolysis minimal until 5–6 weeks. Complete absorption 60–90 days	Mild	Not advised for use in tissues which require prolonged approximation under stress	General surgical use where absorbable sutures required, e.g. gut anastomoses, vascular ligatures. Has become the 'workhorse' suture for many applications in most general surgical practices, including undyed for subcuticular wound closures. Ophthalmic surgery	8/0–2 with needles; 5/0–2 without needles
Polyglyconate	Monofilament Dyed or undyed	Copolymer of glycolic acid and trimethylene carbonate	Approximately 70% remains at 2 weeks Approximately 55% remains at 3 weeks	Hydrolysis minimal until 8–9 weeks. Complete absorption by 180 days	Mild	Not advised for use in tissues which require prolonged approximation under stress	Popular in some centres as an alternative to Vicryl and PDS	7/0–2 with needles
Polyglycolic acid	Braided multifilament Dyed or undyed Coated or uncoated	Polymer of polyglycolic acid. Available with coating of inert, absorbable surfactant poloxamer 188 to enhance surface smoothness 87% excreted in urine within 3 days	Approximately 40% remains at 1 week Approximately 20% remains at 3 weeks	Hydrolysis minimal at 2 weeks, significant at 4 weeks. Complete absorption 60–90 days	Minimal	Not advised for use in tissues which require prolonged approximation under stress	Uses as for other absorbable sutures, in particular where slightly longer wound support is required	9/0–2 with needles; 9/0–2 without needles
Polydioxanone (PDS)	Monofilament Dyed or undyed	Polyester polymer	Approximately 70% remains at 2 weeks Approximately 50% remains at 4 weeks Approximately 14% remains at 8 weeks	Hydrolysis minimal at 90 days Complete absorption at 180 days	Mild	Not for use in association with heart valves or synthetic grafts, or in situations in which prolonged tissue approximation under stress is required	Uses as for other absorbable sutures, in particular where slightly longer wound support is required	Polydioxanone suture (PDS) 10/0–2 with needles
Polyglycaprone	Monofilament	Copolymer of glycolite and caprolactone	21 days maximum	90–120 days	Mild	No use for extended support	Subcuticular in skin, ligation, gastrointestinal and muscle surgery	8/0–2 with needles

Suture techniques

There are four frequently used suture techniques.

1. **Interrupted sutures**. Interrupted sutures require the needle to be inserted at right angles to the incision and then to pass through both aspects of the suture line and exit again at right angles (Figure 4.5). It is important for the needle to be rotated through the tissues rather than to be dragged through for fear of unnecessarily enlarging the needle hole. As a guide, the distance from the entry point of the needle to the edge of the wound should be approximately the same as the depth of the tissue being sutured, and each successive suture should be placed at twice this distance apart (Figure 4.6). Each suture should reach into the depths of the wound and be placed at right angles to the axis of the wound. In linear wounds, it is sometimes easier to insert the middle suture first and then to complete the closure by successively inserting sutures, halving the remaining deficits in the wound length.
2. **Continuous sutures**. For a continuous suture, the first suture is inserted in an identical manner to an interrupted suture, but the rest of the sutures are inserted in a continuous manner until the far end of the wound is reached (Figure 4.7). Each throw of the continuous suture should be inserted at right angles to the wound and this will mean that the externally observed suture material will usually lie diagonal to the axis of the wound. It is important to have an assistant who will follow the suture, keeping it at the same tension in order to avoid either purse stringing the wound by too much tension, or leaving the suture material too slack. There is more danger of producing too much tension by using too little suture length than there is of leaving the suture line too lax. Postoperative oedema will often take up any slack in the suture material. At the far end of the wound, this suture line should be secured either by using an Aberdeen knot or by tying the free end to the loop of the last suture to be inserted.
3. **Mattress sutures**. Mattress sutures may be either vertical or horizontal and tend to be used to produce either eversion or inversion of a wound edge (Figure 4.8). The initial suture is inserted as for an interrupted suture, but then the needle either moves horizontally or vertically and traverses both edges of the wound once again. Such sutures are very useful in producing accurate approximation of wound edges, especially when the edges to be anastomosed are irregular in depth or disposition.
4. **Subcuticular suture**. This technique is used in skin where a cosmetic appearance is important and where the skin edges may be approximated easily (Figure 4.9). The suture material used may be either absorbable or non-absorbable. For non-absorbable sutures, the ends may be secured by means of a collar and bead, or tied loosely over the wound. When absorbable sutures are used, the ends may be secured using a buried knot. Small bites of the subcuticular tissues are

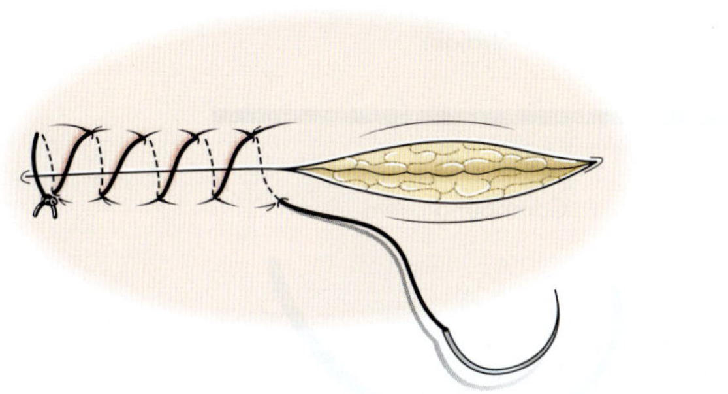

Figure 4.7 Continuous suture technique. Reproduced with permission from Royal College of Surgeons of England. *The intercollegiate basic surgical skills course participants handbook*, edns 1–4. London: RCS.

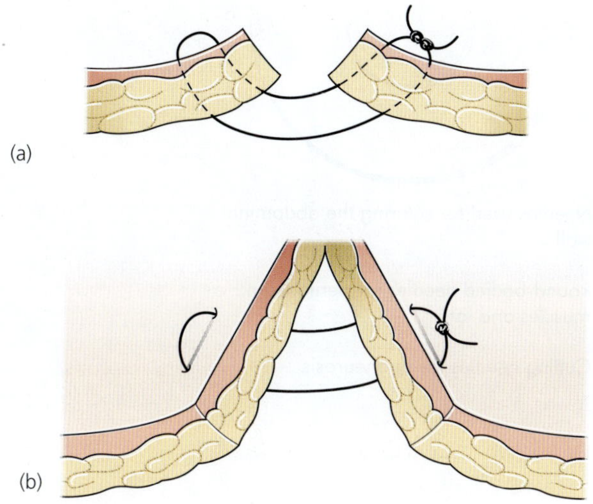

Figure 4.8 Mattress suture techniques. Reproduced with permission from Royal College of Surgeons of England. *The intercollegiate basic surgical skills course participants handbook*, edns 1–4. London: RCS.

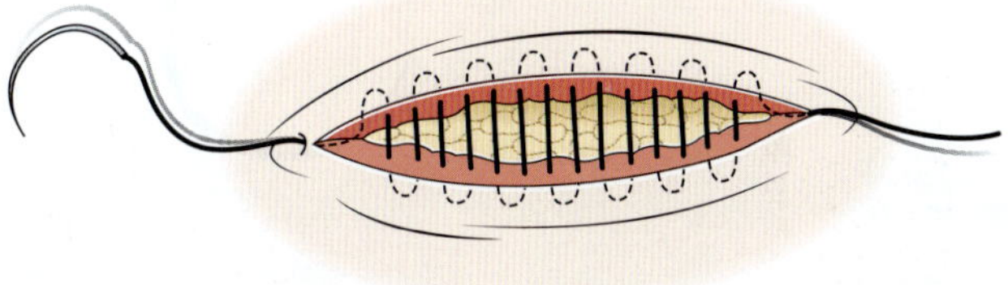

Figure 4.9 Subcuticular suture technique. Reproduced with permission from Royal College of Surgeons of England. *The intercollegiate basic surgical skills course participants handbook*, edns 1–4. London: RCS.

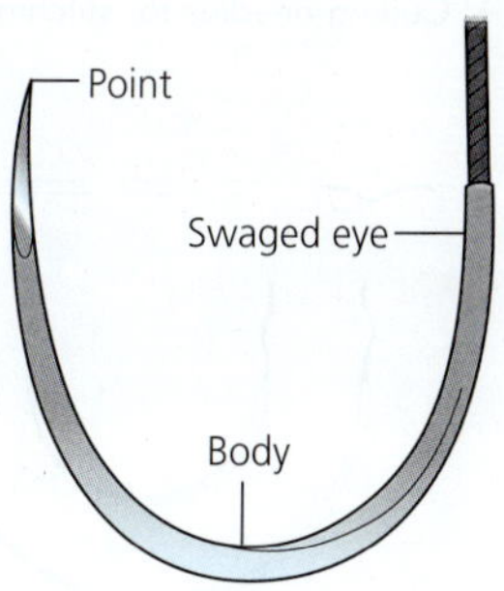

Figure 4.10 The basic parts of a needle. Reproduced with permission from Royal College of Surgeons of England. *The intercollegiate basic surgical skills course participants handbook*, edns 1–4. London: RCS.

taken on alternate sites of the wound and then gently pulled together thus approximating the wound edges without the risk of the cross-hatched markings of interrupted sutures.

Needles

In the past, needles had eyes in them and suture material had to be loaded into them, which was not only time consuming, but it meant that the needle holes in tissues were considerably larger than the suture material being used. Currently, needles are eyeless or 'atraumatic' with the suture material embedded within the shank of the needle. The needle has three main parts (Figure 4.10):

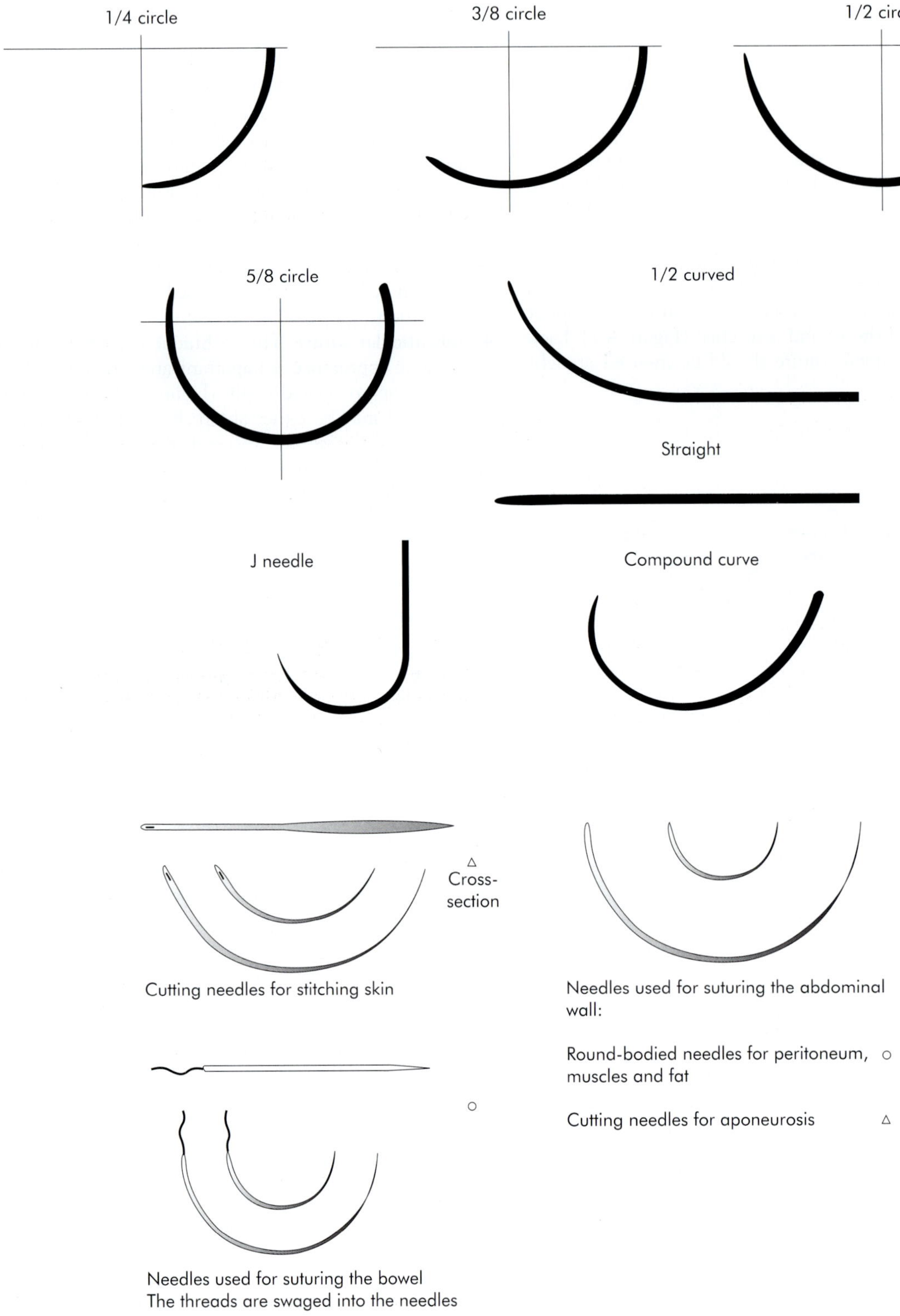

Figure 4.11 Types of needle.

1 Shank
2 Body
3 Point.

The needle should be grasped by the needle holder approximately one-third of the way back from the rear of the needle avoiding both the shank and the point.

The body of the needle is either round, triangular or flattened. Round-bodied needles gradually taper to a point, while triangular needles have cutting edges along all three sides. The actual point of the needle can be round with a tapered end, conventional cutting which has the cutting edge facing the inside of the needle's curvature, or reversed cutting in which the cutting edge is on the outside (Figure 4.11). Round-bodied needles are designed to separate tissue fibres rather than cut through them and are commonly used in intestinal and cardiovascular surgery. Cutting needles are used where tough or dense tissue needs to be sutured, such as skin and fascia. Blunt-ended needles are now being advocated in certain situations, such as closure of the abdominal wall, in order to diminish the risk of needle-stick injuries in this era of virally transmitted disorders.

The choice of needle shape tends to be dictated by the accessibility of the tissue to be sutured, and the more confined the operative space, the more curved the needle. Hand-held straight needles may be used on skin, although today it is advocated that needle holders should be used in all cases to reduce the risk of needle-stick injuries. Half circle needles are commonly utilised in the gastrointestinal tract, while J-shaped needles, quarter circle needles and compound curvature needles are used in special situations such as the vagina, eye and oral cavity, respectively. The size of the needle tends to correspond with the gauge of the suture material, although it is possible to get similar sutures with differing needle sizes.

Knotting techniques

Knot tying is one of the most fundamental techniques in surgery and yet is often poorly performed. The principles behind a secure knot are poorly understood by many surgeons and sadly a poorly constructed knot may thus jeopardise an otherwise successful surgical procedure. The general principles behind knot tying include:

- The knot must be tied firmly, but without strangulating the tissues.
- The knot must be unable to slip or unravel.
- The knot must be as small as possible to minimise the amount of foreign material.
- The knot must be tightened without exerting any tension or pressure on the tissues being ligated, i.e. the knot should be bedded down carefully, only exerting pressure against counter-pressure from the index finger or thumb.
- During tying, the suture material must not be 'sawed' as this weakens the thread.
- The suture material must be laid square during tying, otherwise tension during tightening may cause breakage or fracture of the thread.
- When tying an instrument knot, the thread should only be grasped at the free end, as gripping the thread with artery forceps or needle holders can damage the material and again result in breakage or fracture.
- The standard surgical knot is the reef knot (Figure 4.12), with a third throw for security, although with monofilament sutures such as for vascular surgery, six to eight throws are required for security.
- A granny knot involves two throws of the same type of throw and is a slip knot. It may be useful in achieving the right tension in certain circumstances, but must be followed by a standard reef knot to ensure security.
- When added security is required, a surgeon's knot using a two-throw technique is advisable to prevent slippage.
- When using a continuous suture technique, an Aberdeen knot may be used for the final knot. The free end of the suture is partially pulled through the final loop several times before being pulled through a final time completely prior to cutting.
- When the suture is cut after knotting, the ends should be left about 1–2 mm long to prevent unraveling. This is particularly important when using monofilament material.

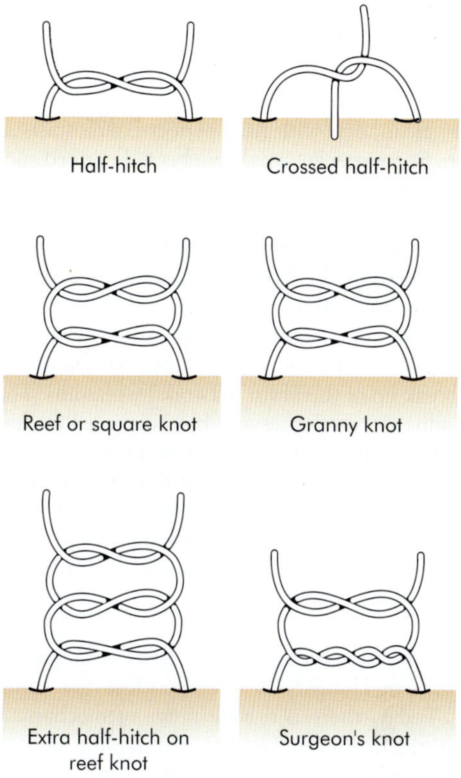

Figure 4.12 Standard knotting formation.

Alternatives to sutures

Many alternatives to standard suture techniques now exist and are in common usage.

Skin adhesive strips

For the skin, self-adhesive tapes or steristrips may be used where there is no tension and not too much moisture, such as after a wide excision of a breast lump. They may also be used to minimise 'spreading' of a scar. Other adhesive polyurethane films, such as Opsite, Tegaderm or Bioclusive, may provide a similar benefit, while such transparent dressings also allow wound inspection and may protect against cross-infection.

Tissue glue

Tissue glue is also available based upon a solution of n-butyl-2-cyanoacrylate monomer. When it is applied to a wound, it polymerises to form a firm adhesive bond, but the wound does need to be clean, dry, with near perfect haemostasis and under no tension. Some specific uses have been described such as closing a laceration on the forehead of a fractious child in Accident and Emergency thus dispensing with local anaesthetic and sutures. Although it is relatively expensive, it is quick to use, does not delay wound healing and is associated with an allegedly low infection rate. Other tissue glues involve fibrin and work on the principles of converting fibrinogen to fibrin by thrombin with crosslinking by Factor XIII, and the addition of aprotinin to slow the break up of the fibrin network by plasmin. This process has good adhesive properties and has been used for haemostasis in the liver and spleen, for dural tears, in ear, nose and throat (ENT) and ophthalmic surgery, to attach skin grafts and also to prevent haemoserous collections under flaps. Fibrin glues have also been used to control gastrointestinal haemorrhage endoscopically, but do not work when the bleeding is brisk.

Staples

Mechanical stapling devices were first used successfully by Hümer Hültl in Hungary in 1908 to close the stomach after resection. Today, there is a wide range of mechanical devices with linear, side-to-side and end-to-end stapling devices that can be used both in the open surgery setting and laparoscopically. Most of these devices are disposable and relatively expensive, but their cost is offset by the saving of operative time and the potential increase in the range of surgery possible (see below).

Clips

Skin clips produce a very neat scar with good wound eversion and a minimal cross-hatching effect. They can be placed faster than suture insertion and have a lower predisposition to infection as they do not penetrate entirely through the wound and do not produce a complete track from one wound edge to the other. However, they can be uncomfortable for the patient and they require a special instrument to remove them. Furthermore, they tend to be a more expensive method for wound closure than simple suture techniques.

Stapling devices

In the gastrointestinal tract, stapling devices tend to apply two rows of staples, offset in relation to each other to produce a sound anastomosis (Figure 4.13). Many of them also simultaneously divide the bowel or tissue that has been stapled while other devices merely insert the staples and the bowel has to be divided separately. For all stapling devices, it is crucial for the surgeon to understand the principles behind each device and to know intimately the mechanism and function of the instrument.

- **End-to-end anastomoses.** Circular stapling devices allow tubes to be joined together and such instruments are in common use in the oesophagus and low rectum. The detached stapling head/anvil is introduced into one end of the bowel, usually being secured within it by means of a purse-string suture. The body of the device is then inserted into the other end of the bowel, either via the rectum for a low rectal anastomosis, or via an enterotomy for an oesophago-jejunostomy, and either the shaft is extended through a small opening in the bowel wall or is secured by a further purse-string suture. The head/anvil is reattached to the shaft and the two ends approximated. Once the device is fully closed as indicated by the green indicator in the window, the device is fired, and after unwinding, the stapler is gently withdrawn. It is important to assess the integrity of the anastomosis by examining the 'doughnuts' of tissue excised for completeness. It is essential that no extraneous tissue is allowed to become interposed between the two bowel walls on closing the stapler.
- **Transverse anastomoses.** These instruments, which come in different sizes, simply provide two rows of staples for a single transverse anastomosis. They are useful for closing bowel ends, and the larger sizes have been used to create gastric tubes and gastric partitioning. One technical point of importance is that the bowel should be divided before the instrument is reopened after firing, as the instrument is designed with a ridge along which to pass a scalpel to ensure the correct length cuff of bowel remains adjacent to the staple line. Down in the pelvis it may be helpful to use such a device with a moveable head (roticulator).
- **Intraluminal anastomoses.** These instruments have two limbs which can be detached. Each limb is introduced into a loop of bowel, the limbs reassembled and the device closed. On firing, two rows of staples are inserted either side of the divided bowel, the division occurring by means of a built-in blade that is activated at the same time as the insertion of staples. Such an instrument may be used in fashioning a gastro-jejunostomy or jejuno-jejunostomy and is used in ileal pouch formation.
- **Other devices.** Other devices are produced that will staple/ligate and divide blood vessels. Skin closure may also be undertaken using hand-held stapling devices rather than individually picking up staples/clips and inserting them as described above. Many of the intestinal stapling devices are now adapted to be inserted down cannulae during laparoscopic surgery, and although they look very different, the principles of function are identical to the open surgery variety.

THE PRINCIPLES OF ANASTOMOSES

Bowel anastomoses

The word anastomosis comes from the Greek 'ανα', without, and 'στομα', a mouth, reflecting the join of a tubular viscus (bowel) or vessel (usually arteries) after a resection or bypass procedure. Prior to the nineteenth century, intestinal surgery was limited to exteriorisation by means of a stoma or closure of simple lacerations. Lembert then described his seromuscular suture technique for bowel anastomosis in 1826, while Senn advocated a two-layer technique for closure. Kocher's method utilised a two-layer anastomosis, first a continuous all-layer suture using catgut, then an inverting continuous (or interrupted) seromuscular layer suture using silk, which became the mainstay of bowel anatomoses for many years (Figure 4.14). However, Halsted favoured a one-layer extramucosal closure, and this was subsequently advocated by Matheson as it was felt to cause the least tissue necrosis or luminal narrowing (Figure 4.15). This techniqe has now become

Hümer Hültl, surgeon, St Stephen's Hospital, Budapest, Hungary, described his gastric stapler in 1908.
Antoine Lembert, 1802–1851, surgeon, Hôtel Dieu, Paris, France.
Nicolas Senn, 1844–1908, Professor of Surgery, Rush Medical College, Chicago, IL, USA.
Emil Theodor Kocher, 1841–1917, Professor of Surgery, Berne, Switzerland. In 1909, he was awarded the Nobel Prize for Physiology or Medicine for his work on the thyroid.
William Stewart Halsted, 1852–1922, Professor of Surgery, Johns Hopkins Hospital Medical School, Baltimore, MD, USA.
Norman Alistair Matheson, 1907–1966, formerly surgeon, Aberdeen Royal Infirmary, UK.

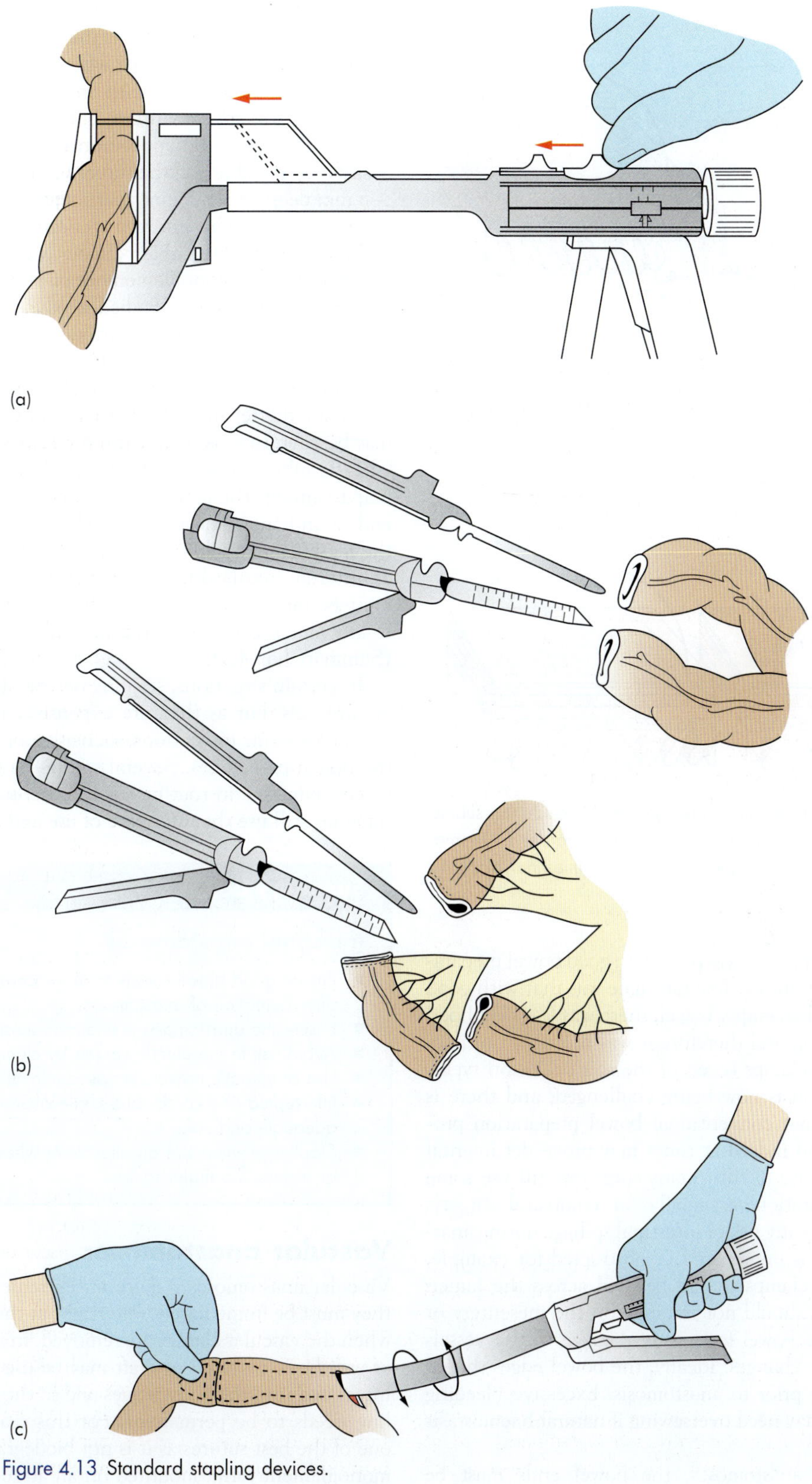

Figure 4.13 Standard stapling devices.

widely accepted, although it is essential that this is not confused with a seromuscular suture technique. The extramucosal suture must include the submucosa as this has a high collagen content and is the most stable suture layer in all sections of the gastrointestinal tract. There are several prospective randomised trials between two-layer and single-layer anastomoses demonstrating that there is probably little to choose between these techniques, provided basic essentials as highlighted in Summary box 4.3 are observed. However, catgut and silk have been replaced by synthetic, usually absorbable, polymers.

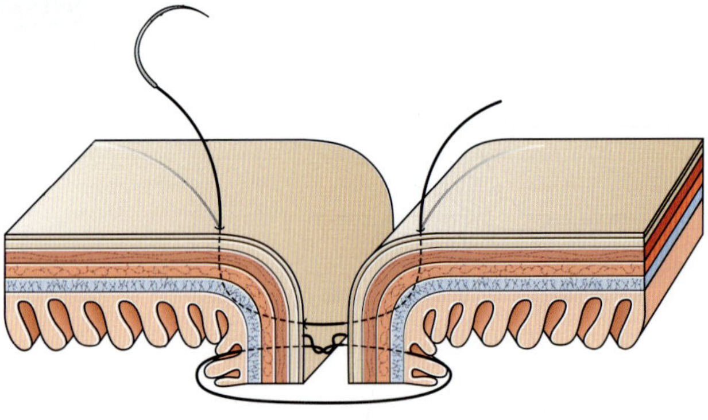

Figure 4.14 Standard two-layer bowel anastomosis. Reproduced with permission from Kocher T, Harder F, Thomas WEG (eds). *Anastomosis techniques in the gastrointestinal tract*, 1st edn. Wollerau: Covidien, 2007.

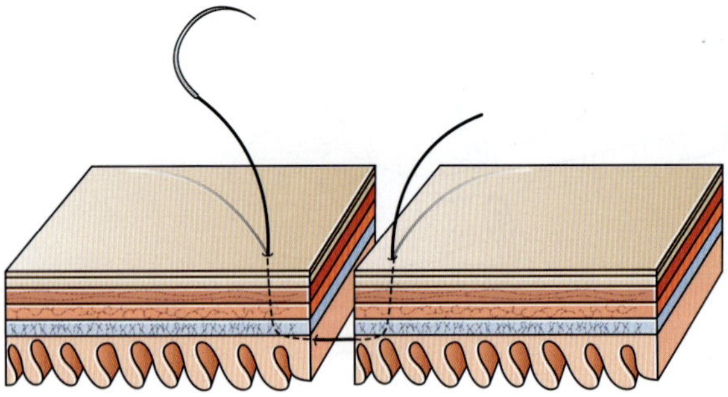

Figure 4.15 Extramucosal technique taking care to include the submucosa. Reproduced with permission from Kocher T, Harder F, Thomas WEG (eds). *Anastomosis techniques in the gastrointestinal tract*, 1st edn. Wollerau: Covidien, 2007.

In the past, great emphasis was placed on good bowel preparation prior to any anastomosis. The rationale was that with good bowel preparation and an empty bowel, there was less likelihood of faecal contamination and therefore it was probably not necessary to apply bowel clamps (even of the soft occlusion type). However, this tradition is now being challenged, and there is evidence to suggest that conventional bowel preparation provides little benefit, and indeed at times may prove detrimental to the outcome. In spite of this, many surgeons still use some form of bowel preparation, especially for colorectal surgery. Furthermore, if there is any risk of intestinal spillage during anastomosis, when bowel is unprepared or obstructed for example, atraumatic intestinal clamps should be used across the lumen of the bowel. Clamps should not impinge on the mesentery or the vasculature of the bowel for fear of damage to the vessels resulting in ischaemic changes. Ideally, the bowel edges should be pink and bleeding prior to anastomosis. Excessive bleeding from the bowel wall may need oversewing if natural haemostasis is inadequate.

For all intestinal anastomoses, the bowel ends must be brought together without tension. Stay sutures, which avoid the need for tissue forceps, are invaluable for displaying the bowel ends and help with the accurate alignment of the bowel and the placement of the sutures. If the anastomosis is being undertaken on mobile bowel, the anterior wall layer of sutures can be inserted, either in a continuous or interrupted manner, and then the bowel rotated and the posterior wall sutured in an identical manner to the anterior wall. As the mesenteric edge of the bowel is the most difficult, especially when a fatty mesentery is present, this angle should be dealt with first, with the final sutures being inserted at the antimesenteric border which is far more accessible and visible. The apposition of bowel edges should be as accurate as possible and the suture bites should be approximately 3–5 mm deep and 3–5 mm apart depending on the thickness of the bowel wall. The suture materials should be of 2/0–3/0 size and made of an absorbable polymer, which can be braided (e.g. polyglactin), or monofilament (e.g. polydioxanone), mounted on an atraumatic round-bodied needle. Braided, coated sutures are the easiest to handle and knot.

It is crucial to make sure that only bowel of similar diameter is brought together to form an end-to-end anastomosis. In cases of major size discrepancy, a side-to-side or end-to-side anastomosis may be safer. In cases where the size discrepancy is not marked, a Cheatle split (making a cut into the antimesenteric border) may help to enlarge the lumen of distal, collapsed bowel and allow an end-to-end anastomosis to be fashioned. After all anastomoses, the mesentery should always be closed to avoid the later risk of an internal hernia through a persistent mesenteric defect. Care must be taken during closure of this defect to prevent damage to any mesenteric vessels running in the edge of the mesentery (Summary box 4.3).

In certain situations, stapling devices are used to fashion the anastomosis, but as they are expensive, most surgeons reserve them for specific indications, such as oesophageal, rectal and gastric pouch procedures. Several studies have shown them not to be cost effective in routine small bowel surgery, although many surgeons still use them for ease of use and to save time.

Summary box 4.3

Intestinal anastomoses

- Ensure good blood supply to both bowel ends before and after formation of anastomosis.
- Ensure the anastomosis is under no tension.
- Avoid risk to mesenteric vessels by clamps or sutures.
- Use atraumatic bowel clamps to minimise contamination.
- Interrupted and continuous single-layer suture techniques are adequate and safe.
- Stapling devices are an alternative when speed is required or access is a major factor.

Vascular anastomoses

Vascular anastomoses require an extremely accurate closure as they must be immediately watertight at the end of the operation when the vascular clamps are removed. In many cases, some form of prosthetic material or graft may be used which will never be integrated into the body tissues and so the integrity of the suture line needs to be permanent. For this reason, polypropylene is one of the best sutures as it is not biodegradable. It is used in its monofilament form, mounted on an atraumatic, curved, round-bodied needle. Knot security is important, and as polypropylene is monofilament and the anastomosis often depends on one final knot, several throws (between six and eight) of a well-laid reef knot are required. The suture line must be regular and watertight with a smooth intimal surface to minimise the risk of thrombosis and embolus, as well as to avoid any leakage. Suture size depends

Sir George Lenthal Cheatle, 1865–1951, surgeon, King's College Hospital, London, UK.

on vessel calibre: 2/0 is suitable for the aorta, 4/0 for the femoral artery and 6/0 for the popliteal to distal arteries. Microvascular anastomoses are made using a loupe and an interrupted suture down to 10/0 size.

All vessel walls must be treated with great care avoiding causing any damage to the intima. If any significant manipulation is necessary, atraumatic forceps (such as DeBakey's) are utilised. Vascular clamps should be applied with great care, particularly for calcified vessels, and in some cases encircling rubber loops or intraluminal balloon catheters may be less traumatic for control. Vessels should always be sewn with the needle moving from within to without on the downstream edge of the vessel to avoid creating an intimal flap and to fix any atherosclerotic plaque. The tip of the needle should be inserted at right angles to the surface of the intima and the curve of the needle followed to prevent vessel trauma. The assistant should 'follow' by keeping the suture taut, and once the closure is complete, the distal clamp is released first, before the final watertight knot is made. This allows backflow to clear any clot or air from the anastomosis. The proximal clamp can then be released, a process which minimises the risk of distal embolus. Suture bites should be placed an equal distance apart, with the bite size dependent on the vessel diameter. Care needs to be taken to avoid damaging the suture, which should not be gripped by any surgical instrument. All haemostats that are used to hold any suture material should be shod with soft rubber to prevent suture material damage.

A transverse arteriotomy is less likely to stenose following closure than a longitudinal arteriotomy, but may not give adequate access, and a longitudinal arteriotomy is easier to make. Therefore, a vein patch can be used if there is any danger of stenosis or doubt about the size of the lumen (Figure 4.16). The suture line can be started at the apex of the arteriotomy with a double-ended suture, and then carried down each side with the final knot being placed at the midpoint of the vein patch graft, and not at the far end. The suture should go from outside to inside on the graft and from inside to outside on the artery, again to minimise the risk of intimal flap formation.

When prosthetic material or grafts are used, similar non-absorbable monofilament sutures are used with the same in–out technique to ensure eversion of the graft edge and a smooth intimal surface. Again the needle should go from outside to inside on the graft and from inside to outside on the artery. Double-ended sutures make the procedures easier (Summary box 4.4).

DRAINS

Drains are inserted to allow fluid or air that might collect at an operation site or in a wound to drain freely to the surface. The fluid to be drained may include blood, serum, pus, urine, faeces,

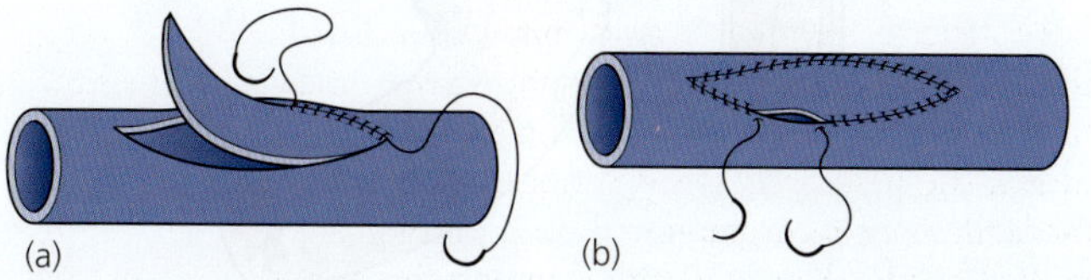

Figure 4.16 Arteriotomy being closed by vein patch. Technique involves a double armed suture ensuring that the final knot is half way along one side of the arteriotomy. Reproduced with permission from Royal College of Surgeons of England. *The intercollegiate basic surgical skills course participants handbook*, edns 1–4. London: RCS.

Summary box 4.4

Vascular anastomosis

- Non-absorbable monofilament suture material should be used, e.g. polypropylene.
- A smooth intimal suture line is essential.
- Knots require multiple throws in order to ensure security.
- The suture must pass from within outwards on the downflow aspect of the anastomosis.

bile or lymph. Drains may also allow wound irrigation in certain specific circumstances. The adequate drainage of fluid collections prevents the development of cavities or spaces that may delay wound healing. Their use can be regarded as prophylactic in elective surgery and therapeutic in emergency surgery. Three basic principles apply in the use of drains:

1 Open drains that utilise the principle of gravity
2 Semi-open drains that work on the principle of the capillary effect
3 Closed drains systems that utilise suction.

They may be placed through the wound or through a separate incision, although it has been clearly shown that placing them through the wound leads to an increased risk of wound infection. With regard to the indications for drainage, in the past drains were in common use ever since Lawson Tait in 1887 suggested 'when in doubt drain!' However, this edict has come under strong criticism recently and the value and use of drains has been the subject of close scrutiny, and their use still remains controversial.

Protagonists suggest that the use of drains may:

- remove any intraperitoneal or wound collection of ascites, serum, bile, chyle, pancreatic or intestinal secretion;
- act as a signal for any postoperative haemorrhage or anastomotic leakage;
- provide a track for later drainage.

However, the antagonists claim that the presence of a drain may:

- increase intra-abdominal and wound infections;
- increase anastomotic insufficiency;
- increase abdominal pain;
- increase hospital stay;
- decrease pulmonary function.

In reality, the use of drains currently tends to depend on a surgeon's individual preference. There are randomised controlled trails suggesting that their use in gastric, duodenal, small bowel, appendix and biliary surgery is unnecessary, and may cause more problems than benefits, and this is now reflected in current practice. There are also randomised controlled trials to suggest that they are also not required in colorectal, liver and pancreatic surgery and yet in today's practice the majority of surgeons will still utilise drains in these forms of surgery. The only area of alimentary tract surgery where drains are still routinely advocated is for oesophageal surgery, although even here the evidence is low with the level of evidence being only 5 and the level of recommendation being 'D' (i.e. based on expert opinion).

Specialist use of drains

There are certain clinical situations where specialist forms of drainage are required.

Michael Ellis DeBakey, b. 1908, Professor of Surgery, Baylor University, Houston, TX, USA.
Robert Lawson Tait, surgeon, Birmingham, UK, 1845–1899.

Chest drains

These are indicated for a pneumothorax, pleural effusion, haemothorax or to prevent the collection of fluid or air after thoracotomy. Once the drain has been inserted, it should be connected to an underwater sealed drain (Figure 4.17). This system allows air to leave the pleural cavity, but cannot draw it back in with the negative pressure that is created in the intrathoracic cavity. During the respiratory process, it should be checked that the meniscus of the fluid is swinging to ensure that the tube is not blocked. Suction can be applied to the venting tube at the bottle whenever there is significant drainage of fluid or air expected. Between 10 and 20 mm of mercury are adequate to obtain a gentle flow of bubbles from the chest cavity.

T-tube drains

After exploration of the common bile duct, a T-tube (Figure 4.18) may be inserted into the duct which allows bile to drain while the sphincter of Oddi is in spasm postoperatively. Once the sphincter relaxes, bile drains normally down the bile duct and into the duodenum. To assist choleresis, it is often advisable to convert the lumen of the limb of the T into a gutter, which also facilitates removal.

Guided drainage

For many intra-abdominal collections or abscesses, drains may be inserted under ultrasound or computed tomography (CT) control. In order for such drains to remain in site, the end is often fashioned with a pigtail to discourage inadvertent removal.

Removal of drains

A drain should be removed as soon as it is no longer required, as if left in, it can itself predispose to fluid collections as a result of tissue reaction. Indeed there is evidence that by 7 days only 20 per cent of drains are still functioning. It should be stressed how important it is to define the objective of each individual drain and to ensure that once that objective has been met, the drain is removed. If a drain is used at all, the following principles may apply:

- Drains put in to cover perioperative bleeding may usually be removed after 24 hours, e.g. thyroidectomy.
- Drains put in to drain serous collections usually can be removed after 5 days, e.g. mastectomy.
- Drains put in because of infection should be left until the infection is subsiding or the drainage is minimal.
- Drains put in to cover colorectal anastomoses should be removed at about 5–7 days. However, it should be stressed that in no way does a drain prevent any intestinal leakage, but merely may assist any such leakage to drain externally rather than to produce life-threatening peritonitis.
- Common bile duct T-tubes should remain in for 10 days. However, once the T-tube cholangiogram has shown that there is free flow of bile into the duodenum and that there are no retained stones, some surgeons like to clamp the T-tube prior to removal. The 10-day period is required to minimise the risk of biliary peritonitis after removal.
- Any suction drain should have the suction taken off prior to removal of the drain.
- During removal of a chest drain, the patient should be asked to breathe in and hold his breath, thus doing a Valsalva manoeuvre. In this way, no air is sucked into the pleural

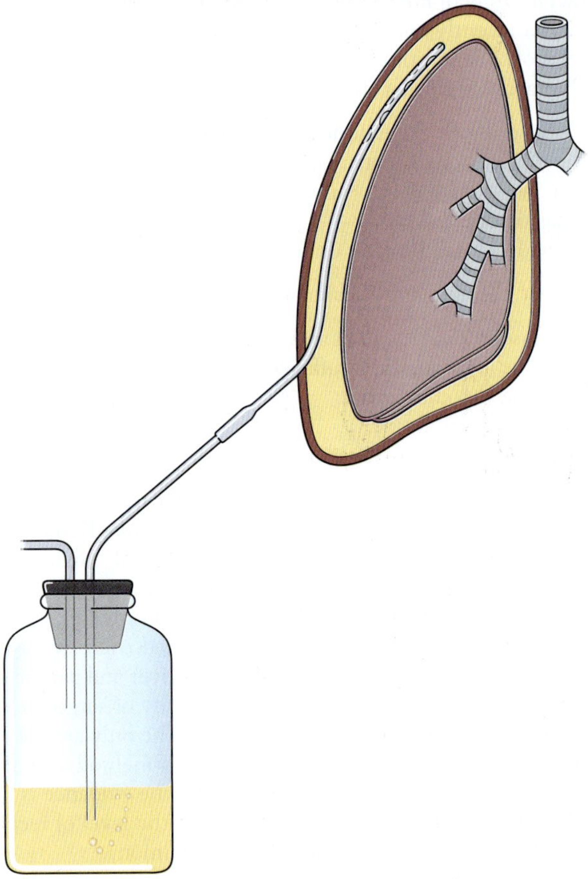

Figure 4.17 Underwater seal chest drain. Reproduced with permission from Thomas WEG. Basic principles. In: Kingsnorth A, Majid A (eds). *Principles of surgical practice*. London: Greenwich Medical, 2001.

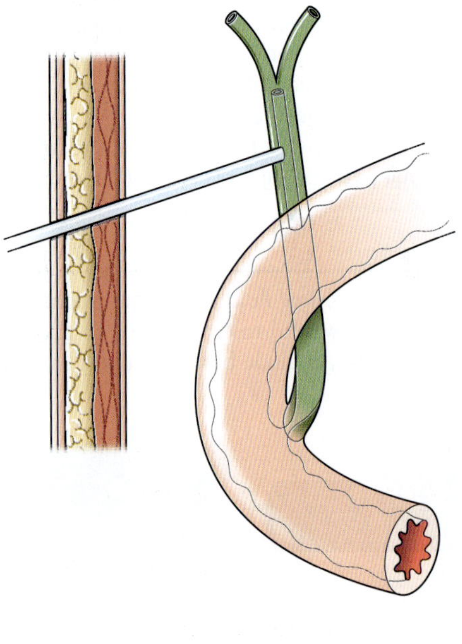

Figure 4.18 T tube. Reproduced with permission from Thomas WEG. Basic principles. In: Kingsnorth A, Majid A (eds). *Principles of surgical practice*. London: Greenwich Medical, 2001.

Ruggero Oddi, Italian physician, 1864–1913.
Antonio Maria Valsalva, Italian physician and anatomist, 1666–1723.

cavity as the tube is removed. Once the drain is out, a previously inserted purse-string suture should be tied.

THE PRINCIPLES OF DIATHERMY: ELECTROSURGERY

For many years, short wave diathermy has proved a most valuable and versatile aid to surgical technique. Its most common use is in securing haemostasis by means of coagulation, but by varying the strength or wave form of the current produced, it can also result in a cutting effect. Both these effects have been used in open surgery, as well as in laparoscopic surgery or down intraluminal endoscopes as in transurethral resection of the prostate. However, although diathermy is a valuable surgical tool, many accidents have occurred due to surgeons being unaware of, or not fully understanding, the principles of its use. Most accidents are avoidable if the diathermy or electrocautery is used with care. It is therefore vital for a surgeon to have a sound understanding of the principles and practice of diathermy, and how to avoid complications.

The principle of diathermy

When an electrical current passes through a conductor, some of its energy appears as heat. The heat produced depends on:

- the intensity of the current;
- the wave form of the current;
- the electrical property of the tissues through which the current passes;
- the relative sizes of the two electrodes.

There are two basic types of diathermy system in use, monopolar diathermy and bipolar diathermy (Figure 4.19). In monopolar diathermy, which is the most commonly used form, an alternating current is produced by a suitable generator and passed to the patient via an active electrode which has a very small surface area. The current then passes through the tissues and returns via a very large surface plate (the indifferent electrode) back to the earth pole of the generator. As the surface area of contact of the active electrode is small in comparison to the indifferent electrode, the concentrated powerful current produces heat at the operative site. However, the large surface area electrode of the patient plate spreads the returning current over a wide surface area, so it is less concentrated and produces little heat.

In bipolar diathermy, the two active electrodes are usually represented by the limbs of a pair of diathermy forceps. Both forceps ends are therefore active and current flows between them and only the tissue held between the limbs of the forceps heats up. This form of diathermy is used when it is essential that the surrounding tissue should be free from either the risk of being burned or having current passed through them.

The effects of diathermy

Diathermy can be used for three purposes:

1 Coagulation: the sealing of blood vessels.
2 Fulguration: the destructive coagulation of tissues with charring.
3 Cutting: used to divide tissues during bloodless surgery.

In **coagulation**, a heating effect leads to cell death by dehydration and protein denaturation. Bleeding is therefore stopped by a combination of the distortion of the walls of the blood vessel,

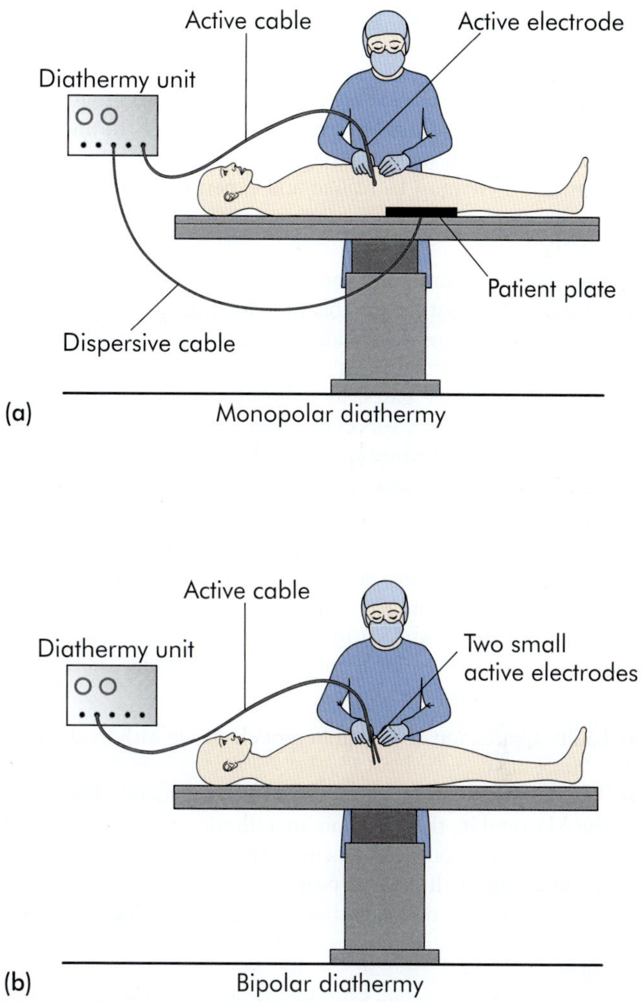

Figure 4.19 The principles of diathermy. (a) Monopolar diathermy. (b) Bipolar diathermy. Reproduced with permission from Royal College of Surgeons of England. *The intercollegiate basic surgical skills course participants handbook*, edns 1–4. London: RCS.

coagulation of the plasma proteins, dried and shrunken dead tissue and stimulation of the clotting mechanism. In an ideal situation, intracellular temperatures should not reach boiling during coagulation, because if it does an unwanted cutting effect may be experienced.

Cutting occurs when sufficient heat is applied to the tissue to cause cell water to explode into steam. The cut current is a continuous wave form and the monopolar diathermy is most effective when the active electrode is held a very short distance from the tissues. This allows an electrical discharge to arc across the gap creating a series of sparks which produce the high temperatures needed for cutting.

In **fulguration**, the diathermy matching is set to coagulation and a higher effective voltage is used to make larger sparks jump an air gap thus fulgurating the tissues. This can continue until carbonisation or charring occurs. The voltage and power output can be varied by adjusting the duration of bursts of current, as well as its intensity to give a combination of both cutting and coagulation. This is known as blended current and provides both forms of diathermy activity.

Complications of diathermy

Electrocution

Today, diathermy machines are manufactured to very high safety standards which minimise the risk of any part of the machine becoming live with mains current. However, as with any such instrument, there must be regular and expert servicing.

Explosion

Sparks from the diathermy can ignite any volatile or inflammable gas or fluid within the theatre. Alcohol-based skin preparations can catch fire if they are allowed to pool on or around the patient. Furthermore, diathermy should not be used in the presence of explosive gases, including those which may occur naturally in the colon, especially after certain forms of bowel preparation, such as mannitol, which has now been banned for this use for this very reason.

Burns

These are the most common type of diathermy accidents in both open and endoscopic surgery. They occur when the current flows in some way other than that in which the surgeon intended and are far more common in monopolar than bipolar diathermy. These may occur as a result of:

- Faulty application of the indifferent electrode with inadequate contact area.
- The patient being earthed by touching any metal object, e.g. the Mayo table, the bar of an anaesthetic screen, an exposed metal arm rest or a leg touching the metal stirrups used in maintaining the lithotomy position.
- Faulty insulation of the diathermy leads, either due to cracked insulation or instruments such as towel clips pinching the cable.
- Inadvertent activity such as the accidental activation of the foot pedal, or accidental contact of the active electrode with other metal instruments, such as retractors, instruments or towel clips.

Channelling

Heat is produced wherever the current intensity is greatest. Normally, this would be at the tip of the active electrode, but if current passes up a narrow channel or pedicle to the active electrode, enough heat may be generated within this channel or pedicle to coagulate the tissues. This can prove disastrous, for example,

- coagulation of the penis in a child undergoing circumcision;
- coagulation of the spermatic cord when the electrode is applied to the testis.

In such situations, diathermy should not be used, or if it is necessary, then bipolar diathermy should be employed.

Pacemakers

Diathermy currents can interfere with the working of a pacemaker with its obvious potential danger to the patient's health. Modern pacemakers are designed to be inhibited by high frequency interference, so that the patient may receive no pacing stimulation at all while the diathermy is in use. Certain demand pacemakers may revert to the fixed rate of pacing and therefore it would be important for the anaesthetist to have a magnet available so that these can be reset if necessary. In most cases, it is therefore wise to undertake precautions and to use bipolar diathermy wherever possible. If monopolar diathermy is required, then the patient plate should be sited as far away from the pacemaker as possible so that the path of the current does not pass through the heart or the vicinity of the pacemaker. Monitoring of the heart rate should be undertaken throughout the operation and a defibrillator should always be available in case a dysrhythmia develops at any time.

Laparoscopic surgery

Diathermy burns are a particular hazard of laparoscopic surgery due to the nature of the visibility of the instrumentation and the actual structure of the instruments used. Such burns may occur by:

- Diathermy of the wrong structure because of lack of clarity of vision or misidentification.
- Faulty insulation of any of the laparoscopic instruments or equipment.
- Intraperitoneal contact of the diathermy with another metal instrument while activating the pedal.
- Inadvertent activation of the pedal while the diathermy tip is out of vision of the camera.
- Retained heat in the diathermy tip touching susceptible structures, such as bowel.
- Capacitance coupling (Figure 4.20). This is a phenomenon in which a capacitor is created by having an insulator sandwiched between two metal electrodes. This can be created in situations where there is a metal laparoscopic port and the diathermy hook is passed through it. The insulation of the diathermy hook acts as the sandwiched insulator and by means of electromagnetic induction, the diathermy current flowing through the hook can induce a current in the metal port, which can potentially damage intraperitoneal structures. In most cases, this current is dissipated from the metal port through the abdominal wall, but if a plastic cuff is used, this dissipation of current does not occur and the danger of capacitance coupling is significantly increased. Therefore, metal ports should never be used with a plastic cuff. The danger of capacitance coupling can be prevented by using entirely plastic ports.

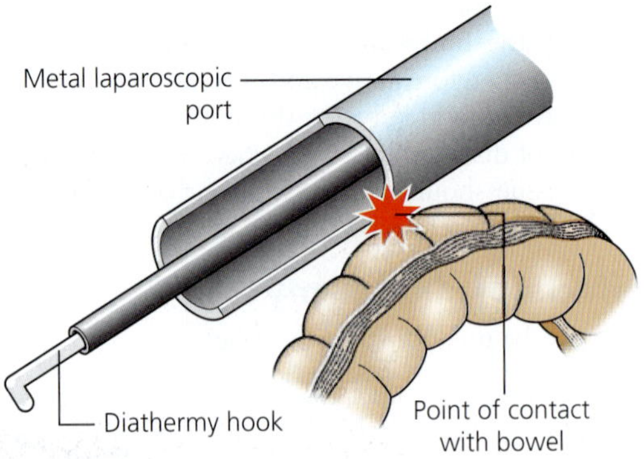

Figure 4.20 Capacitance coupling during laparoscopic surgery. Reproduced with permission from Royal College of Surgeons of England. *The intercollegiate basic surgical skills course participants handbook*, edns 1–4. London: RCS.

THE PRINCIPLES OF LIGASURE

'Ligasure' tissue fusion technology is a vessel sealing system that is used in both open and laparoscopic surgery. It actually fuses the vessel walls to create a permanent seal and is in wide use in a range of surgical specialties, including gynaecology, colorectal, urology and general surgery. It uses a combination of pressure and energy to create vessel fusion which can withstand up to three times the normal systolic pressure.

New technology of the ligasure system involves advanced monopolar technology that uses the body's own collagen and elastin to both seal and divide, allowing surgeons to reduce instrument handling when dissecting, ligating and grasping – a valuable asset particularly during laparoscopic surgery. The feedback sensing technology incorporated in the instrument is designed to manage the energy delivery in a precise manner and results in an automatic discontinuation of energy once the seal is complete, thus removing any concern that the surgeon has to use guesswork as to when the seal is complete. The newer instruments actively monitor tissue impedance and provide a real-time adjustment of the energy being delivered. Using this technology, ligasure can seal vessels of up to 7 mm diameter, with an average seal time of 2–4 seconds, as well as pedicles, tissue bundles and lymphatics with a consistent controlled and predictable effect on tissue, including less dessication.

Therefore, the new Ligasure Advance™ can dissect, seal and divide and was designed to be the only tool that a surgeon would need. However, it is relatively expensive to use compared to some of the competing technology.

THE PRINCIPLES OF THE 'HARMONIC SCALPEL'

The harmonic scalpel is an instrument that uses ultrasound technology to cut tissues while simultaneously sealing them. It utilises a hand-held ultrasound transducer and scalpel which is controlled by a hand switch or foot pedal. During use, the scalpel vibrates in the 20 000–50 000 Hz range and cuts through tissues, effecting haemostasis by sealing vessels and tissues by means of protein denaturation caused by vibration rather than heat (in a similar manner to whisking an egg white). It provides cutting precision, even through thickened scar tissue, and visibility is enhanced due to less smoke being created by this system during use compared to routine electrosurgery. However, the harmonic scalpel does take longer to cut and coagulate tissues than diathermy, and while diathermy can be used to coagulate a bleeding vessel at any time, the harmonic scalpel can only coagulate as it cuts. It is claimed that patients experience less swelling, bleeding and bruising after the use of the harmonic scalpel than when a conventional scalpel is used, and blood vessels are sealed with a much lower temperature than conventional diathermy and so there is less thermal damage to adjacent tissue, with less charring and dessication. Furthermore, it is suggested that the use of the harmonic scalpel reduces operative time and recovery is thus enhanced. Currently, the harmonic scalpel is in common use during laparoscopic procedures, as well as open surgery, such as thyroidectomy and several plastic surgery operations, e.g. cosmetic breast surgery.

FURTHER READING

Royal College of Surgeons of England. *Intercollegiate basic surgical skills course (participant handbook)*, 4th edn. London: Royal College of Surgeons of England, 2007.

Jenkins TPN. The burst abdominal wound: a mechanical approach. *Br Med J* 1976; **131**: 130–40.

Kirk RM. *Basic surgical techniques*, 6th edn. Edinburgh: Churchill Livingstone, 2010.

Eugen (Janö) Alexander Pölya, 1876–1944, Surgeon, St Stephen's Hospital, Budapest, Hungary.
Henri Albert Charles Antoine Hartmann, 1860–1952, Professor of Clinical Surgery, The Faculty of Medicine, The University of Paris, France.
Gaston Michel, 1874–1937, French surgeon.
Frank Gregory Connell, 1875–1968, Professor of Surgery, Rush Medical College, Chicago, IL, USA.

CHAPTER

5 Surgical infection

LEARNING OBJECTIVES

To understand:

- The factors that determine whether a wound will become infected
- The classification of sources of infection and their severity
- The indications for and choice of prophylactic antibiotics
- The characteristics of the common surgical pathogens and their sensitivities
- The spectrum of commonly used antibiotics in surgery and the principles of therapy
- The misuse of antibiotic therapy with the risk of resistance (such as methicillin-resistant *Staphylococcus aureus* (MRSA)) and emergence (such as *Clostridium difficile* enteritis)

To learn:

- Koch's postulates
- The management of abscesses

To appreciate:

- The importance of aseptic and antiseptic techniques and delayed primary or secondary closure in contaminated wounds

To be aware of:

- The causes of reduced resistance to infection (host response)

To know:

- The definitions of infection, particularly at surgical sites
- What basic precautions to take to avoid surgically relevant health care-associated infections

PHYSIOLOGY AND PRESENTATION

Background

Surgical infection, particularly surgical site infection (SSI), has always been a major complication of surgery and trauma and has been documented for 4000–5000 years. The Egyptians had some concepts about infection as they were able to prevent putrefaction, testified by mummification skills. Their medical papyruses also describe the use of salves and antiseptics to prevent SSIs. This 'prophylaxis' had also been known earlier by the Assyrians, although less well documented. It was described again independently by the Greeks. The Hippocratic teachings described the use of antimicrobials, such as wine and vinegar, which were widely used to irrigate open, infected wounds before delayed primary or secondary wound closure. A belief common to all these civilisations, and indeed even later to the Romans, was that, whenever pus localised in an infected wound, it needed to be drained.

Galen recognised that this localisation of infection (suppuration) in wounds, inflicted in the gladiatorial arena, often heralded recovery, particularly after drainage (*pus bonum et laudabile*). Sadly, this dictum was misunderstood by many later healers, who thought that it was the production of pus that was desirable. Until well into the Middle Ages, some practitioners promoted suppuration in wounds by the application of noxious substances, including faeces, in the misguided belief that healing could not occur without pus formation. Theodoric of Cervia, Ambroise Paré and Guy de Chauliac observed that clean wounds, closed primarily, could heal without infection or suppuration.

The understanding of the causes of infection came in the nineteenth century. Microbes had been seen under the microscope, but Koch laid down the first definition of infective disease (Koch's postulates; Summary box 5.1). Koch's postulates do not cover every eventuality though. Organisms of low virulence may not cause disease in normal hosts but may be responsible for disease in immunocompromised hosts. Some hosts may develop

Hippocrates was a Greek physician, and by common consent 'The Father of Medicine'. He was born on the Greek island of Cos off Turkey about 460 bc and probably died in 375 bc. He lived to be about 109 years of age in an era when the life expectancy was about 32 years.

Galen, 130–200, a Roman physician, who commenced practice as surgeon to the gladiators at Pergamum (now Bregama in Turkey) and later became personal physician to the Emperor Marcus Aurelius and to two of his successors. He was a prolific writer on many subjects, among them anatomy, medicine, pathology and philosophy. His work affected medical thinking for 15 centuries after his death. (Gladiator is Latin for 'swordsman'.)

Theodoric of Cervia. Theodoric, 1210–1298, who was Bishop of Cervia, published a book on surgery about 1267.
Ambroise Paré, 1510–1590, a French military surgeon, who also worked at the Hotel Dieu, Paris, France.
Guy de Chauliac, ?1298–1368, was physician and chaplain to Pope Clement VI at Avignon, France. He was the author of *Chirurgia Magna* which was published about 1363.

subclinical disease and yet still be a carrier of the organism capable of infecting others. Also, not every organism that causes disease can be grown in culture, the commonly quoted one being *Mycobacterium leprae* which causes leprosy.

Summary box 5.1

Koch's postulates proving whether a given organism is the cause of a given disease

- It must be found in every case
- It should be possible to isolate it from the host and grow it in culture
- It should reproduce the disease when injected into another healthy host
- It should be recovered from an experimentally infected host

The Austrian obstetrician Ignac Semmelweis showed that puerperal sepsis could be reduced from over 10 per cent to under 2 per cent by the simple act of hand washing between cases, particularly between post-mortem examinations and the delivery suite. He was ignored by his contemporaries.

Louis Pasteur recognised through his germ theory that micro-organisms were responsible for infecting humans and causing disease. Joseph Lister applied this knowledge to the reduction of colonising organisms in compound fractures by using antiseptics. The principles of antiseptic surgery were soon enhanced with aseptic surgery at the turn of the century. As well as killing the bacteria on the skin before surgical incision (antiseptic technique), the conditions under which the operation was performed were kept free of bacteria (aseptic technique). This technique is still employed in modern operating theatres.

The concept of a 'magic bullet' (*Zauberkugel*) that could kill microbes but not their host became a reality with the discovery of sulphonamide chemotherapy in the mid-twentieth century. The discovery of the antibiotic penicillin is attributed to Alexander Fleming in 1928, but it was not isolated for clinical use until 1941 by Florey and Chain. The first patient to receive penicillin was Police Constable Alexander in Oxford. He scratched the side of his mouth while pruning roses and developed abscesses of the face and eyes leading to a severe staphylococcal bacteraemia. He responded to treatment, made a partial recovery before the penicillin ran out, then relapsed and died. Since then, there has been a proliferation of antibiotics with broad-spectrum activity and antibiotics today remain the mainstay of antimicrobial therapy.

Many staphylococci today have become resistant to penicillin. Often bacteria develop resistance through the acquisition of β-lactamases, which break up the β-lactam ring present in the molecular structure of many antibiotics. The acquisition of extended spectrum β-lactamases (ESBLs) is an increasing concern in some Gram-negative organisms that cause urinary tract infections because it is difficult to find an antibiotic effective against them. In addition, there is increasing concern about the rising resistance of many other bacteria to antibiotics, in particular the emergence of methicillin-resistant *Staphylococcus aureus* (MRSA) and glycopeptide-resistant enterococci (GRE), which are also relevant in general surgical practice.

The introduction of antibiotics for prophylaxis and for treatment, together with advances in anaesthesia and critical care medicine, has made possible surgery that would not previously have been considered. Faecal peritonitis is no longer inevitably fatal, and incisions made in the presence of such contamination can heal primarily without infection in 80–90 per cent of patients with appropriate antibiotic therapy. Despite this, it is common practice in many countries to delay wound closure in patients in whom the wound is known to be contaminated or dirty. Waiting for the wound to granulate and then performing a delayed primary or secondary closure may be considered a better option (Summary box 5.2).

Summary box 5.2

Advances in the control of infection in surgery

- Aseptic operating theatre techniques have enhanced the use of antiseptics
- Antibiotics have reduced postoperative infection rates after elective and emergency surgery
- Delayed primary, or secondary, closure remains useful in contaminated wounds

Surgical site infection in patients who have contaminated wounds, who are immunosuppressed or undergoing prosthetic surgery, is now the exception rather than the rule since the introduction of prophylactic antibiotics. The evidence for this is of the highest level. The value of prophylactic antibiotics in clean, non-prosthetic surgery remains controversial, although SSI rates after such surgery is high when judged by close, unbiased, post-discharge surveillance, using strict definitions.

PHYSIOLOGY

Microorganisms are normally prevented from causing infection in tissues by intact epithelial surfaces, most notably the skin. These surfaces are broken down by trauma or surgery. In addition to these mechanical barriers, there are other protective mechanisms, which can be divided into:

- **chemical**: low gastric pH
- **humoral**: antibodies, complement and opsonins
- **cellular**: phagocytic cells, macrophages, polymorphonuclear cells and killer lymphocytes.

All these natural mechanisms may be compromised by surgical intervention and treatment.

Reduced resistance to infection has several causes (Summary box 5.3).

Joseph Lister (Lord Lister), 1827–1912, Professor of Surgery, Glasgow (1860–1869), Edinburgh (1869–1877) and King's College Hospital, London, UK (1877–1892). He was the first to show the relation between microbial infection and surgical sepsis. He associated Pasteur's observations on fermentation with sepsis and, using a carbolic dressing and spray, introduced the 'antiseptic principle' which revolutionised surgery. Asepsis in surgery has now replaced antisepsis but the dangers of sepsis are still very much with us.

Sir Ernst Boris Chain, Professor of Biochemistry, Imperial College, London, UK. Fleming, Florey and Chain shared the 1945 Nobel Prize for Physiology or Medicine for their work on penicillin.

Antony von Leeuwenhoek of Delft, The Netherlands, invented the microscope, and was the first to see bacteria in 1875. He himself made more than 400 microscopes.

Robert Koch, 1843–1910, Professor of Hygiene and Bacteriology, Berlin, Germany, stated his 'Postulates' in 1882.

Ignac Semmelweis, 1818–1865, Professor of Obstetrics, Budapest, Hungary.

Louis Pasteur, 1822–1895, was a French chemist, bacteriologist and immunologist who was Professor of Chemistry at the Sorbonne, Paris, France.

Sir Alexander Fleming, 1881–1955, Professor of Bacteriology, St Mary's Hospital, London, UK, discovered *Penicillium notatum* in 1928.

Howard Walter Florey (Lord Florey of Adelaide), 1898–1968, Professor of Pathology, The University of Oxford, Oxford, UK.

Summary box 5.3

Causes of reduced host resistance to infection

- Metabolic: malnutrition (including obesity), diabetes, uraemia, jaundice
- Disseminated disease: cancer and acquired immunodeficiency syndrome (AIDS)
- Iatrogenic: radiotherapy, chemotherapy, steroids

Host response is weakened by malnutrition, which can be recognised clinically, and most easily, as recent rapid weight loss that can be present even in the presence of obesity. Metabolic diseases such as diabetes mellitus, uraemia and jaundice, disseminated malignancy and acquired immune deficiency syndrome (AIDS) are other contributors to infection and a poor healing response, as are iatrogenic causes including the immunosuppression caused by radiotherapy, chemotherapy or steroids (Summary box 5.4, and Figures 5.1 and 5.2).

When enteral feeding is suspended during the perioperative period, and particularly with underlying disease such as cancer, immunosuppression, shock or sepsis, bacteria (particularly aerobic Gram-negative bacilli) tend to colonise the normally sterile upper gastrointestinal tract. They may then translocate to the mesenteric nodes and cause the release of endotoxins (lipopolysaccharide in bacterial cell walls), which can be one cause of a harmful systemic inflammatory response through the excessive release of proinflammatory cytokines and activation of macrophages (Figure 5.3). In the circumstances of reduced host resistance to infection, microorganisms that are not normally pathogenic may start to behave as pathogens. This is known as opportunistic infection. Opportunistic infection with fungi is an example, particularly when prolonged and changing antibiotic regimens have been used.

The chance of developing an SSI after surgery is also determined by the pathogenicity of the organisms present and by the size of the bacterial inoculum. Devitalised tissue, excessive dead space or haematoma, all the results of poor surgical technique, increase the chances of infection. The same applies to foreign materials of any kind, including sutures and drains. If there is a silk suture in tissue, the critical number of organisms needed to start an infection is reduced logarithmically. Silk should not be used to close skin as it causes suture abscesses for this reason. These principles are important to an understanding of how best to prevent infection in surgical practice (Summary box 5.5).

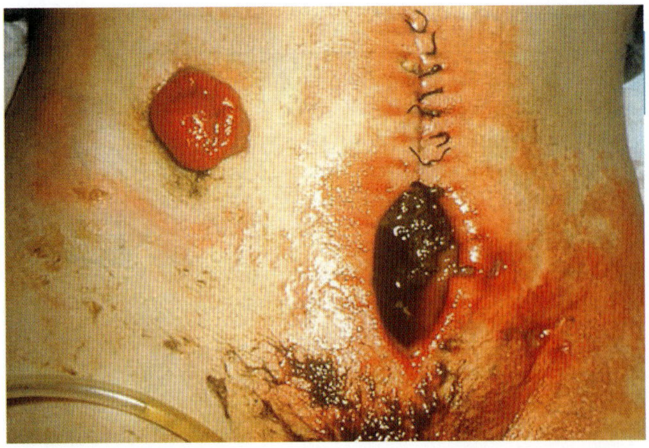

Figure 5.1 Major wound infection and delayed healing presenting as a faecal fistula in a patient with Crohn's disease.

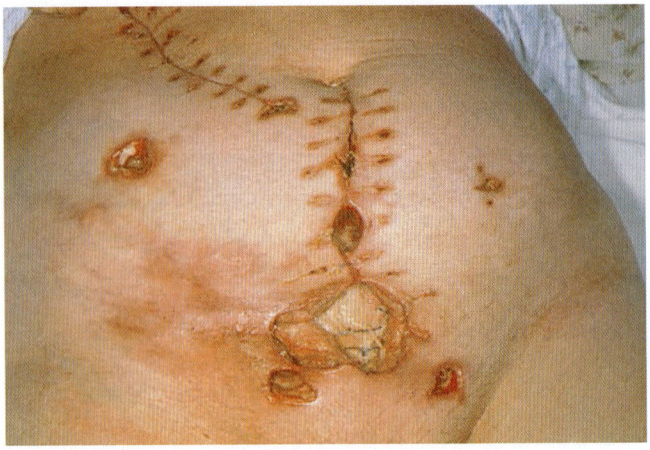

Figure 5.2 Delayed healing relating to infection in a patient on high-dose steroids.

Summary box 5.4

Risk factors for increased risk of wound infection

- Malnutrition (obesity, weight loss)
- Metabolic disease (diabetes, uraemia, jaundice)
- Immunosuppression (cancer, AIDS, steroids, chemotherapy and radiotherapy)
- Colonisation and translocation in the gastrointestinal tract
- Poor perfusion (systemic shock or local ischaemia)
- Foreign body material
- Poor surgical technique (dead space, haematoma)

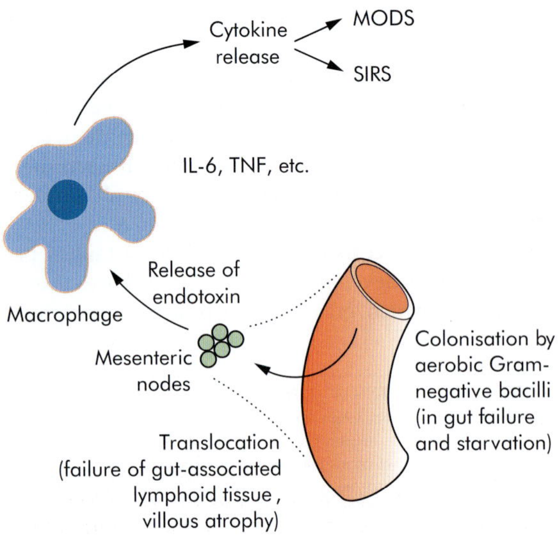

Figure 5.3 Gut failure, colonisation and translocation related to the development of multiple organ dysfunction syndrome (MODS) and systemic inflammatory response syndrome (SIRS). IL, interleukin; TNF, tumour necrosis factor.

> **Summary box 5.5**
>
> **Factors that determine whether a wound will become infected**
>
> - Host response
> - Virulence and inoculum of infective agent
> - Vascularity and health of tissue being invaded (including local ischaemia as well as systemic shock)
> - Presence of dead or foreign tissue
> - Presence of antibiotics during the 'decisive period'

There is a delay before host defences can become mobilised after a breach in an epithelial surface, whether caused by trauma or surgery. The acute inflammatory, humoral and cellular defences take up to 4 hours to be mobilised. This is called the 'decisive period', and it is the time when the invading bacteria may become established in the tissues. Strategies aimed at preventing infection from taking a hold become ineffective after this time period. It is therefore logical that prophylactic antibiotics should be given to cover this period and that they could be decisive in preventing an infection from developing. The tissue levels of antibiotics should be above the minimum inhibitory concentration (MIC_{90}) for the pathogens likely to be encountered.

Local and systemic presentation

The infection of a wound can be defined as the invasion of organisms through tissues following a breakdown of local and systemic host defences, leading to cellulitis, lymphangitis, abscess and bacteraemia. The infection of most surgical wounds is referred to as superficial surgical site infection (SSSI). The other categories include deep SSI (infection in the deeper musculofascial layers) and organ space infection (such as an abdominal abscess after an anastomotic leak).

Pathogens resist host defences by releasing toxins, which favour their spread, and this is enhanced in anaerobic or frankly necrotic wound tissue. *Clostridium perfringens*, which is responsible for gas gangrene, releases proteases such as hyaluronidase, lecithinase and haemolysin, which allow it to spread through the tissues. Resistance to antibiotics can be acquired by previously sensitive bacteria by transfer through plasmids.

The human body harbours approximately 10^{14} organisms. They can be released into tissues by surgery, contamination being most severe when a hollow viscus perforates (e.g. faecal peritonitis following a diverticular perforation). Any infection that follows surgery may be termed primary or secondary (Summary box 5.6).

> **Summary box 5.6**
>
> **Classification of sources of infection**
>
> - Primary: present in or on the host and so acquired from an endogenous source (such as an SSSI following contamination of the wound from a perforated appendix)
> - Secondary or exogenous (HAI): acquired from a source outside the body such as the operating theatre (inadequate air filtration, poor antisepsis) or the ward (e.g. poor hand washing compliance)

Infection that follows surgery or admission to hospital is termed health care-associated infection (HAI). There are four main groups: respiratory infections (including ventilator-associated pneumonia), urinary tract infections (mostly related to urinary catheters), bacteraemia (mostly related to indwelling vascular catheters) and SSIs.

MAJOR AND MINOR SURGICAL SITE INFECTIONS

A major SSI is defined as a wound that either discharges significant quantities of pus spontaneously or needs a secondary procedure to drain it (Figure 5.4). The patient may have systemic signs, such as tachycardia, pyrexia and a raised white count (Summary box 5.7).

> **Summary box 5.7**
>
> **Major wound infections**
>
> - Significant quantity of pus
> - Delayed return home
> - Patients are systemically ill

Minor wound infections may discharge pus or infected serous fluid but should not be associated with excessive discomfort, systemic signs or delay in return home (Figure 5.5). The differentiation between major and minor and the definition of SSI is important in audit or trials of antibiotic prophylaxis. There are scoring systems for the severity of wound infection, which are particularly useful in surveillance and research. Examples are the Southampton (Table 5.1) and ASEPSIS systems (Table 5.2).

Accurate surveillance can only be achieved using trained, unbiased and blinded assessors. Most include surveillance for a 30-day postoperative period. The US Centers for Disease Control (CDC) definition insists on a 30-day follow-up period for non-prosthetic surgery and one year after implanted hip and knee surgery.

Types of localised infection

Abscess

An abscess presents all the clinical features of acute inflamma-

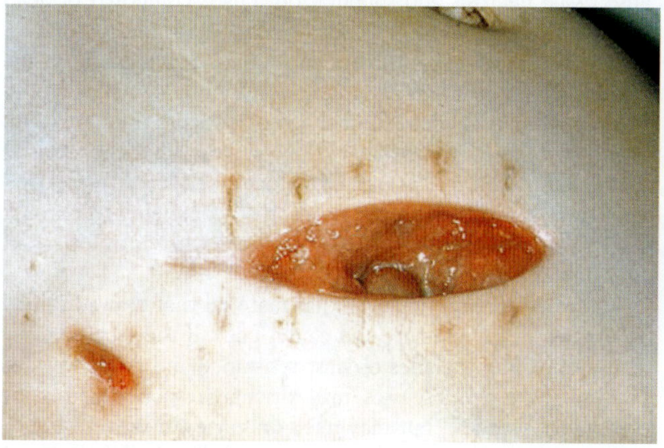

Figure 5.4 Major wound infection with superficial skin dehiscence.

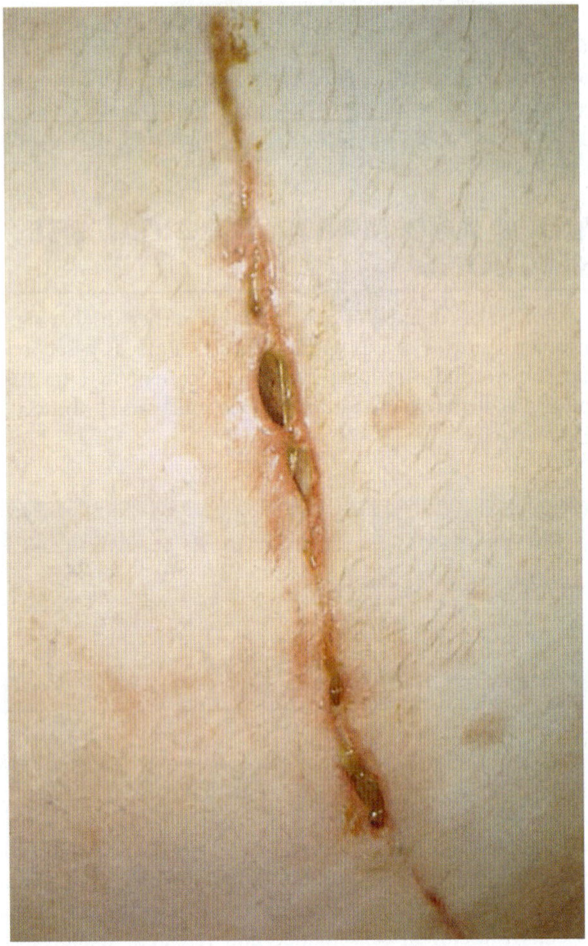

Figure 5.5 Minor wound infection that settled spontaneously without antibiotics.

tion originally described by Celsus: **calor** (heat), **rubor** (redness), **dolour** (pain) and **tumour** (swelling). To these can be added **functio laesa** (loss of function: if it hurts, the infected part is not used). They usually follow a puncture wound of some kind, which may have been forgotten, as well as surgery, but can be metastatic in all tissues following bacteraemia.

Pyogenic organisms, predominantly *Staphylococcus aureus*, cause tissue necrosis and suppuration. Pus is composed of dead and dying white blood cells that release damaging cytokines, oxygen free radicals and other molecules. An abscess is surrounded by an acute inflammatory response composed of a fibrinous exudate, oedema and the cells of acute inflammation. Granulation tissue (macrophages, angiogenesis and fibroblasts) forms later around the suppurative process and leads to collagen deposition. If it is not drained or resorbed completely, a chronic abscess may result. If it is partly sterilised with antibiotics, an antibioma may form.

Abscesses contain hyperosmolar material that draws in fluid. This increases the pressure and causes pain. If they spread, they usually track along planes of least resistance and point towards the skin. Wound abscesses may discharge spontaneously by tracking to a surface, but may need drainage through a surgical incision. Most abscesses relating to surgical wounds take 7–10 days to form after surgery. As many as 75 per cent of SSIs present after the patient has left hospital and may thus be overlooked by the surgical team. Their cost and management, which may be inadequate, is transferred to primary care (Summary box 5.8).

Table 5.1 Southampton wound grading system.

Grade	Appearance
0	Normal healing
I	Normal healing with mild bruising or erythema
Ia	Some bruising
Ib	Considerable bruising
Ic	Mild erythema
II	Erythema plus other signs of inflammation
IIa	At one point
IIb	Around sutures
IIc	Along wound
IId	Around wound
III	Clear or haemoserous discharge
IIIa	At one point only (≤2 cm)
IIIb	Along wound (>2 cm)
IIIc	Large volume
IIId	Prolonged (>3 days)
Major complication	
IV	Pus
IVa	At one point only (≤2 cm)
IVb	Along wound (>2 cm)
V	Deep or severe wound infection with or without tissue breakdown; haematoma requiring aspiration

Table 5.2 The ASEPSIS wound score.

Criterion	Points
Additional treatment	0
Antibiotics for wound infection	10
Drainage of pus under local anaesthesia	5
Debridement of wound under general anaesthesia	10
Serous discharge[a]	Daily 0–5
Erythema[a]	Daily 0–5
Purulent exudate[a]	Daily 0–10
Separation of deep tissues[a]	Daily 0–10
Isolation of bacteria from wound	10
Stay as inpatient prolonged over 14 days as result of wound infection	5

[a] Scored for 5 of the first 7 days only, the remainder being scored if present in the first two months.

Aulus Aurelius Cornelius Celsus, 25 BC to AD 50, a Roman surgeon. He was the author of *De Re Medico Libri Octo*.

Summary box 5.8

Abscesses

- Abscesses need drainage
- Modern imaging techniques may allow guided aspiration
- Antibiotics are indicated if the abscess is not localised (e.g. evidence of cellulitis) or the cavity is not left open to drain freely
- Healing by secondary intention is encouraged

Abscess cavities need cleaning out after incision and drainage and are traditionally encouraged to heal by secondary intention. When the cavity is left open to drain freely, there is no need for antibiotic therapy as well. Antibiotics should be used if the abscess cavity is closed after drainage, but the cavity should not be closed if there is any risk of retained loculi or foreign material. Thus a perianal abscess can be incised and drained, the walls curretted and the skin closed with good results using appropriate antibiotic therapy, but a pilonidal abscess has a higher recurrence risk after such treatment because a nidus of hair may remain in the subcutaneous tissue adjacent to the abscess. Some small breast abscesses can be managed by simple needle aspiration of the pus and antibiotic therapy.

Persistent chronic abscesses may lead to sinus or fistula formation. In a chronic abscess, lymphocytes and plasma cells are seen. There is tissue sequestration and later calcification may occur. Certain organisms are associated with chronicity, sinus and fistula formation. Common ones are *Mycobacterium* and *Actinomyces*. They should not be forgotten when these complications occur and persist.

Perianastomotic contamination may be the cause of an abscess but, in the abdomen, abscesses are more usually the result of anastomotic leakage. An abscess in a deep cavity, such as the pleura or peritoneum, may be difficult to diagnose or locate even when there is strong clinical suspicion that it is present (Figure 5.6). Plain or contrast radiographs may not be helpful, but ultrasonography, computed tomography (CT), magnetic resonance imaging (MRI) and isotope scans are all useful and may allow guided aspiration without the need for surgical intervention.

Cellulitis and lymphangitis

Cellulitis is the non-suppurative invasive infection of tissues. There is poor localisation in addition to the cardinal signs of inflammation. Spreading infection presenting in surgical practice is typically caused by organisms such as β-haemolytic streptococci (Figure 5.7), staphylococci (Figure 5.8) and *C. perfringens*. Tissue destruction, gangrene and ulceration may follow, which are caused by release of proteases.

Systemic signs (the old-fashioned term toxaemia) are common, with chills, fever and rigors. These follow the release of toxins into the circulation, which stimulate a cytokine-mediated systemic inflammatory response even though blood cultures are negative.

Lymphangitis is part of a similar process and presents as painful red streaks in affected lymphatics. Cellulitis is usually located at the point of injury and subsequent tissue infection. Lymphangitis is often accompanied by painful lymph node groups in the related drainage area (Summary box 5.9).

Summary box 5.9

Cellulitis and lymphangitis

- Non-suppurative, poorly localised
- Commonly caused by streptococci, staphylococci or clostridia
- Blood cultures are often negative

SYSTEMIC INFLAMMATORY RESPONSE SYNDROME AND MULTIPLE ORGAN DYSFUNCTION SYNDROME

Systemic inflammatory response syndrome (SIRS) is a systemic manifestation of sepsis, although the syndrome may also be caused by multiple trauma, burns or pancreatitis without infection. Serious infection, such as secondary peritonitis, may lead to SIRS through the release of lipopolysaccharide endotoxin from the walls of dying Gram-negative bacilli (mainly *Escherichia coli*) or other bacteria or fungi. This and other toxins stimulate the release of cytokines from macrophages (Figure 5.3). SIRS should not be confused with bacteraemia although the two may coexist (see Table 5.3).

Septic manifestations and multiple organ dysfunction syndrome (MODS) in SIRS are mediated by the release of proinflammatory cytokines such as interleukin-1 (IL-1) and tumour necrosis factor alpha (TNFα). These cytokines stimulate neu-

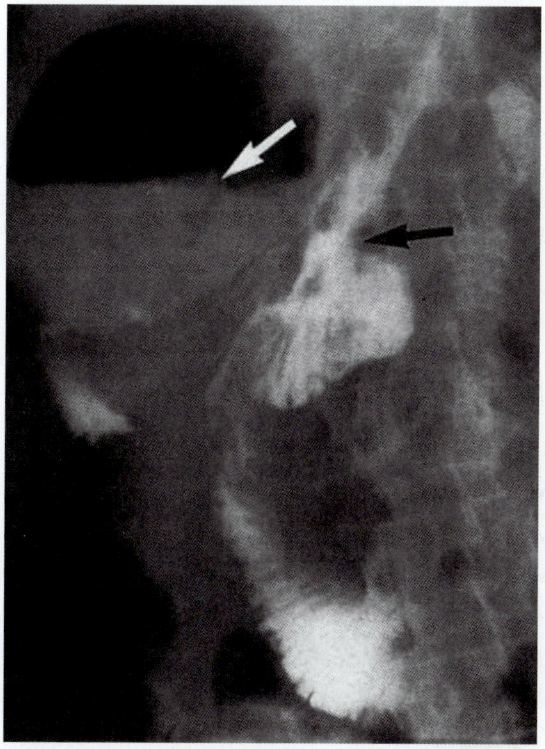

Figure 5.6 Plain radiograph showing a subphrenic abscess with a gas/fluid level (white arrow). Gastrografin is seen leaking from the oesophagojejunal anastomosis (after gastrectomy) towards the abscess (black arrow).

Theodor Escherich, 1857–1911, Professor of Paediatrics, Vienna, Austria, discovered the *Bacterium coli commune* in 1886.

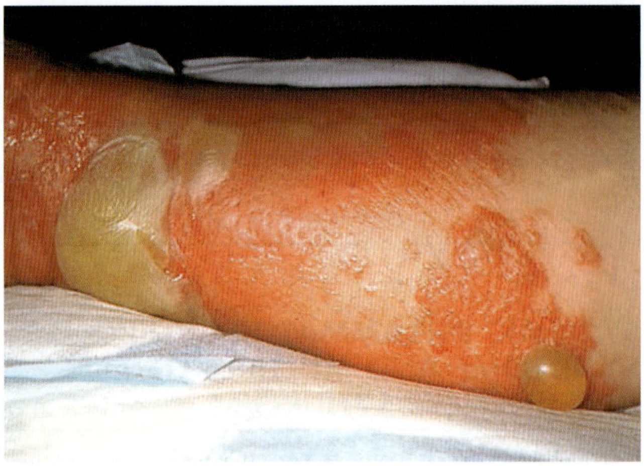

Figure 5.7 Streptococcal cellulitis of the leg following a minor puncture wound.

trophil adhesion to endothelial surfaces adjacent to the source of infection and cause them to migrate through the blood vessel wall by chemotaxis. A respiratory burst occurs within such activated neutrophils, releasing lysosomal enzymes, oxidants and free radicals, which are involved in killing the invading bacteria but which may also damage adjacent cells. Coagulation, complement and fibrinolytic pathways are also stimulated as part of the normal inflammatory response. This response is usually beneficial to the host and is an important aspect of normal tissue repair and wound healing. In the presence of severe sepsis or bacteraemia, this response may become harmful to the host if it occurs in excess, when it is known as SIRS. There are high circulating levels of cytokines and activated neutrophils which stimulate fever, tachycardia and tachypnoea. The activated neutrophils adhere to vascular endothelium in key organs remote from the source of infection and damage it, leading to increased vascular permeability, which in turn leads to cellular damage within the organs, which become dysfunctional and give rise to the clinical picture of MODS. In its most severe form, MODS may progress into multiple system organ failure (MSOF). Respiratory, cardiac, intestinal, renal and liver failure ensue in combination with

Table 5.3 Definitions of systemic inflammatory response syndrome (SIRS) and sepsis.

SIRS
Two of:
hyperthermia (>38°C) or hypothermia (<36°C)
tachycardia (>90/min, no β-blockers) or tachypnoea (>20/min)
white cell count >12 × 10^9/l or <4 × 10^9/l
Sepsis is SIRS with a documented infection
Severe sepsis or sepsis syndrome is sepsis with evidence of one or more organ failures (respiratory (acute respiratory distress syndrome), cardiovascular (septic shock follows compromise of cardiac function and fall in peripheral vascular resistance), renal (usually acute tubular necrosis), hepatic, blood coagulation systems or central nervous system)

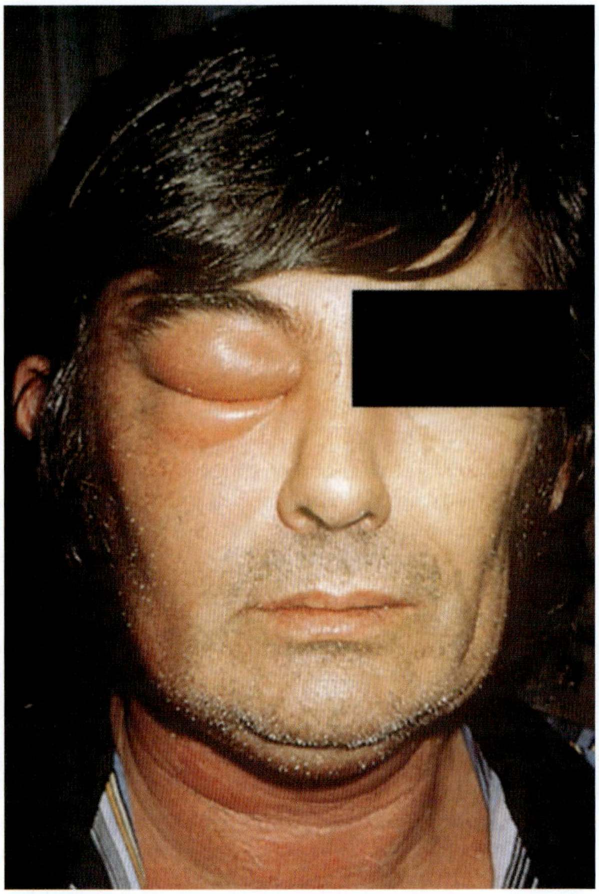

Figure 5.8 Staphylococcal cellulitis of the face and orbit following severe infection of an epidermoid cyst of the scalp.

circulatory failure and shock. In this state, the body's resistance to infection is reduced and a vicious cycle develops where the more organs that fail, the more likely it becomes that death will follow despite all that a modern intensive care unit can do for organ support (Summary box 5.10).

Summary box 5.10

Definitions of infected states

- SSI is an infected wound or deep organ space
- SIRS is the body's systemic response to severe infection
- MODS is the effect that SIRS produces systemically
- MSOF is the end stage of uncontrolled MODS

Bacteraemia and sepsis

Bacteraemia is unusual following superficial SSIs but common after anastomotic breakdown (deep space SSI). It is usually transient and can follow procedures undertaken through infected tissues (particularly instrumentation in infected bile or urine). It may also occur through bacterial colonisation of indwelling intravenous cannulae. Bacteraemia is important when a prosthesis has been implanted, as infection of the prosthesis can occur. Sepsis accompanied by MODS may follow anastomotic breakdown. Aerobic Gram-negative bacilli are mainly responsible, but *S. aureus* and fungi may be involved, particularly after the use of broad-spectrum antibiotics (Summary box 5.11).

Summary box 5.11

Bacteraemia and sepsis

- Sepsis is common after anastomotic breakdown
- Bacteraemia is dangerous if the patient has a prosthesis
- Sepsis may be associated with MODS

Specific wound infections

Gas gangrene

This is caused by *C. perfringens*. These Gram-positive, anaerobic, spore-bearing bacilli are widely found in nature, particularly in soil and faeces. This is relevant to military and traumatic surgery and colorectal operations. Patients who are immunocompromised, diabetic or have malignant disease are at greater risk, particularly if they have wounds containing necrotic or foreign material, resulting in anaerobic conditions. Military wounds provide an ideal environment as the kinetic energy of high-velocity missiles or shrapnel causes extensive tissue damage. The cavitation which follows passage of a missile through the tissues causes a 'sucking' entry wound, leaving clothing and environmental soiling in the wound in addition to devascularised tissue. Gas gangrene wound infections are associated with severe local wound pain and crepitus (gas in the tissues, which may also be noted on plain radiographs). The wound produces a thin, brown, sweet-smelling exudate, in which Gram staining will reveal bacteria. Oedema and spreading gangrene follow the release of collagenase, hyaluronidase, other proteases and alpha toxin. Early systemic complications with circulatory collapse and MSOF follow if prompt action is not taken (Summary box 5.12).

Antibiotic prophylaxis should always be considered in patients at risk, especially when amputations are performed for peripheral vascular disease with open necrotic ulceration. Once gas gangrene infection is established, large doses of intravenous penicillin and aggressive debridement of affected tissues are required.

Summary box 5.12

Gas gangrene

- Caused by *C. perfringens*
- Gas and smell are characteristic
- Immunocompromised patients are most at risk
- Antibiotic prophylaxis is essential when performing amputations to remove dead tissue

Clostridium tetani

This is another anaerobic, terminal spore-bearing, Gram-positive bacterium that can cause tetanus following implantation into tissues or a wound (which may have been trivial or unrecognised and forgotten). The spores are widespread in soil and manure, and so the infection is more common in traumatic civilian or military wounds. The signs and symptoms of tetanus are mediated by the release of the exotoxin tetanospasmin, which affects myoneural junctions and the motor neurones of the anterior horn of the spinal cord. A short prodromal period, which has a poor prognosis, leads to spasms in the distribution of the short motor nerves of the face followed by the development of severe generalised motor spasms including opsithotonus, respiratory arrest and death. A longer prodromal period of 4–5 weeks is associated with a milder form of the disease. The entry wound may show a localised small area of cellulitis; exudate or aspiration may give a sample that can be stained to show the presence of Gram-positive rods. Prophylaxis with tetanus toxoid is the best preventative treatment but, in an established infection, minor debridement of the wound may need to be performed and antibiotic treatment with benzylpenicillin provided in addition. Relaxants may also be required, and the patient may require ventilation in severe forms, which may be associated with a high mortality. The use of antitoxin using human immunoglobulin ought to be considered for both at-risk wounds and established infection.

The toxoid is a formalin-attenuated vaccine and should be given in three separate doses to give protection for a five-year period, after which a single five-yearly booster confers immunity. It should be given to all patients with open traumatic wounds who are not immunised. At-risk wounds are those that present late, when there is devitalisation of tissue or when there is soiling. For these wounds, a booster of toxoid should be given or, if not immunised at all, a three-dose course, together with prophylactic benzylpenicillin; however, the use of antitoxin is controversial because of the risk of toxicity and allergy.

Synergistic spreading gangrene (synonym: subdermal gangrene, necrotising fasciitis)

This condition is not caused by clostridia. A mixed pattern of organisms is responsible: coliforms, staphylococci, *Bacteroides* spp., anaerobic streptococci and peptostreptococci have all been implicated, acting in synergy. Abdominal wall infections are known as Meleney's synergistic hospital gangrene and scrotal infection as Fournier's gangrene (Figure 5.9). Patients are almost always immunocompromised with conditions such as diabetes mellitus. The wound initiating the infection may have been minor, but severely contaminated wounds are more likely to be the cause. Severe wound pain, signs of spreading inflammation with crepitus and smell are all signs of the infection spreading. Untreated, it will lead to widespread gangrene and MSOF. The subdermal spread of gangrene is always much more extensive than appears from initial examination. Broad-spectrum antibiotic therapy must be combined with aggressive circulatory support. Locally, there should be wide excision of necrotic tissue and laying open of affected areas. The debridement may need to be extensive, and patients who survive may need large areas of skin grafting.

TREATMENT OF SURGICAL INFECTION

Now that patients are discharged more quickly after surgery and many procedures are performed as day cases, many SSIs are missed by the surgical team unless they undertake a prolonged and carefully audited follow up with primary care doctors. Suppurative wound infections take 7–10 days to develop, and even cellulitis around wounds caused by invasive organisms (such as the β-haemolytic *Streptococcus*) takes 3–4 days to develop. Major surgical infections with systemic signs (Figure 5.10), evidence of spreading infection, cellulitis or bacteraemia need treatment with appropriate antibiotics. The choice may need to be empirical initially but is best based on culture and sensitivities of isolates harvested at surgery. Although the identification of organisms in surgical infections is necessary for audit and wound surveillance purposes, it is usually 2–3 days before sensitivities are known (Figures 5.11 and 5.12). It is illogical to withhold antibiotics until these are available but, if clinical response is poor by the time sensitivities are known, then antibiotics can be changed. This is unusual if the empirical choice of antibiotics is sensible; change of antibiotics promotes resistance and risks complications, such as *C. difficile* enteritis.

If an infected wound is under tension, or there is clear evidence of suppuration, sutures or clips need to be removed, with curettage if necessary, to allow pus to drain adequately. There is no evidence that subcuticular continuous skin closure contributes to or prevents suppuration. In severely contaminated wounds, such as an incision made for drainage of an abscess, it is logical to leave the skin open. Delayed primary or secondary suture can be undertaken when the wound is clean and granulating (Figures 5.13 and 5.14). Leaving wounds open after a 'dirty' operation, such as laparotomy for faecal peritonitis, is not practised as widely in the UK as in the US or mainland Europe (Summary box 5.13).

Summary box 5.13

Surgical incisions through infected or contaminated tissues

- When possible, tissue or pus for culture should be taken before antibiotic cover is started
- The choice of antibiotics is empirical until sensitivities are available
- Wounds are best managed by delayed primary or secondary closure

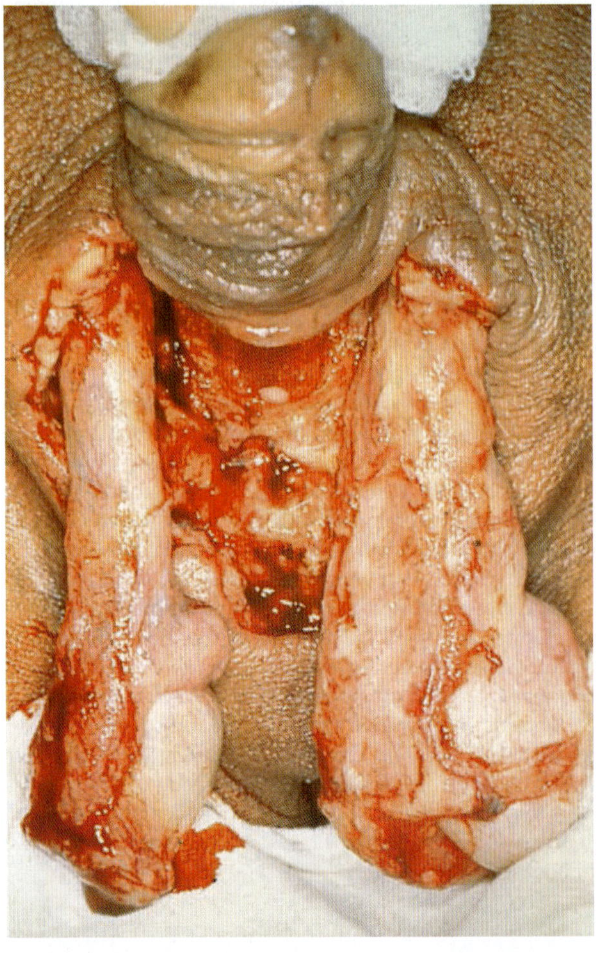

Figure 5.9 A classic presentation of Fournier's gangrene of the scrotum with 'shameful exposure of the testes' following excision of the gangrenous skin.

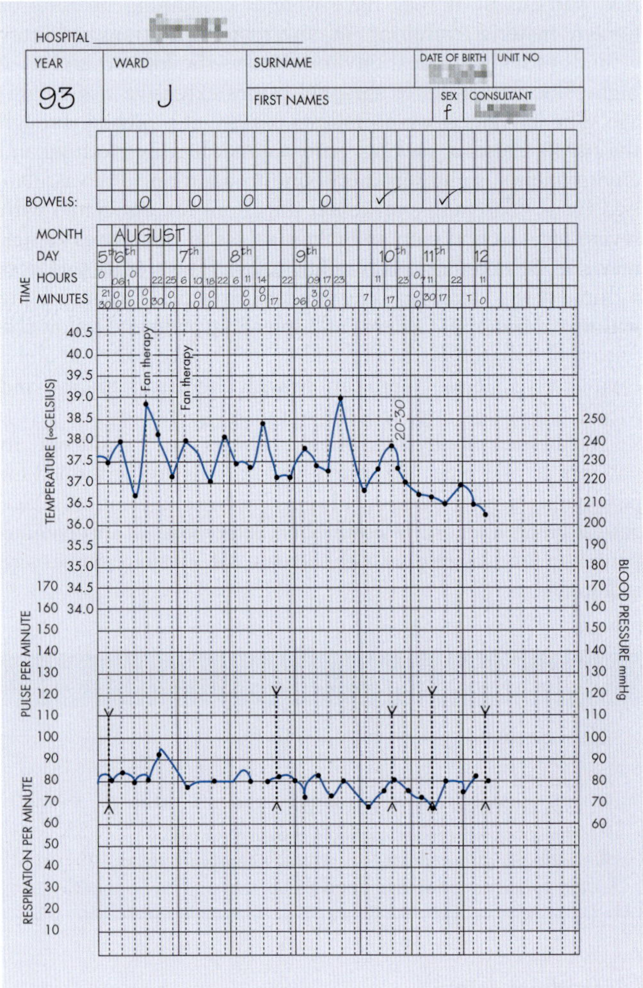

Figure 5.10 Classic swinging pyrexia related to a perianastomotic wound abscess that settled spontaneously on antibiotic therapy.

Frank Lamont Meleney, 1889–1963, Professor of Clinical Surgery, Columbia University, New York, NY, USA.
Jean Alfred Fournier, 1832–1915, syphilologist, the founder of the Venereal and Dermatological Clinic, Hôpital St Louis, Paris, France.

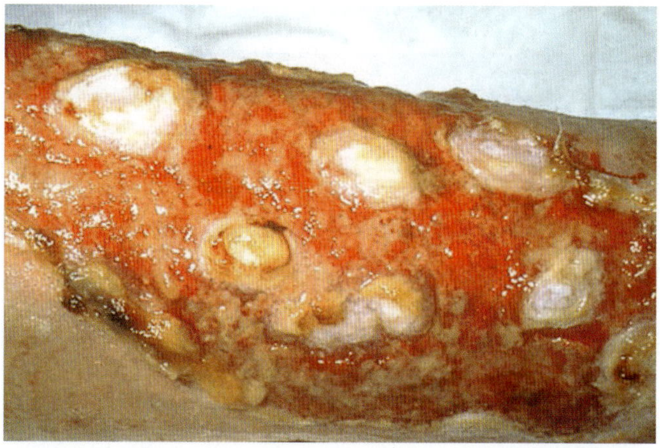

Figure 5.11 Mixed streptococcal infection of a skin graft with very poor 'take'.

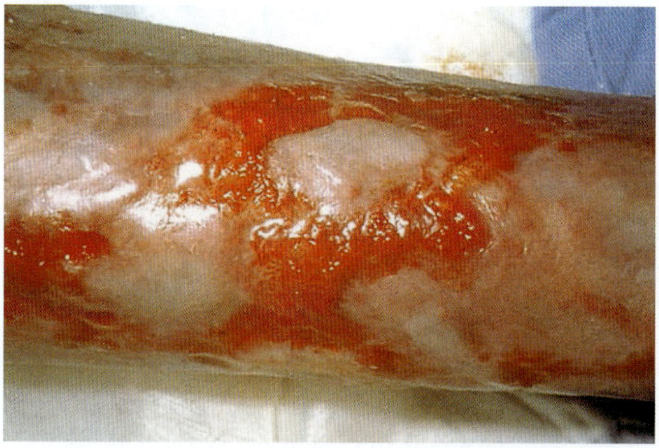

Figure 5.12 After 5–6 days of antibiotics, the infection shown in Figure 5.11 is under control, and the skin grafts are clearly viable.

When taking pus from infected wounds, specimens should be sent fresh for microbiological culture. Swabs should be placed in transport medium, but the larger the volume of pus sent, the more likely is the accurate identification of the organism involved. Providing the microbiologist with as much information as possible and discussing the results with him or her gives the best chance of the most appropriate antibiotic treatment. If bacteraemia is suspected, but results are negative, then repeat specimens for blood culture may need to be taken.

A rapid report on infective material can be based on an immediate Gram stain. Aerobic and anaerobic culture on conventional media allows sensitivities to be assessed by disc diffusion. Measurements of minimum inhibitory antibiotic concentrations (MIC_{90} in mg/L), together with measurements of endotoxin and cytokine levels, are usually only needed for research studies.

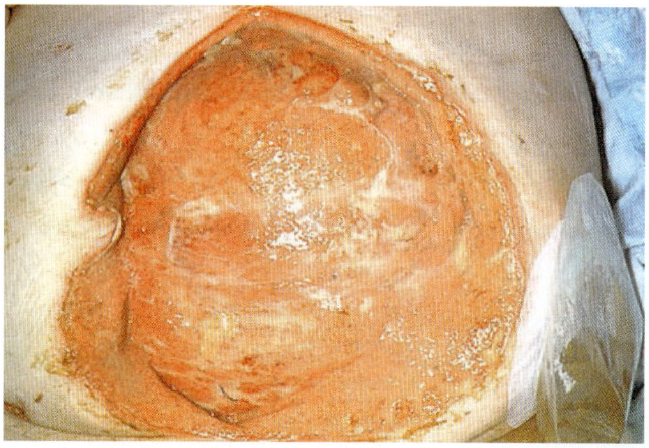

Figure 5.13 Skin layers left open to granulate after laparotomy for faecal peritonitis. The wound is clean and ready for secondary closure.

Many dressings are now available for use in wound care. These are listed in Table 5.4. Polymeric films are used as incision drapes and also to cover sutured wounds, but are not indicated for use in wound infections. Agents that can be used to help debride open infected wounds and others to absorb excessive exudate or to encourage epithelialisation and the formation of granulation tissue are also listed (Figure 5.15). Most contribute to the ideal moist wound environment, and there are others that provide an antibacterial to the wound. There is now a plethora of dressings containing silver or povidone–iodine antiseptics, but the use of topical antibiotics should be avoided because of the risks of allergy and resistance. Topical antiseptics inhibit epithelial ingrowth and should only be used on superficial wounds for a short period to clear infection from heavily contaminated wounds.

Prophylaxis

Prophylactic antibiotics

If antibiotics are given to prevent infection after surgery or instrumentation, they should be used when local wound defences are not established (the decisive period). Ideally, maximal blood and tissue levels should be present at the time at which the first incision is made and before contamination occurs. Intravenous administration at induction of anaesthesia is optimal. In long operations or when there is excessive blood loss or when unexpected contamination occurs, antibiotics may be repeated at 4-hourly intervals during the surgery, as tissue antibiotic levels often fall faster than serum levels. There is no evidence that further doses of antibiotics after surgery are of any value in prophylaxis against infection and the practice can only encourage the development of antibiotic resistance. The choice of an antibiotic depends on the expected spectrum of organisms likely to be encountered, the cost and local hospital policies, which are based on experience of local resistance trends (Summary box 5.14).

Table 5.4 Surgical dressings.

Type	Name (example)	Indications and comments
Debriding agents	Benoxyl–benzoic acid Aserbine–benzoic acid Variclene–lactic acid	Used only in necrotic sloughing skin ulcers. Provide acidic environment. Claimed to enhance healing with debriding action
Enzymatic agents	Varidase–streptokinase/streptodornase	Activate fibrinolysis and liquefy pus on chronic skin ulcers
Bead dressings	Debrisan	Remove bacteria and excess moisture by capillary action in deep granulating wounds. Antimicrobials
	Iodosorb	May be added but with questionable topical benefit
	Other paste dressings	
Polymeric films	Opsite Bioclusive Tegaderm	Primary adhesive transparent dressing for sutured wounds or donor sites
Foams	Silastic (elastomer)	Elastomeric dressing can be shaped to fit deep cavities and granulating wounds. Absorbent and non-adherent
	Lyofoam Allevyn	
Hydrogels	Geliperm Intrasite	Maintain moist environment. Polymers can absorb exudate or antiseptics (but adding antiseptics is of doubtful benefit). Semi-permeable, allow gas exchange
Hydrocolloids	Comfeel Granuflex	Complete occlusion. Promote epithelialisation and granulation tissue. Maintain moisture without gaseous exchange across them
Fibrous polymers	Kaltostat Sorbsan	Absorptive alginate dressings. Derived from natural (seaweed) source Like polymeric hydrocolloids and hydrogels, they can be used to pack deep wounds
Biological membranes	Porcine skin, amnion	Used for superficial chronic skin ulcers. No proven advantage
Simple miscellaneous	Gauzes: viscose/cotton with non-adherent coating (Melolin) Tulles: non-adherent paraffin impregnation	Simple absorptive dressings only used as secondary dressings to absorb exudate. Added antimicrobials probably confer no benefit. Added charcoal absorbents may reduce swelling. Relatively cheap but of questionable effectiveness

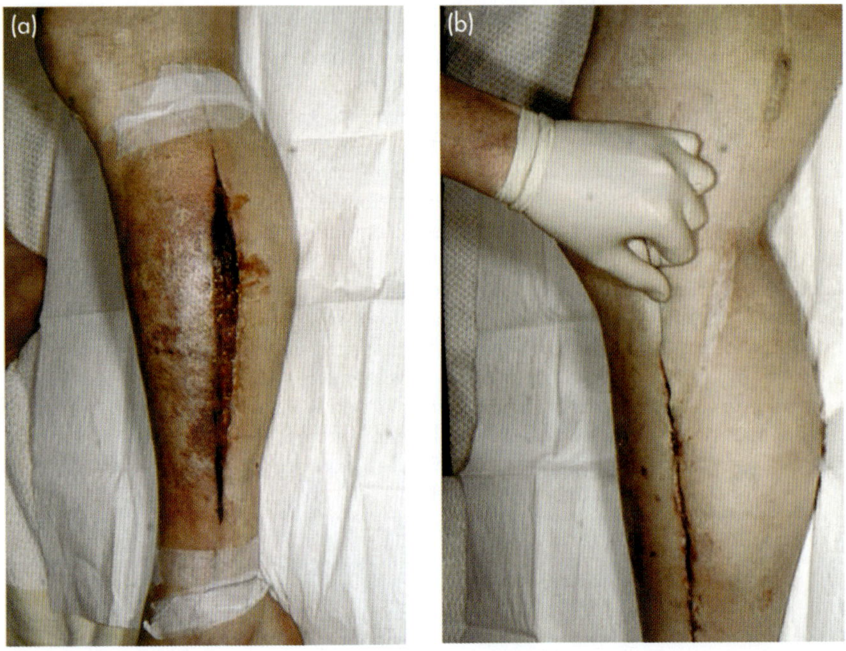

Figure 5.14 Delayed primary closure of fasciotomy wound.

Table 5.5 Suggested prophylactic regimens for operations at risk.

Type of surgery	Organisms encountered	Prophylactic regimen suggested
Vascular	*Staphylococcus epidermidis* (or MRCNS) *S. aureus* (or MRSA) Aerobic Gram-negative bacilli (AGNB)	One dose of augmentin with or without gentamicin, vancomycin or rifampicin if MRCNS/MRSA a risk
Orthopaedic	*S. epidermidis/aureus*	One dose of augmentin
Oesophagogastric	Enterobacteriaceae Enterococci (including anaerobic/viridans streptococci)	One dose of a second-generation cephalosporin and metronidazole in severe contamination
Biliary	Enterobacteriaceae (mainly *Escherichia coli*) Enterococci (including *Streptococcus faecalis*)	One dose of a second-generation cephalosporin
Small bowel	Enterobacteriaceae Anaerobes (mainly *Bacteroides*)	One dose of a second-generation cephalosporin with or without metronidazole
Appendix/colorectal	Enterobacteriaceae Anaerobes (mainly *Bacteroides*)	One dose of a second-generation cephalosporin (or gentamicin) with metronidazole (the use of oral, poorly absorbed antibiotics is controversial)

MRCNS, multiply resistant coagulase-negative staphylococci; MRSA, methicillin-resistant *Staphylococcus aureus*.

Summary box 5.14

Choice of antibiotics for prophylaxis

- Empirical cover against expected pathogens with local hospital guidelines
- Single-shot intravenous administration at induction of anaesthesia
- Repeat only during long operations or if there is excessive blood loss
- Continue as therapy if there is unexpected contamination or if a prosthetic is implanted in a patient with a septic source
- Benzylpenicillin should be used if Clostridium gas gangrene infection is a possibility
- Patients with heart valve disease or a prosthesis should be protected from bacteraemia caused by dental work, urethral instrumentation or visceral surgery

The use of the newer, broad-spectrum antibiotics for prophylaxis should be avoided. Table 5.5 gives some examples of prophylaxis that can be used in elective surgical operations.

Patients with known valvular disease of the heart (or with any implanted vascular or orthopaedic prosthesis) should have prophylactic antibiotics during dental, urological or open viscus surgery. Single doses of broad-spectrum penicillin, for example amoxicillin, orally or intravenously administered, are sufficient for dental surgery. In urological instrumentation, a single dose of gentamycin is often used.

Preoperative preparation

Short preoperative hospital stay lowers the risk of acquiring MRSA, multiply resistant coagulase-negative staphylococci (MRCNS) and other organisms and the acquisition of HAIs. Medical and nursing staff should always wash their hands after any patient contact. Alcoholic hand gels can act as a substitute for hand washing, but do not destroy the spores of *C. difficile*, which may cause pseudomembranous colitis, especially in immunocompromised patients or those whose gut flora is suppressed by antibiotic therapy. Although the need for clean hospitals, emphasised by the media, is logical, the 'clean your hands campaign' is beginning to result in falls in the incidence of HAIs. Staff with open, infected skin lesions should not enter the operating theatre. Ideally, neither should patients, especially if they are having a prosthesis implanted. Antiseptic baths (usually chlorhexidine) are popular in Europe, but there is no hard evidence for their value in reducing wound infections. Preoperative skin shaving should be undertaken in the operating theatre immediately before surgery as the SSI rate after clean wound surgery may be doubled if it is performed the night before; minor skin injury enhances superficial bacterial colonisation. Cream depilation is messy and hair clipping is best, with the lowest rate of infection (Summary box 5.15).

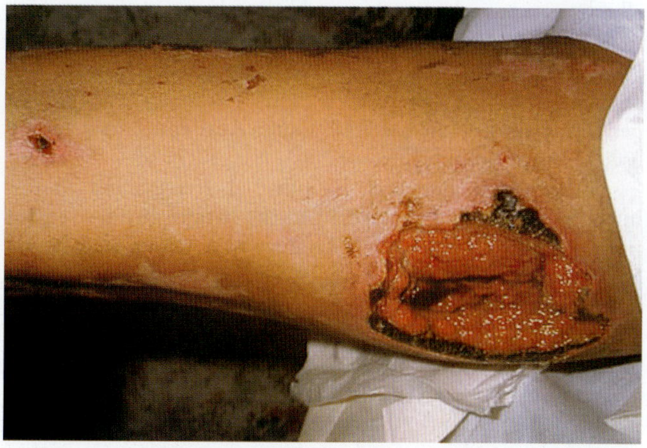

Figure 5.15 Infected animal bite/wound of the upper thigh, treated by open therapy following virulent staphylococcal infection. Deep cavity wounds such as this can be debrided and kept moist with many of the modern dressings listed in Table 5.4.

Table 5.6 Classification of antiseptics commonly used in general surgical practice.

Name	Presentation	Uses	Comments
Chlorhexidine (Hibiscrub)	Alcoholic 0.5% Aqueous 4%	Skin preparation Skin preparation. Surgical scrub in dilute solutions in open wounds	Has cumulative effect. Effective against Gram-positive organisms and relatively stable in the presence of pus and body fluids
Povidone–iodine (Betadine)	Alcoholic 10% Aqueous 7.5%	Skin preparation Skin preparation. Surgical scrub in dilute solutions in open wounds	Safe, fast-acting, broad spectrum. Some sporicidal activity. Anti-fungal iodine is not free but combined with polyvinylpyrrolidone (povidone)
Cetrimide (Savlon)	Aqueous	Hand washing Instrument and surface cleaning	*Pseudomonas* spp. may grow in stored contaminated solutions. Ammonium compounds have good detergent action (surface-active agent)
Alcohols	70% ethyl, isopropyl	Skin preparation	Should be reserved for use as disinfectants
Hypochlorites	Aqueous preparations (Eusol, Milton, Chloramine T)	Instrument and surface cleaning (debriding agent in open wounds?)	Toxic to tissues
Hexachlorophane	Aqueous bisphenol	Skin preparation Hand washing	Has action against Gram-negative organisms

Summary box 5.15

Avoiding surgical site infections

- Staff should always wash their hands between patients
- Length of patient stay should be kept to a minimum
- Preoperative shaving should be done immediately before surgery
- Antiseptic skin preparation should be standardised
- Attention to theatre technique and discipline
- Avoid hypothermia perioperatively and ensure supplemental oxygenation in recovery

Scrubbing and skin preparation

For the first operation of the day, aqueous antiseptics should be used for hand washing, and the scrub should include the nails. Subsequent scrubbing should merely involve washing to the elbows, as repeated extensive scrubbing releases more organisms than it removes.

One application of an alcoholic antiseptic is adequate for skin preparation of the operative site. This leads to a more than 95 per cent reduction in bacterial count. Antiseptics in common use are listed in Table 5.6.

Theatre technique and discipline also contribute to low infection rates. Numbers of staff in the theatre and movement in and out of theatre should be kept to a minimum. Careful and regular surveillance is needed to ensure the quality of theatre ventilation, instrument sterilisation and aseptic technique. Operator skill in gentle manipulation and dissection of tissues is much more difficult to audit, but dead spaces and haematomas should be avoided and the use of diathermy kept to a minimum. There is no evidence that drains, incision drapes or wound guards help to reduce wound infection.

There is the highest level of evidence-based medicine that the perioperative avoidance of hypothermia and supplemental oxygen during recovery can significantly reduce the rate of SSIs.

Postoperative care of wounds

Similar attention to standards is needed in the postoperative care of wounds. Secondary (exogenous) SSIs, as well as other HAIs, can be related to poor hospital standards. For example, outbreaks of MRSA infections are rare but serious. The presence of this organism in wounds, and the number of MRSA bacteraemias, can be a marker of inadequate postoperative wound care, and it can be very difficult and expensive to screen for, identify and eradicate.

Careful audit should lead to changes in practice, and follow up should ensure that audit loops are closed. It is critical that surgeons manage their own audit; league tables kept by non-medical or related personnel must be accurate. Scoring systems are useful in audit but, in general, have only been used in wound infection research (Tables 5.2 and 5.3). Nevertheless, accurate audit ought to involve the use of trained, blinded observers in post-discharge surveillance of all HAIs, using validated and reproducible definitions.

CLASSIFICATION OF SURGICAL WOUNDS

Potential for infection

The best measure of wound contamination at the end of an operation is to sample tissue in the wound edge. The theoretical degree of contamination, proposed by the National Research Council (USA) over 40 years ago, relates well to infection rates (Table 5.7). When wounds are heavily contaminated or when an incision is made into an abscess, therapeutic antibiotics may be justified. In these cases, infection rates of more than 15 per cent are expected. There is undisputed evidence that prophylactic antibiotics are effective in clean-contaminated and contaminated operations. Infection rates after non-prosthetic clean surgery may be higher than expected when carefully audited by post-discharge surveillance. Breast surgery, for example, is associated with a high risk of infection, or wound complications, which may be interpreted

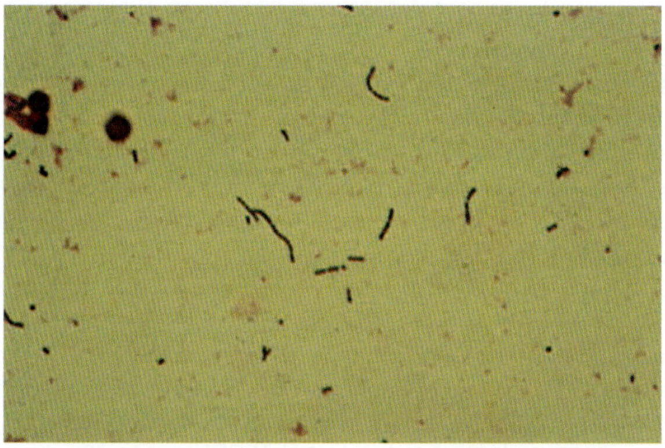

Figure 5.16 Streptococci.

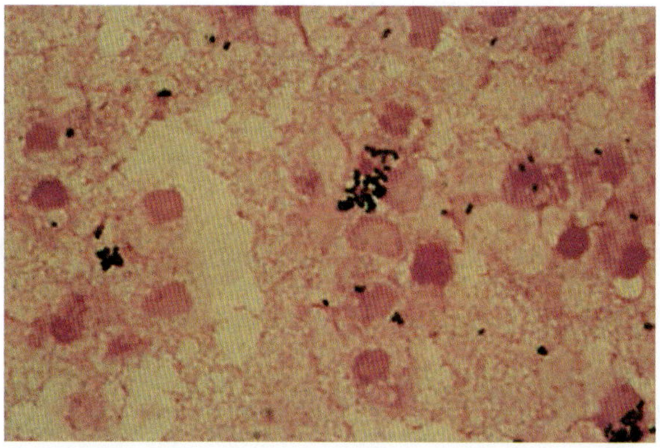

Figure 5.17 Staphylococcal pus.

Table 5.7 Surgical site infection (SSI) rates relating to wound contamination.

Type of surgery	Infection rate (%)	Rate before prophylaxis
Clean (no viscus opened)	1–2	The same
Clean-contaminated (viscus opened, minimal spillage)	<10	Gastric surgery up to 30% Biliary surgery up to 20%
Contaminated (open viscus with spillage or inflammatory disease)	15–20	Variable but up to 60%
Dirty (pus or perforation, or incision through an abscess)	<40	Up to 60% or more

as a failure to heal and related to a high body mass index (BMI). The value of antibiotic prophylaxis is controversial in non-prosthetic clean surgery, with most trials showing no clear benefit.

BACTERIA INVOLVED IN SURGICAL INFECTION

Streptococci

Streptococci form chains and are Gram positive on staining (Figure 5.16). The most important is the β-haemolytic *Streptococcus*, which resides in the pharynx of 5–10 per cent of the population. In the Lancefield A–G carbohydrate antigens classification, it is the group A *Streptococcus*, also called *Streptococcus pyogenes*, that is the most pathogenic. It has the ability to spread, causing cellulitis, and to cause tissue destruction through the release of enzymes such as streptolysin, streptokinase and streptodornase.

Streptococcus faecalis is an enterococcus in Lancefield group D. It is often found in synergy with other organisms, as is the γ-haemolytic *Streptococcus* and *Peptostreptococcus*, which is an anaerobe.

Both *Streptococcus pyogenes* and *Streptococcus faecalis* may be involved in wound infection after large bowel surgery, but the α-haemolytic *Streptococcus viridans* is not associated with wound infections.

All the streptococci remain sensitive to penicillin and erythromycin. The cephalosporins are a suitable alternative in patients who are allergic to penicillin.

Staphylococci

Staphylococci form clumps and are Gram positive (Figure 5.17). *Staphylococcus aureus* is the most important pathogen in this group and is found in the nasopharynx of up to 15 per cent of the population. It can cause exogenous suppuration in wounds (and implanted prostheses). Strains resistant to antibiotics (e.g. MRSA) can cause epidemics and more severe infection. It is controversial but, if MRSA infection is found in a hospital, all doctors, nurses and patients may need to be swabbed so that carriers can be identified and treated. In parts of northern Europe, the prevalence of MRSA infections has been kept at very low levels using 'search and destroy' methods, which use these screening techniques and the isolation or treatment of carriers. Patients found to be positive on screening may be denied access to hospital. Some MRSA strains are now also resistant to vancomycin. Local policies on the management of MRSA depend on the prevalence of MRSA, the type of hospital or clinical specialty and the availability of facilities. Widespread swabbing, ward closures, isolation of patients and disinfection of wards all have to be carefully considered and involve all groups of practitioners. They may be expensive but necessary options.

Infections are usually suppurative and localised (see above under Abscess). Most hospital *Staphylococcus aureus* strains are now β-lactamase producers and are resistant to penicillin, but most strains (MRSA) remain sensitive to flucloxacillin, vancomycin, aminoglycosides, some cephalosporins and fusidic acid (used in osteomyelitis). There are several novel and innovative antibiotics becoming available that have high activity against resistant strains. Some have the advantage of good oral activity (linezolid), some have a wide spectrum (tigecycline), have good activity in bacteraemia (daptomycin) but are relatively expen-

The name Eusol is derived from Edinburgh University solution of lime.

Rebecca Graighill Lancefield, 1895–1981, an American bacteriologist, classified streptococci in 1933.

sive, and some have side effects involving marrow, hepatic and renal toxicity. Their use is justified but needs to be controlled by tight local policies and guidelines that involve clinical microbiologists.

Staphylococcus epidermidis (previously *Staphylococcus albus*), also known as coagulase-negative staphylococci (CNS), was regarded as a commensal but is now recognised as a major threat in prosthetic (vascular and orthopaedic) surgery and in indwelling vascular catheters. They can be multiply resistant (MRCNS) to many antibiotics and represent an important cause of HAI.

Clostridia

Clostridial organisms are Gram-positive, obligate anaerobes, which produce resistant spores (Figure 5.18). *C. perfringens* is the cause of gas gangrene, and *C. tetani* causes tetanus after implantation into tissues or a wound (see above under Specific wound infections).

C. difficile is the cause of pseudomembranous colitis. This is another HAI, now more common than the incidence of MRSA bacteraemia, which is caused by the overuse of antibiotics. The quinolones, such as ciprofloxacin, seem to be most implicated, but the inappropriate sequential use of several antibiotics puts patients most at risk, particularly in elderly or immunocompromised patients. The key symptom of bloody diarrhoea can occur in small epidemics through poor hygiene. In its most severe form, colitis may lead to perforation and the need for emergency colectomy, with an associated high mortality. Treatment involves resuscitation and antibiotic therapy with metronidazole or vancomycin. The fibrinous exudate is typical and differentiates the colitis from other inflammatory diseases; the laboratory recognition of the toxin is an early accurate diagnostic test.

Aerobic Gram-negative bacilli

These bacilli are normal inhabitants of the large bowel. *E. coli* and *Klebsiella* spp. are lactose fermenting; *Proteus* is non-lactose fermenting. Most organisms in this group act in synergy with *Bacteroides* to cause SSIs after bowel operations (in particular, appendicitis, diverticulitis and peritonitis). *E. coli* is a major cause of the HAI of urinary tract infection, although most aerobic Gram-negative bacilli (AGNB) may be involved, particularly in relation to urinary catheterisation. There is increasing concern about the development of ESBLs in many of this group of bacteria, which confer resistance to many antibiotics, particularly cephalosporins.

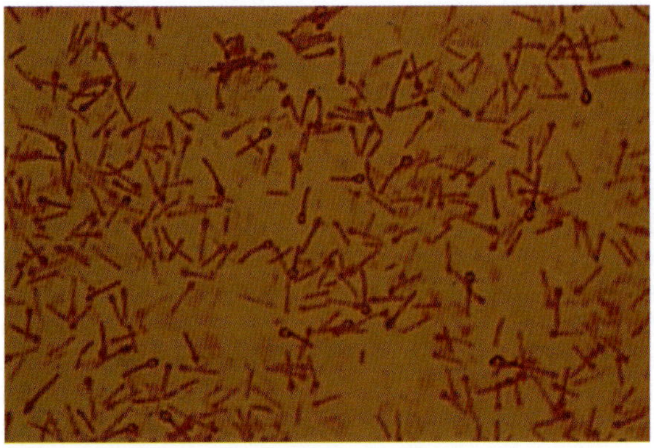

Figure 5.18 *Clostridium tetani* (drumstick spores).

Pseudomonas spp. tend to colonise burns and tracheostomy wounds, as well as the urinary tract. Once *Pseudomonas* has colonised wards and intensive care units, it may be difficult to eradicate. Surveillance of cross-infection is important in outbreaks. Hospital strains become resistant to β-lactamase as resistance can be transferred by plasmids. Wound infections need antibiotic therapy only when there is progressive or spreading infection with systemic signs. The aminoglycosides are effective, but some cephalosporins and penicillin may not be. Many of the carbapenems (e.g. meropenem) are useful in severe infections, whereas the quinolones have been made ineffective through their overuse and the development of ESBLs.

Bacteroides

Bacteroides are non-spore-bearing, strict anaerobes that colonise the large bowel, vagina and oropharynx. *Bacteroides fragilis* is the principal organism that acts in synergy with AGNB to cause SSIs, including intra-abdominal abscesses, after colorectal or gynaecological surgery. They are sensitive to the imidazoles (e.g. metronidazole) and some cephalosporins (e.g. cefotaxime).

PRINCIPLES OF ANTIMICROBIAL TREATMENT

Antimicrobials may be used to prevent (see above under Prophylaxis) or treat established surgical infection (Summary box 5.16).

Summary box 5.16

Principles for the use of antibiotic therapy

- Antibiotics do not replace surgical drainage of infection
- Only spreading infection or signs of systemic infection justifies the use of antibiotics
- Whenever possible, the organism and sensitivity should be determined

The use of antibiotics for the treatment of established surgical infection ideally requires recognition and determination of the sensitivities of the causative organisms. Antibiotic therapy should not be held back if it is indicated, the choice being empirical and later modified depending on microbiological findings. However, once antibiotics have been administered, the clinical picture may become confused and, if a patient's condition does not rapidly improve, the opportunity to make a precise diagnosis may have been lost. It is unusual to have to treat SSIs with antibiotics, unless there is evidence of spreading infection, bacteraemia or systemic complications (SIRS and MODS). The appropriate treatment of localised SSIs is interventional radiological drainage of pus or open drainage and debridement.

Theodor Albrecht Edwin Klebs, 1834–1913, Professor of Bacteriology successively at Prague, Czechoslovakia; Zurich, Switzerland; and The Rush Medical College, Chicago, IL, USA.

There are two approaches to antibiotic treatment:

1 A **narrow-spectrum antibiotic** may be used to treat a known sensitive infection; for example, MRSA (which may be isolated from pus) is usually sensitive to vancomycin or teicoplanin, but not flucloxacillin.
2 **Combinations of broad-spectrum antibiotics** can be used when the organism is not known or when it is suspected that several bacteria, acting in synergy, may be responsible for the infection. For example, during and following emergency surgery requiring the opening of perforated or ischaemic bowel, any of the gut organisms may be responsible for subsequent peritoneal or bacteraemic infection. In this case, a triple-therapy combination of broad-spectrum penicillin (such as ampicillin or mezlocillin) with an aminoglycoside (such as gentamicin) and metronidazole, may be used per- and postoperatively to support the patient's own body defences.

An alternative to the penicillins is a cephalosporin, e.g. cefuroxime. Other alternatives are piperacillin and tazobactam in combination or monotherapy using a carbapenem. The use of such broad-spectrum antibiotic strategies should be guided by specialist microbiological advice.

In surgical units in which resistant *Pseudomonas* or other Gram-negative species (such as *Klebsiella*) have become 'resident opportunists', it may be necessary to rotate anti-pseudomonal and anti-Gram-negative antibiotic therapy (Summary box 5.17).

Summary box 5.17

Treatment of commensals that have become opportunist pathogens

- They are likely to have multiple antibiotic resistance
- It may be necessary to rotate antibiotics

The use of these routines, subsequent wound infection and the alternation of combinations of chemotherapy should be monitored by the infection control team and local hospital protocols. In treating patients who have surgical infection with systemic signs (SIRS and MODS), a failure to respond to antibiotics may indicate that there has been a failure of infection source control. If response is poor after 3–4 days, there should be a re-evaluation with a review of charts and further investigations requested to exclude the development or persistence of infection such as a collection of pus.

New antibiotics should be used with caution and, wherever possible, sensitivities should first be obtained. There are certain general rules on which the choice of antibiotics may be based. For example, it is unusual for *Pseudomonas aeruginosa* to be found as a primary infecting organism unless the patient has had surgical or hospital treatment. Local antibiotic sensitivity patterns vary from centre to centre and from country to country, and the sensitivity patterns of common pathogens should be known to the hospital microbiologist who should be involved.

ANTIBIOTICS USED IN TREATMENT AND PROPHYLAXIS OF SURGICAL INFECTION

Antimicrobials may be produced by living organisms (antibiotics) or by synthetic methods. Some are bactericidal, e.g. penicillins and aminoglycosides, and others are bacteriostatic, e.g. tetracycline and erythromycin. In general, penicillins act upon the bacterial cell wall and are most effective against bacteria that are multiplying and synthesising new cell wall materials. The aminoglycosides act at the ribosomal level, preventing or distorting the production of proteins required to maintain the integrity of the enzymes in the bacterial cell. Hospital and Formulary guidelines should be consulted for doses and monitoring of antibiotic therapy.

Penicillin

Benzylpenicillin has proved most effective against Gram-positive pathogens, including most streptococci, the clostridia and some of the staphylococci that do not produce β-lactamase. It is still effective against *Actinomyces*, which is a rare cause of chronic wound infection, and may be used specifically to treat spreading streptococcal infections. Penicillin is valuable even if other antibiotics are required as part of multiple therapy for a mixed infection. All serious infections, e.g. gas gangrene, require high-dose intravenous benzylpenicillin.

Flucloxacillin

This is a β-lactamase-resistant penicillin and is therefore of use in treating most community-acquired staphylococcal infections, but it has poor activity against other pathogens.

Ampicillin and amoxicillin

These β-lactam penicillins can be taken orally or may be given parenterally. Both are effective against Enterobacteriaceae, *Enterococcus faecalis* and the majority of group D streptococci, but not species of *Klebsiella* or pseudomonads. Their use is now rare as there are more effective alternatives.

Mezlocillin and azlocillin

These are ureidopenicillins with good activity against species of *Enterobacter* and *Klebsiella*. Azlocillin is effective against *Pseudomonas*. Each has some activity against *Bacteroides* and enterococci, but all are susceptible to β-lactamases. Combined with an aminoglycoside, mezlocillin is a valuable treatment for severe mixed infections, particularly those caused by Gram-negative organisms in immunocompromised patients.

Clavulanic acid is available combined with amoxicillin (Augmentin) and can be taken orally. This anti-β-lactamase protects amoxicillin from inactivation by β-lactamase-producing bacteria. It is of value in treating infections caused by *Klebsiella* strains and β-lactamase-producing *E. coli* but is not active against *Pseudomonas* spp. It can be used for localised cellulitis or superficial staphylococcal infections and infected human and animal bites. It is available for oral or intravenous therapy.

Cephalosporins

There are several β-lactamase-susceptible cephalosporins that are of value in surgical practice: cefuroxime, cefotaxime and ceftazidime are widely used. The first two are most effective in intra-abdominal skin and soft-tissue infections, being active against *Staphylococcus aureus* and most Enterobacteriaceae. As a group, the enterococci (*Streptococcus faecalis*) are not sensitive to the cephalosporins. Ceftazidime, although active against the Gram-negative organisms and *S. aureus*, is also effective against *P. aeruginosa*. These cephalosporins may be combined with an aminoglycoside, such as gentamicin, and an imidazole, such as metronidazole, if anaerobic cover is needed. Newer cephalosporins may be effective against organisms such as MRSA, but their spectra are usually limited.

Aminoglycosides

Gentamicin and tobramycin have similar activity and are effective against Gram-negative Enterobacteriaceae. Gentamicin is effective against many strains of *Pseudomonas*, although resistance has been recognised. All aminoglycosides are inactive against anaerobes and streptococci. Serum levels immediately before and 1 hour after intramuscular injection must be taken 48 hours after the start of therapy, and dosage should be modified to satisfy peak and trough levels. Ototoxicity and nephrotoxicity may follow sustained high toxic levels. These antibiotics have a marked post-antibiotic effect, and single, large doses are effective and may be safer. Use needs to be discussed with the microbiologist, and local policies should be observed.

Vancomycin

This glycopeptide is most active against Gram-positive bacteria and has proved to be effective against MRSA, although vancomycin resistance is increasingly being reported. However, it is ototoxic and nephrotoxic, so serum levels should be monitored. It is effective against *C. difficile* in cases of pseudomembranous colitis.

Imidazoles

Metronidazole is the most widely used member of the imidazole group and is active against all anaerobic bacteria. It is particularly safe and may be administered orally, rectally or intravenously. Infections caused by anaerobic cocci and strains of *Bacteroides* and clostridia can be treated, or prevented, by its use. Metronidazole is useful for the prophylaxis and treatment of anaerobic infections after abdominal, colorectal and pelvic surgery.

Carbapenems

Meropenem, ertapenem and imipenem are members of the carbapenems. They are stable to β-lactamase, have useful broad-spectrum anaerobic as well as Gram-positive activity and are effective for the treatment of resistant organisms, such as ESBL-resistant urinary tract infections or serious mixed-spectrum abdominal infections (peritonitis).

Quinolones

Quinolones, such as ciprofloxacin, were active against a wide spectrum of organisms. Their widespread use has been related to the development of resistant organisms, and their role in treating surgical infection is limited.

HUMAN IMMUNODEFICIENCY VIRUS, AIDS AND THE SURGEON

The type I human immunodeficiency virus (HIV) is one of the viruses of surgical importance as it can be transmitted by body fluids, particularly blood. It is a retrovirus that has become increasingly prevalent through sexual transmission, both homo- and heterosexual, in intravenous drug addiction, through infected blood in treating haemophiliacs, in particular, and in sub-Saharan Africans. The risk in surgery is probably mostly through 'needle stick' injury during operations.

After exposure, the virus binds to CD4 receptors with a subsequent loss of $CD4^+$ cells, T-helper cells and other cells involved in cell-mediated immunity, antibody production and delayed hypersensitivity. Macrophages and gut-associated lymphoid tissue (GALT) are also affected. The risk of opportunistic infections (such as *Pneumocystis carinii* pneumonia, tuberculosis and cytomegalovirus) and neoplasms (such as Kaposi's sarcoma and lymphoma) is thereby increased.

In the early weeks after HIV infection, there may be a flu-like illness and, during the phase of seroconversion, patients present the greatest risk of HIV transmission. It is during these early phases that drug treatment, highly active anti-retroviral therapy (HAART), is most effective through the ability of these drugs to inhibit reverse transcriptase and protease synthesis, which are the principal mechanisms through which HIV can progress. Within two years, untreated HIV can progress to AIDS in 25–35 per cent of patients, which is considered to be fatal.

Involvement of surgeons with HIV patients (universal precautions)

Patients may present to surgeons for operative treatment if they have a surgical disease and they are known to be infected or 'at risk', or because they need surgical intervention related to their illness for vascular access or a biopsy when they are known to have HIV infection or AIDS. Universal precautions have been drawn up by the CDC in the United States and largely adopted by the NHS in the UK (in summary):

- when there is a risk of splashing, particularly with power tools, use of a full face mask ideally, or protective spectacles;
- use of fully waterproof, disposable gowns and drapes, particularly during seroconversion;
- boots to be worn, not clogs, to avoid injury from dropped sharps;
- double gloving needed (a larger size on the inside is more comfortable);
- allow only essential personnel in theatre;
- avoid unnecessary movement in theatre;
- respect is required for sharps, with passage in a kidney dish;
- a slow meticulous operative technique is needed with minimised bleeding.

After contamination

Needle-stick injuries are most common on the non-dominant index finger during operative surgery. Hollow needle injury carries the greatest risk of HIV transmission. The injured part should be washed under running water and the incident reported. Local policies dictate whether post-exposure HAART should be given. Occupational advice is required after high-risk

Sub-Saharan Africans come from that part of the African continent which lies south of the Sahara Desert.

exposure together with the need for HIV testing and the option for continuation in an operative specialty.

FURTHER READING

Cohen J, Powderly WG, Opal SM. *Infectious diseases*. St Louis, MO: Mosby, 2010.

Fraise AP, Bradley C. *Ayliffe's control of healthcare associated infection: a practical handbook*. London: Hodder Arnold, 2009.

Fry DE. *Surgical infections*. Boston, MA: Little, Brown & Co, 1995.

Goering R, Dockrell H, Zuckerman M *et al. Mims' medical microbiology*, 4th edn. St Louis, MO: Mosby, 2007.

Greenwood D, Slack RCB, Peutherer JF, Barer MR. *Medical microbiology: a guide to microbial infections: pathogenesis, immunity, laboratory diagnosis and control*. Edinburgh: Churchill Livingstone, 2007.

Howard RJ, Simmons RL. *Surgical infectious diseases*, 3rd edn. East Norwalk, CT: Allyn & Bacon, 1995.

Kumar V, Abbas A, Aster J. *Robbins and Cotran pathologic basis of disease*, 8th edn. Philadelphia, PA: Saunders Elsevier, 2009.

Majno G. *The healing hand. Man and wound in the ancient world*. Cambridge, MA: Harvard University Press, 1991.

Mandell GL, Bennett JE, Dolin R. *Principles and practice of infectious diseases*. Edinburgh: Churchill Livingstone, 2004.

Torok E, Moran E, Cooke F. *Oxford handbook of infectious diseases and microbiology*. Oxford: Oxford University Press, 2009.

Williams JD, Taylor EW. *Infection in surgical practice*. London: Hodder Arnold, 2003.

CHAPTER

6 Surgery in the tropics

LEARNING OBJECTIVES

To be aware of:

- The common surgical conditions that occur in the tropics

To appreciate:

- That many patients do not seek medical help until late in the course of the disease

To know:

- The emergency presentations of the various conditions as patients in developing countries do not seek treatment until they are very ill

To be able to:

- Diagnose and treat these conditions, particularly as emergencies, because of the ease of global travel, visitors from the tropics would mostly present as an emergency in Western hospitals

To realise:

- That ideal management needs good teamwork between the surgeon, physician, radiologist, pathologist and microbiologist. In case of doubt in a difficult situation, there should be no hesitation in seeking help from London School of Hygiene and Tropical Medicine or Liverpool School of Tropical Medicine, the nation's foremost tropical medicine institutions.

INTRODUCTION

Most surgical conditions in the tropics are associated with parasitic infestations. With the ease of international travel, diseases that are common in the tropics and developing countries may be seen in the UK, especially presenting as emergencies.

This section deals with the conditions that a surgeon might occasionally encounter in a visitor to these shores. The life cycles of the parasites will not be dealt with. For academic interest readers are, however, advised to refer to the 24th edition of this book should they wish details of the parasitology. The principles of surgical treatment are dealt with in the appropriate sections although, for operative details, referral to a relevant textbook is advised.

AMOEBIASIS

Introduction

Amoebiasis is caused by *Entamoeba histolytica*. The disease is common in the Indian subcontinent, Africa and parts of Central and South America where almost half the population is infected. The majority remain asymptomatic carriers. The mode of infection is via the faeco-oral route, and the disease occurs as a result of substandard hygiene and sanitation; therefore the population from the poorer socioeconomic strata are more vulnerable. Amoebic liver abscess, the most common extraintestinal manifestation, occurs in less than 10 per cent of the infected population and, in endemic areas, is much more common than pyogenic abscess. Patients who are immunocompromised and alcoholics are more susceptible to infection.

Pathogenesis

The organism enters the gut through food or water contaminated with the cyst. In the small bowel, the cysts hatch, and a large number of trophozoites are released and carried to the colon where flask-shaped ulcers form in the submucosa. The trophozoites multiply, ultimately forming cysts, which enter the portal circulation or are passed in the faeces as an infective form that infects other humans as a result of insanitary conditions.

Having entered the portal circulation, the trophozoites are filtered and trapped in the interlobular veins of the liver. They multiply in the portal triads causing focal infarction of hepatocytes and liquefactive necrosis as a result of proteolytic enzymes produced by the trophozoites. The areas of necrosis eventually coalesce to form the abscess cavity. The term 'amoebic hepatitis' is used to describe the microscopic picture in the absence of macroscopic abscess, a differentiation only in theory as the medical treatment is the same.

The right lobe is involved in 80 per cent of cases, the left in 10 per cent and the rest are multiple. Involvement of the right lobe of the liver is more common possibly because blood from the superior mesenteric vein runs on a straighter course through the portal vein into the larger lobe. The abscesses are most common high in the diaphragmatic surface of the right lobe. This may cause pulmonary symptoms and chest complications. The abscess cavity contains chocolate-coloured, odourless, 'anchovy sauce'-like fluid that is a mixture of necrotic liver tissue and blood. There may be secondary infection of the abscess. This causes the pus to smell. While pus in the abscess is sterile unless secondarily infected, trophozoites may be found in the abscess wall in a minority of cases. Untreated abscesses are likely to rupture.

Chronic infection of the large bowel may result in a granulomatous lesion along the large bowel, most commonly seen in the caecum, called an amoeboma (Summary box 6.1).

Summary box 6.1

Amoebiasis – pathology

- *Entamoeba histolytica* is the most common pathogenic amoeba in man
- The vast majority of carriers are asymptomatic
- Insanitary conditions and poor personal hygiene encourage transmission of the infection
- In the small intestine, the parasite hatches into trophozoites, which invade the submucosa producing flask-shaped ulcers
- In the portal circulation, the parasite causes liquefactive necrosis in the liver producing an abscess. This is the most common extraintestinal manifestation
- The majority of abscesses occur in the right lobe of the liver
- A mass in the course of the large bowel may indicate an amoeboma

Clinical features

The typical patient with amoebic liver abscess is a young adult male with a history of insidious onset of non-specific symptoms such as abdominal pain, anorexia, fever, night sweats, malaise, cough and weight loss; these symptoms gradually progress to more specific symptoms of pain in the right upper abdomen and right shoulder tip, hiccoughs and a non-productive cough. A past history of bloody diarrhoea or travel to an endemic area raises the index of suspicion.

Examination reveals a patient who is toxic and anaemic. The patient will have upper abdominal rigidity, tender hepatomegaly, tender and bulging intercostal spaces, overlying skin oedema, a pleural effusion and basal pneumonitis – the last feature is usually a late manifestation. Occasionally, a tinge of jaundice or ascites may be present. Rarely, the patient may present as an emergency due to the effects of rupture into the peritoneal, pleural or pericardial cavity.

Amoeboma

This is a chronic granuloma arising in the large bowel, most commonly seen in the caecum. It is prone to occur in long-standing amoebic infection that has been treated intermittently with drugs without completion of a full course, a situation that arises from indiscriminate self-medication, particularly in developing countries.

This can easily be mistaken for a carcinoma. An amoeboma should be suspected when a patient from an endemic area with generalised ill health and pyrexia has a mass in the right iliac fossa with a history of blood-stained mucoid diarrhoea. Such a patient is highly unlikely to have a carcinoma as altered bowel habit is not a feature of right-sided colonic carcinoma.

Investigations

The haematological and biochemical investigations reflect the presence of a chronic infective process: anaemia, leukocytosis, raised inflammatory markers – erythrocyte sedimentation rate (ESR) and C-reactive protein (CRP) – hypoalbuminaemia and deranged liver function tests, particularly elevated alkaline phosphatase.

Serological tests are more specific, with the majority of patients showing antibodies in serum. These can be detected by tests for complement fixation, indirect haemagglutination (IHA), indirect immunofluorescence and enzyme-linked immunosorbent assay (ELISA). They are extremely useful in detecting acute infection in non-endemic areas. IHA has a very high sensitivity rate in acute amoebic liver abscess in non-endemic regions and remains elevated for some time. The persistence of antibodies in a large majority of the population in endemic areas precludes its use there as a diagnostic investigation. In these cases, tests such as counter-immunoelectrophoresis are more useful for detecting acute infection.

An outpatient rigid sigmoidoscopy (using a disposable instrument) can be very useful, particularly if the patient complains of bloody mucoid diarrhoea. Most amoebic ulcers occur in the rectosigmoid and are therefore within reach of the sigmoidoscope; shallow skip lesions and 'flask-shaped' or 'collar-stud' undermined ulcers may be seen, and can be biopsied or scrapings can be taken along with mucus for immediate microscopic examination. The presence of trophozoites distinguishes the condition from ulcerative colitis.

Imaging techniques

On ultrasound, an abscess cavity in the liver is seen as a hypoechoic or anechoic lesion with ill-defined borders; internal echoes suggest necrotic material or debris (Figure 6.1). The investigation is very accurate and is used for aspiration, both diagnostic and therapeutic. Where there is doubt about the diagnosis, a computed tomography (CT) scan may be helpful (Figure 6.2).

Diagnostic aspiration is of limited value except for establishing the typical colour of the aspirate, which is sterile and odourless unless it is secondarily infected.

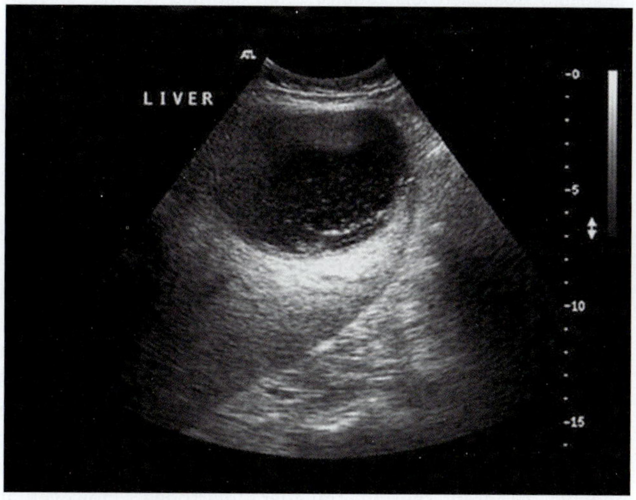

Figure 6.1 Ultrasound of the liver showing a large amoebic liver abscess with necrotic tissue in the right lobe.

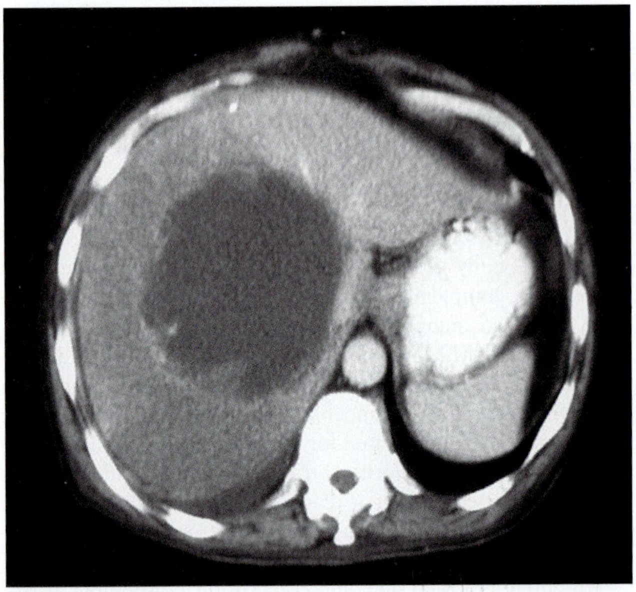

Figure 6.2 Computed tomographic scan showing an amoebic liver abscess in the right lobe.

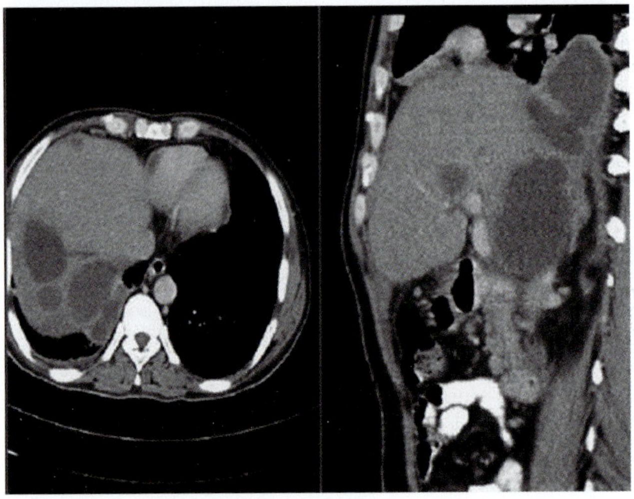

Figure 6.3 Computed tomographic scans showing multiple amoebic liver abscesses with extension into the chest.

A CT scan may show a raised right hemidiaphragm, a pleural effusion and evidence of pneumonitis (Figure 6.3).

An 'apple-core' deformity on barium enema would arouse suspicion of a carcinoma. A colonoscopy and biopsy are mandatory as the radiological and macroscopic appearance may be indistinguishable from a carcinoma. In doubtful cases, vigorous medical treatment is given, and the patient's colon is imaged again in 3–4 weeks, as these masses are known to regress completely on a full course of drug therapy. If symptoms persist even partially following full medical treatment in a patient who has recently returned from an endemic area, a colonic carcinoma must be excluded forthwith. This is because a dormant colonic carcinoma may become apparent as a result of infestation with amoebic dysentery causing 'traveller's diarrhoea'. However, it must be borne in mind that an amoeboma and carcinoma can coexist (Summary box 6.2).

Summary box 6.2

Diagnostic pointers for infection with *Entamoeba histolytica*

- Bloody mucoid diarrhoea in a patient from an endemic area or following a recent visit to such a country
- Upper abdominal pain, fever, cough, malaise
- In chronic cases, a mass in the right iliac fossa = amoeboma
- Sigmoidoscopy shows typical ulcers – biopsy and scraping may be diagnostic
- Serological tests are highly sensitive and specific outside endemic areas
- Ultrasound and CT scans are the imaging methods of choice

Treatment

Medical treatment is very effective and should be the first choice in the elective situation, with surgery being reserved for complications. Metronidazole and tinidazole are the effective drugs. After treatment with metronidazole and tinidazole, diloxanide furoate, which is not effective against hepatic infestation, is used for 10 days to destroy any intestinal amoebae.

Aspiration is carried out when imminent rupture of an abscess is expected. Aspiration also helps in the penetration of metronidazole, and so reduces the morbidity when carried out with drug treatment in a patient with a large abscess. If there is evidence of secondary infection, appropriate drug treatment is added. The threshold for aspirating an abscess in the left lobe is lower because of its predilection for rupturing into the pericardium.

Surgical treatment should be reserved for the complications of rupture into the pleural (usually the right side), peritoneal or pericardial cavities. Resuscitation, drainage and appropriate lavage with vigorous medical treatment are the key principles. In the large bowel, severe haemorrhage and toxic megacolon are rare complications. In these patients, the general principles of a surgical emergency apply. Resuscitation is followed by resection of bowel with exteriorisation. Then the patient is given vigorous supportive therapy. All such cases are managed in the intensive care unit as would any patient with toxic megacolon whatever the cause.

An amoeboma that has not regressed after full medical treatment should be managed with a colonic resection, particularly if cancer cannot be excluded (Summary box 6.3).

Summary box 6.3

Amoebiasis – treatment

- Medical treatment is very effective
- In large abscesses, repeated aspiration is combined with drug treatment
- Surgical treatment is reserved for complications such as rupture into the pleural, peritoneal or pericardial cavities
- Acute toxic megacolon and severe haemorrhage are intestinal complications that are treated with intensive supportive therapy followed by resection and exteriorisation
- When an amoeboma is suspected in a colonic mass, cancer should be excluded by appropriate imaging and biopsy

ASCARIS LUMBRICOIDES (ROUNDWORM)

Introduction

Ascaris lumbricoides, commonly called the roundworm, is the most common intestinal nematode to infest humans and affects a quarter of the world's population. The parasite causes pulmonary symptoms as a larva and intestinal symptoms as an adult worm.

Pathology and life cycle

The eggs can survive in a hostile environment for a long time. The hot and humid conditions in the tropics are ideally suited for the eggs to turn into embryos. The fertilised eggs are present in soil contaminated with infected faeces. Faeco-oral contamination causes human infection.

As the eggs are ingested, the released larvae travel to the liver via the portal system and then through the systemic circulation to reach the lung. The process of maturation takes up to 8 weeks. The developed larvae reach the alveoli, are coughed up, swallowed and continue their maturation in the small intestine. Sometimes, the young worm migrates from the tracheobronchial tree into the oesophagus, thus finding its way into the gastrointestinal tract, from where it can migrate to the common bile duct or pancreatic duct. The mature female, once in the small bowel, produces innumerable eggs that are fertilised and thereafter excreted in the stool to perpetuate the life cycle. Eggs in the biliary tract can form a nidus for a stone.

Clinical features

The larval stage in the lungs causes pulmonary symptoms – dry cough, chest pain, dyspnoea and fever – referred to as Loeffler's syndrome. The adult worm can grow up to 45 cm long. Its presence in the small intestine causes malnutrition, failure to thrive and abdominal pain. Worms that migrate into the common bile duct can produce ascending cholangitis and obstructive jaundice, while features of acute pancreatitis may be caused by a worm in the pancreatic duct.

Small intestinal obstruction can occur, particularly in children, due to a bolus of adult worms incarcerated in the terminal ileum. This is a surgical emergency. Rarely, perforation of the small bowel may occur from ischaemic pressure necrosis from the bolus of worms.

A high index of suspicion is necessary so as not to miss the diagnosis. If a person from a tropical developing country, or one who has recently returned after spending some time in an endemic area, presents with pulmonary, gastrointestinal, hepatobiliary and pancreatic symptoms, ascariasis infestation should be high on the list of possible diagnoses.

Investigations

Increase in the eosinophil count is common, in keeping with most parasitic infestations. Stool examination may show ova. Sputum or bronchoscopic washings may show Charcot–Leyden crystals or the larvae.

Chest x-ray may show fluffy exudates in Loeffler's syndrome. A barium meal and follow-through may show a bolus of worms in the ileum or lying freely within the small bowel (Figure 6.4). An ultrasound may show a worm in the common bile duct (Figure 6.5) or pancreatic duct. On magnetic resonance cholangiopancreatography (MRCP), an adult worm may be seen in the common bile duct in a patient presenting with features of obstructive jaundice (Figure 6.6) (Summary box 6.4).

> **Summary box 6.4**
>
> **Ascariasis – pathogenesis**
>
> - It is the most common intestinal nematode affecting humans
> - Typically found in a humid atmosphere and poor sanitary conditions; hence is seen in the tropics and developing countries
> - Larvae cause pulmonary symptoms; adult worms cause gastrointestinal, biliary and pancreatic symptoms
> - Distal ileal obstruction due to bolus of worms; ascending cholangitis and obstructive jaundice from infestation of the common bile duct
> - Acute pancreatitis when a worm is lodged in the pancreatic duct
> - Perforation of the small bowel is rare

Treatment

The pulmonary phase of the disease is usually self-limiting and requires symptomatic treatment only. For intestinal disease, patients should ideally be under the care of a physician for treatment with anthelmintic drugs. Certain drugs may cause rapid death of the adult worms and, if there are many worms in the terminal ileum, the treatment may actually precipitate acute intestinal obstruction from a bolus of dead worms. Children who present with features of intermittent or subacute obstruction should be given a trial of conservative management in the form of intravenous fluids, nasogastric suction and hypertonic saline enemas. The last of these helps to disentangle the bolus of worms and also increases intestinal motility.

Surgery is reserved for complications such as intestinal obstruction that has not resolved on a conservative regimen, and when perforation is suspected. At laparotomy, the bolus of worms in the terminal ileum is milked through the ileocaecal valve into the colon for natural passage in the stool. Postoperatively, hypertonic saline enemas may help in the extrusion of the worms. Strictures, gangrenous areas or perforations need resection and anastomosis. If the bowel wall is healthy, enterotomy and removal of the worms may be performed (Figure 6.7).

As a result of perforation due to roundworm, the parasites may be found lying free in the peritoneal cavity. The site of perforation may be brought out as an ileostomy because, in the presence of a large number of worms, closure or an anastomosis may be at risk of breakdown from the activity of the worms. Exteriorisation, although the ideal operation in severe sepsis, is unfortunately sometimes not done because of the reluctance on the part of the patient to accept such a procedure as good stoma care is not always available and follow up inadequate in developing countries. In such circumstances, resection of the diseased ileum, closure of the distal bowel and end-to-side ileotransverse anastomosis is a good alternative.

When a patient is operated upon as an emergency for a suspected complication of roundworm infestation, the actual diagnosis at operation may turn out to be acute appendicitis, typhoid perforation or tuberculous stricture, and the presence of roundworms is an incidental finding. Such a patient requires the appropriate surgery depending upon the pathology.

Wilhelm Loeffler, 1887–1972, Professor of Medicine, Zurich, Switzerland.
Jean Martin Charcot, 1825–1893, physician, La Salpêtrière, Paris, France.
Ernst von Leyden, 1832–1910, Professor of Medicine, Berlin, Germany.

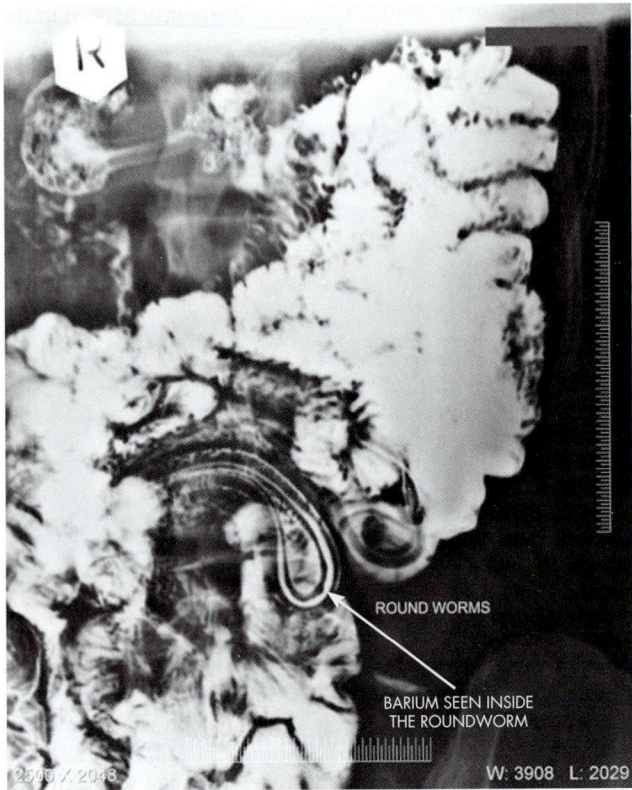

Figure 6.4 Barium meal and follow-through showing roundworms in the course of the small bowel with barium seen inside the worms in an 18-year-old patient who presented with bouts of colicky abdominal pain and bilious vomiting, which settled with conservative management (courtesy of Dr P Bhattacharaya, Kolkata, India).

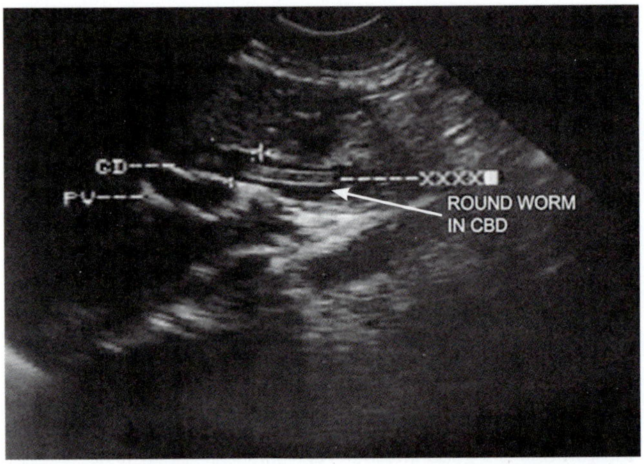

Figure 6.5 Ultrasound scan showing a roundworm in the common bile duct (CBD). The patient presented with obstructive jaundice and had asymptomatic gallstones. On endoscopic retrograde cholangiopancreatography (ERCP), part of the worm was seen outside the ampulla in the duodenum and was removed through the endoscope. Subsequent laparoscopic cholecystectomy was uneventful.

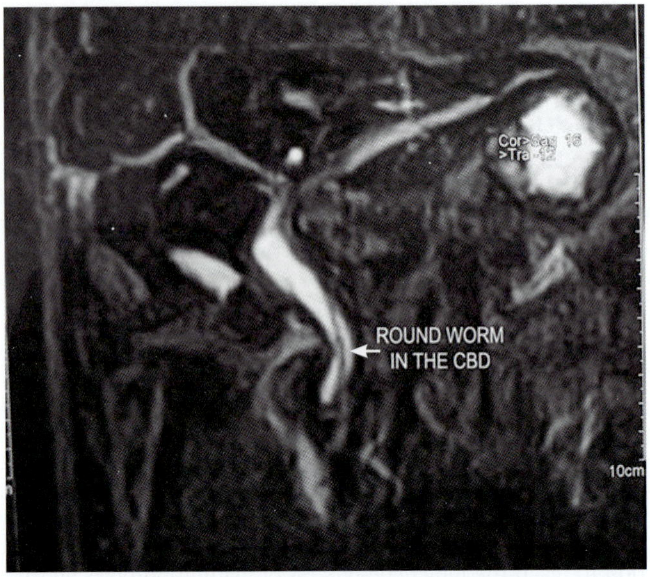

Figure 6.6 Magnetic resonance cholangiopancreatography (MRCP) showing a roundworm in the common bile duct (CBD). The worm could not be removed endoscopically. The patient underwent an open cholecystectomy and exploration of the CBD.

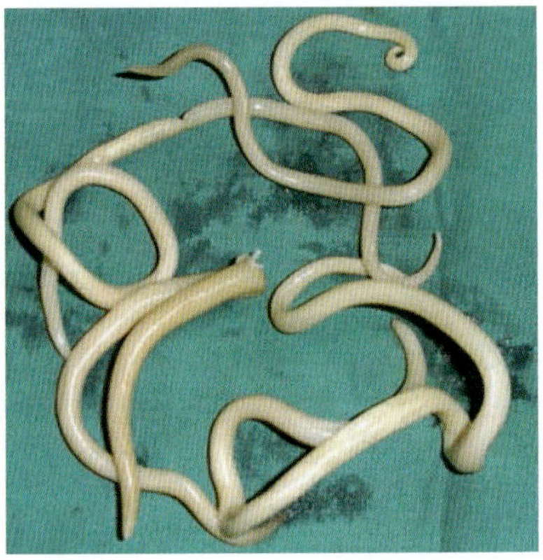

Figure 6.7 Roundworms removed at laparotomy in a 16-year-old patient who presented with acute intestinal obstruction (courtesy of the Pathology Museum, Calcutta Medical Research Institute, Kolkata, India).

Common bile duct or pancreatic duct obstruction from a roundworm can be treated by endoscopic removal, failing which open exploration of the common bile duct is necessary. Cholecystectomy is also carried out. A full course of anti-parasitic treatment must follow any surgical intervention (Summary box 6.5).

Summary box 6.5

Ascariasis – diagnosis and management

- Barium meal and follow-through will show worms scattered in the small bowel
- Ultrasound may show worms in the common bile duct and pancreatic duct
- Conservative management with anthelmintics is the first line of treatment even in obstruction
- Surgery is a last resort – various options are available

ASIATIC CHOLANGIOHEPATITIS

Introduction

This disease, also called oriental cholangiohepatitis, is caused by infestation of the hepatobiliary system by *Clonorchis sinensis*. It has a high incidence in the tropical regions of South East Asia, particularly among those living in the major sea ports and river estuaries. The organism, which is a type of liver fluke, resides in snails and fish that act as intermediate hosts. Ingestion of infected fish and snails when eaten raw or partly cooked causes the infection in humans and other fish-eating mammals, which are the definitive hosts.

Pathology

In humans, the parasite matures into the adult worm in the intrahepatic biliary radicles where they may reside for many years. The intrahepatic bile ducts are dilated with epithelial hyperplasia and periductal fibrosis. These changes may lead to dysplasia causing cholangiocarcinoma – the most serious complication of this parasitic infestation.

The eggs or dead worms may form a nidus for stone formation in the gall bladder or common bile duct, which becomes thickened and much dilated in the late stages. Intrahepatic bile duct stones are also caused by the parasite producing mucin-rich bile. The dilated intrahepatic bile ducts may lead to cholangitis, liver abscess and hepatitis.

Diagnosis

The disease may remain dormant for many years. Clinical features are non-specific, such as fever, malaise, anorexia and upper abdominal discomfort. The complete clinical picture can consist of fever with rigors due to ascending cholangitis, obstructive jaundice due to stones, biliary colic and pruritis. Acute pancreatitis may occur because of obstruction of the pancreatic duct by an adult worm. If any person or an emigrant to the West from an endemic area complains of symptoms of biliary tract disease, *Clonorchis* infestation should be considered in the differential diagnosis.

In advanced cases, liver function tests are abnormal. Confirmation of the condition is by examination of stool or duodenal aspirate, which may show the eggs or adult worms. Ultrasound scan findings can be characteristic, showing the uniform dilatation of small peripheral intrahepatic bile ducts with only minimal dilatation of the common hepatic and common bile ducts, although the latter are much more dilated when the obstruction is caused by stones. The thickened duct walls show increased echogenicity and non-shadowing echogenic foci in the bile ducts representing the worms or eggs. Endoscopic retrograde cholangiopancreatography (ERCP) will confirm these findings (Summary box 6.6).

Summary box 6.6

Asiatic cholangiohepatitis – pathogenesis and diagnosis

- Occurs in the Far Eastern tropical zones
- Causative parasite is *Clonorchis sinensis*
- Produces bile duct hyperplasia, intrahepatic duct dilatation and stones
- Increases the risk of cholangiocarcinoma
- May remain dormant for many years
- When active, there are biliary tract symptoms in a generally unwell patient
- Stool examination for eggs or worms is diagnostic
- Ultrasound scan of hepatobiliary system and ERCP are also diagnostic

Treatment

Praziquantel and albendazole are the drugs of choice. However, the surgeon faces a challenge when there are stones not only in the gall bladder but also in the common bile duct. Cholecystectomy with exploration of the common bile duct is performed when indicated. Repeated washouts are necessary during the exploration, as the common bile duct is dilated and contains stones, biliary debris, sludge and mud. This should be followed by choledochoduodenostomy. As this is a disease with a prolonged and relapsing course, some surgeons prefer to do a choledochojejunostomy to a Roux loop. The Roux loop is brought up to the abdominal wall, referred to as 'an access loop', which allows the interventional radiologist to deal with any future stones.

As a public health measure, people who have emigrated to the West from an endemic area should be offered screening for *Clonorchis* infestation in the form of ultrasound of the hepatobiliary system. This condition can be diagnosed and treated and even cured when it is in its subclinical form. Most importantly, the risk of developing the dreadful disease of cholangiocarcinoma is eliminated (Summary box 6.7).

Summary box 6.7

Asiatic cholangiohepatitis – treatment

- Medical treatment can be curative in the early stages
- Surgical treatment is cholecystectomy, exploration of the common bile duct and some form of biliary–enteric bypass
- Prevention – consider offering hepatobiliary ultrasound as a screening procedure to recently arrived migrants to the West from endemic areas

FILARIASIS

Introduction

Filariasis is mainly caused by the parasite *Wuchereria bancrofti* carried by the mosquito. A variant of the parasite called *Brugia malayi* and *B. timori* is responsible for causing the disease in about 10 per cent of sufferers. The condition affects more than 90 million people worldwide, two-thirds of whom live in India, China and Indonesia. According to the World Health Organization (WHO), filariasis is the second most common cause, after leprosy, of long-term disability.

Once bitten by the mosquito, the matured eggs enter the human circulation to hatch and grow into adult worms; the process of maturation takes about one year. The adult worms mainly colonise the lymphatic system.

Cesar Roux, 1857–1934, Professor of Surgery and Gynaecology, Lausanne, Switzerland, described this method of forming a jejunal conduit in 1908.

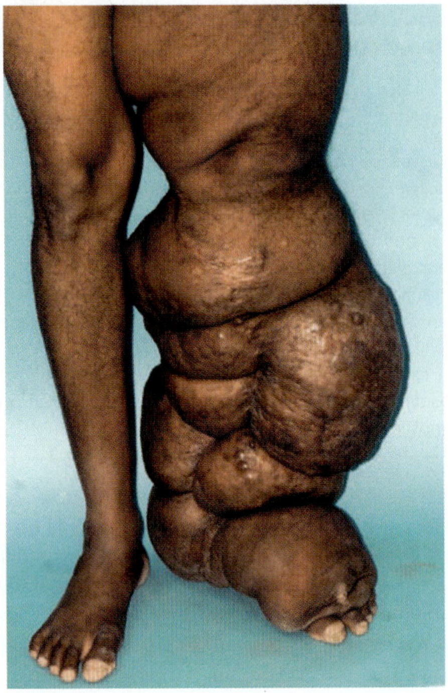

Figure 6.8 Left lower limb filariasis – elephantiasis (courtesy of Professor Ahmed Hassan Fahal, Khartoum, Sudan).

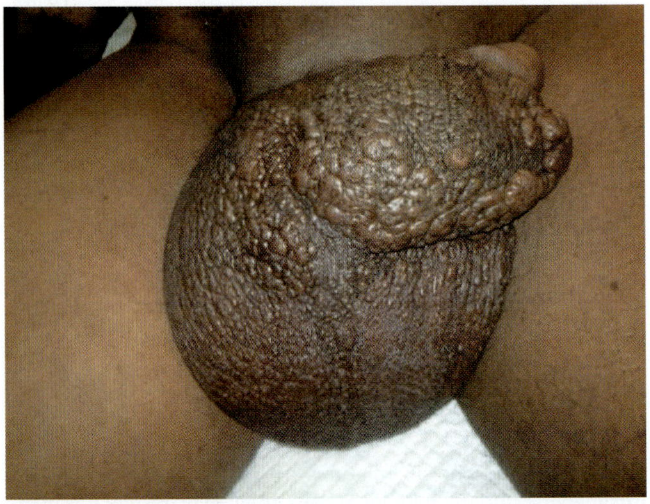

Figure 6.9 Filariasis of the scrotum (courtesy of Professor Ahmed Hassan Fahal, Khartoum, Sudan).

Diagnosis

It is mainly males who are affected because females, in general, cover a greater part of their bodies, thus making them less prone to mosquito bites. In the acute presentation, there are episodic attacks of fever with lymphadenitis and lymphangitis.

Occasionally, adult worms may be felt subcutaneously. Chronic manifestations appear after repeated acute attacks over several years. The adult worms cause lymphatic obstruction resulting in massive lower limb oedema. Obstruction to the cutaneous lymphatics causes skin thickening, not unlike the 'peau d'orange' appearance in breast cancer, thus exacerbating the limb swelling. Secondary streptococcal infection is common. Recurrent attacks of lymphangitis cause fibrosis of the lymph channels, resulting in a grossly swollen limb with thickened skin producing the condition of elephantiasis (Figure 6.8). Bilateral lower limb filariasis is often associated with scrotal and penile elephantiasis. Early on, there may be a hydrocoele underlying scrotal filariasis (Figure 6.9).

Chyluria and chylous ascites may occur. A mild form of the disease can affect the respiratory tract, causing dry cough, and is referred to as tropical pulmonary eosinophilia. The condition of filariasis is clinically very obvious, and thus investigations in the full-blown case are superfluous. Eosinophilia is common, and a nocturnal peripheral blood smear may show the immature forms or microfilariae. The parasite may also be seen in chylous urine, ascites and hydrocoele fluid.

Treatment

Medical treatment with diethylcarbamazine is very effective in the early stages before the gross deformities of elephantiasis have developed. In the early stages of limb swelling, intermittent pneumatic compression helps, but the treatment has to be repeated over a prolonged period.

A hydrocoele is treated by the usual operation of excision and eversion of the sac with, if necessary, excision of redundant skin. Operations for reducing the size of the limb are hardly ever done these days because the procedures are rarely successful (Summary box 6.8).

Summary box 6.8

Filariasis

- Caused by *Wuchereria bancrofti* that is carried by the mosquito
- Lymphatics are mainly affected, resulting in gross limb swelling
- Eosinophilia; immature worms seen in a nocturnal peripheral blood smear
- Gross forms of the disease cause a great deal of disability and misery
- Early cases are very amenable to medical treatment
- Intermittent pneumatic compression gives some relief
- The value of various surgical procedures is largely unproven

HYDATID DISEASE

Introduction and pathology

Commonly called dog tape worm, hydatid disease is caused by *Ecchinococcus granulosus*. While it is common in the tropics, in the UK, the occasional patient may come from a rural sheep-farming community.

The dog is the definitive host and, as a pet, is the most common source of infection transmitted to the intermediate hosts – humans, sheep and cattle. In the dog, the adult worm reaches the small intestine, and the eggs are passed in the faeces. These eggs are highly resistant to extremes of temperature and may survive for long periods. In the dog's intestine, the cyst

Otto Eduard Heinrich Wucherer, 1820–1873, a German physician who practised in Brazil, South America.
Peau d'orange is French for 'orange skin'.
Joseph Bancroft, 1836–1894, an English physician who worked in Australia.

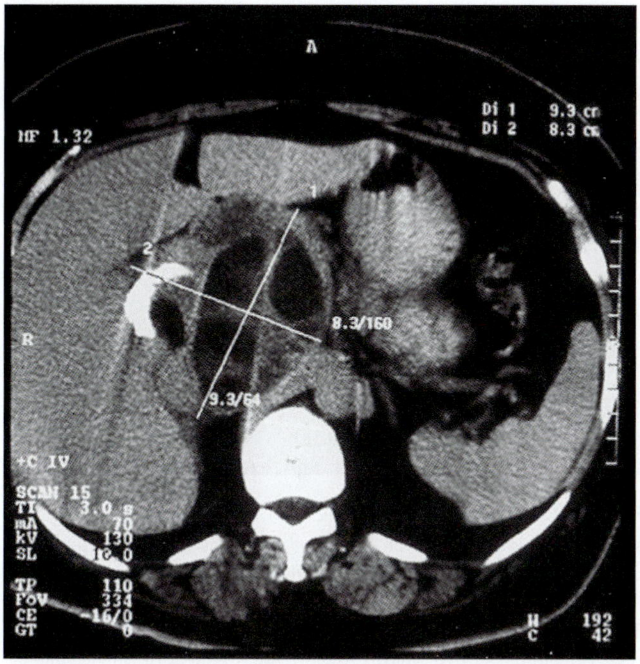

Figure 6.10 Computed tomographic scan showing a hydatid cyst of the pancreas. A differential diagnosis of hydatid cyst or a tumour was considered. At exploration, the patient was found to have a hydatid cyst, which was excised followed by a 30-month treatment with albendazole. The patient remains free of disease.

wall is digested, allowing the protoscolices to develop into adult worms. Close contact with the infected dog causes contamination by the oral route, with the ovum thus gaining entry into the human gastrointestinal tract.

The cyst is characterised by three layers, an outer **pericyst** derived from compressed host organ tissues, an intermediate hyaline **ectocyst** which is non-infective and an inner **endocyst** that is the germinal membrane and contains viable parasites which can separate forming daughter cysts. A variant of the disease occurs in colder climates caused by *Echinococcus multilocularis*, in which the cyst spreads from the outset by actual invasion rather than expansion.

Classification

In 2003, the WHO Informal Working Group on Echinococcosis (WHO-IWGE) proposed a standardised ultrasound classification based on the status of activity of the cyst. This is universally accepted, particularly because it helps to decide on the appropriate management. Three groups have been recognised:

Group 1: Active group – cysts larger than 2 cm and often fertile

Group 2: Transition group – cysts starting to degenerate and entering a transitional stage because of host resistance or treatment, but may contain viable protoscolices

Group 3: Inactive group – degenerated, partially or totally calcified cysts; unlikely to contain viable protoscolices.

Clinical features

As the parasite can colonise virtually every organ in the body, the condition can be protean in its presentation. When a sheep farmer, who is otherwise healthy, complains of a gradually enlarging painful mass in the right upper quadrant with the physical findings of a liver swelling, a hydatid liver cyst should be considered. The liver is the organ most often affected. The lung is the next most common. The parasite can affect any organ (Figures 6.10 and 6.11) or several organs in the same patient (Figure 6.12).

The disease may be asymptomatic and discovered coinciden-

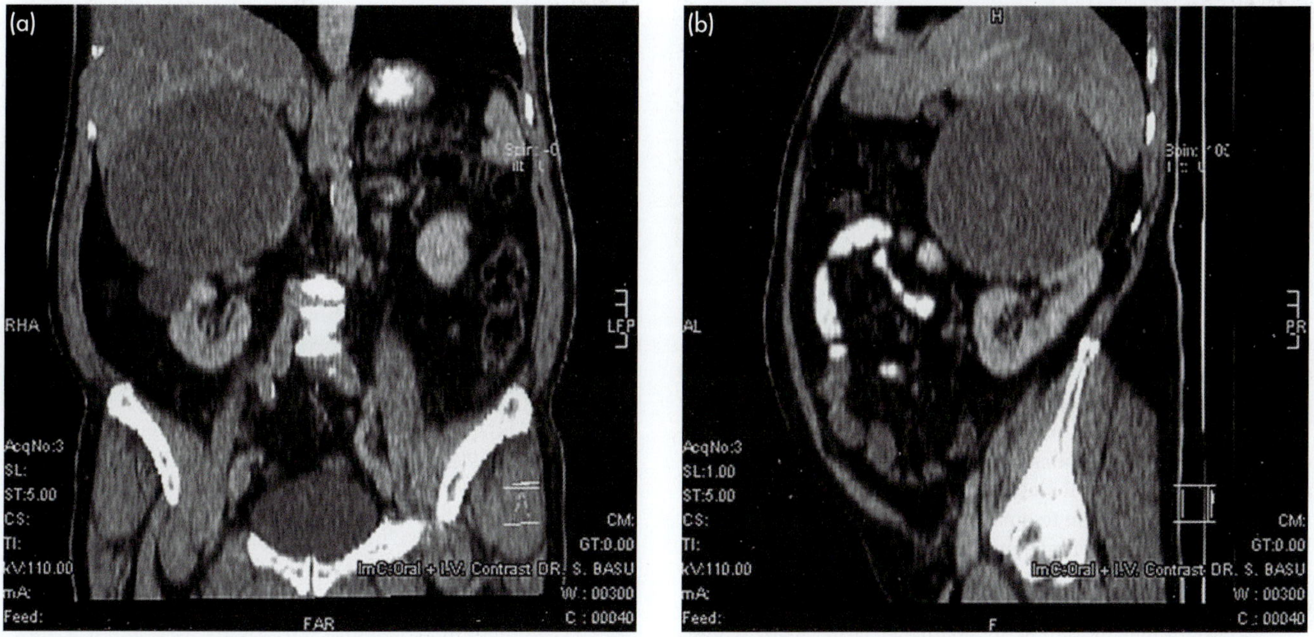

Figure 6.11 Anteroposterior (a) and lateral (b) views of computed tomographic scans showing a large hydatid cyst of the right adrenal gland. The patient presented with a mass in the right loin and underwent an adrenalectomy (courtesy of Dr P Bhattacharaya, Kolkata, India).

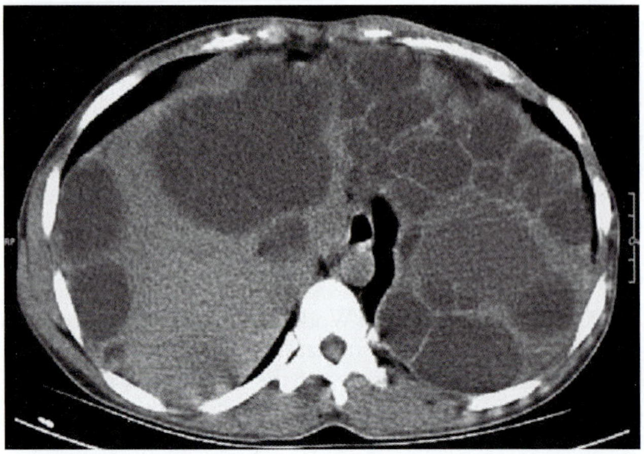

Figure 6.12 Computed tomographic scan showing disseminated hydatid cysts of the abdomen. The patient was started on albendazole and lost to follow up (courtesy of Dr P Bhattacharaya, Kolkata, India).

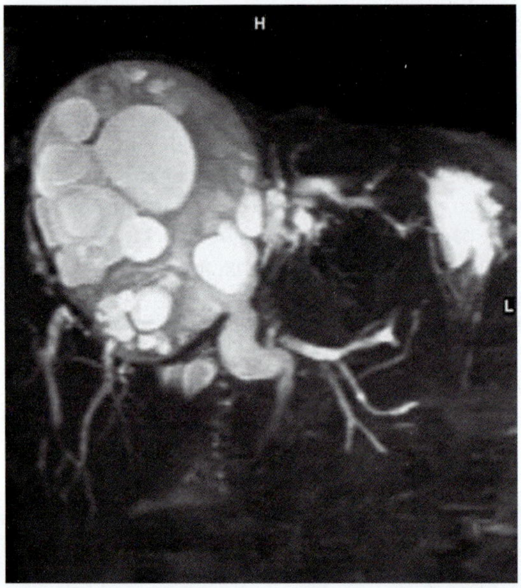

Figure 6.13 Magnetic resonance cholangiopancreatography (MRCP) showing a large hepatic hydatid cyst with daughter cysts communicating with the common bile duct causing obstruction and dilatation of the entire biliary tree (courtesy of Dr B Agarwal, New Delhi, India).

tally at post-mortem or when an ultrasound or CT scan is done for some other condition. Symptomatic disease presents with a swelling causing pressure effects. Thus, a hepatic lesion causes dull pain from stretching of the liver capsule, and a pulmonary lesion, if large enough, causes dyspnoea. Daughter cysts may communicate with the biliary tree causing obstructive jaundice and all the usual clinical features associated with it in addition to symptoms attributable to a parasitic infestation (Figure 6.13). Features of raised intracranial pressure or unexplained headaches in a patient from a sheep-rearing community should raise the suspicion of a cerebral hydatid cyst.

The patient may present as an emergency with severe abdominal pain following minor trauma when the CT scan may be diagnostic (Figure 6.14). Rarely, a patient may present as an emergency with features of anaphylactic shock without any obvious cause. Such a patient may subsequently cough up white material that contains scolices that have travelled into the tracheobronchial tree from rupture of a hepatic hydatid on the diaphragmatic surface of the liver.

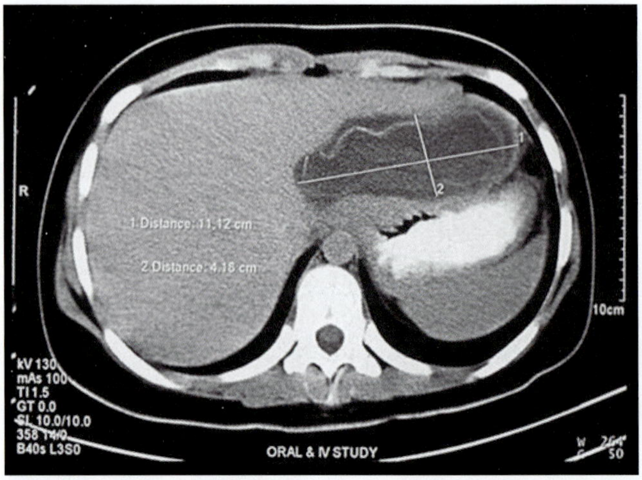

Figure 6.14 Computed tomographic (CT) scan of the upper abdomen showing a hypodense lesion of the left lobe of the liver; the periphery of the lesion shows a double edge. This is the lamellar membrane of the hydatid cyst that separated after trivial injury. The patient was a 14-year-old girl who developed a rash and pain in the upper abdomen after dancing. The rash settled down after a course of antihistamines. The CT scan was done 2 weeks later for persisting upper abdominal pain.

Diagnosis

There should be a high index of suspicion. Investigations show a raised eosinophil count; serological tests such as ELISA and immunoelectrophoresis point towards the diagnosis. Ultrasound and CT scan are the investigations of choice. The CT scan shows a smooth space-occupying lesion with several septa. An ultrasound of the biliary tract may show abnormality in the gall bladder and bile ducts. Hydatid infestation of the biliary system should then be suspected. Ultimately, the diagnosis is made by a combination of good history and clinical examination supplemented by serology and radiological imaging techniques (Summary box 6.9).

Summary box 6.9

Hydatid disease – diagnosis

- In the UK, the usual sufferer is a sheep farmer
- While any organ may be involved, the liver is by far the most commonly affected
- Elective clinical presentation is usually in the form of a painful lump arising from the liver
- Anaphylactic shock due to rupture of the hydatid cyst is the emergency presentation
- CT scan is the best imaging modality – the diagnostic feature is a space-occupying lesion with a smooth outline with septa

Treatment

Here, the treatment of hepatic hydatid is outlined as the liver is most commonly affected, but the same general principles apply whichever organ is involved.

These patients should be treated in a tertiary unit where good teamwork between an expert hepatobiliary surgeon, an experienced physician and an interventional radiologist is available. Surgical treatment by minimal access therapy is best summarised by the mnemonic PAIR (puncture, aspiration, injection and reaspiration). This is done after adequate drug treatment with albendazole, although praziquantel has also been used, both these drugs being available only on a 'named patient' basis.

Whether the patient is treated only medically or in combination with surgery will depend upon the clinical group (which gives an idea as to its activity), the number of cysts and their anatomical position. Radical total or partial pericystectomy with omentoplasty or hepatic segmentectomy (especially if the lesion is in a peripheral part of the liver) are some of the surgical options. During the operation, scolicidal agents are used, such as hypertonic saline (15–20 per cent), ethanol (75–95 per cent) or 1 per cent povidone iodine, although some use a 10 per cent solution. This may cause sclerosing cholangitis if biliary radicles are in communication with the cyst wall. A laparoscopic approach to these procedures is being tried.

Obviously, cysts in other organs need to be treated in accordance with the actual anatomical site along with the general principles described. An asymptomatic cyst which is inactive (group 3) may just be observed (Summary box 6.10).

Summary box 6.10

Hydatid cyst of the liver – treatment

- Ideally managed in a tertiary unit by a multidisciplinary team of hepatobiliary surgeon, physician and interventional radiologist
- Leave asymptomatic and inactive cysts alone – monitor size by ultrasound
- Active cysts should first be treated by a full course of albendazole
- Several procedures are available – PAIR, pericystectomy with omentoplasty and hepatic segmentectomy; it is important to choose the most appropriate option for the particular patient and organ involved
- Increasingly, a laparoscopic approach is being tried

Pulmonary hydatid disease

The lung is the second most common organ affected after the liver. The size of the cyst can vary from being very small to a considerable size. The right lung and lower lobes are slightly more often involved. The cyst is usually single, although multiple cysts do occur and concomitant hydatid cysts in other organs like the liver are not unknown. The condition may be silent and found incidentally. Symptomatic patients present with cough, expectoration, fever, chest pain and sometimes haemoptysis. Silent cysts may present as an emergency due to rupture or an allergic reaction.

Uncomplicated cysts present as rounded or oval lesions on chest x-ray. Erosion of the bronchioles results in air being introduced between the pericyst and the laminated membrane and gives a fine radiolucent crescent, the 'meniscus or crescent sign' (Figure 6.15). This is often regarded as a sign of impending rupture. When the cyst ruptures, the crumpled collapsed endocyst floats in the residual fluid giving rise to the 'water-lily' sign on CT scan (Figure 6.16). Rupture into the pleural cavity results in pleural effusion. CT scan defines the pathology in greater detail.

The mainstay of treatment of hydatidosis of the lung is surgery. Medical treatment is less successful and considered when surgery is not possible because of poor general condition or diffuse

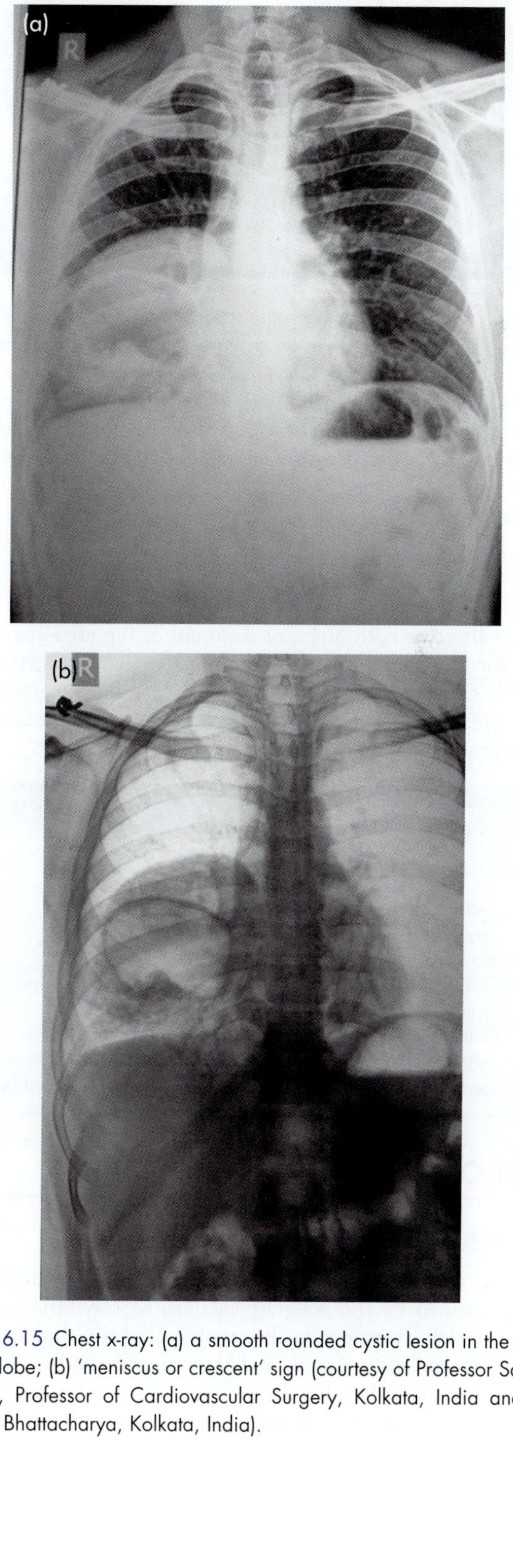

Figure 6.15 Chest x-ray: (a) a smooth rounded cystic lesion in the right lower lobe; (b) 'meniscus or crescent' sign (courtesy of Professor Saibal Gupta, Professor of Cardiovascular Surgery, Kolkata, India and Dr Rupak Bhattacharya, Kolkata, India).

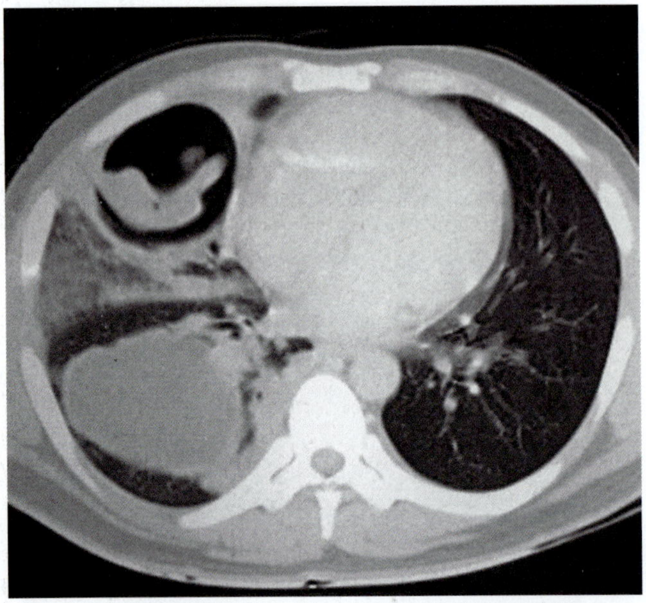

Figure 6.16 Computed tomographic scan showing the 'water-lily' sign. A young mountaineer, while on a high altitude trip, complained of sudden shortness of breath, cough, copious expectoration consisting of clear fluid and flaky material. At first thought to be due to pulmonary oedema, it turned out to be a ruptured hydatid cyst, which was successfully treated by surgery (courtesy of Professor Saibal Gupta, Professor of Cardiovascular Surgery, Kolkata, India and Dr Rupak Bhattacharya, Kolkata, India).

disease affecting both lungs, or recurrent or ruptured cysts. The principle of surgery is to preserve as much of viable lung tissue as possible. The exact procedure can vary: cystotomy, capittonage (suturing together the walls), pericystectomy, segmentectomy or occasionally pneumonectomy (Summary box 6.11).

Summary box 6.11

Pulmonary hydatid disease

- Second most common organ involved
- Size of the cyst has a wide variation
- May present as an incidental finding
- Clinical presentation may be elective or emergency due to rupture
- Plain x-ray shows 'meniscus or crescent' sign; CT shows 'water-lily' sign
- Ideal treatment is surgical – various choices are available

LEPROSY

Introduction

Leprosy, also called Hansen's disease, is a chronic infectious disease caused by the acid-fast bacillus, *Mycobacterium leprae*, that is widely prevalent in the tropics. Globally, India, Brazil, Nepal, Mozambique, Angola and Myanmar (Burma) account for 91 per cent of all the cases; India alone accounts for 78 per cent of the world's disease. Patients suffer not only from the primary effects of the disease but also from social discrimination, sadly compounded by the inappropriate term 'leper' for one afflicted with this disease.

Only close contact over a long time of several years causes the disease to spread. Ignorance of this fact on the part of the general public results in ostracism from social stigma. History records that in the distant past sufferers were made to wear cow bells so that other people could avoid them. The use of the term 'leper', still used metaphorically to denote an outcast, does not help to break down the social barriers that continue to exist against the sufferer.

Pathology

The bacillus inhabits the colder parts of the body – hence found in the nasal mucosa and skin in the region of the ears thus involving the facial nerve as it exits from the stylomastoid foramen. The disease is transmitted from the nasal secretions of a patient, the infection being contracted in childhood or early adolescence. After an incubation period of several years, the disease presents with skin, upper respiratory or neurological manifestations. The bacillus is acid fast but weakly so compared with *Mycobacterium tuberculosis*.

The disease is broadly classified into two groups – lepromatous and tuberculoid. In lepromatous leprosy, there is widespread dissemination of abundant bacilli in the tissues with macrophages and a few lymphocytes. This is a reflection of the poor immune response, resulting in depleted host resistance from the patient. In tuberculoid leprosy, on the other hand, the patient shows a strong immune response with scant bacilli in the tissues, epithelioid granulomas, numerous lymphocytes and giant cells. The tissue damage is inversely proportional to the host's immune response. There are various grades of the disease between the two main spectra (Summary box 6.12).

Summary box 6.12

***Mycobacterium leprae* – pathology**

- Leprosy is a chronic curable infection caused by *Mycobacterium leprae*
- It occurs mainly in tropical regions and developing countries
- The majority of cases are located in the Indian subcontinent
- Transmission is through nasal secretions, the bacillus inhabiting the colder parts of the body
- It is attributed to poor hygiene and insanitary conditions
- The incubation period is several years
- The initial infection occurs in childhood
- Lepromatous leprosy denotes a poor host immune reaction
- Tuberculoid leprosy occurs when host resistance is stronger than virulence of the organism

Clinical features and diagnosis

The disease is slowly progressive and affects the skin, upper respiratory tract and peripheral nerves. In tuberculoid leprosy, the damage to tissues occurs early and is localised to one part of the body with limited deformity of that organ. Neural involvement

Robert Greenhill Cochrane, 1899–1985, a medical missionary who became an international authority on leprosy; he devoted his time to leprosy patients in South East Asia, partcularly India.

Owing to the stigma attached to the word 'leper', RG Cochrane suggested that the best name for **leprosy** is Hansen's disease.
Gerhard Henrik Armauer Hansen, 1841–1912, a physician in charge of a leper hospital near Bergen, Norway.

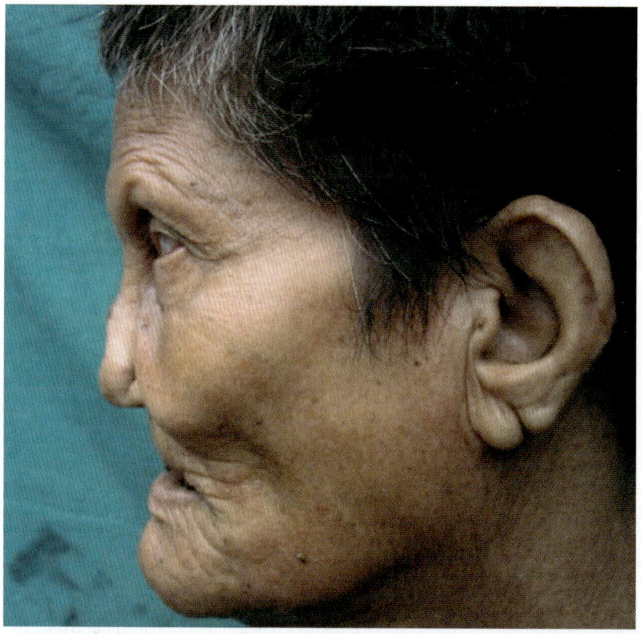

Figure 6.17 Lateral view of the face showing collapse of the nasal bridge due to destruction of nasal cartilage by leprosy.

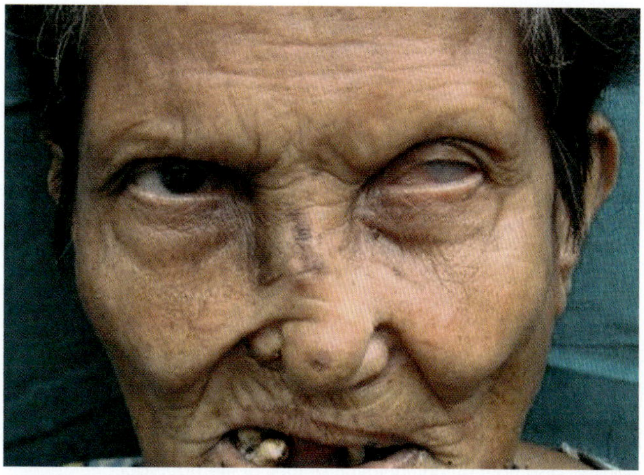

Figure 6.18 Frontal view of the face showing eye changes in leprosy – paralysis of orbicularis oculi and loss of eyebrows.

is characterised by thickening of the nerves, which are tender. There may be asymmetrical well-defined anaesthetic hypopigmented or erythematous macules with elevated edges and a dry and rough surface – lesions called leprids. In lepromatous leprosy, the disease is symmetrical and extensive. Cutaneous involvement occurs in the form of several pale macules that form plaques and nodules called lepromas. The deformities produced are divided into primary, which are caused by leprosy or its reactions, and secondary, resulting from effects such as anaesthesia of the hands and feet.

Nodular lesions on the face in the acute phase of the lepromatous variety are known as 'leonine facies' (looking like a lion). Later, there is wrinkling of the skin giving an aged appearance to a young individual. There is loss of the eyebrows and destruction of the lateral cartilages and septum of the nose with collapse of the nasal bridge and lifting of the tip of the nose (Figure 6.17). There may be paralysis of the branches of the facial nerve in the bony canal or of the zygomatic branch. Blindness may be attributed to exposure keratitis or iridocyclitis. Paralysis of the orbicularis oculi causes incomplete closure of the eye, epiphora and conjunctivitis (Figure 6.18). The hands are typically clawed (Figure 6.19) because of involvement of the ulnar nerve at the elbow and the median nerve at the wrist. Anaesthesia of the hands makes these patients vulnerable to frequent burns and injuries. Similarly, clawing of the toes (Figure 6.20) occurs as a result of involvement of the posterior tibial nerve. When the lateral popliteal nerve is affected, it leads to foot drop, and the nerve can be felt to be thickened behind the upper end of the fibula. Anaesthesia of the feet predisposes to trophic ulceration

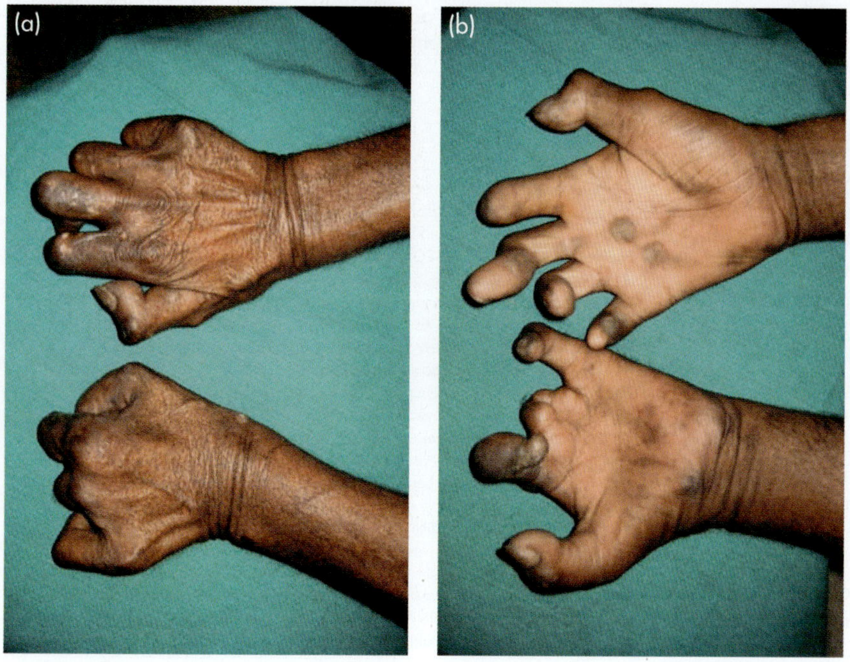

Figure 6.19 (a and b) Typical bilateral claw hand from leprosy due to involvement of the ulnar and median nerves.

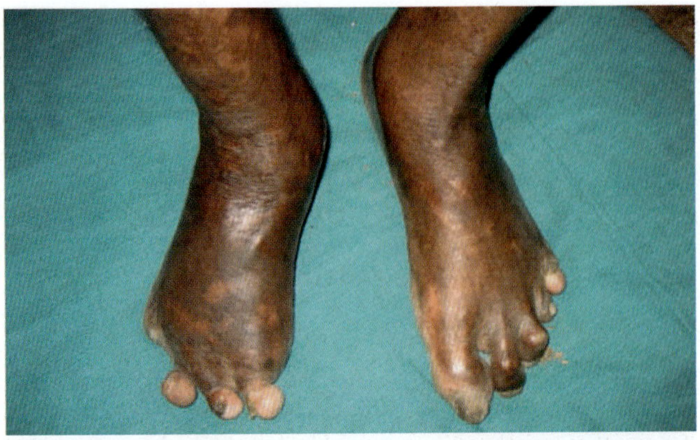

Figure 6.20 Claw toes from involvement of the posterior tibial nerve by leprosy; also note autoamputation of toes of the right foot.

(Figure 6.21), chronic infection, contraction and autoamputation. Involvement of the testes causes atrophy, which in turn results in gynaecomastia (Figure 6.22). Confirmation of the diagnosis is obtained by a skin smear or skin biopsy, which shows the classical histological and microbiological features (Summary box 6.13).

Summary box 6.13

Leprosy – diagnosis

- Typical clinical features and awareness of the disease should help to make a diagnosis
- The face has an aged look about it with collapse of the nasal bridge and eye changes
- Thickened peripheral nerves, patches of anaesthetic skin, claw hands, foot drop and trophic ulcers are characteristic
- Microbiological examination of the acid-fast bacillus and typical histology on skin biopsy are confirmatory

Treatment

A herbal derivative from the seeds of *Hydrocarpus wightiana* called chalmoogra oil was the mainstay of treatment with some success until the advent of dapsone (diamino-diphenyl sulphone). Dapsone, one of the principal drugs, was a derivative of prontosil red. This is used according to the WHO guidelines along with rifampicin and clofazimine. During treatment, the patient may develop acute manifestations. These are controlled with steroids. Multiple drug therapy for 12 months is the key to treatment. A team approach between an infectious diseases specialist, plastic surgeon, ophthalmologist, hand and orthopaedic surgeon is important.

Surgical treatment is indicated in advanced stages of the disease for functional disability of limbs, cosmetic disfigurement of the face and visual problems. These entail major reconstructive surgery, the domain of the plastic surgeon. Deformities of the hands and feet require various forms of tendon transfer, which need to be carried out by specialist hand or orthopaedic surgeons.

The general surgeon may be called upon to treat a patient when the deformity is so advanced that it requires amputation, or when abscesses need to be drained as an emergency.

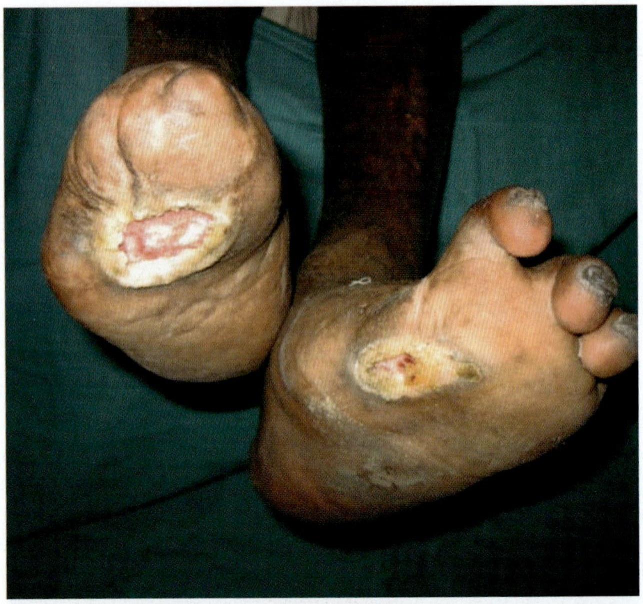

Figure 6.21 Bilateral trophic ulceration of the feet due to anaesthesia of the soles resulting from leprosy; also note claw toes on the left foot.

All surgical procedures obviously need to be done under antileprosy drug treatment. This is best achieved by a team approach. Educating the patients about the dreadful sequelae of the disease so that they seek medical help early is important. It is also necessary to educate the general public that patients suffering from the disease should not be made social outcasts (Summary box 6.14).

Summary box 6.14

Leprosy – treatment

- Multiple drug therapy for a year
- Team approach
- Surgical reconstruction requires the expertise of a hand surgeon, orthopaedic surgeon and plastic surgeon
- Education of the patient and general public should be the keystone in prevention

Gerhard Domagk, 1895–1964, German physician, Lecturer in Pathologic Anatomy, University of Munster, Germany, discovered prontosil in 1935, for which he was awarded the Nobel Prize for Physiology or Medicine in 1939.
Paul Wilson Brand, 1914–2003, born to missionary parents in Southern India, qualified London 1943 CBE, FRCS. He himself was a dedicated missionary who was 'an extraordinary gifted orthopaedic surgeon who straightened crooked hands and unravelled the riddle of leprosy.' As a pioneer in tendon transfer techniques, he established and practised initially in New Life Center, Vellore, South India and Schieffelin Leprosy Research Centre, Karigiri, South India. Initially he trained as a carpenter and builder and maintained that his training as a carpenter helped him in his expertise in tendon transplantation. He later moved to Louisiana State University, Baton Rouge, LA, where he continued his work and finally to Seattle as Emeritus Professor of Orthopaedics in the University of Washington, Seattle, USA.
Margaret Brand, alongside her husband, Paul Brand, also contributed immensely to leprosy patients by concentrating on research to prevent blindness in leprosy. She became known as 'the woman who first helped lepers to see'.
Frank Tovey OBE (b.1921), another English surgeon. At about the same time (1951–1967) in Southern India in the state of Mysore, as a general surgeon, also performed extensive tendon transfers, facial and other reconstructive surgery on leprosy patients; in this he was helped by his wife, Winifred, who organised the physiotherapy and rehabilitation of the patients and established village diagnostic and treatment centres.

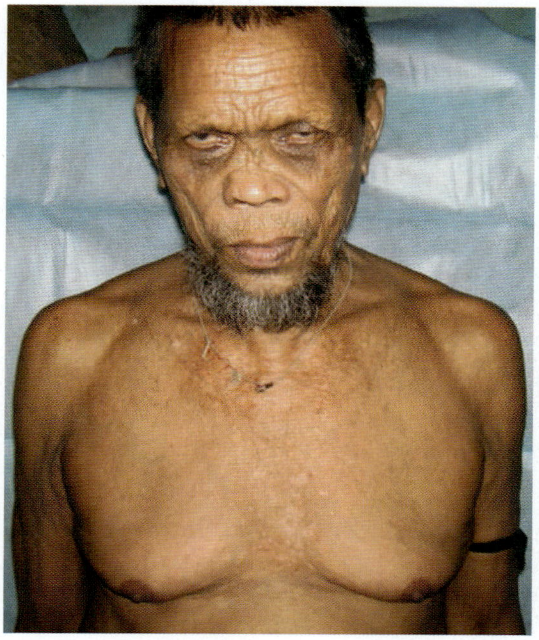

Figure 6.22 Typical leonine facies in leprosy and gynaecomastia in leprosy.

MYCETOMA

(This section has been contributed by Professor Ahmed Hassan Fahal MBBS, FRCS, FRCSI, MD, MS, FRCP(Lond) Professor of Surgery, University of Khartoum, Khartoum, Sudan)

Introduction

Mycetoma is a chronic specific, granulomatous, progressive, destructive inflammatory disease, which involves subcutaneous tissues spreading to the skin and deeper structures. The causative organism may be true fungi when the condition is called eumycetoma; when caused by bacteria it is called actinomycetoma. The pathognomonic feature is the triad of painless subcutaneous mass, multiple sinuses and seropurulent discharge. It causes tissue destruction, deformity, disability and death in extreme cases.

Epidemiology and pathogenesis

The condition predominently occurs in the 'mycetoma belt' that lies between the latitudes 15° south and 30° north comprising the countries of Sudan, Somalia, Senegal, India, Yemen, Mexico, Venezuela, Columbia, Argentina and a few others. The route of infection is inoculation of the organism that is resident in the soil through a traumatised area. Although in the vast majority there is no history of trauma, the portal of entry is always an area of minor unrecognised trauma in a bare-footed individual walking in a terrain full of thorns. Hence the foot is the most common site affected. Mycetoma is not contagious.

Once the granuloma forms it increases in size, the overlying skin becomes stretched, smooth, shiny, and attached to the lesion. Areas of hypo or hyperpigmentation sometimes develop. Eventually it invades the deeper structures. This is usually gradual and delayed in eumycetoma. In actinomycetoma, invasion to deeper tissues occurs earlier and is more extensive. The tendons and the nerves are spared until late in the disease. This may explain the rarity of neurological and trophic changes even in patients with long-standing disease. Trophic changes are rare because the blood supply is adequate (Summary box 6.15).

Summary box 6.15

Mycetoma – pathogenesis

- Mostly occurs in the 'mycetoma belt'
- There are two types – eumycetoma and actinomycetoma
- Caused by fungi or bacteria entering through a site of trauma which may not be apparent; hence foot most commonly affected
- Produces a chronic, specific, granulomatous, progressive, destructive inflammatory lesion
- Results in tissue destruction, deformity, disability and sometimes death

Clinical presentation

As mycetoma is painless, presentation is late in the majority. It presents as a slowly progressive, painless, subcutaneous swelling commonly at the site of presumed trauma. The swelling is variable in its physical characteristics: firm and rounded, soft and lobulated, rarely cystic and is often mobile. Multiple secondary nodules may evolve; they may suppurate and drain through multiple sinus tracts. The sinuses may close transiently after discharge during the active phase of the disease. Fresh adjacent sinuses may open while some of the old ones may heal completely. They coalesce and form abscesses, the discharge being serous, serosanguinous or purulent. During the active phase of the disease the sinuses discharge grains, the colour of which can be black, yellow, white or red depending upon the organism. Pain may supervene when there is secondary bacterial infection.

In some patients there may be areas of local hyperhidrosis over the lesion. This may be due to sympathetic overactivity or increased local temperature due to raised arterial blood flow caused by the chronic inflammation. In the majority of patients, the regional lymph nodes are small and shotty. Lymphadenopathy is common. This may be due to secondary bacterial infection, lymphatic spread of mycetoma or a local immune response to the disease.

The common sites affected are those that come into contact with soil during daily activities: foot in 70 per cent (Figure 6.23) and hand in 12 per cent (Figure 6.24). In endemic areas, the

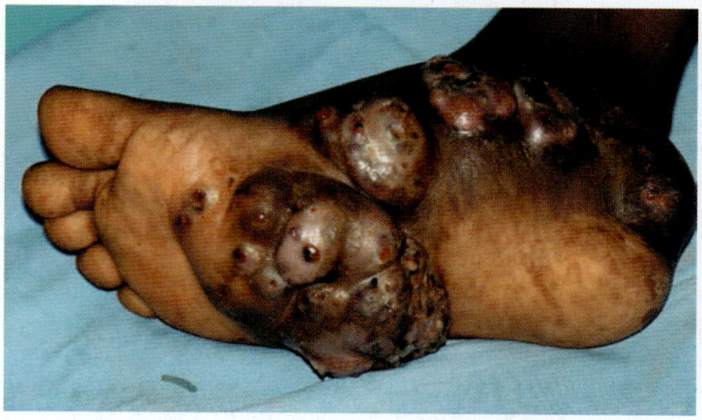

Figure 6.23 Mycetoma of foot.

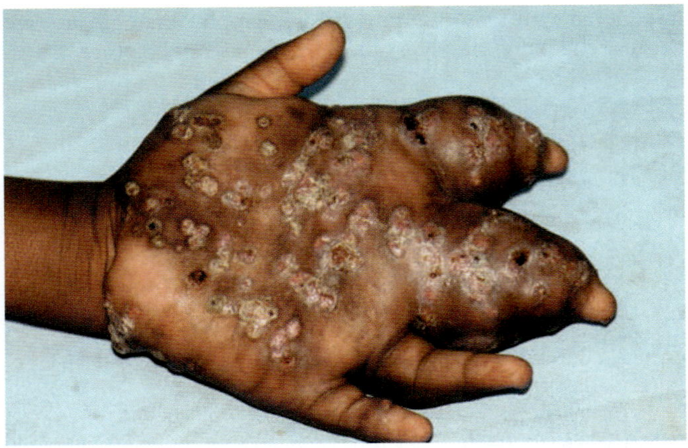

Figure 6.24 Mycetoma of hand.

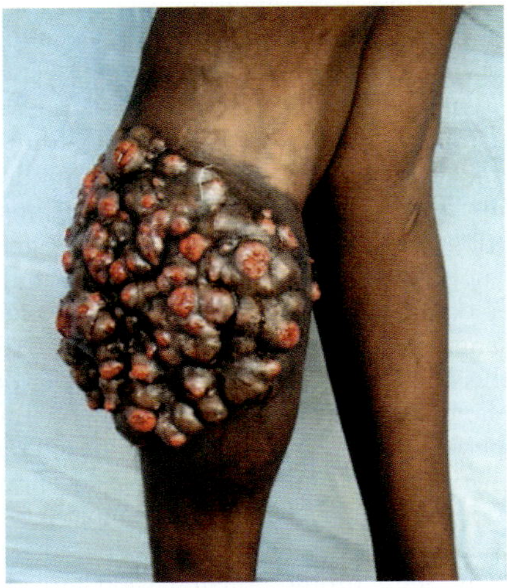

Figure 6.25 Mycetoma of knee.

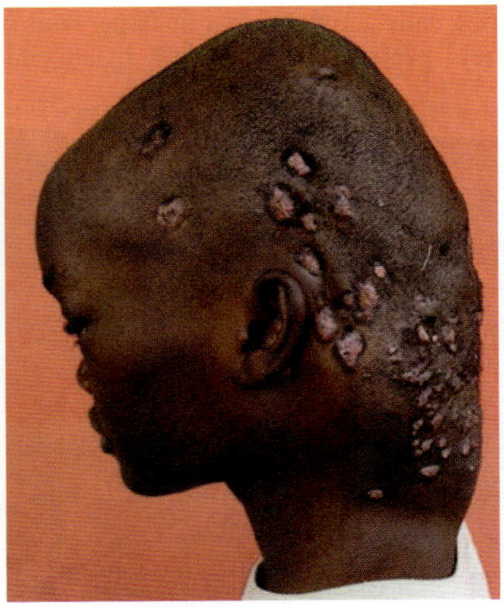

Figure 6.26 Actinomycetoma of head and neck.

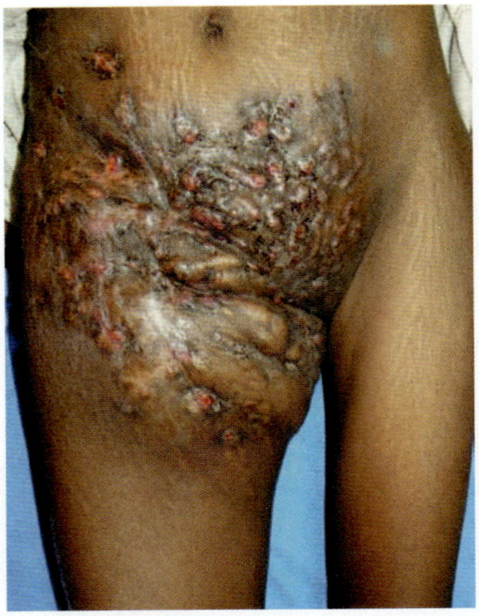

Fibure 6.27 Extensive satellite inguinal actinomycetoma from primary foot lesion involving anterior abdominal wall and perineum.

knee (Figure 6.25), arm, leg, head and neck (Figure 6.26), thigh and perineum (Figure 6.27) can be involved. Rare sites are chest, abdominal wall, facial bones, mandible, testes, paranasal sinuses and eye.

The condition remains localised; constitutional disturbances are a sign of secondary bacterial infection. Cachexia and anaemia from malnutrition and sepsis may be seen in late cases. It can be fatal, especially in cases of cranial mycetoma.

Spread

Local spread occurs predominantly along tissue planes. The organism multiplies forming colonies which spread along the fascial planes to skin and underlying structures. Lymphatic spread occurs to the regional lymph nodes. During the active phase of the disease, these lymphatic satellites may suppurate and discharge. Lymphatic spread is more common in actinomycetoma and its incidence is augmented by repeated inadequate surgical excision; lymphadenopathy may also be due to secondary bacterial infection. Spread by blood stream can occur.

The apparent clinical features of mycetoma are not always a reliable indicator of the extent and spread of the disease. Some small lesions with few sinuses may have many deep connecting tracts, through which the disease can spread quite extensively; therefore, surgery in mycetoma under local anaesthesia is contraindicated.

Differential diagnosis

Mycetoma should be distinguished from Kaposi's sarcoma, malignant melanoma, fibroma and foreign body (thorn) granuloma. In an x-ray the presence of bone destruction in the absence of sinuses is suggestive of tuberculosis. The radiological features of advanced mycetoma are similar to primary osteogenic sarcoma. Primary osseous mycetoma is to be differentiated from chronic osteomyelitis, osteoclastoma, bone cysts and syphilitic osteitis.

Moritz Kaposi, 1837–1902, Hungarian born, Professor of Dermatology, University of Vienna, Austria. Was born to a Jewish family, originally his surname was Kohn. When he converted to Catholicism in 1871, he changed his surname to Kaposi. He described the sarcoma in 1872. The viral cause was discovered in 1994.

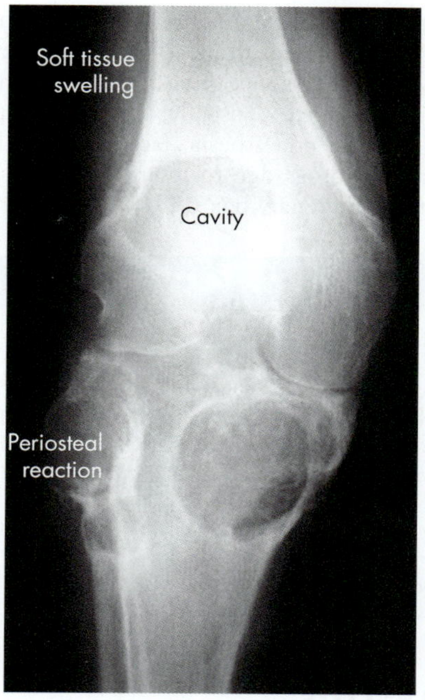

Figure 6.28 Plain x-ray of knee showing multiple large cavities involving the lower femur, upper tibia and fibula with well-defined margins and periosteal reaction typical of eumycetoma.

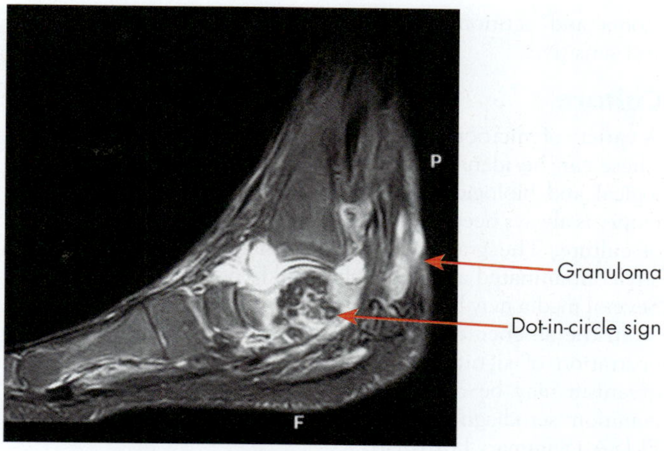

Figure 6.29 Magnetic resonance imaging of foot showing multiple lesions of high signal intensity, which indicates granuloma, interspersed within a low-intensity matrix which is the fibrous tissue and the 'dot-in-circle sign', which indicates the presence of grains.

In endemic areas the dictum should be 'any subcutaneous swelling must be considered a mycetoma until proven otherwise'.

Diagnosis

Several imaging techniques are available to confirm the diagnosis: plain x-ray, ultrasound, CT scan and magnetic resonance imaging (MRI).

Plain x-ray

In the early stages, soft tissue shadow which may be multiple may be seen with calcification and obliteration of the fascial planes. As the disease progresses, the cortex may be compressed from outside by the granuloma leading to bone scalloping. Periosteal reaction with new bone spicules may create a sun-ray appearance and Codman's triangle, not unlike in osteogenic sarcoma (Figure 6.28). Late in the disease, there may be multiple punched-out cavities throughout the bone.

Ultrasound

Ultrasound can differentiate between eumycetoma and actinomycetoma as well as between mycetoma and other conditions. In eumycetoma, the grains produce numerous sharp bright hyper-reflective echoes. There are multiple thick-walled cavities with absence of acoustic enhancement. In actinomycetoma, the findings are similar but the grains are less distinct. The size and extent of the lesion can be accurately determined ultrasonically, a finding useful in planning surgical treatment.

MRI

This helps to assess bone destruction, periosteal reaction and particularly soft tissue involvement (Figure 6.29). MRI usually shows multiple 2–5 mm lesions of high signal intensity which indicates the granuloma, interspersed within a low-intensity matrix denoting the fibrous tissue. The 'dot-in-circle sign', which indicates the presence of grains, is highly characteristic.

CT scan

CT findings in mycetoma are not specific but are helpful to detect early bone involvement.

Histopathological diagnosis

Deep biopsy is obtained under general or regional anaesthesia although the chance of local spread is high. The biopsy should be adequate, contain grains and should be fixed immediately in 10 per cent formal saline.

Three types of host tissue reaction occur against the organism. In Type I, the grains are usually surrounded by a layer of polymorphonuclear leukocytes. The innermost neutrophils are closely attached to the surface of the grain, sometimes invading the grain causing its fragmentation. The hyphae and cement substance disappear and only remnants of brown pigmented cement are left behind. Outside the zone of neutrophils there is granulation tissue containing macrophages, lymphocytes, plasma cells and few neutrophils. The mononuclear cells increase in number towards the periphery of the lesion. The outermost zone of the lesion consists of fibrous tissue.

In Type II tissue reaction, the neutrophils largely disappear and are replaced by macrophages and multinucleated giant cells which engulf grain material. This consists largely of pigmented cement substance although hyphae are sometimes identified. Type III reaction is characterised by the formation of a well-organised epithelioid granuloma with Langhan's type giant cells. The centre of the granuloma sometimes contains remnants of fungal material.

Fine needle aspiration cytology

Fine needle aspiration cytology (FNAC) can yield an accurate diagnosis and helps in distinguishing between eumyc-

Ernest Codman, 1869–1940, American surgeon. This appearance can be seen in osteosarcoma, Ewing's sarcoma and subperosteal abscess and haematoma.
Theodor Langhans, 1839–1915, Professor of Pathological Anatomy, University of Berne, Switzerland.

etoma and actinomycetoma. The technique is simple, rapid and sensitive.

Culture

A variety of microorganisms are capable of producing mycetoma. These can be identified by their textural description, morphological and biological activities in pure culture. Deep surgical biopsy is always needed to obtain the grains which are the source of culture. The grains extracted through the sinuses are usually contaminated and not viable and hence should be avoided. Several media may be used to isolate and grow these organisms.

In the absence of the classical triad of mycetoma, the demonstration of significant antibody titres against the causative organism may be of diagnostic value and for follow up. The common serodiagnostic tests are immunoelectrophoresis and ELISA (Summary box 6.16).

Summary box 6.16

Mycetoma – diagnosis

- Usually presents late as it is painless
- Triad of painless subcutaneous mass, multiple sinuses and seropurulent discharge
- Clinical picture may be deceptive as there may be deep-seated extension
- May spread to lymph nodes
- Can be confused with Kaposi's sarcoma
- Radiologically can be mistaken for osteosarcoma
- MRI shows typical 'dot-in-circle' sign
- Open biopsy and FNAC will be confirmatory

Management

Ideally, this should be a team effort between the physician and the surgeon. In actinomycetoma, combined drug therapy with amikacin sulphate and co-trimoxazole in the form of cycles is the treatment of choice. Amoxicillin–clavulanic acid, rifampacin, sulphonamides, gentamicin and kanamycin are used as a second line of treatment. Long-term drug treatment is beset with serious side effects.

In eumycetoma, ketoconazole, intraconazole and voriconazole are the drugs of choice. They may need to be used for up to a year. Use of these drugs should be closely monitored by the physician for side effects. While not being curative, these drugs help to localise the disease by forming thickly encapsulated lesions which are then amenable to surgical excision. Medical treatment for both types of mycetoma must continue until the patient is cured and also in the postoperative period.

Surgical treatment

Surgery is indicated in small localized lesions, resistance to medical treatment or for better response after medical treatment in patients with massive disease. Excision may need to be much more extensive than suggested at first on clinical appearance because the disease may extend to deeper planes which are not clinically apparent. The surgical options are wide local and debulking excisions and amputations. Amputation, used as a life-saving procedure, is indicated in advanced mycetoma refractory to medical treatment with severe secondary bacterial infection.The amputation rate is 10–25 per cent.

Postoperative medical treatment should continue for an adequate period to prevent recurrence. The recurrence rate varies from 25 to 50 per cent. This can be local or distant to regional lymph nodes. Recurrence is usually due to inadequate surgical excision, use of local anaesthesia, lack of surgical experience, non-compliance of drugs due to financial reasons and lack of health education (Summary box 6.17).

Summary box 6.17

Mycetoma – management

- Ideally combined management by physician and surgeon
- Medical treatment with appropriate long-term antibiotics
- In large lesions medical treatment to reduce the size followed by excision
- Beware of serious drug side effects
- Surgery in the form of wide excision and amputation as a life-saving procedure
- High recurrence rate

POLIOMYELITIS

Introduction

Poliomyelitis is an enteroviral infection that sadly still affects children in developing countries – this is in spite of effective vaccination having been universally available for several decades. The virus enters the body by inhalation or ingestion. Clinically, the disease manifests itself in a wide spectrum of symptoms – from a few days of mild fever and headache to the extreme variety consisting of extensive paralysis of the bulbar form that may not be compatible with life because of involvement of the respiratory and pharyngeal muscles.

Diagnosis

The disease targets the anterior horn cells causing lower motor neurone paralysis. Muscles of the lower limb are affected twice as frequently as those of the upper limb (Figures 6.30 and 6.31).

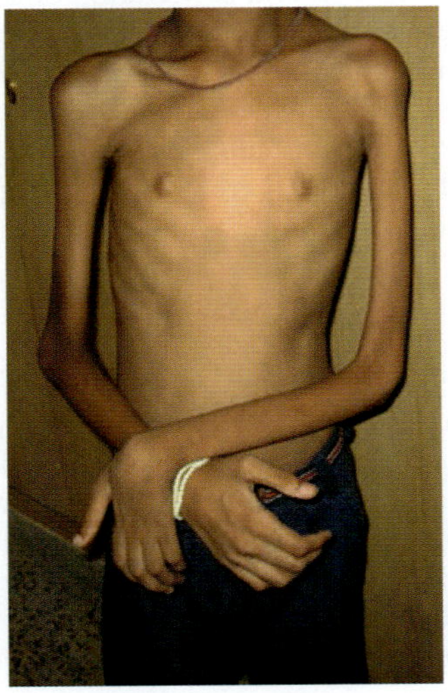

Figure 6.30 Polio affecting predominantly the upper limb muscles with wasting of the intercostal muscles.

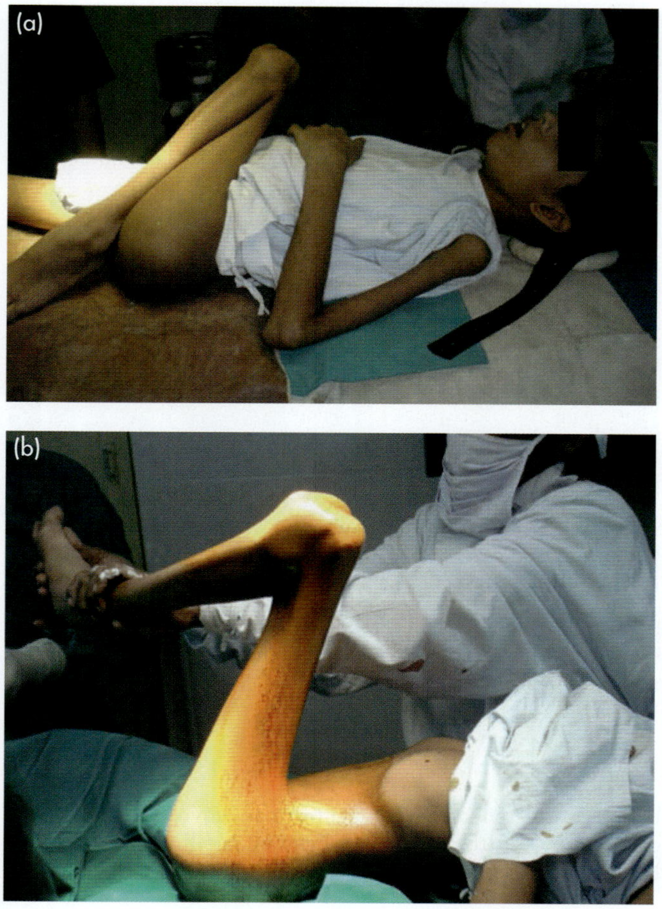

Figure 6.31 (a and b) A 12-year-old patient with polio showing marked wasting of the left upper arm muscles with flexion contractures of the left knee and hip; there is equinus deformity of the foot (courtesy of Dr SM Lakhotia and Dr PK Jain, Kolkata, India).

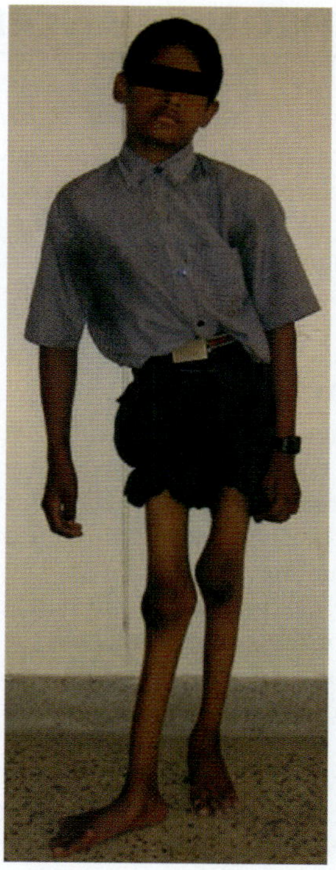

Figure 6.32 A young patient with polio showing paralysis of the lower limb and paraspinal muscles causing marked scoliosis and a deformed pelvis.

Fortunately, only 1–2 per cent of sufferers develop paralytic symptoms but, when they do occur, the disability causes much misery (Figure 6.32). When a patient develops fever with muscle weakness, Guillain–Barré syndrome needs to be excluded. The latter has sensory symptoms and signs, and cerebrospinal fluid (CSF) analysis should help to differentiate between the two conditions.

Management

Surgical management is directed mainly towards the rehabilitation of the patient who has residual paralysis, the operations being tailored to that particular individual's disability. Children especially may show improvement in their muscle function for up to two years after the onset of the illness. Thereafter, many patients learn to manage their disability by incorporating various manoeuvres ('trick movements') into their daily life. The surgeon must be cautious in considering such a patient for any form of surgery.

Surgical treatment in the chronic form of the disease is the domain of a highly specialised orthopaedic surgeon who needs to work closely with the physiotherapist both in assessing and rehabilitating the patient. Operations are only considered after a very careful and detailed assessment of the patient's needs. A multidisciplinary team consisting of the orthopaedic surgeon, neurologist, physiotherapist, orthotist and the family, should decide upon the need for and advisability of any surgical procedure (Summary box 6.18).

A description of the operations for the various disabilities is beyond the scope of this book. The reader should therefore seek surgical details in a specialist textbook. In 2012, WHO has declared India a polio-free country.

Summary box 6.18

Poliomyelitis

- A viral illness that is preventable
- Presents with protean manifestations of fever, headache and muscular paralysis without sensory loss, more frequently affecting the lower limbs
- Treatment is mainly medical and supportive in the early stages
- Surgery should only be undertaken after very careful assessment as most patients learn to live with their disabilities
- Surgery is considered for the various types of paralysis in the form of tendon transfers and arthrodesis, which is the domain of a specialised orthopaedic surgeon

Georges Guillain, 1876–1961, Professor of Neurology, The Faculty of Medicine, Paris, France.
Jean Alexandre Barré, 1880–1967, Professor of Neurology, Strasbourg, France.
Guillain and Barré described this condition in a joint paper in 1916 while serving as Medical Officers in the French Army during the First World War.

TROPICAL CHRONIC PANCREATITIS

Introduction

Tropical chronic pancreatitis is a disease affecting the younger generation from poor socioeconomic strata in developing countries, seen mostly in southern India. The aetiology remains obscure with malnutrition, dietary, familial and genetic factors being possible causes. Alcohol ingestion does not play a part in the aetiology.

Aetiology and pathology

Cassava (tapioca) is a root vegetable that is readily available and inexpensive and is therefore consumed as a staple diet by people from a poor background. It contains derivatives of cyanide that are detoxified in the liver by sulphur-containing amino acids. The less well-off among the population lack such amino acids in the diet. This results in cyanogen toxicity causing the disease. Several members of the same family have been known to suffer from this condition; this strengthens the theory that cassava toxicity is an important cause because family members eat the same food.

Macroscopically, the pancreas is firm and nodular with extensive periductal fibrosis, with intraductal calcium carbonate stones of different sizes and shapes that may show branches and resemble a staghorn. The ducts are dilated. Microscopically, fibrosis is the predominant feature – intralobular, interlobular and periductal – with plasma cell and lymphocyte infiltration. There is a high incidence of pancreatic cancer in these patients (Summary box 6.19).

Summary box 6.19

Pathology of tropical chronic pancreatitis

- Almost exclusively occurs in developing countries and is due to malnutrition; alcohol is not a cause
- Cassava ingestion is regarded as an aetiological factor because of its high content of cyanide compounds
- Dilatation of pancreatic ducts with large intraductal stones
- Fibrosis of the pancreas
- A high incidence of pancreatic cancer in those affected by the disease

Diagnosis

The patient, usually male, is almost always below the age of 40 years and from a poor background. The clinical presentation is abdominal pain, thirst, polyuria and features of gross pancreatic insufficiency causing steatorrhoea and malnutrition. The patient looks ill and emaciated.

Initial routine blood and urine tests confirm that the patient has type 1 diabetes mellitus. This is known as fibrocalculous pancreatic diabetes, a label that is aptly descriptive of the typical pathological changes. Serum amylase is usually normal; in an acute exacerbation, it may be elevated. A plain abdominal x-ray shows typical pancreatic calcification in the form of discrete stones in the duct (Figure 6.33). Ultrasound and CT scanning of the pancreas confirm the diagnosis. An ERCP as an investigation should only be done when the procedure is also being considered as a therapeutic manoeuvre for removal of ductal stones in the pancreatic head by papillotomy (Summary box 6.20).

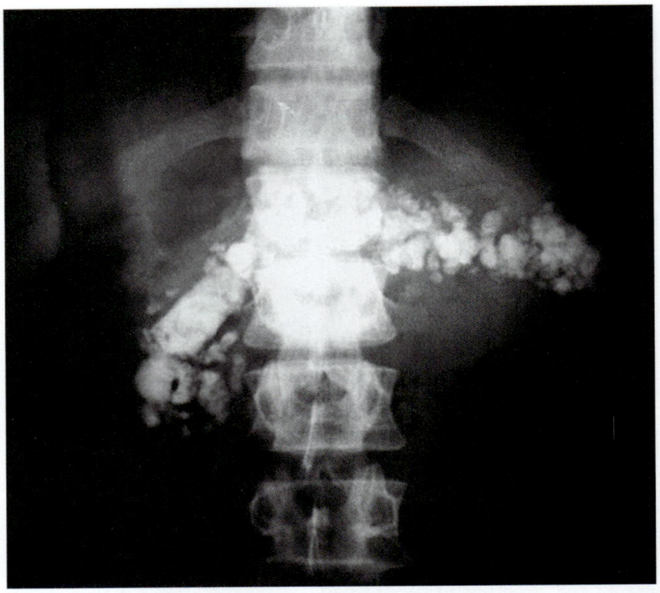

Figure 6.33 Plain x-ray of the abdomen showing large stones along the main pancreatic duct typical of tropical chronic pancreatitis (courtesy of Dr V Mohan, Chennai, India).

Summary box 6.20

Diagnosis of tropical chronic pancreatitis

- The usual sufferer is a type 1 diabetic under 40 years of age
- Serum amylase may be elevated in an acute exacerbation
- Plain x-ray shows stones along the pancreatic duct
- Ultrasound and CT scan of the pancreas confirm the diagnosis
- ERCP may be used as a supplementary investigation and a therapeutic procedure

Treatment

The treatment is mainly medical with exocrine support using pancreatic enzymes, treatment of diabetes with insulin and the management of malnutrition. Treatment of pain should be along the lines of the usual analgesic ladder: non-opioids, followed by weak and then strong opioids and, finally, referral to a pain clinic.

Surgical treatment is necessary for intractable pain, particularly when there are stones in a dilated duct. Removal of the stones, with a side-to-side pancreaticojejunostomy to a Roux loop, is the procedure of choice. As most patients are young, pancreatic resection is only very rarely considered, and then only as a last resort, when all available methods of pain relief have been exhausted (Summary box 6.21).

Summary box 6.21

Treatment of tropical chronic pancreatitis

- Mainly medical – pain relief, insulin for diabetes and pancreatic supplements for malnutrition
- Surgery is reserved for intractable pain
- Procedures are side-to-side pancreaticojejunostomy; resection in extreme cases

TUBERCULOSIS

While tuberculosis can affect all systems in the body, in the tropical developing world the surgeon is most often faced with tuberculosis affecting the cervical lymph nodes and the small intestine. Therefore in this chapter, tuberculous cervical lymphadenitis and tuberculosis of the small bowel will be described.

TUBERCULOUS CERVICAL LYMPHADENITIS

Introduction

This is common in the Indian subcontinent. A young person who has recently arrived in the UK from an endemic area, presenting with cervical lymphadenopathy, should be diagnosed as having tuberculous lymphadenitis unless otherwise proven. With acquired immune deficiency syndrome (AIDS) being globally prevalent, this is not as rare in the West in the indigenous population as it used to be.

Diagnosis

Any of the cervical group of lymph nodes (jugulodigastric, submandibular, supraclavicular, posterior triangle) can be involved.

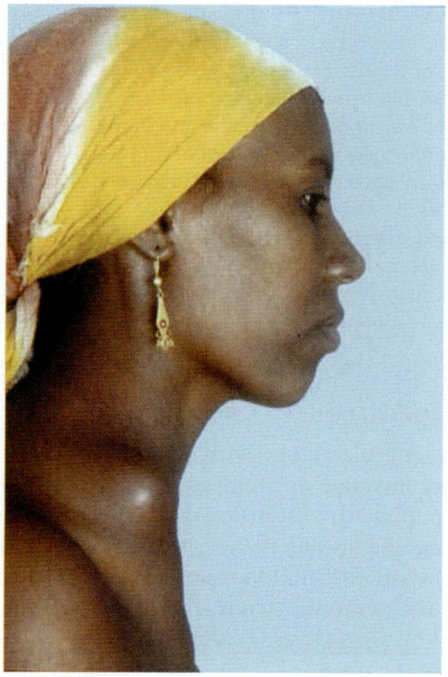

Figure 6.34 Cervical tuberculous cold abscess about to burst (courtesy of Professor Ahmed Hassan Fahal, Khartoum, Sudan).

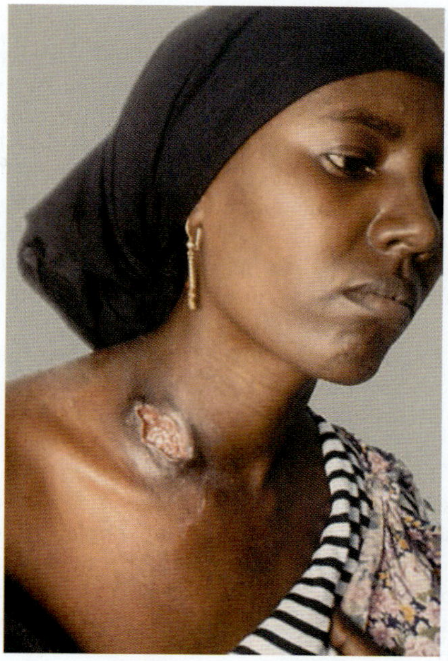

Figure 6.35 Cervical tuberculous sinus with typical overhanging edges (courtesy of Professor Ahmed Hassan Fahal, Khartoum, Sudan).

The patient has the usual general manifestations of tuberculosis: evening pyrexia, cough (maybe from pulmonary tuberculosis), malaise, and if the sufferer is a child, failure to thrive is a significant finding. Locally there will be regional lymphadenopathy where the lymph nodes may be matted; in late stages, a cold abscess may form – a painless, fluctuant, mass, not warm; significantly, there are no signs of inflammation (Figure 6.34), hence called a 'cold abscess'. This is a clinical manifestation of underlying caseation.

Left untreated, the cold abscess initially deep to the deep fascia now bursts through into the space just beneath the superficial fascia. This produces a bilocular mass with cross fluctuation. This is called a 'collar-stud' abscess. Eventually, this may burst through the skin discharging pus and forming a tuberculous sinus (Figure 6.35). The latter typically has watery discharge with undermined edges (Summary box 6.22).

Summary box 6.22

Tuberculous cervical lymphadenitis

- This is a common condition at any age
- Matted lymphnodal mass is the typical clinical feature
- In later stages the mass may be cystic denoting an abscess
- The abscess denotes underlying caseation and does not show any features of inflammation – hence called cold abscess
- Ultimately the abscess may burst forming a sinus
- Diagnosis is clinched by culture of pus and biopsy of the lymph node
- Involvement of other systems must be excluded
- Treatment is mainly medical

Collar-stud abscess is so called because it resembles a collar stud (which has two parts) used in shirts with detachable collars, now largely out of fashion.

Investigations

Raised ESR and CRP, low haemoglobin and a positive Mantoux test are usual, although the last is not significant in a patient from an endemic area. The Mantoux test (tuberculin skin test), although in use for over a hundred years, has now been superseded by interferon gamma (IFN-γ) release assays. This is an *in vitro* blood test of cellular immune response. Antigens unique to *Mycobacterium tuberculosis* are used to stimulate and measure T-cell release of IFN-γ. This helps to earmark patients who have latent or subclinical tuberculosis and thus benefit from treatment.

Sputum for culture and sensitivity (the result may take several weeks) and staining by the Ziehl–Neelsen method for acid-fast bacilli (the result is obtained much earlier) should also be done.

Specific investigations include aspiration of the pus in a cold abscess for culture and sensitivity. If the mass is still in the early stages of adenitis, excision biopsy should be done. Here, part of the lymph nodes should be sent fresh and unfixed to the laboratory who should be warned of the arrival of the specimen so that the tissue can be appropriately processed immediately.

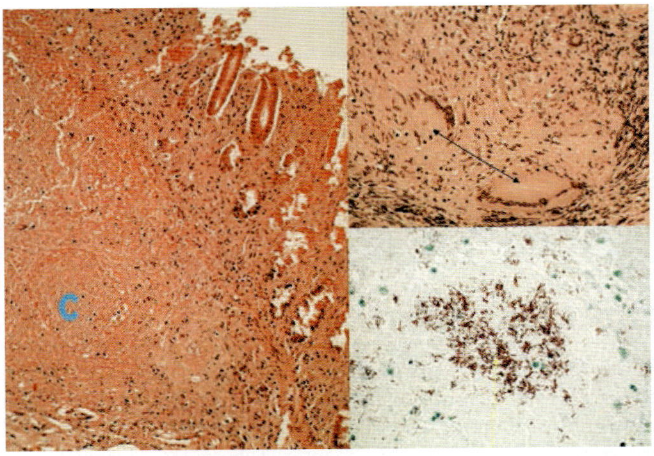

Figure 6.36 Histology of ileocaecal tuberculosis. C: caseation. Black arrows show epithelioid granuloma with multi-nucleated giant cells. Yellow arrow shows acid-fast bacilli on Ziehl–Neelsen staining. (Courtesy of Dr Rosslyn Rankin, Raigmore Hospital, Inverness, Scotland.)

Treatment

This must be a combined management between the physician and the surgeon. Tuberculous infection at other sites must be excluded and suitably managed. Medical treatment is the mainstay. The reader is asked to refer to details of medical treatment in an appropriate source.

TUBERCULOSIS OF SMALL INTESTINE

Introduction

Infection by *Mycobacterium tuberculosis* is common in the tropics. In these days of international travel and increased migration to the UK, tuberculosis in general and intestinal tuberculosis in particular are no longer clinical curiosities in the West. Any patient, particularly one who has recently arrived from an endemic area and who has features of generalised ill health and altered bowel habit, should arouse the suspicion of intestinal tuberculosis. The increased incidence of human immunodeficiency virus (HIV) infection worldwide has also made tuberculosis more common.

Pathology

When a patient with pulmonary tuberculosis swallows infected sputum, the organism colonises the lymphatics of the terminal ileum, causing transverse ulcers with typical undermined edges. The serosa is usually studded with tubercles. Histology shows caseating granuloma with giant cells (Figure 6.36). This pathological entity, referred to as the ulcerative type, denotes a severe form of the disease in which the virulence of the organism overwhelms host resistance.

The other variety, called the hyperplastic type, occurs when host resistance has the upper hand over the virulence of the organism. It is caused by the drinking of infected milk. There is a marked inflammatory reaction causing hyperplasia and thickening of the terminal ileum because of its abundance of lymphoid follicles, thus causing narrowing of the lumen and obstruction. In both types there may be marked mesenteric lymphadenopathy. Macroscopically, this type may be confused with Crohn's disease. The small intestine shows areas of stricture and fibrosis most pronounced at the terminal ileum (Figure 6.37). As a result, there is shortening of the bowel with the caecum being pulled up into a subhepatic position (Summary box 6.23).

Summary box 6.23

Tuberculosis – pathology

- Increasingly being seen in the UK, mostly among immigrants
- Two types are recognised – ulcerative and hyperplastic
- The ulcerative type occurs when the virulence of the organism is greater than the host defence
- The opposite occurs in the hyperplastic type
- Small bowel strictures are common in the hyperplastic type, mainly affecting the ileocaecal area
- In the ulcerative type, the bowel serosa is studded with tubercles
- Localised areas of ascites occur in the form of cocoons
- The lungs and other organs, particularly of the genitourinary system, may also be involved simultaneously

Clinical features

Patients present electively with weight loss, chronic cough, malaise, evening rise in temperature with sweating, vague abdominal pain with distension and alternating constipation and diarrhoea. As an emergency, they present with features of distal small bowel obstruction from strictures of the small bowel, particularly the terminal ileum. Rarely, a patient may present

Burrill Bernard Crohn, 1884–1983, gastroenterologist, Mount Sinai Hospital, New York, NY, USA, described regional ileitis in 1932 along with Leon Ginzburg and Gordon Oppenheimer.

Charles Mantoux, 1877–1947, physician, Le Cannet, Alpes Maritimes, France, described the intradermal tuberculin skin test in 1908.
Franz Heinrich Paul Ziehl, 1859–1926, neurologist, Lubeck, Germany.
Friedrich Carl Adolf Neelsen, 1854–1894, pathologist, Prosector, the Stadt-Krankenhaus, Dresden, Germany.

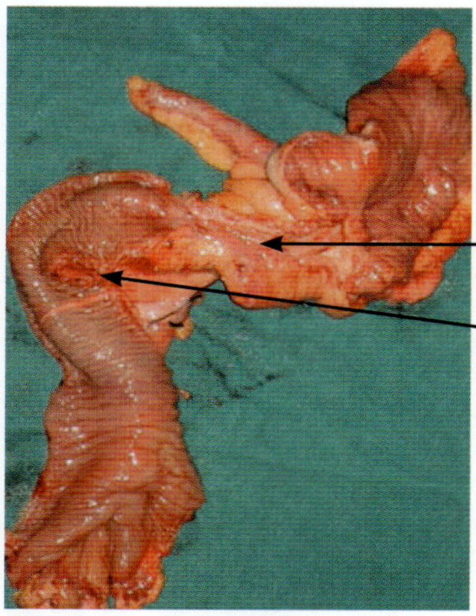

Figure 6.37 Emergency limited ileocolic resection: specimen showing tuberculous stricture in the terminal ileum and perforation of a transverse ulcer just proximal to the stricture.

with features of peritonitis from perforation of a tuberculous ulcer in the small bowel (Figure 6.37).

Examination shows a chronically ill patient with a 'doughy' feel to the abdomen from areas of localised ascites. In the hyperplastic type, a mass may be felt in the right iliac fossa. In addition, some patients may present with fistula-in-ano, which is typically multiple with undermined edges and watery discharge.

As this is a disease mainly seen in developing countries, patients may present late as an emergency from intestinal obstruction. Abdominal pain and distension, constipation and bilious and faeculent vomiting are typical of such a patient who is *in extremis*.

There may be features of other system involvement, such as the genitourinary tract, when the patient complains of frequency of micturition. Clinical examination does not show any abnormality. The genitourinary tract should then be investigated (Summary box 6.24).

Summary box 6.24

Tuberculosis – clinical features

- Intestinal tuberculosis should be suspected in any patient from an endemic area who presents with weight loss, malaise, evening fever, cough, alternating constipation and diarrhoea and intermittent abdominal pain with distension
- The abdomen has a doughy feel; a mass may be found in the right iliac fossa
- The emergency patient presents with features of distal small bowel obstruction – abdominal pain, distension, bilious and faeculent vomiting
- Peritonitis from a perforated tuberculous ulcer in the small bowel can be another emergency presentation

Investigations

General investigations are the same as those for suspected tuberculosis anywhere in the body. They have been detailed in the previous section.

A barium meal and follow-through (or small bowel enema) shows strictures of the small bowel, particularly the ileum, typically with a high subhepatic caecum with the narrow ileum entering the caecum directly from below upwards in a straight line rather than at an angle (Figures 6.38 and 6.39a). Laparoscopy reveals the typical picture of tubercles on the bowel serosa, multiple strictures, a high caecum, enlarged lymph nodes, areas of caseation and ascites. Culture of the ascitic fluid may be helpful. A chest x-ray is essential (Figure 6.39b).

If the patient complains of urinary symptoms, urine is sent for microscopy and culture; the finding of sterile pyuria should alert

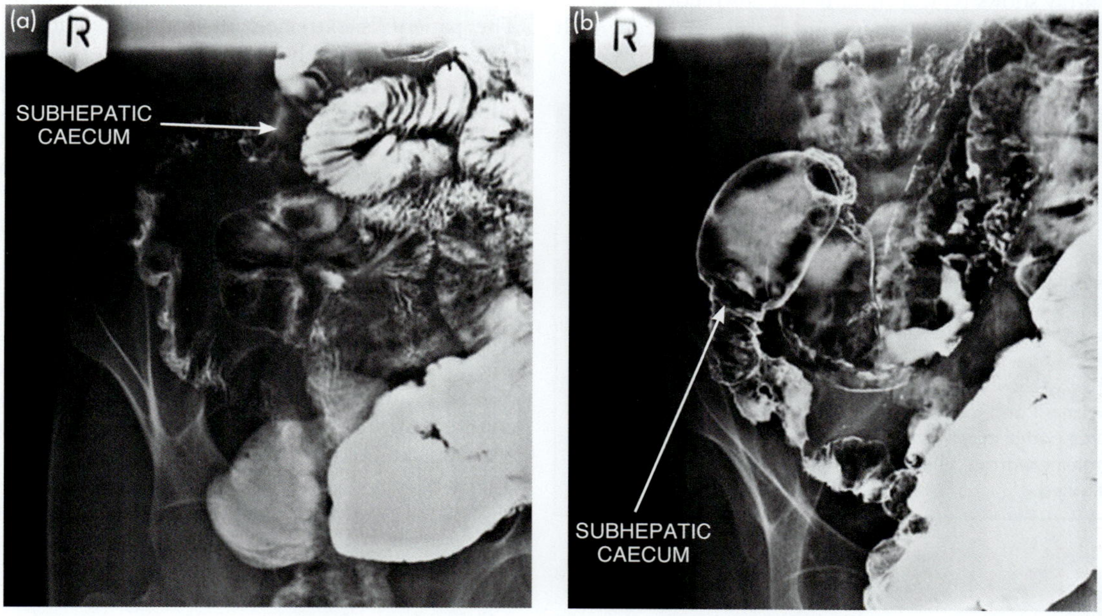

Figure 6.38 (a and b) Series of a barium meal and follow-through showing strictures in the ileum with the caecum pulled up into a subhepatic position.

PART 1 | PRINCIPLES

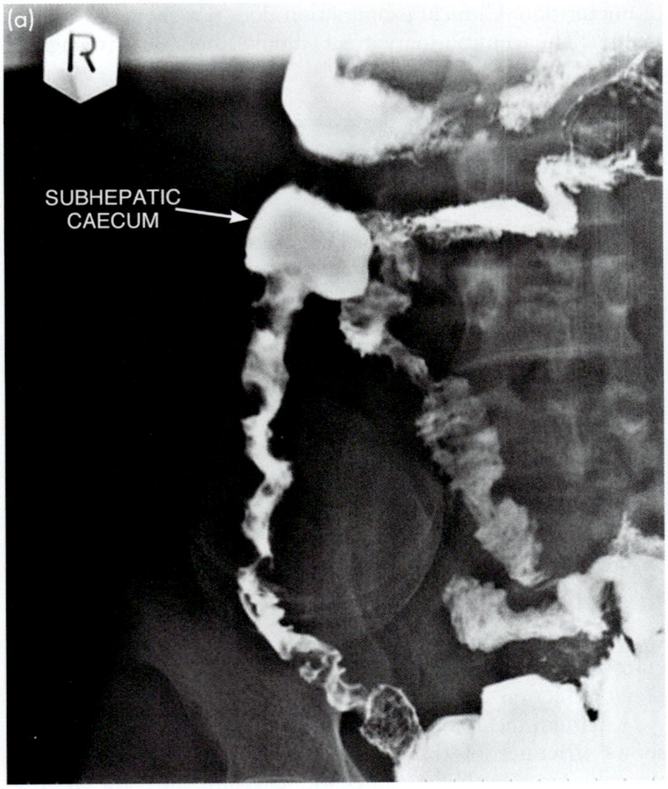

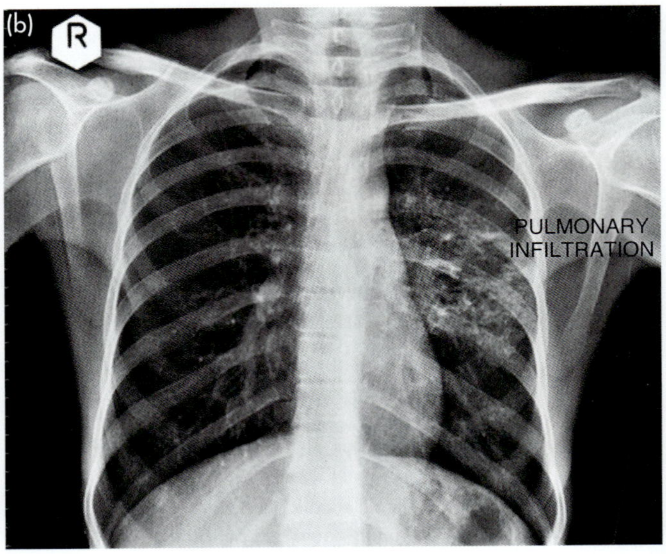

Figure 6.39 Barium meal and follow-through (a) and chest x-ray (b) in a patient with extensive intestinal and pulmonary tuberculosis, showing ileal strictures with high caecum and pulmonary infiltration.

the clinician to the possibility of tuberculosis of the urinary tract, when the appropriate investigations should be done. A flexible cystoscopy would be very useful in the presence of sterile pyuria. A contracted bladder ('thimble' bladder) with ureteric orifices that are in-drawn ('golf-hole' ureter) may be seen; these changes are due to fibrosis.

In the patient presenting as an abdominal emergency, urea and electrolytes show evidence of gross dehydration. Plain abdominal x-ray shows typical small bowel obstruction – valvulae conniventes of dilated jejunum and featureless ileum with evidence of fluid between the loops (Summary box 6.25).

Summary box 6.25

Intestinal tuberculosis – investigations

- Raised inflammatory markers, anaemia and positive sputum culture
- Interferon-gamma release assays for subclinical infection is done
- Ultrasound of the abdomen may show localised areas of ascites
- Chest x-ray shows pulmonary infiltration
- Barium meal and follow-through shows multiple small bowel strictures particularly in the ileum with a subhepatic caecum
- If symptoms warrant, the genitourinary tract is also investigated

Treatment

On completion of medical treatment, the patient's small bowel is reimaged to look for significant strictures. If the patient has features of subacute intermittent obstruction, bowel resection, in the form of limited ileocolic resection (Figure 6.37) with anastomosis between the terminal ileum and ascending colon, strictureplasty or right hemicolectomy, is performed as deemed appropriate. The surgical principles and options in the elective patient are very similar to those for Crohn's disease.

The emergency patient presents a great challenge. Such a patient is usually from a poor socioeconomic background, hence the late presentation of acute, distal, small bowel obstruction. The patient is extremely ill from dehydration, malnutrition, anaemia and probably active pulmonary tuberculosis. Vigorous resuscitation should precede the operation. At laparotomy, the minimum life-saving procedure is carried out, such as a side-to-side ileotransverse anastomosis for a terminal ileal stricture. If the general condition of the patient permits, a one-stage resection and anastomosis may be performed.

Thereafter, the patient should ideally be under the combined care of the physician and surgeon for a full course of anti-tuberculous chemotherapy and improvement in nutritional status; this may require three to six months of care. The patient who had a simple bypass procedure is reassessed and, when the disease is no longer active (as evidenced by return to normal of inflammatory markers, weight gain, negative sputum culture), an elective right hemicolectomy is done. This may be supplemented with strictureplasty for short strictures at intervals.

Perforation is treated by thorough resuscitation followed by resection of the affected segment. Anastomosis is performed provided it is regarded as safe to do so when peritoneal contamination is minimal and widespread disease is not encountered; otherwise, as a first stage, resection and exteriorisation is done followed by restoration of bowel continuity as a second stage later on after a full course of anti-tuberculous chemotherapy and improvement in nutritional status (Summary box 6.26).

Summary box 6.26

Tuberculosis – treatment

- Patients should ideally be under the combined care of a physician and surgeon
- Vigorous supportive and full drug treatment is mandatory in all cases
- Symptomatic strictures are treated by the appropriate resection, e.g. local ileocolic resection or strictureplasty as an elective procedure once the disease is completely under control
- Acute intestinal obstruction from distal ileal stricture is treated by thorough resuscitation followed by side-to-side ileotransverse bypass
- Once the patient has recovered with medical treatment, then the second-stage definitive procedure of right hemicolectomy is done to remove the blind loop
- One-stage resection and anastomosis can be considered if the patient's general condition permits
- Perforation is treated by appropriate local resection and anastomosis or exteriorisation if the condition of the patient is very poor; this is later followed by restoration of bowel continuity after the patient has fully recovered with anti-tuberculous chemotherapy

TYPHOID

Introduction

Typhoid fever is caused by *Salmonella typhi*, also called the typhoid bacillus. This is a Gram-negative organism. Like most infections occurring in developing countries in the tropics, the organism gains entry into the human gastrointestinal tract as a result of poor hygiene and inadequate sanitation. It is a disease normally managed by physicians, but the surgeon is called upon to treat the patient with typhoid fever because of perforation of a typhoid ulcer.

Pathology

Following ingestion of contaminated food or water, the organism colonises the Peyer's patches in the terminal ileum causing hyperplasia of the lymphoid follicles followed by necrosis and ulceration. The microscopic picture shows erythrophagocytosis with histiocytic proliferation (Figure 6.40). If the patient is left untreated or inadequately treated, the ulcers may lead to perforation and bleeding. The bowel may perforate at several sites including the large bowel.

Diagnosis

A typical patient is from an endemic area or who has recently visited such a country and suffers from a high temperature for 2–3 weeks. The patient may be toxic with abdominal distension from paralytic ileus. The patient may have melaena due to haemorrhage from a typhoid ulcer; this can lead to hypovolaemia.

Blood and stool cultures confirm the nature of the infection and exclude malaria. Although obsolete in the UK, the Widal test is still done in the Indian subcontinent. The test looks for the presence of agglutinins to O and H antigens of *Salmonella typhi* and *paratyphi* in the patient's serum. In endemic areas, laboratory facilities may sometimes be limited. Certain other tests have been developed which identify sensitive and specific markers for typhoid fever. Practical and cheap kits are available for their rapid detection that need no special expertise and equipment. These are Multi-Test Dip-S-Ticks to detect immunoglobulin G (IgG), Tubex to detect immunoglobulin M (IgM) and TyphiDot to detect IgG and IgM. These tests are particularly valuable when blood cultures are negative (due to pre-hospital treatment or self-medication with antibiotics) or facilities for such an investigation are not available.

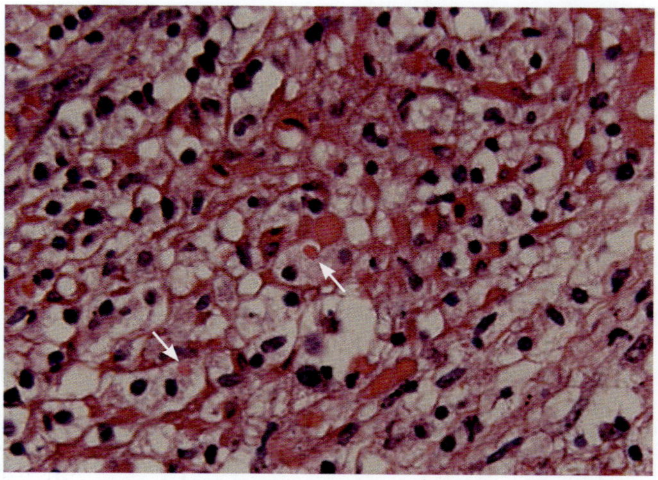

Figure 6.40 Histology of enteric perforation of the small intestine showing erythrophagocytosis (arrows) with predominantly histiocytic proliferation (courtesy of Dr AK Mandal, New Delhi, India).

In the second or third week of the illness, if there is severe generalised abdominal pain, this heralds a perforated typhoid ulcer. The patient, who is already very ill, deteriorates further with classical features of peritonitis. An erect chest x-ray or a lateral decubitus film (in the very ill, as they usually are) will show free gas in the peritoneal cavity. In fact, any patient being treated for typhoid fever who shows a sudden deterioration accompanied by abdominal signs should be considered to have a typhoid perforation until proven otherwise (Summary box 6.27).

Summary box 6.27

Diagnosis of bowel perforation secondary to typhoid

- The patient presents in, or has recently visited, an endemic area
- The patient has persistent high temperature and is very toxic
- Positive blood or stool cultures for *Salmonella typhi* and the patient is already on treatment for typhoid
- After the second week, signs of peritonitis usually denote perforation, which is confirmed by the presence of free gas seen on x-ray

Daniel Elmer Salmon, 1850–1914, Veterinary Pathologist, Chief of the Bureau of Animal Industry, Washington DC, USA.
Johann Conrad Peyer, 1653–1712, Professor of Logic, Rhetoric and Medicine, Schaffhausen, Switzerland, described the lymph follicles in the intestine in 1677.
Georges Fernand Isidore Widal, 1862–1929, Professor of Internal Pathology, and later of Clinical Medicine, Faculty of Medicine, Paris, France. He developed the test in 1896 to diagnose typhoid fever.

Treatment

Vigorous resuscitation with intravenous fluids and antibiotics in an intensive care unit gives the best chance of stabilising the patient's condition. Metronidazole, cephalosporins and gentamicin are used in combination. Chloramphenicol, despite its potential side effect of aplastic anaemia, is still used occasionally in developing countries. Laparotomy is then carried out.

Several surgical options are available, and the most appropriate operative procedure should be chosen judiciously depending upon the general condition of the patient, the site of perforation, the number of perforations and the degree of peritoneal soiling. The alternatives are closure of the perforation (Figure 6.41) after freshening the edges, wedge resection of the ulcer area and closure, resection of bowel with or without anastomosis (exteriorisation), closure of the perforation and side-to-side ileotransverse anastomosis, ileostomy or colostomy where the perforated bowel is exteriorised after refashioning the edges. After closing an ileal perforation, the surgeon should look for other sites of perforation or necrotic patches in the small or large bowel that might imminently perforate, and deal with them appropriately. Thorough peritoneal lavage is essential. The linea alba is closed leaving the rest of the abdominal wound open for delayed closure, as wound infection is almost inevitable and dehiscence not uncommon. In the presence of rampant infection, laparostomy may be a good alternative.

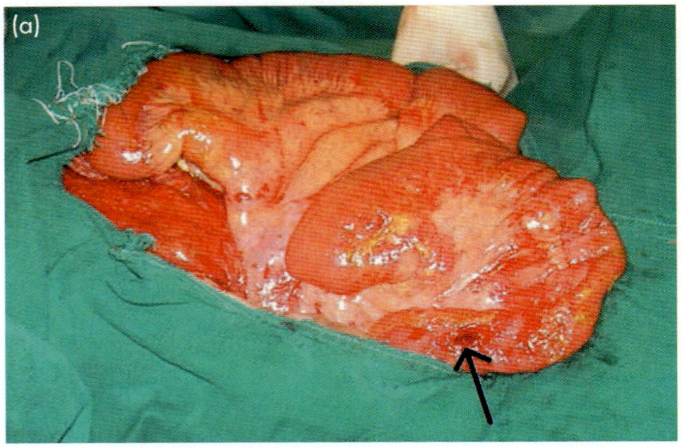

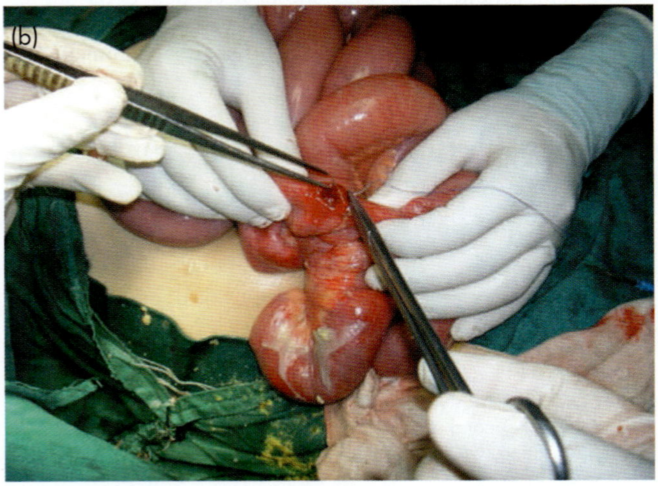

Figure 6.41 (a and b) Typhoid perforation of the terminal ileum.

When a typhoid perforation occurs within the first week of illness, the prognosis is better than if it occurs after the second or third week because, in the early stages, the patient is less nutritionally compromised and the body's defences are more robust. Furthermore, the shorter the interval between diagnosis and operation, the better is the prognosis (Summary box 6.28).

Summary box 6.28

Treatment of bowel perforation from typhoid

- Manage in intensive care
- Resuscitate and give intravenous antibiotics
- Laparotomy – choice of various procedures
- Most common site of perforation is the terminal ileum
- Having found a perforation, always look for others
- In the very ill patient, consider some form of exteriorisation
- Close the peritoneum and leave the wound open for secondary closure

FURTHER READING

Adeniran JO, Taiwo JO, Abdur-Raham LO. Salmonella intestinal perforation (27 perforations in one patient, 14 perforations in another): are the goal posts changing? *J Indian Assoc Pediatr Surg* 2005; **10**: 248–51.

Aziz M, Qadir A, Aziz M, Faizullah. Prognostic factors in typhoid perforation. *J Coll Phys Surg Pakistan* 2005; **15**: 704–7.

Barman KK, Premlatha G, Mohan V. Tropical chronic pancreatitis. *Postgrad Med J* 2003; **79**: 606–15.

Barnes SA, Lillemore KD. Liver abscess and hydatid disease. In: Zinner NJ, Schwartz I, Ellis H (eds). *Maingot's abdominal operations*, 10th edn, Vol. 2. New York: Appleton and Lange, 1997: 1527–45.

Chiodini P. Parasitic infections. In: Russell RCG, Williams NS, Bulstrode CJK (eds). *Bailey & Love's short practice of surgery*, 24th edn. London: Arnold, 2004: 146–74.

Choi BI, Han JK, Hong ST, Lee KH. Clonorchiasis and cholangiocarcinoma: etiologic relationship and imaging diagnosis. *Clin Microbiol Rev* 2004; **17**: 540–52.

Fahal AH. Management of mycetoma. *Expert Rev Dermat* 2010; **5**: 87–93.

Fahal AH. *Mycetoma: clinico-pathological monograph*. University of Khartoum Press, Khartoum, 2006.

Hassan MA, Fahal AH. Mycetoma. In: Kamil R, Lumby J (eds). *Tropical surgery*. London: Westminster Publications Ltd. 2004: 786–790.

Olsen SJ, Pruckler J, Bibb W *et al*. Evaluation of rapid diagnostic tests for typhoid fever. *J Clin Microbiol* 2004; **42**: 1885–9.

Manjula Y, Kate V, Ananthakrishnan N. Evaluation of sequential intermittent pneumatic compression for filarial lymphoedema. *Natl Med J India* 2002; **15**: 192–4.

Steinberg R, Davies J, Millar AJ *et al*. Unusual intestinal sequelae after operations for *Ascaris lumbricoides* infestation. *Paediatr Surg Int* 2003; **19**: 85–7.

Wani RA, Parray FQ, Bhat NA *et al*. Non-traumatic terminal ileal perforation. *World J Emerg Surg* 2006; **10**: 1–7.

WHO Informal Working Group. International classification of ultrasound images in cystic echinococcosis for application in clinical and field epidemiological settings. *Acta Trop* 2003; **85**: 253–61.

World Health Organization. Leprosy – global situation. *Wkly Epidemiol Rec* 2000; **75**: 225–32.

World Health Organization. The World Health Report – bridging the gaps. *World Health Forum* 1995; **16**: 377–85.

CHAPTER 7

Principles of laparoscopic and robotic surgery

LEARNING OBJECTIVES

To understand:
- The principles of laparoscopic and robotic surgery
- The advantages and disadvantages of such surgery
- The safety issues and indications for laparoscopic and robotic surgery
- The principles of postoperative care

DEFINITION

Minimal access surgery is a marriage of modern technology and surgical innovation that aims to accomplish surgical therapeutic goals with minimal somatic and psychological trauma. This type of surgery has reduced wound access trauma, as well as being less disfiguring than conventional techniques. With increasing experience, it offers cost-effectiveness both to health services and to employers by shortening operating times, shortening hospital stays and allowing faster recuperation.

EXTENT OF MINIMAL ACCESS SURGERY

Minimal access surgery has crossed all traditional boundaries of specialties and disciplines. Shared, borrowed and overlapping technologies and information are encouraging a multidisciplinary approach that serves the whole patient, rather than a specific organ system. Broadly speaking, minimal access techniques can be categorised as follows.

Laparoscopy

A rigid endoscope (laparoscope) is introduced through a port into the peritoneal cavity. This is insufflated with carbon dioxide to produce a pneumoperitoneum. Further ports are inserted to enable instrument access and their use for dissection (Figure 7.1). There is little doubt that laparoscopic cholecystectomy has revolutionised the surgical management of cholelithiasis and has become the mainstay of management of uncomplicated gallstone disease. With improved instrumentation, advanced procedures, such as laparoscopic colectomies for malignancy, previously regarded as controversial, have also become fully accepted. There has been an increasing evidence base showing the short-term benefits of laparoscopic surgery over open surgery with regards to postoperative pain, length of stay, earlier return to normal activities, but maintaining equivalence of the benefits of the long-term outcomes, such as oncological quality and cancer-related survival.

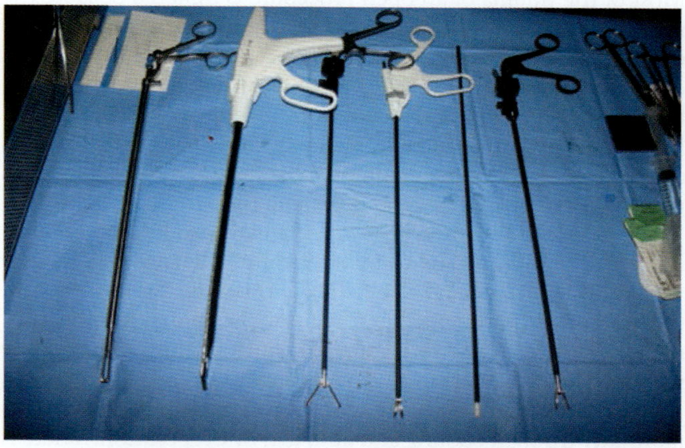

Figure 7.1 Basic laparoscopic instruments (photo courtesy of Daniel Leff).

Thoracoscopy

A rigid endoscope is introduced through an incision in the chest to gain access to the thoracic contents. Usually there is no requirement for gas insufflation as the operating space is held open by the rigidity of the thoracic cavity.

Endoluminal endoscopy

Flexible or rigid endoscopes are introduced into hollow organs or systems, such as the urinary tract, upper or lower gastrointestinal tract, and respiratory and vascular systems (see Chapter 14).

Perivisceral endoscopy

Body planes can be accessed even in the absence of a natural cavity. Examples are mediastinoscopy, retroperitoneoscopy and retroperitoneal approaches to the kidney, aorta and lumbar sympathetic chain. Extraperitoneal approaches to the retroperitoneal organs, as well as hernia repair, are now becoming increasingly commonplace, further decreasing morbidity associated with visceral peritoneal manipulation. Other, more recent, examples include subfascial ligation of incompetent perforating veins in varicose vein surgery.

Arthroscopy and intra-articular joint surgery

Orthopaedic surgeons have long used arthroscopic access to the knee and have now moved their attention to other joints, including the shoulder, wrist, elbow and hip.

Combined approach

The diseased organ is visualised and treated by an assortment of endoluminal and extraluminal endoscopes and other imaging devices.

SURGICAL TRAUMA IN OPEN, LAPAROSCOPIC AND ROBOTIC SURGERY

Most of the trauma of an open procedure is inflicted because the surgeon must have a wound that is large enough to give adequate exposure for safe dissection at the target site. The wound is often the cause of morbidity, including infection, dehiscence, bleeding, herniation and nerve entrapment. Wound pain prolongs recovery time and, by reducing mobility, contributes to an increased incidence of pulmonary atelectasis, chest infection, paralytic ileus and deep venous thrombosis.

Mechanical and human retractors cause additional trauma. Body wall retractors tend to inflict localised damage that may be as painful as the wound itself. In contrast, during laparoscopy, the retraction is provided by the low-pressure pneumoperitoneum, giving a diffuse force applied gently and evenly over the whole body wall, causing minimal trauma.

Exposure of any body cavity to the atmosphere also causes morbidity through cooling and fluid loss by evaporation. There is also evidence to suggest that the incidence of post-surgical adhesions has been reduced by the use of the laparoscope because there is less damage to delicate serosal coverings. In handling intestinal loops, the surgeon and assistant disturb the peristaltic activity of the gut and provoke adynamic ileus.

Minimal access surgery has many advantages, such as a reduction in the trauma of access and exposure and an improvement in visualisation (Summary box 7.1).

Summary box 7.1

Advantages of minimal access surgery

- Decrease in wound size
- Reduction in wound infection, dehiscence, bleeding, herniation and nerve entrapment
- Decrease in wound pain
- Improved mobility
- Decreased wound trauma
- Decreased heat loss
- Improved vision

LIMITATIONS OF MINIMAL ACCESS SURGERY

Despite its many advantages, minimal access surgery has its limitations. To perform minimal access surgery with safety, the surgeon must operate remote from the surgical field, using an imaging system that provides a two-dimensional representation of the operative site. The endoscope offers a whole new anatomical landscape, which the surgeon must learn to navigate without the usual clues that make it easy to judge depth. The instruments are longer and sometimes more complex to use than those commonly used in open surgery. This results in the novice being faced with significant problems of hand–eye coordination.

Some of the procedures performed by these new approaches are more technically demanding and are slower to perform and often have a more difficult learning curve as tactile feedback to the surgeon is lost. Indeed, on occasion, a minimally invasive operation is so technically demanding that both patient and surgeon are better served by conversion to an open procedure. Unfortunately, there seems to be a sense of shame associated with conversion, which is quite unjustified. It is vital for surgeons and patients to appreciate that the decision to close or convert to an open operation is not a complication but, instead, usually implies sound surgical judgement.

Another problem occurs when there is intraoperative arterial bleeding. Haemostasis may be very difficult to achieve endoscopically because blood obscures the field of vision and there is a significant reduction of the image quality owing to light absorption.

Another disadvantage of laparoscopic surgery is the loss of tactile feedback; this is an area of ongoing research in haptics and biofeedback systems. Early work suggested that laparoscopic ultrasonography might be a substitute for the need to 'feel' in intraoperative decision-making. The rapid progress in advanced laparoscopic techniques, including biliary tract exploration and surgery for malignancies, has provided a strong impetus for the development of laparoscopic ultrasound. Now more developed over the last decade, this technique already has advantages that far outweigh its disadvantages.

In more advanced techniques, large pieces of resected tissue, such as the lung or colon, may have to be extracted from the body cavity. Occasionally, the extirpated tissue may be removed through a nearby natural orifice, such as the rectum, or the mouth. At other times, a novel route may be employed. For instance, a benign colonic specimen may be extracted through an incision in the vault of the vagina. Several innovative tube systems have been shown to facilitate this extraction. Although tissue 'morcellators, mincers and liquidisers' can be used in some circumstances, they have the disadvantage of reducing the amount of information available to the pathologist. Previous reports of tumour implantation in the locations of port sites raised important questions about the future of the laparoscopic treatment of malignancy, but large-scale trials have shown this claim to be false. Although emerging evidence from large-scale international prospective trials implicate surgical skill as an important aetiological factor, it is important to consider the biological implications of minimally invasive strategies on the tumours. The use of carbon dioxide and helium as insufflants causes locoregional hypoxia and may also change pH. The resultant modulation of spilled tumour cell behaviour is only now being elucidated.

Hand-assisted laparoscopic surgery is a well-developed technique. It involves the intra-abdominal placement of a hand or forearm through a minilaparotomy incision, while pneumoperitoneum is maintained. In this way, the surgeon's hand can be used as in an open procedure. It can be used to palpate organs or tumours, reflect organs atraumatically, retract structures, identify vessels, dissect bluntly along a tissue plane and provide finger pressure to bleeding points, while proximal control is achieved. In addition, several reports have suggested that this approach is more economical than a totally laparoscopic approach, reducing both the number of laparoscopic ports and the number of instruments required. Some advocates of the technique claim that it is also easier to learn and perform than totally laparoscopic approaches, and that there may be increased patient safety.

There is a growing need for improvement in dissection techniques in laparoscopic surgery and, specifically, for improving the safe use of electrosurgery and lasers. Ultrasonic dissection, tissue fusion devices and tissue removal have been utilised by a growing number of specialties for several years. The adaptation of the technology to laparoscopic surgery grew out of the search for alternative, possibly safer, methods of dissection. The current units combine the functions of three or four separate instruments, reducing the need for instrument exchanges during a procedure. This flexibility, combined with the ability to provide a clean, smoke-free field, improves safety while shortening operating times.

Although dramatic cost savings are possible with laparoscopic cholecystectomy, the position was less clear-cut with other procedures initially. There is another factor that may complicate the computation of the cost–benefit ratio. A significant rise in the rate of cholecystectomy followed the introduction of the laparoscopic approach as the threshold for referring patients for surgery lowered. The increase in the number of procedures performed has led to an overall increase in the cost of treating symptomatic gallstones.

Three-dimensional imaging systems are available, but remain expensive and currently are not commonplace. Stereoscopic imaging for laparoscopy is still progressing. Future improvements in these systems will greatly enhance manipulative ability in critical procedures, such as knot tying and dissection of closely underlying tissues. There are, however, some drawbacks, such as reduced display brightness and interference with normal vision because of the need to wear specially designed glasses for some systems. It is likely that brighter projection displays will be developed, at increased cost. However, the need to wear glasses will not be easily overcome.

Looking further to the future, it is evident that the continuing reductions in the costs of elaborate image-processing techniques will result in a wide range of transformed presentations becoming available. It will ultimately be possible for a surgeon to call up any view of the operative region that is accessible to a camera and present it stereoscopically in any size or orientation, superimposed on past images taken in other modalities. Such augmented reality systems are being developed at present, but are currently in relative infancy. It is for the medical community to decide which of these many potential imaginative techniques will contribute most to effective surgical procedures (Summary box 7.2).

Summary box 7.2

Limitations of minimal access surgery

- Reliance on remote vision and operating
- Loss of tactile feedback
- Dependence on hand–eye coordination
- Difficulty with haemostasis
- Reliance on new techniques
- Extraction of large specimens

ROBOTIC SURGERY

A robot is a mechanical device that performs automated physical tasks according to direct human supervision, a predefined program or a set of general guidelines using artificial intelligence techniques. In terms of surgery, robots have been used to assist surgeons during procedures. This has been primarily in the form of automated camera systems and telemanipulator systems, thus resulting in the creation of a human–machine interface.

Even though laparoscopic surgery has progressed greatly over the last two decades, there are limitations. These include the restriction to two-dimensional views, reduced degrees of freedom of movement, little or no tactile feedback and ergonomically difficult positions for the surgeon. Such problems undoubtedly affect surgical precision. This has led to interest in robotic master–slave systems (where the surgeon is the master, i.e. the operator, and the robot is the slave). Such devices have been under trial during the last ten years. They offer many benefits, which have arisen as a result of new technology in lenses, cameras and computer software. The advantages are two-fold: first for the patient (as for laparoscopic surgery, Summary box 7.1) and second for the surgeon. The advantages for the surgeon include better visualisation (higher magnification) with stereoscopic views; elimination of hand tremor allowing greater precision; improved manoeuvring as a result of the 'robotic wrist', which allows seven degrees of freedom; and the fact that large external movements of the surgical hands can be scaled down and transformed to limited internal movements of the 'robotic hands', extending the surgical ability to perform complex technical tasks in a limited space. Also, the surgeon is able to work in an ergonomic environment with less stress and achieve higher levels of concentration. The computer may also be able to compensate for the beating movement of the heart, making it unnecessary to stop the heart during cardiothoracic surgery. There may also be less need for assistance once surgery is under way.

Many surgical specialties have embraced the progression of robot-assisted techniques, including general surgery, cardiothoracic surgery, urology, orthopaedics, ear, nose and throat (ENT) surgery and paediatric surgery. Specialities that use microsurgical techniques will particularly benefit in the future.

There are different robotic systems available (see Figures 7.2, 7.3, 7.4 and 7.5). Robotic camera systems include AESOP (Computer Motion, Goleta, CA, USA) and EndoAssist (Armstrong Healthcare, High Wycombe, UK). Telerobotic manipulators include the da Vinci (Intuitive Surgical, Menlo Park, CA, USA) and ZEUS (Computer Motion) manipulators. Finally, telerobotics and telementoring has been combined in systems such as SOCRATES (Computer Motion). All of these systems offer different advantages to the operating surgeon,

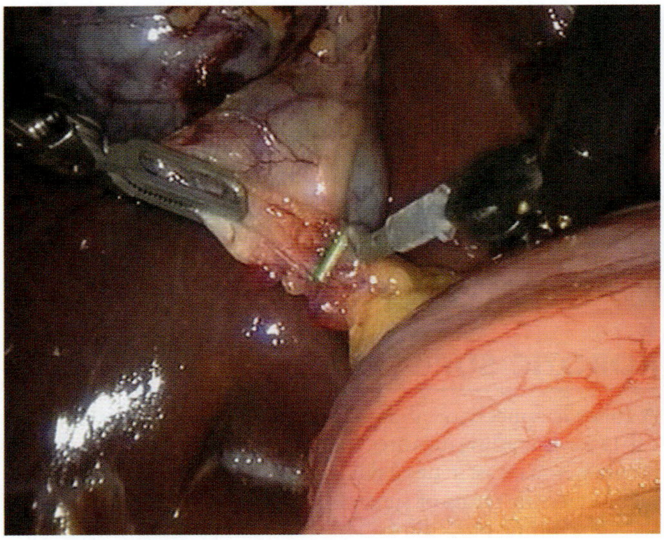

Figure 7.2 da Vinci manipulators used during robotic laparoscopic cholecystectomy. This demonstrates the robotic grasper holding and retracting the gall bladder neck, while the robotic hook is used to free the overlying omentum on the gall bladder and cystic duct (courtesy of the Department of Biosurgery and Surgical Technology, Imperial College, London).

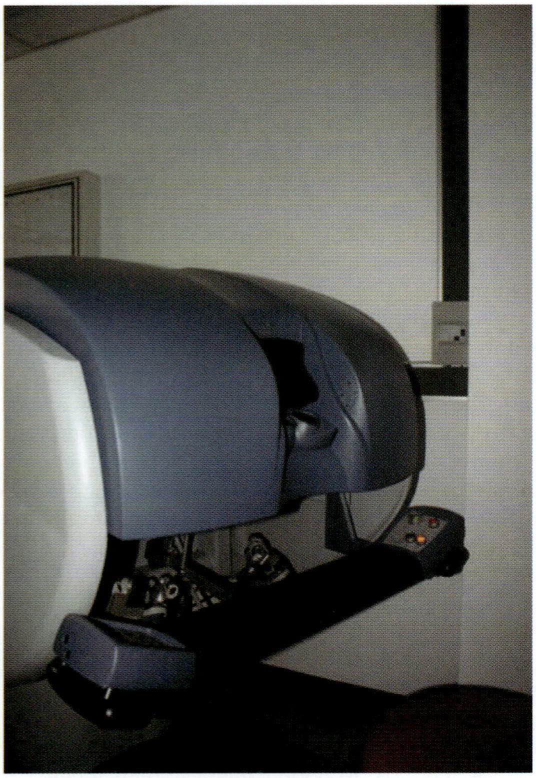

Figure 7.3 da Vinci console (photo courtesy of Daniel Leff).

ranging from reducing the need for assistants and providing better ergonomic operating positions to providing experienced guidance from surgeons not physically present in the operating theatre.

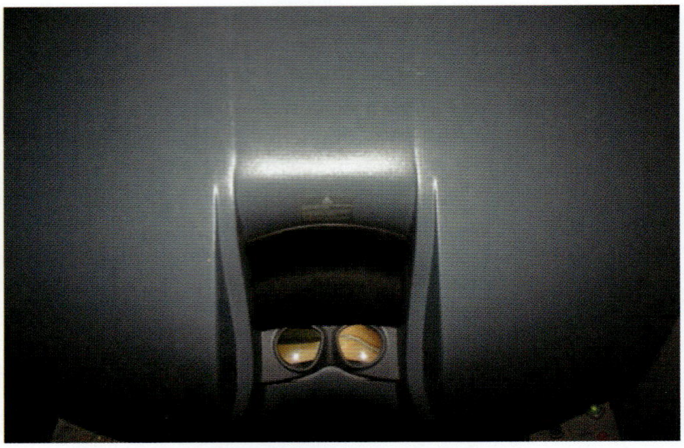

Figure 7.4 da Vinci console, binocular viewer (photo courtesy of Daniel Leff).

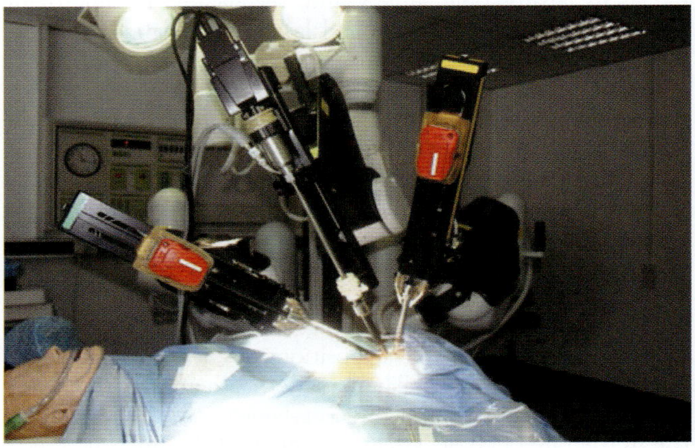

Figure 7.5 Slave unit: da Vinci arms set up in a virtual operating theatre (photo courtesy of Daniel Leff).

PREOPERATIVE EVALUATION

Preparation of the patient

Although the patient may be in hospital for a shorter period, careful preoperative management is essential to minimise morbidity.

History

Patients must be fit for general anaesthesia and open operation if necessary. Potential coagulation disorders (e.g. associated with cirrhosis) are particularly dangerous in laparoscopic surgery. As adhesions may cause problems, previous abdominal operations or peritonitis should be documented.

Examination

Routine preoperative physical examination is required as for any major operation. Although, in general, laparoscopic surgery allows quicker recovery, it may involve longer operating times and the establishment of the pneumoperitoneum may provoke cardiac arrhythmias. Severe chronic obstructive airways disease and ischaemic heart disease may be contraindications to the laparoscopic approach.

Particular attention should be paid to the presence or absence of jaundice, abdominal scars, palpable masses or tenderness.

Moderate obesity does not increase operative difficulty significantly, but massive obesity may make pneumoperitoneum difficult and standard instrumentation may be too short. Access may prove difficult in very thin patients, especially those with severe kyphosis.

Premedication

Premedication is the responsibility of the anaesthetist, with whom coexisting medical problems should be discussed.

Prophylaxis against thromboembolism

Venous stasis induced by the reverse Trendelenburg position during laparoscopic surgery may be a particular risk factor for deep vein thrombosis, as is a lengthy operation and the obesity of many patients. Subcutaneous low molecular weight heparin and antithromboembolic stockings should be used routinely in addition to pneumatic leggings during the operation. Patients already taking warfarin for other reasons should have this stopped temporarily or converted to intravenous heparin, depending on the underlying condition, as it is not safe to perform laparoscopic surgery in the presence of a significant coagulation deficit.

Urinary catheters and nasogastric tubes

In the early days of laparoscopic surgery, routine bladder catheterisation and nasogastric intubation were advised. Most surgeons now omit these, but it remains essential to check that the patient is fasted and has recently emptied the bladder, particularly before the blind insertion of a Verres needle. However, currently, most general surgeons prefer the direct cut-down technique into the abdomen for the introduction of the first port for the establishment of the pneumoperitoneum (Hasson technique). More recently, direct optical entry has been used especially in the setting of bariatric surgery.

Informed consent

The basis of many complaints and much litigation in surgery, especially laparoscopic surgery, relates to the issue of informed consent. It is essential that the patient understands the nature of the procedure, the risks involved and, when appropriate, the alternatives that are available. A locally prepared explanatory booklet concerning the laparoscopic procedure to be undertaken is extremely useful.

In an elective case, a full discussion of the proposed operation should take place in the outpatient department with a surgeon of appropriate seniority, preferably the operating surgeon, before the decision is made to operate. On admission, it is the responsibility of the operating surgeon and anaesthetist to ensure that the patient has been fully counselled, although the actual witnessing of the consent form may have been delegated. The patient should understand what laparoscopic surgery involves and that there is a risk of conversion to open operation. If known, this risk should be quantified, for example the increased risk with acute cholecystitis or in the presence of extensive upper abdominal adhesions. The conversion rate will also vary with the experience and practice of the surgeon. Common complications should be mentioned, such as shoulder tip pain and minor surgical emphysema, as well as rare but serious complications, including injury to the bile ducts and visceral injury from trocar insertion or diathermy.

A few patients may insist on having an open procedure (probably influenced by accounts of mishaps) and the surgeon should be prepared to offer this, although most will opt for laparoscopy if the surgeon has extensive experience and an impressive safety record.

When obtaining consent for robotic surgery, patients should be offered appropriate literature so that they are able to provide fully informed consent. As these procedures are still not routine, this should be carried out by the operating surgeon and, if the procedure is in the context of a clinical trial, the appropriate ethical approval and subsequent paperwork should be available to the patient before signing the consent form (Summary box 7.3).

Summary box 7.3

Preparation for laparoscopic or robotic surgery

- Overall fitness: cardiac arrhythmia, emphysema, medications, allergies
- Previous surgery: scars, adhesions
- Body habitus: obesity, skeletal deformity
- Normal coagulation
- Thromboprophylaxis
- Informed consent

Preparation is very similar to that for open surgery and aims to ensure that:

- The patient is fit for the procedure.
- The patient is fully informed and has consented.
- Operative difficulty is predicted when possible.
- Appropriate theatre time and facilities are available (especially important for robotic cases).

THEATRE SET UP AND TOOLS

Operating theatre design, construction and layout is key to its smooth running on a daily basis. Originally, the video and diathermy equipment and other key tools used in laparoscopic surgery were moved around on stacks, taking up valuable floor space and cluttering up the theatre environment, which was not always ergonomic for the operating team. New theatres are designed with moveable booms that come down from the ceiling; these are easy to place and do not have long leads or wires trailing behind them (Figure 7.6). The equipment consists of at least two high-resolution LCD monitors (and, more recently, high definition (HD) monitors for even clearer images), the laparoscopic kit for maintaining pneumoperitoneum and the audiovisual kit. The advent of DVD and other digital recording equipment has also led to these being incorporated into the rigs so that cases can be recorded with ease. This is further facilitated by cameras being inserted into the light handles of the main overhead lights so that open surgery can also be recorded without distracting the surgeons.

Image quality is vital to the success of laparoscopic surgery. New camera and lens technology allows the use of smaller cameras. Many centres now use 5-mm laparoscopes routinely. Automatic focusing and charge-coupled devices (CCDs) are used to detect different levels of brightness and adjust for the best image possible. Flat panel monitors with HD images are used to give the surgeon the best views possible and three-dimensional technology is now starting to be used for visualisation more

Janos Verres, 1903–1979, chest physician and chief of the Department of Internal Medicine, The Regional Hospital, Kapuvar, Hungary.
Harrith Hasson, Professor of Gynaecology, Chicago, IL, USA.

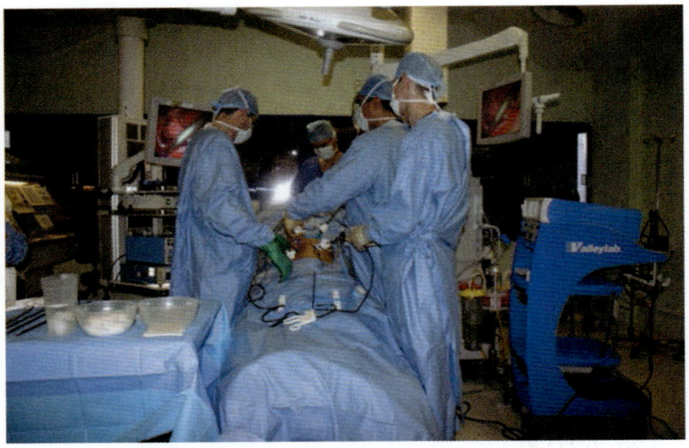

Figure 7.6 Modern laparoscopic theatre set up (photo courtesy of Daniel Leff).

routinely in some centres. The usability of the kit has also improved; touch screen panels and even voice-activated systems are now available on the market.

As minimally invasive and robotic procedures have become routine in some institutions, the dedicated theatre team for such procedures has also evolved. Surgeons and anaesthetists, as well as scrub and circulating nurses, have become familiar with working with the equipment and each other. The efficient working of the team is crucial to high-quality surgery and quick yet safe turnover times. Laparoscopic tools have also changed. Disposable equipment is more readily available, which does unfortunately increase the cost of the surgery. However, easy to use, ergonomically designed and reliable surgical tools are essential for laparoscopic and robotic surgery. Simple designs for new laparoscopic ports are now being studied, with the aim of reducing the incidence of port-site hernias; see-through (optical) ports that allow the surgeon to cut down through the abdomen while observing the layers through the cameras, and new light sources within the abdomen may be simple ideas that affect surgical technique in the near future.

GENERAL INTRAOPERATIVE PRINCIPLES

Laparoscopic cholecystectomy is now the 'gold standard' for operative treatment of symptomatic gallstone disease. The main negative aspect of the technique is the increased incidence of bile duct injury compared with open cholecystectomy. Better understanding of the mechanisms of injury, coupled with proper training, will avoid most of these errors. The following sections highlight the important technical steps that should be taken during any form of laparoscopic surgery to avoid complications.

Creating a pneumoperitoneum

There are two methods for creation of a pneumoperitoneum: open and closed. The closed method involves blind puncture using a Verres needle. Although this method is fast and relatively safe, there is a small but significant potential for intestinal or vascular injury on introduction of the needle or first trocar. The routine use of the open technique for creating a pneumoperitoneum avoids the morbidity related to a blind puncture. To achieve this, a 1-cm vertical or transverse incision is made at the level of the umbilicus. Two small retractors are used to dissect bluntly the subcutaneous fat and expose the midline fascia. Two sutures are inserted each side of the midline incision, followed by the creation of a 1-cm opening in the fascia. Free penetration into the abdominal cavity is confirmed by the gentle introduction of a finger. Finally, a Hasson trocar (or other blunt-tip trocar) is inserted and anchored with the fascial sutures (Figure 7.7). The open technique may initially appear time-consuming and even cumbersome; however, with practice, it is quick, efficient and safe overall. Optical entry to the abdomen under direct vision using optical ports (especially in bariatric surgery) is gaining favour with many laparoscopic surgeons. This allows quick and safe entry to the peritoneal cavity using bladeless see-through trocars that allow the different layer to be dissected through using the laparoscope within an optical port to be inserted into the abdomen.

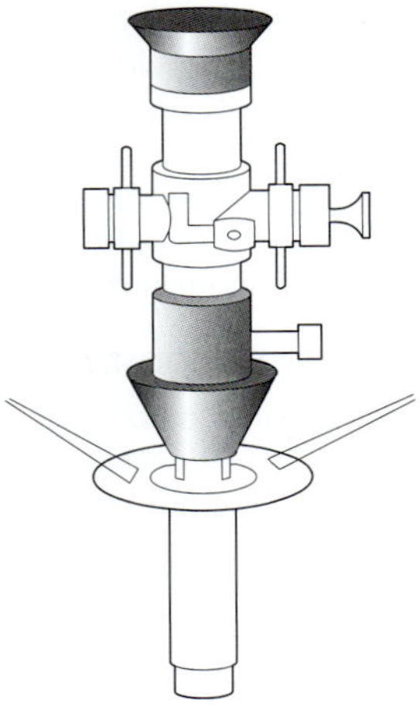

Figure 7.7 Open technique with Hasson port. Apply safe principles of closed technique.

Preoperative problems

Previous abdominal surgery

Previous abdominal surgery is no longer a contraindication to laparoscopic surgery, but preoperative evaluation is necessary to assess the type and location of surgical scars. As mentioned earlier, the open technique for insertion of the first trocar is safer. Before trocar insertion, the introduction of a fingertip helps to ascertain penetration into the peritoneal cavity and also allows adhesions to be gently removed from the entry site. After the tip of the cannula has been introduced, a laparoscope is used as a blunt dissector to tease adhesions gently away and form a tunnel towards the quadrant where the operation is to take place. This step is accomplished by a careful pushing and twisting motion under direct vision. With experience, the surgeon learns to differentiate visually between thick adhesions that may contain bowel and should be avoided and thin adhesions that would lead to a window into a free area of the peritoneal cavity (Figure 7.8).

Obesity

Laparoscopic and robotic surgery have proved to be safe and effective procedures in the obese population. In fact, some procedures are less difficult than their open counterparts for the

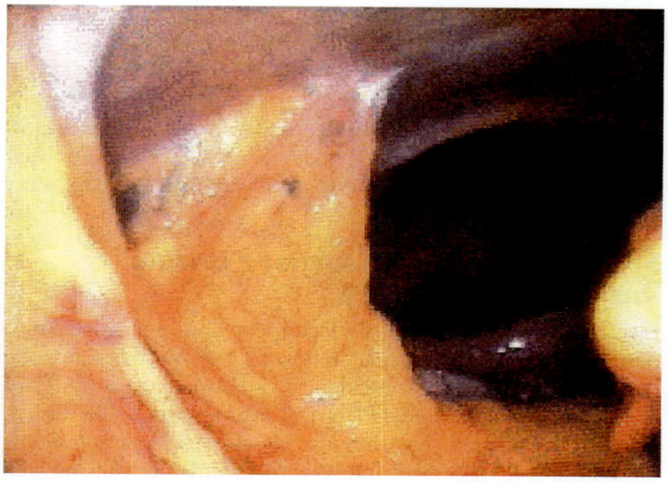

Figure 7.8 Intra-abdominal adhesion.

morbidly obese patient, e.g. in bariatic surgery. Technical difficulties occur, however, in obtaining pneumoperitoneum, reaching the operative region adequately and achieving adequate exposure in the presence of an obese colon. Increased thickness of the subcutaneous fat makes insufflation of the abdominal cavity more difficult. With the closed technique, a larger Verres needle is often required for morbidly obese patients. Pulling the skin up for fixation of the soft tissues is better accomplished with towel clamps. Only moderate force should be used to avoid separating the skin farther away from the fascia. The needle should be passed at nearly a right angle to the skin and preferably above the umbilicus where the peritoneum is more firmly fixed to the midline. The open technique of inserting a Hasson trocar is easier and safer for obese patients, but technically demanding in morbidly obese patients, where optical entry is now more commonplace. The main difficulty is reaching the fascia. A larger skin incision (1–3 cm), starting at the umbilicus and extending superiorly, may facilitate this. To reach the operative area adequately, the location of some of the ports has to be modified and, in some instances, larger and longer instruments are necessary. When the length of the laparoscope appears to be insufficient to reach the operative area adequately, the initial midline port should be placed nearer to the operative field. Recently, the use of optical port entry for laparoscopic bariatric surgery has revolutionised port entry for morbid obesity cases.

Operative problems

Intraoperative perforation of the gall bladder

Perforation of the gall bladder is more common with the laparoscopic technique than with the open technique (see also Chapter 67). Some authors have reported an incidence of up to 30 per cent, but it does not appear to be a factor in increasing the early postoperative morbidity. However, it is well known that bile is not a sterile fluid and bacteria can be present in the absence of cholecystitis. Unless the perforation is small, closure with endoloops or endoclips should be attempted to avoid contamination prior to extraction which should be with the use of an endobag. If there is stone spillage, every attempt must be made to collect and extract the stones and if there is a possibility of stones retained in the peritoneum, then an ultrasound should be arranged 6 weeks postoperatively to assess a collection around a stone and the patient should be informed of this outcome postoperatively.

Bleeding

In some of the larger series, bleeding has been the most common cause for conversion to an open procedure. Bleeding plays a more important role in laparoscopic surgery because of factors inherent to the technique. These include a limited field that can easily be obscured by relatively small amounts of blood, magnification that makes small arterial bleeding appear to be a significant haemorrhage and light absorption that obscures the visual field.

How to avoid bleeding

As in any surgical procedure the best way to handle intraoperative bleeding is to prevent it from happening. This can usually be accomplished by identifying patients at high risk of bleeding, having a clear understanding of the laparoscopic anatomy and employing careful surgical technique.

Risk factors that predispose to increased bleeding include:

- cirrhosis;
- inflammatory conditions (acute cholecystitis, diverticulitis);
- patients on clopidogrel and or dipyridamole
- coagulation defects: these are contraindications to a laparoscopic procedure.

Bleeding from a major vessel

Damage to a large vessel requires immediate assessment of the magnitude and type of bleeding. When the bleeding vessel is identified, a fine-tip grasper can be used to grasp it and apply either electrocautery or a clip, depending on its size. When the vessel is not identified early and a pool of blood forms, compression should be applied immediately with a blunt instrument, a cotton swab (ENT or mastoid swab) or with the adjacent organ. Good suction and irrigation are of utmost importance. Once the area has been cleaned, pressure should be released gradually to identify the site of bleeding. Insertion of an extra port may be required to achieve adequate exposure and at the same time to enable the concomitant use of a suction device and an insulated grasper. Although most of the bleeding vessels can be controlled laparoscopically, judgement should be used in deciding when not to prolong bleeding, but to convert to an open procedure at an early stage. Surgicell or other clot-promoting strips, or tissue glues may also be used laparoscopically to aid haemostasis. If at any stage bleeding is difficult to stem laparoscopically, then there should be no delay to convert to open in the interests of patient safety.

Bleeding from the gall bladder bed

Bleeding from the gall bladder bed can usually be prevented by performing the dissection in the correct plane. When a bleeding site appears during detachment of the gall bladder, the dissection should be carried a little farther to adequately expose the bleeding point. Once this step has been performed, direct application of electrocautery usually controls the bleeding. If bleeding persists, indirect application of electrocautery is useful because it avoids detachment of the formed crust. This procedure is accomplished by applying pressure to the bleeding point with a blunt, insulated grasper and then applying electrocoagulation by touching this grasper with a second insulated grasper that is connected to the electrocautery device. One must be careful to keep all conducting surfaces of the graspers within the visual field while applying the electrocautery current.

Bleeding from a trocar site

Bleeding from the trocar sites is usually controlled by applying upwards and lateral pressure with the trocar itself. Considerable bleeding may occur if the falciform ligament is impaled with the substernal trocar or if one of the epigastric vessels is injured. If significant continuous bleeding from the falciform ligament occurs, haemostasis is achieved by percutaneously inserting a large, straight needle at one side of the ligament. A monofilament suture attached to the needle is passed into the abdominal cavity and the needle is exited at the other side of the ligament using a grasper (Figure 7.9). The loop is suspended and compression is achieved. Maintaining compression throughout the procedure usually suffices. After the procedure has been completed, the loop is removed under direct laparoscopic visualisation to ensure complete haemostasis. When significant continuous bleeding from the abdominal wall occurs, haemostasis can be accomplished either by pressure or by suturing the bleeding site. Pressure can be applied using a Foley balloon catheter. The catheter is introduced into the abdominal cavity through the bleeding trocar site wound, the balloon is inflated and traction is placed on the catheter, which is bolstered in place to keep it under tension. The catheter is left *in situ* for 24 hours and then removed. Although this method is successful in achieving haemostasis, the authors favour direct suturing of the bleeding vessel. This manoeuvre is accomplished by extending the skin incision by 3 mm at both ends of the bleeding trocar site wound. Two figure-of-eight sutures are placed in the path of the vessel at both ends of the wound. Devices such as the EndoClose may also be used to apply transabdominal sutures under direct laparoscopic view to close port sites that bleed.

Evacuation of blood clots

The best way of dealing with blood clots is to avoid them. As mentioned, careful dissection and identification of the cystic artery and its branches, as well as identifying and carrying out dissection of the gall bladder in the correct plane, help to prevent bleeding from the cystic vessels and the hepatic bed. Nevertheless, clot formation takes place when unsuspected bleeding occurs or when inflammation is severe and a clear plane is not present between the gall bladder and the hepatic bed. The routine use of 5000–7000 units of heparin per litre of irrigation fluid helps to avoid the formation of clots. When extra bleeding is foreseen, a small pool of irrigation fluid can be kept in the operative field to prevent clot formation. After clots have formed, a large bore suction device should be used for their retrieval. Care should be taken to avoid suctioning in proximity to placed clips.

Principles of electrosurgery during laparoscopic surgery

Electrosurgical injuries during laparoscopy are potentially serious. The vast majority occur following the use of monopolar diathermy. The overall incidence is between one and two cases per 1000 operations. Electrical injuries are usually unrecognised at the time that they occur, with patients commonly presenting 3–7 days after injury with complaints of fever and abdominal pain. As these injuries usually present late, the reasons for their occurrence are largely speculative. The main theories are: (1) inadvertent touching or grasping of tissue during current application; (2) direct coupling between a portion of bowel and a metal instrument that is touching the activated probe (Figure 7.10); (3) insulation breaks in the electrodes; (4) direct sparking to bowel from the diathermy probe; and (5) current passage to the bowel from recently coagulated, electrically isolated tissue. Bipolar diathermy is safer and should be used in preference to monopolar diathermy, especially in anatomically crowded areas. If monopolar diathermy is to be used, important safety measures include attainment of a perfect visual image, avoiding excessive current application and meticulous attention to insulation. Alternative methods of performing dissection, such as the use of ultrasonic devices, may improve safety.

Postoperative care

The postoperative care of patients after laparoscopic surgery is generally straightforward with a low incidence of pain or other problems. The most common routine postoperative symptoms are a dull upper abdominal pain, nausea and pain around the shoulders (referred from the diaphragm). There has been some suggestion that the instillation of local anaesthetic to the operating site and into the suprahepatic space, or even leaving 1 litre of normal

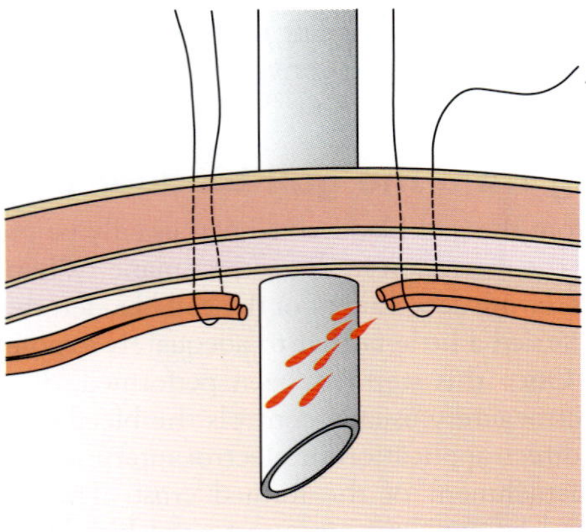

Figure 7.9 Port-side bleeding controlled with sutures.

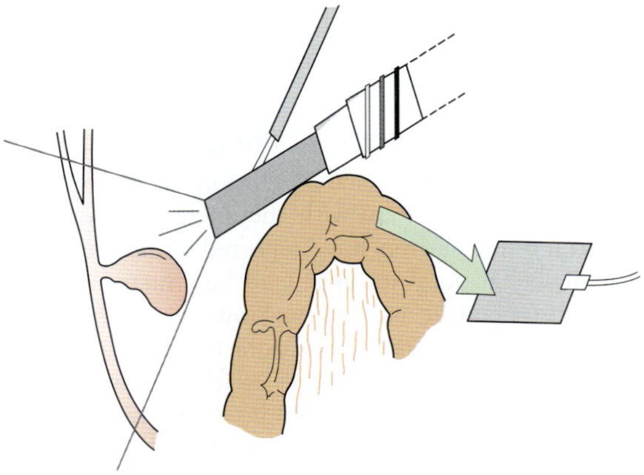

Figure 7.10 Direct coupling between bowel and laparoscope, which is touching the activated probe.

Frederic Eugene Basil Foley, 1891–1966, urologist, Ankher Hospital, St Paul, MN, USA.

saline in the peritoneum, serves to further decrease postoperative pain. It is a good general rule that if the patient develops a fever or tachycardia or complains of severe pain at the operation site, something is wrong and close observation is necessary. In this case, routine investigation should include a full blood count, C reactive protein (CRP) measurement, liver function tests, an amylase test and, probably, an ultrasound scan of the upper abdomen to detect fluid collections. If bile duct leakage is suspected, endoscopic retrograde cholangiopancreatography (ERCP) may be needed. If in doubt, relaparoscopy or laparotomy should be performed earlier rather than later. Death following technical errors in laparoscopic cholecystectomy has often been associated with a long delay in deciding to re-explore the abdomen.

In the absence of problems, patients should be fit for discharge within 24 hours. They should be given instructions to telephone the unit or their general practitioner and to return to the hospital if they are not making satisfactory progress.

Nausea

About half of patients experience some degree of nausea after laparoscopic surgery and rarely this is severe. It usually responds to an antiemetic, such as ondansetron, and settles within 12–24 hours. It is made worse by opiate analgesics and these should be avoided.

Shoulder tip pain

The patient should be warned about this preoperatively and told that the pain is referred from the diaphragm and not due to a local problem in the shoulders. It can be at its worst 24 hours after the operation. It usually settles within 2–3 days and is relieved by simple analgesics, such as paracetamol.

Abdominal pain

Pain in one or other of the port site wounds is not uncommon and is worse if there is haematoma formation. It usually settles very rapidly. Increasing pain after 2–3 days may be a sign of infection and, with concomitant signs, antibiotic therapy is occasionally required. Occasionally, herniation through a port may account for localised pain and this can sometimes be due to a Richter's hernia, such that the patient exhibits no sign of intestinal obstruction. Successful laparoscopic surgery should not cause the patients increasing or undue pain. If there are any clinical concerns postoperatively due to worsening pain, tachycardia and or pyrexia, senior review with a view to imaging, or increasingly commonly relaparoscopy, should be considered.

Analgesia

A 100-mg diclofenac suppository may be given at the time of the operation. It is important that the patient provides separate consent for this if the suppository is to be administered peroperatively. Suppositories may be administered a further two or three times postoperatively for relief of more severe pain. Otherwise, 500–1000 mg of paracetamol 4-hourly usually suffices (orally or if more pain, intravenously). Opiate analgesics cause nausea and should be avoided unless the pain is very severe. In this case, suspect a postoperative complication (as above). The majority of patients require between one and four doses of 1 g of paracetamol postoperatively. Severe pain after routine laparoscopic cases, should warn the clinician that there may be an iatrogenic or surgical cause of this pain that may need further investigation with blood tests, imaging and even relaparoscopy.

Orogastric tube

An orogastric tube may be placed during the operation if the stomach is distended and obscuring the view. It is not necessary in all cases. It should be removed as soon as the operation is over and before the patient regains consciousness. This is more routinely used in bariatrics and oesophagogastric surgery, where a larger, 32F or 34F tube is used.

Oral fluids

There is no significant ileus after laparoscopic surgery, except in resectional procedures, such as colectomy or small bowel resection. Patients can start taking oral fluids as soon as they are conscious; they usually do so 4–6 hours after the end of the operation.

Oral feeding

Provided that the patient has an appetite, a light meal can be taken 4–6 hours after the operation. Some patients remain slightly nauseated at this stage, but almost all eat a normal breakfast on the morning after the operation.

Patients will require advice about what they can eat at home. They should be told that they can eat a normal diet but should avoid excess. It seems sensible to avoid high-fat meals for the first week, although there is no clear evidence that this is necessary.

Urinary catheter

If a urinary catheter has been placed in the bladder during the operation, it should be removed before the patient regains consciousness. The patient should be warned of the possibility and symptoms of postoperative cystitis and told to seek advice in the unlikely event of this occurring.

Drains

Some surgeons drain the abdomen at the end of laparoscopic cholecystectomy, although this is controversial. If a drain is placed to vent the remaining gas and peritoneal fluid, it should be removed within 1 hour of the operation. If it has been placed because of excessive hepatic bleeding or bile leakage it should be removed when that problem has resolved, usually after 12–24 hours. Continued blood loss from a drain is an indication for re-exploration of the abdomen (Summary box 7.4).

Summary box 7.4

Surgical principles

- Meticulous care in the creation of a pneumoperitoneum
- Controlled dissection of adhesions
- Adequate exposure of operative field
- Avoidance and control of bleeding
- Avoidance of organ injury
- Avoidance of diathermy damage
- Vigilance in the postoperative period

DISCHARGE FROM HOSPITAL

Most surgeons discharge a significant proportion of their laparoscopic cholecystectomy patients on the day of surgery, but some are kept in overnight and discharged the following morning. Patients should not be discharged until they are seen to be comfortable, passed urine and eating and drinking satisfactorily. They should be told that if they develop abdominal pain or other severe symptoms then they should return to the hospital or to their general practitioner. Even for more major cases, including procedures such as laparoscopic anterior resection, some units have demonstrated a safe and feasible protocol for a 23-hour stay.

Skin sutures

If non-absorbable sutures or skin staples have been used they can be removed from the port sites after 7 days.

Mobility and convalescence

Patients can get out of bed to go to the toilet as soon as they have recovered from the anaesthetic and they should be encouraged to do so. Such movements are remarkably pain free when compared with the mobility achieved after an open operation. Similarly, patients can cough actively and clear bronchial secretions, and this helps to diminish the incidence of chest infections. Many patients are able to walk out of hospital on the evening of their operation and almost all are fully mobile by the following morning. Thereafter, the postoperative recovery is variable. Some patients prefer to take things quietly for the first 2–3 days, interspersing increasing exercise with rest. After the third day, patients will have undertaken increasing amounts of activity. The average return to work is about 10 days.

THE PRINCIPLES OF COMMON LAPAROSCOPIC PROCEDURES

The principles of common laparoscopic procedures are described in the appropriate chapters:

- laparoscopic cholecystectomy (Chapter 63);
- laparoscopic inguinal hernia repair (Chapter 57);
- laparoscopic antireflux surgery (Chapter 59);
- laparoscopic appendicectomy (Chapter 67).
- laparoscopic bariatric surgery (Chapter 64)
- laparoscopic colectomy/anterior resection (Chapters 69 and 72)
- laparoscopic upper gastrointestinal (GI) surgery (Chapters 62, 63 and 64)

Other elective laparoscopic or minimally invasive procedures that are becoming more widely utilised in certain specialist centres include:

- colectomy;
- gastrectomy
- splenectomy;
- nephrectomy;
- adrenalectomy;
- prostatectomy;
- thyroid and parathyroid surgery;
- aortic aneurysm surgery;
- single-vessel coronary artery bypass surgery;
- video-assisted thorascopic surgery (VATS);
- laparoscopic hernia surgery (inguinal, femoral, paraumbilical, incisional).

Laparoscopy has also been used in certain emergency situations (in stable patients) in the hands of experienced laparoscopic surgeons. These may include diagnostic laparoscopy, repair of a perforated duodenal ulcer, laparoscopic appendicectomy, treatment of intestinal obstruction secondary to adhesions, strangulated hernia repairs and, also, the laparoscopic evaluation of stable trauma patients.

Procedures that have been carried out using robotically assisted minimally invasive surgery include all of those listed above. Currently, robotic surgery still has certain disadvantages:

- increased cost;
- increased set up of the system and operating time;
- socioeconomic implications;
- significant risk of conversion to conventional techniques;
- prolonged learning curve;
- multiple repositioning of the arms can cause trauma;
- haemostasis;
- collision of the robotic arms in extreme positions.

Until these are overcome, by continued development of the technology and the drive of surgeons to progress in the field, robotically assisted surgery will not be commonplace. However, the potential for such systems is immense and continued research and clinical trials will pave the way for future generations of surgeons and patients alike.

FURTHER DEVELOPMENTS THAT HAVE MADE MINIMALLY INVASIVE SURGERY EVEN LESS INVASIVE

Single incision laparoscopic surgery

Laparoscopy has reduced the trauma from surgery compared to open techniques and is now used routinely for benign and oncological surgery in many centres. However, there is continued work on how to reduce the trauma and scarring from the incisions used in laparoscopic surgery as multiple port sites are needed for most procedures. Natural orifice translumenal endoscopic surgery (NOTES) (see below) addresses this but at present, the safety of the transgastric route is not sufficient for the routine use of this approach to surgery. Advanced laparoscopists have therefore turned to focussing on the single incision for open entry via the umbilicus as an alternative. Single incision laparoscopic surgery (SILS) is a technique adopted by some surgeons to insert all the instrumentation via a single incision, through a multiple channel port via the umbilicus to carry out the procedure. The benefit is that only one incision, through a natural scar (the umbilicus), is made therefore these procedures are virtually 'scarless'. Second, less port sites around the abdomen have the potential for less pain, less risk of port site bleeding and reduced incidence of port site hernia. This technique has many other synonyms, including laparoendoscopic single site surgery (LESS) and single port access (SPA) surgery among many others. It does require specially manufactured multichannel ports and often roticulating instruments. There has been an explosion of activity in SILS procedures in the last few years and in some units, laparoscopic cholecystectomies and hernias are routinely started as SILS cases. However, the clinical benefit for this technique which has a difficult and steep learning curve is still awaited from randomised trials being carried out internationally. Non-randomised data have shown understandably better cosmetic outcomes and even less pain in the immediate postoperative period, however, this needs to be further corroborated with randomised data.

Natural orifice translumenal endoscopic surgery

This technique, whereby surgeons enter the peritoneal cavity via endoscopic puncture of a hollow viscus, has been much publicised in recent years. Transvaginal NOTES cholecystectomies have been performed in humans successfully, but most still use hybrid procedures for safety reasons with direct laparoscopic guidance. The closure of the visceral puncture site is the issue that really has prevented widespread uptake of this technique, as transgastric and transcolonic closure of peritoneal entry sites in a routinely safe way is not yet perfected. Also, the equipment needed has significant cost and requires a large number of practitioners in the team at present. Nevertheless, it has much promise to be a technique for truely scarless surgery in the future and much research is being carried out on this field which is less widely adpoted at present compared to SILS.

THE FUTURE

Although there is no doubt that minimal access surgery has changed the practice of surgeons, it has not changed the nature of disease. The basic principles of good surgery still apply, including appropriate case selection, excellent exposure, adequate retraction and a high level of technical expertise. If a procedure makes no sense with conventional access, it will make no sense with a laparoscopic approach. Laparoscopic and robotic surgery training is key to allow the specialty to progress. The pioneers of yesterday have to teach the surgeons of tomorrow not only the technical and dextrous skills required, but also the decision-making and innovative skills necessary for the field to continue to evolve. Training is often perceived as difficult, as trainers have less control over the trainees at the time of surgery and case loads may be smaller, especially in centres where laparoscopic and robotic procedures are not common. However, trainees now rightly expect exposure to these procedures and training systems should be adaptable for international exposure so that these techniques can be disseminated worldwide.

Improvements in instrumentation, the continued progress of robotic surgery and the development of structured training programmes are the key to the future of minimal access surgery. The use of robots in surgery has increased dramatically in the last decade. Indeed, robots are now available not only for assisting in surgery, but also for aiding in the perioperative management of surgical patients. The remote presence systems (In Touch Health, Santa Barbara, CA, USA; Figures 7.11 and 7.12) allow clinicians to assess patients in real time and interact with them while they are not on site or even if in a different continent. Continued advances in related technologies, such as computer science, will allow the incorporation of augmented reality systems alongside robotic systems to enhance surgical precision in image-guided surgery. Endoluminal robotic surgery is in its infancy, but systems are being developed that will enable navigation within the colon to allow surgery on lesions in spaces that are accessible from the outside without an exterior incision being made. The advent of nanotechnology will also bring about much change in surgery. Miniaturisation will be possible, potentially allowing surgery at a cellular level to be carried out.

At present, work has already started on single-port laparoscopy (see above under Single incision laparoscopic surgery), in which a single port may act as a camera and have unfolding instruments open up once they are inside the peritoneum to perform the surgery, therefore reducing the number of port sites needed. Extensive research is also being carried out in the field of NOTES. Minimising the potential contamination of the peritoneum and the ability to carry out a safe closure of the peritoneal entry site are the main technical challenges of this type of minimally invasive and essentially 'scarless' or 'incisionless' surgery.

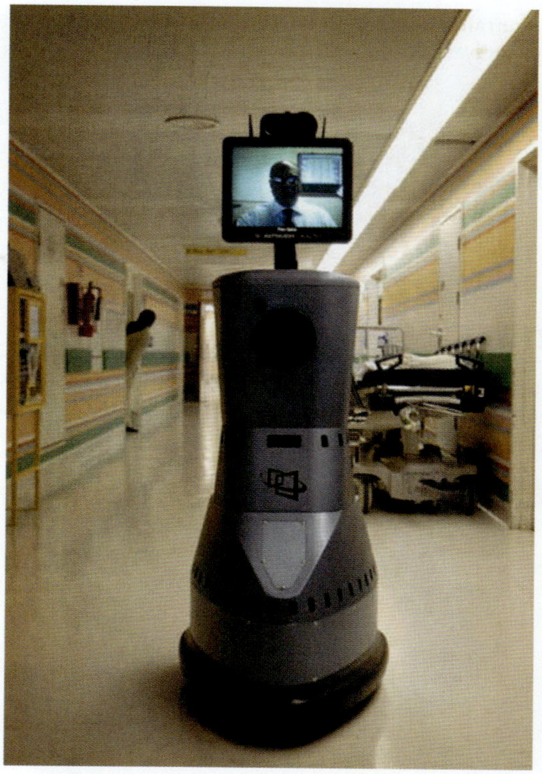

Figure 7.11 Remote presence robot (courtesy of the Department of Biosurgery and Surgical Technology, Imperial College, London).

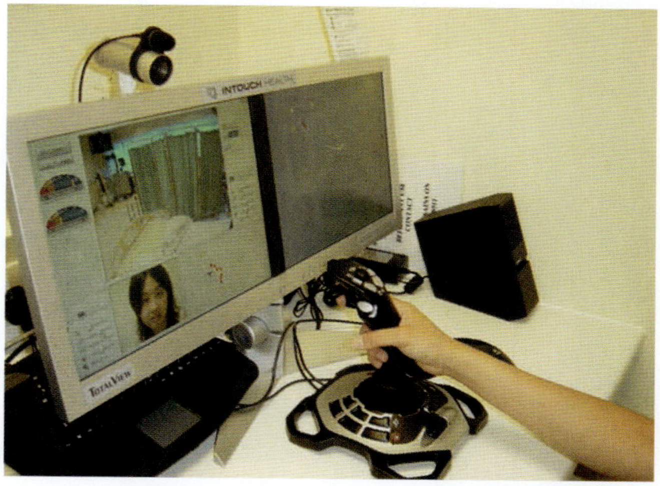

Figure 7.12 Remote presence console (courtesy of the Department of Biosurgery and Surgical Technology, Imperial College, London).

It is certain that there is much that is new in minimal access surgery. Only time will tell how much of what is new is truly better.

The cleaner and gentler the act of operation, the less the patient suffers, the smoother and quicker his convalescence, the more exquisite his healed wound.

Berkeley George Andrew Moynihan (1920)

FURTHER READING

Ballantyne GH, Marescaux J, Giulianotti PC (eds). *Primer of robotic and telerobotic surgery*. Philadelphia, PA: Lippincott Williams & Wilkins, 2004.

Chow AG, Purkayastha S, Zacharakis E, Paraskeva P. Single-incision laparoscopic surgery for right hemicolectomy. *Arch Surg* 2011; **146**: 183–6.

Chow A, Purkayastha S, Aziz O *et al.* Single-incision laparoscopic surgery for cholecystectomy: a retrospective comparison with 4-port laparoscopic cholecystectomy. *Arch Surg* 2010; **145**: 1187–91.

Chow A, Purkayastha S, Paraskeva P. Appendicectomy and cholecystectomy using single-incision laparoscopic surgery (SILS): the first UK experience. *Surg Innov* 2009; **16**: 211–7.

Chow A, Purkayastha S, Aziz O, Paraskeva P. Single-incision laparoscopic surgery for cholecystectomy: an evolving technique. *Surg Endosc* 2010; **24**: 709–14.

Gill IS, Sung GT, Ballantyne GH (eds). Robotics in surgery. *Surg Clin N Am* 2003; **83**: 15–16.

Purkayastha S, Athanasiou T, Casula R, Darzi A. Robotic surgery: a review. *Hosp Med* 2004; **65**: 153–9.

Berkley George Andrew Moynihan (Lord Moynihan of Leeds), 1855–1936, Professor of Clinical Surgery, The University of Leeds, Leeds, UK.

CHAPTER 8

Principles of paediatric surgery

LEARNING OBJECTIVES

To recognize and learn:
- The important differences between adults and children which have clinical implications
- The principles of trauma management in children
- How to safely prescribe perioperative fluids in children
- How to avoid the pitfalls that lead to a missed or delayed diagnosis for common emergency conditions
- A collection of congenital malformations managed by neonatal surgeons that may present later to general surgeons
- The common safeguarding issues in children and know how to proceed if abuse is suspected

INTRODUCTION

Premature and term neonates differ in their anatomy, physiology, neurology, psychology, pathology and pharmacology, just as infants differ from school-age children and adolescents from adults (Table 8.1). These differences underpin the principles of paediatric surgery. A few examples appear in Table 8.2 and in Figure 8.1, but are not exhaustive.

A knowledge of teratology is fundamental to paediatric surgery, but since some anomalies first present to adult services (e.g. duplications, malrotation) this knowledge can occasionally pay dividends to surgeons dealing with adults. Adult surgical services also need to cater for the transitional needs of those graduating to adulthood, sometimes after complex paediatric surgical attention. Generally, children escape the comorbidities of degenerative diseases, but lifestyle problems, such as obesity, drug abuse and sexually transmitted diseases are no longer rare.

We start with three important areas: (1) thermoregulation, (2) airway and (3) fluid management, and then outline trauma, some common problems in older children, a collection of neonatal surgical conditions, oncology and safeguarding children.

Table 8.1 Common terms.

Preterm	<37 completed weeks' gestation
Full term	Between 37 and 42 completed weeks of gestation
Neonate	Newborn baby up to 28 days of age
Infant	Up to 1 year of age
Child	All ages up to 16 years, but often divided into preschool child (usually <5 years), child and adolescent (puberty up to 16 years)

Table 8.2 Some example differences between adults and children.

Facts	Infants and small children have a wide abdomen, a broad costal margin and a shallow pelvis
	The edge of the liver comes below the costal margin and the bladder is largely intra-abdominal
	The ribs are more horizontal and are flexible
	The umbilicus is relatively low lying
Implications	Transverse supraumbilical incisions give greater access than vertical midline ones for open surgery
	Trauma (including surgical access) can easily damage the liver or bladder
	The geometry of the ribs means that ventilation requires greater diaphragmatic movement. Their flexibility means that rib fractures are rare and often a sign of abuse
	A stoma in the lower abdomen of a neonate must be carefully sited for its bag not to interfere with the umbilicus

MAINTAINING TEMPERATURE

In comparison with older children, infants have less subcutaneous fat, immature vasomotor control, greater heat loss from pulmonary evaporation, and their surface area to weight ratio is higher. These need to be considered when managing sick children in the accident and emergency department, anaesthetic room or operating theatre. These environments must be warm

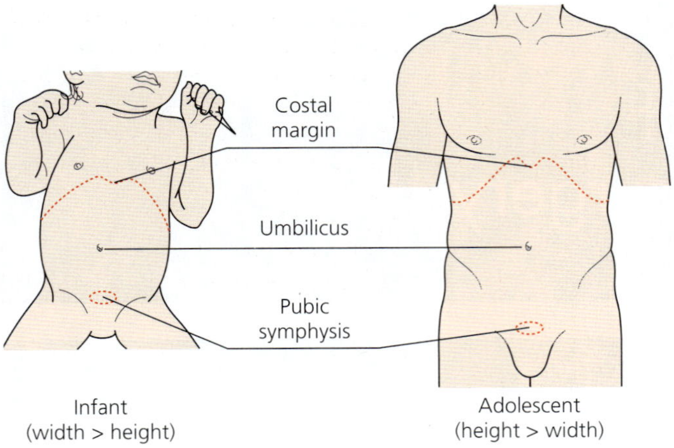

Figure 8.1 Topographical differences in the abdomen.

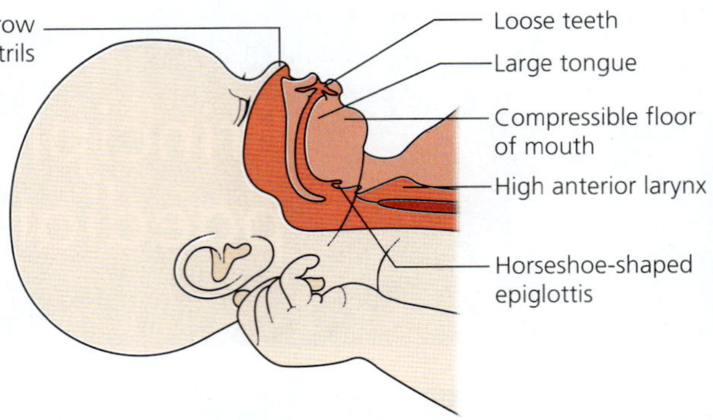

Figure 8.2 Summary of upper airway anatomy in an infant.

and the infant's head (20 per cent of surface area compared with 9 per cent in an adult) should be insulated. Infusions are warmed, and respiratory gases both warmed and humidified. The core temperature is monitored and safe direct warming is needed for lengthy operations.

AIRWAY

There are a number of differences in the airway and these have clinical implications (see Figure 8.2). The infant's large head and short neck predispose to flexion. The large tongue can obstruct the airway when unconscious and impede the airway and laryngoscopy. The epiglottis projects posteriorly and the larynx is high, favouring a straight-bladed laryngoscope in those under one year of age. Uncuffed tubes are preferred as the cricoid ring is the narrowest area (compared with the larynx in an adult) and this is covered in loose epithelium that is easily irritated and damage can result in subglottic stenosis.

PERIOPERATIVE FLUIDS IN CHILDREN

Before prescribing fluids (or drugs), the child's weight must be known, their vital signs and their fluid and electrolyte requirements should be considered in relation to normal values and ranges (see Table 8.3). Dehydration is difficult to assess: moderate dehydration (5 per cent loss of total body water) may manifest in poor urine output, dry mouth, and sunken eyes and fontanelle; severe dehydration (>10 per cent) in decreased skin turgor, drowsiness, tachycardia and poor capillary refill (>2 s) and signs of hypovolaemia.

Children develop hyponatraemic encephalopathy at higher sodium levels than adults because they have a higher brain–skull ratio. A few children have had symptomatic hyponatraemic encephalopathy attributable to poor prescription and monitoring of fluids, some have died and others have permanent neurological disability. Problems have arisen when (1) hypotonic maintenance fluids (e.g. 0.18 per cent saline), have been inappropriately given to resuscitate or replace losses or (2) maintenance fluids have been given in excess (three to five times that required).

Table 8.3 Basic paediatric data.

(a) Weight

Age	Weight (kg)
Term neonate	3.5
1 year	10
5 years	20
10 years	30

(b) Vital signs

Age (years)	Heart rate (bpm)	Systolic blood pressure (mmHg)	Respiratory rate (b/min)
<1	110–160	70–90	30–40
2–5	90–140	80–100	25–30
5–12	80–120	90–110	20–25

(c) Maintenance fluid requirements

Weight	Daily fluid requirement (mL/kg/day)	(mL/kg/hour)
Neonate	120–150	5
Older child:		
First 10 kg	100	4
Second 10 kg	50	2
Each subsequent kg	20	1

(d) Maintenance electrolyte requirements

Weight	Sodium (mmol/kg/day)	Potassium (mmol/kg/day)	Energy (kcal/kg/day)
<10 kg	2–4	1.5–2.5	110
>10 kg	1–2	0.5–1.0	40–75

Approximate guide: weight (kg) = 2 × (age in years +4), or use a Broselow tape which estimates the weight from the height.
Systolic blood pressure = 80 + (age in years × 2) mmHg.
Circulating blood volume = 80 mL/kg (90 mL/kg in infants).

Tonicity and osmolarity

The term 'isotonic' is now considered in relation to the tonicity of the electrolyte components of fluids. Thus, isosmolar fluids such as 0.18 per cent saline with 4 per cent glucose and hyperosmolar fluids such as 0.45 per cent saline with 5 per cent glucose are now considered 'hypotonic' because the glucose is ignored. The National Patient Safety Agency (NPSA) in 2007 instructed that all stocks of 0.18 per cent saline with 4 per cent glucose be removed from non-specialised areas to reduce the risks of hyponatraemia from inappropriate prescription.

Prescribing intravenous fluids

The four reasons for prescribing fluids are detailed in Summary box 8.1. The body's response to stress is to hold on to water and this promotes hyponatraemia. The stresses that drive the non-osmotic retention of water include trauma, head injury, chest infections and the postoperative state. Restricting maintenance fluids to 70 per cent is thus appropriate for 24 hours after major surgery. The liberation of the fluid rate is guided by the results of daily electrolyte levels. Urine output will often be reduced after major surgery, but a common response to this can be to inappropriately increase maintenance fluid. A bolus of fluid is only appropriate if hypovolaemia is evident and needs correction.

In the surgical setting, **hyponatraemia** is usually a consequence of too much free water and **not** insufficient sodium. If mild and asymptomatic (e.g. 130 mmol/L) then fluid restriction is appropriate. If symptomatic with headache, lethargy or seizures and the Na level is <125 mmol/L, a rapid infusion of 4 per cent hypertonic saline is needed and paediatric intensive care unit (PICU) admission.

Summary box 8.1

Fluids in children

Fluids are given intravenously for four reasons:

- Circulatory support in resuscitating vascular collapse. (Given as a bolus of 10 or 20 mL/kg over periods up to 20 minutes with close monitoring of the response. Can be repeated up to 40 mL/kg, then seek urgent help)
  - 0.9 per cent saline
  - Blood
  - 4.5 per cent albumin
  - Colloid
- Replacement of previous fluid and electrolyte deficits. (Given over a longer period up to 48 hours with clinical and biochemical review)
  - 0.9 per cent saline + 0.15 per cent KCl
  - Hartmann's solution
- Replacement of ongoing losses (or a fluid tailored to the losses, e.g. 4.5 per cent albumin if protein loss is great. Replace losses mL for mL)
  - 0.9 per cent saline + 0.15 per cent KCl
  - Hartmann's solution
- Maintenance outside neonatal period (hypotonic 0.18 per cent saline should not be used outside the neonatal period)
  - 0.45 per cent saline + 0.15 per cent KCl in 2.5–5 per cent glucose
  - Hartmann's ± glucose
  - 0.9 per cent saline + 0.15 per cent KCl ± glucose
- Maintenance in the neonate
  - In term neonates in the first 48 hours of life, 10 per cent glucose at 60 mL/kg per day
  - Sodium 0.18 per cent and potassium 0.15 per cent are added on day 2
  - From day 3, around 4–5 mL/kg per hour or 100–120 mL/kg per day
    - Preterm babies or those <2 kg may require 180 mL/kg/day of fluid
  - Consider impaired gluconeogenesis: monitor and keep glucose above 2.6 mmol/L

HISTORY AND EXAMINATION

Time, patience and a genuine interest will help to establish a good rapport with the child and their parents or carers. An opportunistic rather than a systematic approach to the history and examination may be needed, but appropriate areas must be covered. Do not forget to explore perinatal problems and the family and social background. Children should be told what to expect from an examination, investigation or surgical procedure in terms that they can understand. Fear, anxiety and pain can be reduced by involving the parents and by looking after the child in an appropriate environment. General health concerns are best discussed with a paediatrician.

OPERATIVE SURGERY

A well-prepared patient who has not been excessively starved (Summary box 8.2), with appropriate consent, is anaesthetised in a child-friendly anaesthetic room. Surgery demands meticulous and gentle technique, strict haemostasis, fine suture materials and often magnification aids. Basic principles apply: maintaining well-vascularised tissues, avoiding tension, minimising tissue necrosis and contamination. The intestine can be anastomosed with single-layer interrupted extramucosal sutures. Abdominal wounds are closed with absorbable sutures using a layered or a mass closure. Wound dehiscence is rare and usually the result of poor technique. Clean skin incisions are best closed with absorbable subcuticular sutures. Endoscopic minimally invasive approaches can be used at all ages to achieve the same advantages as in adults, but instruments and insufflation pressures must be tailored to the size of the child. Postoperatively, children recover swiftly. Analgesia must be adequate and appropriate, recognising the potential for respiratory depression with opioids. Appropriately trained staff monitor the airway, vital signs, oxygen saturation, fluid balance, temperature, pain control and glucose levels during recovery (Summary box 8.3).

Summary box 8.2

Starvation instructions

- Two hours for clear fluids
- Four hours for breast milk
- Six hours for solids

Summary box 8.3

Surgical technique in children

- Gentle tissue handling
- Abdominal incisions can be closed with absorbable sutures
- Bowel can be anastomosed with interrupted single-layer extramucosal sutures
- Skin can be closed with absorbable subcuticular sutures

Stomas are necessary in some children. A gastrostomy may be required for nutritional support, particularly in the neurologically disabled child. Temporary intestinal stomas are used in the management of anorectal malformations, necrotising enterocolitis and Hirschsprung's disease. Infants with a proximal stoma and high losses frequently require salt or bicarbonate supplements to avoid deficits, which can cause poor weight gain and acidosis.

Surgeons who operate on children should consider the long-term outcomes of surgical disease and its treatment during maturation and adult life. For example, ileal resection in the neonate may later be complicated by vitamin B12 deficiency, malabsorption of fat-soluble vitamins, gallstones, renal oxalate stones and perianastomotic ulceration. Long-term concerns include the impact on continence, fertility, sexual activity, psychosocial adaptation, and the potential risk of late malignancy (e.g. undescended testis, choledochal cyst, duplication cysts).

PAEDIATRIC TRAUMA

Trauma remains a leading cause of death in children and adolescents worldwide. Many of these deaths are avoidable if prompt treatment is given well. Surgeons should attend the Advanced Trauma Life Support (ATLS) programme which covers trauma in children. Some of the important differences for children follow:

- Avoid overextension of the neck which can obstruct the airway.
- Use a Broselow tape if the weight is not known.
- Blood pressure is often normal until >25 per cent of the circulating blood volume is lost.
- Cardiorespiratory arrest is usually due to hypoxia and not vascular disease.
- Diagnostic peritoneal lavage is obsolete in children.

Resuscitation

For information related to fluids, see Summary box 8.1. High-flow oxygen is required if there is cardiorespiratory compromise, and endotracheal intubation and ventilation are required if oxygenation is inadequate or to control a flail chest or in children with a serious head injury (Glasgow Coma Score ≤8). Seriously injured children require two large peripheral intravenous cannulae. The long saphenous at the ankle, femoral, external jugular and, in babies, scalp veins can be used. Central venous access should only be attempted by an expert. Intraosseous infusion however, is straightforward and particularly useful in children (Figure 8.3).

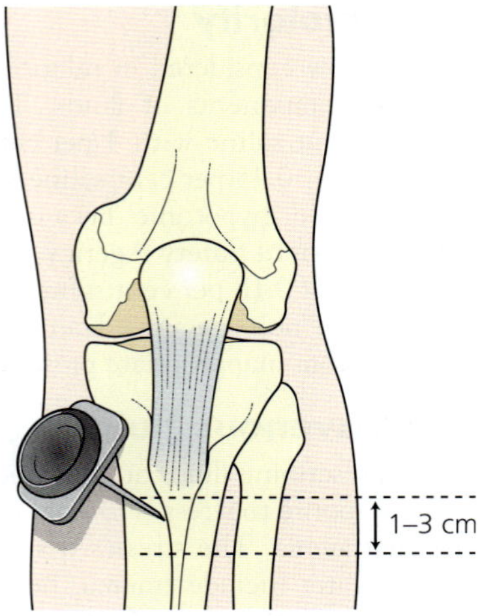

Figure 8.3 The intraosseous needle is inserted into the medullary cavity of the proximal tibia about 1–3 cm below the tibial tuberosity.

A major spinal cord injury can be present in a child without radiographic abnormalities. After major trauma, a cervical spine injury should be assumed and the neck immobilised until cross-sectional imaging 'clears' the spine. Other considerations include intravenous analgesia and, in the unconscious or ventilated child or those with major abdominal injuries, a nasogastric tube (orogastric if suspicion of a basal skull fracture) and a urethral catheter (if no evidence of a urethral injury).

Secondary survey and emergency management

Chest trauma

Children have elastic ribs that rarely fracture but deformation causes lung contusions. A major thoracic injury may exist despite a normal chest radiograph. The airway is secured, oxygen is given and hypovolaemia is corrected. A tension pneumothorax should be suspected clinically before the chest x-ray is requested and immediate needle thoracocentesis (second intercostal space, mid-clavicular line) performed. A chest drain is then placed (fifth intercostal space, mid-axillary line). Massive haemothorax needs a chest drain. Cardiac tamponade may follow blunt or penetrating injury and requires emergency needle pericardiocentesis. Diaphragmatic rupture after blunt abdominal trauma is detected by chest radiography or computed tomography (CT) scan; surgical repair is undertaken once the patient is stable (Figure 8.4).

Abdomen

Blunt trauma is more common than penetrating trauma. The liver and spleen are more vulnerable in children being less well protected by the rib cage. The abdomen is inspected for patterned bruising from seatbelts (Figure 8.5) or tyres. Compression will have been against the rigid skeleton. Intra-abdominal or intrathoracic bleeding should be considered promptly in the shocked child if external bleeding has not been profuse. Plasma amylase levels may be normal despite pancreatic injury (Figure 8.6).

The **Glasgow Coma Score** was introduced in 1977 by William Bryan Jennet, Professor of Neurosurgery, and Graham Michael Teasdale, a neurosurgeon at the University Department of Neurosurgery at the Institute of Neurological Sciences, The Southern General Hospital, Glasgow, UK. Professor Teasdale was later knighted and became President of the Royal College of Physicians and Surgeons of Glasgow.

PART 1 | PRINCIPLES

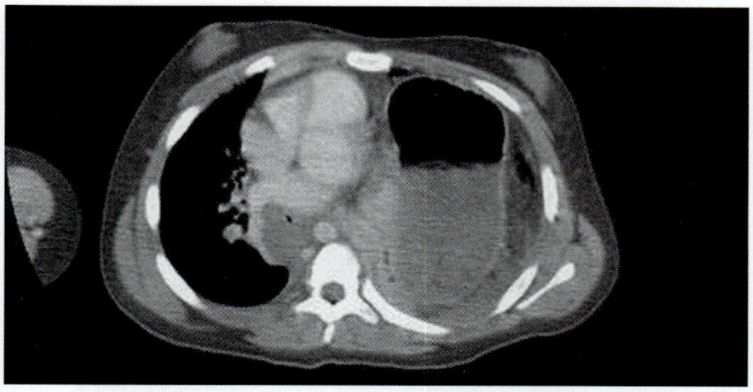

Figure 8.4 Traumatic diaphragmatic rupture.

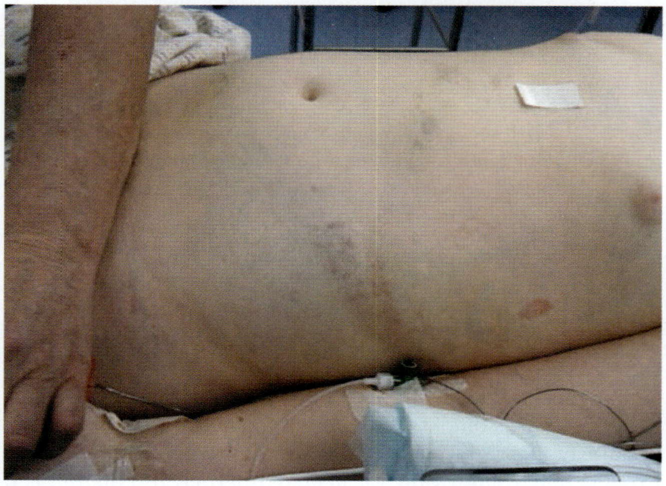

Figure 8.5 Bruises from a lap belt.

Imaging

Focused assessment with sonography for trauma (FAST) looks for fluid in the perihepatic and hepatorenal space, the perisplenic area, the pelvis and the pericardium. It has a role in children but it does not detect solid organ injuries nor replace CT. In the haemodynamically stable child, a CT scan with intravenous contrast is required (Figure 8.7).

Bowel perforation or deep penetrating trauma require a laparoscopy or laparotomy. Isolated blunt splenic and/or liver injuries identified on a CT scan can be safely and effectively managed non-operatively (Summary box 8.4) in the majority of children, so avoiding surgery and the long-term risks of splenectomy.

Summary box 8.4

Requirements for successful non-operative management of isolated blunt liver or spleen trauma

- Haemodynamic stability after resuscitation with no more than 60 mL/kg of fluid
- A good-quality computed tomographic scan
- No evidence of hollow visceral injury
- Close monitoring and the immediate availability of surgical expertise and facilities

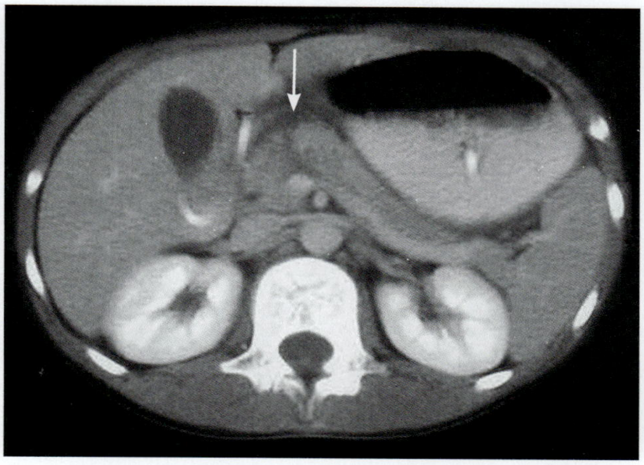

Figure 8.6 Abdominal computed tomographic scan showing a transection through the neck of the pancreas (arrow) from a bicycle handlebar injury.

Ongoing intra-abdominal bleeding requires a laparotomy, though angiography and arterial embolisation can be useful in some. Bile leaks are uncommon and can usually be managed by an interventional radiological technique. Uncomplicated unoperated cases of liver/spleen trauma can be discharged after 5–7, days but activity is restricted for 3–6 weeks and contact sports avoided for between two and three months. Blunt renal trauma can be managed conservatively, but an acutely non-functioning kidney following abdominal trauma may need urgent exploration with a view to revascularisation.

Summary box 8.5

Paediatric trauma

- Use Advanced Trauma Life Support (ATLS) principles
- Overextension of the neck will compromise the airway
- Cervical spine injury can be present without radiographic signs
- Intraosseous vascular access is helpful in small children
- Lung contusion can occur without rib fractures
- Patterned skin bruising suggests underlying organ injury
- In a stable child, abdominal injuries are best assessed by computed tomography
- Isolated liver or splenic injury can usually be managed non-operatively

Patterns of injury

- Lap belts: the small intestine or lumbar spine.
- Bicycle handlebars: pancreatic, duodenal or liver trauma (Figure 8.6).
- Straddle injuries: the urethra and pelvis.
- Run-over injuries: severe crushing of the chest, and/or abdomen and/or pelvis.

The main principles for managing trauma in children appear in Summary box 8.5.

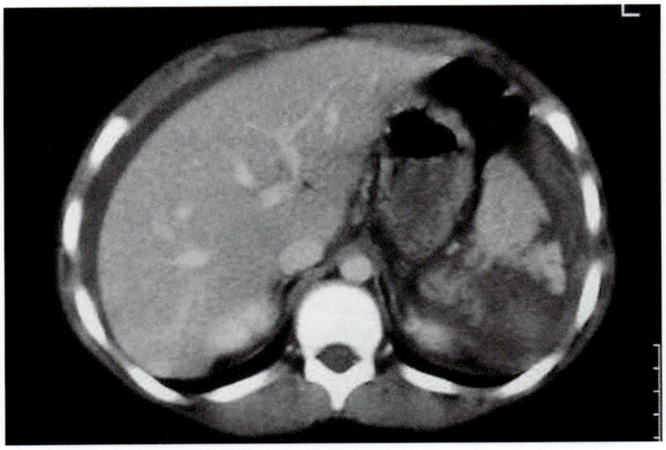

Figure 8.7 Abdominal computed tomographic scan after intravenous contrast in an 11-year-old boy showing a ruptured spleen (successfully managed non-operatively).

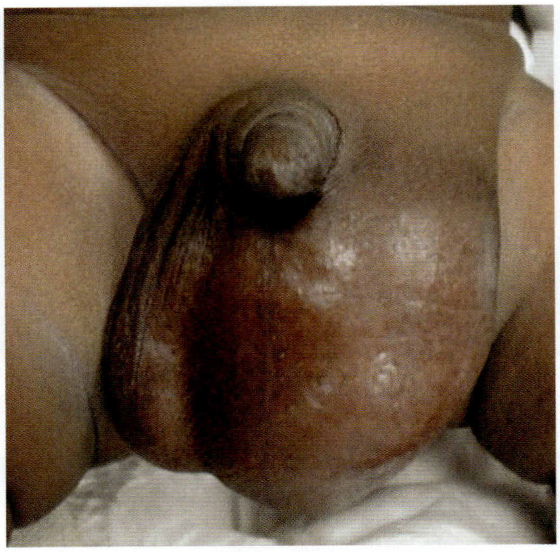

Figure 8.9 A left inguinal swelling. Clinical examination is needed to confidently distinguish a hydrocoele from an inguinal hernia.

COMMON PAEDIATRIC SURGICAL CONDITIONS

Inguinoscrotal disorders

Most genital abnormalities in boys are the result of abnormal development. The testis develops from the urogenital ridge on the posterior abdominal wall. Gonadal induction to form a testis is regulated by genes on the Y chromosome. In the abdominal descent, the testis migrates towards the internal ring, guided by mesenchymal tissue (gubernaculum). Descent into the scrotum is mediated by testosterone from the fetal testis. A tongue of peritoneum precedes the migrating testis through the inguinal canal; this is the processus vaginalis. This peritoneal pouch normally becomes obliterated after birth, but failure to do so leads to the development of an inguinal hernia or hydrocoele (Figure 8.8).

Inguinal hernias

Inguinal hernias in children are almost always indirect and due to a patent processus vaginalis. They are more frequent in boys, especially if premature. An inguinal hernia will develop in at least one in 50 boys and about 15 per cent are bilateral. Rarely, bilateral inguinal hernias in a phenotypic girl may be the presenting feature of androgen insensitivity syndrome (testicular feminisation) and the hernia sac may then contain a testis.

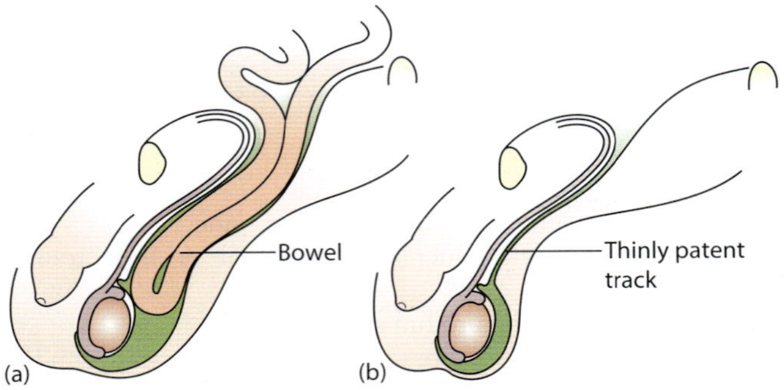

Figure 8.8 (a) Inguinal hernia and (b) hydrocoele in children are the result of incomplete obliteration of the processus vaginalis.

An inguinal hernia typically causes an intermittent swelling in the groin or scrotum on crying or straining (Figure 8.9). Unless an inguinal swelling is observed, the diagnosis relies on the history and the presence of palpable thickening of the spermatic cord (or round ligament in girls). Some inguinal hernias present as a firm, tender, irreducible lump in the groin or scrotum because of incarceration at the external ring. The infant may be irritable and vomit. Most incarcerated hernias in children can be successfully reduced by sustained gentle compression ('taxis') aided by cautious analgesia. Repair is delayed for 24 hours to let the oedema settle. If truly irreducible, emergency surgery is required because of the risk of vascular compromise to the bowel, ovary or testis.

Inguinal herniotomy is performed via an inguinal skin crease incision, opening Scarpa's fascia and then the external oblique. The cremaster is cut and, through an initially small opening, the cord grasped and gently delivered. The vas and vessels are separated from the sac which is then divided and proximally ligated. Outside the neonatal period, inguinal herniotomy is treated as day-case surgery (Summary box 8.6).

Summary box 8.6

Inguinal hernias

- More common in premature boys
- 15 per cent bilateral
- Indirect with a patent processus vaginalis
- Groin lump that appears on straining or crying
- Incarcerated inguinal hernias can usually be reduced with gentle pressure
- In infants, they can transilluminate like a hydrocoele making the test redundant when the distinction is difficult
- If reduction is impossible, emergency surgery is needed
- Infants need repair promptly to prevent the risk of strangulation
- The hernial sac is isolated, ligated and divided

Hydrocoeles

A patent processus vaginalis may allow only peritoneal fluid to track down around the testis to form a hydrocoele. Hydrocoeles are unilateral or bilateral, asymptomatic, non-tender scrotal swellings. They may be tense or lax, but typically transilluminate. The majority resolve spontaneously as the processus continues to obliterate, but surgical ligation is recommended in boys older than three years of age.

Undescended testes are palpable or impalpable

At birth, about 4 per cent of full-term boys have unilateral or bilateral undescended testes, but by one year of age it is <1 per cent and it changes little thereafter. The incidence is higher in preterm infants because the testis descends through the inguinal canal during the third trimester. A normal testis reaches the base of the scrotum with a good length of cord above it. Testes cannot be palpated in the inguinal canal, but can be milked from there into the superficial pouch (**palpable undescended testis**) or in to the scrotum with a good length of cord (normal). A **retractile testis** can be manipulated into the base of the scrotum without tension, but is pulled up by the cremaster muscle. With time, retractile testes reside permanently in the scrotum; however, follow up is advisable as, rarely, the testis ascends into the inguinal canal. The **ascending testis** needs an orchidopexy. An **ectopic** testis lies outside its normal line of descent, often in the perineum (Summary box 8.7).

Summary box 8.7

The undescended testis

- A retractile testis reaches the base of the scrotum, but retracts
- An undescended testis may be palpable or impalpable
- An ectopic testis lies outside the normal line of descent
- Palpable undescended testes undergo a single stage orchidopexy
- Impalpable undescended testes usually require a two stage orchidopexy
- Orchidopexy around one year of age improves fertility and may reduce the risk of malignancy

A palpable undescended testis should undergo a day-case orchidopexy around one year of age. The testis is mobilised through an inguinal incision, preserving the vas deferens and testicular vessels. The associated patent processus vaginalis is ligated and divided, and the testis is placed in a subdartos scrotal pouch.

Impalpable undescended testes are either absent or located in the abdomen or inguinal canal. There is no benefit from imaging and these are best managed with a laparoscopy (Figure 8.10) and usually a staged approach.

The benefits of orchidopexy include:

- **Fertility**. To optimise spermatogenesis, the testis needs to be in the scrotum below body temperature at a young age. Orchidopexy around one year of age is currently recommended. Fertility after orchidopexy for a unilateral undescended testis is near normal. Men with a history of bilateral intra-abdominal testes are often infertile.
- **Malignancy**. Undescended testes are histologically abnormal and at an increased risk of malignancy. The greatest risk is for bilateral intra-abdominal testes. Early orchidopexy for a unilateral undescended testis may reduce the risk, but this is not proven.
- **Cosmetic and psychological**. In an older boy, a prosthetic testis can be inserted to replace an absent one.

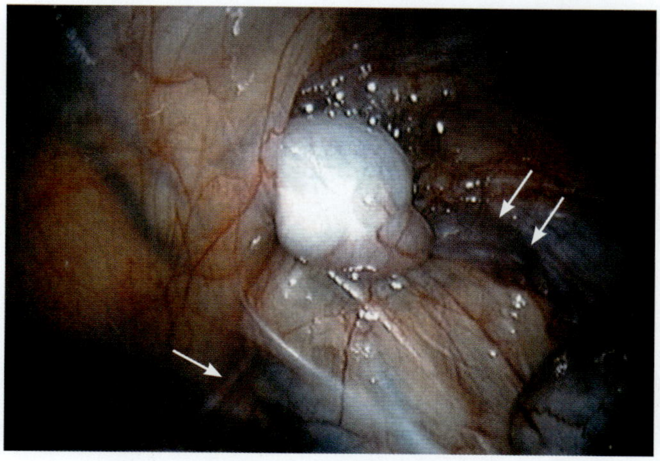

Figure 8.10 Laparoscopic view of a right-sided intra-abdominal testis visible at the internal ring. Vas (single arrow) and testicular vessels (double arrow).

The acute scrotum

Testicular torsion is most common in adolescents, but may occur at any age, including in the perinatal period. The pain is not always scrotal and may be felt in the groin or lower abdomen. Oedema and erythema of the scrotal skin can be absent. Sometimes there is a history of previous transient episodes. Torsion of the testis must be relieved within 6–8 hours of the onset of symptoms for there to be a good chance of testicular salvage. At operation, viability of the testis is assessed after derotation. If salvageable, three-point fixation of both testes with non-absorbable sutures is performed. Expert assessment of testicular blood flow by colour Doppler ultrasound may help in the differential diagnosis, but the scrotum must be explored urgently if torsion cannot be excluded.

Torsion of a testicular or epididymal appendage characteristically affects boys just before puberty (Figure 8.11), possibly because of enlargement of the hydatid in response to gonadotrophins. A hydatid of Morgagni is an embryological remnant found on the upper pole of the testis or epididymis. The pain often increases over a day or two. Occasionally, the torted hydatid can be felt or seen (blue dot sign). Excision of the appendage leads to rapid resolution of symptoms. Viral or bacterial **epididymo-orchitis** may cause an acute scrotum in infants and toddlers, but the diagnosis is often only made after scrotal exploration. Other conditions that rarely cause acute scrotal symptoms and signs include idiopathic scrotal oedema (typically painless, erythematous scrotal swelling in a young boy extending from the scrotum into the groin and towards the anus), an

Giovanni Batista Morgagni, 1682–1771, Professor of Anatomy, Padua, Italy for 59 years. He is regarded as 'The Founder of Morbid Anatomy'.

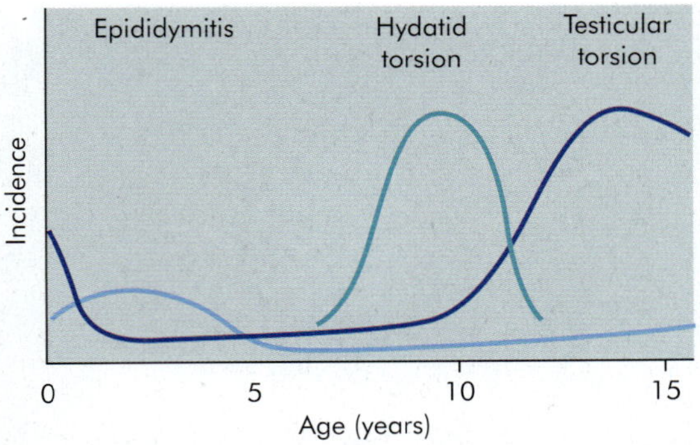

Figure 8.11 Acute scrotal pathology at different ages.

incarcerated inguinal hernia, vasculitis or a scrotal haematoma (Summary box 8.8).

Summary box 8.8

Diagnosis and treatment of the acute scrotum

- Torsion of the testis must be assumed until proven otherwise
- Testicular torsion can present with acute inguinal or abdominal pain
- Urgent surgical exploration is crucial if testicular torsion cannot be excluded
- Torsion of a testicular appendage usually occurs just before puberty
- An incarcerated inguinal hernia must be considered in the differential diagnosis

The penis

Hypospadias

In hypospadias, seen in 1:300 boys, the urethra opens proximally and ventrally. Most commonly, the opening is just proximal to the glans, but it can open on the penile shaft or onto the perineum. It is attributed to failure of complete urethral tubularisation in the fetus. The foreskin is deficient ventrally and there is a variable degree of chordee (a ventral curvature of the penis most apparent on erection) (Figure 8.12). Glanular hypospadias needs correction for cosmetic reasons but more proximal anomalies interfere with micturition and erection. In a newborn with severe hypospadias and bilateral undescended testes, disorders of sexual development (DSD) should be considered. A distal hypospadias is usually repaired before two years of age in one or two stages. Proximal varieties require complex staged procedures. Surgery aims to achieve a terminal urethral meatus so that the boy can stand to micturate with a normal stream, a straight erection and a penis that looks normal. Ritual circumcision is contraindicated in infants with hypospadias because the foreskin is often required for the reconstruction.

The foreskin and circumcision

At birth, the foreskin is adherent to the glans penis. These adhesions separate spontaneously with time, allowing the foreskin to become retractile. At one year of age, about 50 per cent of boys have a non-retractile foreskin. By four years, this has declined to 10 per cent and by 16 years to just 1 per cent. Ballooning of the normal non-retractile foreskin on micturition brings many young boys to doctors and explanation and reassurance are required, but no operation. Gentle retraction of the foreskin at bath times helps to maintain hygiene, but forcible retraction should never be attempted. The presence of preputial adhesions, when the foreskin remains partially adherent to the glans, is normal and resolves spontaneously.

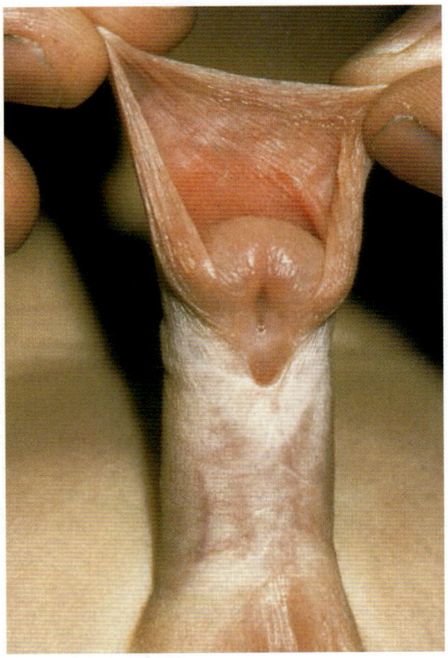

Figure 8.12 Hypospadias: note the hooded foreskin and the ventral meatus.

Circumcision has been an important tradition in Jewish, Muslim and other cultures. Proponents observe that circumcision reduces the incidence of urinary tract infection in infant boys; however, circumcision is not without risk of significant morbidity. The medical indications for circumcision are:

- **Phimosis**. This term is often wrongly applied to describe a normal, non-retractile foreskin. True phimosis is seen as a whitish scarring of the foreskin and is rare before five years of age (Figure 8.13). It is caused by a localised skin disease known as balanitis xerotica obliterans (BXO), which also affects the glans penis and can cause urethral meatal stenosis.
- **Recurrent balanoposthitis**. A single episode of inflammation of the foreskin, sometimes with a purulent discharge, is not uncommon and usually resolves spontaneously; antibiotics are sometimes needed. Recurrent attacks are unusual but may be an indication for circumcision.
- **Recurrent urinary tract infection**. Circumcision is occasionally justified in boys with an abnormal upper urinary tract anomaly and recurrent urinary infection. It may also help boys with spina bifida who need to perform clean intermittent urethral catheterisation.

An emerging but controversial indication for circumcision is in the prevention of sexually acquired human immunodeficiency virus (HIV) infection in communities where this is common; large clinical trials have shown that circumcision reduces the risk of HIV transmission.

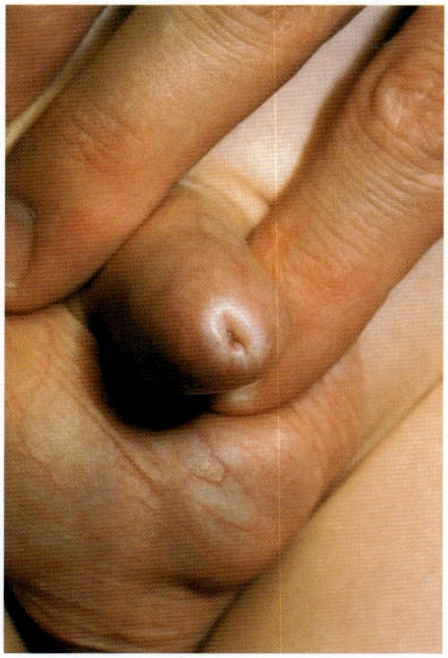

Figure 8.13 True phimosis from balanitis xerotica obliterans.

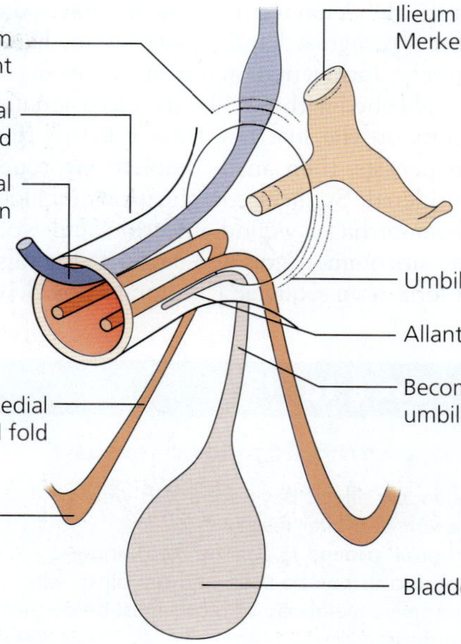

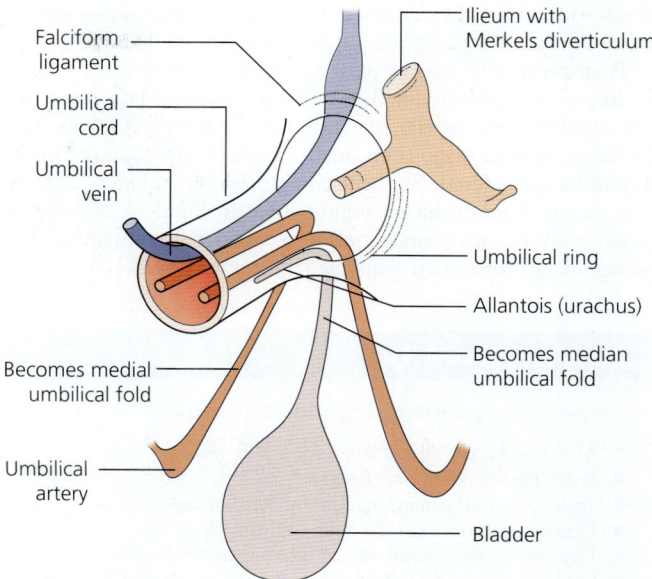

Figure 8.14 Structures at the umbilicus.

Circumcision for medical reasons is best performed under general anaesthesia. A long-acting local anaesthetic regional block can be given to reduce postoperative pain. Circumcision is not a trivial operation; bleeding and infection are well-recognised complications and more serious hazards, such as injury to the glans, may occur if the procedure is not carried out well (Summary box 8.9).

Summary box 8.9

Circumcision

- Medical indications are balanitis xerotica obliterans and recurrent balanoposthitis, paraphimosis, scarring from trauma
- Circumcision is not indicated for an otherwise healthy non-retractile foreskin
- Complications include bleeding, poor cosmesis (too much or too little skin removed) and trauma to the glans or urethra

Midline hernias

In the embryo, the umbilical ring is a relatively large defect in the ventral abdominal wall transmitting several structures that connect the fetus to the placenta (Figure 8.14). An umbilical hernia is common and caused by incomplete closure of the umbilical ring; incarceration is very rare. Most umbilical hernias resolve spontaneously by four years of age. Supraumbilical hernias are through defects in the linea alba just above the umbilical ring and these do not close, but are still repaired at around four years of age. Epigastric hernias are defects higher still that allow a small amount of preperitoneal fat to prolapse. They are repaired if symptomatic.

Infantile hypertrophic pyloric stenosis

Infantile hypertrophic pyloric stenosis (IHPS) presents with non-bilious projectile vomiting between 2 and 8 weeks of age and is only rarely seen after 13 weeks. It is easily distinguished from many other serious causes of vomiting, such as infections, because the baby is particularly hungry. IHPS is a progressive condition and a detailed history helps distinguish it from the more common gastro-oesophageal reflux (GOR) which is commonly seen in infancy. In the UK, it affects 1:300 infants with a male to female ratio of 4:1. However, if a girl has IHPS her offspring have a high chance of developing it, suggesting a genetic predisposition.

The non-bilious nature is stressed here to contrast the condition with the **bilious vomiting** of the potentially life-threatening malrotation and volvulus seen occasionally in neonates.

IHPS can be diagnosed clinically. During a test feed, there is visible gastric peristalsis passing from left to right across the upper abdomen and in a relaxed baby the pyloric 'tumour' is palpable as an 'olive' in the right upper quadrant. The diagnosis can be confirmed by an ultrasound, which shows the thickened pyloric muscle. IHPS is readily treated by surgery but the infant must be adequately rehydrated and the hypochloraemic-hypokalaemic alkalosis corrected; this may take 48 hours. In most babies, the dehydration and alkalosis can be corrected by giving 150–180 mL/kg per day of 0.45 per cent saline with 0.15 per cent KCl in 5 per cent glucose. Oral feeding is discontinued and the stomach emptied with an 8–10 Fr nasogastric tube; ongoing gastric losses should be replaced with normal saline containing potassium chloride.

Ramstedt's pyloromyotomy is performed through an incision around the umbilicus. The pyloric tumour is delivered by gentle traction on the stomach. A serosal incision is made and the tumour spread (Figure 8.15). The end result should be an intact bulging submucosa from duodenal fornix to gastric antrum.

Wilhelm Conrad Ramstedt, 1867–1963, surgeon, The Rafaelklinik, Münster, Germany, performed his first pyloromyotomy in 1911.

Perforation of the duodenal fornix is uncommon and not serious provided that it is recognised and repaired immediately.

Postoperatively, intravenous fluids are continued until oral feeding is re-established within 24 hours. Occasionally, the baby has small vomits on the first few feeds but this resolves after 72 hours. If it persists, then an incomplete myotomy or GOR should be considered. Surgical complications include duodenal perforation, haemorrhage, wound infection and wound dehiscence – all are uncommon and avoidable. Pyloromyotomy has no significant long-term sequelae (Summary box 8.10).

Summary box 8.10

Infantile hypertrophic pyloric stenosis

- Most commonly affects boys aged 2–8 weeks
- Projectile vomiting after feeds
- Test feed or ultrasound to confirm the diagnosis
- Gastric peristalsis can be seen and an 'olive' felt
- Hypochloraemic metabolic alkalosis must be corrected before surgery
- Pyloromyotomy splits the hypertrophied muscle leaving the mucosa intact

Other common or serious causes of vomiting in infancy are shown in Table 8.4.

Gastro-oesophageal reflux is common and tends to resolve spontaneously with maturity. Persistent symptoms respond to thickened feeds and anti-reflux medication. Complications, such as failure to thrive or respiratory problems, demand further investigation and, in some cases, fundoplication.

Table 8.4 Vomiting in infancy.

Bile-stained	Neonate	Intestinal malrotation with volvulus
		Duodenal atresia/stenosis (Down syndrome, antenatal diagnosis)
		Jejunal/ileal atresia (often isolated anomalies)
		Hirschsprung's disease
		Anorectal malformations
		Meconium ileus (cystic fibrosis)
		Necrotising enterocolitis (an acquired condition in the premature)
		Incarcerated inguinal hernia
	Older infant	Intestinal malrotation with volvulus
		Intussusception (often non-bilious initially)
		Incarcerated inguinal hernia
Non-bilious	Infantile hypertrophic pyloric stenosis	
	Gastro-oesophageal reflux	
	Feeding difficulties (technique/volume)	
	Non-specific marker of illness, e.g. infection (urinary tract infection, meningitis, gastroenteritis, respiratory, metabolic disorder, raised intracranial pressure, congenital adrenal hyperplasia)	

Intussusception

Most intussusceptions (Figure 8.16) in children are seen from two months to two years of age. They are life-threatening. Intussusception typically causes a strangulating bowel obstruction, which can progress to gangrene and perforation. Intussusception is classified according to the site of the intussusceptum and intussuscipiens. In children, more than 80 per cent are ileocolic, beginning several centimetres proximal to the ileocaecal valve with their apex found in the ascending or transverse colon.

In the majority, the cause is hyperplasia of Peyer's patches (lymphoid tissue), which may be secondary to a viral infection. In 10 per cent of children, intussusception is secondary to a pathological lead point, such as a Meckel's diverticulum, enteric

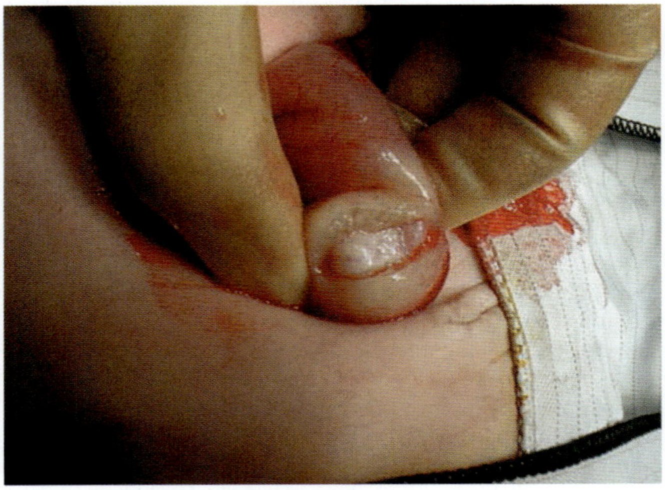

Figure 8.15 Pyloromyotomy for infantile hypertrophic pyloric stenosis.

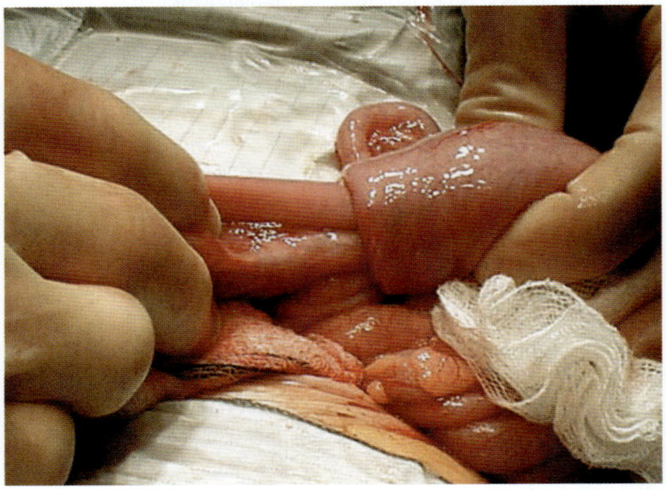

Figure 8.16 Ileocolic intussusception causing small bowel obstruction.

duplication cyst or even a small bowel lymphoma. Such cases are more likely in children over the age of two years and in those with recurrent intussusception.

Classically, a previously healthy infant presents with colicky pain and vomiting (milk, then bile). Between episodes, the child initially appears well. Later, they may pass a 'redcurrant jelly' stool. Clinical signs include dehydration, abdominal distension and a palpable sausage-shaped mass in the right upper quadrant. Rectal examination may reveal blood or rarely the apex of an intussusceptum (Summary box 8.11).

Summary box 8.11

Presentation of intussusception

- Bilious vomiting in an infant is a sign of intestinal obstruction until proved otherwise
- Intussusception classically presents with colicky pain and vomiting
- Intussusception should be considered in any infant with bloody stools
- Age range is between 2 and 24 months of age

A plain radiograph is rarely requested but if done it commonly shows signs of small bowel obstruction and a soft-tissue opacity. Diagnosis is confirmed on an abdominal ultrasound. After resuscitation with intravenous fluids, broad-spectrum antibiotics and nasogastric drainage, non-operative reduction is attempted using an air enema (Figure 8.17). Successful reduction is recognised if air flows into the small bowel, together with later resolution of symptoms and signs. An air enema is contraindicated if there is peritonitis, perforation or shock. More than 70 per cent of intussusceptions can be reduced non-operatively. Strangulated bowel and pathological lead points are unlikely to reduce. Perforation of the colon during pneumatic reduction is a recognised hazard, but is rare. Recurrent intussusception occurs in up to 5 per cent of patients after non-operative reduction (Summary box 8.12).

If an operative reduction is needed, this is usually performed open. The intussusception is milked distally by gentle compression from its apex. Both the intussusceptum and the intussuscipiens are inspected for areas of non-viability. An irreducible intussusception or one complicated by infarction or a pathological lead point requires resection and primary anastomosis.

Summary box 8.12

Management of intussusception

- Bowel infarction will result without treatment
- Most are ileocolic
- Diagnosis can be confirmed by ultrasound scan
- Fluid and electrolyte resuscitation is essential
- Most intussusceptions can be reduced non-operatively using an air enema
- If there are signs of peritonitis or perforation, then an emergency operation is needed

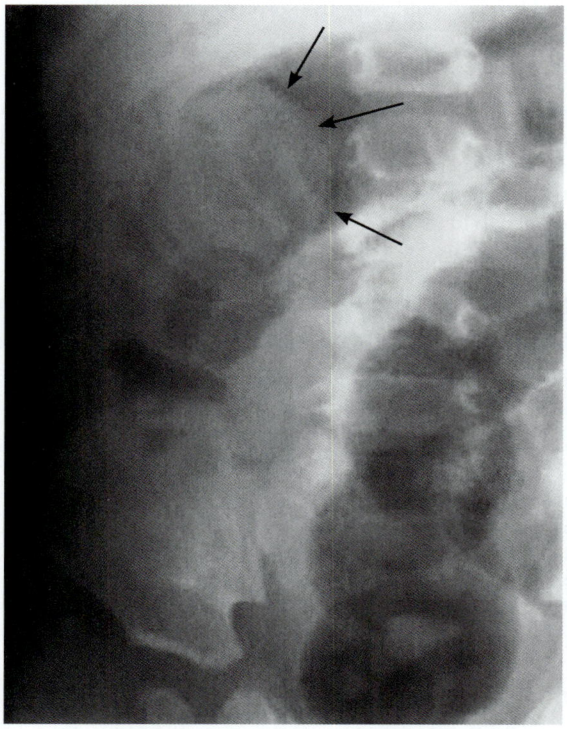

Figure 8.17 Air enema reduction of an intussusception (the arrows mark the soft tissue shadow of the intussusceptum).

Acute abdominal pain in children over three years of age

Between one-third and one-half of children admitted to hospital with acute abdominal pain have non-specific abdominal pain (NSAP). Another one-third have acute appendicitis. Relatively benign conditions, such as constipation and urinary tract infection (UTI), account for most of the remainder. A small proportion of children have more serious pathology.

History and examination

Time and patience are required to accurately evaluate the child with acute abdominal pain. The child may be frightened and the parents worried. Young children find it difficult to accurately describe or localise abdominal pain, but can often give a good history. The abdomen, genitalia, chest, throat and neck are examined. The abdomen may need reassessment after analgesia and a number of reviews. A gentle abdominal examination of the sleeping toddler, before removing their clothes, may reveal tenderness, guarding or a mass. Rectal examination is only performed if a pelvic appendicitis is suspected and should be by the surgeon whose decision will be altered by the findings. **Active observation** acknowledges that a definitive diagnosis is not always possible when the patient is first seen. The surgeon reassesses the child after a few hours whilst rehydrating with intravenous fluids or allowing clear fluids and simple analgesics. This approach reduces the need for investigations and can reduce the negative appendicectomy rate to as low as 4 per cent (Summary box 8.13).

Peter Ferry Jones, 1920–2009, Professor of Clinical Surgery, The University of Aberdeen, Aberdeen, UK.

Summary box 8.13

Work up of children with acute abdominal pain

- A careful history and examination and active observation are paramount
- Routine tests include full blood count (FBC), C-reactive protein (CRP), urine analysis, microscopy and culture
- Other tests may be helpful after a period of observation: abdominal ultrasound scan (can diagnose pelvic and urinary tract pathology, intussusception and other conditions)
- Occasionally helpful tests: a plain supine abdominal radiograph (particularly in the preschool child with pain and vomiting), computed tomography scan in complex patients
- Selective specific investigations: blood culture, stool culture, plasma amylase, diagnostic laparoscopy

Acute non-specific abdominal pain

The clinical features of NSAP are similar to acute appendicitis, but the pain is poorly localised, not aggravated by movement and rarely accompanied by guarding. The site and severity of maximum tenderness often vary during the course of repeated examinations. Symptoms are typically self-limiting within 48 hours. The aetiology of non-specific abdominal pain in children is obscure, but viral infections and transient intussusception account for some cases. Viral infections can cause reactive lymphadenopathy, fever and diffuse abdominal pain. In some children, recurrent acute abdominal pain can be organic or sometimes an expression of underlying psychosocial problems or abuse.

Acute appendicitis and its pitfalls

Classically, there is anorexia and a few episodes of vomiting with central abdominal pain which settles in the right iliac fossa. In early acute appendicitis, there is a fever of 37.3–38.4°C and localised tenderness. Finding persistent guarding in the right iliac fossa on repeated examination is the key to making the diagnosis and distinguishing it from NSAP which usually resolves over 24 to 48 hours. NSAP does not have persistent guarding. Acute appendicitis is a clinical diagnosis and investigations may help, but cannot replace regular expert clinical review. The pitfalls include wrongly making the diagnosis of gastroenteritis when there are loose stools or attributing pain on micturition and pyuria to a UTI. Both of these can occur when there is a pelvic appendicitis or a pelvic collection. Consider also referred pain from a possible right lower lobe pneumonia and remember that if antibiotics have been given the signs may be subdued and presentation can be delayed. The diagnosis can be difficult in those under five years of age. However, many patients under the age of five present with a perforated appendix, not because the diagnosis is made late but rather the omentum is less well developed and inflammation is not well contained. The treatment starts with resuscitation with intravenous fluids, analgesia and broad-spectrum antibiotics. Appendicectomy can be performed laparoscopically or through a muscle-splitting right iliac fossa incision. An appendix mass in a child who is not obstructed may respond to conservative management with antibiotics and an interval appendicectomy can be considered 6 weeks later (Summary box 8.14).

Summary box 8.14

Acute appendicitis

- Anorexia, vomiting, low-grade fever
- Tenderness and guarding in the right iliac fossa
- Exclude referred pain from right lower lobe pneumonia
- Take special care in the preschool child
- Surgery is the treatment of choice after resuscitation and antibiotics

Other causes of acute abdominal pain in children

- **Intestinal obstruction**. Consider intussusception, inguinal hernia, adhesions and secondary to a Meckel's diverticulum.
- **Constipation**. Often over-diagnosed as a cause of acute abdominal pain, particularly as the plain x-ray of a dehydrated ill child frequently shows faecal loading. Constipation is more often a cause of acute abdominal pain in a child who has been treated for Hirschsprung's disease or an anorectal malformation.
- **Urinary tract disorders**. Urinary tract infection is an uncommon cause of acute abdominal pain. Urinary symptoms, fever and vomiting tend to predominate. Urinalysis, microscopy and culture are useful, but a sterile pyuria may accompany acute appendicitis. Boys with pelviureteric junction obstruction can present with acute or recurrent abdominal pain and no urinary symptoms.
- **Gastroenteritis**. May cause colicky abdominal pain. Onset of pain before the diarrhoea and the presence of lower abdominal tenderness should raise the suspicion of appendicitis.
- **Tropical diseases**. Ascariasis, typhoid and amoebiasis can cause acute abdominal pain.

There are numerous rarer causes of acute abdominal pain in children including Henoch–Schönlein purpura, sickle cell disease, primary peritonitis, acute pancreatitis, biliary colic, testicular torsion, gynaecological pathology (e.g. ovarian cysts and tumours, pelvic inflammatory disease, haematometrocolpos) and urinary stone disease (Summary box 8.15).

Summary box 8.15

Rare causes of acute abdominal pain in children

- Obstruction from intussusception, adhesions, Meckel's diverticulum or an inguinal hernia
- Constipation
- Urinary tract disorders
- Gastroenteritis
- Ascariasis
- Typhoid

Urinary tract infection

Urinary tract infections in children may be due to a urinary tract abnormality which may carry a risk of developing renal scarring from ascending infection. Infection and obstruction

Eduard Heinrich Henoch, 1820–1910, Professor of Diseases of Children, Berlin, Germany, described this form of purpura in 1868.
Johann Lucas Schönlein, 1793–1864, Professor of Medicine, Berlin, Germany, published his description of this form of purpura in 1837.

is particularly hazardous. Older children complain of dysuria and frequency, whereas infants present with vomiting, fever and/or poor feeding. Urine specimens from children are easily contaminated during collection and results must be interpreted with care. A proven infection is investigated by an ultrasound scan. Micturating cystography and radioisotope renography are helpful in excluding vesicoureteric reflux and renal scarring. Treatment aims to relieve symptoms, correct causes and prevent renal scarring. Vesicoureteric reflux may resolve spontaneously, some may need antibiotic prophylaxis or, in a very small number of cases, an endoscopic treatment or a reimplantation of the ureter.

Children with **neuropathic bladders** (e.g. spina bifida) are at risk of secondary upper renal tract complications. Management of these children must take into account their dexterity and motivation. An adequate capacity, low-pressure bladder can frequently be managed by clean intermittent catheterisation, but a high pressure bladder is hazardous and other strategies, such as bladder augmentation, may be necessary. Some of these children empty their bladder via a non-refluxing catheterisable channel fashioned from the appendix, the bowel or a redundant ureter interposed between the abdominal wall and bladder (Mitrofanoff).

Anorectal problems

Constipation

The passage of hard or infrequent stools is common in children in the West. Severe constipation may be secondary to an anal fissure, Hirschsprung's disease, an anorectal malformation or a neuropathic bowel. A detailed history and examination of the abdomen, anus and spine will identify most causes. Rectal examination and plain abdominal radiography may be helpful in severe cases. In the absence of specific underlying pathology, the child is best managed jointly with a paediatrician using a combination of diet, extra fluids, reward systems, laxatives and, in some cases, psychological intervention.

Rectal prolapse

Mucosal rectal prolapse can occur in toddlers and is exacerbated by straining or squatting on a potty. It is typically intermittent and frequently self-limiting. Rarely, it may be secondary to cystic fibrosis or spinal dysraphism. The differential diagnosis includes a prolapsing rectal polyp. Underlying factors such as constipation should be treated. Recurrent symptomatic prolapse usually responds to injection sclerotherapy. Strapping the buttocks is ineffective.

Rectal bleeding

Unlike in adults, malignancy is an exceptionally rare cause of rectal bleeding. In newborns, the life-threatening causes are malrotation and necrotising enterocolitis and in older infants and children, intussusception. The quantities of blood loss are small, but the conditions serious. Other causes include anal fissures, juvenile polyps (Figure 8.18) and certain gastroenteritides (e.g. *Campylobacter* infection).

The four-year-old patient who presents with an Hb of 4 gm/dL will most likely have bled profusely from an ulcer adjacent to a Meckel's diverticulum containing ectopic gastric mucosa (Figure 8.19). A technetium scan may confirm the presence of

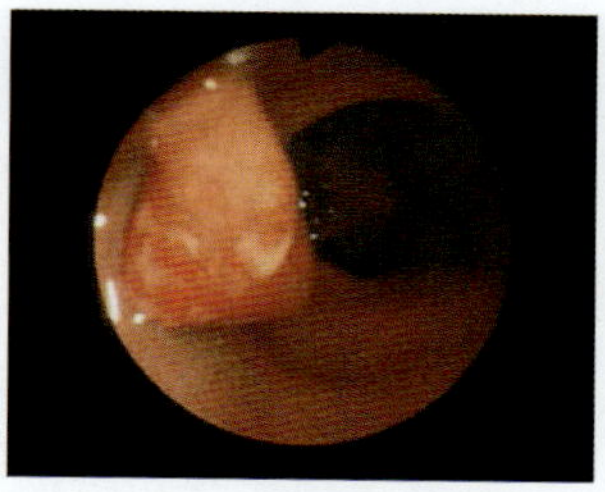

Figure 8.18 Colonic juvenile polyp: these are typically pedunculated.

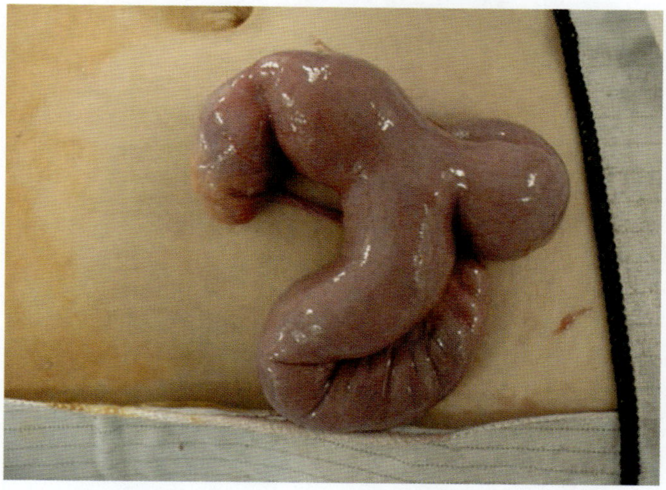

Figure 8.19 Meckel's diverticulum containing ectopic gastric mucosa.

ectopic gastric mucosa (Figure 8.20). A Meckel's diverticulum may also be complicated by an obstructing band between the diverticulum and the umbilicus, diverticulitis, intussusception, intestinal volvulus or perforation.

Swallowed or inhaled foreign bodies

Coins are the most frequently swallowed foreign bodies in children. Once beyond the cardia, they are usually passed in a few days. A plain radiograph of the abdomen, chest and neck should establish the site of radio-opaque objects. Oesophageal objects can be removed endoscopically under general anaesthesia. Button batteries must be removed within hours. If they remain in the oesophagus they can cause gastrointestinal perforation into the trachea. Batteries in the stomach are either removed urgently or followed very closely with repeat x-rays over a couple of days. The need to remove sharp objects depends on their size, the age of the child and their position in the gut. Ingested magnets can cause entero-enteric fistulae when they fix to one another in adjacent loops of bowel.

Inhaled foreign bodies cause sudden-onset coughing and stridor. If there is worsening dyspnoea or signs of hypoxia, then the infant should be given back blows in a head-down position. A Heimlich manoeuvre can be used in older children. A foreign body is suggested by: a unilateral wheeze, decreased transmitted breath sounds and a hyperinflated lung from air trapping on an expiratory chest x-ray (Figure 8.21). A rigid bronchoscopy with a ventilating bronchoscope and appropriate optical forceps are needed to assess and remove objects (Summary box 8.16).

Paul Mitrofanoff, born 1934, Professor of Paediatric Surgery, Rouen, France.
Henry J Heimlich, born 1920, thoracic surgeon, Xavier University, Cincinnati, OH, USA.

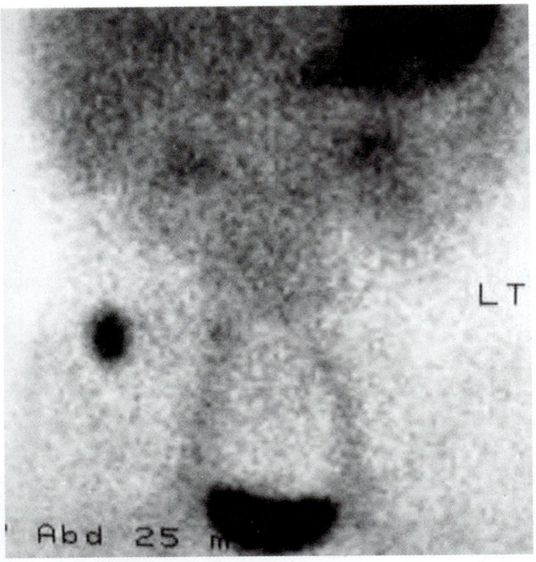

Figure 8.20 A positive Meckel's scan.

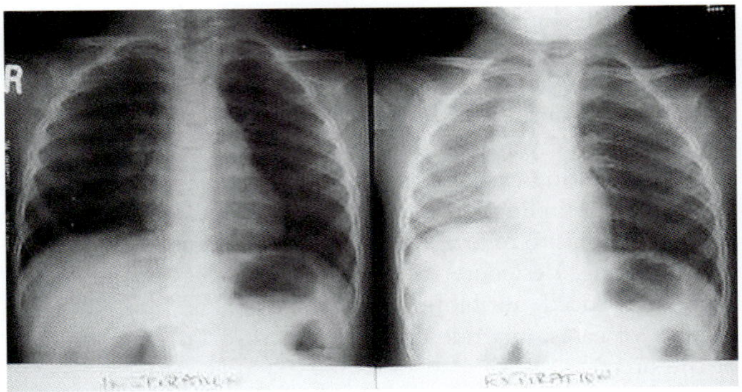

Figure 8.21 An inspiratory (left) and expiratory (right) chest radiograph demonstrating left-sided pulmonary air trapping after inhalation of a radiolucent foreign body.

Summary box 8.16

Swallowed and inhaled objects

- Most swallowed objects pass spontaneously
- Batteries need watching – they must pass quickly if their contents are not to leak
- Objects jammed in the airway or oesophagus need removing promptly

CONGENITAL MALFORMATIONS

Around 2 per cent of babies are born with one or more major structural anomalies caused by genetic defects or teratogenic insults. Some are diagnosed antenatally and surgeons are involved in prenatal counselling. Termination of pregnancy or a planned delivery in a specialist centre are options for severe malformations. Prenatal diagnosis may include checking the karyotype (e.g. Down syndrome (trisomy 21)) or testing for genetic disorders, such as cystic fibrosis.

The incidence of congenital malformations is variable (Table 8.5). Some examples relevant to the general surgeon are briefly outlined in the following sections.

Oesophageal atresia

A blind proximal pouch with a distal tracheo-oesophageal fistula is the most common type (Figure 8.22). Affected infants present soon after birth with drooling and cyanotic episodes on attempting to feed. There may have been polyhydramnios due to failure to swallow amniotic fluid. The diagnosis is confirmed when a nasogastric tube goes no further than the upper oesophageal pouch on the chest x-ray and abdominal gas signifies the tracheo-oesophageal fistula (Figure 8.22). Associated anomalies are common and include cardiac, renal and skeletal defects. Repair is usually via a right-sided extrapleural thoracotomy within a day or two of birth. The fistula is divided and the tracheal side closed. The oesophageal ends are then anastomosed. Postoperative complications include anastomotic leak, stricture, recurrent fistula formation and gastro-oesophageal reflux. Infants with pure oesophageal atresia and no tracheo-oesophageal fistula are usually best managed by a temporary gastrostomy and delayed primary repair or an oesophageal replacement. Except for very-low-birth weight babies and those with major congenital heart disease, most infants with repaired oesophageal atresia have a good prognosis.

John Langdon Haydon Down (sometimes given as Langdon-Down), 1838–1896, physician, The London Hospital, London, UK, published *'Observations on an ethnic classification of idiots'* in 1866.

Congenital diaphragmatic hernia

Typically in congenital diaphragmatic hernia (CDH), there is a left-sided posterolateral diaphragmatic defect allowing herniation of abdominal viscera into the chest (Figure 8.23). Many are detected antenatally and the prognosis relates to the severity of the associated pulmonary hypoplasia. Despite intensive respiratory support or extracorporeal membrane oxygenation (ECMO), up to 30 per cent of babies with a CDH die from res-

Table 8.5 Incidence of selected malformations.

	Abnormality	Incidence
Thoracic	Congenital diaphragmatic hernia	1:3000
	Oesophageal atresia/tracheo-oesophageal fistula	1:3500
Cardiac	Congenital heart disease	1:150
Gastrointestinal	Gastroschisis	1:7500
	Hirschsprung's disease	1:5000
	Anorectal malformations	1:4–5000
Hepatobiliary	Biliary atresia	1:17 000
	Choledochal cyst	1:50 000
Urogenital	Hypospadias	1:300
	Pelviureteric junction dysfunction	1:1000

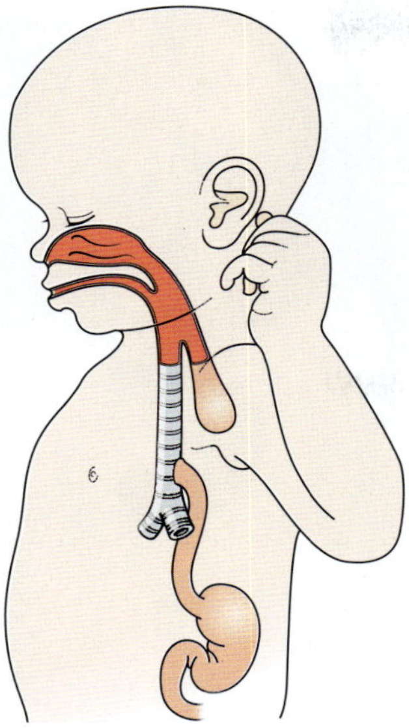

Figure 8.22 Oesophageal atresia with a distal tracheo-oesophageal fistula.

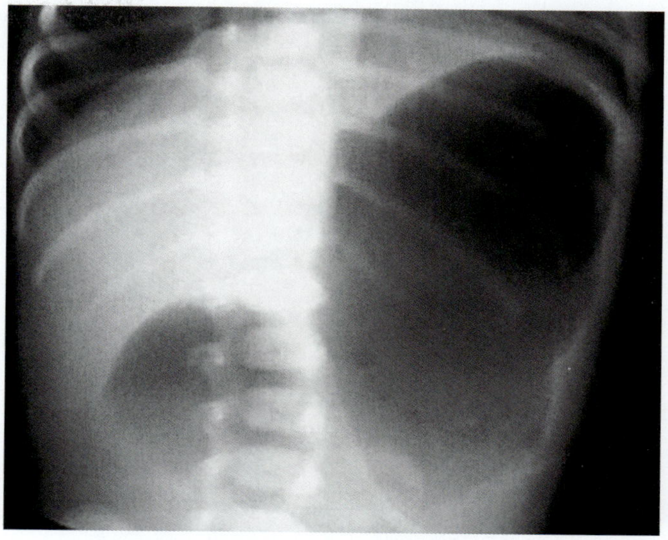

Figure 8.24 Neonatal abdominal x-ray showing the 'double bubble' of duodenal atresia.

piratory failure. If the baby can be stabilised, the diaphragmatic defect is repaired. Small diaphragmatic hernias may present with respiratory or gastrointestinal symptoms in later childhood.

Intestinal atresias

Duodenal atresia may take the form of a membrane or the proximal and distal duodenum may be completely separated. Prenatal ultrasound finds a 'double bubble' in the fetal abdomen with polyhydramnios. There is an association with Down syndrome. Postnatally, there is bilious vomiting if the atresia is distal to the ampulla. A plain abdominal x-ray also shows the double bubble (Figure 8.24). Repair is by duodenoduodenostomy (Figure 8.25). Occasionally, there is a duodenal membrane with a modest central perforation, which may delay symptoms until later childhood.

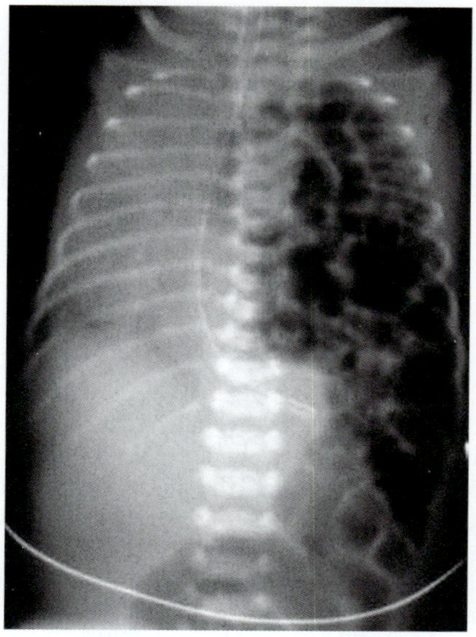

Figure 8.23 Left-sided congenital diaphragmatic hernia.

Jejunal/ileal atresia varies from an obstructing membrane through to widely separated blind-ended bowel ends associated with a mesenteric defect. Small bowel atresias may be single or multiple and are probably secondary to a prenatal vascular or mechanical insult causing sterile infarction of a segment of gut. They present with intestinal obstruction soon after birth. The proximal bowel is often extremely dilated and needs to be tapered or excised prior to anastomosis to the distal bowel (Figure 8.26).

Meconium ileus is a cause of intestinal obstruction from inspissated meconium in the terminal ileum in neonates, most of whom have cystic fibrosis. Meconium is a sterile mixture of epithelial cells, mucin and bile. Babies with uncomplicated meconium ileus (no associated atresia, volvulus or perforation) can sometimes be managed with hyperosmolar contrast enemas to clear the meconium.

Meconium peritonitis is consequent upon a fetal intestinal perforation. The baby is born with a firm, distended, discoloured abdomen and signs of obstruction. An abdominal x-ray shows dilated intestinal loops and areas of calcification. Occasionally, the perforation has resolved spontaneously before birth, but most neonates with meconium peritonitis will need surgery.

Intestinal malrotation. By the 12th week of gestation, the mid-gut has returned to the fetal abdomen from the extra-embryonic coelom and has begun rotating counterclockwise around the superior mesenteric artery axis. In classical **intestinal malrotation**, this process fails; the duodenojejunal flexure lies to the right of the midline and the caecum is central, creating a narrow base for the small bowel mesentery, which predisposes to mid-gut volvulus (Figure 8.27). Malrotation with volvulus is life-threatening and typically presents with bilious vomiting. Bile-stained vomiting in the infant is a sign of intestinal obstruction until proved otherwise.

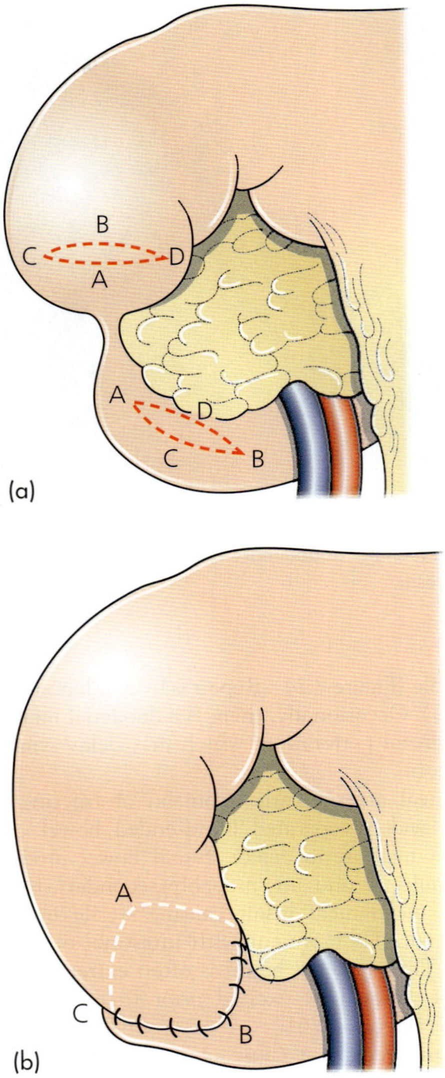

Figure 8.25 (a) Duodenal atresia and (b) the incisions (A–D) used to repair it.

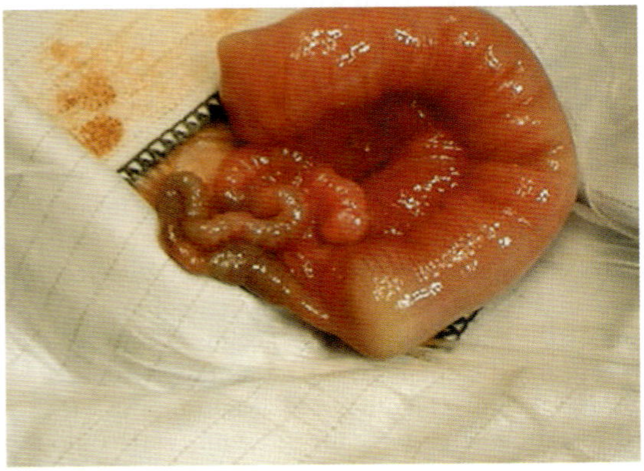

Figure 8.26 Small bowel atresia.

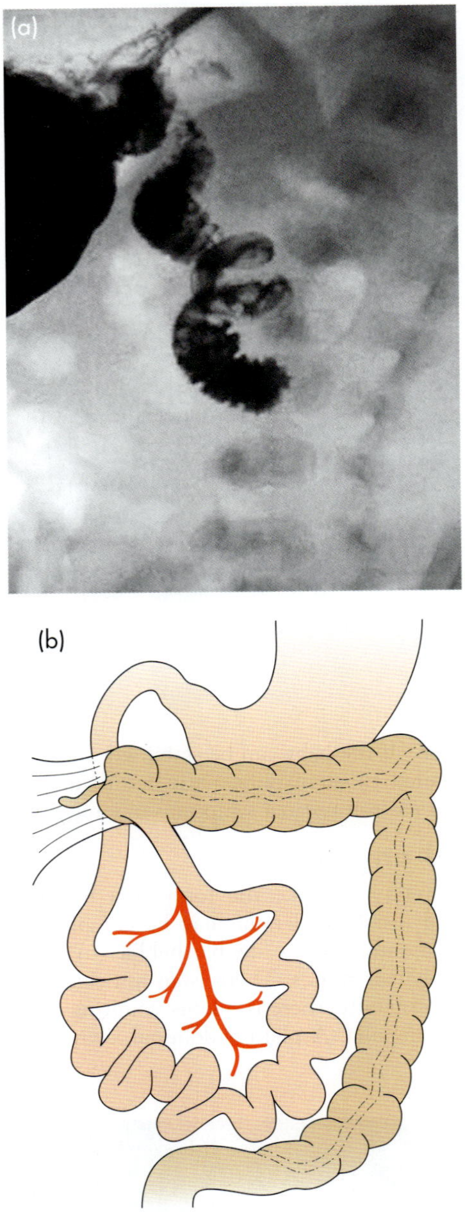

Figure 8.27 (a) Contrast showing malrotation with a volvulus. (b) The narrow origin of the small bowel mesentery predisposes to mid-gut volvulus.

As the gut strangulates, the baby may pass blood-stained stools and becomes progressively more ill. An upper gastrointestinal contrast study confirms the malrotation (Figure 8.27). Resuscitation and urgent surgery are needed to untwist the volvulus, widen the base of the small bowel mesentery, straighten the duodenum and position the bowel in a non-rotated position with the small bowel on the right and the colon on the left (Ladd's procedure). The appendix is usually removed to avoid leaving it in an abnormal site within the abdomen.

William Edward Ladd, 1880–1967, Professor of Child Surgery, The University of Harvard, Boston, MA, USA.

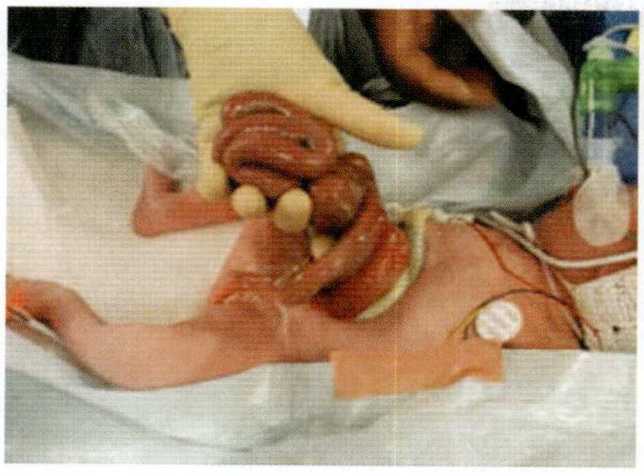

Figure 8.28 A newborn infant with gastroschisis.

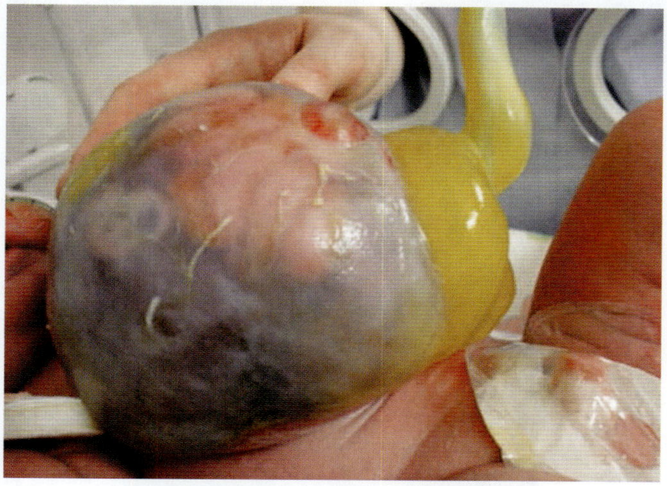

Figure 8.29 Exomphalos major.

Abdominal wall defects

Gastroschisis is now the most common anomaly in babies born to mothers under 20 years of age. The fetal gut prolapses through a defect to the right of the umbilicus. At birth, the bowel is non-rotated, foreshortened and covered by a fibrinous peel (Figure 8.28). After reduction of the bowel, which may need to be staged using a silo, and closure of the defect, gastroschisis has a good prognosis, although gut dysmotility delays recovery. Some infants have an intestinal atresia and some boys have undescended testes but other anomalies are rare.

Exomphalos is quite a different anomaly in which the intestines and sometimes the liver are covered with a membranous sac from which the umbilical cord arises (Figure 8.29). It may be associated with chromosomal or cardiac anomalies.

Biliary atresia

In biliary atresia, the extrahepatic bile ducts are occluded causing obstructive jaundice (conjugated hyper-bilirubinaemia) and progressive liver fibrosis in early infancy. It should be considered if jaundice persists after 2 weeks of age. Fat malabsorption can lead to a coagulopathy correctable with vitamin K. An abdominal ultrasound scan may show a small gall bladder and no visible bile ducts and a biliary radionuclide scan may show no excretion. A liver biopsy may show proliferation of small bile ducts. It is treated by a Kasai porto-enterostomy in which the occluded extrahepatic bile ducts are excised and a jejunal Roux loop anastomosed to the hepatic hilum. Effective drainage is more likely with surgery before 8 weeks of age and may obviate the subsequent need for liver transplantation.

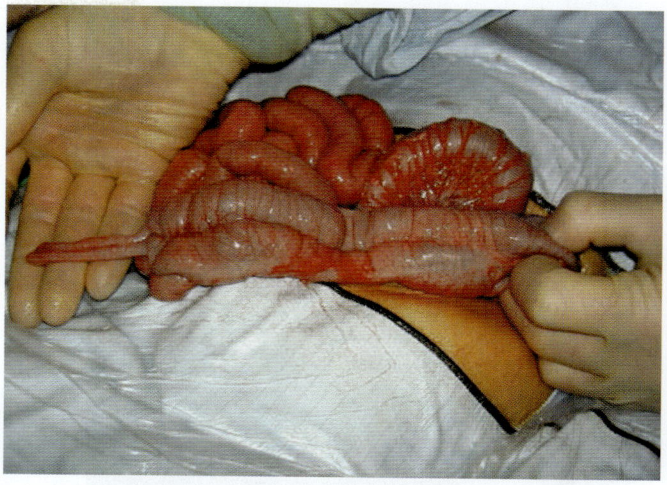

Figure 8.30 A duplicated colon.

Alimentary tract duplications

Alimentary tract duplications are rare. They are usually single, variable in size, and spherical or tubular. Most are located on the mesenteric border of the intestine. Typically, they are lined by alimentary tract mucosa and share a common smooth muscle wall and blood supply with the adjacent bowel, with which they may communicate. Duplications can contain heterotopic gastric mucosa and be associated with spinal anomalies. Most duplications present in infancy or early childhood with intestinal obstruction, haemorrhage, intussusception or perforation (Figure 8.30). Rarely, they present in adults and sometimes with a malignancy which has been reported more often with rectal duplication cysts. Complete excision is the treatment of choice.

Hirschsprung's disease

Hirschsprung's disease is characterised by the congenital absence of intramural ganglion cells (aganglionosis) and the presence of hypertrophic nerves in the distal large bowel. The absence of ganglion cells is due to a failure of migration of vagal neural crest cells into the developing gut. The affected gut is in spasm causing a functional bowel obstruction. The aganglionosis is restricted to the rectum and sigmoid colon in 75 per cent of patients (short segment), involves the proximal colon in 15 per cent (long segment) and affects the entire colon and a portion of terminal ileum in 10 per cent (total colonic aganglionosis). A transition zone exists between the dilated, proximal, normally innervated bowel and the narrow, distal aganglionic segment.

Hirschsprung's disease may be familial or associated with Down syndrome or other genetic disorders. Gene mutations

Michael R Harrison, born 1943, Chief of Paediatric Surgery, San Francisco, CA, USA. A pioneer of fetal surgery.
Morio Kasai, 1922–2008, formerly Professor of Surgery, The University of Tokyo, Tokyo, Japan.
Harald Hirschsprung, 1830–1916, physician, The Queen Louise Hospital for Children, Copenhagen, Denmark, described congenital megacolon in 1887.

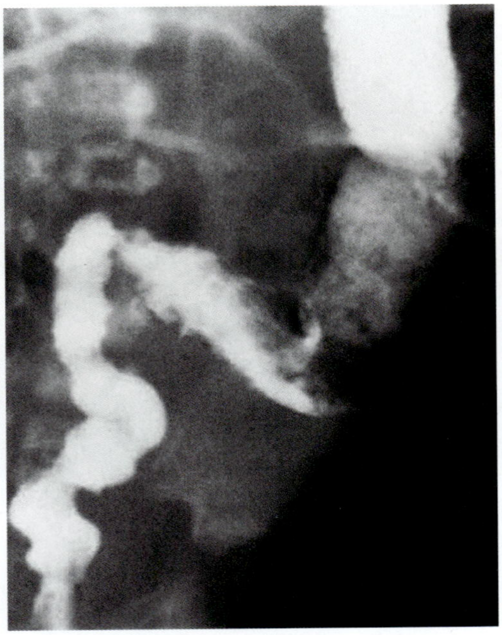

Figure 8.31 Barium enema in an infant showing a 'transition zone' in the proximal sigmoid colon between the dilated proximal normally innervated bowel and the contracted aganglionic rectum.

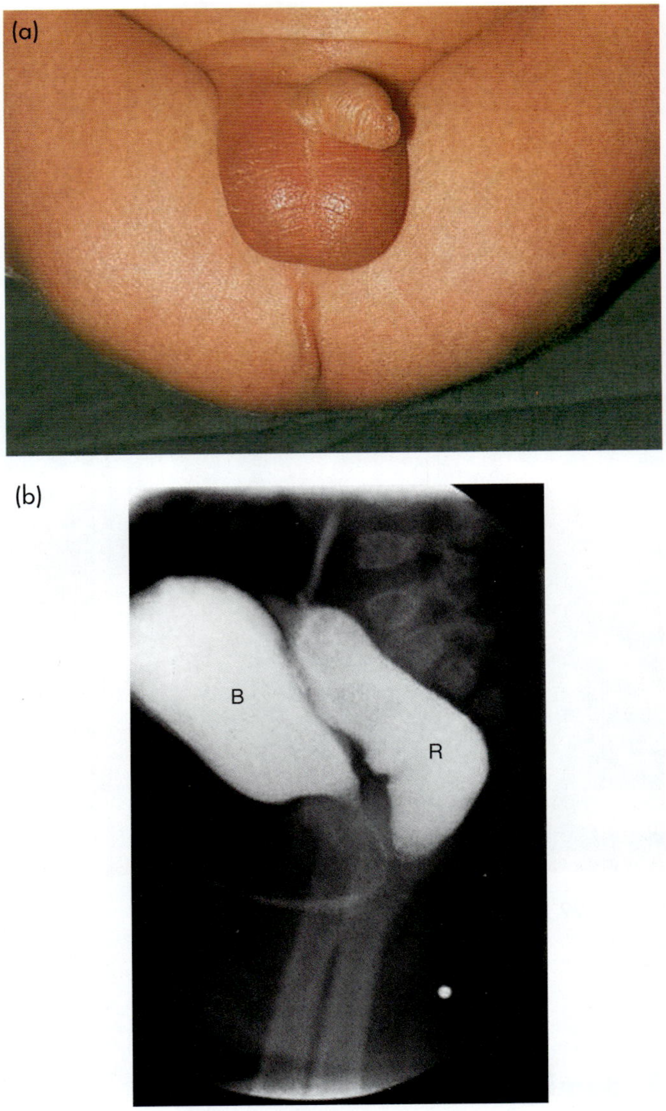

Figure 8.32 (a) An imperforate anus in a neonate associated with (b) a rectourethral fistula, visible on a contrast study performed via a sigmoid colostomy. The bladder is filled with contrast via the fistula and the radio-opaque dot has been placed on the infant's perineum over the normal site of the anus. B, bladder; R, rectum.

have been identified on chromosome 10 (involving the *RET* proto-oncogene) and on chromosome 13 in some patients. Hirschsprung's disease typically presents in the neonatal period with delayed passage of meconium, abdominal distension and bilious vomiting, but it may not be diagnosed until later in childhood or even adult life, when it manifests as severe chronic constipation. Enterocolitis is a potentially fatal complication of the disease.

The diagnosis requires an adequate rectal biopsy and an experienced pathologist. A contrast enema may show the narrow aganglionic segment, a cone and the dilated proximal bowel (Figure 8.31). Surgery aims to remove the aganglionic segment and 'pull-through' ganglionic bowel to the anus (e.g. Swenson, Duhamel, Soave and transanal procedures) and can be done in a single stage or in several stages after first establishing a proximal stoma in normally innervated bowel. Most patients achieve good bowel control, but a significant minority experience residual constipation and/or faecal incontinence or further enterocolitis.

Anorectal malformations

The anus is either imperforate or replaced by a fistula which does not pass through the muscle complex and opens away from the specialised skin which represents the true anal site. The sacrum and genitourinary tract are often abnormal. In boys, there may be a rectoperineal fistula, but the most common anomaly is an imperforate anus with a rectobulbar urethral fistula (Figure 8.32). In girls, the most common anomalies are a fistula opening in the posterior vestibule behind the vagina or on the perineum. Cloacal malformations, in which the rectum and genitourinary tract share a common outflow channel, are also seen in girls. Where there is a fistula, meconium can be passed and the diagnosis can be delayed for months because the perineum has not been inspected carefully. Most low malformations are treated by an anoplasty soon after birth. Higher, more complex defects need a temporary colostomy, detailed investigation and then reconstructive surgery. Functional outcome is related to the type of malformation (low defects are associated with constipation, higher defects with faecal incontinence) and the integrity of the sacrum and pelvic muscles. For children with residual intractable faecal incontinence, antegrade colonic enemas administered via a catheterisable appendicostomy (Figure 8.33) (the Malone/

Orvar Swenson, born 1909, Professor of Surgery, Northern University, Chicago, IL, USA.
Bernard George Duhamel, 1917–1996, Professor of Surgery, Hopital St. Denis, Paris, France.
F Soave, twentieth century Italian paediatric surgeon.

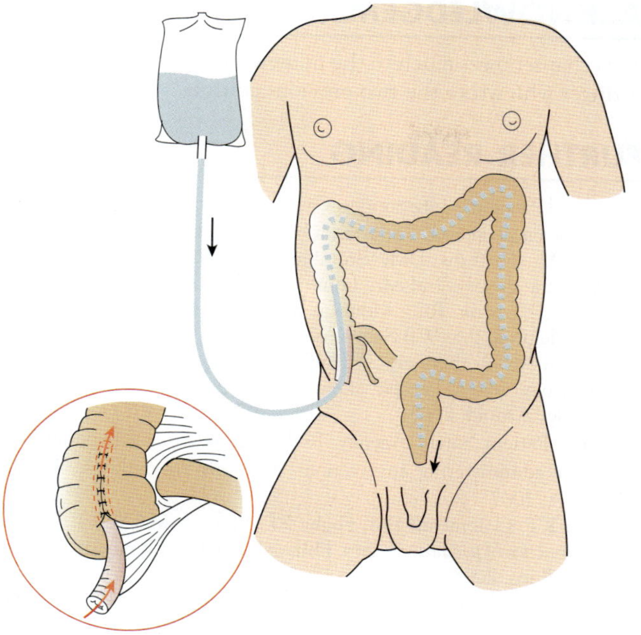

Figure 8.33 Appendicostomy for the delivery of antegrade colonic enemas.

ACE procedure) enable the child to achieve social continence. Causes of intestinal obstruction are summarised below (Summary box 8.17).

Summary box 8.17

Congenital causes of intestinal obstruction

- Intestinal atresia: may be multiple
- Cystic fibrosis: can present with intestinal obstruction from inspissated meconium
- Intestinal malrotation: predisposes to potentially lethal midgut volvulus
- Alimentary tract duplications: may present with obstruction, haemorrhage or intussusception
- Hirschsprung's disease: typically presents with delay in passing meconium after birth
- Anorectal malformations

Urinary tract malformations

Many of these malformations are now detected by prenatal ultrasound scan. Others present in childhood with urinary infection, obstruction or an abdominal mass. Urinary tract disorders in children are investigated by urine microscopy and culture, ultrasound scan, assessment of renal function and a combination of radioisotope renography (uptake and excretion), contrast radiology and endoscopy.

In many infants, prenatally diagnosed mild to moderate hydronephrosis resolves spontaneously. Those with more significant pelviureteric junction obstruction may be asymptomatic or present in later childhood with urinary tract infection or loin pain. Pyeloplasty is indicated for symptoms or impaired

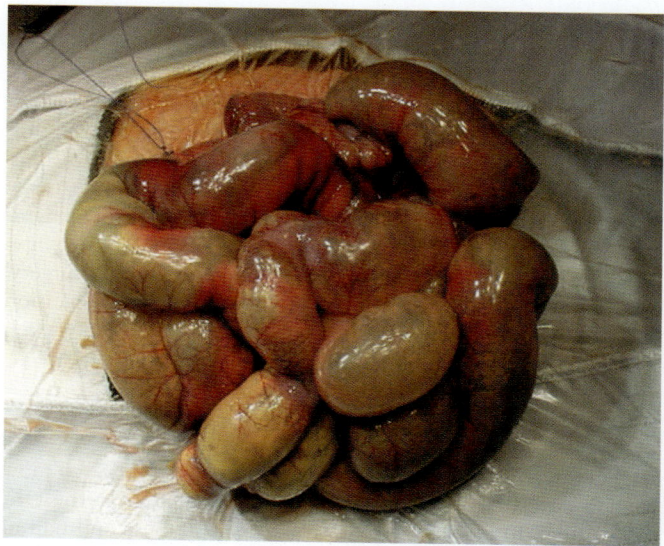

Figure 8.34 Operative appearance of neonatal necrotising enterocolitis.

renal function. In boys, partial membranous obstruction in the posterior urethra (valves) can cause a severe prenatal obstructive uropathy. This condition demands urgent investigation and treatment soon after birth to preserve bladder and kidney function. Renal failure develops in about one-third of affected boys despite early endoscopic ablation of the obstructing valves. Other congenital urinary tract malformations include ureteric abnormalities (e.g. duplex, ureterocoele, vesicoureteric reflux), multicystic dysplastic kidney and bladder exstrophy.

Necrotising enterocolitis is an acquired inflammatory condition of the neonatal gut, mostly affecting premature infants. Immaturity, formula feeds (breast milk is protective), bacterial infection and impaired gut blood flow are implicated in the pathogenesis. The neonate becomes septic with abdominal distension, bloody stools and bilious aspirates. Patchy or extensive pneumatosis intestinalis progresses to necrosis and perforation (Figure 8.34). It commonly affects the terminal ileum and colon. Small intestinal loss can be sufficient to cause severe intestinal failure. Milder cases respond to antibiotics, gut rest and parenteral nutrition, but severe cases need an urgent laparotomy. The mortality remains over 30 per cent.

PAEDIATRIC SURGICAL ONCOLOGY

Although less common in children than adults, neoplasms are a leading cause of death (along with trauma) in those over one year of age. In the western countries, leukaemia, central nervous system (CNS) tumours, lymphomas, neuroblastomas and nephroblastomas account for most paediatric malignancies. Neuroblastoma and nephroblastoma are among the more common solid abdominal tumours. The prognoses for these cancers have improved after numerous multicentre trials.

Neuroblastoma is a malignancy of neuroblasts in the adrenal medulla or sympathetic ganglia and typically presents as an abdominal or paravertebral mass. These cells metastasise to lymph nodes, bone and the liver, and they raise urinary catecholamine levels. Small localised tumours are excised. More advanced tumours require surgery after chemotherapy. Survival relates to tumour biology and stage (>90 per cent for small localised tumours, <50 per cent for advanced tumours).

Wilms' tumour (nephroblastoma) is a malignant renal tumour derived from embryonal cells; it typically affects children aged from one to four years. A mutation in the Wilms' tumour suppressor gene (*WT1*) is responsible for some cases. It usually presents as an abdominal mass. The tumour extends into the renal vein and vena cava and metastasises to lymph nodes and lungs. Treatment is with chemotherapy and surgery. Survival depends on tumour spread, completeness of excision and the histological appearance, but exceeds 70 per cent even with advanced tumours.

SAFEGUARDING

All staff must be able to recognise abuse and neglect, and know the law and their local child safeguarding contacts. In the UK, three children die each week from neglect or abuse and half of these are at the hands of their parents. One per cent of accident and emergency attendances are from abuse. Consider abuse if any of the following are present:

- bruises away from bony prominences (face, back, abdomen, arms, buttocks, ears and hands);
- bruises in clusters or in the pattern of an implement;
- multiple injuries at different stages of healing;
- different types of injury (e.g. soft tissue, burns or scalds, cuts and bruises);
- rib fractures; bite marks (it is difficult to distinguish adult from child bites, but adult bites are associated with fatal abuse);
- significant delay between the injury and seeking medical advice;
- an inconsistent or vague history;
- inappropriate parental behaviour.

ACKNOWLEDGEMENTS

This chapter owes much to the framework laid by Professor Mark Stringer who wrote the two previous editions.

FURTHER READING

Advanced Paediatric Life Support Group. *Advanced paediatric life support. The practical approach*, 8th edn. Oxford: Blackwell Publishing, 2011.

Burge DM, Griffiths DM, Steinbrecher HA, Wheeler RA (eds). *Paediatric surgery*, 2nd edn. London: Hodder Arnold, 2005.

Gearhart JP, Rink RC, Mouriquand PDE (eds). *Pediatric urology*. Philadelphia, PA: WB Saunders, 2007.

Najmaldin AS, Rothenberg S, Crabbe DCG, Beasley S (eds). *Operative endoscopy and endoscopic surgery in infants and children*. London: Hodder Arnold, 2005.

National Patient Safety Agency. Reducing the risk of hyponatraemia when administering intravenous infusions to children. London: NPSA, 2007.

Oldham KT, Colombani PM, Foglia RP, Skinner MA (eds). *Principles and practice of pediatric surgery*. Philadelphia, PA: Lippincott Williams & Wilkins, 2005.

Parikh D, Crabbe D, Auldist A, Rothenberg S (eds). *Pediatric thoracic surgery*. Berlin: Springer, 2009.

Puri P, Hollwarth ME (eds). *Pediatric surgery: diagnosis and management*. New York: Springer, 2009.

Sinha CK, Davenport M. *Handbook of pediatric surgery*. London: Springer, 2009.

Spitz L, Coran AG (eds). *Rob and Smith's Operative surgery. Pediatric surgery*, 6th edn. London: Hodder Arnold, 2006.

Stringer MD, Oldham KT, Mouriquand PDE (eds). *Pediatric surgery and urology: long-term outcomes*, 2nd edn. New York: Cambridge University Press, 2006.

Max Wilms, 1867–1918, Professor of Surgery, Heidelberg, Germany.
John W Broviac, formerly nephrologist, University of Washington, Washington DC, USA.
Robert O Hickman, formerly nephrologist, University of Washington, Washington DC, USA.

CHAPTER 9

Principles of oncology

LEARNING OBJECTIVES

To understand:
- The biological nature of cancer
- The principles of cancer prevention and early detection

To appreciate:
- The principles of cancer aetiology and the major known causative factors
- The likely shape of future developments in cancer management
- The multidisciplinary management of cancer
- The principles of palliative care

WHAT IS CANCER?

History

The name 'cancer' comes from the Greek and Latin words for a crab, and refers to the claw-like blood vessels extending over the surface of an advanced breast cancer.

The study of cancer has always been part of clinical medicine: theories have moved from divine intervention, through the humours, and are now firmly based on the cellular origin of cancer. Rudolf Virchow is credited with being the first to demonstrate that cancer is a disease of cells that progresses as a result of abnormal proliferation encapsulated by his famous dictum '*omnis cellula e cellula*' (every cell from a cell). In 1914, Theodor Boveri pointed out the importance of chromosomal abnormalities in cancer cells and, by the 1940s, Oswald Avery had shown that DNA was the genetic material within the chromosomes. In 1953, the key discovery by Watson and Crick of the structure of DNA paved the way for the study of what has become known as the molecular biology of cancer enabling us to investigate, and, in some cases, understand, the biochemical mechanisms whereby cancer cells are formed and which mediate their abnormal behaviour.

The psychopath within

Cancer cells are psychopaths. They have no respect for the rights of other cells. They violate the democratic principles of normal cellular organisation. Their proliferation is uncontrolled; their ability to spread is unbounded. Their inexorable, relentless progress destroys first the tissue and then the person.

In order to behave in such an unprincipled fashion, cells have to acquire a number of characteristics before they are fully malignant. No one characteristic is sufficient, and not all characteristics are necessary. These features, based on an article by Hanahan and Weinberg, are given in Summary box 9.1.

> **Summary box 9.1**
>
> **Malignant transformation**
>
> - Establish an autonomous lineage:
>   - resist signals that inhibit growth
>   - acquire independence from signals stimulating growth
> - Obtain immortality
> - Evade apoptosis
> - Acquire angiogenic competence
> - Acquire the ability to invade
> - Acquire the ability to disseminate and implant
> - Evade detection/elimination
> - Genomic instability
> - Jettison excess baggage
> - Subvert communication to and from the environment/milieu
> - Develop ability to change energy metabolism

Establish an autonomous lineage

This involves developing independence from the normal signals that control supply and demand. The healing of a wound is a physiological process; the cellular response is exquisitely coordinated so that proliferation occurs when it is needed and ceases

Francis Harry Compton Crick, 1916–2004, a British molecular biologist who worked at the Cavendish Laboratory, Cambridge, UK and later at the Salk Institute, San Diego, CA, USA. Watson and Crick shared the 1962 Nobel Prize for Physiology or Medicine with Maurice Hugh Frederick Wilkins, 1916–2004, of King's College, London.

Rudolf Ludwig Carl Virchow, 1821–1902, Professor of Pathology, Berlin, Germany.
Theodor Heinrich Boveri, 1862–1913, Professor of Zoology and Comparative Anatomy, Wurzburg, Germany.
Oswald Theodore Avery, 1877–1955, a bacteriologist at the Rockefeller Institute, New York, NY, USA.
James Dewey Watson, born 1928, an American biologist who worked at Cambridge, UK, and later became Director of the Cold Spring Harbor Laboratory, New York, NY, USA.
Douglas Hanahan, born 1951, American biologist and director of the Swiss Institute for Experimental Cancer Research (ISREC), Lausanne, Switzerland.
Robert A Weinberg, born 1942, The Whitehead Institute of Biomedical Research and Department of Biology, The Massachusetts Institute of Technology, Cambridge, MA, USA.

when it is no longer required. The whole process is controlled by a series of signals telling cells when to divide and when not to divide. Cancer cells escape from this normal system of checks and balances: they grow and proliferate in the absence of external stimuli regardless of signals telling them not to do so. Oncogenes, an aberrant form of normal cellular genes, are a key factor in this process. They were originally identified as sequences within the genome of viruses that could cause cancer and initially thought to be viral in origin but, surprisingly, turned out to be parts of the normal genome that were hitch-hiking between cells, using the virus as a vector. Viral oncogenes (v-*onc*) had sequence homology with normal cellular genes (c-*onc*) and are now presumed to be mutated versions of genes concerned with normal cellular husbandry. The implication of this is that we all carry within us genetic sequences that, through mutation, can turn into active oncogenes and thereby cause malignant transformation.

Obtain immortality

According to the Hayflick hypothesis, normal cells are permitted to undergo only a finite number of divisions. For humans, this number is between 40 and 60. The limitation is imposed by the progressive shortening of the end of the chromosome (the telomere) that occurs each time a cell divides. Telomeric shortening is like a molecular clock and, when its time is up, the lineage will die out. Cancer cells can use the enzyme telomerase to rebuild the telomere at each cell division, so there is no telomeric shortening and the lineage will never die out. The cancer cell has achieved immortality.

Evade apoptosis

Apoptosis is a form of programmed cell death which occurs as the direct result of internal cellular events instructing the cell to die, rather than external events. Unlike necrosis, apoptosis is an orderly process. The cell dismantles itself neatly for disposal (Figure 9.1). There is a minimal inflammatory response. Apoptosis is a physiological process rediscovered in 1972 and named from the Greek αηοητωσιξ, meaning the act of falling. Cells that find themselves in the wrong place normally die by apoptosis and this is an important self-regulatory mechanism in growth and development. Genes, such as *p53*, that can activate apoptosis function as tumour suppressor genes. Loss of function in a tumour suppressor gene will contribute to malignant transformation. Cancer cells will be able to evade apoptosis, which means that the wrong cells can be in the wrong places at the wrong times.

Acquire angiogenic competence

A mass of tumour cells cannot, in the absence of a blood supply, grow beyond a diameter of about 1 mm. This places a severe restriction on the capabilities of the tumour: it cannot grow much larger or spread widely within the body. If, however, the mass of tumour cells is able to attract or construct a blood supply, then it may then quit its dormant state and behave in a far more aggressive fashion. The ability of a tumour to form blood vessels is termed 'angiogenic competence' and is a key feature of malignant transformation.

Leonard Hayflick, born 1928, while working at the Wistar Institute in Philadelphia in 1962, he noted that normal mammalian cells growing in culture had a limited, rather than an indefinite, capacity for self-replication.

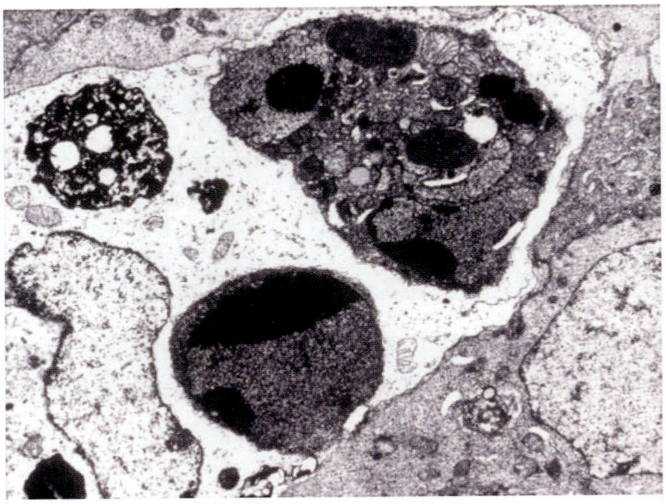

Figure 9.1 Electron micrograph of apoptotic bodies engulfed by a macrophage.

Acquire the ability to invade

Cancer cells have no respect for the structure of normal tissues. They acquire the ability to breach the basement membrane and thus gain direct access to blood and lymph vessels using three main mechanisms to facilitate invasion: (1) they cause a rise in the interstitial pressure within a tissue; (2) they secrete enzymes that dissolve extracellular matrix; and (3) they acquire motility. Unrestrained proliferation and a lack of contact inhibition enable cancer cells to exert pressure directly on the surrounding tissue and push themselves beyond normal limits. They secrete collagenases and proteases that chemically dissolve any extracellular boundaries that would otherwise limit their spread through tissues and by modulating the expression of cell surface molecules called integrins, are able to detach themselves from the extracellular matrix. The abnormal integrins associated with malignancy can also transmit signals from the environment to the cytoplasm and nucleus of the cancer cells ('outside-in signalling'), and these signals can induce increased motility.

Acquire the ability to disseminate and implant

Once cancer cells gain access to vascular and lymphovascular spaces, they have acquired the potential to use the body's natural transport mechanisms to distribute themselves throughout the body, although this will not, of itself, cause tumours to develop at distant sites. They also need to acquire the ability to implant. As Paget pointed out over a century ago, there is a crucial relationship here between the seed (the tumour cell) and the soil (the distant tissue). Most of the cancer cells discharged into the circulation probably do not form viable metastases: circulating cancer cells can be identified in patients who never develop clinical evidence of metastatic disease. Clumping may be important in permitting metastases: outer cells protecting inner cells from immunological attack. These outer protective cells may, on occasion, be normal lymphocytes.

Cancer can spread in this embolic fashion, but also when individual cells migrate and implant. Whether spread occurs in groups or individually, the cells still have to cross the vascular endothelium (and basement membrane) to gain access to the tissue itself. Cancer cells probably implant themselves in distant tissues by exploiting, and subverting, the normal inflammatory response. By expressing inflammatory cytokines, the cancer cells can fool the endothelium of the host tissue into becoming activated and allowing cancer cells access to the extravascular space. Activated endothelium expresses receptors that bind to integrins and selectins on the surface of leukocytes, and this allows the leukocytes to move across the endothelial barrier.

Evade detection/elimination

Cancer cells are simultaneously both 'self' and 'not self'. Although derived from normal cells ('self'), they are, in terms of their genetic make up, behaviour and characteristics, foreign ('not self'). As such, they ought to provoke an immune response and be eliminated and it is entirely possible that malignant transformation is a more frequent event than the emergence of clinical cancer. The possible role of the immune system in eliminating nascent cancers was proposed by Paul Ehrlich in 1909 and revisited by both Sir Frank McFarlane Burnet and Lewis Thomas in the late 1950s. Cancer cells, or at least those that give rise to clinical disease, appear to gain the ability to escape detection by the immune system. This may be by suppressing the expression of tumour-associated antigens, or it may be through actively coopting one part of the immune system to help the tumour to escape detection by other parts of the immune surveillance system.

Genomic instability

A cancer is a genetic ferment. Cells are dividing without proper checks and balances. Mutations are arising all the time and some, particularly those in tumour suppressor genes, may have the ability to encourage the development and persistence of further mutations. This gives rise to the phenomenon of genomic instability – as it evolves, a cancer contains an increasing variety and number of genetic aberrations: the greater the number of such abnormalities, the greater the chance of increasingly deviant behaviour.

Jettison excess baggage

Cancer cells are geared to excessive and remorseless proliferation. They do not need to develop or retain those specialised functions that make them good cellular citizens. They can therefore afford to repress or permanently lose those genes that control such functions. This may bring some short-term advantages. The longer-term disadvantage is that what is today superfluous may, tomorrow, be essential. This can leave cancer cells vulnerable to external stress and may, in part, explain why some cancer treatments work.

Subvert communication to and from the environment/milieu

Providing false information is a classic military strategy. Degrading the command and control systems of the enemy is an essential component of modern warfare. Cancer cells almost certainly use similar tactics in their battle for control over their host. Given the complexity of communication between and within cells, this is not an easy statement to prove or disprove. Nor does it offer any easy targets for therapeutic manipulation.

Develop ability to change energy metabolism

Blood flow in tumours is often sporadic and unreliable. As a result, cancer cells may have to spend prolonged periods starved of oxygen – in a state of relative hypoxia. Compared to the corresponding normal cells, some cancer cells may be better able to survive in hypoxic conditions. This ability may enable tumours to grow and develop despite an impoverished blood supply. Cancer cells can alter their metabolism even when oxygen is abundant, they break down glucose but do not, as normal cells would do, send the resulting pyruvate to the mitochondria for conversion, in an oxygen-dependent process, to carbon dioxide. This is the phenomenon of aerobic glycolysis, or the Warburg effect and leads to the production of lactate. In an act of symbiosis, lactate-producing cancer cells may provide lactate for adjacent cancer cells which are then able to use it, via the citric acid cycle, for energy production. This cooperation is similar to that which occurs in skeletal muscle during exercise.

Malignant transformation

The characteristics of the cancer cell arise as a result of mutation. Only very rarely is a single mutation sufficient to cause cancer; multiple mutations are usually required. Colorectal cancer provides the classical example of how multiple mutations are necessary for the complete transformation from normal to malignant cell. Vogelstein and colleagues identified the genes required and also postulated not only that it is necessary to have mutations in all the relevant genes, but also that these mutations must be acquired in a specific sequence.

Cancer is usually regarded as a clonal disease. Once a cell has arisen with all the mutations necessary to make it fully malignant, it is capable of giving rise to an infinite number of identical cells, each of which is fully malignant. These cells divide, invade, metastasise and destroy but, ultimately, each is the direct descendant of that original, primordial, transformed cell. There is certainly evidence, mostly from haematological malignancies,

Stephen Paget, 1855–1926, surgeon, The West London Hospital, London, UK. Paget's 'seed and soil' hypothesis is contained in his paper 'The distribution of secondary growths in cancer of the breast', in the *Lancet*, 1889.
Paul Ehrlich, 1854–1915, Professor of Hygiene, The University of Berlin, and later Director of The Institute for Infectious Diseases, Berlin, Germany. In 1908, he shared the Nobel Prize for Physiology or Medicine with **Elie Metchnikoff**, 1845–1916, 'in recognition of his work on immunity'. Metchnikoff was Professor of Zoology at Odessa in Russia, and later worked at the Pasteur Institute in Paris, France.

Sir Frank McFarlane Burnett, 1899–1985, an Australian virologist, at the Walter and Eliza Hall Institute, Melbourne, Australia. Burnett shared the 1960 Nobel Prize for Physiology or Medicine with **Sir Peter Brian Medawar**, 1915–1987, Jodrell Professor of Zoology, University College, London, UK, 'for their discovery of acquired immunological tolerance'.
Otto Warburg, 1883–1970, chemist, Director of the Kaiser Wilhelm Institute for Cell Physiology, Berlin-Dahlem. Awarded the Nobel Prize for Physiology or Medicine in 1931 for 'his discovery of the nature and mode of action of the respiratory enzyme'.

Lewis Thomas, 1913–1993, an American pathologist and immunologist, who became President of the Sloan Kettering Memorial Institute, New York, NY, USA.
Bert Vogelstein, born 1949, molecular biologist, Johns Hopkins Hospital, Baltimore, MD, USA.

to support the view that tumours are monoclonal in origin, but recent evidence challenges the universality of this assumption. Some cancers may arise from more than one clone of cells. Epigenetic modification refers to hereditable changes in DNA that are not related to the nucleotide sequence of the molecule. Epigenetic modification may give rise to distinct cancer cell lineages with differing biological properties. The interactions between cells from each lineage and the tissue within which such cells find themselves may determine the overall clinical behaviour of a tumour.

Two mechanisms may help to sustain and accelerate the process of malignant transformation: genomic instability and tumour-related inflammation.

Genomic instability

If a tumour is a genetic ferment, then there is abundant opportunity for mutations to occur in the DNA of tumour cells, some of these mutations (for example, those occurring in tumour suppressor genes) may themselves be capable of facilitating the persistence of further mutations and so the pace of malignant transformation can be accelerated.

Tumour-related inflammation

If a tumour provokes an inflammatory response, then the cytokines and other factors produced as a result of that response may act to promote and sustain malignant transformation. Growth factors, mutagenic ROS (reactive oxygen species), angiogenic factors, anti-apoptotic factors, may all be produced as part of an inflammatory process and all may contribute to the progression of a tumour.

A recurring theme in the molecular biology of cancer is that systems and pathways can behave unpredictably – activation may sometimes promote, and sometimes inhibit, growth and transformation. This has important implications for therapy – treatments designed to inhibit the growth and spread of cancer may, occasionally, have precisely the opposite effect. The most consistent feature of cancer is its lack of consistency.

The growth of a tumour

If it is accepted that a cancer starts from a single transformed cell, then it is possible, using straightforward arithmetic, to describe the progression from a single cell to a mass of cells large enough to kill the host. The division of a cell produces two daughter cells. The relationship 2^n will describe the number of cells produced after n generations of division. There are between 10^{13} and 10^{14} cells in a typical human being. A tumour 10 mm in diameter will contain about 10^9 cells. As $2^{30} = 10^9$, this implies that it would take 30 generations to reach the threshold of clinical detectability and, as $2^{45} = 3 \times 10^{13}$, fewer than 15 subsequent generations to produce a tumour that, through sheer bulk alone, would be fatal. This is an oversimplification because cell loss is a feature of many tumours and, for squamous cancers, as many as 99 per cent of the cells produced may be lost, mainly by exfoliation. It will, in the presence of cell loss, take many cellular divisions to produce a clinically evident tumour – abundant opportunity for further mutations to occur during the preclinical phase of tumour growth. The growth of a typical human tumour can be described by an exponential relationship, the doubling time of which increases exponentially – so-called Gompertzian growth (Figure 9.2). This Gompertzian pattern has several important implications for the diagnosis and treatment of cancer (Summary box 9.2).

Summary box 9.2

Clinical implications of Gompertzian growth

- The majority of the growth of a tumour occurs before it is clinically detectable
- By the time they are detected, tumours have passed the period of most rapid growth, that period when they might be most sensitive to anti-proliferative drugs
- There has been plenty of time, before diagnosis, for individual cells to detach, invade, implant and form distant metastases – in many patients cancer may, at presentation, be a systemic disase.
- 'Early tumours' are genetically old: plenty of time for mutations to have occurred, mutations that might confer spontaneous drug resistance (a probability greatly increased by the existence of cell loss)
- The rate of regression of a tumour will depend upon its age (the Norton–Simon hypothesis extends this: the rate of regression of a tumour will depend upon its growth rate at the time of treatment)

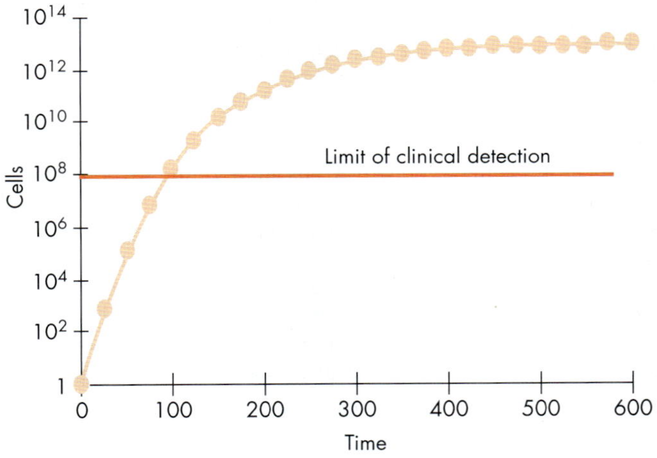

Figure 9.2 The Gompertzian curve describing the growth of a typical tumour. In its early stages, growth is exponential but, as the tumour grows, the growth rate slows. This decrease in growth rate probably arises because of difficulties with nutrition and oxygenation. The tumour cells are in competition: not only with the tissues of the host, but also with each other.

Benjamin Gompertz, 1779–1865, an insurance actuary who was interested in calculating annuities. To do this, he needed to describe mathematically the relationship between life-expectancy and age. He was able to do this using the function that bears his name. The Gompertzian function provides an excellent fit to data points plotting tumour size against time.

THE CAUSES OF CANCER

The interplay between nature and nurture

Both inheritance and environment are important determinants of cancer development. Although environmental factors have been implicated in more than 80 per cent of cases, this still leaves plenty of scope for the role of genetic inheritance: not just the 20 per cent of tumours for which there is no clear environmental contribution but also, as environment alone can rarely cause cancer, the genetic contribution to the 80 per cent of tumours to which environmental factors contribute.

Knowledge about the causes of cancer can be used to design appropriate strategies for prevention or earlier diagnosis. As more is discovered about the genes associated with cancer, genetic testing and counselling will play an increasing role in its prevention. These considerations are incorporated into Table 9.1 on the inherited cancer syndromes, and Table 9.2 on the environmental contribution to cancer.

Table 9.1 Inherited syndromes associated with cancer.

Syndrome	Gene(s) implicated	Inheritance	Associated tumours and abnormalities	Strategies for prevention/early diagnosis
Familial adenomatous polyposis (FAP)/ Gardner syndrome	*APC* gene	D	Colorectal cancer under the age of 25 years Papillary carcinoma of the thyroid Cancer of the ampulla of Vater Hepatoblastomas Primary brain tumours (Turcot's syndrome) Osteomas of the jaw CHRPE (congenital hypertrophy of the retinal pigment epithelium)	Prophylactic panproctocolectomy
Hereditary non-polyposis colorectal cancer (HNPCC)	DNA mismatch repair genes (*MLH1*, *MSH2*, *MSH6*)	D	Colorectal cancer (typically in the 40s and 50s)	Surveillance colonoscopies/ polypectomies Non-steroidal anti-inflammatory drugs
HNPCC1	*MSH2*		Endometrium, stomach, hepatobiliary (Lynch's syndrome 1)	
HNPCC2	*MLH1*			
HNPCC3	*PMS1*			
Peutz–Jeghers syndrome	*STK11*	D	Bowel cancer, breast cancer, freckles round the mouth	Surveillance colonoscopy, mammography
Cowden's syndrome	*PTEN*	D	Multiple hamartomas of skin, breast and mucus membranes Breast cancer Neuroendocrine tumours Endometrial cancer, thyroid cancer	Active surveillance
Retinoblastoma	*RB*	D	Retinoblastoma Pinealoma Osteosarcoma	Surveillance of the uninvolved eye
Multiple endocrine neoplasia (MEN) type 1	*Menin*	D	Parathyroid tumours Islet cell tumours Pituitary tumours	Awareness of associations and paying attention to relevant symptoms
MEN type 2A	*RET*	D	Medullary carcinoma of the thyroid Phaeochromocytoma Parathyroid tumours	Regular screening of blood pressure, serum calcitonin and urinary catecholamines Prophylactic thyroidectomy

Eldon J Gardner, born 1909, Professor of Zoology, Utah State University, Salt Lake City, UT, USA.
Abraham Vater, 1684–1751, Professor of Anatomy and Botany, and later of Pathology and Therapeutics, Wittenburg, Germany.
Jacques Turcot, born 1914, surgeon, Hôtel Dieu de Quebec Hospital, Quebec, Canada.
Henry T Lynch, born 1928, oncologist, Chairman of the Department of Preventive Medicine, Creighton School of Medicine, California, USA.
John Law Augustine Peutz, 1886–1968, Chief Specialist for Internal Medicine, St John's Hospital, The Hague, The Netherlands.
Harold Joseph Jeghers, 1904–1990, Professor of Internal Medicine, The New Jersey College of Medicine and Dentistry, Jersey City, NJ, USA.
One of the few clinical syndromes named after the patient rather than the clinician, **Rachel Cowden** was, in 1963, the first patient described with the syndrome. She died from breast cancer at the age of 20.

Table 9.1 Inherited syndromes associated with cancer – *continued.*

Syndrome	Gene(s) implicated	Inheritance	Associated tumours and abnormalities	Strategies for prevention/early diagnosis
MEN type 2b	*RET*	D	Medullary carcinoma of the thyroid Phaeochromocytoma Mucosal neuromas Ganglioneuromas of the gut	Regular screening of blood pressure, serum calcitonin and urinary catecholamines Prophylactic thyroidectomy
Li–Fraumeni syndrome	*p53*	D	Sarcomas Leukaemia Osteosarcomas Brain tumours Adrenocortical carcinomas	Very difficult, as the pattern of tumours is so heterogeneous and varies from patient to patient
Familial breast cancer	*BRCA1*, *BRCA2*	D	Breast cancer Ovarian cancer Papillary serous carcinoma of the peritoneum Prostate cancer	Screening mammography Pelvic ultrasound Prostate-specific antigen in males Prophylactic mastectomy Prophylactic oophorectomy
Familial cutaneous malignant melanoma	*CDNK2A*, *CDK4*	D	Cutaneous malignant melanoma	Avoid exposure to sunlight, careful surveillance
Basal cell naevus syndrome (Gorlin)	*PTCH*	D	Basal cell carcinomas Medulloblastoma Bifid ribs	Careful surveillance, awareness of diagnosis (look for bifid ribs on x-ray)
Von Hippel–Lindau syndrome	*VHL*	D	Renal cancer Phaeochromocytoma Haemangiomas of the cerebellum and retina	Urinary catecholamines
Neurofibromatosis type 1	*NF1*	D	Astrocytomas Primitive neuroectodermal tumours Optic gliomas Multiple neurofibromas	A difficult problem; maintain a high index of suspicion concerning any rapid changes in the growth or character of any nodule
Neurofibromatosis type 2	*NF2*	D	Acoustic neuromas Spinal tumours Meningiomas Multiple neurofibromas	
Xeroderma pigmentosum	Deficient nucleotide excision repair (*XPA, B, C*)	R	Skin sensitive to sunlight; early onset of cutaneous carcinomas (SCCs, BCCs)	Avoidance of sun exposure Active surveillance and early treatment Retinoids for chemoprevention
Ataxia telangiectasia	*AT*	R	Progressive cerebellar ataxia Leukaemia Lymphoma Breast Melanoma Upper gastrointestinal	Active surveillance
Bloom's syndrome	*BLM helicase*	R	Sensitivity to UV light Leukaemia Lymphoma	Active surveillance

BCC, basal cell carcinoma; D, dominant; R, recessive; SCC, squamous cell carcinoma; UV, ultraviolet.

Frederick P Li, born 1940, Professor of Medicine, Harvard University Medical School, Boston, MA, USA.
Joseph F Fraumeni, born 1933, Director of Cancer Epidemiology and Genetics, The National Cancer Institute, Bethesda, MD, USA.
Robert Gorlin, 1923–2006, Professor of Dentistry, The University of Minnesota, Minneapolis, MN, USA.
Eugen von Hippel, 1867–1939, Professor of Ophthalmology, Göttingen, Germany.
Arvid Lindau, 1892–1958, Professor of Pathology, Lund, Sweden.
David Bloom, born 1892, a dermatologist at the Skin and Cancer Clinic, New York University, New York, NY, USA, described the syndrome in 1954.

Table 9.2 Environmental causes of cancer (and suggested measures for reducing their impact).

Environmental/behavioural factor			Associated tumours	Strategy for prevention/early diagnosis
Tobacco			Lung cancer Head and neck cancer	Ban tobacco Ban smoking in public places Punitive taxes on tobacco
Alcohol			Head and neck cancer Oesophageal cancer Hepatoma	Avoid excess alcohol Surveillance of high-risk individuals
UV exposure			Melanoma Non-melanoma skin cancer	Avoid excessive sun exposure, avoid sunbeds
Ionising radiation			Leukaemia Breast Lymphoma Thyroid	Limit medical exposures to the absolute minimum; safety precautions at nuclear facilities; monitor radiation workers
Viral infections	HPV		Cervix Penis	Avoid unprotected sex Vaccination
	HIV		Kaposi's sarcoma Lymphomas Germ cell tumours Anal cancer	Avoid unprotected sex Anti-retroviral therapy
	Hepatitis B		Hepatoma	Avoid contaminated injections/infusions Vaccination
Other infections	Bilharzia		Bladder cancer	Treatment of infection Cystoscopic surveillance
	Helicobacter pylori		Stomach cancer	Eradication therapy
Inhaled particles	Asbestos		Mesothelioma	Protection of exposed workers
	Wood dust		Paranasal sinus cancers	Protection of exposed workers
Chemicals	Environmental pollutants/chemicals used in industry		Angiosarcoma (vinyl chloride) Bladder cancer (aniline dyes, vulcanisation of rubber) Lung, nasal cavity (nickel) Skin (arsenic) Lung (beryllium, cadmium, chromium) All sites (dioxins)	Protection of exposed workers; avoid chemical discharge and spillages
	Medical	Alkylating agents used in cytotoxic chemotherapy	Leukaemia Lymphoma Lung cancer	Avoid overtreatment; only combine drugs with ionising radiation when absolutely necessary
		Immunosuppressive treatment	Kaposi's sarcoma	As low a dose as possible, for as short a period as possible
		Stilbestrol	Adenocarcinoma of the vagina in daughters of treated mothers	Use of stilbestrol curtailed
		Tamoxifen	Endometrial cancer	Biopsy if patient on tamoxifen develops uterine bleeding
Fungal and plant toxins	Aflatoxins		Hepatoma	Appropriate food storage, screen for fungal contamination of foodstuffs

Table 9.2 Environmental causes of cancer (and suggested measures for reducing their impact) – *continued.*

Environmental/behavioural factor	Associated tumours	Strategy for prevention/early diagnosis
Obesity/lack of physical exercise	Breast Endometrium Kidney Colon Oesophagus	Maintain ideal body weight, regular exercise

HIV, human immunodeficiency virus; HPV, human papillomavirus; UV, ultraviolet.

THE MANAGEMENT OF CANCER

Management is more than treatment

The traditional approach to cancer concentrates on diagnosis and active treatment. This is a very limited view that, in terms of the public health, may not have served society well. It implies a fatalistic attitude to the occurrence of cancer and an assumption that, once active treatment is complete, there is little more do be done. Prevention is forgotten and rehabilitation ignored. Cancer management can be considered as taking place along two axes: one an axis of scale, from the individual to the world population; the other based on the unnatural history of the disease, from prevention to rehabilitation or palliative care (see Figure 9.3).

Prevention

Table 9.2 summarises the approaches that can be used in the prevention of cancer. In 1998, Sir Richard Doll estimated that 30 per cent of cancer deaths were due to tobacco use and that up to 50 per cent of cancer deaths were related to diet. Even allowing for overlap (smokers often have a poor diet), these are impressive figures and add some perspective to the often inflated claims made for the achievements of cancer treatment. Doll estimated that cancers related to occupation accounted for less than 4 per cent of cancer deaths, and that environmental pollution accounted for less than 5 per cent of deaths.

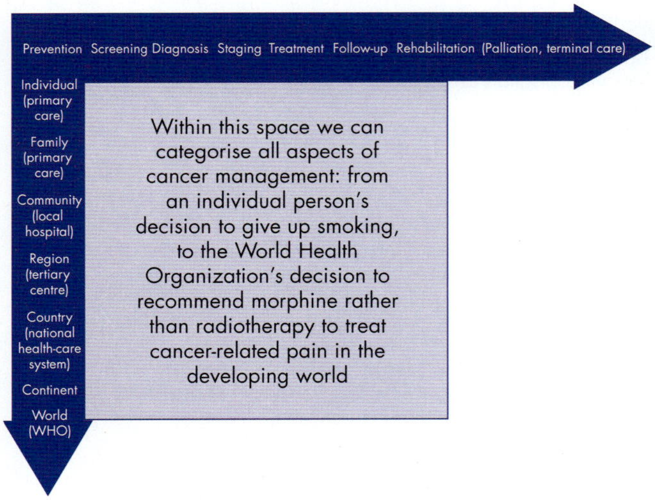

Figure 9.3 The management of cancer spans the natural history of the disease and all humankind, from the individual to the population of the world. WHO, World Health Organization.

Sir William Richard Shaboe Doll, 1912–2005, Regius Professor of Medicine, Oxford University, Oxford, UK, and Sir Austin Bradford Hill, Professor of Medical Statistics, The London School of Hygiene and Tropical Medicine, London, UK, published one of the definitive reports linking smoking to lung cancer in 1950.

Screening

Screening involves the detection of disease in an asymptomatic population in order to improve outcomes by early diagnosis. It follows that a successful screening programme must achieve early diagnosis, and that the disease in question has a better outcome when treated at an early stage. The criteria that must be fulfilled for the disease, screening test and the screening programme itself are given in Summary box 9.3.

Summary box 9.3

Criteria for screening

- The disease
  - Recognisable early stage
  - Treatment at an early stage more effective than at a later stage
  - Sufficiently common to warrant screening
- The test
  - Sensitive and specific
  - Acceptable to the screened population
  - Safe
  - Inexpensive
- The programme
  - Adequate diagnostic facilities for those with a positive test
  - High-quality treatment for screen-detected disease to minimise morbidity and mortality
  - Screening repeated at intervals if the disease is of insidious onset
  - Benefit must outweigh physical and psychological harm

Merely to prove that screening picks up disease at an early stage, and that the outcome is better for patients with screen-detected disease than for those who present with symptoms, is an insufficient criterion for the success of a screening programme. This is because of inherent biases in screening (lead time bias, selection bias and length bias), which make screen-detected disease appear to be associated with better outcomes than symptomatic disease. Lead time bias describes the phenomenon whereby early detection of a disease will always prolong survival from the time of diagnosis when compared with disease picked up at a later stage in its development whether or not the screening process has altered the progression of the tumour (Figure 9.4). Selection bias describes the finding that individuals who accept an invitation for screening are, in general, healthier than those who do not. It follows that individuals with screen-detected disease will tend, independently of the condition for which screening is being performed, to live longer. Length bias is brought about by the fact that slow-growing tumours are likely to be picked up by screening, whereas fast-growing tumours are likely to arise and produce symptoms in between screening rounds. Thus, screen-detected tumours will tend to be less aggressive than symptomatic tumours. Because of these biases, it is essential to carry out population-based randomised controlled trials and to compare mortality rate in a whole population offered screening (including those who refuse to be screened and those who develop cancer after a negative test) with mortality rate in a population that has not been offered screening.

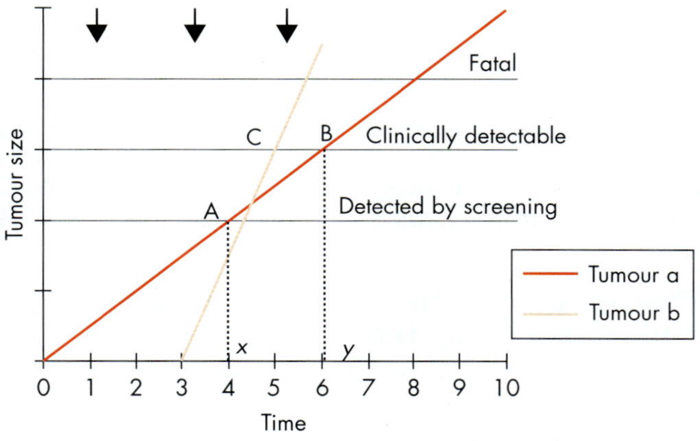

Figure 9.4 Lead time and length bias. Tumour 'a' is a steadily growing tumour; its progress is uninfluenced by any treatment. The arrows indicate the timing of tests in a screening programme. The horizontal lines indicate three thresholds: detectability by screening; clinical detectability; and death due to tumour progression. Point A indicates the time at which the tumour would be diagnosed in a screening programme and point B indicates the time at which the tumour would be diagnosed clinically, that is in the absence of any screening programme. If the date of diagnosis is used as the start time for measuring survival, then it is clear that, in the absence of any effect from treatment, the screening programme will artefactually add to the survival time. The amount of 'increased' survival is equal to $y - x$ years, in this example, just over two years. This artefactual inflation of survival time is referred to as lead time bias. Tumour 'b' is a rapidly growing tumour; again, its progress is uninfluenced by treatment. It grows so rapidly that, in the interval between two screening tests, it can cross both the threshold for detectability by screening and that of clinical detectability. It will continue to progress rapidly after diagnosis, and the measured survival time will be short. This phenomenon, whereby those tumours that are 'missed' by the screening programme are associated with decreased survival, is called length bias.

This research design has been applied to both breast cancer and colorectal cancer: in both cases, there was reduction in disease-specific mortality.

Diagnosis and classification

Accurate diagnosis is the key to the successful management of cancer. Diagnosis lies at the heart of the epidemiology of cancer; if there is an inaccurate picture of the pattern of a disease, reliable inferences about its distribution and causes cannot be drawn. Precise diagnosis is crucial to the choice of correct therapy; the wrong operation, no matter how superbly performed, is useless. An unequivocal diagnosis is the key to an accurate prognosis. Only rarely can a diagnosis of cancer confidently be made in the absence of tissue for pathological or cytological examination. Cancer is a disease of cells and, for accurate diagnosis, the abnormal cells need to be seen. Different tumours are classified in different ways: most squamous epithelial tumours are simply classed as well (G1), moderate (G2) or poorly (G3) differentiated (Figure 9.5). Adenocarcinomas are also often classified as G1, 2 or 3, but prostate cancer is an exception with widespread use of the Gleason system. The Gleason system grades prostate cancer according to the degree of differentiation of the two most prevalent architectural patterns. The final score is the sum of the two grades and can vary from 2 (1 + 1) to 10 (5 + 5), with the higher scores indicating poorer prognosis. The management of malignant lymphomas is based firmly upon histopathological classification: the first distinction is between Hodgkin's lymphoma (HL) and non-Hodgkin's lymphoma (NHL). Each of these main types of lymphoma is then subclassified according to a different scheme. The World Health Organization/Revised European–American Lymphoma (WHO/REAL) system classifies Hodgkin's lymphoma into classical HL (nodular sclerosis HL; mixed cellularity HL; lymphocyte depletion HL; lymphocyte-rich classical HL) and nodular lymphocyte-predominant HL. The WHO/REAL classification of NHL is considerably more complex and recognises 27 distinct pathological subtypes. It is perhaps no coincidence that the non-surgical treatment of lymphomas is, by and large, more successful than the non-surgical treatment of solid tumours. This suggests that precise and accurate subtyping of tumours enables appropriate selection of treatment and, in turn, this is associated with better outcome.

Investigation and staging

It is not sufficient simply to know what a cancer is; it is imperative to know its site and extent. If it is localised, then locoregional treatments such as surgery and radiation therapy may be curative. If the disease is widespread, then, although such local interventions may contribute to cure, they will be insufficient, and systemic treatment, for example with drugs or hormones, will be required. Staging is the process whereby the extent of disease is mapped out. Formerly, staging was a fairly crude process, but nowadays it is a highly sophisticated process, heavily reliant on the technology of modern imaging. These technological advances bring with them the implication that patients staged as having localised disease in 2012 are not comparable to patients described in 1985 as having localised disease. Many of these latter patients would have had occult metastatic disease detected had they been imaged using current technology. This

Donald F Gleason, born 1920, pathologist, The University of Minnesota, Minneapolis, MN, USA.
Thomas Hodgkin, 1798–1866, Curator of the Museum and Demonstrator of Morbid Anatomy, Guy's Hospital, London, UK, described lymphadenoma in 1832.

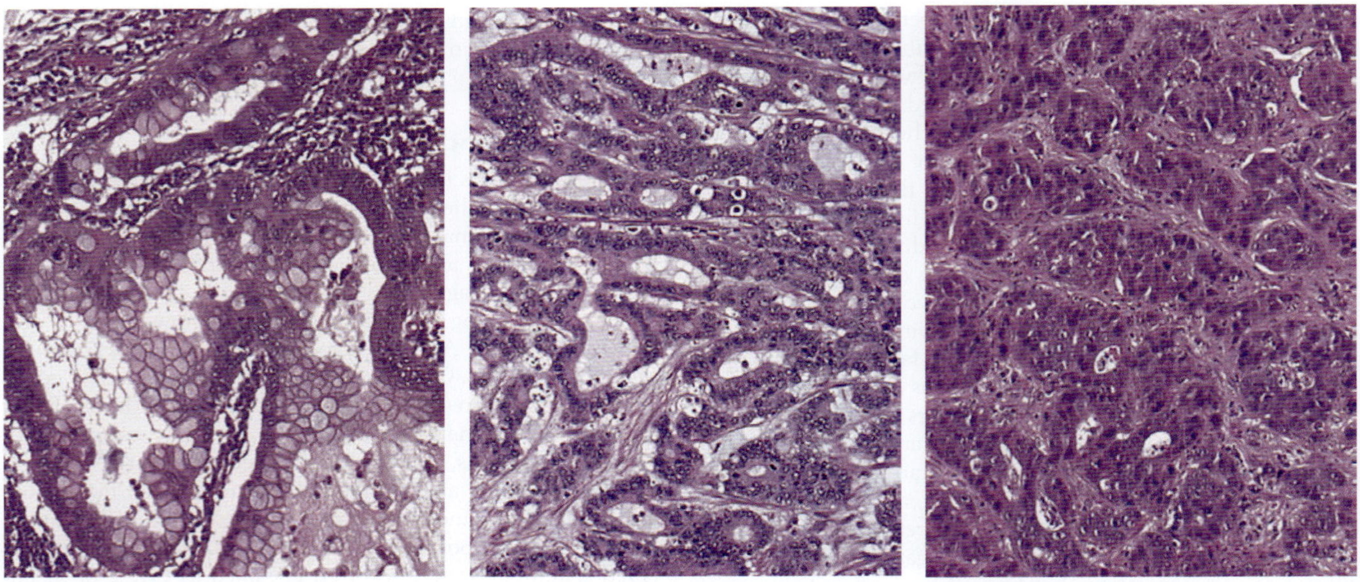

Figure 9.5 Three carcinomas showing different degrees of differentiation. Left to right: well-differentiated, moderately differentiated and poorly differentiated.

leads to the paradox of stage shift, also named the Will Rogers phenomenon by Alvan Feinstein. A change in staging system, or in the techniques used to provide baseline information concerning staging, can produce 'benefits' to patients at all stages of the disease. These benefits are, however, entirely artefactual and depend simply upon patients in each stage being enriched by patients with improved prognosis. The important cross-check to protect against being misled by stage shift is that the prognosis for the entire group (i.e. all stages pooled) has not been changed. Table 9.3 shows a worked example of stage shift.

The International Union against Cancer (UICC) is responsible for the TNM (tumour, nodes, metastases) staging system for cancer. This system is compatible with, and relates to, the American Joint Committee on Cancer (AJCC) system for stage grouping of cancer. Examples of clinicopathological staging systems for colon cancer are shown in Tables 9.4 and 9.5.

Therapeutic decision making and the multidisciplinary team

As the management of cancer becomes more complex, it becomes impossible for any individual clinician to have the intellectual and technical competence that is necessary to manage all the patients presenting with a particular type of

Table 9.3 Stage shift.

Before new staging test				After new staging test				
Stage	Distribution (per cent)	Cure rate (per cent)	Number cured	Stage	Distribution (per cent)	Cure rate (per cent)	Number cured	'Improvement' in cure rate (per cent)
I	70	90	63	I	50	94	47	4
II	10	80	8	II	10	80	8	0
III	10	80	8	III	10	80	8	0
IV	10	50	5	IV	30	70	21	20
All	100		84	All	100		84	0

The cure rate improves in both stage I and stage IV, and there is no change in cure rates for stage II and stage III, after the introduction of a new staging investigation. The overall cure rate is, however, unchanged.

Alvan Feinstein, 1926–2001, American Clinician and Epidemiologist.
Will Rogers (properly William Penn Adair Rogers), 1879–1935, American Actor, Humorist and Wit.
There is much confusion about the use of the terms '**multidisciplinary**' and '**multiprofessional**': we use 'multidisciplinary' to imply the presence of various medically qualified specialists (pathologists, radiologists, etc.) and 'multiprofessional' implies the presence of specialists from non-medical backgrounds (nurses, social workers, radiographers).

Table 9.4 Staging of colorectal cancer.

TNM	
TX, Primary tumour cannot be assessed	
T0, No evidence of primary tumour	
Tis, Intraepithelial or intramucosal carcinoma	
T1, Tumour invades submucosa	
T2, Tumour invades muscularis propria	
T3, Tumour invades through the muscularis propria into the subserosa or into retroperitoneal (pericolic or perirectal) tissues	
	a, Minimal invasion: <1 mm beyond muscularis
	b, Slight invasion: 1–5 mm beyond muscularis
	c, Moderate invasion: >5–15 mm beyond muscularis
	d, Extensive invasion: >15 mm beyond muscularis
T4, Tumour directly invades beyond bowel	
	a, Direct invasion into other organs or structures
	b, Perforates visceral peritoneum
NX, Regional lymph nodes cannot be assessed	
N0, No metastases in regional nodes	
N1, Metastases in 1–3 regional lymph nodes	
N2, Metastases in ≥4 regional lymph nodes	
MX, Not possible to assess the presence of distant metastases	
M0, No distant metastases	
M1, Distant metastases present	

Table 9.5 Relationships between staging systems for colorectal cancer.

TNM	AJCC	Dukes	Modified Astler–Coller
TisN0M0	0	–	–
T1N0M0	I	A	A
T2N0M0	I	A	B1
T3N0M0	IIA	B	B2
T4N0M0	IIB	B	B3
T1 or T2 N1M0	IIIA	C	C1
T3 or T4 N1M0	IIIB	C	C2, C3
Any T N2M0	IIIC	C	C1, C2, C3
Any T Any N M1	IV	D	–

tumour. The formation of multidisciplinary teams represents an attempt to make certain that each and every patient with a particular type of cancer is managed appropriately. Teams should not only be multidisciplinary, they should be multiprofessional (Summary box 9.4).

Summary box 9.4

Members of the multiprofessional team

- Site-specialist surgeon
- Surgical oncologist
- Plastic and reconstructive surgeon
- Clinical oncologist/radiotherapist
- Medical oncologist
- Diagnostic radiologist
- Pathologist
- Speech therapist
- Physiotherapist
- Prosthetist
- Clinical nurse specialist (rehabilitation, supportive care)
- Palliative care nurse (symptom control, palliation)
- Social worker/counsellor
- Medical secretary/administrator
- Audit and information coordinator

The advantages and disadvantages of multidisciplinary teams are summarised in Table 9.6.

Principles of cancer surgery

For most solid tumours, surgery remains the definitive treatment and the only realistic hope of cure. However, surgery has several

Vernon B Astler, surgeon, The Medical School of the University of Michigan, Ann Arbor, MI, USA.
Frederick A Coller, pathologist, The Medical School of the University of Michigan, Ann Arbor, MI, USA.
Cuthbert Esquire Dukes, 1890–1977, pathologist, St Mark's Hospital, London, UK.

Table 9.6 The advantages and disadvantages of the multidisciplinary team.

Advantages	Disadvantages
Open debate concerning management	An opportunity for rampant egotism and showing off
Patient has the advantage of many simultaneous opinions from many different specialties	Less confident and less articulate members of the team may not be able to express their views, even though their views may be extremely important
Decision making is open, transparent and explicit	May degenerate into a rubber-stamping exercise in which the class solutions implied by guidelines are unthinkingly applied to disparate individuals
Team members educate each other	Decisions are made in the absence of patients and their carers: the commodification of the person
A useful educational experience for trainees and students	Clinicians are able to avoid having to take responsibility for their decisions and their actions: the figleaf of 'corporate responsibility'
	Time-consuming and resource intensive: takes busy clinicians away from clinical practice for hours at a time

roles in cancer treatment including diagnosis, removal of primary disease, removal of metastatic disease, palliation, prevention and reconstruction.

Diagnosis and staging

In most cases, the diagnosis of cancer has been made before definitive surgery is carried out but, occasionally, a surgical procedure is required to make the diagnosis. This is particularly true of patients with malignant ascites where laparoscopy has an important role in obtaining tissue for diagnosis. Laparoscopy is also widely used for the staging of intra-abdominal malignancy, particularly oesophageal and gastric cancer. By this means, it is often possible to diagnose widespread peritoneal disease and small liver metastases that may have been missed on cross-sectional imaging. Laparoscopic ultrasound is a particularly useful adjunct for the diagnosis of intrahepatic metastases. Other examples in which surgery is central to the diagnosis of cancer include orchidectomy where a patient is suspected of having testicular cancer and lymph node biopsy in a patient with lymphoma. Recently, sentinel node biopsy in melanoma and breast cancer has attracted a great deal of interest. Here, a radiolabelled colloid is injected into or around the primary tumour, and the regional lymph nodes are scanned with a gamma camera that will pinpoint the lymph node nearest to the tumour. This lymph node can then be removed for histological diagnosis. Until recently, staging laparotomy was an important aspect of the staging of lymphomas but, with more accurate cross-sectional imaging and the much more widespread use of chemotherapy, this practice is now largely redundant.

Removal of primary disease

Radical surgery for cancer involves removal of the primary tumour and as much of the surrounding tissue and lymph node drainage as possible in order not only to ensure local control but also to prevent spread of the tumour through the lymphatics. Although the principle of local control is still extremely important, it is now recognised that ultraradical surgery probably has little effect on the development of metastatic disease, as evidenced by the randomised trials of radical versus simple mastectomy for breast cancer. It is important, however, to appreciate that high-quality, meticulous surgery taking care not to disrupt the primary tumour at the time of excision is of the utmost importance in obtaining a cure in localised disease and preventing local recurrence.

Removal of metastatic disease

In certain circumstances, surgery for metastatic disease may be appropriate. This is particularly true for liver metastases arising from colorectal cancer where successful resection of all detectable disease can lead to long-term survival in about one-third of patients. With multiple liver metastases, it may still be possible to take a surgical approach by using *in situ* ablation with cryotherapy or radiofrequency energy. Another situation where surgery may be of value is pulmonary resection for isolated lung metastases, particularly from renal cell carcinoma.

Palliation

In many cases, surgery is not appropriate for cure but may be extremely valuable for palliation. A good example is the patient with a symptomatic primary tumour who also has distant metastases. In this case, removal of the primary may improve the patient's quality of life, but will have little effect on the ultimate outcome. Other examples include bypass procedures, such as an ileotransverse anastomosis to alleviate symptoms of obstruction caused by an inoperable caecal cancer or bypassing an unresectable carcinoma at the head of the pancreas by cholecysto- or choledochojejunostomy to alleviate jaundice.

Principles underlying the non-surgical treatment of cancer

The relationship between dose and response and the principle of selective toxicity

Non-surgical treatments, in common with surgery, have the potential to cause harm as well as benefit. Surgery is difficult to quantify; it is hard to describe a mastectomy in units of measure.

Both drugs and radiation can be expressed in reproducible units: milligrams in the case of drugs; Grays (Gy) in the case of radiation. Thus, in contrast to surgery, it is possible to construct dose–response relationships for both the benefits (such as tumour cure rate) and harms (such as tissue damage that is both severe and permanent) associated with non-surgical interventions. These curves (see Figure 9.6) have the same general shape: they are sigmoidal. The practical consequence of this is that, over a relatively narrow dose range, we move from failure to success, from tolerability to disaster. In theory, it is possible to calculate an optimal dose for treating each tumour using dose–response curves: the dose is that which is associated with the maximal probability of an uncomplicated cure. Lying behind the concept of the probability of an uncomplicated cure is the principle of selective toxicity: the treatment should be selectively toxic to the tumour and, as far as possible, should spare the normal tissues from damage. It is this simple principle that underpins both the selection of agents used to treat cancer and the schedules employed to deliver them. Although the graphical representations of the relationships between dose, response and the probability of uncomplicated cure are conceptually simple and intuitively appealing, they are, in clinical practice, impractical. The construction of full dose–response curves for all possible combinations of tumours and normal tissues is neither feasible nor ethical. Reliance, when it comes to defining optimal doses and schedules, must be on incomplete clinical data and a knowledge of the general shape of the relationship between dose and response.

Louis Harold Gray, 1905–1965, director, The British Empire Cancer Campaign Research Unit in Radiobiology, Mount Vernon Hospital, Northwood, Middlesex, UK. A Gray (Gy) is the SI unit for the absorbed dose of ionising radiation.

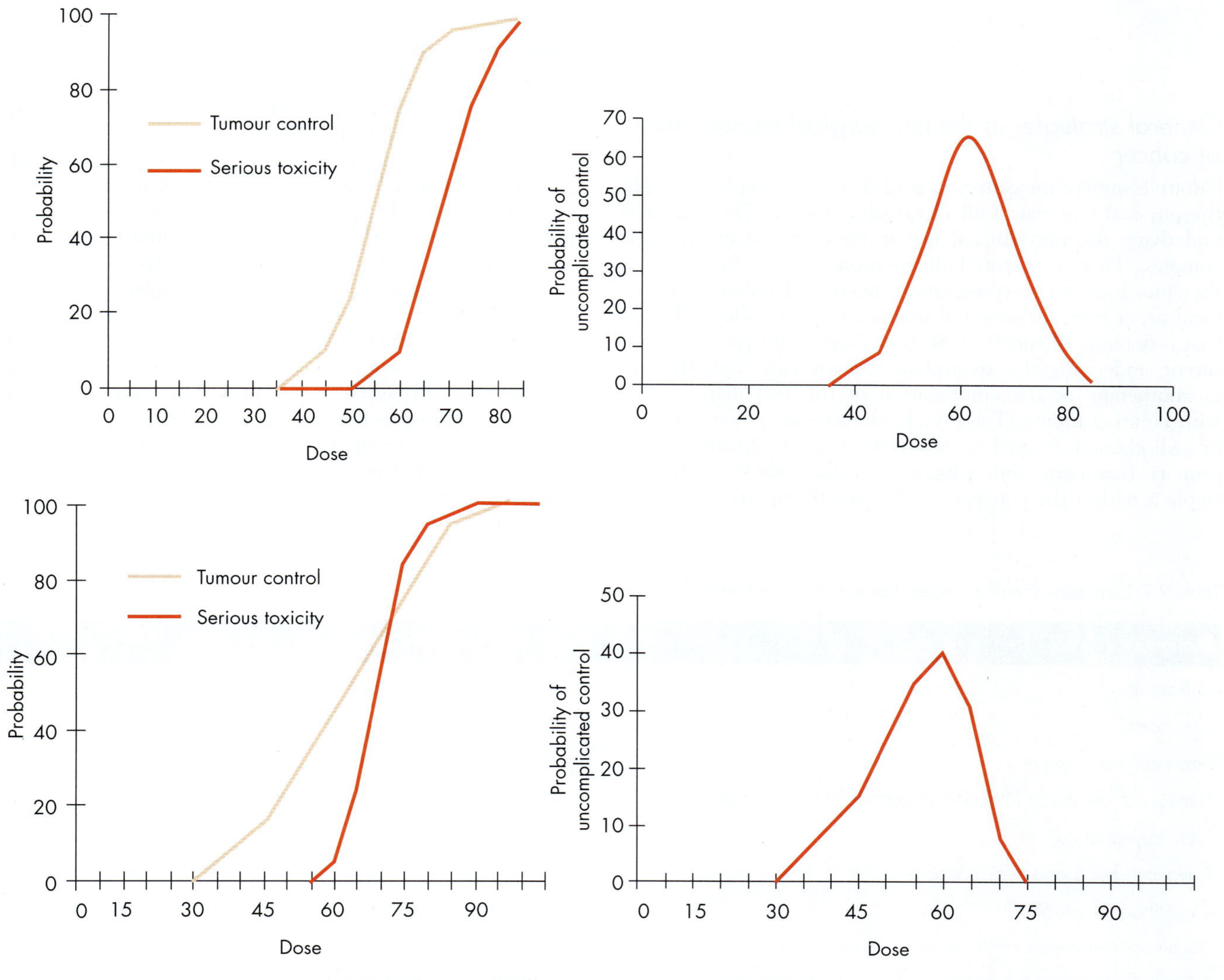

Figure 9.6 A schematic illustration of the relationship between dose, response and the probability of uncomplicated cure. The upper figures show ideal circumstances with steep dose–response relationships for both normal tissue damage and tumour control. The lower figures show something more like the real world. The dose–response relationship for tumour control is flatter, because tumours are heterogeneous and, consequently, the probability of uncomplicated cure is lower – even for the optimal dose (40 per cent in the lower figure compared with 70 per cent in the upper figure).

in situ is Latin for 'in the place'.

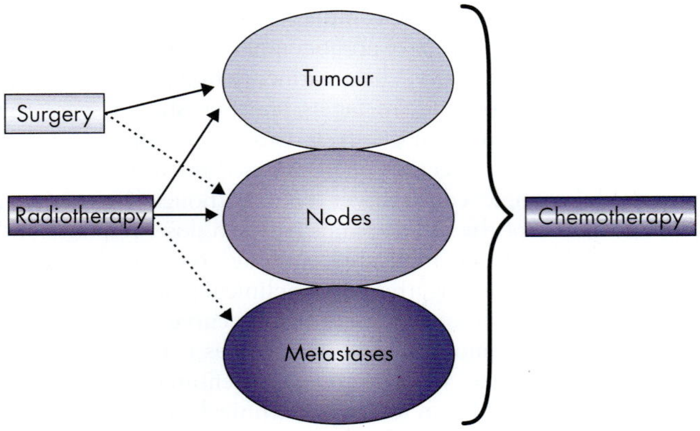

Figure 9.7 Schematic diagram to show the spatial scope of cancer treatments. Chemotherapy is systemic; surgery is mainly a local treatment. Radiotherapy is usually local or locoregional, but can, as in radioiodine therapy for thyroid cancer, be systemic.

General strategies in the non-surgical management of cancer

Curative surgery for cancer is guided by one simple principle: the physical removal of all identifiable disease. The principles underlying the non-surgical management of cancer are more complex. First, the spatial distribution of the effects of our therapies have to be considered: surgery and radiotherapy are local or, at best, locoregional treatments; drugs offer a therapy that is systemic (Figure 9.7). Second, there is the question of the intent underlying the treatment. Occasionally, radiotherapy, chemotherapy or the combination of the two may be used with curative intent (Table 9.7). More usually, chemotherapy or radiotherapy is used to lower the risk of recurrence after primary treatment with surgery, so-called adjuvant therapy. Implicit within the concept of adjuvant therapy is the realisation that much of what is done is unnecessary or futile, or both. The need for adjuvant therapy, to treat the risk that residual disease might be present after apparently curative surgery, is an acknowledgement of the current inability to detect or predict, with sufficient precision, the presence of residual disease. It also explains why the incremental benefits from adjuvant treatments are so small and why the existence of these benefits can only be proven using randomised controlled trials, including many thousands of patients. As illustrated in Figures 9.8 and 9.9, our current approach to the selection of patients for post-surgical adjuvant treatment is both intellectually impoverished and inefficient. Patients may be far better off if, rather than so much time and effort having been invested in attempting to discover new 'cures' for cancer, equivalent resources had been devoted to devising clinically useful tests to detect residual cancer cells persisting after apparently successful initial therapy. Had this been the case, we might now be better able to distinguish between those patients with systemic disease at presentation and those with truly localised disease.

Radiotherapy

Within a month of their discovery in 1895, x-rays were being used to treat cancer. Despite over 100 years of use and despite some outstanding clinical achievements, it is still not known how best to use radiation to treat cancer. In part this is because it is not known precisely how radiation treatment affects tumours or normal tissues. Until about 20 years ago, it was assumed that the biological effects of radiation resulted from radiation-induced damage to the DNA of dividing cells. Nowadays, it is known that, although this undoubtedly explains some of the biological effects of radiation, it does not provide a full explanation. Radiation can, both directly and indirectly, influence gene expression: over 100 radiation-inducible effects on gene expression have now been described. These changes in gene expression are responsible for a considerable proportion of the biological effects of radiation upon tumours and normal tissues. In this sense, radiotherapy is a precisely targeted form of gene therapy for cancer.

Table 9.7 Examples of malignancies that may be cured without the need for surgical excision.

Malignancy	Potentially curative treatment
Leukaemia	Chemotherapy (±radiotherapy)
Lymphoma	Chemotherapy (±radiotherapy)
Small cell lung cancer	Chemotherapy (±radiotherapy)
Tumours of childhood (rhabdomyosarcoma, Wilms' tumour)	Chemotherapy (±radiotherapy)
Early laryngeal cancer	Radiotherapy
Advanced head and neck cancer	Chemoradiation (synchronous chemotherapy and radiotherapy)
Oesophageal cancer	Chemoradiation (synchronous chemotherapy and radiotherapy)
Squamous cell cancer of the anus	Chemoradiation (synchronous chemotherapy and radiotherapy)
Advanced cancer of the cervix	Radiotherapy (±chemotherapy)
Medulloblastoma	Radiotherapy (±chemotherapy)
Skin tumours (BCC, SCC)	Radiotherapy

BCC, basal cell carcinoma; SCC, squamous cell carcinoma.

Max Wilms, 1867–1918, Professor of Surgery, Heidelberg, Germany.
Hubert Rodney ('Rod') Withers, Professor of Radiation Oncology at the University of California, Los Angeles.

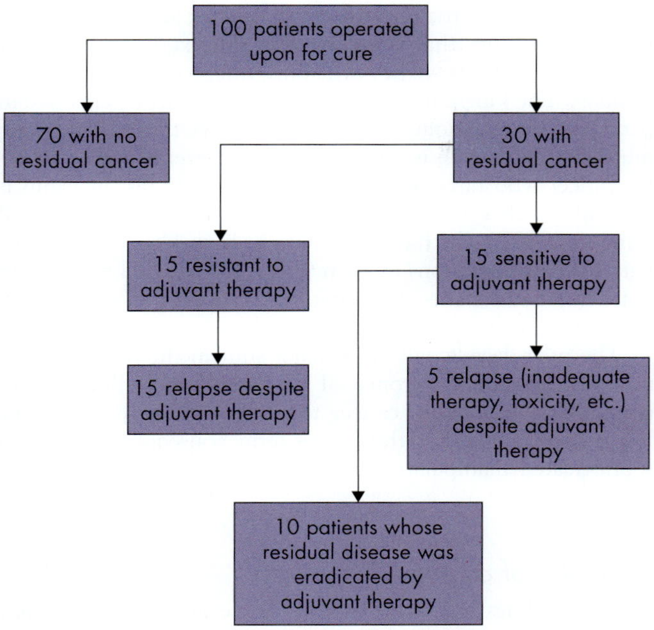

Net benefits		
Futile therapy	20%	90% treated inappropriately
Unnecessary therapy	70%	
Beneficial therapy	10%	10% treated appropriately
No therapy	0%	

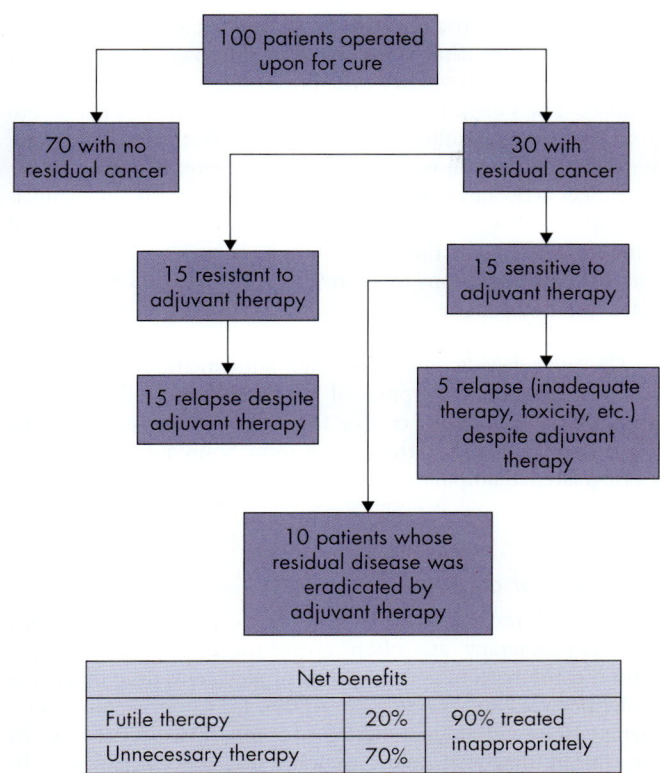

Figure 9.8 The concept of adjuvant therapy.

The practicalities of radiation therapy are reasonably straightforward: define the target to treat; design the optimal technical set up to provide uniform irradiation of that target; and choose that schedule of treatment that delivers radiation to that target so as to maximise the therapeutic ratio (Figure 9.10). One of the main problems with assessing a therapeutic ratio for a given schedule of radiation is that there is a dissociation between the acute effects on normal tissues and the late damage. The acute reaction is not a reliable guide to the adverse consequences of treatment in the longer term. As the late effects following irradiation can take over 20 years to develop, this poses an obvious difficulty: if the radiation schedule is changed, it will be known within two or three years whether or not the new schedule has improved tumour control; it may, however, be two decades before it is known, with any degree of certainty, whether the new technique is safe. Fractionated radiotherapy selectively spares late, as opposed to immediate, effects. For any given total dose, the smaller the dose per treatment (the larger the number of fractions), the less severe the late effects will be. The problem is that the greater the number of fractions of daily treatment, the longer the overall treatment time and the greater the opportunity for the tumour to proliferate during treatment. All fractionation is a compromise. Thirty years ago, Withers defined the four Rs of radiotherapy (see Summary box 9.5); subsequently, a fifth 'R' (intrinsic **r**adiosensitivity) has been added. The clinical practice of radiation oncology operates within the limits defined by these five Rs.

Chemotherapy and biological therapies

Selective toxicity is the fundamental principle underlying the use of chemotherapy in clinical practice. The importance of the principle is further emphasised by the fact that, by itself, chemotherapy is rarely sufficient to cure cancer. Chemotherapy is often (in effect, if not intent) a palliative rather than a cura-

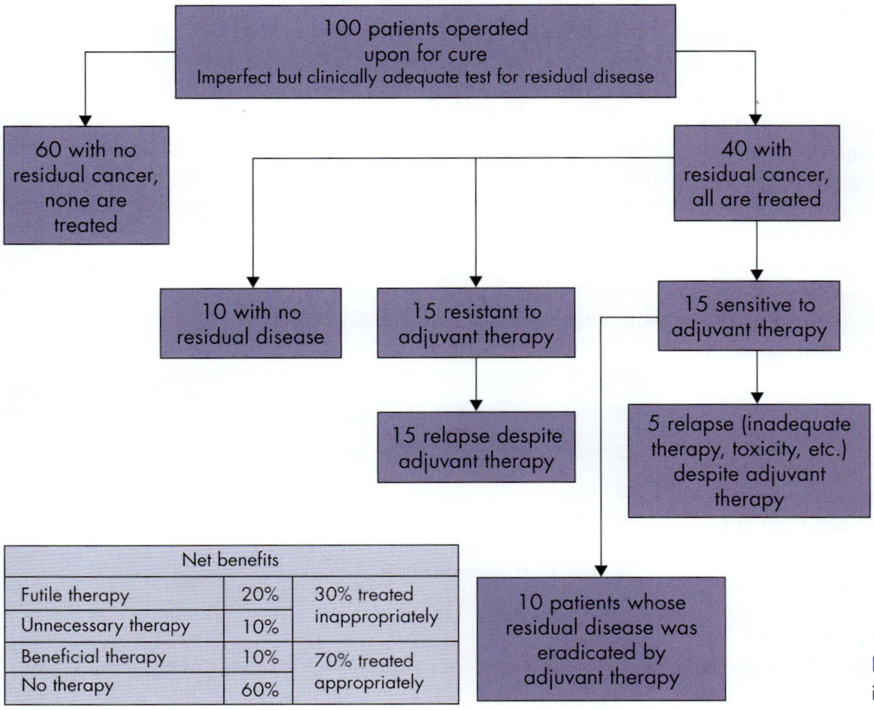

Net benefits		
Futile therapy	20%	30% treated inappropriately
Unnecessary therapy	10%	
Beneficial therapy	10%	70% treated appropriately
No therapy	60%	

Figure 9.9 The concept of adjuvant therapy and testing for minimal residual disease.

Summary box 9.5

The five Rs of radiotherapy

- **Repair**. If given sufficient time between fractional doses of radiation, cells will repair the radiation-induced damage. Repair half-times are typically 3–6 hours. Fractionation offers a means whereby any differentials in repair capacity between tumour and normal cells may be exploited.
- **Reoxygenation**. Hypoxic cells are relatively radioresistant compared with well-oxygenated cells. Normal tissues are well oxygenated; tumours are often hypoxic. This is an obvious therapeutic disadvantage.
- **Repopulation**. As radiotherapy kills cancer cells, rapid proliferation of tumour cells is stimulated. Thus, during protracted treatment, production of cells by the tumour may equal, or even exceed, radiation-induced cell loss. It is thus better that the overall treatment time is as short as possible.
- **Redistribution**. The sensitivity of cells to radiation varies according to their position within the cell cycle. This may lead to a degree of synchronisation of cellular division within the tumour: ideally, fractions of radiotherapy should be timed to coincide with vulnerable phases of the cell cycle (late G2 and M).
- **Radiosensitivity**. Low-dose rate irradiation experiments demonstrate that cells derived from tumours differ in their intrinsic sensitivity to radiation. Some cells are so intrinsically resistant to treatment that no clinically viable schedule of radiation therapy would eliminate them. Conversely, some cells may be so sensitive that virtually any schedule would be successful – the majority of cells will lie somewhere between these extremes.

tive intervention. As such, its use should be influenced by the cardinal principle of palliative treatment: treatment aimed at relieving symptoms should not, itself, produce unacceptable symptoms. The cure of a disease should not be more grievous than its endurance. There are now over 95 different drugs licensed by the US Food and Drug Administration (FDA) for the treatment of cancer. Of these, over 65 per cent are cytotoxic drugs, 15 per cent are hormonal therapies and 15 per cent are designed to interact with specific molecular targets – so-called targeted therapies. Over 50 per cent of these agents have been licensed since 1990: in terms of potential progress, achievement over the past 15 years has equalled that of the previous 40 years. There are now many more options than there were 20 years ago and, perhaps more importantly, lessons have been learnt about how better to deploy resources. The classes of cytotoxic drugs, their mode of action and clinical indications are summarised in Table 9.8.

The newer 'targeted' therapies available for treating cancer present particular dilemmas. They offer modest prolongation of survival, often with minimal toxicity, but at considerable financial cost. When compared with conventional therapies, these drugs typically cost over £50 000 (US$94 000) per quality-adjusted life-year gained and, when overall resources are limited, they may be considered unaffordable. Table 9.9 puts into context the cost-effectiveness of various clinical interventions. The current cost of targeted therapies should not obscure their importance: they represent the first attempts to translate advances in molecular biology into clinical practice. The discoveries of the mid-twentieth century are finally bearing fruit. One feature that is emerging is the exquisite selectivity of these treatments – they will only target specific subsets of tumours. The kinase inhibitor PLX4032 will only be effective in patients with melanoma whose tumours have the V600E BRAF mutation; cetuximab is only effective in patients with colorectal cancer who have wild-type (non-mutated) ras; imatinib is particularly effective in patients with gastrointestinal stromal tumours (GIST) who have mutations in exon 11 of the *Kit* gene, patients with mutations in exon 9 may still respond to imatinib but will require higher doses, patients without mutations in *Kit* are far less likely to respond to imatinib.

The next decade will see a major shift in the medical management of cancer – from cell destruction to cellular reprogramming. As a result, cancer therapies are likely to become less acutely toxic, but the longer-term consequences of such sophisticated manipulations may be uncertain and unpredictable.

Principles of combined treatment

Cytotoxic drugs are rarely used as single agents; radiotherapy and chemotherapy are often given together. The rationale behind combination, as opposed to single-agent, drug therapy is straightforward and is analogous to that for combined antibiotic therapy: it is a strategy designed to combat drug resistance. By the time of diagnosis, many tumours will contain cancer cells that, through spontaneous mutation, have acquired resistance to cytotoxic drugs. Unlike antibiotic resistance, there is no need for previous exposure to the drug. Spontaneous mutation rates are high enough to allow chance to permit the development, and subsequent expansion, of clones of cells resistant to drugs to which they have never been exposed. If drugs were used as single agents, then the further expansion of these *de novo* resistant subclones would limit cure. The problem can be mitigated by combining drugs from the outset.

The choice of drugs for combination therapy is based upon three main principles: (1) use drugs active against the disease in question; (2) use drugs with distinct modes of action; and (3) use drugs with non-overlapping toxicities. By using drugs with different biological effects, for example by combining an anti-metabolite with an agent that actively damages DNA, it may be possible to obtain a truly synergistic effect. It is inadvisable to combine drugs with similar adverse effects: combining two highly myelosuppressive drugs may produce an unacceptably high risk of neutropenic sepsis. Where possible, combinations should be based upon a consideration of the toxicity profiles of the drugs concerned (Summary box 9.6).

Summary box 9.6

Basic principles of combined therapy

- Use effective agents
- Use agents with different modes of action (synergy)
- Use agents with non-overlapping toxicities
- Consider spatial cooperation

In considering the combination of radiotherapy and chemotherapy, radiation could be considered as just another drug.

A **synergistic effect** is one in which the damage caused by giving the agents together is greater than the damage caused when the drugs are given separately.

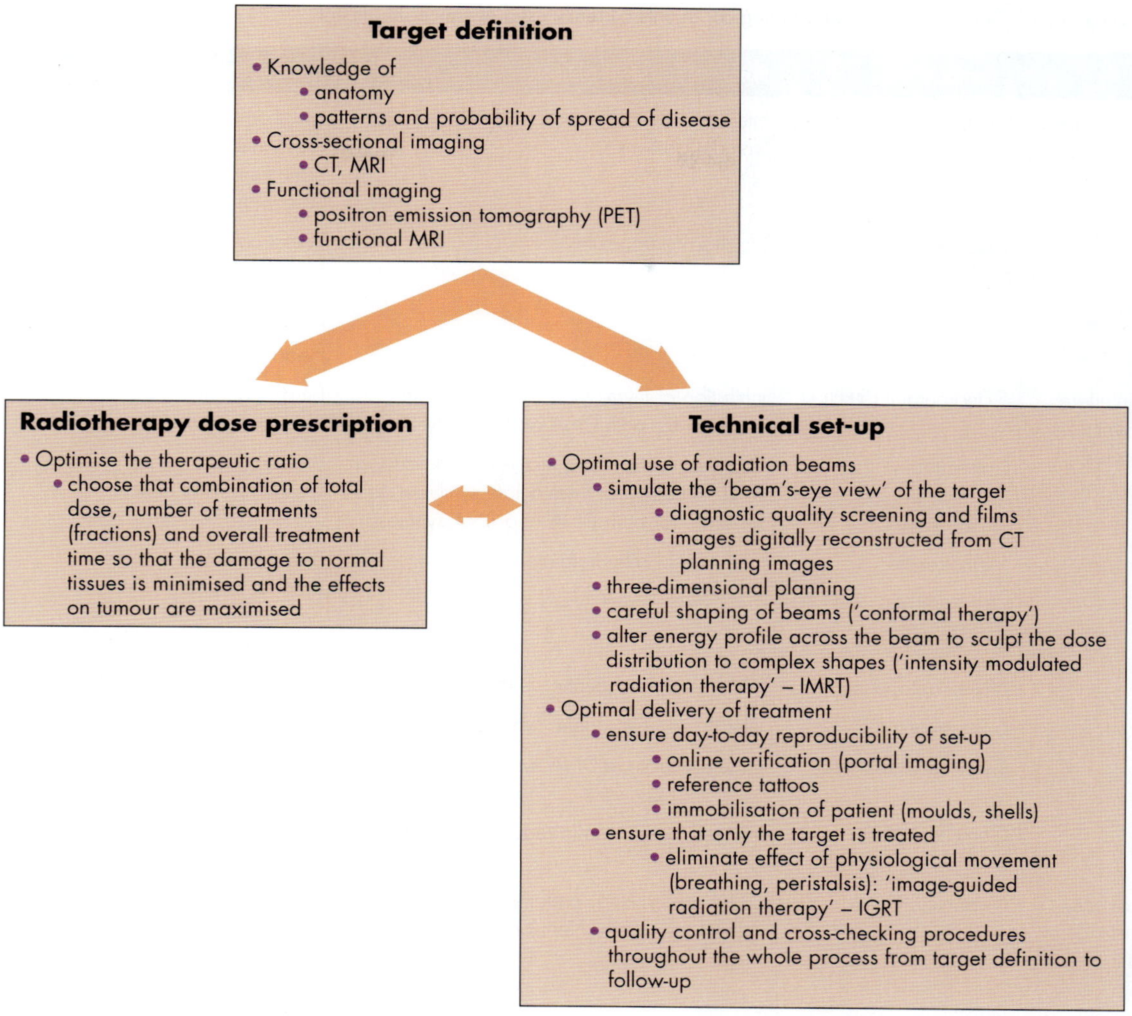

Figure 9.10 The processes involved in clinical radiotherapy. CT, computed tomography; MRI, magnetic resonance imaging.

There is, in addition to synergy and toxicity, another factor to consider in the combination of drugs and radiation – the concept of spatial cooperation. Chemotherapy is a systemic treatment; radiotherapy is not, but it is able to reach sites, such as the central nervous system and testis, which drugs may not reach effectively. This is why, for example, in patients treated primarily with chemotherapy for leukaemias, lymphomas and small cell lung cancer, prophylactic cranial irradiation is part of the treatment protocol.

Palliative therapy

The distinction between palliative and curative treatment is not always clear cut and will become increasingly blurred as professional and public attitudes towards the management of cancer change. Ten years ago, cancer was perceived as a disease that was either cured or not; patients either lived or died. There was little appreciation that, for many patients, cancer might be a chronic disease. Nowadays, many of the so-called curative treatments are simply elegant exercises in growth delay. Five-year survival is not necessarily tantamount to cure. With the development of targeted therapies that regulate, rather than eradicate, cancer, this situation is likely to continue. The aim of treatment will be growth control rather than the extirpation of every last cancer cell. Patients will live with their cancers, perhaps for years. They will die with cancer, but not necessarily of cancer. Against this background, the distinction between curative and palliative therapy seems somewhat arbitrary, nevertheless the control and relief of symptoms is crucial to the successful management of patients with cancer. Much of the fear associated with cancer is due to past failures to control symptoms.

Patients fear the symptoms, distress and disruption associated with cancer almost as much as they fear the disease itself. Palliative treatment has as its goal the relief of symptoms. Sometimes, this will involve treating the underlying problem, as with palliative radiotherapy for bone metastases. Sometimes, it may be inappropriate to treat the cancer itself, but that does not imply that there is nothing more to be done; there may be better ways to assuage the distress and discomfort caused by the tumour. Palliative medicine in the twenty-first century is about far more than optimal control of pain: its scope is wide, its impact immense (Table 9.10). The most important factor in the successful palliative management of a patient with cancer is

Table 9.8 A summary of chemotherapeutic and biological agents currently used in cancer treatment.

Class	Examples	Putative mode of action	Tumour types that may be sensitive to drug
Drugs that interfere with mitosis	Vincristine, vinblastine	Interfere with the formation of microtubules: 'spindle poisons'	Lymphomas Leukaemias Brain tumours Sarcomas
	Taxanes: taxol, paclitaxel	Stabilise microtubules	Breast cancer Non-small cell lung cancer Ovarian cancer Prostate cancer Head and neck cancer
Drugs that interfere with DNA synthesis (anti-metabolites)	5-Fluorouracil (5-FU)	Inhibition of thymidylate synthase, false substrate for both DNA and RNA synthesis	Breast cancer Gastrointestinal cancer
	Capecitabine	Orally active prodrug that is metabolised to 5-FU. Inhibition of thymidylate synthase, false substrate for both DNA and RNA synthesis	Breast cancer Gastrointestinal cancer
	Methotrexate	Inhibition of dihydrofolate reductase	Breast cancer Bladder cancer Lymphomas Cervix cancer
	6-Mercaptopurine	Inhibits *de novo* purine synthesis	Leukaemias
	6-Thioguanine	Inhibits *de novo* purine synthesis	Leukaemias
	Cytosine arabinoside	False substrate in DNA synthesis	Leukaemias Lymphomas
	Gemcitabine	Inhibits ribonucleotide reductase	Non-small cell lung cancer Pancreatic cancer
Drugs that directly damage DNA or interfere with its function	Mitomycin C	DNA cross-linking, preferentially active at sites of low oxygen tension (a bioreductive drug)	Anal cancer Bladder cancer Gastric cancer Head and neck cancer Rectal cancer
	Cisplatinum	Forms adducts between DNA strands and interferes with replication	Germ cell tumours Ovarian cancer Non-small cell lung cancer Head and neck cancer Oesophageal cancer
	Carboplatin	Forms adducts between DNA strands and interferes with replication	Germ cell tumours Ovarian cancer Non-small cell lung cancer Head and neck cancer
	Oxaliplatin	Forms adducts between DNA strands and interferes with replication	Colorectal cancer
	Doxorubicin	Intercalates between DNA strands and interferes with replication	Breast cancer Lymphomas Sarcomas Kaposi's sarcoma
	Cyclophosphamide	A prodrug converted via hepatic cytochrome p450 to phosphoramide mustard; causes DNA crosslinks	Breast cancer Lymphomas Sarcomas
	Ifosfamide	Related to cyclophosphamide, causes DNA crosslinks	Small cell lung cancer Sarcomas
	Bleomycin	DNA strand breakage via formation of metal complex	Germ cell tumours Lymphomas

Table 9.8 A summary of chemotherapeutic and biological agents currently used in cancer treatment – *continued.*

Class	Examples	Putative mode of action	Tumour types that may be sensitive to drug
Drugs that directly damage DNA or interfere with its function – *continued*	Irinotecan	Inhibits topoisomerase 1 and thereby prevents the DNA from unwinding and repairing during replication	Colorectal cancer
	Etoposide	Inhibits topoisomerase 2; prevents the DNA from unwinding and repairing during replication	Small cell lung cancer Germ cell tumours Lymphomas
	Trabectedin	Binds to minor groove of the DNA double helix and inhibits transcription	Soft tissue sarcoma
	Dacarbazine	A nitrosourea that requires activation by hepatic cytochrome p450. Methylates guanine residues in DNA	Brain tumours Sarcoma Melanoma
	Temozolomide	A nitrosourea but, unlike dacarbazine, does not require activation by hepatic cytochrome p450. Methylates guanine residues in DNA	Glioblastoma multiforme Melanoma
	Actinomycin D	Intercalation between DNA strands, DNA strand breaks	Rhabdomyosarcoma Wilms' tumour
Hormones	Tamoxifen	Blocks oestrogen receptors	Breast cancer
	Anastrazole	An aromatase inhibitor that blocks post-menopausal (non-ovarian) oestrogen production	Breast cancer
	Exemestane	An aromatase inhibitor that blocks post-menopausal (non-ovarian) oestrogen production	Breast cancer
	Letrozole	An aromatase inhibitor that blocks post-menopausal (non-ovarian) oestrogen production	Breast cancer
	Leuprolide	Analogue of gonadotrophin-releasing hormone; continued use produces downregulation of the anterior pituitary with a consequent fall in testosterone levels	Prostate cancer
	Goserelin	Analogue of gonadotrophin-releasing hormone; continued use produces downregulation of the anterior pituitary with a consequent fall in testosterone levels	Prostate cancer
	Buserelin	Analogue of gonadotrophin-releasing hormone; continued use produces downregulation of the anterior pituitary with a consequent fall in testosterone levels	Prostate cancer
	Cabergoline	Blocks prolactin release, a long-acting dopamine agonist	Prolactin-secreting pituitary tumours
	Bromocriptine	Dopamine agonist, blocks stimulation of the anterior pituitary	Pituitary tumours
	Cyproterone acetate	Blocks the effect of androgens	Prostate cancer
	Flutamide	Blocks the effect of androgens	Prostate cancer
	Nilutamide	Blocks the effect of androgens	Prostate cancer
	Bicalutamide	Blocks the effect of androgens	Prostate cancer
Inhibitors of tyrosine kinases	Gefitinib	Inhibits EGFR tyrosine kinase	Non-small cell lung cancer

Table 9.8 A summary of chemotherapeutic and biological agents currently used in cancer treatment – *continued*.

Class	Examples	Putative mode of action	Tumour types that may be sensitive to drug
Inhibitors of tyrosine kinases – *continued*	Imatinib	Blocks the ability of mutant BCR-ABL fusion protein to bind ATP	Chronic myeloid leukaemia
		Inhibition of mutant c-KIT	Gastrointestinal stromal tumours (GIST)
	Erlotinib	Inhibits EGFR tyrosine kinase	Non-small cell lung cancer Pancreatic cancer
	Sunitinib	Promiscuous tyrosine kinase inhibitor (PDGFR, VEGFR, cKit, FLT3)	Renal cancer GIST refractory to imatinib
	Lapatinib	Inhibits tyrosine kinases associated with EGFR and HER	Breast cancer
	Crizotinib	Inhibits ALK and cMET receptor tyrosine kinases	Lung cancer, Neuroblastoma, Lymphoma
	Pazopanib	Promiscuous tyrosine kinase inhibitor – VEGFRs, PDGFR, cKit	Renal cancer
	Sorafenib	Promiscuous tyrosine kinase inhibitor (PDGFR, VEGFR, cKit, FLT3)	Renal cancer, Thyroid cancer
	Dasatinib	BCR-ABL TKI	CML
Protease inhibitors	Bortezomib	Interferes with proteasomal degradation of regulatory proteins; in particular, prevents NF kappa B from preventing apoptosis	Multiple myeloma
Differentiating agents	All *trans*-retinoic acid	Induces terminal differentiation	Acute promyelocytic leukaemia
Farnesyl transferase inhibitors	Lonafarnib	Inhibition of farnesyl transferase and consequent inactivation of *ras*-dependent signal transduction	Leukaemia
	Tipifarnib	Inhibition of farnesyl transferase and consequent inactivation of *ras*-dependent signal transduction	Acute leukaemia Myelodysplastic syndrome
BRAF kinase inhibitor	PLX4032	Blocks MAP kinase pathway	Melanoma
Histone deacetylase inhibitors (HDACi)	Vorinostat	Inhibition of HDAC	Cutaneous T-cell lymphoma
mTOR inhibitors	Temsirolimus	Inhibits mTOR	Renal cancer
	Everolimus	Inhibits mTOR	Mantle-cell lymphoma, Renal cancer
Antibodies directed to cell surface antigens	Trastuzumab	Antibody directed against HER2 receptor	Breast cancer
	Cetuximab	Antibody directed against EGFR receptor	Colorectal cancer Head and neck cancer
	Bevacizumab	Antibody directed against VEGFR	Colorectal cancer
	Rituximab	Antibody against CD20 antigen	Lymphomas
	Alemtuzumab	Antibody against CD52 antigen	Lymphomas
Inducers of apoptosis	Arsenic trioxide	Induces apoptosis by caspase inhibition, inhibition of nitric oxide	Acute promyelocytic leukaemia
Immunological mediators	Interferon alpha-2b	Activates macrophages, increases the cytotoxicity of T lymphocytes, inhibits cell division (and viral replication)	Renal carcinoma Melanoma Hairy cell leukaemia
	Thalidomide	Anti-inflammatory, stimulates T cells, anti-angiogenic	Myeloma

Table 9.8 A summary of chemotherapeutic and biological agents currently used in cancer treatment – *continued*.

Class	Examples	Putative mode of action	Tumour types that may be sensitive to drug
Immunological mediators – *continued*	Ipilimumab	A monoclonal antibody that blocks cytotoxic T-lymphocyte antigen-4 and acts as a potentiator of T-cell mediated anti-tumour responses	Melanoma

CML, chronic myeloid leukaemia; EGFR, epidermal growth factor receptor; FLT3, FMS-like tyrosine kinase; mTOR , mammalian target of rapamycin; NF, nuclear factor; PDGFR, platelet-derived growth factor receptor; TKI, tyrosine kinase inhibitor; VEGFR, vascular endothelial growth factor receptor.

Table 9.9 Estimates of cost-effectiveness for a selection of interventions

Intervention	Approximate cost per QALY in 2005 US$
Universal antenatal screening for HIV	30 725
Laparoscopic inguinal hernia repair versus expectant management in adults with inguinal hernia	660
Annual mammograms from age 40 (cost per QALY over and above screening every 2 years aged 50 to 70)	145 160
Annual CT chest screening for lung cancer in a 60-year-old male ex-smoker versus no screening	2.6 million
Erlotinib versus usual care in the treatment of relapsed non-small cell lung cancer	75 750
Trabectedin versus best supportive care for advanced soft tissue sarcoma	96 000
Smoking cessation programme implemented at the time of surgery for lung cancer	16 400
Stroke unit care versus usual care in survivors of acute stroke	1750
Adjuvant radiotherapy for T1 breast cancer: whole breast radiotherapy (long course) versus short course partial breast irradiation	630 000
Adding trastuzumab to adjuvant chemotherapy for HER2 receptor-positive breast cancer	18 900
Adding trastuzumab to conventional chemotherapy for advanced gastric cancer	80 000
Sunitinib compared with interferon for metastatic renal cancer	52 500
^{18}FDG-PET-CT in the follow up of non-small cell lung cancer patients after radical radiotherapy with or without chemotherapy	91 500
Letrazole vs. tamoxifen in the first-line management of post-menopausal women with advanced breast cancer	130 000

Calculations are based on sources identified via the CEA register (https://research.tufts-nemc.org/cear4/default.aspx), last accessed March 21, 2011
QALY, quality adjusted life year

early referral. Transition between curative and palliative modes of management should be seamless.

End-of-life care

End-of-life care is distinct from palliative care. Patients treated palliatively may survive for many years; end-of-life care concerns the last few months of a patient's life. Many issues, such as symptom control, are common to both but there are also problems that are specific to the sense of approaching death. These may include a heightened sense of spiritual need, profound fear and the specific needs of those who are facing bereavement. The concept of the 'good death' has been embedded in many cultures over many centuries. Health-care professionals deal with many deaths and sometimes forget that the patient who hopes for a 'good death' has only one chance to get it right. This is why end-of-life care is worth considering in its own right and not as a mere appendage to palliative care. Some of the issues unique to end-of-life care are summarised in Summary box 9.7.

Summary box 9.7

End of life issues

- Appropriateness of active intervention
- Euthanasia
- Physician-assisted suicide
- Living wills
- Bereavement
- Spirituality
- Support to allow death at home
- The problem of the medicalisation of death

Table 9.10 An outline of the domains and interventions included within palliative and supportive care.

Type of support	
Symptom assessment	Pain, anorexia, fatigue, dyspnoea, etc. Treatment-related toxicity
Quality of life assessment	
Symptom relief	Drugs Surgery Radiotherapy Complementary therapies Acupuncture Homeopathy Aromatherapy, etc.
Psychosocial interventions	Psychological support Relaxation techniques Cognitive behavioural therapy Counselling Group therapy Music therapy Emotional support
Physical and practical support	Physiotherapy Occupational therapy Speech therapy
Information and knowledge	Macmillan Maggie's centres
Nutritional support	Dietary advice Nutritional supplements
Social support	Patients Relatives and carers
Financial support	Ensure uptake of entitlements Grants from charities, e.g. Macmillan Cancer Relief
Spiritual support	

FURTHER READING

Bailar JC, Gornik HL Cancer undefeated. *N Engl J Med* 1997; **336**: 1569–74.

Barcellos-Hoff MH. It takes a tissue to make a tumor: epigenetics, cancer and the microenvironment. *J Mammary Gland Biol Neoplasia* 2001; **6**: 213–21.

Capasso LL Antiquity of cancer. *Int J Cancer* 2005; **113**: 2–13.

Doll R. Epidemiological evidence of the effects of behaviour and the environment on the risk of human cancer. *Rec Res Cancer Res* 1998; **154**: 3–21.

Feinberg AP, Ohlsson R, Henikoff S. The epigenetic progenitor origin of human cancer. *Nature Rev Genet* 2006; **7**: 21–33.

Feinstein AR, Sosin DM, Well CK. The Will Rogers phenomenon. Stage migration and new diagnostic techniques as a source of misleading statistics for survival in cancer. *N Engl J Med* 1985; **312**: 1604–8.

Hanahan D, Weinberg RA. Hallmarks of cancer: the next generation. *Cell* 2011; **144**: 646–74.

Kerr JF, Wyllie AH, Currie AR. Apoptosis: a basic biological phenomenon with wide-ranging implications in tissue kinetics. *Br J Cancer* 1972; **26**: 239–57.

Vogelstein B, Kinzler KW. Cancer genes and the pathways they control. *Nature Med* 2004; **10**: 789–99.

CHAPTER 10

Surgical audit and clinical research

LEARNING OBJECTIVES

To understand:

- The planning and conduct of audit and research
- How to write up a project
- How to review a journal article and determine its value

INTRODUCTION

It is essential for a surgeon to understand the educational and legal framework in which he or she works. The agenda for medical education and clinical governance requires surgeons to expand their skills to encompass audit and clinical research capabilities as useful tools for continued outcome measurement, service improvement and innovations for the benefit of patient care.

The aim of this chapter is to enable improvements in patient experience as a result of a successful audit cycle or by recognising the need for clinical research to determine a new and innovative way of treatment. It will also show how to keep track of personal clinical results. In addition, much clinical work is tedious and repetitive. Rigorous evaluation of even the most simple techniques and conditions can help to keep a surgeon stimulated throughout a long career and ensure good outcomes for patients, with cost benefits to the provider and a benefit to society as a whole.

Large numbers of clinical papers appear in the surgical literature every year. Many are flawed, and it is important that a surgeon has the skills to examine publications critically. The best way to develop a critical understanding of the research and audit undertaken by others is to perform studies of one's own. The hardest part of audit and research is writing it up, and the hardest article to write is the first. This chapter also contains the information required to write a surgical paper and to evaluate the publications of others.

AUDIT OR RESEARCH?

Health professionals are expected to undertake audit and service evaluation as part of quality assurance. These usually involve minimal additional risk, burden or intrusion for participants. It is important to determine at an early stage whether a project is audit or research, and sometimes that is not as easy as it seems. The decision will determine the framework in which the study is undertaken. In the UK, the National Research Ethics Service has developed helpful guidance for the definition of research, audit, service evaluation and public health surveillance. Although developed as national guidance, it is a useful guide to decision-making generally (www.nres.npsa.nhs.uk/applications/is-your-project-research/) (Table 10.1).

AUDIT AND SERVICE EVALUATION

Clinical audit is a process used by clinicians who seek to improve patient care. The process involves comparing aspects of care (structure, process and outcome) against explicit criteria and defined standards. Keeping track of personal outcome data and contributing to a clinical database ensures that a surgeon's own performance is monitored continuously and can be compared with a national dataset to ensure compliance with agreed standards. It is also an essential component of revalidation for the individual surgeon in the UK. If the care falls short of the criteria chosen, some change in the way that care is organised should be proposed. This change may be required at one of many levels. It might be an individual who needs training or surgical equipment that needs replacing. At times, the change may need to take place at the team level. Sometimes, the only appropriate action is change at an institutional level (e.g. a new antibiotic policy), regional level (provision of a tertiary referral centre) or, indeed, national level (screening programmes and health education campaigns).

Essentially, two types of audit may be encountered: national audits (e.g. in the UK, the National Institute for Health and Clinical Excellence (NICE)) and local/hospital audits. Both are designed to improve the quality of care. In an ideal world, national audits should be driven by needs identified in local and hospital-based audits that are closest to the patient. For example, hospital topics are often identified at the departmental morbidity and mortality meetings, where issues related to patient care are discussed. The reporting process might identify a possible national issue, and a national audit could be designed to be completed by the local audit department and surgical teams. The Vascular Society of Great Britain and Ireland is working continually with all its members in an evaluation of process and outcomes for major vascular operations. This is driven by

Table 10.1 Research, audit or service evaluation?

Research	Clinical audit	Service evaluation
The attempt to derive generalisable new knowledge including studies that aim to generate hypotheses as well as studies that aim to test them	Designed and conducted to produce information to inform the delivery of best care	Designed and conducted solely to define or judge current care
Quantitative research – designed to test a hypothesis	Designed to answer the question: 'Does this service reach a predetermined standard?'	Designed to answer the question: 'What standard does this service achieve?'
Qualitative research – identifies/explores themes following established methodology		
Addresses clearly defined questions, aims and objectives	Measures against a standard	Measures current service without reference to a standard
Quantitative research – may involve evaluating or comparing interventions, particularly new ones	Involves an intervention in use only. (The choice of treatment is that of the clinician and patient according to guidance, professional standards and/or patient preference)	Involves an intervention in use only. (The choice of treatment is that of the clinician and patient according to guidance, professional standards and/or patient preference)
Qualitative research – usually involves studying how interventions and relationships are experienced		
Usually involves collecting data that are additional to those for routine care, but may include data collected routinely. May involve treatments, samples or investigations additional to routine care	Usually involves analysis of existing data, but may include administration of simple interviews or questionnaires	Usually involves analysis of existing data, but may include administration of simple interviews or questionnaires
Quantitative research – study design may involve allocating patients to intervention groups	No allocation to interventions: the health professional and patient have chosen intervention before clinical audit	No allocation to intervention: the health professional and patient have chosen intervention before service evaluation
Qualitative research uses a clearly defined sampling framework underpinned by conceptual or theoretical justifications		
May involve randomisation	No randomisation	No randomisation

Although any of the above may raise ethical issues, under current guidance, research requires ethics committee review, whereas audit and service evaluation do not. Advice (in the UK) from National Research Ethics Service (www.nres.npsa.nhs.uk/).
Based on information by the National Research Ethics Service.

a Quality Improvement Programme (www.aaaqip.org.uk) that was originally designed to feedback outcomes in aortic surgery to individual units, but which has been extended to include other high risk vascular procedures, such as carotid endarterectomy and leg amputation. Issues that are of local importance are addressed within the local hospital or hospital trusts (in the UK).

Audits are formal processes that require a structure. The following steps are essential to establish an audit cycle:

1 Define the audit question in a multidisciplinary team.
2 Identify the body of evidence and current standards.
3 Design the audit to measure performance against agreed standards based on strong evidence. Seek appropriate advice (local audit department in UK).
4 Measure over an agreed interval.
5 Analyse results and compare performance against agreed standards.
6 Undertake gap analysis:
   a. If all standards are reached, reaudit after an agreed interval.
   b. If there is a need for improvement, identify possible interventions such as training, and agree with the involved parties.
7 Reaudit.

Research study

During the design of the audit project, it might become apparent that there is a limited body of evidence available. In this case, the study should be structured as a research proposal. Research is designed to generate new knowledge and might involve testing a new treatment or regimen.

IDENTIFYING A RESEARCH TOPIC

The hardest part of research is to come up with a good idea. Once an idea has been formed, or a question asked, it needs to be transformed into a hypothesis. It is helpful to approach surgeons who regularly publish articles and who have a special interest in the surgical area being considered. As ideas are suggested, keep thinking whether the question posed really matters. Spend some time refining the question because this is probably the most important part of the study. Choosing the wrong topic at this stage can lead to many wasted hours. Once a topic has been identified, do not rush into the study. It is worth spending considerable time investigating the subject in question. The worst possible outcome is to find at the end of a long arduous study that the research has already been done.

First port of call for information is the internet (with assistance as needed from a medical library). Look for current articles about the proposed research; review articles and meta-analyses can be particularly helpful. At this stage, most clinicians go to an electronic library and perform a database search. It is very important to learn how to do an accurate and efficient search as early as possible. Details are beyond the scope of this chapter, but most librarians will help out if a little interest and enthusiasm is shown. Current techniques involve searching on Medline or other collected databases such as Google Scholar, but as electronic information advances and the web becomes more user friendly, new search strategies may emerge. Collections of reviews are becoming available – the Cochrane Collaboration brings together evidence-based medical information and is available in most libraries (Table 10.2).

Once a stack of articles on the subject has been obtained, it is important that these are carefully perused. Don't just read the abstract on Medline! If the proposed project is still looking good after some thorough reading, it is worth further discussion with colleagues who have written a paper on a similar subject. All scientists are flattered by interest in their work. Now it should be possible to start to plan the research project.

PROJECT DESIGN

During the first phase, it is important to keep in the mind some important questions (Summary box 10.1).

Summary box 10.1

Questions to answer before undertaking research

- Why do the study?
- Will it answer a useful question?
- Is it practical?
- Can it be accomplished in the available time and with the available resources?
- What findings are expected?
- What are the research governance requirements?
- What are the ethical issues?
- What impact could it have?

Time spent carefully designing a potential project is never wasted. There are many different types of scientific study. The design used depends on the study. A randomised controlled trial (RCT) is regarded as one of the best methods of scientific research, however that much surgical practice has been advanced through other different types of study such as those listed in Table 10.3. For example, testing a new type of operation often requires a pilot study to assess feasibility that is then followed by a formal RCT. The introduction of innovative surgical techniques may require novel handling, and recomendations have been made by the IDEAL collaborators (see Further reading).

Research can be qualitative or quantitative. Quantitative

Table 10.2 Electronic information sites.

Database	Producer	Coverage	Availability[a]
Pubmed (www.ncbi.nlm.nih.gov/pubmed/)	US National Library of Medicine (NLM)	PubMed comprises more than 20 million citations for biomedical literature from MEDLINE, life science journals, and online books	Internet
Pubmed Central (www.pubmedcentral.nih.gov/)	US National Institutes of Health (NIH) free digital archive	Digital archive of biomedical and life sciences journal literature	Internet
EMBASE (http://embase.com/)	EMBASE	Providing extensive coverage of peer-reviewed biomedical literature, along with indexing, searching and information management tools	Subscription
CINAHL (www.ebscohost.com/cinahl/)	CINAHL is owned and operated by EBSCO Publishing	Cumulated index to nursing and allied health literature	Subscription
CochraneCollaboration and Library (www.cochrane.co.uk)	International network of people helping healthcare providers, policy makers, patients, their advocates and carers, make well-informed decisions about human health care	Preparing, updating and promoting the accessibility of Cochrane Reviews published online in *The Cochrane Library*	Internet

[a]Licensed to many organisations who provide their own interface. Main providers offering a pay-as-you-go service can be found: www.ovid.com or www.silverplatter.com.

The Cochrane Collaboration was formed in 1993 and named after Archibald Leman Cochrane, 1909–1988, Director of the Medical Research Council Epidemiology Unit, Cardiff, and later the first President of the Faculty of Community Medicine (now the Faculty of Public Health) of the Royal College of Physicians of London, UK.

Table 10.3 Types of study.

Type of study	Definition
Observational	Evaluation of condition or treatment in a defined population
	Retrospective: analysing past events
	Prospective: collecting data contemporaneously
Case–control	Series of patients with a particular disease or condition compared with matched control patients
Cross-sectional	Measurements made on a single occasion, not looking at the whole population, but selecting a small similar group and expanding results
Longitudinal	Measurements are taken over a period of time, not looking at the whole population, but selecting a small similar group and expanding results
Experimental	Two or more treatments are compared. Allocation to treatment groups is under the control of the researcher
Randomised	Two randomly allocated treatments
Randomised controlled	Includes a control group with standard treatment

research allows hard facts to speak for themselves. A medical condition is analysed systematically using hard, objective end points such as death or major complications, which should be clearly defined. In qualitative research, data often come from patient narratives, and the psychosocial impact of the disease and its treatment are analysed, for example narratives from patients with breast cancer. These kinds of data are often collected using quality-of-life measurements. A variety of different quality-of-life questionnaires exist to suit several different clinical situations. Much of the best research is both quantitative and qualitative.

Research should be focused according to national (and international) strategies. As finances for health care are always limited, it is important to consider including a cost–benefit analysis in any major area of research so that the value of the proposed intervention or change in treatment can be assessed. 'Best Research for Best Health' provided a National Health Service (NHS) research strategy for England and Wales that has resulted in the successful set up of the National Institute for Health Research (NIHR). NIHR provides the framework through which the Department of Health maintains and manages the research, research staff and research infrastructure of the NHS in England (www.nihr.ac.uk/Pages/default.aspx).

Sample size

Calculating the number of patients required to perform a satisfactory investigation is an important prerequisite to the study. An incorrect sample size is probably the most frequent reason for research being invalid. Often, surgical trials are marred by the possibility of error caused by the inadequate number of patients investigated.

- **Type I error**. Benefit is perceived when really there is none (false positive)
- **Type II error**. Benefit is missed when it was there to be found (false negative)

Calculating the number of patients required in the study can overcome this bias. Unfortunately, it often reveals that a larger number of patients is needed for the study than can possibly be obtained from available resources. This often means expanding enrolment by using a multicentre study. There is no point in embarking on a trial if it will never be possible to recruit an adequate population to answer the research question. More patients will need to be randomised than the final sample size to take into account patients who die, drop out or are lost to follow up.

The following is an example calculation for a study to recruit patients into two groups. In order to calculate a sample size, it is common practice to set the level of power for the study at 80 per cent with a 5 per cent significance level. This means that, if there is a difference between study groups, there is an 80 per cent chance of detecting it. Based on previous studies, realistic expectations of differences between groups should be used to calculate the sample size. The formula below uses the figures of a reduction in event rate from 30 to 10 per cent (e.g. a new treatment expected to reduce the complication rate such as wound infection from 30 per cent = r to 10 per cent = s).

$$8 \times \frac{[r(100 - r) + s(100 - s)]}{(r - s)^2}$$

$$\text{e.g. } 8 \times \frac{[30(100 - 30) + 10(100 - 10)]}{(30 - 10)^2}$$

$$= 60 \text{ needed in each group}$$

Eliminating bias

It is important to imagine how a study could be invalidated by thinking of things that could go wrong. One way to eliminate any bias inherent in the data collection is to have observers or recorders who do not know which treatment has been used (blinded observer). It might also be possible to ensure that the patient is unaware of the treatment allocation (single blind). In the best randomised studies, neither patient nor researcher is aware of which therapy has been used until after the study has finished (double blind). Randomised trials are essential for testing new drugs. In practice, however, in some surgical trials, randomisation may not be possible or ethical.

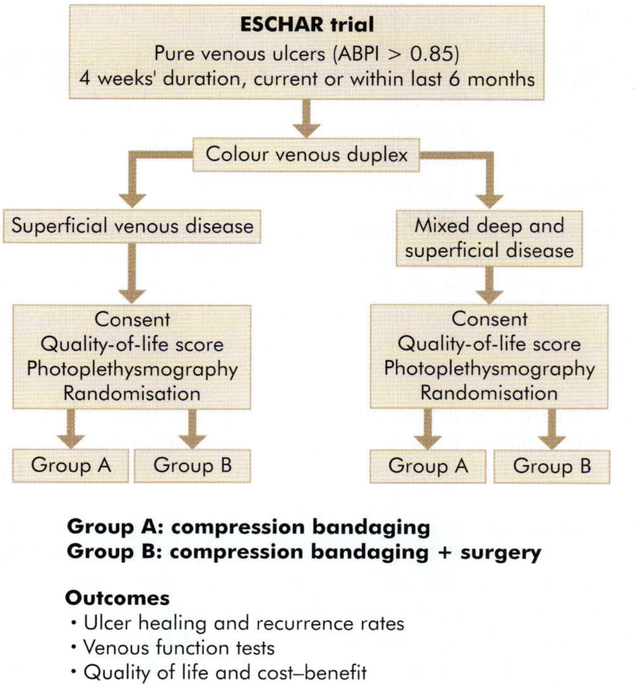

Figure 10.1 ESCHAR trial: completed in Gloucestershire, UK (Gohel MS *et al. British Journal of Surgery* 2005; **92**: 291–7. Copyright British Journal of Surgery Society Ltd. Permission is granted by John Wiley & Sons Ltd on behalf of the BJSS Ltd.) ABPI, ankle–brachial pressure index.

Study protocol

Now that the question to pose has been decided, and it has been checked that sufficient patients will be available to enrol into the study, it is time to prepare the detail of the trial. At this stage, a study protocol should be constructed to define the research strategy. It should contain a paragraph on the background of the proposed study, the aims and objectives, a clear methodology, definitions of population and sample sizes and methods of proposed analysis. It should include the patient numbers, inclusion and exclusion criteria and the timescale for the work. At this stage, it is useful to construct a flow diagram giving a clear summary of the research protocol and its requirements (Figure 10.1). It is helpful to imagine the paper that will be written about the study, before it is performed. This may prevent errors in data collection.

When a study is planned, sufficient time should be reserved at the beginning for fund-raising and obtaining ethical, regulatory and NHS R&D or other management approvals. Time for data analysis and preparation of publication needs to be included in funding applications. The cost of any non-routine investigations and extra treatments should be identified and covered by the research grant.

A data collection form should be designed or a computer collection package developed. If data are collected on computer, appropriate safeguards for privacy and confidentiality will be necessary to comply with legislation on data protection. Any form of data collection needs to be quality assured. The quality assurance process will include training, as well as monitoring and checking a certain sample of the data. At the end of data collection and analysis, a final database with all data should be locked and kept for future reference in a safe location. A data archiving policy via a data controller needs to be in place.

It is important to ensure the cooperation of any other specialties or clinicians who will be involved in the study and to agree on the sharing of responsibility for the trial. This will also help to prevent disagreement about who takes the credit once a study is ready for presentation and publication.

Regulatory framework

In the UK, the implementation of the research governance framework by the Department of Health provides a framwork that enhances the integrity of your study and includes requirements for sponsorship by an institution to ensure the following: peer review, independent ethics review, compliance with data protection principles, financial probity, dissemination and management of intellectual property.

Peer review

Once the protocol is finalised, formal peer review is needed. In the UK, evidence of peer review will be needed before submitting an application to an ethics committee and for hospital trust approval.

- If the research is part of a university course, the university should undertake this review.
- Surgeons working for the NHS can arrange their own peer review by experts who are not connected with the study. Alternatively, most Research and Development Support Units (NHS) will give guidance through the review process.
- Funders of research will usually undertake their own independent peer review. There is usually feedback from this process that often gives valuable advice about the study.

Ethics

In the first instance, common sense is the best guide to whether or not a study is ethical. It is still important to seek advice from an ethics committee whenever research is contemplated.

In the UK, the requirement is that a NHS Research Ethics Committee (NHS REC) provides an independent ethical review of all health and social care research if it involves patients, carers, NHS staff and NHS premises (www.dh.gov.uk/assetRoot/04/12/24/27/04122427.pdf). In addition, the NHS REC provides an ethical review for studies that involve relevant material in line with the Human Tissue Act (www.legislation.gov.uk/ukpga/2004/30/contents) and studies that might involve participants that might lack capacity in line with the Mental Capacity Act (www.legislation.gov.uk/ukpga/2005/9/contents).

The application for NHS REC review should be made using the Integrated Research Administration System (IRAS) (www.myresearchproject.org.uk/SignIn.aspx). IRAS is a single system for applying for the permissions and approvals for health and social care/community care research in the UK. It enables regulatory and governance requirements to be met while entering the information about the project once, instead of duplicating information in separate application forms for:

- Administration of Radioactive Substances Advisory Committee (ARSAC)
- Gene Therapy Advisory Committee (GTAC)
- Medicines and Healthcare products Regulatory Agency (MHRA)
- Ministry of Justice

- NHS/HSC R&D offices
- NRES/NHS/HSC Research Ethics Committees
- National Information Governance Board (NIGB)
- National Offender Management Service (NOMS)
- Social Care Research Ethics Committee.

Once all relevant forms and associated study documentation have been completed, guidance provided by the National Research Ethics Service should be followed for submission of the request for ethical review (www.nres.npsa.nhs.uk/applications/).

If the study does not require review by an NHS REC, the need for an independent ethical review should still be considered. Universities have developed their own ethical review infrastructure and this will be institute and location specific. For collaborative research, local ethical review should be obtained where possible and developing a local ethics infrastructure should be considered if it does not already exist. Duplication of ethical review should be avoided where possible.

Ethics committees prefer to see fully developed trial protocols, but it is often possible to get some preliminary advice from the committee chair. Ethics committee forms may seem long and detailed, but it is important that these are filled in correctly. All dealings with ethics committees should be intelligent and courteous. It is important to attend the meeting at which the study will be discussed, if invited, as it provides a forum for direct communication in relation to the study. It can save time as possible concerns of the ethics committee can be addressed immediately, avoiding lengthy correspondence.

Regulatory approvals

In the case of clinical trials, the European Union Clinical Trial Directive applies and is regulated by the Medicines and Health Care products Regulatory Agency (MHRA) in the UK (www.mhra.gov.uk/Howweregulate/index.htm). A clinical trial should be registered with the European Clinical Trials Database (www.eudract.emea.europa.eu) or one of the other free databases (www.clinicaltrials.gov) before applying to the MHRA for a Clinical Trial Authorisation. This can be a complicated and trying process, and support should be sought from the investigators' employing institution. Editors of the major surgical journals now agree that all clinical trials should have been registered before an article relating to a trial can be published. All studies undertaken in the NHS will need NHS R&D management approval. Studies involving animals require approval from statutory licensing authorities. Do not embark on the study until the correct approval has been granted.

STATISTICAL ANALYSIS

Both audit and research commonly require statistical analysis. Many surgeons find the statistical analysis of a project the most difficult part. It is also the most commonly criticised part of papers written by clinicians.

There are many useful books about statistics which can be consulted (see Further reading); if in any doubt, a statistician will be pleased to give assistance. Statisticians like to be consulted before research or audit has been conducted rather than being presented with the data at the end; they often give helpful advice over study design.

The following terms are frequently used when summarising statistical data:

- **Mean**: the result of dividing the total by the number of observations (the average);
- **Median**: the middle value with equal numbers of observations above and below – used for numerical or ranked data;
- **Mode**: the value with the highest frequency observed – used for nominal data collection;
- **Range**: the largest to the smallest value.

The most important decision for analysis is whether the distribution of results is normal, i.e. parametric or non-parametric. Normally distributed data have a symmetrical, bell-shaped curve, and the mean, median and mode all lie at the same value. The type of data collected determines which statistical test should be used.

1 Numerical and normally distributed (e.g. blood pressure) – use unpaired *t*-test to compare two groups, or paired *t*-test to assess whether a variable has changed between two time points.
2 Numerical but not normally distributed (e.g. tumour size) – use Mann–Whitney *U*-test to compare two groups, or a Wilcoxon signed rank test to assess whether a variable has increased/stayed the same/decreased between two time points.
3 Categorical (e.g. admitted or not admitted to an intensive care unit) – can use chi-squared test to compare two groups.

(Please note: the use of any other tests may benefit from professional advice.)

Confidence intervals are the best guide to the possible range in which the true differences are likely to lie. A confidence interval that includes zero usually implies a lack of statistical significance.

Scientists usually employ probability (*p*-values) to describe statistical chance. A p-value <0.05 is commonly taken to imply a true difference. It is important not to forget that $p = 0.05$ simply means there is only a 1:20 chance that the differences between the variables would have happened by chance when in fact there is no real difference. If enough variables are examined in any study, significant differences will occur simply by chance. Trials with multiple end points or variables require more sophisticated analysis to determine the significance of individual risk factors. Univariable or multivariable logistic regression analysis techniques may be appropriate.

Statistics simply deal with the chance that observations between populations are different and should be treated with caution. Clinical results should show clear differences. If statistics are required to demonstrate differences between results, it is possible that they are unlikely to have major clinical significance.

Computer software packages available

Statistical computer packages offer a quick way of analysing descriptive statistics, such as mean, median and range, as well as the most commonly used statistical tests, such as the chi-squared test. Various packages are available commercially and are useful tools in data analysis.

ANALYSING A SCIENTIFIC ARTICLE

The simplest way to analyse an article from a scientific journal is to look at the checklist of requirements for good scientific research. A group of scientists and editors developed

Table 10.4 Checklist for authors.

Heading	Sub-heading	Descriptor
Title		Identify as randomised trial
Abstract		Structured format
Introduction		Prospectively defined hypotheses, clinical objective
Methods	Protocol	Study population
		Intervention, timing
		Primary and secondary outcome
		Statistical rationale
		Stopping rules
	Assignment	Unit of randomisation
		Method: allocation schedule
	Masking (blinding)	
Results	Participant flow and follow up	Trial profile, flow diagram
	Analysis	Estimated effect of intervention
		Summary data with appropriate inferential statistics
		Protocol deviation
Comment		Specific interpretation of study
		Sources of bias
		External validity
		General interpretation

From the CONSORT statement: *Journal of the American Medical Association* 1996; **276**: 637–9.

the CONSORT (Consolidated Standards of Reporting Trials) statement to improve the quality of reporting of RCTs. Looking in detail at the study design is often the best way of deciding whether a trial is any good. The CONSORT document includes a checklist for the conduct of good randomised trials (Table 10.4). Often, clinicians overlook biases that others find obvious to detect, which can have a profound influence on the outcome of any study. Even the randomised design does not always guarantee quality, and a core component of systematic review is the grading of trial quality; several scoring systems have been developed, e.g. Jadad Score. Recent guidelines have been published formalising the methods of systematic review and meta-analysis (PRISMA guidelines), and most surgical journals will now only accept articles that follow the rules.

PRESENTING AND PUBLISHING AN ARTICLE

There is no point in conducting a research or audit project and then leaving the results unreported. Even when results are negative, they are worth distributing; no project if properly conducted is worthless. Under-reporting of negative outcomes causes a systematic bias in the literature in favour of positive trials. Most studies do not provide dramatic results, and few surgeons publish seminal articles.

The key to both presentation and publication is to decide on the message, and then aim for an appropriate forum. Large important randomised studies or national audits merit presentation at national meetings and publication in international journals. Small observational studies and audits are more often accepted for presentation at regional or hospital meetings and for publication in smaller specialist journals. Help and advice from clinicians familiar with presentation and publication are invaluable at this stage. The most important piece of advice is to follow the instructions for journal submission accurately. Most international meetings will accept presentations eagerly (especially by poster) as this increases the attendance at a conference.

Most surgeons publish research in peer-reviewed journals. The work that is submitted is checked anonymously by other surgeons before publication. If in doubt about whether to submit to a journal, many editors will give advice about the suitability of an article for submission to their journal.

Convention dictates that articles are submitted in IMRAD form (introduction, methods, results and discussion). Increasingly, electronic publication and the internet may change the face of scientific publication and, in the next decade, these restrictions on style may disappear. For now, the IMRAD format remains inviolable. The length of an article is important: a paper should be as long as the size of the message. Readers of large randomised multicentre trials wish to know as much detail about the study as possible; reports on small negative trials should be brief.

- **Introduction.** This should always be short. A brief background of the study should be presented and then the aims of the trial or audit outlined.
- **Methods.** The methodology and study design should be given in detail. It is important to own up to any biases. Any new techniques or investigations should be detailed in full; if they are common practice or have been described elsewhere, this should be referenced instead of described.
- **Results.** Results are almost always best shown diagrammatically using tables and figures if possible. Results shown in the form of a diagram need not then be duplicated in the text.
- **Discussion.** It is important not to repeat the introduction or reiterate the results in this section. The study should be interpreted intelligently, and any suggestions for future studies or changes in management should be made. It is important not to indulge in flights of fantasy or wild imagination about future possibilities; most journal editors will delete these. Recently, a standard format for the discussion section has been promoted, and journals such as the *British Medical Journal* are keen that authors use it.
- **References.** This section should include all relevant papers recording previous studies on the subject in question. The number should reflect the size of the message and the importance of the work. The reference section does not usually have to be exhaustive, but should include up-to-date articles. Remember to present the references in the style of the journal of submission.

EVIDENCE-BASED SURGERY

Surgical practice has been considered an art: ask 50 surgeons how to manage a patient and one will probably get 50 different answers. There is so much clinical information available that no surgeon can know it all. Evidence-based surgery is a move to find the best ways of managing patients using clinical evidence from collected studies. It was estimated that sufficient evidence to justify routine myocardial thrombolysis for heart attacks was available years before the randomised clinical studies that finally made it clinically acceptable. No-one had gathered all the available information together. Centres such as the Cochrane Collaboration have been collecting randomised trials and reviews to provide up-to-date information for clinicians. The Cochrane Library presently includes a database of systematic reviews, reviews of surgical effectiveness and a register of controlled trials. The *British Journal of Surgery* has been collecting surgical randomised trials on its website archive for ten years (www.bjs.co.uk). There are now almost 1500 annotated references that can be a valuable resource for scientific authors. As evidence accumulates, it is expected that this will gradually smooth out the differences between clinicians as the best way of managing patients becomes more obvious. Collecting published evidence together and analysing it often requires reviews of multiple randomised trials. These meta-analyses involve complex statistical analyses designed to interpret multiple findings and synthesise the results of multiple studies. There exist standard formats for the presentation of meta-analyses described in the PRISMA guidelines (produced after a conference that was convened to address standards for improving the quality of reporting of meta-analysis of clinical RCTs).

FURTHER READING

Altman DG. *Statistics with confidence*. London: BMJ Publishing Group, 2002.

Brown RA, Swanson Beck J. *Medical statistics on personal computers*. Plymouth: BMJ Publishing Group, 1994.

Greenhalgh T. *How to read a paper: the basiscs of evidence based medicine*. London: BMJ Publishing Group, 2010.

Institute of Medicine. *Guidelines for clinical practice: from development to use*. Washington, DC: National Academic Press, 1992.

Kelson M. *Promoting patient involvement in clinical audit*. London: London College of Health and the Clinical Outcomes Group, 1998.

Kirkwood BR. *Essentials of medical statistics*, 2nd edn. Oxford: Blackwell Publishing, 2003.

Lyratzopoulos G, Patrick H, Campbell WB. Registers needed for new interventional procedures. *Lancet* 2008; **371**: 1734–6.

McCulloch P, Altman DG, Campbell WB *et al*. No surgical innovation without evaluation: the IDEAL recommendations. *Lancet* 2009; **374**: 1105–12.

Moher D, Cooke DJ, Eastwood S *et al*. Improving the quality of reports of meta-analyses of randomised controlled trials: the QUORUM statement. *Lancet* 1999; **354**: 1896–900.

Moher D, Liberati A, Tetzlaff J *et al*. The PRISMA Group. Preferred reporting items for systematic reviews and meta-analyses: the PRISMA statement. *Open Medicine* 2009; **3**: 123–30.

Morrell C, Harvey G. *The clinical audit handbook*. London: Baillière Tindall, 1999.

Schein M, Farndon JR, Fingerhut A. *A surgeon's guide to writing and publishing*. Kemberton, Shropshire: TFM Publishing, 2001.

Smith R. *The trouble with medical journals*. London: RSM Press, 2006.

Swinscow TDV. *Statistics at square one*, 9th edn. London: BMJ Publishing Group, 1996.

Walshe K. Adverse events in health care: issues in measurement. *Quality in Health Care* 2000; **9**: 47–52.

Whitman B, Ginham R, Perkins M, Langley D. The Human Tissue Act 2004. Reflections on recent changes of regulatory affairs in the United Kingdom. *Journal of Research Administration* 2008; **2**: 91–9.

ON-LINE RESOURCES

Clinical Evidence: www.clinicalevidence.com

Cochrane Library: www.cochrane.org/index.htm

Consolidated Standards of Reporting Trials: http://www.consort-statement.org/consort-statement/

National Institute for Health and Clinical Excellence (NICE): www.nice.org.uk

National Research Ethics Service: http://www.nres.npsa.nhs.uk/

Scottish Intercollegiate Guideline Network (SIGN): www.sign.ac.uk

Integrated Research Administration System: https://www.myresearchproject.org.uk/SignIn.aspx

CHAPTER 11

Surgical ethics and law

LEARNING OBJECTIVES

To understand:

- The importance of autonomy in good surgical practice
- The moral and legal boundaries and practical difficulties of informed consent
- Good practice in making decisions about the withdrawal of life-sustaining treatment
- The importance and boundaries of confidentiality in surgical practice
- The importance of appropriate regulation in surgical research
- The importance of rigorous training and maintenance of good practice standards

INTRODUCTION

This chapter incorporates references to English common and statute law. Nevertheless, these legal and ethical principles have much in common with many other jurisdictions across the world.

Surgery, ethics and law go hand in hand. In any other arena of public or private life, if someone deliberately cuts another person, draws blood, causes pain, leaves scars and disrupts everyday activity, then the likely result will be a criminal charge. If the person dies as a result, the charge could be manslaughter or even murder. Self-evidently, the difference between the criminal and the surgeon is that their intentions differ. While a criminal intentionally (or recklessly) inflicts harm, the surgeon's intention is limited to the treatment of illness. Any harm that ensues is either unintentional, or is necessary (such as an incision), to facilitate treatment.

Patients submit to surgery because they trust their surgeons. What should consent entail in practice and what should surgeons do when patients need help but are unable or unwilling to agree to it? When patients do consent to treatment, surgeons are provided with a wide discretion. The end result may be cure, but disfigurement, disability and death may also result. How should such surgical 'power' be regulated to reinforce the trust of patients; and to ensure that surgeons practise to an acceptable professional standard? Are there circumstances, in the public interest, in which it is acceptable to sacrifice the trust of individual patients through revealing information that was communicated in what patients believed to be conditions of strict privacy?

These questions about what constitutes good professional practice concern medical ethics and law relating to consent, confidentiality, and the underlying concept of personal autonomy.

In addition, these principles need to be applied to surgical activities, including professional matters relating to governance, regulation and the process of revalidation, in its different guises around the world. Surgical training is starting to embrace the 'basic science' of surgical law, to offer surgeons assistance in the resolution of such ethical dilemmas. This chapter is evidence of that process.

RESPECT FOR AUTONOMY

Surgeons have a duty of care towards their human patients which goes beyond just protecting their life and health. Their additional duty of care is to respect the autonomy of their patients and their ability to make choices about their treatments, and to evaluate potential outcomes in light of other life plans. Such respect is particularly important for surgeons because, without it, the trust between them and their patients may be compromised, along with the success of the surgical care provided. We are careful enough in everyday life about whom we allow to touch us; and to see us unclothed. It is hardly surprising that many people feel strongly about exercising the same control over a potentially hazardous activity, such as surgery.

For all these reasons, there is a wide moral and legal consensus that patients have the right to exercise choice over their surgical care. In this context, a right should be interpreted as a claim that can be made on the surgeon. The surgeon, therefore, accepts the strict duty to respect the patient's choice, regardless of personal preferences. Thus, to the degree that patients have a right to make choices about proposed surgical treatment, it then follows that they should be allowed to refuse treatments that they do not want, even when surgeons think that they are wrong. For example, patients can even refuse surgical treatment that will save their lives, either at present or in the future, through the formulation of advance decisions specifying the types of life-saving treatments that they do not wish to have, notwithstanding that they may later become incompetent to refuse them.

INFORMED CONSENT

In surgical practice, respect for autonomy translates into the clinical duty to obtain informed consent before the commencement of treatment.

It is easy to underestimate the gap in understanding between a surgeon and his or her patient. How many patients would recognise that unilateral eye surgery might lead to contralateral blindness? The risks and side effects of many operations are not intuitive, and the surgeon is not in the position to guess how the patient's plans for employment, leisure and family life may be inadvertently affected by a forseeable complication. A budding Olympic gymnast might choose to forgo surgery on a quiescent posterior triangle lesion if they knew the potential consequences of division of the accessory nerve. That is why patients need to be informed, beforehand, so they can choose whether to take the risk.

To establish valid consent to treatment, patients need to be given appropriate and accurate information. In England and Wales, the Department of Health's Reference Guide to Consent should be consulted.

Such information should include:

- the condition and the reasons why it warrants surgery;
- the type of surgery proposed and how it might correct the condition;
- the anticipated prognosis and expected side effects of the proposed surgery;
- the unexpected hazards of the proposed surgery;
- any alternative and potentially successful treatments other than the proposed surgery;
- the consequences of no treatment at all.

With such information, patients can link their clinical prospects with the management of other aspects of their life and the lives of others for whom they may be morally and/or professionally responsible. Good professional practice dictates that obtaining informed consent should occur in circumstances that are designed to maximise the chances of patients understanding what is said about their condition and proposed treatment, as well as giving them an opportunity to ask questions and express anxieties.

Where possible:

- a quiet venue for discussion should be found;
- written material in the patient's preferred language should be provided to supplement verbal communication, together with diagrams where appropriate;
- patients should be given time and help to come to their own decision;
- the person obtaining the consent should ideally be the surgeon who will carry out the treatment. It should not be – as is sometimes the case – a junior member of staff who has never conducted such a procedure and thus may not have enough understanding to counsel the patient properly.

Good communication skills go hand in hand with properly obtaining informed consent for surgery. It is not good enough just to go through the motions of providing patients with the information required for considered choice. Attention must be paid to:

- whether or not the patient has understood what has been stated;
- avoiding overly technical language in descriptions and explanations;
- the provision of translators for patients whose first language is not English;
- asking patients if they have further questions.

When there is any doubt about their understanding, surgeons should ask patients questions about what has supposedly been communicated to see if they can explain the information in question for themselves.

Surgeons have a legal, as well as a moral, obligation to obtain consent for treatment based on appropriate disclosure. Failure to do so could result in one of two civil proceedings, assuming the absence of criminal intent. First, in law, intentionally to touch another person without their consent is a battery, remembering that we are usually touched by strangers as a consequence of accidental contact. Surgeons have a legal obligation to give the conscious and competent patient sufficient information 'in broad terms' about the surgical treatment being proposed and why. If the patient agrees to proceed, no other treatment should ordinarily be administered without further explicit consent.

Negligence is the second legal action that might be brought against a surgeon for not obtaining appropriate consent to treatment. Patients may have been given enough information about what is surgically proposed to agree to be touched in the ways suggested. However, surgeons may still be in breach of their professional duty if they do not provide sufficient information about the risks that patients will encounter through such treatment. Although standards of how much information should be provided about risks vary between nations, as a matter of good practice, surgeons should inform patients of the hazards that any reasonable person in the position of the patient would wish to know. In English law, this level of disclosure has been most recently reviewed in the case of *Chester* v. *Afshar*.

Finally, surgeons now understand that, when they obtain consent to proceed with treatment, then patients are expected to sign a consent form of some kind. The detail of such forms can differ, but they often contain very little of the information supposedly communicated to the patient who signed it. Partly for this reason, the process of formally obtaining consent can become overly focused on obtaining the signature of patients rather than ensuring that appropriate types and amounts of information have been provided, and have been understood.

Both professionally and legally, it is important for surgeons to understand that a signed consent form is not proof that valid consent has been properly obtained. It is simply a piece of evidence that consent may have been attempted. Even when they have provided their signature, patients can and do deny that appropriate information has been communicated or that the communication was effective. Surgeons are therefore well advised to make brief notes of what they have said to patients about their proposed treatments, especially information about significant risks. These notes should be placed in the patient's clinical record. In addition, information sheets describing the generic risks, benefits and complications associated with the proposed procedure can be provided.

PRACTICAL APPLICATION

Thus far, we have examined the moral and legal reasons why the duty of surgeons to respect the autonomy of patients translates into the specific responsibility to obtain informed consent to treatment. For consent to be valid, patients must:

- be competent to give it – be able to understand, remember and deliberate about whatever information is provided to them about treatment choices, and to communicate those choices;
- not be coerced into decisions that reflect the preferences of others rather than themselves;
- be given sufficient information for these choices to be based on an accurate understanding of reasons for and against proceeding with specific treatments.

Surgical care would grind to a halt if it were always necessary to obtain explicit informed consent every time a patient is touched in the context of their care. Fortunately, it is an elementary step merely to ask the patient whether they mind being examined – the usual response will be acceptance. This simple transaction illustrates that the legal and ethical 'rules' that govern a surgeon are often no more than an expression of good clinical practice; in this case, politeness.

Some patients will not be able to give consent because of temporary incapacity. This may result from their presenting illness or intoxication; or an unanticipated situation may be encountered midway through a general anaesthetic. The moral and legal rules that govern such situations are clear. The doctrine of medical necessity enables the surgeon, in an emergency, to save life and prevent permanent disability, operating without consent. This is employed daily, where unconsious emergency patients undergo surgery to save 'life and limb'. No consent has been provided, and none is required, providing the treatment is in the patient's best interests.

However, if the patient has made a legally valid advance decision refusing treatment of the specific kind required, their decision must be honoured, providing it is applicable to the current clinical situation. Where possible, surgery on patients who are temporarily incapacitated should be postponed until their capacity is restored, and they are able to give informed consent or refusal for themselves.

Surgeons must take care to respect the distinction between procedures that are necessary to prevent death or irremediable harm, and those that are done merely out of convenience. If the patient consents only to a dilatation and currettage, do not consider performing an additional hysterectomy 'in her best interests', simply because she is anaesthetised.

Consent may be made impossible by incompetence of other kinds. In the case of children, parents or someone with parental responsibility are ordinarily required to provide consent on their behalf. This said, surgeons should:

- take care to explain to children what is being surgically proposed and why;
- always consult with children about their response;
- where possible, take the child's views into account and note that even young children can be competent to consent to treatment provided that they too can understand, remember, deliberate about and believe information relevant to their clinical condition.

When such *Gillick* competence is present, under English law, children can provide their own consent to surgical care, although they cannot unconditionally refuse it until they are 18 years old. These provisions illustrate the importance of respecting as much autonomy as is present among child patients and remembering that, for the purposes of consent to medical treatment, they may be just as autonomous as adults.

If competence is severely compromised by psychiatric illness or mental handicap, other moral and legal provisions hold. If patients lack the autonomy to choose how to protect themselves as regards the consequences of their illness then others charged with protecting them must assume the responsibility. Yet care must be taken not to abuse this duty. Even when such patients have been legally detained for compulsory psychiatric care, it does not follow that such patients are unable to provide consent for surgical care. Their competence should be assumed and consent should be sought. If it is established with the help of their carers that such patients are also incompetent to provide consent for surgery and that they are at risk of death or serious and permanent disability, then therapy can proceed in their best interests. However, if treatment can be postponed, then this should be done until, as a result of their psychiatric care, patients become able either to consent or to refuse. If this recovery is not predicted, then legal steps may be taken to make elective surgery lawful. As with children, respect should always be shown for as much autonomy as is present.

In adult patients who are permanently incapacitated, and thus unable to provide consent for surgery, the doctrine of necessity obtains, and surgery can proceed in an emergency to save life, to prevent serious and permanent injury. Elective treatment for less grave complaints can also be provided, and in England and Wales is done so under the auspices of the Mental Capacity Act 2005. The associated Code of Practice guides the surgeon in matters of capacity and disclosure; and in dealing with those who have taken steps to influence their treatment, anticipating the time that they will have lost their capacity. These arrangements may manifest either in documentary form, as Advance Decisions; or in person, in the form of persons appointed with a Lasting Power of Attorney.

It is not possible for relatives of incompetent adult patients to sign consent forms for surgery on their behalf. Indeed, to make such requests can be a disservice to relatives, who may feel an unjustified sense of responsibility if the surgery fails. This said, relatives play a vital role in providing background information about the patient, allowing the clinician to assess and then determine what treatment is in the best interests of the patient.

MATTERS OF LIFE AND DEATH

It has been noted that the right of a competent adult to consent to and refuse treatment is unlimited, including the refusal of life-sustaining treatment. Probably the example of this most familiar to surgeons is Jehovah's Witnesses, who may refuse blood transfusions at the risk of their own lives.

There will be some circumstances in which sustaining the life and health of incompetent patients is judged to be inappropriate. They are no longer able to be consulted; and may not have expressed a view about what their wishes would be in such circumstances. Here, if possible after discussion and consensus with the next of kin, a decision may be made to withhold or to withdraw life-sustaining treatment on behalf of the incompetent

A **Jehovah's Witness** is a member of a millenarian fundamentalist Christian sect founded in America in 1884. They have their own translation of the Bible which they interpret literally.

patient. The fact that such decisions can be seen as omissions to act does not excuse surgeons from morally and legally having to reconcile them with their ordinary duty of care. Ultimately, this can only be done through arguing that such omissions to sustain life are in the patient's best interests.

The determination of best interests in these circumstances will rely on one of three objective criteria, over and above the subjective perception by the surgeon that the quality of life of the patient is poor. There is no obligation to provide or to continue life-sustaining treatment:

- If doing so is futile, when clinical consensus dictates that it will not achieve the goal of extending life. Thought of in this way, judgements about futility exclude considering the patient's quality of life; and thus can be difficult to justify as long as treatment might stand even a very small chance of success.
- If a patient is imminently and irreversibly close to death – in such circumstances, it would not be in the patient's best interests to prolong life slightly (e.g. through the application of intensive care) when, again, there is no hope of any sustained success. Declining needlessly to interfere with the process of a dignified death can be just as caring as the provision of curative therapy.
- If a patient is so permanently and seriously brain damaged that, lacking awareness of themselves or others, they will never be able to engage in any form of self-directed activity. The argument here is backed up by morally and legally reasoning that further treatment other than effective palliation cannot be in the best interests of the patient as it will provide them with no benefit.

When any of these principles are employed to justify an omission to provide or to continue life-sustaining treatment, the circumstances should be carefully recorded in the patient's medical record, along with a note of another senior clinician's agreement.

Finally, surgeons will sometimes find themselves in charge of the palliative care of patients whose pain is increasingly difficult to control. There may come a point in the management of such pain when effective palliation is possible at the risk of shortening a patient's life because of the respiratory effects of the palliative drugs. In such circumstances, surgeons can with legal justification administer a dose that might be dangerous (although experts in palliative care are sceptical that this is ever necessary with appropriate training). In any case, the argument employed to justify such action refers to its 'double effect': that both the relief of pain and death might follow from such an action. Intentional killing (active euthanasia) is rejected as unlawful malpractice throughout most of the world. A foreseeably lethal analgesic dose is thus regarded as appropriate only when it is solely motivated by palliative intent; and this motivation can be documented.

TRANSPLANTATION

The law and ethics of organ transplantation require more space than this chapter allows. In common with other nations, the United Kingdom has a statutory framework for transplantation, but even among this small group of nations, there is no unanimity of legislation, thus rules for deceased and live donor transplants differ. In general, the rules for defining a dead donor; for compensating a living donor; and for legitimising a market in organs differ widely. It is strongly recommended that you refer to the rules within your own jurisdiction.

CONFIDENTIALITY

Respect for autonomy does not entail only the right of competent patients to consent to treatment. Their autonomous right extends to control over their confidential information, and surgeons must to respect their privacy, not communicate information revealed in the course of treatment to anyone else without consent. Generally speaking, such respect means that surgeons must not discuss clinical matters with relatives, friends, employers and others unless the patient explicitly agrees. To do otherwise is regarded by all the regulatory bodies of medicine and surgery as a grave offence, incurring harsh penalties. For breaches of confidentiality are not only abuses of human dignity, they again undermine the trust between surgeon and patient on which successful surgery and the professional reputations of surgeons depend.

Important as respect for confidentiality is, however, it is not absolute. Surgeons are allowed to communicate private information to other professionals who are part of the healthcare team – provided that the information has a direct bearing on treatment. Here, it is argued that patients have given their implied consent to such communication when they explicitly consent to a treatment plan. Whether implied consent can ever be valid is a matter for public debate, as government attempts to apply the doctrine to tissue donation and access to electronic health records.

Patients cannot expect strict adherence to the principle of confidentiality if it poses a serious threat to the health and safety of others. There will be some circumstances in which confidentiality either must or may be breached in the public interest. For example, it must be breached as a result of court orders or in relation to the requirements of public health legislation. Confidentiality may be waived in the interests of preventing serious crime or to protect the safety of other known individuals who are at risk of serious harm.

RESEARCH

As part of their duty to protect life and health to an acceptable professional standard, surgeons have a subsidiary responsibility to strive to improve operative techniques through research, to assure themselves and their patients that the care proposed is the best that is currently possible. Yet, there is moral tension between the duty to act in the best interests of individual patients and the duty to improve surgical standards through exposing patients to the unknown risks that any form of research inevitably entails.

The willingness to expose patients to such risks may be further increased by the professional and academic pressures on many surgeons to maintain a high research profile in their work. For this reason, surgeons (and physicians, who face the same dilemmas) now accept that their research must be externally regulated to ensure that patients give their informed consent, that any known risks to patients are far outweighed by the potential benefits, and that other forms of protection for the patient are in place (e.g. proper indemnity) in case they are unexpectedly harmed. The administration of such regulation is through research ethics committees, and surgeons should not participate in research that has not been approved by such bodies. Equally, special provisions will apply to research involving incompetent patients who cannot provide consent to participate and research ethics committees will evaluate specific proposals with great care.

In practice, it is not always clear as to what constitutes 'research' that should be subjected to regulation, as compared with a minor innovation dictated by the contingencies of a particular clinical situation. Surgeons must always ask themselves in such circumstances whether or not the innovation in question falls within the boundaries of standard procedures in which they are trained. If so, what may be a new technique for them will count not as research but as an incremental improvement in personal practice. Nevertheless, major innovations in operative procedure are scrutinised by national regulatory authorities; in the United Kingdom, by the National Institute for Clinical Healthcare Excellence. This process of scrutiny has been designed to ensure that the innovation is safe, efficacious and cost-effective. It is regarded (by the NHS) as a mandatory step when introducing a new interventional procedure.

Equally, surgeons know that exigencies of operative surgery sometimes demand a novel and hitherto undescribed manoeuvre to get the surgeon (and their patient) out of trouble. Providing your solution is necessary, proportionate to the circumstances, performed in good faith and would pass the scrutiny of your peers as reasonable, it is unlikely that any subsequent criticism of your actions could be sustained.

If a proposed innovation passes the criteria for research, it should be approved by a research ethics committee. Such surgical research should also be subject to a clinical trial designed to ensure that findings about outcomes are systematically compared with the best available treatment and that favourable results are not the result of arbitrary factors (e.g. unusual surgical skill among researchers) that cannot be replicated.

MAINTAINING STANDARDS OF EXCELLENCE

To optimise success in protecting life and health to an acceptable standard, surgeons must only offer specialised treatment in which they have been properly trained. To do so will entail sustained further education throughout a surgeon's career in the wake of new surgical procedures. While training, surgery should be practised only under appropriate supervision by someone who has appropriate levels of skill. Such skill can be demonstrated only through appropriate clinical audit, to which all surgeons should regularly submit their results. When these results are unacceptable, no further surgical work of that kind should continue unless further training is undergone under the supervision of someone whose success rates are satisfactory. To do otherwise would be to place the interest of the surgeon above that of their patient, an imbalance that is never morally or professionally appropriate.

Surgeons also have a duty to monitor the performance of their colleagues. To know that a fellow surgeon is exposing patients to unacceptable levels of potential harm and to do nothing about it is to incur some responsibility for such harm when it occurs. Surgical teams and the institutions in which they function should have clear protocols for exposing unacceptable professional performance and helping colleagues to understand the danger to which they may expose patients. If necessary, offending surgeons must be stopped from practising until they can undergo further appropriate training and counselling. Too often, such danger has had to be reported by individuals whose anxieties have not been properly heeded and who have then been professionally pilloried rather than acknowleged for their contribution to patient safety. Those who participate in closing ranks, and ostracism, share the moral responsibility for any resulting harm to patients.

CONCLUSION

Surgeons have a combination of duties to their patients: to protect life and health, and to respect autonomy; both to an acceptable professional standard. The specific duties of surgeons are shown to follow from these: reasonable practice concerning informed consent, confidentiality, decisions not to provide, or to omit, life-sustaining care, surgical research and the maintenance of good professional standards. The final duty of surgical care is to exercise all these general and specific responsibilities with fairness and justice, and without arbitrary prejudice. Now, at least partly either enshrined in statute or echoed in the English common law, these duties closely reflect the guidance of the General Medical Council.

The conduct of ethical surgery illustrates good citizenship: protecting the vulnerable and respecting human dignity; and equality. To the extent that the practice of individual surgeons is a reflection of such sustained conduct, they deserve the civil respect which they often receive. To the extent that it is not, they should not practise the honourable profession of surgery.

FURTHER READING

Beauchamp T, Childress J. *Principles of biomedical ethics*. London: Oxford University Press, 1994.

British Medical Association. *Medical ethics today*, 2nd edn. London: BMJ Books, 2004.

Chester v. *Afshar* [2004] UKHL 41.

Department of Constitutional Affairs. *Mental Capacity Act 2005 Code of Practice*. London: The Stationery Office, 2007.

Department of Health. *Reference guide to consent for examination or treatment*, 2nd edn. London: DoH, 2009.

Department of Health. *Confidentiality: NHS Code of Practice. Supplementary guidance: public interest disclosures*. London: DoH, 2010.

General Medical Council. *Seeking patients' consent: the ethical considerations*. London: GMC, 1998.

General Medical Council. *Withholding and withdrawing life prolonging treatments: good practice in decision making*. London: GMC, 2002.

General Medical Council. *Confidentiality: protecting and providing information*. Available from: http://gmc-uk.org/guidance/current/library/confidentiality.asp.

General Medical Council. *Good medical practice*. London: GMC, 2006.

General Medical Council. *0–18 years: guidance for all doctors*. London: GMC, 2007.

General Medical Council. *Confidentiality*. London: GMC, 2009.

Mason JK, Laurie GT. *Mason and McCall Smith's law and medical ethics*, 8th edn. Oxford: Oxford University Press, 2011.

McCullough LB, Jones JW, Brody BA (eds). *Surgical ethics*. New York: Oxford University Press, 1998.

Nair R, Holroyd DJ (eds). *Oxford handbook of surgical consent*. Oxford: Oxford University Press, 2012.

Royal College of Surgeons. *Good surgical practice*. London: RCS, 2002.

Senate of Surgery of Great Britain and Ireland. *The surgeon's duty of care: guidance for surgeons on ethical and legal issues*. London: RCS, 1997.

Wheeler RA. Gillick or Fraser? A plea for consistency over competence in children. *BMJ* 2006; **332**: 807.

Wheeler RA. Presumed or implied, it's not consent. *Clin Risk* 2010; **16**: 1–2.

Woodcock T. Surgical research in the United Kingdom. *Ann Roy Coll Surg* 2009; **91**: 188–91.

Woodcock T. Law and medical ethics in organ transplantation surgery. *Ann Roy Coll Surg* 2010: **92**: 282–5.

CHAPTER 12

Patient safety

LEARNING OBJECTIVES

To learn:

- The importance of patient safety and the scale of the problem
- Medical errors, their range and definition
- Models for understanding how adverse events and near misses occur
- Patient safety strategies and solutions
- Applying the science of patient safety to practice
- Patient safety principles that are specific to the surgeon
- Dealing with the 'second victim' of a medical error

INTRODUCTION

Medicine will never be a risk-free enterprise. From the beginning of training, doctors are taught that errors are unacceptable and that the philosophy of *primum non nocere* (first, do no harm) should permeate all aspects of treatment. Yet, worldwide, despite all the improvements in treatment and investment in technologies, training and services, there remains the challenge of dealing with unsafe practices, incompetent healthcare professionals, poor governance of healthcare service delivery, errors in diagnosis and treatment and noncompliance with accepted standards.

When errors do occur there continues to be a lack of adequate systems in place to ensure that all those affected are informed and cared for, and that there is a process of analysis and learning to uncover the cause and prevent recurrence of such events. Patient safety has become an established healthcare discipline in its own right thus formalizing approaches to these inadequacies, directing research and offering solutions for the future.

THE PREVALENCE OF ADVERSE HEALTHCARE EVENTS

The aviation and nuclear industries have a much better safety record than healthcare. This became abundantly clear when, in 1999, the Institute of Medicine of the National Academy of Sciences released a report, *To Err is Human: Building a Safer Health System*, that drew widespread attention to the alarming statistics that there were between 44 000 and 98 000 preventable deaths annually due to medical error in American hospitals with some 7000 preventable deaths related to medication errors alone. This experience has been found to be similar in other developed countries and was emphasised by the Bristol Royal Infirmary Inquiry of 2001 into a series of unacceptable paediatric cardiac surgical deaths. The World Health Organization estimates that, even in advanced hospital settings, one in ten patients receiving healthcare will suffer preventable harm.

The financial burden of unsafe care globally is also compelling resulting as it does in prolonged hospitalization, loss of income, disability and litigation costing many billions of dollars every year.

In the decade or more since the Institute of Medicine report there have been many initiatives to improve patient safety. Some interventions have been shown to reduce errors but many have still not been rigorously evaluated. Overall, it remains unclear whether efforts to reduce errors at national, regional and local levels have yet translated into significant improvements in the safe care of patients. This situation is unlikely to improve significantly while the reporting of adverse events remains low.

COMMON CAUSES OF ADVERSE HEALTHCARE EVENTS

Most medical care entails some level of risk to the patient either from their underlying condition or its treatment which, of itself, may lead to recognised complications or side effects. These episodes are different from **patient safety incidents** which have been described as preventable events or circumstances that could have, or did, result in unnecessary harm to the patient. This might be an adverse event, near miss and no-harm event (Table 12.1).

The most frequent contributing factors that lead to patient safety incidents are listed in Table 12.2. Of these, inadequate communication between healthcare staff, or between medical staff and their patients or family members, ranks highest in frequency.

UNDERSTANDING PATIENT SAFETY INCIDENTS

Understanding the concepts underlying patient safety incidents is useful because it helps to anticipate situations that are likely to

Table 12.1 Patient safety incidents.

Definitions	
An adverse event	An incident which results in harm to the patient
A near miss	An incident that could have resulted in unwanted consequences but did not, either by chance or through a timely intervention preventing the event from reaching the patient
A no-harm event	An incident that occurs and reaches the patient but results in no injury to the patient. Harm is avoided by chance or due to mitigating circumstances

Table 12.2 Factors that contribute to patient safety incidents.

Human factors	Inadequate patient assessment; delays or errors in diagnosis Failure to use or interpret appropriate tests Error in performance of an operation, treatment or test Inadequate monitoring or follow up of treatment Deficiencies in training or experience Fatigue, overwork, time pressures Personal or psychological factors, e.g. depression or drug abuse Patient or working environment variation Lack of recognition of the dangers of medical errors
System failures	Poor communication between healthcare providers Inadequate staffing levels Disconnected reporting systems or over-reliance on automated systems Lack of coordination at handovers Drug similarities Environment design, infrastructure Equipment failure, due to lack of parts or skilled operators Cost-cutting measures by hospitals Inadequate systems to report and review patient safety incidents
Medical complexity	Advanced and new technologies Potent drugs, their side effects and interactions Working environments – intensive care, operating theatres

lead to errors and highlights the areas where preventative action can be taken.

The problem of error can be viewed in two ways – from a person approach or from a system approach.

The person approach

Human performance principles tell us that humans are fallible and that errors can occur through doing the wrong thing – errors of commission; failure to act – errors of omission; or errors of execution – doing the right thing incorrectly. These principles also tell us that, by understanding the reasons why adverse events and near misses occur and by applying the lessons learnt from past events, future errors can be prevented. However, for most errors the person approach on its own tends to blame the individual and restricts learning.

The system approach

Health systems add complex organisational structures to human fallibility thus substantially increasing the potential for errors. A systems approach to error recognises that adverse events rarely have a single isolated cause and that they are best addressed by examining why the system failed rather than who made the mistake. James Reason, former Professor of Psychology at Manchester University, has stated that, 'We cannot change the human condition but we can change the conditions under which people work so as to make error less provoking'.

Heinrich's safety pyramid

Developed in 1931, Heinrich's safety pyramid theorised that unsafe acts or near misses lead to minor injuries and over time to a major injury. The accident pyramid proposes that for every 300 near misses there are 29 minor injuries and one major injury (Figure 12.1). **Risk assessment**, which is a step in risk management that calculates the value of risk related to a situation or hazard, has shown us that, what prevents patients from being hurt, is not only by reducing the number of mistakes but rather by increasing the number of defences set up against the consequences of mistakes. The key message is that near misses provide the best data about the reliability of safety systems. It is, therefore, most important to report near misses as well as adverse events to ensure that defences against adverse events are built and sustained.

Swiss cheese model

Reason's theory of accident causation, often referred to as the Swiss cheese model, is as well known in the aviation and nuclear power industries as it is in healthcare. His model takes Heinrich's concept forward and proposes the notion of **active failures** – acts that are committed by those at the coal face such as slip-ups, lapses or mistakes, and **latent conditions** – created by decisions taken at a higher level within the organisation leading, for example, to staff shortages or time pressures.

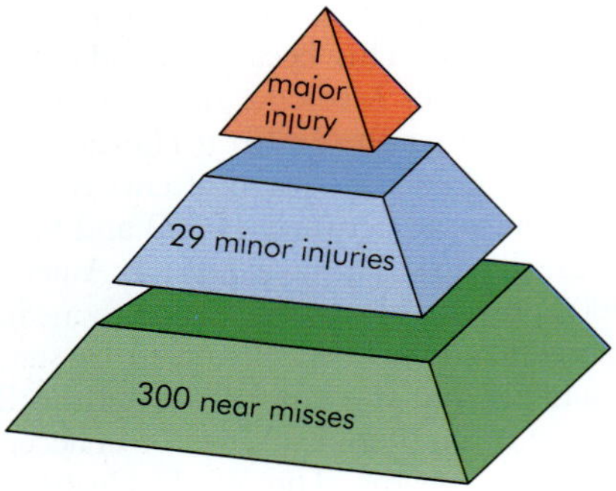

Figure 12.1 Heinrich's pyramid.

Herbert William Heinrich, 1886–1962, Assistant Superintendent, Engineering and Inspection Division of Travellers Insurance Co., Hartford, Connecticut, USA. He was a pioneer in industrial safety and developed his pyramid in 1931 when he published the book *Industrial Accident Prevention: A Scientific Approach*.

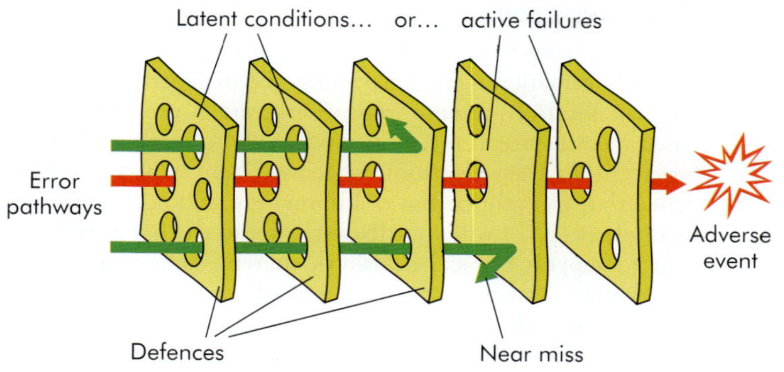

Figure 12.2 Reason's Swiss cheese model.

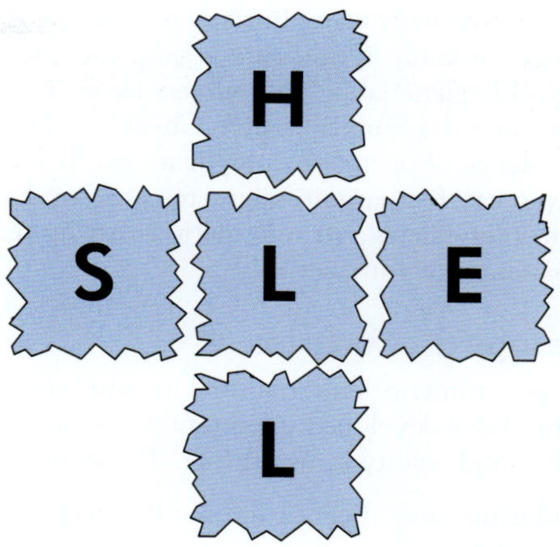

Figure 12.3 SHELL model.

Reason hypothesised that all organisations operating in potentially harmful environments tend to build up defences against potential damage and that these defences can be broken down by active failures or latent conditions. Although latent conditions are not harmful in themselves, they lie dormant within the system before combining with active failures to bypass the defences.

The defences in this model are represented as slices of Swiss cheese. This is because, instead of being intact, they are, in reality, full of holes or defects which represent either active failures or latent conditions. What is more, these gaps in the defences may not be static but can open and close and change position over time. Danger arises when a set of holes line up for a brief window allowing a potential hazard to become a fully blown accident. Each slice of cheese or defence is an opportunity to prevent an accident and the more slices there are and the fewer holes the less likely it is that an accident will occur or harm be done to a patient (Figure 12.2).

While healthcare workers are often at the sharp end of an error they are also often error catchers. It is the clinician's responsibility to observe, discuss and highlight latent conditions before adverse events occur and ensure the appropriate defences are in place.

SHELL model

Human factors is the study of the interrelationship between humans, the tools they work with and the environment in which they work. Working with this concept the SHELL model, developed in aviation, is designed to help understand the conditions that lead to adverse events.

The SHELL concept is named after the initial letters of its components – **Software**, **Hardware**, **Environment** and **Liveware** (Figure 12.3). In the centre of the model is the human operator, or the Liveware, represented by 'L'. This may be any individual whose job is relevant to patient care. It is the most flexible component in the system but may be unpredictable due to individual factors, such as personality, motivation, stress tolerance, skills, knowledge and attitudes. To overcome these intrinsic limitations the interface with the other components of the SHELL model must be adapted and matched to the Liveware component for optimum performance.

The first interface, the Liveware–Hardware has much to do with the ergonomic design of medical devices such that they should make it difficult for an operator to make a mistake.

The Liveware–Software interface encompasses the non-physical aspects of the system, such as manuals, checklists and computer programs. An adequate Liveware–Software interface should produce a situation where procedural omissions are difficult to make.

The Liveware–Environment interface may include stressors in the physical environment that have to be coped with, such as noise, poor acoustics and overcrowding.

The Liveware–Liveware interface is the interface of interpersonal communication. It embraces concepts, such as team coordination, conflict resolution and the continuity of information flow in the care of patients.

In the SHELL model diagram the edges of the blocks are uneven. This is to illustrate that the interdependent components are constantly changing and will never match perfectly. Human factors are concerned with minimising the mismatch between the different components (Summary box 12.1).

Summary box 12.1

Understanding patient safety incidents

- Errors can be viewed from a person-centred or system approach
- The majority of near misses or adverse events are due to system factors
- Understanding why these errors occur and applying the lessons learnt will prevent future injuries to patients
- It is important to report all near misses or adverse events so that we can constantly learn from mistakes
- Error models can help us understand the factors that cause near misses and adverse events and also direct us to where our defences against harm need to be improved

STRATEGIES FOR PATIENT SAFETY

International

Safety is everybody's business. Since the Institute of Medicine report, the World Health Organization has adopted a strong

James T Reason, contemporary, Professor of Psychology, University of Manchester, proposed in 1990 'The Swiss Cheese Model of Accident Causation'.

leadership role with many initiatives aimed at addressing safety challenges, notably 'Clean care is safer care', to ensure sustainable hand hygiene; and, 'Safe surgery saves lives', a programme that includes the Surgical Safety Checklist aimed at decreasing the incidence of operative complications. It has also identified priority areas for patient safety research and has introduced 'patient safety alerts', an information-sharing resource to learn from patient safety incidents.

Developed countries

Many governments and national organisations in developed countries have developed important strategies aimed at delivering safety and quality in healthcare. These include:

- regulating and licensing of physicians and healthcare institutions;
- developing and adopting policies for patient safety and quality improvement;
- providing patient safety education programmes;
- instituting national clinical audits;
- reporting (and learning from) adverse events;
- setting up agencies to resolve concerns about the practice of doctors by providing case and incident management services.

Developing countries

Developing countries share many aspirations and similar challenges with developed countries. However, they also face issues that are different and require different strategies. The probability of a patient being harmed in hospital is higher with, for example, the risk of healthcare-associated infection being as much as 20 times higher than in developed countries. At least 50 per cent of medical equipment in developing countries is unusable or only partly usable and often the equipment is not used due to lack of parts or necessary skills. In some countries, the proportion of injections given with syringes or needles reused without sterilisation is as high as 70 per cent. Each year, unsafe injections cause 1.3 million deaths, primarily due to transmission of hepatitis B virus, hepatitis C virus and HIV. Clearly, these issues need to be met with a specific range of initiatives.

Institutional or hospital

Team working and training

In order to decrease errors and increase patient safety many medical team training programmes have now been developed internationally, often based on **crew resource management** (CRM) programmes, the team training strategy used in the aviation industry. This kind of training heightens safety awareness, improves communication and decision-making behaviours and has been shown to both reduce errors and surgical mortality. Some of these programmes are domain-specific (such as in anaesthesia); others are multidisciplinary (emergency department or operating room based); some rely on state of the art simulators (critical care); others rely primarily on classroom instruction.

Motivated and well-prepared healthcare workers who are educated and trained to work together can reduce risks to patients, themselves and their colleagues, especially if they manage incidents positively and make the most of opportunities to learn from adverse events and near misses. Increasingly, healthcare institutions will have to provide this kind of educational support for their workforce.

Using information technology

A major barrier to providing quality care to patients is the way health information is collected and stored in paper-based records often in locations remote from where care is provided. Paper-based record systems are more susceptible to errors and permit fewer checks than electronic systems. There is now good evidence that the routine use of information and communication technology (ICT) will contribute greatly to the use of real-time data to support clinical decisions, thereby supporting healthcare workers and patients to more easily access reliable health information and reduce medical errors. Good examples include computerised patient records and physician order entry systems for medication prescribing.

Redesigning systems and processes

Improvements in healthcare are likely only if the systems and processes are designed to eliminate small contributory errors across a wide range of care processes. Attempts at radical system redesign in order to improve quality and safety across an organisation, which are relatively common in industry, have so far been infrequent in healthcare. Perhaps the most successful example of system redesign in industrial settings has been the Toyota Production System, or **'Lean'** methodology which, in essence, involves the elimination of waste through continuous improvement with waste including anything that does not give customer value.

In healthcare, the customer is the patient and reducing waste includes eliminating error. In medical settings, there is good evidence of the benefits of 'Lean' in improving efficiency, reducing costs and improving patient satisfaction as well as potentially reducing error (Summary box 12.2).

Summary box 12.2

Strategies for patient safety

- The WHO has established a number of international initiatives for patient safety
- Various national approaches are being undertaken by countries in the developed world
- In developing countries patient safety issues are more acute due to a lack of resource, and face different challenges
- Hospitals or institutions that will offer the greatest patient safety systems in the future will include those that foster team working, maximise the use of information technology and are prepared to realign their systems and processes

PATIENT SAFETY AT THE COALFACE

Communicating openly with patients and their carers and obtaining consent

A patient-centred approach by medical staff, with involvement of patients and their carers as partners is now recognised as being of fundamental importance. There are better treatment outcomes and fewer errors when there is good communication while poor communication is a common reason for patients taking legal actions.

Involving patients in and respecting their right to make decisions about their care and treatment is crucial. Explaining risk is

Table 12.3 Information to be provided when seeking consent for surgery.

Details and uncertainties of the diagnosis
The purpose and details of the proposed surgery
Known possible side effects and potential complications
The likely prognosis
Other options for treatment, including the option not to treat
Explanation of the likely benefits and probabilities of success for each option
The name of the doctor who will have overall responsibility
A reminder that the patient can change his or her mind at any time

a difficult but important part of good communication. It requires skill to explain the potential for harm of a procedure so that it is fully understood because patients vary in their perception and understanding; and it is often difficult to assess the trade-offs between harm and benefit.

Obtaining consent for surgery requires that surgeons provide information to help patients to understand the positives and negatives of their various treatment options (Table 12.3). If only for the purposes of defending claims, hospitals invariably make signed consent mandatory. However, patients should be allowed to make these informed decisions without coercion or manipulation. Consent should be obtained by someone who is capable of performing the surgery and this should be taken when the patient is fully aware, especially in the non-urgent situation, well before the surgical procedure (see also Chapter 11).

Communicating honestly with patients after an adverse event, or **open disclosure**, includes a full explanation of what happened, the potential consequences, and what will be done to fix the problem. Safe care also involves taking care of the patient after the event, ensuring that the problem does not happen again, and a sincere offer of regret or apology, as appropriate.

Professional behaviour and maintaining fitness to practice

Professionalism is an important component of patient safety. This embraces those attitudes and behaviours that serve the patient's best interests above and beyond other considerations. Organisations responsible for maintaining ethical standards include professionalism as one of those standards by which healthcare workers are judged.

Fitness to work or practice – **competence** – refers not just to knowledge and skills but also to the attitudes required to be able to carry out one's duties. Monitoring their fitness for work is the responsibility of each individual and also their employers and professional organisations. Healthcare workers are now required to have transparent systems in place to identify, monitor and assist them to maintain their competence. **Credentialing** is one way that is used to ensure that clinicians are adequately prepared to safely treat patients with particular problems or to undertake defined procedures.

Reporting adverse events and near misses

Adverse events and near misses go unreported for many reasons including a fear of blame and the potential for litigation. **Clinical risk management** is a specific task, based upon risk identification, analysis and control of events, carried out within a 'blame-free' environment. Data collected from these episodes should be collated and learnt from at an institutional level and by uploading to a national database. Doctors should be familiar with the systems that operate within their own working environment.

Complaints from a patient or carer often highlight a problem that, when analysed, provides opportunities for reducing adverse events and near misses. Poor communication is often the cause and knowing how to manage complaints is an important part of providing better healthcare. There is wide acceptance for the need for complaints to be made easily and effectively, such that now, more and more **patient advocacy** units provide a range of options for resolving complaints including the provision of information, mediation, and the setting up of conciliation meetings between the parties.

Staff communication, understanding the work environment and working well within it

Nowhere is team working more important than in managing the flow of information within healthcare. Poor communication can lead to misinformation to patients and staff, delays in diagnosis, treatment and discharge as well as in failures to follow up on test results. On the other hand, good team work, good communication and continuity of care reduce errors and improve patient care.

Stress, tiredness and mental fatigue in the workplace are significant occupational health and safety risks in healthcare. There is good evidence linking tiredness with medical errors. Fatigue can also affect well-being by causing depression, anxiety and confusion, all of which negatively impact on clinician performance. Organisations and individuals each bear the responsibility for managing working environments and practices so as to reduce fatigue and stress.

Prescribing safely

Prescribing medication is common to almost all strands of medical practice and patients are vulnerable to mistakes being made in any one of the many steps involved in the ordering, dispensing and administration of medications (Summary box 12.3). Accuracy requires that all steps are correctly executed. Unfortunately, medication errors are common and their many causes include:

- poor assessment or inadequate knowledge of patients and their clinical conditions;
- inadequate knowledge of the medications;
- dosage calculation errors;
- illegible hand writing;
- confusion regarding the name or the mixing up of medications.

PATIENT SAFETY AND THE SURGEON

Surgery is one of the most complex health interventions to deliver. More than 100 million people worldwide require surgical treatment every year for different reasons. Problems associated with surgical safety in developed countries account for half of the avoidable adverse events that result in death or disability.

The 'more than one cause' theory of accident causation can be aptly applied to many aspects of surgical patient care during

> **Summary box 12.3**
>
> **Patient safety at the coalface requires**
>
> - Communicating well with patients and their carers
> - Professionalism, as another essential component of patient safety
> - Clinical risk management and patient advocacy and their roles in adverse events and patient complaints
> - Team working and information flow as well as managing the work environment
> - Recognising the pitfalls to safe prescribing

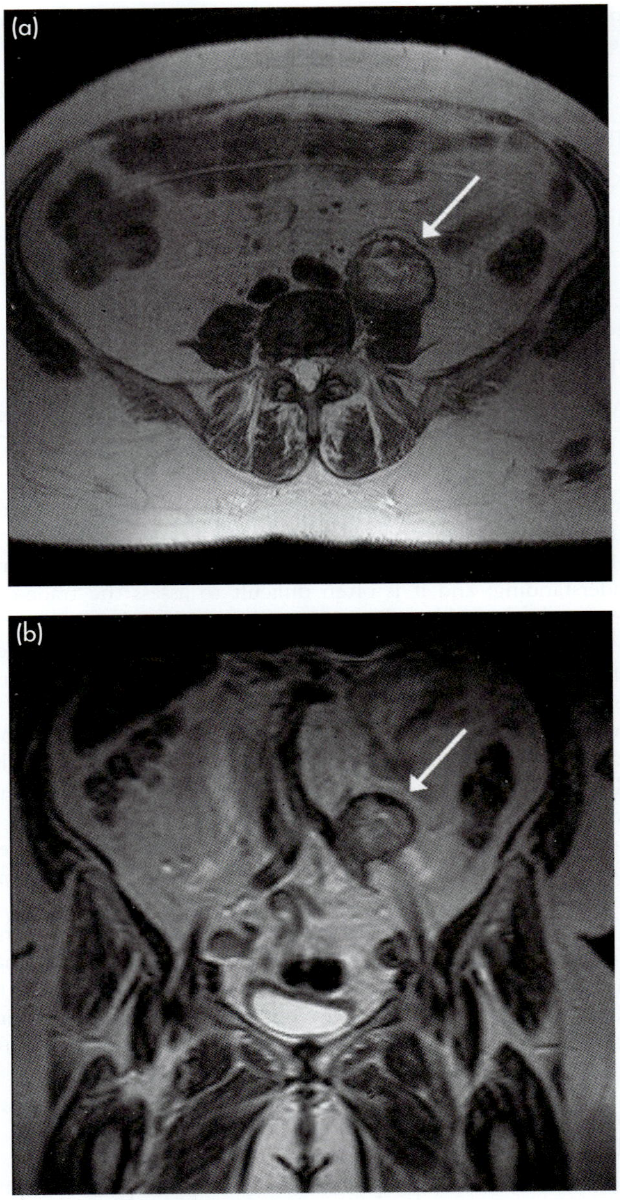

Figure 12.4 Axial and coronal magnetic resonance images demonstrating a well-defined abdominal mass with whorled stripes in fluid-filled central cavity. (Arrows) This 60-year-old woman had had an abdominal hysterectomy ten years previously and presented with a pyrexia and flank pain. The cause was due to the late presentation of a retained surgical swab.

the perioperative period. Cuschieri and others have described surgical **coalface errors** as those that can potentially be committed by surgeons during the care of their patients and include:

- diagnostic and management errors;
- resuscitation errors;
- prophylaxis errors;
- prescription/parenteral administration errors;
- situation awareness, identification and teamwork errors;
- technical and operative errors.

Situation awareness – identifying teamwork errors

Operating rooms have been described as 'among the most complex political, social, and cultural structures that exist, full of ritual, drama, hierarchy, and too often conflict'. In such an environment, systems should seek to prevent error by improving workplace preparedness and by incorporating defences so as to reduce human error or minimise its consequence. Well recognised and potential errors include:

- the wrong patient in the operating room;
- surgery performed on the wrong side or site;
- the wrong procedure performed;
- failure to communicate changes in the patient's condition;
- disagreements about proceeding;
- retained instruments or swabs (Figure 12.4).

All these events are catastrophic for the patient and almost invariably occur through a lack of communication. This means that all theatre staff should follow protocols and be familiar with the underlying principles supporting a uniform approach to caring for patients.

Checklists

Checklists in the operating theatre environment are now accepted as standard safety protocols since the 'Safe Surgery Saves Lives' Study Group at the World Health Organization published their results. The use of a perioperative surgical safety checklist in eight hospitals around the world was associated with a reduction in major complications from 11.0 per cent before, to 7.0 per cent after, the introduction of the checklist.

The surgical safety checklist identifies specific checks to be carried out at three obligatory time points (Figure 12.5). The items are not intended to be comprehensive and additions and modifications are encouraged.

We now know that the benefits of standardisation of surgical processes need not be limited to the operating room; several studies have shown that the majority of surgical errors (53–70 per cent) occur outside the operating room, before or after surgery, and that a more substantial improvement in safety can be achieved by targeting the entire surgical pathway.

There is no question that checklists are tools that improve outcomes. However, there are some important considerations. Checklists are suited to solving specific kinds of problems, but not others. Even in comparison to aviation, managing patients involves an enormous amount of coordinated, time-pressured decision-making, and potential delays. Checklists are simple reminders of what to do, and unless they are coupled with

Surgical safety checklist (first edition)

Before induction of anaesthesia

SIGN IN

- ☐ Patient has confirmed
  - identity
  - site
  - procedure
  - consent
- ☐ Site marked/not applicable
- ☐ Anaesthesia safety check completed
- ☐ Pulse oximeter on patient and fuctioning

Does patient have a:

Known allergy?
- ☐ No
- ☐ Yes

Difficult airway/aspiration risk?
- ☐ No
- ☐ Yes, and equipment/assistance available

Risk of >500ml blood loss (7ml/kg in children)?
- ☐ No
- ☐ Yes, and adequate intravenous access and fluids planned

Before skin incision

TIME OUT

- ☐ Confirm all team members have introduced themselves by name and role
- ☐ Surgeon, anaesthesia professional and nurse verbally confirm
  - patient
  - site
  - procedure

Anticipated critical events
- ☐ Surgeon reviews: what are the critical or unexpected steps, operative duration, anticipated blood loss?
- ☐ Anaesthesia team reviews: are there any patient-specific concerns?
- ☐ Nursing team reviews: has sterility (including indicator results) been confirmed? are there equipment issues or any concerns?

Has antibiotic prophylaxis been given within the last 60 minutes?
- ☐ Yes
- ☐ Not applicable

Is essential imaging displayed?
- ☐ Yes
- ☐ Not applicable

Before patient leaves operating room

SIGN OUT

Nurse verbally confirms with the team:
- ☐ The name of the procedure recorded
- ☐ That instrument, sponge and needle counts are correct (or not applicable)
- ☐ How the specimen is labelled (including patient name)
- ☐ Whether there are any equipment problems to be addressed
- ☐ Surgeon, anaesthesia professional and nurse review the key concerns for recovery and management of this patient

Figure 12.5 WHO Surgical Safety Checklist.

attitude change and efforts to remove barriers to actually using them, they will have limited impact. Finally, if one begins to believe that safety is simple and that all it requires is a checklist, there is a danger of abandoning other important efforts to achieve safer, higher quality care.

Technical and operative errors

In surgery, the person rather than systems approach emphasizes the accountability of the surgeon who, unlike colleagues in other medical disciplines, when operating, is the treatment.

During a surgical procedure, for example, there may be a specific action that, of itself, may be the error, such as the inadvertent cutting of the common bile duct during a cholecystectomy (Figure 12.6). The practical value of this kind of interpretation is that, provided latent conditions are excluded, it gives a sense of responsibility to surgeons and it may also help to point to the most effective pathway for remediation, by counselling or retraining, as against reassessing the system and putting in place further safeguards.

Central to operative performance is proficiency which is an acquired state, honed by sound teaching, practice and repetition, by which a surgeon consistently performs operations with good outcomes. In cognitive psychology, high surgical proficiency is a state of automatic unconscious processing, with the execution being effortless, intuitive and untiring; as opposed to non-proficient execution which is characterized by conscious control processing requiring constant attention and resulting in slow, deliberate execution and inducing fatigue. The transition from one state to the other is better known as the 'learning curve'. This should not carry negative connotations for trainee surgeons who might be at the conscious processing stage but still perform a perfectly good operation although it might take longer and be more tiring.

Failures in operative technique include:

- cognitive errors of judgement, such as failure or late conversion of a difficult laparoscopic procedure into an open one;
- procedural, when the steps of an operation are not followed, or omitted;
- executional, when, for example, too much force is used which may result in damage that may or may not have consequences;
- misinterpretation, which is unique to minimal access surgery and is a function of the misreading of a two-dimensional image;
- misuse of instrumentation, such as with energised dissection modalities, for example, diathermy;
- missed iatrogenic injury either at the time of surgery or diagnosed late.

CARING FOR THE SECOND VICTIM

The first victim of an adverse event is the patient and their family. Doctors do not purposely set out to injure patients but when it does happen due to an error they may experience a range of emotions including distress, shame, guilt, fear and depression. To that extent they can be regarded as a 'second victim'. Indeed, the wound to the second victim may at times be profound, leading to physical and psychological disturbances. These problems can last many months or years, especially in cases of severe disablement or death. Under such circumstances it is easy to see how a doctor's distress can lead to further deficits in patient care.

Coping with the impact of error can be challenging and the 'second' victim requires management. Doctors often find it difficult to admit to and cope with mistakes or resort to employee support systems. Dysfunctional coping strategies include denial, blaming others or refusal to discuss the issue.

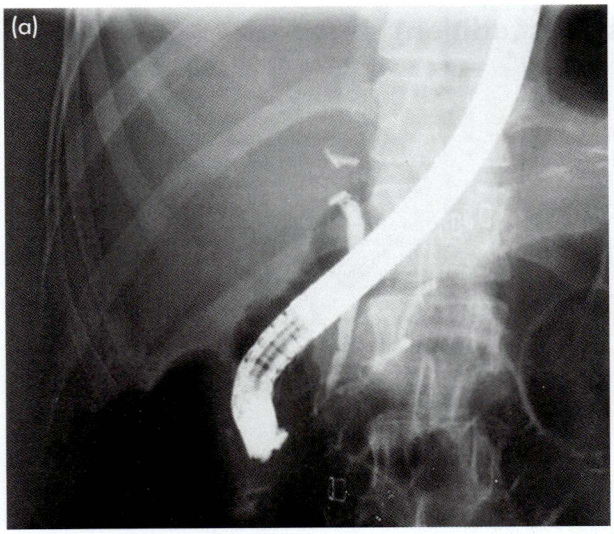

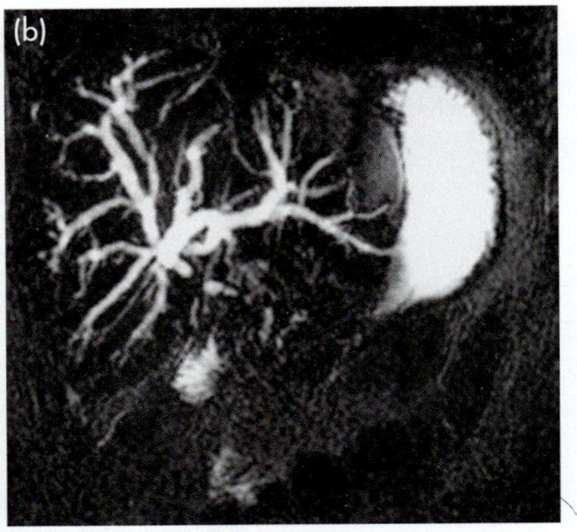

Figure 12.6 Radiograph showing an iatrogenic bile duct injury.

There are two recognised and helpful management strategies. The first is the problem-focused strategy which includes attempting to deal with the problem itself and this might include accepting responsibility for the mistake or disclosing the error and apologising to the patient. The second is the emotion-focused strategy which takes in attempts to deal with the negative emotions aroused by the problem. Here it is important that the second victim opens up lines of communication and it is equally important that professional colleagues show compassion and empathy by sensing difficulty or poor coping, providing a sounding board and by offering advice and support (Summary box 12.4).

Summary box 12.4

Patient safety and the surgeon and caring for the second victim

- Errors that can be made by surgeons in their overall management of patients
- Errors that occur in the operating theatre and how they can be mitigated
- The role of checklists in patient safety
- Performance proficiency and understanding technical and operative failures
- The 'second victim' in medical error and how this situation can be best managed

FURTHER READING

Cuschieri A. Reducing errors in the operating room; surgical proficiency and quality assurance of execution. *Surg Endosc* 2005; **19**: 1022–7.

De Vries EJ, Prins HA, Crolla R *et al.* Effect of a comprehensive surgical safety system on patient outcomes. *N Engl J Med* 2010; **363**: 1928–37.

Haynes AB, Weiser TG, Berry WR *et al.* A surgical safety checklist to reduce morbidity and mortality in a global population. *N Engl J Med* 2009; **360**: 491–19.

Kohn LT, Corrigan JM, Donaldson MS (eds). *To err is human – building a safer health system.* Washington DC: National Academies Press, 2000: 312.

Kumar S. *Fatal care – survive in the US Health system.* Minneapolis, MN: IGI Press, 2008.

McCulloch P, Kreckler S, New S *et al.* Effect of a 'Lean' intervention to improve safety processes and outcomes on a surgical emergency unit. *BMJ* 2010; **341**: c5469.

Molloy GJ, O'Boyle CA. The SHELL model: a useful tool for analyzing and teaching the contribution of human factors to medical error. *Acad Med* 2005; **80**: 152–4.

Neily J, Mills PD, Young-Xu Y *et al.* Association between implementation of a medical team training program and surgical mortality. *JAMA* 2010; **304**: 1693–1700.

Reason J. Human error: models and management. *BMJ* 2000; **320**: 768–70.

PART

2 Investigation and diagnosis

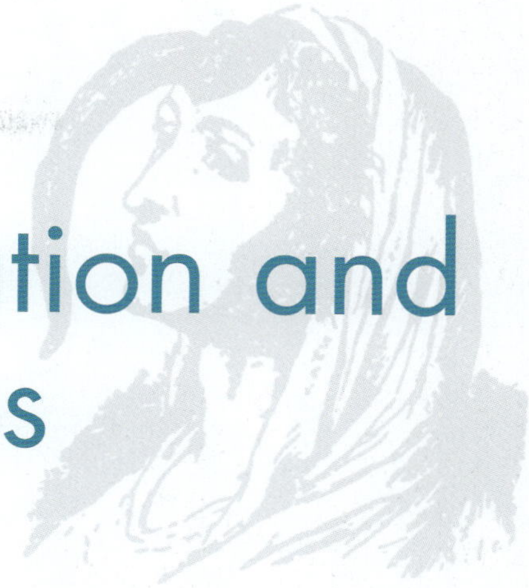

CHAPTER 13

Diagnostic imaging

LEARNING OBJECTIVES

To understand:

- The advantages of good working relationships and close collaboration with the imaging department in planning appropriate investigations
- The basic principles of radiation protection and know the law in relation to the use of ionising radiation
- The principles of different imaging techniques and their advantages and disadvantages in different clinical scenarios

INTRODUCTION

Appropriate surgical management of the patient relies on correct diagnosis. While clinical symptoms and signs may provide a firm diagnosis in some cases, other conditions will require the use of supplementary investigations including imaging techniques. The number and scope of imaging techniques available to the surgeon have dramatically increased within a generation from a time when radiographs alone were the mainstay of investigation. The development of ultrasound and colour Doppler, computed tomography (CT) and magnetic resonance imaging (MRI) has enabled the surgeon to make increasingly confident diagnoses and has reduced the need for diagnostic surgical techniques such as explorative laparotomy. Faced with such a plethora of imaging to choose from, it is important that the patient is not sent on a journey through multiple unnecessary examinations.

As a basic principle, the simplest, cheapest test should be chosen that it is hoped will answer the clinical question. This necessitates knowledge of the potential complications and diagnostic limitations of the various methods. For example, in a patient presenting with the clinical features of biliary colic, an ultrasound examination alone may give enough information to enable appropriate surgical management. In more complex cases, it may be more efficient to opt for a single, more expensive investigation, such as CT, rather than embarking on multiple simpler and cheaper investigations that may not yield the answer. The choice of technique is often dictated by equipment availability, expertise and cost, as well as the clinical presentation. However, it must be emphasised that, not infrequently, the most valuable investigation is a prior radiograph; this not only reduces the cost and the amount of radiation a patient receives but very often improves patient care.

HOW TO REQUEST IMAGING

Best practice depends on close collaboration between the radiologist and the referrer and must take into account local expertise and access to facilities. When requesting imaging, consider what it is that you want to know from the investigation. Give a provisional diagnosis or state the clinical problem. If there is uncertainty over the best method to answer the clinical problem, then discussion with a radiologist is always worthwhile, informally or within the context of a clinicoradiological meeting or a multidisciplinary team (MDT) meeting.

As well as the basic demographic information stored on the radiology information system (RIS), it is important to provide relevant past medical history, e.g. diabetes, epilepsy, renal failure, allergies and anticoagulation, all of which can affect which contrast agent can be given safely, and the date of the last menses in women of childbearing potential.

INTERPRETING IMAGES

Complex imaging may best be left to radiologists to interpret, but the clinician should be able to examine radiographs to exclude major abnormalities. The plain radiograph can be systematically examined using the system in Summary box 13.1.

The systematic approach to examining a radiograph varies according to the part of the body being imaged. For instance, for a radiograph of an extremity, the alignment, the cortices and the medullary cavity of the individual bones, the joints and the soft tissues all need to be assessed on each view. You should develop, learn and practise your own method for ensuring that you study all of these in each case. This will take a long time when you start, but speed comes with practice.

Summary box 13.1

A simple system for checking radiographs

Label	Name of patient
Site	Date of examination
	Side (check marker)
	What part is the film centred on?
	Does the film cover the whole area required?
	Is there more than one view?
Quality	Is the penetration appropriate?
Compare	How have the appearances changed from previous images?
Conclude	Is the diagnosis clear?
	Is further imaging needed?

HAZARDS OF IMAGING

Contrast media

There has been a dramatic increase in the use of contrast agents in recent years, mainly related to the increasing use of CT. Potential problems include allergic reaction and nephrotoxicity. The newer low-osmolality contrast media (LOCM) are 5–10 times safer than the older higher-osmolality agents. Reactions are rare: serious reactions occur in about 1:2500 cases and life-threatening reactions in about 1:25 000 cases. The risk of sudden death, however, has not changed with the new agents. Local policies for dealing with patients at increased risk vary between departments and, indeed, between countries. A recent publication from the Royal College of Radiologists (RCR) in the UK does not recommend routine steroid prophylaxis for patients at increased risk of allergic reaction, but rather the use of a LOCM and observation of the patient for 30 minutes after injection with the intravenous cannula still *in situ*, as most serious reactions occur shortly after injection. Guidelines from the European Society of Uroradiology (ESUR), however, continue to advocate the use of steroids.

In patients with diabetes or renal impairment, a recent creatinine level should be available. The radiologist should be informed of any history of renal impairment, as all contrast media are nephrotoxic in patients with impaired renal function. The risks and benefits of contrast administration need to be carefully assessed in these patients and, if contrast is given, the patient should be well hydrated and the lowest dose of a LOCM should be given. The British RCR does not recommend the routine use of *N*-acetylcysteine for renal protection.

Concerns about lactic acidosis in patients on metformin receiving contrast led to various recommendations for stopping the metformin. The latest RCR recommendations are that it can be continued in patients receiving 100 mL or less of intravenous contrast (which is the case for the majority of CT examinations) who are thought to have normal renal function. Other patients, including those who have intra-arterial contrast for angiography, should be discussed with the radiologist.

Gadolinium-containing contrast agents are used in MRI examinations. Allergic reactions to these agents are rare; mild reactions may occur in around 1:200 patients, with severe reactions in around 1:10 000 patients. However, they can be nephrotoxic in patients with pre-existing renal failure. In addition, they are associated with a risk of nephrogenic systemic fibrosis (NSF), a serious life-threatening condition whereby connective tissue forms in the skin causing it to become coarse and hard. NSF may also affect other organs, including joints, muscle, liver and heart. High risk gadolinium-containing contrast agents are contraindicated in severe renal failure, in neonates and in the perioperative period of liver transplantation, and are not recommended in pregnancy.

HAZARDS OF IONISING RADIATION

The majority of ionising radiation comes from natural sources on the earth and cosmic rays, and this makes up the background radiation. However, medical exposure accounts for around 15 per cent of the total received by humans. The effects of ionising radiation can be broadly divided into two groups. The first group comprises predictable, dose-dependent tissue effects and includes, for example, the development of cataracts in the lens of the eye. These effects are important for those chronically exposed to radiation, including those using image intensifiers regularly. The second group comprises the all or nothing effects such as the development of cancer (termed stochastic). These effects are not dose dependent, but increase in likelihood with increased radiation dose.

The risk of radiation-induced cancer for plain films of the chest or extremities is very small, of the order of 1:1 000 000. However, that risk rises considerably for high-dose examinations such as CT of the abdomen or pelvis, where the estimated lifetime excess risk of cancer increases to the order of 1:1000. Use of CT has increased dramatically in the last 20 years, with a 12-fold increase in the UK, and it has been estimated that up to 30 per cent of these examinations may be unnecessary. Obviously, the risk of such examinations has to be balanced against the benefit to the patient in terms of increased diagnostic yield, and must also be viewed in the context that the lifetime risk of cancer for people generally is about 1:3. Nevertheless, the increased risk is important since it is iatrogenic and applied to a large population. Therefore, techniques that do not use ionising radiation, such as ultrasound and MRI, should be carefully considered as alternatives, particularly in children and young people.

CURRENT LEGISLATION

In the UK, the Ionising Radiation (Medical Exposure) Regulations (IRMER) introduced in 2000 impose on the radiologist the duty to the patient to make sure that all studies involving radiation (plain radiographs, CT and nuclear medicine) are performed appropriately and to the highest standards. Inappropriate use of radiation is a criminal offence, so investigations involving radiation need careful consideration in order to prevent wasteful use of radiology (Summary box 13.2).

Summary box 13.3 gives a summary of the responsibilities of both the radiologist and the referrer.

The RCR has published a book, *Making the Best Use of a Department of Clinical Radiology* (6th edition, 2012), which has been adopted in many European countries. Local rules and guidelines are in place to deal with particular circumstances. Table 13.1, showing the radiation doses for common procedures, is taken from this publication.

Summary box 13.2

Wasteful use of radiology

Results unlikely to affect patient management	
Positive finding unlikely	
Anticipated finding probably irrelevant for management	Do I need it?
Investigating too often	
Before disease could be expected to have progressed or resolved	Do I need it now?
Repeating investigations done previously	
Other hospital (?)	
GP (?)	Has it been done already?
Failing to provide adequate information	
Therefore wrong test performed or essential view omitted	Have I explained the problem?
Requesting wrong investigation	
Discuss with radiologist	Is this the best test?
Over-investigating	Are too many investigations being performed?

After: *Making the Best Use of a Department of Clinical Radiology*, 6th edn. Royal College of Radiologists, 2007.

Summary box 13.3

Responsibilities

- Radiologists have a legal responsibility to keep imaging as safe as possible
- The referrer has a duty to balance risk against benefit
- The referrer must provide adequate clinical details to allow justification of the examination
- Avoid using portable (mobile) x-ray machines whenever practical
- Take all precautions when using an image intensifier
- The gonads, eyes and thyroid are especially vulnerable to radiation and should be protected

There are special considerations for portable and fluoroscopy units. The longer an operator keeps the fluoroscopy unit running, the higher the dose of radiation to all in the vicinity. Portable x-ray machines and fluoroscopic imaging equipment use much more radiation to achieve the same result. The staff, and patients in the next bed, are at risk when portable equipment is used. The result is also of lower quality, so portable x-ray machines should not be used unless absolutely necessary.

When using the image intensifier, lead aprons, thyroid shields, lead glasses and radiation badges should always be worn. Pregnancy in the female patient or staff must be excluded.

DIAGNOSTIC IMAGING

Basic principles of imaging methods

Conventional radiography

Despite the fact that it is over a hundred years since the discovery of x-rays by Roentgen in 1895, conventional radiography continues to play a central role in the diagnostic pathway of many acute surgical problems and particularly in chest disease, trauma and orthopaedics.

X-rays emitted from an x-ray source are absorbed to varying degrees by different materials and tissues and therefore cause different degrees of blackening of radiographic film, resulting in a radiographic image. This differential absorption is dependent partly on the density and the atomic number of different substances. In general, higher-density tissues result in a greater reduction in the number of x-ray photons and reduce the amount of blackening caused by those photons. In terms of conventional radiographs, a large difference in tissue structure and density is required before an appreciable difference is manifested radiographically. The different densities visible consist of air, fat, soft tissue, bone and mineralisation, and metal. Different soft tissues cannot be reliably distinguished as, in broad terms, they possess similar quantities of water (Figure 13.1). Manipulation of x-ray systems and x-ray energies, as used in circumstances such as mammography, may allow better differentiation between some soft-tissue structures.

Despite this inherent lack of soft-tissue contrast, conventional radiography has many advantages. It is cheap, universally available, easily reproducible and comparable with prior examinations and, in many instances, has a relatively low dose of ionising radiation in contrast to more complex examinations. However, injudicious repeat radiography, particularly of the abdomen, pelvis and spine, can easily result in doses similar to CT.

The lack of soft-tissue contrast allows little assessment of the internal architecture of many abdominal organs. To obviate

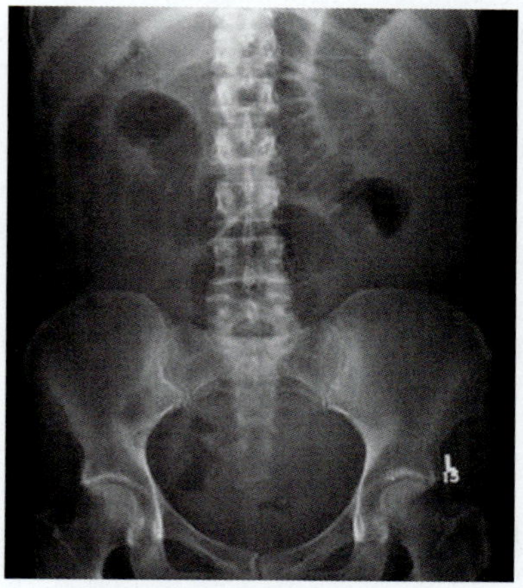

Figure 13.1 Supine abdominal radiograph of a patient with small bowel obstruction demonstrating multiple dilated small bowel loops. The different densities visible are air (within the bowel), bones, soft tissues and fat. The different soft tissues, subcutaneous and intra-abdominal, cannot be differentiated.

Wilhelm Conrad Roentgen, 1845–1923, Professor of Physics, Wurtzburg (1888–1900), and then at Munich, Germany. He was awarded the Nobel Prize for Physics in 1901 for his work on x-rays.

Table 13.1 Typical effective doses from diagnostic medical exposure in the 2000s.

Diagnostic procedure	Typical effective dose (mSv)	Equivalent no. of chest radiographs	Approximately equivalent period of natural background radiation[a]
Radiographic examinations			
Limbs and joints (except hip)	<0.01	<0.5	<1.5 days
Chest (single posteroanterior film)	0.02	1	3 days
Skull	0.07	3.5	11 days
Thoracic spine	0.7	35	4 months
Lumbar spine	1.3	65	7 months
Hip	0.3	15	7 weeks
Pelvis	0.7	35	4 months
Abdomen	1.0	50	6 months
Intravenous urography (IVU)	2.5	125	14 months
Barium swallow	1.5	75	8 months
Barium meal	3	150	16 months
Barium follow-through	3	150	16 months
Barium enema	7	350	3.2 years
CT head	2.3	115	1 year
CT chest	8	400	3.6 years
CT abdomen or pelvis	10	500	4.5 years
Radionuclide studies			
Lung ventilation (^{133}Xe)	0.3	15	7 weeks
Lung perfusion (^{99m}Tc)	1	50	6 months
Kidney (^{99m}Tc)	1	50	6 months
Thyroid (^{99m}Tc)	1	50	6 months
Bone (^{99m}Tc)	4	200	1.8 years
Dynamic cardiac (^{99m}Tc)	6	300	2.7 years
PET head (18F-FDG)	5	250	2.3 years

[a]UK average background radiation = 2.2 mSv per year; regional averages range from 1.5 to 7.5 mSv.
18F-FDG, 18F-2-fluoro-2-deoxy-D-glucose; CT, computed tomography; ^{99m}Tc, ^{99m}technetium; PET, positron emission tomography.
From *Making the Best Use of a Department of Clinical Radiology*, 6th edn. Royal College of Radiologists, 2007. By kind permission.

this problem, techniques employing the administration of contrast material combined with radiography have long been used. These techniques include intravenous urography and barium examinations (Figure 13.2). In intravenous urography (IVU), intravenous administration of iodinated contrast material initially results in opacification of the renal parenchyma, followed by opacification of the pelvicalyceal system, ureters and bladder, allowing identification of pelvicalyceal morphology and filling defects (Figure 13.3). Iodinated contrast material may even be instilled retrogradely into the bladder per urethra and combined with radiographs obtained during micturition to allow the assessment of the lower urinary tract.

A further modification of conventional x-rays uses fluorescent screens to allow real-time monitoring of organs and structures as opposed to the 'snapshot' images obtained with radiographs. This is used to follow the passage of barium through the bowel, obtaining dedicated images at specific points of interest only. Motility of the bowel can also be assessed in this way. Fluoroscopy is used extensively in interventional radiology and, in particular, in vascular intervention by allowing real-time assessment of the passage of intravascular iodinated contrast and the acquisition of multiple images per second to diagnose intravascular lesions and to guide treatment. Naturally, with the more sustained use of ionising radiation, the cumulative doses tend to be greater than obtaining a conventional radiograph.

Ultrasound

Ultrasound is the second most common method of imaging. It relies on high-frequency sound waves generated by a transducer containing piezoelectric material. The generated sound waves are reflected by tissue interfaces and, by ascertaining the time taken for a pulse to return and the direction of a pulse, it is possible to form an image. Medical ultrasound uses frequencies in the range 3–20 MHz. The higher the frequency of the ultrasound wave, the greater the resolution of the image, but the less depth of view from the skin. Consequently, abdominal imaging uses transducers with a frequency of 3–7 MHz, while higher-frequency transducers are used for superficial structures, such as musculoskeletal and breast ultrasound. Dedicated transducers have also been developed for endocavitary ultrasound such as transvaginal scanning and transrectal ultrasound of the prostate, allowing high-frequency scanning of organs by reducing the distance between the probe and the organ of interest (Figure 13.4). A further application of dedicated probes has been in the field of

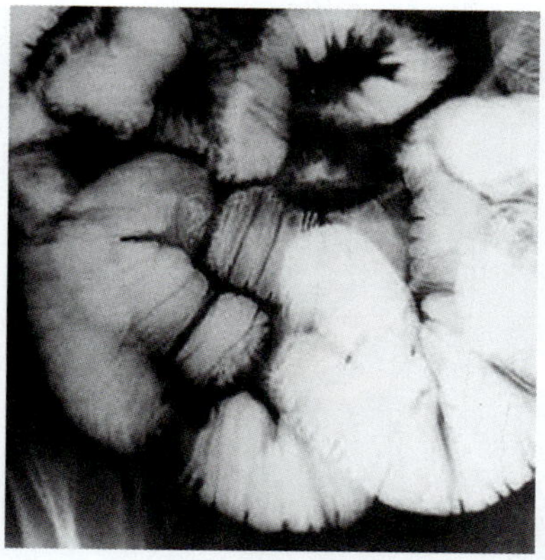

Figure 13.2 Barium examination of the small bowel demonstrates a focal short segment stricture of the distal ileum in a patient with Crohn's disease.

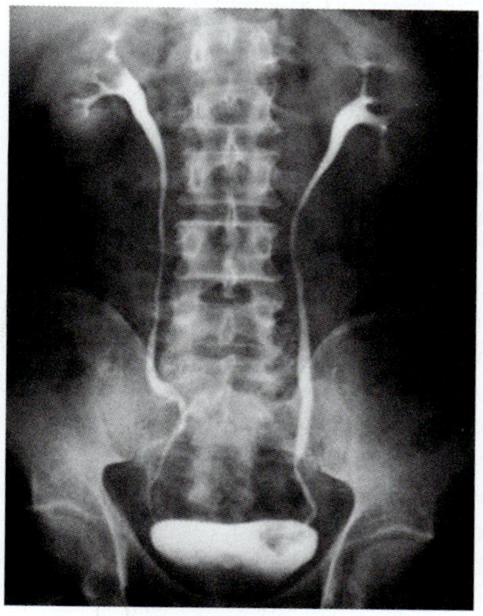

Figure 13.3 Intravenous urogram in a patient with macroscopic haematuria. There are focal irregular filling defects in the left side of the bladder and the right renal pelvis, consistent with multifocal transitional cell carcinomas.

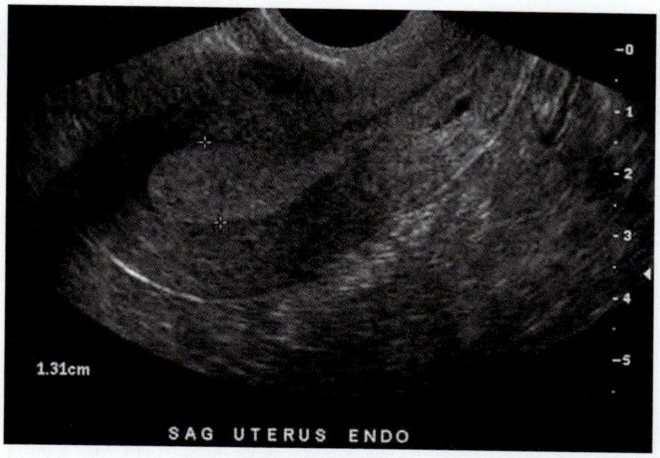

Figure 13.4 Longitudinal transvaginal ultrasound scan of the uterus demonstrating thickening of the endometrium in a patient during the secretory phase of the menstrual cycle.

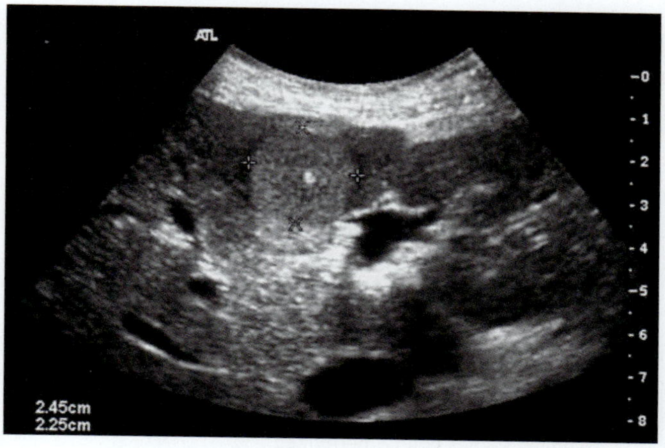

Figure 13.5 Transverse ultrasound image of the liver in a patient with colorectal cancer shows a solitary liver metastasis.

endoscopic ultrasound, allowing exquisite imaging of the wall of a hollow viscus and the adjacent organs such as the gastric wall and the pancreas.

Reflection of an ultrasound wave from moving objects such as red blood cells causes a change in the frequency of the ultrasound wave. By measuring this frequency change, it is possible to calculate the speed and direction of the movement. This principle forms the basis of Doppler ultrasound, whereby velocities within major vessels as well as smaller vessels in organs such as the liver and the kidneys can be measured. Doppler imaging is widely used in the assessment of arterial and venous disease, in which stenotic lesions cause an alteration in the normal velocity. Furthermore, diffuse parenchymal diseases, such as cirrhosis, may cause an alteration in the normal Doppler signal of the affected organ.

The advantages of ultrasound are that it is cheap and easily available. It is the first-line investigation of choice for assessment of the liver, the biliary tree and the renal tract (Figures 13.5 and 13.6). Ultrasound is also the imaging method of choice in obstetric assessment and gynaecological disease. High-frequency transducers have made ultrasound the best imaging technique for the evaluation of thyroid and testicular disorders in terms of both diffuse disease and focal mass lesions. It is also an invaluable tool for guiding needle placement in interventional procedures such as biopsies and drainages, allowing direct real-time visualisation of the needle during the procedure.

Ligament, tendon and muscle injuries are also probably best imaged in the first instance by ultrasound (Figure 13.7). The ability to stress ligaments and to allow tendons to move during the investigation gives an extra dimension, which greatly improves its diagnostic value. The use of 'panoramic' or 'extended field of view' ultrasound (Figure 13.8) provides images that are more easily interpreted by an observer not performing the examination, and are of particular assistance to surgeons planning a procedure. Ultrasound will demonstrate most foreign bodies in soft tissues, including those that are not radio-opaque.

The disadvantages of ultrasound are that it is highly operator dependent, and most of the information is gained during the actual process of scanning as opposed to reviewing the static images. Another drawback is that the ultrasound wave is

Christian Johann Doppler, 1803–1853, Professor of Experimental Physics, Vienna, Austria, enunciated the 'Doppler Principle' in 1842.

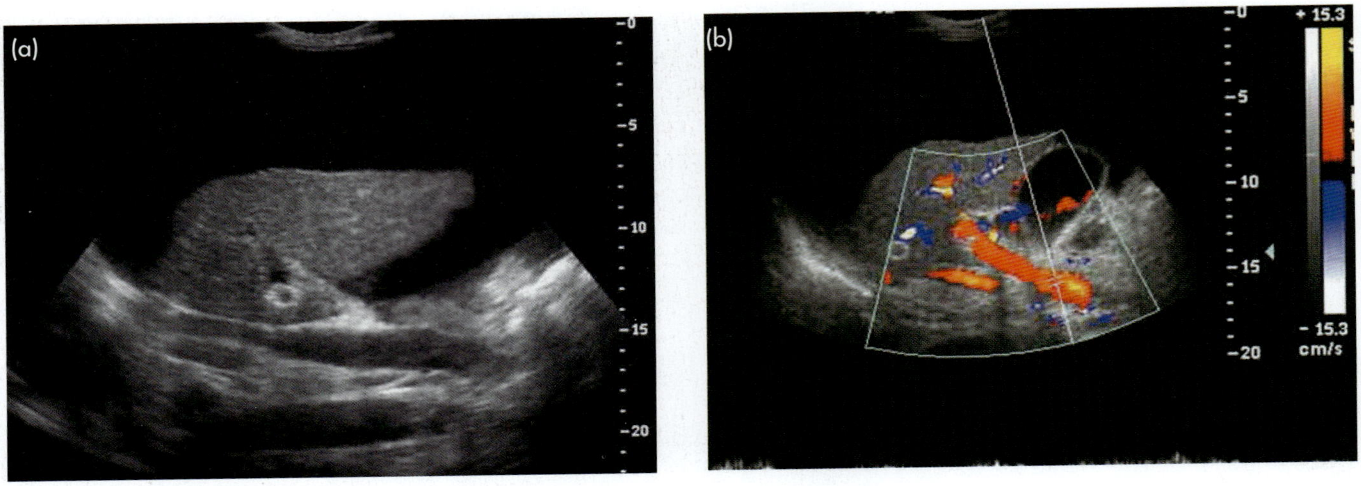

Figure 13.6 Sagittal ultrasound image of the liver (a) in a patient with cirrhosis demonstrates nodularity of the liver surface and extensive ascites. Doppler ultrasound (b) illustrates portal vein flow with a normal direction.

highly attenuated by air and bone and, thus, little information is gained with regard to tissues beyond bony or air-filled structures; alternative techniques may be required to image these areas (Summary box 13.4).

Summary box 13.4

Ultrasound

Strengths
- No radiation
- Inexpensive
- Allows interaction with patients
- Superb soft-tissue resolution in the near field
- Dynamic studies can be performed
- First-line investigation for hepatic, biliary and renal disease
- Endocavitary ultrasound for gynaecological and prostate disorders
- Excellent resolution for breast, thyroid and testis imaging
- Good for soft tissue, including tendons and ligaments
- Excellent for cysts and foreign bodies
- Doppler studies allow assessment of blood flow
- Good real-time imaging to guide interventional biopsies and drainages

Weaknesses
- Interpretation only possible during the examination
- Long learning curve for some areas of expertise
- Resolution dependent on the machine available
- Images cannot be reliably reviewed away from the patient

Computed tomography

There has been a great deal of development in CT technology over the last 30 years from the initial conventional CT scanners through to helical or spiral scanners and the current multi-detector machines. CT scanners consist of a gantry containing the x-ray tube, filters and detectors, which revolve around the patient, acquiring information at different angles and projections. This information is then mathematically reconstructed to produce a two-dimensional grey-scale image of a slice through the body. This technique overcomes the problem of superimposition of different structures, which is inherent in conventional radiography. Improvements in gantry design, advances in detector technology using more sensitive detectors and an increase in the number of detectors have resulted in an increase in spatial resolution as well as the speed at which the images are acquired. In early CT scanners, the table on which the patient was positioned moved in between the gantry revolution to allow imaging of an adjacent slice. Modern scanners allow for continuous movement of the table and the patient during the gantry revolution, thus greatly reducing the scan time. With modern equipment, it is now not only possible to obtain images of the chest, abdomen and pelvis in under 20 seconds, but these axial images can be reformatted in multiple planes with practically no degradation in image quality.

In addition, CT has a far higher contrast resolution than plain radiographs, allowing the assessment of tissues with similar attenuation characteristics. As with radiographs, the natural contrast of tissues is further augmented by the use of intravenous

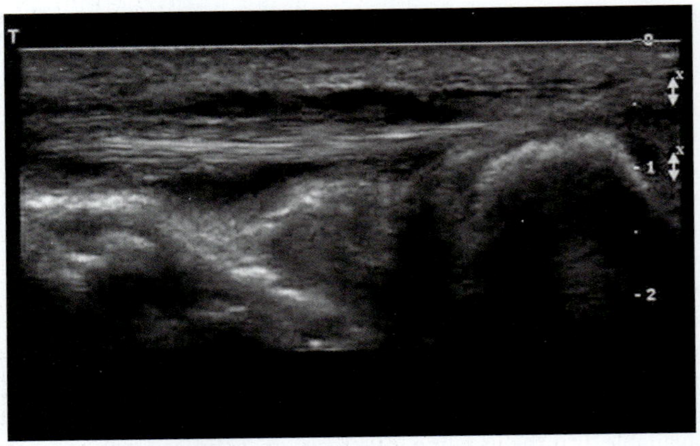

Figure 13.7 Ultrasound of the dorsal surface of the wrist shows the normal fibrillar pattern of the extensor tendons. There is increased fluid within the tendon sheath in this patient with extensor tenosynovitis.

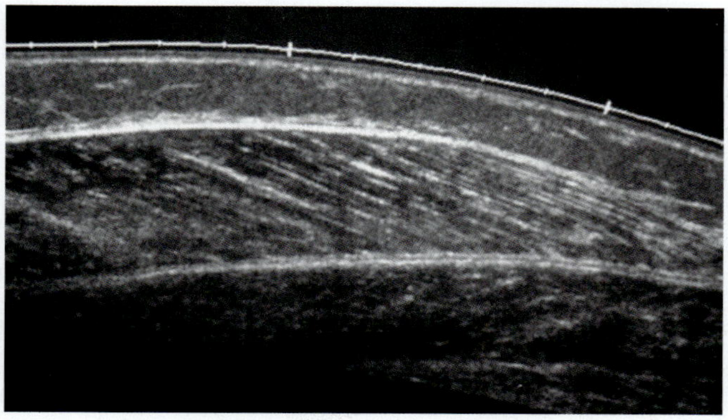

Figure 13.8 Panoramic ultrasound of the calf. The normal muscle fibres and the fascia can be identified over an area measuring approximately 12 cm.

contrast medium. Rapid scanning of a volume of tissue also allows the scans to be performed at different phases of enhancement, which is advantageous in identifying different diseases. For instance, very early scanning during the arterial phase is ideally suited to the examination of the arterial tree and hypervascular liver lesions, whereas scanning performed after a delay may be better suited to the identification of other solid organ pathology such as renal masses. Furthermore, it is possible to obtain scans during several phases including the arterial and venous phases in the same patient, which may aid in the identification and characterisation of lesions.

CT is widely used in thoracic, abdominal (Figure 13.9), neurological (Figure 13.10), musculoskeletal (Figure 13.11) and trauma imaging. The thinner collimation and improved spatial resolution have also resulted in the development of newer techniques such as CT angiography, virtual colonoscopy and virtual bronchoscopy. Furthermore, three-dimensional images can be reconstructed from the raw data to aid in surgical planning. The disadvantage of CT compared with ultrasound and conventional

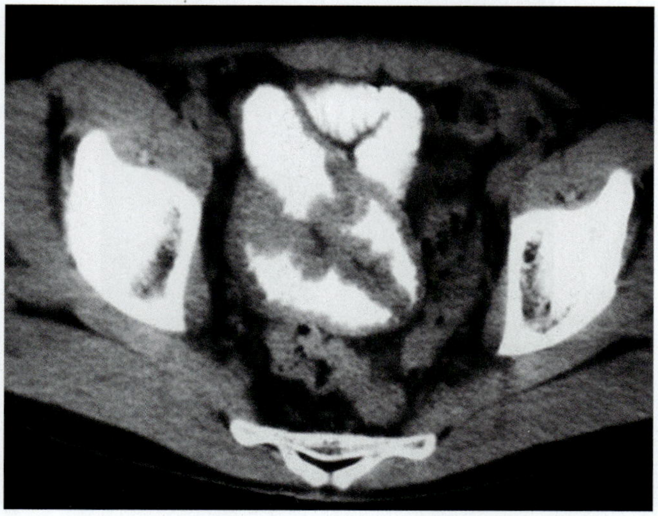

Figure 13.9 Axial computed tomography scan through the pelvis with oral contrast administration illustrates loops of distal ileum with mural thickening in a patient with Crohn's disease.

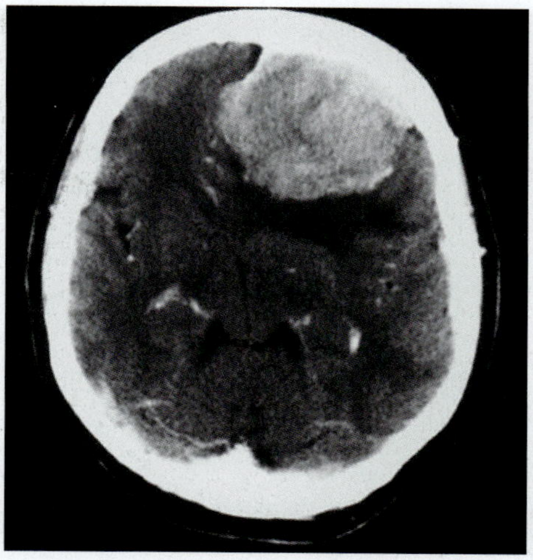

Figure 13.10 Axial computed tomography scan of the head following intravenous contrast demonstrates a large mass lesion in the left frontal region in a patient with a large left frontal meningioma.

radiography lies largely in the increased costs and the far higher doses of ionising radiation. For instance, a CT scan of the abdomen and pelvis has a radiation dose equivalent to approximately 500 chest radiographs (Summary box 13.5).

Summary box 13.5

Computed tomography

Strengths

- High spatial and contrast resolution
- Contrast resolution enhanced by imaging in arterial and/or venous phases
- Rapid acquisition of images in one breath-hold
- Imaging of choice for the detection of pulmonary masses
- Allows global assessment of the abdomen and pelvis
- Excellent for liver, pancreatic, renal and bowel pathology
- Three-dimensional reconstruction allows complex fracture imaging
- Multiplanar reconstruction and three-dimensional imaging, e.g. CT angiography and colonoscopy

Weaknesses

- High radiation dose
- Poor soft-tissue resolution of the peripheries and superficial structures
- Patient needs to be able to lie flat and still

Magnetic resonance imaging

Over the last 20 years, MRI has become an integral part of the imaging arsenal with ever-expanding indications. MRI relies on the fact that nuclei containing an odd number of protons or electrons have a characteristic motion in a magnetic field (precession) and produce a magnetic moment as a result of this motion. In a strong uniform magnetic field such as an MRI scanner, these nuclei align themselves with the main magnetic field and result in a net magnetic moment. A brief radiofrequency pulse is then applied to alter the motion of the nuclei. Once the

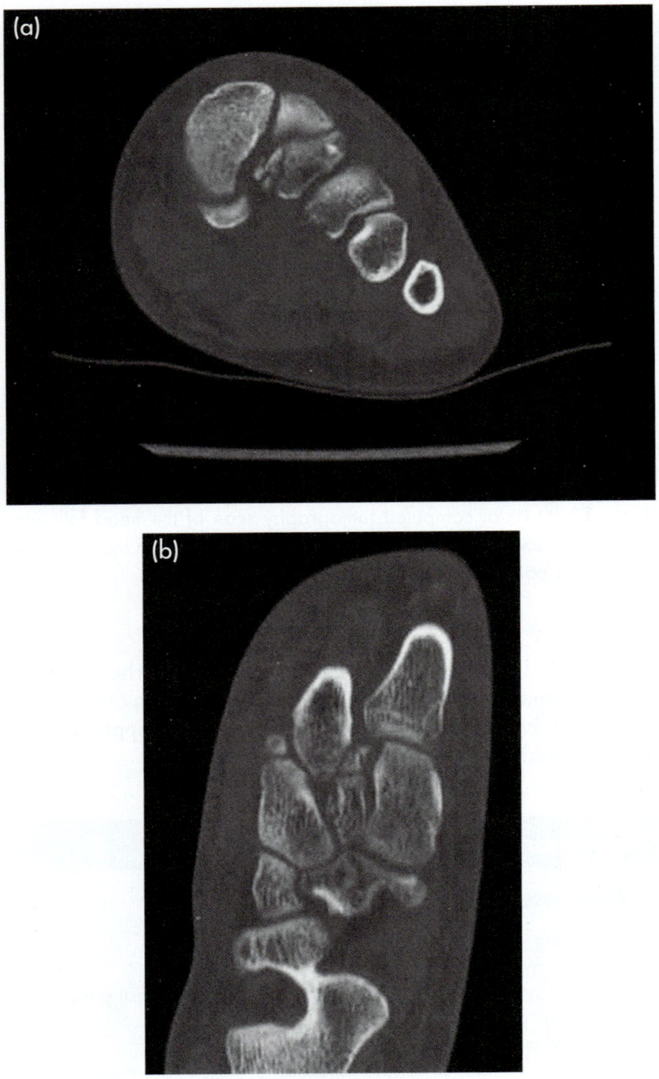

Figure 13.11 Coronal computed tomography (a) and axial reformats (b) of the foot in a patient involved in a road traffic accident demonstrates Lisfranc fracture dislocation with a comminuted fracture of the base of the second metatarsal.

radiofrequency pulse is removed, the nuclei realign themselves with the main magnetic field (relaxation) and in the process emit a radiofrequency signal that can be recorded, spatially encoded and used to construct a grey-scale image. The specific tissue characteristics define the manner and rate at which the nuclei relax. This relaxation is measured in two ways, referred to as the T1 and T2 relaxation times. The relaxation times and the proton density determine the signal from a specific tissue.

There are a large number of imaging sequences that can be used by applying radiofrequency pulses of different strengths and durations. The image characteristic and signal intensity from different tissues are governed by the pulse sequence employed and whether it is T1 weighted or T2 weighted. For instance, fat, methaemoglobin and mucinous fluid are bright on T1-weighted images, whereas water and thus most pathological processes, which tend to increase tissue water content, are bright on T2-weighted images. Cortical bone, air, haemosiderin and ferromagnetic materials are of very low signal on all pulse sequences. In general, T1-weighted images are superior in the delineation of anatomy, while T2-weighted images tend to highlight pathology better. For added tissue contrast, intravenous gadolinium may be administered. Other more specific contrast media are also available for liver, bowel and lymph node imaging.

MRI's exquisite contrast resolution, coupled with a lack of ionising radiation, is very attractive in imaging, particularly of tissues that have relatively little natural contrast. MRI also has the advantage of multiplanar imaging, as images can be acquired in any plane prescribed. It has traditionally been used extensively in the assessment of intracranial, spinal and musculoskeletal disorders (Figures 13.12, 13.13 and 13.14), allowing a

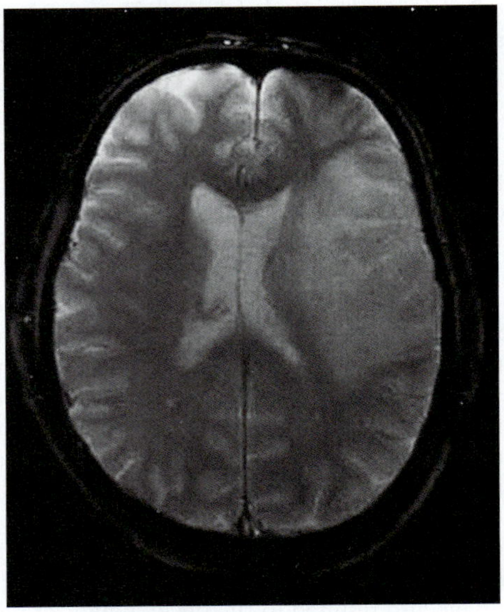

Figure 13.12 T2-weighted axial magnetic resonance imaging scan of the head in a patient with a large left-sided oligodendroglioma.

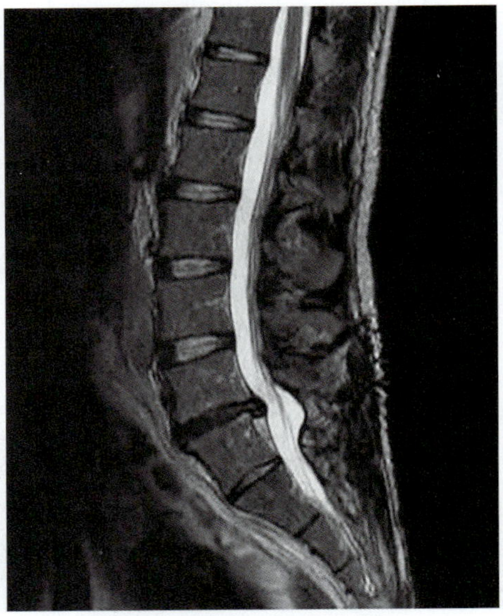

Figure 13.13 Sagittal T2-weighted magnetic resonance imaging scan of the lumbar spine demonstrates disc herniation in a patient with acute back pain.

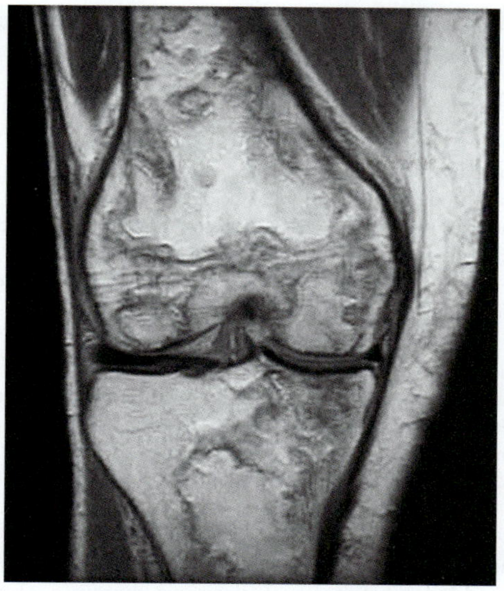

Figure 13.14 Coronal magnetic resonance imaging scan of the knee demonstrating extensive serpiginous areas of altered signal intensity in the distal femur and proximal tibia in a patient with bone infarcts secondary to oral corticosteroids.

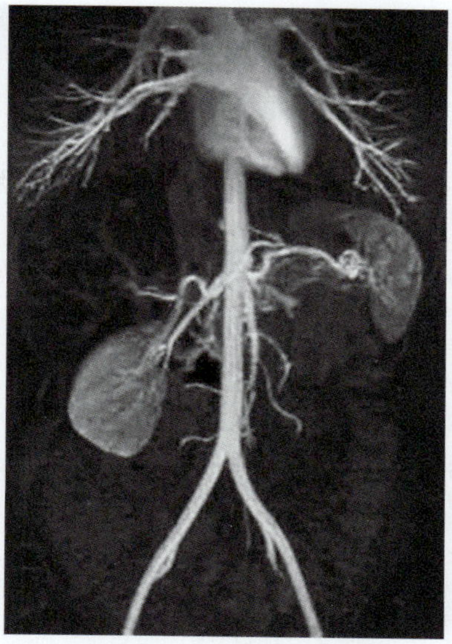

Figure 13.16 Maximum intensity projection image from a magnetic resonance angiogram demonstrating the abdominal aorta, common and external iliac arteries as well as parts of the pulmonary, mesenteric and renal vasculature.

global assessment of bony and soft-tissue structures. More recent developments have resulted in new indications and applications. Today, MRI is commonly used in oncological imaging, such as staging of rectal carcinoma and gynaecological malignancies, identification and characterisation of hepatic masses, assessment of the biliary tree (magnetic resonance cholangiopancreatography (MRCP) (Figure 13.15)) and cardiac imaging. Techniques have also been developed which allow non-invasive angiography of the cranial and peripheral circulation (MR angiography) (Figure 13.16).

However, the availability of MRI is still relatively limited in comparison with other imaging techniques, and it is time-consuming with respect to image acquisition and interpretation. Images are easily degraded by motion, including respiratory and

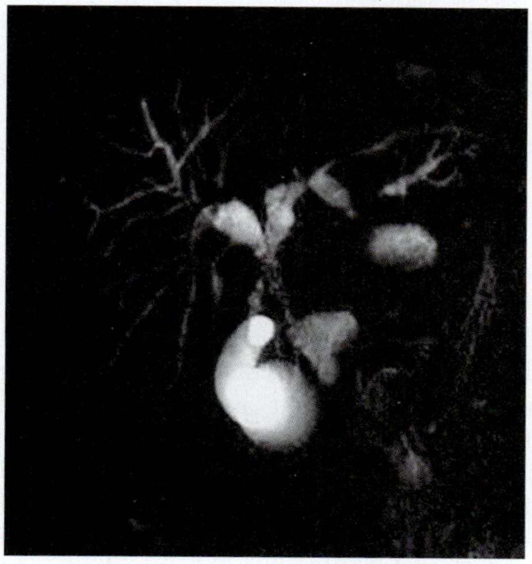

Figure 13.15 Magnetic resonance cholangiopancreatography demonstrating dilated central intrahepatic bile ducts and a stricture of the common bile duct in a patient with obstructive jaundice and cholangiocarcinoma.

cardiac motion. The use of respiratory and cardiac gating can minimise this, although bowel peristalsis can still be a problem. The long acquisition times require a cooperative patient who can lie very still, which can be difficult especially in claustrophobic individuals or those in pain. Furthermore, because of the use of high-strength magnetic fields, patients with some metallic implants, such as some aneurysm clips and prosthetic heart valves, and those with implanted electronic devices, such as pacemakers and defibrillators, cannot be examined. Some newer implants may, however, be MRI compatible, and patients with joint replacements can be studied safely (Summary box 13.6).

Nuclear medicine

In other imaging techniques using ionising radiation such as CT and conventional radiography, the individual is exposed to ionising radiation from an external source and the radiation transmitted through the patient is recorded. In nuclear medicine, however, a radioactive element or radionuclide such as technetium, gallium, thallium or iodine is administered to the patient as part of a radiopharmaceutical agent, and a detector such as a gamma camera is then used to record and localise the emission from the patient, thus forming the image. The radionuclide is chosen and coupled with other compounds such that it is distributed and taken up in the tissues of interest. Therefore, a variety of radionuclides are required for imaging of different tissues. Nuclear medicine also differs from other means of imaging, which are largely anatomically based, as it also provides functional information.

Radionuclide imaging is widely used in bone imaging with very high sensitivity for assessing metastatic disease, metabolic bone disease, established arthropathies and occult infection and traumatic injuries (Figure 13.17), although many of these applications are being replaced by MRI. In genitourinary disease, dynamic imaging can be performed to assess renal perfusion and function including obstruction, investigate renovascular hypertension and evaluate renal transplants. Radionuclide imaging

Jacques Lisfranc de St. Martin, 1790–1847, Professor of Surgery and Operative Medicine, Paris, France.

Summary box 13.6

Magnetic resonance imaging

Strengths
- No ionising radiation
- Excellent soft-tissue contrast
- Best imaging technique for
  - Intracranial lesions
  - Spine
  - Bone marrow and joint lesions

Evolving use
- Staging
- MRCP
- MR angiography
- Breast malignancy
- Pelvic malignancy
- Cardiac imaging

Weaknesses
- Absolute contraindications
  - Ocular metallic foreign bodies
  - Pacemakers
  - Cochlear implants
  - Cranial aneurysm clips
- Relative contraindications
  - First trimester of pregnancy
  - Claustrophobia
- Long scan times so patients may not be able to keep still, especially if in pain
- Limited availability
- Expensive

is also commonly used in thyroid and parathyroid disorders, ischaemic cardiac disease, detection of pulmonary emboli and assessment of occult infection and inflammatory bowel disease.

Positron emission tomography (PET) is an extension of nuclear medicine, in which a positron-emitting substance such as 18F is tagged and used to assess tissue metabolic characteristics. The most commonly used radiolabelled tracer is 18F-2-fluoro-2-deoxy-D-glucose (FDG), although other tracers can also be used in order to assess metabolic functions such as oxygen and glucose consumption and blood flow. Radioisotope decay causes the emission of a positron, which subsequently, within a few millimetres, collides with and annihilates an electron to produce a pair of annihilation photons. The drawbacks have been high cost, very limited availability and relatively low spatial resolution. The last of these has been addressed by PET/CT systems combining simultaneous PET imaging and CT, allowing the two sets of images to be registered so that the anatomical location of the abnormality can be localised more precisely (Summary box 13.7).

Summary box 13.7

Radionuclide imaging

Strengths
- Allows functional imaging
- Allows imaging of the whole body
- Bone scan has a high sensitivity for metastatic bone disease, fractures and infection
- PET scanning is valuable in the detection of metastatic cancer

Weaknesses
- Specific agents are required for specific indications
- Often non-specific and an abnormal result may require further imaging
- Generally poor spatial resolution

IMAGING IN ORTHOPAEDIC SURGERY

Introduction

Imaging is an intricate part of musculoskeletal diagnosis, and image-guided, minimally invasive techniques also play a major role in treatment. In broad terms, radiographs are the best method of looking for bony lesions or injuries, MRI shows bone marrow disease, muscle tendon and soft-tissue disorders, and ultrasound has better resolution than MRI for small structures, with the added advantage of showing dynamic changes. CT enables visualisation of the fine detail of bony structures, clarifying abnormalities seen on plain radiographs (Summary box 13.8).

There are occasions when a combination of techniques will be important, and due consideration should be given to reducing the ionising radiation burden to the patient, using ultrasound and MRI as primary investigations whenever appropriate.

Summary box 13.8

Types of imaging

- Radiographs are the best first-line test for bone lesions and fractures
- MRI is good for diagnosing bone marrow disease, occult fractures and tendon and soft-tissue disorders
- CT enables visualisation of the fine detail of bony structures
- CT gives the best three-dimensional information on fractures
- Ultrasound has better resolution in accessible soft tissues and can be used dynamically
- Ultrasound is the best method of distinguishing solid from cystic lesions
- Ultrasound is the only method for locating non-metallic foreign bodies
- Ultrasound is the best method for detecting muscle hernias

Skeletal trauma

Musculoskeletal trauma is best imaged by an initial plain radiograph. All skeletal radiographs should be taken from two different angles, usually at right angles to each other. This is important in trauma because a fracture or dislocation may not be visible on a single view (Figure 13.18). Occasionally, and in specific locations such as the scaphoid, more than two views are routinely performed. If this fails to make a clear diagnosis, or if there is suspicion of soft-tissue injuries, then cross-sectional studies are indicated.

In the spine, CT is a normal second-line investigation, but this is best performed with reference to good-quality radiographs, including oblique views if necessary (Summary box 13.9).

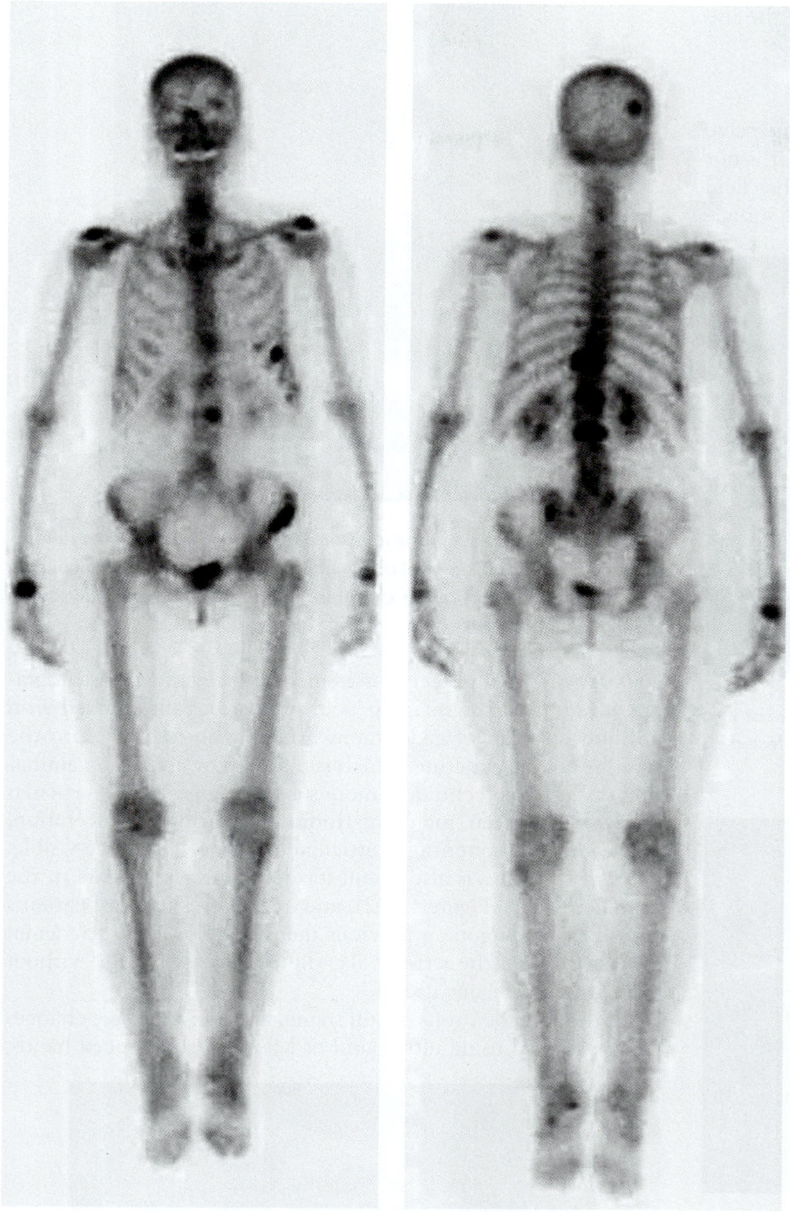

Figure 13.17 Bone scintigraphy in a patient with carcinoma of the breast illustrating bony metastatic deposits involving multiple vertebrae, the skull, pelvis and ribs.

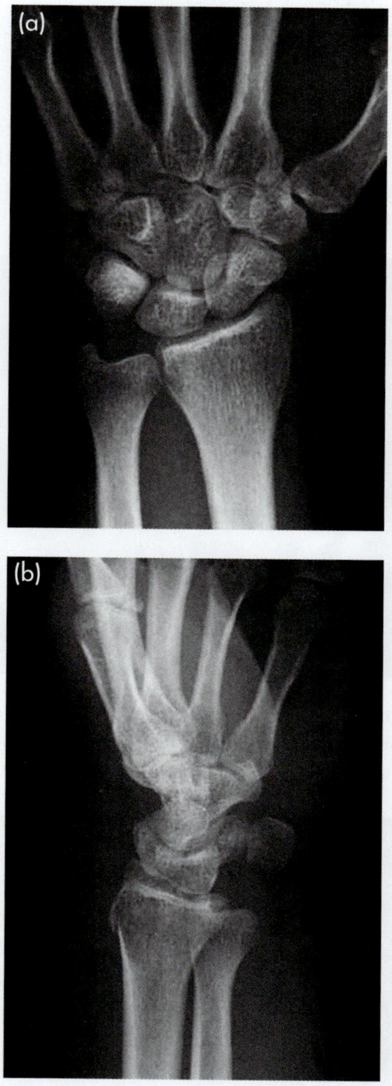

Figure 13.18 Anteroposterior radiograph of the wrist (a) in a patient following a fall does not show an acute bony injury. It is only on the second view (b) that a fracture of the dorsal cortex of the distal radius is visualised.

Summary box 13.9

Trauma imaging

- Initial imaging is radiography
- At least two views are needed
- Use CT for spine, intra-articular or occult fractures

Axial CT images alone may fail to diagnose some fractures, so three-dimensional reformatting is important to prevent errors. Sections should be thin, but care must be taken not to cover too wide an area, as the radiation burden may be excessive, particularly with multislice CT.

Degenerative disease

Synovitis

Radiographs are usually the first-line imaging investigation performed for the examination of joints. Typical changes of a degenerative or an erosive arthropathy are well known and understood. However, early arthropathy will be missed on radiographs and, with the advent of disease-modifying drugs, it is important to detect early synovitis before it is even apparent on clinical examination. Gadolinium diethyl triamine pentaacetic (DTPA)-enhanced MRI is the most sensitive method for detecting synovial thickening of numerous joints, but ultrasound is also sensitive, albeit more laborious to perform. Ultrasound shows effusions and synovial thickening clearly, and shows the increased blood flow around the affected joints without the use of contrast agents (Figures 13.19 and 13.20).

Articular cartilage damage

Articular surface disease is difficult to detect using non-invasive techniques. MRI is probably the best method, although it is not sensitive to early chondral changes (Figure 13.21). Higher field strength magnets (3 Tesla and above) with dedicated surface coils provide more precise assessment; however, MR arthrography is currently the imaging 'gold standard'. Saline mixed with a dilute quantity of gadolinium DTPA is introduced into the joint by needle puncture, which is followed by an MRI examination. Using this technique, more subtle changes in the articular surface can be seen, including thinning, fissuring and ulceration. However, early softening of articular cartilage will not be visible. MR arthrography is also useful for detecting labral tears in the shoulder or hip (Figure 13.22), and in the assessment of patients who have undergone a previous meniscectomy. The triangular fibrocartilage of the wrist is also difficult to assess fully without arthrography (Figure 13.23).

In the shoulder, rotator cuff trauma and degenerative changes can be studied using ultrasound or MRI. In experienced hands,

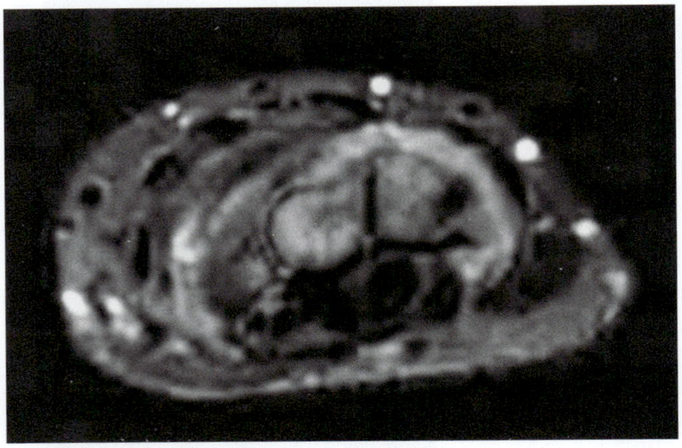

Figure 13.19 Axial T2-weighted fat-suppressed image of the wrist in a patient with rheumatoid arthritis demonstrating synovitis manifested as increased signal dorsal to the carpal bones.

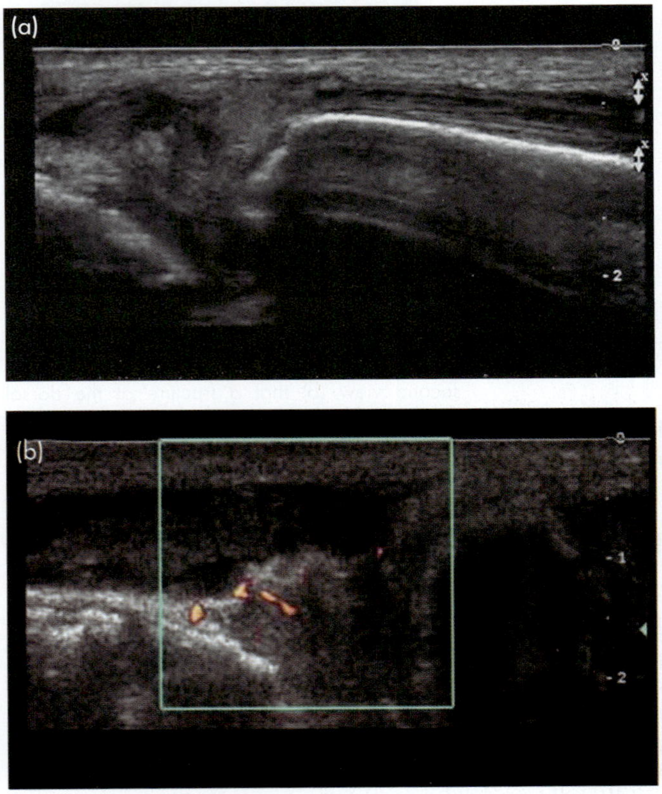

Figure 13.20 Ultrasound of the wrist (a) shows thickening of tissues on the dorsal aspect of the radiocarpal joint. (b) There is increased flow on power Doppler ultrasound in this patient with wrist synovitis and rheumatoid arthritis.

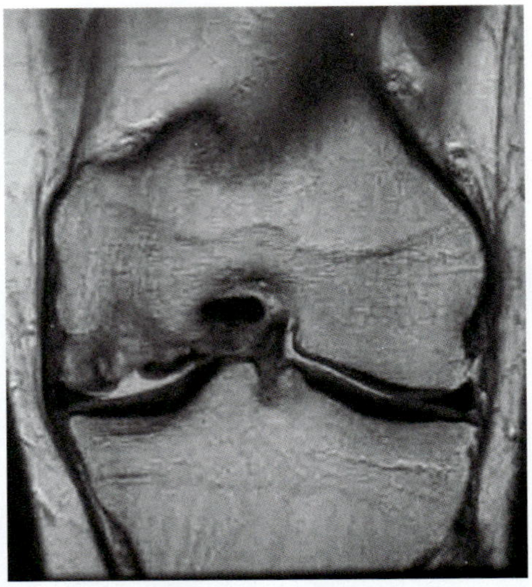

Figure 13.21 Coronal magnetic resonance imaging of the knee demonstrates a focal osteochondral abnormality of the medial femoral condyle with full-thickness loss of the articular cartilage and abnormality of the subchondral bone.

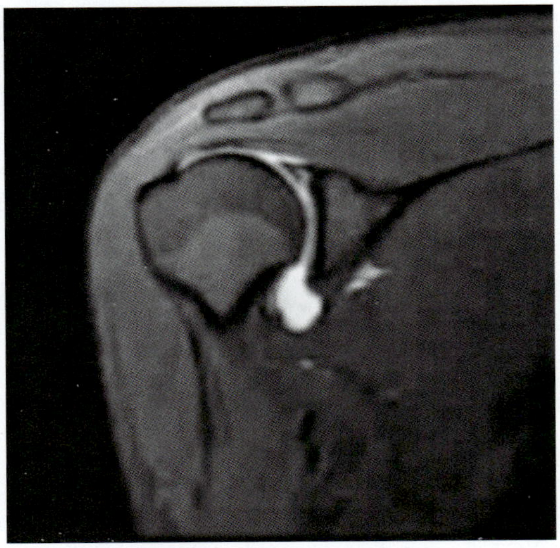

Figure 13.22 Coronal oblique T1-weighted fat-suppressed image of the right shoulder following intra-articular injection of diluted gadolinium demonstrates imbibition of the gadolinium mixture into the superior labrum in a patient with superior labrum anterior posterior (SLAP) tear.

Nikola Tesla, 1856–1943, an American physicist and electrical engineer who worked for the Westinghouse Company. A Tesla is the SI unit of magnetic flux density.

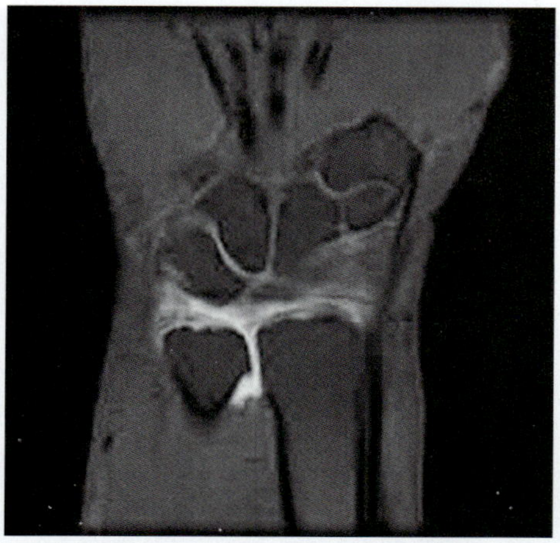

Figure 13.23 Coronal T1-weighted fat-suppressed image following injection of diluted gadolinium mixture into the radiocarpal joint shows extension of gadolinium into the distal radioulnar joint through a tear in the triangular fibrocartilage.

ultrasound has a higher accuracy rate, because image resolution is better and because the mechanical integrity of the cuff can be tested by dynamically stressing it (Figure 13.24). MRI has the advantage of being able to show abnormalities in the subcortical bone.

In the majority of arthropathies and degenerative disorders, serial imaging is useful. Changes in films taken weeks or months apart are far easier to see and interpret than from a single snapshot study (Summary box 13.10).

Summary box 13.10

Imaging techniques for joint disease

- Radiographs are good for assessing established articular disease
- Synovitis can be detected using ultrasound or contrast-enhanced MRI
- Early damage to articular cartilage is difficult to image by conventional methods
- Rotator cuff lesions are best studied using ultrasound or MRI
- Destructive lesions are best studied first on plain radiographs
- MRI is best for staging tumours
- Biopsy can be guided by fluoroscopy, CT or ultrasound

Aggressive bone disease

The radiograph is the first imaging technique for destructive lesions in bones. There is considerable experience in the interpretation of these films, especially with regard to whether the lesion is benign or malignant (Figure 13.25).

Radiographs are also vital in the assessment of soft-tissue calcification in tumours of muscle, tendon and subcutaneous fat. When a lesion is detected, there needs to be an early decision as to whether this is benign or malignant. If there is a suspicion of malignancy on the radiograph, or any uncertainty, then local staging is indicated. This is best performed by MRI for both bone and soft-tissue lesions (Figure 13.26). At this stage, it is likely that a biopsy will be indicated, and preferably under image guidance. Soft-tissue and bone biopsy needles may be guided by CT, ultrasound or interventional MRI systems. The route of puncture should avoid vital structures and must be agreed with the surgeon, who will perform local excision if the lesion proves to be malignant. Care should be taken to avoid contaminating other compartments. In all circumstances, samples are best sent for both histopathological and microbiological examination. It may be difficult to tell on imaging whether or not a lesion is infected, and histology often provides a clear diagnosis in inflammatory conditions. Bone scintigraphy is useful in detecting whether a lesion is solitary or multiple, although whole-body MRI is becoming available (Summary box 13.11).

Summary box 13.11

Imaging of aggressive lesions in bone

- Plain radiographs are important as a first investigation
- MRI is best for local staging
- Bone scintigraphy or whole-body MRI for solitary or multiple lesion determination
- CT detects lung metastases
- Fluoroscopy, CT, MRI or ultrasound can be used to guide the biopsy

Mass lesions

Mass lesions in muscle and soft tissue are examined by ultrasound, which can be diagnostic in the majority of cases, thereby avoiding the need for further imaging. This is most often the case when a lesion is purely cystic and, as most soft-tissue masses are cysts, ultrasound is a very effective screening test. There are occasions when no mass lesion is found at the site of concern, and then reassurance can be offered. If the ultrasound examination is normal, this effectively excludes soft-tissue neoplasia. A reasonable protocol is to perform ultrasound on all palpable

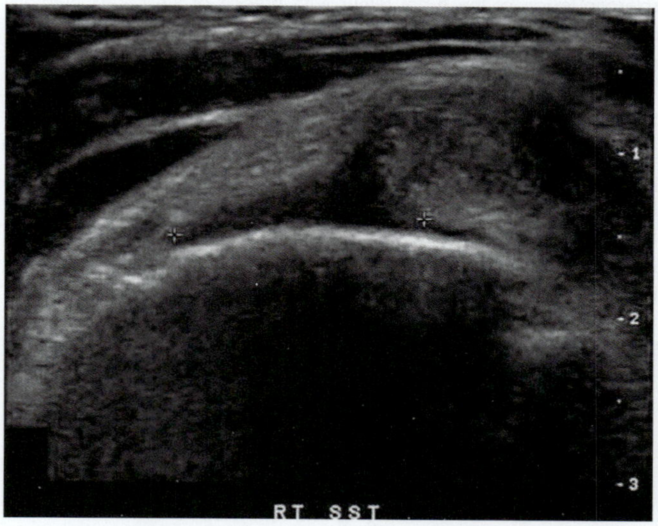

Figure 13.24 Ultrasound of the supraspinatus tendon identifies a partial tear of the tendon, which is predominantly articular sided but with a component that is nearly full thickness.

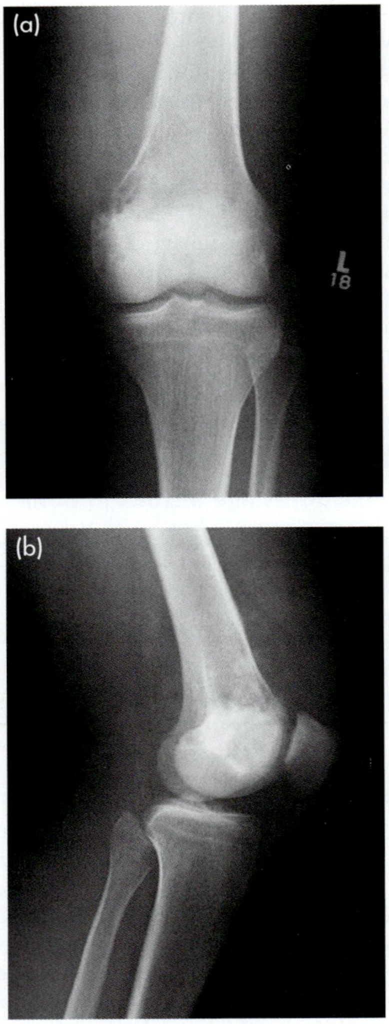

Figure 13.25 Anteroposterior (a) and lateral (b) radiographs of the left knee in a young patient with knee pain. There is a mixed lucent and sclerotic lesion of the distal femur with breach of the cortex medially and soft-tissue extension seen anteriorly and posteriorly. The location and appearances are consistent with osteosarcoma.

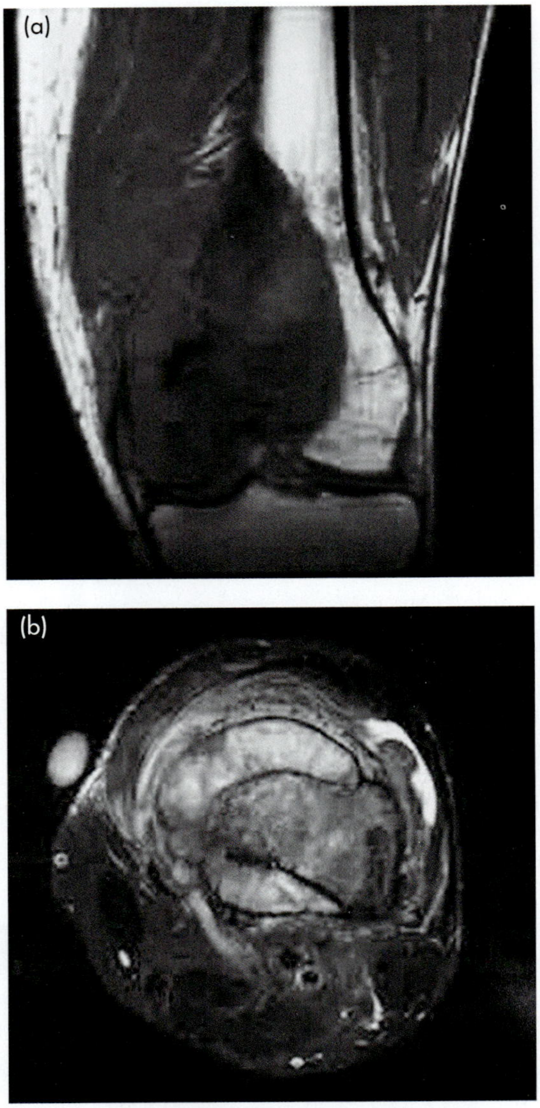

Figure 13.26 Coronal T1- (a) and axial T2-weighted fat-suppressed (b) images through the distal femur of the patient in Figure 13.25 illustrates the bony area involved, the soft-tissue extent of the tumour and the relationship of the neurovascular structures to the mass.

'lesions' to exclude cysts, and on patients without any identifiable mass, and to proceed to MRI only when there is a solid or partly solid element to an unidentifiable lesion. Tumour vascularity is best assessed by Doppler ultrasound. It can be studied by intravenous gadolinium DTPA-enhanced MRI; however, this is a more expensive and invasive technique, providing no more information than Doppler ultrasound (Summary box 13.12).

Summary box 13.12

Imaging of soft-tissue lesions

- Ultrasound is the best for screening; it is often the only imaging required
- MRI is best for local staging and follow up
- Doppler ultrasound can assess vascularity cheaply and effectively
- Ultrasound is useful for biopsy

Infection

In the early stages of joint infection, the plain films may be normal, but they should still be performed to exclude bony erosions, in case a painful joint is the first sign of an arthropathy. Ultrasound examination is the easiest and most accurate method of assessing joint effusions, although, when an effusion is identified, it is not possible to discriminate between blood and pus. Aspiration guided by ultrasound is the best method of making this distinction. MRI may be required to assess early articular cartilage and bone involvement.

Radiographs should also be used to examine patients with suspected osteomyelitis. Although they may not detect early infection, they will demonstrate or exclude bony destruction, calcification and sequestrum formation. CT may be needed to give a cross-sectional view, in order to assess the extent of bony sequestrum.

MRI is perhaps the most sensitive method for detecting early disease and is the preferred technique to define the activity and extent of infection, as it shows not only the bony involvement but also the extent of oedema and soft-tissue involvement (Figure 13.27). Abscesses may be detected or excluded, and subperiosteal oedema is readily visible. MRI can be used as a staging procedure to plan treatment, including surgical intervention. Serial examinations can be used to follow the response to intravenous antibiotics and are very useful in the management of complex osteomyelitis. In cases of negative or equivocal MRI, nuclear medicine techniques such as bone scintigraphy can be very sensitive, and specialised studies using tracers such as gallium citrate or indium-labelled white cells increase specificity (Summary box 13.13).

Summary box 13.13

Imaging of potentially infected bone and joint

- Plain radiographs may be needed to exclude bone erosion
- Ultrasound is sensitive for an effusion, periosteal collections and superficial abscesses and can be used for guided aspiration
- CT is useful in established infection to look for sequestrum
- MRI is useful to define the activity of osteomyelitis, early infection and soft-tissue collections
- Bone scans are sensitive but of low specificity
- Complex nuclear medicine studies are useful in negative MR examinations or equivocal cases

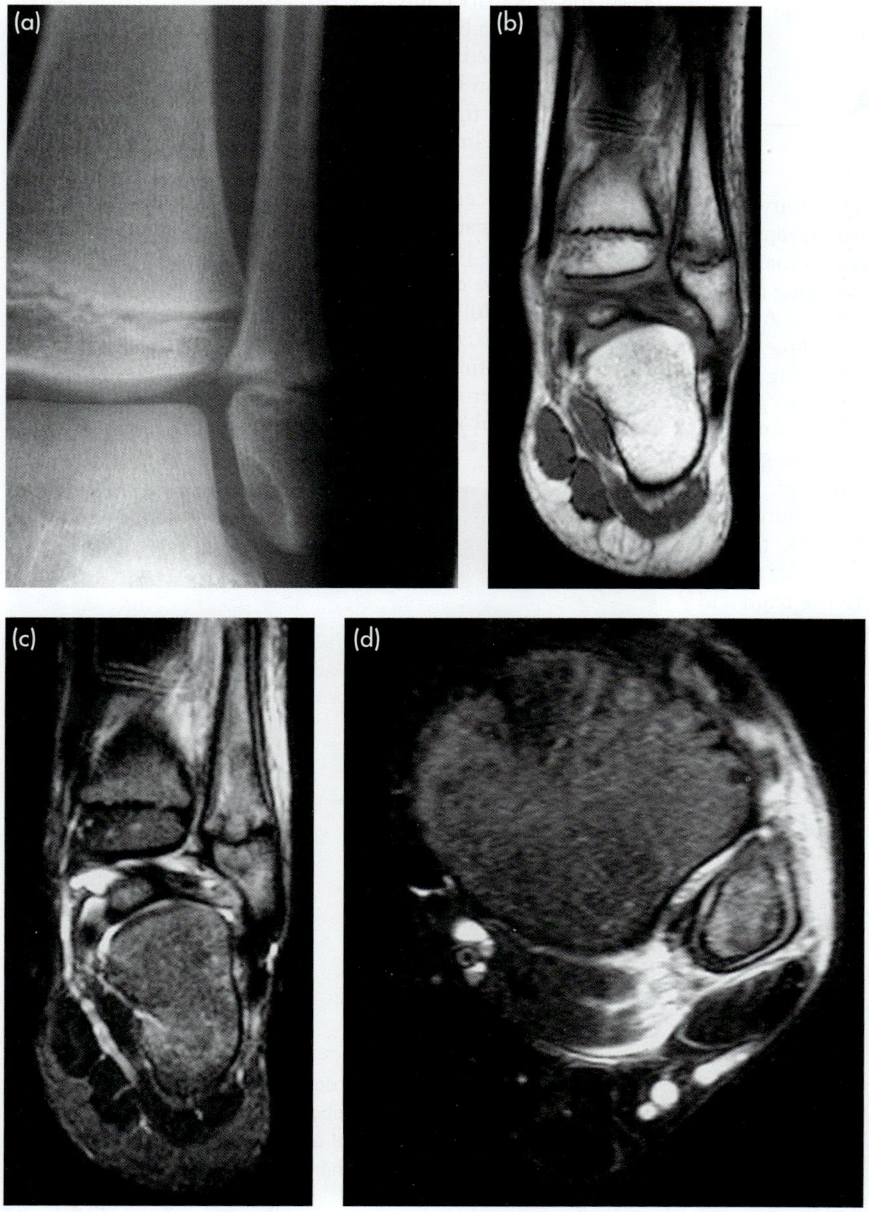

Figure 13.27 (a) The plain films of this 13-year-old are close to normal. On close inspection, there is a fine periosteal reaction on the fibula. (b) The coronal T1-weighted magnetic resonance image shows little more, but (c) the coronal fast STIR (short tau inversion recovery) images and (d) axial T2 fast spin echo with fat suppression show the oedema in bone as white and the extensive periosteal fluid with soft-tissue inflammation. The diagnosis is acute osteomyelitis.

Metabolic bone disease

Plain radiographs should be the first images of patients with metabolic bone disease. They may detect the subperiosteal erosions in hyperparathyroidism or, more commonly, the osteopenia in osteoporosis, but they cannot be used to quantify osteoporosis. The apparent density of the bone on the film is linked to the penetration of the rays, among other variables, as well as to the bone density. If a quantitative method is needed, however, bone mineral density using dual x-ray absorptiometry (DEXA) is the most accurate and practical. However, fractures will cause erroneously high readings, and they tend to occur in the vertebrae used for DEXA measurements. Quantitative CT is an alternative technique, although this is less readily available. Ultrasound transmission measurement in the extremities has its advocates, as it arguably measures factors that better represent the strength of bone rather than its density. Its limitations are that it cannot be used to study the vertebrae or hip, and these are the sites where osteoporotic fractures occur most frequently. MRI may be useful in detecting fractures and is an essential prerequisite to percutaneous vertebroplasty.

IMAGING IN MAJOR TRAUMA

Introduction

Trauma remains a major cause of mortality and morbidity in all age groups. Presented with a multiply injured patient, rapid and effective investigation and treatment are required to maximise the chances of survival and to reduce morbidity. Imaging plays a major role in this assessment and in guiding treatment. As with the clinical assessment, imaging is carried out according to the principles of primary and secondary surveys, identifying major life-threatening injuries of the airway, respiratory system and circulation before a more detailed and typically time-consuming assessment of other injures. At no point should imaging delay the treatment of immediately life-threatening injuries. As in other settings, the quickest and least invasive examinations should be performed first. A radiologist present in the trauma room at the time of patient assessment is able to rapidly evaluate the radiographs, relay this information back to the team and guide further imaging, which may include further plain films, CT, ultrasound and MRI.

Plain radiographs

Conventional radiography allows rapid assessment of the major injuries and can be carried out in the trauma room while the patient is clinically assessed and treated. Despite the time constraints, the number of staff involved and the restricted mobility of the patient, high-quality images can be routinely obtained with due care and attention.

There is no routine set of radiographs to be obtained, and the decision is based on the mechanism of injury, the stability of the patient's condition and whether the patient is intubated. The most commonly performed initial radiographs are a chest radiograph, a single anteroposterior view of the pelvis and a cervical spine series.

The supine chest radiograph should encompass an area from the lung apices to the costophrenic recesses and include the ribs laterally. Chest radiographs give valuable information in both blunt and penetrating trauma. Evaluation of the radiograph should be undertaken in a systematic manner to minimise the chances of missing an injury. In the first instance, the position of line and tubes including the endotracheal tube should be assessed followed by assessment of the central airways. Following this, the lungs should be evaluated for abnormal focal areas of opacification, which may represent aspiration, haemorrhage, haematoma or oedema as well as more diffuse opacification reflecting a pleural collection. Alternatively, relative focal or unilateral lucency may reflect a pneumothorax in the supine position. Evaluation of the mediastinum should include its position, which may be altered by tension pneumothoraces or large collections, as well as its contour, an alteration of which may reflect a mediastinal haematoma due to aortic or spinal injury. Finally, the skeleton and the soft tissue should be carefully examined for rib, vertebral, scapular and limb fractures as well as evidence of surgical emphysema and paraspinal haematomas (Figure 13.28).

Pelvic radiographs are also commonly performed to screen for and assess fractures of the bony pelvis. The image should include the iliac crests in their totality and extend inferiorly to below the lesser trochanters. When assessing the film, the alignment of the sacroiliac joints and the symphysis pubis should be carefully examined, as some fractures, especially those of the sacral arcades, can be very subtle on the pelvic radiograph. The presence of pubic fractures raises the possibility of urethral injury and should alert clinicians to exercise caution with bladder catheterisation (Figure 13.29).

The utility of cervical spine x-rays depends on the consciousness level of the patient and the presence of distracting injuries. In fully conscious patients with an isolated neck injury, clinical assessment can be used to guide the need for x-rays. In patients with distracting injuries and/or altered consciousness, including intubated patients, radiography is required. Typically, in patients who are not intubated, at least three views are performed including an anteroposterior view, an open mouth odontoid peg view and a lateral view extending down to the cervicothoracic

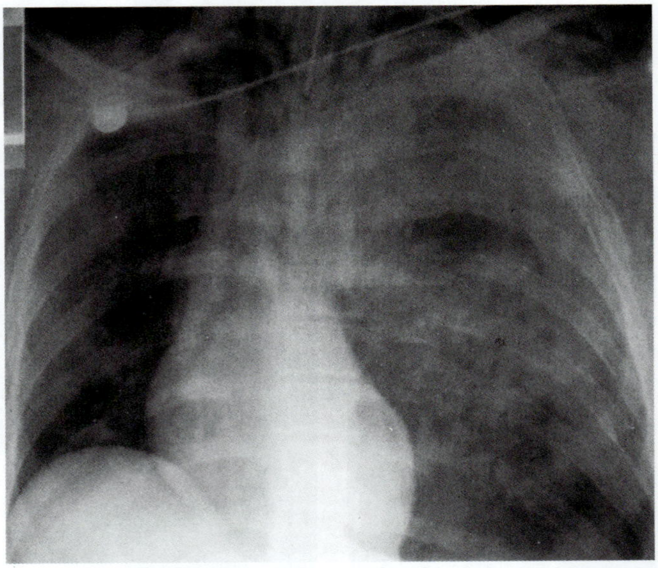

Figure 13.28 Supine chest radiograph of a patient involved in a road traffic accident. The patient is intubated. There are multiple left-sided rib fractures and extensive surgical emphysema. Depression of the left hemidiaphragm and mediastinal shift to the right suggest that there is a tension pneumothorax present.

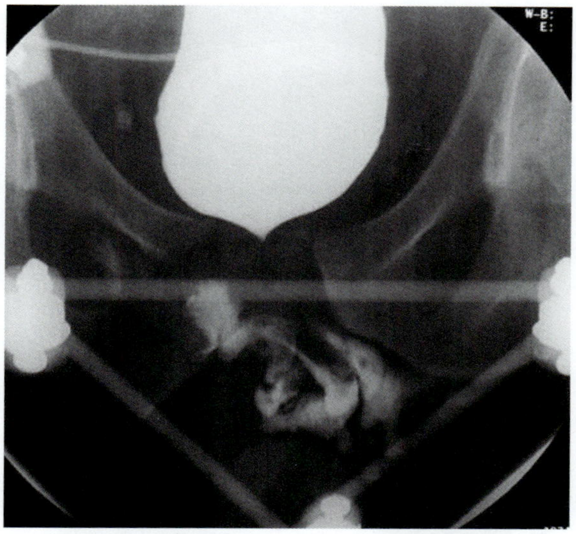

Figure 13.29 Retrograde urethrogram in a patient who sustained extensive pelvic fractures following a fall. The pelvic injuries have been stabilised using an external fixation device. The urethrogram identifies extensive injury to the urethra with extravasation of contrast.

junction. These may be supplemented with trauma oblique views in which the tube is rotated rather than the patient. In intubated individuals, open mouth views cannot be performed, and soft-tissue assessment is impaired by the presence of the endotracheal tube, so CT should be used to supplement an initial lateral radiograph (Figure 13.30). When fractures are identified or when the radiographs do not fully examine the cervicothoracic junction, CT is indicated. If the patient is to undergo emergency CT examination for head or chest indications, a good-quality multidetector CT study using thin sections and both coronal and sagittal reconstructions may be used to replace radiographs. CT may also be indicated when the radiographs appear normal but the nature of the injury or the clinical circumstances strongly suggest that the cervical spine may be injured.

Further radiographs of the thoracic and lumbar spine and the peripheral skeleton may be required depending on the clinical setting. As with all skeletal radiographs, two perpendicular views are required for adequate assessment. Radiographs of the skull or facial bones have no role in the immediate assessment of the multitrauma individual except for immediate localisation of a penetrating object.

Ultrasound

Ultrasound has an evolving role in the assessment of acutely traumatised patients. The main current roles of ultrasound include the assessment of intraperitoneal fluid and haemopericardium (focused assessment with sonography for trauma, FAST), the evaluation of pneumothoraces in supine patients and in guiding intervention.

FAST ultrasound is a limited examination directed to look for intraperitoneal fluid or pericardial injury as a marker of underlying injury. This avoids the invasiveness of diagnostic peritoneal lavage. In the presence of free intraperitoneal fluid and an unstable patient, the ultrasound allows the trauma surgeon to explore the abdomen as a cause of blood loss. In the presence of fluid and a haemodynamically stable individual, further assessment by way

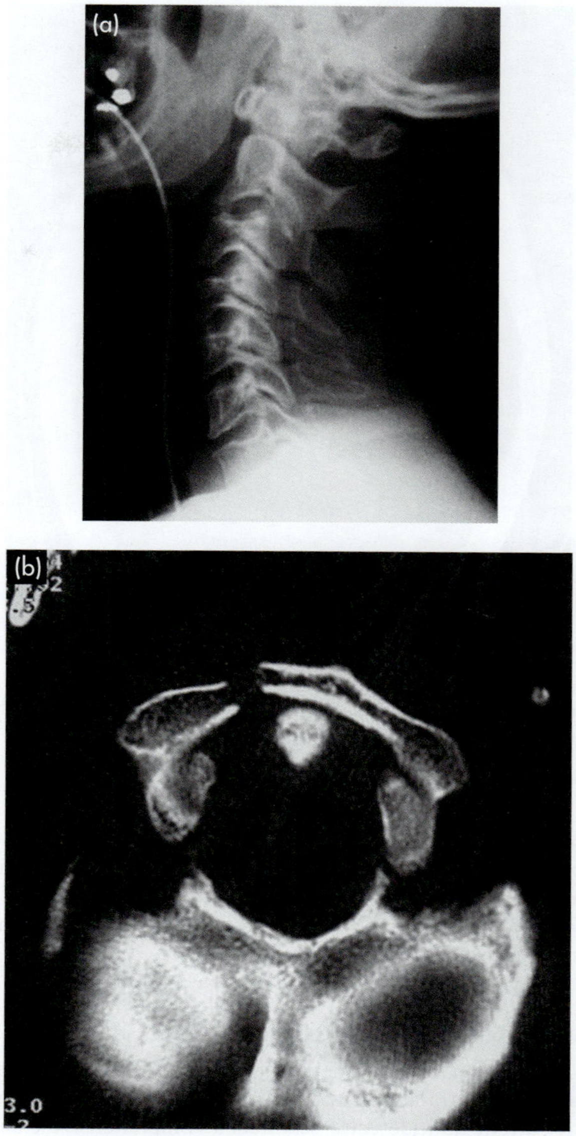

Figure 13.30 Lateral view of the cervical spine (a) fails to demonstrate the cervicothoracic junction. In addition, there appears to be a break in the posterior arch of C1. Computed tomography of the cervical spine (b) demonstrated a fracture of the anterior arch as well as the posterior arch of C1.

of CT can be performed. However, it is important to realise that ultrasound has limitations in the identification of free fluid. This includes obscuration of fluid by bowel gas or extensive surgical emphysema. More organised haematoma may be more difficult to visualise. It must also be emphasised that the principal role of ultrasound is not to identify the primary solid organ injury, although this may be visualised. Occasionally, a second ultrasound scan may show free fluid in the presence of an initially negative FAST scan.

The detection of a pneumothorax on a supine radiograph can be very difficult. Ultrasound examination may be used to identify a radiographically occult pneumothorax. With a high-resolution linear probe, the pleura can be visualised as an echogenic stripe,

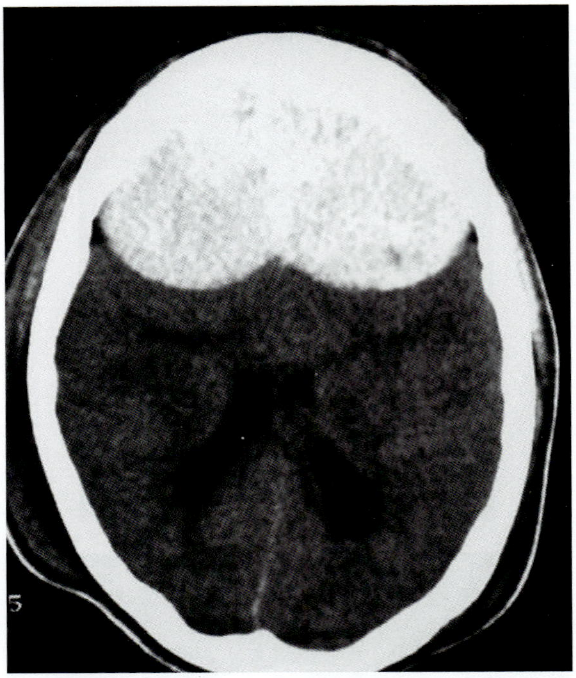

Figure 13.31 Computed tomography of the head in a patient with head injury shows bilateral large frontal extradural collections.

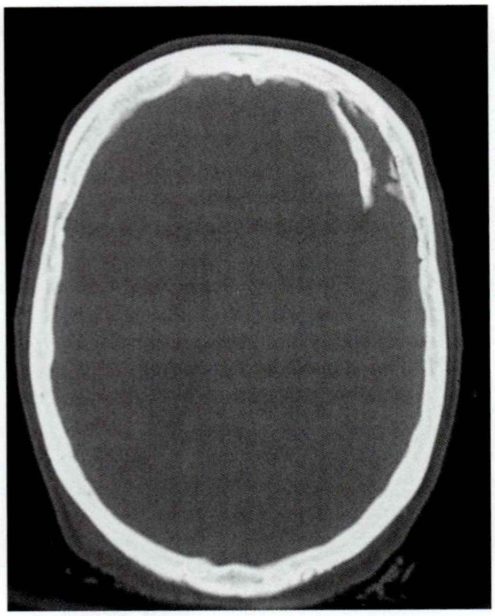

Figure 13.32 Computed tomography of the head following head trauma shows a skull fracture with a large depressed component.

and its motion with respiration can also be assessed. In the presence of a pneumothorax, the sliding motion of the pleura is lost. Ultrasound may also be used to detect a haemothorax or haemopericardium.

Finally, ultrasound may be of value in guiding the placement of an intravascular line by direct visualisation of the vessels. This can be especially advantageous in shocked patients.

Computed tomography

CT is the main imaging method for the investigation of intracranial and intra-abdominal injuries and vertebral fractures. With current multidetector scanners a comprehensive examination of the head, spine, chest, abdomen and pelvis can be completed in less than 5 minutes. However, much more time is taken up in transferring the patient and the associated monitoring equipment onto the scanner. Therefore, the total time can be in excess of 30 minutes, and CT should be reserved for individuals whose condition is stable.

CT examination of the head is accurate in identifying treatable intracranial injuries (Figures 13.31 and 13.32) and should not be delayed by radiography of peripheral injuries, as there is declining success in cases of intracranial collection when treated after the initial 3–4 hours. In comparison, identification of more widespread injuries, such as diffuse axonal injury, is relatively poor. Examination of facial injuries and cervical spine fractures can also be carried out at the same time as this only adds seconds to the examination. There is evidence that CT of the abdomen and pelvis is of benefit in multiple trauma when there is a head injury, as it often shows unexpected abnormalities, and this may affect the immediate management, especially if the patient deteriorates.

Chest CT with intravenous contrast agent is valuable in identifying vascular and lung injuries and is the most accurate way of demonstrating haemothorax and pneumothorax. The position of chest drains can be identified, allowing adjustment of position if necessary. Abdominal and pelvic CT is usually undertaken as an extension to the chest CT. If an abdominal examination is performed, the pelvis should be included to avoid missing pelvic injuries and free pelvic fluid. CT is an excellent means of identifying hepatic, splenic (Figure 13.33) and renal injuries. Delayed examination after the administration of intravenous contrast agents allows assessment of the pelvicalyceal system in cases of renal trauma. Pancreatic and duodenal injuries may also be identified, but detection of these injuries may be more problematic. Using CT, the accuracy of detection of bowel or mesenteric injuries is less than it is for solid organ injury, and these injuries should be suspected when there is free intraperitoneal fluid without an identifiable cause (Figure 13.34).

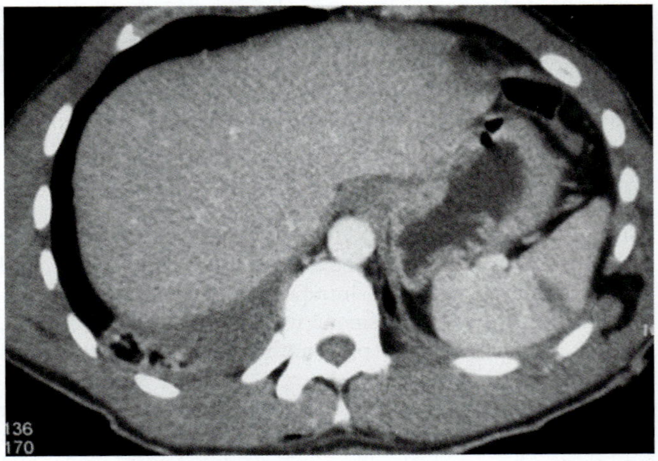

Figure 13.33 Post-contrast abdominal computed tomography of a patient following blunt abdominal trauma shows a splenic laceration with herniation of mesenteric fat. A right-sided pleural collection is also evident.

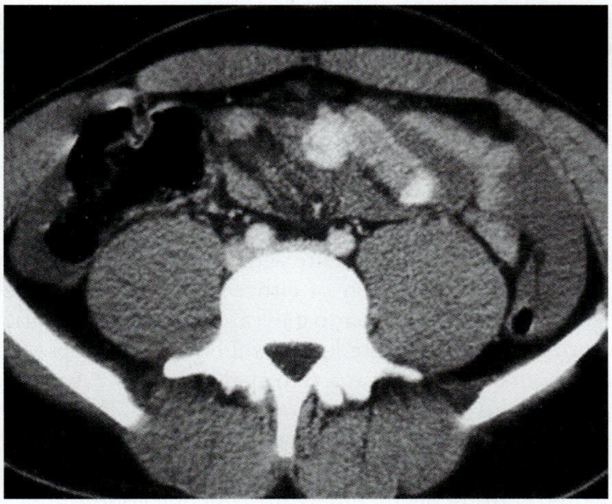

Figure 13.34 Post-intravenous contrast computed tomography examination in a patient with a penetrating abdominal injury and mesenteric tear shows free fluid in the flanks and active extravasation of contrast centrally.

The image data may be reconstructed into thinner slices for the diagnosis of injuries to the thoracic and lumbar spine and for the better delineation of pelvic and acetabular fractures. Multidetector machines will be optimal for this purpose but, with older CT scanners, additional dedicated thin sections may be required for adequate examination. Complex intra-articular fractures of the peripheral skeleton, such as calcaneal and tibial plateau fractures, may be usefully examined by dedicated thin-section studies provided this does not delay the treatment of other more serious injuries (Figure 13.35). CT angiography may be used to demonstrate vascular injuries in the limbs in those with penetrating injuries or complex displaced fractures.

Magnetic resonance imaging

The value of immediate MRI in trauma is relatively limited and is largely confined to the imaging of spinal injuries (Figure 13.36).

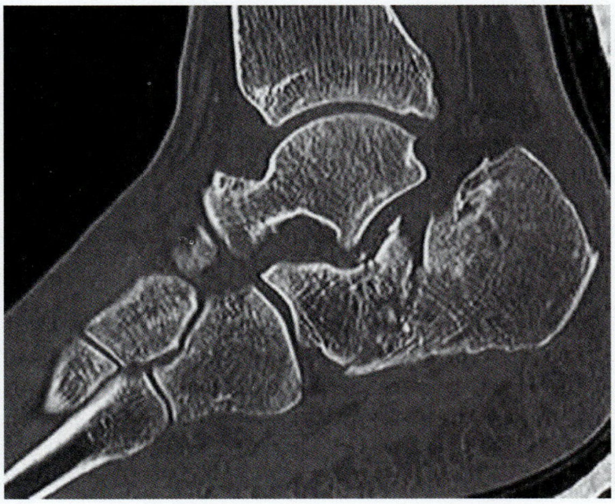

Figure 13.35 Sagittal reformats of computed tomography of the calcaneus in a patient following a fall illustrate a comminuted calcaneal fracture with intra-articular extension into the posterior facet of the subtalar joint.

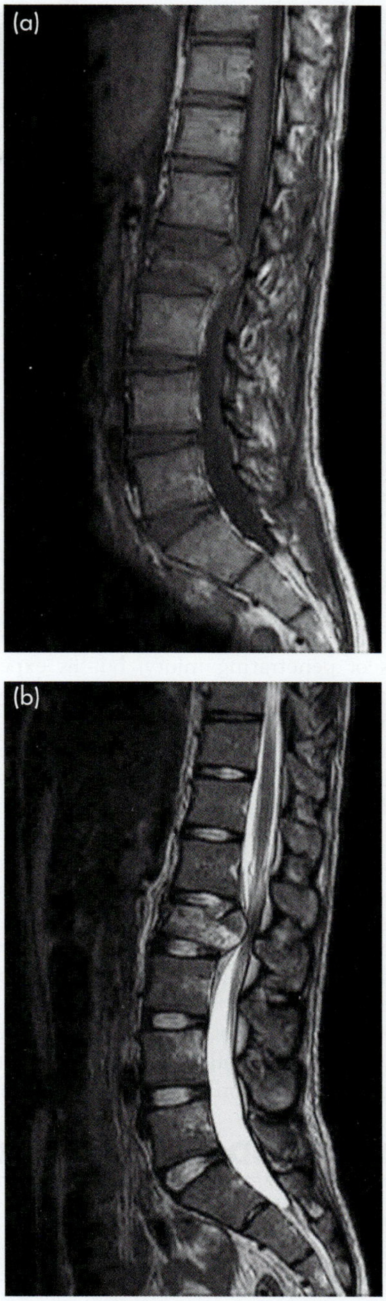

Figure 13.36 Sagittal T1-weighted (a) and T2-weighted (b) magnetic resonance imaging of the spine demonstrates a burst fracture of L2 causing neural compression.

Access to urgent MRI is not widely available, and there are major practical problems in imaging patients who require ventilation or monitoring. MRI is therefore only practical in stable patients. All monitoring equipment must be MRI compatible, and ventilation support should be undertaken by staff skilled and experienced in these techniques as applied to the MRI environment. MRI may be used to diagnose injuries of the spinal cord and associated perispinal haematomas in patients with neurological signs or symptoms. MRI can supplement CT in spinal injuries by imaging soft-tissue injuries to the longitudinal and interspinous ligaments. MRI is mandatory in patients in whom there is facetal dislocation if surgical reduction is being considered to minimise the risk of displacing soft-tissue or disc material into the spinal canal during reduction procedures. Subtle fractures may be difficult to identify, particularly if they are old, but an acute injury is normally identified by the surrounding oedema. Bony abnormities should be reviewed using CT, as fracture lines are hard to identify with MRI and unstable injuries may be overlooked. In the less acute setting, MRI may also be used to assess diffuse axonal injuries, with an accuracy exceeding CT.

Vascular interventional radiology

Angiography has been used for both the diagnosis and treatment of vascular injuries in the trauma patient. With the development and refinement of CT angiography techniques, the diagnostic role of interventional radiology may become more limited. Already, CT has a diagnostic accuracy similar to that of formal angiograms in patients with suspected aortic injuries, with the latter reserved for cases where CT has been suboptimal, doubt exists about the diagnosis or stent grafting is being considered. At present, peripheral angiograms are still performed, particularly in cases of penetrating injury, but as experience grows with CT peripheral angiography, this will probably become the preferred technique.

Endovascular techniques play an important role in the treatment of acute solid organ injuries, and the interventional radiologist should be consulted early in the decision-making process. Using coaxial catheter systems and a variety of available embolic agents such as soluble gelatine sponge and microcoils, selective embolisation and reduction of blood flow to the injured segment can be achieved without causing infarction. Selective embolisation techniques are also suitable for the treatment of patients with pelvic fractures with ongoing blood loss and volume issues. With penetrating and non-penetrating extremity trauma, balloon occlusion and embolisation may be employed to control haemorrhage, while the application of stent grafts can aid in re-establishing the circulation to the affected extremity.

IMAGING IN ABDOMINAL SURGERY

The acute abdomen

The term 'acute abdomen' encompasses many diverse entities.

IMAGING IN COMMON SURGICAL CLINICAL SCENARIOS

In this section the roles of different radiological modalities in common surgical scenarios are discussed with a brief rationale behind their use and typical appearances of various pathological processes.

Bowel obstruction

The plain abdominal radiograph is a useful tool in diagnosing bowel obstruction. Small bowel obstruction can generally be distinguished from large bowel obstruction by virtue of the following: small bowel lies centrally in the abdomen while large bowel lies peripherally, the valvulae conniventes (folds) of the small bowel traverse the entire width of the lumen while the haustra of the large bowel do not, and the calibre of the small bowel is typically less than the large, even when obstructed (typical measurements in obstruction: small bowel 3.5–5 cm, large bowel 5–8 cm).

However, it must be stressed that a normal plain radiograph does not exclude an obstruction and if there is persistent concern further imaging is indicated and CT is the modality of choice having largely superseded the contrast follow-through or enema, particularly in the acute setting. The key to diagnosis of a mechanical obstruction of either small or large bowel on CT, and differentiation from paralytic ileus, is identification of a transition zone from dilated proximal bowel to collapsed distal bowel. In small bowel obstruction if no obvious cause such as a mass, volvulus or intussusception is identified, then the most likely aetiology is adhesional. There is no need to give oral contrast for a suspected bowel obstruction CT as fluid in the lumen is a natural contrast agent and in any case oral contrast may well not reach the point of obstruction by the time of the scan. CT is also invaluable to diagnose complications of bowel obstruction such as perforation and ischaemia.

Perforation

The erect chest x-ray (CXR) is the ideal first test for hollow organ perforation and as little as 10–20 mL of free air can be detected under the diaphragm, with the following caveats (Figures 13.37 and 13.38): about 10 minutes should be left between sitting the patient upright to allow air time to rise, the free air must be sought under the right hemidiaphragm to prevent misinterpretation of the gastric air bubble and the reviewer must be able to recognise Chilaiditi's syndrome, the harmless and asymptomatic interposition of large bowel between the liver and diaphragm. Caution must also be exercised in interpreting any free air in the context of recent abdominal surgery as air can persist for up to 5–7 days in the peritoneal cavity.

If the erect CXR is equivocal or a possible walled-off perforation is suspected, a CT is the optimal modality, which may show tiny quantities of free air but may also show the cause,

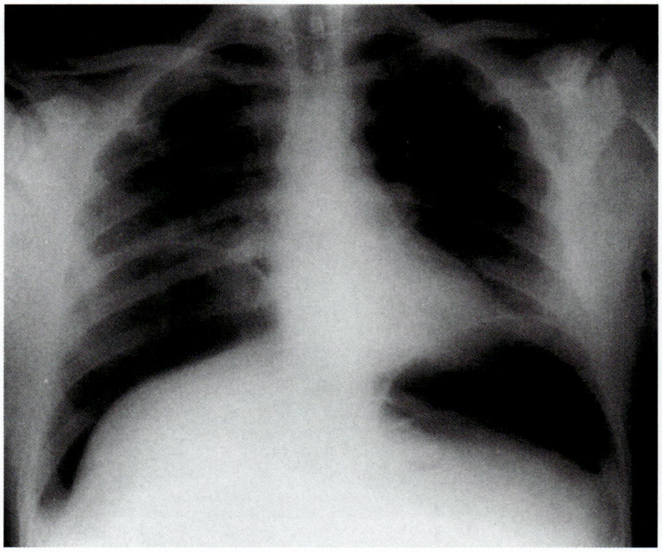

Figure 13.37 Erect chest radiograph showing marked bilateral elevation of the hemidiaphragms with a large volume of subdiaphragmatic free gas.

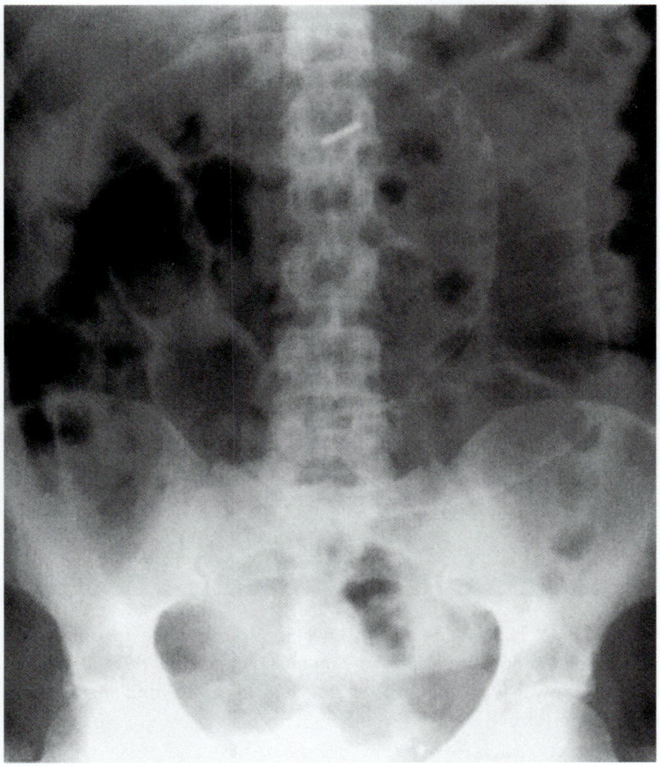

Figure 13.38 Pneumoperitoneum. The presence of free intraperitoneal air outlines the bowel so that both sides of the bowel wall can be seen (Rigler's sign).

e.g. peptic ulcer, diverticulitis or a neoplastic lesion. As with suspected obstruction, oral or rectal contrast is unnecessary if perforation is suspected as making the diagnosis should prompt appropriate management even if the precise site of perforation is not identified. Also, it cannot be overstressed that if there is any possibility of a leak from the gastrointestinal tract (including an anastomotic leak after surgery), then the use of barium is absolutely contraindicated as it can induce a serious and potentially fatal peritonitis.

Ischaemia/infarction

The most useful test when bowel ischaemia or infarction is suspected is a CT scan. Intravenous contrast administration is essential to look for thrombus/embolus in the mesenteric vessels, though ischaemia due to low flow states can still occur in their absence. Ischaemia can be a difficult diagnosis to make radiologically but is suspected, in the appropriate clinical context, by bowel wall thickening, submucosal oedema and free fluid between the folds of the mesentery (particularly if haemorrhagic). Ischaemia must be strongly suspected if these findings are seen in association with a closed loop obstruction or strangulated hernia. Ischaemic colitis typically affects the 'watershed area', which is the junction of the areas supplied by the superior and inferior mesenteric arteries, typically in the region of the splenic flexure.

When bowel wall ischaemia proceeds to transmural infarction, the diagnosis is usually more straightforward with evidence of pneumatosis (air in the bowel wall) typically identified. The air in the bowel wall can then track into mesenteric veins and thence to the portal vein, a CT sign of grave prognostic significance in an adult as it implies widespread and relatively long-standing bowel infarction.

Gastrointestinal haemorrhage

The aetiology of acute gastrointestinal haemorrhage varies between the upper gastrointestinal tract (GIT) (common causes including peptic ulcer disease, varices and Mallory Weiss tears) and the lower GIT (common causes including angiodysplasia, diverticular haemorrhage and neoplastic lesions). While endoscopy is a useful first-line investigation for both, in refractory or occult gastrointestinal (GI) haemorrhage radiology can also contribute to diagnosis and management. Nuclear medicine scans using radioisotope-labelled red blood cells are useful when bleeding is intermittent. An increasingly popular investigation is a CT mesenteric angiogram. Non-contrast scans to look for bright blood in the bowel lumen should be supplemented with scans in the arterial phase to assess for a blush due to active extravasation, and portal venous phase to optimise detection of wall thickening and masses and to look for sites of venous bleeding. If non-invasive imaging is effective, catheter angiography can be used to embolise a bleeding point, though it is occasionally used as a diagnostic test should other tests be negative.

Inflammatory processes

Appendicitis

Historically, a straightforward clinical diagnosis of appendicitis obviated any need for imaging, but with the proven accuracy of available modalities imaging has become increasingly popular to reduce negative appendicectomy rates and to make alternative diagnoses. While a plain radiograph may demonstrate a calcified appendicolith in the right iliac fossa, it is insufficiently sensitive or specific to be reliable. In children ultrasound is the best test, to reduce radiation exposure and due to typically favourable body habitus. This also applies to females of childbearing age, again to reduce radiation exposure, but also as the symptoms may be mimicked by gynaecological pathology, such as ectopic pregnancy, haemorrhagic ovarian cyst and tubo-ovarian abscess, all diagnoses best made with ultrasound. The definitive exclusion of appendicitis, however, hinges on the identification of a normal appendix, measuring less than 6 mm diameter. Retrocaecal appendicitis can readily escape detection with ultrasound and thus CT is the next modality of choice and indeed frequently the first requested in most adults (Figure 13.39). The diagnosis of appendicitis on CT requires the identification of a thickened appendix (>7 mm), with periappendiceal inflammatory change as evidenced by stranding in the surrounding fat. Other signs which may be sought include free fluid, thickening of the caecal pole, possible localised small bowel ileus and right iliac fossa lymphadenopathy. Both CT and ultrasound can also identify collections if an inflamed appendix ruptures and can be used to guide percutaneous drainage as a bridge to definitive surgery.

Diverticulitis

Inflammation of an obstructed diverticulum typically presents with left iliac fossa pain and pyrexia (Figure 13.40). While some authors have promoted the use of focused ultrasound for this indication, in general it is best diagnosed with a CT scan. The typical CT appearance is of pericolic inflammatory change

Leo George Rigler, 1896–1979, an American radiologist, described the double wall sign in pneumoperitoneum.

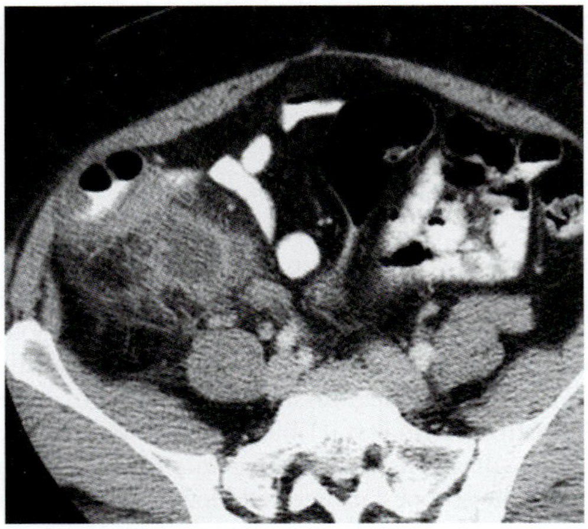

Figure 13.39 Computed tomography scan. Acute appendicitis. Note the thickening of the caecal wall with a periappendiceal fluid collection indicating an appendix abscess.

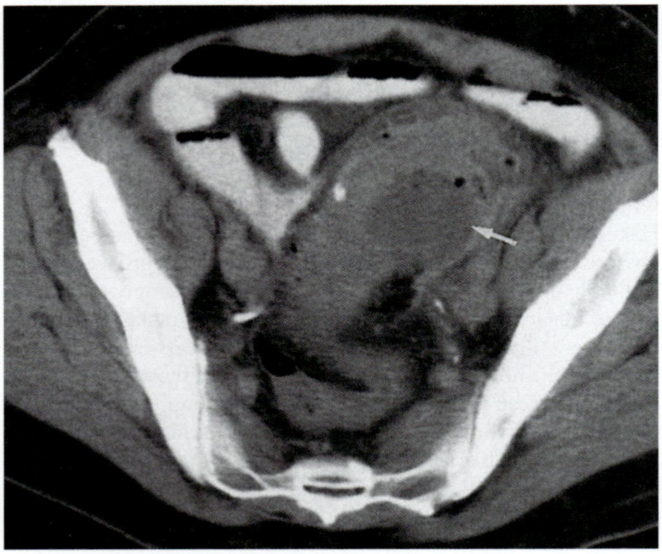

Figure 13.40 Computed tomography scan showing a segment of thickened sigmoid colon with a paracolic abscess (arrow) in a patient with diverticulitis.

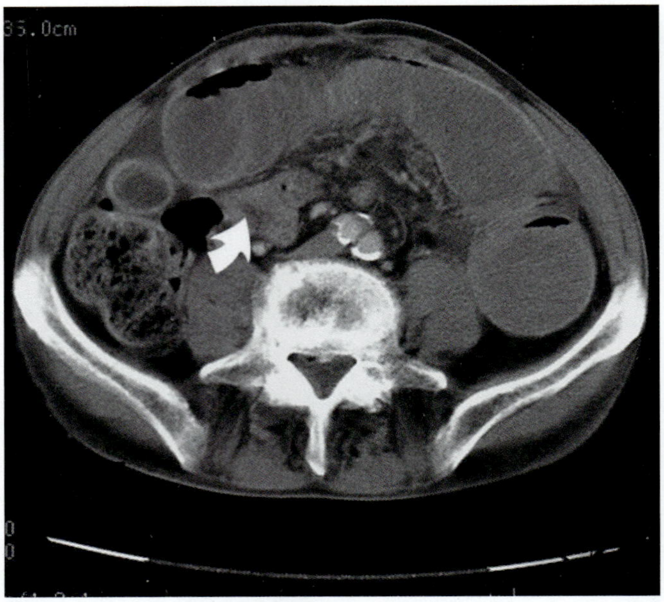

Figure 13.41 High-grade small bowel obstruction due to adhesions. Computed tomography scan showing multiple, dilated, fluid-filled loops of small bowel with collapsed distal ileal loops beyond the point of obstruction (arrow).

around a diverticulum, most commonly in the sigmoid colon. Complications of diverticulitis include perforation, abscess formation, fistulation to adjacent structures and strictures in the bowel; CT is also the modality of choice to identify these, and as with appendicitis can be used to guide percutaneous abscess drainage as a bridge to definitive surgery (Figure 13.41).

Inflammatory bowel disease

The diagnosis of inflammatory bowel disease is made histologically though a barium study of the small bowel, either a follow-through (where barium is ingested orally) or enteroclysis (where dilute barium is infused via an NJ tube) is often used as a screening tool if symptoms are vague. If the diagnosis of Crohn's disease is established, barium studies are useful to demonstrate the extent of disease, particularly to demonstrate the length and number of strictures if surgery is planned, although increasingly this role is being superseded by MRI enterography, which entails an abdominopelvic MRI scan after ingestion of an agent such as lactulose or mannitol to distend the small bowel. The other obvious advantage of MRI is the lack of radiation, particularly relevant in young patients with Crohn's disease who often undergo multiple imaging studies over their lifetime, and for this reason it is gaining in popularity for inflammatory bowel disease follow up.

An acute flare up may also require imaging, and an ultrasound is usually a good first test to look for dilated bowel loops and any abscess, though CT may ultimately be required as gas-filled bowel loops can obscure visualisation of an abscess on ultrasound. MRI is the imaging modality of choice to assess perianal fistulae and abscesses.

Acute pancreatitis

As with acute appendicitis, when the diagnosis is straightforward clinically there may be no need for imaging, though increasingly it is used to confirm the diagnosis, to assess the severity of the process and to look for complications. While ultrasound may show gallstones and can demonstrate an enlarged pancreas with peripancreatic fluid and inflammatory changes, the optimal modality is CT. CT performed too early in the course of the attack, e.g. in the first 12 hours, can be equivocal and the optimal timing of imaging is 48–72 hours.

In mild acute pancreatitis, CT may be normal or may show an enlarged oedematous gland, but in more severe attacks other findings which should be sought include peripancreatic fluid collections, vascular complications such as arterial pseudoaneurysm formation or venous thrombosis and necrosis either of the gland itself or of the surrounding fat. Necrosis typically develops 48–72 hours after the onset of symptoms, and is manifest on CT as lack of enhancement of the necrotic areas.

CT with intravenous contrast is therefore essential to look for necrosis, which is potentially catastrophic particularly if it becomes infected. While CT is not always reliable to diagnose infected necrosis it is suggested by bubbles of air in the necrotic segment. As with other intra-abdominal inflammatory processes, either ultrasound or more usually CT can be used to guide percutaneous drainage of inflammatory fluid collections.

Acute cholecystitis/biliary colic/jaundice

While acute cholecystitis is usually due to mechanical obstruction of the cystic duct or gallbladder neck by a gallstone, acute acalculous cholecystitis can occur in critically ill patients from a number of causes. In any case ultrasound is the modality of choice should this diagnosis be suspected, and the classic diagnostic features are of gallbladder distension with wall thickening (>3 mm). A gallstone obstructing the gallbladder neck or cystic duct may be visualised; alternatively, in acalculous cholecystitis sludge may be seen layering in the gallbladder lumen. Associated signs include pericholecystic fluid and hyperaemia on Doppler examination. Ultrasonographic Murphy's sign refers to tenderness over the gallbladder when pressure is applied while scanning and is a supportive finding in making the diagnosis. As a second-line investigation CT is also accurate for this condition, demonstrating similar signs of gallbladder distension and wall thickening with surrounding inflammatory changes. CT is also useful to diagnose complications such as gangrenous cholecystitis, gallbladder perforation and emphysematous cholecystitis, which may necessitate emergency cholecystectomy. If cross-sectional studies are equivocal, hepatobiliary scintigraphy can be useful, with the diagnosis of acute cholecystitis suggested by non-visualisation of the gallbladder 3 hours after radioisotope administration.

A frequent limitation of ultrasound is failure to visualise the common bile duct throughout its length due to overlying bowel gas, and elective cholecystectomy was typically accompanied by bile duct exploration to look for duct calculi. Increasingly, however, MRCP has been shown to be highly accurate in excluding bile duct calculi before surgery.

Ultrasound is also a useful first-line investigation for jaundice of unknown cause as it can demonstrate duct dilatation and gallstones. If a definitive cause is not shown with ultrasound, or a mass is identified but its precise nature and extent is uncertain, CT is indicated to look for common causes including stones, cholangiocarcinoma and pancreatic carcinoma. CT can not only identify malignant lesions but can also demonstrate the extent of local infiltration and the presence of metastases to determine potential resectability. If the ducts are of normal calibre in a jaundiced patient, liver biopsy should be considered.

Renal colic

The historical methods of imaging for renal colic all have their limitations. Plain film radiography may not demonstrate all calculi, will not show renal tract obstruction and is unreliable for alternative diagnoses. IVU necessitates the administration of intravenous contrast and, if a level of obstruction is sought, delayed films up to 8 hours after injection may be required; it also will not provide alternative diagnoses. Ultrasound will demonstrate hydronephrosis and hydroureter, and calculi in the kidneys and either the proximal or distal ureters can usually be identified as echogenic foci with posterior acoustic shadowing; however, the ureter from just below the kidneys to the pelvis is usually obscured by bowel gas which significantly impairs stone detection.

For these reasons the optimal investigation is now CT KUB, a non-contrast, low dose (2–3 MSv if a low mA scan is performed, equivalent to the dose from a limited IVU series) scan from the upper poles of the kidneys to the pubic symphisis. Contrast administration, either orally or intravenously, is not employed as it does not aid stone detection and may even impair it. Stones are readily identified as high attenuation (typically calcific) foci, and the secondary signs of acute ureteric obstruction may also be seen, including hydronephrosis and hydroureter, renal enlargement and perinephric fat stranding. The most common sites for stones to be seen are at the areas of ureteric narrowing, namely the pelvi-ureteric junction, the pelvic brim and vesico-ureteric junction. CT also offers unrivalled capability for making alternative diagnoses when compared with other modalities.

Abdominal aortic aneurym

If a pulsatile mass is felt in the abdomen and the diagnosis of a possible abdominal aortic aneuryism (AAA) is suspected, ultrasound is a useful modality and provided the aorta is not obscured by bowel gas an aneurysm can usually reliably be excluded. If, however, ultrasound visualisation is suboptimal and the diagnosis is as a result equivocal, or if an aneurysm is identified and information regarding the extent and exact size is required, for example for surgical or endovascular repair planning, CT angiography is indicated, with the aorta typically scanned from the arch to the pubic symphisis in the arterial phase after intravenous contrast. MR angiography is a useful alternative if iodinated contrast is contraindicated.

In the case of suspected aneurysm rupture, provided the patient is sufficiently haemodynamically stable to undergo CT, CT angiography should be urgently performed and supplemented by a non-enhanced initial scan which is useful to look for retroperitoneal haematoma, which is typically of relatively high attenuation compared to the blood in the lumen on a non-contrast scan.

IMAGING IN ONCOLOGY

Modern surgical treatment of cancer requires an understanding of tumour staging systems, as in many instances the tumour stage will define appropriate management. The development of stage-dependent treatment protocols involving neoadjuvant chemotherapy and preoperative radiotherapy relies on the ability of imaging to determine stage accurately before surgical and pathological staging. Once a diagnosis of cancer has been established, often by percutaneous or endoscopic biopsy, new imaging techniques can considerably improve the ability to define the extent of tumour, although the pathological specimen remains the 'gold standard'. Many staging systems are based on the tumour–node–metastasis (TNM) classification.

Tumour

In most published studies, cross-sectional imaging techniques (CT, ultrasound, MRI) are more accurate in staging advanced (T3, T4) than early (T1, T2) diseases, and the staging of early disease remains a challenge. In gut tumours, endoscopic ultrasound is more accurate than CT or MRI in the local staging of early disease (T1 and T2) by virtue of its ability to demonstrate the layered structure of the bowel wall and the depth of tumour

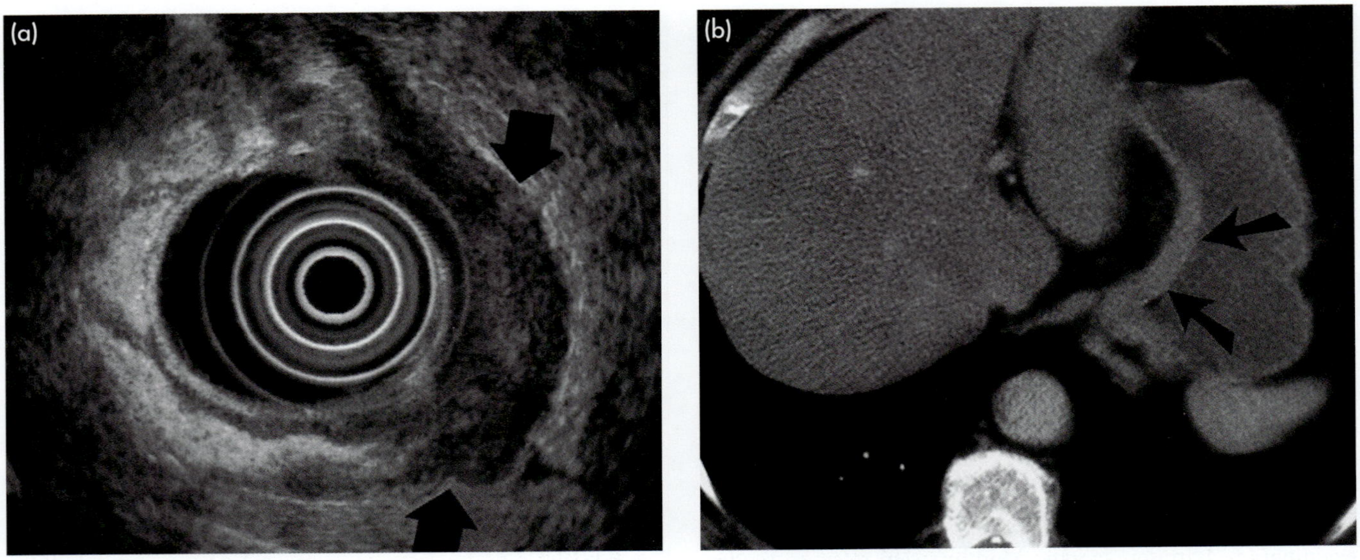

Figure 13.42 (a) Echo endoscopy in gastric cancer. The hypoechoic tumour (arrows) is destroying the layered structure of the gastric wall and extending out beyond the serosa. (b) Computed tomography scan demonstrates thickening and enhancement of the gastric wall in the same area (arrows). The stomach is distended with water to provide low-density contrast.

penetration (Figure 13.42). Developments in MRI may also improve the staging accuracy of early disease. MRI is extremely valuable in bone and soft-tissue tumour staging and in intracranial and spinal disease.

Nodes

Accurate assessment of nodal involvement remains a challenge for imaging. Most imaging techniques rely purely on size criteria to demonstrate lymph node involvement, with no possibility of identifying micrometastases in normal-sized nodes. A size criterion of 8–10 mm is often adopted, but it is not usually possible to distinguish benign reactive nodes from infiltrated nodes. This is a particular problem in patients with intrathoracic neoplasms, in whom enlarged benign reactive mediastinal nodes are common. The echo characteristics of nodes at endoscopic ultrasound have been used in many centres to increase the accuracy of nodal staging, and nodal sampling is possible via either mediastinoscopy or transoesophageal biopsy under endoscopic ultrasound control. New radioisotope techniques are being developed using radiolabelled monoclonal antibodies against tumour antigens, which may increase the detection of nodal involvement by demonstrating micrometastases in non-enlarged nodes. There are current clinical studies of new MRI contrast agents that may identify tumour-infiltrated nodes.

Metastases

The demonstration of metastatic disease will usually significantly affect surgical management. Modern cross-sectional imaging has greatly improved the detection of metastases, but occult lesions will be overlooked in between 10 and 30 per cent of patients. CT is the most sensitive technique for the detection of lung deposits, although the decision to perform CT will depend on the site of the primary tumour, its likelihood of intrapulmonary spread and the effect on staging and subsequent therapy of the demonstration of intrapulmonary deposits.

Ultrasound and CT are most frequently used to detect liver metastases. Contrast-enhanced CT can detect most lesions greater than 1 cm, although accuracy rates vary with the technique used and range from 70 to 90 per cent. Recent studies suggest that MRI may be more accurate than CT in demonstrating metastatic disease. Although enhanced CT is used in most centres for screening for liver deposits, CT-AP (CT with arterial portography), which requires contrast injection via the superior mesenteric artery, is considered by many to be the most accurate technique for staging liver metastases if surgical resection is being considered. However, thin-section multislice CT with arterial and portal venous phase scanning is likely to replace this. Preoperative identification of the segment of the liver involved can be determined by translation of the segmental surgical anatomy, as defined by Couinaud, to the cross-sectional CT images (Figure 13.43).

The technique of PET/CT is becoming a powerful tool in oncological imaging. This functional and anatomical imaging technique reflects tumour metabolism and allows the detection of otherwise occult metastases. The most common indications for PET/CT have been staging of lymphoma, lung cancer, particularly non-small cell lung cancer, and preoperative assessment of potentially resectable liver metastases such as colorectal carcinoma metastases.

Intraoperative ultrasound is an additional method of staging that provides superb high-resolution imaging of subcentimetre liver nodules that may not be palpable at surgery. This is often used immediately prior to resection of liver metastases.

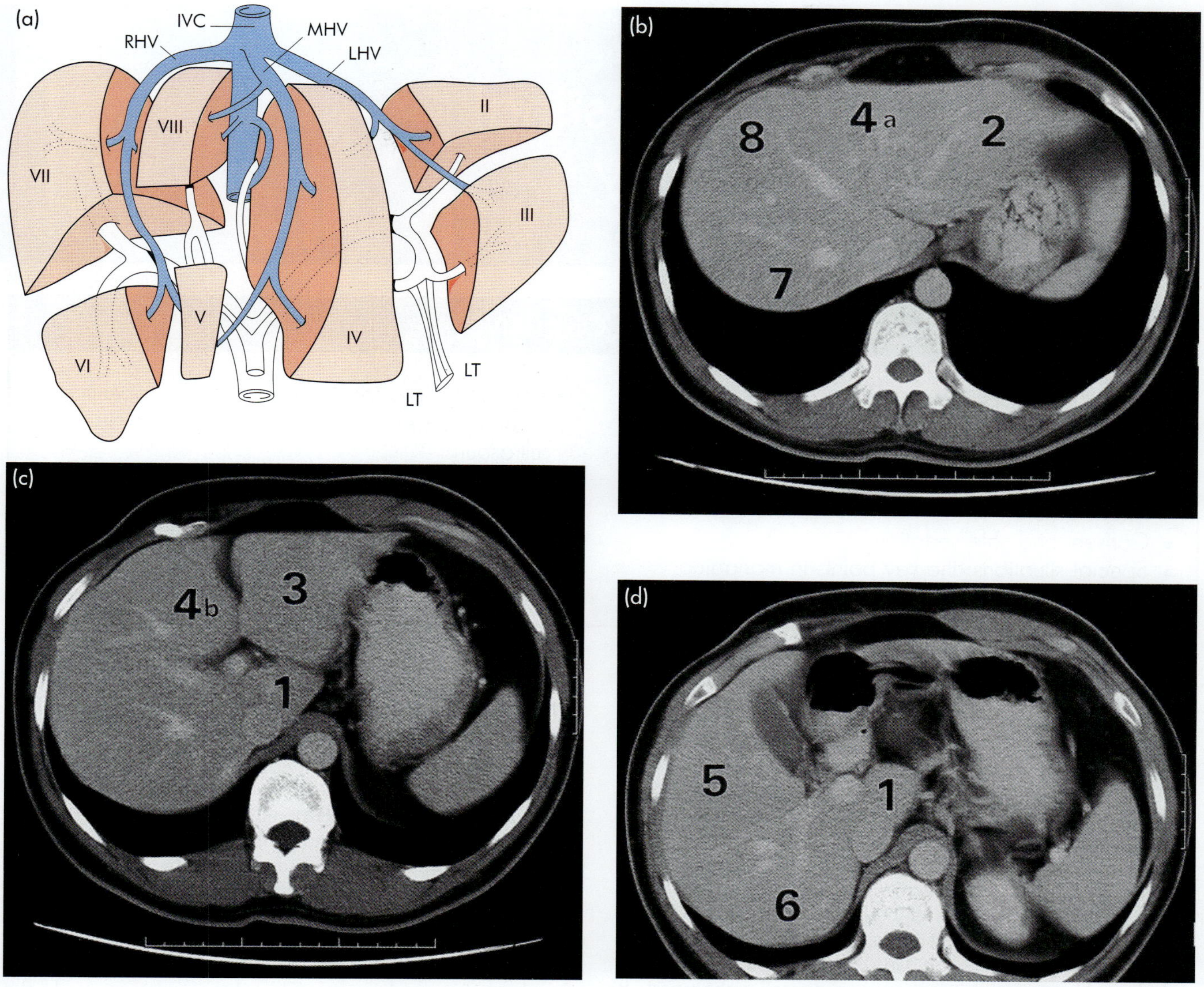

Figure 13.43 (a) Surgical lobes of the liver (after Couinaud). IVC, inferior vena cava; LHV, left hepatic vein; LT, ligamentum teres; MHV, middle hepatic vein; RHV, right hepatic vein. (b) Segmental anatomy on computed tomography scan at the level of the hepatic veins. (c) Segmental anatomy at the level of the portal veins. (d) Segmental anatomy below the level of the portal veins.

FURTHER READING

Adam A, Dixon AK (eds). *Grainger and Allison's diagnostic radiology: a textbook of medical imaging*, 5th edn. London: Churchill Livingstone, 2007.

Armstrong P, Wastie M (eds). *A concise textbook of radiology*. London: Arnold, 2001.

Grainger RG, Allison DJ, Dixon AK (eds). *Grainger and Allison's diagnostic radiology: a textbook of medical imaging*, 4th edn. London: Harcourt Publishers, 2001.

iRefer. *Making the best use of a department of clinical radiology: guidelines for doctors*, 6th edn. London: Royal College of Radiologists, 2012.

Krishnam MS, Curtis J (eds). *Emergency radiology*. New York: Cambridge Medicine, 2010.

Pope T, Bloem HL, Beltran J *et al. Imaging of the musculoskeletal system*. Oxford: Saunders, 2008.

Royal College of Radiologists. *Making the best use of a department of clinical radiology: guidelines for doctors*, 6th edn. London: Royal College of Radiologists, 2007.

Shuman WP. CT of blunt abdominal trauma in adults. *Radiology* 1997; **205**: 297–306.

CHAPTER 14

Gastrointestinal endoscopy

LEARNING OBJECTIVES

To gain an understanding of:

- The role of endoscopy as a diagnostic and therapeutic tool
- The basic organisation of an endoscopy unit and its equipment
- Consent and safe sedation
- Special situations: the key points in managing endoscopy in high-risk patients
- The indications for diagnostic and therapeutic endoscopic procedures including endoscopic ultrasound
- The recognition and management of complications
- Novel techniques for endoscoping the small bowel
- Advances in diagnostic ability

INTRODUCTION

The gastrointestinal tract has a myriad of functions, such as digestion, absorption and excretion, as well as the synthesis of an array of hormones, growth factors and cytokines. In addition, a complex enteric nervous system has evolved to control its function and communicate with the central and peripheral nervous systems. Finally, as the gastrointestinal tract contains the largest sources of foreign antigens to which the body is exposed, it houses well-developed arms of both the innate and acquired immune system. Therefore, it is not surprising that malfunction or infection of this complex organ results in a wide spectrum of pathology. However, its importance in disease pathogenesis is matched only by its inaccessibility to traditional examination.

Few discoveries in medicine have contributed more to the practice of gastroenterology than the development of diagnostic and therapeutic endoscopy. Although spectacular advances in radiology have occurred recently with the introduction of multislice spiral computed tomography (CT) and magnetic resonance imaging (MRI), the ability to take targeted mucosal biopsies remains a unique strength of endoscopy. Historically, radiological techniques were required to image areas of jejunum and ileum inaccessible to the standard endoscope; however, the introduction of both capsule endoscopy and single/double-balloon enteroscopy allows both diagnostic and therapeutic access to the entire gastrointestinal tract. Image enhancement with techniques such as chromoendoscopy, magnification endoscopy and narrow band imaging allow increased resolution at the mucosal level and increase diagnostic yield. Endoscopic ultrasound can examine all layers of the intestinal wall as well as extraintestinal structures. Finally, experimental techniques such as confocal laser endomicroscopy give resolution at a level compatible with standard histology. The advances in the diagnostic accuracy of endoscopy lend themselves to disease surveillance for specific patient groups as well as population screening for gastrointestinal malignancy. Likewise, there has been a rapid expansion in the therapeutic capability of endoscopy with both luminal and extraintestinal surgery being performed via endoscopic access.

As in all areas of interventional practice, competent endoscopists must match a thorough grounding in anatomy and physiology with a clear understanding of the capabilities and limitations of the rapidly advancing techniques available. Perhaps most importantly they must appreciate all aspects of patient care including pre-procedural management, communication before and during the procedure and the management of endoscopic complications. This chapter aims to guide the reader through these areas in addition to providing an introduction to the breadth of procedures that are currently performed.

HISTORY OF ENDOSCOPY

Over the last 50 years, endoscopy has become a most powerful diagnostic and therapeutic tool. However, its development required two obvious but formidable barriers to be overcome. First, the gastrointestinal tract is rather long and tortuous and, second, no natural light shines through the available orifices! Therefore, successful visualisation of anything beyond the distal extremities requires a flexible instrument with an intrinsic light source that can transmit images to the operator. The illumination issue was solved in 1879 by Thomas Edison, but 25 years

Thomas Alva Edison, 1847–1931, American physicist and inventor of Menlo Park, NJ, USA, produced the first carbon filament electric light bulb in 1879. His major innovation was the first industrial research laboratory called Menlo Park (1876–1881) and therefore he was called 'The Genius of Menlo Park'. He held the world record of 1093 patents for invention. He was such a poor student that a schoolmaster called him 'addled'. At this, his mother was so furious that she took him out of school and taught him at home.

elapsed before a light source was incorporated into the primitive rigid endoscopes available at that time. The first approach to gastrointestinal tortuosity was an instrument with articulated lenses and prisms, proposed by Hoffmann in 1911. Again, approximately two decades elapsed before this concept was incorporated into a semiflexible gastroscope by Wolf, a fabricator of medical instruments, and Schindler, a physician.

The real breakthrough was the discovery that images could be transmitted using flexible quartz fibres. Although this was first described in the late 1920s, it was not until 1954 that Hopkins built a model of a flexible fibre imaging device. The availability of highly transparent optical quality glass led to the development in 1958 of the first flexible fibreoptic gastroscope by Larry Curtiss, a graduate student in physics, and Basil Hirschowitz, a trainee in gastroenterology. Over the next 30 years, the fibrescope evolved to allow examination of the upper gastrointestinal tract, the biliary system and the colon. In parallel with advances in diagnostic ability, a range of therapeutic procedures was developed (Table 14.1). Although the fibreoptic endoscope has been the workhorse of many endoscopy units over the last three decades, its obsolescence was guaranteed by the invention of the charge coupled device (CCD) in the 1960s, which allowed the creation of a digital electronic image, permitting endoscopic images to be processed by a computer and transmitted to television screens. Thus the modern endoscope was born (Figure 14.1).

History does not sit still, and endoscopic evolution will continue with the replacement of much diagnostic endoscopy with capsule endoscopy and virtual imaging. Enhanced resolution using chromoendoscopy, and even histological grade images, have increased the diagnostic yield of surveillance procedures. Endoscopic ultrasound allows diagnosis and therapy to extend beyond the mucosal surface of the intestine. Traditional endoscopy will therefore become increasingly therapeutic and historical divisions between medicine, radiology and surgery will become progressively blurred. As the complexity of the procedures increases, the distinction between specialist and general endoscopists will become more definite. This reinforces the need for all endoscopic practitioners to have a detailed understanding of the units in which they work and the instruments that they use.

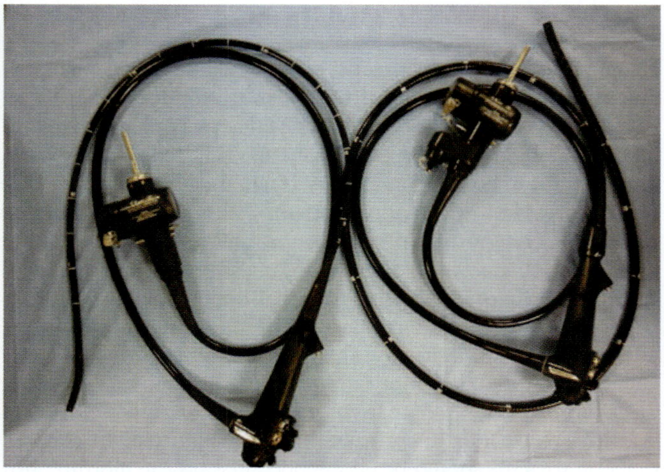

Figure 14.1 Photograph of standard gastroscope and colonoscope.

Table 14.1 Historical landmarks of gastrointestinal endoscopy.

1958	Development of fibreoptic gastroscope
1968	Endoscopic retrograde pancreatography
1969	Colonoscopic polypectomy
1970	Endoscopic retrograde cholangiography
1974	Endoscopic sphincterotomy (with bile duct stone extraction)
1979	Percutaneous endoscopic gastrostomy
1980	Endoscopic injection sclerotherapy
1980	Endoscopic ultrasonography
1983	Electronic (charge coupled device) endoscope
1985	Endoscopic control of upper gastrointestinal bleeding
1990	Endoscopic variceal ligation
1996	Introduction of self-expanding metal stents
2008	Endomicroscopy delivers histological mucosal definition

THE MODERN ENDOSCOPY UNIT

Organisation

A well-designed endoscopy unit staffed by trained endoscopy nurses and dedicated administrative staff is essential to support good endoscopic practice and training. Clinical governance with regular appraisal and assessment of performance should be a routine process embedded within the unit philosophy. Endoscopist training demands particular attention, with a transparent process of skills- and theory-based education centred on practical experience and dedicated training courses. Experienced supervision of all trainee endoscopists is essential until competency has been obtained and assessed by an appropriately validated technique such as direct observation of practical skills (DOPS) and review of procedure logbooks. However, all endoscopists should keep an ongoing log to record diagnostic and therapeutic procedure numbers and markers of competency such as colonoscopy completion rates, polyp detection rates, mean sedation use and complication rates. Central to this is an efficient data management system that provides outcome analysis for all aspects of endoscopy including adherence to guidelines, near misses, patient satisfaction, decontamination processes and scope tracking, as well as the more obvious completion and complication rates.

Equipment

A full description of all available endoscopic equipment is beyond the scope of this chapter. However, each unit should have a sufficient range of endoscopes, processors and accessories as dictated by the local case mix and sufficient endoscope numbers to ensure smooth service provision. These should include both forward- and lateral-viewing gastroscopes, an enteroscope for proximal small bowel visualisation and a range of adult and paediatric colonoscopes to aid examination of both redundant and fixed colons. Dedicated small bowel centres require capsule endoscopy and a single/double-balloon enteroscope for ileojejunal visualisation and therapeutics. Larger centres will require linear and radial endoscopic ultrasound, particularly if they specialise in gastrointestinal and hepatobiliary malignancy. An electrosurgical unit is the cornerstone of many therapeutic procedures and this may be supplemented by an argon plasma

Harold Horace Hopkins, 1918–1994, Professor of Applied Optics, The University of Reading, Reading, UK.
Basil I Hirschowitz, Professor of Medicine, Birmingham, AL, USA.

coagulation unit and laser units for advanced therapeutics in specialised centres.

Instrument decontamination

Endoscopes will not withstand steam-based autoclaving and therefore require high-level disinfection between cases to prevent transmission of infection. Although accessories may be autoclaved, best practice requires the use of disposable single use items whenever possible. All equipment should be decontaminated to an identical standard whether for use on immunocompromised/infected patients or not. This process involves two equally important stages: first, removal of physical debris from the internal and external surfaces of the instrument and, second, chemical neutralisation of all microbiological agents. A variety of agents are available and endoscopists should familiarise themselves with the agent in use in their department. The British Society of Gastroenterology has developed guidelines for decontamination of endoscopes (www.bsg.org.uk/images/stories/docs/clinical/guidelines/endoscopy/decontamination_2008.pdf). Key points in endoscope decontamination are shown in Summary box 14.1.

Summary box 14.1

Disinfection of endoscopes

- All channels must be brushed and irrigated throughout the disinfection process
- All instruments and accessories should be traceable to each use, patient and cleaning cycle
- All staff should be trained and protected (particularly if glutaraldehyde is used in view of its immune-sensitising properties)
- Regular monitoring of disinfectant power and microbiological contamination should be performed

There are currently no reliable means of decontaminating scopes from contact with prion-associated conditions such as new variant Creutzfeldt–Jakob disease (nvCJD). Endoscopy should be avoided in patients thought to be at risk of this condition, as instruments may require quarantine until the diagnosis can be excluded (which is often only possible post-mortem). In many countries, previously exposed endoscopes are available if a patient with suspected nvCJD requires endoscopy. Sheathed biopsy forceps are now being developed to allow samples to be taken from high-risk individuals without compromising the endoscope.

CONSENT IN ENDOSCOPY

Approximately 1 per cent of medical negligence claims in the USA relate to the practice of endoscopy. Many of these could have been avoided by a careful explanation of the procedure, including an honest discussion of the risks and benefits. Therefore, obtaining informed consent is a cornerstone of good endoscopic practice. It preserves a patient's autonomy, facilitates communication and acts as a shield against future complaints and claims of malpractice.

The most important aspect of the consent procedure is that a patient understands the nature, purpose and risk of a particular procedure. Current guidelines would suggest that a patient should be informed of minor adverse events with a risk of more than 10 per cent and serious events with an incidence of more than 0.5 per cent. The key risks of endoscopy are summarised in Summary box 14.2. The 2008 British Society of Gastroenterology guidelines for consent can be found using the link www.bsg.org.uk/images/stories/docs/clinical/guidelines/endoscopy/consent08.pdf

Summary box 14.2

The risks of endoscopy

- Sedation related cardiorespiratory complications
- Damage to dentition
- Aspiration
- Perforation or haemorrhage after endoscopic dilatation/therapeutic endoscopic ultrasound
- Perforation, infection and aspiration after percutaneous endoscopic gastrostomy insertion
- Perforation or haemorrhage after flexible sigmoidoscopy/colonoscopy with polypectomy
- Pancreatitis, cholangitis, perforation or bleeding after endoscopic retrograde cholangiopancreatography

SAFE SEDATION

If performed competently, the majority of diagnostic endoscopy and colonoscopy can be performed without sedation or with pharyngeal anaesthesia alone. However, therapeutic procedures may cause pain and patients are often anxious; thus in most countries sedation and analgesia are offered to achieve a state of conscious sedation (**not** anaesthesia). Medication-induced respiratory depression in elderly patients or those with comorbidities is the greatest cause of endoscopy-related mortality and, therefore, safe sedation practices are essential. The involvement of anaesthetists to advise on appropriate protocols is recommended (Summary box 14.3). Endoscopy in certain situations (particularly paediatric endoscopy) requires general anaesthetic – this should only be undertaken by appropriately trained staff with adequate equipment available.

ENDOSCOPY IN DIABETIC PATIENTS

As approximately 2 per cent of the population is diabetic, managing glycaemic control before and after endoscopy is an essential aspect of endoscopic practice. Factors influencing management include the type of diabetes, the procedure that is planned, the preparation/recovery time, and the history of diabetic control in the individual patient. Thus, a poorly controlled insulin-dependent diabetic undergoing colonoscopy will require more input than a type 2 diabetic on oral hypoglycaemic medication undergoing upper gastrointestinal endoscopy. All patients should bring their own medication to the unit and should be advised not to drive in case there is an alteration in their glycaemic control. The majority of patients can be managed using clear protocols on an outpatient basis; however, elderly patients and those with brittle control should be admitted. In general, diabetic patients should be endoscoped first on the morning list. In complex cases the diabetic team should be involved.

Hans Gerhard Creutzfeldt, 1885–1964, a neurologist, of Kiel, Germany.
Alfons Marie Jakob, 1884–1931, a neurologist of Hamburg, Germany.

Summary box 14.3

Sedation in endoscopy

- Pharyngeal anaesthesia may increase the risk of aspiration in sedated patients
- Comorbidities must be identified so that sedation can be individualised
- All sedated patients require secure intravenous access
- Benzodiazepines reach their maximum effect 15–20 min after administration – doses should be titrated carefully, particularly in the elderly or those with comorbidities
- Co-administration of opiates and benzodiazepines has a synergistic effect – opiates should be given first and doses need to be reduced
- The use of supplementary oxygen is essential in all sedated patients
- Sedated patients require pulse oximetry to monitor oxygen saturation; high-risk patients or those undergoing high-risk procedures also require blood pressure and electrocardiogram monitoring
- A trained assistant should be responsible for patient monitoring throughout the procedure
- Resuscitation equipment and sedation reversal agents must be readily available
- The use of anaesthetic agents such as propofol for complex procedures requires specialist training
- The half-life of benzodiazepines is 4–24 hours – appropriate recovery and monitoring is essential. Post-procedural consultations may not be remembered, and patients must be advised not to drink alcohol or drive for 24 hours

ANTIBIOTIC PROPHYLAXIS

The majority of endoscopy can be performed safely without the need for routine antibiotic prophylaxis. However, given that certain endoscopic procedures are associated with a significant bacteraemia (Table 14.2), there are several specific situations where antibiotic cover is required to prevent either bacterial endocarditis, infection of surgical prostheses or systemic sepsis. In general, the risk of infection relates to the level of bacteraemia and the risk of the underlying medical condition. Traditionally, patients with a previous history of endocarditis or a metallic heart valve received antibiotic prophylaxis for all endoscopic procedures, and many national guidelines still reflect this. However, UK guidelines have recently changed in response to the low reported incidence of infective endocarditis in this patient group undergoing endoscopy (www.bsg.org.uk/images/stories/docs/clinical/guidelines/endoscopy/prophylaxis_09.pdf). Patients with severe neutropenia may also require antibiotic prophylaxis for endoscopy. The antibiotic regime used will depend on local guidelines. Procedures such as endoscopic percutaneous gastrostomy are associated with a significant incidence of infection, particularly if inserted for malignancy. There is excellent evidence that antibiotic prophylaxis reduces this complication and a single intravenous injection of coamoxiclav should be administered before the procedure. Ciprofloxacin is routinely used during endoscopic manipulation of an obstructed biliary tree in which it is unlikely that complete drainage will be achieved or there is significant comorbidity. Finally, patients

Table 14.2 Approximate incidence of bacteraemia in immunocompetent individuals following various procedures involving the gastrointestinal tract.

Procedure	Incidence of bacteraemia (%)[a]
Rectal digital examination	4
Proctoscopy	5
Barium enema	11
Tooth brushing	25
Dental extraction	30–60
Colonoscopy	2–4
Diagnostic upper gastrointestinal endoscopy	4
Sigmoidoscopy	6–9
ERCP (no duct occlusion)	6
ERCP (duct occluded)	11
Oesophageal varices band ligation	6
Oesophageal varices sclerotherapy	10–50[b]
Oesophageal dilatation/prosthesis	34–54
Oesophageal laser therapy	35
EUS ± fine needle aspirate	0–6

[a]Summary of published data.
[b]Higher after emergency than after elective management.
ERCP, endoscopic retrograde cholangiopancreatography; EUS, endoscopic ultrasound.

with chronic liver disease and ascites undergoing variceal sclerotherapy should receive antibiotic prophylaxis to prevent bacterial peritonitis.

ANTICOAGULATION IN PATIENTS UNDERGOING ENDOSCOPY

Many patients undergoing endoscopy may be taking medication that interferes with normal haemostasis, such as warfarin, heparin, clopidogrel or aspirin. The key points to remember when managing anticoagulants in patients undergoing endoscopy are given in Summary box 14.4.

Summary box 14.4

Managing anticoagulants in patients undergoing endoscopy

It is important to recognise and understand:

- The risk of complications related to the underlying gastrointestinal disease from anticoagulant therapy
- The risk of haemorrhage related to an endoscopic procedure in the setting of anticoagulant therapy
- The risk of a thromboembolic/ischaemic event related to interruptions of anticoagulant therapy

Gastrointestinal bleeding in the anticoagulated patient

The risk of clinically significant gastrointestinal bleeding in patients on warfarin is increased, particularly in patients with a past history of similar events, if the international normalised ratio (INR) is above the therapeutic range or if they are taking concomitant aspirin/non-steroidal anti-inflammatory drugs (NSAIDs). In these situations the risk of reversing the anticoagulation must be weighed against the risk of ongoing haemorrhage. If complete reversal is not appropriate, correction of the INR to approximately 1.5 is usually sufficient to allow endoscopic diagnosis and therapy. Anticoagulation can be resumed 24 hours after successful endoscopic therapy. If rapid resumption of anticoagulation is required, intravenous heparin should be used.

Elective endoscopy in the anticoagulated patient

Endoscopic procedures vary in their potential to produce significant or uncontrolled bleeding. Diagnostic oesophagogastroduodenoscopy (OGD), colonoscopy, enteroscopy and endoscopic retrograde cholangiopancreatography (ERCP) without sphincterotomy are considered low risk, as is mucosal biopsy. High-risk procedures include colonoscopic polypectomy (1–2.5 per cent), gastric polypectomy (4 per cent), laser ablation of tumour (6 per cent), endoscopic sphincterotomy (2.5–5 per cent) and procedures with the potential to produce bleeding that is inaccessible or uncontrollable by endoscopic means, such as dilatation of benign or malignant strictures, percutaneous gastrostomy insertion and endoscopic ultrasound (EUS)-guided fine-needle aspiration. Likewise, the probability of a thromboembolic complication during temporary cessation of anticoagulant therapy depends on the underlying medical condition (see Table 14.3 and Summary box 14.5).

Table 14.3 The risk of a thromboembolic event varies according to the underlying medical condition.

Condition	Risk
Atrial fibrillation with valvular heart disease	High
Mechanical mitral valve	High
Mechanical valve and previous thromboembolic event	High
Deep vein thrombosis	Low
Uncomplicated atrial fibrillation	Low
Bioprosthetic valve	Low
Mechanical aortic valve	Low

Aspirin, non-steroidal anti-inflammatory drugs and anti-platelet therapies

Aspirin and NSAIDs inhibit platelet cyclo-oxygenase resulting in suppression of thromboxane A2-induced platelet aggregation. Limited published data do not suggest an increased bleeding risk in patients taking standard doses and, therefore, there is no need to discontinue therapy before endoscopic procedures. Increasing evidence suggests an increased risk of bleeding after high-risk endoscopic procedures in patients taking clopidogrel and ticlodipine. However, there is also a high risk of acute myocardial infarction or death if clopidogrel is discontinued early after coronary stent insertion, which may extend to one year post-procedure. Therefore, clopidogrel should not be discontinued in this situation without discussion with a cardiologist. If clopidogrel therapy needs to be discontinued prior to an endoscopic procedure this should be limited to a maximum of 5 days as the risk of stent thrombosis increases after this interval.

Summary box 14.5

Recommendations concerning anticoagulant management

Low-risk procedures
- No adjustment to anticoagulation required
- Check INR 1 week before procedure
- Avoid elective procedures when anticoagulation is above the therapeutic range

High-risk procedure in a patient with a low-risk condition
- Discontinue warfarin 5 days before the procedure
- Check INR on day of procedure to ensure <1.5
- Restart warfarin 24 hours after procedure if uncomplicated and recheck INR in one week

High-risk procedure in a patient with a high-risk condition
- Discontinue warfarin 5 days before the procedure
- Start low molecular weight heparin 2 days after stopping warfarin
- Check INR on day of procedure to ensure <1.5
- Omit LMWH on day of procedure
- Warfarin may be resumed the night of the procedure
- LMWH should be continued until INR adequate
- The decision to administer intravenous heparin should be individualised

UPPER GASTROINTESTINAL ENDOSCOPY

OGD is the most commonly performed endoscopic procedure. Excellent visualisation of the oesophagus, gastro-oesophageal junction, stomach, duodenal bulb and second part of the duodenum can be obtained (Figure 14.2). Retroversion of the gastroscope in the stomach is essential to obtain complete views of the gastric cardia and fundus (Figure 14.2). Traditional forward-viewing endoscopes do not adequately visualise the ampulla, and a side-viewing scope should be used if this is essential. Likewise, although it is possible to reach the third part of the duodenum with a standard 120-cm instrument, a longer enteroscope is required if views beyond the ligament of Treitz are required. In addition to clear mucosal views, diagnostic endoscopy allows mucosal biopsies to be taken, which may either undergo processing for histological examination or be used for near-patient detection of *Helicobacter pylori* infection using a commercial urease-based kit. In addition, brushings may be taken for cytology and aspirates for microbiological culture.

Indications for oesophagogastroduodenoscopy

A full assessment of the role of OGD is outside the scope of this chapter. It will vary with local circumstances and the availability of alternative diagnostic techniques. OGD is usually appropriate when a patient's symptoms are persistent despite appropriate empirical therapy or are associated with warning signs such as intractable vomiting, anaemia, weight loss, dysphagia or bleeding. It is also part of the diagnostic work-up for patients with anaemia, symptoms of malabsorption and chronic diarrhoea. However, increasing ease of access to OGD with the availability of 'open access' endoscopy has resulted in a significant number of unnecessary procedures being performed in young patients with

Wenzel Treitz, 1819–1872, Professor of Pathology, Prague, The Czech Republic.

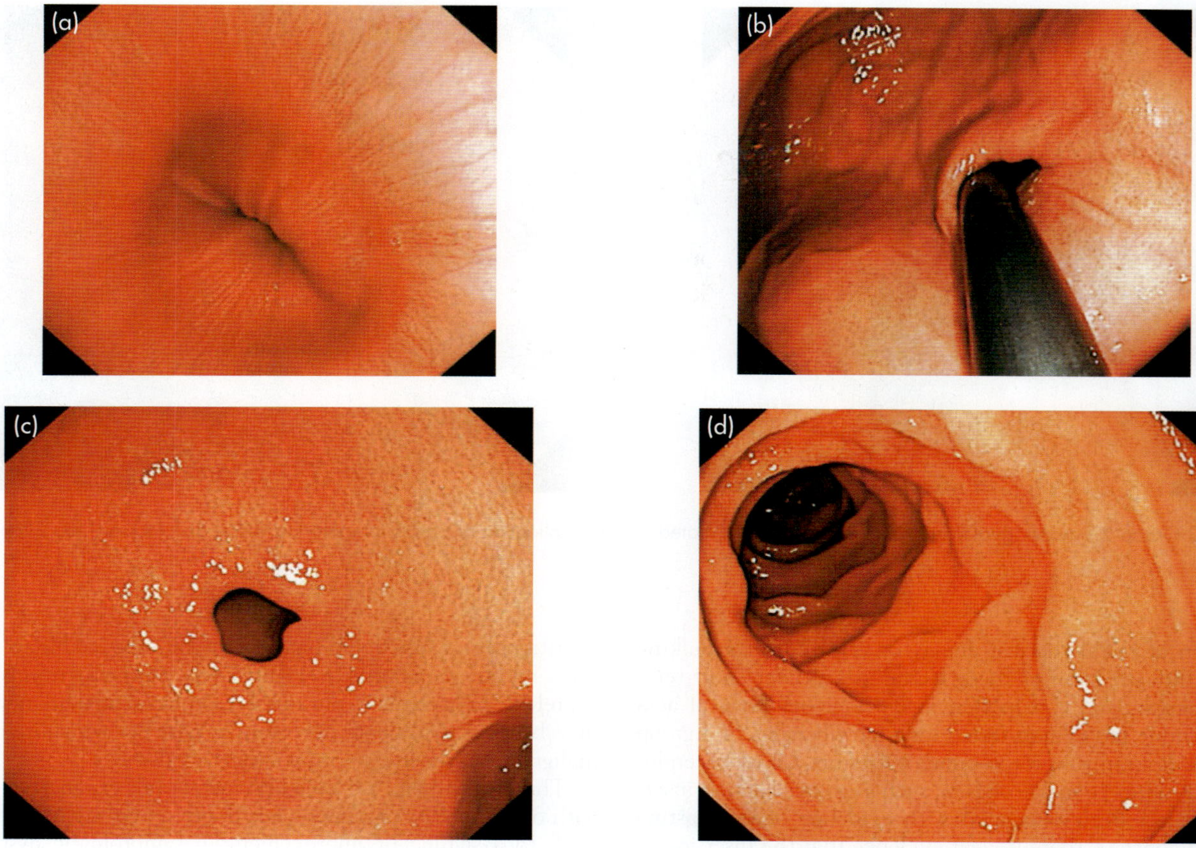

Figure 14.2 A normal upper gastrointestinal endoscopy showing the gastro-oesophageal junction (a), the gastric fundus in the 'J' position (b), the gastric antrum (c) and the second part of the duodenum (d).

dyspepsia or gastro-oesophageal reflux disease (GORD). This has led to a number of international gastroenterology societies proposing guidelines for the management of dyspepsia/GORD, including the empirical use of acid suppression and non-invasive *H. pylori* tests, such as urease breath tests and serology (e.g. the National Institute for Health and Clinical Excellence guidelines on dyspepsia: www.nice.org.uk/CG017NICEguideline). In addition to the role of OGD in diagnosis, it is also commonly used in the surveillance of neoplasia development in high-risk patient groups. Whereas there is consensus about its role in genetic conditions such as familial adenomatous polyposis and Peutz–Jeghers syndrome, controversy remains about the role and frequency of endoscopic surveillance in premalignant conditions such as Barrett's oesophagus and gastric intestinal metaplasia.

Therapeutic oesophagogastroduodenoscopy

Increasing technological advances have revolutionised the therapeutic applications of upper gastrointestinal endoscopy. However, appropriate patient selection and monitoring is essential to minimise complications. The most common therapeutic endoscopic procedure performed as an emergency is the control of upper gastrointestinal haemorrhage of any aetiology. Band ligation has replaced sclerotherapy in the management of oesophageal varices (Figure 14.3), whereas sclerotherapy using thrombin-based glues can be used to control blood loss from gastric varices. Injection sclerotherapy with adrenaline coupled with a second haemostatic technique, such as heater probe vessel obliteration or haemoclip application, remains the technique of choice for a peptic ulcer with an active arterial spurt or stigmata of recent haemorrhage (Figure 14.4). This should be followed by 72 hours of intravenous proton pump inhibition in all cases. Chronic blood loss from angioectasia is most safely treated with argon plasma coagulation because of the controlled depth of burn compared with alternative thermal techniques (Figure 14.5).

Benign oesophageal and pyloric strictures may be dilated under direct vision with 'through the scope' (TTS) balloon dilators or the more traditional guidewire-based systems such as Savary–Guillard bougie dilators (Figure 14.6). Intractable disease can be treated by the insertion of a removable stent. Likewise, the lower oesophageal sphincter hypertension associated with achalasia can be reduced by pneumatic balloon dilatation, although the procedure may need to be repeated every few years and the large (2–3 cm) balloons required are associated with a significantly increased risk of perforation. An alternative is the injection of botulinum toxin, which has a considerably more favourable side-effect profile but a shorter duration of benefit.

There are an increasing number of endoscopic techniques available to reduce gastro-oesophageal reflux that rely on tightening the loose gastro-oesophageal junction by plication, the

John Law Augustine Peutz, 1886–1968, Chief Specialist for Internal Medicine, St. John's Hospital, The Hague, The Netherlands.
Harold Joseph Jeghers, 1904–1990, Professor of Internal Medicine, New Jersey College of Medicine and Dentistry, Jersey City, NJ, USA.
Norman Rupert Barrett, 1903–1979, surgeon, St. Thomas's Hospital, London, UK.

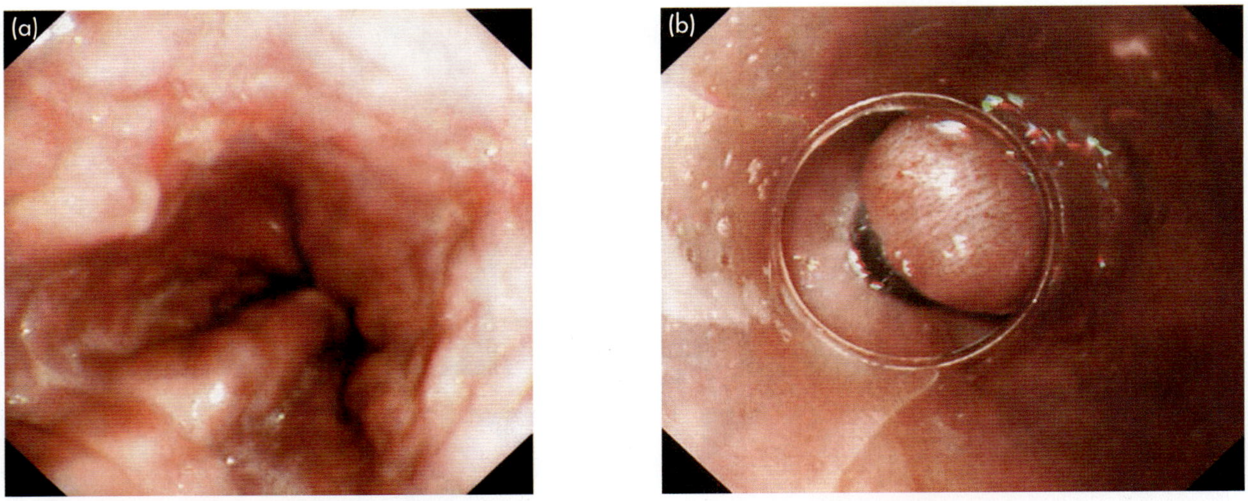

Figure 14.3 Grade 2 oesophageal varices (a), which can be treated by the application of bands to ligate the vessel and reduce blood flow (b).

application of radial thermal energy or injection of a bulking agent. Although many of these techniques deliver short-term clinical benefits and a reduction in 24-hour oesophageal acid exposure, none has demonstrated long-term benefits in a group of patients resistant to proton pump inhibitors. Likewise, endoscopic techniques to tackle obesity, such as gastric balloon insertion, have not been associated with evidence of long-lasting benefit. In contrast, there is clear evidence that the insertion of a percutaneous endoscopic gastrostomy (PEG) tube enhances nutritional and functional outcome in patients unable to maintain oral nutritional intake (Figure 14.7). PEG insertion is often a prelude to treatment of complex orofacial malignancy, and may be used to support nutrition in patients with alternative malignant, degenerative or inflammatory diseases.

The deployment of 'memory metal' self-expanding stents with or without a covering sheath inserted over a stiff guidewire leads to a significant improvement in symptomatic dysphagia and quality of life in patients with malignant oesophageal and

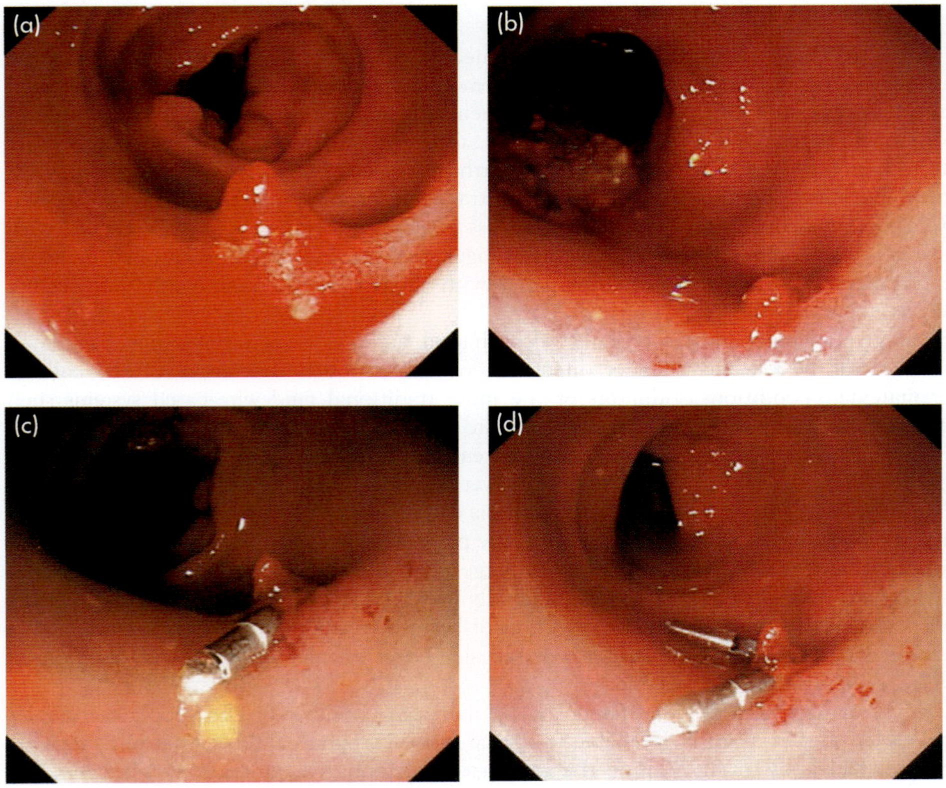

Figure 14.4 A gastric ulcer with active bleeding (a) is initially treated with adrenaline injection to achieve haemostasis (b). Two haemoclips are then applied to prevent re-bleeding (c and d).

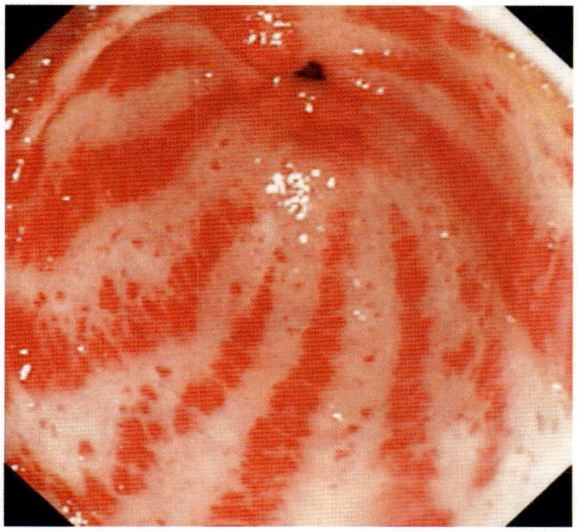

Figure 14.5 The classic appearance of gastric antral vascular ectasia (GAVE), which is often treated with argon plasma coagulation.

gastric outlet obstruction (Figure 14.8). Covered stents are the mainstay of treatment for benign or malignant tracheo-oesophageal fistulae. However, the area of greatest progress over the last few years has been in the endoscopic management of early oesophageal and gastric neoplasia with endoscopic mucosal resection (EMR) and the destruction of areas of high-grade dysplasia (HGD) using either EMR (Figure 14.9) or photodynamic therapy. However, long-term follow-up studies are required to ensure that the endoscopic ablation of areas of HGD has an impact on the progression to cancer.

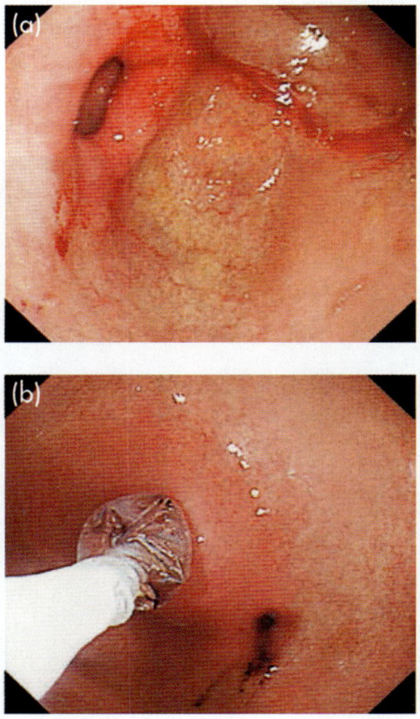

Figure 14.6 A pyloric stricture (a) can be dilated using a 'through the scope' balloon under direct vision to minimise complications (b).

Complications of diagnostic and therapeutic oesophagogastroduodenoscopy

Diagnostic upper gastrointestinal endoscopy is a safe procedure with minimal morbidity as long as appropriate patient selection and safe sedation practices are embedded in the unit policy. The mortality rate is estimated to be less than 1:10 000, with a complication rate of approximately 1:1000. As mentioned above, the majority of adverse events relate to sedation and patient comorbidity. Particular caution should be exercised in patients with recent unstable cardiac ischaemia and respiratory compromise. Perforation can occur at any point in the upper gastrointestinal tract, including the oropharynx. It is rare during diagnostic procedures and is often associated with inexperience. Perforation is more common in therapeutic endoscopy, particularly oesophageal dilatation and EMR for early malignancy. Early diagnosis significantly improves outcome and thus all staff must be alert to the symptoms (Summary box 14.6).

Summary box 14.6

Symptoms of endoscopic oesophageal perforation

- Neck/chest pain
- Dysphagia/drooling saliva
- Abdominal pain
- Increasing tachycardia
- Hypotension
- Surgical emphysema

Prompt management includes radiological assessment using CT/water-soluble contrast studies, strict nil by mouth, intravenous fluids and antibiotics, and early review by an experienced upper gastrointestinal surgeon.

ENDOSCOPIC ASSESSMENT OF THE SMALL BOWEL

Introduction and indications

The requirement to visualise, biopsy and treat the small bowel is far less than in the stomach, biliary tree or colon, resulting in a time lag in technological advances. The most frequent indication is the investigation of gastrointestinal blood loss, which may present with either recurrent iron deficiency anaemia (occult haemorrhage) or recurrent overt blood loss per rectum (cryptic haemorrhage) in a patient with normal OGD (with duodenal biopsies) and colonoscopy. Other indications include the investigation of malabsorption; the exclusion of cryptic small bowel inflammation such as Crohn's disease in patients with diarrhoea/abdominal pain and evidence of an inflammatory response; targeting lesions seen on radiological investigations; and surveillance for neoplasia in patients with inherited polyposis syndromes.

A standard enteroscope is able to reach and biopsy lesions detected in the proximal small bowel; however, even in the most experienced hands this is limited to approximately 100 cm distal to the pylorus, although the use of a stiffening overtube

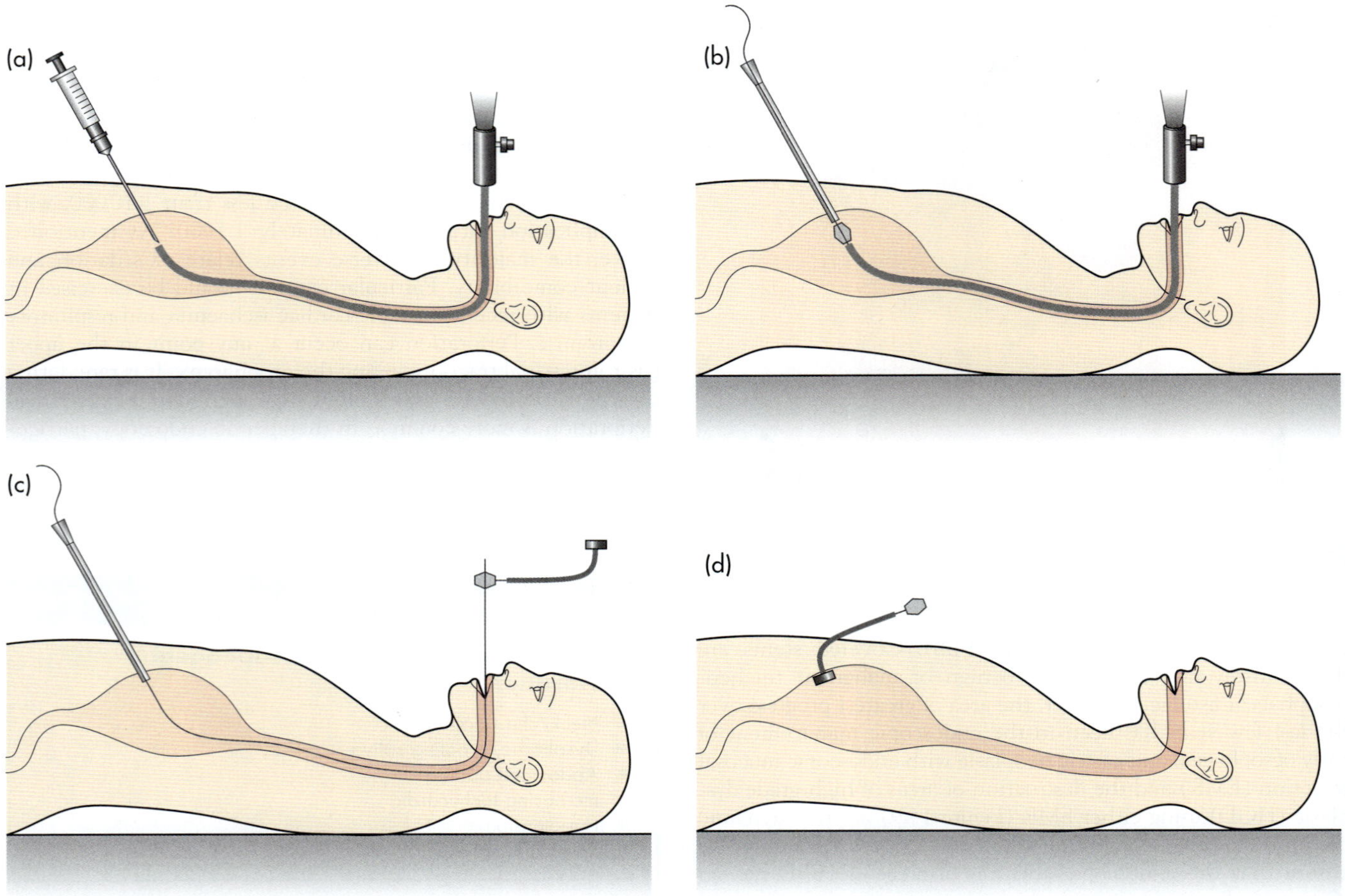

Figure 14.7 A schematic diagram of percutaneous endoscopic gastrostomy insertion. A standard endoscopy is performed to ensure that there are no contraindications to gastrostomy insertion. The stomach is insufflated with air and a direct percutaneous needle puncture made at a point where the stomach abuts the abdominal wall. Lignocaine is infused on withdrawal (a). A trochar is inserted and a wire passed into the stomach, which can be caught with a snare (b). The scope is withdrawn, pulling the wire out through the mouth, at which point it is attached to the gastrostomy tube (c). The gastrostomy is pulled through into the stomach and out through the track created by the trochar insertion (d).

may increase this somewhat. The procedure takes approximately 45 minutes and may be uncomfortable, requiring high doses of sedation with the attendant increased risk of perforation and sedation-related morbidity. Sonde endoscopy, in theory, has the potential to examine the entire small bowel. In this procedure a long thin endoscope is inserted transnasally into the stomach and pushed through the pylorus with a gastroscope passed through the mouth. It is carried distally by peristalsis, which propels a balloon inflated at the tip. The technique has several limitations including a long examination time (6–8 hours), patient discomfort, the danger of perforation and the inability to perform therapeutic procedures. For these reasons it is not widely performed and will soon become obsolete.

Therefore, until recently, barium follow-through or enteroclysis were the most effective imaging modalities to visualise the distal duodenum, jejunum and ileum. Obviously these techniques do not give true mucosal views, and outside specialist centres their decreasing use has led to diminished expertise and a reduced diagnostic yield. There have been rapid advances in axial radiological techniques such as MRI and CT enteroclysis, which demonstrate excellent diagnostic accuracy in this area

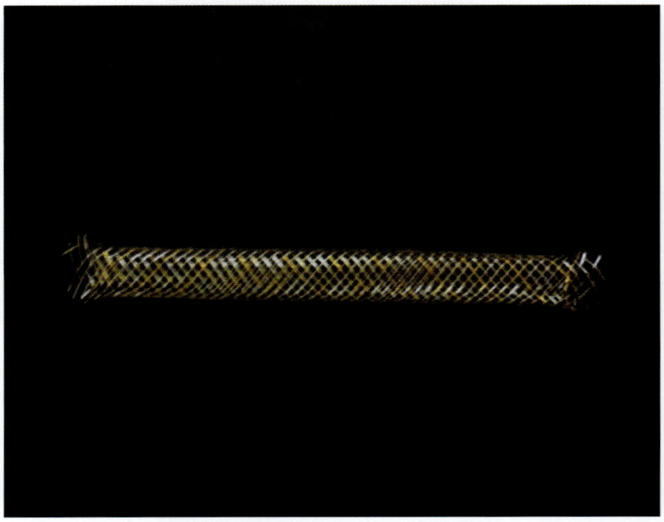

Figure 14.8 A self-expanding metal stent may be used to alleviate symptoms relating to malignant oesophageal strictures.

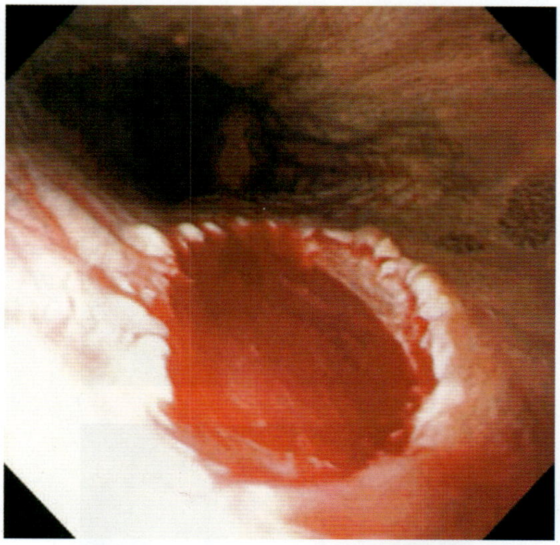

Figure 14.9 Novel upper gastrointestinal therapeutic uses of oesophagogastroduodenoscopy include the use of endoscopic mucosal resection to remove early gastric cancer leaving a clean base.

(see Chapter 13). However, although these techniques may yield information about vascularity and bowel wall thickening, they do not allow direct mucosal views, have no biopsy capability and have limited scope in terms of therapeutics. Until recently, if an area of interest was outside the reach of a standard enteroscope, direct access via enterotomy under either laparoscopic or open surgery was required. Two major clinical advances over the last 2–3 years have revolutionised small bowel diagnosis and therapeutics. First, the development of the capsule endoscope allows diagnostic mucosal views of the entire small bowel to be obtained with minimal discomfort in unsedated patients. Second, the novel technique of single/double-balloon enteroscopy allows endoscopic access to the entire small bowel for biopsy and therapeutics (Table 14.4).

Capsule endoscopy

The prototype capsule endoscope was developed at the Royal London Hospital in the UK by Professor Paul Swain. Several companies have developed different systems for routine clinical use, but the basic principles remain identical. The technique requires three main components: an ingestible capsule, a portable data recorder and a workstation equipped with image-processing software. The capsule consists of an optical dome and lens, two light-emitting diodes, a processor, a battery, a transmitter and an antenna encased in a resistant coat the size of a large vitamin pill (Figure 14.10). It acquires video images during natural propulsion through the digestive system that it transmits via a digital radiofrequency communication channel to the recorder unit worn outside the body; this also contains sensors which allow basic localisation of the site of image capture within the abdomen. Upon completion of the examination, the physician transfers the accumulated data to the workstation for interpretation via a high-capacity digital link. The workstation is a modified personal computer required for off-line data storage, interpretation and analysis of the acquired images, and report generation.

The small bowel capsule provides good visualisation from mouth to colon with a high diagnostic yield. It compares favourably with the 'gold standard' techniques for the localisation of cryptic and occult gastrointestinal bleeding and the diagnosis of small bowel Crohn's disease. Use of the capsule endoscope is contraindicated in patients with known small bowel strictures in which it may impact, resulting in acute obstruction requiring retrieval at laparotomy or via laparoscopy. Severe gastroparesis and pseudo-obstruction are also relative contraindications to its use. Some units advocate a barium follow-through to exclude stricturing disease in all patients before capsule endoscopy. An alternative is to use a 'dummy' patency capsule that can be tracked via a hand-held device or conventional radiology as it passes through the intestine; it dissolves after 40 hours if it becomes impacted. Technology in this field is rapidly advancing with capsule systems designed to image the oesophagus and colon nearing the market. Prototype capsules that can be directed, take biopsies and deliver thermal therapy to angioectasia are in development.

Table 14.4 Comparison of the advantages and disadvantages of the currently available modalities to endoscope the small intestine.

Technique	Advantages	Disadvantages
Traditional enteroscopy	Simple technique with wide availability Full range of therapeutics available Performed under sedation	Some discomfort Can only access proximal small bowel
Capsule endoscopy	Able to visualise the entire small bowel Preferable for patients No sedation Painless	No biopsies Not controllable and no accurate localisation Variable transit Incomplete studies due to battery life Not suitable for patients with strictures Large capsule to swallow
Double/single-balloon enteroscopy	Able to visualise the entire small bowel Full range of therapeutics	Requires sedation/general anaesthesia Patient discomfort May take 3–4 hours; may require admission Specialist centres only Complications include perforation

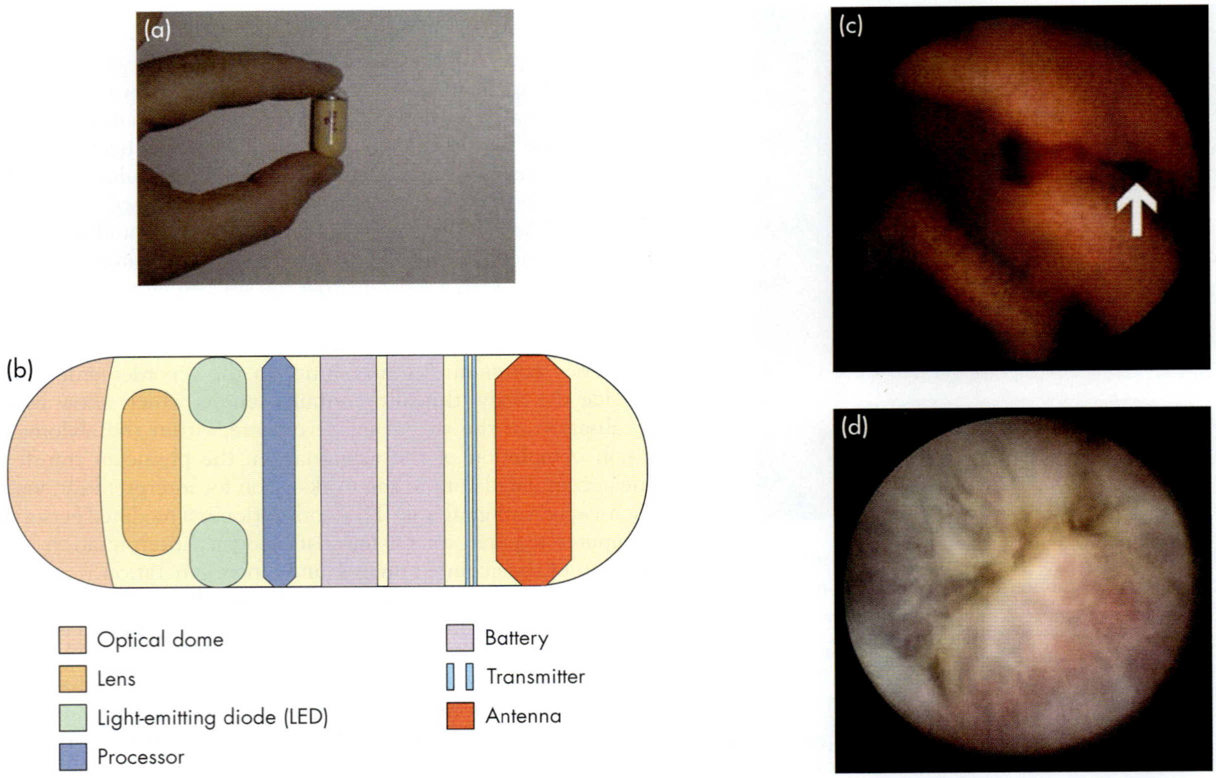

Figure 14.10 Complete diagnostic visualisation of the small bowel can be achieved with capsule endoscopy (a). The structure of the capsule is shown in (b). Clear mucosal pictures can be achieved here showing angioectasias (arrow) (c) and small bowel Crohn's disease (d).

Single/double-balloon enteroscopy

This technique allows the direct visualisation of and therapeutic intervention for the entire small bowel and may be attempted via either the oral or rectal route. Double-balloon enteroscopy was developed in 2001 in Japan; it involves the use of a thin enteroscope and an overtube, which are both fitted with a balloon. The procedure is usually carried out under general anaesthesia, but may be undertaken with the use of conscious sedation. The enteroscope and overtube are inserted through either the mouth or anus and steered to the proximal duodenum/terminal ileum in the conventional manner. Following this the endoscope is advanced a small distance in front of the overtube and the balloon at the end is inflated. Using the assistance of friction at the interface between the enteroscope and intestinal wall, the small bowel is accordioned back to the overtube. The overtube balloon is then deployed and the enteroscope balloon is deflated.

The process is then continued until the entire small bowel is visualised (Figure 14.11). In single-balloon enteroscopy, developed more recently, an enteroscope and overtube are used, but only the overtube has a balloon attached. A full range of therapeutics including diagnostic biopsy, polypectomy, argon

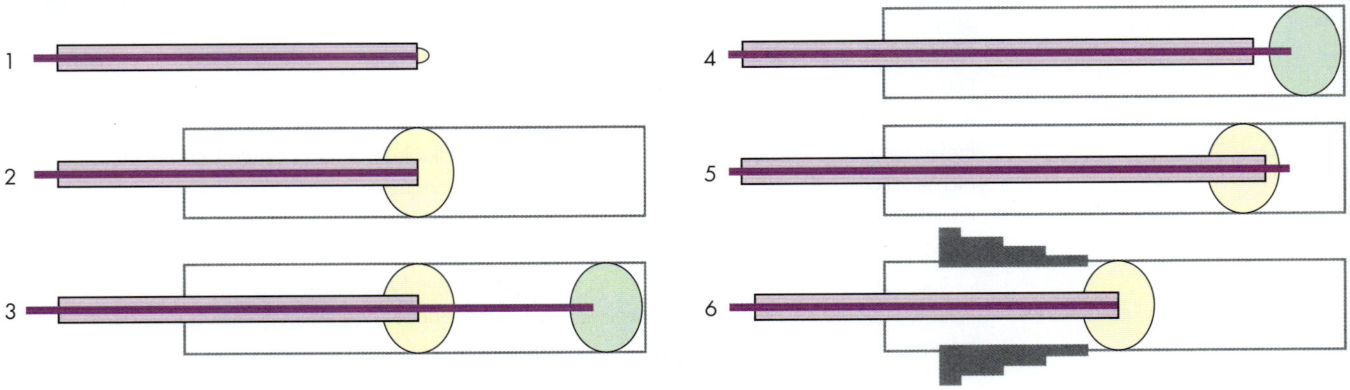

Figure 14.11 The technique of double-balloon enteroscopy is performed with an adapted enteroscope and overtube, both of which have inflatable balloons at their tip.

Christopher Paul Swain, contemporary, Professor of Gastroenterology, The Royal London Hospital, London, UK.

plasma coagulation and stent insertion are available for balloon enteroscopy. Some experts advocate routine capsule endoscopy before balloon enteroscopy in an attempt to localise any lesions and plan whether oral or rectal access is more appropriate. The indications for single/double-balloon endoscopy are given in Summary box 14.7.

Summary box 14.7

Current established indications for single/double-balloon endoscopy

- Bleeding from the gastrointestinal tract of obscure cause
- Iron deficiency anaemia with normal colonoscopy and gastroscopy
- Visualisation of and therapeutic intervention for abnormalities seen on traditional small bowel imaging/capsule endoscopy

ENDOSCOPIC RETROGRADE CHOLANGIOPANCREATOGRAPHY

This procedure involves the use of a side-viewing duodenoscope, which is passed through the pylorus and into the second part of the duodenum to visualise the papilla. This is then cannulated, either directly with a catheter or with the help of a guidewire (Figure 14.12). Occasionally, a small pre-cut is required to gain access. By altering the angle of approach one can selectively cannulate the pancreatic duct or biliary tree, which is then visualised under fluoroscopy after contrast injection. The significant range of complications associated with this procedure and improvements in radiological imaging using magnetic resonance cholangiopancreatography (MRCP) have rendered much diagnostic ERCP obsolete, and thus most procedures are currently performed for therapeutic purposes. There is still a role for accessing cytology/biopsy specimens.

Therapeutic endoscopic retrograde cholangiopancreatography

It is essential to ensure that patients have appropriate assessment prior to therapeutic ERCP, which is associated with a significant morbidity and occasional mortality. All patients require routine blood screening including a clotting screen. Assessment of respiratory and cardiovascular comorbidity is essential. Patients with an obstructed biliary system require antibiotic prophylaxis. The use of supplementary oxygen and both cardiac and oxygen saturation monitoring during the procedure are essential because of the high levels of sedation that are often required. The most common indication for therapeutic ERCP is the relief of biliary obstruction due to gallstone disease and benign or malignant biliary strictures. The pre-procedural diagnosis can be confirmed by contrast injection, which will clearly differentiate the filling defects associated with gallstones and the luminal narrowing of a stricture. If there is likely to be a delay in relieving an obstructed system, percutaneous drainage may be required.

The cornerstone of gallstone retrieval is an adequate biliary sphincterotomy, which is normally performed over a well-positioned guidewire using a sphincterotome connected to an electrosurgical unit. Most gallstones less than 1 cm in diameter will pass spontaneously in the days and weeks following a sphincterotomy, but most endoscopists prefer to ensure duct clearance at the initial procedure to reduce the risk of impaction, cholangitis or pancreatitis. This can be achieved by trawling the duct using a balloon catheter or by extraction using a wire basket. If standard techniques fail, large or awkwardly placed stones can be crushed using mechanical lithotripsy. If adequate stone extraction cannot be achieved at the initial ERCP it is imperative to ensure biliary drainage with the placement of a removable plastic stent while alternative options are considered. These include surgery, endoscopically directed shockwaves under direct choledochoscopic vision using a mother and baby scope, and extracorporeal shockwave lithotripsy with subsequent ERCP to remove stone fragments.

Dilation of benign biliary strictures uses balloon catheters similar to those used in angioplasty inserted over a guidewire under fluoroscopic control. It is traditional to insert a temporary plastic stent to maintain drainage as several attempts at dilatation may be required. Self-expanding metal stents are most commonly used for the palliation of malignant biliary obstruction and are also normally inserted after a modest sphincterotomy. Correct stent placement can normally be confirmed by a flow of bile after release and by the presence of air in the biliary tree on follow-up plain abdominal radiographs. Stent malfunction, associated with recurrent or persistent biochemical cholestasis, may be due to poor initial stent position, stent migration, blockage with blood clot or debris, or tumour in-growth. A repeat procedure is required to assess the cause, which can usually be remedied by the insertion of a second stent through the original one.

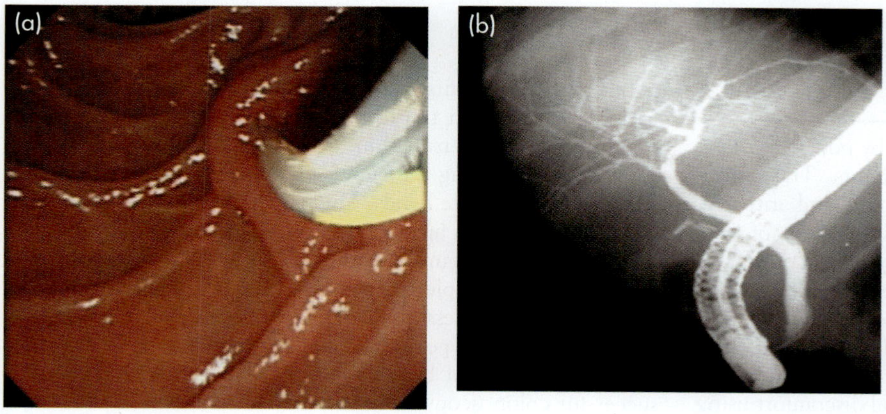

Figure 14.12 During endoscopic retrograde cholangiopancreatography a side-viewing duodenoscope is positioned opposite the papilla, which can then be cannulated using either a catheter or a guidewire (a). Contrast is injected to achieve a cholangiogram (b).

Ruggero Oddi, 1845–1906, physiologist, Perugia, who later worked in Rome, Italy.

In addition to the standard techniques discussed above, ERCP is also used for pancreatic disease and the assessment of biliary dysmotility (sphincter of Oddi dysfunction) using manometry in specialist centres. Indications include pancreatic stone extraction, the dilatation of pancreatic duct strictures and the transgastric drainage of pancreatic pseudocysts. To minimise the risks of subsequent pancreatitis, pancreatic sphincterotomy is most safely performed after the placement of a temporary pancreatic stent to prevent stasis within the pancreatic duct.

Complications associated with endoscopic retrograde cholangiopancreatography

The same risks associated with other endoscopic procedures also apply to patients undergoing ERCP, but risks may be increased because of the increased patient frailty and high sedation levels required. Complications specific to ERCP include duodenal perforation (1.3 per cent)/haemorrhage (1.4 per cent) after scope insertion or sphincterotomy, pancreatitis (4.3 per cent) and sepsis (3–30 per cent); the mortality rate approaches 1 per cent. It is important to remember that post-sphincterotomy complications may be retroperitoneal and, therefore, CT scanning is essential in patients with pain, tachycardia or hypotension post-procedure. Although normally mild, post-ERCP pancreatitis can be severe with extensive pancreatic necrosis and a significant mortality rate. Many trials have assessed pharmacological strategies to reduce the incidence of pancreatitis, particularly in high-risk patients (Table 14.5). There is some evidence for the use of periprocedural nitroglycerine or rectal NSAIDs after a high-risk procedure.

Table 14.5 Risk factors for post-ERCP pancreatitis.

Definite	Suspected SOD
	Young age
	Normal bilirubin
	Prior ERCP-related pancreatitis
	Difficult cannulation
	Pancreatic duct contrast injection
	Pancreatic sphincterotomy
	Balloon dilatation of biliary sphincter
Possible	Female sex
	Low volume of ERCPs performed
	Absent CBD stone

CBD, common bile duct; ERCP, endoscopic retrograde cholangiopancreatography; SOD, sphincter of Oddi dysfunction.

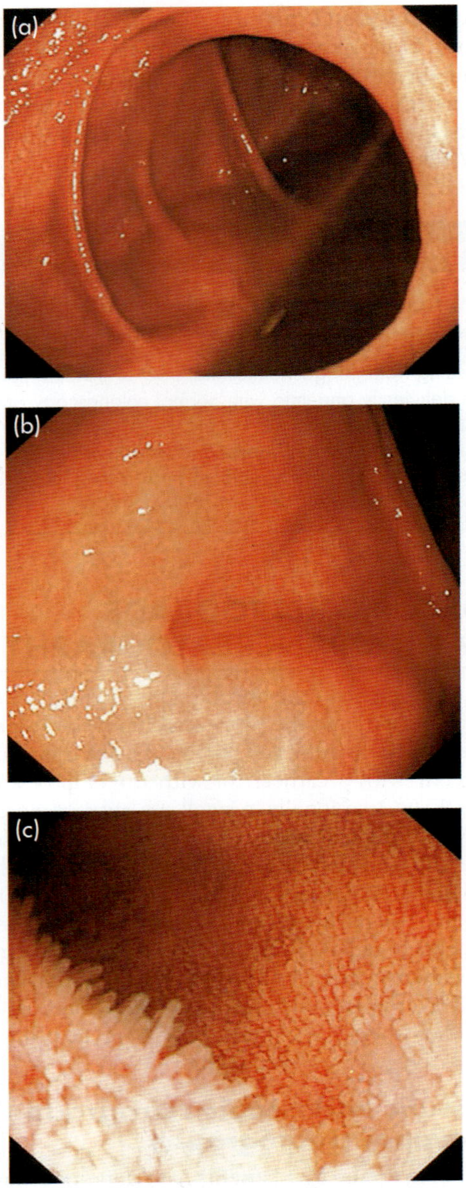

Figure 14.13 The caecal pole may not be easy to identify (a) and, therefore, the endoscopist should confirm complete colonoscopy by visualising the appendix orifice (b) or preferably intubating the terminal ileum (c), which demonstrates villi and Peyer's patches.

COLONOSCOPY

Early attempts at colonoscopy were hindered by poor technique and the limitations of the available instruments. The ability to steer an endoscope around the entire colon and into the terminal ileum was made possible by the development of fully flexible colonoscopes with greater than 90° angulation of the tip. Advances in bowel preparation have enhanced mucosal visualisation during the examination. Two key revelations about the practical performance of colonoscopy have allowed skilled operatives to achieve a greater than 95 per cent caecal intubation rate and frequent ileal intubation with minimal discomfort using light sedation. The first is that continued inward pressure of the endoscope results in the formation of loops within the mobile sigmoid and transverse colon, decreasing angulation control at the tip and removing the beneficial effect of shaft torque to aid steering around acute bends. The second is that pulling back the scope regularly with appropriate torque to ensure a straight passage through the sigmoid colon and around the splenic flexure greatly aids the completion of right-sided examination. Targeted abdominal hand pressure to prevent loops in a mobile colon and regular patient position change to enhance mucosal views and remove residual bowel content are also important aids to successful colonoscopy. It is essential that caecal intubation is confirmed to avoid missing pathology by incorrectly assuming that the caecal pole has been reached. The landmarks may not be clear and, therefore, visualisation of the appendix orifice or preferably terminal ileal intubation is necessary to confirm a complete colonoscopy (Figure 14.13).

Mucosal biopsies may either be targeted to areas of abnormality or random to exclude microscopic colitis in a patient with chronic diarrhoea but a macroscopically normal mucosa. Despite the increasing sophistication of radiological techniques to assess the colon, such as CT colonography, the ability to biopsy areas of abnormality and resect polyps will ensure that colonoscopy remains the most appropriate investigation for the majority of patients (Summary box 14.8). Several countries, including the USA and the UK, have recently introduced colorectal cancer (CRC) screening programmes in the asymptomatic population once they reach a predetermined age. The goal is to increase the number of early-stage CRCs detected and hence decrease mortality, as well as to identify and remove adenomatous polyps and prevent the onset of disease. There is ongoing debate about the relevant benefits of different screening modalities including colonoscopy, CT colonography, flexible sigmoidoscopy and biannual/one-off faecal occult blood testing with colonoscopy only in positive patients. Whichever modality is used, colonoscopy is essential to resect any polyps identified and biopsy unresectable lesions.

Summary box 14.8

Indications for colonoscopy

- Rectal bleeding with looser or more frequent stools ± abdominal pain related to bowel actions
- Iron deficiency anaemia (after biochemical confirmation ± negative coeliac serology): oesophagogastroduodenoscopy and colonoscopy together
- Right iliac fossa mass if ultrasound is suggestive of colonic origin
- Change in bowel habit associated with fever/elevated inflammatory response
- Chronic diarrhoea (>6 weeks) after sigmoidoscopy/rectal biopsy and negative coeliac serology
- Follow up of colorectal cancer and polyps
- Screening of patients with a family history of colorectal cancer
- Assessment/removal of a lesion seen on radiological examination
- Assessment of ulcerative colitis/Crohn's extent and activity
- Surveillance of inflammatory bowel disease
- Surveillance of acromegaly/ureterosigmoidostomy

Therapeutic colonoscopy

The most common therapeutic procedure performed at colonoscopy is the resection of colonic polyps (Figure 14.14). Retrieved specimens can be assessed for risk factors for neoplastic progression and an appropriate surveillance strategy determined (www.bsg.org.uk/images/stories/docs/clinical/guidelines/endoscopy/ccs_10.pdf). Small polyps up to 5 mm should be removed by cheese-wiring with a 'cold' snare. Hot biopsy is a technique in which the tip of a small pedunculated polyp is grasped between diathermy biopsy forceps and tented away from the bowel wall. A brief burst of monopolar current is used to coagulate the stalk, allowing the polyp to be removed. This is rarely performed in current practice due to an increased risk of immediate and delayed thermal damage to the bowel wall, particularly in the right colon. Larger polyps with a defined stalk can be resected using snare polypectomy with coagulating current either *en bloc* or piecemeal depending on their size (Figure 14.14). Post-polypectomy bleeding can be prevented by the application of haemoclips or an endoloop to the polyp stalk. Sessile polyps extending over several centimetres can be removed by endoscopic mucosal resection, which involves lifting the polyp away

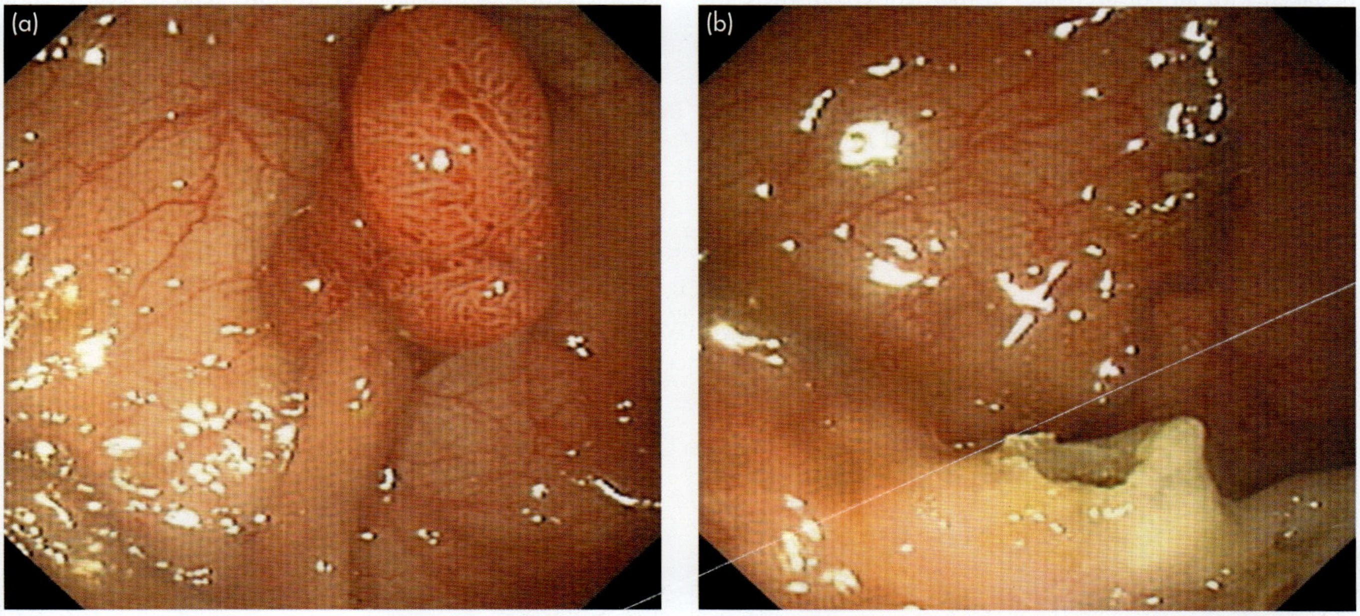

Figure 14.14 Colonoscopy is the most appropriate investigation to detect colonic polyps (a), which can be removed by snare polypectomy during the same procedure leaving a clean polyp base (b).

Johann Conrad Peyer, 1653–1712, Professor of Logic, Rhetoric and Medicine, Schaffhausen, Switzerland, described the lymph follicles in the intestine in 1677.

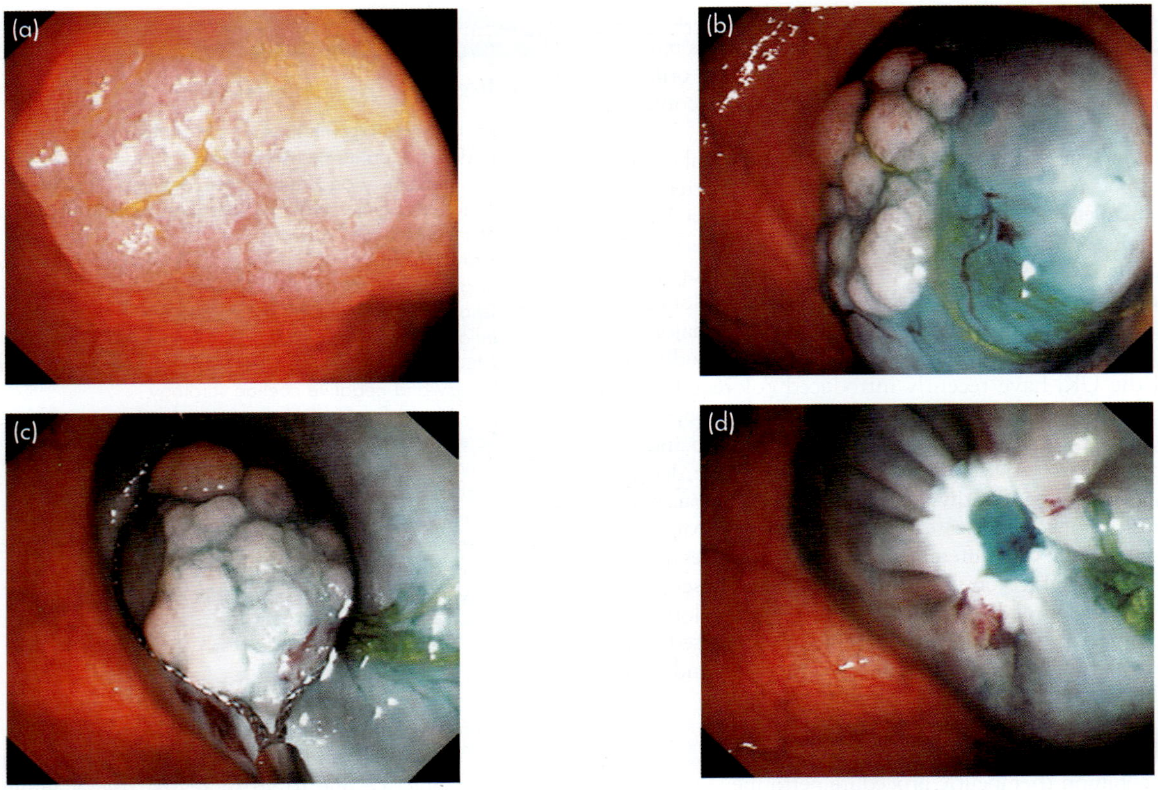

Figure 14.15 Large sessile polyps (a) can be removed by endoscopic mucosal resection. First the polyp is raised on a bed of injected saline containing dye (b). This ensures that there is no submucosal invasion and protects from transmural perforation. A snare is closed around the polyp (c), which is then resected leaving a clean excision base (d).

from the muscularis propria with a submucosal injection of saline to prevent iatrogenic perforation (Figure 14.15). Any residual polyp is obliterated with argon plasma coagulation. Care should be taken with all polypectomies in the right colon where the wall may only be 2–3 mm thick. Removal of large or extensive flat polyps should only be attempted by appropriately trained endoscopists.

Argon plasma coagulation (APC) and alternative thermal therapies such as heater probes are also used in the treatment of symptomatic angioectasias of the colon (Figure 14.16). Laser photocoagulation may be used to debulk colonic tumours not suitable for resection. As with benign oesophageal strictures, TTS balloons can be used to dilate short (less than 5 cm) colonic strictures. The dilatation of surgical anastomoses gives the most durable benefit as inflammatory strictures tend to recur even if intramucosal steroids are injected at the time of the dilatation.

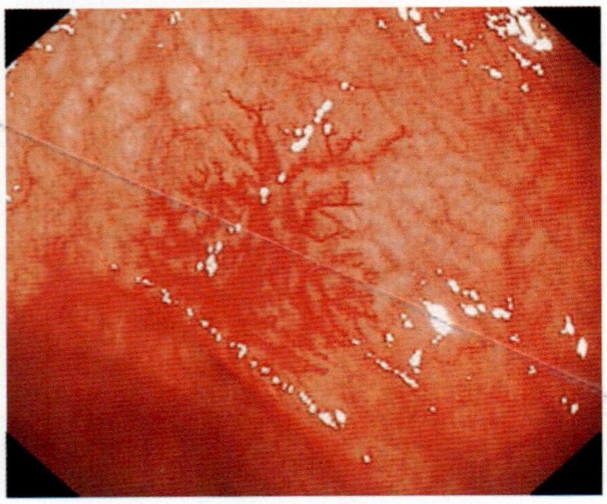

Figure 14.16 A large angioectasia of the colon. If this results in symptomatic anaemia, it should be obliterated with argon plasma coagulation.

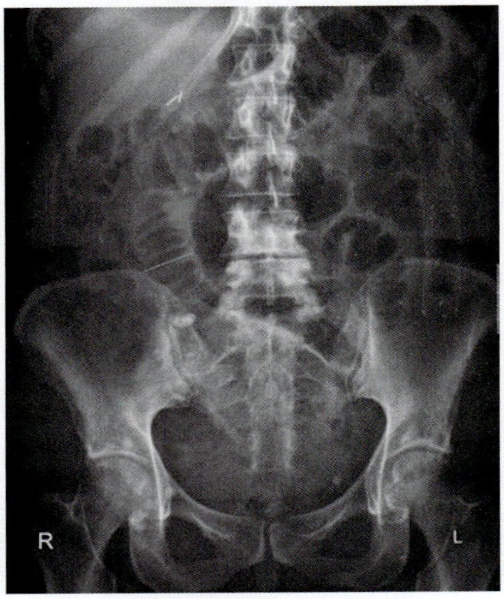

Figure 14.17 Malignant colonic obstruction can be palliated or temporarily relieved by insertion of a self-expanding metal stent.

en bloc is French for 'in a block'.

Finally, the colonoscopic placement of self-expanding metal stents may provide excellent palliation of inoperable malignant strictures (Figure 14.17) and may also play an invaluable role in decompressing an obstructed colon to allow planned as opposed to emergency surgery.

Complications of colonoscopy

Complications during routine diagnostic colonoscopy by an experienced colonoscopist are rare, although perforations have been reported as a result of excessive shaft tip pressure and with excessive air insufflation in severe diverticular disease. Total colonoscopy is contraindicated in the presence of severe colitis; a limited unprepped examination and careful mucosal biopsy only should be performed. Polypectomy is associated with a well-documented rate of perforation (approximately 1 per cent) and haemorrhage (1–2 per cent). Immediate haemorrhage should be managed by re-snaring the polyp stalk where possible and applying tamponade for several minutes followed by careful coagulation if this is unsuccessful. Submucosal adrenaline injection and the deployment of haemoclips are alternatives if this is not possible. Delayed haemorrhage may occur 1–14 days post-polypectomy and can normally be managed by conservative observation. Transfusion may occasionally be required, but repeat colonoscopy is rarely necessary. If recognised at the time of polypectomy, small perforations should be closed using clips and the patient admitted for observation. Symptoms of abdominal pain and cardiovascular compromise after a polypectomy should alert one to the risk of delayed perforation. Patients should be kept nil by mouth and receive intravenous resuscitation and antibiotics. Prompt assessment with plain radiography and a CT scan will often distinguish between a frank perforation and a transmural burn with associated localised peritonitis (the post-polypectomy syndrome). Assessment by an experienced colorectal surgeon is essential, as surgery is often the most appropriate course of action.

ENDOSCOPIC ULTRASOUND

One key disadvantage of conventional endoscopy is that the views are limited to the mucosal surface and it is therefore not possible to diagnose submucosal or extraintestinal pathology.

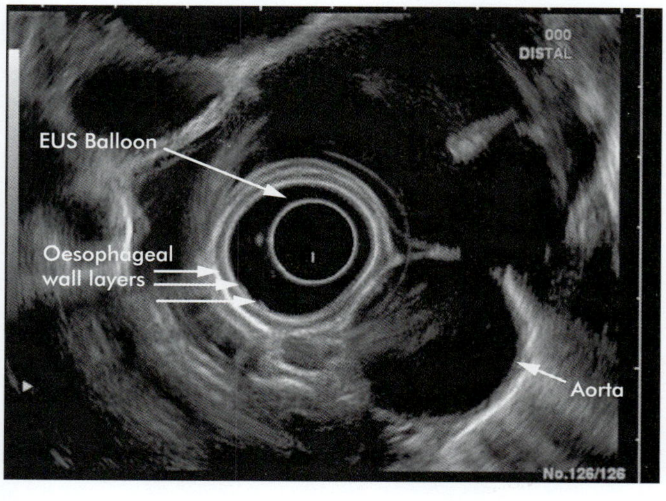

Figure 14.18 Layers of the intestinal wall.

These limitations can be overcome using endoscopic ultrasound which combines the traditional mucosal image with a separate ultrasound view that clearly depicts the intestinal layers (Figure 14.18) and proximate extraintestinal structures. Its use has revolutionised the staging and management of upper gastrointestinal and hepatobiliary malignancy, as the depth of invasion of a tumour can be accurately assessed at the same time that a biopsy is taken to confirm diagnosis (Figure 14.19). It allows sampling of paraoesophageal and coeliac lymph nodes and drainage of peripancreatic abscess or pseudocysts. The availability of linear and radial probes allows diagnosis and therapy to be appropriately targeted. Its use requires dedicated training and in some centres EUS is performed by an endoscopist working alongside a radiologist. Due to the width and lack of flexibility of the endoultrasound scope, as well as the duration of complex therapeutic procedures, sedation is normally required, and some units perform tests using propofol-based anaesthesia. The main indications for endoscopic ultrasound are listed in Table 14.6. All patients undergoing therapeutic endoscopic ultrasound require a normal coagulation screen. Complications include oversedation and oesophageal perforation during diagnostic procedures and haemorrhage/perforation during therapeutic procedures.

Table 14.6 Indications for endoscopic ultrasound.

Diagnostic	Staging of oesophageal/gastric malignancy
	Staging of hepatobiliary malignancy
	Diagnosis of choledoccal microlithiasis
Therapeutic	Biopsy of paraoesophageal lymph nodes
	Biopsy of submucosal upper gastrointestinal lesions
	Biopsy of pancreaticobiliary mass
	Biopsy of portal lymphadenopathy
	Transgastric drainage of pancreatic pseudocyst

FUTURE DIRECTIONS IN ENDOSCOPY

Chromoendoscopy, narrow band imaging and high resolution magnification endoscopy

The ability to enhance lesion detection and achieve near-perfect discrimination of pathology without the need for histology is a common theme of several active areas of endoscopic development. The goal is to allow accurate discrimination of dysplasia grade in areas of Barrett's oesophagus or quiescent ulcerative colitis and to aid polyp detection and the recognition of early gastric and colorectal cancer. The most widely available technique is chromoendoscopy, which involves the topical application of stains or pigments to improve tissue localisation, characterisation or diagnosis. Several agents have been described, which can broadly be categorised as absorptive (vital) stains such as methylene blue, contrast (reactive) stains such as indigo carmine, and those used for tattooing such as India ink. Narrow band imaging (NBI) relies on an optical filter technology that radically improves the visibility of capillaries, veins and other subtle tissue structures by optimising the absorbance and scattering characteristics of light. NBI uses two discrete bands of light: one blue at 415 nm and one green at 540 nm. Narrow band blue light displays superficial capillary networks whereas

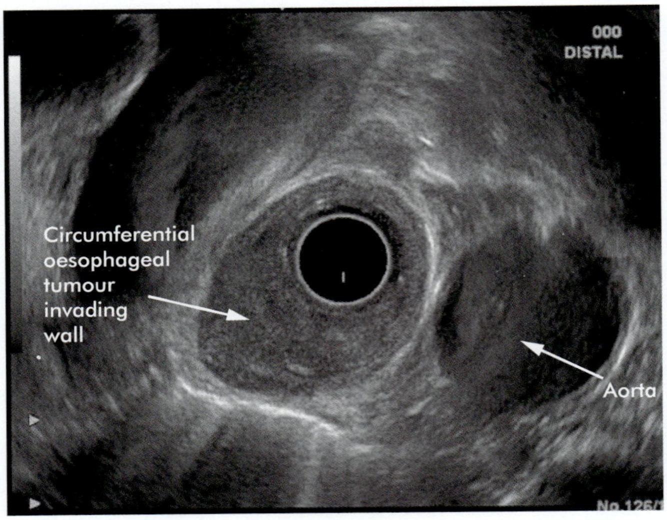

Figure 14.19 Endoscopic ultrasound image of an oesophageal tumour invading into the wall.

green light displays sub-epithelial vessels; when combined they offer an extremely high contrast image of the tissue surface. Autofluorescence images can also be used to increase a lesion's discrimination. Finally, high-resolution magnifying endoscopy may be used alone or in combination with one of the above techniques to achieve near-cellular definition of the mucosa (Figure 14.20). New directions for the future include the use of confocal endomicroscopy to achieve histological images at the time of the endoscopic procedure.

CONCLUSIONS

Over the last 30 years endoscopy has become an integral part of the diagnostic work-up of patients with gastrointestinal disease. Whereas advances in radiology may obviate the need for some diagnostic procedures (routine OGD and ERCP), the ability to take mucosal biopsies will ensure that it retains a vital role. Moreover, ongoing advances in technology, such as magnifying endoscopy and chromoendoscopy, are able to give near-histological quality definition to allow near-patient diagnosis. There have also been major advances in the range of conditions that are amenable to endoscopic therapy; such therapy may have substantially lower associated morbidity rates than traditional surgical approaches. However, as the scope of procedures widens and the age range/comorbidities of the patients increases, it is beholden to the endoscopist to ensure that he or she adheres to appropriate governance/consent and sedation practice to minimise complications.

FURTHER READING

Cotton P, Williams C. *Practical gastrointestinal endoscopy*, 6th edn. Oxford: Blackwell Science, 2009.

Lieberman DA. Clinical practice. Screening for colorectal cancer. *N Engl J Med* 2009; **361**: 1179–87.

Saunders BP. Polyp management. In: Phillips RKS, Clark S (eds). *Frontiers in colorectal surgery*. Shrewsbury: TFM, 2005.

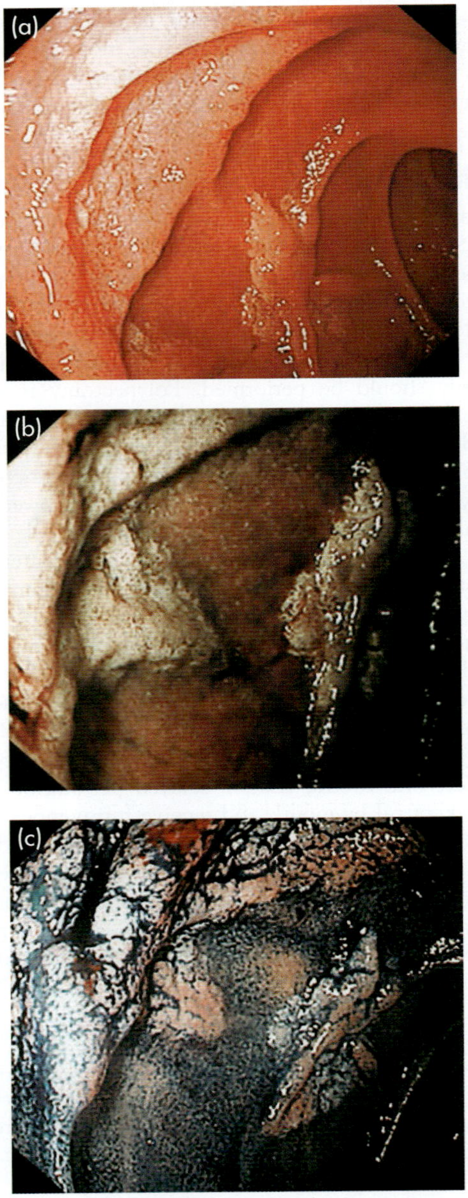

Figure 14.20 Endoscopic diagnostic accuracy can be improved by novel endoscopic techniques. This duodenal adenoma can be seen with conventional white light (a), but its full extent is more clearly delineated using narrow band imaging (b) or chromoendoscopy with indigo carmine (c).

CHAPTER
15 Tissue diagnosis

LEARNING OBJECTIVES

To understand:
- The value and limitations of tissue diagnosis
- How tissue samples are processed
- The role of histology, cytology and the autopsy

To be aware of:
- The role of additional techniques used in clinical practice, including special stains, immunohistochemistry and molecular methods
- The principles of microscopic diagnosis, particularly of neoplasia
- The importance of clinicopathological correlation
- Relevant management issues

INTRODUCTION

For centuries, tissue diagnosis was restricted to macroscopic examination of autopsy material and a limited range of surgical specimens. Microscopic examination of human tissue from autopsies and surgical procedures was introduced in the nineteenth century. Analysis of tissue samples is now an integral part of clinical management. Tissue diagnosis is usually the responsibility of a histopathologist (or 'pathologist'), who is a medically qualified practitioner. The specialty now known as histopathology (or sometimes cellular pathology) encompasses histopathology, cytopathology and autopsy work and is heavily dependent on microscopy.

In the UK, the nature of the histopathologist's work has changed since the 1960s. There has been a steady increase in biopsy numbers, partly because of flexible endoscopy. Many resection specimens are assessed with management and prognosis in mind, the diagnosis having been made preoperatively. Screening programmes have had a major impact. New techniques have improved the quality and value of histopathological assessment, while autopsies have steadily decreased in number. Published minimum standards for the assessment of a specimen, e.g. a cancer resection, are often in place. In addition, histopathologists are increasingly involved in multidisciplinary patient management meetings.

A modern histopathology department is usually located in a medium-sized or large hospital. Typically, more than 80 per cent of specimens are from the gastrointestinal tract, gynaecological tract or skin. In line with clinical services, highly specialised work, e.g. neuropathology, is confined to major regional centres.

Summary box 15.1

Reasons for tissue analysis

- To make a new diagnosis
- To confirm a suspected or established clinical diagnosis
- To exclude additional diagnoses
- To assist with prognosis
- To help plan management
- Audit

REASONS FOR ASSESSMENT OF TISSUE

There are several reasons for tissue analysis (Summary box 15.1). A new diagnosis may be made, e.g. squamous cell carcinoma, or a known diagnosis confirmed. Microscopic clues may be found, e.g. granulomatous inflammation. Additional expected or unexpected diagnoses may be made. For example, biopsies from a patient with inflammatory bowel disease are taken to confirm the diagnosis and exclude dysplasia but might reveal additional findings, e.g. cytomegalovirus. An appendix removed for appendicitis could contain an incidental carcinoid tumour. Tissue analysis also helps to determine treatment and prognosis. For example, a liver biopsy from a patient with chronic viral hepatitis is not taken to make the diagnosis but instead helps to determine therapy, exclude other diseases (e.g. steatohepatitis) and exclude complications of chronic liver disease (e.g. neoplasia). The pathologist's assessment of resections also helps surgeons to audit their performance.

A tissue sample does not necessarily represent the entire patient. The interpretation of microscopic changes may be considerably enhanced by correlation with the macroscopic findings and the clinical picture. Accordingly, a request form with adequate clinical details should accompany all specimens. Essential details include site of biopsy, date of birth, gender, medications, relevant risk factors and past medical history.

TISSUE SPECIMENS

Routine tissue specimens received by a histopathology department include those intended for histopathological analysis and those for cytopathological assessment (Summary box 15.2). Sometimes these two areas overlap.

> **Summary box 15.2**
>
> **Common types of tissue sample**
>
> - Histology
>   - Formalin-fixed tissue
>   - Biopsy
>   - Mucosal
>   - Punch
>   - Needle (core)
>   - Currettings
>   - Excision
>   - Resection
>   - Small
>   - Large
>   - Fresh tissue (usually for frozen section)
> - Cytology
>   - Cervical
>   - Washings, brushings, scrapes
>   - Fine-needle aspirate (FNA)
>   - Fluids/sputum

Histology

Specimens for histology are arbitrarily classified as biopsies and resections, although the word 'biopsy' can refer to any tissue sample. Types of biopsy include punch biopsy, needle core biopsy and mucosal biopsy. An excision biopsy serves as both a diagnostic biopsy and a small resection. Samples for routine histology are immediately placed in a fixative, usually formalin (10 per cent formaldehyde), to preserve morphology.

Cytology

Cytological specimens can be obtained from many sites using a variety of approaches. Some are easy to obtain, e.g. urine and sputum, whereas others require more intervention.

A conventional cervical smear is obtained by sampling the cervical transformation zone with a brush/broom. Bronchial aspirates, washings and brushings, and gastrointestinal and biliary brushings sample a relatively wide area and may therefore be useful for the diagnosis of neoplasia. Fine-needle aspiration (FNA) cytology may sample accessible sites such as the breast, thyroid and superficial lymph nodes, while FNA from deeper and less accessible structures, e.g. liver, pancreas, kidney and lung, is usually assisted by ultrasound or computed tomography (CT) guidance. Ultrasound-guided transbronchial FNA may be used for mediastinal masses and transmucosal FNA for submucosal gastrointestinal lesions or perivisceral lesions. Fluids may be submitted directly to the laboratory for cytological assessment.

Fresh tissue

The most common indication for submission of a fresh tissue sample (i.e. without fixative) is rapid frozen section diagnosis, but other indications are microbiological assessment, electron microscopy, chemical analyses (e.g. quantification of iron) and various types of molecular pathological analysis. Before fixing a histology or cytology specimen, the operator should ask whether any of these investigations might be useful.

Risk management

Safety and risk management are priorities in the laboratory. Any risk of contamination by transmissible infection, e.g. hepatitis B virus, HIV, must be minimised by the use of warning labels, especially when fresh tissue is being submitted. Formalin kills many micro-organisms, but any risk of infection should still be notified. Also, formalin itself is toxic to the eyes and skin. Accordingly, leaking or faulty specimen containers should be discarded. Containers must be labelled with the patient's details to avoid errors of identity (Figure 15.1).

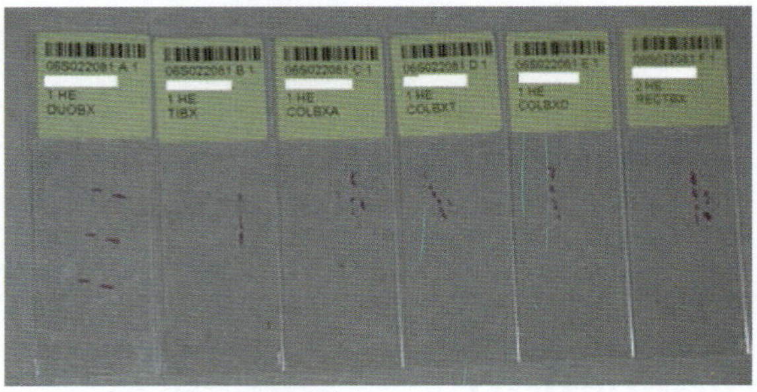

Figure 15.1 Sections on glass slides stained with haematoxylin and eosin (H&E). Each slide has a unique specimen identifying number (06S022081), a letter corresponding to the biopsy site (A1–F1) and a site label (e.g. DUOBX for duodenal biopsy).

SPECIMEN PROCESSING

Histology specimen

On arrival in the histopathology department, specimens are given a unique number and submitted for macroscopic assessment and sampling ('cut up'). The largest specimens are opened (e.g. bowel) or sliced (e.g. uterus) and left to fix in formalin for at least 1 day (Figure 15.2a–c). Once fixed and in a suitable condition for cutting, a text description of the specimen and any visible lesion is made. Representative samples ('blocks') are taken from any specimen too large to be processed whole (Figure 15.3). This is usually done by a histopathologist, especially if a case is complex, but sometimes by non-medical staff. A local or national protocol for sampling is often followed. For example, samples from most types of cancer include resection margins, tumour, lymph nodes, non-neoplastic tissue, and any other abnormal areas. Coloured inks may be used to identify resection margins and surfaces (Figure 15.4a and b).

Specimens, or samples from specimens, are placed in plastic cassettes (Figure 15.5), and then embedded in paraffin wax while in the cassette to make a tissue block (Figure 15.6). Sections with a thickness of approximately 5 μm (microns) are cut from the block using a microtome (Figure 15.7). The sections are placed on a glass slide and stained with haematoxylin and eosin (H&E) (Figure 15.1). This work is done by trained staff, known in the UK as biomedical scientists (BMSs). High

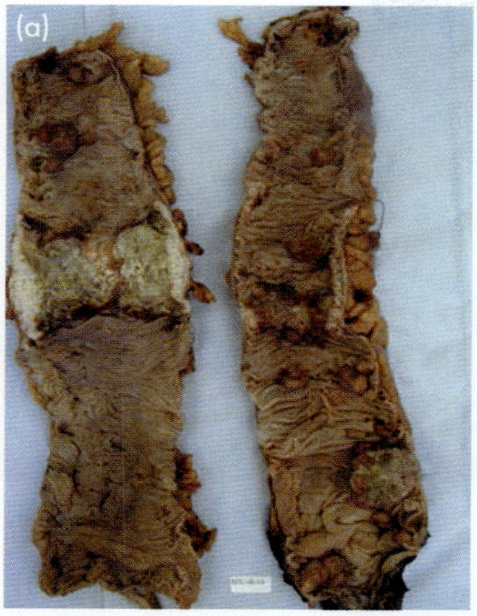

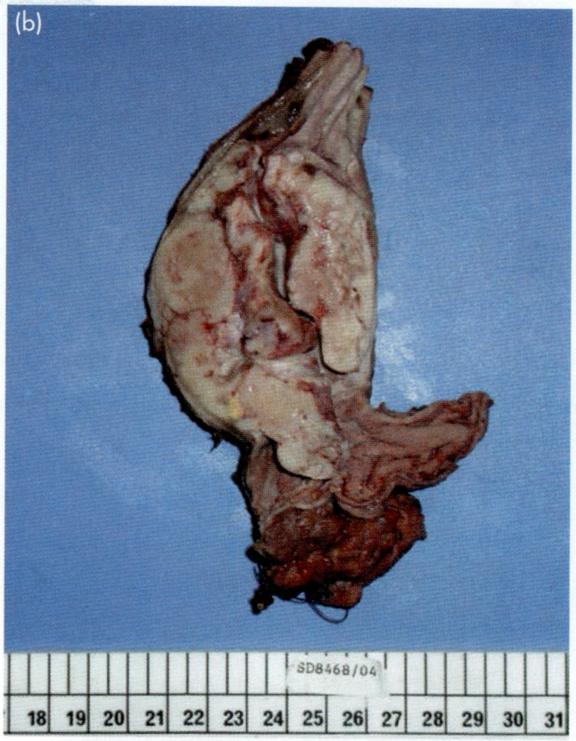

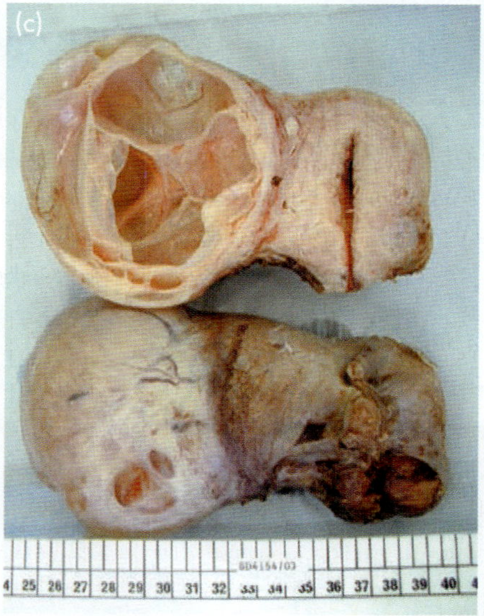

Figure 15.2 (a) A colon from a patient with familial adenomatous polyposis has been opened longitudinally to allow fixation. Multiple polyps and a carcinoma are seen. (b) An oesophagogastrectomy containing a distal oesophageal tumour has been opened and sliced to allow fixation. (c) A uterus and an adjacent cystic lesion have been bisected with a knife to allow fixation (all figures courtesy of Dr J Chin Aleong, Barts and the London NHS Trust, United Kingdom).

standards are necessary because a poorly cut section may have various artefacts, such as lines and folds, which impede accurate assessment. H&E as the first line stain has stood the test of time, probably because it is inexpensive, safe, fast, reliable, familiar and informative.

The stained sections are examined with a microscope (Figure 15.8) by a histopathologist, who correlates the histological features with the clinical details and with the macroscopic description. After any appropriate further studies, the pathologist writes a report which may be entered onto a computer system (Summary box 15.3).

FROZEN SECTION SPECIMEN

Frozen section diagnosis is useful when a rapid answer is necessary. Surgeons are the main users of this service. A fresh tissue sample (i.e. not fixed in formalin) is frozen quickly on a portable metal chuck or similar device, and sections are cut and stained within a few minutes. There are several disadvantages (Summary box 15.4). Fresh tissue carries a higher risk of infection than fixed tissue. The quality of a frozen section slide is inferior to that of routinely processed material, reducing the accuracy and precision of diagnosis. Small samples are required. In addition, certain types of tissue, e.g. fat, are difficult to process. Furthermore, frozen sections are time-consuming and disruptive for the histopathology department.

Summary box 15.3

Histological processing: sequence of events

- Biopsy or resection specimen received
- Description made
- Specimen sampled (unless small enough to submit in its entirety)
- Specimen or samples placed in cassette(s)
- Paraffin wax block(s) made
- 5-µm sections cut
- Sections put on glass slides
- Sections stained with H&E
- Histopathologist examines slides
- Histology compared with clinical and macroscopic findings
- Further studies if necessary
- Report entered onto computer system
- Report authorised or signed

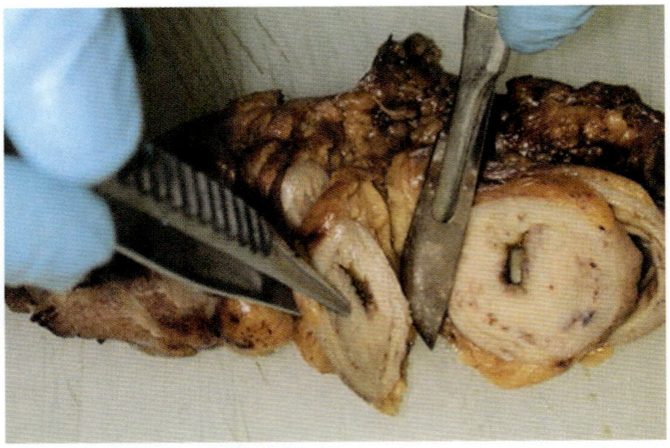

Figure 15.3 A scalpel is used to take a sample from a resection specimen.

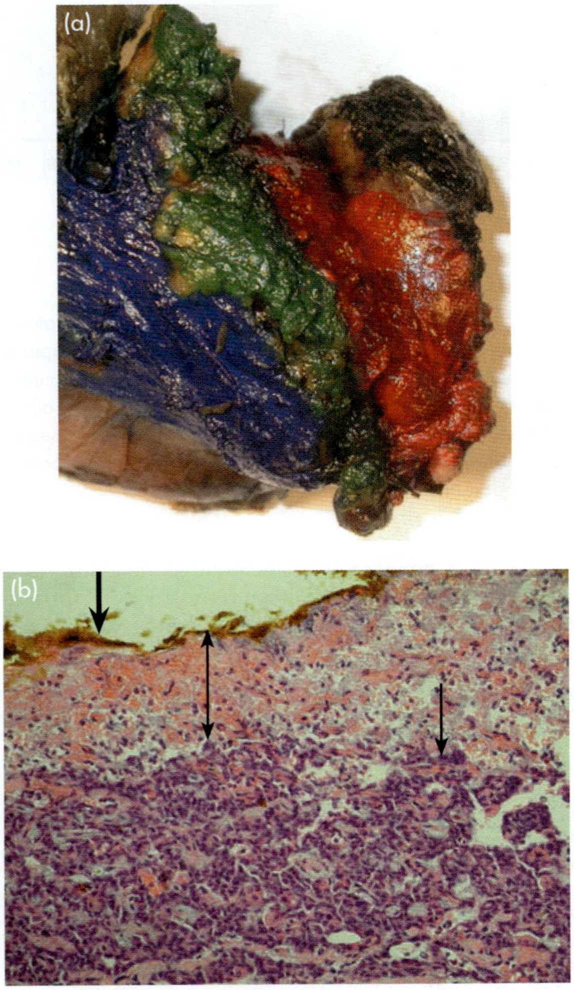

Figure 15.4 (a) An unopened pancreatoduodenectomy specimen (posterior view). Four inks of different colours have been painted onto various resection margins and external surfaces. (b) Yellow ink on the edge of a histology section (thick arrow). Tumour (thin arrow) lies close to the surface. The distance between the tumour and a surface or a resection margin can be measured (double-headed arrow).

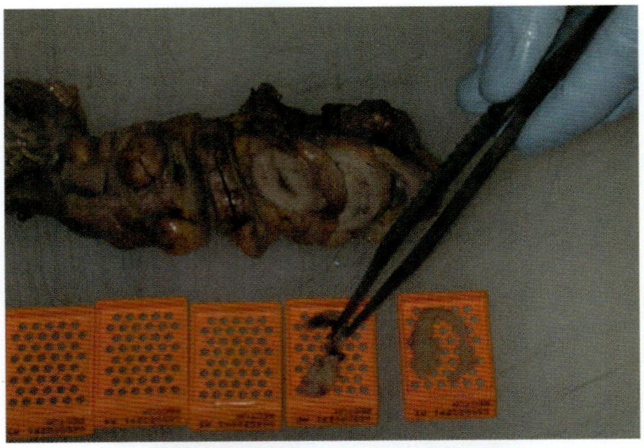

Figure 15.5 A tissue sample from a resection specimen is placed in a cassette.

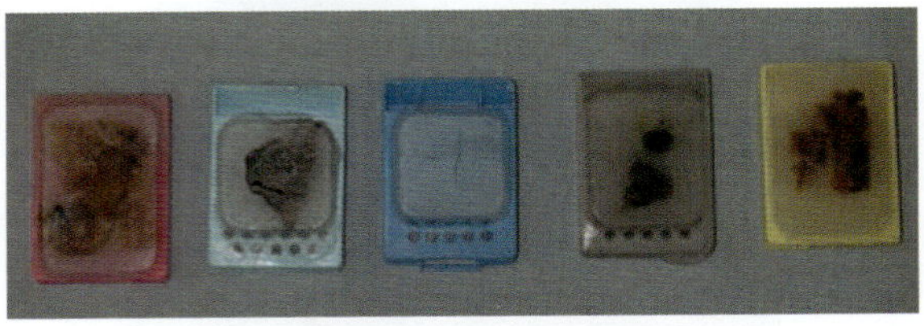

Figure 15.6 Paraffin wax blocks. Cassettes of different colours allow specimens to be organised into groups.

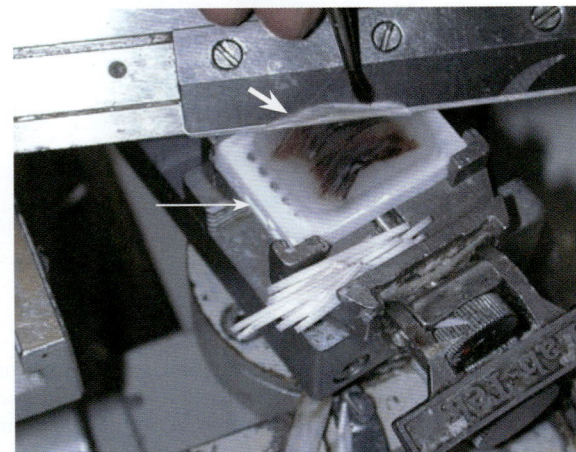

Figure 15.7 A section (thick arrow) being cut from a paraffin wax block (thin arrow) with a microtome.

Summary box 15.4

Frozen section: advantages and disadvantages

Advantages
- Quick diagnosis

Disadvantages
- Labour intensive
- Disruptive
- Risk of infection
- Poorer quality sections
- Small sample required
- Some tissue types difficult to process

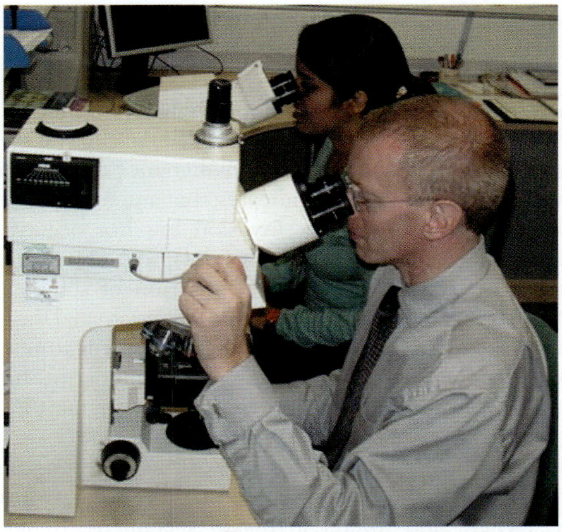

Figure 15.8 A double-headed microscope allows a consultant histopathologist and a trainee to view a slide simultaneously.

Cytology specimen

Many samples for cytology can be smeared immediately onto glass slides, fixed (usually in alcohol) or air dried, and stained immediately or later. Several slides are usually produced, some of which are stained with a Papanicolaou (Pap) stain and some with another method such as May–Grünwald–Giemsa (MGG) or Romanowsky. Pap stain is regarded as the preferred stain for fixed specimens while MGG is better for air-dried material. Often the sample will be stained with both. Cervical smears are usually stained with a Pap stain only (Figure 15.9). There has been a move towards liquid-based thin-layer technology for many samples. For liquid-based cytology, the sampling device is usually washed in a liquid medium and the material obtained is then processed in the laboratory using purpose-built equipment.

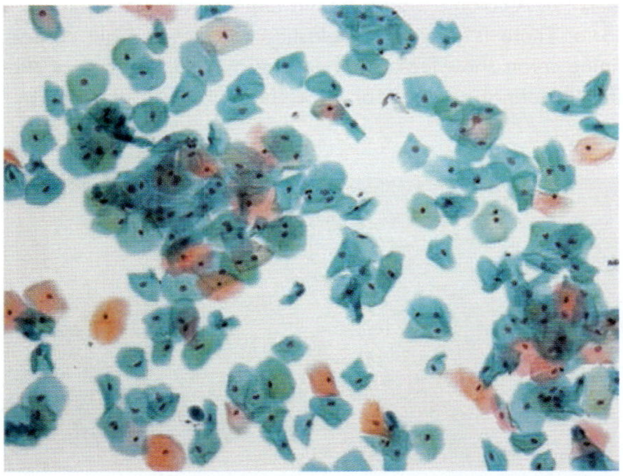

Figure 15.9 A cervical smear stained with a Papanicolaou stain. Numerous cells are present (courtesy of Professor MT Sheaff, Barts and the London NHS Trust).

George Nicholas Papanicolaou, 1883–1962, Professor of Anatomy, Cornell University, New York, NY, USA, reported on the value of cervical smears in the diagnosis of carcinoma of the uterus in 1941.

Storage

Resection specimens are generally stored for about 4–6 weeks. Tissue blocks are retained for as long as space permits, e.g. 30 years, while glass slides might be retained for a shorter time, e.g. 10 years. Fresh tissue can be frozen and stored. Stored tissue may be useful for future clinical review, teaching, audit or research. In many countries, the subsequent use of stored tissue for non-clinical purposes is now subject to legal constraints.

PRINCIPLES OF MICROSCOPIC DIAGNOSIS

Diagnosis of malignancy

The main histological criteria for malignancy are metastasis, invasion, architectural changes and cytological features (Summary box 15.5).

Summary box 15.5

Microscopic features of malignancy

- Metastasis
- Invasion
  - Of surrounding tissue
  - Vascular
  - Perineural
- Architectural abnormalities
- Necrosis
- Numerous mitotic figures
- Atypical mitotic figures
- Nuclear abnormalities
  - Pleomorphism
  - Enlargement
  - Hyperchromaticity
  - Chromatin clumping
- Nucleolar enlargement and multiplicity

Metastasis (most often to lymph nodes or liver) is diagnostic of malignancy. Invasion of surrounding structures, perineural invasion (Figure 15.10) and vascular invasion (Figure 15.11) strongly suggest malignancy. Other microscopic features seen in

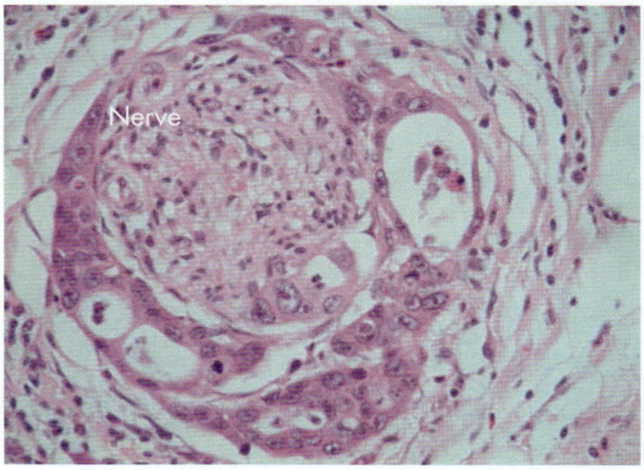

Figure 15.10 Perineural invasion. A nerve is almost completely surrounded by adenocarcinoma.

Richard May, born 1863, a physician of München, Germany.
Ludwig Grünwald, born 1863, an otolaryngologist of München, Germany.
Gustav Giemsa, 1867–1948, a bacteriologist who became Privatdozent in Chemotherapy, at The University of Hamburg, Hamburg, Germany.
Dimiti Leonidovich Romanovsky, 1861–1921, Professor of Medicine, St. Petersburg, Russia.

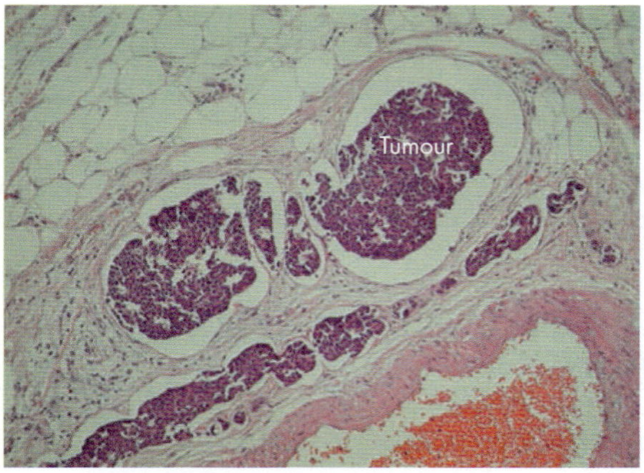

Figure 15.11 Vascular invasion. Aggregates of carcinoma cells are present within blood vessels. The tumour is poorly differentiated.

malignancy include architectural derangement, an increased number of mitotic figures, atypical mitoses, and necrosis (tissue death) (Figure 15.12). Microscopic changes at the cellular level (cytological changes) include nuclear enlargement, an increased nuclear:cytoplasmic ratio, nuclear pleomorphism (variation in shape) and nuclear hyperchromasia (dark colour) (Figure 15.13a). Multiplicity, irregularity and enlargement of nucleoli may also be seen (Figure 15.13b).

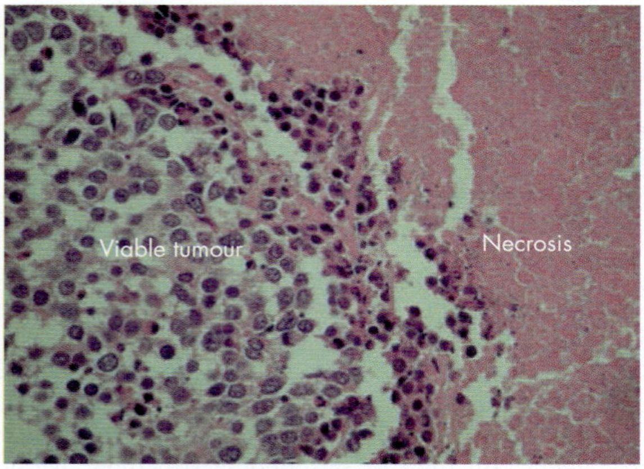

Figure 15.12 An area of necrosis in a poorly differentiated carcinoma.

The criteria for a diagnosis of malignancy are influenced by the site and type of tissue. In general, epithelial cells must invade beyond their normal boundaries for malignancy to be diagnosed. The term 'dysplasia' usually indicates that microscopic features of carcinoma are present but invasion has not occurred, e.g. cervical intraepithelial neoplasia (CIN), colorectal dysplasia (Figure 15.14). However, the categorisation of some types of non-epithelial tumour (e.g. lymphoid, mesenchymal) as malignant may rely on cytological and architectural features rather than on invasiveness. In some cases, e.g. endocrine tumours, histological distinction between benign and malignant is impossible.

There are various causes of a false-positive diagnosis of malignancy. These include contamination of a specimen with tumour from elsewhere and interchanging of specimens. In addition, many conditions can mimic malignancy histologically. The risk of interpretative error by the histopathologist is reduced by

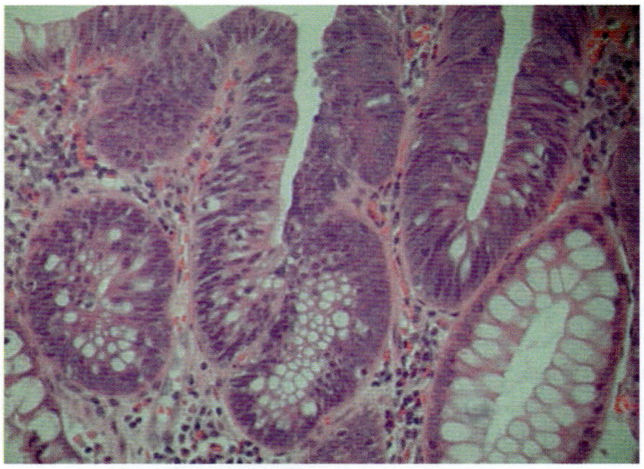

Figure 15.14 A colonic biopsy from a tubular adenoma with low-grade dysplasia. There is one non-dysplastic crypt (lower right corner). The remaining crypts show features of dysplasia, including nuclear stratification (multilayering) and nuclear hyperchromaticity (dark colour).

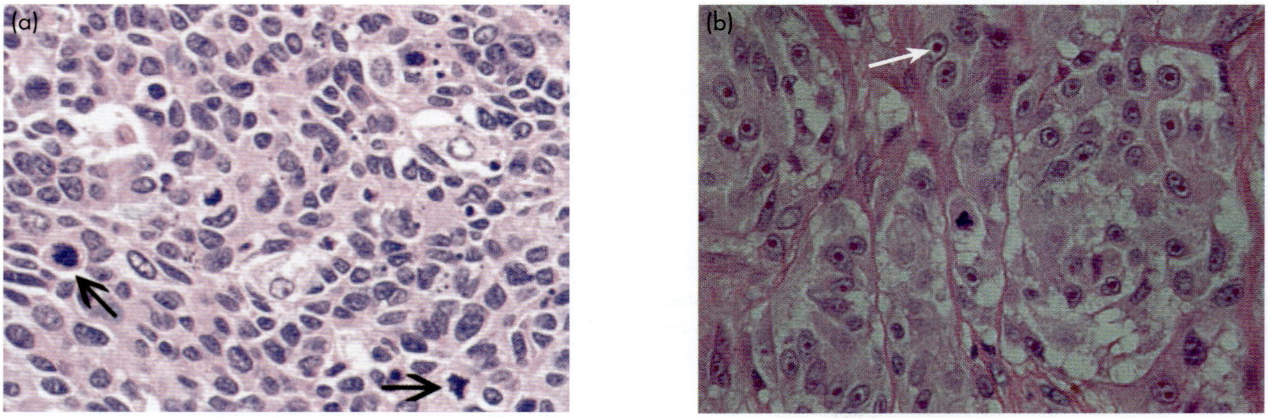

Figure 15.13 Cytological features of malignancy. (a) A high grade neuroendocrine carcinoma showing nuclear pleomorphism (variation in shape) and variation in nuclear size. There are several mitotic figures (arrows). (b) A malignant melanoma showing nuclear pleomorphism and prominent nucleoli (arrow) (courtesy of Dr E Husain, Aberdeen Royal Infirmary, UK).

thorough training, regular updating, discussion of difficult cases with colleagues, and avoidance of excessive workloads. The surgeon also helps to minimise such errors by supplying adequate clinical details. For example, a history of radiotherapy is essential because radiation effect can mimic malignancy. The histological changes in regenerating tissue, e.g. next to an ulcer, may also resemble malignancy (Summary box 15.6).

Summary box 15.6

Causes of false-positive diagnoses of malignancy

- Interchanged samples
- Contamination
- Interpretative error
- Treatment-induced change
- Ulceration

Histological types of malignancy

A malignant tumour showing features of epithelial differentiation, and typically arising in an epithelial layer, is a carcinoma. Other important types of malignancy include malignant melanoma (melanocytes) (Figure 15.13b), lymphoma (lymphoid cells) and sarcoma (mesenchymal cells). In most cases, further subclassification is possible. For example, a carcinoma can be classified as squamous cell carcinoma (which shows keratinisation) (Figure 15.15), adenocarcinoma (which shows tubule formation and/or mucin production) (Figure 15.16), neuroendocrine carcinoma/small cell carcinoma (Figure 15.13a) (usually requiring immunohistochemical confirmation), clear cell carcinoma (Figure 15.17), or one of many other types.

Prognostic factors for tumours

Tissue assessment is important for prognosis. Stage is generally the most important prognostic factor for carcinomas. The commonly used and internationally accepted Union Internationale Contre le Cancer (UICC) staging scheme depends heavily on the histopathological TNM category (pTNM), although the M (metastasis) category is usually evaluated clinically. Grade may also be prognostic and is usually determined microscopically.

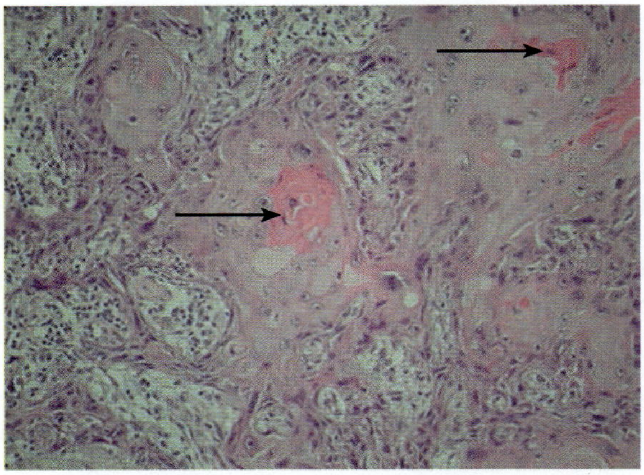

Figure 15.15 A well-differentiated squamous cell carcinoma. Irregular nests of squamous cells with foci of keratinisation (arrows).

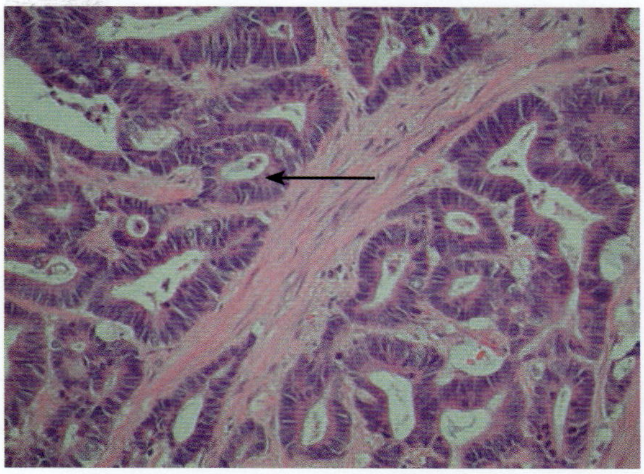

Figure 15.16 A well-differentiated adenocarcinoma. Gland formation (arrow) is obvious.

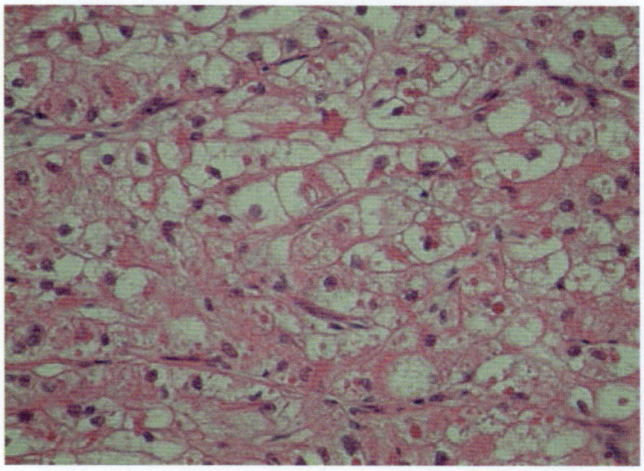

Figure 15.17 A metastatic clear cell carcinoma, composed of sheets of cells with clear cytoplasm. A tumour with this appearance is most likely to be of renal origin.

Low-grade/well-differentiated tumours resemble their normal tissue counterparts (Figures 15.15 and 15.16), whereas high-grade/poorly differentiated tumours do not (Figures 15.11 and 15.12). Other histological features associated with a poor prognosis include vascular invasion (Figure 15.11), perineural invasion (Figure 15.10) and positive resection margins. These factors differ in their prognostic value between tumour types and sites.

Inflammatory conditions

Acute inflammation is characterised by neutrophils (polymorphonuclear leukocytes) (Figure 15.18), and chronic inflammation by lymphocytes and plasma cells. Other inflammatory cells include eosinophils (Figure 15.19), mast cells and histiocytes. Granulomas (i.e. collections of epithelioid histiocytes) (Figure 15.20a and b) raise the possibility of mycobacterial infection, fungal infection, sarcoid, and a reaction to foreign material, among numerous other possible causes. Eosinophils in large numbers may reflect parasitic infection or allergy. Interpretation depends heavily on the site and clinical setting.

Other microscopic changes

Other abnormalities are also detectable by microscopy. Histopathologists may use specific terms for these changes. For

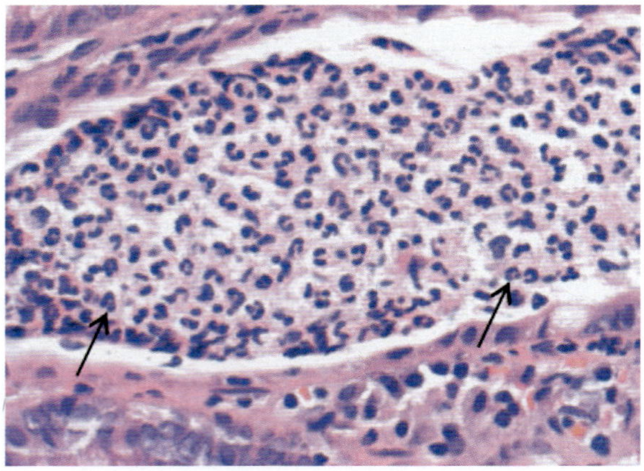

Figure 15.18 An acute inflammatory process characterised by numerous neutrophils. Note the typical multilobated nuclei in many cells (arrows).

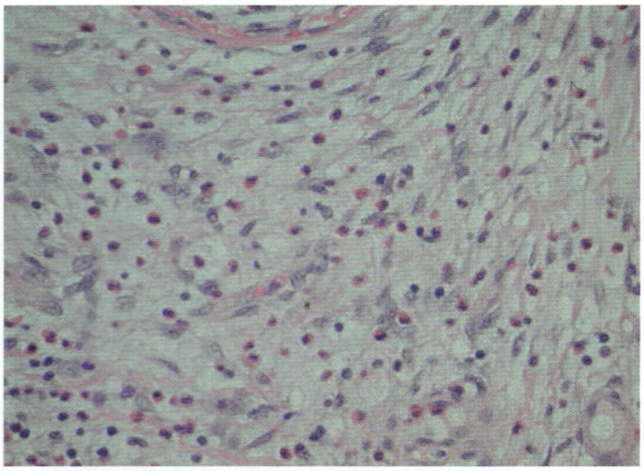

Figure 15.19 An inflammatory lesion in which eosinophils, characterised by bright red cytoplasm, are predominant.

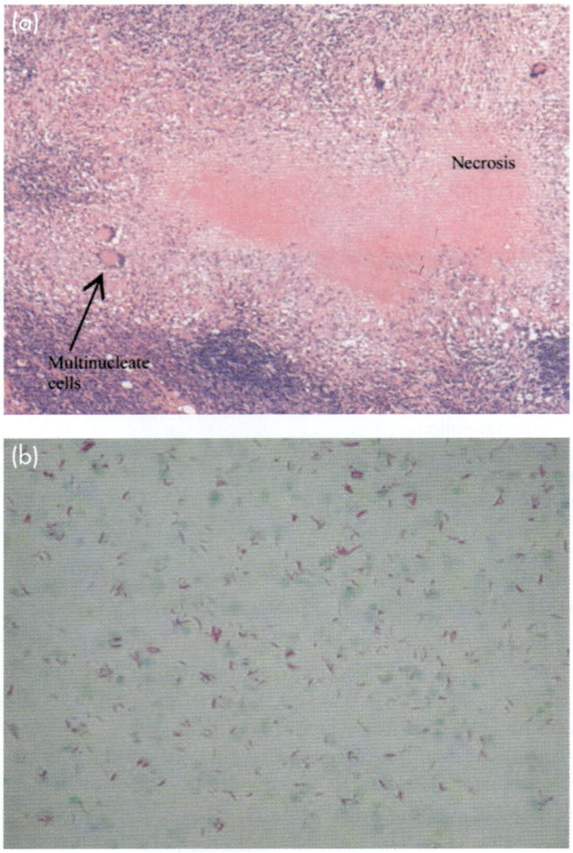

Figure 15.20 (a) A granuloma with necrosis, suggesting tuberculosis. Multinucleate giant cells of Langhan's type are also present (arrow). (b) A Ziehl–Neelsen stain (different case) shows numerous acid-fast bacilli.

example, hyperplasia means an increase in cell number while hypertrophy refers to an increase in cell size. Atrophy encompasses a reduction in cell number and/or cell size. Metaplasia describes the change from one mature cell type to another, e.g. columnar metaplasia in the oesophagus (Barrett's oesophagus) where squamous epithelium is replaced by gastric or intestinal type epithelium. Necrosis refers to cell or tissue death.

ASSESSMENT

Light microscopy

Most tissue assessment depends on conventional light microscopy. Microscopes have several lenses with various powers of magnification, typically ranging from ×20 to ×400 or more. A low-power lens allows a sample to be scanned and its overall architecture to be assessed, while a high-power lens allows a closer and more detailed view (Figure 15.21a and b). A teaching arm and a camera can be attached to most microscopes (Figure 15.8). Polarisation can be used to detect foreign material (e.g. sutures) or to assess a special stain (e.g. Congo red).

Histological assessment

In a histological preparation, the microscopic structure of the tissue is preserved, allowing direct visualisation of architecture. Accordingly, the pathologist can see not only the characteristics of the cells that form the tissue, but also the way in which these cells are related to one another and the way in which different tissue compartments are arranged.

Cytological assessment

A cytological preparation consists of a sample of cells. Architecture cannot be determined, because intact tissue is absent or sparse (Figures 15.9 and 15.22a and b). Therefore, assessment relies mainly on the characteristics of the cells themselves. Accordingly, it may be difficult to diagnose malignancy because many of the criteria, particularly invasiveness, cannot be assessed. However, cytology has several potential advantages over histology (Summary box 15.7). A wider area may be sampled, and obtaining a specimen may be easier and less traumatic. Processing times are usually shorter and costs lower. Also, non-medical staff can be trained to report the cases, particularly cervical smears (Figure 15.9).

Screening

Screening programmes aim to detect and treat pre-malignant tissue changes, e.g. dysplasia, or early stage malignancy (rather than advanced disease). They may rely on cytology, histology or both. The largest is the cervical cancer programme, which uses cytology initially, with biopsy and histology follow up if

Norman Rupert Barrett, 1903–1979, surgeon, St Thomas's Hospital, London, UK.

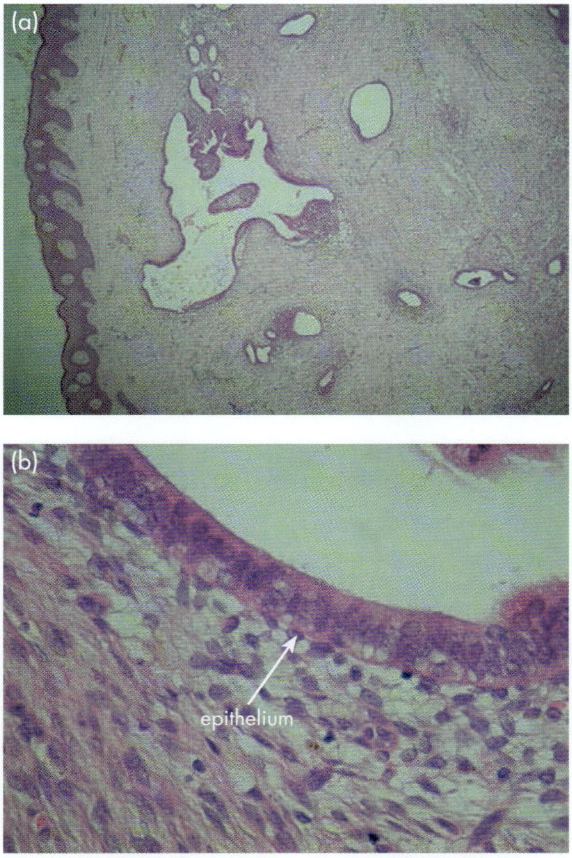

Figure 15.21 (a) Low-power view of an umbilical nodule. Glands are distributed irregularly through the tissue. (b) High-power view shows benign columnar epithelium lining the glands, favouring endometriosis over carcinoma.

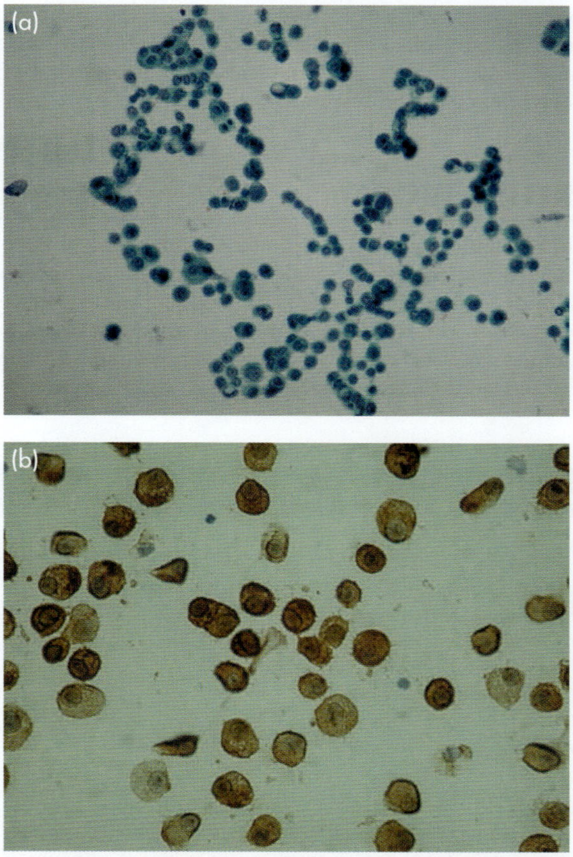

Figure 15.22 (a) A cytology preparation of a pleural effusion. Numerous cells with atypical features are present. (b) Immunohistochemistry shows positive staining for carcinoembryonic antigen (CEA), favouring carcinoma over mesothelioma

Summary box 15.7

Cytology compared with histology

Advantages
- Wider area may be sampled
- Sampling may be less invasive
- Fast
- Cheap
- Can be interpreted by non-medical staff

Disadvantages
- Cannot assess tissue architecture
- Less amenable to further studies

appropriate. The breast cancer screening programmes may use cytology and/or histology, while the bowel cancer screening programmes and screening for cancer in ulcerative colitis rely on histology.

Specimen adequacy

There are several possible reasons for an inadequate specimen (Summary box 15.8). The operator may fail to sample the intended organ or lesion, or may take too few samples to detect a heterogeneous abnormality. A sample from the centre of a necrotic or ulcerated lesion might include no viable tissue. Superficial biopsies from a carcinoma may fail to distinguish dysplasia (Figure 15.14) from invasive carcinoma. Cautery and crush artefact are sometimes severe enough to impede assessment. Cytology samples which have been spread too thickly can be uninterpretable.

Summary box 15.8

Reasons for an inadequate sample

Histology and cytology
- Failure to sample the intended organ or lesion
- Sample too limited
- Non-viable tissue

Histology
- Sample too superficial
- Cautery artefact
- Crush artefact

Cytology
- Thick smear

Deeper levels and extra blocks

The pathologist may request 'deeper levels', whereby the BMS cuts further into the paraffin block to obtain further sections. For example, deeper levels of an atypical but non-invasive epithelial lesion might show foci of invasion, allowing carcinoma to be diagnosed. Extra blocks may be taken if a specimen has been sampled inadequately, e.g. if insufficient lymph nodes have been retrieved from a cancer resection specimen.

FURTHER WORK

Further diagnostic work is performed on a minority of histology specimens, and includes special stains and immunohistochemistry. *In situ* hybridisation, electron microscopy and polymerase chain reaction (PCR)-based methods are used less often. Some techniques can also be applied to cytology specimens (Summary box 15.9, Figure 15.22a and b).

Summary box 15.9

Additional techniques

- Special stains
- Immunohistochemistry
- *In situ* hybridisation
- Fluorescence *in situ* hybridisation (FISH)
- PCR-based techniques
- Electron microscopy

SPECIAL STAINS

A 'special stain' is a stain that is not routine. Immunohistochemical stains are conventionally excluded from this category. Some special stains demonstrate normal substances in increased quantities or in abnormal locations. The periodic acid–Schiff (PAS) stain demonstrates both glycogen and mucin, whereas a diastase periodic acid–Schiff (D-PAS) stain demonstrates mucin, e.g. in an adenocarcinoma. Perls Prussian blue stain demonstrates iron accumulation (Figure 15.23a and b), e.g. in haemochromatosis. A reticulin stain helps to demonstrate fibrosis (Figure 15.24a and b). Elastic stains also show fibrosis and can highlight blood vessels by outlining their elastic laminae. Special stains can also reveal the accumulation of abnormal substances, e.g. a Congo red stain for amyloid (Summary box 15.10).

Summary box 15.10

Common special stains

- PAS: glycogen, fungi
- D-PAS: mucin
- Perls Prussian blue: iron
- Reticulin: reticulin fibres, fibrosis
- van Gieson: collagen
- Congo red: amyloid
- Ziehl–Neelsen: mycobacteria

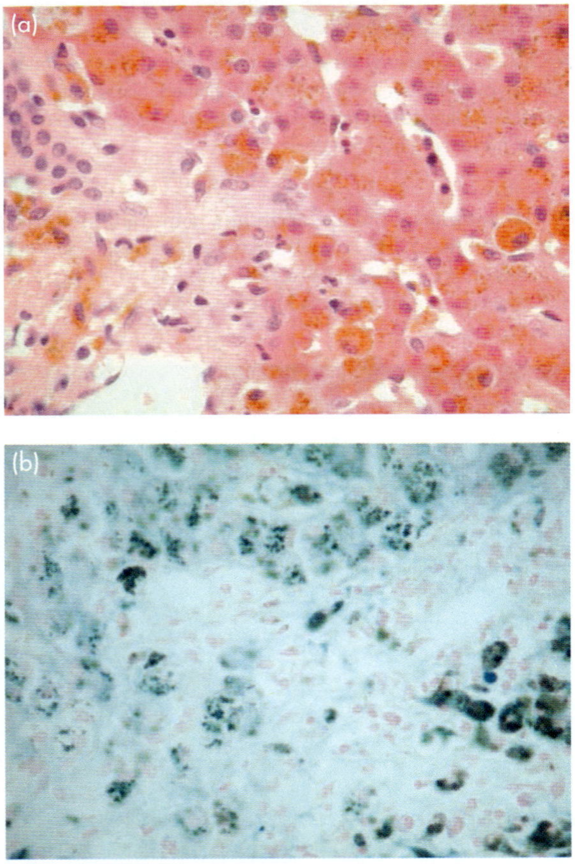

Figure 15.23 (a) Brown pigment in a biopsy. (b) A Perls stain is positive, indicating that the pigment is iron.

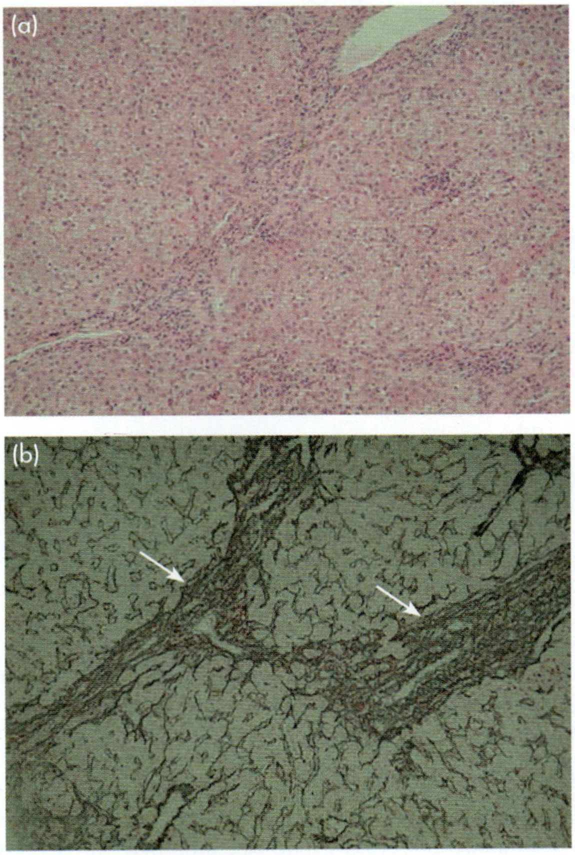

Figure 15.24 (a) A liver biopsy stained with haematoxylin and eosin (H&E) in which the severity of fibrosis cannot be determined. (b) A reticulin stain demonstrates fibrous bridges (arrows).

Hugo Schiff, 1834–1915, a German biochemist who worked in Florence, Italy.
Max Perls, 1843–1881, a pathologist of Giesen, Germany.
Congo red is sodium diphenylbisazobisnaphthylamine sulphonate.

Special stains are also useful for the diagnosis of infection. For example, a Ziehl–Neelsen stain demonstrates acid-fast bacilli, particularly mycobacteria, by staining them bright red in a blue background (Figure 15.20a and b). Mycobacteria cannot be seen on H&E slides. Other micro-organisms that may be detectable on H&E but are easier to see with a special stain include fungi (PAS or Grocott stain), protozoa (Giemsa stain) and spirochaetes (Warthin–Starry stain).

IMMUNOHISTOCHEMISTRY

Immunohistochemistry, which was introduced in the 1970s, has had a major impact on histopathological diagnosis. This technique detects a specific antigen using an antibody. The antibody is labelled with a dye and when bound to its target antigen is seen in the tissue section as a coloured stain, often brown (Figure 15.25). This allows the presence, tissue distribution and cellular localisation of an antigen to be determined. Immunohistochemistry can be applied to fixed and frozen tissue and to cytological preparations (Figure 15.22b). It is specific, safe, quick and relatively inexpensive. However, false-positive results can result from non-specific staining or from cross-reaction with similar antigens.

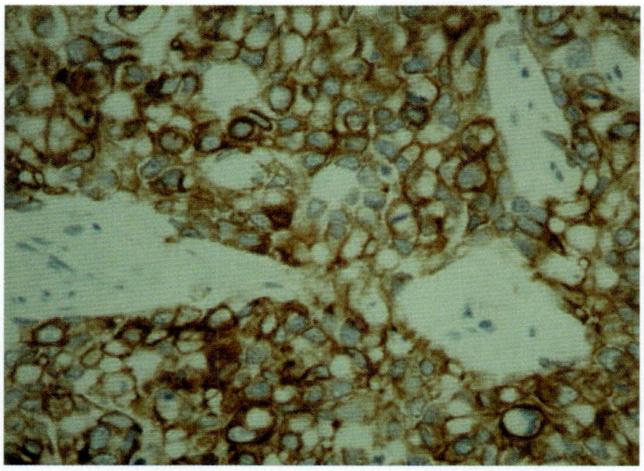

Figure 15.25 Diffuse immunohistochemical staining (brown) for a pancytokeratin marker in a malignancy, favouring carcinoma over other tumours.

Immunohistochemistry: tumour pathology

Immunohistochemistry has multiple applications in tumour pathology, including determination of cell type/direction of differentiation and elucidation of site of origin. Immunohistochemistry may also help to confirm neoplasia, determine the selection of treatment and refine prognostic predictions (Summary box 15.11).

Various immunohistochemical stains are used to detect cell type. Cytokeratins are expressed by epithelial cells. Cytokeratin positivity favours carcinoma (Figure 15.25) over other malignancies. Lymphoid markers include the panlymphoid marker CD45, the T-cell marker CD3 and the B-cell marker CD20. Markers of melanocytic differentiation include S100, MelanA and HMB45. Chromogranin, synaptophysin and CD56 stain neuroendocrine tumours such as carcinoid and small cell carcinoma. A gastrointestinal stromal tumour (GIST) typically expresses CD117 (Figure 15.26a and b) and DOG-1. Endothelial cell markers

Summary box 15.11

Some immunohistochemical stains used for tumours

- Cell type/site of origin:
  - Epithelial (carcinoma): cytokeratins
  - Lymphoid (lymphoma): CD45, CD3, CD20
  - Melanocytic (melanoma): S100
  - Neuroendocrine: synaptophysin, chromogranin
  - Vascular: CD31
  - Myoid: desmin, actin
- Site of origin/cell type:
  - Prostate: prostate-specific antigen (PSA)
  - Lung: thyroid transcription factor-1 (TTF-1)
  - Thyroid: thyroglobulin
  - Colorectum: cytokeratin 20 (CK20), CDX2
  - Liver: HepPar
  - Gastrointestinal stromal tumour (GIST): CD117, DOG-1
- Prognosis and treatment:
  - Breast carcinoma: receptors (ER, PR, HER2)
  - Endocrine tumours: Ki67 proliferative index

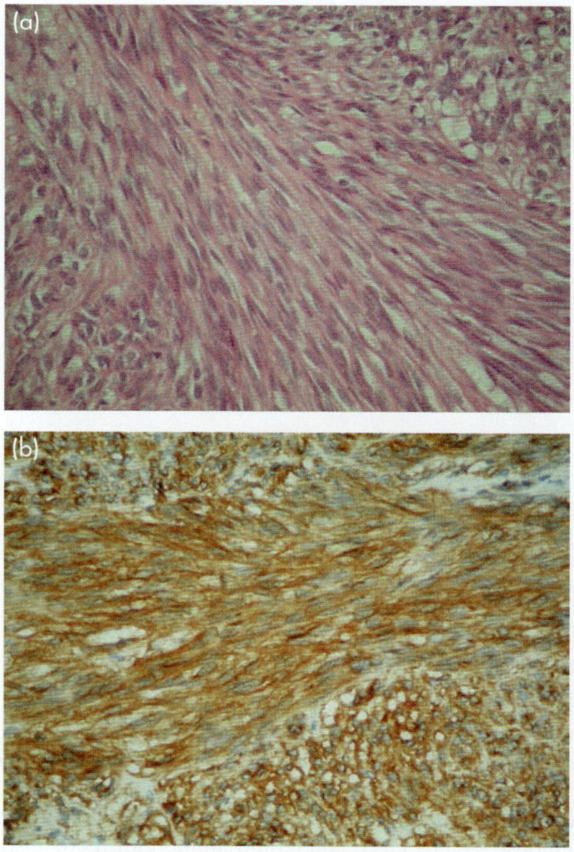

Figure 15.26 (a) A metastatic tumour composed of spindle cells. Gastrointestinal stromal tumour (GIST) was suspected. (b) Positive immunohistochemistry for CD117, confirming GIST.

Ira Thompson van Gieson, 1866–1913, an American neuropathologist, described this stain in 1889.
Aldred Scott Warthin, 1866–1931, Professor of Pathology, The University of Michigan, Ann Arbor, MI, USA.

include CD31, which may highlight vascular invasion or confirm a diagnosis of vascular neoplasia.

The site of origin of a metastatic tumour may be suggested by H&E appearances. For example, a clear cell carcinoma (Figure 15.17) is most likely to be of renal origin while an adenocarcinoma has several possible sources. Immunostains may provide further information. Some are highly specific, e.g. prostate-specific antigen (PSA) and thyroglobulin. Others are somewhat less specific, e.g. thyroid transcription factor-1 (TTF-1), which favours bronchogenic origin; HepPar, which favours hepatocellular origin; and cytokeratin 20 and CDX2 which are typically expressed by colorectal carcinoma. Carcinoembryonic antigen (CEA) is seen in several types of carcinoma (Figure 15.22a and b), while CA125 is a marker for ovarian and other gynaecological tumours. However, some tumours (especially poorly differentiated examples) do not conform to the typical patterns. Therefore, the clinical picture and imaging results must always be taken into account.

Less often, immunohistochemistry is used to help confirm malignancy. For example, light chain restriction (expression of only one immunoglobulin light chain) in lymphoid proliferations suggests clonality and favours neoplasia.

Immunohistochemistry may also play a role in the selection of treatment and in predicting prognosis. For example, carcinomas of the breast are routinely assessed for oestrogen receptor (ER), progesterone receptor (PR) and HER2 status, while lymphomas are typically subjected to a comprehensive panel of markers. Assessment of the Ki67 proliferative index enhances the management of endocrine tumours and some other neoplasms (Figure 15.27).

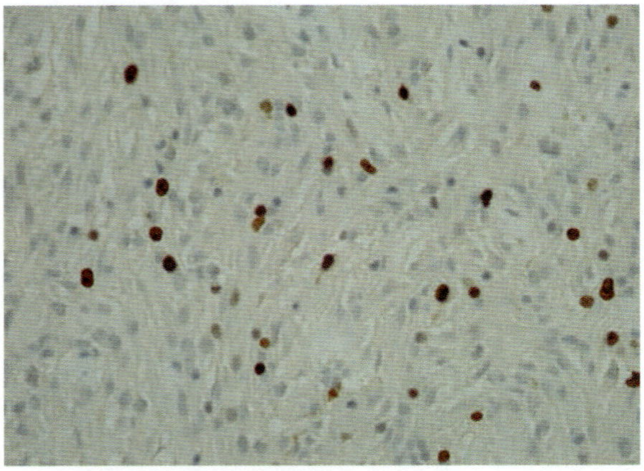

Figure 15.27 Immunohistochemistry for Ki67. The proliferative index is approximately 10 per cent.

Immunohistochemistry: infections and other applications

There are antibodies to many infective agents, including cytomegalovirus (CMV), Epstein–Barr virus (EBV), herpes simplex virus, human herpes virus 8 (HHV8), hepatitis B virus and *Helicobacter pylori*. Some of these, e.g. EBV and HHV8, cannot be demonstrated by H&E and require immunohistochemistry or other techniques for their detection.

Immunohistochemistry can also be used to study immunoglobulin and complement expression (e.g. in lymphomas or renal biopsies), to assess the abnormal accumulation of various proteins such as alpha-1-antitrypsin (A1AT), to characterise amyloid, and to screen for mismatch repair gene mutations (Summary box 15.12).

Summary box 15.12

Uses of immunohistochemistry

- Cell type
- Neoplasia:
  - Differentiation
  - Determination of site of origin
  - Confirmation of neoplasia
  - Selection of treatment
  - Screening for mutations
  - Prognosis
- Micro-organisms
- Other:
  - Amyloid
  - Immunoglobulins
  - Complement

ELECTRON MICROSCOPY

Electron microscopy allows tissue to be visualised at very high magnification, e.g. ×1000 to ×500 000. It may help to decide the lineage of a non-neoplastic or neoplastic cell in difficult cases, and may help to determine the nature of abnormal deposits, e.g. in renal disease. Unfortunately, it is time-consuming, labour intensive and expensive, and is now used very selectively.

IN SITU HYBRIDISATION

In situ hybridisation (ISH) uses a labelled oligonucleotide probe targeted at a specific RNA or DNA sequence. It can be performed on fixed or fresh tissue sections, allowing the presence or absence of a particular sequence and its location to be determined. Viral genomes, e.g. EBV (Figure 15.28), CMV and human papillomavirus, can be detected using this approach.

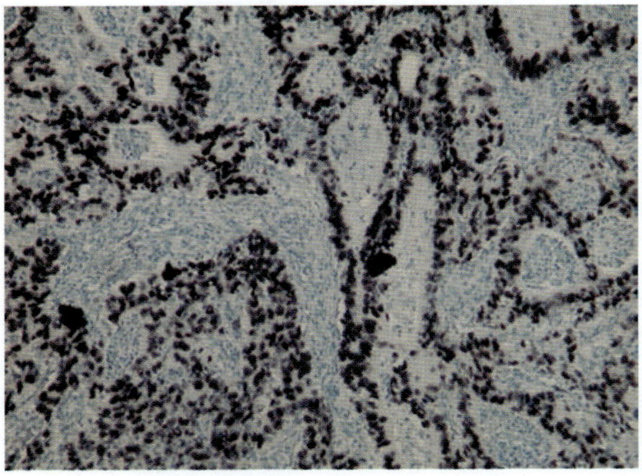

Figure 15.28 *In situ* hybridisation for Epstein–Barr virus (EBV) showing extensive nuclear positivity (black nuclei) in a gastric adenocarcinoma.

Michael Anthony Epstein, born 1921, formerly Professor of Pathology, the University of Bristol, Bristol, UK.
Yvonne Barr, born 1931, a virologist who emigrated to Australia. Epstein and Barr discovered this virus in 1964.

Interphase cytogenetics

This technique is relatively safe and fast and has largely replaced conventional cytogenetics for the analysis of chromosomal changes. It relies mainly on fluorescent *in situ* hybridisation (FISH) (named after the probe's fluorescent label), but also silver *in situ* hybridisation (SISH) and other methods. Fresh and fixed histological material and cytological preparations can be used, the latter typically yielding better results. The probe can target centromeres in order to assess numerical or structural chromosomal abnormalities or can target specific genes.

The technique is used (alongside immunohistochemistry) to detect HER2 amplification in breast cancer and, more recently, in advanced gastric cancer. The results inform the selection of therapy. Other uses include detection of chromosomal gains, losses, and translocations in tumours (e.g. haematological malignancies) and non-neoplastic conditions (e.g. trisomy 23) and loss of specific gene regions in tumours (e.g. 1p and 19q in oligodendrogliomas). Some of these changes can also be detected using PCR, which is more expensive.

POLYMERASE CHAIN REACTION-BASED AND RELATED TECHNIQUES

The PCR amplifies DNA, yielding millions of copies from a single copy of a selected target. The amplified DNA is detected using various techniques, e.g. electrophoresis. RNA can also be amplified, using the technique of reverse transcriptase polymerase chain reaction (RT-PCR). PCR is highly sensitive, fast and safe. However, it is expensive and has a high chance of contamination with DNA from outside sources. PCR can be performed on non-tissue samples (e.g. peripheral blood) and on homogenised fresh tissue. DNA or RNA extracted from formalin fixed tissue may be of lower quality but is also widely used. PCR has many clinical applications, particularly the detection of gene mutations and amplifications and the confirmation of clonality in tumours (Summary box 15.13).

Summary box 15.13

Clinical applications of PCR to tissue samples

- Mutational analysis
- Clonality
- Loss of heterozygosity
- Chromosomal abnormalities
- Detection of micro-organisms

Detection of mutations

Mutational analysis includes screening methods and direct sequencing. Direct sequencing for mutations requires DNA, which has usually been amplified using PCR.

A germline mutation may predispose a patient to a specific disease or tumour. If the mutation is known, a sample of blood or tissue can be used to test patients and screen their families for the disease. For example, most patients with hereditary haemochromatosis are homozygous for a mutation of the *HFE* gene. Another example is colorectal carcinoma which can harbour germline or sporadic mutations of the *APC* gene (Figure 15.29) or of mismatch repair genes (MLH1, MSH2, MSH6, PMS2). Immunohistochemistry on fixed tumour tissue can be used to screen for mismatch repair gene defects (Figure 15.30), allowing

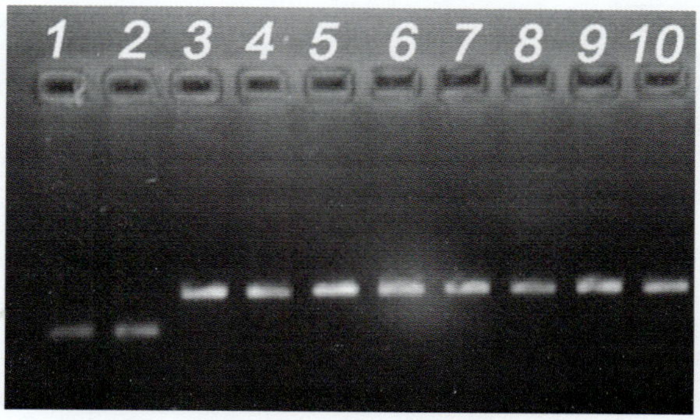

Figure 15.29 Mutation analysis of the *APC* gene. Several different tumours have been tested for mutation of the *APC* gene by polymerase chain reaction (PCR). Samples 1 and 2 (colorectal cancers) show loss of part of the *APC* gene resulting in smaller sized PCR products. All samples underwent sequence analysis, and point mutations (resulting in sequence change without loss of DNA) were identified in samples 5 and 7 (also colorectal cancers) (courtesy of Professor M Ilyas, Nottingham University, UK).

(a)

(b)

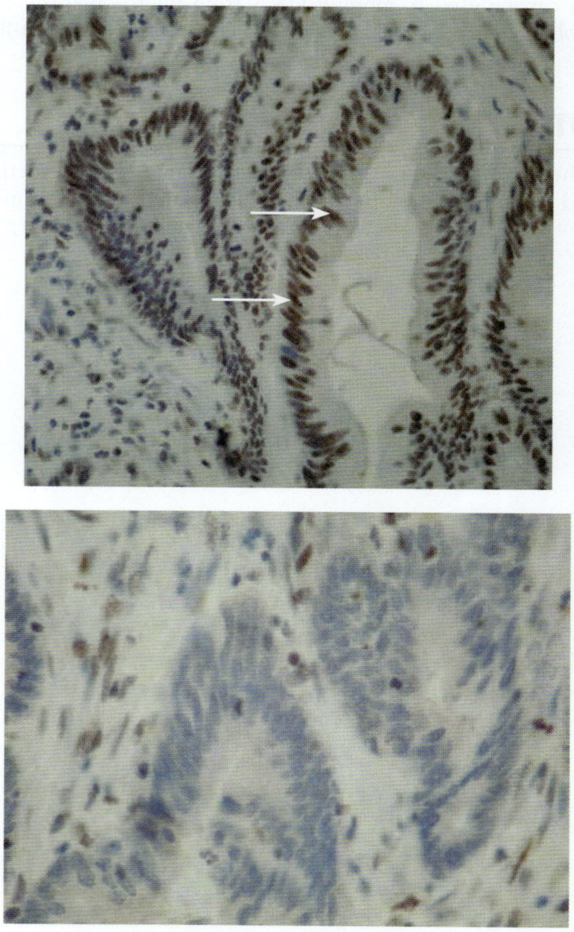

Figure 15.30 Immunohistochemical screening for mismatch repair gene mutations in a carcinoma. (a) Nuclear MLH1 expression is retained (arrows showing positively staining brown neoplastic nuclei). (b) In contrast, MSH2 expression is lost, suggesting a mismatch repair gene abnormality.

Eugen von Hippel, 1867–1939, Professor of Ophthalmology, Göttingen, Germany.
Arvid Lindau, 1892–1958, Professor of Pathology, Lund, Sweden.

a subsequent decision about direct sequencing and family screening to be made.

Analysis of mutations in tumour tissue can also enhance treatment plans. For example, detection and characterisation of KIT and PDGFRA gene mutations in GIST can help confirm the diagnosis, refine prognostic predictions, and assist with selection of drug therapy for advanced lesions. K-RAS mutational analysis in metastatic colorectal carcinoma may help predict response to anti-EGFR chemotherapy.

Clonality

Clonal immunoglobulin heavy chain (IgH) gene rearrangements in B-cell proliferations and clonal T-cell receptor gene rearrangements in T-cell proliferations favour lymphoma over reactive proliferations. These rearrangements can be detected using PCR.

Loss of heterozygosity

PCR-based methods are the most reliable for detection of loss of heterozygosity. FISH can yield similar information and is quicker and cheaper.

Micro-organisms

PCR can be used to amplify DNA from micro-organisms, e.g. *Mycobacterium tuberculosis*. It can be performed on formalin-fixed tissue, but the reliability of this approach is variable.

AUTOPSY

In the past, advances in medical knowledge were sometimes based on autopsy findings. Autopsies remain very useful for medical education and audit. In the UK, there are two types of autopsy. The first is the coroner's post-mortem, when the coroner has decided that there is a legal need to establish the cause of death. The second is the hospital autopsy, which requires relatives' consent. This type occurs less frequently now than in the past. In most cases, all organs are examined. Tissue may be retained for further examination if appropriate and if permitted by ethical guidelines.

SUMMARY

Analysis of tissue has played a steadily more important role in clinical management over the past few decades. Accordingly, pathologists work more closely with surgeons and their teams than ever before, and the interaction is greatly enhanced when the surgeon appreciates the value and limitations of tissue diagnosis.

ACKNOWLEDGEMENT

The author is grateful to Professor MT Sheaff for assistance with the sections on cytology.

FURTHER READING

Kumar V, Abbas AK, Fausto N, Aster JC. *Robbins and Cotran. Pathologic basis of disease*, 8th edn. Philadelphia: Saunders Elsevier, 2010.
Rosai J (ed.). *Rosai and Ackerman's surgical pathology*, 10th edn. Philadelphia: Mosby Elsevier, 2011.

PART

3 Perioperative care

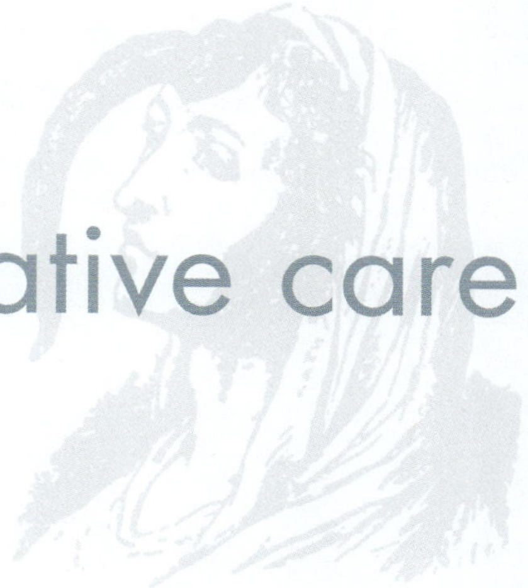

CHAPTER 16

Preoperative preparation

LEARNING OBJECTIVES

To be able:
- To organise preoperative care and the operating list

To understand:
- Surgical, medical and anaesthetic aspects of assessment
- How to optimise the patient's condition
- How to take consent
- How to organise an operating list

INTRODUCTION

Many patients requiring inpatient elective procedures arrive in hospital on the day of surgery. Therefore a 'preoperative assessment' clinic may be the only opportunity to gather all information, optimise comorbidities, and then organise anaesthetic, surgical and postoperative care before surgery actually takes place.

First, a history should be taken, examination performed and the relevant investigations ordered. Focus should then turn to the specific problems uncovered. All sources of information should be exploited including the patient, the general practioner (GP) and hospital records. GPs can offer valuable help by monitoring chronic conditions, adjusting medications, facilitating weight reduction, as well as encouraging the patient to take exercise and stop smoking.

Patients with severe comorbidities should be referred to the relevant specialist to quantify the risks and to take appropriate measures to minimise operative morbidity. Surgery cannot be made risk free, but risks must be known so that the patient can make an informed decision. Patients should be given advice on when they should be nil by mouth (NBM) and what to do about regular medications and premedication.

Finally, a plan for the operating list should be drawn up and all those involved in making the list run smoothly should be informed (Summary box 16.1).

Summary box 16.1

Preoperative plan for the best patient outcomes

- Gather and record all relevant information
- Optimise patient condition
- Choose surgery that offers minimal risk and maximum benefit
- Anticipate and plan for adverse events
- Inform everyone concerned

PATIENT ASSESSMENT

The aim of a structured assessment is to learn to look actively for risks and manage them so as to enable surgery to go ahead safely. Assessment is done by the surgical, nursing team and/or anaesthetic team at outpatient or inpatient setting.

History taking

A standard history should be taken focusing on the patient's hopes and expectations (open questions and then listen), then on specific questions aimed at clarifying the diagnosis and severity of symptoms (closed questions). A set of fixed questions are needed to determine 'fitness' for surgery. Surgery-specific symptoms (including features not present), onset, duration and exacerbating and relieving factors should also be documented.

For each system a relevant history should be taken, noting what problems have occurred and when (Table 16.1). These should include a cardiovascular history focusing on high blood pressure, chest pains, palpitations, syncope, dyspnoea and poor exercise tolerance. Similarly, respiratory problems should be explored further if there is history of smoking, productive cough, wheeze, dyspnoea, hoarseness of voice or stridor present. Increasing severity of symptoms generally indicates worsening of the condition.

The history of past surgery and anaesthesia can reveal problems that may present during current hospitalisation (e.g. intra-abdominal adhesions and suxamethonium apnoea). The use of recreational drugs and alcohol consumption should be noted as they are known to be associated with adverse outcomes. Check for allergies and risk factors for deep vein thrombosis (DVT). Social history, ability to communicate and mobility are important in planning rehabilitation after surgery (Summary box 16.2).

Table 16.1 Key topics in past medical history.

Cardiovascular	Ischaemic heart disease: angina, **myocardial infarction**
	Hypertension
	Heart failure
	Dysrhythmia
	Peripheral vascular disease
	Deep vein thrombosis and pulmonary embolism
Respiratory	Chronic obstructive pulmonary disease
	Asthma
	Respiratory infections
Gastrointestinal	Peptic ulcer disease and gastro-oesophageal reflux
	Liver disease
Genitourinary tract	Urinary tract infection
	Renal dysfunction
Neurological	Epilepsy
	Cerebrovascular accidents and transient ischaemic attacks
	Psychiatric disorders
	Cognitive function
Endocrine/metabolic	Diabetes
	Thyroid dysfunction
	Phaeochromocytoma
	Porphyria
Locomotor system	Osteoarthritis
	Inflammatory arthropathy, such as rheumatoid arthritis
Other	Human immunodeficiency virus
	Hepatitis
	Tuberculosis
	Malignancy
	Allergy
Previous surgery	**Problems encountered**
	Family history of problems with anaesthesia

Those in bold font need recording even when negative.

Summary box 16.2

Principles of history taking

- Listen: What is the problem? (Open questions)
- Clarify: What does the patient expect? (Closed questions)
- Narrow: Differential diagnosis (Focused questions)
- Fitness: Comorbidities (Fixed questions)

Examination

Patients should be treated with respect and dignity, receive a clear explanation of the examination undertaken and kept as comfortable as possible (Table 16.2). A chaperone should always be present, especially for intimate examinations.

Table 16.2 Medical examination.

General	Anaemia, jaundice, cyanosis, nutritional status, sources of infection (teeth, feet, leg ulcers)
Cardiovascular	Pulse, blood pressure, heart sounds, bruits, peripheral oedema
Respiratory	Respiratory rate and effort, chest expansion and percussion note, breath sounds, oxygen saturation
Gastrointestinal	Abdominal masses, ascites, bowel sounds, hernia, genitalia
Neurological	Consciousness level, cognitive function, sensation, muscle power, tone and reflexes
Airway assessment	

Along with routine cardiovascular examination one should look specifically for evidence of cardiac failure (raised jugular venous pressure (JVP), fine crackles, gallop rhythm), peripheral vascular disease (loss of peripheral pulses, ulcerations) and valvular heart disease with characteristic murmurs (e.g. ejection systolic in aortic stenosis, pansystolic in tricuspid regurgitation and mid-diastolic murmur in mitral stenosis heard at the respective area on auscultation) in symptomatic patients.

Presence of a high respiratory rate, reduced air entry, crepitations and ronchi indicate respiratory problems. History of dyspnoea along with examination findings of tachycardia, raised JVP, tricuspid regurgitation, hepatomegaly and oedema of the feet will indicate severe respiratory disease with pulmonary hypertension and right ventricular failure (Summary box 16.3).

Summary box 16.3

Examination

- General: Positive findings even if not related to the proposed procedure should be explored
- Surgery related: Type and site of surgery, complications which have occurred due to underlying pathology
- Systemic: Comorbidities and their severity
- Specific: For example, suitability for positioning during surgery

Examination specific to surgery

At preoperative assessment, the clinical findings, site, side, specific imaging or investigation findings related to the pathology for which the surgery is proposed should be noted. Suitability of the patient for the proposed surgical option and vice versa should also be assessed. For example, laparoscopic procedures are less invasive and are therefore preferred in most. However not all patients can tolerate a pneumoperitoneum, head-down positioning, etc.

Surgery puts the patient's life 'at risk' and so the benefit of the procedure should outweigh the risk of surgery. Type of surgery along with patient comorbidities determine perioperative risks, for example perioperative mortality in major surgery, such as that of aortic aneurysm repair in the UK is 4–5 per cent.

Sources of potential bacteraemia can compromise surgical results especially if artificial material is implanted, such as in joint replacement surgery or arterial grafting. Check for and treat infections in the preoperative period (e.g. infected toes, pressure sores, teeth and urine; screen the patients for methicillin-resistant *Staphylococcus aureus* colonisation).

Investigations

Minor and intermediate surgery generally requires no routine investigations unless the patient has comorbidities. The UK National Institute of Health and Clinical Excellence (NICE) guidelines lay out the investigations needed for various categories of surgery (Summary box 16.4).

Summary box 16.4

Investigations needed

- Type of surgery: Major surgery can lead to organ system dysfunction so needs most investigations
- Patient: For example, sickle cell test for patient with Afro-Caribbean origin
- Comorbidities: For example, peak flow rates for severe asthmatics

- **Full blood count.** A full blood count (FBC) is needed for major operations, in the elderly and in those with anaemia or pathology with ongoing blood loss. A sickle cell test is needed in any patient of Afro-Caribbean origin.
- **Urea and electrolytes.** Urea and electrolytes (U&E) are needed before all major operations, in most patients over 60 years of age especially with cardiovascular, renal and endocrine disease or if significant blood loss is anticipated. It is also needed in those on medications which affect electrolyte levels, e.g. steroids, diuretics, digoxin, NSAIDs (non-steroidal anti-inflammatory drugs), intravenous fluid or nutrition therapy.
- **Electrocardiography.** Electrocardiography (ECG) is required for those patients aged over 60 years, cardiovascular, renal and cerebrovascular involvement, diabetes and in those with severe respiratory problems.
- **Clotting screen.** If a patient has a history suggestive of bleeding diathesis, liver disease, eclampsia, cholestasis or has a family history of bleeding disorder, or is on antithrombotic or anticoagulant agents, then coagulation screening will be needed. However, the effects of antiplatelet agents, low molecular weight heparins and newer agents affecting factor Xa cannot be measured by routine laboratory tests.
- **Chest radiography.** A chest x-ray is not required unless the patient has a significant cardiac history, cardiac failure, severe chronic obstructive pulmonary disease (COPD), acute respiratory symptoms, pulmonary cancer, metastasis or effusions, or is at risk of tuberculosis.
- **Urinalysis.** Dipstick testing of urine should be performed on all patients to detect urinary infection, biliuria, glycosuria and inappropriate osmolality.
- **β-Human chorionic gonadotrophin.** Pregnancy needs to be ruled out in all women of childbearing age.
- **Blood glucose and HbA1c.** These should be performed in patients with diabetes mellitus and endocrine problems. HbA1c indicates how well diabetes has been controlled over a longer duration.
- **Arterial blood gases.** This test allows detailed assessment of severe respiratory conditions and acid–base disturbances.
- **Liver function tests.** These are indicated in patients with jaundice, known or suspected hepatitis, cirrhosis, malignancy or patients with poor nutritional reserves.
- **Other investigations.** Further relevant investigations should be undertaken to assess capacity of specific organ system and risks associated. Specialist radiological views and recent imaging are sometimes required. If imaging is going to be needed during surgery then this needs to be planned in advance.

SPECIFIC PREOPERATIVE PROBLEMS, REFERRALS AND MANAGEMENT

Specific medical problems encountered during preoperative assessment should be corrected to the best possible level. Many patients with severe disease will need to be referred to specialists; the referral letter should include all the details including history, examination and investigation results (Summary box 16.5).

Summary box 16.5

Preoperative management of patients with systemic disease

- Capacity: Baseline organ function capacity should be assessed
- Optimisation: Medication, lifestyle changes, specialist referral will improve organ capacity
- Alternative: Minimally impacting procedure, appropriate postoperative care will improve outcomes
- Theatre preparations: Timing, teamwork, special instruments and equipment

Cardiovascular disease

Patients who can climb a flight of stairs without getting short of breath or having chest pain, or indeed stopping have a lower risk of perioperative morbidity and mortality of cardiovascular origin than those who cannot.

At preoperative assessment, it is important to identify the patients who have a high perioperative risk of myocardial infarction (MI) and make appropriate arrangements to reduce this risk. These patients include those who have suffered coronary artery disease, congestive cardiac failure, arrhythmias, severe peripheral vascular disease, cerebrovascular disease or renal failure, especially if they are undergoing intra-abdominal or intrathoracic surgery.

In patients with ischaemic heart disease (IHD), the left ventricular status can be evaluated using a stress test. The test has a high negative predictive value and a low positive predictive value. In other words, if the test is negative, then the patient is unlikely to have IHD and if it is positive the chances of the patient actually having IHD is not high.

For patients with symptomatic valvular heart disease or poor left ventricular function, an echocardiography should be performed. Pressure gradients across the valves, dimensions of the chambers and contractility can be determined using echocardiography; an ejection fraction of less than 30 per cent is associated with poor patient outcomes.

Cardiopulmonary exercise testing when performed provides a non-invasive assessment of combined pulmonary, cardiac and circulatory function.

The patient should be referred to a cardiologist if:

- A murmur is heard and the patient is symptomatic.
- The patient is known to have poor left ventricular function or cardiomegaly.
- Ischaemic changes can be seen on ECG even if patient is not symptomatic (silent MI).
- There is an abnormal rhythm on the ECG, tachy/bradycardia or a heart block that may lead to cardiovascular compromise.

Hypertension, ischaemic heart disease and stents

Prior to elective surgery, blood pressure should be controlled to near 160/90 mmHg. If a new antihypertensive is introduced, a stabilisation period of at least 2 weeks should be allowed.

Patients with angina which is not well controlled should be investigated further by a cardiologist (Figure 16.1). Some of these patients may need thrombolysis, percutaneous coronary balloon angioplasty, statins, coronary artery bypass surgery or coronary stenting prior to non-cardiac surgery.

Elective surgery should be postponed for three to six months after a proven myocardial infarct to reduce the risk of perioperative reinfarction.

Patients may have had coronary stents inserted for IHD and should be asked about effectiveness of the treatment, concurrent antiplatelet medications, e.g. clopidrogel and/or aspirin. Risk of stent thrombosis with consequences of MI and death is reduced if elective surgery is delayed until after dual antiplatelet therapy is stopped (about 6 weeks after bare metal and 12 months after drug-eluting stent insertion).

If surgery cannot be postponed and the risk of significant perioperative bleeding is low, the dual antiplatelet therapy can be continued during surgery. If surgery poses a significant risk (spinal, intracranial, cardiac, posterior chamber of eye and prostate surgery), clopidrogel may be stopped and aspirin continued, however, cardiology opinion will need to be sought.

Most long-term cardiac medications should be continued over the perioperative period. Ongoing treatment with beta-blockers and statins is known to reduce perioperative morbidity and mortality.

Dysrhythmias

In patients with atrial fibrillation, beta-blockers, digoxin or calcium channel blockers should be started preoperatively (or continued if the patient is already on the treatment) in order to control the rate and possibly rhythm. Cardiac output can increase by 15 per cent if sinus rhythm is restored. This reduces the risk of perioperative myocardial ischaemia and infarction. Warfarin in patients with atrial fibrillation should be stopped 5 days preoperatively to achieve an INR (international normalised ratio) of 1.5 or less, which is safe for most surgery; an alternative anticoagulation is not required in the perioperative period.

Implanted pacemaker and cardiac defibrillator checks and appropriate reprogramming should be done preoperatively. Bipolar diathermy activity during surgery may be sensed by the pacemaker as ventricular fibrillation. Therefore, cardioversion and overpace modes may be turned off (switch on after surgery) or converted to 'ventricle paced, not sensed with no response to sensing' (VOO) mode especially if bipolar diathermy cannot be used.

Symptomatic heart blocks and asymptomatic second- (Mobitz II) and third-degree heart blocks, if discovered at preoperative assessment clinic, will need cardiology consultation and temporary pacemaker insertion.

Figures 16.2 and 16.3 illustrate two cases requiring preoperative optimisation.

Valvular heart disease

While anaesthetic management is altered to achieve haemodynamic stability in moderate valvular diseases, the patients with severe aortic and mitral stenosis may benefit from valvuloplasty before undergoing elective non-cardiac surgery. Appropriate referral to anaesthetist and cardiologists should be made.

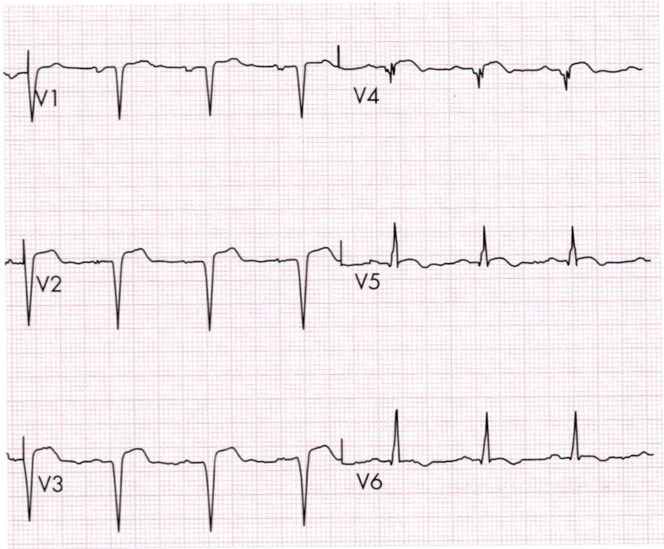

Figure 16.1 Preoperative electrocardiogram of a patient who complained of chest pain the previous day showing recent transmural anterior myocardial infarction with Q waves and ST elevation.

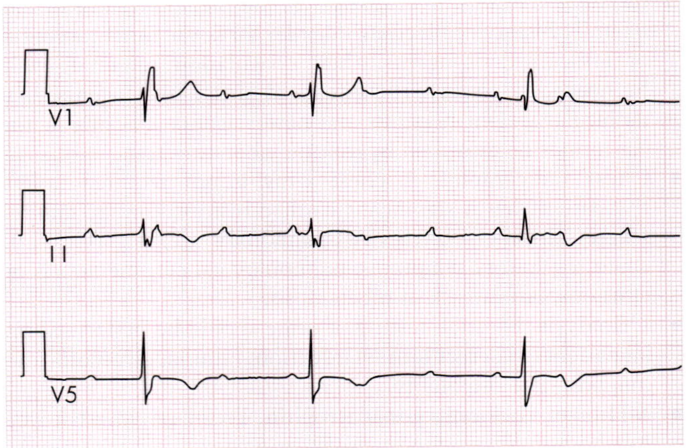

Figure 16.2 Routine preoperative electrocardiogram in an 83-year-old patient with no symptoms other than lethargy for the last three months. This shows complete heart block with dissociated P waves and QRS complexes, requiring preoperative pacing.

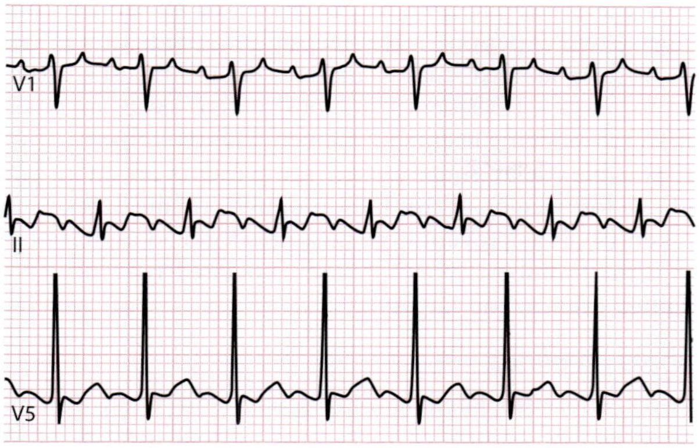

Figure 16.3 Atrial flutter.

In patients with mechanical heart valves, warfarin needs to be stopped for 5 days before surgery, and an infusion of unfractionated heparin started when the INR falls below 1.5. The activated partial thromboplastin time (APTT) should be monitored to keep it at 1.5 times normal and the infusion is then stopped 2 hours before surgery. Heparin and warfarin should be started in the postoperative period and heparin is stopped when the full effect of warfarin is realised.

Anaemia and blood transfusion

Patients found to be anaemic at preoperative assessment should be treated with iron and vitamin supplements. Chronic anaemia is well tolerated in the perioperative period; however, if the patient is undergoing a major procedure, preoperative transfusion may be considered below a haemoglobin level of 8 g/dL. If excessive bleeding is expected, then a preoperative 'group and save' should be performed and an appropriate number of units of blood crossmatched.

Jehovah's Witness patients usually refuse blood transfusion; the legal document as to which blood and products they will accept or refuse should be made available and abided by (e.g. cell salvage, reinfusion from drains may be acceptable).

Respiratory disease

The patient's current respiratory status should be compared with their 'normal state'. Note should be made of regular treatment, records of peak expiratory flow rates (PEFR), use of steroids, home oxygen and continuous positive airway pressure (CPAP) ventilation; check for evidence of right heart failure.

Encourage the patients to be compliant with the medications, take exercise and a balanced diet, and stop smoking.

Administration of regular medications with an additional dose of bronchodilators given just prior to surgery will reduce the chances of untoward events. Patients taking more than 10 mg of prednisolone and undergoing high-risk surgery will need perioperative steroid supplements.

Regional anaesthetic techniques and less invasive surgical options should be considered in severe cases. Elective surgery should be postponed until acute exacerbations are treated.

Refer the patient to respiratory physicians if:

- There is a severe disease or significant deterioration from usual condition.
- Major surgery is planned in a patient with significant respiratory comorbidities.
- Right heart failure is present: dyspnoea, fatigue, tricuspid regurgitation, hepatomegaly and oedema of the feet.
- The patient is young with COPD (indicates a rare and life-threatening condition).

Pulmonary function tests will indicate the type and severity of the disease, as well as response to the treatment.

Smoking

Information should be provided to indicate perioperative risks associated with smoking. Stopping smoking reduces carbon monoxide levels and the patient is better able to clear sputum.

Asthma

It is important to establish the severity of the asthma, precipitating causes, frequency of bronchodilator and steroid use, PEFR (peak expiratory flow rate) and any previous intensive care unit admissions. Patients should continue to use their regular inhalers until the start of anaesthesia. Brittle asthmatics may also need extra steroid cover.

Chronic obstructive pulmonary disease

Patients on steroid treatment, or oxygen therapy, or who have a forced expiratory volume in the first second (FEV1) less than 30 per cent of predicted value (for age, weight and height) have severe disease and may have respiratory failure in the postoperative period. Preoperative chest x-ray or scans are useful in patients with known emphysematous bullae, pulmonary cancer, metastasis or effusions. Patients with significant COPD who are undergoing major surgery will need to be referred to the respiratory physicians for optimisation of their condition.

An arterial blood gas analysis may also be useful as it can give an indication of carbon dioxide retention. This is associated with an increased risk of perioperative respiratory complications.

Infection

Elective surgery should be postponed if the patient has a chest infection. It should be treated with antibiotics and physiotherapy and the operation rescheduled after 4–6 weeks.

Gastrointestinal disease

Nil by mouth and regular medications

Patients are advised not to take solids within 6 hours and clear fluids (isotonic drinks and water) within 2 hours before anaesthetic to avoid the risk of acid aspiration syndrome. Infants are allowed a clear drink up to 2 hours, mother's milk up to 3 hours and cow or formula milk up to 6 hours before anaesthetic.

If the surgery is delayed, oral (until 2 hours of surgery) or intravenous fluids should be started especially in the vulnerable groups of patients, e.g. children, elderly and diabetics.

Patients can continue to take their specified routine medications with sips of water in the nil by mouth period.

Regurgitation risk

Patients with hiatus hernia, obesity, pregnancy and diabetes are at high risk of pulmonary aspiration even if they have been NBM before elective surgery. Clear antacids, H2-receptor blockers, e.g.

> A **Jehovah's Witness** is a member of a millenarian fundamentalist Christian sect founded in America in 1884. They have their own translation of the Bible which they interpret literally and do not allow blood transfusion.

ranitidine or proton pump inhibitors, e.g. omeprazole, may be given at the appropriate time in the preoperative period.

Liver disease

In patients with liver disease, the cause of the disease needs to be known, as well as any evidence of clotting problems, renal involvement, and encephalopathy. Elective surgery should be postponed until any acute episode has settled (e.g. cholangitis). The blood tests which need to be performed are liver function tests, coagulation, blood glucose, urea and electrolyte levels. The presence of ascitis, oesophageal varices, hypoalbuminaemia, sodium and water retention should be noted as all these can influence choice and outcomes of anaesthesia and surgery.

Genitourinary disease

Renal disease

Underlying conditions leading to chronic renal failure, such as diabetes mellitus, hypertension and ischaemic heart disease, should be stabilised before elective surgery. Appropriate measures should be taken to treat acidosis, hypocalcaemia and hyperkalaemia of greater than 6 mmol/L. Arrangements should be made to continue peritoneal or haemodialysis until a few hours before surgery. After the final dialysis before surgery, a blood sample should be sent for FBC and U&E.

Chronic renal failure patients often suffer chronic microcytic anaemic that is well tolerated, therefore preoperative blood transfusion is usually not necessary.

Acute renal failure can present with acute surgical problems, for example bowel obstruction needing emergency surgery. In such patients, simultaneous medical and surgical treatment and critical care unit support will be needed in the perioperative period.

Urinary tract infection

Uncomplicated urinary infections are common in women, while outflow uropathy with chronically infected urine is common in men. These infections should be treated before embarking on elective surgery where infection carries dire consequences, e.g. joint replacement. For emergency procedures, antibiotics should be started and care taken to ensure that the patient maintains a good urine output before, during and after surgery.

Endocrine and metabolic disorders

Malnutrition

Body mass index (BMI) is weight in kilograms divided by height in metres squared. A BMI of less than 18.5 indicates nutritional impairment and a BMI of less than 15 is associated with significant hospital mortality. Nutritional support for a minimum of 2 weeks before surgery is required to have any impact on subsequent morbidity.

If a patient is unlikely to be able to eat for a significant period, arrangements should be made by the preoperative assessment team to start nutritional support in the immediate postoperative phase.

Obesity

Morbid obesity is defined as BMI of more than 35 and is associated with increased risk of postoperative complications. Patients should be made aware of risks involved and advised on healthy eating and taking regular exercise.

Associated sleep apnoea can be predicted by using a clinical scoring system of perioperative sleep apnoea prediction (P-SAP) score or sleep apnoea studies. Patients should be asked to continue to use a CPAP device for obstructive sleep apnoea and cholesterol-reducing agents in the perioperative phase.

If possible, delay surgery until the patients are more active and have lost weight. If this fails, prophylactic measures need to be taken (such as preventative measures for acid aspiration and deep vein thrombosis (DVT)) and associated risks need to be explained prior to the surgery.

Diabetes mellitus

Diabetes and associated cardiovascular and renal complications should be controlled to as near normal level as possible before embarking on elective surgery. Any history of hyper- and hypoglycaemic episodes, and hospital admissions, should be noted. HbA1c levels should be checked. Lipid-lowering medication should be started in patients who are in a high-risk group of cardiovascular complications of diabetes.

Patients with diabetes should be first on the operating list and if they are operated on in the morning advised to omit the morning dose of medication and breakfast. Though tight control of blood sugar is not needed, the patient's blood sugar levels should be checked every 2 hours. For those on the afternoon list, breakfast can be given with half their regular dose of insulin (or full-dose oral anti-diabetic agents) and then managed with regular blood sugar checks as above. An intravenous insulin sliding scale should be started for insulin-dependent diabetes mellitus undergoing major surgery or if blood sugar is difficult to control for other reasons.

Adrenocortical suppression

Patients receiving oral adrenocortical steroids should be asked about the dose and duration of the medication in view of supplementation with extra doses of steroids perioperatively to avoid an Addisonian crisis.

Coagulation disorders

Thrombophilia

Patients with a strong family history or previous personal history of thrombosis should be identified. They will need thromboprophylaxis in the perioperative period (Table 16.3).

The progesterone-only pill should be continued, however, the risks of continuing the combined pill (slight increased risk of significant thrombosis) should be weighed against the risks of an unplanned pregnancy. Hormone replacement therapy (HRT) should be stopped 6 weeks prior to surgery.

Patients with a low risk of thromboembolism can be given thromboembolism-deterrent stockings to wear during the perioperative period. High-risk patients with a history of recurrent DVT, pulmonary embolism (PE) and arterial thrombosis will be on warfarin. This should be stopped before surgery and replaced by low molecular weight heparin or factor Xa inhibitors. Each hospital has guidelines which advise what type of DVT prophylaxis should be used for each type of surgery.

Neurological and psychiatric disorders

In patients with a history of stroke, pre-existing neurological deficit should be recorded. These patients may be on antiplatelet agents or anticoagulants. If it is felt that the neurological

Thomas Addison, 1795–1860, physician, Guy's Hospital, London, UK, described the effects of the disease of the suprarenal capsules in 1849.

Table 16.3 Risk factors for thrombosis.

Age >60 years
Obesity: body mass index (BMI) >30 kg/m^2
Trauma or surgery (especially of the abdomen, pelvis and lower limbs), anaesthesia >90 minutes
Reduced mobility for more than 3 days
Pregnancy/puerperium
Varicose veins with phlebitis
Drugs, e.g. oestrogen contraceptive, hormone replacement therapy (HRT), smoking
Known active cancer or on treatment, significant medical comorbidities, critical care admission
Family/personal history of thrombosis, e.g. deficiencies in antithrombin III, protein S and C

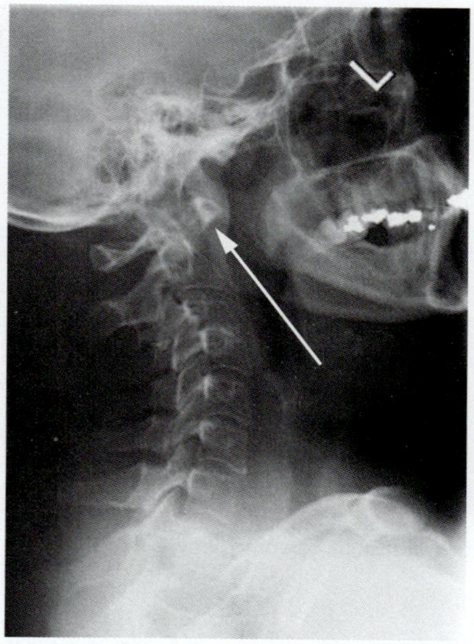

Figure 16.5 Flexion view in the same patient as in Figure 16.4. Note the huge increase in the atlantodens interval, implying significant instability at this level.

and cardiovascular thrombotic risks are low, antiplatelet agents should be withdrawn (7 days for aspirin, 10 days for clopidogrel). If the thrombotic risks are perceived to be high and the patient is undergoing surgery with a high risk of bleeding, aspirin alone should be continued.

Anticonvulsant and antiparkinson medication is continued perioperatively to help early mobilisation of the patient.

Lithium should be stopped 24 hours prior to surgery; blood levels should be measured to exclude toxicity. The anaesthetist should be informed if patients are on psychiatric medications such as tricyclic antidepressants or monoamine oxidase inhibitors, as these may interact with anaesthetic drugs.

Musculoskeletal and other disorders

Rheumatoid arthritis can lead to unstable cervical spine with the possibility of spinal cord injury during intubation. Therefore, flexion and extension lateral cervical spine x-rays should be obtained (Figures 16.4 and 16.5).

Assessment of severity of renal, cardiac valvular and pericardial involvement, as well as restrictive lung disease, should be carried out. Rheumatologists will advise on steroids and disease-modifying drugs so as to balance immunosuppression (chance of infections) against the need to stabilise the disease perioperatively (stopping disease-modifying drugs can lead to flare up of the disease).

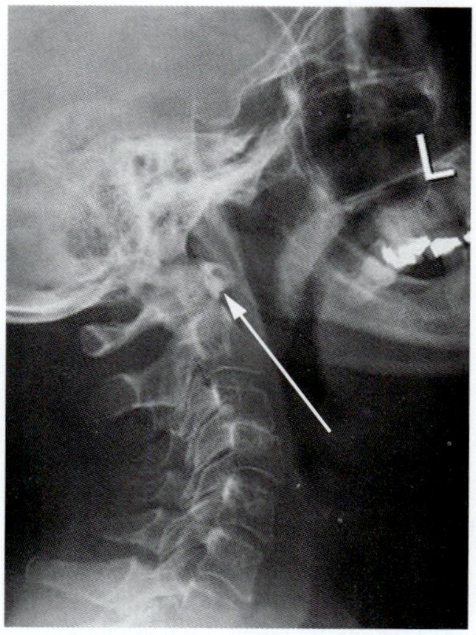

Figure 16.4 Extension view of cervical spine in patient with rheumatoid arthritis.

In ankylosing spondylitis patients in addition to the problems discussed above, techniques of spinal or epidural anaesthesia are often challenging. Patients with systemic lupus erythematosis may exhibit a hypercoagulable state along with airway difficulties.

Airway assessment

The ability to intubate the trachea and oxygenate the patient are basic and crucial skills of the anaesthetist. The ease or difficulty in performing airway manoeuvres can be predicted by simple examination findings of full mouth opening (modified Mallampati class), jaw protrusion, neck movement and thyromental distance. The Samsoon and Young modified Mallampati test is performed with the clinician sitting in front of the patient, with the patient's mouth open and tongue protruding (Figure 16.6). The higher the grade, the higher the risk in obtaining and securing an airway (Table 16.4). Look for loose teeth, obvious tumours, scars, infections, obesity, thickness of the neck, etc., which will indicate difficulty in obtaining the airway. When more than one of the above tests is positive, the chances of experiencing difficulty in obtaining and securing the airway become greater.

Table 16.4 Airway assessment (Samsoon and Young modified Mallampati test).

Fauces, pillars, soft palate and uvula seen	Grade 1
Fauces, soft palate with some part of uvula seen	Grade 2
Soft palate seen	Grade 3
Hard palate only seen	Grade 4

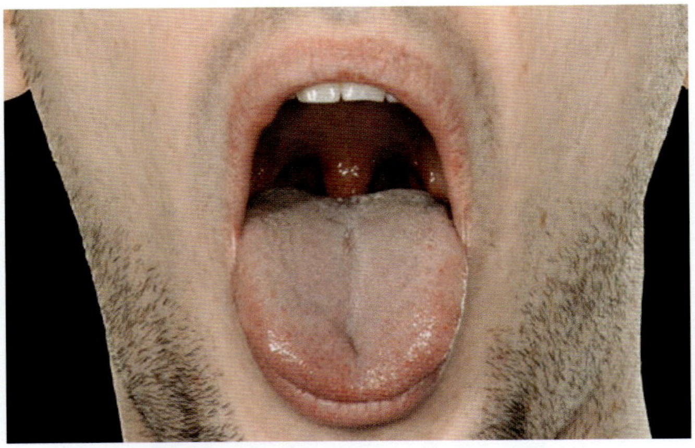

Figure 16.6 Normal mouth opening view.

Preoperative assessment in emergency surgery

In urgent or emergency surgery, the principles of preoperative assessment should be the same as in elective surgery, except that the opportunity to optimise the condition is limited by time constraints. Medical assessment and treatments should be started (e.g. according to the Advanced Trauma Life Support (ATLS) guidelines) even if there is no time to complete those before the surgical procedure is started. Some risks may be reduced, but some may persist and whenever possible these need to be explained to the patient (Summary box 16.6).

Summary box 16.6

Preoperative assessment for emergency surgery

- Start: Similar principles to that for elective surgery
- Constraints: Time, facilities available
- Consent: May not be possible in life-saving emergencies
- Organisational efforts: For example, local/national algorithms for treatment of multi-trauma patient

RISK ASSESSMENT AND CONSENT

All life- or limb-threatening complications and all complications with an incidence of 1 per cent or more should be discussed with the patient (Table 16.5). The risk of death doubles with every seven years of adult life lived. The presence of peripheral vascular disease, stroke, heart failure, myocardial infarction or renal failure each independently increases the risk of death by about 1.5 times the baseline. The risks of the surgical procedure itself are then to be added on separately.

Valid consent implies that it is given voluntarily by a competent and informed person who is not under duress (see LED TO REASON in Table 16.6) . In emergency situations or in an unconscious patient, consent may not be obtained and the procedure carried out 'in the best interests of the patient'.

Adults are presumed to have capacity to consent unless there is contrary evidence. For adults who are not deemed competent to give consent, treatment can still proceed in their best interests by filling in an inability to consent form. Those under 16 years who demonstrate the ability to appreciate the risks and benefits fully are deemed competent. This is known as Gillick competence (Summary box 16.7).

Table 16.5 Perioperative teams.

Ward, theatre and specialist nursing staff
Anaesthetic and surgical teams
Radiology, pathology involvement
Rehabilitation and social care workers
Specific personnel in individual cases

Summary box 16.7

Risk assessment and consent

- Risks: Related to the comorbidities, anaesthesia and surgery
- Explain: Advantages, side effects, prognosis
- Language: Simple, use daily life comparisons to explain risks
- Consents: Valid consent is necessary except in life-saving circumstances

ARRANGING THE THEATRE LIST

The date, place and time of operation should be matched with availability of personnel. Appropriate equipment and instruments should be made available. The operating list should be distributed as early as possible to all staff who are involved in making the list run smoothly (Table 16.5).

Prioritise patients, e.g. children and diabetic patients should be placed at the beginning of the list; life- and limb-threatening surgery should take priority; cancer patients need to be treated early.

Table 16.6 Taking a comprehensive consent (acronym LED TO REASON).

Lead in	Introduce yourself and identify the patient
Explore	How much does the patient know
Diagnosis	Why the operation is being proposed
Treatment	Explain whether the treatment proposed is in accordance with protocols and if not why not
Options	Discuss all the options including that of doing nothing, use lay language
Results	Explain likely outcome in terms of pain, mobility, work, diet and return to normal activities
Eventualities	For example, the possibility of needing to remove the testicle in a hernia operation
Adverse events	Myocardial infarction, stroke and embolus, bleeding and specific damage
Sound mind	Ask if they have understood
Open question	Check if further clarification is needed
Notes	Document everything discussed and agreed

FURTHER READING

Howard-Alpe GM, de Bono J, Hudsmith L *et al.* Coronary artery stents and non-cardiac surgery. *Br J Anaesth* 2007; **98**: 560–74.

Mental Capacity Act [2005] UK.

National Institute for Health and Clinical Excellence. CG3 preoperative tests: NICE guideline, June 2003.

Ramachandran SK, Kheterpal S, Consens F *et al.* Derivation and validation of a simple perioperative sleep apnea prediction score. *Anesth Analg* 2010; **110**: 1007–15.

van Veen JJ, Spahn DR, Makris M. Routine preoperative coagulation test: an outdated practice? *Br J Anaesth* 2011; **106**: 1–3.

CHAPTER 17

Anaesthesia and pain relief

LEARNING OBJECTIVES

To gain an understanding of:

- Techniques of anaesthesia and airway maintenance
- Methods of providing pain relief
- Local and regional anaesthesia techniques
- The management of chronic pain and pain from malignant disease

HISTORY

Anaesthesia, as we know it today was first successfully demonstrated by William Morton, a local dentist, at the Massachusetts General Hospital in Boston, USA on October 16, 1846 when he administered ether to Gilbert Abbot for operation on a vascular tumour on his neck. Earlier, Horace Wells had successfully used nitrous oxide in 1844 for painless extraction of teeth.

Simpson at Edinburgh University overcame some of the technical difficulties of ether administration by introducing chloroform. The benefits of anaesthesia were then universally recognised and antagonism by religious leaders was countered when Queen Victoria accepted chloroform from John Snow during the birth of Prince Leopold in 1853.

KEY PRINCIPLES OF ANAESTHESIA

Optimum patient care is dependent on a collaborative approach from anaesthetic and surgical teams. The importance of multidisciplinary collaboration has been clearly demonstrated by national audits such as the *Confidential Enquiries in Perioperative Deaths (CEPOD)* and *Enquiries into Maternal Deaths UK*. These audits have led to changes in clinical and non-clinical practice to improve morbidity and mortality.

The use of a set of safety checklists in the operating theatre in the form of the *WHO Surgical Safety Checklist* has shown a reduction in incidence of perioperative untoward events.

The role of the modern anaesthetist has evolved from just being responsible for the patient in the operating suite into a 'perioperative physician' who optimises the patient for surgery, assessing and minimising risk, cares for them during the operation, and then manages both pain and homeostasis in the postoperative period (Table 17.1) (Summary box 17.1).

Summary box 17.1

Ground rules for anaesthesia

- Safe surgery is achieved by close teamwork between surgeon and anaesthetist
- Safety checklists make sure that things are not forgotten
- Risk assessment allows the best strategy to be chosen
- Anaesthetists are extending their care into the pre- and postoperative phase

Table 17.1 Key features of commonly used intravenous anaesthetic agents.

Propofol (di-isopropyl phenol)	Smooth induction, better haemodynamic stability, blunting of autonomic reflexes and ability to use as a continuous infusion
Thiopentone (barbiturate)	Rapid induction, myocardial depression. Reduced metabolic rate and lowering of intracranial pressure is useful in neurosurgical patients, but drop in blood pressure can have detrimental effects
Etomidate (steroid derivative)	Good haemodynamic stability, brief duration of action, but concern over adrenocortical depression
Ketamine (phencyclidine derivative)	Preservation of blood pressure and respiratory reflexes together with excellent analgesia makes it an ideal choice for field anaesthesia. Emergence delirium is associated with administration of ketamine

William Thomas Gren Morton, 1819–1868, a dentist who practised in Boston, MA, USA.
John Collins Warren, 1778–1856, Professor of Anatomy and Surgery, The Harvard Medical School, Boston, MA, USA.
Robert Liston, 1794–1847, surgeon, University College Hospital, London, UK.
Sir James Young Simpson, 1811–1870, Professor of Midwifery, Edinburgh, UK.
Alexandrina Victoria, Queen of the United Kingdom of Great Britain and Ireland, 1837–1901.
John Snow, 1813–1858, a general practitioner of London, UK, who was one of the pioneers of anaesthesia.
Prince Leopold, 1853–1884, who later became Duke of Albany, was the eighth of Queen Victoria's nine children, and her fourth son.

PREPARATION FOR ANAESTHESIA

In cooperation with the anaesthetist, a surgeon's job is to perform a thorough preoperative assessment which recognises medical and anaesthetic risk factors, and facilitates the optimisation of the patient's condition.

A careful preassessment, multidisciplinary approach, standardised care pathway with a carefully chosen anaesthetic and analgesic technique is the cornerstone of 'enhanced recovery programmes', which were introduced recently across the surgical specialities.

GENERAL ANAESTHESIA

General anaesthesia is commonly described as the triad of unconsciousness, analgesia and muscle relaxation (Summary box 17.2).

Summary box 17.2

The general anaesthetic triad

- Amnesia: loss of awareness
- Analgesia: pain relief
- Muscle relaxation

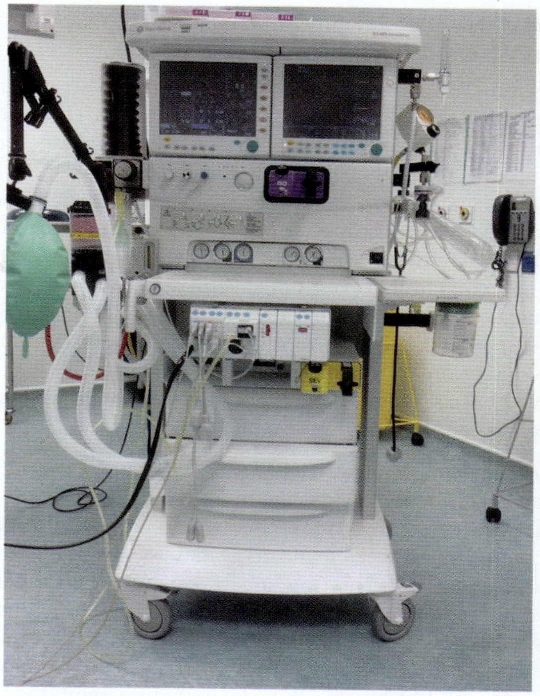

Figure 17.1 Anaesthetic machine.

Induction of general anaesthesia is most frequently done by intravenous agents. Propofol has replaced thiopentone as the most widely used induction agent and can be used for maintenance of anaesthesia. Other infrequently used intravenous agents include etomidate and ketamine. Newer agents based on benzodiazepine receptor agonist, etomidate derivatives and fospropofol are still in the experimental stage.

Inhalational induction using agents such as non-pungent sevoflurane is useful in children, needle-phobic adults and those in whom a difficult airway is anticipated. These patients will have a higher risk of developing airway obstruction (Figure 17.1).

Rapid sequence induction (RSI) using a predetermined dose of intravenous anaesthetic agent together with rapidly acting muscle relaxant is used in those with high risk of regurgitation in order to secure the airway quickly. Commonly needed in emergency surgery, it is also a technique of choice in any non-emergency surgery in a patient with delayed emptying of stomach.

Total intravenous anaesthesia (TIVA) is becoming popular following the introduction of propofol and ultra-short acting opioid remifentanil. The lack of a cumulative effect, better haemodynamic stability, excellent recovery profile and concerns over the environmental effects of inhalational agents have made TIVA an attractive choice. TIVA is routinely used in neurosurgery, in airway laser surgery, during cardiopulmonary bypass and for day-case anaesthesia (Figure 17.2) (Summary box 17.3).

Maintenance of anaesthesia, on the other hand, can be done using continuous infusion of intravenous agent (propofol) or inhaled vapour such as isoflurane, sevoflurane or desflurane.

The use of nitrous oxide is declining despite its analgesic and weak anaesthetic properties due to concerns over postoperative nausea and vomiting. It also increases the size of the air bubble causing adverse effects, for example in eye, ear and abdominal surgery. Finally, it is possibly mutagenic and is a powerful greenhouse gas.

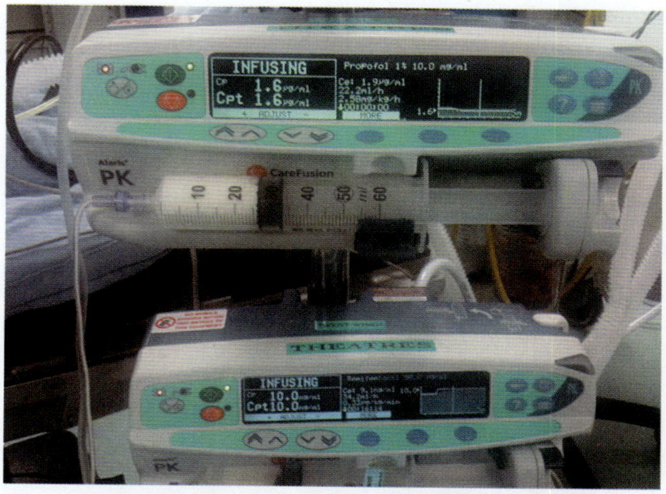

Figure 17.2 Total intravenous anaesthesia (TIVA) pumps in use.

Summary box 17.3

Special terms in anaesthesia

- Rapid sequence induction (RSI) is a technique that allows the airway to be rapidly secured. It is used when there is a high risk of regurgitation that may lead to pulmonary aspiration
- Total intravenous anaesthesia (TIVA) is becoming increasingly popular

Arthur Ernest Guedel, 1883–1956, Clinical Professor of Anaesthesiology, University of Southern California, Los Angeles, CA, USA.
Sir Ivan Whiteside Magill, 1888–1986, anaesthetist, The Westminster Hospital, London, UK.

Management of airway during anaesthesia

Loss of muscle tone as a result of general anaesthesia means that the patient can no longer keep their airway open. Therefore, the patients need their airway maintained for them. The use of muscle relaxants will mean that they will also be unable to breathe for themselves and so will require artificial ventilation. Head tilt, chin lift and jaw thrust manoeuvres along with adjuncts such as oropharyngeal airways are used to facilitate bag-mask ventilation, while induction agents exert full effect. Laryngeal mask airway or endotracheal tube is then inserted and the patient is allowed to breathe spontaneously or is ventilated during the procedure.

The addition of a cuff to the endotracheal tube facilitates positive pressure ventilation and protects the lungs from aspiration of regurgitated gastric contents.

- **Laryngeal mask airway (LMA).** Developed by Dr Archie Brain in the UK, the mask with an inflatable cuff is inserted via the mouth and produces a seal around the glottic opening, providing a very reliable means of maintaining the airway. Its placement is less irritating and less traumatic to a patient's airway than endotracheal intubation. The technique can be easily taught to non-anaesthetists and paramedics and can be used as an emergency airway management tool. Several varieties of LMA are available including reinforced, I-gel and an intubating LMA that aids endotracheal intubation (Figure 17.3).
- **Difficult intubation.** Endotracheal intubation is feasible in most patients, but in a certain proportion of patients this may be difficult or impossible; if compounded by inability to ventilate the patient by bag-mask, the consequences can be catastrophic hypoxia. Many devices have been developed to aid intubation if difficulty is anticipated and protocols have been created by specialised societies to deal with such situations. The gold standard for intubation in difficult situations is the use of the fibreoptic intubating bronchoscope, facilitated by topical local anaesthetic in awake patients or using general anaesthesia. The anaesthetist places the endotracheal tube in the trachea by threading the tube over the bronchoscope and so places the tube in the trachea under direct bronchoscopic vision (Figures 17.4, 17.5 and 17.6).

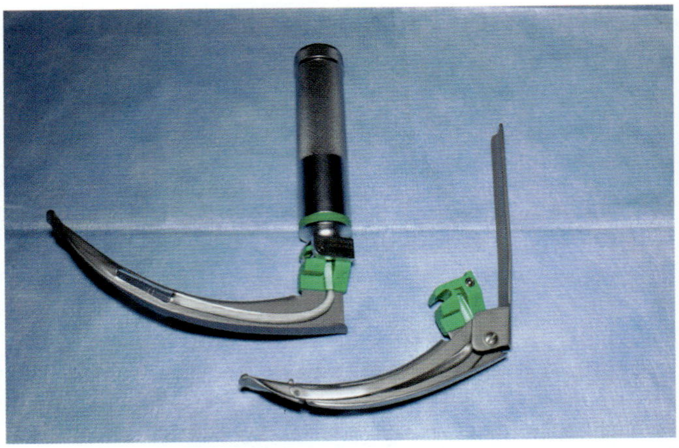

Figure 17.4 The Macintosh laryngoscope with a standard blade (left) and McCoy's modification of the Macintosh blade (right).

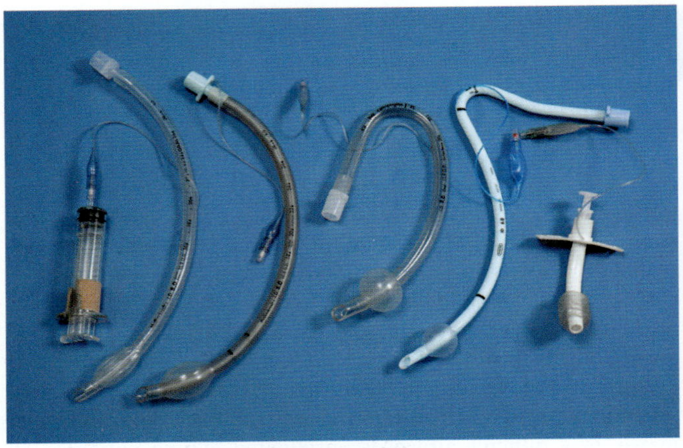

Figure 17.5 Endotracheal devices. From left to right: an uncut orotracheal tube; reinforced orotracheal tube; oral version of an RAE (Ring, Adair and Elwyn) preformed tube; nasal version of an RAE preformed tube; tracheostomy tube.

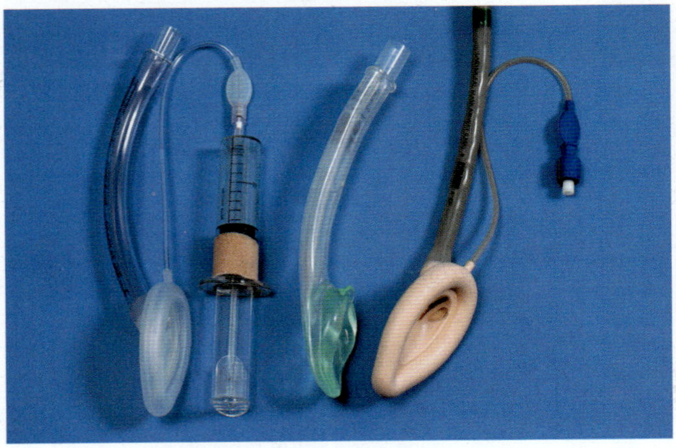

Figure 17.3 The laryngeal mask airway. The laryngeal mask airway (left), I-gel airway (centre) and reinforced laryngeal mask airway (right).

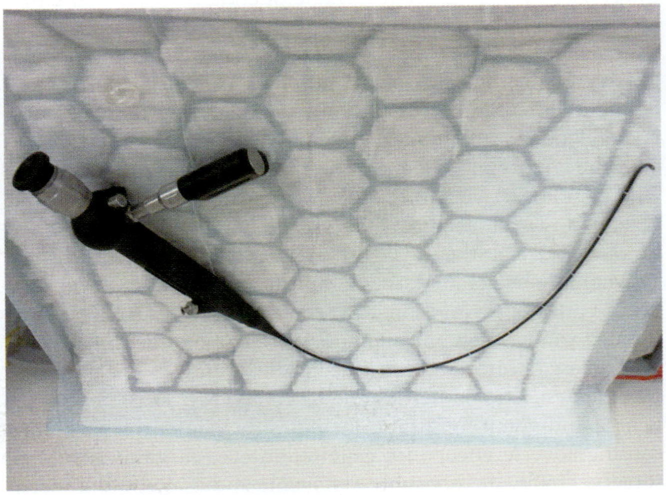

Figure 17.6 Fibreoptic intubating bronchoscope.

Archibald Ian Jeremy Brain, formerly anaesthetist, The Royal Berkshire Hospital, Reading, UK.
Sir Robert Reynolds Macintosh, 1897–1989, Nuffield Professor of Anaesthetics, The University of Oxford, Oxford, UK.
The RAE tube takes its name from the initials of the surnames of the people who introduced it, Wallace Harold Ring, John Adair and Richard Elwyn.

Double-lumen tubes and endobronchial tubes are used in procedures such as thoracoscopic, pulmonary and oesophageal surgery to allow collapse of one lung (while ventilating the other) for ease of surgery. Their use is also essential to isolate the healthy lung in pyopneumothorax and in case of bronchopleural fistula.

Ventilating bronchoscope and endobronchial catheters can be used to maintain oxygenation during laryngotracheal surgery or bronchoscopy by using intermittent jets of oxygen (Summary boxes 17.4 and 17.5).

Summary box 17.4

Techniques for maintaining an airway

- Chin lift and jaw thrust: suitable for short term when no aid available
- Guedel airway: holds tongue forward but does not prevent aspiration
- Laryngeal mask: easy insertion, reliable airway, allows ventilation
- Endotracheal intubation: secure and protected airway

Summary box 17.5

Complications of intubation

- Failed intubation
- Accidental bronchial intubation
- Trauma to teeth, pharynx and larynx
- Aspiration of gastric contents during intubation
- Disconnection, blockage, kinking of tube
- Delayed tracheal stenosis

Muscle relaxation and artificial ventilation

Pharmacological blockade of neuromuscular transmission provides relaxation of muscles allowing easy surgical access, but the patient requires artificial ventilation.

Neuromuscular blocking agents are broadly classified into depolarising and non-depolarising groups according to their mode of action.

Suxamethonium is the most commonly used depolarising agent. It binds to the nicotinic acetylcholine receptors resulting in opening of the cation channel leading to depolarisation and rapid relaxation of muscles. Despite its adverse effects, such as hyperkalaemia, muscle pain, anaphylaxis and potentially life-threatening malignant hyperthermia, suxamethonium is still widely used because of its quick onset and short duration of action. These properties are useful where rapid endotracheal intubation is necessary to protect the patient's airway or short duration surgery is performed.

Non-depolarising muscle relaxants act by competitive blockade of postsynaptic receptors at the neuromuscular junction. They provide longer, predictable activity, but require careful monitoring, appropriate timing and reversal of their action by agents, such as neostigmine and sugammadex, at the end of the procedure. A peripheral nerve stimulator is routinely used to monitor the depth of neuromuscular block and also to confirm satisfactory recovery of muscle power prior to extubation (Table 17.2).

Table 17.2 Properties of commonly used muscle relaxants.

Suxamethonium	Quickest onset, very short duration, spontaneous recovery. Ideal for rapid intubation and for short procedures	Muscle pain, hyperkalaemia, prolonged apnoea and life-threatening malignant hyperthermia
Vecuronium	Long-acting, minimal cardiovascular effect and less allergic reaction	Dependent on hepatic metabolism and renal clearance, hence caution if hepatic and renal impairment
Atracurium	Intermediate acting. Non-enzymatic Hoffmann degradation. Suitable in renal and hepatic failure	Histamine release and allergic reactions
Rocuronium	Rapid onset, intermediate action. Suitable for rapid intubation. Rapid reversal possible using Sugammadex	Allergic reaction. Excreted unchanged via bile and urine

Ventilation during anaesthesia

Mechanical ventilation is required when the patient's spontaneous ventilation is inadequate or when the patient is not breathing because of the effects of the anaesthetic, analgesic agents or muscle relaxants.

In volume control ventilation, a preset volume is delivered by the machine irrespective of the airway pressure. The pressure generated will be in part dependent on the resistance and compliance of the airway. In laparoscopic surgery requiring the Trendelenburg position (the patient is positioned head down), and in morbidly obese patients and those with lung disease, this may result in excessive pressures being developed, which may lead to barotrauma (pneumothorax).

In pressure control mode, the ventilator generates flow until a preset pressure is reached. The actual tidal volume delivered is variable and depends on airway resistance, intra-abdominal pressure and the degree of relaxation.

Positive end expiratory pressure (PEEP) is often applied to help maintain functional residual capacity (FRC). This avoids lung collapse by opening collapsed alveoli, and maintains a greater area of gas exchange so reducing vascular shunting (Summary box 17.6).

Summary box 17.6

Intermittent positive pressure ventilation

- Volume controlled which ensures adequate gas entry, but risks high pressure damage
- Pressure controlled which avoids high pressure damage but risks inadequate ventilation
- Positive end expiratory pressure (PEEP) reduces alveolar collapse and reduces vascular shunting so improving perfusion

Giovanni Batista Venturi, 1746–1822, Professor of Physics, The University of Modena, Modena, Italy.

Monitoring and care during anaesthesia

A minimum basic monitoring of cardiovascular parameters is required during surgery. This includes:

- Vascular
  - electrocardiogram (ECG)
  - blood pressure
- Adequacy of ventilation:
  - inspired oxygen concentration
  - oxygen saturation by pulse oximetry
  - end tidal carbon dioxide concentration.

Monitors of temperature, ventilation parameters and delivery of anaesthetic agents are also routinely used, while measurement of urine output and central venous pressure are recommended for major surgery.

Anaesthesia for day case surgery

This is discussed in Chapter 22.

LOCAL ANAESTHESIA

Local anaesthetic drugs may be used to provide anaesthesia and analgesia as a sole agent or as adjuncts to general anaesthesia. Available techniques include topical anaesthesia, local infiltration, regional nerve blocks and central neuroaxial blocks (spinal and epidural anaesthesia) (Table 17.3).

Local anaesthesia techniques can lead to complications that may be local like infection or haematoma, or systemic due to overdose or accidental intravascular injection. The systemic effects of local anaesthetic agents are dose dependent and manifest as cardiovascular (cardiac arrhythmia, cardiac arrest) or neurological (depressed consciousness, convulsions). Prilocaine overdose causes methaemoglobinaemia while bupivacaine overdose causes treatment-resistant ventricular arrhythmia and cardiac arrest.

The addition of adrenaline to local anaesthetic solutions hastens onset, prolongs duration of action and permits a higher upper dose limit. The use of adrenaline is contraindicated in patients with cardiovascular disease, those taking tricyclic and monoamine oxidase inhibitors, and in end-arterial locations.

Appropriately skilled personnel, resuscitation equipment and oxygen should always be available with local anaesthetic use because of the potential risks of life-threatening complications.

Regional anaesthesia

Regional anaesthesia involves central neuroaxial or peripheral nerve or plexus blocks. It has a clear advantage where general anaesthesia carries a higher risk of morbidity and mortality, such as in patients with debilitating respiratory and cardiovascular disease and obstetric cases. It also provides excellent pain relief in the postoperative period reducing the need for analgesics, such as opioids.

As with general anaesthesia obtaining venous access, monitoring vital parameters should be performed during regional anaesthesia.

Localising nerves using anatomical landmarks and eliciting paraesthesia alone carries a high risk of nerve damage, intravascular injection, and has a lower success rate. The use of nerve stimulators to localise nerves improves success rate and reduces risks. Ultrasound-guided regional anaesthesia allows the visualisation of nerves and the spread of local anaesthetics enabling use of a smaller dose of local anaesthetic agents with improved success rates and safety (Summary box 17.7).

Summary box 17.7

Types of anaesthesia

- General anaesthesia may be more acceptable to the patient
- Regional anaesthesia has major advantages in obstetrics and patients with respiratory compromise
- Local blocks have been transformed by nerve stimulators and ultrasound guidance
- All require full resuscitation and monitoring equipment to be available

Common local anaesthesia techniques

Topical anaesthesia

- **EMLA (eutectic mixture of local anesthetics)**. This is a mixture of lignocaine and prilocaine for application to the skin for venepuncture in children.
- **Cocaine**. It may be called Mofatt's solution and used in nasal surgery for anaesthesia and vasoconstriction.
- **Lignocaine 4%**. Spray to anaesthetise the airway during awake fibreoptic intubation.

Nerve blocks

- Interscalene block for shoulder surgery produces excellent postoperative analgesia. Complications include phrenic nerve block, Horner's syndrome, as well as accidental intravascular and spinal injection.
- Axillary brachial plexus block can be used as the sole anaesthetic technique for upper limb surgery (Figure 17.7).
- Femoral and sciatic nerve blocks are often used for anaesthesia and analgesia for lower limb surgery.

Transversusabdominis plane block

The transversusabdominis plane (TAP) block is growing rapidly in popularity. The technique has been shown to provide

Table 17.3 The common local anaesthetic drugs.

Name	Maximum dose	Comments
Lignocaine	3 mg/kg (7 mg/kg with adrenaline)	Early onset, short acting, good sensory block
Bupivacaine	2 mg/kg	Long-lasting, more cardiotoxic, must never be used intravenously
Prilocaine	6 mg/kg (9 mg/kg with adrenaline)	Least systemic toxicity, causes methaemoglobinaemia
Ropivacaine	3–4 mg/kg (225 mg)	Less cardiotoxic, greater sensory–motor separation
Levobupivaciane	2 mg/kg	Isomer of bupivacaine with less cardiotoxic properties

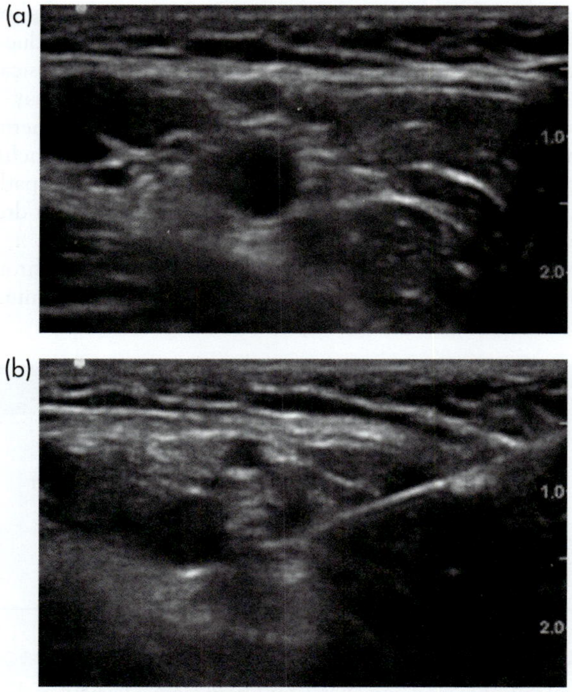

Figure 17.7 (a,b) Ultrasonic scans of brachial plexus block.

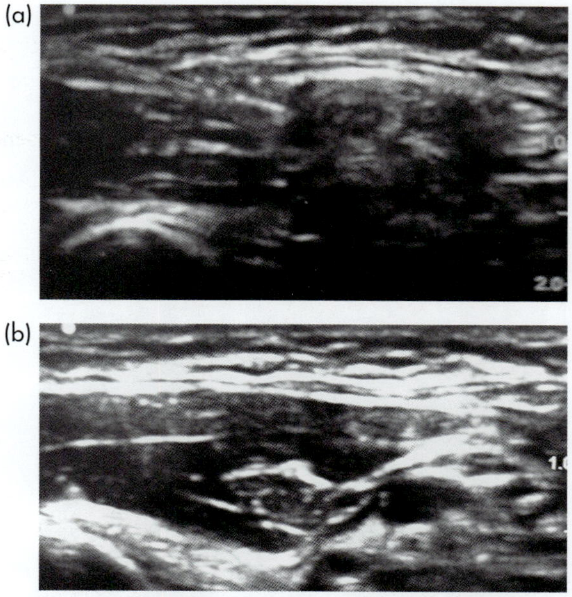

Figure 17.8 (a,b) Ultrasonic scans of lateral abdominal wall and the spread of local anaesthetics.

effective analgesia after a wide range of abdominal surgery. The T6–L1 segmental nerves enter the Triangle of Petit just medial to the anterior axillary line. Injection of local anaesthetic into the fascial plane between the internal oblique and transversus abdominis muscles allows a block of all these nerves, and excellent anaesthesia of the anterior abdominal wall (Figure 17.8).

Intravenous regional anaesthesia (Bier's block)

Bier's block produces excellent anaesthesia for short surgery, particularly for the upper limb (e.g. carpal tunnel release). Exsanguination using an Esmarch bandage, inflation of proximal cuff of the double tourniquet is followed by intravenous injection of prilocaine into the vein on the back of the hand that is being operated on. After 5–10 minutes, the distal cuff of the tourniquet is inflated and then the proximal one deflated. Even if surgery is finished, the tourniquet should be left inflated until the local anaesthetic has bound to tissues (20 minutes) so that release of local anaesthetic into the systemic circulation does not occur. Lignocaine can be used with caution (consider safe dose and time of tourniquet inflation), but bupivacaine should never be used for Bier's block.

Spinal anaesthesia

Spinal anaesthesia alone, in combination with general anaesthesia or sedation is used extensively for lower limb, obstetric and pelvic surgery. Injection of a 'single shot' local anaesthetic agent intrathecally produces intense and rapid block for surgery. Addition of opioids provides prolonged postoperative analgesia, but carries the risk of late respiratory depression.

Autonomic sympathetic blockade produces hypotension, particularly if the level of block is above T10. Caution is needed in patients with hypovolaemia and cardiovascular disease.

The incidence of dural puncture headache can be minimised by limiting the number of punctures and use of fine bore pencil tip needles designed to split rather than cut the dura.

Epidural anaesthesia

Epidural anaesthesia is slower in onset than spinal, but has the advantage of prolonged analgesia by multiple dosing or continuous infusion through a catheter placed in the epidural space. Being slower in onset, the resulting hypotension from sympathetic blockade can be better controlled and can reduce blood loss.

Continuous infusion (with a patient-controlled bolus) of weak local anaesthetic combined with opioids (such as fentanyl) is routinely used for postoperative analgesia. Placement of an epidural catheter in the high thoracic region provides excellent analgesia for a wide variety of upper abdominal and thoracic surgical operations enabling early mobilisation and reducing respiratory complications.

Epidural anaesthesia is technically more difficult than spinal anaesthesia with a higher failure rate and carries the risk of nerve damage, spinal injuries, accidental spinal injection of large volume of local anaesthetics and risk of infection and epidural haematoma (Figures 17.9 and 17.10) (Summary box 17.8).

Summary box 17.8

Local anaesthetics

- EMLA cream for children needing injections
- Regional and nerve blocks for limb surgery
- Spinal anaesthesia offers quick onset and short duration of anaesthesia
- Epidurals are more difficult, but can then be topped up postoperatively and used as continuous infusion

Edward Boyce Tuohy, 1908–1959, Professor of Anaesthesiology, Georgetown Medical Center, Washington DC (1947–1952) and later at the University of Southern California Medical School, Los Angeles, CA, USA.

August Karl Gustav Bier, 1861–1949, Professor of Surgery, Bonn (1903–1907) and Berlin, Germany (1907–1932).
Ralph J Huber, 1890–1953, a dentist in Seattle, WA, USA.
Ralph Douglas Kenneth Reye, 1912–1977, Director of Pathology, The Royal Alexandra Hospital for Children, Sydney, NSW, Australia, described this syndrome in 1963.

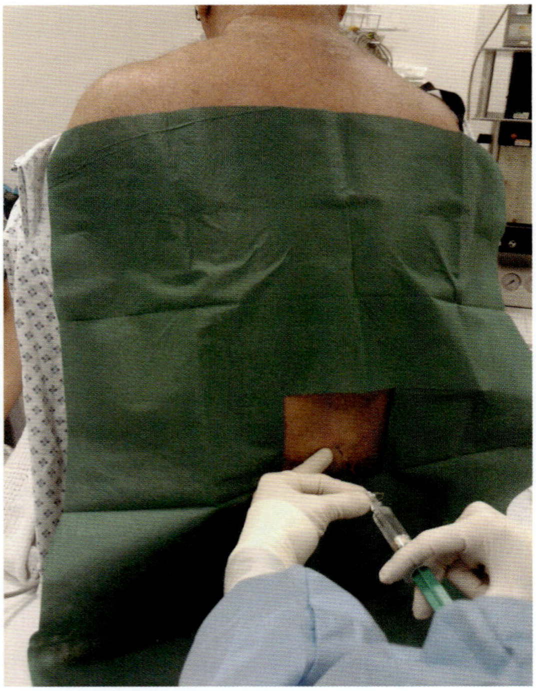

Figure 17.9 Patient positioned for epidural/spinal anaesthesia.

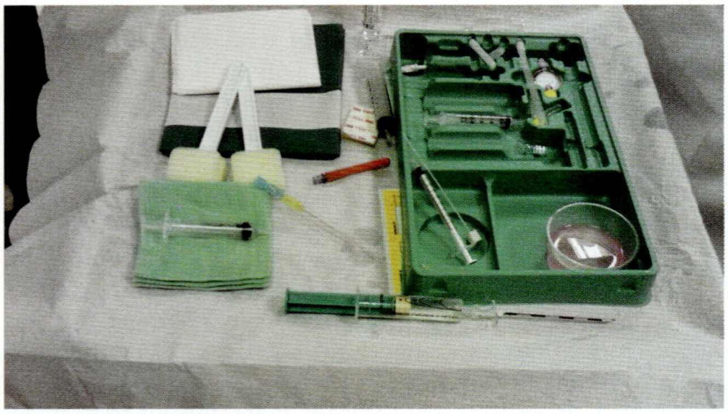

Figure 17.10 Equipment for epidural/spinal anaesthesia.

Chronic pain management

In surgical practice, the patient with chronic pain may present for treatment of the cause (e.g. pancreatitis, malignancy) or concomitant benign pathology. Acute pain after surgery may progress to chronic pain and is believed to be due to inadequate treatment of acute pain itself.

Chronic pain may be of several types:

- **Nociceptive pain** may result from musculoskeletal disorders or cancer activating cutaneous nociceptors (pain receptors). Prolonged ischaemic or inflammatory processes result in sensitisation of peripheral nociceptors and altered activity in the central nervous system leading to exaggerated responses in the dorsal horn of the spinal cord. The widened area of hyperalgesia and increased sensitivity (allodynia) has been attributed to the increased transmission in the central nervous system.
- **Neuropathic (or neurogenic) pain** is dysfunction in peripheral or central nerves (excluding the 'physiological' pain due to noxious stimulation of the nerve terminals). It is classically of a 'burning', 'shooting' or 'stabbing' type and may be associated with allodynia, numbness and diminished thermal sensation. It is poorly responsive to opioids. Examples include trigeminal neuralgia, postherpetic and diabetic neuropathy. Monoaminergic, tricyclic inhibitors and anticonvulsant drugs are the mainstay of treatment.
- **Psychogenic pain** is associated with depressive illness; chronic pain and the illness may exacerbate each other (Summary box 17.9).

Summary box 17.9

Types of pain

- Nociceptive pain arises from inflammation and ischaemia
- Neuropathic pain arises from a dysfunction in the central nervous system
- Psychogenic pain is modified by the mental state of the patient

Chronic pain control in benign disease

Surgical patients may have persistent pain from a variety of disorders including chronic inflammatory disease, recurrent infection, degenerative bone or joint disease, nerve injury and sympathetic dystrophy. This may result from persistent excitation of the nociceptive pathways causing spontaneous firing of pain signals at N-methyl-D-aspartate receptors in the ascending pathways. This pain does not respond to opiates or neuroablative surgery.

Amputation of limbs may result in phantom limb pain, the likelihood is increased if the limb was painful before surgery. Continuous regional local anaesthetic blockade (epidural or brachial plexus) established before operation and continued postoperatively for a few days, is believed to effectively reduce the risk of phantom limb pain (Summary box 17.10).

- **Local anaesthetic and steroid injections** can be effective around an inflamed nerve and they reduce the cycle of constant pain transmission with consequent muscle spasm. Epidural injections are used for the pain of nerve root irritation associated with minor disc prolapse along with active physiotherapy to promote mobility.
- **Nerve stimulation procedures** such as acupuncture, transcutaneous nerve stimulation, and spinal cord stimulators increase endorphin production in the central nervous system. Nerve decompression craniotomy rather than percutaneous coagulation of the ganglion is now performed for trigeminal neuralgia.

Summary box 17.10

Pain control in benign disease

- Bring pain under control before amputation to avoid phantom pain
- Local anaesthetic and steroid injected around a nerve may reduce muscle spasm
- Transcutaneous nerve stimulators (TNS) modify pain by increasing endorphin production
- Trigeminal neuralgia responds to decompression of the nerve

Drugs in chronic non-malignant pain

Paracetamol and the non-steroidal anti-inflammatory drugs (NSAID) are the mainstay of musculoskeletal pain treatment. The tricyclic antidepressant drugs and anticonvulsant agents are often useful for the pain of nerve injury, although side effects can prove troublesome and reduce compliance. Both pregabalin and gabapentin reduce spontaneous neuronal activity and are now used for managing the neuropathic chronic pain. In more severe and debilitating non-malignant chronic pain, opioid analgesic drugs are used in slow release oral preparations of morphine and oxycodone, and transcutaneous patches delivering fentanyl and buprenorphine. Combinations of drugs often prove useful to achieve the optimum of efficacy with minimal side effects.

Treatment of pain dependent on sympathetic nervous system activity

Even minor trauma and surgery (often of a limb) can provoke chronic burning pain, allodynia, trophic changes and resultant disuse due to excessive sympathetic adrenergic activity inducing vasconstriction and abnormal nociceptive transmission.

Management may include a test response to systemic α-adrenergic blockade using intravenous phentolamine and/or local anaesthetic injection of stellate ganglion or lumbar sympathetic chain. Percutaneous chemical lumbar sympathectomy with phenol/local anaesthetic is used for relief of rest pain in advanced ischaemic disease of the legs. It has an added advantage as it assists in the healing of ischaemic ulcers by improving peripheral blood flow.

Pain control in malignant disease

Pain is a common symptom associated with cancer, more so during the advanced stages. In intractable pain, the underlying principle of treatment is to encourage independence of the patient and an active life in spite of the symptom. The World Health Organization's booklet advises use of a 'pain step ladder':

- First step. **Simple analgesics**: aspirin, paracetamol, non-steroidal anti-inflammatory agents, tricyclic drugs or anticonvulsant drugs.
- Second step. **Intermediate strength opioids**: codeine, tramadol or dextropropoxyphene.
- Third step. **Strong opioids**: morphine (pethidine has now been withdrawn).

Oral opiate analgesia is necessary when the less powerful analgesic agents no longer control pain on movement, or enable the patient to sleep. Fear that the patient may develop an addiction to opiates is usually not justified in malignant disease. It is also important to distinguish between the addiction and dependence; the former being a psychosocial phenomenon while the latter is a pure physiological response to a given drug. Some patients experience 'breakthrough pain' (acute, excruciating and incapacitating), which occurs either spontaneously or in relation to a specific predictable or unpredictable trigger, experienced by patients who have relatively stable and adequately controlled background pain.

Oral morphine, often used for chronic pain, can be prescribed in short-acting liquid or tablet form and should be administered regularly every 4 hours until an adequate dose of drug has been titrated to control the pain over 24 hours. Once this is established, the daily dose can be divided into two separate administrations of enteric-coated, slow-release morphine tablets (MST morphine) every 12 hours. Additional short-acting opioids (morphine/fentanyl) can then be used to cover episodes of breakthrough pain. Nausea treated using anti-emetic agents does not usually persist, but constipation is a frequent and persistent complication requiring regular prevention with laxatives.

Infusion of subcutaneous, intravenous, intrathecal or epidural opiate drugs

The infusion of opiates is necessary if a patient is unable to take oral drugs. Subcutaneous infusion of diamorphine is simple and effective to administer. Epidural infusions of diamorphine with an external pump can be used on mobile patients. Intrathecal infusions with pumps programmed by external computer are used, however, there is a possibility of developing infection with catastrophic effects. Intravenous narcotic agents may be reserved for acute crises, such as pathological fractures.

Neurolytic techniques in cancer pain

These should only be used if the life expectancy is limited and the diagnosis is certain. The useful procedures are:

- Subcostal phenol injection for a rib metastasis.
- Coeliac plexus neurolytic block with alcohol for pain of pancreatic, gastric or hepatic cancer.
- Intrathecal neurolytic injection of hyperbaric phenol.
- Percutaneous anterolateral cordotomy divides the spinothalamic ascending pain pathway. It is a highly effective technique in experienced hands, selectively eliminating pain and temperature sensation in a specific limited area.

Alternative strategies include:

- The development of anti-pituitary hormone drugs, such as tamoxifen and cyproterone, enables effective pharmacological therapy for the pain of widespread metastases instead of pituitary ablation surgery.
- Palliative radiotherapy can be most beneficial for the relief of pain in metastatic disease.
- Adjuvant drugs, such as corticosteroids to reduce cerebral oedema or inflammation around a tumour, may be useful in symptom control. Tricyclic antidepressants, anticonvulsants and flecainide are also used to reduce the pain of nerve injury (Summary box 17.11).

In the management of chronic pain, a multidisciplinary approach by a team of medical and nursing staff working with psychologists, physiotherapists and occupational therapists can often achieve much more benefit than the use of powerful drugs. Pain management programmes lay out a logical structure for this.

Summary box 17.11

Options for controlling severe pain in malignant disease

- Oral morphine using slow-release, enteric-coated tablets
- Slow infusion of opiates subcutaneously, by epidural, or intrathecally
- Neurolysis for patients with limited life expectancy
- Palliative hormone, radiotherapy, or steroids control pain from swelling

FURTHER READING

Aitkenhead AR, Smith G, Rowbotham DJ. *Textbook of anaesthesia*, 5th edn. Edinburgh: Churchill Livingstone Elsevier, 2007.

Rawal N (ed.). *Management of acute and chronic pain*. London: BMJ Books, 1998.

Sneyd JR. Recent advances in intravenous anaesthesia. *Br J Anaesth* 2004; **93**: 725–36.

Wildsmith I, Armitage EN (eds). *Principles and practice of regional anaesthesia*. Edinburgh: Churchill Livingstone, 1990.

CHAPTER

18

Care in the operating room

LEARNING OBJECTIVES

To understand:

- How to prepare a patient for theatre
- The importance of the World Health Organization checklist and its components
- How to reduce intraoperative risks of positioning, venous thromboembolism, infection and hypothermia, by using appropriate monitoring and equipment.
- The operating theatre environment and how to behave in it, including scrubbing up, the role of the assistant and how to write an operation note.

'First do no harm.'

Hippocrates

PREOPERATIVE PREPARATION IMMEDIATELY BEFORE SURGERY

Patient preparation

Both the operating surgeon and the anaesthetist should see the patient prior to surgery. The patient's identity and the proposed surgery should be confirmed. After explaining the risks and benefits to the patient, valid consent for surgery should be obtained. There should be an opportunity for questions, and the patient should have adequate time to make their decision (see LED TO REASON Table 16.6). Any changes in the patient's condition since listing for surgery should be noted, and a check made for any contraindications to elective surgery, e.g. intercurrent illness or remote site infection. In procedures that may cause neurovascular complications, the preoperative neurovascular status should be assessed and documented. Check that all relevant results and imaging are available, and that the side or area to be operated on is marked with an arrow at or near to the incision site.

Theatre team preparation

Preoperative planning should cover all aspects of the surgical process. Close communication and coordination between preoperative departments and operating theatres allows timely preparation and improves efficiency and safety in the operating theatre.

Every hospital will have a policy for booking and scheduling of elective and emergency theatre cases.

The theatre list should have a header with the date, time and details of the theatre, surgeon and anaesthetist. For each operation, the patient's name and hospital number, preoperative ward, operation title and site of surgery should be recorded. Additional information may include the need for specialised equipment or implants, instrument sets, use of a specific operating table, patient positioning, availability of blood products and need for postoperative higher dependency care.

Up-to-date information about the operating lists must be available to all personnel including patients, ward staff, porters, theatre and recovery staff. Lists should be scheduled to meet the needs of the patient, theatre team and staff in other disciplines. For example, infectious patients should be listed last to avoid delays from theatre contamination. Children and diabetic patients will need to go first.

Support services, e.g. radiology for intraoperative imaging, haematology for blood products, cell salvage and pathology for frozen sections, should also be informed and be available. A good operation list contains all the relevant information and is distributed on time to everyone involved so that there are 'no surprises' for anyone (Summary box 18.1).

Summary box 18.1

Before theatre

- Patient must be seen by anaesthetist and operating surgeon preoperatively
- Communicate early with theatre team regarding specific requirements
- Arrange theatre list appropriately for the case-mix and resources available

IN THEATRE

Surgical safety checklist

In 2008, the World Health Organization (WHO) published guidelines of recommended practices to reduce the rate of preventable surgical complications and death worldwide. A core set of checks have been incorporated into the WHO surgical safety checklist, which should be completed for every patient undergoing a surgical procedure. In the UK, a five-step process is used to improve theatre team communication and to verify and check essential care interventions (Summary box 18.2).

Summary box 18.2

WHO Surgical Safety Checklist: UK process

- Step 1: Prelist briefing
- Step 2: Sign in
- Step 3: Time out
- Step 4: Sign out
- Step 5: Postlist debriefing

Prelist briefing

A short meeting before the start of the operating list provides an opportunity for the theatre team to introduce themselves, share information about potential safety problems and highlight concerns about specific patients to ensure smooth running of the list. For example, patient issues such as positioning, allergies and imaging, anticipated surgical complications, last minute list order changes and the need for antibiotics and thromboembolism prophylaxis may be discussed at this time.

Sign in

The sign in checklist should be read out prior to induction of anaesthesia:

- Has the patient confirmed their identity, site of surgery, procedure and consent?
- Is the surgical site marked?
- Is the anaesthesia machine and medication check complete?
- Does the patient have a known allergy?
- Does the patient have a difficult airway risk or risk of aspiration?
- Does the patient have a risk of >500 mL blood loss (7 mL/kg in children) and if yes, is adequate intravenous access and fluid/blood replacement planned?

Other preoperative checks may vary between institutions, but include ensuring removal of dentures and jewellery, and confirming any implanted metalwork.

Antibiotics

To prevent surgical site infection, patients should receive appropriate antibiotics, using local guidelines, less than an hour before surgical incision. Antibiotic prophylaxis should be given to patients before clean surgery involving insertion of a prosthesis or implant, clean-contaminated surgery or contaminated surgery. Antibiotic prophylaxis should not be used routinely for clean, non-prosthetic surgery. Prophylactic antibiotics should be discontinued within 24 hours of surgery.

Venous thromboembolism

All patients should be risk-assessed preoperatively for venous thromboembolism (VTE). Patients should not be allowed to become dehydrated perioperatively. In theatre, mechanical and pharmacological VTE prophylaxis can be used.

Mechanical methods include:

- anti-embolism graduated compression stockings;
- foot impulse devices;
- intermittent pneumatic compression devices.

The choice of pharmacological VTE agents depends on local policies and individual patient factors, including comorbidities (such as renal failure).

Regional anaesthesia (spinal or epidural) carries a lower risk of VTE than general anaesthesia. If used, plan the timing of pharmacological VTE prophylaxis to minimise the risk of spinal haematoma.

Monitoring

The most important 'monitor' is the presence of a trained, dedicated individual to observe the patient throughout anaesthesia. However, minimum monitoring standards apply in several countries worldwide and their guidance should be followed.

Operating theatre environment

Ventilation

The aim of the air flow system is to prevent airborne microorganisms entering the surgical wound. After filtration, air is introduced at ceiling height and exhausted near the floor with at least 20 air changes per hour. The operating theatre is maintained at positive pressure relative to surroundings. Keeping doors closed and limiting the movement of personnel in and out of theatre will reduce the risk of surgical site infection.

Laminar air flow provides 100–300 air changes per hour and is used in some centres for surgery involving implants, e.g. joint replacements, to avoid airborne infection.

Humidity and temperature

Theatre temperature should be acceptable for the patient and theatre staff. Ideal working temperatures for surgeons are 19–20°C, but patients may develop hypothermia below 21°C. Temperatures of 20–24°C are acceptable with a relative humidity of 50–60 per cent to protect against electrostatic charges.

Patient transfer and positioning

Both transfer and positioning should be performed carefully under the supervision of the anaesthetist and surgeon. These precautions are essential under general anaesthesia as the patient will be immobile and unable to communicate problems; the patient receiving local or regional anaesthesia should also feel comfortable.

Transfer

Patient transfer is coordinated by the anaesthetist, who protects airway devices and other connections during the move. A variety of manual handling aids are used (sliding boards and low-friction sliding sheets) to reduce risks to staff and patient; universal precautions should be maintained by everyone (Figure 18.1).

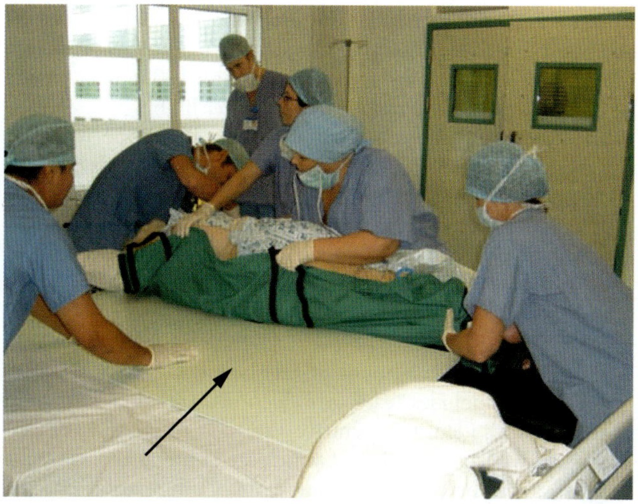

Figure 18.1 Patient transfer. Enough personnel are available to undertake the transfer. The anaesthetist supervises and protects the head, neck and airway. The patient is rolled and a sliding board (arrow) is placed under the patient and undersheet or canvas, which will allow the patient to slide across to the bed in a controlled fashion. Care is being taken by all of the team members to protect the whole patient.

Positioning

The plan for intraoperative positioning should be communicated to the entire team as it may require specific accessories, such as arm supports, to be available; anaesthetic management may also be affected. Stability of the patient on the table should be ensured using straps and/or solid supports, particularly where anything other than supine positioning is anticipated.

Pressure and stretch injuries resulting from poor positioning are common. High-risk groups include the elderly, the cachectic or the obese. High-risk areas should be checked and padded prior to starting surgery. During lengthy operations, movement of non-involved limbs may be necessary to relieve pressure (Summary box 18.3).

Summary box 18.3

Pressure areas which must be given special consideration

- The skin over bony prominences
- Nerves in superficial courses, e.g. common peroneal nerve (take care with placement of the calves in leg supports)
- Nerves at risk of stretch injury, e.g. brachial plexus (head should be neutral where possible)
- Areas at risk of developing a compartment syndrome
- Eye protection: eyes should be protected from direct pressure (particularly in the prone position), corneal abrasion and splash injuries. Ointment, or eye closure with tape and/or eye pads may be used

In addition, in order to avoid electrical injury, no part of the patient should be in contact with any metal other than the diathermy plate. If radiological imaging is to be used intraoperatively, the patient could be protected with lead shielding and a radiolucent table used.

Finally, the awake patient should be comfortable. A pillow under the knees often relieves the aching low back pain associated with lying supine.

Equipment

Following the induction of anaesthesia, any remaining equipment should be set up, including diathermy, tourniquet and urethral catheterisation, if indicated.

Diathermy

If monopolar diathermy is to be used, the diathermy dispersal electrode must be applied to an appropriate site, which should be:

- clean and dry, free of hair;
- situated over well-perfused muscle mass, avoiding bony prominences, scar tissue, areas distal to tourniquets and implanted metalwork;
- as close to the operative site as feasible;
- checked at the end of surgery for injury.

The patient should not be in contact with any earthed metal appliance. Special consideration must be given to the risks of monopolar diathermy if the patient has implanted devices which may be affected by the current (including pacemakers, implantable defibrillators, cochlear implants and spinal cord stimulators).

Tourniquets

A tourniquet may be used to improve visibility at surgery and to reduce blood loss (Figure 18.2).

The complications of using a tourniquet include neurovascular compression and skin injury due to direct compression, chemical burns from the liberal application of skin preparation fluid which then leaks under the tourniquet, and distal ischaemic/reperfusion injury (Summary box 18.4).

Summary box 18.4

Application of tourniquet

- Appropriate size should be selected
- Apply as proximally as possible
- Apply padding to site without creases
- Apply tightly enough to avoid slippage, but not so tightly as to impede exsanguination
- Exsanguinate the limb prior to inflating the tourniquet using elevation, an Esmarch bandage or a roll cylinder
- When the tourniquet is inflated, the time must be noted
- When the tourniquet is removed, the site should be inspected for damage and the limb for return of circulation. This should be recorded in the notes (with the time)

The precautions which should be taken to avoid these injuries are:

- tourniquet use to be avoided in high-risk patients (including those with sickle cell disease and peripheral vascular disease);
- padding to be used under the tourniquet and tape to prevent fluid leaking underneath it;

Johann Friedrich August von Esmarch, 1823–1965, Professor of Clinical Surgery, Kiel, Germany, devised this type of bandage while working as a military surgeon during the Franco-Prussian war (1870–1871) and described its use in 1873.

Charles Bingham Penrose, 1862–1925, Professor of Gynaecology, The University of Pennsylvania, Philadelphia, PA, USA described this type of drain in 1890.

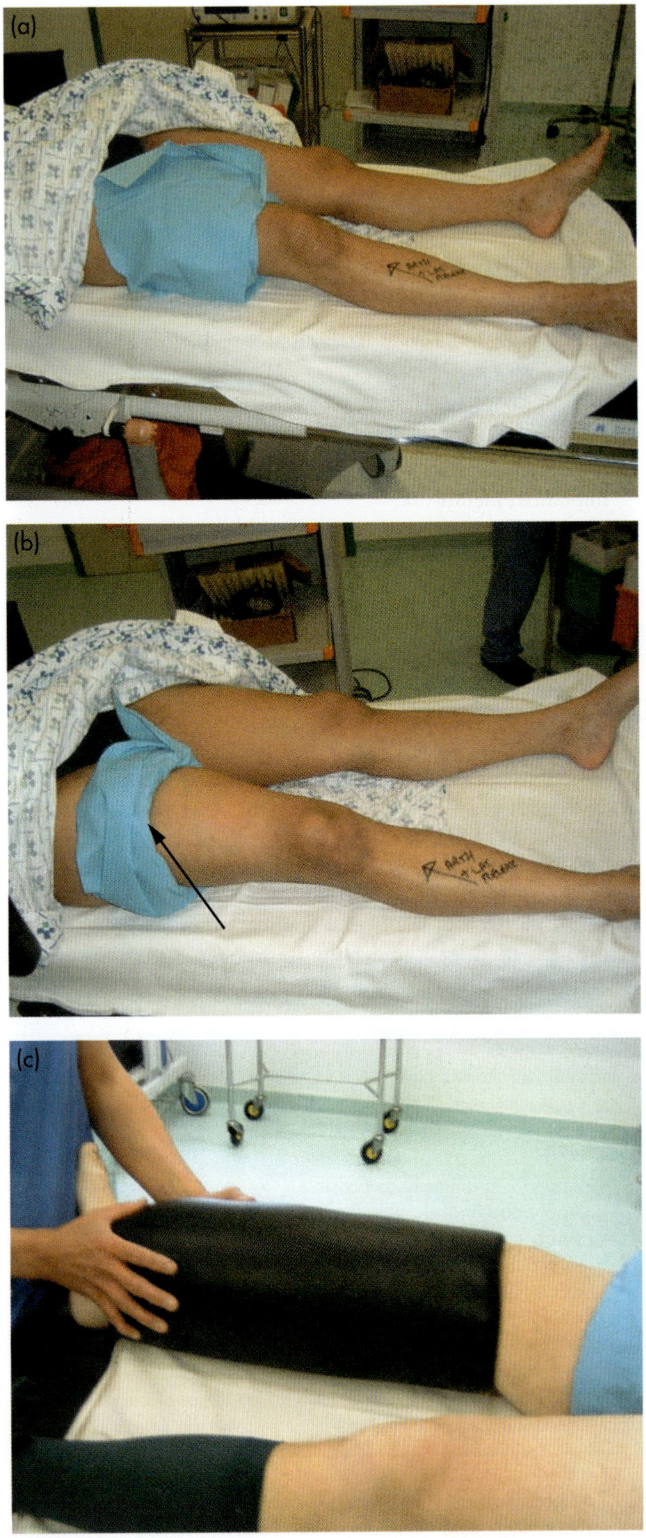

Figure 18.2 Tourniquet and tourniquet dressing. (a) Poor placement, too low – interfering with operative field. (b) Optimal placement of the tourniquet using a single-use tourniquet cover, which protects the skin under the tourniquet and has an adhesive strip to prevent ingress of preparation solution (arrow). This tourniquet is less likely to slip and provides a much larger skin preparation field, important as the patient is undergoing knee surgery. (c) Rhys-Davies exsanguinator.

- minimum cuff pressures required for adequate operating conditions to be used: the standard is to set the pressure a constant amount above systolic pressure, 100 mmHg for the upper limb and 150 mmHg for the lower limb;
- use of a tourniquet clock: the surgeon should be informed when 1 hour of 'tourniquet time' has elapsed. It may be appropriate at this point to consider letting the tourniquet down for a short period before reinflating, if more than a few minutes' extra tourniquet time is required. Total tourniquet time should not exceed 1.5 hours.

'Time out'

This must be performed immediately before the surgical procedure starts: it includes team introductions, verbal confirmation of the patient's identity, operative site and procedure to be performed, as well as discussion of anticipated critical events by the surgeon, anaesthetist and nursing team. Confirmation of antibiotic prophylaxis and review of essential imaging (if required) is carried out at this stage.

Specific additional checks including the areas outlined below may be included according to local adaptations of the checklist.

Temperature control

Patients undergoing anaesthesia and surgery lose heat rapidly from radiation to the environment, latent heat of evaporation from exposed wet organs in body cavities or from cleaning fluids applied to the body surface, exposure to cold intravenous fluids and anaesthetic gases. The patient's ability to compensate for these losses is also impaired (reduced metabolic heat production, limited vasoconstriction and the loss of behavioural responses).

The measures which will limit the development of intraoperative hypothermia include the use of forced air warming blankets, warmed intravenous and irrigation fluids, increasing the operating room ambient temperature and minimising exposure of the patient.

Hair removal

This may be necessary over the operative field to facilitate exposure (for incision, suturing and dressing application) or the diathermy plate site (to maximise plate contact with skin). Surgical site infections may be reduced if hair is clipped rather than shaved; there is a lack of evidence to determine whether the timing or location of hair removal affects the incidence of wound infection.

Glycaemic control

The blood glucose needs careful monitoring and controlling in the diabetic patient. Hyperglycaemia perioperatively may increase the incidence of postoperative wound infection. If unrecognised, hypoglycaemia may lead to seizures and death.

Infection control

Asepsis and universal precautions

Cross-infection between patients or between staff member and patient (in either direction) is potentially disastrous and every effort must be made to minimise this risk. In addition to some of the specific areas considered below, universal precautions should be taken in every case involving exposure to body fluids. These include the following:

- protective non-porous gloves, eyewear, mask, apron for staff;

The late Noel C Rhys-Davies, clinical assistant in orthopaedics, Yeovil District Hospital, in 1985, described his exsanguinator with Anne T Stotter, orthopaedic surgeon, St Mary's Hospital, Harrow Road, London.

- safe sharps handling techniques and adequate provision of sharps bins;
- staff vaccination for hepatitis B;
- staff with infected wounds or active dermatitis should not work in theatre.

In particular, surgeons handling sharp instruments are responsible for placing them in a safe container (bowl or tray) for transfer, one at a time.

Scrubbing up

The risk of transfer of microbes between staff and patients is minimised by meticulous 'scrubbing up' (washing hands and arms and putting on gown and gloves) (Figures 18.3 and 18.4) (Summary box 18.5).

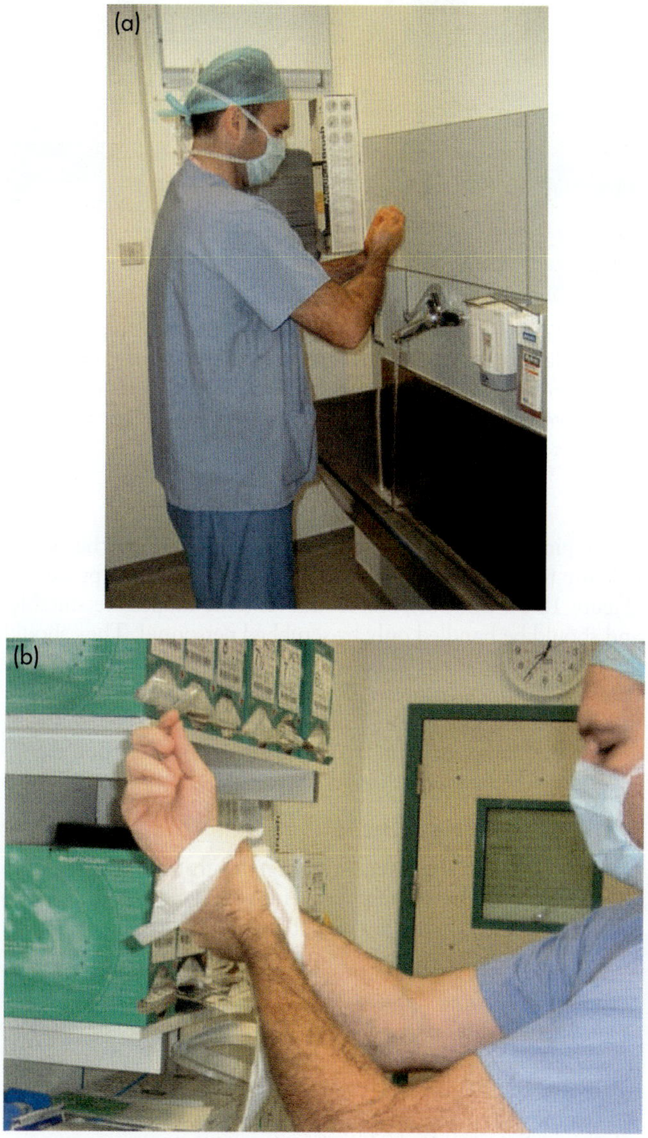

Figure 18.3 (a,b) Scrubbing up.

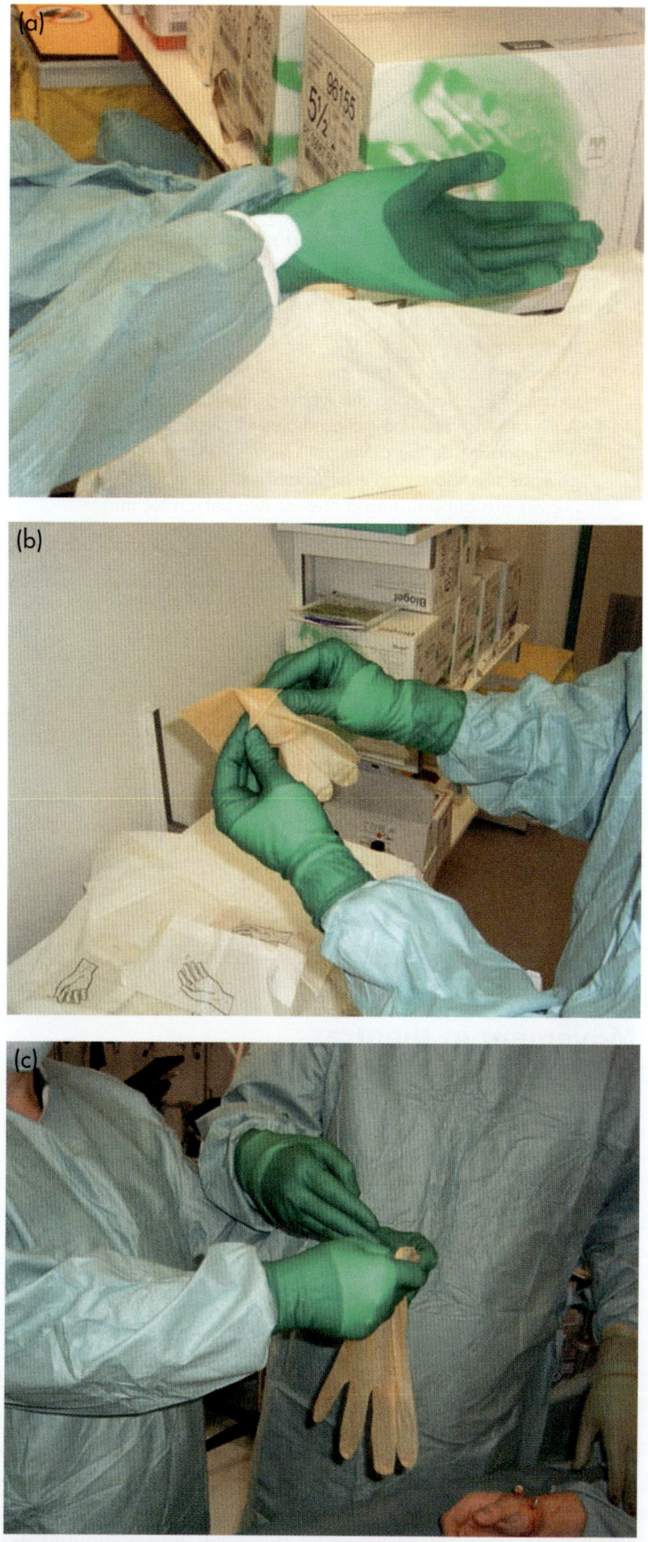

Figure 18.4 Gloving techniques. (a) The initial gloving occurs with the hands covered by the gown. The first glove is then placed on to the palmar surface and pulled into position. (b) The double gloving technique, with minimal touch technique. (c) The closed two-person gloving technique; the glove being held open by one person for the second to insert their hand into the glove.

Summary box 18.5

Scrubbing up

- Hat, mask and eye protection should be worn and jewellery should be removed prior to scrubbing
- Nails and deep skin creases are cleaned for 1–2 minutes using a brush
- Hands and forearms are washed systematically three times, the hands being held above the level of the elbows throughout
- Hands and arms are dried from distal to proximal using a sterile towel
- The folded gown is lifted away from the trolley and allowed to unfold (inside facing the wearer), while the top is held
- Arms are inserted into the armholes simultaneously, hands remaining inside the gown until gloves are donned: the gown is secured by an unscrubbed staff member
- Gloves are put on using a one- or two-person technique: from this point on, hands remain above waist level at all times.

Standard scrub solutions include:

- 2 per cent chlorhexidine (effective for more than 4 hours, potent against Gram-positive and -negative organisms, some viruses, less effective against the tubercle bacillus);
- 7.5 per cent povidone-iodine (duration of effect shorter, highly bactericidal, fungicidal and viricidal; some effect against spores and good anti-tubercle effect);
- alcohols (highly effective against all but spores and inexpensive).

Allergic reactions are recognised to both chlorhexidine and iodine solutions.

Movement in theatre

Scrubbed personnel should:

- keep their hands and arms on the operating table where possible;
- keep their hands away from their faces;
- touch only sterile items or areas;
- watch the sterile fields to avoid contamination;
- not lean over unsterile fields;
- pass each other back-to-back or front-to-front.

Unscrubbed personnel should:

- touch only unsterile items or areas;
- face and observe a sterile area when passing it to be sure that they do not touch it;
- avoid walking between the patient and trays;
- minimise activity near the sterile field.

Instrument trays are prepared by the scrub nurse; supplies are brought to the sterile team members by the non-sterile circulating nurse who opens the outside wrappers and passes the item to the scrub nurse.

Prepping and draping the patient

'Pre-prep' may be indicated where there is visible debris to be removed; it consists of washing the skin with soapy disinfectant, then water or saline, then surgical disinfectant (Figure 18.5). Patients undergoing elective surgery may instead shower on the day of surgery with a soapy disinfectant.

Skin preparation should include the surgical site and a wide area around it, starting from the incision site and working away from it. Contaminated areas (groin, perineum, axilla) should be covered last. Two coats are usually used and the solutions are similar to those used for scrubbing up (see above). Care should be taken to avoid using excessive amounts of prep solution. This leads to pooling which can cause a chemical burn or ignite in the presence of a spark.

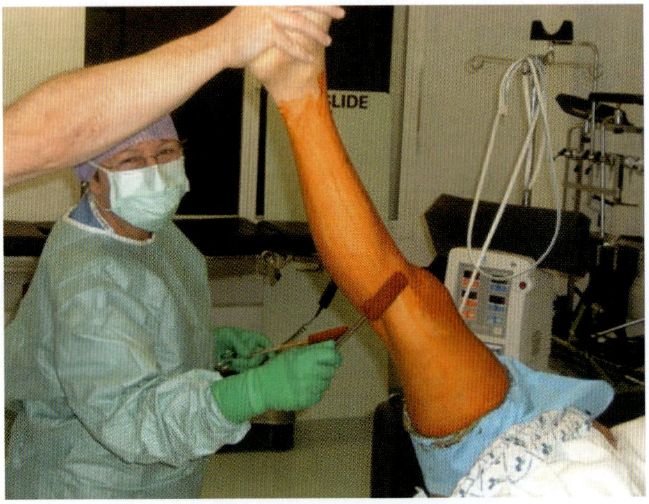

Figure 18.5 Prepping (skin preparation) and draping. Application of skin disinfectant solution to skin. Note that this is the second coat being applied to the posterior aspect of the leg. The leg holder is standing away from the scrub nurse and should be gloved. For this operation, the foot is not being prepped.

Draping aims to create a protective zone around the operative site to avoid contamination of items used for the procedure (Figure 18.6). Both disposable and reusable drapes are suitable, and should be handled only by scrubbed personnel. They should be sited to allow full access to the incision (or any possible extension). Once in place, they should not be disturbed. Skin immediately around the incision site may also be covered with a self-adhesive transparent drape. Diathermy and suction equipment are attached to the drape.

Role of the assistant

Surgical assistants are frequently surgeons in training. They are therefore in theatre to help the senior surgeon and to learn as much as possible (Summary box 18.6).

- **Preparation**. Assistants should review the anatomy and the operation before surgery so that they can anticipate and understand the actions of the senior surgeon. They should start scrubbing first, having checked that the patient is ready for theatre.
- **Training**. Trainees should write important steps of proposed operation in brief on a board in the operating theatre.
- **At surgery**. The assistant should try to provide the surgeon with the best access possible by placing and holding retractors and showing the surgeon the field where they are working.

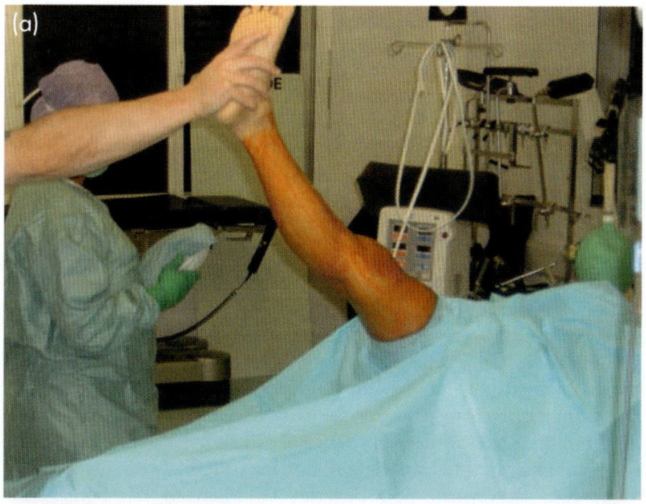

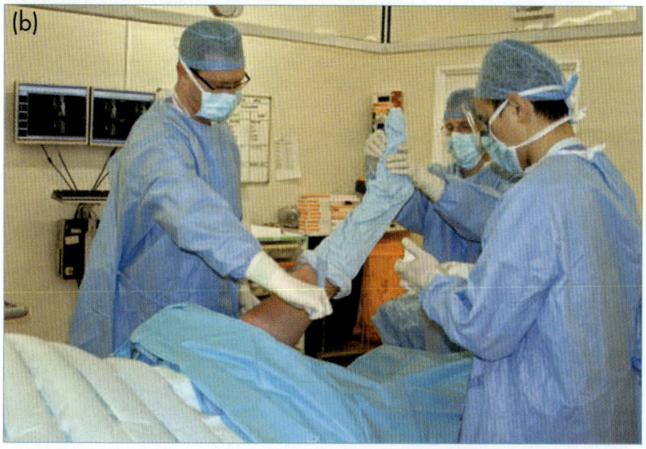

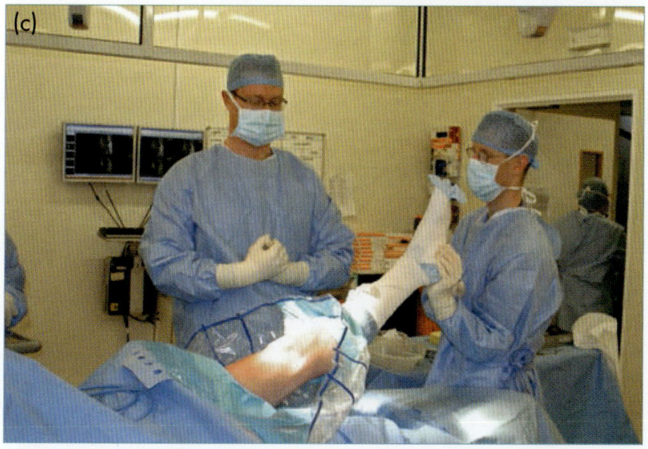

Figure 18.6 (a) A waterproof underdrape is applied with adhesive edges. A sterile waterproof stockingette is about to be applied by the scrub nurse, initially on to the forefoot with the unscrubbed assistant supporting the heel. The unsterile assistant will then move away carefully from the operating table. All of these drapes are disposable. (b) The stockingettes applied. (c) The final drapes are placed over the stockingettes, the operation sites are covered with clear adhesive and a sterile bandage is used to secure the stockingettes. Some surgeons will prep the feet entirely before draping. Note also the hand position of the surgeon.

Instruments and retractors should always be asked for by name.

- **After surgery**. The assistant should help transfer the patient safely off the table and may write the operative note. They should keep a log of all operations attended and what they have learnt from each case.

Summary box 18.6

In theatre

- The WHO checklist is a universal tool to improve patient safety and should be completed for every patient coming to theatre
- Risks to the patient are minimised by appropriate antibiotic and venous thromboembolism (VTE) prophylaxis, monitoring, careful positioning, temperature, glycaemic and infection control
- The operating theatre environment should be optimised with regard to lighting, ventilation, humidity and temperature
- Additional equipment, such as diathermy and tourniquets, should be used while recognising their potential complications
- Theatre etiquette including scrubbing, prepping and draping and personnel movement is designed to minimise cross-infection

POSTOPERATIVE CARE

'Sign out'

Before any personnel leave theatre, the WHO 'sign out' checks should be completed. These include checking that the procedure has been recorded, that instrument and swab counts are correct, that there have been no equipment problems requiring further action and the key concerns for recovery recorded for the staff taking over care of the patient (Summary box 18.7).

Summary box 18.7

Postoperative care

- The 'sign out' process and postlist briefing complete the WHO checklist
- The operation note should be completed at the time of surgery and contain full patient, personnel and operative information
- Clear postoperative instructions are vital

Writing the operation note

The following information should be included:

- Patient details (name, date of birth, hospital number, address, ward)
- Date and start/finish times of the operation
- Location of the operation
- Name of the operation
- Surgeon, assistant and anaesthetist
- Anaesthetic type
- Patient position and set up

- If applicable, tourniquet use (location and time), antibiotics given, catheterisation, skin prep used and draping method
- Operative information:
  - incision and approach
  - findings
  - procedure (illustrate if appropriate)
  - complications or untoward events
  - implants used
  - closure and suture material used
  - dressing
- Postoperative instructions:
  - observations and frequency
  - possible complications and required action
  - specific treatment, e.g. intravenous fluids
  - time line for normal recovery (when to mobilise, when to resume oral intake, physiotherapy, dressing changes, etc.)
  - discharge and follow-up details (including instruction for sutures, casts, etc.).

FURTHER READING

Association of Anaesthetists of Great Britain and Ireland. *Recommendations for standards of monitoring during anaesthesia and recovery*, 4th edn. London: AAGBI, 2007.

Knight DJW, Mahajan RP. Patient positioning in anaesthesia. Continuing education in anaesthesia. *Crit Care Pain* 2004; **4**: 160–3.

National Institute for Health and Clinical Excellence. Inadvertent perioperative hypothermia – the management of inadvertent perioperative hypothermia in adults. NICE clinical guideline 65, 2008. Available from: www.nice.org.uk/CG65.

National Institute for Health and Clinical Excellence. Surgical site infection. Prevention and treatment of surgical site infection. London: NICE, 2008.

National Institute for Health and Clinical Excellence. Venous thromboembolism: reducing the risk. Reducing the risk of venous thromboembolism (deep vein thrombosis and pulmonary embolism) in patients admitted to hospital. London: NICE, 2010.

Rigby KA, Palfreyman SSJ, Beverley C, Michaels JA. Surgery for varicose veins: use of tourniquet. *Cochrane Database Syst Rev* 2002; (**4**): CD001486.

Tanner J, Woodings D, Moncaster K. Preoperative hair removal to reduce surgical site infection. *Cochrane Database Syst Rev* 2006; (**3**): CD004122.

World Alliance for Patient Safety. *WHO guidelines for safe surgery*. Geneva: World Health Organization, 2008.

CHAPTER 19

Perioperative management of the high-risk surgical patient

LEARNING OBJECTIVES

To understand:

- Factors that place patients at a high risk of complications
- Importance of identifying the high-risk patient
- Role of preoptimisation in minimising risk
- Importance of critical care in management

INTRODUCTION

In modern day medicine, the majority of patients enjoy a safe and uneventful recovery following surgery. There remains, however, a subgroup at higher risk of morbidity and mortality after surgery. Operative mortality is more meaningfully expressed in terms of deaths occurring during surgery and up to 28–30 days after surgery. The overall 30-day mortality risk for operative procedures in Western Europe is 0.7–1.85 per cent, but this figure includes the high-risk patient population. Seventy per cent of all elective procedures have a mortality risk of less than 1 per cent, the high-risk group has a mortality risk in excess of 5 per cent and when the risk exceeds 20 per cent, patients are said to be at 'extremely high risk' (Figure 19.1). It is estimated that the high-risk group accounts for about 12.5 per cent of all surgical procedures and more than 80 per cent of deaths.

What causes these patients to be at a high risk of death and complications after surgery? After surgery tissue destruction, blood loss, fluid shifts, changes in temperature, pain and anxiety result in increased demands for oxygen delivery to the tissues. This demand increases from an average of 110 mL/m^2 per minute at rest to 170 mL/m^2 per minute in the postoperative period. Most patients meet this increase in demand by increasing their cardiac output and tissue oxygen extraction. Failure to meet these demands as a result of a limited cardiorespiratory reserve, can lead to myocardial ischaemia and multiorgan failure. These account for the majority of predictable surgical morbidity and mortality. Cardiac and respiratory problems contribute equally to this.

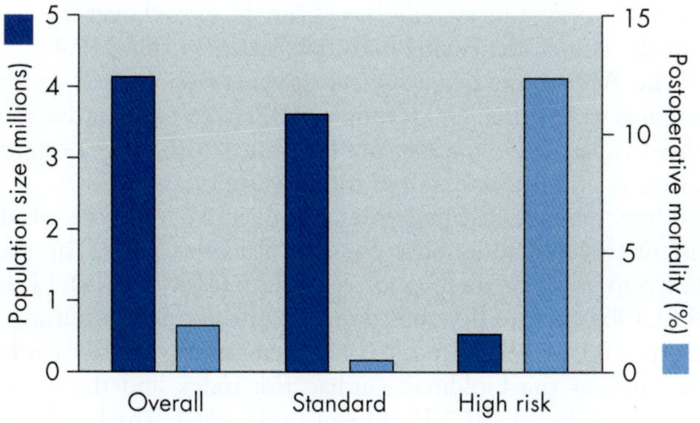

Figure 19.1 Size and mortality rates for different populations of surgical patients.

CLASSIFICATION OF RISK

Risk after surgery is a complex interaction of multiple factors which can be classified into patient and surgical factors (Table 19.1). The elderly, though not independently at higher risk, not only suffer more cardiac, pulmonary and renal disease, but also require surgery four times as often as the rest of the population.

The type of surgery contributes independently, but patient factors are probably more important as shown by the mortality rates of patients in different categories of fitness (Table 19.2). This risk increases if the surgery is performed as an emergency. Often, the underlying condition necessitating surgery itself may be associated with an increased risk of complications. For example, a patient with severe peripheral vascular disease resulting from heavy smoking, may need a femoral-popliteal bypass graft and can be expected also to have significant chronic obstructive pulmonary disease (COPD) and ischaemic heart disease (IHD).

Moreover, when mortality by type of surgery is adjusted for patient risk factors, the apparent hierarchy of surgical risk may change. The average mortality risk for an individual patient undergoing thoracic surgery, for example, is likely to be higher than the average risk for that same patient undergoing vascular surgery. Complications associated with the latter are nevertheless more frequent because vascular patients have greater medical risk factors (Table 19.3).

The typical high-risk patient is the elderly patient with coexisting conditions, such as IHD and/or COPD, undergoing major surgery. The risk would increase if the surgery is performed as an emergency.

Table 19.1 Factors that predispose patients to a high risk of morbidity and mortality.

Patient factors	History of severe cardiac disease (ischaemic heart disease (IHD), myocardial infarction (MI), cardiac failure)
	Severe respiratory disease (chronic obstructive pulmonary disease (COPD), respiratory failure)
	Aged >70 years with limited physiological reserve in one or more vital organs
	Metabolic disease (renal failure, poorly controlled diabetes)
	Morbid obesity
	Late stage vascular disease
	Poor nutrition
Surgical factors	Prolonged duration of surgery (>1.5 hours)
	Extensive surgery (e.g. oesophagectomy, gastrectomy)
	Type of surgery (thoracic, abdominal, vascular)
	Emergency surgery (e.g. perforated viscus, gangrenous bowel, gastrointestinal bleeding)
	Acute massive blood loss (>2.5 litres)
	Septicaemia (positive blood cultures or septic focus)
	Severe multiple trauma e.g. >3 organs or >2 systems or ≥2 body cavities open

Adapted from criteria outlined by Shoemaker and colleagues and Mangano and colleagues.

Table 19.2 Operative mortality by ASA (American Society of Anesthesiologists) grade.

ASA grade	Description	30-day mortality (%)
I	Healthy	0.1
II	Mild systemic disease, no functional limitation	1
III	Severe systemic disease, definite functional limitation	4
IV	Severe systemic disease, constant threat to life	20
V	Moribund patient unlikely to survive 24 hours with or without operation	90
E	Emergency operation	–

Table 19.3 The effect of adjustment for patient factors on surgery-specific operative mortality (modified from Noordzij *et al.*, 2010).

Type of surgery	Unadjusted 30-day mortality (% (rank))	Adjusted 30-day mortality (% (rank))
Vascular	6.0 (1)	1.0 (5)
Thoracic	3.4 (2)	2.3 (1)
Abdominal	2.7 (3)	1.8 (2)
Cardiac	2.7 (4)	1.1 (4)
Neurosurgery	1.7 (5)	1.6 (3)
Orthopaedic	1.3 (6)	0.5 (7)
ENT	0.9 (7)	0.7 (6)
Urology	0.8 (8)	0.4 (8)
Gynaecology	0.1 (9)	0.2 (9)
Breast	0.7 (10)	0.1 (10)

GENERAL PRINCIPLES OF MANAGEMENT

The key to managing these patients is the identification of risk, the accurate estimation of that risk and the work done to minimise it.

Realistic estimates of risk are the cornerstone of informed patient consent. The patient and the surgeon may choose a less extensive or even a non-surgical option where risks of the definitive procedure are deemed to be too high or unacceptable. Senior staff, both surgical and anaesthetic, should be involved in these cases from the start and surgery should be performed during normal working hours wherever possible.

Depending on particular comorbidities, it may be possible for a patient's underlying conditions to be improved by optimising their medical therapy. Additional physiological optimisation may take the form of measures to minimise myocardial ischaemia or measures to improve oxygen delivery to the other major organs, depending on the prevailing risks. Optimisation before surgery can be more effective in a critical care environment and patients may need to be admitted to a high dependency unit (HDU) or intensive treatment unit (ITU) preoperatively. The likelihood of the high-risk patient requiring postoperative critical care should be discussed with the duty critical care physician.

Identification of patients who will benefit most from these additional considerations is important not only for the improvement of outcomes, but also the effective allocation of resources. Emergency surgery is associated with higher risks because by its very nature, there is less time and opportunity to organise these additional levels of care (Summary box 19.1).

Summary box 19.1

A practical approach to perioperative care for the high-risk patient

- Identify the high-risk patient
- Assess the level of risk
- Detailed preoperative assessment
- Optimise medical management
- Intraoperative considerations
- Consider specific strategies, e.g. β-blockade or goal-directed therapy
- Consider admission to a critical care facility postoperatively

Identification of the high-risk patient

A number of scoring systems have been developed over the years with the aim of identifying high-risk patients (Table 19.4).

The ASA (American Society of Anesthesiologists) scoring system is widely used and is simple and related to operative mortality (Table 19.2), but does not take into account age or nature of surgery and is prone to user interpretation.

More may be gleaned from a subjective estimate of the patient's overall functional physical fitness as judged by their ability to tolerate metabolic equivalent tasks (METs) (Table 19.5). Objective indices based on weighted scores pertaining to surgery and comorbidity have been created to stratify cardiac risk, such as the Goldman cardiac risk index and the revised cardiac risk index (RCRI) of Lee (Table 19.6), which although designed to predict cardiac morbidity, may also be used to stratify the risk of mortality.

Lee Goldman, born 1948, Dean of Health Sciences and Medicine, Columbia University, New York, USA, since 2006. He developed his Index in 1977.
Thomas H Lee, contemporary, Professor of Medicine, Harvard Medical School, Professor of Health Policy and Management, Harvard School of Public Health, Boston, Mass., USA.

Table 19.4 Risk scoring systems.

ASA is simple, but subject to user interpretation
MET measures exercise tolerance related to daily living
RCRI used to predict cardiac risk for non-cardiac surgery
POSSUM can only be used postoperatively and better for some types of surgery, e.g. colorectal, vascular
CPET is non-invasive, objective and becoming increasingly popular

ASA, American Society of Anesthesiologists; CPET, cardiopulmonary exercise testing; MET, metabolic equivalent of task; RCRI, revised cardiac risk index; POSSUM, Physiologic and Operative Severity Score for the enUmeration of Mortality and Morbidity.

Table 19.5 Metabolic equivalent of task (MET).

1 MET = 3.5 mL O_2/kg per minute (oxygen consumption by 40 year, 70 kg man at rest)
1 MET = eating and dressing
4 MET = climbing two flights of stairs
6 MET = short run
>10 MET = able to participate in strenuous sport
Patients who can exercise at 4 METS or above have lower risk of perioperative mortality

Table 19.6 The revised cardiac risk index of Lee.

Number of risk factors	Risk of major cardiac complications (%)
Risk of complications according to number of risk factors	
0	0.4
1	0.9
2	7.0
3+	11
Risk factors	
History of ischaemic heart disease	
History of compensated or prior heart failure	
History of cerebrovascular disease	
Diabetes mellitus	
Renal insufficiency (creatinine > 177 μmol/litre)	
High risk surgery	

Another widely used scoring system is POSSUM (Physiologic and Operative Severity Score for the enUmeration of Mortality and Morbidity) for predicting all-cause mortality in postoperative critical care patients, as well as non-cardiac morbidity. POSSUM can, however, only be calculated after surgery and appears to be more useful for some types of surgery than others.

In recent years, cardiopulmonary exercise testing (CPET) has become a popular screening tool to identify high-risk patients. O_2 consumption and CO_2 production of the subject are measured while they undergo a 10-minute period of incrementally demanding exercise (usually on a cycle ergometer) up to their maximally tolerated level (Figure 19.2).

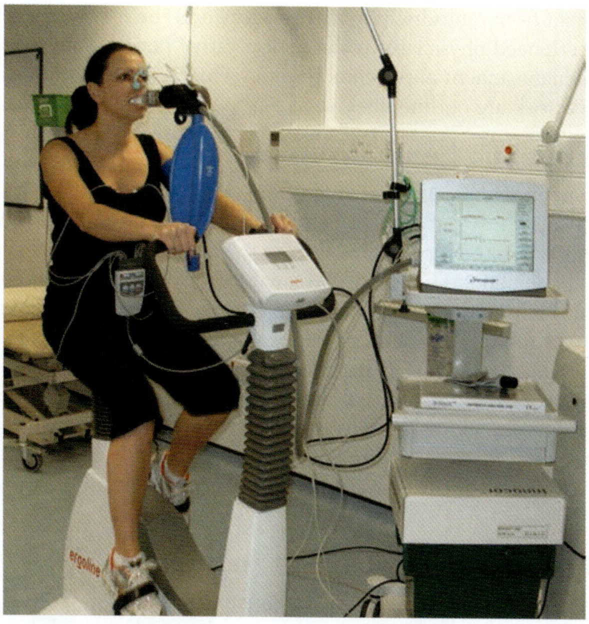

Figure 19.2 Cardiopulmonary exercise testing (CPET).

CPET is based on the principle that when a subject's delivery of O_2 to active tissues becomes inadequate, anaerobic metabolism begins; lactate is buffered by bicarbonate and the resulting CO_2 increases out of proportion to the escalation in physical difficulty and O_2 consumption. The 'anaerobic threshold' (AT) is the O_2 consumption in mL/kg per minute above which this occurs. Peak oxygen consumption (VO_2) is also measured. They are the end product of a subject's combined respiratory, cardiac, vascular and musculoskeletal fitness, and subjects with either an AT below a somewhat arbitrary cut-off of 11 and a VO_2 below 15 mL/kg per minute are at higher risk of morbidity and mortality after surgery (Summary box 19.2).

Summary box 19.2

Risk scoring systems

- ASA is simple but subject to user interpretation
- RCRI used to predict cardiac risk for non-cardiac surgery
- POSSUM can only be used postoperatively and is better for some surgery e.g. colorectal, vascular
- CEPT is a non-invasive and objective method

Optimise medical management of coexisting diseases and intraoperative considerations

The medical management of all coexisting disease processes should be reviewed and optimised. The actions taken may be simple measures, such as stopping smoking, reducing alcohol intake, losing weight, improving nutrition and/or haemoglobin levels. In some cases, there will be a need for more complex investigations, review of medication or even consideration of further surgery. Patients scheduled for abdominal aortic aneurysm (AAA) repair surgery for example, frequently require carotid duplex scans. If the scans reveal a significant blockage and a high risk of perioperative stroke, a carotid endarterectomy may be indicated prior to AAA repair. All high-risk patients benefit from multidisciplinary team care and the involvement of experienced physicians in the perioperative period. The impact and management of the comorbidities which commonly contribute to risk are outlined below.

Ischaemic heart disease

Perioperative myocardial infarction (MI) is associated with a high mortality (15–25 per cent). Ischaemia and ultimately MI occur when the supply of oxygen to the myocardium is exceeded by its demand. This situation can be precipitated by hypotension, tachycardia and procoagulant states (of which the inflammatory response to surgery is an example).

Preparation of these patients for surgery should be aimed at optimising their myocardial oxygen supply and demand ratio and so minimise the risk of myocardial ischaemia developing. This work may involve further investigations or even the decision to postpone non-cardiac surgery for three to six months after an MI.

Minimising myocardial ischaemia

Anaesthesia techniques that dampen the stress response to surgery (especially minimising pain) and provide a good degree of cardiac stability should be used. Anaesthesia should avoid tachycardia, systolic hypertension and diastolic hypotension and may be aided by use of invasive arterial blood pressure monitoring to facilitate this. Blood loss must be accurately monitored and haemoglobin maintained at a level suitable for the patient's cardiac risk factors. Perioperative use of β-blockers may be considered, but this is controversial and is discussed below under Prophylactic β-blockade.

Troponin testing allows early diagnosis of perioperative MIs, but there are limited reperfusion options due to risk of bleeding from the surgical site. Admission to a HDU should be considered for patients with IHD and supplemental oxygen therapy continued for 3 to 4 days (Summary box 19.3).

Summary box 19.3

Minimising myocardial ischaemia

- Anaesthesia should avoid tachycardia, hypertension and hypotension
- Pain control is important
- Oxygen supplementation is advisable for 3–4 days postoperatively
- Perioperative β-blockade should be considered
- Elective postoperative critical care admission should be considered

Cardiac failure

Left ventricular failure is the end result of several conditions including IHD, hypertension, cardiomyopathies and valve dysfunction. Decompensated heart failure puts patients at a risk of multiorgan failure and those with ejection fractions of less than 35 per cent and in whom the failure is undiagnosed or its severity underestimated are at the highest risk. The patient's functional capacity needs to be assessed and surgery may have to be delayed for investigations such as an echocardiogram and/or for optimisation of medical therapy. Drugs used in chronic heart failure have significant implications for perioperative care and β-blockers and probably ACE inhibitors (unless renal perfusion is to be significantly affected) should be continued. Anaesthesia should ensure minimal myocardial depression and change in afterload during surgery. Arrhythmias must be rapidly brought under control, particularly atrial fibrillation (AF), and correcting any electrolyte imbalance is crucial in this respect. Invasive monitoring of trends in central venous and arterial pressure monitoring may help management, particularly when large fluid shifts are expected to occur.

Respiratory failure

Surgery, particularly open abdominal procedures under general anaesthesia result in changes to respiratory physiology. The functional residual capacity of the lungs is reduced. This combined with respiratory depressant effects of residual anaesthetic agents, the patient's limited mobility, and pain from surgery causes atelectasis (failure of gas exchange due to alveolar collapse) and predisposes patients to postoperative respiratory infection. Together with other complications, including bronchospasm, pneumothorax and acute respiratory distress syndrome (ARDS), these contribute as much to morbidity and length of hospital stay as cardiac complications. Respiratory failure defined as a PaO_2 <8 kPa in air, PaO_2/FiO_2 <40 kPa or inability to extubate a patient 48 hours after surgery, is by far the most significant of these and is associated with a mortality of 27–40 per cent.

Again, as with cardiac risk management, it may be necessary to postpone surgery to allow medical optimisation or consider a non-operative option. Preoperatively, bronchodilator therapy will be required in those with reversible obstructive airway disease and steroids may need to be started or increased. Nutritional status should be optimised and albumin levels corrected. Physiotherapy for postural drainage and deep breathing exercises or incentive spirometry should be considered for patients at increased risk of respiratory complications. General anaesthesia is associated with more respiratory complications and so regional techniques should be considered where possible in these patients. Hypoxaemia and CO_2 retention leading to the need for reintubation is better avoided in those at risk, by delaying extubation until analgesia, hydration and acid–base status have been corrected. Patients may benefit from ITU admission and this needs planning. Application of non-invasive respiratory support (Figure 19.3) may allow certain patients to be extubated earlier (Summary box 19.4).

Summary box 19.4

Optimising perioperative respiratory function

- Preoperative pulmonary function needs testing to assess functional status
- Consider bronchodilator ± steroid therapy
- Arrange pre- and postoperative chest physiotherapy and breathing exercises
- Consider regional anaesthesia
- Give good quality pain relief
- Use non-invasive ventilation strategies

Other comorbidities

Acute renal failure, chronic kidney disease, diabetes, peripheral vascular disease and liver dysfunction are some of the medical conditions that contribute to risk and need to be optimised.

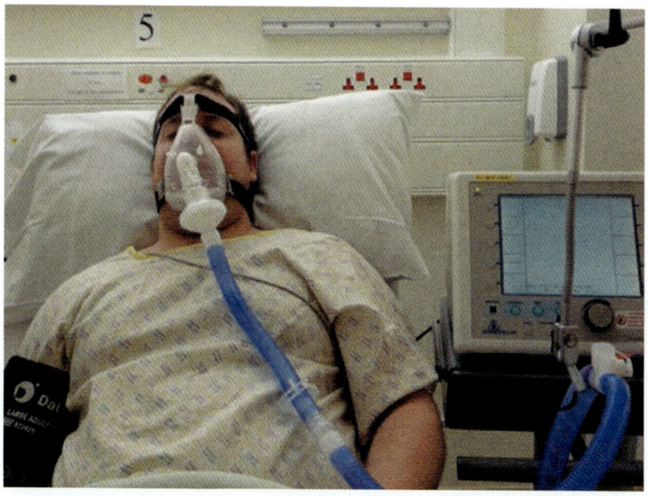

Figure 19.3 Non-invasive ventilation.

SPECIFIC STRATEGIES

Prophylactic β-blockade

A number of studies have considered the prophylactic use of nitrates, calcium channel blockers and β-blockers for patients at high risk of perioperative myocardial ischaemia. With the exception of β-blockade, none of these therapies has resulted in an improvement in outcome.

'POISE', a large randomised trial, looked at the use of β-blockers in the 'at risk' group undergoing non-cardiac surgery. They found that perioperative β-blockers lead to reduced deaths and MIs combined, but increased risk of hypotension, strokes and deaths overall. Patients already on β-blockers should continue taking them in the perioperative period. When β-blockers are added preoperatively, they must be titrated to heart rate and blood pressure over at least a week before surgery. Recent European guidelines may be used to determine which patients may benefit from preoperative β-blockade (see Further reading).

Goal-directed therapy

Persistent inadequate tissue perfusion is a major factor in the development of perioperative organ failure. High-risk patients who survive without multiorgan failure are known to have higher cardiac indices (CI) and oxygen delivery (DO_2) than those who die. This led to the concept of goal-directed therapy (GDT). The aim of GDT is to manipulate a patient's physiology to achieve targets that are associated with an improved outcome (CI >4.5 L/m^2 per minute, DO_2 >600 mL/m^2 per minute) using intravenous fluids and inotropes directed by measurements of cardiac output (CO).

For many years, the pulmonary artery catheter (PAC) was used to measure CO and facilitate GDT. However, it is an invasive technique associated with risks of arrhythmia, catheter knotting and pulmonary artery rupture. Thus, the need for critical care support was imperative while using PAC with subsequent resource implications.

Today, PAC has been replaced by less invasive devices to measure cardiac output, such as oesophageal Doppler, lithium dilution and pulse contour analysis equipment. The oesophageal Doppler device measures blood velocity in the aorta and then calculates the CO (Figure 19.4). Single values are inaccurate,

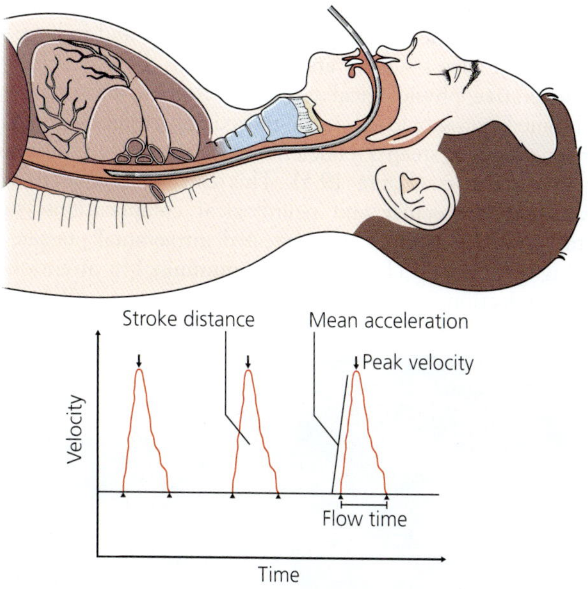

Figure 19.4 Oesophageal Doppler.

but as a device to monitor trends it is useful to rapidly detect CO changes in response to fluid administration. The administration of intravenous fluids to Doppler-guided targets compared to conventional replacement has been shown to reduce complications in cardiac, orthopaedic and abdominal surgery.

Some patients may need therapy with inotropes and/or vasopressors along with fluid administration. However, vasopressors increase myocardial oxygen demand and are not suitable in all patients. In addition to the above treatment, titrated doses of β-blockers can benefit those with a prevailing risk of ischaemia. Evidence is now emerging that GDT may have benefits if commenced intraoperatively and even postoperatively (Summary box 19.5).

Summary box 19.5

Specific strategies

- Initiation of perioperative β-blockade remains controversial
- Patients already taking β-blockers must continue their medication
- Less invasive modalities of CO measurement have largely superseded the PAC
- Fluids guided by GDT can reduce complications from surgery
- Inotropes and/or vasopressors are still required in many high-risk patients

MINIMISING THE IMPACT OF SURGICAL RISK FACTORS

There are situations where a choice of surgical techniques exists and which may be significantly influenced by patient risk factors. Some techniques are not primarily high-risk, but may become so in unsuitable patients. Laparoscopic surgery, for example, has come of age as a preferred technique for patients predisposed to postoperative respiratory complications, but its effect on cardiac physiology means the same may not apply to patients at risk of cardiac complications. The expanding demand and indications for minimal access surgery are now pushing the boundaries of intraoperative physiological tolerance. Robotic prostatectomy and some laparoscopic colorectal procedures, require a pneumoperitoneum with steep Trendelenburg (head down) positioning for several hours (Figure 19.5). This can be associated with adverse cardiovascular and neurological complications, such as myocardial ischaemia and increased intracranial pressure in the high-risk group. This risk may be minimised by attention to patient selection.

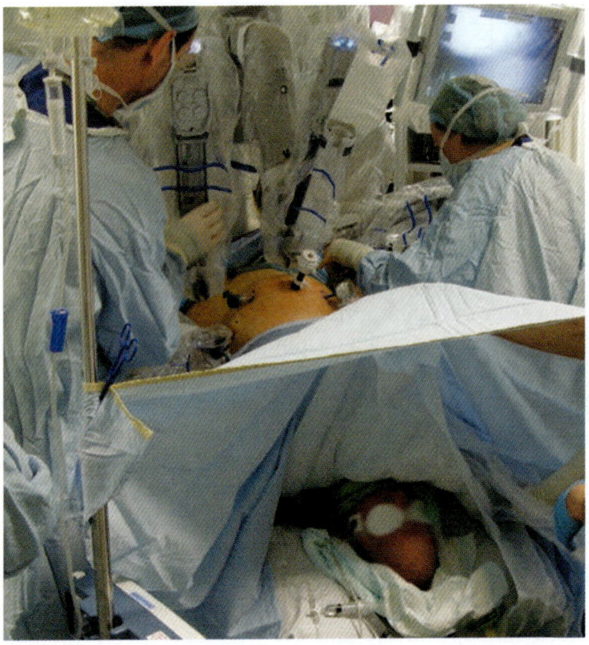

Figure 19.5 Robotic surgery.

ROLE OF CRITICAL CARE AND OUTREACH SERVICES

Optimal care in the high-risk group should be extended to include postoperative support which for a majority of these patients means admission to a critical care bed. Reports from the National Confidential Enquiry into Patient Outcome and Death (NCEPOD) show that the majority of postoperative deaths in the UK occur more than 5 days after surgery. Admission to a critical care unit allows for early intervention and a level of care that is difficult to deliver in the ward environment during this crucial period (Figure 19.6). The high-risk surgical population accounts for 80 per cent of postoperative deaths, but only about 15–30 per cent of high-risk surgical patients are admitted to a critical care unit at any time following surgery. One study which compared surgical mortality in the UK and the United States found an observed mortality of 10 per cent in the UK as compared to 2 per cent in the United States. It is suggested that the difference may be related to the provision of critical care services, with 10 critical care beds per 100 000 population in the UK compared to 30 in the United States.

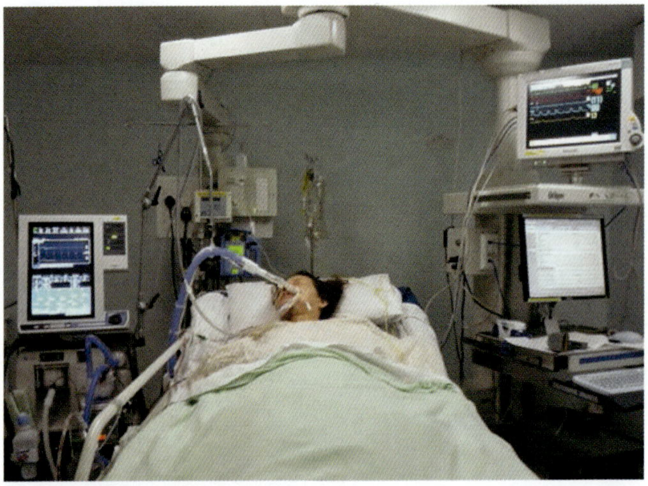

Figure 19.6 A high-risk patient admitted to the intensive care unit postoperatively.

In the last decade, the role of critical care has been expanded to the concept of 'critical care without walls'. The intensive care outreach services (ICORS) grew from a recognition that there were many patients in the hospital who are at risk of being critically ill and early identification of these patients could allow for early intervention. The outreach team functions to bridge the gap between critical care unit and ward.

SUMMARY

The majority of postoperative complications and deaths after surgery occur in the high-risk population. In most instances, mortality results ultimately either from a cardiac event or multiorgan dysfunction secondary to a severe deficiency in tissue oxygen delivery. Increased awareness along with improved systems for the identification of the high-risk surgical patient are important, as today novel treatment strategies offer the prospect of significant improvements in outcome. A multidisciplinary team approach is crucial to successful management.

FURTHER READING

Boyd O, Jackson N. How is risk defined in high-risk surgical patient management? *Crit Care* 2005; **9**: 390–6.

Fleisher LA, Beckman JA, Buller CE *et al.* ACCF/AHA focused update on perioperative beta blockade. *J Am Coll Cardiol* 2009; **54**: 2102–28.

Giglio MT, Marucci M, Testini M, Brienza N. Goal-directed haemodynamic therapy and gastrointestinal complications in major surgery: a meta-analysis of randomised controlled trials. *Br J Anaesth* 2009; **103**: 637–46.

Poldermans D, Bax JJ, Boersma E *et al.* Guidelines for pre-operative cardiac risk assessment and perioperative cardiac management in non-cardiac surgery: the Task Force for Preoperative Cardiac Risk Assessment and Perioperative Cardiac Management in Non-cardiac Surgery of the European Society of Cardiology (ESC) and European Society of Anaesthesiology (ESA). *Eur Heart J* 2009; **30**: 2769–812.

CHAPTER 20

Nutrition and fluid therapy

LEARNING OBJECTIVES

To understand:

- The causes and consequences of malnutrition in the surgical patient
- Fluid and electrolyte requirements in the pre- and postoperative patient
- The nutritional requirements of surgical patients and the nutritional consequences of intestinal resection
- The different methods of providing nutritional support and their complications

INTRODUCTION

Malnutrition is common. It occurs in about 30 per cent of surgical patients with gastrointestinal disease and in up to 60 per cent of those in whom hospital stay has been prolonged because of postoperative complications. It is frequently unrecognised and consequently patients often do not receive appropriate support. There is a substantial body of evidence to show that patients who suffer starvation or have signs of malnutrition have a higher risk of complications and an increased risk of death in comparison with patients who have adequate nutritional reserves.

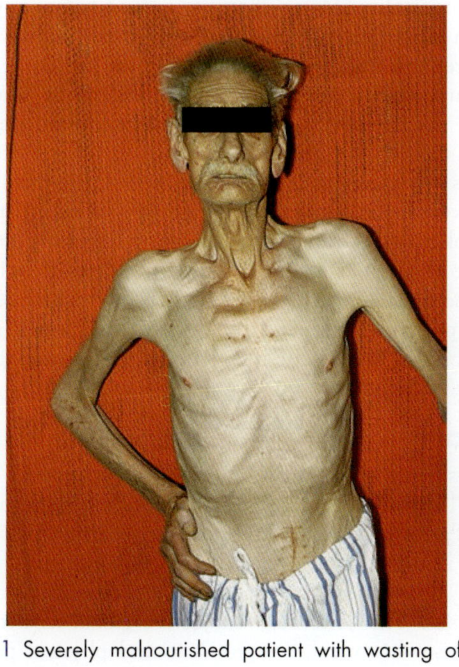

Figure 20.1 Severely malnourished patient with wasting of fat and muscle.

Long-standing protein–calorie malnutrition is easy to recognise (Figure 20.1). Short-term undernutrition, although less easily recognised, frequently occurs in association with critical illness, major trauma, burns or surgery, and also impacts on patient recovery. The aim of nutritional support is to identify those patients at risk of malnutrition and to ensure that their nutritional requirements are met by the most appropriate route and in a way that minimises complications.

PHYSIOLOGY

Metabolic response to starvation

After a short fast lasting 12 hours or less, most food from the last meal will have been absorbed. Plasma insulin levels fall and glucagon levels rise, which facilitates the conversion of 200 g of liver glycogen into glucose. The liver, therefore, becomes an organ of glucose production under fasting conditions. Many organs, including brain tissue, red and white blood cells and the renal medulla, can initially utilise only glucose for their metabolic needs. Additional stores of glycogen exist in muscle (500 g), but these cannot be utilised directly. Muscle glycogen is broken down (glycogenolysis) and converted to lactate, which is then exported to the liver where it is converted to glucose (Cori cycle). With increasing duration of fasting (>24 hours), glycogen stores are depleted and *de novo* glucose production from non-carbohydrate precursors (gluconeogenesis) takes place, predominantly in the liver. Most of this glucose is derived from the breakdown of amino acids, particularly glutamine and alanine as

Carl Ferdinand Cori, 1896–1984, Professor of Pharmacology and later Biochemistry, Washington University Medical School, St Louis, MI, USA and his wife Gerty Theresa Cori, 1896–1957, also Professor of Biochemistry at the Washington University Medical School. In 1947, the Coris were awarded a share of the Nobel Prize for Physiology or Medicine for their discovery of how glycogen is catalytically converted.

de novo is Latin for 'from the beginning'.

a result of catabolism of skeletal muscle (up to 75 g per day). This protein catabolism in simple starvation is readily reversed with the provision of exogenous glucose.

With more prolonged fasting there is an increased reliance on fat oxidation to meet energy requirements. Increased breakdown of fat stores occurs, providing glycerol, which can be converted to glucose, and fatty acids, which can be used as a tissue fuel by almost all of the body's tissues. Hepatic production of ketones from fatty acids is facilitated by low insulin levels and, after 48–72 hours of fasting, the central nervous system may adapt to using ketone bodies as their primary fuel source. This conversion to a 'fat fuel economy' reduces the need for muscle breakdown by up to 55 g per day.

Another important adaptive response to starvation is a significant reduction in the resting energy expenditure, possibly mediated by a decline in the conversion of inactive thyroxine (T4) to active tri-iodothyronine (T3). Despite these adaptive responses, there remains an obligatory glucose requirement of about 200 g per day, even under conditions of prolonged fasting (Summary box 20.1).

Summary box 20.1

Metabolic response to starvation

- Low plasma insulin
- High plasma glucagon
- Hepatic glycogenolysis
- Protein catabolism
- Hepatic gluconeogenesis
- Lipolysis: mobilisation of fat stores (increased fat oxidation)– overall decrease in protein and carbohydrate oxidation
- Adaptive ketogenesis
- Reduction in resting energy expenditure (from approximately 25–30 kcal/kg per day to 15–20 kcal/kg per day

Hepatic production of ketones from fatty acids is facilitated by low insulin levels and, after 48–72 hours of fasting, the central nervous system may adapt to using ketone bodies as their primary fuel source.

Metabolic response to trauma and sepsis

This is described in full in Chapter 1 and summarised in Summary box 20.2.

Summary box 20.2

Metabolic response to trauma and sepsis

- Increased counter-regulatory hormones: adrenaline, noradrenaline, cortisol, glucagon and growth hormone
- Increased energy requirements (up to 40 kcal/kg per day)
- Increased nitrogen requirements
- Insulin resistance and glucose intolerance
- Preferential oxidation of lipids
- Increased gluconeogenesis and protein catabolism
- Loss of adaptive ketogenesis
- Fluid retention with associated hypoalbuminaemia

From a nutritional point of view, two factors deserve emphasis. First, in contrast to simple starvation, patients with trauma have impaired formation of ketones and the breakdown of protein to synthesise glucose (gluconeogenesis) cannot be entirely prevented by the administration of glucose. Second, although it is generally accepted that the metabolic response to trauma and sepsis is always associated with 'hypermetabolism' or hypercatabolism', these terms are ill defined and do not indicate the need for very high-energy intakes. There is no evidence to show that the provision of high-energy intakes is associated with an amelioration of the catabolic process and it may indeed be harmful.

NUTRITIONAL ASSESSMENT

Laboratory techniques

There is no single biochemical measurement that reliably identifies malnutrition. Albumin is not a measure of nutritional status. Although a low serum albumin level (<30 g/L) is an indicator of poor prognosis, hypoalbuminaemia invariably occurs because of alterations in body fluid composition and because of increased capillary permeability related to ongoing sepsis. Malnutrition is associated with defective immune function, and measurement of lymphocyte count and skin testing for delayed hypersensitivity frequently reveal abnormalities in malnourished patients. Immunity is not, however, a precise or reliable indicator of nutritional status, nor is it a practical method in routine clinical practice.

Body weight and anthropometry

A simple method of assessing nutritional status is to estimate weight loss. Measured body weight is compared with ideal body weight obtained from tables or from the patient's usual or premorbid weight. Unintentional weight loss of more than 10 per cent of a patient's weight in the preceding six months is a good prognostic indicator of poor outcome. Body weight is frequently corrected for height, allowing calculation of the body mass index (BMI, defined as body weight in kilograms divided by height in metres squared). A BMI of less than 18.5 indicates nutritional impairment and a BMI below 15 is associated with significant hospital mortality. Major changes in fluid balance, which are common in critically ill patients, may make body weight and BMI unreliable indicators of nutritional status.

Anthropometric techniques incorporating measurements of skinfold thicknesses and mid-arm circumference permit estimations of body fat and muscle mass, and these are indirect measures of energy and protein stores. These measurements are, however, insufficiently accurate in individual patients to permit planning of nutritional support regimens. Similarly, use of bioelectrical impedence analysis (BIA) permits estimation of intra- and extracellular fluid volumes. These techniques are only useful if performed frequently on a sequential basis in individual patients. All of these techniques are significantly impaired by the presence of oedema.

Clinical

The possibility of malnutrition should form part of the work up of all patients. A clinical assessment of nutritional status involves a focused history and physical examination, an assessment of risk of malabsorption or inadequate dietary intake and selected laboratory tests aimed at detecting specific nutrient deficiencies. This is termed 'subjective global assessment' and encompasses historical, symptomatic and physical parameters. Recently, the British Association of Parenteral and Enteral Nutrition introduced a malnutrition universal screening tool

(MUST), which is a five-step screening tool to identify adults who are malnourished or at risk of undernutrition (Figure 20.2).

FLUID AND ELECTROLYTES

Fluid intake is derived from both exogenous (consumed liquids) and endogenous (released during oxidation of solid foodstuffs) fluids. The average daily water balance of a healthy adult is shown in Table 20.1.

Fluid losses occur by four routes:

1 **Lungs**. About 400 mL of water is lost in expired air each 24 hours. This is increased in dry atmospheres or in patients with a tracheostomy, emphasising the importance of humidification of inspired air.
2 **Skin**. In a temperate climate, skin (i.e. sweat) losses are between 600 and 1000 mL/day.
3 **Faeces**. Between 60 and 150 mL of water are lost daily in patients with normal bowel function.
4 **Urine**. The normal urine output is approximately 1500 mL/day and, provided that the kidneys are healthy, the specific gravity of urine bears a direct relationship to volume. A minimum urine output of 400 mL/day is required to excrete the end products of protein metabolism.

Table 20.1 Average daily water balance of a healthy adult in a temperate climate (70 kg).

Output	Volume (mL)	Intake	Volume (mL)
Urine	1500	Water from beverage	200
Insensible losses	900	Water from food	1000
Faeces	100	Water from oxidation	300

Maintenance fluid requirements are calculated approximately from an estimation of insensible and obligatory losses. Various formulae are available for calculating fluid replacement based on a patient's weight or surface area. For example, 30–40 mL/kg gives an estimate of daily requirements.

The following are the approximate daily requirements of some electrolytes in adults:

- sodium: 50–90 mM/day;
- potassium: 50 mM/day;
- calcium: 5 mM/day;
- magnesium: 1 mM/day.

The nature and type of fluid replacement therapy will be determined by individual patient needs. The composition of some commonly used solutions is shown in Table 20.2.

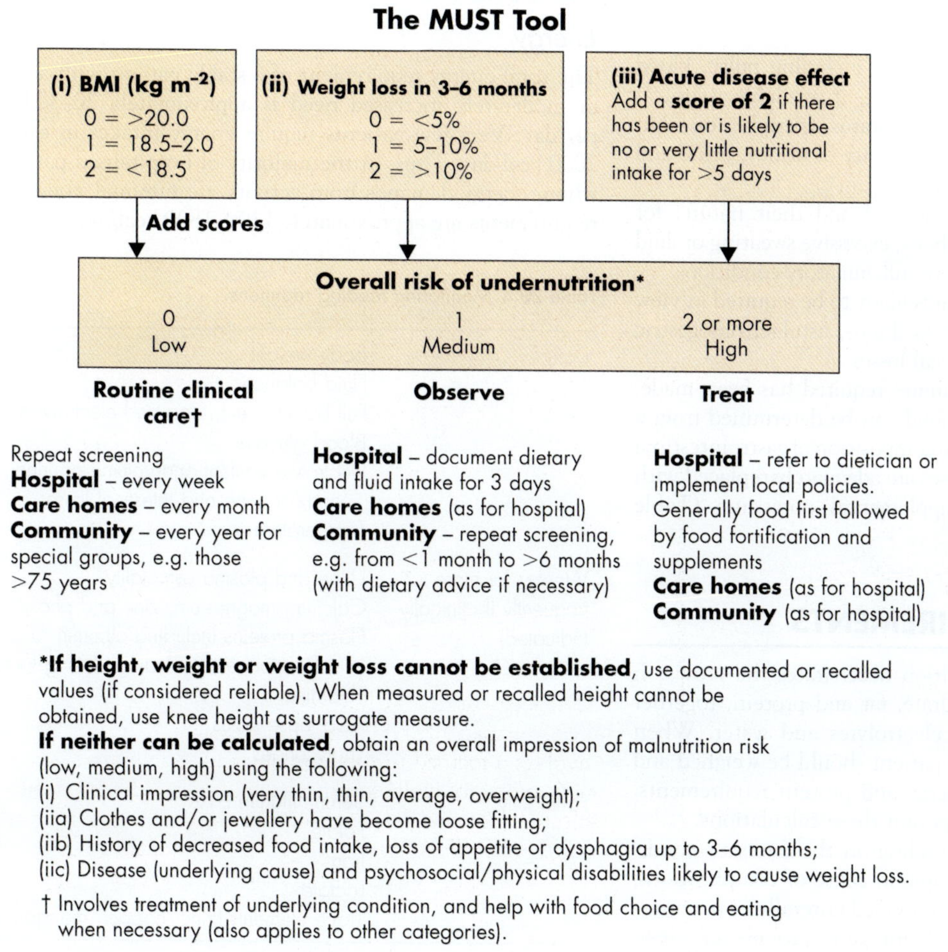
The MUST Tool
(i) BMI (kg m⁻²)
0 = >20.0
1 = 18.5–2.0
2 = <18.5
(ii) Weight loss in 3–6 months
0 = <5%
1 = 5–10%
2 = >10%
(iii) Acute disease effect
Add a score of 2 if there has been or is likely to be no or very little nutritional intake for >5 days
Add scores
Overall risk of undernutrition*
0 Low
1 Medium
2 or more High
Routine clinical care†
Observe
Treat
Repeat screening
Hospital – every week
Care homes – every month
Community – every year for special groups, e.g. those >75 years
Hospital – document dietary and fluid intake for 3 days
Care homes (as for hospital)
Community – repeat screening, e.g. from <1 month to >6 months (with dietary advice if necessary)
Hospital – refer to dietician or implement local policies.
Generally food first followed by food fortification and supplements
Care homes (as for hospital)
Community (as for hospital)
*If height, weight or weight loss cannot be established, use documented or recalled values (if considered reliable). When measured or recalled height cannot be obtained, use knee height as surrogate measure.
If neither can be calculated, obtain an overall impression of malnutrition risk (low, medium, high) using the following:
(i) Clinical impression (very thin, thin, average, overweight);
(iia) Clothes and/or jewellery have become loose fitting;
(iib) History of decreased food intake, loss of appetite or dysphagia up to 3–6 months;
(iic) Disease (underlying cause) and psychosocial/physical disabilities likely to cause weight loss.
† Involves treatment of underlying condition, and help with food choice and eating when necessary (also applies to other categories).

Figure 20.2 The malnutrition universal screening tool (MUST) for adults (adapted from Elia M (ed.). *The MUST Report. Development and use of the 'malnutrition universal screening tool' (MUST) for adults*. A report by the Malnutrition Advisory Group of the British Association for Parenteral and Enteral Nutrition. Report No. 152, 2003, ISBN 1 899467 70X).

Marinos Elia, contemporary, Head of the Adult Clinical Nutrition Group, The Medical Research Council, Cambridge, UK.

Table 20.2 Composition of crystalloid and colloid solutions (mmol/L).

Solution	Na	K	Ca	Cl	Lactate	Colloid
Hartmann's	131	5	2	111	29	
Normal saline (0.9% NaCl)	154	154				
Dextrose saline (4% dextrose in 0.18% saline)	30	30				
Gelofusine	150	150				Gelatin 4%
Haemacel	145	5.1	<1	145		Polygelin 75g/L
Hetastarch						Hydroxyethyl starch 6%

Note that Hartmann's solution also contains lactate 29 mmol/L. Dextrose solutions are also commonly employed. These provide water replacement without any electrolytes and with modest calorie supplements (1 litre of 5 per cent dextrose contains 400 kcal). A typical daily maintenance fluid regimen would consist of a combination of 5 per cent dextrose with either Hartmann's or normal saline to a volume of 2 litres.

There has been much controversy in the literature regarding the respective merits of crystalloid versus colloid replacement. There is no consensus on this topic and the usual advice is to replace like with like. If the haematocrit is below 21 per cent, blood transfusion may be required. There is increasing recognition, however, that albumin infusions are of little value.

In addition to maintenance requirements, 'replacement' fluids are required to correct pre-existing deficiencies and 'supplemental' fluids are required to compensate for anticipated additional intestinal or other losses. The nature and volumes of these fluids are determined by:

- A careful assessment of the patient including pulse, blood pressure and central venous pressure, if available. Clinical examination to assess hydration status (peripheries, skin turgor, urine output and specific gravity of urine), urine and serum electrolytes and haematocrit.
- Estimation of losses already incurred and their nature: for example, vomiting, ileus, diarrhoea, excessive sweating or fluid losses from burns or other serious inflammatory conditions.
- Estimation of supplemental fluids likely to be required in view of anticipated future losses from drains, fistulae, nasogastric tubes or abnormal urine or faecal losses.
- When an estimate of the volumes required has been made, the appropriate replacement fluid can be determined from a consideration of the electrolyte composition of gastrointestinal secretions. Most intestinal losses are adequately replaced with normal saline containing supplemental potassium (Table 20.3).

NUTRITIONAL REQUIREMENTS

Total enteral or parenteral nutrition necessitates the provision of the macronutrients, carbohydrate, fat and protein, together with vitamins, trace elements, electrolytes and water. When planning a feeding regimen, the patient should be weighed and an assessment made of daily energy and protein requirements. Standard tables are available to permit these calculations.

Daily needs may change depending on the patient's condition. Overfeeding is the most common cause of complications, regardless of whether nutrition is provided enterally or parenterally. It is essential to monitor daily intake to provide an assessment of tolerance. Failure to do so is the most common reason for inadequate nutrition. In addition, regular biochemical monitoring is mandatory (Table 20.4).

Table 20.3 Composition of gastrointestinal secretions (mmol/L).

	Na	K	Cl	HCO_3
Saliva	10	25	10	30
Stomach	50	15	110	–
Duodenum	140	5	100	–
Ileum	140	5	100	30
Pancreas	140	5	75	115
Bile	140	5	100	35

Macronutrient requirements

Energy

The total energy requirement of a stable patient with a normal or moderately increased need is approximately 20–30 kcal/kg per day. Very few patients require energy intakes in excess of 2000 kcal/day. Thus, in the majority of hospitalised patients in whom energy demands from activity are minimal, total energy requirements are approximately 1300–1800 kcal/day.

Table 20.4 Monitoring feeding regimens.

Daily	Body weight Fluid balance Full blood count, urea and electrolytes Blood glucose Electrolyte content and volume of urine and/or urine and intestinal losses Temperature
Weekly (or more frequently if clinically indicated)	Urine and plasma osmolality Calcium, magnesium, zinc and phosphate Plasma proteins including albumin Liver function tests including clotting factors Thiamine Acid–base status Triglycerides
Fortnightly	Serum vitamin B12 Folate Iron Lactate Trace elements (zinc, copper, manganese)

Alexis Frank Hartmann, 1898–1964, paediatrician, St Louis, MO, USA.

Carbohydrate

There is an obligatory glucose requirement to meet the needs of the central nervous system and certain haematopoietic cells, which is equivalent to about 2 g/kg per day. In addition, there is a physiological maximum to the amount of glucose that can be oxidised, which is approximately 4 mg/kg per minute (equivalent to about 1500 kcal/day in a 70-kg person), with the non-oxidised glucose being primarily converted to fat. However, optimal utilisation of energy during nutritional support is ensured by avoiding the infusion of glucose at rates approximating physiological maximums. Plasma glucose levels provide an indication of tolerance. Avoid hyperglycaemia. Provide energy as mixtures of glucose and fat. Glucose is the preferred carbohydrate source.

Fat

Dietary fat is composed of triglycerides of predominantly four long-chain fatty acids. There are two saturated fatty acids (palmitic (C16) and stearic (C18)) and two unsaturated fatty acids (oleic (C18 with one double bond) and linoleic (C18 with two double bonds)). In addition, smaller amounts of linolenic acid (C18 with three double bonds) and medium-chain fatty acids (C6–C10) are contained in the diet.

The unsaturated fatty acids, linoleic and linolenic acid, are considered essential because they cannot be synthesised *in vivo* from non-dietary sources. Both soybean and sunflower oil emulsions are rich sources of linoleic acid and provision of only 1 litre of emulsion per week avoids deficiency. Soybean emulsions contain approximately 7 per cent alpha-linolenic acid (an omega-3 fatty acid). The provision of fat as a soybean oil-based emulsion on a regular basis will obviate the risk of essential fatty acid deficiency.

Safe and non-toxic fat emulsions based upon long-chain triglycerides (LCTs) have been commercially available for over 30 years. These emulsions provide a calorically dense product (9 kcal/g) and are now routinely used to supplement the provision of non-protein calories during parenteral nutrition. Energy during parenteral nutrition should be given as a mixture of fat together with glucose. There is no evidence to suggest that any particular ratio of glucose to fat is optimal as long as under all conditions the basal requirements for glucose (100–200 g/day) and essential fatty acids (100–200 g/week) are met. This 'dual energy' supply minimises metabolic complications during parenteral nutrition, reduces fluid retention, enhances substrate utilisation (particularly in the septic patient) and is associated with reduced carbon dioxide production.

Concerns have been expressed about the possible immunosuppressive effects of LCT emulsions. These are more likely to occur if the recommended infusion rates (0.15 g/kg per hour) are exceeded. Nonetheless, these concerns have prompted the development of newer emulsions based upon medium-chain triglycerides, omega-3 fatty acids and, most recently, structured triglycerides, which combine long- and medium-chain triglycerides in the same emulsion. The evidence of clinical benefit for these emulsions compared with conventional LCTs is tenuous, particularly if infusion rates are appropriate and hypertriglyceridaemia is avoided.

Protein

The basic requirement for nitrogen in patients without pre-existing malnutrition and without metabolic stress is 0.10–0.15 g/kg per day. In hypermetabolic patients, the nitrogen requirements increase to 0.20–0.25 g/kg per day. Although there may be a minority of patients in whom the requirements are higher, such as after acute weight loss when the objective of therapy is long-term repletion of lean body mass, there is little evidence that the provision of nitrogen in excess of 14 g/day is beneficial.

Vitamins, minerals and trace elements

Whatever the method of feeding, these are all essential components of nutritional regimens. The water-soluble vitamins B and C act as coenzymes in collagen formation and wound healing. Postoperatively, the vitamin C requirement increases to 60–80 mg/day. Supplemental vitamin B12 is often indicated in patients who have undergone intestinal resection or gastric surgery and in those with a history of alcohol dependence. Absorption of the fat-soluble vitamins A, D, E and K is reduced in steatorrhoea and the absence of bile.

Sodium, potassium and phosphate are all subject to significant losses, particularly in patients with diarrhoeal illness. Their levels need daily monitoring and appropriate replacement.

Trace elements may also act as cofactors for metabolic processes. Normally, trace element requirements are met by the delivery of food to the gut and so patients on long-term parenteral nutrition are at particular risk of depletion. Magnesium, zinc and iron levels may all be decreased as part of the inflammatory response. Supplementation is necessary to optimise utilisation of amino acids and to avoid refeeding syndrome.

FLUID AND NUTRITIONAL CONSEQUENCES OF INTESTINAL RESECTION

Up to 50 per cent of the small intestine can be surgically removed or bypassed without permanent deleterious effects. With extensive resection (<150 cm of remaining small intestine), metabolic and nutritional consequences arise, resulting in the disease entity known as short bowel syndrome. The clinical presentation of patients with short bowel syndrome is dependent upon the nature and extent of intestinal resection.

Small bowel motility

Small bowel motility is three times slower in the ileum than in the jejunum. In addition, the ileocaecal valve may slow transit. The adult small bowel receives 5–6 litres of endogenous secretions and 2–3 litres of exogenous fluids per day. Most of this is reabsorbed in the small bowel. In the jejunum, the cellular junctions are leaky and jejunal contents are always isotonic. Fluid absorption in this region of bowel is inefficient compared with the ileum. It has been estimated that the efficiency of water absorption is 44 and 70 per cent of the ingested load in the jejunum and ileum, respectively. The corresponding figures for sodium are 13 and 72 per cent, respectively. It can be seen, therefore, that the ileum is critical in the conservation of fluid and electrolytes (Table 20.5).

Ileum

The ileum is the only site of absorption of vitamin B12 and bile salts. Bile salts are essential for the absorption of fats and fat-soluble vitamins. The enterohepatic circulation of bile salts is critical to maintain the bile salt pool. Following resection of

in vivo is Latin for 'in a living thing'.

the ileum, the loss of bile salts increases and is not met by an increase in synthesis. Depletion of the bile salt pool results in fat malabsorption. In addition, loss of bile salts into the colon affects colonic mucosa, causing a reduction in salt and water absorption, which increases stool losses.

Colon

Transit times in the colon vary between 24 and 150 hours. The efficiency of water and salt absorption in the colon exceeds 90 per cent. Another important colonic function is the fermentation of carbohydrates to produce short-chain fatty acids. These have two important functions: first, they enhance water and salt absorption from the colon and, second, they are trophic to the colonocyte.

Effects of resection

Resection of proximal jejunum results in no significant alterations in fluid and electrolyte levels as the ileum and colon can adapt to absorb the increased fluid and electrolyte load. Absorption of nutrients occurs throughout the small bowel and resection of jejunum alone results in the ileum taking over this lost function. In this situation, there is no malabsorption.

Resection of ileum results in a significant enhancement of gastric motility and acceleration of intestinal transit. Following ileal resection, the colon receives a much larger volume of fluid and electrolytes and it also receives bile salts, which reduce its ability to absorb salt and water, resulting in diarrhoea. Even the loss of 100 cm of ileum causes steatorrhoea, which may necessitate the administration of oral cholestyramine to bind bile salts. With larger resections (>100 cm) dietary fat restriction may be necessary. Regular parenteral vitamin B12 is required.

The most challenging patients are those with short bowel syndrome who have had in excess of 200 cm of small bowel resected together with colectomy. These patients will usually have a jejunostomy. They are conveniently divided into two groups termed 'net absorbers' and 'net secretors'. Absorbers characteristically have more than 100 cm of residual jejunum and they absorb more water and sodium from the diet than passes through the stoma. These patients can be managed without supplementary parenteral fluids.

Secretors usually have less than 100 cm of residual jejunum and lose more water and sodium from their stoma than they take by mouth. These patients require supplements. Their usual daily jejunostomy output may exceed 4 litres per 24 hours. The sodium content of jejunostomy losses or other high-output fistulae is about 90 mmol/L. Jejunal mucosa is leaky and rapid sodium fluxes occur across it. If water or any solution with a sodium concentration of less than 90 mmol/L is consumed, there is a net efflux of sodium from the plasma into the bowel lumen. It is therefore inappropriate to encourage patients with high-output jejunostomies (secretors) to drink large amounts of oral hypotonic solutions. Treatment begins with restricting the total amount of hypotonic fluids (water, tea, juices, etc.) consumed to less than a litre a day. Patients should be encouraged to take glucose and saline replacement solutions, which have a sodium concentration of at least 90 mmol/L. The World Health Organization (WHO) cholera solution has a sodium concentration of 90 mmol/L and is commonly used.

Complications of short bowel syndrome include peptic ulceration related to gastric hypersecretion, cholelithiasis because of interruption of the enterohepatic cycle of bile salts, and hyperoxaluria as a result of the increased absorption of oxalate in the colon predisposing to renal stones. Some patients with short bowel syndrome develop a syndrome of slurred speech, ataxia and altered affect. The cause of this syndrome is fermentation of malabsorbed carbohydrates in the colon to D-lactate and absorption of this metabolite. Treatment necessitates the use of a low carbohydrate diet.

Anti-secretory drugs reduce the amount of fluid secreted from the stomach, liver and pancreas. These include H2-receptor antagonists, proton pump inhibitors and the somatostatin analogue octreotide. Octreotide also reduces gastrointestinal motility. Anti-motility drugs include loperamide and codeinephosphate, which also decrease water and sodium output from the stoma by about 20 per cent.

ARTIFICIAL NUTRITIONAL SUPPORT

The indications for nutritional support are simple. Any patient who has sustained 5–7 days of inadequate intake or who is anticipated to have no intake for this period should be considered for nutritional support. The periods may be less in patients with pre-existing malnutrition. This concept is important because it emphasises that the provision of nutritional support is not specific to certain conditions or diseases. Although patients with Crohn's disease or pancreatitis, or those who have undergone gastrointestinal resections, may frequently require nutritional support, it is the fact that they have had inadequate intakes for defined periods that is the indication rather than the specific disease process.

Enteral nutrition

The term 'enteral feeding' means delivery of nutrients into the gastrointestinal tract. The alimentary tract should be used whenever possible. This can be achieved with oral supplements (sip

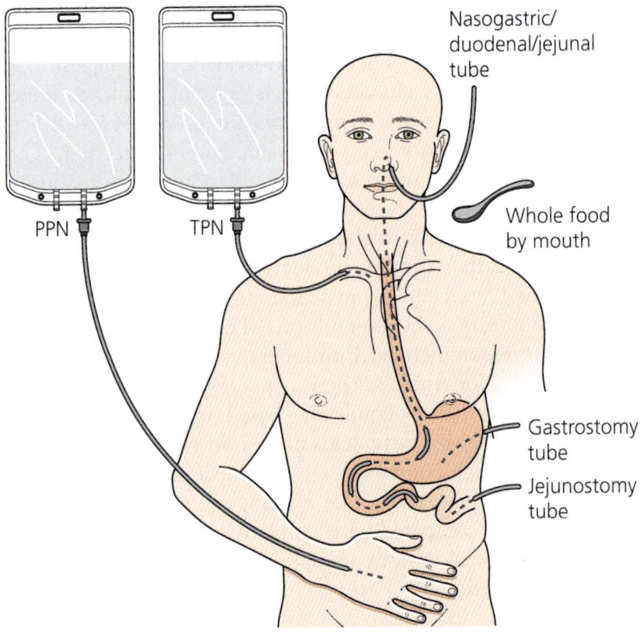

Figure 20.3 Techniques used for adjuvant nutritional support. PPN, partial parenteral nutrition; TPN, total parenteral nutrition. Redrawn with permission from Rick Tharp, rxkinetics.com.

feeding) or with a variety of tube-feeding techniques delivering food into the stomach, duodenum or jejunum.

A variety of nutrient formulations is available for enteral feeding. These vary with respect to energy content, osmolarity, fat and nitrogen content and nutrient complexity; most contain up to 1–2 kcal/mL and up to 0.6 g/mL of protein. Polymeric feeds contain intact protein and hence require digestion, whereas monomeric/elemental feeds contain nitrogen in the form of either free amino acids or, in some cases, peptides. These are less palatable and are used much less frequently than in previous years. Newer feeding formulations are available that include glutamine and fibre to optimise intestinal nutrition or immunonutrients such as arginine and fish oils, but these are expensive and their use is controversial.

Sip feeding

Commercially available supplementary sip feeds are used in patients who can drink but whose appetites are impaired or in whom adequate intakes cannot be maintained with *ad libitum* intakes. These feeds typically provide 200 kcal and 2 g of nitrogen per 200 mL carton. There is good evidence to demonstrate that these sip-feeding techniques are associated with a significant overall increase in calorie and nitrogen intakes without detriment to spontaneous nutrition. The evidence that these techniques improve patient outcomes is less convincing.

Tube-feeding techniques

Enteral nutrition can be achieved using conventional nasogastric tubes (Ryle's), fine-bore feeding tubes inserted into the stomach, surgical or percutaneous endoscopic gastrostomy (PEG) or, finally, post-pyloric feeding utilising nasojejunal tubes or various types of jejunostomy. The choice of method will be determined by local circumstances and preference in many patients. Whichever method is adopted, it is important that tube feeding is supervised by an experienced dietician who will calculate the patient's requirements and aim to achieve these within 2–3 days of the instigation of feeds. Conventionally, 20–30 mL are administered per hour initially, gradually increasing to goal rates within 48–72 hours. In most units, feeding is discontinued for 4–5 hours overnight to allow gastric pH to return to normal. There is some evidence that this might reduce the incidence of nosocomial pneumonia and aspiration. There is good evidence to confirm that feeding protocols optimise the tolerance of enteral nutrition. In these, aspirates are performed on a regular basis and if they exceed 200 mL in any 2-hour period, then feeding is temporarily discontinued.

Tube blockage is common. All tubes should be flushed with water at least twice daily. If a build up of solidified diet occurs, instillation into the tube of agents such as chymotrypsin or papain may salvage a partially obstructed tube. Guidewires should not be used to clear blockages as these may perforate the tube and cause contiguous damage.

Nasogastric tubes are appropriate in a majority of patients. If feeding is maintained for more than a week or so, a fine-bore feeding tube is preferable and is likely to cause fewer gastric and oesophageal erosions. These are usually made from soft polyurethane or silicone elastomer and have an internal diameter of <3 mm.

John Alfred Ryle, 1889–1950, Regius Professor of Medicine, Cambridge University and later Professor of Social Medicine, Oxford University, Oxford, UK, introduced the Ryle's tube in 1921.

Fine-bore tube insertion

The patient should be semi-recumbent. The introducer wire is lubricated and inserted into the fine-bore tube (Figure 20.4). The tube is passed through the nose and into the stomach via the nasopharynx and oesophagus. The wire is withdrawn and the tube is taped to the patient. There is a small risk of malposition into a bronchus or of causing pneumothorax. The position of the tube should be checked using plain abdominal radiography (Figure 20.5). Alternatively, 5 mL of air can be injected and a stethoscope used to confirm bubbling from the stomach. Confirmation of position by pH testing is possible but limited by the difficulty of obtaining a fluid aspirate with narrow lumen tubes.

Gastrostomy

The placement of a tube through the abdominal wall directly into the stomach is termed 'gastrostomy'. Historically, these were created surgically at the time of laparotomy. Today, the majority are performed by percutaneous insertion under endoscopic control using local anaesthesia, known as PEG (percutaneous endoscopic gastrostomy) tubes (Figure 20.6).

Two methods of PEG are commonly used. The first is called the 'direct-stab' technique in which the endoscope is passed and the stomach filled with air. The endoscopist then watches a cannula entering the stomach having been inserted directly through the anterior abdominal wall. A guidewire is then passed through the cannula into the stomach. A gastrostomy tube (commercially available) may then be introduced into the stomach through a 'peel away' sheath. The alternative technique is the transoral or push-through technique, whereby a guidewire or suture is brought out of the stomach by the endoscope after

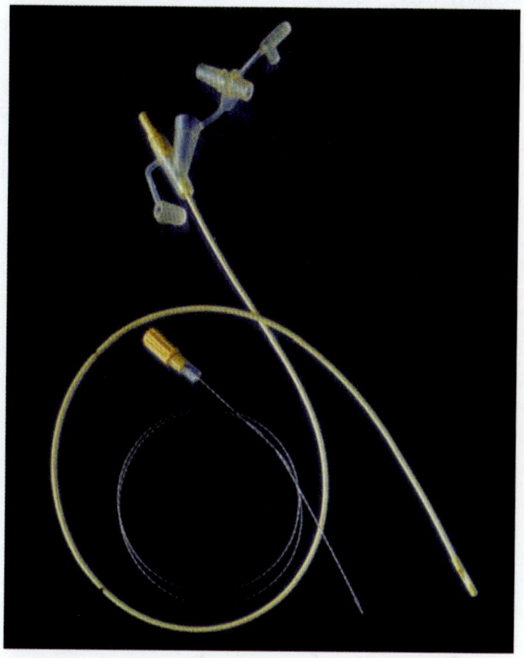

Figure 20.4 A fine-bore feeding tube with its guidewire.

ad libitum is Latin for 'freely or as much as you wish'.

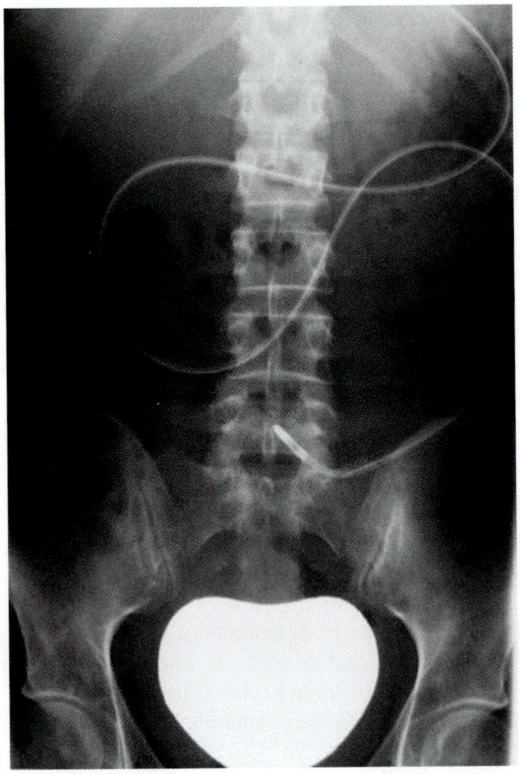

Figure 20.5 Radiograph of a tube similar to that in Figure 20.4 inserted beyond the duodenojejunal flexure.

transabdominal percutaneous insertion and is either attached to a gastrostomy tube or the tube is pushed over a guidewire. The abdominal end of the wire is then pulled, advancing the gastrostomy tube through the oesophagus and into the stomach. Continued pulling abuts it up against the abdominal wall.

If patients require enteral nutrition for prolonged periods (4–6 weeks), then PEG is preferable to an indwelling nasogastric tube; this minimises the traumatic complications related to indwelling tubes. PEG does have procedure-specific complications, although these are uncommon. Necrotising fasciitis and intra-abdominal wall abscesses have been recorded. Sepsis around the PEG site is more common and may necessitate systemic antibiotics or repositioning. A persistent gastric fistula can occur on removal of a PEG if it has been in place for prolonged periods and epithelialisation of the tract has occurred. This necessitates surgical closure.

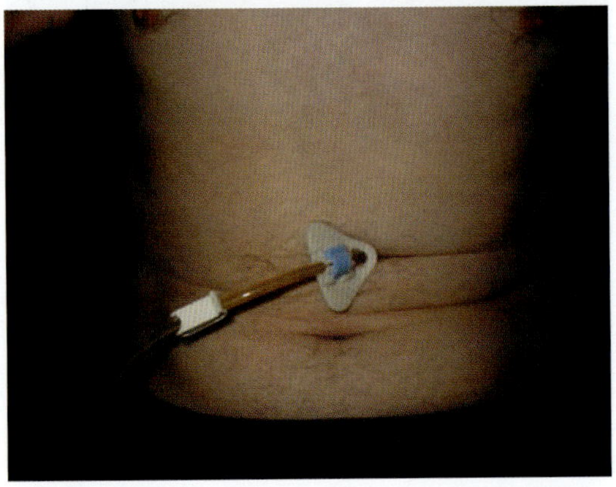

Figure 20.6 Percutaneous endoscopic gastrostomy tube.

Jejunostomy

In recent years, the use of jejunal feeding has become increasingly popular. This can be achieved using nasojejunal tubes or by placement of needle jejunostomy at the time of laparotomy. Some authorities advocate the use of jejunostomies on the basis that post-pyloric feeding may be associated with a reduction in aspiration or enhanced tolerance of enteral nutrition. In particular, there are many advocates of jejunostomies in patients with severe pancreatitis, in whom a degree of gastric outlet obstruction may be present, related to the oedematous head of pancreas. In most patients it is appropriate to commence with conventional nasogastric feeding and progress to post-pyloric feeding if the former is unsuccessful.

Nasojejunal tubes often necessitate the use of fluoroscopy or endoscopy to achieve placement, which may delay commencement of feeding. Surgical jejunostomies, even using commercially available needle-insertion techniques, do involve creating a defect in the jejunum, which can leak or be associated with tube displacement; both of these complications result in peritonitis.

Complications

Most complications of enteral nutrition can be avoided with careful attention to detail and appropriate infusion rates. Patients should be nursed semi-recumbent to reduce the possibility of aspiration. Complications can be divided into those resulting from intubation of the gastrointestinal tract and those related to nutrient delivery. The former are more frequent with more invasive means of gaining access to the intestinal tract (see above under Enteral nutrition). The latter include diarrhoea, bloating and vomiting. Diarrhoea occurs in more than 30 per cent of patients receiving enteral nutrition and is particularly common in the critically ill. Up to 60 per cent of patients in intensive care units may fail to receive their targeted intakes. There is no evidence that the incidence of diarrhoea and bloating is reduced by the use of half-strength feeds. It is important to introduce normal feeds at a reduced rate according to patient tolerance. Metabolic complications associated with excessive feeding are uncommon in enterally fed patients. There have been reports of nosocomial enteric infections associated with contamination of feeds, which should be kept in sealed containers at 4°C and discarded once opened. In all patients, it is essential to monitor intakes accurately as target intakes are often not achieved with enteral nutrition.

The complications of enteral nutrition are summarised in Summary box 20.3.

Parenteral nutrition

Total parenteral nutrition (TPN) is defined as the provision of all nutritional requirements by means of the intravenous route and without the use of the gastrointestinal tract.

Parenteral nutrition is indicated when energy and protein needs cannot be met by the enteral administration of these substrates. The most frequent clinical indications relate to those patients who have undergone massive resection of the small intestine, who have intestinal fistula or who have prolonged intestinal failure for other reasons.

Summary box 20.3

Complications of enteral nutrition

- Tube-related
  - Malposition
  - Displacement
  - Blockage
  - Breakage/leakage
  - Local complications (e.g. erosion of skin/mucosa)
- Gastrointestinal
  - Diarrhoea
  - Bloating, nausea, vomiting
  - Abdominal cramps
  - Aspiration
  - Constipation
- Metabolic/biochemical
  - Electrolyte disorders
  - Vitamin, mineral, trace element deficiencies
  - Drug interactions
- Infective
  - Exogenous (handling contamination)
  - Endogenous (patient)

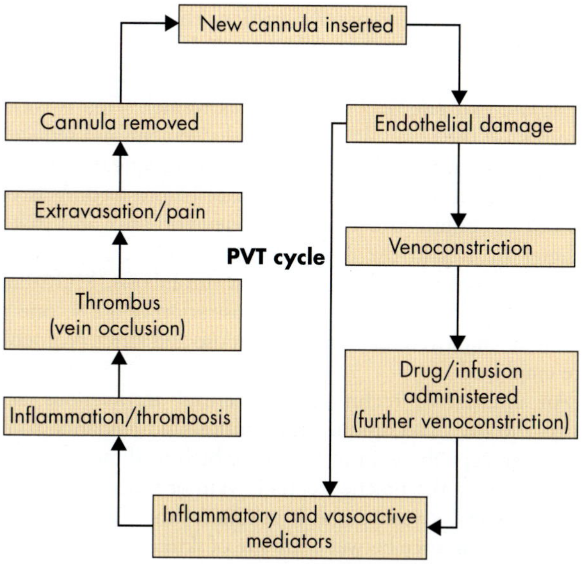

Figure 20.7 Cycle of causes of peripheral vein thrombophlebitis (PVT) (after Payne-James J, Grimble G, Silk D (eds). *Artificial nutrition support in clinical practice*, 2nd edn. London, Greenwich Medical Media, 2001).

Route of delivery: peripheral or central venous access

TPN can be administered either by a catheter inserted in the central vein or via a peripheral line. In the early days of parenteral nutrition, the only energy source available was hypertonic glucose, which, being hypertonic, had to be given into a central vein to avoid thrombophlebitis. In the second half of the last century, there were a number of important developments that have influenced the administration of parenteral nutrition. These include the identification of safe and non-toxic fat emulsions that are isotonic; pharmaceutical developments that permit carbohydrates, fats and amino acids to be mixed in single containers; and a recognition that the provision of energy during parenteral nutrition should be a mixture of glucose and fat and that energy requirements are rarely in excess of 2000 kcal/day (25–30 kcal/kg per day). These changes enabled the development of peripheral parenteral nutrition.

Peripheral

Peripheral feeding is appropriate for short-term feeding of up to 2 weeks. Access can be achieved either by means of a dedicated catheter inserted into a peripheral vein and manoeuvred into the central venous system (peripherally inserted central venous catheter (PICC) line) or by using a conventional short cannula in the wrist veins. The former method has the advantage of minimising inconvenience to the patient and clinician. PICC lines have a mean duration of survival of 7 days. The disadvantage is that when thrombophlebitis occurs, the vein is irrevocably destroyed. In the alternative approach, intravenous nutrients are administered through a short cannula in wrist veins, infusing the patient's nutritional requirements on a cyclical basis over 12 hours. The cannula is then removed and resited in the contralateral arm. Peripheral parenteral nutrition has the advantage that it avoids the complications associated with central venous administration, but suffers the disadvantage that it is limited by the development of thrombophlebitis (Figure 20.7). Peripheral feeding is not indicated if patients already have an indwelling central venous line or in those in whom long-term feeding is anticipated.

Central

When the central venous route is chosen, the catheter can be inserted via the subclavian or internal or external jugular vein. There is good evidence to show that the safest means of establishing central venous access is by insertion of lines under ultrasound guidance; however, this will not be practicable for all cases. Most intensive care physicians and anaesthetists favour cannulation of internal or external jugular veins as these vessels are easily accessible. They suffer the disadvantage that the exit site is situated inconveniently on the side of the neck, where repeated movements result in disruption of the dressing with the attendant risk of sepsis. The infraclavicular subclavian approach is more suitable for feeding as the catheter then lies flat on the chest wall, which optimises nursing care (Figure 20.8).

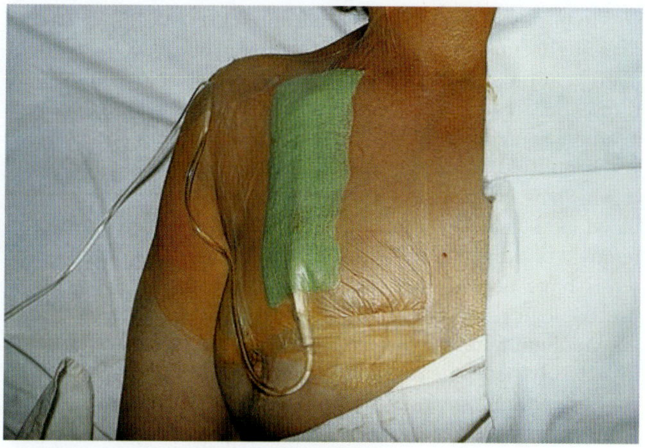

Figure 20.8 Infraclavicular subclavian line.

For longer-term parenteral nutrition, Hickman lines are preferable. These are often inserted by a radiologist with fluoroscopic guidance or ultrasound. They incorporate a small cuff, which sits at the exit site of a subcutaneous tunnel. This is thought to minimise the possibility of line dislodgement and reduce the possibility of line sepsis. Whichever technique is employed, a post-insertion chest x-ray is essential before feeding is commenced to confirm the absence of pneumothorax and that the catheter tip lies in the distal superior vena cava to minimise the risk of central venous or cardiac thrombosis. Multi-lumen catheters can be used for the administration of TPN; one port should be employed for that sole purpose and strict protocols of care employed.

An alternative technique for central intravenous access allows the PICC technique under ultrasound guidance to cannulate the cephalic vein in the arm which facilitates passage of a catheter into the bracheocephalic vein or superior vena cava. This has many advantages as it minimises the risks of insertion and ensures distance between the site of skin entry and the tip of the catheter. Thrombophlebitis, however, can occur.

Complications of parenteral nutrition

The commencement of TPN may precipitate or accentuate underlying nutrient deficiency by encouraging anabolism. Common metabolic complications include fluid overload, hyperglycaemia, abnormalities of liver function and vitamin deficiencies. Fluid overload can be avoided by daily weighing of the patient. A weight change of >1 kg/day normally indicates fluid retention. Hyperglycaemia is common because of insulin resistance in critically ill patients. Even modest rates of glucose administration may be associated with hyperglycaemia. Hyperglycaemic patients undergoing surgery are known to run a substantially higher risk of infectious complications.

Abnormalities of liver enzymes are common in patients who are receiving TPN. Although the precise mechanisms are unclear, intrahepatic cholestasis may occur and hepatic steatosis and hepatomegaly have been reported. Reducing the fat content or infusion of fat-free TPN may be required. If liver enzymes continue to deteriorate, TPN should be temporarily discontinued. In addition, overfeeding is a major factor in hepatic and other metabolic complications associated with TPN. Supplemental parenteral glutamine during parental nutrition should be considered, particularly in the critically ill patient.

Catheter-related sepsis occurs in 3–14 per cent of patients. It may occur at the time of line insertion or afterwards by migration of skin bacteria along the external catheter surface. Some studies suggest that manoeuvring of the catheter hub due to frequent manipulation is a common cause. Contamination of the infusate is rare. Seeding on the catheter at the time of bacteraemia from a remote source may also cause catheter infection.

Diagnosis of catheter-related sepsis requires that the same organism is grown from the catheter tip as is recovered from blood and that the clinical features of infection resolve on removal of the catheter. Traditional methods of confirming line sepsis have necessitated removal of the line with subsequent bacteriological assessment. An alternative approach is to use an endoluminal brush passed down the catheter and withdrawn into a polythene sheath. The brush tip is cultured at the same time as performing blood cultures. Catheter sepsis is confirmed if identical organisms are cultured from brush and blood. A second alternative is to culture blood withdrawn through the catheter and compare this with peripheral blood cultures. If the colony count from the catheter sample is five or more times higher than that from peripheral blood then line sepsis is probable.

The complications of parenteral nutrition are summarised in Summary box 20.4.

Summary box 20.4

Complications of parenteral nutrition

- Related to nutrient deficiency
  - Hypoglycaemia/hypocalcaemia/hypophosphataemia/hypomagnesaemia (refeeding syndrome)
  - Chronic deficiency syndromes (essential fatty acids, zinc, mineral and trace elements)
- Related to overfeeding
  - Excess glucose: hyperglycaemia, hyperosmolar dehydration, hepatic steatosis, hypercapnia, increased sympathetic activity, fluid retention, electrolyte abnormalities
  - Excess fat: hypercholesterolaemia and formation of lipoprotein X, hypertriglyceridaemia, hypersensitivity reactions
  - Excess amino acids: hyperchloraemic metabolic acidosis, hypercalcaemia, aminoacidaemia, uraemia
- Related to sepsis
  - Catheter-related sepsis
  - Possible increased predisposition to systemic sepsis
- Related to line
  - On insertion: pneumothorax, damage to adjacent artery, air embolism, thoracic duct damage, cardiac perforation or tamponade, pleural effusion, hydromediastinum
  - Long-term use: occlusion, venous thrombosis

Refeeding syndrome

This syndrome is characterised by severe fluid and electrolyte shifts in malnourished patients undergoing refeeding. It can occur with either enteral or parenteral nutrition, but is more common with the latter. It results in hypophosphataemia, hypocalcaemia and hypomagnesaemia. These electrolyte disorders can result in altered myocardial function, arrhythmias, deteriorating respiratory function, liver dysfunction, seizures, confusion, coma, tetany and death. Patients at risk include those with alcohol dependency, those suffering severe malnutrition, anorexics and those who have undergone prolonged periods of fasting. Treatment involves matching intakes with requirements and assiduously avoiding overfeeding. Calorie delivery should be increased slowly and vitamins administered regularly. Hypophosphataemia and hypomagnesaemia require treatment.

Nutrition support teams

Multidisciplinary nutrition teams ensure cost-effective and safe nutritional support, irrespective of how this is administered. The incidence of catheter-related sepsis is significantly reduced.

John Jason Payne-James, contemporary forensic physician and medical writer, Leigh-on-Sea, Essex, UK.
Robert O Hickman, formerly nephrologist, The University of Washington, WA, USA.

SUMMARY

Fluid therapy and nutritional support are fundamental to good surgical practice. Accurate fluid administration demands an understanding of maintenance requirements and an appreciation of the consequences of surgical disease on fluid losses. This requires knowledge of the consequences of surgical intervention and, in particular, intestinal resection. Malnutrition is common in hospital patients. All patients who have sustained or who are likely to sustain 7 days of inadequate oral intake should be considered for nutritional support. This may be dietetic advice alone, sip feeding or enteral or parenteral nutrition. These are not mutually exclusive. The success or otherwise of nutritional support should be determined by tolerance to nutrients provided and nutritional end points, such as weight. It is unrealistic to expect nutritional support to alter the natural history of disease. It is imperative that nutrition-related morbidity is kept to a minimum. This necessitates the appropriate selection of feeding method, careful assessment of fluid, energy and protein requirements, which are regularly monitored, and the avoidance of overfeeding.

ACKNOWLEDGEMENTS

With thanks to Marcel Gatt, FRCS, who provided some illustrations and helped with proofreading the text.

FURTHER READING

British Association Parenteral and Enteral Nutrition. BAPEN. Available from: (www.bapen.org.uk/res_pub.html).

Gibney M, Elia M, Ljungqvist O, Dowsett J (eds). *Clinical nutrition*. The Nutrition Society Textbook Series. Oxford: Blackwell Sciences, 2005.

Nightingale J. *Intestinal failure*. London: Greenwich Medical Media, 2001.

CHAPTER

21 Postoperative care

LEARNING OBJECTIVES

To understand:

- The system of postoperative care
- How to recognise and treat postoperative complications
- The principles of enhanced recovery
- The system for discharging patients

INTRODUCTION

The aim of postoperative care is to provide the patient with as quick, painless and safe recovery from surgery as possible. Trainees should acquire knowledge and skills to manage surgical, as well as medical, postoperative problems.

GENERAL MANAGEMENT

The immediate postoperative period: recovery room

The theatre team should formally hand over the care of the patient to the recovery staff. The information provided should include the patient's name, age, the surgical procedure, existing medical problems, allergies, the anaesthetic and analgesics given, fluid replacement, blood loss, urine output, any surgical and anaesthetic problems encountered or expected.

Patient's vital parameters, consciousness, pain and hydration status are monitored in the recovery room and supportive treatment is given (Figure 21.1). Specific monitoring, such as Doppler flow for a free flap, observations like neurological evaluation and laboratory tests such as blood gas analysis may also be requested where necessary (Summary box 21.1).

Summary box 21.1

Postoperative period

- All anaesthetised patients should be recovered in a recovery room.
- All vital parameters should be monitored and documented.
- Treat pain and nausea/vomiting.
- Watch for complications.

The patient can be discharged from the recovery room when they fulfil the following criteria:

- Patient is fully conscious.
- Respiration and oxygenation are satisfactory.
- Patient is normothermic, not in pain nor nauseous.
- Cardiovascular parameters are stable.
- Oxygen, fluids and analgesics have been prescribed.
- There are no concerns related to the surgical procedure.

SYSTEM-SPECIFIC POSTOPERATIVE COMPLICATIONS

The presentation of complications may be similar for more than one underlying condition. Shortness of breath can be due to respiratory or cardiac problems, abdominal pain can be due to surgical causes or sepsis, while chest pain may be present in cardiac, respiratory and even in gastrointestinal problems.

Respiratory complications

The most common respiratory complications in the recovery room are hypoxaemia, hypercapnia and aspiration. Pneumonia and pulmonary embolism tend to appear later in the postoperative period.

Postoperative hypoxia

Hypoxia is defined as an oxygen saturation of less than 90 per cent. Hypoxia may present as shortness of breath or agitation or as upper airway obstruction (absence of air movement, seesaw motion of chest, suprasternal recession) or cyanosis or as a combination of any of the above.

Hypoxia in the postoperative period may occur due to a variety of reasons, for example:

- Upper airway obstruction due to the residual effect of general anaesthesia, secretions or wound haematoma after neck surgery.
- Laryngeal oedema from traumatic tracheal intubation, recurrent laryngeal nerve palsy and tracheal collapse after thyroid surgery.
- Hypoventilation related to anaesthesia or surgery.
- Atelectasis and pneumonia especially after upper abdominal and thoracic surgery (Figure 21.2).
- Pulmonary oedema of cardiac origin or related to fluid overload.

Christian Johann Doppler, 1803–1853, Professor of Experimental Physics, Vienna, Austria, enunciated the 'Doppler Principle' in 1842.

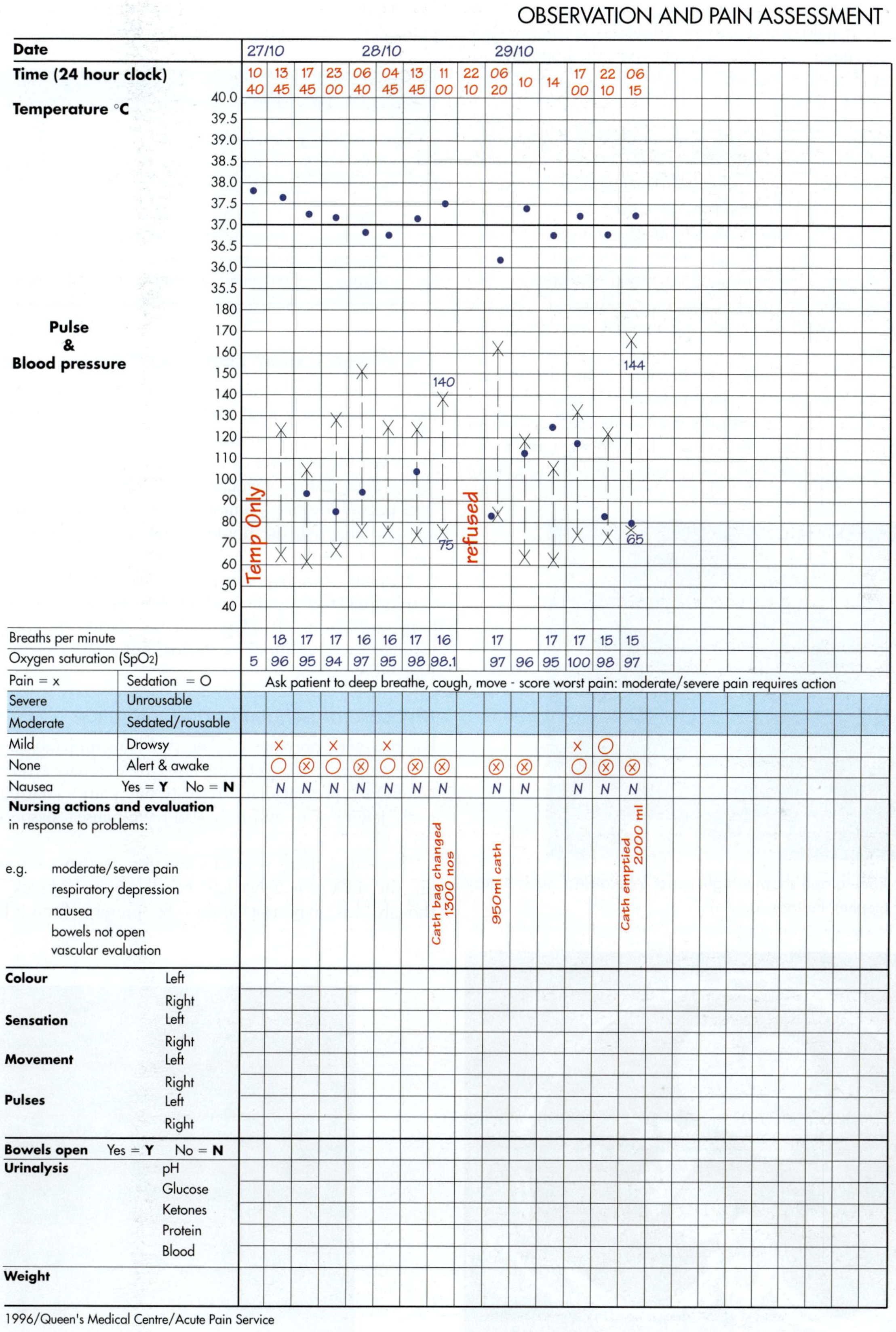

OBSERVATION AND PAIN ASSESSMENT
Date
27/10
28/10
29/10
Time (24 hour clock)
10 40 | 13 45 | 17 45 | 23 00 | 06 40 | 04 45 | 13 45 | 11 00 | 22 10 | 06 20 | 10 | 14 | 17 00 | 22 10 | 06 15
Temperature °C
40.0 39.5 39.0 38.5 38.0 37.5 37.0 36.5 36.0 35.5
Pulse & Blood pressure
180 170 160 150 140 130 120 110 100 90 80 70 60 50 40
Temp Only
refused
140
75
144
65
Breaths per minute
18 17 17 16 16 17 16 17 17 17 15 15
Oxygen saturation (SpO2)
5 96 95 94 97 95 98 98.1 97 96 95 100 98 97
Pain = x
Sedation = O
Ask patient to deep breathe, cough, move - score worst pain: moderate/severe pain requires action
Severe
Unrousable
Moderate
Sedated/rousable
Mild
Drowsy
None
Alert & awake
Nausea
Yes = Y
No = N
N N N N N N N N N N N N
Nursing actions and evaluation
in response to problems:
e.g.
moderate/severe pain
respiratory depression
nausea
bowels not open
vascular evaluation
Cath bag changed 1300 mls
950ml cath
Cath emptied 2000 ml
Colour
Left
Right
Sensation
Left
Right
Movement
Left
Right
Pulses
Left
Right
Bowels open
Yes = Y
No = N
Urinalysis
pH
Glucose
Ketones
Protein
Blood
Weight
1996/Queen's Medical Centre/Acute Pain Service

Figure 21.1 Postoperative nursing chart showing various monitoring parameters.

- Pulmonary embolism: this often presents with the sudden onset of chest pain and shortness of breath. In the presence of a large embolism, there will be systemic hypotension, pulmonary hypertension and an elevated central venous pressure (CVP) (Figure 21.3).

In obese patients or in those with acute or chronic lung disease, hypoxia develops more quickly.

Patients with hypoxia or imminent signs should be treated urgently. If the patient is breathing spontaneously administer oxygen at 15 L/min, using a non-rebreathing mask. A head tilt, chin lift or jaw thrust should relieve obstruction related to reduced muscle tone. Suctioning of any blood or secretions and insertion of an oropharyngeal airway may be needed. Call the anaesthetist as tracheal intubation and manual ventilation may also be needed.

Neck wound haematoma can become a life-threatening emergency, and must be evacuated immediately under local or general anaesthetic. Along with the immediate management of hypoxia, appropriate antibiotics, chest physiotherapy and bronchodilators will be needed to treat pneumonia. In the case of pulmonary oedema, diuretics should be started and a cardiology opinion should be sought (Summary box 21.2).

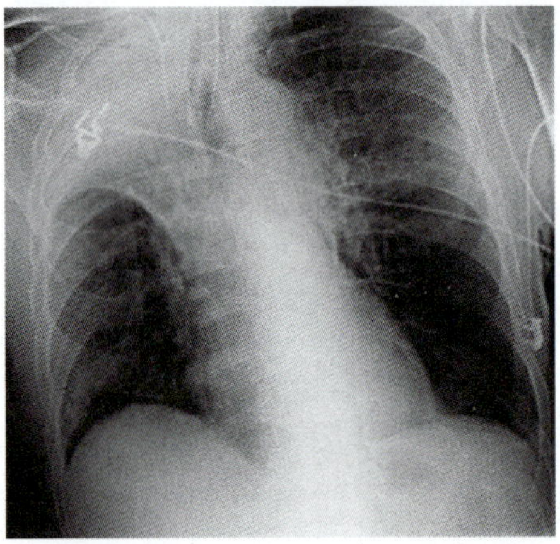

Figure 21.2 Radiograph showing right upper lobe atelectasis (courtesy of Professor Stephen Eustace, Dublin).

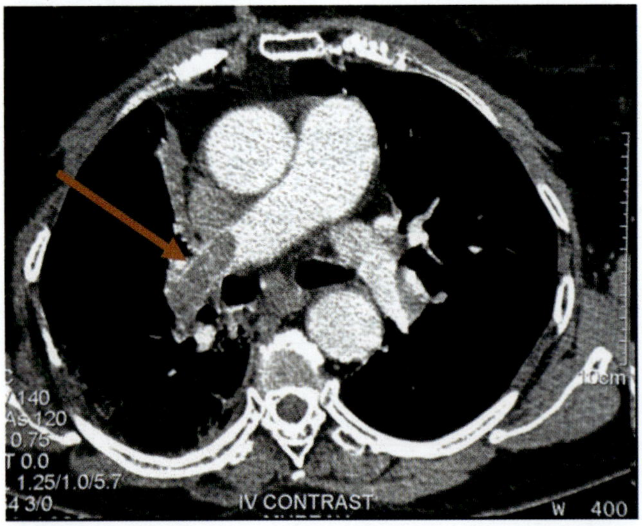

Figure 21.3 Computed tomography (CT) scan showing pulmonary artery blood embolism (arrow) (courtesy of Professor Stephen Eustace, Dublin).

Summary box 21.2

Respiratory complications

- Respiratory complications can occur either immediately or a few days later on the ward.
- Obese, smokers and those with chronic lung conditions are more likely to have respiratory complications.
- Early intervention and multidisciplinary involvement can prevent life threatening respiratory complications.

Cardiovascular complications

Hypotension in the immediate postoperative period may be due to inadequate fluid replacement, vasodilatation from subarachnoid and epidural anaesthesia or rewarming of the patient. However, other causes of hypotension such as surgical bleeding, sepsis, arrhythmias, myocardial infarction, cardiac failure, tension pneumothorax, pulmonary embolism, pericardial tamponade and anaphylaxis should be also sought (Figures 21.4, 21.5 and 21.6).

Patients with hypotension are likely to have cold clammy extremities, tachycardia and a low urine output ≤0.5 mL/kg per hour and low CVP. Hypovolaemia should be corrected with intravenous crystalloid or colloid infusions (see below under Bleeding).

Myocardial ischaemia and infarction

Patients with previous cardiac problems undergoing major surgery are at risk of developing an acute coronary syndrome. They commonly present with retrosternal pain radiating into the neck, jaw or arms and may also have nausea, dyspnoea or syncope.

Typically, there is a ST-elevation in two continuous leads on the ECG or new left bundle branch block (STEMI), though this may not always be present (non-ST-elevation

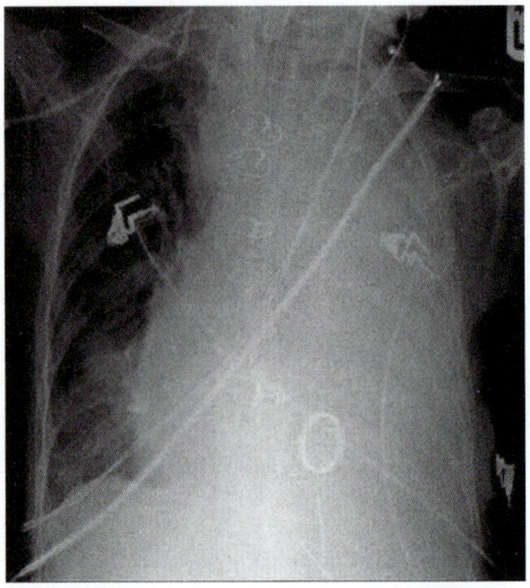

Figure 21.4 Radiograph showing lower left lobe consolidation (courtesy of Professor Stephen Eustace, Dublin).

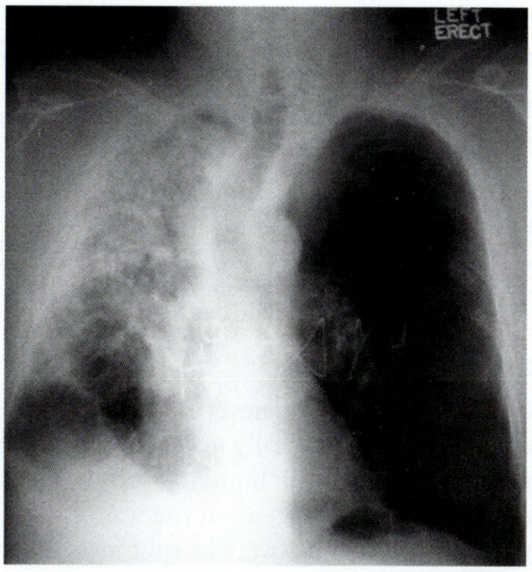

Figure 21.5 Radiograph showing classical *Staphylococcus aureus* pneumonia (courtesy of Professor Stephen Eustace, Dublin).

myocardial infarction (NSTEMI)). However, serum troponin levels will be high in both types of MI (myocardial ischaemia and myocardial infarction). Start treatment with oxygen, glyceryl trinitrate, morphine and aspirin and involve a cardiologist. Beta-blockers and/or calcium antagonists may be started to reduce further episodes of ischaemia. Cardiologists may start coronary reperfusion therapy for STEMI in the form of primary percutaneous coronary intervention or thrombolysis. However, these should be discussed first with a senior due to the risk of bleeding after major surgery.

Arrhythmias

Arrhythmia in the postoperative period can cause hypotension and ischaemia. Therefore, these patients will need to be continuously monitored. Treatment should be delivered according to the Resuscitation Council peri-arrest guidelines, correcting underlying causes including acid-base and electrolyte imbalance, hypoxia and hypercapnia (Summary box 21.3).

Summary box 21.3

Cardiovascular complications

- Hypotension in the postoperative period can be multifactorial
- Arrhythmias can be prevented and corrected by treating hypotension and electrolyte imbalance
- Arrhythmias and myocardial ischaemia/infarction will need management with the help of cardiologists

Tachycardia (sinus or supraventricular) may be caused by anxiety, pain, MI, hypovolaemia, sepsis or hypoxia in the postoperative period. Correct any underlying causes of the dysrhythmia and control the heart rate with beta-blockers, amiodarone or cardioversion.

Sinus bradycardia may be normal in athletes, but it may also be associated with hypoxia, preoperative beta-blockers, digoxin and increased intracranial pressure. If the heart rate is 40 bpm or less, glycopyrrolate 0.2–0.4 mg or atropine 0.6 mg should be given intravenously and the patient reviewed.

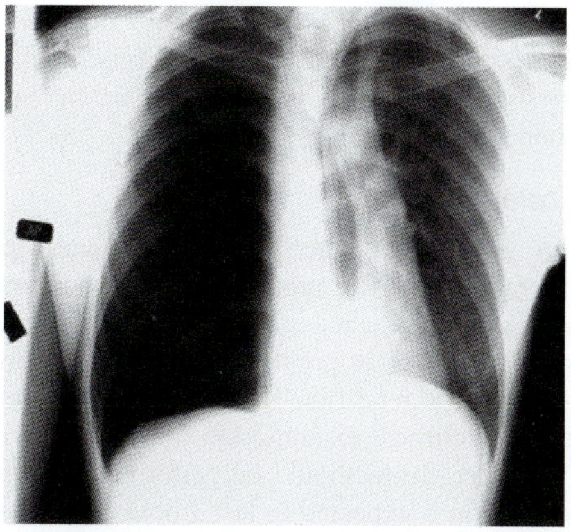

Figure 21.6 Radiograph showing a right tension pneumothorax with tracheal deviation to the left (courtesy of Professor Stephen Eustace, Dublin).

Renal and urinary complications

Acute renal failure

About a quarter of cases of hospital-acquired renal failure occur in the perioperative period and are associated with high mortality especially after cardiac and major vascular surgery (Table 21.1). Patients with known chronic renal disease, diabetes, liver failure, peripheral vascular disease and cardiac failure are at high risk. Perioperative events such as sepsis, bleeding, hypovolaemia, rhabdomyolysis or abdominal compartmental syndrome can all precipitate acute renal failure (Summary box 21.4).

Table 21.1 Common causes of acute renal failure.

Prerenal	Hypotension Hypovolaemia
Renal	Nephrotoxic drugs (gentamicin, diuretics, nonsteroidal anti-inflammatory agents) Surgery involving renal vessels Myoglobinuria Sepsis
Postrenal	Ureteric injury Blocked urethral catheter

Summary box 21.4

Renal and urinary complications

- Postoperative renal failure is associated with high mortality.
- Prophylactic measures to prevent renal failure should be taken in high risk cases.
- Urinary retention and infection are a common problem postoperatively.

If urine output is less than 0.5 mL/kg per hour for 6 hours, check that the catheter is not blocked, correct hypovolaemia, correct metabolic and electrolyte disturbances, and stop nephrotoxic drugs. Stage I of kidney failure is associated with a rise in serum creatinine levels to more than 1.5 times baseline or a greater than 25 per cent decrease in GFR (glomerular filtration rate); aggressive treatment should be started at this early stage to avoid further damage.

Urinary retention

Inability to void after surgery is common with pelvic and perineal operations or after procedures performed under spinal anaesthesia. Pain, fluid deficiency, problems in accessing urinals and bed pans, and lack of privacy on wards may contribute to the problem of urine retention. The diagnosis of retention may be confirmed by clinical examination and by using ultrasound imaging. Catheterisation should be performed prophylactically when an operation is expected to last 3 hours or longer or when large volumes of fluid are administered.

Urinary infection

Urinary infection is one of the most commonly acquired infections in the postoperative period. Patients may present with dysuria and/or pyrexia. Immunocompromised patients, diabetics and those patients with a history of urinary retention are known to be at higher risk. Treatment involves adequate hydration, proper bladder drainage and antibiotics depending on the sensitivity of the microorganisms.

COMPLICATIONS RELATED TO SPECIFIC SURGICAL SPECIALTIES

Abdominal surgery

The abdomen should be examined daily for excessive distension, tenderness or drainage from wounds or drain sites. In certain operations, such as those for intestinal obstruction, oesophageal and gastric procedures (but not in lower intestinal operations), a nasogastric tube may be used. It is of particular value in those patients suffering from ileus or a marked level of altered consciousness who are therefore liable to aspirate.

Paralytic ileus

Paralytic ileus may present with nausea, vomiting, loss of appetite, bowel distension and absence of flatus or bowel movements. Following laparotomy, gastrointestinal motility temporarily decreases. Treatment is usually supportive with maintenance of adequate hydration and electrolyte levels. However, intestinal complications may present as prolonged ileus and so should be actively sought and treated.

Return of function of the intestine occurs in the following order: small bowel, large bowel and then stomach. This pattern allows the passage of faeces despite continuing lack of stomach emptying and, therefore, vomiting may continue even when the lower bowel has already started functioning normally.

Localised infection

An abscess may present with persistent abdominal pain, focal tenderness and a spiking fever. The patient may have a prolonged ileus. If the abscess is deep-seated, these symptoms may be absent. The patient will have a neutrophilic leukocytosis and may have positive blood cultures. An ultrasound or computed tomography (CT) scan of the abdomen should identify any suspicious collection and will identify the subphrenic abscess which can otherwise be difficult to find (Summary box 21.5).

Summary box 21.5

The main complications after abdominal surgery

- Paralytic ileus
- Bleeding or abscess
- Anastomotic leakage

Orthopaedic surgery

In patients who have undergone open reduction and internal fixation of fractures, and especially if a tourniquet has been used, the neurovascular status of the limb must be checked every half an hour first in recovery and then on the ward for at least a further 4 hours. Plasters should always be split for the first 24 hours (or until swelling starts to reduce) and the nurses given instructions to check and record distal circulation every 4 hours. If the patient has an external fixator, the pin sites should be checked daily for signs of infection.

Radiographs are taken after the operation to check that the implants are correctly positioned and that fractures remain reduced.

Patients with compartment syndrome complain of pain out of proportion to that expected. It is not relieved by simple analgesics. Passive stretching of the muscles in the affected compartment produces severe pain. The limb is usually swollen and tense and, in the later stages, there may be altered sensation distally. Distal pulses are only lost at a very late stage and so their presence does not exclude a compartment syndrome. Intracompartmental pressure studies are not reliable so should only be used in the unconscious patient. If there is any possibility that a patient might have a compartment syndrome then all circumferential dressings should be removed at once. If there is no immediate improvement in the pain, then a fasciotomy should be performed. The diagnosis is a clinical one and is made on suspicion not certainty (Summary box 21.6).

Summary box 21.6

Compartment syndrome

- Severe/greater than expected pain unresponsive to analgesia
- The earliest sign is pain on passive stretching of muscles in the affected compartment
- Paralysis, paraesthesia and pulselessness are very late signs

Neck surgery

Patients having neck surgery, e.g. thyroid surgery, must be observed for accumulation of blood in the wound, which may cause rapid asphyxia. A check also needs to be made pre- and postoperatively for damage to the recurrent laryngeal nerve. The findings must be recorded in the medical notes.

Thoracic surgery

Fluid intake should be restricted in patients undergoing a lobectomy or pneumonectomy as they are susceptible to fluid overload in the first 24–48 hours postoperatively. Chest drains require regular review. If the fluid in a chest drain swings then the drain has been inserted correctly in the pleural cavity. If the chest drain continues to bubble, then a bronchopleural fistula probably exists. A haemothorax or pleural effusion (Figure 21.4) will reveal itself as a prolonged loss of blood or fluid, respectively, into the drain. Cardiac patients require continuous electrocardiography monitoring postoperatively (Figures 21.5, 21.6 and 21.7).

Neurosurgery

Postoperatively, the patient should be kept under close observation. A rise in intracranial pressure may be signalled by a deterioration in the state of consciousness, as well as by the appearance of new neurological signs. Some patients may have an intracranial monitoring device to allow for more sensitive monitoring.

Vascular surgery

The patency of grafts and anastomoses in patients with femoropopliteal bypasses and abdominal aneurysmal repairs needs to be checked by regular clinical assessment of the limbs and by Doppler ultrasound in the postoperative phase.

Plastic surgery

The viability of flaps is crucial and the perfusion needs to be monitored regularly. The blood supply may be compromised by position, dressings or collection of fluids or blood beneath the flap.

Urology

Catheter patency must be checked regularly following urological surgery. In patients who have undergone transurethral resection of the prostate (TURP), continuous bladder irrigation may be used, and pulmonary oedema may develop if a large amount of irrigation fluid is absorbed into the circulation.

GENERAL POSTOPERATIVE PROBLEMS AND MANAGEMENT

Pain

This is discussed in Chapter 17.

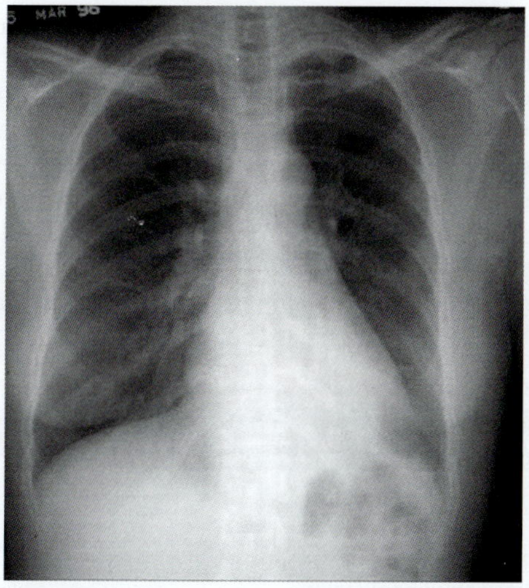

Figure 21.7 Radiograph showing a bilateral pleural effusion (courtesy of Professor Stephen Eustace, Dublin).

Fluid and nutrition

This is covered in Chapter 19.

Nausea and vomiting

Postoperative nausea and vomiting (PONV) can precipitate bleeding and dehiscence of wounds by dislodging the clots and bursting suture lines. In neurosurgical patients, it may precipitate raised intracranial pressure with disastrous effects.

Women, non-smokers or those who have a past history of PONV, motion sickness or migraine are known to have a higher risk of developing PONV. Use of volatile anaesthetic agents, opioids and nitrous oxide add to the risk. Duration and type of surgery also affect the incidence of PONV.

Adequate treatment of pain, anxiety, hypotension and dehydration will minimise the risk of the patient developing PONV. Administer antiemetics that work at different sites, such as HT3 receptor antagonists (e.g. ondansetron), steroids (e.g. dexamethasone), phenothiazines (e.g. prochlorperazine), antihistamines (e.g. cyclizine). At least one antiemetic should be given on a regular basis in the high risk group of patients and a second one written up to be given when needed.

Bleeding

The patient's blood pressure, pulse, urine output, dressings and drains should be checked regularly in the first 24 hours after surgery. If bleeding is more than expected for a given procedure, then pressure should be applied to the site and blood samples should be sent for blood count, coagulation profile and crossmatch. Fluid resuscitation should also be started. Ultrasound or CT scan may need to be arranged to determine the size and extent of the haematoma. If immediate control of bleeding is essential, the patient may be taken back to the operating theatre. If surgical haemostasis is not successful using conventional methods, haemostatic dressings or surgical glue may be tried. The radiological embolisation of bleeding vessels can also prove useful.

All hospitals should have a 'major haemorrhage protocol' in place. The consultant surgeon, anaesthetist and haematologist should all be informed early about unstable patients.

In a patient with postoperative bleeding, oxygenation and fluid resuscitation should be continued, and blood or blood products given if the haemoglobin concentration is less than 8 g/dL. Serum fibrinogen levels below 1 g/L or a prothrombin time (PT) and activated partial thromboplastin time (APTT) greater than 1.5 times normal levels indicate the need for fresh frozen plasma, cryoprecipitate and fibrinogen concentrates. The platelet count should be maintained above 75×10^9/L.

The risks versus the benefits of blood transfusion should be weighed, especially if only one or two units are to be transfused.

Incompatible transfusion causes an acute haemolytic transfusion reaction. The patient may present with fever, chills and rigors, tachycardia, urticaria, body pain, respiratory distress or sudden cardiovascular collapse. If a transfusion reaction is suspected, then the transfusion should be stopped immediately, the patient resuscitated and the blood sent back to the blood bank for retesting.

Blood transfusion can lead to acute fluid overload, hyperkalaemia, severe allergic reaction or anaphylaxis, acute lung injury and delayed haemolytic reaction caused by Kidd and Rh antibodies. Transmission of hepatitis B, C, A, human immunodeficiency virus, cytomegalovirus and variant Creutzfeldt–Jakob disease are also possible (Summary box 21.7).

Summary box 21.7

Postoperative bleeding

- All hospitals should have a major haemorrhage protocol in place
- Need to transfuse blood in the absence of continued bleeding in patients with Hb >8 g/dL should be weighed against the risks
- Minor bleeding in an airway can have a catastrophic effect.

Deep vein thrombosis

Patients suffering postoperative deep vein thrombosis (DVT) may present with calf pain, swelling, warmth, redness and engorged veins. However, most will show no physical signs. On palpation, the muscle may be tender and there is a positive Homans' sign (calf pain on dorsiflexion of the foot), but this test is neither sensitive nor specific.

Venography or duplex Doppler ultrasound is used to assess flow and the presence of thromboses. If a significant DVT is found (one that extends above the knee), treatment with intravenous heparin initially, followed by longer-term warfarin, should be started. In some patients with a large DVT, a caval filter may be required to decrease the possibility of pulmonary embolism.

Most hospitals have a DVT prophylaxis protocol. This may include the use of stockings, calf pumps and pharmacological agents, such as low molecular weight heparin. No method of prophylaxis is foolproof and they all have their own complications, and so an optimal strategy needs to be developed, which is individualised to the patient and the operation that they are receiving (Table 21.2).

Table 21.2 Stratification of risk of deep vein thrombosis.

Low	Medium	High
Maxillofacial surgery	Inguinal hernia repair	Pelvic elective and trauma surgery
Neurosurgery	Abdominal surgery	Total knee and hip replacement
Cardiothoracic surgery	Gynaecological surgery	
	Urological surgery	

Hypothermia and shivering

Anaesthesia induces loss of thermoregulatory control. Exposure of skin and organs to a cold operating environment, volatile skin preparation (which cool by evaporation), and the infusion of cold i.v. fluids all lead to hypothermia. This, in turn, leads to increased cardiac morbidity, a hypocoagulable state, shivering with imbalance of oxygen supply and demand, and immune function impairment with the possibility of wound infection. Active warming devices should be used to treat hypothermia as appropriate.

Fever

About 40 per cent of patients develop pyrexia after major surgery; however, in most cases no cause is found. The inflammatory response to surgical trauma may manifest itself as fever, and so pyrexia does not necessarily imply sepsis. However, in all patients with a pyrexia, a focus of infection should be sought.

The causes of a raised temperature postoperatively include:

- days 2–5: atelectasis of the lung;
- days 3–5: superficial and deep wound infection;
- day 5: chest infection, urinary tract infection and thrombophlebitis;
- >5 days: wound infection, anastomotic leakage, intracavitary collections and abscesses;
- DVTs, transfusion reactions, wound haematomas, atelectasis and drug reactions, may also cause pyrexia of non-infective origin.

Patients with a persistent pyrexia need a thorough review. Relevant investigations include full blood count, urine culture, sputum microscopy and blood cultures (Summary box 21.8).

Summary box 21.8

Fever

- A very common problem postoperatively
- Consider problems in the lung, urine and wound

Prophylaxis against infection

In patients who have had foreign material inserted during the operation, including a hip or knee prosthesis in orthopaedic surgery or aortic valves in cardiovascular surgery, up to three doses of a prophylactic antibiotic should be administered, usually one dose 30 minutes before 'knife to skin' and two postoperatively. Bacteria can be incorporated into the biofilm that forms on the surface of the implant, where they are protected from antibiotics and from the natural defences of the body; prophylactic antibiotics appear to reduce the risk of any contamination developing into infection by destroying bacteria before they are incorporated into the biofilm.

Pressure sores

These occur as a result of friction or persisting pressure on soft tissues. They particularly affect the pressure points of a recumbent patient, including the sacrum, greater trochanter and heels. Risk factors are poor nutritional status, dehydration and lack of mobility and also include the use of a nerve block anaesthesia technique. Early mobilisation prevents pressure sores, while those who are unable to turn in bed should be turned every 30 minutes to prevent pressure sores from developing. High-risk patients may be nursed on an air filter mattress, which automatically relieves the pressure areas (Summary box 21.9).

Summary box 21.9

Preventing pressure sores

- Recognise patients at risk
- Address nutritional status
- Keep patients mobile or regularly turned if bed-bound

John Homans, 1877–1954, Professor of Clinical Surgery, Harvard Medical School, Boston, MA, USA.

Confusional state

Acute confusional states can occur on recovery from anaesthesia (postoperative delirium (POD)) or a few days after surgery. The overall incidence of POD is 5–15 per cent, but is higher in the elderly with hip fractures and is associated with increased morbidity and mortality (Table 21.3).

Table 21.3 Causes of confusion.

	Cause
Renal	Renal failure/uraemia
	Hyponatraemia and electrolyte disorders
	Urinary tract infection
	Urinary retention
Respiratory	Hypoxia, e.g. chest infection
	Atelectasis
Cardiovascular	Pulmonary embolism
	Dehydration
	Septic shock
	Myocardial infarction
	Chronic heart failure
	Arrhythmia
Drugs	Opiates, including heroin
	Hypnotics
	Cocaine
	Alcohol withdrawal
	Hypoglycaemia
Neurological	Epilepsy
	Encephalopathy
	Head injury
	Cerebrovascular accident
Idiopathic (rare)	Hypothyroidism
	Hyperthyroidism
	Addison's disease

Confusion may present as anxiety, incoherent speech, clouding of consciousness or destructive behaviour, e.g. pulling out of cannulae.

Risk factors for POD include pre-existing cognitive impairment (dementia), use of narcotics, benzodiazepines, alcohol (and withdrawal from it), severe illness, renal impairment and depression. Precipitating factors include use of physical restraints, addition of new medications, electrolyte and fluid abnormalities, intraoperative blood loss and admission to an intensive care unit.

Treating the underlying medical problems, involving relatives or friends who are known to the patient, and pain control will all be valuable. As a last option, haloperidol may be given in titrating doses.

Drains

Drains are used to prevent accumulation of blood, serosanguinous or purulent fluid or to allow the early diagnosis of a leaking surgical anastomosis. In clean surgery, such as joint replacement, blood collected in drains can be transfused back into the patient provided that an adequate volume (>150 mL) is collected rapidly (<12 hours) and that a specifically designed drain and filter system is used.

The use of surgical drains has decreased in recent years as the evidence for their benefits has been questioned. They can result in complications, such as trauma to surrounding tissues, and act as a conduit for infection. The quantity and character of drain fluid can be used to identify any abdominal complication, such as fluid leakage (e.g. bile or pancreatic fluid) or bleeding. This lost fluid should be replaced with additional intravenous fluids with the same electrolyte contents. Continued loss of blood through the drain should be investigated for the source.

Drains should be removed as soon as possible and certainly once the drainage has stopped or become less than 25 mL/day.

Wound care

Within hours of the wound being closed, the dead space fills up with an inflammatory exudate. Within 48 hours of closure, a layer of epidermal cells from the wound edge bridges the gap. So, sterile dressings applied in theatre should not be removed before this time.

Wounds should be inspected only if there is any concern about their condition or the dressing needs changing. Inspection of the wound should be performed under sterile conditions. If the wound looks inflamed, a wound swab may need to be taken and sent for Gram staining and culture. Infected wounds and hematoma may need treatment with antibiotics or even a wound washout. Samples obtained at this time should be sent for bacteriology (before any antibiotics are given), any dead tissue excised and bleeding vessels identified and closed off. The wound should be packed if it is contaminated or if any nonviable tissue remains. The patient should return to theatre every 24–48 hours for further cleaning until the wound is clean enough to close.

Skin sutures or clips are usually removed between 6 and 10 days after surgery. The period can be shorter in wounds on the face or neck, and are left longer if incision has been closed under tension. If the wound is healing satisfactorily, then the patient may be allowed to shower one week after surgery. Wound healing is delayed in patients who are malnourished, or have vitamin A and C deficiency. Steroids also inhibit the adequate healing of wounds as they inhibit protein synthesis and fibroblast proliferation. Diabetes, particularly if uncontrolled, also has a deleterious effect on wound healing.

Wound dehiscence

Wound dehiscence is disruption of any or all of the layers in a wound. Dehiscence may occur in up to 3 per cent of abdominal wounds and is very distressing to the patient.

Wound dehiscence most commonly occurs from the 5th to the 8th postoperative day when the strength of the wound is at its weakest. It may herald an underlying abscess and usually presents with a serosanguinous discharge. The patient may have felt a popping sensation during straining or coughing. Most patients will need to return to the operating theatre for resuturing. In some patients, it may be appropriate to leave the wound open and treat with dressings or vacuum-assisted closure (VAC) pumps (Summary box 21.10).

Thomas Addison, 1795–1860, physician, Guy's Hospital. London, UK, described the effects of disease of the suprarenal capsules in 1849.
Arthur Ernest Guedel, 1883–1956, Clinical Professor of Anaesthesiology, University of Southern California, Los Angeles, CA, USA

Summary box 21.10

Risk factors in wound dehiscence

General
- Malnourishment
- Diabetes
- Obesity
- Renal failure
- Jaundice
- Sepsis
- Cancer
- Treatment with steroids

Local
- Inadequate or poor closure of wound
- Poor local wound healing, e.g. because of infection, haematoma or seroma
- Increased intra-abdominal pressure, e.g. in postoperative patients suffering from chronic obstructive airway disease, during excessive coughing

Enhanced recovery

Enhanced recovery is an approach to the perioperative care of patients undergoing surgery. It is designed to speed clinical recovery of the patient, and reduce the cost and the length of stay of the patient in the hospital.

It is achieved by optimising the health of the patient before surgery and then delivering evidence-based best care in the perioperative period.

Postoperative strategies for enhanced recovery include:

- Early planned physiotherapy and mobilisation.
- Early oral hydration and nourishment.
- Good pain control using regular paracetamol with nonsteroidal anti-inflammatory drugs (NSAIDs). Epidurals and nerve blocks are managed by acute pain teams.
- Discharge planning is started before the patient is even admitted to hospital and involves support from stoma care nurses, physiotherapists and other community care workers.

Early mobilisation is encouraged to reduce the risks of DVT, urinary retention, atelectasis, pressure sores and faecal impaction. Telephone follow up is carried out to make sure that the patient is recovering well once discharged.

DISCHARGE OF PATIENTS

Patients discharged home need a 'discharge letter' detailing the postoperative plan. The discharge letter should include details of the final diagnosis, the treatment and any complications that may have occurred. There should be advice for referring the patient back to hospital and indications for readmission if specific problems do occur. The GP should be informed of the subsequent care plan including follow up, physiotherapy and other support needed. Pathology results should be included if available and the basis of these in the subsequent care plan should be described along with the prognosis if appropriate (Summary box 21.11).

Summary box 21.11

Discharge letter

- Diagnosis
- Treatment
- Laboratory results
- Complications
- Discharge plan
- Support needed
- Follow up

Follow up in clinic

Patients should only be reviewed in clinic when a key decision on management needs to be made. The findings and the care plan agreed with the patient at the clinic appointment should be included in a letter to the patient's GP, as well as in a clear handwritten entry in the notes. This should include advice on how to recognise the onset of complications and what to do if there is concern. Patients should be discharged from clinic as soon as their GPs or they themselves can manage their care.

FURTHER READING

Burkitt G, Quick C, Gatt D. *Essential surgery*, 2nd edn. Oxford: Churchill Livingstone, 1995.

Cuschieri A, Grace PA. *Clinical surgery*. Oxford: Blackwell, 2003.

Gan TJ, Meyer TA, Apfel CC *et al.* Society for Ambulatory Anesthesia guidelines for the management of postoperative nausea and vomiting. *Anesth Analg* 2007; **105**: 1615–28.

Grace PA, Borley N. *Surgery at a glance*. Oxford: Blackwell, 2006.

Intensive Care Society website. Levels of critical care for adult patients. Available from: www.ics.ac.uk/intensive_care_professional/standards_and_guidelines/levels_of_critical_care_for_adult_patients.

CHAPTER

22 Day case surgery

LEARNING OBJECTIVES

To understand:

- The concept of the day-surgery pathway
- The importance of patient selection and preoperative assessment
- Basic principles of anaesthesia for day surgery
- The spectrum of surgical procedures suitable for day surgery
- Postoperative management and discharge arrangements

DAY SURGERY PATHWAY

Day surgery offers advantages for health-care delivery around the world and so rates have steadily increased in both developed and developing countries. The increase in day surgery popularity is due to both patient preference and financial considerations. The removal of an overnight stay provides significant savings to the hospital. The original concept of day surgery was the admission and discharge of a patient for a specific procedure within the 12-hour working day. Where a patient requires an overnight admission, then the term '23-hour stay' should be used (Summary box 22.1).

Summary box 22.1

Definition of terms used in ambulatory surgery

- Outpatient surgery: not admitted to a ward facility
- Procedure room surgery: surgery not requiring full sterile theatre facilities
- Day or same-day surgery: admitted and discharged within the 12-hour day
- Overnight stay: 23-hour admission with early morning discharge
- Short-stay surgery: admission of up to 72 hours

Day surgery is a patient pathway, not a surgical procedure and extends from first patient contact to final discharge (Figure 22.1). Success in day surgery requires each component of the pathway to be safe and efficient and to be performed in sequence. Unplanned overnight admissions are minimised by ensuring that:

- the patient is informed and fit for the procedure;
- the procedure itself is achievable as a day case; and
- the home environment can support a postoperative patient.

SELECTION CRITERIA

Stand-alone day surgery facilities can safely perform minor and intermediate procedures, but if they lack overnight beds then the surgery undertaken and the selection criteria will need to be conservative to minimise the risk of unplanned overnight admissions requiring transfer of the patient to the parent hospital. Advanced day surgery procedures with an increased likelihood of an unplanned admission are best performed where overnight beds are available. Procedures which carry an increased intraoperative risk of complications and operations on more challenging patients are best managed in a hospital-integrated unit with the immediate availability of support services.

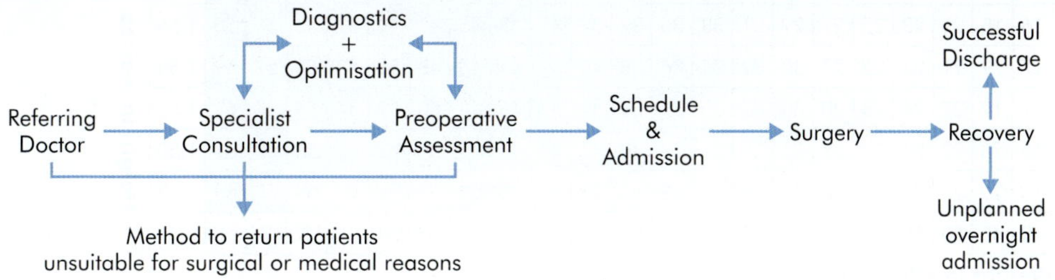

Figure 22.1 Day-surgery pathway.

James H Nicoll, 1864–1921, paediatric surgeon from Glasgow, Scotland, who specialised in pyloric stenosis and spina bifida, and pioneered the 'Glasgow dispensary', where his work earned him the title of 'Father of Day Surgery'. He was made Legion of Honour France.

Medical criteria

Age

There is no upper age limit. Healthy patient physiological status is a better determinant of day surgery success.

Comorbidity

Units traditionally use the American Society of Anesthesiologists (ASA) classification which is a crude evaluation of chronic health (Table 22.1). Stand-alone units often confine their criteria to ASA I and II patients, while ASA III patients are more suitable for hospital-integrated units. Patients with significant respiratory or cardiovascular disease should be reviewed by an anaesthetist before being accepted for day surgery. Historically many patients who are fit but hypertensive have been incorrectly excluded from day surgery. Current published evidence does not support cancellation when blood pressure is below 180/110.

Table 22.1 The American Society of Anaesthesiologists Physical Status Classification.

Classification	
1	A normal healthy patient
2	A patient with mild systemic disease
3	A patient with severe systemic disease
4	A patient with severe systemic disease that is a constant threat to life
5	A moribund patient who is not expected to survive without the operation

Reproduced with permission from: American Society of Anaesthesiologists (1963).

Obesity

The body mass index (BMI) is calculated as weight in kilograms divided by the square of height in metres (kg/m^2) and obesity is defined as a BMI >30 (Figure 22.2). Traditional guidelines are conservative about obesity due to fears of intra- and postoperative complications. Although there is an increased incidence of non-serious respiratory complications intraoperatively and in the immediate postoperative recovery period, the course of these patients is otherwise uneventful. They should, however, be managed by experienced medical and nursing staff. Hypertension, congestive cardiac failure and sleep apnoea are all more common in patients with morbid obesity, but in selected and optimised patients, a BMI up to 40 for surface procedures and 38 for laparoscopic procedures are acceptable in advanced units.

Weight in kilograms

Height in metres	40	45	50	55	60	65	70	75	80	85	90	95	100	105	110	115	120	125	130	135	140	Height in metres
1.92	11	12	14	15	16	18	19	20	22	23	24	26	27	28	30	31	33	34	35	37	38	1.92
1.90	11	12	14	15	17	18	19	21	22	24	25	26	28	29	30	32	33	35	36	37	39	1.90
1.88	11	13	14	16	17	18	20	21	23	24	25	27	28	30	31	33	34	35	37	38	40	1.88
1.86	12	13	14	16	17	19	20	22	23	25	26	27	29	30	32	33	35	36	38	39	40	1.86
1.84	12	13	15	16	18	19	21	22	24	25	27	28	30	31	32	34	35	37	38	40	41	1.84
1.82	12	14	15	17	18	20	21	23	24	26	27	29	30	32	33	35	36	38	39	41	42	1.82
1.80	12	14	15	17	19	20	22	23	25	26	28	29	31	32	34	35	37	39	40	42	43	1.80
1.78	13	14	16	17	19	21	22	24	25	27	28	30	32	33	35	36	38	39	41	43	44	1.78
1.76	13	15	16	18	19	21	23	24	26	27	29	31	32	34	36	37	39	40	42	44	45	1.76
1.74	13	15	17	18	20	21	23	25	26	28	30	31	33	35	36	38	40	41	43	45	46	1.74
1.72	14	15	17	19	20	22	24	25	27	29	30	32	34	35	37	39	41	42	44	46	47	1.72
1.70	14	16	17	19	21	22	24	26	28	29	31	33	35	36	38	40	42	43	45	47	48	1.70
1.68	14	16	18	19	21	23	25	27	28	30	32	34	35	37	39	41	43	44	46	48	50	1.68
1.66	15	16	18	20	22	24	25	27	29	31	33	34	36	38	40	42	44	45	47	49	51	1.66
1.64	15	17	19	20	22	24	26	28	30	32	33	35	37	39	41	43	45	46	48	50	52	1.64
1.62	15	17	19	21	23	25	27	29	30	32	34	36	38	40	42	44	46	48	50	51	53	1.62
1.60	16	18	20	21	23	25	27	29	31	33	35	37	39	41	43	45	47	49	51	53	55	1.60
1.58	16	18	20	22	24	26	28	30	32	34	36	38	40	42	44	46	48	50	52	54	56	1.58
1.56	16	18	21	23	25	27	29	31	33	35	37	39	41	43	45	47	49	51	53	55	58	1.56
1.54	17	19	21	23	25	27	30	32	34	36	38	40	42	44	46	48	51	53	55	57	59	1.54
1.52	17	19	22	24	26	28	30	32	35	37	39	41	43	45	48	50	52	54	56	58	61	1.52
1.50	18	20	22	24	27	29	31	33	36	38	40	42	44	47	49	51	53	56	58	60	62	1.50
1.48	18	21	23	25	27	30	32	34	37	39	41	43	46	48	50	53	55	57	59	62	64	1.48
	40	45	50	55	60	65	70	75	80	85	90	95	100	105	110	115	120	125	130	135	140	

Weight in kilograms

21	BMI 20–25
25	BMI 25–30
32	BMI 30–35
37	BMI 35–40
41	BMI >40

Figure 22.2 Body mass index calculator.

Adolphe Quetelet, 1796–1874, Belgian mathematician, astronomer and statistician who was the pioneer in establishing the criteria of obesity that became known as the Quetelet Index. In 1972 Ancel Keys (1904–2004), an American Scientist from the University of Minnesota and an expert on human nutrition, public health and epidemiology, named it the Body Mass Index.

Social criteria

Safe and comfortable discharge home requires the patient to be accompanied by a responsible and physically able adult to remain with them overnight. Home circumstances require appropriate toilet facilities and the means of contacting the hospital should complications occur. A journey time to home of an hour or less is advocated, but the comfort of the journey rather than the time involved is more relevant.

Surgical criteria

Patients undergoing procedures up to 2 hours in duration can safely undergo day surgery with modern anaesthetic techniques. The degree of surgical trauma is an important determinant of success therefore entry to abdominal and thoracic cavities should be confined to minimal access techniques. Whatever the procedure, the main requirement is that there is suitable control of pain and the ability to drink and eat in a reasonable timescale (Summary box 22.2).

Summary box 22.2

Selection criteria for day surgery

- Medical: use physiological rather than chronological age
  ASA status over II requires careful review
  Provided that the BMI is under 40, this alone is not a contraindication
- Social: a responsible adult carer must be available for first 24 hours
  home conditions need to be suitable
  ability to contact hospital in an emergency
- Surgical: operations up to 2 hours
  recognised day-surgery procedures
  ability to eat and drink within reasonable timescale.

PREOPERATIVE ASSESSMENT

The evaluation and optimisation of a patient's fitness for surgery is known as preoperative assessment and is best performed by a specialist nursing team with support from an anaesthetist with an interest in day surgery. The assessment should be performed early in the pathway to allow time to optimise health problems before surgery. The consultation consists of a basic health screen to include the measurement of BMI, blood pressure and an assessment of past medical history with current medication recorded. Appropriate investigations are performed to ensure the patient is fit for surgery. The patient and/or their carer should be given verbal and written information regarding admission, operation and discharge (Summary box 22.3).

Summary box 22.3

Preoperative assessment

- On all day-surgery patients
- Early in the patient pathway
- By a specialist nursing team with anaesthetic support

PERIOPERATIVE MANAGEMENT

Scheduling

With dedicated day surgery lists, major procedures should be scheduled early on morning lists to allow maximum recovery time. When the list is in the afternoon, the allocation of local or regional anaesthetic cases later in the day helps reduce unplanned overnight admissions following general anaesthesia. When mixed lists of day and inpatient cases are planned, then day cases should go first. Where complex inpatient surgery is undertaken, the mixing of day and inpatient cases is not advisable. The complex case may be inappropriately delayed if the day case is scheduled first and conversely if the day-case patient is scheduled later, it may result in cancellation or an unplanned overnight admission for the day case.

Anaesthesia and analgesia

Successful day-surgery anaesthesia requires a multimodal approach to analgesia, while ensuring patients are given optimal dosages of anaesthetic agent. The agents used matter less than the skill of the person providing anaesthesia.

Multimodal analgesia starts in the preoperative period and unless contraindicated, patients should receive full oral doses of paracetamol and a nonsteroidal anti-inflammatory drug (NSAID), such as ibuprofen. Intraoperative anaesthesia can be maintained by any of the traditional inhalational agents. TIVA (total intravenous anaesthesia) techniques using propofol are also popular and offer the advantage of reduced postoperative nausea and vomiting (PONV). The use of intraoperative analgesia will depend on the procedure being performed. When available, the anaesthetist should use short-acting opioids (fentanyl, alfentanil). Careful use of these agents can minimise the incidence of PONV. Where the choice is limited to morphine, this should be used in small doses (under 0.1 mg/kg) to minimise sedation and PONV. Wherever possible, a long-acting local anaesthetic agent, such as bupivacaine, should be injected into wounds by the surgeon.

Pain levels should be routinely assessed in the postoperative recovery area. Further doses of paracetamol, fentanyl or low doses of morphine can be used to ensure that patients are comfortable prior to return to the ward (Summary box 22.4).

Summary box 22.4

Optimal analgesia and anaesthesia

- Multimodal analgesia with paracetamol and nonsteroidal anti-inflammatory drug (NSAID) (if not contraindicated) should be given preoperatively
- Use long-acting local anaesthetic infiltration of the surgical wound
- Careful dosing of inhalational or intravenous agents should be used to maintain anaesthesia
- Avoid long-acting opioids, such as morphine, to reduce the incidence of sedation and postoperative nausea and vomiting (PONV)

Postoperative complications

The range of postoperative complications is no different from normal surgery. However, the fact that the patient will be discharged home within a few hours of surgery requires proactive monitoring after surgery. Haemorrhage is dealt with later in the chapter. Nausea and vomiting is not uncommon and should be managed actively to maximise successful discharge (Figure 22.3). Inadequate recovery from anaesthesia, uncontrolled nausea and vomiting and inadequate pain control are the most common anaesthetic related causes of postoperative admission.

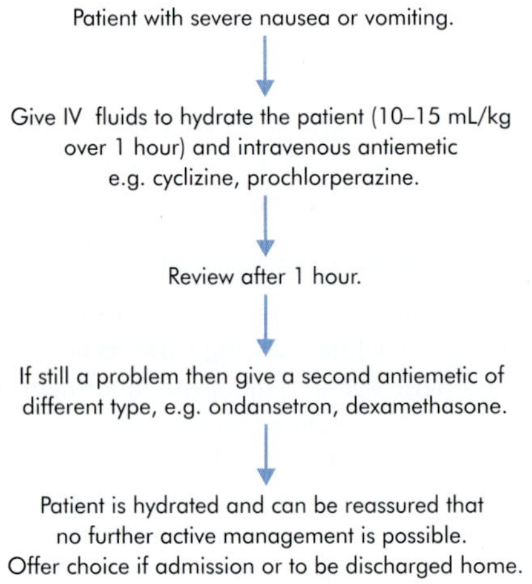

Figure 22.3 Active management of postoperative nausea and vomiting (PONV).

SURGERY

For some surgical specialties, over 90 per cent of their elective workload can be achieved in day surgery. As a result, teaching and training now routinely occurs on day-surgery lists, but requires structure and close supervision. As the spectrum of procedures has increased and become more challenging, there has been a culture change among surgeons to increase their involvement in day surgery. This is important because safe and efficient day surgery demands the competence and skill of an experienced surgeon. Some surgeons have concerns regarding patient safety after discharge. The risk of postoperative haemorrhage occurring once the patient has returned home following tonsillectomy or laparoscopic surgery is often stated as a major reason to keep the patient in hospital overnight. Reactionary haemorrhage commonly occurs in the first 4–6 hours after surgery, but the patient is unlikely to have been discharged home within this time period. It may be caused by slippage of a ligature, displacement of blood clot, cessation of vasospasm, after coughing or increased mobility. Secondary haemorrhage is defined as occurring at least 24 hours after surgery, but usually presents several days later, as it is due to postoperative infection. Thus, even if the patient had stayed overnight, these postoperative bleeds are still likely to occur once the patient has returned home (Summary box 22.5).

Good surgical technique requires minimal tissue traction or tension and good haemostasis. In day surgery, these attributes are even more important (Summary box 22.6). The number and variety of surgical procedures performed on a day-case basis is increasing year on year. Many developments have been pioneered by individual surgeons in isolated centres and their expertise has yet to spread to mainstream surgery. Volume procedures in general surgery where the British Association of Day Surgery considers at least 40 per cent of procedures can be performed on a day-case basis are shown in Table 22.2.

Summary box 22.5

Surgical haemorrhage

- Reactionary: occurs 4–6 hours after surgery and is caused by ligature slippage, clot displacement or cessation of vasospasm, after mobilisation or coughing
- Secondary: occurs more than 24 hours after surgery and is due to infection eroding a vessel

Summary box 22.6

Requirements for successful day surgery

- Minimal access techniques
- Good haemostasis
- Avoidance of unnecessary tissue handling or tension

Table 22.2 Volume procedures where 40 per cent or more should be performed on a day-case basis.

Surgery	
Abdominal	Excisional/treatment of anal lesions, haemorrhoidectomy, primary and recurrent inguinal/femoral herniae, laparoscopic cholecystectomy, laparoscopic fundoplication, pilonidal sinus surgery
Breast	Excision/biopsy breast lesion, sentinel node excision
Genitourinary	Laser prostatectomy, orchidectomy, circumcision, excision of hydrocoele/varicocoele/epididymis
Orthopaedic	Dupuytren's fasciectomy, carpal tunnel release, therapeutic arthroscopy of knee or shoulder, bunion operations, removal of metalwork
Vascular	Varicose vein procedures, thoracoscopic sympathectomy

Reproduced with permission from British Association of Day Surgery (2009).

DISCHARGE

The assessment of when a patient is fit for discharge is best performed by trained day-surgery nurses using strict discharge criteria (Table 22.3). While postoperative review by the surgical team is encouraged, the discharge should not be delayed by failure of their timely attendance. A suitable supply of analgesics for the management of pain should be provided. Paracetamol, NSAIDs and codeine form the basis of the drugs available in many countries.

Table 22.3 Discharge criteria.

Vital signs stable for at least 1 hour
Correct orientation as to time, place and person
Adequate pain control with supply of oral analgesia
Understands how to use oral analgesia supplied
Ability to dress and walk, where appropriate
Minimal nausea, vomiting or dizziness
Has taken oral fluids
Minimal bleeding or wound drainage
Has passed urine (if appropriate)
Has a responsible adult to take them home
Has a carer at home for the next 24 hours
Written and verbal instructions given about postoperative care
Knows when to come back for follow up (if appropriate)
Emergency contact number supplied

FURTHER READING

Jakobsson J. *Anaesthesia for day case surgery*. Oxford: Oxford University Press, 2009.

Lemos P, Jarrett P, Philip B (eds). *Day surgery: development and practice*. Porto: Clássica Artes Gráficas, 2006.

Thomas WEG, Senninger N (eds). *Short stay surgery*. New York: Springer, 2008.

PART 4

Trauma

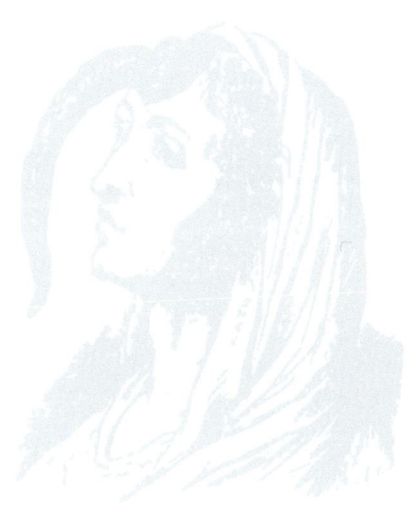

CHAPTER

23 Introduction to trauma

LEARNING OBJECTIVES

To gain an understanding of:

- The importance of time in trauma management
- How to assess a trauma problem
- How to respond to a trauma problem
- The value of planning

WHAT IS TRAUMA?

Trauma is the study of medical problems associated with physical injury. The injury is the adverse effect of a physical force upon a person. There are a variety of forces that can lead to injury, including thermal, ionising radiation and chemical. However, the force involved in most injuries is mechanical. The subject of trauma therefore centres upon the deleterious effects of kinetic energy on the human frame. In the next group of chapters we will explore trauma from a variety of perspectives related to different specialties. In this introduction, we will look at the aspects that bind the whole topic together.

THE SCALE OF THE PROBLEM

Trauma is recognised as a serious public health problem. In fact, it is the leading cause of death and disability in the first four decades of life and is the third most common cause of death overall.

Millions of people are killed or disabled by injury each year. Of the 5 million people killed as a result of injuries in 2000, approximately 1.2 million people died of road traffic injuries, 815 000 from suicide and 520 000 from homicides. In the UK, the accidental and deliberate injury standardised death rate (SDR) is 27.28 deaths over all ages per 100 000 inhabitants per year. Hundreds of thousands who survive their injuries experience long-term or permanent disabilities, time lost from work or family responsibilities, costly medical expenses, profound change in lifestyle, pain and suffering, regardless of gender, race or economic status. An injury affects more than just the injured person; it affects everyone who is involved in the injured person's life. The importance of the modern epidemic of motor vehicle accidents (MVA) to the global epidemic of violent injury cannot be overstated.

Trauma is not just related to high-energy transfer in road accidents or to violence. The elderly fall victim makes up the most common group to be admitted to hospital following injury in the UK. Fragility fractures represent an increasing load on health services. About 70 000 patients suffer a proximal femoral fracture each year in the UK. About 30 per cent of those over the age of 65 years who suffer a proximal femoral fracture will die within a year of the incident, and most of the others will have diminished independence and mobility. It can be appreciated that this represents a huge burden on the health services and society in general.

The great majority of injuries are not life- or limb-threatening. Here the challenge is not only to treat the minor injuries, but also to differentiate between those injuries that have some important aspects and those that are genuinely straightforward. For instance, in children, one must always be alert to the potential for non-accidental injury (NAI). There is a chilling statistic that in 66 per cent of cases when children die as the result of abuse there has been some previous relevant contact with a health professional or social services. In all age groups, we need to be wary of pathological fractures; here the more important problem may not be the injury itself, but the underlying disease process (Summary box 23.1).

Summary box 23.1

Trauma: the scale of the problem

- Trauma is the major cause of death in the young
- Fragility fractures are an increasing burden
- Look beyond the obvious in trauma management

THE MANAGEMENT OF TRAUMA

We learn how to manage trauma based on evidence, extrapolation from principle and by copying. All of our actions should have a purpose, for those based on evidence or principle this is frequently apparent. However, our actions based on mimicry and protocol may have less obvious foundations. While this may help to reduce delay when under pressure, we should also attempt to understand why we are carrying them out.

The importance of time

An identifying feature in the study of trauma is time. At time zero, the person/patient is at their normal baseline. There is then some interaction with an external force leading to injury. The subsequent development of pathology, the response of the body by way of compensation and healing, and the external responses by health professionals all have a timeline. The timeline may be used to compare and consider the progress from time zero to other significant events or deadlines that follow.

Figure 23.1 depicts an estimate of the periods of time that may elapse from time zero to death or irretrievable damage for various injuries. It reflects the fact that some problems tend to lead to earlier death than others. An obstructed airway, a tension pneumothorax, an extradural haematoma or an ischaemic limb will all tend to progress along a characteristic timeline after the moment of initial injury if left untreated. This creates an 'imperative of time' that shapes and provides a basis for the hierarchy of our initial medical response to the injured patient. Thus, an obstructed airway will need emergency initial management at the scene of the accident. An ischaemic limb may be dealt with urgently once the patient has reached a definitive treatment centre. The ATLS (Advanced Trauma Life Support) system defines an order of priorities given by ABCD; that is **a**irway, **b**reathing, **c**irculation and **d**isability (neurology). This is founded upon this time dependence.

To this raw diagram of the time from injury to death or irretrievable damage may be added other components. These are the time to understand or assess the nature of the problem and the time to respond effectively to that which has been discovered. Each of these will take a finite length of time and this is shown schematically for a generic condition in Figure 23.2. It can be seen that in this example there is adequate time for an orderly process of all the stages of assessment followed by a response before irretrievable damage or death.

The block of time allocated to assessment may be broken down further. Understanding and assessing the nature of the problem usually hinges on diagnosing the injury. An injury may be found by careful physical examination or need special investigation before it is discovered. It therefore becomes obvious at different points on its timeline. An example is an evolving extradural haematoma: the initial skull fracture may be visible on radiography or computed tomography (CT); as the haematoma develops it will first be visible on CT; later, it will be suspected on careful clinical examination; and, finally, it will become clinically very obvious. This is represented in Figure 23.3a.

The next feature to add to the timeline is the response time. Once an obstructed airway is identified, the response time to carry out a life-saving simple airway manoeuvre may be a matter of seconds. Thus, even at the stage when the diagnosis is clinically obvious, there may still be time to resolve the problem before irretrievable damage occurs. However, when dealing with an extradural haemorrhage, the average response time from identification of the problem to surgical resolution may be measured in hours. This may seem an unduly long time, but bringing the patient to an operating theatre with a neurosurgeon takes time to arrange, as seen in Figure 23.3b. If we now combine the various features of a timeline for the single condition of extradural haematoma, difficulties become apparent. In Figure 23.3c, it is seen that if the response is only initiated once the diagnosis has become obvious, then there may be insufficient time left to resolve the problem before death intervenes. This seems to suggest that we need to initiate a response to a problem before we are sure of its existence if we are to save the patient's life. This apparent paradox will be explored further. However, for the moment it can be likened to the need to identify a cancer at an early stage to give the best chance of successful treatment. A common approach to such a problem is to screen the at-risk population, and the same principle applies in the management of trauma.

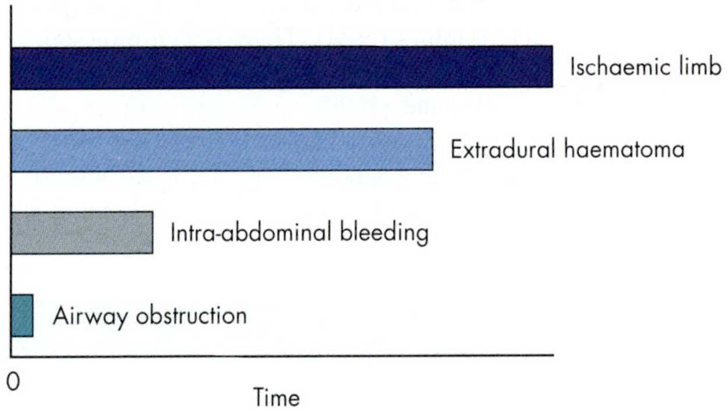

Figure 23.1 Estimated time from incident to death or irretrievable damage for various conditions.

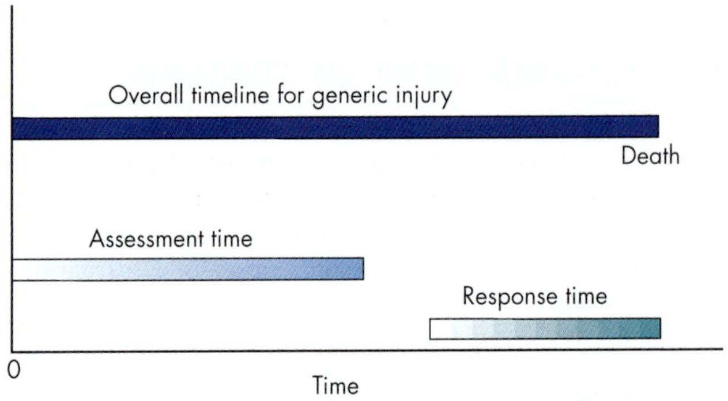

Figure 23.2 Diagrammatic representation of the relationship between assessment and response times. In this example, there is time to assess and respond effectively before death.

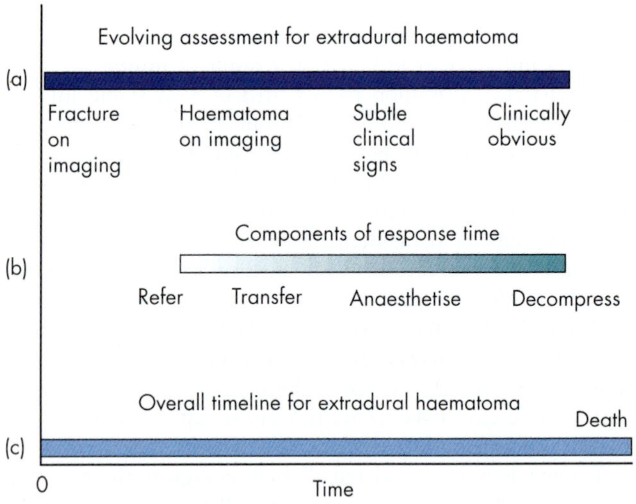

Figure 23.3 Diagrammatic representation of the relationship between assessment and response times for extradural haematoma. (a) The stages of assessment; (b) the components of the response and (c) the overall time from incident to death. It can be seen that relying on obvious clinical signs gives insufficient time to respond effectively.

George Quentin Chance, formerly Director of Diagnostic Radiology, Derby Group of Hospitals, Derbyshire, England.

As we will see, much of the medical preparation and planning related to trauma is aimed at reducing the diagnosis time and the response time so that they will fit into the time available before death or irretrievable damage. To revise the meanings of these terms, the diagnosis time is the time between injury and recognition of the problem and the response time is the time that elapses between identifying the problem and effective intervention being completed. We can reduce these times by using a practised, protocol-driven approach to the initial stages of the management of an injured patient. We must still think, but it does mean that we can have a pre-existing structure upon which to build those thought processes. This allows us to move forward more rapidly. This structured initial approach allows for more straightforward teamwork, standardisation of the equipment required and confidence in a difficult situation.

The pressure of time determines the manner in which we deal with the multiply-injured patient. The normal sequence of history, examination, provisional diagnosis, special investigations, diagnosis and management plan is not appropriate under this pressure. When dealing with the multiply-injured, a quite different approach is needed. As will be seen, the primary survey used in ATLS combines the identification of life-threatening problems with their management. It has evolved to improve the chances of the necessary actions being taken within the time available. The system has to allow for diagnosis to be made and response completed within the timeline for the injuries sustained. Increasingly, special investigations are being lavished on the multiply-injured patient with the aim of trying to reduce further the delay to accurate diagnosis.

The model of a timeline need not be restricted to the multiply-injured patient. The role of time when dealing with an elderly person who has been injured is still present, but is frequently ignored. In these cases, there may be hidden urgent issues. Thus, when dealing with the elderly, we too readily label a patient with the most obvious problem (such as a hip fracture) without performing the vital initial physiological triage. The patient may often have a primary cardiac, respiratory or neurological problem that has resulted in a fall and the response to this may be the most urgent issue. Therefore, the timeline is not only relevant to the acute and obviously urgent clinical issues. As noted at the beginning of this chapter, a timeline may be used to compare and consider the progress from time zero to other significant events or deadlines that follow. In this case, the response time to arrange a discharge from hospital for the elderly patient may be critically protracted. Figure 23.4 demonstrates that, with such a long response time, to allow for discharge at the appropriate clinical time the social planning needs to commence almost at the time of admission. This is well before it would seem clinically reasonable, but to achieve an efficient system, it can be seen to be necessary. This approach allows an emergency unit to get as close as is possible to the practice of an effective elective unit where discharge plans are made before the patient is admitted.

Time also plays a part in how we deal with more minor injuries. There is a need and expectation that these patients will be dealt with rapidly; however, there is then a danger, especially with inexperienced doctors, that corners will be cut and problems missed. Focusing on the important issues without risking missing problems is a difficult skill. Although not all patients will be seen by more than one doctor, another health professional, usually a nurse, will see them and their observations should not be ignored. A common safety net for the front-line medical staff is that all x-rays of patients discharged are independently reviewed by a radiologist. Should their findings differ from those in the clinical record, the patient can be recalled and reassessed.

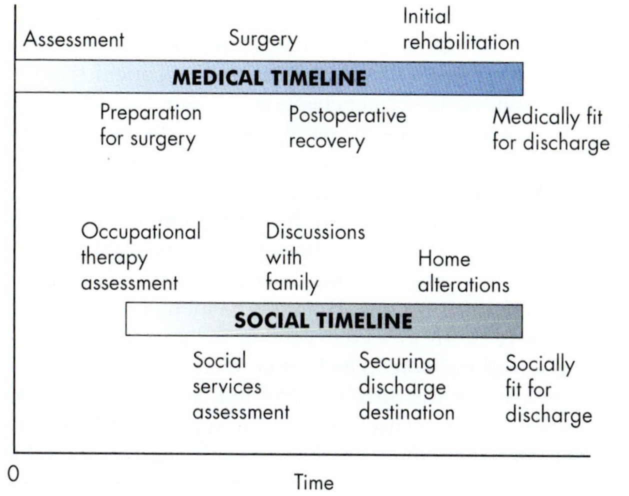

Figure 23.4 Social and medical timelines for an elderly patient with a proximal femoral fracture. Discharge can only occur when both are complete.

Timelines reveal that things change. As a consequence, reassessment can be of vital importance. An observation, an x-ray or a blood test are only snapshots in time. Repeated observation will reveal trends that may make a diagnosis more straightforward. Modern monitoring allows this continuing vigilance to be carried out more straightforwardly. Graphical recording of results in a single place makes trends easier to follow.

Although the pressure and relevance of time shapes our response to the injured, it should not be allowed to degrade it (Summary box 23.2).

Summary box 23.2

The importance of time

- Time pressure shapes our management of trauma
- There is a finite time to assess
- There is a finite time to respond
- For success, these must fit into the available time before irretrievable damage or death

ASSESSMENT AND RESPONSE

The breakdown of our approach to the injured into two components of assessment and response has been introduced. Although the two concepts overlap and intertwine, it is helpful to explore them separately.

The assessment of trauma

At time zero, a person in their baseline condition comes together with an external force to produce injury. Understanding this relationship between the patient, the mechanism of injury and the injury produced is the key to understanding the problem that has to be solved. This is helpful both when making a diagnosis and treatment plan for an individual, and also for structuring the thinking of the management of trauma in general. The relationship can be expressed simply as: mechanism + patient = injury.

The nature of these components may be quite obvious (overt) or in some way hidden (covert). We need to convert everything to the overt. We can only treat what we have found; we can only resolve the problems that we have identified.

A tidy relationship between the mechanism, the patient and the resulting injury is often obvious. A previously healthy 40-year-old man falling vertically 2 metres and landing on his feet may sustain an os calcis fracture. From this position of understanding, we can move swiftly forward to confirm and treat. In many cases, there is something more to find out or to understand.

It may be that the three variables just do not add up to form a complete picture. This failure of the relationship is not real but apparent. If the three variables do not fit together something has probably been misjudged, and the factor that is causing the failure of the clinical picture to 'add up' must be sought. It may be that some aspect of the injury has not yet been discovered, the mechanism suggested may not be genuine or there may be some aspect of the patient before the injury of which one is unaware (Summary box 23.3). To expand on this theme, we will explore how to use the available information to best effect.

Summary box 23.3

The assessment of trauma

- Use all of the information: mechanism, patient and injury
- Allow the obvious features to be a guide to the less obvious
- If the equation does not add up, look for more reasons

Mechanisms

Mechanisms may be blunt or penetrating. One of the easiest of these to understand is the incision caused by a knife. We are used to knives both at home when we eat and as surgeons when we operate. A knife has a sharp edge that may cut tissues with which it makes contact; these effects are easily appreciated because they happen in a timescale that we understand. A knife damages only what it can reach. A good history of the length of blade coupled with an entry point allows for a potential pattern of injury to be imagined and then individual components to be confirmed or excluded by examination, special investigation or wound exploration (Table 23.1).

Thus, an incisional injury over an extremity is readily evaluated as long as the relevant anatomy is known. The distal perfusion, peripheral nerve function and tendon and muscle function can all be assessed by clinical examination. However, should joint penetration be a possibility then the problem is different. Understanding the timeline is of value. The consequences of a septic arthritis are severe and if treatment is delayed until the condition is clinically obvious, then it may be too late to prevent permanent damage. Therefore, the diagnosis of joint penetration needs to be excluded by screening the at-risk group. If a large joint is involved, for example the knee, an algorithm such as that in Figure 23.5 can help identify those joints that need formal exploration. One component of this algorithm is to fill the joint until tense with sterile saline and watch whether fluid leaks through the traumatic wound. This will show whether the joint has been penetrated. If the joint has been breached, a

Table 23.1 Examples of patterns of injury.

Mechanism	Obvious features	Covert injuries
Left-sided impact from road traffic accident	Lateral compression of the pelvis	Splenic rupture
	Left-sided pneumothorax	Extradural haematoma
Flexion distraction (lap belt)	Chance fracture of the lumbar spine	Duodenal rupture
	Dislocated knee	Popliteal artery disruption
	Head injury	Cervical spine fracture
Electrocution	Burn on hand and collapse	Posterior dislocation of the shoulder
Dashboard impact	Knee wound	Posterior dislocation of the hip

formal procedure in an operating theatre is required. This action is now therapeutic and not exploratory.

In assessing the effects of an incisional mechanism over the torso, the first step is again to decide which structures are at risk. This may seem simple, but it is not always easy to determine the direction that a blade has entered. The anatomy can also be confusing; it is worth recalling that the abdominal contents extend higher than normally expected, up to the level of the fifth rib in expiration. A notable feature of stab injuries is that they are often eminently treatable; even cardiac injuries can be treated with a realistic chance of success if identified early (Summary box 23.4).

Penetrating injuries caused by firearms are not so easily understood as incisional injuries. A low-velocity projectile behaves

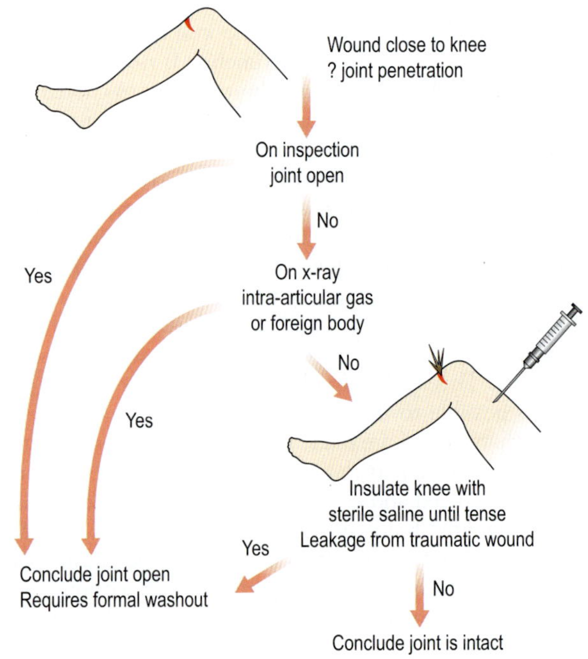

Figure 23.5 Algorithm for assessing a wound that has potentially entered a joint.

Summary box 23.4

Incisional injuries

- Require knowledge of anatomy
- The abdominal contents extend high into the chest
- Even cardiac injuries are treatable if recognised early and treated quickly

more or less like a stabbing injury. However, as the velocity increases, the energy increases in line with $E = ½mv^2$; as the amount of energy increases, the ability of the system to dissipate that introduced energy in a simple way is overcome. In the case of high-velocity projectiles, the result is not like anything we are familiar with in day-to-day life. Furthermore, these projectiles are deliberately designed to produce particular results: some are designed to kill, whereas others are designed to maim but not kill. In a military conflict, it is more disabling and demoralising to your opponent's forces if individuals do not die but consume resources in their treatment and protection.

The high-velocity bullet crushes particles of the human body in its pathway and produces lateral acceleration away from the point of impact. This motion of the tissue particles away from their original position produces a cavity. Two types of cavity are produced: (1) a permanent cavity – one that remains after the initial impact; (2) a temporary cavity – one that lasts for milliseconds, and may no longer be apparent during the physical examination of the wounded. This temporary cavitation can extend well beyond the boundaries of the apparent injury. High-speed photography shows the dramatic nature of the temporary deformation, which happens on a very rapid timescale (Figure 23.6). Awareness of this phenomenon will encourage the treating surgeon to perform an adequate exploration and, if appropriate, a more radical wound excision than would otherwise be used (Summary box 23.5).

Summary box 23.5

Firearm injuries

- Low-velocity bullets behave like knife injuries
- High-velocity bullets cause cavitation
- The temporary cavity is large and draws in foreign materials
- The permanent cavity is smaller and gives no clue to the extent of damage

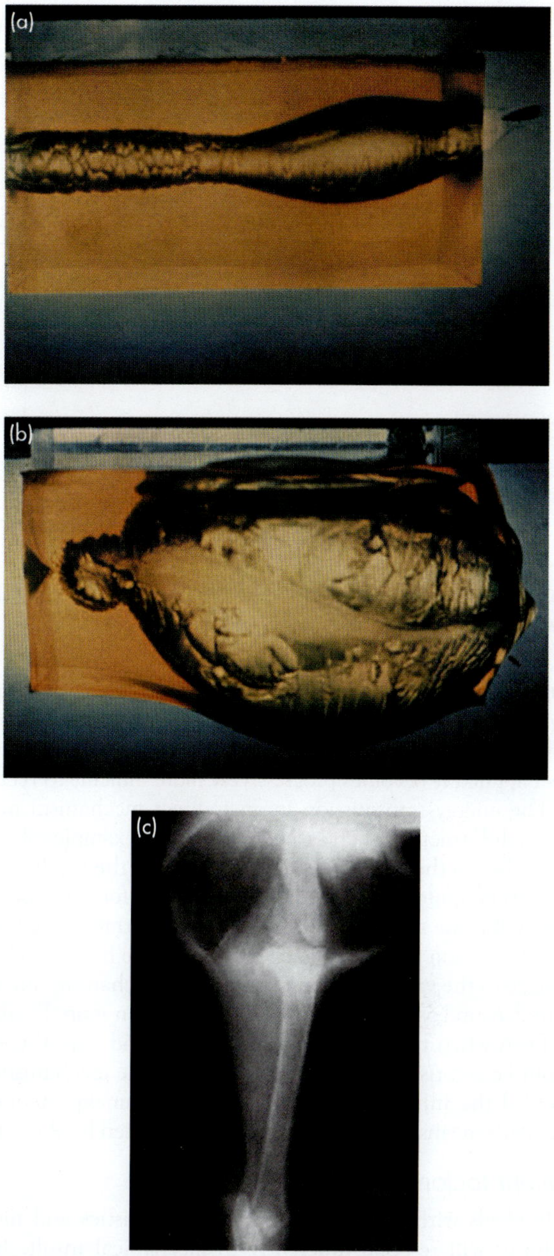

Figure 23.6 A projectile passing through a gelatin block. (a) Low energy transfer; (b) High energy transfer. (c) The effect of high energy transfer on tissues. Photographs courtesy of Professor J Ryan.

A blunt mechanism of injury can be considered as direct or indirect. A direct mechanism is when the damage occurs at or close to the site of impact. An indirect mechanism is when the damage occurs at a distant site after transmission of that force. The following examples, in which two different mechanisms leading to fracture of the ulna are considered, may help to understand this. Should an attacker strike with a strong stick, the victim may protect their head by raising their arm. The blow will then fall on the ulna. This may cause an isolated fracture of that bone generally called a 'nightstick fracture' (a nightstick being a weapon of enforcement carried by the police). This is clearly a direct injury. All of the injury is concentrated at the site of application of the force; the soft tissues may be bruised, contused or lacerated at the site. A different situation occurs if a person falls on an outstretched hand. This may lead to a fracture of the ulna, but here the mechanism is indirect. The force has been transmitted through the body's tissues to a site at some distance from its application. It is unlikely that an ulnar fracture would occur in isolation in such circumstances and the 'associated injuries' should be sought. In this instance, the associated injury is often a dislocation of the radial head, the whole injury complex being called a Monteggia fracture dislocation. These injuries are demonstrated diagrammatically in Figure 23.7. The injury is often missed and the consequences are severe in the growing child. Thus, we should always evaluate the elbow fully (radiologically and clinically) in an apparently 'isolated' ulnar fracture, especially if the mechanism was indirect, usually a fall

Giovanni Batista Monteggia, 1762–1815, Professor of Anatomy and Surgery, Ospedale Maggoire, Milan, Italy.

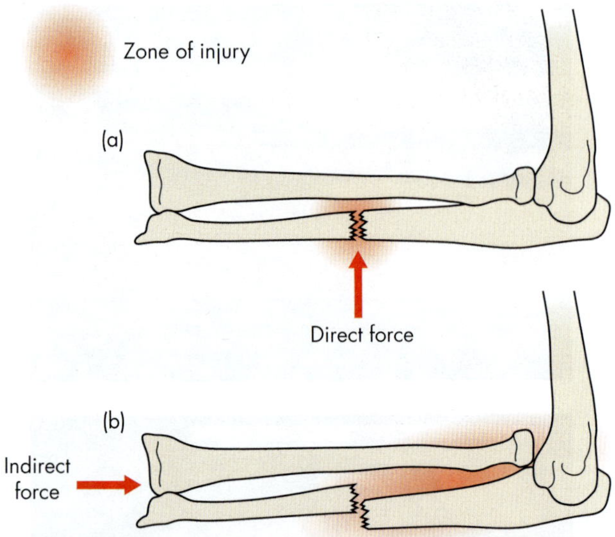

Figure 23.7 Two examples of a fracture of the ulna. (a) A nightstick fracture from a direct blow. (b) A Monteggia fracture from an indirect force.

onto the hand. The timeline in these circumstances is not pressing. The injury can be adequately treated for some weeks after it occurs, but once the diagnosis has been missed and the wrong label applied it becomes progressively more difficult to rectify.

The energy transmission in an indirect mechanism may be via a solid structure, such as a bone, as in the examples above, or it may be via the soft tissues or fluid. Some of the resulting injuries can be quite unexpected. A compressive force to the abdomen will cause a rise in pressure that may be transmitted by the vascular system. A sudden back pressure at the heart can lead to damage to the valves. The results of direct mechanisms are easier to understand as the damaging effects are often more localised.

Even when the patient was alert before and after the event, it can be surprisingly difficult to be sure of the mechanism as it affected the injured part. The rapidity and unexpectedness of accidents means that precision in history is often hard to obtain.

Patient factors

Individuals with different physical characteristics and medical histories will respond differently to mechanical insult. In the standard history taken, a quick categorisation of a patient is normally carried out.

As we take a history, we intuitively group patients to assess the nature of their likely injuries. Children, adults and the elderly are three obvious separate groups. We anticipate different injuries in these different groups even if the mechanism is the same. A torus fracture, a Colles fracture, or fractured hip may each result from a simple fall.

Similarly knowing a patient is on anticoagulants, has osteogenesis imperfecta, has a previous total knee replacement or has known metastatic disease guides assessment.

Obvious injuries

Some injuries are so obvious that they may present before any mechanism or patient details are known. It may therefore be the presence of one overt injury that leads to the search for another; the obvious injury is being used just as a history would in other circumstances. The most obvious injuries will be those that are visible externally. It is for this reason that there is an E at the end of ABCDE in the ATLS system: E is for exposure – look for the clues.

If a wound suggests a penetrating injury then thought should be given to the underlying structures at risk. A contusion over the knee of a driver suggests a dashboard injury. Finger-shaped bruises on a child's arms suggest non-accidental injury (NAI).

A good example of a minor but obvious injury helping in a timeline is singed facial hair. This sign is often associated with carbonaceous sputum and suggests inhalational burns. Calling an anaesthetic colleague when singed nasal hair is first noted is far better than a crash call 15 minutes later when laryngeal oedema obstructs the airway of a patient with an inhalational burn.

Exposing the patient comes readily to those dealing with trauma. The perils of not exposing the patient were demonstrated in an infamous case in the UK. A patient already in hospital for another problem had 'collapsed' by the phone within the hospital and was dealt with by the cardiac arrest team. The patient responded poorly to treatment and it was only some time later that the bullet was noticed on the chest x-ray. Following this, the bullet wound in the victim's back was found. A helpful adage borrowed from radiology is that 'unless you are very lucky you only find what you look for'.

Hidden factors

Mechanisms

Sometimes, when the normal relationship of 'mechanism + patient = injury' does not seem to hold, the hidden information may be in the mechanism. The most obvious examples are in situations in which there has been a deliberate attempt to mislead.

Conscious sensible patients reporting their own injuries will generally tell the truth; however, sometimes to protect themselves or others they may fabricate a mechanism. The risk here is that if the mechanism is incorrect, the wrong pattern of injuries may be anticipated. Thus, the man who fell from 6 metres when in some illegal activity does not help achieve an accurate diagnosis if he reports the mechanism as a twist to his ankle from a stumble. Similarly, if it is not admitted that an injury results from an assault, then no action can reasonably be taken to help protect that person from further aggression. This situation is most commonly encountered when the patient is the victim of abuse within a relationship. The patient should be given the opportunity to tell their story, but it should not always be believed.

More commonly, the problem of a hidden mechanism arises when the patient is unable to give their own history. A very young child or an elderly person is both physically and mentally vulnerable. They may have been physically abused, but be unable to report it. In these circumstances, the mechanism of injury may have been criminal. A list of some of the factors that should make one suspicious of the history and suspect that NAI has occurred is given below:

- history clearly inconsistent with the injuries sustained;
- changing history;
- aggressive behaviour of carers at interview;
- injuries of different ages;
- posterior rib injuries;
- long bone fractures in a pre-ambulatory child.

The interests of the patient are paramount and so we need to

Abraham Colles, 1773–1843, Professor of Surgery, The Royal College of Surgeons in Ireland, and surgeon, Dr Steven's Hospital, Dublin, Ireland. At the age of 28 years, he was elected as President of the College and described his fracture in 1814. In view of his major contributions, he was awarded a baronetcy in 1839, which he declined.

not only identify injuries that need treatment, but also protect patients from further harm. The timeline of importance here is that which has shown that 66 per cent of children who die as the result of abuse have been in contact with a health or social work professional before the fatal episode. We have already accepted that to adequately treat an extradural haematoma, we must respond to subtle indicators in the history and physical examination to allow our response to begin early enough to be effective. An analogous situation applies with child abuse – if we ignore the early signs, we may be too late to prevent the later episode in which real harm is done. NAI is a very difficult problem to deal with. As clinicians we are more comfortable trying to help everyone; acting to police a situation does not come naturally.

In some criminal situations, the nature of any overt injuries may provide important evidence of the mechanism. Such evidence may be affected by our medical assessment and treatment. Although we should not compromise the medical management of an injured person, it is folly not to bear in mind at every stage that the victim of an assault may need good forensic evidence at some later date to convict their assailant. Indeed, the injured victim of an assault may later become a murder victim (Summary box 23.6).

Summary box 23.6

Covert mechanisms

- Patients usually tell the truth, but may not if criminal activity is involved
- Fear of abuse may prevent vulnerable patients telling the truth
- If a non-accidental injury (NAI) is suspected, you have a responsibility to take action
- Patients likely to have covert medical problems need careful checking even if their injury appears to have a simple mechanical cause

Patients

When the mechanism and the injury are obvious but inconsistent, it may be that there is something previously unknown about the patient to discover. Most commonly, this is a pre-existing pathology. Thus, a healthy adult who breaks their femur following a trivial insult may well have had a pathological weakness of the bone, such as a neoplasm. Thoughtless treatment of this as a simple fracture, without tissue diagnosis, staging, etc., may result in entirely inappropriate treatment with unnecessary loss of limb or life.

Injury in the older patient may be the manifestation of general health problems. The obvious injury may be the fractured proximal femur, the hidden patient factor may be the transient ischaemic attack or abnormal cardiac rhythm that caused the fall. Rather like the practice of the secondary survey looking for covert injury in the polytraumatised patient, a medical secondary survey is required as a screen in the elderly.

Injuries

Looking for the hidden injury when deduction has failed can follow two methods:

1 the look everywhere approach;
2 the focused exclusion approach.

1 **The look everywhere approach.** One of the mainstays of trauma evaluation has been the secondary survey. The essence is that once the initial life-saving manoeuvres have been completed you look everywhere for further injury. This detailed examination may take place shortly after admission, the following morning on the ward round or sometimes a week later when the patient first regains consciousness. As its name suggests, the look everywhere secondary survey comes later in the sequence of the ATLS approach. However, the emphasis placed on the timeline at the beginning of this chapter and the need for early diagnosis is leading to a different approach to the traditional 'look everywhere' one. The ATLS system has included a plain pelvic and a chest x-ray as part of the primary survey. This may confirm a clinical diagnosis, but is also a screening tool to identify injuries that may progress to a clinical problem; the response to that injury can then be initiated earlier. The threshold for using more generalised investigations such as CT scanning, ultrasound, cardiac echo and magnetic resonance imaging (MRI) to check for these covert injuries is progressively being lowered. Some emergency departments now have CT scanners in their resuscitation rooms. A head-to-pelvis CT scan is being used to replace the early plain radiographs of the chest and the pelvis. A CT scan is more sensitive and specific and its use to identify injury before the clinical signs become obvious is certain to improve patient care.
2 **The focused exclusion approach.** Some important injuries or conditions are for some reason missed on a surprisingly regular basis. This suggests that a normal deductive approach is not always adequate. Classic examples are scaphoid fractures, perilunate dislocations, posterior dislocations of the shoulder and tarso-metatarsal dislocations.

Therefore, if such injuries are suspected or possibly present they should be positively excluded by focused history, examination and investigation (Summary box 23.7).

Summary box 23.7

Trauma assessment

- Know the timelines for important diagnoses
- Prioritise the assessment accordingly
- Positively exclude critical diagnoses
- If required, screen at-risk patients before clinical signs are apparent

The response to trauma

Once an assessment has been made based on the factors of mechanism, patient and injury discussed above, the response must be planned and executed. At the same time, the patient will have an evolving response to injury. On the positive side, physiological compensatory and reserve mechanisms will be recruited and healing processes will be initiated. Countering this, there may be progressive pathophysiological responses, the consumption of limited resources and decompensation.

The patient's response to injury

The patient's own homeostatic mechanisms will respond to the injury and there will be physiological and pathophysiological changes. In the light of this evolution of responses, we may alter the nature or the timing of our interventions.

A simple example is body temperature. A drop in body temperature is common after injury; this may be due to exposure, inactivity, damp, blood loss or loss of vasomotor control. The body's own thermoregulatory mechanisms may not be able to resolve the problem and so we must be prepared to support that role – body temperature should be monitored and heat loss prevented as required. It may not be possible to do this adequately in an operating theatre during a surgical procedure.

Similarly, oxygenation can be monitored and support may be given by way of increased inspired oxygen or different modes of ventilation.

The response to blood loss is not only an evolving situation for an individual patient, but our response to it also changes. The patient calls on compensatory mechanisms when blood is lost. As long as organ perfusion is adequate, low blood pressure is not a problem in its own right. The body has a finite resource of clotting factors and the injured lung does not tolerate excess fluid. The combination of these factors has led to a tendency to draw back from large-scale early fluid replacement with a crystalloid. Instead, the emphasis is placed on identifying and stopping the source of bleeding. The patient also mounts a generalised immunological response to trauma. This has an impact on their ability to tolerate surgical interventions. There is growing evidence that procedures should be timed and staged to better fit the conditions created by the patient's systemic immune response.

The medical response to injury

Initial management

The structure of ATLS is discussed in Chapter 22. Reducing the elapsed time from injury to useful intervention is critical for some patients. Preparation can aid this process. When a department is made aware of the impending arrival of a seriously injured patient, a decision needs to be made as to whether to call the 'trauma team'; this will allow a trained team of nurses and doctors to be waiting to meet the patient. While waiting, equipment is made ready, a leader is identified and each team member is given a role. Protective clothing will be needed: gloves to protect from fluids and lead aprons to protect from x-rays.

For the medical and nursing staff, the beginning of the patient's pathway can become familiar just like any routine journey and, thus, planning becomes less complex. However, if wasteful delays are to be avoided, alternatives need to be available if for some reason the routine cannot be followed. Anticipating and dealing with potential rate-limiting steps in the patient's journey will allow delays to be avoided and further reduce the response time. The component of the response that will be the rate-limiting step will depend on local, as well as general circumstances. Examples of causes of delay are obtaining a CT scan, getting the patient into an operating theatre or obtaining a necessary specialist opinion. Such steps that can potentially bring the progress of the patient to a halt need to be addressed early and sometimes in a way that may seem out of the normal sequence. This is one of the major roles of the team leader who should have an overview and be able to foresee and pre-empt problems. Whenever a system is protocol driven, someone should be in a position to take the responsibility to break protocol if required to keep the overall process flowing.

Having a practised common pathway can be disadvantageous; a patient with the wrong 'label' may go along the wrong pathway. We all have to be wary of labelling. Should two patients with identical histories and injuries arrive in an emergency department with one on a spine board and the other in a chair, the former will be treated as if more severely injured when in fact that may not be the case. We must make our own judgements on reasonable evidence and not just rely on the labels (in this case, the cervical collars) applied by others.

Labelling is most frequently a dangerous problem in the elderly. A patient with an obviously short externally rotated leg may be quickly given the label 'NOF' (fracture neck of femur). There are a number of problems with this practice. The focus is now on the orthopaedic label rather than the whole patient. The incorrect label may mask the fact that the patient could be dying. The patient may have fallen as a consequence of a cardiac arrhythmia or other comorbidity; the early labelling may therefore send the patient off on entirely the wrong pathway. All vulnerable patients should have a physiological triage to avoid such problems. This means assessing the airway, respiratory rate, blood pressure, pulse rate and consciousness. All of these assessments are more important, even in the elderly, than the presence of a fractured hip.

Beyond the first hour

The primary survey of ATLS encourages the identification and treatment of life-threatening problems. Once these have been addressed, there may be other problems that require intervention. The timing and order of these interventions is a matter of judgement. There has been an evolution in the approach to the management of polytrauma. It has been variously said that a patient may be 'too sick to operate on' or that they may be 'too sick *not* to operate on'. The work of Bone in particular has promoted the concept of early definitive stabilisation of long bone fractures to allow better control of the pathophysiology of trauma. Others have highlighted the need in some circumstances for limited early intervention, sometimes called 'damage control surgery'. This is followed by definitive treatment when the patient is better able to tolerate it. In orthopaedic trauma, the debate has focused on whether long bone fractures should be fixed temporarily or definitively. In general surgery, the question is whether the abdomen should be definitively treated or packed. Any patient needing a sequence of interventions, e.g. laparotomy, femoral nailing, tibial nailing, should have the most important done first. Thus, if there needs to be a break in the procedures for any reason, the most important interventions will have been completed. As each component of a sequence of procedures nears its end, a decision needs to be made whether it is safe or appropriate to proceed to the next stage. Monitoring of core temperature, coagulation, base excess, etc., will allow this decision to be made on rational grounds. When necessary the patient can then be transferred to the more controlled environment of an intensive care unit and return for definitive surgery when physiologically and immunologically better able to tolerate it; this may be hours or days later.

A useful adjunct is to record the treatment plan on a whiteboard in the operating theatre. This informs others of the intended pathway of treatment so that preparations can be made. An example of such a tactic is shown in Figure 23.8. Note the alternative pathway that exists should the patient's general condition require a shorter procedure, when the femur

Nicholas Andry, 1658–1742, was born in Lyon, France. He was a priest originally and taught theology before becoming a doctor. His expertise was in parasitology and orthopaedics. His illustration of a bent tree being supported by a stake to encourage it to grow straight symbolises the art and practice of orthopaedics worldwide.

can be temporarily stabilised with an external fixator rather than definitively fixed with a nail.

LOCAL PROTOCOLS AND GUIDELINES

A general guideline, such as ATLS, deals with some aspects of patient management and is used in many institutions. However, hospitals generally have individual policies to guide or direct decision making in smaller areas of practice. Examples are prophylaxis against infection and thromboembolism, the use of steroids in spinal injury and clearance of the cervical spine. These represent the efforts of individuals within an institution to plan for common and foreseeable circumstances. These protocols allow for easier and quicker decision making. Their application should protect the patient and, in an increasingly litigious world, the doctor as well.

'Clearing' of the spine is a practice that has particular relevance to trauma. The early policy for managing the spine in polytrauma patients is straightforward; it can be summarised as 'suspect and protect'. This approach is widely employed, and so very many patients have their spine protected. However, this is a precautionary approach and at some stage one has to have a strategy for discontinuing protection, or 'clearing' the spine in those patients in whom protection is not required. In the event that it is not possible to exclude spinal injury on clinical grounds, the managing clinicians may request clearance on radiological grounds. An example of such a policy for clearing the spine is given in Table 23.2.

Record-keeping for the injured patient is both important and difficult. It is often said that trends in a patient's condition are more important than isolated observations. Because an injured patient may be cared for by a large number of individuals, trends can only become apparent by reference to the sequential recorded notes. If each individual clinician records their observations in an 'individual' manner, it becomes very difficult to identify trends. Adoption of the Glasgow Coma Scale to monitor the level of consciousness demonstrates the advantage of using a consistent system of recording observations. Such sequential observations, especially when displayed on a single chart, demonstrate trends. The clinical evolution of a problem, such as raised intracranial pressure secondary to an extradural haematoma is then easier to identify (Summary box 23.8).

Summary box 23.8

The response to trauma

- Guidelines and protocols speed and streamline management
- Pre-empt time-limiting steps to avoid delay
- Respond to the evolving condition of the patient
- Use charts to plot trends

Table 23.2 An example of a policy for clearing the spine in the obtunded patient.

Cervical spine	Fine-quality computed tomography (CT) scans of C0–T4, reformatted and assessed in the axial, sagittal and coronal planes Powers ratio to assess the atlanto-occipital junction
Thoracolumbar spine (T4 distally)	Either good-quality anteroposterior and lateral plain films or CT scans reformatted and assessed in the anteroposterior, lateral and axial planes

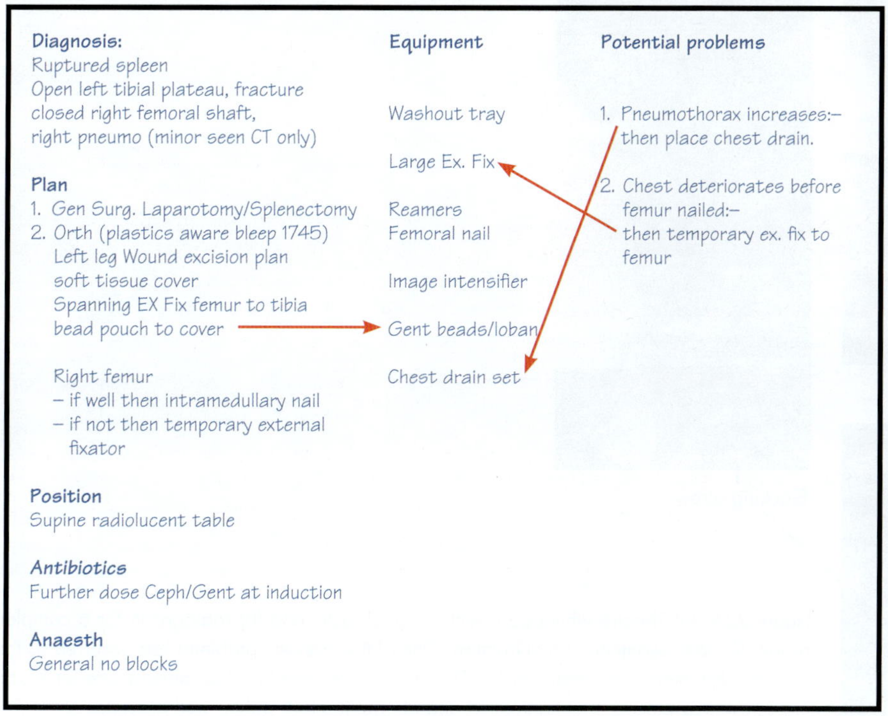

Figure 23.8 An example of a surgical tactic on a whiteboard in the operating theatre.

Planning an individual operation

The central part of a surgeon's work is operating. Dealing with injuries is not repetitive and so thought and planning are required. Even when an individual surgeon is involved in performing the surgery, care is delivered as part of a team. It is good practice to think through the plan for the operating theatre. Mental rehearsal of a procedure may allow potential hazards to be predicted and avoided. For example,

- As the procedure is planned, it may become apparent that the proposed surgical approach will not allow the access required. In a whiteboard exercise, this can readily be altered. This cannot be done so easily if the first time this problem is appreciated is after the skin has been cut.
- It may be decided in planning that another surgeon is better suited to perform a particular procedure.

The use of the whiteboard in theatre, discussed earlier in the context of multiple injuries, is equally applicable for the isolated injury. An example of a surgical tactic for a segmental tibial fracture is given in Figure 23.9. This not only helps the surgeon, but also informs others. The position of the patient, the surgical approach, position of the image intensifier, method of fracture reduction and instruments required, and method of fixation and implants required are all noted. Theatre staff, anaesthetic staff and radiographers can all see what is intended and it can also act as a teaching aid. A trainee may be asked to complete the whiteboard plan; they then have to commit to a plan of action and not just drift along. An important addition to the planned progress of the procedure is a list of potential problems or hazards. The strategies that will be used to deal with these problems should they arise can then be considered and prepared for (Summary box 23.9).

Summary box 23.9

Planning an individual operation

- Plan procedures before performing them
- Commit a plan to paper
- Share the surgical plan by use of a whiteboard

(a)

Diagnosis	Equipment	Problems/solutions
Open segmental fracture left tibia Procedure – Excise wound with plastics – Plan soft tissue cover – Secure nail entry point – Ream segment through traumatic wound – Statically lock nail – Dress wound with a bead pouch – Continue antibiotics until definitive soft-tissue cover	– Radiolucent table – Tourniquet (during wound excision) – Soft tissue tray – Washout tray 9 litres washout – Reamers – Cannulated tibial IM nail In reserve external fixator/long plates	– Segment viable but too narrow to nail/proceed to bridge plate or ex. fix depending on soft tissue – Segment non-viable/remove segment place temp ex. fix with view to subsequent Illizarov transport – On passing nail malalignment of proximal fragment/remove nail and place blocking screw

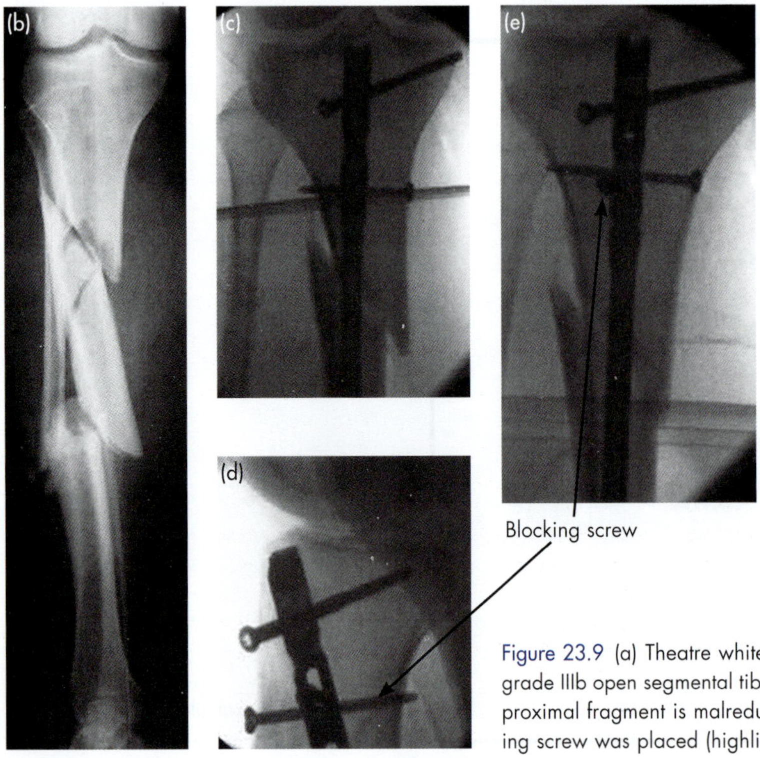

Figure 23.9 (a) Theatre whiteboard with surgical tactic and (b) radiograph for a complex grade IIIb open segmental tibial fracture. One of the foreseen problems has occurred as the proximal fragment is malreduced (c). The nail was removed and an anteroposterior blocking screw was placed (highlighted) (d and e). The fracture is then well reduced.

The response to the mechanism of injury (injury prevention)

When assessing the 'mechanism + patient = injury' relationship, it is easy for the doctor to focus on managing the injury; however, the mechanism of injury can also be addressed, that is we should aim to prevent rather than just treat injury.

When a mechanism of injury becomes particularly prevalent or has serious consequences, it is prudent to take steps to either remove the mechanism or reduce the consequences.

Accidents occur in a variety of places: the home, the workplace and the roads are the most common. The strategy and motivation for prevention varies from place to place. Within the workplace there is legislation to protect employees and a tendency for an injured employee to sue the employer. Thus, although some work environments are naturally dangerous, many advances in safety have been made. Within the home, legislation has little effect on behaviour. The safety of the structure of a home may be influenced by building regulations, but the thrust is on education of the individual. It is difficult to educate adults to behave more safely and so accidents in the home remain very common. Road safety is a contentious issue. The safe management of the kinetic energy of travel would seem to be a straightforward physical problem. Great advances have been made in the technology of motor vehicles to protect drivers. Restricting speed, separating vehicles travelling in different directions and segregating motor vehicles from vulnerable road users, such as pedestrians, are not popular measures (Summary box 23.10).

Summary box 23.10

Response to the mechanism of injury

- The saying that 'prevention is better than cure' is true
- Legislation and education are required
- Prevent further abuse by responding to the initial clues

The response to patient factors

Another approach to injury prevention is to alter the patient. This particularly applies to the epidemic of injuries in the elderly. Falls are the most common mechanism of injury, so one can try to address the cause or the effects of falls. Fall prevention clinics are now common. The at-risk patients are assessed and remediable causes of falls are addressed. Postural hypotension, transient ischaemic attacks and arrhythmias can be identified and treated.

Elderly people will continue to fall, so we can try to minimise the effect of the fall. Schemes, such as using hip protector pads to cushion a fall, have been tried with limited success. The area most likely to expand and give results is that of strengthening the skeleton. Identifying those at risk of osteoporosis, screening them and then treating appropriately offers a hope of reducing the incidence of low energy fractures. There was initial scepticism about the expense of such treatments and the potentially huge number of people who would require them. It is now accepted that treatment targeted appropriately will be cost-effective by reducing later fractures with the consequent costs of hospitalisation, morbidity and mortality.

Another of the patient factors discussed earlier is when injury occurs in pathological tissues, the common example being a fracture of a bone with a neoplastic deposit. This should influence management in one of two ways. When there is a doubt as to whether the tumour is a primary or secondary, it is important to think before treatment. Injudicious operative management of a fracture associated with a primary deposit may prejudice proper tumour management; when the situation allows, a proper opinion should be obtained. When dealing with obvious secondary deposits, the situation is quite different. Aggressive surgical management is often justified to allow an early return to function. A patient with a limited life expectancy should not spend long periods of time rehabilitating (Summary box 23.11).

Summary box 23.11

Response to patient factors

- Pre-empt injury with the use of fall prevention clinics
- Carry out targeted osteoporosis treatment
- Do not treat thoughtlessly an injury that is possibly secondary to a primary neoplasm

CONCLUSION

Trauma is usually the adverse consequence of a mechanical force on a patient. The prime importance of time in trauma care needs to be appreciated. At time zero, there is a relationship between the mechanism, the patient and the injury. The components of this relationship should fit together in a rational manner. When this rational fit is not apparent, great care should be taken to look for hidden injuries, pre-existing pathology or some deliberate deception in the given history.

There is a timeline that progresses from the moment of injury. Prompt understanding of the problems is key in allowing an early reaction. It may not be possible to wait for overt clinical signs and so diagnoses should be positively sought and in some circumstances patients screened. There is a minimum response time to initiate and complete the interventions to deal with the problems. Preparation can reduce this response time. Knowledge of realistic response times is important, because only then does the clinician know the real urgency of initiating action.

When presented with an injured patient, the early management is largely protocol driven. As more details become known and the patient moves towards definitive care, a more individual plan is made. This plan coordinates the different specialties and should be flexible to allow for evolving pathology. Someone should be responsible for the patient.

Trauma does not just consist of care of the young injured. Increasingly, the injured patient will be elderly. The team involved needs to reflect the needs of these elderly patients.

Trauma need not only be addressed by tackling the injury itself. Preventative measures should be employed when particular mechanisms can be identified as being common or important causes of injury. For example, prophylactic measures may reduce the propensity for individuals to fall or reduce the consequences of those falls when they occur.

The following chapters in this section will look further at these principles as applied to specific regions or surgical disciplines (Summary box 23.12).

Summary box 23.12

Conclusion

- The management of trauma is dependent upon time
- Multiple specialties may be involved, but do not lose sight of the overall problem
- Planning increases the chances of success

CHAPTER 24

Early assessment and management of trauma

LEARNING OBJECTIVES

To identify:
- The sequence of priorities in the early assessment of the injured patient

To learn:
- The principle of triage in immediate management of the injured patient
- The concepts of injury recognition prediction based on the mechanism and energy of injury

To apply:
- The principles of primary and secondary surveys in the assessment and management of trauma
- Techniques for the initial resuscitative and definitive care aspects of trauma

To be able to perform:
- The necessary protocols to allow early stabilization of the patient leading on to definitive care

To recognize:
- Patients whose management should differ from the normal

EPIDEMIOLOGY

Trauma is the most common cause of death between the ages of one and 44 years worldwide. By 2020, it is estimated that more than 10 per cent of people will die from trauma. In addition to mortality, injuries have the potential to cause many other long-term health problems, with serious consequences for individuals, families, communities and health-care systems. Subsequently, this represents a significant drain on resources. The economic impact of trauma and injury is huge globally, with some figures quoted in the region of $500 billion annually.

INTRODUCTION

Much effort has gone into trying to improve trauma care, with the most recent in the UK being the introduction of specialist regional 'level one' trauma centres, where all the required facilities and subspecialties are available on site to deal with multiply-injured patients.

It is the initial assessment that is probably the most important factor in the subsequent outcome of the trauma patient, as it is at this stage that a subsequent care pathway and protocol is formed for definitive treatment.

The Advanced Trauma Life Support (ATLS) principles were introduced into practice in the late 1970s, and have since revolutionised the management of trauma (Summary box 24.1).

Once the attending clinician is versed in the structure and protocol of the ATLS philosophy, it becomes very easy to apply this to any trauma event, regardless of the nature and severity of the injuries.

Summary box 24.1

The steps in the Advanced Trauma Life Support (ATLS) philosophy

- Primary survey with simultaneous resuscitation: identify and treat what is killing the patient
- Secondary survey: proceed to identify all other injuries
- Definitive care: develop a definitive management plan

MECHANISMS OF TRAUMA

Trauma can be classified in type by causation and by effect (see Table 24.1).

Table 24.1 Types of injury.

Blunt, e.g. car bonnet
Penetrating, e.g. knife
Blast, e.g. bomb
Crush, e.g. building collapse
Thermal

Blunt trauma

The most common cause of blunt trauma is the motor vehicle accident (MVA). Speed is a critical factor: a 10 per cent increase in impact speed translates to a 40 per cent rise in the case fatality. Ejection from a vehicle is associated with a significantly greater incidence of severe injury. The use of seatbelts reduces the risk of death or serious injury for front-seat occupants by approximately 45 per cent (Figure 24.1). Although seatbelts reduce mortality overall, they can cause a specific pattern of internal injuries. Patients with seatbelt marks have been found to have a four-fold increase in thoracic trauma and an eight-fold increase in intra-abdominal trauma compared with those without seatbelt marks (Figure 24.2 and Summary box 24.2).

Summary box 24.2

Energy and injury prevention

- A 10 per cent increase in speed of impact increases pedestrian fatality risk by 40 per cent
- Seatbelts reduce the risk of injury in a vehicle by 45 per cent

In direct frontal MVAs, airbags provide a reduced risk of fatality of approximately 30 per cent. However, airbags themselves may also cause specific patterns of injury. In order to reduce the risk of airbag-induced injury, children younger than 12 years should be properly restrained in the back seat. Infants (aged <1 year) in rear-facing child safety seats should never ride in the front seat of a vehicle fitted with an activated passenger-side airbag.

Motorcyclists experience a significantly higher mortality rate than the occupants of cars, and fractures of the lower extremities are also more common in this group.

Penetrating trauma

Although the incidence of penetrating injuries is increasing, such injuries are less common in the UK compared with other countries. Important factors include the proximity of the underlying viscera to the path of the penetrating object, and the velocity of the missile. The distance from the weapon to the wound may give important information regarding the energy of the injury and therefore predict internal damage.

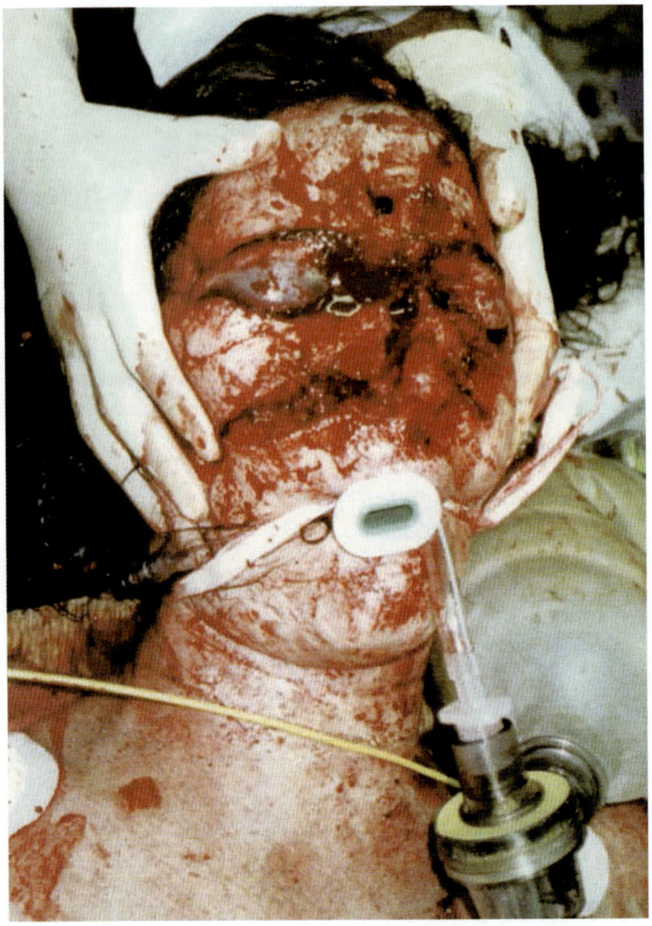

Figure 24.1 Unrestrained driver with severe craniofacial injury (courtesy of Johannesburg Hospital Trauma Unit).

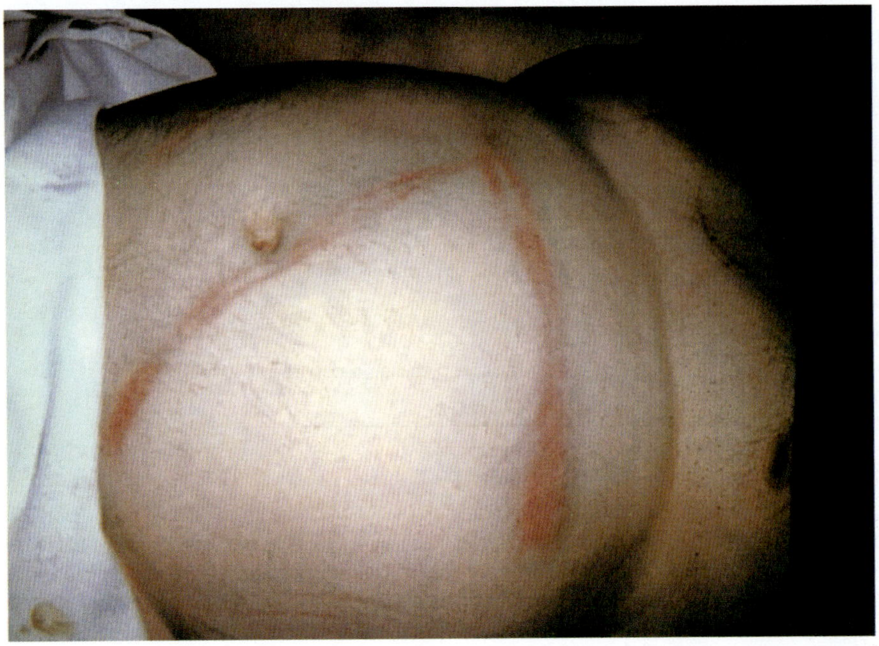

Figure 24.2 Seatbelt mark after motor vehicle accident (courtesy of Johannesburg Hospital Trauma Unit).

Blast injury

Terrorism is now a global phenomenon. It is conceivable that civilian as well as military surgeons will be exposed to patients injured in explosions.

Crush injury

See Chapter 32 on disaster surgery.

Thermal injury

See Chapter 30 on burns.

Alcohol and drugs

Alcohol and other forms of substance abuse are major associated factors in all forms of trauma. Drivers with illegal blood alcohol levels account for nearly one-third of non-fatal injuries, and half of driver deaths. Injury to drunken pedestrians shows an even greater correlation with alcohol.

ASSESSMENT AND MANAGEMENT OF THE SERIOUSLY INJURED

Following major trauma, there is a well described 'trimodal distribution of death'.

The three 'peaks' as follows:

1 **Immediate**, 50 per cent of all deaths. These are probably not possible to save. They are usually the result of massive head injury or severe cardio-pulmonary insult.
2 **Early**, within the first few hours. These will result from a failure of oxygenation of tissue either because oxygen is not getting into the body (airway or breathing problem), or because the circulation has failed and so oxygen cannot be delivered to the tissues.
3 **Late**, 20 per cent of deaths. Usually from multiple organ failure and sepsis, influenced by inadequate early resuscitation and care.

The ATLS principles are aimed primarily at the 'early' group of patients. They try to optimise the speed and accuracy of the initial assessment and management, and so reduce subsequent morbidity and mortality.

The multidisciplinary team approach

A team approach is important for achieving the best possible outcome for traumatised patients. The 'trauma team' should be assembled and organised prior to patient arrival, with a nominated leader, and each team member should be assigned a specific role. Clear and concise communication among the team members is essential. Support staff such as radiographers, laboratory technicians and porters should also be immediately available.

PRIMARY SURVEY AND RESUSCITATION

The initial management of the traumatised patient must first consist of a rapid primary evaluation and resuscitation of vital functions as soon as abnormalities are detected. Only when the patient has been stabilised and the team are content with the primary survey is a more detailed secondary assessment carried out. The primary survey comprises the fundamental principles of the ATLS system, the 'ABCDE' of trauma care (Summary box 24.3).

Summary box 24.3

ABCDE of trauma care

- **A**, Airway with cervical spine protection
- **B**, Breathing and ventilation
- **C**, Circulation with haemorrhage control
- **D**, Disability: neurological status
- **E**, Exposure: completely undress the patient and assess for other injuries

Airway with cervical spine protection

In every trauma situation, the patient's airway is of paramount importance, and hence this is assessed first. If there is a vocal response from the patient, then the airway cannot be immediately compromised. Ensuring a patent airway may require simple measures, such as clearing the mouth and suction, or manoeuvres such as a jaw thrust or chin lift. If the airway is compromised again as soon as the chin lift or jaw thrust are relaxed, then a nasopharyngeal or Guedel airway should be used, provided that the patient will tolerate it.

In the case of severe head trauma, where the patient is unconscious (a Glasgow Coma Score (GCS) of 8 or less), then a definitive airway (such as endotracheal intubation) may be required.

It is important to suspect that every patient who has had significant trauma (especially to the head) has a cervical spine injury until proven otherwise. Therefore, throughout the initial assessment, the cervical spine must be immobilized providing that this is not impairing their safety or their airway. This is either performed manually, with in-line immobilization techniques, or with the traditional collar, sandbags and tape. Any efforts to maintain airway patency must also bear in mind the safety of the potentially unstable cervical spine (Summary box 24.4).

Summary box 24.4

Airway assessment

- Ensure cervical spine immobilization and check for vocal response
- Clear mouth and airway if obvious foreign bodies
- Jaw trust and chin lift, if required
- Consider airway adjuncts
- If Glasgow Coma Score ≤ 8, consider a definitive airway

Breathing and ventilation

Oxygen should be administered to all trauma patients, using a high concentration mask with a reservoir. Ventilation requires an adequately functioning chest wall, lungs and diaphragm, and each must be systematically evaluated. A check should be made for signs of surgical emphysema, dilatation of the neck veins, asymmetry of the chest wall, excessive respiratory effort and abnormal rate. Your findings should be recorded, as it is a change

The Glasgow Coma Score was introduced in 1977 by William Bryan Jennet, Professor of Neurosurgery and Graham Michael Teasdale, a neurosurgeon at the University Department of Neurosurgery at the Institute of Neurological Sciences, The Southern General Hospital, Glasgow, UK. Professor Teasdale was later knighted and became President of the Royal College of Physicians and Surgeons of Glasgow.

Arthur Ernest Guedel, 1883–1956, Clinical Professor of Anaesthesiology, University of Southern California, Los Angeles, CA, USA.

in these parameters which may be more useful in determining emergency treatment than any absolute finding. Percussion and auscultation should be performed on both the front and back of the chest wall after log rolling.

Tension pneumothorax, a flail chest with contusion, a massive haemothorax and an open pneumothorax are examples of life-threatening injuries that must be identified and treated in the primary survey. Critical findings include the tracheal deviation, absence of or asymmetry of breath sounds, hyper-resonance (consistent with tension pneumothorax) or dullness to percussion (haemothorax). However, these signs are often not as easy to pick up in the emergency room as they are to learn in a textbook. Therefore, the diagnosis must be assumed in any patient whose oxygenation is deteriorating despite a patent airway and a good ventilator effort. A tension pneumothorax should be immediately decompressed with the insertion of a needle into the second intercostal space, midclavicular line. This can then be followed by definitive chest drain insertion at an appropriate time. Open chest wounds should be occluded with a three-sided dressing, then an intercostal drain is inserted through a separate incision. If there is evidence of massive haemothorax (>1.5 L of blood), this may lead to severe respiratory compromise, cardiac tamponade and compression of the affected lung. Inserting a chest drain to drain the blood without any accompanying effort to control the haemorrhage may lead to a rapid and terminal deterioration in the patient's condition (Summary box 24.5).

Summary box 24.5

Breathing

- Give 100 per cent oxygen at high flow
- Inspect/percuss and auscultate chest
- Check for tension pneumothorax and immediately decompress if suspected
- Insert chest drain for haemothorax/pneumothorax
- Major vessel bleeding within the chest needs to be controlled

Circulation and control of bleeding

Assessment here centres on three critical clinical observations:

1. **Conscious level.** If this is impaired or altered, in the absence of obvious head injury, one must assume that the patient has lost a significant amount of blood and that cerebral perfusion has become compromised.
2. **Skin colour.** A patient with pink skin and warm peripheries is rarely critically hypovolaemic, and the converse is true for a pale, ashen, grey-looking patient with ominous signs of hypovolaemia.
3. **Pulse.** A full, slow, regular peripheral pulse is usually the sign of relative normovolaemia, whereas a rapid, thready pulse or, worse still, one that is not peripherally palpable is a grave sign of hypovolaemic shock, and blood volume must be rapidly restored.

While the primary survey is being carried out, other team members should be securing two large-bore cannulae for intravenous access. Fluid resuscitation should be titrated against the patient's response to the initial fluid challenge and their vital signs. Potential sites for major blood loss include the chest cavity, the abdomen, the pelvis and long bone fractures. Each of these must be examined in turn. Surgical intervention may ultimately be required to control haemorrhage (Summary box 24.6).

Summary box 24.6

Circulation

- Check pulse and blood pressure
- Secure two large-bore cannulae, take bloods and commence fluid resuscitation
- Examine for evidence of blood loss and treat accordingly

Disability

The neurological status of the patient should be rapidly assessed. The pupils are monitored for size and reactivity, and a GCS measured. This should be repeated regularly as the test is quick to perform and once again it is change in the score which is more important in determining how treatment is going than one isolated measurement. Other than severe head injury, other reversible causes of an altered level of consciousness include hypovolaemia, hypoglycaemia, alcohol and drug abuse. These must all be excluded or treated during the initial assessment.

Exposure

The patient must be fully exposed and examined front and back using a carefully controlled log roll. Spinal alignment must be maintained during this procedure with in-line traction. Hypothermia can be rapid following trauma, and warming air blankets are vitally important in the resuscitative phase.

Adjuncts to the primary survey

At the same time as intravenous access is secured, blood should taken for haematological and biochemical analysis. A 'group and save' and cross-match should also be requested. Additional monitoring should be attached to the patient, including a blood pressure cuff, 12-lead electrocardiography (ECG) monitoring and pulse oximetry. Arterial blood gas sampling gives a very quick idea of oxygenation, ventilation, and electrolyte imbalance. Additional adjuncts include a nasogastric tube, urinary catheter and a 'trauma series' of radiographs. Other, more specialised forms of imaging, such as ultrasound, computed tomography (CT) and angiography, should be considered once the patient's condition is seen to be stable after the initial assessment and resuscitation (Summary box 24.7).

Summary box 24.7

Adjuncts to the primary survey

- Blood tests – full blood count, urea and electrolytes, clotting screen, glucose, toxicology, cross-match
- ECG, pulse oximetry, arterial blood gas (ABG)
- Two wide-bore cannulae for intravenous fluids
- Urinary and gastric catheters
- Radiographs of the cervical spine, chest and pelvis

SECONDARY SURVEY

The secondary survey does not begin until after the primary survey has been completed, and all potentially life-threatening injuries have been dealt with. In the case of a severely injured patient, for example, the secondary survey may not commence until the patient has returned from the operating theatre, having had life-saving surgery for primary survey 'ABCDE' problems.

The purpose of the secondary survey is to identify all other injuries and perform a more thorough 'head to toe' examination. If possible, it is here that the patient's history is reviewed. The 'AMPLE' mnemonic from the ATLS group is helpful here (Summary box 24.8).

Summary box 24.8

Review of patient's history (AMPLE)

- **A**llergy
- **M**edication, including tetanus status
- **P**ast medical history
- **L**ast meal
- **E**vents of the incident

Secondary survey physical examination

Examine each region of the body for signs of injury, bony instability and tenderness to palpation.

- **Head and face**. Evaluate the head for penetrating injuries and depressed fractures, and any evidence of bleeding or discharge from the ears suggestive of a basal skull fracture (Chapter 25). Check the face for maxillofacial fractures and ocular injury. Inspect the mouth, mandible, zygoma, nose and ears. Exclude midfacial injury and potential airway compromise (Chapter 27).
- **Neck**. Inspect and palpate the cervical spine anteriorly and posteriorly for haematomas, crepitus, tenderness and evidence of steps on palpation. The spine is held immobilised until formally cleared clinically and radiographically (Chapter 26).
- **Chest**. Review the primary survey and perform full palpation and auscultation of the chest wall. Palpate the entire chest wall including the clavicle, sternum and ribs.
- **Neurological**. Examine the GCS regularly. Perform a full neurological examination if the patient's condition allows. Any evidence of sensory and motor disturbance requires full spinal immobilisation and urgent review by the neurosurgeons or spinal orthopaedic surgeons with imaging as appropriate.
- **Abdomen and pelvis**. Inspect for distension, bruising or penetrating wounds. Inspect and palpate for tenderness and signs of peritonism. Palpate the iliac crests for pain which might indicate pelvic instability, resulting from ring fractures. Inspect the perineum for evidence of ecchymosis or bleeding. A rectal examination is needed to assess tone, prostate level and to look for bleeding (Chapter 28).
- **Extremities**. It is often here that attention is diverted immediately when a dramatic injury to the limbs presents itself (Figure 24.3). It is important to note that, unless there is severe haemorrhage, the injury to the limb is not immediately life threatening and focus must be maintained on the primary survey and 'ABCDE' sequence. Obviously, deformed limbs should be manipulated into as near anatomical alignment as possible, remembering to document the distal neurovascular status before and after the intervention.
- **Log roll**. Once the patient has been evaluated anteriorly, a log roll should be performed to inspect the back. One member of the team is responsible for maintaining in-line spinal stabilisation (usually the anaesthetist when the patient is intubated.) Three other trained staff hold the patient steady through the turn. Inspect and palpate the entire spine from occiput to sacrum, looking and feeling for tenderness and bony abnormalities. Identify any penetrating injuries or exit wounds from gunshot injuries and cover these once they have been photographed. Percuss, palpate and auscultate the posterior chest wall.

Re-evaluation

This cannot be stressed enough. It is an integral process in the initial assessment of major trauma and should not stop once the patient leaves the emergency room. Continuous monitoring is invaluable here, especially of the vital signs and urinary output.

It is also very important to stress that, should the patient's condition change at any time during the initial assessment, then the primary survey must be repeated from the beginning, since additional life-threatening injuries may be declaring themselves.

Definitive care and transfer

Definitive care will be discussed in subsequent chapters, but it is important to recognise that there should be as little delay as possible in reaching this stage where initial resuscitation and assessment has been completed. It has increasingly been recognised that early transfer to an appropriate care facility is the most important contributor to successful outcome. When it becomes mandatory to transfer the patient from the initial receiving hospital, the patient must be haemodynamically and cardiovascularly stable. An experienced anaesthetist should accompany the patient, the airway should be secured as necessary. Life-saving surgery may need to be performed prior to transfer for other injuries. This is called 'damage control surgery' (Chapter 32).

SPECIAL SUBGROUP CONSIDERATIONS

The initial management of any traumatised individual initially follows the same methodical 'ABCDE' pathway. However, there are three very important subgroups which require special consideration: the paediatric, the elderly and the pregnant. Each will be considered separately, highlighting the differences in initial assessment and management.

Paediatric trauma

Injury is the leading cause of mortality among children and adolescents. Children have a smaller body mass and, therefore, there may be a greater force applied per unit surface area for a given injury. The energy is transmitted to a body with less fat, less connective tissue and an immature skeleton; therefore, injuries to more than one organ are more frequent. As the surface area to body volume ratio of children is high, thermal energy loss is higher and hypothermia is a higher risk.

Airway and cervical spine control

As with any traumatised patient, control of the airway is the first priority. Anatomically, children differ from adults in that they have a smaller and more anteriorly positioned and funnel-shaped larynx, floppy epiglottis, short trachea and large tongue. Nasotracheal intubation in children younger than nine years

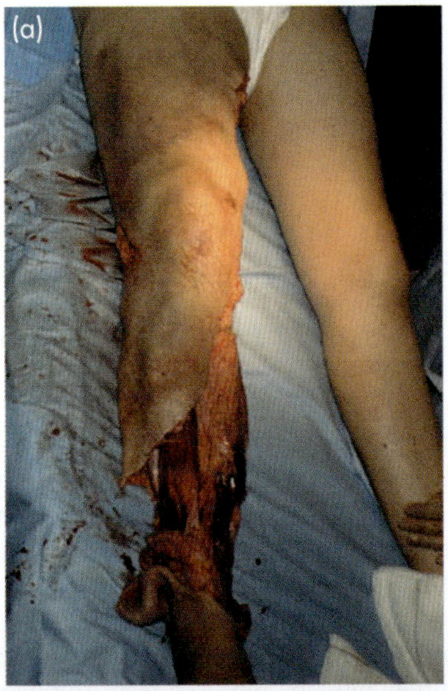

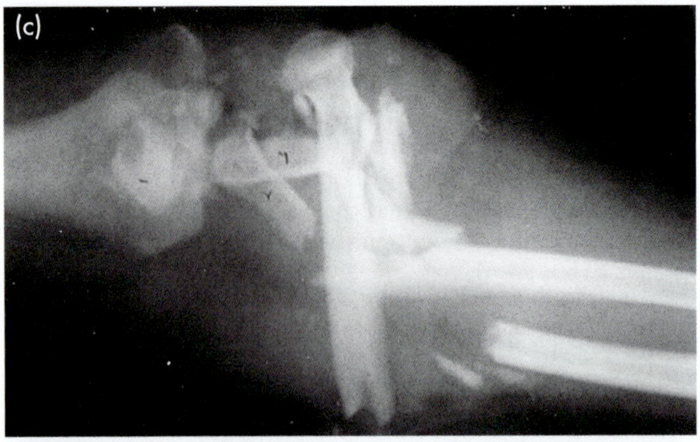

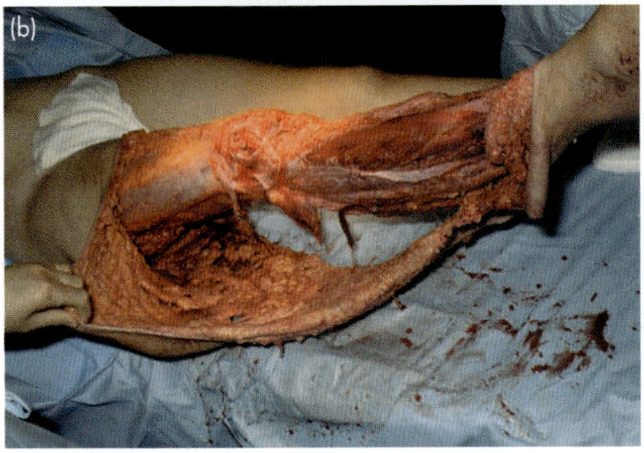

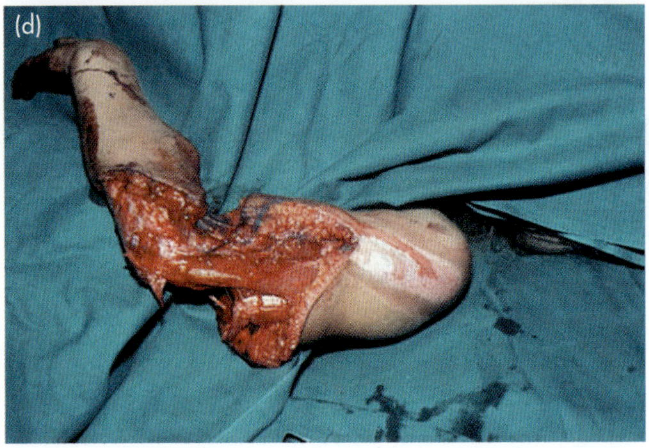

Figure 24.3 (a–d) Severe degloving injuries to the upper and lower limbs following a high-speed road traffic accident. The initial appearance and severity of the injury should not detract from following the important Advanced Trauma Life Support (ATLS) sequence in evaluating and treating immediate life-threatening injuries.

should not be performed because of the possibility of damage to the cranial vault and to the fragile soft tissues causing bleeding. With respect to a definitive airway, cuffed tubes are rarely indicated for children less than nine years of age because of the delicate structures within the airway and the fact that the cricoid ring provides an adequate seal. It should also be remembered that in children, the trachea is relatively short, and care should be taken not to intubate the right main bronchus.

Breathing and ventilatory control

The respiratory rate in the child decreases with age. Infants require 40–60 breaths per minute, whereas the older child has a rate of 20 breaths per minute (Table 24.2). Hypoxia is a common cause of cardiorespiratory arrest; however, before this, hypoventilation causes a respiratory acidosis, which is the most common acid–base disturbance in the injured child. Correction must be through adequate and controlled ventilation. Flail chest and aortic rupture are uncommon in children due to the elastic nature and resilience of the underlying structures. Pulmonary contusions are not evident in the early chest x-ray, but as before, re-evaluation is necessary for the following 24–48 hours.

Circulation with haemorrhage control

Vital signs vary with age (Table 24.2). Due to the greater physiological capacity and ability of children to compensate for fluid loss, hypotension is a very late and ominous sign of hypovolae-

Table 24.2 Paediatric vital signs.

Normal vital signs by age	Pulse (beats per min)	Systolic blood pressure (mmHg)	Respiratory rate (breaths per min)
Infant (<1 year)	160	80	40
Preschool (<5 years)	140	90	30
Adolescent (>10 years)	120	100	20

mic shock. Once they have become hypotensive, deterioration can be rapid and fatal. If intravenous access has failed after two attempts, consideration should be given to intraosseous access, especially in children younger than six years of age. The uninjured proximal tibia is the ideal route or, alternatively, the distal femur.

Disability

Head injury is the most common cause of disability and death among children in trauma. The principles of assessment and management are similar to those in the adult population with strict avoidance of hypoxia and hypovolaemia. Diffuse axonal injury is more common in children than in adults, who have a higher incidence of intracranial mass lesions.

Exposure

As mentioned above, surface area to volume ratios make children particularly vulnerable to environmental changes, especially hypothermia. Overhead lamps or heaters, warming blankets and warmed intravenous fluids and blood are often necessary (Figure 24.4).

Paediatric secondary survey

This is essentially similar to the head to toe examination described for adults. Consideration must be given to the fact that the liver and spleen are the most common organs to be injured in the abdomen. A number of specific visceral injuries are more common in children:

- duodenal haematoma or pancreatic injury: secondary to a bicycle handlebar striking the right upper quadrant relatively unprotected by an underdeveloped anterior abdominal musculature;
- small bowel perforation and mesenteric injuries;
- bladder injury: more common due to pelvic shallowness (Table 24.3);
- restraint from a lap belt (less common now) results in enteric disruption, especially if there is an associated 'chance' fracture of the lumbar spine.

Child abuse

Whenever managing paediatric trauma, non-accidental injury (NAI) must always be considered. It is our responsibility as health-care professionals to safeguard these children and prevent them from further harm. There are certain features from both the history and examination that may point towards NAI, and early identification and alerting of child protection authorities is essential (see Table 24.4).

Trauma in the elderly population

Trauma in the elderly population presents many challenges for the treating physicians due to the fragility of the patient's physiological status and comorbidities. It does not require high-velocity or high-energy trauma to put the elderly life at risk following injury. An elderly patient may only be surviving with just enough physiological reserve, and any injury, no matter how insignificant, may prove fatal (Figure 24.5). Initial assessment and, more importantly, management has to be even more meticulous in this subgroup of patients.

Airway and cervical spine control

This is the same for the elderly as it is in the normal population. However, one should watch for dentition status, nasopharyngeal

Table 24.3 Urine output by age in the paediatric population.

Age	Optimal urine output
Infant (<1 year)	2 mL/kg per hour
Preschool (1–5 years)	1.5 mL/kg per hour
Child–adolescent (6–16 years)	1 mL/kg per hour

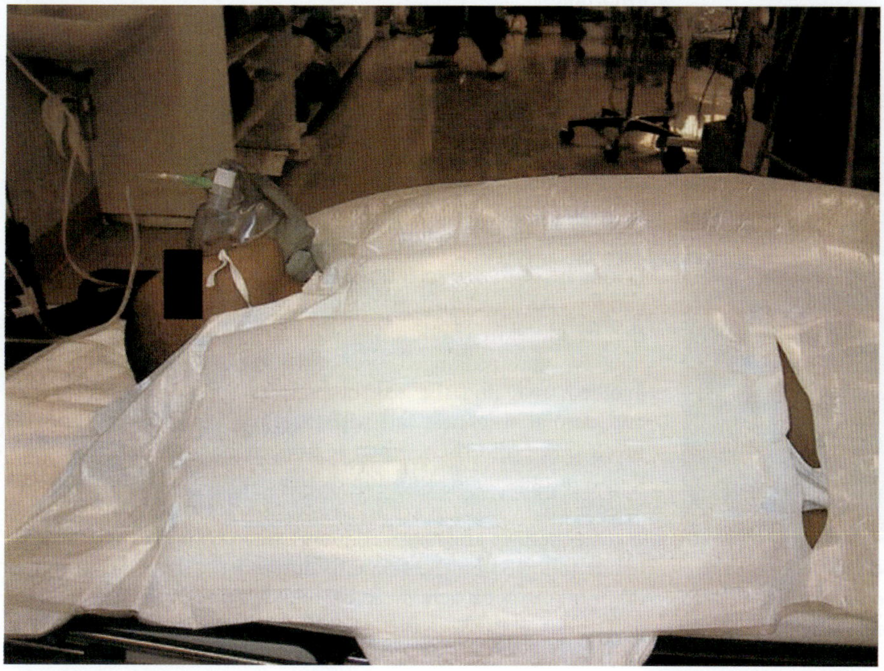

Figure 24.4 External warming blanket (courtesy of Johannesburg Hospital Trauma Unit).

Table 24.4 Markers for non-accidental injury

Repeated hospital visits for minor injuries
Late presentations and multiple visits to different hospitals
Vague or inconsistent history from the child's parent or guardian and the child
Withdrawn behaviour of the child with resistance to examination
History of abuse in a sibling
Bite marks, finger marks, belt marks or cigarette burns
Multiple fractures of different ages
Perineal injury
Intracranial haemorrhage without a history of motor vehicle accident

fragility as in children, macroglossia and cervical spine and temporomandibular joint arthritis. Stiffness in the cervical spine may make the usual airway clearing measures difficult.

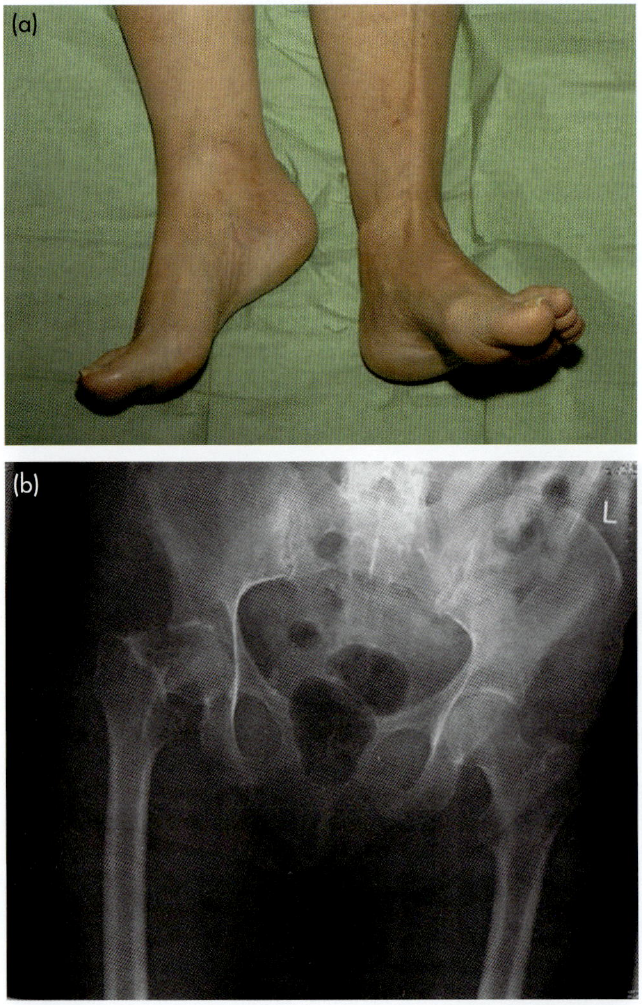

Figure 24.5 Classical shortened externally rotated right lower limb of a subcapital fractured neck of femur – it should be emphasised that this represents a significant major trauma in this vulnerable group of elderly individuals.

Breathing and ventilation

In patients with a known history of chronic obstructive airways disease, it may be prudent to consider early intubation and ventilation because of their instability in maintaining respiratory drive. However, it should also be remembered that they may prove very difficult to extubate too. Mortality rates following chest injuries in the elderly are higher; rib fractures and pulmonary contusion are not well tolerated. Pulmonary complications, such as atelectasis, pneumonia and pulmonary oedema, occur with great frequency.

Circulation

By the age of 65 years, nearly half of the population has some coronary artery stenosis. Cardiac reserve and maximum potential heart rate decreases with age and, therefore, it may be difficult to detect ongoing hypovolaemic shock. Furthermore, many of the elderly population may be taking cardiac medication that may mask a compensatory tachycardia following trauma, e.g. beta-blockers. Urinary response also changes with age; the elderly kidney is also more susceptible to damage from hypovolaemia, medications and other nephrotoxins. Retroperitoneal haemorrhage may occur from relatively minor pelvic or hip fractures, and a patient who fails to stabilise after fluid resuscitation may require prompt angiography and embolisation. Prompt treatment or transfer to an appropriate facility may be life-saving.

Disability

Cerebral atrophy is common with increasing age. This leads to increased space within the cranium and therefore some protection from contusion. Pre-existing medical conditions may be a cause of confusion in the elderly, making assessment of head injury difficult. This is where a change in conscious state between two observations is more useful than a single measurement. Osteoporosis can lead to increased risk of spinal fractures after even very minor injury. Spinal injury may also be more common because of pre-existing stiffness and spinal stenosis. This rigidity predisposes the patient to central and anterior cord syndromes.

Exposure

Reduced thermoregulatory ability is well documented in the elderly. It is important that, as in children, the elderly patient is protected from the effects of hypothermia during the initial assessment and management.

Secondary survey in the elderly

A full head to toe examination needs to be undertaken after careful 'AMPLE' history-taking (where possible). Owing to the friable skin condition, spinal injury should be ruled out quickly, and prolonged use of the spinal board should be avoided, reducing the risk of pressure sores. Skin vascularity and dermal thickness fall with age, so skin is more likely to break down and then, when it does, it heals badly. It is commonly a musculoskeletal injury that the patient presents with after a fall, usually a consequence of pre-existing osteoporosis or osteopenia. The most common fracture is in the proximal femur followed by the humerus and wrist. Above all, a multidisciplinary approach must be adopted including the patient and their relatives if the definitive treatment plans are to be successful.

Trauma in pregnancy

For the purposes of trauma management, pregnancy must be considered and excluded in all women of child-bearing age. Anatomic and physiological changes must be considered when assessing and resuscitating a pregnant woman. The trauma team in this situation should include both an obstetrician for early assessment of the fetus, and potentially a paediatrician. The fundamental principles of the ATLS system remain the same and although there are two patients, the best chance of a favourable outcome for the foetus, is with optimal resuscitation of the mother.

During the primary survey, the uterus of the third trimester pregnant patient should be manually displaced to the left side in order to take pressure off the inferior vena cava. This promotes venous return to the heart and increasing cardiac output in a potentially shocked state. Due to the increased intravascular volume in pregnancy, these patients can lose significant amounts of blood before they display the usual signs of hypovolaemia. This is important to understand and recognize since the mother may appear relatively stable while the fetus is in distress due to a lack of placental perfusion.

The potential for fetomaternal haemorrhage must always be considered in the traumatized pregnant patient, since only a minor haemorrhage could result in the sensitization of a Rhesus negative mother. Therefore, all Rh-negative patients should be administered Rh immunoglobulin when there is a concern about potential fetomaternal haemorrhage.

SUMMARY

Trauma is a massive and growing worldwide health burden. Despite injury prevention strategies, a significant number of the world's population will be exposed to or involved in trauma. In the initial assessment and management of these patients, it is demonstrated that the ATLS approach is still the most reproducible protocol for a successful outcome. A team approach must be utilised, and good organisation of the system leads to very real reductions in mortality and morbidity globally. The paediatric and elderly are special groups of individuals who have unique inherent differences that must be recognised but, essentially, the framework for assessment remains the same. It is only through education and training that truly significant inroads can be made into this hugely debilitating and resource-intensive 'disease'.

FURTHER READING

American College of Surgeons' Committee on Trauma. *Advanced trauma life support course*. Chicago, IL: American College of Surgeons, 2008.

Jacobs D. Special considerations in geriatric injury. *Curr Opin Crit Care* 2003; **9**: 535–9.

Jacobs D, Plaisier B, Barie P, Hammond J. Practice management guidelines for geriatric trauma: the EAST Practice Management Guidelines Work Group. *J Trauma* 2003; **54**: 391–416.

Peden M, McGee K, Sharma G. *The injury chart book: a graphical overview of the global burden of injuries*. Geneva: World Health Organization, 2002.

Velmahos GC, Jindal A, Chan LS *et al*. Insignificant mechanism of injury: not to be taken lightly. *J Am Coll Surg* 2001; **192**: 147–52.

Website addresses

American Association for the Surgery of Trauma: www.aast.org.
Eastern Association for the Surgery of Trauma: www.east.org.
Trauma.org: www.trauma.org.
American Orthopedic Trauma Association: www.ota.org.

CHAPTER 25

Emergency neurosurgery

LEARNING OBJECTIVES

To understand:
- The physiology of cerebral blood flow and the pathophysiology of raised intracranial pressure
- The management of head injury and prevention of secondary brain injury
- The diagnosis and management of spontaneous intracranial bleeding including subarachnoid haemorrhage

PHYSIOLOGY AND PATHOPHYSIOLOGY

Cerebral blood flow

The brain is dependent on continuous cerebral bloodflow for oxygen and glucose delivery, and hence survival. Normal cerebral blood flow (CBF) is about 55 mL/minute for every 100 g of brain tissue. Ischaemia results when this rate drops below 20 mL/min, and even lower levels will result in infarction unless promptly corrected.

The flow rate is related to cerebral perfusion pressure (CPP), the difference between mean arterial pressure (MAP) and intracranial pressure (ICP): CPP (75–105 mmHg) = MAP (90–110 mmHg) – ICP (5–15 mmHg).

Typical normal values are given in parentheses. In fact, in the normal brain, variations in vascular tone maintain a constant CBF across a range of MAP between 50 and 150 mmHg, and a corresponding range of CPP, a process termed 'cerebral autoregulation'. The limits of this range are elevated in patients with chronic hypertension.

Neurosurgical emergencies, especially head injury, lead to brain swelling, bleeding and hydrocephalus. The common pathophysiological pathway is then elevated ICP and reduced CPP and CBF.

Other factors which may compromise CBF include the failure of autoregulation which follows brain insult, and vasospasm after aneurysm rupture (see below under Aneurysmal subarachnoid haemorrhage).

ICP and the Monro Kellie doctrine

Alexander Monro observed in 1783 that the cranium is a 'rigid box' containing a 'nearly incompressible brain'. Therefore any expansion in the contents, especially haematoma and brain swelling, may be initially accommodated by exclusion of fluid components, venous blood and cerebrospinal fluid (CSF). Further expansion is associated with an exponential rise in intracranial pressure (see Figure 25.1). The result is hypoperfusion and herniation.

Herniation syndromes

The rapid increase in intracranial pressure which accompanies the exhaustion of compensation mechanisms ultimately results in herniation of brain tissue. The uncus of the temporal lobe may herniate over the tentorium resulting in pupil abnormalities (see below under Pupils), usually occurring first on the side of any expanding haematoma. Cerebellar tonsillar herniation through the foramen magnum compresses medullary vasomotor and respiratory centres, classically producing Cushing's triad of hypertension, bradycardia and irregular respiration (Summary box 25.1).

Summary box 25.1

Intracranial pressure

- Perfusion of the brain with oxygenated blood is critical for its survival
- Cerebral perfusion pressure is the difference between mean arterial pressure and intracranial pressure
- Cerebral perfusion is kept constant across a range of perfusion pressures by the process of autoregulation
- Autoregulation is compromised in the injured brain

HEAD INJURY

Epidemiology

Head injury accounts for 3–4 per cent of emergency department attendances, with around 1500 cases per 100 000 population per year in the UK. Of these, 300 per 100 000 require admission, 15 to a neurosurgical unit. Annual mortality attributable to head injury is estimated at nine per 100 000, and it remains

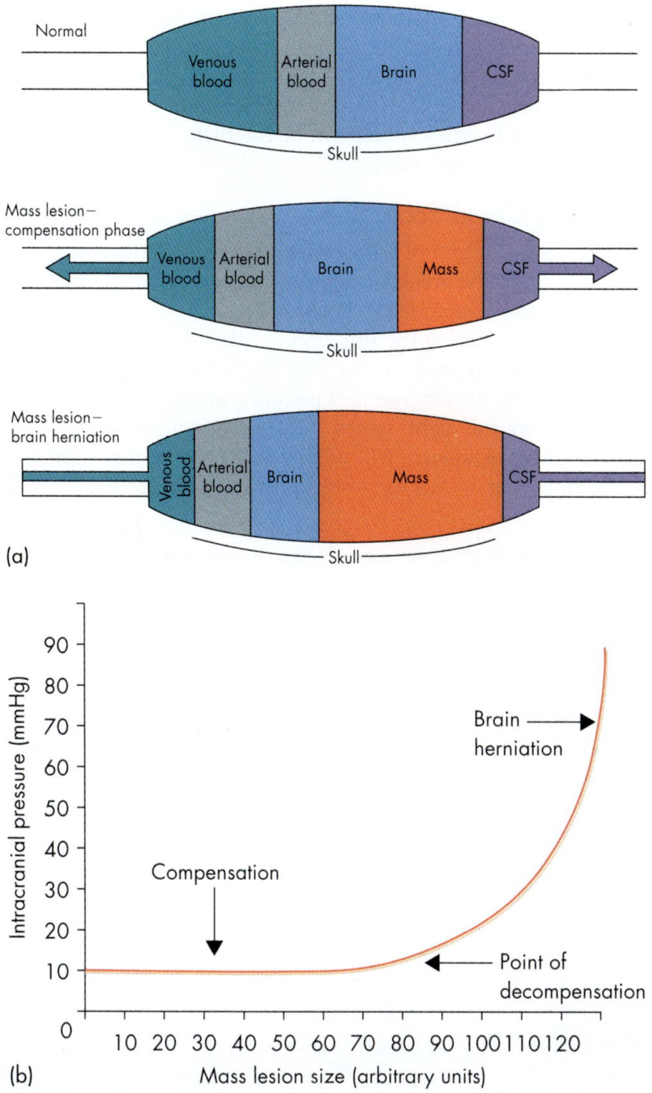

Figure 25.1 (a, b) Initially, compensation for this expansion within the cranium is compensated for by displacement of CSF and venous blood. When this mechanism has no further reserve capacity, the intracranial pressure increases rapidly. The result is hypoperfusion and herniation.

the leading cause of death and disability from childhood to early middle age.

Risk factors include male sex, recreational drugs (including alcohol and substance abuse) and youth, with a peak at 15–30 years of age. This latter factor contributes to the overwhelming social and economic impact of head injuries, with an estimated 2 per cent of the US population suffering long-term disability as a result of head injury.

Road traffic accidents are the leading cause of head injury, being responsible for up to 50 per cent of cases. Other common mechanisms of injury include falls and assault. There is significant geographical variation, for example firearms are the third leading cause in the US.

Initial evaluation and management

Resuscitation is performed according to Advanced Trauma Life Support (ATLS) guidelines, beginning with management of the airway and cervical spine control (see Chapter 24).

History

Vital information may need to be obtained from paramedics and observers when the patient is unable to give a full history (as is usually the case).

Mechanism

Head injuries arising from high energy mechanisms of injury, such as a fall from a height or a high-speed road accident. This makes multisystem injury (especially to the spine) likely so a full search should be made for these (see Chapter 24). In the case of road traffic accidents in particular, extraction time and evidence of hypoxia or haemodynamic instability at the scene is important information to obtain from the paramedics. The possibility that a fall or crash may have resulted from a prior medical problem, such as myocardial infarction, hypoglycaemia or subarachnoid haemorrhage, should be borne in mind when trying to get a full history (Summary box 25.2).

Summary box 25.2

The history in head injury

- Bystanders and paramedics may give vital information on the:
  - pre-injury state (fits, alcohol, chest pain)
  - energy involved in the injury (speed of vehicles, height fallen)
  - conscious state and haemodynamic stability of the patient after the accident
  - length of time taken for extrication
- The length of retro- and antegrade amnesia are useful for grading severity
- Check the medication history, especially anticoagulants

Neurological progression

A specific check should be made for any loss of consciousness at the time of injury, and its duration. The Glasgow Coma Score (GCS) and pupil responses at the scene and on arrival in Accident and Emergency should be obtained and documented. They should also be checked regularly thereafter. It cannot be overemphasised that deterioration in GCS is an important index of developing, and potentially reversible, secondary injury. It is also useful to assess the extent of amnesia, retrograde (events prior to the injury) and anterograde (events afterwards). If the patient was intubated at the scene of the accident, it is valuable to know whether the patient was moving all four limbs before this?

Other history

Obtain details of the patient's medical background, including allergies and normal medications. Of particular note here are antiplatelet agents, potentially requiring platelet transfusion especially if surgery is needed, and anticoagulants, which may need reversal.

Examination: primary survey

The primary survey is performed as normal (see Chapter 29). The priority in any resuscitation is to ensure uninterrupted perfusion of the brain with oxygenated blood. This is especially true after a head injury given the disturbance to intracranial autoregulation and the sensitivity of the primary injured brain tissue to further insult. Bleeding from scalp lacerations may require management as part of the primary survey, as the blood loss can be substantial and on-going.

Check the responsiveness of the pupils, conscious level and for any gross focal neurological deficits. Blood glucose level should also be measured as early as possible as hypoglycaemia is very dangerous and eminently reversible (Summary box 25.3).

Summary box 25.3

The primary survey in head injury

- Ensure adequate oxygenation and circulation
- Check pupil size and response and Glasgow Coma Score as soon as possible
- Check for focal neurological deficits before intubation if possible
- Check blood sugar for hypoglycaemia

Pupils

The pupil size should be recorded in millimetres, and reactivity documented as present, sluggish or absent. Uncal herniation (Figure 25.2) can compress the third nerve, compromising the parasympathetic supply to the pupil, so that unopposed sympathetic activity produces an enlarged and sluggish pupil, which then, if the compression continues, becomes fixed and dilated. However, an abnormal pupil size and response may reflect pathology anywhere in the eye or the reflex loop made up by the optic nerve, the oculomotor nerve, and the brainstem. Direct ocular trauma or nerve injury in association with a skull base fracture can cause mydriasis (dilated pupil) present from the time of injury. Pre-existing discrepancy in pupil size (anisocoria), as a result of Holmes-Adie pupil or cataracts for example, may also complicate assessment.

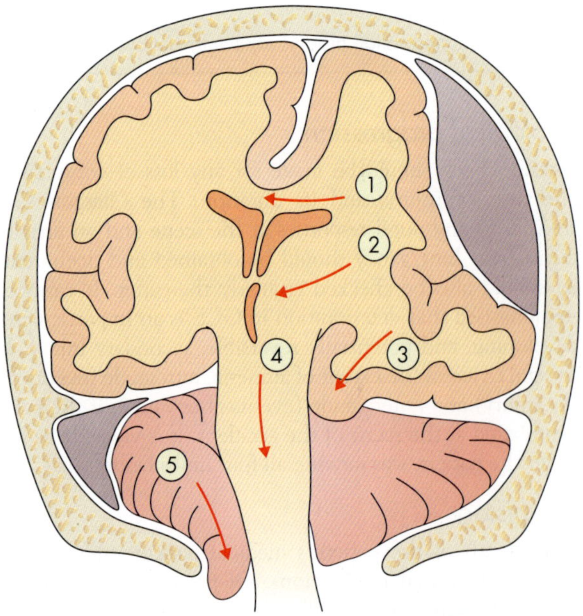

Figure 25.2 Brain herniation. Herniation of the cingulate gyrus under the falx cerebri is called 'subfalcine herniation' (1). Herniation is associated with midline shift (2). Herniation of the uncus of the temporal lobe (3) is associated with compression of the ipsilateral third nerve. Central herniation (4) and tonsillar herniation (5) are associated with compression of brainstem structures.

Glasgow Coma Score

The GCS is the sum of scores on three components as detailed in Table 25.1. The breakdown of the GCS into eye opening, verbal and motor components should always be recorded and used when communicating the situation to other doctors. Remember that the score represents the best performance elicited, so a patient flexing in response to a painful stimulus on the left and localising on the right scores 'M5'. A sternal or supraorbital rub, or trapezius squeeze will usually be an appropriate stimulus. Remember that 3/15 is the lowest possible GCS score!

Table 25.1 Head injury severity: clinical classification.

Eyes open	Spontaneously	4
	To verbal command	3
	To painful stimulus	2
	Do not open	1
Verbal	Normal oriented conversation	5
	Confused	4
	Inappropriate/words only	3
	Sounds only	2
	No sounds	1
	Intubated patient	T
Motor	Obeys commands	6
	Localises to pain	5
	Withdrawal/flexion	4
	Abnormal flexion	3
	Extension	2
	No motor response	1

Neurological deficit

Gross focal neurological deficits, such as paraplegia, may be evident at the primary survey, and an assessment to exclude such deficit should be carried out, especially if the patient is to be intubated so that subsequent examination will be impossible. Detailed neurological examination is included in the secondary survey.

Examination: secondary survey

A full secondary survey will be required. Particular attention must be paid to the head, neck and spine.

Head

Examination of the head should include inspection and palpation of the scalp for evidence of subgaleal haematoma and scalp lacerations, which may bleed profusely, and potentially overlie fractures. Examine the face for evidence of fractures, especially to the orbital rim, zygoma and maxilla. Clinical evidence of a skull base fracture may include Battle's sign (bruising over the mastoid, see Figure 25.3), and 'racoon' or 'panda' eyes (bilateral periorbital bruising). Haemotympanum, or overt bleeding from

Sir Gordon Morgon Holmes, 1876–1965, physician, The National Hospital for Nervous Diseases, Queen's Square, London, UK.
William John Adie, 1886–1935, physician, The National Hospital for Nervous Diseases, Queen's Square, London, UK.

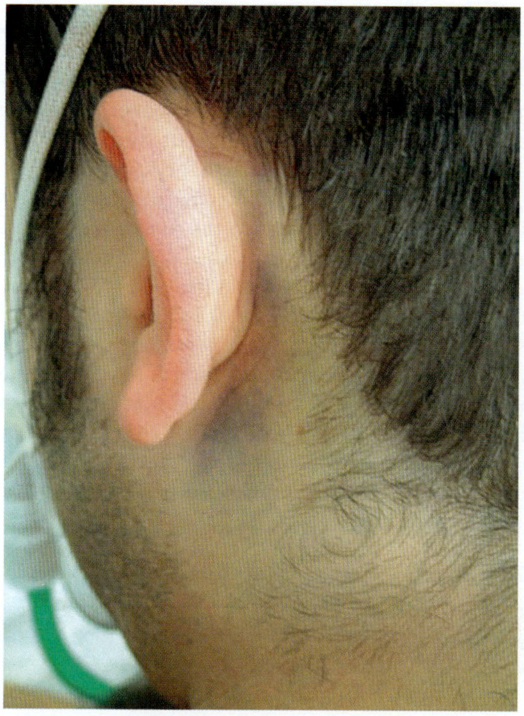

Figure 25.3 Battle's sign. A skull base fracture may be associated with bruising over the mastoid process.

the ear if the tympanic membrane has ruptured, and CSF rhinorrhoea or otorrhoea (clear cerebro spinal fluid usually mixed with blood coming from the nose or the ear) are also highly suggestive of a fracture of the base of the skull.

A complete examination of the cranial nerves will reveal, for example, facial or vestibulo-cochlear nerve damage associated with skull base fracture. Midbrain or brainstem dysfunction may produce gaze paresis (inability of eye to look across beyond the midline), dysconjugate gaze (inability of the eyes to work together), or roving eye movements. Inspect the conjunctiva and cornea of the eyes, and the retina using an ophthalmoscope, looking for hyphaema (blood in the anterior chamber of the eye), papilloedema or retinal detachment. Blood in the mouth may be due to tongue-biting at seizure or at the time of trauma.

The GCS and pupil status, assessed as part of the primary survey, require re-evaluation at the secondary survey and regularly thereafter (Summary box 25.4).

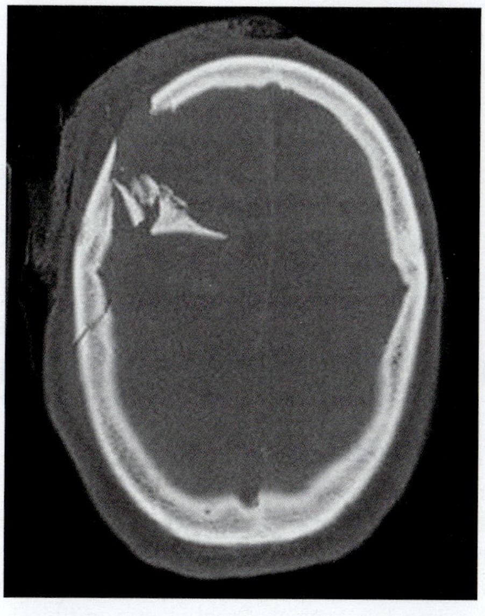

Figure 25.4 A right frontal comminuted depressed skull fracture, with a linear undisplaced fracture of the right parietal bone visible posteriorly.

Summary box 25.4

Examination of the head (secondary survey)

- Look and feel over the whole skull and face for cuts, bruises and fractures
- Check for fractured base of skull by looking for blood in the ears, nose or mouth and Battle's sign
- Check the cranial nerves
- Check the eyes for movement and for damage to the orbit itself

Neck and spine

In moderate or severe traumatic brain injury (TBI), there is an associated cervical spine fracture in around 10 per cent of cases. Therefore, cervical spine injury must be presumed in the context of head injury until actively excluded. In a high energy mechanism, such as road traffic accident or fall from a height, thoracic and lumbar spine injuries must also be excluded. Plain x-rays are of limited value in excluding significant cervical spine injury. Even computed tomography (CT) imaging does not exclude the possibility of significant ligamentous injury. Therefore, where possible, these patients should be managed in a hard collar until their spine can be cleared clinically.

A peripheral nerve examination with documentation of limb tone, power, reflexes and sensation needs to be performed early to identify spinal pathology. This is especially important in patients who may subsequently be intubated and ventilated when this assessment will no longer be possible. Obtunded (partially conscious) patients should move all four limbs in response to an appropriate painful stimulus.

The patient will need to be log-rolled to palpate for thoracic or lumbar deformity, and any cervical collar should be removed at this stage to allow palpation of the cervical spine, before it is then replaced again. If there is associated spinal injury, a thoracic sensory level is much more easily established by sensory examination on the back. A per rectal examination is also performed at log-roll, assessing for anal tone, sensation in the awake patient, and anal wink (sphincter seen to contract in response to a pinprick stimulus). Priapism is a strong predictor of severe cord injury even in intubated patients (Summary box 25.5).

CLASSIFICATION OF SEVERITY AND TYPE OF HEAD INJURY

Glasgow Coma Score

Severity of head injury is classified according to the Glasgow Coma Score (Table 25.1), as it is the GCS – and in particular the motor score – that is the best predictor of neurological outcome. On-going impaired conscious level, beyond isolated

William Henry Battle, 1855–1936, surgeon, St Thomas's Hospital, London, UK.
A racoon is a small mammal native to North and Central America which has a pale face with dark rings round its eyes.

Summary box 25.5

Examination of the whole patient in head injury

- Cervical spine injury is common in patients with head injuries
- Even obtunded patients should move all four limbs
- Check and record power, tone and sensation in the peripheral nerves
- Log roll to check the whole spine for steps and tenderness
- Perform a rectal examination to check for anal tone and anal wink
- Check for priapism

confusion and amnesia, implies a moderate injury and coma suggests a severe injury.

Important aspects of injury

Head injuries can be divided into three categories which overlap and in which more than one may be present in a patient. These are diffuse (the brain has been shaken), blunt (a direct non-penetrating blow) and penetrating (the cranium has been breached). Rapid deceleration often produces shearing of axons (diffuse axonal injury) and coup–contrecoup contusions (see below under Cerebral contusions). Penetrating injuries can be classified as low velocity or high velocity. The cavitation caused by high velocity injuries is especially damaging to the brain. Skull fractures can be open or closed. If intracranial air can be seen on the x-ray, then the dura has been breached too. Fractures may be linear (when they can be difficult to see on x-ray) or comminuted when they may also be depressed. Fractured base of skull may present with bleeding from the eyes, ears nose or mouth or with rhinorrhoea (CSF leaking from the nose).

Intracranial haematoma

Haemorrhage within the cranium occurs in four main sites: extradural, subdural, subarachnoid and intraparenchymal. Each has a characteristic cause, presentation and treatment, which will be discussed below. However, a common characteristic is that all cause a rise in intracranial pressure, which may compromise perfusion of the brain. Minimising the secondary injury by making sure that the patient is well oxygenated and that their blood pressure is within normal limits is important in the early management of these cases (Summary box 25.6).

Summary box 25.6

Classification of traumatic head injuries

- Scalp: open and closed (beware air under the dura)
- Skull site: vault and base of skull
- Skull type: linear, comminuted and depressed
- Intracranial bleeding: extradural, subdural, subarachnoid and intraparenchymal
- Brain tissue causes: diffuse, blunt (direct, coup–contrecoup) and penetrating

MANAGEMENT OF MINOR AND MILD HEAD INJURY

In general, patients without on-going deficits can safely be discharged from the emergency department, provided they meet the criteria listed (Table 25.2). An observation period of a few hours is advisable, especially where there is history of loss of consciousness at the time of injury: this avoids discharge during the 'lucid interval' which may precede delayed deterioration due to an expanding intracranial haematoma.

Patients who do not meet all the discharge criteria will need admission for a further period of observation, and in this case it may be more economical to perform a CT to allow safe early discharge in this group. In the UK, the National Institute for Health and Clinical Excellence (NICE) also recommends CT imaging in patients with a persistent reduced conscious level, focal deficits, suspected fractures or risk factors for intracranial bleed (see Table 25.3).

Table 25.2 Discharge criteria in minor and mild head injury.

GCS 15/15 with no focal deficits
Normal CT brain if indicated (see below)
Patient not under the influence of alcohol or drugs
Patient accompanied by a responsible adult
Verbal and written head injury advice: seek medical attention if:
• Persistent/worsening headache despite analgesia
• Persistent vomiting
• Drowsiness
• Visual disturbance
• Limb weakness or numbness

CT, computed tomography; GCS, Glasgow Coma Scale.

Table 25.3 National Institute for Health and Clinical Excellence (NICE) guidelines for computed tomography (CT) in head injury.

GCS <13 at any point
GCS 13 or 14 at 2 hours
Focal neurological deficit
Suspected open, depressed or basal skull fracture
More than one episode of vomiting
Any patient with a mild head injury over the age of 65 years or with a coagulopathy, for instance warfarin use, should be scanned urgently
Dangerous mechanism or injury or antegrade amnesia >30 minutes warrants CT within 8 hours

SURGICAL ASPECTS OF HEAD INJURY

Skull fractures

Closed linear fractures are managed conservatively, with primary closure of associated wounds where possible. Skull base fractures may be complicated by CSF leak, pituitary dysfunction, arterial dissection or cranial nerve deficits, with anosmia, facial palsy or hearing loss typical. Prophylactic antibiotics are not usually required, even in the case of CSF leak, which generally resolves spontaneously without the need for craniotomy and repair. Blind nasogastric tube placement is contraindicated in these patients.

Fractures which involve the air sinuses may be managed as open fractures, using broad spectrum antibiotics with or without exploration.

Depressed skull fractures involve inward displacement of a bone fragment by at least the thickness of the skull (Figures 25.4 and 25.5). They occur when small objects hit the skull at high velocity. They are usually compound (open) fractures, and are associated with a high incidence of infection, neurological deficit and late-onset epilepsy.

Most compound fractures will require exploration, debridement and elevation of the fragment. Prophylactic treatment with a course of broad spectrum antibiotics is normal practice (Summary box 25.7).

Summary box 25.7

Management of head injuries

- Early discharge if NICE criteria are met
- Scalp wounds need closure
- Significant depressed fractures need elevating, antibiotics and antiepileptics
- Skull base fractures may may be associated with CSF leak. Pneumococcus vaccination is valuable, but prophylactic antibiotics are not usually indicated

Extradural haematoma

Extradural haematoma (Figure 25.6) is a neurosurgical emergency. It results from rupture of an artery, vein or venous sinus, in association with a skull fracture. Typically, it is damage to the middle meningeal artery under the thin temporal bone. A low energy injury mechanism, perhaps with brief loss of consciousness, is sufficient to start the extradural bleeding. The patient may then present in the subsequent lucid interval with headache, but without any neurological deficit. At this stage, the increase in the intracranial volume is not yet causing a significant rise in intracranial pressure because compensation is occurring. However, once the limits of compensation have been reached after as long as some hours (see Monro Kellie doctrine) rapid deterioration follows. There is contralateral hemiparesis, reduced conscious level and ipsilateral pupillary dilatation, the cardinal signs of brain compression and herniation. Although this classical presentation occurs in only one third of cases, it emphasises the potential for rapid avoidable secondary brain injury in patients with minimal primary injury.

On CT, extradural haematomas appear as a lentiform (lens-shaped or biconvex) hyperdense lesion between skull and brain, constrained by the adherence of the dura to the skull. Mass effect may be evident, with compression of surrounding brain and midline shift. Areas of mixed density suggest active bleeding. A skull fracture will usually be evident (Summary box 25.8).

Extradural haematoma requires immediate transfer to the most accessible neurosurgical facility, for immediate evacuation in deteriorating or comatose patients or those with large bleeds, and for close observation with serial imaging in all cases.

Overall mortality is around 10–20 per cent, but is considerably lower in isolated extradural haematoma.

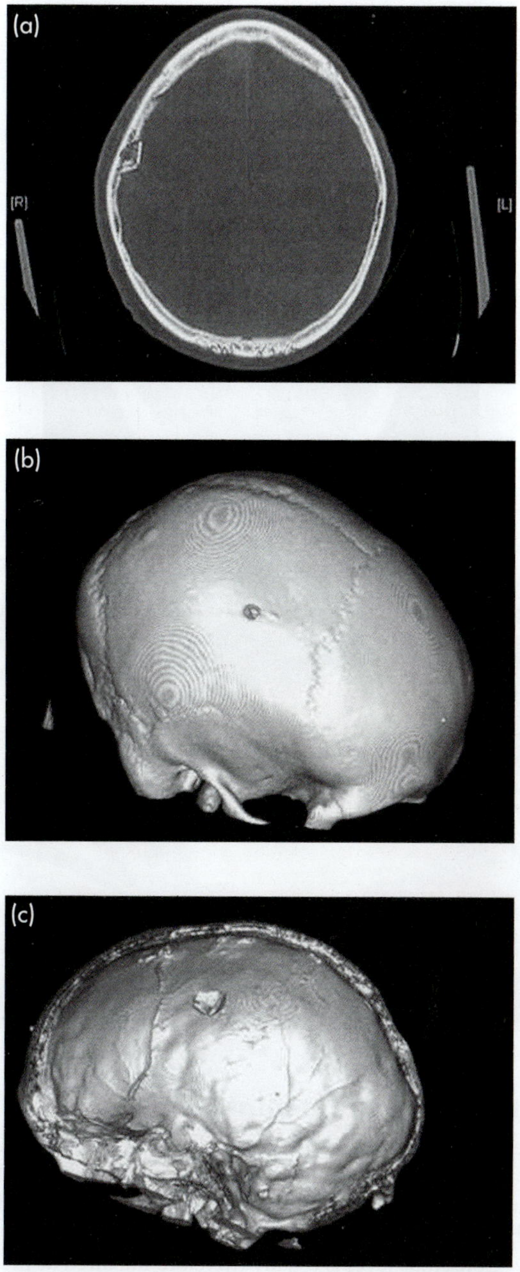

Figure 25.5 (a–c) A small depressed skull fracture of the parietal bone visible on axial bone windows (a), visualized on bone vault reconstructions (b) and with an underlying breach of dura (c).

Summary box 25.8

Extradural haemorrhage

- Can occur in the context of apparently minor trauma
- Isolated extradural haematoma may manifest as sudden deterioration following a lucid interval
- Lentiform lesion on computed tomography
- Require immediate transfer to a neurosurgical unit for decision on evacuation

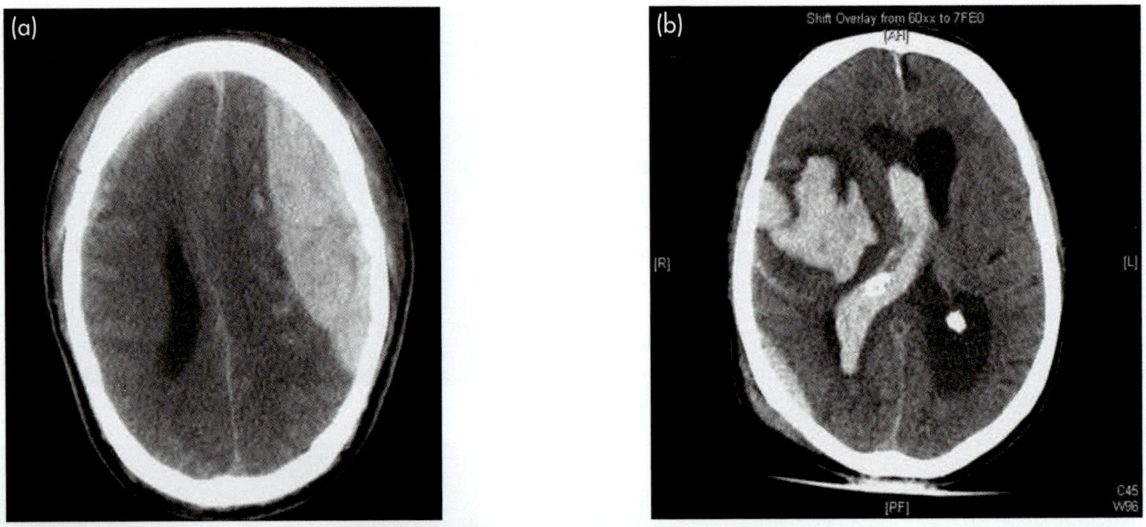

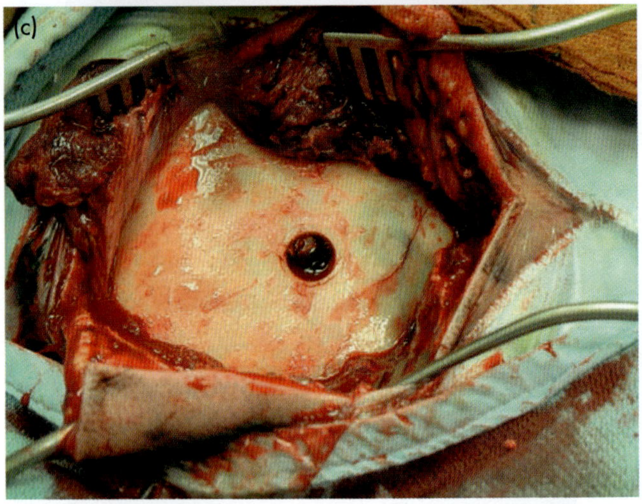

Figure 25.6 (a) A large left extradural haematoma (note the biconvex shape) exerts a mass effect; a smaller right acute subdural haematoma is also evident. (b) Right frontal intracerebral haematoma extending into the lateral ventricle is evident. There is a small right posterior extradural haematoma, and traumatic subarachnoid bleeding in the sulci of the right hemisphere. (c) A surgical temporal bone exposure showing a linear skull fracture with underlying extradural haematoma visible through a burr hole.

Acute subdural haematoma

Acute subdural bleeding arises from rupture of cortical vessels. In contrast to extradural haematoma (and chronic subdural haematoma), acute subdural haematoma is usually associated with a high energy injury mechanism and significant primary brain injury. Conscious level is usually therefore impaired at presentation, but may deteriorate further as the haematoma expands. Since the dura is not adherent to the brain as it is to the skull, subdural blood is free to expand across the brain surface giving a diffuse concave appearance (Figures 25.6a and 25.7a).

Acute subdural bleeds of significant size or with significant associated midline shift require evacuation, and the cumulative mortality in this group is about 50 per cent. Smaller bleeds in neurologically stable patients may be managed conservatively, with ICP monitoring, in a neurosurgical unit (Summary box 25.9).

Summary box 25.9

Subdural haemorrhage

- Relatively severe trauma
- No lucid interval
- Diffuse concave lesion on computed tomography
- Require immediate transfer to a neurosurgical unit for decision on evacuation
- 50 per cent mortality

Chronic subdural haematoma

The epidemiology and presentation are completely different from acute subdural haematoma. The patient is generally elderly, may be taking antiplatelet or anticoagulant medications, and there is usually a history of a recent fall, or falls. Cerebral atrophy commonly found in the elderly is believed to stretch bridging veins. These can then rupture after only minor trauma, bleed, and then tamponade (stop bleeding due to the pressure which has been produced by the bleed). Subsequent degradation of the blood clot over days or weeks leads to osmotic expansion. It is this which produces the mass effect. Presenting features, just as for any expanding intracranial mass, include pressure symptoms, especially headache and drowsiness, neurological deficit and seizures. In this group, it is important to exclude coexisting electrolyte disturbance and infections, which may be contributory. Imaging reveals diffuse hypodensity overlying the brain surface. Recent bleeding may be isodense or hyperdense, and mixed density can indicate an acute-on-chronic subdural haematoma (Figure 25.7b).

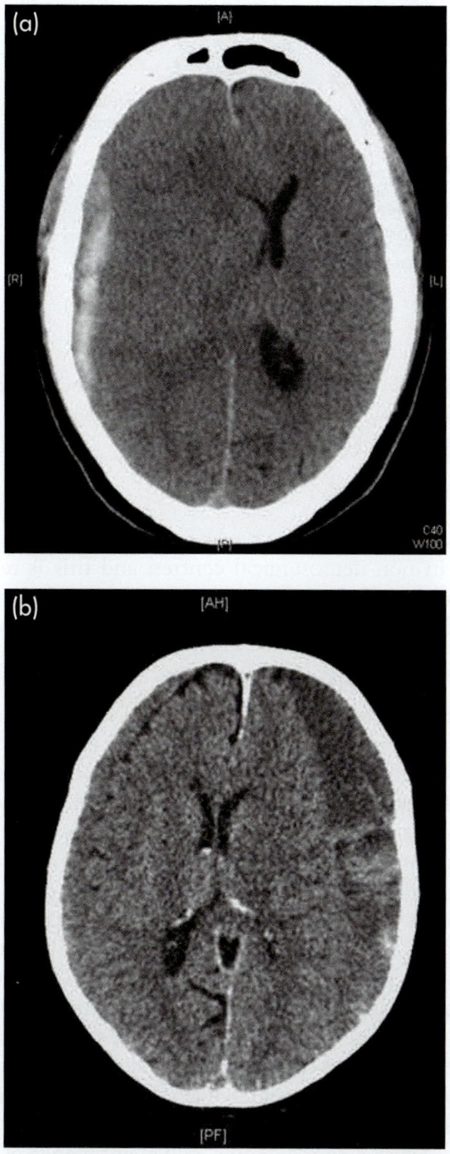

Figure 25.7 (a) Right-sided acute subdural haematoma (hyperdense). The substantial midline shift reflects brain swelling as well as bleeding: this is a high energy injury. (b) Bilateral subdural haematomas: the left is mixed density, the hypodense material representing old blood and the higher density indicating more recent bleeding, probably loculated so requiring a craniotomy to evacuate. The bleed on the right is isodense, indicating intermediate age.

Drainage is performed using burr holes, often under local anaesthetic (especially in elderly patients who present a substantial anaesthetic risk). Urgency is dictated by the clinical condition of the patient. If clinically stable, a delay of 7–10 days to allow platelet function to normalise after withdrawal of aspirin may be considered. Anticoagulation should be reversed either by administration of vitamin K, or urgently by transfusion of recombinant clotting factors in patients who have deteriorated acutely. Occasionally, acute-on-chronic bleeds with residual solid clot or septations require a craniotomy for adequate clot evacuation (Summary box 25.10).

Summary box 25.10

Chronic subdural haemorrhage

- Occurs in the elderly, especially those on anticoagulants
- May take days or weeks to develop
- Diffuse hypodense lesion on computed tomography
- Evacuation may be delayed until clotting has been improved

Traumatic subarachnoid haemorrhage

Trauma is the most common cause of subarachnoid haemorrhage (Figures 25.6b and 25.8), and this is managed conservatively. It is not usually associated with significant vasospasm, which characterises aneurysmal subarachnoid haemorrhage (see below under Aneurysmal subarachnoid haemorrhage). The possibility of spontaneous subarachnoid haemorrhage actually leading to collapse and so causing a head injury needs to be borne in mind and formal or CT angiography may be required to exclude this.

Cerebral contusions

Contusions are common and are found predominantly where the brain is in contact with the irregularly ridged inside of the skull, i.e at the inferior frontal lobes and temporal poles. 'Coup–contrecoup' injury describes contusion of the brain on the skull at the site of impact combined with contusion elsewhere sustained as the brain rebounds from the initial impact. Contusions appear heterogenous on CT, reflecting their composition of injured brain matter interspersed with acute blood (Figure 25.8). Contusions rarely require surgical intervention, but may warrant delayed evacuation to reduce mass effect.

Diffuse axonal injury

This is a form of primary brain injury, seen in the high energy accidents, and which usually renders the patient comatose. It is strictly a pathological diagnosis made at post-mortem, but

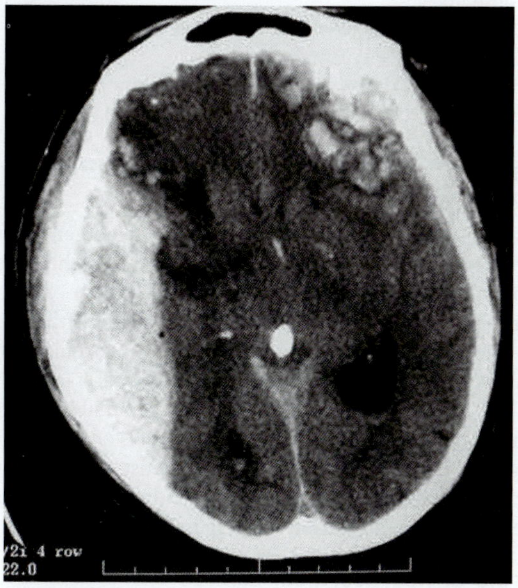

Figure 25.8 A large right extradural haematoma is evident. There are widespread cerebral contusions most prominent in the left frontal lobe. There is traumatic subarachnoid blood in the third and lateral ventricles.

haemorrhagic foci in the corpus callosum and dorsolateral rostral brainstem on CT may be suggestive, although the CT often appears normal.

Arterial dissection

Cerebral arterial dissection occurs spontaneously or in the context of trauma, which may be as trivial as nose-blowing or coughing. In the hours after significant trauma, dissection of the carotid extracranially, or at the skull base in association with fractures, is most common. It presents with headache, neck pain and focal ischaemic deficits, due to occlusion by mural haematoma, thrombus and thromboembolism. Intracranial dissection often affects the vertebral artery and may result in subarachnoid bleeding.

Development of a delayed deficit, especially in the context of a skull base fracture involving the carotid canal, should prompt urgent investigation and treatment. Carotid dissection is generally managed with anticoagulation, but vertebral dissection with subarachnoid haemorrhage usually requires surgical or endovascular intervention.

Non-accidental injury

Head injury in children and vulnerable adults may be due to abuse. Significant findings include delayed presentation, injuries of disparate age, retinal haemorrhages, bilateral chronic subdural haematomas, multiple skull fractures and neurological injury without external signs of trauma (Summary box 25.11).

Summary box 25.11

Types of brain injury

- Apparent traumatic subarachnoid haemorrhage may actually be a spontaneous subarachnoid haemorrhage which then led to the fall
- Diffuse axonal injury results from high energy injury
- Carotid dissection may be a delayed complication of skull base fracture
- Non-accidental injury in children: beware delayed presentation

Ongoing management: prevention of secondary injury

Following initial resuscitation and any emergency surgery required for systemic pathology and intracranial haematomas, the patient will require on-going management directed at minimizing secondary brain injury. This occurs in the minutes, hours and days following primary injury, as a result of factors summarised in Figure 25.9. Unlike the primary injury which describes the diffuse axonal injury and intracranial bleeding with which the patient presents, secondary injury is often preventable through avoidance of hypoxia and hypotension, and control of intracranial pressure. Unchecked, secondary injury leads to a further cycle of deterioration (see Figure 25.9).

The role of neurosurgical centres

Early discussion of patients and imaging with the regional neurosurgical service is advisable. UK Trauma Audit and Research Network data show higher mortality in patients with severe TBI

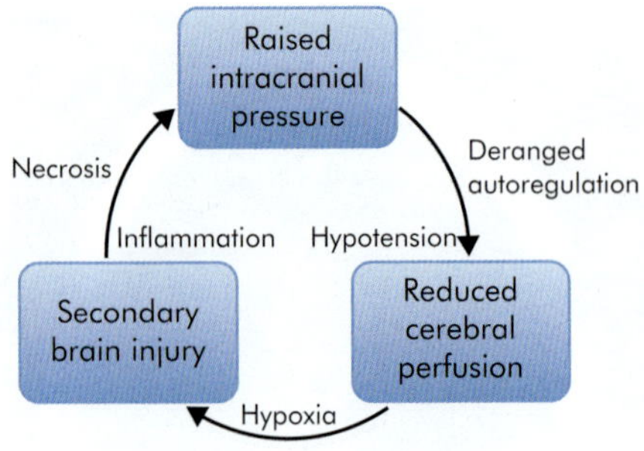

Figure 25.9 Brain swelling and mass lesions contribute to raised intracranial pressure, which compromises perfusion, leading to secondary brain injury and further swelling.

managed in non-neurosurgical centres, and this is reflected in NICE guidelines, which recommend early transfer irrespective of the need for surgery.

Control of intracranial pressure

Intubation and ventilation is required early in the management of severe brain injury for airway control. It is often required in moderate brain injury to facilitate the safe management and transfer of unstable and frequently agitated patients and in order to control intracranial pressure. Sedating the patient prevents clinical assessment of intracranial pressure by monitoring of GCS and focal neurological signs, leaving only pupil responses as a guide. It is therefore important that intracranial pressure monitoring is instituted as soon as possible to guide pressure management. This is typically achieved using a bolt ICP monitor, or else an external ventricular drain inserted into the lateral ventricle which also allows drainage of CSF for pressure control. The patient will need measurements of coagulation parameters, platelet count, and CT head available prior to insertion of the probe. A sustained rise of intracranial pressure over 20–25 mmHg is associated with a poor outcome, and maintenance of a cerebral perfusion pressure of at least 60 mmHg is important in preventing secondary injury.

The hierarchy of management strategies for controlling intracranial pressure is set out in Figure 25.10.

Initial measures

Initial measures include positioning the head up 20–30° (reverse Trendelenburg positioning by tilt of the whole bed if the spine has not been cleared). The cervical collar should be loose enough so that it does not restrict venous return. Ventilation is regulated to achieve normocapnia: hypocapnia may be used to achieve transient ICP control in the short term, but the cerebral vasoconstriction which results can produce hypoperfusion and eventual further secondary brain injury. Sedation using a combination of opiates and barbiturates at escalating doses and with boluses to coincide with turns and suctioning will assist in control (Table 25.4).

Friedrich Trendelenburg, 1844–1924, Professor of Surgery successively at Rostock (1875–1882), Bonn (1882–1895), Leipzig (1895–1911), Germany. The Trendelenburg position was first described in 1885.

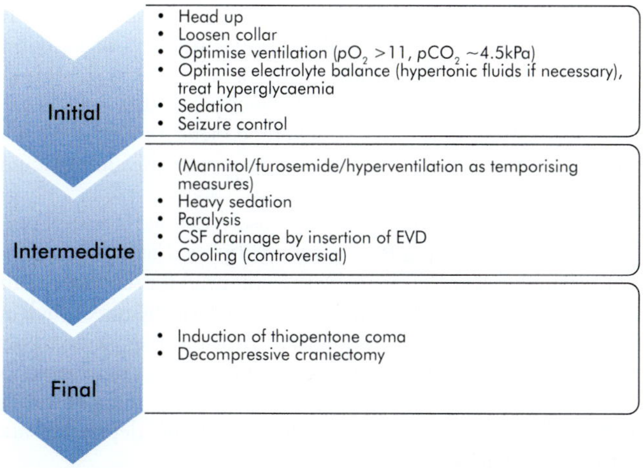

Initial
• Head up
• Loosen collar
• Optimise ventilation (pO_2 >11, pCO_2 ~4.5kPa)
• Optimise electrolyte balance (hypertonic fluids if necessary), treat hyperglycaemia
• Sedation
• Seizure control
Intermediate
• (Mannitol/furosemide/hyperventilation as temporising measures)
• Heavy sedation
• Paralysis
• CSF drainage by insertion of EVD
• Cooling (controversial)
Final
• Induction of thiopentone coma
• Decompressive craniectomy

Figure 25.10 A hierarchy of intracranial pressure management strategies in ventilated head injury patients. CSF, cerebrospinal fluid; EVD, external ventricular drainage.

Table 25.4 Key parameters to maintain in head-injured patients on intensive care.

pCO_2 = 4.5–5.0 kPa
pO_2>11 kPa
MAP = 80–90 mmHg
ICP <20 mmHg
CPP >60 mmHg
[Na+] >140 mmol/L
[K+] >4 mmol/L

Intermediate measures

Where initial measures fail adequately to control ICP, sedation may be escalated and supplemented with paralysis. External ventricular CSF drainage represents a useful adjunct to physiological compensation.

Mannitol can be administered to control ICP temporarily. This is helpful where there is evidence of herniation, such as development of a dilated unresponsive pupil during transfer. 100 mL of 20 per cent mannitol is a typical bolus. Repeated or excessive use is counterproductive because it is an osmotic diuretic and produces hypovolaemia and hypotension. This will compromise cerebral perfusion. Administration of mannitol necessitates catheterising the patient to monitor fluid balance.

Pyrexia increases brain oxygen requirements and cell damage, and so should be avoided. Active induction of therapeutic hypothermia is effective in controlling intracranial pressure, but predisposes to complications including sepsis and coagulopathy so that its overall benefit is not firmly established.

Final measures

Decompressive craniectomy (Figure 25.11) involves removal of a portion of the skull vault and opening of the underlying dura, so that brain swelling can occur without the pressure increases predicted by the Monro Kellie doctrine. Generally, a unilateral or bifrontal decompressive craniectomy is performed, with the bone flap placed subcutaneously in the abdomen, then replaced (cranioplasty) weeks or months later.

Summary box 25.12

On-going management of significant head injury

- The patient should be intubated and ventilated with adequate sedation and pressure monitoring
- The goal of ongoing management is to minimise secondary brain injury
- Key parameters include oxygenation and ventilation, blood pressure and ICP, and electrolyte balance. Pyrexia should be actively controlled
- A hierarchy of management strategies exists to achieve control of intracranial pressure (Figure 25.10)

An alternative strategy for managing uncontrolled intracranial hypertension is induction of thiopentone coma. This carries a high risk of complications and results in the loss of normal EEG activity and pupil responses, compromising ongoing evaluation of the patient.

A multicentre randomised control trial with the aim of establishing the relative effectiveness of these interventions, the Randomised Evaluation of Surgery with Craniectomy for Uncontrollable Elevation of Intra-Cranial Pressure (RESCUE-ICP), is underway (Summary box 25.12).

Pituitary dysfunction: endocrine and metabolic management

Electrolyte imbalance is common in TBI, and contributes to brain swelling and to causing seizures. Diverse mechanisms are involved. Cerebral salt wasting, a poorly understood form of excretory dysregulation in association with brain insult, leads to volume depletion and hyponatraemia.The syndrome of inappropriate antidiuretic hormone (SIADH) leads to water retention

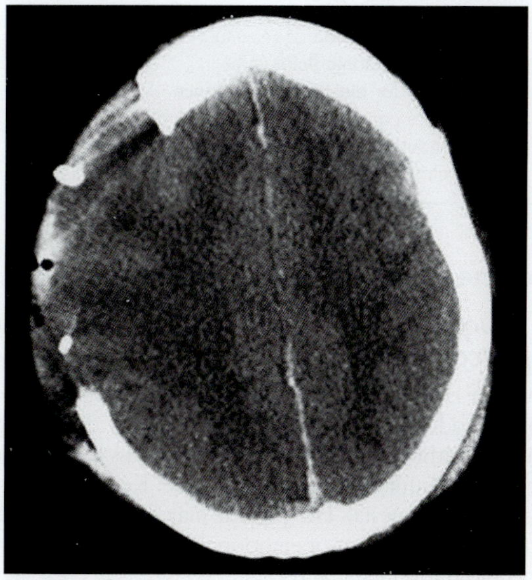

Figure 25.11 Decompressive craniectomy. A right-sided decompressive craniectomy has been performed allowing the swollen right hemisphere to herniate through the skull defect. This procedure can help to control raised intracranial pressure. The bone flap can be stored and replaced at a later date.

and hyponatraemia in the context of pituitary damage. This is of particular concern in head injury since low serum osmotic pressure can contribute to brain swelling, so hypotonic fluids are avoided in this setting. Conversely, antidiuretic hormone (ADH) secretion may be compromised in the context of trauma, producing diabetes insipidus resulting in hypernatraemia. This may be managed with boluses of desmopressin in consultation with endocrine specialists.

All aspects of pituitary function may be compromised in the setting of TBI. Routine screening of pituitary hormone levels and liaison with endocrinology is an important aspect of optimal medical management.

Note that routine, rather than directed, administration of corticosteroids in severe head injury is associated with increased mortality and is not recommended.

Seizures

Seizures may occur early (within 7 days) or late. The cumulative probability is between 2 per cent (mild TBI) and 60 per cent (severe TBI with exacerbating features). Risk factors include injury severity, especially the presence of ICH, and depressed skull fractures and tears of the dura.

Antiepileptics, typically phenytoin, are administered prophylactically to patients at high risk of seizures.

Nutrition

Enteral nutrition is preferred to intravenous parenteral nutrition on grounds of cost and associated complications, and should be commenced within 72 hours of injury. Prokinetics (e.g. metaclopramide, erythromycin) can be administered to promote absorption (Summary box 25.13).

Summary box 25.13

Investigations and prophylactic measures in significant head injury

- Check pituitary function
- Do not give hypotonic fluids
- Monitor daily for electrolyte imbalance
- Antiepileptics can be used prophylactically
- Steroids should not be given routinely
- Enteral nutrition should be started within 72 hours

Outcomes and sequelae

Mild injury: concussion, second impact syndrome and postconcussive syndrome

Concussion is defined as alteration of consciousness as a result of closed head injury, but is generally used in describing mild head injury without imaging abnormalities: loss of consciousness at the time of injury is not a prerequisite. Key features include confusion and amnesia. The patient may be easily distractable, forgetful, slow to interact or emotionally labile. Gait disturbance and incoordination may be seen.

It is claimed that while symptomatic following a head injury, patients may be especially vulnerable to repeat impacts. It is proposed that in the context of disordered cerebral autoregulation, a second minor injury may trigger a form of malignant cerebral oedema refractory to treatment. Although the existence of the syndrome is disputed, and it is certainly rare, it should be considered in advice to individuals engaged in sports or activities carrying a risk of further injury: symptomatic players should not return to play. After a very mild concussion, they should not play again that day; after a severe concussion, they should refrain for the rest of that season (see www.headinjury.com/sports.htm#guidelines).

Postconcussive syndrome is a loosely defined constellation of symptoms, persisting for a prolonged period after injury, and exacerbated in some patients by the potential for secondary gain (compensation). Patients may report somatic features, such as headache, dizziness and disorders of hearing and vision. They may also suffer a variety of neurocognitive and neuropsychological disturbances, including difficulty with concentration and recall, insomnia, emotional lability, fatigue, depression and personality change.

Moderate and severe injury

The long-term sequelae of significant brain injury are likely to include many of the somatic and neurocognitive problems described above, combined with the effect of deficits attributable directly to the primary and secondary injury sustained. Rehabilitation represents a complex and prolonged challenge, requiring multidisciplinary coordination. The Glasgow Outcome Score is used to quantify the degree of recovery achieved after head injury, especially for research purposes, and is detailed in Table 25.5. Good recovery implies independence and potential to return to work rather than a full return to previous capacity (Summary box 25.14).

Table 25.5 Glasgow Outcome Score (GOS).

Good recovery	5
Moderate disability	4
Severe disability	3
Persistent vegetative state	2
Dead	1

Summary box 25.14

Outcomes of a head injury

- Post-concussion syndrome gives persisting headaches and problems in concentrating
- Players concussed when playing sport should not return immediately to the field
- Good recovery is not necessarily a return to normal; it may be independent living

ANEURYSMAL SUBARACHNOID HAEMORRHAGE

'Spontaneous' aneurysmal subarachnoid haemorrhage (SAH) is due to the rupture of an aneurysm in about 80 per cent of cases. In addition to saccular aneurysms discussed below, aneurysms may develop due to infective infiltration of arterial walls in the context of bacteraemia (mycotic aneurysm). This may occur following intravenous drug use or infective endocarditis. Pseudoaneurysms may also develop after trauma or after surgery.

Epidemiology

Berry aneurysms of the circle of Willis develop at branch points in the arterial tree associated with turbulent blood flow (Figure 25.12).

Aneurysmal bleeding has an incidence of 10–15 per 100 000 population per year. Risk factors include age, female sex, hypertension, smoking, cocaine abuse and a family history with two first-degree relatives affected. A range of genetic disorders, in particular adult polycystic kidney disease, fibromuscular dysplasia, neurofibromatosis type 1, Ehlers-Danlos and Marfan syndromes, are known to predispose patients to this condition.

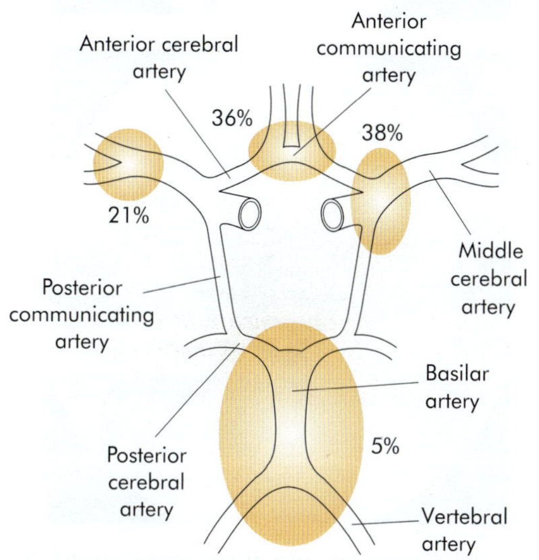

Figure 25.12 Main sites of intracranial supraclinoid aneurysms.

Clinical features

Approximately one third of subarachnoid haemorrhages are incorrectly diagnosed at initial presentation. They are then at high risk of succumbing to early complications, especially a rebleed.

The typical presentation of a subarachnoid haemorrhage includes a 'thunderclap' headache, which is both sudden and severe and is outside the patient's normal experience. Some patients describe prodromal headaches preceding the event, potentially representing aneurysm growth or subclinical bleeds. The sudden onset occurs commonly but not exclusively during exertion, and may be associated with seizure (10 per cent), unresponsiveness (50 per cent) and vomiting (70 per cent). Sometimes it is difficult to establish whether SAH has caused a fall, or whether a fall with head injury is responsible for the SAH.

Neurological examination may be normal ('good clinical grade', see Table 25.6), or the patient may have focal deficits and an impaired conscious level ('poor grade'). The World Federation of Neurosurgical Societies (WFNS) grading of subarachnoid haemorrhage is measured against the condition of the patient after resuscitation rather than at the time of the onset of symptoms (ictus). Often patients are referred to as 'good grade' (WFNS 1-3) or 'poor grade' (WFNS 4 and 5) patients. A painful third nerve palsy points to compression from a posterior communicating artery aneurysm. Meningitic features of neck stiffness and photophobia often develop over hours. Intraocular haemorrhages, classically subhyaloid, may be visible on fundoscopy. The combination of subarachnoid haemorrhage and vitreous haemorrhage is known as Terson syndrome and occurs in 15–20 per cent of patients. Papilloedema should be sought, but may not be evident early in the course of a developing hydrocephalus (Summary box 25.15).

Table 25.6 World Federation of Neurological Surgeons Grading of subarachnoid haemorrhage.

Grade	Glasgow Coma Scale	Focal deficits[a]
I	15	–
II	13–14	–
III	13–14	+
IV	7–12	±
V	3–9	±

[a]Focal deficit = dysphasia or limb weakness.

Summary box 25.15

Subarachnoid haemorrhage

- Most develop from a saccular aneurysm
- They are most common at junctions of the circle of Willis
- Presentation is a thunderclap headache often during exertion
- If neurological examination is normal, the prognosis is good
- Computed tomography (CT) is the investigation of choice

Investigation

CT scan is the imaging of first choice, and, when performed within 12 hours of ictus, will confirm bleeding in more than 98 per cent of cases. This makes a diagnostic lumbar puncture unnecessary (Figure 25.13).

The sensitivity of CT scan, however, deteriorates to less than 50 per cent at 1 week after a bleed. In light of this, patients with a suggestive history and negative CT scan will require lumbar

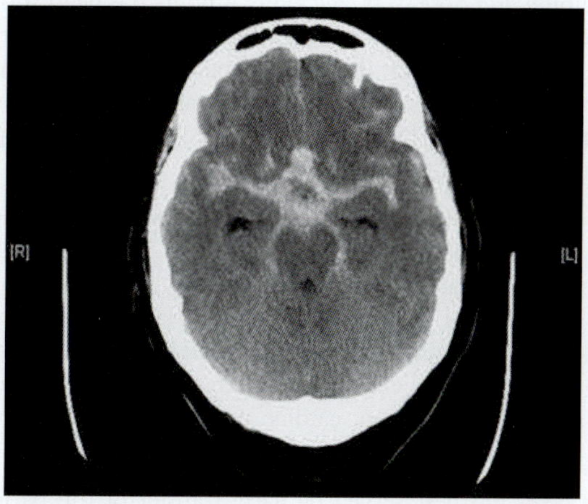

Figure 25.13 Diffuse subarachnoid bleeding from a ruptured anterior communicating artery aneurysm extends to the prepontine and ambient cisterns around the brainstem, and into both Sylvian fissures.

puncture, especially where presentation is delayed. The CSF supernatant should be analysed by spectrophotometry (visual inspection is not reliable) for the spectra of haemoglobin breakdown products oxyhaemoglobin and bilirubin. These are clearly detectable in samples taken at least 6 and preferably 12 hours after subarachnoid haemorrhage, but not in CSF mixed with fresh blood due to traumatic puncture and analysed immediately. Failure to exclude subarachnoid haemorrhage with an appropriate delayed lumbar puncture may necessitate formal cerebral angiography, and the risks this entails.

Catheter angiography generally involves access to both vertebral and carotid arteries through the femoral artery under local anaesthetic. This allows visualisation of the vascular anatomy by injection of contrast medium with simultaneous x-ray screening (Figures 25.14 and 25.15). The serious potential risks include ischaemic stroke or arterial dissection (1–2 per cent), and renal failure or allergic reactions attributable to contrast.

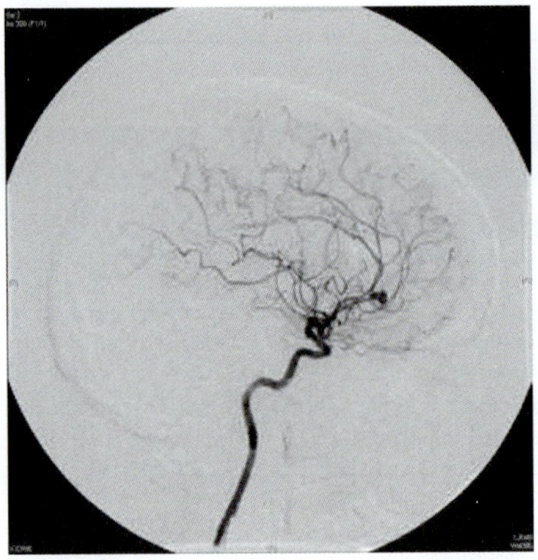

Figure 25.14 There is a small saccular aneurysm of the pericallosal branch of the anterior cerebral artery.

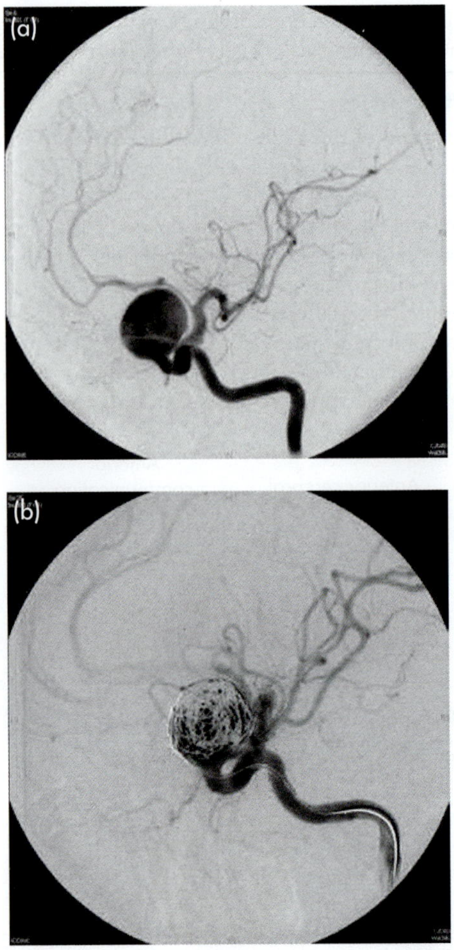

Figure 25.15 (a) A giant aneurysm of the internal carotid; (b) angiographic embolisation (coiling) of the giant aneurysm. Note the single displaced coil passing into the distal ICA (internal carotid artery) and then the MCA (middle cerebral artery).

Management

Patients should be placed on bed rest with hourly neurological observations. They require strict input–output monitoring and intravenous fluid replacement with normal saline initially. Oral nimodipine at a dose of 60 mg every 4 hours has been shown to reduce the rate of poor outcome associated with delayed neurological ischaemic deficit due to cerebral vasospasm. Analgesics, laxatives, antiemetics, gastric protection and compression stockings are also likely to be necessary. After resuscitation, the priorities in subarachnoid haemorrhage are:

- to prevent rebleeding by identifying and controlling any underlying lesion;
- to recognise and manage:
  - neurological complications, especially vasospasm (or delayed ischaemic neurologic deficit) and hydrocephalus;
  - systemic complications, including electrolyte imbalance, severe hypertension, cardiac infarct and arrhythmia, and neurogenic pulmonary oedema.

These goals are best served by early transfer of the patient to a neurosurgical centre. In elderly patients with a poor WFNS grade, a decision to offer only supportive management may be appropriate.

Prevention of rebleed

CT angiography (CTA) has a high sensitivity for aneurysms and arteriovenous malformations (AVMs), but digital subtraction angiography (DSA) remains the gold standard.

Aneurysms demonstrated may be removed from the circulation surgically by craniotomy and 'clipping', or by endovascular embolization, also known as 'coiling'. Sometimes, mesh stents may also be used to help secure the metal coils within the aneurysm sac as part of this procedure. Class 1 evidence suggesting a lower risk of poor outcomes, at least for small anterior circulation aneurysms, has driven the uptake of coiling. However, a surgical approach remains necessary or preferable in many cases. A rebleed risk of 4 per cent in the first 24 hours, then 1.5 per cent per day thereafter is quoted for aneurysms, and 80 per cent of patients who rebleed have an eventual poor outcome. For this reason, and to permit optimal management of complications discussed later, the current consensus favours early intervention, despite the surgical challenges presented by brain swelling and blood load (Summary box 25.16).

Identification and management of complications

After subarachnoid haemorrhage, even initially good grade patients may deteriorate rapidly due to reversible neurological

Summary box 25.16

Treatment of subarachnoid haemorrhage

- Early securing of the responsible aneurysm reduces the risk of rebleed and is necessary for management of later vasospasm
- Endovascular treatment ('coiling') is generally preferred over craniotomy and clipping for aneurysms amenable to this approach
- 'Good grade' patients commonly suffer poor outcomes, primarily as a result of cerebral vasospasm

or systemic complications. They should be managed in a neurosurgical unit, and will require careful neurological observation, on a high dependency unit where possible. The approach to a patient who has deteriorated should follow standard principles of resuscitation, with consideration paid to the high incidence of electrolyte imbalance, cardiac infarcts and arrhythmias, and neurogenic pulmonary oedema in this group. Neurological deterioration should prompt a repeat scan to exclude evidence of rebleeding and of hydrocephalus. This is typically the communicating type, which is a common sequel of haemorrhage. Where these complications are not demonstrated, deterioration is often attributable to delayed ischaemic neurological deficit (DNID), which commonly develops 3–10 days after aneurysmal haemorrhage and can progress rapidly to infarction. The process is attributed to cerebral vasospasm in response to, and correlating with, the blood load. This process can be visualised angiographically, and the velocity of blood flow in the cerebral vasculature, measured using transcranial Doppler ultrasound (TCDs), provides an indirect assessment of the degree of stenosis. Outcomes are optimised by the prophylactic administration of nimodipine and maintenance of fluid volume, typically with 2.5–3 L/day of normal saline. In established vasospasm, the goal is to maintain cerebral perfusion. Practically this involves maintaining mean arterial pressure with aggressive fluid replacement and inotropes. This is done by the administration of fluid and inotropes. This strategy would risk rerupturing an unsecured underlying aneurysm, a factor weighing in favour of early clipping or coiling. Hyponatraemia is a frequent complication of subarachnoid haemorrhage, attributed to cerebral salt wasting in the context of fluid depletion, and otherwise to the syndrome of inappropriate antidiuretic hormone secretion. This is associated with a higher incidence of DNID, and practical management, irrespective of the underlying pathology, is based on sodium replacement, with hypertonic infusions if necessary. Fluid restriction is not appropriate in these patients since this risks further compromising perfusion (Summary box 25.17).

Summary box 25.17

Complications of subarachnoid haemorrhage

- Electrolyte imbalance, cardiac arrhythmias and neurogenic pulmonary oedema are common
- Neurological deterioration may indicate a communicating hydrocephalus
- Delayed ischaemic neurological deficit (DNID) is attributed to vasospasm of the cerebral vasculature typically developing 3–10 days post ictus. It is the main cause of poor outcome in good grade subarachnoid patients
- After securing the aneurysm, perfusion can be maintained in the context of vasospasm by artificial elevation of the arterial blood pressure

Prognosis

Overall survival of subarachnoid haemorrhage is about 50 per cent and one third of survivors remain dependent. Only 50 per cent of WFNS grade 1 patients return to work. Treated aneurysms can regrow and rebleed, especially after coiling, so that a program of surveillance is necessary.

A distinct subgroup of SAH patients suffer bleeds confined to the basal cisterns anterior to the midbrain and pons, without an underlying lesion evident on angiogram. This is termed 'perimesencephalic SAH', and is believed to represent venous bleeding. It has an excellent prognosis.

Unruptured aneurysms represent a thorny management problem: incidentally detected small anterior circulation aneurysms represent a minimal bleeding risk. Screening, even in high risk groups, is therefore of questionable benefit.

OTHER SPONTANEOUS INTRACRANIAL HAEMORRHAGE

Intracerebral haemorrhage

Intracerebral haemorrhage may be spontaneous or traumatic. The former accounts for a 10–15 per cent of strokes and has a mortality of 40 per cent at one year. The majority occur in the context of hypertension or amyloid angiopathy, or as a complication of ischaemic stroke. Coagulation disorders, especially patients being treated with warfarin, are a major risk factor (Summary box 25.18).

Summary box 25.18

Intracerebral haemorrhage

- These account for 10–15 per cent of strokes
- The presentation, as for ischaemic stroke, may include focal neurological deficit with or without decreased conscious level
- High blood pressure may be chronic so should only be reduced with care
- Diagnosis is by computed tomography
- Anticoagulants should be reversed at once
- Craniotomy and evacuation is especially useful in young patients

Patients typically present with sudden focal deficit and reduced conscious level. Following initial resuscitation, these patients will require CT scan to establish the diagnosis, and the size and position of the bleed (Figure 25.16). They require reversal of anticoagulation, on-going hourly neurological observations and blood pressure monitoring. High blood pressure may be longstanding and associated with adaptations to autoregulation, so attempts at lowering it acutely with intravenous antihypertensives should be made only if the values are very high (e.g. MAP >130 mmHg).

Craniotomy and evacuation is used to alleviate raised intracranial pressure, just as it can be in a subgroup of patients with ischaemic strokes in the posterior fossa or in the middle cerebral artery territory. Surgery has no role in addressing focal deficits corresponding to direct damage from the bleed itself. Young patients with haematomas close to the cortical surface, demonstrating progressive neurological deterioration, represent good surgical candidates. Posterior fossa clot is also a strong indication for surgery because of the potential for rapid deterioration due to brainstem compression and hydrocephalus. A substantial minority of intracerebral bleeds are attributable to focal vascular lesions, and this must be considered when planning any surgery.

Vascular malformations

Vascular malformations are usually congenital in origin, with certain key exceptions discussed below. They may present with headaches, pulsatile tinnitus, seizures or focal deficit, or else acutely with rupture and haemorrhage.

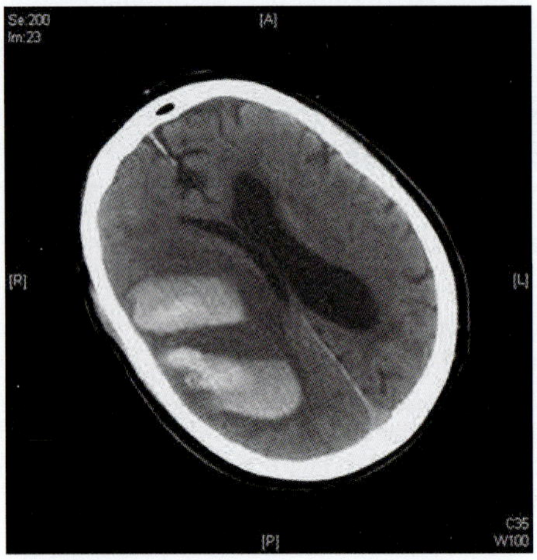

Figure 25.16 Large acute intracerebral haemorrhages in the right frontal and parietal lobes are evident, with surrounding oedema and midline shift.

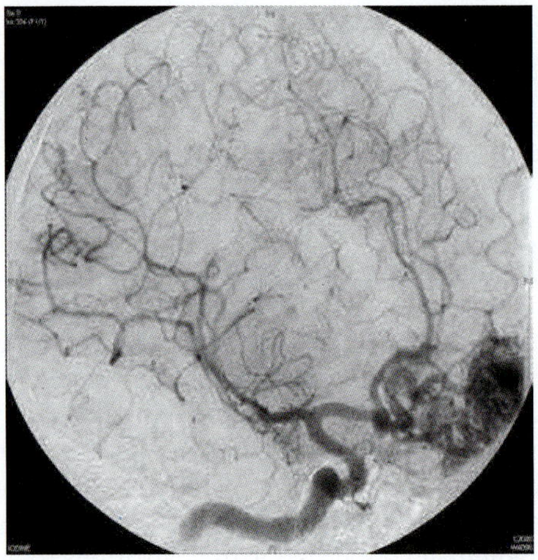

Figure 25.17 An arteriovenous malformation supplied by the anterior cerebral, middle cerebral and middle meningeal arteries is demonstrated at the 4 o'clock position in this angiogram.

Arteriovenous malformations are responsible for about 10 per cent of subarachnoid haemorrhages. Vessels and calcification may be apparent on CT or magnetic resonance imaging (MRI), and the lesion is confirmed on angiography (Figure 25.17).

When AVMs present with bleeding, there is an approximate 4 per cent risk of rebleed per annum. The risk is particularly high in the first 6 weeks, and where the bleed is from an aneurysm related to the AVM. This fact often weighs against treatment by radiosurgery, which typically takes more than one year to achieve complete occlusion, but may nevertheless be applied to some small, deep AVMs. Endovascular embolisation, with tissue glue, is often a useful first-line therapy, but carries significant risks and rarely achieves complete and permanent obliteration. Most patients will therefore ultimately require craniotomy, taking into account the risks of deficit associated with operation. These may be predicted using the Spetzler–Martin grading system, which is based on the size of the lesion, the eloquence of adjacent brain, and the pattern of venous drainage.

Vein of Galen malformations are AVMs feeding into an embryological venous remnant dorsal to the brainstem presenting in childhood. High-flow malformations may cause cardiac failure. They may be treated by embolisation.

Dural arteriovenous fistulae (DAVFs) are shunts between dural arteries and veins or sinuses. They are proposed to arise as a result of vessel remodelling in response to dural sinus thrombosis and subsequent recanalisation. They may present with subarachnoid, intracerebral or subdural bleeding, or with headache and pulsatile tinnitus. A carotid cavernous fistula is a spontaneous or traumatic DAVF between the internal carotid artery and surrounding cavernous sinus, typically producing eye pain, ocular muscle palsies and exophthalmos. Angiography is diagnostic.

Cavernomas (Figure 25.18) are venous anomalies, demonstrated on MRI, but not with angiography, which may require operation if they cause progressive deficits, intractable epilepsy or recurrent bleeding.

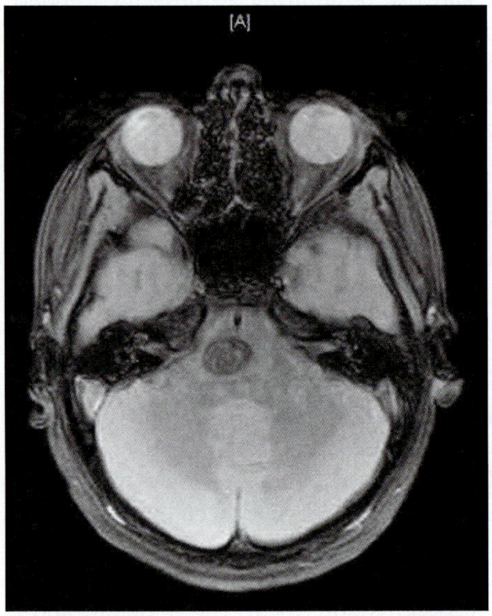

Figure 25.18 A brainstem cavernoma.

Related lesions, usually clinically silent, include developmental venous anomalies (DVAs) and capillary telangectasia.

SUMMARY

The guiding principle of management for neurosurgical emergencies is the prevention of secondary injury by ensuring satisfactory brain perfusion. This demands immediate attention to blood pressure and oxygenation, as reflected in the ATLS resuscitation algorithms, as well as intracranial pressure management. Early imaging to identify treatable pathology and timely discussion with the local Neurosurgery Centre are key to outcome.

ACKNOWLEDGEMENTS

The authors are indebted to John Leach, Consultant Neurosurgeon, Salford Hospital, Manchester, for his contributions to the structure and content of this chapter.

> No head injury is too slight to neglect, or too severe to be despaired of
>
> *Hippocrates*

CHAPTER

26 Neck and spine

LEARNING OBJECTIVES

To be familiar with:
- The accurate assessment of spinal trauma
- The pathophysiology and types of spinal cord injury
- The basic management of spinal trauma and the major pitfalls
- The prognosis of spinal cord injury, factors affecting functional outcome, and common associated complications

EPIDEMIOLOGY OF SPINAL CORD INJURY

The incidence of spinal cord injury ranges between 27 and 47 cases per million per year. Road traffic accidents remain the leading cause of spinal cord injuries worldwide. Males in the third decade of life are the most likely group to sustain serious spinal cord injury.

EVOLUTION OF THE MANAGEMENT OF SPINAL CORD INJURY

There is clear evidence to show that fewer complications, decreased length of stay, and improved patient outcome occur in patients treated in specialised spinal centres (Summary box 26.1).

Summary box 26.1

Spinal cord injury

- Incidence of spinal cord injury remains constant
- Outcome is improved in regional/national spinal cord injury centres

ANATOMY OF THE SPINE AND SPINAL CORD

Spinal column anatomy

The vertebral column is composed of a series of motion segments (Figure 26.1). A motion segment consists of two adjacent vertebrae, their intervertebral disc and ligamentous restraints (Figure 26.2).

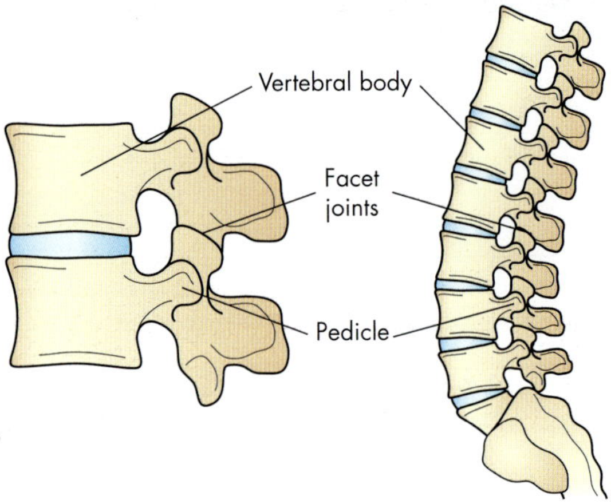

Figure 26.1 The spinal motion segment.

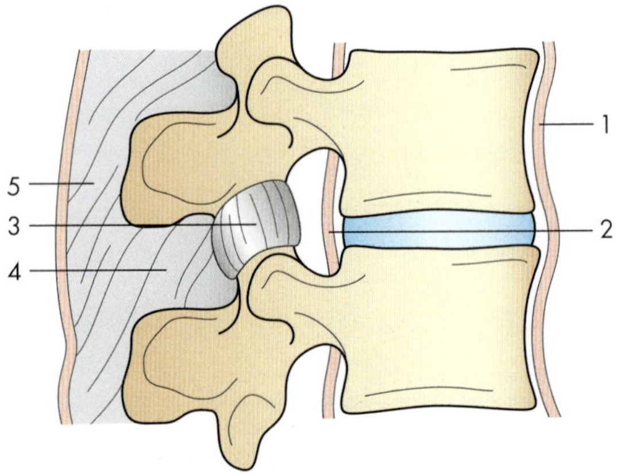

Figure 26.2 Ligamentous spinal restraints. (1) Anterior longitudinal ligament, (2) intervertebral disc and posterior longitudinal ligament, (3) facet joint capsule, (4) interspinous ligament, (5) supraspinous ligament.

Regional variations

Upper cervical spine anatomy is designed to facilitate motion (Figure 26.3), and stability here is dependent on ligamentous restraints (Figure 26.4). Vertebral anatomy from C3 to C7 is similar. The cervicothoracic junction is a transitional zone from mobile to fixed and is thus prone to injury. It may be difficult to visualise this area on x-ray (Figure 26.5).

The thoracolumbar junction is also prone to injury and is the most common area of injury outside the cervical spine (Figure 26.6).

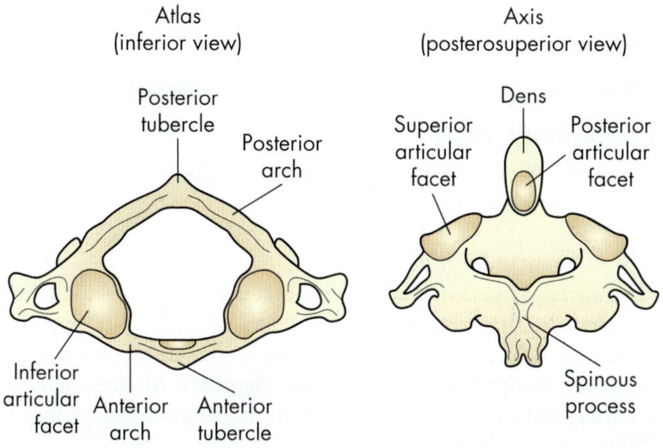

Figure 26.3 Atlantoaxial bony anatomy.

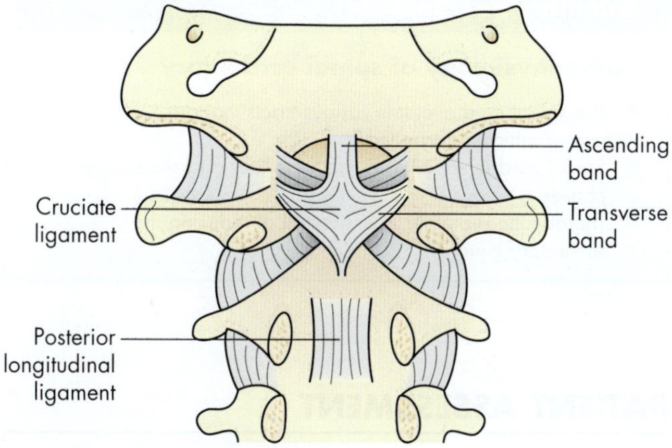

Figure 26.4 Atlantoaxial ligaments.

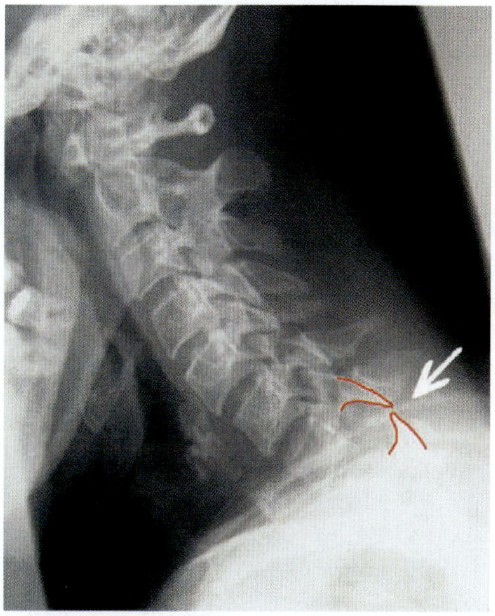

Figure 26.5 Cervicothoracic facet subluxation (easily missed with inadequate x-rays).

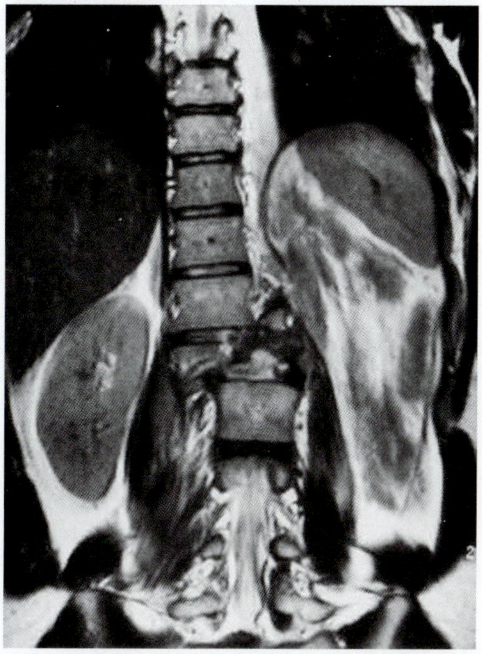

Figure 26.6 Coronal T2-weighted magnetic resonance image demonstrating a fracture dislocation at the thoracolumbar junction.

The three column concept of spinal stability

The spinal column can be divided into three columns: anterior, middle and posterior (Figure 26.7). When all three columns are injured the spine is unstable. Instability may also exist in some two-column injuries (Summary box 26.2).

Summary box 26.2

Spinal column anatomy

- Upper cervical spine stability is dependent on ligamentous restraints
- The cervicothoracic and thoracolumbar junctions are prone to injury

Spinal neuroanatomy

The spinal cord extends from the foramen magnum to the T12/L1 junction where it ends as the conus medullaris (Figure 26.8). Below this level lies the cauda equina. Figure 26.9 illustrates a cross-section of the spinal cord. The lateral spinothalamic tracts transmit the sensation of pain and temperature, the lateral corticospinal tracts are responsible for motor function, and the posterior columns transmit, position, vibration and deep pressure sensation.

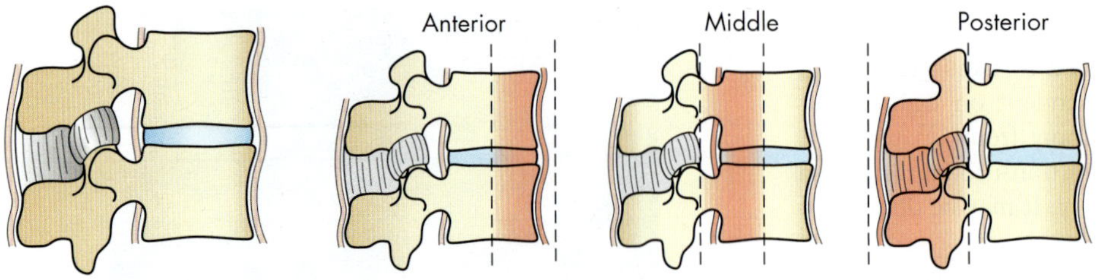

Figure 26.7 The three-column model of spinal stability.

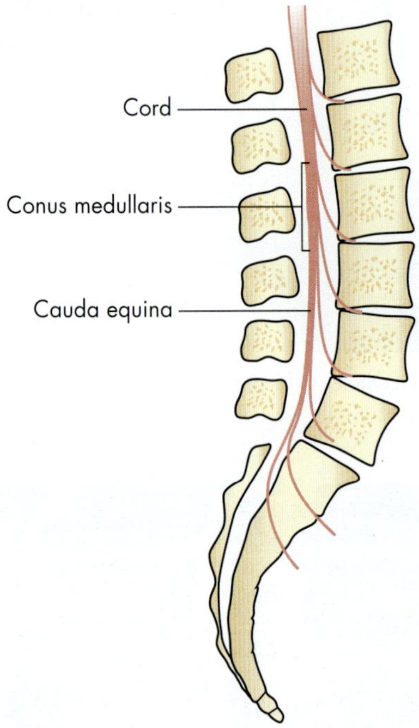

Figure 26.8 The spinal cord ends at T12/L1 at the conus medullaris which gives rise to the cauda equina.

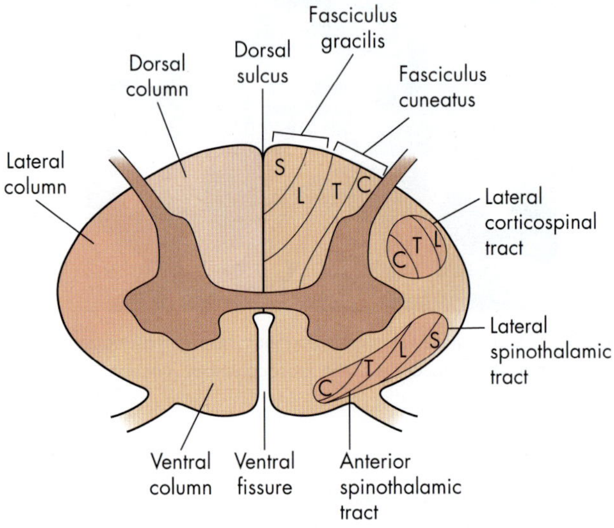

Figure 26.9 A cross-section of the spinal cord.

The spinothalamic tracts cross to the opposite side of the spinal cord within three levels of entering the cord. In contrast, the corticospinal tracts and the posterior columns decussate proximally at the craniocervical level. The tracts are topographically arranged; proximal body function is represented centrally with distal body function arranged peripherally.

Pathophysiology of spinal cord injury

The primary injury

This is the direct insult to the neural elements and occurs at the time of the initial injury.

The secondary injury

Haemorrhage, oedema and ischaemia results in a biochemical cascade that causes the secondary injury. This may be accentuated by hypotension, hypoxia, spinal instability and/or persistent compression of the neural elements. Management of a spinal cord injury must focus on minimising secondary injury (Summary box 26.3).

Summary box 26.3

Pathophysiology of spinal cord injury

- The spinal cord contains various tracts that are topographically arranged
- Spinal cord injury involves both primary and secondary phases
- Therapeutic strategies are directed at reducing the secondary injury

PATIENT ASSESSMENT

Basic points

Advanced Trauma Life Support (ATLS) principles apply in all cases (Chapter 23). The spine should initially be immobilised on the assumption that every trauma patient has a spinal injury until proven otherwise (Figure 26.10). The finding of a spinal injury makes it more likely (not less) that there will be a second injury at another level.

Spinal boards lead to skin breakdown in insensate patients, and are very uncomfortable for those with normal sensation. Therefore, they are for very short-term use only (Figure 26.11).

The unconscious patient

Definitive clearance of the spine may not be possible in the initial stages and spinal immobilisation should then be maintained, until magnetic resonance imaging (MRI) or equivalent can be used to rule out an unstable spinal injury (Summary box 26.4).

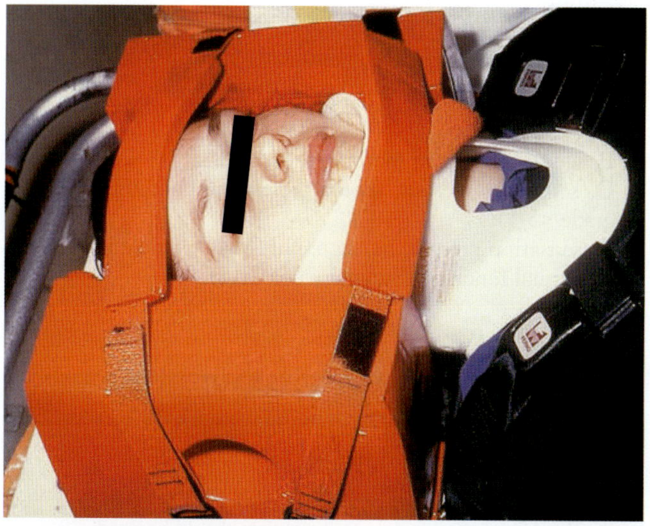

Figure 26.10 Spinal immobilisation.

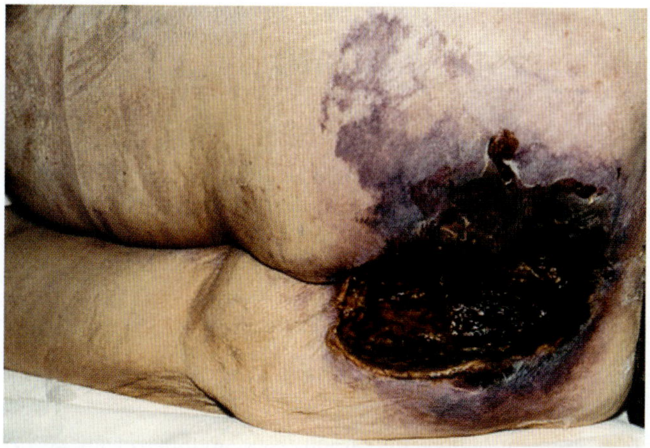

Figure 26.11 Pressure sores and ulcers may develop rapidly in insensate patients.

Summary box 26.4

Patient assessment

- Use Advanced Trauma Life Support (ATLS) principles in all cases of spinal injury
- In polytrauma cases, suspect a spinal injury
- A second spinal injury at a remote level may be present in 10 per cent of cases
- Spinal boards cause pressure sores

PERTINENT HISTORY

The mechanism and velocity of injury should be determined at an early stage. A check for the presence of spinal pain should be made. The onset and duration of neurological symptoms should also be recorded.

PHYSICAL EXAMINATION

Initial assessment

The primary survey always takes precedence, followed by careful systems examination, paying particular attention to the abdomen and chest. Spinal cord injury may mask signs of intra-abdominal injury.

Identification of shock

Three categories of shock may occur in spinal trauma:

1. **Hypovolaemic shock**. Hypotension with tachycardia and cold clammy peripheries. This is most often due to haemorrhage. It should be treated with appropriate resuscitation.
2. **Neurogenic shock**. This presents with hypotension, a normal heart rate or bradycardia and warm peripheries. This is due to unopposed vagal tone resulting from cervical spinal cord injury above the level of sympathetic outflow (C7/T1). It should be treated with inotropic support, and care should be taken to avoid fluid overload.
3. **Spinal shock**. There is initial loss of all neurological function below the level of the injury. It is characterised by paralysis, hypotonia and areflexia. It usually lasts 24 hours following spinal cord injury. Once it has resolved the bulbocavernosus reflex (Figure 26.12) returns.

Spinal examination

The entire spine must be palpated and the overlying skin inspected. A formal spinal log roll must be performed to achieve this (Figure 26.13). Significant swelling, tenderness, palpable steps or gaps suggest a spinal injury. Wounds may be part of penetrating trauma. Seat belt marks on the abdomen and chest must be noted, as these suggest a high energy accident.

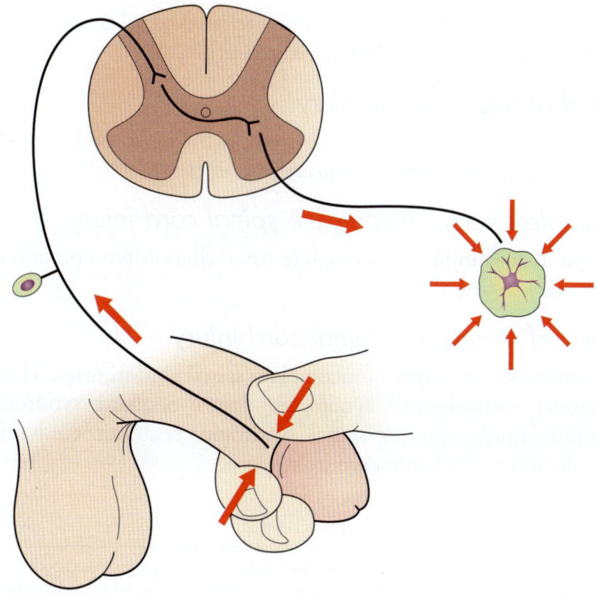

Figure 26.12 The bulbocavernosus reflex (this can be elicited in females by traction on the Foley catheter).

Eugene Basil Foley, 1891–1966, urologist, Anker Hospital, St Louis, MN, USA.

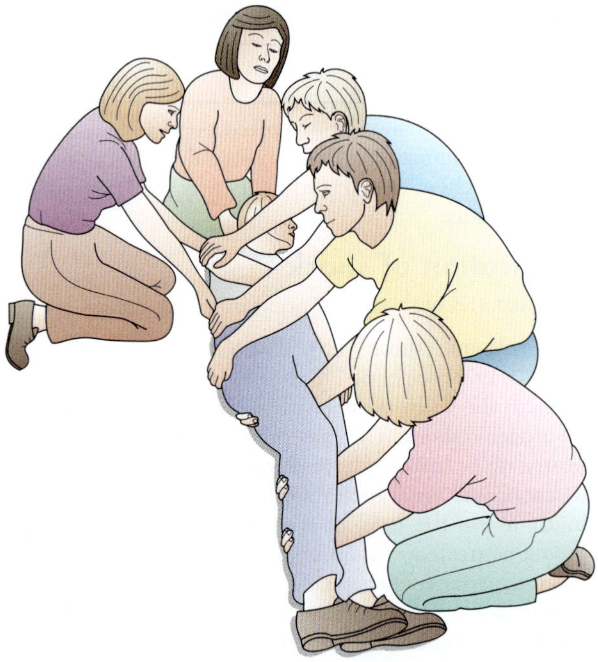

Figure 26.13 Spinal log roll.

Neurological examination

The American Spinal Injury Association (ASIA) neurological evaluation system (Figure 26.14) is an internationally accepted method of neurological evaluation.

Motor function is assessed using the Medical Research Council (MRC) grading system (0–5) in key muscle groups (Figure 26.14). A motor score can then be calculated (maximum 100).

Sensory function (light touch and pin prick) is assessed using the dermatomal map (Figure 26.14). A total sensory score is then calculated.

Rectal examination is performed to assess anal tone, voluntary anal contraction and perianal sensation.

Level of neurological injury

The level of neurological injury is simply the most caudal neurological level with normal neurological function.

Complete versus incomplete spinal cord injury

A spinal cord injury is incomplete when there is preservation of perianal sensation.

Type of incomplete spinal cord injury

There are several types of incomplete spinal cord injuries. These include: central cord syndrome, Brown-Séquard syndrome (hemisection), anterior spinal syndrome, posterior cord syndrome and cauda equina syndrome.

Charles Edward Brown-Séquard, 1817–1894, was a physiologist and neurologist who held a number of academic posts. He came from Mauritius and in his dotage reported enhanced sexual prowess after treating himself with extract of monkey testis. Some therefore think of him as the father of endocrinology.

Level of neurological impairment

The ASIA neurological impairment scale is based on the Frankel classification of spinal cord injury:

- **A**, complete;
- **B**, sensation present motor absent;
- **C**, sensation present, motor present but not useful (MRC grade <3/5);
- **D**, sensation present, motor useful (MRC grade ≥3/5);
- **E**, normal function (Summary box 26.5).

Summary box 26.5

Physical examination

- There are three types of shock following spinal cord injury
- The ASIA neurological scoring system should be used
- Functional motor power is grade 3/5 or higher

DIAGNOSTIC IMAGING

Plain radiographs

A full cervical spine series includes anteroposterior and lateral views of the whole cervical spine, and open mouth views. However, in many trauma centres computed tomography (CT) scanning, with sagittal reformats, is considered more accurate. This modality is particularly useful in visualising the cervicothoracic junction and in surveying the entire spine.

A system for evaluation of the lateral cervical spine x-ray

1 Assessment of prevertebral soft tissue swelling (Figure 26.15)
2 Assess sagittal alignment using three imaginary lines (Figure 26.16)
3 Assess for instability (Figure 26.17):
   a 3.5 mm of sagittal translation;
   b Sagittal angulation of >11° (compared to adjacent level).

Computed tomography

CT scanning with two-dimensional reconstruction remains the most sensitive imaging modality in spinal trauma (Figure 26.18).

Magnetic resonance imaging

MRI is indicated in cases with neurological deficit and where assessment of ligamentous structures is important (Figure 26.19) (Summary box 26.6).

Summary box 26.6

Diagnostic imaging of spinal injuries

- Clear visualisation of the cervicothoracic junction is mandatory
- Plain cervical spine radiographs fail to identity 15 per cent of injuries

Hans Ludwing Frankel, formerly clinical director, The National Spinal Injuries Centre, Stoke Mandeville, UK.

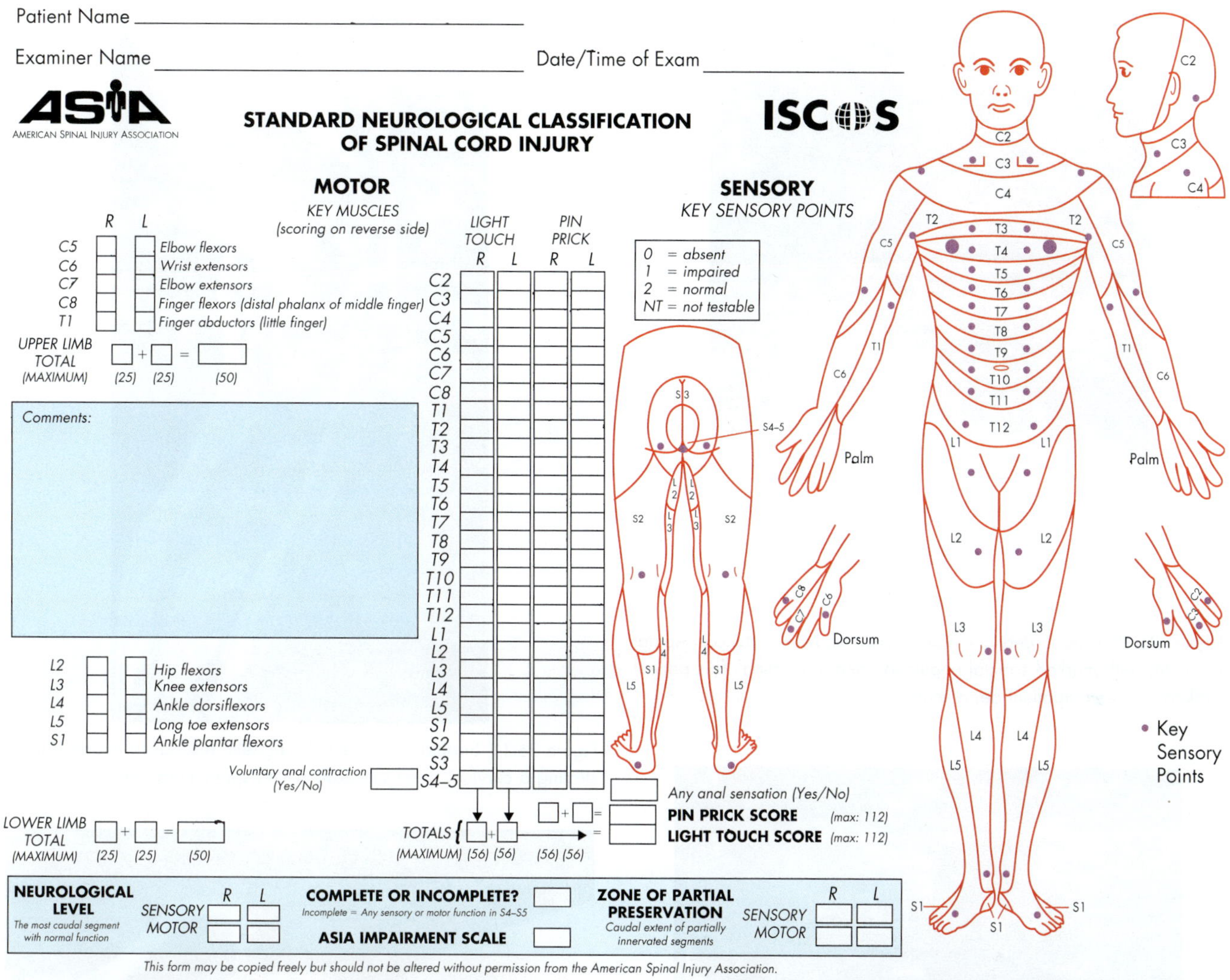
Patient Name
Examiner Name
Date/Time of Exam
ASIA
AMERICAN SPINAL INJURY ASSOCIATION
STANDARD NEUROLOGICAL CLASSIFICATION OF SPINAL CORD INJURY
ISCOS
MOTOR
KEY MUSCLES
(scoring on reverse side)
R L
C5 Elbow flexors
C6 Wrist extensors
C7 Elbow extensors
C8 Finger flexors (distal phalanx of middle finger)
T1 Finger abductors (little finger)
UPPER LIMB TOTAL (MAXIMUM) (25) (25) (50)
Comments:
L2 Hip flexors
L3 Knee extensors
L4 Ankle dorsiflexors
L5 Long toe extensors
S1 Ankle plantar flexors
Voluntary anal contraction (Yes/No)
LOWER LIMB TOTAL (MAXIMUM) (25) (25) (50)
LIGHT TOUCH R L
PIN PRICK R L
C2 C3 C4 C5 C6 C7 C8 T1 T2 T3 T4 T5 T6 T7 T8 T9 T10 T11 T12 L1 L2 L3 L4 L5 S1 S2 S3 S4–5
TOTALS (MAXIMUM) (56) (56) (56) (56)
SENSORY
KEY SENSORY POINTS
0 = absent
1 = impaired
2 = normal
NT = not testable
Any anal sensation (Yes/No)
PIN PRICK SCORE (max: 112)
LIGHT TOUCH SCORE (max: 112)
Palm
Dorsum
Key Sensory Points
NEUROLOGICAL LEVEL
The most caudal segment with normal function
SENSORY
MOTOR
R L
COMPLETE OR INCOMPLETE?
Incomplete = Any sensory or motor function in S4–S5
ASIA IMPAIRMENT SCALE
ZONE OF PARTIAL PRESERVATION
Caudal extent of partially innervated segments
SENSORY
MOTOR
This form may be copied freely but should not be altered without permission from the American Spinal Injury Association.

Figure 26.14 American Spinal Injury Association neurological evaluation.

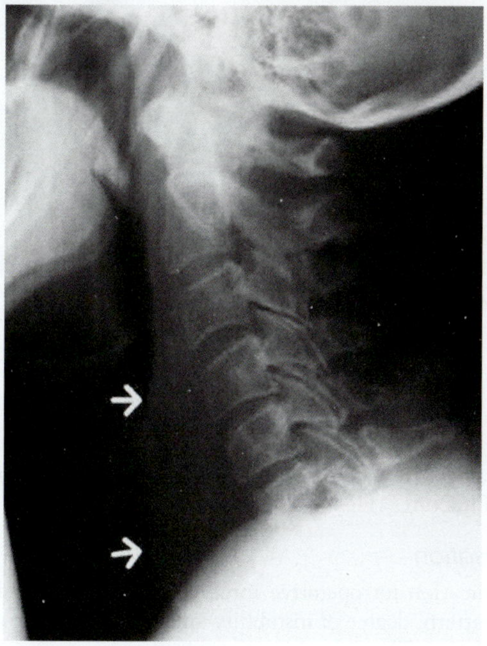

Figure 26.15 Large prevertebral haematoma.

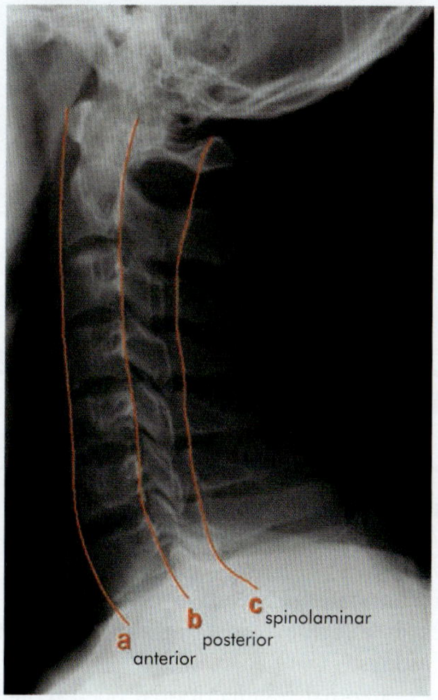

Figure 26.16 The anterior, posterior and spinolaminar lines are useful in identifying anterior translation on lateral x-rays of the neck.

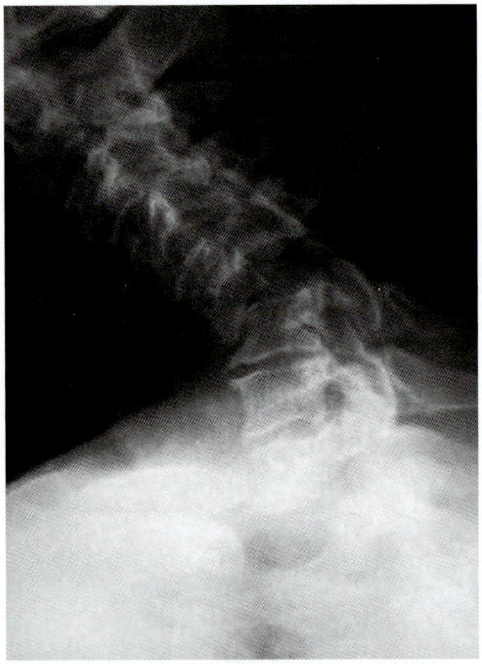

Figure 26.17 Lateral cervical spine x-ray showing obvious spinal instability with marked sagittal angulation and translation. This patient walked into the outpatient department.

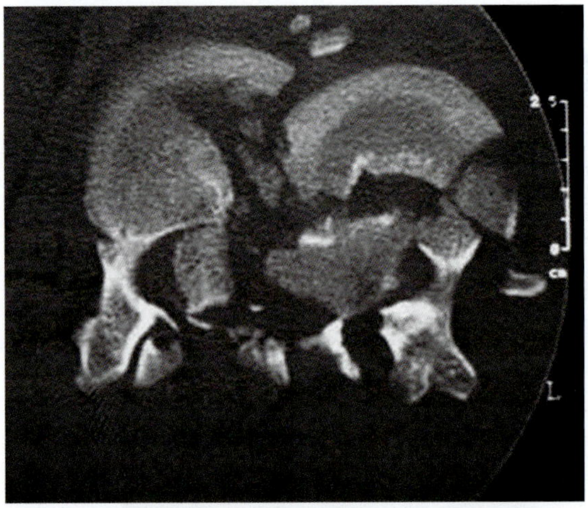

Figure 26.18 Axial computed tomography scan demonstrating a thoracolumbar fracture dislocation.

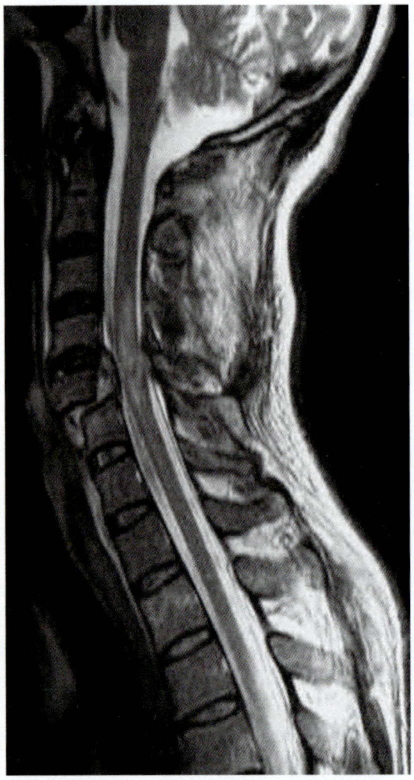

Figure 26.19 Sagittal T2-weighted magnetic resonance image demonstrating a cervical spine subluxation and spinal cord contusion.

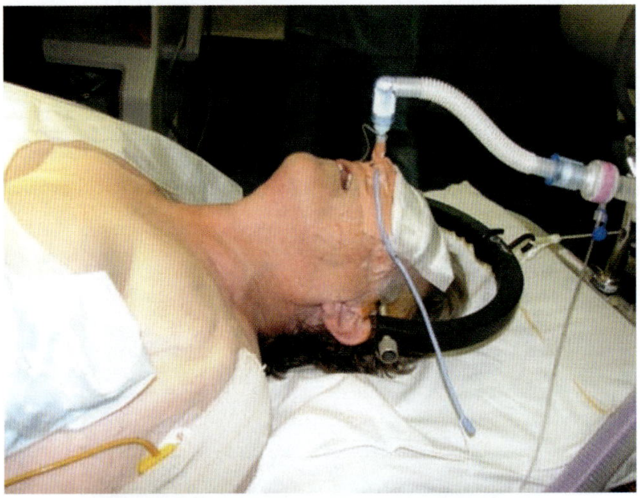

Figure 26.20 Skeletal traction using skull tongs.

CLASSIFICATION AND MANAGEMENT OF SPINAL AND SPINAL CORD INJURIES

Basic managenent principles

Spinal realignment

In cases of cervical spine subluxation or dislocation, skeletal traction is necessary to achieve anatomical realignment. This is done using skull tongs (Figure 26.20).

In many cases of spinal trauma, formal open reduction and stabilisation using internal fixation is also required (Figure 26.21).

A halo brace can be used to hold a closed realignment of cervical fractures (Figure 26.22).

Stabilisation

The indication for operative intervention is influenced by the injury pattern, degree of instability and the presence of a neurological deficit. The only absolute indication for surgery in spinal trauma is deteriorating neurological function.

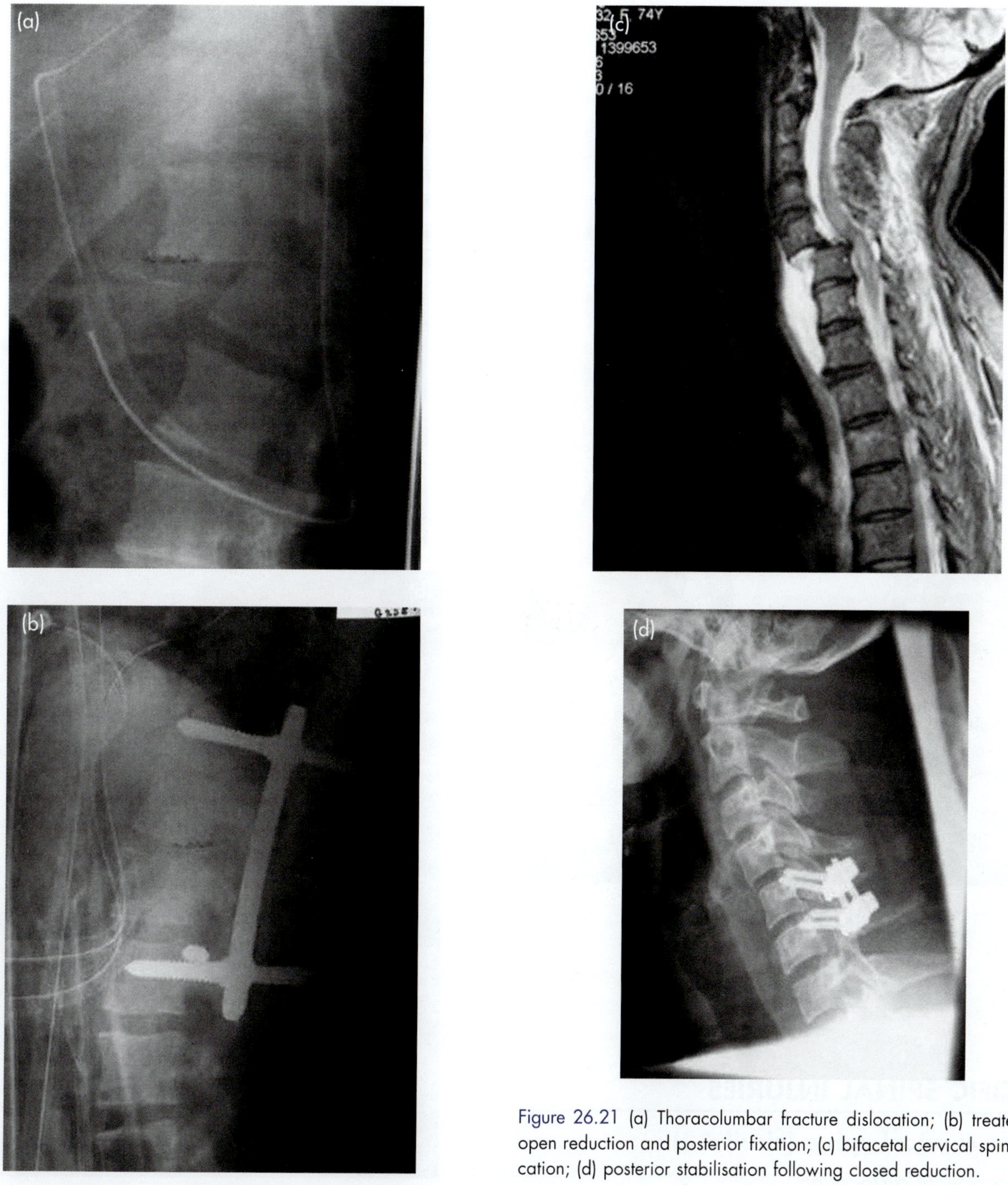

Figure 26.21 (a) Thoracolumbar fracture dislocation; (b) treated with open reduction and posterior fixation; (c) bifacetal cervical spine dislocation; (d) posterior stabilisation following closed reduction.

Decompression of the neural elements

Decompression involves spinal realignment and/or direct decompression of the neural elements (Figure 26.23). The timing of surgery in spinal cord trauma remains controversial.

Corticosteroids

Many spinal trauma centres no longer use steroids in cases of spinal cord injury due to lack of evidence to support efficacy (Summary box 26.7).

Summary box 26.7

Management of spinal trauma

- Neurological deficit determines management
- Deteriorating neurological status requires surgical intervention
- Corticosteroids are ineffective

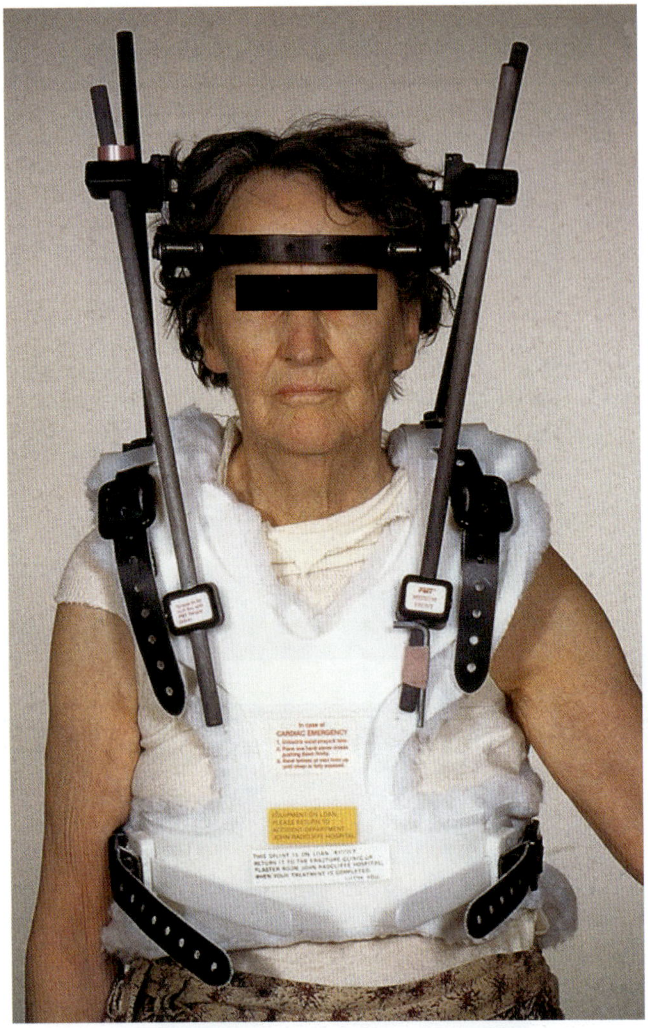

Figure 26.22 External immobilisation using a halo jacket.

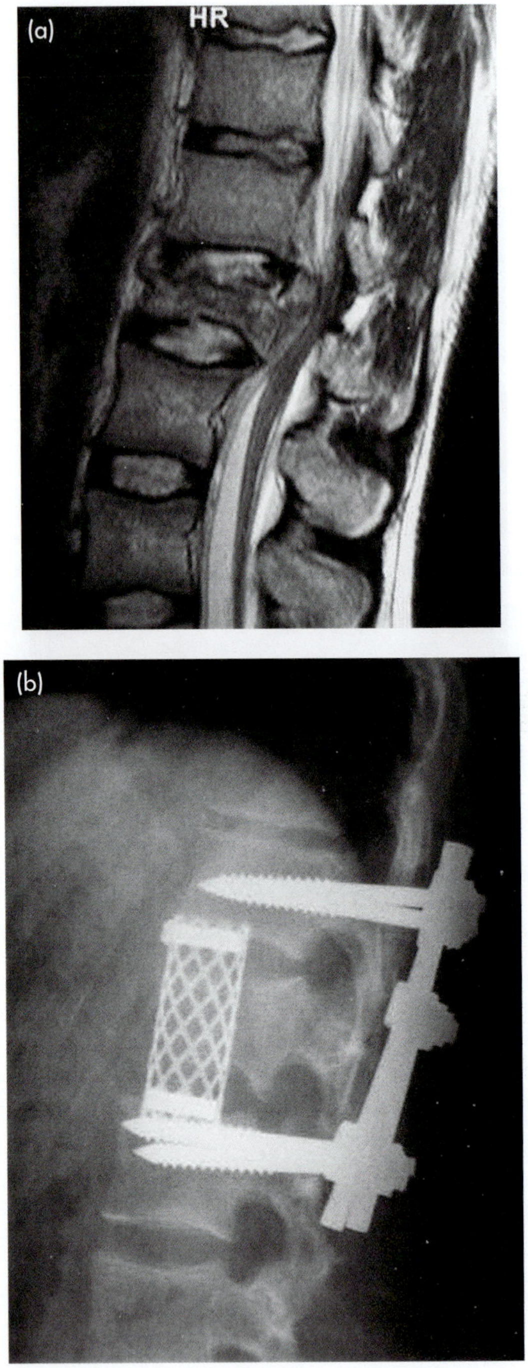

Figure 26.23 (a) Sagittal T2-weighted magnetic resonance image showing an L1 burst fracture and neural compression; (b) treated with combined anterior and posterior surgery.

SPECIFIC SPINAL INJURIES

Upper cervical spine (skull–C2)

Craniocervical dislocation

This injury is usually caused by high energy trauma and is often fatal. The dislocation may be anterior, posterior or vertical (Figure 26.24). Power's ratio (Figure 26.25) is used to assess skull translation.

Atlantoaxial instability

This is uncommon and either resolves spontaneously or with traction. Isolated, traumatic transverse ligament rupture leading to C1/2 instability is uncommon and is treated with posterior C1/2 fusion (Figure 26.26).

Occipital condyle fracture

This is a stable injury often associated with head injuries, and is best treated in a hard collar for 8 weeks.

Jefferson fractures (C1 ring)

These injuries are associated with axial loading of the cervical spine and may be stable or unstable (Figure 26.27a). Associated

Sir Geoffrey Jefferson, 1886–1961, Professor of Neurosurgery, University of Manchester, UK. He became the UK's first Professor of Neurosurgery in 1939. In 1947, he was elected a Fellow of The Royal Society, a rare distinction for a practising surgeon. Although he became a neurosurgeon, he performed the first successful embolectomy in England in 1925 at Salford Royal Hospital.

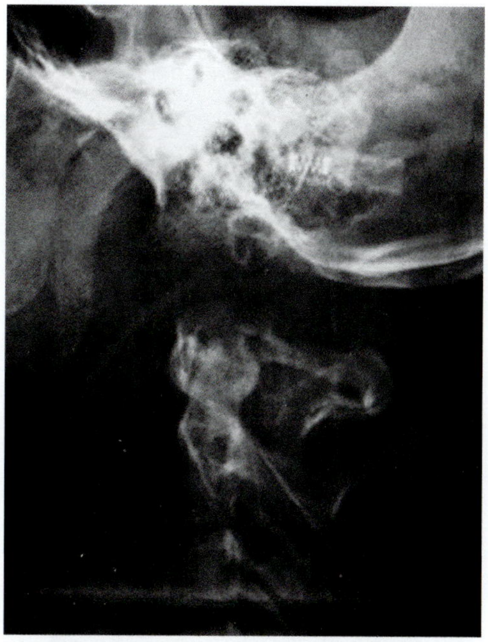

Figure 26.24 Vertical occipitocervical dislocation.

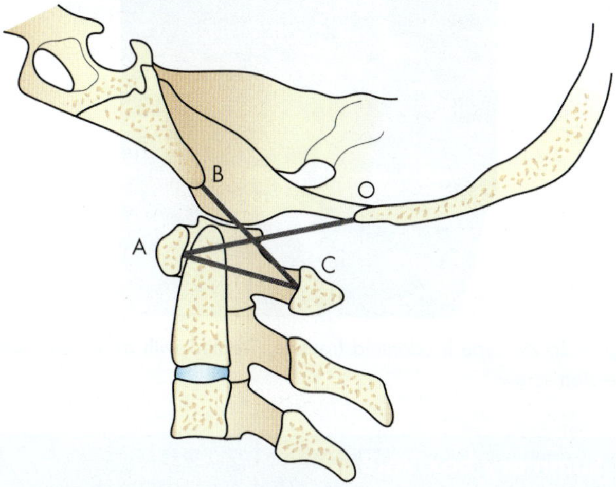

Figure 26.25 Power's ratio. BC/OA ≥1 indicates anterior translation, ≤0.75 indicates posterior translation.

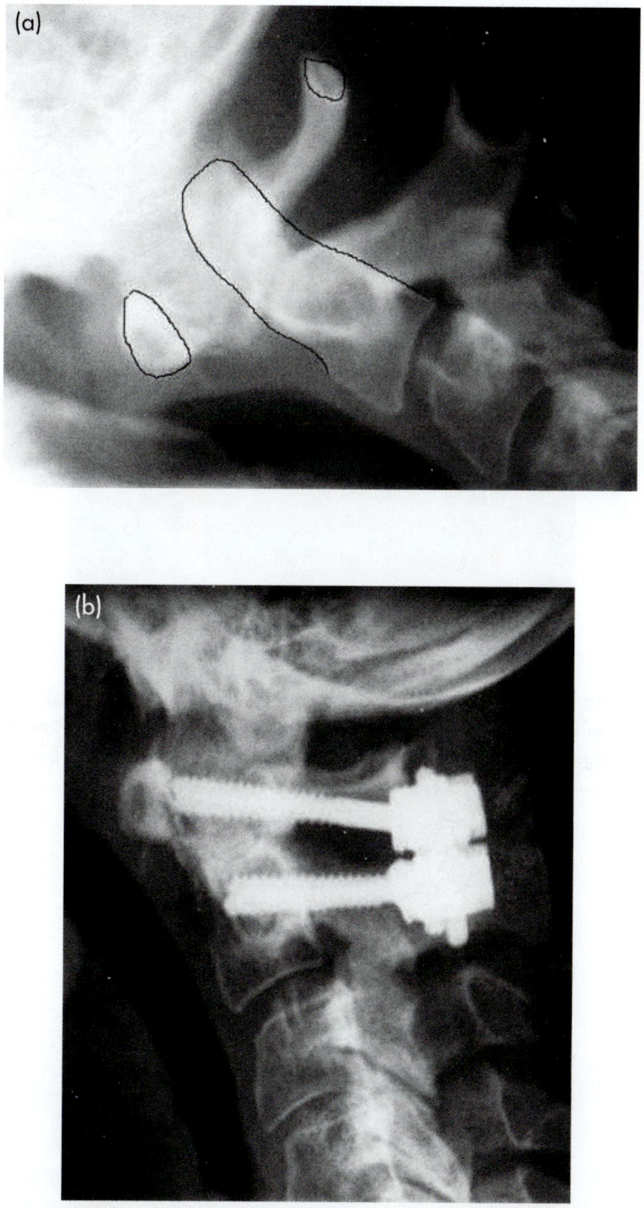

Figure 26.26 (a) Atlantoaxial subluxation. (b) C1/2 posterior fusion using C1 lateral mass and C2 pedicle screws.

transverse ligament rupture may occur (Figure 26.27b). Most are treated non-operatively in a collar or halo brace.

Odontoid fractures

There are three types of Odontoid peg fracture (Figure 26.28). Neurological injury is rare. The majority of acute injuries are treated non-operatively in a halo jacket or hard collar for three months. Internal fixation with an anterior compression screw is indicated in displaced fractures (Figure 26.29).

Posterior C1/2 fusion is required in cases of non-union.

Hangman's fracture

The Hangman's fracture is a traumatic spondylolisthesis of C2 on C3. There are four types with varying degrees of instability (Figure 26.30). Those with significant displacement or associated facet dislocation are treated operatively, usually with posterior stabilisation.

Subaxial cervical spine (C3–C7)

The pattern of lower cervical spine injury depends on the mechanism of trauma. These include wedge (hyperflexion), burst (axial compression), tear-drop fractures (hyperextension) and facet subluxation/dislocation (rotation and hyperflexion). The more severe injuries are accompanied by spinal cord injury (Figure 26.31a). Operative intervention may be required to decompress the spinal cord and stabilize the spine with internal fixation (Figure 26.31b).

Facet subluxation/dislocation ranges in severity from minor instability to complete dislocation with spinal cord injury (Figure 26.32) (Summary box 26.8).

Barry Powers, contemporary, Chief and Clinical Professor of Radiology, Duplin General Hospital, Kenansville, NC, USA, described his ratio in 1979.

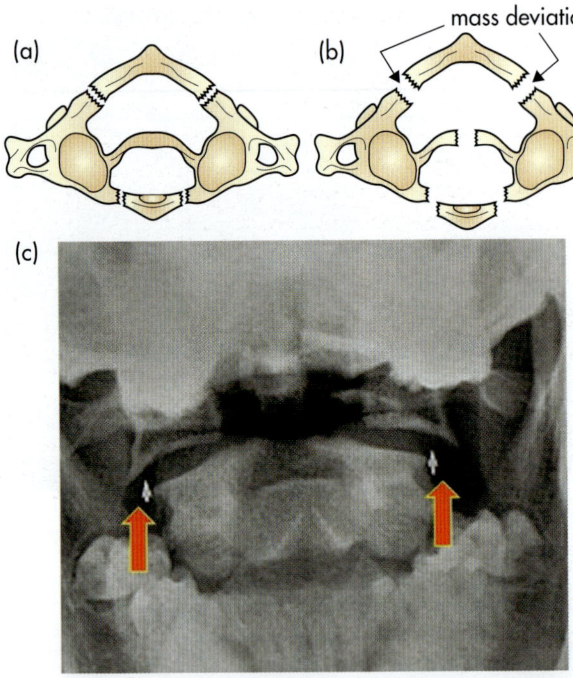

Figure 26.27 Stable (a) versus unstable (b) Jefferson's fracture of C1. Open mouth view of C1/2 demonstrating C1 lateral mass deviation. Rupture of the transverse ligament is present when the combined lateral mass deviation exceeds 6.9 mm.

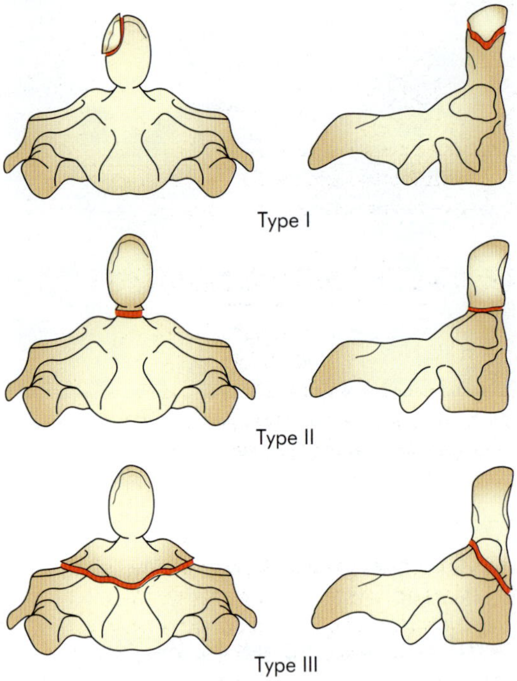

Figure 26.28 Types of odontoid fracture.

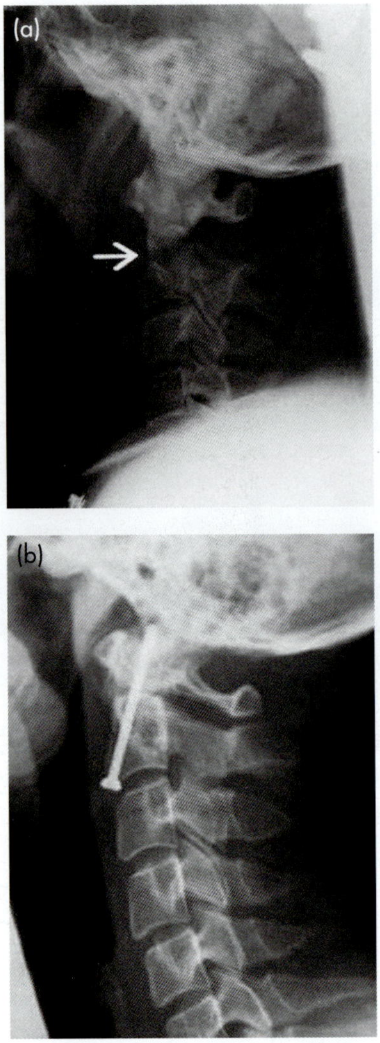

Figure 26.29 Type II odontoid fracture. Treated with an anterior compression screw.

Summary box 26.8

Cervical spine injuries

- The majority of upper cervical spinal injuries are treated non-operatively
- Spinal cord injury is more commonly associated with subaxial cervical spinal injuries

Thoracic and thoracolumbar fractures

The system developed by the AO (*Arbeitsgemeinschaft fűr Osteosynthesefragen*) can be used to classify these fractures. There are three main injury types (A, B and C) with increasing instability and risk of neurological injury. Type A fractures involve the vertebral body. Type B injuries have additional distraction/disruption of the posterior elements and type C injuries are rotational. The majority of type B and type C injuries require surgical stabilization.

Thoracic spine (T1–T10)

Osteoporotic wedge compression fractures in the elderly are the most common injury in this group. Symptomatic fractures can be treated with percutaneous bone cement augmentation, known as vertebroplasty or kyphoplasty (Figure 26.33).

In trauma cases, unstable fractures are associated with significant energy transfer to the patient and may be associated with major internal injuries, such as pulmonary contusion and spinal cord injury. The combination of thoracic spine disruption and

AO (*Arbeitsgemeinschaft fűr Osteosynthesefragen*) which may be translated from the German as 'Working Party on Problems of Bone Repair'.

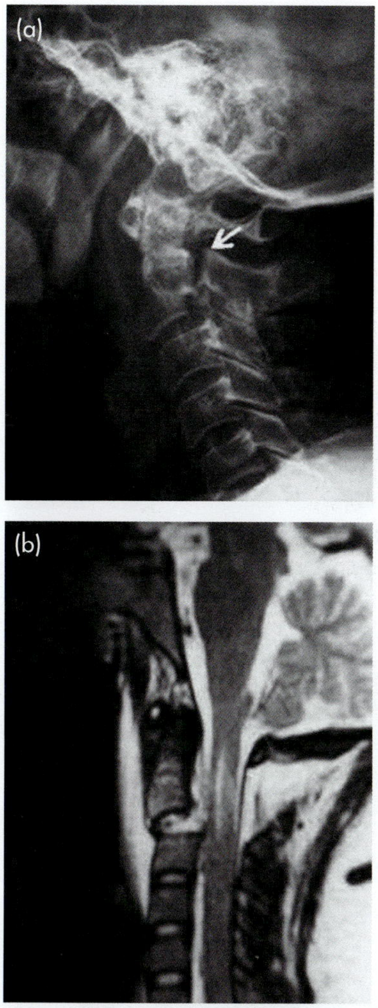

Figure 26.30 (a) Hangman's fractures of C2 with minimal forward translation. (b) C2/3 subluxation with spinal cord contusion.

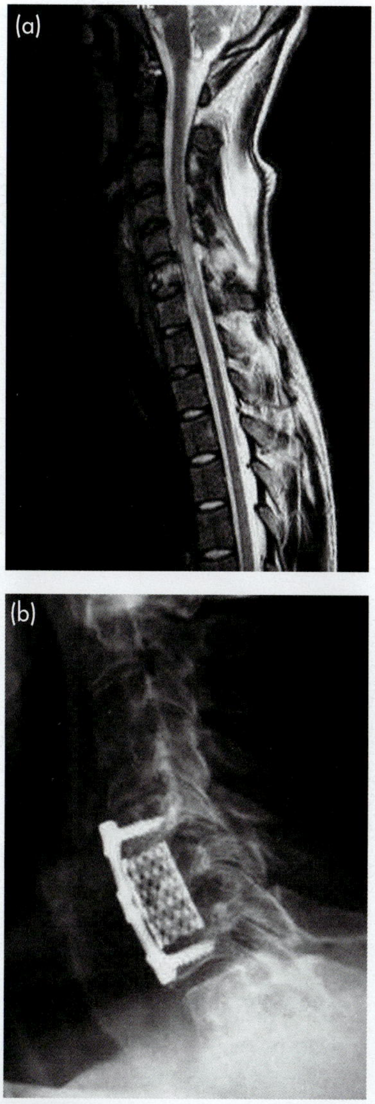

Figure 26.31 (a) Cervical burst fracture with spinal cord contusion. (b) Treated by anterior decompression and reconstruction.

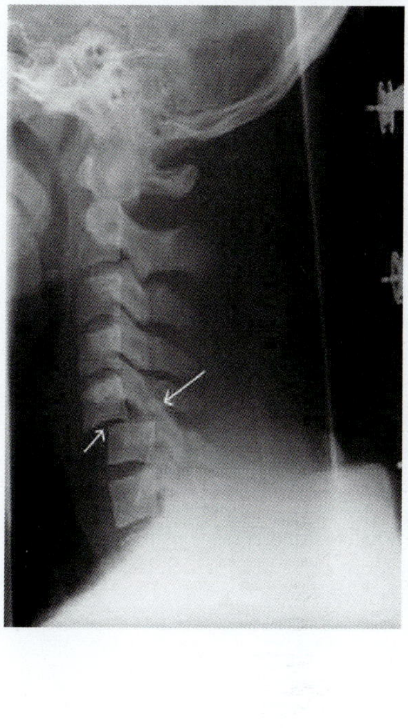

Figure 26.32 C5/6 bifacetal dislocation.

a sternal fracture (Figure 26.34) also carries a significant risk of aortic rupture. Multiple posterior rib fractures and rib dislocations above and below a thoracic spinal injury signify a major rotational injury to the chest and are associated with vascular injury and significant pulmonary contusion (Figure 26.35).

Multimodality diagnostic imaging is recommended. Surgery is appropriate in almost all unstable thoracic injuries.

Thoracolumbar spinal fractures (T11–S1)

The thoracolumbar junction is especially prone to injury. This can vary from a minor wedge fracture to spinal dislocation (Figure 26.36). Burst fractures are comminuted fractures of the vertebral body. Usually the distance between the pedicles is widened and bone fragments are retropulsed into the spinal canal (Figure 26.37). The surgical approach can be anterior, posterior or combined. For burst fractures with neurological compromise, an anterior approach with vertebral corpectomy, canal clearance and anterior reconstruction (Figure 26.38) is often used.

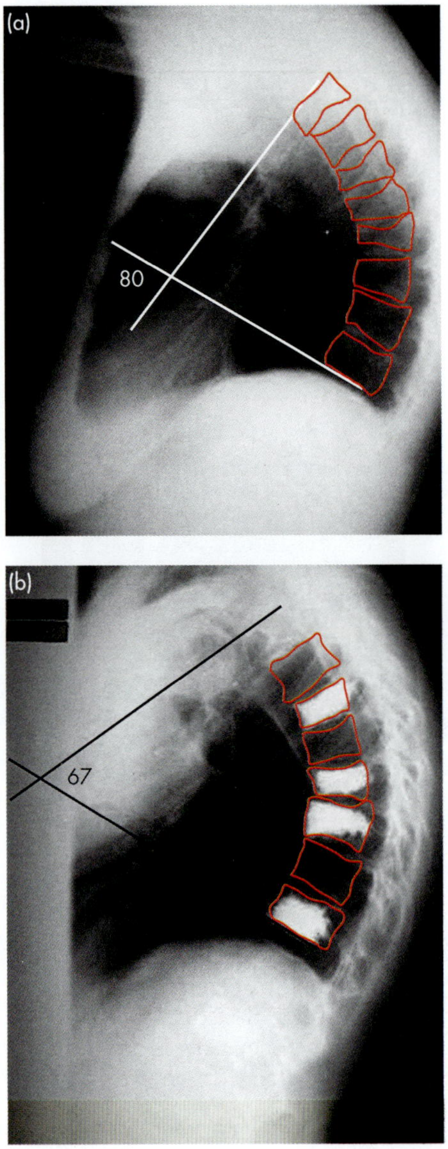

Figure 26.33 (a) Lateral x-ray showing multiple osteoporotic compression fractures. (b) Reduction in thoracic kyphotic deformity following four level kyphoplasty.

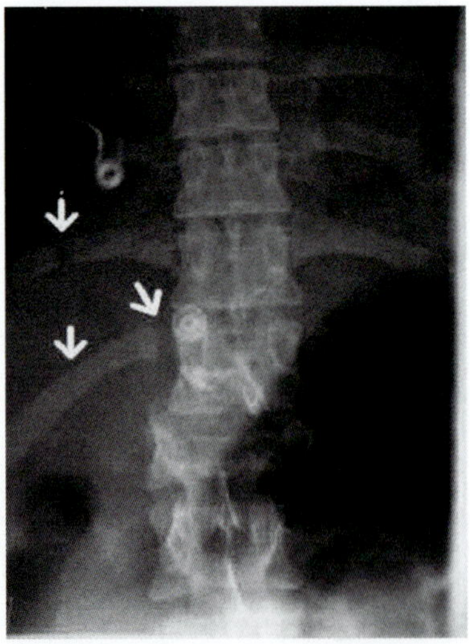

Figure 26.35 Rotational (type C) injury at the thoracolumbar junction. Note rib fractures and dislocation, and presence of chest tube.

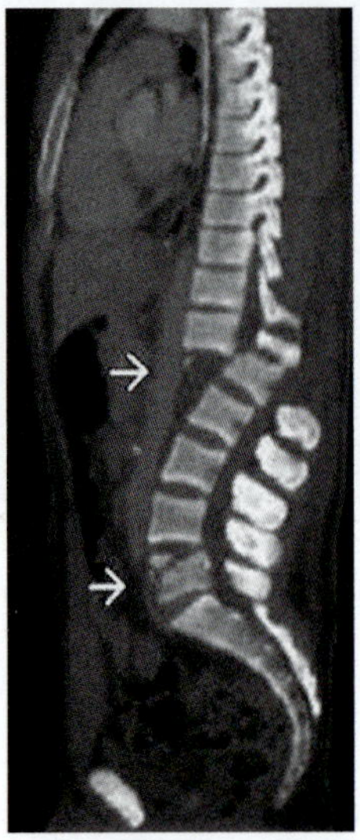

Figure 26.36 Total spinal sagittal computed tomographic reconstruction demonstrating a thoracolumbar fracture dislocation and fracture of L5.

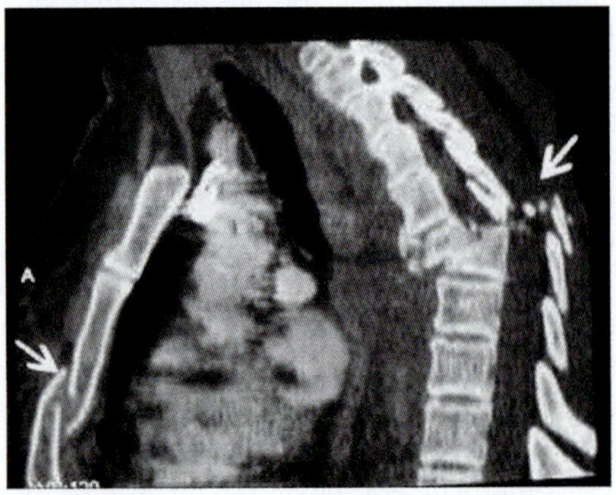

Figure 26.34 Sagittal computed tomographic reconstruction showing an upper thoracic spine fracture dislocation and associated sternal fracture.

Chance fractures are flexion–distraction injuries of the thoracolumbar junction and are classically associated with the use of lap belts (Figure 26.39). Duodenal, pancreatic and/or aortic rupture, are also associated with these injuries (Summary box 26.9).

Summary box 26.9

Thoracic and thoracolumbar fractures

- Unstable thoracic spine fractures and thoracolumbar flexion–distraction injuries are commonly associated with vascular and/or visceral injuries

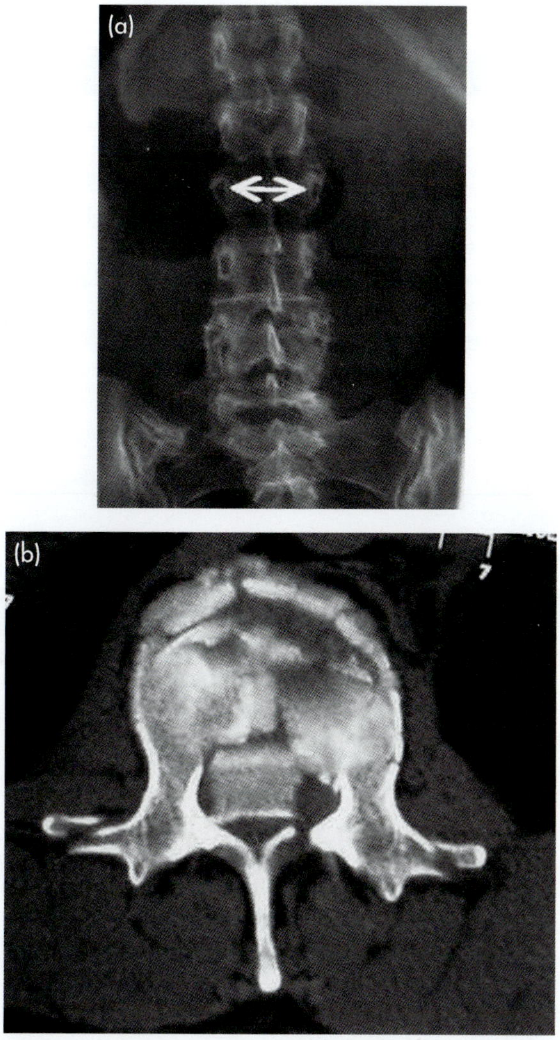

Figure 26.37 Lumbar burst fracture with increase in interpedicular distance (a) and spinal canal compromise (b).

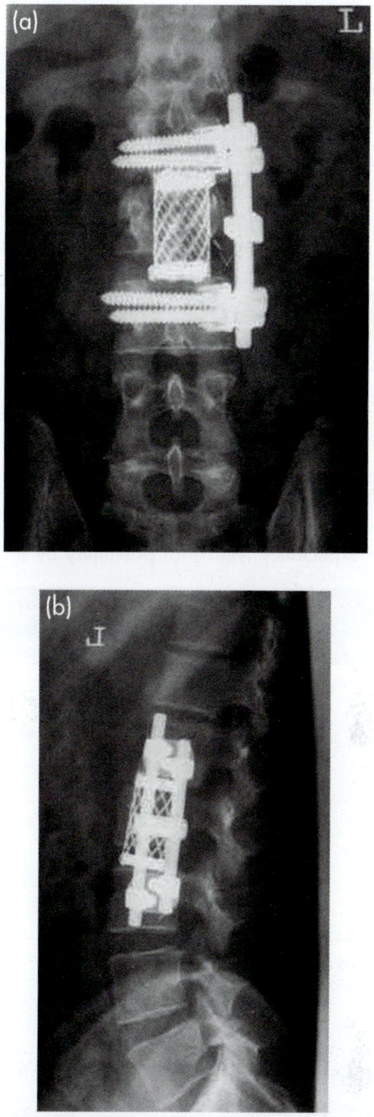

Figure 26.38 Anterior spinal reconstruction for a lumbar burst fracture.

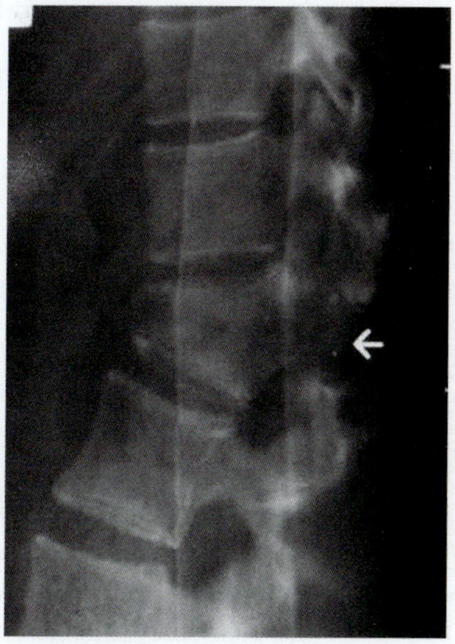

Figure 26.39 A bony Chance fracture at the thoracolumbar junction secondary to a lap belt injury.

REHABILITATION AND PATIENT OUTCOME

The goal of spinal cord injury rehabilitation focuses on maximising the remaining neurological function. The level of neurological impairment determines functional outcome (Table 26.1).

Prognosis of spinal cord injury

Despite continuing improvements in patient care, life expectancy remains reduced (Table 26.2).

The prognosis for neurological recovery is strongly influenced by the pattern of initial injury, the completeness of the cord injury and the age at the time of injury.

Complications associated with spinal cord injury

Pain and spasticity

Neurogenic pain is common. Once reflex activity returns following cord injury, spasticity may occur and can be problematic.

Table 26.1 Expected functional outcome versus level of cervical spinal cord injury.

Level of Injury	Functional goal
C3–C4	Power wheelchair with mouth or chin control. Verbalise care, communicate through adaptive equipment. May be ventilator dependent
C5	Power wheelchair, dress upper body, self-feed with aids, wash face with assistance
C6	Propel power wheelchair, possibly push manual wheelchair, transfer with assistance, dress upper body (lower body with assistance), self-groom with aids, bladder/bowel care with assistance, self-feed with splints, able to drive
C7	Manual wheelchair, independent transfer, dressing (with aids), feeding, bathing, self-care. Bladder and bowel care with assistance
C8–T4	Independent with most activities of daily living, and bowel and bladder care
T5–T12	As above, but with more ease. Independent with all self-care
L1–L5	Independent. Walk with short or long leg braces
S1–S5	Independent, able to walk if able to push off (S1) (may need brace). Bladder, bowel and sexual function may remain compromised

Table 26.2 Life expectancy (years) for post-injury by severity of injury and age at injury.

Age at injury	No SCI	Motor functional at any level	Para	Low tetra (C5–C8)	High tetra (C1-C4)	Ventilator-dependent at any level
(a) For people who survive the first 24 hours						
20	58.4	52.8	45.6	40.6	36.1	16.6
40	39.5	34.3	28.0	23.8	20.2	7.1
60	22.2	17.9	13.1	10.2	7.9	1.4
(b) For people surviving at least one year post-injury						
20	58.4	53.3	46.3	41.7	37.9	23.3
40	39.5	34.8	28.6	24.7	21.6	11.1
60	22.2	18.3	13.5	10.8	8.8	3.1

SCI, spinal cord injury.

Intrathecal infusion of baclofen may be required in resistant cases.

Autonomic dysreflexia

This is a paroxysmal syndrome of hypertension, hypohydrosis (above level of injury), bradycardia, flushing and headache in response to noxious visceral and other stimuli. It is most commonly triggered by bladder distension or rectal loading from faecal impaction.

Neurological deterioration

Post-traumatic syringomyelia may cause late (>3 months post-injury) neurological deterioration and occurs in 3–5 per cent of spinal cord injury cases. Increase in pain and/or spasticity, ascending loss of sensation and deep tendon reflexes are suspicious and warrant early MRI assessment. Expanding cavities require neurosurgical intervention.

Thromboembolic events

Deep vein thrombosis (DVT) occurs in 30 per cent of spinal cord-injured patients. Fatal pulmonary embolus is reported in 1–2 per cent of cases. Therefore, prophylaxis with low molecular heparin is recommended.

Osteoporosis, heterotopic ossification and contaractures

Disuse osteoporosis is an inevitable consequence of spinal cord injury, and fragility fractures may occur. Heterotopic ossification may affect hips, knees, shoulders and elbows. It occurs in 25 per cent of spinal cord-injured patients. Surgery is appropriate in selected cases. Soft tissue contractures around joints may occur due to spasticity, but can be avoided by appropriate physical therapy, positioning and splinting.

FURTHER READING

Aebi M, Thalgott JS, Webb JK. *AO ASIF principles in spine surgery.* Berlin: Springer-Verlag, 1998.

Bridwell KH, DeWald RL (eds). *The textbook of spinal surgery.* Philadelphia: Lippincott-Raven, 1997.

British Orthopaedic Association. The initial care and transfer of patients with spinal cord injuries, 2006. Available from: www.sbns.org/rcsed/RCSEdDocuments/DocumentsView.aspx?tabID=0&ItemID=31562&MId=4607&wversion=Staging.

Cotler JM, Simson MJ, An HS *et al.* (eds). *Surgery of spinal trauma.* Philadelphia: Lippincott, Williams and Wilkins, 2000.

Fardon DF, Herzog RJ, Mink JH *et al.* (eds). *Orthopaedic knowledge update – spine.* Rosemont, IL: American Academy of Orthopaedic Surgeons, 1997.

Focus issue. Spinal trauma. *Spine* 2006; **31**(11S): S1–104.

CHAPTER

27 Maxillofacial trauma

LEARNING OBJECTIVES

To be able to:
- Recognise the life-threatening nature of facial injuries through compromise of the airway and associated head and spinal injuries

To have:
- A methodology for examining facial injuries

To know:
- The classification of facial fractures

To understand:
- The diagnosis and management of fractures of the middle third of the facial skeleton and the mandible

To appreciate:
- The importance of careful cleaning and accurate suturing of facial lacerations

INTRODUCTION

An unscarred face is important to the well-being of the individual, and thus all injuries, however trivial, should be treated thoughtfully and sympathetically, with every effort made to produce an optimal outcome. In addition, even trivial blows to the face may:

- cause injuries which compromise the airway;
- directly or indirectly cause a head injury;
- cause injuries to the cervical spine.

EPIDEMIOLOGY

Injuries to the orofacial soft tissues and facial skeleton commonly result from sporting activities, accidents and intentional violence.

There is significant variation in the aetiological causes of orofacial injuries in different parts of the world and this affects their incidence:

- **Social factors**. Interpersonal violence has steadily increased and in many countries is now the most common cause of orofacial injuries. This increase is noticed to a greater extent in conurbations and urban areas. It is often fuelled by alcohol excess.
- **Climatic factors**. The arrival of snow and freezing weather during the winter, and increased traffic volume and interpersonal violence during the warmer months of the year often produce seasonal variations in the incidence of injuries.
- **Road traffic accidents**. Legislation and improved vehicular design have lessened the number of injuries presenting as a result of road traffic accidents. Air bag provision, seat belts, laminated windscreens and drink/drive laws have all helped in reducing orofacial injuries in the developed world. However, the enforcing of lower speed limits has not, as yet, been shown to reduce injuries.

CLINICAL EFFECTS

The mouth and nasal passages form part of the upper aerodigestive tract. Lacerations and fractures of the facial skeleton may give rise to immediate or delayed respiratory obstruction. Immediate obstruction may arise from inhalation of tooth fragments, accumulation of blood and secretions, and loss of control of the tongue in the unconscious or semiconscious patient. Patients with facial injuries should not be allowed to lie supine. They should be nursed in the semiprone position (Figure 27.1) with the head supported on the bent arm. Damaged teeth, blood and secretions can then fall out of the mouth and gravity pulls the tongue forward. As the patient is manoeuvred into the correct nursing position, the neck should be supported and held in a neutral position – a protective collar is advisable until a fracture of the cervical spine has been excluded. An intracranial injury should always be considered as a possibility, however minor the injury to the face.

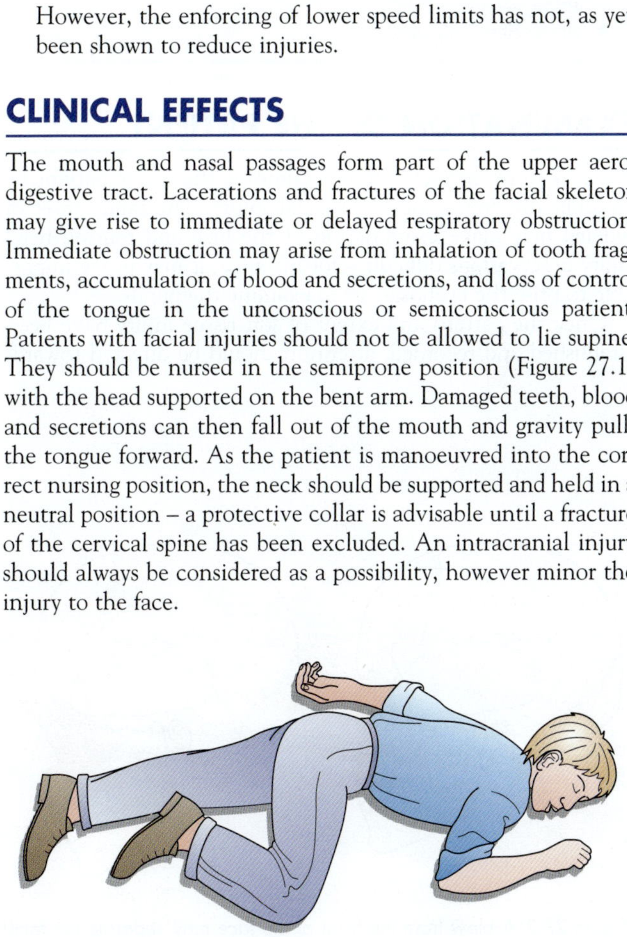

Figure 27.1 The patient should be nursed in the semiprone position to allow secretions, blood and foreign bodies to fall from the mouth.

Initial haemorrhage after a facial injury can be dramatic, but sustained bleeding is unusual. The most likely cause of circulatory failure in a facial injury is the accompanying skeletal fractures or a ruptured viscus. These should always be actively sought in the shocked patient.

Oedema is a particular feature of all fractures of the facial skeleton and tends to develop within 60–90 minutes. Thus, a patient with a shattered face may appear to have a good airway immediately after the injury, but then swelling of the tongue, facial and pharyngeal tissues may then cause respiratory compromise. This is especially important when the middle third of the face is involved. In Le Fort III fractures (see below under The middle third), the maxilla may be thrust downwards and backwards along the base of the skull. As it does so, the posterior teeth of the upper and lower jaws contact prematurely and the mouth is held open (Figure 27.2) giving the impression of a good airway. However, as oedema develops, the soft palate and tongue may swell to meet, and close the pharyngeal airway. This leads to respiratory distress and even obstruction (Figure 27.3) (Summary box 27.1).

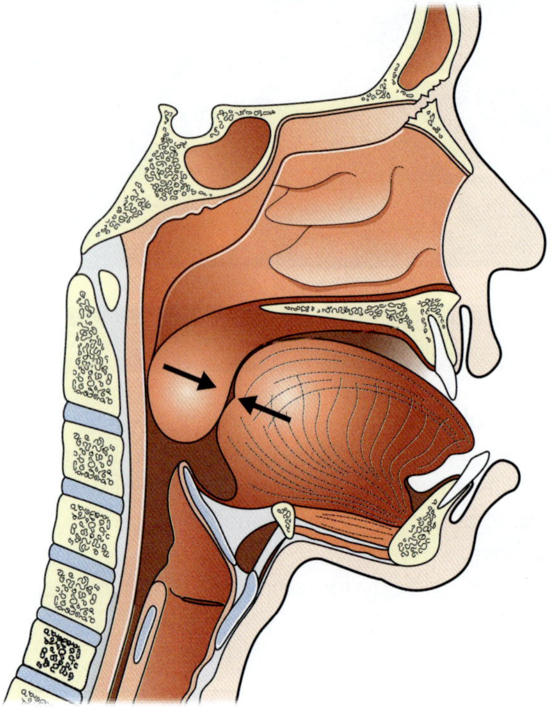

Figure 27.3 Loss of nasopharyngeal space and odema of the soft palate and tongue may close off the airway in severe maxillofacial injuries, 2–3 hours after injury.

Summary box 27.1

Facial injuries

- Are potentially life-threatening
- May be associated with injuries to the brain and cervical spine
- Are cosmetically very important

EXAMINATION OF THE PATIENT

It is easy to be distracted from examining the whole patient by the dramatic appearance of a facial injury. The rapid onset of oedema may make examination of the face and routine head injury observations difficult – for instance, it may prove impossible to prise the eyelids apart to examine the pupils.

Once the pattern and extent of soft tissue injury have been established and recorded, attention should be directed towards the hard tissues. Regardless of the apparent site of the injury, the whole head should be examined visually and by palpation starting with the vault of the skull. The face should be examined from in front. Any asymmetry should be noted, although oedema may make this difficult. Gentle palpation gives the most information in searching for step deformities. Tenderness over sites of known weakness and potential for fracture (see below under Fractures of the facial skeleton) is a very good guide to the possibility of there being an underlying fracture. A good system is to examine from above downwards – checking first the supraorbital and infraorbital ridges, the nasal bridge and then the zygomas, including the arches. The mandible should then be examined starting at the condyles bilaterally and then following the posterior and lower border of the mandible as far as the midline. The majority of middle third injuries are accompanied by some degree of epistaxis (except isolated zygomatic arch fractures) and Le Fort II and III injuries frequently have a cerebrospinal fluid (CSF) leak with CSF rhinorrhoea. A particularly useful sign in the fractured zygoma is the frequent subconjunctival haemorrhage, which will often be found to have no posterior limit when the patient is asked to look to the other side (Figure 27.4).

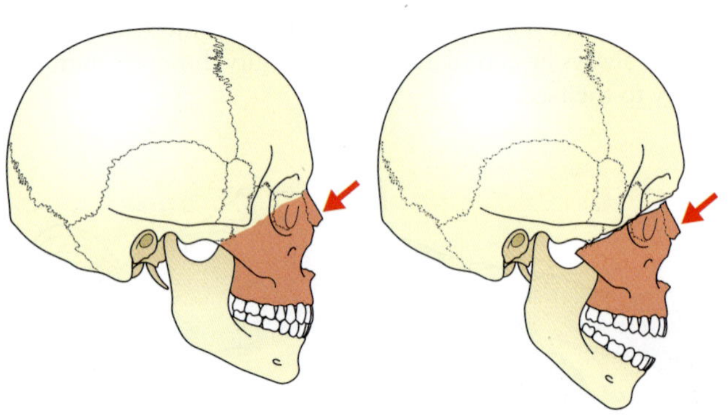

Figure 27.2 A blow from the front of the face may separate the facial skeleton from the base of the skull and thrust it downwards and backwards.

The patient should then be examined intraorally with good illumination, taking note of the occlusion. The maxillary and mandibular dentition normally 'fit' together even if the occlu-

René Le Fort, 1869–1951, was a French surgeon who classified facial fractures after macabre research in which he dropped rocks and other heavy objects on the faces of cadavers.
Thomas Brian Gunning, 1813–1889, American dentist.

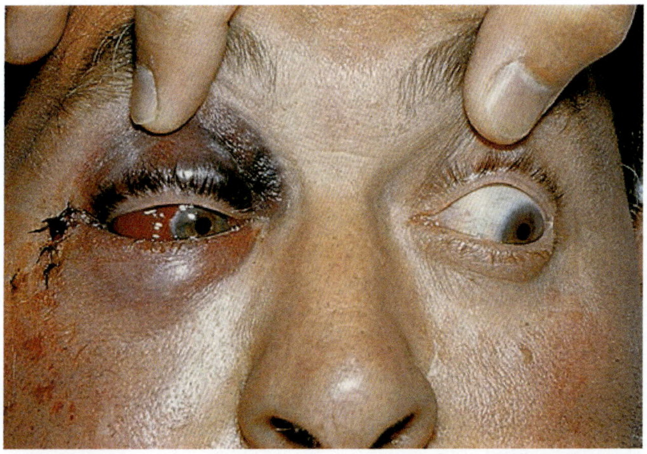

Figure 27.4 Fractures of the zygoma may often be associated with subconjunctival haemorrhage. This example shows no posterior border to the haemorrhage as the patient looks away from the side of the fracture.

sion is naturally irregular – if they do not, a fracture of the jaws may be suspected. All fractures involving the alveolus (the tooth-bearing portion of the jaw in the dentate patient) tear the gingivae and are compound into the mouth (Figure 27.5). A haematoma in the floor of the mouth is an indication of a fracture of the mandible, particularly in patients with no teeth of their own. The alignment of the teeth should be noted and any missing or broken teeth and dental restorations/prostheses should be carefully recorded. The occlusal plane must be examined for the presence of step defects. These indicate a likely fracture of the underlying bone. The patient should be asked to bring the teeth together, so that any occlusal anomalies may be observed. In some cases, independent movement of the fragments may also be detected. Jaw movement should be tested: deviation from the midline at rest or on opening suggests a fracture of the side to which the jaw is deviating.

If a fracture of the maxilla is suspected, then the maxillary dental arch should be grasped between the index finger and thumb of one hand in the incisor region, while the other is placed on the forehead. If the maxilla is fractured, gentle pressure forward and backward, or side to side, will reveal movement between the examining hands. With the mandible, gentle manipulation across the suspected site of a fracture will produce 'springing' if a fracture is present.

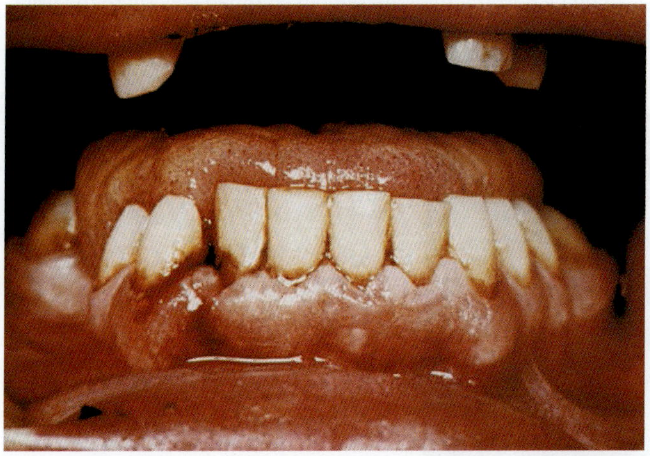

Figure 27.5 A fracture of the right parasymphysis of the mandible, demonstrating a tear of the gingivae in the lower right lateral incisor/canine region.

Lacerations of the oral mucosa may occur independently of hard tissue injuries, and can often involve the buccal mucous membrane and tongue. Degloving lacerations most commonly involve the labial sulcus and the body of the mandible. Tongue injuries require careful assessment, as the depth of lacerations is often underestimated and may be a source for significant haemorrhage, which may be delayed. Palatal lacerations tend to occur in young children who fall on to objects held in the oral cavity, especially pens and pencils. With such a history, the possibility of a retained foreign body must be considered.

Checking for intact nerves

Paraesthesia suggests a fracture proximally along the course of the nerve. Thus, paraesthesia of the cheek and upper lip suggests a fracture involving the infraorbital foramen or floor of the orbit, while paraesthesia of the lower lip suggests a fracture of the mandibular body. Facial palsy may indicate damage to the branches of the facial nerve involved in facial lacerations. This is common in penetrating wounds of the parotid gland. In the absence of lacerations, facial palsy may indicate a fractured temporal bone.

Check visual acuity in both eyes. This may be difficult in the oedematous patient with marked periorbital oedema, but a pen torch shone directly through the lids will confirm gross optic nerve function. Where possible, pupil size and reflexes to light should be observed and recorded, as should eye movements. Check for diplopia by asking the patient to follow the light of a pen torch through a full range. Diplopia can occur with damage to the thin orbital plates of bone, particularly the floor of the orbit or from damage to the III, IV or VI cranial nerves.

All findings should be recorded accurately, preferably with diagrams to include measurements of lacerations, abrasions and areas of tissue loss. Photographs of the initial injury can be very helpful if litigation is likely to follow (Summary box 27.2).

Summary box 27.2

Examination of facial injuries

- Commence with lacerations and soft tissue injuries
- Systematically examine bones, including the occiput and cranial vault
- Check dental occlusion and palpate the mouth
- Examine cranial nerves

ADDITIONAL INVESTIGATIONS

Radiological investigations

Table 27.1 demonstrates the regularly used radiographic views utilised in the diagnosis of maxillofacial injuries. Coronal computed tomography (CT) scanning has superseded tomographic views in the diagnosis of orbital floor fractures, and coronal and axial CT scanning is often the choice of radiographic investigation in the more complex middle third fractures (Figure 27.6). A chest radiograph is indicated if there is any suggestion of inhalation of dental fragments or dental prostheses. It should be

Table 27.1 Radiological views for specific fractures.

Site of fracture	Radiographs
Mandible: body and ramus	OPT, lateral obliques, lower occlusal, PA mandible
Mandible: condyles	OPT, PA mandible with mouth open, Toller transpharyngeal views
Maxilla	OM 15° and 30°, lateral facial bones
Zygomatic complex	OM 15° and 30°, submentovertex
Orbital blow-outs	OM 15° and 30° and tomograms
Nasal bones	Lateral nasal bones, occipitofrontal
Frontal bones	Lateral skull, occipitofrontal

OM, posteroanterioroccipitomental; OPT, orthopantomogram; PA posteroanterior.

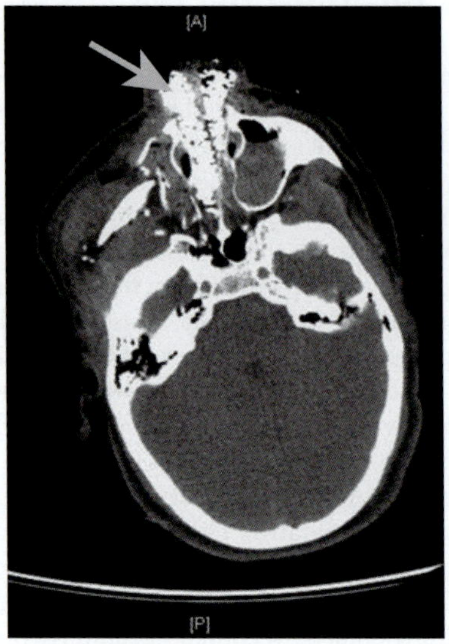

Figure 27.6 Computed tomographic (CT) scan showing a comminuted fracture of the right maxilla and zygomatic complex (nasal pack in place).

remembered, however, that polymethylmethacrylate (PMMA) used in the construction of dentures is not radiopaque and so may not be visible on plain radiographs.

Posteroanterior occipitomental radiographs are the optimum initial radiographs to illustrate the site and displacement of a middle third fracture. A panoramic oral radiograph, or orthopantomogram (Figure 27.7), is the radiograph of choice for the mandible as it shows the whole bone from condyle to condyle.

FRACTURES OF THE FACIAL SKELETON

Fractures of the facial skeleton may be divided into those of the upper third (above the eyebrows), the middle third (above the mouth) and the lower third (the mandible). Fractures tend to occur through points of weakness – the sutures and foramina – and in thin unsupported bone.

The upper third

The patterns of fracture of the skull tend to be related to the site and type of trauma (sharp or blunt), but there are points of weakness in the skull, mainly involving the frontal sinuses and the supraorbital ridges.

The middle third

In 1911, Rene Le Fort classified fractures according to patterns which he created on cadavers using various degrees of force. The Le Fort classification is still used extensively today (Figure 27.8).

The **Le Fort I** fracture effectively separates the alveolus and palate from the facial skeleton above. The fracture line runs through points of weakness from the nasal piriform aperture, through the lateral and medial walls of the maxillary sinus, running posteriorly to include the lower part of the pterygoid plates.

The **Le Fort II** fracture is pyramidal in shape. The fracture involves the orbit, running through the bridge of the nose and the ethmoids whose cribriform plate may be fractured. It continues to the medial part of the infraorbital rim and often through the infraorbital foramen. It continues posteriorly to the pterygoid plates at the back through the lateral wall of the maxillary antrum at a higher level than the **Le Fort I**.

The **Le Fort III** fracture effectively separates the facial skeleton from the base of the skull – the fracture lines run high through the nasal bridge, septum and ethmoids. This creates the potential for dural tear and CSF leak. It then passes irregularly through the bones of the orbit to the frontozygomatic suture. The zygomatic arch fractures and the facial skeleton are separated from the bones above at a high level through the lateral wall of the maxillary sinus and the pterygoid plates.

The Le Fort fractures are seldom confined exactly to the original classification and combinations of any of the above fractures may occur.

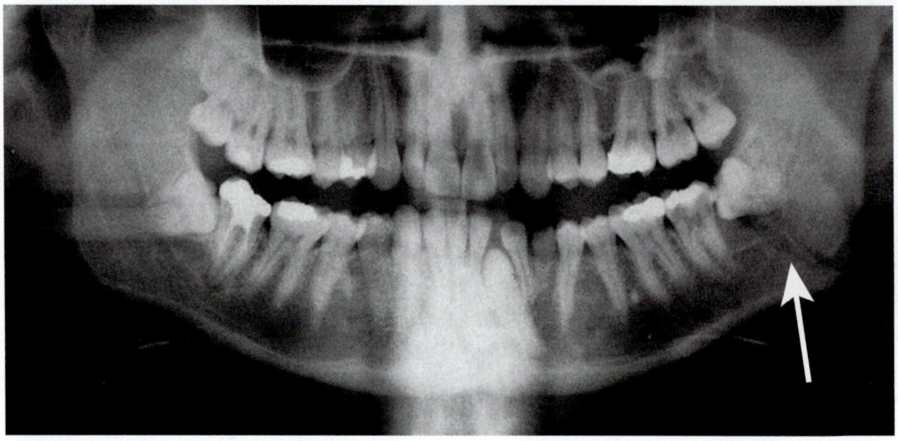

Figure 27.7 An orthopantomogram demonstrating a fracture of the left angle of the mandible.

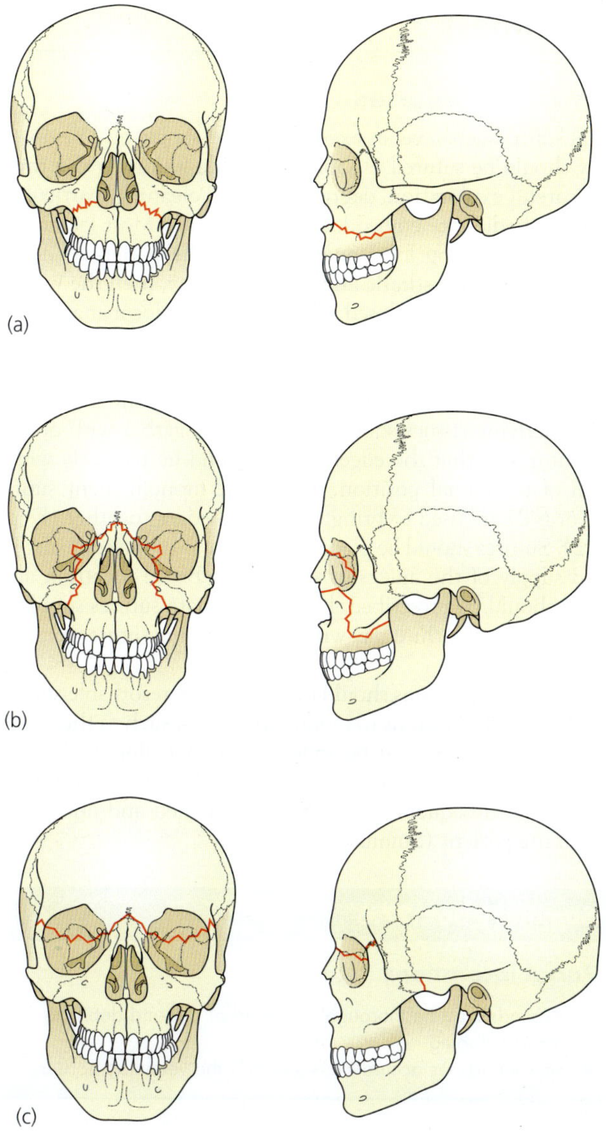

Figure 27.8 Maxillary fractures as classified by Le Fort. (a) Le Fort I; (b) Le Fort II; (c) Le Fort III.

Fracture of the zygomatic complex

This is the most common fracture of the middle third of the face, apart from the nose. The fractures occur through points of weakness: the infraorbital margin, the frontozygomatic suture, the zygomatic arch and the anterior and lateral wall of the maxillary sinus. Tears of the antral mucosa may lead to epistaxis on the affected side and damage to the infraorbital nerve may cause paraesthesia in its sensory distribution (Summary box 27.3).

Summary box 27.3

Fractures of the zygomatic complex

- Damage to the infraorbital nerve is common, causing numbness of the cheek

Blow-out fractures of the orbit

Direct blunt trauma to the globe of the eye may push it back within the orbit. The globe is a fairly robust structure and as it is thrust backwards, the weakest plate of bone, most commonly the orbital floor, fractures and the orbital contents herniate down into the maxillary antrum. This soft tissue herniation may trap the inferior oblique and inferior rectus muscles, leading to failure of the eye to rotate upwards. Enophthalmos and diplopia can follow, although initially both may be concealed by oedema. Paraesthesia in the distribution of the infraorbital nerve may be an important clue to the blow-out fracture.

There should be a high index of suspicion of any possible orbital blow-out fracture. A coronal CT is the investigation of choice, as significant delay in treatment may be associated with less success than early diagnosis and treatment (Figure 27.9) (Summary box 27.4).

Summary box 27.4

Blow-out fractures of the orbit

- Damage to the infraorbital nerve is common, causing numbness of the cheek
- Any fracture that involves the orbital floor (Le Fort II and zygomatic complex) has the potential for orbital content entrapment

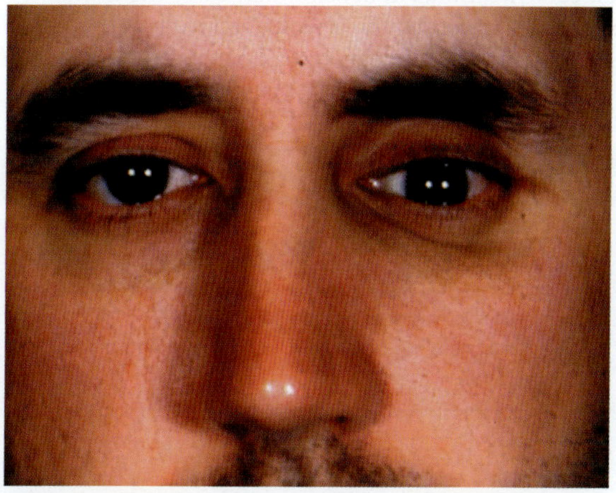

Figure 27.9 Previously undiagnosed left orbital blow-out fracture, presenting three months after the initial injury. Enophthalmos and lowered pupillary level are evident.

Nasoethmoidal complex fractures

Fractures of the nasoethmoidal complex, as opposed to isolated nasal bone fractures, are usually comminuted fractures involving the nasal bones, maxilla, infraorbital rims and the frontal bones. Such injuries can cause significant deformity (Figure 27.10), and due to disruption of the medial canthal ligaments may cause traumatic telecanthus (widened intercanthal distance).

Fractures of the mandible

The condylar neck is the weakest part of the mandible and is the

William Johnson Walsham, 1847–1903, surgeon, St Bartholomew's Hospital, London, UK.
Morris Joseph Asch, 1833–1902, surgeon, New York Eye and Ear Hospital, New York, NY, USA.

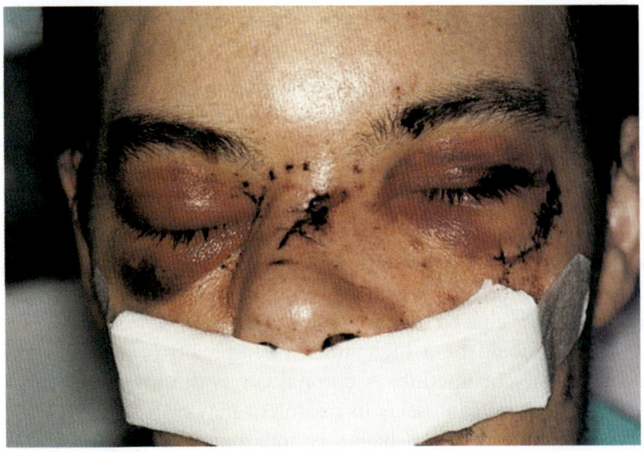

Figure 27.10 Nasoethmoidal complex fracture, demonstrating gross nasal deformity and traumatic telecanthus.

most frequent site of fracture (Figure 27.11), while other fractures tend to occur through unerupted teeth (the impacted wisdom tooth) or where the roots are long (the canine tooth). The mandible may fracture directly at the point of the blow, or indirectly at a point of weakness distant from the original blow. The latter is characteristically seen in the so-called 'guardsman' fracture, where a blow to the chin point may cause a direct fracture of the symphysis or parasymphysis of the lower jaw. Indirect transmission of the kinetic energy causes a unilateral or bilateral fracture of the mandibular condyles. Blows from below may cause the mandible to be thrust upwards fracturing the alveolus and teeth as they strike the maxillary dentition (Summary box 27.5).

Summary box 27.5

Fractures of the mandible

- The condylar neck is the weakest point and the most common site of mandibular fracture
- Indirect transmission of energy may fracture the mandibular condyle(s)

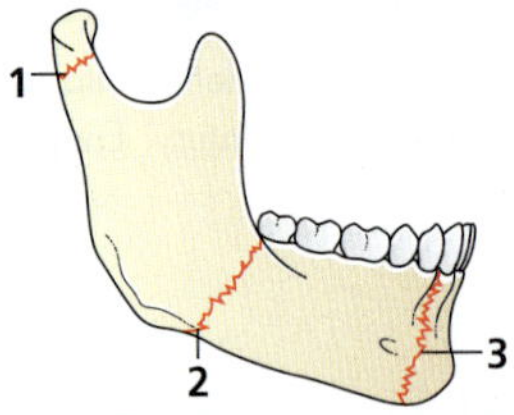

Figure 27.11 The patterns of fracture of the mandible. (1) The neck of the condyle is the most common site, followed by (2) the angle of the mandible through the last tooth. (3) The third point of weakness is in the region of the canine tooth.

A 'guardsman' fracture is so called because it refers to the Queen's Guards who, when they fainted on parade, still held themselves in a position of attention. As a consequence, if they fell forward, the first point of contact with the ground would be the point of the chin. This resulted in a direct fracture of the symphysis/parasymphysis of the mandible, and indirect fractures of both mandibular condyles.

TREATMENT

Soft tissue injuries

Facial soft tissues have an excellent blood supply and heal well. They should be sutured as soon as possible following the injury after careful exploration, debridement and cleaning, particularly if foreign bodies are embedded in the wounds. Most lacerations can be closed using local anaesthesia. If the patient is due to have a general anaesthetic and there is a delay, then the wounds should be temporarily closed in advance, using local anaesthesia.

Great care should be taken to replace tissues accurately, particularly in cosmetically important landmarks, such as the vermilion border of the lips, the eyelids and nasal contours. Muscle and underlying tissues should be brought together with absorbable sutures so that the edges of the wound lie passively within 2 mm of their final position. Then, fine monofilament sutures (5-0 or 6-0) are used to bring the wound edges together (Figure 27.12). Sutures should be placed so as to avoid compromising the blood supply of the apices of small flaps. Broad spectrum antibiotics should be prescribed. Ideally, alternate sutures should be removed from the third day with the remaining sutures removed on the fifth day.

Intraoral lacerations should be closed with resorbable sutures. The depth of lacerations to mobile structures, such as the tongue and soft palate, can easily be underestimated. Failure to close the deeper layers of intraoral lacerations may lead to wound dehiscence. The subsequent scars will be thickened and uncomfortable to the patient (Summary box 27.6).

Summary box 27.6

Facial lacerations

- Wounds must be thoroughly cleaned of dirt and debris to avoid tattooing
- Replace tissues accurately, especially the vermilion border

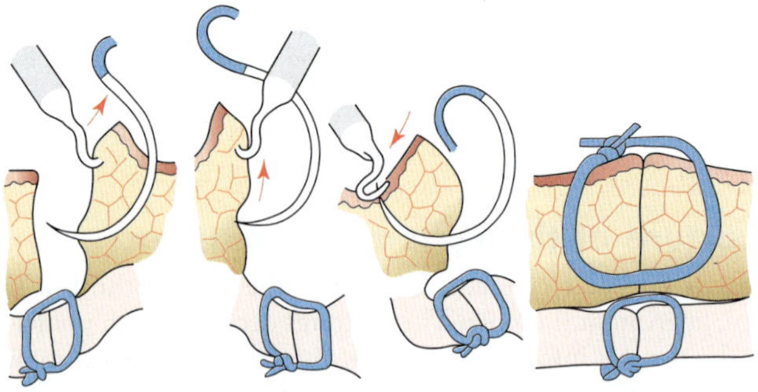

Figure 27.12 Facial wound. The method of skin closure avoiding inversion of the wound edges. The skin suture has a greater bite of deep tissue than at the surface.

Skin loss

Substantial skin and deeper tissue loss can occur as a result of human bite injuries (Figure 27.13), most commonly the nose and ear. Small areas of tissue loss can be closed by careful undermining of the surrounding soft tissues, providing that there is no significant tension on the wound edges and no distortion of the

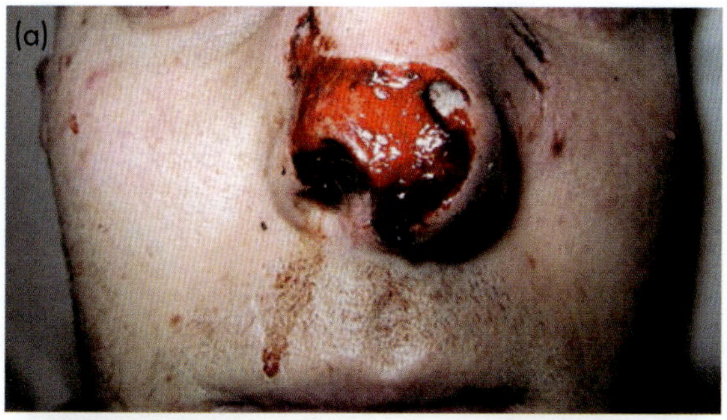

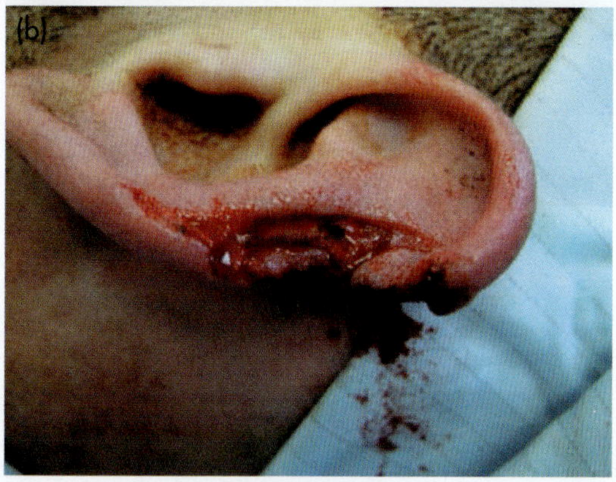

Figure 27.13 Skin and cartilage loss sustained as a result of human bite injuries. (a) Nose; (b) ear.

surrounding tissues or structures. Larger areas of skin loss require careful assessment and planned reconstruction with grafts and local tissue flaps.

Facial nerve injury

The branches of the facial nerve may be severed in the depths of a lateral facial wound. If this is suspected, primary repair should be attempted, particularly where clinical signs suggest that a major division is involved. Locating the divided branches in oedematous and damaged tissue can prove extremely difficult. Proximal and distal flaps in relatively normal adjacent tissue may have to be raised to identify the nerve on each side of the laceration. The severed nerve ends may then be approximated using an operating microscope. Attempt at primary repair should always be undertaken, as secondary repair is generally unsatisfactory (Summary box 27.7).

> **Summary box 27.7**
>
> **Facial nerve injury**
>
> - Primary repair is the most appropriate treatment

Parotid duct

Lacerations in the same vicinity as those which transect the facial nerve may also transect the parotid duct. The suggested management is to insert a fine cannula into the parotid duct from within the mouth and pass it posteriorly until it appears in the wound. The position of the proximal duct should then be identified and this portion passed over the cannula, so approximating the severed portions of the duct. The two portions of the duct are then anastomosed, and the cannula left in position for several days in an attempt to prevent post-anastomotic stricture (Summary box 27.8).

> **Summary box 27.8**
>
> **Parotid duct transection**
>
> - Cannulate from the mouth and anastomose over the stent

The lacrimal apparatus

The nasolacrimal apparatus may be involved in damage to the eyelids and skeletal facial injuries involving the naso-orbital region. The tissues are generally grossly oedematous and the manipulation required to reduce the fractures adds to the difficulty of identifying the cannaliculae. Most surgeons do not attempt repair primarily, but refer to an ophthalmic surgeon if epiphora becomes a problem later, as many heal spontaneously.

Frontal bone fractures

The presence of depressed frontal bone fractures and fractures of the posterior wall of the frontal sinus require neurosurgical collaboration. However, fractures of the anterior wall of the sinus are amenable to maxillofacial techniques for reduction and fixation. Access may be through pre-existing lacerations overlying the area, but excellent access with minimal morbidity is achieved using the bicoronal scalp flap (see below). Bone fragments may then be reduced and fixed using titanium bone plates and screws. Any missing bone should be replaced with bone grafts, thereby avoiding any cosmetic forehead depression postoperatively.

Fractures of the maxilla

The principle of reducing and stabilising fractures of the frontal and facial bones is that the surgeon starts at the top and works down. Where no convenient lacerations exist, fractures of the frontal bone, supraorbital ridge and nasal root may be approached through a bicoronal incision, at the vault of the skull, high in the hair line. The incision is taken from just in front of each ear across the vault of the skull. The skin and galea are reflected forwards until the supraorbital ridges are exposed. The supraorbital nerves are identified and freed and the flap extended as required. The nasal bones, lateral orbital rim, frontal bones and zygomatic arches may all be exposed through this approach. The fractured bones may be reduced and fixed by stainless steel wire or titanium mini/microplates, under direct vision. Bone deficiencies in this area may be made up with free, outer cortical cranial bone grafts, with the donor sites available through the bicoronal incision. Where there has been disruption of the medial canthal ligaments, these should be identified and sutured/wired to the opposite side to restore canthal width.

When the stabilisation of the upper part of the face is complete, attention may be turned to the midface. Incisions in the lower eyelid (blepharoplasty incision), lower conjunctival sac or infraorbital region are used to explore fractures of the infraorbital rim. These also give access to the orbital floor and are used to treat orbital blow-out fractures. The fractured rim may be fixed using mini/microplates or wires as above, and the floor of the orbit reconstructed with bone, titanium mesh or alloplastic material.

The lower part of the maxilla is approached through a gingival sulcus incision above the maxillary teeth as far back as the second molar. Fractures are fixed with plates or wires. The dental arch is restored to its original shape as far as possible so that it matches the premorbid occlusion with the mandibular arch. To achieve accurate location, dental arch bars, intermaxillary fixation screws or eyelet wires (see below) may need to be applied. Where this is anticipated, the necessary wiring is undertaken before the main part of the operation is commenced.

The principle of treatment is to restore the maxillary fragments to their original position. To achieve this, usually it is necessary to reduce the maxilla first with Rowe's disimpaction forceps, which grasp the palate between the nasal and palatal mucosa. Considerable force is sometimes required in a series of downward, forwards and sideways movements to mobilise it. After 2–3 weeks, full disimpaction is often impossible (Summary box 27.9).

Summary box 27.9

Fixation of maxillary fractures

- Orbital floor deficiencies may be made up with grafts, titanium mesh or alloplasts
- Intermaxillary fixation may be needed to achieve the correct occlusion

Fractures of the mandible

Fractures of the mandible were traditionally reduced indirectly and then fixed with intermaxillary fixation (IMF). IMF is simply a means of splinting the upper and lower arches of teeth together (Figure 27.14). However, the introduction of maxillofacial fixation systems utilising titanium fixtures has significantly altered the management of patients sustaining maxillofacial fractures. Prior to the introduction of these plating systems, patients would often have their jaws 'wired together' for a period of up to 6 weeks. Now, although patients may be placed in temporary IMF during their operative procedure, it is more often than not released at the end of the procedure when the rigid plate fixation has been applied (Figure 27.15).

Mandibular fractures may be explored through intraoral or extraoral incisions according to the access required. Pre-existing lacerations overlying the mandible may be used to gain access to the fracture (Figure 27.16). To be sure of achieving a correct dental occlusion, it is wise to use temporary intraoperative IMF. There are occasions where, in spite of rigid fixation with titanium miniplates, IMF or elastic traction is still required in the postoperative period. In this event, the IMF is removed during the recovery from anaesthesia, so as not to risk complications involving the airway. The IMF may then be reapplied when the patient has fully recovered from the general anaesthetic.

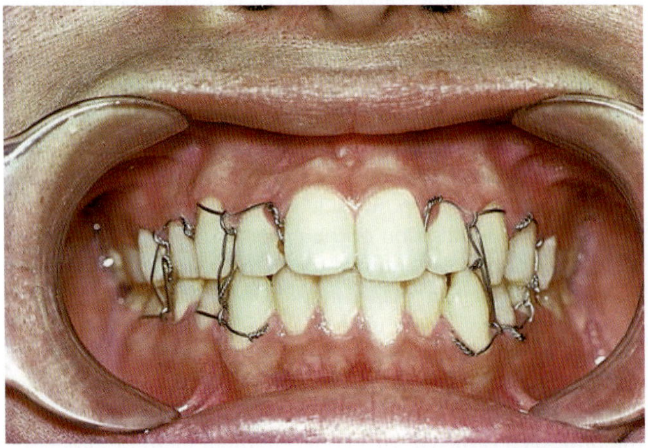

Figure 27.14 Intermaxillary fixation using eyelet wires.

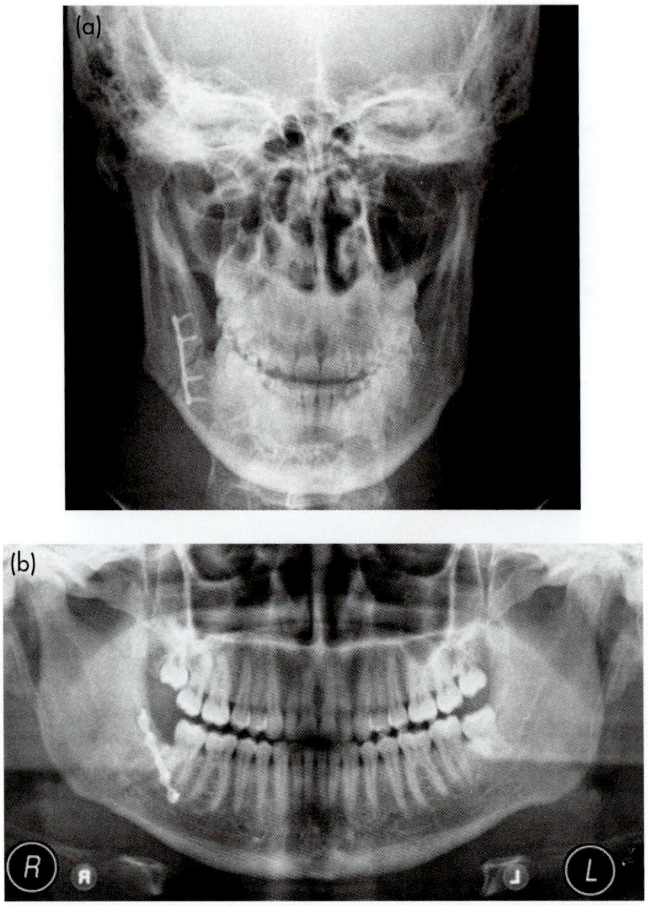

Figure 27.15 A fractured mandible treated by open reduction and fixation using a titanium miniplate. No postoperative intermaxillary fixation (IMF) has been used. (a) Posteroanterior view; (b) orthopantomogram.

Fractures of the edentulous (non-tooth-bearing) mandible are generally reduced and fixed using titanium plates. In the very atrophic mandible, the raising of the periosteum should be kept to a minimum as the blood supply to the jaw may be compromised (Summary box 27.10).

Summary box 27.10

Fixation of the mandible

- Plating has made long term jaw wiring almost redundant

Fractures of the mandibular condyle may cause disturbance of the occlusion with deviation of the mandible to the side of the fracture. In unilateral fractures, which are minimally displaced,

Norman Lester Rowe, 1915–1991, maxillofacial surgeon, Queen Mary's University Hospital, Roehampton, London, UK.

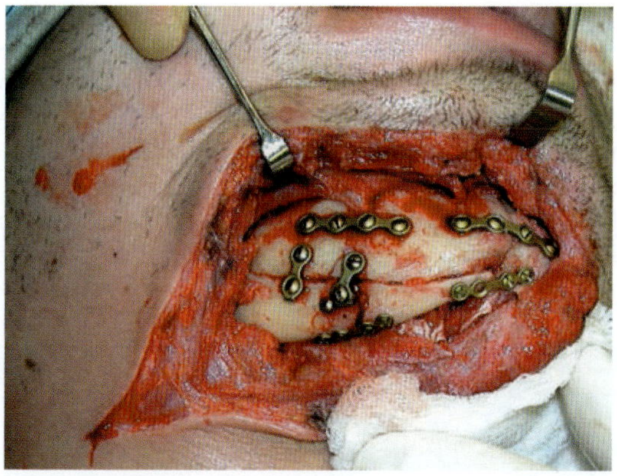

Figure 27.16 Comminuted fracture of the mandible approached through a pre-existing laceration.

this disturbance may not be evident. However, displaced unilateral fractures and bilateral condylar fractures often present with such a disturbance and, as such, constitute an indication for open reduction and fixation of the condylar fractures to prevent the formation of an abnormal occlusion. This malocclusion develops due to the vertical pull of the muscles of mastication shortening the ramus height. The posterior teeth contact first and the anterior teeth remain apart. Functionally and cosmetically, this is undesirable and is difficult to counteract by secondary procedures. It is not adequate to simply fix the mandible in IMF, except in the most minimally displaced malocclusions. Open reduction and fixation of the fractured mandibular condyle within 7–14 days of the original injury is indicated if a significant malocclusion is evident in a unilateral condylar fracture with displacement, or a in a bilateral condylar fracture (Summary box 27.11).

Summary box 27.11

Fixation of mandibular condyles

- If displaced or bilateral, with significant occlusal disturbance, surgical intervention will be required
- Reduction and plating helps prevent anterior open bite

Fractures of the zygomatic complex

Displacement of zygomatic complex fractures is usually in a posterior direction, although it is important to assess the actual displacement by studying the occipitomental radiographs. Most fractures may be reduced by the Gillies temporal approach. This entails an incision in the hairline, superficial to the temporal fossa, about 15 mm long, at 45° to the vertical. It is deepened down to and through the temporalis fascia. A channel is prepared below the fascia and down under the body of the zygoma and arch. A Bristow or Rowe elevator is then inserted beneath the body of the zygoma or arch, according to the site of the fracture. Force is then applied in the opposite direction to the displacement of the fracture. After reduction, the position of the zygoma can be checked by palpating the bony prominences of the zygomatic arch, and the lateral and inferior orbital rims. As all fractures of the zygoma, other than those solely of the arch, involve the orbital floor, it is essential to apply a forced duction test to ensure no limitation of movement of the inferior oblique and inferior rectus muscles. For this to be done, the lower eyelid is retracted and the inferior rectus grabbed in the lower fornix. The globe can then be rotated upwards and should move freely. Any restriction in movement suggests entrapment of the infraorbital soft tissues, and the floor of the orbit should be explored as for a blow-out fracture (see below).

Should the fracture be unstable, open reduction and fixation of the fracture may be necessary. The frontozygomatic suture may be exposed by a small incision just behind the lateral part of the eyebrow and visualised. Displacements may be reduced and fixed with intraosseous wires or bone plates. Occasionally, it is necessary to explore and fix fractures at the infraorbital rim (see above under Fractures of the maxilla), or at the zygomatic buttress intraorally (Summary box 27.12).

Sir Harold Delf Gillies, 1882–1960, plastic surgeon, St Bartholomew's Hospital, London, UK. Born in New Zealand, widely considered the 'father of plastic surgery', started his craft to better the lives of the victims of the First World War. Later, he became a pioneer in gender reassignment (sex change) surgery. When he was finally knighted in 1930 for his wartime work, William Arbuttinot-Lane commented 'Better late than never!'. He excelled in most sports (cricket, rowing, golf) and despite a stiff elbow from a childhood injury was an accomplished painter.

Summary box 27.12

Fixation of fractures of the zygomatic complex

- The arch is elevated
- Ocular tethering should be checked if the fracture involves the orbital floor
- Regular postoperative observations must be made for retrobulbar haemorrhage

All patients who have had operations involving the orbit should have formal eye observations in the postoperative period. The condition of the eye, pupil size and light reaction should be recorded. Occasional complications occur, the most serious of which is a developing retrobulbar haematoma. Increasing proptosis and loss of vision constitute a postoperative emergency requiring immediate action to reduce the pressure of the haematoma.

Orbital blow-out fractures

These fractures are ideally treated within 10–14 days of the original injury. The aim of treatment is to reduce any soft tissue herniation of the periorbita (Figure 27.17), restore the continuity of the orbital floor, and restore any functional deficit of ocular function caused by extraocular muscle dysfunction. The floor of the orbit is approached either through a blepharoplasty incision in the lower eyelid or through the inferior fornix. The infraorbital margin is identified and the periosteum raised, attempting to avoid displacement of the delicate fragments of bone constituting the fracture. The periorbital soft tissues are gently separated from the bone of the fracture and freed so that no trapping or soft tissue herniation into the antrum remains. Defects of the orbital floor may be made up with bone grafts or from a variety of sources, such as titanium mesh or other suitably rigid materials. These materials may be fixed in place with wires, screws or plates (Summary box 27.13).

Walter Rowley Bristow, 1882–1947, orthopaedic surgeon, St Thomas's Hospital, London, UK.
Henri Luc, 1855–1925, otolaryngologist, in Paris, France, described his operation in 1889.
Walter Whitehead, 1840–1913, surgeon, The Royal Infirmary, Manchester, UK. Whitehead's varnish consists of iodoform, benzoin, storax and Tolu balsam in ether.

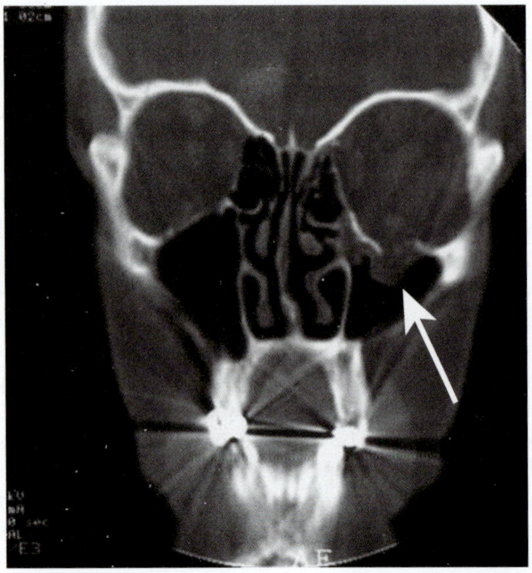

Figure 27.17 Coronal computed tomographic (CT) scan showing a left orbital blow-out fracture, with evident soft-tissue herniation into the maxillary antrum.

Summary box 27.13

Orbital blow-out fractures

- Defects of the orbital floor can be made up with bone graft or with synthetic materials

GENERAL

Fractures of the facial skeleton are almost always compound and prophylactic antibiotics are important. Penicillin/amoxycillin and metronidazole singly or in combination are ideal for those patients who are not allergic to them.

All patients with fractures of the facial skeleton benefit from intraoperative and postoperative dexamethasone, to reduce facial oedema (Summary box 27.14).

Summary box 27.14

General principles in facial fractures

- Prophylactic antibiotics should be given
- Dexamethasone may help to reduce facial oedema

FURTHER READING

Langdon J, Patel M, Ord R, Brennan P (eds). *Operative oral and maxillofacial surgery*, 2nd end. London: Hodder Arnold, 2010.

Ward Booth P, Eppley B, Schmelzeisen R. Maxillofacial trauma and esthetic reconstruction. Edinburgh: Churchill Livingstone, 2003.

Ward Booth P, Schendel SA, Hausamen JE. *Maxillofacial surgery*, 2nd edn. Edinburgh: Churchill Livingstone, 2006.

George Walter Caldwell, 1866–1946, otolaryngologist who practised successively in New York, San Francisco and Los Angeles. He described his operation for suppuration in the maxillary antrum in 1893.

CHAPTER

28

Torso trauma

LEARNING OBJECTIVES

To understand:

- That the management of trauma is based on physiology, as well as anatomy (as in general surgery)
- The gross and surgical anatomy of the chest and abdomen
- The pathophysiology of torso injury
- The strength and weaknesses of clinical assessment in the injured patient
- The use of special investigations and their limitations
- The operative approaches to the thoracic cavity
- The special features of an emergency department thoracotomy for haemorrhage control
- The indications for and techniques of the trauma laparotomy
- The philosophy of damage control surgery

INTRODUCTION

The torso is generally regarded as the area between the neck and the groin, made up of the thorax and abdomen. This is the largest area of the body and is commonly injured. Because injury does not respect anatomical boundaries, division of the body into abdomen and thorax is artificial, and injury to the torso, with its associated physiological consequences, is more appropriate. About 42 per cent of all deaths are the result of brain injury, but some 39 per cent of all trauma deaths are caused by major haemorrhage, usually from torso injury (Figure 28.1).

Although initially injury was treated on an anatomical basis, it has become clear that physiology should be the over-riding consideration, and the driver of successful resuscitation is therefore the preservation of normal physiology. Techniques such as 'damage control resuscitation' and 'damage control surgery' have dramatically improved survival through an understanding of the best techniques required to restore physiological stability (see Chapters 24 and 32).

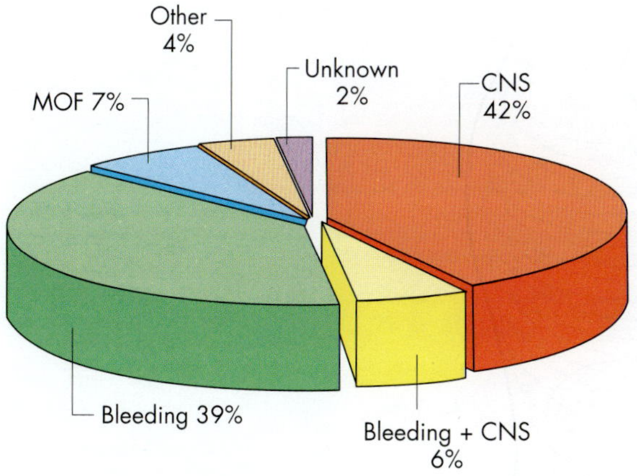

Figure 28.1 Causes of death in trauma. CNS, central nervous system; MOF, multiple organ failure.

INJURY MECHANISMS ASSOCIATED WITH TORSO TRAUMA

Injury often traverses different anatomical zones of the body, affecting structures on both sides of traditional anatomical zones. These zones are known as 'junctional zones'.

Junctional zones

The key junctional zones are:

- between the neck and the thorax;
- between the thorax and the abdomen;
- between the abdomen, the pelvic structures and the groin.

These zones represent surgical challenges in terms of both the diagnosis of the area of injury and the surgical approach, which have to be balanced against the physiological stability of the patient.

Root of the neck

Most injuries affecting the base of the neck also affect the upper mediastinum and thoracic inlet. Choice of access is determined by the need for surgical control of the vascular structures contained within.

The mediastinum

The zone overlying the mediastinum with its major vessels and the heart is also an extremely high-risk area for penetrating wounds. Any wound in this region should immediately raise the suspicion of an associated cardiac or major vascular injury even in the absence of initial gross physical signs.

Diaphragm

The thorax and abdomen are separated by the diaphragm, which is mainly responsible for breathing, and moves during breathing, between the fourth to the eighth interspace. Any penetrating injury of the lower half of the chest may therefore have penetrated the diaphragm and entered the abdomen. Injuries in this junctional zone, therefore, should be managed as if both cavities had been penetrated (Figure 28.2).

Pelvic structures and groin

The pelvis contains a large plexus of vessels, both venous and arterial. Should injury occur, control of haemorrhage can prove to be exceptionally difficult and may require control of both inflow and outflow. This may involve surgical control at the groin of the external iliac and femoral vessels, as well as at the aortic and cava level. Angioembolisation can be a very useful adjunct to treatment.

Retroperitoneum

Injury to the retroperitoneum is often difficult to diagnose, especially in the presence of other injury, when the signs may be masked. Intraperitoneal diagnostic tests (ultrasound and diagnostic peritoneal lavage) may be negative. The best diagnostic modality is the computed tomography (CT) scan, but this requires a physiologically stable patient. The retroperitoneum is divided into three zones (Figure 28.3):

1. Zone 1 (central): central haematomas should always be explored, once proximal and distal vascular control has been obtained.
2. Zone 2 (lateral): lateral haematomas are usually renal in origin and can be managed non-operatively, they may sometimes require angioembolisation.
3. Zone 3 (pelvic): pelvic haematomas are exceptionally difficult to control and, whenever possible, should not be opened; they should be controlled with packing (intra- or extraperitonial) and angioembolisation (Summary box 28.1).

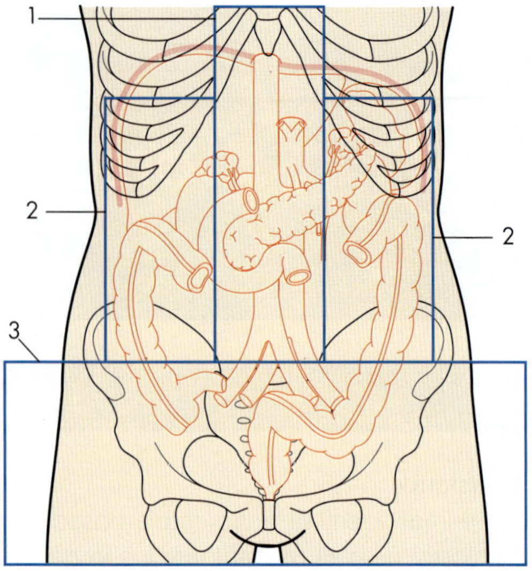

Figure 28.3 The zones of the retroperitoneum. Zone 1, central; zone 2, lateral; zone 3, pelvic.

Summary box 28.1

Junctional zones

- Neck
- Mediastinum
- Diaphragm
- Groin
- Retroperitoneum

CRITICAL PHYSIOLOGY

Resuscitation of all injuries to the chest and abdomen should follow traditional Advanced Trauma Life Support (ATLS) principles (Table 28.1 and see Chapter 24).

Bleeding is the major problem for diagnosis. This may be obvious at the time of evaluation; however, in the young fit individual, bleeding into the chest and abdomen may only produce subtle changes in vital measures and therefore be difficult to assess (Table 28.2). Bleeding occurs from five major sites: 'one on the floor and four more':

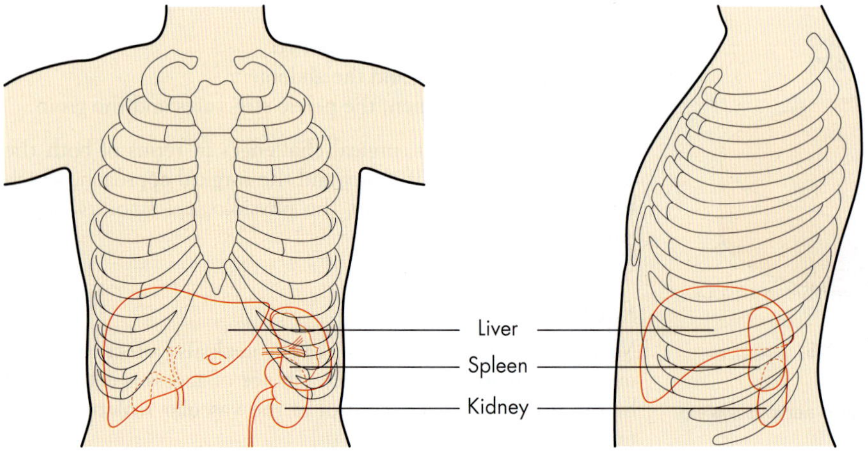

Figure 28.2 The extent of the abdomen.

1 external (i.e. skin);
2 chest;
3 abdomen;
4 pelvis;
5 extremities (e.g. fractures).

Although obvious injury may be present, traditional indicators (such as pulse rate) are unreliable in young patients. A normal pulse for a middle-aged patient may be a significantly raised pulse for a young fit person.

Table 28.1 Advanced Trauma Life Support (ATLS) principles of resuscitation.

A	Airway
B	Breathing
C	Circulation
D	Disability (neurology)
E	Environment and exposure

Table 28.2 Clinical indicators of potential ongoing bleeding in torso trauma.

Physiological	Increasing respiratory rate
	Increasing pulse rate
	Falling blood pressure
	Rising serum lactate
Anatomical	Visible bleeding
	Injury in close proximity to major vessels
	Penetrating injury with a retained missile

THORACIC INJURY

Thoracic injury accounts for 25 per cent of all severe injuries. In a further 25 per cent, it may be a significant contributor to the subsequent death of the patient. In most of these patients, the cause of death is haemorrhage.

Chest injuries are often life-threatening, either in their own right or in conjunction with other system injuries. About 80 per cent of patients with chest injury can be managed non-operatively. The key to a good outcome is early physiological resuscitation followed by a correct diagnosis.

Investigation

Routine investigation in the emergency department of injury to the chest is based on clinical examination, supplemented by chest radiography. Ultrasound can be used to differentiate between contusion and the actual presence of blood. A chest tube can be a diagnostic procedure, as well as a therapeutic one, and the benefits of insertion often outweigh the risks.

The pitfalls of investigation are:

- failure to auscultate both front and back (an inflated lung will 'float' on a haemothorax, so auscultation from the front may sound normal);
- failure to pass a nasogastric tube if rupture of the diaphragm is suspected;
- pursuing radiological investigation (radiography or CT scan) instead of resuscitation in the unstable patient.

Computed tomography scan

The CT scan has become the principal and most reliable examination for major injury in thoracic trauma. Scanning with contrast allows for three-dimensional reconstruction of the chest and abdomen, as well as of the bony skeleton. In blunt chest trauma, the CT scan will allow the definition of fractures, as well as showing haematomas, pneumothoraces and pulmonary contusion. In penetrating trauma, the scan may show the track or presence of the missile and allow the proper planning of definitive surgery.

CT scanning has replaced angiography as the diagnostic modality of choice for the assessment of the thoracic aorta (Summary box 28.2).

Summary box 28.2

Investigation of chest injuries

- Directly or indirectly involved in 50 per cent of trauma deaths in the United States.
- Eighty per cent can be managed non-operatively
- A chest radiograph is the investigation of first choice
- A spiral computed tomography scan provides rapid diagnoses in the chest and abdomen
- A chest drain can be diagnostic as well as therapeutic

Management

Most patients who have suffered penetrating injury to the chest can be managed with appropriate resuscitation and drainage of haematoma.

If a sucking chest wound is present, this should not be fully closed but should be covered with a piece of plastic, closed on three sides, to form a one-way valve, and thereafter an underwater chest drain should be inserted remote from the wound. No attempt should be made to close a sucking chest wound until controlled drainage has been achieved, in case a stable open pneumothorax is converted into an unstable tension pneumothorax.

In blunt injury, most bleeding occurs from the intercostal or internal mammary vessels and it is relatively rare for these to require surgery. If bleeding does not stop spontaneously, the vessels can be tied off or encircled. In blunt chest compressive injury, there is injury to the ribs and frequently to the underlying structures as well, with an associated lung contusion (Summary box 28.3).

Summary box 28.3

Closed management of chest injuries

- About 80 per cent of chest injuries can be managed closed
- If there is an open wound, insert a chest drain
- Do not close a sucking chest wound until a drain is in place
- If bleeding persists, the chest will need to be opened

The patient *in extremis* with exsanguinating chest haemorrhage will be discussed in the section below under Emergency thoracotomy.

Life-threatening injuries can be remembered as the 'deadly dozen'. Six are immediately life-threatening and should be sought during the primary survey and six are potentially life-threatening and should be detected during the secondary survey (Table 28.3).

Table 28.3 The 'deadly dozen' threats to life from chest injury.

Immediately life threatening	Airway obstruction
	Tension pneumothorax
	Pericardial tamponade
	Open pneumothorax
	Massive haemothorax
	Flail chest
Potentially life threatening	Aortic injuries
	Trachcobronchial injuries
	Myocardial contusion
	Rupture of diaphragm
	Oesophageal injuries
	Pulmonary contusion

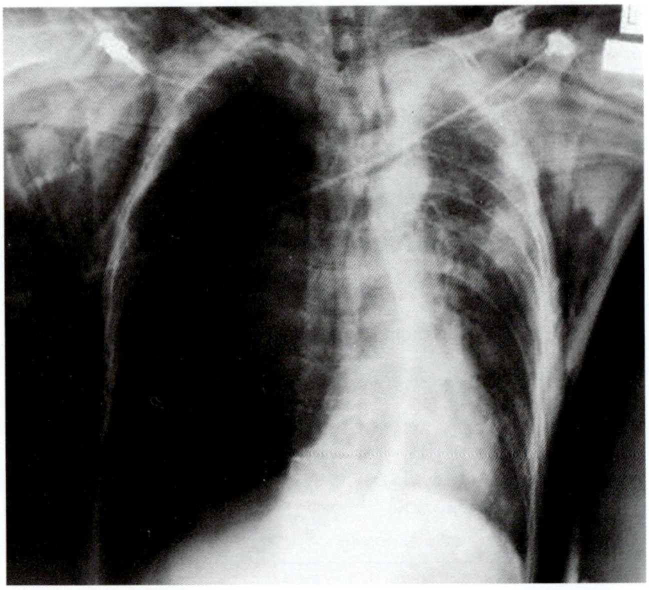

Figure 28.4 Radiological appearance of a tension pneumothorax.

Efficient initial assessment should focus on identifying and correcting the immediate threats to life. A high index of suspicion must be maintained thereafter to diagnose the potential threats to life as their symptoms and signs can be very subtle. Early consultation and referral to a trauma centre is advised in cases of doubt.

Immediate life-threatening injuries

Airway obstruction

Early intubation is very important, particularly in cases of neck haematoma or possible airway oedema. Airway distortion can be insidious and progressive and can make delayed intubation more difficult if not impossible.

Tension pneumothorax

A tension pneumothorax develops when a 'one-way valve' air leak occurs either from the lung or through the chest wall. Air is sucked into the thoracic cavity without any means of escape, completely collapsing then compressing the affected lung. The mediastinum is displaced to the opposite side, decreasing venous return and compressing the opposite lung.

The most common causes are penetrating chest trauma, blunt chest trauma with parenchymal lung injury and air leak that did not spontaneously close, iatrogenic lung punctures (e.g. due to subclavian central venepuncture) and mechanical positive pressure ventilation.

The clinical presentation is dramatic. The patient is increasingly panicky with tachypnoea, dyspnoea and distended neck veins (similar to pericardial tamponade). Clinical examination may reveal tracheal deviation. This is a late finding and is not necessary to clinically confirm diagnosis. There will also be hyper-resonance and absent breath sounds over the affected hemithorax. Tension pneumothorax is a clinical diagnosis and treatment should never be delayed by waiting for radiological confirmation (Figure 28.4).

Treatment consists of immediate decompression, initially by rapid insertion of a large-bore needle into the second intercostal space in the midclavicular line of the affected hemithorax, and then followed by insertion of a chest tube through the fifth intercostal space in the anterior axillary line.

Pericardial tamponade

Pericardial tamponade needs to be differentiated from a tension pneumothorax in the shocked patient with distended neck veins. It is most commonly the result of penetrating trauma. Accumulation of a relatively small amount of blood into the non-distensible pericardial sac can produce physiological obstruction of the heart. All patients with penetrating injury anywhere near the heart plus shock must be considered to have a cardiac injury until proven otherwise. Classically, the presentation consists of venous pressure elevation, decline in arterial pressure with tachycardia, and muffled heart sounds. A high index of suspicion and further diagnostic investigations will be needed to make the diagnosis is those cases which are not clinically obvious. This includes chest radiography looking for an enlarged heart shadow or a cardiac ultrasound showing fluid in the pericardial sac. A central line should be inserted checking for a rising central venous pressure. However, in cases in which major bleeding from other sites has taken place, the neck veins may be flat.

Needle pericardiocentesis may allow the aspiration of a few millilitres of blood and this, along with rapid volume resuscitation to increase preload, can buy enough time to move the patient to the operating room. However, in penetrating injury to the heart, there is usually a substantial clot in the pericardium, which may prevent aspiration. A dry pericardiocentesis proves only that there is a 'clot' on both ends of the needle! Pericardiocentesis has a high potential for iatrogenic injury to the heart and it should at the most be regarded as a desperate temporising measure in a transport situation (under electrocardiogram (ECG) control). The correct immediate treatment of tamponade is operative (sternotomy or left thoracotomy), with repair of the heart in the operating theatre if time allows or otherwise in the emergency room (Summary box 28.4).

> **Summary box 28.4**
>
> **Pericardial tamponade**
>
> - The presentation is similar to a tension pneumothorax: deteriorating cyanosis tachycardia and agitation
> - Ultrasound is diagnostic
> - The central venous pressure may not be elevated if the circulating volume is depleted, e.g. because of other injuries
> - Pericardiocentesis is a temporising measure only with a high complication rate and is not a substitute for immediate operative intervention

Open pneumothorax ('sucking chest wound')

This is due to a large open defect in the chest (>3 cm), leading to equilibration between intrathoracic and atmospheric pressure. Air accumulates in the hemithorax (rather than in the lung) with each inspiration, leading to profound hypoventilation on the affected side and hypoxia. Signs and symptoms are usually proportionate to the size of the defect. If there is a valvular effect, increasing amounts of air in the pleura will result in a tension pneumothorax (see above under Tension pneumothorax).

Initial management consists of promptly closing the defect with a sterile occlusive plastic dressing (e.g. Opsite®), taped on three sides to act as a flutter-type valve. A chest tube is inserted as soon as possible in a site remote from the injury site. Definitive treatment may warrant formal debridement and closure, and early referral.

The following points are important in the management of an open pneumothorax:

- a common problem is using too small a tube: a 28FG or larger tube should be used in an adult;
- If the lung does not reinflate, the drain should be placed on low-pressure (5 cm water) suction;
- a second drain is sometimes necessary (but see below under Tracheobronchial injuries);
- physiotherapy and active mobilisation should begin as soon as possible.

Massive haemothorax

The most common cause of massive haemothorax in blunt injury is continuing bleeding from torn intercostal vessels or occasionally from the internal mammary artery.

Accumulation of blood in a hemithorax can significantly compromise respiratory efforts, compressing the lung and preventing adequate ventilation. Presentation is with haemorrhagic shock, flat neck veins, unilateral absence of breath sounds and dullness to percussion. The treatment consists of correcting the hypovolaemic shock, insertion of an intercostal drain and, in some cases, intubation.

Blood in the pleural space should be removed as completely and rapidly as possible to prevent ongoing bleeding, empyema or a late fibrothorax. Clamping a chest drain to tamponade a massive haemothorax is usually not helpful.

Initial drainage of more than 1500 mL of blood or ongoing haemorrhage of more than 200 mL/hour over 3–4 hours is generally considered an indication for urgent thoracotomy.

Flail chest

This condition usually results from blunt trauma associated with multiple rib fractures, and is defined as three or more ribs fractured in two or more places. The blunt force required to disrupt the integrity of the thoracic cage typically produces an underlying pulmonary contusion as well. The diagnosis is made clinically, not by radiography. On inspiration, the loose segment of the chest wall is displaced inwards and therefore less air moves into the lungs. To confirm the diagnosis, the chest wall can be observed for paradoxical motion of a chest wall segment during respiration and during coughing. Voluntary splinting of the chest wall occurs as a result of pain, so mechanically impaired chest wall movement and the associated lung contusion all contribute to the hypoxia. There is a high risk of developing a pneumothorax or haemothorax.

Traditionally, mechanical ventilation was used to 'internally splint' the chest, but had a price in terms of intensive care unit resources and ventilation-dependent morbidity. Currently, treatment consists of oxygen administration, adequate analgesia (including opiates) and physiotherapy. If a chest tube is *in situ*, intrapleural local analgesia can be used as well. Ventilation is reserved for cases developing respiratory failure despite adequate analgesia and oxygen. Surgery to stabilise the flail chest may be useful in a selected group of patients with isolated or severe chest injury and pulmonary contusion.

Potentially life-threatening injuries

Thoracic aortic disruption

Traumatic aortic rupture is a common cause of sudden death after an automobile collision or fall from a great height. The vessel is relatively fixed distal to the ligamentum arteriosum, just distal to the origin of the left subclavian artery. The shear forces from a sudden impact disrupt the intima and media. If the adventitia is intact, the patient may remain stable. For the subgroup of immediate survivors, salvage is frequently possible if aortic rupture is identified and treated early. It should be clinically suspected in patients with asymmetry of upper or upper and lower extremity blood pressure, widened pulse pressure and chest wall contusion. Erect chest radiography can also suggest thoracic aortic disruption, the most common radiological finding being a widened mediastinum (Figure 28.5). The diagnosis is confirmed by a CT scan of the mediastinum (Figure 28.6) or possibly by transoesophageal echocardiography.

Initially, management consists of control of the systolic arterial blood pressure (to less than 100 mmHg). Thereafter, an endovascular intra-aortic stent (Figure 28.7) can be placed or the tear can be operatively repaired by direct repair or excision and grafting using a Dacron graft.

Tracheobronchial injuries

Severe subcutaneous emphysema with respiratory compromise can suggest tracheobronchial disruption. A chest drain placed on the affected side will reveal a large air leak and the collapsed lung may fail to re-expand. If after insertion of a second drain the lung fails to re-expand, referral to a trauma centre is advised.

Bronchoscopy is diagnostic. Treatment involves intubation of the unaffected bronchus followed by operative repair.

Blunt myocardial injury

Significant blunt cardiac injury that causes haemodynamic instability is rare. Blunt myocardial injury should be suspected in any patient sustaining blunt trauma who develops early ECG abnormalities.

in situ is Latin for 'in place'.

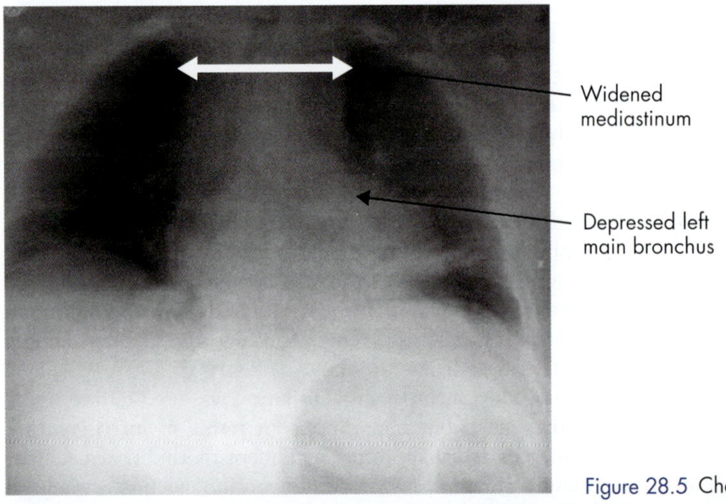

Figure 28.5 Chest radiograph showing a widened mediastinum.

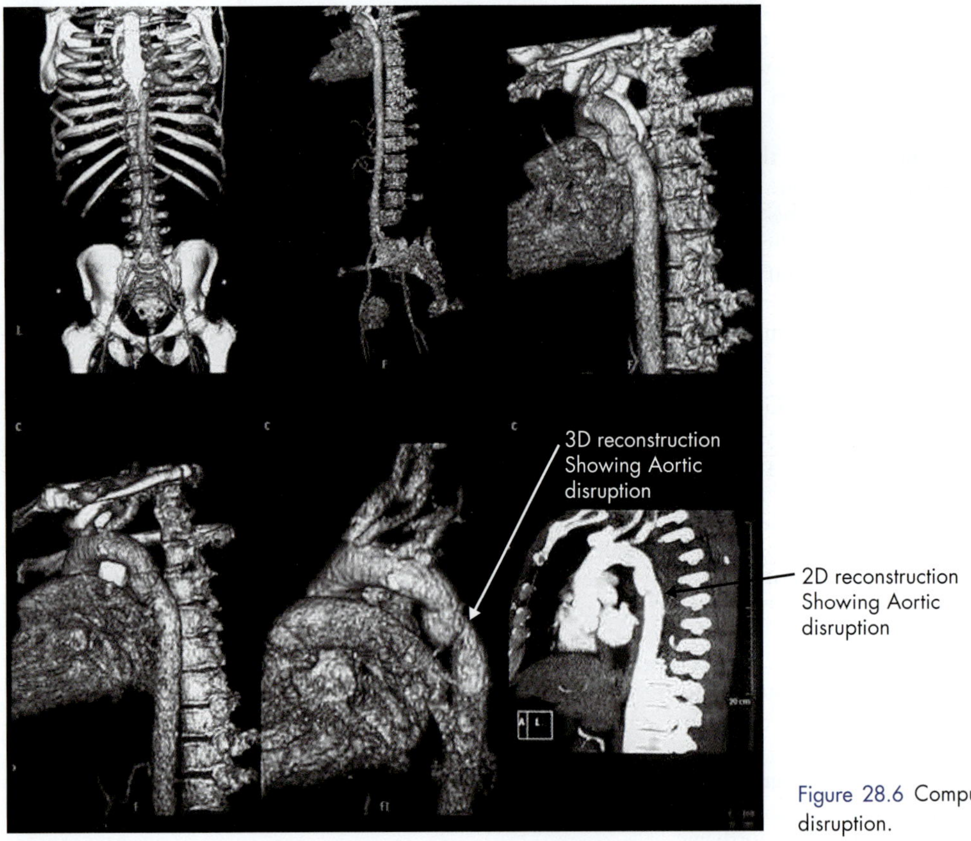

Figure 28.6 Computed tomography scan showing aortic disruption.

Two-dimensional echocardiography may show wall motion abnormalities. A transoesophageal echocardiogram may also be helpful. There is very little evidence that enzyme estimations have any place in diagnosis.

All patients with myocardial contusion diagnosed by conduction abnormalities are at risk of developing sudden dysrhythmias and should be closely monitored.

Diaphragmatic injuries

Any penetrating injury below the fifth intercostal space should raise suspicion of diaphragmatic penetration and, therefore, injury to the abdominal contents.

Blunt injury to the diaphragm is usually caused by a compressive force applied to the pelvis and abdomen. The diaphragmatic rupture is usually large, with herniation of the abdominal contents into the chest. Diagnosis of blunt diaphragmatic rupture is missed even more often than penetrating injuries in the acute phase.

Most diaphragmatic injuries are silent and the presenting features are those of injury to the surrounding organs. There is no single standard investigation. Chest radiography after placement of a nasogastric tube may be helpful (as this may show the stomach herniated into the chest). Contrast studies of the upper or lower gastrointestinal tract, CT scan and diagnostic peritoneal

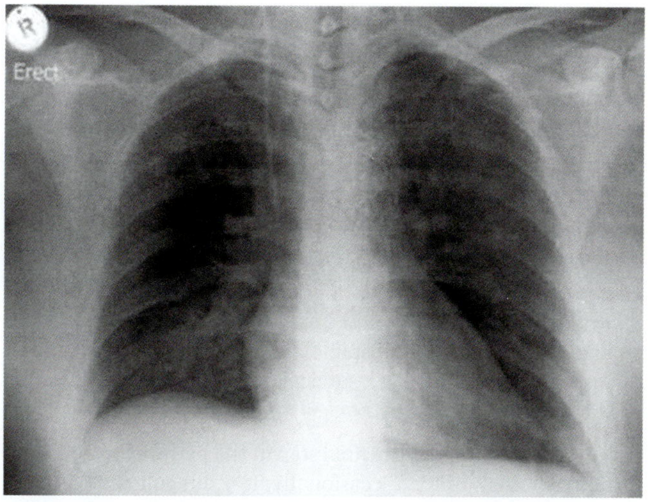

Figure 28.7 Aortic tear showing presence of stent.

lavage all lack positive or negative predictive value. The most accurate evaluation is by video-assisted thoracoscopy (VATS) or laparoscopy, the latter offering the advantage of allowing the surgeon to proceed to a repair and additional evaluation of the abdominal organs (Summary box 28.5).

Summary box 28.5

Blunt injuries

- Rupture of the diaphragm is easily missed
- Myocardial injury must be suspected if there are abnormal ECG changes
- Mortality rises rapidly with delay in diagnosis of oesophageal rupture
- In severe pulmonary contusion ventilation may be needed

Operative repair is recommended in all cases. All penetrating diaphragmatic injury must be repaired via the abdomen and not the chest, to rule out penetrating hollow viscus injury.

The thorax is at negative pressure and the abdomen is at positive pressure. A late complication of rupture of the diaphragm is herniation of the abdominal contents into the chest. Strangulation of any of the contents can then occur, and the patients have a high mortality rate.

Oesophageal injury

Most oesophageal injuries result from penetrating trauma; blunt injury is rare. A high index of suspicion is required. The patient can present with odynophagia (pain on swallowing foods or fluids), subcutaneous or mediastinal emphysema, pleural effusion, air in the retro-oesophageal space and unexplained fever. Mediastinal and deep cervical emphysema are evidence of an aerodigestive injury until proven otherwise.

The mortality rate rises exponentially if treatment is delayed. A combination of oesophagogram in the decubitus position and oesophagoscopy confirm the diagnosis in the great majority of cases. The treatment is operative repair and drainage.

Pulmonary contusion

Pulmonary contusion occurs following blunt trauma, usually underneath a flail segment or fractured ribs. This is a very common, potentially lethal injury and the major cause of hypoxaemia after blunt trauma.

The natural progression of pulmonary contusion is worsening hypoxemia for the first 24–48 hours. The chest radiography findings are typically delayed. Contrast CT scanning can be confirmatory. Haemoptysis or blood in the endotracheal tube is a sign of pulmonary contusion.

In mild contusion, the treatment is oxygen administration, aggressive pulmonary toilet and adequate analgesia. In more severe cases, mechanical ventilation is necessary. Normovolaemia is critical for adequate tissue perfusion and fluid restriction is not advised.

Continuing blood loss

The first principle of all care is to assess and treat the patient according to the physiology. Initial blood loss of more than 1500 mL indicates the potential for class III shock, and any ongoing bleeding must be dealt with surgically, as soon as possible. Similarly, an ongoing blood loss of more than 200 mL/hour for 3 consecutive hours requires resuscitative surgery to stop the bleeding.

EMERGENCY THORACOTOMY

Emergency thoracic surgery is an essential part of the armamentarium of any surgeon dealing with major trauma. A timely thoracotomy for the correct indications can be the key step in saving an injured patient's life.

Indications for thoracotomy include the need to perform:

- internal cardiac massage;
- control of haemorrhage from injury to the heart or lung;
- control of intrathoracic haemorrhage from other causes;
- control of massive air leak.

The clinical decision as to whether a casualty requires an emergency department thoracotomy (EDT) or can be transferred to the operating theatre can be complex. It is far better to perform a thoracotomy in the operating theatre, either through an anterolateral approach or a median sternotomy, with good light and assistance, and the potential for autotransfusion or bypass, than it is to attempt heroic emergency surgery in the resuscitation area. However, if the patient is *in extremis* with a falling systolic blood pressure, there is no choice but to proceed immediately with a left anterolateral thoracotomy. In certain circumstances, when care is futile, it may not need to be performed at all. A resuscitation room thoracotomy following blunt trauma has limited indications and is rarely successful.

Emergency department thoracotomy

EDT should be reserved for those patients suffering penetrating injury in whom signs of life are still present. Patients who have received cardiopulmonary resuscitation (CPR) in the prehospital phase of their care are unlikely to survive, and electrical activity must be present. The survival rates for EDT in patients with penetrating trauma in whom the blood pressure is falling despite adequate resuscitation are shown in Table 28.4.

It is important to make a distinction between:

- immediate thoracotomy in the emergency department for the control of haemorrhage, cardiac tamponade, or for internal cardiac massage;

Table 28.4 Survival rates for thoracotomy in patients with penetrating trauma.

Blood pressure despite resuscitation	Survival (%)
>60 mmHg	60
>40 mmHg	30
<40 mmHg	3

- planned thoracotomy for definitive correction of the problem: this usually takes place in the more controlled environment of the operating theatre.

In certain situations, EDT is considered futile:

- CPR in the absence of endotracheal intubation for more than 5 minutes;
- CPR for more than 10 minutes (with or without endotracheal intubation);
- blunt trauma when there have been no signs of life at scene (see above).

Planned emergency thoracotomy

Planned emergency thoracotomy implies an emergency thoracotomy performed as a planned procedure in the operating room, directed at the management of a specific injury. As such, the approach chosen is dependent on the indication for surgery and the organ injured (Table 28.5). Some organs are best approached through a median sternotomy.

Otherwise, the thoracotomy may be right- or left-sided, and these may be joined, producing the so-called 'clamshell incision'. This gives excellent exposure for any surgeon who is not routinely entering the chest.

Posterolateral thoracotomy is not generally used in the emergency situation because of the difficulties in positioning the patient.

Table 28.5 Different approaches to the contents of the chest cavity.

Approach	Best for
Left anterolateral thoracotomy	Left lung and lung hilum
	Thoracic aorta
	Origin of left subclavian artery
	Left side of heart
	Lower oesophagus
Right anterolateral thoracotomy	Right lung and lung hilum
	Azygos veins
	Superior vena cava
	Infracardiac inferior vena cava
	Upper oesophagus
	Thoracic trachea
Median sternotomy	Anterior aspect of heart
	Anterior mediastinum
	Ascending aorta and arch of aorta
	Pulmonary arteries
	Carina of the trachea

ABDOMINAL INJURY

Patients who have suffered abdominal trauma can generally be classified into the following categories based on their physiological condition after initial resuscitation:

- Haemodynamically 'normal': investigation can be completed before treatment is planned.
- Haemodynamically 'stable': investigation is more limited. It is aimed at establishing whether the patient can be managed non-operatively, whether angioembolisation can be used, or whether surgery is required.
- Haemodynamically 'unstable': investigations need to be suspended as immediate surgical correction of the bleeding is required.

A trauma laparotomy is the final step in the pathway to delineate intra-abdominal injury. Occasionally, it is difficult to determine the source of bleeding in the shocked multiply-injured patient. If doubt still exists, especially in the presence of other injuries, a laparotomy may still be the safest option.

Investigation

Investigations are driven by the cardiovascular status of the patient. In torso trauma, the best and most sensitive modality is a CT scan with intravenous contrast; however, in the unstable patient, this is generally not possible.

In patients with penetrating injury, metal markers (e.g. bent paper clips) should be placed on all external wounds before plain films are taken, irrespective of the area being radiographed, as this allows an assessment of the trajectory and helps to correlate the number of holes and the number of missiles which can be seen within the patient. This will help determine whether two holes are indicative of one missile passing through the patient, or two missiles, both retained internally (Figure 28.8).

The patient's physiology must be assessed at regular intervals and, if there as an indication that the patient is still actively bleeding, then the source must be found. Blood loss into the abdomen can be subtle and there may be no clear clinical signs.

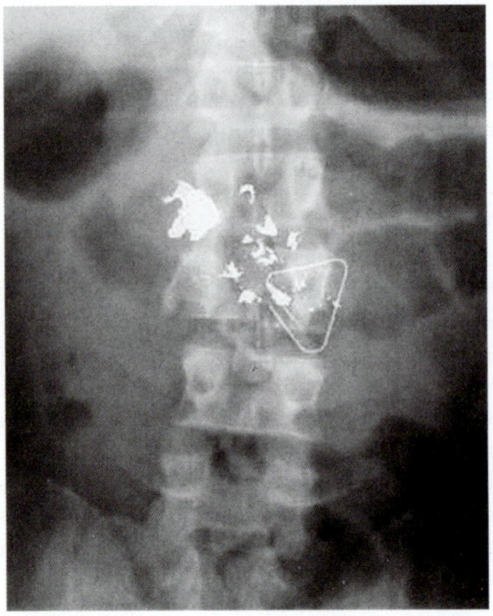

Figure 28.8 Abdominal radiograph of a gunshot wound showing bullet markers.

Blood is not an irritant and does not initially cause any abdominal pain. Distension is subjective, and a drop in the blood pressure may be a very late sign in a young fit patient. Examination in unstable patients should take place either in the emergency department or in the operating theatre if the patient is deteriorating rapidly.

Focused abdominal sonar for trauma

Focused abdominal sonar for trauma (FAST) is a technique whereby ultrasound (sonar) imaging is used to assess the torso for the presence of free blood, either in the abdominal cavity or in the pericardium. The technique therefore focuses on six areas: the pericardium, the areas around the liver and the spleen, the left and right pericolic gutters, and the peritoneal space in the pelvis. There should be no attempt to determine the nature or extent of the specific injury. FAST is usually a rapid, reproducible, portable and non-invasive bedside test, and can be performed at the same time as resuscitation. FAST is accurate at detecting >100 mL of free blood; however, it is very operator- and experience-dependent and, especially if the patient is very obese or the bowel is full of gas, it may be unreliable. Hollow viscus injury is difficult to diagnose, even in experienced hands, and has a low sensitivity (29–35 per cent) for organ injury without haemoperitoneum. FAST is also unreliable for excluding injury in penetrating trauma. If there is doubt, the FAST examination should be repeated (Summary box 28.6).

Summary box 28.6

Focused abdominal sonar for trauma

- It detects free fluid in the abdomen or pericardium
- It will not reliably detect less than 100 mL of free blood
- It does not identify injury to hollow viscus
- It cannot reliably exclude injury in penetrating trauma
- It may need repeating or supplementing with other investigations

Extensions of the FAST technique to include assessment of the chest for haemothorax and pneumothorax, as well as assessment of the extremities, depend on the experience of the operator and are not yet widely accepted.

Diagnostic peritoneal lavage

Diagnostic peritoneal lavage (DPL) is a test used to assess the presence of blood in the abdomen. A gastric tube is placed to empty the stomach and a urinary catheter is inserted to drain the bladder.

A cannula is inserted below the umbilicus, directed caudally and posteriorly. The cannula is aspirated for blood (>10 mL is deemed as positive) and, following this, 1000 mL of warmed Ringer's lactate solution is allowed to run into the abdomen and is then drained out. The presence of >100 000 red cells/μL or >500 white cells/μL is deemed positive (this is equivalent to 20 mL of free blood in the abdominal cavity). In the absence of laboratory facilities, a urine dipstick may be useful. Drainage of lavage fluid via a chest drain indicates penetration of the diaphragm.

Although DPL has largely been replaced by FAST (see above under Focused abdominal sonar for trauma), it remains the standard in many institutions where FAST is not available or is unreliable. DPL is especially useful in the hypotensive, unstable patient with multiple injuries as a means of excluding intra-abdominal bleeding.

Computed tomography

CT has become the 'gold standard' for the intra-abdominal diagnosis of injury in the stable patient. The scan should be performed using intravenous contrast. CT is sensitive for blood, and individual organ injury, as well as for retroperitoneal injury. An entirely normal abdominal CT is usually sufficient to exclude injury.

The following points are important when performing CT:

- Despite its tremendous value, it remains an inappropriate investigation for unstable patients.
- If duodenal injury is suspected from the mechanism of injury, oral contrast may be helpful.
- If rectal and distal colonic injury is suspected in the absence of blood on rectal examination, rectal contrast may be helpful.

Diagnostic laparoscopy

Diagnostic laparoscopy (DL) or thoracoscopy may be a valuable screening investigation in stable patients with penetrating trauma, to detect or exclude peritoneal penetration and/or diaphragmatic injury.

In most institutions, evidence of penetration requires a laparotomy to evaluate organ injury, as it is difficult to exclude all intra-abdominal injuries laparoscopically. When used in this role DL reduces the non-therapeutic laparotomy rate. DL is not a substitute for open laparotomy, especially in the presence of haemoperitoneum or contamination.

INDIVIDUAL ORGAN INJURY

Liver

Blunt liver trauma occurs as a result of direct injury. The liver is a solid organ and compressive forces can easily burst the liver substance. The liver is usually compressed between the impacting object and the rib cage or vertebral column. Most injuries are relatively minor and can be managed non-operatively. Many are not even suspected at the time.

Penetrating trauma to the liver is relatively common. Bullets have a shock wave and when they pass through a solid structure, such as the liver, they cause significant damage some distance from the actual track of the bullet. Not all penetrating wounds require operative management and a number may stop bleeding spontaneously.

In the stable patient, CT is the investigation of choice. It provides information on the liver injury itself, as well as on injuries to the adjoining major vascular and biliary structures. Close proximity injury and injury in which there is a suggestion of a vascular component should be reimaged, as there is a significant risk of the development of subsequent ischaemia.

Liver injury can be graded and managed using the American Association for the Surgery of Trauma (AAST) Organ Injury Scale (OIS) (www.aast.org/injury).

Management

The operative management of liver injuries can be summarised as 'the four Ps':

1 push;

2 Pringle;
3 plug;
4 pack.

At laparotomy, the liver is reconstituted as best as possible in its normal position and bleeding is controlled by direct compression (push). The inflow from the portal triad is controlled by a Pringle's manoeuvre, with direct compression of the portal triad, either digitally or using a soft clamp (Figure 28.9). This has the effect of reducing arterial and portal venous inflow into the liver, although it does not control the backflow from the inferior vena cava and hepatic veins. Any holes due to penetrating injury can be plugged directly and, after controlling any arterial bleeding, the liver can then be packed (see below under Damage control surgery).

Bleeding points should be controlled locally when possible and such patients should subsequently undergo angioembolisation. It is not usually necessary to suture penetrating injuries of the liver. If there has been direct damage to the hepatic artery, it can be tied off. Damage to the portal vein must be repaired, as tying off the portal vein carries a greater than 50 per cent mortality rate. If it is not technically feasible to repair the vein at the time of surgery, it should be shunted and the patient referred to a specialist centre. A closed suction drainage system must be left *in situ* following hepatic surgery.

Penetrating injuries and deep tracts can be plugged using silicone tubing or a Sengstaken–Blakemore tube.

Finally, the liver can be definitively packed, restoring the anatomy as closely as possible. Placing omentum into cracks in the liver is not recommended (Summary box 28.7).

Biliary injuries

Isolated traumatic biliary injuries are rare, occur mainly from penetrating trauma, and often occur in association with injuries to other structures that lie in close proximity. The common bile duct can be repaired over a T-tube or drained and referred to appropriate care as part of damage control.

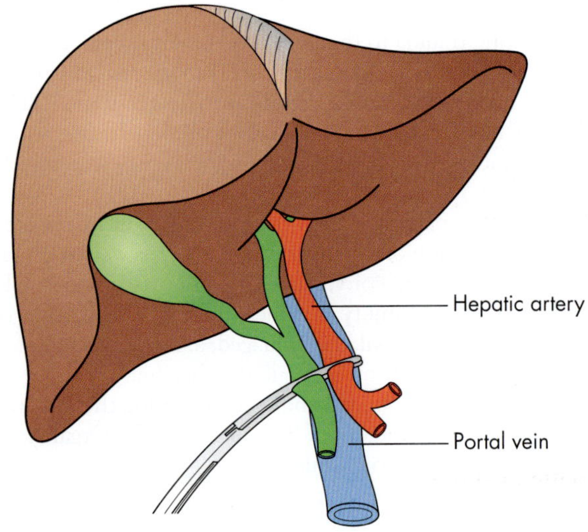

Figure 28.9 The Pringle manoeuvre.

Summary box 28.7

Liver trauma

- Blunt trauma occurs as the result of direct compression
- Penetrating trauma of the upper abdomen or lower thorax can damage the liver
- Computed tomography scanning is the investigation of choice, but only in the stable patient
- Surgical management consists of push, Pringle, plug and pack
- The hepatic artery can be tied off, but not the portal vein (stent)
- Closed suction should always be used

Spleen

Splenic injury occurs from direct blunt trauma. Most isolated splenic injuries, especially in children, can be managed nonoperatively. However, in adults, especially in the presence of other injury, age >55 years, or physiological instability, splenectomy should be considered. The spleen can be packed, repaired or placed in a mesh bag. Splenectomy may be a safer option, especially in the unstable patient with multiple potential sites of bleeding and who is >55 years of age, due to risk of rebleed. In certain situations, selective angioembolisation of the spleen can play a role.

Following splenectomy, there are significant though transient changes to blood physiology. The platelet and white count rises and may mimic sepsis.

Pancreas

Most pancreatic injury occurs as a result of blunt trauma. The major problem is that of diagnosis, because the pancreas is a retroperitoneal organ. CT remains the mainstay of accurate diagnosis. Amylase estimation is only relatively sensitive.

Classically, the pancreas should be treated with conservative surgery and closed suction drainage. Injuries are treated according to the OIS system of the AAST. Injuries to the tail are treated by closed suction drainage, with distal pancreatectomy if the duct is involved. Proximal injuries (to the right of the superior mesenteric artery) are treated as conservatively as possible, although partial pancreatectomy may be necessary. The pylorus can be temporarily closed (pyloric exclusion) in association with a gastric drainage procedure. A Whipple's procedure (pancreaticoduodenectomy) is rarely needed and should not be performed in the emergency situation because of the very high associated mortality rate. A damage control procedure with packing and drainage should be performed and the patient referred for definitive surgery once stabilised.

Stomach

Most stomach injuries are caused by penetrating trauma. Blood may be present and is diagnostic if found in the nasogastric tube.

Surgical repair is required but great care must be taken to examine the stomach fully, as an injury to the front of the stomach can be expected to have an 'exit' wound elsewhere on the organ.

Duodenum

Duodenal injury is frequently associated with injuries to the

James Hogarth Pringle, 1863–1941, Australian-born surgeon, Royal Infirmary, Glasgow, UK.
Robert William Sengstaken, born 1923, surgeon, Garden City, NY, USA.
Arthur Hendley Blakemore, 1897–1970, Associate Professor of Surgery, The College of Physicians and Surgeons, Columbia University, New York, NY, USA.
Allen Oldfather Whipple, 1881–1963, Valentine Mott Professor of Surgery, The College of Physicians and Surgeons, Columbia University, New York, NY, USA.

adjoining pancreas. Like the pancreas, the duodenum lies retroperitoneally and so injuries are hidden and only discovered late or at laparotomy performed for other reasons. The only sign may be gas in the periduodenal tissue seen at CT.

Smaller injuries can be repaired primarily. Major injuries and those also involving the head of the pancreas should undergo initial damage control surgery and be referred for definitive care.

Small bowel

The small bowel is frequently injured as a result of blunt trauma. The individual loops may be trapped, causing high-pressure rupture of a loop or tearing of the mesentery.

Small bowel injuries need urgent repair. Haemorrhage control takes priority and these wounds can be temporarily controlled with simple sutures. The small bowel can also be temporarily occluded until haemorrhage control has been achieved. In blunt trauma, the mesenteric vessels damage, and the bowel ischaemia which results, may dictate the extent of a resection. Resections should be carefully planned to limit the loss of viable small bowel but should be weighed against an excessive number of repairs or anastomoses. Haematomas in the small bowel mesenteric border need to be explored to rule out perforation. With low-energy wounds, primary repair can be performed after debridement of any dead tissue, whereas more destructive wounds associated with military-type weapons require resection and anastomosis.

Colon

Injuries to the colon from blunt injury are relatively infrequent, and are a more frequent penetrating injury. If relatively little contamination is present and the viability is satisfactory, such wounds can be repaired primarily. If, however, there is extensive contamination, the patient is physiologically unstable, or the bowel is of doubtful viability, then the colon can be closed off and a defunctioning colostomy formed.

Rectum

Only 5 per cent of colon injuries involve the rectum. These are generally from a penetrating injury, although occasionally the rectum may be damaged following fracture of the pelvis. Digital rectal examination will reveal the presence of blood, which is evidence of colorectal injury. These injuries are often associated with bladder and proximal urethral injury.

With intraperitoneal injuries, the rectum is managed as for colonic injuries. Full-thickness extraperitoneal rectal injuries should be managed with either a diverting end-colostomy and closure of the distal end (Hartmann's procedure) or a loop colostomy. Presacral drainage is generally no longer used.

Renal and urological tract injury

In the stable patient, CT scanning with contrast is the investigation of choice.

For assessment of bladder injury, a cystogram should be performed. A minimum of 400 mL of contrast is instilled into the bladder via a urethral catheter. The large volume is essential because a small volume may not produce a leak from a small bladder injury once the cystic muscle has contracted. It is important to assess the films as follows:

- with two views: anteroposterior and lateral;
- on two occasions: full and post-micturition.

Generally, renal injury is managed non-operatively unless the patient is unstable. The kidney can be angioembolised if required.

Ureteric injury is rare and is generally due to penetrating injury. Most ureters can be repaired or diverted if necessary.

Intraperitoneal ruptures of the bladder, usually from direct blunt injury, will require surgical repair. Extraperitoneal ruptures are usually associated with a fracture of the pelvis and will heal with adequate urine drainage (Summary box 28.8).

Summary box 28.8

Injuries to structures in the abdomen

- In children, splenic injury can be managed non-operatively
- Duodenal injuries are associated with pancreatic damage
- Small bowel injuries need urgent repair
- Large bowel injuries can be resected and stapled off
- Rectal injuries may be best managed initially with a defunctioning colostomy
- Kidney and urinary tract damage is best diagnosed with enhanced computed tomography scanning
- Intra-abdominal bladder tears need formal repair and drainage

ABDOMINAL COMPARTMENT SYNDROME AND THE OPEN ABDOMEN

Raised intra-abdominal pressure has far-reaching consequences for the patient; the syndrome that results is known as abdominal compartment syndrome (ACS). ACS is a major cause of morbidity and mortality in the critically ill patient and its early recognition is essential (Table 28.6).

In all cases of abdominal trauma in which the development of ACS in the immediate postoperative phase is considered a risk, the abdomen should be left open and managed as for damage control surgery.

DAMAGE CONTROL

Following major injury, protracted surgery in the physiologically unstable patient can in itself prove fatal. Patients with the 'deadly triad' of hypothermia, acidosis and coagulopathy are those at highest risk. 'Damage control' or 'damage limitation surgery' is a concept that originated from naval strategy, whereby a ship which has been damaged may have minimal repairs needed to prevent it from sinking, while definitive repairs wait until it has reached port.

The minimum surgery needed to stabilise the patient's condition may be the safest course until the physiological derangement can be corrected. Damage control surgery is restricted to only two goals:

1 stopping any active surgical bleeding;
2 controlling any contamination.

Once these goals have been achieved, then the operation is suspended and the abdomen temporarily closed. The patient's resuscitation then continues in the intensive care unit. Once the physiology has been corrected, the patient warmed and the coagulopathy corrected, the patient is returned to the operating theatre for any definitive surgery.

Henri Albert Charles Antoine Hartmann, 1860–1952, Professor of Clinical Surgery, Faculty of Medicine, University of Paris, France.

Table 28.6 Effect of raised intra-abdominal pressure on individual organ function.

Organ	Effect
Renal	Increase in renal vascular resistance leading to a reduction in glomerular filtration rate and impaired renal function
Cardiovascular	Decrease in venous return resulting in decreased cardiac output because of both a reduction in preload and an increase in afterload
Respiratory	Increased ventilation pressures because of splinting of the diaphragm, decreased lung compliance and increased airway pressures
Visceral perfusion	Reduction in visceral perfusion
Intracranial effects	Severe rises in intracranial pressures

Damage control resuscitation

The concept of damage control has been broadened to include the techniques used in resuscitation as well as in surgery. The time in the emergency department is minimised and the majority of resuscitation of the patient is carried out in the operating room and not in the resuscitation bay (Table 28.7). The resuscitation is individualised through repeated point of care (POC) testing of haemoglobin, acidosis (pH and lactate) and thrombo-elastography to assess clotting, and is therefore directed towards the early delivery of biologically active colloids, clotting products, and whole blood in order to buy time. The physiological disturbances that are associated with the downward spiral of acidosis, coagulopathy and hypothermia in these serious injuries are predicted and attempts are made to avoid them rather than react to them.

Damage control surgery

The decision that damage control surgery is the appropriate course should be made early (Table 28.8) and allows the whole surgical and anaesthetic team to work together to limit the time in surgery and the earliest possible admission of the patient to the intensive care unit. Damage control is a staged process.

The initial focus is haemorrhage control, followed by control and limitation of contamination, achieved using a range of abbreviated techniques including simple ligation of bleeding vessels, shunting of major arteries and veins, drainage, temporary stapling off of bowel, and therapeutic packing.

Following the above, the abdomen is closed in a temporary fashion using a sheet of plastic (e.g. Opsite) over the bowel, an intermediate pack to allow suction, and a further sheet of adherent plastic drape to the skin to form a watertight and airtight seal. Suction is applied to the intermediate pack area to collect abdominal fluid. This technique is known as the 'Vacpac' or 'Opsite sandwich' (Figure 28.10).

Table 28.7 The stages of damage control surgery.

Stage	
I	Patient selection
II	Control of haemorrhage and control of contamination
III	Resuscitation continued in the intensive care unit
IV	Definitive surgery
V	Abdominal closure

Table 28.8 Indications for damage control surgery.

Anatomical	Inability to achieve haemostasis
	Complex abdominal injury, e.g. liver and pancreas
	Combined vascular, solid and hollow organ injury, e.g. aortic or caval injury
	Inaccessible major venous injury, e.g. retrohepatic vena cava
	Demand for non-operative control of other injuries, e.g. fractured pelvis
	Anticipated need for a time-consuming procedure
Physiological (decline of physiological reserve)	Temperature <34°C
	pH <7.2
	Serum lactate >5 mmol/L (N (normal) <2.5 mmol/L)
	Prothrombin time (PT) >16 s
	Partial thromboplastin time (PTT) >60 s
	>10 units blood transfused
	Systolic blood pressure <90 mmHg for >60 min
Environmental	Operating time >60 min
	Inability to approximate the abdominal incision
	Desire to reassess the intra-abdominal contents (directed relook)

As soon as control has been achieved, the patient is transferred to the intensive care unit where resuscitation is continued.

The next stage following damage control surgery and physiological stabilisation is definitive surgery. The team should aim to perform definitive anastomoses, vascular reconstruction and closure of the body cavity within 24–72 hours of injury. However, this must be individualised to the patient, the response to critical care resuscitation, and the progression of injury complexes.

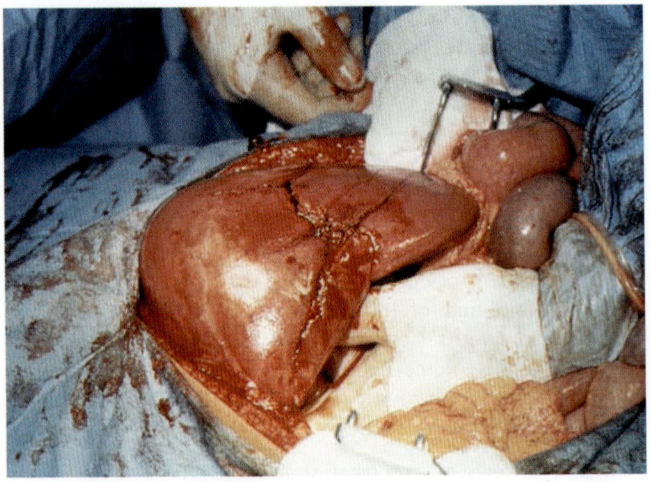

Figure 28.10 Abdominal closure following damage control surgery.

The abdomen is closed as soon as possible, bearing in mind the risks of ACS. The closure is not without its own morbidity. Successful closure may require aggressive off-loading of fluid and even haemofiltration to achieve this, if the patient will tolerate it. The best situation is closure of the abdominal fascia, or, if this cannot be achieved, then skin closure only. Occasionally, mesh closure can be used, with skin grafting over the mesh and subsequent abdominal wall reconstruction.

Thoracic damage control is conceptually based on the same philosophy. This is that haemorrhage control and focused surgical procedures minimise further surgical insult, and lead to improved survival in the unstable trauma patient. The aim is to control bleeding and limit air leaks using the fastest procedures available to minimise the operative time.

The indications and techniques for emergency thoracotomy have already been described.

Damage control applies equally to the extremities. In this case, it is shunting of blood vessels, identifying and marking damaged structures, such as nerves, fasciotomy and removal of contaminated tissue which are the main tasks. Subsequent definitive management can be carried out at a later stage (Summary box 28.9).

Summary box 28.9

Damage control surgery

- Resuscitation is carried out in the operating theatre using biologically active fluids
- The surgery performed is the minimum needed to stabilise the patient
- The aims of surgery are to control haemorrhage and limit contamination
- Secondary surgery is aimed at definitive repair

INTERVENTIONAL RADIOLOGY

Interventional radiology can be useful in the management of torso trauma as both an investigative and a therapeutic tool for patients with vascular injury. Angioembolisation following demonstration of ongoing bleeding in splenic and renal injury is a valuable technique.

NON-OPERATIVE MANAGEMENT

Non-operative management is universally preferred for the management of solid organ injury in haemodynamically stable children. Non-operative management of solid abdominal organ injury has rapidly gained acceptance in the management of adults as well. A stable patient and accurate CT imaging are prerequisites for this approach. Failure of non-operative management is uncommon and typically occurs within the first 12 hours after injury. Therefore, if correctly selected, the vast majority of these patients will avoid surgery, require less blood transfusion, and sustain fewer complications than operated patients.

Antibiotics in torso trauma

There is no level 1 evidence to recommend the use of antibiotics for the insertion of chest drains. However, they should be used in all cases of penetrating abdominal trauma.

FURTHER READING

American Association for the Surgery of Trauma. Organ injury scaling system. Last accessed February 2011. Available from www.aast.org.

American College of Surgeons. *Advanced trauma life support course manual for doctors*. Chicago, IL: American College of Surgeons, 2008.

Boffard KD (ed.). *Definitive surgery of trauma care*, 3rd edn. London: Hodder Arnold, 2011.

Eastern Association for the Surgery of Trauma. Guidelines for practice management: evidence-based guidelines. 4a: Blunt aortic injury; 4b: Blunt myocardial injury; 4c: Evaluation of blunt abdominal trauma; 4d: Non-operative management of liver and spleen; 4e: Penetrating intraperitoneal colon injuries; 4f: Pain management in blunt thoracic trauma; 4g: Prophylactic antibiotics in penetrating abdominal trauma; 4h: Prophylactic antibiotics in tube thoracostomy. Last accessed 2011. Available from www.east.org.

Moore EE, Feliciano DV, Mattox LK (eds). *Trauma*, 6th edn. New York: McGraw Hill, 2008.

World Society for Abdominal Compartment Syndrome. Abdominal compartment syndrome. Last accessed February 2011. Available from www.wsacs.org.

CHAPTER 29

Extremity trauma

LEARNING OBJECTIVES

To gain an understanding of:

- How to identify whether an injury exists
- The important injuries not to miss
- The principles of the description and classification of fractures
- The range of available treatments
- How to select an appropriate treatment

INTRODUCTION

The objective when treating any injured person is to restore maximum function with minimum risk. So, the first duty is to identify and treat any immediate threats to life. Following the Advanced Trauma Life Support (ATLS) system (see Chapter 24), management of skeletal injuries starts after the primary survey and initial resuscitation have been completed. Very occasionally, the haemorrhage associated with a fracture may be life-threatening. For example, a pelvic injury may require urgent stabilisation, or a major open fracture needs direct pressure to control blood loss.

DIAGNOSIS, DESCRIPTION AND CLASSIFICATION OF INJURY

Missing an injury can be serious, both medically and legally. Table 29.1 contains a list of injuries which are notoriously easy to miss.

Assessment: history and examination

The mechanism of injury and the patient's description of their symptoms will give the first clues to the injuries which are likely to be found. However, if the trauma was severe enough to cause one injury, then there was enough energy to cause more injuries. Therefore, the identification of one injury is not a reason for satisfaction; it is a warning to search for others. Injuries occur in patterns, e.g. a dislocated knee is often associated with a vascular injury, and a head injury may be accompanied by and mask a fractured cervical spine. In 15 per cent of cases in which a spinal fracture has been identified, there is another spinal injury at a separate site. A repeat examination on the 'morning after' ward round is a time for a further secondary survey to search for occult injuries.

In the multiply-injured or obtunded patient, it may not be possible to obtain a history. In this case, a top-to-toe clinical examination in the secondary survey is even more important than usual. The patient's pre-injury condition needs to be checked as this may limit recovery.

Table 29.1 Extremity injuries which are notorious for being missed.

Posterior dislocation of the shoulder
Lateral condylar mass fracture of the distal humerus
Perilunate dislocation
Scaphoid fracture
Tarsometatarsal fracture dislocation
Compartment syndrome
Vascular injury with knee dislocation
Talar neck fracture
Slipped upper femoral epiphysis
Achilles tendon rupture

Principles of investigation

A summary of the available methods of investigation is given in Table 29.2.

For almost 100 years, the mainstay of the orthopaedic surgeon's investigation has been the plain radiograph. Radiographs should include orthogonal views (two views at 90° separation) and, for long bones, should show the joints above and below the

Sir John Charnley, 1911–1982, Professor of Orthopaedic Surgery, the University of Manchester, Manchester, UK. He pioneered the hip replacement operation. In 1962, he moved his practice to Wrightington Hospital, Appley Bridge, which became a place of pilgrimage for young orthopaedic surgeons from all over the world wishing to specialise in hip replacement. In the same hospital, the John Charnley Research Institute was opened by his wife in 1992. In September 2010, the Royal Mail issued a series of stamps commemorating medical breakthroughs. The 60p stamp featured John Charnley's hip replacement operation as an x-ray.

Hugh Owen Thomas, 1834–1891, a general practitioner of Liverpool, UK. He is regarded as the 'founder of orthopaedic surgery', although never holding a hospital appointment preferring to treat patients in their own homes. He introduced the Thomas splint in 1875.

Gavriil Abramovich Ilizarov, 1921–1993, orthopaedic surgeon, Kurgan, Western Siberia, Russia. He did not attend school until he was 11 years old as his family was too poor to buy him shoes.

Sir Isaac Newton, 1642–1727, Lucasian Professor of Mathematics, Cambridge University, Cambridge, UK.

Table 29.2 Investigation modalities.

Modality	Good for	Problems
Plain radiographs	Fractures and dislocations. Easily available	Radiation. Not good for soft tissues
Computed tomography	Bony spinal injury Global view in polytrauma Planning treatment of complex fractures	Radiation dose. Availability. Safety in severe injuries
Ultrasound scan	Soft-tissue injuries	Operator dependency
Magnetic resonance imaging	Soft-tissue problems and fractures	Availability and expensive Difficult to use in the ventilated patient
Bone scan	Stress fractures and tumours	Radiation dose
Fluoroscopy	Checking progress of surgery	Small field of view Quality Image distortion

injury. Other imaging modalities are now being used more frequently. Computed tomography (CT) scans are invaluable for defining more complex patterns of a fracture, particularly adjacent to a joint. They are now also being used for the global assessment of the multiply-injured person. As scan acquisition times decrease and physiological monitoring improves, the dangers for the multiply-injured patient of being isolated in a scanner are reduced and the benefits of accurate diagnosis increased. Ultrasound is used to assess soft-tissue structures, e.g. Achilles tendon or rotator cuff injuries. Magnetic resonance imaging (MRI) is used primarily to show soft-tissue injury, particularly around the knee. Injuries with a reputation for being missed, such as a posterior dislocation of the shoulder (Figure 29.1), should be actively sought whenever there is any chance that they may be present (Summary box 29.1).

Summary box 29.1

Finding an injury

- Look specifically for 'easily missed injuries'
- Re-examine the multiply injured patient

Achilles, the Greek hero was the son of Peleus and Thetis. When he was a child, his mother dipped him in the Styx, one of the rivers of the Underworld so that he should be invulnerable in battle. The heel by which she held him did not get wet, and was, therefore, not protected. Achilles died from a wound in the heel received at the seige of Troy.

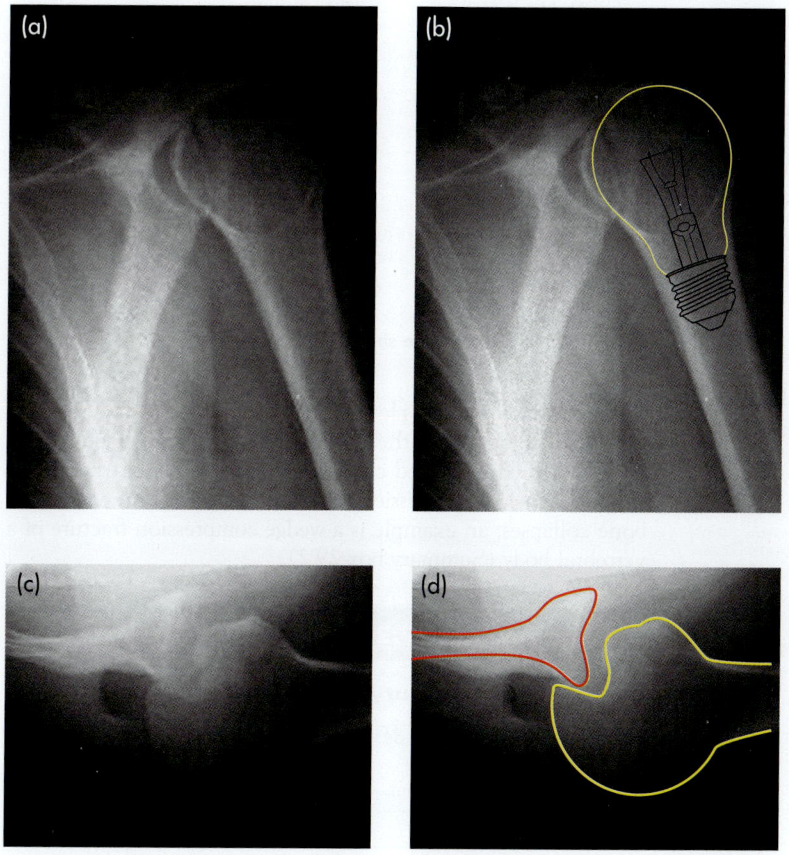

Figure 29.1 Posterior dislocation of the shoulder. (a) Anteroposterior view; (b) origin of the light bulb sign; (c) axial projection demonstrating how much easier it is to visualise the injury on this view; (d) axial projection highlighting this point and further demonstrating the impacted fracture in the humeral head, or Hill–Sachs lesion.

DESCRIPTION AND CLASSIFICATION OF MUSCULOSKELETAL INJURY

Description of injury

The soft-tissue injury

There are two components of soft-tissue injury that need to be identified: the degree of damage to the soft-tissue envelope around the fracture and the integrity of the important structures passing through the area, primarily the arteries and nerves. A fracture is defined as open when the haematoma associated with it is exposed by a breach in an epithelial surface; this is usually skin, but is sometimes mucous membrane of the bowel or vagina. When there is such a wound, it should be described in plain terms, e.g. 'a ragged 6-cm laceration over the anterior aspect of the midshaft of the left tibia with contused skin edges, but no gross contamination'. To minimise contamination, the wound, with a scale beside it, should be photographed and then covered. It should not be disturbed again until definitive treatment is given in an operating theatre.

Even if there is no wound, the damage to the soft-tissue envelope will need describing. There may still be bruising, swelling, contusion, tissue shearing or crushing. Severe soft-tissue swelling may make it wise to delay surgery.

Injuries to arteries and nerves

Major arterial injuries may be limb or life threatening. Distal neurovascular status should always be checked and recorded, especially if there is penetrating trauma, a dislocation or a displaced fracture. This record should be specific, e.g. 'dorsalis pedis present' or 'capillary refill <2 s', not just 'neurovascularly intact'. The warm ischaemia time should be kept to below 4 hours. If the level of the injury is clinically obvious, it is best to proceed immediately to treatment; on-table arteriography can be obtained later if required.

Nerve injuries should be identified and recorded. It is important that if operative treatment of a fracture is planned, the preoperative neurological status is recorded. As with the vascular examination, the findings should be recorded in such a way that they can be interpreted without ambiguity.

Compartment syndrome

Compartment syndrome is discussed in Chapter 32.

The bony injury

The terminology used in this description is illustrated in Figure 29.2. Figure 29.3 shows 'a 45° oblique fracture at the junction of the proximal and middle thirds of the right tibia with an associated fibular fracture'. A good description needs the following components:

- name the injured bone;
- give the region of the bone;
- is the fracture simple or multifragmentary;
- describe the direction of the fracture line: transverse, oblique or spiral;
- are the fragments displaced or undisplaced;
- if displaced, describe the alignment, length and rotation;
- note any evidence of pre-existing pathology;
- any associated joint dislocation.

In adults, the fracture line is generally complete, i.e. it extends through both cortices. However, in children, the fracture line may be incomplete as the bone is plastic. These fractures are called torus (ring-shaped crumpling) and greenstick (buckling) (Figure 29.4). Compression fractures occur when cancellous bone collapses; an example is a wedge compression fracture of a vertebral body (Summary box 29.2).

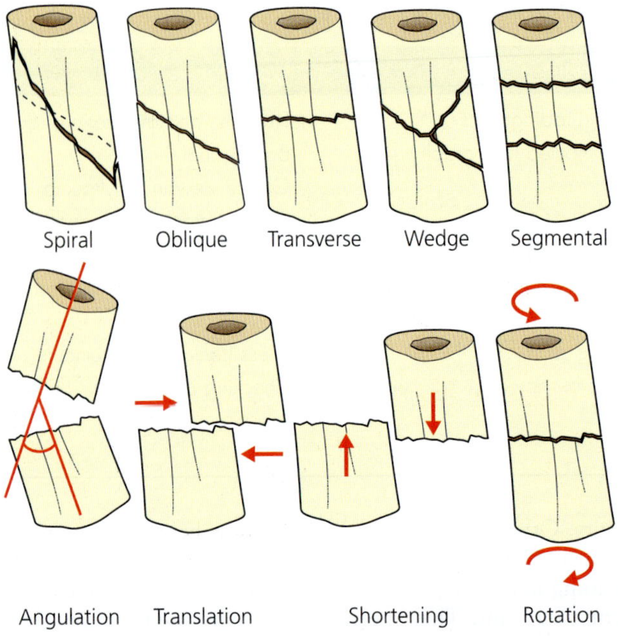

Figure 29.2 Descriptive terms for fractures.

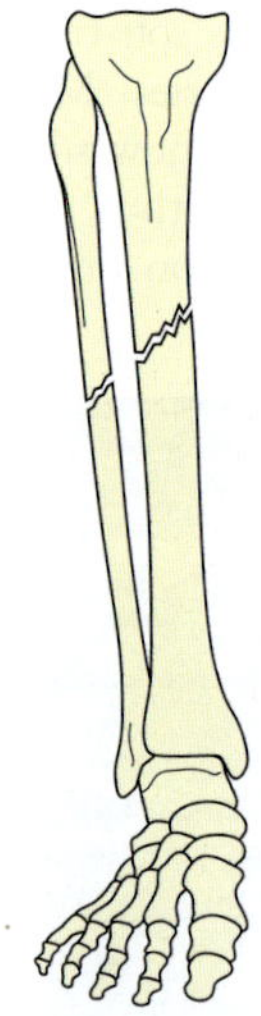

Figure 29.3 Fracture of the shaft of the tibia.

Summary box 29.2

Describing an injury

Use plain language to describe:

- Location
- Soft-tissue component
- Bony injury

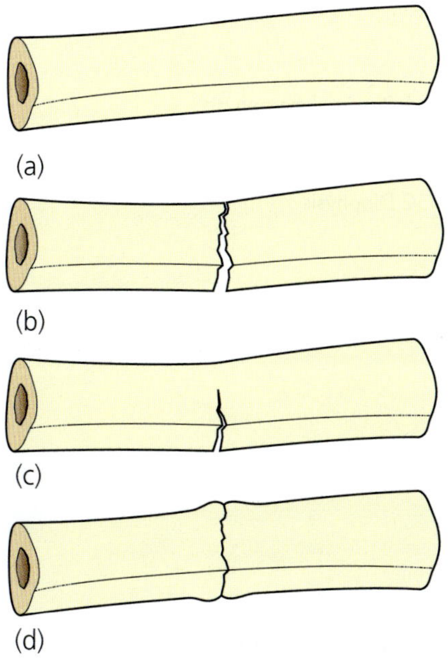

Figure 29.4 Types of bony injury. (a) Uninjured bone; (b) adult transverse fracture failure across the whole bone; (c) greenstick fracture; the bone has failed on the tension side; (d) torus or buckle fracture; the bone has failed on the compression side.

Classification of injury

Soft-tissue injury

Despite the emphasis placed upon management of the soft tissues, it remains common practice that unless it is an open injury the soft-tissue component of an injury is described and not classified (Summary box 29.3).

> **Summary box 29.3**
>
> **The value of classification**
>
> - Encourages and directs evaluation of the injury
> - Assists planning of treatment
> - Guides prognosis
> - Results in easier data retrieval
> - Allows comparison with the results of other surgeons

Open injuries are generally classified; the system most commonly used is that of Gustilo and Anderson, where the grade of the injury is not determined by the size of the wound alone: thus, a high-energy fracture with a <1-cm wound is a grade III fracture. This means that the injury cannot be finally classified until its full extent is assessed on completion of the initial wound excision. The classification is summarised in Table 29.3.

Bony injury in adults

The AO (*Arbeitsgemeinschaft für Osteosynthesefragen*, literally Working Party on Problems of Bone repair) system provides a principle-based comprehensive classification of fractures. The system is organised to identify the site and nature of a fracture. Initially, the site is identified by two numbers: the first records

Table 29.3 Gustilo and Anderson open fracture classification.

Type	
I	A low energy open fracture with a wound less than 1 cm long and clean
II	An open fracture with a laceration more than 1 cm long without extensive soft tissue damage, flaps or avulsion
III	Characterised by high energy injury irrespective of the size of the wound. Extensive damage to soft tissues, including muscles, skin, and neurovascular structures, and a high degree of contamination. Multifragmentary and unstable fractures
Subgroups of type III	
A	Adequate soft tissue cover of a fractured bone after stabilisation
B	Inadequate soft tissue cover of a fractured bone after stabilisation, i.e. flap coverage required
C	Open fracture associated with an arterial injury requiring repair

Source: Gustilo RB, Mendoza RM, Williams DN. Problems in the management of type III (severe) open fractures: a new classification of type III open fractures. *J Trauma* 1984; **24**: 742–6.

which bone is involved and the second which segment of that bone (Figure 29.5). The classified fracture is recorded as an alphanumeric; for instance, the tibial fracture described at the beginning of this section is a 42A2. The '4' and the '2' are simply shorthand for the tibial shaft. The letter begins to define the nature of the fracture as shown in Figure 29.6; in this case it is a simple or 'A-type' diaphyseal fracture. The final number given refines the record of the fracture pattern; for a simple diaphyseal fracture '1' represents a spiral, '2' an oblique and '3' a transverse fracture. The system goes into further detail but this requires reference to the AO classification book (see Further reading).

Growth plate injuries

The weakest area of a child's bone is the epiphyseal plate and fractures are common here. The physis contains cells that are responsible for longitudinal bone growth. Damage may lead to growth arrest, especially if a bridge of bone (bony bar) forms between the epiphysis and metaphysis.

The classification of Salter and Harris is used to describe the nature of the epiphyseal injury. These patterns of injury are shown in Figure 29.7 and a description of the types and their characteristics is given below:

- Type I, a transverse fracture along the line of the physis; the growing zone is not usually injured so there is no growth disturbance. This fracture is common.
- Type II, similar to a type 1 injury, but the fracture line deviates off into the metaphysis at one end, producing a metaphyseal fragment; this fracture seldom affects growth. This fracture is very common.
- Type III passes along the physis and then deviates into the epiphysis (intra-articular); rarely results in significant

Robert Bruce Salter, 1924–2010, Professor of Orthopaedic Surgery, The University of Toronto, Ontario, Canada. A pioneer in the field of paediatric orthopaedic surgery; received international awards for medical science and the Distinguished Achievement for Orthopaedic Research award.

Ramon Balgoa Gustilo, surgeon, Hennepin County Medical Center, Minneapolis, MN, USA.
John T Anderson, surgeon, Hennepin Medical Center, Minneapolis, MA, USA.

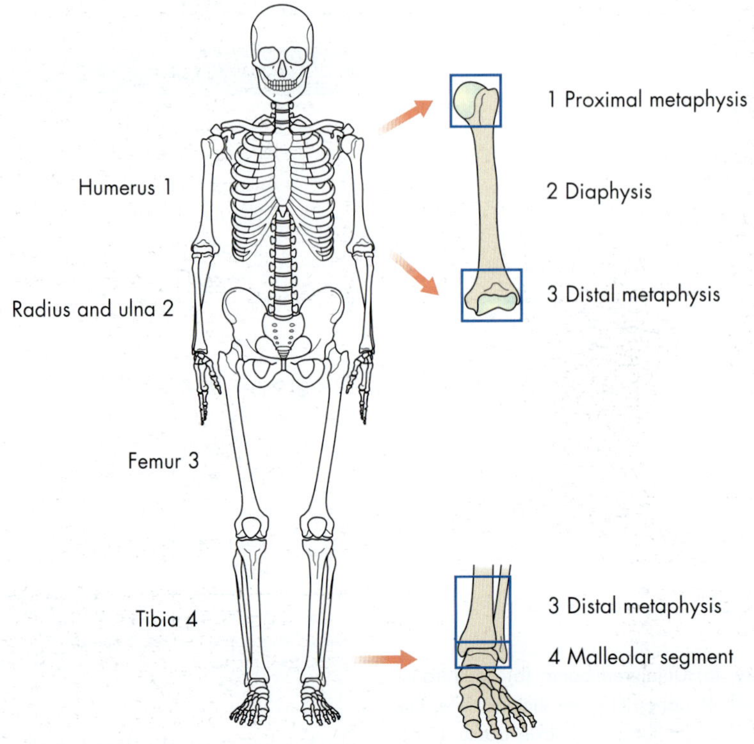

Figure 29.5 The AO classification system: the first two numbers specify the site of the fracture.

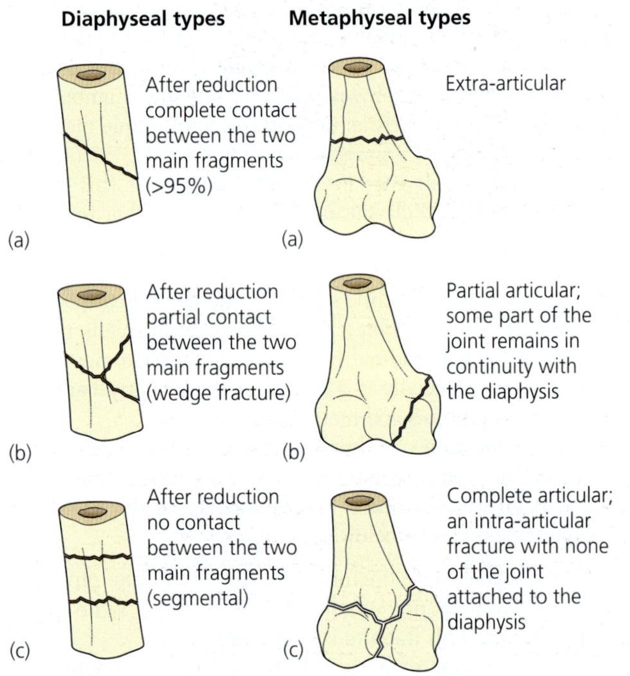

Figure 29.6 The AO classification system: the letter defines the nature of the fracture.

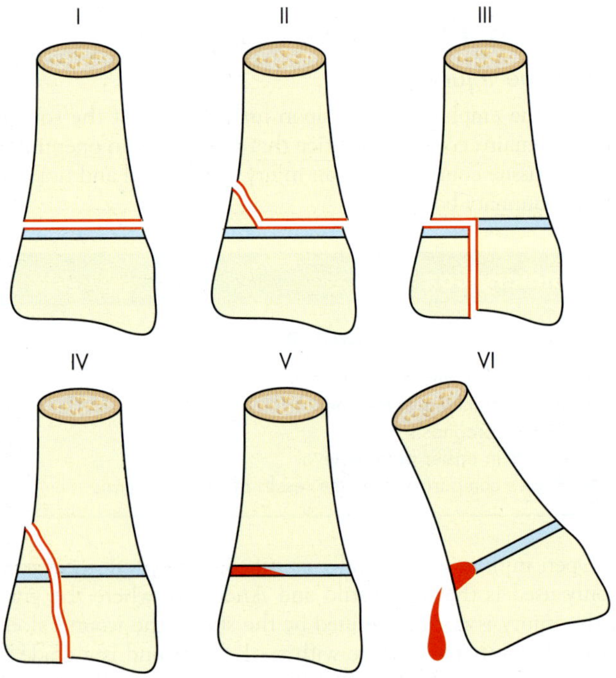

Figure 29.7 The Salter–Harris classification of growth plate injuries.

deformity, but can lead to joint incongruity. This fracture is not common.

- Type IV crosses the physis passing from the epiphysis into the metaphysis; if displaced it interferes with the growing layer of cartilage cells so can cause premature focal fusion of the physis followed by deformity. This fracture is not common.
- Type V, a crush injury of the physis; associated with growth disturbances at the physis. Diagnosis may be difficult as the radiograph may look normal; however, premature closure of the physis reveals the diagnosis. This fracture is rare.

WR Harris, formerly Professor of Orthopaedic Surgery, The University of Toronto, Ontario, Canada.

- Type VI, rare injury consisting of an injury to the perichondral structures by direct trauma, e.g. heat or chemical (Summary box 29.3).

THE RESPONSE TO INJURY

The natural history of a fracture is that the broken bone will heal. However, it may be slow (delayed union) or even fail to unite (non-union), or unite in a poor position (malunion).

Bone healing

Fractures heal by indirect or direct mechanisms:

- **Indirect (secondary) bone healing.** This occurs with a callus precursor and is referred to as enchondral ossification. It tends to occur when the bone ends are not perfectly aligned and when there is some movement at the fracture site during the healing process. Such secondary bone healing is broadly characterised by three main phases: (1) inflammation, (2) repair with callus formation and (3) remodelling of immature woven bone to mature lamellar bone. It may be thought of as the natural way for a bone to heal and takes only weeks to complete.
- **Direct (primary) bone healing.** This occurs without callus formation. It is part of the normal process of remodelling with cutting cones crossing the fracture and new lamellar bone being laid down behind them. It tends to occur when the fracture ends are closely opposed and there is no relative movement between them. This occurs after rigid internal fixation of fractures and takes up to a year to complete.

If fixation of a fracture achieves absolute stability between the fragments, direct healing occurs. This process is slow, but if the construct is strong then the patient can return to most activities quickly and well before the fracture has healed. The amount of movement which occurs between the fracture fragments depends both upon the surgical construct and also on the amount of load applied.

Bone union is not just dependent upon mechanical factors. The healing tissues require an adequate blood supply. At the time of surgery, care must be taken to minimise disruption to the blood supply of the healing tissues.

Adverse outcomes

Malunion

Malunion is when the bone unites in an incorrect position. As a guide, an articular step should not be greater than the thickness of the articular cartilage (2 mm) or premature arthritis will result. In the lower limb, angulation or rotation should not exceed 5°. Visible deformity is seldom acceptable, and malrotation can be very disabling.

Non-union

Non-union of a fracture may be defined as failure to show progressive clinical or radiographic signs of healing. The principle types of non-union are atrophic, hypertrophic and infected. These can be secondary to failure of biology and/or mechanical environment and patient factors (smoking). In atrophic non-union, the problem is often poor blood supply. The fracture gap is filled by fibrous tissue and the bone fragments remain mobile. Hypertrophic union usually occurs when there is excessive movement at the fracture site, leading to abundant periosteal bone formation. If stability is improved, union is likely.

Infected non-union

Infected non-union merits a separate mention as it is a potentially catastrophic complication. Its treatment is often prolonged, multistaged and can result in loss of the limb. This is why the top priority in open fractures is to prevent contamination from becoming infection.

Delayed union

Delayed union is the term used to describe a fracture that has not healed in the expected time. Fractures in children tend to heal more rapidly than fractures in adults, and upper limb fractures can heal more quickly than lower limb fractures. Fractures in children may unite (the bone ends stick together) within 2–3 weeks and consolidate in 4–6 weeks. Femoral fractures in adults may take 12 weeks to unite and 24 weeks until they are as strong as they were before (consolidation) (Summary box 29.4).

> **Summary box 29.4**
>
> **Fracture healing**
>
> - **Mechanics.** Movement and strain determines whether bone healing is indirect or direct
> - **Biology.** The blood supply needs to be intact or atrophic non-union will result
> - **Infection.** Must be avoided at all costs

Understanding outcome

Table 29.4 lists the potential advantages and disadvantages of the range of treatments available for a fracture.

PRINCIPLES OF FRACTURE MANAGEMENT

When planning fracture treatments, the first principle is to consider whether any intervention is necessary; many fractures require only symptomatic treatment. The interventional management of the bony injury has two components: reduction and stabilisation.

Reduction

A fracture can be reduced using closed or open methods. Manipulating a fracture by a closed technique, i.e. without surgically exposing the bone, is an art. The key is to utilise the remaining soft tissues, especially the intact periosteum on the concave side of the fracture; they will tend to guide the bony fragments. The most elegant way of obtaining a good reduction is to reverse the mechanism of the injury. The sequence of injury and reversal is illustrated in Figure 29.8.

At open operation, the bony fragments can be manipulated just as in a closed reduction; it is easier to do because the bony fragments can be watched. The fragments can also be moved by applying clamps directly to the bone. The adequacy of the reduction with a simple fracture pattern can be judged by direct reference to the fracture fragments themselves, just as when solving a simple jigsaw. With more complex fracture patterns, exposure of all of the individual fragments may devitalise them

Table 29.4 Risks and benefits of fracture treatment.

Benefits	Risks
Pain relief	Anaesthesia
Prevention of infection	Introduction of infection
Restoration of anatomy	Damage to soft tissues and neurovascular structures
Early movement of the limb	
Early movement of the patient	Devitalising bone
Improved function	Need for implant removal
Reduced risk of secondary arthritis	Financial cost (cost of treatment)
Financial cost (time off work)	

and so reduction is assessed indirectly by restoring the overall position of the limb. The assessment of the adequacy of fracture reduction may be made by direct viewing of the fracture ends with the naked eye at open operation. Otherwise, the shape of the limb can simply be compared with the opposite side. Reference to Figure 29.2 demonstrates that the fracture with rotational deformity is difficult to depict graphically and for the same reason is often not noticed on radiography or at open surgery. However, merely looking at the whole limb and comparing it with the normal side generally reveals whether the rotational reduction is adequate (Summary box 29.5).

Summary box 29.5

Reduction

- Reduction has two components: reducing the fragments and assessing adequacy of reduction
- Reduction can be performed open or closed
- The principle is to reverse the movement which created the fracture
- Over-angulation allows the intact periosteum to guide the fragments into position

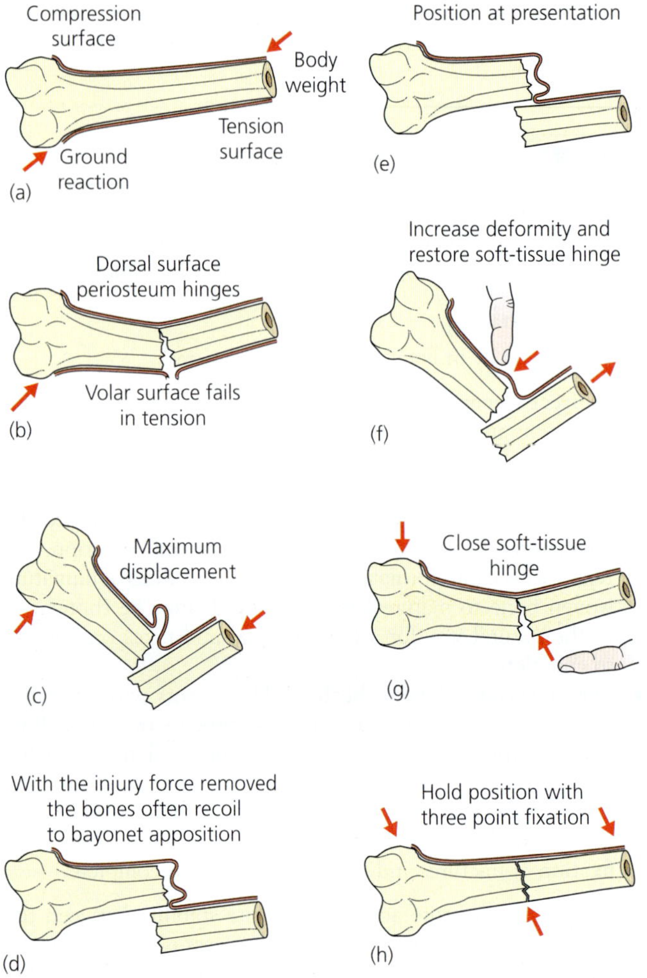

Figure 29.8 (a–d) Representation of how the mechanism of injury causes the bony and soft-tissue injury. (e–h) Representation of how the residual mechanical properties of the tissues may be used to effect and hold a reduction.

Stabilisation

When a fracture has been reduced it needs to be held or stabilised while healing progresses.

When choosing a technique of stabilisation, the aim is to:

- optimise the biological and mechanical environment to create the most favourable conditions possible for fracture healing;
- minimise the period of disability by speeding healing or creating stability so that function can be allowed during healing.

Absolute stability is generally achieved by precise reduction and compression of the fracture ends. No displacement should occur during the loading permitted in the postoperative period. This provides the environment for direct bone healing. In contrast, **relative stability** will produce a situation that allows some movement in proportion to the load applied. This stimulates callus formation and quick secondary bone healing. Figure 29.9 shows some of the configurations that can be used to achieve relative and absolute stability. Simple fracture patterns allow absolute stability to be obtained; in the more complex fracture patterns, the biological cost of achieving precise reduction (for example, soft-tissue stripping) may outweigh the advantages of struggling to obtain absolute stability.

Methods used for stabilising a fracture

Casting and splinting

A cast may be plaster of Paris or fibreglass. Immediately following a fracture, there may be significant soft-tissue swelling. If the risk of a compartment syndrome is to be avoided, only a backslab (or a split plaster) should be applied until the swelling has peaked out. Even then, the patient may need to be admitted for a period of observation, or instructions given to the patient and family to follow in the event of compromise to the circulation of the limb.

In an unstable fracture (as in Figure 29.9), the cast should be moulded to stabilise the fracture using a so-called 'three-point fixation'. A plaster achieving this will appear crooked; this leads to the adage that 'if you want a straight bone then you need a bent plaster' (Figure 29.10).

The advantages and disadvantages of casting and splinting are described in Table 29.5.

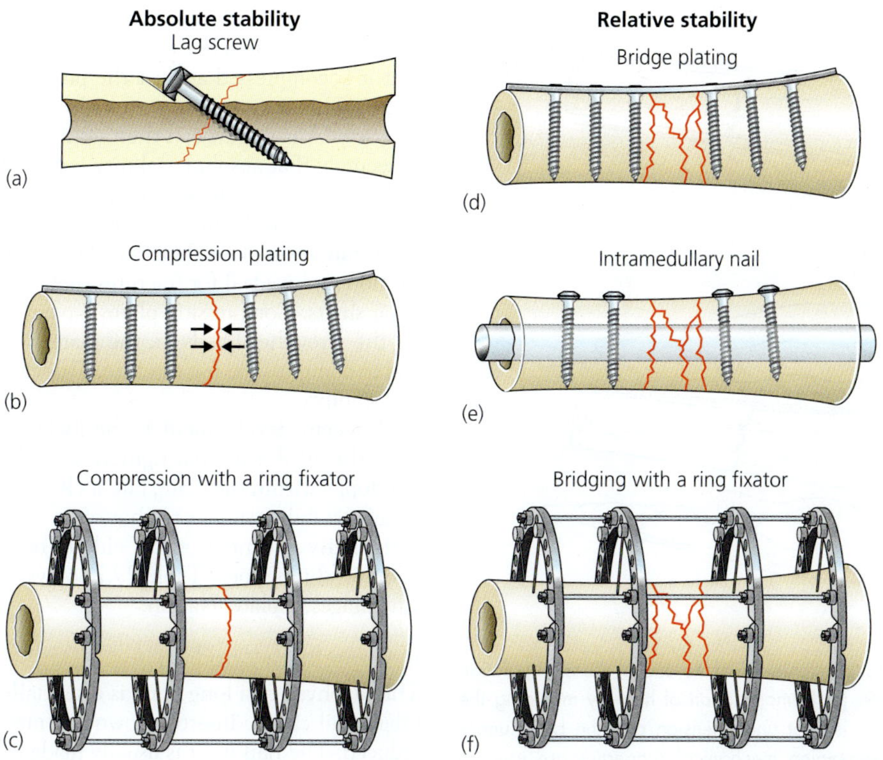

Figure 29.9 How absolute and relative stability can be achieved. The same implants may be used to achieve different mechanical effects.

Traction

Traction is the process of putting a stetching force on a limb to pull a fracture straight. The advantages and disadvantages of traction are given in Table 29.6. It relies on the integrity of the surrounding soft tissues (especially the periosteum) to create the tension which forces the fracture fragments to line up straight. Traction splints are still often used for temporary stabilization of a fracture. The Thomas splint for transporting a patient with a fractured femur is a typical example of static traction, creating tension between two fixed points (Figure 29.11a). Hamilton Russel traction is an example of dynamic traction where the pull is exerted by a system of weights. This tension is balanced against the patient's own body weight, which provides the opposing force but allows the patient to move around in bed (Figure 29.11b).

Traction can be applied either using the skin (skin traction) or by direct coupling to the bone with pins or wires (skeletal traction). The simplest practical example of traction is the use of a collar and cuff to treat a proximal humeral fracture. As long as the patient is upright, the weight of the elbow and forearm provides the traction. More complex systems of weights, counterweights and pulleys can be used to provide the appropriate force required to maintain alignment of a lower limb fracture. The concept of a controlled and uncontrolled fragment is helpful; failure to understand this can lead to failure of traction.

Open reduction and internal fixation

Open reduction and internal fixation (ORIF) is the term used to describe the operation of reducing a fracture under direct vision and then applying plates, screws, wires or intramedullary nails to hold the reduction.

Table 29.5 Advantages and disadvantages of casting and splinting.

Advantages	No wound
	No interference with fracture site
	Cheap
	Adjustable
	No implants to remove
Disadvantages	Limited access to the soft tissues
	Cumbersome (particularly in the elderly)
	Interferes with function
	Poor mechanical stability
	'Plaster disease'

Table 29.6 Advantages and disadvantages of traction.

Advantages	No wound in zone of injury
	No interference with fracture site
	Materials cheap
	Adjustable
Disadvantages	Restricts mobility of patient
	Expensive in hospital time
	Skin pressure complications
	Pin site infection
	Thromboembolic complications

Plaster of Paris is a white crystalline powder, calcium sulphate hemihydrate $CaSO_4\ 0.5H_2O$, which sets hard when water is added to it.

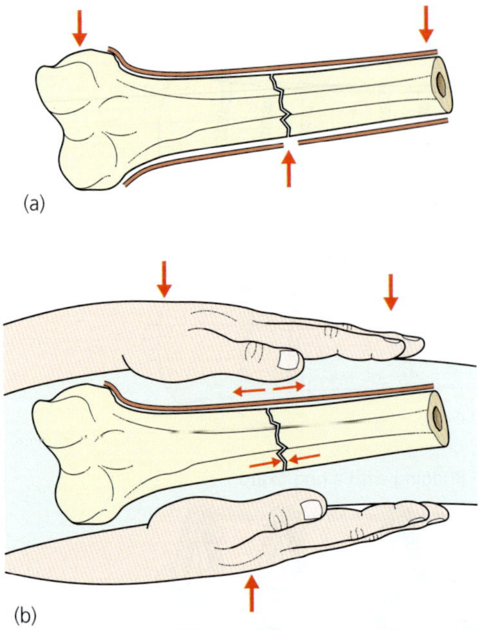

Figure 29.10 (a) The position achieved at the end of the manipulation described in Figure 29.9. (b) Demonstration of how by moulding the cast the intact periosteum is kept under tension and the bone under compression; thus, the remaining mechanical properties are used to achieve stability.

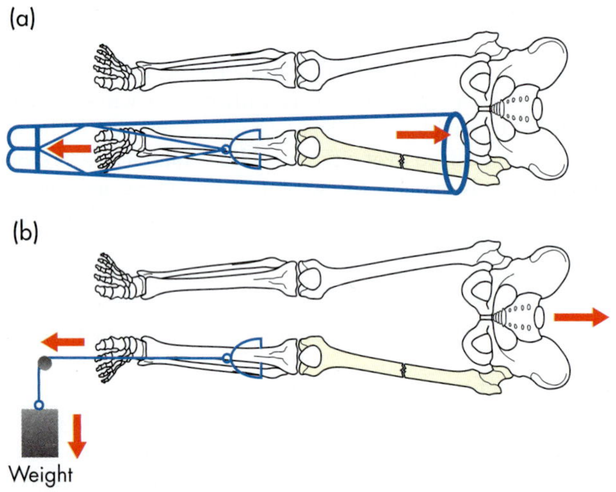

Figure 29.11 (a) Static traction with a Thomas splint. The force and counterforce are contained within a static system. The load is applied to the patient through the tibial traction pin via a cord tightened with a Spanish windlass. The counterforce is applied through pressure by the splint on the ischial tuberosity. (b) A dynamic system in which the load is applied by weights suspended from the tibial pin and the counterforce is the patient's own weight.

Plates and screws

A lag screw is used to compress two things together. This is achieved by drilling the hole under the screw head in the proximal fragment to a diameter which is greater than can be grasped by the threads of the screw. This allows the screw to slide down this hole until the head of the screw impacts against the sides of this hole. The hole in the distal fragment is smaller so that the thread of the screw grips its walls. Further turning of the screw then results in the screw thread pulling the distal fragment in, so that it is compressed against the proximal fragment (see Figure 29.9a). This is especially useful when a fracture can be reduced precisely. A lag screw can then hold the two fragments together so securely that absolute stability is provided. A single lag screw will provide absolute stability, but may not provide a strong durable fixation. If this is the case, then it may be protected by a neutralisation plate. This is a classic method of stable internal fixation and is ideal for fractures such as those of the radial and ulnar shafts. Compression plates have oval screw holes in them. As the screw head beds in, the plate is forced to slide sideways and to compress the fracture site. This can improve bone contact and stability.

A recent development is the locking plate. Here the screw has a threaded head that tightens into the plate. The screws are not floppy within the plate, but 'lock' when tightened. This gives angular stability similar to that of an external fixator and seems particularly advantageous in elderly bone and at metaphyseal/diaphyseal junctions. Table 29.7 shows the advantages and disadvantages of plate fixation.

Intramedullary nailing

The diaphysis of a long bone is essentially a tube. An intramedullary nail can be inserted down the medulla to hold a fracture reduced. The nail itself is usually made of steel or titanium, and may be solid, hollow or slotted in cross-section. To extend the range of fractures suitable for stabilisation, nails are now made with drill holes at either end; this allows locking of the nail to the bone with further screws to control both rotation and length.

Thin nails can be inserted without reaming or heavier nails can be inserted after reaming. There are pros and cons to both techniques. Table 29.8 summarises this debate.

Standard nails are not suitable for the growing bone where they would transgress and damage a growth plate. The advantages and disadvantages of intramedullary nailing are described in Table 29.9.

External fixation

In external fixation, each side of the fracture is connected to the main fixator which lies outside the patient. The connection of the frame to the bone is via either half-pins (that is, stiff metal rods typically 5–6 mm in diameter) or tensioned wires (typi-

Table 29.7 Advantages and disadvantages of plate and screw fixation.

Advantages	Can be used when anatomical reduction is required
	Allows early mobilisation
	Can provide absolute or relative stability
Disadvantages	May interfere with fracture site
	Periosteal/soft-tissue damage
	Does not normally allow for immediate load-bearing
	Potential for infection
	Metalwork complications
	?Need for plate removal

Table 29.8 A comparison of reamed versus unreamed nailing (an assumption is that nails used unreamed are usually thinner than those used reamed)

	Reamed IMN	Unreamed IMN
Insertion time	Longer	Quicker
Time to union	Shorter	Longer
Size of implant	Larger	Smaller
Reduction of distal fractures	Easier	More difficult
Strength of construct	More	Less

IMN, intramedullary nail.

Table 29.9 Advantages and disadvantages of intramedullary nailing.

Advantages	Minimally invasive
	Early weight-bearing
	Less periosteal damage than open reduction and internal fixation
	Seldom need removal
Disadvantages	Increased risk of fat emboli/chest complications
	Infection difficult to treat
	Difficult to remove if broken

cally 1.8 mm in diameter), which are then secured to the frame by clamps (see Figure 29.9c). External fixators are quick and relatively simple to apply. A further great advantage of external fixation is that it can be used even if there is soft tissue loss and bone is exposed. Plastic surgeons can work on providing soft tissue cover while the fracture remains stable (Table 29.10). A third advantage of external fixators is that it is possible to modify the mechanical environment of the fracture (compressing, distracting and correcting alignment) without needing to subject the patient to further surgery.

The prime disadvantage of an external fixator is the 'pin sites', i.e. the point where the pins or wires penetrate the skin. These pin sites require care as they may become infected or tether soft tissues, thereby interfering with function.

Specific indications for external fixators include:

- emergency stabilisation of a long bone fracture in the polytrauma patient thought too unwell to have other interventions, 'damage control orthopaedics';
- stabilisation of a dislocated joint after reduction, e.g. a spanning fixator across the knee joint while the vascular surgeons repair an arterial injury with a knee dislocation;
- complex periarticular fractures, temporary stabilisation to allow the soft tissues to settle before definitive fixation, e.g. a distal tibial (pilon) fracture;
- fractures associated with infection;
- treating fractures with bone loss.

A Kirschner wire (also called a K-wire) is a thin, flexible wire made of stainless steel. Transfixing wires can be passed percutaneously to keep fracture fragments reduced. They are cheap and often quick and simple to use. They have been used extensively around the hand and wrist as definitive fixation. Another common use of wires is for temporary fixation intraoperatively. Thus, a provisional reduction can be held with wires while the more definitive and robust fixation is applied. Some of their uses are shown in Table 29.11.

Flexible wire is also used in fracture fixation. Both patella and olecranon fractures can be fixed using a 'figure-of-eight' tension band. This is a dynamic fixation such that, when a predictable load is applied to the bone, compression across the fracture site is actually increased.

Complications of K-wires are pin-track infection, wire breakage, loss of fixation and migration of the wire. Migration of a wire is a potentially serious problem and, as a consequence, their use in some areas is ill advised. K-wires placed around the clavicle have been known to migrate, penetrating the thoracic cavity and even the heart.

Arthroplasty

Prosthetic replacements may be used for treating articular fractures or those in which avascular necrosis is inevitable (e.g. the subcapital fractured neck of femur). In the proximal humerus, a multifragmentary fracture that is considered unsalvageable by internal fixation methods can be treated with a shoulder hemiarthroplasty.

Table 29.10 Advantages and disadvantages of external fixation.

Advantages	No interference with fracture site
	Adjustable after application: alignment; biomechanics
	Soft tissues accessible for plastic surgery
	Rapid stabilisation of fracture
	Hardware easy to remove
Disadvantages	Pin site infection
	Interferes with plastic surgical procedures
	Soft-tissue tethering
	Cumbersome for the patient

Table 29.11 Indications for K-wire insertion.

Temporary fixation
Definitive fixation – with small fracture fragments (e.g. wrist fractures and hand injuries)
Tension band wiring (fractures of the patella and olecranon)
Temporary immobilisation of a small joint

MANAGEMENT BY TYPE AND REGION

Table 29.12 gives some of the general indications for operative stabilisation. Two simple questions to ask of a fracture are: 'Does it need to be reduced?' and 'Does it need to be held?'

Diaphyseal fractures

The diaphysis is composed predominantly of a tube of dense cortical bone. Fracture treatment is aimed at restoring function by achieving bony union with correction of the length, alignment and rotation. In many diaphyseal fractures, if the bone heals with the adjacent joints in their normal relationship, the anatomical reduction of the fracture fragments at the fracture site is of secondary importance. This is demonstrated in Figure 29.12, which shows C-type fractures treated in this way.

Martin Kirschner, 1879–1942, Professor of Surgery, Heidelberg, Germany, introduced the use of skeletal traction wires in 1909.

Table 29.12 Indications for surgery in limb trauma (the main indication is that operation will produce a better outcome; the principles are given below).

A fracture requiring treatment that is unsuitable for non-operative measures
Open fractures
Failed non-operative management
Multiple injuries
Pathological or impending pathological fractures
Displaced intra-articular fractures
Fractures through the growth plate, where arrest is possible (Salter–Harris type III–V)
Avulsion fractures that compromise the functional integrity of a ligament/tendon around a joint (e.g. olecranon fracture)
Established non-unions or malunions

Femoral shaft fractures

The anatomy of the proximal femur allows easy access to the medullary canal for inserting an intramedullary device nail. A statically locked intramedullary nail is suitable for the vast majority of adult femoral shaft fractures irrespective of their pattern. With an isolated femoral shaft fracture, the patient can be expected to mobilise rapidly postoperatively and may only be hospitalised for a few days.

Traction was traditionally used as the definitive treatment for these fractures and treatment took 12–16 weeks. Now traction is only used as a first aid measure to provide pain relief and maintain length while transferring a patient to definitive care.

Tibial shaft fractures

When the fracture is sufficiently stable, generally an A-type pattern, casting is the safest and cheapest choice. A full-leg cast is applied immediately and split to the skin. Once the risk of compartment syndrome has passed, the cast is closed. By 4 weeks, it can generally be changed to a moulded, patella tendon-bearing, below-knee cast. This allows the knee to move. Cast treatment requires frequent and careful monitoring and there should be no hesitation in changing the cast should the reduction be deteriorating. To correct minor deformity in a controlled and comfortable manner, the cast may be wedged.

Surgery to a tibial shaft fracture is often indicated either as a result of instability (B- or C-type fractures) or because the patient also has other injuries. Currently, intramedullary nailing is the most frequent choice of treatment, but there is a high incidence of anterior knee pain following this operation, and so it should be used with caution in those patients who have to kneel. Malunion is common in nailed fractures of the proximal tibial shaft; so plating is a better option for fractures which are closer to the metaphysis. External fixation remains a good option for a wide range of tibial shaft fractures. The subcutaneous position of the tibia makes pin placement and pin site care relatively straightforward.

Humeral shaft fractures

In humeral shaft fractures, the maintenance of limb length and alignment is nowhere near as important as in the leg. Thus, the majority of humeral shaft fractures can be treated non-operatively with a simple protective functional brace and a collar and cuff. This is the safest and cheapest option. The indications for operative management include an open fracture, the presence of other injuries such as head injury, multiple injuries, ipsilateral arm fractures and failed non-operative management. In these circumstances, fixation and stability can be achieved by either plating or intramedullary nailing. The rate of non-union is significantly higher when nailing the humerus than when nailing the femur or tibia; thus, plating is generally the treatment of choice. Figure 29.13 shows a plated B-type diaphyseal fracture. Should the need for fixation be combined with signs of radial nerve damage, plating has the advantage of allowing exploration of the nerve.

Radius and ulna

Although the radius and ulna appear outwardly similar to other long bones, they can best be visualised as the two components of a large joint. Their relationship requires precise anatomical restoration if they are to function normally in supination and pronation. This precision is best and most easily achieved by open reduction and plate fixation (Summary box 29.6).

Summary box 29.6

Diaphyseal fractures

- Restore length, alignment and rotation
- Consider whether primary or secondary bone healing is the objective
- Radius and ulna need precise reduction to function

Metaphyseal fractures

Fractures in the metaphyseal region are classified as A-type if they are extra-articular, B-type if they are partial articular and C-type if they are complete articular.

In an A-type fracture, the joint surfaces remain intact, so congruity is not an issue. Therefore, the problem may be thought of as being similar to that of treating a diaphyseal fracture; however, there are two differences that need attention. First, the injury and the subsequent treatment, being close to a joint, are more liable to cause joint stiffness. Second, the bone on either side of the fracture is not of a similar type or quality. It is generally easier to obtain a mechanical hold on the diaphyseal bone of the shaft than on the spongy bone of the metaphysis; thus the quality of fixation may be imbalanced. This imbalance in fixation is even more apparent when dealing with osteoporotic bone and can easily lead to fixation failure.

With B- and C-type fractures, the joint surfaces themselves are involved. Thus, in addition to providing stability and overall alignment, the congruity of the joint surface is also important.

In an A-type metaphyseal fracture, the emphasis is on maintaining length, alignment and rotation, while allowing continued function. This requires sound fixation as demonstrated in Figure 29.14. In this instance, the fixation has been achieved with a plate and screws, but it could equally have been carried out with an external fixator.

In a B-type partial articular fracture joint, congruity is the prime objective. This can often be maintained with relatively lightweight fixation as the load borne by the metalware itself is

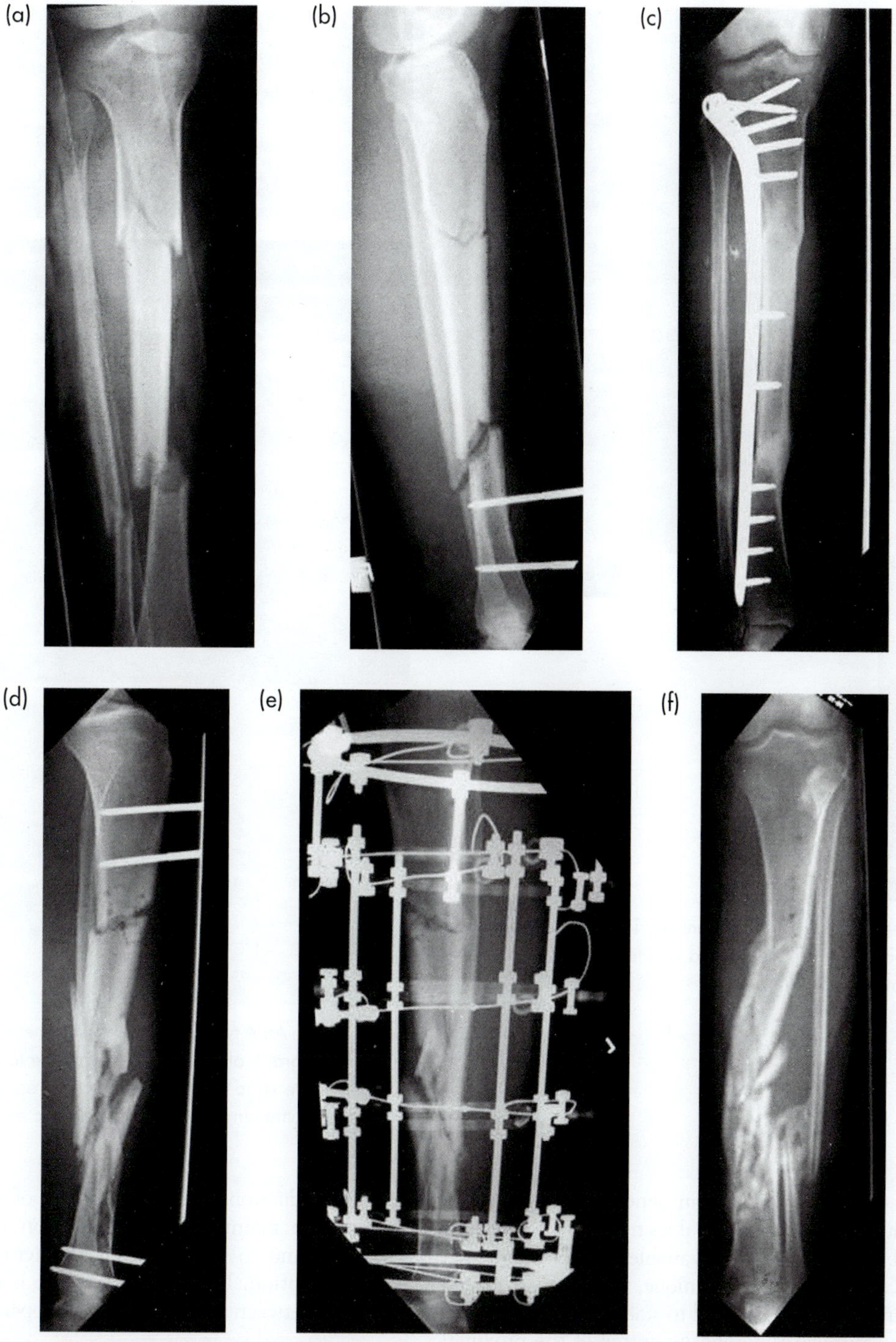

Figure 29.12 (a) and (d) are C-type or segmental tibial fractures. Each was a high-energy injury. (b) and (e) show a temporary spanning external fixator applied in each case. (c) and (f) show definitive relative stability was achieved with different methods of bridging fixation. Healing was by indirect means in both cases. Despite irregularities at the fracture sites the overall position was satisfactory and function was good.

low (Figure 29.15). B-type fractures, when they require surgery, are nearly always treated with screws, or screws and plates.

The C-type or complete articular fracture combines both of these features. They need joint congruity and bone alignment. This is demonstrated in the tibial plateau in Figure 29.16. The articular component of the fracture is generally held with screws, allowing for interfragmental compression. The metaphyseal component of the fracture may be held as in the A-type fracture, with plates and screws or an external fixator.

Distal radial fractures

Because of the frequency of their occurrence, distal radial fractures deserve separate mention. The common fractures in this area are A-type, i.e. extra-articular. The Colles fracture

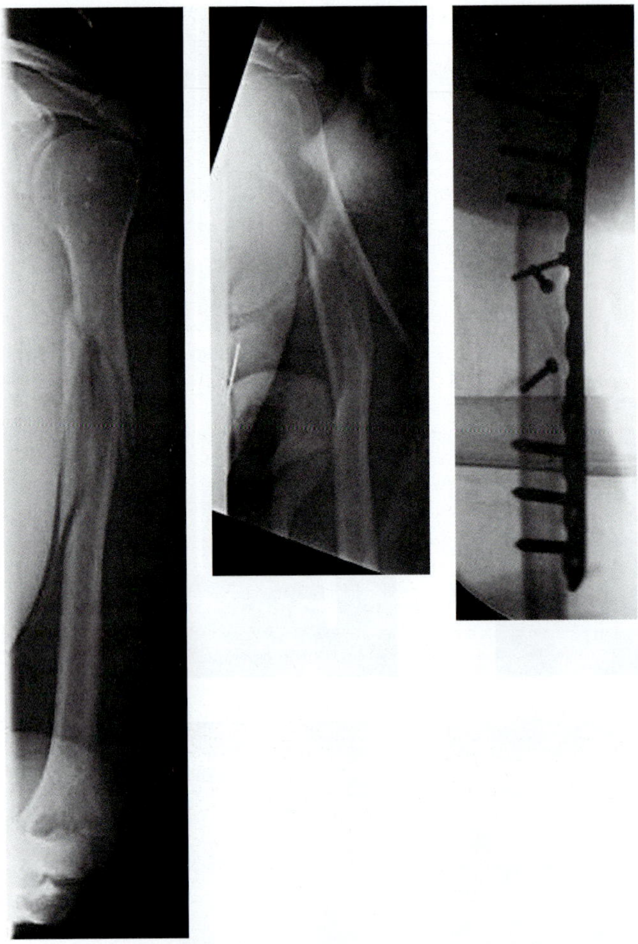

Figure 29.13 A B-type humeral shaft fracture. This fracture could not be controlled by non-operative means and was treated with lag screws protected by a plate.

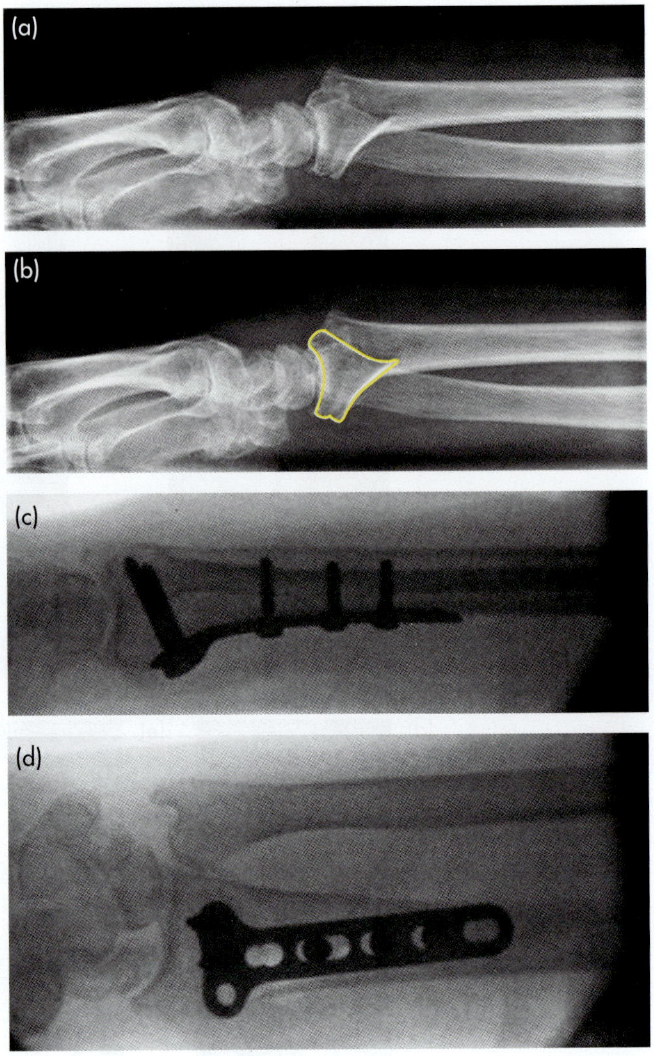

Figure 29.14 An A-type or extra-articular metaphyseal fracture. A plain lateral radiograph of this Smith-type fracture (a and b). Fracture fixed to a plate. There is no interfragmental compression. The plate is pushing against or buttressing the distal fragment (c and d).

with dorsal and radial angulation can generally be treated by manipulation and casting. When this does not provide sufficient stability, a useful technique to have available is intrafocal wiring, popularised by Kapandji. In this technique, the wires are placed through the fracture site, then angled to stabilise the distal fragment and secured through the opposite cortex of the proximal fragment (Figure 29.17).

When the displacement is in the opposite direction, i.e. volar, the so-called Smith's fracture, stability is difficult to achieve by casting, and so plating is generally employed.

When there is significant articular displacement of a distal radial fracture, formal open reduction and fixation with plates and screws is being performed in a very similar fashion to dealing with a tibial plateau fracture, but with smaller implants.

Ankle fractures

The eventual functional outcome of ankle fractures depends upon the position of union. Thus, if the fracture is stable, it requires only symptomatic treatment. An unstable ankle fracture requires reduction and maintenance of reduction until bony union. The maintenance of reduction is more reliable with operation and so in the younger patient this is generally the preferred option. In the elderly, there is no clear evidence for choosing between operative and non-operative management.

Managing fractures in the skeletally immature

Many injuries are dealt with in an analogous way in the child and the adult; however, there are naturally differences. As discussed in Chapter 23, there needs to be constant vigilance for evidence of non-accidental injury.

Children's fractures heal more rapidly than those of adults. Remodelling is also possible, so a position which may not be acceptable in an adult may turn out to give a good result in a child. The nearer the fracture is to the growth plate, the greater the remodelling capacity. Deformity is more acceptable in the plane of motion of the adjacent joint. Remodelling is greatest at the ends of the bone that contribute most to longitudinal

Robert William Smith, 1807–1873, Professor of Surgery, Trinity College, Dublin, Ireland, described the reverse Colles fracture in 1847.

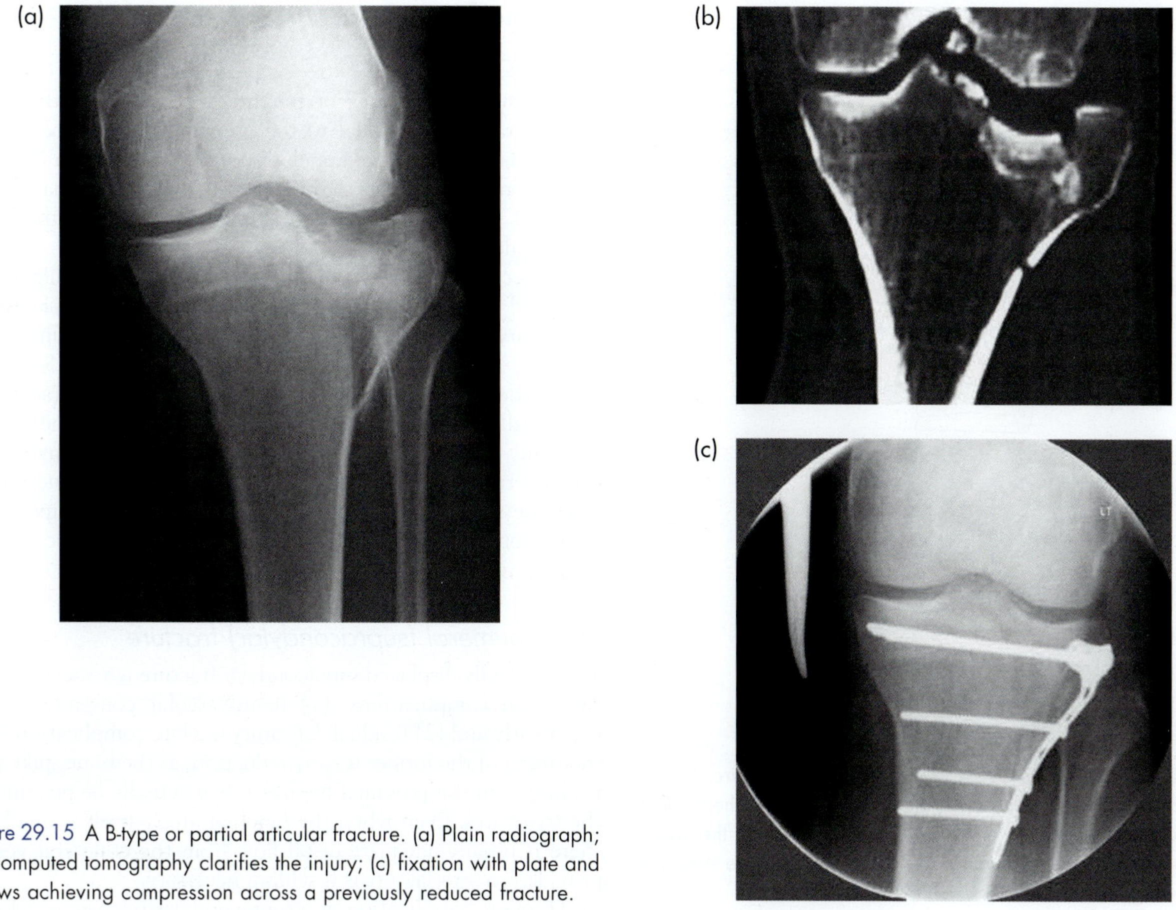

Figure 29.15 A B-type or partial articular fracture. (a) Plain radiograph; (b) computed tomography clarifies the injury; (c) fixation with plate and screws achieving compression across a previously reduced fracture.

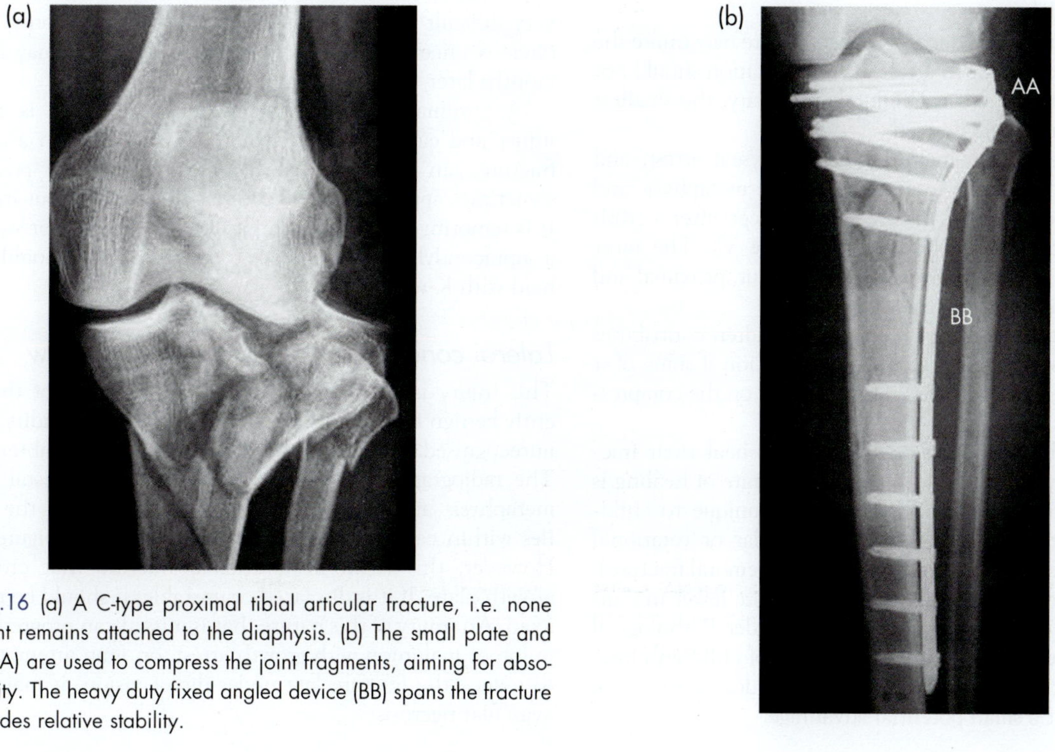

Figure 29.16 (a) A C-type proximal tibial articular fracture, i.e. none of the joint remains attached to the diaphysis. (b) The small plate and screws (AA) are used to compress the joint fragments, aiming for absolute stability. The heavy duty fixed angled device (BB) spans the fracture and provides relative stability.

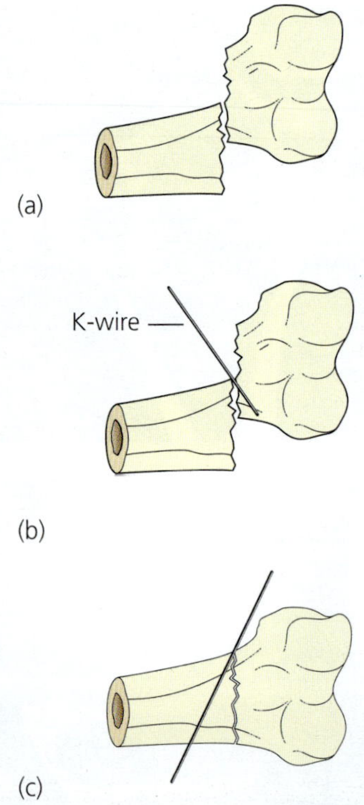

Figure 29.17 (a) A displaced distal radial fracture. (b) A wire is introduced percutaneously by hand through the fracture site. (c) The fracture is manipulated into a reduced position (not levered using the wire). Once reduced, the wire is advanced under power into the opposite cortex, securing the reduction.

growth. For example, fractures at the distal femur have more potential to remodel than proximal femoral fractures. Significant remodelling is also expected at the proximal humerus (70 per cent of longitudinal growth). Young children have the greatest capacity to remodel.

Repeated attempts to reduce a physeal fracture may injure the physis, and so lead to growth arrest. Internal fixation should not cross the physis, but if this is absolutely necessary, the smallest and smoothest pin should be used.

Trauma is the most common cause of physeal arrest, and occurs when a bony bridge forms between the metaphysis and epiphysis. Complete arrest is most commonly seen after a crush injury to the growth plate (Salter-Harris type V). The most common area for growth arrest is the distal femur, proximal and distal tibia and the distal radius.

The thicker and stronger periosteum in children contributes both to fracture stability and to fracture reduction if some of it (known as the 'periosteal hinge') remains intact on the compression side of the fracture.

Children rarely experience non-union and heal their fractures more rapidly than adults. In general, the rate of healing is inversely proportional to age. Complications unique to childhood include growth arrest, progressive angular or rotational deformity and overgrowth of a long bone (post-femoral fracture).

The indications for operative intervention are fewer in children than adults (see Figure 29.26c below under Pathological failure). The generally benign natural history of children's fractures means that the risk of complications often does not balance favourably against a small potential advantage.

Specific injuries

Distal radial fracture

The most common area of fracture in children is the distal radius. Fractures proximal to the growth plate may be treated symptomatically or by manipulation under anaesthesia (MUA). There is no clear rule as to the amount of deformity that can be accepted. As puberty approaches, fractures should be treated as for the adult.

A special case is when the distal radial fracture is sufficiently displaced to require manipulation while the ulna itself is intact. Secondary redisplacement is common under these circumstances and it is advisable to hold the radius with primary K-wiring. When the growth plate is involved in a distal radial fracture, it is generally a Salter-Harris type I or II injury. MUA and casting is usually adequate and growth disturbance is uncommon after primary treatment; however, should the fracture reduction be lost, one should try not to proceed to a second manipulation. The second manipulation is much more likely to cause damage to the physis and subsequent growth problems.

Distal humeral (supracondylar) fracture

The markedly displaced supracondylar fracture is associated with two main complications: (1) neurovascular compromise may occur early and (2) residual deformity is a late complication. The treatment of the former is early reduction, as the bone spike protruding from the proximal fragment may actually be pressing on the structures. Even when the brachial artery itself is involved, there is usually adequate distal flow from the collateral vessels provided so arterial repair is seldom necessary.

The late complication of a supracondylar fracture is deformity. This is due not to an interference with growth (the fracture is proximal to the growth plate), but to poor initial reduction or loss of reduction. As noted above, deformity in the plane of the adjacent joint tends to correct satisfactorily. It is the varus/valgus angulatory deformity that is critical at the elbow. This is very difficult to assess initially as the deformity only becomes obvious once full extension is regained, which may be many months later.

A minimally displaced supracondylar fracture is a benign injury and can be treated symptomatically. When a displaced fracture can be manipulated into a satisfactory position, it sometimes appears stable as soon as the elbow is put in flexion. It is tempting to leave this injury in a flexed cast for stability. If a supracondylar fracture needs to be reduced, it should then be held with K-wires.

Lateral condylar mass fracture of the elbow

This injury is easily missed and is an example of the apparently benign injury that may have significant morbidity if it goes unrecognised. Clinically, the clue is localised lateral tenderness. The radiograph may show just a flake off the distal humeral metaphysis above the capitellum as the bulk of the fracture lies within cartilage which has not yet ossified (Figure 29.18). However, this is an intra-articular fracture that crosses the growth plate. If it is displaced or unstable, it should be primarily fixed. An injury of this nature that is missed can progress to non-union or malunion with growth arrest, or, if an attempt is made to reduce the fracture late under direct vision, it may develop avascular necrosis.

Slipped upper femoral epiphysis

This injury is readily missed. A painful hip in a child approaching puberty should arouse suspicion. The injury can be diagnosed on plain radiography as seen in Figure 29.19. When treated in its early stages, the outcome is excellent; if it progresses to a more severe slip, then the outcome is poor. It is frequently bilateral.

Femoral shaft fracture

Femoral shaft fractures in children can be managed with traction as the short time to union makes this a reasonable choice providing that there is not an accompanying head injury or other long bone fracture. With children under 12–15 kg, simple gallows traction is appropriate. Here the legs are suspended vertically with the buttocks just off the bed. This maintains an adequate position for the fracture, and nappy changes are straightforward. With older children, operative fixation has become more attractive. Standard intramedullary nailing poses a risk to the proximal growth plate and should be avoided in girls below 12 years and boys below 14 years. Flexible intramedullary nails may be placed to avoid the growth plate (Figure 29.20).

Tibial shaft fracture

In a child with an unstable tibial fracture that is not amenable to cast management, external fixation, elastic nailing and plating are all reasonable options (Summary box 29.7).

Summary box 29.7

Fractures in the skeletally immature

- Do not forget non-accidental injury
- Be reluctant to remanipulate a physeal injury
- Elastic nails are a significant step forward in fracture treatment in children
- Not many fractures require operative intervention in children

Osteoporotic fractures

In osteoporosis, there is a decrease in bone mass and strength. Eventually, a relatively minor accident can cause a fracture (fragility fracture). These fractures, occurring mainly in the elderly, constitute the bulk of the orthopaedic trauma workload of a UK hospital. The elderly have less capacity to tolerate an injured limb and, thus, it is often not possible for them to partially weight-bear. Therefore, if treatment is to allow them to function, fixation must be able to tolerate full weight-bearing.

Internal fixation in osteoporotic bone remains a challenge. The hold of screws inserted into the bone is often poor. This leads to 'backing out' of the screws and subsequent loss of fracture reduction. Locking plates may help to overcome this problem. In a locking plate construction, the integrity of the structure depends also upon the tightness of the screw in the plate rather than just the tightness of the screw in the bone (Figure 29.21b).

The need for early restoration of function in the elderly makes intervention more attractive, although care must be taken because of wound healing problems.

Intra-articular fractures

It is not always necessary to obtain a perfect anatomical reduction of an intra-articular fracture in an elderly osteoporotic patient, and it is even more difficult to hold it. The long-term complication of post-traumatic arthritis is of relatively less importance in the elderly. Thus, in dealing with a tibial plateau fracture in an older patient, the object of operative fixation is different from that in the younger person; it is primarily stability and not congruity that is required. The first stage of an operation to treat a tibial plateau fracture in the elderly is an examination under anaesthesia. If the joint is stable, then there is no indication for operative treatment even though there may be joint incongruity. When a reconstruction is required, bone grafting

(a)

(b)

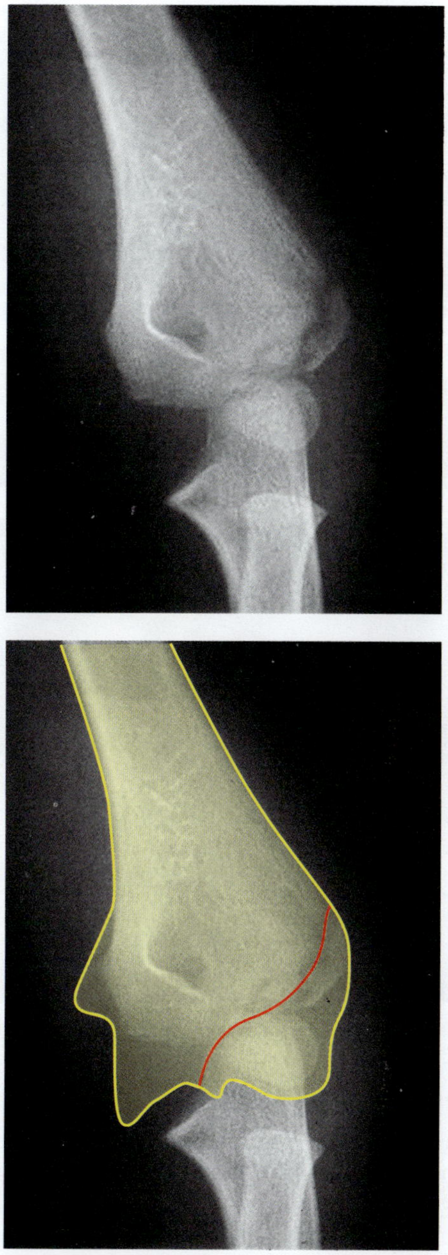

Figure 29.18 Lateral condylar mass fracture. (a) Plain radiograph showing the metaphyseal fracture. (b) The yellow shows the shape of the distal humerus including the cartilaginous analogue, and the red shows the true extent of the injury, i.e. a significant intra-articular fracture.

(a)

(b)

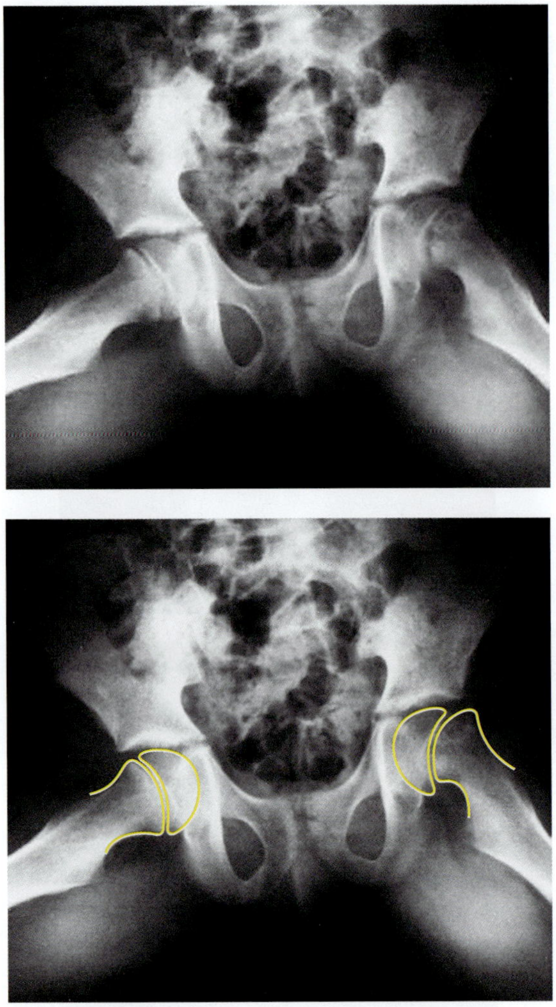

Figure 29.19 Slipped left upper femoral epiphysis. (a) Plain radiograph; (b) the injury highlighted.

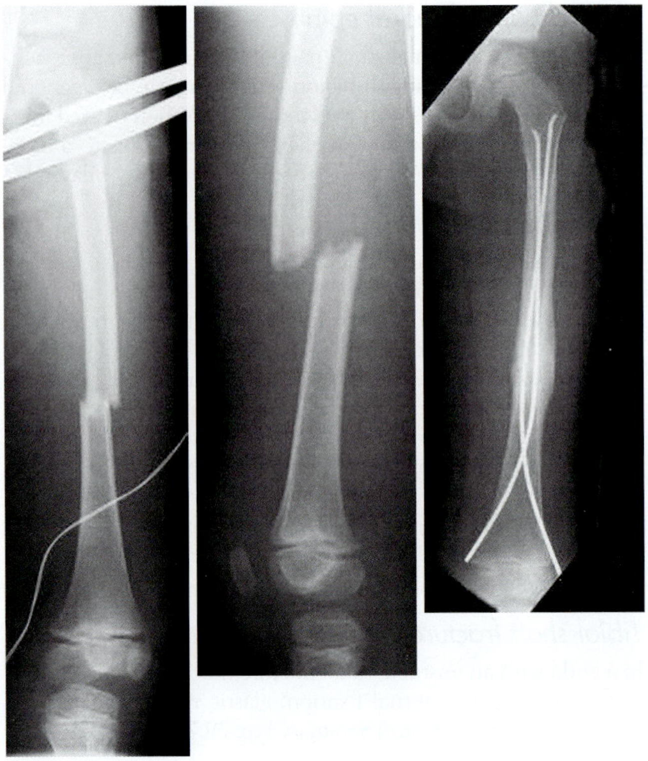

Figure 29.20 Femoral shaft fracture in a child, which has been stabilised with elastic nails.

may be needed as the patient's bone will be crushed. Figure 29.22a shows a case in which bone substitute has been used to help support the reduced joint surface.

Proximal femoral fractures

Proximal femoral fractures fall into two groups: extracapsular and intracapsular. The blood supply to the femoral head and neck travels down through the hip capsule and then back up the femoral neck. Fractures of the femoral neck inside the capsule (intracapsular or subcapital) are liable to sever the blood supply to the head of the femur and so need to be treated differently to those outside the capsule.

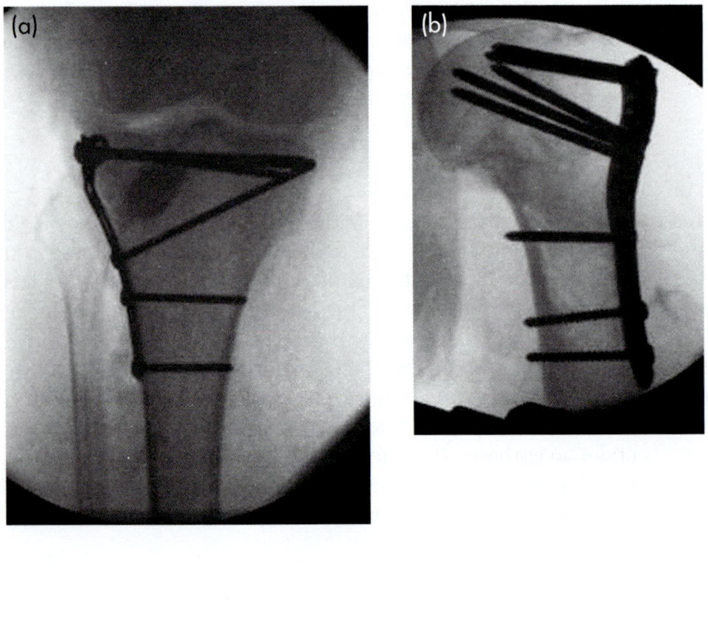

Figure 29.21 Variations in fixation technique suited to osteoporotic bone. (a) Norian bone substitute has been injected to support the lateral tibial plateau in the partial articular fracture. (b) A locking plate in a proximal humerus. The screws are threaded into the plate to make a fixed-angle device.

Extracapsular fracture

Biological fixation principles are used to fix this type of fracture. Indirect reduction using a traction table is followed by fixation with a dynamic hip screw (DHS) placed using an image intensifier. The dynamic nature of the implant (the screw slides on the plate) allows the fragments to impact together when the patient walks, as shown in Figure 29.22. This stimulates healing while improving stability and protects the femoral head from penetration by the implant.

Intracapsular fracture

Most patients presenting with an intracapsular (subcapital) fractured neck of femur are elderly and osteoporotic. Early mobilisation offers their best chance of sustaining such independence as they have. However, if the fracture has displaced, then the femoral head will be likely to have lost its blood supply. Fixing it back in place will be fruitless as the bone is dead (avascular necrosis) Therefore, the treatment of choice is to simply replace the compromised femoral head with an artificial head (a hemi-arthoplasty). This treatment is not ideal in younger patients, where the chances of the femoral head being viable is much higher, especially if the fracture is relatively undisplaced (Summary box 29.8). The alternatives for the younger patient are:

- attempt to reduce and fix the fracture holding with screws placed under image intensifier control. Some of these fixations will be successful, but if they fail a total hip replacement is the salvage option.

or

- to perform a primary total hip replacement. This is a mechanically sounder but a more extensive procedure and has a limited life span before it will need revising.

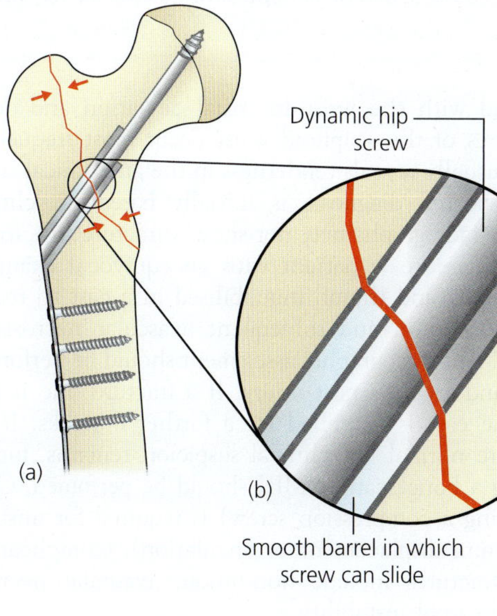

Figure 29.22 (a) A dynamic hip screw for fixing a trochanteric proximal femoral fracture. This allows for compression at the fracture site on load-bearing and protects the femoral head from penetration by the screw when the osteoporotic bone settles. (b) Insert to show the sliding screw in the barrel.

Summary box 29.8

Osteoporotic fractures

- Fragility fractures in the elderly are the most common cause of trauma admission
- The elderly do not tolerate immobility so need secure fixation to allow early mobilisation
- Inter-trochanteric fractures need a dynamic hip screw for an unstable fracture
- Subcapital fractures usually need a hemi-arthroplasty as the blood supply of the femoral head is lost

Injuries to the foot and hand

Foot injuries

Calcaneal fractures

The os calcis is the largest and most frequently fractured hindfoot bone. The most common cause of injury is a fall from a height. Associated injuries include lumbar spine and lower extremity fractures, which occur in 10–20 per cent of cases. Plain radiographs do not clearly show the degree of damage, and CT is necessary for a proper evaluation. Figure 29.23 shows an intra-articular fracture of the os calcis. When accurate reduction and fixation is achieved, surgery is valuable in improving function and reducing pain. However, a good reduction is often difficult to achieve, and the results are then no better than treating the fracture in plaster.

Talus fractures and dislocations

The talus consists of three parts (head, neck and body). It articulates superiorly with the distal tibia and inferiorly with the calcaneus and navicular. The talus has no muscular or tendinous attachments and therefore its blood supply is tenuous. Talar neck fractures are the most common injury and are usually high energy (historically termed 'aviator's astragalus'). A significant complication of this fracture is avascular necrosis of the talus. The goal of treatment is anatomical reduction and stable fixation, as this is thought to reduce the risk of osteonecrosis. Hawkins' sign can be seen approximately 6–8 weeks after injury on plain radiographs. This appears as subchondral lucency of the talar dome, which signifies bony reabsorption. This can only occur if the bone is viable.

Tarsometatarsal (Lisfranc) joint injuries

The tarsometatarsal joint is a very strong weight-bearing structure. It requires significant force to injure it. Poorly treated injuries of this joint can give rise to long-term debilitating symptoms. Once suspected, the injury is then confirmed on plain radiography and delineated further with CT. The treatment of the displaced injury is open reduction and internal fixation.

Achilles tendon rupture

Up to 20 per cent of these injuries are missed at initial presentation. The typical history of a sensation of being kicked behind the ankle while playing sport is frequently given. Sometimes, there is a palpable gap. Simmonds' test (squeezing the calf to produce passive plantar flexion of the ankle) is usually positive.

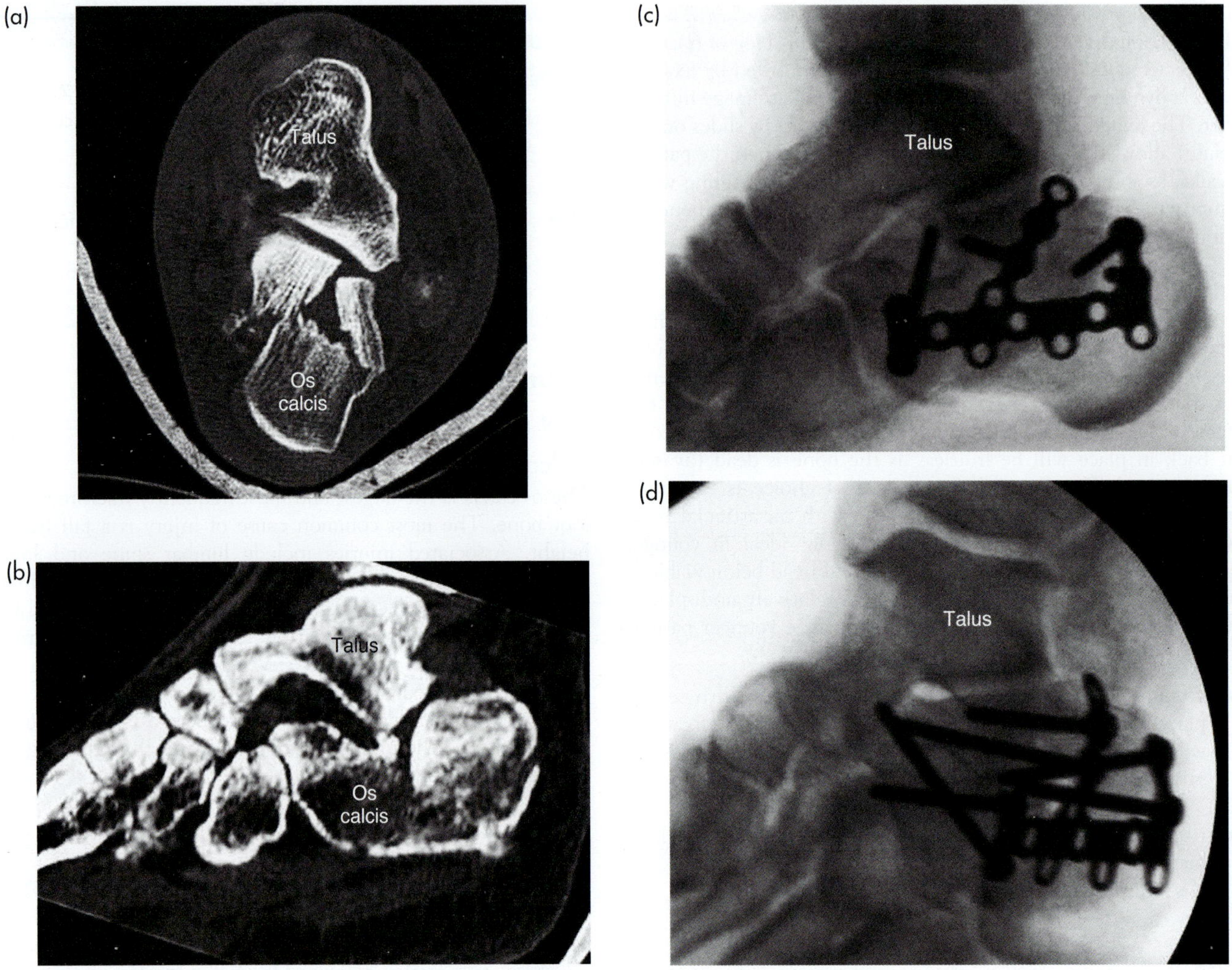

Figure 29.23 Axial (a) and sagittal (b) views of a displaced intra-articular fracture of the os calcis. (c and d) Intraoperative views of the reconstruction. Both the overall shape and the articular surface have been restored.

The differential diagnosis is an intra-substance tear of the gastrocnemius muscle. In this case, Simmond's test is painful and negative (the foot moves with calf pressure). The diagnosis is confirmed using ultrasound. If the gap separating the torn ends is small, the patient can be treated with serial plasters (starting in equinus and bringing the ankle up to neutral). In patients with a wider gap (>5 mm), a percutaneous repair can be performed.

Hand injuries

Scaphoid fracture

The scaphoid is made up of the proximal and distal poles, a tubercle and the waist. The proximal pole is completely intra-articular and receives all of its blood supply from the distal branches of the radial artery. This enters the scaphoid in a retrograde fashion (distal to proximal). Therefore, fractures across the waist of the scaphoid are most at risk of non-union or avascular necrosis. In contrast, distal pole fractures tend to heal without problems. Figure 29.24 shows a scaphoid fracture and demonstrates how awkward it can be to make the diagnosis on standard anteroposterior and lateral views of the wrist.

The scaphoid is the most commonly injured carpal bone. The mechanism of injury is typically a fall onto the outstretched hand with the wrist in radial deviation and dorsiflexed. Fractures of the scaphoid waist occur most frequently. Examination usually reveals tenderness in the anatomical snuffbox. The suspected diagnosis is initially based on clinical findings. Plain radiographs may not show a fracture line for up to 10 days. Therefore, a patient with an equivocal examination has the wrist and thumb immobilised in a cast to reduce the risk of non-union and subsequent avascular necrosis. A repeat clinical and radiographic assessment should be performed between 10 and 14 days post-injury. If a fracture line is now seen, then the cast is reapplied for a further 6 weeks. If the radiographs are normal but clinical suspicion remains, further imaging using a bone scan or MRI should be perfomed. Open reduction (using a compression screw) is required for unstable fractures (>1 mm displacement or angulation). Complications of scaphoid fractures include non-union, avascular necrosis, malunion and carpal instability.

Lunate dislocation

The lunate forms a part of the proximal row of the carpus with the scaphoid and triquetrum. Articulating with the radius, this row forms the radiocarpal joint.

Jacques Lisfranc de St Martin, 1790–1847, Professor of Surgery and Operative Medicine, Paris, France.
Franklin Adin Simmonds, 1911–1983, orthopaedic surgeon, The Rowley Bristow Hospital, Pyrford, UK.

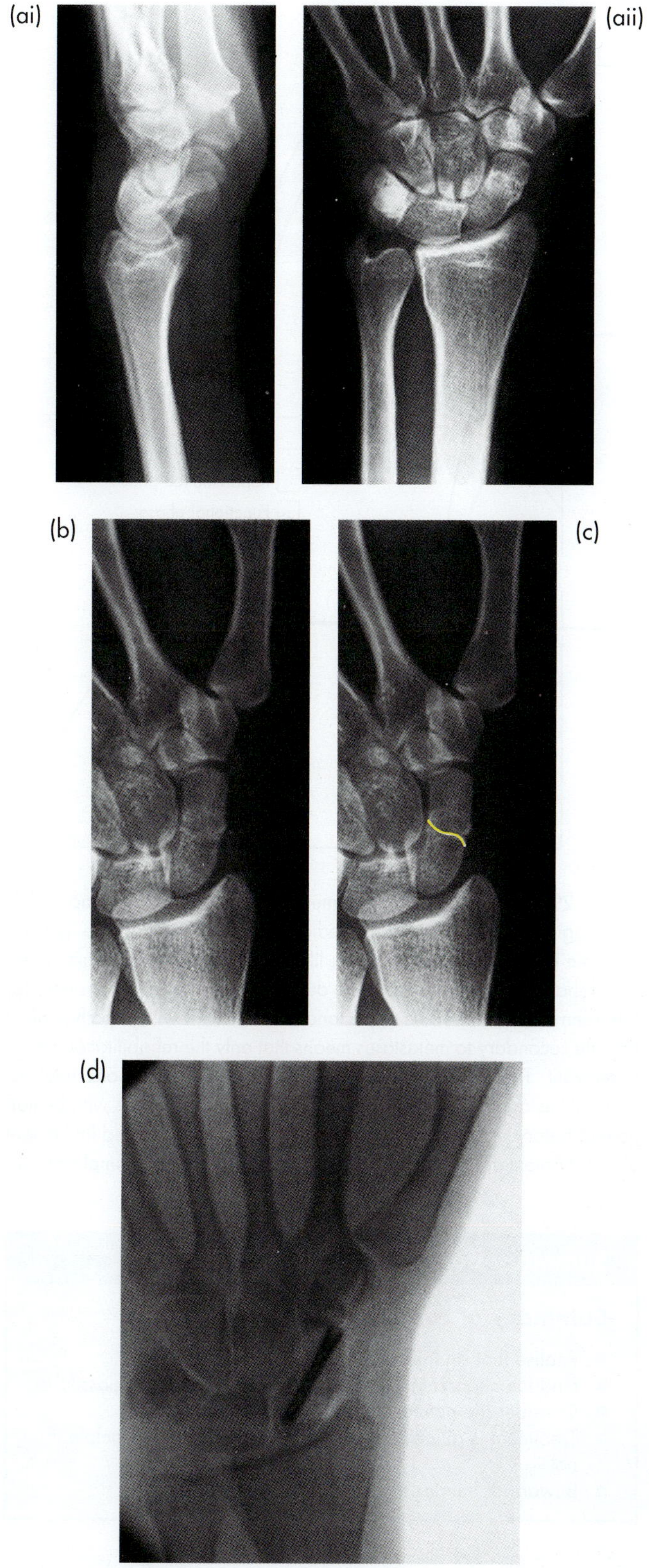

Figure 29.24 Scaphoid fracture. (a) Anteroposterior and lateral views in which the injury is difficult to see. (b and c) Oblique views with the fracture line highlighted. (d) In this case of a young patient, the fracture was treated with early fixation.

The lunate resides in the concavity of the lunate fossa of the distal radius. Interosseus ligaments hold it to the adjacent scaphoid and triquetrum.

Perilunate dislocations are often unrecognised. Clinical examination reveals significant swelling of the entire carpus. In the absence of a fracture on x-ray, this is diagnostic of carpal dissociation. The diagnosis is made with plain radiographs, but these can be difficult to interpret (Figure 29.25); the lateral view demonstrates the 'spilled tea cup sign' with volar tilt of the lunate. Acute injuries may be initially treated with closed reduction and casting. Irreducible or unstable injuries require open reduction and stabilisation with K-wires. Note that associated injuries, such as scaphoid and radial styloid fractures, as well as median nerve injury, should be excluded.

Thumb metacarpophalangeal ulnar collateral ligament

The integrity of this ligament is important for effective lateral key pinch. Injury to the ulnar collateral ligament is commonly referred to as 'gamekeeper's thumb' or 'skier's thumb', and is caused by the thumb being forced laterally away from the rest of the hand. Tenderness is located on the ulnar aspect of the metacarpophalangeal joint. To assess the integrity of the ligament, perform a stress test.

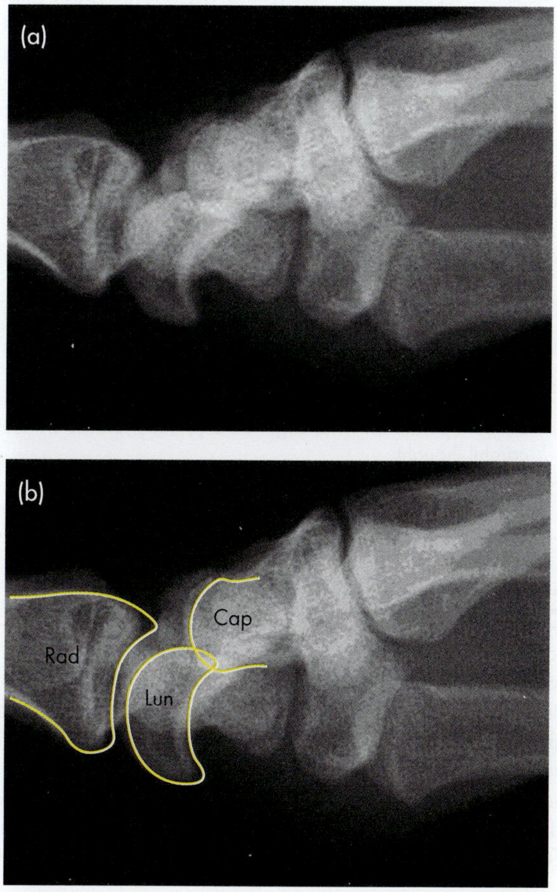

Figure 29.25 Perilunate dislocation. (a) A plain lateral radiograph of the wrist. (b) The outline of the perilunate dislocation is highlighted. Cap, capitate; Lun, lunate; Rad, radius.

Cast immobilisation can be used in the treatment of partial tears with a good endpoint. A complete tear with instability (excessive opening of the joint when compared with the other side), or a displaced fracture, requires open repair as the ends of the ruptured ligament may become separated by the aponeurosis of adductor pollicis so that natural healing cannot take place (Stener lesion).

Pathological failure

When abnormal bone gives way under normal load, this is referred to as a pathological fracture. Examples include primary bone tumours and bony metastases, osteomyelitis, metabolic bone disease (osteomalacia, Paget's disease, osteoporosis) and haematopoietic disease (myeloma, lymphoma, leukaemia).

The typical history is of a minor trauma. This alerts the surgeon to the possibility of an underlying bony pathology. Blood tests, a chest radiograph and full-length views of the fractured bone are essential. A bone scan is the most sensitive detector of skeletal disease.

In a patient with a primary bone tumour, treatment must be planned to avoid disseminating the disease (see Chapter 39). In a patient who has multiple metastases and whose life span is limited, treatment is aimed at regaining immediate mobility and relief of pain. As can be seen in Figure 29.26, there is a clear rationale for aggressive treatment to restore function despite the risks. The goals of surgical treatment are to reduce pain and to splint the bone so that the patient can use it. Femoral, tibial and humeral fractures are nailed where possible. Some juxta-articular fractures that would require protection if treated with ORIF and bone grafting may be mobilised earlier if bone cement is substituted for the graft. Prophylactic stabilisation should be considered in patients with metastases where there has been cortical bone destruction of ≥50 per cent or a femoral lesion longer than 2.5 cm, pathological fracture of the lesser trochanter and persistent pain after irradiation (Summary box 29.9).

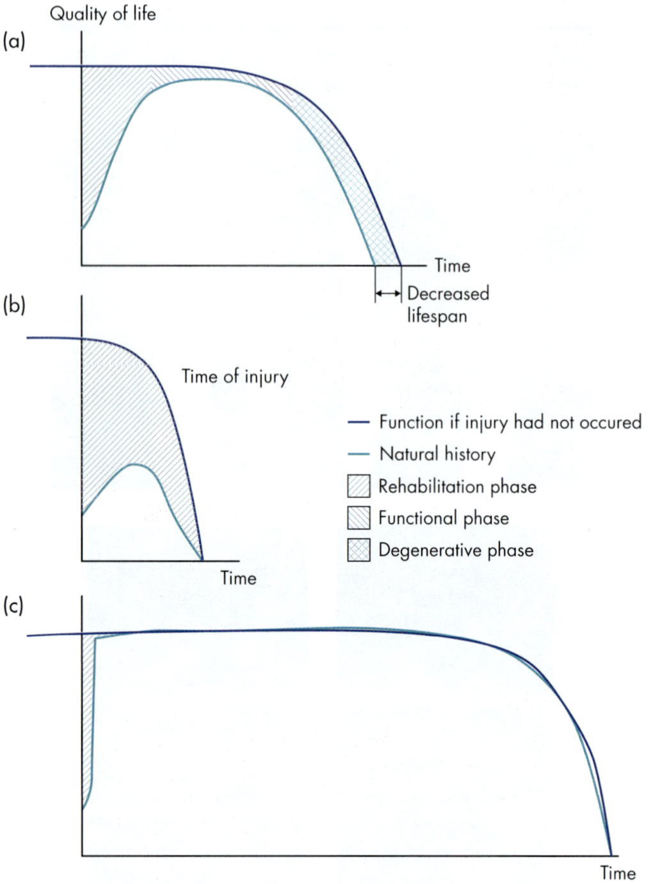

Figure 29.26 Comparative outcome curves for a normal adult (a), pathological fracture (b) and paediatric fracture (c). (a) The generic outcome curve for a patient with a life expectancy of >20 years. There is a rehabilitation, functional and degenerative phase to consider. (b) It is seen that the short life expectancy of a patient with a pathological fracture secondary to metastases means that only the rehabilitation phase is relevant. The patient must be able to function before bone healing. This justifies aggressive treatment. (c) The paediatric fracture with benign natural history. Any marginal early gain has to be considered in the light of great potential for long-term detriment should there be complications.

Summary box 29.9

Pathological failure

- Do not operate on what might be a primary tumour without careful thought
- Fractures through secondary tumours are treated aggressively to optimise early function

CONCLUSION

The management of extremity trauma is in theory quite straightforward. The first step is to realise that an injury exists as a missed injury cannot be treated. The injury then needs to be understood; this generally involves description and classification. When there is clear evidence as to the best method of treatment for a particular injury, this should be followed. When such evidence is lacking, as is generally the case, the treatment of fractures is generally principle based (Summary box 29.10).

Summary box 29.10

Summary of extremity trauma

- Realise that an injury exists
- Find the characteristics of the injury, describe and classify it
- Consider the natural history of the injury
- Treatment is guided by outcome if known or by principle if not
- Beware of injuries that are 'easily missed'

FURTHER READING

Bone LR, Johnson KD, Weight J, Scheinberg RJ. Early versus delayed stabilization of femoral fractures. *J Bone Joint Surg* 1989; **71A**: 336–40.

Charnley J. *The closed treatment of common fractures*. Edinburgh: E&S Livingstone, 1950.

Gustilo RB, Anderson JT. Prevention of infection in the treatment of 1025 open fractures of long bones. *J Bone Joint Surg* 1976; **8A**: 453–8.

Mast J, Jakob R, Ganz R. *Planning and reduction technique in fracture surgery*. Berlin: Springer-Verlag, 1989.

Muller ME, Nazarian S, Koch P. *The AO classification of fractures*. Schatzker J (trans). Berlin: Springer-Verlag, 1988.

Sir James Paget, 1814–1899, surgeon, St Bartholomew's Hospital, London, UK.

CHAPTER

30 Burns

LEARNING OBJECTIVES

To assess:
- The area and depth of burns

To understand:
- Methods for calculating the rate and quantity of fluids to be given
- Techniques for treating burns and the patient
- The pathophysiology of electrical and chemical burns

INTRODUCTION

The incidence of burn injury varies greatly between cultures. In the United Kingdom (with its population of 65 million), each year around 175 000 people visit accident and emergency (A&E) departments suffering from burns, of whom about 13 000 need to be admitted. About 1000 have severe burns requiring fluid resuscitation, and half of the victims are under 16 years of age.

The majority of burns in children are scalds caused by accidents with kettles, pans, hot drinks and bath water. Among adolescent patients, the burns are usually caused by young males experimenting with matches and flammable liquids. In adults, scalds are not uncommon, but are less frequent than flame burns. Most electrical and chemical injuries occur in adults. Cold and radiation are very rare causes of burns. Associated conditions in adults, such as mental disease (attempted suicide or assault), epilepsy and alcohol or drug abuse, are underlying factors in as many as 80 per cent of patients with burns admitted to hospital in some populations.

Legislation, health promotion and appliance design have reduced the incidence of burns, with regulations regarding flame-retardant clothes and furniture, the promotion of smoke alarms, the design of cookers and gas fires, the almost universal use of cordless kettles and the education of parents to keep their hot water thermostat to 60°C all playing their part (Summary box 30.1).

Summary box 30.1

Prevention of burns

A significant proportion of burns can be prevented by:
- Implementing good health and safety regulations
- Educating the public
- Introducing of effective legislation

The last 50 years have seen great strides made to reduce both morbidity and mortality from burn injuries. The coming years will see a better understanding of the control of physiology along with improvements in reconstruction and rehabilitation.

A large burn injury will have a significant effect on the patient's family and friends and the patient's future. The importance of multidisciplinary care needs to be stressed for the adequate and effective care of the burn patient.

THE PATHOPHYSIOLOGY OF BURN INJURY

Burns cause damage in a number of different ways, but by far the most common organ affected is the skin. However, burns can also damage the airway and lungs, with life-threatening consequences. Airway injuries occur when the face and neck are burned. Respiratory system injuries usually occur if a person is trapped in a burning vehicle, house, car or aeroplane and is forced to inhale the hot and poisonous gases (Summary box 30.2).

Summary box 30.2

Warning signs of burns to the respiratory system

- Burns around the face and neck
- A history of being trapped in a burning room
- Change in voice
- Stridor

INJURY TO THE AIRWAY AND LUNGS

Physical burn injury to the airway above the larynx

The hot gases can physically burn the nose, mouth, tongue, palate and larynx. Once burned, the linings of these structures will start to swell. After a few hours, they may start to interfere with the larynx and may completely block the airway if action is not taken to secure an airway (Summary box 30.3).

Summary box 30.3

Dangers of smoke, hot gas or steam inhalation

- Inhaled hot gases can cause supraglottic airway burns and laryngeal oedema
- Inhaled steam can cause subglottic burns and loss of respiratory epithelium
- Inhaled smoke particles can cause chemical alveolitis and respiratory failure
- Inhaled poisons, such as carbon monoxide, can cause metabolic poisoning
- Full-thickness burns to the chest can cause mechanical blockage to rib movement

Physical burn injury to the airway below the larynx

This is a rare injury as the heat exchange mechanisms in the supraglottic airway are usually able safely to absorb the heat from hot air. However, steam has a large latent heat of evaporation and can cause thermal damage to the lower airway. In such injuries, the respiratory epithelium rapidly swells and detaches from the bronchial tree. This creates casts, which can block the main upper airway.

Metabolic poisoning

There are many poisonous gases that can be given off in a fire, the most common being carbon monoxide, a product of incomplete combustion that is often produced by fires in enclosed spaces. This is the usual cause of a person being found with altered consciousness at the scene of a fire. Carbon monoxide binds to haemoglobin with an affinity 240 times greater than that of oxygen and therefore blocks the transport of oxygen. Levels of carboxyhaemoglobin in the bloodstream can be measured. Concentrations above 10 per cent are dangerous and need treatment with pure oxygen for more than 24 hours. Death occurs with concentrations around 60 per cent.

Another metabolic toxin produced in house fires is hydrogen cyanide, which causes a metabolic acidosis by interfering with mitochondrial respiration.

Inhalational injury

Inhalational injury is caused by the minute particles within thick smoke, which, because of their small size, are not filtered by the upper airway, but are carried down to the lung parenchyma. They stick to the moist lining, causing an intense reaction in the alveoli. This chemical pneumonitis causes oedema within the alveolar sacs and decreasing gaseous exchange over the ensuing 24 hours (Figure 30.1), and often gives rise to a bacterial pneumonia. Its presence or absence has a very significant effect on the mortality of any burn patient.

Mechanical block on rib movement

Burned skin is very thick and stiff, and this can physically stop the ribs moving if there is a large full-thickness burn across the chest.

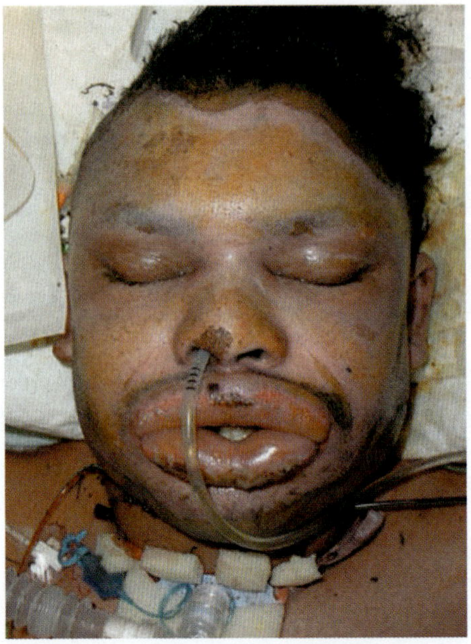

Figure 30.1 The swelling that occurs with inflammation due to burns.

INFLAMMATION AND CIRCULATORY CHANGES

The dangers to the airway and respiration described above are readily apparent, but the cause of circulatory changes following a burn are more complex. The changes occur because burned skin activates a web of inflammatory cascades. The release of neuropeptides and the activation of complement are initiated by the stimulation of pain fibres and the alteration of proteins by heat. The activation of Hageman factor initiates a number of protease-driven cascades, altering the arachidonic acid, thrombin and kallikrein pathways.

At a cellular level, complement causes the degranulation of mast cells and coats the proteins altered by the burn. This attracts neutrophils, which also degranulate, with the release of large quantities of free radicals and proteases. These can, in turn, cause further damage to the tissue. Mast cells also release primary cytokines such as tumour necrosis factor alpha (TNF-α). These act as chemotactic agents to inflammatory cells and cause the subsequent release of many secondary cytokines. These inflammatory factors alter the permeability of blood vessels such that intravascular fluid escapes. The increase in permeability is such that large protein molecules can also now escape with ease. The damaged collagen and these extravasated proteins increase the oncotic pressure within the burned tissue, further increasing the flow of water from the intravascular to the extravascular space (Figure 30.2).

The overall effect of these changes is to produce a net flow of water, solutes and proteins from the intravascular to the extravascular space. This flow occurs over the first 36 hours after the injury, but does not include red blood cells. In a small burn, this reaction is small and localised but, as the burn size approaches 10–15 per cent of total body surface area (TBSA), the loss of intravascular fluid can cause a level of circulatory shock. Furthermore, once the area increases to 25 per cent of TBSA, the inflammatory reaction causes fluid loss in vessels remote from the burn injury. This is why such importance is

John Hageman was a 37-year-old railroad brakeman in whom this factor deficiency was discovered by Dr Oscar Ratnoff in 1955.

(a)

(b)

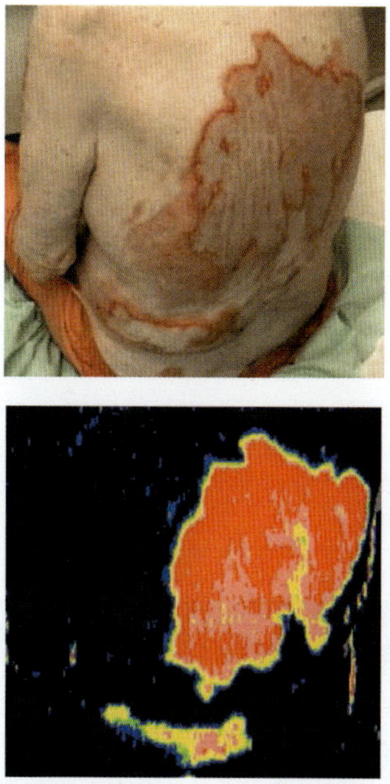

Figure 30.2 A scald burn (a) and its laser doppler image (b) showing burn depth. Red and pink areas are superficial burns, which should heal with conservative dressings.

attached to measuring the TBSA involved in any burn. It dictates the size of inflammatory reaction and therefore the amount of fluid needed to control shock (Summary box 30.4).

Summary box 30.4

The shock reaction after burns

- Burns produce an inflammatory reaction
- This leads to vastly increased vascular permeability
- Water, solutes and proteins move from the intra- to the extravascular space
- The volume of fluid lost is directly proportional to the area of the burn
- Above 15 per cent of surface area, the loss of fluid produces shock

OTHER LIFE-THREATENING EVENTS WITH MAJOR BURNS

The immune system and infection

The inflammatory changes caused by the burn have an effect on the patient's immune system. Cell-mediated immunity is significantly reduced in large burns, leaving them more susceptible to bacterial and fungal infections. There are many potential sources of infection, especially from the burn wound and from the lung if this is injured, but also from any central venous lines, tracheostomies or urinary catheters present.

Changes to the intestine

The inflammatory stimulus and shock can cause microvascular damage and ischaemia to the gut mucosa. This reduces gut motility and can prevent the absorption of food. Failure of enteral feeding in a patient with a large burn is a life-threatening complication. This process also increases the translocation of gut bacteria, which can become an important source of infection in large burns. Gut mucosal swelling, gastric stasis and peritoneal oedema can also cause abdominal compartment syndrome, which splints the diaphragm and increases the airway pressures needed for respiration.

Danger to peripheral circulation

In full-thickness burns, the collagen fibres are coagulated. The normal elasticity of the skin is lost. A circumferential full-thickness burn to a limb acts as a tourniquet as the limb swells. If untreated, this will progress to limb-threatening ischaemia (Summary box 30.5).

Summary box 30.5

Other complications of burns

- Infection from the burn site, lungs, gut, lines and catheters
- Malabsorption from the gut
- Circumferential burns may compromise circulation to a limb

IMMEDIATE CARE OF THE BURN PATIENT

Pre-hospital care

The principles of pre-hospital care are:

- **Ensure rescuer safety.** This is particularly important in house fires and in the case of electrical and chemical injuries.
- **Stop the burning process.** Stop, drop and roll is a good method of extinguishing fire burning on a person.
- **Check for other injuries.** A standard ABC (airway, breathing, circulation) check followed by a rapid secondary survey will ensure that no other significant injuries are missed. Patients burned in explosions or even escaping from fires may have head or spine injuries and other life-threatening problems.
- **Cool the burn wound.** This provides analgesia and slows the delayed microvascular damage that can occur after a burn injury. Cooling should occur for a minimum of 10 minutes and is effective up to 1 hour after the burn injury. It is a particularly important first aid step in partial-thickness burns, especially scalds. In temperate climates, cooling should be at about 15°C, and hypothermia must be avoided.
- **Give oxygen.** Anyone involved in a fire in an enclosed space should receive oxygen, especially if there is an altered consciousness level.
- **Elevate.** Sitting a patient up with a burned airway may prove life-saving in the event of a delay in transfer to hospital care. Elevation of burned limbs will reduce swelling and discomfort.

Hospital care

The principles of managing an acute burn injury are the same as in any acute trauma case:

- A, Airway control
- B, Breathing and ventilation
- C, Circulation
- D, Disability – neurological status
- E, Exposure with environmental control
- F, Fluid resuscitation.

The possibility of injury additional to the burn must be sought both clinically and from the history, and treated appropriately. The major determinants of severity of any burn injury are the percentage of TBSA that is burned, the presence of an inhalation injury and the depth of the burn (Summary box 30.6).

Not all burned patients will need to be admitted to a burns unit, but the main criteria are given in Table 30.1.

Summary box 30.6

Major determinants of the outcome of a burn

- Percentage surface area involved
- Depth of burns
- Presence of an inhalational injury

Airway

The burned airway creates problems for the patient by swelling and, if not managed proactively, can completely occlude the upper airway. The treatment is to secure the airway with an endotracheal tube until the swelling has subsided, which is usually after about 48 hours. The symptoms of laryngeal oedema, such as change in voice, stridor, anxiety and respiratory difficulty, are very late symptoms. Intubation at this point is often difficult or impossible owing to swelling, so acute cricothyroidotomy equipment must be at hand when intubating patients with a delayed diagnosis of airway burn. Because of this, early intubation of suspected airway burn is the treatment of choice in such patients. The time-frame from burn to airway occlusion is usually between 4 and 24 hours, so there is time to make a sensible decision with senior staff and allow an experienced anaesthetist to intubate the patient (Summary box 30.7).

Summary box 30.7

Initial management of the burned airway

- Early elective intubation is safest
- Delay can make intubation very difficult because of swelling
- Be ready to perform an emergency cricothyroidotomy, if intubation is delayed

The key in the management of airway burn is the history and early signs, rather than the symptoms. The history is of inhalation of hot gases such as in a house or car fire. Clues on examination include blisters on the hard palate, burned nasal mucosa and loss of all the hair in the nose (the anterior hairs are often burned), but perhaps the most valuable signs are the presence of deep burns around the mouth and in the neck (Summary box 30.8).

Table 30.1 The criteria for acute admission to a burns unit.

Suspected airway or inhalational injury
Any burn likely to require fluid resuscitation
Any burn likely to require surgery
Patients with burns of any significance to the hands, face, feet or perineum
Patients whose psychiatric or social background makes it inadvisable to send them home
Any suspicion of non-accidental injury
Any burn in a patient at the extremes of age
Any burn with associated potentially serious sequelae, including high-tension electrical burns and concentrated hydrofluoric acid burns

Summary box 30.8

Recognition of the potentially burned airway

- A history of being trapped in the presence of smoke or hot gases
- Burns on the palate or nasal mucosa, or loss of all the hairs in the nose
- Deep burns around the mouth and neck

Breathing

Inhalational injury

Time is also a factor; anyone trapped in a fire for more than a couple of minutes must be observed for signs of smoke inhalation. Other signs that raise suspicion are the presence of soot in the nose and the oropharynx and a chest radiograph showing patchy consolidation.

The clinical features are a progressive increase in respiratory effort and rate, rising pulse, anxiety and confusion and decreasing oxygen saturation. These symptoms may not be apparent immediately and can take 24 hours to 5 days to develop.

Treatment starts as soon as this injury is suspected and the airway is secure. Physiotherapy, nebulisers and warm humidified oxygen are all useful. The patient's progress should be monitored using respiratory rate, together with blood gas measurements. If the situation deteriorates, continuous or intermittent positive pressure may be used with a mask or T-piece. In the severest cases, intubation and management in an intensive care unit will be needed.

The key, therefore, in the management of inhalational injury is to suspect it from the history, institute early management and observe carefully for deterioration.

Thermal burn injury to the lower airway

These rare injuries can occur with steam injuries. Their management is supportive and the same as that for an inhalational injury.

Metabolic poisoning

Any history of a fire within an enclosed space and any history of altered consciousness are important clues to metabolic poisoning. Blood gases must be measured immediately if poisoning is a possibility. Carboxyhaemoglobin levels raised above 10 per cent must be treated with high inspired oxygen for 24 hours to speed its displacement from haemoglobin. Metabolic acidosis is a feature of this and other forms of poisoning.

Once again, the key to diagnosing these injuries is suspicion from the history. Blood gas measurement will confirm the diagnosis. The treatment is oxygen.

Mechanical block to breathing

Any mechanical block to breathing from the eschar of a significant full-thickness burn on the chest wall is obvious from the examination. There will also be carbon dioxide retention and high inspiratory pressures if the patient is ventilated. The treatment is to make some scoring cuts through the burned skin to allow the chest to expand (escharotomy). The nerves have been destroyed in the skin, and this procedure is not painful for the patient.

ASSESSMENT OF THE BURN WOUND

Assessing size

Burn size needs to be formally assessed in a controlled environment. This allows the area to be exposed and any soot or debris washed off. Care should be taken not to cause hypothermia during this stage. In the case of smaller burns or patches of burn, the best measurement is to cut a piece of clean paper the size of the patient's whole hand (digits and palm), which represents 1 per cent TBSA, and match this to the area. Another accurate way of measuring the size of burns is to draw the burn on a Lund and Browder chart (Figure 30.3), which maps out the percentage TBSA of sections of our anatomy. It also takes into account different proportional body surface area in children according to age. The rule of nines, which states that each upper limb is 9 per cent TBSA, each lower limb 18 per cent, the torso 18 per cent each side and the head and neck 9 per cent, can be used as a rough guide to TBSA outside the hospital environment (Summary box 30.9).

Summary box 30.9

Assessing the area of a burn

- The patient's whole hand is 1 per cent TBSA, and is a useful guide in small burns
- The Lund and Browder chart is useful in larger burns
- The rule of nines is adequate for a first approximation only

Assessing depth from the history

The first indication of burn depth comes from the history (Table 30.2). The burning of human skin is temperature- and time-dependent. It takes 6 hours for skin maintained at 44°C to suffer irreversible changes, but a surface temperature of 70°C for 1 s is all that is needed to produce epidermal destruction. Taking an example of hot water at 65°C: exposure for 45 s will produce a full-thickness burn, for 15 s a deep partial-thickness burn and for 7 s a superficial partial-thickness burn (Summary box 31.10).

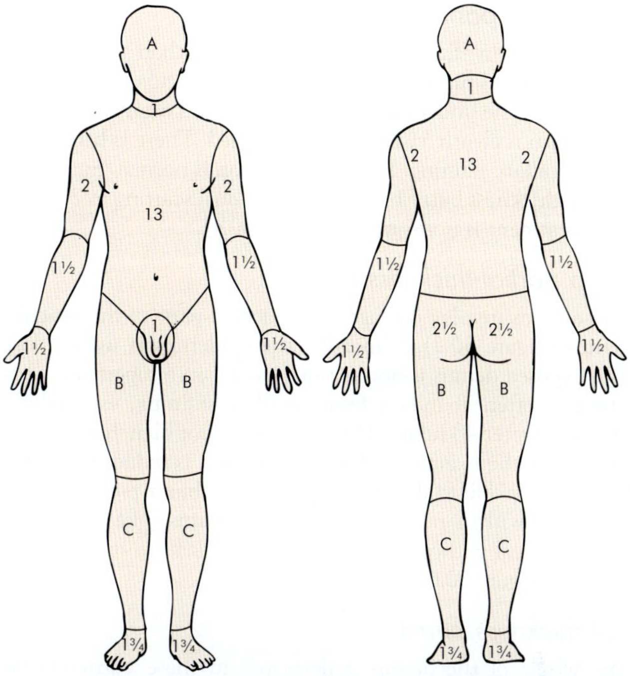

Relative percentage of area affected by growth

Age in years	0	1	5	10	15	Adult
A Head	9	8	6	5	4	3
B Thigh	2	3	4	4	4	4
C leg	2	2	3	3	3	3

Figure 30.3 The Lund and Browder chart.

Table 30.2 Causes of burns and their likely depth.

Cause of burn	Probable depth of burn
Scald	Superficial, but with deep dermal patches in the absence of good first aid. Will be deep in a young infant
Fat burns	Deep dermal
Flame burns	Mixed deep dermal and full thickness
Alkali burns, including cement	Often deep dermal or full thickness
Acid burns	Weak concentrations superficial; strong concentrations deep dermal
Electrical contact burn	Full thickness

Summary box 30.10

Assessing the depth of a burn

- The history is important – temperature, time and burning material
- Superficial burns have capillary filling
- Deep partial-thickness burns do not blanch, but have some sensation
- Full-thickness burns feel leathery and have no sensation

Superficial partial-thickness burns

The damage in these burns goes no deeper than the papillary dermis. The clinical features are blistering and/or loss of the epidermis. The underlying dermis is pink and moist. The capillary return is clearly visible when blanched. There is little or no fixed capillary staining. Pinprick sensation is normal. Superficial partial-thickness burns heal without residual scarring in 2 weeks. The treatment is non-surgical (Figure 30.4).

Deep partial-thickness burn

These burns involve damage to the deeper parts of the reticular dermis (Figure 30.5). Clinically, the epidermis is usually lost. The exposed dermis is not as moist as that in a superficial burn. There is often abundant fixed capillary staining, especially if examined after 48 hours. The colour does not blanch with pressure under the examiner's finger. Sensation is reduced, and the patient is unable to distinguish sharp from blunt pressure when examined with a needle. Deep dermal burns take 3 or more weeks to heal without surgery and usually lead to hypertrophic scarring (Figure 30.6).

Full-thickness burns

The whole of the dermis is destroyed in these burns (Figure 30.7). Clinically, they have a hard, leathery feel. The appearance can vary from that similar to the patient's normal skin to charred black, depending upon the intensity of the heat. There is no capillary return. Often, thrombosed vessels can be seen under the skin. These burns are completely anaesthetised: a needle can be stuck deep into the dermis without any pain or bleeding.

FLUID RESUSCITATION

The principle of fluid resuscitation is that the intravascular volume must be maintained following a burn in order to provide sufficient circulation to perfuse not only the essential visceral organs such as the brain, kidneys and gut, but also the peripheral tissues, especially the damaged skin (Summary box 30.11).

Intravenous resuscitation is appropriate for any child with a burn greater than 10 per cent TBSA. The figure is 15 per cent TBSA for adults. In some parts of the world, intravenous resuscitation is commenced only with burns that approach 30 per cent TBSA. If oral resuscitation is to be commenced, it is important that the water given is not salt free. It is rarely possible to undergo significant diuresis in the first 24 hours in view of the stress hormones that are present. Hyponatraemia and water intoxication can be fatal. It is therefore appropriate to give oral rehydration with a solution such as Dioralyte®.

The resuscitation volume is relatively constant in proportion to the area of the body burned and, therefore, there are formulae that calculate the approximate volume of fluid needed for the

Summary box 30.11

Fluids for resuscitation

- In children with burns over 10 per cent TBSA and adults with burns over 15 per cent TBSA, consider the need for intravenous fluid resuscitation
- If oral fluids are to be used, salt must be added
- Fluids needed can be calculated from a standard formula
- The key is to monitor urine output

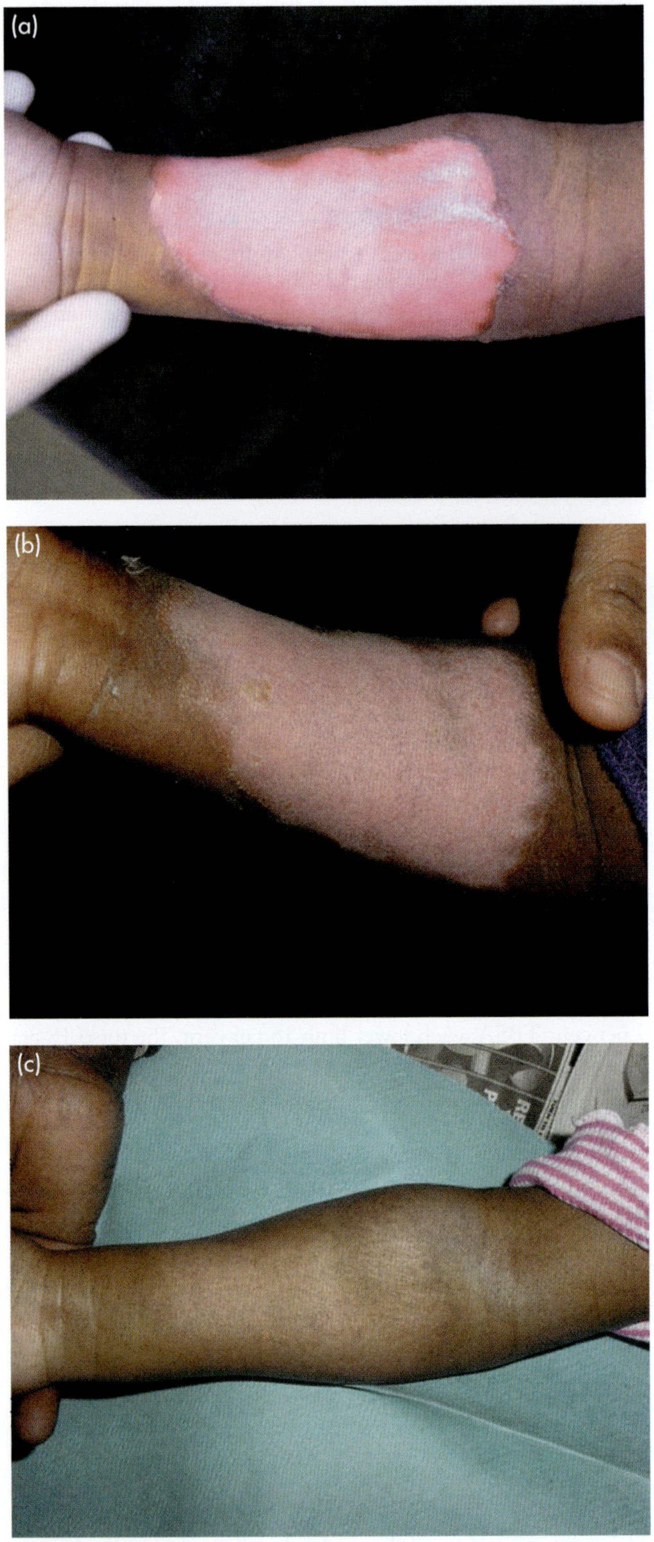

Figure 30.4 (a) A superficial partial-thickness scald 24 hours after injury. The dermis is pink and blanches to pressure. (b) At 2 weeks, the wound is healed but lacks pigment. (c) At three months, the pigment is returning.

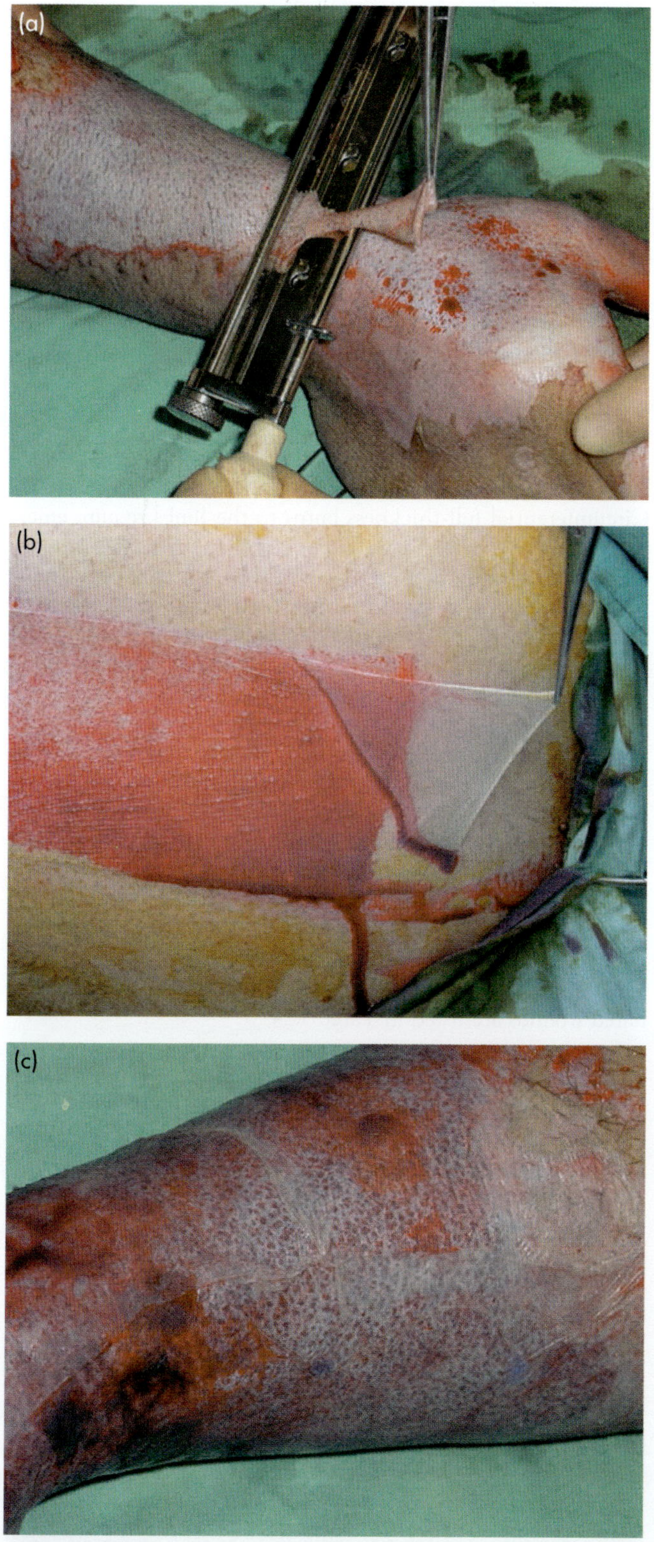

Figure 30.5 (a) A deep dermal burn undergoing tangential shaving. The dead dermis is removed layer by layer until healthy bleeding is seen. The burn is pale because it was dressed with silver sulphadiazine cream, but no blanching was visible under this layer. The patient was unable to differentiate between pressure from the sharp and blunt ends of a needle. (b) A thin, split-thickness graft harvested from the thigh. (c) The thin graft is placed in the dermal remnants. The rete pegs can be seen between the remnants of the dermis through the graft.

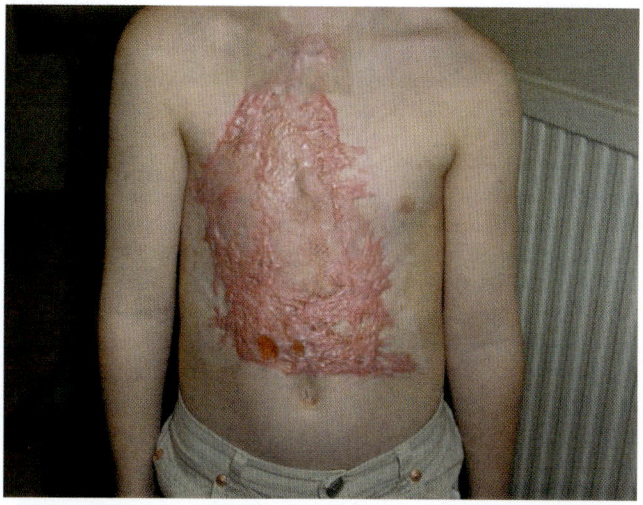

Figure 30.6 Hypertrophic scarring following a deep dermal burn.

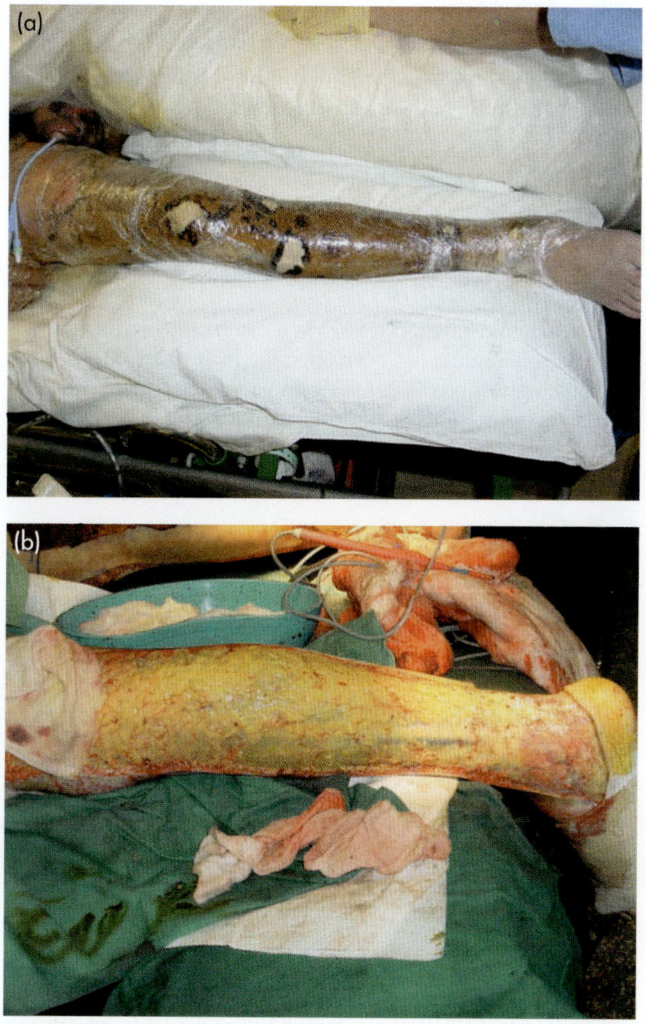

Figure 30.7 (a) A full-thickness burn on admission just prior to escharotomy. The wound is wrapped in cling film while in transit. The patient's facial burn is shown in Figure 30.10. (b) Excision of the same full-thickness burn, down to healthy fat.

resuscitation of a patient of a given body weight with a given percentage of the body burned. These regimens follow the fluid loss, which is at its maximum in the first 8 hours and slows, such that, by 24–36 hours, the patient can be maintained on his or her normal daily requirements.

There are three types of fluid used. The most common is Ringer's lactate or Hartmann's solution; some centres use human albumin solution or fresh-frozen plasma, and some centres use hypertonic saline.

Perhaps the simplest and most widely used formula is the Parkland formula. This calculates the fluid to be replaced in the first 24 hours by the following formula: total percentage body surface area × weight (kg) × 4 = volume (mL). Half this volume is given in the first 8 hours and the second half is given in the subsequent 16 hours.

Crystalloid resuscitation

Ringer's lactate is the most commonly used crystalloid. Crystalloids are said to be as effective as colloids for maintaining intravascular volume. They are also significantly less expensive. Another reason for the use of crystalloids is that even large protein molecules leak out of capillaries following burn injury; however, non-burnt capillaries continue to sieve proteins virtually normally.

In children, maintenance fluid must also be given. This is normally dextrose–saline given as follows:

- 100 mL/kg for 24 hours for the first 10 kg;
- 50 mL/kg for the next 10 kg;
- 20 mL/kg for 24 hours for each kilogram over 20 kg body weight.

Hypertonic saline

Human albumin solution (HAS) is a commonly used colloid.

Hypertonic saline has been effective in treating burns shock for many years. It produces hyperosmolarity and hypernatraemia. This reduces the shift of intracellular water to the extracellular space. Advantages include less tissue oedema and a resultant decrease in escharotomies and intubations.

Colloid resuscitation

Plasma proteins are responsible for the inward oncotic pressure that counteracts the outward capillary hydrostatic pressure. Without proteins, plasma volumes would not be maintained as there would be oedema. Proteins should be given after the first 12 hours of burn because, before this time, the massive fluid shifts cause proteins to leak out of the cells.

The most common colloid-based formula is the Muir and Barclay formula:

- 0.5 × percentage body surface area burnt × weight = one portion;
- periods of 4/4/4, 6/6 and 12 hours, respectively;
- one portion to be given in each period.

Monitoring of resuscitation

The key to monitoring of resuscitation is urine output. Urine output should be between 0.5 and 1.0 mL/kg body weight per hour. If the urine output is below this, the infusion rate should be increased by 50 per cent. If the urine output is inadequate and the patient is showing signs of hypoperfusion (restlessness with tachycardia, cool peripheries and a high haematocrit), then a bolus of 10 mL/kg body weight should be given. It is important that patients are not overresuscitated, and urine output in excess of 2 mL/kg body weight per hour should signal a decrease in the rate of infusion.

Other measures of tissue perfusion such as acid–base balance are appropriate in larger, more complex burns, and a haematocrit measurement is a useful tool in confirming suspected under- or overhydration. Those with cardiac dysfunction, acute or chronic, may well need more exact measurement of filling pressure, preferably by transoesophageal ultrasound or with the more invasive central line.

TREATING THE BURN WOUND

Escharotomy

Circumferential full-thickness burns to the limbs require emergency surgery (Figure 30.8). The tourniquet effect of this injury is easily treated by incising the whole length of full-thickness burns. This should be done in the mid-axial line, avoiding major nerves (Table 30.3). One should remember that an escharotomy can cause a large amount of blood loss; therefore, adequate blood should be available for transfusion if required.

Thereafter, the management of the burn wound remains the same, irrespective of the size of the injury. The burn needs to be cleaned, and the size and depth need to be assessed. Full thickness burns and deep partial-thickness burns that will require operative treatment will need to be dressed with an antibacterial dressing to delay the onset of colonisation of the wound.

Full-thickness burns and obvious deep dermal wounds

The four most common dressings for full-thickness and contaminated wounds are listed in Table 30.4.

Dressings with nanocrystalline silver

- **Silver sulphadiazine cream (1 per cent).** This gives broad-spectrum prophylaxis against bacterial colonisation and is particularly effective against *Pseudomonas aeruginosa* and also methicillin-resistant *Staphylococcus aureus*.

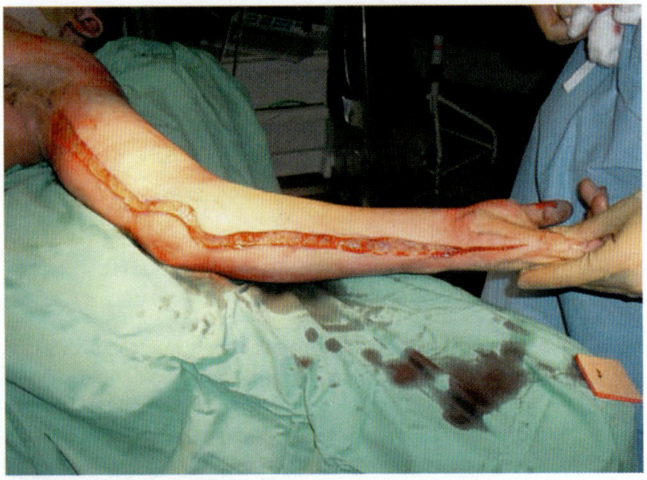

Figure 30.8 A full-thickness burn to the upper limb with a mid-axial escharotomy. The soot and debris have been washed off.

Alexis Frank Hartmann, 1898–1964, paediatrician, St Louis, MO, USA.
Thomas Laird Barclay, d. 2007, formerly plastic surgeon, The Royal Infirmary, Bradford, UK.
Ian Fraser Kerr Muir, 1921–2008, formerly plastic surgeon, Aberdeen Royal Infirmary, Aberdeen, UK. Referred to as 'a gentle giant of plastic surgery'.

Table 30.3 Key features of escharotomy placement.

Upper limb	Mid-axial, anterior to the elbow medially to avoid the ulnar nerve
Hand	Midline in the digits. Release muscle compartments if tight. Best done in theatre and with an experienced surgeon
Lower limb	Mid-axial. Posterior to the ankle medially to avoid the saphenous vein
Chest	Down the chest lateral to the nipples, across the chest below the clavicle and across the chest at the level of the xiphisternum
General rules	Extend the wound beyond the deep burn Diathermy any significant bleeding vessels Apply haemostatic dressing and elevate the limb postoperatively

Table 30.4 Options for topical treatment of deep burns.

1% silver sulphadiazine cream
0.5% silver nitrate solution
Mafenide acetate cream
Serum nitrate, silver sulphadiazine and cerium nitrate

- **Silver nitrate solution (0.5 per cent)**. Again, this is highly effective as a prophylaxis against *Pseudomonas* colonisation, but it is not as active as silver sulphadiazine cream against some of the Gram-negative aerobes. The other disadvantage of this solution is that it needs to be changed or the wounds resoaked every 2–4 hours. It also produces black staining of all the furniture surrounding the patient.
- **Mafenide acetate cream**. This is popular, especially in the United States, but is painful to apply. It is usually used as a 5 per cent topical solution, but has been associated with metabolic acidosis.
- **Silver sulphadiazine and cerium nitrate**. This is also a very useful burn dressing, especially for full-thickness burns. It induces a hard effect on the burned skin and has been shown in certain instances, especially in elderly patients, to reduce some of the cell-mediated immunosuppression that occurs in burns. Cerium nitrate forms a sterile eschar and is specially useful in treating burns when a conservative treatment option has been chosen. Cerium nitrate has also been shown to boost cell-mediated immunity in these patients.

Superficial partial-thickness wounds and mixed-depth wounds

Around the world, a wide variety of substances are used to treat these wounds, from honey or boiled potato peel to synthetic biological dressings with live cultured fibroblasts within the matrix. This is testament to the fact that superficial partial-thickness burns will heal almost irrespective of the dressing. Thus, the key lies with dressings that are easy to apply, non-painful, reduce pain, simple to manage and locally available. The choice of dressings does, however, become crucial in the case of burns that border on being deep dermal (Figure 30.9). Here, the choice of dressing can make the difference between scar and no scar and/or operation and no operation. Some of the options for dressing choice are described below.

If the wound is heavily contaminated as a result of the accident, then it is prudent to clean the wound formally under a general anaesthetic. With more chronic contamination, silver sulphadiazine cream dressing for 2 or 3 days is very effective and can be changed to a dressing that is more efficient at promoting healing after this period.

The simplest method of treating a superficial wound is by exposure. The initial exudate needs to be managed by frequent changes of clean linen around the patient but, after a few days, a dry eschar forms, which then separates as the wound epithelialises. This is often used in hot climates and for small burns on the face. However, this method is painful and requires an intensive amount of nursing support. A variation on this theme is to cover

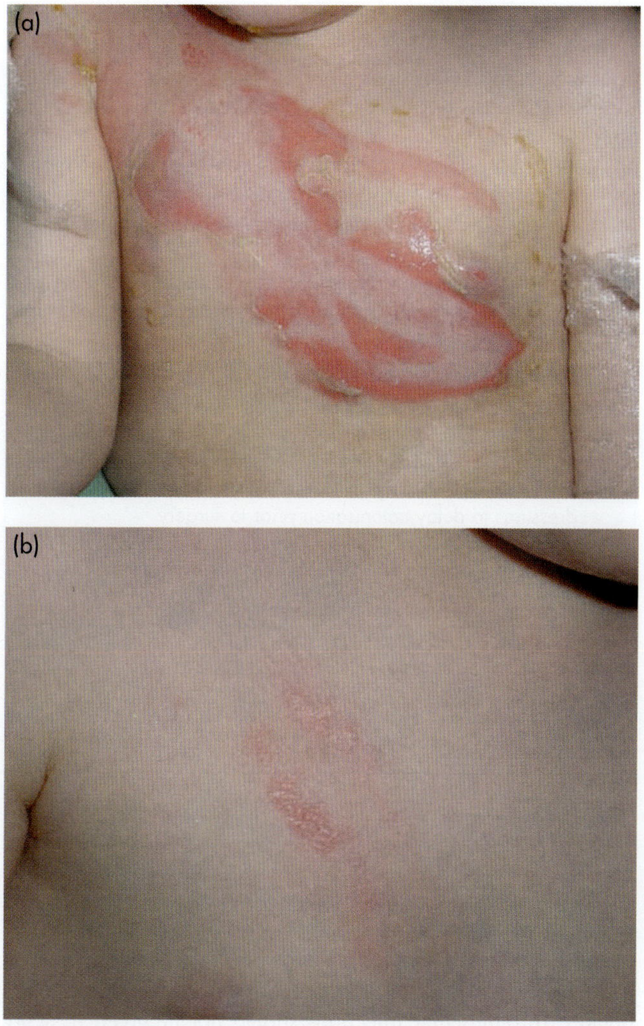

Figure 30.9 (a) A scald to the chest from boiling water, mainly superficial but in some areas close to being deep dermal. This was treated with a hydrocolloid dressing. (b) There are two tiny areas of hypertrophy indicating how close the burn was to being deep dermal. The good first aid this patient received probably made a difference to the outcome.

the wound with a permeable wound dressing, such as Mefix® or Fixamol®. This allows the wounds to dry but, because it is a covering, it avoids the problems of the wound adhering to the sheets and clothes. A similar method of managing these types of burn is to place a Vaseline-impregnated gauze (with or without an antiseptic, such as chlorhexidine) over the wound. An alternative is a fenestrated silicone sheet (e.g. Mepitel®). These can then be backed with swabs to absorb the exudate. The Vaseline gauze or silicone layer is used to prevent the swabs adhering to the wound and reduces the stiffness of the dry eschar, preventing it from cracking so easily. The swabs need to be changed after the first 48 hours as they are often soaked. After that, they can be left for longer.

More interactive dressings include hydrocolloids and biological dressings. Hydrocolloid dressings need to be changed every 3–5 days. They are particularly useful in mixed-depth burns as the high protease levels under the occlusive dressings aid with the debridement of the deeper areas of burn. They also provide a moist environment, which is good for epithelialisation. Duoderm® is a hydrocolloid dressing. There is good evidence for its value in burns.

Biological, synthetic (e.g. Biobrane®) and natural (e.g. amniotic membranes) dressings also provide good healing environments and do not need to be changed. They are ideal for one-stop management of superficial burns, being easy to apply and comfortable. However, they will become detached if applied to deep dermal wounds as the eschar needs to separate. They are therefore not as useful in mixed-depth wounds (Summary box 30.12).

Early debridement and grafting is the key to effectively treating deep partial- and full-thickness burns in a majority of cases.

Summary box 30.12

Principles of dressings for burns

- Full-thickness and deep dermal burns need antibacterial dressings to delay colonisation prior to surgery
- Superficial burns will heal and need simple dressings
- An optimal healing environment can make a difference to outcome in borderline depth burns

ADDITIONAL ASPECTS OF TREATING THE BURNED PATIENT

Analgesia

Acute

Analgesia is a vital part of burns management. Small burns, especially superficial burns, respond well to simple oral analgesia, paracetamol and non-steroidal anti-inflammatory drugs. Topical cooling is especially soothing. Large burns require intravenous opiates. Intramuscular injections should not be given in acute burns over 10 per cent of TBSA, as absorption is unpredictable and dangerous.

Subacute

In patients with large burns, continuous analgesia is required, beginning with infusions and continuing with oral tablets, such as slow-release morphine. Powerful, short-acting analgesia should be administered before dressing changes. Administration may require an anaesthetist, as in the case of general anaesthesia or midazolam and ketamine, or less intensive supervision, as in the case of morphine and nitrous oxide.

Energy balance and nutrition

One of the most important aspects in treating burns patients is nutrition. Any adult with a burn greater than 15 per cent (10 per cent in children) of TBSA has an increased nutritional requirement. All patients with burns of 20 per cent of TBSA or greater should receive a nasogastric tube. (Feeding should start within 6 hours of the injury to reduce gut mucosal damage.) A number of different formulae are available to calculate the energy requirements of patients (Summary box 30.13).

Summary box 30.13

Nutrition in burns patients

- Burns patients need extra feeding
- A nasogastric tube should be used in all patients with burns over 15 per cent of TBSA
- Removing the burn and achieving healing stops the catabolic drive

Burn injuries are catabolic in the acute episode. Successful management of the patient's energy balance involves a number of strategies. The catabolic drive continues while the wound remains unhealed and, therefore, rapid excision of the burn and stable coverage of the wound are the most significant factors in reversing this. Obligatory energy utilisation must be reduced to a minimum by keeping the patient warm with good environmental control. The excess energy requirements must be provided for and the nutritional balance monitored by measuring weight and nitrogen balance (see Table 30.5).

Monitoring and control of infection

Patients with major burns are immunocompromised, having large portals of entry to pathogenic and opportunistic bacteria and fungi via the burn wound (Summary box 30.14). They have compromised local defences in the lungs and gut due to oedema, and usually have monitoring lines and catheters, which themselves represent portals for infection.

Table 30.5 Commonly used feeding formulae.

Curreri formula	Age 16–59 years: (25)W + (40)TBSA
	Age 60+ years: (20)W + (65)TBSA
Sutherland formula	Children: 60 kcal/kg + 35 kcal%TBSA
	Adults: 20 kcal/kg + 70 kcal%TBSA
Protein needs	Greatest nitrogen losses between days 5 and 10
	20% of kilocalories should be provided by proteins
Davies formula	Children: 3 g/kg + 1 g%TBSA
	Adults: 1 g/kg + 3 g%TBSA

TBSA, total body surface area.

Summary box 30.14

Infection control in burns patients

- Burns patients are immunocompromised
- They are susceptible to infection from many routes
- Sterile precautions must be rigorous
- Swabs should be taken regularly
- A rise in white blood cell count, thrombocytosis and increased catabolism are warnings of infection

Control of infection begins with policies on hand-washing and other cross-contamination prevention measures. Bacteriological surveillance of the wound, catheter tips and sputum helps to build a picture of the patient's flora. If there are signs of infection, then further cultures need to be taken and antibiotics started. This is often initially on a best guess basis, hence the usefulness of prior surveillance; close liaison with a bacteriologist is essential. In patients with large burns that remain catabolic, the core temperature is usually reset by the hypothalamus above 37°C. Significant temperatures are those above 38.5°C, but often other signs of infection are more useful to the clinician. These include significant rise or fall in the white cell count, thrombocytosis, increasing signs of catabolism and decreasing clinical status of the patient.

Nursing care

Burns patients require particularly intensive nursing care. Nurses are the primary effectors of many decisions that directly affect healing. Bandaged hands and joints which are stiff and painful need careful coaxing. Personal hygiene, baths and showers all become time-consuming and painful, but are vital parts of the patient's physiotherapy. Their success or failure has a powerful psychological impact on the patient and his or her family.

Physiotherapy

All burns cause swelling, especially burns to the hands. Elevation, splintage and exercise reduce swelling and improve the final outcome. The physiotherapy needs to be started on day 1, so that the message can be reinforced on a daily basis.

Psychological

A major burn is an overwhelming event, outside the normal experience, which overwhelms the patient's coping ability, suspends the patient's sense of safety and causes post-traumatic reactions. These are normal and usually self-limiting, receding as the patient heals. The features of this intensity of experience are of intrusive reactions, arousal reactions and avoidance reactions.

SURGERY FOR THE ACUTE BURN WOUND

Any deep partial-thickness and full-thickness burns, except those that are less than about 4 cm^2, need surgery. Any burn of indeterminate depth should be reassessed after 48 hours. This is because burns that initially appear superficial may well deepen over that time. Delayed microvascular injury is especially common in scalds (Summary box 30.15).

Summary box 30.15

Surgical treatment of deep burns

- Deep dermal burns need tangential shaving and split-skin grafting
- All but the smallest full-thickness burns need surgery
- The anaesthetist needs to be ready for significant blood loss
- Topical adrenaline reduces bleeding
- All burnt tissue needs to be excised
- Stable cover, permanent or temporary, should be applied at once to reduce burn load

The essence of burns surgery is control. First and foremost, the anaesthetist needs good control of the patient. A wide-bore cannula should be used and the patient's blood pressure must be monitored adequately. If a large excision is considered, then an arterial line (to monitor blood pressure) and a central venous pressure monitor are needed. The anaesthetist also needs measurements and control of the acid–base balance, clotting time and haemoglobin levels. The core temperature of the patient must not drop below 36°C, otherwise clotting irregularities will be compounded.

For most burn excisions, subcutaneous injection of a dilute solution of adrenaline 1:1 000 000 or 1:500 000 and tourniquet control are important for controlling blood loss.

In deep dermal burns, the top layer of dead dermis is shaved off until punctate bleeding is observed and the dermis can be seen to be free of any small thrombosed vessels (Figure 30.5a). A topical solution of 1:500 000 adrenaline also helps to reduce bleeding, as does the application of the skin graft. The use of a tourniquet during burn excisions in the limbs helps to decrease blood loss and maintain control.

Full-thickness burns require full-thickness excision of the skin (Figure 30.5b). In certain circumstances, it is appropriate to go down to the fascia but, in most cases, the burn excision is down to viable fat. Wherever possible, a skin graft should be applied immediately. With very large burns, the use of synthetic dermis or homografts provides temporary stable coverage and will allow complete excision of the wound and thus reduce the burn load on the patient.

Postoperative management of these patients obviously requires careful evaluation of fluid balance and levels of haemoglobin. The outer dressings will quickly be soaked through with serum and will need to be changed on a regular basis to reduce the bacterial load within the dressing.

Physiotherapy and splints are important in maintaining range of movement and reducing joint contracture. Elevation of the appropriate limbs is important. The hand must be splinted in a position of function after grafting, although the graft needs to

The Guinea Pig Club. Sir Archibald McIndoe (1900–1960), born in New Zealand, was appointed in 1938 as consultant plastic surgeon to the Royal Air Force. He trained with his cousin, Sir Harold Gillies, another internationally reputed plastic surgeon. McIndoe became world famous for his pioneering work on Battle of Britain pilots who were badly burnt. His work on these airmen, who needed several operations, and using his innovative technical and psychological methods, was the start of a life-long service. The young fighter pilots were therefore referred to as 'guinea pigs' – thus was formed The Guinea Pig Club. McIndoe referred to his patients as 'the boys' who in turn called him 'the boss' or 'the maestro'. To this day, some of the members of the Guinea Pig Club from all over the world still meet on an annual basis in Sussex. McIndoe founded the British Association of Plastic Surgeons (BAPS).

be applied in the position of maximal stretch. Knees are best splinted in extension, axillae in abduction. Supervised movement by the physiotherapists, usually under direct vision of any affected joints, should begin after about 5 days.

Delayed reconstruction and scar management

Delayed reconstruction of burn injuries is common for large full-thickness burns. In the early healing period, acute contractures around the eye need particular attention. Eyelids must be grafted at the first sign of difficulty in closing the eyelids, and this must be done before the patient has any symptoms of exposure keratitis (Figure 30.10). Other areas that require early intervention are any contracture causing significant loss of range of movement of a joint. This is particularly important in the hand and axilla (Summary box 30.16).

Summary box 30.16

Delayed reconstruction of burns

- Eyelids must be treated before exposure keratitis arises
- Transposition flaps and Z-plasties with or without tissue expansion are useful
- Full-thickness grafts and free flaps may be needed for large or difficult areas
- Hypertrophy is treated with pressure garments
- Pharmacological treatment of itch is important

An established contracture can be treated in a number of ways. Burn alopecia is best treated with tissue expansion of the unburned hair-bearing skin. Tissue expansion is also a useful technique for isolated burns and other areas with adjacent normal skin. Z-plasty is useful in the situation in which there is a single band and a transposition flap is useful in wider bands of scarring (Figure 30.11). In areas of circumferential or very broad areas of scarring, the only real treatment is incision and replacement with tissue. By far the best tissue for replacement is from either a full-thickness graft or vascularised tissue as in a free flap. Occasionally, the situation requires the less ideal covering of split skin, possibly with an artificial dermis, such as Integra® (Figure 30.12). These last two options require prolonged scar management after their use.

Hypertrophy of many scars will respond to pressure garments. These need to be worn for a period of 6–18 months. Where it is difficult to apply pressure with pressure garments, or with smaller areas of hypertrophy, silicone patches will speed scar maturation, as will intralesional injection of steroid. Itching and dermatitis in burn scar areas are common. Pharmacological treatment of itch is an essential adjunct to therapy.

MINOR BURNS/OUTPATIENT BURNS

Local burn wound care

Blisters

Whether to remove blisters or leave them intact has been the subject of much debate. Proponents of blister removal quote laboratory studies which show that blister fluid depresses immune function, slowing down chemotaxis and intracellular killing and also acting as a medium for bacterial growth.

Conversely, other authors advocate leaving blisters intact as they form a sterile stratum spongiosum. Leaving a ruptured blister is not advised.

Initial cleaning of the burn wound

Washing the burn wound with chlorhexidine solution is ideal for this purpose.

Topical agents

For initial management of minor burns that are superficial or partial thickness, dressings with a non-adherent material, such as Vaseline-impregnated gauze or Mepitel are often sufficient. These dressings are left in place for 5 days. These burns, by definition, should be healed after 7–10 days. Various topical creams and ointments have been used for the treatment of minor burns. All published comparative data show no advantage of these agents over petroleum gauze.

Silver sulphadiazine (1 per cent) or Flamazine® is the most commonly used topical agent. However, it should be avoided in pregnant women, nursing mothers and infants less than two months of age because of the increased possibility of kernicterus in these patients.

Dressing the minor burn wound

The aims of dressing are to decrease wound pain and to protect and isolate the burn wound. The small superficial burn requires Vaseline gauze or another non-adherent dressing, such as Mepitel, as the first layer. Following this, gauze or Kerlix® is wrapped around with sufficient tightness to keep the dressing intact, but not to impede the circulation. This is further wrapped with bandage. It is important to realise that bulkiness of dressings in the minor burn wound depends upon the amount of wound discharge. A special case is burns of the hands where dressings should be minimised so as not to impede mobilisation and physiotherapy.

Synthetic burn wound dressings are popular as they:

- decrease pain associated with dressings;
- improve healing times;
- decrease outpatient appointments;
- lower overall costs.

Biobrane is a bilaminar dressing made up of an inner layer of knitted nylon threads coated with porcine collagen and an outer layer of rubberised silicone impervious to gases, but not to fluids and bacteria. Wounds to be dressed with Biobrane should be carefully selected. Burn wounds should be fresh (less than 24 hours), sensate, show capillary blanching and refill. Biobrane® should be applied to the wound after removal of all blisters. It should be checked at 48 hours for adherence and any signs of infection. It should be removed if any sign of infection is found.

Duoderm or hydrocolloid dressings are not bulky, help in healing and can be kept in place for 48–72 hours. They provide a moist environment, which helps in re-epithelialisation of the burn wound.

Healing of burn wounds

Burns that are being managed conservatively should be healed within 3 weeks. If there are no signs of re-epithelialisation in this time, the wound requires debridement and grafting.

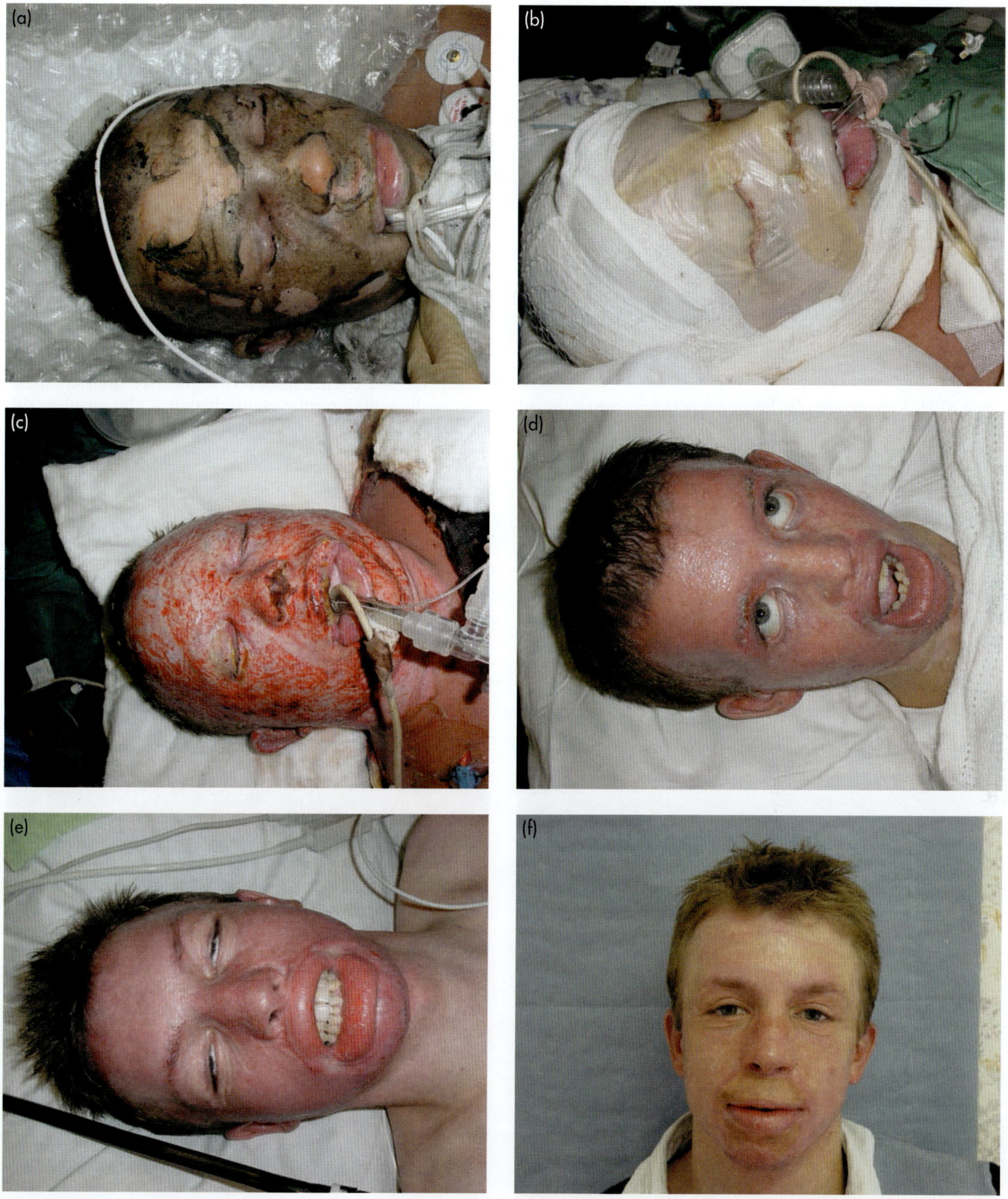

Figure 30.10 (a) A mixed superficial and deep burn to the face after a petrol explosion. The patient's airway was protected prior to transfer. He has an orogastric tube and feeding has commenced. (b) The face dressed with a hydrocolloid dressing. The endotracheal tube is wired to the teeth. (c) Day 6, the swelling is still present. (d) Six weeks after injury. With the mouth wide open, the lower eyelids are pulled down, demonstrating the intrinsic and extrinsic shortening of the eyelids. (e) Three months after injury. The eyelids have been grafted but note the contracture of the lips. (f) Six months after injury. The patient has had grafts to the upper and lower lips.

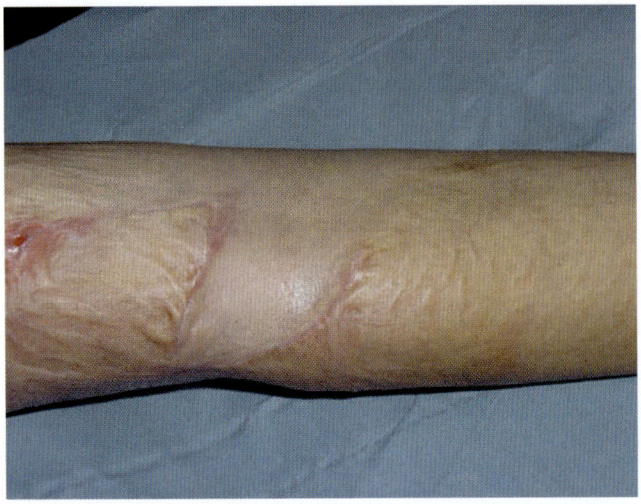

Figure 30.11 A transposition flap bringing normal skin across a scarred elbow.

Infection

Infection in the minor burn should be tackled very aggressively as it is known to convert a superficial burn to a partial-thickness burn and a partial- to a deep partial-thickness burn, respectively. It should be managed using a combination of topical and systemic agents. Debridement and skin grafting should also be considered.

Itching

Most burn patients have itchy wounds. Histamine and various endopeptides are said to be the causative factors of itching. Antihistamines, analgesics, moisturising creams, aloe vera and antibiotics have all been tried with varying degrees of success.

Traumatic blisters

The healed burn wound is prone to getting traumatic blisters because the new epithelium is very fragile. Non-adherent dressings usually suffice; regular moisturisation is also useful in this condition.

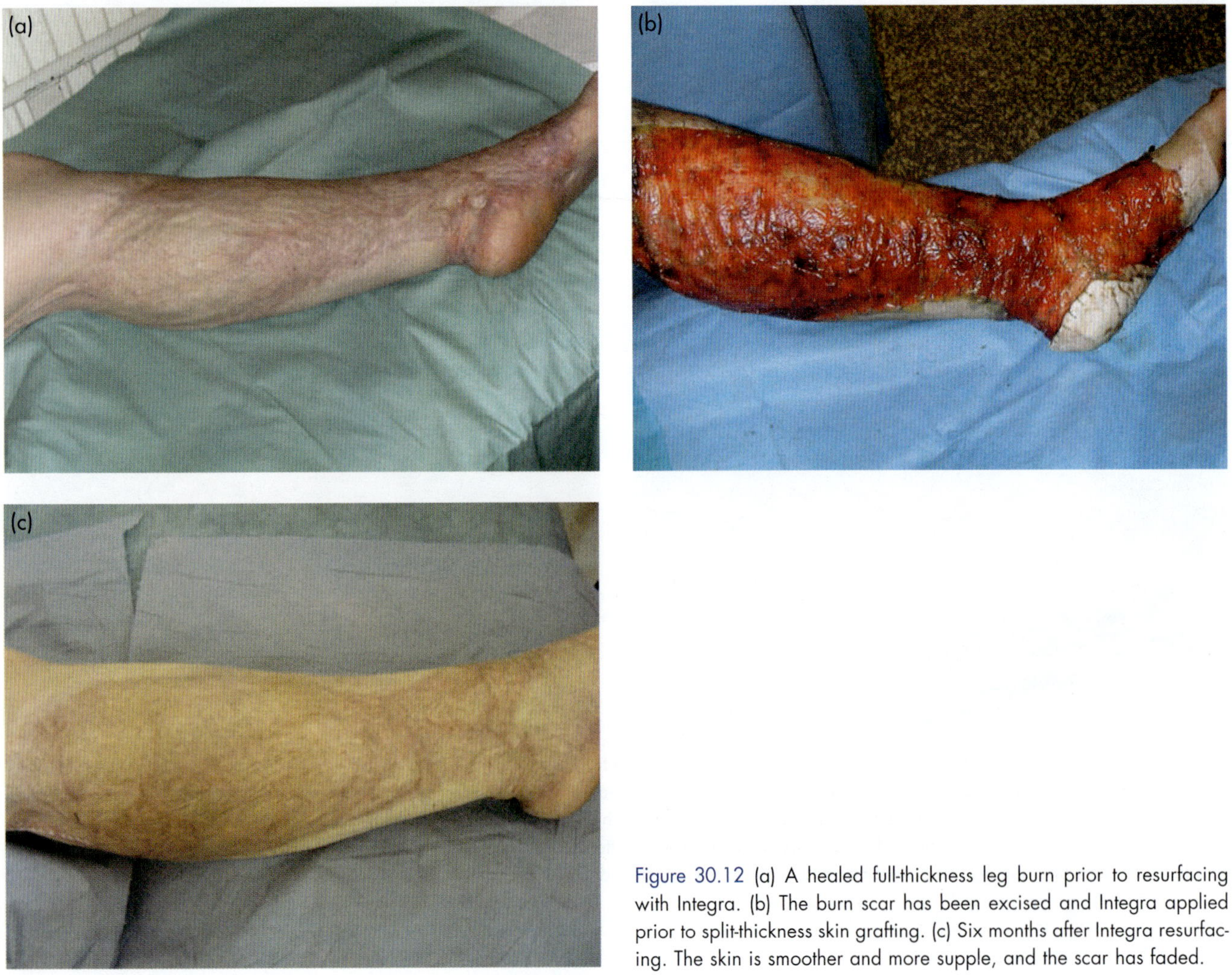

Figure 30.12 (a) A healed full-thickness leg burn prior to resurfacing with Integra. (b) The burn scar has been excised and Integra applied prior to split-thickness skin grafting. (c) Six months after Integra resurfacing. The skin is smoother and more supple, and the scar has faded.

NON-THERMAL BURN INJURY

Electrical injuries

Electrical injuries are usually divided into low- and high-voltage injuries, the threshold being 1000 V (Summary box 30.17).

> **Summary box 30.17**
>
> **Electrical burns**
>
> - Low-voltage injuries cause small, localised, deep burns
> - They can cause cardiac arrest through pacing interruption without significant direct myocardial damage
> - High-voltage injuries damage by flash (external burn) and conduction (internal burn)
> - Myocardium may be directly damaged without pacing interruption
> - Limbs may need fasciotomies or amputation
> - Look for and treat acidosis and myoglobinuria

Low-tension injuries

Low-tension or domestic appliance injuries do not have enough energy to cause destruction to significant amounts of subcutaneous tissues when the current passes through the body. The resistance is too great. The entry and exit points, normally in the fingers, suffer small deep burns; these may cause underlying tendon and nerve damage, but there will be little damage between. The alternating current creates a tetany within the muscles, and thus patients often describe how they were unable to release the device until the power was turned off. The main danger with these injuries is from the alternating current interfering with normal cardiac pacing. This can cause cardiac arrest. The electricity itself does not usually cause significant underlying myocardial damage, so resuscitation, if successful, should be lasting.

High-tension injuries

High-tension electrical injuries can be caused by one of three sources of damage: the flash, the flame and the current itself.

When a high-tension line is earthed, enormous energy is released as the current travels from the line to the earth. It can arc over the patient, causing a flash burn. The extremely rapid heating of the air causes an explosion that often propels the victim backwards. The key here is that the current travelled from the line to the earth directly and not through the patient. The flash, however, can go on to ignite the patient's clothes and so cause a normal flame burn.

In accidents with overhead lines, the patient often acts as the conduction rod to earth. In these injuries, there is enough current to cause damage to the subcutaneous tissues and muscles. The entry and exit points are damaged but, importantly, the current can cause huge amounts of subcutaneous damage between these two points. These can be extremely serious injuries.

The damage to the underlying muscles in the affected limb can cause the rapid onset of compartment syndrome. The release of the myoglobins will cause myoglobinuria and subsequent renal dysfunction. Therefore, during the resuscitation of these patients, efforts must be made to maintain a high urine output of up to 2 mL/kg body weight per hour. Severe acidosis is common in large electrical burns and may require boluses of bicarbonate. These patients are also at risk of myocardial damage as a result of direct muscle damage rather than by interference with cardiac pacing. This gives rise to significant electrocardiogram changes, with raised cardiac enzymes. If there is significant damage, there is rapid onset of heart failure. In the case of a severe injury through a limb, primary amputation is sometimes the most effective management (Figure 30.13).

Chemical injuries

There are over 70 000 different chemicals in regular use within industry. Occasionally, these cause burns. Ultimately, there are two aspects to a chemical injury. The first is the physical destruction of the skin and the second is any poisoning caused by systemic absorption (Summary box 30.18).

> **Summary box 30.18**
>
> **Chemical burns**
>
> - Damage is from corrosion and poisoning
> - Copious lavage with water helps in most cases
> - Then identify the chemical and assess the risks of absorption

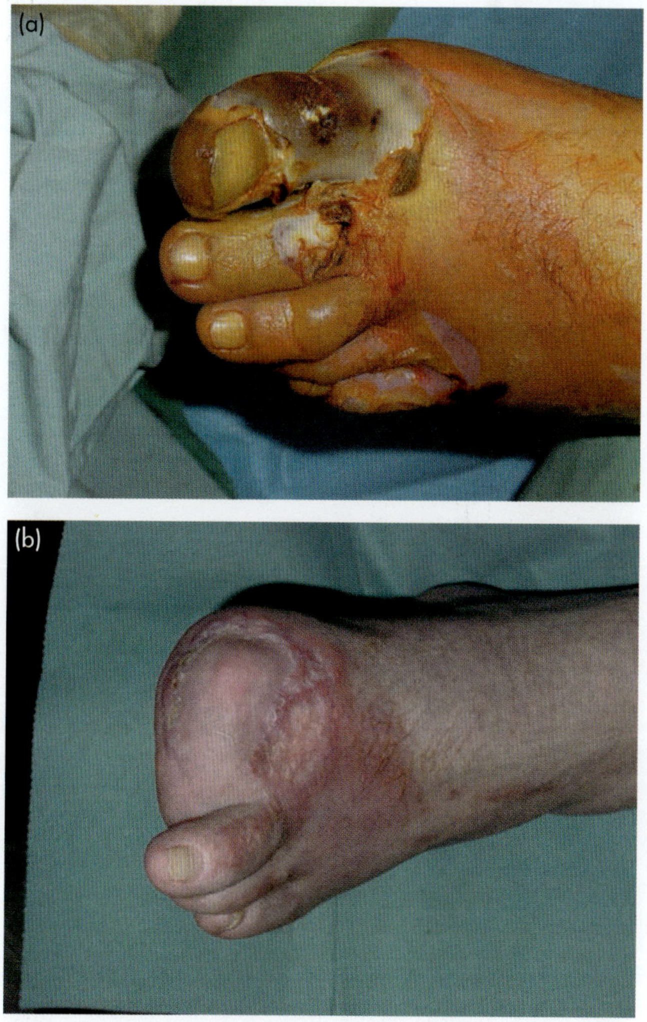

Figure 30.13 (a) An exit wound of a high-tension injury, with a dead big toe and significant damage to the medial portion of the second toe. (b) Amputation and cover with the lateral portion of the second toe.

The initial management of any chemical injury is copious lavage with water. There are only a handful of chemicals for which water is not helpful, for example phosphorus, which is a component of some military devices, and elemental sodium, which is occasionally present in laboratory explosions. These substances need to be physically removed with forceps; however, it is extremely rare that any medical practitioner will encounter these in his or her lifetime. The more common injuries are caused by either acids or alkalis. Alkalis are usually the more destructive and are especially dangerous if they have come into contact with the eyes. After copious lavage, the next step in the management of any chemical injury is to identify the chemical and its concentration and to elucidate whether there is any underlying threat to the patient's life if absorbed systemically.

One acid that is a common cause of acid burns is hydrofluoric acid. Burns affecting the fingers and caused by dilute acid are relatively common. The initial management is with calcium gluconate gel topically; however, severe burns or burns to large areas of the hand can be subsequently treated with Bier's blocks containing calcium gluconate 10 per cent gel. If the patient has been burnt with a concentration greater than 50 per cent, the threat of hypocalcaemia and subsequent arrhythmias then becomes high, and this is an indication for acute early excision. It is best not to split-skin graft these hydrofluoric acid wounds initially, but to do this at a delayed stage.

Ionising radiation injury

These injuries can be divided into groups depending on whether radiation exposure was to the whole body or localised. The management of localised radiation damage is usually conservative until the true extent of the tissue injury is apparent. Should this damage have caused an ulcer, then excision and coverage with vascularised tissue is required.

Whole-body radiation causes a large number of symptoms. The dose of radiation either is or is not lethal. A patient who has suffered whole-body irradiation and is suffering from acute desquamation of the skin has received a lethal dose of radiation, which can cause a particularly slow and unpleasant death. Non-lethal radiation has a number of systemic effects related to the gut mucosa and immune system dysfunction. Other than giving iodine tablets, the management of these injuries is supportive (Summary box 30.19).

Summary box 30.19

Radiation burns

- Local burns causing ulceration need excision and vascularised flap cover, usually with free flaps
- Systemic overdose needs supportive treatment

Cold injuries

Cold injuries are principally divided into two types: acute cold injuries from industrial accidents and frostbite.

Exposure to liquid nitrogen and other such liquids will cause epidermal and dermal destruction. The tissue is more resistant to cold injury than to heat injury, and the inflammatory reaction is not as marked. The assessment of depth of injury is more difficult, so it is rare to make the decision for surgery early.

Frostbite injuries affect the peripheries in cold climates. The initial treatment is with rapid rewarming in a bath at 42°C. The cold injury produces delayed microvascular damage similar to that of cardiac reperfusion injury. The level of damage is difficult to assess, and surgery usually does not play a role in its management, which is conservative, until there is absolute demarcation of the level of injury.

FURTHER READING

British Burns Association. *Emergency management of burns*, 8th edn. UK Course Pre-reading. British Burns Association, 2004.

Herndon D (ed.). *Total burn care*, 3rd edn. Philadelphia, PA: Saunders and Elsevier, 2007.

Pape S, Judkins K, Settle J. *Burns: the first five days*, 2nd edn. Romford: Smith and Nephew, 2000.

August Karl Gustav Bier, 1861–1949, Professor of Surgery, Berlin, Germany.

CHAPTER 31

Plastic and reconstructive surgery

LEARNING OBJECTIVES

To understand:
- The spectrum of plastic surgical techniques used to restore bodily form and function
- The relevant anatomy and physiology of tissues used in reconstruction
- The various skin grafts and how to use them appropriately
- The principles and use of flaps
- How to use plastic surgery to manage difficult and complex tissue loss

HISTORICAL CONTEXT

Reconstructive plastic (from the ancient Greek *plassein*, to mould or shape – also the stem for our modern use of the materials termed 'plastics') surgery involves using various techniques to restore form and function to the body when tissues have been damaged by injury, cancer or congenital loss. Its origins can be traced back to ancient Egypt, with wound care depicted in hieroglyphs on papyrus, to India in the sixth century BC, where Sushruta described using the forehead flap to reconstruct a nose, and to Al-Zahrawi, the tenth-century Islamic surgical scholar from Cordoba. Modern techniques were developed after the First World War, especially with Sir Harold Gillies' work on reconstructing facial injuries (Figure 31.1), which was enabled by new safe anaesthetic intubation (Sir Ivan Magill). Later in the twentieth century, renewed understanding of detailed soft tissue anatomy led to an explosion in the use of new flaps, which with microsurgical methods, craniofacial surgery and tissue expansion resulted in an entirely new set of techniques becoming available to surgeons for reconstructing parts.

Today, the need for reconstructive plastic surgery, especially in developing nations, has never been greater. Road, war and domestic injury inflict life-diminishing effects, which plastic surgery can reduce. The reconstructive surgeon's 'toolbox' is now very diverse and will continue to grow in order to address problem wounds and tissue defects, which arise as modern medical care is more successful in treating cancer, preserving life into old age and salvaging victims of trauma.

Sushruta, regarded as the father of modern surgery, lived in the Indian city of Kashi (now called Banaras) in 600BC (while the exact period is unclear, most scholars maintain that he practised between 600 and 1000BC). A large part of his practice was plastic surgery in the form of rhinoplasty carried out on criminals who had their noses amputated as a punishment for their crimes. His medical pursuits were recorde d in '*Sushsruta Samhita* (compendum)'.

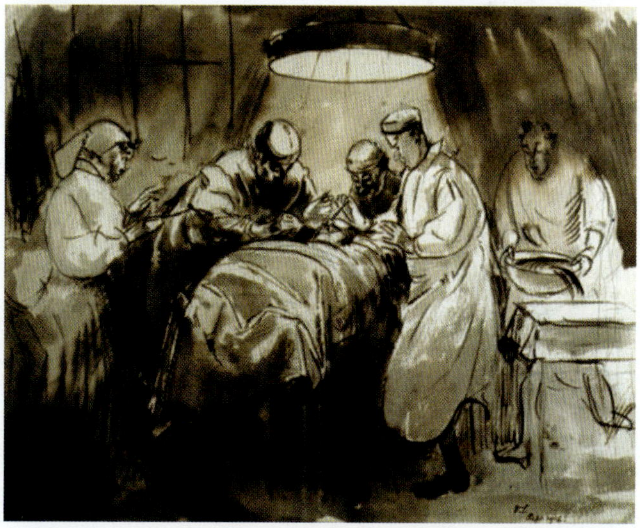

Figure 31.1 Sir Harold Gillies operating during the First World War – 'the birth of plastic surgery'. Picture by Henry Tonks (by kind permission of the Royal College of Surgeons of England).

ANATOMY RELATED TO RECONSTRUCTIVE SURGERY

Skin

The surface of the skin is important as a biological layer for homeostasis. Restoring the skin surface is therefore critical even if the underlying structures can await later reconstruction. Epidermis regenerates from deeper follicular elements, with the most superficial layer losing vascularity and acting as a barrier to fluid loss and providing important protection against invasion by microorganisms. (Epidermal keratinocytes can be artificially cultured *in vitro* and are used in some wound management systems.)

The depth of the dermis and the amounts of elastin and skin

Sir Ivan Whiteside Magill, 1888–1986, anaesthetist, Westminister Hospital, London, UK.
Henry Tonks, 1862–1937, commenced a career in surgery, but abandoned it for art and became, from 1917 to 1930, Slade Professor at the Westminster School of Art, London, UK.

adnexal elements, such as sweat glands and hair follicles, vary depending on the functional requirements of the area concerned. This means that some areas are much more vulnerable to injury than others, e.g. the fine flexible elastic skin of the eyelid rapidly suffers a full-thickness burn after a flash burn, whereas thick back skin suffers only a partial loss after the same flash burn.

Skin vascularity is derived from fine perforating vessels that run through underlying muscles or through fascial septal layers, and then horizontally in a subcutaneous plane from which capillaries branch (Figure 31.2). Nerves run axially out from major trunks and are less well defined than most perforating blood vessels.

When local, random-pattern skin flaps are raised, they are lifted at the subcutaneous level and are nourished by the subdermal plexus of blood vessels. However, this plexus can only survive a limited distance from the more substantial arterial branches running in the fascial, septal or muscle-perforating planes. Understanding the anatomy of different parts of the skin and tissues to be moved is a key element of successful plastic surgery.

Without skin, wounds heal by **secondary intention** with fibrosis and contracture (Figure 31.3), and underlying structures are vulnerable to necrosis, chronic infection and dysfunction.

Graft anatomy

Split-thickness skin grafts

Split-thickness skin grafts are harvested by taking all of the epidermis together with some dermis, leaving the remaining dermis behind to heal the donor site. The thicker the dermis that is taken (seen by more brisk punctate bleeding at the donor site; Figure 31.4), the more durable will be the graft once healed (although it might take longer and require more care), but also the more difficult will be donor site healing (Summary box 31.1).

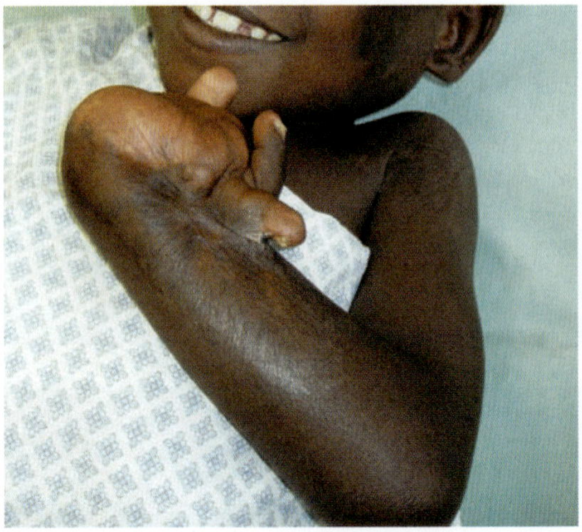

Figure 31.3 A severely contracted hand following burn to the dorsal aspect.

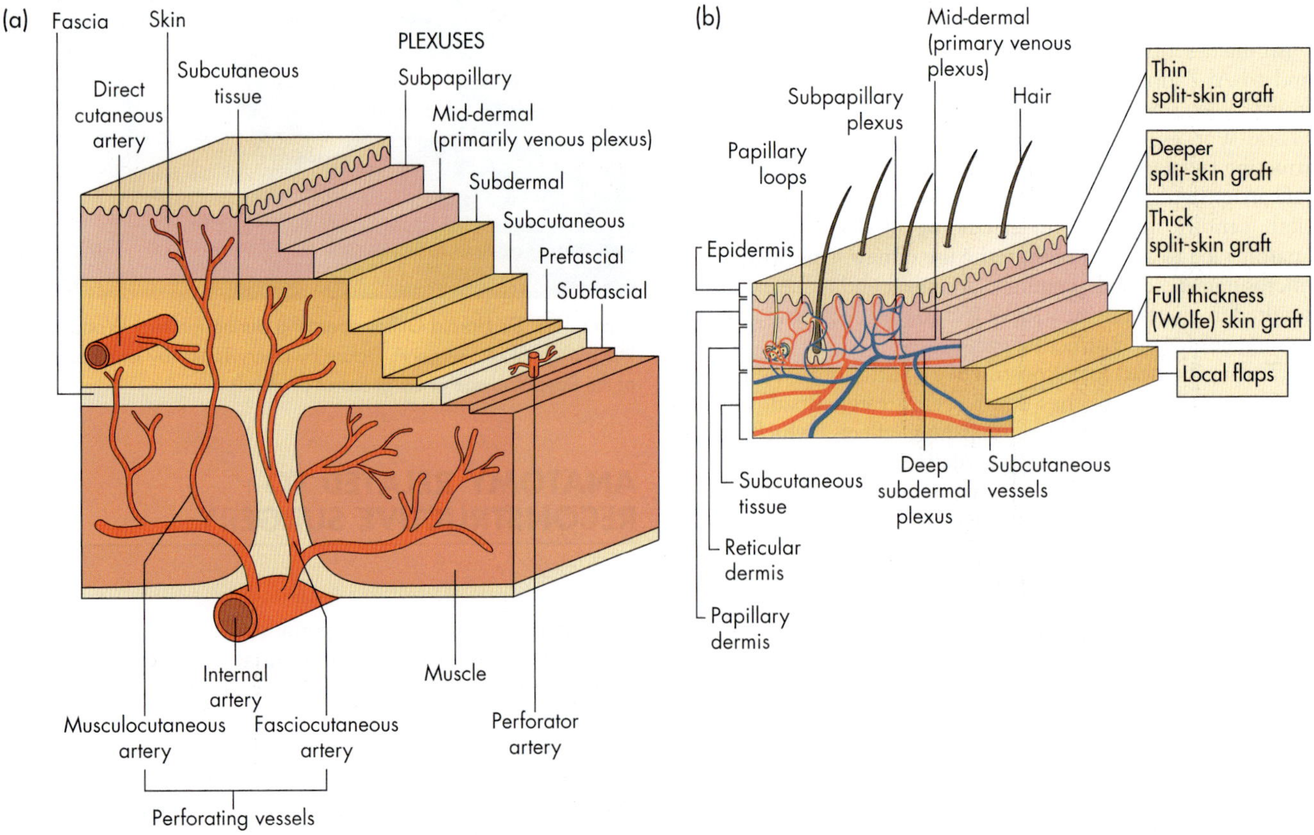

Figure 31.2 Diagram of skin anatomy with vascular plexus.

in vitro is Latin for 'in the glass'.

Summary box 31.1

Split-thickness skin grafts

- Thicker knife-gap settings give rise to fewer but brisker bleeding points on the donor site.
- Thicker grafts heal with less contracture and are more durable.
- Thinner donor sites heal better.
- Grafts are hairless and do not sweat (these structures are not transferred).

Full-thickness skin grafts

Full-thickness grafts are harvested to incorporate the whole dermis, with the underlying fat trimmed away – unless elements of fat (or even cartilage as well) are deliberately left attached to form a **composite graft**. Full-thickness and composite grafts require the most careful handling and postoperative nursing to help ensure that they 'take' in their transplanted site.

How does a skin graft survive?

Split-thickness skin grafts survive initially by **imbibition** of plasma from the wound bed; after 48 hours, fine anastomotic connections are made, which lead to **inosculation** of blood. Capillary ingrowth then completes the healing process with fibroblast maturation. Because only tissues that produce granulation will support a graft, it is usually contraindicated to use grafts to cover exposed tendons, cartilage or cortical bone.

Skin grafts inevitably contract, with the extent of contracture determined by the amount of dermis taken with the graft and the level of postoperative splintage and physiotherapy applied to the grafted site.

CLASSIFICATION

The reconstructive toolbox

Plastic surgery offers a variety of techniques to address clinical problems. Sometimes, a problem is managed using a 'ladder' approach, with the simplest methods being used first and only moving to more complex methods when absolutely necessary. However, this is frequently not the ideal approach for best outcomes. If resources permit, it is often more cost-effective and better functionally for the patient to begin with a more complex treatment, with other easier managements held in reserve as 'lifeboats'. Plastic surgeons now prefer to think of the range of options available as a toolbox from which they can take the most appropriate method to solve a problem, taking into account available skill, resources and the consequences of failure.

The scope of plastic surgery

The tools of reconstruction are used for a wide range of conditions:

- trauma:
  - soft-tissue loss (skin, tendons, nerves, muscle);
  - hand and lower limb injury;
  - faciomaxillary;
  - burns;
- cancer:
  - skin, head and neck, breast, soft tissue sarcoma;
- congenital:
  - clefts and craniofacial malformations;
  - skin, giant naevi, vascular malformations;
  - urogenital;
  - hand and limb malformations;
- miscellaneous:
  - Bell's (facial) palsy;
  - pressure sores;
  - aesthetic surgery;
  - chest wall reconstruction.

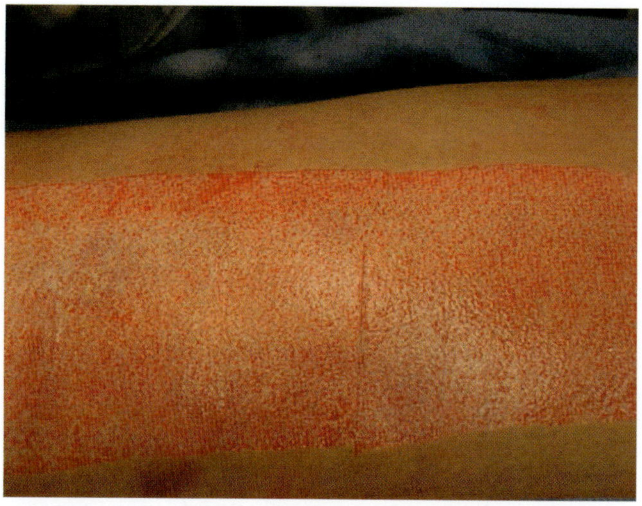

Figure 31.4 Fine punctate bleeding from a split-thickness skin graft donor site.

A few key principles that can also be applied to other surgical specialties should be observed. In many reconstructions, success depends upon good rapid wound healing, which itself depends upon attention to detail from the surgeon. Adequate debridement, careful technique, gentle handling of tissues and consideration of blood supply are all key factors that influence outcome (Table 31.1).

The placement of incisions can be critical, especially in reducing the appearance of scars on the face and in areas of tension. When possible, incisions should lie in the lines of minimal tension (described by Langer, but frequently different from those originally noted) (Figure 31.5).

Table 31.1 Plastic surgery principles.

Optimise wound by adequate debridement or resection
Wound or flap must have a good blood supply to heal
Place scars carefully – 'lines of election'[a]
Replace defect with similar tissue – 'like with like'[b]
Observe meticulous surgical technique
Remember donor site 'cost'

[a]Lines of election – analogous to Langer's lines of minimal skin tension.
[b]Millard DR. *Principalization of plastic surgery*. Boston: Little & Brown, 1986.

Grafts

Grafts are tissues that are transferred without their blood supply, which therefore have to revascularise once they are in a new site. They include the following:

Sir Charles Bell, 1774–1842, surgeon, Middlesex Hospital, London, UK and from 1835 until his death, Professor of Surgery, the University of Edinburgh, Edinburgh, UK.
Karl Ritter von Edenberg Langer, 1819–1887, Professor of Anatomy, Vienna, Austria described these lines in 1862.

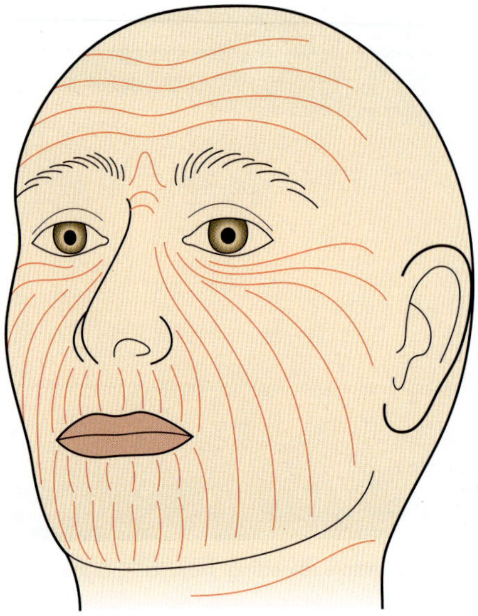

Figure 31.5 Lines of relaxed skin tension.

- **Split-thickness skin grafts (of varying thickness).** These are sometimes called Thiersch grafts. They are used to cover all sizes of wound, are of limited durability and will contract. They may be used to provide valuable temporary wound closure before better cosmetic secondary correction after rehabilitation.
- **Full-thickness skin grafts (Wolfe grafts).** Used for smaller areas of skin replacement where good elastic skin that will not contract is required (such as fingers, eyelids, facial parts).
- **Composite skin grafts (usually skin and fat, or skin and cartilage).** Often taken from the ear margin and useful for rebuilding missing elements of nose, eyelids and fingertips.
- **Nerve grafts.** Usually taken from the sural nerve, but smaller cutaneous nerves may be used.
- **Tendon grafts.** Usually taken from the palmaris longus or plantaris tendon (runs just anteromedial to the Achilles tendon) and used for injury loss or nerve damage correction.

Flaps

Flaps are tissues that are transferred with a blood supply. They therefore have the advantage of bringing vascularity to the new area. Flaps can be raised to consist of any specific tissue; for skin flaps the following will illustrate the types that exist (Figure 31.6):

- **Random flaps.** Three sides of a rectangle, bearing no specific relationship to where the blood supply enters; the length to breadth ratio is no more than 1.5:1. This pattern can be lengthened by 'delaying' the flap, a process in which the cuts are partially made and the flap is part lifted at a first operation; it is then replaced, thus 'training' the blood supply from a single border of the rectangle. At a second procedure, it is raised further and finally transferred.
- **Axial flaps.** Much longer flaps, based on known blood vessels supplying the skin. This technique was rediscovered in the 1960s and 1970s and enables many long thin flaps to be safely moved across large distances.
- **Pedicled/islanded flaps.** The axial blood supply of these flaps means that they can be swung round on a stalk or even fully 'islanded' so that the business end of the skin being transferred can have the pedicle buried (Figure 31.7).
- **Free flaps.** The blood supply has been isolated, disconnected and then reconnected using microsurgery at the new site (Figure 31.8).
- **Composite flaps.** Various tissues are transferred together, often skin with bone or muscle (osseocutaneous or myocutaneous flaps, respectively).

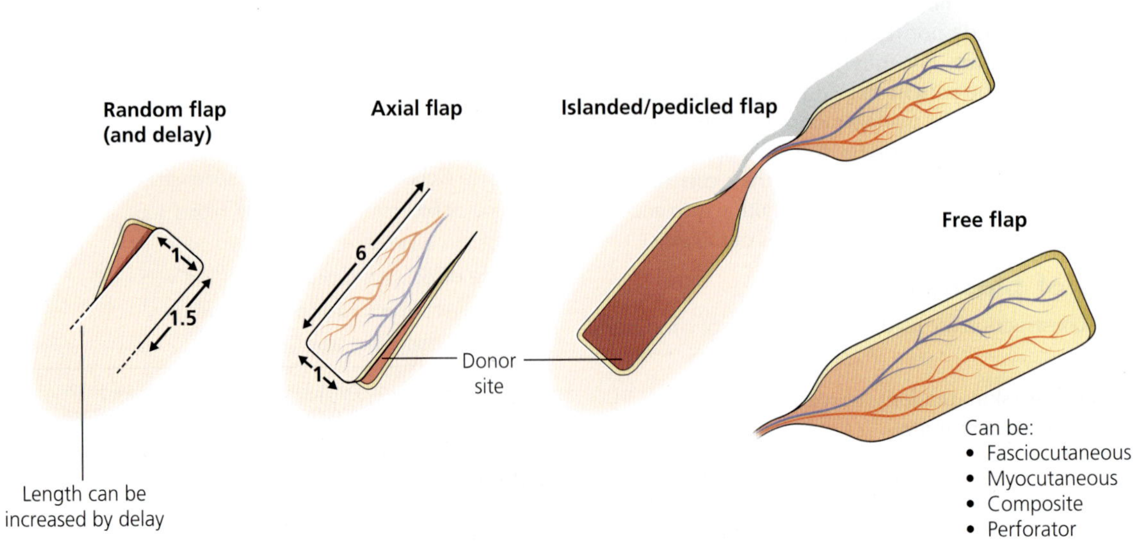

Figure 31.6 Skin flaps, from simple to complex.

Karl Thiersch, 1822–1895, Professor of Surgery, Leipzig, Germany. He was a pioneer of free skin grafts and described his method of skin grafting in 1874.
John Reissburg Wolfe, 1824–1904, ophthalmic surgeon, Glasgow, UK, described full thickness skin grafts in 1875 and in the same year used forearm skin to construct an eyelid.

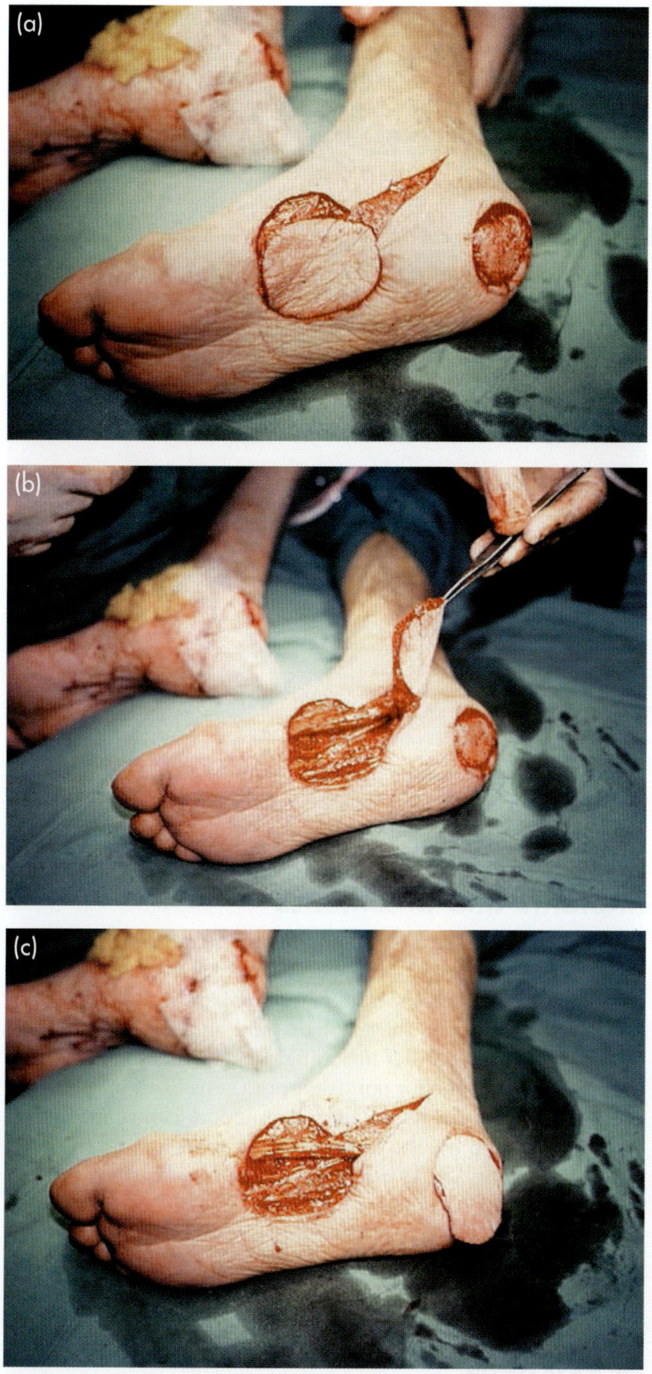

Figure 31.7 (a–c) Islanded pedicled flap used from instep to resurface heel defect.

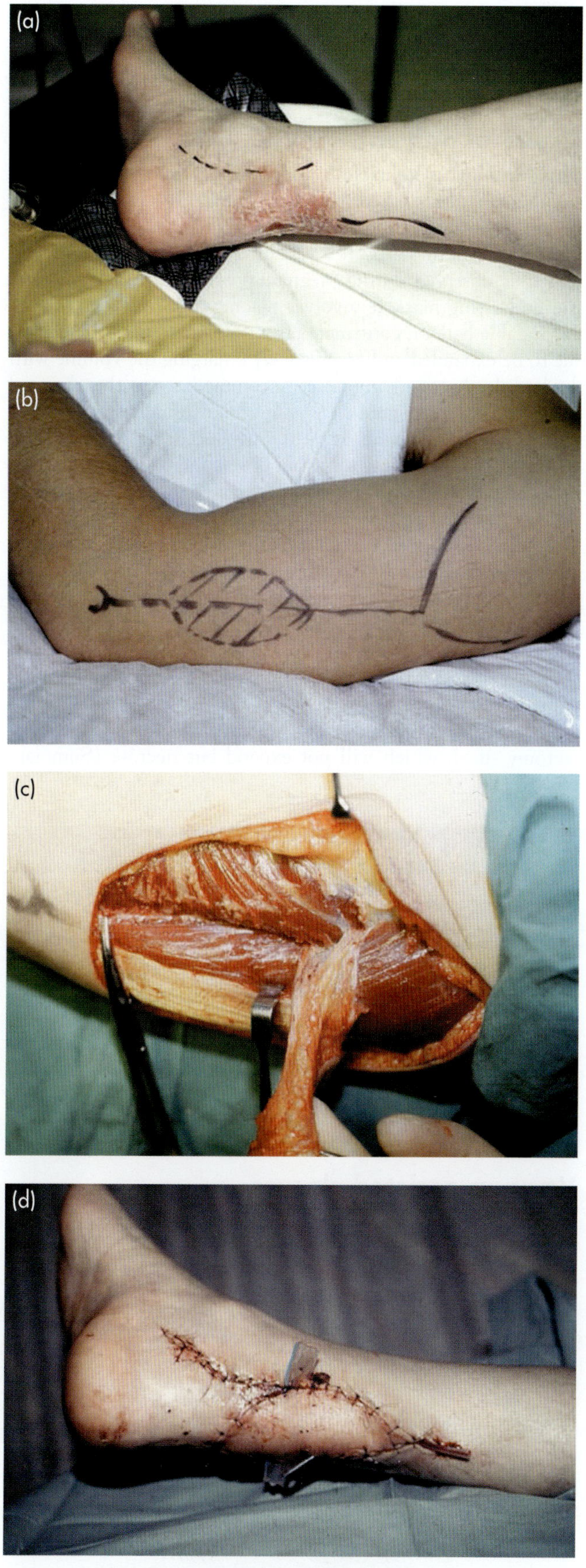

Figure 31.8 (a–d) Free lateral arm fasciocutaneous flap used to resurface a tendo Achilles defect.

- **Perforator flaps**. This description refers to a whole new subgroup of axial flaps in which tissues are isolated on small perforating vessels that run from more major blood vessels to supply the surface.

Skin substitutes

One solution to the problem presented by major skin loss with inadequate skin donor sites has been to use artificially engineered skin substitutes. These vary from thin sheets of autologous keratinocytes, to artificial collagen matrices with embedded fibroblasts and a keratinocyte sheet covering. They are costly, but are becoming widely used, and it is likely that tissue-engineered products will continue to be developed in an attempt to solve difficult reconstructive problems.

Tissue expansion

This technique is valuable in using 'local' tissue for reconstruction. The natural ability of tissue to expand has been harnessed clinically since the experiments of Austad and the clinical work of Radovan in the 1970s. It is a technique borrowed from nature, and it is observed during pregnancy when skin expands over the underlying mass. It involves placing a device – usually an expandable balloon constructed from silicone – beneath the tissue to be expanded and progressively enlarging the volume with fluid while the overlying tissue accommodates to the changed vascular pressure (Figure 31.9). The fluid (usually sterile saline coloured blue in Figure 31.9) is introduced via a self-sealing port attached to a filling tube that enters the balloon. It may be introduced as frequently as can be tolerated by the patient until the tissues are stretched enough to be used for reconstruction. The tissues expanded do not hypertrophy, but there are major changes in the collagen structure.

The process is time-consuming, although it can be very valuable in problematic cases. It is invaluable for sharing remaining areas of scalp hair after severe burns, removing major congenital skin naevi and restoring full-thickness skin over previously grafted limb wounds.

It must never be used under irradiated tissues (such as mastectomy sites), which will not expand but necrose (Summary box 31.2).

Summary box 31.2

Tissue expansion

Advantages
- Well-vascularised tissue
- Tissue next to defect, so likely to be of similar consistency
- Good colour match

Disadvantages
- Multiple expansion episodes (sometimes painful)
- Cost of device
- High incidence of infection and extrusion (especially limbs)

Vacuum-assisted closure

The use of negative pressure applied to a tissue defect has positive effects on wound closure, as well as making difficult and complex wounds more manageable during the early stages of granulation.

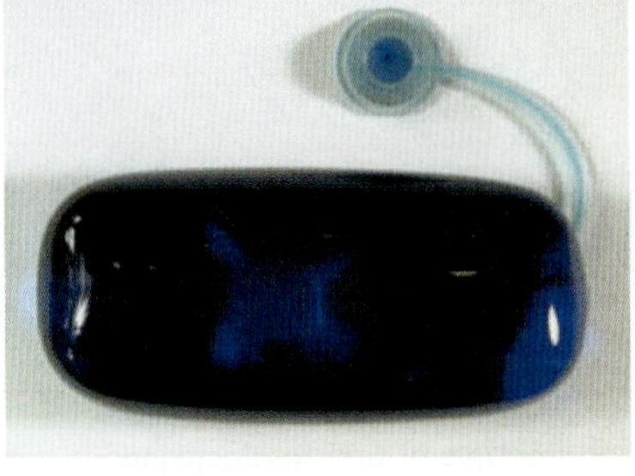

Figure 31.9 Tissue expander.

Exudate is removed and the suction pressure affects angiogenesis and tissue regeneration. The technique can be applied as part of early wound management before definitive surgical closure has been planned, or in some cases to avoid the need for surgery altogether. The foam sponge dressing is connected by a tube to a negative pressure pump that can be controlled to give intermittent suction (Figure 31.10).

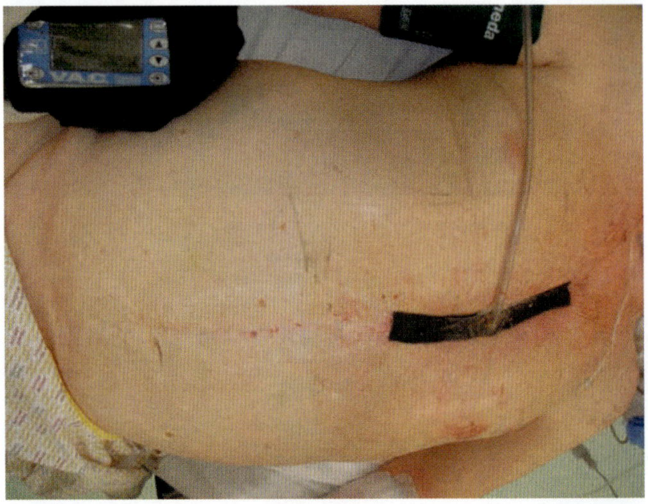

Figure 31.10 VAC™ device used to temporarily close a sternal dehiscence prior to definitive debridement and flap cover.

Implants and prosthetics

Many tissue deficiencies cannot be adequately reconstructed with autologous tissue, however sophisticated the technique used. In such circumstances, implants are part of the reconstructive surgical 'toolbox'; they include solid and soft silicone materials, many forms of filler including collagen and polymers, and osseointegratable anchor points for prosthesis fixation.

The use of fat harvested using liposuction, centrifuged down and washed, then used to inject deficient areas around the body is now commonplace. It is a form of graft transfer since the cellular fluid regains vascularity in the host tissue. It is used for restoring contour deficits after injury and tumour treatment, as well as for cosmetic deformities.

ASSESSMENT AND DIAGNOSTIC PLANNING

Formation of a definitive treatment plan, carefully considering all available options for care with the whole of the patient's needs in mind, is a vital component of wise plastic surgical practice. This is never more so than when managing major trauma cases in the acute setting or when planning major cancer management, which might be staged over a period of treatments and procedures. If the reconstructive surgeon can be involved in early wound debridement and incisions, vital flap pedicles can be protected and the functional and cosmetic outcome made optimal. This pattern of shared team care has become the norm in many units demonstrating good outcomes from major trauma salvage.

The initial assessment of wounds involves adequate removal of devitalised tissue, assessment of which vital structures will need reconstruction immediately and which might be better reconstructed later, and assessment of the degree of contamination involved, which will require further cleaning. Further planning will include the definitive soft-tissue cover of the wound and functional rehabilitation with full psychosocial rehabilitation.

TREATMENT AND COMPLICATIONS

Split-thickness skin grafts

Split-thickness skin grafts are taken with either hand-held (Figure 31.11) or powered skin knives (Figure 31.12). The most used donor site is the thigh, with the buttock preferable in children and cosmetically sensitive individuals. For larger grafts, almost any flat surface can be harvested, including the scalp if shaved (a very good and useful donor site). The thickness of the graft harvested, ease of graft 'take' and donor site healing must be weighed against the lack of durability of thin split-thickness skin grafts.

Split grafts can be perforated to allow exudates to escape and improve 'take'; they can be further meshed to allow expansion (Figure 31.13). This is carried out on a device that cuts a series of slits along the skin, allowing it to expand from a ratio of anything from 1:1.5 to about 1:6.

Grafts will only take on a bed on which they can become vascularised. Preparation of the wound bed is therefore an essential part of a successful graft (Figure 31.14). Graft failure is commonly caused by pus, exudate or residual dead tissue beneath the skin, haematoma or shearing forces. A clean healthy wound bed with a meshed graft tied in place to stop movement will encourage success. The group A β-haemolytic *Streptococcus* can destroy split grafts completely (and also convert a donor site to a full-thickness defect) and so the presence of this micro-organism is a contraindication to grafting.

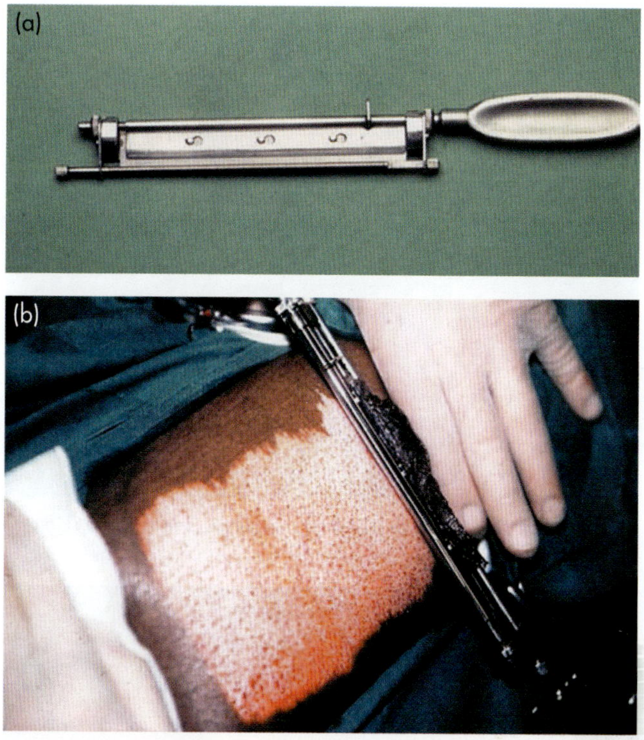

Figure 31.11 Hand-held skin knife (a) and harvesting skin with hand-held knife (b).

Full-thickness skin grafts

Small dermal grafts (Wolfe grafts) can be taken from behind the ear, the groin creases and the neck, with easy direct closure of the donor site. Older people can sustain larger harvests because of skin laxity. Large full-thickness skin graft use is uncommon

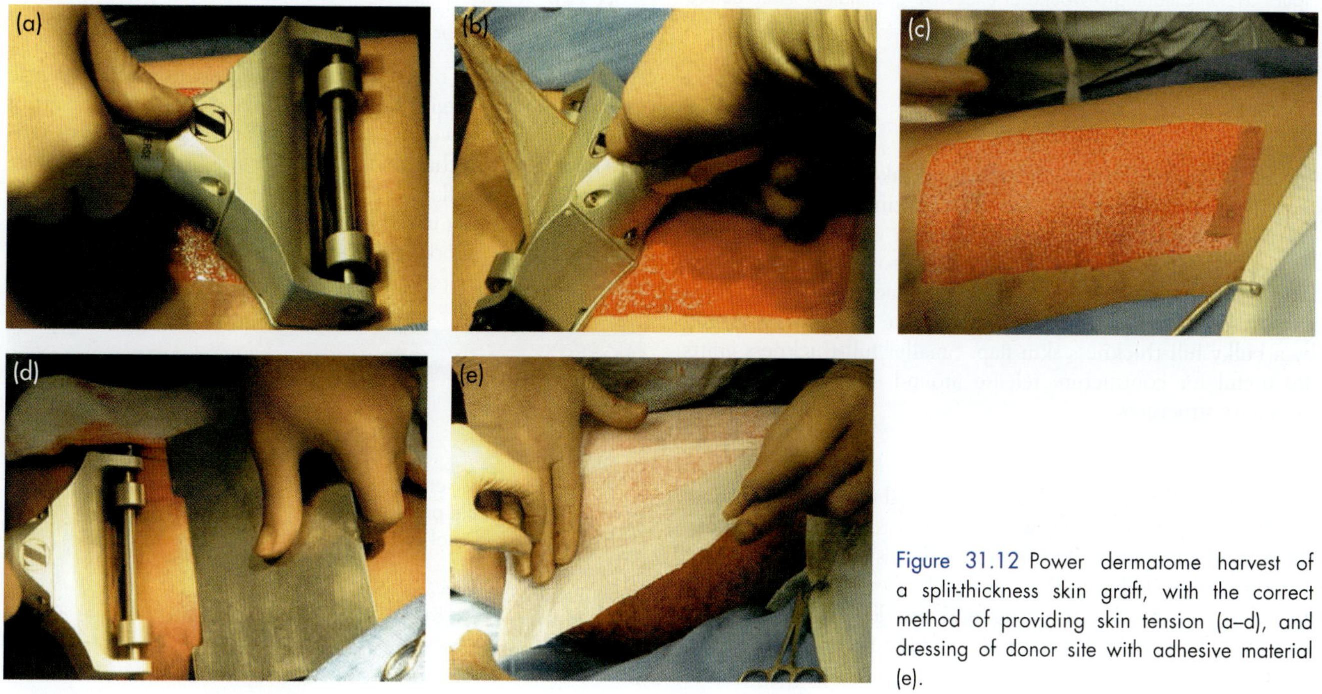

Figure 31.12 Power dermatome harvest of a split-thickness skin graft, with the correct method of providing skin tension (a–d), and dressing of donor site with adhesive material (e).

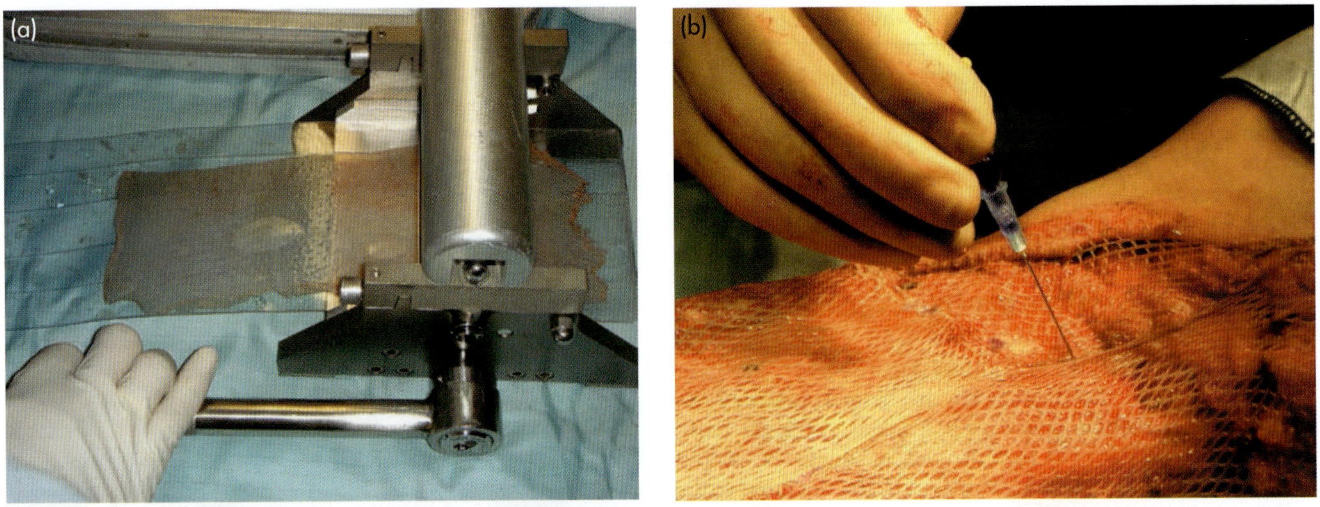

Figure 31.13 Split-thickness skin graft mesher (a) and meshed skin applied to wound (b).

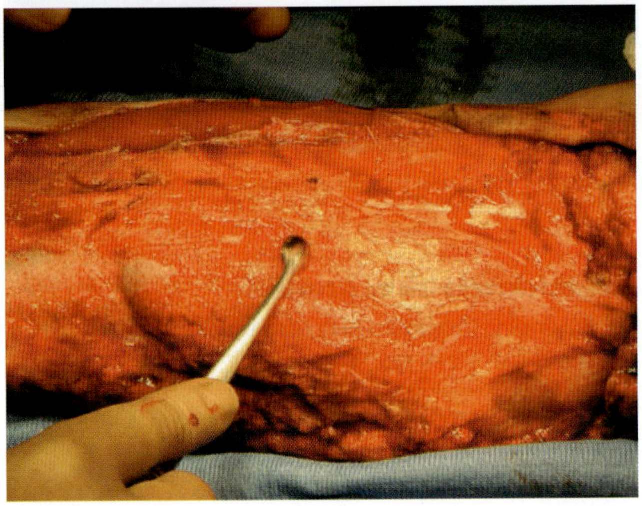

Figure 31.14 Cleaning a wound of excessive granulation tissue before grafting.

and requires great care to obtain a good take. Large donor sites require secondary split-thickness skin grafting. Major secondary burn contractures of the face and flexion creases can achieve remarkable functional and cosmetic improvement using such large grafts, particularly as the remaining facial muscle function can still produce a more natural appearance than when covered by a bulky full-thickness skin flap. Smaller full-thickness grafts are useful for contracture release around sensitive facial and extremity structures.

Technique

The shape of the graft needed is drawn and copied onto a small template (paper or cloth), which is used to transfer the same shape to the donor site. Full-thickness skin is cut; grafts take best if additional underlying fat is removed, after which the graft is applied with normal skin tension and tied down with a pressure dressing. The graft will remain vulnerable to shearing forces for several weeks after application.

Flaps

Local flaps

A local flap is raised next to a tissue defect in order to reconstruct it. Basic patterns include (Figure 31.15):

- **Transposition flap**. The most basic design, leaving a graftable donor site (Figure 31.16);
- **Z-plasty**. For lengthening scars or tissues;
- **Rhomboid flap**. For cheek, temple, back and flat surface defects;
- **Rotation flap**. For convex surfaces;
- **Advancement flap**. For flexor surfaces; may need triangles excised at the base to make it work (commonly called Burow's triangles);
- **V-to-Y advancement**. Commonly used for fingertips and extremities;
- **Bilobed flap**. For convex surfaces, especially the nose (Figure 31.17);
- **Bipedicle flap**. For eyelids, rarely elsewhere.

All flaps must be raised in the subcutaneous plane. Gentle undercutting of margins helps to close the donor site. The art of making local flaps work is to pull available local spare lax skin into the defect, so that the scar when closed sits in a good 'line of election'. Local flaps are usually not based on specific blood vessels, but are very useful in head and neck and smaller defect reconstructions. Good planning is essential to gain the best result from these flaps (Summary box 31.3).

Summary box 31.3

Local flaps

Benefits
- Best local cosmetic tissue match
- Often a simple procedure
- Local or regional anaesthesia option

Disadvantages
- Possible local tissue shortage
- Scarring may exacerbate the condition
- Surgeon may compromise local resection

Karl August von Burow, 1809–1974, surgeon, Konigsberg, Germany.

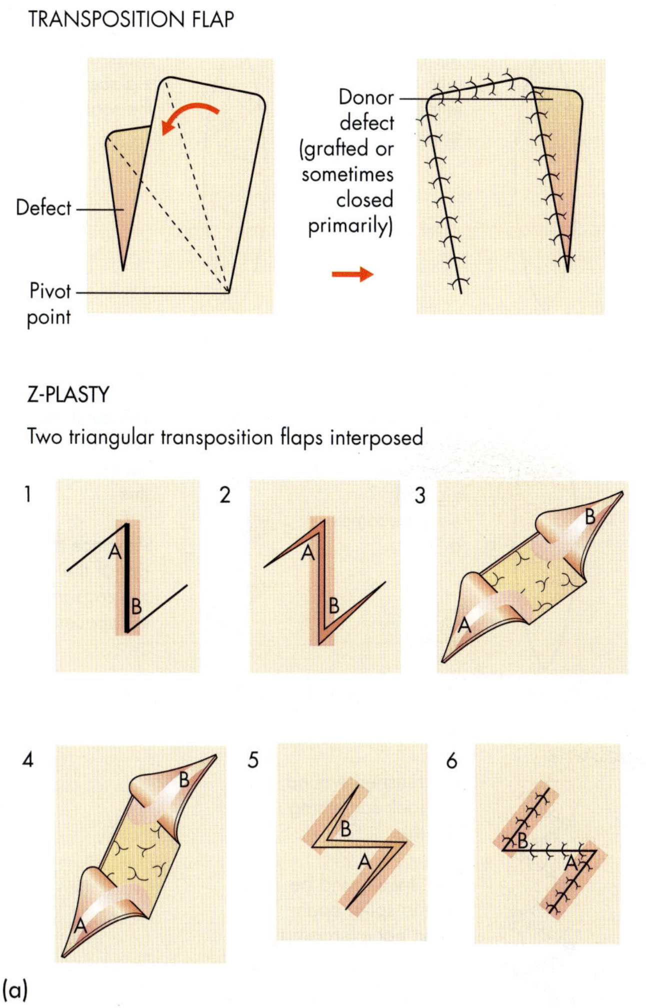
TRANSPOSITION FLAP
Donor defect (grafted or sometimes closed primarily)
Defect
Pivot point
Z-PLASTY
Two triangular transposition flaps interposed
1
2
3
4
5
6
A
B
(a)

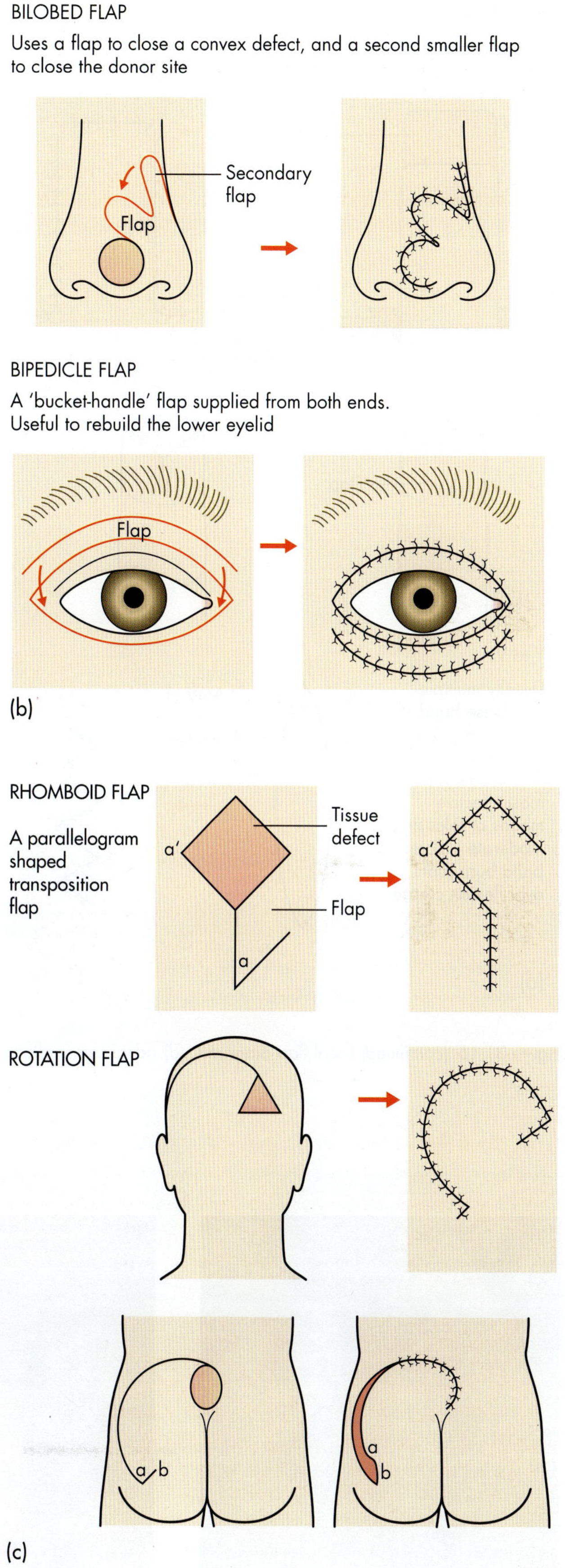
BILOBED FLAP
Uses a flap to close a convex defect, and a second smaller flap to close the donor site
Secondary flap
Flap
BIPEDICLE FLAP
A 'bucket-handle' flap supplied from both ends.
Useful to rebuild the lower eyelid
Flap
(b)
RHOMBOID FLAP
A parallelogram shaped transposition flap
Tissue defect
Flap
a'
a
ROTATION FLAP
a
b
(c)

Figure 31.15 Local flap diagrams. (a) Transposition and Z-plasty flaps; (b) bilobed and bipedicled flaps; (c) rhomboid and rotation flaps. *(continued opposite)*

Combined local flaps

In some circumstances, such as burn contracture release, local flaps can usefully be combined to import surplus tissue from a wide area adjacent to a scar or defect that needs removal. Examples are the W-plasty and the multiple Y-to-V plasty, which is a very versatile means of releasing an isolated band scar contracture over a flexion crease (Figure 31.18).

Distant flaps

To repair defects in which local tissue is inadequate, distant flaps can be moved on long pedicles that contain the blood supply. The pedicle may be buried beneath the skin to create an island flap or left above the skin and formed into a tube.

The most common means of moving flaps long distances while still attached are with a long muscular pedicle that contains a dominant blood supply (a myocutaneous flap) (Figure 31.19) or with a long fascial layer that likewise contains a major septal blood supply (a fasciocutaneous flap) (Figure 31.20). These flaps can carry large composite skin parts for reconstruction very great distances, e.g. from the abdomen to the chest (for

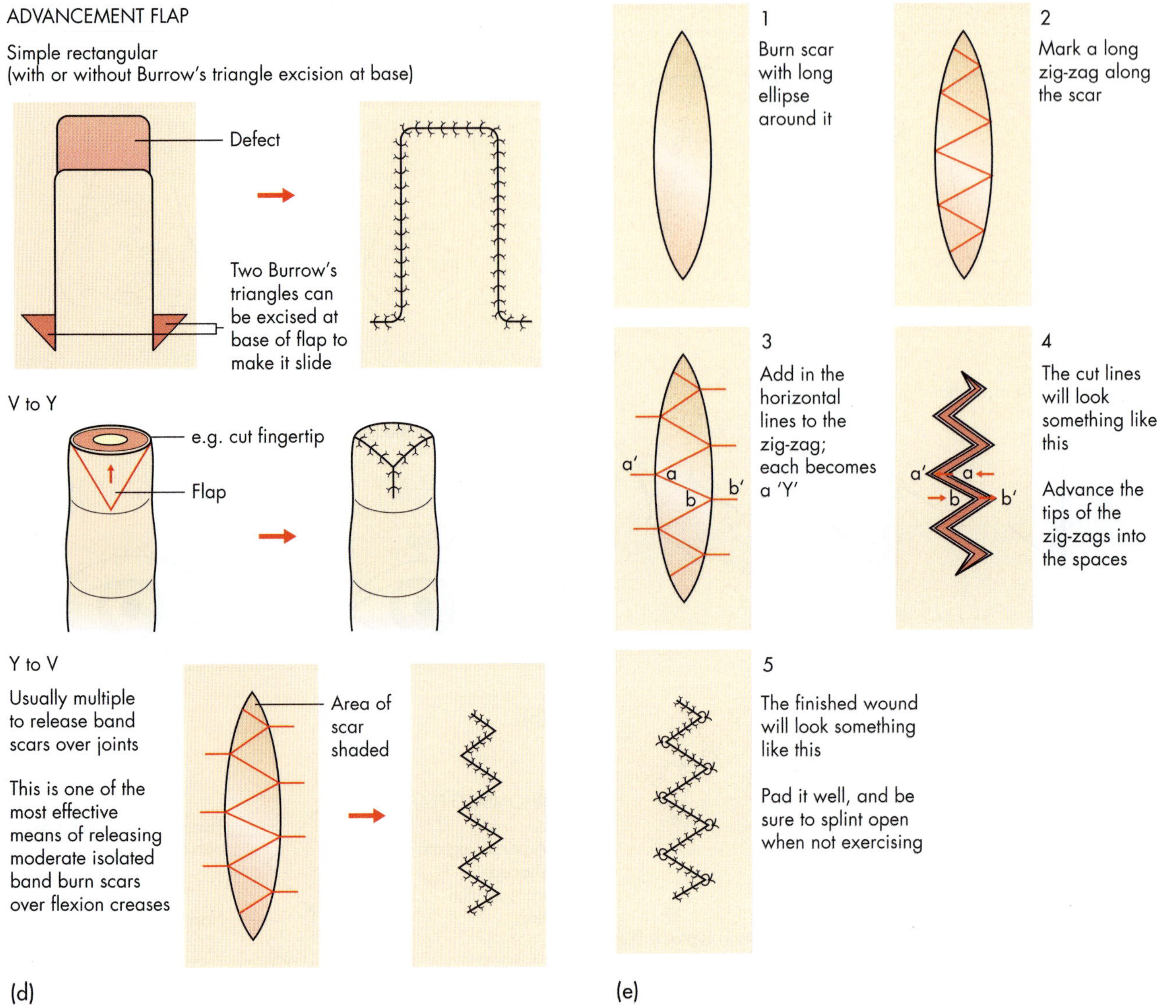

ADVANCEMENT FLAP
Simple rectangular
(with or without Burrow's triangle excision at base)
Defect
Two Burrow's triangles can be excised at base of flap to make it slide
V to Y
e.g. cut fingertip
Flap
Y to V
Usually multiple to release band scars over joints
This is one of the most effective means of releasing moderate isolated band burn scars over flexion creases
Area of scar shaded
(d)
1
Burn scar with long ellipse around it
2
Mark a long zig-zag along the scar
3
Add in the horizontal lines to the zig-zag; each becomes a 'Y'
a'
a
b
b'
4
The cut lines will look something like this
Advance the tips of the zig-zags into the spaces
5
The finished wound will look something like this
Pad it well, and be sure to splint open when not exercising
(e)

Figure 31.15 (*continued*) Local flap diagrams. (d) advancement flaps; (e) multiple Y-to-V plasty for burn scar.

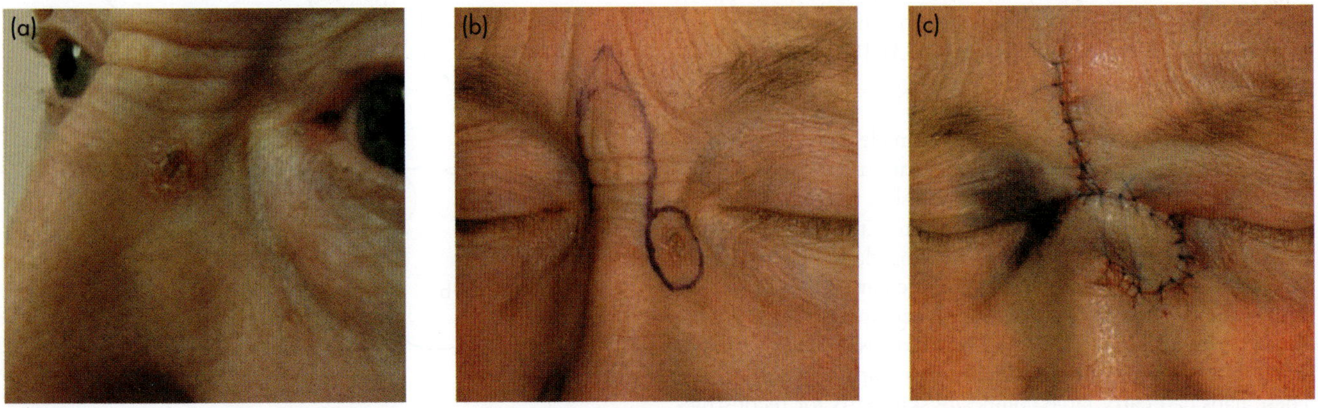

(a)
(b)
(c)

Figure 31.16 (a–c) Example of transposition flap (in this case from glabellar area to inner canthal defect) (*continued overleaf*)

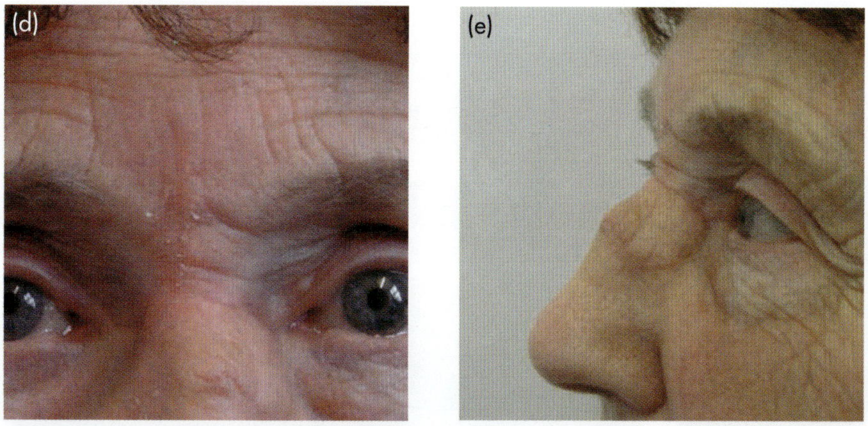

Figure 31.16 (*continued*) (d and e) appearance at one month post-transfer.

breast reconstruction), from the chest to the face (for oral cancer reconstruction) and from the calf to the knee.

There are a vast number of carefully described myocutaneous and fasciocutaneous flaps throughout the body, all of which are based on known blood vessels. They are reliable when the anatomy of the blood supply is known by the surgeon and the skin is raised carefully in continuity with the underlying fascia or muscle, through which the small perforating vessels run to supply the piece of skin that is being transferred. They are the 'workhorse' of plastic surgery worldwide because they do not require complex equipment to raise them and they can solve the majority of reconstructive problems.

Microsurgery and perforator flaps

With fine instruments and materials, it has become commonplace to be able to disconnect the blood supply of the flap from its donor site and reconnect it in a distant place using the operating microscope.

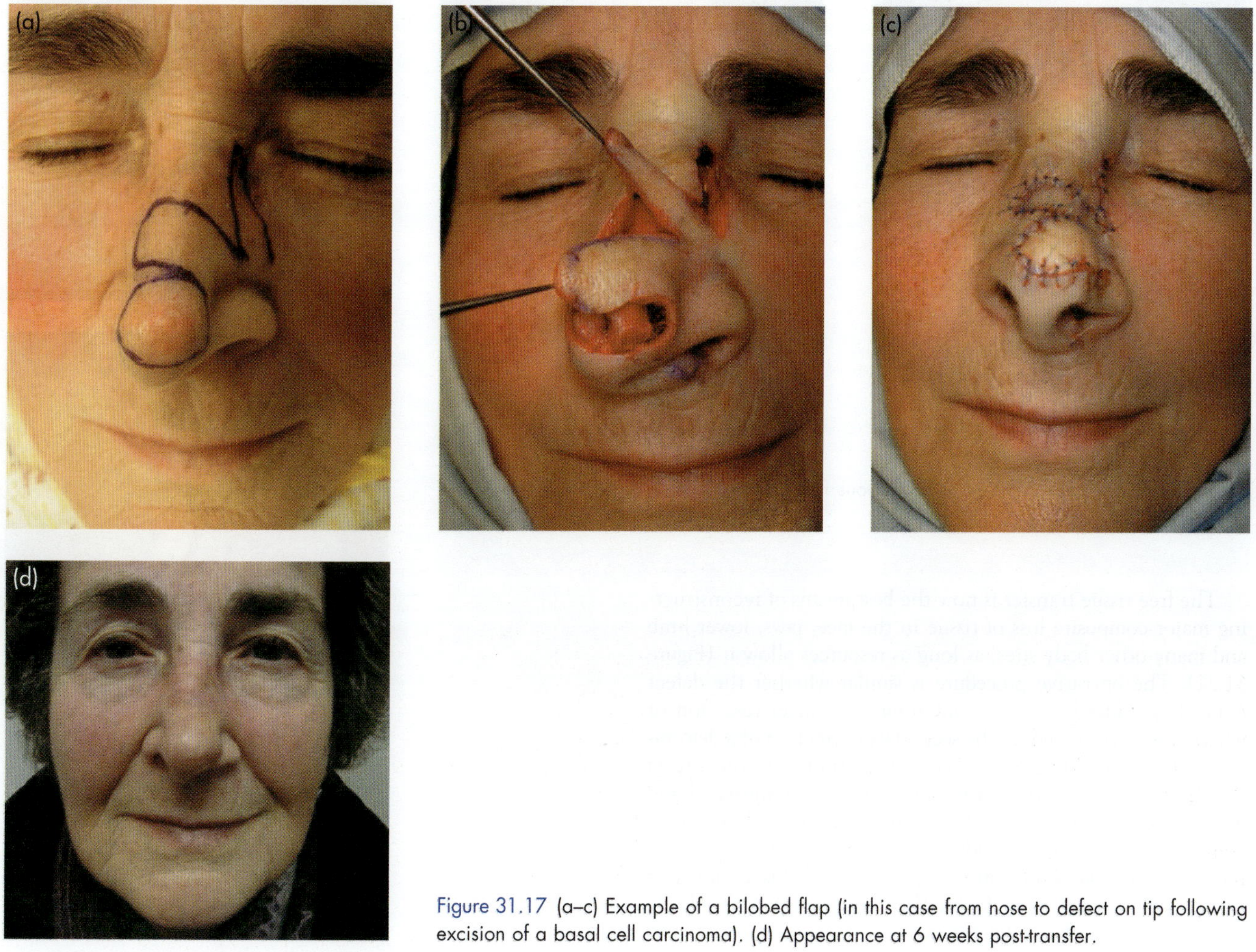

Figure 31.17 (a–c) Example of a bilobed flap (in this case from nose to defect on tip following excision of a basal cell carcinoma). (d) Appearance at 6 weeks post-transfer.

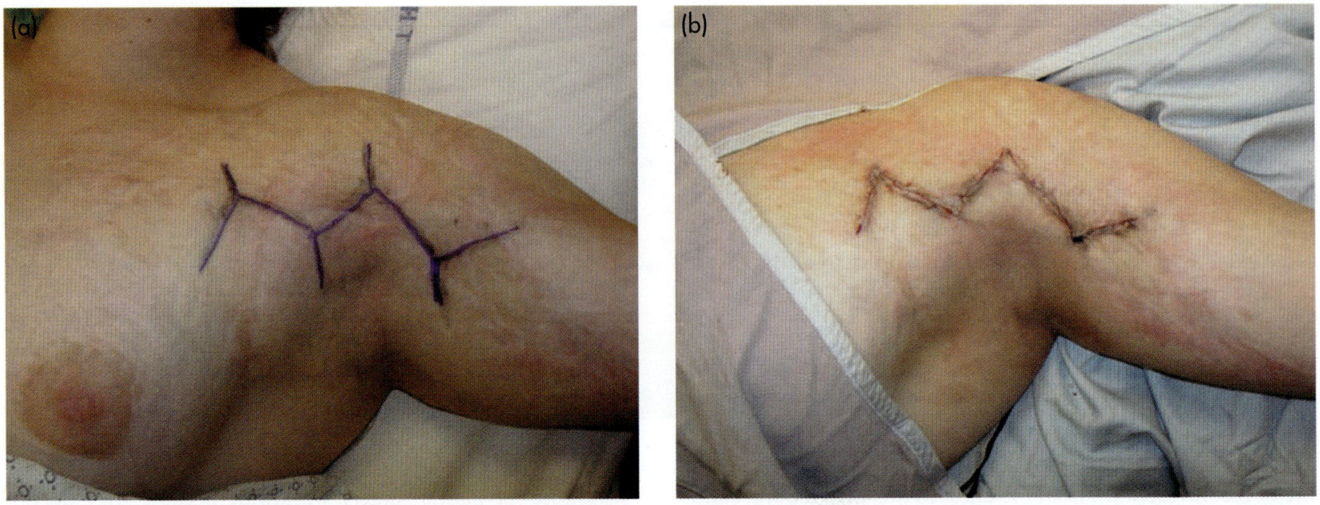

Figure 31.18 (a and b) Y-to-V flap to release axillary contracture.

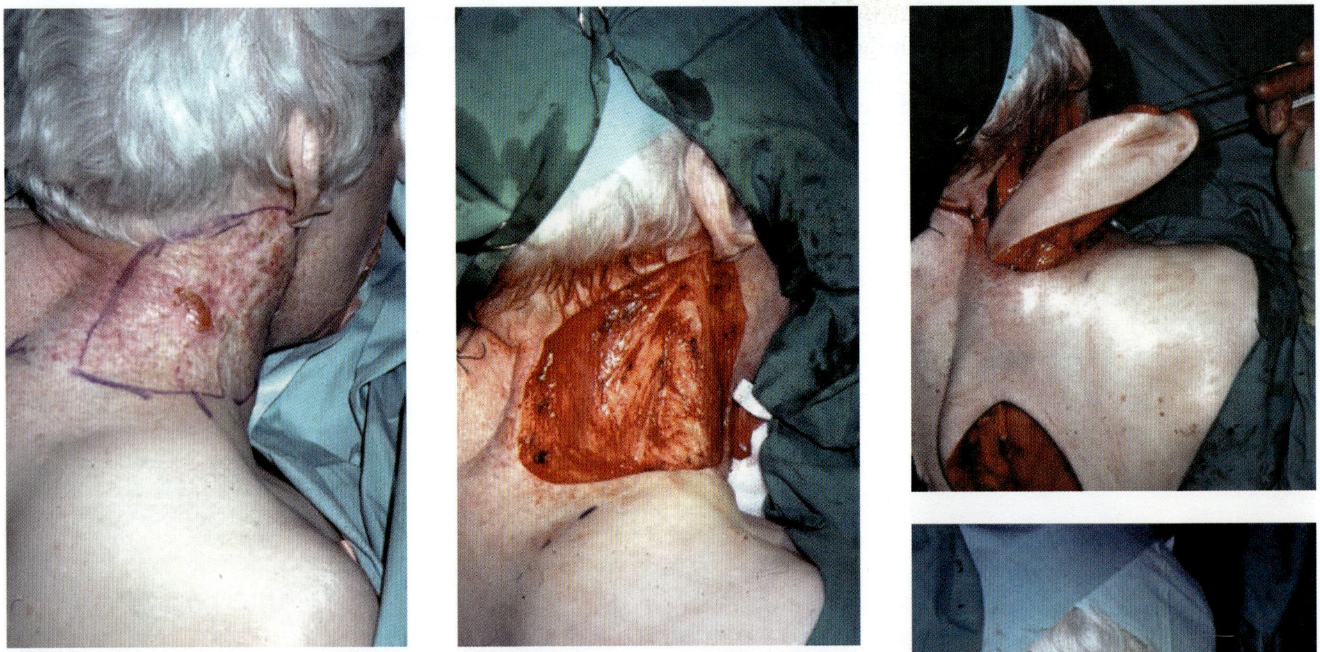

Figure 31.19 Trapezius pedicled myocutaneous flap to an area of recurrent squamous carcinoma in neck.

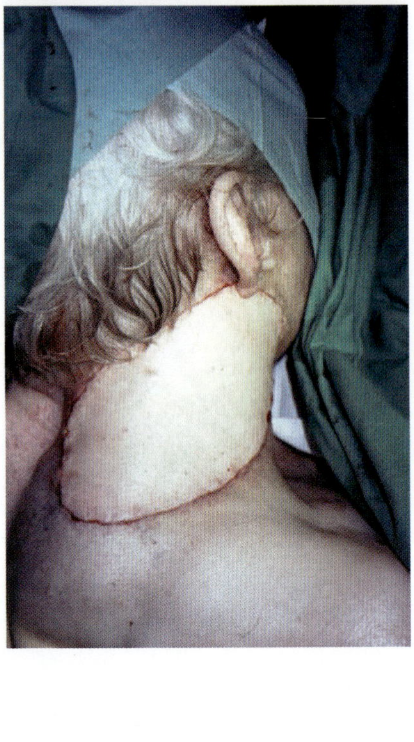

The free tissue transfer is now the best means of reconstructing major composite loss of tissue in the face, jaws, lower limb and many other body sites, as long as resources allow it (Figure 31.21). The operative procedure is similar whether the defect is newly produced from a recent injury or cancer resection or whether it is to be used for the secondary correction of a deformity, such as rebuilding a mastectomy deformity. At the site of the defect, the surgeon must be sure that all contaminated and dead tissue has been thoroughly cleared and cleaned, a process commonly described as debridement, although that term strictly refers to the release of constricting tissue. If this removal of poorly viable tissue is in doubt, then consideration should be given to delaying the reconstruction.

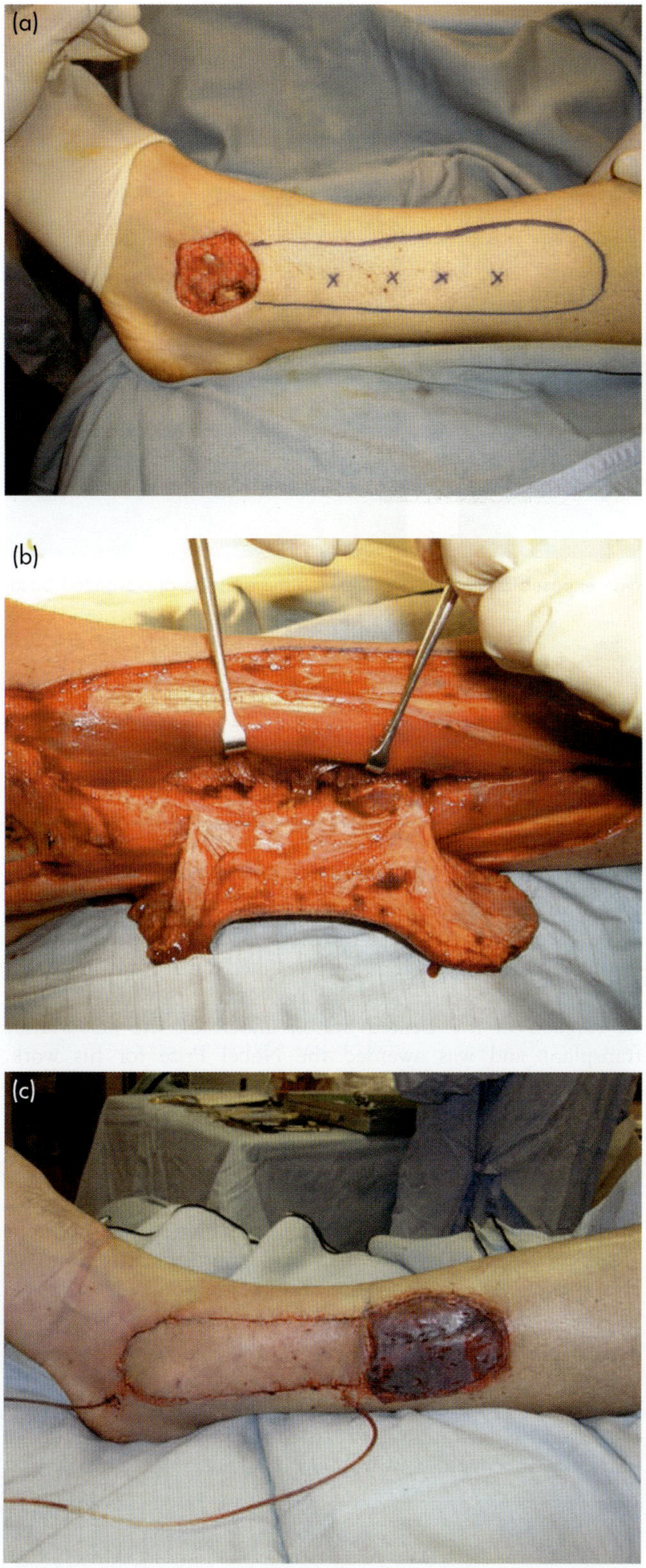

Figure 31.20 (a) Defect at ankle with the flap to be transferred outlined and the position of the perforating vessels (identified with hand-held Doppler device) marked with crosses; (b) flap raised with preserved septal perforators to skin paddle clearly visible; (c) flap rotated into position to cover the defect; proximal donor defect covered with a split-thickness skin graft (case courtesy of Mr David Johnson FRCS(Plast)).

The surgeon must then find a suitable blood supply for the tissue transfer at the site to be reconstructed. A good arterial flow in and venous return out, without external tissue pressure (such as from surrounding wound induration), is of paramount importance in achieving a successful transfer. The flap is then raised (Table 31.2) and transferred using magnification (Figure 31.22). Free muscle transfers should be reanastomosed within 1–2 hours if possible; fasciocutanous flaps are more robust and can survive slightly greater ischaemic times (Summary box 31.4).

Summary box 31.4

Free tissue transfer (or free flap)

Advantages
- Being able to select exactly the best tissue to move
- Only takes what is necessary
- Minimises donor site morbidity

Disadvantages
- More complex surgical technique
- Failure involves total loss of all transferred tissue
- Usually takes more time unless the surgeon is experienced

Table 31.2 Common free tissue transfer donor sites.

Muscle only	Latissimus dorsi
	Rectus abdominis
	Gracilis
Myocutaneous	Latissimus dorsi
	Transverse rectus abdominis
Fasciocutaneous	Radial forearm flap
	Scapular
	Lateral arm
	Anterolateral thigh
	Groin
Osseous	Fibula (may be cutaneous as well)
	Forearm (taking sliver of radius bone)
	Iliac crest
Fascial	Temporoparietal
Miscellaneous	Jejunum – for oesophageal reconstruction
	Pectoralis minor – for facial reanimation
	Omentum – for chest wall and limb defects

Recent developments have led to surgeons dissecting distant flaps free from the carrier muscle or fascia, to reduce the donor morbidity further. These distant 'perforator' flaps increase the flexibility of the use of the flap tissue while reducing donor site problems. Future flap design is moving towards individualised flaps customised in freestyle fashion for the specific reconstructive requirement demanded.

Care of flaps and monitoring

After a flap has been moved, it should be observed for tissue colour, warmth and turgor, and be pressed to assess blanching and capillary refill time. Loss of arterial inflow results in pale, cold, flaccid tissue; loss of venous outflow results in blue conges-

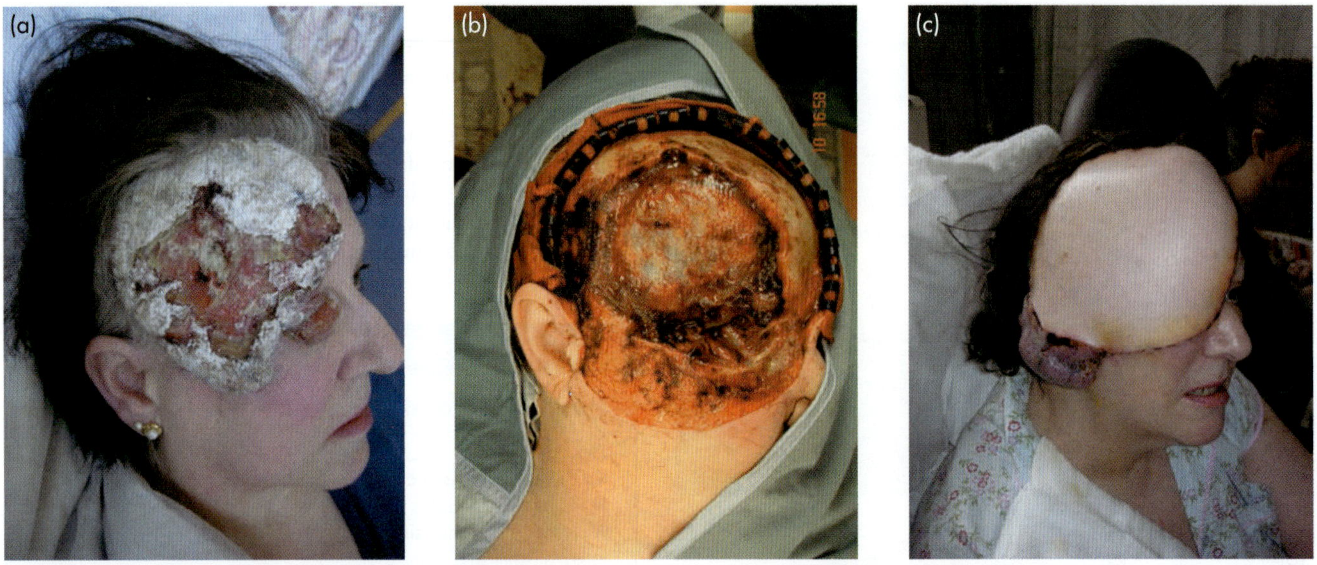

Figure 31.21 (a–c) Large myocutaneous free flap (latissimus dorsi) to cover an exposed cranial defect following the excision of advanced basal cell carcinoma (case courtesy of Mr David Johnson FRCS(Plast)).

tion, increased turgor, rapid capillary refill and initially a warm flap. In a pedicled flap, such venous congestion may be relieved by releasing suture tension; applying leeches to suck out excess venous blood is a last resort when no other means of restoring venous drainage can be obtained.

The most common causes of flap failure are:

- poor anatomical knowledge when raising the flap (such that the blood supply is deficient from the start);
- flap inset with too much tension;
- local sepsis or a septicaemic patient;
- the dressing applied too tightly around the pedicle;
- microsurgical failure in free flap surgery (usually caused by problems with surgical technique)
- tobacco smoking by patient.

'Wet, warm and comfortable'

The best advice for postoperative flap care for major tissue transfers is to keep the patient 'wet, warm and comfortable'. This means that the patient should be well hydrated with a hyperdynamic circulation, a very warm body temperature and well-controlled analgesia to reduce catecholamine output.

Reconstructing complex areas

Certain areas, such as the eyelids, nose, lips, ears, genitalia, fingers, breast and intraoral structures, often require a combination of methods to produce the most functional and acceptable outcome for the patient. Planning such reconstruction involves considering each cosmetic subunit involved in the defect and bringing the best tissue to rebuild it. An example is the Indian forehead rhinoplasty of Sushruta, which involves transposition of a pedicled fasciocutaneous flap from forehead to nose, with the donor site usually thin skin grafted, but occasionally closed primarily in small flaps. It remains the finest means of transporting cosmetically correct tissue to the nose.

FUTURE TRENDS

Vascularised composite allografting

Plastic surgeons have long sought to use transplanted tissue to solve the problems posed by the most severe tissue defects. Esser, in the early twentieth century, pioneered much innovative surgery and urged research into this area. Later, Joe Murray, a plastic surgeon in the United States, undertook the first kidney transplant and was awarded the Nobel Prize for his work. Improved understanding of immunology and means of tolerance induction are now leading to the use of transplanted composite tissues for the most intractable cases of loss of tissue following injury and cancer. Limb transplantation in cases of multiple loss (especially following war injury) is becoming accepted practice in centres where all aspects of care including ethical considerations have been addressed. It is likely that sophisticated tolerance induction for donor-specific transplantation will be possible within the next decade, and lead to a rapid increase in the use of such procedures.

Tissue and bioengineering

Improved understanding of tissue behaviour is leading to numerous innovations in wound manipulation using biological

Johannes Fredericus Samuel Esser, 1877–1946 born in Leyden, Netherlands. A Dutch plastic surgeon who pioneered reconstructive surgery on soldiers wounded in the First World War. He is thought to have coined the term 'stent' in 1917 to describe his use of a dental impression compound invented in 1856 by the English dentist Charles Stent (1807–1885) to create a form for facial reconstruction.

Joseph E Murray, born 1919, Professor Emeritus of Plastic Surgery, Harvard University Medical School, Boston, MA, USA. He shared the 1990 Nobel Prize for Physiology or Medicine with E Donnall Thomas for his work on organ and cell transplantation. Murray's interest in transplantation began during his military service in the Second World War. The early experiences with skin transplantation for burns in pilots formed the basis for Murray's interest in solid organ transplantation. He performed the world's first kidney transplantation in identical twins in Peter Brent Brigham Hospital, Boston in 1954.

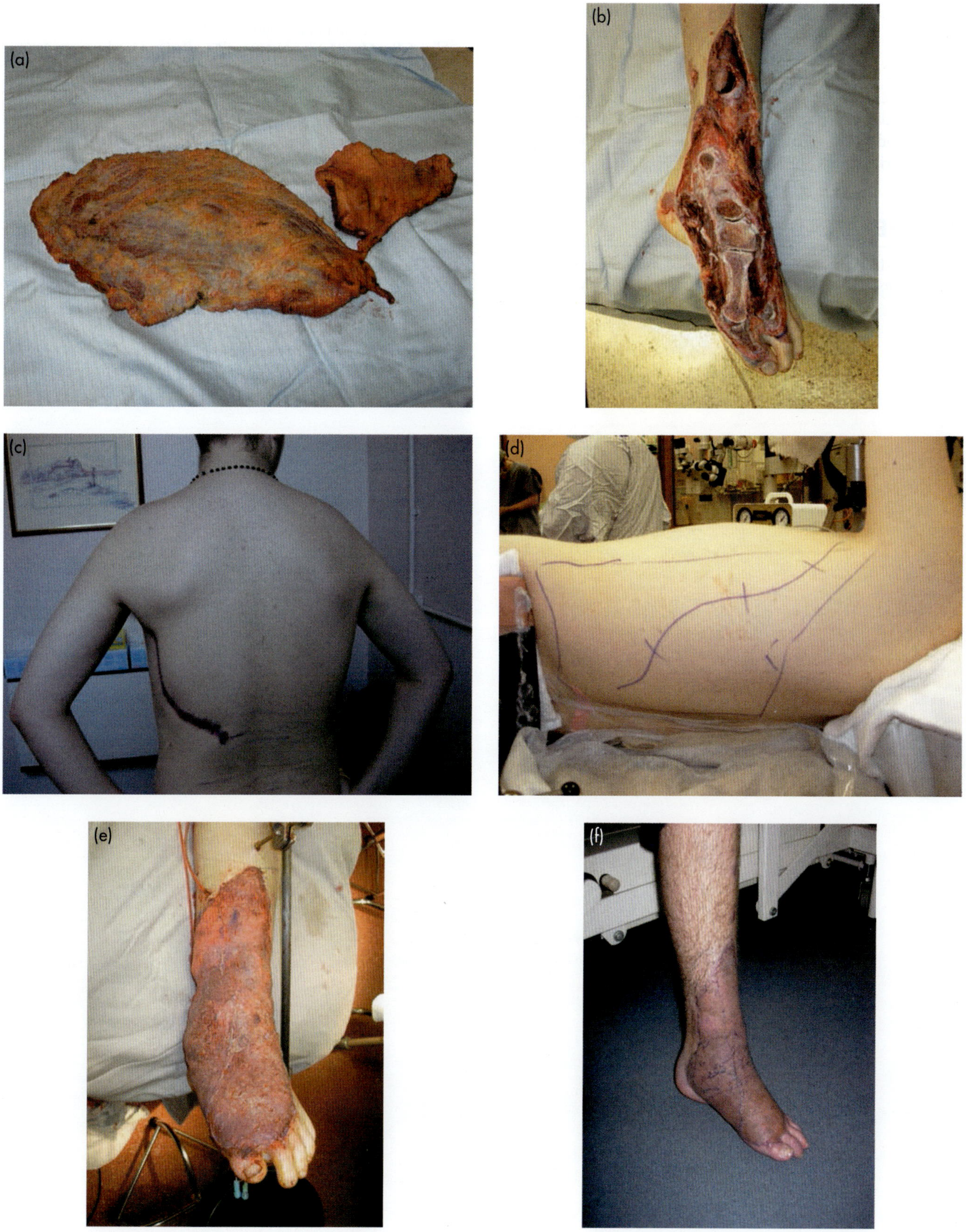

Figure 31.22 Large 'chimeric flap' of latissimus dorsi and serratus anterior muscles (a) to cover a complex open wound of the foot and ankle (b), illustrating the donor site (c and d) and fully covered defect (e and f) (case courtesy of Mr David Johnson FRCS(Plast)).

mechanisms. Tissue-engineered biological substitutes for tendon, nerve, larynx and other vital structures are becoming established, and will greatly influence the spectrum of reconstructive procedures in the coming years.

Novel polymers and biologically tolerated materials are also being developed to act as nerve conduits, facial muscle substitutes and self-inflating expansion devices. The interface of new material science with reconstructive surgery is still in its infancy.

FURTHER READING

Achauer BM, Erikson E, Guruyon R *et al.* (eds). *Plastic surgery indications, operations and outcomes*, vols 1–5. St Louis: Mosby, 2000.

Cormack GC, Lamberty BGH. *The arterial anatomy of skin flaps*. Edinburgh: Churchill Livingstone, 1986.

Geddes CR, Morris SF, Neligan PC. Perforator flaps: evolution, classification, and applications. *Ann Plastic Surg* 2003; **50**: 90–9.

Koshima I, Soeda S. Inferior epigastric artery skin flaps without rectus abdominis muscle. *Br J Plastic Surg* 1989; **42**: 645–8.

MacGregor AD, MacGregor IA. *Fundamental techniques in plastic surgery*, 10th edn. Edinburgh: Churchill Livingstone, 2000.

Mathes SJ. *Plastic surgery*, vols 1–8. Philadelphia: WB Saunders, 2006.

Mustarde JC, Jackson IT. *Plastic surgery in infancy and childhood*. Edinburgh: Churchill Livingstone, 1988.

Nabri IA. El Zahrawi (936–1013 AD), the father of operative surgery. *Ann R Coll Surg Engl* 1983; **65**: 132–4.

Serafin D. *Atlas of microsurgical composite tissue transplantation*. Philadelphia: WB Saunders, 1996.

CHAPTER

32 Disaster surgery

LEARNING OBJECTIVES

To recognise and understand:

- The common features of various disasters
- The principles behind the organisation of the relief effort and of triage in treatment and evacuation
- The role and limitations of field hospitals
- The features of conditions peculiar to disaster situations and their treatment

INTRODUCTION

Natural disasters such as floods and earthquakes provide a constant reminder of the awesome power and capricious nature of our planet. The depletion of the ozone layer and global warming mean that the future may hold in store natural events that will be even greater in magnitude than any of the ones that we have experienced before. Alongside the ravages of nature is our own propensity to damage our fellow man. National conflicts and ideological differences have not lessened over the millennia and the resultant 'unnatural disasters' have the potential to rival the natural ones in enormity and the impact on human life. The spectre of terrorist attacks constantly haunts security organisations and health-care providers.

COMMON FEATURES OF MAJOR DISASTERS

Any event that results in the loss of human life is disastrous, but most accidents, such as aeroplane and train crashes, are limited in the number of people involved. Conversely, earthquakes, tsunamis and nuclear explosions leave in their wake massive destruction over large areas, which may transcend national boundaries. All the apparatus of a society that responds to such disasters (the civil administration, emergency services, fire brigades and hospitals) may themselves also be crippled (Figure 32.1). Large numbers of people may require immediate shelter, clean water and food before medical care can be considered.

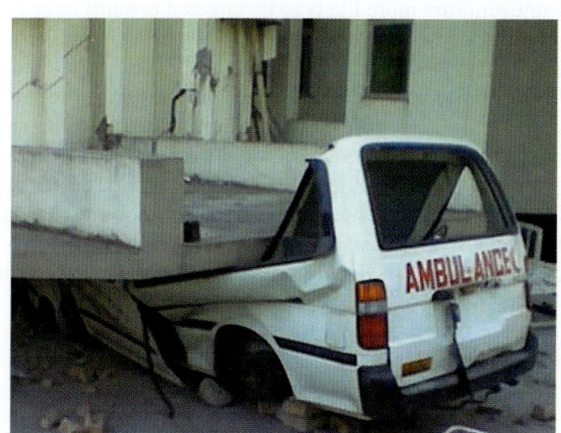

Figure 32.1 Damage to emergency medical services.

A breakdown of communication is inevitable and is accompanied by widespread panic and a disruption of civil order. Access to the disaster area may be limited because of the destruction of bridges, road and rail links (Summary box 32.1).

Summary box 32.1

Common features of major disasters

- Massive casualties
- Damage to infrastructure
- A large number of people requiring shelter
- Panic and uncertainty among the population
- Limited access to the area
- Breakdown of communication

FACTORS INFLUENCING RELIEF EFFORTS AND PROVISION OF MEDICAL AID

Communication is the critical factor that enables the authorities to respond quickly and appropriately. Wireless technology and satellite imagery have revolutionised the way in which real-time information can be obtained (Figure 32.2). Even so, there is an inevitable lag period between the occurrence of the disaster and the response from the establishment.

The location of the disaster area, whether rural or urban, has a significant bearing on relief efforts. Terrorist attacks and

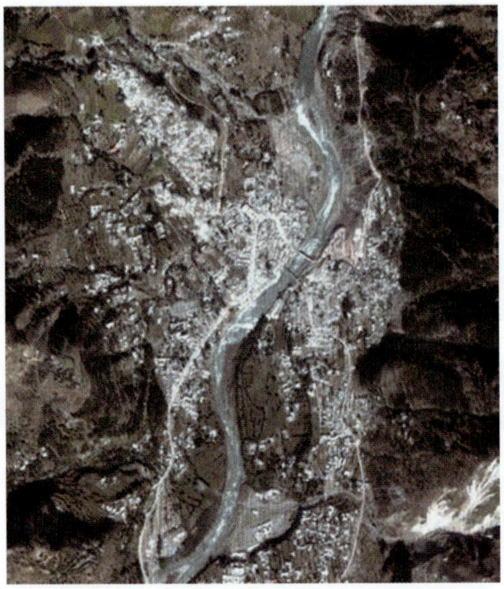

Figure 32.2 Satellite image showing destruction of a bridge as a result of flood.

nuclear events are more likely to be targeted towards large population centres where emergency and medical services are better developed. However, these areas are also densely populated and may have limited access by road and air. Natural disasters can strike anywhere, but can be particularly difficult to manage if they occur in remote areas because relief efforts are hampered by geographical isolation and the lack of a suitable infrastructure.

The time-frame in which a disaster occurs also has an impact on the relief efforts. Earthquakes and blasts unleash havoc in fractions of a second, but floods and hurricanes may continue for several days and nuclear fallout can damage the ecosystem for years to come. Another important factor is the state of development of the country; disasters in the developing world can seldom be managed without significant outside assistance (Summary box 32.2).

Summary box 32.2

Factors influencing rescue and relief efforts

- Status of communications
- Location, whether rural or urban
- Accessibility of the location
- Time-frame in which disaster occurs
- Economic state of development of the area

SEQUENCE OF RELIEF EFFORTS AFTER A DISASTER

Establishing a chain of command

Many countries have organisations that deal with disasters, such as the Federal Emergency Management Authority (FEMA) in the United States. In others, an ad-hoc administrative hierarchy is established to coordinate the efforts of the teams participating in relief efforts. The actual organisation that deals with a particular disaster will depend upon the circumstances, but the principles are similar (Figure 32.3).

Damage assessment

The first objective in disaster management is an accurate assessment of the damage and the number of casualties. All sources

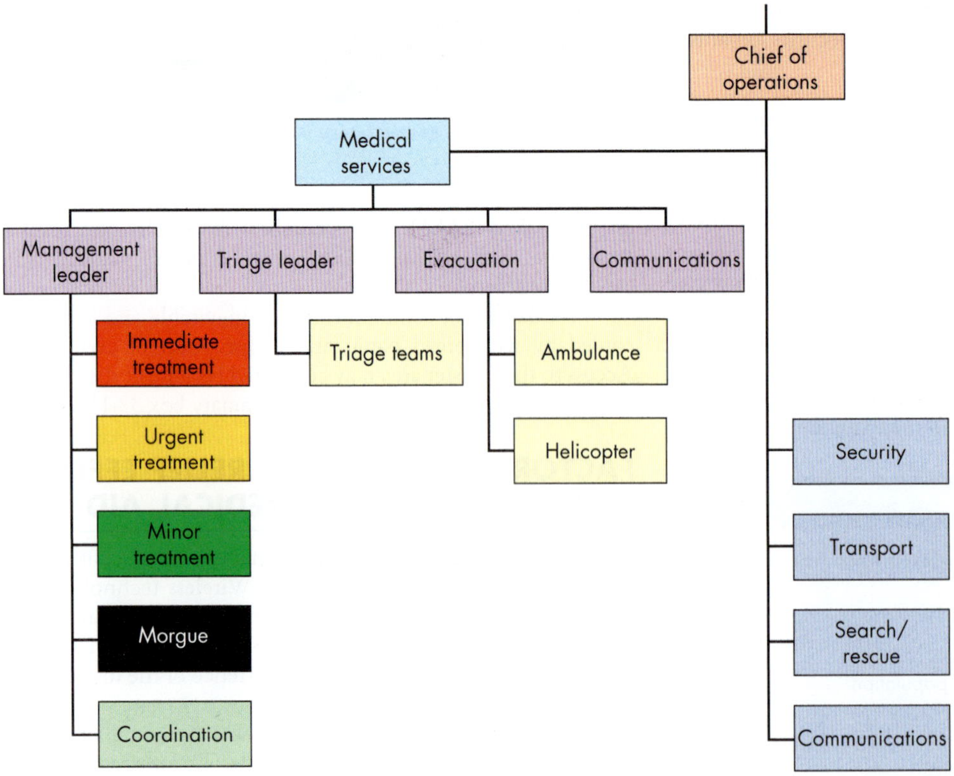

Figure 32.3 Organisation chart for disaster management.

of information must be employed, not just the official channels. The 24-hour news services are frequently the first on the scene and can be an important source of information.

Mobilising resources

The next step is mobilisation of human and material resources appropriate to the size and nature of the disaster. Although all modes of transport available need to be considered, helicopters provide the quickest access for the first responders (Figure 32.4). The teams who make up the initial response must include experienced staff who can assess the situation and have the authority to take immediate decisions and organise further assistance.

Rescue operation

Early coordination of the rescue effort allows optimal use of limited resources. Rescue teams from the outside can complement local volunteers who are familiar with the area. The first priority is to prevent further damage from occurring, both to people and to the infrastructure. Fires should be put out, people moved away from falling debris and well-meaning non-professionals stopped from embarking on hazardous rescue efforts.

The types of injuries encountered by rescue workers depends upon the delay between the onset of the disaster and their arrival. Patients with head injuries and abdominal and thoracic trauma will either have been treated or have succumbed to their injuries within 48–72 hours of a disaster. After the first 2 weeks, the only casualties requiring treatment are those with complex limb trauma, and infected wounds (Figure 32.5).

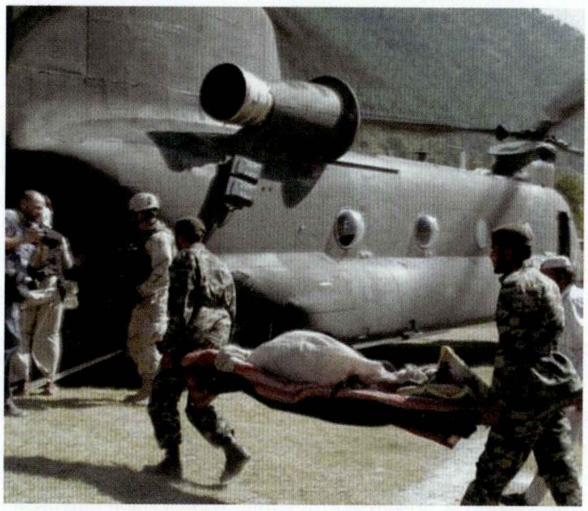

Figure 32.4 Heli-evacuation.

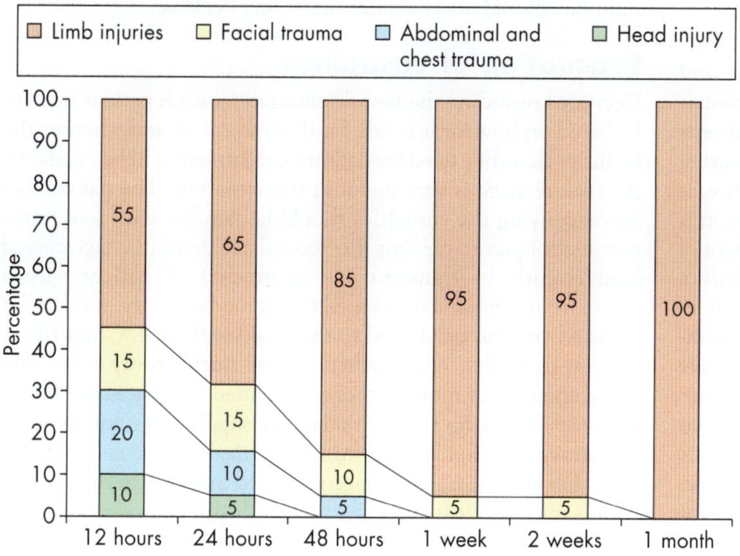

Figure 32.5 Time-line showing the type of injuries encountered at different times in a disaster.

Coordination with relief agencies

A laudable aspect of globalisation is the outpouring of help from governments and non-governmental organisations (NGO) in response to a disaster on the other side of the world. Some, like Rescue and Preparedness in Disasters (RAPID), deal with search and rescue whereas others, like the International Committee of the Red Cross (ICRC) and Oxfam, provide general disaster-related relief (Figure 32.6). United Nations (UN) agencies, such as the World Health Organization (WHO), the World Food Programme (WFP) and the UN High Commissioner for Refugees (UNHCR) deal with medical care, food provision and refugees, respectively. Coordinating the efforts of these organisations is essential for optimal results, as medical aid in isolation is inadequate without the simultaneous provision of safe drinking water, food, clothing and shelter. Rescue teams should be prepared to be self-sufficient and not rely on the local infrastructure, which will be stretched to the limit if not completely destroyed (Summary box 32.3).

Summary box 32.3

Sequence of the relief effort in major disasters

- Establish chain of command
- Set up lines of communication
- Carry out damage assessment
- Mobilise resources
- Initiate rescue operation
- Triage casualties
- Start emergency treatment
- Arrange evacuation
- Start definitive management

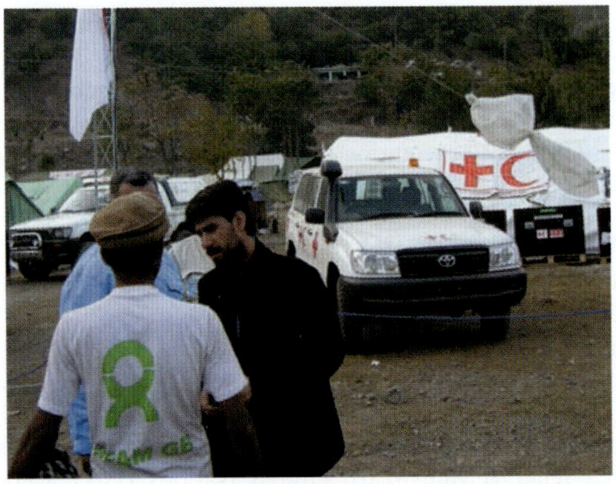

Figure 32.6 Oxfam and the International Committee of the Red Cross provide generalised relief.

Safety of the helpers

Rescue and relief workers are a diverse group of volunteers and may have little experience of dealing with the breakdown in civil order that occurs in the wake of disasters. It is not uncommon to encounter mobs looting stores of food and other essentials, especially if help has arrived late. This results in injuries, occasionally serious, to personnel trying to provide an equitable distribution of goods. It is therefore imperative that the local authorities make it a point to safeguard the lives and property of aid workers to allow them to work without duress and fear.

Dealing with the media

Disasters act like a magnet for the news media and, in today's world of 24-hour news coverage, it exerts a powerful influence in shaping public opinion. It is frequently accused of dramatising situations and emphasising the inadequacies of the relief effort. Aid workers may find dealing with the media difficult as their priorities are rightly different. Nevertheless, it is essential to establish a working relationship between the two groups. With careful handling, the media can become a powerful ally and play a constructive role in identifying problems, galvanising aid and keeping the public informed.

Triage

Derived from the French verb '*trier*', triage means 'to sort' and has been the cornerstone of the management of mass casualties since the Napoleonic Wars. It aims to identify the patients who will benefit the most by being treated the earliest, ensuring the greatest good for the greatest number. In a broader sense, it determines who will be treated first, what mode of evacuation is best and which medical facility is optimal for the management of the patient. Numerous studies show that only 10–15 per cent of disaster casualties are serious enough to require hospitalisation. By sorting out the minor injuries, triage lessens the immediate burden on medical facilities. Deciding who should receive priority when faced with hundreds of seriously injured victims is a daunting prospect. Senior doctors tend to believe that their services are better utilised in the actual management of patients, rather than in triage. This is a mistake and it is crucial that this task be undertaken by someone senior, who has the training and experience, and authority to make these critical decisions.

To keep pace with the changing clinical picture of an injured person, triage needs to be undertaken at several levels, i.e. in the field, before evacuation and at the hospital.

Triage areas

For efficient triage, the injured need to be brought together into any undamaged structures that can shelter a large number of wounded. Examples are school buildings and stadia. A good water supply, lighting and ease of access are useful. Separate areas should be reserved for patient holding, emergency treatment and decontamination (in the event of discharge of hazardous materials). An area should also be designated to serve as a morgue, preferably a little removed from the holding and treatment areas.

Practical triage

Emergency life-saving measures should proceed alongside triage and actually help the decision-making process. The assessment and restoration of airway, breathing and circulation are critical and are discussed in Chapter 24. A simple visual check of the injuries of each casualty is notoriously unreliable. Vital signs and a general physical examination should be combined with a brief history taken by a paramedic, or volunteer worker if one is available.

Documentation for triage

Accurate documentation is an inseparable part of triage and should include basic patient data, vital signs with timing, brief details of injuries (preferably on a diagram) and treatment given. In addition, a system of colour-coded tags attached to the patient's wrist or around the neck should be employed by the emergency medical services. The colour denotes the degree of urgency with which a patient requires treatment (Figure 32.7).

Triage categories

All methods of triage use simple criteria based on vital signs. A rapid clinical assessment should be made taking into account the patient's ability to walk, their mental status and the presence or absence of ventilation or capillary perfusion. A commonly used four-tier system is presented in Table 32.1. Triage carries serious consequences, especially for patients who are consigned to the unsalvageable category. It should be carried out with compassion, but should also be quick, clear and decisive.

Evacuation of casualties

Decisions regarding the best destination for each patient need to be based on how far it is safe for them to travel and whether the facilities that they need for definitive treatment will be available. A quick retriage is very useful in this situation. The paramedics accompanying the casualties should be familiar with safe transport techniques to prevent the 'second accident' (damage caused inadvertently by transport and treatment). A patient with a spinal injury should be strapped to a spine board, the hard collar adjusted and the head fixed to the board with tape. Chest tubes, urinary catheters, endotracheal tubes, tracheotomy tubes and intravenous lines must be properly secured. For patients obliged to travel for a long time, an adequate supply of essentials, such as intravenous fluids, dressings, pain medication and oxygen, must be arranged. For unaccompanied minor children, their details must be clearly documented and social services informed (Summary box 32.4).

Triage is the earliest example of clinical risk management. This is done on the basis of need so that resources can be allocated by good prioritisation. The process was first used in 1792 by Baron Dominique Jean Larrey, Surgeon in Chief to Napoleon's Imperial Guard. The concept of triage emerged from the French Service de Sante so that resources could be used to the optimum – "most for the most".

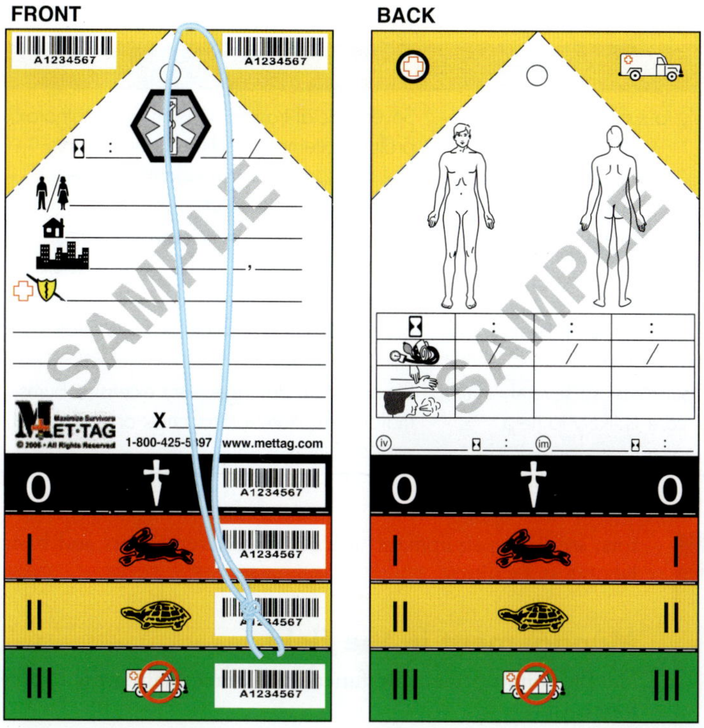

(a)

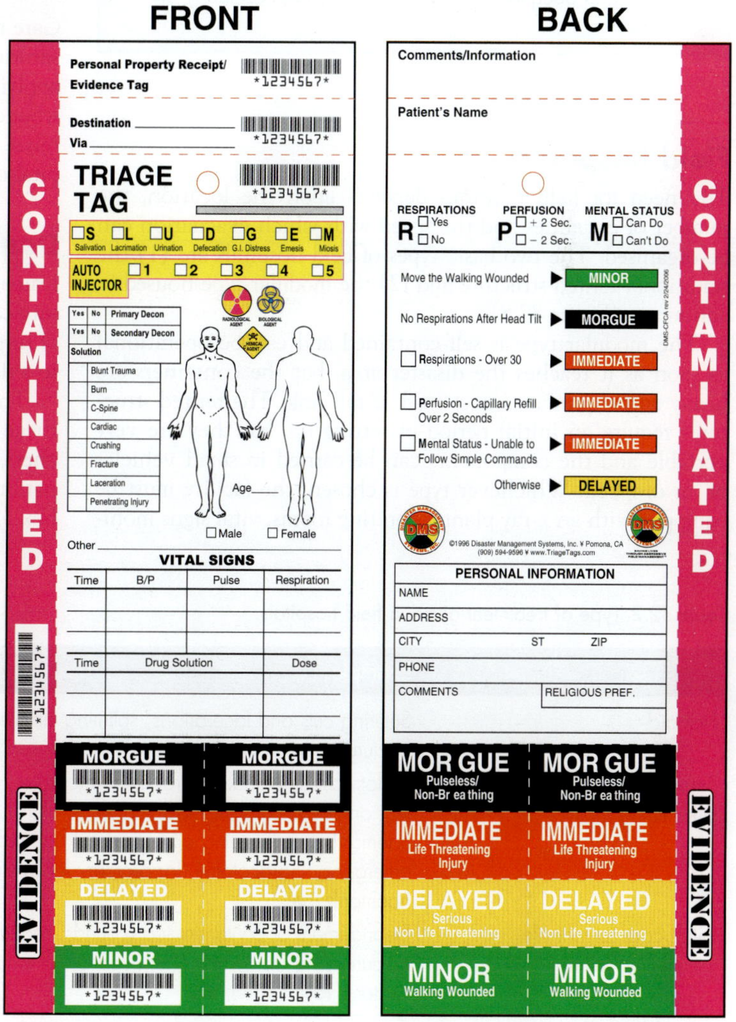

Figure 32.7 Triage tags. (a) Courtesy of TACDA and METTAG products, American Civil Defense Association. (b) Courtesy of Disaster Management Systems.

(b)

Table 32.1 Triage categories.

Priority	Colour	Medical need	Clinical status	Examples
First (I)	Red	Immediate	Critical, but likely to survive if treatment given early	Severe facial trauma, tension pneumothorax, profuse external bleeding, haemothorax, flail chest, major intra-abdominal bleed, extradural haematomas
Second (II)	Yellow	Urgent	Critical, likely to survive if treatment given within hours	Compound fractures, degloving injuries, ruptured abdominal viscus, pelvic fractures, spinal injuries
Third (III)	Green	Non-urgent	Stable, likely to survive even if treatment is delayed for hours to days	Simple fractures, sprains, minor lacerations
Last (0)	Black	Unsalvageable	Not breathing, pulseless, so severely injured that no medical care is likely to help	Severe brain damage, very extensive burns, major disruption/loss of chest or abdominal wall structures

Summary box 32.4

Essentials of casualty evacuation

- Retriage to upgrade priorities among the injured
- Select appropriate medical facilities for transfer
- Choose appropriate means of transport
- Prevent the 'second accident' during transfer
- Ensure an adequate supply of materials to accompany the patient

Field hospitals

The need for field hospitals depends upon the location, the number of casualties and the speed with which evacuation can be organised. The two basic types of field hospitals are (1) the traditional tented structure and (2) the modular type housed in containers (Figure 32.8).

The modular type is self-contained and can be operational as soon as it reaches the disaster area, but the containers are heavy and require an intact road or rail link. The tented structures require an initial period of setting up, but they are very portable and the components can be carried in small vehicles or air dropped. Whichever type is chosen, the facility must be equipped with an x-ray plant, operating rooms, vital signs monitors, sterilising equipment, a blood bank, ventilators and basic laboratory facilities.

Management in the field

Field hospitals principally function in three main areas (Table 32.2).

First aid

Care for patients with minor injuries involves cleaning wounds, suturing lacerations, splinting simple fractures and sprains, and applying bandages to cuts and bruises. Most of these 'walking wounded' can be sent away with antibiotics and simple pain relief. They can be asked to arrange follow up at their usual hospital or the field hospital.

Damage control surgery

Damage control surgery is the concept that in the temporary surgical facility closest to the injured, only the minimum amount of surgery should be performed to allow safe transfer of a patient to a definitive treating facility (see also Chapter 28).

This will include ensuring that the airway is secure, haemorrhage is under control, compartments are decompressed in the chest, skull, abdomen and limb compartments, and any contamination is prevented from developing into infection (Summary box 32.5).

Table 32.2 Type of treatment given in field hospitals.

	Examples	Further
First aid	Suturing cuts and lacerations, splinting simple fractures	Review at local hospital
Emergency care for life-threatening injuries	Endotracheal intubation, tracheotomy, relieving tension pneumothorax, stopping external haemorrhage, relieving an extradural haematoma, emergency thoracotomy/laparotomy for internal haemorrhage	After damage control surgery, transfer patients to base hospitals once stable
Initial care for non-life-threatening injuries	Debridement of contaminated wounds, reduction of fractures and dislocations, application of external fixators, vascular repairs	Transfer patients to base hospitals for definitive management

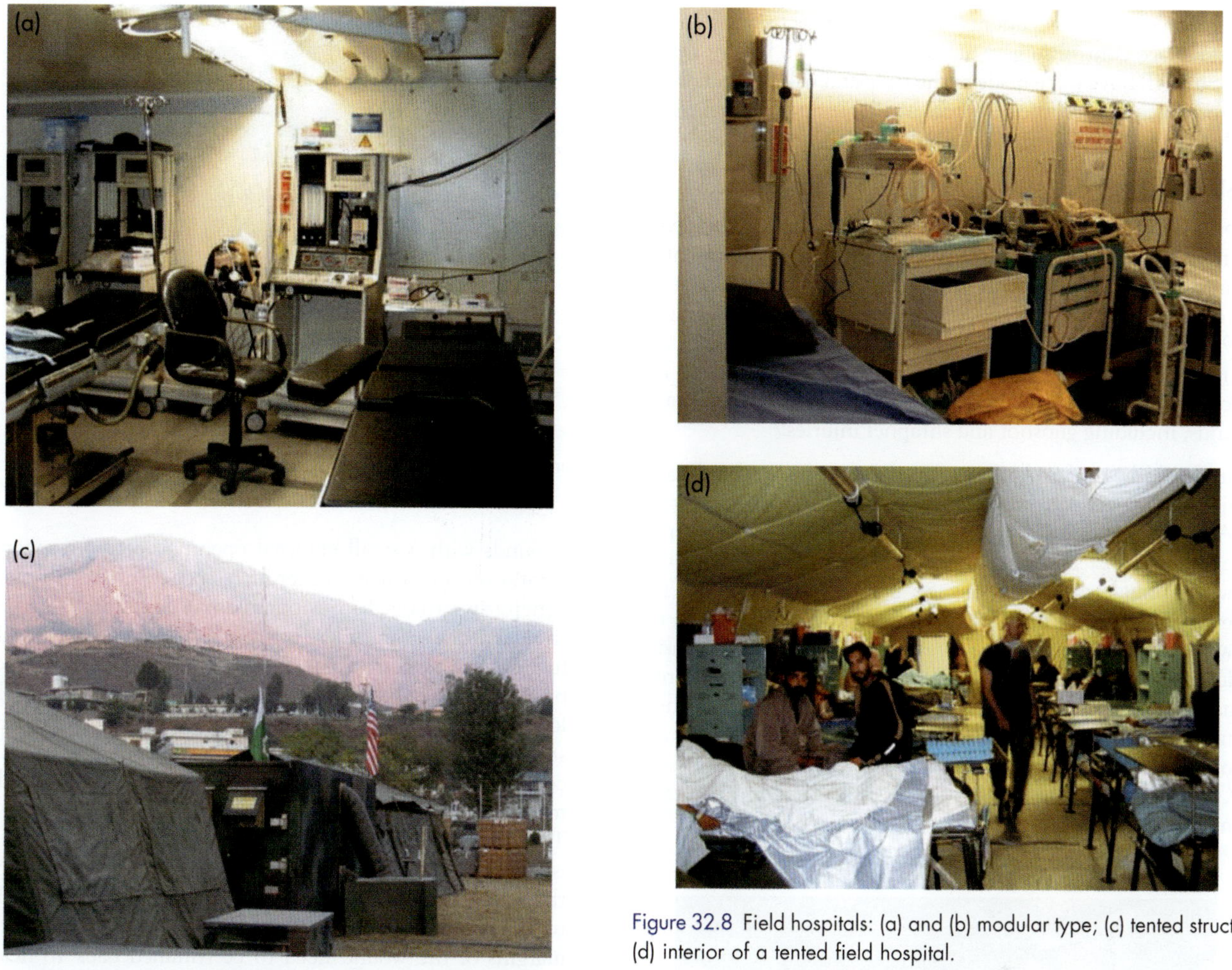

Figure 32.8 Field hospitals: (a) and (b) modular type; (c) tented structure; (d) interior of a tented field hospital.

Summary box 32.5

Principles of damage control surgery

- Do the minimum needed to allow safe transfer to definitive facility
- Take actions which prevent deterioration of that patient during transfer
- Secure the airway (tracheostomy?)
- Control bleeding (craniotomy, laparotomy, thoracotomy, repair major limb vessels?)
- Prevent pressure build up (burr holes, chest drain, laparotomy, fasciotomy?)
- Prevent infection by extensile exposure and removing dead and contaminated tissue

Emergency care for immediate life-threatening injuries

There are many patients who may be saved by relatively simple measures provided that these are taken urgently. Endotracheal intubation and tracheotomy may be needed to provide a secure airway. A needle thoracocentesis will relieve a tension pneumothorax, and a chest drain will be needed before a patient with a significant chest injury is transferred by air. An open pneumothorax should be closed. A clam-shell thoracotomy can be used by all surgeons to open a chest rapidly when dealing with cardiac tamponard or major vessel damage in the thorax (Chapter 28). A laparotomy may be needed to isolate loops of bowel with penetrating injuries (simply staple across the bowel each side of the perforation). Excision and reanastomosis of damaged bowel can be left for definitive surgery later. If the abdomen is opened, it is probably best left open and covered with a sterile plastic sheet, during transfer to definitive care (Opsite closure). This will prevent the development of abdominal compartment syndrome, as well as saving time. Burr-holes will be needed if intracranial pressure is rising and is thought to be the result of an extradural haemorrhage, but a flap should not be raised (see Chapter 25). Damaged major vessels to limbs should be repaired if possible. Faciotomies will be needed for muscle compartments which are swelling from injury or from reperfusion. Amputation for clearly devitalised limbs and gas gangrene should be undertaken at field hospitals as delay will be fatal.

Initial care for non-life-threatening injuries

Many patients present with serious injuries that require complex, prolonged care. Compound limb fractures, degloving injuries, dislocations of major joints, major facial injuries and complex hand injuries all fall into this category. These patients will need specialised care requiring transfer to the appropriate facility. Replantations of amputated limbs and other extensive reconstructive procedures should not be attempted in field hospitals as they are time consuming and divert resources and personnel to the treatment of a few patients. The decision as to what constitutes damage control surgery and what should be left for definitive care will have to be made at the time and will depend on the number of casualties, the resources available and the logistics of transport to a definitive care facility.

Debridement

Debridement has come to mean more than simply the laying open of tissues. It plays a crucial part in the management of trauma. Wounds sustained in disasters are often heavily contaminated, containing foreign bodies and non-viable tissues (Figure 32.9). Debridement reduces the chances of anaerobic and necrotising infections and can prevent systemic sepsis. The following principles of debridement apply to all contaminated wounds, including gunshot and shrapnel injuries:

- It should be undertaken in a sterile environment with good lighting by surgeons who are well versed in trauma surgery.
- After the administration of anaesthesia, the first step is opening and cleaning of the injured area by copious irrigation with normal saline. Pulse lavage, if available, is ideal for this but a large syringe can also be used (Figure 32.10). Next, the wound is palpated and all foreign matter is lifted out using forceps. In-driven dirt is best removed using a nail brush as even small particles of retained dirt result in permanent tattooing. Dirt intimately enmeshed in the soft tissues can only be removed by excision of those contaminated tissues. Open joints should be thoroughly irrigated and all foreign material removed.

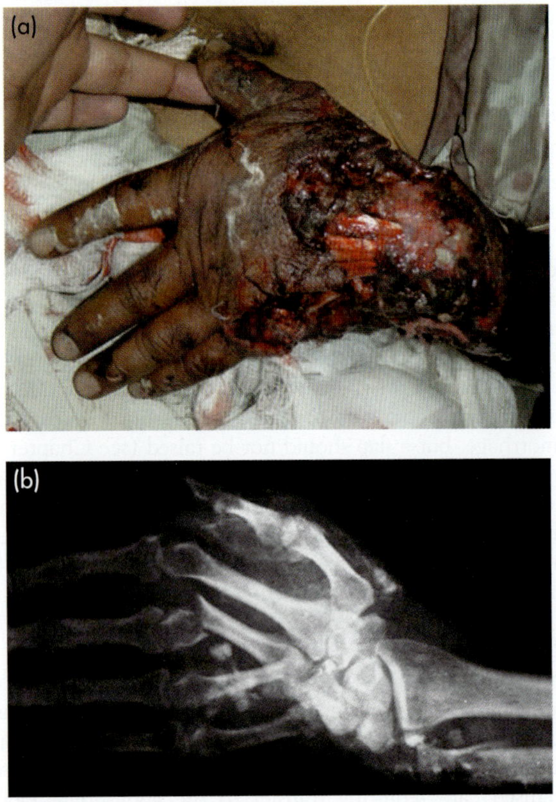

Figure 32.9 Gross contamination typically seen in wounds sustained in disasters. The radiograph shows numerous radio-opaque foreign bodies in the soft tissues.

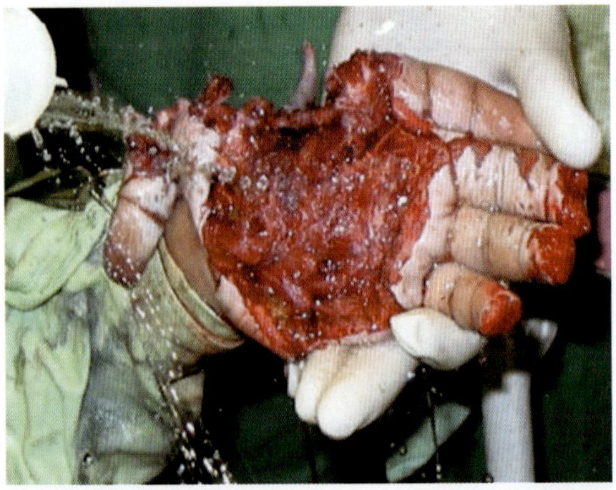

Figure 32.10 Lavage with normal saline to decontaminate a wound.

- Wounds with a small external opening but more extensive cavitation (firearm and other high-impact injuries) should be generously enlarged in a longitudinal direction (along with the deep fascia) in order to gain better access, and to allow full decompression of the underlying muscles. This should preferably be carried out under tourniquet to reduce blood loss. This extensile exposure helps to visualise the damaged structures and allows the surgeon to gain proximal and distal control of vascular injuries, and to identify severed ends of major nerves and tendons.
- The next step is excision of all dead and devitalised tissue. It is advisable at this stage to let down the tourniquet to check the vascularity of the tissues. Skin excision should be kept to a minimum as it is quite resistant to trauma and only the margins of the wound need to be trimmed back to healthy bleeding edges. Removal of devitalised muscle is important and should be undertaken generously. Muscle that is pale or dark in colour, has a soft consistency, does not contract on pinching, and does not bleed on cutting is definitely non-viable and must be removed if the risk of gangrene is to be minimised. Small pieces of crushed bone lying free should be removed. Large segments of bone that retain some soft-tissue attachment should be left undisturbed. In patients with traumatic amputations, the bone ends are tidied, the skin and muscle edges trimmed to the lowest level possible and the wound left open.
- In patients with associated fractures, skeletal stabilisation should be obtained before embarking on any repairs. External fixators are invaluable for this and make wound management much easier (Figure 32.11).
- In major trauma in the acute setting, only vascular repairs are justified. For lacerated vessels, the ends are trimmed and an anastomosis performed. In the case of loss of substance of the vessel wall a vein patch or reversed vein graft may be employed. Silicone tubing may be used as a temporary bypass (stent) while vascular repair is being carried out in patients with critically compromised distal circulation.
- Nerves and tendons should not be dissected out, nor any attempt made at definitive repair in wounds with tissue devitalisation and gross oedema, as it leads to poor results. The key structures should simply be identified and the edges trimmed and tagged with non-absorbable sutures to facilitate repair during subsequent exploration.

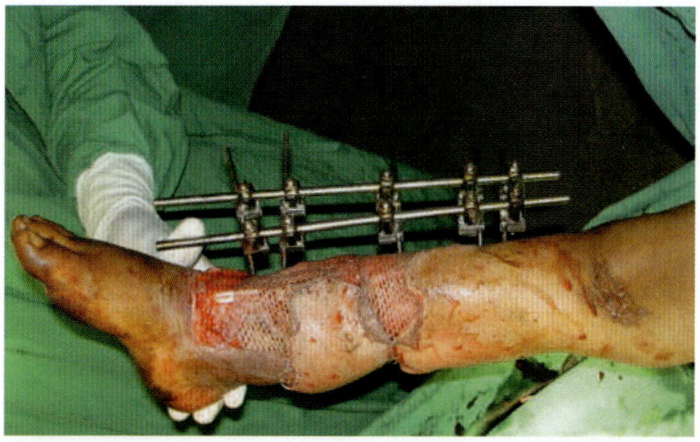

Figure 32.11 External fixators provide skeletal stabilisation and allow easy management of the soft tissues.

- Wounds sustained in disasters are heavily contaminated and therefore are not suitable for primary closure. However, blood vessels (whether repaired or simply exposed) and exposed joint surfaces need to be covered. This can be achieved by loosely tacking adjoining muscle over the exposed area. The wound is then covered with fluffed gauze and sterile cotton and the extremity splinted with a plaster of Paris slab, even if there is no fracture. For the upper extremity, elevation with a drip stand and, for the lower limb, elevation on a couple of pillows are important to reduce oedema.
- Broad-spectrum antibiotics, such as third-generation cephalosporins, are started prophylactically and continued for 5–7 days.
- The wound should be reinspected at 24–48 hours to assess the viability of the tissues and the distal circulation. The wounds are closed between the fourth and sixth day if there is no infection. Tension should be avoided and you should not hesitate to use partial thickness skin grafts to obtain cover. Skin staplers are particularly useful and save time when dealing with large numbers of casualties.
- In wounds with gross infection, no attempt at closure is made until infection is eradicated. These wounds are re-explored to make sure that there are no residual foreign bodies or devitalised tissue. Surface swabs are not useful, but tissue should be taken for microbiological culture. Vacuum-assisted closure (Vac-Pac) has emerged as a very useful tool for irregular and deeply cavitating wounds. It utilises low-pressure suction to evacuate exudate, promote granulation tissue and reduce the size of the wound (Figure 32.12). Once the wounds are free from infection secondary closure can be undertaken (Summary box 32.6).

Summary box 32.6

Principles of debridement and initial wound care

- Obtain generous exposure through skin and fascia
- Identify neurovascular bundles
- Excise devitalised tissue
- Remove foreign bodies
- Repair major vessels
- Obtain skeletal stabilisation with external fixators
- Only tag tendons and nerves which have been cut
- Leave the wound open and delay primary closure
- Avoid tight dressings
- Elevate the injured limb

DEFINITIVE MANAGEMENT

Definitive management is undertaken at major hospitals. They should be given as much notice as possible as to the expected number of casualties so that the staff are prepared. The hospitals to which casualties are sent should be selected on the basis of the facilities available and the number of injured that they can handle. The actual number of beds available is seldom a good guide to capacity, as the ancillary resources required for trauma patients are more than for the typical case mix of a hospital. A rule of thumb is that only half the bed strength of a hospital can be utilised to provide optimum trauma care in an emergency situation.

Hospital reorganisation

In hospitals receiving mass casualties during disasters, some reorganisation of services is unavoidable. This includes transferring patients with non-urgent conditions to other facilities, augmenting surgical services, reorganising the specialist rota and redesignating medical wards as surgical care areas to accommodate the patient load. A quick check of hospital inventories should be undertaken to ensure availability of essential equipment and medicines. An appeal for blood donations should be broadcast.

SPECIFIC ISSUES

There is no injury that is peculiar to disasters. Destruction of buildings and explosions can produce the whole spectrum of external injuries from minor cuts to extensive degloving,

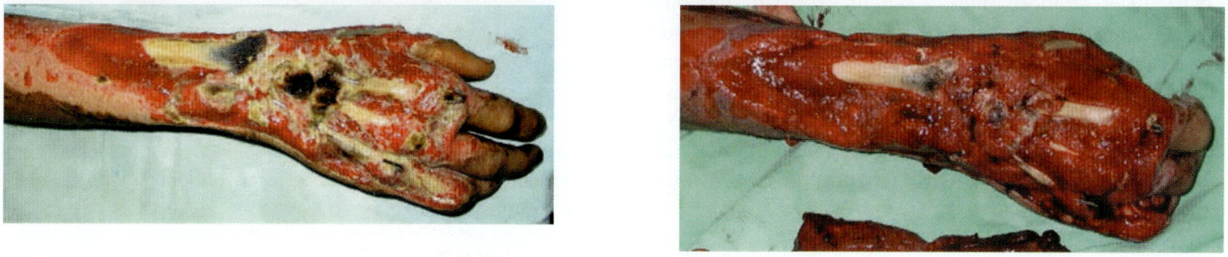

Figure 32.12 Use of low-pressure vacuum therapy in preparing a wound for secondary closure.

compound fractures and amputations. Internal organ damage is frequent and, unless immediate help is available, this accounts for the major share of early mortality figures. People trapped under fallen buildings may suffer crush injuries and crush syndrome if the duration is prolonged. Those near an explosion can suffer injury to the lungs and abdominal viscera, as well as burns, because of the heat of the blast.

Crush injuries and missile injuries cause extensive tissue damage and gross contamination, both favourable conditions for anaerobic and microaerophilic infections.

Limb salvage

The Mangled Extremity Severity Score (MESS) and its modifications are useful in making a judgement about limb salvage. In the past, extensive tissue loss, neurovascular damage and loss of long fragments of bone were all considered indications for amputation. Currently, with the use of microvascular flaps, wounds of any dimension can be covered with healthy tissue in a single stage. If performed in time, vascular repairs can salvage most acutely ischaemic limbs. Distraction osteogenesis and vascularised bone transfers can restore bony continuity in all but the most massive bone losses. In view of these developments the indications for amputation in trauma have undergone a paradigm shift and the majority of patients who reach a tertiary-care facility within 24 hours are candidates for limb salvage (Figure 32.13). This assumes that debridement and, if required, vascular repairs have been performed in a field medical facility. Restoration of vascular continuity is the critical issue. A limb is unlikely to survive if vascular repairs of major limb vessels has been delayed for more than 4–6 hours.

Facial injuries

The management of facial injuries follows the same general principles of debridement and delayed closure as already outlined. Because of the functional and cosmetic importance of facial structures, skin and soft-tissue excisions are kept to a minimum. There is a robust blood supply to the face and the ability to counter infection is therefore very high. Even in patients who present late with gross contamination, a careful debridement followed by delayed primary closure can lead to good results (Figure 32.14).

Tetanus

This potentially fatal condition, also called 'lockjaw', is caused by *Clostridium tetani*, a Gram-positive spore-forming bacillus occurring naturally in the intestines of humans and animals and in the soil. It enters the body through a wound and replicates, thriving on the anaerobic conditions present in devitalised tissues. It produces tetanospasmin, a potent exotoxin that binds to the neuromuscular junctions of the central nervous system neurones, rendering them incapable of neurotransmitter release. This leads to failure of inhibition of motor reflex responses to sensory stimulation. The result is generalised contractions of agonist and antagonist muscles causing tetanic spasms. The median incubation period is 7 days, ranging from 4 to 14 days (Summary 32.7).

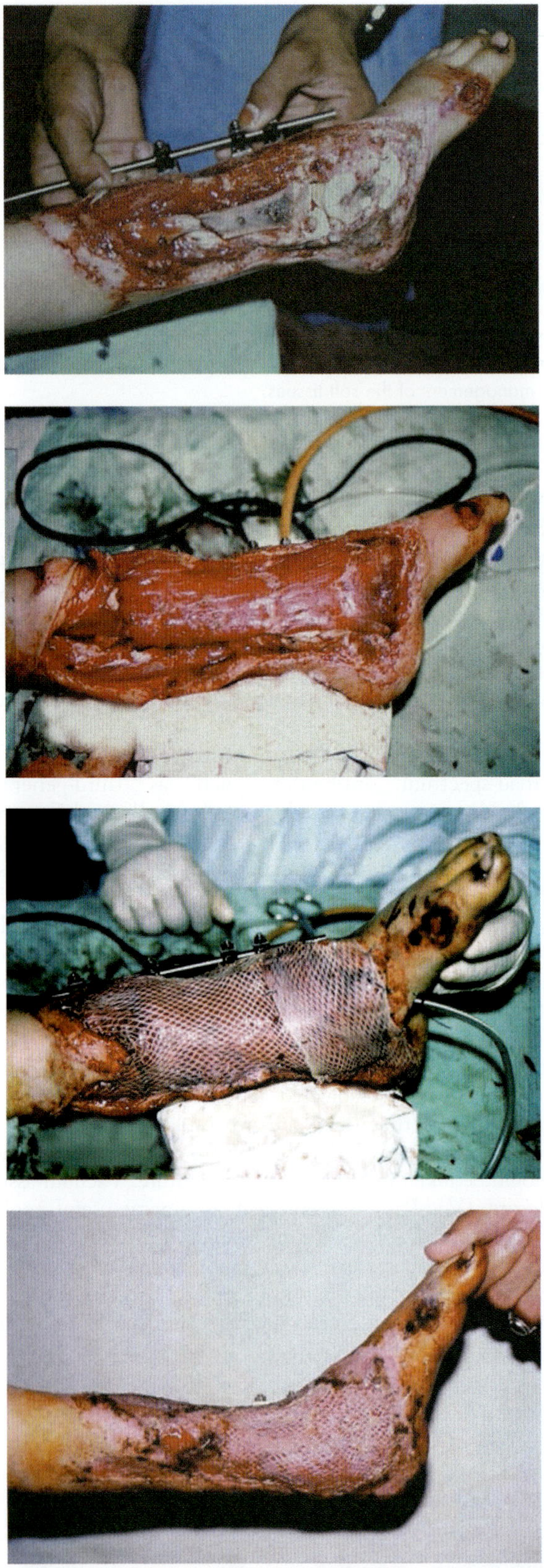

Figure 32.13 Badly traumatised lower limb. Reconstruction has been performed using a microvascular rectus abdominis flap covered with a skin graft.

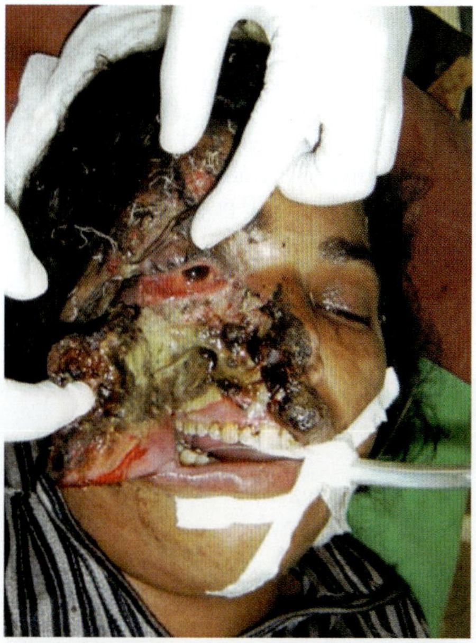

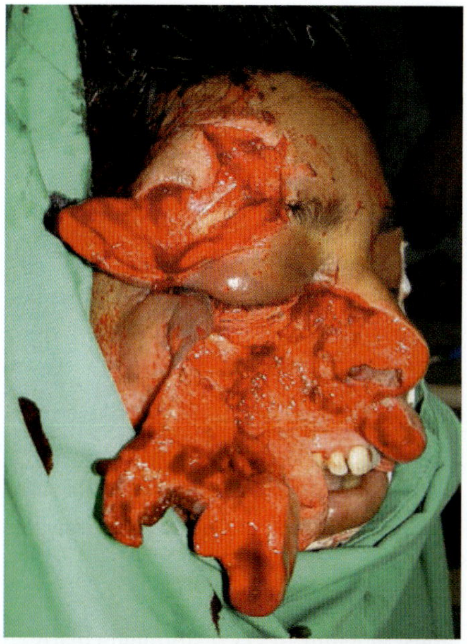

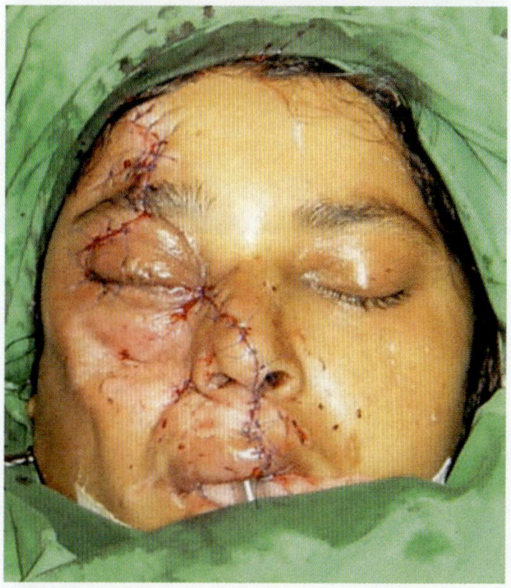

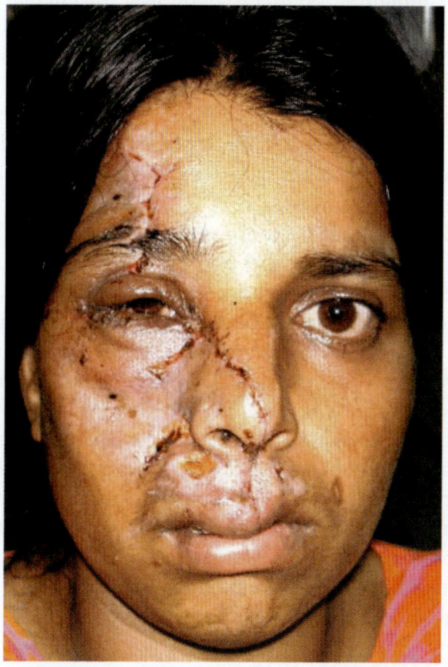

Figure 32.14 Late-presenting facial injury with gross contamination. A thorough debridement followed by delayed primary closure has yielded good results.

Summary box 32.7

Tetanus

- Caused by *Clostridium tetani*
- Spores are present in the soil
- Thrives in dead or contaminated tissue
- Produce tetanospasmin, an exotoxin
- Produces spasm of muscles
- Make sure patients are immunised
- For heavily contaminated wound, give anti-tetanus globulin

Early symptoms are painful spasms of the masseter and facial muscles resulting in the classical risus sardonicus (Figure 32.15). The spasms spread to involve the muscles of respiration and the laryngeal musculature. Spasms of the paravertebral and extensor limb musculature produce opisthotonus, an arching of the whole body. Laryngeal muscle spasm leads to apnoea and, if prolonged, to asphyxia and respiratory arrest. The spasms can be brought on by the slightest of sensory stimulus. They may be sustained and severe enough to produce long-bone fractures and joint dislocations.

The diagnosis is obvious once it is fully manifest. There are three aspects of management:

- **Prevention**. Wounds contaminated with soil are likely to harbour the tetanus spores, and active immunisation is indicated by administering 0.5 mL of tetanus toxoid intramuscularly. Patients with gross contamination of deeply cavitating wounds should also receive 250–500 units of human

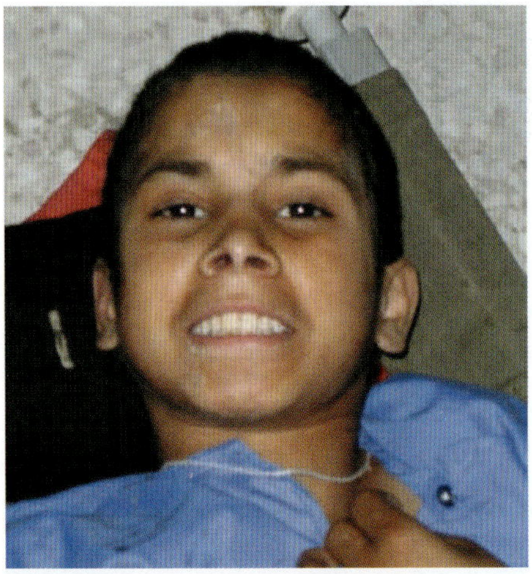

Figure 32.15 Risus sardonicus of 'lockjaw' (courtesy of Dr Samira Ajmal FRCS).

anti-tetanus globulin (ATG) intramuscularly to provide passive immunisation and to neutralise the circulating toxin. In full-blown clinical tetanus, 3000–10 000 units of ATG should be administered. Wound manipulation should be avoided for 2–3 hours after ATG administration to minimise tetanospasmin release.

- **Local wound care**. This includes a thorough wound debridement to eliminate the anaerobic environment. Intravenous administration of 10–24 × 106 units per day of penicillin G should be continued for 10–14 days. The wound should be closed using the delayed primary or secondary closure techniques (see above under Debridement).
- **Supportive care for established disease**. These patients are nursed in an intensive care unit (ICU) environment, free from strong sensory stimuli. Unnecessary manipulations are avoided. Diazepam is useful in preventing the onset of spasms but if these become frequent and sustained the patient should be paralysed, intubated and placed on a ventilator. The patient is then gradually weaned off the ventilator under cover of anticonvulsants. The overall mortality rate is around 45 per cent, prognosis being determined by the incubation period and the time from the first symptom to the first tetanic spasm. In general, shorter intervals indicate a poorer prognosis.

Necrotising fasciitis

Necrotising fasciitis is a dangerous and rapidly spreading infection of the fascial planes leading to necrosis of the subcutaneous tissues and overlying skin. It is caused by β-haemolytic streptococci and, occasionally, *Staphylococcus aureus*, but may take the form of a polymicrobial infection associated with other aerobic and anaerobic pathogens, including *Bacteroides*, *Clostridium*, *Proteus*, *Pseudomonas* and *Klebsiella*. It is termed Fournier's gangrene when it affects the perineal area, and Meleney's synergistic gangrene when it involves the abdominal wall. The underlying pathology is identical wherever it occurs and includes acute inflammatory infiltrate, extensive necrosis, oedema and thrombosis of the microvasculature. The area becomes oedematous, painful and very tender. The skin turns dusky blue and black secondary to the progressive underlying thrombosis and necrosis (Figure 32.16). The area may develop bullae and progress to overt cutaneous gangrene with subcutaneous emphysema. It spreads to contiguous areas but occasionally also produces skip lesions that later coalesce. It is accompanied by fever and severe generalised toxicity. Renal failure may occur as a result of hypovolaemia and cardiovascular collapse caused by septic shock. The rate of progression can catch the unwary by surprise and unless aggressively treated it leads to serious consequences with a mortality rate approaching 70 per cent (Summary box 32.8).

The diagnosis is usually made on clinical grounds. Creatinine kinase levels may show enormous elevation and biopsy of the fascial layers will confirm the diagnosis. Patients should

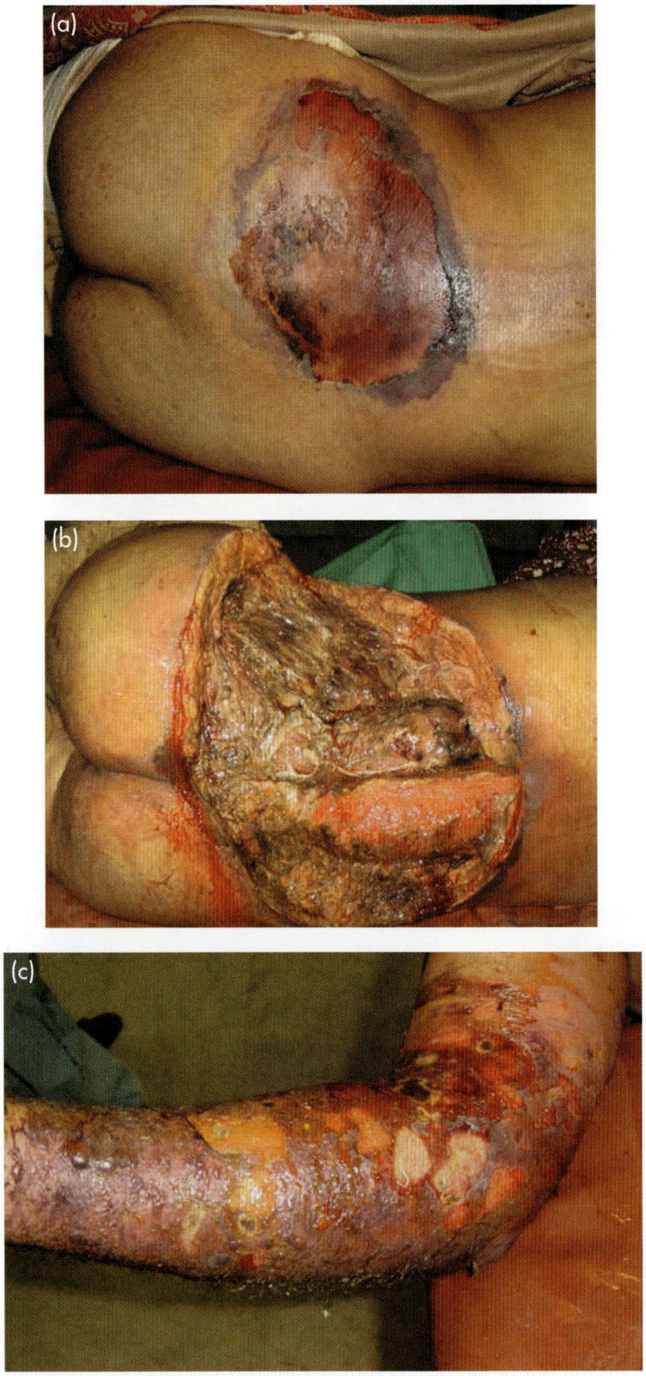

Figure 32.16 (a) Necrotising fasciitis at presentation and (b) rapid progression seen after 24 hours. (c) Typical bullae and induration.

Theodor Albrecht Edwin Klebs, 1834–1913, Professor of Bacteriology successively at Prague, Czechoslovakia, Zurich, Switzerland and then Rush Medical College, Chicago, IL, USA.
Frank Lamont Meleney, 1889–1963, Professor of Clinical Surgery, Columbia University, New York, NY, USA.
Jean Alfred Fournier, 1832–1915, syphilologist, the founder of the Venereal and Dermatological Clinic, Hospital St Louis, Paris, France.

Summary box 32.8

Necrotising fasciitis

- Caused by beta-haemolytic strep or is polymicrobial
- Also called Fournier's or Meleney's gangrene
- Progress is rapid and renal failure is an early complication
- Treat with radical surgical excision repeated every 24 hours
- Give oxygen and penicillin

be admitted to the ICU and treated aggressively with careful monitoring of volume derangements and cardiac status. Oxygen supplementation is beneficial and endotracheal intubation is required in patients unable to maintain their airway.

High-dose penicillin G along with broad-spectrum antibiotics, such as third-generation cephalosporins and metronidazole, should be given intravenously until the patient's toxicity abates. The cornerstone of management is surgical excision of the necrotic tissue. The fascial planes are opened with ease as the infection produces inflammatory degloving and the yellowish-green necrotic fascia is visible. Devitalised tissue should be removed generously, preferably going beyond the area of induration. This can lead to profuse bleeding and it is wise to have blood already cross-matched. The wound is lightly packed with fluffed gauze and then dressed. This process should be continued on a daily basis as the necrosis is prone to spread beyond the edges of the excised wound. In patients who survive, this results in a large wound, which will require skin grafting or flap coverage.

Recently, the role of hyperbaric oxygen (HBO) has become more established. It is claimed that it is bactericidal, improves neutrophil function and promotes wound healing. The patient is placed in a high-pressure chamber and 100 per cent oxygen administered at a pressure of 2–3 atmospheres. Studies have shown a reduction in mortality rate in patients treated with HBO (9–20 per cent) compared with patients who did not receive HBO (30–50 per cent). The main limitation to its use is availability of the pressure chamber.

Gas gangrene

Gas gangrene is a dreaded consequence of inadequately treated missile wounds, crushing injuries and high-voltage electrical injuries. It is a rapidly progressive, potentially fatal condition characterised by widespread necrosis of the muscles and subsequent soft-tissue destruction. The common causative organism is *Clostridium perfringens*, a spore-forming, Gram-positive saprophyte that flourishes in anaerobic conditions. Other organisms implicated in gas gangrene include *C. bifermentans*, *C. septicum* and *C. sporogenes*. They are present in the soil and have also been isolated from the human gastrointestinal tract and female genital tract. Non-clostridial gas-producing organisms, such as coliforms, have also been isolated in 60–85 per cent of cases of gas gangrene (Summary box 32.9).

Clostridium perfringens produces many exotoxins, but their exact role is unclear. Alpha-toxin, the most important, is a lecithinase, which destroys red and white blood cells, platelets, fibroblasts and muscle cells. The phi-toxin produces myocardial suppression while the kappa-toxin is responsible for the destruction of connective tissue and blood vessels.

Wounds which have become contaminated with clostridial spores then become infected if devitalised tissue, foreign bodies or premature wound closure provide the anaerobic conditions necessary for spore germination. The usual incubation period is <24 hours, but it can range from 1 hour to 6 weeks. A vicious cycle of tissue destruction is initiated by rapidly multiplying bacteria and locally and systemically acting exotoxins. Locally, this results in spreading necrosis of muscle and thrombosis of blood vessels while progressive oedema further compromises the blood supply. The typical feature of this condition is the production of gas (composed of nitrogen, hydrogen sulphide and carbon dioxide) that spreads along the muscle planes. Systemically, the exotoxins cause severe haemolysis and, combined with the local effects, this leads to the rapid progression of the disease, hypotension, shock, renal failure and acute respiratory distress syndrome (ARDS).

Summary box 32.9

Gas gangrene

- Caused by *Clostridium perfringens*
- Spores are present in the soil
- Thrives in anaerobic conditions and produces many exotoxins
- Treat with radical and regular surgical excision
- Give oxygen and penicillin
- Early amputation may be life-saving

The earliest symptom is acute onset of pain that increases in severity as the myonecrosis progresses. The limb swells up and the wound exudes a serosanguinous discharge. The skin is involved secondary to underlying muscle necrosis, turning brown and progressing to a blue-black colour with the appearance of haemorrhagic bullae (Figure 32.17). The characteristic sickly sweet odour and soft tissue crepitus caused by gas production appear with established infection, but the absence of either does not exclude the diagnosis. These local signs are accompanied by pyrexia, a tachycardia disproportionate to body temperature, tachypnoea and alteration in mental status.

The diagnosis is made on the basis of history and clinical features: a peripheral blood smear may suggest haemolysis; a Gram stain of the exudate reveals large Gram-positive bacilli without neutrophils; and the biochemical profile may show metabolic acidosis and renal failure. Radiography can visualise gas in the soft tissues and computed tomography (CT) scans are useful in patients with chest and abdominal involvement.

Patients should be admitted to the ICU and treated

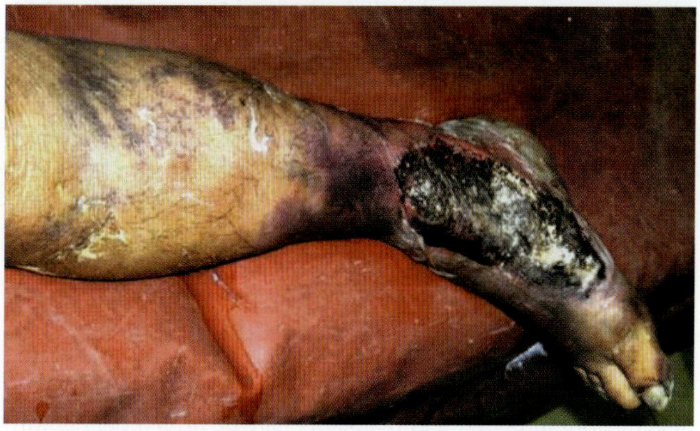

Figure 32.17 Typical picture of spreading gas gangrene caused by crush injury.

aggressively with careful monitoring. High-dose penicillin G and clindamycin, along with third-generation cephalosporins, should be given intravenously until the patient's toxicity abates. The mainstay of management is early surgical excision of the necrotic tissue. The muscle planes are opened through generous longitudinal incisions and all devitalised tissue is removed, going beyond the area of induration. Excision should be continued daily until the process of necrosis has stopped spreading. In established gas gangrene with systemic toxicity, amputation of the involved extremity is life saving and should not be delayed. No attempt is made at closure, amputation stumps are left open and the wound is lightly packed with saline-soaked gauze and then dressed.

The role of HBO is not as clear as in necrotising fasciitis, but it is recommended in severe cases if the facilities are available.

Blast injuries

Mechanism of explosive blast injury

The explosive pressure accompanying the bursting of bombs or shells ruptures their casing and imparts a high velocity to the fragments. These can cause even more devastating injury to the tissues than bullets. In addition, all explosions are accompanied by a complex blast wave composed of a blast pressure wave (dynamic overpressure) and the mass movement of air (blast wind). A mass movement of air from the rapid expansion of gases at the centre of the explosion displaces air at supersonic speed. This results in injury patterns ranging from traumatic amputation to total body disruption. When a blast pressure wave hits the body, the force of the impact sets up a series of stress waves that are capable of internal injury, particularly at air–fluid interfaces. Thus, injury to the ear, lungs, heart and, to a lesser extent, the gastrointestinal tract is notable (Summary box 32.10).

Summary box 32.10

Blast injuries

- Each fragment is a high velocity missile
- The blast wave hits air–fluid interfaces and bursts them
- Explore and fully excise each wound as all are likely to be heavily contaminated

General management of blast injuries

The structures injured by the primary blast wave, in order of prevalence, are the middle ear, the lungs and the bowel. However, the most common urgent clinical problem in survivors are penetrating injuries caused by blast-energised debris and fragments of the exploding device. Many of those exposed to a blast will have blunt, blast and thermal injuries in addition to more obvious penetrating wounds. The deafness of blast victims caused by tympanic membrane rupture makes communication difficult and may complicate early assessment. Here, the primary survey and resuscitation phases of a system such as Advanced Trauma and Life Support (ATLS) are particularly apt. The management of penetrating wounds differs little from that of missile wounds referred to earlier. The soft-tissue wounds are usually heavily contaminated and fragments may be driven deeply into adjacent tissue planes opened up by the force of the explosion. In blast injuries, one cannot be sure of complete wound excision and it is imperative that wounds should be left open at the end of the initial operation and delayed primary closure performed.

Crush injury and syndrome

A crush injury occurs when a body part is subjected to a high degree of force or pressure, usually after being squeezed between two heavy or immobile objects. Damage related to a crush injury includes lacerations, fractures, bleeding, bruising, compartment syndrome and crush syndrome. It can have disastrous consequences on local tissues with extensive destruction and devitalisation (Figure 32.18).

Crush syndrome

The association between crush injury, rhabdomyolysis and acute renal failure was first reported in victims trapped during the 'London Blitz'. It is seen in earthquake and mining accident survivors and in battlefield casualties. Prolonged crushing of muscle leads to a reperfusion injury when the casualty is rescued. This releases myoglobin and vasoactive mediators into the circulation. It also sequesters many litres of fluid, reducing the effective intravascular volume and resulting in renal vasoconstriction and ischaemia. The myoglobinuria leads to renal failure from tubular obstruction (Summary box 32.11).

Summary box 32.11

Crush syndrome

- Arises as a result of reperfusion
- Renal failure from myoglobinuria is a complication
- A late fasciotomy may make things worse not better

The treatment of crushed casualties should begin as soon as they are discovered. Rescuers must be alert to the presence of associated injuries (Figure 32.19). Aggressive volume-loading of patients, preferably before extrication, is the best treatment. After provision of first aid and starting intravenous fluids the patient should be catheterised to measure urine output. In adults, a saline infusion of 1000–1500 mL/hour should be initiated. Alkalinisation of the urine increases the solubility of acid haematin in urine and aids its excretion. This should be continued until myoglobin is no longer detectable in the urine. Mannitol administration can reduce the reperfusion component of this injury. Once a flow of urine is observed, a mannitol–alkaline diuresis of up to 8 litres/day should be maintained, keeping the urinary pH greater than 6.5. A late fasciotomy when it is obvious that the muscles of that compartment must be dead is only likely to cause a massive release of myoglobin, as well as potentially introducing infection into dead tissue. It therefore best not to perform a fasciotomy in cases where entrapment has occurred for over 12 hours.

Intensive care is required with close attention to fluid balance and renal dialysis if required.

Compartment syndrome

A compartment syndrome develops when the pressure within a muscle compartment starts to rise as a result of trauma. This

The London Blitz is the name given to the German air raids on London between September 7, 1940 and May 17, 1941, during which it is estimated that more than 15 000 people were killed. Blitz is short for *Blitzkrieg*, the German for 'lightning war'.

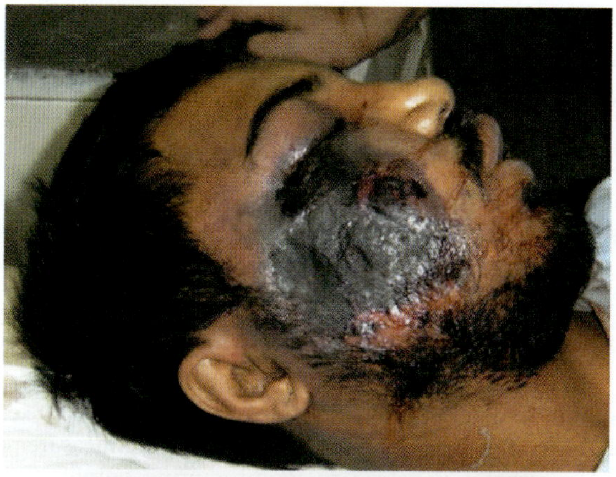

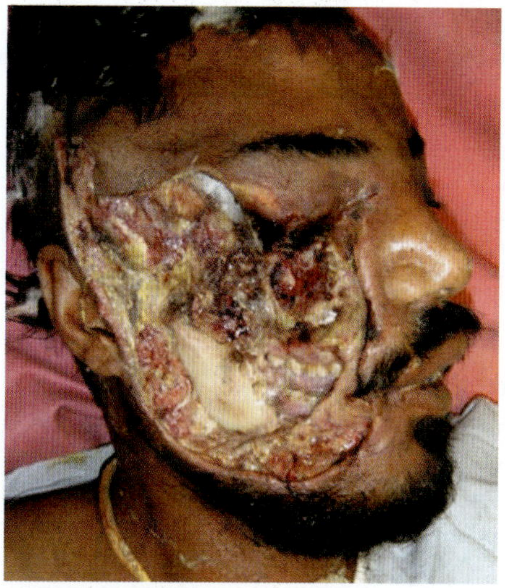

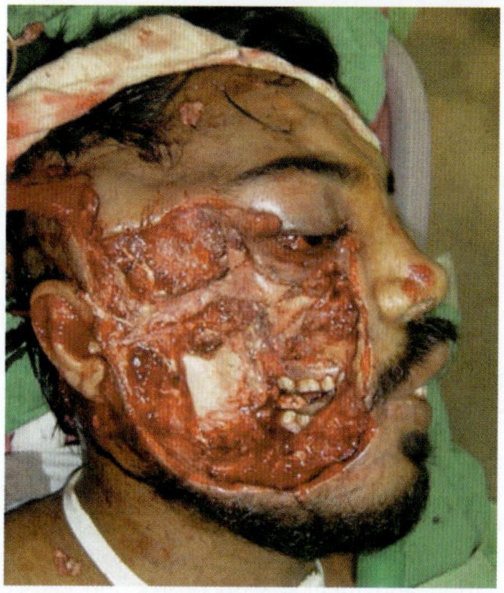

Figure 32.18 Extensive crush injury in a man trapped in a fallen house. The depth to which the soft tissues have been devitalised is seen clearly.

normally only occurs in muscles enclosed in a fascia, such as the muscles of the calf and forearm, and the intrinsic muscles of the hand and foot. It is less likely to occur in an open fracture, as the integrity of the fascial compartment is breached. An overly tight bandage or plaster, haemorrhage from a closed fracture,

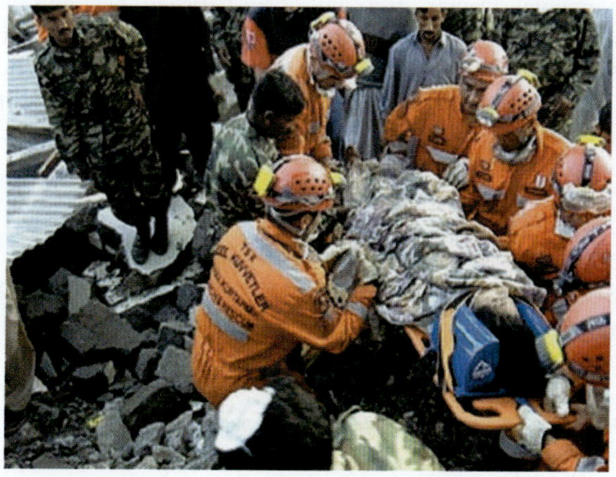

Figure 32.19 Rescuers must be prepared for injuries to the spine. Treatment of crush syndrome should start before extrication.

or severe blunt trauma to the muscle leads to a rise in pressure in the compartment until it exceeds venous drainage pressure. The thin-walled veins then collapse under the raised external pressure, and they no longer allow blood to leave the compartment. If the pressure in the compartment is not relieved, it will then rise to mean arterial pressure and perfusion of the muscle will cease. It is important to note that at this stage the distal pulses will still be palpable, though some patients may develop early paraesthesias in the extremity. However, passive stretching of the affected muscle will cause extreme pain and this is diagnostic of the condition. It is at this stage that the situation is still salvageable. Removal of any constricting bandage or plaster, and then if necessary a fasciotomy, will relieve the pressure and perfusion of the muscle will restart. If the condition is left unrelieved then any nerves passing through that compartment will cease to function (distal numbness) and in the final stages even the distal pulses may be lost. The muscle will die and then undergo fibrosis and shortening, producing a Volkmann's ischaemic contracture. Pressure studies are not reliable and if in doubt perform a fasciotomy. Intracompartmental pressure measurements should only be used for diagnosis in the unconscious patient where the classic sign of extreme pain on passive stretching cannot be elicited. Closure of the wound will need to be delayed (Summary box 32.12).

Summary box 32.12

Compartment syndrome

- Most common in a closed fracture or soft-tissue crush injury
- Pain on passive extension of the muscles is diagnostic
- Intracompartmental pressure studies are not reliable
- If there is any suspicion, then fasciotomy must be performed early

Summary box 32.13

Hypothermia

- Occurs commonly after trauma
- Diagnosed by rectal temperature of 35°C or less
- Rewarming should be passive
- Cardiac arrhhthmias and clotting disorders are likely in severe cases
- Continue resuscitation until the patient has been rewarmed

Hypothermia

Hypothermia is a major cause of morbidity and mortality during disasters in cold regions and at high altitudes. It develops rapidly if the individual is immersed in water, covered with wet clothing or exposed to windy conditions. The body responds to cold temperatures by peripheral vasoconstriction as a result of catecholamine release. Shivering is caused by increased tone of the musculature. If the body temperature continues to fall, the body's metabolism declines, and bradycardia with hypoventilation develops. The risk of ventricular fibrillation increases at temperatures below 28°C (82.4°F), and the clotting mechanism is also compromised in hypothermia.

In mild hypothermia, symptoms are vague, including dizziness, lethargy, joint stiffness and nausea. The skin becomes pale and the patient may exhibit confusion and impaired judgement, which progresses to uncoordinated movements and slurred speech. In severe hypothermia, the mental status is further impaired, leading to hallucinations, stupor and coma. Cardiac arrest usually occurs at 20°C (68°F).

The diagnosis is based on a history of exposure and is confirmed by finding a rectal temperatures of 35°C (95°) or less. The principles of treatment in the field include preventing further heat loss, restoring the core temperature and avoiding ventricular fibrillation.

The patient should be moved into dry shelter and wet clothing removed. A fire should be built or a stove lit to increase the temperature of the surroundings. No fluids should be given by mouth and the patient should be warmed passively. This is a safe and simple method of treating mild hypothermia and often the only choice in the field. The patient is covered with blankets or a sleeping bag and rewarmed for 24 hours at a room temperature of 25–33°C (77–91.4°F). Blood volume should be expanded using crystalloid solutions (warmed to 45°C/111°F). In adults, 300–500 mL should be administered rapidly, with the subsequent rate of infusion adjusted according to the blood pressure and urine output.

Severe hypothermia (<28°C/82.4°) should be treated as a life-threatening emergency. If the patient is breathing, humidified oxygen (10 litres/minute) should be administered using a non-rebreathing mask. If the patient is not breathing, ventilation should be initiated with an Ambu® bag connected to a humidified, heated oxygen delivery system. Supplemental oxygen is necessary to prevent hypoxia, reduce the risk of ventricular fibrillation and treat pulmonary oedema (Summary box 32.13).

Even after prolonged cardiac arrest, resuscitation is possible, and patients should not be declared dead until they are first rewarmed. If the patient is still not breathing, endotracheal intubation should be undertaken to maintain the airway. External cardiac compression must be continued in pulseless patients for some time. A central line or a venous cut-down should be established to administer warm fluids and for pressure measurements. A Foley catheter is passed to monitor urine output. Cardiac arrhythmias represent an immediate threat to life, but most revert spontaneously with rewarming. At core body temperatures below 30°C (86°F), the heart is usually unresponsive to defibrillation and inotropic agents, so medications are best withheld until rewarming has been achieved.

In severe hypothermia, active rewarming is required, which involves the internal or external addition of heat to the body: externally by heating blankets and warm water immersion; internally by heated humidified inhalation, peritoneal dialysis, haemodialysis or extracorporeal bypass.

Frost bite and immersion injuries (Trench foot)

Frost-bite occurs when a part of the body freezes. The cells are disrupted and the tissue dies. It is in effect a 'cold' burn and can be categorized according to the depth that it affects in the same way as a conventional burn. Other mechanisms are also at play in its causation and include vasoconstriction caused by cold, capillary sludging and reperfusion injury with the release of free radicals which occurs on rewarming the part. It can occur in fingers, toes, cheeks, the tip of the nose and the ears. When frozen, the tissue feels hard and cannot be indented. Immersion injury is a cold injury which does not involve actual freezing of the tissue and is commonly caused by prolonged immersion in cold water (hence 'trench foot'). The patient may also be hypothermic. Warming should be gentle as the heat used may actually cause a burn. Rehydration with warm fluids and use of non-steroidal anti-inflammatory drugs (NSAID), like ibuprofen, are beneficial. Demarcation will occur between dead and viable tissue and at this stage no surgery should be undertaken as there is often considerable deep recovery. The injured area should be kept clean and dry and every effort made to prevent further injury to it, as well as to prevent infection. Definitive surgery to excise dead tissue can be left for many months (Summary box 32.14).

Summary box 32.14

Frostbite

- Can be superficial or deep like a burn
- Rewarm gently
- Allow demarcation to occur naturally
- Protect against further trauma and infection

Frederick Eugene Basil Foley, 1891–1966, urologist, Ankher Hospital, St Paul, MN, USA.

HANDING OVER

Follow up and secondary problems

The medical aspect of disaster management does not involve a single short-term effort. It requires a long-term commitment and involvement of various disciplines. Because of the large numbers of casualties, the initial treatment received by patients is directed towards the anatomical restoration of damaged structures. This does not always translate into good functional results. There are therefore numerous patients who will need secondary procedures, such as nerve, tendon and bone grafts, release of contractures and treatment of chronic infection (osteomyelitis). This second wave of patients is encountered three to six months following a major catastrophe and appropriate arrangements should be made to deal with this.

Designated centres

Initially, the casualties seen in major disasters may be scattered among many hospitals. After the first few weeks most of the acute problems have been dealt with and only those patients who require longer-term treatment remain. At this point, it is advisable to designate a particular hospital as a centre for patients with spinal cord injuries and complex limb trauma, who require combined orthopaedic and plastic surgical care along with rehabilitation. It concentrates resources and expertise and makes it easier to follow up these patients.

DISASTER PLANS

Disasters are unforeseen events and planning for them may seem paradoxical. It has, however, been shown that disaster planning not only works but also saves lives. Disaster planning is a wide field but a résumé of the important aspects follows.

Establishment of a national level disaster management organisation

This is the first step in the planning for disasters. Most developed countries already have such an agency, which can formulate policy at the national level and has the infrastructure to react quickly when the need arises.

Anticipating disasters

Areas near active volcanoes and geological fault lines are at risk from seismic disturbances, whereas regions along major rivers are liable to flood. The urban centres of all countries are now potential targets for terrorist attacks. It is important to not only carry out threat assessments, but also, if possible, set up an early warning system (Summary box 32.15).

Summary box 32.15

Disaster planning

- Disaster can be anticipated and should be prepared for
- Evacuation of a whole population may be a best option
- Coordination between military, police, fire, ambulance and medical services is important

Evacuation planning

Evacuation of large population centres as a prelude to or in the wake of an impending disaster is a complex exercise. Yet it may be the most prudent course of action to remove as many people as possible from harm's way. Clear identification of exit routes must be determined and communicated to the populations at risk.

Organisation of emergency services

Emergency services such as the fire brigade, police and ambulance service must have definite roles and areas of responsibility assigned to them to ensure a smooth and coordinated response during a crisis. Members of these teams must be included in the planning phase to ensure that the final plan is practicable and reflects the situation on the ground.

Medical planning

Identification of hospitals able to take large numbers of casualties and the location of areas that can be used for patient holding and triage in case of mass casualties is very important. Hospitals that offer specialised services should be identified and their role during a major crisis made clear. Suitable hospitals in the surrounding areas must be designated as overflow hospitals in the eventuality of a very large volume of patients.

FURTHER READING

Der Heide EA. *Disaster response: principles of preparedness and coordination.* St Louis, MO: Mosby, 1989.

Hogan DE, Burstein JL. *Disaster medicine*, 2nd edn. Philadelphia, PA: Lippincott, Williams & Wilkins, 2007.

Huskjum H, Gilbert M, Wisborg T. *Save lives save limbs – life support for victims of mines, wars and accidents.* Malaysia: Third World Network, 2000.

Mattox K, Feliciano DV, Moore EE (eds). *Trauma*, 6th edn. New York: McGraw Hill, 2008.

Website

Center for Excellence in Disaster Management and Humanitarian Assistance. http://coe-dmha.org/.

PART

5 Elective orthopaedics

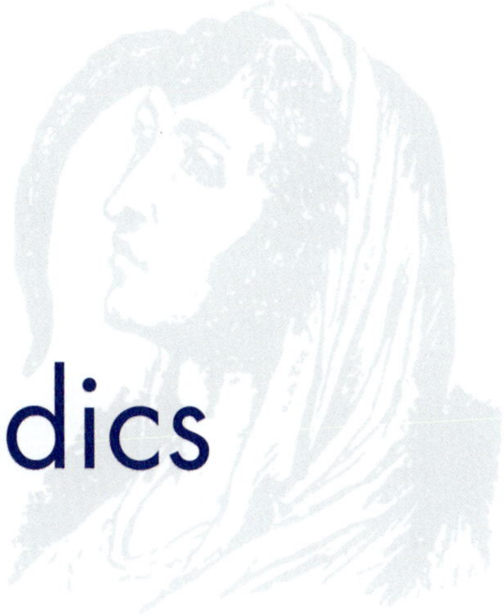

CHAPTER 33

History taking and clinical examination in musculoskeletal disease

LEARNING OBJECTIVES

To understand how to:

- Take a general orthopaedic history
- Perform a systematic examination of each region of the musculoskeletal system

INTRODUCTION

The components of the musculoskeletal system include the bones, joints, ligaments, muscles and tendons as well as the neurological and vascular structures. A simple system allows a concise yet comprehensive history to be taken and a reliable examination to be performed, which will reveal all of the common as well as the more rare but dangerous musculoskeletal problems that are likely to be encountered in clinical practice.

HISTORY

Introduction

- Introduce yourself and check the patient's name and date of birth.
- Explain what you are going to do, obtain verbal consent and ensure that the patient is comfortable.

Take a history

- **Presenting complaint**. Start with an open-ended question. Ask the patient to 'explain what the problem is' in their own words, and ask the patient what their hopes and expectations are from the interview.
- **History of the presenting complaint** ('the three Ws'). When did you first notice the problem? What were you doing when it started? Was is sudden or did it develop gradually?
- **Associated symptoms**. Ask about the following: pain; swelling; instability – 'giving way'; mechanical symptoms (e.g. locking, clicking, clunking); loss of power; altered sensation.
- **Functional impairment**. Ask whether the patient is having difficulties performing activities of daily living: upper limb, e.g. personal hygiene, feeding; lower limb, e.g. putting on shoes and socks, standing, walking and climbing stairs.
- **Past medical history** (PMH). Check for comorbid conditions which may affect the patient's fitness for an anaesthetic, e.g. diabetes, asthma, previous heart attack or stroke. Check for any previous problems with anaesthetics.
- **Past relevant surgical procedures**.
- **Drug history**. Ask about the following in particular: anticoagulants, steroids, aspirin, immunosuppressants, oral contraceptive pill and hormone replacement therapy.
- **Social history**. Tailor questions to the patient's condition: patient's age; hand dominance; employment status; dependents; alcohol; smoking and hobbies; home help; accommodation – own house, residential or nursing home; use of walking aids; mental test score assessment (Summary box 33.1).

Summary box 33.1

Taking a history

- Introduce yourself and put the patient at ease
- Explain what you are doing and ensure that the patient agrees
- Start with an open question for patient's agenda
- Check for history of presenting complaint and associated symptoms
- Ask about functional impairment
- Check past medical history and relevant surgical history
- Check drug and social history

MUSCULOSKETETAL EXAMINATION

General principles

Apley described a useful and systematic approach to clinical examination. This approach is divided into three parts:

Ernest William Hey Groves, 1872–1944, Professor of Surgery at Bristol. Born in India, he was one of the pioneers of orthopaedic surgery and a great pupil of Sir Robert Jones. Although an orthopaedic surgeon, in his early days, he was consulted by a lady with backache. He correctly diagnosed the cause of the backache to be an ovarian cyst. The lady insisted that Hey Groves should remove the cyst himself. With the help of his wife, a nurse, he successfully removed the cyst in an improvised room at his home. He was the founder member of the *British Journal of Surgery*.

Alan Graham Apley, 1914–1996, Director of Orthopaedic Surgery, St Thomas' Hospital, London, UK. As a consultant also at Rowley Bristow Orthopaedic Hospital, he conducted the most popular orthopaedic postgraduate course for the FRCS examination in Pyrford, Surrey, which became internationally known as the 'Pyrford Orthopaedic Course'.

1 look;
2 feel;
3 move.

Look

The inspection begins as soon as you enter the examination room. Look for any walking aids. Remember to look at the whole patient and not just at the joint of interest. For example:

- look at the hands for rheumatoid arthritis;
- look at the eyes for Horner's syndrome;
- look for any obvious upper or lower limb or spinal deformity.

Gait

The gait cycle is all of the activity between the initial contact of the foot with the ground and the succeeding initial contact of the same limb. There are two main stages: the stance phase (60 per cent) and the swing phase (40 per cent). Ask the patient to stand, and inspect from the front, side and back. Then, ask the patient to walk using any walking aids. Some of the types of limp that might be present are described in Table 33.1.

Focused inspection

Adequately expose the joint above and below. Expose the opposite limb for comparison. Make sure that the patient is comfortable. It may be easier for you and the patient if they remain standing for the first part of the examination. When a couch is used, make sure that it is in the centre of the room (not against the wall) so that you can work on both sides of the patient.

Remember that all joints are covered by an envelope of soft tissues and skin. Look at the skin for:

- surgical scars;
- bruising (may indicate recent injury or a bleeding disorder);
- erythema (e.g. cellulitis);
- ulcers (e.g. arterial, vascular or neuropathic);
- rashes;
- sinuses (e.g. secondary to osteomyelitis);
- hair loss and the presence or absence of sweating;
- pigmentations or raised lesion (e.g. café-au-lait spots or neurofibromas).

Look at the soft tissues for:
- swelling (e.g. may indicate a joint effusion);
- lumps (consider which tissue layer they are arising from);
- muscle wasting (e.g. may be secondary to disuse atrophy, neuropathy);
- muscle fasciculation (lower motor neurone pathology).

Look at the bones for:
- abnormal limb alignment – comparison with the other side may be helpful;
- deformity.

Feel

Ask the patient if they have any areas of tenderness. Ensure that you do not cause the patient pain – watch their face as you feel. It may be easier (especially with children) to feel the normal side first.

Skin

The aim of sensory testing is to establish a pattern of sensory loss. Look for a dermatomal (may indicate spinal root or peripheral nerve pathology) or glove and stocking distribution (may indicate a neuropathy, e.g. diabetes).

Perform a screening test by lightly stroking both limbs. Record whether the patient feels a difference. If none is noticed there is no need to spend more time on the neurological examination. If there is a difference, then a full neurological examination should now be performed.

Soft tissues

- Tenderness: Try to determine the actual anatomical structure from which the pain arises (e.g. subcutaneous fat, bursae, nerves, arteries).
- Lumps and effusions: Determine the characteristics of any lump or effusion using Table 33.2 as a guide.
- Pulses: Palpate the distal pulses (or capillary return) of the limb. Recording distal neurovascular status both before and after surgery is important. Absence of distal pulses is an

Friedrich Trendelenburg, 1844–1924, Professor of Surgery successively at Rostock (1875–1882), Bonn (1882–1895), Leipzig (1895–1911), Germany. The Trendelenburg position was first described in 1885.

Table 33.1 Types of limp.

Cause	Pathogenesis	Presentation
Long	Osteoarthitis (in other leg)	Head dips. Cadence dash/dash
Incoordinated	Cerebral palsy	Head moves everywhere. No regular cadence
Muscle weakness	Osteoarthritis hip	Head moves from side to side (windscreen wiper)
Pain	Osteoarthritis hip	Head dips. Cadence dot/dash
Stiff	Arthrodesis hip	Head rocks too and fro
Limp	**Pathology**	
Antalgic	Hip joint arthritis	
Trendelenburg	Weakness of hip abductors	
High-stepping gait	Foot drop secondary to common peroneal nerve palsy	
Spastic	Cerebral palsy	
Ataxic	Cerebellar pathology	

Johann Friedrich Horner, 1831–1886, Professor of Ophthalmology, Zurich, Switzerland, described this syndrome in 1869.

Table 33.2 Swelling – an acronym for history and examination of a lump.

Start	Did it appear after trauma or gradually on its own?
Where	Anatomical site and layer (skin, fat, muscle); does it move in relation to these?
External features	Size, surface and definition of margins
Lymph nodes	Are the local ones enlarged?
Liquid	Is it fluctuant? Can it be transilluminated?
Internal features	Is it hard? Is it tender?
Noise	Is there a thrill? Is there a bruit?
General	Examination of the whole patient for general lumps

absolute contraindication to elective surgery in that limb. Acute loss of circulation to a limb is a surgical emergency.

Bone

Palpate the contours of the joint and assess for tenderness. For superficial joints, such as the knee, the joint line can be felt and checked for lumps and tenderness.

Move

There are three stages to assessing movement. The words used to describe a particular movement are shown in Table 33.3.

Table 33.3 Terminology used to describe the direction of movement.

Flexion	Forward or anterior movement of the trunk or limb
Lateral flexion	Bending of the forward-facing head and trunk to either side
Extension	Backward or posterior movement
Abduction	A movement away from the midline of the body
Adduction	A movement towards the midline of the body
Internal rotation	Rotation towards the midline of the body
External rotation	Rotation away from the midline
Supination	Movement of the forearm so that the palm faces anteriorly
Pronation	Movement of the forearm so that the palm faces posteriorly
Circumduction	A combination of flexion, abduction, extension and adduction without rotation
Inversion	Movement of the foot that directs the sole of the foot medially
Eversion	Movement of the foot that directs the sole of the foot laterally
Retraction	Backwards movement of the head, jaw or shoulders

- **Active**. Ask the patient to move the joint within the limits of their pain.
- **Passive**. Move the joint yourself. Record the range of movement in 'degrees' (a goniometer may be helpful). Comparison of active and passive range allows the three causes of loss of range of movement to be distinguished. In limitation caused by pain or stiffness the ranges are the same but one is painful. In weakness passive range is greater than active.
- **Stability**. Stability has a static and a dynamic component: static tests assess the integrity of the ligaments and joint (bone) surfaces; dynamic tests assess the integrity and functions of the muscles and tendons. Ask the patient to actively move the joint through its range of motion while you try to stop the movement. Record power using the Medical Research Council (MRC) grading system as illustrated in Table 33.4. Consider the muscles that drive each movement, the peripheral nerves that supply them and the nerve root values (Table 33.5).

Table 33.4 The Medical Research Council grading system of muscle power.

Grade	Description
0	No movement
1	Flicker of movement
2	Active movement with gravity elimination
3	Active movement against gravity
4	Active movement against resistance but power less than full
5	Normal power

In the following sections, in addition to the approach of 'Look, Feel, Move', we have included details of special tests for each joint as well as neurological examination of the limb. The peripheral nerve examination comprises sensory and motor testing, reflexes, tone and coordination and proprioception (Summary box 33.2).

Summary box 33.2

Musculoskeletal examination

- Introduce yourself and put the patient at ease
- Assess the gait
- Look
- Feel
- Move
- Special tests
- Neurological examination
- Pulses

CLINICAL EXAMINATION OF THE SPINE

The spinal column consists of 33 vertebrae with 23 intervertebral discs. This is supported by numerous ligaments and paraspinal muscles.

Table 33.5 Peripheral nerves.

Root level	Sensation	Motor	Reflex
C5	Lateral upper arm	Deltoid	Biceps
C6	Lateral forearm	Wrist extension	Brachioradialis
C7	Middle finger	Triceps	Triceps
C8	Little finger	Finger flexors	–
T1	Medial forearm	Interossei	–
L1	Anterior thigh	Psoas	–
L2	Anterior thigh/groin	Quadriceps	–
L3	Anterior and lateral thigh	Quadriceps	–
L4	Medial leg and foot	Tibialis anterior	Knee jerk
L5	Lateral leg and first dorsal web space	Extensor hallucis longus	–
S1	Lateral and plantar foot	Gastrocnemius/perineals	Achilles
S2–S4	Perianal	Bladder and foot intrinsics	–

When observed from the front (coronal plane) with the patient standing and the hips and knees fully extended, the head should be centred over the sacrum. A 'plumb line' dropped from the spinous process of C7 should fall through the gluteal crease (Figure 33.1). If it falls to either side of the cleft, lateral tilt of the spine is present. The ear, shoulder and greater trochanter of the hip should lie in the same vertical plane. When the patient is observed from the side, assess the four physiological sagittal plane curves (cervical and lumbar lordosis, and the thoracic and sacral kyphosis) (Figure 33.2).

Cervical spine

Look

Ensure that the shoulders, back muscles and scapulae can be seen. Look for muscle wasting and asymmetry of the neck creases and check that the shoulders are level and that there is a normal cervical lordosis (range 20–40°).

Feel

Stand behind the patient and support the patient's chin:

- **Soft tissues**. Feel for spasm of the paraspinal muscles.
- **Bone**. Palpate the spinous processes (tenderness and alignment); the spinous processes of C7 (vertebra prominens) and T1 are usually large and are easily palpable at the base of the neck.

Move

Motion occurs in three planes: flexion/extension, bending and rotation (Figure 33.3):

- **Flexion (45°)/extension (55°)**. Ask the patient to bend their neck forwards – place the chin on the chest. Measure the distance from the chin to the sternum. Ask the patient to extend their neck by looking up at the ceiling.
- **Right/left bending (40°)**. Ask the patient to lay their ear on their ipsilateral shoulder.
- **Right/left rotation (70°)**. Ask the patient to look over each shoulder while not moving the chest wall.

Neurological

Focus your examination on the C5 to T1 nerve roots. These supply the upper extremities (Figure 33.4).

Thoracic spine

Pathology commonly presents with pain and deformity. The thoracic spine is normally convex with a gentle kyphosis (normal range 20–45°).

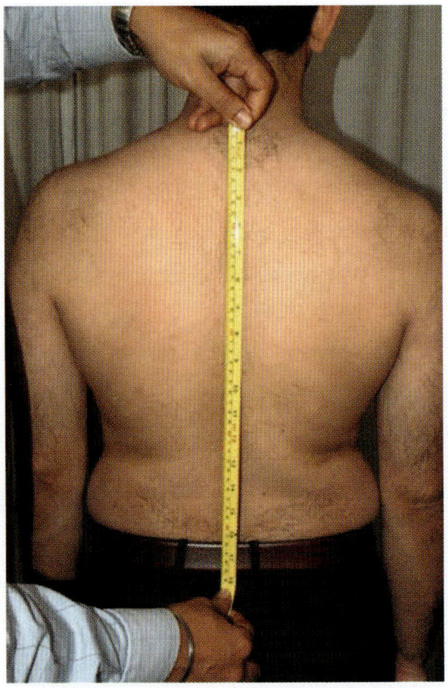

Figure 33.1 Plumb line.

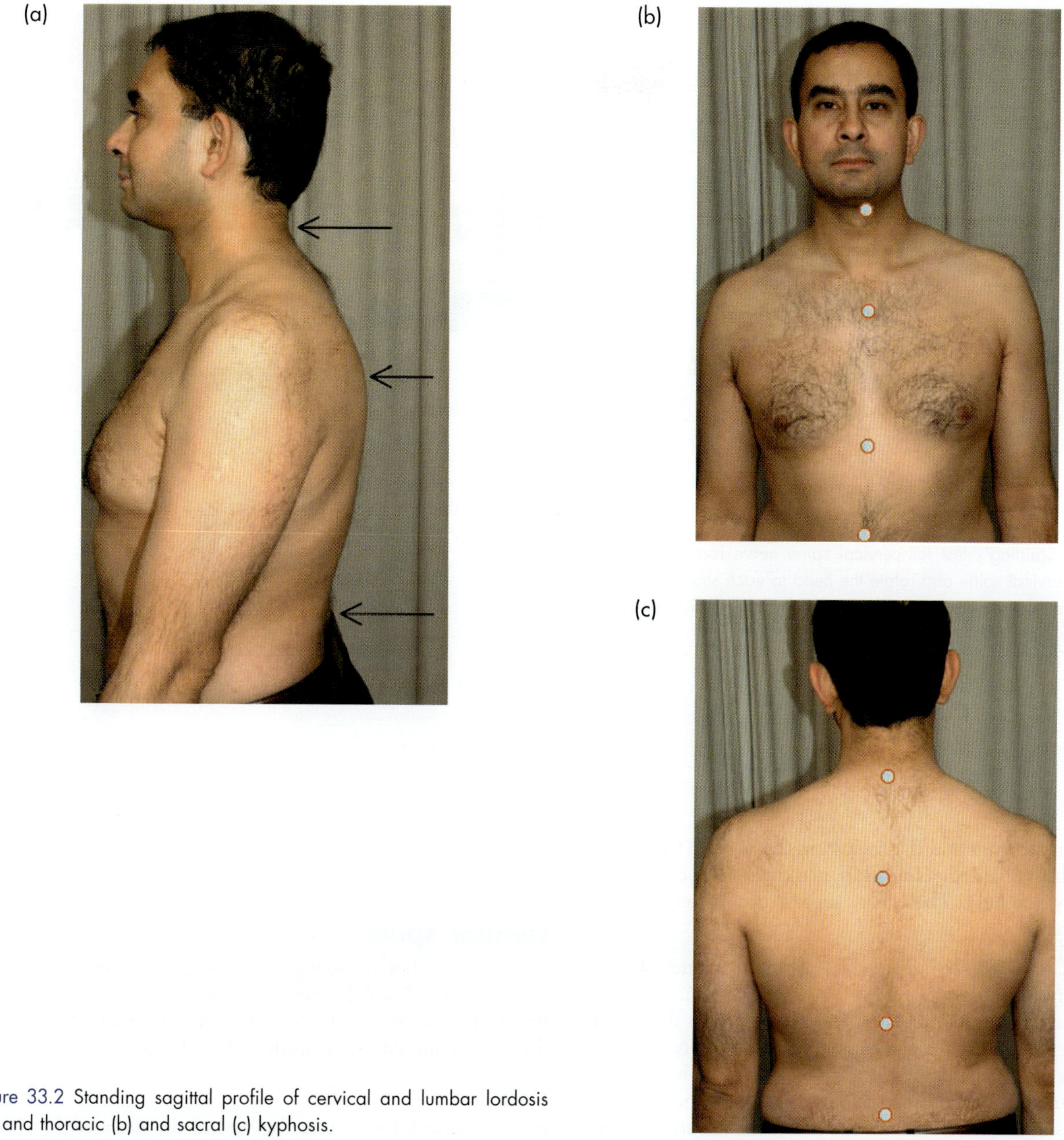

Figure 33.2 Standing sagittal profile of cervical and lumbar lordosis (a), and thoracic (b) and sacral (c) kyphosis.

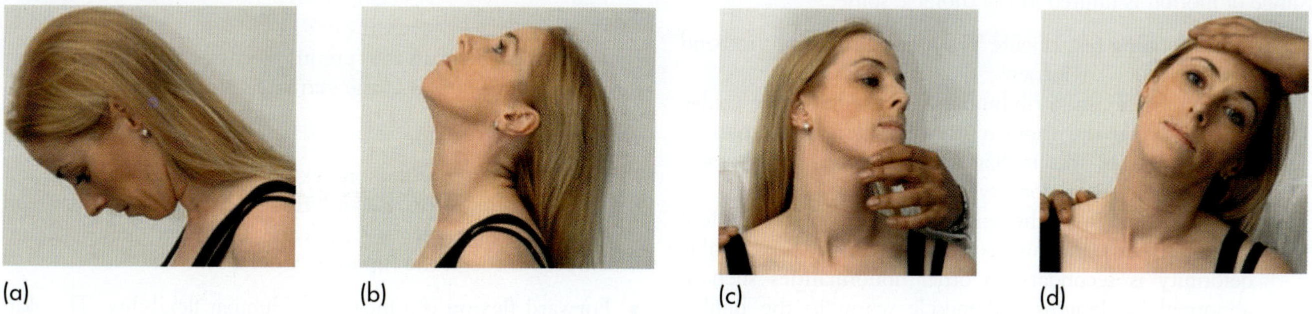

Figure 33.3 Cervical spine flexion/extension (a and b), rotation (c) and bending (d).

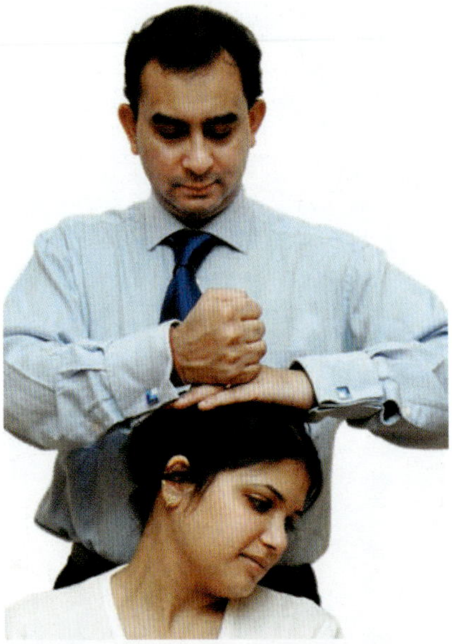

Figure 33.4 Spurling's test for cervical spine nerve root entrapment. Extend the cervical spine and rotate the head to each shoulder in turn. The presence of a shooting pain down the arm may indicate cervical nerve root compression.

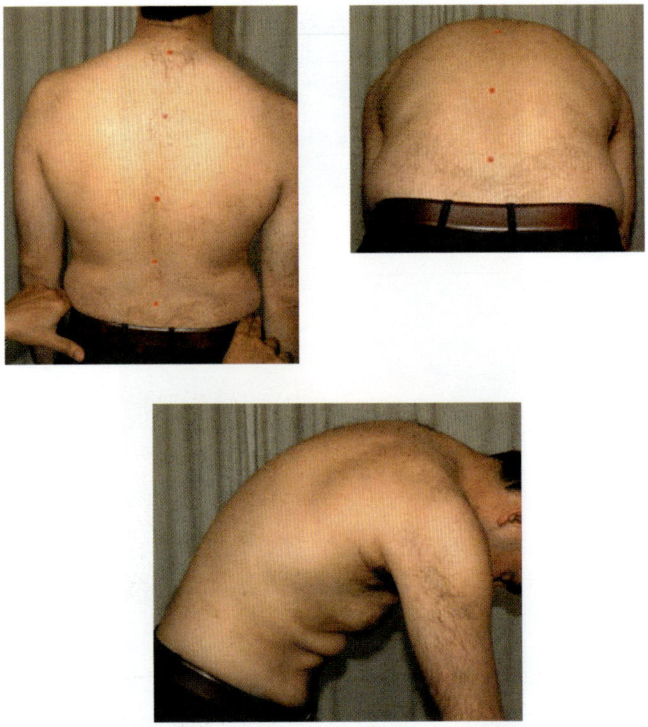

Figure 33.5 Forward bending test.

Look

Ensure that the front and the back from the neck to the gluteal cleft can be visualised. Note skin markings (e.g. café-au-lait spots, hairy patches). These may suggest occult neurology or bony pathology.

- Front: Check for asymmetry of the shoulder and rib cage suggesting scoliosis.
- Back: Look for a difference in the height of the iliac crests (pelvic tilt). Assess for coronal plane deformity, such as scoliosis (lateral curvature of the thoracic spine with rotation). A rib hump suggesting a structural scoliosis may be visible.
- Side: Assess for sagittal plane deformity, such as an increased kyphosis.

Feel

Palpate with one hand supporting the patient's pelvis.

Move

Range of motion is limited in the thoracic spine:

- **Forward bending test** (Figure 33.5). Ask the patient to bend forwards to touch their toes:
  - structural scoliosis: a rib hump will increase in size (bulge posteriorly on the thoracic convex side) as the patient bends forwards; this is diagnostic of idiopathic thoracic scoliosis (rotatory deformity);
  - functional scoliosis: the spine straightens as the patient bends forwards and no rib hump is visible; this flexible deformity is secondary to other abnormalities such as abnormal leg lengths and muscle spasm in the lumbar region.
- **Lateral bending** can be used to assess the flexibility of a scoliosis. Radiographs are taken in this position to supplement the assessment.

Lumbar spine

Examination should include the pelvis, hips, lower limbs, gait and peripheral vascular system as well as the lumbar region. Irritation of nerves in the lumbar spine can mimic problems in the lower limb. Always consider referred pain.

Look

- Back: Check the skin at the base of the spine for hairy tufts and dimples (underlying spina bifida). Prominence of the spinal muscles on one side may be the result of muscle spasm secondary to pain.
- Side: The lumbar spine has a smooth concavity known as the lumbar lordosis (normal range is 40–60°). Muscle spasm is a cause of loss of the normal lordosis.

Feel

Feel for any 'step-off' in the spinous processes. This may indicate forward slippage of one of the vertebrae on another.

Move

Movement occurs in flexion, extension, lateral bending and rotation (Figure 33.6). Record the motion in each plane in degrees. Remember that a significant portion of lumbar flexion is achieved through the hip joint.

- **Forward flexion** is a measure of lumbar flexibility. The skin of the lumbar spine stretches as the patient bends forwards.

(a)

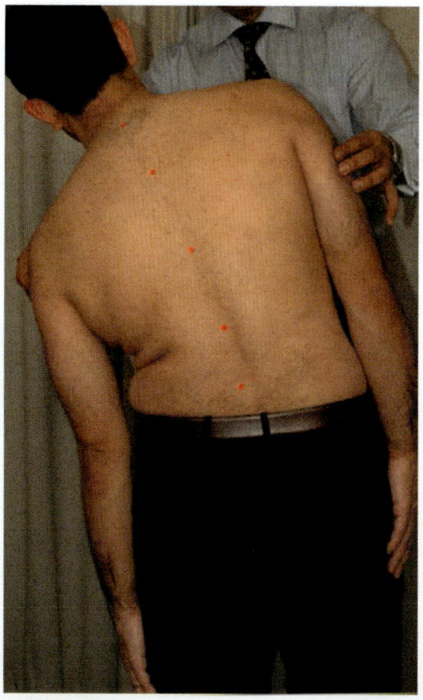

(b)

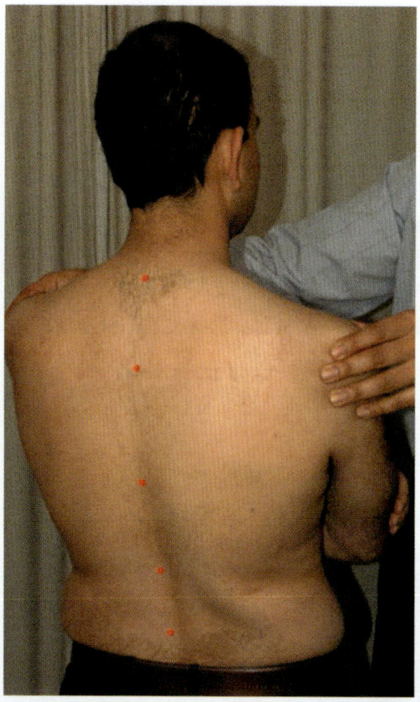

Figure 33.6 Lumbar flexion/extension, lateral bending (a) and rotation (b).

To measure flexion, place the tip of your thumb over the T12–L1 junction and the tip of your index finger of the same hand over the lumbosacral junction. Ask the patient to bend forwards and touch the toes (normal range 40–60°). Measure the distance by which your thumb and the tip of your index finger separate.

- **Lateral bending**. Ask the patient to slide their right hand down the outer side of their right leg and then their left hand down the outside of their left leg. Note the distance that each hand moves down that side of the thigh.
- **Rotation**. Stand behind the patient and hold their pelvis still with both hands. Ask the patient to twist around and look over their shoulder. Note the angle that the shoulder girdle forms with the pelvis (range 3–18°).

Special tests

- **Lasègue's straight leg raise test** (Figure 33.7). This test increases tension along the sciatic nerve (L5 and S1 nerve roots). With the patient supine, elevate the leg with the knee bent to check pain-free movement of the hip. Then, straighten the knee and note the angle which the hamstrings allow the hip to flex. Finally, allow the hip to extend until tension is removed from the hamstring muscles and then the ankle is dorsiflexed firmly, tugging on the sciatic nerve. If the patient experiences pain running down the leg, then the test is positive.
- **Contralateral stretch test**. Elevate the asymptomatic leg; if pain is reproduced in the other leg the test is considered positive (Summary box 33.3).

Charles Ernest Lasègue, 1816–1863, Professor of Medicine, The University of Paris, and Physician, La Salpêtrière, Paris, France. This test was described by Lasègue's student, who named it after his teacher.

Summary box 33.3

Spine examination

Inspection of the standing patient
- From the front and back (coronal plane)
- From the side (saggittal plane)

Palpation
- Palpation of the posterior bony elements and the paraspinal muscles

Move
- Assess flexion, extension, lateral rotation and bending

Neurological
- Assess sensation, tone, power, reflexes, proprioception and coordination

Special tests
- Spurling's test
- Forward bending test
- Lasègue's straight leg test
- Contralateral stretch test

CLINICAL EXAMINATION OF THE HAND AND WRIST

The hand and wrist should be thought of as one functional unit. The muscles may be divided into extrinsic (the muscle bellies in the forearm) and intrinsic (origins and insertions within the hand alone). The 'flexors' (volar side) flex the wrist and fingers and the 'extensors' (dorsal surface) extend the digits and fingers.

Look

Inspect the posture of both hands. A nerve lesion will produce a specific resting position (e.g. an ulnar nerve lesion will produce clawing of the little and ring fingers).

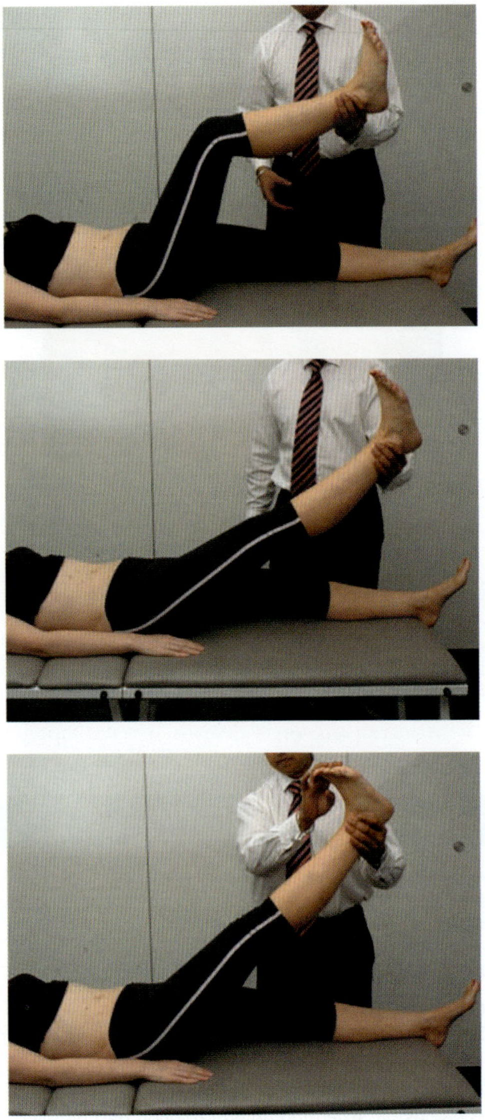

Figure 33.7 Lasègue's straight leg test.

Table 33.6 Patterns of muscle wasting in the hand.

Thenar wasting	Median nerve palsy (C8)
Hypothenar wasting	Ulnar nerve palsy (T1)
Intrinsic wasting	Ulnar nerve palsy (T1)

(a)

(b)

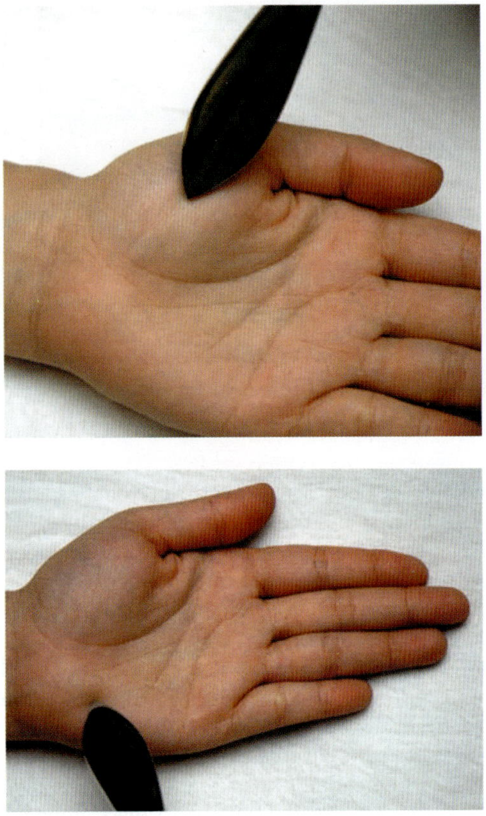

Figure 33.8 Thenar (a) and hypothenar (b) wasting.

- **Skin**. Assess for scars, discolouration (café-au-lait spots, erythema) and loss of hair. The nails may reveal systemic disease (e.g. psoriatic pitting). Look for tight bands in the palm (Dupuytren's contracture). Loss of sweating is seen in complex regional pain syndrome.
- **Soft tissue**. Centrally located swellings at the wrist may indicate a ganglion arising from the wrist joint itself; de Quervain's tenosynovitis may present with a swelling around the radial styloid.
- Check for thenar, hypothenar (Figure 33.8) and intrinsic muscle wasting. To assess thenar eminence wasting, place the hands side by side with the thumbs upwards and look down and compare the thenar regions. Patterns of muscle wasting are shown in Table 33.6.
- **Bones**. Look for bony deformity (dinner fork deformity, Colles' fracture). Typical bony deformities are described in Table 33.7.

Feel

- **Skin**. If there is any question of abnormal sensation on a simple stroke test comparing both sides, proceed to the two-point discrimination test using the sharp ends of a paper clip. Record the minimum distance between the tips of the paper clip at which the patient is able to recognise two points. Table 33.8 describes the anatomical region supplied by the median, ulnar and radial nerves.
- **Pen sliding test**. To assess the absence or presence of sweating, slide a pen along the radial border of the index finger. If the pen slides smoothly, this may indicate loss of sweating.
- **Soft tissue**:
  - blood vessels: check the radial and ulnar artery pulses; assess the capillary refill time, which is normally less than 2 seconds; Allen's test should also be performed before surgery (Table 33.9 and Figure 33.9);

Baron Guillaume Dupuytren, 1777–1835, Surgeon Hôtel Dieu, Paris, France, described the condition in 1831.
Friedrich Joseph de Quervain, 1868–1940, Professor of Surgery, Berne, Switzerland, described this form of tenosynovitis in 1895.
William Heberden (Snr), 1710–1801, a physician who practised first in Cambridge and later in London, UK.
Charles Jacques Bouchard, 1837–1915, physician, Dean of the Faculty of Medicine, Paris, France.
Boutonnière is French for 'button-hole'.

Table 33.7 Bony deformities of the hand.

Anatomical site	Name	Association
Distal interphalangeal joint (DIPJ)	Heberden's nodes	Osteoarthritis
Proximal interphalangeal joint (PIPJ)	Bouchard's node	Osteoarthritis
Hyperextension of the metacarpophalangeal joint (MCPJ), flexion of the PIPJ and hyperextension of the DIPJ	Boutonnière deformity	Rheumatoid arthritis
Hyperextension of the MCPJ and PIPJ and flexion of the DIPJ	Swan neck deformity	Rheumatoid arthritis
Flexion of the MCPJ with hyperextension of the interphalangeal joint	Z deformity of the thumb	Rheumatoid arthritis
Subluxation of the MCPJ	Ulnar drift	Rheumatoid arthritis

Table 33.8 Sensory distribution of the nerve supply to the hand.

Nerve	Sensory distribution
Ulnar	Little finger and ulnar half of the ring finger
Median	Thumb, index, middle and radial half of the ring finger
Radial	Base of the thumb on the dorsum of the hand

  - nerves: compressive neuropathies are most commonly seen affecting the median nerve (see Tinel's (Figure 33.10a) and Phalen's (Figure 33.10b) test in Table 33.9);
  - palmar fascia: feel for palmar thickening and skin pits; long finger-like structures (cords), most commonly affecting the ring and little fingers, are suggestive of Dupuytren's disease.
- **Bones**. Palpate from the radial to the ulnar side of the wrist joint. In the trauma setting, palpate the anatomical snuff box (Figure 33.11). A fracture of the scaphoid may cause tenderness.

The scaphoid tubercle, pisiform and the hook of hamate are all palpable on the volar aspect of the wrist.

Move

The wrist can be moved into flexion and extension, and ulnar and radial deviation.

- **Wrist**. Extension is tested by asking the patient to push the hands together into a 'prayer' position (Figure 33.12a). If there is loss of extension, the palms will not meet and/or one forearm will be dropped. Palmar flexion is tested in a similar fashion but with the hands pointing down and the back of the hands in contact (Figure 33.12b). Ulnar and radial deviation are tested by taking the patient's hand in your own and moving the hand into these directions.
- **Hand**. A general screening assessment is to ask the patient to roll up their fingers from full extension to full flexion. This will reveal a trigger finger.

Extensors and flexors

Asking the patient to grip two of your fingers in their fist tests the power of the extensors of the wrist (radial nerve) because they are needed to brace the wrist. It also tests the power of the flexors in the forearm (median nerve). Asking the patient then to extend and spread their fingers apart against resistance tests the intrinsic muscles of the hand (mainly the ulnar nerve).

George S Phalen, contemporary, orthopaedic surgeon and Chief of Hand Surgery, The Cleveland Clinic, Cleveland, OH, USA. He helped to establish the American Society for Surgery of the Hand.

Table 33.9 Special hand tests.

Test	Technique	Significance
Allen's test	Elevate the hand and apply digital pressure on the radial and ulnar arteries to occlude them. Ask the patient to make a fist several times. The tips of the finger should go pale. Release each artery in turn and observe the return of colour	Tests the adequacy of the blood supply to the hand from the radial and ulnar arteries and the arcade between them
Tinel's test	Tap over the nerve of interest. Tingling may indicate nerve compression	Identifies compression of a peripheral nerve
Phalen's test	Place the wrist in maximum flexion with the elbows extended	Compression of the medial nerve causes paraesthesia
Froment's sign	Ask the patient to grip a sheet of paper between the index finger and thumb of both hands. Grip the paper yourself similarly. Ask the patient to resist as you attempt to pull the paper away	A positive test indicated by flexion of the thumb interphalangeal joint suggests weakness of the adductor pollicis muscle supplied by the ulnar nerve. Recruitment of the median nerve-innervated flexor pollici brevis explains the thumb posture

Edgar van Nuys Allen, 1900–1961, Professor of Medicine, The Mayo Clinic, Rochester, MN, USA.
Jules Tinel, 1879–1952, Physician, Hôpital Beaujon, Paris, France.

(a)
(b)
(c)

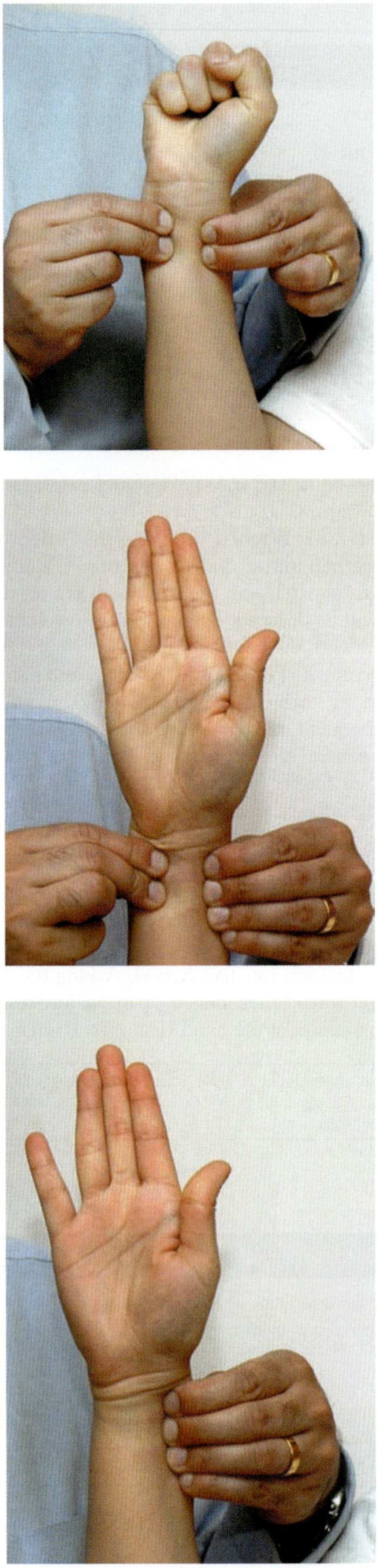

Figure 33.9 (a–c) Performing Allen's test.

(a)
(b)

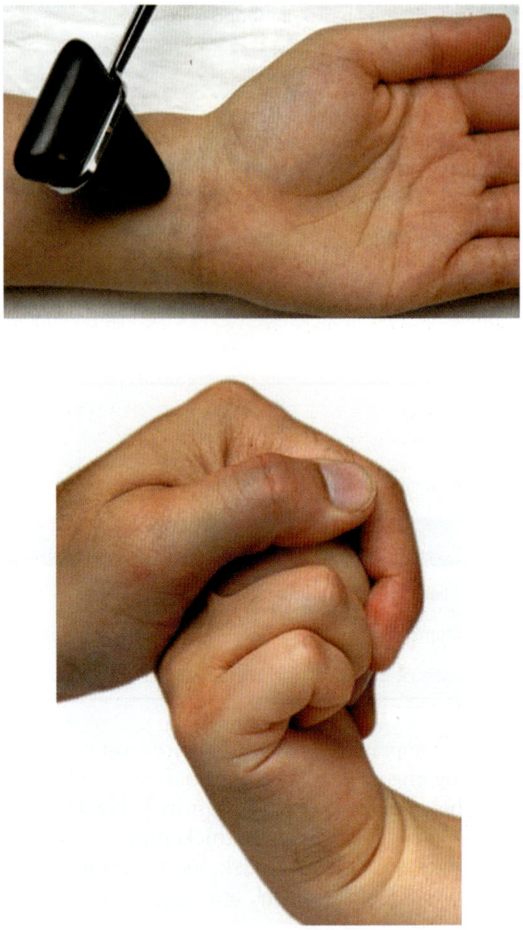

Figure 33.10 (a) Tinel's test; (b) Phalen's test.

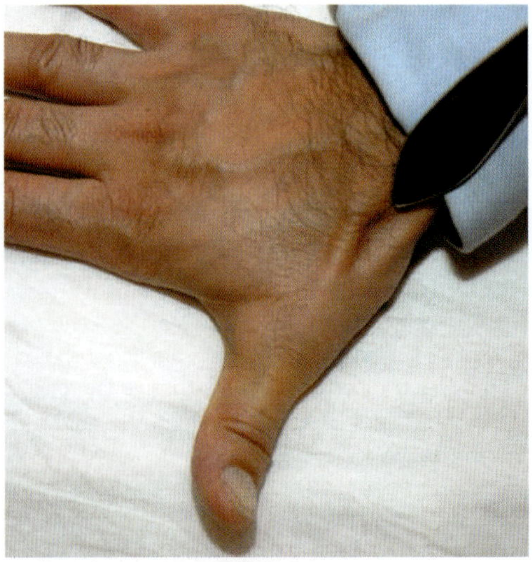

Figure 33.11 Palpating the anatomical snuff box between the tendons of extensor pollicis longus and abductor pollicis brevis.

Finger flexors

- **Superficialis tendon test**. The flexor digitorum profundus (FDP) usually has one muscle belly from which tendons to all of the fingers arise. The FDP can be immobilised by holding all of the fingers (except the one being examined) in extension; this allows the superficialis tendon to be tested in isolation. If the test finger is able to flex, despite profundus being immobilised, then the superficialis tendon to that finger is working. Repeat the test for the other fingers individually (Figure 33.13).

Other muscles

- **Thenar eminence**:
  - The abductor pollicis brevis, opponens pollicis and flexor pollicis brevis can be tested together by opposing the thumb to the little finger.
  - The flexor pollicis longus which is supplied by the anterior interosseus nerve (branch of the median nerve) can be tested by asking the patient to bring the tips of the thumb and index finger together (the 'OK' sign – Figure 33.14).
  - The integrity of the extensor pollicis longus tendon is tested by asking the patient to lift the thumb off a table with the palm flat on the table (Figure 33.15).
- **Adductor pollicis**: Test using Froment's sign (see Table 33.9 and Figure 33.16).

Thumb abductor pollicis brevis

This muscle is supplied by the median nerve. With the hand lying flat on a table with the palm facing upwards, ask the patient to raise the thumb towards the ceiling. Ask the patient to resist as you push the thumb back towards the palm (Figure 33.17) (Summary box 33.4).

(a)

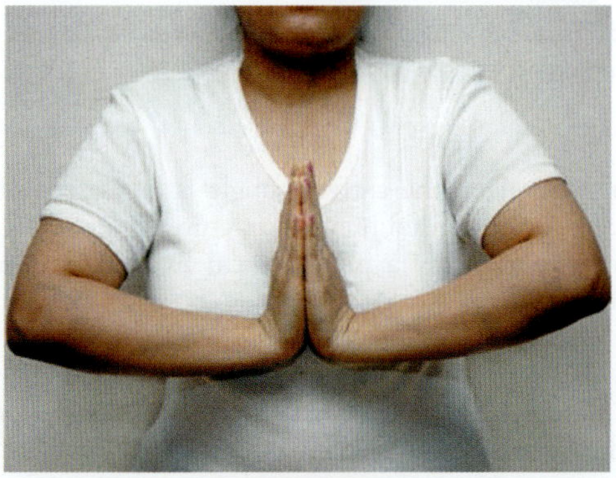

(b)

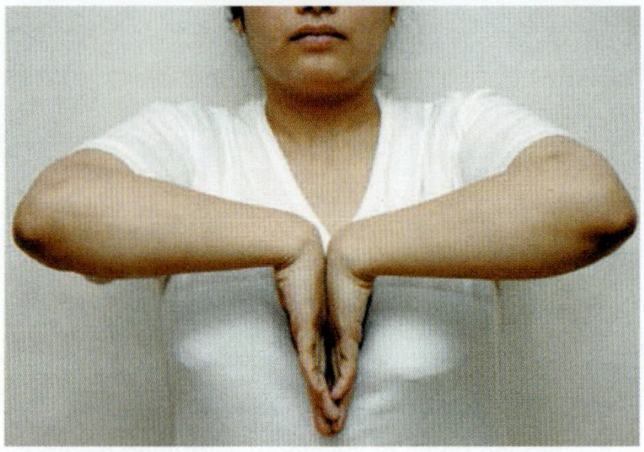

Figure 33.12 Testing the range of (a) wrist extension; (b) wrist flexion.

(a)

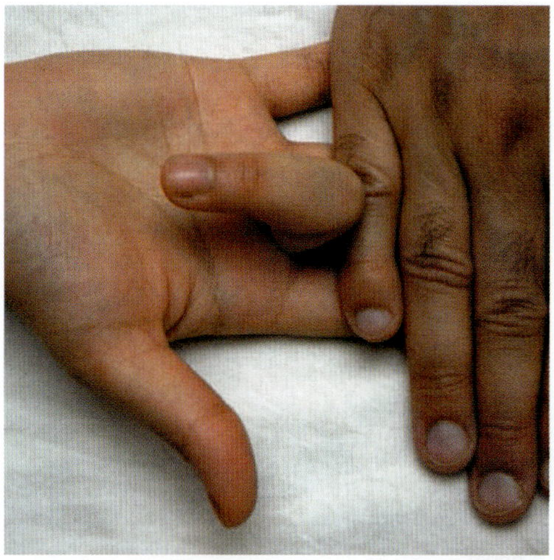

(b)

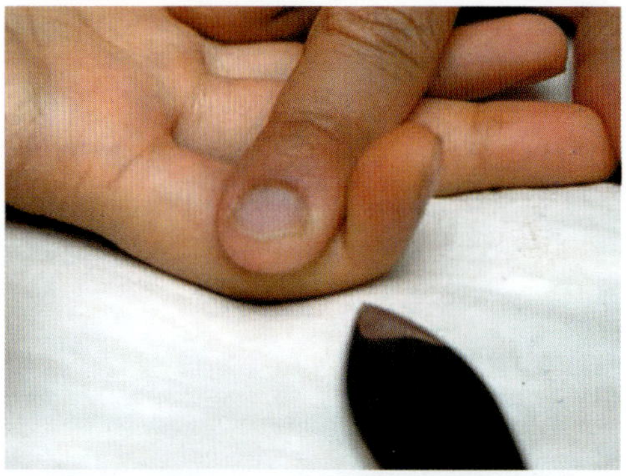

Figure 33.13 Testing the (a) flexor digitorum superficialis; (b) flexor digitorum profundus.

> **Summary box 33.4**
>
> **Hand and wrist examination**
>
> Inspection of the standing patient
> - Dorsum and palm – asymmetry, deformity, muscle wasting
>
> Inspection of the supine patient
> - Skin, scars, soft tissues
> - Palpation of bony structures and joints of the hand
>
> Movements
> - Wrist – flexion and extension, ulnar and radial deviation
> - Hand – thumb movements, metatarsophalangeal joints and small joints of the hand
>
> Special tests
> - Allen's test
> - Tinel's and Phalen's test for the median nerve
> - Froment's sign
> - Finkelstein's test

Jules Froment, 1878–1946, Professor of Clinical Medicine, Lyons, France.

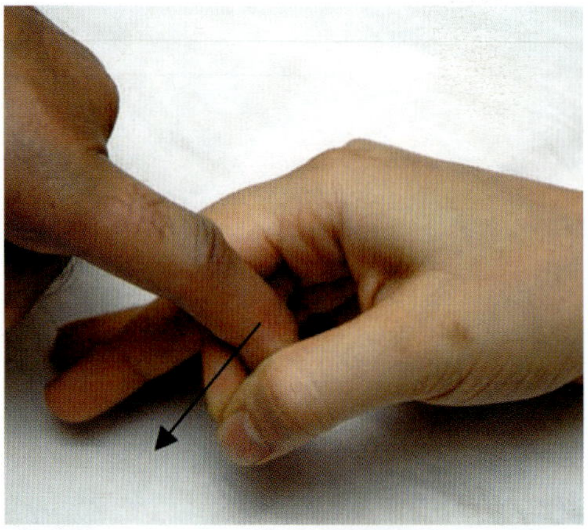

Figure 33.14 Test for flexor pollicis longus supplied by the anterior interosseus nerve.

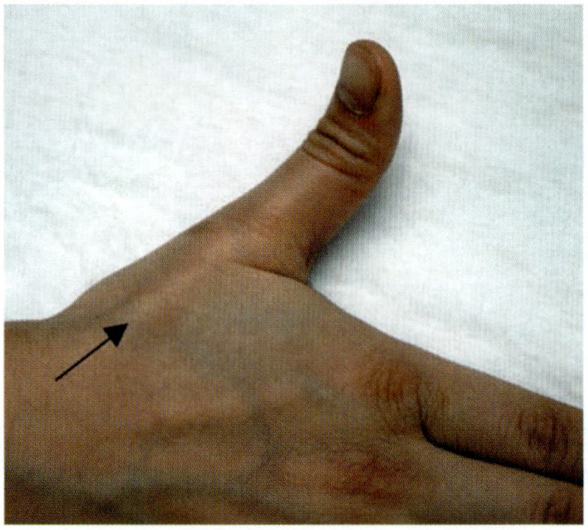

Figure 33.15 Testing the integrity of extensor pollicis longus.

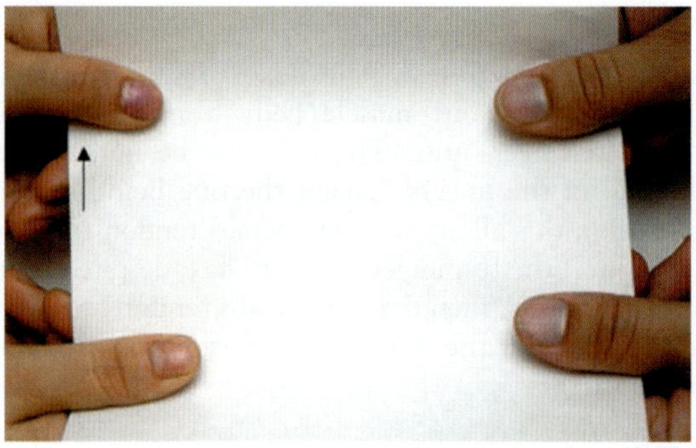

Figure 33.16 Froment's sign; the arrow illustrates the flexed posture of the thumb interphalangeal joint, indicating weakness of the ulnar nerve-innervated adductor pollicis muscle.

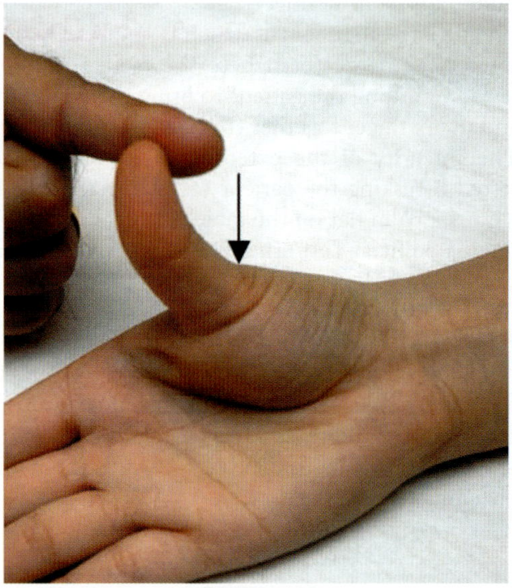

Figure 33.17 Testing the power of the abductor pollicis brevis supplied by the median nerve.

CLINICAL EXAMINATION OF THE ELBOW

The elbow is a hinge joint formed by the articulation of the ulna and radius with the humerus.

Look

- **Skin**. Check the extensor surface for signs of psoriasis.
- **Soft tissues**. Look for any swellings, e.g. olecranon bursa, rheumatoid nodules, gouty tophi.
- **Muscle wasting**. Examine the biceps and triceps muscle bulk. Note that compression of the ulnar nerve at the elbow leads to wasting distally in the hypothenar eminence and intrinsic muscles of the hand – assess the hand for the presence of clawing and wasting.
- **Bone**. With the elbow in extension, look at the axis between the upper arm and forearm. There is a physiological valgus ('carrying angle') of 9–14° (2–3° greater in women) (Figure 33.18). This angle allows the elbow to be tucked into the waist depression above the iliac crest:
  - cubitus varus (gun-stock deformity): the carrying angle is reversed, secondary to a malunited supracondylar fracture;
  - cubitus valgus: the carrying angle is increased, caused by malunion of a distal humeral fracture;
  - there is normally a physiological hyperextension of the elbow (5°).

Feel

- **Soft tissues**. An effusion may be elicited by performing a crossfluctuation test. The ulnar nerve can be rolled under

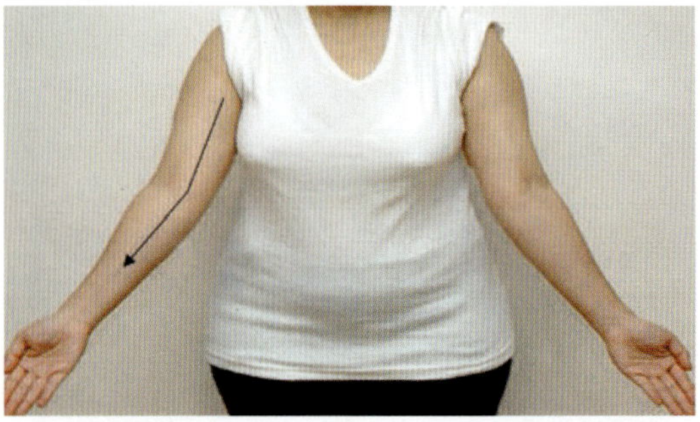

Figure 33.18 Carrying angle of the elbow illustrating the normal cubitus valgus.

your fingers placed between the medial epicondyle and the olecranon. Test the distal sensation in the hand (especially in the distribution of the ulna nerve) and assess the vascular status.

- **Bones**. The three palpation landmarks are the medial and lateral epicondyles and the apex of the olecranon. These form an equilateral triangle when the elbow is flexed to 90°. The radial head is palpated with the examiner's thumb while the other hand pronates and supinates the forearm. On the medial side, palpate the medial epicondyle. Posteriorly, palpate the olecranon fossa.

Move

- **Flexion–extension**. The normal range is from −5° (slight hyperextension) to 150°. Ask the patient to bend the elbow from the fully straight position (Figure 33.19).
- **Pronation and supination**. With the elbows at 90° and the palms facing upwards (full supination), ask the patient to turn the forearm so that the dorsum of the hand faces upwards (full pronation) (Figure 33.20). The normal values are 70° pronation and 90° supination.

Special tests and diagnoses

Tennis elbow and golfer's elbow

These are inflammatory processes of the tendons that attach the large muscle mass of the forearm to the lateral or medial epicondyle.

- **Medial epicondylitis (synonym = golfer's elbow)**. The medial epicondyle is the common origin of the forearm flexors and the pronator muscle. Palpate the medial epicondyle for tenderness. The diagnostic test is resisted wrist flexion, which reproduces the pain over the medial epicondyle.
- **Lateral epicondylitis (synonym = tennis elbow)**. The lateral epicondyle is the common origin of the forearm extensors. Palpate for tenderness – usually just distal (5–10 mm) to the epicondyle near the origin of the extensor carpi radialis brevis muscle. Wrist extension against resistance with the elbow extended should provoke the patient's symptoms (Summary box 33.5).

(a)
(b)

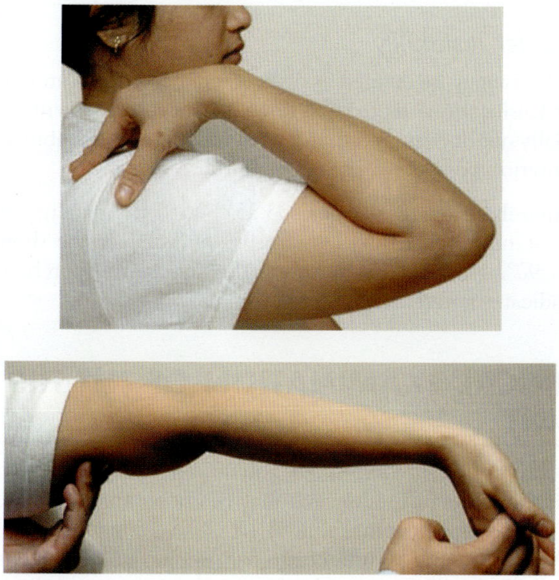

Figure 33.19 (a) Elbow flexion; (b) elbow extension.

(a)
(b)
(c)

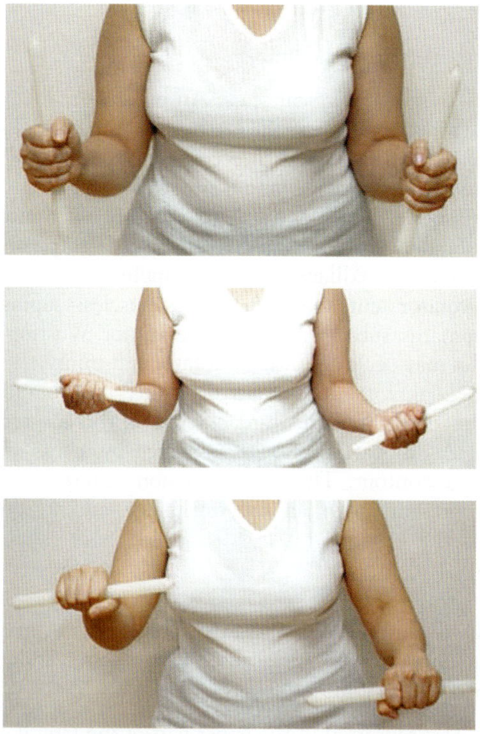

Figure 33.20 Testing forearm rotation: (a) mid-prone position; (b) full supination; (c) full pronation.

> **Summary box 33.5**
>
> **Elbow examination**
>
> Inspection of the standing patient
> - Front – asymmetry, carrying angle, deformity
> - Back – olecranon fossa
>
> Inspection of the supine patient
> - Skin, scars, soft tissues, deformity
> - Palpation of bony structures
>
> Movements
> - Flexion and extension, pronation and supination
>
> Special tests
> - Tennis and golfer's elbow
> - Stability testing
> - Ulnar nerve compression
> - Biceps tendon power

CLINICAL EXAMINATION OF THE SHOULDER

Pain arising from the shoulder joint may be felt anterolaterally. Referred pain may present from the cervical spine, heart, mediastinum and the diaphragm.

Look

Assess the attitude of the limb.

- **Skin**. Check for surgical scars. An anterior scar is used for the deltopectoral approach. At the side, the deltoid splitting approach and lateral arthroscopic portals may be seen. Posteriorly, arthroscopic portal sites can be seen.
- **Soft tissues**. Wasting of the deltoid muscle is commonly seen after shoulder dislocation when there is a temporary loss of function of the axillary nerve that supplies it.
- **The rotator cuff** comprises four muscles: supraspinatus, infraspinatus, subscapularis and teres minor. Wasting of these muscles may occur following a rotator cuff injury.
- **Bone**. Look for any obvious deformity or prominence. A fracture of the middle third clavicle is the most common cause. A dislocation may be suspected by a loss of normal shoulder contour. The more common anterior dislocation often presents with an anterior bulge and a squared-off shoulder.

Feel

Generalised pain in the shoulder may arise from the neck or the shoulder joint itself. More localised pain is often indicative of acromioclavicular joint pathology.

- **Skin**. Test sensation in the upper part of the lateral aspect of the arm ('regimental badge area') (Figure 33.21). Loss may indicate damage to the axillary nerve (following shoulder dislocation).
- **Bones**. Palpate the acromioclavicular and sternoclavicular joints and the clavicle.

Move

Differentiate between movements of the shoulder joint and scapulothoracic movement of the scapula on the chest wall. Patients with a painful shoulder will commonly move from the scapulothoracic joint. Stabilise the scapula by placing the thumb over the coracoid process and the fingers of the same hand over the spine of the scapula. Start in the 'neutral position' with the arms by the side, elbows extended and the palm facing forwards. Note any pain throughout the range of movement (Figure 33.22).

- **Forward flexion**. Ask the patient to raise their hands in front to touch the ceiling while keeping the elbows extended (0–180°).
- **Extension**. Ask the patient to extend both arms behind (0–30°).
- **Abduction**. Shoulder abduction involves the glenohumeral joint and scapulothoracic movement. The first 60° of movement is mainly at the glenohumeral joint. Beyond this the scapula begins to rotate on the thorax and final movements are almost entirely scapulothoracic. Raise the arms sideways until the fingers point to the ceiling (180°).
- **Adduction**. Ask the patient to touch their other shoulder tip.
- **Internal rotation**. Ask the patient to touch their back with the dorsum of the hand and to raise their hand up the back as high as possible (normal range is thoracic spine level T7–9).
- **External rotation**. With the arms by the sides, bend the elbow to 90° and rotate the forearms to the mid-prone position. Ask the patient to separate their hands as much as possible (0–40°).

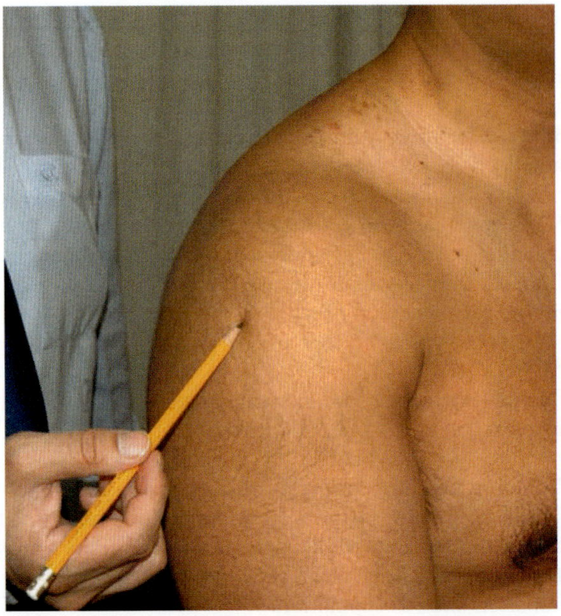

Figure 33.21 The area of skin supplied by the axillary nerve – the 'regimental badge area'.

Special tests and diagnoses

Impingement syndrome

This is impairment of rotator cuff function within the subacromial bursa. It may lead to inflammation (tendinitis) or a partial- or full-thickness tear. Impingement is characterised by pain and weakness on abduction and internal rotation.

- **Painful arc test** (Figure 33.23). Ask the patient to abduct their arms from their sides. The presence of pain from 60° to 120° is positive.
- **Jobe's test (empty can)** (Figure 33.24). Ask the patient to abduct the arm to 90° elevation in the scapula plane with full internal rotation (empty can position). Ask the patient to resist downward pressure. The presence of pain is a positive test.

Shoulder instability

Instability may be defined as a shoulder that slips in and out of joint (dislocation) more than once or twice, or frequently slips partially out of joint and then returns on its own. Instability can be anterior, posterior, inferior or multidirectional.

- **Apprehension test** (Figure 33.25). With the patient supine or standing, flex the elbow to 90° and abduct the shoulder to 90°. Now externally rotate the shoulder. Apprehension indicates anterior instability (Summary box 33.6).

CLINICAL EXAMINATION OF THE HIP JOINT

The hip is a synovium-lined ball and socket joint. Typical clinical diseases of the hip that may be encountered in children and adults are shown in Table 33.10.

A patient complaining of hip pain should undergo a careful examination of the spine, abdomen, pelvis, groin and thigh. In addition, consider a gynaecological examination in women.

(a)

(c)

(d)

(b)

(e)

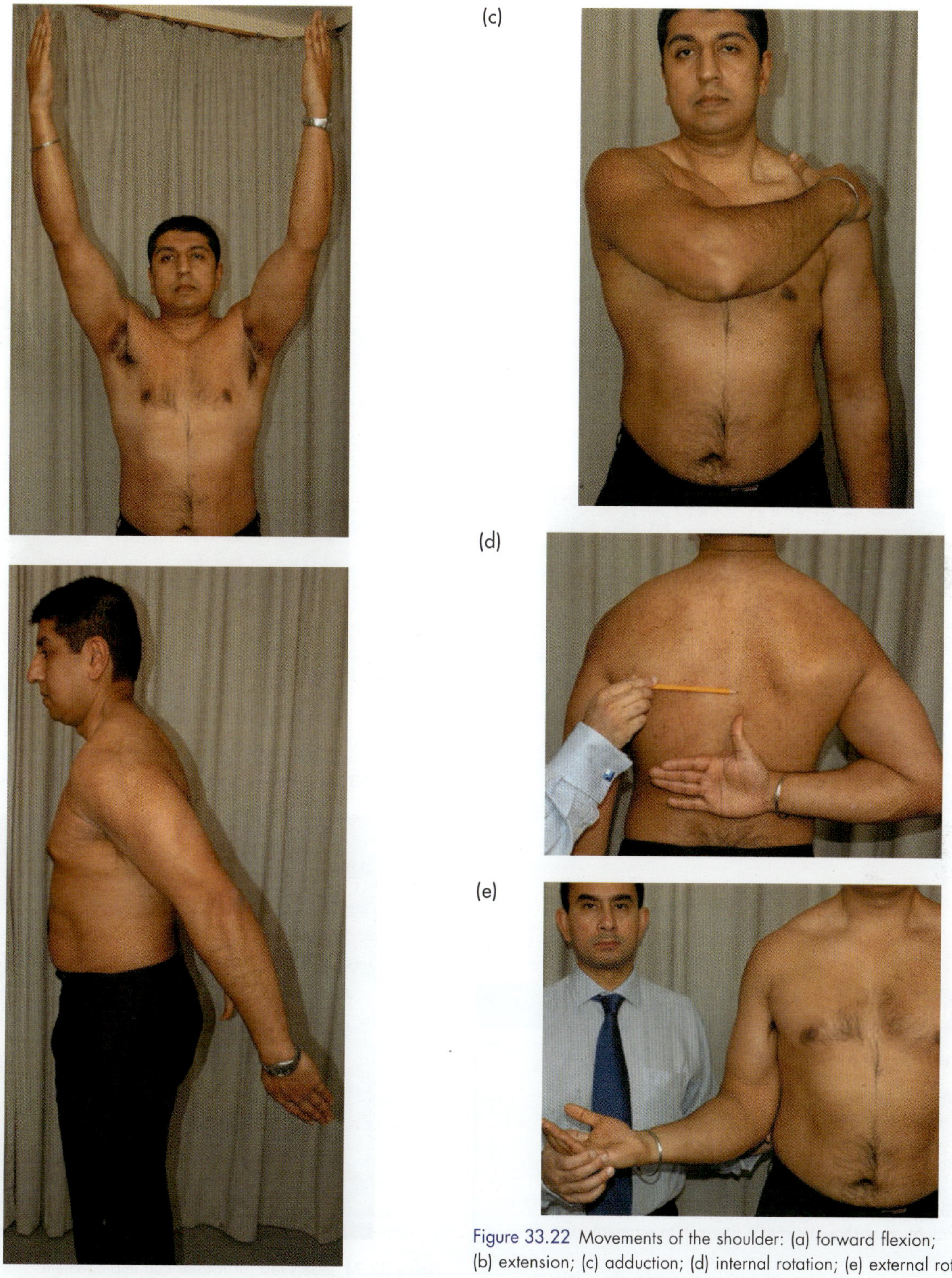

Figure 33.22 Movements of the shoulder: (a) forward flexion; (b) extension; (c) adduction; (d) internal rotation; (e) external rotation.

Look

With the patient standing, look at the front, side and back of the hip. Look around the room for walking aids and heel raises in the shoes.

- **Skin**. Look for scars and sinuses.
- **Soft tissues**. Muscle wasting may be present as a consequence of hip arthritis or primary muscle or neurological disease.
- **Bone**. Look at the posture of the limb and assess for adduction deformity; fixed adduction may be present in severe osteoarthritis and cerebral palsy, and makes the leg appear short because the pelvis is tilted (apparent shortening).

Feel

- **Soft tissues**. Tenderness overlying the greater trochanter may suggest trochanteric bursitis or an abductor enthesopathy.

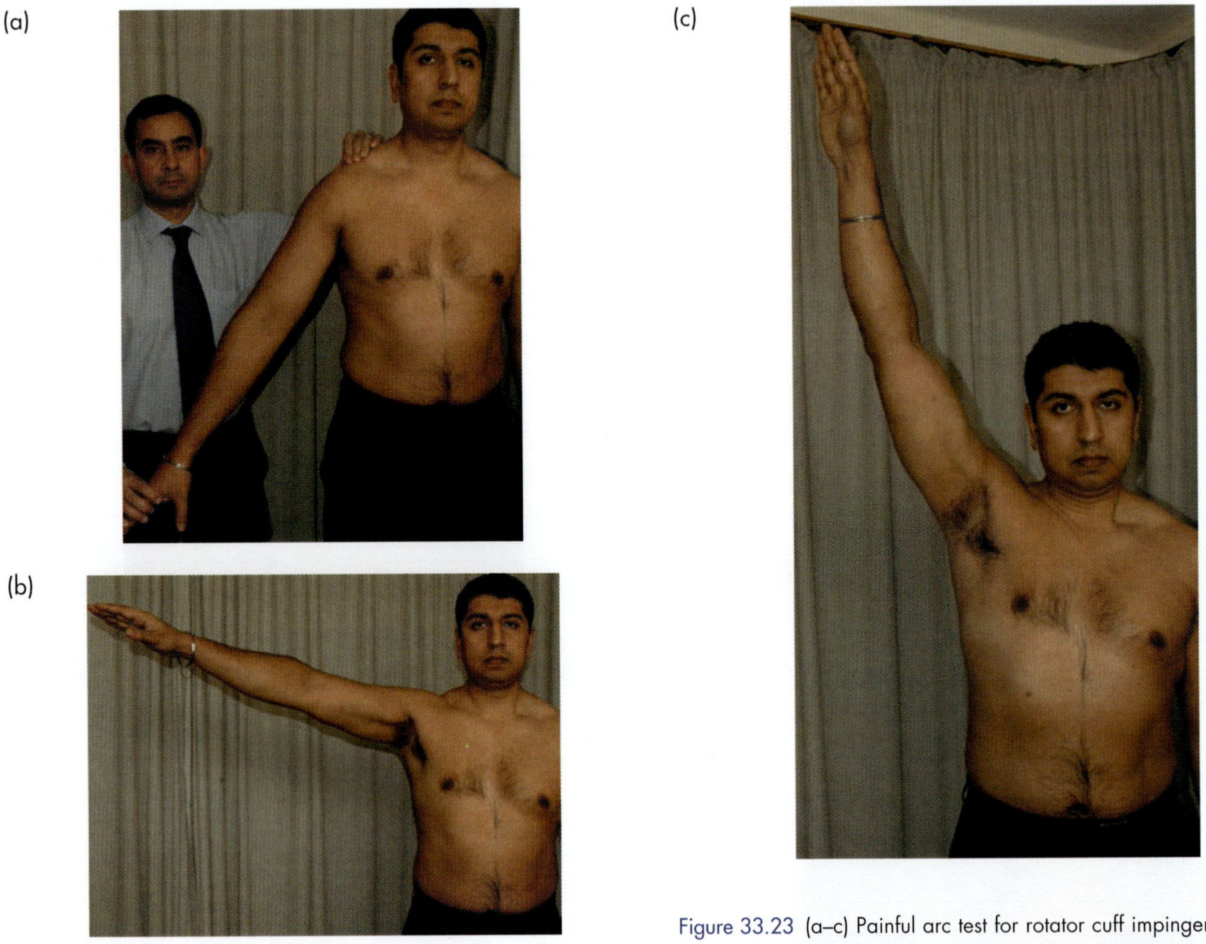

Figure 33.23 (a–c) Painful arc test for rotator cuff impingement.

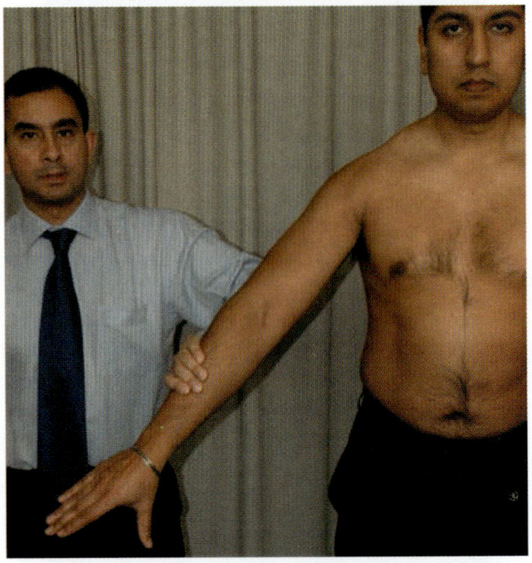

Figure 33.24 Jobe's test for rotator cuff impingement.

> **Summary box 33.6**
>
> **Shoulder examination**
>
> Inspection of the standing patient
> - Front – asymmetry, deformity
> - Side – muscle wasting
> - Back – muscle wasting, scapula
>
> Inspection of the supine patient
> - Skin, scars, soft tissues, deformity
> - Palpation of shoulder girdle (sternum to scapula)
>
> Movements
> - Flexion and extension, abduction and adduction, internal and external rotation
>
> Special tests
> - Impingement syndrome – painful arc, Jobe's test, Hawkins' test
> - Shoulder instability – apprehension, relocation test, sulcus sign
> - Rotator cuff assessment
> - Acromioclavicular joint pathology
> - Frozen shoulder versus glenohumeral osteoarthritis

Move

The hip joint can be moved into flexion, extension, abduction and adduction and internal and external rotation (Figure 33.26). True hip movement ends when the pelvis begins to move. To detect true hip movement, simultaneously place a finger/hand on the anterior superior iliac spine (ASIS) contralateral to the hip being examined. Remember to compare both sides.

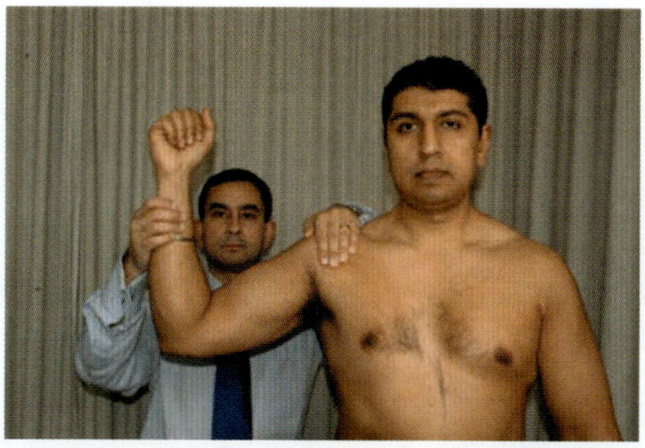

Figure 33.25 Anterior apprehension test for anterior shoulder instability.

Passive movement

Hip flexion and extension (120–0°)

The patient is asked to lie on their back and then roll themselves into a ball, flexing the hips and the spine fully. A comparison of the flexion of the two hips can be made in this position. The patient is then asked to hold onto the knee of the 'bad' leg with both hands (thereby fixing the pelvis in flexion) and the other leg is allowed to extend down onto the couch. A note is made of any fixed flexion deformity (inability of the thigh to come down onto the couch). This 'good' hip is then returned to full flexion and the patient grasps that knee while dropping the other 'bad' hip into extension. This modified Thomas's test is the most comfortable and accurate way of measuring flexion and extension of the hip, minimising movement of the painful hip (Figure 33.27).

Rotation

- **Internal rotation (45°)**. With the hip flexed to 45° and the knee in 90° of flexion, hold the front of the knee with one hand and the foot with the other. Internally rotate the hip (the foot goes outwards), then externally rotate the hip (the foot goes in). The angle that the tibia makes with the vertical indicates the range of movement. Pain at the extremes of movement suggest inflammation in the hip.
- **Abduction (40°)**. The hip should be abducted by moving the leg away from the midline with the other hand on the patient's pelvis to detect any tilt in the pelvis.

Special tests

- **Trendelenburg test** (Figure 33.28). Face the patient and ask them to place their hands on the palm of your hands for support. Then ask them to stand first on one leg, then the other. Increased pressure from the opposite hand as they take weight through the weak hip indicates a positive Trendelenburg test.
- Leg length discrepancy (LLD). The inequality may be in the hip joint, femur, tibia, ankle or foot or a combination of these. The pathology may be from the bone being too short or too long (Summary box 33.7). When assessing LLD, square the pelvis. If that is not possible then place both legs in the same position. For example, if there is an adduction deformity present in the affected leg, place the good leg in the same degree of adduction. LLD can be caused by a real difference in the leg lengths (the bones are different lengths) or by a deformity that makes the leg appear short because the pelvis must be tilted to get the leg onto the ground. The first is called 'real' LLD. The second is called 'apparent' LLD. Both are real to the patient but the cause and therefore the treatment are different. The LLD apparent to the patient can also be measured using wooden blocks placed under the patient's 'short' leg until the patient feels level.

Hugh Owen Thomas, 1834–1891, general practitioner, Liverpool, UK. He is regarded as the founder of orthopaedic surgery although never holding a hospital appointment, preferring to treat patients in their own homes. He introduced the Thomas splint in 1875.

Table 33.10 Common clinical diseases of the hip in children and adults.

Children	Adults
Developmental dysplasia of the hip	Primary osteoarthritis
Transient synovitis of the hip	Secondary osteoarthritis
Perthe's disease	Inflammatory arthritis
Septic arthritis and osteomyelitis	Avascular necrosis
Slipped capital femoral epiphysis	Labral tears
Juvenile idiopathic arthritis	Referred pain

Summary box 33.7

Common causes of limb length inequality in the hip

- Osteoarthritis
- Hip fracture
- Hip dislocation
- Hip dysplasia
- Avascular necrosis
- Fixed flexion deformity

- **Gait**. Hip disease can present with an altered gait pattern. The common types of abnormal gait are described in Table 33.11 (Summary box 33.8).

Table 33.11 Common limps observed in hip disease.

Gait pattern	Description
Weak: Trendelenburg	May lead to pelvic sway or tilt. The patient swings the body over the weak hip to stay in balance when it is weight bearing
Painful: antalgic	The rhythm is dot–dash, with a short period spent on the painful limb
Unbalanced: broad-based	May be caused by ataxia, e.g. cerebellar pathology. The rhythm also tends to be disordered
Loss of muscle control: high-stepping	May be due to loss of proprioception or a drop foot. This leads to difficulty in clearing the toes during the swing phase and the patient compensates by externally rotating the leg and flexing the hip and knee
Deformity: in-toeing	Can be caused by persistent femoral anteversion. The foot may catch on the back of the calf of the weight-bearing leg, tripping the patient

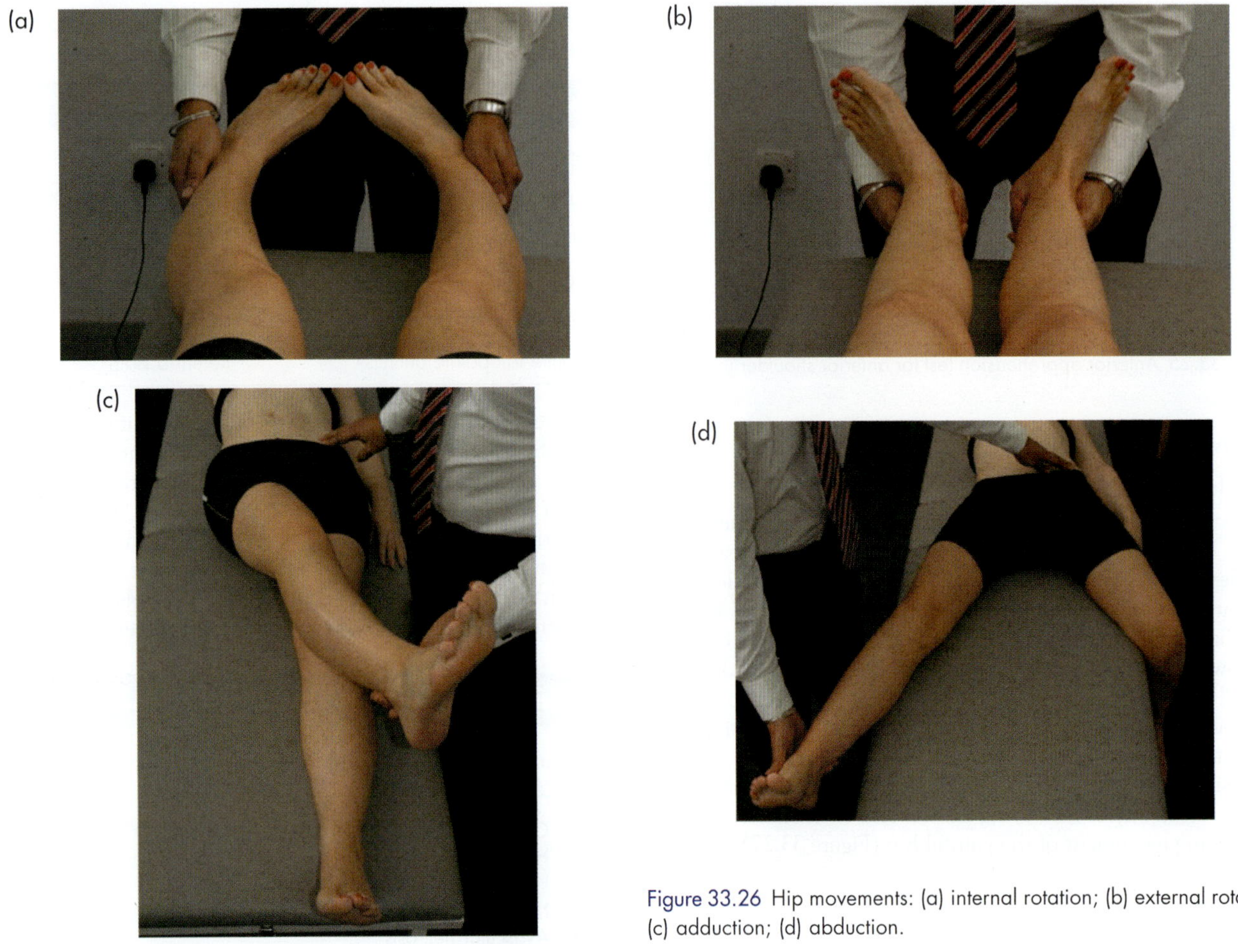

Figure 33.26 Hip movements: (a) internal rotation; (b) external rotation; (c) adduction; (d) abduction.

Summary box 33.8

Hip examination

Inspection of the standing patient

- Front – pelvic tilt, rotational deformity
- Side – lumbar lordosis
- Back – pelvic tilt, scoliosis, gluteal wasting
- Gait – Trendelenburg, antalgic

Inspection of the supine patient

- Skin, scars, soft tissues, deformity
- Palpation of the anterior joint line, adductor origin, greater trochanter, ischial tuberosity

Movements

- Flexion and extension
- Abduction and adduction
- Internal and external rotation

Special tests

- Thomas's test
- Leg length assessment – real/apparent
- Trendelenburg test
- Snapping hip
- Impingement tests

- **Impingement test**. To assess for femoroacetabular impingement, perform two tests: hip flexion at greater than 90° combined with some adduction and internal rotation (FADIR test). The second test is placing the hip into flexion, full adduction and external rotation. A positive test is indicated by pain.

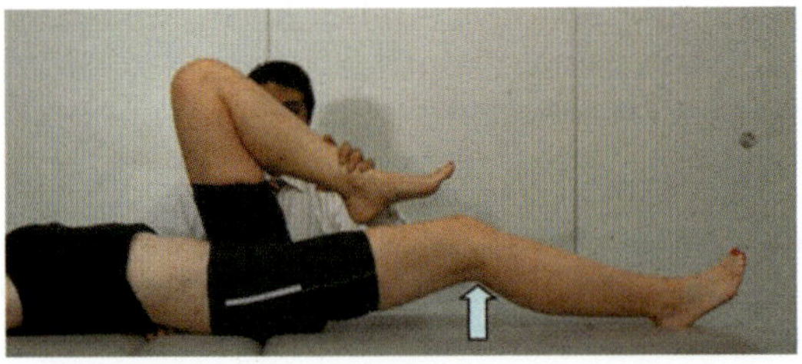

Figure 33.27 Modified Thomas's test for assessing a fixed flexion deformity. A fixed flexion deformity of the right hip is indicated by an inability to fully straighten the right leg (arrow).

CLINICAL EXAMINATION OF THE KNEE

The knee is a synovial hinged joint. There are three compartments: medial, lateral and patellofemoral. The quadriceps, quadriceps tendon, patella, patella tendon and tibial tuberosity comprise the extensor mechanism of the knee.

The anterior cruciate ligament (ACL) provides primary restraint to anterior displacement of the tibia. The posterior cruciate ligament (PCL) provides posterior restraint of the tibia. The medial collateral ligament (MCL) resists valgus and external rotation forces whereas the lateral collateral ligament (LCL) resists varus forces.

(a)

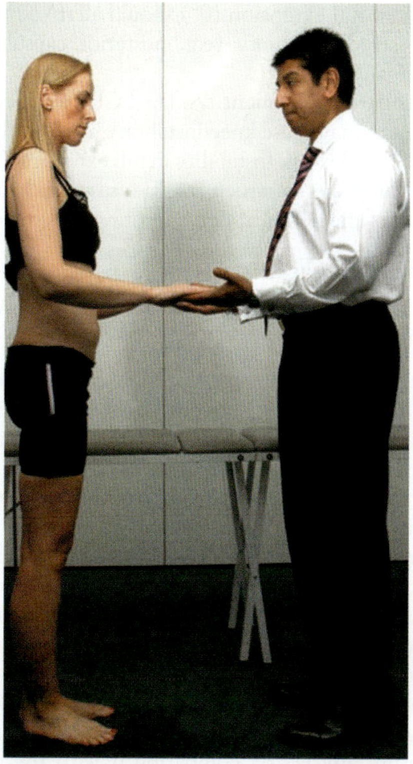

(b)

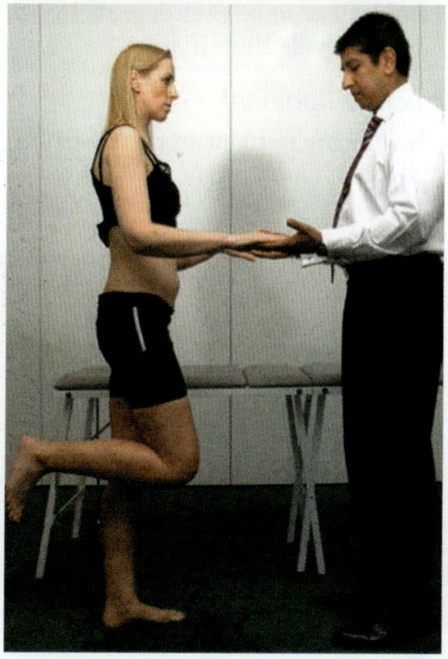

Figure 33.28 (a, b) Trendelenburg test.

Look

Look at the front, sides and back of both knees and for any walking or mobility aids or external appliances.

- **Skin**. Check for scars.
- **Soft tissues**. Look for wasting of the quadriceps and swelling in front of and behind the knee.
- **Bone**. Look for overall alignment (varus or valgus deformity). Measure the intermalleolar distance if a valgus deformity is present. With varus deformity, measure the distance between the medial aspect of both knees. From the side of the knee look for fixed flexion or recurvatum (hyperextension).

Gait

Look for antalgic gait (osteoarthritis) and varus thrust (collapse of the knee into more varus as weight is taken on that leg).

Feel

- **Soft tissue**. Feel the tendons for quadriceps and patellar tendon rupture.
- **Fluid displacement or stroke test**. First empty the medial side of the knee by stroking any fluid up from the medial side into the suprapatella pouch. Then place your hand on the superior aspect of the suprapatellar pouch and move it inferiorly, attempting to displace any fluid into the knee joint. Maintain your hand at the level of the superior pole of the patella. Now look to see if the normal gutters on either side of the knee are less noticeable because of fluid distension. Stroke the back of your hand over either gutter in turn. Look at the opposite gutter to see if there is cross-filling.
- **Patellar tap test**. This test is used when a large effusion is present. Place one hand on either side of the patella and, with the other hand, push down on the patella. With an effusion, fluctuance is present as the patella moves towards the joint.
- **Bone**. Feel the tibial tuberosity, inferior pole of the patella, patella facets, origin and insertion of the knee ligaments and joint line (medial and lateral). Remember to palpate for any popliteal swellings. Note the height of the patella.

Move

The knee moves principally in flexion (0–135°) and extension (from 0 to −10°) (Figure 33.29). Assess hyperextension by placing one of your hands on the anterior aspect of the distal femur. Now lift the distal tibia with the other hand. Measure the angle or the height that the heel can be lifted off the couch before the knee starts to move.

Perform a lag test to assess the integrity of the extensor mechanism. The patient is asked to lift the whole leg up off the bed (10°) with the knee straight. They are then asked to bend the knee and then try to straighten it again with the leg still held in the air. If they are unable to restraighten the knee they have a positive lag. This indicates significant weakness of the quadriceps mechanism.

In the presence of an apparent fixed flexion deformity of the knee (seen in osteoarthritis), decide if this is arising from the knee or hip joint. To differentiate, sit the patient up with the knees hanging over the edge of the couch; this obliterates the effect of any hip flexion deformity. Passively try to extend the knee fully. With a flexion deformity of the knee, this is not possible.

Special tests

Collateral ligaments

To assess the ligaments, place the leg under your arm. Flex the knee to 10° (not more) to relax the posterior capsule (the MCL and LCL are taut in full extension and lax in flexion). Stress each ligament in turn by applying a valgus or varus force. With your index fingers simultaneously palpate over the collateral ligaments. Assess for signs of instability (excessive opening of the joint). The quality of the end point should be noted (is it firm or spongy?). Compare both sides (Figure 33.30).

(a)

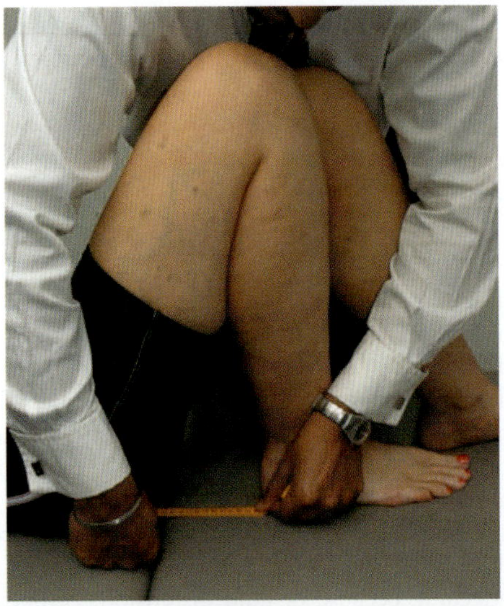

(b)

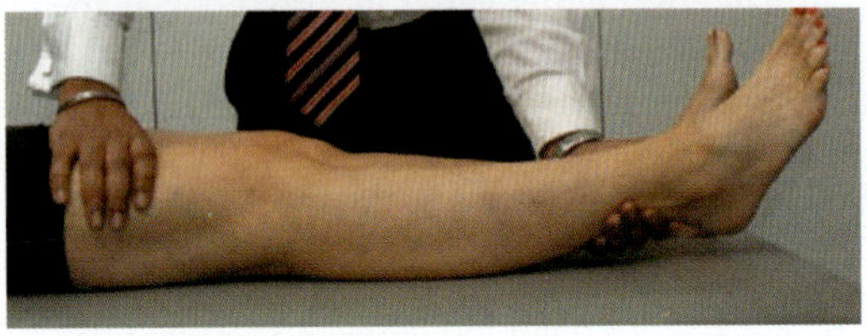

Figure 33.29 (a) Knee flexion and (b) extension.

- **Medial collateral ligament**. A lax MCL or deficient lateral compartment may cause knee instability when applying a valgus stress. It is important to note that the valgus stress test should be applied with the knee in 30° of flexion. Valgus instability in full extension (0°) should alert you to a possible posterior structure injury (e.g. posterior capsule, posterior cruciate ligament).
- **Lateral collateral ligament**. A lax LCL or deficient medial compartment may cause knee instability when applying a varus stress in 10° of flexion. Instability in full extension (0°) suggests injury to the posterior structures. In a suspected lateral injury, evaluation of the peroneal nerve must be performed.

Anterior cruciate ligament

The most sensitive test for evaluation of the ACL is the Lachmann test.

- **The Lachmann test** (Figure 33.31). Flex the knee to 15–30° and pull the proximal tibia gently forwards. Excessive laxity may indicate rupture of the ACL. Anterior translation of the tibia associated with a soft or no end point is a positive test. The test may be negative in chronic ruptures as the ACL stump can scar to the PCL.
- **Anterior draw test** (Figure 33.32a). Flex both knees to 90° and look for a posterior sag (compare the height of the tibial tuberosities looking from the side). This may indicate an injury to the PCL. Stabilise the feet by sitting on them. Now place your hands around the proximal and posterior aspect of the tibia. With your index fingers, push up the hamstrings to encourage them to relax. Now draw the tibia gently forwards and measure any laxity, comparing it with the other knee. The degree of laxity can be graded: grade I (0–5 mm), grade II (5–10 mm) and grade III (>10 mm).

Posterior cruciate ligament

The PCL is the primary restraint to posterior tibial translation between 30 and 90° of knee flexion. At 90°, the PCL accepts 95

(a)

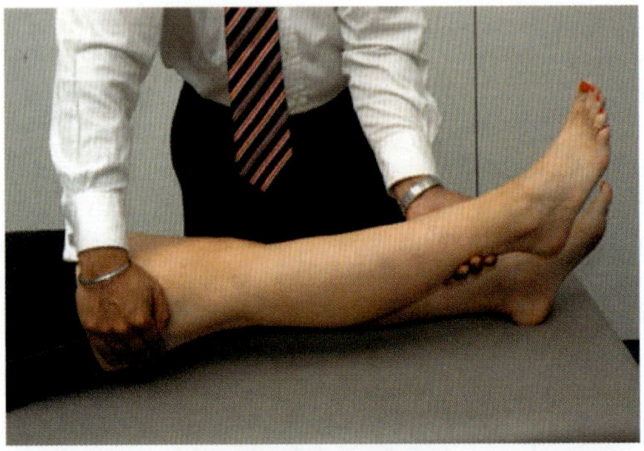

(b)

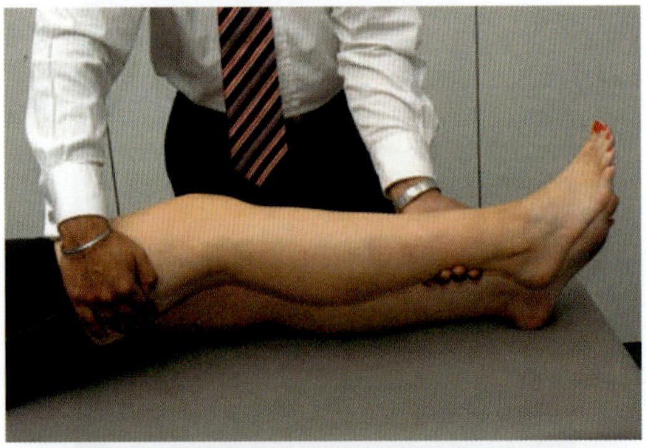

(c)

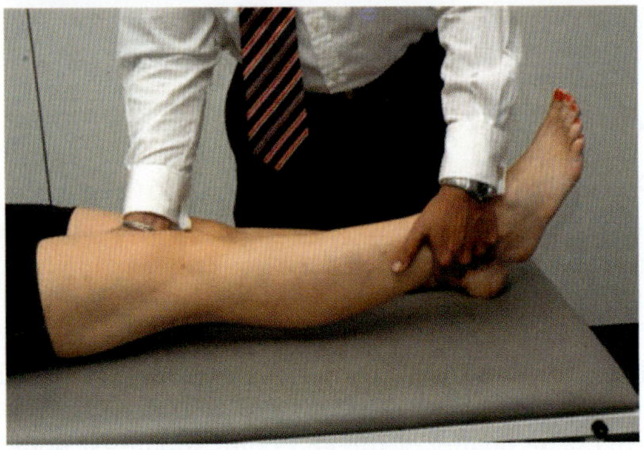

(d)

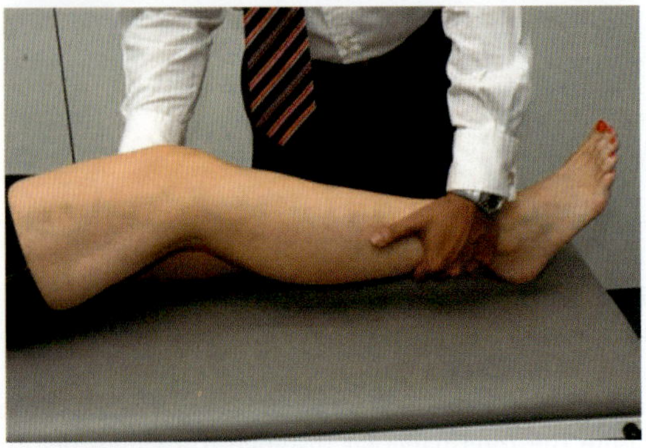

Figure 33.30 Assessing the medial (a, b) and lateral (c, d) collateral ligaments.

per cent of the posterior translational forces. Isolated PCL injuries are graded by the degree of posterior translation of the tibia with the knee in 90° of flexion. Look for a posterior sag with the knees flexed to 90°. The posterior draw test is the most reliable clinical test for a PCL injury.

- **Posterior draw test** (Figure 33.32b). Perform the test with the knee flexed to 90°. Push the anterior aspect of the proximal tibia posteriorly and compare any laxity with the other side. If more than 10 mm of posterior tibial translation is noted at 30 and/or 90° of knee flexion, a combined PCL and posterolateral corner injury may be present. An evaluation of the competency of the posterolateral corner is necessary.

Menisci

The presence of palpable joint line tenderness is the most sensitive clinical examination test for a meniscal tear. Flex the knee to 90° and palpate the joint line using your thumb and index finger. Note any areas of tenderness. The well-known tests for meniscal tears (McMurray's test and Apley's grind test) are unreliable and so are not described here. In the Thessaly test, the patient stands on the bad leg, rotating their body to twist the knee. This test is performed with the knee flexed first to 25° and then 45°. Pain and giving way is diagnostic of a meniscal tear. (You may need to support the patient by holding their hands during this test, if they are not to fall.)

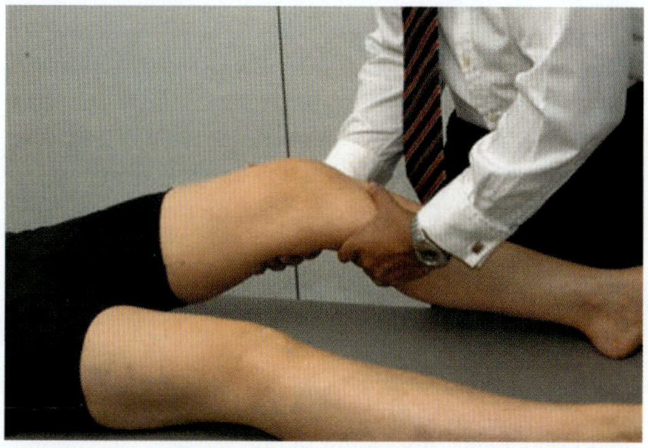

Figure 33.31 Lachmann's test: flex the knee to 15–30° and pull the proximal tibia forwards.

(a)

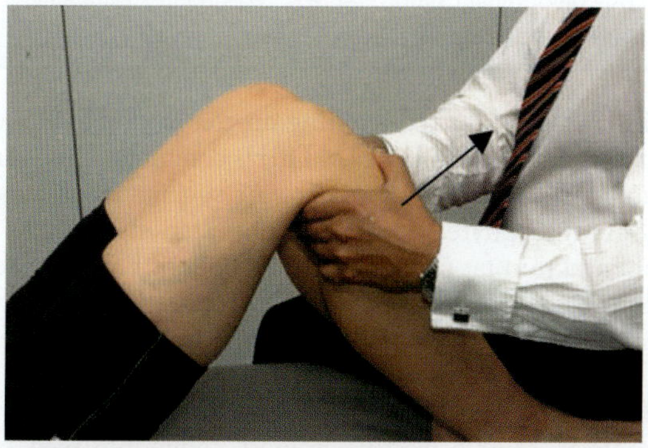

(b)

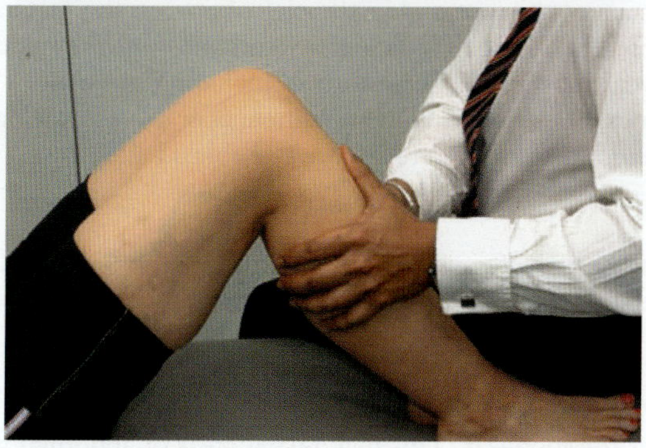

Figure 33.32 (a) Anterior draw test for anterior cruciate ligament stability; (b) posterior draw test for posterior cruciate ligament stability.

Patellofemoral joint

The patella normally enters the trochlea from a lateral position and becomes centralised with increasing knee flexion, travelling in a 'J' pattern.

- **Patellar tracking** (Figure 33.33). Sit the patient and ask them to let their legs hang off the end of the couch with the knees flexed to 90°. Ask the patient to slowly extend the knee to full extension. Toward the end of extension, look for lateral subluxation of the patella ('J' sign). This indicates maltracking.
- **Patellar apprehension (Fairbank's) test (for instability).** Attempt to laterally displace the patella with the knee in extension. Patients with instability contract their quadriceps muscle or complain of pain. With the patient supine and the quadriceps relaxed, flex the knee to 30° while trying to push the patella laterally. With instability the patient may react with apprehension. In addition, the quadriceps muscle may contract in an attempt to realign the patella.

Patellar tendon

The patellar tendon serves as the distal extent of the extensor mechanism. Rupture usually occurs at the osseotendinous junction. This results in an inability to actively perform and maintain full knee extension. A rupture presents with diffuse swelling in the anterior knee. A high-riding patella (patella alta) is present secondary to the unopposed pull of the quadriceps muscle. A defect in the tendon is usually palpable. When the rupture extends through the medial and lateral retinaculae, active extension is lost (Summary box 33.9).

Summary box 33.9

Knee examination

Inspection of the standing patient
- Front – alignment (varus/valgus/rotational deformity), muscle bulk
- Side – fixed flexion deformity
- Back – popliteal swellings, hamstrings
- Gait – antalgic, high stepping gait (foot drop), varus thrust

Inspection of the supine patient
- Skin, scars, soft tissues, deformity
- Palpation of the extensor mechanism, medial and lateral joint lines and collateral ligaments, hamstrings, tibial tuberosity, fibular head

Movements
- Flexion and extension

Special tests
- Patellar apprehension test and extensor mechanism
- Cruciate ligaments
- Collateral ligaments
- Menisci

Thomas Porter McMurray, 1887–1949, Professor of Orthopaedic Surgery, Liverpool University, Liverpool, UK.
Sir Harold Arthur Thomas Fairbank, 1876–1961, orthopaedic surgeon, King's College Hospital, London, UK.

(a)

(b)

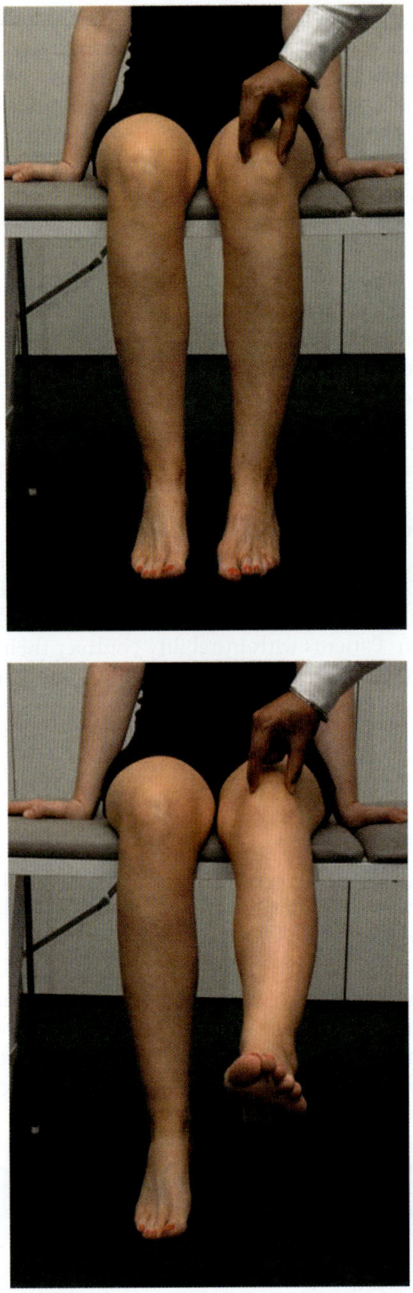

Figure 33.33 (a, b) Patellar tracking.

CLINICAL EXAMINATION OF THE FOOT AND ANKLE

The foot can be divided into three parts: the hindfoot (calcaneus, talus), the midfoot (navicular, cuboids, cuneiforms) and the forefoot (metatarsals and phalanges).

Look

Ask the patient to stand and assess the overall limb alignment. Assess pelvic obliquity, limb length discrepancy (and its level), valgus/varus deformities of the knee and rotational alignment. Check for contractures of the hips and knees, Now focus your attention on the foot itself:

- **Foot shape.** Assess the overall shape of the forefoot from the front. From the side, look for the normal medial arch (Figure 33.34a). The hindfoot is best appreciated from behind. Now look at the vertical relationship between the Achilles tendon and the calcaneus (normal heel valgus of 5–7°). Look from behind and count the number of toes that can be seen. The 'too many toes' sign demonstrates increased forefoot abduction (pes planus (flat foot)) and a splayed forefoot. Foot shapes that may be encountered include neutral foot (no overall deformity), skew foot (hindfoot valgus and forefoot adduction), metatarsus adductus (neutral hindfoot and adduction of the metatarsus), pes planus (collapse of the medial arch) and pes cavus or high arch (increased medial arch). The possible causes of pes planus and pes cavus are shown in Summary boxes 33.10 and 33.11, respectively.

Summary box 33.10

Causes of pes planus

- Normal variant
- Hyperlaxity syndrome, e.g. Marfan's syndrome
- Tarsal coalition – rigid and painful flat foot (Figure 33.39a)
- Tibial posterior dysfunction

Summary box 33.11

Causes of pes cavus (Figure 33.34b)

- Spinal anomalies, e.g. spina bifida
- Hereditary sensorimotor neuropathies, such as Charcot–Marie–Tooth disease
- Charcot foot (e.g. neuropathic foot)
- Post-compartment syndrome (e.g. Volkmann's ischaemic contracture)

- **Skin.** A bunion or red swelling on the medial aspect of the metatarsophalangeal joint (MTPJ) is common. This is an area of inflamed skin with an underlying subcutaneous bursa and a joint osteophyte. Systemic manifestations include gouty tophi and thin fat pads under the metatarsal heads as seen in rheumatoid arthritis. Corns are callosities which form where toes rub against the inside of shoes. Remember to assess the appearance of the nails.
- **Soft tissues.** Swelling may indicate soft tissue or joint pathology. Muscle wasting is most commonly seen on the dorsum of the foot and in the clefts between the metatarsals. If present, a full neurological examination of the upper and lower limbs should be performed including the spine.
- **Bones.** Look for any bony prominences or exostoses. Common forefoot deformities are shown in Table 33.12.

Gait

Look for a high stepping gait (foot drop), painful (antalgic) gait (ankle and foot joint pain) and a short propulsive phase (forefoot pain).

Footwear

Inspect the footwear. This may reveal areas of abnormal weight bearing. With normal wear of the sole, a corner is typically worn off the posterolateral aspect of the heel (heel strike). In addition,

(a)

(b)

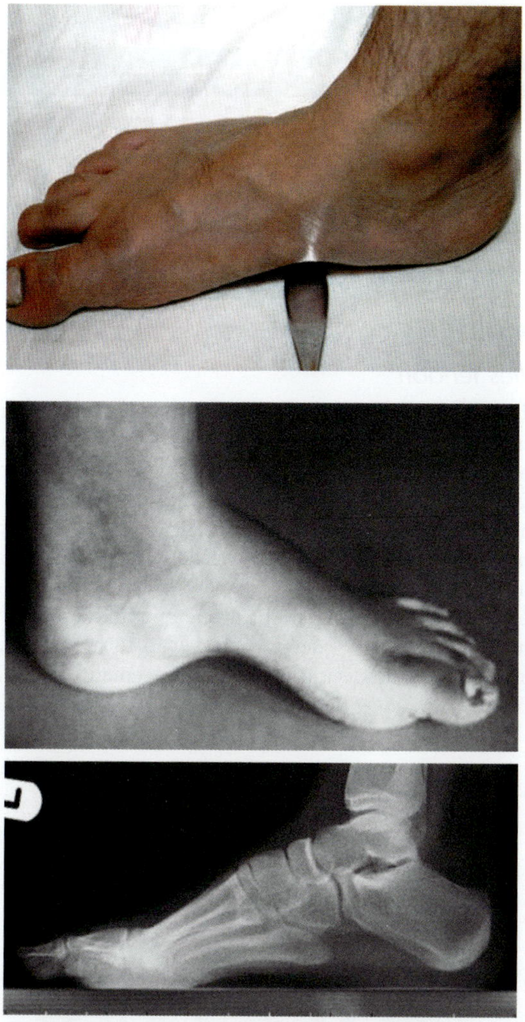

Figure 33.34 (a) Normal medial longitudinal arch of the foot. (b) Clinical and radiological appearance of pes cavus.

there may be a circular wear pattern under the ball of the big toe (toe-off phase).

- External appearance: Look at the materials used, the metal supports and heel raise, depth and width.
- Internal appearance: Look at the insoles, arch supports and heel cups.

Feel

- **Skin**. Reduced sensation in a glove and stocking distribution is seen with diabetes.
- **Soft tissues**. The posterior tibial and the dorsal pedis pulses should be identified (Figure 33.35). Palpate the tibialis anterior tendon and the long extensor tendons on the dorsum of the foot. From the back, palpate the Achilles tendon. Palpate the peroneal tendons from the lateral side and the tibialis posterior tendon from the medial side. The sinus tarsi can be assessed. This is an anatomical space bounded by the talus and calcaneus and is recognisable as a soft-tissue depression anterior to the lateral malleolus. It is filled with fat and the extensor digitorum brevis muscle. Sinus tarsi syndrome may occur. This may be caused by injury to the interosseous talocalcaneal ligament or the subtalar joint. There is pain and tenderness over the sinus tarsi with subjective hindfoot instability. The pain is characteristically relieved by local anaesthetic injection.
- **Bones**. Feel for deformity, bony prominences and loose bodies:
  - ankle joint: the medial and lateral malleoli, anterior and posterior joint line, lateral gutter and ligament complex, the syndesmosis (front of the ankle), medial gutter and medial ligament complex;
  - subtalar joint: palpate each facet;
  - midtarsal joints: the talonavicular and calcaneocuboid joints;
  - tarsometatarsal joints (TMTJ): note that the second TMTJ is several millimetres proximal to the others; movement is minimal in the second ray, limited in the third ray, moderate in the fourth and fifth rays and very variable in the first ray.
- Specific structures to palpate:
  - calcaneus (heel bone): the most common cause of pain is plantar fasciitis; this may present with numbness, burning and electric shock sensations, which are worse in the morning and improve as the day goes on; identify the exact point of tenderness;
  - tendons: examine for contracture of the Achilles tendon insertion and the peroneal or tibialis posterior tendons;
  - head of talus: invert and evert the patient's foot;
  - sustentaculum tali: palpate one fingerbreadth below the medial malleolus; this important structure serves as an attachment for the spring ligament;
  - cuneiforms (medial, middle and lateral), MTPJs, web spaces and all the forefoot bones.

Move

The movements of the foot and ankle are linked via the ankle, subtalar and midfoot joints. Remember the acronyms PAED – **p**ronation, **a**bduction, **e**version and **d**orsiflexion – and SAPI – **s**upination, **a**dduction, **p**lantarflexion and **i**nversion. These are the two common general foot deformities.

Ankle (Figure 33.36)

- **Dorsiflexion**. Test dorsiflexion with the knee both flexed and extended. If restriction is greater with the knee extended than flexed, the contracture is principally in the gastrocnemius. Restriction that is equal in all knee positions is caused by a contracture principally of the soleus.
- **Plantarflexion**. Ask the patient to touch the floor with their foot (15°). Weakness suggests injury to the Achilles tendon or pathology affecting the S1 nerve root.

Subtalar joint (Figures 33.37 and 33.38)

Hold the talar neck and ask the patient to move their heel from side to side. Repeat using a hand on the heel to move the joint and apply a varus and valgus stress while feeling for movements of the talus. Holding the talus as opposed to the tibia isolates subtalar from ankle motion. (Normal range is 5° in each direction.)

Pierre Marie, 1853–1940, Neurologist, Hospice de Bicêtre, Paris, France, later became Professor of Pathological Anatomy in the Faculty of Medicine, and finally, in 1918, Professor of Neurology.
Howard Henry Tooth, 1856–1925, Physician, St Bartholomew's Hospital and the National Hospital for Nervous Diseases, Queen's Square, London, UK, described peroneal muscular atrophy in 1886, independently of Charcot and Marie.

Antoine Bernard-Jean Marfan, 1858–1942, physician, Hôpital des Infants-Malades, Paris, France, described this syndrome in 1896.
Jean Martin Charcot, 1825–1893, physician, La Salpêtrière, Paris, France.

Table 33.12 Common forefoot deformities.

Deformity	Metatarsophalangeal joint	Proximal interphalangeal joint	Distal interphalangeal joint
Claw toe	Hyperextension	Flexion	Flexion
Hammer toe	Normal	Flexion	Flexion
Mallet toe	Normal	Normal	Flexion
Hallux valgus or varus	Valgus or varus position	Normal	–

(a)

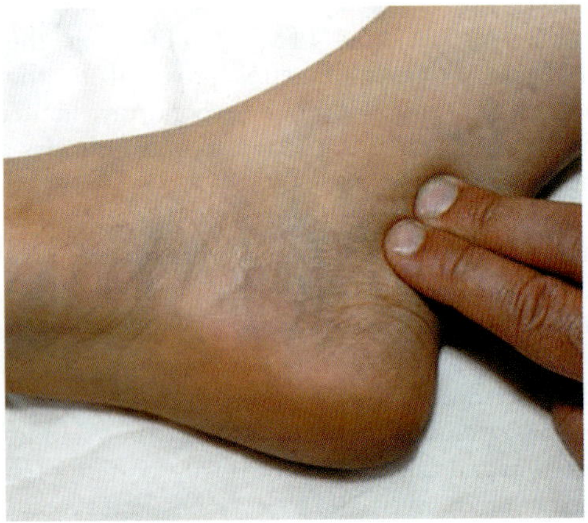

(b)

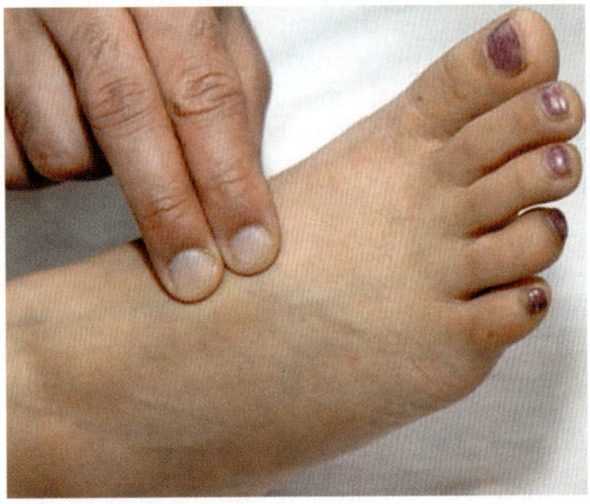

Figure 33.35 (a) Palpation of the posterior tibial pulse; (b) palpation of the dorsalis pedis pulse.

- **Inversion**. Ask the patient to move their foot in towards them.
- **Eversion**. Ask the patient to move their foot out to the side.

Midtarsal joint

Hold the heel with one hand and move the forefoot medially (adduction = 20°) and laterally (abduction = 10°) with the other hand.

Tarsometatarsal joint

Hold the midfoot and manipulate each metatarsal up and down to estimate the passive range of movement.

Metatarsophalangeal joint

Test extension (70–90°) by asking the patient to lift the toes to the ceiling and test flexion (45°) by pointing the toes to the floor. Normal toe-off requires 35–40° of dorsiflexion.

Special tests

Achilles tendon

Feel the gastrocnemius and soleus bellies and the whole length of the tendon for gaps (rupture), tenderness or swelling. Also identify the posterolateral (Haglund's) prominence of the calcaneus and palpate the retro-Achilles bursa.

The best test for integrity of the tendon is the **Thompson's** or **Simmonds' test**. Do not be misled by the patient's ability to stand on tiptoes – some people can do this using their long toe flexors alone. Lie the patient prone and allow the calves to rest on your forearms. Squeeze each calf in turn and watch for movement at the ankle joint. Lack of movement may indicate a rupture.

(a)

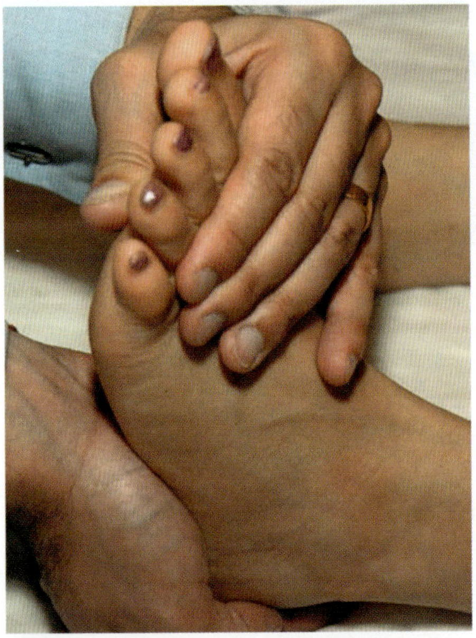

(b)

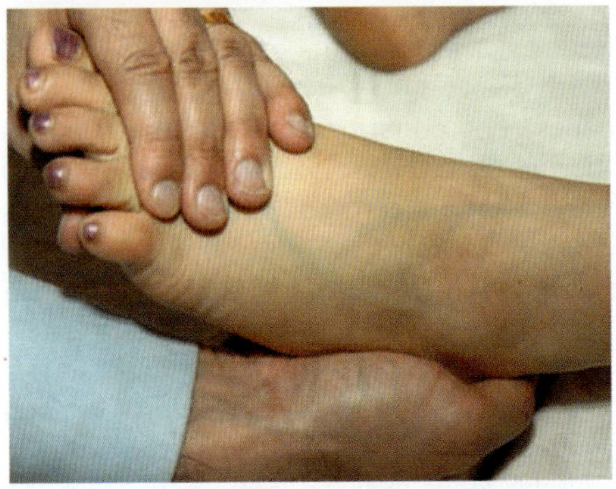

Figure 33.36 (a) Ankle dorsiflexion and (b) ankle plantarflexion.

Subtalar joint flexibility

Ask the patient to stand on their toes and observe the heel from behind; the heel moves normally from valgus to varus indicating flexibility. The **Coleman's block test** is used to assess the flexibility of the subtalar joint. Ask the patient to stand on a 2-cm block with the great toe over the medial edge, resting on the floor. Now look from behind. If the hindfoot varus remains, the subtalar joint is fixed. If it corrects to valgus, the joint is mobile (Figure 33.38).

Flat foot flexibility

Use the Windlass and Jack's test to distinguish a flexible from a fixed flat foot (Figure 33.39):

- **Windlass test**. Ask the patient to stand on their toes and observe the arch of the foot on the medial aspect. As soon as the patient stands on their toes, the arch forms. Failure of this indicates a fixed flat foot.
- **Jack's test**. With the patient standing, lift up the great toe. The arch should form in the flexible flat foot.

Ankle stability

Trauma to the ankle is a common cause of instability. Accurate assessment may be difficult in the acute setting because of pain.

- **Anterior draw test**. With the foot resting over the bed, hold the heel with one hand and the front of the tibia with the other. Move the heel forwards on the fixed tibia. Compare with the other side. Instability of the syndesmosis may be palpable (Figure 33.40).
- **Squeeze test for distal tibiofibular stability**. Compress the proximal calf. Pain at the ankle may indicate separation of the distal fibula from the tibia.
- **Tilt test**. Hold the talus at the neck rather than the heel so that you can be sure that any tilt is in the ankle and not the subtalar joint.

Tarsometatarsal joint stability

Stability can be assessed by pushing each joint up and down. Standing lateral radiographs may be used in addition.

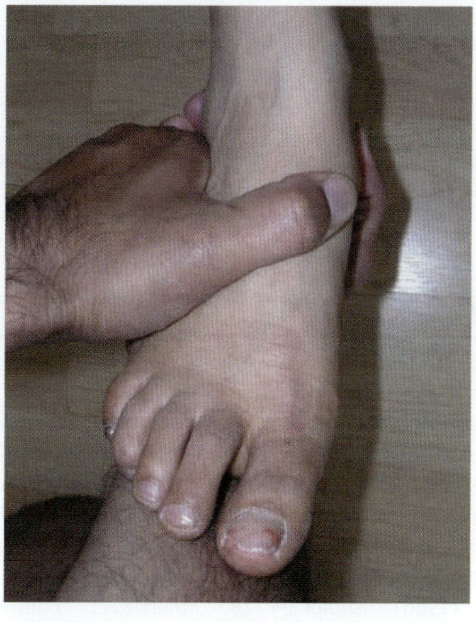

Figure 33.37 Testing subtalar joint motion.

Tibialis anterior

Ask the patient to walk on their heels with their feet inverted; the tibialis anterior tendon can be seen. With the patient's feet resting over the edge of the couch, ask the patient to actively dorsiflex and invert their foot to reach your hand. Palpate the tibialis anterior muscle.

Tibialis posterior

Pathology of the tibialis posterior typically presents with posteromedial ankle pain, swelling and gradual onset of a flat foot. When assessing the tendon, look for swelling along its course, a flat foot with heel valgus, the 'too many toes' sign and prominence of the talar head. Palpate for tenderness, swelling or gaps in the tendon. To test integrity:

- Ask the patient to perform a single foot tiptoe test on both sides. The inability to lift the affected heel off the ground is suggestive of a tibialis posterior tendon injury or insufficiency.
- To test strength, position the foot in the plantarflexed and inverted position. Ask the patient to hold this position while you push against their foot.

Dorsiflexors

Tendinitis of the long toe dorsiflexors usually presents in athletes. Pain affects gait in the early contact phase. Palpate for swelling, gaps or any tenderness. Ask the patient to move the foot into dorsiflexion and to hold this position while you push the foot down.

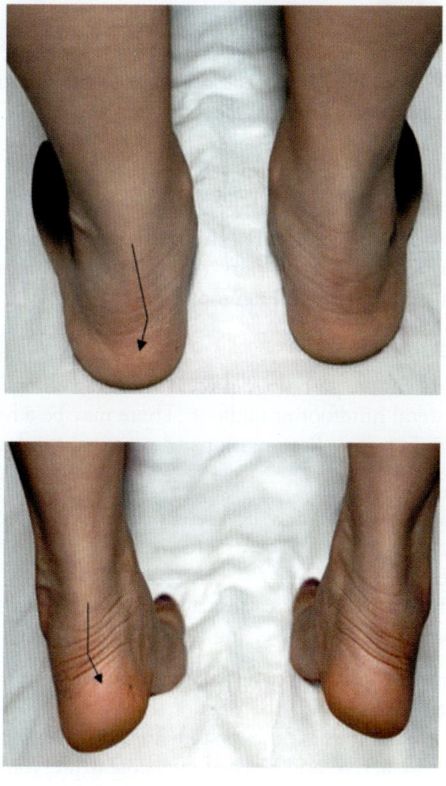

Figure 33.38 Testing subtalar joint flexibility.

Patrik Haglund, 1870–1937, Swedish orthopaedic surgeon.
Frankin Adin Simmonds, 1911–1983, Orthopaedic Surgeon, The Rowley Bristow Hospital, Pyrford, Surrey, UK.

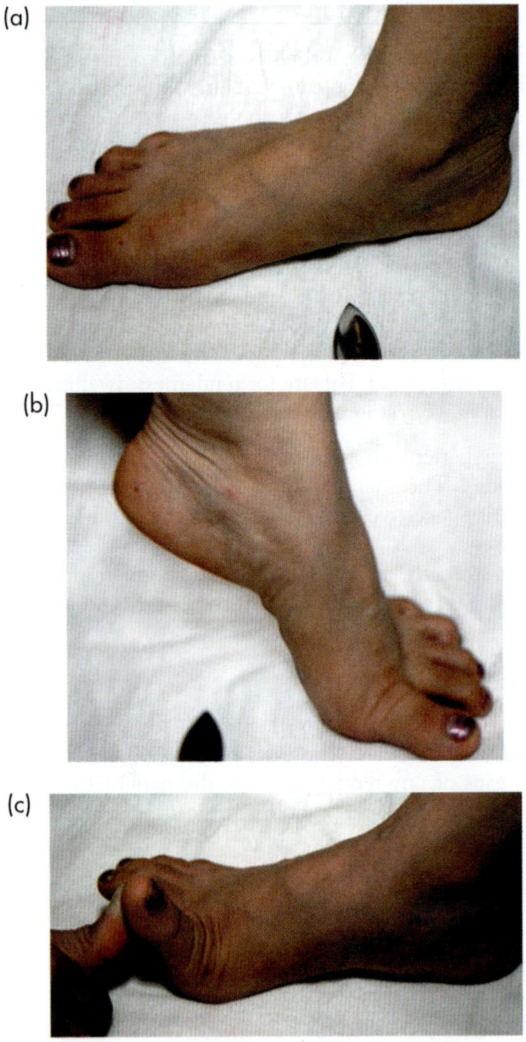

Figure 33.39 (a) Flat foot appearance with a reduced medial longitudinal arch; (b) Windlass test; (c) Jack's test.

Inability to dorsiflex the foot is referred to as foot drop. Causes include stroke, spinal injury, spinal stenosis or disc prolapse, peripheral nerve injury (e.g. sciatic, common and deep peroneal) or a peripheral neuropathy.

Peroneals

Peroneal tendon pathology presents with swelling and/or pain of the lateral hindfoot or midfoot. There may be a history of the ankle 'giving way'. Presentations of peroneal tendon pathology include:

- 'peroneal spasm': may be seen in tarsal coalition; here, the muscles are usually contracted secondary to the hindfoot valgus;
- peroneal tendon dislocation: attempt to dislocate the tendons by dorsiflexing and everting the foot.

The peroneus longus may be palpated just before it crosses under the foot to insert onto the base of the first metatarsal. Ask the patient to plantarflex the first metatarsal. Test strength and integrity by active and resisted eversion while you palpate the tendons for swelling, tenderness or gaps.

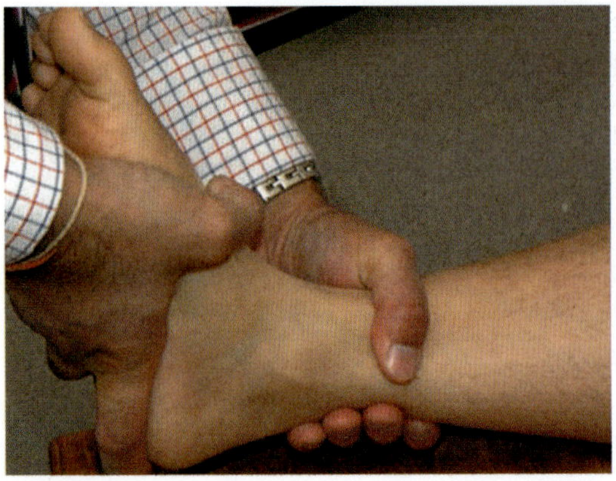

Figure 33.40 Anterior draw test.

Morton's neuroma

This condition represents thickening of the tissue that surrounds the digital nerve leading to the toes as the nerve passes under the ligament connecting the metatarsals in the forefoot. It is most frequent between the third and fourth toes. A neuroma presents with burning pain in the ball of the foot that radiates to the involved toes. The condition is difficult to diagnose and requires a high index of suspicion. Palpate in the web space between the symptomatic toes for a mass. Compression of the metatarsals may elicit a 'click' between the bones (Molders' click) (Summary box 33.12).

Summary box 33.12

Ankle and foot examination

Inspection of the standing patient
- Front – alignment, foot shape and deformity
- Side – medial arch
- Back – heel position
- Gait – antalgic, high stepping gait (foot drop)

Inspection of the supine patient
- Skin, scars, soft tissues, bony deformity
- Palpation of the ankle, subtalar, midfoot and forefoot joints

Movements
- Dorsiflexion, plantarflexion, inversion, eversion

Special tests
- Flexibility of the subtalar joint and a flat foot
- Joint stability, Morton's neuroma
- Tendons – tibialis posterior and anterior, Achilles tendon, peroneals and dorsiflexors

FURTHER READING

Aitken McCrae D. *Hugh Owen Thomas: his principles and practice*. London: Oxford University Press, 1935.

Ganz R, Parvizi J, Beck M *et al.* Femoroacetabular impingement: a cause for osteoarthritis of the hip. *Clin Orthop* 2003; **217**: 112–20.

Miller MD, Bergfeld JA, Fowler PJ *et al.* The posterior cruciate ligament injured knee: principles of evaluation and treatment. *Instr Course Lect* 1999; **48**: 199–207.

Neer CS. Impingement lesions. *Clin Orthop* 1983; **173**: 70–7.

Rang M. (1966) *Anthology of orthopaedics*. Edinburgh: E&S Livingstone, 1966: 139–43.

Thomas George Morton, 1835–1903, surgeon, The Pennsylvania Hospital, Philadelphia, PA, USA.

CHAPTER 34 Sports medicine and sports injuries

LEARNING OBJECTIVES

To understand:
- The important issues behind a patient's sporting injury in the context of taking a history

To know:
- The common sports injuries
- The appropriate ways of imaging to confirm or refute a diagnosis

To assess:
- The patient and offer treatment and rehabilitation plans

INTRODUCTION

Regular physical exercise is integral to the body staying healthy. However, stressing the human body to its limits may lead to injury. Sports medicine is the science of understanding how these injuries can be avoided, recognised when they do occur, and then treated appropriately. Sports injuries are, in principle, the same as other injuries. The major difference can be in the expectation of the patients. The injuries can be classified into three broad groups. Acute extrinsic injuries are those which arise from a direct external blow. These are commonly wounds, bruises and fractures. Acute intrinsic injuries result from failure of a patient's structures as a result of excessive loading. Examples are tendon ruptures, avulsion fractures and ligament injuries. Chronic injuries are those with an insidious or unknown onset, commonly inflammation or failure secondary to repetitive loading. Examples are inflammation of the Achilles tendon and stress fractures (Summary box 34.1).

Summary box 34.1

Types of sports injury

- Acute extrinsic – caused by direct external blow (bruises)
- Acute intrinsic – internal failure secondary to excessive external force (ligament tear)
- Chronic – repetitive and stress injuries

DIAGNOSIS OF SPORTS INJURIES

There are some additional questions which need to be asked in the history when treating a patient with a sports injury:

1. How was the injury sustained?
2. What type of sport or training were they undertaking; mixed training or only one type of sport?
3. Have they had a previous injury? When was this and what rehabilitation have they had?
4. What were they aiming for in the way of competitions or level of sport that they performed before the injury?
5. Do they now want to compete again or are they considering retiring?

The examination should follow the system described in Chapter 26.

TENDON DISEASE

Tendons can become weak and/or painful as a result of physical damage or as a result of inflammation of the tendon sheath around them (peritendonitis).

Tendon injury is either due to overload (the strength of the tendon being exceeded by the force applied) or to overuse (where there is repetitive low level load to the tendon) leading to fatigue and failure. In this case the patient may present with inflammation rather than rupture.

Overuse injuries

Internal factors

Overuse injury can be precipitated in a tendon by decreased oxygen supply, decreased nutrition, hormonal changes, chronic inflammation and ageing.

External factors

A change in the environment (new running surface), or worn out equipment (old running shoes), may both bring about an overuse injury as can excessive training when the patient is not fit enough to tolerate it.

In younger patients, the weakest area of a tendon is the apophyseal attachment. In adults, the musculotendinous junction is more liable to injury. In adolescents, the common sites of injury are tendon insertions. Examples are the anterior superior iliac spine (origin of Sartorius), the anterior inferior iliac spine (rectus femoris), the lesser trochanter of the femur (iliopsoas) and the ischial tuberosity (hamstrings) (Summary box 34.2).

Summary box 34.2

Problems with tendons

- Rupture due to excessive loads
- Pain and inflammation due to repetitive or abnormal loading

MUSCLE INJURY

Muscle injuries can be classified into a sprain, partial tear, complete tear or re-tear (if there has been previous injury). Most will heal spontaneously but may leave a painless defect in the muscle belly.

LIGAMENTS

Ligament injuries are acute intrinsic injuries and can be graded according to their severity (Table 34.1).

Table 34.1 Ligament injuries graded according to severity.

Grade	Description
0	Normal ligament
1	No increase in joint laxity but there is tenderness around the injured ligament
2	Partial disruption of the ligament fibres with increased joint laxity, and a soft end point
3	Complete disruption of the ligament. There is a marked increase in joint laxity with no end point clinically

In the acute phase it may be difficult to assess the ligament injury thoroughly. Once the acute injury has settled then any difference in laxity when comparing the two sides is diagnostic. However, the laxity of ligaments varies dramatically between patients and with age, so absolute measurements are not reliable. Grade 1 and 2 ligament injuries can be treated with pain relief, splinting and gentle mobilisation to avoid stiffness. Grade 3 injuries may require surgical repair to bring together the torn ends of the ligament (Summary box 34.3).

Summary box 34.3

Ligament injuries

- Difficult to assess in the acute phase
- Use the opposite side for comparison
- Surgical repair may be needed for complete disruption

BURSAE

Bursae are found between the joints and overlying tissues or muscles and tendons and are small fluid-filled endothelium-lined sacks. They decrease frictional forces between structures, but can become inflamed. The most commonly affected sites are over the first metatarsal phalangeal joint (bunion), in front of the patella (housemaid's knee) and behind the elbow (olecranon bursa). They can become inflamed or even infected. If they fail to settle with appropriate treatment then they can be surgically excised.

BONE FRACTURES AND STRESS FRACTURES

True fractures can be encountered in any sport, but the fracture type found more commonly in sportsmen and women is a stress fracture. This is caused by multiple repetitions of moderate loads. Clinically, these lesions give poorly localised pain, which is worse on exercise. They are more common in runners, especially women who may have reduced bone density. The most common sites for stress fractures are the metatarsals and the tibia.

INJURIES ASSOCIATED WITH INDIVIDUAL SPORTS

Golf

The shoulder and back are the most common sites of overuse injuries. Golfer's elbow or medial epicondylitis is due to a common flexor origin tendinosis. It does not just occur in golfers.

Tennis

Tennis elbow is inflammation of the common extensor origin.

Partial ruptures of the calf muscles, especially the medial head of the gastrocnemius are also found in tennis players (called tennis leg), and in other sports requiring sudden extreme acceleration.

Rowing

The common problems with rowing are rib fractures and intercostal muscle tears and tendon problems such as intersection syndrome (a tendinosis where the first and second extensor tendon compartments cross) (Figures 34.1 and 34.2).

Football

The main injuries are fractures, groin injuries, muscle tears and twisting injuries to the knees and ankles leading to ligament tears (Figures 34.3 and 34.4). Injuries specific to football include turf toe and neuromas to the deep peroneal nerve due

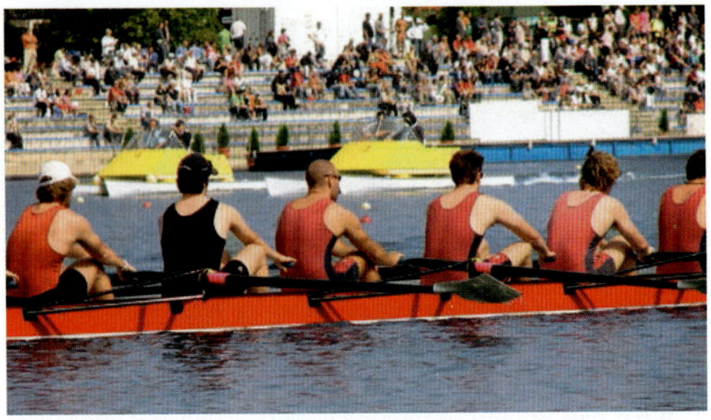

Figure 34.1 Rowers in action at a regatta (© Vladislav Gagic–Fotolia).

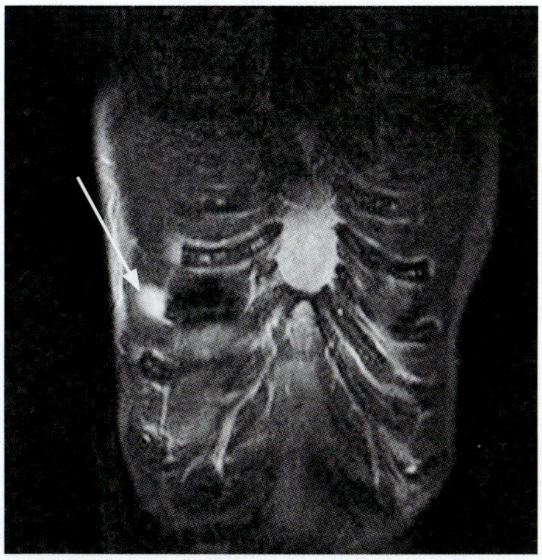

Figure 34.2 Coronal magnetic resonance imaging of the chest showing an intercostal muscle injury in a rower.

to repetitive trauma from kicking the football. Goalkeepers get wrist and hand injuries, including occult scaphoid fractures.

Rugby

This is a high intensity contact sport so injuries include concussion due to head trauma, neck injuries including fractures to the cervical spine, muscle tears, shoulder, acromiocalvicular joint and finger injuries including dislocation of the phalanges and tendon injuries e.g Rugger jersey finger – where there is injury to the flexor profundus tendon.

Javelin throwers

Javelin throwers get injuries due to abnormal stresses on the elbow similar to those seen in baseball. This causes abnormalities of the ulnar collateral ligament and capitellum.

Swimming

Shoulder injuries are more common in swimmers, especially in those performing the crawl or the butterfly stroke as these can lead to impingement syndromes (rotator cuff tendinosis and tears).

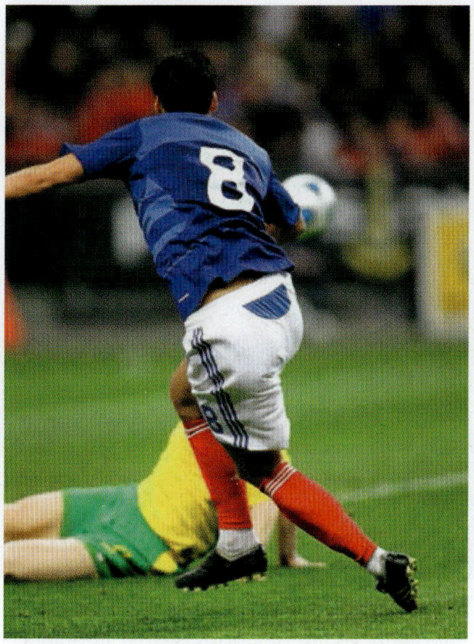

Figure 34.3 A footballer in action (© lilufoto–Fotolia).

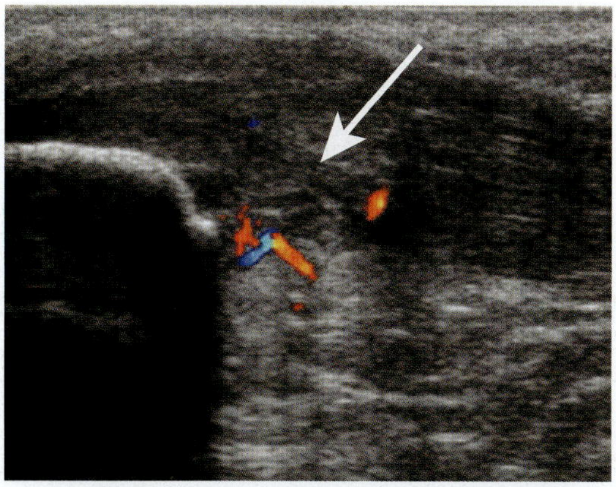

Figure 34.4 Ultrasound showing a patellar tendinosis with neovascularisation in a footballer.

Volleyball, netball and basketball

Hand injuries are common, as is patellar tendinopathy and internal derangements of the ankle and knee.

Ballet dancing

Ballet dancers get problems with posterior impingement of the ankle and tendinopathy of the flexor hallucis longus tendon when working on pointe (tip-toe) (Figures 34.5 and 34.6). Stress fractures are also found in female ballet dancers due to the abnormal stresses. Male ballet dancers are prone to back and shoulder injuries due to carrying ballerinas.

Young dancers often complain of clicking and pain around the hip which may be due to iliopsoas tendinopathy.

Snowboarders and skiers

Both sports have the full range of injuries associated with a high speed sport (Figure 34.7). The rigid high boots used by skiers protect the ankle, but increase the loads transmitted up the limb, risking fracture of the tibia, and ligament disruption of the knee (especially the anterior cruciate) (Figure 34.8). Novice snowboarders get wrist fractures.

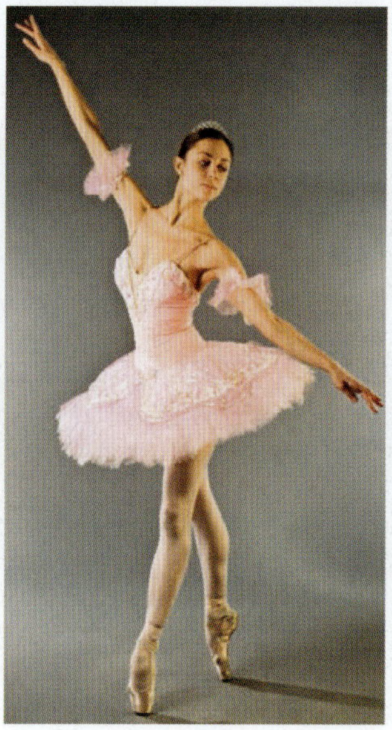

Figure 34.5 Ballet dancer on pointe (© Zoja–Fotolia).

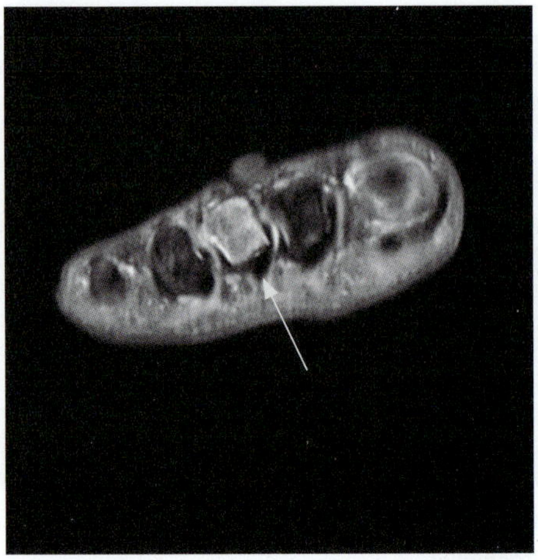

Figure 34.6 Magnetic resonance imaging STIR (short TI inversion recovery) sequence showing a stress injury to a metatarsal (arrow).

Martial arts: judo, karate and taekwondo

All are associated with acute extrinsic injuries (direct blows), and acute intrinsic injuries (failure of ligaments and other structures due to sudden excessive loads).

Weight training

Weight training tends to produce the third type of sports injury (chronic) with problems with the shoulders and carpal tunnel syndrome and the spine.

Kayaking

There are problems with the forearm and posterior interosseous nerve compression.

Marathon runners

Problems include iliotibial band syndrome and stress fractures in the feet and shins.

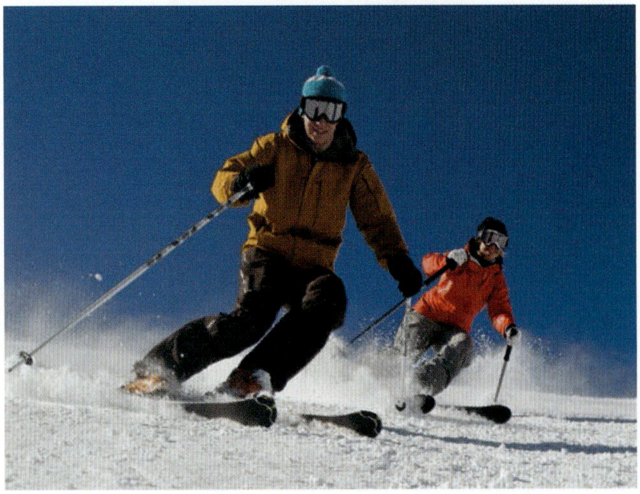

Figure 34.7 Skiers in action (©Alexander Rochau–Fotolia).

INJURIES ACCORDING TO REGION OF SYMPTOMS

Pelvis, hip and thigh injuries

- Thigh bruise (Charley Horse, corked thigh or helmet thigh): These occur in all contact sports and can be both large and painful. They require prolonged rest as they are slow to settle and can rebleed. A pseudo-tumour may develop. Surgical drainage should be avoided if at all possible as it can lead to infection of the haematoma.
- Quadriceps tears: These most commonly occur in the rectus femoris muscle. They may be due to a direct blow, but more commonly they are due to twisting injury and they occur along the aponeurosis of the rectus femoris, which is a weak point where the two muscle bellies join.
- Complete quadriceps rupture is less common, but may occur when kicking balls or in older patients. The patient can often perform a straight leg raise due to trick manoeuvres. However, they cannot restraighten the raised leg (quadriceps lag). Surgical repair is not usually needed.
- Hamstring injury commonly occurs due to twisting injuries following sudden and maximal muscle contraction. The injuries most commonly occur in the biceps femoris tendon, but can occur in the semimembranosis and to a lesser degree semitendinosis.

Groin pain

This is a very difficult area to assess as referred pain to the groin can come from many sources. These include:

- the hip, (labral tears, and osteoarthritis)
- adductor tendon injuries
- stress fractures of the femur, pubis or stress fractures of the femoral neck
- hernias (these may be small and include femoral and obturator hernias)

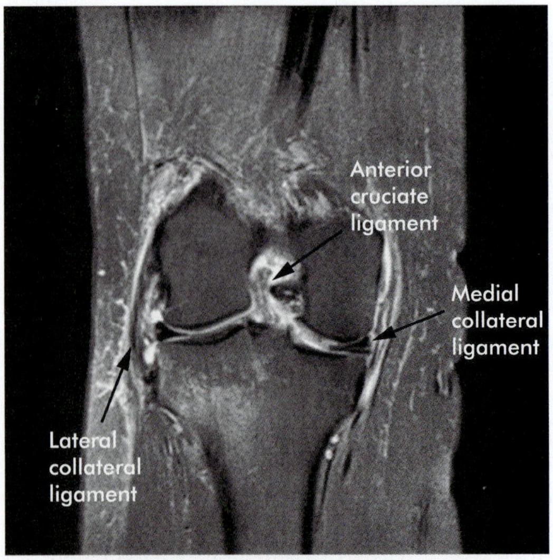

Figure 34.8 Knee magnetic resonance imaging showing a significant skiing injury with tears of the anterior cruciate ligament, medial collateral ligament and lateral collateral ligament.

- tumours
- sexually transmitted diseases
- gynaecological and urinary problems
- referred pain from the lumbar spine.

Adductor tendon injuries produce localised tenderness over the adductor origin.

A labral tear of the hip will cause clicking and pain.

Knee injury

Acute

Knee injuries are common in contact sports, and as a result of studded boots applying excessive loads to the knee in rapid turning. If the patient cannot continue playing and the knee swells immediately then there is likely to be blood in the knee. The most likely causes are a tear of the anterior cruciate ligament, dislocation of the patella (which usually relocates again immediately), and an intra-articular fracture (there will be marrow fat globules visible in the aspirate).

If the patient continues to play and the knee swells later, then the diagnosis is more likely to be a tear of a meniscus and the fluid aspirated will be clear. The early diagnosis of a knee injury is very difficult as the knee is too painful to examine. Aspiration of any effusion, using full sterile precautions, followed by early physiotherapy to maintain quads strength will allow most acute injuries to settle.

Patellar dislocation is more common in the hyper-mobile patient and in contact sports. If it has not already relocated, straightening the knee allows it to relocate.

Subsequent diagnosis

Patients who have had a patellar dislocation will have a patellar apprehension sign (see Chapter 31).

True locking is caused by a loose body in the knee (osteochondritis dissecans), or a torn meniscus. The patient will be moving normally at the time (unlike pseudo-locking) and will suddenly find that they are unable to straighten or even bend the knee. After a period of 'jiggling' the knee they may be able to release the block and move normally again. The Thessaly test is said to have high sensitivity and specificity for this condition (see Chapter 33) but the MacMurray test does not, so is no longer included. Imaging should be performed in locked knees as clinical assessment is difficult and an arthroscopy may not be needed.

If the meniscal tear is peripheral (where there is a blood supply) then meniscal repair should be undertaken.

Giving way can be caused by weakness, pain or instability. Weakness will usually be the result of quadriceps wasting secondary to the injury and is best treated with physiotherapy.

Patellofemoral pain can arise spontaneously in adolescents, but can also arise after a knee injury when the vastus medialis wastes rapidly, and the patella starts to mal-track. Clinically the patient will give a history of finding it difficult to descend stairs and experience severe pain and giving way when trying to move the knee after a period when it has been held still (pseudo-locking). Once again, physiotherapy is the treatment of choice.

Instability may be the result of disruption of the anterior cruciate ligament with or without medial collateral ligament damage. The knee will give way on twisting or turning, and on examination the pivot shift test will be positive and reproduce the patient's symptoms (see Chapter 33).

If physiotherapy fails to build the patient's muscles enough to stabilise the knee (it often does succeed) then reconstruction of the cruciate ligament must be considered, using a synthetic graft or a length of tendon transferred from elsewhere (Summary box 34.4).

Summary box 34.4

Knee injuries

- Very difficult to examine in the acute stage
- Effusions should be aspirated and early physiotherapy started
- Patella dislocations will have a positive apprehension sign
- Cruciate reconstruction should only be undertaken once the patient has been given a trial of physiotherapy

Iliotibial band syndrome is due to a friction injury of the iliotibial band both proximally over the greater trochanter and distally over the tibia. It occurs most commonly in long distance runners, such as marathon runners, and occurs proximally in females and distally as it extends over the lateral femoral epicondyle in males. If it does not respond to stretching and rest then sometimes steroid injections can help.

Ankle injury

Ankle sprains are the most common cause of morbidity. Most of these injuries occur due to inversion, when the lateral ligament complex and fibula and lateral talus can be injured. Eversion or abduction injuries are much less common and will cause trauma to the medial ligament complex.

The ankle should only be x-rayed if the Ottawa ankle rules are fulfilled as otherwise the likelihood of a fracture is very low. The Ottawa ankle rules are:

- bone tenderness along the distal 6 cm of the posterior margin of the lateral malleolus;
- bone tenderness along the distal 6 cm of the posterior margin or at the tip of the medial malleolus;
- inability to weight bear at the time of the accident or at the time of examination.

Ankle dislocations should be reduced immediately as otherwise necrosis of the tented skin will occur.

Sprains of the ankle should be treated with analgesia, ice and elevation, then a physiotherapy programme started to reintroduce proprioception to the ankle. If this is not done, repeat injuries are more likely.

In adolescents, the peroneal tendon retinaculum can be torn. This leads to a subluxing peroneal tendon, with a painful flicking sensation over the lateral malleolus. In younger patients this is best treated by immobilisation for a month, but if this does not resolve the problem then surgical intervention may be needed (Summary box 34.5).

The Achilles tendon is a common site for tendinosis due to repetitive trauma. There is a fusiform swelling of the central tendon.

Tendon rupture classically occurs in middle-aged squash and badminton players. Simmonds' or Thompson's test is usually diagnostic (see Chapter 33). The tendon can be allowed to heal in plaster with the foot plantar flexed to bring the tendon ends

Summary box 34.5

Ankle injuries

- Dislocated ankles should be reduced immediately
- X-rays should only be performed if the Ottawa ankle rules are fulfilled
- Physiotherapy to rebuild proprioception reduces the risk of recurrence
- In Achilles tendon rupture Simmonds' test is positive

into contact. This takes several months. Alternatively, a surgical repair can be attempted. This apposes the ends and so should speed return to function, but risks compromising the blood supply to the tendon ends and so delays healing.

Foot injuries

Turf toe is pain, swelling and stiffness in the first metatarsophalangeal joint due to rupture of the plantar plate and injury to the joint capsule following hyperextension of the toe. Treatment is symptomatic.

Stress fractures are a common source of pain in marathon runners. These cause localised pain over a metatarsal on pressure and running. They can be identified by magnetic resonance imaging (MRI) or ultrasound. Navicular stress fractures are difficult to detect clinically and MRI should be performed in unexplained pain. Prolonged rest is the best treatment.

Shoulder and upper limb injuries

Shoulder dislocations occur in contact sports such as rugby. Almost all are anterior. Those who dislocate for the first time should be treated with intensive physiotherapy and rehabilitation. However, over half will have significant anatomical damage (tear of the labrum) (Figure 34.9) and will go on to become recurrent dislocators. In these cases, surgical stabilisation (either open or arthroscopic) is the only treatment.

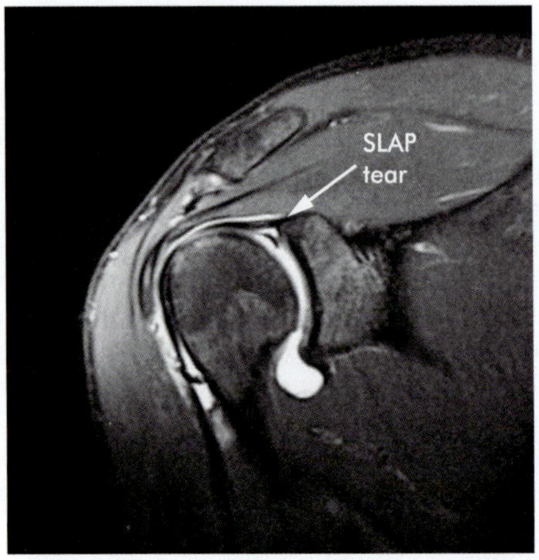

Figure 34.9 A magnetic resonance arthrogram of the shoulder showing a labral SLAP (superior labrum anterior posterior) tear in a rugby player.

Shoulder instability can also result from overuse. This happens with throwing sports and also sports such as gymnastics, tennis serves and squash.

Tendinosis of the rotator cuff can also occur with overuse in patients who perform overhead sports repetitively, such as tennis players and cricket bowlers. Overload leads to impingement and then inflammation. Subacromial subdeltoid bursitis will cause pain radiating down the arm and to the wrist. This can be worse at night. Impingement can be significant in the overhead position and the patient may have difficulty combing their hair. The supraspinatus tendon can also tear either secondary to impingement or after an acute injury. In the younger athlete this should be repaired surgically.

The acromioclavicular joint can be injured by direct impact in wrestlers, rugby and cyclists. Treatment is usually symptomatic as surgical repair is not easy. If osteoarthritis develops in the joint, the distal end of the clavicle can be excised (Summary box 34.6).

Summary box 34.6

Shoulder injuries

- Anterior dislocations are initially treated with physiotherapy
- Recurrent dislocations will require surgical stabilisation
- Overuse injuries are common in throwing sports
- Rotator cuff impingement is common
- Torn rotator cuffs should be repaired in young patients

Biceps injuries can occur at the long head of biceps proximally and the distal biceps tendon in weightlifters and wrestlers, but can also occur as part of a significant rotator cuff injury proximally where the rotator cuff can be torn from the supraspinatus across the anterior interval and into the subscapularis tendon. There is no treatment needed.

Arm and hand injuries

Medial and lateral epicondylitis are discussed above (Figure 34.10). There is no reliable treatment apart from symptomatic support.

De Quervain's tenosynovitis occurs in repetitive injuries involving the fingers.

Skiers (or gamekeeper's) thumb occurs where the proximal phalanx of the thumb is forced radially in a fall. The ulnar collateral ligament of the thumb at the level of the metacarpophalangeal joint is damaged. If it is avulsed the aponeurosis of the abductor pollicis brevis can become interposed (a Stener lesion) and so surgical intervention is the only option if this lesion is to repair. Mallet fingers or baseball fingers occur when there is a rupture of the distal insertion of the extensor tendon into the distal phalanx. This can be treated conservatively with a mallet splint.

The radial slips of the extensor tendon can be torn at the level of the metacarpophalangeal joints in boxing injuries and here the retinaculum needs reattaching surgically.

Disruption of the flexor tendon pulleys in the hand occurs in climbers, and leads to bow stringing of the flexor tendons. If this occurs, then surgical intervention is needed (Summary box 34.7).

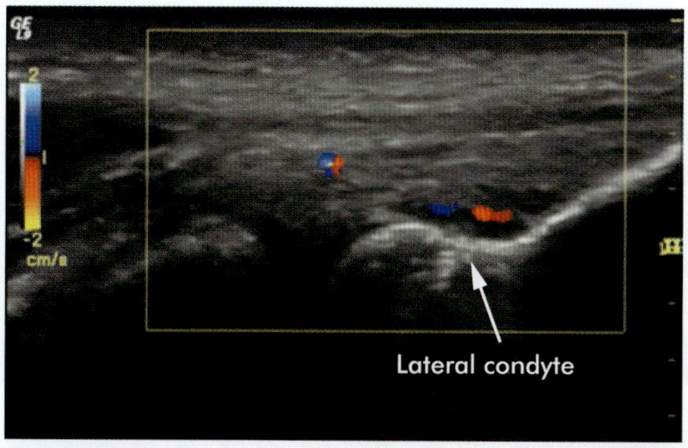

Figure 34.10 An ultrasound of the common extensor origin at the elbow showing a tendinosis with neovascularisation.

Summary box 34.7

Arm and hand injuries

- Medial and lateral epicondylitis should be treated symptomatically
- Ulna collateral ligament injuries of the thumb require surgical repair
- Flexor tendon pulley injuries require surgical repair

TREATMENT OF INJURIES

In the acute phases of a sports injury PRICE describes the treatment plan:

- Protect
- Rest
- Ice
- Compression
- Elevation.

In the initial phase of an injury, non-steroidal anti-inflammatory drugs are thought to slow healing, but may reduce pain and oedema. This is especially true in fracture healing. Paracetamol and codeine have less of an effect on injury healing and can also help with pain relief.

When prescribing any drugs it is important to be aware of the World Anti-Doping Agency (WADA) guidelines on doping for athletes as some substances can be banned in competition and training. Spot checks are performed on athletes so they need to adhere to this throughout the year. A prohibited list is available on the WADA website (www.wada-ama.org).

If steroids are needed to help with the continued rehabilitation then a TUE or temporary use exemption certificate needs to be given to the athlete so that if they are spot checked for drugs they will not be disqualified.

After an initial period of rest, passive movements should be started, followed by more active movements as healing occurs. Physiotherapy is an essential part of rehabilitation and close liaison between the sports doctor and the coach are needed in getting an athlete back to their sport. Steroid treatment should not be used around the Achilles tendon (advice from NICE (National Institute for Health and Clinical Excellence) and the British National Formulary.

Some patients develop myositis ossificans after a muscle haematoma. This presents itself as increasing swelling and pain. It can also be treated by Indomethacin which helps prevent further formation. It resolves naturally.

FURTHER READING

Brukner P, Khan K. *Clinical sports medicine*, 3rd revised edn. Sydney: McGraw Hill Sports Medicine, 2009.

Hutson M, Speed C. *Sports Injuries*. Oxford: Oxford Press, 2011.

Madden C, Putukian M, oung CC, McCarty E. *Netter's sports medicine*. Philadelphia, PA: Saunders Elsevier, 2010.

Peterson L, Renstrom P. *Sports injuries: their prevention and treatment*. London: Martin Dunitz, 2005.

CHAPTER
35 The spine

LEARNING OBJECTIVES

To learn:
- The salient features relating to the history and examination of the spine
- The investigations commonly used in the field of spinal disorders
- The treatment principles for common conditions affecting the spine

EPIDEMIOLOGY

The lifetime prevalence of low back pain has been reported at between 60 and 80 per cent. By contrast, the lifetime prevalence of true sciatica is between 2 and 4 per cent. It is generally accepted that 90 per cent of acute low back pain episodes settle, allowing return to work within 6 weeks. However, some 5–7 per cent of the population aged between 45 and 64 years will report back problems as a 'chronic sickness' . Up to 70 per cent of acute episodes of sciatica resolve within three months (Summary box 35.1).

Summary box 35.1

Epidemiology

- Low back pain is extremely common
- Ninety per cent of acute low back pain episodes settle within 6 weeks
- Sciatica is much less frequent
- Seventy per cent of acute sciatic episodes settle within three months

CLINICAL ANATOMY

The normal cervical lordosis measures between 35 and 45°. The normal lumbar lordosis is between 40 and 80° (mean 60°) and decreases with age. Most lumbar lordosis occurs between L4 and S1. The normal thoracic kyphosis is between 20 and 50° (mean 35°) and increases with age. When standing, the normal sagittal vertical axis (sagittal plumb-line) falls from the odontoid process through the C7–T1 disc space and crosses the spinal column at the T12–L1 disc space, before reaching the posterosuperior corner of the S1 vertebral body. For an energy efficient posture, cervical and lumbar lordosis will balance thoracic kyphosis.

The spinal canal is formed behind the articulated vertebral body by the posterior elements of the vertebral column and can be divided into a central portion and two lateral portions. The central portion is occupied by the thecal sac containing the spinal cord which terminates behind the body of L1. The lateral portions contain the nerve roots.

The spinal nerve roots comprise eight cervical, twelve thoracic, five lumbar, five sacral and one coccygeal. Dorsal and ventral roots join to form spinal nerves.The ventral root and the dorsal root ganglion lie within the intervertebral foramen. This foramen is bounded superiorly and inferiorly by pedicles, anteriorly by the disc and posteriorly by the facet joint. Degenerative changes in these structures may lead to neural compromise. Laminar overlap within the lumbar spine decreases from L1 to S1 so that, at the L5–S1 level, access to the intervertebral disc requires less bone removal than a more proximal level.

The blood supply of the spinal cord is derived from the vertebral, deep cervical, intercostal and lumbar arteries. The arteries of the spinal cord include the anterior spinal artery and two posterior spinal arteries, with the anterior spinal artery supplying the majority of the vascular supply to the spinal cord. The radicular artery of Adamkiewicz makes a major contribution to the anterior spinal artery, supplying the lower spinal cord. It originates on the left in 80 per cent of people, usually accompanying the ventral root of T9, T10 or T11, but can originate anywhere from T5 to L5. Ligation of this important artery may lead to critical ischaemia of the spinal cord. Ligating segmental vessels over the midpoint of the vertebral body will minimise the risk of injury to this important artery during anterior approaches to the spine.

PATIENT HISTORY

The most common reasons for referral to a spinal clinic include pain and spinal deformity. A detailed history of the pain including site, type, severity, duration, frequency and aggravating

Albert Adamkiewicz, 1850–1921, Professor of Pathology, The University of Krakow (Cracow), Poland, described the arterial supply of the spinal cord in 1882.

factors should be sought. Has there been any history of trauma? Is the pain present at night? Is there associated pain in the upper limbs (brachalgia) or lower limbs (sciatica)? Is there associated numbness, tingling, weakness, or difficulty with gait? Is there a family history of ankylosing spondylitis or rheumatoid arthritis? Are there concurrent medical conditions such as diabetes, peripheral vascular diseases, osteoarthritis of the hip or previous malignancies? Are there systemic symptoms such as unexplained weight loss, chills or fever? Table 35.1 lists the commonly accepted 'red flags' that allow diagnostic triage into those with serious pathology of the spine (such as fractures, tumours, infection or cauda equina syndrome) and those without serious pathology.

Table 35.1 'Red flags': when present in patients with back pain, red flags suggest the likelihood of serious underlying pathology.

Age <20 years or >50 years
Recent significant trauma
History of malignant disease
Unexplained weight loss
Constitutional symptoms (fever, chills)
Immunosuppression (intravenous drug abuse, prolonged corticosteroid use)
Severe or progressive sensory alteration or motor weakness
Acute difficulty with micturition (painless retention)
Numbness in perineum or buttocks and/or faecal incontinence

Pain may be arising from the spine, but non-spinal causes of pain must also be considered (Table 35.2). Patients should always be asked about the presence of perineal numbness (saddle area) and/or difficulties passing urine or faeces, as these symptoms may indicate a cauda equina syndrome (Table 35.3).

Table 35.2 Non-spinal causes of low back pain; referred pain.

Respiratory, e.g.mesothelioma
Vascular, e.g. abdominal aortic aneurysm
Renal, e.g. pyelonephritis
Gastrointestinal, e.g. peptic ulcer, pancreatitis
Urogenital, e.g. testicular, ovarian or prostatic carcinoma

Patients should be asked whether the pain is interfering with their ability to work. What treatment has the patient already tried and how effective were these treatments, e.g. analgesics, exercise, physiotherapy or spinal injections? Pending litigation or workers' compensation claims may have a negative prognostic effect on future treatments and therefore should be enquired about.

Spinal deformities, e.g. scoliosis and kyphosis are generally painless in children, but may become symptomatic in adult life. How quickly has the spinal deformity progressed? It is important to assess skeletal maturity and whether the child has gone through a recent growth spurt? Has menstruation commenced in the female or has the voice dropped in the male?

Table 35.3 Cauda equina syndrome.

Low back pain
Uni- or bilateral sciatica
Saddle anaesthesia
Motor weakness in the lower extremities
Variable rectal and urinary symptoms

PHYSICAL EXAMINATION

The patient should be undressed and posture should be evaluated in both the frontal and sagittal plane. Shoulder or waist asymmetry suggests the presence of scoliosis. The Adams' forward bend test will accentuate trunk asymmetry and allow appreciation of rib or loin prominence on the convex side of the curve. The skin should be examined for cutaneous neurofibromata, café-au-lait patches or axillary freckles commonly present in neurofibromatosis. Neurological examination should include abdominal reflexes. Leg lengths should be measured. In the case of kyphosis, the sagittal alignment and forward gaze should be assessed.

William Adams described the forward bending test for scoliosis in 1865. His understanding of the nature of the rotational element of scoliosis was given by a post-mortem he performed on an eminent surgeon and geologist, Gideon Mantell. The clinical history of Dr Mantell is well documented.

Palpation is useful to locate specific areas of tenderness. Ranges of motion should be assessed. The normal range of motion in the cervical spine is 45° of flexion, 55° of extension, 70° of rotation and 40° lateral bend. The normal range of motion in the lumbar spine is 40–60° of flexion, 20–35° of extension, 15–20° lateral bending and 3–18° of rotation. Schober's test is a simple clinical test to evaluate spinal mobility. A tape measure is used to mark the skin midway between the posterior superior iliac crests and at points 10 cm proximal and 5 cm distal to this mark while the patient is standing. The patient is then asked to bend forward as far as possible and the distance between the two points is measured with the patient in the flexed position. Normally one would expect to see an increase of at least 5 cm between the two points in the erect and flexed positions.

Neurological examination of the upper and lower limbs will focus on tone, power, coordination, reflexes, sensation and gait (Tables 35.4 and 35.5). A rectal examination should be performed if there is any concern about cauda equina integrity. The superficial abdominal reflex is an upper motor neurone reflex. It is performed by stroking one of four abdominal quadrants in succession. The umbilicus should move towards the quadrant that was stroked. The reflex should be symmetric from side to side. Asymmetry suggests intraspinal pathology (Summary box 35.2).

Myelopathy or upper motor neurone (UMN) lesions are suggested by spasticity, motor weakness, hyper-reflexia, a positive Hoffmann's sign (if the middle finger is flicked into extension,

Table 35.4 Neurological evaluation of the upper limb.

Neurological level	Motor	Sensation	Reflex
C5	Deltoid	Lateral arm	Biceps
C6	Wrist extensors and extensor carpi radialis longus	Lateral forearm	Brachioradialis
C7	Triceps	Middle finger	Triceps
C8	Long finger flexors	Medial forearm	No reflex
T1	Interosseus muscles	Medial arm	No reflex

Table 35.5 Neurological evaluation of the lower limb.

Neurological level	Motor	Sensation	Reflex
L2	Hip flexion	Anterior thigh, groin	No reflex
L3	Knee extension	Anterior and lateral thigh	Patellar (L3, 4)
L4	Ankle dorsiflexion	Medial leg and foot	Patellar (L3, 4)
L5	Extensor hallucis longus	Lateral leg and foot	No reflex
S1	Ankle plantarflexion	Lateral foot and little toe	Achilles

the thumb and other fingers flex briskly), up-going Babinski response, patellar and ankle clonus. Typical signs of radiculopathy (lower motor neurone (LMN) lesion) include sensory loss, motor weakness, flaccid paralysis, muscle atrophy, loss of reflexes and muscle fasciculation.

The straight leg raise test is performed with the patient in the supine position. The leg is elevated with the knee straight to increase tension along the L5 and S1 nerve roots. The test is positive if the leg elevation provokes radicular pain. Lasègue's sign denotes radicular pain aggravated by ankle dorsiflexion. The femoral stretch test is performed with the patient in the prone position by extending the hip and flexing the knee. This creates tension on the L2, L3 and L4 nerve roots. The femoral nerve stretch test is considered positive if radicular pain occurs in the anterior thigh region during the test.

The examination should include, where appropriate, examination of the shoulder, hip, knee, sacroiliac joint and vascular system, as dual pathology is common in the ageing community.

Waddell developed and validated a series of signs and tests that have proved helpful in identifying individuals who are magnifying or exaggerating symptoms, possibly for secondary gain (Table 35.6) (Summary box 35.3).

INVESTIGATIONS

The most common diagnostic imaging tests used to evaluate spinal disorders include plain radiographs, magnetic resonance imaging (MRI), computed tomography (CT), CT myelography and isotope bone scanning. These investigations are extremely sensitive, but relatively non-specific. For example, at least one-third of asymptomatic patients have been noted to have 'abnormalities' on MRI scans. All investigations must therefore be carefully correlated with the clinical findings.

Table 35.6 Non-organic physical signs in low back pain.

Tenderness	Superficial or non-anatomical
Simulation tests	Axial loading or rotation
Distraction tests	Variable straight leg raises
Regional disturbances	Non-anatomical sensory or motor loss
Over-reaction	Grimacing, muscle tremor, etc.

Summary box 35.2

Upper motor neurone lesion characterised by:

- Increased tone – spastic
- Hyper-reflexia
- Muscle spasms
- Motor weakness
- Disuse atrophy
- Positive Hoffman's sign
- Ankle and patellar clonus
- Upgoing plantar response

Summary box 35.3

Lower motor neurone lesion characterised by:

- Decreased tone – flaccid
- Hyporeflexia
- Denervation fasciculations
- Motor weakness
- Sensory loss
- Severe atrophy
- Downgoing plantar response

Johann Hoffmann, 1857–1919, Professor of Neurology, Heidelberg, Germany.
Joseph Francis Felix Babinski, 1857–1932, neurologist, Hôpital de la Pitie, Paris, France.

Plain radiographs

It is not appropriate to order spine radiographs for every patient presenting with neck or low back pain. Patients with red flag signs or symptoms and those who have not responded to conservative treatment require imaging, but most units in developed countries would use MRI initially rather than x-rays. Standing radiographs of the whole spine are important for the full assessment of scoliosis. Radiographs cannot diagnose early-stage tumour or infection, because significant bone destruction (between 40 and 60 per cent of bone mass) must occur before a radiographic abnormality is detected.

Magnetic resonance imaging

This allows detailed visualisation of the thecal sac, spinal cord, epidural space, intervertebral disc, nerve roots, paraspinal soft tissues and bone marrow. It is contraindicated for patients with pacemakers, some drug pumps or spinal cord stimulators.

Computed tomography

This investigation is the best test for bone anatomy. Three-dimensional reconstructions are often useful for the assessment of congenital spinal deformity.

Bone scintigraphy

Isotope bone scanning is a highly sensitive, but non-specific test useful for screening of the skeletal system for metastatic disease, discitis or vertebral body osteomyelitis, or to assess the relative activity of bone lesions such as pars interarticulares defects or a pseudarthrosis. In the case of multiple myeloma or purely lytic metastases, the bone scan may not show increased activity as these tumours may not stimulate a significant osteoblastic response.

Bone densitometry

Bone density and osteoporosis can be measured using dual-energy x-ray absorptiometry (DEXA).

Provocative discography

This involves the injection of a radio-opaque contrast agent into a presumed degenerated and painful disc in the conscious patient as a preoperative test to elucidate the source of pain before considering spinal fusion or disc replacement (Figure 35.1).

Facet joint injections

For patients with facet joint arthropathy, x-ray-guided local anaesthetic and steroid injections may be both diagnostic and therapeutic.

Foraminal epidural steroid injections

For patients with radiculopathy due to a prolapsed intervertebral disc or lateral recess stenosis, a targeted foraminal epidural steroid injection of local anaesthetic and steroid may provide important diagnostic information and have a lasting therapeutic effect.

Spinal biopsy

CT-guided or open biopsy is often performed to obtain tissue for diagnostic study in cases of suspected tumour and/or infection.

DEGENERATIVE CONDITIONS OF THE SPINE

Cervical radiculopathy

Patients present with neck and arm pain (brachalgia), paraesthesia and motor weakness in the distribution of the compromised nerve root (radiculopathy). This may be caused by disc herniation or degenerative stenosis.

Symptoms often respond to conservative treatment including physiotherapy and medication for neuropathic pain (amitriptyline, gabapentin or pregabalin) or fluoroscopically guided foraminal epidural steroid injections of local anaesthetic and steroid. Intractable pain or functional neurological deficit is an indication for surgical intervention. Surgical options include anterior cervical discectomy (with or without the application of a cervical spine locking plate), posterior laminoforaminotomy or cervical total disc replacement.

Cervical myelopathy

Degenerative change in the cervical spine leading to spinal cord compression is the most common cause of cervical myelopathy in patients over 55 years of age (Figure 35.2). Lower motor neurone changes occur at the level of the lesion, with atrophy of the upper extremity muscles, particularly the intrinsic muscles of the hands. Upper motor neurone findings are noted below the level of the lesion and may involve both upper and lower extremities. If surgery is considered appropriate then an anterior or posterior decompression will be needed.

Thoracic disc herniation

Thoracic disc herniations that require surgical intervention are rare, accounting for less than 2 per cent of all discectomy procedures. Typically, the patient presents with axial pain, radiculopathy or myelopathy. Conservative treatment including non-steroidal anti-inflammatory drugs, physiotherapy and general fitness improvement should be tried initially. If required, thoracic discectomy may be performed via a thoracotomy or, for a soft disc prolapse, via a thoracoscopic approach.

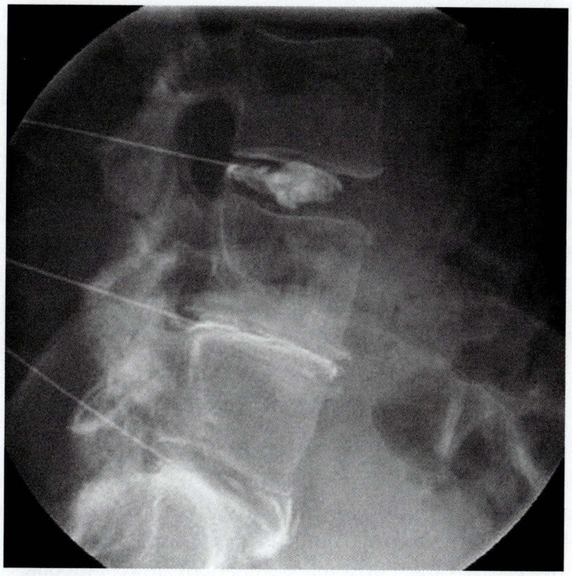

Figure 35.1 Three level discography.

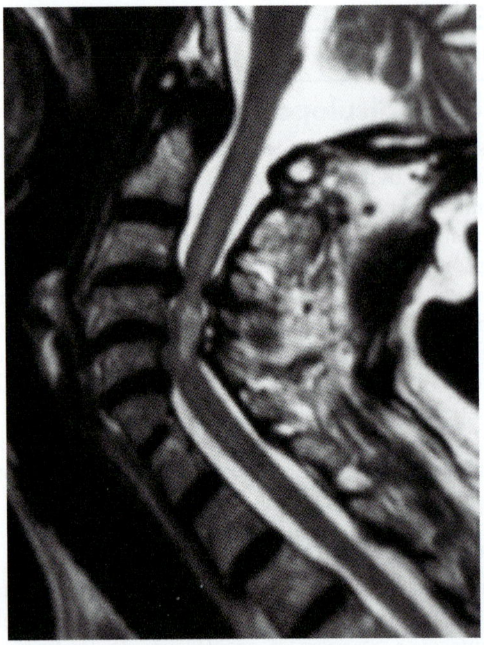

Figure 35.2 Cervical myelopathy. Magnetic resonance image showing a block fusion at C6/7 with adjacent level degenerative changes and compromise of the spinal cord at C3/4, C4/5 and C5/6. Signal change was noted within the cord, particularly at the C4/5 level.

Cauda equina syndrome

Cauda equina syndrome (CES) is rare, accounting for only 2–6 per cent of all lumbar disc herniations. It presents most commonly in the 20–45 year age group with some or all of the following symptoms: low back pain, unilateral or bilateral sciatica, lower limb motor weakness, sensory abnormalities including saddle anaesthesia, bladder dysfunction (painless retention in early stages, overflow incontinence in later stages), sexual and bowel dysfunction. CES may result from acute or chronic compression of the cauda equina nerve roots. The most frequent cause is a massive central lumbar disc protrusion at L4/5; other causes include lumbar fractures, postoperative epidural haematoma, spinal stenosis, spinal tumours, and occlusion of the lumbar arteries by dissection or aneurysm of the abdominal aorta.

Nerve roots within the cauda equina nerve roots lack epineurium and perineurium, and only have a thin endoneurium root sheath making them more susceptible to compression forces when compared to peripheral nerves. The syndrome can result in permanent motor deficit, bladder, bowel and sexual dysfunction. It represents a true spinal emergency and requires urgent surgical decompression. The outcome for patients who undergo surgical decompression within 24 hours of the onset of loss of bladder or bowel control is significantly better compared to those that undergo surgery beyond this 24-hour period (Summary box 35.4).

Lumbar disc herniation

Symptomatic lumbar disc herniation occurs during the lifetime of approximately 2–4 per cent of the population. Risk factors include family history, male gender, age (30–50 years), heavy lifting or twisting, stressful occupation, lower income and cigarette smoking.

Summary box 35.4

Cauda equina syndrome

- Most common presenting symptoms: perineal numbness, painless urinary retention and faecal incontinence
- Urgent investigation with magnetic resonance imaging is required for all suspected cases
- Confirmed cauda equina syndrome requires surgical decompression within 24 hours to achieve optimum outcomes

Over 90 per cent of lumbar disc herniations occur at the L4–5 or L5–S1 levels (Figure 35.3). A posterolateral disc protrusion will affect the traversing root, e.g. an L4–L5 disc protrusion affects the L5 nerve root. A far-lateral disc protrusion (extraforaminal) will affect the exiting nerve root, e.g. a far-lateral L5–S1

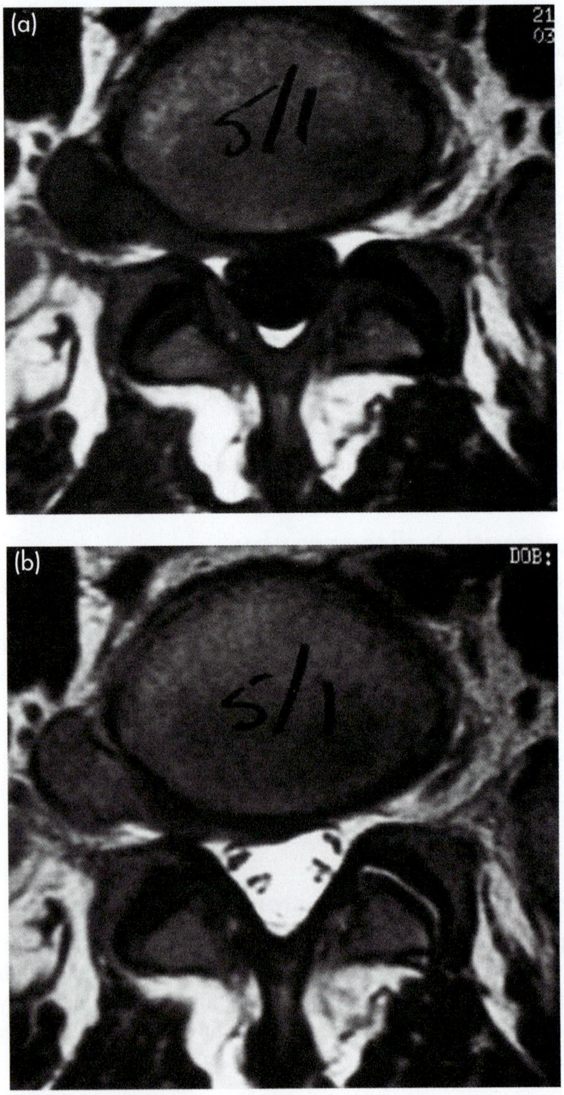

Figure 35.3 Far-lateral disc prolapse at L5/S1. A right-sided far-lateral disc protrusion is noted at L5/S1 on the T1-weighted (a) and the T2-weighted (b) magnetic resonance imaging scan. The patient presented with an L5 radiculopathy.

disc protrusion affects the L5 nerve root. Symptoms typically commence with a period of back pain followed by sciatica. There may be paraesthesia, motor weakness, loss of reflexes and a reduction in straight leg raise.

For simple sciatica, a period of 6–12 weeks of conservative treatment is advised. Up to 70 per cent of patients will settle within this period. Transforaminal epidural steroid injections may be helpful. Microdiscectomy is the standard surgical intervention for those in whom conservative treatment has failed. The procedure is carried out in the prone position with radiographic confirmation of the correct level. Loupes with a headlight or use of the operating microscope greatly facilitate the procedure. A 3–5 cm incision is made with a unilateral take down of the multifidus. The spinal canal is entered via removal of the ligamentum flavum under the lamina. The thecal sac and traversing nerve root are identified. The dura and nerve root are retracted medially and the offending disc prolapse incised via a transverse annulotomy. The disc fragment is removed and the disc space cleared of any remaining nuclear material with rongeurs and multiple washouts of the disc space. The wound is closed. Patients are generally discharged the next morning.

Spinal stenosis

Spinal stenosis may be defined as any type of narrowing of the spinal canal, nerve root canal or intervertebral foramen. The resultant nerve root compression leads to nerve root ischaemia presenting with back, buttock or leg pain provoked by exercise. Spinal stenosis may be congenital as is the case in achondroplasia or acquired as is the case for degenerative types (commonly presenting between 50 and 70 years of age). The narrowing is caused by facet joint hypertrophy, disc bulge and ligamentum flavum thickening.

Symptoms of spinal claudication can be distinguished from vascular claudication because they are frequently associated with neurological symptoms, are often worse in extension, and pedal pulses are present on clinical examination. Symptoms progress in approximately 20–33 per cent of patients who receive no treatment. The condition may be treated successfully by surgical decompression with preservation of the facet joints (Summary box 35.5).

Summary box 35.5

Spinal stenosis

- Extremely common condition in the 50–70 year age group
- Classic symptoms: back, buttock, thigh and calf pain
- Provoked by walking and extended posture
- Relieved by flexed posture
- Symptoms progress in up to one-third of untreated patients

Discogenic low back pain

Discogenic low back pain has been defined as a continuum of diagnostic categories (internal disc disruption, degenerative disc disease, segmental instability) reflecting various stages of degenerative pathology affecting the intervertebral disc. Not all degenerate discs are painful. Patients typically present with chronic relapsing episodes of low back pain between the ages of 40 and 60 years old.

A recent study has compared rehabilitation with spinal fusion for discogenic pain. Both groups reported reductions in disability with the authors strongly recommending a course of rehabilitation before surgical intervention. For those who fail to improve with conservative measures, provocative lumbar discography (Figure 35.1) may help to identify the source of pain, and surgery in the form of lumbar fusion (Figure 35.4) or lumbar disc replacement (Figure 35.5) may be considered. Spondylolysis and spondylolisthesis

Spondylolysis

This is a unilateral or bilateral defect in the region of the pars interarticularis without vertebral slippage. The incidence is reported at approximately 6 per cent by the age of 14 years, but much higher in the young athletic population. Many cases remain asymptomatic.The diagnosis is difficult with x-rays. SPECT (single photon emission computed tomography), reverse gantry CT and MRI scans are helpful. Treatment involves rest, non-steroidal anti-inflammatory medication, activity modification and a lumbosacral orthosis. For patients who remain symptomatic despite an adequate trial of non-operative care, surgery in the form of a direct repair of the pseudarthrosis by a Buck's fusion may be indicated (Summary box 35.6).

Summary box 35.6

Spondylolysis

- Incidence general population 6 per cent by 14 years
- Incidence athletic population 15–47 per cent
- May be complete asymptomatic/incidental finding on x-ray
- Difficult to image, but magnetic resonance imaging proving more useful
- Conservative treatment: activity modification, anti-lordotic brace
- Surgical treatment: direct repair preserving motion or spinal fusion if associated disc degeneration

Spondylolisthesis

Spondylolisthesis is a forward slippage of the vertebral body engendered by a break in the continuity or elongation of the pars interarticularis and present in 4 per cent of the adult population (Figure 35.6). Spondylolisthesis can be classified into six types by causation (Table 35.7), or by the degree of slip (Table 35.8).

For progressive slips in skeletally immature patients (less than 18 years old), those patients with intractable low back or radicular pain, or neurological symptoms, surgery may be indicated. For low-grade slips (Meyerding I and II) fusion *in situ* is the procedure of choice. If there is objective evidence of neural compression (e.g. weakness of extensor hallucis longis), a spinal decompression should be performed at the same time. For high-grade slips (Meyerding III and IV), opinion is divided on whether to reduce the slip first and then fuse, or simply to fuse *in situ*.

TUMOURS OF THE SPINE

Metastatic tumours

These are the most common tumours affecting the spine, accounting for 98 per cent of all spine lesions. The most common malignancies that metastasise to the spine are shown

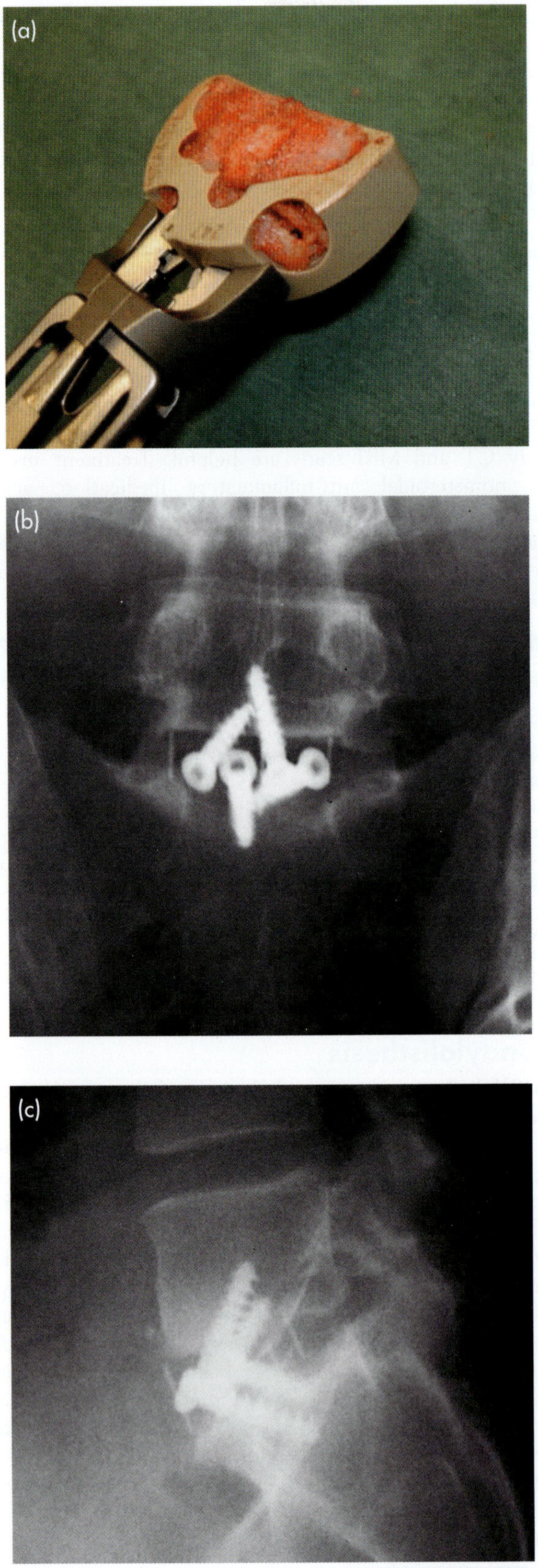

Figure 35.4 Anterior lumbar interbody fusion. The PEEK (poly-ethyl-ethyl-ketone) cage has been packed with bone graft prior to insertion (a); (b) and (c) show the anteroposterior and lateral postoperative radiographs, respectively.

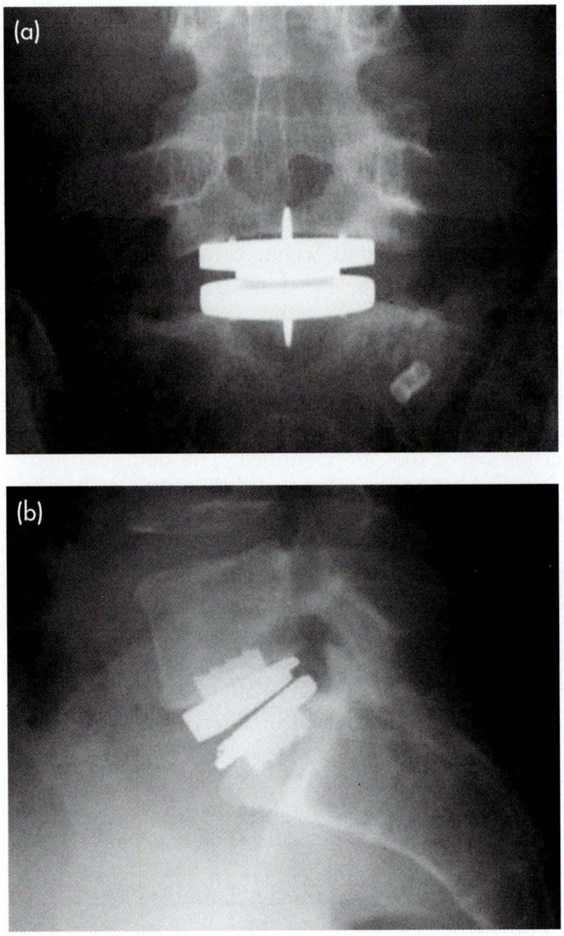

Figure 35.5 Lumbar total disc replacement. (a) Anteroposterior radiograph with 30° of cranial inclination. (b) Lateral radiograph with the implant appropriately positioned.

in Table 35.9. Red flags picked up on history or examination will alert the clinician to this possible diagnosis.

Over 80 per cent of patients with spinal metastases present with progressive pain, and only 20 per cent present with spinal cord compression. Useful investigations include full blood count (FBC), urea and electrolytes, liver function tests, calcium erythrocyte sedimentation rate (ESR), C-reactive protein (CRP), prostate-specific antigen (PSA), serum protein electrophoresis, thyroid function tests (where a thyroid mass has been palpated) and nutritional indices. Plain radiographs may show an absent pedicle ('winking owl' sign), vertebral cortical erosion and/or vertebral collapse. Whole spine MRI will detect most metastases. Most metastases are osteoblastic and will show up on bone scintigraphy; however, osteolytic lesions such as multiple myeloma and hypernephroma may not show up on an isotope bone scan. Metastases from the prostate may be sclerotic. Biopsies may be obtained via a percutaneous CT-guided method or open biopsy.

Treatment options include orthotics, steroids (dexamethasone), radiotherapy, chemotherapy, hormonal therapy, surgery or a combination of any of the above. Radiotherapy promotes reossification of the vertebral body and reduces tumour load. It can be very effective for reducing 'bone pain'.

Table 35.7 The Wiltse classification of spondylolisthesis.

Type 1	Dysplastic	Associated with congenital deficiency of the L5–S1 articulation
Type 2	Isthmic	Associated with a lesion of the pars interarticulares. Three subtypes: 2A: lytic defect of the pars 2B: elongated or attenuated pars 2C: acute pars fracture
Type 3	Degenerative spondylolisthesis	Segmental instability due to disc degeneration and facet arthrosis
Type 4	Traumatic	Acute fracture in the region of the posterior elements, other than the pars interarticulares
Type 5	Pathological	Generalised bone disease resulting in attenuation of the pars (e.g. metabolic, neoplastic)
Type 6	Post-surgical	After decompression of the lumbar spine

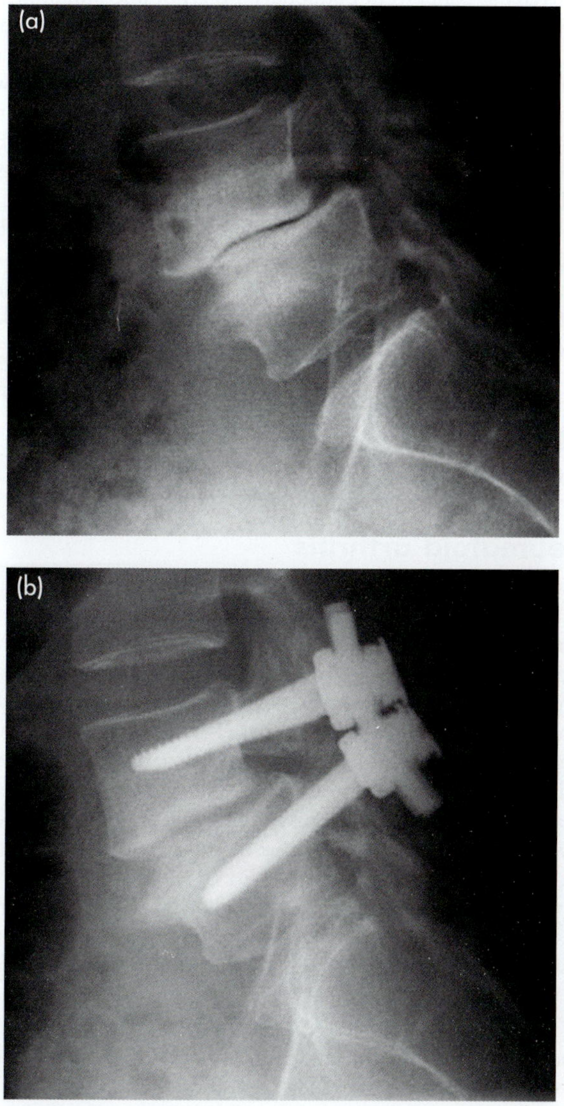

Figure 35.6 Lytic spondylolisthesis L4/L5. (a) Lateral radiograph showing a Meyerding grade I spondylolisthesis. The patient underwent a decompression and instrumented fusion *in situ* (b).

Table 35.8 The Meyerding classification for the degree of slip of spondylolisthesis.

Grade	Per cent
I	1–25
II	26–50
III	51–75
IV	76–100

Table 35.9 Commonest malignancies that metastasise to the spine and their frequency.

Malignancy	Frequency (per cent)
Breast	21
Lung	14
Prostate	7.5
Renal	5
Gastrointestinal	5
Thyroid	2.5

Lymphoma, breast, lung and prostate metastases are highly radiosensitive. Gastrointestinal adenocarcinoma, metastatic melanoma, thyroid and renal carcinoma are radioresistant. Small cell carcinoma of the lung, Ewing's sarcoma, thyroid carcinoma, breast carcinoma and neuroblastoma are usually sensitive to chemotherapy and should have chemotherapeutic agents as the first-line management. Adenocarcinoma of the lung is resistant to chemotherapy. Prostate metastases may respond well to anti-androgenic hormone medication.

Extensive reconstructive tumour surgery should be reserved for those patients whose life expectancy exceeds three months. For patients with malignant spinal cord compression, the combination of decompressive surgery with stabilisation and postoperative radiotherapy has been shown to be superior in outcome when compared to radiotherapy alone. In one randomised trial, surgery and radiotherapy permitted most patients to remain ambulatory for the remainder of their lives, whereas patients treated with radiotherapy alone spent a large proportion of their remaining time as paraplegics (Summary box 35.7).

James Ewing, 1866–1943, Professor of Pathology, Cornell University Medical College, New York, NY, USA, described this type of sarcoma in 1921.

Summary box 35.7

Metastatic tumours of the spine

- Most common presentation is progressive spinal pain
- Magnetic resonance imaging of whole spine will detect most metastases
- Surgery is indicated for instability pain, progressive deformity or neurological deficit

Primary spine tumours

These may be benign, intermediate or malignant. These are discussed further in Chapter 39.

Benign tumours tend to occur in the posterior elements (Figure 35.7); malignant tumours (Figure 35.8) tend to involve the vertebral body.

Intradural tumours

These are rare. They may be intramedullary (within the substance of the cord) or extramedullary (outside the cord). Most are extramedullary and benign; the most common are meningiomas and neurofibromas. They are discussed in Chapter 39.

INFECTIONS OF THE SPINE

Pyogenic infections

Pyogenic vertebral osteomyelitis is primarily a lesion of the disc and its osseous margins (Figure 35.9). The most common method by which an organism spreads to the spine is via the haematogenous route. The disc is nearly always involved in pyogenic vertebral infection. In contrast, granulomatous infection, such as tuberculosis, typically does not involve the disc space.

Risk factors for pyogenic vertebral osteomyelitis include advancing age, intravenous drug abuse, diabetes, renal failure, recent infections and trauma. *Staphylococcus aureus* accounts for 30–55 per cent of the infections. Gram-negative organisms such as *Escherichia coli*, *Pseudomonas* species and *Proteus* species are associated with recent genitourinary infections and intravenous drug abuse. Anaerobic infections are uncommon, but may be seen in diabetic patients and after penetrating trauma.

The principles of treatment of bone infection are discussed in Chapter 40.

Operative intervention should be considered for:

- an open biopsy (when a closed biopsy has failed);
- failure of medical management (persistent pain, elevated ESR);
- drainage of abscesses;
- decompression of spinal cord compression;
- correction of progressive spinal deformity;
- stabilisation of progressive spinal instability.

Epidural abscess

This condition is often a surgical emergency. The majority of cases occur within the thoracic spine. Without treatment, neurological deficit including paralysis may develop.

Tuberculosis

Spinal tuberculosis is still unfortunately common in developing countries. Any patient, usually from a lower socio-economic background, complaining of backache associated with constitutional symptoms such as weight loss, evening pyrexia, cough and malaise should alert one to the possibility of spinal tuberculosis (Pott's disease).

On examination there will be tenderness of the spine over the affected segment. In advanced cases the patient may have a soft fluctuant mass in the right iliac fossa and femoral triangle, the mass exhibiting cross-fluctuation. This would be classical of a cold abscess tracking along the psoas sheath; the patient may be oblivious to its presence. The pathology would be in the lumbar or lower thoracic vertebrae. When the thoracic vertebrae are affected there may be collapse in advanced cases giving rise to a kyphosis (gibbus).

Investigations would show a rise in inflammatory markers (ESR and CRP) and anaemia; sputum is sent for culture and sensitivity as concurrent pulmonary TB is not uncommon. Chest x-ray may show pulmonary TB; spinal x-ray would show vertebral collapse with a para-spinal soft tissue shadow (cold abscess) with absence of psoas shadow. Aspiration of a cold abscess with staining for acid-fast bacilli and culture and sensitivity (this may take a few weeks) is essential. It is important to exclude TB in other sites such as the gastrointestinal and genitourinary systems. MRI and CT scans are also helpful.

Once diagnosed, the patient should be closely managed by a chest physician and spinal surgeon. Full anti-tuberculous chemotherapy and spinal immobilisation is the mainstay of treatment. For further details of treatment, the reader is advised to look up more specialised sources.

INFLAMMATORY SPONDYLOARTHROPATHY

Rheumatoid arthritis

Between 33 and 50 per cent of patients develop atlanto-axial subluxation (AAS) within five years of diagnosis of rheumatoid arthritis. Some 2–10 per cent of patients with AAS develop myelopathy over the next ten years. Once diagnosed with myelopathy, 50 per cent of patients die within one year. Approximately 20 per cent of patients develop symptomatic subaxial disease. Neurological symptoms may occur as a result of direct compression by bone or soft tissue or from neural ischaemia. Care needs to be taken with these patients whenever they require surgery. The degree of subluxation may need to be checked by performing flexion and extension x-rays, and the theatre staff (especially the anaesthetist) need to be warned to take special care especially with intubation. The indications for surgery to stabilise the cervical spine are given in Table 35.10.

Ankylosing spondylitis

Should a patient with ankylosing spondylitis (AS) present following trauma, a high index of suspicion for occult fractures should be present. It is common for AS patients to develop epidural haematomas with subtle neurological deficit.

Patients with a significant fixed flexion deformity at the cervicothoracic junction ('chin-on-chest' deformity), limited forward gaze, eating and swallowing difficulties may be treated with a closing wedge osteotomy at the cervicothoracic junction (Figure 35.10). Extension osteotomies can also be performed in the thoracic and lumbar spine.

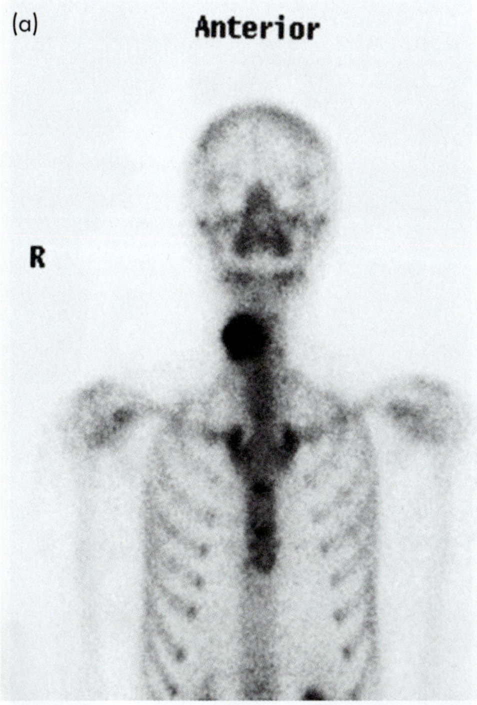

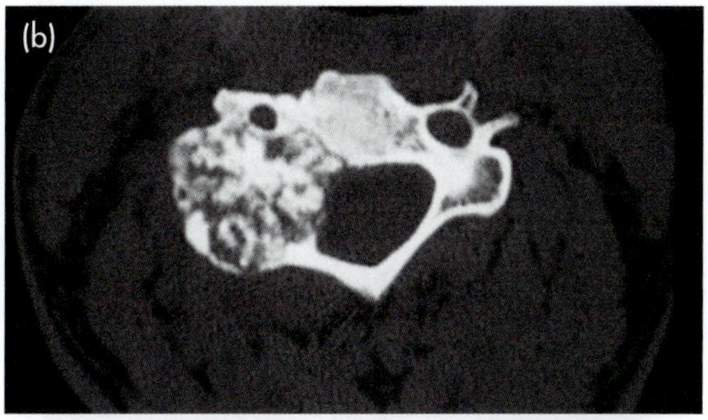

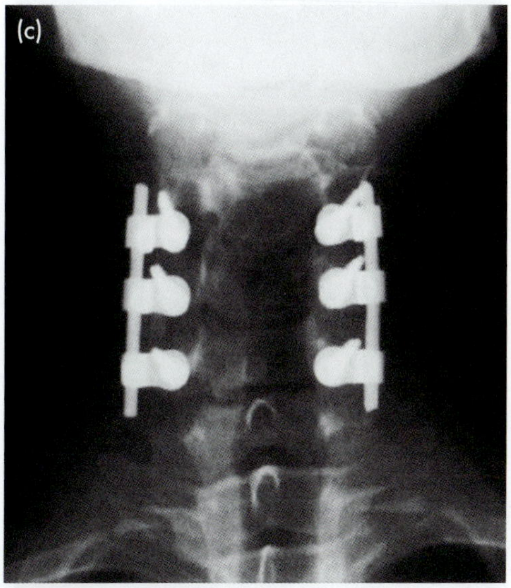

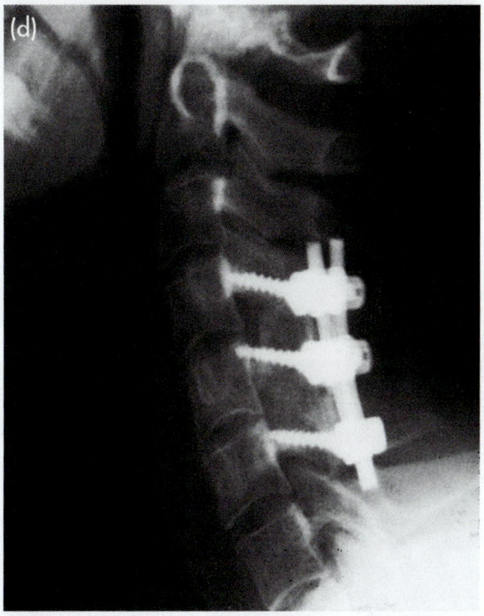

Figure 35.7 Osteoblastoma arising from the posterior elements of the fifth cervical vertebra. This 21-year-old man presented with severe unremitting neck pain. An isotope bone scan (a) demonstrated increased uptake in C5. An axial computed tomography scan (b) further delineated the expansive lesion. The tumour was successfully removed with the aid of an intraoperative gamma probe to confirm complete excision. (c) and (d) show the postoperative anteroposterior and lateral radiographs, respectively, following reconstruction with a tricortical bone graft, lateral mass screws and rods.

Table 35.10 Recommendations for spinal surgery in rheumatoid arthritis.

Atlantoaxial subluxation (AAS) with a posterior atlantodental interval (PADI) of 14 mm or less
AAS with at least 5 mm of basilar invagination
Subaxial subluxation with a sagittal canal diameter of 14 mm or less

SPINAL DEFORMITY

Spinal deformity may be categorised into a coronal plane deformity (scoliosis) or a sagittal plane deformity (kyphosis and lordosis.). Further classification may be made on the basis of aetiology into congenital, neuromuscular, idiopathic or syndromic. Appropriate radiographs for the assessment of scoliosis include a full posteroanterior and lateral standing spine. When surgery is contemplated, supine lateral bending radiographs are performed to assess the flexibility of the curve(s). Curve magnitude is measured in degrees and known as the Cobb angle. The criterion for diagnosis of scoliosis is a Cobb angle of 10° or more. The causes of scoliosis are given in Table 35.11.

Congenital scoliosis

This is caused by vertebral anomalies that produce a frontal plane growth asymmetry. The anomalies are present at birth,

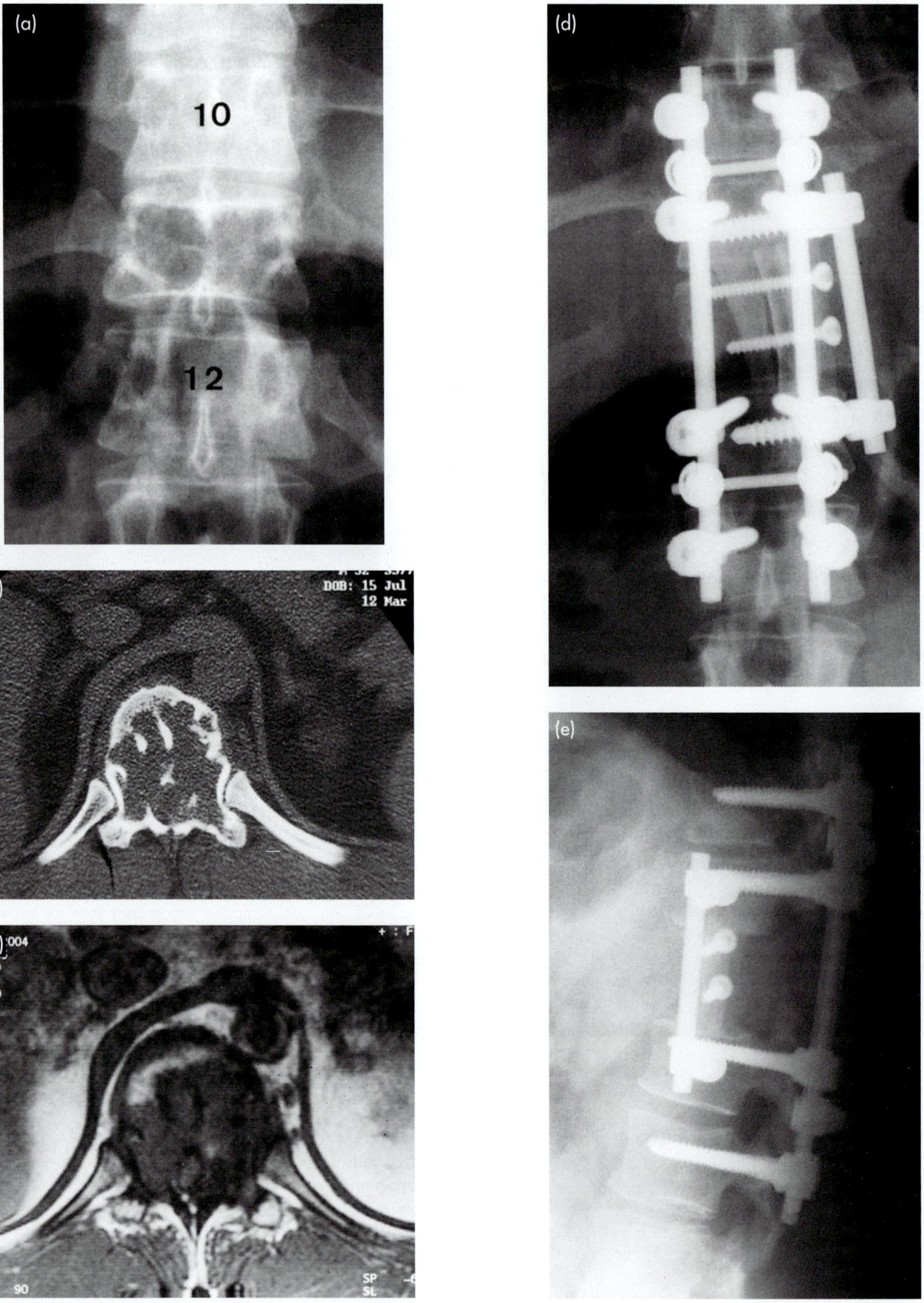

Figure 35.8 Haemangioendothelioma arising from the body of the 11th thoracic vertebra. This 34-year-old man presented with signs of spinal cord compression and severe pain in the lower thoracic region.The anteroposterior radiograph (a) demonstrated loss of both pedicles at T11. Axial computed tomography (b) confirmed a lytic lesion. Magnetic resonance imaging (c) demonstrated spinal cord compression on the axial T1-weighted scan. The patient underwent a staged posterior stabilisation, total en bloc spondylectomy and anterior column reconstruction. (d) and (e) show the postoperative anteroposterior and lateral radiographs, respectively.

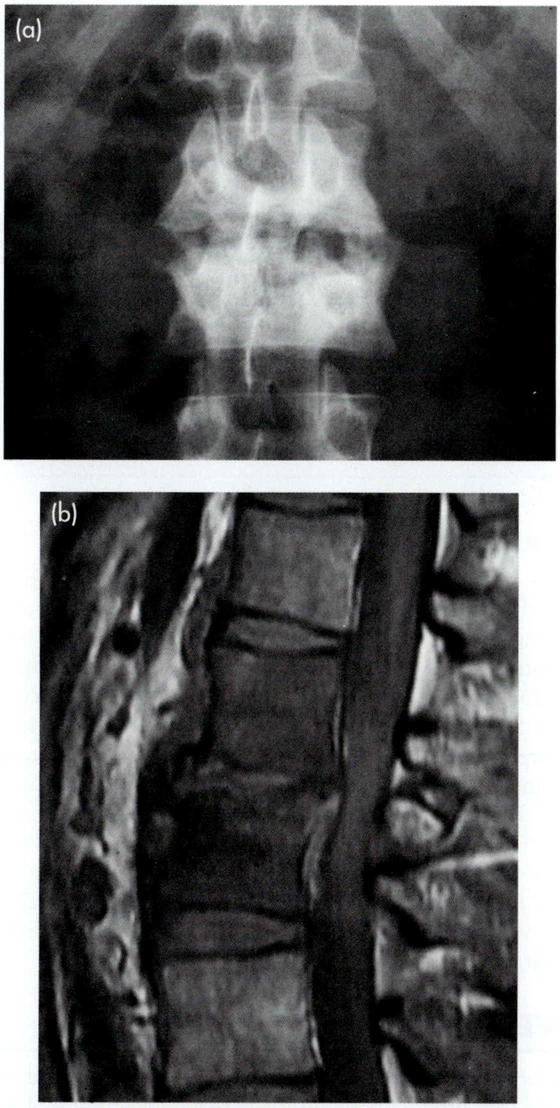

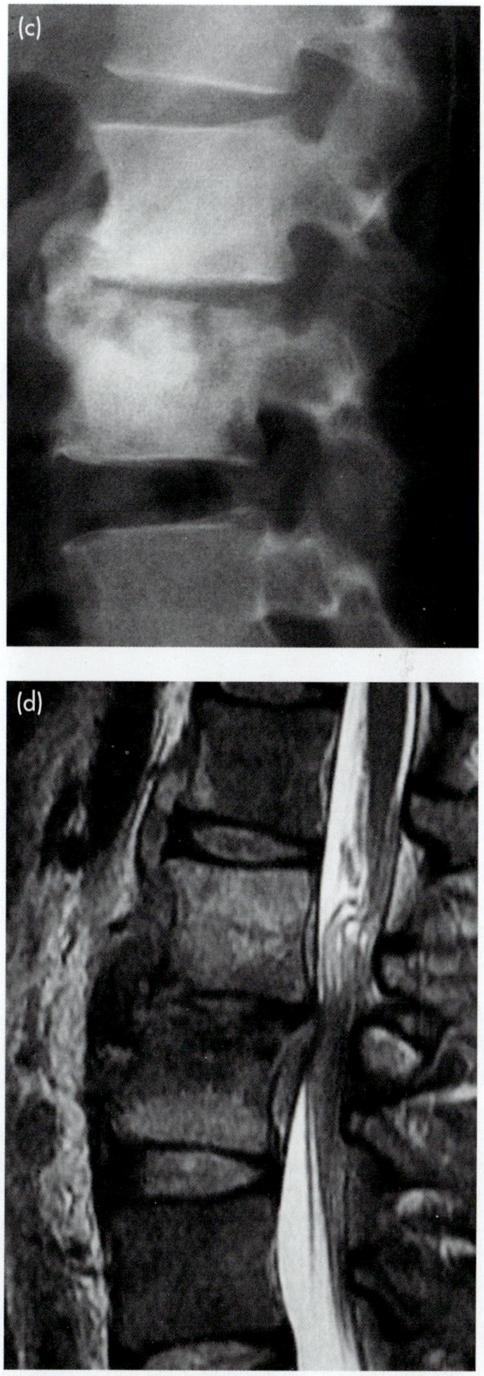

Figure 35.9 Discitis and vertebral body osteomyelitis arising from the lumbar L2/3 disc. A 46-year-old man presented with back pain, fever, malaise and night sweats. Anteroposterior (a) and lateral (b) radiographs revealed loss of disc space and sclerosis. Magnetic resonance imaging revealed decreased signal in the vertebral body and disc on T1-weighted scan (c) and increased signal in the vertebral body and disc on T2-weighted scan (d). The man underwent a biopsy under general anaesthetic. The causative organism was identified as *Staphylococcus aureus*. He was successfully treated with intravenous antibiotics and an orthosis.

Table 35.11 Aetiology of scoliosis.

Congenital
Neuromuscular
Idiopathic
Syndrome related

but the curvature may take years to be clinically evident. Close observation of spinal growth is required until skeletal maturity is reached. Brace treatment is ineffective for the primary structural curves, which are often short and rigid, but it may have a role in the control of compensatory curves. For progressive curves, surgical options include growing rod constructs, hemivertebra excison, correction and fusion or posterior instrumented correction and fusion.

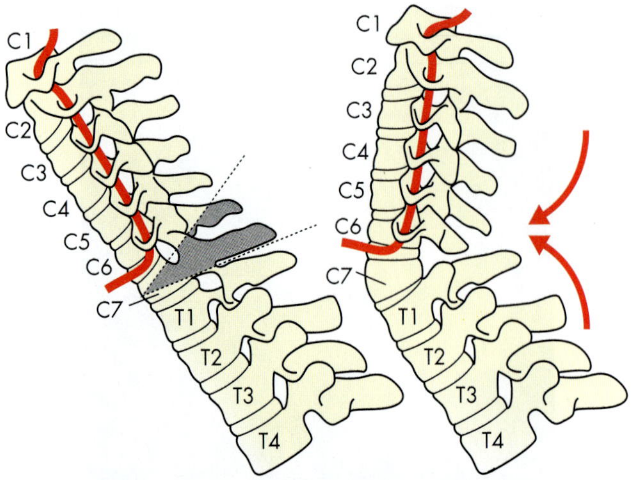

Figure 35.10 Cervical osteotomy for correction of cervicothoracic kyphosis. Planned resection lateral view for closing wedge osteotomy (left) and lateral view after closure of the osteotomy (right).

Neuromuscular scoliosis

This may be due to neuropathic disorders, such as cerebral palsy, spinocerebellar degeneration, syringomyelia, quadriplegia, spinal muscular atrophy and poliomyelitis, or myopathic disorders, such as Duchenne muscular dystrophy and myotonic dystrophy. There is good evidence that stabilisation of the spine in children with Duchenne muscular dystrophy who are able to walk (before respiratory compromise is too severe to preclude a general anaesthetic), may increase their lifespan by several years.

Idiopathic scoliosis

Idiopathic scoliosis can be divided into early onset (before eight years of age) (Figure 35.11) and late onset (after eight years of age; typical adolescent idiopathic scoliosis) (Figure 35.12). The distinction is important, as the number of alveoli in the lung does not increase after the age of eight years. Patients with severe curves in the early-onset group may develop cor pulmonale and right ventricular failure resulting in premature death. Adolescent idiopathic scoliosis is associated with a normal or near-normal life expectancy.

The prevalence of curves with a Cobb angle greater than 10° is between 0.5 and 3 per cent. The prevalence of curves greater than 30° is between 1.5 and 3 per 1000. Risk factors for progression include female gender, remaining skeletal growth, curve location and curve magnitude. Not all curves stabilise when skeletal maturity is reached. In long-term studies, 68 per cent experienced curve progression; the most marked progression of 1° per year was observed in thoracic curves between 50 and 75°.

Idiopathic curves of less than 25° are monitored with clinical and radiographic examination. In growing children (pre-menarchal) with curves between 20 and 29°, a brace may be indicated. Bracing is used to prevent curve progression and generally does not lead to permanent curve improvement. Curves beyond 45° are not amenable to brace treatment.

Surgery in the form of corrective instrumentation and spinal fusion is indicated for curve progression beyond 40°, truncal imbalance and unacceptable cosmesis. During surgery, continuous electrical spinal cord monitoring is used in the form of somatosensory-evoked potentials and, more recently, motor-evoked potentials to minimise the risk of neurological damage. The risk of neurological injury is 0.4 per cent (1:250) (Summary box 35.8).

Summary box 35.8

Spinal deformity

- Congenital scoliosis: rigid curves do not respond to brace treatment
- Neuromuscular scoliosis: timely surgery may prolong life
- Early onset scoliosis: (<8 years old) has potential to impair lung function

Scheuermann's kyphosis

In this condition typically there is wedging of the seventh to tenth thoracic vertebrae. The patient presents with backache. The incidence has been estimated at 1–8 per cent of the population, and is more common in males. Physiotherapy may be useful. Bracing for skeletally immature patients with kyphosis up to 65° may be effective in arresting progression. Indications for surgery include pain (apical or low back pain produced by compensatory hyperlordosis), progressive deformity greater than 70°, unacceptable cosmesis, and neurological and cardiac pulmonary compromise. If surgery is contemplated, it may require anterior release followed by posterior correction and fusion. Increasingly, posterior chevron osteotomies carried out at the time of posterior instrumentation may prevent the need for the initial anterior release.

DEVELOPMENTAL ABNORMALITIES

Developmental abnormalities of the spine and spinal cord can be divided into primary bony disorders (e.g. congenital scoliosis as discussed above) and primary neurological disorders (e.g. spina bifida, Arnold–Chiari malformation and spinal dysraphism).

Spina bifida

Spinal bifida is caused by a failure of fusion of the vertebral arches and possibly the underlying neural tube. Spina bifida cystica has an incidence of 1:300 live births and is associated with hydrocephalus. It is now decreasing as a consequence of folic acid supplementation, antenatal ultrasound and the measurement of alpha-fetoprotein levels. There are two basic types:

- **Meningocele**: The meninges herniate through the bony defect and are covered by skin.
- **Myelomeningocele**: The roof of the defect is formed by exposed neural tissue with 75 per cent of cases developing hydrocephalus.

A meningocele with good-quality skin over the defect may be treated conservatively. A meningocele with a more prominent sac can be excised at 3–6 months. The management of myelomeningocele is more controversial. Enthusiasm for closing all defects has been replaced by a more selective approach with the recognition that it was inappropriate to operate on children with

Holger Werfel Scheuermann, 1877–1960, radiologist, The Municipal Hospital, Sundby, Copenhagen, Denmark, described juvenile kyphosis in 1920.

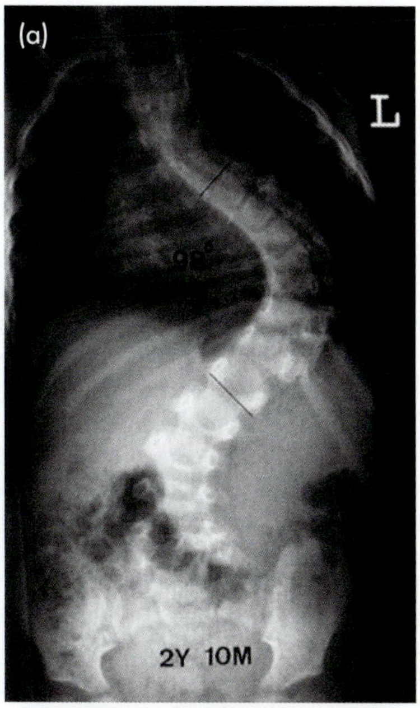

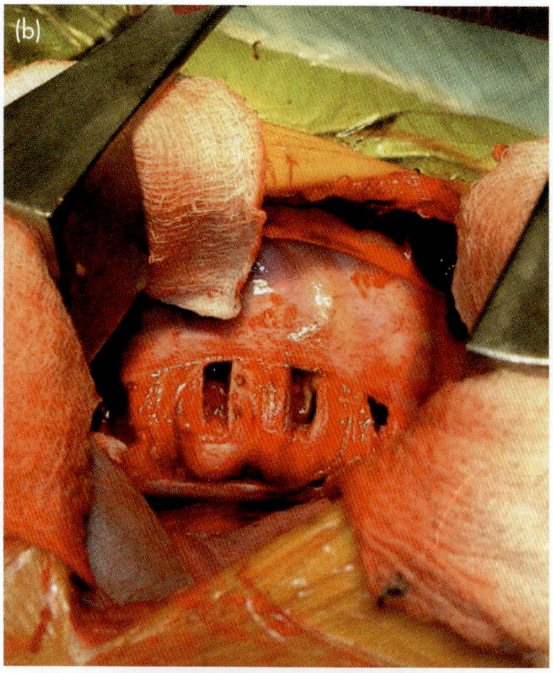

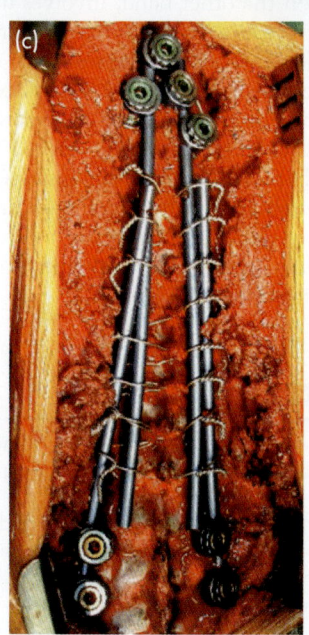

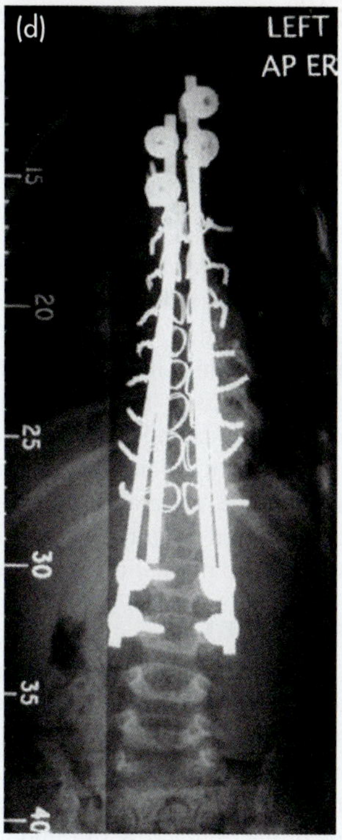

Figure 35.11 Early-onset idiopathic scoliosis. The anteroposterior standing radiograph (a) demonstrates a Cobb angle of 98° and dextrocardia. This 34-month-old boy underwent a convex hemiepiphysiodesis over the apical four discs (b), followed by posterior Luque trolley instrumentation without fusion to correct the spinal deformity and allow continued growth (c and d).

Hans Chiari, 1851–1916, an Austrian, Professor of Pathological Anatomy at German University in Prague, first described these hindbrain malformations between 1891 and 1896 as four types.
Julius Arnold, 1835–1915, German pathologist born in Zurich, Professor of Pathological Anatomy, Heidelberg, Germany, described this malformation in an infant in 1894. In 1907 Dr Arnold's students coined the eponym 'Arnold–Chiari malformation' in their honour. Some refer this condition specifically to the Type 2 variety.

severe hydrocephalus, a large open defect and no distal neurological function. The majority of these children die in their first year if closure is not attempted. With antibiotics, early surgical closure and shunts to prevent hydrocephalus, half the children who survive the first 24 hours will reach school age, but long-term problems remain, including skin, neuromuscular scoliosis, bone and joint deformity and the complications associated with a neuropathic bladder.

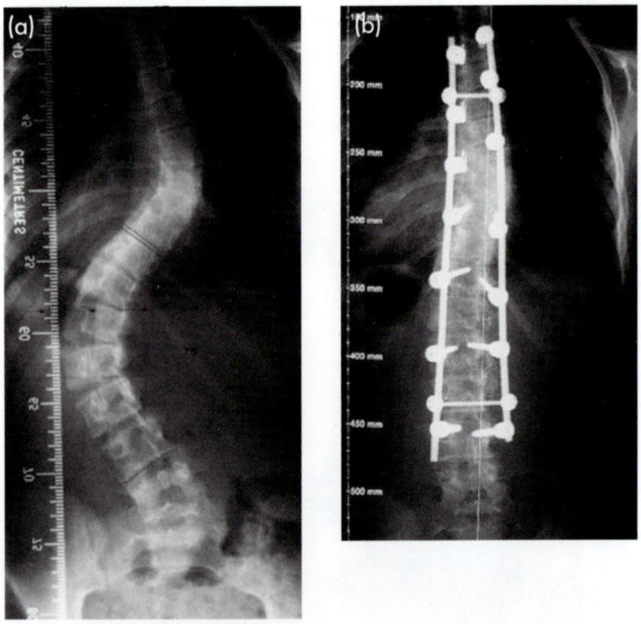

Figure 35.12 Late-onset idiopathic scoliosis. This 15-year-old girl had a progressive scoliosis with unacceptable cosmesis. The standing radiograph (a) demonstrated a right thoracic curve with a Cobb angle of 59° and a left thoracolumbar curve of 75°. Both curves were flexible on supine bending films. She underwent a posterior correction and instrumented fusion from T4 to L4 (b).

Arnold–Chiari malformation

Arnold–Chiari malformation occurs when the medulla oblongata and the cerebellar tonsils extend through the foramen magnum into the cervical spinal canal, causing pressure on the lower medulla. Hydrocephalus and impaired neurological function are common, and there is a strong association with spina bifida and syringomyelia. Symptoms may include headache, vomiting, visual disturbances, mental impairment, cerebellar ataxia, sensory disturbances or paralysis. Management consists of decompressing the foramen magnum and, usually, the posterior arch of the atlas to restore normal cerebrospinal fluid flow.

Spinal dysraphism

This is a group of disorders arising from abnormal embryological formation of tissues: all are associated with a progressive neurological deficit as the result of cord tethering and traction or cord compression. There is a strong association with spina bifida.

In diastematomyelia, there is an abnormal bony or cartilaginous spur projecting across the middle of the vertebral canal, dividing the dural tube and spinal cord in two. Between 50 and 70 per cent of patients have a skin naevus, dimple or hairy patch when the spine is examined. Surgical release of the tethering has variable results.

Syringomyelia

Patients may present with sensory disturbance, weakness of the hands, loss of pain and temperature sensation or progressive kyphoscoliosis. It is associated with Arnold–Chiari malformation and spinal cord tumours. Where syringomyelia is associated with an Arnold–Chiari malformation and scoliosis, a posterior cranial fossa decompression should be carried out first to resolve the syringomyelia. The scoliosis may then be corrected at a later date.

METABOLIC BONE DISEASES AFFECTING THE SPINE

Osteoporosis

Patients with osteoporosis may present with pain after minimal trauma or loss of height and an exaggerated thoracic kyphosis. Medications used to prevent and treat osteoporosis include the bisphosphonates (alendronate, risedronate), oestrogen or hormone replacement therapy and calcitonin.

Patients with painful thoracic fractures may be treated with short-term bed rest, analgesics and a spinal orthosis. If the back is still painful 6 weeks after the injury, patients may be considered for vertebroplasty or kyphoplasty. Vertebroplasty involves the injection of polymethyl methacrylate (PMMA) bone cement under pressure into the vertebral body under fluoroscopic guidance. The goal of the procedure is to stabilise the spine and decrease pain associated with compression fractures.

Kyphoplasty, on the other hand, involves inserting bilateral bone tamps with balloons into the vertebral body. These are inflated under fluoroscopic control with the bone tamp re-expanding the body, elevating the end-plates to reduce the fracture deformity. The balloons are then deflated and removed, and PMMA is placed into the cavity created by the balloons. The goals of kyphoplasty are spinal stabilisation, pain relief and restoration of vertebral body height. Significant complications have been reported, including nerve root injury and spinal cord injury resulting from cement extravasation along with cement embolism, infection and hypotension.

FURTHER READING

Debnath UK, Freeman BJ, Gregory P *et al.* Clinical outcome and return to sport after the surgical treatment of spondylolysis in young athletes. *J Bone Joint Surg Br* 2003; **85**: 244–9.

Fairbank J, Frost H, Wilson-McDonald J *et al.* Randomised controlled trial to compare surgical stabilisation of the lumbar spine with an intensive rehabilitation programme for patients with chronic low back pain: The MRC spine stabilisation trial. *BMJ* 2005; **330**: 1233–8.

Fritzell P, Hägg O, Wessperg P, Nordwall A. Volvo award in clinical science: lumbar fusion versus non-surgical treatment for chronic low back pain. A multi-centre randomised controlled trial from the Swedish lumbar spine study group. *Spine* 2001; **26**: 2521–34.

Gardner A, Gardner E, Morley T. Cauda equina syndrome: a review of the current clinical and medico-legal position. *Eur Spine J* 2011; **20**: 690–7.

Patchell RA, Tibb PA, Regine WF *et al.* Direct decompressive surgical resection in the treatment of spinal cord compression caused by metastatic cancer: a randomised trial. *Lancet* 2005; **366**: 643–8.

Tokala DP, Lam KS, Freeman BJ, Webb JK. C7 decancellisation closing wedge osteotomy for the correction of fixed cervico-thoracic kyphosis. *Eur Spine J* 2007; **16**: 1471–8.

Waddell G, McCulloch JA, Kummel ED *et al.* Volvo award in clinical science: non-organic physical signs in low-back pain. *Spine* 1979; **5**: 117–25.

Wiltse LL, Newman PH, Macnab I. Classification of spondylosis and spondylolisthesis. *Clin Orthop* 1976; **117**: 23–9.

CHAPTER 36

Upper limb – pathology, assessment and management

LEARNING OBJECTIVES

To understand:
- Anatomy and physiology relevant to upper limb pathology

To be able to explain:
- The diagnosis and treatment of common upper limb conditions

SHOULDER GIRDLE

Anatomy and function

The shoulder moves around the sternoclavicular joint, controlled and limited by muscles crossing between the thorax, scapula and humerus. The glenohumeral joint is controlled by the deltoid and rotator cuff muscles (subscapularis, supraspinatus, infraspinatus and teres minor). The scapula is integral to shoulder motion by both gliding and rotating on the posterior surface of the thorax (Figure 36.1).

Congenital abnormalities

Sprengel's shoulder

The most common congenital abnormality is due to abnormal scapular descent from its embryonic midcervical position. Presentation is a high, small, rotated scapula with connection to the cervical spine by a bony bar, fibrous band or an omovertebral body (Figure 36.2). Other congenital deformities are rib abnormalities, and cervical or thoracic scoliosis including Klippel–Feil syndrome (congenital fusion of cervical vertebrae).

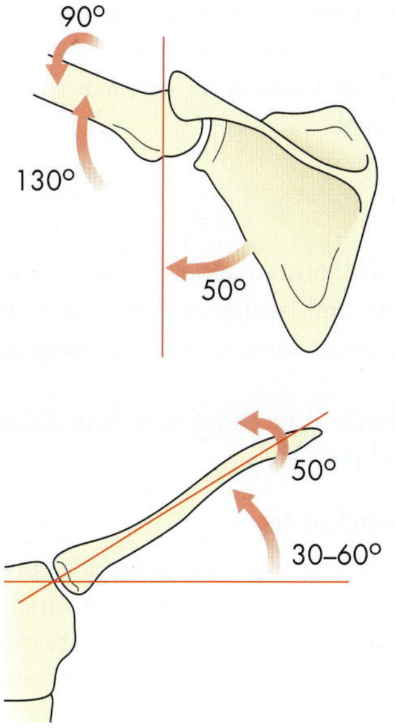

Figure 36.1 Relative motion of the elements of the shoulder girdle.

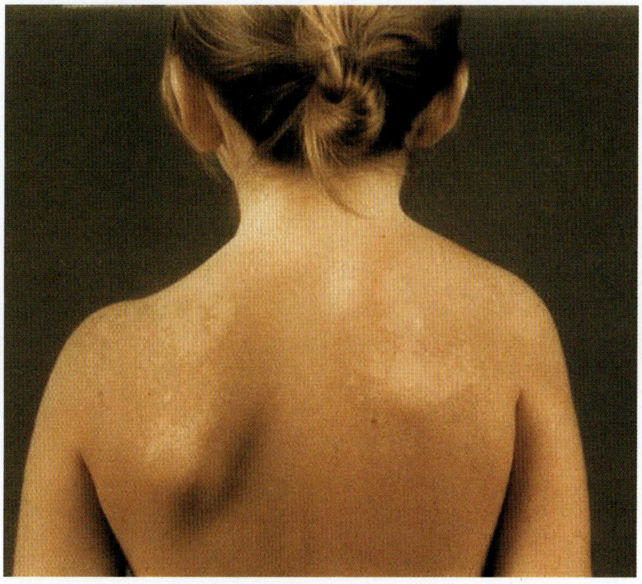
Figure 36.2 Sprengel's shoulder (right) of a four-year-old girl.

Otto Gerhard Karl Sprengel, 1852–1915, surgeon, Grossherzogliches Krankenhaus (the Grand Ducal Hospital), Brunswick, Germany, described congenital high scapula in 1891.
Maurice Kippel, 1858–1942, neurologist, Hôpital Tenon, Paris, France.
André Feil, 1889–?, neurologist, Paris, France.
Kippel and Feil described this condition in a joint paper in 1912.
Charles Sumner Neer II, orthopaedic surgeon, Columbia-Presbyterian Medical Center, New York, NY, USA.

Acquired abnormalities

History

Patients usually associate the onset of their symptoms with an unusual event (trauma or excessive activity) even though the causation may not be as clear as the patient thinks. Even so, the onset (sudden or gradual) and duration are important as is the age of the patient and their occupation. Pain presenting in the shoulder (or anywhere in the upper limb) can arise from the nerves of the neck, so the history should include questions about neck problems.

Examination

If the patient can localise the source of the pain to an exact point in the shoulder, then the problem is unlikely to be referred from the neck. Tests for inflammation and impingement involve trying to reproduce the pain by loading the limb in the position which creates the problem (Hawkin's test for impingement, see Figure 36.3). Tests for tears in structures such as the rotator cuff look specifically for weakness, while apprehension tests check for instability (such as shoulder dislocation).

Investigations

X-rays are only of limited value because most lesions in the shoulder involve damage to the soft tissues. However, a reduced subacromial space and an acromial spur may be clearly visible in rotator cuff damage (Figure 36.4).

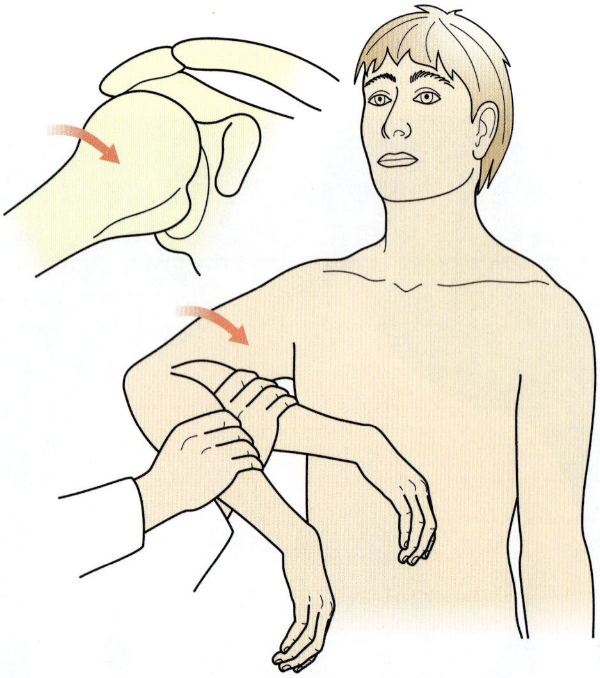

Figure 36.3 Hawkin's impingement test. Impingement pain is reproduced when the shoulder is internally rotated with 90° of forward flexion, thereby locating the greater tuberosity underneath the acromion.

(a) (b)

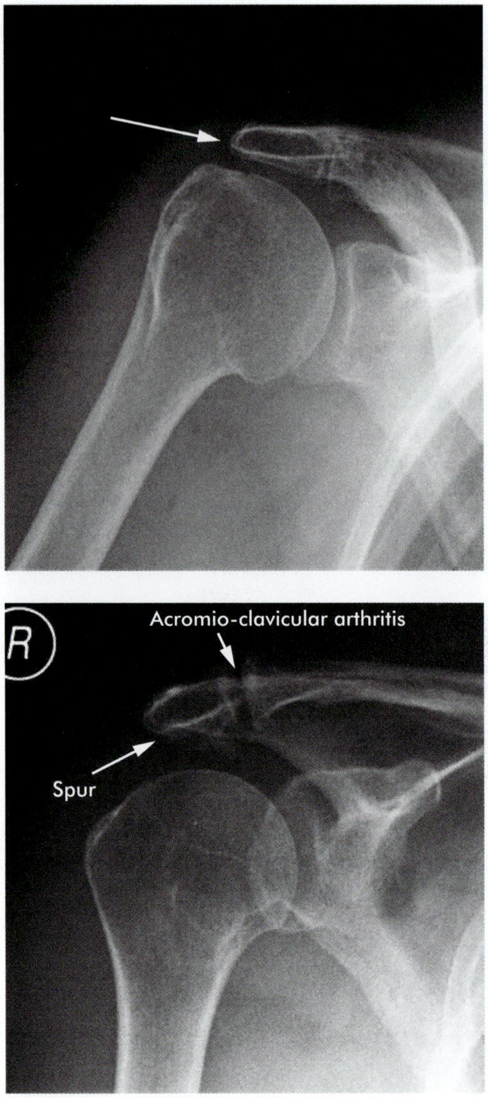

Figure 36.4 (a) Radiograph showing sclerosis on the undersurface of the acromion and the greater tuberosity with reduced subacromial space. (b) Radiograph showing an acromial spur and arthritis of the acromioclavicular joint.

Both ultrasound and magnetic resonance imaging (MRI) allow the integrity and health of the rotator cuff to be checked, and the integrity of the labrum of the glenohumeral joint (Figure 36.5).

Local anaesthetic injections may help localise the source of inflammation and pain.

Rotator cuff tendonitis

The rotator cuff moves in a confined space between the humeral head, the acromion and the coracoacromial (CA) ligament. Even a trivial injury can start a progression of inflammation, swelling and pain, which in turn causes impingement. The impingement then causes further swelling and pain and a vicious circle is set up. The likelihood of tendonitis developing is increased by a beak of bone which tends to appear beneath the acromion with age (Figure 36.6). The result is a painful arc

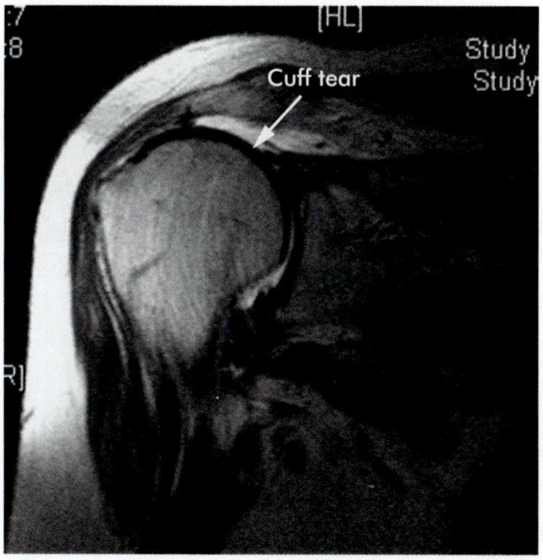

Figure 36.5 Magnetic resonance imaging showing a retracted cuff tear.

of movement for the patient which corresponds to the position where the inflamed segment of the supraspinatus tendon jams under the subacromial beak. The examiner may find that although the patient cannot lift their arm through this segment (because of the pain), passively lifting the arm for the patient enables them to continue with pain-free movement once the impingement is past (Figure 36.7).

Treatment

Injection of steroid into the inflamed area may break the cycle of inflammation and impingement (Figure 36.8), but arthroscopic removal of the subacromial beak and of the CA ligament (if it is impinging) should give good relief of symptoms (Figure 36.9) (Summary boxes 36.1 and 36.2).

Summary box 36.1

Rotator cuff tendonitis

- Tendonitis produces weakness secondary to pain (often a painful arc)
- A tendon tear produces weakness which is only secondarily painful
- Injection of local anaesthetic can be diagnostic

Summary box 36.2

Treatment of subacromial impingement

- Non-operative treatment includes injections
- Surgery indicated if symptoms persist beyond six months
- Surgery decompresses the rotator cuff

Rotator cuff tears

The rotator cuff also has a poor blood supply and is subject to degenerative changes which weaken it with age. This means that tears are more common in the elderly and at any age are unlikely to repair spontaneously. Tears usually begin at the anterolateral edge of the supraspinatus, and progress posteriorly to involve the infraspinatus and teres minor, tendons. This creates a bare area over the greater tuberosity, as the torn cuff retracts medially (Figure 36.10).

History

In the younger patient the onset is often relatively major trauma, e.g. saving a fall by hanging onto the rung of a ladder, but in the elderly the onset may follow a painful period of tendonitis or even apparently occur spontaneously.

Examination

The patient may have a mixed picture of tendonitis and of a tear, but if the pain is removed by injection of local anaesthetic the weakness will persist. Symptomatic tears are associated with pain, weakness, limited active abduction, cuff muscle wasting and hunching of the shoulder when attempting abduction (Figure 36.11).

Investigation

Tears are classified as small (less than 1 cm), intermediate (2–4 cm) and large (more than 5 cm).

Treatment

Treatment depends on the patient's age, lifestyle and severity of symptoms. Arthroscopic or open repair with subacromial decompression can be considered for all tears, but is likely to give a much better and useful result in the young than in the old. It may not be possible to suture large tears due to loss of muscle contractility, and then complex surgery, e.g. tendon transfers, patch grafts or reverse joint replacement (Figure 36.12) will need to be considered (Summary box 36.3).

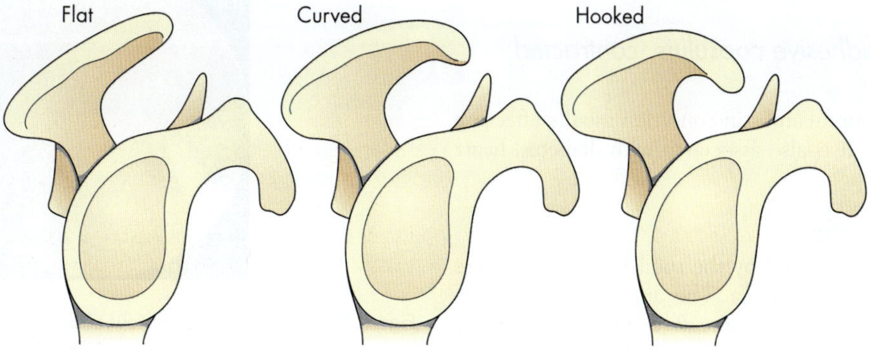

Figure 36.6 The three most common acromial morphologies.

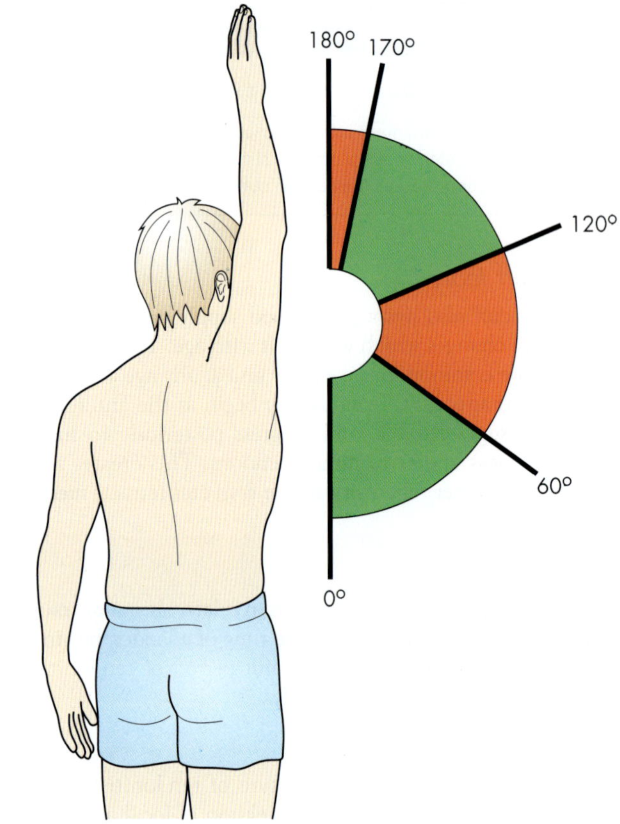

Figure 36.7 Arcs of shoulder girdle motion with subacromial impingement pain between 60 and 120° of abduction, and acromioclavicular joint pain between 170 and 180°.

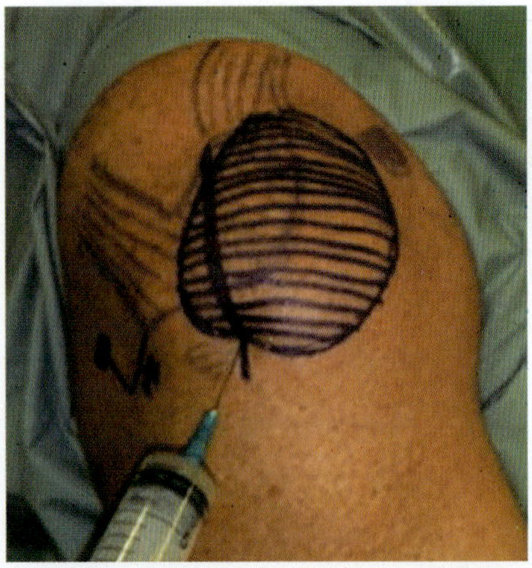

Figure 36.8 Technique of administering an injection into the subacromial bursa.

Summary box 36.3

Rotator cuff tears

- Occur in older age group
- Twenty to forty per cent of 40–50 year olds have asymptomatic rotator cuff tears
- Fifty per cent of 70 year olds have an asymptomatic tear
- Subacromial decompression is important for pain relief following cuff repair
- Acute tears present with little pain but profound weakness
- Early repair gives good results

Frozen shoulder (adhesive capsulitis, contracted shoulder)

This is an idiopathic painful and stiff condition usually affecting females in their fifties. It is also associated with diabetes, heart or thyroid disease.

History and examination

Frozen shoulder is characterised by the sudden onset of severe pain and may follow minor trauma. The differential diagnoses are infection, fractures and rotator cuff tears. Initially there is severe pain but this improves with time; however, there is global loss of active and passive movements limited by pain. The pathognomonic sign is a loss of external rotation. X-rays are normal.

Treatment

The clinical course can run over one to three years and is divided into painful, stiffening and thawing phases. If untreated, frozen shoulder will usually resolve, and the majority of patients are left with no functional problems. In the first phase of the condition, treatment is pain relief. Corticosteroids can also be injected locally. Despite the pain, the patient should be encouraged to perform as much active and passive movement as they can. Surgical release of the tight capsule can produce some pain relief in the early stages and is also indicated for prolonged stiffness.

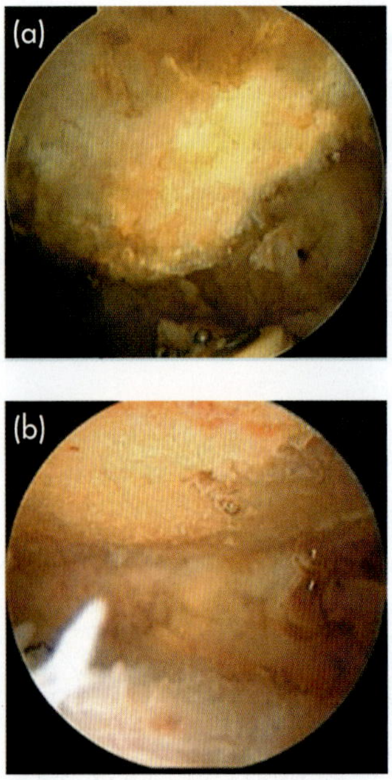

Figure 36.9 (a) Arthroscopic view of an acromial spur. (b) Arthroscopic view after the acromial spur has been removed and the cuff decompressed.

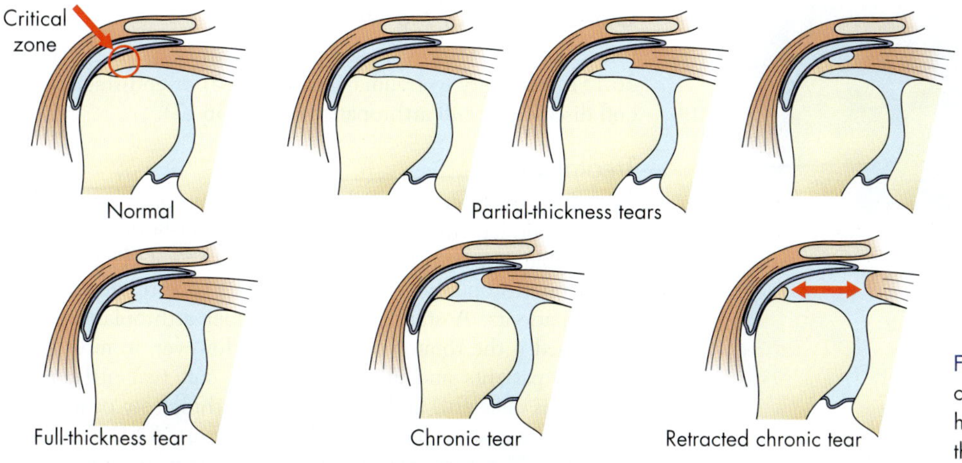

Figure 36.10 Various stages of rotator cuff tear. Initial partial-thickness tears have the potential to progress to full thickness and retracted tears.

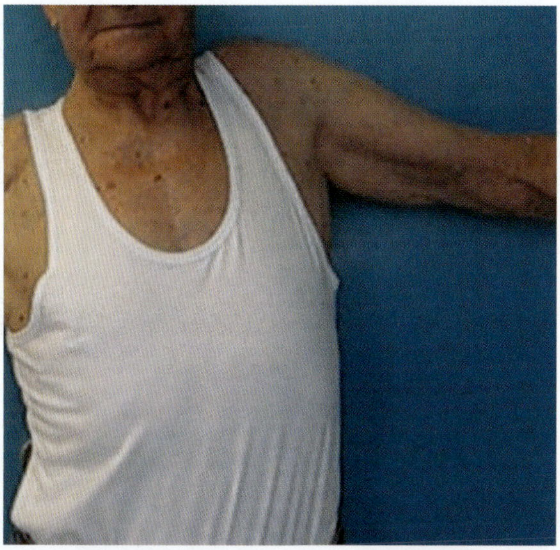

Figure 36.11 A 75-year-old man with a >5 cm retracted cuff tear attempting to abduct his shoulder, which is limited, by lack of balanced motor power, below 60°.

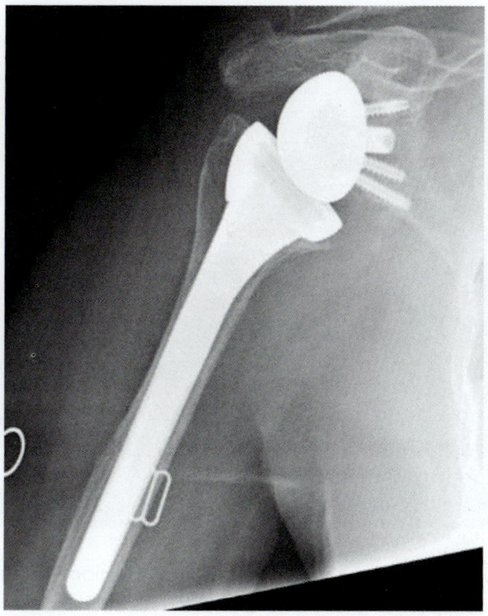

Figure 36.12 Reverse geometry total shoulder replacement.

Manipulation under anaesthesia or arthroscopic saline distension of the joint with release of the rotator cuff interval is also felt to reduce pain and improve mobility (Summary box 36.4).

Summary box 36.4

Frozen shoulder (adhesive capsulitis)

- Predominantly occurs in females in their fifties
- Spontaneous onset
- Produces severe pain followed by reduced shoulder motion
- Spontaneous resolution can occur over one to three years
- Differential diagnoses: calcific tendonitis and rotator cuff tear
- Injections, distension with saline and surgical release may all help

Calcific tendinitis

Calcium deposition within the supraspinatus tendon is believed to be part of a degenerative process, or the consequence of a partial degenerative tear of the tendon.

History and examination

There is severe, rapid onset shoulder pain with painful restricted motion. However, in contrast to adhesive capsulitis, external rotation is possible. Subacromial calcific deposits can be seen on plain radiographs (Figure 36.13).

Treatment

Subacromial corticosteroid injections may help. The condition is often self-limiting, with resorption of the calcium deposits. Surgery for resistant cases includes arthroscopic or open subacromial decompression and excision of the calcific deposits.

Arthritis of the shoulder

Rheumatoid arthritis

The glenohumeral joint is commonly involved in rheumatoid arthritis (Figure 36.14). Usually, there is osteoporosis, destruction of the articular cartilage and synovial proliferation with

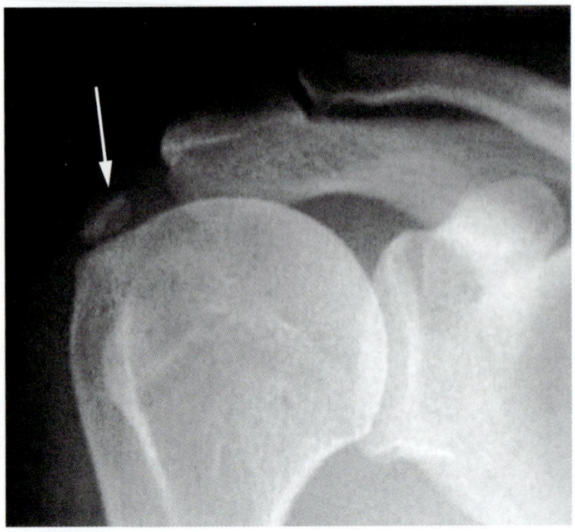

Figure 36.13 Radiograph demonstrating calcific tendonitis.

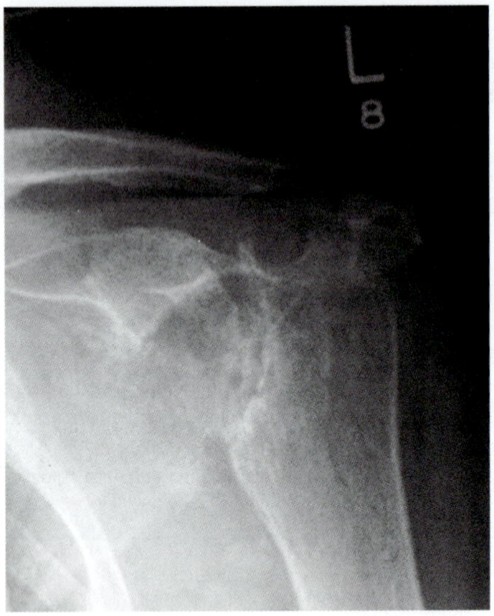

Figure 36.14 Rheumatoid arthritis of the shoulder.

pannus formation. The rotator cuff is weakened and frequently tears. Arthroscopic synovectomy may slow the progress of the joint destruction and lead to a reduction in pain and improvement in range of movement. Intra-articular steroid injections may also be helpful. Shoulder replacement is complicated by poor bone stock and damage to the stabilising structures around the shoulder, especially the rotator cuff. The patient should only expect a reduction in pain. Any increase in range of movement is a bonus (Summary box 36.5).

Summary box 36.5

Shoulder problems in rheumatoid arthritis

- Arthroscopic synovectomy is effective
- Rotator cuff tears are common
- Glenohumeral joint replacement improves pain but motion to a lesser degree

Osteoarthritis of the shoulder

Glenohumeral joint osteoarthritis is either primary (Figure 36.15), secondary to trauma (Figure 36.16) or end-stage rotator cuff disease, i.e. cuff arthropathy (Figure 36.17).

Treatment

If medical treatment has failed, the surgical options are arthroscopic debridement or joint arthroplasty. Debridement is not predictable, but both total shoulder replacement (Figure 36.18) and hemiarthroplasty (Figure 36.19) have good results in appropriate patients. A standard total shoulder arthroplasty can be performed if the rotator cuff is intact. However, in most osteoarthritis patients and all patients with cuff tear arthropathy, the cuff is deficient, and either a hemiarthroplasty or a reverse polarity total shoulder arthroplasty (Figure 36.12) should be used. Shoulder arthroplasty is an effective pain-relieving procedure, but less predictable in restoring motion, especially above shoulder level.

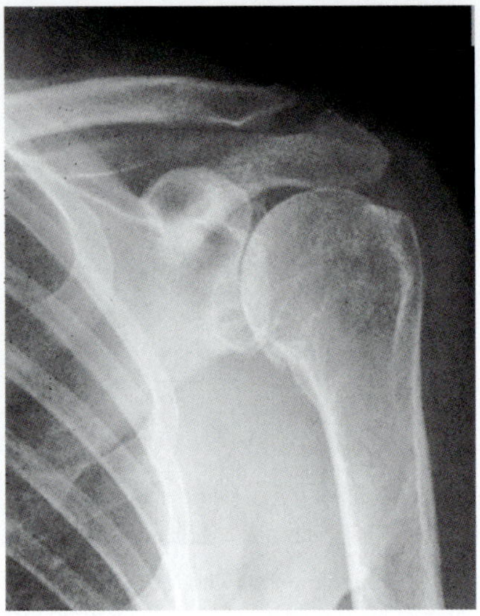

Figure 36.15 Osteoarthritis of the glenohumeral joint.

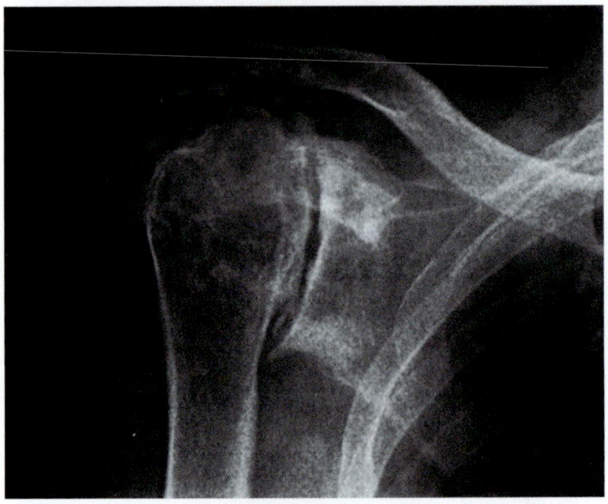

Figure 36.16 Post-traumatic arthritis with malunion of the proximal humerus, collapse of the humeral head, subchondral sclerosis and osteophytes.

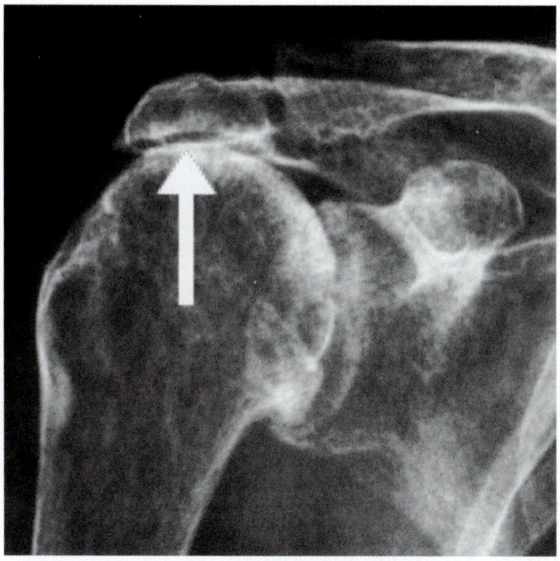

Figure 36.17 A massive cuff tear that has led to superior migration of the humeral head and secondary osteoarthritis of the glenohumeral joint.

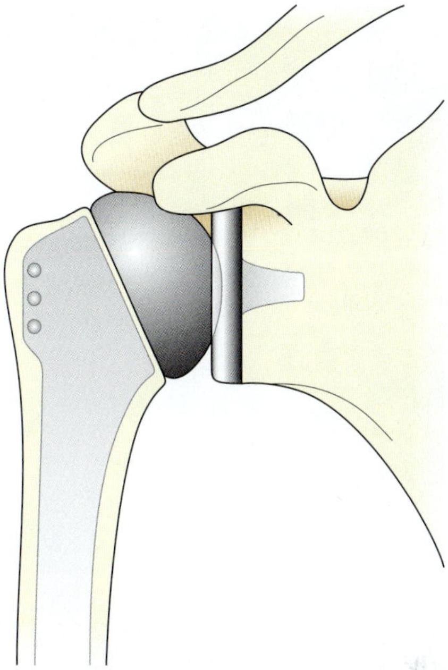

Figure 36.18 Total shoulder replacement done for osteoarthritis. An intact rotator cuff is essential.

Arthrodesis of the joint is an alternative in younger patients with a history of sepsis or neurological problems (Figure 36.20). Patients retain a moderate range of movement at the shoulder, as a result of scapulothoracic motion (Summary box 36.6).

Summary box 36.6

Arthritis of the shoulder

- Severe cases are treated with hemiarthroplasty or total shoulder arthroplasty
- Total shoulder replacements should not be performed if the rotator cuff is deficient
- Pain relief is good following arthroplasty though improvement in range of motion is less predictable
- Glenohumeral arthrodesis is an option in the young or those with a history of sepsis
- Post-arthrodesis motion is fair but is entirely scapulothoracic

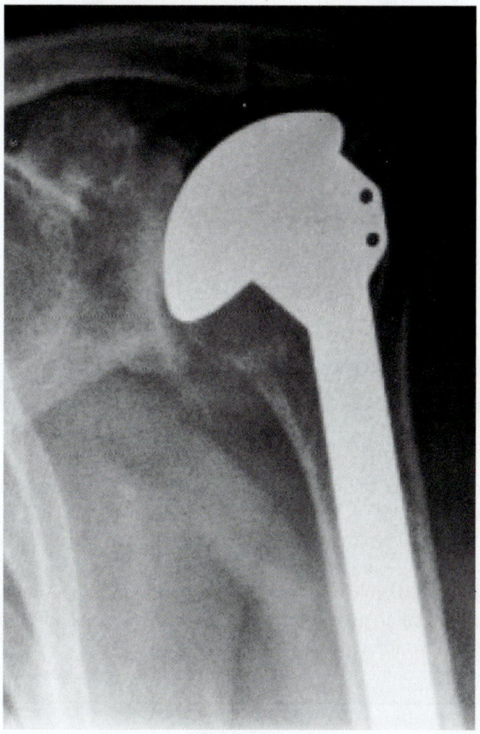

Figure 36.19 Shoulder hemiarthroplasty is performed for arthritis if there is a deficient rotator cuff.

Acromioclavicular joint arthritis

Acromioclavicular joint (ACJ) arthritis is common and is often asymptomatic, noted as an incidental finding on x-ray (Figure 36.4b). Symptoms typically arise in males aged 20–50 years. Inferior osteophytes can impinge on the underlying rotator cuff.

History and examination

There is frequently a history of trauma to the ACJ. Pain is activity related. There is prominence of the lateral end of the clavicle. The joint line is tender. Flexing and adducting the arm to place the hand behind the opposite shoulder reproduces pain. If symptoms are related to inferior osteophytes, impingement symptoms and signs are also present.

Treatment

An intra-articular corticosteroid injection will usually help. Surgery involves arthroscopic or open excision of the lateral 0.5–1 cm of the clavicle (Figure 36.21). This gives good pain relief. In patients with symptoms, which are predominantly impingement, arthroscopic removal of the osteophytes should be performed (Summary box 36.7).

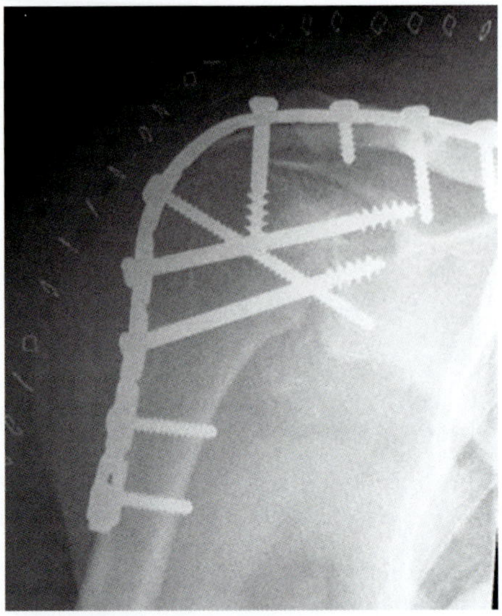

Figure 36.20 Arthrodesis of the shoulder.

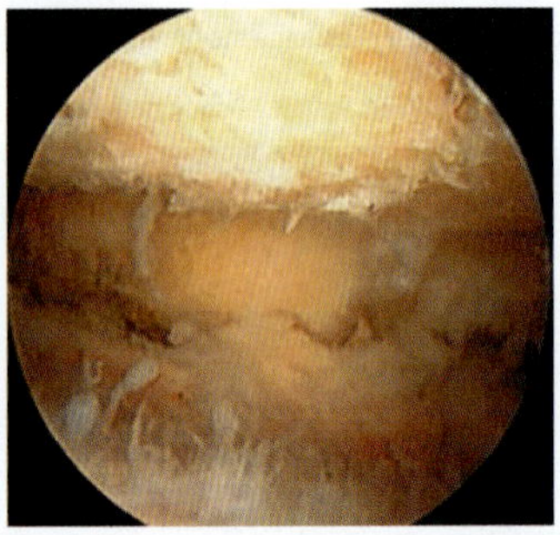

Figure 36.21 Arthroscopic end-on view of the clavicle after excision of its distal end.

Summary box 36.7

Acromioclavicular joint problems

- Acromioclavicular joint arthritis is common and may be asymptomatic
- It becomes symptomatic secondary to trauma or repetitive overload
- Inferior clavicular osteophytes can impinge on the cuff
- Intra-articular steroid and local anaesthetic injection may relieve symptoms
- Excision of the lateral end of the clavicle gives good results

Long head of biceps tendon rupture

Rupture of the long head of biceps usually occurs in the elderly, and is due to abrasion of the tendon in the bicipital groove. It is associated with rotator cuff tears. Most patients present with few symptoms, although they often seek advice because of the bulge they notice in their arm.

History and examination

Patients feel a sense of 'something giving way' in front of the shoulder. The upper arm is bruised, and elbow flexion produces a swelling in the front and middle of the arm. The lump will be permanent and is initially tender. Power is diminished (Figure 36.22).

Treatment

Reassurance that pain and bruising will resolve is sufficient. Power improves over several months and surgery (biceps tenodesis) is not needed.

Dislocation of the shoulder and instability of the glenohumeral joint

Three broad groups of shoulder instability exist:

- Traumatic: unidirectional; involuntary; surgery is usually successful
- Atraumatic: multidirectional, painful; involuntary; responds to surgery
- Habitual: voluntary with ligament laxity, painless; surgery usually contraindicated.

Recurrent traumatic instability

History

Traumatic shoulder dislocation is the most common of all dislocations, usually first presenting in patients under 25 years of age. Usually, the shoulder dislocates anteroinferiorly. Initially, there is a notable traumatic event. Subsequent dislocations require less force. The shoulder may sublux or actually dislocate (complete separation of the joint surfaces).

Examination

On examination the shoulder has a full range of motion, but with forced abduction and external rotation, the patient experiences apprehension (a sense of impending doom!) (Figure 36.23).

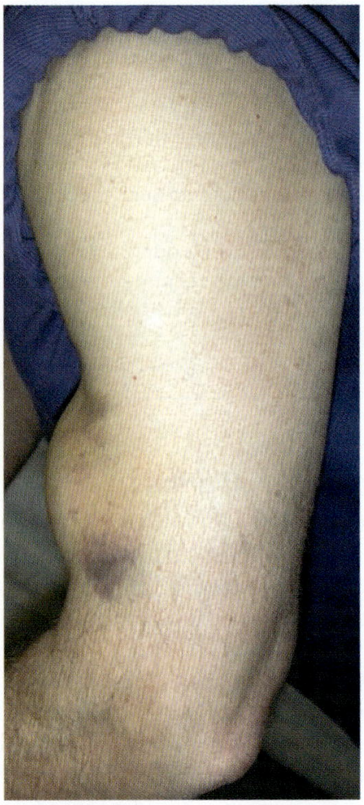

Figure 36.22 Bruising and change in the upper arm shape due to rupture of the long head of biceps.

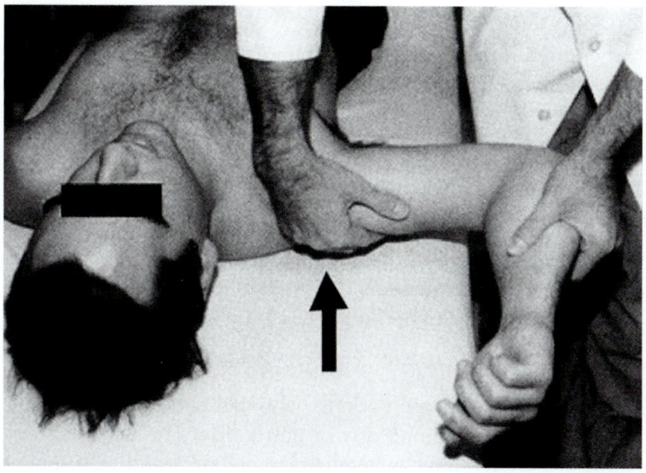

Figure 36.23 Apprehension test for anterior instability.

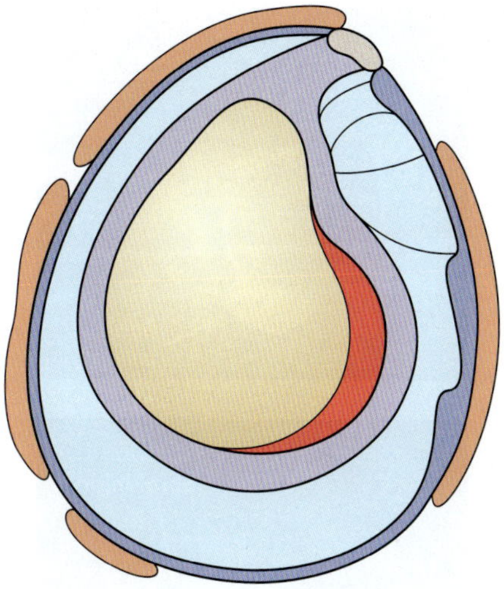

Figure 36.25 An end-on view of the glenoid labrum, demonstrating anteroinferior labral detachment (red) with the rotator cuff muscles (brown), long head of biceps tendon and labrum (blue).

Investigations

On ultrasound or MR arthrogram, detachment of the anteroinferior labrum (Bankart lesion) and damage to the humeral head (Hill–Sachs lesion) can often be seen (Figures 36.24, 36.25 and 36.26).

Treatment

The relative indications for surgery are repeated dislocations which are interfering with the patient's quality of life. An absolute indication for surgery is when dislocations occur when the patient is asleep. Anterior instability requires arthroscopic or open repair of the Bankart defect with tightening of the capsule, and produces good results in 90–95 per cent of patients. Bony defects may have to be grafted. For the less common recurrent posterior instability, repair of the damaged labrum and tightening of the posterior capsule is needed (Summary box 36.8).

Summary box 36.8

Recurrent traumatic shoulder instability

- An appreciable force leads to the first dislocation or subluxation
- Subsequent dislocations/subluxations require less force
- The most common direction of dislocation is anteroinferior
- There is a positive apprehension sign
- Surgical treatment repairs the labral lesion and tightens the capsule

Posterior dislocation of the shoulder

This is a rare event but is easy to miss. The clue is in the history as the patient will have either had an electric shock, an epileptic fit, or have been subject to severe restraint when their arm has been forced up their back (a half-nelson).

The patient will be in severe pain and if they are psychotic (and this is why they are being restrained) then they will be difficult to examine. For the same reason, the radiographer may only be able to get an anteroposterior view of the shoulder, and on this view, the shoulder looks normal to the unwary (Figure 36.27). It is the high 'index of suspicion' from the history which gives the best chance of making the diagnosis.

Treatment

This dislocation is frequently difficult to reduce as the posterior margin of the acromion is embedded in the humeral head, so that open reduction is needed.

Atraumatic instability

History

There is usually no history of an initial injury. Instability may be multidirectional and the shoulder usually only subluxes rather than dislocates. The patient is often able to reduce the shoulder without assistance.

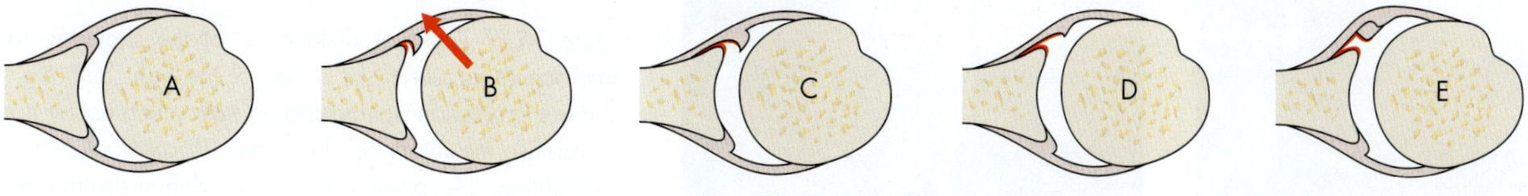

Figure 36.24 Schematic representation of Bankart's lesion that forms a spectrum of pathology from minor labral detachment (B) to large detachments with glenoid rim fractures (bony Bankart; E).

Arthur Sydney Blundell Bankart, 1879–1951, orthopaedic surgeon, The Middlexsex Hospital, London, UK.

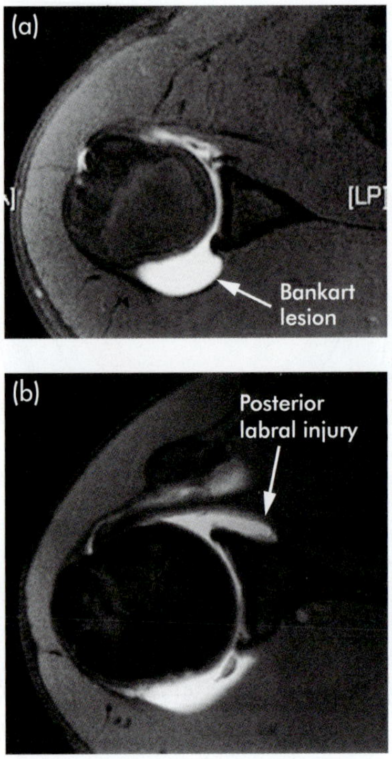

Figure 36.26 (a) Magnetic resonance arthrogram showing anterior Bankart lesion. (b) Magnetic resonance arthrogram showing posterior labral injury.

Examination

Generalised ligament laxity is common. Apprehension tests are positive, but often in more than one direction. Anterior and posterior drawing of the humeral head allows laxity to be tested (Figure 36.28).

Treatment

Specialist physiotherapy should be tried first in these patients, aiming to improve both the proprioception and strength of the muscles around the shoulder. If this fails then surgery is needed to perform capsular tightening.

Habitual dislocation

Habitual dislocators are patients who can sublux the shoulder at will, either anteroinferiorly or posteriorly. The manoeuvre is painless. Patients have generalised joint laxity and may sublux the shoulder as a 'party trick'.

Patients should be told to stop subluxing the shoulder, and the capsule will tighten naturally. Surgery is associated with high failure rate and should be avoided.

DISORDERS OF THE ELBOW

Anatomy and function

The elbow joint allows flexion and extension as well as making up the proximal part of the radioulnar joint which permits

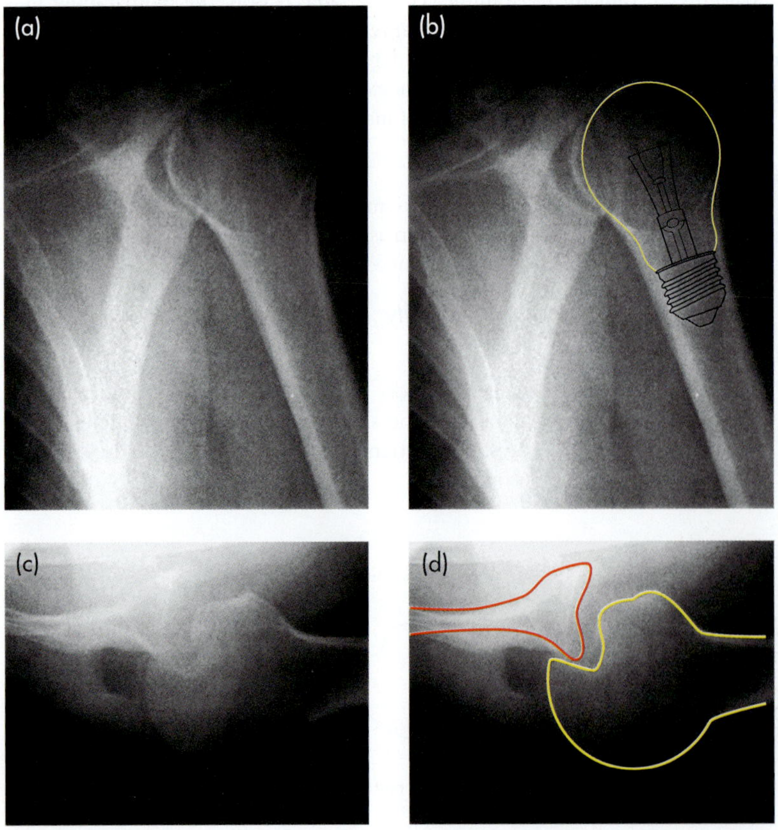

Figure 36.27 Posterior dislocation of the shoulder. (a) Anteroposterior view; (b) origin of the light bulb sign; (c) axial projection demonstrating how much easier it is to visualise the injury on this view; (d) axial projection highlighting this point and further demonstrating the impacted fracture in the humeral head, or Hill–Sachs lesion.

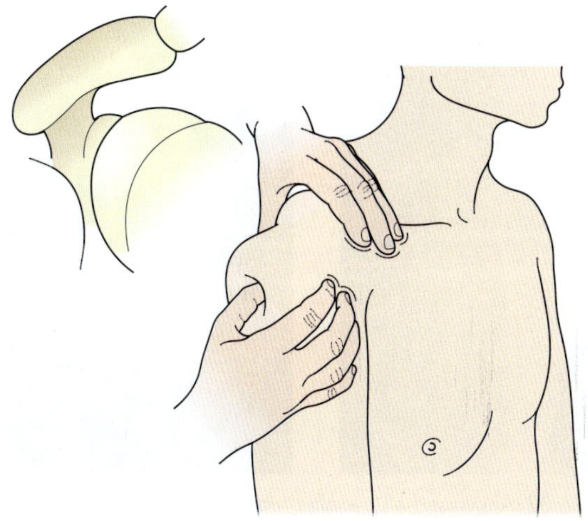

Figure 36.28 Generalised laxity can be appreciated by drawing the humeral head in anterior and posterior direction. A sulcus will be produced under the acromion if the humerus is drawn inferiorly (sulcus sign).

pronation and supination of the forearm. The brachial artery passes immediately in front of the joint, while the ulna nerve passes lateral to the medial epicondyle immediately behind it.

Tennis elbow (lateral epicondylitis) and golfer's elbow (medial epicondylitis)

These are discussed in Chapter 34.

Arthritis of the elbow

Rheumatoid arthritis

Surgery is required, especially in end-stage disease. Arthroscopic or open radial head excision and synovectomy is effective for painful, restricted pronation and supination. Elbow arthroplasty is effective for pain relief and functional restoration (Figure 36.29).

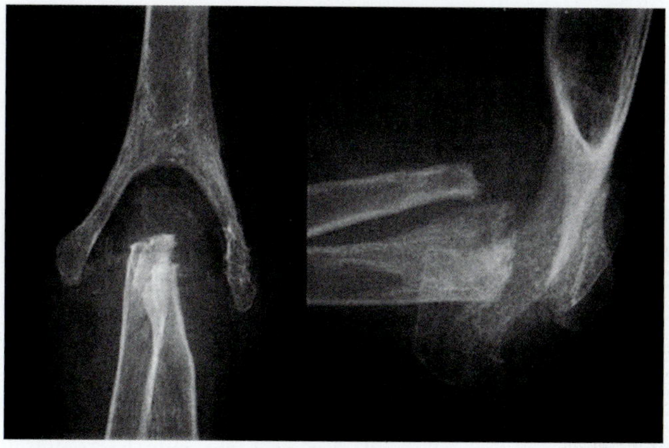

Figure 36.29 Typical end stage unstable and destroyed rheumatoid elbow.

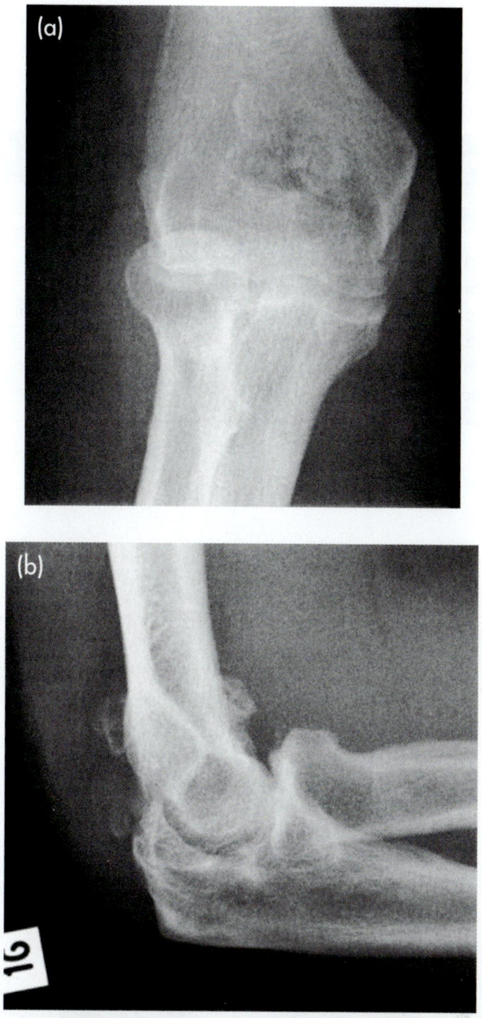

Figure 36.30 (a and b) X-rays showing osteoarthritis of the elbow joint.

Osteoarthritis

Osteoarthritis of the elbow is usually primary (Figure 36.30) or secondary to trauma.

History

Typical patients are middle-aged males in manual occupations. Symptoms are pain, locking, crepitus and painful motion with loss of extension. Ulnar nerve entrapment symptoms may be present.

Examination

There is usually loss of extension and restriction of flexion. Pronation and supination tends to be spared in comparison with rheumatoid arthritis.

Treatment

Surgery should be considered only if medical treatment fails. Arthrodesis is the treatment of choice for those performing heavy manual work, as a joint replacement will not survive long under heavy loading. Surgical debridement alleviates pain and increases range of motion in earlier stages. Prosthetic joint arthroplasty provides a more predictable symptomatic relief (Figures 36.31 and 36.32) (Summary box 36.9).

Summary box 36.9

Arthritis of the elbow

- Excision of the radial head improves pain and pro-supination in rheumatoid arthritis
- Total elbow replacement gives good results in rheumatoid and low demand patients
- Arthrodesis is the better option in a high demand manual labourer

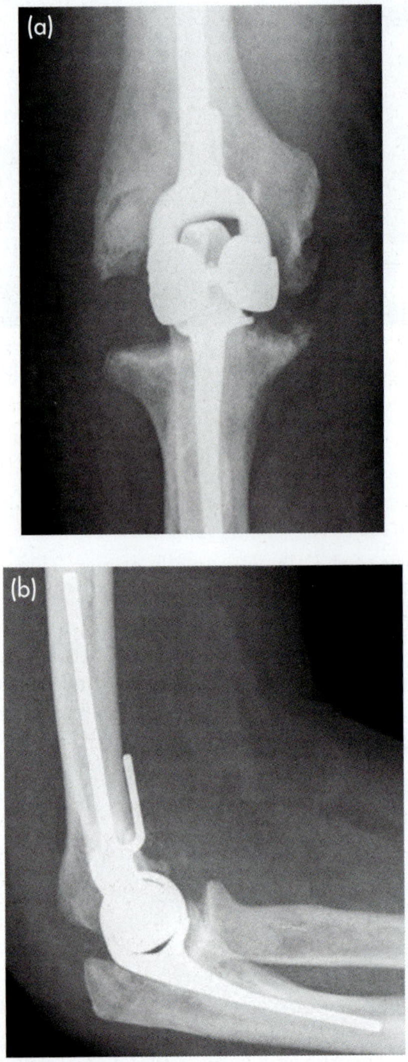

Figure 36.31 (a and b) Linked total elbow replacement.

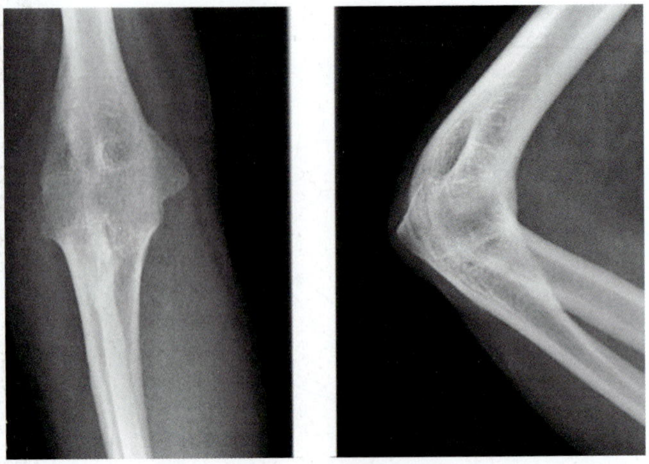

Figure 36.32 Ankylosed elbow after tuberculosis.

Loose bodies in the elbow

The common causes are osteoarthritis, osteochondritis dissecans in the young (Figure 36.33) and synovial chondromatosis (Figure 36.34). Patients describe sudden pain and locking, and need to manipulate the elbow for relief. Plain radiographs will usually confirm the diagnosis (Figure 36.35). Arthroscopic clearance of the joint produces good results (Figure 36.36).

Olecranon bursitis

This is a relatively common disorder where the elbow becomes red, warm, swollen and painful. Initially, septic arthritis may be suspected. However, on examination, signs and symptoms are confined to the back of the elbow (Figure 36.37) and movement within an arc of 30–130° is possible. Most cases settle with anti-inflammatories. If the patient is pyrexial, antibiotics should be given. Formal drainage of the bursa is indicated if purulent material is present.

Chronic bursitis may be associated with calcific nodules of the bursal lining (Figure 36.38). These can be excised if they prove troublesome.

Ulnar nerve compression

Compression of the ulnar nerves occurs around the elbow at the junction of the arcade of Struthers and also the medial intermuscular septum as the nerve passes into the posterior compartment of the distal humerus. It can also occur under the medial epicondyle or as the nerve passes between the heads of the flexor carpi ulnaris (Figure 36.39).

History and examination

Patients describe tingling/numbness in little and ring fingers. A positive Tinel's sign is usually present at the compression site, with wasting and weakness of the intrinsic muscles of the hand (Figure 36.40). Foment's sign will be positive due to weakness of the adductor pollicis (Figure 36.41). Nerve conduction studies have an unpredictable diagnostic value in the early stages. X-rays may confirm medial osteophytes.

Treatment

Splints preventing elbow flexion at night may be useful. If symptoms persist, surgery including simple nerve decompression (most cases), partial medial epicondylectomy, and/or anterior

Emil Theodor Kocher, 1841–1917, Professor of Surgery, Berne, Switzerland. In 1909 he was awarded the Nobel Prize for Physiology or Medicine for his work on the thyroid.
Sir John Struthers, 1823–1899, Professor of Anatomy, University of Aberdeen, Aberdeen, UK.

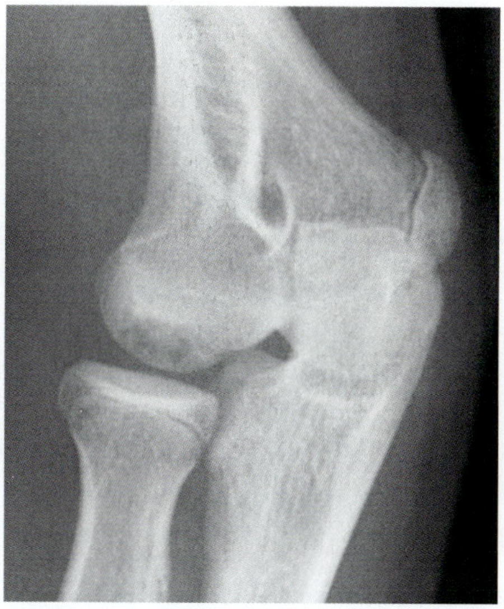

Figure 36.33 Osteochondritis dessicans of the capitellum (Panner's disease).

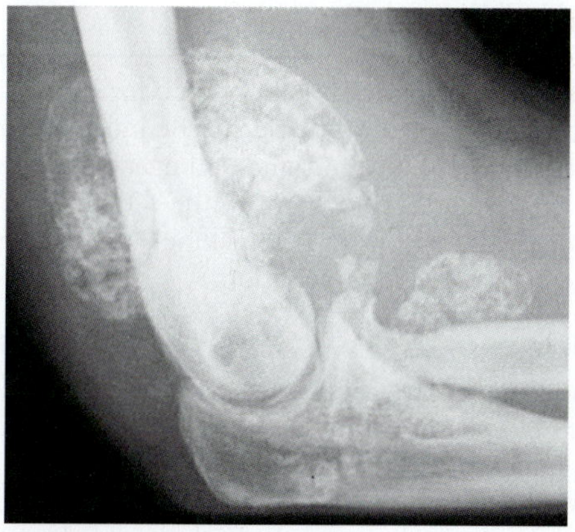

Figure 36.34 Synovial chondromatosis.

transposition of the nerve can be performed. Transposition is necessary in cases of valgus deformity or if the nerve is unstable after decompression (Summary box 36.10).

Summary box 36.10

Other common elbow problems

- Loose bodies cause locking and can be removed arthroscopically
- If the ulnar nerve is compressed weakness and wasting will be seen in the hands
- Simple decompression is usually successful

TUMOURS OF THE UPPER LIMB

Tumours are discussed in Chapter 39.

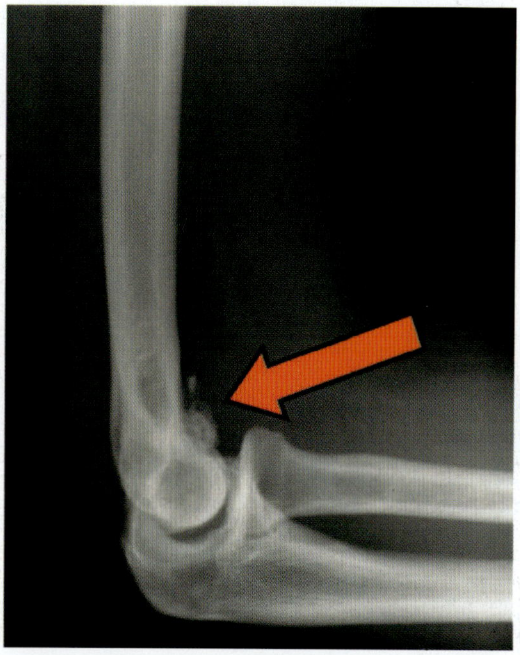

Figure 36.35 X-rays showing loose bodies in the elbow.

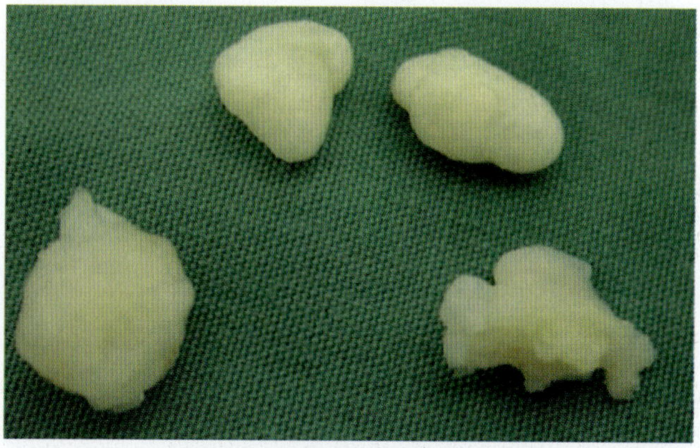

Figure 36.36 Loose bodies removed arthroscopically from patient in Figure 36.35.

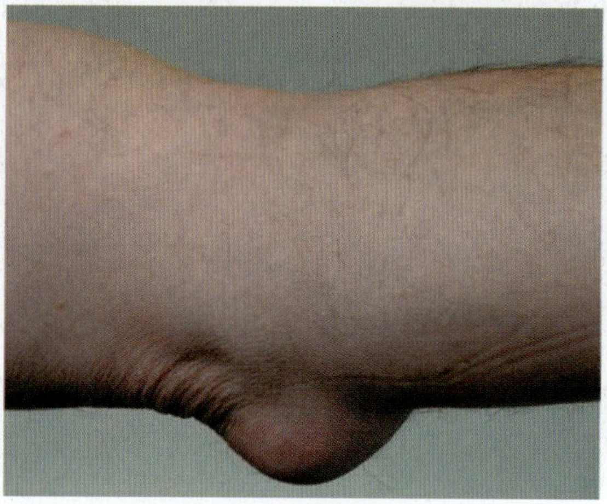

Figure 36.37 Olecranon bursitis.

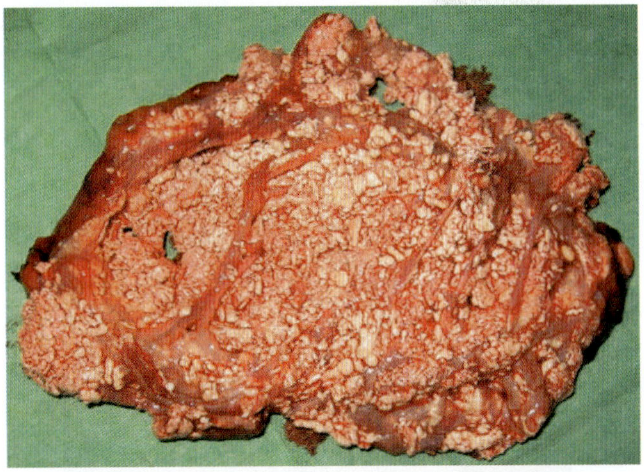

Figure 36.38 Large chronic olecranon bursa with dense calcific deposit.

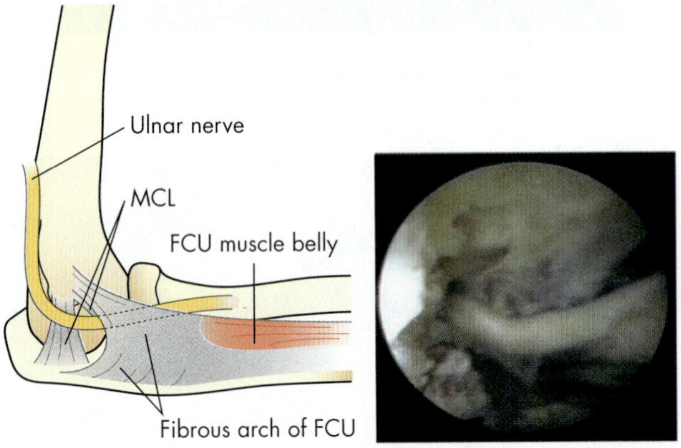

Figure 36.39 Anatomy of the cubital tunnel site for ulnar nerve compression, with a view of arthroscopic ulnar nerve decompression (inset). FCU, flexor carpi ulnaris; MCL, medial collateral ligament.

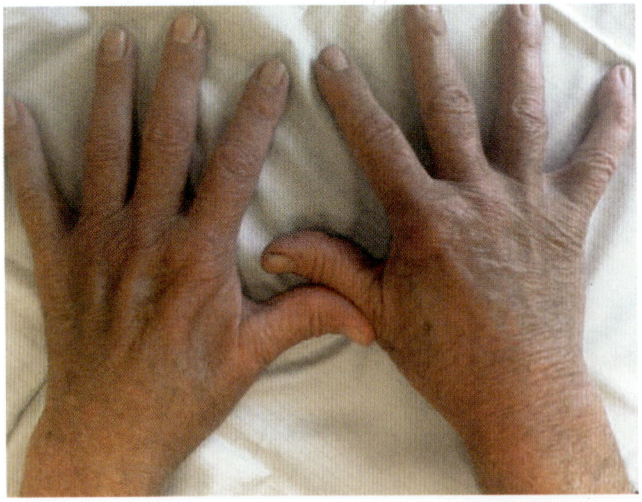

Figure 36.40 Intrinsic muscle wasting due to ulnar neuropathy.

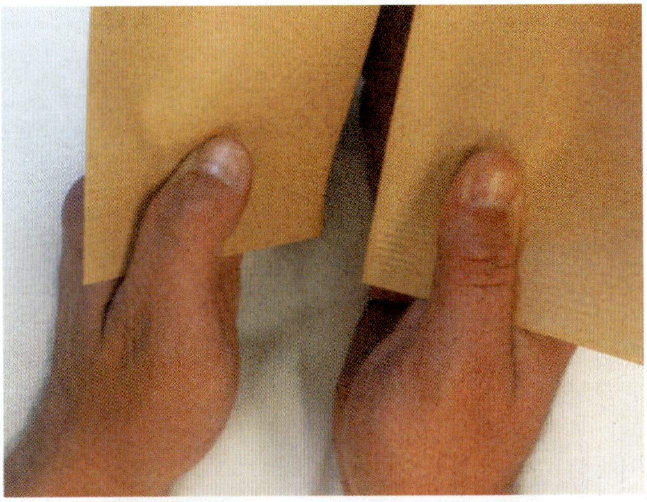

Figure 36.41 Foment's sign tests the adductor pollicis. Patient is asked to hold a piece of paper in a side pinch between the thumb and the index finger. The examiner attempts to pull the paper out. Due to weakness of the adductor pollicus the patient will compensate by flexing the flexor pollicis longus that is supplied by the anterior interosseous nerve.

HAND

The index finger works against the thumb for a fine pinch grip; the thumb can press against the side of the index finger for a key grip; the tip of the index and middle fingers provides a tripod pinch; all fingers curl for hook grip while the little and ring fingers provide the most power when making a fist. A stable wrist is required to allow good hand function.

Clinical history and physical examination

The occupation, sports and recreation (especially music) and hand dominance are all important information needed when treating a hand problem.

The examination of the hand should assess sensation, movement, power and coordination. A check should also be made for the rotational malalignment of the digits (Figure 36.42).

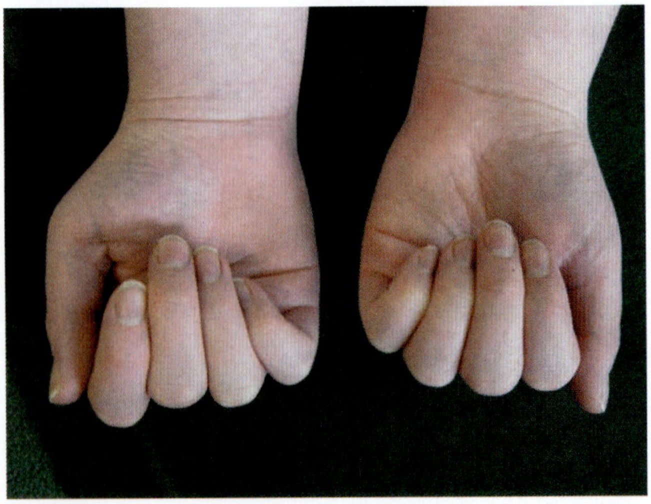

Figure 36.42 Rotational deformity of the little finger.

Investigations

Radiographs assess for arthritis or tumours. Electrophysiological studies may be required to assess nerve function. MRI is useful for diagnosing avascular necrosis and ligament injuries.

Hand swelling and stiffness

Swelling followed by stiffness is the arch enemy of hand rehabilitation. The hand will swell after injury, surgery or infection. In response the wrist flexes and then there is compensatory metacarpophalangeal joints' extension and interphalangeal flexion. If action is not taken this position will become permanent as collateral ligaments shrink and tissues fibrose. Hand elevation to reduce swelling, splintage in position of safety to prevent collateral shortening ('Edinburgh' position described by James – full extension of the proximal and distal inter-phalangeal joints, and flexion to 90° of the metacarpal-phalangeal joint) and early mobilisation prevent permanent stiffness (Summary box 36.11).

Summary box 36.11

General principles of treatment

Avoid swelling and stiffness by:

- Elevation – reduce swelling
- Splintage – avoid contractures
- Movement – pump away swelling and encourage suppleness

Thumb ulnar collateral ligament injury

Chronic thumb overuse leads to stretching of the ulnar collateral ligament and instability (gamekeeper's thumb). The ligament can also rupture acutely if the thumb is forcibly abducted (skier's thumb). If valgus stress causes significant opening of the joint on the ulnar side then the ligament needs to be repaired surgically as the torn end can become trapped behind the adductor aponeurosis (Figure 36.43).

Triangular fibrocartilage complex

The triangular fibrocartilage is a complex consisting of the ulnocarpal ligaments and a meniscus form. It is continuous with dorsal and volar wrist capsules and stabilises the distal radioulnar joint. It can undergo traumatic or degenerative tears, presenting with ulna-sided wrist pain and distal radioulnar instability. An MR arthrogram and wrist arthroscopy aid diagnosis (Figure 36.44). Peripheral tears of the triangular fibrocartilage complex (TFCC) can be repaired (open or arthroscopically) while central degenerative tears are arthroscopically debrided.

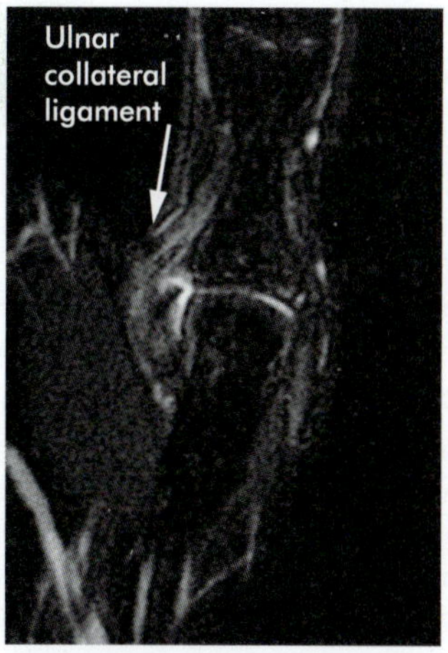

Figure 36.43 Magnetic resonance imaging shows rupture of the ulnar collateral ligament of the thumb (skier's thumb).

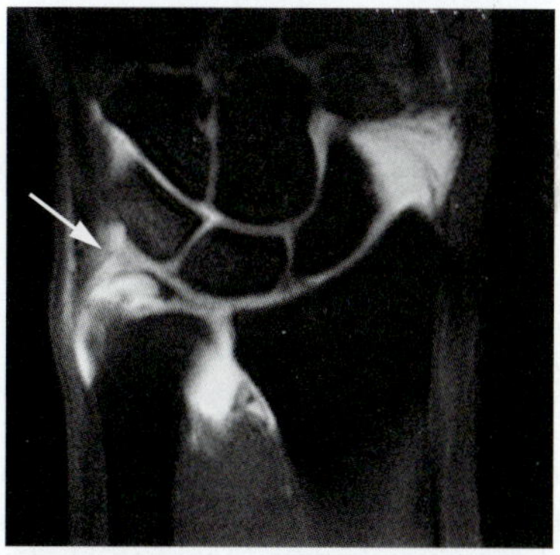

Figure 36.44 Magnetic resonance imaging arthrogram showing peripheral detachment of the triangular fibrocartilage complex (TFCC).

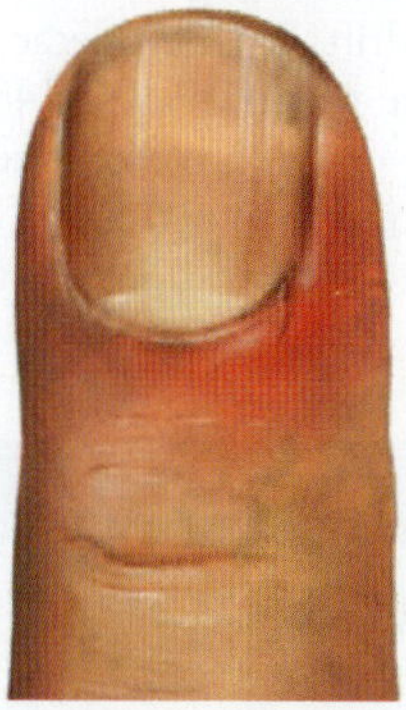

Figure 36.45 Acute paronychia.

Infections

Paronychia

Nail bed infection is the most common hand infection (Figure 36.45). After initial inflammation, pus accumulates beside the nail. It is best treated with incision and drainage, partial nail removal and antibiotics.

Felon

A felon is an abscess between the specialised fingertip septae in the distal pulp. It causes intense fingertip pain. It may lead to terminal phalangeal osteomyelitis. Incision and drainage covered by intravenous antibiotics is recommended.

Flexor tendon sheath infection

Flexor tendon sheath infections present as a painful, swollen, flexed finger. There is extreme pain with passive extension, tenderness along the tendon sheath and symmetric swelling (Kanavel's signs). Treatment is by closed sheath irrigation by a catheter or open drainage and intravenous antibiotics. If infection is untreated, tendon adhesion and necrosis occur. Infection can spread proximally, damaging the whole hand (Summary box 36.12).

John Ivor Pulsford James, 1913–2001, Professor of Orthopaedic Surgery, the University of Edinburgh, Edinburgh, UK.

Summary box 36.12

Treatment of hand infections

- Elevate, splint and give intravenous antibiotics
- Surgical drainage should include tendon sheath irrigation
- Early mobilisation

Mycobacterial infections

Tuberculosis may involve the tenosynovium, joints or bone. The most dramatic form is the compound palmar ganglion, with synovial swelling, proximal and distal to the transverse carpal ligament. Diagnosis is made by taking a biopsy. Synovectomy should be performed and the patient treated with the appropriate antibiotics.

Deep fascial space infections

These infections occur in the palm but may be limited to a web space. The whole hand becomes swollen and tender, as pus collects on either side of the septum. Treatment is incision and drainage with thorough washout of the wound. It is important that all deep spaces are opened and incision on both dorsal and volar sides of the hand may be needed.

Arthritis

Rheumatoid arthritis

Rheumatoid arthritis presents with classic symptoms: morning stiffness, symmetrical arthritis, hand deformities and rheumatoid nodules. Diagnostic criteria include seropositive rheumatoid factor and radiographic changes (Table 36.1). The rheumatoid synovitis (pannus) destroys ligaments, tendons and joints, producing pain, deformity and loss of function. Typical rheumatoid deformities in the hand include boutonnière (Figure 36.46), swan neck (Figure 36.47) and ulnar drift of the metacarpophalangeal joints with radial drift of the wrist (Figure 36.48). Activities such as thumb pinch and the opening of jars stress the weakened ligaments and become impossible to perform. The treatment should be dictated by pain and disability, not deformity (Summary box 36.13).

Summary box 36.13

Manifestations in rheumatoid arthritis

- Fingers: swan neck, boutonnière
- Extensor tendon rupture
- Flexor tendon rupture
- Flexor synovitis
- Metacarpophalangeal joints: flexion, ulnar deviation, subluxation, dislocation
- Wrist: radial deviation, carpal supination, prominent ulna head, extensor tenosynovitis

Management

The primary indications for surgery are: (1) pain relief; (2) functional improvement; (3) prevent disease progression; and (4) cosmesis. Patients may require many surgical procedures and a helpful axiom is to start proximally and work distally alternating

Table 36.1 Radiographic differences between rheumatoid and osteoarthritis.

Rheumatoid arthritis	Osteoarthritis
Periarticular osteoporosis/ subchondral erosions	Subchondral sclerosis and cysts
Periarticular soft-tissue swelling	Less pronounced swelling
Joint space narrowing	Joint space narrowing
Marginal erosions	Marginal osteophytes
Joint deformity/malalignment	Less pronounced deformities
Ankylosis	Less common ankylosis

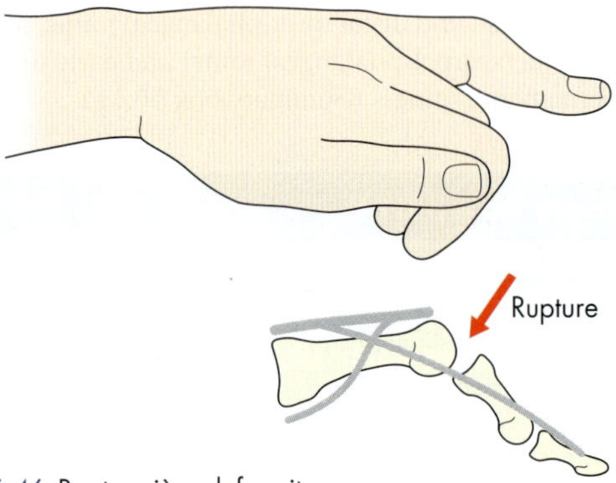

Figure 36.46 Boutonnière deformity.

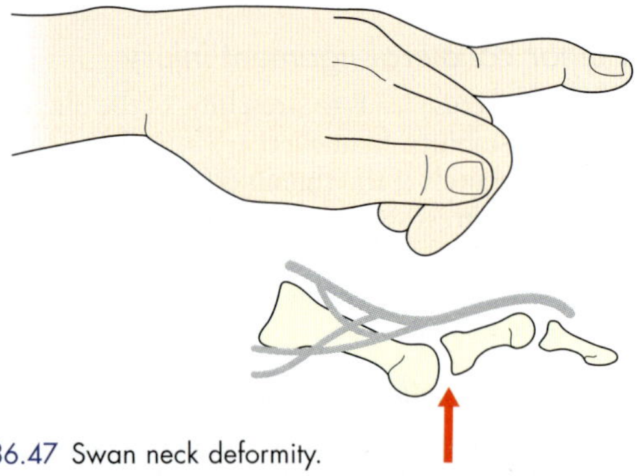

Figure 36.47 Swan neck deformity.

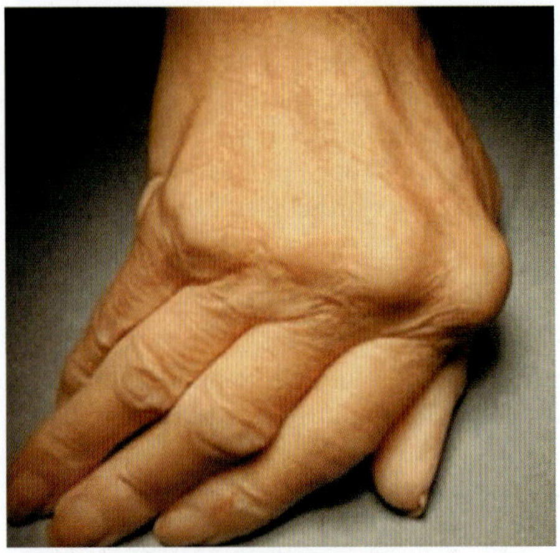

Figure 36.48 Rheumatoid hand showing ulnar drift at the metacarpophalangeal joints.

Boutonnière is French for 'button-hole'.

between motion sacrificing and sparing procedures. The various procedures which can be considered are:

1 Synovectomy: improves pain, increases function and prevents tendon rupture, trigger digits and nerve compression (Carpal tunnel syndrome).
2 Distal ulna excision: reduces pain, prevents extensor tendon rupture or protects repaired extensor tendons. Distal ulna excision leads to instability and so in the young patient ulna head arthroplasty is preferred.
3 Arthrodesis of the wrist, thumb and some of the smaller joints: gives good pain relief, and creates a stable axis against which other parts can function.
4 Metacarpophalangeal and interphalangeal joint replacement: provides pain relief and functional improvement. Total wrist arthroplasty will also provide good pain relief and motion (Figure 36.49).
5 Tendon reconstructions: some ruptured tendons cause significant morbidity (Figure 36.50), often treated either by a tendon transfer or a local joint fusion.

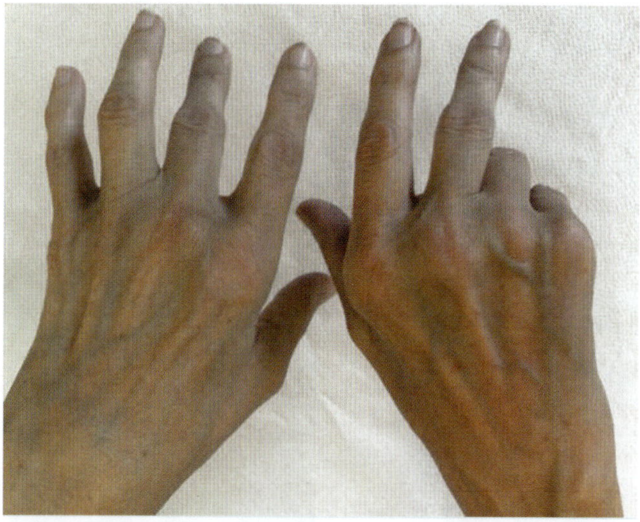

Figure 36.50 Rupture of the extensor tendons to the little and ring fingers.

Osteoarthritis

Wrist

The radiocarpal joint can develop primary or secondary osteoarthritis (after intra-articular trauma and infection). If conservative measures have failed then operative management includes limited or total wrist arthrodesis and total wrist replacement.

Hand

Females are more commonly affected than males. The commonly affected joints are the distal interphalangeal (Heberden's nodes), proximal interphalangeal (Bouchard's nodes) and the thumb carpometacarpal joints (Figure 36.51). Symptoms rarely correlate with the appearance clinically or radiographically. Treatment includes splinting, therapy and steroid injections. Surgical options include arthrodesis for distal interphalangeal (DIP) and proximal interphalangeal (PIP) joints (Figure 36.52), joint replacement (PIP and metacarpophalangeal joints) and excision arthroplasty (excision of trapezium for thumb carpometacarpal joint). Joint arthrodesis eliminates pain at the expense of motion, but function is often well preserved.

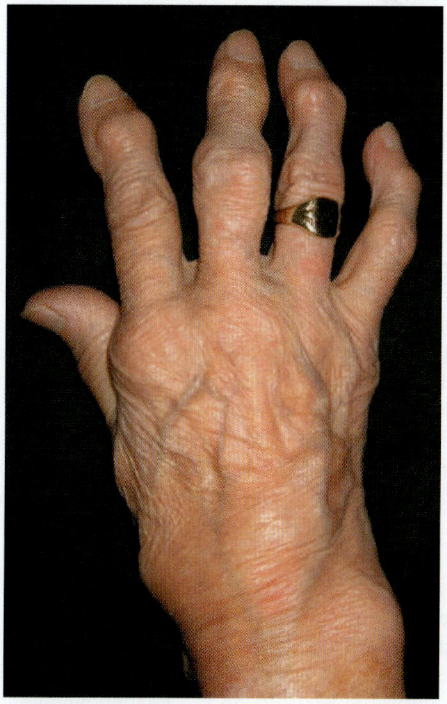

Figure 36.51 Hand deformities secondary to osteoarthritis.

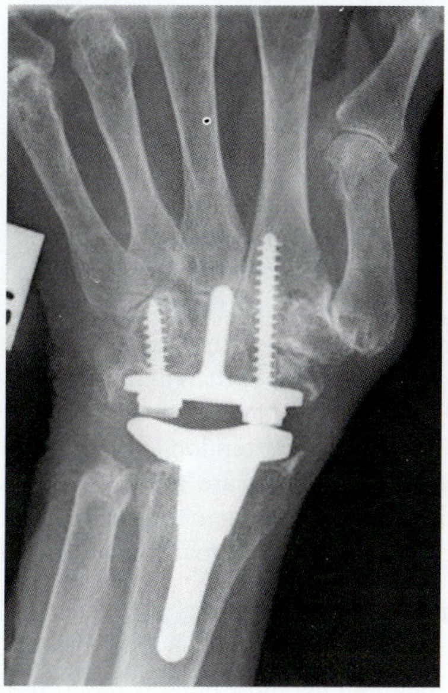

Figure 36.49 Total wrist replacement.

Other forms of arthritis in the hand

Psoriasis especially affects the DIP joints. It is asymmetrical and causes fusiform swelling of the digits and nail changes. Gout causes pain, joint redness, occasional tophi, and can be difficult to differentiate from septic arthritis. Serum urate and negative microscopic birefringence of joint aspirated sodium urate crystals are diagnostic.

William Heberden (Snr), 1710–1801, a physician who practised first in Cambridge and from 1748 in London, UK, described these nodes in 1802.
Charles Jacques Bouchard, 1837–1915, physician, Dean of the Faculty of Medicine, Paris, France.

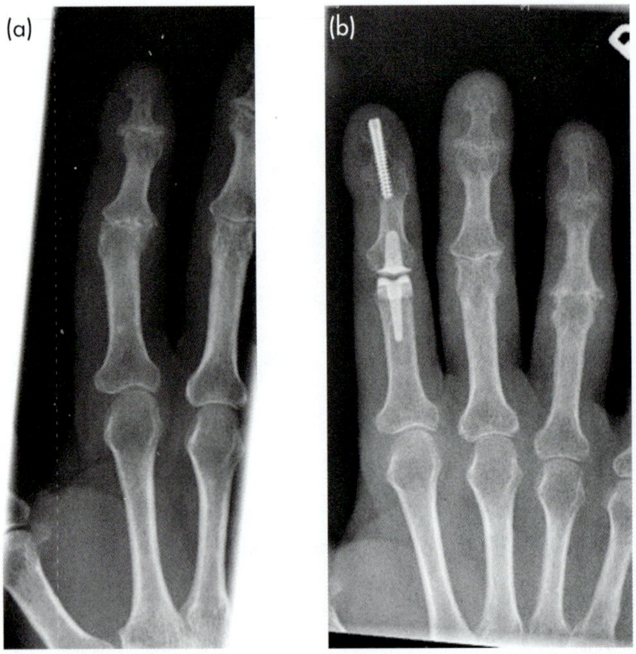

Figure 36.52 X-rays of the distal interphalangeal and proximal interphalangeal joints treated with arthrodesis (a) and joint replacement (b).

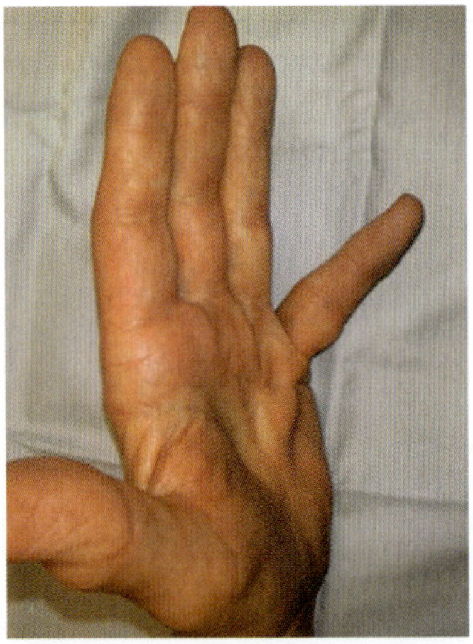

Figure 36.53 Dupuytren's contracture.

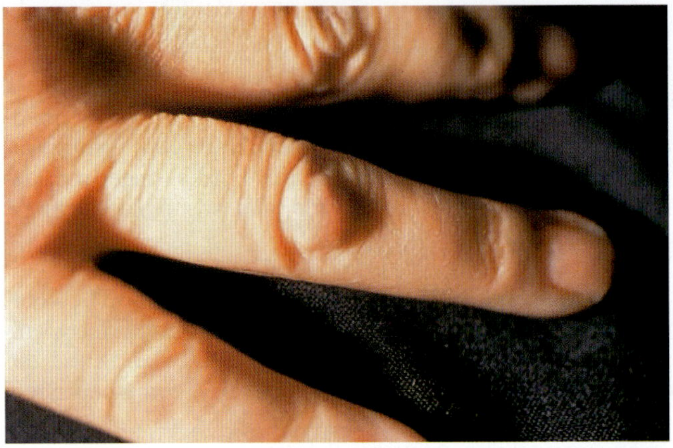

Figure 36.54 Garrod's knuckle pads.

Dupuytren's contracture

Dupuytren's contracture is an autosomal dominant condition, common in northern Europe, predominantly in men in the fifth to seventh decades of life. It is associated with smoking, trauma, epilepsy, AIDS, hypothyroidism and alcoholic cirrhosis. It also appears very frequently as a clinical case in British surgical exams! The characteristic features are palmar nodules, skin puckering, cords of the palm and digits, and flexion contractures of the digits (Figure 36.53). It is most common on the ulna side of the hand. Garrod's knuckle pads (thickened skin on dorsum of proximal interphalangeal joint) are another feature visible on examination (Figure 36.54). It can also produce cords in the penis which cause it to become curved (Peyronie's disease) and may also produce plantar thickening (Ledderhose's disease). Surgery is indicated when the patient cannot put their hand flat on the table due to deformity or when flexion contracture develops in the PIP joint. Great care should be taken during surgery to avoid damage to the digital nerves which may be trapped in the fibrous tissue. At the end of surgery, it may not be possible to obtain closure of the skin, and so healing may have to be by secondary intention.

In the late stage of the disease, a fixed contracture of the metacarpal phalangeal and proximal phalangeal joints may develop. In these cases, excision of the fibrous bands will produce no improvement in the condition, and if the contracted finger is preventing useful function of the hand, then an amputation may have to be considered (Summary box 36.14).

Summary box 36.14

Dupuytren's contracture

- Autosomal dominant inheritance (trait)
- Fibroblastic hyperplasia with resultant skin nodules, cords and deformities
- Surgical management is indicated if hand cannot be placed flat
- Fixed flexion deformities mean that amputation is the only surgical option

Tendon disorders

Trigger digit

Triggering occurs in the fingers or in the thumb as a result of a size mismatch between the flexor tendon and sheath (usually at A1 pulley) in which it runs.

The patient complains of painful locking of the finger either in extension or in flexion or both. There is a palpable nodule in the tendon. Management is a steroid injection into the sheath, and if this fails then surgical tendon sheath (A1 pulley) release should be performed, taking care not to cut too much of the pulley and create bowstringing of the flexor tendon. Trigger digits can occur in infants and usually resolve spontaneously.

De Quervain's disease

De Quervain's disease is caused by tenosynovitis of the abductor pollicis longus and extensor pollicis brevis in the first dorsal

Baron Guillaume Dupuytren, 1777–1835, surgeon, Hôtel Dieu, Paris, France, described this condition in 1831.
Sir Archibald Edward Garrod, 1857–1936, Regius Professor of Medicine, the University of Oxford, Oxford, UK described this condition in 1893.
Francois de la Peyronie, 1678–1747, surgeon to King Louis XIV of France and founder of the Royal Academy of Surgery, Paris, France.
Georg Ledderhose, 1855–1925, a German surgeon, described this disease in 1894.

wrist compartment. It is predominantly seen in middle-aged females, and is associated with pregnancy (new mother's wrist), and inflammatory arthritis. The clinical features are radial wrist pain, tenderness, swelling (Figure 36.55) and a positive Finkelstein's test (pain with wrist and thumb in ulnar deviation while the thumb is fully flexed). The management options are non-steroidal anti-inflammatories, splintage, steroid injection and surgical release of the extensor retinaculum of the first dorsal compartment.

Compressive neuropathies

Median nerve (carpal tunnel syndrome)

The majority of cases of carpal tunnel syndrome are idiopathic. It is associated with diabetes, thyroid disorders, aloholism, amyloidosis, inflammatory arthritis, pregnancy and obesity.

History

The patient presents with tingling and infrequently numbness in the radial three and a half fingers. Patients also complain of being woken at night with pain and that hanging their hand out of the bed provides relief. They may also complain of clumsiness when picking up small objects or carrying heavy ones.

On examination

Wasting of the thenar eminence is visible (Figure 36.56) and there is sometimes weakness of the abductor pollicis brevis. This is frequently bilateral. The tests for carpal tunnel compression are described in Chapter 33 but the most reliable are: (1) Tinel's – percussion over the carpal tunnel and (2) Phalen's test – reproduction of paraesthesia with full wrist flexion. Electrophysiological studies can confirm diagnosis with evidence of slowing of nerve conduction through the carpal tunnel. Non-operative treatment includes night splintage of the wrist in extension, and steroid injections. If surgery is required the median nerve is surgically decompressed by incising the roof of the tunnel (transverse carpal ligament) either open or through a small arthroscope (Summary box 36.15).

Summary box 36.15

Carpal tunnel syndrome

- Night pain is common and relieved by shaking the hand
- Thenar wasting is an advanced sign
- Tinel's and Phalen's tests are useful
- Treatment includes splints and surgical decompression

Ulnar nerve (Guyon's tunnel syndrome)

Ulnar nerve compression in Guyon's canal can lead to tingling and numbness in the ring and little fingers with hypothenar wasting. There is preservation of the dorsal sensations over the little and ring finger. Compression is due to a ganglion, ulnar artery aneurysm or a fracture of the hook of hamate.

Avascular necrosis of carpal bones

Idiopathic avascular necrosis of the lunate (Keinböck's disease) or scaphoid (Preiser's disease) can occur (Figure 36.57). The clinical presentation is of wrist pain and the diagnosis can be confirmed with x-rays and MRI. The natural history of the condition leads to collapse of the carpal bones and subsequent

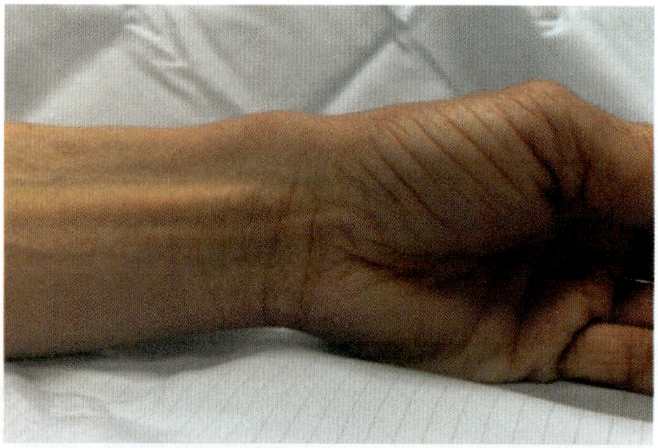

Figure 36.55 De Quervain's disease.

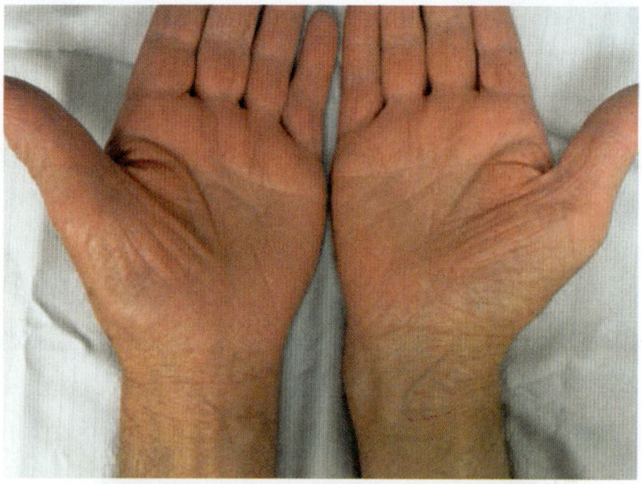

Figure 36.56 Thenar muscle wasting in carpal tunnel syndrome.

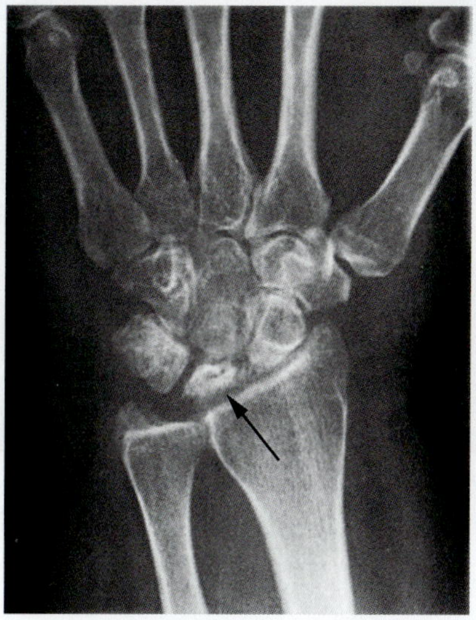

Figure 36.57 Avascular necrosis of the lunate (Keinbock's).

George S Phalen, contemporary, orthopaedic surgeon and Chief of Hand Surgery, The Cleveland Clinic, Cleveland, OH, USA. He helped to establish the American Society for Surgery of the Hand.

Fritz de Quervain, 1868–1940, Professor of Surgery, Berne, Switzerland, described this form of tenosynovitis in 1895.
Jean Casimir Felix Guyon, 1831–1920, Professor of Genito-urinary Surgery, Paris, France.
Robert Keinböck, 1871–1953, Professor of Radiology, Vienna, Austria, described this condition in 1910.

arthritis of the carpus which may be best treated with a fusion of the wrist. This will at least give a strong and painless wrist. The limitation in movement produces a disability which is not as great as might be expected.

Ganglion cysts

Ganglion cysts are the most common cause of a swelling in the hand and are found most often on the dorsum (Figure 36.58), the volar (Figure 36.59) side of the wrist, over the dorsum of the DIP joint (myxoid cyst) or within the flexor tendon sheath at the base of the finger (seed ganglion). The dorsal and volar wrist ganglions can cause discomfort. The swellings are smooth, fluctuant and transilluminable. Mucus cysts can frequently discharge and cause nail changes (Figure 36.60). Seed ganglions can be painful when gripping. Aspiration or surgical excision can be considered. Patients should be informed regarding possible recurrence.

Congenital malformations

There are many congenital malformations of the upper limb and these are discussed in Chapter 41.

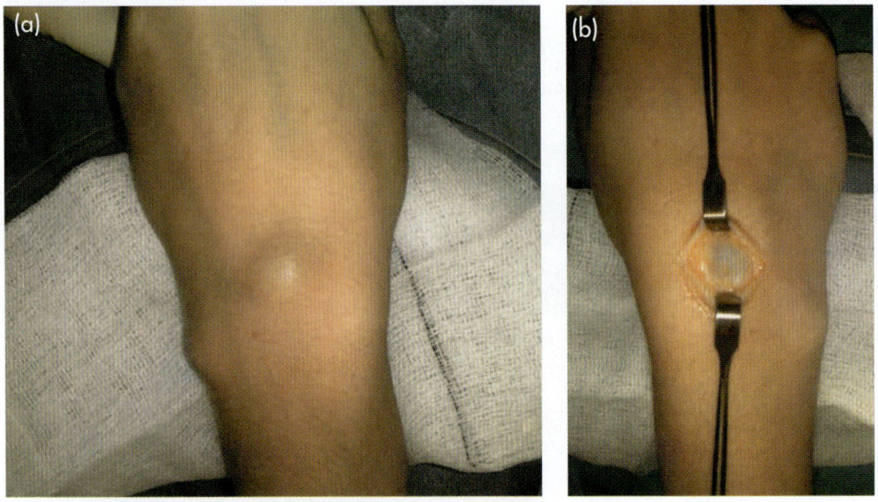

Figure 36.58 (a) Clinical and (b) surgical appearance of dorsal wrist ganglion.

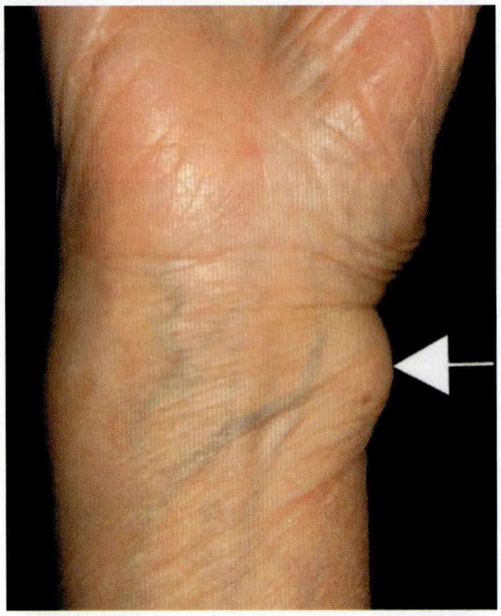

Figure 36.59 Volar wrist ganglion.

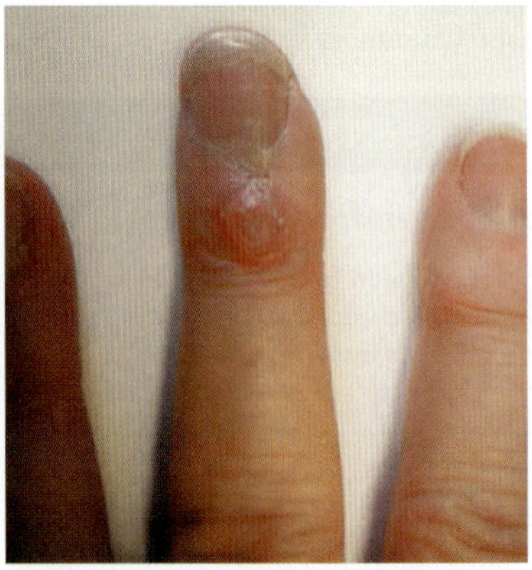

Figure 36.60 Myxoid cyst with changes in the nail.

CHAPTER

37 Hip and knee

LEARNING OBJECTIVES

To understand:

- The anatomy and biomechanics of the hip and knee and its clinical implications
- The clinical presentation, aetiology and management of common hip and knee pathologies
- The principles of joint replacement including guidelines about deep vein thrombosis prevention
- The advances in surgical practice in this field

THE HIP JOINT

Applied anatomy

The hip is a ball and socket joint formed by the head of the femur and the cup-shaped acetabulum (Latin – little vinegar cup) (Figure 37.1). The joint allows a considerable range of movement in different planes but is still inherently stable because of both its bony anatomy and the static (ligaments) and dynamic (muscle) stabilisers. The static stabilisers are composed of the ligaments (iliofemoral and pubofemoral ligaments anteriorly and the ischiofemoral ligament posteriorly), the joint capsule and the labrum, whereas the muscles running across the joint (short external rotator muscles posteriorly, the iliopsoas anteriorly and the hip abductors laterally) constitute the dynamic stabilisers. The acetabular labrum is a fibrocartilagenous structure which is triangular in cross section and attached to the rim of the acetabulum except at its base where it is replaced by the transverse ligament. It helps in deepening the socket thereby enhancing stability. It also acts as a fluid seal and thereby helps improve joint lubrication. The femoral head derives its blood supply mainly from the retinacular branches of the medial circumflex femoral artery and there is a small contribution from the artery of the ligamentum teres (Summary box 37.1).

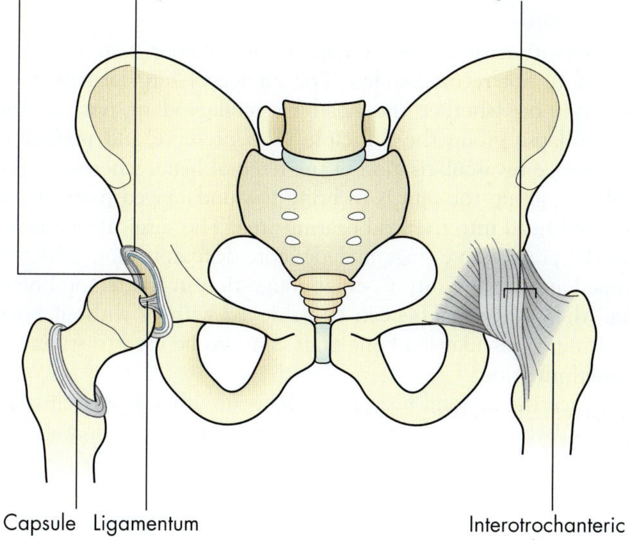

Figure 37.1 Anatomy of the hip joint.

Summary box 37.1

Anatomy

- The hip joint is a ball and socket joint, which is stabilised by static and dynamic stabilisers
- Static stabilisers include the capsule, ligaments and labrum
- Dynamic stabilisers consist of the muscles acting across the joint
- Blood supply to the femoral head is mainly derived from the medial circumflex femoral artery

Biomechanics of the hip joint

Kinetic analysis reveals that forces as high as eight times body weight can be exerted across the hip joint during activities of daily living and this is primarily the result of contraction of muscles crossing the joint. The abductors, because of their insertion on the greater trochanter, help in supporting the pelvis when the patient stands on one leg and thereby form the basis of a Trendelenburg test (Figure 37.2) (Summary box 37.2).

Friedrich Trendelenburg, 1844–1924, Professor of Surgery successively at Rostock (1875–1882), Bonn (1882–1895), Leipzig (1895–1911), Germany. The Trendelenburg position was first described in 1885.

Summary box 37.2

Forces going through the hip joint

- Lifting leg from bed – one and a half times body weight
- Standing on one leg – three times body weight
- Running and jumping – ten times body weight

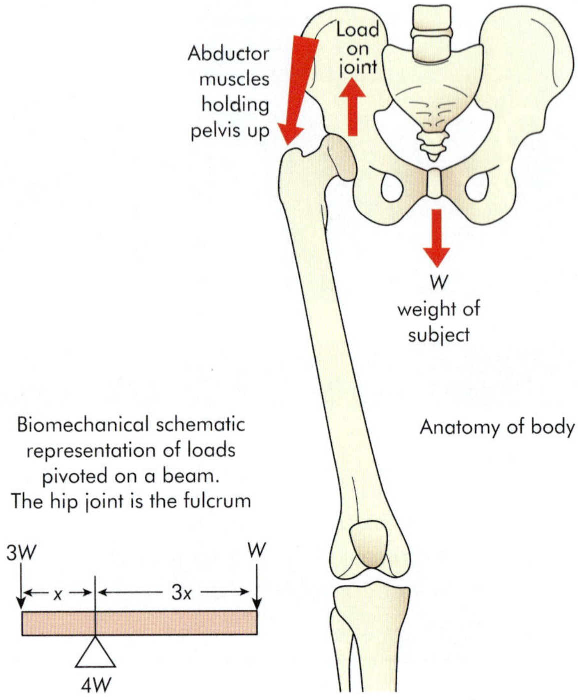

Figure 37.2 Load on the hip joint when subject (weighing W) stands on one leg. Hopping increases the load from 4 to 10 W.

Conditions affecting the hip joint

Common hip pathologies in the paediatric age group and secondary to trauma are covered in Chapters 41 and 29, respectively. This chapter focuses on the acquired pathological conditions in the adult.

Avascular necrosis

Avascular necrosis (AVN) or osteonecrosis of the femoral head occurs because of an interruption in the blood supply to the femoral head, which causes bone death. This leads to collapse of the femoral head causing secondary osteoarthritis subsequently. AVN can be primary (idiopathic) or secondary to other pathology (Table 37.1).

Table 37.1 Aetiology of avascular necrosis of the femoral head.

Sickle cell disease
Haemoglobinopathies
Caisson disease ('the bends' in divers)
Hyperlipidaemia
Systemic lupus erythematosus
Gaucher's disease
Chronic liver disease
Antiphospholipid antibody syndrome
Radiotherapy
Chemotherapy
Human immunodeficiency virus
Hypercoagulable states (protein C and protein S deficiency)
Steroids
Alcohol excess
Idiopathic (see Perthes' disease, Chapter 41)

Clinical features

Avascular necrosis usually affects men aged from 35 to 45 years and is bilateral in over 50 per cent of patients. The patient is frequently asymptomatic in the early stages. As the disease progresses the patient may complain of an ache in the groin, walk with a limp and clinical examination may reveal limitation of movement.

Investigations

A weight-bearing anteroposterior (AP) radiograph of the pelvis along with a lateral radiograph will show the classical features of AVN including increased sclerosis in the early stages, the crescent sign indicating subchondral bone resorption. In the late stages there may be flattening indicating a segmental head collapse (Figure 37.3). However, radiographs may be normal in the early stages of the disease and, therefore, the most sensitive and specific way of investigating these patients is with magnetic resonance imaging (MRI). MRI allows accurate assessment of the extent of involvement and can also identify associated bone marrow changes. This helps in early diagnosis and prediction of prognosis (Figure 37.4). In 1985, Ficat classified the disease into five stages. In 1995, Steinberg modified this classification into seven stages based upon the type of radiological change on MRI and radiography (Table 37.2). Stages I–IV are further divided into A, B or C depending upon the extent of involvement of the femoral head.

Treatment

Conservative treatment usually leads to poor results and is therefore not recommended. The choice of surgical treatment depends on whether the head has collapsed or not. In the pre-collapse group the principle is to preserve and preferably encourage revascularisation of the femoral head, whereas in the collapse group the aim is to bring the undamaged parts of the femoral head into the load bearing area. The surgical treatment for the pre-collapse stage includes core decompression, which is aimed at relieving intravascular congestion in the femoral head and thereby pain. This can be achieved with or without bone grafting; a vascularised bone graft can also be used to stimulate bone formation.

Once the femoral head has collapsed, either a femoral osteotomy (which aims to transfer the weight-bearing area of the

A **caisson** is a watertight chamber used to protect construction workers during the building of underwater structures. Caisson disease (also called decompression sickness or bends) occurs in construction workers when they leave the compressed atmosphere in the caisson and are rapidly brought up to enter normal atmospheric conditions.

Philippe Charles Ernest Gaucher, 1854–1918, Physician, Hôpital St Louis, Paris, France, described familial splenic anaemia in 1882.

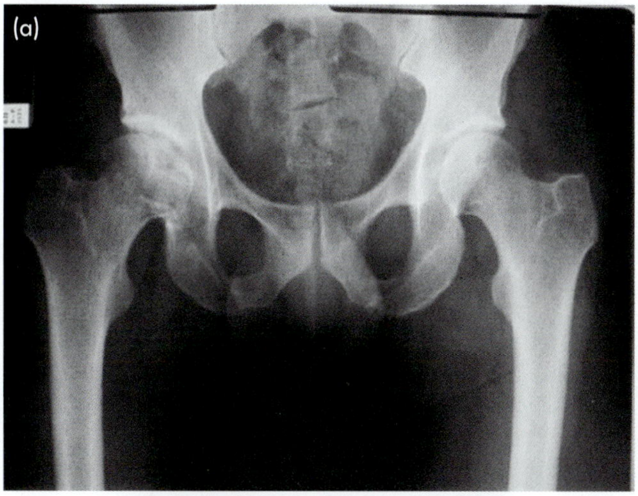

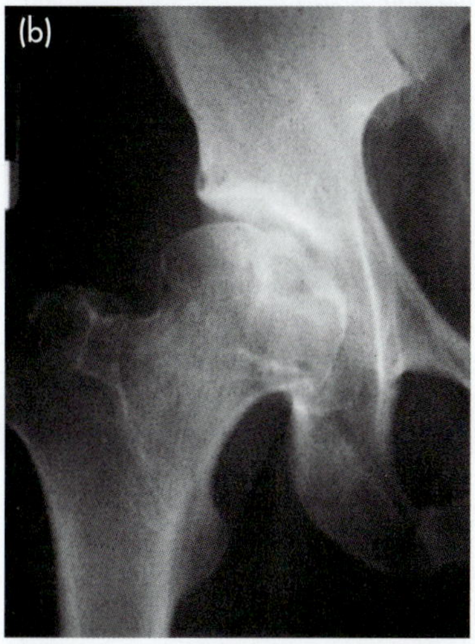

Figure 37.3 (a and b) Radiological appearance of avascular necrosis of the femoral head.

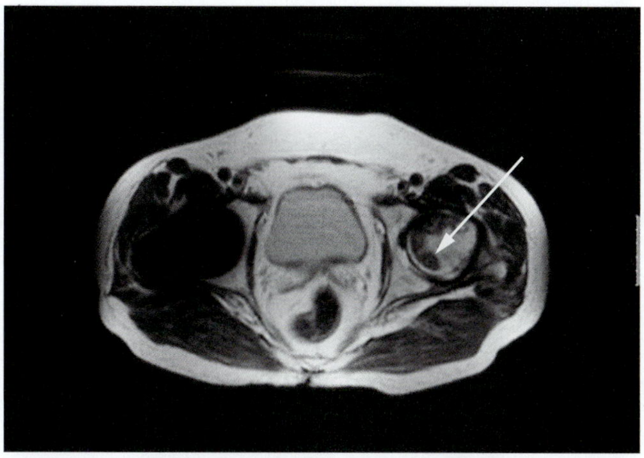

Figure 37.4 Magnetic resonance imaging scan of the hip joint showing avascular necrosis and the extent of involvement of the femoral head.

Summary box 37.3

Avascular necrosis of the femoral head

- Patients can be asymptomatic in the early stages and therefore a high index of suspicion is necessary for initial diagnosis
- Magnetic resonance scans are needed for early diagnosis
- Treatment is based upon whether the patient presents before or after the femoral head has collapsed
- In the pre-collapse stage treatement focuses on revascularisation
- In the collapsed stage the aim is to replace the damaged joint surface
- Prognosis is dependent upon the extent of head involvement

femoral head and thereby protect the collapsed segment), or a joint replacement (if degenerative changes have set in) is the preferred option. The choice is resurfacing arthroplasty (Figure 37.5) or a total joint replacement (Figure 37.6) (Summary box 37.3).

Table 37.2 Steinberg's classification of avascular necrosis of the femoral head.

Stage	Description
0	Normal or non-diagnostic radiograph, bone scan or MRI
I	Normal radiograph, abnormal MRI or bone scan
II	Sclerosis and cysts
III	Subchondral collapse, crescent sign
IV	Flattening of the head, normal acetabulum
V	Acetabular involvement
VI	Obliteration of joint space

MRI, magnetic resonance imaging.

Osteoarthritis

Introduction and aetiology

Osteoarthritis (OA) is termed as primary when no predisposing cause can be found and traumatic is when it develops after an insult to the hip joint. A multitude of factors including genetic, biochemical and mechanical influences have been implicated in the development of primary OA. The exact mechanism for the development of primary OA remains unknown and it is therefore termed idiopathic. Recently, femoroacetabular impingement (FAI) has been proposed as an aetiological factor responsible for the development of primary OA. The causes of OA of the hip are given in Table 37.3.

Clinical features

Osteoarthritis of the hip affects 10–25 per cent of those over the age of 65 years. The most consistent symptoms are groin pain and limitation of movement. The pain may also radiate down to the knee joint, and in some cases the only presenting feature may be a painful knee. In the early stages of the disease, pain is activity-related but as the disease progresses the patient also complains of pain at rest. The patient frequently complains of

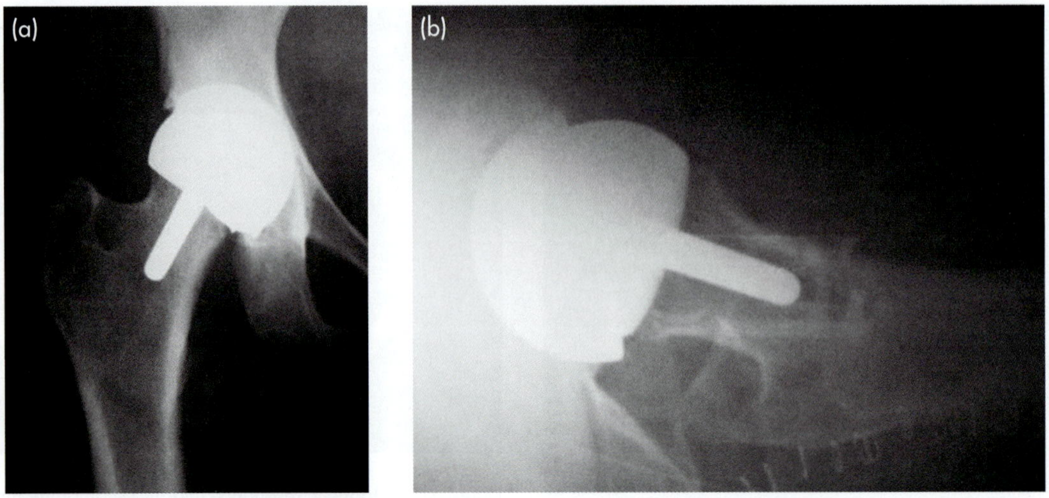

Figure 37.5 Anteroposterior (a) and lateral (b) radiographs of the hip showing a resurfacing arthroplasty.

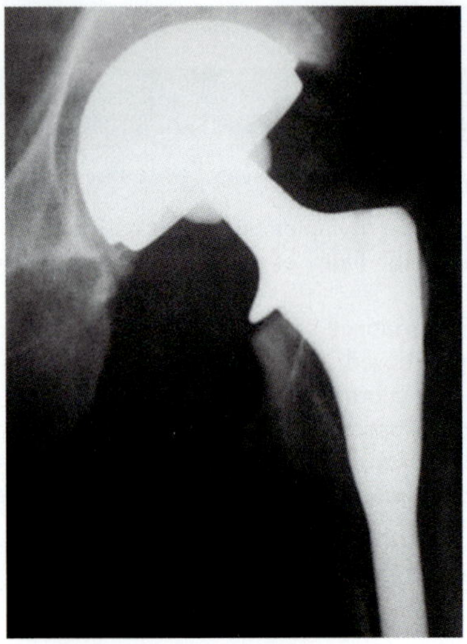

Figure 37.6 Radiograph showing an uncemented total hip replacement *in situ*.

Table 37.3 Aetiology of osteoarthritis.

Primary
Cause unknown, termed idiopathic
Femoroacetabular impingement implicated as a possible cause
Secondary
Trauma
Avascular necrosis
Inflammatory arthropathy (e.g. rheumatoid arthritis)
Perthes' disease
Developmental dysplasia of the hip
Slipped capital femoral epiphysis
Septic arthritis

night pain and may also find it difficult to get into a comfortable position while sleeping. Functionally, most have difficulty in putting on their shoes/socks and getting into and out of a bath or a car. As the pain increases, the joint gradually loses its movement because of muscle spasm, capsular contracture and osteophyte formation.

Clinical examination may reveal gluteal muscle wasting. There may also be a limp with a positive Trendelenburg sign. Leg length discrepancy (usually shortening) and limitation of movement, particularly internal rotation, are consistent features. Many patients present with a fixed flexion deformity. This is best elicited by a modified Thomas' test (see Chapter 33).

Investigations

The characteristic features on x-ray are: (1) a reduction of joint space, (2) sclerosis in the periarticular bone, (3) subchondral cysts and (4) osteophyte formation (Figure 37.7). Eventually, a collapsed femoral head may also be evident.

Treatment

There is no specific pharmacological therapy for osteoarthritis; however, conservative treatment with non-steroidal anti-inflammatories, regular exercise, physiotherapy and modification of lifestyle with loss of weight does help. Patients should also be encouraged to use walking aids (usually a walking stick in the opposite hand to offload the affected joint).

The indications for surgery are relentless pain, limitation of lifestyle and activities of daily living, and failure of conservative treatment. The surgical options include an arthrodesis (fusion), an osteotomy (realignment) or a joint replacement.

More and more joint replacements are now being performed. The indications are based on limitation of lifestyle and individual needs, thereby making it a truly life-improving operation (Summary box 37.4).

Inflammatory arthritis

The hip joint can also be affected by inflammatory arthritides; however, these are not as common as OA. This group includes rheumatoid arthritis, ankylosing spondylitis, gout and chondrocalcinosis, juvenile rheumatoid arthritis and systemic lupus erythematosus.

Georg Clemens Perthes, 1869–1927, Professor of Surgery, Tubingen, Germany, described osteochondritis of the femoral capital epiphysis in 1910.

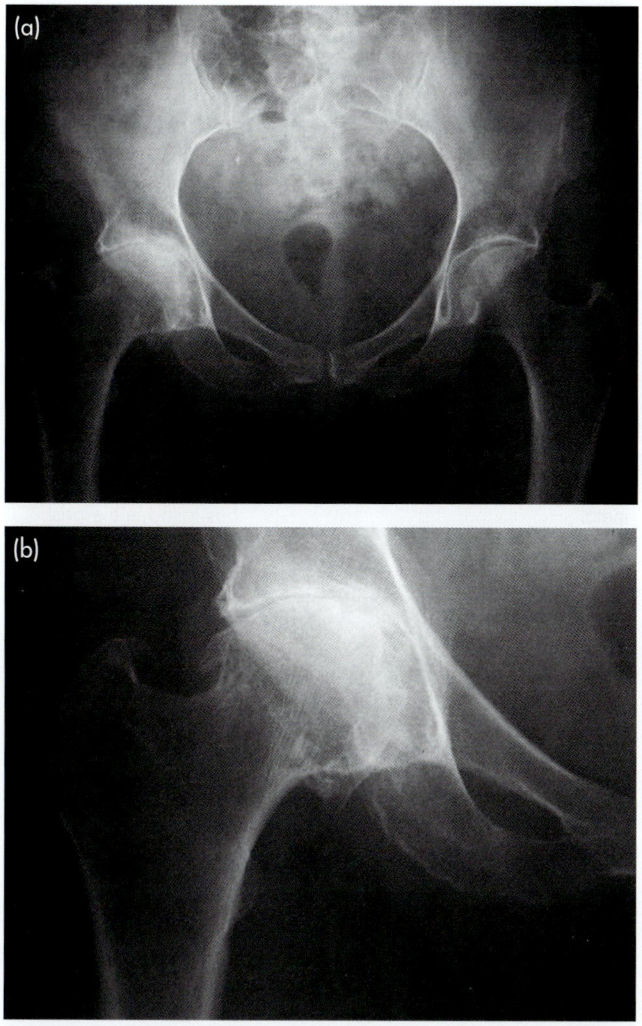

Figure 37.7 Anteroposterior (a) and enlarged anteroposterior (b) radiographs of the hip joint showing osteoarthritis.

Summary box 37.4

Osteoarthritis of the hip

- Osteoarthritis is a non-inflammatory condition leading to progressive damage of the articular cartilage
- The most consistent features are groin pain and limitation of movement
- Characteristic radiological findings include reduction of joint space, joint-line sclerosis, subchondral cysts and osteophyte formation
- Conservative treatment includes walking aids, non-steroidal analgesics and physiotherapy
- Surgical options include osteotomy, arthrodesis or a joint replacement

Surgical procedures

Osteotomies around the hip

The goal of an osteotomy around the hip is to redistribute forces evenly across the joint, thereby eliminating excessive point loading. This can be achieved by performing an osteotomy on the femoral or the acetabular side, depending upon the desired goal, e.g. an excessive valgus neck–shaft angle and an uncovered femoral head on the lateral aspect can be corrected by carrying out a varus femoral osteotomy. Similarly, a redirection osteotomy on the acetabular side can also be performed to improve coverage of the femoral head. The common indications for an osteotomy around the hip include:

- developmental dysplasia of the hip;
- Perthes' disease;
- OA in a young patient;
- slipped upper femoral epiphysis;
- AVN.

Ideally, an osteotomy should be considered in a young patient who maintains a good range of movement of the hip and radiographs show a reasonable amount of joint space. Thorough preoperative planning is essential to assess whether the desired position can be achieved postoperatively. Three-dimensional computed tomography (CT) scans may be helpful for appropriate preoperative planning.

Arthrodesis of the hip

Arthrodesis or fusion of the hip is an uncommon operation. It is generally reserved for young patients with severe osteoarthritis who have heavy manual jobs and in whom joint replacements would fail fairly quickly. The aim is to achieve a painless joint by fusing it in a functional position, which is about 30° of flexion, 15° of external rotation and 5° of abduction. This can be achieved by an intra-articular dynamic hip screw or by an extra-articular plate with screws.

Several problems can occur following an arthrodesis, including altered gait and excessive loading of the ipsilateral knee, the contralateral hip and the spine. Degenerative change in these joints in the long term is the rule rather than the exception.

Joint replacement

Over 70 000 total hip replacements are performed annually in the UK. The results of surgery are encouraging. In good hands, up to 95 per cent of patients will have a well-functioning hip replacement at ten years after surgery. In the best series, 85 per cent will still be functioning at 20 years, although many are still in place only because the patients are too old and infirm for them to be revised. Following surgery, pain is reduced, mobility increases and sleep as well as social and sexual function is improved. Nevertheless, with the ever increasing number of patients with joint replacements, the number of patients whose replacement has failed or worn out and who now want a revision, or even a re-revision, is rising rapidly.

Principles and design of hip replacements

Any joint replacement should be biocompatible and made of inert materials. It should be well fixed to the host tissue and the design should incorporate features to allow a good range of movement and stability. The bearing surfaces should produce minimal friction (to prevent early loosening), and the material released from the bearing surface should be non-toxic. It should remove the minimum amount of the patient's bone, so that revision is possible, and it should create a biomechanically stable joint. Finally, any joint implanted should ideally outlive the patient and be cost effective (Summary box 37.5).

Summary box 37.5

Features of an ideal joint replacement

- Biocompatible
- Well fixed to the host tissue, stable and allowing a good range of movement
- Bearing surfaces should be designed to minimise friction
- Material released from the bearings should be non-toxic
- Remove the minimum amount of bone
- Produce mechanical stability
- Should ideally outlive the patient

Materials for the femoral component

Most of the implants available currently are made of cobalt–chrome alloy or stainless steel or titanium. Metal implants are able to withstand high loads, are relatively inert and can be manufactured easily. However, they do pose problems in terms of ion release if they are used as bearing surfaces. Also, corrosion can be a cause for concern if two dissimilar metals are used.

Bearing surfaces (the acetabular cup)

The total hip replacement (THR) designed by Charnley uses a joint surface of metal on high-density polyethylene. This is described as a hard-on-soft bearing surface and has a low coefficient of friction. High-density polyethylene has good shock-absorbing properties but does wear slowly over the years, producing small particles that can stimulate an inflammatory response in the joint, which then leads to aseptic loosening of the joint. The activated macrophages resorb bone and may also stimulate osteoclasts to do the same. There has, therefore, been a move towards using bearing surfaces with a lower wear rate, such as metal on metal or ceramic on ceramic. Although the wear rate of these newer bearing surfaces is less than conventional metal-on-polyethylene articulations, the wear particles are smaller (nano rather than micro) and there is increasing evidence that these implants are less forgiving than conventional metal on polyethylene THRs when surgical technique is suboptimal. Ceramic femoral heads bearing on polyethylene cups have far lower friction, but ceramic femoral heads on ceramic acetabular cups have the lowest friction of all. However, they are expensive to manufacture and produce small-sized wear particles. A summary of the advantages and disadvantages of each bearing surface is provided in Table 37.4.

Fixation of implants

Artificial joints must bed securely into the bones each side of the joint so that the implant does not work loose. This can be achieved with the help of cement or biological interdigitation between the prosthesis and bone (Table 37.5).

Sir John Charnley, 1911–1982, Professor of Orthopaedic Surgery, University of Manchester, Manchester, UK. He pioneered the hip replacement operation. The first hip replacements he made were from a hard plastic (Bakelite). They all broke within a year but the patients were so happy during that year that he was encouraged to persevere with new designs including high density polyethylene. In 1962 he moved his practice to Wrightington Hospital, Appley Bridge, which became a place of pilgrimage for young orthopaedic surgeons from all over the world wishing to specialise in hip replacement. In the same hospital, The John Charnley Research Institute was opened by his wife in 1992. In September 2010, the Royal Mail issued a series of stamps commemorating medical breakthroughs. The 60 pence stamp featured John Charnley's hip replacement operation as an x-ray.

Table 37.4 Bearing surfaces.

Type of bearing	Advantages	Disadvantages
Metal on polyethylene	Proven efficacy; easy to manufacture; cheap	High friction; high wear rates; wear particles excite an inflammatory response, which leads to osteolysis
Ceramic on polyethylene	Lower friction	Expensive; ceramic fracture can be a problem
Ceramic on ceramic	Low friction	Very expensive; ceramic can fracture, squeaking
Metal on metal	Lowest friction	Bad reputation as has failed in the past; metal ion release is a problem; expensive

Table 37.5 Fixation of implants.

Method of fixation	Advantages	Disadvantages
Cemented	Implant does not need to fit cavity exactly; well-proven results	Cement gets hot; fragments may cause third-body wear and stimulate aseptic loosening; difficult to remove at revision; non-biological and static fixation
Uncemented	No cement needed; fixation more secure; dynamic and biological fixation	Fit must be perfect; osseous integration does not always work; expensive

Traditionally, hip replacements were fixed into a bed of polymethyl methacrylate (PMMA) cement (Figure 37.8a). The cement acts as a grout (spacer) and not as a glue between the implant and the bone. In the majority of cases, it gives an excellent outcome. As the cement sets during surgery, some of the monomer is released into the patient's bloodstream. This can cause a drop in blood pressure.

On the other hand, biological fixation can be achieved by providing a rough surface on the prosthesis or by coating the surface of the prosthesis with hydroxyapatite, an osteoconductive agent, to encourage bone to bond to the prosthesis (Figure 37.8b). These cementless devices are increasingly used although they can be associated with higher implant costs, increased risk of intraoperative fracture and difficulty in removing them if revision surgery is needed.

Surgical approaches to the hip, postoperative course and complications

The operation can be performed via a posterior approach, an anterolateral or Hardinge approach, a trochanteric osteotomy or an anterior approach (Table 37.6). Each approach has its own advantages and disadvantages. There is also a move towards minimally invasive surgery and shortening the size of the incision. The proponents of this concept have described a two-incision approach wherein the femoral component is inserted via a small incision around the greater trochanter and the acetabular component via an incision in the groin. Although the concept is attractive, no long-term benefits have been conclusively shown in hip surgery over the conventional technique. Eventually, whichever approach is taken, it is essential to be able to implant a prosthesis that has the correct offset, a correct centre of rotation, the correct component orientation and which equalises leg lengths and carries a minimal risk.

Table 37.6 Surgical approaches to the hip.

Surgical approach	Anatomical interval and muscle
Posterior	Along the fibres of the gluteus maximus
Anterolateral/ Hardinge	Parts of the gluteus medius and minimus are reflected off the greater trochanter
Anterior	Interval is developed between the sartorius and rectus femoris and the tensor fascia lata
Trochanteric	A trochanteric osteotomy is required

The postoperative course involves a 3–7-day stay in hospital where the physiotherapist encourages the patient to mobilise safely and independently, avoiding any movements which might lead to a dislocation (Figure 37.9). Before discharge, the occupational therapist assesses the patient's home circumstances and arranges for any modifications that may be required to assist the patient, e.g. a raised toilet seat. Follow-up visits are arranged at 6 weeks and at one year post-surgery. Although hip replacement is a fairly successful and safe procedure, it does have associated complications. A comprehensive list of complications is given in Table 37.7.

Table 37.7 Complications of total hip replacement.

Intraoperative complications
Nerve injury – sciatic, femoral and obturator
Vascular injury – femoral vein and artery
Femoral fracture
Fragments of cement left in joint
Postoperative complications
Deep vein thrombosis and pulmonary embolism
Infection
Dislocation (Figure 37.9)
Leg length inequality
Heterotopic ossification
Implant loosening

Deep vein thrombosis (DVT) is relatively common if no precautions are taken to reduce this risk. Use of regional anaesthesia and early postoperative mobilisation are invaluable in reducing this risk. In addition, either mechanical devices (thromboembolic deterrent (TED) stockings or foot pumps) or medication (low molecular weight heparin or warfarin or oral anticoagulants) are commonly prescribed for a period of 4–6 weeks after surgery to reduce the risk of DVT.

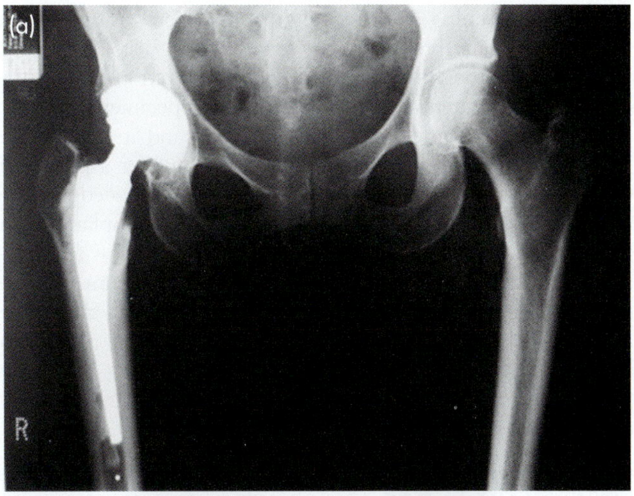

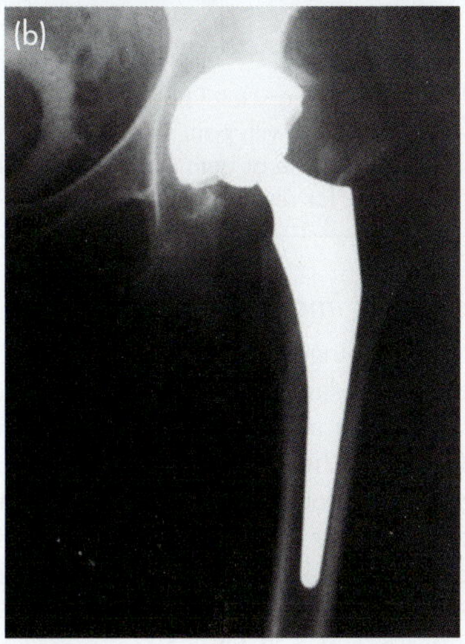

Figure 37.8 Radiographs of a cemented (a) and non-cemented (b) femoral component.

Revision total hip replacement

Revision of a total hip replacement is required if the patient is symptomatic secondary to failure of the implant by loosening (Figure 37.10), recurrent dislocations or a periprosthetic fracture. Loosening of the implant can occur because of an infection or as a result of aseptic osteolysis caused by an inflammatory response secondary to particle wear.

In the initial stages of loosening the patient complains of pain, which is experienced mainly on weight-bearing. A history of infection in the immediate postoperative period may suggest infection as a cause of premature implant loosening. The infection is likely to be low-grade with *Staphylococcus epidermidis* multiplying slowly within a glycocalyx coating, so normal measures of infection such as a raised C-reactive protein may be equivocal.

If the loosening is secondary to infection, a two-staged revision is usually preferred. The first stage consists of implant removal, a thorough debridement and implantation of an antibiotic-loaded cement spacer. Multiple deep specimens are sent for bacteriology to determine the organism and its sensitivity. The patient is put onto appropriate antibiotics for a period of 6 weeks or more. At the second stage of the procedure, the cement spacer is removed and a new prosthesis implanted. In the case of aseptic loosening, revision is performed as a single-stage procedure. If there has been a significant amount of bone loss, bone grafting may be required and the patient should be advised of this preoperatively. The results following a revision hip replacement are not as good as those following a primary total hip replacement, and the rate of complications, especially dislocation, is also higher (Summary box 37.6).

Summary box 37.6

Revision total hip replacement

- Needed when the primary total hip replacement fails
- Patients usually present with pain on weight bearing
- Aseptic loosening of one or both components is the most frequent indication for revision

Femoroacetabular impingement

Femoroacetabular impingement has increasingly been recognised as a cause of secondary hip OA. The non-spherical portion of the femoral head is assumed to exert abnormal shear and compressive forces on the corresponding portion of the acetabular cartilage on vigorous hip flexion with internal rotation. Patients typically present with groin pain and MRI arthrogram typically reveals acetabular rim lesions and aberrant femoral head morphology.

Two distinct types of FAI have been described – cam and pincer, although many patients have a mixed picture with both morphologies occurring simultaneously. Pincer impingement is a result of anterior overcoverage or retroversion of the acetabulum while cam impingement is secondary to abnormal morphology of the femoral head/neck junction. Treatment options for FAI depend on patient symptoms and vary from conservative treatment to hip arthroscopy to address labral pathology and impingement to periacetabular osteotomy.

THE KNEE

Applied anatomy

The knee joint is a synovial hinge joint. It consists of two tibiofemoral joints (condyloid) and the patellofemoral joint (sellar or saddle shaped). Its shape makes the joint inherently unstable, but stability is achieved by a combination of static (ligaments) and dynamic stabilisers (muscles acting across the joint).

Interposed between the tibial and femoral condyles are the medial and lateral menisci. These fibrocartilaginous structures aid shock absorption, increase the area over which load is taken and have a role in AP stability (Figure 37.11). Medial meniscal tears are three times more common than those in the more mobile lateral meniscus. The outer third of the meniscus is vascular and so can be repaired allowing tears to heal.

The medial and lateral collateral ligaments are the primary restraints to valgus and varus stress, respectively. The medial collateral ligament is a broad, flat ligament and is composed of a superficial and a deep layer. The deep layer is attached to the medial meniscus. The lateral collateral ligament is a simple cord-like structure.

The cruciate ligaments are vital for AP stability. Each cruciate ligament comprises two bundles. The anterior cruciate ligament (ACL) is composed of an anteromedial bundle that is tight in flexion and a posterolateral bundle that is tight in extension. The posterior cruciate ligament (PCL) has an anterolateral bundle (tight in flexion) and a posteromedial portion (tight in extension). The ACL and PCL prevent anterior and posterior translation of the tibia on the femur, respectively.

The knee has bursae surrounding it which can become inflamed and infected (Summary box 37.7).

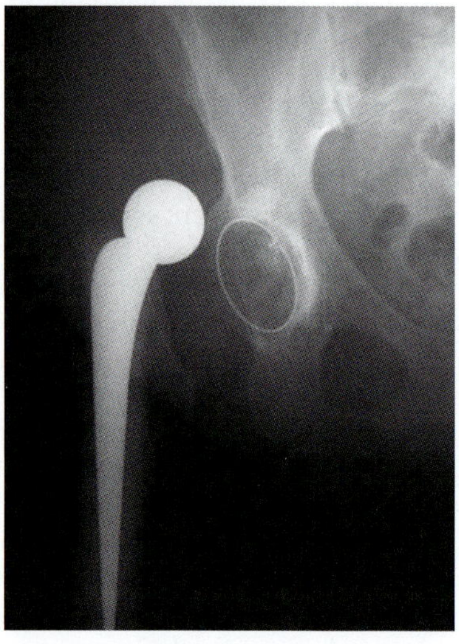

Figure 37.9 Dislocation of the hip.

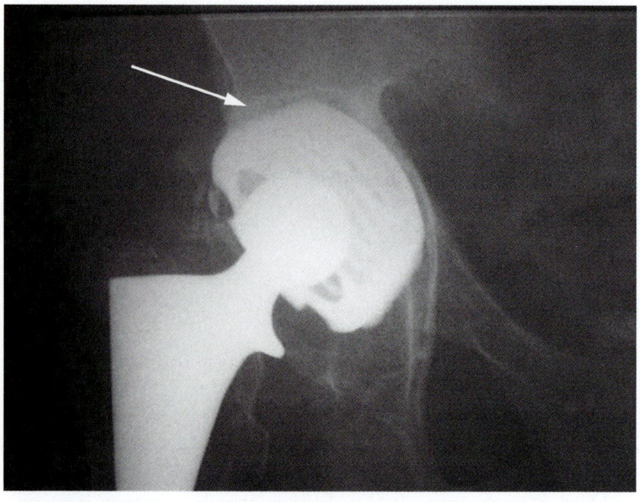

Figure 37.10 Acetabular loosening.

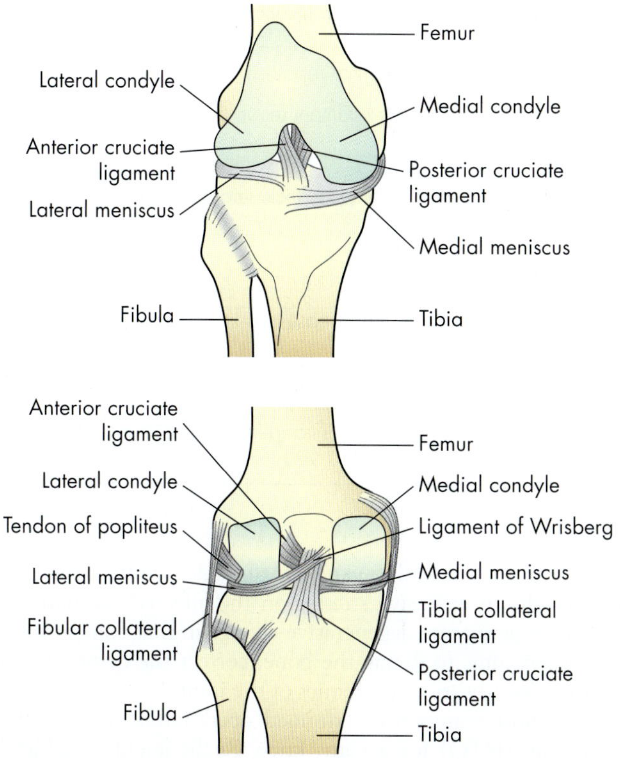

Figure 37.11 Anatomy of the knee joint.

> **Summary box 37.7**
>
> **Anatomy of the knee joint**
>
> - Complex synovial hinge joint
> - The shape of the joint surfaces makes it inherently unstable
> - The static stabilisers are the joint capsule, menisci, cruciate and collateral ligaments
> - The dynamic stabilisers are the quadriceps and hamstring muscles

Biomechanics

Axes of the lower limb

The mechanical axis of the lower limb runs from the centre of the femoral head, through the intercondylar notch of the knee to the centre of the ankle joint. The angle between the anatomical and mechanical axes of the femur is called the valgus angle (usually 5–7°) (Figure 37.12).

Kinematics and kinetics

Knee motion is predominately in the sagittal plane. A limited degree of rotation also occurs and increases as knee flexion increases. The normal range of motion is between 5° of hyperextension and 135° of flexion. MRI of cadaveric knees has revealed that during knee flexion, a combination of rolling and sliding of the femur on the tibia.

The biomechanical role of the patella is to function as a pulley for the quadriceps. It increases the power of the quadriceps by increasing the lever arm. It has the thickest articular cartilage in the body and is designed to withstand loads as high as 20 times body weight when jumping (Summary box 37.8).

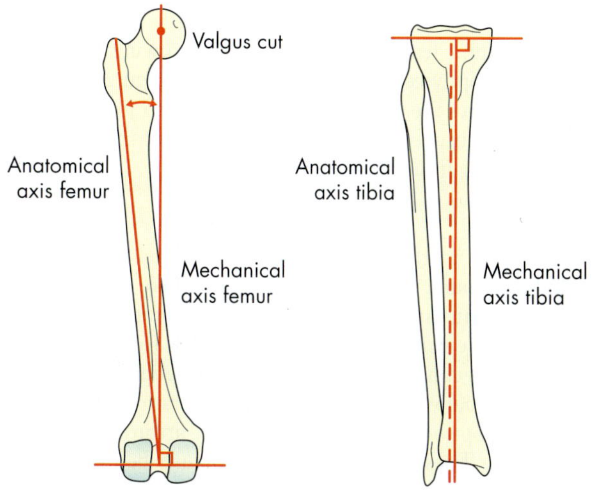

Figure 37.12 Axes of the lower limb. Anatomical and mechanical axes are coincident. Adapted from Miller, M. *Review of Orthopaedics*, 4th edn. 2004, Elsevier, Philadelphia. By kind permission of the publishers.

> **Summary box 37.8**
>
> **Biomechanics of the knee joint**
>
> - An artificial knee joint must have the joint surface parallel with the ground, and with the load transmitted equally between the condyles
> - Knee motion is mainly in the sagittal plane with minimal rotation
> - The patella acts as a pulley, increasing the lever arm of the quadriceps
> - Loads of up to 20 times body weight are transmitted across the patella when jumping

Conditions affecting the knee joint

Osteoarthritis

Osteoarthritis commonly affects the knee joint. Females are affected more often than their male counterparts and more than 3 per cent of women aged over 75 years are affected. OA can be either primary (idiopathic) or secondary.

Clinical features

Pain is the chief symptom, made worse with use. With patellofemoral involvement, pain is worse on stairs. As the disease progresses exercise tolerance diminishes, pain becomes constant (disturbing sleep) and patients will become increasingly reliant on walking aids, and may even become housebound in severe cases.

Clinical examination reveals a limp where they spend a short time on the painful limb and drop their centre of gravity (bob their head) as they try to minimise the weight that they are taking through this limb. In osteoarthritic patients the deformity is usually varus with bone loss on the medial side, while in rheumatoid patients valgus deformity is commonplace. An effusion is frequently present and movement is restricted, particularly extension. Crepitus can be both palpable and audible.

Investigations

The radiographic features are joint space narrowing, subchondral sclerosis, osteophytes and subchondral cysts (Figure 37.13).

Some centres are increasingly using MRI to judge both articular cartilage involvement and the integrity of the ACL with a view to guiding future surgical intervention.

Treatment

Non-operative methods are the first line of treatment. Patients should be encouraged to lose weight, undertake regular exercise to prevent joint stiffness and use anti-inflammatory medication. Walking aids (e.g. a stick) may be beneficial. Intra-articular steroid injections can provide long-term pain relief, but if repeated often may actually cause more rapid degeneration of the joint.

Surgical options include osteotomy, arthrodesis or knee replacement. These are all discussed in turn below (Summary box 37.9).

Summary box 37.9

Knee osteoarthritis

- More common in females
- Can be primary (idiopathic) or secondary (e.g. post-traumatic)
- Main symptom is pain made worse by use
- Examination reveals swelling, and reduced range of motion with or without deformity
- The four key radiographic features are: joint-space narrowing, subchondral sclerosis and cysts and osteophytes
- Treatment is non-operative initially. Knee replacement is reserved for end-stage disease

Surgical procedures in the knee

Knee arthroscopy

Knee arthroscopy can be used in the diagnosis and treatment of articular cartilage defects, meniscal and ligament injuries. Arthroscopic washout/debridement for end-stage OA is a controversial area with varying support among orthopaedic surgeons; however, half of patients report short-term symptomatic improvement.

There are a number of other indications for knee arthroscopy summarised in Table 37.8.

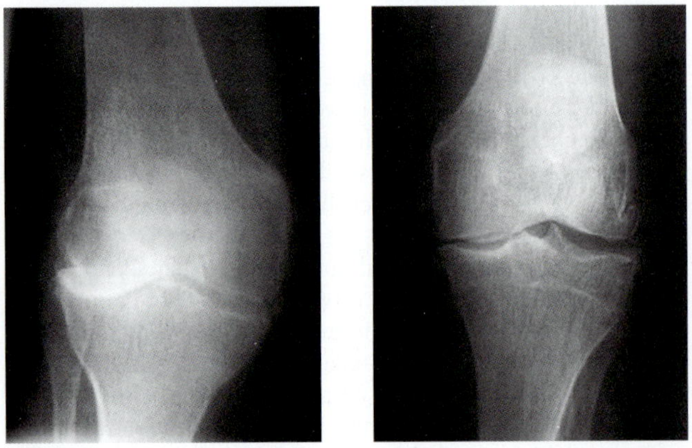

Figure 37.13 Osteoarthritis of the knee.

Table 37.8 Indications for knee arthroscopy.

Torn meniscus – for resection or repair
Anterior/posterior cruciate ligament reconstruction
Loose body removal
Cartilage regeneration techniques including microfracture
Septic arthritis – for washout
Inflammatory arthritis – synovectomy
Osteoarthritis – 'staging' the disease, resection of degenerate meniscus and washout
Diagnosis of unexplained knee pain
Tibial plateau fractures; allows intraoperative assessment of the articular surface

Osteotomy

Osteoarthritis can lead to varus or valgus deformity of the knee. This results in excessive stresses on the affected compartment leading to premature degenerative change in that compartment. Osteotomy aims to divide the bone, correct the deformity and alter the load-bearing mechanics of the joint.

The most commonly performed operation is a high tibial osteotomy (HTO) for a varus knee. Realignment is achieved with either an opening-wedge medial HTO or a closing-wedge lateral HTO. In valgus knees with relatively mild deformity (less than 12°) a varus-producing HTO on the medial side can be performed. A deformity of 12° or more requires distal femoral varus osteotomy.

The ideal patient for osteotomy is a young and active, well-motivated individual with disease limited to one compartment.

Knee arthrodesis

The most common indication for knee arthrodesis is a failed total knee replacement. Other indications include uncontrollable sepsis, neuropathic joint, post-traumatic arthritis in a young patient or disruption of the extensor mechanism. The ideal position of fusion is 7° of valgus and 15° of flexion. Arthrodesis is performed using either a custom-made intramedullary nail or an extramedullary technique such as an external fixator.

Knee replacement

There are three compartments within the knee: medial and lateral tibiofemoral and patellofemoral. Osteoarthritis may affect these individually or collectively. The medial compartment is most commonly affected producing a varus deformity. For single compartment disease a unicompartmental replacement may be used while in tricompartmental disease a total knee replacement (TKR) is indicated.

Knee replacement can be regarded as a resurfacing procedure in which the tibial and femoral articular surfaces are replaced with metal and the menisci by a tough polyethylene insert.

The main indication for knee replacement is pain, especially when combined with deformity and instability. Knee replacement should be reserved until a patient's quality of life is significantly impaired.

Unicompartmental knee replacement

The natural history of osteoarthritis reveals that in 92 per cent of cases the disease begins in the medial compartment alone. This was the basis for the development of the medial unicompartmental knee replacement (UKR) which is available in either fixed or mobile bearing forms (Figure 37.14). A number of series report ten-year survival figures of over 90 per cent for UKR.

Prerequisites to undertake medial UKR include intact ligaments (especially ACL), disease limited to one compartment and varus/flexion deformities not more than 15°. The operation is now performed using minimally invasive techniques through a quadriceps-sparing incision. Advantages over TKR include more rapid recovery, shorter hospital stay and preservation of knee kinematics. It is a bone preserving procedure which, if it fails, allows straightforward conversion to TKR.

Lateral UKR is performed for lateral compartment disease; numbers are far less than medial UKR partly owing to a reported dislocation rate of 10 per cent.

Patellofemoral replacement is also performed, but again numbers are low in view of the scarcity of patients with isolated patellofemoral disease, and the unproven nature of the procedure.

Total knee replacement

Natural knee motion is complex. It involves translation and rotation about each of the x, y and z axes (six degrees of freedom). It has proved very difficult to reproduce this natural motion in TKRs (Figure 37.15). In comparison to total hip replacement, patients with TKR find it hard to forget they have a knee replacement. Consequently, patient satisfaction is lower with TKR.

There are three types of TKR currently used: unconstrained, constrained-non-hinged and constrained-hinged. Almost all primary TKRs are unconstrained while the constrained types are used in revision total knee replacement when there may be significant bone loss and ligament deficiency.

The more constrained the implant the greater the force transmitted to the implant–cement–bone interface therefore increasing the risk of loosening.

The main aim of TKR is to create a mechanical axis (weight-bearing line) which passes through the centre of the femoral head, knee and ankle. The joint line should then be perpendicular to the mechanical axis. It should also be parallel with the ground. If the correct size of implants are used and exactly the right amount of bone is cut away from both the tibia and the femur, then the new joint surface will be placed exactly where the patient's original surface had been before disease supervened. The collateral ligaments will then provide stability without constraint and ensure the patella will track correctly on the femur (Summary box 37.10).

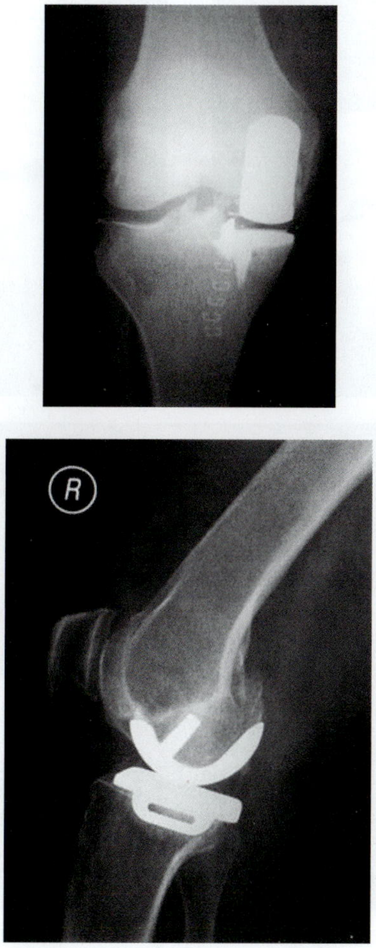

Figure 37.14 Unicompartmental knee replacement.

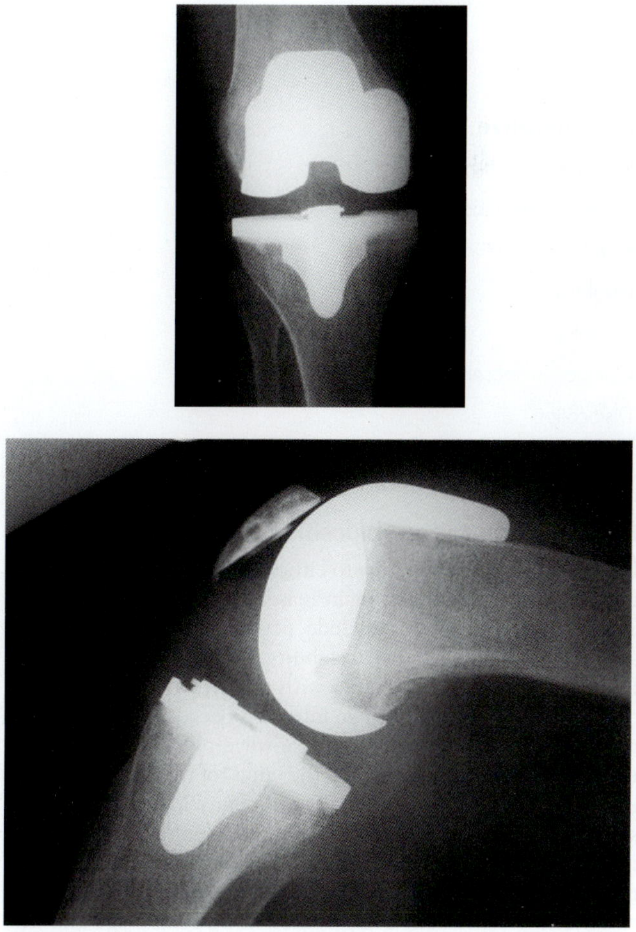

Figure 37.15 Total knee replacement.

Summary box 37.10

Aims of total knee replacement

- Mechanical axis through centre of knee
- Joint line perpendicular to mechanical axis
- Balance collateral ligaments
- Ensure patellofemoral joint tracks normally

Postoperatively, patients require intensive physiotherapy to regain quadriceps strength and to achieve full extension. In addition, they need at least 90° knee flexion to enable them to sit comfortably. The average length of hospital stay is between 5 and 7 days.

Complications

Complications following TKR can be broadly classified into intraoperative and postoperative (Table 37.9).

Table 37.9 Complications of total knee replacement.

Intraoperative
Misplacement of implants leading to instability or stiffness, or pain
Nerve or vessel injury including tourniquet damage
Fracture
Patellar tendon avulsion
Malalignment
Fat embolism
Postoperative
Infection
Deep vein thrombosis/pulmonary embolism
Pain/stiffness
Instability
Osteolysis
Component loosening
Dislocation

Revision total knee replacement

Implant loosening secondary to either infection or polyethylene-induced osteolysis are the main reasons for performing revision TKR. Other indications include periprosthetic fracture, malalignment (Figure 37.16), instability and patella maltracking. Regardless of the indication, as with any type of revision procedure it is important to exclude infection because this often warrants a two-stage rather than single-stage procedure. Although more technically challenging, the aims of revision TKR are no different to primary TKR, that is to provide a well-aligned, stable and pain-free knee. The revision burden of hips and knees is increasing with time and more complex revisions need to be performed as the patients are living longer, along with the primary joint replacement being offered at a younger age and in a more active patient.

Anterior cruciate ligament injury

The ACL is the most commonly injured ligament in the knee. It most commonly results from pivoting injuries in high energy contact sport (see Chapter 34) and may be associated with an audible 'pop' and immediate swelling, with the patient being 'carried off'. The injury rate is higher among females than males.

Some controversy exists concerning the incidence of secondary OA in ACL-deficient versus reconstructed knees. However, chronic ACL deficiency is clearly linked with an increased incidence of complex meniscal tears and chondral injury.

Investigation

MRI of the knee is useful for confirming the ACL injury but also for excluding the involvement of other structures, including menisci, PCL and collateral ligaments, chondral surfaces and posterolateral corner.

Treatment

Some patients may decide that they have adequate stability in the knee once they have been through a full rehabilitation programme. Surgical reconstruction of the ACL should only be undertaken in those patients who have a full range of knee motion and good hamstring/quadriceps function preoperatively as otherwise results are poor.

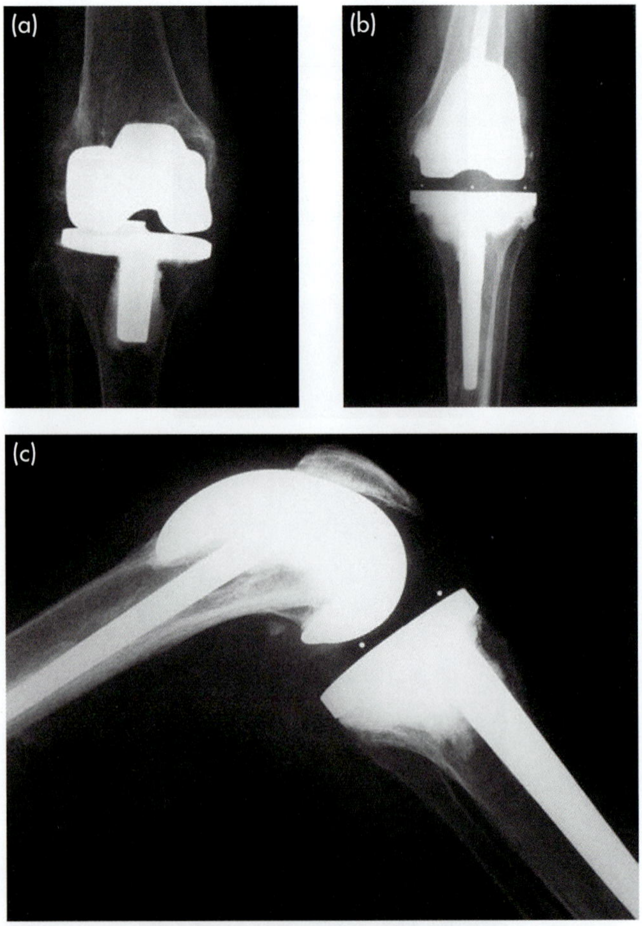

Figure 37.16 Radiographs of a malaligned knee (a) and a well-aligned revised knee (b and c).

An isolated ACL injury is most commonly treated with an arthroscopic intra-articular reconstruction. Graft can be bone–patella, tendon–bone or four-strand hamstring autograft. Postoperative rehabilitation programmes are crucial to a favourable outcome.

Complications following ACL surgery are usually a result of incorrect tunnel placement (femoral tunnel too anterior limits knee flexion) and early surgery. Graft re-rupture rate is approximately 1 per cent per year.

FURTHER READING

Bulstrode C, Buckwalter J, Carr A *et al. Oxford textbook of trauma and orthopaedics*. Oxford: Oxford University Press, 2002.

Miller MD. *Review of orthopaedics*, 5th edn. Philadelphia, PA: Saunders, 2008.

Solomon L, Warwick DJ, Nayagam S.*Apley's concise system of orthopaedics and fractures*, 3rd edn. London: Hodder Arnold, 2005.

Ramachandran M. *Basic orthopaedic sciences, the Stanmore guide*. London: Hodder Arnold, 2007.

CHAPTER 38

Foot and ankle

LEARNING OBJECTIVES

To understand:

- The basic anatomy and biomechanics of the foot and ankle
- The common problems affecting the foot and ankle in each age group
- The principles behind the treatment of each condition, be it conservative or surgical
- The significance of progressive neurological diseases

ANATOMY

There are 25/26 main bones in the foot (seven tarsal bones, five metatarsals and 13/14 phalanges) plus the two sesamoids of the hallux and a variable number of other sesamoid and accessory bones.

Movements at the ankle joint are mainly dorsiflexion and plantarflexion but, because the talus is wider anteriorly than posteriorly, dorsiflexion of the ankle leads to external rotation of the fibula at the syndesmosis. This means that the foot externally rotates with dorsiflexion and internally rotates with plantarflexion.

Stability is conferred upon the ankle by the shape of the medial, lateral and posterior malleoli and the integrity of the medial and lateral ligaments and the inferior tibiofibular ligaments.

The subtalar joint is divided into anterior, middle and posterior facets and, along with the talonavicular and calcaneocuboid joints, makes up the triple joint complex. These joints are responsible for inversion and eversion of the hind and midfoot. Most of this movement occurs at the talonavicular joint.

The second tarsometatarsal joint is recessed relative to the first and third and acts as a 'keystone'. Disruption of this joint (Lisfranc's injury) leads to loss of the transverse arch and an acquired flat foot.

The lower leg is divided into four compartments:

1 the superficial posterior – gastrocnemius, soleus and plantaris;
2 the deep posterior – tibialis posterior, flexor digitorum longus and flexor hallucis longus;
3 the lateral – peroneus brevis and peroneus longus;
4 the anterior – tibialis anterior, extensor hallucis longus, extensor digitorum longus and peroneus tertius.

There is only one muscle on the dorsum of the foot, the extensor digitorum brevis. The muscles on the plantar aspect of the foot are divided into four layers, the first being the most superficial. The plantar fascia is a very important structure that takes its origin from the heel and inserts into the bases of the proximal phalanges of the toes. At toe-off, the fascia tightens and accentuates the medial plantar arch and helps provide a rigid lever arm, the so-called 'windlass mechanism'.

The blood supply of the foot is from the anterior tibial, the posterior tibial and the peroneal arteries. The following nerves supply sensation to the foot: posterior tibial, saphenous, sural, superficial and deep peroneal (Figure 38.1) (Summary box 38.1).

Summary box 38.1

Anatomy of the foot

- There are 26 major bones in the foot
- There are four layers of muscles in the sole of the foot
- The blood supply of the foot is from the anterior and posterior tibial arteries plus the peroneal artery

BIOMECHANICS

The walking cycle is divided into the stance (60 per cent) and swing (40 per cent) phases. The stance phase is divided into three intervals: (1) heel strike to foot flat; (2) foot flat until the body passes over the ankle; and (3) ankle joint plantarflexion to toe-off. During walking up to 12 per cent of the gait cycle is spent with both feet in the stance phase but with running there is a period when neither foot is in contact with the ground, the 'float' phase. During running the cycle time is shortened but the forces generated are very much increased (Summary box 38.2).

Examination

The examination of the foot is described in Chapter 33. The patient should be watched walking and both the foot and the footwear of the patient need examining when looking for abnormal load and wear.

Jacques Lisfranc, 1790–1847, Professor of Surgery and Operative Medicine, Paris, France.

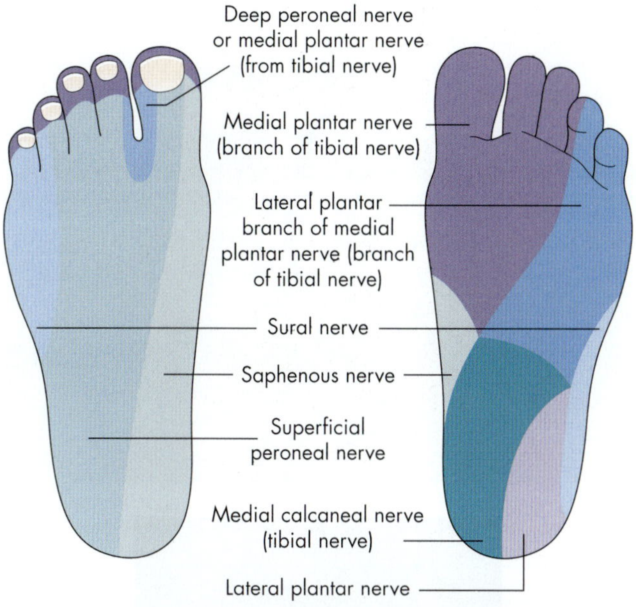

Figure 38.1 Cutaneous nerve supply of the foot. Courtesy of Bartleby.com.

Summary box 38.2

Biomechanics

- The gait cycle is divided into swing and stance phases
- Running generates increased forces, shortens the gait cycle and has a float phase when neither foot touches the ground

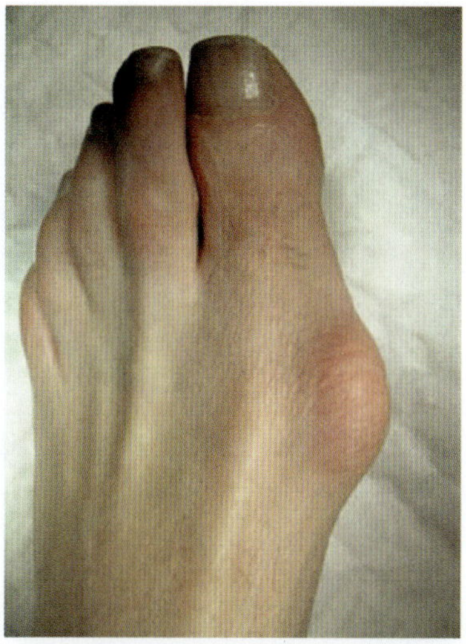

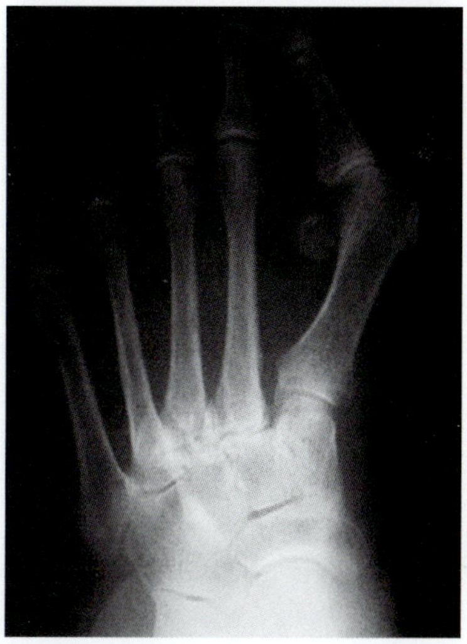

Figure 38.2 Hallux valgus and bunion.

PAEDIATRIC CONDITIONS

These are discussed in Chapter 41.

PATHOLOGY IN THE ADULT

The forefoot

Hallux valgus

Hallux valgus is deviation of the big toe away from the midline, i.e. towards the lesser toes, and is usually associated with a bunion, a swelling made up of both bone and bursa on the medial aspect of the first metatarsal head (Figure 38.2). It is a common condition that affects women more than men, and which is often bilateral. It is believed that the tendency to hallux valgus is inherited and that fully enclosed shoes accelerate the development of the condition.

With increasing deformity the first ray becomes defunctioned, and overload of the second metatarsophalangeal (MTP) joint results in pain and swelling with a prominent callosity beneath the second MTP joint and eventually hammering of the second toe.

The non-operative treatment of hallux valgus is unlikely to be acceptable to the younger patient as it involves relieving the load on the toe by use of an ugly shoe with a wide toe box. However, although hallux valgus may be merely a cosmetic problem, the fact that it is likely to progress makes surgical intervention reasonable provided that the patient realises that recovery can take from 6 to 12 months and that the surgery is not without risk.

For mild deformities a distal osteotomy (e.g. chevron) is usually adequate. For moderate deformities the surgeon is more likely to use a shaft (e.g. Scarf/Ludloff, Figure 38.3) or a basal (proximal chevron or crescentic) osteotomy. Severe deformities can be corrected by shaft and basal osteotomies but sometimes a fusion of the first tarsometatarsal joint (modified Lapidus) or a first MTP joint fusion can be effective. Basal osteotomies/fusions have a higher risk of abnomal elevation/depression of the rays resulting in overload of the rest of the forefoot. However, they do allow a massive correction. They are best stabilised using plates.

Operations such as a Keller's excision arthroplasty, where the proximal third of the proximal phalanx is excised, serve to defunction the toe and sesamoids and are reserved for low-demand high-risk patients where there is a high risk that healing of an osteotomy might fail.

The complications of surgery are infection, cutaneous nerve damage, recurrence/overcorrection of deformity, stiffness and overload of the second MTP joint (transfer lesion), and

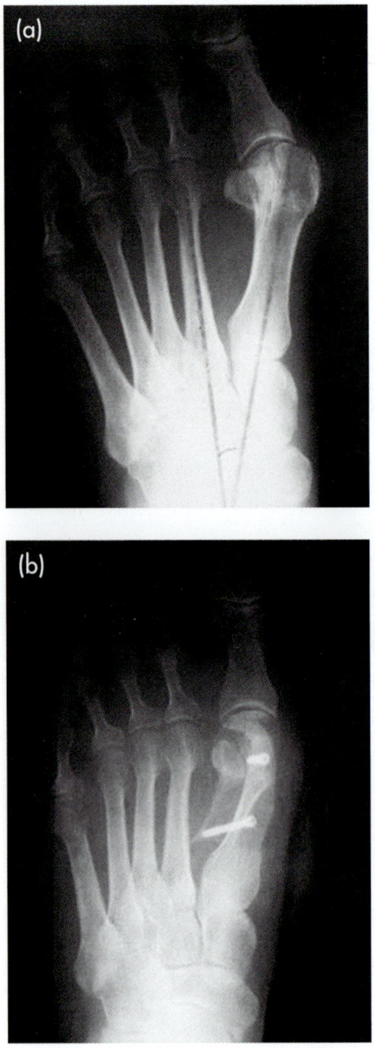

Figure 38.3 Pre- (a) and postoperative (b) radiographs of a Scarf osteotomy.

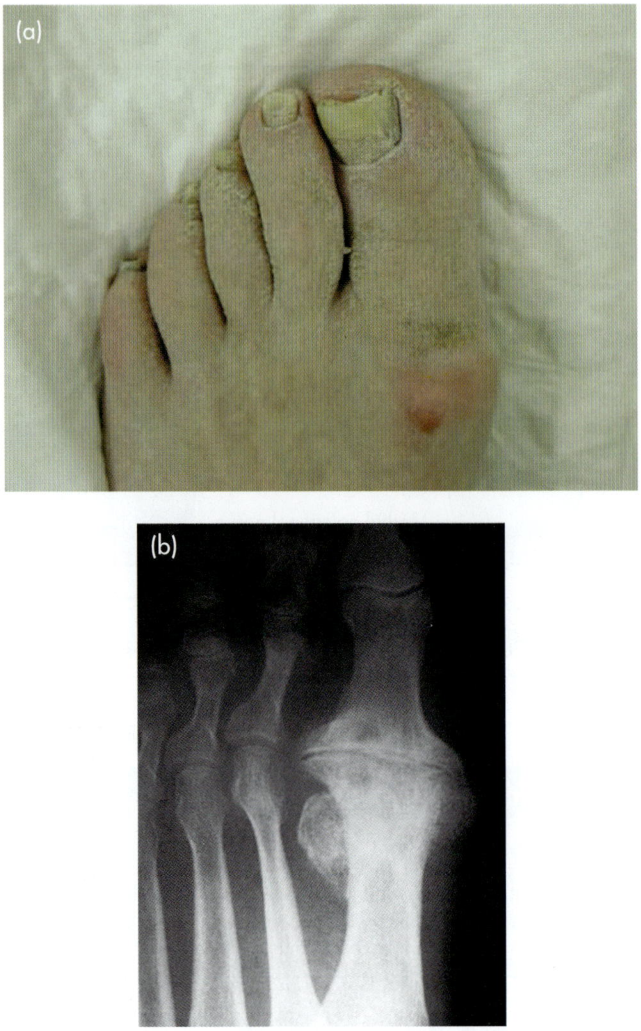

Figure 38.4 Clinical (a) and radiographic (b) appearances of hallux rigidus.

10 per cent of patients have reservations about their outcome. Occasionally, patients develop early arthritis following surgery and require revision to fusion (Summary box 38.3).

Hallux rigidus

Hallux rigidus is a painful condition of the hallux MTP joint characterised by loss of motion especially in dorsiflexion and osteophyte formation on the dorsum and sides of the joint (Figure 38.4).

In adults there is often a history of trauma or repetitive microtrauma (sport) but, occasionally, there is a strong family history of the condition. Gout and rheumatological conditions may present in this way. Patients complain of stiffness and pain on weight-bearing.

The most effective non-operative treatment is provision of a stiff-soled shoe with a deep toe box or a rocker-soled shoe which are now available in high-street shops.

The mainstays of surgical management are injection/manipulation, cheilectomy (a radical debridement and excision of the part of the joint blocking movement) fusion and interposition arthroplasty (Keller's-type procedure).

Fusion is for the severely affected and is an effective means of abolishing pain. A fusion will still usually allow sports participation (Summary box 38.4).

Summary box 38.3

Hallux valgus

- Bunions affect women more than men
- Patients with hallux valgus have inherited a tendency to develop the condition
- Not all patients need surgery
- The choice of operation is determined by the severity of the deformity and presence or otherwise of any arthritis

Sesamoid problems

Management includes offloading with orthotics and injections of steroids.

Lesser toe deformities

Non-operative treatment involves appropriate padding and footwear modification. For symptomatic flexible deformities soft-tissue surgery, such as flexor/extensor tenotomies ± capsulotomy

William Lordan Keller, 1874–1959, Head of the Department of Surgery, the Walter Reed Hospital, Washington, DC, USA, described this operation in 1904.

Summary box 38.4

Hallux rigidus

- Hallux rigidus can affect adolescents as well as adults
- Stiff-soled shoes with a deep toe box are the most comfortable type of shoe
- Cheilectomy and fusion are the mainstays of surgical treatment

is usually adequate but for fixed deformities bony procedures are required, such as interposition arthroplasty, fusion or excision arthroplasty.

Freiberg's disease

Freiberg's disease is an ischaemic necrosis of the epiphysis, resulting in pain and swelling of the joint (Figure 38.5). It will often settle with rest. Excision of the whole head should never be performed.

Morton's neuroma and metatarsalgia

Metatarsalgia usually occurs secondary to joint problems or irritation of a nerve. Morton's neuroma is a painful condition which in most cases arises from compression of the common digital nerve between the third and fourth metatarsal heads.

Diagnosis is confirmed by ultrasound. Non-operative treatments include advice about footwear, an orthosis (pre-metatarsal dome) to splay the metatarsal heads or an injection of steroids for short-term relief.

Surgery involves resection (the affected toes will be permanently partly numb if the nerve is removed) (Summary box 38.5).

Summary box 38.5

Morton's neuroma

- Morton's neuroma most commonly affects the third web space
- Surgical excision of a neuroma is often successful but guided injections form the mainstay of treatment for most

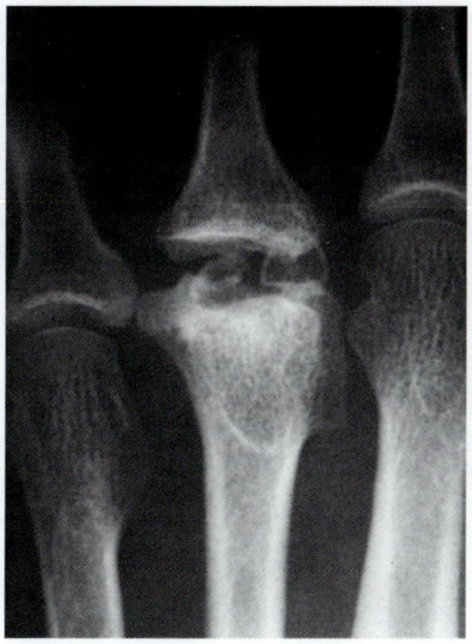

Figure 38.5 Freiberg's disease.

Midfoot and hindfoot

The hindfoot comprises the talus and calcaneum. The midfoot comprises the remaining tarsal bones as far as the tarsometatarsal joints.

Arthritis

In the majority of cases pain will be the reason for the patient seeking help. On examination there is usually joint-line tenderness.

If a foot is swollen and deformed but relatively painless, there is likely to be an underlying neuropathy and urgent investigation and protection is required (Charcot foot).

Non-operative treatments include offloading painful areas, physiotherapy and intra-articular steroids. Surgery is reserved for those patients who fail non-operative treatment and involves fusion of the affected joints.

Ankle arthritis

The definitive operative treatment for arthritis of the ankle will usually be in the form of arthrodesis (fusion); this is often carried out via an open approach but arthroscopic ankle and triple arthrodesis are now established procedures and have better outcomes, more rapid recovery and fewer complications. Such techniques are mandatory in the presence of poor soft-tissue envelope or in the presence of a clotting diathesis. Ankle replacements are now available but the results are not as reliable.

The advantage of fusion is it has a known track record, good outcomes (90 per cent plus do well) and minimal morbidity, especially with modern arthroscopic techniques, but not all do well with fusion. Function following isolated fusion is virtually normal for most patients and this is probably due to increased mobility at other joints. However, this may precipitate arthralgia elsewhere.

Hindfoot (excluding ankle) arthritis

The triple complex refers to the subtalar (talocalcaneal), calcaneocuboid and talonavicular joints. These joints are often affected by arthritis. Treatment options are limited and if simple measures have failed, a fusion should be performed. Smokers and diabetics have a massively increased non-union rate for all foot fusion procedures and should be warned of this when they give consent.

Ankle with other hindfoot arthritis

If surgical input is required then one option is to do one set of joints and then see how the patient fares. Secondary surgery to the other joints can then be performed only if required. The alternative is to treat all joints at once. Modern techniques now use third-generation hindfoot fusion nails which fuse both ankle and subtalar joints and are inserted with an open or arthroscopic fusion technique.

A pantalar fusion is quite disabling but may be necessary in rheumatological patients with deformities/stress fractures, failed arthroplasty with subtalar joint involvement or avascular necrosis (AVN) collapse of talus.

Midfoot arthritis

The aetiology is usually not known but the risk factors include microtrauma, rheumatological causes, flat foot, Lisfranc or similar injuries (which may have been missed), Charcot and cavus

Albert Henry Freiberg, Professor of Orthopaedic Surgery, University of Cincinnati, Cincinnati, OH, USA, gave his account of this condition in 1926.
Thomas George Morton, 1835–1903, surgeon, the Pennsylvania Hospital, Philadelphia, PA, USA, described this condition in 1876.

foot. Patients are best managed non-operatively with orthotics, shoes, analgesia and modifications of their lifestyle.

Inflammatory joint conditions

It is important to remember that knee deformity must be addressed before corrective hindfoot surgery is undertaken.

Rheumatological presentations in the foot

The early presentations of rheumatological disease may be with synovitis of the lesser MTP joints and widespread small joint disease, often in association with enthesopathy such as plantar fasciitis or Achilles tendonosis. However, the classic deformity is of hallux valgus with or without hallux rigidus deformity and subluxation or even dislocation of the lesser MTP joints.

The patient may present with a bunion and prominent lesser metatarsal heads which can often be felt to be dislocated on clinical examination, and are painful to palpation.

Excision of the metatarsal heads produces an almost instantaneous and gratifying relief of pain. If a plantar approach is used an ellipse of skin can be excised to move the metatarsal padding back over the end of the metatarsal. While most surgeons avoid scars on the plantar aspect of the foot wherever possible, this is one procedure when the results are good.

Midfoot

Rheumatological disease may also affect the midfoot and here the outcome is usually just pain and stiffness. Options are limited to injections and fusion surgery if non-operative measures have failed.

Hindfoot and ankle

Rheumatological disease also affects the hindfoot and ankle. Many patients require surgical hindfoot fusions.

The options for the ankle are discussed in the arthritis section. The rheumatological diseases also affect soft tissues. Patients are more prone to developing enthesopathy, tendinitis and tendonosis and even tendon rupture.

The Achilles tendon should never be injected with steroid for fear of rupture and similarly the tibialis anterior and tibialis posterior tendons are risky for injection (Summary box 38.6).

Summary box 38.6

Midfoot and hindfoot

- Joint disorders are degenerative or inflammatory
- The mainstay of surgical treatment remains fusion although ankle replacements are becoming more successful
- Rheumatoid arthritis must be medically controlled as well as possible before surgery
- Knee deformities should be corrected before tackling foot problems

Tendon disorders

Tenosynovitis occurs as a result of injury or overuse or is secondary to inflammatory joint conditions. Rest, anti-inflammatory medication and physiotherapy are often helpful but, in inflammatory conditions, tenosynovectomy may be required.

The tendons most commonly affected by degeneration are the Achilles (Figure 38.6), tibialis posterior and peroneii (brevis more than longus).

Ruptured Achilles tendon

The Achilles tendon rupture is more frequent in the 40–50-year-old age group who are undertaking vigorous sport after a long period away from such activities. Many patients do not suffer the acute rupture classically described in all textbooks and many seem to have a series of micro tears that gradually lead to total rupture. Studies have shown that elderly patients with Achilles rupture regained 70–90 per cent of normal power with no treatment whatsoever when reviewed at one year and, for many patients, this is enough to allow them to return to normal function.

Non-operative options include a sprung ankle–foot orthotic (AFO) ankle brace.

Peroneal tendon problems

The peroneal tendons may develop a tendinosis, may sublux or may become involved in an inflammatory process with or without bony overgrowth at the inferior retinaculum (Figure 38.7). An associated varus heel will amplify the problem and will need addressing with an appropriate reconstruction/osteotomy or fusion.

Peroneal tendon subluxation can occur spontaneously or after injury. It may be associated with the groove at the back of the fibula being too shallow to contain the peroneal tendons, but may just be secondary to a superior retinaculum tear. The patient may be able to demonstrate a tendon subluxation over the fibula. Surgical repair is usually required and involves deepening of the groove.

Ankle instability

Most people who sustain an ankle sprain will recover, particularly if they receive prompt physiotherapy. However, some individuals develop significant instability. On examination an unstable ankle due to ligament disruption will show a marked 'anterior draw' sign.

If physiotherapy is unsuccessful at resolving the problem, a reconstruction may be needed with ligament augmentation.

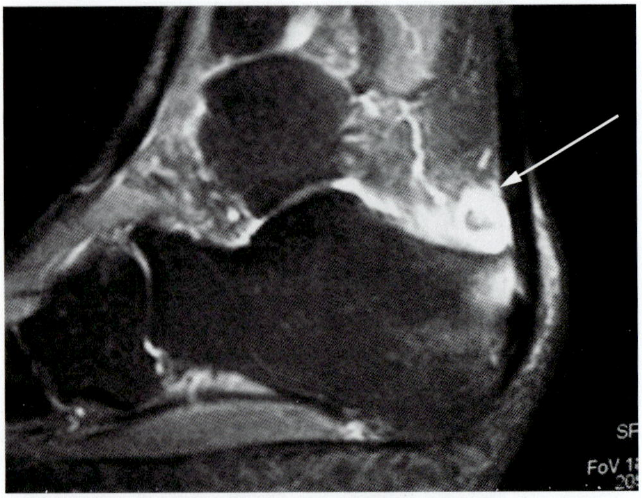

Figure 38.6 Insertional Achilles tendinitis.

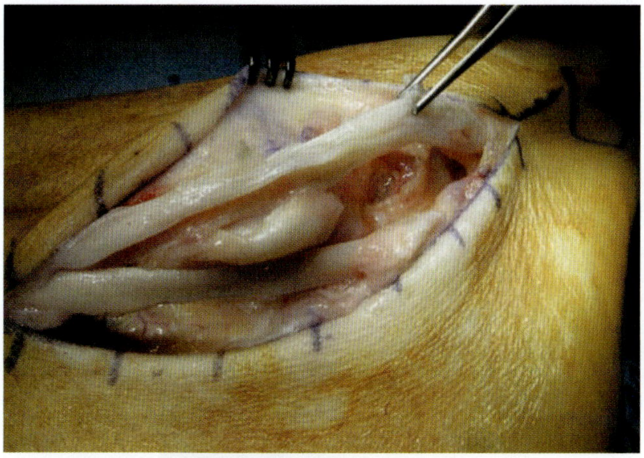

Figure 38.7 Split and degenerate peroneus brevis.

Osteochondral lesion of the talus

Patients with persistent pain in the ankle following an injury should be suspected of having an osteochondral lesion. Juveniles seem to have a high spontaneous recovery rate and surgery should not be necessary.

Synovitis

Many patients have ongoing pain following the ankle injury that is simply due to synovitis within the ankle joint. This may be treated non-operatively with an injection of steroid or may require surgical debridement.

Pes cavus

The development of unilateral pes cavus is likely to be arising from an upper motor neurone lesion so an appropriate neurological examination should be performed.

Pes cavus is usually bilateral and most cases will be associated with an underlying neurological condition, the most common being Charcot–Marie–Tooth disease. These patients may present with characteristic progressive small muscle wasting, thin calf musculature, hand symptoms, aches and pains, and cavovarus feet. Examination may show early loss of vibration sense. Precise diagnosis is confirmed with nerve conduction studies.

The key deforming force is always relative preservation of the tib post tendon. Surgical correction of deformity is often required. The principal goal of treatment is to obtain a foot which can be placed flat on the ground, and with the power of the muscles around the ankle in balance. It will be necessary to transfer or release the tib post tendon. The most commonly performed procedure is to transfer the tib post to the dorsolateral side of the foot, followed by lateralising of the heel with an osteotomy (Summary box 38.7).

Summary box 38.7

Pes cavus

- Pes cavus needs neurological investigation
- About 80 per cent of cases of pes cavus are associated with a neurological disease
- The most common cause is Charcot–Marie–Tooth disease
- Unilateral pes cavus – think diastematomyelia/tumour

Acquired flat foot

There is a wide range of normal appearances of adult feet. Pathological causes of a flat foot include:

- tibialis posterior tendon dysfunction;
- tarsometatarsal arthritis/injury (Figure 38.8);
- Charcot neuroarthropathy, e.g. diabetes;
- inflammatory/degenerative arthritis of the subtalar/talonavicular/naviculo-cuneiform joints;
- spring ligament rupture;
- tarsal coalition.

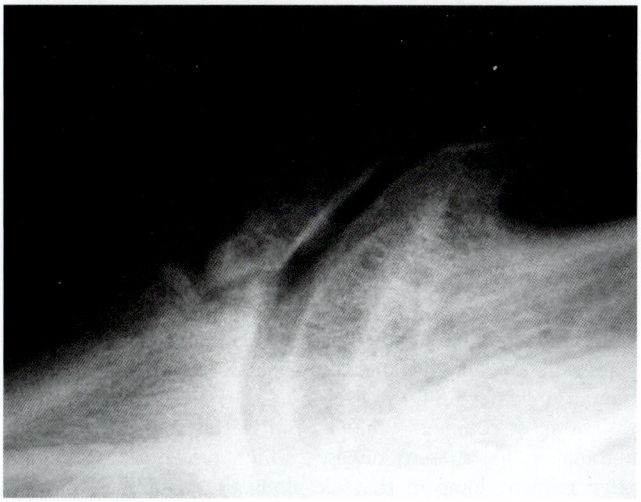

Figure 38.8 Tarsometatarsal arthritis.

Acquired adult flat foot

The tibialis posterior tendon tends to fail in overweight individuals and those who have flat feet. Often, after unaccustomed exercise, the tendon swells and is painful. The diagnosis is rarely made early. The condition occurs mainly in women and the key test is that the patient cannot stand on tiptoe on that leg alone. Many individuals will require surgical treatment in the form of a medial displacement calcaneal osteotomy, flexor digitorum longus or flexor hallucis longus tendon transfer and spring ligament repair. Failure to treat this condition can lead to spectacular deformity (Figure 38.9). An acute traumatic flat foot may develop in young athletes and military recruits after traumatic injury; here the injury is an isolated spring ligament tear and early surgery is needed to effect a repair (Summary box 38.8).

Summary box 38.8

Acquired flat foot

- Tibialis posterior tendon dysfunction and tarsometatarsal OA are common causes of an acquired flat foot
- Orthoses, rest and non-steroidal anti-inflammatory drugs (NSAIDs) can help with symptomatic relief
- Surgery is a major undertaking but often highly successful at achieving symptomatic relief

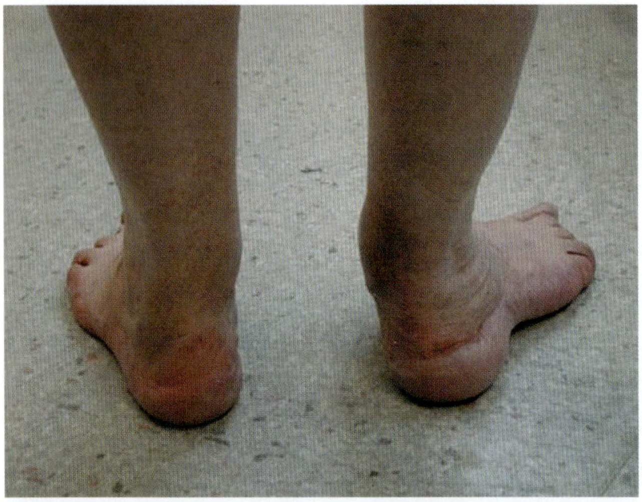

Figure 38.9 A tibialis posterior tendon-deficient foot.

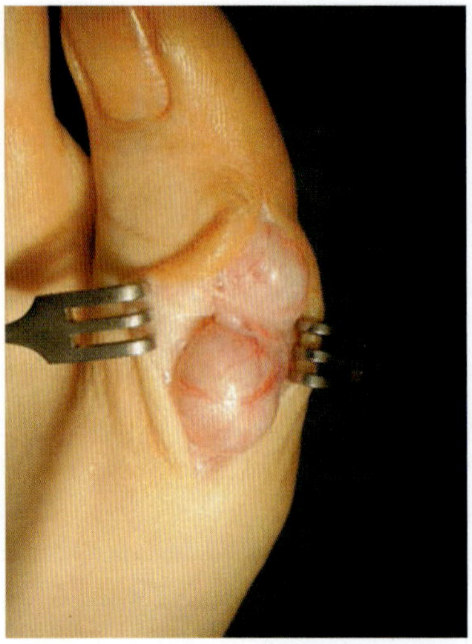

Figure 38.10 Angioleiomyoma of the hallux.

Tumours

The three most common benign tumours of the foot are ganglia, giant cell tumour and angioleiomyomas (Figure 38.10); these tumours may need surgical excision.

The most common 'tumour' seen in the foot is the plantar fibroma or 'lederhosens disease', which presents as a painful often growing lump in the sole along the plantar fascia. The condition is linked to Dupytren's and Peyronie's disease. Surgery is not helpful.

Infection

Septic arthritis in the foot or ankle is rare; when it occurs it usually follows a surgical procedure but it can also arise as a result of haematogenous spread. Treatment is immediate surgical drainage and administration of appropriate high-dosage antibiotics once cultures are obtained. The most common causative organism is *Staphylococcus aureus* with methicillin-resistant *S. aureus* (MRSA) becoming more common. Even with prompt treatment chondrolysis often occurs and subsequent degenerative changes develop rapidly.

In immunocompromised patients opportunistic infections can arise and, in diabetics, failure to treat with debridement can lead to amputation. It is important to realise that x-rays in the early stages of infection are usually normal and that diagnosis is made on clinical suspicion and with blood tests and more sophisticated imaging such as magnetic resonance imaging (MRI) or bone scanning.

Tuberculosis can affect the foot and is associated with major bony damage; it responds surprisingly well to debridement and appropriate anti-tuberculous therapy (Figure 38.11).

Diabetes

Diabetics have foot problems secondary to neuropathy and microvascular changes. They are at increased risk of infection and ulceration, and trauma (sometimes trivial) can lead to collapse of the foot, also known as Charcot neuroarthropathy (Figure 38.12).

Ulceration can lead to major morbidity and amputation (Figure 38.13). Ulcers need to be treated and, when ulcer healing has occurred, the aim should be to keep the foot ulcer free.

Charcot

Charcot is a disease whereby patients develop a neuropathic destruction of the joints. It is often described as painless but actually the majority of patients have some pain. In the Western world, diabetes is the biggest cause but in the rest of the world leprosy is also important. However, any other neurological condition can cause this condition.

Charcot disease often presents with a hot swollen, red extremity and is often misdiagnosed as cellulitis, gout, fracture or deep vein thrombosis (DVT), and a great many present late because of the difficulty in diagnosis. If there is no history of skin damage, infection is unlikely, but MRI and even biopsy can help differentiate between infection and Charcot. There are three stages to the process of Charcot neuroarthropathy, which takes up to 18

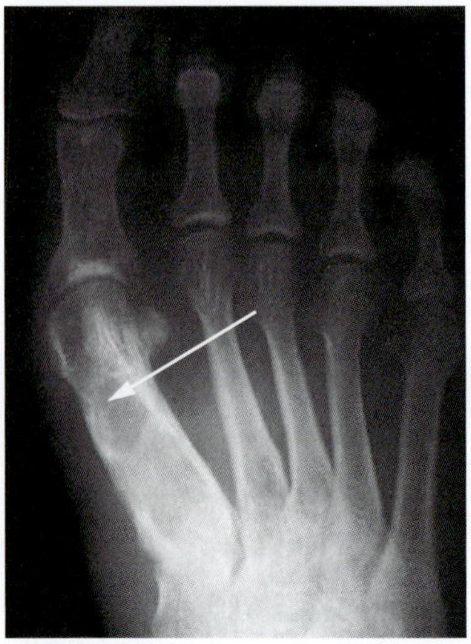

Figure 38.11 Tuberculosis of the foot.

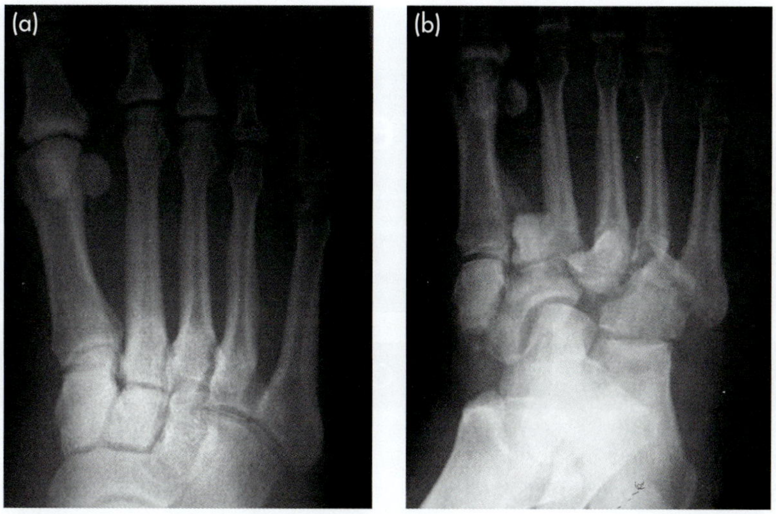

Figure 38.12 Charcot foot. Radiographs taken at the time of a trivial injury (a) and 6 weeks later (b).

months to run its course: stage I, fragmentation; stage II, coalescence; and stage III, bone consolidation. The principle of treatment throughout is to maintain a foot-shaped foot to prevent late pressure ulcers. The acute Charcot foot requires appropriate splintage in a Charcot retaining orthotic walker (CROW) or a total contact cast (TCC), but many surgeons offer an aggressive early surgical approach. Surgical options include early stabilisation to prevent deformity or late reconstruction or removal of bony prominences to prevent ulceration (Summary box 38.9).

Summary box 38.9

Diabetes

Diabetics are prone to infection because of:
- Peripheral neuropathy
- Peripheral vascular disease
- Impaired resistance to infection

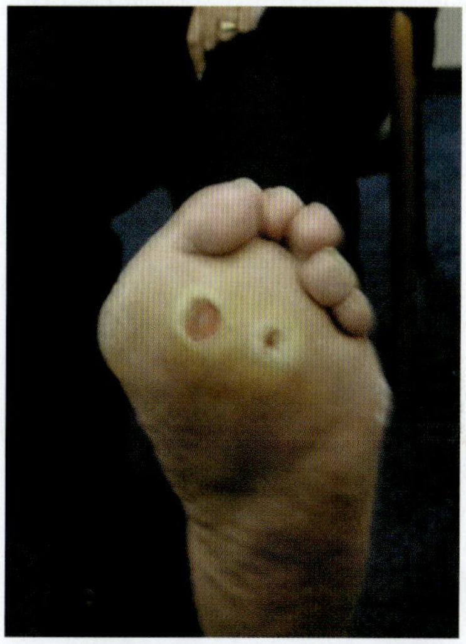

Figure 38.13 Diabetic foot ulcer.

Entrapment neuropathies

Any nerve supplying the foot can become entrapped and result in pain, and treatment often requires surgical decompression. Tarsal tunnel syndrome is much rarer than carpal tunnel syndrome in the hand.

Heel pain

The most common cause of heel pain is plantar fasciitis. Pain is located inferomedially within the heel and is worst first thing in the morning and after periods of rest. The majority of cases settle within 18 months and surgery is rarely required or successful.

FURTHER READING

Bulstrode C, Buckwalter J, Carr A *et al. Oxford textbook of trauma and orthopaedics*. Oxford: Oxford University Press, 2002.
Miller MD. *Review of orthopaedics*, 4th edn. Philadelphia, PA: Saunders, 2004.
Solomon L, Warwick DJ, Nayagam S. *Apley's concise system of orthopaedics and fractures*, 3rd edn. London: Hodder Arnold, 2005.

CHAPTER 39

Musculoskeletal tumours

LEARNING OBJECTIVES

- List the symptoms and signs which suggest the presence of a benign or malignant musculoskeletal tumour
- Recognise that a suspicious lesion should be referred to a centre of excellence for staging, biopsy and multidisciplinary assessment
- Understand why staging should be completed before biopsy
- Explain why a diagnosis is required before treatment
- Understand the principles of taking a biopsy
- Describe the principles of surgical treatment of musculoskeletal tumours
- List the aims of surgical treatment in metastatic disease
- How to manage a pathological fracture or impending fracture
- Recognise when a lesion is at risk of pathological fracture

The most common malignant bone tumours are metastases (Figure 39.1). Due to advances in oncological treatment, the number of patients presenting with skeletal failure due to metastatic disease is increasing. The most common tumours that metastasise to bone are breast, prostate, lung, kidney and thyroid carcinomas (Figure 39.2).

Multiple myeloma (Figure 39.3) is a malignant neoplasm arising from the plasma cells in the bone marrow. It is usually multicentric. If the condition is solitary it is called plasmacytoma.

Malignant primary sarcomas of bone are very rare. The most common of these is osteosarcoma (Figure 39.4). Osteosarcoma has two incidence peaks, one in adolescence, the other later in life, arising in patients with Paget's disease and those who have

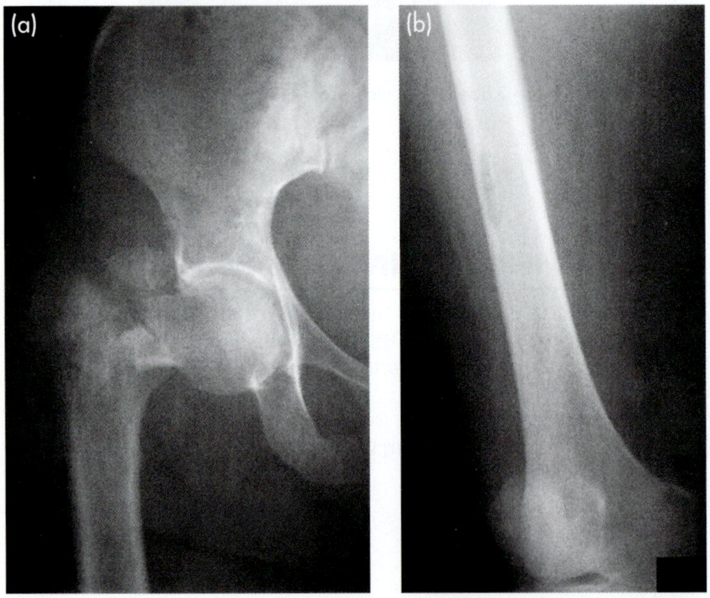

Figure 39.1 (a) Pathological fracture of the proximal femur through metastatic breast carcinoma. (b) X-rays of the whole femur show a further, more distal metastatic deposit.

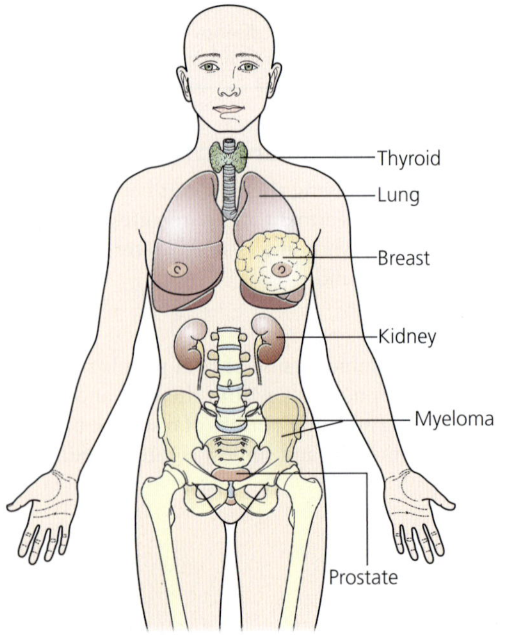

Figure 39.2 Malignant tumours commonly metastasising to bone.

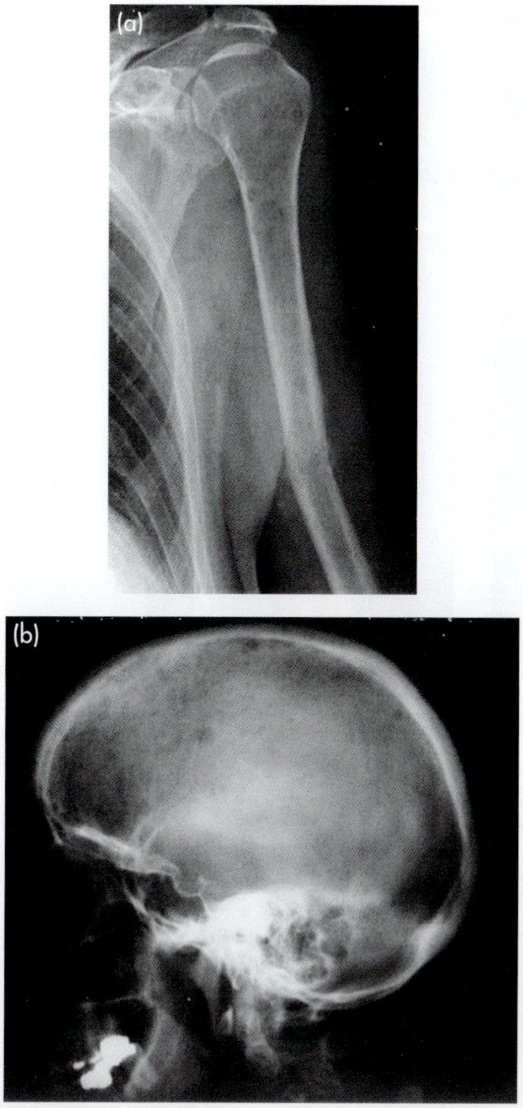

Figure 39.3 (a) Multiple myeloma affecting the left humerus with a pathological fracture. (b) Multiple myeloma with multiple deposits in the skull.

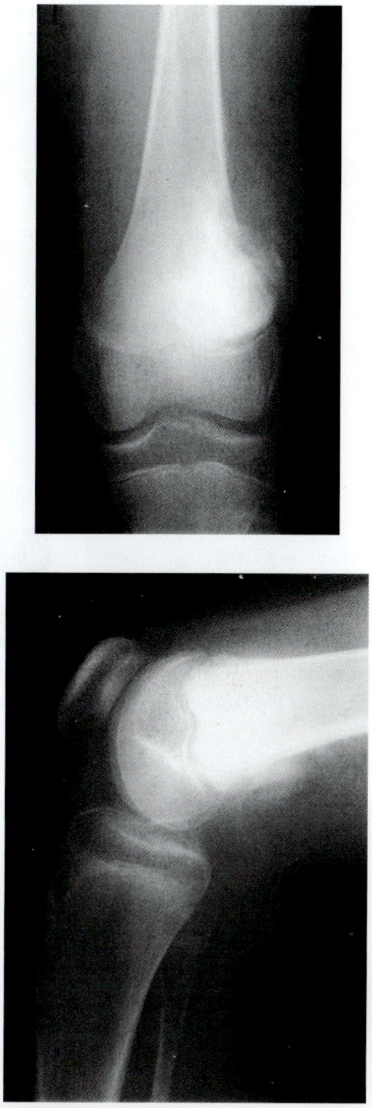

Figure 39.4 Sclerotic osteosarcoma of the distal femur in a child.

had previous radiotherapy. Chondrosarcoma (Figures 39.5, 39.6 and 39.7) and Ewing's sarcoma (Figure 39.8) make up most of the rest. Ewing's sarcoma occurs in adolescence, while the incidence of chondrosarcoma increases from middle age onwards.

Some conditions are associated with an increased likelihood of developing malignant disease in bone and/or cartilage (Table 39.1).

Soft tissue tumours are also quite rare and most are benign, with only one in a hundred being malignant (Figure 39.9).

Malignant tumours usually metastasise to bone by means of haematogenous spread. The spine is the third most common site for metastases, after the lung and liver. Although most patients with systemic cancer will have metastatic disease in the spine before they die, only 10 per cent are symptomatic.

Tumour cells metastasise to the spine via Batson's venous plexus. These retroperitoneal veins have no valves and allow retrograde embolisatic spread to the spine and proximal long bones (Figure 39.10).

Metastases can be lytic, sclerotic or mixed. Lytic metastases usually arise from tumours that are vascular. However, they can also occur in very aggressive, destructive tumours with no healing response from the bone. Sclerotic lesions are commonly from the prostate.

BONE TUMOURS

Bone tumours are classified according to the tissue of origin. These include:

- metastases – may show histological features of their tissue of origin;
- haemopoietic tumours – e.g. myeloma;
- osteogenic tumours – e.g. osteosarcoma;
- chondrogenic tumours – e.g. chondrosarcoma;
- others – e.g. Ewing's sarcoma.

Sir James Paget, 1814–1899, surgeon, St Bartholomew's Hospital, London, UK, described osteitis deformans in 1877.
James Ewing, 1866–1943, Professor of Pathology, The Cornell University Medical College, New York, NY, USA, described this type of sarcoma in 1921.
Oscar V Batson, 1894–1979, an American otolaryngologist.

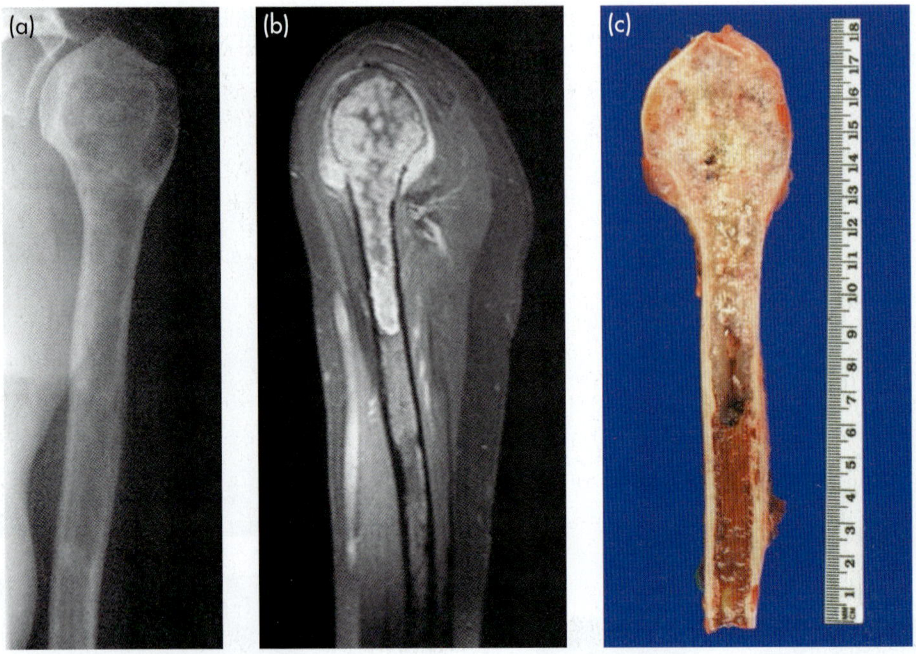

Figure 39.5 (a) Chondrosarcoma of the proximal humerus with multiple calcifications. (b) Magnetic resonance imaging scan showing extensive involvement. (c) Excised chondrosarcoma of the proximal humerus.

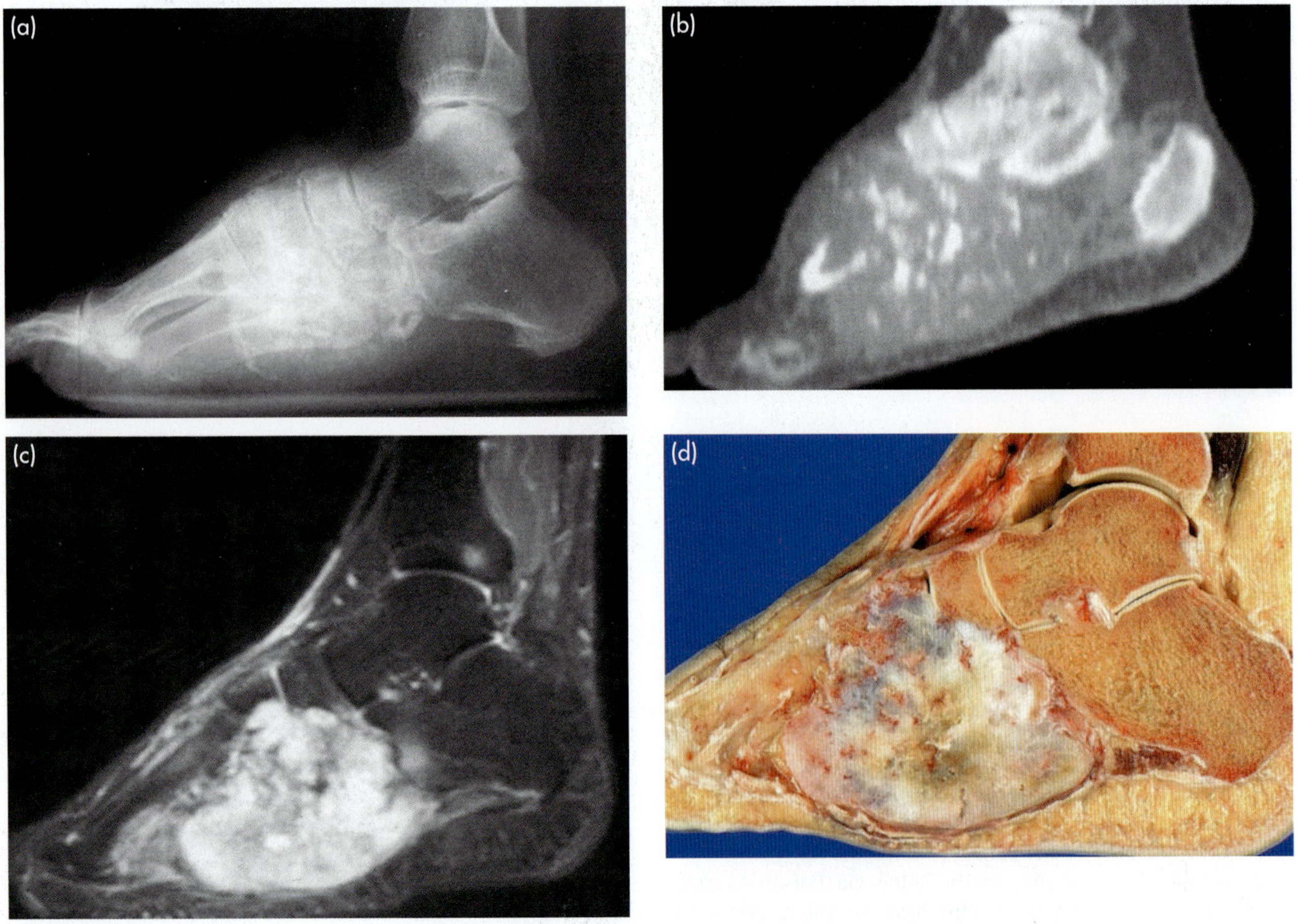

Figure 39.6 (a) Chondrosarcoma of the foot. (b) Computed tomography scan reconstruction showing multiple calcifications. (c) T2-weighted magnetic resonance imaging scan shows high signal in chondrosarcoma. (d) Excised chondrosarcoma of the foot.

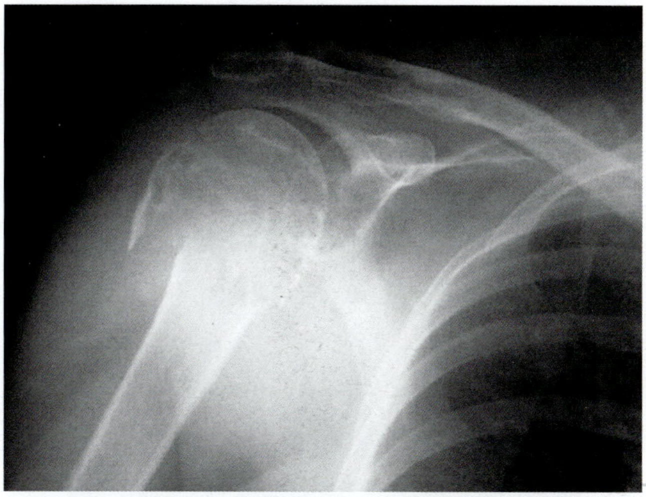

Figure 39.7 Pathological fracture through a primary chondrosarcoma of the proximal humerus.

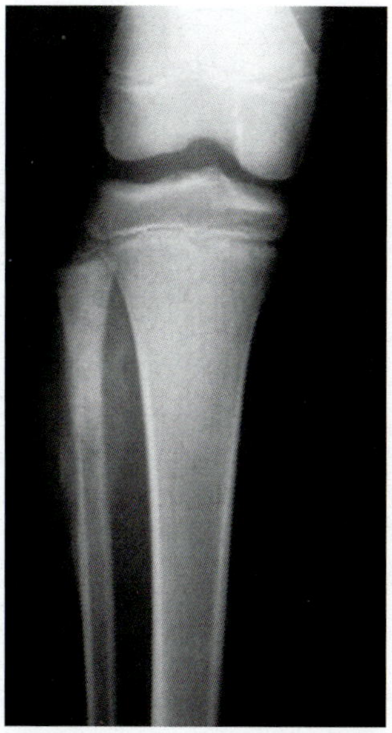

Figure 39.8 Ewing's sarcoma of the proximal fibula. The tumour is metadiaphyseal in location with a periosteal reaction and subtle onion-skinning.

Table 39.1 Conditions associated with an increased risk of malignant disease in bone and cartilage.

High risk	Moderate risk	Low risk
Maffucci syndrome (enchondromatosis and angiomas of soft tissue)	Diaphyseal aclasia (multiple osteochondromas)	Chronic osteomyelitis
Ollier's disease (enchondromatosis)	Polyostotic Paget's disease	Osteonecrosis
Familial retinoblastoma syndrome	Radiation osteitis	Fibrous dysplasia, osteogenesis imperfecta, osteoblastoma and chondroblastoma

METASTASES

The vast majority of tumours spreading to the skeleton are carcinomas; but not infrequently the primary tumour is never found.

Metastases are rare in children, but can occur from neuroblastoma, rhabdomyosarcoma and clear cell carcinoma of the kidney (Summary boxes 39.1 and 39.2).

Summary box 39.1

Most common bone metastases (93 per cent)

- Breast
- Prostate
- Lung
- Renal
- Thyroid

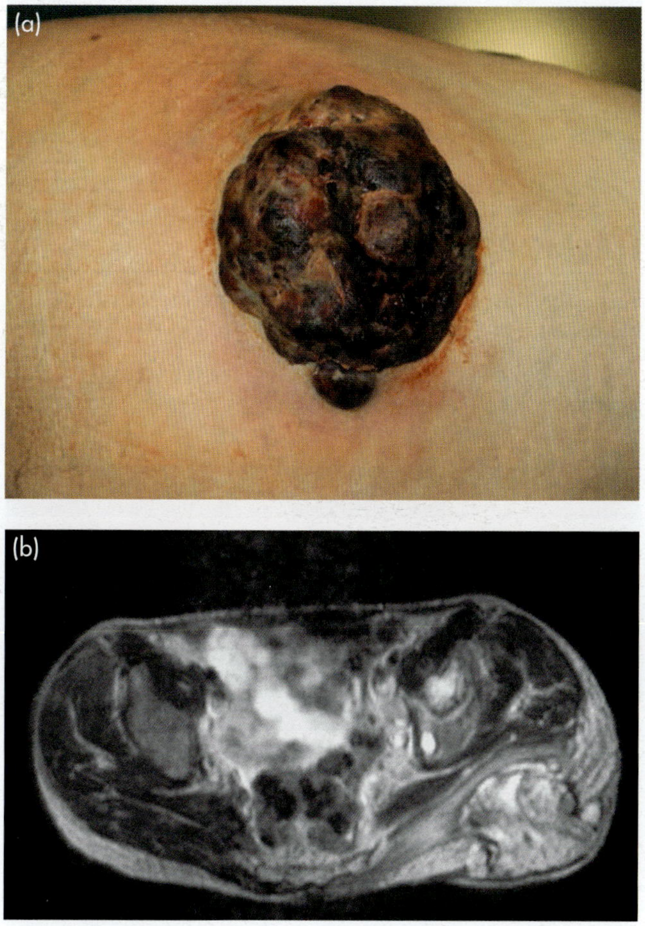

Figure 39.9 (a) Large, fungating soft-tissue sarcoma of the buttock. (b) Magnetic resonance imaging confirmed its extent.

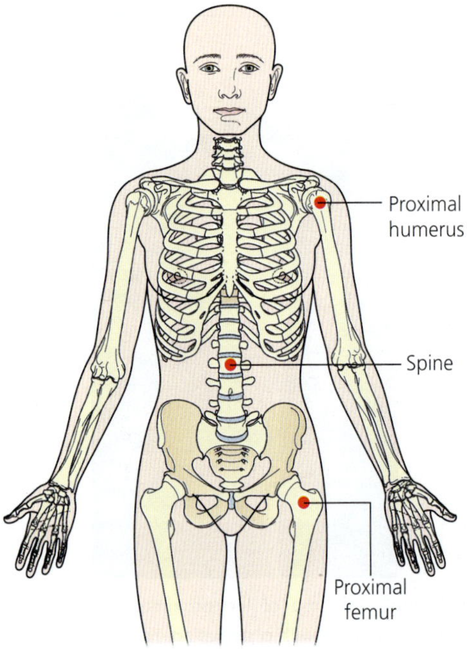

Figure 39.10 Common sites of metastatic bone disease.

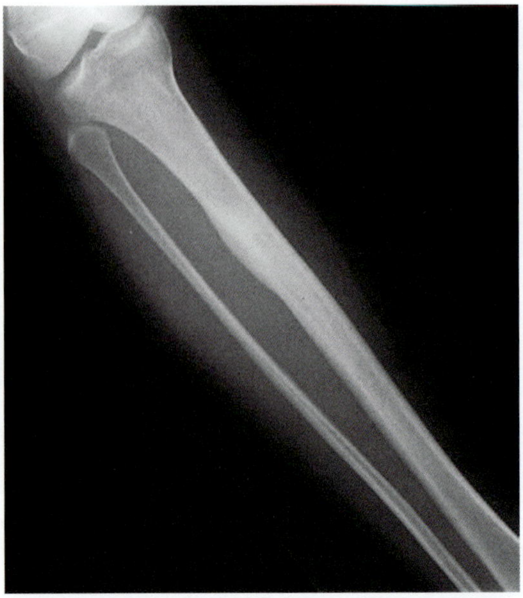

Figure 39.11 X-ray showing an osteoid osteoma of the tibial diaphysis with reactive bone formation.

Summary box 39.2

Most common sites of bone metastases

- Spine
- Proximal femur
- Proximal humerus

HAEMOPOIETIC TUMOURS

There are no benign neoplasms of the haemopoietic system. Malignant tumours can be divided into two groups:

1 solitary plasmacytoma/multiple myeloma (Figure 39.2);
2 lymphomas; malignant neoplasm of the lymphoid cells (Summary box 39.3).

Summary box 39.3

Malignant bone tumours

- Plasmacytoma – solitary form of multiple myeloma
- Osteosarcoma – often secondary to Paget's disease and radiotherapy
- Chondrosarcoma
- Ewing's sarcoma

OSTEOGENIC TUMOURS

These tumours produce osteoid or bony matrix.

Osteoid osteoma (Figures 39.11 and 39.12) is a benign bone-forming lesion which is small but very painful. Usually, symptoms occur at night and are typically relieved by anti-inflammatories. Children and adolescents are frequently affected. They can occur in any bone but are common in the proximal femur.

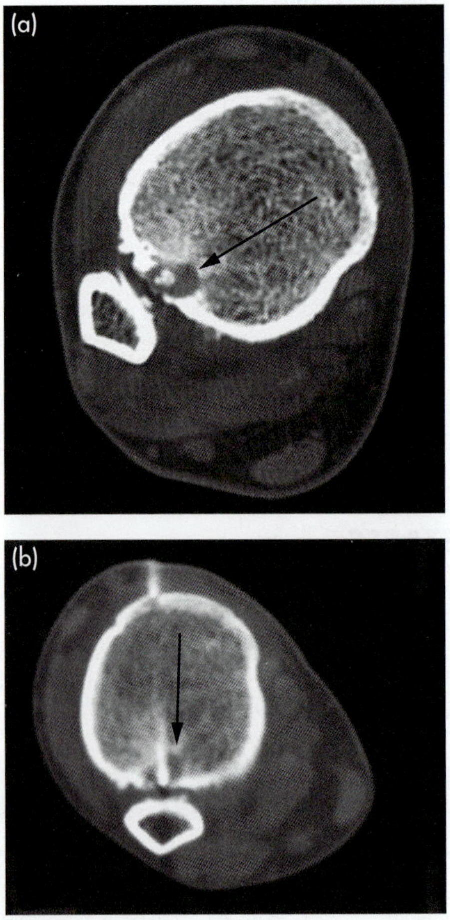

Figure 39.12 (a) Axial computed tomography (CT) scan showing an osteoid osteoma nidus in the distal tibia. (b) CT-guided radiofrequency thermocoagulation of an osteoid osteoma of the distal tibia. The scan shows the electrode *in situ*.

Osteoid osteomas are usually diaphyseal in location and give rise to a dense cortical reaction (Figure 39.11). Osteoblastoma is the larger more aggressive counterpart of osteoid osteoma that commonly occurs in the spine.

Osteosarcoma (Figures 39.3 and 39.4) is most common in the distal femur, followed by proximal tibia, proximal humerus and distal tibia.

Radiologically and histologically the tumour can be sclerotic (Figure 39.3), chondroblastic, teleangiectic and other more unusual histological forms. Usually, osteosarcomas are intraosseous, but they can also arise from the surface of the bone. Paraosteal osteosarcoma (Figure 39.13) is a low grade osteosarcoma that arises from the surface of the bone. It frequently affects the distal femur and proximal tibia. The clinical symptoms are often mild and long-standing (Summary box 39.4).

Summary box 39.4

Tumours producing bone

- Osteoid osteoma – small painful; produce dense cortical reaction
- Osteoblastoma – larger and more aggressive than osteoid osteoma
- Osteosarcoma – malignant; most commonest in lower femur and upper tibia

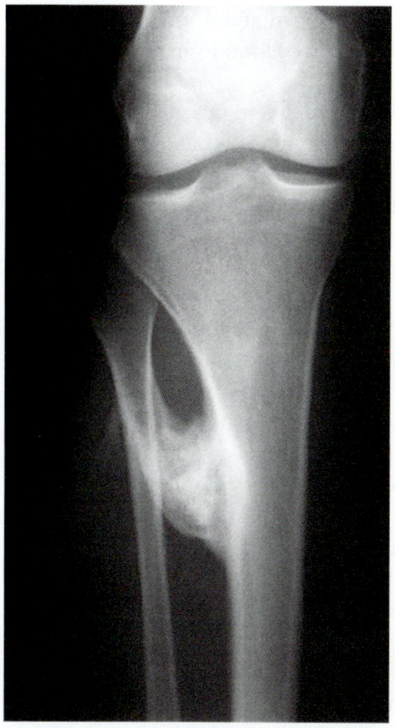

Figure 39.14 Pedunculated osteochondromas of the proximal fibula with pseudarthrosis. Osteochondromas always grow away from the physis and are in continuity with the intramedullary cavity of the bone it arises from.

CHONDROGENIC TUMOURS

These tumours produce chondroid matrix. The biological spectrum of these tumours ranges from very benign to highly malignant.

Osteochondroma (Figures 39.14 and 39.15) is a benign cartilage capped bony projection. It is thought to originate from the physis. The bony projection is always growing away from the joint; towards the diaphyseal region of the bone. It has no structures attached to it. Osteochondromas can be pedunculated or sessile. The stalk or base is always continuous with the intramedullary cavity of the bone. They are usually solitary, but can be multiple (Figure 39.16) in diaphyseal aclasia (autosomal dominant inheritance). Complications include mechanical symptoms, nerve impingement, vascular pseudoaneurysm, fracture and infarction. Increasing size or pain, particularly after skeletal maturity, is concerning and may indicate malignant

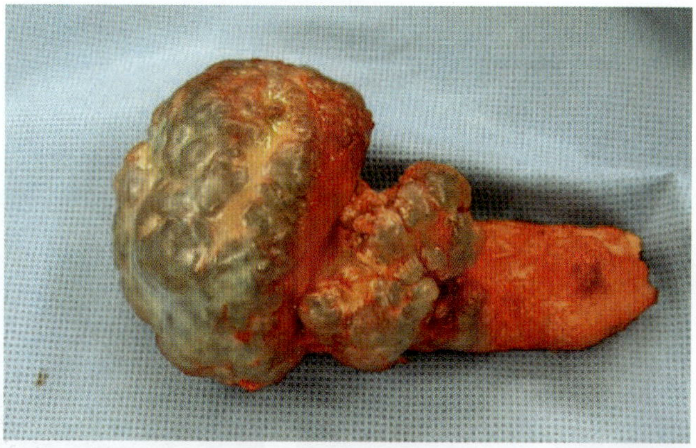

Figure 39.15 Excised pedunculated osteochondroma showing cartilage cap.

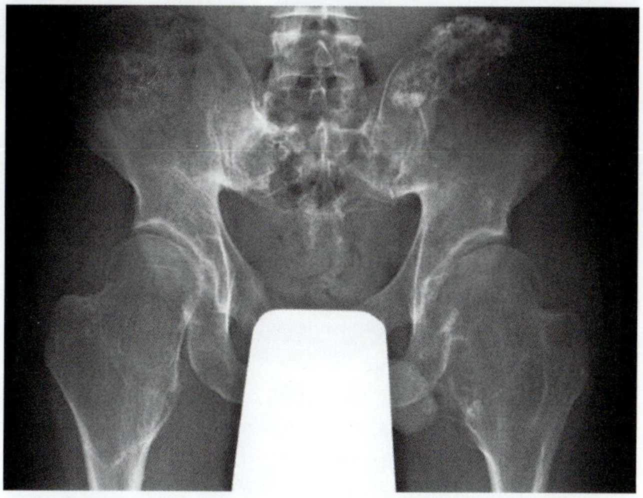

Figure 39.16 Multiple osteochondromas in diaphyseal aclasia.

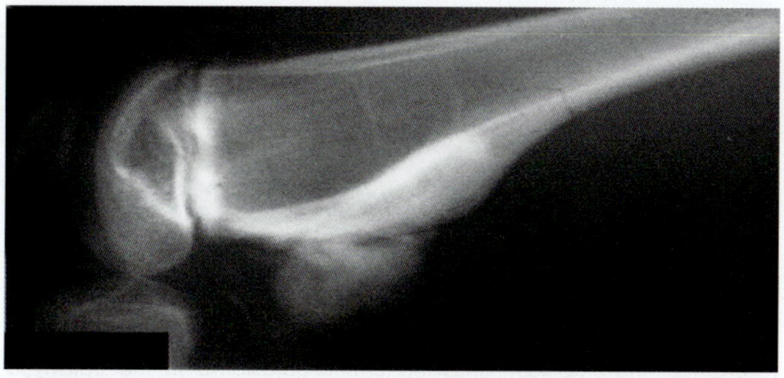

Figure 39.13 Paraosteal osteosarcoma of the distal femur in an unusually young patient. There is no continuity between the tumour and the intramedullary cavity of the femur.

transformation. The incidence of malignant transformation is less than 1 per cent in solitary osteochondromas and 1–3 per cent in diaphyseal aclasia.

Enchondroma (Figure 39.17) is a benign cartilaginous neoplasm within the intramedullary cavity of bone. Approximately 50 per cent are in the hands and feet. Enchondroma is the most common bone tumour in the hand. A large proportion of these tumours are entirely asymptomatic, and diagnosis is often incidental. They can present with pain, swelling or pathological fracture.

Patchy calcification, expansion and scalloping can be visible on the x-rays, but some are only diagnosed on magnetic resonance (MR) scan.

Ollier's disease is a developmental condition characterised by multiple enchondromas. In Maffucci syndrome, the multiple enchondromas are associated with multiple angiomas. Malignant transformation to chondrosarcoma can occur in approximately 20 per cent of patients with Ollier's disease and is almost inevitable in patients with Maffucci syndrome.

Chondroblastoma (Figure 39.18) is a benign cartilage producing tumour that occurs in the epiphysis of children. It is most common around the knee. Pain is often severe with associated inflammation and possibly joint effusion. Radiologically, there is

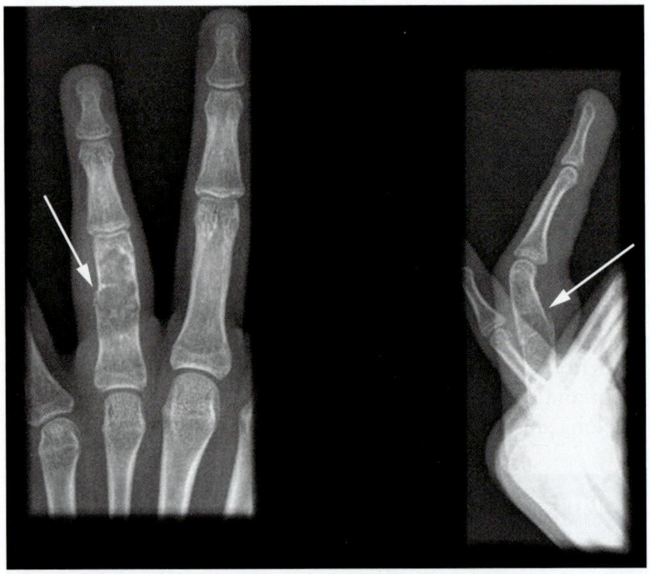

Figure 39.17 Calcification and pathological fracture in a benign enchondroma of the proximal phalanx of the ring finger.

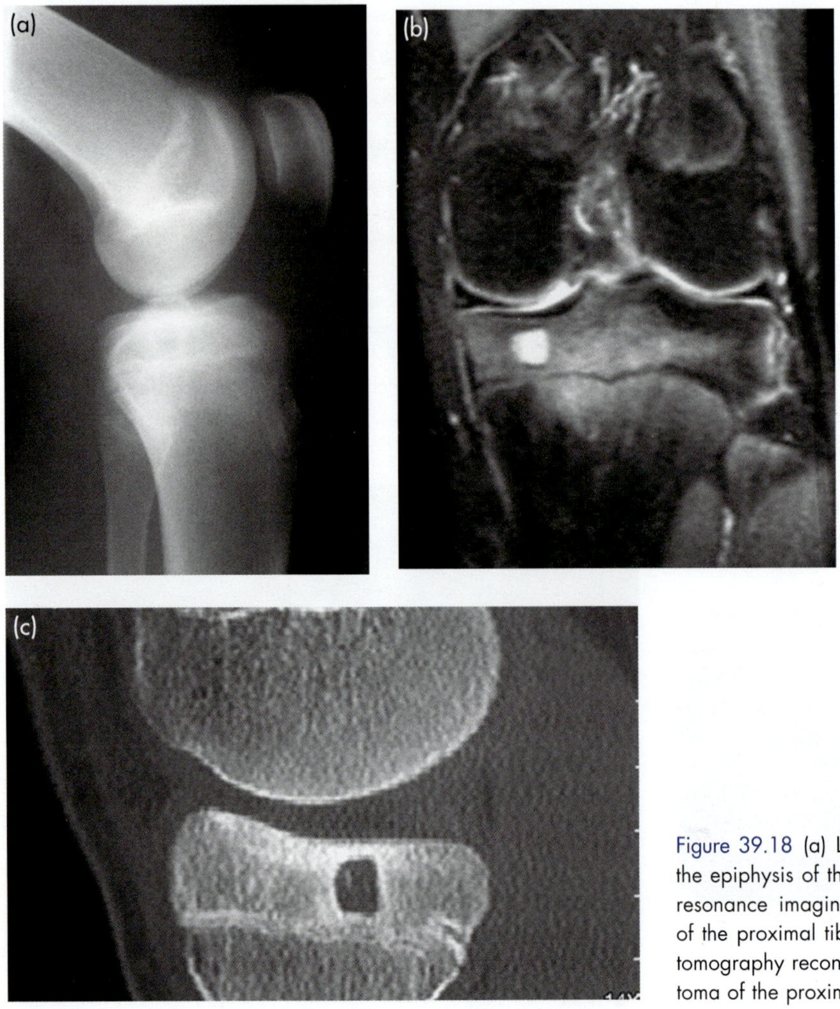

Figure 39.18 (a) Lateral x-ray with barely visible chondroblastoma in the epiphysis of the proximal tibia. (b) Coronal T2-weighted magnetic resonance imaging scan showing chondroblastoma in the epiphysis of the proximal tibia with surrounding oedema. (c) Sagittal computed tomography reconstruction showing calcification within a chondroblastoma of the proximal tibial epiphysis.

Angelo Maffucci, 1845–1903, Professor of Surgery, Lyons, France described enchondromatosis in 1899.

an often barely visible lytic lesion in the centre of the epiphysis. The diagnosis is often missed, and bone scan can aid in the localization of the lesion.

Chondrosarcoma (Figures 39.5, 39.6 and 39.7) is a malignant tumour with cartilage differentiation. The biological spectrum is very wide; it ranges from very low grade lesions to highly aggressive dedifferentiated tumours. Clinically, the presenting symptom is pain and/or swelling. Symptoms are often long-standing. Radiological and pathological correlation is particularly important in the evaluation of this condition. Clear cell chondrosarcoma is a rare form of chondrosarcoma that occurs in the epiphysis (Figure 39.19 and Summary box 39.5).

Summary box 39.5

Tumours producing cartilage

- Osteochondroma – cartilage capped; grows away from physis
- Enchondroma – inside bone; most common in hands and feet
- Chondroblastoma – in epiphyses of adolescents
- Chondrosarcoma – of varying malignancy

OTHERS

Simple bone cyst, or unicameral bone cyst (Figure 39.20), is a membrane-lined cavity filled with serous fluid. It usually occurs in proximal long bones of children.

Aneurysmal bone cyst (Figure 39.21) is a benign cystic lesion of bone consisting of blood-filled spaces separated by fibrous septa. The lesion is much more aggressive than a simple bone cyst and often presents with pain and swelling. Plain x-rays show commonly aggressive features with eccentric expansion of the cortex and an open physis. Scans often show multiple fluid levels (Figure 39.20).

Giant cell tumour of bone (Figure 39.22) is a benign aggressive tumour with large osteoclast-like giant cells. It usually occurs between the ages of 20 and 45, when the physes have closed. Giant cell tumour typically affects the epiphysis of long bones, especially around the knee, proximal humerus and distal radius.

Eosinophilic granuloma is a rare neoplasm of Langerhans cells (Figure 39.23). It can be unifocal (eosinophilic granuloma), multifocal (Hand–Schuller–Christian disease) or disseminated (Letterer–Siwe disease). There is a predilection for the skull and diaphyses of long bones. In the spine it can present with collapse, known as vertebra plana. X-rays can appear aggressive and similar to Ewing's sarcoma.

Fibrous dysplasia (Figure 39.24) is a benign fibro-osseous lesion that can be monostotic or polyostotic. It usually affects the long bones, ribs and skull. Patients can present with pain, swelling and or fracture. Hip fractures can produce a shepherd's crook deformity. Radiologically, there is often expansion and a ground glass appearance. Cysts may well be present.

Ewing's sarcoma (Figure 39.8) is a round cell sarcoma of bone. It tends to arise in the diaphyses of long bones or the pelvis. Patients usually present with a painful mass and may have general symptoms with fever, anaemia and increased erythrocyte sedimentation rate (ESR). Radiologically, the bone appears moth-eaten and may show an 'onion-skin' periosteal reaction. There is often significant inflammation with oedema on the MR scan.

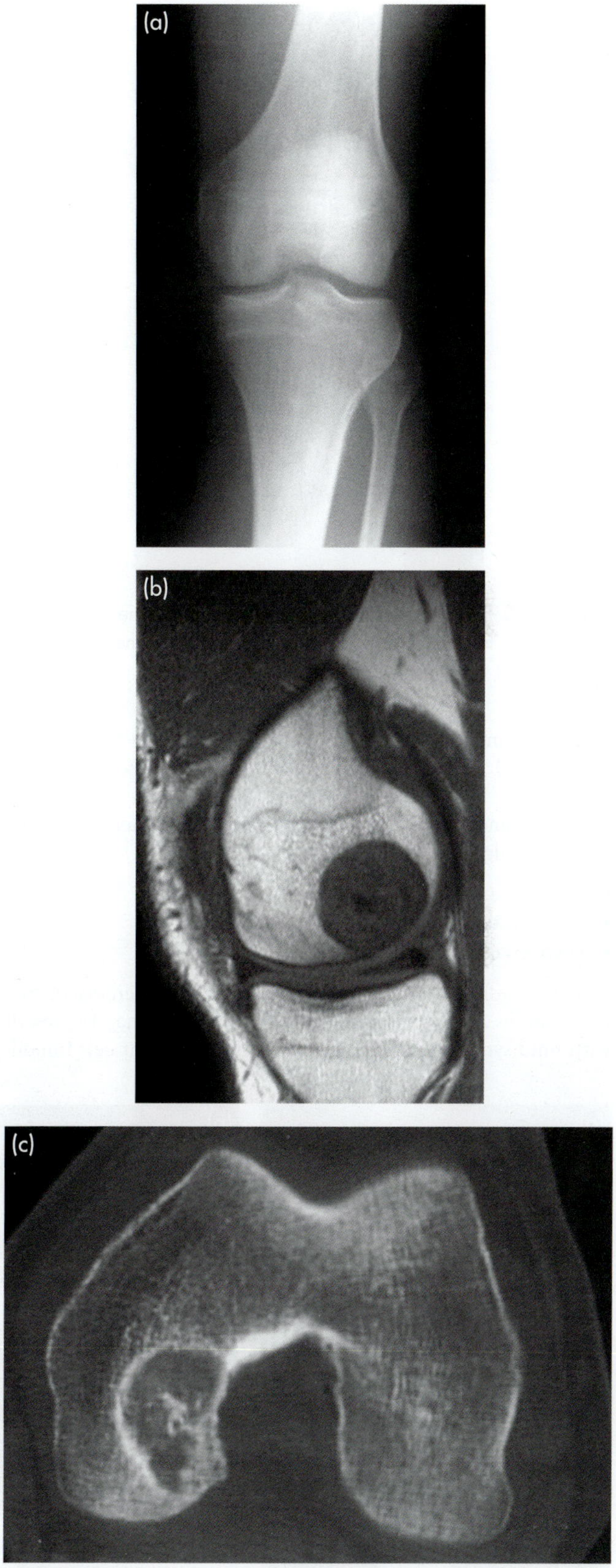

Figure 39.19 (a) Clear cell chondrosarcoma of the medial femoral condyle. (b) Sagittal T1-weighted magnetic resonance imaging scan showing clear cell chondrosarcoma in the medial femoral condyle. (c) Computed tomography scan reconstruction shows calcification within the lesion.

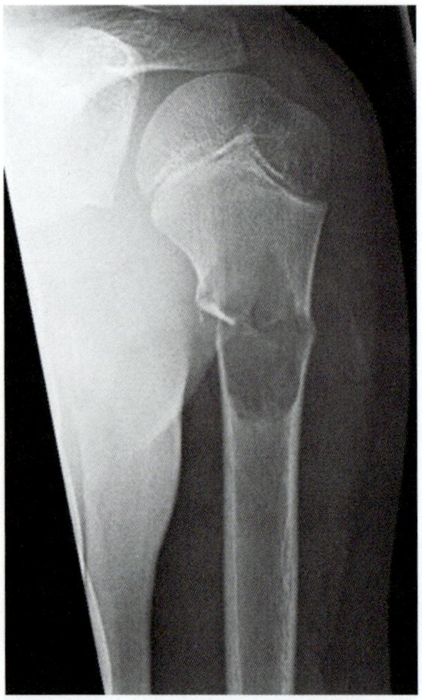

Figure 39.20 Pathological fracture through a simple bone cyst with the pathognomic fallen leaf sign. The fracture healed and the cyst consolidated without operative intervention.

Table 39.2 Classication of bone tumours by site.

Tumour and site		
Diaphyseal	Metaphyseal	Epiphyseal
Eosinophil granuloma	Most	Chondroblastoma
Osteoid osteoma		Intra-articular osteoid osteoma
Fibrous dysplasia		Giant cell tumour (physis closed)
Adamantinoma		Clear cell chondrosarcoma
Ewing's sarcoma		

Table 39.3 Common diaphyseal bone tumours according to age.

Age	Most common diaphyseal tumour
<10	Eosinophil granuloma
Teenage	Ewing's sarcoma
Adult	Lymphoma
>60	Metastasis/myeloma

Bone tumours can also be classified according to their site (Table 39.2). Epiphyseal tumours are likely to be benign (Table 39.3).

Bone tumours are usually staged using the Enneking staging system. Benign tumours are staged as:

- latent (i.e. osteochondroma);
- active (i.e. osteoid osteoma);
- aggressive (i.e. giant cell tumour).

Latent lesions are usually asymptomatic and often discovered incidentally. Active lesions, such as osteoid osteoma, do present with mild symptoms and continue to grow. A giant cell tumour is an example of an aggressive lesion. Aggressive lesions tend to grow rapidly.

For malignant tumours, the Enneking system combines stage and grade of a tumour (Table 39.4).

The compartment is the bone that is involved with the tumour. A tumour is extracompartmental when the tumour has breached the cortex of the bone as visible on plain x-rays. Most bone tumours are Enneking stage 2B at diagnosis (Summary boxes 39.6 and 39.7).

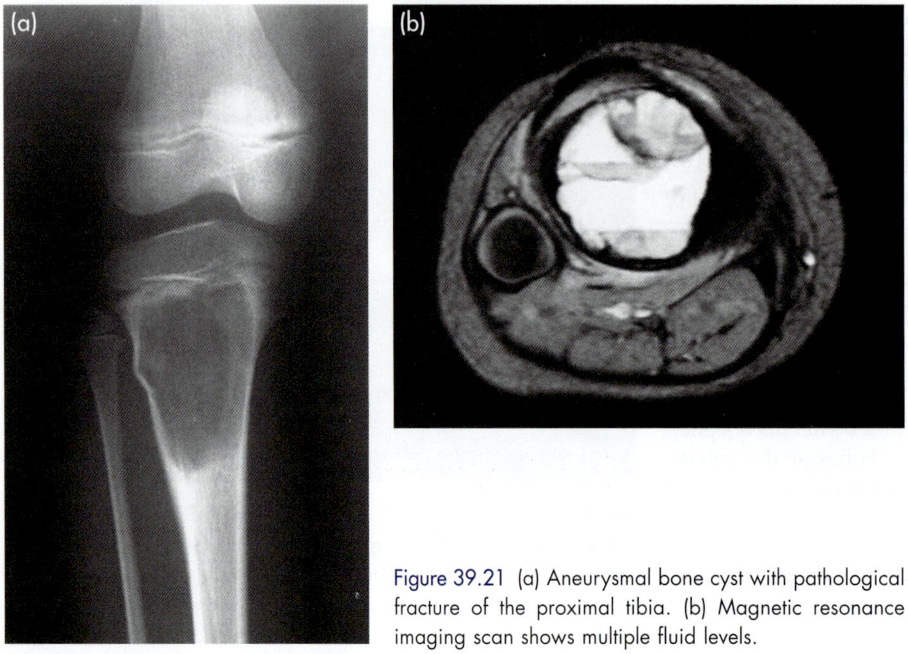

Figure 39.21 (a) Aneurysmal bone cyst with pathological fracture of the proximal tibia. (b) Magnetic resonance imaging scan shows multiple fluid levels.

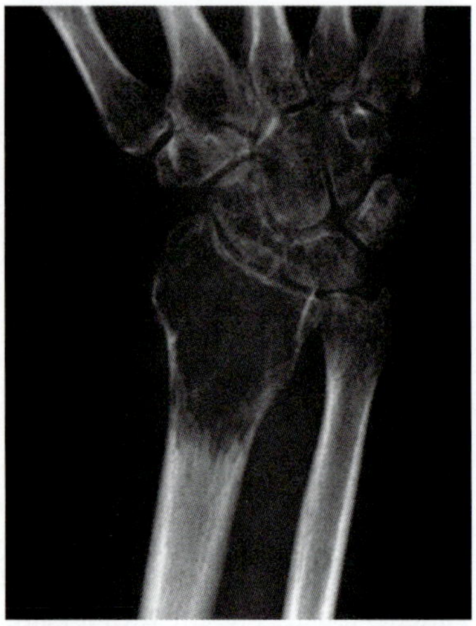

Figure 39.22 Giant cell tumour of the distal radius.

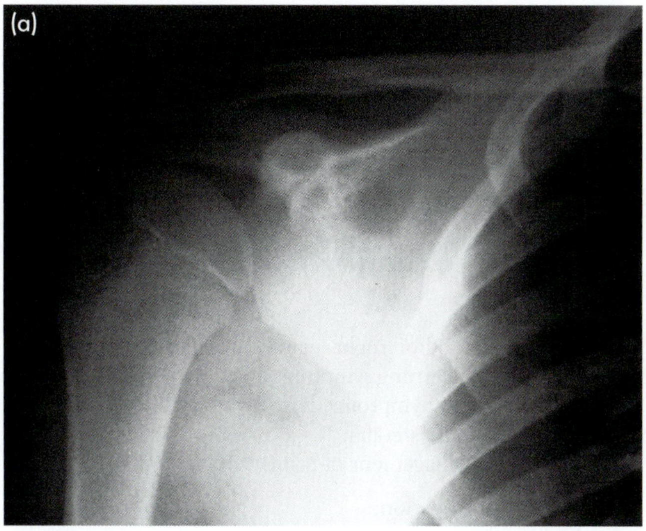

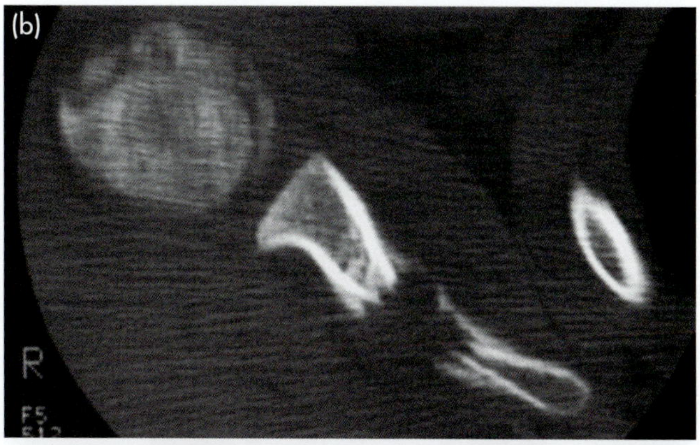

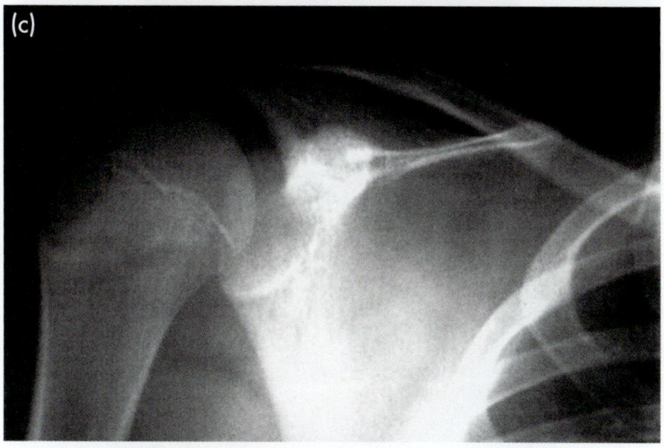

Figure 39.23 (a) Eosinophilic granuloma of the scapula. (b) Computed tomography scan shows a 'punched-out' lesion. (c) Spontaneous resolution.

Table 39.4 The Enneking staging system for bone tumours.

Enneking staging of bone tumours		
Low grade	Intra compartmental	1A
	Extra compartmental	1B
High grade	Intra comp artmental	2A
	Extra compartmental	2B
Any grade	Metastases	3

Summary box 39.6

Other bone tumours

- Simple bone cyst – proximal long bones of children
- Aneurysmal bone cyst – more aggressive, expanding
- Giant cell tumour – found in epiphyses around the knee
- Fibrous dysplasia – may be multiple; found in long bones, ribs and skull
- Ewing's – round cell sarcoma; patients may have fever and anaemia

Summary box 39.7

Warning signs – bone tumour

- Non-mechanical bone pain
- Especially around the knee in young adolescents
- Concerning x-rays

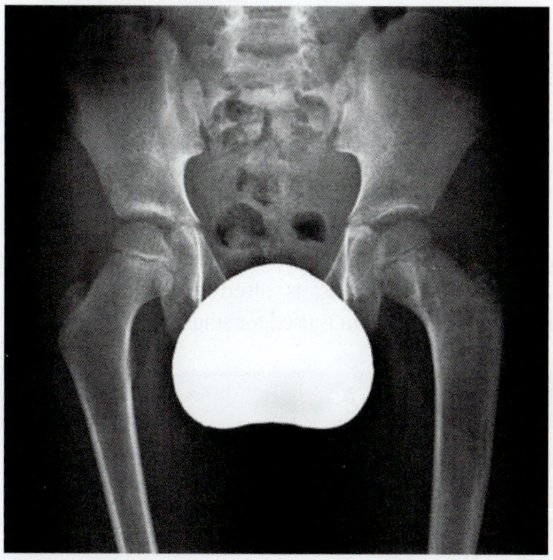

Figure 39.24 Fibrous dysplasia affecting the left proximal femur. There is expansion of the bone with a ground glass appearance.

SOFT TISSUE TUMOURS

These tumours are also classified according to the cell of origin. Most types have a benign and malignant counterpart (i.e. lipoma (Figure 39.25) and liposarcoma). The biological spectrum of these tumours is wide and full multidisciplinary assessment essential to make a correct diagnosis.

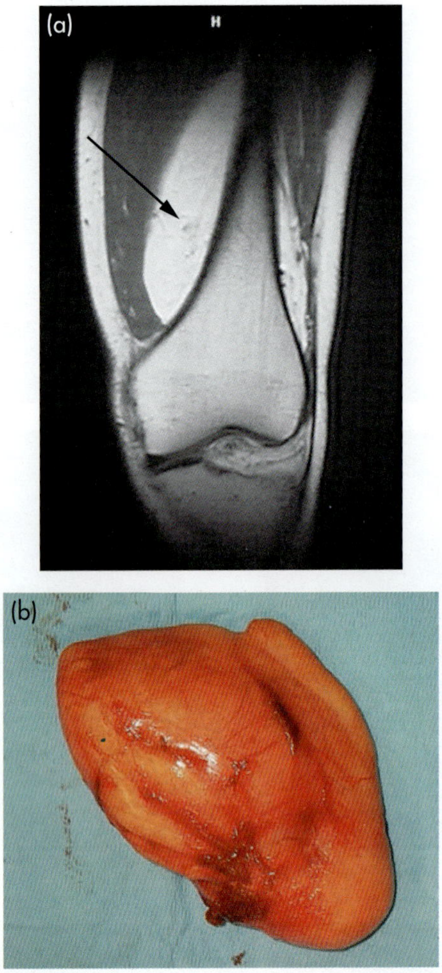

Figure 39.25 (a) Coronal T1-weighted magnetic resonance imaging scan showing a benign lipoma deep to the quadriceps muscle. (b) Excised benign lipoma.

The Trojani system, based on tumour differentiation, mitotic count and tumour necrosis, is often used to grade soft tissue tumours. The TNM system is used for staging (Summary box 39.8).

Summary box 39.8

Warning signs – soft tissue tumour

- Larger than 5 cm
- Increasing in size
- Painful
- Deep to the fascia
- Recurrence after previous excision

HISTORY AND EXAMINATION/ INVESTIGATIONS/DIAGNOSIS INCLUDING DIFFERENTIAL

In the assessment of musculoskeletal tumours, a multidisciplinary approach that allows clinical, radiological and pathological correlation is essential to establish a correct diagnosis. Treatment of primary bone and soft tissue tumours should only take place in an institution that has a full multidisciplinary team (centre of excellence).

When a musculoskeletal tumour is suspected:

- Stop
- Think
- Stage.

History and examination

Bone tumours

Non-mechanical and/or night pain, particularly in the young adolescent, are concerning symptoms and a primary bone tumour should be suspected. Symptoms that resolve with aspirin are suggestive of an osteoid osteoma.

Principles of management of primary bone tumours:

- high index of suspicion;
- early referral to a tumour centre;
- careful imaging studies;
- biopsy after completion of imaging investigations;
- minimally invasive technique for biopsy;
- multidisciplinary approach to management.

Patients with a past medical history of malignancy who present with back pain should be considered to have metastatic disease until proven otherwise. Plain x-rays of the spine and routine blood tests are the minimum that is required.

For metastatic disease of bone:

- the extent of metastases is best demonstrated on bone scan;
- prophylactic treatment of any impending fracture should be considered;
- radiotherapy and internal fixation improves pain and quality of life;
- beware the 'solitary' metastasis. This could be a primary bone tumour and full staging, including biopsy, is required.

Multiple myeloma (Figure 39.2) is the most common primary malignancy of bone in adults:

- It should be considered in all patients with back pain over 65 years of age
- Back pain with an ESR >100 mm/hour is multiple myeloma until proven otherwise
- Monoclonal gammopathy is diagnostic
- Elevated urinary and serum Bence Jones proteins are diagnostic.

Soft tissue tumours

Soft tissue swellings are common and the vast majority are benign. Symptoms and signs that suggest malignant disease are:

- pain;
- size: larger than 5 cm and/or increasing;
- position: deep to fascia;
- behaviour: recurrence after previous excision (whatever the pathology).

Each of these factors has a 25 per cent risk of malignancy.

Staging

Primary musculoskeletal tumours should be staged according to local and distant features:

Henry Bence Jones, 1813–1873, physician, St George's Hospital, London, UK.

- Local
  - Plain x-rays of the whole affected bone or soft tissue lesion (Figure 39.1);
  - MRI whole affected bone or soft tissue lesion
  - computed tomography (CT) scan;
  - ultrasound scan (for soft tissue tumours only).
- Distant
  - blood tests: including blood count, ESR, profile, calcium and myeloma screen;
  - plain x-rays of the chest;
  - CT scan of the lungs;
  - bone scan (for bone tumours only);
  - ultrasound scan abdomen (if renal metastasis is a possibility).

For bone tumours, plain film x-rays are the most informative, but appropriate scans are required for further confirmation and staging.

Imaging should always include the whole of the affected bone to look for satellite lesions and skip metastases. Satellite lesions occur within, while skip lesions occur beyond the reactive zone of the tumour.

Both primary bone sarcomas and soft tissue sarcomas commonly metastasise to the lungs and a CT scan is an essential part of the staging.

Patients who present with a lytic bone lesion could have a renal primary and an ultrasound scan of the kidneys is advised. Biopsy without this could result in unexpected massive blood loss (Summary box 39.9).

Summary box 39.9

Staging

- Plain x-ray is most informative for bone tumours
- Always image the whole bone in case of skip lesions
- CT of the lung detects lung metastases
- Lytic lesions require ultrasound abdomen to check for a renal primary

Biopsy

A biopsy is performed only when the staging process is completed. This should be carried out in the centre performing the definitive surgical procedure.

Image-guided biopsies have a higher diagnostic accuracy as areas of radiological concern can be targeted. If image-guided biopsy is performed, close discussion between radiologist and surgeon is required to ascertain that the correct biopsy route is used. It is essential that the biopsy track is excised at the time of definitive surgery (Figures 39.26 and 39.27).

Biopsies for bone tumours are usually taken using a Jamshidi needle (Figure 39.28), while Trucut needles are preferred for soft tissue tumours.

Principles of biopsy

- A tourniquet can be used; but exsanguination should be avoided as this can release tumour cells in the circulation.
- Use longitudinal incisions that are part of an extensile approach.
- Do not cross compartments.
- Biopsy track will have to be excised at the time of definitive surgery (Summary box 39.10).

Summary box 39.10

Biopsy

- Only biopsy once staging is completed
- Biopsy should be performed at the centre undertaking the main surgery
- Image-guided biopsy is more reliable
- The biopsy track must be excised at definitive surgery
- Jamshidi needles for bone, Trucut needles for soft tissues

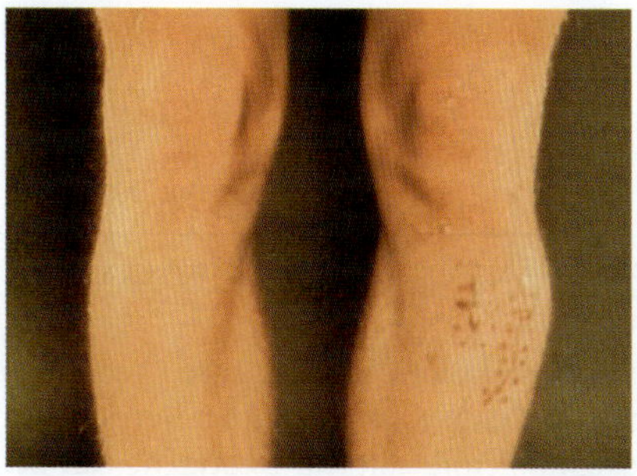

Figure 39.26 Poorly placed biopsies, making subsequent surgical excision of the track impossible.

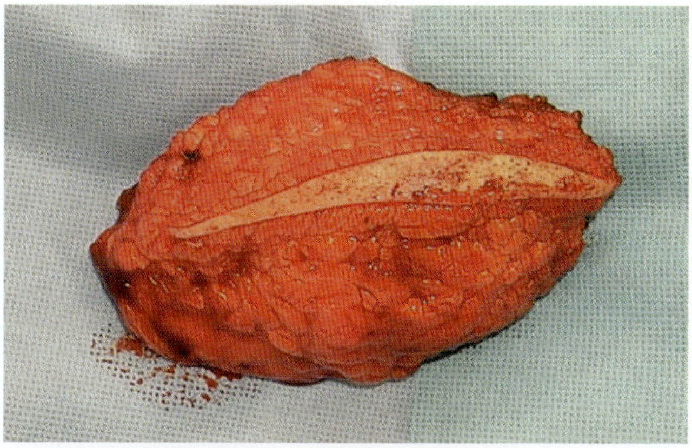

Figure 39.27 *En bloc* excised tumour and biopsy track.

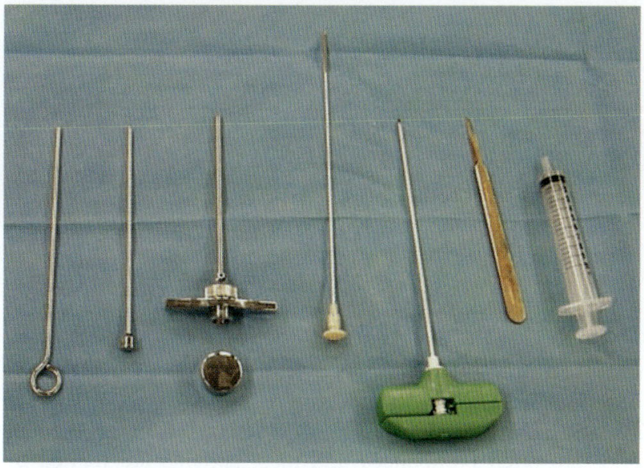

Figure 39.28 Bone biopsy instruments.

Assessment

The assessment of any bone or soft tissue lesion can be divided into three phases. The first two phases can be performed in a district general hospital, but the third phase is best carried out in a tumour treatment centre (Table 39.5).

Table 39.5 The three phases of assessment of lesions.

Phase 1 (within 24 hours)	Phase 2 (within first week)	Phase 3 (at tumour centre)
History and examination	Bone scan	CT-scan lesion
Bloods	Ultrasound scan abdomen	MRI-scan lesion
X-ray whole bone	CT-scan chest	Biopsy
Chest x-ray		

CT, computed tomography; MRI, magnetic resonance imaging.

Patients with metastatic disease often require resuscitation for electrolyte imbalance, anaemia, cardiorespiratory problems or hypercalcaemia before surgical treatment can be considered. Hypercalcaemia can be treated effectively with fluid resuscitation and pamidronates.

The risk of pathological fracture needs to be assessed. This is best assessed using the Mirel score (Table 39.6).

Table 39.6 The Mirels scoring system for risk of pathological fracture.

	Score		
	1	2	3
Site	Upper limb	Lower limb	Peritrochanter
Pain	Mild	Moderate	Functional
Size	<1/3	1/3–2/3	>2/3
Lesion	Blastic	Mixed	Lytic

Score >8, high risk of fracture – urgent prophylactic treatment needed; score <7, low risk of fracture – stabilization of the bone not immediately needed.

TREATMENT/PROGNOSIS/ COMPLICATIONS

Primary bone tumours

Most latent and active benign bone tumours are treated by intralesional curettage. Packing of the cavity with graft of bone substitutes is usually not required.

Simple bone cysts can heal following pathological fracture and an initial observant approach following fracture is best. If the cyst persists following union of the fracture, a variety of treatments including injection with steroid or bone marrow and surgical curettage have been described.

Osteoid osteomas can resolve spontaneously. However, symptoms are often pronounced and most patients are treated by CT-guided thermocoagulation.

Large or more rapidly growing benign bone tumours might require more extensive surgical excision and reconstruction.

Malignant primary bone tumours require a more aggressive approach. Osteosarcoma and Ewing's sarcoma are treated with neoadjuvant chemotherapy and surgery. Chondrosarcomas are not sensitive to chemotherapy or radiotherapy and treatment is surgical.

The surgical options for malignant primary bone tumours are:

- amputation or van Ness rotationplasty;
- excision alone (for dispensable bones);
- excision and replacement with graft or prosthesis.

If surgery excision is undertaken it is important for the biopsy track to be excised 'en bloc' with the surgical specimen to avoid local recurrence through the biopsy track.

Following excision the resection margins can be classed as in Table 39.7.

In most cases, limb salvage with excision and reconstruction is possible (Figure 39.29). Only a minority of cases have neurovascular invasion and require amputation. Limb salvage, as compared to amputation, has a slightly higher rate of local recurrence. However, no difference in overall survival has been demonstrated (Summary boxes 39.11 and 39.12).

Table 39.7 Classification of surgical resection margins.

Surgical margins	
Intralesional	Resection through the lesion
Marginal	Resection through the reactive zone of the tumour
Wide	Resection outside the reactive zone of the tumour
Radical	Excising the whole affected compartment

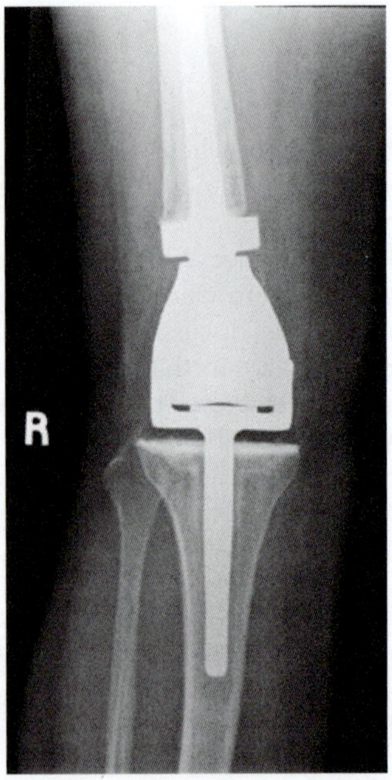

Figure 39.29 Endoprosthetic replacement of the distal femur.

en bloc is French for 'in a block'.

Summary box 39.11

Treatment – benign bone tumours

- Benign lesions can be simply curetted
- CT-guided thermocoagulation is used for osteoid osteoma
- Large benign tumours may require reconstruction

Summary box 39.12

Treatment – malignant bone tumours

- Osteosarcomas and Ewing's sarcoma require neoadjuvant chemotherapy
- Chondrosarcomas are insensitive to radiotherapy or chemotherapy
- Most malignant tumours can be treated with limb salvage
- There is no difference in survival between amputation and limb salvage

Metastatic bone tumours

Surgical treatment in patients with metastatic bone disease is palliative. This should be kept in mind when planning treatment. Surgery is unable to lengthen life in patients with metastatic bone disease, but can shorten it.

Spinal surgery may be required for stabilisation of the spine and/or decompression of patients with (impending) cord compression.

Surgery in the peripheral skeleton is mainly for treatment of (impending) pathological fracture.

Renal metastases tend to be very vascular and massive blood loss can be encountered during surgery. Therefore, preoperative embolisation should be considered just before surgery to prevent blood loss (Figure 39.30).

Treatment of myeloma is mainly haematological. Surgical treatment is only required for complications such as fracture and spinal cord compression. Solitary plasmacytoma is an exception and surgical excision is usually advised.

Patients with a previous history of malignancy may present with a (solitary) bony lesion or pathological fracture. It should not be assumed that this is a metastatic lesion. Prior to planning surgical treatment it is important to ascertain the diagnosis is correct. Staging including biopsy will be required to exclude a malignant primary bone tumour.

Prior to planning surgical treatment for patients with metastatic bone disease it is important to have an assessment of:

- survival
  - prognosis of the primary tumour (Figure 39.31)
- quality of life
- medical fitness
- biomechanical/risk of fracture
- single or multiple bone lesions
- response to adjuvant treatment such as radiotherapy and hormonal treatment
- radiotherapy can be administered pre- or postoperatively.

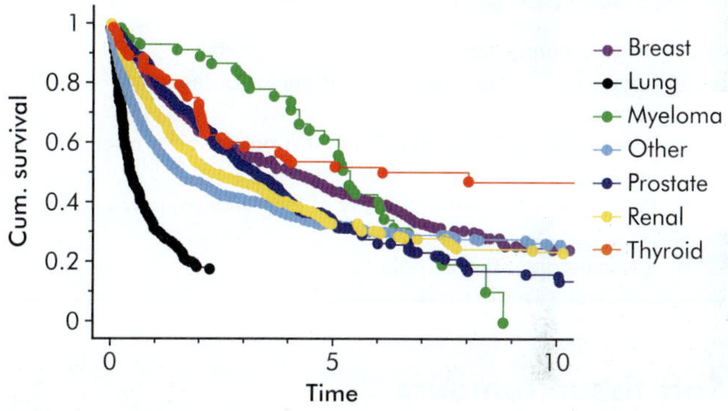

Figure 39.31 Survival curves of patients who present with bony metastasis.

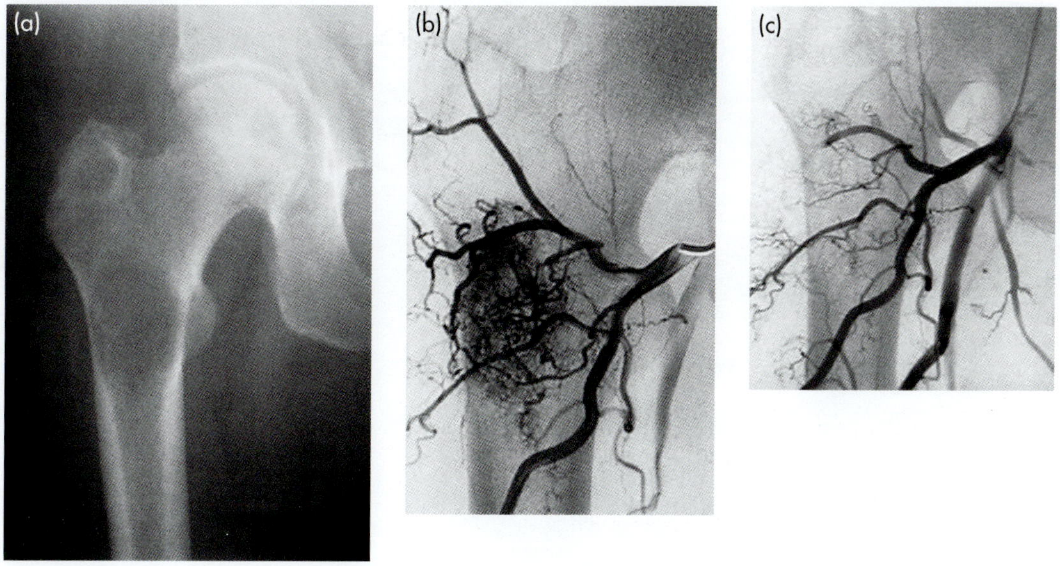

Figure 39.30 (a) Lytic metastasis of renal cell carcinoma. (b) Angiogram shows increased vascularity. (c) Following embolisation.

It is difficult to give strict guidelines for the surgical management of patients with metastatic bone disease. However, when a prolonged disease-free interval is expected, prosthetic replacement is usually preferred to intramedullary nailing. Particularly in patients with a longer life expectancy, a high failure rate is associated with internal fixation of pathological fractures.

Prior to surgical treatment it is essential to stabilise the patient's medical condition. Pamidronates can have a dramatic effect and might make surgery unnecessary.

Epiphyseal and metaphyseal lesions are best treated with prosthetic replacement; while diaphyseal lesions are usually best treated with an intramedullary nail. In the shoulder, prosthetic replacements have a poor function and internal fixation usually gives the best results. However, in hip lesions the best treatment usually is joint replacement.

Solitary breast and renal metastases can have a prolonged disease-free survival so excision and replacement rather than fixation should be the treatment of choice (Summary box 39.13).

Summary box 39.13

Treatment of bone metastases

- Surgery cannot lengthen life but may shorten it
- Spines may need stabilising and nerves or the cord decompressing
- Long bones will need stabilising if a pathological fracture is imminent
- Patients who have a possibility of long survival may need a prosthesis
- Radiotherapy relieves pain

Soft tissue tumours

Malignant soft tissue tumours are preferably excised with as wide a margin as possible. As in bone tumours, it is important for the biopsy track to be excised *en bloc* with the surgical specimen (Figure 39.27). The skin might require reconstruction with a split skin graft or skin flap. In general, skin flaps are preferred as they allow for early administration of radiotherapy. Following surgical excision of high grade soft tissue sarcomas, adjuvant radiotherapy should be considered. Preoperative radiotherapy can also have good results, but there is a risk of wound healing problems following surgery. Chemotherapy has a limited role in the treatment of soft tissue sarcomas.

ACKNOWLEDGEMENTS

Parts of this chapter were previously published in the 24th edition of this book under the title Diseases of Bones and Joints, written by Tony Berendt and Martin McNally. Their material has been added to and updated by the new authors. Diagrams have been drawn from sketches by Mr Andy Biggs, RJAH Orthopaedic Hospital, Oswestry.

FURTHER READING

Cool P, Grimer R. Pathological fractures of the extremities. *Trauma* 2000; **2**: 101–11.

Cool P, Grimer R, Rees R. Surveillance in patients with sarcoma of the extremities. *Eur J Surg Oncol* 2005; **31**: 1020–4.

Enneking WF, Spanier SS, Goodman MA. A system for the surgical staging of musculoskeletal sarcoma. *Clin Orthop Relat Res* 1980; **153**: 106–20.

Fletcher CDM, Unni KK, Mertens F (eds). *World Health Organisation classification of tumours. Pathology and genetics tumours of soft tissue and bone.* IARC Press: Lyon, 2002.

Mankin HJ, Lange TA, Spanier SS. The hazards of biopsy in patients with malignant primary bone and soft tissue tumors. *J Bone Joint Surg* 1982; **64-A**: 1121–7.

Mirels H. Metastatic disease in long bones. *Clin Orthop* 1989: **249**: 256–64.

Wedin R, Bauer HC. Surgical treatment of skeletal metastatic lesions of the proximal femur: endoprosthesis or reconstruction nail? *J Bone Joint Surg Br* 2005; **87**: 1653–7.

CHAPTER

40 Infection of the bones and joints

LEARNING OBJECTIVES

To understand:
- Characteristic features in the history and examination of infection of bone and joint
- Treatment of infection of bone and joint

INTRODUCTION

Osteomyelitis is an old disease, identified in dinosaur bones, early hominids and skeletons from ancient civilisations. It can present acutely with major systemic upset, local inflammation and purulence, or insidiously, with gradual bone destruction, variable symptoms and prolonged chronicity.

The pattern of bone infection is changing. Worldwide, childhood acute haematogenous osteomyelitis and septic arthritis are common, with chronic disease following inadequate initial management. In the developed world, bone infection is now mostly seen after injury or surgery (contiguous focus osteomyelitis) and is often implant-related (Figure 40.1). The high number of patients with comorbidities (diabetes, peripheral vascular disease, immunocompromise), more frequent bone and joint surgery and longer population survival have produced a group of patients with increased susceptibility to infection. The incidence of bone and joint infection is likely to increase in the future.

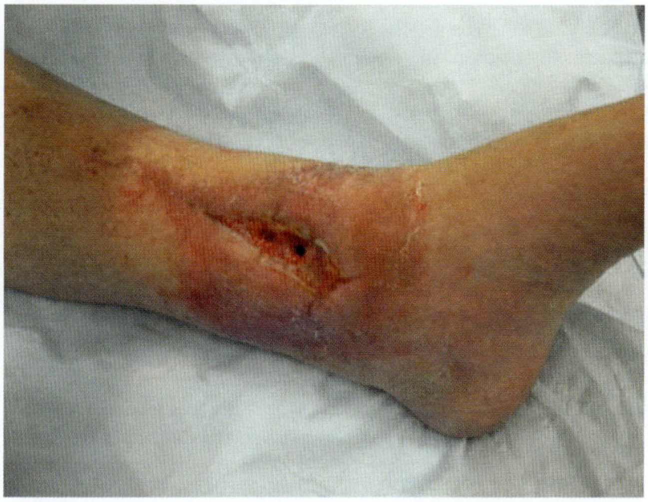

Figure 40.1 Osteomyelitis of the distal tibia after a fracture with sinus formation and surrounding skin infection.

General principles: pathology

Acute osteomyelitis occurs when pathogenic bacteria cause inflammation in the bone and surrounding tissues. The medullary bone may form abscesses and the infection may track through the cortex to form periosteal elevation and soft-tissue extension. This process will devascularise the bone causing bone death which is the characteristic feature of chronic osteomyelitis (Summary box 40.1).

Summary box 40.1

Epidemiology of bone infection

- Bone and joint infections from haematogenous spread are now less common
- The increased use of implants for joint replacement and fracture fixation are a new source
- Immunocompromised patients, e.g. diabetes are another increasing source

Many bacteria can adhere to dead bone or implant surfaces, forming a complex community enveloped in a polysaccharide matrix, known as a biofilm. These bacteria alter their metabolic state, becoming resistant to the host immune system and to antibiotics.

The infected bone reacts to the infection by separating off dead fragments of bone (sequestration) and forming sinuses to drain pus and discharge small bone fragments. New bone is laid down around the infection from the periosteum (involucrum) (Figure 40.2).

In septic arthritis, infection may follow direct ingress of bacteria after injury or surgery, or may result from discharge of an adjacent acute osteomyelitis into the joint. In neonates or the elderly, bacteraemia may infect a previously normal joint. Toxins and lytic enzymes from bacteria cause early damage to articular cartilage (Summary box 40.2).

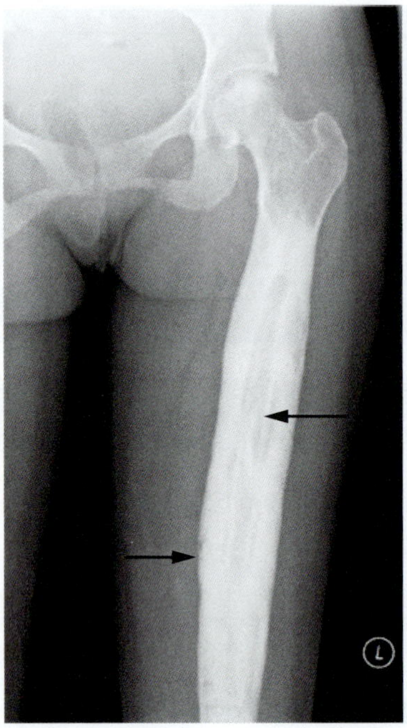

Figure 40.2 X-ray of chronic infection of the femur with a large central sequestrum and well-developed involucrum.

Summary box 40.2

Pathology of bone infection

- Bacteria infecting bone form a protective bio-film
- Infected bone dies and forms a sequestrum
- The periosteum around lays down new bone – an involucrum

General principles: microbiology

Virulent Gram-positive organisms, particularly *Staphylococcus aureus*, are the most common cause of bone or joint infection in native tissue. However, once prosthetic material is implanted, a wide range of organisms can be involved. This includes organisms with low virulence that are usually considered skin commensals, such as coagulase-negative staphylococci and propionibacteria (Table 40.1).

General principles: diagnosis

Clinical

Diagnosis is predominantly clinical with confirmation using other diagnostic tests.

Table 40.1 Organisms most commonly involved in bone and joint infection.

Gram-positive	*Staphylococcus aureus* (most common across all settings)	
	Coagulase-negative staphylococci (in implant-associated infections)	
	Streptococci	*Strep. pneumonia*
		Beta-haemolytic streptococci
		Strep. viridans (in implant-associated infection)
Gram-negative	Enterobacteriaceae	*Escherichia coli* (especially at extremes of age)
		Klebsiella species
		Salmonella species (associated with sickle cell disease)
	Pseudomonas species	
	Haemophilus species	*H. influenzae* (consider in non-immunised children)
	Neisseria species	*N. meningitides*
		N. gonorrhoeae (consider risk factors for sexually transmitted infection)
Others	Anaerobes	
	Fungi	(cause infection in immunocompromised hosts)
	Mycobacteria	*Mycobacterium tuberculosis*
		Atypical mycobacteria
Mixed	Any combination of the above	
'Culture negative'	No growth from cultures, but diagnosis of infection made on clinical/radiological/histopathological grounds	

Biomarkers

Raised inflammatory markers (erythrocyte sedimentation rate (ESR), C-reactive protein (CRP) and white cell count (WCC)) are characteristic of acute infection, but they are neither sensitive nor specific. These tests cannot rule in or rule out infection.

Imaging

Plain x-rays can only detect extensive bone loss, and cannot be relied on, especially in early disease. Plain x-rays are useful in evaluating implant loosening and progression of chronic disease.

Ultrasonography is ideal for identifying soft-tissue collections and can be used to guide bone biopsy and aspiration.

Computed tomography (CT) scans are helpful in assessing bone union of infected fractures. Small sequestra and cortical erosions are best seen with CT (Figure 40.3a).

Isotope bone scans are of very limited value as they are non-specific.

Magnetic resonance imaging (MRI) is the investigation of choice. It is highly sensitive and specific, showing all components of the disease (Figure 40.3b) (Summary box 40.3).

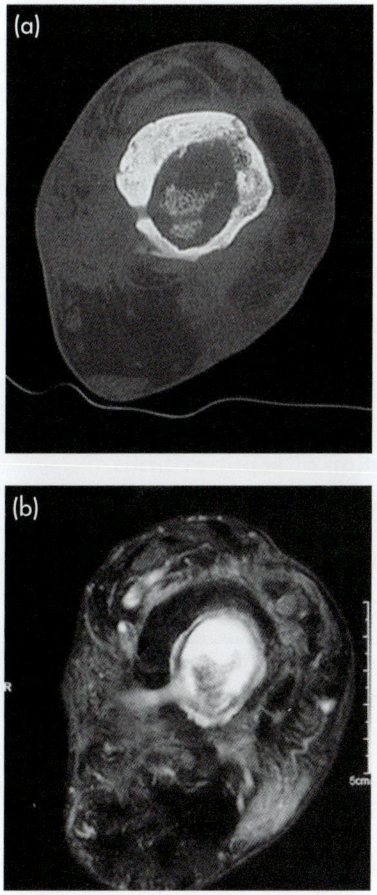

Figure 40.3 (a) Transverse computed tomography (CT) scan of femur with central sequestrum, sinus and cortical bone erosion. (b) Magnetic resonance imaging (MRI) scan of the same femur with better resolution of medullary infection and soft-tissue involvement.

Summary box 40.3

Investigations in bone infection

- ESR and CRP are neither sensitive nor specific in making a diagnosis of bone infection
- X-ray can only identify major bone loss
- Ultrasound is valuable for identifying collections of pus
- MRI is the investigation of choice in bone infection

Tissue sampling

Superficial samples and swabs from wounds or spontaneously draining pus are unreliable, since the organisms colonising the surface may bear no relation to those causing the invasive infection in the deeper tissues and bone. Microbiological samples may be falsely negative if antibiotics are given first. The histological diagnosis of infection (rather than other sources of inflammation) depends on identifying a neutrophilic infiltrate. However, such an infiltrate may be patchy and so histological studies are incompletely sensitive. Synovial tissue samples are particularly important in producing a higher diagnostic yield for infection with mycobacteria or fungi.

In complex infections, particularly those involving prosthetic material, multiple biopsy samples are needed to help determine whether organisms such as coagulase-negative staphylococci are likely to be the causative pathogens, or whether they are simply contaminants from the skin. This distinction cannot be made on a single sample, but the growth of an indistinguishable organism from three or more culture samples is 94 per cent specific for infection (Summary box 40.4).

Summary box 40.4

Identifying the organism in osteomyelitis

- Superficial swabs are of no value in identifying the organism involved
- If the patient is on antibiotics specimens may give a false negative
- A neutrophil infiltrate on histology is diagnostic of infection
- Multiple biopsy specimens are needed for reliable diagnosis

General principles: surgical management

Successful surgical treatment relies on the delivery of a few basic principles. These are:

- Preoperative
  - Patient assessment and clinical staging of disease
  - Full discussion of all treatment options with potential complications
  - Diagnostic tests for general health
  - Optimisation of patients and treatment of comorbidities
- Operative
  - Exposure for multiple, deep bone sampling
  - Excision of all affected tissue
  - Intravenous antibiotics after sampling
  - Bone stabilisation, if necessary
  - Dead space management
  - Soft-tissue cover which may include plastic surgery

- Postoperative
  - Functional rehabilitation
  - Continued antimicrobial therapy guided by culture results

General principles: antibiotic choice

If possible, patients should stop antibiotics 2 weeks before biopsy or surgery.

It is essential that patients with septic shock receive prompt empiric antibiotic therapy. However, whenever possible antibiotics should be delayed until microbiological samples have been taken (especially when prosthetic material is involved). When delay would be unsafe, blood cultures, local aspiration of pus or radiologically guided biopsy may give valuable culture material prior to starting antibiotics (Summary box 40.5).

Summary box 40.5

Treatment of osteomyelitis

- Septic shock needs treatment without delay with antibiotics chosen empirically
- Otherwise the start of antibiotics should be delayed until specimens have been taken
- In elective surgery for osteomyelitis antibiotics should be stopped 2 weeks in advance

Local guidelines should be followed, but in general hospitals recommend a 'community acquired' level of cover using agents such as co-amoxiclav. Antibiotics to cover resistant Gram-positive organisms (e.g. vancomycin for MRSA) are considered if there has been prior hospital exposure, and antibiotics to cover resistant Gram-negatives (e.g. meropenem for Pseudomonas) are considered in settings such as severe diabetic foot infection. Prolonged intravenous antibiotic courses (i.e. 4–6 weeks of treatment) are usually recommended for bone infection, but there is little evidence to support this (Summary box 40.6).

Summary box 40.6

Antibiotics in osteomyelitis

- Follow local guidelines
- Amoxiclav is good for community-acquired infections
- Vancomycin is better for hospital-acquired MRSA
- Meropenem may be needed for Pseudomonas

NATIVE JOINT SEPTIC ARTHRITIS

Epidemiology

Bacterial infection of native joints occurs at an estimated incidence of 4–10 per 100 000 population per year in Western Europe, with higher rates in association with socioeconomic deprivation and in developing countries. The condition most characteristically affects patients at extremes of age, and in the context of an underlying joint abnormality or immunocompromise (see Summary box 40.7).

Summary box 40.7

Risk factors for septic arthritis

- Extremes of age
- Underlying joint abnormality, especially rheumatoid arthritis
- Immunocompromise (e.g. diabetes mellitus, HIV infection, immunosuppressive therapy)
- Joint instrumentation (e.g. steroid injection, arthroscopy)
- Intravenous drug abuse
- Indwelling central venous catheter
- Bacteraemia (especially *Staphylococcus aureus*)

Clinical features

Most patients present with an acute or subacute history of a single hot, swollen, painful joint. The joint is held immobile in the 'position of comfort', and there is severe pain if any attempt is made to move the affected joint actively or passively. In children and adults, the knee joint is most frequently affected; in neonates, the hip. Fever and other systemic signs are usually present, but their absence does not rule out the diagnosis, especially in adults where there may be no fever or only a low grade one.

Diagnosis

Aspiration and/or biopsy of intra-articular fluid or tissue will allow a Gram stain to be performed (although this is positive in only about one-third of infected cases), and then culture of a causative organism (positive in 80–90 per cent). However, results are delayed by the time taken to grow and identify the organism in the laboratory. The number of white cells seen is not diagnostic of sepsis, and crystals may be seen in infected joints as well as gout or pseudo-gout. The delay in obtaining a positive culture result, and the limited sensitivity and specificity of direct microscopy and Gram stain, should not delay early treatment for the infection. The decision to perform a surgical washout and give antibiotics should be based on the clinical picture (Summary box 40.8).

Summary box 40.8

Presentation of septic arthritis

- Children may be toxic and febrile but adults may only have a low-grade fever
- The joint is swollen and held in a characteristic position of comfort
- Any movement causes extreme pain

Management

Medical management

Antibiotics are usually given for 3–6 weeks (of which the first 2 weeks are commonly given intravenously).

Surgical management

Medical treatment alone is rarely indicated in joint sepsis. Prompt surgical drainage is a priority in order to avoid further damage to the joint (Figure 40.4a,b) In general, open washout is preferred to arthroscopic washout, depending on the joint involved. Chronic sepsis may lead to destruction of the joint and

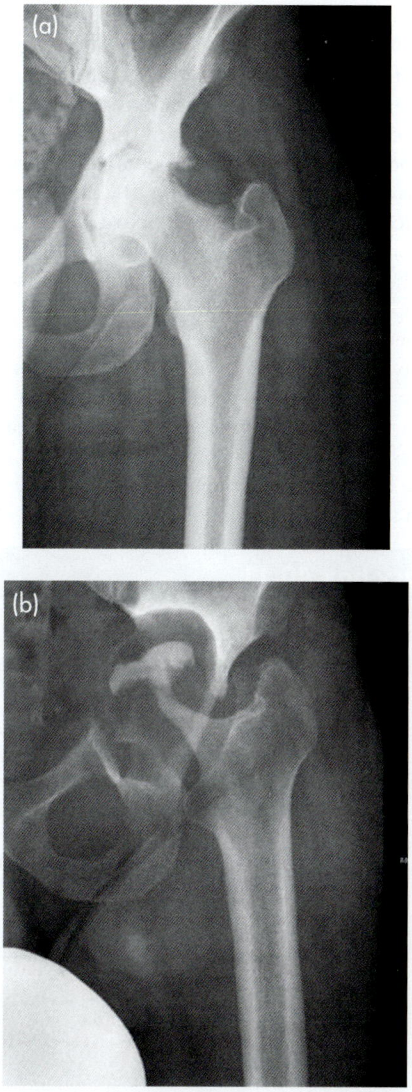

Figure 40.4 (a) Septic arthritis of the hip in an intravenous drug user. This was untreated for several weeks resulting in destruction of the joint surface. (b) The same hip after nine months without treatment. The proximal femur and acetabulum have been grossly eroded by infection.

excision arthroplasty may be required. Subsequent joint replacement or fusion should only be considered when the infection has been completely cleared (Summary box 40.9).

IMPLANT-RELATED INFECTION

Epidemiology

The incidence of prosthetic joint infection in the UK is now <1 per cent per joint per year, with hips at slightly higher risk than knees. These rates appear to have fallen with improved operative practice and the recent introduction of surgical 'care bundles'. Risk factors include obesity, skin disease, comorbidity, prolonged or complicated surgery, revision surgery, fracture and postoperative wound infections.

Infection may follow internal fixation in up to 25 per cent of open tibial fractures.

Summary box 40.9

Native joint septic arthritis

- Most common at extremes of age, in patients with rheumatoid arthritis, and in association with immunocompromise
- Most commonly affects hips in neonates, and knees in adults and children
- Commonest pathogen is *Staphylococcus aureus*
- Joints should be aspirated for microbiology before starting antibiotics
- Management is prompt joint washout, followed by 3–6 weeks of antibiotics
- Gram stains are poorly predictive of infection and should not delay surgery.

Clinical features

Prosthetic joint infection may present with a discharging wound, cellulitis, pain, inflammation and swelling. Late infections are more likely to present with an indolent clinical syndrome of joint discomfort or mechanical dysfunction ('start-up' symptoms are particularly characteristic), with or without a discharging sinus. These presentations have led some to classify prosthetic joint infection into early (<3 months after implantation), intermediate (3–12 months) or chronic (>12 months).

Diagnosis

Plain radiographs may show features of loosening of a chronically infected prosthesis, and ultrasound may identify associated collections.

Multiple surgical specimens should be sent for culture (see 'General principles: diagnosis'), and it is most convenient to obtain these at the time of revision surgery or open debridement (Summary box 40.10).

Summary box 40.10

Implant-related septic arthritis

- The incidence in good units after joint replacement is now below 1 per cent
- Incidence after internal fixation of open tibial fractures remains as high as 25 per cent
- Late infection may present with low-grade symptoms (grumbling pain and start-up stiffness)
- X-rays may show lucency around the implant
- Multiple specimens need to be taken at surgery for reliable diagnosis

Management

A multidisciplinary approach is required, including orthopaedics, plastic surgery, infectious diseases, associated healthcare professionals, and, not least, the patient's understanding and views regarding their condition.

The choice of management strategy can be categorised as:

- salvage of an infected implant or
- removal of the infected implant with or without reimplantation.

Some groups have used the timing of presentation to determine this (i.e. salvage for early infection, but removal and revision for late infection). Others regard any firmly fixed implant as potentially salvageable, irrespective of the timing (and there are now several case series suggesting that this is feasible). However, it is agreed that loose infected implants should always be removed (Figure 40.5a,b) Furthermore, it is essential to achieve soft-tissue cover of bone and prosthetic material. This may be difficult around the knee, requiring local muscle flaps and the involvement of a plastic surgical team.

Management options can be divided into the following broad approaches:

- Debridement, antibiotics and implant retention (DAIR): can only be undertaken if the prosthesis is well-fixed. The surrounding infected soft tissue and bone must be fully excised and modular components exchanged. This cannot be achieved by arthroscopic surgery. Good soft-tissue cover is essential. Following debridement, the patient is treated with long-term antibiotics (frequently 6 weeks of intravenous therapy followed by six months or more of oral suppression).
- Two-stage joint revision surgery: a thorough excision is undertaken and all cement and loose foreign material is removed. An antibiotic-impregnated spacer may be implanted (which may be articulating). This is a temporary measure and cannot withstand full weight-bearing. The patient is treated with oral or intravenous antibiotics, most commonly for 6 weeks. A new prosthesis is implanted after the course of antibiotics has been completed. Re-revision surgery for infection has a higher failure rate than a first revision, and so early referral to a specialist centre should be considered.
- Single-stage joint revision surgery: the procedure is the same as above, but removal and reimplantation are undertaken in the same operating session. Some centres consider single-stage revisions when less florid signs of infection are present (i.e. absence of collections or sinus tracts), or for frail patients for whom the risk of a second operation is higher. There are no trial data comparing outcomes with the two-stage approach.
- Joint removal or fusion: for patients who have intolerable symptoms (either pain, or profuse discharge), but for whom the surgical strategies outlined above are technically not possible or are ruled out by comorbid conditions, removal of the prosthesis without reimplantation may palliate symptoms. An example is the Girdlestone hip arthroplasty. Amputation may be necessary for knee or ankle implants.
- Suppressive therapy with antibiotics: in patients who are not medically fit for any operative intervention, or who choose to decline all surgical options, long-term treatment with antibiotics may help to suppress the symptoms of infection. There are limited data, but anecdotally the success rate of this approach seems low (Summary box 40.11).

Summary box 40.11

Prosthetic joint infection

- Well-fixed prostheses may be debrided and retained
- Loose prostheses must be removed
- Replacement can be made at the initial surgery (one stage) or after a delay to allow infection to be eradicated with a course of antibiotics (two stage)
- Multiple surgical samples are crucial for identifying a pathogen
- Thorough excision of infected tissue is a key determinant of outcome
- Long-term antibiotics may be used for patients who are not suitable for major revision surgery

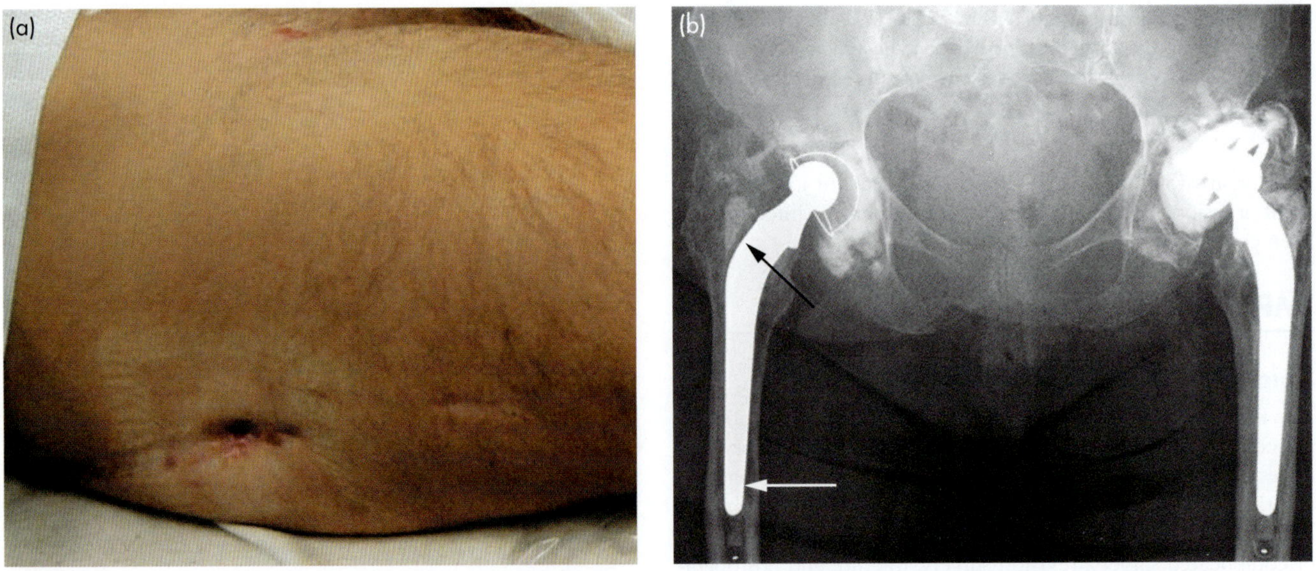

Figure 40.5 (a) Sinus draining from the scar over the lateral side of the hip. This patient had a total hip replacement 14 years before which had been complicated by a wound haematoma and infection. (b) X-ray of both hips of the same patient. Both hips are loose but only the right side has definite infection.

Gathorne Robert Girdlestone, 1881–1950, Nuffield Professor of Orthopaedics, The University of Oxford, Oxford, UK.

INFECTION FOLLOWING FRACTURE FIXATION

Many of the principles outlined above can be applied to infections associated with metalwork used to fix fractures. Strategies which retain well-fixed implants need to achieve fracture union, at which point removal of the metalwork simplifies managing the infection. A course of oral antibiotics is unlikely to eradicate infection, but may allow fracture healing. The infection can then be addressed with implant removal.

If there is doubt about fracture stability, the implant should be removed and an external fixator applied after excision of the infected tissue. These cases may produce major reconstructive challenges (Figure 40.6a–d).

ACUTE OSTEOMYELITIS

This presents like septic arthritis with a short history of pain, limb swelling, loss of function and systemic upset. In young children, a fever and refusal to weight-bear may be the only clues.

Diagnosis

In the early phase (2–3 days), x-rays may be normal but MRI will show bone oedema and periosteal elevation. After 5–7 days, plain x-ray may show subtle abnormality with osteopenia and periosteal new bone formation. WCC and CRP are often abnormal in the early phase. Treatment should not be delayed pending investigations.

Management

Acute osteomyelitis can be treated with antibiotics alone, when the diagnosis is made within 2–3 days of onset of symptoms, there is no dead bone on imaging and there is no adjacent septic arthritis. Blood cultures are taken and high-dose intravenous antibiotics, active against *Staphylococcus aureus*, *Streptococci* and Gram-negative rods such as *Escherichia coli* are given. Cephalosporins, co-amoxiclav or a combination of flucloxacillin and gentamicin may be used.

The limb should be splinted and good analgesia given. Intravenous antibiotics are usually converted to oral therapy after cultures and continued for at least 4 weeks.

If the patient does not respond rapidly, the limb deteriorates or there is imaging evidence of progression of disease, surgery is indicated to prevent bone destruction and the onset of chronic osteomyelitis.

With prompt treatment, acute bone infection has a good prognosis with a 90 per cent cure rate. Failure to treat adequately produces chronicity, with recurrent infection over many years. In

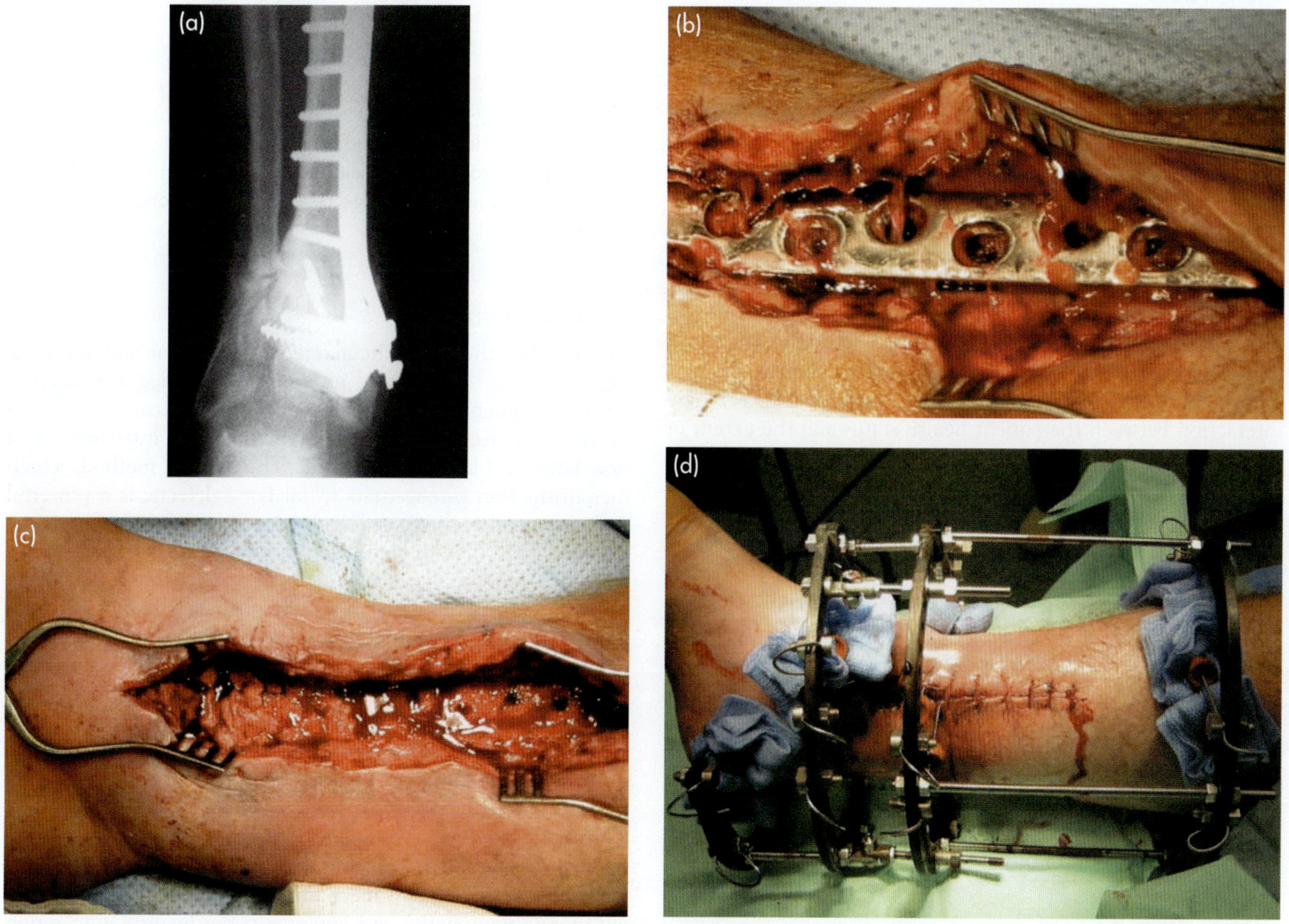

Figure 40.6 (a) X-ray of a complex distal tibia fracture which was internally fixed but complicated by deep infection. (b) At operation, the plate was loose and grossly infected. (c) The plate and all infected tissue was excised. The defect at the lower end was filled with an absorbable collagen antibiotic carrier. (d) The bone was stabilised with an Ilizarov circular external fixator.

children, the adjacent growth plates and joints may be affected with subsequent deformity and joint destruction (Summary box 40.12).

> **Summary box 40.12**
>
> **Acute osteomyelitis**
>
> - Presents in children with toxaemia, fever and unwillingness to move the limb
> - X-rays are normal for up to 1 week so are of no value in making an early diagnosis
> - WBC and CRP are usually raised
> - Early diagnosis is treated with high-dose i.v. antibiotics
> - Late diagnosis and failure of medical treatment requires surgical debridement

CHRONIC OSTEOMYELITIS

This is a serious condition which may affect the patient for decades. It often occurs in those with multiple comorbidities which must be managed with the infection. Chronic bone infection is best treated within a dedicated multidisciplinary team.

Diagnosis

Plain x-rays can delineate soft-tissue swelling, subperiosteal reaction, bone destruction and sequestra. CT scans are good for cortical bone imaging and for planning surgical excision. MRI is the imaging test of choice. It can be adversely affected by metal implants and can overestimate the extent of infection when there is widespread reactive oedema. Blood tests are often normal in chronic osteomyelitis.

Management

The Cierny and Mader classification helps to define the features of the infection in the bone (four stages) and to relate this to the general condition of the patient. Patients can be divided into three physiologic 'host types' (A, no concurrent disease; B, compromised host; C, severe comorbidity preventing surgery). The interaction between the patient health status and the extent of the bone infection has been shown to be prognostic in outcome after surgery.

Stage 1 (medullary)

Only cancellous bone is involved. Excision of the dead bone can be carried out by intramedullary reaming or by windowing the cortex. The resulting defect may be filled with antibiotic-loaded cement beads or absorbable pellets. Structural stability is rarely affected.

Stage 2 (superficial)

Only the cortical bone is involved and this requires excision. It often follows skin ulceration and there may be large skin defects which require complete excision and local or free muscle flaps. If more than one-third of the cortical circumference is excised, splintage is essential, usually with external fixation to prevent fracture. Secondary bone grafting may be needed.

> **George Cierny III**, contemporary, Medical Director, Department of Hyperbaric Medicine, St Joseph's Hospital, Atlanta, Georgia, USA.
> **Jon T Mader**, 1944–2002, formerly Department of the Marine Biomedical Institute, Division of Infectious Diseases, The University of Texas Medical Branch, Galveston, USA.
> Cierny and Mader described the classification in: Cierny G, Mader JT, Pennick JJ. A clinical staging for adult osteomyelitis. Contemp Orthop 1985; 10: 17–37.

Stage 3 (localized)

There is a limited area of dead cortical bone with medullary infection. Radical excision is required, and filling the defect and providing soft-tissue cover may be a challenge. Staged reconstruction may be necessary with cancellous bone grafting (Figure 40.7).

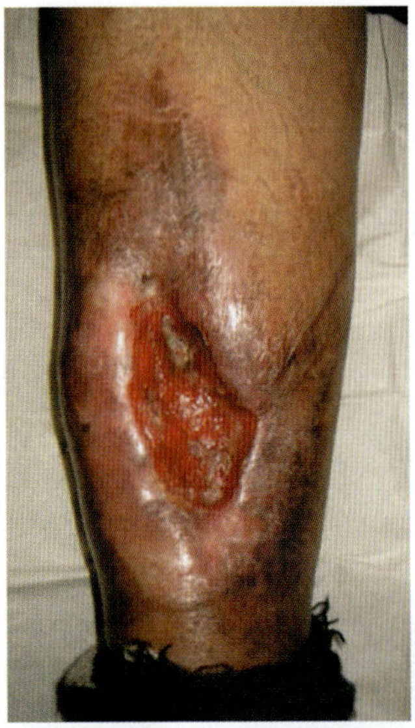

Figure 40.7 This large ulcer had been present for 30 years with underlying stage 3 chronic osteomyelitis. Biopsy of the skin edge revealed a squamous cell carcinoma; a rare complication of a long-standing sinus (Marjolijn's ulcer).

Stage 4 (diffuse)

This involves the entire circumference of the bone and surrounding soft tissue. All infected non-unions are stage 4. Resection must be segmental and stabilisation in an external fixator will be required. Reconstruction will involve the introduction of new bone and healthy soft tissue. The Ilizarov method, which uses distraction osteogenesis to fill bone defects, is a powerful and successful technique. It can be combined with free tissue transfer. This allows reconstruction to proceed in parallel with rehabilitation.

After surgery, patients should be given antibiotics. In total segmental excision of infection, a short course may be indicated but in most chronic infections, 6–12 weeks is often advised. In infected fractures, antibiotics should continue until fracture union (Summary box 40.13).

DIABETIC FOOT INFECTION

The incidence of foot complications among patients with diabetes is 1–2 per cent per year, due to the combined influence of vascular insufficiency, mechanical disruption, peripheral and autonomic neuropathy and impaired tissue healing. Ulceration of the calcaneum and bones of the forefoot, especially the great toe and first metatarsal head, is common, leading to deep extension and osteomyelitis (Figure 40.8).

Gavril Abramovich Ilizarov, 1921–1992, pioneered this approach in Siberia in the 1950s in the management of osteomyelitis, fractures and limb deformities.

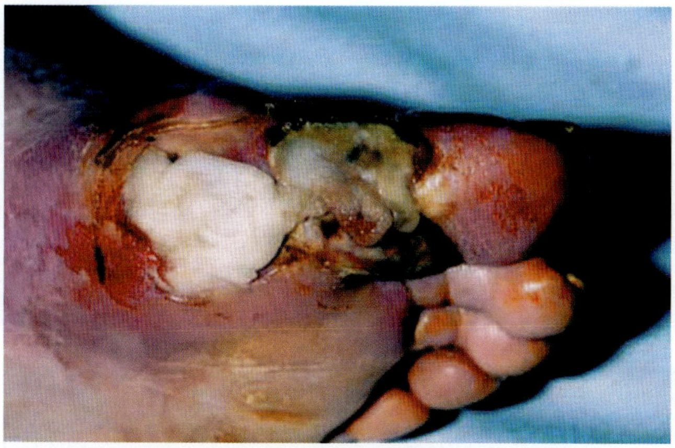

Figure 40.8 A severe diabetic foot infection, with marked infection, necrosis and soft-tissue loss. The patient was neuropathic but not ischaemic and it was possible to salvage a functional foot by 'filleting' the hallux and using the soft tissues to cover the defect.

Summary box 40.13

Osteomyelitis

- Acute infection must be treated rapidly to prevent morbidity
- Haematogenous infection most commonly affects long bones in children and the spine in adults
- MRI gives the best assessment of acute and chronic disease
- Chronic disease requires specialist surgery with excision, stabilisation and reconstruction
- Following surgery, antibiotic therapy is typically continued for 6 weeks

MRI is the most sensitive imaging modality for diagnosis of bone involvement. In severe infections antibiotic therapy should be guided by the results of culture of bone or tissue samples obtained surgically or radiologically. However, limited disease has a good prognosis, and in the absence of risk factors for resistant organisms (including prior treatment), empiric treatment can be justified.

Surgical debridement is required for collections, necrotic areas or more extensive osteomyelitis. Thought should be given to distinguishing superficial osteitis (stage 2 disease) resulting from loss of soft tissue cover (often in association with vascular compromise) from more extensive bone involvement. In the former, biopsy and antibiotic therapy may be of limited importance and improving vascular sufficiency and relieving pressure with appropriate footwear much more important. Vascular compromise should be considered a relative contraindication to a surgical approach, and amputation may not be an easy option as wound healing will be poor (Summary box 40.14).

Summary box 40.14

Diabetic foot infection

- The most important risk factor for osteomyelitis is the presence of a foot ulcer
- Bone biopsy for culture is the criterion standard for assessment, but may not be necessary in mild disease
- In severe disease, surgical debridement of collections and/or necrotic tissue is required, followed by antibiotics tailored according to culture results

MUSCULOSKELETAL INFECTION CAUSED BY MYCOBACTERIA

Tuberculous arthritis/osteomyelitis had become uncommon in the UK, but remains prevalent in the developing world. There is now a resurgence in the developed world as a consequence of immigration, immunocompromise and drug addiction. The usual organism is *Mycobacterium tuberculosis*. Around half of all cases affect the spine, typically manifesting as paradiscal infection but also causing discitis and vertebral osteomyelitis. Native joint infection typically presents with monoarticular pain in a weight-bearing joint. Surgery may be crucial to facilitate synovial biopsy for diagnosis by culture and histopathology, as well as to decompress the spinal cord and debride infected tissue. When the mycobacteria are sensitive to antimicrobials the prognosis for microbiological cure is good.

FURTHER READING

Mathews CJ, Weston VC, Jones A *et al.* Bacterial septic arthritis in adults. *Lancet* 2010; **375**: 846–55.

Matthews PC, Berendt AR, McNally MA, Byren I. Diagnosis and management of prosthetic joint infection. *BMJ* 2009; **338**: 1378–83.

Matthews PC, Berendt AR, Lipsky BA. Clinical management of diabetic foot infection: diagnostics, therapeutics and the future. *Expert Rev Anti Infect Ther* 2007; **5**: 117–27.

McNally MA, Nagarajah K. Osteomyelitis. *Orthop Trauma* 2010; **24**: 416–29.

Lew DP, Waldvogel FA. Osteomyelitis. *Lancet* 2004; **364**: 369–79.

CHAPTER

41 Paediatric orthopaedics

LEARNING OBJECTIVES

To be familiar with:

- Normal and abnormal development of the musculoskeletal system
- Normal variants versus pathological deformity
- Diagnosis and treatment of developmental hip dysplasia
- Presentation and management of other childhood hip conditions
- Management of clubfoot
- Problems associated with musculoskeletal infection in childhood

INTRODUCTION

Immature skeletons heal rapidly and can remodel with growth but physeal injury or muscle imbalance can lead to progressive deformity. The conservative treatment of common conditions, such as developmental dysplasia of the hip (DDH) combines the child's remodelling ability with an understanding of the Heuter–Volkmann principle and Wolff's law (Summary box 41.1): improving the biomechanical environment reverses abnormal growth. In contrast, in conditions such as Blount's disease, growth plate damage leads to asymmetrical growth and deformity. Advances in genetics and molecular science may improve our understanding of certain conditions and suggest new avenues of treatment.

Summary box 41.1

Laws governing the remodelling of bone

Heuter–Volkmann principle

- Compressive forces inhibit growth
- Tensile forces stimulate growth

Wolff's law

- Bone deposition and resorption depends on the stresses applied

DEVELOPMENT OF THE MUSCULOSKELETAL SYSTEM

The upper limb bud forms on the lateral wall of the embryo 4 weeks after fertilisation, followed promptly by the lower limb bud. By two months' gestation, differentiation of the limb elements is complete. Most congenital limb anomalies arise during this second month.

Three intercoordinated signalling centres control limb development. The apical ectodermal ridge (AER) guides mesodermal differentiation in a proximal-to-distal direction and controls digit formation. The zone of polarising activity (ZPA) directs anteroposterior limb development via the sonic hedgehog protein. The Wnt signalling centre develops dorsoventral axis configuration and limb alignment.

Certain limb anomalies are directly related to alterations in these centres. In experiments it is found that removal of the AER leads to a truncated limb, similar to a congenital amputation, and prevents interdigital necrosis. This results in syndactyly.

An error during fetal limb development may disturb the formation of other organs. Thus some limb anomalies are associated with systemic disorders which may be life-threatening (Summary box 41.2).

Summary box 41.2

Development of the musculoskeletal system

- Occurs 4–8 weeks after fertilisation
- AER controls proximal-to-distal differentiation and interdigital necrosis
- ZPA directs posterior-to-anterior differentiation
- Wnt influences dorsal-to-ventral differentiation

NORMAL VARIANTS

There are common normal variants which cause parental concern. These are intoeing, bowlegs, knock-knees and flatfeet: if they are symmetrical, symptom-free and supple, they require no intervention. There is often a family history of similar complaints. If the child fails to achieve their developmental milestones or there are functional problems, further investigation and help may be required.

Richard von Volkmann, 1830–1889, Professor of Surgery, Halle, Germany.
Julius Wolff, 1836–1902, Professor of Orthopaedic Surgery, Berlin, Germany.
Walter Putnam Blount, 1900–1992, Professor of Orthopaedic Surgery, Marquette University, Milwaukee, WI, USA, described this condition in 1937.

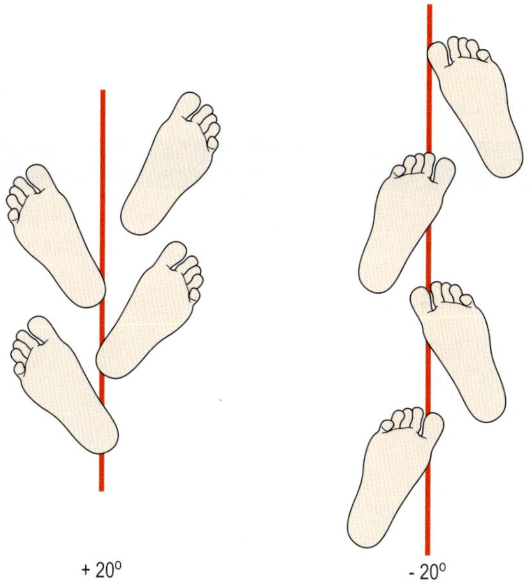

Figure 41.1 Foot progression angle: a positive angle is caused by an extoeing gait, a negative angle by an intoeing gait.

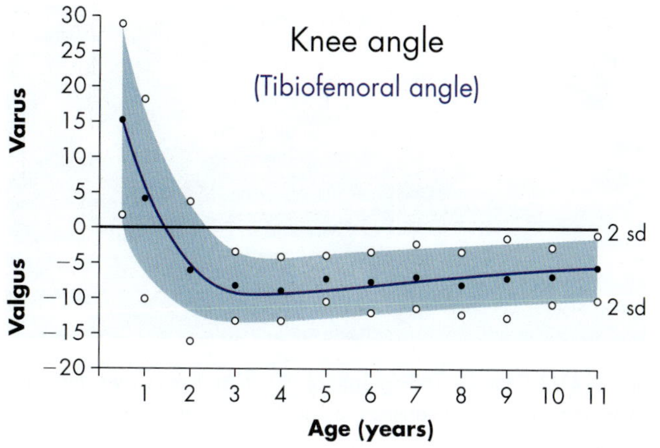

Figure 41.2 Graph to show the normal tendency of limb alignment to change from varus to valgus with growth.

Intoeing gait

Intoeing is defined as a negative foot progression angle. It can result from one or more lower limb torsional anomalies (Figure 41.1 and Table 41.1).

Persistent femoral anteversion presents clinically with excessive internal rotation at the hip joint. All femurs are anteverted at birth but spontaneous correction occurs because as the femur lengthens it also rotates. If by 12–13 years a significant deformity persists associated with functional difficulties, corrective osteotomy may be justified. Compensatory external tibial torsion may develop.

Internal tibial torsion is assessed by the foot/thigh angle and is commonly associated with physiological tibia vara in infants. Spontaneous correction can be expected by age 4, as the tibia also rotates as it grows.

Metatarsus varus is usually flexible; spontaneous correction occurs in 90 per cent of children by the age of 2–4 years. For the more rigid foot, stretching, corrective plasters or straight-last shoes may help. Surgical release is rarely indicated.

Table 41.1 Common sites and causes of intoeing gait in childhood.

Site	Cause
Femur/hip	Persistent femoral neck anteversion
Tibia	Internal tibial torsion
Foot	Metatarsus varus

Other abnormalities of gait

Toe-walking is a phase in normal gait development. If the gait does not mature to a heel–toe pattern by the age of three years, physiotherapy may help, and older children benefit from surgical lengthening of contracted gastrocsoleus complexes. If toe-walking starts after walking age, a spinal or neuromuscular aetiology such as a tethered cord or a muscular dystrophy must be considered.

Extoeing is less common than intoeing but may result from relative femoral retroversion, external tibial torsion or flexible flat feet. The young child may be late walking because of poor balance associated with the foot posture. This condition improves with growth/time.

Knock-knees and bowlegs

Normal children's leg shape changes dramatically over time. All children start life with bowlegs, often accompanied by tibial torsion. By the age of 2–3 years they have developed knock-knees, which regress towards the normal adult tibiofemoral angle of 7° valgus by the age of 7 (Figure 41.2).

Traditionally, the intercondylar or intermalleolar distance is used to quantify the deformity, rather than measuring the angle. This is not very accurate. Further investigation is needed when the deformity is severe, asymmetrical or symptomatic. The most common pathological causes are previous trauma, rickets or a skeletal dysplasia.

Flat foot

Before development of the medial longitudinal arch, all children (<3 years) have flat feet. Only 15 per cent of adults have flat feet so the natural history is for improvement, influenced by both familial and racial factors.

The painless, flexible flat foot needs no treatment. Orthoses do not alter the natural history but can alleviate symptoms if they arise. All flat feet have a flattened medial arch with a valgus heel but the two major types should be distinguished from each other (Table 41.2).

The symptomatic, rigid flat foot is usually the result of a tarsal coalition or inflammation and requires appropriate medical or surgical treatment (Figure 41.3) (Summary box 41.3).

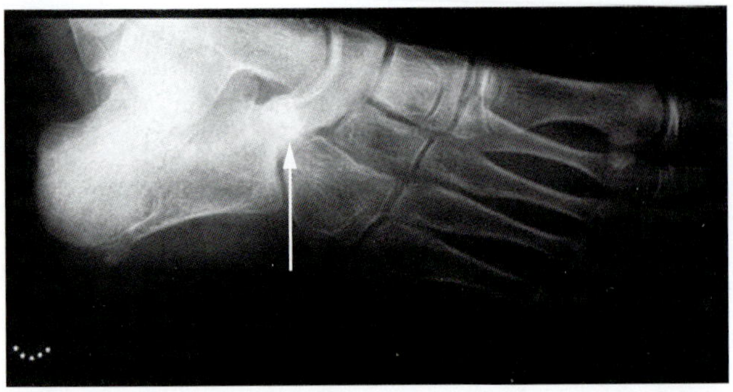

Figure 41.3 Oblique radiograph of the foot that shows the most common form of tarsal coalition, a calcaneonavicular bar.

Table 41.2 Flat feet.

Types	Characteristics
Flexible	On tiptoe the arch is restored and the heel corrects into varus; subtalar joint movements are full and pain free
Rigid	On tiptoe the arch fails to return; subtalar joint movements are restricted and often painful

Summary box 41.3

Normal variants

- Intoeing or extoeing may be caused by excessive foot deformity, tibial or femoral torsion
- Neurological abnormalities must be excluded in toe walkers
- Children's legs are often bowed until age 2 and then knock-kneed until age 6 or 7
- Flexible, pain-free flat feet do not need treatment

Postural abnormalities

Many babies are subjected to moulding pressures *in utero*. At birth they have 'postural abnormalities' such as torticollis, calcaneovalgus feet and plagiocephaly, which improve with time and stretching exercises.

CONGENITAL AND DEVELOPMENTAL ABNORMALITIES OF THE SKELETON

Although many skeletal abnormalities are identified antenatally or at birth, others only become apparent with growth. Skeletal disorders are often linked to soft-tissue abnormalities; the presence of a skin dimple or the presence of a vascular malformation should be a warning sign (see Table 41.3).

Many anomalies require little treatment and cause minimal functional disability whereas others, such as proximal femoral focal deficiency and radial club hand, pose considerable challenges. In these cases the functional and cosmetic needs of the child and family must be balanced against available resources and expertise. Despite advances in limb reconstruction techniques, there is little high quality evidence-based data from skeletally mature patients to support their widespread use. In the meantime, considerable advances are occurring with amputation prosthetics.

Table 41.3 Classification of congenital limb malformations.

Category	Example
Failure of formation of parts	
Transverse	Congenital amputation
Longitudinal	Fibular hemimelia
Failure of differentiation	Vertebral body fusion; syndactyly
Duplication	Extra digits
Overgrowth	Gigantism; macrodactyly
Undergrowth	
Congenital constriction band syndrome	Often affects hands/feet with poor formation of the digits
Generalised skeletal abnormalities	Skeletal dysplasia, e.g. achondroplasia

Generalised skeletal dysplasias

Achondroplasia

Achondroplasia is caused by a defect in the *FGFR3* (fibroblast growth factor receptor 3) gene that affects enchondral bone formation. Patients present with a disproportionate short stature (disproportionate means that the limbs are shorter than the trunk) and classic clinical and radiographic features (Figure 41.4). Underdevelopment of the foramen magnum and spinal stenosis can cause neurological difficulties. Correction of limb alignment may be necessary and limb lengthening techniques are used in some countries.

Hereditary multiple exostoses – diaphyseal aclasis

Exostoses grow as the child grows and may cause cosmetic or functional difficulties that justify excision. Differential growth between the paired bones of the lower arm and leg can lead to joint deformity, exacerbated by the physeal distortion secondary to altered mechanical forces. Such growth abnormalities are predictable and treatment is designed to prevent deformity from developing (Figure 41.5).

Enchondromas

Abnormal ossification of the physeal cartilage columns may be the precursor of these cartilaginous masses, and can be seen on x-ray because they are ossified (see Chapter 39).

Fibrous dysplasia

This common disorder is often a chance finding on x-ray and probably results from a somatic mutation causing defective bone formation, see also Chapter 39 (Figure 41.6 and Summary box 41.4).

METABOLIC BONE DISEASE

Rickets

In all types of rickets, the primary problem is inadequate

Louis Xavier Edouard Léopold Ollier, 1830–1900, Professor of Surgery, Lyons, France, described enchondromatosis in 1899.
Angelo Maffucci, 1845–1903, Professor of Pathological Anatomy, Pisa, Italy, described this syndrome in 1881.

Summary box 41.4

Congenital and developmental abnormalities of the skeleton

- Achondroplasia affects endochondral ossification and presents with disproportionate dwarfism
- Exostoses may cause cosmetic or functional problems
- Patients with Ollier's disease (multiple enchondromatosis) often have lesions in the hand and feet

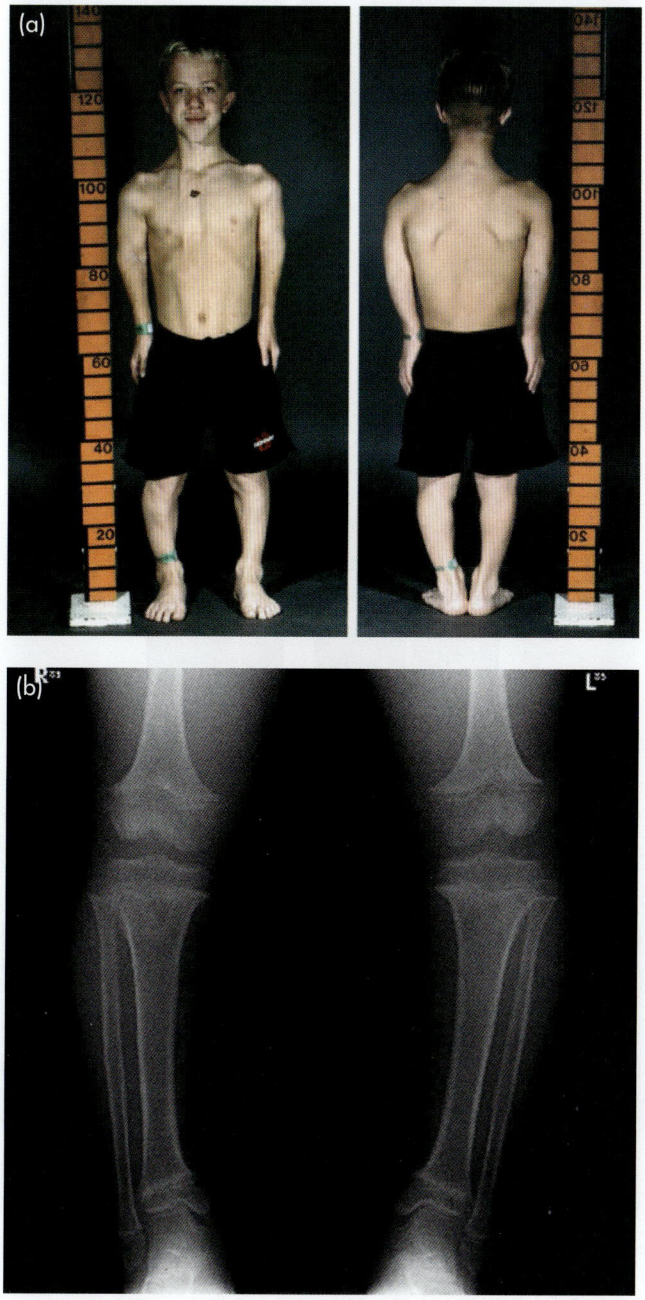

Figure 41.4 Achondroplasia. (a) Clinical photograph of a child with achondroplasia. (b) X-ray of the lower limb of a child with achondroplasia showing short limbs, widened metaphyses and a varus deformity of the distal tibia.

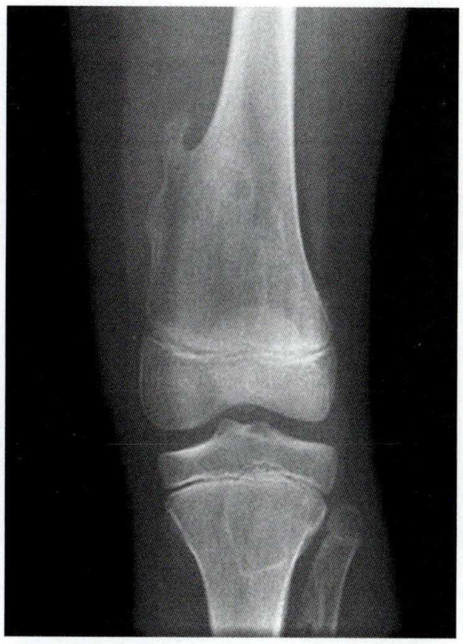

Figure 41.5 X-ray of the knee showing multiple broad-based osteochondromas.

mineralisation of growing bone (Table 41.4). In severe cases, skeletal deformities, with classic radiographic features, affect every physis (Figure 41.7). Medical treatment improves mineralisation. Correction of the deformity then occurs with growth. Surgery may be necessary for the management of pathological fractures or to correct mechanical misalignment once the medical condition has been controlled.

Table 41.4 Common causes of rickets.

Nutritional	Reduced intake of vitamin D and calcium
Environmental	Inadequate exposure to sunlight
Gastrointestinal disease	Crohn's disease, gluten-sensitive enteropathy
Genetic	X-linked hypophosphataemia
Renal disease	End-stage renal failure, renal tubular anomalies
	Secondary hyperparathyroidism changes may be present

Osteogenesis imperfecta (brittle bone disease)

Osteogenesis imperfecta (OI) represents a spectrum of conditions linked by a qualitative and/or quantitative malfunction of collagen production. Many specific genetic defects have been identified; most caused by mutations in the collagen genes. The bone may break easily but it heals promptly and well. All structures that contain collagen may be affected. This accounts for the ligamentous laxity, blue sclerae and poor teeth found in some phenotypes.

Cyclical bisphosphonate treatment decreases bone resorption and bone turnover. This reduces bone pain and the fracture rate, which in turn improves weight-bearing mobility and bone strength (Figure 41.8).

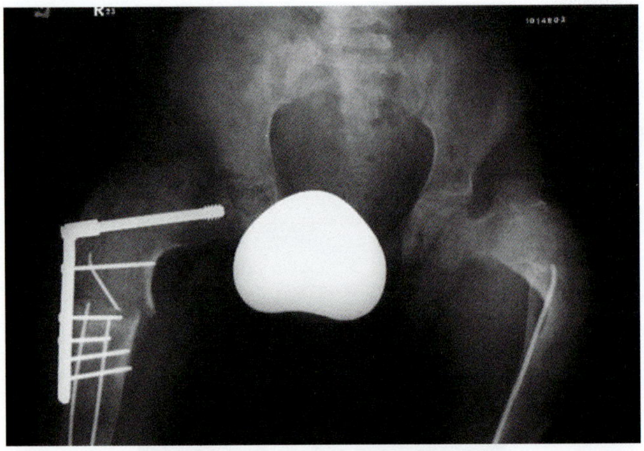

Figure 41.6 The diaphyseal lesions of fibrous dysplasia classically have a 'ground glass' appearance and, if extensive, may be associated with angular deformity or pathological fracture.

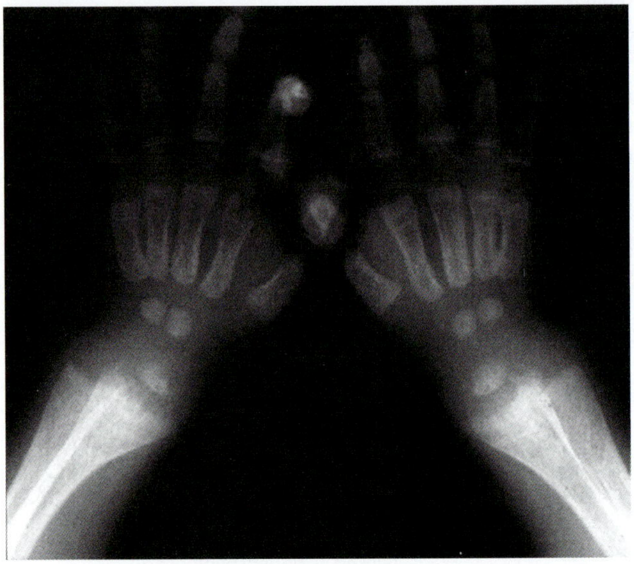

Figure 41.7 X-rays, which are characteristic of rickets, show widened physes with cupped, flared metaphyses.

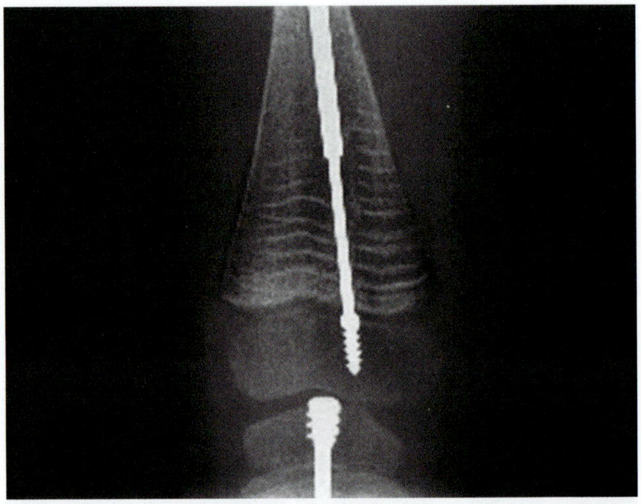

Figure 41.8 X-ray of a child with osteogenesis imperfecta who has been treated with cyclical bisphosphonates. Multiple growth lines are visible in addition to an intramedullary device.

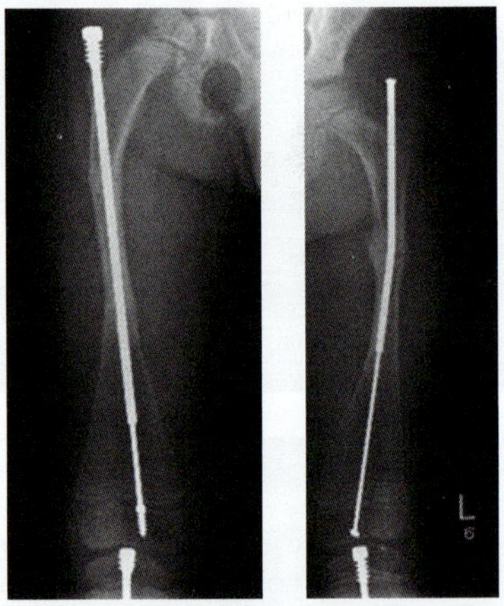

Figure 41.9 X-ray of two adolescent femora showing different types of intramedullary alignment device *in situ*.

Following fracture, care must be taken to minimise disuse osteoporosis and to maintain bone alignment. Treatment options range from simple casting techniques to more specialised surgical procedures to correct/maintain limb alignment while allowing growth (Figure 41.9 and Summary box 41.5).

Summary box 41.5

Metabolic bone disease

- Rickets from nutritional or other causes, is characterised by failure of bone mineralisation
- In OI there is defective type I collagen production
- In severe forms of OI, frequent fractures lead to progressive deformity: Bisphosphonate treatment may reduce the fracture rate

ABNORMALITIES OF THE HIP

Developmental dysplasia of the hip

DDH defines the spectrum of hip instability ranging from the hip that is in joint but has a shallow (dysplastic) acetabulum and may be 'pushed out' (Barlow positive) to the dislocated hip that is irreducible (Ortolani negative). These tests are described below. The associated clinical picture varies with the pathology and the age at presentation: neonatal hips may be unstable, a toddler may limp, adolescents may experience exercise-induced pain and an adult may have pain secondary to degenerative arthritis.

Incidence

The incidence of neonatal instability is 1–2:1000 live births whereas that of true dislocation is ~2:1000 live births, many hips stabilise spontaneously.

Thomas Geoffrey Barlow, 1915–1975, orthopaedic surgeon, Salford Royal Hospital and Hope Hospital, Salford, UK.
Marius Ortolani, orthopaedic surgeon, Instituto Provinciale Per L'Infanzia di Ferrara, Italy, described this test in 1937.

Aetiology of DDH

- Gender: DDH is five times more common in girls than boys, possibly related to hormonal factors causing temporary joint laxity.
- Breech presentation: DDH is present in ≤20 per cent of breech babies, particularly with the extended breech position.
- Birth order: DDH is more common in firstborns and in the left hip because of the common fetal position in a tight primigravid uterus where movement is restricted.
- Oligohydramnios: Restricts fetal movement. The presence of other postural deformities (torticollis and metatarsus adductus) raises the possibility of DDH.
- Family history: A positive family history significantly increases the risk of DDH. This may reflect faulty acetabular development or excessive ligamentous laxity.

DDH is often found in association with generalised syndromes or neuromuscular conditions. These teratologic hips are usually resistant to surgical intervention and the child's overall condition and prognosis must be considered when planning treatment.

Diagnosis

Neonates

Clinical assessment

All neonates are screened for limitation of hip abduction and instability. The hips are examined again at 6 weeks. The knees and hips are flexed and the thigh held by the examiner with the thumb along the medial aspect and a finger behind the greater trochanter. The hips are abducted gently: if abduction is limited, the hip may be dislocated. The examiner's finger then lifts the greater trochanter upwards; a soft clunk – the Ortolani test – with improved hip abduction, signifies hip reduction (Figure 41.10a). If the hip does abduct fully, then the leg is adducted while downward pressure is applied to the knee with the examiner's thumb and palm: an unstable hip may dislocate or sublux – the Barlow test (Figure 41.10b). With an irreducible hip there is no clunk of reduction but there will be limitation of abduction. Bilateral dislocation may be missed as abduction is symmetrical and abduction may be normal when there is ligamentous laxity.

Ultrasound assessment

Ultrasonography defines the anatomy and the stability of the hip joint. It is used to monitor early treatment (Figure 41.11) or as a screening tool (universally or just for 'at risk' patients). Ideally, screening scans should be performed between 4 and 6 weeks of age and, when necessary, treatment started promptly. It should not be forgotten that the sonographic appearances of most hips improve (become less dysplastic) spontaneously as the child grows. X-rays are used to evaluate dysplasia from four to five months of age, but are of limited value in the newborn because no ossific nucleus is visible so the position of the hip cannot be seen. The appearance of the femoral ossific nucleus is also often delayed in DDH (Figure 41.12).

Infants

Hip checks, looking for limitation of abduction in flexion and limb shortening, are part of routine developmental monitoring.

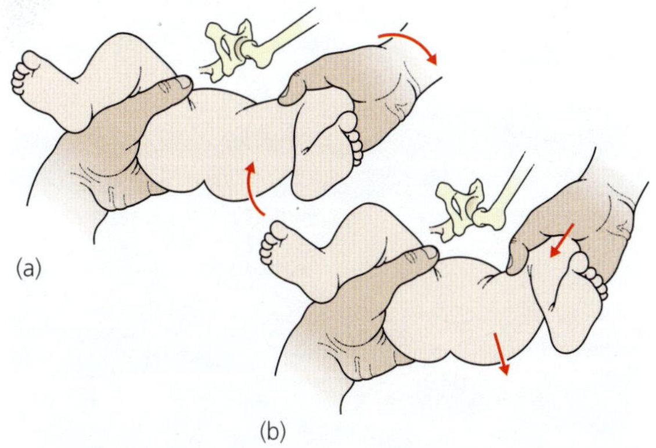

Figure 41.10 Line diagram illustrating the Ortolani (a) and Barlow (b) tests for developmental dysplasia of the hip.

Child

Children present with a limp and sometimes with unilateral tiptoeing because the affected leg is short. It is also externally rotated. Abduction in flexion is limited and there may be an extra thigh crease. The signs may be subtle and easily missed in an unsteady toddler. If both hips are affected there will be a waddling gait and a lumbar lordosis.

Adolescent/adult

Discomfort after exercise is common but the pain may be in the knee. X-rays show dysplasia, subluxation or degenerative change (Summary box 41.6).

Summary box 41.6

Diagnosis of DDH

- All neonates are screened clinically (Barlow and Ortolani tests), at birth and at 6 weeks
- Ultrasound is used to monitor hip stability/anatomy and as a screening test in 'at-risk' babies
- X-ray is useful from four months onwards
- Older children present with a limp or tiptoe walking

Management

When diagnosed early, conservative treatment is usually successful, but after walking age surgery is required. The objective is to obtain a stable, congruous reduction of the femoral head into the acetabulum while avoiding damage to the capital epiphysis (avascular necrosis) or to the growth plate which causes stiffness, coxa vara and shortening.

Neonate

Due to ligamentous laxity, some normal hips are unstable initially. Most stabilise within the first few weeks of life and do not need treatment.

Hips that remain unstable or are dislocated at rest are treated with harnesses or splints that maintain hip reduction in the position of abduction and flexion. Most harnesses (Figure 41.13) allow controlled movement while splints hold the hips more rigidly and so may carry a greater risk of avascular necrosis. If

Sophus von Rosen, orthopaedic surgeon, Malmo General Hospital, Malmo, Sweden.

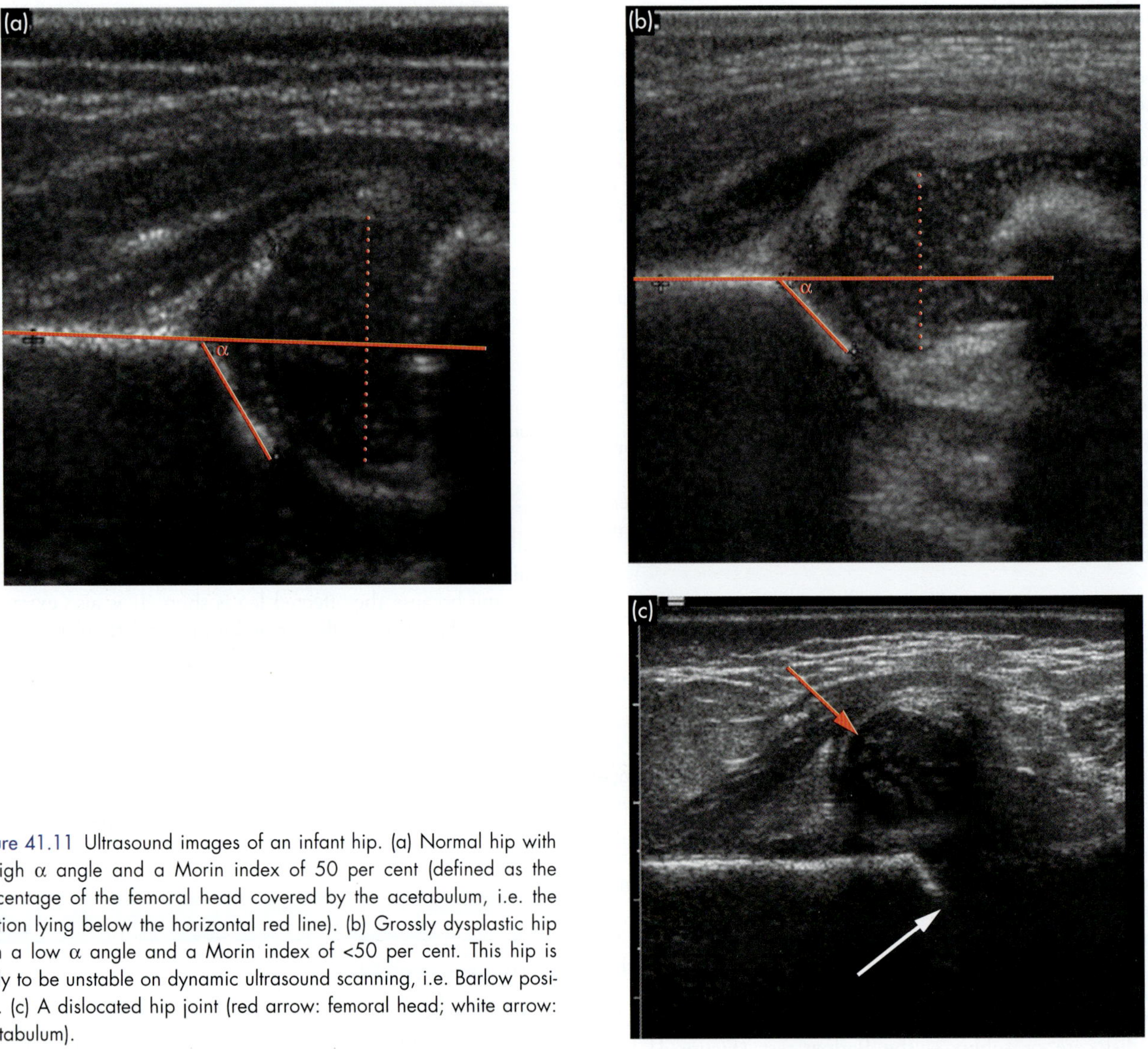

Figure 41.11 Ultrasound images of an infant hip. (a) Normal hip with a high α angle and a Morin index of 50 per cent (defined as the percentage of the femoral head covered by the acetabulum, i.e. the portion lying below the horizontal red line). (b) Grossly dysplastic hip with a low α angle and a Morin index of <50 per cent. This hip is likely to be unstable on dynamic ultrasound scanning, i.e. Barlow positive. (c) A dislocated hip joint (red arrow: femoral head; white arrow: acetabulum).

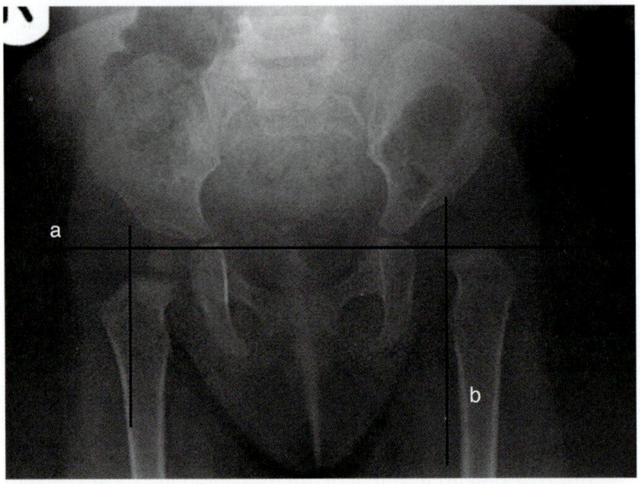

Figure 41.12 Anteroposterior pelvic x-ray showing Hilgenreiner's line (a) and Perkins' line (b). The femoral head (ossific nucleus) of a normal hip lies in the inner lower quadrant. The right hip is normal, the left hip has developmental dysplasia of the hip.

the hips fail to relocate or stabilise then non-operative treatment should be discontinued.

Infant

Successful treatment using a harness is unusual after the age of 4–6 months. For the late-presenting hip or the hip that fails conservative treatment, an examination under anaesthetic may result in a closed reduction. The arthrogram shows whether a concentric reduction is present and, if not, it will indicate which structures are blocking reduction. Apsoas/adductor release can be performed as necessary. A closed reduction will need to be held reduced with a hip spica cast for several months.

If the hip is irreducible or can only be held reduced in an extreme position with a small safe zone, then treatment must be abandoned and an open reduction considered via a medial or anterior approach (Summary box 41.7).

Toddler and young child

The older the child, the less likely it is that reduction by closed methods will succeed (Figure 41.14). The traditional approach is then to carry out open reduction via an anterior approach

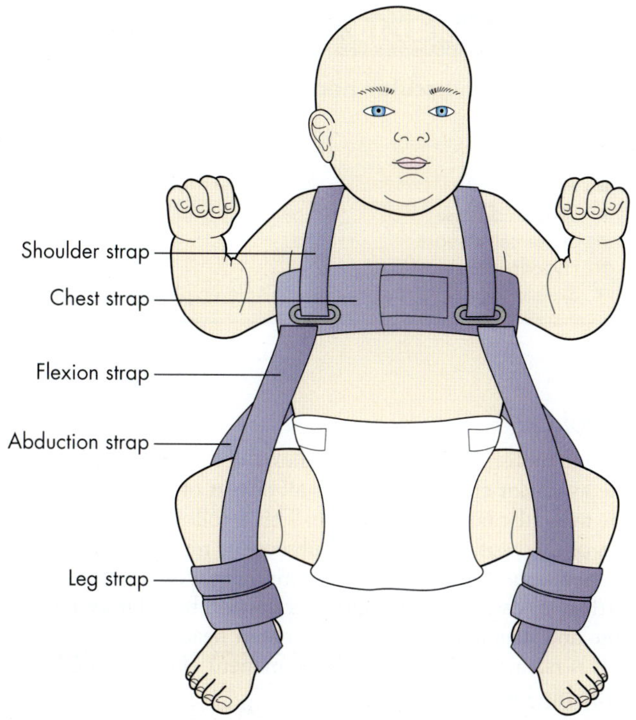

Figure 41.13 The anterior strap of the Pavlik harness controls hip flexion whereas the posterior strap limits adduction and encourages abduction.

Summary box 41.7

Management of early DDH

- Many hips that are unstable in the first few days of life do not need treatment
- Up to 4–6 months, a harness or splint is effective treatment
- In older babies, closed reduction is sometimes possible
- For failed closed treatment, open surgical reduction is required

around the age of 9–12 months. A pelvic osteotomy may be required to reorientate or close down the acetabulum and femoral shortening or derotation osteotomies are often required to improve stability. Earlier surgery via the medial approach can be considered but no additional surgery, such as capsulorraphy or bony realignment can be performed through that incision.

Older child

In the older child a similar approach is necessary but pelvic and femoral realignment will always be needed, and the results tend to be less rewarding. Surgery is often avoided in children over the age of 6–8 years in bilateral cases and the age of 8–10 in unilateral cases.

Adolescent and young adult

These hips are often subluxed rather than truly dislocated. On investigation, the hip may be reducible and the joint can be recreated with a combination of pelvic and femoral osteotomies. For the irreducible hip, acetabular augmentation may reduce symptoms and delay the onset of degenerative change (Summary box 41.8).

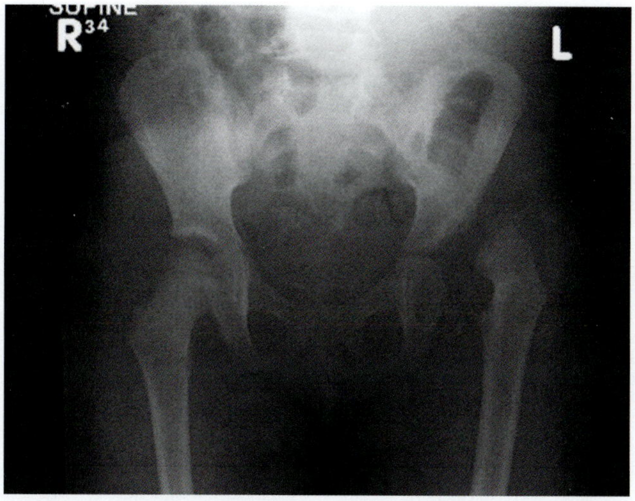

Figure 41.14 Anteroposterior pelvic x-ray showing acetabular dysplasia with subluxation (developmental dysplasia of the hip) of the left hip. This child presented at the age of 4.

Summary box 41.8

Management of late-presenting DDH

- The older the child, the more likely it is that they will need surgery
- Femoral osteotomy can stabilise the hip and reduce pressure on the femoral head
- Pelvic osteotomy redirects or reshapes the acetabulum
- Acetabular remodelling decreases after the age of 3–4 years
- Avascular necrosis is a risk of DDH treatment

Secondary procedures and complications

Regular follow up ensures that the hip development is monitored. Acetabular remodelling may be assessed objectively by measuring the acetabular index or the centre-edge angle (Figure 41.15).

If the acetabulum does not improve, a variety of pelvic osteotomies can be considered. Avascular necrosis (AVN) with overgrowth of the greater trochanter can cause a Trendelenburg limp and distal transfer of the trochanter may help. Occasionally, a leg length difference needs treatment. There is also an increased risk of osteoarthritis which may need arthroplasty later in life.

Legg–Calvé–Perthes' disease

Incidence and aetiology

This rare condition, characterised by the development of AVN of the proximal femoral epiphysis, affects boys predominantly between the ages of 4 and 8 years. Ten per cent develop bilateral disease. Although the aetiology is unclear, several factors have been implicated (Summary box 41.9). There are also other causes of AVN of the femoral head (Summary box 41.10).

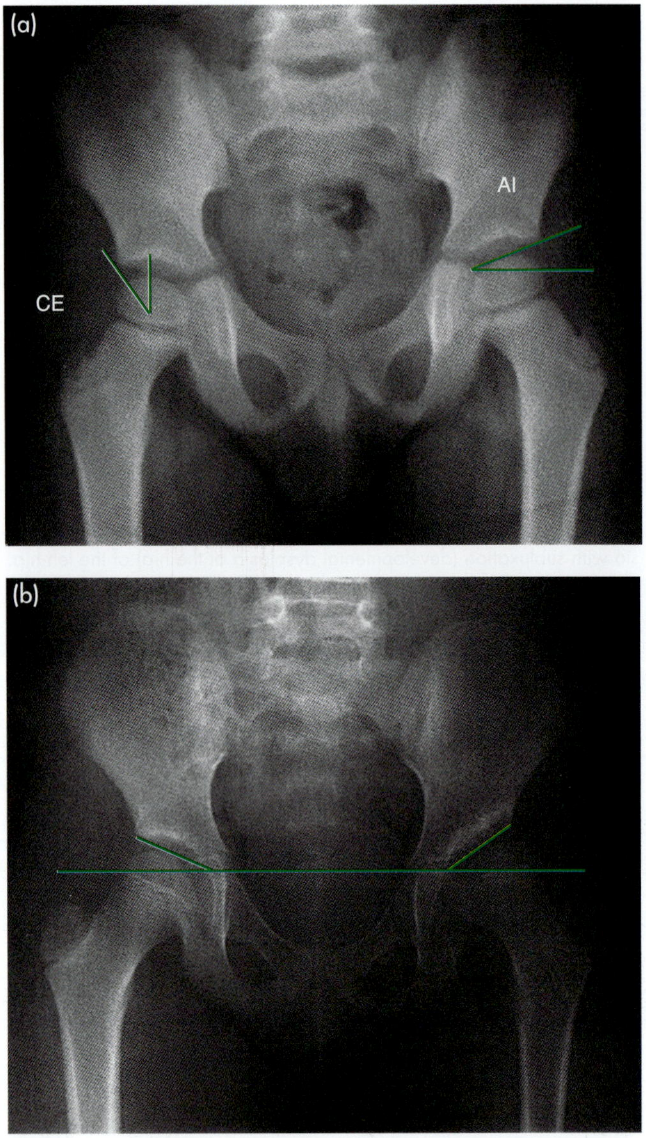

Figure 41.15 Anteroposterior pelvic radiographs demonstrating the acetabular index (AI) and the centre-edge (CE) angle. (a) Normal hips; (b) the left hip shows residual dysplasia. The AI is increased compared with the normal right hip. The left CE angle would be smaller than the right too but is has not been measured on this x-ray.

Summary box 41.9

Factors implicated in the pathogenesis of Perthes' disease

- Low birthweight
- High birth order
- Delayed bone age
- Low socioeconomic status

Summary box 41.10

Causes of avascular necrosis of the femoral head

- Steroids
- Infection
- Perthes' disease
- Sickle cell disease
- Hypothyroidism
- Skeletal dysplasia – classically multiple epiphyseal dysplasia

Pathology

Once established the process follows a well-described course. The avascular change may affect all or part of the femoral head. The avascular bone may collapse. This is followed by fragmentation of the ossific nucleus and subsequent revascularisation and regeneration ('healing') of the bony epiphysis; in this respect Perthes' disease is a self-limiting condition but, during the collapse and fragmentation phases, femoral head deformity occurs. This is not reversible and has a permanent effect on the health of the hip joint.

Diagnosis

The history, clinical examination and anteroposterior and 'frog' lateral x-rays of the pelvis make the diagnosis. An intermittently painful hip (or knee) with a limp and restriction of hip movements requires investigation. The x-ray features vary with the disease stage and may not correlate with the clinical condition (Figure 41.16). MRI can be helpful.

AVN of the femoral head may be due to other causes and a differential diagnosis should be considered, particularly when changes are bilateral.

Management

Treatment aims to minimise femoral head deformity, and thus the likelihood of secondary acetabular dysplasia. This is achieved by maintaining a good range of joint movement, with some restriction in activity level, and using analgesia and physiotherapy as required. The routine use of crutches and/or wheelchairs are discouraged because they promote a flexion/adduction posture. Recent evidence suggests that brace management on its own does not alter the natural history of the condition.

The role of operative treatment is controversial. Surgery can be performed early to prevent deformity secondary to femoral head collapse or late to 'salvage' a poor mechanical situation when deformity is limiting movement (Table 41.5). Joint distraction (arthrodiastasis) may preserve joint movement and maintain femoral head height but has not gained popularity.

Not all hips with deformity require 'salvage' surgery: young children, with more time to remodel, have a better prognosis as the secondary acetabular changes result in an aspherical but congruent joint. Long-term follow up may be required to deal with mechanical symptoms caused by loose osteochondral fragments, a Trendelenburg gait secondary to trochanteric overgrowth or a short-leg gait. Degenerative change may occur in adult life.

Other conditions (all eponymous) also show x-ray changes of AVN (Table 41.6).

Arthur Thornton Legg, 1874–1939, orthopaedic surgeon, The Children's Hospital, Boston, MA, USA.
Jacques Calvé, 1875–1927, orthopaedic surgeon, La Fondation Franco-Americaine, Berck Plage, Pas-de-Calais, France.
Georg Clemens Perthes, 1869–1927, Professor of Surgery, Tübingen, Germany.
Legg, Calvé and Perthes all described osteochondritis of the head of the femur independently in 1910.

Table 41.5 A guide to some of the surgical options available for the management of Perthes' disease.

Timing	Type of procedure	Comments	Aim
Early	Femoral osteotomy Innominate osteotomy Shelf acetabuloplasty	Varus and derotation	To cover ('contain') the vulnerable femoral head
Intermediate	Arthrodiastasis	Hinged distraction to allow movement	To reduce deforming pressures on the femoral head
Late	Femoral osteotomy Cheilectomy Arthrotomy Trochanteric epiphyseodesis	Valgus and extension To remove osteochondral fragments	To improve joint congruity and hence function; to improve joint mechanics
Contralateral limb	Distal femoral epiphyseodesis		To improve leg length discrepancy and reduce effects on hip joint mechanics

Again, the x-ray changes 'heal' but the change in shape of the affected bone may lead to secondary joint stiffness and loss of function (Summary box 41.11).

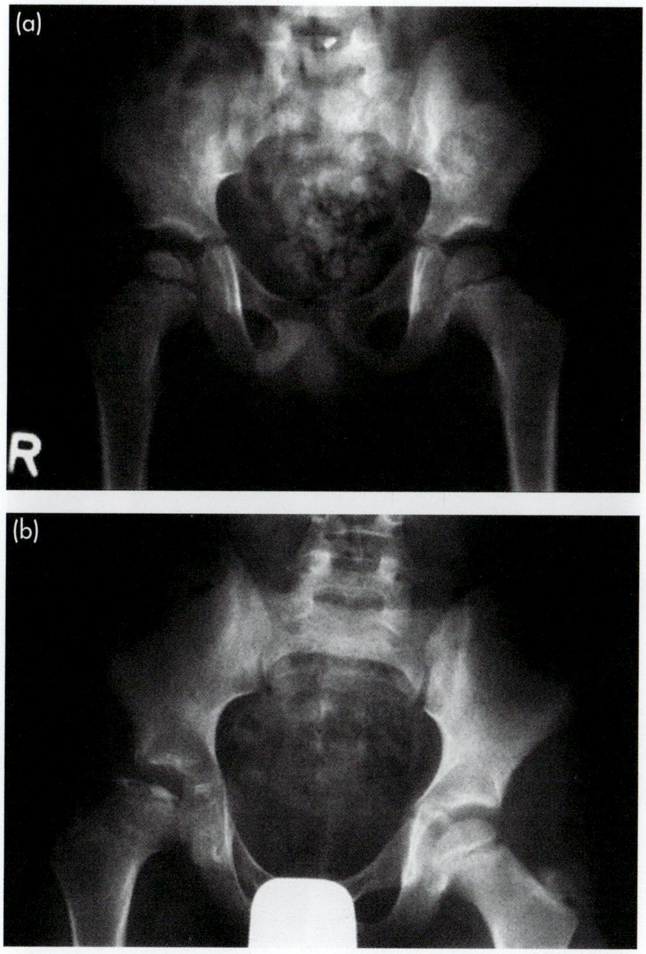

Figure 41.16 Anteroposterior pelvic x-rays of Perthes' disease demonstrating whole head involvement. (a) Right-sided disease; the process is in an early phase. The area of dense necrotic bone is visible (b). There has been collapse and fragmentation.

Summary box 41.11

Legg–Calvé–Perthes' disease

- Most common in boys aged 4–8 years
- AVN leads to femoral head collapse, healing occurs with the return of the blood supply
- Management aims to maintain femoral head sphericity
- Treatment may be non-surgical (to maximise range of movement) or surgical (for containment or 'salvage')
- The prognosis is better in younger children who have more remodelling potential

Table 41.6 Other conditions (commonly classified as osteochondroses) in which the x-ray appearance is of avascular necrosis.

Condition	Affected bone
Keinbock's disease	Lunate
Panner's disease	Capitellum of the humerus
Freiberg's disease	Metatarsal head – usually the second
Köhler's disease	Navicular

Slip of the upper (capital) femoral epiphysis

The physis connects the proximal femoral epiphysis (the femoral head) to the metaphysis (femoral neck). In certain physiological or pathological conditions a 'stress fracture' through the physis allows the epiphysis to displace as it would with an intracapsular femoral neck fracture, so the leg lies short and externally rotated. There is painful limitation of hip movement. Hilton's law, which states that a joint is supplied by the same nerves as the muscles that move the joint, explains why many children present with knee pain although the pathology is in the hip.

Incidence and aetiology

Slip of the upper (capital) femoral epiphysis (SUFE or SCFE) is rare with an incidence of ~5:100 000 population. Boys are

Robert Kienbock, 1871–1953, Professor of Radiology, Vienna, Austria, described this condition in 1910.

affected most commonly: the peak incidence is related to the start of puberty, hence it is earlier in girls. As a result of growth stimulated by hormonal changes, the strength of the growth plate, its resistance to shear and its orientation are reduced. The hip is therefore 'at risk' and normal forces, exacerbated by obesity and repetitive minor trauma, precipitate a slip. Other conditions, such as hypothyroidism, renal failure and previous radiotherapy treatment (local or to the pituitary region) also increase the risk.

Diagnosis

The diagnosis is suggested by the history and examination and confirmed on plain x-ray (Figure 41.17). Displacement is often more obvious on a lateral view. Indeed it can easily be missed by the unwary clinician if only the anteroposterior (AP) view is checked.

Classification

Slip severity can be graded on the lateral x-ray (Table 41.7) or classified according to the onset of symptoms: acute, chronic or acute-on-chronic.

Table 41.7 Grading of the severity of slip of the upper (capital) femoral epiphysis.

Slip severity	Metaphysis uncovered (%)
Mild	<33
Moderate	33–66
Severe	>66

Management

Following an acute episode the patient is often unable to weight-bear and the slip is considered to be unstable by the Loder classification. Displacement is often moderate or severe. This situation is essentially equivalent to a displaced intracapsular femoral neck fracture. This means that an acute unstable SUFE is an emergency. The AVN risk is considerable but is reduced by prompt screw fixation that stabilises the 'fracture' (Figure 41.18). Gentle repositioning of the femoral head often occurs inadvertently with the reduction of muscle spasm that accompanies the anaesthetic. To be effective such treatment must take place within 24 hours of injury. If delayed, the AVN rate increases.

With chronic slips the patient is usually able to weight-bear, albeit with pain, and the slip is considered stable. Screw or pin fixation *in situ* relieves pain and often improves the range of movement but a permanent restriction of movement will be present with limitation of flexion, internal rotation and adduction (Figure 41.19). The leg will also always be slightly short.

In the acute-on-chronic case, repositioning of the acute element of the slip may be feasible. In the severe slip it may be impossible to place a screw in a satisfactory position in the epiphysis, even by starting anteriorly on the neck. In addition, once healed, there may be significant, persistent deformity leading to restriction of joint movement. In these cases a realignment osteotomy may be considered. As with all osteotomies, the closer the correction is to the site of deformity, the better the outcome; however, in this situation, the risks of AVN or chondrolysis may

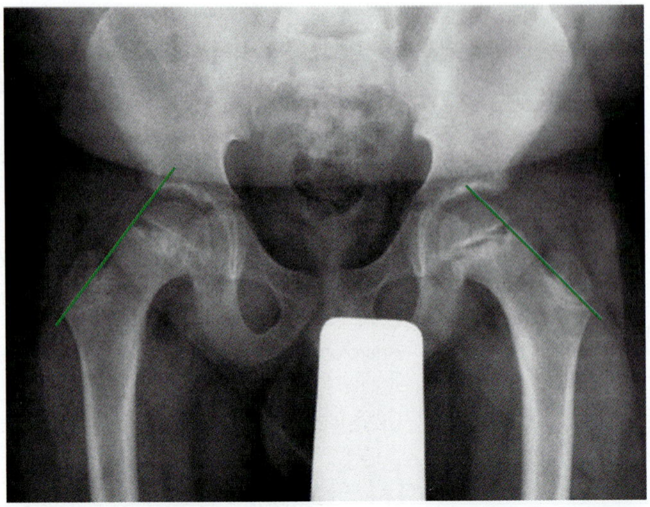

Figure 41.17 Anteroposterior pelvic x-ray demonstrating a mild slip of the upper (capital) femoral epiphysis on the right side. A line drawn along the upper margin of the femoral neck should transect the femoral head (left side) – if it does not do so (right side) a slip is present. There are many other x-ray features that help confirm the diagnosis but the changes are often subtle.

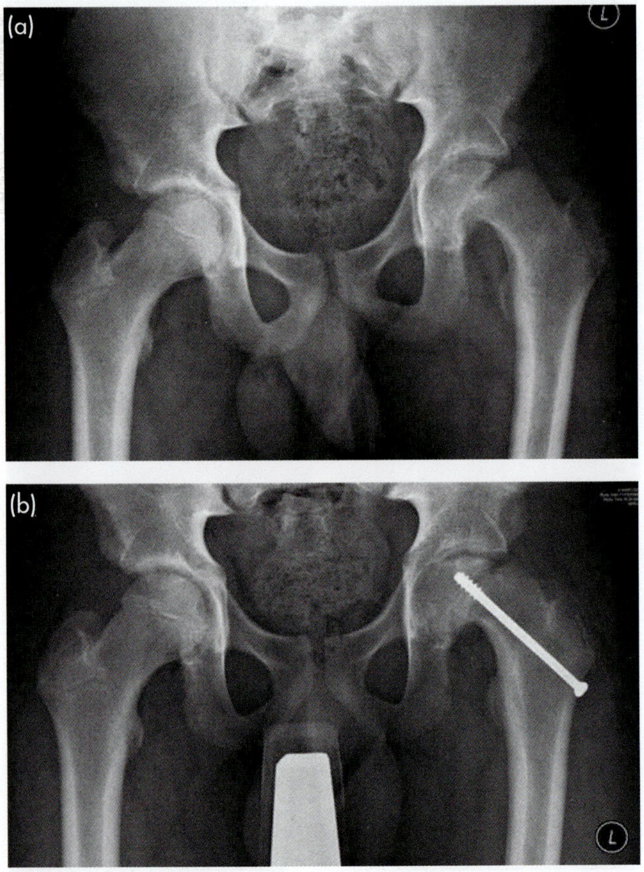

Figure 41.18 Anteroposterior pelvic x-ray showing a left-sided acute severe unstable slip of the upper (capital) femoral epiphysis. (a) At presentation; (b) following partial repositioning and fixation with a cannulated screw.

John Hilton, 1805–1878, surgeon, Guy's Hospital, London, UK.
Randall Loder, Professor of Orthopaedic Surgery, Philadelphia, PA, USA.

be unacceptably high, and so an intertrochanteric osteotomy could be considered. Bilateral slips do occur and prophylactic pinning of the normal but 'at-risk' hip may be indicated (Summary box 41.12).

Summary box 41.12

Slip of the upper (capital) femoral epiphysis

- Occurs in prepubertal children, mainly boys
- Often presents with knee pain and the leg may be short and externally rotated
- Classification may be according to the severity of slip, whether acute or chronic, or whether stable or unstable – all affect the prognosis
- Most slips are pinned *in situ* with a single screw into the centre of the epiphysis
- Avascular necrosis is the most feared complication of both the condition and its treatment

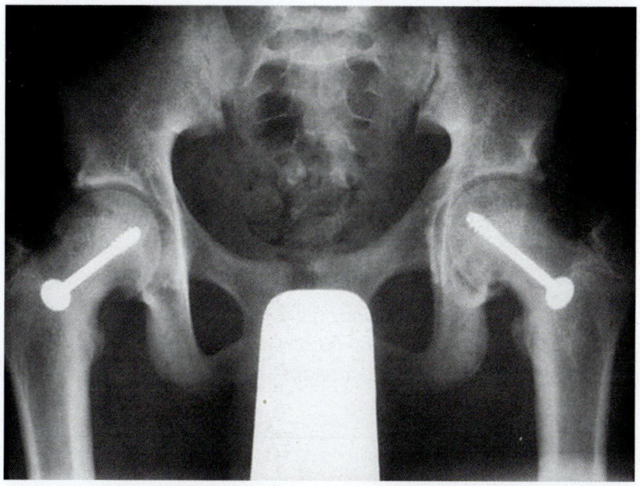

Figure 41.19 Anteroposterior x-ray showing screw fixation *in situ* of a case of bilateral chronic slip of the upper (capital) femoral epiphysis. Note the position of the screw entry point on the anterior femoral neck.

ABNORMALITIES OF THE KNEE AND LOWER LEG

Many knee problems are self-limiting. Others require surgical consideration to reduce the risk of later degenerative change.

Osteochondritis dissecans

Osteochondritis dissecans (OCD) most commonly affects the knee. An osteochondral fragment becomes partially or completely separated from the joint surface. Magnetic resonance imaging (MRI) is the best way of showing the lesion. In mild cases, or those treated early with rest and activity modification, the osteochondral fragment may remain attached and heal. If it detaches, partially or completely, mechanical symptoms necessitate treatment either to encourage bone healing via fixation of the fragment or to remove a loose body. Younger children have a better prognosis.

Discoid meniscus

This invariably affects the lateral meniscus which is abnormally thick and covers most of the tibial plateau. The child presents with a painful clunk on knee extension. MRI is usually diagnostic. Surgery is indicated for relief of pain or mechanical symptoms.

Anterior knee pain

In adolescents the extensor mechanism of the knee is a common site of knee pain.

Osgood–Schlatter disease is a traction apophysitis of the patellar tendon insertion. Pain, tenderness and swelling at the tibial tubercle, exacerbated by exercise, are diagnostic and x-rays are unnecessary. Treatment is relative rest and analgesia and the condition resolves once the apophysis has fused.

Patellofemoral pain is common and often attributed to a degree of patellar maltracking. As for patellar instability, treatment starts with physiotherapy to develop the quadriceps muscles, and to correct any wasting which may have occurred as a result of the pain. There are a multitude of operations described to improve the 'postulated mal-tracking', but as is so often the case in surgery when there is a large choice of operations, none work reliably and so surgery is rarely appropriate.

Fibular hemimelia

In fibula hemimelia there is a congenital failure of formation of the lateral 'column' of the lower leg (Figure 41.20 and Table 41.8).

Management is tailored to the severity of the deficiency. Treatment options range from a shoe raise, through multiple episodes of limb equalisation surgery to amputation for the worst cases. An early prediction of the leg length discrepancy at maturity allows a realistic treatment plan to be devised for the patient.

Table 41.8 Classical x-ray features of fibula hemimelia.

Foot and ankle	Absent lateral rays; tarsal coalition; ball and socket ankle joint
Lower leg	Absent or deficient fibula; tibial bow
Knee	Absent cruciate ligaments; deficient lateral femoral condyle
Femur	Relative hypoplasia
Limb length and alignment	Short; external rotation ± valgus

Blount's disease

The aetiology of this disordered growth in the posteromedial proximal tibial physis is unknown. The infantile form is more common in Afro-Caribbeans but the adolescent-onset disease affects all ethnic origins. The child presents with progressive and often severe tibia vara with significant intoeing. The x-ray features are diagnostic (Figure 41.21).

Treatment is surgical: following correction of limb alignment via an osteotomy, an epiphyseodesis of the remaining physis may be necessary to prevent recurrence with subsequent limb length equalisation surgery as required.

Robert Bailey Osgood, 1873–1956, Professor of Orthopaedic Surgery, Harvard University Medical School, Boston, MA, USA.
Carl Schlatter, 1864–1934, Professor of Surgery, Zurich, Switzerland.
Osgood and Schlatter described osteochondritis of the tibial tubercle independently in 1903.

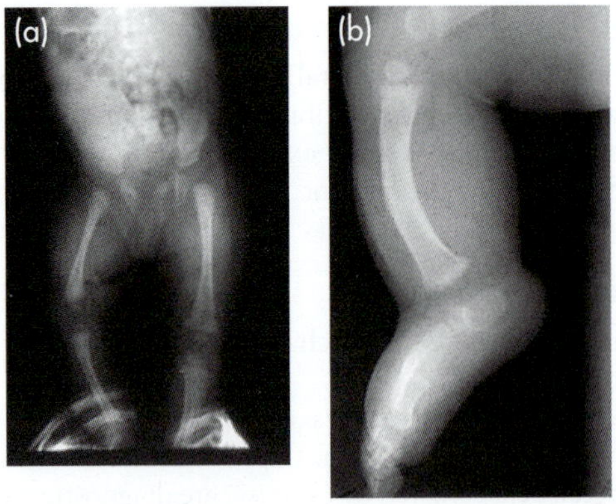

Figure 41.20 Anteroposterior (a) and lateral (b) x-rays of two lower limbs showing some of the features of a fibular hemimelia: absent fifth ray in the foot, absent fibula and deformed tibia.

Congenital pseudarthrosis of the tibia

This rare condition presents clinically with an anterolateral bow of the tibia with or without a fracture. Classic x-ray changes are noted and 50 per cent are associated with neurofibromatosis. Once fractured, the tibia is reluctant to heal. Long-term orthotic treatment may be necessary, with subsequent surgical procedures designed to obtain bony union and restore leg length (Summary box 41.13).

Summary box 41.13

Abnormalities of the knee and lower leg

- Osteochondritis dissecans – better prognosis in children than adults
- Discoid meniscus – usually lateral, may require surgery
- Anterior knee pain – treatment almost always conservative
- Fibular hemimelia – associated with abnormalities from the foot proximally (foot worse than hip)
- Blount's disease – clinically, a sharp proximal tibial angulation
- Congenital pseudarthrosis of the tibia – anterolateral bowing

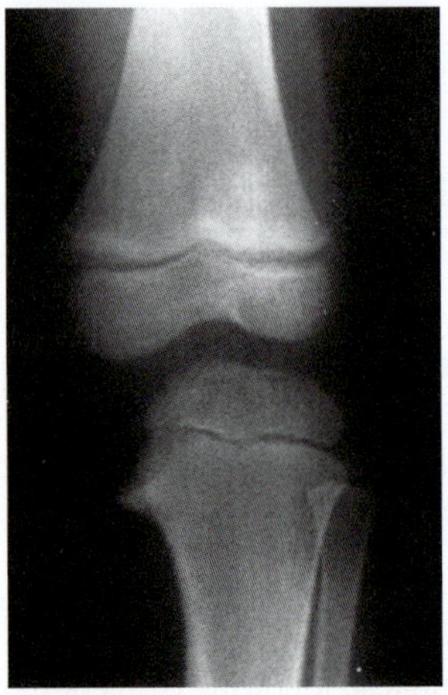

Figure 41.21 Anteroposterior x-ray of the left knee demonstrating changes compatible with Blount's disease affecting the posteromedial tibial physis with changes in both the epiphysis and the metaphysis.

ABNORMALITIES OF THE FOOT AND ANKLE

Parents are often concerned that minor foot abnormalities will cause their child to be clumsy or slow. This is rarely the case, so reassurance is a cornerstone in the management of abnormalities of the foot and ankle in children.

Congenital talipes equinovarus (the 'clubfoot')

The clubfoot is deformed in three planes (Figure 41.22). In true congenital talipes equinovarus (CTEV) the deformity is fixed. Intrauterine moulding can cause an identical pattern of deformity that is postural and therefore correctable.

Incidence and aetiology

The reported incidence varies from one to six cases per 1000 live births, depending on racial differences. It is more common in boys and bilateral in approximately 50 per cent of cases. A family history is common but inheritance is multifactorial. Most cases are idiopathic but the outcome varies with the aetiology so it is important to consider the cause when planning treatment (Table 41.9).

Table 41.9 Several different types of clubfoot are recognised.

Type	Example
Postural	
Idiopathic	
Neuromuscular	Spina bifida; arthrogryposis; spinal cord anomalies – considered in feet that resist treatment or relapse
Syndromic	Trisomy 15

Pathology

The talonavicular joint is subluxed with the navicular displaced medially with respect to a deformed talar head and

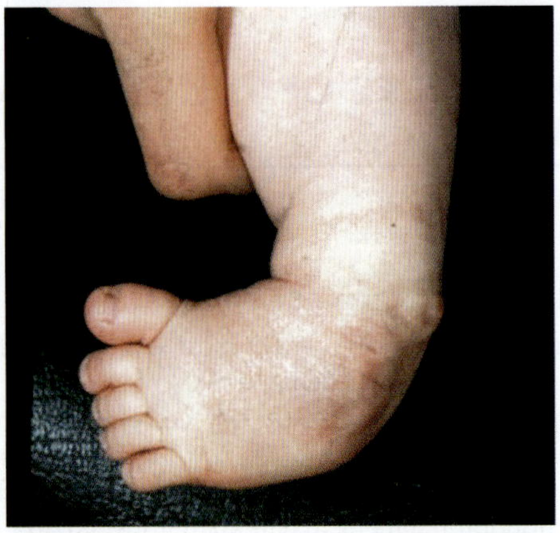

Figure 41.22 Anteroposterior photograph of a foot showing the classic deformities associated with a clubfoot. The hindfoot is in equinus and varus, there is midfoot cavus and the forefoot lies adducted and apparently supinated, although actually pronated relative to the hindfoot.

neck. Ligaments, particularly the calcaneofibular ligament, and tendon sheaths, such as the posterior tibial tendon sheath, are shortened and thickened and contain contractile myofibroblasts. The gastrocsoleus and posterior tibial muscles are smaller than normal, with reduced myofibrils and increased connective tissue, possibly because of a local neuromuscular abnormality. The vascular supply via the dorsalis pedis may be diminished. It remains unclear which abnormalities are primary and which occur as the deformity develops.

Clinical assessment

It should be possible to distinguish the postural clubfoot from the structural (rigid) foot soon after birth.

The postural clubfoot may require physiotherapy with stretching or casting, but can soon be manipulated into a 'normal' position of 45° of abduction and full dorsiflexion with the calcaneus well down in the heel pad. Medial creases are minimal and posterior creases shallow and multiple.

The structural clubfoot has fixed deformity with elements of equinus, varus and supination and cannot be corrected beyond neutral. Cavus is often marked. The heel feels 'empty' as the calcaneus is held up by the shortened tendo Achilles. There is a deep medial and single posterior crease.

All children with structural clubfoot deformity have a small calf and foot and some tibial shortening. Children should be examined carefully for neurological signs of intraspinal pathology.

Both Pirani and Dimeglio have developed scoring systems based on foot appearance in the position of maximal correction which predict treatment response and progress (Summary box 41.14).

Family counselling

The diagnosis of CTEV may be made during an antenatal ultrasound: counselling is limited by uncertainty as to the severity of the problem but the parents can be reassured that their child will walk, run and play with his/her peers.

Summary box 41.14

Clubfoot

- Multiplanar deformity: hindfoot equinus and varus, forefoot adduction and supination with a plantarflexed first ray
- Incidence is 1–6:1000 live births, more common in boys and with a familial tendency
- Most cases are idiopathic but neuromuscular causes include spina bifida and arthrogryposis
- Scoring systems (Pirani/Dimeglio) are used to assess the severity

Treatment

Ponseti method

The method described by Ponseti corrects foot deformity in 95 per cent of cases without the need for a formal surgical release. The technique has been introduced successfully worldwide. Treatment commences within a few days of birth. A specific series of manoeuvres, followed by a series of well-moulded above-knee plaster casts results in gradual correction of the deformity (Figure 41.23). The head of the talus is the fulcrum around which the rest of the foot swivels. After the forefoot has been corrected, most feet (about 80 per cent) require a percutaneous Achilles tenotomy in order to dorsiflex the foot satisfactorily.

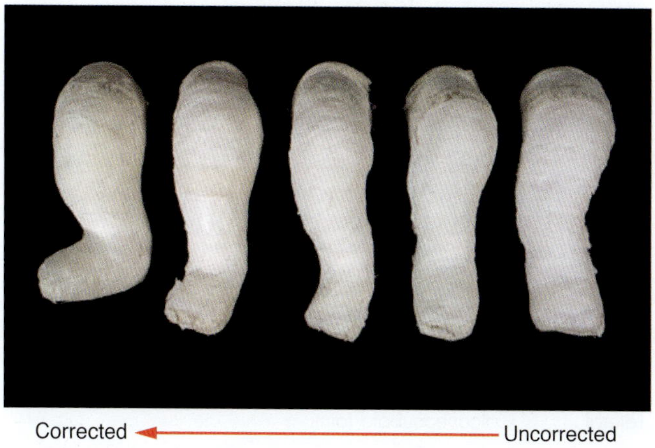

Figure 41.23 A photograph of a series of casts documenting the stepwise correction of the foot deformity with the Ponseti method of serial manipulation and casting.

Once corrected, the foot position is maintained by a foot abduction orthosis (FAO) that holds the foot in external rotation and slight dorsiflexion. The FAO is worn full-time for three months and at 'night and nap-time' for up to four years. Poor compliance with the FAO is associated with a higher relapse rate. Recurrent deformity can be treated with further plasters, but a tibialis anterior tendon transfer may be required around the age of 2.5–4 years for dynamic supination.

Feet treated with the Ponseti method are less stiff, less likely to be painful and less subject to overcorrection than those treated surgically. The Ponseti method is significantly better than other reported conservative regimes.

Surgical treatment

When conservative treatment fails, surgical intervention is required, ideally before walking age.

Surgical release is generally performed 'à la carte', with sequential release of the pathologically tight structures via either a Turco incision or the Cincinnati incision to reduce the subluxed joints (Table 41.10). Stabilisation may require the use of temporary Kirschner wires. Deformity correction should not be compromised by wound closure and the Cincinnati incision can be left to heal by secondary intention if necessary.

Postoperative casting is followed by splinting and physiotherapy as required. Good or excellent results are reported in 60–80 per cent of children treated surgically but stiffness and over- or undercorrection are common complications.

Surgery for residual or recurrent deformity is often difficult and requires a careful assessment of the forefoot, hindfoot and tibial torsion. Surgical procedures may involve further soft-tissue releases or tendon transfers but, in the presence of fixed deformity, bony correction is often necessary. The foot becomes progressively stiffer with each surgical intervention (Summary box 41.15).

Other foot and ankle conditions

Most postural deformities such as metatarsus adductus and calcaneovalgus feet improve spontaneously.

Congenital vertical talus (CVT) is rare and often associated

Ignacio Ponseti, 2010, professor at Iowa, USA.
Martin Kirschner, 1879–1942, Professor of Surgery, Heidelberg, Germany, introduced the use of skeletal traction wires in 1909.

Table 41.10 The four stages of a peritalar release that might be required for the correction of a severe clubfoot deformity.

Site	Structures requiring lengthening or release
Posterior	Tendo Achilles Ankle and subtalar joints Calcaneofibular ligament Posterior elements of the peroneal tendon sheaths
Medial	Abductor hallucis Tibialis posterior Talonavicular joint Toe flexors
Lateral	Calcaneocuboid joint
Plantar	Plantar ligaments Plantar fascia
Protect	Neurovascular bundle Talocalcaneal interosseous ligament (if possible)

Summary box 41.15

Treatment of clubfoot

- The Ponseti method of serial casting is successful in 95 per cent of feet, avoiding formal surgical release although percutaneous tenotomy is usually required
- The standard sequence is elevation of the first ray, gradual forefront abduction to 60° and, finally, dorsiflexion, usually following Achilles tenotomy
- Tibialis anterior transfer can be used to correct dynamic supination in older children
- Surgical release may need to address posterior, medial, plantar and lateral structures, and will result in a stiffer foot than one treated conservatively

with neuromuscular conditions such as arthrogryposis and spinal dysraphism. Clinically, there is a stiff 'rocker-bottom' foot with dorsal dislocation of the navicular on the talus (Figure 41.24). Correction is surgical although a 'reverse' Ponseti method with a limited surgical approach is showing good early results.

In **tarsal coalition** there is failure of segmentation of adjacent tarsal bones. School-age children present with hindfoot pain and recurrent ankle sprains. The stiff subtalar joint cannot accommodate uneven ground. The most common coalitions are talocalcaneal and calcaneonavicular (see Figure 41.3). X-ray, computed tomography (CT) or MR may be required to confirm the diagnosis. Treatment is initially conservative but, if the coalition requires surgical excision, this should be carried out before significant degenerative changes develop.

Curly toes that are flexed and medially deviated are common, often familial and rarely need treatment. Strapping is ineffective. Flexor tenotomy is used when there are symptoms.

Other causes of foot pain in children include osteochondroses (see Table 41.6):

- Köhler's disease: presents with dorsal forefoot pain and swelling in young children. The navicular appears to suffer a spontaneous avascular necrosis and collapses. The alarming radiological appearances resolve spontaneously and without sequelae.

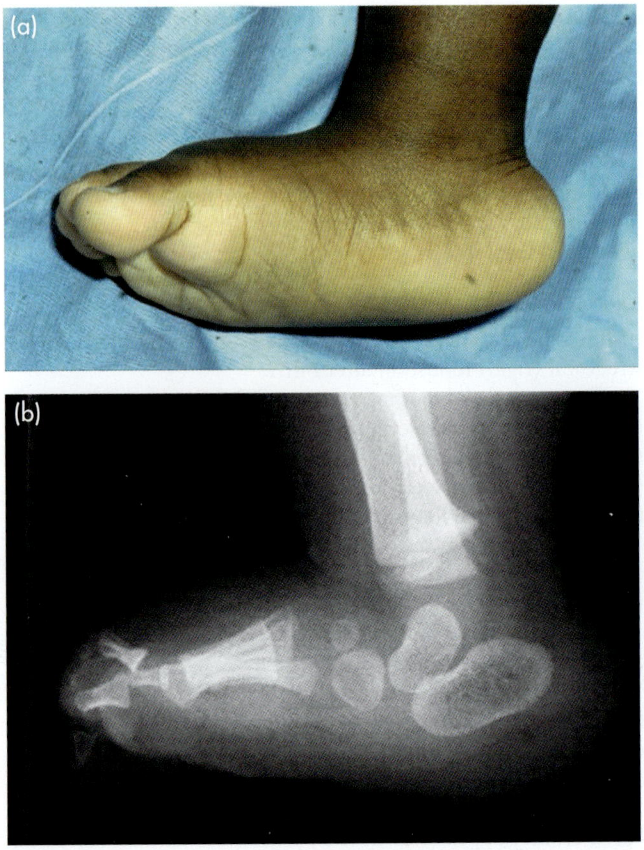

Figure 41.24 Congenital vertical talus. (a) Lateral photograph demonstrating a 'rocker-bottom foot'. (b) Lateral x-ray showing hindfoot equinus and suggesting dorsal subluxation of the non-ossified navicular and forefoot with respect to the head of the talus.

- Sever's disease (enthesopathy of the calcaneal apophysis): presents with heel pain related to activity. Tightness in the calf muscle complex may be a contributing factor.
- Freiberg's osteochondrosis: presents with forefoot pain and avascular change in the second metatarsal head. It may be asymptomatic and present as an incidental finding on x-ray. Symptomatic bony spurs and osteochondral fragments may need excision (Summary box 41.16).

Summary box 41.16

Other foot and ankle conditions

- Congenital vertical talus – presents as 'rocker-bottom' foot
- Tarsal coalition – presents as a stiff, painful flat foot
- Curly toes are common – most do not need treatment
- Osteochondroses - almost always self-limiting

ABNORMALITIES OF THE UPPER LIMB

Minor finger abnormalities are common (Table 41.11) and frequently require surgical intervention. Comfort and function are more important than appearance.

Function is also the most important consideration when managing more extensive upper limb abnormalities. Treatment

Alban Köhler, 1874–1947, radiologist of Wiesbaden, Germany, described this disease in 1908.
James Warren Sever, 1878–1964, orthopaedic surgeon, The Children's Hospital, Boston, MA, USA, described apophysitis of the os calcis in 1912.
Albert Henry Freiberg, 1869–1940, Professor of Orthopaedic Surgery, The University of Cincinnati, Cincinnati, OH, USA, described this disease in 1926.

is delayed until hand dominance is established and it is clear what problems a specific deformity is causing a given child. Children are very adaptable and cope with disabilities much more readily than their parents/doctors expect.

Table 41.11 Common minor congenital anomalies affecting the hand.

Anomaly	Definition	Treatment
Extra/accessory digits		Excise/amputate when necessary
Syndactyly	Failure of separation of digits	Separation with/without skin grafting for functional or cosmetic reasons
Trigger thumb (digit)		Release of the A1 pulley of the flexor tendon sheath
Clinodactyly (usually the fifth digit)	Abnormal angulation of the digit in the radioulnar plane	Surgical treatment of the delta phalanx if deformity progressive or interfering with hand function
Camptodactyly (usually the fifth digit)	Fixed flexion deformity of proximal interphalangeal joint	Splinting/physiotherapy; surgery rarely indicated

Radial club hand

This longitudinal failure of formation is commonly associated with other malformations, for example as part of the VACTERL syndrome (abnormal vertebrae, anus, cardiovascular system, trachea, oesophagus, renal system and limb buds). The clinical problem depends, most specifically, on whether the thumb is present and functional (Figure 41.25). Treatment is a balance of conservative measures including physiotherapy and splinting, and judicious surgery to centralise and stabilise the hand and wrist on the single bone forearm. Thumb reconstruction may be technically challenging. In later childhood, forearm lengthening may be considered.

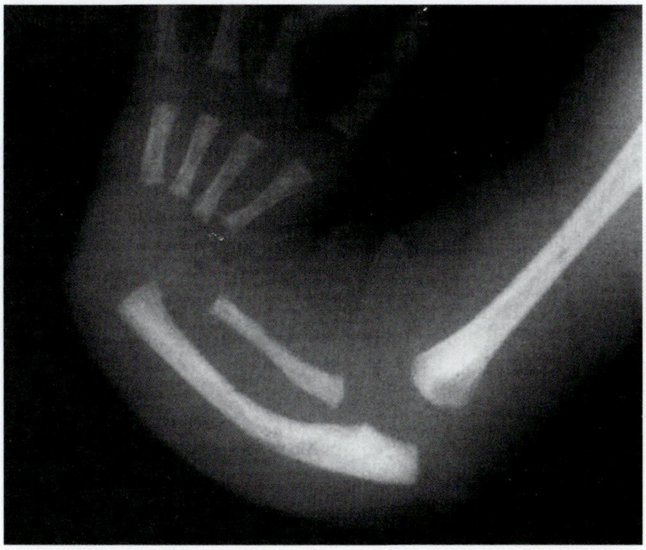

Figure 41.25 Anteroposterior x-ray of a radial club hand demonstrating a short radius, a deformed ulna and an absent thumb.

Radioulnar synostosis

Failure of proximal separation of the embryonic radius and ulna means that the forearm cannot pronate and supinate. The hand is in a fixed position and the child presents if this results in a functional problem. Osteotomy of the forearm bones can change the fixed position (from pronation to neutral) but does not restore movement.

Congenital radial head dislocation

The dislocation is usually posterolateral compared with the classic traumatic anterior dislocation (Figure 41.26). Some restriction of elbow joint movement and forearm rotation is noted along with discomfort on activity. Radial head excision may be required (Summary box 41.17).

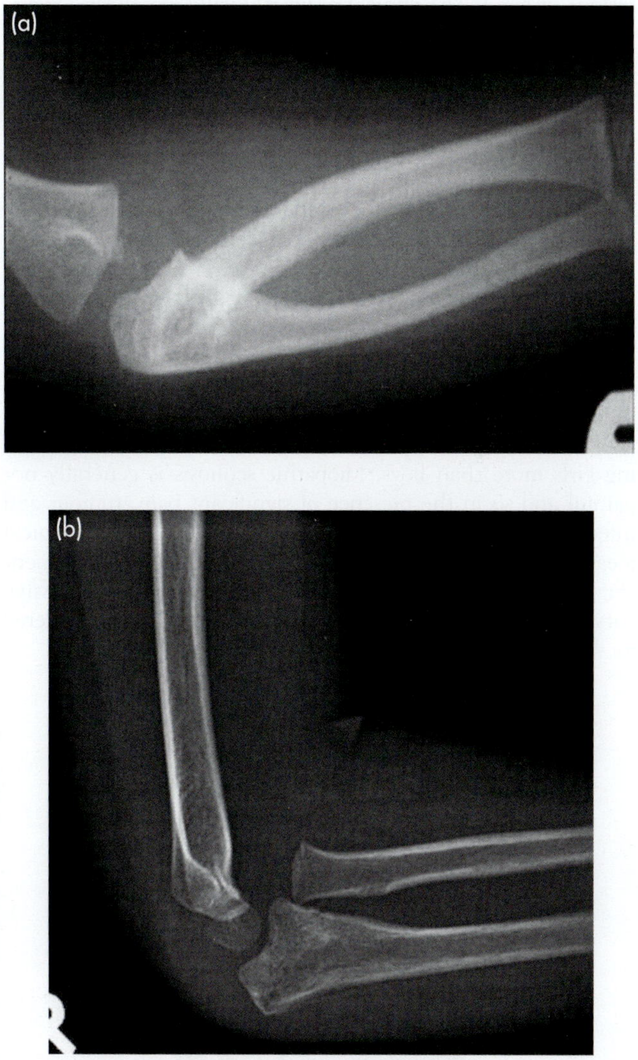

Figure 41.26 Radial head dislocation. (a) Lateral x-ray of a forearm showing a proximal radioulnar synostosis with a congenital posterolateral dislocation of the radial head. Note the underdeveloped radial head and neck and compare with. (b) Lateral x-ray of a traumatic anterior dislocation of the radial head with a normal appearance to the head and neck and a deformity in the proximal ulna.

Giovanni Battista Monteggia, 1762–1815, Professor of Anatomy and Surgery, Ospedale Maggiore, Milan, Italy.

Summary box 41.17

Upper limb abnormalities

- Radial club hand is frequently associated with other congenital anomalies, for example the VACTERL or Holt–Oram syndromes
- Radioulnar synostosis presents with a fixed forearm position in childhood
- Congenital radial head dislocation is usually posterolateral

SPINAL DEFORMITIES AND BACK PAIN

Congenital deformities

Congenital vertebral deformities are either failures of formation (a hemivertebra) or of segmentation (unilateral or bilateral fusions or bars). The clinical result is usually a scoliosis (Figure 41.27). Treatment should be based on the potential for curve progression. When a kyphosis develops, progressive neurological deficit is common. Bracing is ineffective for congenital vertebral deformities.

Scoliosis

The term 'scoliosis' describes spinal deformity in three planes: lateral curvature is the most obvious deformity while the rotational component is most apparent in forward flexion when the rib asymmetry creates a 'rib hump' (Figure 41.28). The cause may be idiopathic, neuromuscular, syndrome-related or congenital. Both the aetiology and the age of onset affect the natural history (Table 41.12). In general, the earlier the onset, the more likely the deformity is to be progressive.

The adolescent idiopathic curve is the most common, affecting girls more than boys. Idiopathic scoliosis is generally not painful and so in the presence of significant pain, tumour and infection must be excluded. The Cobb angle is a radiological measurement that defines severity and helps to guide treatment (Figure 41.29). Curves <20° do not need treatment, progressive curves of 25–40° may be braced, and those >40° are considered for surgery (Summary box 41.18).

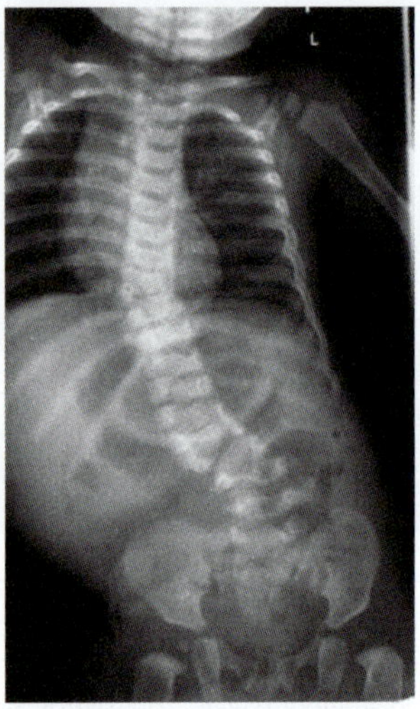

Figure 41.27 Anteroposterior x-ray of the spine demonstrating multiple congenital vertebral anomalies including hemivertebrae.

Table 41.12 Classification of idiopathic scoliosis.

Type	Age of onset
Infantile	0–3 years
Juvenile	4–10 years
Adolescent	11–18 years
Adult	Onset at maturity

Summary box 41.18

Scoliosis

- Multiplanar deformity includes an unsightly rotational component
- Aetiology may be congenital (underlying bony malformation), neuromuscular, syndromic or idiopathic
- A leg length discrepancy causes a postural scoliosis
- Adolescent idiopathic scoliosis is the most common structural scoliosis
- Back pain associated with scoliosis may be due to infection or tumour
- Treatment depends on the severity and likelihood of curve progression – it varies from observation, through bracing, to surgery

Kyphosis

When a kyphosis exceeds the normal 20–50°, the cause may be postural or structural. Structural kyphosis is commonly secondary to Scheuermann's disease, presenting as a progressive adolescent kyphosis characterised radiologically by ≥5° vertebral wedging at three adjacent levels and end-plate changes. The aetiology is unknown. Treatment ranges from physiotherapy and bracing to surgery, depending on severity, progression and symptoms.

Spondylolisthesis

Spondylolysis defines a defect in the pars interarticularis of the vertebra. There are six types: congenital (dysplastic facet joints), isthmic (weak or elongated pars), degenerative, post-traumatic, pathological or post-surgical. Spondylolisthesis occurs when the upper vertebra slips forward on the lower; it is graded according

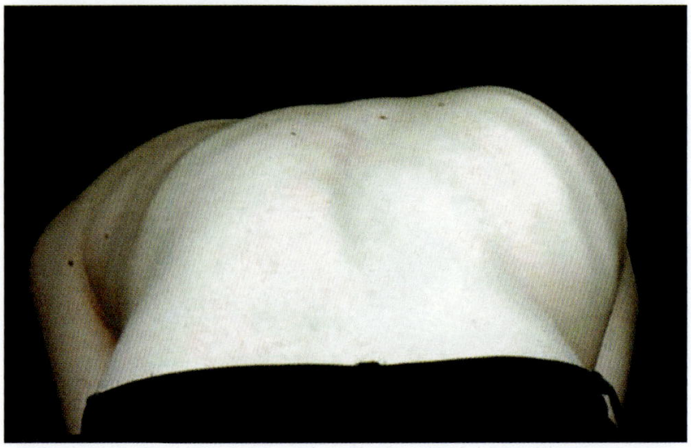

Figure 41.28 Clinical photograph of the Adam's forward bend test that demonstrates the presence of a rib hump and the level of the curve.

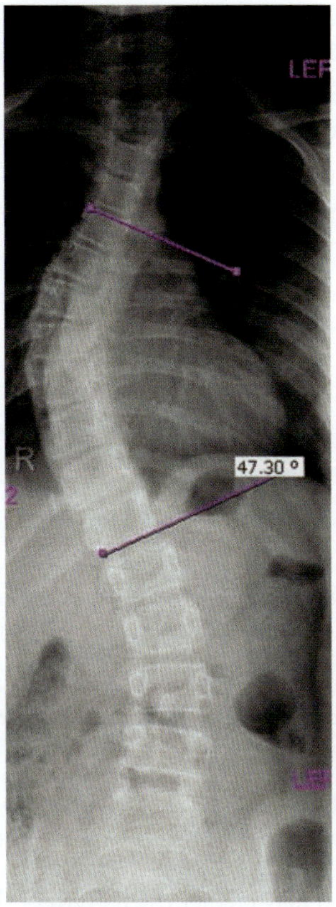

Figure 41.29 Anteroposterior x-ray of a spine with a scoliosis (right thoracic), with a Cobb angle of 47°.

to the percentage slip, measured by relating the slipped vertebra to the one below (Table 41.13).

Mild slips are often asymptomatic and do not require treatment. Treatment (physiotherapy, bracing and surgery) depends on the degree of slip and symptoms; mechanical back pain may respond to conservative methods but neurological involvement usually requires surgical intervention.

Table 41.13 Classification of spondylolisthesis according to severity of the slip.

Grade	Percentage slip
0	No slip
1	<25%
2	26–50%
3	51–75%
4	>75%
Spondyloptosis	>100% – complete translation

Torticollis

In torticollis the head is tilted toward and rotated away from the tight sternocleidomastoid muscle.

Congenital torticollis is usually secondary to intrauterine moulding but may present with fixed sternocleidomastoid contracture or with a palpable 'tumour' within the muscle. There is a strong correlation with DDH. Most cases resolve with stretching but persistent cases develop facial asymmetry and require surgical release of the sternocleidomastoid at one or both ends.

Acquired torticollis is less common and may be caused by gastro-oesophageal reflux, posterior fossa tumour/other regional abnormality, inflammation/infection, ocular problems or atlanto-axial rotatory subluxation.

Back pain

Children report back pain less frequently than adults although >50 per cent will have had an episode by late adolescence. Back pain in a child is a 'red flag' for serious spinal pathology but if mild, intermittent or occurring only on strenuous activity, it is usually self-limiting (Summary box 41.19).

Summary box 41.19

'Red flag' symptoms and signs for spinal pathology

- Systemic illness, fever or weight loss
- Progressive neurological deficit
- Unrelenting or night pain
- Spinal deformity

All these require urgent further investigation with a full blood count (FBC), erythrocyte sedimentation rate (ESR) and C-reactive protein (CRP), plain x-ray and MRI or other appropriate imaging. Other causes of back pain include intra-abdominal, renal and systemic pathology, and all must be considered. Physiotherapy encourages symptomatic improvement (Summary box 41.20).

Summary box 41.20

Other spinal conditions

- Excessive kyphosis may be caused by Scheuermann's disease
- Spondylolisthesis is forward slip of one vertebra on another; it may cause mechanical and, rarely, neurological symptoms
- Torticollis may be congenital and usually responds to stretching of the fibrosed sternocleidomastoid muscle. Acquired torticollis may be due to one of several significant pathologies
- Back pain with red flag symptoms and signs requires urgent investigation

NEUROMUSCULAR CONDITIONS

Joint stability and limb function rely on the complex integration of the musculoskeletal and neurological systems. Damage to either leads to one of several conditions linked only by the fact that they are incurable. Management is directed at helping the child cope with their disability, minimising further deterioration and maximising function. It is important to have an understanding of what the damage is and what the future holds.

Spina bifida and polio are classic lower motor neurone lesions whereas cerebral palsy and head injuries affect upper motor

Holger Werfel Scheuermann, 1877–1960, radiologist, The Municipal Hospital, Sundby, Copenhagen, Denmark, described juvenile kyphosis in 1920.

neurones and the higher centres. There are often other disabilities such as blindness, epilepsy and intellectual difficulties to consider.

In children, even if the initial insult to the neuromuscular system is non-progressive, the effects of the insult change with growth. Damage at any level of the neuromuscular system leads to an alteration in tone and muscle imbalance associated with decreased control of movement. Abnormal muscle pull, particularly in combination with the effects of gravity, alters bone growth leading to deformity and joint contracture. Muscles are relatively weak and with body growth and a weight increase, they are no longer strong enough to control a heavier limb, particularly when deformity means they are working at a mechanical disadvantage.

A multidisciplinary approach to management is essential. Good physiotherapists and orthotists will reduce the need for surgical intervention and in the postoperative period they help ensure that the surgical benefits are maximised. In conditions such as Duchenne muscular dystrophy there is substantial evidence for the benefits of certain surgical procedures; however, in other conditions (cerebral palsy) there are fewer such long-term validated studies.

In general, it is important to maintain a full range of joint movement, muscle length and tendon excursion. This is easier to achieve in patients with a flaccid paralysis or low tone. The maintenance of muscle strength is also important. The use of splints, positioning techniques, seating and sleeping systems is common with the aim of preventing fixed contractures.

Surgery has a valuable role in the management of selected patients (Table 41.14).

The surgeon must understand that altering ankle posture may affect knee and hip posture/function and vice versa. The patient must have the intellectual ability and motivation to recover from the surgical procedure. Some of the factors which need to be considered in an holistic approach to the patient are given in Summary box 41.21 (see also Summary box 41.22).

Summary box 41.21

Factors to be considered in the assessment of a neuromuscular disability

- Is the insult to the neurological system progressive or non-progressive?
- Is it located centrally or peripherally?
- Is it general or focal?
- Is it associated with other abnormalities or not?

Summary box 41.22

Principles of treatment of neuromuscular conditions

- A neurological defect, whether progressive or not, may cause progressive deformity as the skeleton grows
- A multidisciplinary approach is essential
- Primary therapy aims to maintain range of movement and prevent fixed contractures with an emphasis on managing tone and position
- Surgery has a limited role in the management of neuromuscular conditions

Cerebral palsy

Cerebral palsy is caused by a non-progressive insult to the developing brain in the perinatal period; in most cases only risk factors, such as prematurity, rather than specific causes, such as hypoxia, can be identified. The effects of cerebral palsy may only become apparent as the child grows and fails to reach expected developmental milestones. At this stage investigations may help with aetiology and may predict the pattern of the cerebral palsy: premature babies may show evidence of periventricular leucomalacia on a brain MRI, which is associated with the development of a spastic diplegia with relative preservation of intellectual function.

In general, the pattern of involvement can be classified according to the anatomical site involved and the effect on muscle tone (Table 41.15). The prognosis for walking can be predicted by identifying evidence of neurological development, i.e. the loss of primitive reflexes.

An important aspect of management is the control of high tone. Tone can be reduced with drugs such as diazepam and baclofen. Alternatively, neuromuscular blockers such as botulinum toxin can bring about a focal reduction in tone by preventing acetylcholine release at the neuromuscular junction. The effect is temporary, giving a 'window' during which the physiotherapists can stretch agonists and strengthen antagonists. It is important to

Table 41.14 General types of surgical procedure that might be considered in the management of a patient with a neuromuscular condition.

Surgical procedure	Aim of treatment
Lengthening of the muscle–tendon unit	Restore joint range (but results in relative muscle weakness)
Tendon transfer	Improve functional movement; rebalance muscle forces, after correction of fixed deformity
Release of joint contracture; correction of bony deformity	Restore mechanical alignment, and allow muscles to work in a more efficient manner
Fuse/stabilise/relocate joints	Improve posture/function Reduce pain
Neurological procedures, e.g. selective dorsal rhizotomy, intrathecal baclofen pumps	Reduce tone
Leg equalisation procedures	Improve lower limb mechanics

Guillaume Benjamin Amand Duchenne (Duchenne de Boulogne), 1806–1875, a neurologist who worked successively in Boulogne and Paris, France, but who never held a hospital appointment.

differentiate between dynamic and fixed contractures; the latter will not respond to tone management or splinting.

Table 41.15 Classification of cerebral palsy with respect to muscle tone and site of involvement.

	Characteristics
Tone	
Low	
High	
Mixed	Often low tone in trunk with high tone in the limbs
Variable	High tone and low tone apparent in the same limb on different occasions
Site	
Hemiplegia	Arm more affected than leg
Diplegia	Legs more affected than arms
Total body involvement	Often significant intellectual impairment

The classic cerebral palsy gait patterns demonstrate flexor spasticity. The child with spastic diplegia has problems at all levels of the lower limb. Single event multilevel surgery (SEMLS) is popular and gait analysis (both observational and computerised) contribute to the patient management planning. Computerised analysis provides objective evidence of joint movement and mechanics in multiple planes (Figure 41.30). Appropriate bone and soft-tissue procedures can then be planned. Botulinum toxin helps with postoperative pain and spasm.

In the child with total body involvement (TBI) and high muscle tone, hip subluxation and eventual dislocation are common but often asymptomatic (Figure 41.31). Current thinking is that symmetry and pelvic position are important so hips should be kept in joint by the simplest means possible with early surgical intervention if necessary. Aggressive management of a spinal deformity will initially concentrate on seating position and subsequently emphasise spinal bracing or surgery.

Overall, it is important to remember what the child's needs will be once they have reached adulthood. Independent mobility and an effective means of communication are two of the most important requirements. Hence, it may not be appropriate to invest time and effort into gaining an upright posture if mobility will be achieved via an electric wheelchair and a hand-controlled car (Summary box 41.23).

Summary box 41.23

Cerebral palsy

- Brain injury is non-progressive
- Classified as hemiplegia, diplegia or TBI
- Tone may be high, low or variable but there is generalised, relative muscle weakness
- In ambulant children, gait analysis may be used to plan surgery or botulinum toxin injections
- In TBI, primary concerns are hip subluxation and spinal deformity

Polio

Despite an effective polio vaccine, this disease still occurs. About 1–2 per cent of patients develop neurological problems when the virus affects the anterior horn cells. Muscle weakness is proportionate to the number of motor units destroyed. Patients often develop trick movements to cope with their muscle weakness and minor joint contractures might actually improve function. Careful assessment before surgery is essential and both the surgeon and the patient must understand the goals of treatment.

Spina bifida

The extent of the disability varies with the level of the lesion: upper motor neurone involvement will produce spasticity while the more classic lower motor neurone lesion will merely produce weakness. Hydrocephalus may contribute to the complexity of the situation. Muscle imbalance leads to secondary joint deformity but the often profound, accompanying sensory disturbance, may affect the choice of surgical and non-surgical options.

Muscular dystrophy

Many types of muscular dystrophy exist that vary in terms of severity and distribution of involvement. Surgical intervention aims to improve quality of life. This is best achieved by operating early to release joint contractures. This will help to maintain walking ability and good spinal posture.

Brachial plexopathy

The obstetric brachial plexus injury is still common with a devastating effect on upper limb function, particularly if antigravity motor activity has not recovered by six months. Neural repair may be necessary in the infant. Later surgical interventions aim to prevent joint contractures and improve function.

INFECTION

Worldwide, bone and joint infection remain frequent causes of significant morbidity.

Septic arthritis

Joint infection is usually secondary to haematogenous spread but direct inoculation does occur, for example during a neonatal venepuncture. Diagnosis can be difficult in the very young and in those presenting with overwhelming sepsis. Neonates, children with immunocompromise and those with sickle cell disease are at increased risk. At the other end of the spectrum, the differentiation between joint sepsis and transient synovitis of the hip can be difficult to make.

Classically, the child presents with pain, fever and a reluctance to use the joint; in the lower limb this implies a reluctance to weight-bear. On examination, local tenderness and painful restriction of movement are apparent and in superficial joints inflammation may be obvious, with joint swelling.

Investigations include FBC, ESR, CRP and blood cultures. Plain x-rays help to exclude other diagnoses and may identify osteomyelitis. Ultrasound scans of deep-seated joints, such as the hip, will identify joint effusions (Figure 41.32). Other investigations such as MRI may be useful but should not be regarded as a necessity: good clinical skills, regular patient review and a high index of suspicion are more valuable. Four clinical predictors can differentiate between septic arthritis and transient synovitis (Summary box 41.24 and Table 41.16).

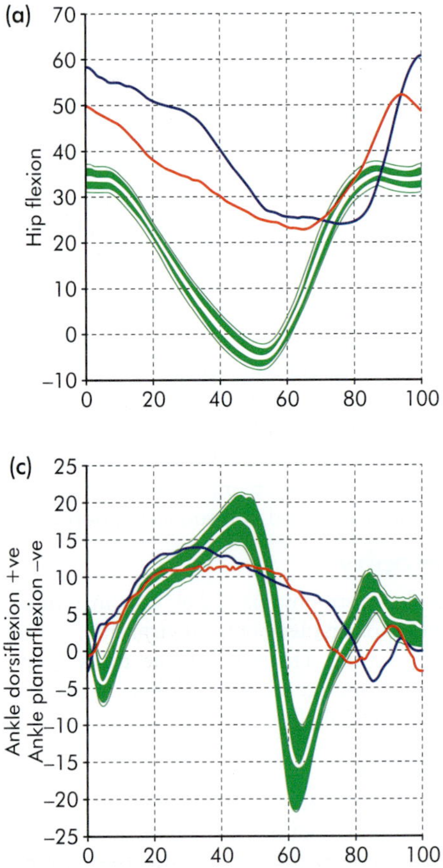

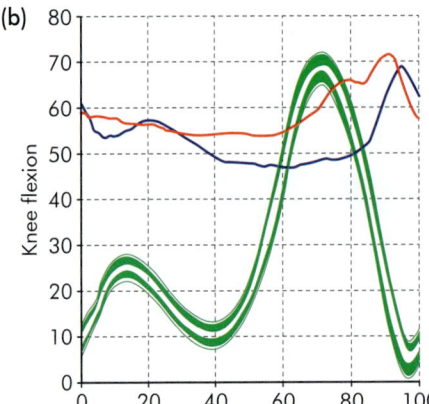

Figure 41.30 Gait analysis graphs such as these demonstrate the normal range of joint movements (green band) at hip (a), knee (b) and ankle (c) during the stance and swing phases of gait. The abnormal joint ranges are shown in red (right leg) and blue (left leg) and demonstrate the excessive hip flexion and lack of knee extension and abnormal ankle function associated with the 'crouch' gait of a child with cerebral palsy.

Summary box 41.24

The clinical predictors of Kocher *et al.* for the diagnosis of a septic joint

- History of fever
- Non-weight-bearing
- Erythrocyte sedimentation rate >40 mm/h
- White cell count >12 × 10^9 µL

Table 41.16 The value of the clinical predictors of Kocher *et al.* in determining the likelihood of the joint being septic.

No. of positive predictors	Predicted probability of joint sepsis
0	<0.2%
1	3.0%
2	40.0%
3	93.1%
4	99.6%

Pus in a joint is destructive: the proteases produced by leukocytes destroy both the collagen matrix of the articular cartilage and the bacteria. AVN may occur secondary to pressure effects or ischaemic infarction. The treatment of a presumed septic arthritis is thus the prompt removal of pus from the joint and appropriate adequate antibiotic therapy. Pain relief and rest are also important

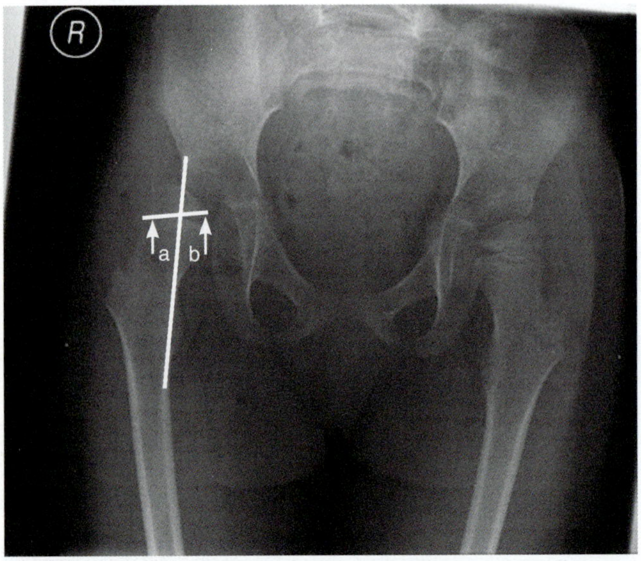

Figure 41.31 Anteroposterior pelvic x-ray of a child with spastic cerebral palsy. Both hips are subluxed. Reimer's migration percentage (a/a + b as a percentage) has been measured as approximately 60 per cent on the right hip.

as are the general health and nutrition of the patient. The joint is aspirated and if pus is confirmed then a formal washout is mandatory; standard teaching states that the joint must be opened, irrigated and free drainage encouraged via the capsulotomy. Recent literature supports repeated aspiration/irrigation via a large-bore cannula or a small arthroscope. Antibiotic usage is guided by the local hospital policy, the source of the infection, the Gram stain and, in due course, the culture and sensitivity of the organism identified. Joint instability, particularly in the hip joint (Figure 41.33a), may require the joint to be splinted in the reduced position while the inflammatory process settles.

The most frequently identified organism is *Staphylococcus aureus*. Streptococcal infection is also common and other organisms are more prevalent in certain age groups, e.g. the neonate, in certain conditions such as sickle cell disease, or in certain countries. The *Haemophilus influenzae* type B (Hib) vaccine has essentially eliminated *Haemophilus influenzae* as a cause of infection.

Improvement is judged clinically and by monitoring the inflammatory markers. Reaccumulation of pus does occur and must be suspected and treated promptly if the child fails to improve (Summary box 41.25).

Summary box 41.25

Septic arthritis

- Diagnosis is difficult in neonates and the immunocompromised
- Typical presentation is pain, fever and a reluctance to move the joint or weight-bear
- Investigations should include FBC, ESR, CRP, blood cultures and appropriate imaging studies, combined with astute clinical skills
- Pus in a joint can destroy articular cartilage and cause avascular necrosis
- Treatment is prompt removal of pus, appropriate antibiotic therapy, pain relief and splintage

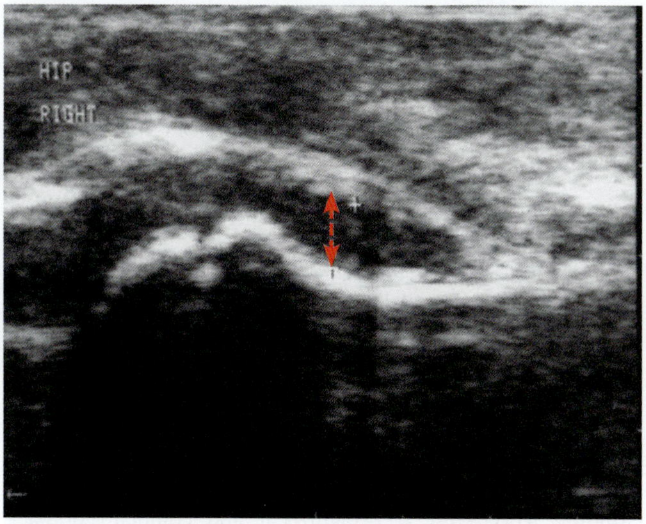

Figure 41.32 Ultrasound scan of a hip joint. A large effusion is distending the joint capsule. The dotted line represents the distance between the femoral neck and the joint capsule.

Osteomyelitis

As with septic arthritis, bone infection is usually caused by haematogenous spread. Infection often occurs in long bones in which the slow vascular flow within the looped vessels of the metaphysis combined with microtrauma is believed to encourage seeding of infection during a bacteraemia (Figure 41.34a). Inflammation follows and, if purulent material develops, the pressure effects of the subsequent abscess will lead to progressive bony destruction. Pus can pass through cortical bone and will then elevate the strong periosteum which may render the cortical bone avascular. As in cases of trauma or tumour, the periosteal elevation is a potent stimulus for new bone formation. In cases of untreated or chronic infection this new bone or involucrum may surround the dead bone, the sequestrum, leading to a 'bone-within-a-bone' appearance (Figure 41.34b).

The presentation and investigation of osteomyelitis is similar to that for joint sepsis. The differentiation between the two may be difficult and a sympathetic joint effusion may occur with

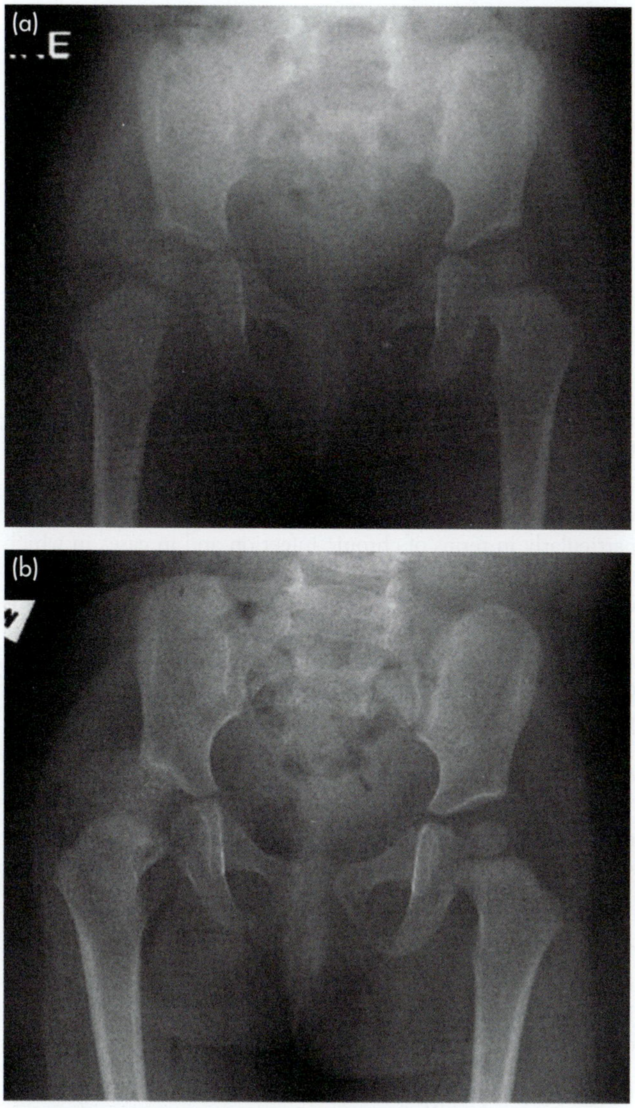

Figure 41.33 Septic arthritis of the right hip. (a) Anteroposterior pelvic x-ray with subtle signs of right hip subluxation. (b) Anteroposterior pelvic x-ray six months later showing destruction of the femoral head secondary to late treatment of a septic joint.

metaphyseal osteomyelitis. Thus, if there are no organisms seen on microscopy of a joint aspirate the possibility of a coexisting osteomyelitis must be considered. The metaphysis of a long bone may be intracapsular and infection may spread easily into the joint once the periosteum is breached. In the neonate, proximal femoral osteomyelitis and septic arthritis are essentially the same condition (Figure 41.34c).

General principles for the management of infection should be followed. Pus needs to be drained but otherwise the treatment is medical. Debate continues over the treatment and indeed whether antibiotics should be parenteral or oral (Summary box 41.26).

Summary box 41.26

Occurrence and treatment principles for bone and soft tissue infection

- Occurs by haematogenous spread, enhanced by microtrauma
- If untreated, new involucrum envelops dead sequestrum
- A joint effusion may be sympathetic or caused by direct spread from the adjacent metaphysis
- Treatment is drainage of pus, when present, appropriate and often prolonged antibiotic therapy, pain relief and splintage
- Rest/splintage of affected limb
- Analgesia
- Surgical drainage of pus
- Appropriate antibiotics via a suitable route and for the correct time
- Treatment of the underlying condition, e.g. nutritional deficiency, sickle cell disease

Complications of bone and joint sepsis

Treated appropriately, most cases of bone and joint sepsis resolve with no sequelae. However, significant complications can occur, particularly in terms of chronic infection and in cases in which there has been damage to the joint and/or the physis and the epiphyseal growth centres. In the neonate, vascular channels pass through the physis, connecting the metaphysis with the epiphysis, and a poorer outcome may ensue (see Figure 41.33b). Orthopaedic follow up should be continued until normal growth patterns are documented.

Meningococcal sepsis

The often debilitating, late orthopaedic sequelae of meningococcal septicaemia are secondary to endotoxin-induced microvascular injury and ischaemic physeal damage.

Tuberculosis

Tuberculosis is still common. The clinical presentation is often insidious, with malaise and weight loss combined with a boggy joint swelling, muscle wasting and joint contractures. Spinal deformity and neurological symptoms are particular problems.

Chronic relapsing/recurrent multifocal osteomyelitis

X-ray features suggest subacute or chronic osteomyelitis but laboratory and histopathological findings are usually non-specific and cultures negative. This is probably an inflammatory rather than an infective condition.

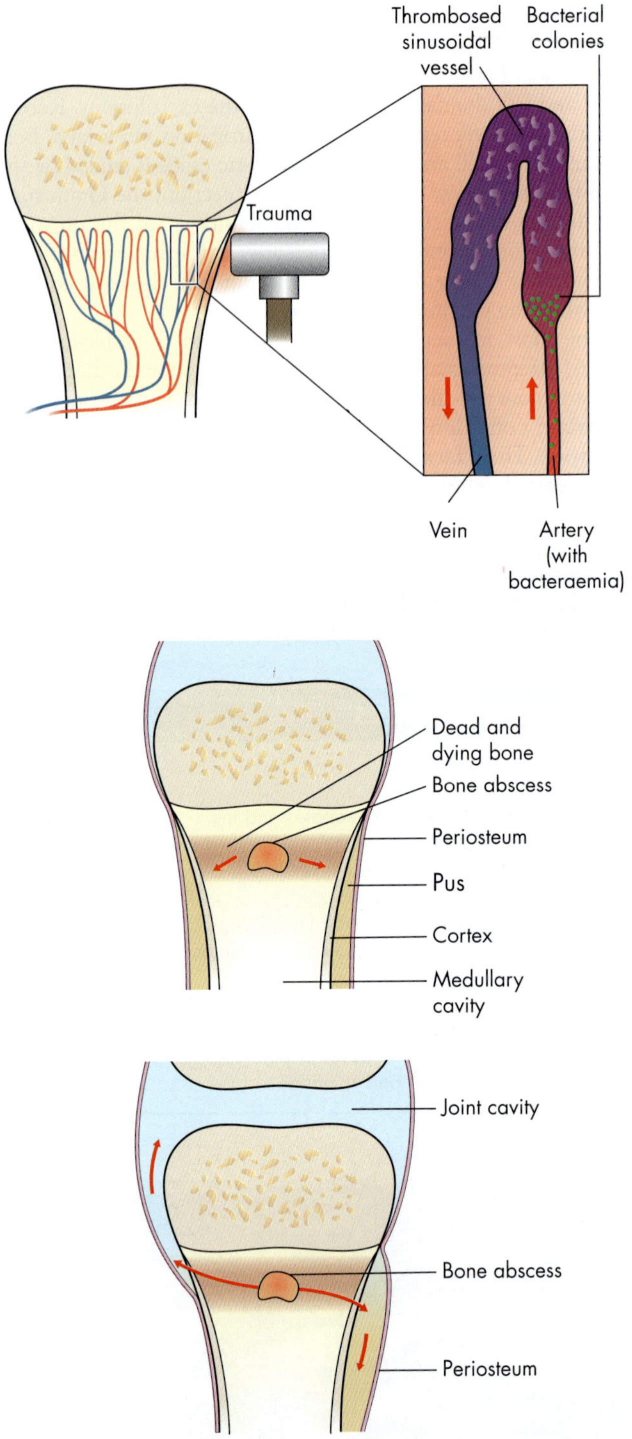

Figure 41.34 Diagrams illustrating the pathology underlying the development of osteomyelitis. The longer the infection goes untreated, the greater the destruction, with the possibility of sequestrum formation and secondary joint infection.

Discitis

Children who refuse to weight-bear and complain of back pain may have discitis. The aetiology of this condition may be infective or inflammatory but if vertebral bodies are involved, infection is assumed.

Brodies's abscess

Chronic infections may present with x-ray features of a sclerotic walled cyst.

CLINICAL DILEMMAS

The limping child

Children may limp because of pain, weakness, deformity or to gain attention: the causes vary from sepsis to a spinal tumour and from a leg length discrepancy to a shoe that rubs. Serious causes must be excluded and the 'surgical sieve' helps identify the most likely diagnoses (Summary box 41.27).

Summary box 41.27

A guide to the clinical assessment of the limping child

- Symptom onset: sudden or gradual?
- Symptom duration
- Concurrent events: recent viral infection, trauma, new shoes, new sport?
- General health: is the child well?

The examination must include all joints and soft tissues and, in addition, a brief neurological examination, measurement of leg length and an assessment of pain at rest or on weight bearing.

Many conditions, such as sepsis and juvenile arthritis, can present at any age but certain hip conditions are more likely in particular age groups (Table 41.17).

Plain x-rays should usually include both anteroposterior and 'frog' lateral views of the pelvis. Always bear in mind the possibility of a tumour; further imaging such as MRI may be required.

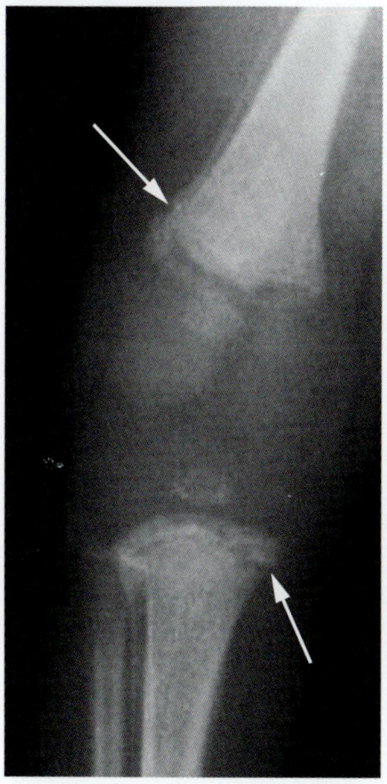

Figure 41.35 Anteroposterior x-ray of a knee showing metaphyseal corner fractures that are often considered to be pathognomonic of non-accidental injury. Non-accidental injury must also be considered in any fracture that presents late or without an adequate explanation.

Summary box 41.28

Factors that raise concern in the clinical assessment of suspected non-accidental injury

History
- Delay in seeking medical advice
- Variable story
- Mechanism inconsistent with injury pattern

Examination
- Unexpected bruising to the buttocks/back of legs
- 'Finger-mark' bruises
- Bruising of various ages
- Burns, deep scratches, etc.

Summary box 41.29

Fracture patterns with a high specificity for NAI

- Corner or bucket-handle metaphyseal fractures
- Multiple fractures at different stages of healing/old fractures
- Scapular fractures
- Posterior rib fractures
- Any fracture in a child below walking age

Table 41.17 Age at presentation of certain hip conditions.

Age (years)	Diagnosis
1–3	Late presenting developmental dysplasia of the hip; sepsis
3–10	Transient synovitis; Perthes' disease
11–15	Slipped upper femoral epiphysis

Non-accidental injury

No child is exempt but some children are at particular risk, including those under three years and those with disabilities. A careful clinical assessment is required (Figure 41.35) (Summary box 41.28). Characteristic patterns should warn the clinician to consider the possibility (Summary box 41.29).

Child abuse occurs in different forms: emotional, physical, sexual and neglect. When suspected it should be discussed with the relevant child protection team. All injuries should be documented carefully. It may be prudent to admit the child until further checks have been made.

FURTHER READING

Benson MKD, Fixsen JA, MacNicol MF (eds). *Children's orthopaedics and fractures*, 3rd edn. London: Harcourt, 2010.

Kocher MS, Mandiga R, Zurakowski D *et al.* Validation of a clinical prediction rule for the differentiation between septic arthritis and transient synovitis of the hip in children. *J Bone Joint Surg Am* 2004; **86–A**: 1629–35.

Loder RT, Richards BS, Shapiro PS *et al.* Acute slipped capital femoral epiphysis: the importance of physeal stability. *J Bone Joint Surg Am* 1993; **75**: 1134–40.

Morrissy RT, Weinstein SL (eds). *Lovell and Winter's pediatric orthopaedics*, vols 1 and 2, 6th edn. Philadelphia, PA: Lippincott, Williams and Wilkins, 2006.

Sir Benjamin Collins Brodie, 1783–1862, surgeon, St. George's Hospital, London, UK, described 'Brodie's Abscess' in 1828.

PART 6
Skin and subcutaneous tissue

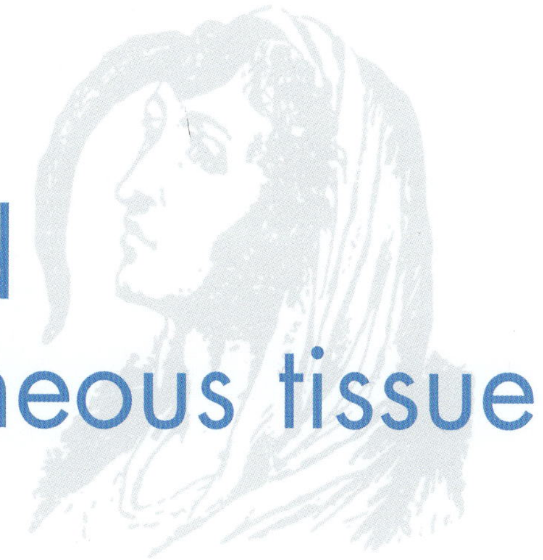

CHAPTER 42

Skin and subcutaneous tissue

LEARNING OBJECTIVES

To understand:
- the structure and functional properties of skin
- the classification of vascular skin lesions

To be aware of:
- the cutaneous manifestations of generalised disease as related to surgery

To know:
- the classification of benign skin tumours
- the management of malignant skin tumours

FUNCTIONAL ANATOMY AND PHYSIOLOGY OF SKIN

Skin can be divided into an outer layer: the epidermis and an inner layer: the dermis. Deep to the dermis is the hypodermis which is composed of subcutaneous fat and remnants of the panniculus carnosus.

Epidermis

The epidermis is composed of keratinised stratified squamous epithelium and can be further subdivided into five layers: the stratum basale (deepest), the stratum spinosum, the stratum granulosum, the stratum lucidum and the stratum corneum (superificial) (Figure 42.1). It accounts for 5 per cent of the total skin (Summary box 42.1).

> **Summary box 42.1**
>
> **Epidermis**
> - Stratum basale
> - Stratum spinosum
> - Stratum granulosum
> - Stratum lucidum
> - Stratum corneum
>
> **Dermis**
> - Papillary layer
> - Reticular layer

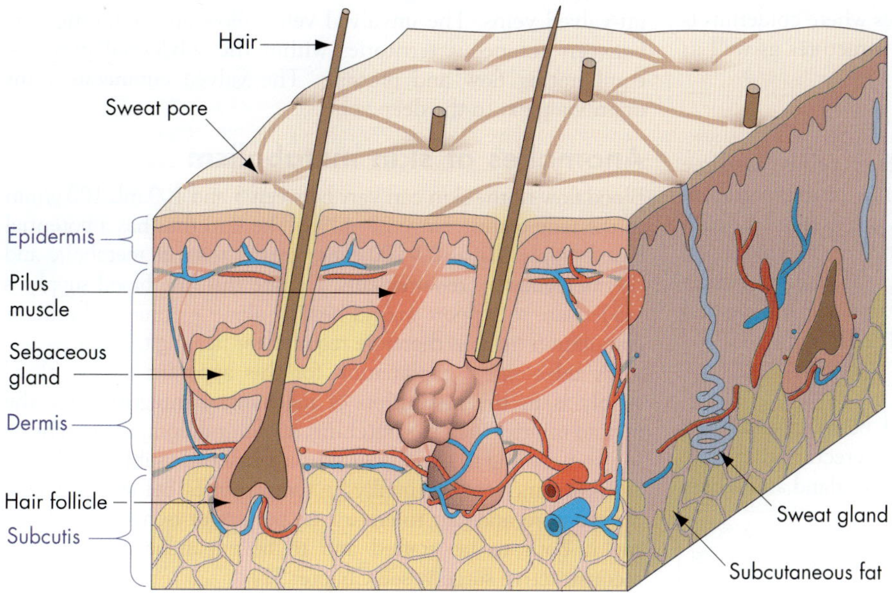

Figure 42.1 Three-dimensional diagram of the structural layers of the skin and its adnexal structures. (Reproduced from Simonsen T, Aarbakke J, Kay I *et al. Illustrated pharmacology for nurses.* London: Hodder Arnold, 2006 with kind permission of the illustrator Roy Lysaa.)

The majority of epidermal cells are keratinocytes arranged in layers. The basal epidermis (stratum basale) also contains melanocytes. Keratinocytes are classified according to their depth in the epidermis and their degree of differentiation. Keratinocytes grow and are replaced via mitoses in the cells of the stratum granulosum as they progress from deep to superficial, losing their nuclei and organelles as they progress upwards before forming the stratum corneum. The other keratinocyte layers in the skin (the strata lucidum; granulosum and spinosum) are variably present according to body site – for instance all three are present in the glaberous skin of the palms and soles of the feet.

Melanocytes are dendritic cells of neural crest origin usually located in the basal epidermis. Each melanocyte synthesises the brown-black pigment melanin, which is transferred via membrane processes to the keratinocytes in the strata granulosum and spinosum. Melanin provides protection against ultraviolet radiation. Ethnic differences in skin colour are determined by variations in the amount, combination and distribution of melanin within the keratinocytes, rather than differences in the number of melanocytes.

Dermis

The dermis comprises 95 per cent of the skin and is structurally divided into two layers. The superficial papillary layer is composed of delicate collagen and elastin fibres in ground substance, into which a capillary and lymphatic network ramifies. The deeper reticular layer is composed of course branching collagen, layered parallel to the skin surface.

The epidermis and dermis meet at the dermoepidermal junction in a three-dimensional wave-like arrangement in which epidermal rete pegs project down and interdigitate with upward-pointing, dermal papillary ridges containing vascular and lymphatic plexi.

The skin also contains specialised cells such as Langerhan's cells, whose role is to engulf antigens and present them to T cells. Merkel cells, Meissner's and Pacinian corpuscles have a role in mechanosensation.

Skin adnexia

Adnexial structures such as hair follicles, sebaceous and sweat glands span both the epidermal and dermal layers and contain some keratinocytes in their ducts. In injuries where epidermis is lost, re-epithelialisation occurs from these structures as well as from the wound margins.

Hair follicles

The human body is covered by fine downy hair (vellus) for three months *in utero*. This is eventually shed before birth, apart from the eyebrows and lashes. Hair which grows out from a hair bulb at the base of a follicle (tubular invaginations of the epidermis) is a shaft of dead keratinised tissue. Strips of smooth muscle (erector pili) are inserted into the wall of the hair follicle and lead to hair elevation in times of stress and cold.

Sebaceous glands

Most are hair follicle appendages situated between each hair follicle and its erector pili muscle. When the erector pili muscle contracts to elevate the hair, it compresses the gland and sebum is released (holocrine secretion). The function of the sebum is to act as a skin lubricant and physical protection barrier.

George Meissner, 1829–1905, successively Professor of Anatomy and Physiology, Basle, Switzerland, Professor of Zoology and Physiology, Freiberg, Germany and Professor of Physiology, Göttingen, Germany.

Sweat glands

Eccrine and apocrine are simple sweat glands that open into pores in hair follicles. Eccrine glands are distributed throughout the entire body surface except on the lips. These glands secrete sweat in response to emotion or as part of thermoregulation. Apocrine glands are found in the axillary and groin areas and become active at puberty. Their secretion, which is characteristically malodourous, varies in response to emotion, hormone secretion and bacterial degradation.

Skin thickness

Skin thickness varies with age and body area. It is thinner in children than in adults in any given region. The dermis is between 15 and 40 times thicker than the epidermis, but starts to thin during the fourth decade as part of the ageing process. The epidermis is thickest on the palms, soles, back and buttocks and thinnest on eyelids (0.5–1 mm on sole of the foot, 0.05–0.09 mm on the eyelid).

Blood supply of the skin

In the last 25 years, the 'angiosome model' has furthered our understanding of the anatomical blood supply of skin and therefore the ability to reconstruct soft tissue defects using vascularised flaps of various tissue compositions. With respect to its blood supply, the body can be envisaged as three-dimensional segments of tissue called angiosomes, each with an arterial supply and a venous drainage. Blood equilibrates and flows between neighbouring angiosomes via 'choke' vessels, which tend to be situated within muscles. Cutaneous arteries, direct branches of segmental arteries (concentrated at the dorsoventral axes and intermuscular septae), perforate the underlying muscles or run directly within fascial layers to the skin from the deep tissues (Figure 42.2).

The blood supply to the skin anastomoses in subfascial, fascial, subdermal, dermal and subepidermal plexi. The epidermis contains no blood vessels so cells there derive nourishment by diffusion.

The venous drainage of the skin is via both valved and un-valved veins. The unvalved veins allow an oscillating flow between cutaneous territories within the subdermal plexus – equilibrating flow and pressure. The valved cutaneous veins drain via plexi to the deep veins.

Anomalies of skin metabolism

Blood flow to the skin can vary between 5 and 100 mL 100 g/min in the temperature range 20–40°C. The skin thus has a potential blood supply that is 20–100 times greater than its metabolic and thermoregulatory requirements. Despite this, the blood supply is inadequate to support wound healing alone – primary closure or granulation tissue is therefore required for healing to occur.

A teleological explanation for this apparent excess blood supply is in the restitution of mechanical integrity after the myriad injuries such as scratching, stretching, compressing, heating and cooling to which our skin is constantly subjected.

Skin functions optimally at temperatures below body core temperature and can tolerate long periods of ischaemia (allowing it both to be grafted and to be expanded and used in reconstructive surgery, see Chapter 31).

Paul Langerhans, 1847–1888, Professor of Pathological Anatomy, Freiberg, Germany.
Friedrich Sigmud Merkel, 1845–1919, Professor of Anatomy successively at Rostock, Koningsberg (now Kaliningrad in Russia) and Göttingen, Germany.
Filippo Pacini, 1812–1883, Professor of Anatomy and Physiology, Florence, Italy.

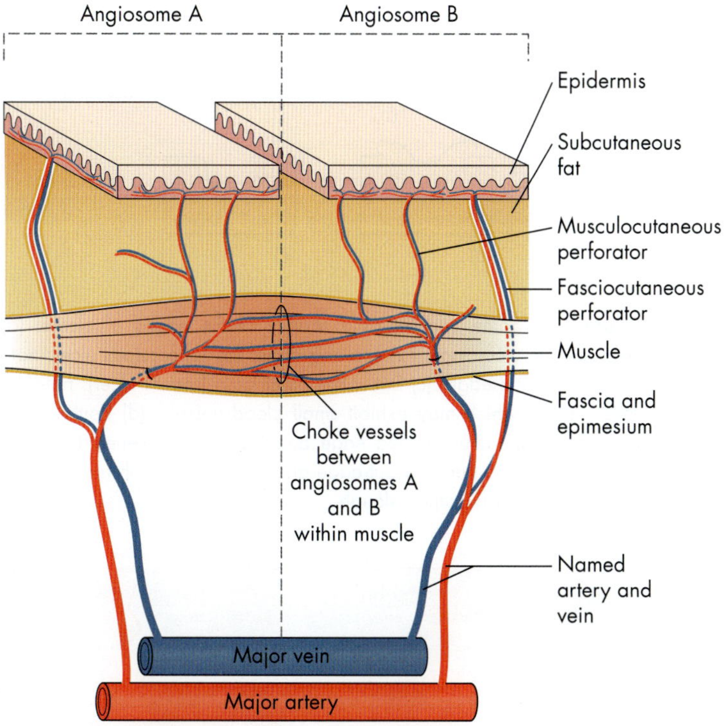

Figure 42.2 Schematic showing two neighbouring angiosomes. Note the choke vessels within the muscle spanning the two cutaneous territories of angiosome A and B – two common examples of myocutaneous flaps which utilise this physiology include the rectus abdominus and the latisimus dorsi flaps.

FUNCTION OF THE SKIN

Human skin and subcutaneous tissue have several important functions (Summary box 42.2).

Summary box 42.2

Function of the skin

- Barrier to the environment: trauma, radiation, pathogens
- Temperature and water homeostasis
- Excretion (e.g. urea, sodium chloride, potassium, water)
- Endocrine and metabolic functions
- Sensory organ for pain, pressure, movement

Skin grafts

Grafts of the skin can be used to reconstruct wounds having been harvested as split (leaving some epidermal components) or full thickness. The process by which a skin graft adheres to and heals a wound is a unique and unnatural process, in which normal wound healing at the recipient site is altered by the presence of the graft. The survival of a skin graft is largely dependent on how fast the graft derives new blood supply from the wound on which it is placed. Until the graft establishes a new blood supply, nutrition is derived by diffusion through the fibrin layer formed between it and the wound bed. After 48–72 hours, a fine capillary network grows into the graft and anastomoses with the native vasculature of the graft. Factors that inhibit this process (haematoma, seroma or bacterial exudates) will decrease the likelihood that the graft will successfully 'take' (see Chapter 31).

Ulcers

An ulcer is a discontinuity of an epithelial surface. It is characterised by progressive destruction of the surface epithelium and a granulating base. Ulcers can be classified as non-specific, specific and malignant (Table 42.1 and Figure 42.3).

Sinus

A sinus is a blind-ending tract that connects a cavity lined with granulation tissue (often an abscess cavity) with an epithelial surface. Sinuses may be congenital or acquired (Table 42.2). Congenital sinuses arise from the remnants of embryonic ducts that persist instead of being obliterated and involuted during embryonic development. Acquired sinuses occur as a result of the presence of a retained foreign body (for example suture material), specific chronic infection (for example tuberculosis (TB) or actinomycosis), malignancy or inadequate drainage of the cavity (Figure 42.4).

Treatment of the sinus is directed at removing the underlying cause. Biopsies should always be taken from the wall of the sinus to exclude malignancy or specific infection.

For specific management of the disease conditions please refer to the appropriate chapter.

Fistula

A fistula is an abnormal communication between two epithelium lined surfaces. This communication or tract may be lined by granulation tissue but may become epithelialised in chronic cases. Fistulas may be congenital or acquired.

Examples of congenital fistula include tracheo-oesophageal and branchial fistulas. Acquired fistulas include fistula in ano, enterocutaneous fistula following Crohn's disease or postoperative anastomotic complications, arteriovenous fistula which may

Table 42.1 Classification of common types of ulcer.

Ulcer	Type
Peptic	Non-specific
Pressure sores (decubitus ulcers) and ischaemic ulcers	Non-specific
Gravitational ulcers – venous insufficiency	Non-specific
Secondary infective – wound infection and abscess drainage	Non-specific
Traumatic ulcers	Non-specific
Neuropathic ulcers – diabetes, tabes dorsalis, leprosy	Non-specific
Iatrogenic – intravenous fluid extravasation	Non-specific
Dermatitis artefacta – self-mutilation	Non-specific
Aphthous	Non-specific
Primary infective – herpes simplex, tuberculosis, fungal, syphilis	Specific
Gastrointestinal tract and skin	Malignant

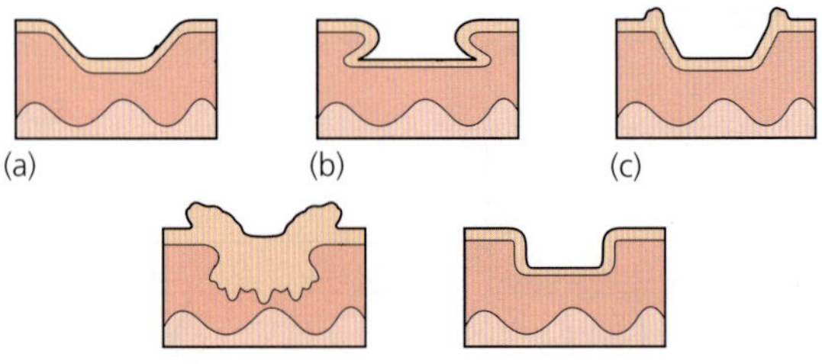

Figure 42.3 Some characteristic shapes of the edges of ulcers. (a) Non-specific ulcer: note the shelving edge. (b) Tuberculous ulcer: note the undermined edge. (c) Basal cell carcinoma (rodent ulcer): note the rolled edge, which may exhibit small blood vessels. (d) Epithelioma: note the heaped-up, everted edge and irregular thickened base. (e) Syphilis: note the punched-out edge and thin base, which may be covered with a 'wash-leather' slough.

Table 42.2 Sinuses.

Congenital	Acquired
Preauricular	Post surgical (abdominal or perineal)
Umbilical	Pilonidal
Urachal	Suture
Coccygeal	TB
Sacral	Actinomycosis
	Osteomyelitis
	Crohn's disease

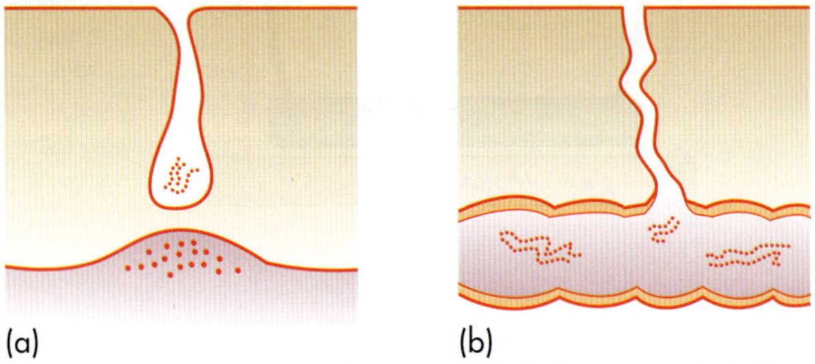

Figure 42.4 A sinus (a) and a fistula (b); both usually arise from a preceding abscess. (a) This is a blind track, in this case a pilondial abscess. (b) This is a track connecting two epithelium-lined surfaces, in this case a colocutaneous fistula from colon to skin.

be traumatic or iatrogenic (for haemodialysis).

Again, management of the fistula is directed to treating the underlying aetiology (see appropriate chapter).

PATHOPHYSIOLOGY OF THE SKIN AND SUBCUTANEOUS TISSUES

Radiation damage

Ultraviolet radiation (UVR) and ionising radiation (IR) damage cellular DNA via the tumour suppressor gene *p53*, inhibiting cellular repair and apoptotic mechanisms. There is also evidence that efferent immune responses are impaired after skin exposure to ultraviolet radiation facilitating neoplasia.

Ultraviolet radiation

UVR is divisible into A, B and C according to wavelength. UVR is the principal cause of skin cancer in all skin types. Its effects are attenuated by melanin and there is an inverse relationship between melanin content and skin susceptibility to UV-induced neoplasia. Some protection is afforded by the stratum corneum, which reflects and refracts UVR and by clothing, protective creams, cloud cover and buildings.

Ionising radiation

The effects of IR are dose and time dependent. The skin with its rapid cellular turnover exhibits signs soon after exposure. High frequency rays cause electron coupling at the molecular level damaging proteins, polysaccharides and lipids.

Infrared radiation

Infrared radiation generates heat with cumulative exposure posing the risk of thermal burns (see Chapter 30).

Congenital/genetic disorders

Neurofibromatosis

There are two distinct neurofibromatosis syndromes where Schwann cells form tumours (Figure 42.5). Each is caused by different genes on different chromosomes. Seventy per cent are

Friedrich Theodor Schwann, 1810–1882, Professor of Anatomy successively at Louvain (1839–1848) and Liege, Belgium (1849–1880). Original researches before the age of 27 laid the foundation of physiology of nerve and muscle. The first to deal with problems related to living matter on a purely physical and chemical basis, and to recognise the cell as the unit of living matter. Discoverer of pepsin, and role of living organisms in fermentation.

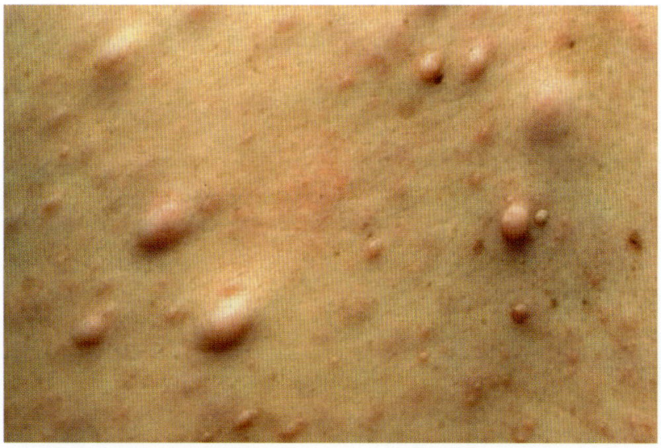

Figure 42.5 Neurofibromatosis (courtesty of St John's Institute for Dermatology, London, UK).

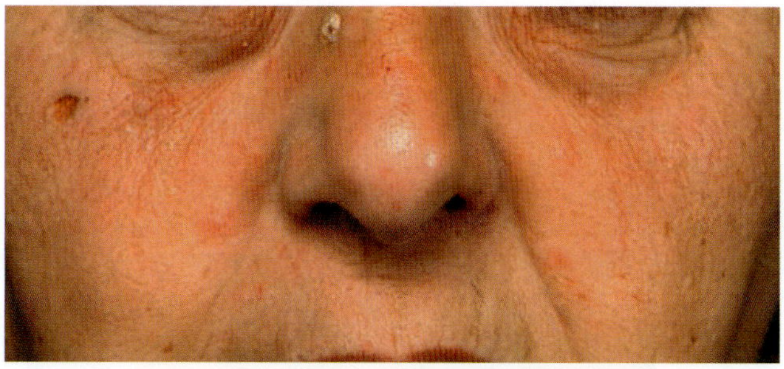

Figure 42.6 Mid-face of a patient with Ferguson–Smith syndrome. Note the two tumours at different stages of development: on the nose and the right cheek (courtesy of St John's Institute for Dermatology, London, UK).

autosomal dominant and 30 per cent arise from sporadic mutations. Neurofibromatosis (NF) 1 or von Recklinghausen's disease is the more common variant, affecting approximately 1:4000 births. It arises from a gene mutation on chromosome 17. Skin manifestations can appear in early life, with the development of more than five smooth-surfaced café-au-lait spots, subcutaneous neurofibromata, armpit or groin freckling and Lisch nodules.

Naevoid basal cell carcinoma (Gorlin's) syndrome

This is an autosomal dominant inherited condition caused by an abnormality in the tumour suppressor gene on chromosome 9q22-31 that codes for the 'patched' protein. Ninety per cent of patients develop multiple basal cell carcinomas. Patients may also exhibit specific phenotypical characteristics including overdeveloped supraorbital ridges, broad nasal roots, hyperteliorism, bifid ribs, scoliosis, brachymetacarpalism, palmar pits and molar odontogenic cysts.

Xeroderma pigmentosum

Described by Kaposi in 1874, this syndrome is caused by an abnormality on the 'patched' gene of chromosome 9q resulting in aberrant nucleotide repair during cellular DNA maintenance. It has an autosomal recessive inheritance confering >2000-fold increase in skin cancer risk. Sufferers have an intolerance to UVR manifested as erythema, pigmentation and photophobia. This leads to premature skin ageing and the development of multiple neoplasms, with most affected individuals dying in early adulthood from metastatic disease (60 per cent mortality by 20 years of age).

Gardner's syndrome

An autosomal dominant disease variant of familial adenomatous polyposis (FAP) is caused by an abnormal gene on chromosome 5. Gardner's syndrome can cause the development of cutaneous pathology such as multiple epidermoid cysts and lipomata.

Ferguson-Smith syndrome

This is a rare, autosomal-dominantly inherited abnormality on chromosome 9q (Figure 42.6). This results in a syndrome that can be traced to a single familial line from western Scotland with affected individuals developing multiple self-healing squamous cell carcinomas.

Cutaneous manifestations of generalised disease

Many diseases have cutaneous manifestations that may present in surgical practice. These include necrobiosis lipoidica, granuloma annulare in diabetes mellitus and pyoderma gangrenosum in inflammatory bowel disease.

Hyperhydrosis

This condition involves excessive eccrine sweating of the palms, soles of the feet, axillae and groins. This can cause functional and social problems, but can be controlled depending on severity, with anti-perspirants or periodic local injections with botulinum toxin A. More resistant cases are treated by laparoscopic cervical sympathectomy.

Lipodystrophy

Lipodystrophy (lipoatrophy) is a localised or generalised loss of fatty tissue which can have primary or secondary causes. It is most commonly seen as a complication of long-term administration of insulin, following treatment of HIV with protease inhibitors or in transplant recipients.

It can be treated in selected cases by autologous fat grafting, injections of poly-L-lactic acid and free tissue transfer.

Inflammatory conditions

Hidradenitis suppurativa

This is a chronic inflammatory disease culminating in suppurative skin abscesses, sinus tracts and scarring (Figure 42.7). It most commonly occurs in the apocrine gland containing skin, namely in the axillary and groin areas. Less common sites include the scalp, breast, chest and perineum.

Hidradenitis suppurativa appears to have a genetic predisposition with variable penetrance, and is strongly associated with obesity and smoking. Women are four times more likely affected than men.

The pathophysiology involves follicular occlusion followed by folliculitis and secondary infection with skin flora (usually *Staphylococcus aureus* and *Propionibacterium acnes*). Clinically, patients develop tender, subcutaneous nodules which may not

Friedrich von Recklinghausen, 1833–1910, Professor of Pathology, Strasbourg, France, described generalised neurofibromatosis in 1882.
Karl Lisch, 1907–1999, ophthalmologist, Wörgl, Austria.
Moritz Kaposi, 1837–1902, Professor of Dermatology, Vienna, Austria.
John Francis Ferguson-Smith, 1888–1978, dermatologist, The Victoria Infirmary, Glasgow, UK.
Eldon J Gardner, 1909–1989, Professor of Zoology, Utah State University, Salt Lake City, UT, USA.

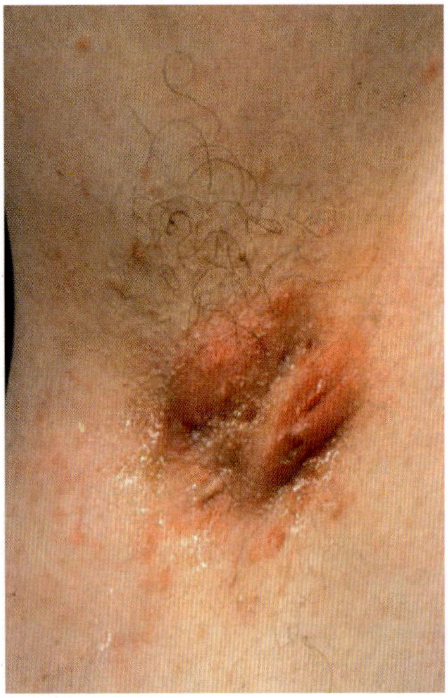

Figure 42.7 Hidradenitis suppurativa affecting the axilla (courtesy of St John's Institute for Dermatology, London, UK).

point and discharge, but which usually progress to cause chronic inflammation and scarring.

Management

Patients should be advised to stop smoking and lose weight where appropriate. Symptoms can be reduced by the use of antiseptic soaps, tea tree oil, non-compressive and aerated underwear.

Medical treatments include topical and oral antibiotics and anti-androgen drugs.

In selected cases, patients may require radical excision of the affected skin and subcutaneous tissue with reconstruction. Healing by secondary intention more frequently leads to contracture and functional impairment than when plastic surgical techniques, such as skin grafting or flap transposition are employed.

Pyoderma gangrenosum

Pyoderma gangrenosum is characterised by cutaneous ulceration with purple undermined edges (Figure 42.8). It is secondary to heightened immunological reactivity, usually from another disease process such as inflammatory bowel disease; rheumatoid arthritis, non-Hodgkin's lymphoma or Wegener's granulomatosis.

Cultures from ulcers often grow Gram-negative streptococci. These skin lesions generally respond to steroids. Surgery is rarely indicated and may exacerbate the condition.

Infections

Skin and soft tissue infections can be localised or spreading, necrotising or non-necrotising. Localised or spreading, non-necrotising infections usually respond to broad-spectrum antibiotics. Localised necrotising infections will need surgical debridement as well as antibiotic therapy. Spreading, necrotising soft tissue infection constitutes a life-threatening surgical emergency, requiring immediate resuscitation, intravenous antibiotic therapy and urgent surgical intervention with radical debridement.

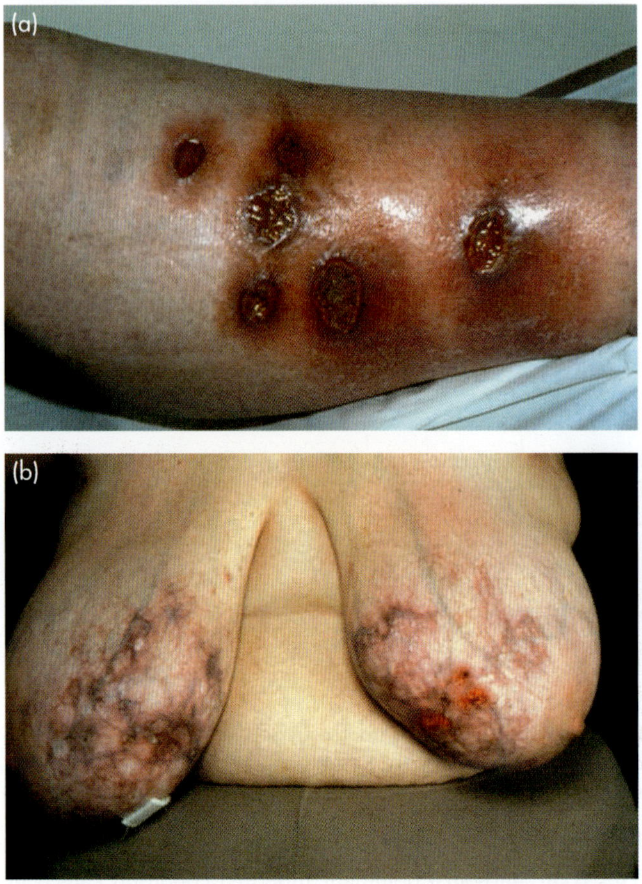

Figure 42.8 Pyoderma gangrenosum affecting the legs (a) and the breasts (b) (courtesy of St John's Institute for Dermatology, London, UK).

Impetigo

Impetigo is a superficial skin infection with staphylococci, streptococci or both (Figure 42.9). It is highly infectious and usually affects children. Impetigo is characterised by blisters that rupture and coalesce to become covered with a honey-coloured crust. Treatment is directed at washing the affected areas and applying topical anti-staphyloccocal treatments, and broad-spectrum oral antibiotics if streptococcal infection is implicated.

Erysipelas

Erysipelas is a sharply demarcated streptococcal infection of the superficial lymphatic vessels, usually associated with broken skin on the face (Figure 42.10). The area affected is erythematous and oedematous. The patient may be febrile and have a leukocytosis. Prompt administration of broad-spectrum antibiotics after swabbing the area for culture and sensitivity is usually all that is necessary.

Cellulitis/lymphangitis

This is a bacterial infection of the skin and subcutaneous tissue that is more generalised than erysipelas (Figure 42.11). It is usually associated with broken skin or pre-existing ulceration. Cellulitis is characterised by an expanding area of erythematous,

Thomas Hodgkin, 1798–1866, Curator of the Museum and Demonstrator of Morbid Anatomy, Guy's Hospital, London, UK.

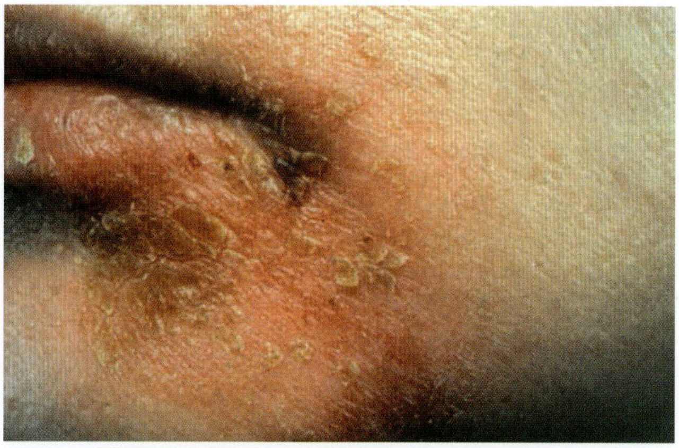

Figure 42.9 Impetigo. Note the honey-coloured crust (courtesy of St John's Institute for Dermatology, London, UK).

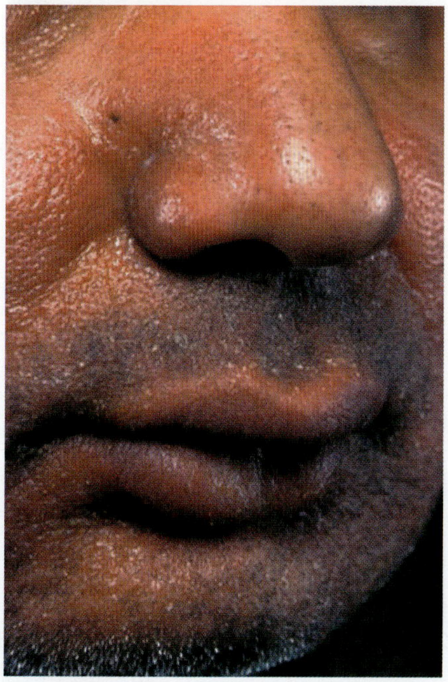

Figure 42.10 Erysipelas (courtesy of St John's Institute for Dermatology, London, UK).

oedematous tissue that is painful and associated with a fever, malaise and leukocytosis. Erythema tracking along lymphatics may be visible (lymphangitis). The most common causative organism is streptococcus. Blood and skin cultures for sensitivity should be taken before prompt administration of broad-spectrum intravenous antibiotics and elevation of the affected extremity.

Necrotising fasciitis

Necrotising fasciitis was first described by Paré in the sixteenth century. Meleney's synergistic gangrene and Fournier's gangrene are all variants of a similar disease process (Summary box 42.3).

Necrotising fasciitis results from a polymicrobial, synergistic infection, most commonly a streptococcal species (group A β haemolytic) in combination with *Staphylococcus*, *Escherichia coli*, *Pseudomonas*, *Proteus*, *Bacteroides* or *Clostridia*. Eighty per cent have a history of previous trauma/infection and over 60 per cent

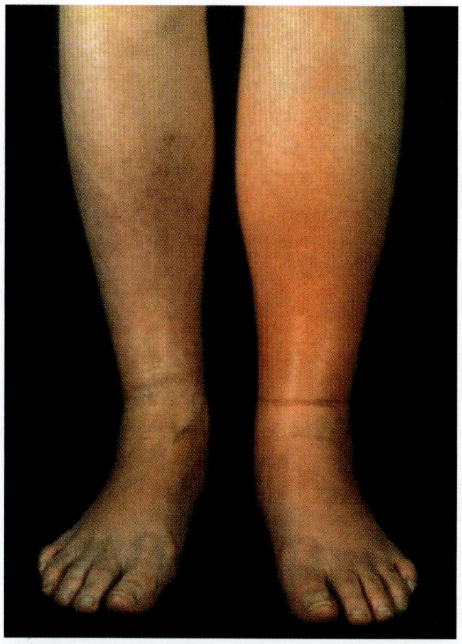

Figure 42.11 Cellulitis affecting the left leg (courtesy of St John's Institute for Dermatology, London, UK).

Summary box 42.3

Necrotising fasciitis

- Surgical emergency
- Polymicrobial synergistic infection
- 80 per cent history of previous trauma or infection
- Rapid progression to septic shock
- Urgent resuscitation, antibiotics and surgical debridement
- Mortality 30–50 per cent

commence in the lower extremities. Predisposing conditions include:

- diabetes;
- smoking;
- penetrating trauma;
- pressure sores;
- immunocompromised states;
- intravenous drug abuse;
- perineal infection (perianal abscess, Bartholin's cysts);
- skin damage/infection (abrasions, bites, boils).

Classical clinical signs include: oedema stretching beyond visible skin erythema; a woody hard texture to the subcutaneous tissues; an inability to distinguish fascial planes and muscle groups on palpation; disproportionate pain in relation to the affected area with associated skin vesicles and soft tissue crepitus (Figure 42.12). Lymphangitis tends to be absent. Early on, patients may be febrile and tachycardic, with a very rapid progression to septic shock. Radiographs should not delay treatment but if taken, they may demonstrate air in the tissues.

Ambrose Paré, 1510–1590, a French military surgeon who also worked at the Hôtel Dieu, Paris, France. He was regarded as the great official royal surgeon for the kings. He devised a dressing of egg white, oil of roses and turpentine which he applied to the wounds of soldiers successfully. He also developed the ligature as a means to stop bleeding.

Frank Lamont Meleney, 1889–1963, Professor of Clinical Surgery, Columbia University, New York, NY, USA.
Jean Alfred Fournier, 1832–1915, syphilologist, founder of the Venereal and Dermatological Clinic, Hôpital St Louis, Paris, France.

Management should commence with urgent fluid resuscitation, monitoring of haemodynamic status and administration of high-dose broad-spectrum intravenous antibiotics. This is a surgical emergency and the diseased area should be debrided as soon as possible until viable, healthy, bleeding tissue is reached. Early re-look and further debridement is advisable together with the use of vacuum-assisted dressings. Early skin grafting in selected cases may minimise protein and fluid losses. Mortality of between 30 and 50 per cent can be expected even with prompt operative intervention.

Purpura fulminans

This is a rare condition in which intravascular thrombosis produces a rapid skin necrosis with haemorrhagic skin infarction. This progresses rapidly to septic shock and disseminated intravascular coagulation. It is usually seen in children, but can occur in adults. It may be sub-divided into three types based on aetiological mechanism.

Acute infectious purpura fulminans

This is the most common form of purpura fulminans and is caused by either an acute bacterial or viral infection (Figure 42.13). *Neisseria meningitidis* and varicella are the most common causal organisms. Acute infectious purpura fulminans causes an acquired protein C deficiency as endotoxins produce an imbalance in the procoagulant and anticoagulant endothelial activity.

Acute infectious purpura fulminans is most common in children under seven years, following an upper respiratory tract infection or in asplenia. Clinically, an initial petechial rash is observed. This develops into confluent ecchymoses and haemorrhagic bullae, which in turn necrose to form well-demarcated lesions that form hard eschars. Extensive tissue loss is common which often culminates in limb amputation. Acute infectious purpura fulminans is associated with a mortality rate of 40–50 per cent, usually a result of multiorgan failure.

Neonatal purpura fulminans

This is an inherited deficiency of protein C and protein S and primarily affects children causing extensive venous thrombosis of the skin and viscera in the first days of life.

Idiopathic purpura fulminans

Usually follows a viral illness after a latent period before the development of the clinical picture of purpura fulminans.

Skin and soft tissue cysts

Milia

These are tiny hard keratin retention cysts seen both in babies and the elderly after chronic sun exposure damage (Figure 42.14).

Epidermal cysts

These are cysts lined with true stratified squamous epithelium derived from the infundibulum of the hair follicle or traumatic inclusion. They are commonly known as sebaceous cysts and are often found on hairy areas of the body, such as the scalp, trunk and face. They are fixed to the skin and usually have a central punctum that is often indentable (Figure 42.15).

Treatment depends on the clinical state of the cyst. When they are inflamed or infected they should be incised and drained initially, and subsequently removed approximately 6 weeks later once the inflammation and induration has subsided. It is important to excise the cyst in its entirety as failure to do so usually results in recurrence.

Meibomian cysts are epidermal cysts found on the free edge of the eyelid. A chronic Meibomian cyst is called a chalazion. Tricholemmal (pilar/pilosebaceous) cysts can be confused with epidermal cysts, except they are derived from the epidermis of the external root sheath of the hair follicle. Ninety per cent are found in the scalp and 70 per cent are multiple.

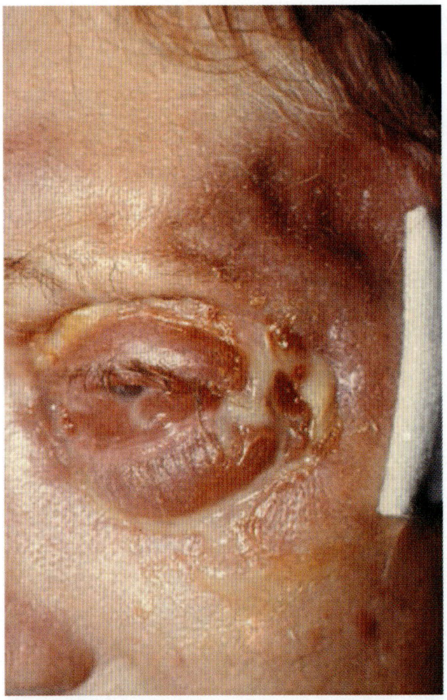

Figure 42.12 Necrotising fasciitis affecting the left orbit and facial skin (courtesy of St John's Institute for Dermatology, London, UK).

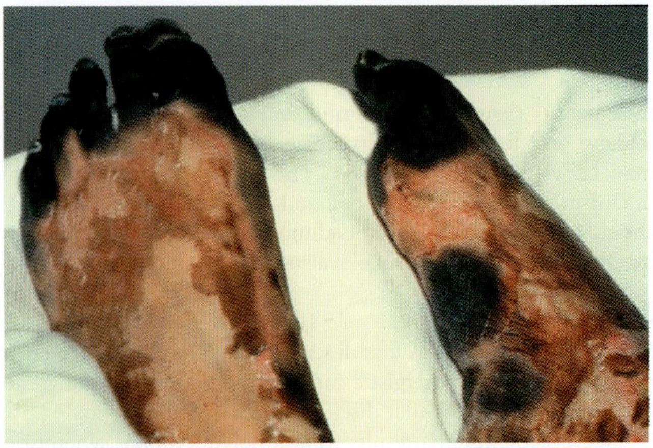

Figure 42.13 Acute infectious purpura fulminans caused by meningococcal septicaemia. Note the sharply demarcated necrotic areas distal to the affected end or perforating arteries with surrounding normal skin (courtesy of St John's Institute for Dermatology, London, UK).

Albert Ludwig Seigmund Neisser, 1855–1916, Director of the Dermatological Institute, Breslau, Germany (now Wroclaw, Poland).
Heinrich Meibom (Meibomius), 1638–1700, Professor of Medicine, History and Poetry, Helmstadt, Germany, described these glands in 1666.

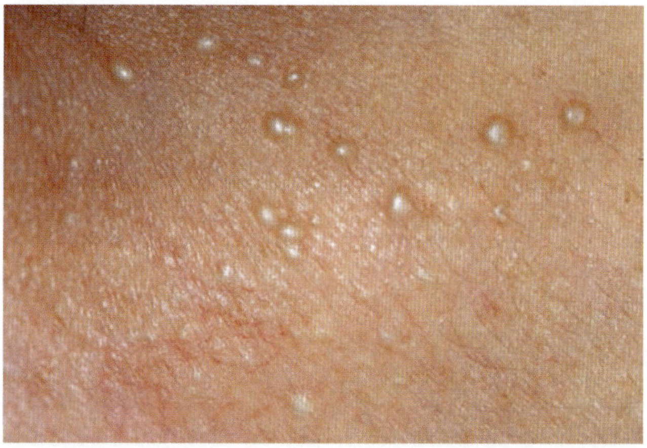

Figure 42.14 Milia (courtesy of St John's Institute for Dermatology, London, UK).

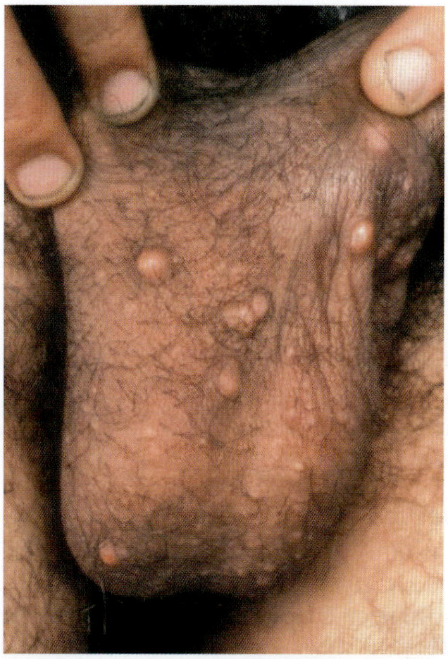

Figure 42.15 Multiple scrotal epidermal cysts (courtesy of St John's Institute for Dermatology, London, UK).

SKIN TUMOURS

Benign lesions

Basal cell papilloma (seborrhoeic keratosis, senile keratosis, verruca senilis)

These are soft warty lesions, which are often pigmented and hyperkeratotic. They are formed from the basal layer of epidermal cells and contain melanocytes. They are one of the most common benign skin tumours in the elderly (Figure 42.16).

Papillary wart (verruca vulgaris)

This is a benign skin tumour arising from infection with the human papilloma virus, which is also responsible for plantar warts and condylomata acuminata.

Freckle (ephilis)

A freckle is an area of skin that contains a normal number of melanocytes, producing an abnormally large number of melanin granules.

Lentigo

Lentigens are small, sharply circumscribed pigmented macules which are a marker for sun damage and some systemic syndromes. Solar lentigenes are more common in fairer skins. An example of a systemic syndrome associated with lentigenes is Peutz–Jeghers syndrome.

Moles/naevi

Melanocytes migrate from the neural crest to the basal epidermis during embryogenesis. When these melanocytes layer in the epidermis they form a simple mole. Melanocytes that aggregate in the dermis or at the dermoepidermal junction are called naevus cells.

Junctional naevus

A junctional naevus is a deeply pigmented macule or papule that occurs commonly in childhood or adolescence (Figure 42.17). It represents a dermoepidermal proliferation of naevus cells, which

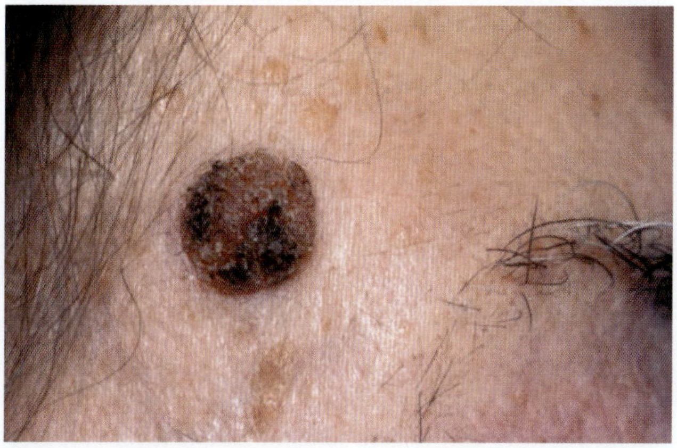

Figure 42.16 Basal cell papilloma (courtesy of St John's Institute for Dermatology, London, UK).

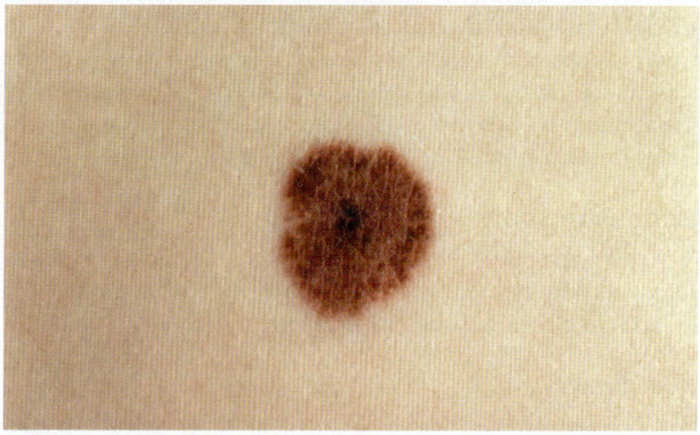

Figure 42.17 Junctional naevus (courtesy of St John's Institute for Dermatology, London, UK).

John Law Augustine Peutz, 1886–1968, Chief Specialist for Internal Medicine, St John's Hospital, The Hague, The Netherlands.
Harold Joseph Jeghers, 1904–1990, Professor of Internal Medicine, New Jersey College of Medicine and Dentistry, Jersey City, NJ, USA.

usually progresses to form a compound or intradermal naevus with advancing age. It may be found on any part of the body but has no malignant potential. Benign mucosal lesions tend to be junctional naevi.

Compound naevus

This is a maculopapular, pigmented lesion that becomes most prominent during adolescence (Figure 42.18). It represents a junctional proliferation of naevus cells with nests and columns in the dermis.

Intradermal naevus

Intradermal naevi are faintly pigmented papules in adults showing no junctional proliferation but a cluster of dermal melanocytes (Figure 42.19).

Spitz naevus

These are reddish brown (occasionally deeply pigmented) nodules previously termed 'juvenile melanoma' (Figure 42.20). They most commonly occur on the face and legs, growing rapidly initially then remaining static. The differential diagnosis is melanoma and excision biopsy is warranted if there is doubt as to the diagnosis.

Spindle cell naevus

Spindle cell naevi are dense black lesions which contain spindle cells and atypical melanocytes at the dermoepidermal junction. They are commonly seen on the thighs and affect women more frequently. They may have malignant potential.

Halo naevus

The halo of depigmentation around any benign naevus represents an antibody response to melanocytes (Figure 42.21). The importance of this depigmentation is that it may also be a feature of a malignant melanoma. A halo naevus is associated with vitiligo.

Café-au-lait spots

These are coffee-coloured macules of variable size (from a few millimetres to 10 cm) (Figure 42.22). Multiple lesions are associated with neurofibromatosis type 1 and McCune–Albright syndrome. They are more common in dark-skinned races.

Naevus spilus

This is also known as speckled lentiginous naevus (Figure 42.23). It is similar in appearance to a café-au-lait spot but with hyperpigmented speckles throughout. It is a benign lesion that is associated with various cutaneous diseases. The mainstay of management is observation and serial photography as malignant transformation is rare.

Mongolian spot

A Mongolian spot is a congenital blue-grey macule found over the sacral skin area (Figure 42.24). Pigmentation initially deepens and then regresses completely by age seven years.

Blue naevus

This is a benign skin lesion that is four times more common in children, typically affecting the extremities and face (Figure 42.25).

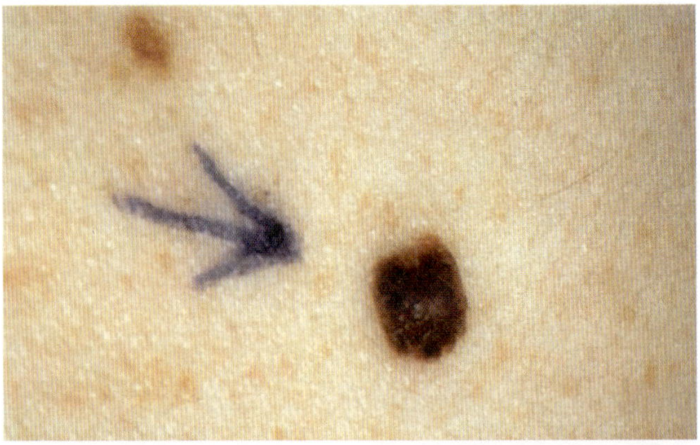

Figure 42.18 Compound naevus (courtesy of St John's Institute for Dermatology, London, UK).

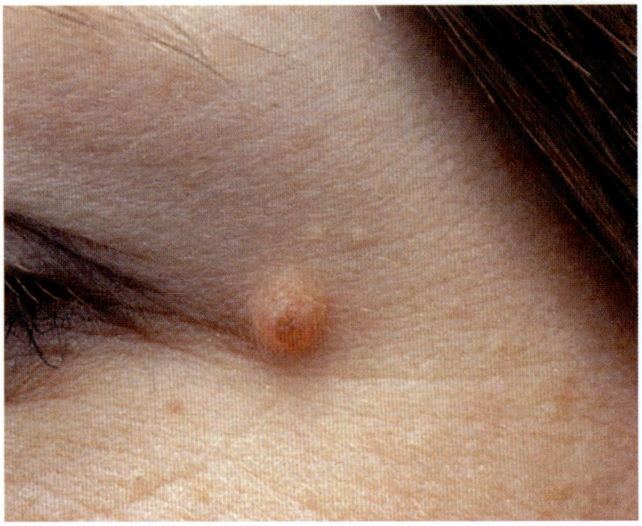

Figure 42.19 Intradermal naevus (courtesy of St John's Institute for Dermatology, London, UK).

Naevi of Ota and Ito

The naevus of Ota is a dermal melanocytic hamartoma with a characteristically blue or grey macule in the trigeminal V_1 and V_2 dermatomes (Figures 42.26 and 42.27). It is four times more common in women and most frequently seen in Oriental and African races.

The Naevus of Ito is characterised by dermal melanocytosis in the shoulder region and can occur simultaneously in a patient with naevus of Ota.

Hair follicles

Trichoepithelioma

These are small skin-coloured nodules most often found in the nasolabial fold. It is clinically and histologically similar to a basal cell carcinoma.

Sophie Spitz, 1910–1956, American pathologist. Dermatopathologist at Sloan-Kettering Cancer Center, published the first case series of 'juvenile melanoma' in 1948. Died at the age of 46 from carcinoma of the colon.

Donovan James McCune, 1902–1976, American paediatrician.
Fuller Albright, 1900–1969, physician, Massachusetts General Hospital, Boston, MA, USA.
Minoru Ito, 1892–1986, Professor of Dermatology, Tohoku University, Sendai, Honshu, Japan.

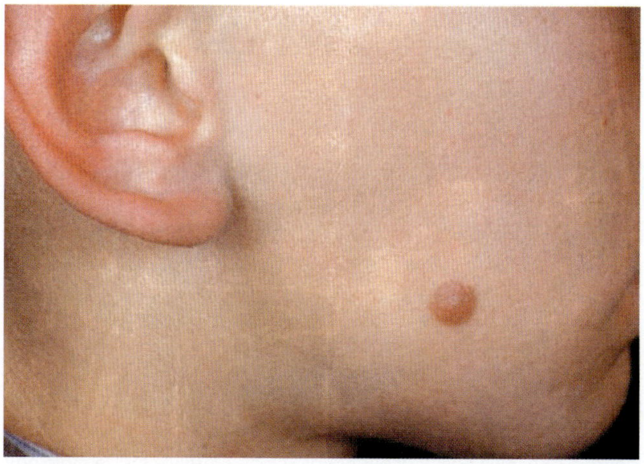

Figure 42.20 Spitz naevus (courtesy of St John's Institute for Dermatology, London, UK).

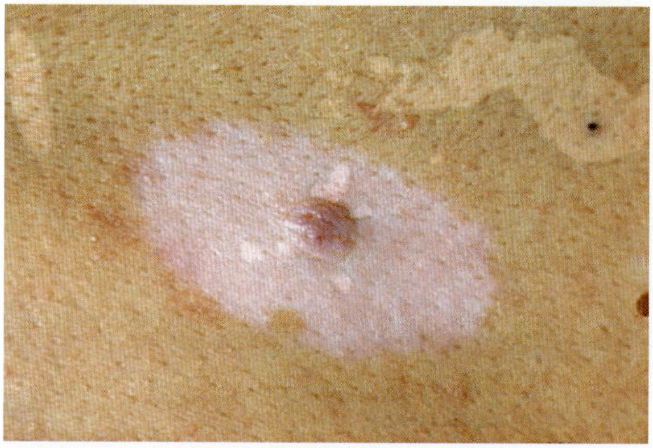

Figure 42.21 Halo naevus (courtesy of St John's Institute for Dermatology, London, UK).

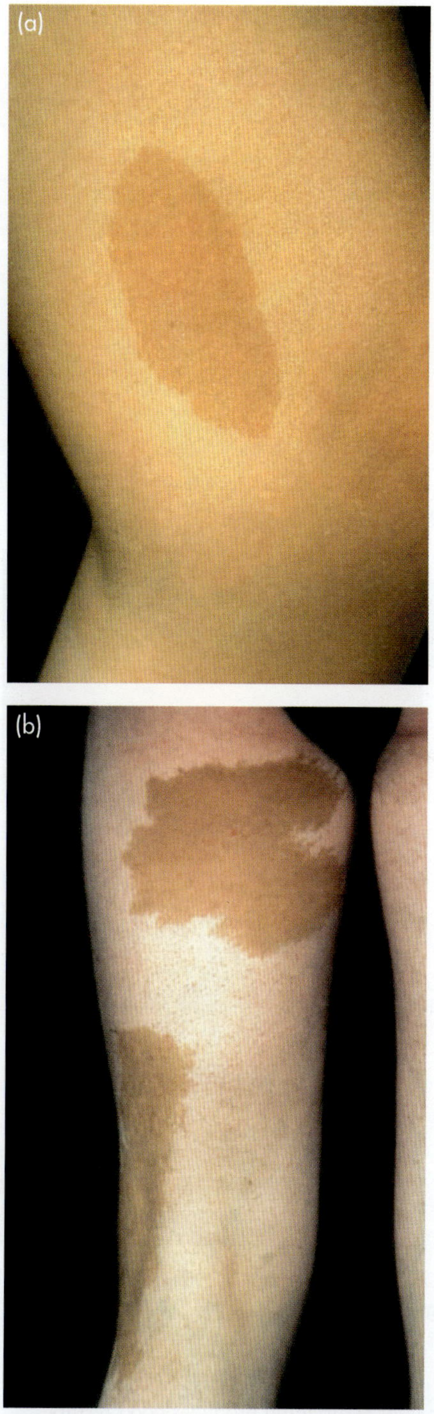

Figure 42.22 Café-au-lait spots. Note the two topographical variants: in (a) the spot has a smooth 'coast of California' border, whereas the upper spot in (b) has an irregular 'coast of Maine' border. Multiple smooth-bordered lesions are commonly associated with syndromes (courtesy of St John's Institute for Dermatology, London, UK).

Pilomatrixoma (calcifying epithelioma of Malherbe)

These are benign tumours of hair matrix cells characterised by basaloid and eosinophilic ghost cells. They commonly calcify and 40 per cent are found in the under-10 age group.

Tricholemmoma (naevus sebaceous of Jadassohn)

Tricholemmoma is a congenital hamartoma with the appearance of a linear verrucous naevus. These are believed to form basal cell carcinomata (BCC) in up to 10 per cent of cases (Figure 42.28).

Adenoma sebaceum (tuberous sclerosis, Bourneville disease)

These are typically red facial papules (angiofibromas) found usually on the nasolabial folds, cheek and chin (Figure 42.29). They form part of the disease process in tuberous sclerosis. These skin lesions usually appear in children less than ten years of age and increase in size and number until adolescence. Cosmetic removal by argon or pulse dye lasers or scalpel is indicated.

Rhinophyma

Rhinophyma is the end-stage sequela of acne rosacea (Figure 42.30). It is a hypertrophy and hyperplasia of the sebaceous glands and tends to affect elderly men (M:F 12:1). Up to 3 per

Josef Jadassohn, 1863–1936, a dermatologist of Breslau, Germany (now Wroclaw, Poland).
Desire M Bourneville, 1840–1909, physician, Le Bicêtre, Paris, France.

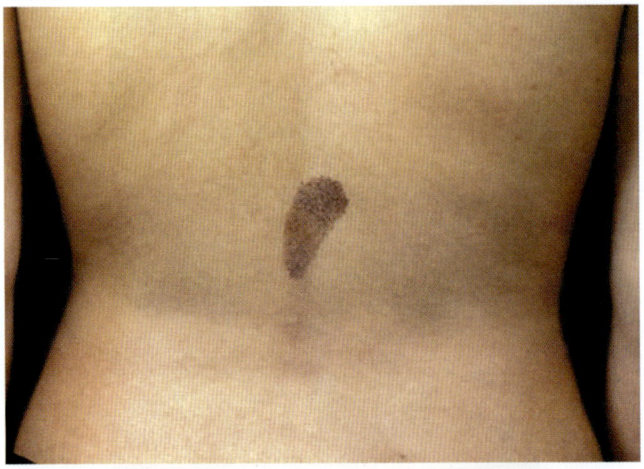

Figure 42.23 Naevus spilus (courtesy of St John's Institute for Dermatology, London, UK).

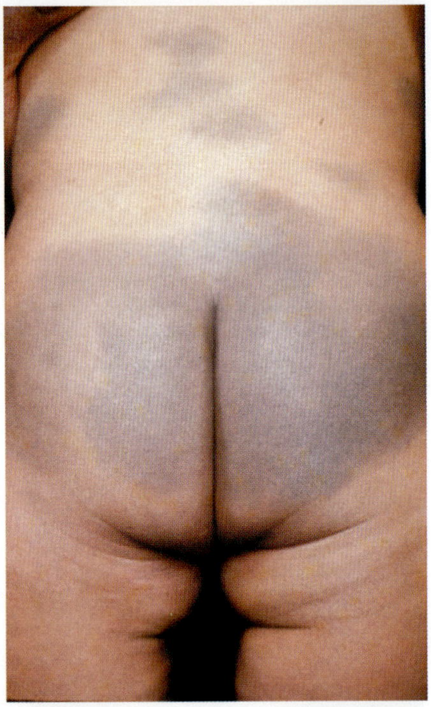

Figure 42.24 Mongolian spot (courtesy of St John's Institute for Dermatology, London, UK).

cent of cases may have an occult BCC. Treatment by dermabrasion or laser resurfacing produces good results.

Sweat glands

Cystadenoma (hydrocystadenomas, hidradenomas)

These are 1–3-cm translucent blue cystic nodules.

Eccrine poroma (papillary syringoma)

These are single raised or pedicled lesions found most often on the palm or sole.

Cylindroma (turban tumour)

A variant of eccrine spiradenoma which can be multiple on the scalp and can coalesce to form a 'turban tumour'.

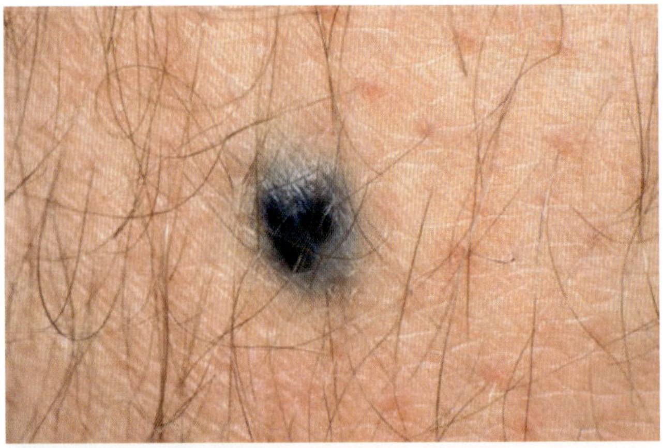

Figure 42.25 Blue naevus (courtesy of St John's Institute for Dermatology, London, UK).

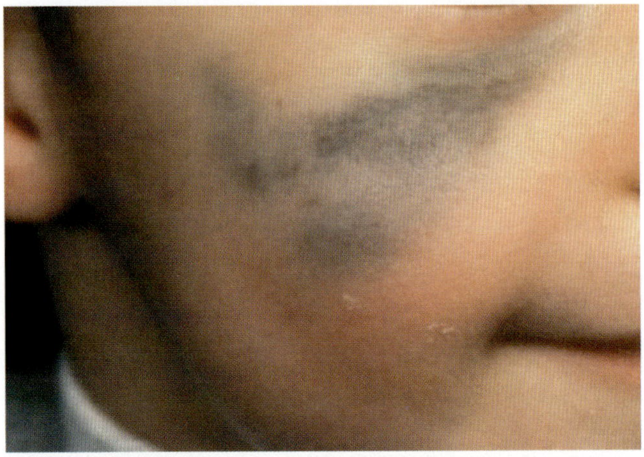

Figure 42.26 Naevus of Ota (courtesy of St John's Institute for Dermatology, London, UK).

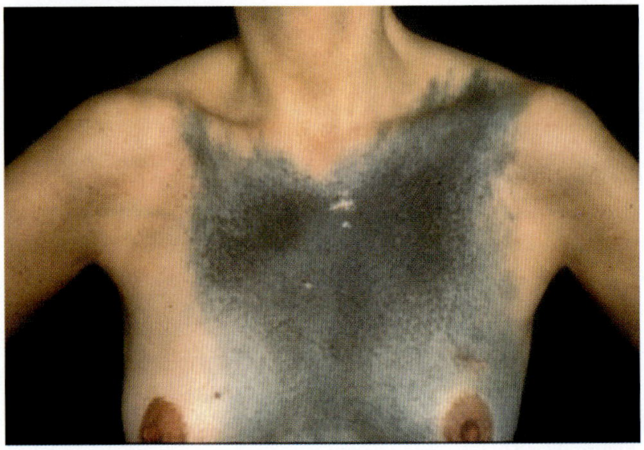

Figure 42.27 Naevus of Ito (courtesy of St John's Institute for Dermatology, London, UK).

Premalignant lesions

Actinic/solar keratosis

These are areas of dyskeratosis and cellular atypia, with subepidermal inflammation, but a normal dermoepidermal junction

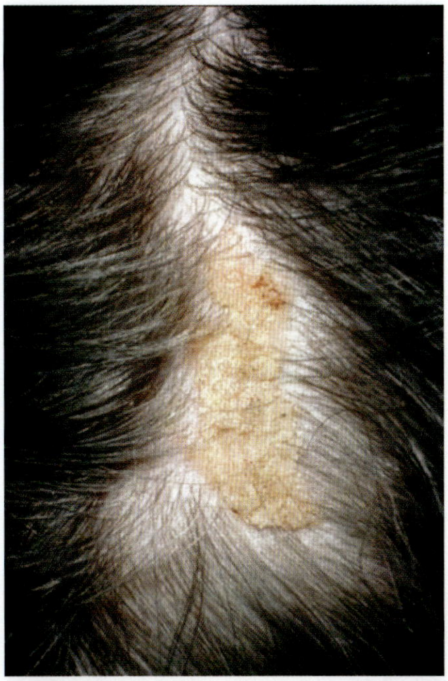

Figure 42.28 Naevus sebaceous of Jadassohn (courtesy of St John's Institute for Dermatology, London, UK).

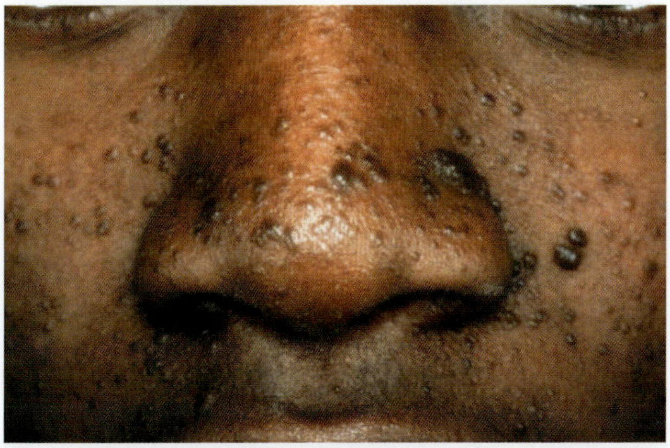

Figure 42.29 Adenoma sebaceum (courtesy of St John's Institute for Dermatology, London, UK).

(Figure 42.31). However, up to 20 per cent go on to form squamous cell carcinomas.

Cutaneous horn

A cutaneous keratin accumulation which by definition has a height greater than its base diameter. Ten per cent will have an underlying squamous cell carcinoma (SCC) (Figure 42.32).

Keratoacanthoma

Classically, this is a symmetrical, cutaneous growth with a central crater filled with a keratin plug (Figure 42.33). It is twice as common in men and is usually found on the face of 50–70 year olds. The aetiology of keratoacanthoma is unclear but may be caused by a papilloma virus in a hair follicle during the growth phase. It has also been associated with smoking and chemical carcinogen exposure.

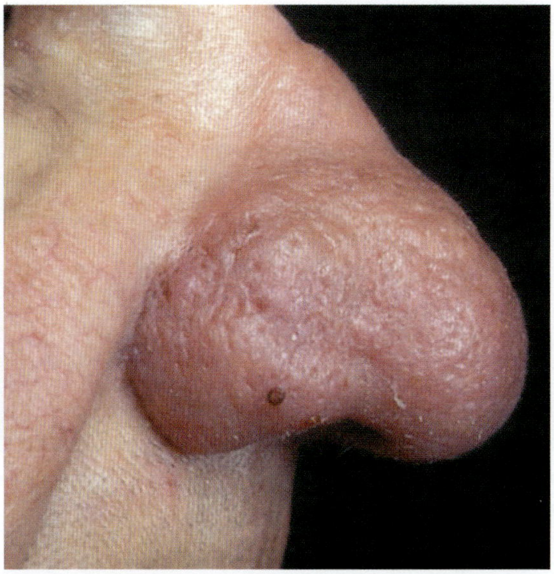

Figure 42.30 Rhinophyma (courtesy of St John's Institute for Dermatology, London, UK).

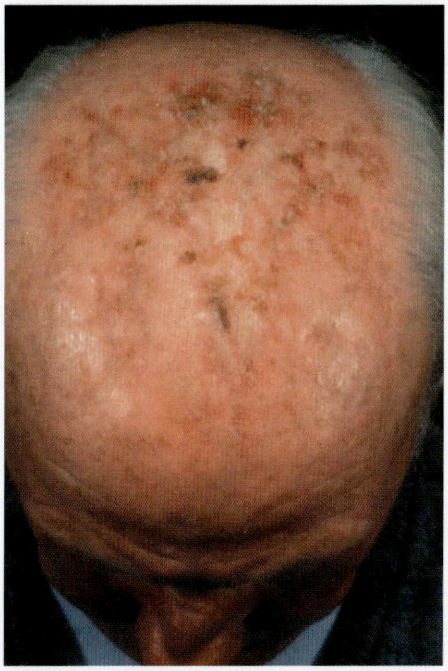

Figure 42.31 Actinic keratosis (courtesy of St John's Institute for Dermatology, London, UK).

Keratoacanthoma can grow to between 1 and 3 cm in a 6-week period and then typically resolve spontaneously over the subsequent six months. Removal of the central keratin plug may speed resolution. Excision is recommended as the differential diagnosis includes anaplastic SCC and the excision scar is often better than that which remains after resolution.

Bowen's disease

Bowen's disease was first described by John T Bowen in 1912. It is a carcinoma *in situ* with between 3 and 11 per cent progressing to SCC (Figure 42.34). It is currently not thought to be a paraneoplastic condition. Chronic solar damage and inorganic

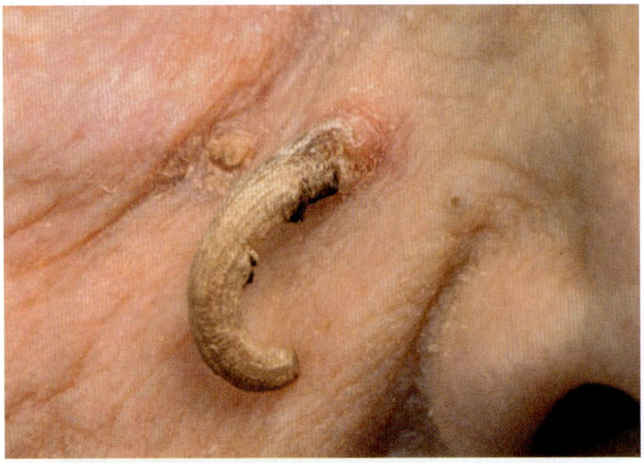

Figure 42.32 Cutaneous horn (courtesy of St John's Institute for Dermatology, London, UK).

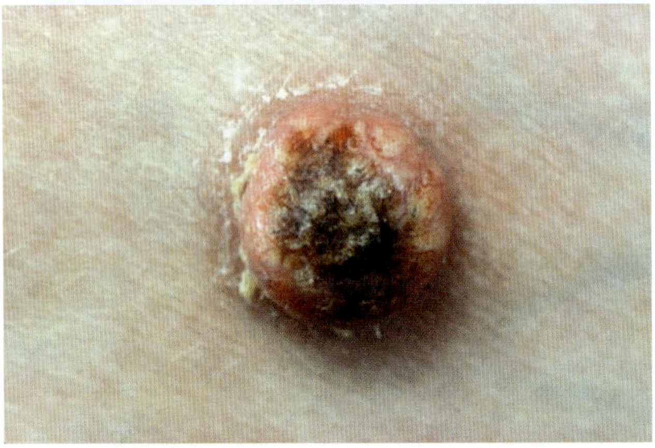

Figure 42.33 Keratocanthoma (courtesy of St John's Institute for Dermatology, London, UK).

arsenic ingestion have been implicated as aetiologic factors in the development of Bowen's disease. The human papilloma virus 16 has also been documented as a cause.

Bowen's disease often presents as a slowly enlarging, erythematous, scaly patch or plaque. It may occur anywhere on the mucocutaneous surface of the body. On the glans penis, it is called erythroplasia of Querat (Figure 42.35).

Topical therapy with 5-fluorouracil or imiquimod are effective treatments. Alternatives include surgical excision with a 4-mm margin or Mohs' micrographic surgery for larger or recurrent lesions.

Extramammary Paget's disease

It is a form of intraepidermal adenocarcinoma, which may occur in the genital, perianal regions or in cutaneous sites rich in apocrine glands such as the axilla (Figure 42.36). Approximately 25 per cent of the cases of extramammary Paget's disease are associated with an underlying *in situ* or invasive neoplasm.

The early skin changes are subtle and may present as an eczematous lesion or intertrigo.

Surgical excision forms the basis of treatment with up to 20 per cent demonstrating invasion on excision.

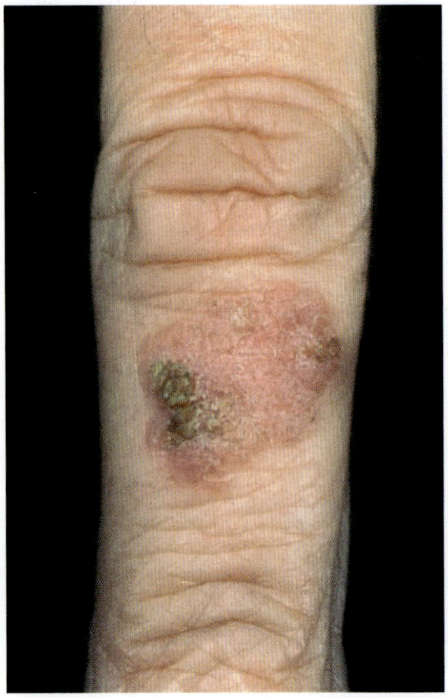

Figure 42.34 Bowen's disease – squamous cell carcinoma *in situ* (courtesy of St John's Institute for Dermatology, London, UK).

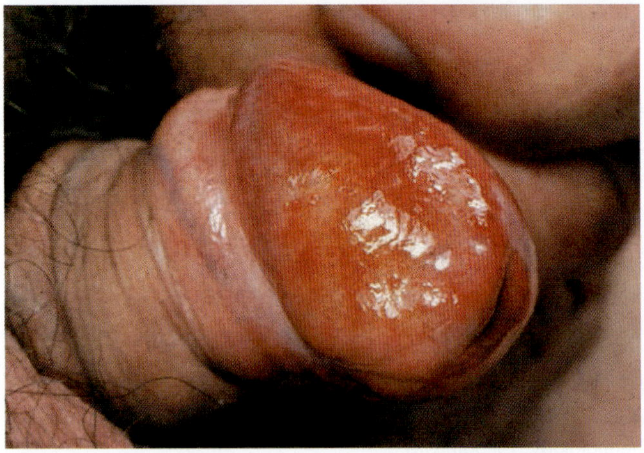

Figure 42.35 Erythroplasia of Queyrat – squamous cell carcinoma *in situ* on the glans penis; also called Paget's disease of the penis (courtesy of St John's Institute for Dermatology, London, UK).

Giant congenital pigmented naevus or giant hairy naevus

The giant congenital pigmented naevus (GCPN) causes a great deal of confusion as its definition and management is contentious. It is a hamartoma of naevo-melanocytes that has a tendency to dermatomal distribution (Figure 42.37). It has a similar histology to compound naevi, but the naevus cells are distributed variably from the epidermis throughout all layers and into the subdermal fat and muscle. There is general agreement that

Frederic E Mohs, 1910–2002, a twentieth century American Surgeon, Physician and General Surgeon, University of Wisconsin, Madison, WI, USA. Developed the Mohs Micrographic Surgical technique in 1938 for cutaneous malignant lesions.

John Templeton Bowen, 1857–1941, Professor of Dermatology, Harvard University Medical School, Boston, MA, USA, described this intradermal precancerous skin lesion in 1912.
August Queyrat, 1856–1933, dermatologist, Paris, France, described this condition in 1911.

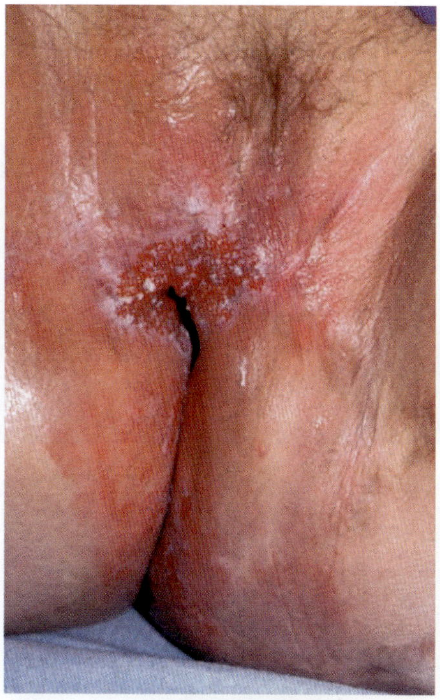

Figure 42.36 Extramammary Paget's disease involving perineum (courtesy of St John's Institute for Dermatology, London, UK).

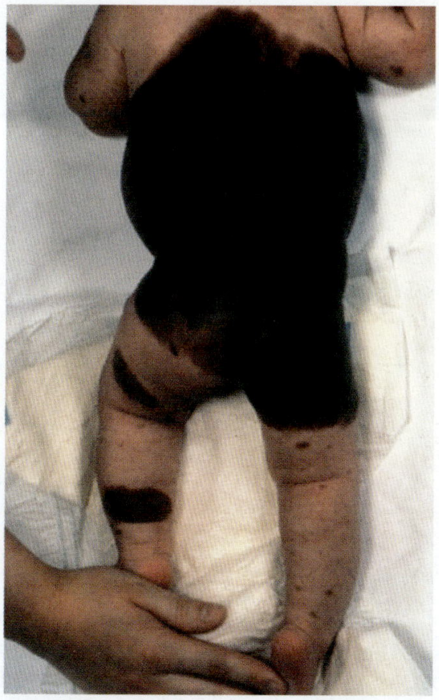

Figure 42.37 Giant congenital pigmented naevus (courtesy of St John's Institute for Dermatology, London, UK).

GCPNs are precursors of melanoma but the magnitude of this risk is unclear largely due to the lack of well-conducted studies and poor classification. A 3–5 per cent lifetime risk of melanoma is quoted. One in three childhood malignant melanomas arise in patients with GCPN but the risk decreases with age with 15 per cent presenting at birth, 62 per cent present by puberty and 99 per cent by 45 years of age.

A multidisciplinary management approach is advocated with initial investigations examining for neurocutaneous melanosis as there may be leptomeningeal involvement. Removal of GCPN should be considered for both aesthetic and oncological reasons.

Dysplastic (atypical) naevus

Dysplastic naevus is an irregular proliferation of atypical melanocytes at the basal layer of epidermis (Figure 42.38). It has variegated pigmentation with irregular borders, measuring more than 5 mm in size. Dysplastic naevus has a familial inheritance and carries a 5–10 per cent risk of forming a superficial spreading melanoma.

Malignant lesions

Basal cell carcinoma

Usually a slow growing, locally invasive malignant tumour of pluripotential epithelial cells arising from basal epidermis and hair follicles, hence affecting the pilosebaceous skin (Summary box 42.4).

Summary box 42.4

Basal cell carcinoma

- Slow growing
- Risk factor – ultraviolet light
- 90 per cent nodular/nodular cystic
- High and low risk basal cell carcinoma

Epidemiology

The strongest predisposing factor to BCC is ultraviolet radiation. The incidence of BCC therefore rises with proximity to the equator, although 33 per cent arise in parts of the body which are not sun exposed. It occurs in the middle aged or elderly with 90 per cent of lesions found on the face above a line from the lobe of the ear to the corner of the mouth. Other predisposing factors include exposure to arsenical compounds, coal tar, aromatic hydrocarbons, ionising radiation and genetic skin cancer syndromes. White-skinned people are almost exclusively

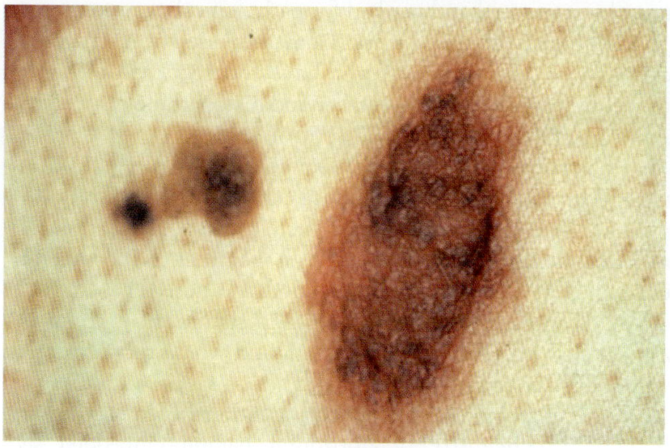

Figure 42.38 Dysplastic naevus (courtesy of St John's Institute for Dermatology, London, UK).

affected. Ninety-five per cent occur between the ages of 40 and 80 years and are more common in men.

Pathogenesis

BCCs have no apparent precursor lesions and their development is proportional to the initial dose of the carcinogen, but not duration of exposure. BCCs rarely metastasise, are hard to culture and resist transplantation. All of this suggests that a multistep mechanism for their development is unlikely, and that mesodermal factors acting as intrinsic promoters coupled with an initiation step is the most likely mechanism.

Macroscopic

BCC can be divided into localised (nodular, nodulocystic, cystic, pigmented and naevoid) and generalised lesions. These lesions can be superficial (multifocal or superficial spreading) or infiltrative (morphoeic, ice pick and cicatrising) (Figure 42.39). Nodular and nodulocystic variants account for 90 per cent of BCC.

Microscopic

Twenty-six histological types have been described. The characteristic finding is of ovoid cells in nests with a single 'palisading' layer. It is only the outer layer of cells that actively divide. This may explain why tumour growth rates are slower than the cell cycle speed would suggest, and why incompletely excised lesions are more aggressive. Morphoeic BCCs synthesise type 4 collagenase and so spread rapidly (Figure 42.40).

Prognosis

There are 'high risk' and 'low risk' BCCs. High risk BCCs are the ones that are large (>2 cm) and located at specific sites (near the eye, nose, ear) and have ill-defined margins. Recurrent tumours and those forming in the presence of immunosuppression are also higher risk.

Management

Treatment can be surgical or non-surgical. Margins should always be assessed and marked under loupe magnification and vary between 2 and 15 mm depending on the macroscopic variant. Where margins are ill-defined, or tissue at a premium (nose, eyes), then either Mohs' micrographic surgery or a two-stage surgical approach with subsequent reconstruction after confirmation of clear margins is advisable. The histological sample must be orientated and marked for pathological examination.

Mohs' micrographic surgery is a method used by dermatological surgeons (dermatologists who have undergone extra training in techniques of cutaneous surgery and histopathology) to excise skin cancer under microscopic control.

It has been demonstrated in suitable skin tumours to minimise recurrence rates and maximise conservation of surrounding normal tissue. This technique is therefore considered the optimal treatment for poorly demarcated, recurrent or incompletely excised BCC (including BCC around the nose, eyes and ears where clearance may be uncertain and significant morbidity is associated with incomplete excision, and where reconstruction with a flap is preferable cosmetically).

Mohs' micrographic surgery (using either frozen section and immunohistochemistry or horizontal paraffin-embedded sections) can also be used for excision of SCC, dermatofibrosarcoma protuberans and lentigo maligna.

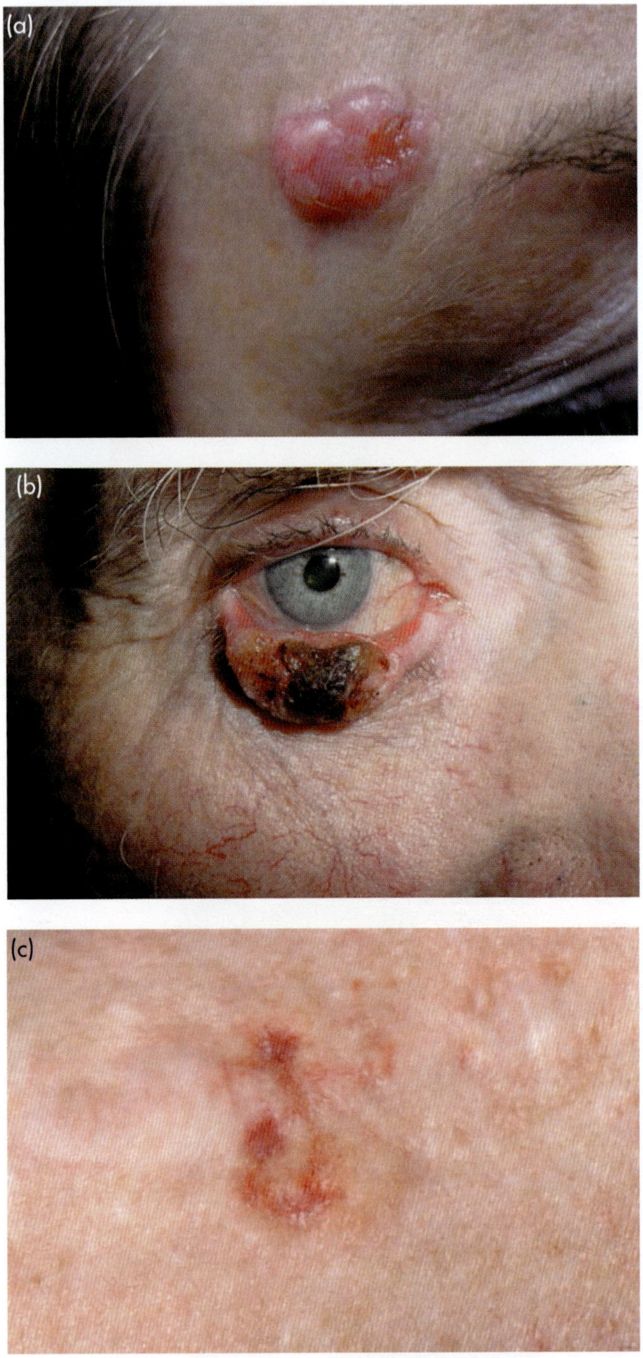

Figure 42.39 (a) A nodulocystic basal carcinoma (BCC). Note the characteristic pearly surface with telangectasia. (b) An ulcerating BCC on the lower eyelid. (c) A recurrent morphoeic BCC ((a) and (b) courtesy of Mr AR Greenbaum; (c) courtesy of St John's Institute for Dermatology, London, UK).

Mohs' micrographic surgery is performed under local anaesthesia (which is one of its limitations) and involves an initial 'saucerising excision' of the primary tumour's gross extent. The sample and the defect are then marked and orientated. A map of the specimen is drawn and characterised using different coloured stains in different quadrants. A histotechnician and a Mohs' surgeon work together, whereby the histotechnician sections the tissue horizontally (including lateral and deep margins

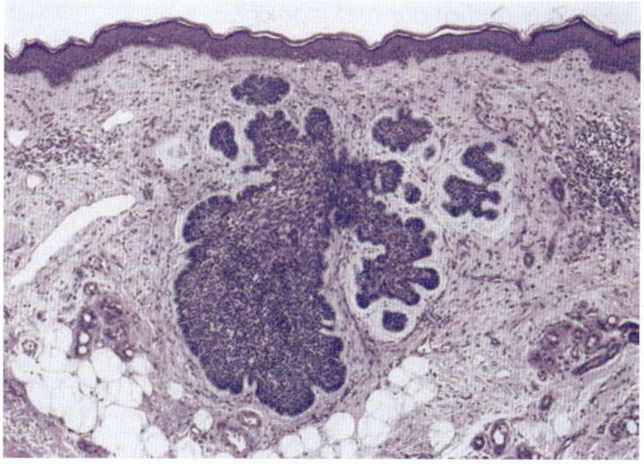

Figure 42.40 A basaloid, epithelial tumour with palisading cells on the periphery of the tumour that sits within a mucinous stroma (courtesy of Dr Catherine di Stefanato, Consultant Dermatopathologist, St John's Institute for Dermatology, London, UK).

in the same slide) and stains it with haematoxylin and eosin. The Mohs' surgeon then examines the slides for the presence of residual tumour and excises more tissue from the relevant parts of the mapped defect as necessary. In theory, the technique offers complete evaluation of the lateral and deep margins of tumour excision and so should thus be dependable. Complete excision rates exceeding 99 per cent are the rule in trained experienced hands.

In the elderly or infirm patients, radiotherapy produces similar recurrence rates to surgery. Superficial tumours can be treated with topical treatments (5-fluorouracil, imquimod) or cryotherapy.

Excision must be complete as there is a 67 per cent recurrence rate if margins are grossly involved and a 33 per cent recurrence rate within two years with microscopic involvement or when reported 'close'. Thus, patients with uncomplicated completely excised lesions can be discharged. Follow up is reserved for patients with tumours in high-risk areas, namely globally sun-damaged skin, syndromes (for example naevoid basal cell carcinoma syndrome) and incomplete excisions in patients who have declined further surgery.

Cutaneous squamous cell carcinoma

SCC is a malignant tumour of keratinising cells of the epidermis or its appendages. It arises from the stratum germinatum of the epidermis and expresses cytokeratins 1 and 10.

Epidemiology

SCC is the second most common form of skin cancer. It is four times less common than BCC and affects the elderly. It is strongly related to cumulative sun exposure and damage, and is twice as common in men and in white-skinned individuals living nearer the equator. SCC is also associated with chronic inflammation (chronic sinus tracts, pre-existing scars, osteomyelitis, burns, vaccination points) and immunosuppression (organ transplant recipients). When an SCC appears in a scar it is known as a Marjolin's ulcer.

The time taken to develop an SCC after radiation exposure is proportional to the wavelength of the radiation. SCC is also caused by chemical carcinogens (arsenicals, tar), and infection with human papilloma virus 5 and 16. There is also evidence that current and previous tobacco use doubles the relative risk of SCC (Summary box 42.5).

Summary box 42.5

Squamous cell carcinoma

- Associated with chronic inflammation
- Invariably ulcerated lesion
- Metastasis in 2 per cent cases

Macroscopic

The appearance of SCC may vary from smooth nodular, verrucous, papillomatous to ulcerating lesions (Figure 42.41). However, all variants will eventually ulcerate as they grow. The ulcers have a characteristic everted edge and are surrounded by inflamed, indurated skin. The differential diagnosis of an SCC are actinic keratosis, BCC, keratoacanthoma, pyoderma gangrenosum and warts.

Microscopic

Characteristic irregular masses of squamous epithelium are noted to proliferate and invade the dermis from the germinal layer (Figure 42.42). This tumour stains positive for cytokeratins 1 and 10. SCC can be histologically graded according to Broders' histological grading. This system describes the proportion of de-differentiated cells (i.e. the ratio of pleomorphic and anaplastic cells:normal cells).

The histopathology report on an SCC should include information on the pathological pattern (e.g. adenoid); the cellular morphology (e.g. spindle); the Broders' grade; the depth of invasion, the presence of any perineural or vascular invasion and the deep and peripheral margin clearance (Table 42.3).

Prognosis

There are several independent prognostic variables for SCC:

1 Invasion:
   a. Depth: the deeper the lesion, the worse the prognosis. For SCC <2 mm, metastasis is highly unlikely; whereas if >6 mm, 15 per cent of SCCs will have metastasised.
   b. Surface size: lesions >2 cm have a worse prognosis than smaller ones.
2 Histological grade: the higher the Broders' grade, the worse the prognosis.
3 Site: SCCs on the lips and ears have higher local recurrence rates than lesions elsewhere and tumours at the extremities fare worse than those on the trunk.
4 Aetiology: SCCs that arise in burn scars, osteomyelitis skin sinuses, chronic ulcers and areas of skin that have been irradiated have a higher metastatic potential.

Albert Compton Broders, 1885–1964, an American pathologist of Minnesota, USA and Chairman of the Department of Surgical Pathology, The Mayo Clinic, Rochester, Minnesota, MN, USA; for one year in 1935 Professor of Surgical Pathology and Director of Cancer Research, University of Virginia, VA, USA. Broders graded rectal cancer in the USA in a manner that Cuthbert Dukes classified them in the UK. A combination of Broders' grading and Dukes' classification gave a more accurate prognosis for rectal carcinoma than either method alone.

Jean-Nicholas Marjolin, 1780–1850, surgeon, Paris, France, described the development of carcinomatous ulcers in scars in 1828.

5 Immunosuppression: SCC will invade further in those with impaired immune response.
6 Tumours with perineural involvement have a worse prognosis and require a wider than usual clearance.

The overall rate of metastasis is 2 per cent for SCC – usually to regional nodes – with a local recurrence rate of 20 per cent.

Management

SCC is a heterogeneous tumour with a malignant behaviour that varies between subtypes. Management must therefore address the need for definitive treatment, the possibility of in-transit metastasis and the tumour's tendency for lymphatic metastasis.

Surgical excision is the only means of providing accurate histology. The margins for primary excision should be tailored to surface size in the first instance. This should ideally be assessed using surgical loupe magnification. A 4-mm clearance margin should be achieved if the SCC measures <2 cm across, and a 1-cm clearance margin if >2 cm.

Ninety-five per cent of local recurrence and regional metastases occur within five years, thus follow up beyond this period is not indicated.

Cutaneous malignant melanoma

Melanoma is a cancer of melanin producing cells and can therefore arise in skin, mucosa, retina and the leptomeninges.

Epidemiology

Cutaneous melanoma is caused largely by exposure to ultraviolet radiation. Its rise in incidence reflects social behaviour and increased recreational activity in the sun among white-skinned races not suited to sun exposure. Although it accounts for less than 5 per cent of skin malignancy, it is responsible for over 75 per cent of skin malignancy related deaths.

Malignant melanoma (MM) accounts for 3 per cent of all malignancy worldwide. It is the most common cancer in young adults (20–39 years) and the most likely cause of cancer-related death.

Distribution between the sexes varies around the world and reflects occupational and recreational exposure to sunlight. Likewise, geographical distribution reflects exposure of white-skinned individuals to sunlight: Auckland in New Zealand currently reports the highest incidence per capita, and before that Brisbane in Australia held that distinction.

Five per cent of all patients with MM will develop a second

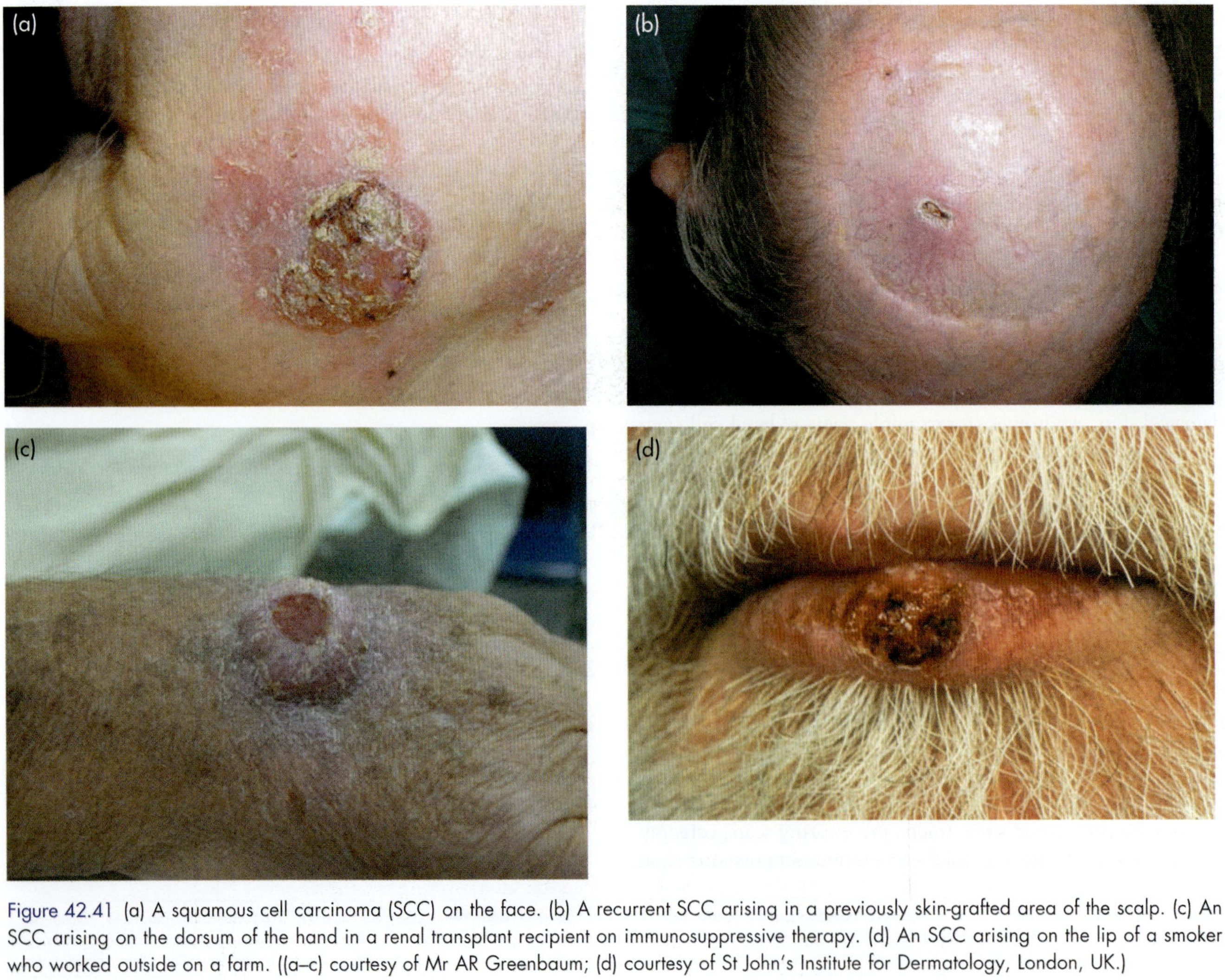

Figure 42.41 (a) A squamous cell carcinoma (SCC) on the face. (b) A recurrent SCC arising in a previously skin-grafted area of the scalp. (c) An SCC arising on the dorsum of the hand in a renal transplant recipient on immunosuppressive therapy. (d) An SCC arising on the lip of a smoker who worked outside on a farm. ((a–c) courtesy of Mr AR Greenbaum; (d) courtesy of St John's Institute for Dermatology, London, UK.)

Table 42.3 TNM classification and staging.

Size	Nodes	Mets	Grade
T_1 = <2 cm	N_0 = no regional nodes	M_0 = no mets	G_1 = low grade
T_2 = 2–5 cm	N_1 = regional nodes	M_1 = distant mets	G_2 = moderately differentiated
T_3 > 5 cm			G_3 = high grade or highly anaplastic
T_4 = muscle or bony invasion			

Stage I = T1, N0, M0; stage II = T2–3, N0, M0; stage III = T4, N0, M0 and any T, N1, M0; stage IV = any T, any N1, M1(+).

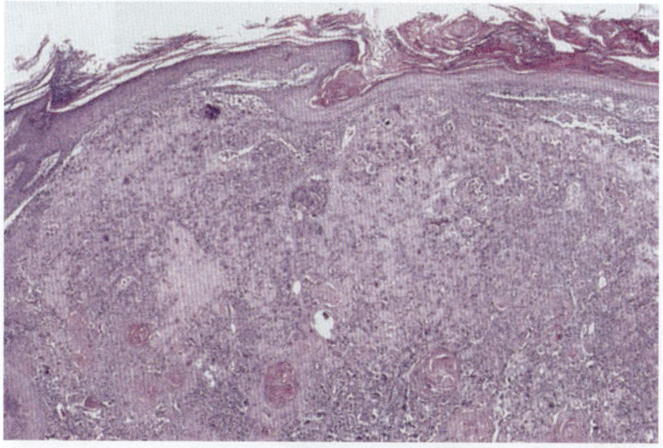

Figure 42.42 An invasive, epidermal keratinising tumour characterised by proliferation of atypical squamous cells with 'horn pearls' (courtesy of Dr Catherine di Stefanato, Consultant Dermatopathologist, St John's Institute for Dermatology, London, UK).

primary melanoma. Seven per cent of MMs present as occult metastases from an unknown primary.

Pathophysiology

UV exposure is the major causal factor for developing MM. Cumulative exposure favours the development of lentigo maligna melanoma (LMM), whereas 'flash fry' exposure – typical of rapidly acquired holiday tans – favours the other morphological variants (Summary box 42.6).

Summary box 42.6

Malignant melanoma

- Rising incidence
- Genetic and acquired risk factors
- Superficial spreading form the most common
- Breslow thickness most important prognostic indicator
- Sentinel node biopsy useful for lymphatic mapping

A small proportion of MMs are genetically mediated, as in xeroderma pigmentosum which increases the relative risk of developing MM to 1000. Immunosuppression secondary to drugs or HIV infection will increase the incidence of MM by 20–30-fold.

The risk factors for developing MM are summarised below:

- Xeroderma pigmentosum (relative risk = 1000)
- Past medical or family history of MM with dysplastic naevi (relative risk = 33–1269)
- Previous melanoma (relative risk = 84)
- High total number of naevi (relative risk = 3.4, if >20 naevi)
- Dysplastic naevi (10 per cent lifetime risk)
- Red hair (relative risk = 3)
- Tendency to freckle (relative risk = 1.9)
- Immune compromised conditions: HIV infection, Hodgkin's disease, cyclosporin A therapy
- Giant congenital pigmented naevus (increased risk)
- History of sunburn – especially in childhood.

Macroscopic

Only 10–20 per cent of MM form in pre-existing naevi, with the remainder arising *de novo* in previously normally pigmented skin. The most likely naevi to form MM are the junctional and compound types.

Macroscopic features in a pre-existing naevus that suggest malignant change are listed in Summary box 42.7.

There are four common macroscopic variants of MM. There are several other notable, but rarer forms.

Summary box 42.7

Macroscopic features in naevi suggestive of malignant melanoma

- Change in size – any adult naevus >6 mm is suspect (for reference a lead pencil diameter is 7 mm) and anything changing to >10 mm is more likely to be malignant than benign
- Shape
- Colour
- Thickness (elevation/nodularity or ulceration)
- Satellite lesions (pigment spreading into surrounding area)
- Tingling/itching/serosanguinous discharge (usually late signs)
- Blood supply: melanomas >1 mm thick have a blood supply which can be found with a hand-held Doppler, so 'Doppler positive' pigmented lesions should be excised

Superficial spreading melanoma

This is the most common type (70 per cent), usually arising in a pre-existent naevus, after several years of slow change, followed by rapid growth in the preceding months before presentation

(Figure 42.43). Typically it is a darker pigmented area in a junctional naevus. Nodularity within superficial spreading melanoma (SSM) heralds the onset of the vertical growth phase.

Nodular melanoma

Nodular melanoma (NM) accounts for 15 per cent of all MM and tends to be more aggressive than SSM, with a shorter clinical onset. These lesions typically arise *de novo* in skin and are more common in men than women, often presenting in middle age and usually on the trunk, head or neck (Figure 42.44). They typically appear as blue/black papules, 1–2 cm in diameter, and because they lack the horizontal growth phase, they tend to be sharply demarcated. Up to 5 per cent are amelanotic.

Lentigo maligna melanoma

Previously also known as Hutchison's melanotic freckle. This variant presents as a slow-growing, variagated brown macule, on the face, neck or hands of the elderly (Figure 42.45). They are positively correlated with prolonged, intense sun exposure, affecting women more than men. They account for between 5 and 10 per cent of MM. LMM are thought to have less metastatic potential than other variants as they take longer to enter a vertical growth phase. Nonetheless, when they have entered the vertical growth phase their metastatic potential is the same as any other melanoma.

Acral lentigious melanoma

Acral lentigious melanoma (ALM) affects the soles of the feet and the palms of the hands. It is rare in white-skinned individuals (2–8 per cent of MM) but is more common in the Afro-Caribbean, Hispanic and Asian populations (35–60 per cent). It usually presents as a flat, irregular macule in later life (Figure 42.46). Twenty-five per cent are amelanotic and may mimic a fungal infection or pyogenic granuloma.

MM under the finger nail is usually SSM rather than ALM. For finger or toe nail lesions it is vital to biopsy the nail matrix rather than just the pigment on the nail plate. A classical feature of a subungual melanoma is Hutchinson's sign. This is nail fold pigmentation which then widens progressively to produce a triangular pigmented macule with associated nail dystrophy. The differential diagnosis is 'benign racial melanonychia', which produces a linear dark streak under a nail in a dark-skinned individual. Malignancy is unlikely if the nail fold is uninvolved.

Miscellaneous

- Amelanotic melanoma (often arising in the gastrointestinal tract and presenting with obstruction, intussusception or as a metastasis from an unknown primary).
- Desmoplastic – mostly found on the head and neck region. It has a propensity for perineural infiltration and often recurs locally if not widely excised. May be amelanotic clinically.

Microscopic

Malignant change occurs in the melanocytes in the basal epidermis, while *in situ*, atypical melanocytes are limited to the dermoepidermal junction and show no evidence of dermal involvement. During the horizontal growth phase, cells spread along the dermoepidermal junction and although they may breach the dermis, their migration is predominantly radial. During the vertical growth phase, the dermis may be invaded.

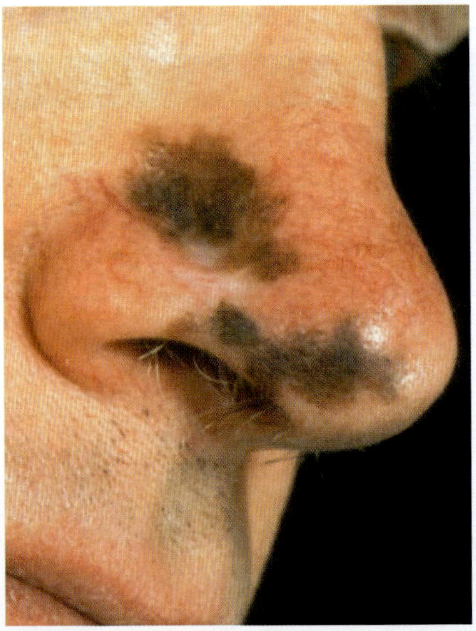

Figure 42.43 Superficial spreading melanoma (courtesy of St John's Institute for Dermatology, London, UK).

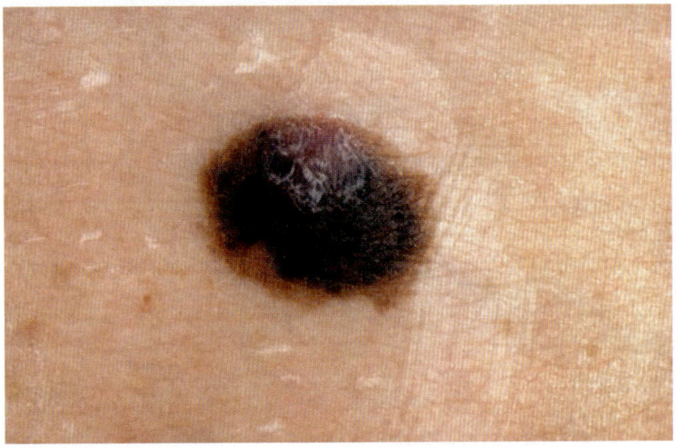

Figure 42.44 Nodular melanoma (courtesy of St John's Institute for Dermatology, London, UK).

The greater the depth of invasion, the greater is the metastatic potential of the tumour.

Management

History and clinical examination should be directed at discovering the primary lesion and identification of local, regional or distant spread. Clinical photography is useful when observation is chosen rather than excision biopsy for definitive histopathological diagnosis. An excision biopsy with a 2–5 mm margin of skin and a cuff of subdermal fat is acceptable. Incision biopsy is occasionally indicated – for instance in large lesions on the face where an excision biopsy of the whole lesion would be disfiguring.

Biopsy and pathological examination provide the first step towards staging melanoma. The Breslow thickness of a melanoma (measured to the nearest 0.1 mm from the granular layer to the

Alexander Breslow, 1928–1980, American pathologist. Pathologist, George Washington University, Washington DC, USA, first reported in 1970 that the prognosis depends upon the thickness of the tumour.

Sir Jonathan Hutchinson, 1828–1913, surgeon, St Bartholomew's Hospital, London, UK.

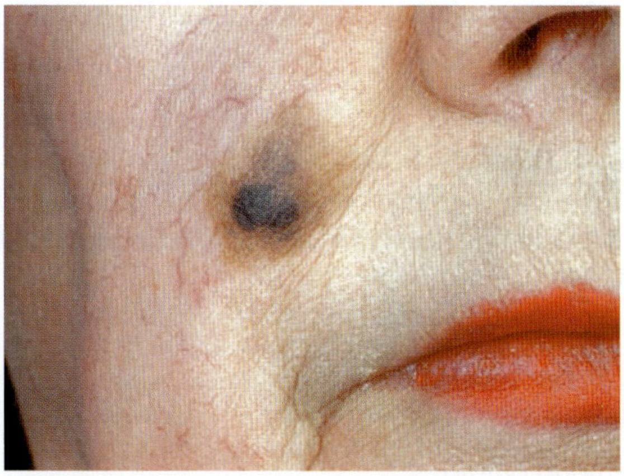

Figure 42.45 Lentigo maligna melanoma (courtesy of St John's Institute for Dermatology, London, UK).

base of tumour) is the most important prognostic indicator in the absence of lymph node metastases. The AJCC staging system then takes lymph node and distant metastases into account (see Table 42.4).

Investigations

Guidelines for staging are controversial. One approach is to aim investigations towards detecting occult disease so as to upstage patients and then treat them accurately and appropriately. Thus, offering sentinel node biopsy to patients with clinical stage II disease is prudent, investigations for stage III disease should be directed to individual clinical presentation.

Local treatment

The treatment for melanoma is surgery. Lentigo maligna (melanoma *in situ*) should be excised completely in most clinical situations because of the risk of it entering the vertical growth phase to become LMM. A complete excision requires no further treatment.

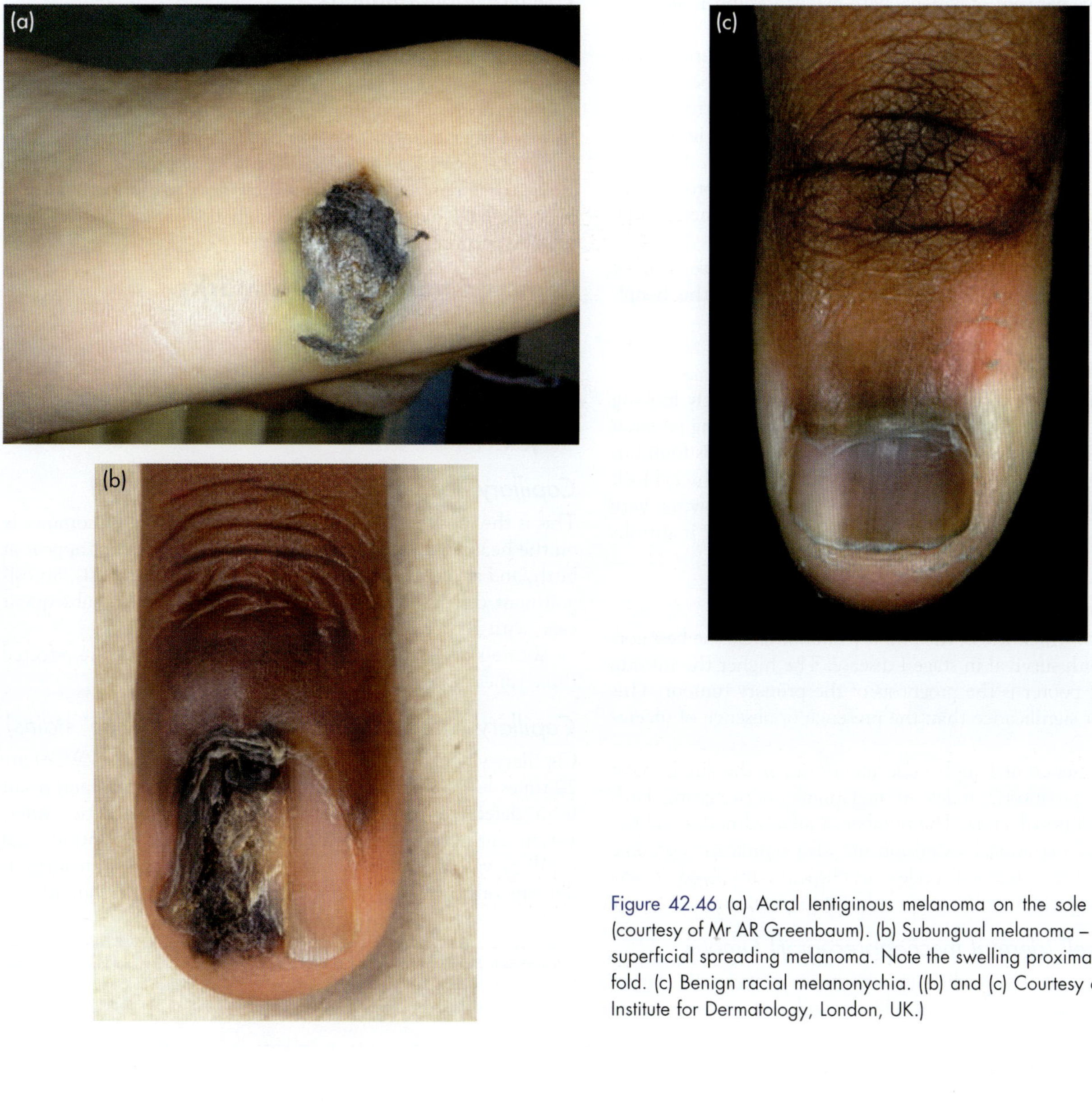

Figure 42.46 (a) Acral lentiginous melanoma on the sole of the foot (courtesy of Mr AR Greenbaum). (b) Subungual melanoma – probably a superficial spreading melanoma. Note the swelling proximal to the nail fold. (c) Benign racial melanonychia. ((b) and (c) Courtesy of St John's Institute for Dermatology, London, UK.)

For melanoma <1 mm deep, wide local excision with a 1 cm margin is sufficient. For deeper lesions, a 2 cm margin is recommended as there is no evidence that wider margins make a difference.

Regional lymph nodes

The likelihood of metastatic spread to regional lymph nodes is proportional to the Breslow thickness of the melanoma. Management of regional lymph nodes has been a contentious topic for well over a century. Some advocate simultaneous elective lymph node clearance at the time of wide excision of the primary melanoma. Ideally, one would like to be able to select for treatment those patients with the highest risk of metastatic spread.

Sentinel node biopsy (SNB) is an investigation based on the fact that lymphatic metastasis proceeds in an orderly fashion and can be predicted by mapping the lymphatic drainage from a primary tumour to the first or 'sentinel' node in the regional lymphatic basin. There is negligible benefit in performing SNB in patients whose primary melanoma is thinner than 1 mm. When SNB is performed according to consensus standards, it is predictive of the regional nodal status in 99 per cent of cases. Seventy-five per cent of patients with metastases in the sentinel nodes will have no other involved regional nodes, so while the current standard approach is to proceed to completion lymphadenectomy, this will overtreat a significant number of sentinel node-positive patients. This might appear a better option than potentially undertreating 20–30 per cent of patients with positive sentinel nodes. Evidence of objective survival benefit from SNB is currently unavailable, but several large prospective clinical trials are in progress to investigate this and meanwhile, SNB remains part of the AJCC staging system.

Current treatment for biopsy positive nodal disease is block dissection of regional lymph nodes to remove all the lymph nodes in that regional basin.

Adjuvant therapy

None is of proven benefit, with clinical trials currently looking at vaccine and interferon treatments. Recent promising research has focused on mutations in the *BRAF* gene, which is found in about 60 per cent of malignant melanoma. Drugs which block the products of the faulty gene are currently showing very promising results in clinical trials with evidence that it shrinks metastatic deposits in patients with stage 4 disease.

Prognosis

The Breslow thickness of the primary tumour offers the best correlation with survival in stage I disease. The higher the mitotic index, the poorer is the prognosis of the primary tumour. This has greater significance than the presence or absence of ulceration.

The presence of lymph node metastases is the single most important prognostic index in melanoma; outweighing both tumour and host factors. The number of affected nodes and the presence of extranodal extension are also significant outcome predictors. Once regional nodes are clinically involved, 70–85 per cent of patients will have occult distant metastases.

Merkel cell (dermal mechanoreceptor) tumour

This is an aggressive malignant tumour of Merkel cells (Figure 42.47). It usually affects the elderly and is four times more common in women than men. Treatment is with wide local excision aiming for a 25–30-mm margin, followed by radiotherapy.

VASCULAR LESIONS

Congenital: haemangiomata and vascular malformations

These can be subclassified biologically into vascular tumours or vascular malformations based on their endothelial characteristics; or radiologically into haemangiomata, vascular and lymphatic malformations based on their vascular dynamics.

Haemangiomata

These are benign endothelial tumours that affect three girls for every boy. Thirty per cent have a herald patch at birth, which then grows rapidly in the first year of life, then slowly involutes over several years with 70 per cent having resolved by seven years of age. Large haemangiomata can trap platelets leading to thrombocytopenia (Kasabach–Merritt syndrome).

Vascular malformations

Vascular malformations affect boys and girls equally and are associated with numerous syndromes. They are invariably present at birth but may be missed if deep to the skin. Vascular malformations subsequently grow in proportion to the child's growth (other than in response to sepsis or hormonal stimulation). Stasis can lead to a localised, consumptive coagulopathy in large venous malformations. Low-flow malformations may cause skeletal hypoplasia, while high flow malformations can cause hypertrophy.

Common vascular birthmarks

Salmon patch

This is a haemangioma that presents as a pinkish macule usually at the nape of neck (Figure 42.48). It is caused by an area of persistent fetal dermal circulation, which usually disappears at one year.

Capillary haemangioma (strawberry naevus)

This is the most common birth mark occurring most commonly on the head and neck (Figure 42.49). Ninety per cent appear at birth, and as a consequence of intravascular thrombosis, fibrosis and mast cell infiltration, 10 per cent resolve each subsequent year, with 70 per cent resolved by seven years of age.

White skin is affected most commonly and girls are affected three times more than boys.

Capillary vascular malformations ('port-wine' stains)

Capillary vascular malformations ('port-wine' stains (PWS)) are 20 times less common than capillary haemangiomata and result from defective maturation of cutaneous sympathetic innervation during embryogenesis leading to localised intradermal capillary vasodilatation (Figure 42.50). They appear at birth as flat, smooth, intensely purple stained areas, most frequently on

Katharine K Merritt, b. 1886, American paediatrician, Department of Paediatrics, the Babies Hospital, Columbia University College of Physicians and Surgeons, New York, NY, USA. Kasabach and Merritt described the condition as a joint paper in 1940.

Haig H Kasabach, 1898–1943, radiologist, the Presbyterian Hospital, New York, NY, USA.

Table 42.4 American Joint Committee on Cancer 2001 staging.

Stage	Primary tumour	Lymph node	Metastases
0	*In situ*	No nodal involvement	No distant metastases
IA	<1 mm, no ulceration		
IB	<1 mm, with ulceration		
	>1 but <2 mm, no ulceration		
IIA	>1 but <2 mm, with ulceration		
	>2 but <4 mm, no ulceration		
IIB	>2 but <4 mm, with ulceration		
	>4 mm, no ulceration		
IIC	>4 mm, with ulceration		
IIIA	Any Breslow, no ulceration	Micrometastasis	
IIIB	Any Breslow, with ulceration	Micrometastasis	
	Any Breslow, no ulceration	≤3 palpable nodes	
	Any Breslow, ± ulceration	In transit metastases/satellites	
IIIC	Any Breslow, with ulceration	≤3 palpable nodes	
	Any Breslow, ± ulceration	≥4 palpable or matted nodes or nodes + in transit metastases	
			M1: skin, subcutaneous or distant
			M2 : lung
			M3 all other sites/or any site +↑[LDH]

LDH, concentration of lactate dehydrogenase.

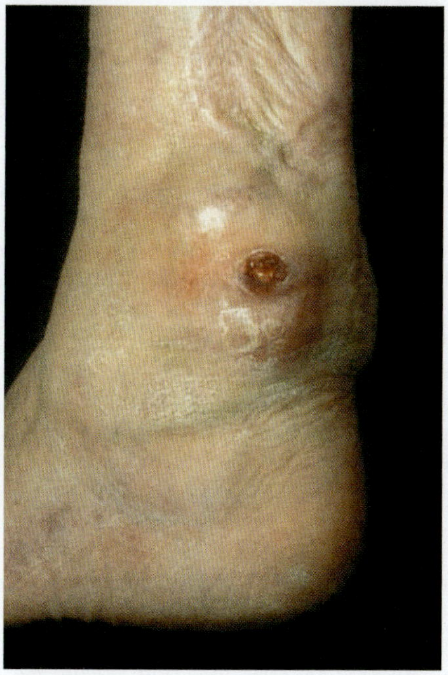

Figure 42.47 Merkel cell tumour (courtesy of St John's Institute for Dermatology, London, UK).

the head and neck, often within the maxillary and mandibular dermatomes of the trigeminal nerve.

Treatment with intense pulsed light and pulse dye laser are successful. PWS may be associated with various syndromes listed below:

- Sturge–Weber syndrome: PWS affecting trigeminal dermatomes; associated with epilepsy, glaucoma secondary to ipsilateral, leptomeningeal angiomatosis, cortical atrophy and visual field defects.
- Klippel–Trenaunay syndrome: PWS on a limb with associated bone and soft tissue hypertrophy and lateral varicose veins when the lower limb is involved. It is called Parkes Weber syndrome if there is an associated arteriovenous malformation.
- Proteus syndrome: PWS and regional gigantism in association with lymphatic (lymphaticovenous) malformation. Hypertrophy is always asymmetrical.

Acquired

Campbell de Morgan spots

These are arteriovenous fistulas at the dermal capillary level in sun exposed skin of older patients (Figure 42.51).

Spider naevi

These are angiomata that appear (and may disappear) spontaneously at puberty or in two-thirds of pregnant women, usually

William Allen Sturge, 1850–1919, physician, The Royal Free Hospital, London, UK.
Frederick Parkes Weber, 1863–1962, physician, The German Hospital, Dalston, London, UK.
Maurice Klippel, 1858–1942, neurologist, La Salpêtrière, Paris, France.
Paul Trenaunay, b. 1875, a French neurologist, Klippel and Trenaunay described the condition as a joint paper in 1900.
Proteus was a minor sea god of Greek mythology, who had the power of prophesy and was able to assume different shapes in order to avoid answering questions.
Campbell Greig de Morgan, 1811–1876, surgeon, the Middlesex Hospital, London UK.

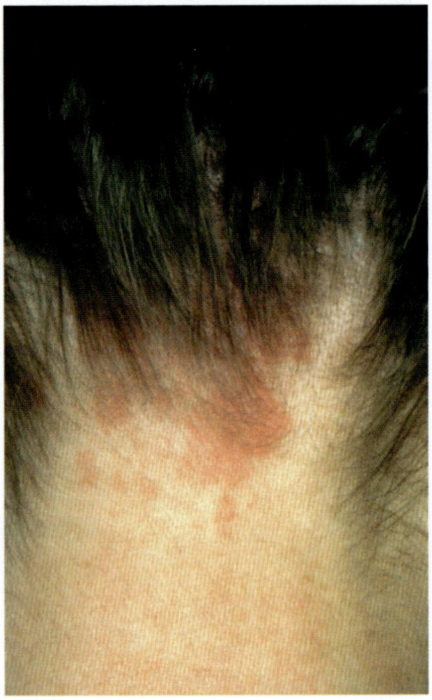

Figure 42.48 Salmon patch (courtesy of St John's Institute for Dermatology, London, UK).

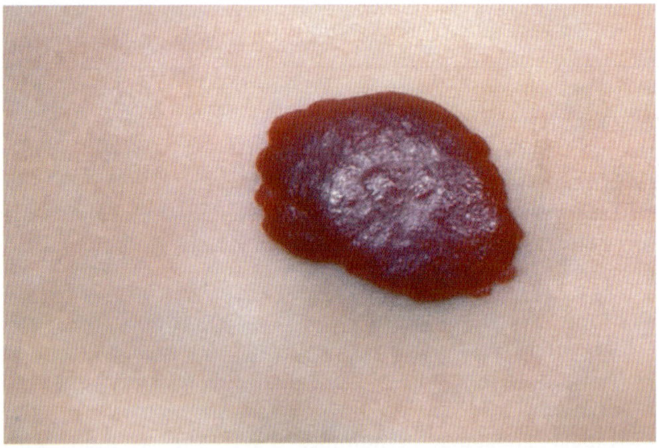

Figure 42.49 Capillary haemangioma (courtesy of St John's Institute for Dermatology, London, UK).

disappearing in the puerperium (Figure 42.52). Spider naevi are also associated with chronic liver disease. They can be treated with intense pulsed light or pulse dye laser.

Pyogenic granuloma

These share many histological characteristics of haemangiomas and are probably a subtype thereof (Figure 42.53).

Most are small (0.5–1.5 cm), raised, pedunculated, soft red nodular lesions showing superficial ulceration and a tendency to bleed after trivial trauma. They should be excised with a minimal margin.

Glomus tumour

These arise from subcutaneous arteriovenous shunts (Sucquet–Hoyer canals) especially in the corium of the nail bed. Typically,

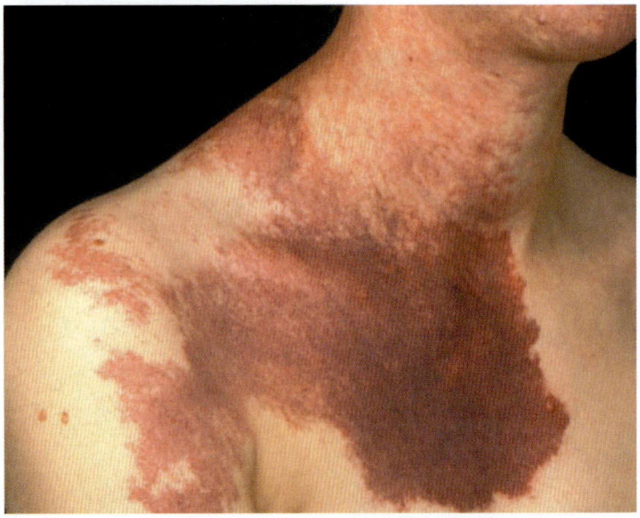

Figure 42.50 'Port-wine' stain (courtesy of St John's Institute for Dermatology, London, UK).

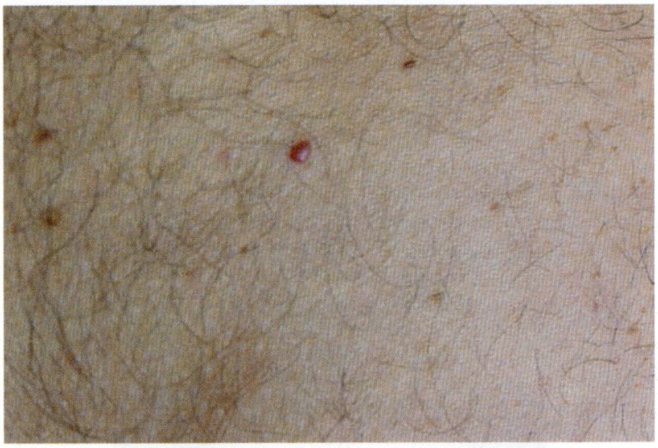

Figure 42.51 Campbell de Morgan spot (courtesy of Mr AR Greenbaum).

it is a small, purple nodule measuring a few millimetres in size which is disproportionately painful in response to insignificant stimuli, including cold exposure (Figure 42.54). Subungual varieties may be invisible causing paroxysmal digital pain.

Angiosarcoma ('malignant angioendothelioma')

Angiosarcoma is a rare, highly malignant tumour arising from the endothelial cells (Figure 42.55). The lymphangiosarcoma variant arises from lymphatic endothelium and can develop in lymphoedematous tissue, particularly an extremity. Proliferation is rapid with early systemic spread.

Kaposi's sarcoma

This is a malignant, proliferative tumour of vascular endothelial cells, which was first described in elderly Jewish men, but is now most commonly associated with immune compromise after transplantation or HIV infection (Figure 42.56). There appears to be a causal link with infection by human herpes virus 8. Kaposi's sarcoma usually starts as a red brown, indurated, plaque-like skin lesion that becomes nodular and then ulcerates. Treatment is with radiotherapy.

JP Sucquet, 1840–1870, an anatomist of Paris, France.
Heinrich Hoyer, 1834–1907, Professor of Histology, Embryology and Anatomy, the Central Medical School, The Polish University, Warsaw, Poland.

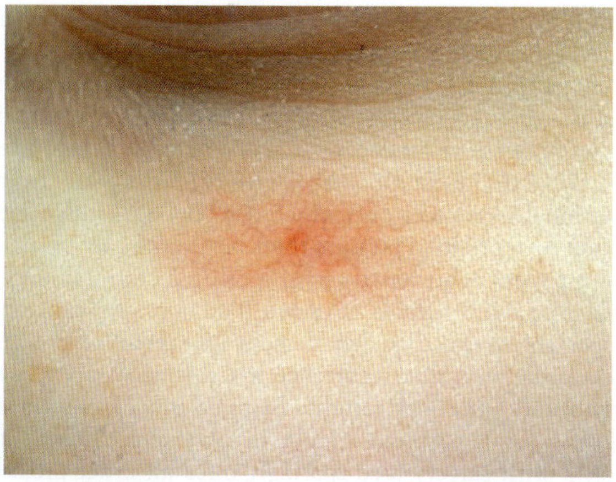

Figure 42.52 Spider naevus (courtesy of St John's Institute for Dermatology, London, UK).

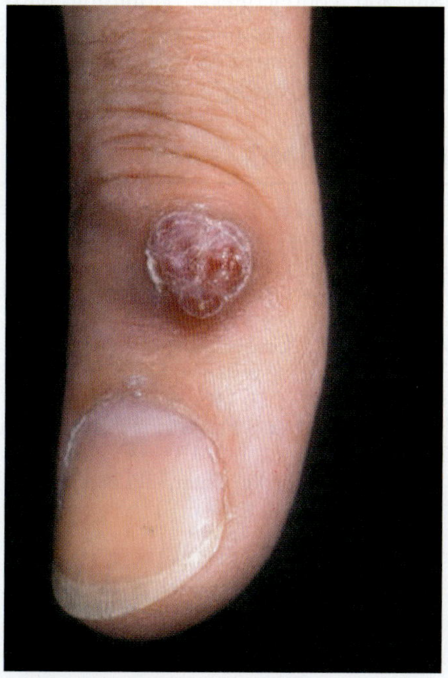

Figure 42.53 Pyogenic granuloma (courtesy of St John's Institute for Dermatology, London, UK).

WOUNDS: CONGENITAL

Cutis aplasia congenita

A rare condition characterised by the congenital absence of epidermis, dermis and, in some cases, subcutaneous tissues, with underlying bony defects in 20 per cent. Lesions may occur on any body surface, but localised scalp agenesis is most frequent.

Treatment depends on the severity of the presentation, but usually involves plastic surgery.

Parry–Romberg disease

An uncommon and poorly understood progressive, hemi-facial atrophy of skin, soft tissue and bone. Its incidence is unknown and its inheritance uncertain, but it affects women more commonly than men.

It commonly starts in a patient's late 20s, but can present in

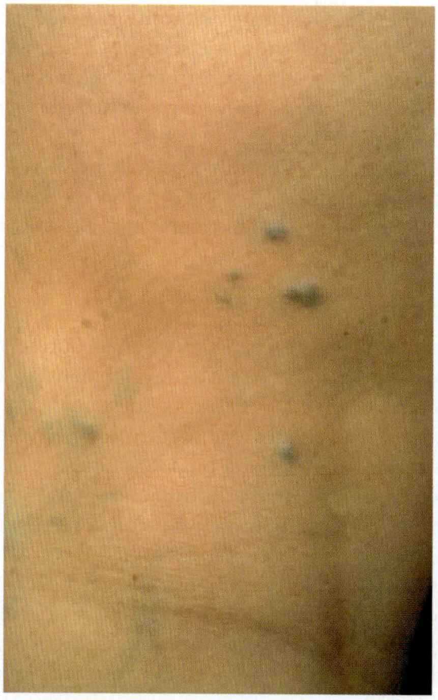

Figure 42.54 Glomus tumour (courtesy of St John's Institute for Dermatology, London, UK).

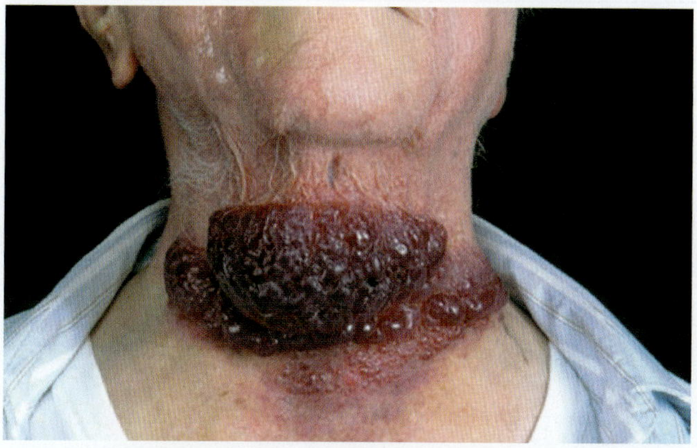

Figure 42.55 Angiosarcoma (courtesy of St John's Institute for Dermatology, London, UK).

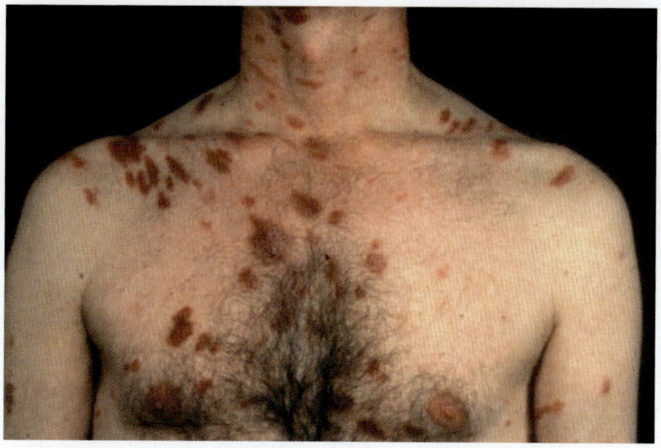

Figure 42.56 Kaposi's sarcoma (courtesy of St John's Institute for Dermatology, London, UK).

Caleb Hillier Parry, 1755–1822, physician, The General Hospital, Bath, UK.
Moritiz Heinrich Romberg, 1795–1873, a German neurologist who was Director of the University Hospital, Berlin, Germany.

childhood, when the resulting deformity is worse because it is magnified by differential growth elsewhere. The most common presentation is confined to lipodystrophy, but mixed atrophy of skin, fat, muscle, cartilage and bone combined result in the classic 'Coup de Sabre' deformity.

The condition is self-limiting, usually by 5–10 years after onset. Once the condition is stable, plastic surgical techniques can be employed alone or in combination to reconstruct an aesthetic contour.

Spina bifida

Failure of closure of the caudal neuropore during the fourth week *in utero* results in incomplete development of some or all of the structural elements posterior to the spinal cord. This can occur anywhere, but is most common in lumbar vertebrae and presents as gross variants: spina bifida occulta in which there is a bony defect without neural protrusion and spina bifida cystica, in which there is herniation of the meninges (meningocoele); spinal cord (myelocoele) or, most commonly, both (menigomyelocoele) and therefore, asymptomatic. Management ideally involves a multidisciplinary approach and is directed towards protecting the spinal cord, preventing cerebrospinal fluid contamination and secondary hydrocephalus and meningitis.

WOUNDS: ACQUIRED

Pressure sores

These begin with tissue necrosis at a pressure point (next to a bony prominence) and develop into a cone shape volume of necrotic loss (with the cone's tip superficial). As many as 10 per cent of acute hospital inpatients will suffer some degree of pressure sores. The majority affect the elderly and patients with spinal injury or decreased sensibility; 80 per cent of paraplegics will get a pressure sore and 8 per cent die as a result.

The pathogenesis of pressure sores revolves around unrelieved pressure: an increase in local tissue pressure above that of perfusion pressure produces ischaemic necrosis that is directly proportional to the duration and degree of pressure and inversely proportional to the area over which it is applied. Muscle and fat are more susceptible to pressure than skin.

In a patient who has no predisposing factors (who developed a sore while unable to move, but normally can move), management is aimed at debridement and repair of the defect on the assumption that recurrence will not occur once normal function and sensibility returns. In the paraplegic, recurrence is likely, so management should involve a multidisciplinary approach with surgery used sparingly once all other predisposing factors have been addressed. Primary treatment involves relieving pressure (special mattress; nursing care; relief of muscle spasm and contractures); optimising nutrition; correcting anaemia; preventing infection and dressings. Surgery involves thorough debridement to promote healing and plastic surgery to reconstruct the defect.

FURTHER READING

Balch CM, Buzaid AC, Soong SJ *et al.* Final version of the American Joint Committee on Cancer staging system for cutaneous melanoma. *J Clin Oncol* 2001; **19**: 3635–48.

Du Vivier A. *Atlas of clinical dermatology*, 3rd edn. Oxford: Churchill Livingstone, 2002.

Johnson TM, Bradford CR, Gruber SB *et al.* Staging workup, sentinel node biopsy, and follow-up tests for melanoma: update of current concepts. *Arch Dermatol* 2004; **140**: 107–13.

McKee PH, Calonje E, Granter S. *Pathology of the skin*, 3rd edn. Oxford: Mosby, 2005.

Weedon D. *Skin pathology*. Oxford: Churchill Livingstone, 2002.

Coup de Sabre is French for a 'sabre cut', a vertical cut across the shoulder from the front to the back.

PART 7 Head and neck

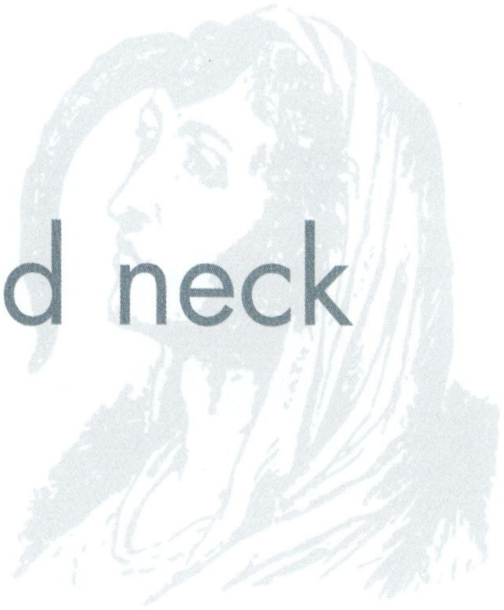

CHAPTER

43 Elective neurosurgery

LEARNING OBJECTIVES

- To review the pathophysiology of raised intracranial pressure (ICP) and to incorporate an understanding of hydrocephalus
- To recognise common presentations of intracranial infection, and know the principles of management
- To appreciate the spectrum of common brain tumours, their presentation, investigation and treatment
- To be familiar with common developmental and other pathologies encountered in paediatric neurosurgical practice
- To understand the indications and approaches available for the management of epilepsy, pain syndromes and movement disorders
- To be aware of other pathology which may be addressed by neurosurgeons, including occlusive vascular disease and peripheral neuropathies
- To note key practical and ethical issues affecting the practice of neurosurgery, including risks of craniotomy, complication rates, Creutzfeldt–Jakob disease (CJD) infection and diagnosis of brainstem death

PRINCIPLES OF PATHOPHYSIOLOGY

Raised intracranial pressure

The pathophysiology of raised intracranial pressure (ICP) is addressed in Chapter 25. In summary, when expanding masses exhaust the limited compensation within the rigid cranium, the Monro–Kellie doctrine predicts a rapid increase in pressure, culminating in compromised perfusion and fatal brainstem herniation (see Chapter 25, Figure 25.2).

In the elective context, masses such as tumours produce raised intracranial pressure directly through their own mass effect, and indirectly through surrounding oedema and obstruction of cerebrospinal fluid (CSF) drainage. Patients may complain of pressure headache, worse in the morning and provoked by bending, lying or straining. Nausea, vomiting and visual disturbance are also early features. Later the mass effect will result in drowsiness and lethargy, and ultimately coma.

Examination may reveal a cranial nerve palsy due to compression. Papilloedema (Figure 43.1) develops slowly, so is not a reliable sign of acute raised ICP.

Parinaud's syndrome results from dorsal midbrain compression, and its features include a loss of upgaze known as 'sun-setting' (Figure 43.2). In infants, the fontanelle is tense and bulging, with an increase in head circumference and bulging scalp veins.

Although the presentation may be subacute, raised ICP requires urgent evaluation and management: delay risks progression to cerebral herniation (see Chapter 25, Figure 25.2) resulting in neurological deficit and death, vision may also deteriorate rapidly and irreversibly (Summary box 43.1).

Summary box 43.1

Raised intracranial pressure

Acutely raised ICP is a neurosurgical emergency. The symptoms are:

- headache
- nausea and vomiting
- diplopia and blurred vision
- drowsiness then coma

Cerebral oedema

Cytotoxic oedema represents neuronal and glial swelling in response to insults such as ischaemia. Vasogenic oedema, by contrast, represents fluid accumulation in the extracellular spaces as a result of capillary leak and breakdown of the blood–brain barrier. It is commonly seen around tumours.

Hydrocephalus

Hydrocephalus refers to an increase in CSF volume and ventricular enlargement due to disturbance of production, flow or reabsorption of CSF.

The total CSF volume is normally about 150 mL. Production from the walls of the ventricles and the choroid plexus is about 20 mL/hour. CSF flows from the lateral ventricles through

Alexander Monro (Secundus), 1733–1817, Professor of Anatomy, Edinburgh, UK.
James Watson Kernohan 1896–1981, pathologist, The Mayo Clinic, Rochester, MN, USA.
Octave Crouzon, 1874–1938, neurologist, La Salpêtrière, Paris, France.
Eugene Apert, 1868–1940, physician, L'hôpital des Enfants-Malades, Paris, France.

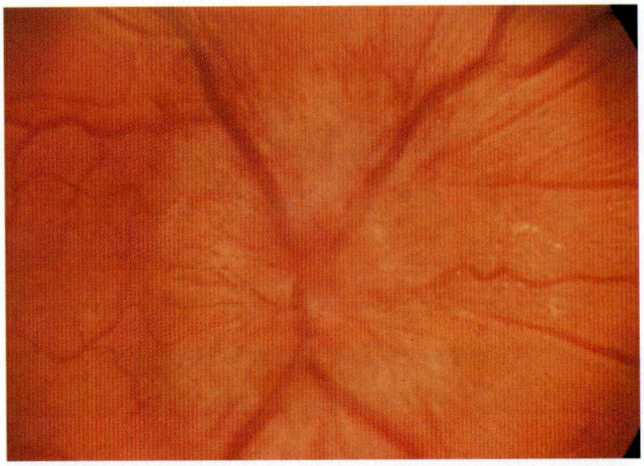

Figure 43.1 Papilloedema showing a swollen optic disc with blurred margins.

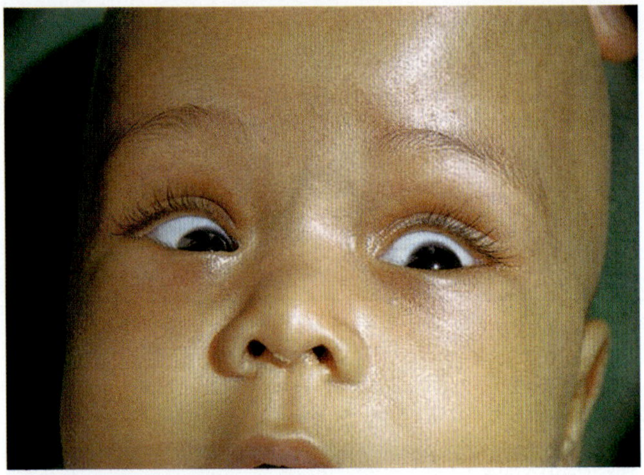

Figure 43.2 Child with 'sun-setting' eye sign due to hydrocephalus.

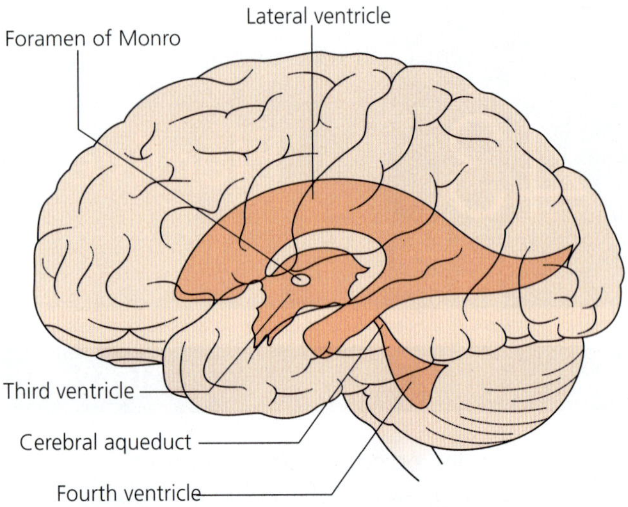

Figure 43.3 'CSF pathways'. Cerebrospinal fluid (CSF) is produced by the choroid plexus of the lateral ventricles, and flows through the foramina of Monro into the midline third ventricle, then through the cerebral aqueduct to the fourth ventricle, before exiting through the foramina of Magendie and Luschka to the subarachnoid space around the brain.

Table 43.1 Aetiology of hydrocephalus.

Obstructive hydrocephalus	Lesions within the ventricle
	Lesions in the ventricular wall
	Lesions distant from the ventricle but with a mass effect
Communicating hydrocephalus	Post-haemorrhagic
	CSF infection
	Raised CSF protein
Excessive CSF production (rare)	Choroid plexus papilloma/carcinoma

CSF, cerebrospinal fluid.

the foramina of Monro to the third ventricle, then down the cerebral aqueduct to the fourth ventricle, where it exits to the subarachnoid space via the midline foramen of Magendie and the lateral foramina of Luschka (Figure 43.3). CSF is reabsorbed into the arachnoid villi along the superior sagittal sinus.

Hydrocephalus may result from an excess of CSF production (in the rare condition of choroid plexus papilloma), from obstruction to circulation (an obstructive hydrocephalus) and from failure of reabsorption (a communicating hydrocephalus) (see Figures 43.4, 43.5 and 43.6). Hydrocephalus ex vacuo describes the ventriculomegaly associated with brain atrophy. Causes of hydrocephalus are listed in Table 43.1.

Disorders of CSF flow with poorly understood pathogenesis manifest in two syndromes, normal pressure hydrocephalus and idiopathic intracranial hypertension (IIH).

1 Normal pressure hydrocephalus. This is an important cause of dementia since it is readily reversible. It typically presents in older patients with the triad of gait disturbance, incontinence and cognitive decline. It may occur *de novo* or on a background of previous brain insults including subarachnoid haemorrhage (SAH), head injury, meningitis and tumour. Ventriculomegaly is evident on imaging, although this is also seen in the context of cortical atrophy due to other dementia pathologies. The CSF pressure at lumbar puncture (LP) is typically normal, but it is believed that intermittent elevations in pressure may be involved in the aetiology. Lumbar infusion testing involves insertion of a fine drain at lumbar puncture, followed by measurement of the CSF pressure changes associated with a fluid challenge administered through this. This allows evaluation of the likely benefit from definitive treatment by shunt insertion.
2 Idiopathic intracranial hypertension. This condition presents with features of raised ICP without an underlying tumour, explaining the old terms for the condition, pseudotumour cerebri or benign intracranial hypertension. This description is misleading, since IIH can progress rapidly to blindness. The patient, typically a young overweight female, describes a headache typical of raised pressure, and visual deterioration.

Francois Magendie, 1783–1855, Professor of Pathology and Physiology, at the College of France, and Physician, Hôtel Dieu, Paris, France.
Hubert von Luschka, 1820–1875, Professor of Anatomy, Tubingen, Germany.

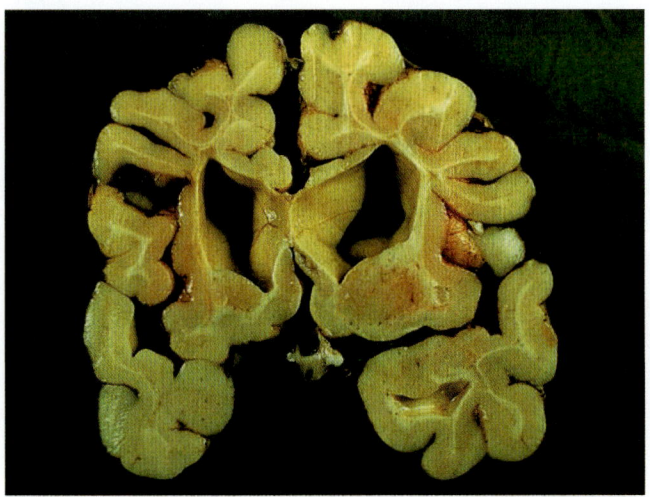

Figure 43.4 Pathological specimen of a hydrocephalic brain.

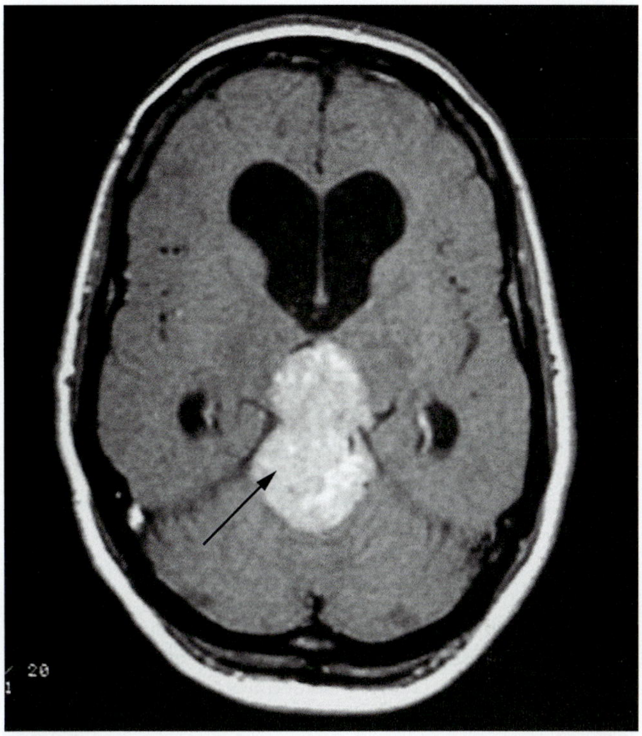

Figure 43.5 Pineal region tumour (arrow) causing obstructive hydrocephalus.

Examination may reveal papilloedema, and occasionally cranial nerve palsies. Imaging is unremarkable, but lumbar puncture demonstrates a raised opening pressure >25 mmHg. The diagnosis is one of exclusion, and the aetiology is not well understood. Impaired CSF resorption may reflect raised venous pressure, either as a result of sinus thrombosis, or secondary to raised intra-abdominal pressure in obese patients. Weight loss and cessation of certain medications including the oral contraceptive pill is often effective. This is combined with medical therapy.

Chronic compensated hydrocephalus is also commonly seen after craniotomy with breach of the ventricles, manifesting as failure to progress or with an overt CSF leak (Summary box 43.2).

Summary box 43.2

Hydrocephalus

- Hydrocephalus describes an increase in CSF volume and ventricular enlargement, often resulting in symptoms of raised ICP
- It may occur as a result of a physical blockage (obstructive hydrocephalus) or due to failure of normal reabsorption (communicating hydrocephalus)

Investigation of raised intracranial pressure

Where raised ICP is suspected, computed tomography (CT) is a first-line investigation to demonstrate hydrocephalus, underlying pathology and to evaluate the degree of mass effect and the patency of the basal cisterns, the spaces surrounding the brainstem. This is key to management since lumbar puncture in the setting of raised intracranial pressure can result in downward herniation of brain structures to replace the fluid drained (Chapter 25, Figure 25.2). Many pathologies, as well as the anatomy relating to potential treatments such as third

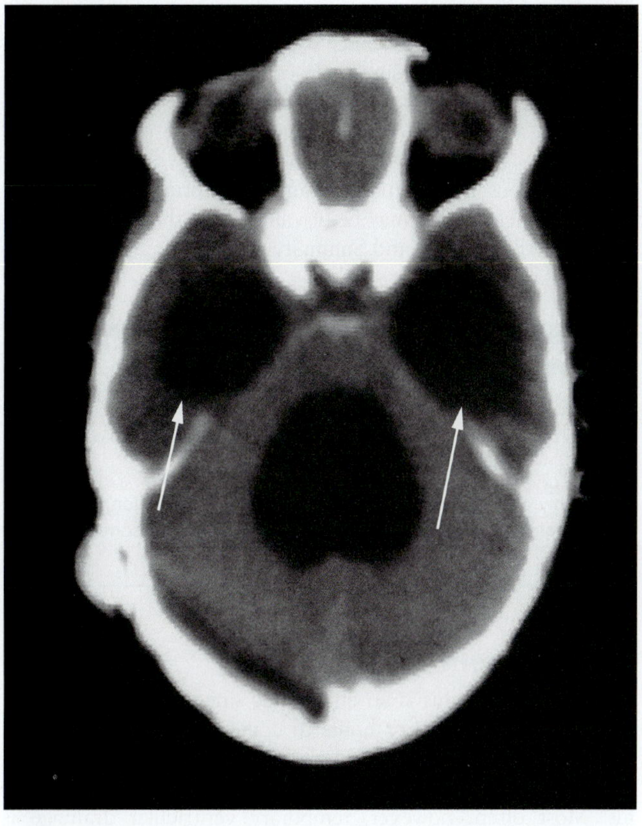

Figure 43.6 Axial computed tomography scan, showing a neonate with hydrocephalus and markedly dilated ventricles. The temporal horns (arrows), normally just visible, are particularly enlarged.

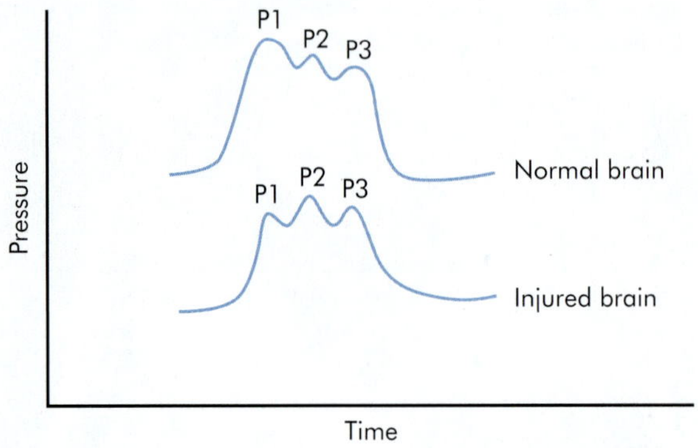

Figure 43.7 The intracranial pressure waveform: The P1 (percussion wave) corresponds to arterial pulsation. Pathologies including normal pressure hydrocephalus and traumatic injury are associated with a prominent P2 (tidal wave), representing reduced brain compliance.

ventriculostomy, may be better visualised on magnetic resonance imaging (MRI).

Lumbar puncture in obstructive hydrocephalus risks herniation of the brainstem and cerebellar tonsils due to the resulting differential pressure changes (sometimes termed 'coning'). For communicating hydrocephalus, lumbar puncture is of diagnostic value, deriving an opening pressure and assessment of the CSF contents. It is also therapeutic – drainage of typically between 10 and 30 mL of CSF, with the goal of halving the opening pressure, can relieve the hydrocephalus at least temporarily.

Lumbar infusion testing involves insertion of a lumbar drain into the thecal sac, then infusion of saline and pressure measurement to establish the resistance to CSF outflow. For example, in the case of normal pressure hydrocephalus, values greater than 14 mmHg/mL per minute can be taken to imply compromised resorption and the potential for good response to shunt insertion.

Continuous intracranial pressure monitoring using an ICP bolt as for head injury may be of value when the diagnosis is in doubt (see Figure 43.7 and Summary box 43.3).

Summary box 43.3

Investigation of raised ICP

- CT is the first line of investigation
- LP can confirm raised ICP and relieve it temporarily, but only after review of the CT to exclude a mass lesion or obstructive hydrocephalus, which might lead to 'coning' at LP

Management

Acute hydrocephalus is an emergency since the condition can progress over minutes or hours to coma and death. It may be relieved by addressing the underlying pathology, for instance by excision of a tumour responsible for an obstructive hydrocephalus. Most often, however, temporary ventricular drainage is required, either as an emergency in an obtunded or deteriorating patient, or as a precaution during definitive surgery considering the possibility for postoperative swelling.

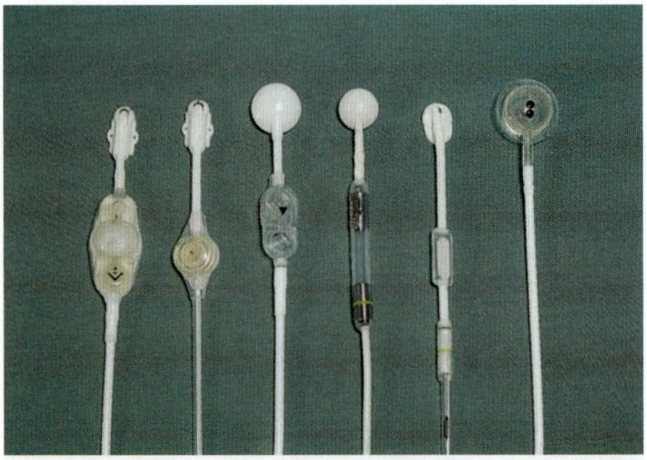

Figure 43.8 Various types of cerebrospinal fluid shunt.

External ventricular drain

External ventricular drains (EVDs) are an effective temporary measure to relieve hydrocephalus. Most commonly they are inserted freehand to the right of midline, anterior to the coronal suture, so that the catheter tip rests adjacent to the foramen of Monro in the lateral ventricle. The catheter is then connected to a drain set such that CSF drains when the ventricular pressure exceeds a threshold typically set at 10–20 mmHg. Intrathecal antibiotics may also be delivered through the EVD.

Ventriculoperitoneal shunts

Ventriculoperitoneal (VP) shunting comprises insertion of a ventricular catheter, which may be antibiotic impregnated, into the frontal or occipital horn of the lateral ventricle, while a distal catheter is tunnelled subcutaneously to the abdomen. Ventriculoatrial and ventriculopleural shunting is also possible. A shunt valve, with an opening pressure which may be high, medium or low, is inserted at the junction of these catheters (see Figure 43.8). Selection of the shunt valve is a balance and must be tailored to each patient: high pressure valves may fail to allow adequate CSF drainage, whereas low pressure valves can overdrain (see below). Flow regulated valves incorporate mechanisms to maintain relatively constant rates of drainage despite a range of pressures across the valve. Other valves feature different opening pressures depending on position, preventing overdrainage on standing for instance. Programmable valves can be adjusted magnetically using a device applied externally over the valve. Valves also typically incorporate a CSF reservoir which allows for sampling.

Shunt complications

Overdrainage can result in low-pressure headaches, which are typically worse on standing. Collapse of the ventricles can cause accumulation of fluid in the subdural space, a subdural hygroma, or bleeding producing a subdural haematoma. The slit ventricle syndrome describes the situation in children treated with shunts, whose ventricles and subarachnoid spaces are underdeveloped, resulting in poor brain compliance. In these patients normal fluctuations in ICP are exaggerated so that coughing and straining may cause symptoms of raised ICP. Any shunt blockage may not be evident on scan as the ventricles fail to enlarge.

Shunts are vulnerable to infection and to blockage, so that 15–20 per cent require replacement within three years. Seventy-five per cent of infection presents within one month, a result of introduction at the time of insertion. Risk factors include very young patients, open myelomeningocoele, long operation time and staff movement in and out of theatre. The shunt is removed, and external CSF drainage or serial LP instituted to cover a course of antibiotic therapy. Once CSF sampling confirms resolution of the infection and a normal protein concentration, a shunt can be inserted at a new site.

The majority of blockages are attributable to cellular and proteinaceous debris especially due to infection, but choroid plexus adhesion or blood clot may also be responsible.

Endoscopic third ventriculostomy

This procedure is especially useful in obstructive hydrocephalus due to aqueduct stenosis. A neuroendoscope is inserted into the frontal horn of the lateral ventricle and then into the third ventricle via the foramen of Monro. The floor of the ventricle is then opened between the mamillary bodies and the pituitary recess. Free drainage between the third ventricle and the adjacent subarachnoid cisterns is then possible, without the infection risk posed by implanted tubing. Reblockage of this route is common, however, and many patients will subsequently require a shunt. Rare but serious complications include damage to the basilar artery, or damage to the fornix resulting in permanent memory impairment (Summary box 43.4).

Summary box 43.4

Treating hydrocephalus

- Temporary CSF diversion can be achieved with an EVD
- In the long term a shunt, usually connecting the lateral ventricles with the peritoneal cavity in the abdomen (VP shunt), is the mainstay of management
- Shunt blockage and infection are common complications

INTRACRANIAL INFECTION

Meningitis and ventriculitis

Meningitis describes inflammation of the meninges of the brain and spinal cord, most commonly and most seriously due to bacterial infection.

Community-acquired bacterial meningitis typically presents with fever, meningism (headache, neck stiffness and photophobia) and deterioration in conscious level. The natural history involves a rapid progression to subpial encephalopathy, venous thrombosis, cerebral oedema and death. Therefore empirical intravenous antibiotic therapy should be commenced as soon as the diagnosis is suspected. Urgent lumbar puncture is required to confirm the diagnosis and ultimately to guide treatment. Since the differential diagnosis of this presentation includes abscess, empyema and subarachnoid haemorrhage, initial CT imaging, where available immediately, is desirable to confirm that lumbar puncture is necessary and safe. A 2007 Cochrane review demonstrated improved mortality and neurological outcome associated with administration of steroids (dexamethasone 0.15 mg/kg up to 10 mg four times daily for 4 days).

The common organisms responsible for spontaneous bacterial meningitis are *Streptococcus pneumonia*, *Haemophilus influenzae* and *Neisseria meningitides*, the latter occurring in sporadic outbreaks. Neonates are susceptible to group B streptococcus, *Escherichia coli* and Listeria.

Meningitis in the context of surgery typically follows a more insidious course, but nonetheless remains a feared complication requiring prompt intervention. Typical organisms are *Staphylococcus aureus*, Enterobacteriaceae, Pseudomonas and Pneumococci.

Meningitis after head injury is common, affecting 25 per cent of patients with base of skull fracture and CSF leak. Repair of the CSF leak may be required, and empirical antibiotics should have activity against commensal nasal organisms including Gram-positive cocci and Gram-negative bacilli in the presence of symptoms/signs of clinical meningitis.

Ventriculitis refers to infection in the ventricles, commonly as a complication of meningitis or due to contamination from a shunt or external drain. Where a drain is present, treatment may include administration of intrathecal antibiotics through it (Summary box 43.5).

Summary box 43.5

Meningitis

- A feared complication of neurosurgery and of head injury
- Clinical diagnosis is supported by CT to exclude other pathology
- CSF samples are taken for glucose and protein assay, and for microscopy and culture
- Treatment, pending identification of an organism, is with broad-spectrum antibiotics

Brain abscess and empyema

Abscesses arise when the brain is exposed directly, for example as a result of fracture or infection of an air sinus, or at surgery. They also result from haematogenous spread, typically in association with respiratory and dental infections, or endocarditis. In 25 per cent of cases, no underlying primary infection is found. The organisms involved are normally bacteria, but immunocompromised hosts in particular are vulnerable to a broad range of pathogens:

- sinus/mastoid infection: aerobic and anaerobic Streptococci; Bacteroides; Enterobacteria; Staphylococci; Pseudomonas;
- haematogenous spread: Bacteroides; Streptococci;
- penetrating trauma: *Staphylococcus aureus*; Clostridium; Bacillus; Enterobacteria;
- food contamination: toxoplasma, pork tapeworm (producing neurocysticercosis);
- immunocompromise e.g. HIV/AIDS: protozoal (e.g toxoplasma), fungal (e.g Cryptococcus), viral (e.g. JC virus producing multifocal leukoencephalopathy) and mycobacterial abscesses are encountered.

Early cerebritis (day 3–5) is characterised by neutrophil infiltration (Figure 43.9). This progresses to a late cerebritis with necrosis, oedema and macrophage recruitment (day 5–14) (Figure 43.10). After this the abscess is walled off by a developing collagenous capsule which matures over weeks and months.

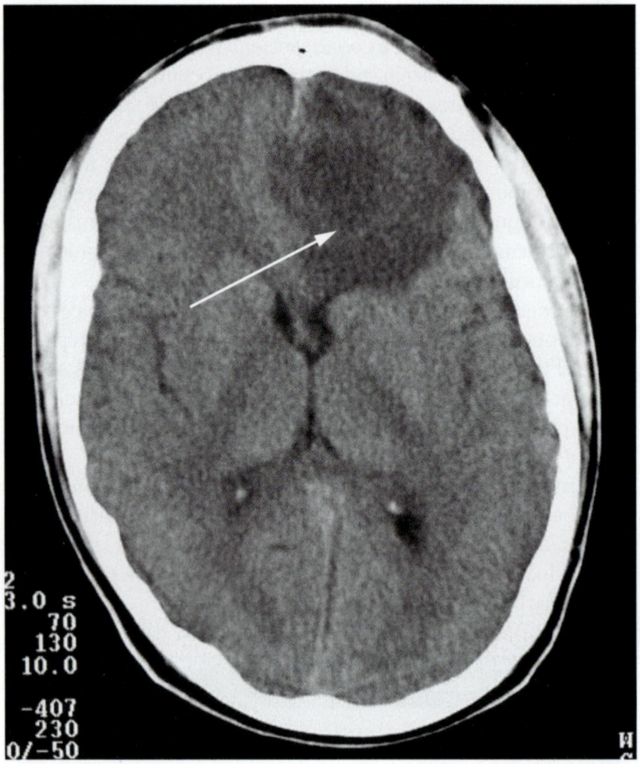

Figure 43.9 Axial computed tomography scan with contrast of a patient with frontal sinusitis and epilepsy, showing a hypodense area of cerebritis in the left frontal region.

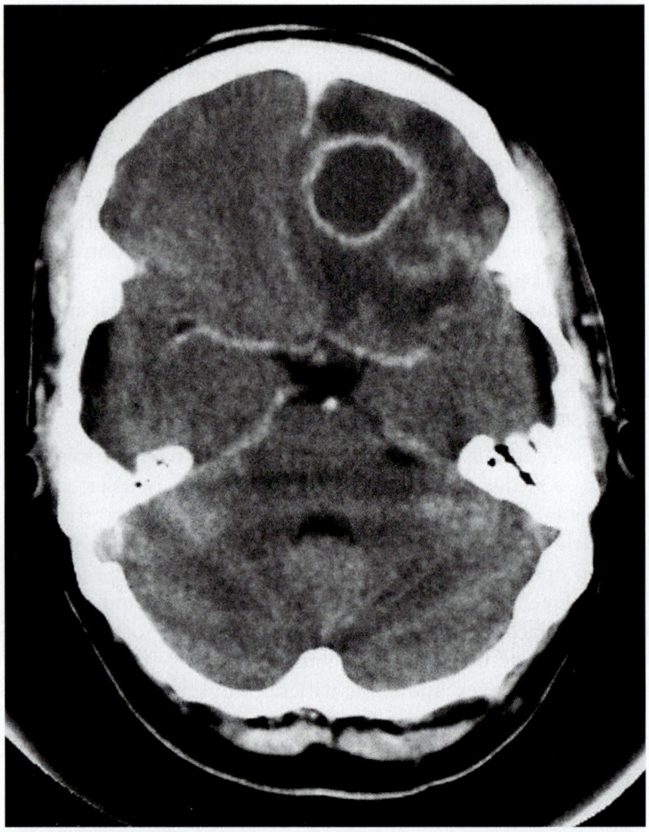

Figure 43.10 Axial computed tomography scan with contrast of the same patient as in Figure 43.9 but 2 weeks later. A ring-enhancing lesion has developed, typical of a pyogenic abscess.

Diagnosis

Patients present with the triad of features associated with mass lesions; these are focal deficits, seizures and raised ICP. A typical history might include fever and malaise, progressing over hours or days to drowsiness and confusion, then focal weakness or seizure. Low-grade pyrexia and equivocal blood markers of inflammation are typical; blood cultures should be obtained at an early stage. CT scan with contrast is the initial imaging modality of choice, and this will demonstrate a well-defined ring-enhancing mass (i.e. the edge enhances on the post-contrast images), typically with a thin smooth wall. The distinction between abscess and tumour can be difficult and has important management implications, since abscesses generally require urgent drainage. Diffusion-weighted MRI is a valuable tool in this context (see Figure 43.11).

Management

The mainstay of management of bacterial abscesses is early surgical drainage, involving needle aspiration through a burrhole with or without image-guidance, or by craniotomy. Intravenous antibiotic therapy is then commenced, using broad-spectrum agents initially then tailoring to the sensitivity of organisms cultured. Treatment should last at least 6 weeks, but a switch to oral therapy may be appropriate after an interval and in consultation with microbiology. Mortality with prompt treatment is about 4 per cent, but if the abscess is allowed to rupture into a ventricle mortality it is over 80 per cent. Up to 50 per cent of patients with brain abscess will develop seizures at some stage, so that prophylactic anticonvulsants should be considered (Summary box 43.6).

Summary box 43.6

Brain abscesses

- Presenting features are those of infection and of intracranial mass lesion
- Imaging reveals a 'ring-enhancing lesion', with tumour usually the main differential
- Early diagnosis, usually followed by drainage, is key for good outcome

Subdural empyema

Subdural empyema refers to an infective collection in the subdural space and may develop as a result of sinusitis, mastoiditis or meningitis, and can complicate trauma or surgery. Figure 43.12 shows a subdural empyema associated with osteomyelitis of the frontal bone and associated scalp swelling, a 'Pott's puffy tumour'. In empyema, pus will generally collect in the parafalcine region and over the convexity, triggering inflammation and thrombosis in the cortical veins which helps to explain the high mortality of 8–12 per cent. Presentation mimics that of meningitis and cerebral abscess; typical CT appearances are of hypodense or isodense subdural collection, with contrast enhancement at the margins, and a degree swelling and midline shift. The empyema may be difficult to visualise, especially on non-contrast CT. Given the risk of herniation, LP should not be performed.

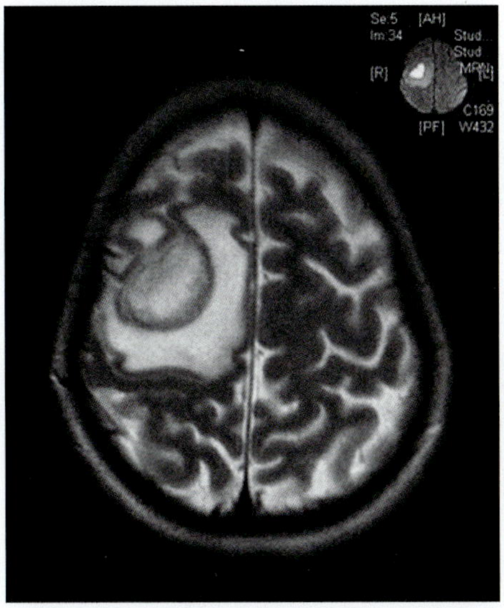

Figure 43.11 The right frontal lesion evident on T2 magnetic resonance imaging (MRI) (main image) exhibits high signal on DWI MRI sequences (top right inset) indicative of restricted diffusion suggestive brain abscess.

Craniotomy or craniectomy allows drainage of the collection and relieves raised ICP and is the treatment of choice. Burrhole drainage, and occasionally intravenous antibiotics without surgical intervention, may also be considered (Summary box 43.7).

Summary box 43.7

Subdural empyema

- Presenting features are similar to those of meningitis or cerebral abscess
- Typically a crescentic collection with a contrast-enhancing rim is evident on CT
- Drainage is the mainstay of treatment

Tuberculosis

Tuberculosis (TB) infection of the central nervous system (CNS) is believed to represent haematogenous spread from primary pulmonary foci. A high index of suspicion is required, especially when population or individual risk factors are present. TB can result in a diverse but overlapping spectrum of pathology, including in the head:

- Tuberculous meningitis – this commonly affects young children; CT demonstrates intense meningeal enhancement, and hydrocephalus is a common sequel.
- Tuberculoma – discrete tumour-like granulomas at the base of the cerebral hemispheres, presenting with mass effect.

Percival Pott, 1714–1788, surgeon, St Bartholomew's Hospital, London, UK, described the 'Puffy Tumour' in 1760. In 1756 he sustained a broken leg after a fall from his horse. As he lay on the ground, he sent a servant to buy a door which acted as a stretcher. While his surgeons were contemplating amputating his leg, he persuaded them to splint the leg instead as a result of which he recovered completely. Although some think that Pott's fracture of the ankle was described after this injury of his, it is not so. He sustained a compound fracture of the femur. Pott was the first to link an environmental factor to the aetiology of cancer when he demonstrated that chimney sweeps developed squamous cell scrotal cancer.

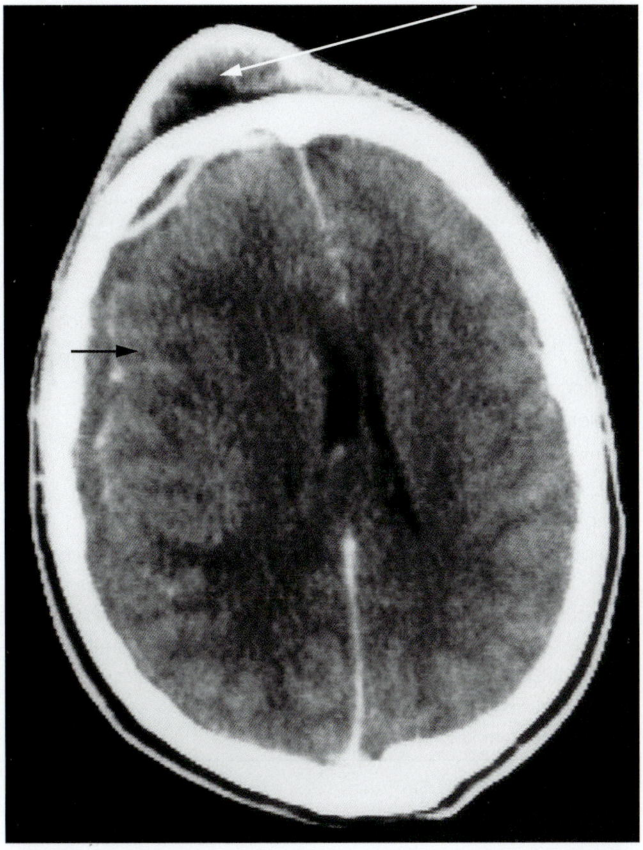

Figure 43.12 Axial computed tomography scan with contrast showing a right hemisphere subdural empyema (short arrow) and a right frontal Pott's puffy tumour (long arrow) (osteomyelitis of the frontal bone).

- Tuberculous abscess – seen predominantly in immunocompromised hosts, this represents progression of a tuberculoma with prominent central caseating necrosis.
- Miliary tuberculosis – describes a diffuse distribution of multiple small tuberculomas through brain substance.

Where the meninges are involved, lymphocytes can be expected to predominate in the CSF, rather than the polymorphs seen with other bacterial meningitides. The increase in protein content and reduction in glucose concentration are also less marked. Ziehl–Neesen staining for myobacteria is frequently negative, and polymerase chain reaction (PCR) testing offers relatively rapid diagnosis compared to culture for acid-fast bacilli which may take weeks. A 20–30 mL CSF sample allows spinning to increase the culture yield.

Management is with anti-tuberculous therapy; hydrocephalus may require shunt insertion.

BRAIN TUMOURS

The term 'brain tumour' applies to a wide array of pathologies, detailed in the extensive World Health Organization (WHO) classification. Many are malignant, but even histologically benign tumours may carry a grave prognosis where they encroach on key structures which also limit surgical access. The most common brain tumour is a metastasis. Primary brain tumours represent 1.5 per cent of all cancers, with an incidence

Table 43.2 World Health Organization classification of brain tumours.

Neuroepithelial tumours	Glioma	Astrocytomas Oligodendrogliomas Ependymoma Choroid plexus tumour
	Pineal tumours	
	Neuronal tumours	Ganglioglioma Gangliocytoma Neuroblastoma
	Medulloblastoma	
Nerve sheath tumours	Vestibular schwannoma	
Meningeal tumours	Meningioma	
Pituitary tumours		
Germ cell tumours	Germinoma	
	Teratoma	
Lymphomas		
Tumour-like malformations	Craniopharyngioma Epidermoid tumours Dermoid tumour Colloid cyst	
Metastatic tumours		
Contiguous extension from regional tumours, e.g. glomus tumour		

of 19 per 100 000 person years. Nevertheless, many, especially glial tumours, present commonly in younger age groups and are incurable, so that they account for disproportionate morbidity and mortality.

Classification

The WHO classifies primary brain tumours on the basis of cell of origin and histological grade (Table 43.2).

The common primary brain tumours are gliomas, meningiomas (15–20 per cent of total), pituitary adenomas (10–15 per cent of total) and vestibular schwannomas.

Grade 1 is applied to 'benign' lesions, while grade 4 implies high grade malignancy.

Aetiology

The common primary brain tumours mentioned above occur sporadically. There is no proven risk due to environmental factors, except for radiation exposure, but genetic abnormalities may also predispose (see Table 43.3).

Table 43.3 Chromosomal abnormalities associated with brain tumours.

Syndrome	Gene defect	Tumour
Neurofibromatosis type 1	Neurofibromin (Chr 17)	Astrocytomas; neurofibromas
Neurofibromatosis type 2	Schwannomin (Chr 22)	Acoustic neuromas (bilateral); meningiomas
Cowden's disease	PTEN (Chr 10)	Astrocytomas
Hereditary non-polyposis colorectal cancer	Multiple	Astrocytomas
Li–Fraumeni syndrome	p53 (Chr 17)	Astrocytomas

Presentation

Most tumours present with one or more features belonging to three cardinal categories: these are seizure, raised ICP and focal neurological deficit. Pituitary adenomas may also present with endocrine disturbance.

Seizures

Seizures are a common presenting feature, especially of low-grade gliomas arising in the cortical hemispheres. Simple partial seizures, involving focal twitching or similar with preserved consciousness, are the rule, but temporal location will commonly produce complex partial seizures, and any seizure may progress to a secondary generalised tonic-clonic fit.

Patients who have had a seizure should be started on an anti-epileptic drug, usually phenytoin or carbamazepine. Therapeutic levels of phenytoin can be achieved rapidly with i.v. loading, but its enzyme-inducing effect can complicate the administration of chemotherapy. Routine prophylaxis in patients with tumours who have no history of seizures is not recommended, although a short course at the time of craniotomy for tumour excision may be warranted.

Raised intracranial pressure

Headache is a presenting feature in only about 50 per cent of patients. It is classically worse in the morning and on straining,

Table 43.4 Patterns of deficit generally associated with certain tumours.

Tumour location	Expected deficit
Pituitary (e.g. pituitary adenoma)	Bitemporal hemianopia; gaze palsies
Cerebellopontine angle (e.g. vestibular schwannoma)	Hearing loss; balance disturbance; tinnitus
Anterior skull base (e.g. olfactory groove meningioma)	Anosmia; ipsilateral optic atrophy; contralateral papilloedema (Foster-Kennedy syndrome)
Occipital (e.g. glioma, metastasis)	Homonymous hemianopia with central sparing
Parietal (dominant hemisphere)	Acalculia; agraphia; left-right disorientation; finger agnosia (Gerstmann syndrome)
Parietal (e.g. glioma)	Sensory inattention; dressing apraxia; astereognosis
Temporal (e.g. glioma)	Memory disturbance; contralateral superior quadrantanopia; dysphasia (dominant hemisphere)
Frontal (e.g. glioma)	Personality change; gait disturbance; urinary incontinence
Brainstem (e.g. brainstem glioma)	Multiple cranial nerve deficits; long tract signs; nystagmus
Posterior fossa (e.g. medulloblastoma)	Ataxia; hydrocephalus

and is accompanied by nausea and vomiting. Pressure effect develops due to tumour mass effect and surrounding oedema, especially in fast-growing metastases and high-grade gliomas (see above under Raised intracranial pressure). Where the differential diagnosis of abscess can be confidently excluded (see above under Brain abscess and empyema), mass effect is controlled initially using high-dose glucocorticoids (e.g. dexamethasone) to reduce swelling. Acute deterioration in this group may represent a developing obstructive hydrocephalus due to compression of CSF drainage pathways (see above under Hydrocephalus), a neurosurgical emergency.

Focal neurological deficit

A focal deficit progressive over time, as opposed to the sudden onset of a vascular accident, is suspicious of tumour. Lesions generally produce characteristic deficits due to local pressure effect, and reflecting location (See Table 43.4 and Summary box 43.8).

Summary box 43.8

Brain tumours

Most brain tumours will present with one or more feature related to the following triad:

- raised ICP
- seizures
- focal deficit

Common brain tumours

Cerebral metastases

Cerebral metastases (Figure 43.13) are the most common intracranial tumours, and affect about one-quarter of cancer sufferers. The tumours of origin and their contribution to the burden of cerebral metastases is detailed in Table 43.5. In general, patients with multiple cerebral metastases are not suitable for surgery. Occasionally, diagnostic biopsy may be warranted where the primary is unknown. In patients with good functional status and well-controlled systemic disease, craniotomy for resection of a single metastasis, and exceptionally up to three metastases, may be considered.

Glioma

These are tumours of glial cell origin, with subtypes including astrocytomas, oligodendrogliomas, ependymomas and mixed tumours. The diagnosis is histological, but imaging often predicts both a glial origin and the grade of tumour (Figure 43.14): MRI with and without contrast is the preferred modality. If the diagnosis is in doubt, a whole-body CT scan and liver function tests may be required to help exclude an extracranial primary. Initial management should generally include steroids to alleviate any mass effect, and anti-epileptics where seizures are a presenting feature, or are likely in view of temporal location. Definitive treatment depends on the likely tumour grade in view of presentation and imaging findings. Gliomas, except for the grade I pilocytic astrocytoma which typically occurs in children, are notable for their diffuse infiltration into surrounding brain, so that recurrence after even macroscopically complete resection is the rule.

Low grade glioma (WHO Grade II) has a peak incidence in the fourth decade of life. Historically a 'watch-and-wait' strategy, with or without initial biopsy to confirm the diagnosis, has been applied. This reflects the natural history of progression to high grade tumour over a variable period, usually several years. The alternative, now more generally favoured, approach is to pursue initial complete macroscopic resection where feasible. However, this is based on limited evidence that progression is delayed and survival prolonged by this approach. Where tumours encroach on eloquent cortex, especially the speech areas of the dominant hemisphere, awake craniotomy allows mapping of function with surface electrodes at operation, to limit resection and minimise postoperative deficit.

High grade gliomas include anaplastic astrocytomas (WHO grade III) and glioblastomas (WHO grade IV), the most common glial tumour (Figure 43.15).

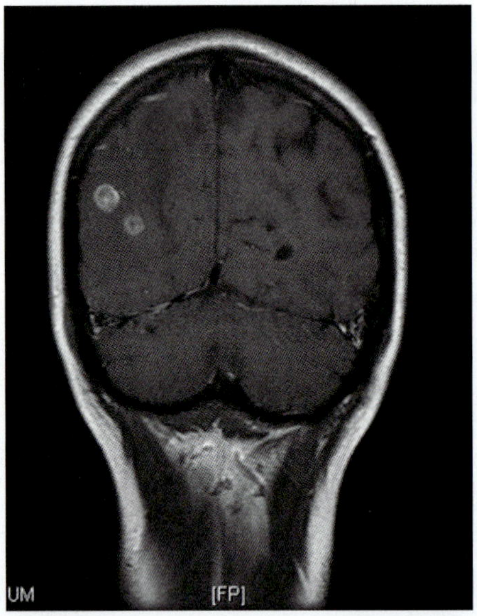

Figure 43.13 T1 magnetic resonance imaging (MRI) with contrast – two right occipital lung metastases are demonstrated. They are well demarcated and enhance with gadolinium contrast.

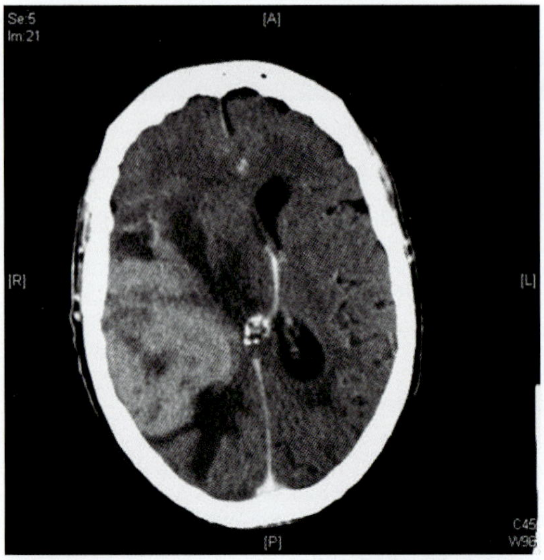

Figure 43.14 Computed tomography (CT) with contrast demonstrates a heterogenous right frontoparietal lesion with mass effect and midline shift, almost certainly a glioblastoma multiforme. A magnetic resonance image with and without contrast will aid evalutation.

Table 43.5 Tissue of origin for brain metastases (approximate).

Origin	Percentage
Lung	40
Breast	15
Melanoma	10
Renal/GU	10
Other Unknown	25

They present *de novo* with peak incidence in the fifth and sixth decades of life respectively, or may represent transformation of previously diagnosed, or clinically silent, low grade gliomas. Active treatment consists of maximal resection, high-dose-focused radiation therapy, and chemotherapy administered locally as carmustine wafers at the time of resection, or systemically with oral temozolomide. Median survival for glioblastoma remains just over 12 months.

Solitary metastasis represents a differential diagnosis for many gliomas, so that a chest x-ray is an important component of the work-up, and if the diagnosis is in significant doubt a whole-body CT and liver function tests to exclude an extracranial primary are required.

Meningioma

Meningiomas are usually benign lesions, although anaplastic variants do occur. They arise from the meninges, and typically present due to mass effect from the tumour, compounded by vasogenic oedema in the adjacent brain and obstructive hydrocephalus where CSF drainage is impaired. Imaging will demonstrate a contrast-enhancing mass distinct from the brain with a dural base (Figure 43.16).

These are generally slow-growing lesions: smaller lesions, perhaps detected incidentally in an elderly patient, may well warrant a 'watch-and-wait' approach. If the lesion is large or positioned so as to impinge on key structures, the patient may require steroids and early surgery. The degree of resection predicts recurrence, with rates of 10 per cent at ten years for total excision with a clear dural margin and 30 per cent at ten years for subtotal excision. Lesions which are difficult to approach surgically may be managed with radiotherapy or stereotactic radiosurgery (Summary box 43.9).

Summary box 43.9

Common brain tumours

- Metastases and gliomas are common tumours arising within brain substance, appearing as 'ring-enhancing' lesions on contrast CT. Surgery is usually life-extending rather than curative
- Meningiomas arise from the meninges around the brain and typically enhance uniformly on contrast CT. Most are benign and amenable to curative resection
- MRI brain is optimal for evaluation of these lesions. Diffusion-weighted sequences help to exclude abscess when glioma or metastasis is suspected
- Where metastasis is suspected, CT of the body may demonstrate the primary lesion and allow staging
- Steroids are administered to control swelling and mass effect in the short term

Pituitary tumours

Most tumours in this region are benign pituitary adenomas, although the differential includes malignant variants, craniopharyngioma, meningioma, aneurysm and Rathke's cleft cyst (Figure 43.17).

Microadenomas are less than 10 mm in size and usually present incidentally or with endocrine effects. Macroadenomas

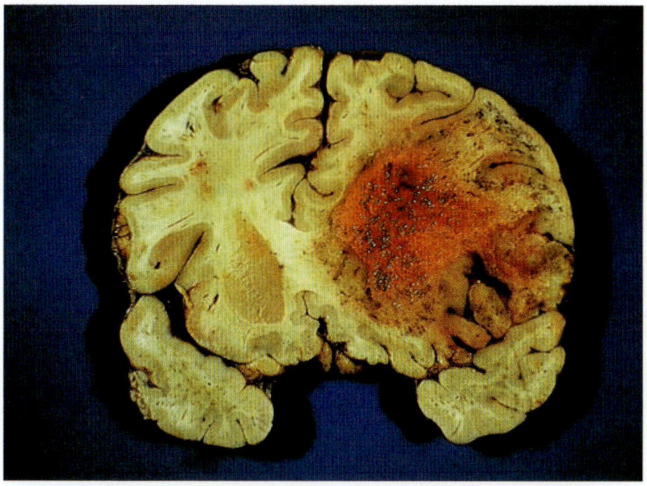

Figure 43.15 Pathological specimen of a glioblastoma multiforme.

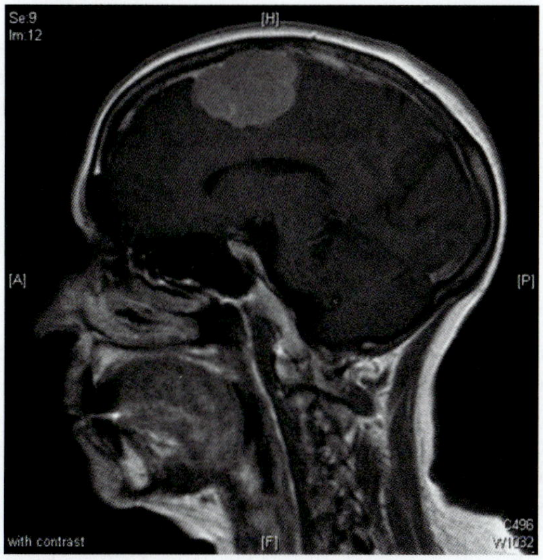

Figure 43.16 On T1 magnetic resonance imaging an extra-axial, durally based lesion is seen to arise in the region of the falx. This is a meningioma.

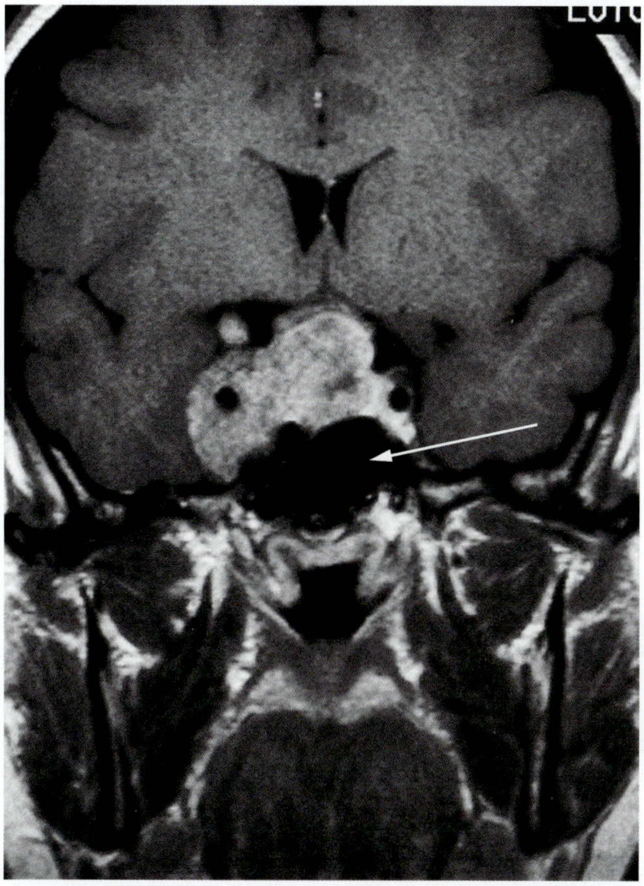

Figure 43.17 Pituitary non-functioning macroadenoma with suprasellar extension and right cavernous sinus invasion.

are larger than 10 mm, and often present with visual field deficits (Figure 43.17). Thirty per cent of adenomas are prolactinomas, 20 per cent are non-functioning, 15 per cent secrete growth hormone and 10 per cent secrete adrenocorticotropic hormone (ACTH).

Features of note in the initial assessment include any history of galactorrhoea (suggestive of prolactinoma), and Cushingoid or acromegalic features pointing to ACTH- or growth hormone-secreting tumours, respectively. Baseline assessment of pituitary function should include serum prolactin, follicle-stimulating hormone and luteinising hormone together with testosterone in males or oestradiol in females, thyroid function tests, and fasting serum growth hormone and cortisol. Preoperative prolactin levels are crucial since prolactinomas may be managed without the need for surgery. The cortisol level is also important, since deficiency must be corrected especially in the perioperative period. Diagnosis of ACTH-secreting tumours can be difficult, and may require the use of specialised tests, such as petrosal sinus sampling and the dexamethasone suppression test.

Effective treatment requires close cooperation between the neurosurgical team and an endocrinologist.

Prolactinomas are managed initially with dopamine agonists, such as bromocryptine and cabergoline. Growth hormone-secreting tumours may also respond to dopamine agonists, or to somatostatin analogues, such as octreotide.

Surgical resection is usually performed by a trans-sphenoidal approach, using a microscope or endoscope. Sometimes large tumours also require a craniotomy. After operation, patients are at risk of CSF leak (3 per cent) and pituitary insufficiency. Diabetes insipidus resulting from manipulation of the pituitary stalk is common in the immediate postoperative period and usually resolves spontaneously. Where it is suspected, the patient will require hourly measurement of urine output, and blood and urine samples for calculation of sodium concentration and osmolality. If confirmed, the condition can be managed with DDAVP (desmopressin) in consultation with endocrinology.

Urgent intervention is generally reserved for patients with deteriorating vision.

Pituitary apoplexy is the syndrome associated with haemorrhagic infarction of a pituitary tumour. It presents with sudden headache, visual loss and ophthalmoplegia with or without impaired conscious level. Intravenous steroids and urgent surgical decompression are required.

Harvey Williams Cushing, 1869–1939, Professor of Surgery, Harvard University Medical School, Boston, MA, USA.

Vestibular schwannoma (acoustic neuroma)

These are nerve sheath tumours arising in the cerebellopontine angle, which present with hearing loss, tinnitus and balance problems. Facial numbness and weakness are less common, while large tumours may present with features of brainstem compression or hydrocephalus. The differential diagnosis includes meningioma, metastasis and epidermoid cyst (Figure 43.18).

Small intracanalicular tumours (within the internal auditory canal) may be managed with surveillance. For intermediate size tumours, radiosurgery is an alternative to operation. Large lesions (>4 cm), especially with brainstem compression, will require excision and consideration of ventriculoperitoneal shunt to relieve hydrocephalus. Translabyrinthine, retrosigmoid and middle fossa approaches are possible, the latter options offering potential preservation of hearing in smaller tumours with some intact function at presentation. In removing larger tumours, it is often impossible to preserve hearing, or indeed facial nerve function.

Brain tumours in children

Brain tumours are the most common solid tumours in children.

Neonates develop predominantly neuroectodermal tumours in supratentorial locations, including subtypes detailed below (see also Summary box 43.10):

- teratoma;
- primitive neuroectodermal tumour (PNET);
- high grade astrocytoma;
- choroid plexus papilloma/carcinoma.

Older children tend to suffer infratentorial tumours, especially:

- medulloblastoma (an infratentorial PNET);
- ependymoma;
- pilocytic astrocytoma.

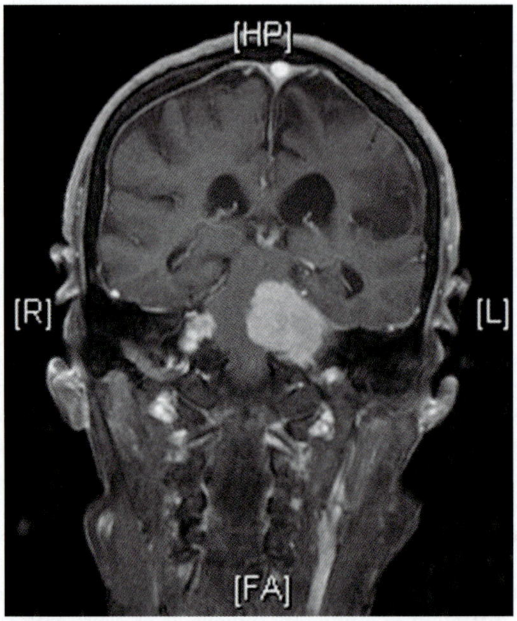

Figure 43.18 The appearances of a meningioma in the left cerebellopontine angle (CPA), with a coexisting vestibular schwannoma in the right CPA.

Summary box 43.10

Other key tumour types

- Pituitary tumours typically present with endocrinological disturbance (microadenomas) or visual deficits due to compression (macroadenomas). Some of these tumours are managed surgically, in close cooperation with endocrinologists
- Vestibular schwannomas (acoustic neuromas) are benign nerve sheath tumours, usually presenting with hearing loss, tinnitus and balance problems. Their proximity to the brainstem allows them to cause significant morbidity and mortality, and can present a major surgical challenge
- A large variety of mostly neuroectodermal brain tumours represent the most common solid organ tumours in children

PAEDIATRIC NEUROSURGERY

Paediatric neurosurgery presents a wide range of isolated and syndrome-associated developmental abnormalities including cysts, neural tube defects and posterior fossa malformations. In general, these present with combinations of developmental delay, seizures, and macrocephaly or hydrocephalus. Early fusion of one or more cranial sutures, craniosynostosis, is also a common neonatal presentation.

Cysts

A number of benign fluid-filled intracranial lesions typically present incidentally, or with mass effect or hydrocephalus. Treatment of symptomatic or enlarging lesions is usually surgical, involving excision, endoscopic fenestration into a cistern or ventricle, or shunting for hydrocephalus.

Cyst types

- Arachnoid cyst – typically middle fossa, CSF enclosed in an envelope of arachnoid mater.
- Colloid cyst – occurs in the roof of the third ventricle, believed to represent embryonic endoderm remnants.
- Dermoid and epidermoid cysts – epithelial lined structures arising from displaced ectodermal remnants, typically in the posterior fossa (midline) and cerebellopontine angle, respectively.
- Porencephalic cysts – brain cavities lined with gliotic white matter, containing CSF in communication with the ventricles or subarachnoid space.

Neural tube defects

Failure of closure of the neural tube is associated with folate deficiency, family history and some anticonvulsants. Prenatal screening, using serum alphaprotein levels and ultrasound, and diagnostic testing, using amniocentesis, are possible. The spectrum of conditions associated with failed closure of the posterior neuropore includes:

- Spina bifida occulta: a congenital absence of a spinous process, without exposure of meninges or neural tissue, but presenting a characteristic shallow hair-covered hollow at the base of the spine. This is common and rarely clinically significant. Sometimes it may be associated with tethered cord syndrome, which involves thickening of the filum terminale, resulting in traction on the cord. Presentation is with progressive deficits, spasticity, bladder dysfunction or scoliosis, and treatment involves surgical exploration and untethering of the cord.

- Meningocoele: a sac of meninges, covered by skin and containing CSF alone, herniates through an anterior or posterior bony defect.
- Myelomeningocoele: a herniating sac of meninges without covering skin contains spinal cord, nerves or both. This is always associated with Chiari II malformation (see below). Open myelomeningocoele presents a high infection risk and requires early surgical repair.
- Lipomyelomeningocoele: adipose tissue adherent to the spinal cord herniates through a bony defect to the sacrolumbar soft tissue. This may be associated with bladder dysfunction and requires surgical relief of the resultant cord tethering.

Failure of closure of the anterior neuropore produces anencephaly, which is uniformly fatal – the spectrum of spinal dysraphisms, however, is replicated in the skull. Cranium bifidum is a failure of fusion, often in the occipital region. This may be associated with herniation of meninges and CSF (meningocoele), and potentially also brain substance (encephalocoele) (Figure 43.19).

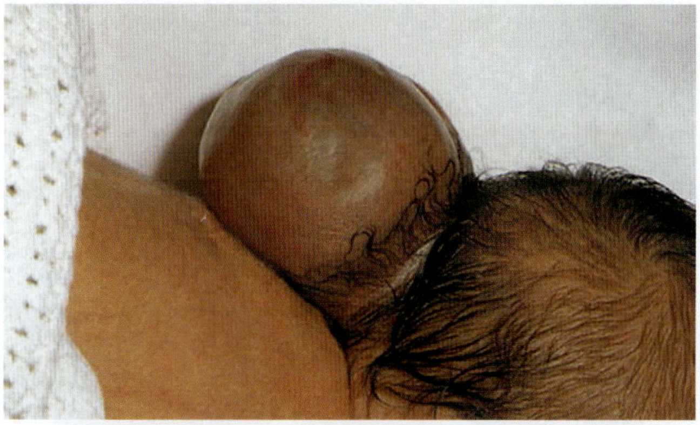

Figure 43.19 An occipital encephalocoele.

Posterior fossa malformations

Chiari malformations involve cerebellar herniation through the foramen magnum:

- Normal: Up to 5 mm of cerebellar tonsillar descent through the foramen magnum
- Chiari I: >5 mm of tonsillar descent: presents typically in young adults with headache and variable neurological disturbance
- Chiari II: descent of the tonsils and vermis: presents in infancy with poor feeding, stridor and apnoeic episodes.

They are often associated with syringomyelia, the presence of a fluid-filled cavity (syrinx) in the spinal cord. Compression of the brainstem and cerebellum, or development of a syrinx, may cause neurological deficits. Shunting and foramen magnum decompression are the mainstay of treatment. Chiari malformations may also present incidentally or with headaches exacerbated by valsalva.

Dandy Walker malformations present in infancy with macrocephaly, developmental delay and hydrocephalus; most patients have associated abnormalities in the CNS and other organ systems. Imaging demonstrates a hypoplastic cerebellar vermis, with the posterior fossa occupied by a large thin-walled cyst. Treatment usually involves shunt placement.

Craniosynostosis

Normal fusion of the coronal, lamdoidal, squamosal and sagittal sutures occurs between six and 12 months of age; others, such as the frontal suture fuse later. Craniosynostosis is the premature fusion of one (simple craniosynostosis) or more (complex craniosynostosis) cranial sutures, preventing growth perpendicular to the suture. This results in a range of skull deformities (see Table 43.6; Figures 43.20 and 43.21) and hydrocephalus. Syndromic craniosynostosis, often associated with abnormalities of the fibroblast growth factor receptor genes, is accompanied by developmental delay and other abnormalities. The surgical treatment aims to correct deformity and prevent development of raised ICP (Summary box 43.11).

Table 43.6 Types of craniosynostosis.

Type	Suture involved	Clinical features
Scaphocephaly	Sagittal suture	Narrow boat-shaped head
Brachycephaly	Coronal suture	Shortened/ broad forehead
Microcephaly	All sutures involved	Small head
Plagiocephaly	Unilateral coronal/ lamdoid suture	Asymmetric skull
Trigonocephaly	Metopic suture	Pointed narrow forehead

Summary box 43.11

Paediatric neurosurgery

Children manifest a range of developmental pathologies requiring neurosurgical management including:

- cysts
- neural tube defects
- posterior fossa abnormalities
- craniosynostosis

In general, intracranial pathologies present with features including developmental delay, seizures, macrocephaly and hydrocephalus.

FUNCTIONAL NEUROSURGERY

Where neurosurgery normally seeks to avoid disturbing neural tissue as far as possible, functional procedures aim to relieve epilepsy, movement disorders or pain by ablation or stimulation.

Epilepsy

Up to 10 per cent of the population will suffer a seizure at some point in their lives, and epilepsy, a syndrome of recurrent unprovoked seizures, represents the most common neurological

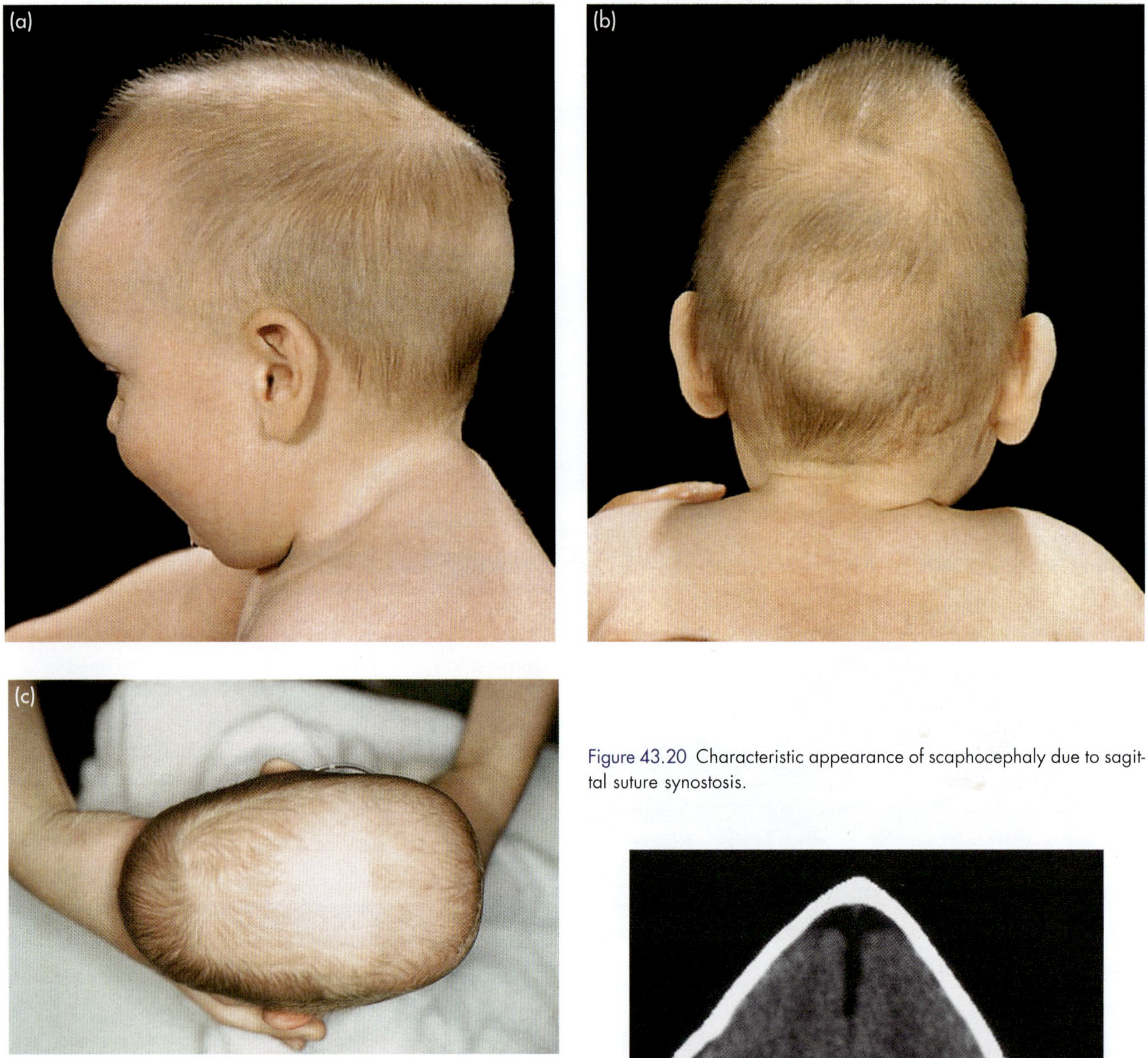

Figure 43.20 Characteristic appearance of scaphocephaly due to sagittal suture synostosis.

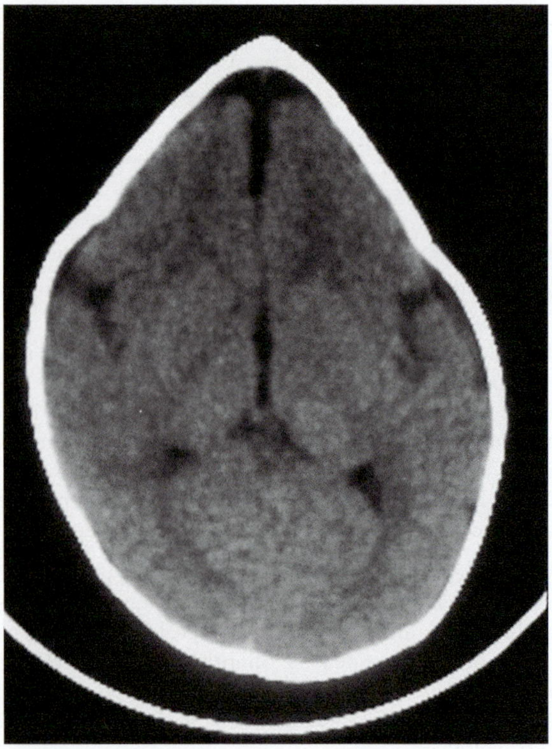

Figure 43.21 Axial computed tomography scan showing severe trigonocephaly due to premature fusion of the metopic suture.

disorder. About 20–30 per cent of patients fail to achieve adequate seizure control with drugs, and many of these focal epilepsies may benefit from surgery. Where a primary lesion, such as a tumour, arteriovenous malformation (AVM) or cavernoma is present, lesionectomy alone may be appropriate. In other cases, the clinical picture including seizure type, focal features and investigation results can be used to identify the seizure focus. Dual pathology refers to the presence of an extrahippocampal lesion plus hippocampal atrophy, important because removal of both the lesion and the atrophic hippocampus is the best surgical approach and should be considered whenever possible.

Investigation

MRI imaging is a mainstay, demonstrating for example reduced hippocampal volume and distorted architecture in mesial temporal sclerosis. Nuclear medicine modalities including single-photon emission computed tomography (SPECT) and positron emission tomography (PET) are sometimes used to demonstrate ictal and inter-ictal metabolic abnormalities.

Electroencephalography (EEG) entails recording from an array of scalp electrodes, and comparison between ictal and inter-ictal recordings. This is especially helpful in lateralising the focus of complex partial seizures in temporal lobe epilepsy, and is combined with video monitoring of the seizure in a videotelemetry suite. A more detailed localisation may be achieved invasively by the preoperative placement of subdural or depth electrodes, preoperatively or by intraoperative electrocorticography (ECoG).

Neuropsychological evaluation is used to evaluate the patient's preoperative function looking for concordant focal impairments, and, using the Wada test where sodium amytal is injected into each internal carotid artery in turn, with simultaneous speech and memory testing to localise function. The aim is to establish language laterality and to confirm that resection on the side of the lesion will not significantly impair verbal memory function.

Surgical management

The seizure focus may be resected, generally where it is in non-eloquent brain, or otherwise a disconnection can be performed. Awake craniotomy, allowing mapping particularly of speech centres, is increasingly employed.

Mesial temporal epilepsy is commonly medically refractory and can be addressed surgically by amygdalohippocampectomy or resection of the temporal lobe including the mesial structures. The extent of resection is limited by the potential for damage to the optic tracts, and to speech areas in the dominant hemisphere. With careful patient selection, cure rates of up to 70 per cent or greater can be achieved.

Functional, or rarely anatomical, hemispherectomy (Figure 43.22) may be performed for specific epilepsy syndromes associated with hemiplegia, such as infantile hemiplegia syndrome. This is usually considered in the early years of life when plasticity and potential for functional recovery is greatest.

Disconnection procedures include corpus callosotomy, used for patients suffering drop attacks, and subpial transections to isolate a seizure focus in eloquent brain from the surrounding cortex.

Vagal nerves stimulators are implanted in severe drug refractory epilepsy, usually in children, and can achieve some success in reducing seizure frequency, although the mechanism is unclear, and is never curative.

Movement disorders

Prior to the advent of levodopa, surgical ablation of the subthalamic nucleus or globus pallidus interna was a mainstay of management for Parkinson's. Inhibition of the action of these centres remains a valuable tool later in the course of the disease as the therapeutic window using levodopa narrows, but this is now generally achieved using deep brain stimulation with electrodes. This offers the advantage of an adjustable and reversible effect, and can be performed bilaterally where equivalent lesioning surgery would likely result in deficits.

Juhn Atsushi Wada, b.1924 Tokyo, appointed as Professor of Neurology, University of British Columbia, Vancouver, Canada in 1956. The test is also known as 'intracarotid sodium amobarbitol' procedure.

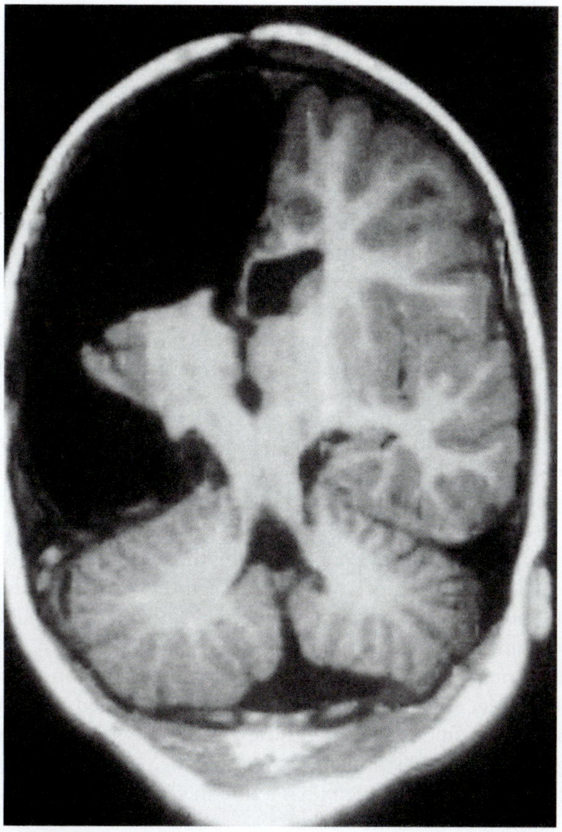

Figure 43.22 Coronal T2-weighted magnetic resonance imaging scan image following an anatomical hemispherectomy.

Deep brain stimulation is also an option for other movement disorders where less invasive approaches are ineffective. These include dystonias, which may be amenable to bilateral stimulation of the globus pallidus interna, and essential tremor where the ventral intermediate nucleus of the thalamus is the target.

Pain syndromes

Neurosurgical approaches to the relief of pain may address the underlying aetiology directly, or may seek to interrupt or modulate the transmission responsible for the pain. The contrasting approaches are demonstrated in the management of trigeminal neuralgia. This manifests, generally in middle age or later, with paroxysmal lancinating pain in the distribution of one or more divisions of the trigeminal nerve. The pain occurs without other neurological disturbance, and may be triggered by trivial stimuli such as eating or brushing the teeth. The pain was first attributed to stimulation of the nerve by an adjacent vascular structure, often the superior cerebellar artery, by Walter Dandy. Occasionally, another primary lesion is responsible; for example, bilateral trigeminal neuralgia in younger patients is suggestive of multiple sclerosis. Where medications, such as gabapentin and carbamazepine cannot achieve control, surgical options include:

- Craniotomy and microvascular decompression: this is designed to address the proposed origin of the neuropathic pain, by applying material between the nerve and adjacent vessel to prevent direct contact and stimulation. It achieves long-lasting relief of symptoms in about 80 per cent of patients,

James Parkinson, 1755–1824, a general practitioner of Shoreditch, London, UK.

but is associated with the standard risks of craniotomy (see below Risks of craniotomy, p. 19) and a significant incidence of cranial nerve deficit.

- Peripheral nerve injections, which can achieve good short-term relief of pain restricted to small areas supplied by terminal branches of the trigeminal.
- Percutaneous Gasserian rhizolysis: this involves needle placement under x-ray guidance at the Gasserian ganglion in Meckel's cave. This permits lesioning of the ganglion by glycerol injection, radiofrequency thermocoagulation or balloon compression, with the aim of disrupting aberrant pain transmission. A similar effect can also be achieved using stereotactic radiosurgery. Facial numbness and late recurrence of pain are common after these procedures.

Treatment of pain elsewhere may also be based on lesioning of nerve tracts. For example, pain related to brachial plexus infiltration or injury may be treated by sectioning the spinothalamic tract (cordotomy), or the dorsal root entry zone (DREZ operation). These approaches are limited by the potential for producing deficits, and especially by the occurrence of deafferentation ('phantom limb') pain syndromes which are particularly unpleasant and difficult to treat.

Electrical stimulation is used to modulate pain transmission; for example, spinal cord stimulators can be applied to a range of pain syndromes, especially those associated with failed spinal surgery. Deep brain stimulation targeting the periaqueductal grey and sensory thalamic nuclei has a role in chronic pain arising in the context of thalamic stroke.

Implanted devices may also be used for intrathecal delivery of opiates for pain control, or baclofen to alleviate spasticity (Summary box 43.12).

Summary box 43.12

Functional neurosurgery

- Intractable epilepsy can be treated surgically by implantation of a vagal nerve stimulator or by resection of one or more seizure foci
- Deep brain stimulation using implanted electrodes has largely replaced lesioning of these structures for management of drug-refractory Parkinson's disease
- Microvascular decompression is offered for trigeminal neuralgia, and other neuropathic pain syndromes may respond to lesioning of nerve tracts

OCCLUSIVE VASCULAR DISEASE

There is class 1 evidence for the role of carotid endarterectomy in reducing the risk of stroke in patients with symptomatic carotid stenosis, and a debatable role for the procedure in patients with no previous transient ischaemic episodes.

In a subgroup of otherwise fit patients with completed posterior fossa or non-dominant middle cerebral artery territory infarcts, there is a role for decompressive craniectomy in the acute setting to manage the brain swelling and raised ICP associated with the infarct.

Moya moya disease is the progressive obliteration of one or both internal carotid arteries, thought to represent an autoimmune process. The development of external carotid circulation collaterals produces the angiographic 'puff of smoke' appearance responsible for this Japanese-derived name. It presents in youth or early middle age with ischaemia or haemorrhage. Untreated, the majority of patients suffer major deficit or die within two years. Ischaemia may be addressed by a variety of bypass techniques, for example by anastomosing the superficial temporal artery (arising from the external carotid) to the middle cerebral artery.

COMPRESSIVE NEUROPATHIES

Carpal tunnel syndrome is a compression neuropathy resulting from entrapment of the median nerve under the flexor retinaculum at the wrist. Risk factors include diabetes, obesity, thyroid disorders and acromegaly. The presentation is usually with paraesthesia in the hand, worse at night. Examination will reveal sensory disturbance in the median nerve distribution – the palmar aspect of the thumb, index and middle fingers, and the radial aspect of the ring finger. The palm itself is relatively spared, reflecting supply by the palmar cutaneous branch passing superficial to the retinaculum. Wasting of the thenar eminence, and weakness of abductor pollicis brevis may also be apparent, and tapping over the carpal tunnel (Tinel's test) or wrist flexion (Phalen's test) may reproduce symptoms. Nerve conduction studies confirm the diagnosis, and management includes wrist splints, steroid injections, and carpal tunnel decompression by division and release of the flexor retinaculum.

A range of related peripheral mononeuropathies, characterised by sensory disturbance, wasting and weakness in the nerve distribution, are investigated using nerve conduction studies, and are typically amenable to surgical decompression. Common examples include:

- Ulnar nerve entrapment at the elbow: the sensory disturbance affects the little finger and ulnar aspect of the ring finger, and wasting of the hypothenar eminence may be evident. Froment's sign is elicited by asking the patient to hold a piece of paper in the first webspace while the examiner attempts to slide it away; the distal phalanx of the thumb is seen to flex, reflecting the use of flexor pollicis longus (anterior interosseous innervated) instead of adductor pollicis (ulnar innervated, so weak).
- Meralgia paraesthetica: the lateral cutaneous nerve of the thigh is compressed under the inguinal ligament, producing sensory disturbance in the lateral thigh.

PRACTICAL AND ETHICAL ISSUES

Creutzfeldt–Jakob disease

CJD is a rare transmissible spongiform encephalopathy producing a rapidly progressive dementia, and is uniformly fatal. The causative agent seems to be a mis-folded protein, a prion, which is not destroyed by conventional sterilisation techniques. UK practice involves undertaking preoperative checks to exclude any risk factors for CJD infection. These include family history,

George S Phalen, contemporary, orthopaedic surgeon and Chief of Hand Surgery, The Cleveland Clinic, Cleveland, OH, USA. He helped to establish the American Society for Surgery of the Hand.

Jules Froment, 1878–1946, Professor of Clinical Medicine, Lyons, France.

receipt of pituitary-derived human growth hormone, cadaveric dura mater grafts, and previous brain or spinal surgery prior to 1997. Where risk factors are present, instruments must be quarantined or destroyed postoperatively.

Risks of craniotomy

The risks associated with craniotomy are important to appreciate in discussing operations with patients and family, and in evaluating patients who deteriorate postoperatively. The figures quoted in brackets will vary significantly between individual procedures and even between centres:

- infection (5 per cent) and wound breakdown;
- intracerebral haemorrhage;
- seizures;
- CSF leak;
- permanent neurological deficit;
- death (1 per cent).

Brainstem death

This is defined as the irreversible loss of cerebral and brainstem function. Brainstem death is legally equivalent to death, and is a pre-condition for the harvesting of organs for transplant from heart-beating donors.

Diagnosis requires:

- identification of the cause of irreversible coma;
- exclusion of reversible causes of coma;
- clinical demonstration of the absence of brainstem function.

In the UK, this entails testing twice, by two clinicians, to demonstrate the absence of:

- response to pain;
- respiratory drive (apnoea despite a *p*CO2 >6.7 kPa);
- pupillary light reflex;
- corneal reflex;
- vestibulo-ocular reflex;
- oculocephalic reflex;
- gag reflex.

FURTHER READING

Greenberg MS. *Handbook of neurosurgery*, 7th edn. New York: Thieme, 2010.

Patten J. *Neurological differential diagnosis*, 2nd edn. New York: Springer, 1994.

Samandouras G. *The neurosurgeon's handbook*. Oxford: Oxford Publishing, 2010.

Ambroise Paré, 1510–1590. He was official surgeon to the Kings: Henry II, Francis II, Charles IX and Henry III. He is considered as one of the fathers of surgery and a modest man who said 'I dressed him and God healed him'.

CHAPTER

44 The eye and orbit

LEARNING OBJECTIVES

To understand and appreciate:

- The common ocular disorders and recognise ophthalmic symptoms and specific signs
- The value of special investigations
- When specialist referral is appropriate

OCULAR ANATOMY

Adnexae

The lids comprise skin, connective tissue, the orbicularis oculi (VIIth cranial nerve) and the tarsal plate, with multiple meibomian glands opening posterior to the lashes and lined with conjunctiva, which is reflected onto the sclera. The upper lid is elevated by the levator muscle (IIIrd cranial nerve) and has a horizontal strip of sympathetically innervated Müller's muscle, giving rise to 2 mm of ptosis in Horner's syndrome. Both lids are attached to the orbital rim by the medial and lateral canthal tendons. Both have a rich vascular supply and are innervated by the V1 division of the trigeminal nerve (Vth cranial nerve) above and the V2 division below.

Lacrimal system

The almond-shaped lacrimal gland lies under the upper outer orbital rim and opens into the upper conjunctival fornix through 10–15 ducts. Tears are swept across the globe by the lids and evaporate or pass into the upper and lower lid puncta, and then into the canaliculi to join the common canaliculus, which passes into the lacrimal sac under the medial canthal tendon. The sac is drained by the nasolacrimal duct into the nose, opening in the inferior meatus under the inferior turbinate.

The globe

The cornea is the 12-mm diameter window of the eye, 0.5 mm thick centrally; its clarity is due to the regular arrangement of collagen bundles and relative dehydration. It merges into the sclera at the corneoscleral junction (the limbus), the insertion of the bulbar conjunctiva. The sclera, which is 1 mm thick, comprises four-fifths of the wall of the eye, and gives attachment to the extraocular muscles. It is perforated by the long and short posterior ciliary arteries and the vortex veins and is contiguous with the optic nerve sheath. The uvea comprises iris, ciliary body and vascular choroid. The optic nerve is continuous with the retina and retinal pigment epithelium. The most sensitive part of the retina, the macula, lies at the posterior pole within the vascular arcade. The biconvex lens and capsule are suspended by the suspensory ligament, over 300 tiny fibres attached to the ciliary muscle. Aqueous humour arises from the ciliary processes, hydrates the vitreous gel, passes through the pupil into the anterior chamber between the iris and the cornea and then drains out through the trabecular meshwork into Schlemm's canal in the drainage angle. The inner retina is supplied by the central retinal artery and drained by the central retinal vein (Figure 44.1).

Orbit

The orbit is four-sided and pyramidal in structure, housing the globe, optic nerve, the four rectus and two oblique muscles, the lacrimal gland, orbital fat, the IIIrd, IVth, Vth and VIth cranial

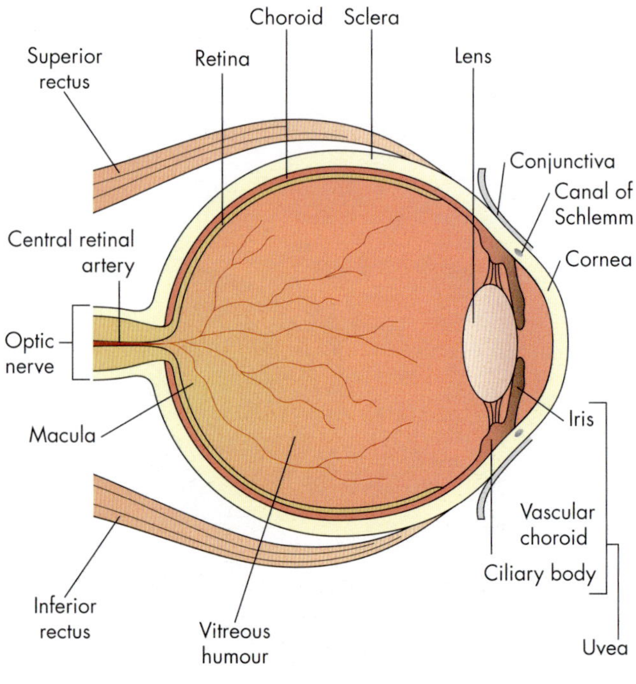

Figure 44.1 Anatomy of the eye.

Johannes Peter Müller, 1801–1858, Professor of Anatomy and Physiology, Berlin, Germany.
Johan Friedrich Horner, 1831–1886, Professor of Ophthalmology, Zurich, Switzerland, described this syndrome in 1869.
Friedrich Schlemm, 1795–1858, Professor of Anatomy, Berlin, Germany.

nerves, the ophthalmic artery with its tributaries and the ophthalmic veins, which anastomose anteriorly with the face and posteriorly with the cranial cavity. Above is the frontal lobe of the brain, temporally the temporal fossa, inferiorly the maxillary sinus and nasally the lacrimal sac and ethmoidal and sphenoidal air sinuses. The optic nerve passes through the optic canal to the chiasm, with other nerves and vessels passing through the superior ophthalmic fissure.

PERIORBITAL AND ORBITAL SWELLINGS

Swellings related to the supraorbital margin

Dermoid cysts

Dermoid cysts are usually external angular cysts although they may occur medially (Figure 44.2). They often cause a bony depression by their pressure and they may have a dumbbell extension into the orbit. They can also erode the orbital plate of the frontal bone to become attached to dura and for this reason it is important to image the area by computed tomography (CT) before excision.

Neurofibromatosis

Neurofibromatosis may also produce swellings above the eye. The diagnosis can usually be confirmed by an examination of the whole body, as there are often multiple lesions. Proptosis can also result (Figure 44.3). Other ophthalmic features may be present.

Swellings of the lids

Meibomian cysts (chalazion)

These are the most common lid swellings (Figure 44.4). A meibomian cyst is a chronic granulomatous inflammation of a meibomian gland. It may occur on either upper or lower lids and presents as a smooth, painless swelling. It can be felt by rolling the cyst on the tarsal plate. It can be distinguished from a stye (hordeolum), which is an infection of a hair follicle and is usually painful. Persistent meibomian cysts are treated by incision and curettage from the conjunctival surface. Styes are treated by antibiotics and local heat.

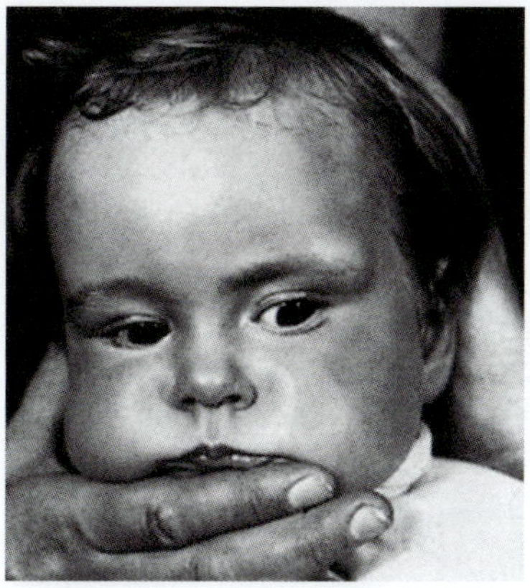

Figure 44.2 External angular dermoid.

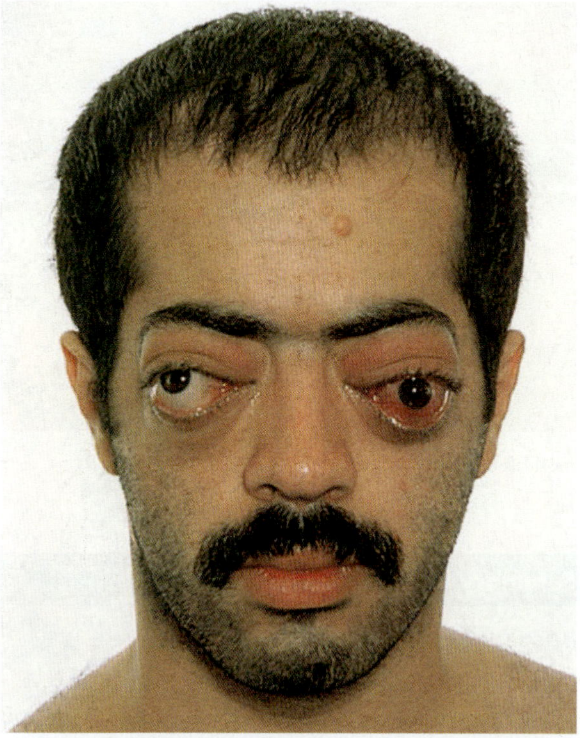

Figure 44.3 Neurofibroma in the orbit with proptosis, and also similar lesions in the forehead.

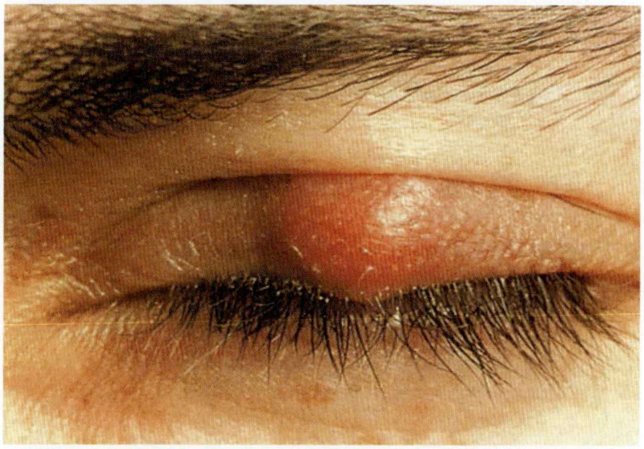

Figure 44.4 Meibomian cyst (courtesy of Mr D Spalton, FRCS).

Basal cell carcinomas (rodent ulcers)

This is the most common malignant tumour of the eyelids (Figure 44.5). It is locally malignant, is more common on the lower lids and usually starts as a small pimple that ulcerates and has raised edges ('rodent ulcer'). It is easily excised in the early stages. Histological confirmation that the excision is complete is required. More extensive lesions may require specialist techniques, such as Mohs' micrographic surgical excision controlled by frozen section. Local radiotherapy or cryotherapy can be carried out; however, recurrence is more common, more aggressive and more difficult to detect (Summary box 44.1).

Frederic E Mohs, 1910–2002, physician and general surgeon, University of Wisconsin, Madison, WI, USA. Developed Mohs' micrographic surgical technique in 1938 for cutaneous malignant lesions.

Heinrich Meibom (Meibomius), 1638–1700, Professor of Medicine, History and Poetry, Helmstadt, Germany, described these glands in 1666.

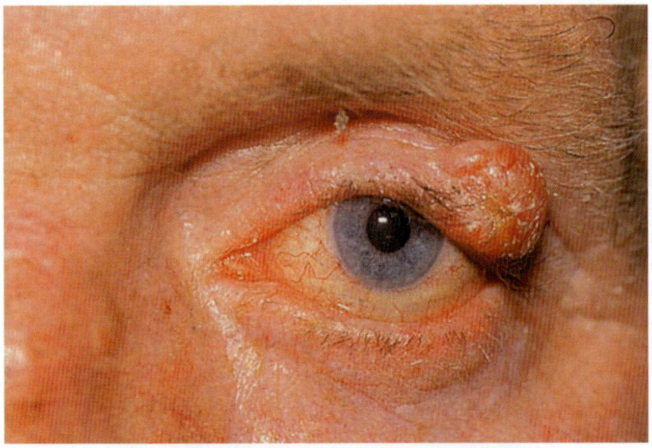

Figure 44.5 Rodent ulcers (courtesy of Mr J Beare, FRCS).

Summary box 44.1

Basal cell carcinomas

- Basal cell carcinomas are the most common malignant eye tumour
- Treatment is by excision with care with histopathological margin control
- All unusual lesions (especially in the elderly) should be biopsied

Other lid swellings

Other types of lid swelling can occur but they are less common. They include sebaceous cysts, papillomas, keratoacanthomas, cysts of Moll (sweat glands) (Figure 44.6) or Zeis (sebaceous glands) and molluscum contagiosum. When molluscum contagiosum occurs on the lid margin, it can give rise to a mild viral chronic keratoconjunctivitis and should be curetted or excised.

Carcinoma of the meibomian glands and rhabdomyosarcomas are rare lesions; they need to be treated by radical excision. Atypical or meibomian cysts that recur should be biopsied.

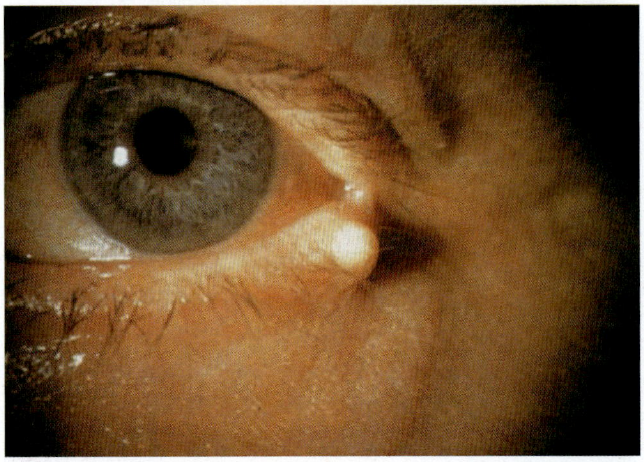

Figure 44.6 Cyst of Moll.

Swellings of the lacrimal system

Lacrimal sac mucocele

This occurs from obstruction of the lacrimal duct beyond the sac and results in a fluctuant swelling that bulges out just below the medial canthus. It can become infected to give rise to a painful tense swelling (acute dacryocystitis). If untreated it may give rise to a fistula. Treatment is by performing a bypass operation between the lacrimal sac and the nose (a dacryocystorrhinostomy (DCR)). Watering of the eye can occur due to eversion of the lower lid (ectropion), which causes loss of contact between the lower punctum and the tear film, or from reflex hypersecretion as a result of irritation of inturning lashes in entropion, and these must be distinguished from a mucocoele.

Lacrimal gland tumours

These are swellings of the lacrimal glands, which lie in the upper lateral aspect of the orbit. Eventually, they lead to impairment of ocular movements and displacement of the globe forwards, downwards and inwards. Pathologically the tumours resemble parotid tumours and they can be pleomorphic adenomas with or without malignant change, carcinomas or mucoepidermoid tumours.

Orbital swellings

Orbital swellings result in displacement of the globe and limitation of movement. A full description of orbital swellings is outside the realm of this text but some of the most common causes include the following:

- **Pseudoproptosis.** This results from a large eyeball, as seen in congenital glaucoma or high myopia.
- **Orbital inflammatory conditions** that result in orbital cellulitis (Figure 44.7).
- **Haemorrhage** after trauma or retrobulbar injection.
- **Neoplasia** affecting the lacrimal gland, the optic nerve, the orbital walls or the nasal sinuses, e.g. glioma (neurofibromatosis) (see Figure 44.3), meningioma and osteoma (Figure 44.8).
- **Dysthyroid exophthalmos** (Figures 44.9, 44.10 and 44.11). This may be unrelated to active thyroid disease but can start after thyroidectomy and may need urgent tarsorrhaphy, large doses of steroids or even orbital lateral wall decompression if the eyeball is threatened by exposure or optic nerve compression. CT and magnetic resonance imaging (MRI) scans are useful in diagnosis.

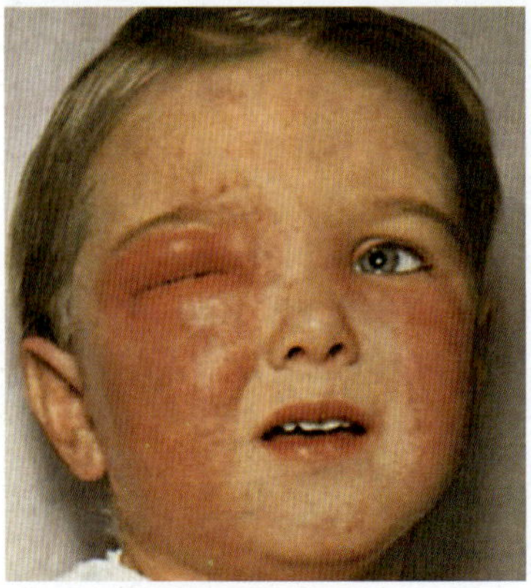

Figure 44.7 Orbital cellulitis.

Jacob Antonius Moll, 1832–1913, ophthalmologist of The Hague, The Netherlands.
Edward Zeis, 1807–1868, Professor of Surgery, Marburg (1844–1850), who later worked at Dresden, Germany, described these glands in 1835.

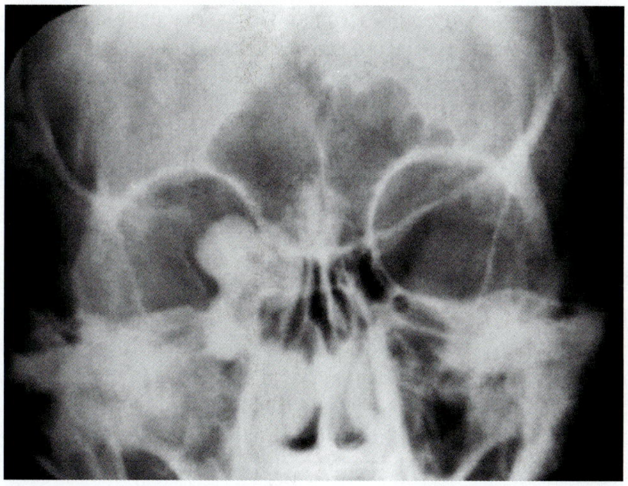

Figure 44.8 Radiograph showing an osteoma on the nasal side of the orbit giving rise to proptosis.

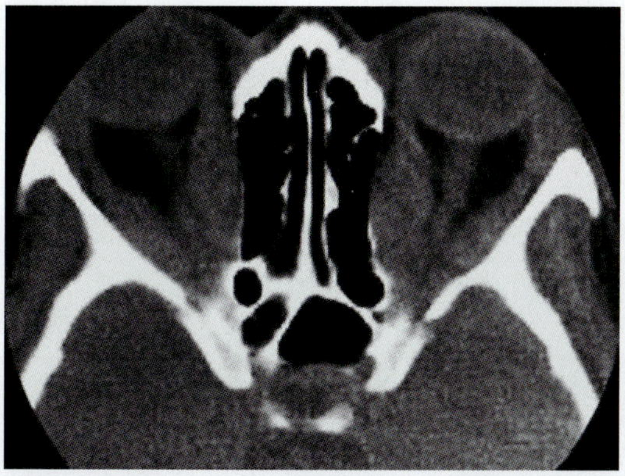

Figure 44.9 Computed tomogram of the orbit in dysthyroid exophthalmos, showing swollen muscles (courtesy of Dr Glyn Lloyd).

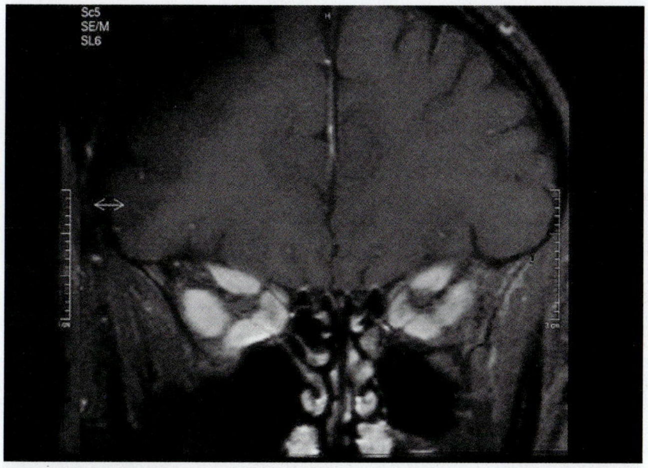

Figure 44.10 Magnetic resonance imaging scan of a coronal view of the orbit, showing enlarged muscles in thyroid disease (courtesy of Dr Juliette Britton).

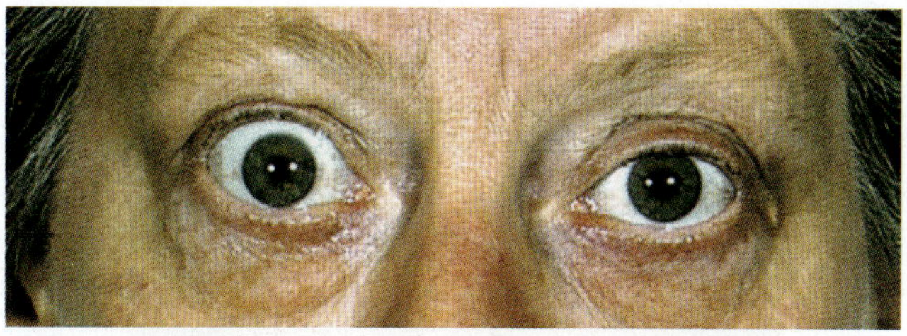

Figure 44.11 Exophthalmos in dysthyroid eye disease.

- **Pseudotumour**, or malignant lymphoma.
- **Haemangiomas** of the orbit (Figure 44.12).
- **Tumour metastases**. These are rare. In children they usually arise from neuroblastomas of the adrenal gland, whereas in adults the oesophagus, stomach, breast and prostate can be sites of primary lesions.

Diagnostic aids

Diagnostic aids include radiography, CT, MRI, ultrasonography and, less commonly, tomography and orbital venography.

Treatment

Treatment is directed to the cause of the lesion if at all possible, taking care to prevent exposure of the eye, diplopia or visual impairment from optic nerve compression.

INTRAOCULAR TUMOURS

Children

Retinoblastoma is a multicentric malignant tumour of the retina, which can be bilateral. Some are sporadic, but many are hereditary. Children with a family history should be carefully monitored from birth. It is often not spotted until the tumour fills the globe and presents as a white reflex in the pupil or as a squint (Figure 44.13). The differential diagnosis includes retinopathy of prematurity, primary hyperplastic vitreous and intraocular infections. If the tumour is large, enucleation may be required, but radiotherapy, cryotherapy, chemotherapy or laser treatment can cure small lesions. Liaison with a paediatric oncologist is essential (Summary box 44.2).

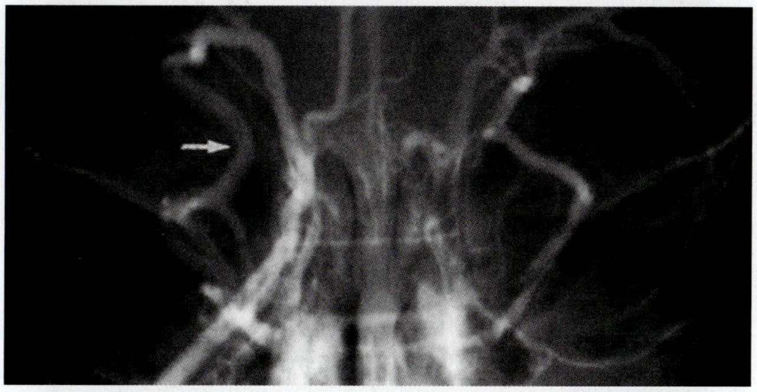

Figure 44.12 Capillary haemangioma in a child. An orbital venogram demonstrates displacement of the second part of the superior ophthalmic vein (arrow) (courtesy of Dr Glyn Lloyd).

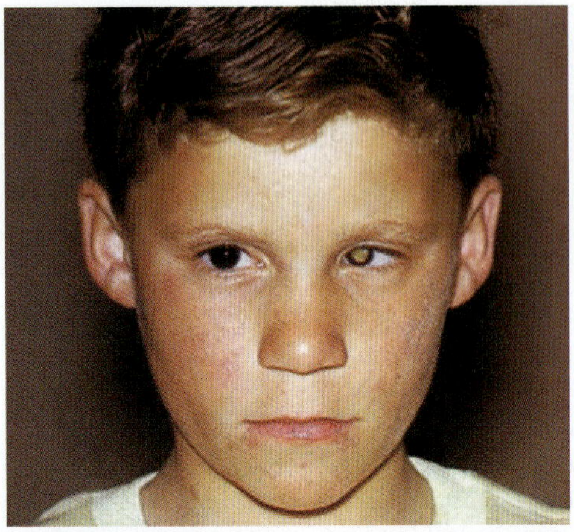

Figure 44.13 Retinoblastoma giving rise to a white pupillary reflex (courtesy of MA Bedford, FRCS).

> **Summary box 44.2**
>
> **Intraocular tumours**
>
> - All children with a squint should have a fundal examination to exclude a retinoblastoma
> - A blind painful eye may hide a melanoma

Adults

Malignant melanoma is the most common tumour and it originates in the pigment cells of the choroid (Figure 44.14), ciliary body or iris. It can present with a reduction in vision, a vitreous haemorrhage or by the chance finding of an elevated pigmented lesion in the eye. Tumour growth is variable but, as a general rule, the more posterior the lesion, the more rapidly progressive it is likely to be. Spread may be delayed for many years; however, the liver is frequently involved, hence the advice 'beware of the patient with a glass eye and an enlarged liver'. Treatment is by light or laser coagulation, radioactive plaque, radiotherapy, enucleation and, in selected cases, local excision using hypotensive anaesthesia. Diagnosis is made by direct observation and/or ultrasound, which shows a solid tumour (Figure 44.15).

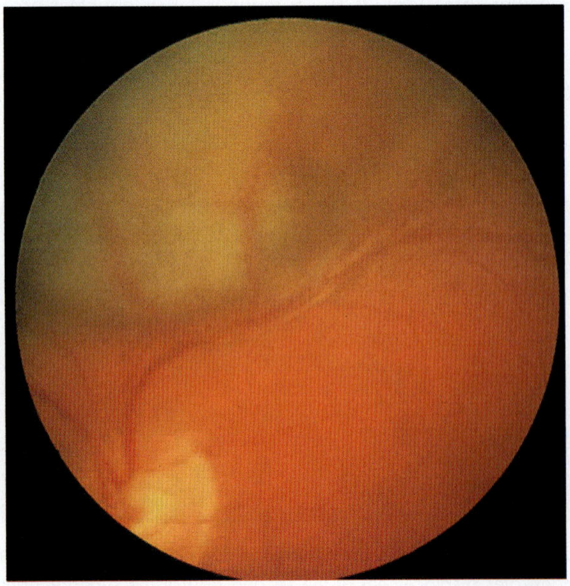

Figure 44.14 Choroidal melanoma.

INJURIES INVOLVING THE EYE AND ADJACENT STRUCTURES

Corneal abrasions and ulceration

The cornea is frequently damaged by direct trauma or by foreign bodies (Figure 44.16). Ulceration can occur with infection or after damage to the facial nerve. Post-herpetic ulceration is common and serious if not treated. Fluorescein instillation illuminated by blue light shows up corneal ulceration at an early stage (Summary box 44.3).

> **Summary box 44.3**
>
> **Corneal abrasions**
>
> - A drop of fluorescein dye illuminated by a blue light reveals even the smallest corneal abrasion

Treatment is by protection (eye pads, tarsorrhaphy or a bandage contact lens) and antibiotics topically and rarely systemically: 0.5 per cent chloramphenicol or ofloxacin eye

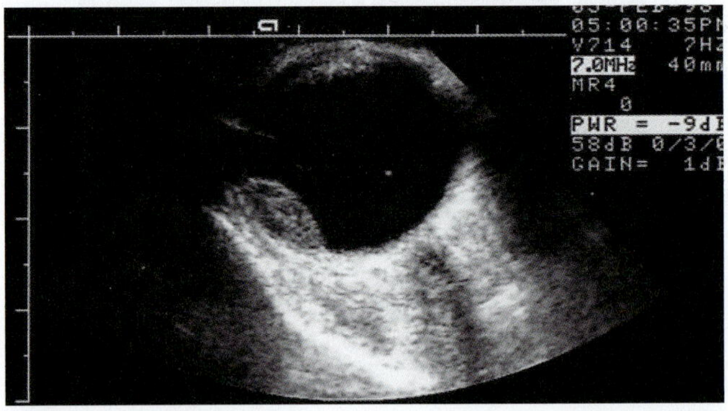

Figure 44.15 B-scan showing choroidal melanoma (courtesy of Dr Marie Reston).

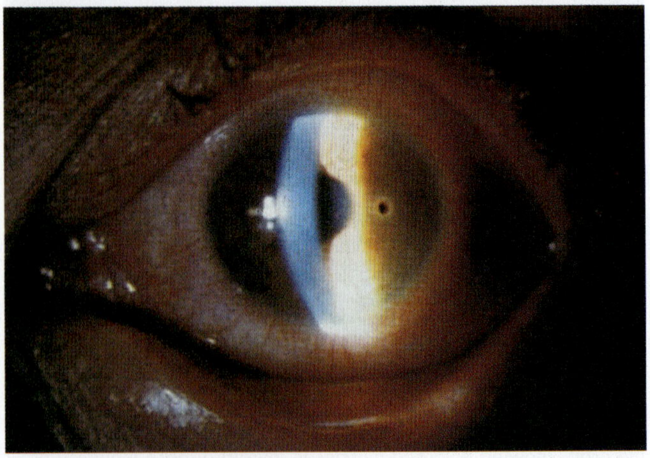

Figure 44.16 Corneal foreign body.

drops are commonly used. The eye is made more comfortable by the use of mydriatics, such as homatropine or cyclopentolate. Herpes simplex dendritite ulcers are treated with aciclovir ointment. In countries in the Far and Middle East, chronic infection with trachoma can cause corneal opacification and blindness. Corneal grafting is the only cure for an opaque cornea. Until recently, full thickness penetrating keratoplasty was the only corneal graft technique. This has largely been replaced by lamellar or partial thickness graft surgery, in a technique termed DSEK or 'Descamets stripping endothelial keratoplasty'. Rarely, osteo-odonto keratoprosthesis can be attempted in very severe cases of opaque corneas that are not suitable for grafting. Acanthamoeba is a rare serious cause of corneal infection. This infection usually follows the use of contact lenses. Specialist management and treatment is recommended.

Blunt injuries to the eye and orbit

The floor of the orbit is its weakest wall and in blunt trauma, such as a blow from a fist, it is often fractured without fractures of the other walls. This is called a blow-out fracture. Clinical signs are enophthalmos, bruising around the orbit, maxillary hypoaesthesia, limitation of upward gaze due to entrapment of the inferior rectus muscle leading to vertical diplopia. This occurs when the extraocular muscles or orbital septa become trapped in the fracture and can be identified as a soft-tissue mass in the antrum on a radiograph (Figure 44.17), although CT scans or tomograms may be necessary. Surgical repair of the orbital floor with freeing of the trapped contents may be necessary if troublesome diplopia persists or enophthalmos is marked. A child with an orbital floor fracture requires urgent assessment as a 'greenstick' fracture can result in ischaemia of a trapped inferior rectus muscle and may require urgent surgery. If an orbital haemorrhage is too extensive to examine the eye, it may be necessary to examine the eye under anaesthesia because there may be a hidden perforation of the globe. Injuries to the lids and lid margins must be repaired, and if the lacrimal canaliculi are damaged they should be repaired if possible, especially the lower canaliculus as 75 per cent of tear drainage goes through it.

Blunt injuries can also cause damage to the optic nerve, which can result in blindness and a total afferent pupillary defect (Figures 44.18 and 44.19).

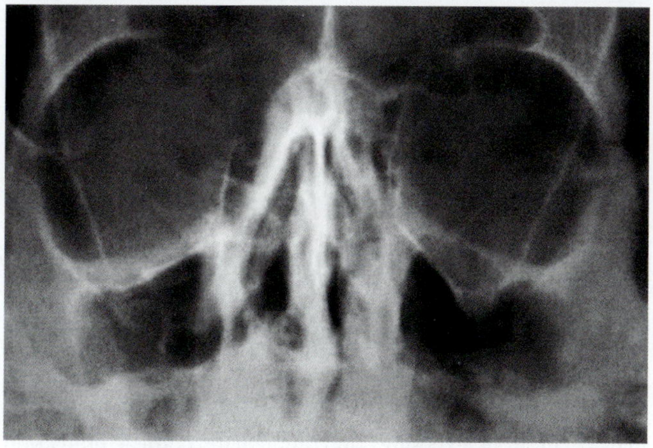

Figure 44.17 Radiograph showing a blow-out fracture of the orbit (left) with soft tissue in the antrum (courtesy of Dr Glyn Lloyd).

Concussion injuries

Concussion injuries of the eye can give rise to several problems, which include the following:

- **Iritis**. Inflammation, treated with topical steroids.
- **Hyphaema** (blood in the anterior chamber) (Figure 44.20). Rest and sedation, particularly in children, are advised because the main danger in this condition is secondary bleeding, resulting in an acute rise in intraocular pressure and blood staining of the cornea. The use of antifibrinolytic agents (ε-aminocaproic acid) has been advocated and, if the pressure rises, surgery to wash out the blood may be necessary.

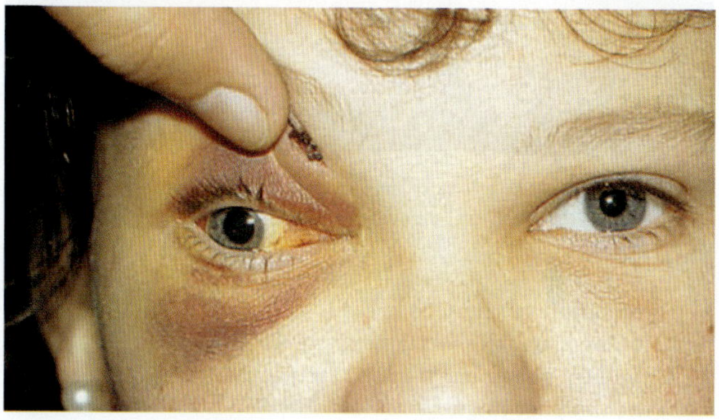

Figure 44.18 Injury from a ski stick into the right brow. Vision reduced to 'no perception of light' (courtesy of J Beare, FRCS).

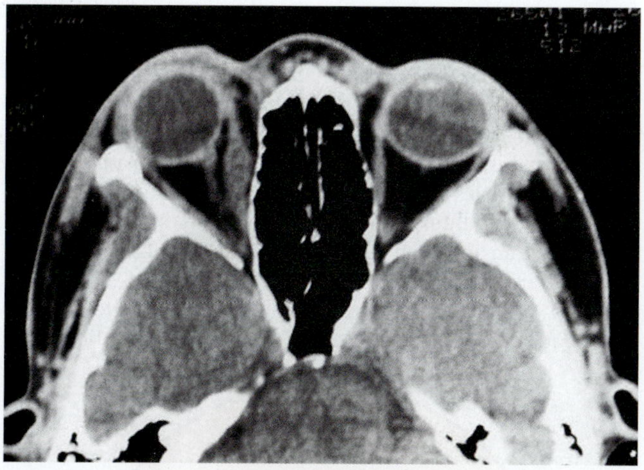

Figure 44.19 Scan of orbit from Figure 44.18 showing a massive swelling of the medial rectus (courtesy of J Beare, FRCS).

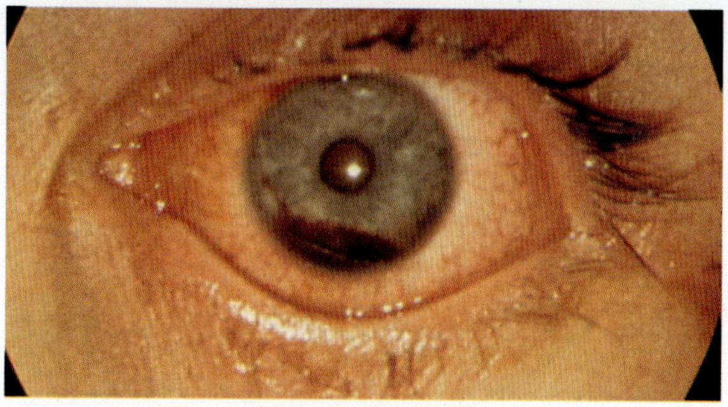

Figure 44.20 Hyphaema. Blood in the vitreous chamber after concussional injury.

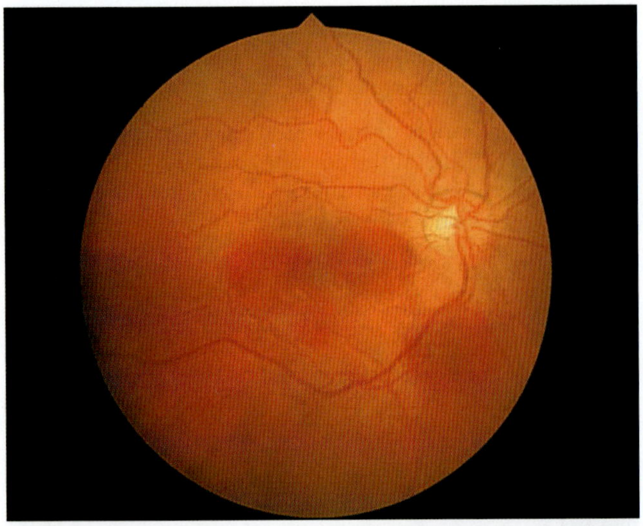

Figure 44.21 Retinal haemorrhage from a cricket bat injury (courtesy of J Beare, FRCS).

- **Subluxation of the lens**. This is suspected if the iris, or part of the iris, 'wobbles' on movement (iridodonesis).
- **Secondary glaucoma**. This is often associated with recession of the drainage angle.
- **Retinal and macular haemorrhages and choroidal tears** (Figure 44.21).
- **Retinal dialysis**. This may lead to a retinal detachment and permanent damage to vision (Figure 44.22).

Penetrating eye injuries

These occur when the globe is penetrated, often in road traffic and other major accidents (Figure 44.23), and also in injuries from sharp instruments. The compulsory wearing of seatbelts in motor vehicles has substantially reduced the incidence of this type of eye injury, by up to 73 per cent in the UK. The presence of an irregular pupil suggests prolapse of the iris and should arouse the suspicion of a penetrating injury. Treatment is prompt primary repair to restore the integrity of the globe. If a perforation is suspected, extensive eye examination should not

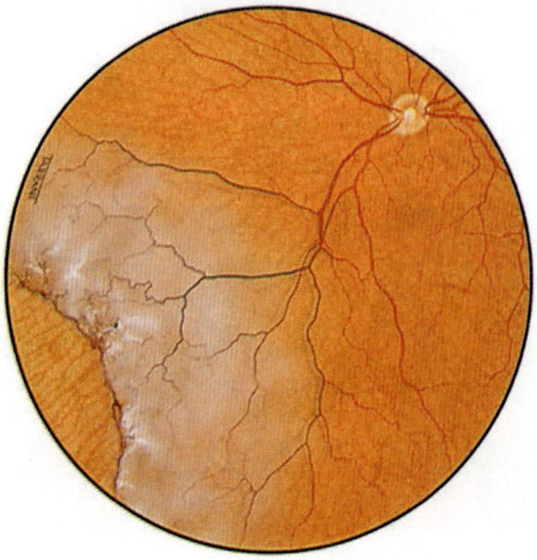

Figure 44.22 Retinal dialysis after concussional injury.

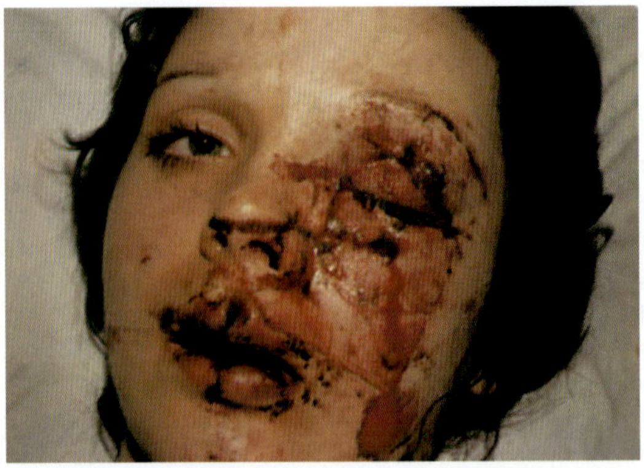

Figure 44.23 Facial lacerations from a windscreen injury. Beware of a perforating eye injury.

be attempted before anaesthesia because this may lead to further extrusion of the intraocular contents. If the fundal view is poor, ultrasonography and orbital imaging are indicated. Secondary corneal grafting, lensectomy and vitrectomy have considerably improved the visual prognosis; these must be done by an experienced eye surgeon. Injuries to the optic nerves must also be excluded in severe accidents.

Intraocular foreign bodies

Intraocular foreign bodies must always be excluded when patients attend the accident and emergency department with an eye injury and a history of working with a hammer and chisel or a history of a potentially high-velocity injury. Radiography of the orbits should always be performed, and ferrous and copper foreign bodies should always be removed, sometimes requiring the use of a magnet. B-scan ultrasonography can also assist in localising foreign bodies when a vitreous haemorrhage or cataract is present. CT can be used, but MRI is contraindicated (Summary box 44.4).

Summary box 44.4

Penetrating eye injuries

- A distorted and irregular pupil warrants the careful exclusion of a penetrating eye injury

Burns

Radiation burns

These occur following exposure to ultraviolet radiation after arc welding or excessive sunlight (snow blindness) and sun lamps. Such burns cause intense gritty burning pain and photophobia as a result of keratitis (corneal inflammation), which starts some hours after exposure. Mydriatic and local steroids with antibiotic drops ease the condition, and healing usually occurs after 24 hours.

Thermal burns

If these involve the full thickness of the lids, corneal scarring may occur from exposure, and immediate corneal protection is necessary. A splash of molten metal may cause marked local necrosis and may lead to permanent corneal scarring. Treatment

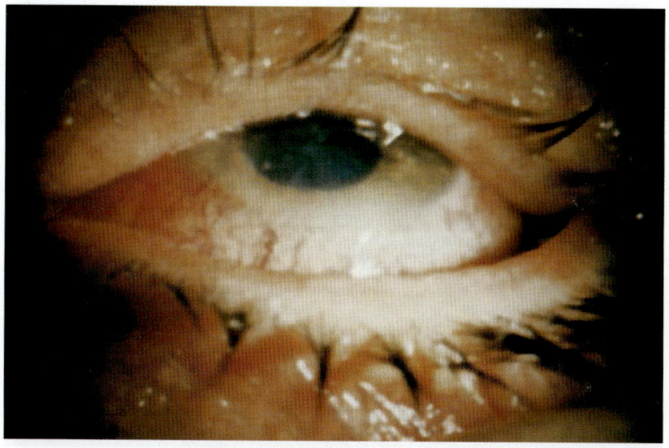

Figure 44.24 Chemical burn showing conjunctival necrosis.

is to remove any debris by irrigation and to instill local atropine, antibiotics and steroids to prevent superadded infection and scarring. Lid reconstruction may be necessary.

Chemical burns

Chemical burns, and especially alkali burns, can be serious because ocular penetration occurs quickly and ischaemic necrosis can result (Figure 44.24). Immediate copious irrigation until the pH is neutral will ensure that the chemical is diluted as much as possible, and all particles should be removed from the fornices. Treatment can then be continued as with thermal burns. Well-fitting goggles should prevent such injuries.

DIFFERENTIAL DIAGNOSIS OF THE ACUTE RED EYE

This is important in the management of minor ocular complaints and the recognition of conditions that require expert attention. Possible causes of the acute red eye include:

- subconjunctival haemorrhage
- conjunctivitis
- keratitis
- uveitis
- episcleritis and scleritis
- acute glaucoma.

Any condition with pain, visual impairment or a pupil abnormality suggests a more serious diagnosis.

Subconjunctival haemorrhage

This presents as a bright-red eye, often noticed incidentally, with only minimal discomfort and normal vision. Causes include coughing, sneezing, minor trauma, hypertension and, rarely, a bleeding disorder. Reassurance and treatment of the underlying cause are required. Most settle within a week, but can recur.

Conjunctivitis

Symptoms are grittiness, redness and discharge. Causes are infective, chemical, allergic or traumatic. In the newborn, it can be serious; gonococcal and chlamydial infection must be excluded. Bacterial conjunctivitis is purulent, usually self-limiting and treated with topical broad-spectrum antibiotics. Chlamydial and

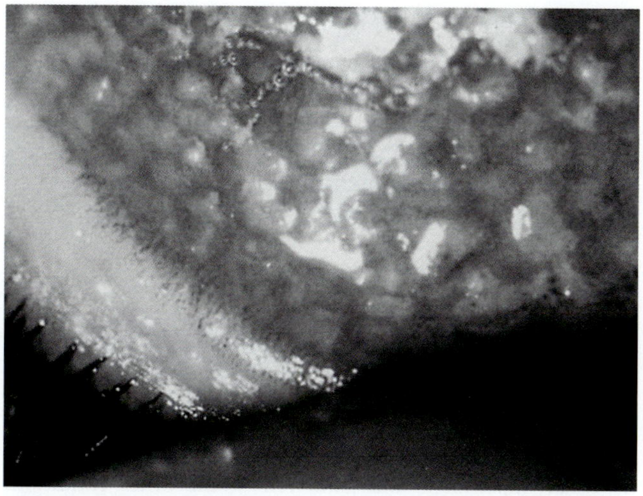

Figure 44.25 Vernal conjunctivitis (spring catarrh) showing cobblestone appearance under the upper lid.

adenovirus infections must be considered. Adenoviral infections are common and usually affect one eye much more in severity and onset, tending to be more watery than sticky, and are often associated with a palpable preauricular gland.

Vernal conjunctivitis (Figure 44.25) is a form of allergic conjunctivitis, characterised by itchy eyes, usually worse in the spring and early summer and often associated with other allergic problems such as hay fever. Clinically, most signs are under the upper lid, which may have a cobblestone appearance instead of a smooth surface.

Giant pupillary conjunctivitis with large papillae under the upper lid may be seen in soft contact lens wearers. This is usually caused by an allergy to the sterilising solutions and lens protein and may be helped by either using a preservative-free solution or using daily-wear disposable lenses.

Kaposi's sarcoma can rarely present like a subconjunctival haemorrhage (Figure 44.26).

Considerable conjunctival and corneal irritation can be caused by the lids turning in (entropion) (Figure 44.27) or turning out (ectropion) (Figures 44.28 and 44.29), and by ingrowing lashes. The lids should be repaired surgically to their normal position.

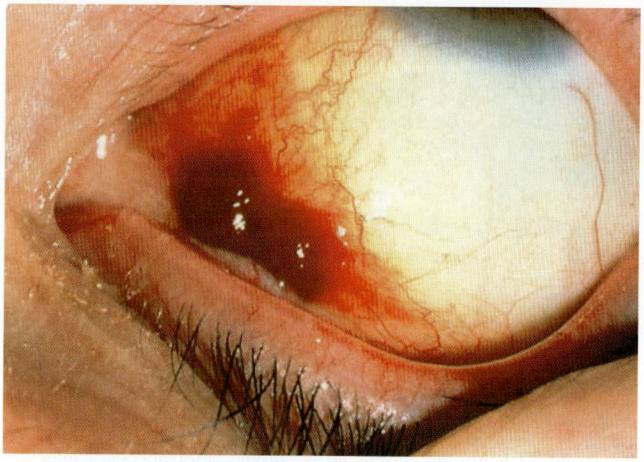

Figure 44.26 Kaposi's sarcoma of conjunctiva.

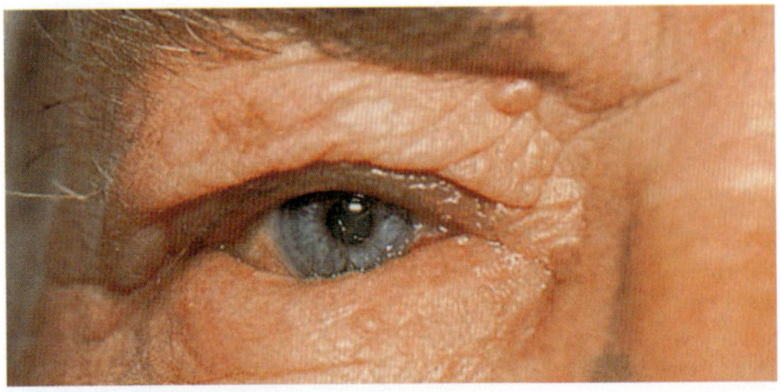

Figure 44.27 Entropion (courtesy of J Beare, FRCS).

Vision is not commonly affected in conjunctivitis but, with some viral infections, a keratitis may be present and result in visual impairment and pain. All of the other conditions described below are painful and usually affect vision.

Keratitis (inflammation of the cornea)

Herpes simplex infection presents as a dendritic (branching) ulcer, shown easily by staining with fluorescein or Bengal Rose. It is treated with aciclovir ointment five times per day. The use of steroid drops must be avoided as this can make the condition much worse (Figure 44.30).

Corneal ulceration may occur as a result of ingrowing lashes or corneal foreign bodies, marginal ulceration and infected abrasions. Infected ulcers can occur in patients wearing soft contact lenses or elderly immunocompromised individuals. Herpes zoster (shingles) may affect the ophthalmic division of the Vth nerve and can give rise to a keratitis and uveitis. It is important to avoid the use of steroid drops until a diagnosis has been made. Local anaesthetic drops should also not be given on a regular basis.

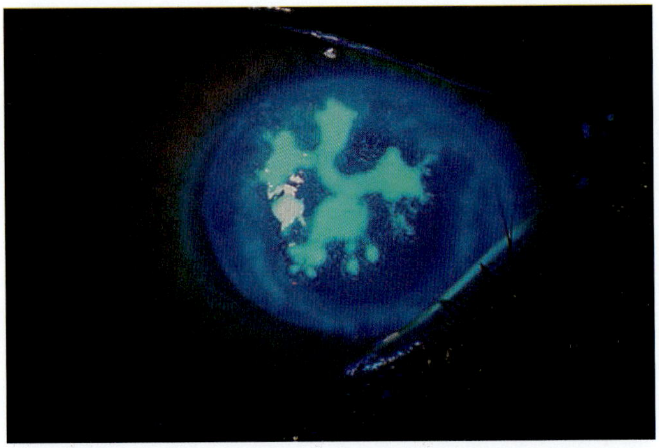

Figure 44.30 Dendritic staining caused by herpes keratitis.

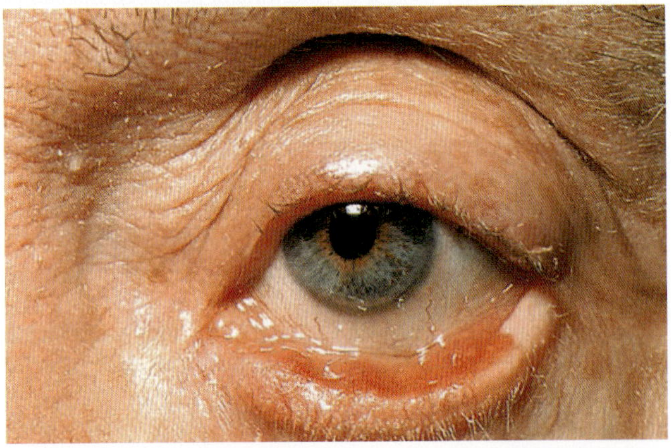

Figure 44.28 Ectropion, lower lid (courtesy of J Beare, FRCS).

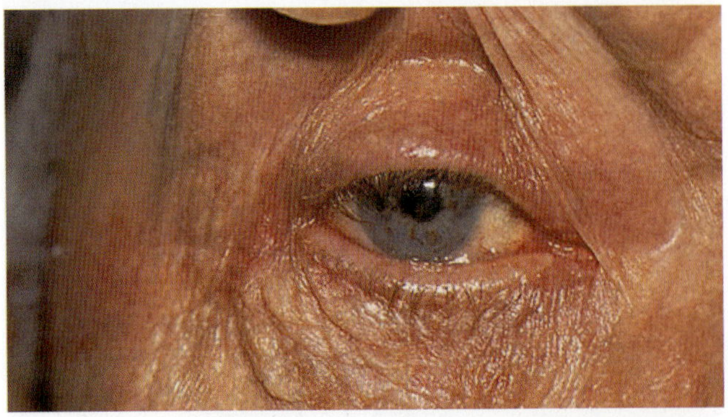

Figure 44.29 Ectropion, upper lid – chronic staphylococcal infection (courtesy of J Beare, FRCS).

Uveitis

This can be anterior (iritis) or, more rarely, posterior. In anterior uveitis, the pupil will be small, sometimes irregular, there is circumcorneal injection and there may be keratic precipitates present on the posterior surface of the cornea. Pain, photophobia and some visual loss are usually present. Posterior uveitis can present with a white eye and blurred vision. It usually takes a chronic course. Granulomatous diseases, Behçet's disease, Reiter's syndrome, toxoplasmosis and cytomegalovirus infection should be excluded. Topical systemic steroids and, sometimes, immunosuppressive drugs are useful in treating these conditions.

Episcleritis and scleritis

Episcleritis or inflammation of the episcleral tissue often occurs as an idiopathic condition (Figure 44.31).

Scleritis is a less common, more serious, condition in which the deeper sclera is involved. There is often an associated uveitis

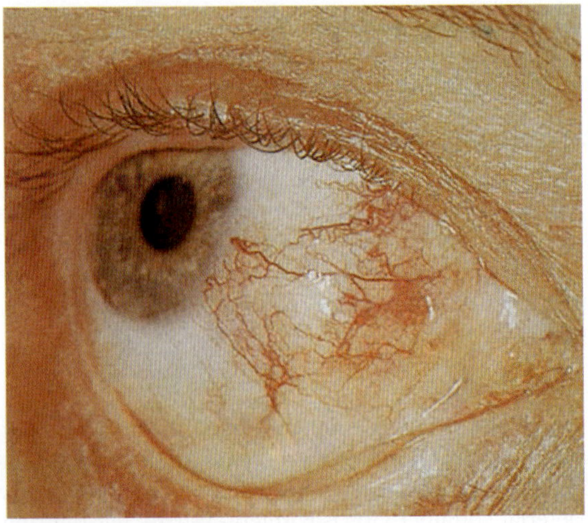

Figure 44.31 Episcleritis.

Bengal Rose (or Rose Bengal) is dichlortetraiodofluorescein.
Hulusi Behçet, 1889–1948, Professor of Dermatology, Istanbul, Turkey, described this disease in 1937.
Hans Conrad Julius Reiter, 1881–1968, President of the Health Service, and Honorary Professor of Hygiene at the University of Berlin, Germany, described this disease in 1916.

and severe pain. Thinning of the sclera may result. Systemic non-steroidal anti-inflammatory drugs (NSAIDs) or steroids may be required to treat the condition adequately.

Scleritis is often associated with severe rheumatoid conditions. The presence of scleritis suggests that there is active systemic disease and it requires systemic work-up including renal function tests.

Acute glaucoma

This usually occurs in older, often hypermetropic, patients. The cornea becomes hazy, the pupil oval, dilated and non-reacting, the vision poor and the eye feels hard. In severe cases, pain may be accompanied by vomiting and the condition can be mistaken for an acute abdominal problem. Tonometry (intraocular pressure measurement) is diagnostic. Urgent treatment to reduce the pressure with pilocarpine, acetazolamide and, if refractory, mannitol should be started, followed by YAG laser iridotomy or surgical iridectomy. The condition is usually bilateral and the second eye usually needs a prophylactic iridotomy at the same time.

Except for a simple conjunctivitis and subconjunctival haemorrhage, which are self-limiting, the management of an acute red eye requires expert treatment and a specialist opinion should be sought. A painful eye with a IIIrd nerve palsy (ptosis, dilated pupil, globe down and out) often signifies an intracranial aneurysm and should be investigated immediately.

PAINLESS LOSS OF VISION

This may occur in one or both eyes, and the visual loss may be transient or permanent. Possible causes are:

- Acute:
  - obstruction of the central retinal artery (Figure 44.32);
  - obstruction of the central retinal vein (Figure 44.33);
  - ischaemic optic neuropathy;
  - migraine and other vascular causes;
  - vitreous and retinal haemorrhages;
  - retinal detachment (Figure 44.34);
  - macular hole, cyst or haemorrhage;
  - cystoid macular oedema, often after surgery;
  - hysterical blindness.
- Chronic:
  - cataract;
  - glaucoma;
  - macular degeneration;
  - diabetic retinopathy;

Specialist help should be sought in any case of loss of vision. The erythrocyte sedimentation rate and C-reactive protein should be measured immediately if cranial arteritis is suspected, and the carotid system should be examined for bruits and other signs of arteriosclerosis in cases of ischaemic optic neuropathy and central retinal artery occlusion. Glaucoma, hypertension, hyperviscosity syndromes and diabetes should be looked for in cases of central vein thrombosis.

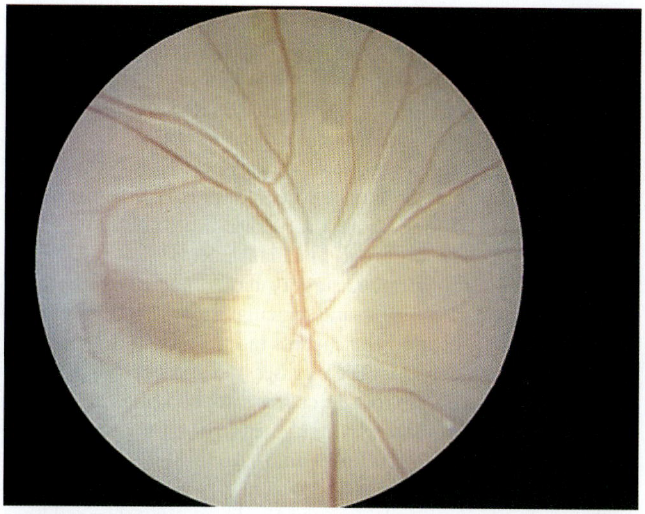

Figure 44.32 Retinal artery occlusion.

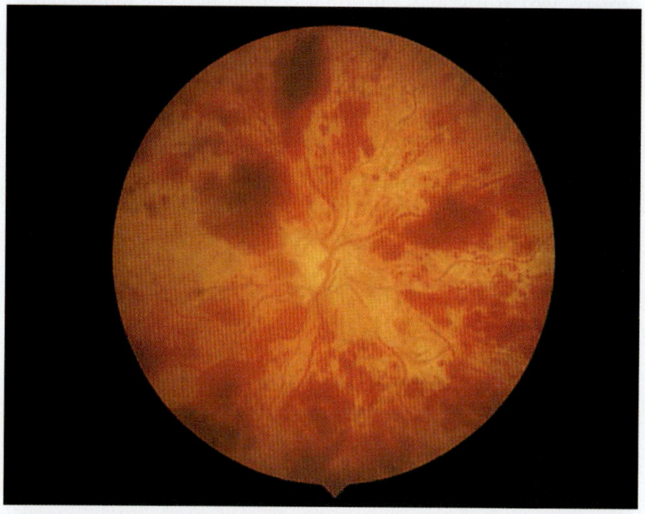

Figure 44.33 Central retinal vein occlusion.

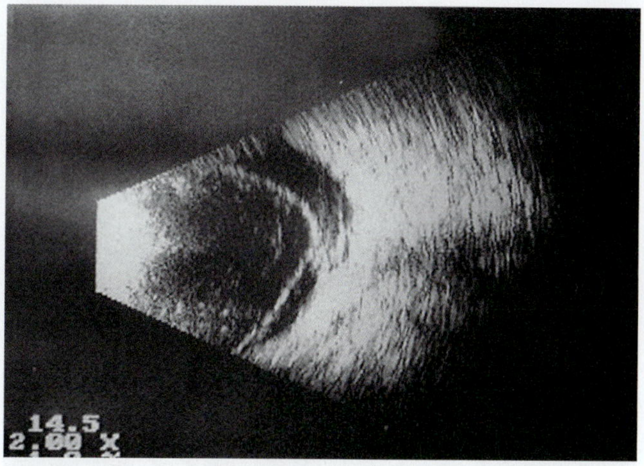

Figure 44.34 B-scan of a retinal detachment.

RECENT DEVELOPMENTS IN EYE SURGERY

In the last three decades, eye surgery has become a microsurgical specialty. Cataract surgery has been transformed by changes in local anaesthesia, implants, phacoemulsification and small-incision surgery, which allow compressible/foldable silicone or acrylic implants to be inserted through a 2-mm incision. The implant power can be more accurately measured by new formulae and the use of A-scan ultrasonography or laser wavefront biometry, and multifocal and accommodative lenses are now available.

There are new treatments for eye disorders that involve abnormal growth of blood vessels in the back of the eye, such as the wet form of age-related macular degeneration. Monoclonal anti-vascular endothelial growth factor (VEGF) antibodies, such as the drug ranibizumab, may be injected directly into the vitreous cavity to reduce new vessel proliferation. Intravitreal steroid injections help to treat cystoid macular oedema.

Developments in vitreous surgery have enabled membranes to be peeled off the retina and macular holes to be repaired. They have also increased the success rate in retinal detachment surgery with the additional use of gases and silicone oil or heavy liquid inserted into the vitreous cavity tamponading the retina.

Some paralytic squints can be helped by the use of adjustable sutures or injections of botulinum toxin into the overacting muscles.

Refractive errors can be treated by the excimer laser. These can be combined with laser *in situ* keratomeilusis (LASIK) surgery, which involves cutting a corneal flap (by femtosecond laser or surgery) and performing the laser surgery at a deeper level. There have been some concerns about defective contrast sensitivity and problems with night vision after laser correction of myopia. Phakic implants have also been used to correct high refractive errors. Corneal topography aids the accuracy of corneal and refractive surgery and the increased use and quality of CT and MRI scans has revolutionised the diagnosis of orbital and intracranial lesions involving the optic pathways (Figures 44.35, 44.36 and 44.37).

Fluorescein angiography, and ocular coherence tomography (OCT) are invaluable in the diagnosis and treatment of macular conditions. The glaucoma detection (GDx) retinal nerve fibre analyser and Heidelberg retinal tomography (HRT) are increasingly used in the diagnosis and management of glaucoma.

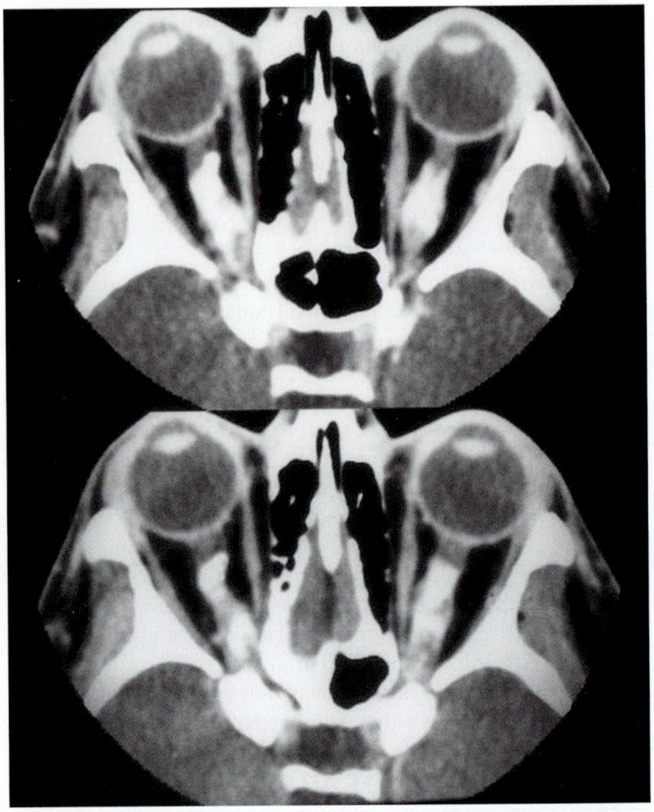

Figure 44.36 High-resolution computed tomography through the orbits showing dense calcification of the optic nerve sheaths typical of optic nerve meningioma (courtesy of Dr Juliette Britton).

LASERS IN OPHTHALMOLOGY

Argon blue–green or diode laser is used to treat the retina in diabetic retinopathy (pan-retinal photocoagulation from proliferative disease or focal treatment for leaky microaneurysms),

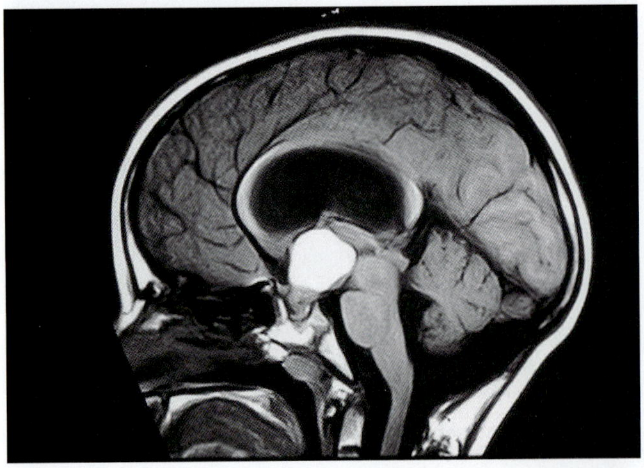

Figure 44.35 Magnetic resonance imaging scan, sagittal view. Craniopharyngioma. The mass in the suprasellar cistern is of high signal intensity because of the proteinaceous fluid that the cyst contains (courtesy of Dr Juliette Britton).

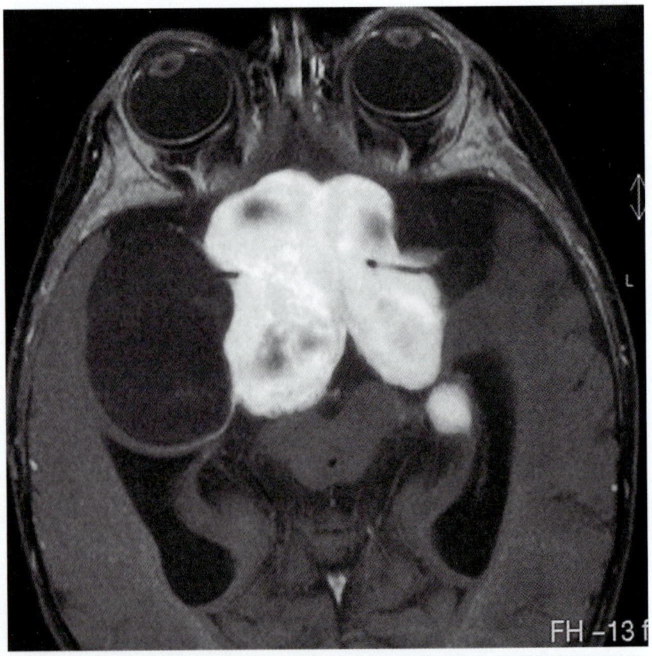

Figure 44.37 Axial enhanced magnetic resonance imaging scan showing a mass involving the optic chiasma and extending down the optic nerves and tracts.

and is also used to close retinal tears or breaks that might lead to retinal detachment.

Argon laser or selective laser trabeculoplasty can be used to open the drainage angle to control elevated intraocular pressure in open angle glaucoma. Trans-scleral diode photocoagulation of the ciliary body is used to treat refactory secondary glaucoma with uncontrolled ocular pressure.

Laser iridotomy with the Nd:YAG laser is used to treat both the affected and fellow eye in acute angle closure glaucoma. The Nd:YAG laser is also used to photodisrupt and clean an opaque posterior capsule which occurs in 5–10 per cent of cases following cataract surgery.

SURGICAL PROCEDURES

Excision of an eyeball/enucleation

Indications include a blind, painful eye, a blind, cosmetically poor eye/intraocular neoplasm and, in cadavers, for use in corneal grafting.

The operation

The speculum is introduced between the lids and opened. The conjunctiva is picked up with toothed forceps and divided completely all round as near as possible to the cornea. Tenon's capsule is entered and each of the four rectus and two oblique muscle tendons is hooked up on a strabismus hook and divided close to the sclera. The speculum is now pressed backwards and the eyeball projects forwards. Blunt scissors, curved on the flat, are insinuated on the inner side of the globe, and these are used to sever the optic nerve. The eyeball can now be drawn forwards with the forceps, and the oblique muscles, together with any other strands of tissue that are still attaching the globe to the orbit, are divided. A swab, moistened with hot water and pressed into the orbit, will control the haemorrhage. If an orbital implant is inserted to give better eye movement, the muscles are sutured to the implant at the appropriate sites. The subconjunctival tissues and conjunctiva are closed in layers.

Evisceration of an eyeball

Evisceration is preferred to excision in endophthalmitis, minimising the risk of orbital and intracranial spread with meningitis. The sclera is transfixed with a pointed knife a little behind the corneosclerotic junction, and the cornea is removed entirely by completing the encircling incision in the sclera. The contents of the globe are then removed with a curette, care being exercised to remove all of the uveal tract. At the end of the operation the interior must appear perfectly white. A ball orbital implant made of acrylic or hydroxyapatite is placed within the orbit behind the sclera to improve the appearance when the artificial eye is fitted.

Incision and curettage of chalazion (meibomian cyst)

The lid margin is everted to allow the application of a meibomian clamp. The ring of the clamp is placed on the palpebral conjunctiva with the granuloma in the centre. An incision is made with a small blade in the axis of the gland. The herniating granulomatous tissue is removed with a curette and the cavity is scraped clean. Recurrent cysts may have to have the cyst wall dissected away with scissors. A biopsy may be necessary in atypical or recurrent cysts to exclude malignant change.

FURTHER READING

Findlay RD, Payne PAG. *The eye in general practice*, 10th edn. Oxford: Butterworth-Heinemann, 1997.

Kanski J, Bowling B. *Clinical ophthalmology: a systematic approach*, 7th edn. Philadelphia, PA: Saunders, 2011.

Kline LB, Bajandas FJ. *Neuro-ophthalmology review manual*, 6th edn. Thorofare, NJ: Slack Incorporated, 2008.

Olver J, Cassidy L. *Ophthalmology at a glance*. Oxford: Blackwell Publishing, 2005.

Wills Eye Hospital. *The Wills eye manual: office and emergency room diagnosis and treatment of eye disease*, 6th edn. Philadelphia, PA: Lippincott Williams & Wilkins, 2012.

Jacques Rene Tenon, 1724–1816, surgeon, La Salpêtrière, Paris, France.

CHAPTER

45

Cleft lip and palate: developmental abnormalities of the face, mouth and jaws

LEARNING OBJECTIVES

To understand:

- The aetiology and classification of cleft lip and palate
- The principles of reconstruction of cleft lip and palate
- The key features of the perioperative care of the child with cleft lip and palate
- The associated complications of cleft lip and palate and their management

INTRODUCTION

Clefts of the lip, alveolus and hard and soft palate are the most common congenital abnormalities of the orofacial structures. They frequently occur as isolated deformities, but can be associated with other medical conditions, particularly congenital heart disease. They are also an associated feature in over 300 recognised syndromes.

All children born with a cleft lip and palate need a thorough paediatric assessment to exclude other congenital abnormalities. In certain circumstances, genetic counselling must be sought if a syndrome is suspected.

INCIDENCE

The incidence of cleft lip and palate is 1:600 live births and of isolated cleft palate is 1:1000 live births. The incidence increases in Oriental groups (1:500) and decreases in the black population (1:2000). The highest incidence reported for cleft lip and palate occurs in the Indian tribes of Montana, USA (1:276).

Although cleft lip and palate is an extremely diverse and variable congenital abnormality, several distinct subgroups exist, namely cleft lip with/without cleft palate (CL/P), cleft palate (CP) alone and submucous cleft palate (SMCP).

The typical distribution of cleft types is:

- cleft lip alone: 15 per cent;
- cleft lip and palate: 45 per cent;
- isolated cleft palate: 40 per cent.

Cleft lip/palate predominates in males, whereas cleft palate alone appears to be more common in females. In unilateral cleft lip, the deformity affects the left side in 60 per cent of cases.

AETIOLOGY

Contemporary opinion on the aetiology of cleft lip and palate is that cleft lip and palate and isolated cleft palate have a genetic predisposition and a contributory environmental component. A family history of cleft lip and palate in which the first-degree relative is affected increases the risk to 1:25 live births. Genetic influence is more significant in cleft lip/palate than cleft palate alone, in which environmental factors exert a greater influence.

Environmental factors implicated in clefting include maternal epilepsy and drugs, e.g. steroids, diazepam and phenytoin. The role of antenatal folic acid supplements in preventing cleft lip and palate remains equivocal.

Although most clefts of the lip and palate occur as an isolated deformity, Pierre Robin sequence remains the most common syndrome. This syndrome comprises isolated cleft palate, retrognathia and a posteriorly displaced tongue (glossoptosis), which is associated with early respiratory and feeding difficulties.

Isolated cleft palate is more commonly associated with a syndrome than cleft lip/palate and cleft lip alone. Over 150 syndromes are associated with cleft lip and palate, although Stickler's (ophthalmic and musculoskeletal abnormalities), Shprintzen's (cardiac anomalies), Down's, Apert's and Treacher Collins' syndromes are most frequently encountered (Summary box 45.1).

Summary box 45.1

Cleft lip and palate

- Associated with other congenital abnormalities
- Incidence varies between races from 1:300 to 1:2000 live births
- Aetiology is both genetic and environmental

Pierre Robin, 1867–1950, professor, The French School of Dentistry, Paris, France, described this syndrome in 1929.
Gunnar B Stickler, 1925–2010, born in Germany, Chair of Section of Paediatrics and later Paediatric Cardiology, The Mayo Clinic, Rochester, MN, USA.
Robert J Shprintzen, born 1946, surgeon, Syracuse, NY, USA.
John Langdon Haydon Down (sometimes given as Langdon-Brown), 1828–1896, physician, The London Hospital, UK, published the classification of aments in 1866.
Eugene Apert, 1868–1940, physician, L'Hopital des Infants-Malades, Paris, France, described this syndrome in 1906.
Edward Treacher Collins, 1862–1932, ophthalmic surgeon, the Royal London Ophthalmic Hospital, and Charing Cross Hospital, London, UK, described this syndrome in 1900.

ANATOMY OF CLEFT LIP AND PALATE

Cleft lip

The abnormalities in cleft lip are the direct consequence of disruption of the muscles of the upper lip and nasolabial region. The facial muscles (Figure 45.1) can be divided into three muscular rings of Delaire: the nasolabial muscle ring surrounds the nasal aperture; the bilabial muscle ring surrounds the oral aperture; and the labiomental muscle ring envelops the lower lip and chin regions.

Unilateral cleft lip

In the unilateral cleft lip, the nasolabial and bilabial muscle rings are disrupted on one side resulting in an asymmetrical deformity involving the external nasal cartilages, nasal septum and anterior maxilla (premaxilla) (Figure 45.2a and b). These deformities influence the mucocutaneous tissues causing a displacement of nasal skin onto the lip and a retraction of labial skin, as well as changes to the vermilion and lip mucosa. All these changes need to be considered in planning the surgical repair of the unilateral cleft lip.

Bilateral cleft lip

In the bilateral cleft lip, the deformity is more profound but symmetrical. The two superior muscular rings are disrupted on both sides producing a flaring of the nose (caused by lack of nasolabial muscle continuity), a protrusive premaxilla and an area of skin in front of the premaxilla devoid of muscle, known as the prolabium (Figure 45.3a and b). As in the unilateral cleft lip, the muscular, cartilaginous and skeletal deformities influence the mucocutaneous tissues, which must be respected in planning the repair of the bilateral cleft lip.

Cleft palate

Embryologically, the **primary** palate consists of all anatomical structures anterior to the incisive foramen, namely the alveolus and upper lip. The **secondary** palate is defined as the remainder of the palate behind the incisive foramen, divided into the hard palate and, more posteriorly, the soft palate.

Cleft palate results in failure of fusion of the two palatine shelves. This failure may be confined to the soft palate alone or involve both hard and soft palate. When the cleft of the hard palate remains attached to the nasal septum and vomer, the cleft is termed **incomplete**. When the nasal septum and vomer are completely separated from the palatine processes, the cleft palate is termed **complete** (Summary box 45.2).

> **Summary box 45.2**
>
> **Types of cleft palate**
>
> - May involve the soft palate or the soft and hard palate
> - It is complete when nasal septum and vomer are separated from the palatine process

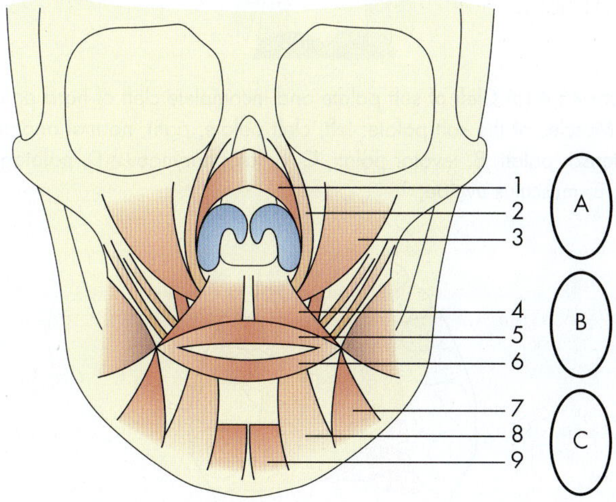

Figure 45.1 The muscle chains of the face: frontal view. The nasal cartilages are represented in blue. A, nasolabial (muscles 1–3); B, bilabial (muscles 4–6); C, labiomental (muscles 7–9); 1, transverse nasalis; 2, levator labii superioris alaeque nasi; 3, levator labii superioris; 4, orbicularis oris (oblique head) – upper lip; 5, orbicularis oris (horizontal head) – upper lip; 6, orbicularis oris – lower lip; 7, depressor anguli oris; 8, depressor labii inferioris; 9, mentalis.

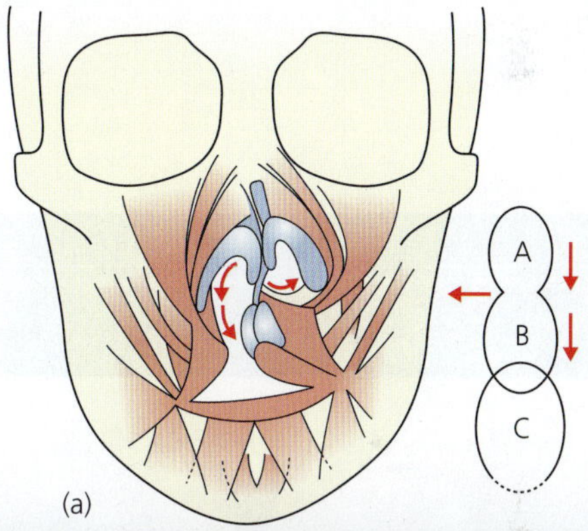

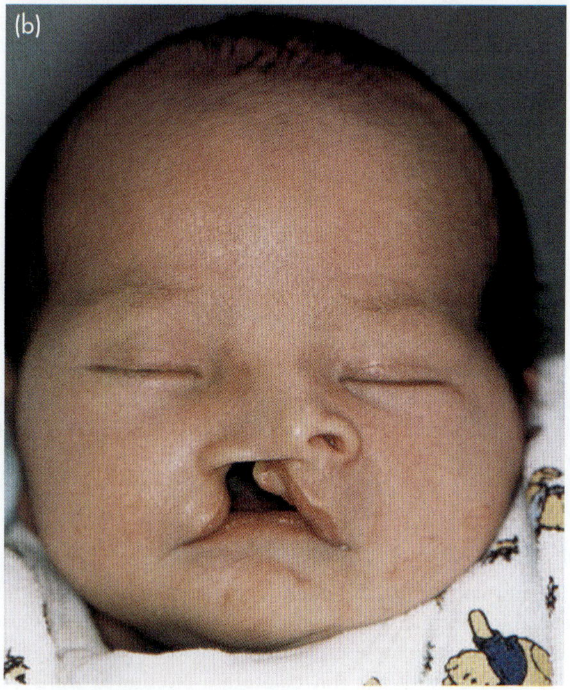

Figure 45.2 (a) Schematic representation of disruption of the nasolabial and bilabial muscle chains in unilateral (left) cleft lip. A, nasolabial; B, bilabial; C, labiomental. (b) Unilateral cleft lip before muscular reconstruction.

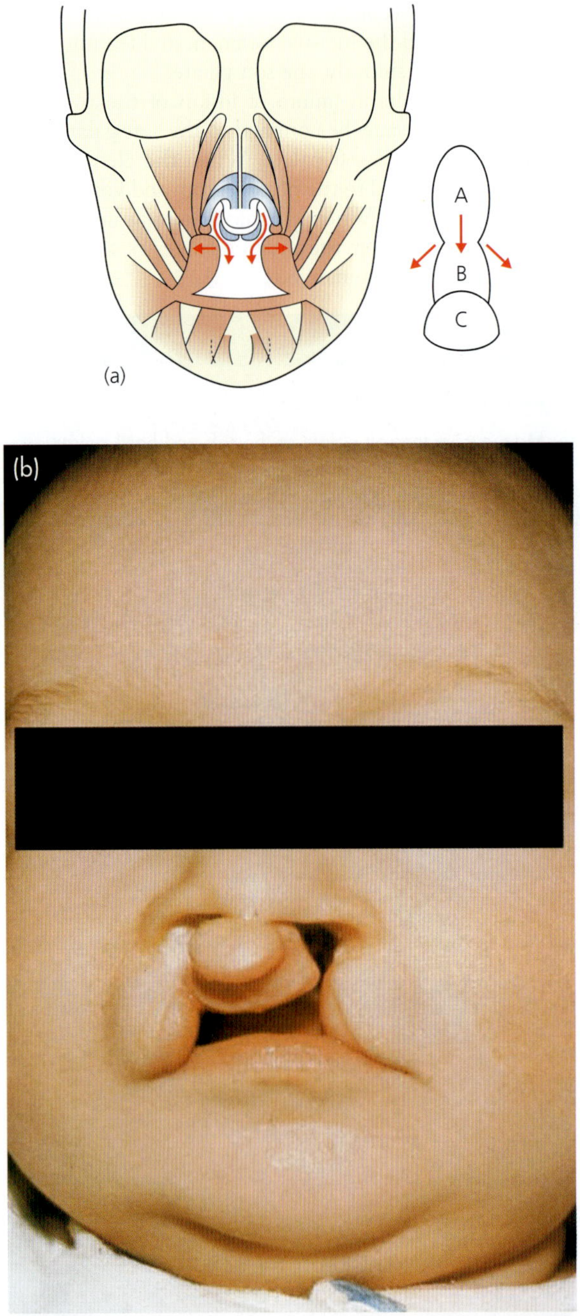

Figure 45.3 (a) Schematic representation of disruption of the nasolabial and bilabial muscle chains in bilateral cleft lip. A, nasolabial; B, bilabial; C, labiomental. (b) Bilateral cleft lip before muscular reconstruction.

Soft palate

In the normal soft palate, closure of the velopharynx, which is essential for normal speech, is achieved by five different muscles functioning in a complete but coordinated fashion. In general, the muscle fibres of the soft palate are orientated transversely with no significant attachment to the hard palate.

In a cleft of the soft palate (Figure 45.4a) the muscle fibres are orientated in an anteroposterior direction, inserting into the posterior edge of the hard palate (Figure 45.4b).

Hard palate

The normal hard palate can be divided into three anatomical and physiological zones (Figure 45.5). The central **palatal fibromucosa** is very thin and lies directly below the floor of nose. The **maxillary fibromucosa** is thick and contains the greater palatine neurovascular bundle. The **gingival fibromucosa** lies more lateral and adjacent to the teeth.

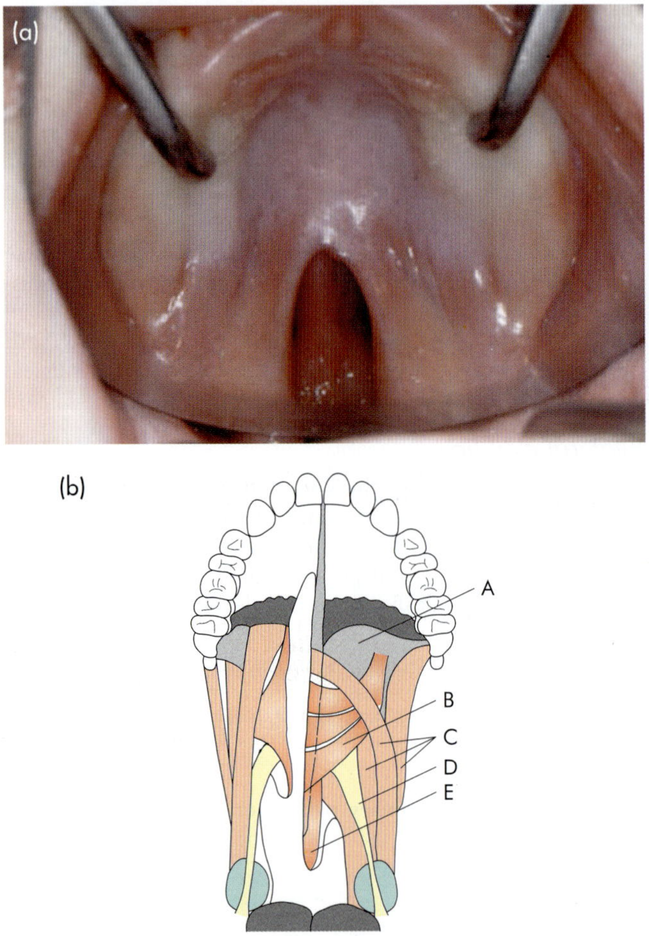

Figure 45.4 (a) Cleft of soft palate and incomplete cleft of hard palate. (b) Muscles of the soft palate: left, cleft palate; right, normal anatomy. A, tensor palati; B, levator palati; C, palatopharyngeus; D, palatoglossus; E, musculus uvulae.

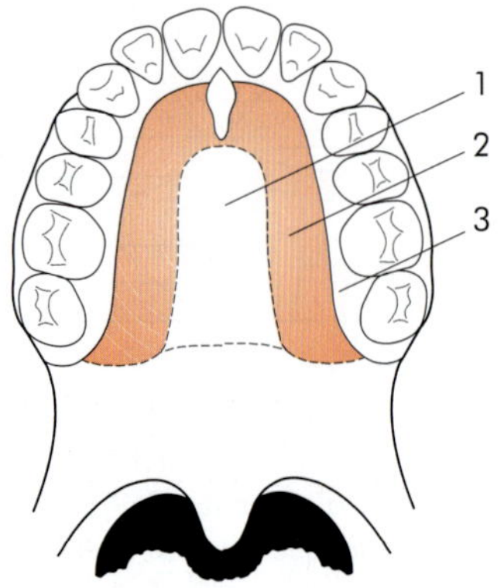

Figure 45.5 The three mucosal zones of the hard palate. 1, palatal fibromucosa; 2, maxillary fibromucosa; 3, gingival fibromucosa.

Jean Delaire, Professor of Stomatology and Maxillofacial Surgery, University of Nantes, Nantes, France from 1960 until 1991.

In performing surgical closure of cleft palate the changes associated with the cleft must be understood to obtain an anatomical and functional repair. In complete cleft palate, the median part of the palatal vault is absent and the palatal fibromucosa is reduced in size. The maxillary and gingival fibromucosa are not modified in thickness, width or position.

CLASSIFICATION

Any classification for such a diverse and varied condition as cleft lip and palate needs to be simple, concise, flexible and exact but graphic. It must be suitable for computerisation but descriptive and morphological. An example of such a classification is the LAHSHAL system, which is able to describe site, size and extent, as well as type of cleft (Figure 45.6).

Complete clefts of the lip, alveolus and hard and soft palate are designated as capitals L, A, H and S, respectively. Incomplete clefts are recorded in lower case letters whereas microform clefts are documented with asterisks. Hence, LAHSHAL is the anatomical paraphrase of a complete bilateral cleft lip and palate. Another example, lahSh, represents an incomplete right unilateral cleft lip and alveolus with a complete cleft of soft palate extending partly onto the hard palate.

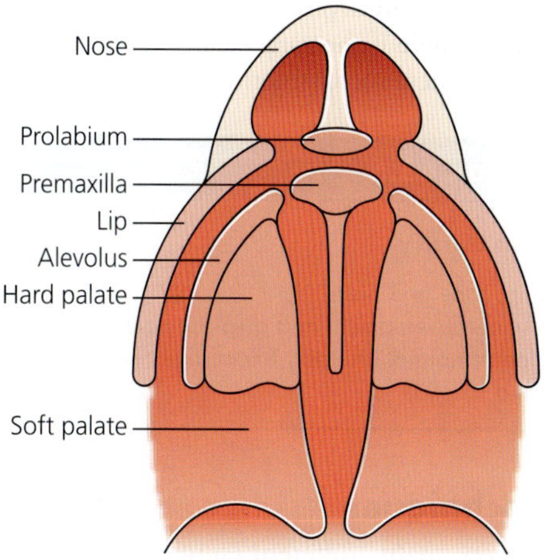

Figure 45.6 LAHSAL: an anatomical representation of cleft lip (L), alveolus (A) and hard (H) and soft palate (S).

PRIMARY MANAGEMENT

Antenatal diagnosis

An antenatal diagnosis of cleft lip, whether unilateral or bilateral, is possible by ultrasound scan after 18 weeks of gestation. Isolated cleft palate cannot be diagnosed by antenatal scan. When an antenatal diagnosis is confirmed, referral to a cleft surgeon is appropriate for counselling to allay fears. Photographs of cleft lip shown to parents 'before and after' surgery are invaluable. Introduction to a parent support group and meeting parents of a child with a similar cleft who has undergone surgery may also be extremely helpful (Summary box 45.3).

> **Summary box 45.3**
>
> **Antenatal diagnosis and counselling**
>
> - All but isolated cleft palate can be diagnosed by ultrasound scan after 18 weeks' gestation
> - Parents will need counselling and support

Feeding

Most babies born with cleft lip and palate feed well and thrive, provided that appropriate advice is given and support is available. Some mothers are successful in breastfeeding, particularly when the cleft is incomplete and confined to the lip. Good feeding patterns can be established with soft bottles (e.g. Mead Johnson) and modified teats (orthodontic, Nuyk). Simple measures, such as enlarging the hole in the teat, often suffice. Feeding plates, constructed from a dental impression of the upper jaw, are rarely necessary to improve feeding. Some babies are provided with an active plate that aims not only to improve feeding but also reduce the width of the cleft lip and palate prior to surgery. The long-term benefit of such a regime remains unproven.

Airway

Major respiratory obstruction is uncommon and occurs exclusively in babies with Pierre Robin sequence. Hypoxic episodes during sleep and feeding can be life-threatening. Intermittent airway obstruction is more frequent and is managed by nursing the baby prone. More severe and persistent airway compromise can be managed by 'retained nasopharyngeal intubation' to maintain the airway. Surgical adhesion of the tongue to the lower lip (labioglossopexy) in the first few days after birth is an alternative but less commonly practised method of management (Summary box 45.4).

> **Summary box 45.4**
>
> **Problems immediately after birth**
>
> - Some babies are able to feed normally but some will need assistance
> - Breathing problems in Pierre Robin sequence may be life-threatening

PRINCIPLES OF CLEFT SURGERY

The ultimate goal in cleft lip and palate management is a patient with a normal appearance of lip, nose and face, whose speech is normal and whose dentition and facial growth fall within the range of normal development.

Surgical techniques are aimed at restoring normal anatomy. With the exception of rare conditions such as holoprosencephaly, there is no true hypoplasia of the tissues involved on either side of the cleft. There is, however, displacement, deformation and underdevelopment of the muscles and facial skeleton. Emphasis is placed on muscular reconstruction of the lip, nose and face, as well as muscles of the soft palate. Normal or near-normal anatomy promotes normal function, thereby encouraging normal growth and development of lip, nose, palate and facial skeleton. An in-depth understanding of the anatomy of the cleft is invaluable if the surgeon is to achieve normal, or near-normal, anatomical reconstruction (Summary box 45.5).

Summary box 45.5

Surgical anatomy

- Normal lip, face and nose
- There is underdevelopment and displacement of the muscles
- Restoration of normal anatomy encourages normal facial growth and function

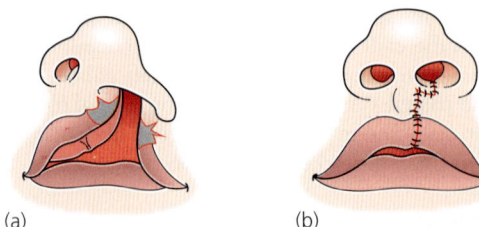

(a) (b)

Figure 45.7 (a and b) Skin incisions (highlighted in red) for left unilateral complete cleft lip (after Delaire).

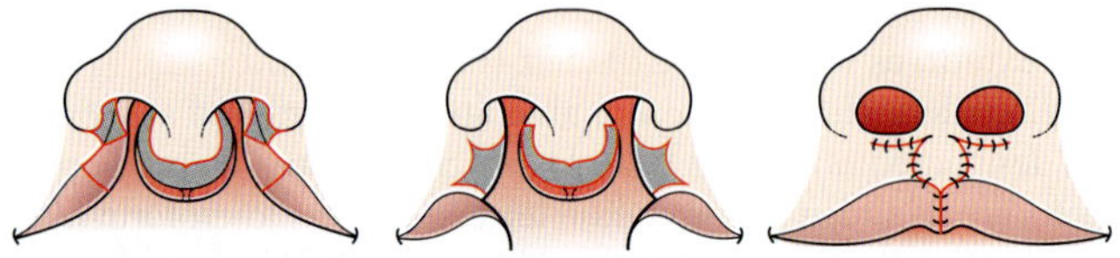

(a) (b) (c)

Figure 45.8 (a–c) Skin incisions for bilateral complete cleft lip, showing the shaded area from Figure 45.7a. Areas for removal of excess mucosa (a) or skin (b) (after Delaire).

Surgical techniques

There have been many different surgical techniques and sequences advocated in cleft lip and palate management. Cleft lip repair is commonly performed between three and six months of age, whereas cleft palate repair is frequently performed between six and 18 months.

The Delaire technique and sequence (Table 45.1) is one of many regimes currently practised.

Cleft lip surgery

Skin incisions (Figures 45.7 and 45.8) are developed to restore displaced tissues, including skin and cartilage, to their normal position, while gaining access to the facial, nasal and lip musculature.

Table 45.1 Timing of primary cleft lip and palate procedures (after Delaire).

Cleft lip alone		
Unilateral (one side)	One operation at 5–6 months	
Bilateral (both sides)	One operation at 4–5 months	
Cleft palate alone		
Soft palate only	One operation at 6 months	
Soft and hard palate	Two operations	Soft palate at 6 months
		Hard palate at 15–18 months
Cleft lip and palate		
Unilateral	Two operations	Cleft lip and soft palate at 5–6 months
		Hard palate and gum pad with or without lip revision at 15–18 months
Bilateral	Two operations	Cleft lip and soft palate at 4–5 months
		Hard palate and gum pad with or without lip revision at 15–18 months

Muscular continuity is achieved by subperiosteal undermining over the anterior maxilla. Nasolabial muscles are anchored to the premaxilla with non-resorbable sutures. Oblique muscles of orbicularis oris are sutured to the base of the anterior nasal spine and cartilaginous nasal septum. Closure of the cleft lip is completed by suturing the horizontal fibres of orbicularis oris to achieve a functioning oral sphincter (Figures 45.9 and 45.10).

When the cleft lip is incomplete (Figures 45.11a and 45.12a), meticulous assessment of the cleft deformity is of paramount importance, as complete muscle disruption may be present leading to nasal and skeletal deformity. Full muscular exposure and reconstruction is imperative in many incomplete clefts if facial symmetry is to be achieved (Figures 45.11b and 45.12b).

Cleft palate surgery

Cleft palate closure can be achieved by one- or two-stage palatoplasty. The surgical principle is mobilisation and reconstruction of the aberrant soft palate musculature (Figure 45.13a and b), together with closure of the residual hard palate cleft by minimal dissection and subsequent scar formation (Figure 45.14a and b). Excess scar formation in the palate adversely affects growth and development of the maxilla. The philosophy of two-stage closure encourages a physiological narrowing of the hard palate cleft to minimise surgical dissection at the time of the second procedure (Summary box 45.6).

Summary box 45.6

Principles of surgery

- Cleft lip surgery attaches and reconnects the muscles around the oral sphincter
- Cleft palate surgery aims to bring together mucosa and muscles with minimal scarring
- Two-stage procedures attempt to minimise dissection

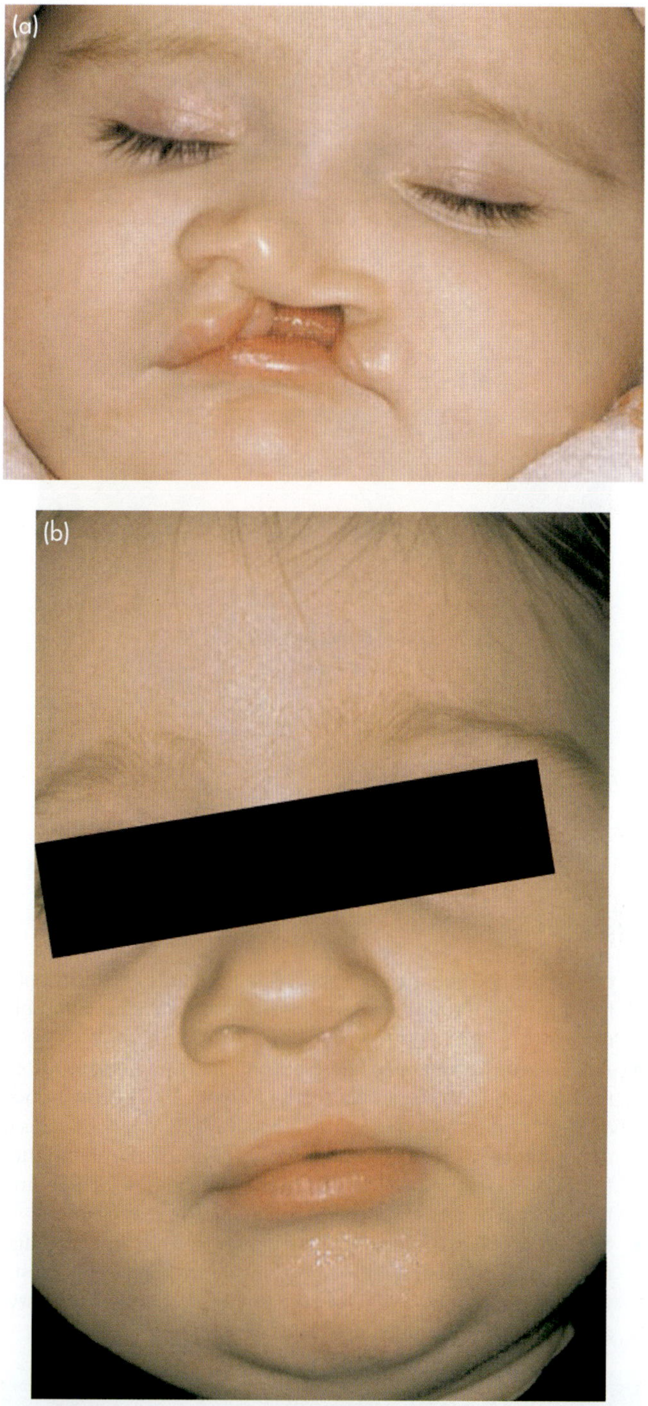

Figure 45.9 Unilateral complete cleft lip before (a) and after (b) muscular reconstruction.

SECONDARY MANAGEMENT

Following primary surgery, regular review by a multidisciplinary team is essential. Many aspects of cleft care require long-term review:

- hearing
- speech
- dental development
- facial growth.

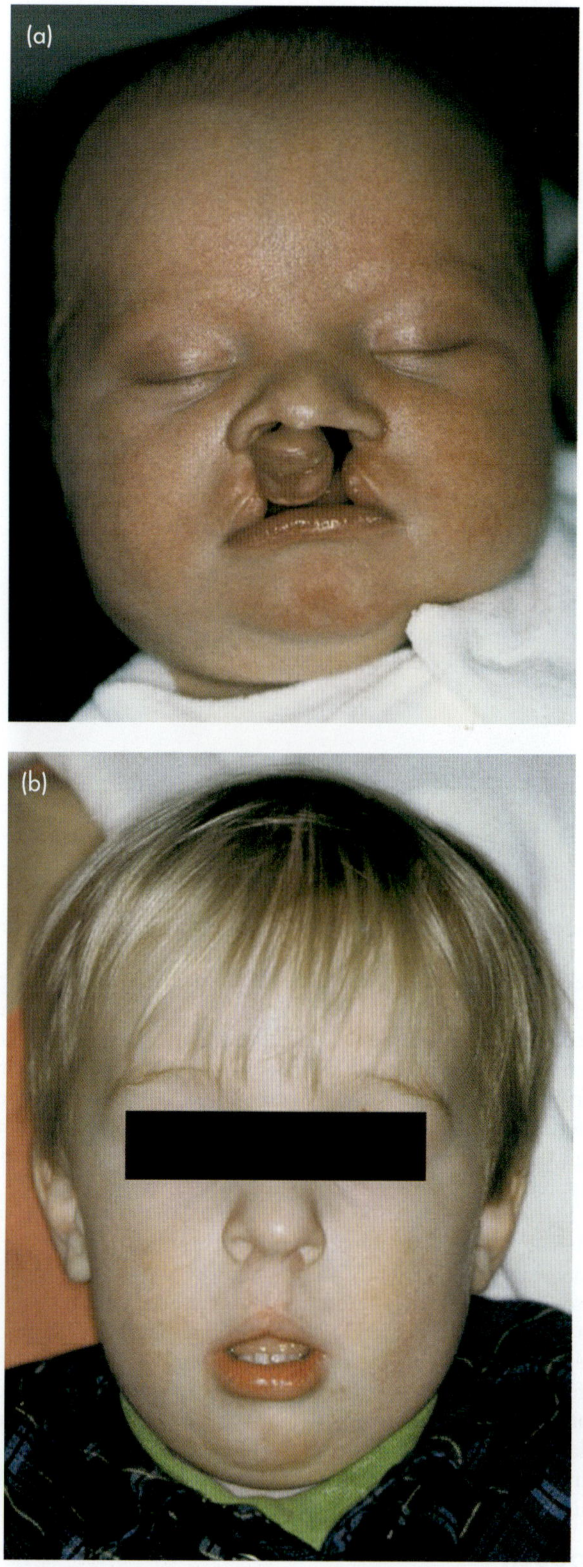

Figure 45.10 Bilateral cleft lip before (a) and after (b) muscular reconstruction.

Hearing

Eustachian tube dysfunction plays a central role in the pathogenesis of otitis media with effusion in babies and children born with a cleft palate. Children with a cleft lip alone exhibit

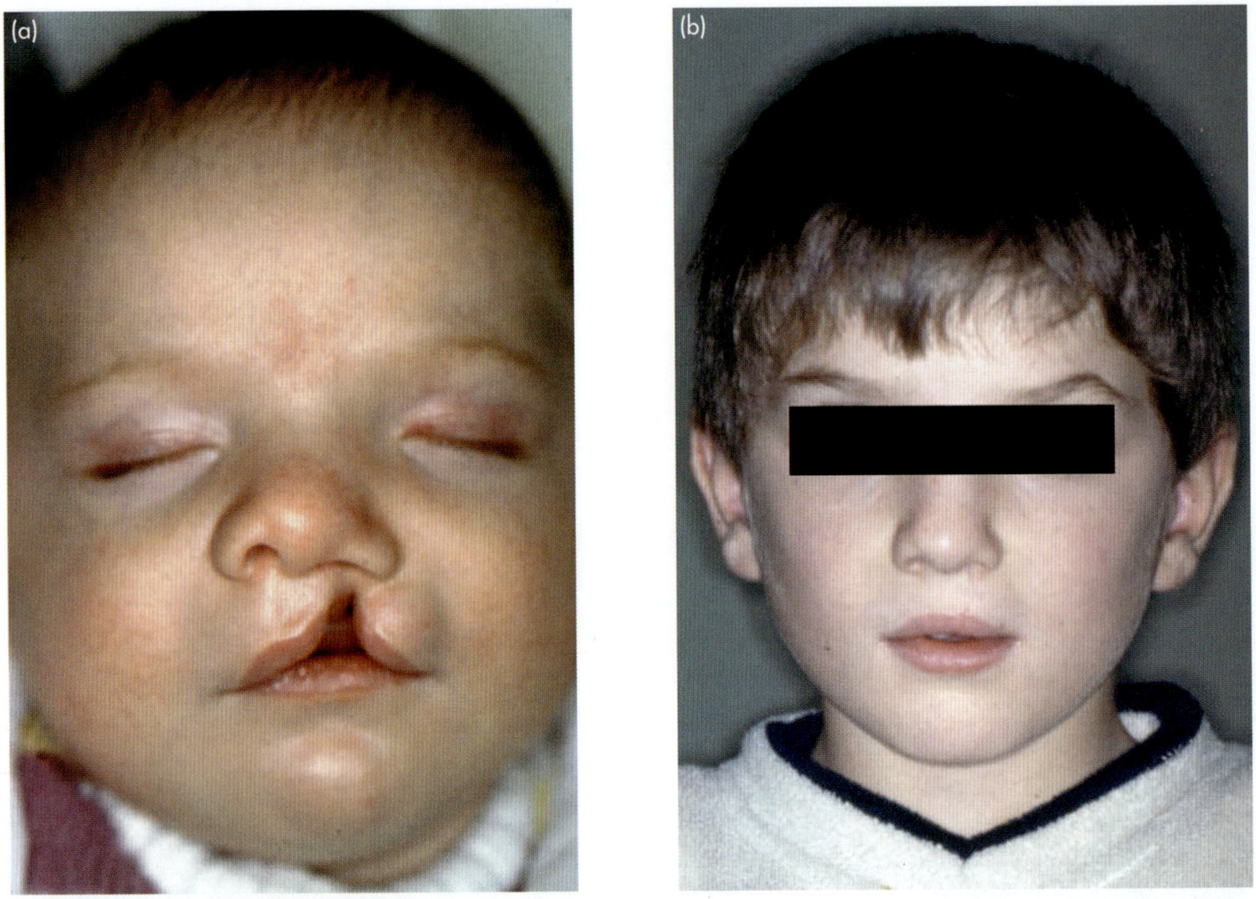

Figure 45.11 Unilateral incomplete cleft lip before (a) and after (b) muscle reconstruction.

the same frequency of otitis media as their age-matched non-cleft counterparts. It has been recently recognised that a child with a craniofacial anomaly including cleft lip and palate is at increased risk of a sensorineural hearing deficit. All children born with a cleft lip and palate should undergo assessment before 12 months of age for **sensorineural and conductive hearing loss** by auditory brainstem responses (ABR) and tympanometry, respectively.

Sensorineural hearing loss is managed with a hearing aid whereas the management of secretory otitis media remains more controversial. Early (6–12 months) prophylactic myringotomy and grommet insertion temporarily eliminates middle ear effusion. Regular audiological testing may be as appropriate, reserving surgery for established secretory otitis media with infection. No firm evidence is available to support the interventional approach over the conservative regime. Nevertheless, the relationship between hearing loss and potential speech problems remains important. Regular audiological assessment during childhood is of utmost importance.

Speech

Initial speech assessment should be performed early (18 months) and repeated regularly to ensure that problems are identified early and managed appropriately.

Common speech problems associated with cleft lip and palate are:

- **Velopharyngeal incompetence**. This is associated with increased nasal airflow and resonance, producing a nasal or 'hypernasal' quality to speech. It frequently reflects poor function of the soft palate associated with inadequate muscle repair.
- **Articulation problems**. These arise either as a compensatory mechanism to overcome velopharyngeal incompetence or, less commonly, are caused by jaw/dental and occlusal abnormalities. Videofluoroscopy, nasal airflow studies (aerophonoscopy) and nasendoscopy are helpful in defining the exact mechanism of the problem, aiding management.
- **Speech problems**. These are managed by speech and language therapy; secondary palatal surgery, either intravelar veloplasty (muscular reconstruction of soft palate) or pharyngoplasty; and speech training devices (Summary box 45.7).

Summary box 45.7

Associated hearing and speech problems

- Higher incidence of sensorineural and conductive hearing loss
- Regular hearing tests are important if speech is to develop normally
- Speech problems may result from airflow problems

Dental

Dental anomalies are common findings in children with cleft lip and/or palate. Various phenomena including delayed tooth development, delayed eruption of teeth and morphological

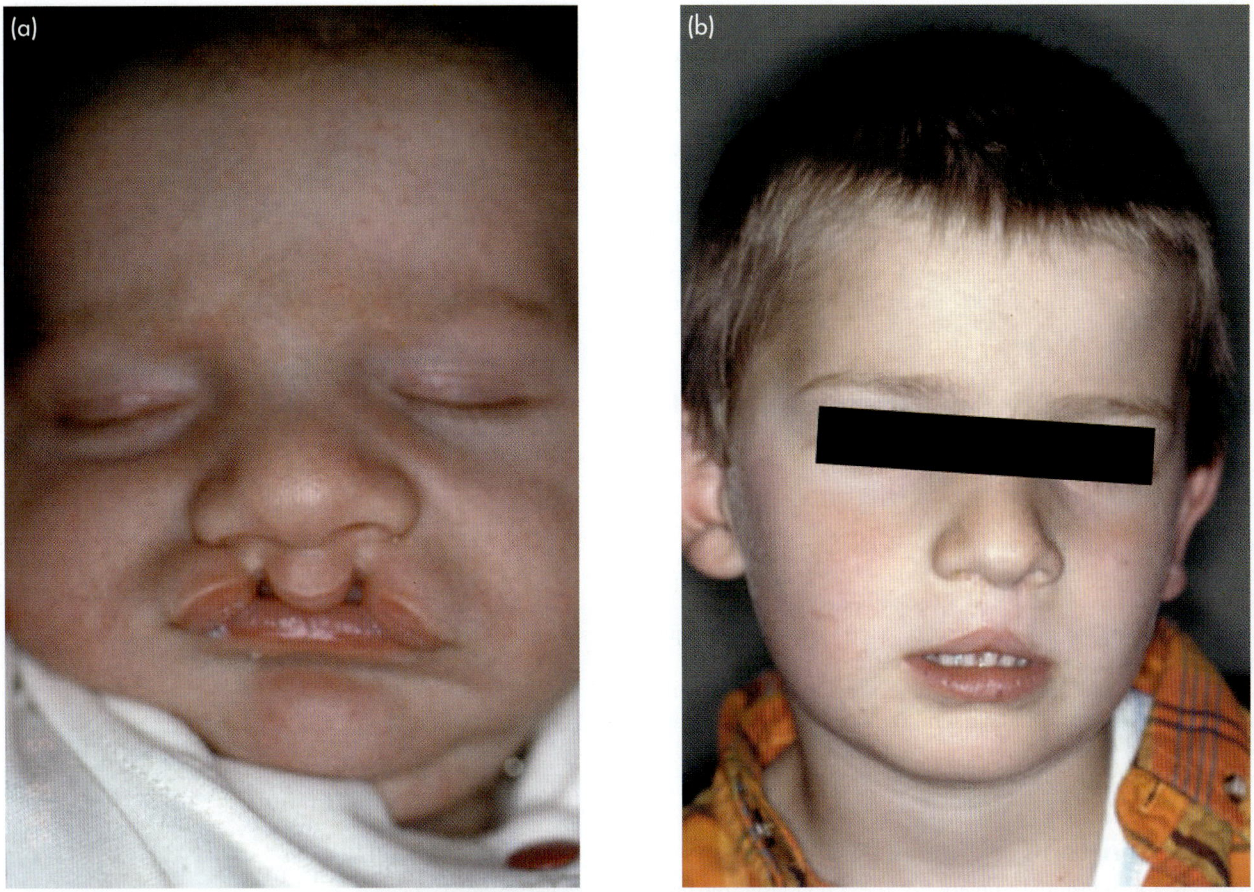

Figure 45.12 Bilateral incomplete cleft lip before (a) and after (b) muscular reconstruction.

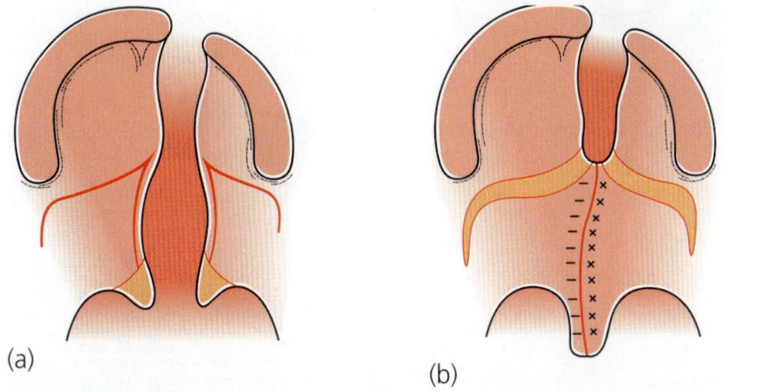

Figure 45.13 (a and b) Method of repair of cleft palate. First-stage palatoplasty to reconstruct muscles of the soft palate. Red lines represent incisions, and orange areas raw surfaces.

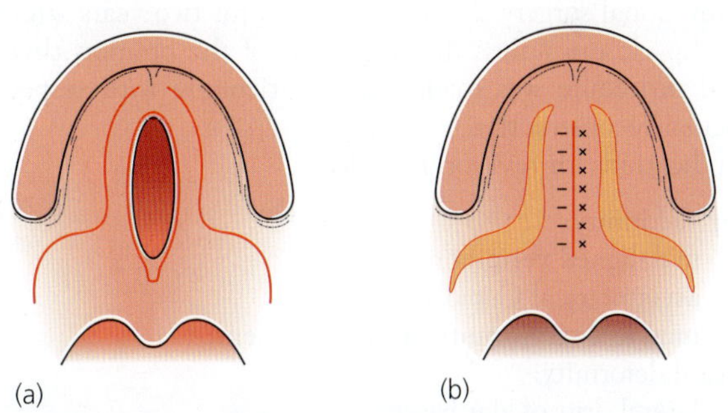

Figure 45.14 (a and b) Schematic representation of closure of the hard palate. Second-stage palatoplasty achieved with two-layered closure. Red lines represent incisions, and orange areas raw surfaces.

abnormalities are well documented. The number of teeth may be reduced (hypodontia) or increased (hyperdontia), occurring most commonly in the region of the cleft alveolus involving the maxillary lateral incisor tooth. These abnormalities can occur in both primary and secondary dentition.

All children with cleft lip and palate should undergo regular dental examination. Dental management should also include preventative measures, such as dietary advice, fluoride supplements and fissure sealants.

A well-maintained and disease-free dentition in childhood is an absolute prerequisite for orthodontic treatment (Summary box 45.8).

Summary box 45.8

Dental problems

- Too many/too few teeth or problems with eruption of teeth are common
- Good dentition is essential for successful reconstructive surgery

Orthodontic management

Many children with cleft lip and palate require orthodontic treatment. Orthodontic treatment is commonly carried out in two phases:

1. Mixed dentition (8–10 years) – to expand the maxillary arches as a prelude to alveolar bone graft.
2. Permanent dentition (14–18 years) – to align the dentition and provide a normal functioning occlusion. This phase of treatment may also include surgical correction of a malpositioned/retrusive maxilla by maxillary osteotomy (Figure 45.15a and b).

Secondary surgery for cleft lip and palate

Good outcome in cleft lip and palate is directly attributable to the quality of the primary surgery. Secondary cleft procedures include:

- cleft lip revision (unilateral and bilateral);
- alveolar bone graft;
- simultaneous lip revision and alveolar bone graft;
- secondary palate procedures, e.g. veloplasty and pharyngoplasty, closure of a palatal fistula;
- dentoalveolar procedures, including transplantation of teeth/insertion of osseointegrated dental implants;
- orthognathic surgery;
- rhinoplasty.

Cleft lip revision

Indications for revisional surgery to the previously repaired cleft lip are dependent on the site and severity of the residual deformity.

Revisional surgery should be delayed for two years after primary lip closure unless the surgeon is of the opinion that the initial procedure was inadequate, particularly with respect to muscular reconstruction.

Indications for revision include:

- lip deformity:
  - malaligned vermilion;
  - asymmetrical Cupid's bow;
  - muscle discontinuity or malalignment;
- nasal deformity:
  - lateral drift of alar base;
  - poor nasal tip projection;
  - deviation of cartilaginous nasal septum into the non-cleft nostril.

Residual nasal deformity is an external manifestation of incomplete reconstruction of the nasolabial muscle ring.

Examples of lip revision are shown in Figures 45.16, 45.17, 45.18 and 45.19 (Summary box 45.9).

Summary box 45.9

Cleft lip revision surgery

- Should be delayed for at least two years after primary surgery
- Aims to improve incomplete primary reconstruction

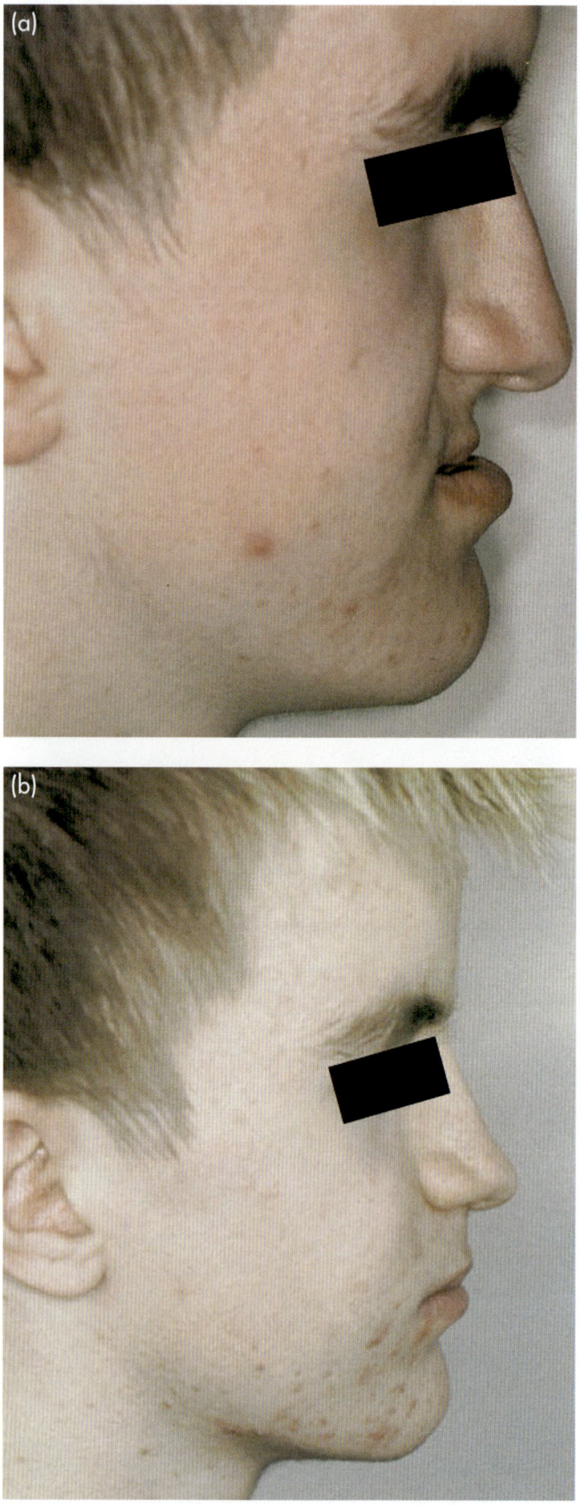

Figure 45.15 Correction of midface retrusion by maxillary advancement osteotomy, before (a) and after (b) surgery.

Alveolar bone grafting

Alveolar bone grafting in a mixed dentition is a well-established procedure for patients with a residual alveolar cleft associated with cleft lip and palate. The rationale for performing alveolar bone grafting includes:

Cupid's Bow. Cupid, the Roman god of love, is often depicted holding a double-curved bow which he uses to shoot arrows into his victims.

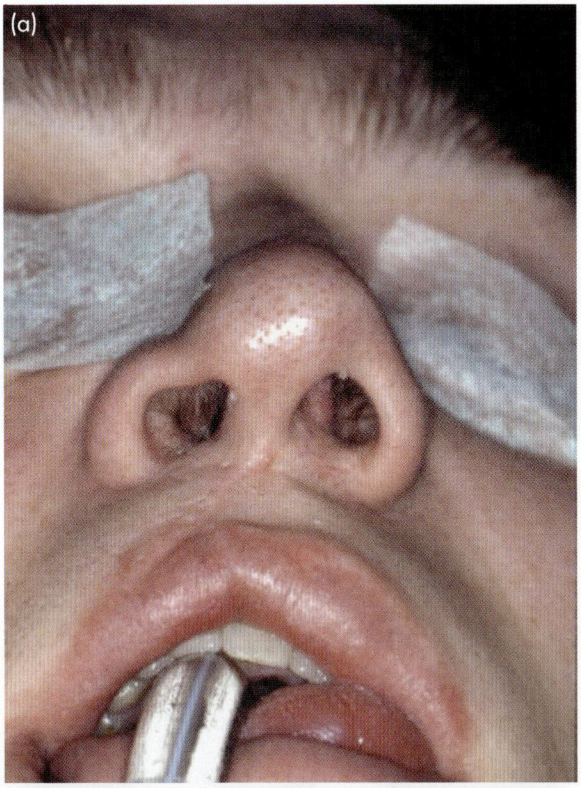

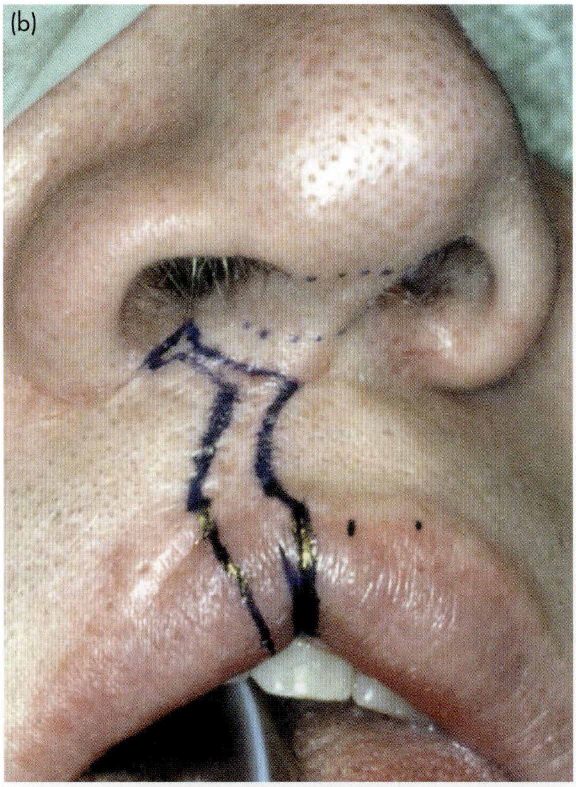

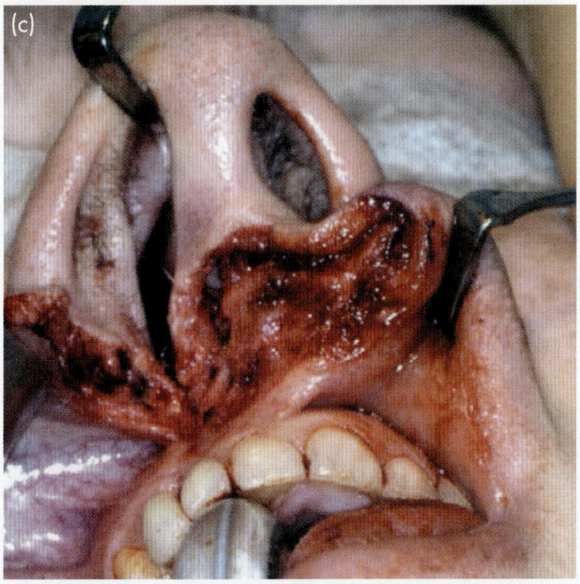

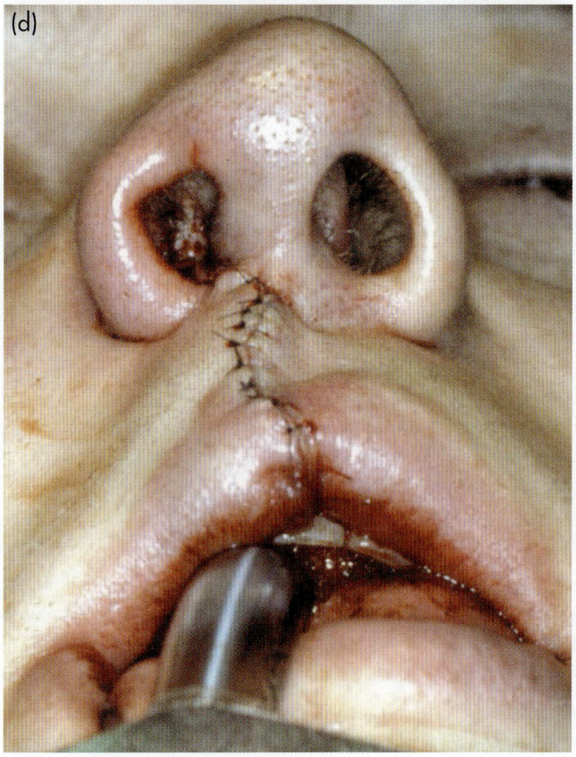

Figure 45.16 (a) Revision of unilateral complete cleft lip, seen from below. (b) Skin incisions. (c) Wide exposure of nasolabial and orbicularis oris muscle. (d) Lip closure highlighting improved nasal symmetry.

- stabilisation of maxillary segments;
- to promote eruption of the canine tooth into the cleft site;
- to enhance bony support of the teeth adjacent to the cleft alveolus;
- to promote closure of the oronasal fistula;
- to close residual fistula of the anterior palate;
- to provide adequate bone stock to receive an osseointegrated dental implant where a tooth is congenitally absent.

Normally, but not universally, patients undergo a period of orthodontic treatment prior to bone grafting. The collapsed maxillary segment is expanded orthodontically to widen the

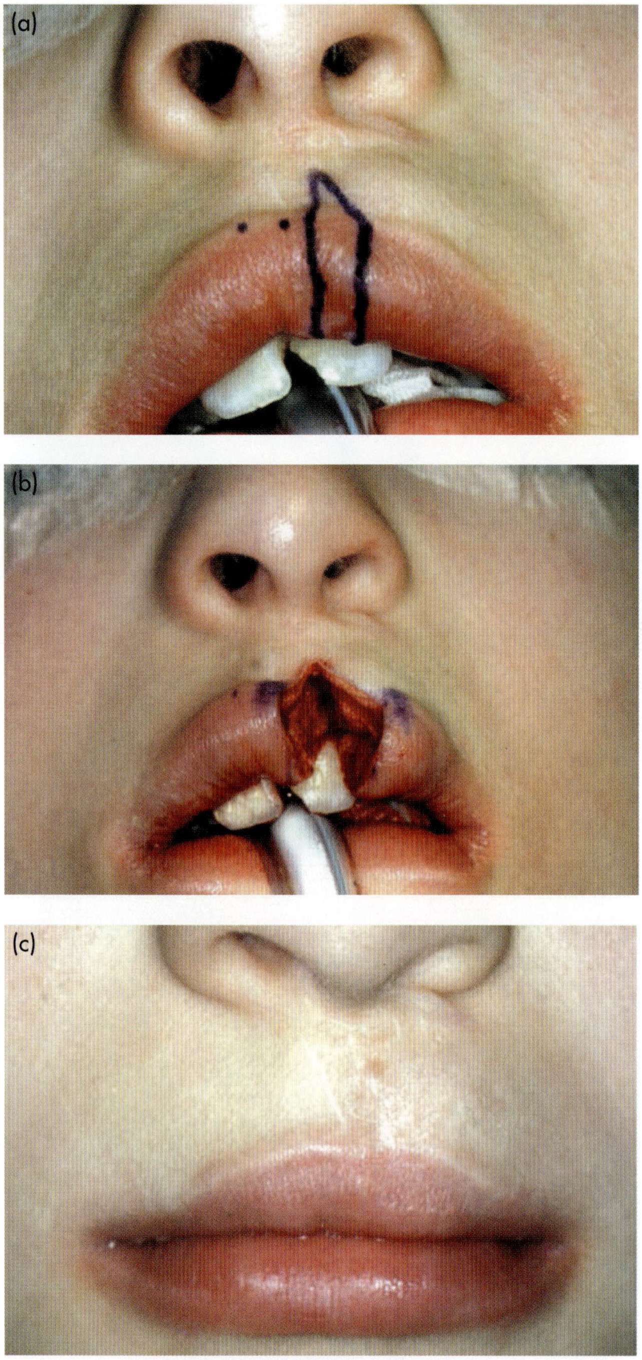

Figure 45.17 (a) Asymmetrical Cupid's bow. Revision of unilateral cleft lip – skin markings. (b) Identification and realignment of orbicularis oris muscle. (c) Postoperative appearance.

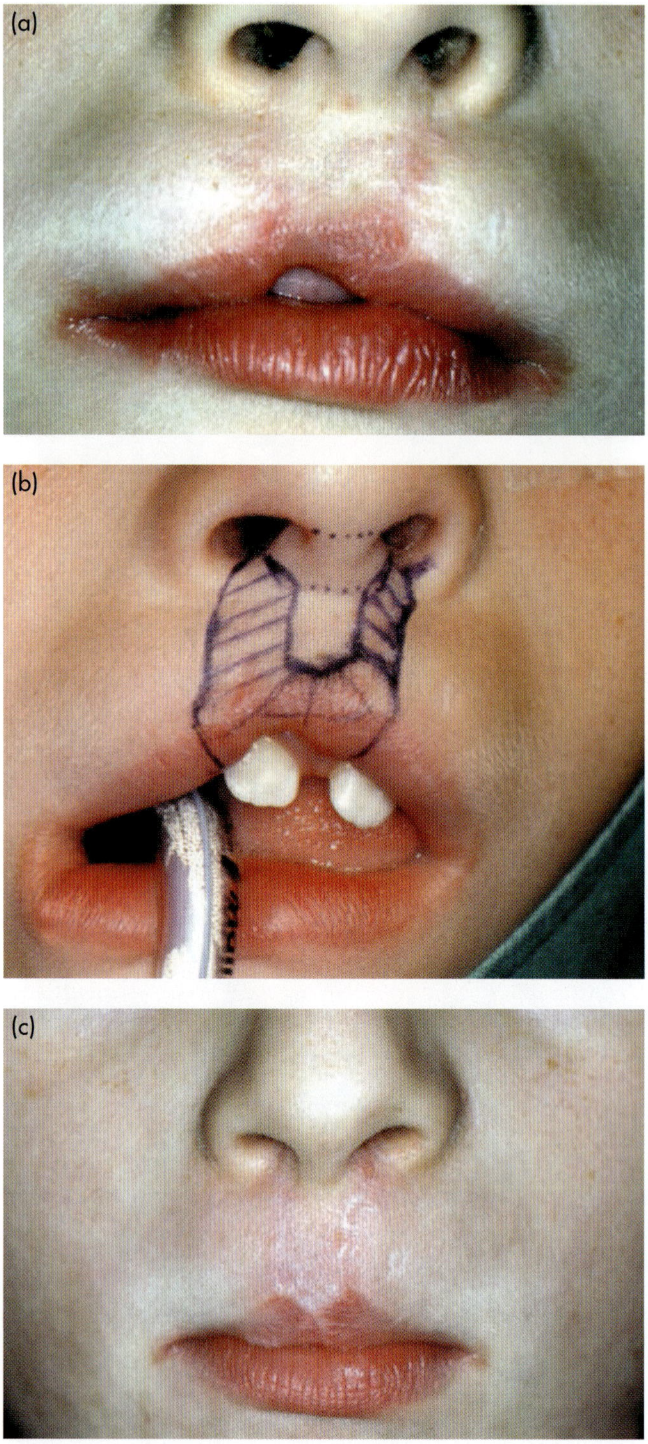

Figure 45.18 (a) Revision of bilateral cleft lip with reconstruction of nasolabial muscles. (b) Skin incisions and development of philtrum. (c) Postoperative view – improved nasal and lip symmetry.

cleft alveolus. The surgery is best performed before the canine tooth erupts (between 8 and 11 years of age). There is a consensus that earlier bone grafting may be beneficial not only for the unerupted canine tooth but also to promote eruption and bony support to the adjacent central and lateral incisor when present. Alveolar bone grafting can also be performed simultaneously with secondary lip revision (Figure 45.20).

Cancellous bone is harvested from either the iliac crest or tibial plateau. This is achieved either through an open approach or preferably through a small incision utilising a trephine. When the defect is very small, alternative bone sites, e.g. mental symphysis, are sometimes advocated. Bone grafting is a highly successful procedure when carried out in experienced hands, with over 90 per cent of patients achieving acceptable interdental alveolar bone height, but it does require the interaction of surgeon and orthodontist. When the lateral incisor is absent and the canine tooth fails to erupt, surgical exposure of the canine

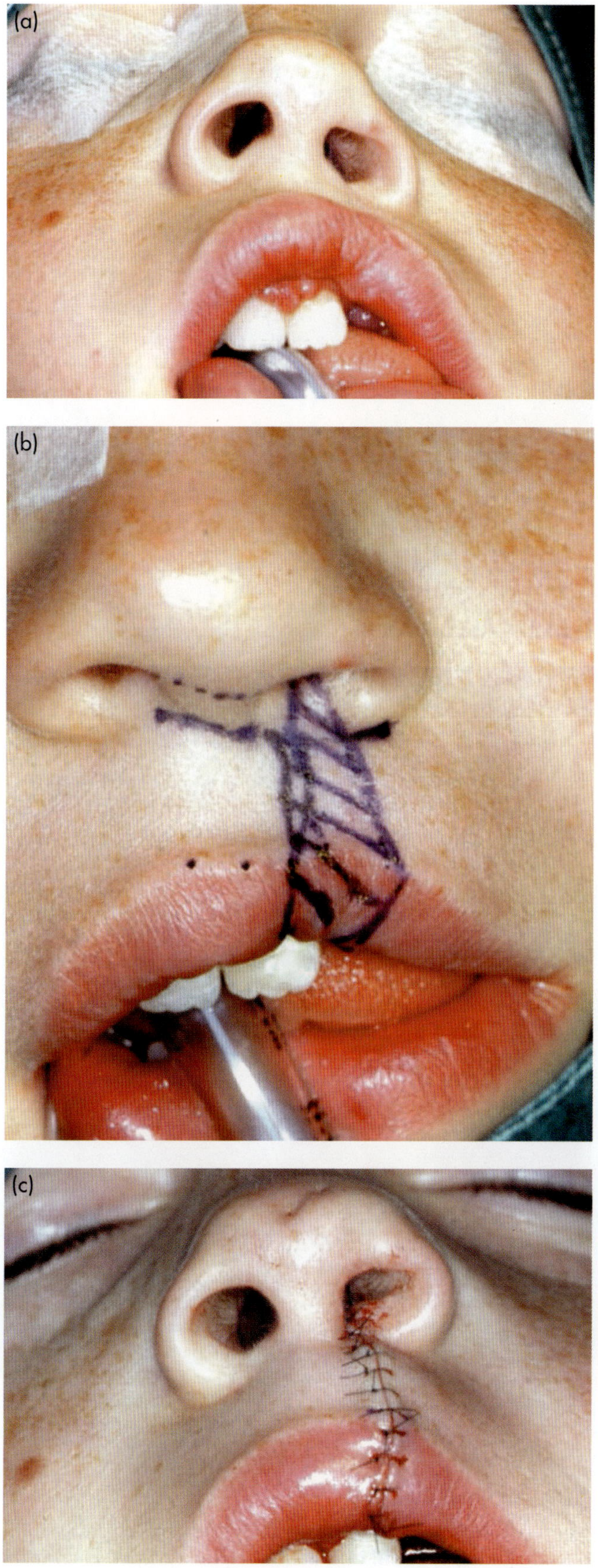

Figure 45.19 (a) Revision of left unilateral cleft lip to correct nasal deformity. (b) Skin incision. (c) Postoperative view.

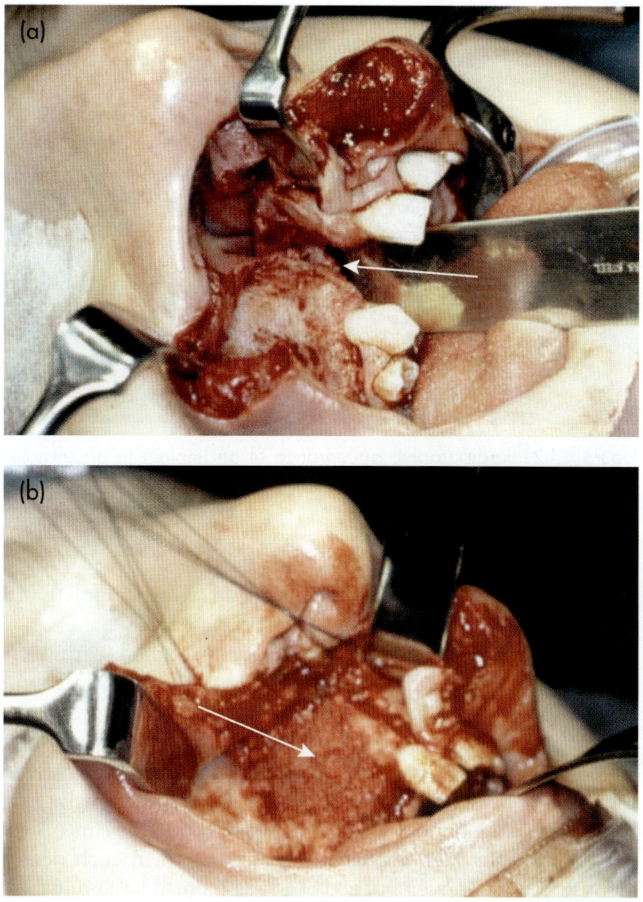

Figure 45.20 (a) Peroperative view of alveolar bone graft demonstrating defect in alveolus (arrow) (simultaneous lip revision). (b) Cancellous bone graft (arrow) packed into defect.

tooth may be required to aid its eruption. It is a fundamental principle that, following alveolar bone grafting, efforts should be made to ensure that a tooth erupts into the alveolar bone graft site. Failure to provide a tooth in the alveolar bone graft site usually results in bony resorption in the long term. This can be overcome by the insertion of an osseointegrated implant into the grafted site, thereby preserving bone stock (Figure 45.21) (Summary box 45.10).

Summary box 45.10

Alveolar bone grafting

- Aimed at stabilising orthodontic treatment
- Promotes normal eruption of canine and other teeth

Orthognathic surgery

Impaired growth of the midface (maxilla) is now attributed to poor and traumatic primary surgery. Surgical techniques must endeavour to minimise scarring, although in many cases patients have a genetic predisposition to poor midfacial growth. Elective maxillary advancement or bimaxillary surgery is often indicated to restore aesthetics and dental occlusal harmony. Orthognathic

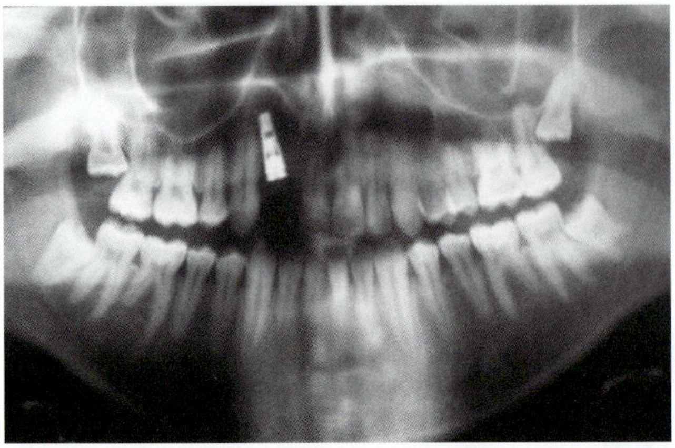

Figure 45.21 Radiographic appearance of an implant in an alveolar bone graft site.

surgery is usually performed when facial growth is complete (16 years in female patients, 19 years in male patients).

The principal dentofacial deformity associated with cleft lip and palate is underdevelopment in both the horizontal and vertical direction of the maxilla. This leads to a pseudoprognathism in late adolescence, which is not correctable by orthodontic fixed-appliance therapy alone. Patients needing orthognathic surgery can be identified as early as ten years old, although planning and treatment does not commence until 14–15 years of age. Treatment with fixed appliances to align teeth in each dental arch is carried out over a period of 18–24 months as a prelude to orthognathic surgery. Orthognathic surgery may require maxillary osteotomy advancement alone (Figure 45.15a and b) or bimaxillary osteotomy and genioplasty (Figure 45.22). Rigid fixation, with or without bone grafting of the maxilla, is essential as cleft lip and palate patients undergoing orthognathic surgery have a high risk of a skeletal relapse as a result of the scarring associated with primary cleft lip and palate surgery.

Open septorhinoplasty

Following revisional cleft lip and palate surgery, orthognathic surgery and alveolar bone grafting, many patients still require definitive surgical nasal correction. In patients with cleft lip and palate, open rhinoplasty is preferred to gain access to the external cartilaginous framework, which is frequently deformed (Figure 45.23). The principal deformity is a collapse of the lower lateral cartilage on the cleft side, together with a dislocation of the cartilaginous septum into the non-cleft nostril. The open method ensures adequate access and repositioning of the cartilaginous framework as a tertiary procedure to improve nasal tip projection, correct septal deformity and relocate alar cartilages. A postauricular onlay graft to the middle crus of the cleft nostril lower lateral cartilage may be required to enhance good nasal tip projection and symmetry (Summary box 45.11).

Summary box 45.11

Deformities requiring nasal reconstruction

- Collapse of the lower lateral cartilage on the cleft side
- Dislocation of cartilaginous septum into the non-cleft nostril

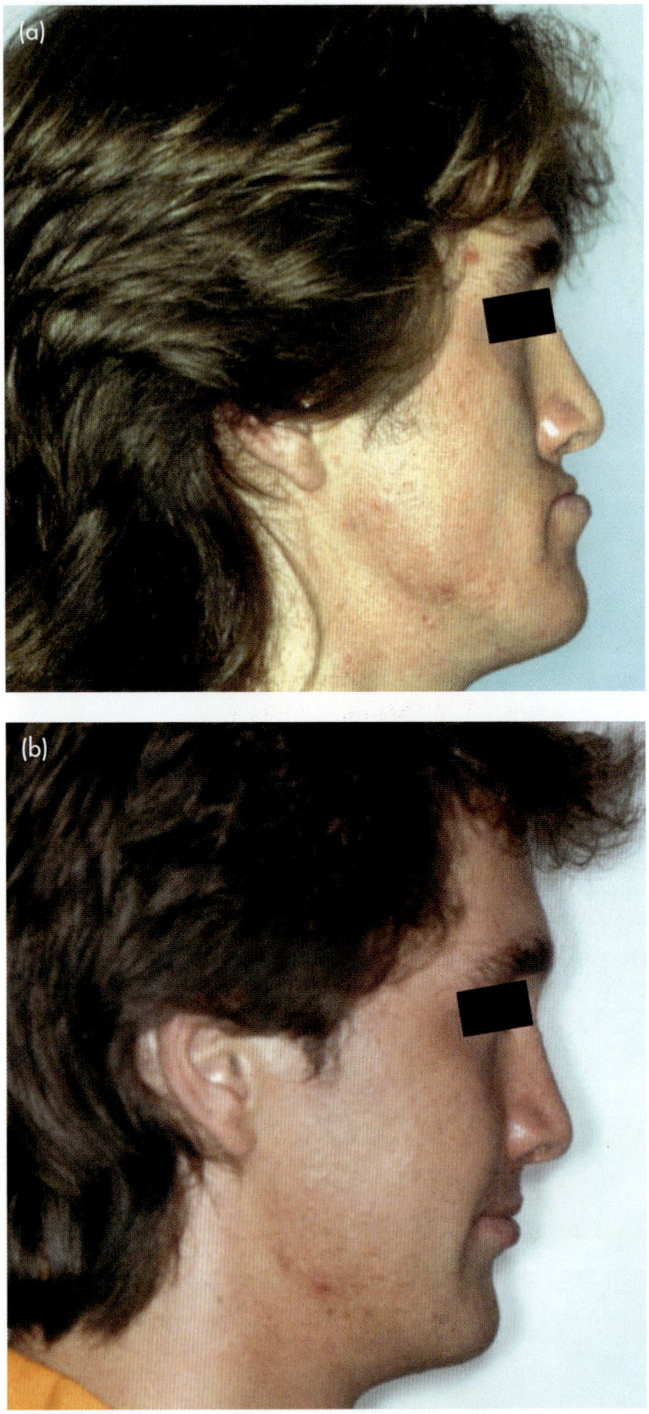

Figure 45.22 (a) Lateral view of an adult a with previously repaired cleft lip and palate demonstrating mandibular prognathism and maxillary retrusion. (b) Postoperative appearance following maxillary advancement and mandibular setback surgery.

Summary

The management of children with cleft lip and palate is complex, requiring the skill of a multidisciplinary team. Each team should include professionals who are appropriately qualified with specialist training, treating an adequate number of patients per year in centralised units. Meticulous record keeping of

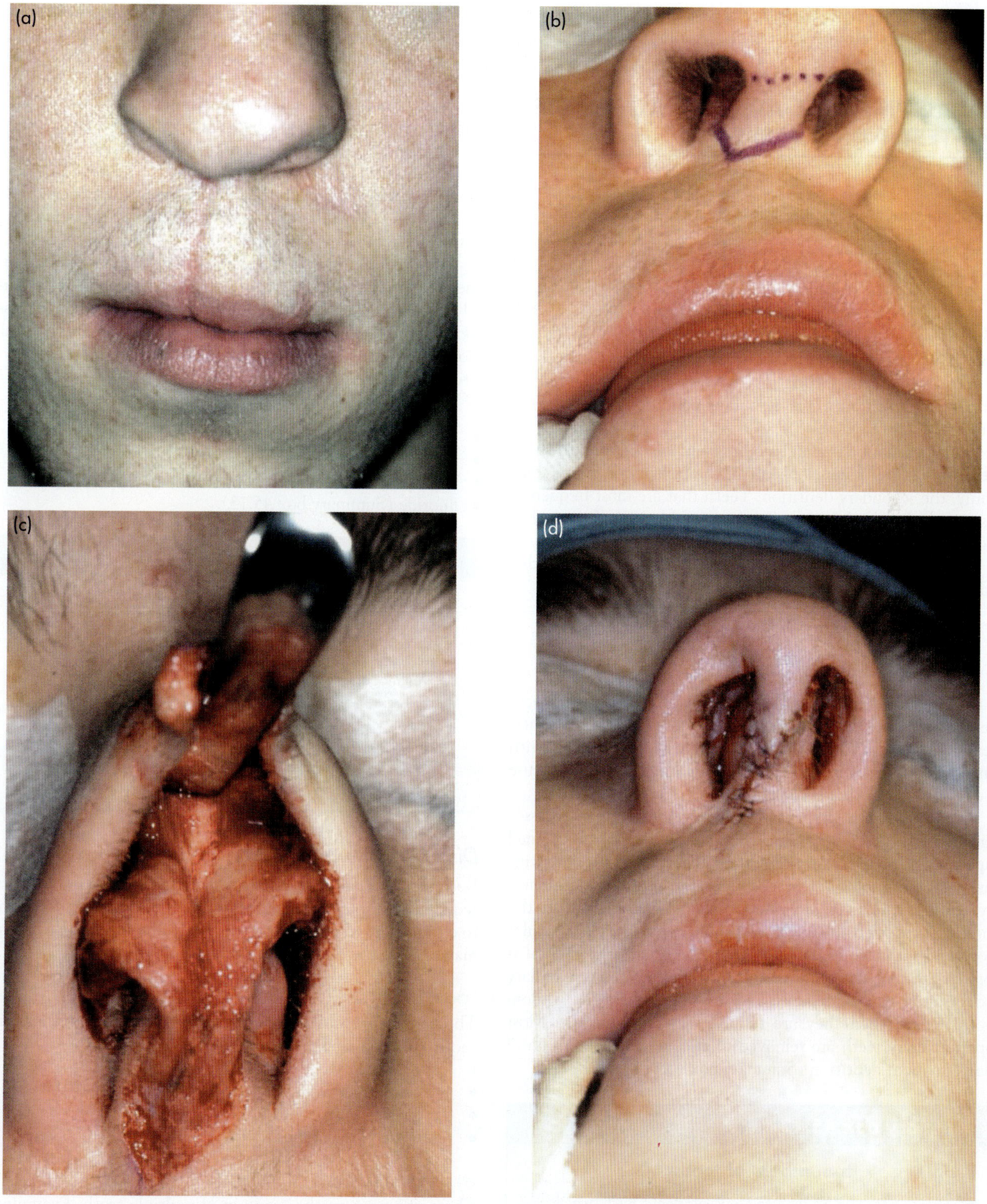

Figure 45.23 (a) Characteristic nasal deformity of a non-functional unilateral cleft lip repair. (b) Incisions for open rhinoplasty. (c) Exposure of the cartilaginous skeleton of the external nose. (d) Repositioning of external nasal cartilages to improve nasal tip projection.

photography, radiology, dental casts and speech recordings are indispensable to permit regular audits and improve outcomes.

DEVELOPMENTAL ABNORMALITIES OF THE TEETH AND JAWS

Teeth

Developmental abnormalities of the teeth can be divided into:

- abnormality in number;
- defects of structure and size;
- disorders of eruption of teeth.

Number

Anodontia is the term that is strictly applied to congenital absence of all teeth, which may involve both deciduous and permanent dentition. This is a rare condition that is often hereditary.

Partial anodontia is a much more common disorder in which there is a failure of development of the primary or, more commonly, the secondary dentition. Teeth that are most frequently absent are the third molars (wisdom teeth), second premolars and maxillary lateral incisor teeth.

Partial anodontia is associated with certain congenital disorders:

- ectodermal dysplasia;
- Down's syndrome;
- cleft lip and palate.

Management of partial anodontia involves prosthetic replacement of the teeth, usually in combination with orthodontic treatment. Congenitally missing teeth can be replaced with removable prostheses, fixed prostheses or, more recently, the use of osseointegrated dental implants.

Additional teeth (**hyperdontia**) can occur alone or in association with other syndromes. Additional teeth are termed **supernumerary** teeth and are often impacted in the jaw with abnormal morphology. The most common site for supernumerary teeth is the maxillary incisor region, particularly in the midline (mesiodens). When additional teeth are of a similar morphology to the normal dentition, the term supplemental is appropriate. Supplemental teeth are common in the maxillary incisor and premolar regions, and less common in the wisdom tooth region when they are termed the fourth molars. Most supernumerary teeth are removed to encourage the eruption of the permanent dentition (Summary box 45.12).

> **Summary box 45.12**
>
> **Problems with numbers of teeth**
>
> - Absent teeth can be replaced with prosthetic teeth, which may involve osseointegrated implants
> - Supernumerary teeth are often impacted and are removed to allow eruption of secondary dentition

Defects of the structure of teeth

Structural changes of the teeth can occur as a consequence of genetic disorders or environmental factors.

Genetic disorders frequently include **amelogenesis imperfecta** and **dentinogenesis imperfecta**, which affect the enamel and dentine of the teeth, respectively. Both of these conditions are characterised by defects in both dentitions, in which all teeth are affected. In amelogenesis imperfecta, the defects are variable and may involve changes in structure (hypoplasia) or in mineralisation (hypocalcification). The loss of enamel leads to rapid attrition of the teeth to gum level in early adolescence. Dentinogenesis imperfecta results in soft dentine associated with short roots. Dentinogenesis imperfecta is strongly associated with osteogenesis imperfecta.

Acquired conditions producing changes in the structure of the teeth may be either local or systemic. Local causes are usually the consequence of trauma to the deciduous predecessor tooth, which interferes with enamel formation (amelogenesis). Common examples of systemic causes that produce tooth structure disruption are:

- measles
- rickets
- hypoparathyroidism
- tetracycline
- fluoride (Summary box 45.13).

> **Summary box 45.13**
>
> **Causes of defects of the structure of teeth**
>
> Congenital
> - Amelogenesis imperfecta
> - Dentinogenesis imperfecta
>
> Acquired local
> - Trauma
>
> Acquired systemic
> - Disease – measles, rickets
> - Drugs – fluoride, tetracycline

Disorders of eruption

Both primary and secondary dentition erupt in a specific sequence, although the timing of eruption does vary from child to child. Delayed eruption of teeth may involve a single tooth or may involve the entire dentition.

Local factors

There are numerous factors that impair the eruption of a single tooth. These include:

- loss of space/overcrowding
- additional teeth
- dentigerous cysts
- retention of deciduous tooth.

Systemic factors

These can prevent the eruption of multiple teeth. Examples of such conditions include:

- metabolic diseases – cretinism and rickets
- osteodystrophies – cleidocranial dysostosis and fibrous dysplasia
- hereditary gingival fibromatosis.

Management of unerupted teeth involves the removal of the obstruction to eruption, including supernumerary teeth, as well as the relief of crowding. Patients with cleidocranial dysostosis should undergo long-term follow up with regular radiographic assessment. Supernumerary teeth, as and when they appear, should be removed to encourage the eruption of permanent dentition in adolescence. Many patients with cleidocranial dysostosis require multiple operations to expose teeth and encourage eruption (Summary box 45.14).

Summary box 45.14

Management of unerupted teeth

- Remove obstruction to eruption
- Surgical exposure if eruption delayed

Jaws

Disproportionate growth between the maxilla and mandible can occur, which results in derangement of the dental occlusion. The occlusion can be classified into three different subtypes:

- class I: a normal relationship of upper and lower incisors and molar dentition;
- class II: the mandibular teeth are placed posterior to the maxillary teeth;
- class III: the mandibular teeth are placed anterior to the maxillary teeth.

This classification is usually, but not invariably, the consequence of aberrant skeletal development of the maxilla and mandible, such that in a class II condition there is usually an underdevelopment of the mandible (mandibular retrognathia), whereas in a class III condition there may be simultaneous overgrowth of the mandible (mandibular prognathism) and underdevelopment of the maxilla (maxillary hypoplasia).

In the Caucasian population, the most common deformity of the facial skeleton is an underdevelopment of the mandible (retrognathia), producing a skeletal class II relationship often associated with excessive vertical growth of the maxilla. Bimaxillary protrusion is rare but is a characteristic of African races.

Condylar hyperplasia is an idiopathic condition seen in patients between 15 and 30 years of age, more common in women than men, in which there is hyperplasia or overgrowth of the neck of the mandibular condyle. This gives an asymmetrical growth to the jaw in both a vertical and horizontal plane.

Facial disproportionate growth is also a characteristic of many syndromes. Examples include:

- Treacher Collins' syndrome
- Crouzon's syndrome
- Apert's syndrome
- Pierre Robin sequence.

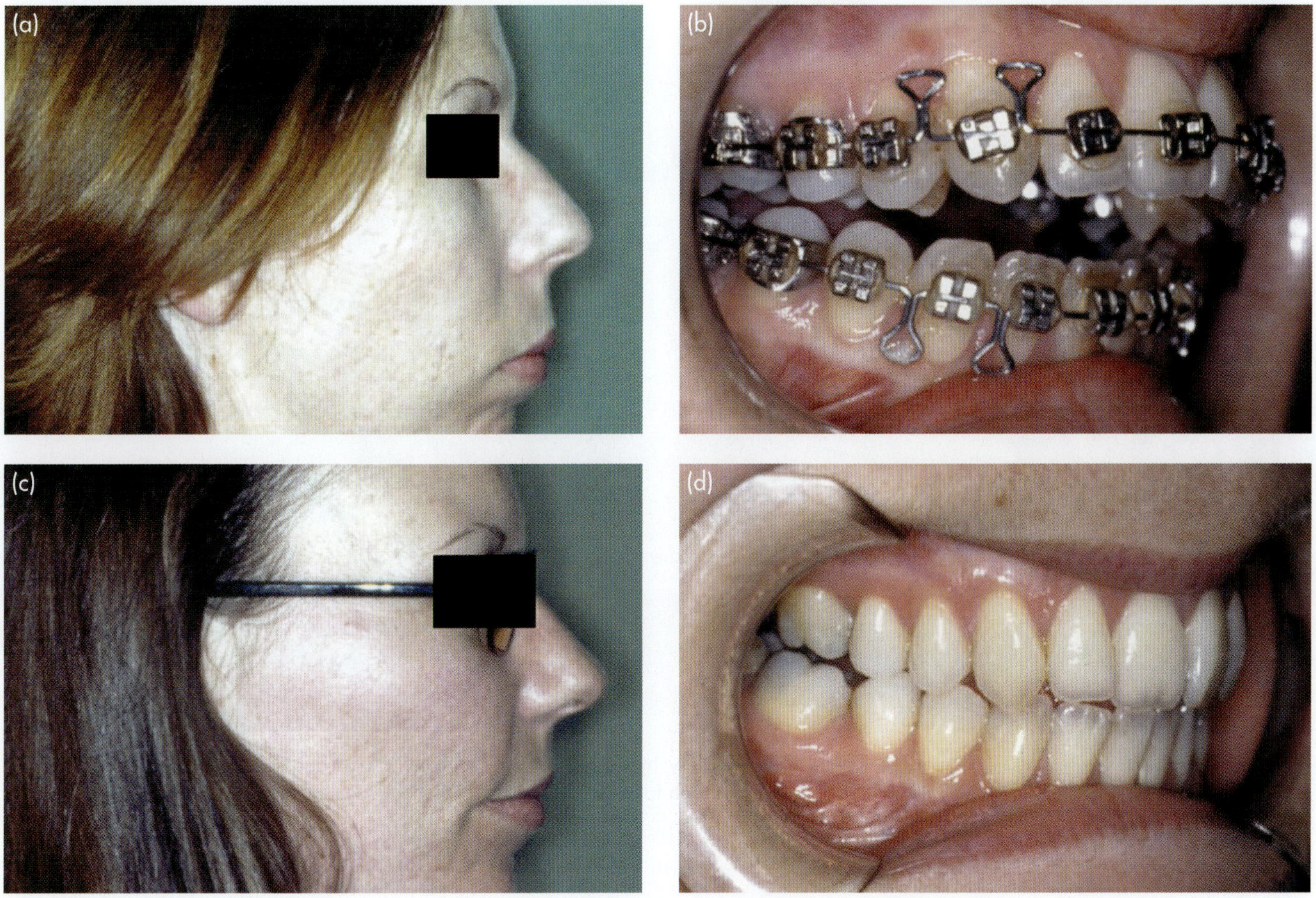

Figure 45.24 (a) Profile of class II relationship with vertical growth of maxilla and mandibular retrognathia. (b) Preoperative occlusion with anterior open bite. (c) Postoperative view following superior repositioning of maxilla, mandibular advancement and genioplasty. (d) Postoperative occlusion.

Octave Crouzon, 1874–1938, physician, La Salpêtrière, Paris, France, described this condition in 1912.

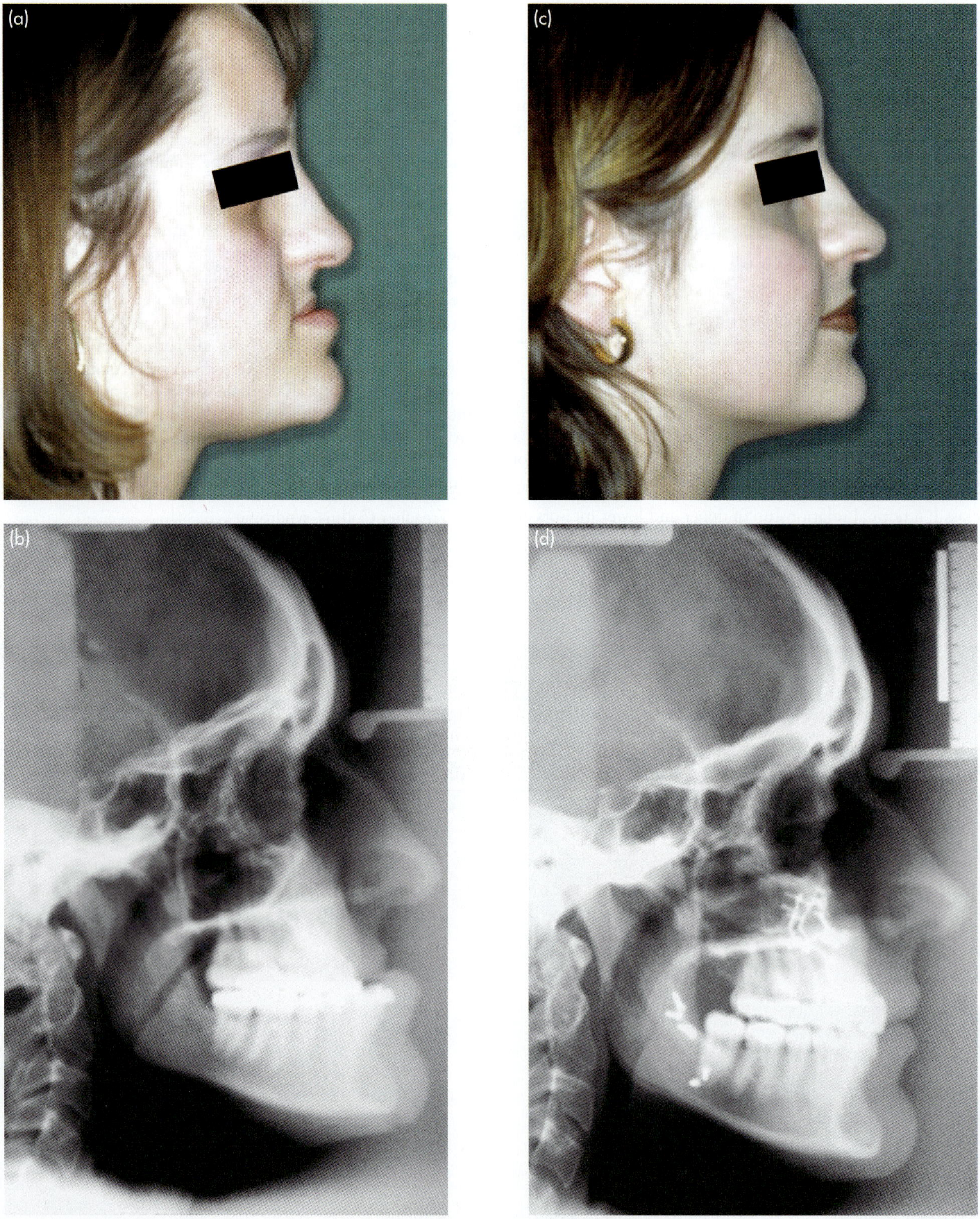

Figure 45.25 (a) Profile of class III skeletal relationship and maxillary hypoplasia and mandibular prognathism. (b) Lateral skull radiograph. (c) Profile following bimaxillary osteotomy. (d) Postoperative radiograph following bimaxillary osteotomy demonstrating internal fixation.

(e)

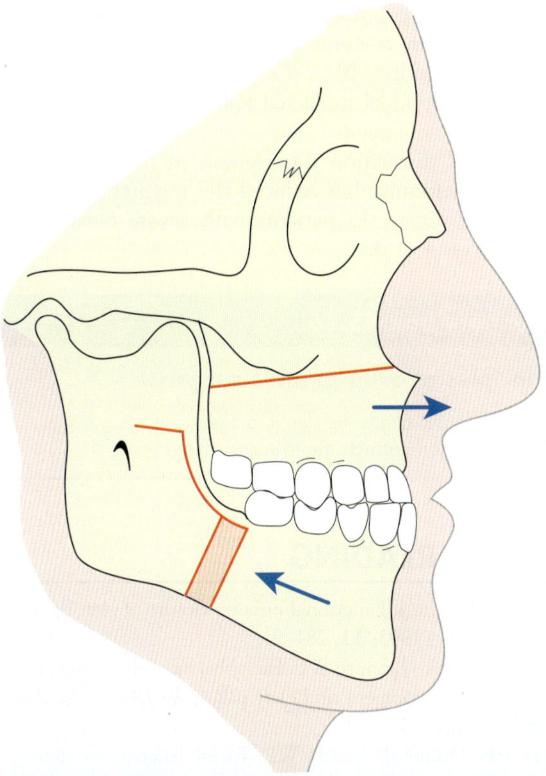

Figure 45.25 *continued* (e) Schematic representation of bimaxillary osteotomy with maxillary advancement and mandibular retrusion.

(a)

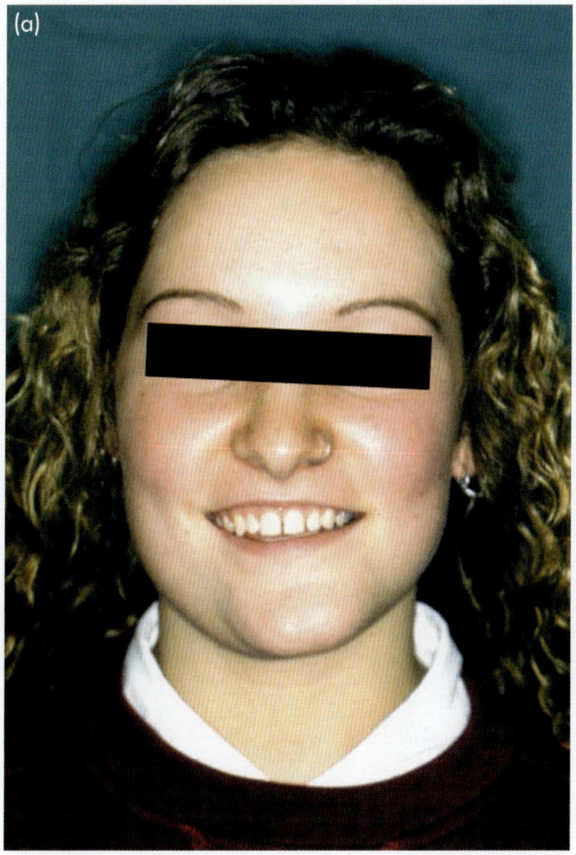

(b)

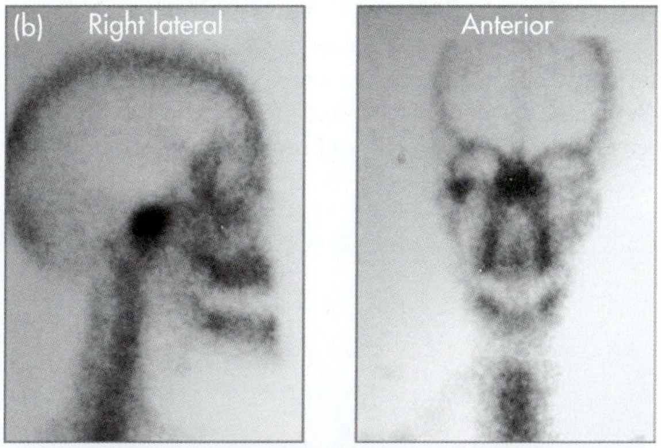

(c)

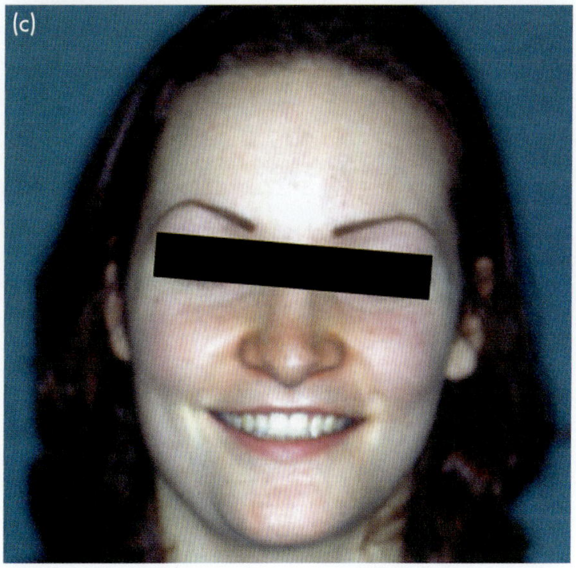

Figure 45.26 (a) Condylar hyperplasia with mandibular asymmetry. (b) Bone scan revealing increased bone activity in the right mandibular condyle. (c) Postoperative appearance following bimaxillary osteotomy to correct facial asymmetry.

Orthognathic surgery

Orthognathic surgery is the term given to the surgical correction of deformities of the jaw. It is usually undertaken in close cooperation between orthodontic and maxillofacial surgeons. Surgery is directed at simultaneously changing the position of both maxilla and mandible at the end of the growth period. This is termed bimaxillary osteotomy. Treatment planning usually commences at the age of 12–13 years, in which the orthodontist aligns the dental arches in correct relation for each jaw. This frequently results in an accentuation of the facial deformity at the end of the orthodontic phase of treatment. Treatment normally takes two years, in which orthognathic surgery is performed towards the end of orthodontic treatment, although orthodontic treatment in the form of fixed appliances usually continues postoperatively for up to six months after surgery. Surgical planning should be meticulous and involves clinical examination and cephalometric assessment in the form of radiograph analysis, as well as study model analysis, working in close cooperation with maxillofacial technologists.

Orthognathic surgery is generally carried out through intraoral incisions, in which the upper and lower jaws are mobilised by achieving osteotomy cuts with saws and drills (Figure 45.24). Following mobilisation of the mandible and maxilla, the jaws are repositioned and held with titanium plates and screws placed through an intraoral approach. This frequently avoids the use of intermaxillary fixation and allows earlier function of the jaws, as well as improved early dietary intake. Examples of orthognathic surgery are shown in Figures 45.25 and 45.26.

Patients with syndromic conditions, such as hemifacial microsomia and Crouzon's and Treacher Collins' syndromes, require the services of a craniofacial surgeon. As these syndromes are extremely rare, management and surgery should only be carried out in designated centres. The principal treatment is to correct the deformity from the cranium downwards, with correction of the cranial deformity within the first three years of life and correction of the residual midfacial and lower facial deformity in childhood and adolescence.

The use of distraction osteogenesis in the management of craniofacial deformity has reduced the requirements for major orthognathic surgery in patients with severe facial deformity (Summary box 45.15).

Summary box 45.15

Principles of orthognathic surgery

- Orthodontist aligns the dental arches
- Surgery then corrects the jaw deformity

FURTHER READING

Markus AF, Delaire J. Functional primary closure of cleft lip. *Br J Oral Maxillofac Surg* 1993; **31**: 281–91.

Markus AF, Delaire J, Smith WP. Facial balance in cleft lip and palate. I: Normal development and cleft palate. *Br J Oral Maxillofac Surg* 1992; **30**: 287–95.

Markus AF, Delaire J, Smith WP. Facial balance in cleft lip and palate. II: Cleft lip and palate and secondary deformities. *Br J Oral Maxillofac Surg* 1992; **30**: 296–304.

Markus AF, Smith WP, Delaire J. Primary closure of cleft palate: a functional approach. *Br J Oral Maxillofac Surg* 1993; **31**: 71–7.

Smith WP, Markus AF, Delaire J. Primary closure of the cleft alveolus: a functional approach. *Br J Oral Maxillofac Surg* 1995; **33**: 156–65.

CHAPTER 46

The nose and sinuses

LEARNING OBJECTIVES

To be familiar with:

- The basic anatomy of the nose and paranasal sinuses
- The principles of managing post-traumatic nasal and septal deformity
- The causes and management of epistaxis
- The diagnosis and management of nasal polyposis
- The clinical features of sinus infection and its treatment and potential complications
- The common sinonasal tumours, their presentation, investigation and principles of treatment

BASIC ANATOMY OF THE NOSE AND PARANASAL SINUSES

The supporting structures of the nose are shown in Figure 46.1. The septum consists of the anterior quadrilateral cartilage, the perpendicular plate of the ethmoid and the vomer (Figure 46.2). The lateral wall of the nasal cavity contains the superior, middle and inferior turbinates (Figure 46.3). Opening onto the lateral nasal wall are the ostea of all of the nasal sinuses, except the sphenoid sinus (Figures 46.4 and 46.5).

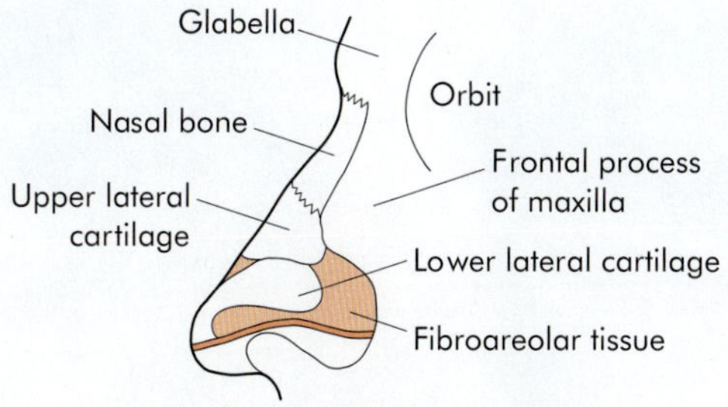

Figure 46.1 The nasal skeleton.

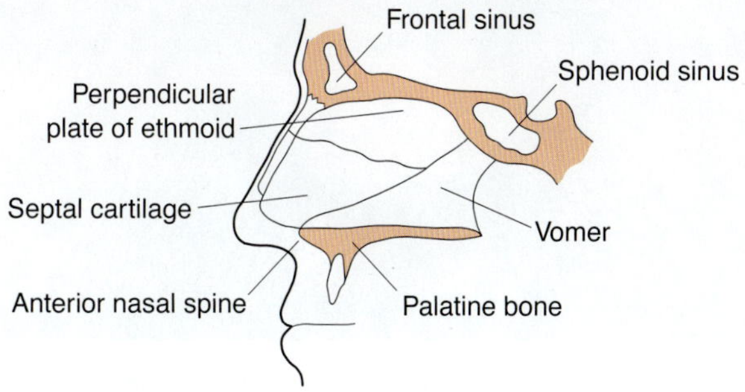

Figure 46.2 The left side of the nasal septum.

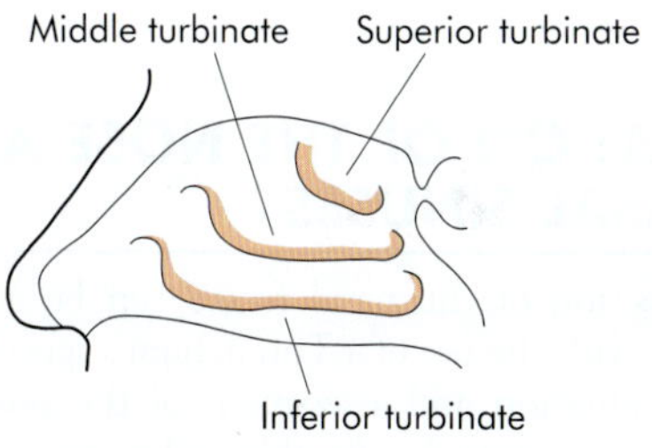

Figure 46.3 The right lateral nasal wall.

The nasal fossae and sinuses receive their blood supply via the external and internal carotid arteries. The external carotid artery supplies the interior of the nose via the maxillary and sphenopalatine arteries. The greater palatine artery supplies the

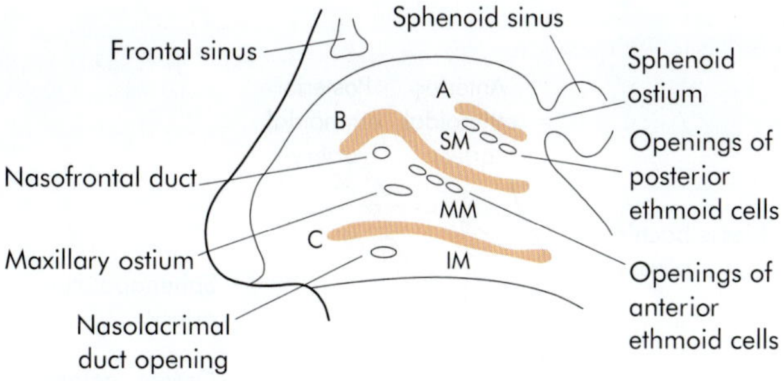

Figure 46.4 The right lateral nasal wall with turbinates removed to show the sinus ostia. A, insertion of superior turbinate; B, insertion of middle turbinate; C, insertion of inferior turbinate; SM, superior meatus; MM, middle meatus; IM, inferior meatus.

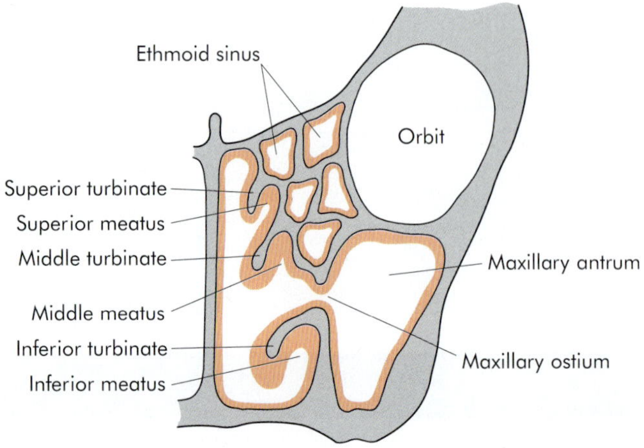

Figure 46.5 Coronal section through the left maxillary and ethmoid sinuses.

anteroinferior septum via the incisive canal. The contribution from the internal carotid artery is via the anterior and posterior ethmoidal arteries, which are branches of the ophthalmic artery (Figure 46.6). All of these arteries anastomose to form a plexus of vessels (Kiesselbach's plexus) on the anterior part of the nasal septum. Venous drainage is via the ophthalmic and facial veins and the pterygoid and pharyngeal plexuses. Intracranial drainage into the cavernous sinus via the ophthalmic vein is of particular clinical importance because of the potential for intracranial spread of nasal sepsis.

EXAMINATION OF THE NOSE AND PARANASAL SINUSES

Internal inspection of the nasal fossae can be achieved to a limited extent with the use of a Thudichum's speculum. A more thorough examination and assessment of the nose is possible with the use of either rigid or flexible endoscopes.

IMAGING OF PARANASAL SINUSES

Plain radiographs are of limited value in the assessment of sinus disease. A minimum of four views, namely occipitomental, occipitofrontal, submentovertical and lateral, are required to demonstrate the paranasal sinuses adequately. Computed tomography (CT) scanning is far superior in demonstrating sinus pathology. Coronal and axial scans are necessary for detailed assessment.

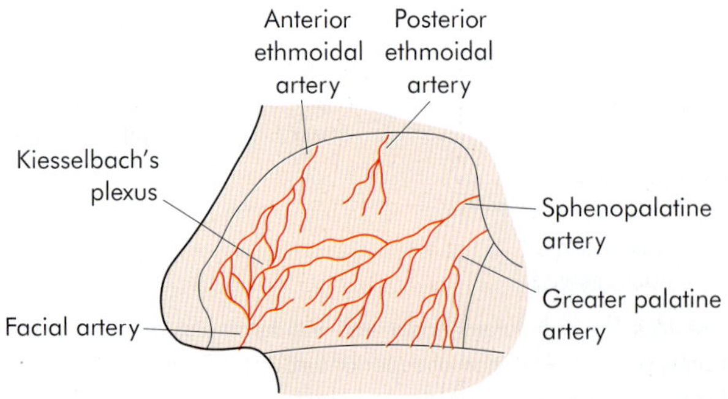

Figure 46.6 Arterial blood supply to the left side of the nasal septum.

TRAUMA TO THE NOSE AND PARANASAL SINUSES

Fracture of the nasal bones

Blunt injury to the nose may fracture the nasal bones (Figure 46.7). The fracture line can extend into the lacrimal bone and tear the anterior ethmoidal artery producing catastrophic haemorrhage. This may be delayed, occurring only as the soft tissue swelling subsides, reducing the tamponade effect on the torn vessel.

Violent trauma to the frontal area of the nose can result in a fracture of the frontal and ethmoid sinuses with potential extension into the anterior cranial fossa. Dural tears and brain injuries, either open or closed, are then at risk from sinonasal ascending infection which may progress to meningitis or brain abscess. Cerebrospinal fluid (CSF) rhinorrhoea is a certain sign of a dural tear.

Management of fractured nasal bones

Fractured nasal bones are often accompanied by extensive overlying soft tissue swelling and bruising, which may hinder the assessment of any underlying bony deformity. Reviewing after 4–5 days when the soft tissue swelling has diminished will allow a better assessment of any deformity. If there is a significant degree of nasal deformity then this can be corrected by manipulation of the nasal bones under local or general anaesthesia. This should be carried out within 10–20 days of the injury while the bony fragments are still mobile.

Septal injury

A blunt injury of moderate force may lead to lateral displacement or deformity of the septal cartilage, restricting the nasal airway. Unlike the nasal bones, the nasal septum cannot be manipulated back into position and requires a formal septoplasty

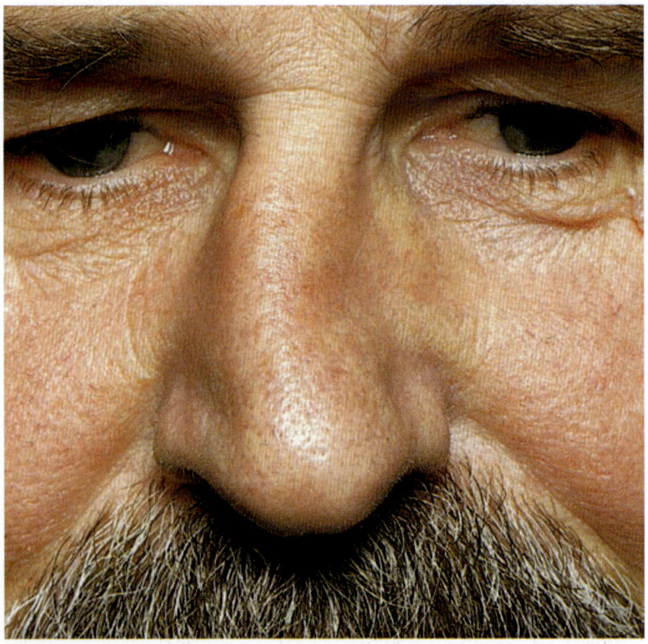

Figure 46.7 Fracture of the nasal bones with displacement of the bony nasal complex to the right side.

Wilhelm Kiesselbach, 1839–1902, Professor of Otology, Erlangen, Germany.
Johann Ludwig Wilhelm Thudichum, 1829–1901, biochemist and general practitioner, London, UK.

procedure to restore the anatomy and the patency of the nasal airways.

Bleeding under the mucoperichondrium of the septum will cause a septal haematoma and nasal obstruction. Untreated, a septal haematoma will progress to abscess formation and ultimately result in necrosis of the septal cartilage and nasal collapse. A septal haematoma should be treated by incision and evacuation of the blood clot, insertion of a small silicone drain and packing of the nasal fossa. A broad-spectrum prophylactic antibiotic should be prescribed (Summary box 46.1).

Summary box 46.1

Nasal trauma

- Do not overlook a septal haematoma
- Displaced nasal bone fractures should be reduced within 10–20 days of injury
- Severe persistent epistaxis after trauma suggests lacrimal bone fracture and injury to the anterior ethmoid artery
- Cerebrospinal fluid rhinorrhoea indicates a fracture involving the frontal or ethmoid sinuses with a dural tear

THE NASAL SEPTUM

Septal deformity

Deviation of the nasal septum may occur naturally or arise as a result of nasal trauma and is readily apparent on anterior rhinoscopy (Figure 46.8). Surgical correction can be achieved by a submucous resection (SMR) of the septum, where the deformed septal cartilage is excised while preserving a dorsal strut. The alternative is a septoplasty procedure during which the septal cartilage is preserved, but the anatomical abnormalities giving rise to its deformity, such as a twisted maxillary crest or inclination of the bony septum, are corrected.

Complications of septal surgery include septal perforation. If too much cartilage is excised in the SMR procedure, loss of support to the dorsum of the nose may result in a supratip depression or drooping of the tip of the nose.

Septal perforation

A hole in the nasal septum causes a turbulent airflow through the nose and a resulting sensation of nasal blockage and extensive nasal crusting. The causes of septal perforation are listed in Summary box 46.2.

Septal perforations seldom heal spontaneously. A great variety of operations have been described to close septal perforations, but none has met with universal success. A more certain

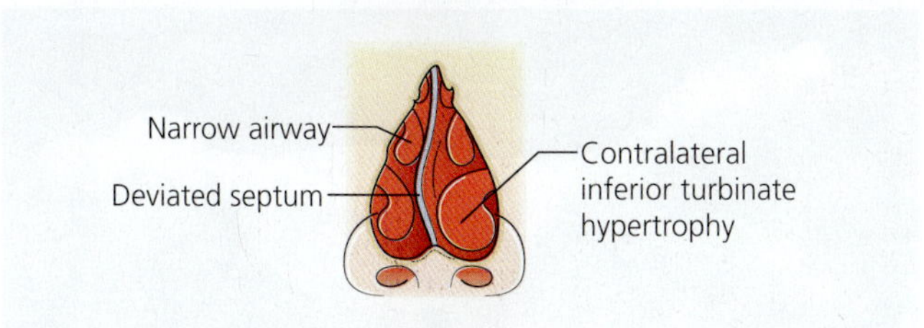

Figure 46.8 Coronal section through the anterior nasal fossae with deviated nasal septum to the right side.

Summary box 46.2

Causes of septal perforations

- Trauma
  - Iatrogenic following septal surgery
  - Nose picking
- Infection
  - Syphilis
  - Tuberculosis
- Vasculitis
  - Wegener's granulomatosis
- Tumours
- Toxins
  - Chrome salts
  - Cocaine
- Idiopathic

option is to occlude the perforation by inserting a Silastic biflanged prosthesis (Figures 46.9 and 46.10).

Wegener's granulomatosis is a systemic idiopathic autoimmune disease affecting the nose, lungs and kidneys. Mucosal granulations on the nasal septum destroy cartilage, producing a septal perforation with saddle deformity of the nose. Laboratory findings include a high erythrocyte sedimentation rate, impaired creatinine clearance and antineutrophil cytoplasmic antibodies (ANCA) in most cases.

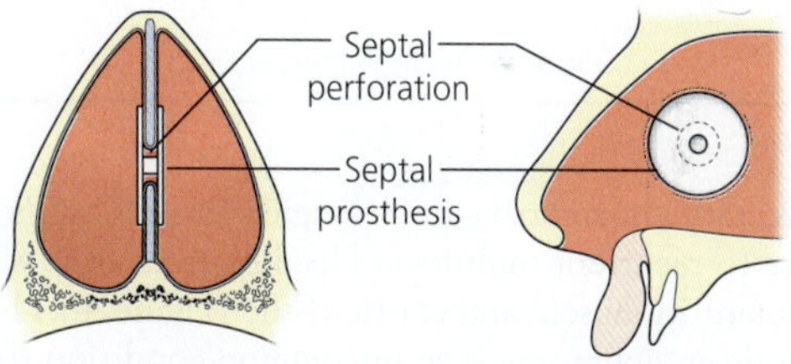

Figure 46.9 Anterior and lateral views of septal perforation occluded with prosthesis.

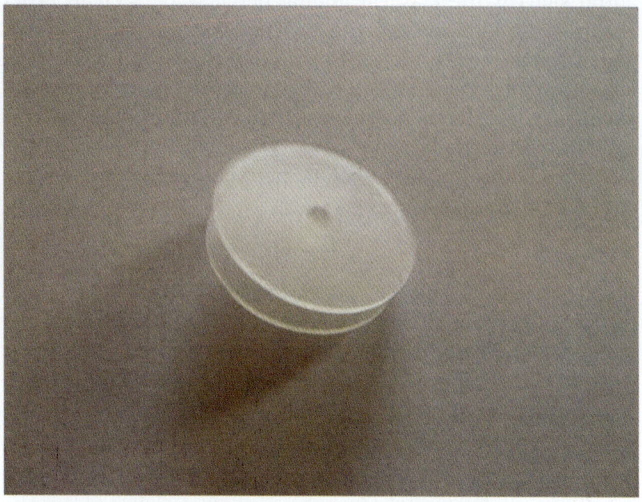

Figure 46.10 Silastic prosthesis for septal perforation.

Friedrich Wegener, 1907–1990, Professor of Pathology, Lübeck, Germany, described this form of granulomatosis in 1939.

EPISTAXIS

The causes of epistaxis are listed in Table 46.1. The most common site of bleeding is from Kiesselbach's plexus in Little's area of the anterior portion of the septum (see Figure 46.6). Anterior bleeding is common in children and young adults as a result of nose blowing or picking. In the elderly, arteriosclerosis and hypertension are the underlying causes of arterial bleeding from the posterior part of the nose.

Table 46.1 Causes of epistaxis.

Local	Nose picking
	Nasal trauma
	Nasal foreign bodies
	Tumours
	Infection
	Granulomatous disorders
	Juvenile angiofibroma
Systemic	Hypertension
	Warfarin therapy
	Aspirin therapy
	Haemophilia
	Von Willebrand's disease
	Leukaemia
	Haemorrhagic telangiectasia

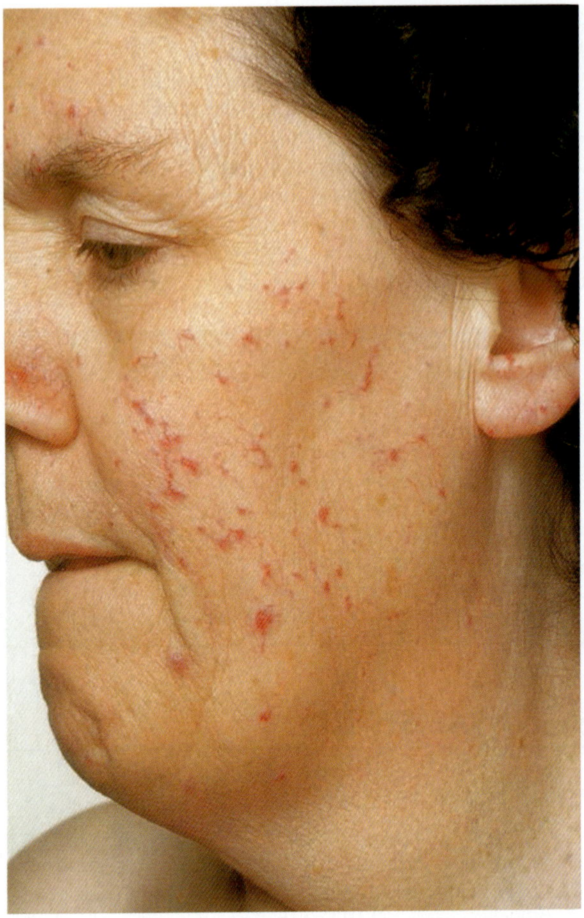

Figure 46.11 Osler's disease showing the multiple telangiectasia.

Hereditary haemorrhagic telangiectasia (Osler's disease) gives rise to recurrent multifocal bleeding from thin-walled vessels deficient in muscle and elastic tissue (Figure 46.11).

Juvenile angiofibroma is an uncommon condition that affects adolescent boys and may lead to massive life-threatening episodes of bleeding. Diagnosis is made with contrast CT scanning or magnetic resonance imaging (MRI). Anterior bowing or indentation of the posterior antral wall (Holman–Miller or antral sign) is the classical finding but may be seen in other expansive lesions in this area. It is a very vascular tumour, which should not be biopsied because of the risk of uncontrollable haemorrhage. Excision is best carried out by a surgeon experienced in the management of the condition. Preoperative embolisation of the feeding blood vessels may help to reduce blood loss during surgery. Sometimes the tumour is managed with radiotherapy.

Management of epistaxis

Bleeding from Kiesselbach's plexus may be controlled by silver nitrate cautery under local anaesthesia. Posterior bleeding, as seen in the elderly, may require anterior nasal packing either with Vaseline-impregnated ribbon gauze or absorbable sponge. An alternative to anterior packing is the use of an inflatable epistaxis balloon catheter (Figure 46.12). The catheter is passed into the nose and the distal balloon is inflated in the nasopharynx to secure it. The proximal balloon, which is sausage shaped, is then inflated within the nasal fossa to compress the bleeding point. Although usually effective, they can be uncomfortable.

Post-nasal packing may be required in refractory cases whereby a gauze pack is positioned in the nasopharynx under general anaesthesia. Endoscopic-assisted cautery or clipping of a posterior bleeding point can be an effective alternative to nasal packing.

For uncontrolled life-threatening epistaxis in which the above methods have proved ineffective, haemostasis is secured by vascular ligation. Depending on the origin of bleeding, it may be necessary to ligate the internal maxillary artery in the pterygopalatine fossa and the anterior and posterior ethmoidal

Sir William Osler, 1849–1919, Professor of Medicine successively at McGill University, Montreal, Canada; the University of Philadelphia, Pennsylvania, PA, and the Johns Hopkins University, Baltimore, MD, USA, finally becoming Regius Professor of Medicine at Oxford University, Oxford, UK in 1904.

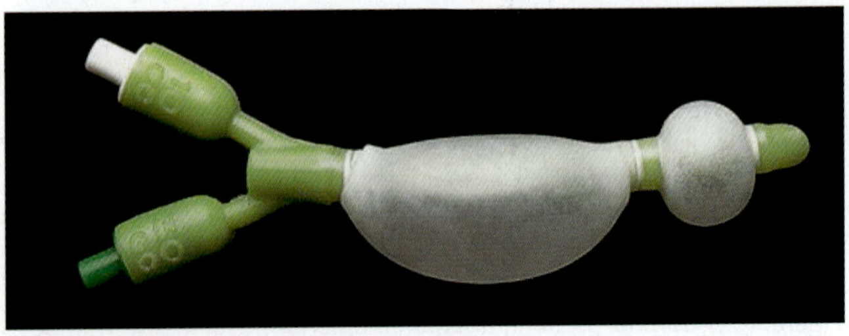

Figure 46.12 Epistaxis balloon catheter.

James Laurence Little, 1836–1885, Professor of Surgery, the University of Vermont, Montpelier, VT, USA.
Erik Adolf von Willebrand, 1870–1949, physician, Diakonissanstaltens Hospital, Helsinki, (Helsingfors), Finland, described hereditary pseudohaemophilia in 1926.

arteries. An alternative measure is external carotid artery ligation above the origin of the lingual artery.

In Osler's disease, anterior nasal packing is best avoided, if at all possible, because it is most likely to lead to further mucosal trauma and bleeding. High-dose oestrogen induces squamous metaplasia of the nasal mucosa and has been used effectively in treating this condition (Summary box 46.3).

Summary box 46.3

Epistaxis

- The most common causes are nose picking, hypertension and anticoagulant therapy
- Young people bleed from the anterior septum – Kiesselbach's plexus
- Elderly people bleed from the posterior part of the nose
- Silver nitrate cautery is used to control anterior bleeding
- Moderate bleeding may require anterior nasal packing
- Severe bleeding may require anterior and posterior nasal packing
- Persistent bleeding may require endoscopic cautery/clipping or arterial ligation

NASAL POLYPS

Pathology

Nasal polyps are benign swellings of the ethmoid sinus mucosa of unknown origin. Histologically, the polyps contain a waterlogged stroma infiltrated with inflammatory cells and eosinophils. The majority of nasal polyps arise from the ethmoid sinuses, with each individual ethmoid air cell giving rise to a single polyp as its swollen mucosal lining prolapses out of the air cell to hang down inside the nasal cavity. Polyps can arise from the other nasal sinuses and a single large polyp arising from the maxillary antrum is referred to as an antrochoanal polyp (Figure 46.13).This usually fills the nose and eventually prolapses posteriorly down into the nasopharynx.

Clinical features

Patients present with nasal obstruction, watery rhinorrhoea, sinus infection and often anosmia. Polyps are easily identifiable within the nose as pale semitransparent grey masses, which are mobile and insensitive when palpated with a fine probe. This allows them to be distinguished from hypertrophied turbinates (Figure 46.14).

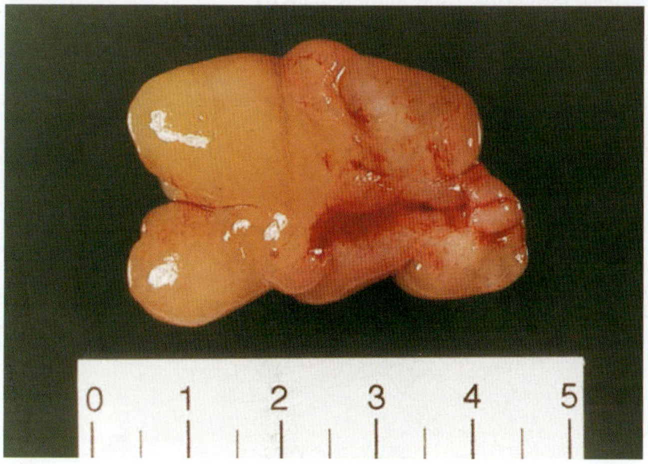

Figure 46.13 Antrochoanal polyp.

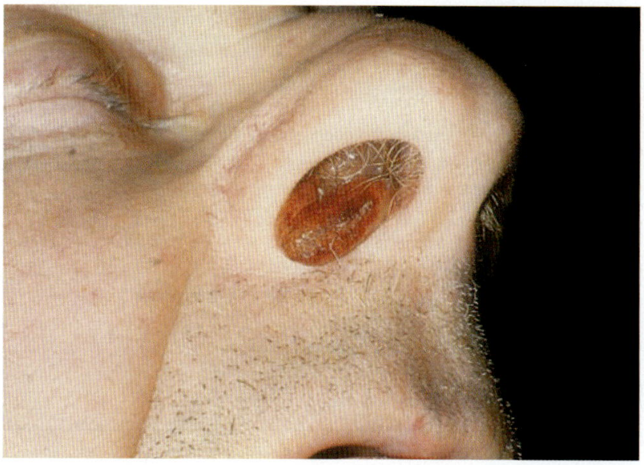

Figure 46.14 Nasal polyp in right nasal vestibule.

Malignancy should be considered in adults with unilateral nasal polyps, whereas in children such polyps must be distinguished from a meningocoele or encephalocoele by high-resolution CT scanning of the anterior cranial fossa. Nasal polyps are unusual in children. However, they do occur in conjunction with cystic fibrosis in 10 per cent of cases.

Management of nasal polyps

Medical treatment with systemic steroids will often reduce the size of nasal polyps and give short-term relief of nasal blockage. Unfortunately, the polyps tend to recur when the treatment stops. Surgical treatment is required in patients with severe nasal obstruction and pansinusitis that is refractory to medical treatment. Polyps may be removed either by avulsion with a nasal snare or endoscopically with a powered nasal microresector (Figure 46.15). After multiple recurrences, ethmoidectomy should be considered (Summary box 46.4).

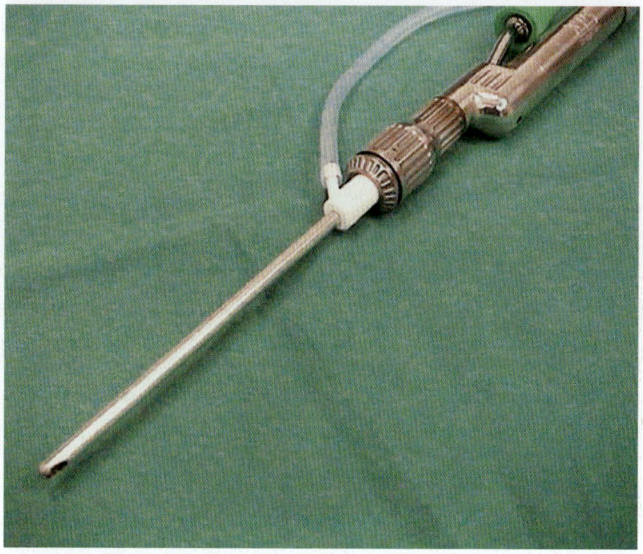

Figure 46.15 Powered nasal microresector.

Summary box 46.4

Nasal polyps

- Polyps are insensitive to touch and are mobile
- Simple polyps are bilateral
- Unilateral nasal polyps should be removed for histology
- Bleeding polyps may indicate malignancy
- Meningocoele and encephalocoele must be excluded in children with polyps
- Polyps can be removed with a snare or a powered microresector
- Recurrent polyps may require ethmoidectomy
- Transitional papilloma may mimic simple nasal polyps
- All polyps should be submitted for histology

MAXILLARY SINUSITIS

Clinical features

Local disorders, such as nasal polyps, deviated nasal septum or upper dental sepsis, may predispose to sinus infection. Patients with persistent maxillary sinusitis have a mucopurulent post-nasal discharge, headache, which is variable in severity and location, facial pain and nasal obstruction. Irritation of the superior alveolar nerve may give rise to referred upper toothache. The nasal mucosa is swollen and bathed in mucopurulent secretions. Plain sinus radiographs may show a fluid level in the antrum or complete opacity (Figure 46.16). About 10 per cent of infections of the maxillary antrum are caused by dental sepsis from anaerobic organisms. The resultant mucopurulent nasal secretion has a foul taste and smell. Complications of maxillary sinusitis include acute orbital cellulitis or osteitis.

Treatment

Adequate penetration of antibiotics into chronically inflamed sinus mucosa is doubtful and, therefore, treatment may need to

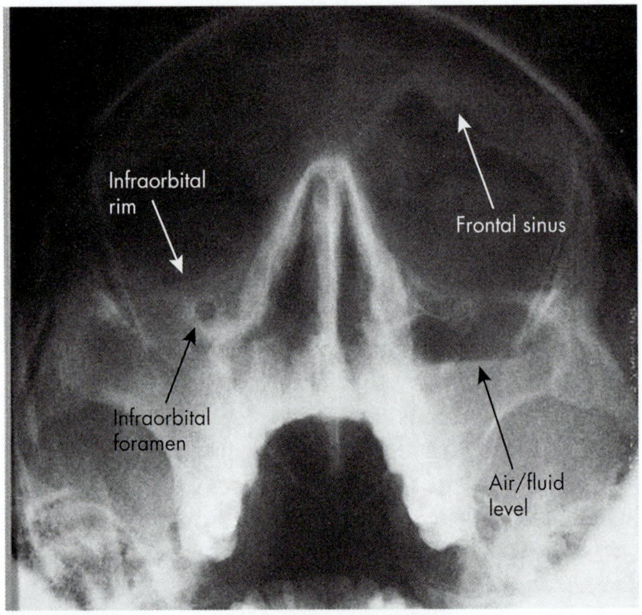

Figure 46.16 Plain radiograph showing the fluid level in the left maxillary antrum and total opacity of the right antrum.

be prolonged. Topical nasal decongestants, such as ephedrine nasal drops, will often encourage the sinus to drain.

Antral lavage under local or general anaesthesia allows confirmation of the diagnosis and provides the opportunity to obtain samples for bacteriology. The antrum is entered through the inferior meatus below the inferior turbinate where the bone separating the antrum from the nasal fossa is extremely thin and can be easily penetrated by a trocar and cannula (Figure 46.17). If infection has caused a significant degree of inflammation and fibrosis of the lining of the antrum, intranasal endoscopic techniques may be employed to create a middle meatal antrostomy or enlarge the natural ostium. Endoscopic nasal surgery allows a more functional approach to diseases of the paranasal sinuses and, as a result, the indications for radical antrostomy are decreasing (Summary box 46.5).

Summary box 46.5

Maxillary sinusitis

- The most common causative organisms are *Streptococcus pneumoniae* and *Haemophilus influenzae*
- Anaerobic infection may result from dental sepsis
- Acute infection should be treated with antibiotics and topical decongestants
- Antral lavage is diagnostic and therapeutic
- Intranasal antrostomy or endoscopic middle meatal antrostomy may be required
- Complications of untreated infection include cellulitis, osteitis and involvement of the orbit

FRONTOETHMOIDAL SINUSITIS

Chronic frontoethmoiditis gives rise to mucopurulent catarrh, frontal headache or a feeling of pressure between the eyes, nasal obstruction and hyposmia. Nasal endoscopy will confirm pus issuing from the middle meatus. The ethmoid sinuses can only be properly assessed radiologically by CT scanning, including coronal as well as axial sections.

Complications include periorbital cellulitis (Figure 46.18). This may progress to cavernous sinus thrombosis and septicaemia. Spread of infection by direct bone penetration or via the diploic vein can give rise to extradural, subdural or frontal lobe abscess formation (Summary box 46.6).

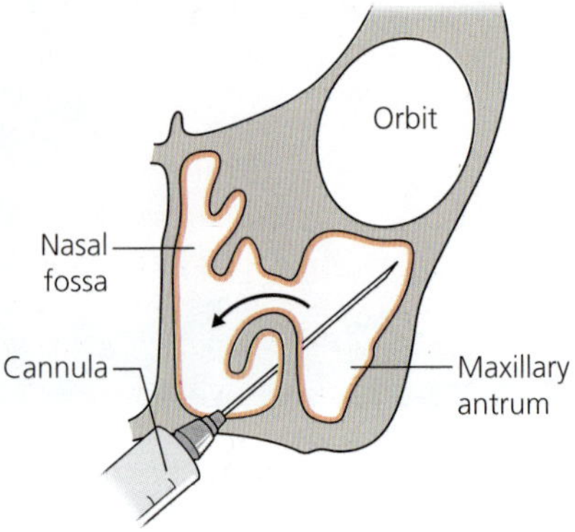

Figure 46.17 Diagram of left maxillary antral lavage.

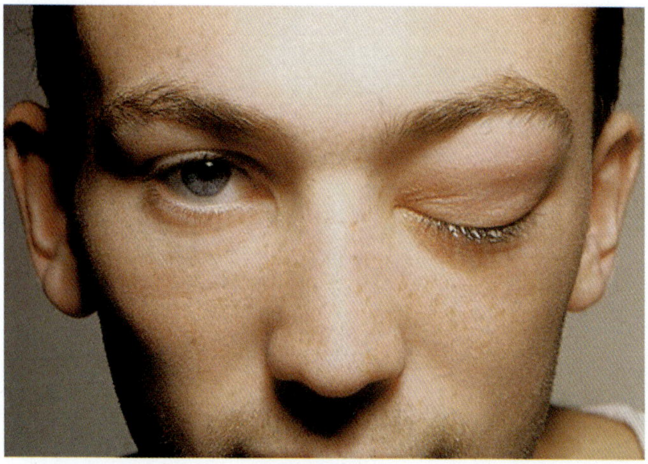

Figure 46.18 Left periorbital cellulitis complicating acute left ethmoiditis.

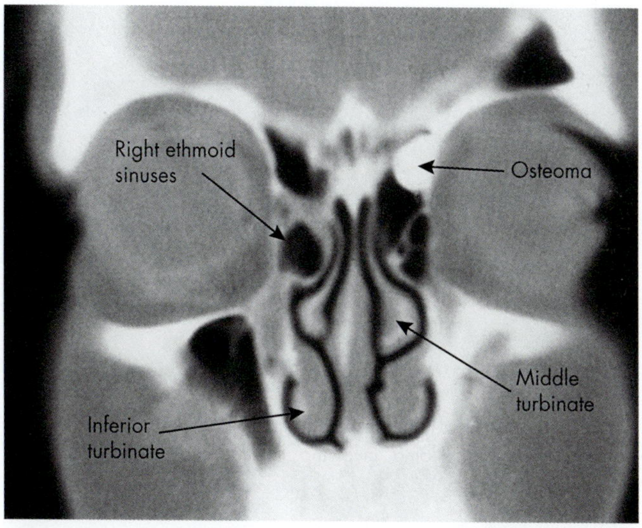

Figure 46.19 Coronal computed tomography scan showing a small osteoma in the right ethmoid sinus adjacent to the orbit.

Summary box 46.6

Frontoethmoiditis

- Assessment is best achieved by CT scanning
- It may require open surgical drainage
- Chronic infection may require an obliterative osteoplastic flap procedure
- Orbital infections may threaten sight
- Intracranial spread may cause meningitis, cerebral abscess or cavernous sinus thrombosis

TUMOURS OF THE NOSE AND SINUSES

Tumours arising in the nasal fossa may present with unilateral nasal obstruction, persistent unilateral anterior rhinorrhoea, post-nasal catarrh, epistaxis, unilateral blood-stained rhinorrhoea, facial swelling or proptosis.

Benign tumours

Simple papillomas or viral warts can grow inside the nasal vestibule. They can be confused with carcinomas and are best excised for histological diagnosis.

Osteomas of the nasal skeleton are not uncommon and are usually detected on radiography as an incidental finding (Figure 46.19). In symptomatic individuals, the osteoma can be removed via the frontal sinus or an external ethmoidectomy.

Transitional cell papillomas can occur both in the nasal cavity and the nasal sinuses. They are sometimes referred to as inverted papillomas because histologically the hyperplastic epithelium inverts into the underlying stroma. The papillomas are covered with transitional epithelium. Calcification within the tumour may be seen on CT scanning along with sclerosis of bone at the margins of the growth (Figure 46.20). Transitional cell papillomas can undergo malignant change.

Malignant tumours

The most common malignant tumours to occur within the nasal cavity and paranasal sinuses are squamous cell carcinoma (Figure 46.21), adenoid cystic carcinoma and adenocarcinoma. Adenocarcinoma has been linked to exposure to hardwood dust in the furniture industry. Adenoid cystic carcinomas arise from minor salivary glands, which can be found in the nose. Suspicious signs of invasion of neighbouring tissues include diplopia, proptosis, loosening of the teeth (Figure 46.22), trismus, cranial nerve palsies and regional lymphadenopathy (Figure 46.23).

Patients with sinus or intranasal malignancy are best managed in a combined clinic where the expertise of ear, nose and throat (ENT) surgeons, maxillofacial surgeons and radiotherapists can be employed (Summary box 46.7).

Summary box 46.7

Tumours of the nose and sinuses

- Unilateral nasal blockage, discharge and bleeding are often presenting symptoms in nasal or sinus tumours
- Osteomas are often asymptomatic
- Transitional cell papilloma is the most common benign tumour – this tumour may undergo malignant change
- Squamous cell carcinoma is the most common malignant tumour
- Almost 50 per cent of sinonasal cancers arise on the lateral nasal wall and 33 per cent in the maxillary antrum
- Multidisciplinary management of malignant sinonasal tumours requires input from ENT surgeons, maxillofacial surgeons and radiotherapists

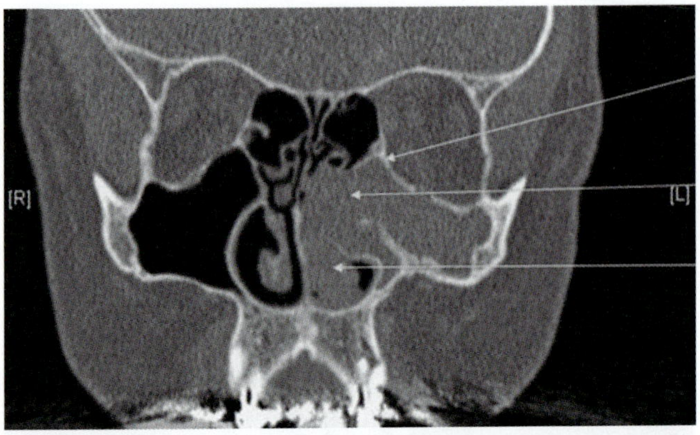

Figure 46.20 Coronal computed tomography scan showing extensive transitional cell papilloma involving the left maxillary antrum and ethmoid sinuses.

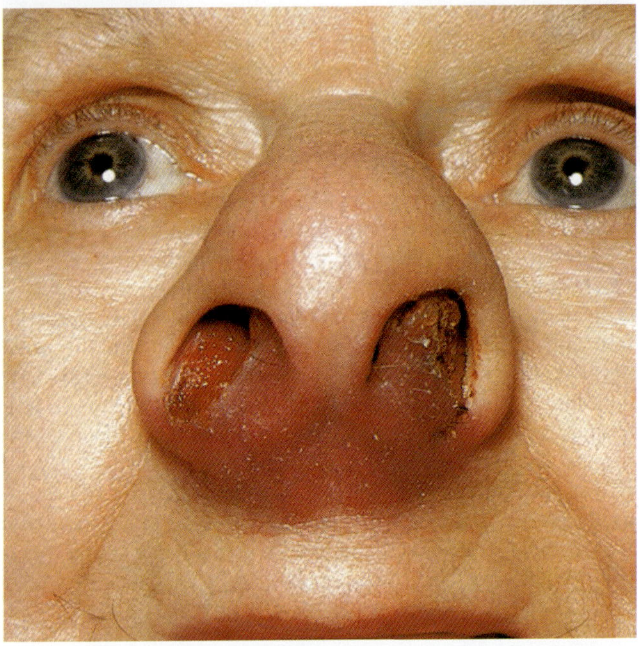

Figure 46.21 Squamous cell carcinoma of the nasal septum.

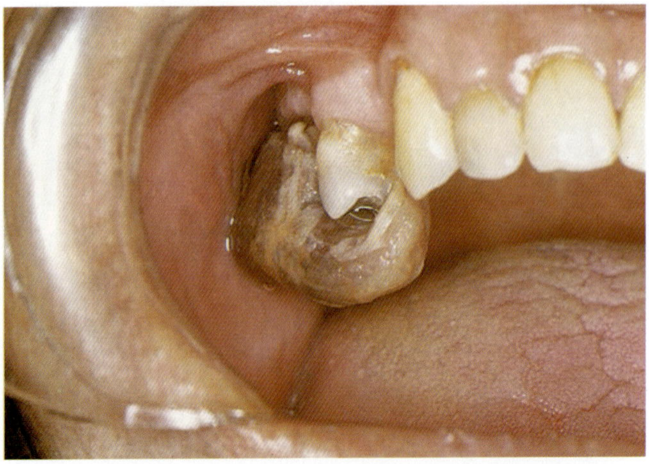

Figure 46.22 Maxillary antral carcinoma presenting through an oroantral fistula.

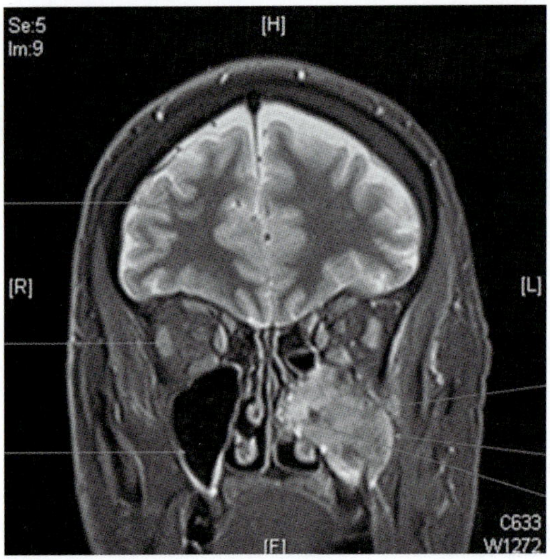

Figure 46.23 Axial computed tomography scan of paranasal sinuses showing extensive left maxillary antral carcinoma invading adjacent structures.

FURTHER READING

Hosemann WG, Weber RK, Keerl RE, Lund VJ (eds). *Minimally invasive endonasal sinus surgery: principles, techniques, results, complications, revision surgery*. New York: Thieme, 2000.

Kennedy DW, Hwang PH (eds). Rhinology: *Diseases of the nose, sinuses, and skull base*. New York: Thieme, 2012.

Lund VJ (ed.). Rhinology, vol. 2. In: Gleeson MJ (ed.). *Scott-Brown's otorhinolaryngology: head and neck surgery*, 7 edn. London: Hodder Arnold, 2008.

CHAPTER

47 The ear

LEARNING OBJECTIVES

To be familiar with:
- The anatomy of the ear
- The conditions of the outer, middle and inner ear
- The examination of the ear including hearing tests

To understand that:
- The outer layer of the tympanic membrane migrates outwards
- The facial nerve can be damaged by trauma and ear disease
- Chronic ear disease can lead to intracranial sepsis
- There are two types of hearing loss: conductive and senorineural

INTRODUCTION

The mammalian ear is an evolutionary masterpiece. Its highly complex 'three-dimensional anatomy' is best learnt by dissecting cadaver temporal bones.

SURGICAL ANATOMY OF THE EAR

The external ear

The external and middle ear develop from the first two branchial arches. The external ear canal is 3 cm in length; the outer two-thirds is cartilage and the inner third is bony. The skin on the lateral surface of the tympanic membrane is highly specialised and migrates outwards along the ear canal. As a result of this migration most people's ears are self-cleaning. The external canal is richly innervated and the skin is tightly bound down to the perichondrium so that swelling in this region results in severe pain.

The lymphatics of the external ear drain to the retroauricular, parotid, retropharyngeal and deep upper cervical lymph nodes.

The tympanic membrane and middle ear

The anatomy of the tympanic membrane and ossicles is shown in Figure 47.1. The relations of the middle ear are important (Figure 47.2).

The tympanic membrane and ossicles act as a transformer system converting vibrations in the air to vibrations within the fluid-filled inner ear.

The inner ear

The inner ear comprises the cochlea and vestibular labyrinth (saccule, utricle and semicircular canals). These structures are embedded in dense bone called the otic capsule.

The cochlea is a minute spiral of two and three-quarter turns. Within this spiral, perilymph and endolymph are partitioned by the thin Reissner's membrane. The endolymph has a high concentration of potassium, similar to intracellular fluid, and the perilymph has a high sodium concentration and communicates with the cerebrospinal fluid (CSF). Maintenance of the ionic gradients is an active process and is essential for neuronal activity.

There are approximately 15 000 hair cells in the human cochlea. They are arranged in rows of inner and outer hair cells. The inner hair cells act as mechanicoelectric transducers, converting the acoustic signal into an electric impulse. The outer hair cells contain contractile proteins and serve to tune the basilar membrane on which they are positioned.

Each inner hair cell responds to a particular frequency of vibration. When stimulated, it depolarises and passes an impulse to the cochlear nuclei in the brainstem.

The vestibular labyrinth consists of the semicircular canals, utricle and saccule and their central connections. The three semicircular canals are arranged in the three planes of space at right angles to each other. Like the auditory system, hair cells are present. In the lateral canals, the hair cells are embedded in a gelatinous cupula. Shearing forces, caused by angular movements of the head, produce hair cell movements and generate action potentials. In the utricle and saccule, the hair cells are embedded in an otoconial membrane that contains particles of calcium carbonate. These respond to changes in linear acceleration and the pull of gravity.

Impulses are carried centrally by the vestibular nerve and connections are made to the spinal cord, cerebellum and external ocular muscles. Its function is to record the position and movements of the head.

The sensory nerve supply

The external ear is supplied by the auriculotemporal branch

Bartolomeo Eustachio (Eustachius), 1513–1574, was appointed physician to the Pope in 1547, and Professor of Anatomy at Rome, Italy, in 1549.
Ernst Reissner, 1824–1878, Professor of Anatomy at Dorpat, and later at Breslau, Germany (now Wroclaw, Poland), described the vestibular membrane of the cochlea in 1851.

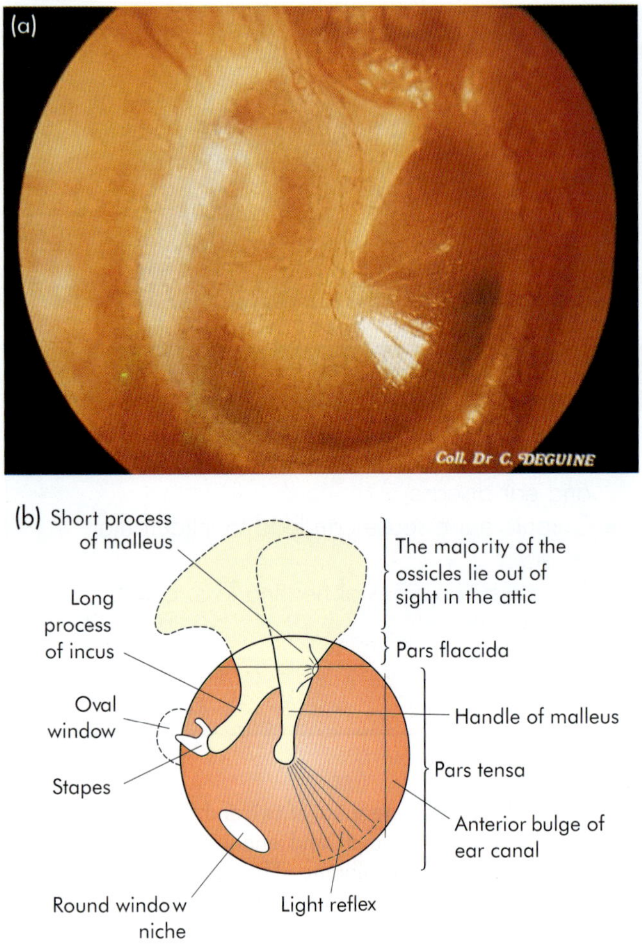

Figure 47.1 (a) Right tympanic membrane and (b) diagram to illustrate anatomy (courtesy of Dr Christian Deguine).

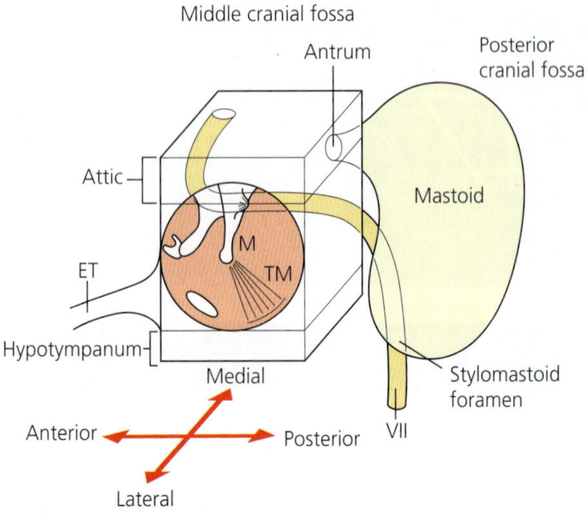

Figure 47.2 Diagram to show the relations of the middle ear (courtesy of Dr Christian Deguine). ET, Eustachian tube; M, malleus; TM, tympanic membrane; VII, facial nerve.

of the trigeminal nerve (Vth) and the greater auricular nerve (C2/3), together with branches of the lesser occipital nerve (C2). The VIIth, IXth and Xth cranial nerves also supply small sensory branches to the external ear. The middle ear is supplied by the glossopharyngeal nerve (IXth).

This complicated and rich sensory innervation means that referred otalgia is common and may originate from the normal area of distribution of any of the above nerves. A classic example is the referred otalgia caused by cancer of the larynx (Summary box 47.1).

Summary box 47.1

Applied anatomy

- The skin on the outer surface of the eardrum migrates outwards so that the ear canal is 'self-cleaning'
- Infection of the middle ear and mastoid can easily spread to the cranial cavity
- The facial nerve pursues a tortuous course through the middle ear
- The ear has a rich sensory innervation so that 'referred otalgia' is common
- Cancer of the larynx can present with otalgia

Taking a thorough history is the most important part of the assessment; the symptoms that need to be enquired after are listed in Table 47.1.

Table 47.1 History-taking.

Earache, pain and itch
Hearing loss
Discharge: type, quantity and smell
Tinnitus
Vertigo
Facial movements
Speech and development (in children)
Past history: head injury, baro- or noise trauma, ototoxics, family history and previous ear surgery

EXAMINATION OF THE EAR

The tools of the trade are shown in Figure 47.3. Examination of the ear is part of the general ear, nose and throat (ENT) examination. The Rinne and Weber tuning fork tests are used to distinguish between a conductive and a sensorineural hearing loss.

In Weber's test, the base of a 256 Hz vibrating tuning fork is placed on the centre of the patient's forehead so that the sound is conducted through the bones of the skull (not air). If the patient hears the sound more clearly in one ear than the other, then there is either a conductive loss in that ear or neurological loss in the opposite ear. Rinne's test then distinguishes between these two possibilities. A 512-Hz tuning fork is placed on the mastoid bone until the patient can no longer 'feel' it vibrating. It is then moved so that its tips are just outside the ear. The patient should now 'hear' the sound again if conduction is normal.

The cranial nerves and especially the function of the facial nerve should be examined.

Friedrich Heinrich Adolf Rinne, 1819–1868, otologist, Göttingen, Germany, described his test in 1855.
Friedrich Eugen Weber-Liel, 1832–1891, otologist, University of Berlin and Jena, Germany. He described the operation of tenotomy of the tensor tympani used for certain forms of partial deafness.

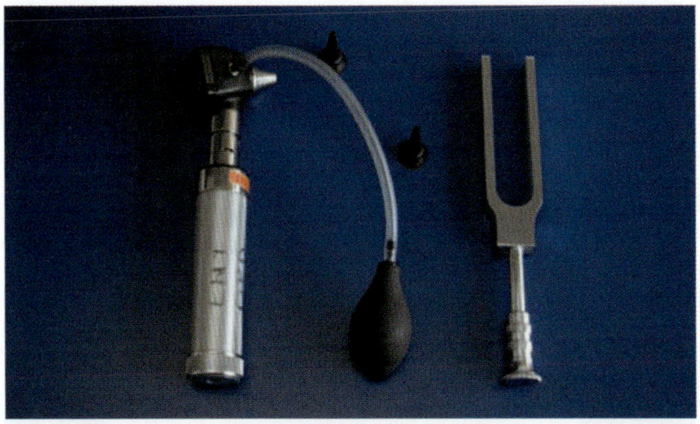

Figure 47.3 Tools of the trade: a fibreoptic otoscope, with pneumatic attachment and a selection of specula. Also a 512-Hz tuning fork.

Although conversational testing can give a useful guide to the level of hearing, pure tone audiometry in a soundproof booth is the best way of establishing the air and bone hearing levels (Figure 47.4). Other common audiological tests include speech audiometry, tympanometry, stapedial reflexes, electric response audiometry, otoacoustic emissions, caloric testing and electronystagmography (see Further reading).

Radiological investigation

Computed tomography (CT) scanning of the temporal bones is routinely used preoperatively to show detailed individual anatomy, as well as alerting the surgeon to anatomical variants. Pus, bone and air are shown well on high-resolution CT (Figure 47.5).

Magnetic resonance imaging (MRI) is better than CT at imaging soft tissue (e.g. facial and auditory nerve) and is the best method for imaging tumours of the acoustic nerves (Figure 47.6).

CONDITIONS OF THE EXTERNAL EAR

Congenital anomalies

See Table 47.2.

Table 47.2 Congenital anomalies of the external ear.

The external and middle ear originate from the first and second branchial arches, but the cochlea is neuroectodermal in origin
An individual can have a congenital abnormality of the pinna and middle ear with a normal cochlea and, therefore, the potential for normal hearing.
Osseointegration allows a prosthetic ear and hearing aid to be attached to the skull

Trauma

A haematoma of the pinna occurs when blood collects under the perichondrium. The cartilage receives its blood supply from the perichondrial layer and will die if the haematoma is not evacuated, resulting in a cauliflower ear. A generous incision under general anaesthetic, with a pressure dressing or compressive sutures and antibiotic cover, is recommended (Figure 47.7).

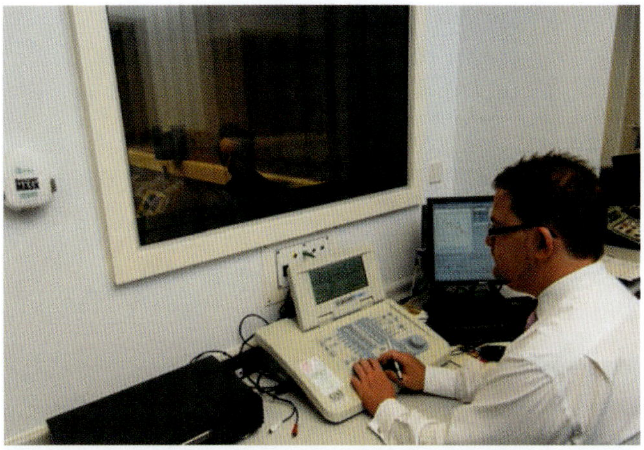

Figure 47.4 Audiometry: the patient sits in a soundproof room and the audiologist presents sounds at different thresholds and records the responses.

Foreign bodies in the ear canal need to be treated with the greatest respect. If an object is not easily removed at the first attempt, it is better to do it with the aid of a microscope and general anaesthesia. An active two-year-old with a bead in the ear can be a formidable opponent (Figure 47.8) (Summary box 47.2).

Summary box 47.2

Trauma of the external ear

- A haematoma of the pinna requires thorough drainage, antibiotics and a compressive dressing or sutures
- Consider general anaesthesia when attempting to remove a foreign body in a young child

Inflammation and infection

Otitis externa is common and consists of generalised inflammation of the skin of the external auditory meatus. The cause is

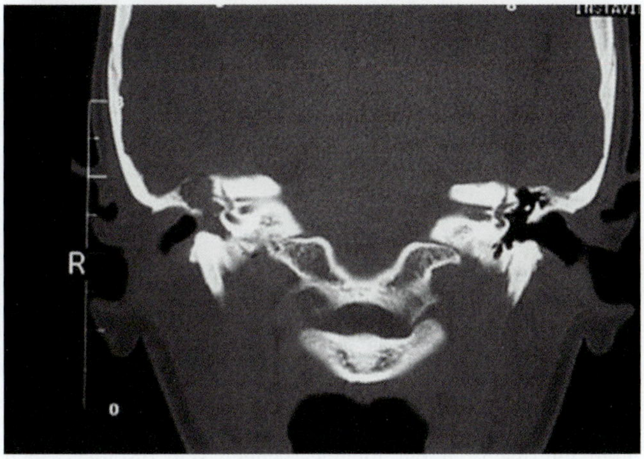

Figure 47.5 The computed tomography scan shows a normal left ear; note the air-filled middle ear and the incus and stapes and the lateral and semicircular canals and internal acoustic meatus (IAM) can be seen. In the right ear, the entire middle ear and mastoid is opaque and filled with soft tissue. This is the typical appearance of cholesteatoma.

Celsus (AD 70) recommended tying the patient on a wooden plank with the affected ear downwards and hitting the plank with a hammer.

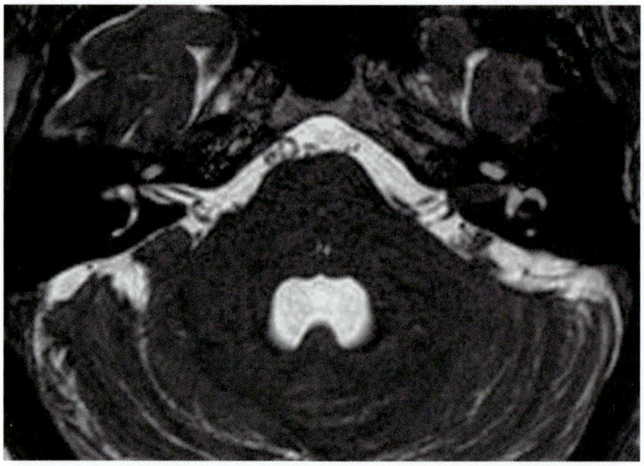

Figure 47.6 A high resolution T2-weighted image at the level of the internal acoustic meatus (IAM) showing an intracannalicular acoustic neuroma (AN) on the left and a normal IAM on the right (courtesy of Dr Peiter Petorius).

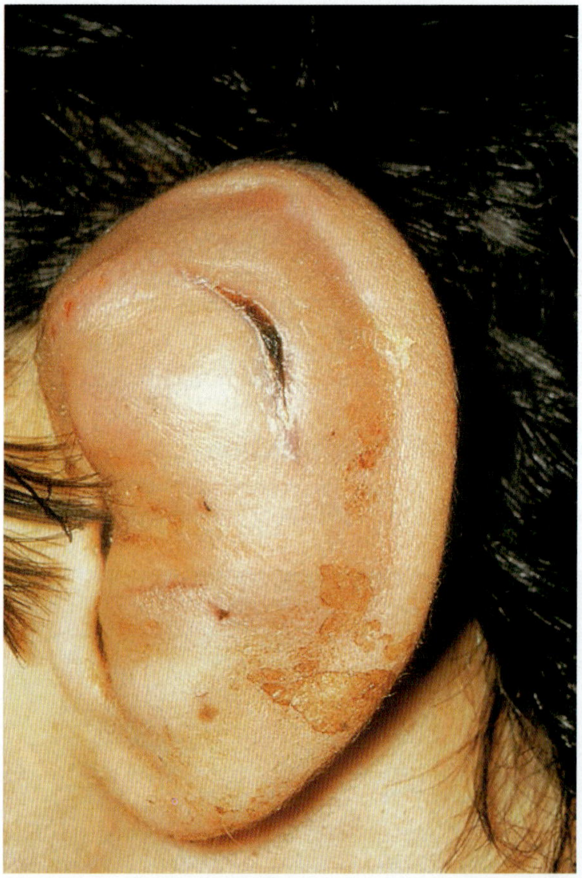

Figure 47.7 Haematoma of the pinna.

often multifactorial but includes general skin disorders, such as psoriasis and eczema, and trauma. Common pathogens are *Pseudomonas* and *Staphylococcus* bacteria, *Candida* and *Aspergillus*. Once the skin of the ear canal becomes oedematous, skin migration stops and debris collects in the ear canal. This acts as a substrate for the pathogens. The hallmark of acute

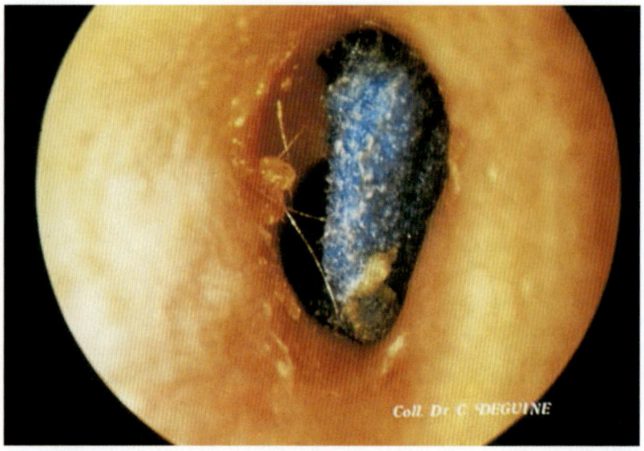

Figure 47.8 A foreign body seen in the ear canal, the removal of which can be a challenge (courtesy of Dr Christian Deguine).

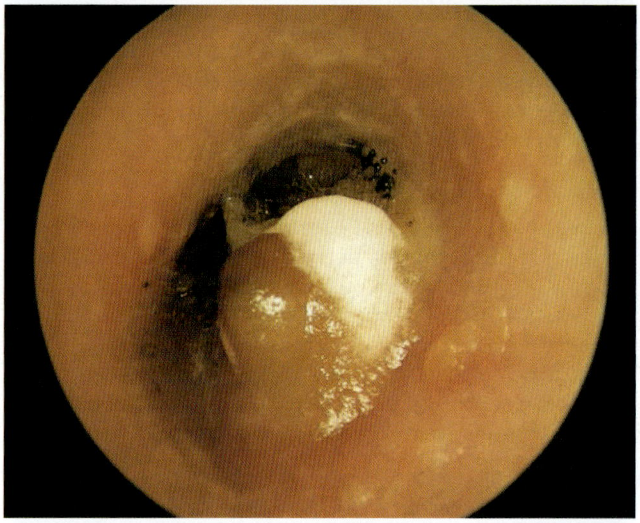

Figure 47.9 Fungal otitis externa; note the presence of hyphae (white) and spores (black).

otitis externa is severe pain. Movement of the pinna elicits pain, which distinguishes it from otitis media.

The initial treatment is with topical antibiotics and steroid ear drops, together with analgesia. If this fails, meticulous removal of the debris with the aid of an operating microscope is required. Fungal infection can be recognised by the presence of hyphae within the canal (Figure 47.9). Fungal infection causes irritation and itch. The treatment is meticulous removal of the fungus and any debris, as well as stopping any concurrent antibiotics. Systemic antibiotics are rarely required for otitis externa but should be used if cellulitis of the pinna occurs (Figure 47.10).

Necrotising otitis externa is a rare but important condition. It presents as a severe, persistent, unilateral otitis externa in an immunocompromised individual. It is important to think of the diagnosis in an elderly diabetic patient. Usually the infecting organism is *Pseudomonas aeruginosa*. Osteomyelitis of the skull base occurs and several cranial nerves (VII, IX, X) may be destroyed by the progressing infection. Intensive systemic antibiotics are required and the disease process should be monitored by high-resolution imaging (Summary box 47.3).

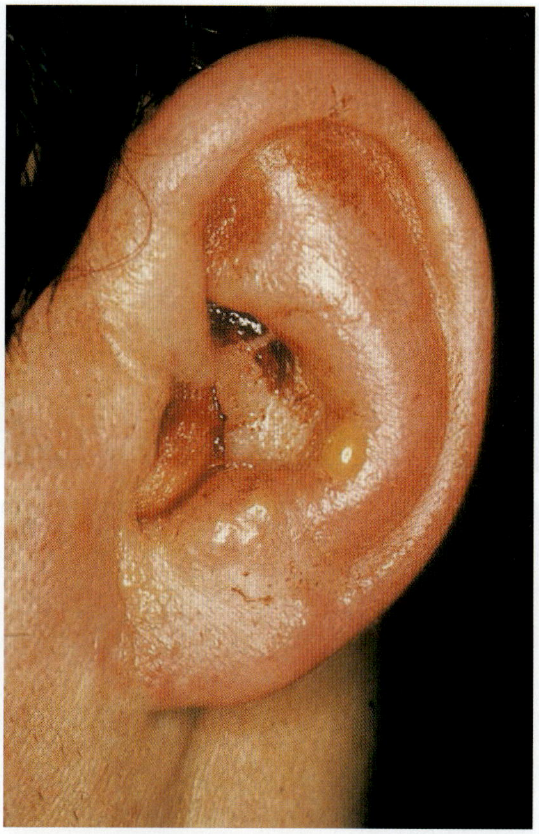

Figure 47.10 Cellulitis of the pinna.

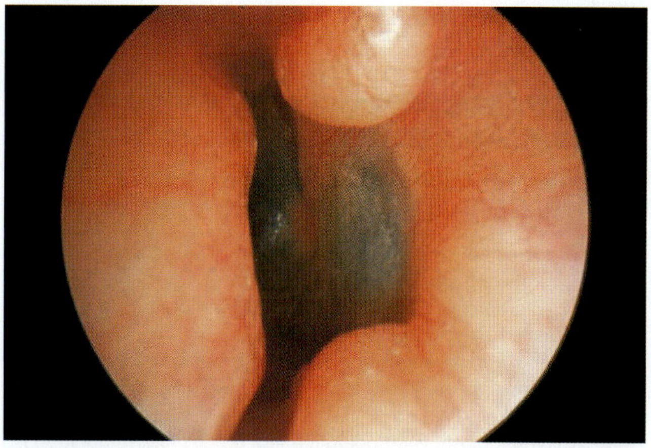

Figure 47.11 Osteomas grow from the bony part of the ear canal in response to cold and so are found in swimmers, surfers and divers. Treatment is only required if the osteomas occlude the ear canal.

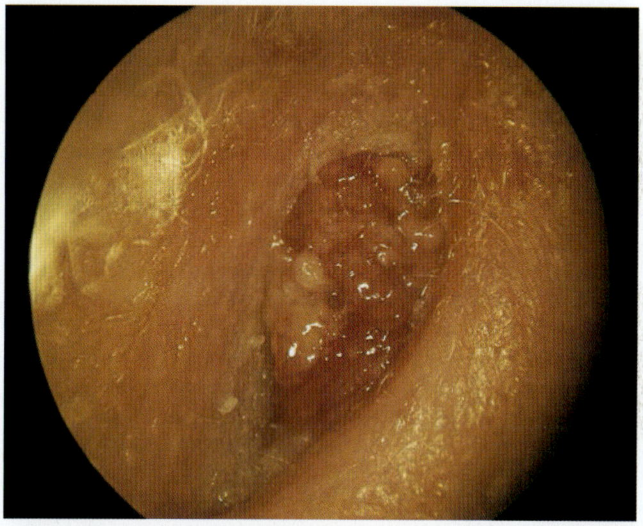

Figure 47.12 Squamous cell carcinomas of the external ear usually originate from the pinna; in this case, the tumour is growing from the canal (courtesy of Mr P Beasley).

Summary box 47.3

Types of otitis externa

- Acute bacterial otitis externa is very common and extremely painful; treat with topical steroids and topical antibiotics
- Systemic antibiotics should be reserved for cellulitis of the pinna
- Chronic otitis externa needs the underlying dermatitis to be treated; application of topical steroid in spirit is recommended
- Fungal otitis externa itches and can be diagnosed by the presence of hyphae and spores; treat with meticulous cleaning and stop antibiotics
- Necrotising otitis externa is a progressive skull base infection that occurs in immunocompromised individuals and can be life-threatening; intensive long-term antibiotic treatment is required

Neoplasms

Benign osteomas arise from the bone of the ear canal in individuals who swim in cold water (Figure 47.11). No treatment is required unless the osteomas obstruct the canal. Other benign tumours include papillomas and adenomas.

Malignant primary tumours of the external ear are either basal cell or squamous cell carcinomas (Figure 47.12). Both may present as ulcerating or crusting lesions that grow slowly and may be ignored by elderly patients. Squamous cell carcinomas metastasise to the parotid and/or neck nodes. The ear canal may be invaded by tumours from the parotid gland and post-nasal space carcinomas, which 'creep' up the Eustachian tube. All resectable malignant tumours of the ear are treated primarily with surgery, with or without the addition of radiation therapy.

CONDITIONS OF THE MIDDLE EAR

Congenital anomalies

Congenital anomalies of the middle ear may be associated with other general congenital deformities. There are a number of branchial arch syndromes, e.g. Pierre Robin's, craniofacial dysostosis, Down's and Treacher Collins' syndromes.

Trauma

Trauma to the middle ear can result in a perforated tympanic membrane (Figure 47.13a). Such perforations usually heal spontaneously (Figure 47.13b). Trauma can also result in ossicular discontinuity and it is usually the incus that is displaced. Tympanoplasty operations are available to reconstruct the damaged ossicular chain and repair the tympanic membrane (Summary box 47.4).

Summary box 47.4

Congenital anomalies and trauma of the middle ear

- Congenital anomalies may be isolated or associated with general congenital deformities
- CT can identify middle ear abnormalities that may be corrected by surgery
- Traumatic perforations of the tympanic membrane usually heal spontaneously, but explosive and welding injuries do not
- A myringoplasty is an operation that repairs the tympanic membrane
- With severe head trauma, the incus can be displaced, which leads to a conductive hearing loss

Suppurative otitis media

Suppurative otitis media is extremely common in childhood and is characterised by purulent fluid in the middle ear. Mastoiditis may be associated with otitis media because the mastoid air cells connect freely with the middle ear space. The tympanic membrane bulges because of pressure from the pus in the middle ear (Figure 47.14). The child suffers extreme pain until the tympanic membrane bursts. The most common infecting organisms are *Streptococcus pneumoniae* and *Haemophilus influenzae*. Appropriate systemic antibiotics should be given for 10 days.

Mastoiditis (Figure 47.15) requires hospital admission and intravenous antibiotics. If the infection does not resolve quickly, a cortical mastoidectomy is required, together with a myringotomy. Mastoiditis can lead to intracranial infection.

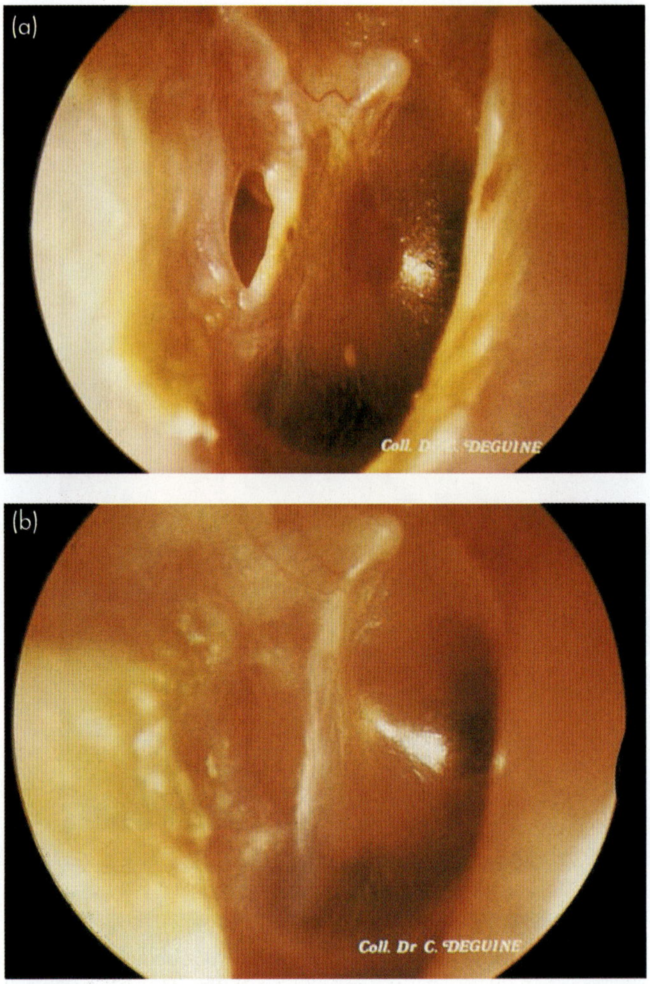

Figure 47.13 (a) Traumatically perforated tympanic membrane. (b) The same tympanic membrane 2 days later (courtesy of Dr Christian Deguine). (Reproduced from O'Donoghue, G.M., Bates, G.J. and Narula, A. (1991) *Clinical ENT*, with permission from Oxford University Press, Oxford.)

Otitis media with effusion (glue ear)

The majority of children experience at least one episode of glue ear. It is primarily thought to be caused by poor Eustachian tube function. Initially, the negative middle ear pressure results in transudation of fluid into the middle ear space (Figure 47.16). If hypoxia continues, a mucoid exudate is produced by the glands within the middle ear mucosa. This sticky exudate is referred to as 'glue ear'.

The following symptoms may be associated with glue ear:

- hearing impairment, which often fluctuates;
- delayed speech;
- behavioural problems;
- recurrent ear infections, which occur because the exudate is an ideal culture medium for micro-organisms;
- reading and learning difficulties at school.

The otoscopic findings with glue ear

The otoscopic findings of exudative glue ear are of a dull drum that is immobile on pneumatic otoscopy. The tympanic membrane is retracted and radial blood vessels may be present (Figure 47.17).

In children first presenting with bilateral glue ear, 50 per cent will be better within 6 weeks. Initially, a 'wait and watch' policy is therefore appropriate. If a bilateral conductive hearing loss persists, the child will miss out on educational opportunities

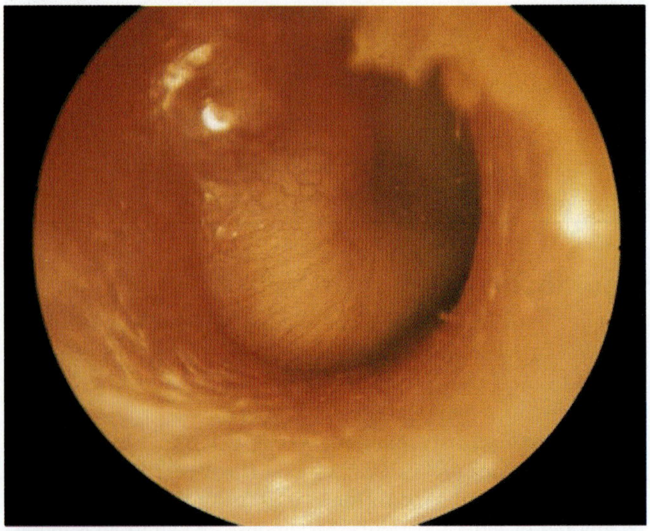

Figure 47.14 Acute otitis media of the left ear; note the bulging tympanic membrane.

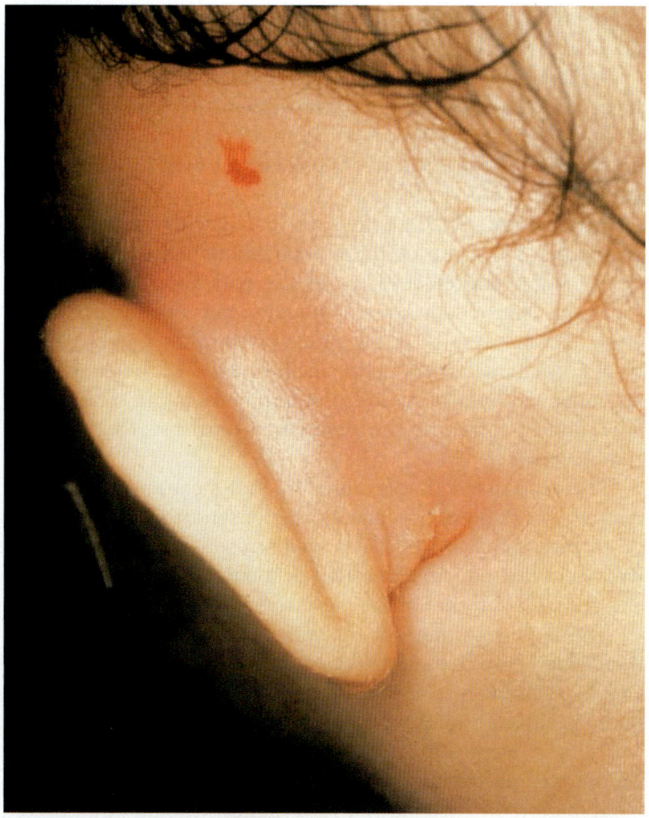

Figure 47.15 Child with acute mastoiditis whose tympanic membrane is shown in Figure 47.14.

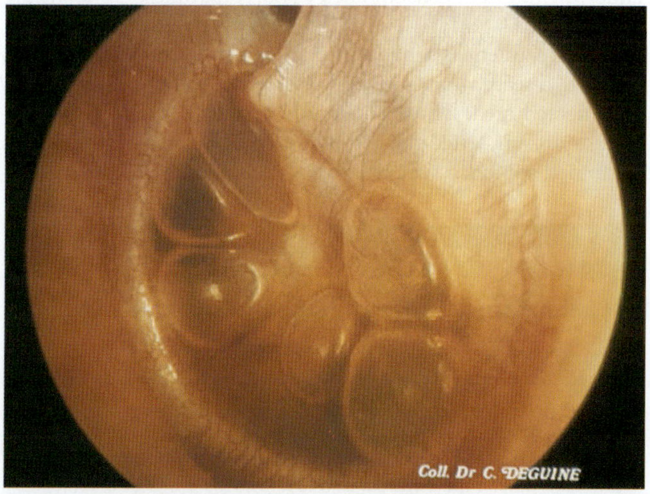

Figure 47.16 The initial serous transudate of glue ear, left ear (courtesy of Dr Christian Deguine). (Reproduced from O'Donoghue, G.M., Bates, G.J. and Narula, A. (1991) *Clinical ENT*, with permission from Oxford University Press, Oxford.)

and may not fulfil his or her academic potential; in these circumstances, treatment is required.

Medical treatment is of limited value. The Otovent® device may improve Eustachian tube function and is worth trying. Insertion of ventilation tubes (grommets) (Figure 47.18) and adenoidectomy are effective. The controversy is not whether surgery works, but when to intervene.

A middle ear effusion in adults is relatively rare and, when

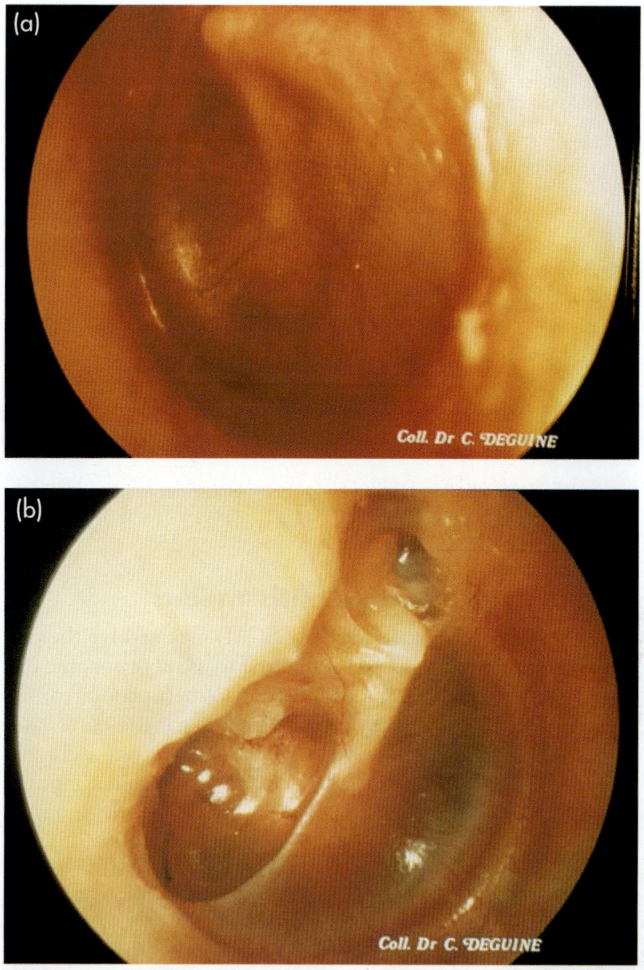

Figure 47.17 (a) Left exudative glue ear. The tympanic membrane is dull and retracted. The light reflex has gone and there are radial blood vessels. The drum does not move with pneumatic otoscopy. (b) Right ear. Advanced exudative glue ear with retraction pockets (courtesy of Dr Christian Deguine). (Reproduced from O'Donoghue, G.M., Bates, G.J. and Narula, A. (1991) *Clinical ENT*, with permission from Oxford University Press, Oxford.)

it occurs, it does not usually last long. The condition is often associated with an upper respiratory tract infection. A persistent unilateral effusion in an adult should always be viewed with suspicion. A nasopharyngeal carcinoma may cause the effusion by blocking the opening of the Eustachian tube in the post-nasal space. This is the most common carcinoma in men in southern China (Summary box 47.5).

Summary box 47.5

Acute suppurative otitis media and glue ear

- Acute suppurative otitis media can progress to mastoiditis
- Glue ear is very common in children and usually resolves without treatment
- Persistent hearing loss and/or recurrent acute otitis media is best treated with grommets and/or an adenoidectomy
- A persistent middle ear effusion in an adult is rare and may be caused by a cancer of the post-nasal space, especially in Chinese and Asian races

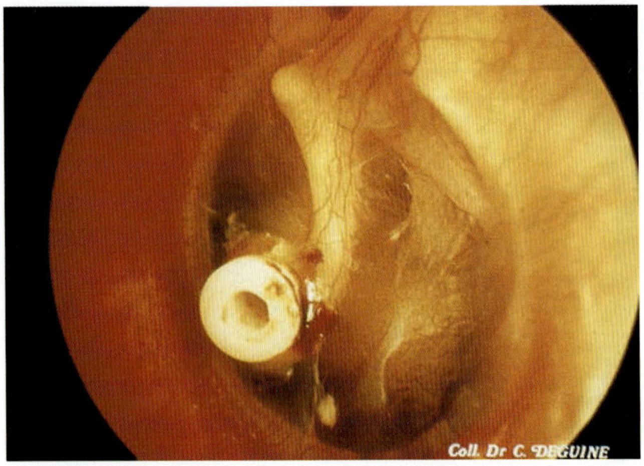

Figure 47.18 Ventilation tube in tympanic membrane, left ear (courtesy of Dr Christian Deguine).

Chronic suppurative otitis media

Chronic suppurative otitis media (CSOM) may involve the pars tensa and the middle ear and is referred to as tubotympanic disease; it results from trauma or infection. When perforated, the tympanic membrane usually repairs itself, but if the outer layer of the tympanic membrane fuses with inner mucosa a chronic perforation results (Figure 47.19). The patient's main symptoms are of an intermittent mucoid discharge associated with a mild conductive hearing loss. It is rare for this type of disease to be associated with intracranial complications.

A diagnosis is made on otoscopy and the tuning forks usually suggest a conductive hearing impairment. The first-line treatment is topical antibiotics and steroid drops and, on occasion, microsuction. If medical treatment fails, it may be necessary to graft the tympanic membrane.

Atticoantral CSOM (often associated with cholesteatoma) is important because of the complications associated with it. A retraction pocket develops in the pars flaccida and, if the squamous epithelium cannot migrate out of this pocket, a cholesteatoma results. A low-grade osteomyelitis gives the discharge its characteristic faecal smell. Invariably, the discharge is accompanied by hearing loss and mild discomfort. The patient may simply put up with these symptoms until a severe complication occurs.

The hearing loss that is caused by cholesteatoma may be conductive as a result of ossicular erosion or sensorineural as a result of cochlea damage. Vestibular symptoms may occur because of erosion of the semicircular canals or the migration of toxins into the vestibule. Erosion of the facial nerve is relatively unusual.

The close proximity of the middle ear and mastoid to the middle and posterior cranial fossae means that intracranial sepsis can result from chronic ear disease. The infection spreads to the dura via emissary veins, which connect the middle ear mucosa to the dura, or by direct extension of the disease through the bone. Meningitis, extradural, subdural or intracerebral abscess, or a combination of these may occur. Diagnosis should be suspected on otoscopy (Figure 47.20). Pus, crusts, granulations or a whitish debris in the attic are hallmarks of the disease. Examination under the microscope, audiometry and, sometimes, CT scanning are indicated.

The treatment is surgical and follows the principle of exposing the disease, excising the disease and then exteriorising the affected area. Three commonly applied operations for this disease are an atticotomy, modified radical mastoidectomy or combined approach tympanoplasty (Summary box 47.6).

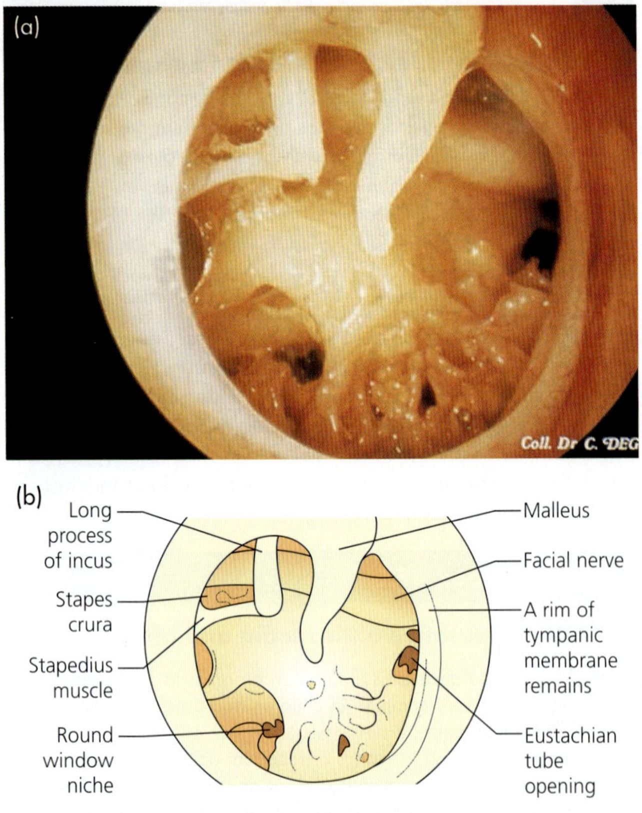

Figure 47.19 (a) Tubotympanic chronic suppurative otitis media showing central perforation, right ear. (b) Anatomy (courtesy of Dr Christian Deguine).

Summary box 47.6

Chronic suppurative middle ear disease

- Tubotympanic CSOM, in which there is a hole in the eardrum and frequently a mucoid discharge; this is seldom serious
- Atticoantral CSOM (cholesteatoma). In this condition, squamous epithelium has invaded a retraction pocket in the attic part of the eardrum and is known as a cholesteatoma. Presents with hearing loss and faecal smell from the ear. It is a common cause of intracranial sepsis

Tuberculous otitis media

This is an important cause of suppuration in many countries. The diagnosis should always be considered in any ear that fails to respond to standard therapy.

Otosclerosis

This is a condition in which new abnormal spongy bone is laid down in the temporal bone. Of particular importance is the bone that is laid down around the footplate of the stapes, which impedes the mobility of the stapes and results in a conductive hearing loss (Figure 47.21). A diagnosis should be suspected in any patient with a conductive hearing loss and a normal tympanic membrane.

A similar type of stapes fixation occurs in osteogenesis imperfecta and is known as van der Hoeve's syndrome. Otosclerosis is often bilateral.

The treatment options are simple reassurance, a hearing aid or a stapedotomy operation (Figure 47.22).

Neoplasms

Middle ear tumours are rare with the most common being a glomus tumour (Figure 47.23). Glomus tumours arise from non-chromaffin paraganglionic tissue. The carotid body tumour arising in the neck is an example of this type of tumour. In the temporal bone, three types of glomus tumour are recognised and classification depends on the location: glomus tympanicum (arising in the middle ear), glomus jugularae (arising next to the jugular bulb) and glomus vagali (skull base).

Pulsatile tinnitus is a classic symptom and the hearing loss that occurs may be either conductive or sensorineural. Palsies of the VIIth, IXth, Xth, XIth and/or XIIth nerves may occur. The classic sign is a cherry-red mass lying behind the tympanic membrane. An audible bruit may be heard with a stethoscope over the temporal bone. The treatment of choice is preoperative embolisation followed by surgical excision. Radiotherapy is also effective.

Squamous cell carcinoma may also occur within the middle ear. It usually presents with deep-seated pain and a blood-stained discharge. Facial paralysis often occurs. Squamous carcinomas usually arise in a chronically discharging ear and can arise in a chronically infected mastoid cavity. Radical surgical excision, with or without radiotherapy, provides the only chance of cure (Summary box 47.7).

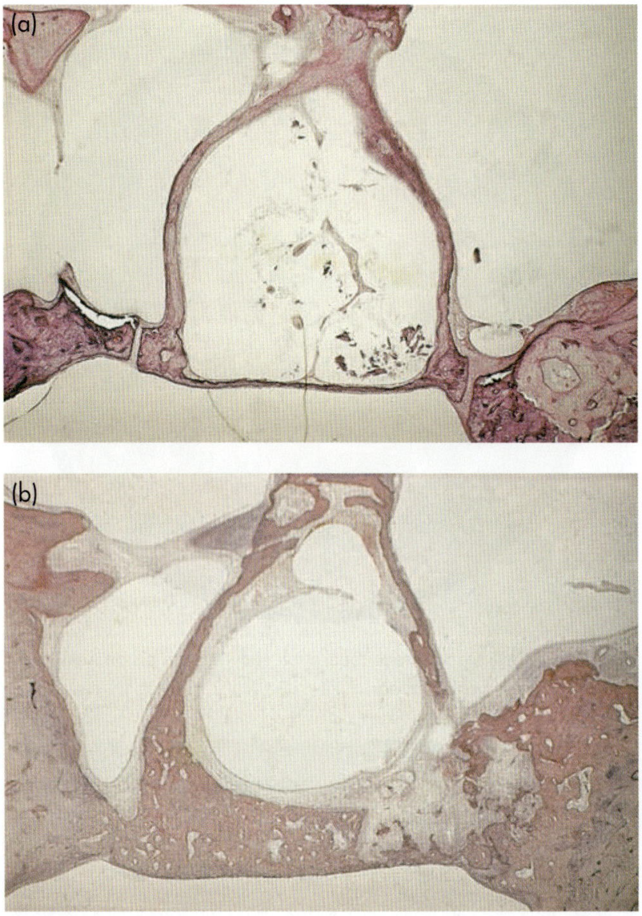

Figure 47.21 Section of normal stapes (a) and section of stapes affected by otosclerosis (b).

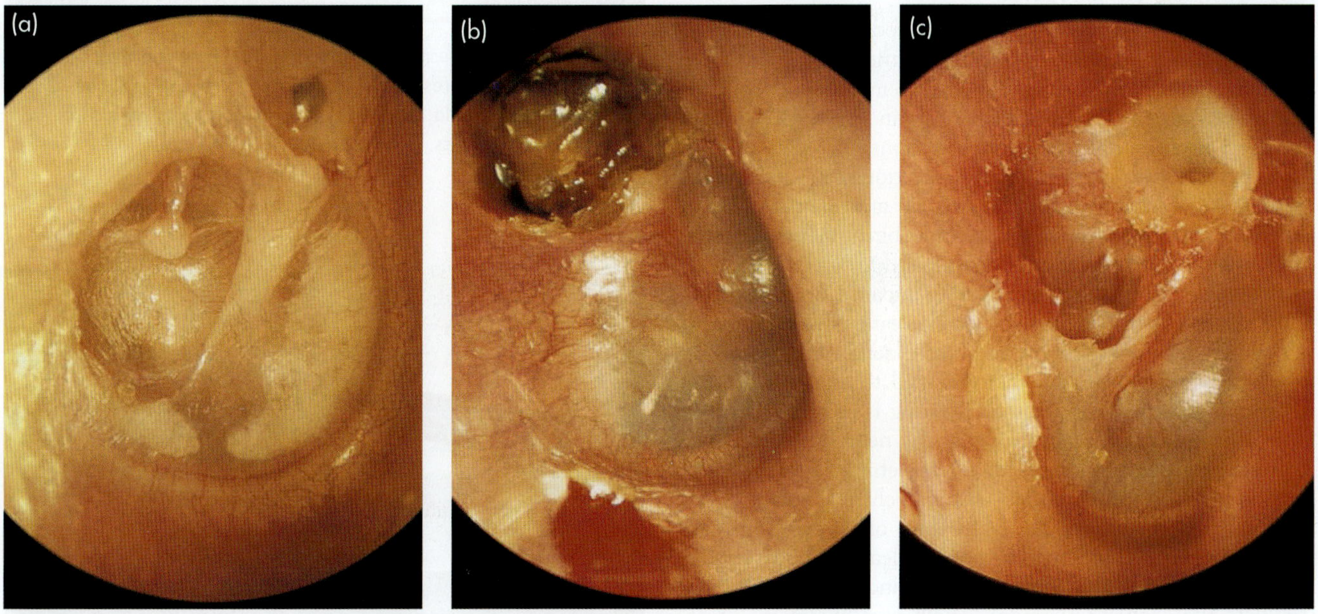

Figure 47.20 (a) Empty attic retraction pocket, right ear. (b) Attic crust covering cholesteatoma, right ear. (c) Attic erosion with cholesteatoma, right ear.

Jan van der Hoeve, 1878–1952, Dutch ophthalmologist, described this syndrome in 1918.

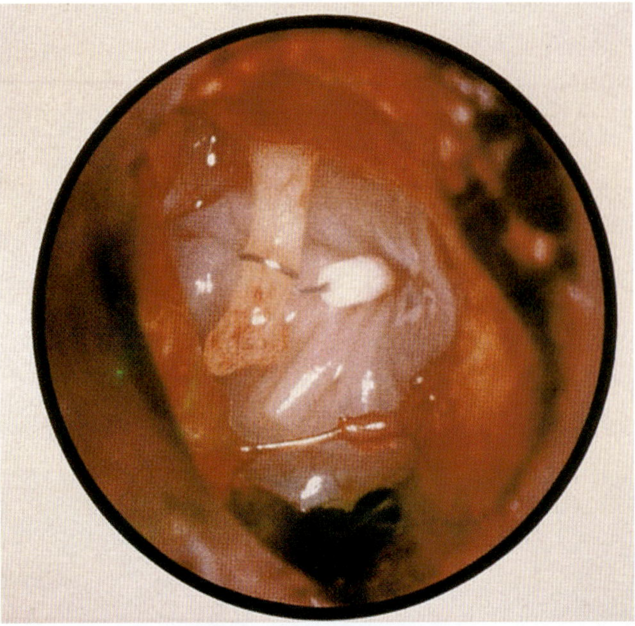

Figure 47.22 The stapedotomy operation showing the piston linking the incus to the vein graft, left ear.

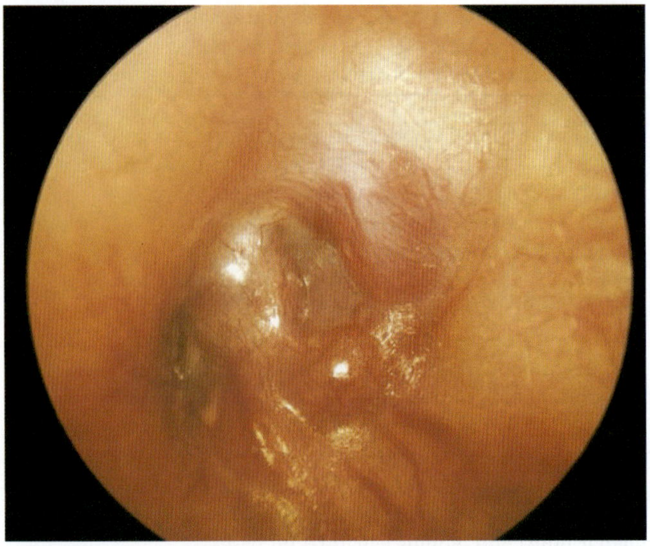

Figure 47.23 Glomus tumour in the middle ear, left ear.

Summary box 47.7

Neoplasms of the middle ear

- Highly vascular glomus tumours are rare and may present with pulsatile tinnitus
- Squamous cell cancer usually presents with pain and facial paralysis

CONDITIONS OF THE INNER EAR

Congenital anomalies

Congenital inner ear disorders may be associated with external or middle ear abnormalities or exist on their own. The most common anomaly is dysplasia of the membranous labyrinth, although dysplasia of the bony labyrinth and even total aplasia of the ear may occur. Intrauterine infections, including rubella, toxoplasmosis and cytomegalovirus infection, can cause inner ear damage. Perinatal hypoxia, jaundice and prematurity are also risk factors for a hearing loss. After birth, meningitis may cause profound sensorineural hearing loss.

If a child's parents suspect a hearing impairment, it is important to believe them, especially when glue ear has been excluded. In children in whom there is a suspicion of sensorineural hearing loss, brainstem-evoked audiometry is used to establish hearing thresholds (Figure 47.24). If some hearing is present, the early fitment of hearing aids can maximise the neural plasticity that is present in the developing brain. If a child has a profound hearing loss, early intervention with a cochlear implant is the ideal solution (Figure 47.25). Most cases of profound sensorineural hearing loss are due to loss of cochlear hair cells, so that an implant inserted through the round window can selectively stimulate the cochlear neurones, which usually remain intact. The results of cochlear implantation are miraculous but it is expensive technology.

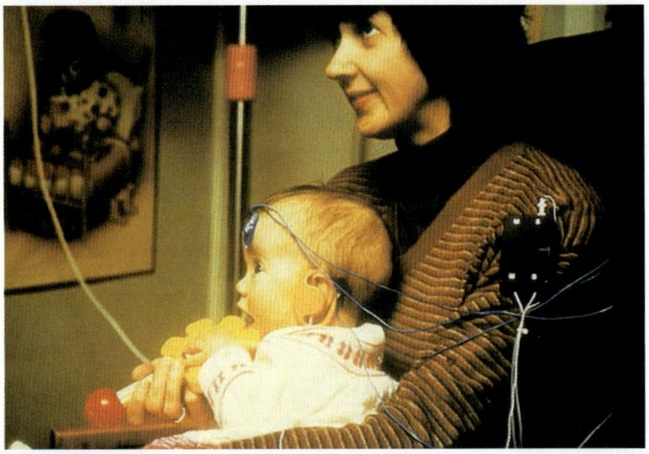

Figure 47.24 Evoked-response audiometry. A simple non-invasive objective test of hearing thresholds. (Reproduced from O'Donoghue, G.M., Bates, G.J. and Narula, A. (1991) *Clinical ENT*, with permission from Oxford University Press, Oxford.)

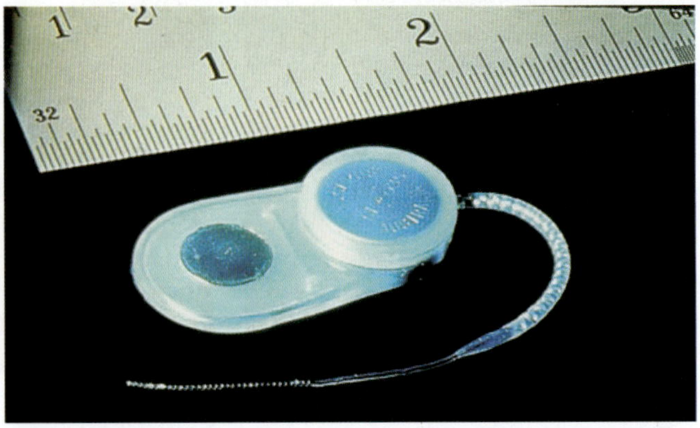

Figure 47.25 Multichannel cochlear implant (Cochlear Corporation).

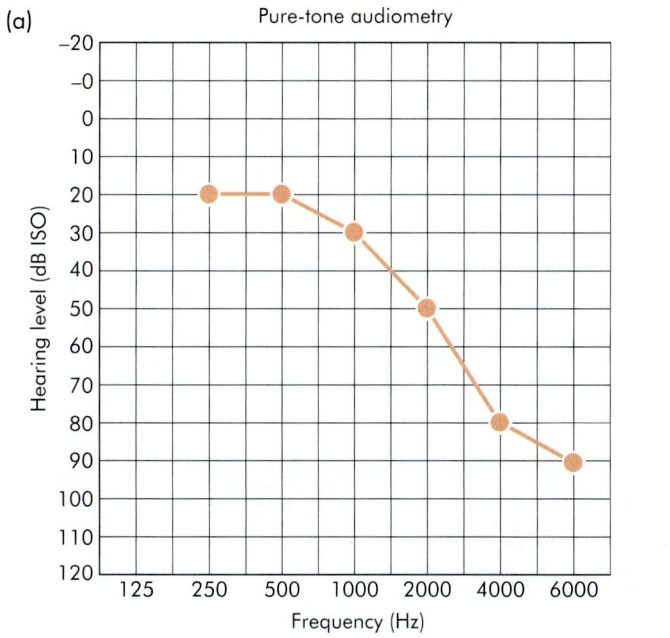

Figure 47.26 Typical audiogram of presbycusis: (a) right ear; (b) left ear.

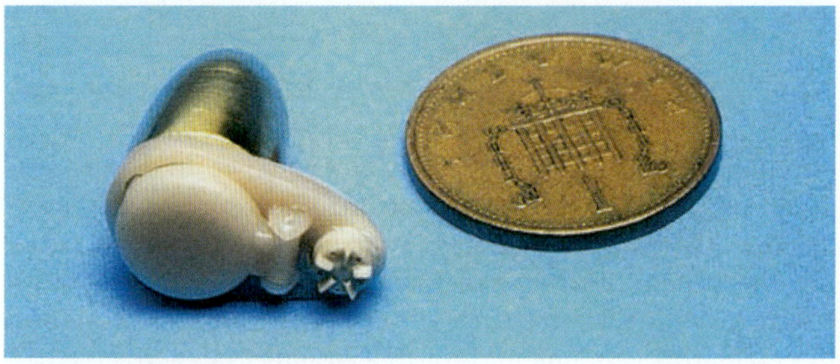

Figure 47.27 A tinnitus masker.

Presbycusis

Presbycusis is characterised by a gradual loss of hearing in both ears, with or without tinnitus. The hearing loss usually affects the higher frequencies and a classical audiogram is shown in Figure 47.26. The consonants of speech lie within the high-frequency range, which makes speech discrimination difficult.

Many patients with presbycusis are concerned that they may lose their hearing completely and they need reassurance. Hearing aid technology has improved dramatically and most patients can benefit.

Tinnitus

Tinnitus is an abnormal noise that appears to come from the ear or within the head. It may have an extrinsic cause, for example the pulsatile tinnitus of a glomus tumour. Usually, however, the tinnitus is generated within the cochlea. Most people will experience tinnitus at some time in their lives. Tinnitus frequently accompanies presbycusis, as well as any other condition that damages the inner ear structures. Most individuals adapt to the presence of tinnitus, but in some patients it proves intrusive. Reassurance and relaxation therapy are highly effective as are hearing aids for patients who also have presbycusis. An ENT surgeon who was a keen fisherman found that he could not hear his tinnitus when fishing next to a waterfall. From this observation, tinnitus maskers were developed (Figure 47.27). A masker provides a similar noise to the tinnitus and 'blanks it out'.

Trauma

Noise exposure

Hair cells within the cochlea are damaged by sudden acoustic trauma (blast injury or gunfire) or prolonged exposure to excessive noise. The sensorineural hearing loss that results is greatest at high frequencies (particularly 4000 Hz) and is often accompanied by tinnitus (Figure 47.28). The law in the UK requires that workers are protected from noise, but in a disco an individual relies on common sense!

Head injury

The otic capsule is the hardest bone in the body but, if trauma to the head is severe, temporal bone fractures may occur. These tend to be either longitudinal (80 per cent) or transverse (20 per cent). Transverse fractures usually involve the labyrinth and lead to a sensorineural hearing loss that is permanent. Profound vertigo occurs initially, followed by gradual compensation. In about 50 per cent of cases, there is an associated facial nerve paralysis.

Drug ototoxicity

Certain drugs differentially affect the cochlea, causing hearing loss and tinnitus, whereas others affect the vestibular system, causing vertigo. Aminoglycosides are well known to be ototoxic, as is *cis*-platinum. Recognition of risk factors, such as poor renal function in patients being treated with aminoglycosides, is most important. Although many topical ear drops contain aminoglycosides, there is little evidence that such topical treatment causes sensorineural hearing loss if used for short periods.

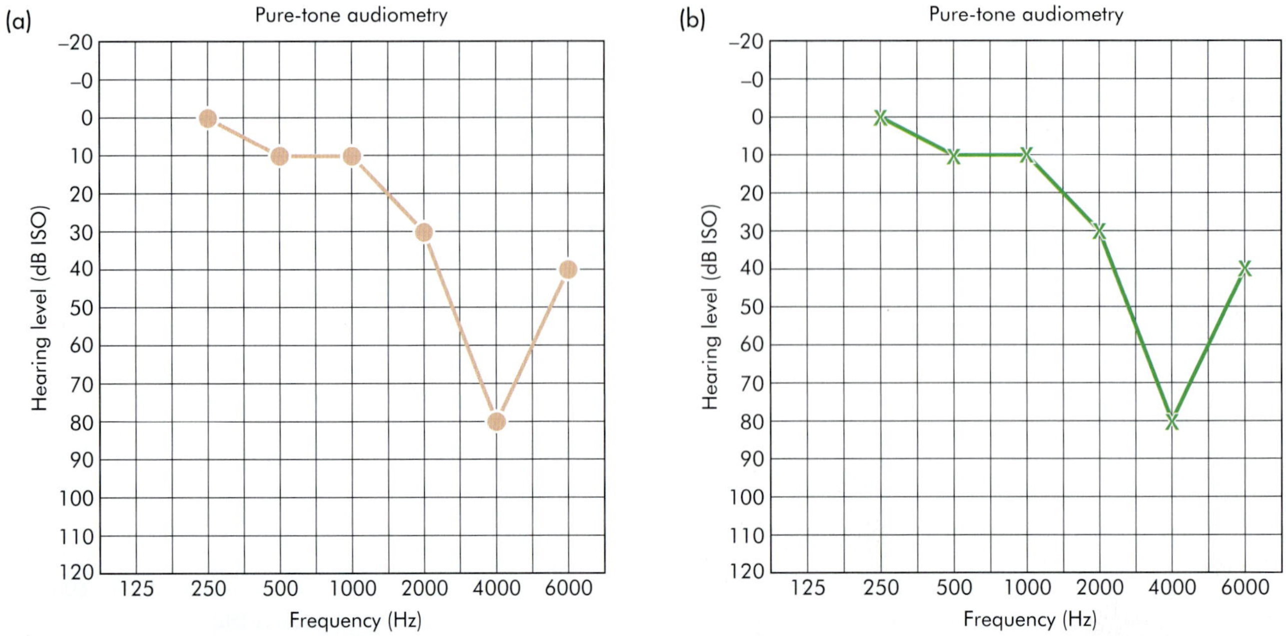

Figure 47.28 A typical audiogram of noise damage: (a) right ear; (b) left ear.

Benign paroxysmal positional vertigo

Benign paroxysmal positional vertigo (BPPV) may follow head or neck trauma. Vertigo is an illusion of movement and BPPV is characterised by intermittent attacks of vertigo that occur when the head is moved in a certain position. Typically, the vertigo only lasts for a few seconds and is not associated with other otological symptoms. Positional testing can evoke nystagmus and helps in the diagnosis of this condition. The condition is usually self-limiting, and special manoeuvres described by Epley help the majority of patients.

Reduction in cochlear blood flow

This is the most likely cause for most cases of sudden onset of severe sensorineural hearing loss. Five per cent of patients with an acoustic neuroma present with sudden sensorineural hearing loss and, therefore, radiological investigation is required to exclude this diagnosis.

Inflammation

Viral infections are thought to account for acute vestibular failure. This condition is characterised by a sudden onset of vertigo. The vertigo is so severe that the patient goes to bed for 5 days. Central compensation then occurs, although recurring episodes of vertigo can occur for up to 18 months.

Menière's disease

The aetiology is not known but the pathology is well documented. There is an excessive accumulation of endolymphatic fluid (hydrops) and it is thought that the distension of the endolymphatic compartment may rupture Reissner's membrane, which leads to mixing of endolymph and perilymph. The condition is characterised by a triad of symptoms: intermittent attacks of vertigo, a fluctuating sensorineural hearing loss and tinnitus. The patient often has a sensation of pressure in the affected ear before an attack. The hearing loss typically affects the lower frequencies. The vertigo characteristically lasts between 30 minutes and 6 hours and is often accompanied by nausea and vomiting. The investigations include pure tone audiometry, electrocochleography and an MRI scan to exclude an acoustic neuroma. Medical treatment with betahistadine and diuretics is effective, with selective destruction of the vestibular labyrinth by percolating gentamicin through a grommet being reserved for resistant cases.

Facial paralysis

Viral infections that involve the facial nerve are one of the most common causes of facial weakness (80 per cent). Bell's palsy results from a viral infection of the facial nerve. The nerve swells and is compressed within the temporal bone. Early treatment with high-dose steroids is appropriate. Not all facial nerve palsies are due to viral infection and a thorough otoneurological examination is required. The facial nerve can be damaged at the cerebellopontine angle, within the internal auditory meatus, within the middle ear, at the skull base and within the parotid gland. It is essential to consider these potential sites of facial nerve damage in any patient with VIIth nerve paralysis (Summary box 47.8).

Summary box 47.8

Facial paralysis

- The facial nerve passes through the middle ear and mastoid
- When considering a paralysis, think 'complete' or 'partial'
- Protect the eye: carry out a full otoneurological examination to find the cause
- If acute, consider steroids and antiviral agents

Prosper Menière, 1799–1862, physician, Institute for Deaf Mutes, Paris, France, described this condition in 1861.
Sir Charles Bell, 1774–1842, surgeon, The Middlesex Hospital, London, UK (1812–1835), and later Professor of Surgery, the University of Edinburgh, Scotland, UK (1836–1842).
John W Epley, contemporary, Director, Portland Otology Clinic, Portland, Oregon, USA, established his clinic in 1975; he developed the Epley manoeuvre for treating benign paroxysmal positional vertigo.

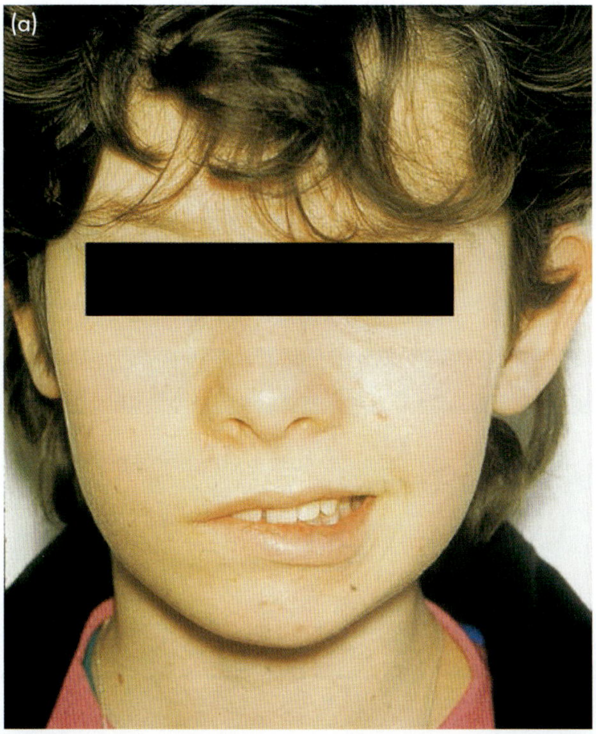

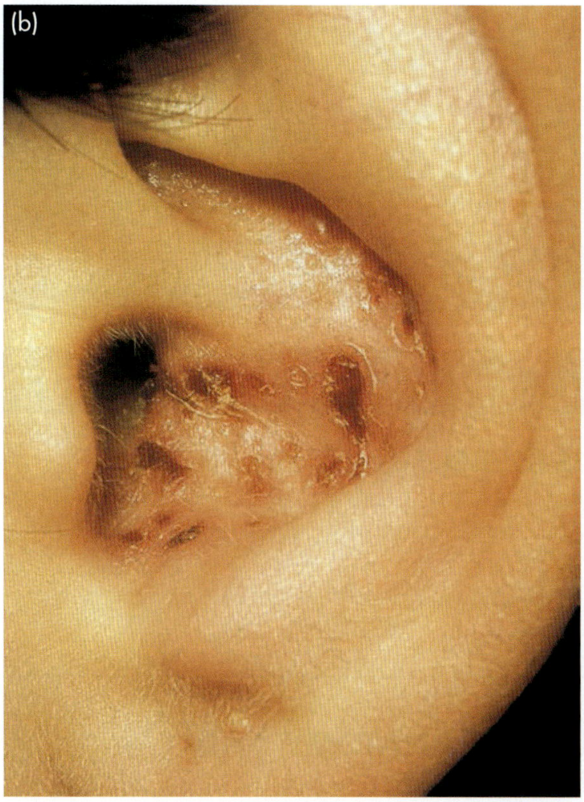

Figure 47.29 Herpes zoster infection of the VIIth (a) and VIIIth (b) nerves with vesicles on the pinna.

Ramsay Hunt syndrome

This is caused by herpes zoster and is characterised by facial paralysis, pain and the appearance of vesicles on the tympanic membrane, ear canal and pinna (Figure 47.29). It is accompanied by vertigo and sensorineural hearing loss (VIIIth nerve). Treatment with aciclovir is effective if given early.

The metabolic causes of inner ear damage

These include diabetes mellitus and thyroid disease, both of which may cause sensorineural hearing loss.

Neoplasms

These are uncommon but can present with sensorineural hearing loss, tinnitus and vertigo. Acoustic neuromas, which are actually schwannomas of the vestibular division of the VIIIth nerve, are the most common, followed by meningiomas. Acoustic neuromas grow slowly and somewhat unpredictably and as they expand can cause cranial nerve palsies, brainstem compression and raised intracranial pressure. The early symptoms are a unilateral sensorineural hearing loss or unilateral tinnitus, or both. It is important to diagnose these tumours early and remove them when they are small. The morbidity and mortality from surgery is directly related to tumour size. If the tumour is removed when it is small, there is an extremely good chance of preserving facial nerve function.

The investigation of choice for detecting acoustic neuromas is MRI. The treatment options include a 'wait and see' policy, which may be appropriate for an elderly patient with minimal symptoms. MRI can be used to monitor the tumour (Summary box 47.9).

Summary box 47.9

Conditions of the inner ear

- Presbycusis is the bilateral high-frequency loss associated with ageing
- Unilateral tinnitus or sensorineural hearing loss needs to be investigated to exclude acoustic neuroma
- Sudden sensorineural hearing loss needs immediate treatment, and radiological investigation in the case of acoustic neuroma
- Menière's disease presents with the triad of sensorineural hearing loss, tinnitus and vertigo

FURTHER READING

Gleeson M (ed.). *Scott-Brown's otorhinolaryngology: Head and neck surgery*, 7th edn. London: Hodder Arnold, 2008.

James Ramsay Hunt, 1874–1937, Professor of Neurology, The Columbia College of Physicians and Surgeons, New York, NY, USA.

CHAPTER 48

Pharynx, larynx and neck

LEARNING OBJECTIVES

To understand:

- The relevant anatomy, physiology, disease processes and investigations of the pharyngolarynx and neck
- The diagnosis and emergency treatment of airway obstruction
- The aetiology, natural history, management and prevention of squamous carcinoma of the upper aerodigestive tract

CLINICAL ANATOMY AND PHYSIOLOGY

The pharynx

The pharynx is a fibromuscular tube forming the upper part of the respiratory and digestive passages. It extends from the base of the skull to the level of the sixth cervical vertebra at the lower border of the cricoid cartilage where it becomes continuous with the oesophagus. It is divided into three parts: the nasopharynx, oropharynx and hypopharynx (Figure 48.1).

Nasopharynx

The nasopharynx lies anterior to the first cervical vertebra and has the openings of the Eustachian tubes in its lateral wall, behind which lie the pharyngeal recesses, the fossae of Rosenmüller. The adenoids are situated submucosally at the junction of the roof and posterior wall of the nasopharynx.

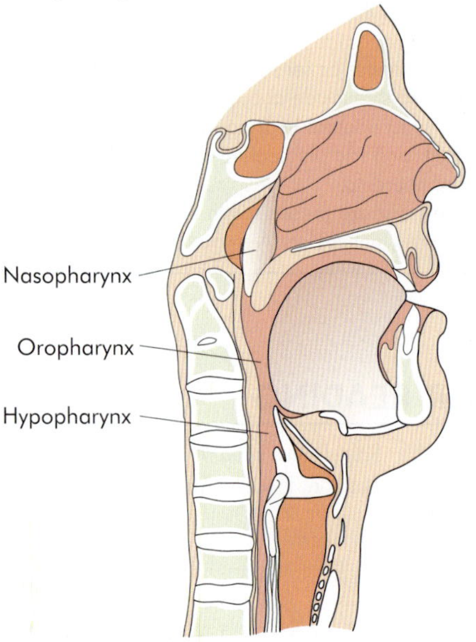

Figure 48.1 The component parts of the pharynx.

Oropharynx

This is bounded above by the soft palate, below by the upper surface of the epiglottis and anteriorly by the anterior faucial pillars. The oropharynx contains the palatine tonsils situated in the lateral wall between the anterior and posterior pillars of the fauces. They are part of the complete ring of lymphoid tissue (Waldeyer's ring) together with the adenoids and lingual tonsils on the posterior third of the tongue. This ring of lymphoid tissue occupying the entry to the air and food passages is constantly exposed to new antigenic stimuli and is an important part of the mucosa-associated lymphoid tissues (MALT), which process antigen and present it to T helper cells and B cells (Figure 48.2).

The tissue of Waldeyer's ring undergoes physiological hypertrophy during early childhood as the child is exposed to

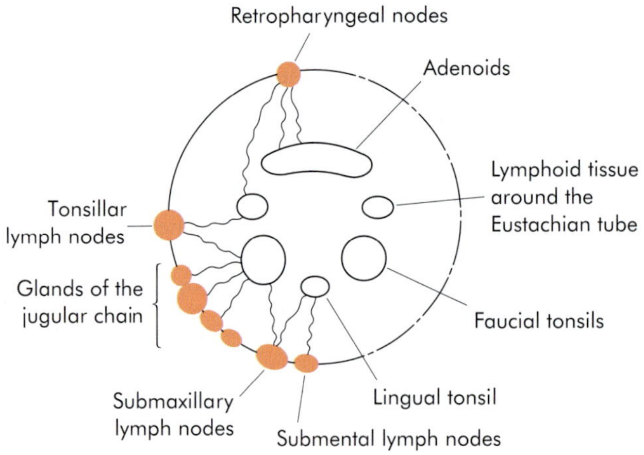

Figure 48.2 Waldeyer's ring.

Johann Christian Rosenmüller, 1771–1820, Professor of Anatomy and Surgery, Leipzig, Germany.
Heinrich Wilhelm Gottfried Waldeyer-Hartz, 1836–1921, Professor of Pathological Anatomy, Berlin, Germany.

increasing amounts of antigenic stimuli, and there is often a similar hypertrophy of the cervical lymph nodes.

It also has an exceptionally good blood supply from the facial artery, which may be closely related to the lower pole, and laterally a plexus of paratonsillar veins, which may be the source of serious venous bleeding following tonsillectomy.

Hypopharynx

The hypopharynx is bounded above and anteriorly by the sloping laryngeal inlet. Its inferior border is the lower border of the cricoid cartilage where it continues into the oesophagus. The hypopharynx is commonly divided into three areas: the pyriform fossae, the posterior pharyngeal wall and the post-cricoid area. The mucosa of these areas is, however, continuous so disease processes, such as squamous carcinoma, can easily involve more than one area and may also spread submucosally. The motor nerve supply of the pharynx and larynx is the vagus nerve.

Understanding of the physiology of normal swallowing and the problems caused by disease has been enhanced in the last two decades by the use of videofluoroscopy in which the passage of a bolus of radio-opaque liquid or solid from the point at which it enters the oral cavity down to its passage within the stomach is examined radiologically. It is considerably more accurate than a barium swallow.

Swallowing is mediated via efferent fibres passing to the medulla oblongata through the second division of the trigeminal nerve (V), glossopharyngeal nerve (IX) and vagus nerve (X) (Figure 48.3). The afferent pathway is from the nucleus ambiguus and is mediated via the glossopharyngeal (IX), vagus (X) and hypoglossal (XII) nerves. Damage to these major cranial nerves at any point along their pathway, by trauma or disease, may cause dysphagia with or without aspiration.

The main function of the larynx is not the production of voice but the protection of the tracheobronchial airway and lungs; it closes completely during swallowing.

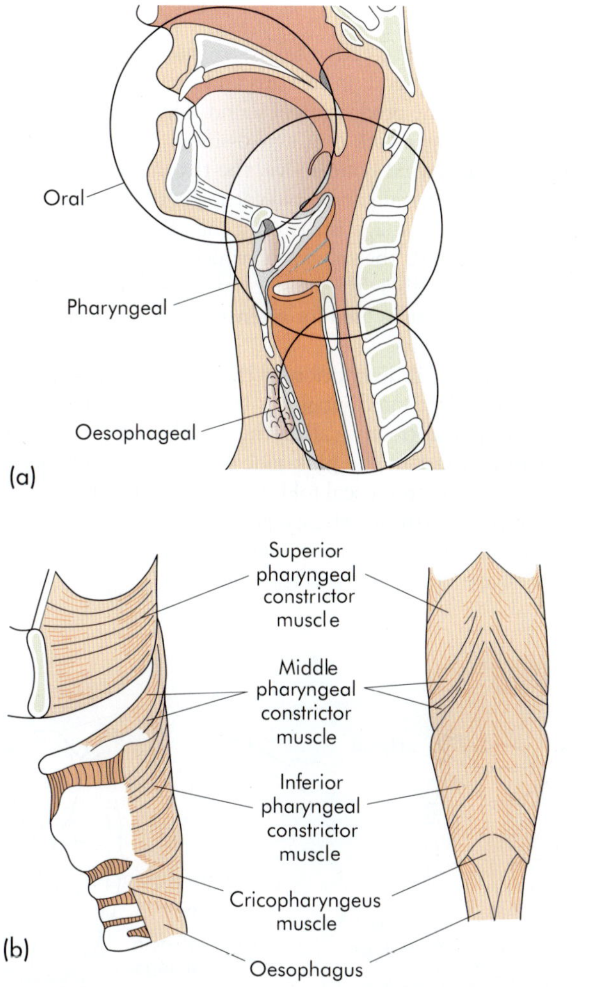

Figure 48.3 The three phases of swallowing (a) and the muscles involved (b).

RELATIONS OF THE PHARYNX

Some of these are illustrated in Figure 48.4.

Parapharyngeal space

This potential space lies lateral to the pharynx and extends from the base of the skull above to the superior mediastinum below. It is occupied by the carotid vessels, internal jugular vein, deep cervical lymph nodes, the last four cranial nerves and the cervical sympathetic trunk.

Infection and suppuration of the cervical lymph node in the parapharyngeal space most commonly occurs from infections of the tonsils or teeth (particularly the third lower molar tooth). It may then spread up to the skull base or down to the paraoesophageal region and superior mediastinum.

Retropharyngeal space

This potential space lies posterior to the pharynx, bounded anteriorly by the posterior pharyngeal wall and its covering buccopharyngeal fascia and posteriorly by the cervical vertebrae and their covering muscles and fascia. It contains the retropharyngeal lymph nodes, which are usually paired lateral nodes but which are separated by a tough median partition that connects the prevertebral with the buccopharyngeal fascia.

These nodes are more developed in infancy and young children, and it is at this age that they are most likely to be involved in inflammatory processes, which, if severe, may affect swallowing and respiration as a consequence of gross swelling and suppuration of the retropharyngeal space.

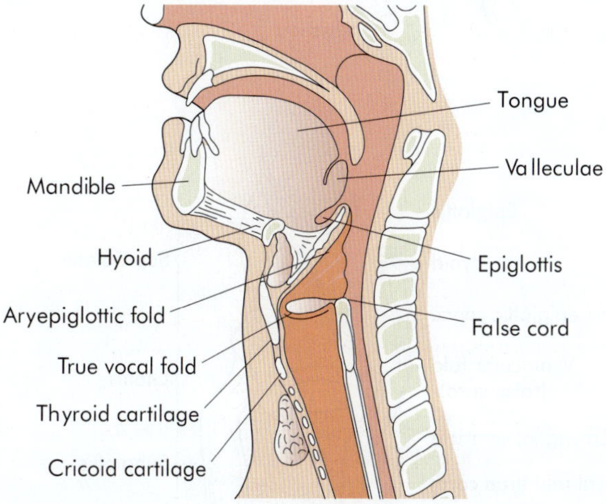

Figure 48.4 Sagittal diagram of upper aerodigestive tract.

Larynx

The larynx is the protective sphincter that closes off the airway during swallowing and, in humans and some other mammals, is responsible for the production of sound. The larynx has a mainly cartilaginous framework that may ossify in later life, and which consists of the hyoid bone above, the thyroid and cricoid cartilages and the intricate arytenoid cartilages posteriorly.

The cricoid cartilage is the only complete ring in the entire airway and bounds the subglottis, which is the narrowest point of the airway. This is the most common site for damage from an endotracheal tube used for intensive care unit ventilation in seriously ill patients.

An anatomical description of the larynx divides it into the supraglottis, glottis and subglottis (Figure 48.5). The true vocal folds (often incorrectly called the vocal cords) are normally white in contrast to the pink mucosa of the rest of the larynx and airway. The true vocal folds meet anteriorly at the midlevel of the thyroid cartilage, whereas posteriorly they are separate and attached to an arytenoid cartilage. This arrangement produces the 'V' shape of the glottis (Figure 48.6).

Nerve supply

The sensory nerve supply to the larynx above the vocal folds is from the superior laryngeal nerve and below the vocal folds is from the recurrent laryngeal nerve. Both these nerves are branches of the vagus nerve (X). The motor nerve supply to the larynx is from the recurrent laryngeal nerve, which is a branch of the vagus nerve and which supplies all intrinsic muscles. Only one of these intrinsic muscles, the posterior cricoarytenoid, abducts the vocal folds during respiration. All other intrinsic muscles adduct the cords. As all of the intrinsic muscles of the larynx are supplied by the recurrent laryngeal nerve, damage to this nerve or to the vagus nerve will cause paralysis of the vocal fold on the side of the damage.

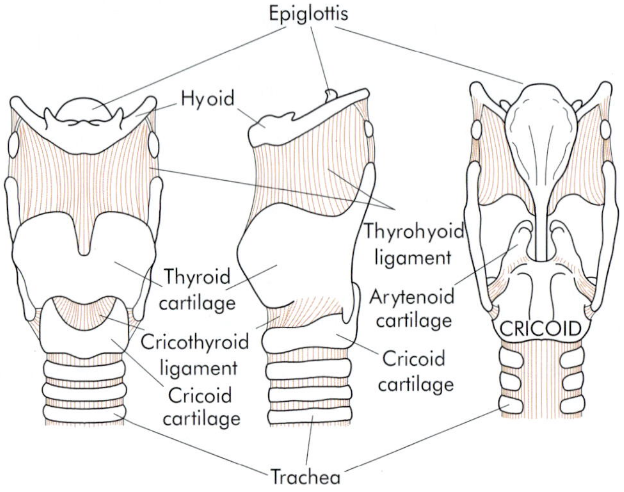

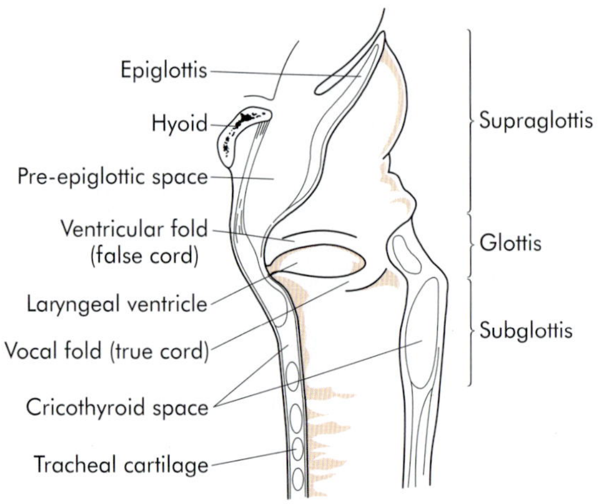

Figure 48.5 Anatomy of the larynx. (Reprinted from Aird's Companion in Surgical Studies, 2nd edn, Burnand, K.G. and Young, A.E. (eds), 1998, Fig. 20.37, with permission from Elsevier.)

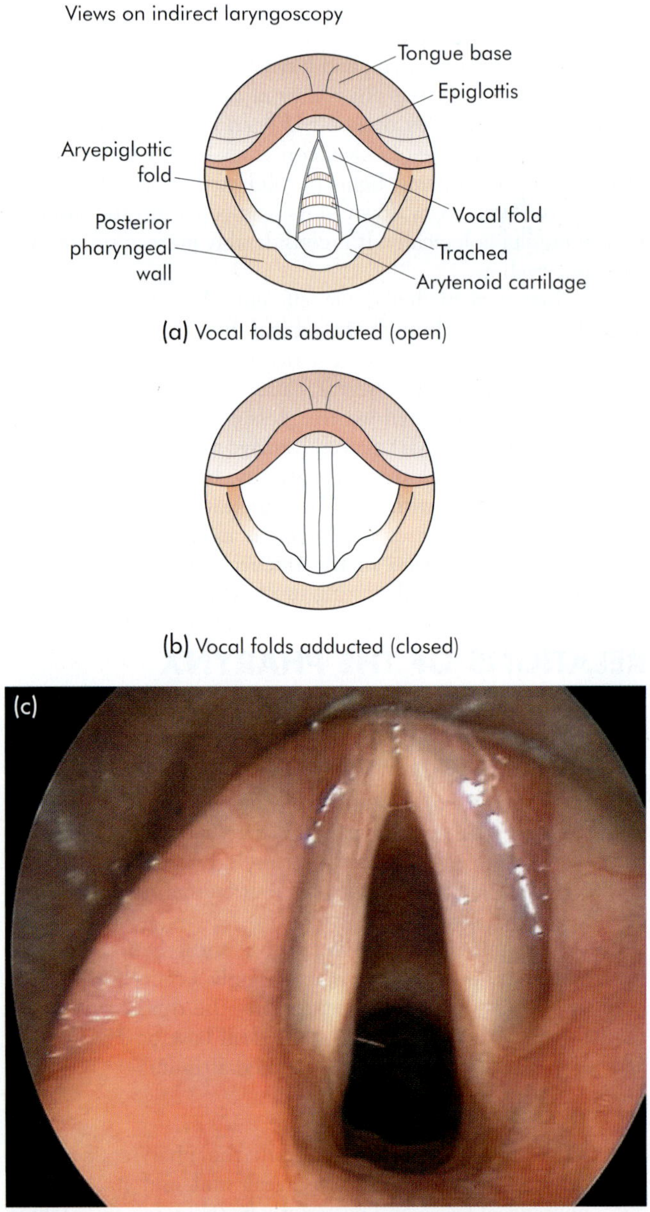

Figure 48.6 A view of the larynx on indirect laryngoscopy: (a) vocal folds abducted; (b) vocal folds adducted. (c) Photograph of normal larynx in abduction. (Adapted from Aird's Companion in Surgical Studies, 2nd edn, Burnand, K.G. and Young, A.E. (eds), 1998, Fig. 20.38, with permission from Elsevier.)

Phonation/speech

The larynx functions by closing the vocal fold against the air being exhaled from the lungs, but the rise in subglottic pressure forces the vocal folds apart slightly for an instant of time with accompanying vibration of the vocal fold epithelium. The opening and closing occurs in rapid sequence to produce a vibrating column of air, which is the source of sound.

Paralysis or disease of the vocal folds or closely associated laryngeal structures will give rise to disturbance of the sound, producing hoarseness.

The functions of the larynx are given in Summary box 48.1.

Summary box 48.1

Functions of the larynx

Protection of the lower respiratory tract by
- Closure of the laryngeal inlet
- Closure of the false cords
- Closure of the glottis
- Cessation of respiration
- Cough reflex

Phonation
- Vocal folds produce sound by quasi-periodic vibration

Respiration
- Control of pressure

Fixation of chest
- Aids lifting, straining and climbing

The neck

The neck is divided into anterior and posterior triangles by the sternocleidomastoid muscle. The anterior triangle extends from the inferior border of the mandible to the sternum below, and is bounded by the midline and the sternocleidomastoid muscle. The posterior triangle extends backwards to the anterior border of the trapezius muscle and inferiorly to the clavicle. The upper part of the anterior triangle is commonly subdivided into the submandibular triangle above the digastric muscle and the submental triangle below. The lymphatic drainage of the head and neck is of considerable clinical importance (Figure 48.7). The most important chain of nodes are the jugular nodes (also called cervical), which run adjacent to the internal jugular vein. The other main groups are the submental, submandibular, pre- and post-auricular, occipital and posterior triangle nodes.

A system of levels is used to describe the location of these neck nodes (Figure 48.8). The upper jugular nodes, level II, which contain the large jugulodigastric node, drain the naso- and oropharynx, including the tonsils, posterolateral aspects of the oral cavity, and the superior aspects of the larynx and pyriform fossae. They are the most common site of enlargement and may be palpated along the anterior border of the sternocleidomastoid muscle.

Metastatic spread of squamous cell carcinoma (80 per cent of head and neck cancer) most commonly occurs with tumours of the nasopharynx, tongue base, tonsil, pyriform fossae and supraglottic larynx. When an enlarged neck node is detected and malignant disease is suspected, these five primary sites must be carefully examined.

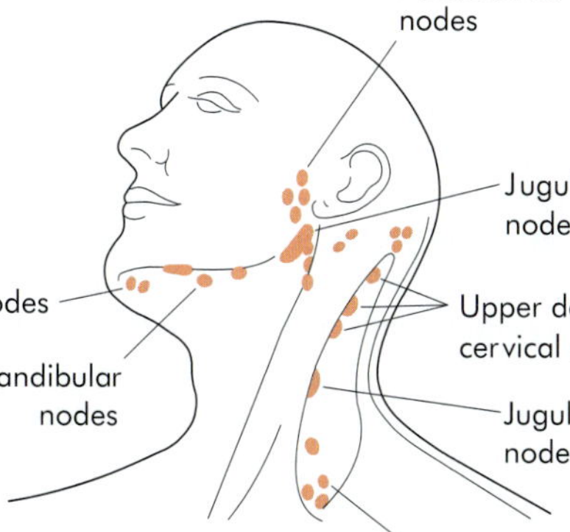

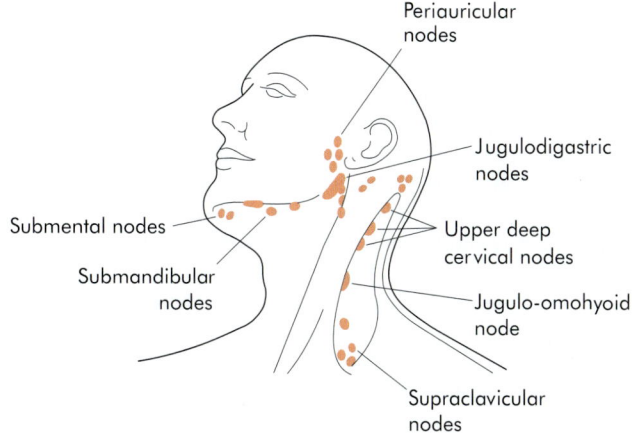

Figure 48.7 Distribution of cervical lymph nodes.

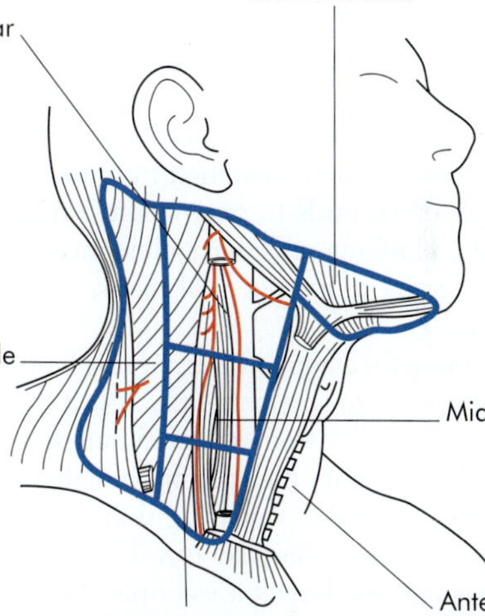

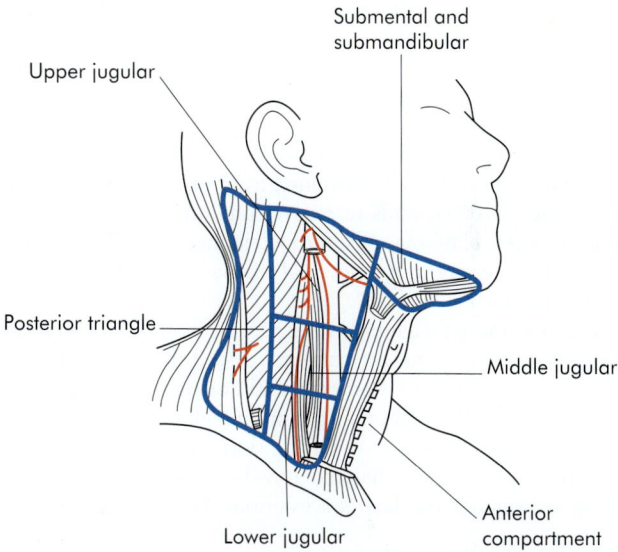

Figure 48.8 The level system for describing location of lymph nodes in the neck. Level I, submental and submandibular group; level II, upper jugular group; level III, middle jugular group; level IV, lower jugular group; level V, posterior triangle group; level VI, anterior compartment group.

CLINICAL EXAMINATION

Pharynx and larynx

Before examination of the pharynx, the oral cavity should be examined with the aid of a good light and tongue depressors. A reflecting mirror on the head or a headband-mounted fibreoptic light source permits use of both hands to hold instruments. Inspection should include the buccal mucosa and lips, the palate, the tongue and floor of the mouth, all surfaces of the teeth and gums, opening and closing of the mouth and dental occlusion. Patients should be asked to elevate the tongue to the roof of the mouth and protrude the tongue to both the right and the left. Palpation may be required using one or two fingers gently intraorally to feel any swellings and this may be combined with extraoral palpation of the submental and submandibular lymph nodes and salivary glands.

Following examination of the oral cavity, the oropharynx is

then inspected with the tongue depressor placed firmly onto the tongue base to depress it inferiorly. The anterior and posterior faucial pillars, the tonsil, retromolar trigone and posterior pharyngeal wall should all be inspected for colour changes, ulceration, pus, foreign bodies and swellings. Even with an experienced examiner, approximately one-third of patients cannot tolerate the depression of the posterior base of tongue without gagging. Pain and trismus as a consequence of pharyngolaryngeal or neck pathology may additionally add to the difficulty of the examination.

Fibreoptic endoscopes passed through the nose or through the mouth, with or without topical anaesthesia, allow high-quality examination of the entire nasopharynx, oropharynx and larynx in almost every patient.

The neck

The patient should be examined sitting with the whole neck exposed so that both clavicles are clearly seen. The neck is inspected from in front and the patient asked to swallow, preferably with the aid of a sip of water. Movements of the larynx and any swelling in the neck are noted. The patient should be asked to protrude the tongue if there is a midline neck swelling. A thyroglossal cyst will move upwards with the tongue protrusion. The patient is then examined from behind with the chin flexed slightly downwards to remove any undue tension in the strap muscles, platysma and sternocleidomastoids. The neck is palpated bilaterally in a sequential manner comparing the two sides of the neck.

On examining for a lump in the neck, it is often helpful to ask the patient to point to the lump first. Ask if the lump is tender. A swelling beneath the sternomastoid muscle may be considerably larger than thought on palpation. If malignancy is suspected (hard, irregular or fixed to overlying skin or to deep structures), inspection of the nasopharynx, tonsils, tongue base, pyriform fossae and supraglottic larynx is essential (Summary box 48.2).

Summary box 48.2

Key points of history and examination

Mouth
- Adequate light source and two spatulas to examine the mouth
- Examine
  - Teeth, gums, gingival sulci
  - Buccal mucosa, opening of parotid duct
  - Floor of mouth
  - Hard and soft palates
  - Retromolar trigone region ('coffin corner')
  - Anterior and posterior faucial pillars, tonsils
  - Posterior pharyngeal wall
  - Tongue (observe full movements)
- Palpate
  - Salivary glands/ducts

Larynx, oropharynx and hypopharynx
- Indirect laryngoscopy
  - Mirror and headlight
- Direct flexible fibreoptic pharyngolaryngoscopy

Nasopharynx
- Rigid Hopkins' rod endoscopy
- Flexible fibreoptic nasendoscopy

Neck
- Inspection
  - Tongue protrusion
  - Observe swallowing
- Palpation
  - If a mass is palpable, evaluate for size, site, shape, consistency, superficial and deep fixation, fluctuation, transillumination, auscultation

INVESTIGATIONS OF THE PHARYNX, LARYNX AND NECK

Plain lateral radiographs

Plain lateral radiographs of the neck and cervical spine may show soft tissue abnormalities; of particular importance is the depth and outline of the prevertebral soft tissue shadow. The outline of the laryngotracheal airway may be a useful guide to the presence of disease in the pharynx and larynx (Figure 48.9).

There should be no air within the upper oesophagus. If air is seen, endoscopy is advised. Radio-opaque foreign bodies may be seen impacted in the pharynx, larynx or upper oesophagus on these radiographs.

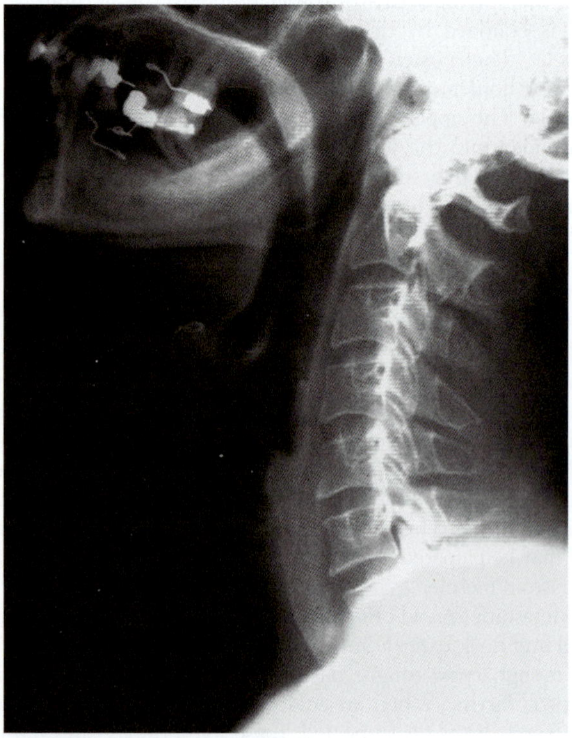

Figure 48.9 Plain lateral radiograph showing normal anatomy.

Barium swallow

Barium liquid video fluoroscopic studies record the movement of a small quantity of radio-opaque liquid and allow detailed evaluation of the oral and pharyngeal phases of swallowing (Figure 48.10).

Computed tomography scanning

Computed tomography (CT) scanning provides much improved demonstration of disease in the pharynx, larynx and neck. Intravenous contrast given at the same time as the CT scan

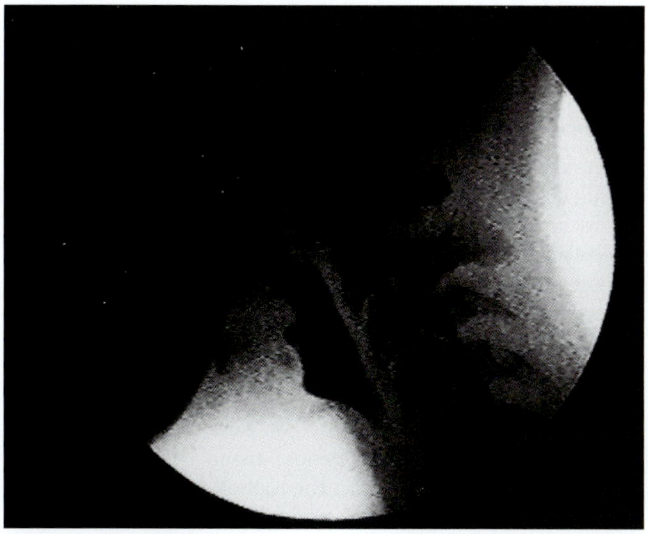

Figure 48.10 Videofluoroscopy image showing liquid barium in the upper pharynx in a normal swallow.

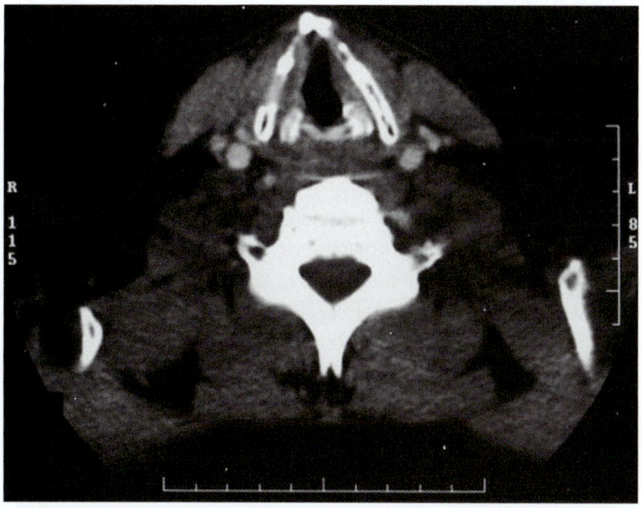

Figure 48.11 Axial computed tomography scan through the larynx at the level of the glottis.

(dynamic scanning) further improves the demonstration of disease in these areas (Figure 48.11).

Other imaging

Magnetic resonance imaging (MRI) may be used to give better soft tissue definition of some diseases, however, bony and cartilaginous structures are less well defined (Figure 48.12). MRI is more vulnerable to movement artefact. Ultrasound scanning can be useful in differentiating solid lesions, e.g. malignant lymph nodes from cystic lesions such as a branchial cyst.

Fine-needle aspiration cytology

This technique can be performed under local anaesthesia. It is useful particularly if a neck lump is thought to be malignant. Increasingly high rates of accurate histological diagnosis are reported and there is no evidence of spread of tumour through the skin track caused by the fine hypodermic needle used with this technique. Flow cytometry should be undertaken if haematological malignancy, such as lymphoma, is suspected. Fine-needle aspiration is considerably aided by ultrasound or CT guidance.

Angiography or digital subtraction vascular imaging

These may be indicated if a vascular lesion, such as a carotid body tumour, is suspected. Angiography may have a therapeutic role to play by facilitating embolisation of the lesion.

Direct pharyngoscopy and laryngoscopy

Examination of the pharynx, larynx and neck under general anaesthesia may be required if there are problems with the routine examination of patients, such as an inadequate view as a result of trismus from pain, poor patient compliance or large obstructive pharyngeal or laryngeal pathology. These examinations may be further aided by the use of an operating microscope or rigid endoscope (Hopkins' rod) (Figure 48.13).

Harold Horace Hopkins, 1918–1994, Professor of Applied Optics, University of Reading, Reading, UK. He invented the rigid rod endoscope (Hopkins' rod, 1954), and contributed to the development of the fibres for flexible endoscopes.

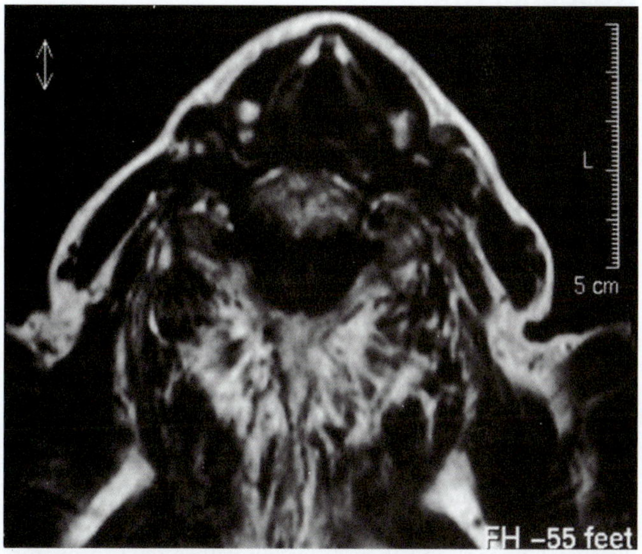

Figure 48.12 Axial magnetic resonance imaging scan at the same level as Figure 48.11.

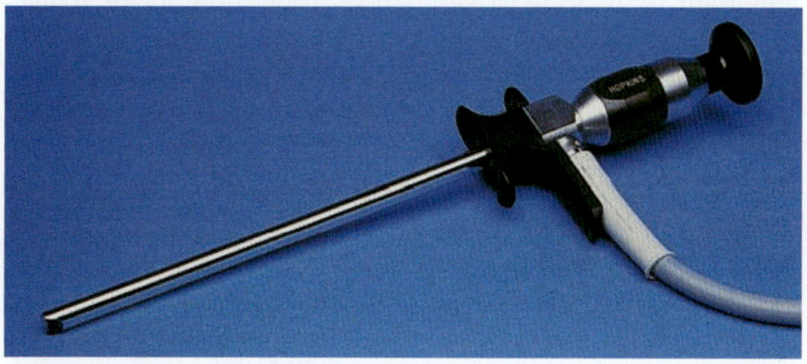

Figure 48.13 A rigid Hopkins' rod or endoscope.

The advantages and disadvantages of laryngeal examination techniques are given in Summary box 48.3.

Summary box 48.3

Advantages and disadvantages of larynx and pharynx examination techniques

Flexible nasendoscopy
- Well-tolerated examination
- Can also examine nasal passages and post-nasal space
- Need fibreoptic light source

Rigid endoscopy
- Can be used with stroboscope for evaluation of voice
- High definition view
- Needs fibreoptic light source
- Bulky and difficult if prominent gag reflex present

Laryngeal mirror
- Does not need fibreoptic light source
- No record of exam, small image

DISEASES OF THE PHARYNX

Nasopharynx

Enlarged adenoid

The most common cause of an enlarged adenoid (there is only one nasopharyngeal adenoid, despite the common use of the term 'adenoids') is physiological hypertrophy. The size of the adenoid alone is not an indication for removal. It is often associated with hypertrophy of the other lymphoid tissues of Waldeyer's ring. If excessive hypertrophy causes blockage of the nasopharynx in association with tonsil hypertrophy, the upper airway may become compromised during sleep causing obstructive sleep apnoea.

Obstructive sleep apnoea

This condition is becoming increasingly diagnosed and is important because it can cause sleep deprivation and secondary cardiac complications. It has been implicated in some cases of sudden infant death syndrome. The most common symptom is snoring, which is typically irregular, with the child actually ceasing respiration (apnoea) and then restarting with a loud inspiratory snort. The child is often restless and may take up strange sleep positions as he or she tries to improve the pharyngeal airway. Surgical removal of the tonsils and adenoid is curative, but it is important to avoid sedative premedications and opiate analgesics postoperatively because they may further depress the child's respiratory drive.

Obstructive sleep apnoea (OSA) may also occur in adults, where the obstruction may result from nasal deformity, a hypertrophic soft palate associated with an altered nasopharyngeal isthmus, obesity and general narrowing of the pharyngeal airway, or supraglottic laryngeal pathology. Initial investigation may include a sleep study, during which measurement of the patient's sleep pattern and arterial oxygenation are undertaken. Continuous positive airways pressure (CPAP) devices may ameliorate OSA by splinting the obstruction open. Surgery may also be indicated, depending on the level(s) of the obstruction.

Hypertrophy of adenoid tissue most commonly occurs between the ages of four and ten, but the adenoid tissue usually undergoes spontaneous atrophy during puberty, although some remnants may persist into adult life (Figure 48.14). The relationship of adenoid enlargement to recurrent secretory otitis media or recurrent acute otitis media is not entirely clear.

Adenoidectomy

Adenoid tissue can be removed alone or in conjunction with a tonsillectomy. The indications for adenoidectomy are:

- obstructive sleep apnoea associated with post-nasal obstruction;
- post-nasal discharge;
- recurrent acute otitis media or prolonged serous otitis media, usually longer than three months' duration;
- recurrent rhinosinusitis.

Removal of the adenoid

Operative technique. The adenoid tissue is removed with a guarded curette pressed against the roof of the nasopharynx and then carried downwards in a moderately firm sweeping movement bringing the excised adenoid into the oropharynx (Figures 48.15 and 48.16). The guard on the curette secures the adenoid and prevents it from dropping inferiorly into the airway. A

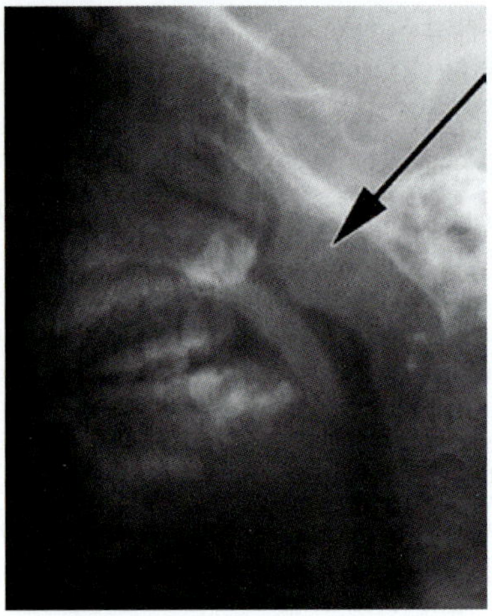

Figure 48.14 Plain lateral radiograph showing a large pad of adenoid tissue (arrow) in the postnasal space.

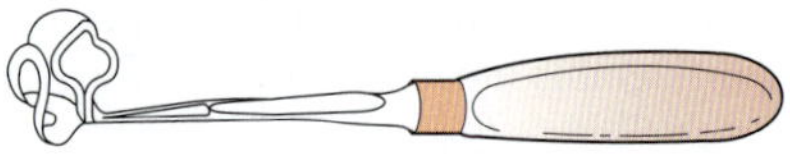

Figure 48.15 St Clair Thomson's adenoid curette.

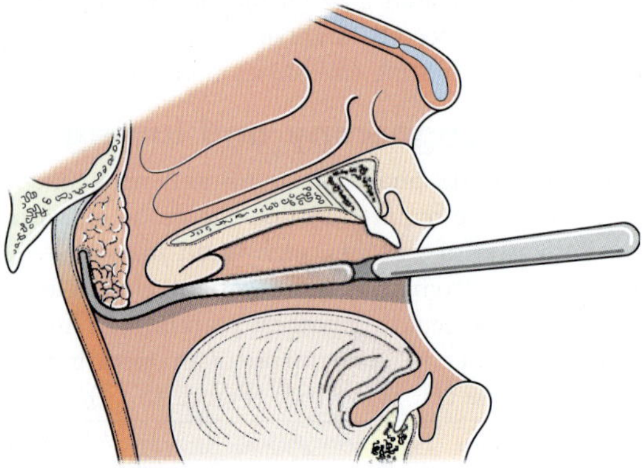

Figure 48.16 Curettage of the adenoid.

post-nasal swab is placed into the nasopharynx until all haemorrhage has ceased. A mirror can be used to guide the direction of the adenoid curette. Alternatively, suction monopolar diathermy may be used to remove adenoid tissue.

Reactionary or secondary haemorrhage during the recovery period may require a nasopharyngeal pack under a further anaesthetic. This can occasionally cause respiratory depression in children and adults, and strict observation is required while the pack is in place.

TUMOURS OF THE NASOPHARYNX

Benign

There are two main types of benign tumour of the nasopharynx: the angiofibroma and the antrochoanal polyp. Both are rare.

Angiofibroma

This tumour is confined to young male patients, most commonly between the ages of 8 and 20 years. It usually causes progressive nasal obstruction, recurrent severe epistaxis, purulent rhinorrhoea and, occasionally, loss of vision because of compression of the optic nerve. Although the tumour is rare, these symptoms in a young male patient should always arouse suspicion. The tumour is most common in northern India, although the reasons for this are unknown. Clinical examination often shows a tumour in the nasal cavity or nasopharynx, but CT scanning best demonstrates the extent of the tumour and its accompanying bony erosion. MRI scanning defines the soft tissue extent and, with these two modern investigations, angiography is rarely indicated. Biopsy should be avoided unless clinical and radiological examinations are not diagnostic because of the risk of bleeding.

Surgical resection requires adequate exposure either through a midfacial approach or lateral rhinotomy (Figures 48.17 and 48.18). Both allow ligation of the feeding maxillary artery. More recently, endoscopic resection has been used for smaller lesions.

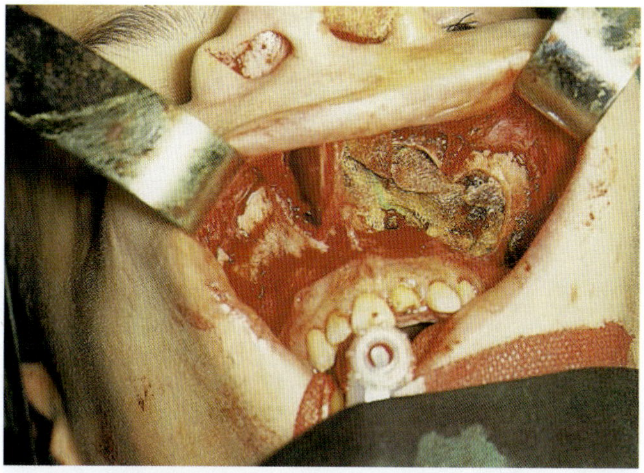

Figure 48.17 Intraoperative photograph showing exposure during a midfacial degloving approach.

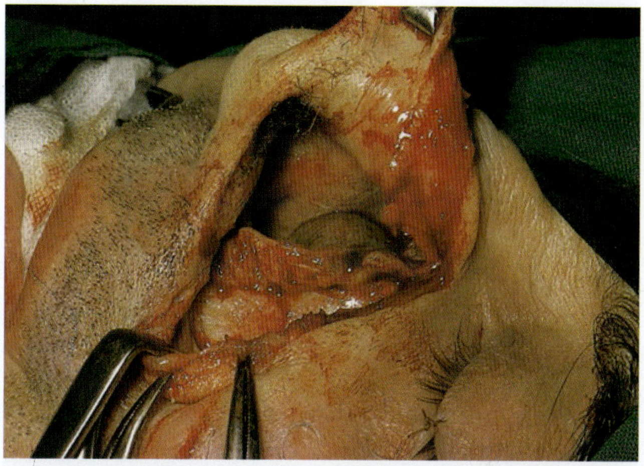

Figure 48.18 Intraoperative photograph showing an incision in lateral rhinotomy.

Antrochoanal polyp

This relatively uncommon lesion is a benign mucosal polyp that arises in the maxillary antrum and prolapses into the nasal cavity where it expands backwards into the nasopharynx and occasionally into the oropharynx (Figures 48.19 and 48.20). It may mimic an angiofibroma from which it is distinguished by its avascularity and pale colour, and its site of origin on endoscopic examination and imaging. It requires complete removal via an endoscopic approach through the middle meatus or, occasionally, a Caldwell–Luc procedure.

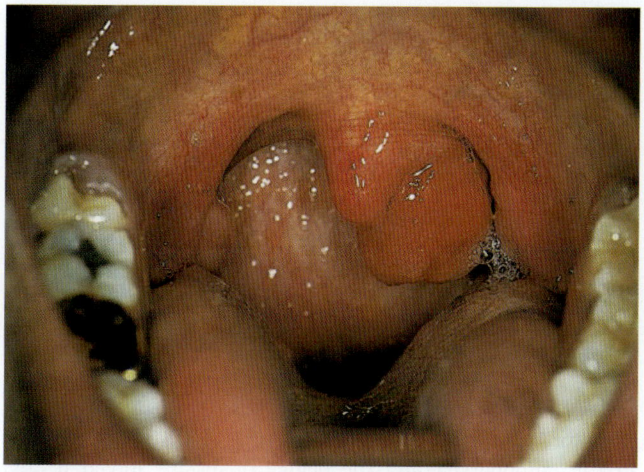

Figure 48.19 Intraoral view showing a fleshy polyp hanging in the oropharynx.

Malignant

Nasopharyngeal carcinoma

Nasopharyngeal carcinomas are usually squamous cell carcinomas and have a very variable incidence. In most parts of the world, the tumour is rare with an annual incidence of one case per 100 000 population; however, among southern Chinese populations the rate is 30–50 cases per 100 000 population.

George Walter Caldwell, 1834–1918, otolaryngologist, who practised successively in New York, San Francisco and Los Angeles, USA, devised this operation for treating suppuration in the maxillary antrum in 1893.

Henri Luc, 1855–1925, otolaryngologist, Paris, France, described his operation in 1889.

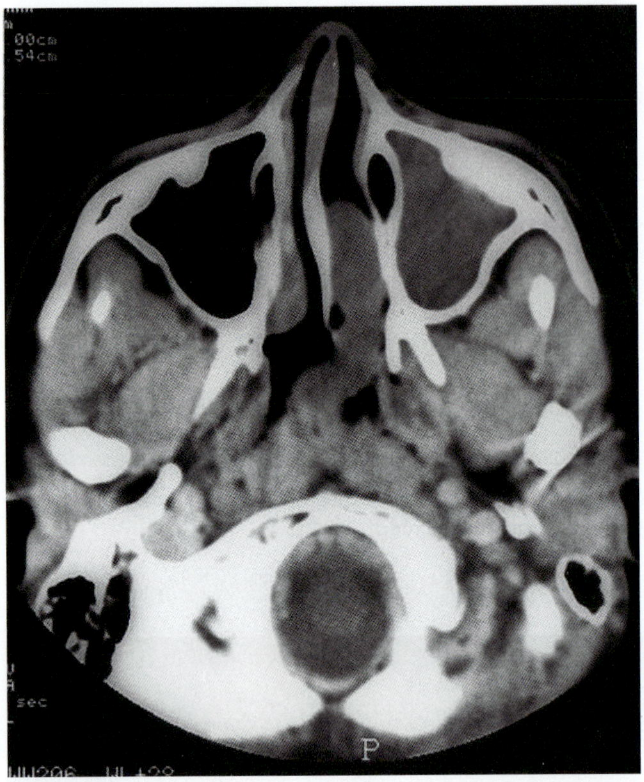

Figure 48.20 Axial computed tomogram of an antrochoanal polyp (as seen in Figure 48.19), with opaque maxillary antrum and a mass in the nasal cavity and nasopharynx.

The aetiology of nasopharyngeal carcinoma is multifactorial. Genetic susceptibility, early infection by the Epstein–Barr virus and consumption of traditional diets, particularly salted fish, are known to contribute (Summary box 48.4).

Summary box 48.4

Aetiological factors in nasopharyngeal carcinoma

- Genetic, e.g. Cantonese
- Infective, e.g. Epstein–Barr virus
- Environmental, e.g. salted fish

The majority of tumours are undifferentiated with a characteristic morphology, comprising over 90 per cent of nasopharyngeal malignancy in endemic areas. Rare epithelial tumours are adenocarcinoma and adenoid cystic carcinoma. B- and T-cell lymphomas also occur in this region and should not be confused with the more common undifferentiated carcinoma. Nasopharyngeal carcinoma has a bimodal distribution with an increased incidence in teenagers and young adults and then again in the 50–60 age group.

Clinical features

Symptoms are closely related to the position of the tumour in the nasopharynx and the degree of distant spread if any. Early symptoms are often minimal and may be ignored by both patient and doctor. Approximately 50 per cent of patients will present with a mass of malignant nodes in the neck, indicating an advanced tumour. This percentage is even higher in patients under 21 years of age. Fine-needle aspiration or a biopsy of a neck node showing undifferentiated carcinoma requires immediate thorough examination of the nasopharynx. In about 5 per cent of patients, the nasopharynx may look normal or minimally asymmetrical but contains submucosal nasopharyngeal carcinoma. A biopsy of the nasopharynx is essential if there is suspicion of nasopharyngeal malignancy. Nasal complaints occur in one-third of patients and aural symptoms of unilateral deafness as a consequence of Eustachian tube obstruction and secretory otitis media occur in approximately 20 per cent. Neurological complications with cranial nerve palsies as a result of disease in the skull base occur relatively late in the disease, but are a poor prognostic factor (Summary box 48.5).

Summary box 48.5

Nasopharyngeal carcinoma: main presenting complaints

Systemic

- Cervical lymphadenopathy

Local

- Unilateral serous otitis media, otalgia
- Nasal obstruction, bloody discharge, epistaxis
- Cranial nerve palsies, especially III–VI then IX–XII

Investigation is by direct inspection with a flexible or rigid nasendoscope and biopsy under topical or general anaesthesia. Serological investigation for Epstein–Barr virus-associated antigenic markers in combination with the clinical and histological examination is valuable for the early detection of disease. Highly sensitive assays for antiviral antibodies together with virus-associated serological markers are useful in early detection. Immunoglobulin (Ig)A antiviral capsid antigen antibody and early antigen antibody have been evaluated in mass surveys in southern China and have been found to be an excellent screening method for the early detection of nasopharyngeal carcinoma in high-risk groups.

Imaging

Imaging is essential for staging and to determine the extent of disease. The investigation of choice is MRI with gadolinium and fat suppression. This allows for assessment of brain parenchyma, cavernous sinus and the closely associated cranial foramina. CT or positron emission tomography (PET) CT of the head, neck and chest has a major role in planning radiotherapy and assessing the response to treatment, diagnosing recurrence and detecting complications.

Treatment

The primary treatment of nasopharyngeal carcinoma is external beam or intensity modulated radiotherapy as the majority of the tumours are radiosensitive undifferentiated squamous cell carcinomas. Elective bilateral external radiotherapy is given to the skull base and neck in all patients, even when no neck nodes are apparent. Chemotherapy in both the adjuvant and neoadjuvant setting remains controversial. Surgery is usually reserved for regional recurrence in the neck. For early disease, three-year disease-free survival rates of more than 75 per cent are common;

however, in advanced disease the results are less good, with three-year disease-free survival rates of 30–50 per cent.

OROPHARYNX

Acute tonsillitis

This common condition is characterised by a sore throat, fever, general malaise, dysphagia, enlarged upper cervical nodes and sometimes referred otalgia. Approximately half the cases are bacterial, the most common cause being a pyogenic group A streptococcus. The remainder are viral and a wide variety of viruses have been implicated, in particular infectious mononucleosis, which may be mistaken for bacterial tonsillitis.

On examination, the tonsils are swollen and erythematous, and yellow or white pustules may be seen on the palatine tonsils, hence the name 'follicular tonsillitis' (Figure 48.21). A throat swab should be taken at the time of examination as well as blood for Paul–Bunnell testing.

Treatment

Paracetamol or similar analgesia may be administered to relieve pain and gargles of glycerol–thymol are soothing. The condition is frequently sensitive to benzyl- or phenyoxymethylpenicillin (penicillin V) and these are given until antibiotic sensitivities are established. Ampicillin is avoided as it may precipitate a rash in patients with infectious mononucleosis. Most cases resolve in a few days.

Quinsy

This is an abscess in the peritonsillar region that causes severe pain and trismus (Figure 48.22). The trismus caused by spasm induced in the pterygoid muscles may make examination difficult but may be overcome by instillation of local anaesthesia into the posterior nasal cavity (anaesthetising the sphenopalatine ganglion) and the oropharynx. Inspection reveals a diffuse swelling of the soft palate just superior to the involved tonsil, displacing the uvula medially. In more advanced cases, pus may be seen pointing underneath the thin mucosa.

Treatment

In the early stages, intravenous broad-spectrum antibiotics may produce resolution. However, if there is frank abscess formation, incision and drainage of the pus can be carried out under local anaesthesia. A small scalpel is best modified by winding a strip of adhesive tape around the blade so that only 1 cm of the blade projects. In teenagers and young adults, the patient sits upright and an incision is made approximately midway between the base of the uvula and the third upper molar tooth (Figure 48.23). This may produce immediate release of pus, but, if not, a dressing forceps is pushed firmly through the incision and, on opening, pus may then be encountered. In small children, general anaesthesia is required.

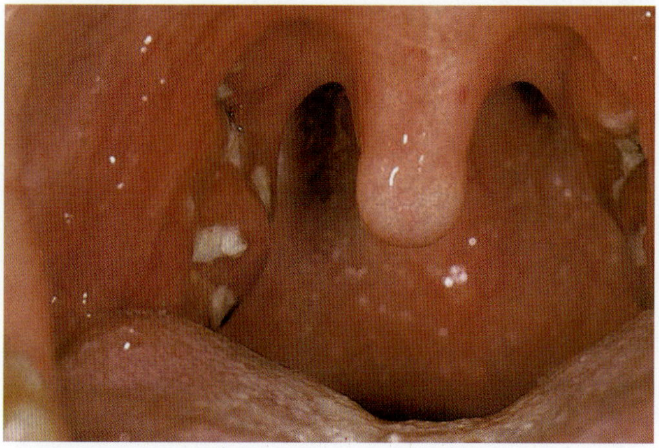

Figure 48.21 Acute follicular tonsillitis.

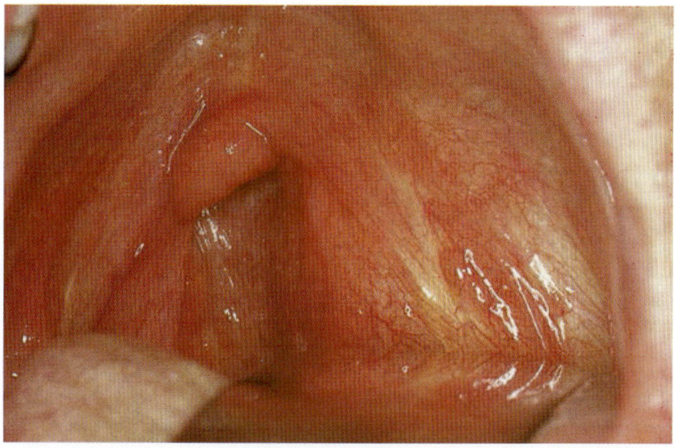

Figure 48.22 Quinsy (peritonsillar abscess).

Chronic tonsillitis

Chronic tonsillitis usually results from repeated attacks of acute tonsillitis in which the tonsils become progressively damaged and provide a reservoir for infective organisms.

Tonsillectomy

Recurrent acute tonsillitis is the most common relative indication for tonsillectomy in children and adolescents, although it is important that these attacks are well documented, frequent and do not simply constitute a minor viral sore throat. Chronic tonsillitis more frequently affects young adults, in whom it is important to establish that chronic mouth breathing secondary to nasal obstruction is not the main problem rather than the tonsils themselves. Absolute indications for tonsillectomy are when the size of the tonsils is contributing to airway obstruction or a malignancy of the tonsils is suspected (Table 48.1).

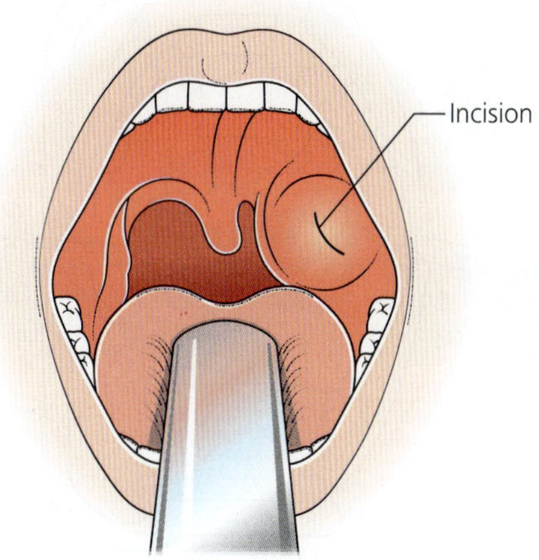

Figure 48.23 Site of incision in peritonsillar abscess.

John Rodman Paul, 1893–1971, Professor of Preventative Medicine, Yale University, New Haven, CT, USA.
Walls Willard Bunnell, 1902–1966, an American physician. Paul and Bunnell described this test in 1932.

Table 48.1 Indications for tonsillectomy.

Absolute	Sleep apnoea, chronic respiratory tract obstruction, cor pulmonale Suspected tonsillar malignancy
Relative	Documented recurrent acute tonsillitis Chronic tonsillitis Peritonsillar abscess (quinsy) Tonsillar asymmetry Tonsillitis resulting in febrile convulsions Diphtheria carriers Systemic disease caused by β-haemolytic *Streptococcus* (nephritis, rheumatic fever)

Ideally, the procedure should be undertaken when the tonsils are not acutely infected, and it is important to discuss factors that may increase the tendency to bleed. Blood transfusion is rarely required, but it is normal practice to type and screen blood for cross-match in children under 15 kg in weight.

Dissection tonsillectomy is carried out under general anaesthesia. The mucosa of the anterior faucial pillar is incised and the tonsil capsule identified. Using blunt dissection, the tonsil is separated from its bed until only a small inferior pedicle is left (Figure 48.24). It is then separated from the lingual tonsil. A tonsil swab is placed in the tonsillar bed and pressure applied for some minutes, following which bleeding points may be controlled by ligature or by bipolar diathermy.

Following surgery, the patient is kept under close observation for any systemic or local evidence of bleeding, with regular pulse and blood pressure measurements and observation to see whether the patient is swallowing excessively (Figure 48.25). Postoperatively, patients are encouraged to eat normally. Paracetamol is preferred to non-steroidal analgesics. Patients are allowed home on the same or following day and are warned that they may experience otalgia as a result of referred pain from the glossopharyngeal nerve and that secondary haemorrhage may occur up to 10 days following the surgery.

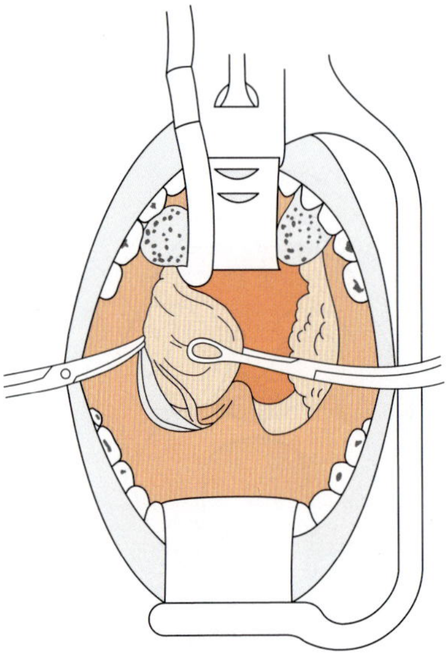

Figure 48.24 Removal of the tonsils.

Haemorrhage is the most common complication in the immediate postoperative period. Local pressure may help in mild cases, but reactionary haemorrhage usually requires return to theatre for definitive treatment, particularly in younger patients. Under general anaesthesia, it may be possible to identify a bleeding spot, but often a more generalised ooze is observed and suturing of the tonsil bed combined with the application of Surgicel and bipolar diathermy is often more successful than attempted placement of ligatures.

Late haemorrhage is generally secondary to infection and patients should be commenced on intravenous antibiotics with aerobic and anaerobic cover. Significant or persistent bleeding may require a further general anaesthetic and undersewing of the surgical bed, which by this time will often be covered with slough and granulation tissue. Postoperative tonsillar haemorrhage is still a serious and life-threatening complication and should not be underestimated, particularly in the younger patient (Summary box 48.6).

Summary box 48.6

Complications of tonsillectomy

- Haemorrhage (immediate or late)
- Infection
- Pain/otalgia
- Postoperative airway obstruction
- Velopharyngeal insufficiency

Parapharyngeal abscess

Parapharyngeal abscess may be confused with a peritonsillar abscess, but the maximal swelling is **behind** the posterior faucial pillar and there may be little oedema of the soft palate. The patient is usually a young child and there may be a severe general malaise. In early cases, admission to hospital and the institution of fluid replacements coupled with intravenous antibiotics may produce resolution. In advanced cases, drainage and intravenous antibiotics are required. With an obvious abscess pointing into the oropharynx, drainage may be carried out with a blunt instrument or the glove finger, but general anaesthesia is frequently required and the expertise of a senior anaesthetist, good illumination and good suction are absolutely essential. A large parapharyngeal abscess may compromise both the airway and swallowing.

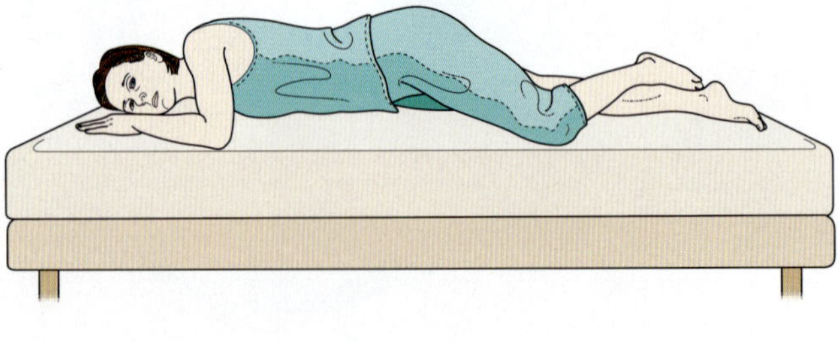

Figure 48.25 Positioning of the patient after tonsillectomy.

Acute retropharyngeal abscess

This is the result of suppuration of the retropharyngeal lymph nodes and, again, is most commonly seen in children, with most cases occurring under one year of age. It is associated with infection of the tonsils, nasopharynx or oropharynx, and is frequently accompanied by severe general malaise, neck rigidity, dysphagia, drooling, a croupy cough, an altered cry and marked dyspnoea.

Dyspnoea may be the prominent symptom and may also be accompanied by febrile convulsions and vomiting. These children should always be carefully examined. Inspection of the posterior wall of the pharynx may show gross swelling and an abscess pointing beneath the thinned mucosa.

In countries where diphtheria still occurs, an acute retropharyngeal abscess may be confused with this, but the presence of the greyish-green membrane aids differentiation. Occasionally, a foreign body, most commonly a fish bone which has perforated the posterior pharyngeal mucosa, will give rise to a retropharyngeal abscess in older children and young adults. Intravenous antibiotics are commenced immediately, but surgical drainage of the abscess is often necessary. It requires experienced anaesthesia because, on induction, care must be taken to avoid rupturing the abscess. The airway is protected by placing the child in a head-down position while a pair of dressing forceps guided by the finger may be thrust into an obvious abscess in the posterior wall and the contents evacuated. On other occasions, an approach anterior and medial to the carotid sheath via a cervical incision may be required.

Chronic retropharyngeal abscess

This condition is now rare and is most commonly the result of an extension of tuberculosis of the cervical spine, which has spread through the anterior longitudinal ligament to reach the retropharyngeal space. In addition to the retropharyngeal swelling seen intraorally, there may be fullness behind the sternocleidomastoid muscle on one side. In contrast to an acute retropharyngeal abscess, this condition occurs almost solely in adults. Radiology usually shows evidence of bone destruction and loss of the normal curvature of the cervical spine. The spine may be quite unstable and undue manipulation may precipitate a neurological event.

A chronic retropharyngeal abscess must not be opened into the mouth, as such a procedure may lead to secondary infection. Drainage of the abscess may not be necessary if suitable treatment of the underlying tuberculosis disease is instituted. If it is necessary, drainage should be carried out through a cervical incision anterior to the sternocleidomastoid muscle with an approach anterior and medial to the carotid sheath to enter the retropharyngeal space. The cavity is opened and suctioned dry after taking biopsy material. Occasionally, surgery is required to decompress the spinal cord if there is a progressive neurological deficit.

Glandular fever (infectious mononucleosis)

This systemic condition is usually caused by the Epstein–Barr virus, but similar features can be caused by cytomegalovirus or toxoplasmosis. The tonsils are typically erythematous with a creamy grey exudate and appear almost confluent, usually symmetrical in contrast to a quinsy. In addition to the discomfort and dysphagia, patients may drool saliva and have respiratory difficulty, particularly on inspiration. They commonly have a high temperature and gross general malaise with other notable cervical or generalised lymphadenopathy. Occasionally, an enlarged spleen or liver may be detected. The condition is most frequent in teenagers and young adults. The diagnosis can be confirmed by serological testing showing a positive Paul–Bunnell test, an absolute and relative lymphocytosis, and the presence of atypical monocytes in the peripheral blood.

Treatment

Analgesia and maintenance of fluid intake are important. A small number of patients require admission to hospital if the airway is compromised and a short course of steroids may be helpful. Antibiotics are of little value and ampicillin is contraindicated because of the frequent appearance of a widespread skin rash. Rarely if the airway is severely compromised, an unhurried elective tracheostomy under local anaesthesia is safer and less traumatic than an emergency intubation. Emergency tonsillectomy is contraindicated because of the generalised pharyngeal oedema and compromised airway.

Human immunodeficiency virus

Acquired immune deficiency syndrome (AIDS) can affect the ear, nose and throat (ENT) system at any point during the disease. The initial seroconversion may present with the symptoms of glandular fever, which is followed by an asymptomatic period of variable length. In the pre-AIDS period, before the full-blown symptoms of the AIDS-related complex, many patients have minor upper respiratory tract symptoms that are often overlooked, such as otitis externa, rhinosinusitis and a non-specific pharyngitis. As the patient moves into the full-blown AIDS-related complex, a persistent, generalised lymphadenopathy is frequently found affecting the cervical nodes, which is usually due to follicular hyperplasia. However, patients may also develop tumours such as Kaposi's sarcoma, sometimes seen in the oral cavity, and high-grade malignant B-cell lymphoma affecting the cervical lymph nodes and nasopharynx. In addition, multiple ulcers may be found in the oral cavity or pharynx associated with herpes infection. Severe candida may affect the oral cavity, pharynx, oesophagus or even larynx, and a hairy leukoplakia may affect the tongue (Figure 48.26).

The globus syndrome

A wide variety of patients experience the feeling of a lump in the throat (from the Latin *globus* = lump). The symptom most commonly affects adults between 30 and 60 years of age. This feeling is not true dysphagia as there is no difficulty in swallowing. Most patients notice the symptom more if they swallow their own saliva, i.e. a forced, dry swallow, rather than when they eat or drink.

The aetiology of this common symptom is unknown, but some patients may have gastro-oesophageal reflux or spasm of their cricopharyngeus muscle.

The original name of 'globus hystericus' is unhelpful and although these patients may be anxious and at times introverted, they nonetheless require full examination to exclude local disease. Radiological and endoscopic investigation may be necessary to exclude an underlying cause.

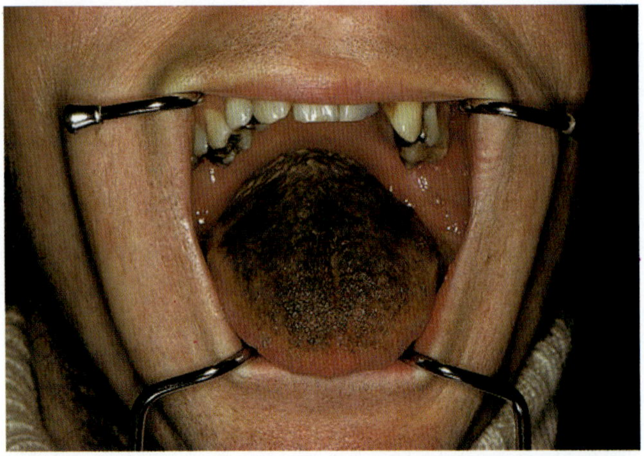

Figure 48.26 Intraoral view showing hairy tongue in a human immunodeficiency virus-positive patient.

Pharyngeal pouch

A pharyngeal pouch is a protrusion of mucosa through Killian's dehiscence, a weak area of the posterior pharyngeal wall between the oblique fibres of the thyropharyngeus and the transverse fibres of cricopharyngeus at the lower end of the inferior constrictor muscle (Figure 48.27). These fibres, along with the circular fibres of the upper oesophagus, form the physiological upper oesophageal sphincter mechanism. Why the pouch forms is not yet clear, even with modern videofluoroscopic and manometric studies. Many patients with pharyngeal pouches have been demonstrated to have normal relaxation of the upper oesophageal sphincter mechanism in relation to swallowing, but others have been shown to have incomplete pharyngeal relaxation, early cricopharyngeal contraction and abnormalities of the pharyngeal contraction wave.

Clinical features

Patients suffering from this condition are commonly more than 60 years of age and it is more common in men than women. As the diverticulum enlarges, patients may experience regurgitation of undigested food, sometimes hours after a meal, particularly if they are bending down or turning over in bed at night. They sometimes wake at night with a feeling of tightness in the throat and a fit of coughing. Occasionally, they may present with recurrent, unexplained chest infections as a result of aspiration of the contents of the pouch. As the pouch increases in size, the patients may notice gurgling noises from the neck on swallowing and the pouch may become large enough to form a visible swelling in the neck.

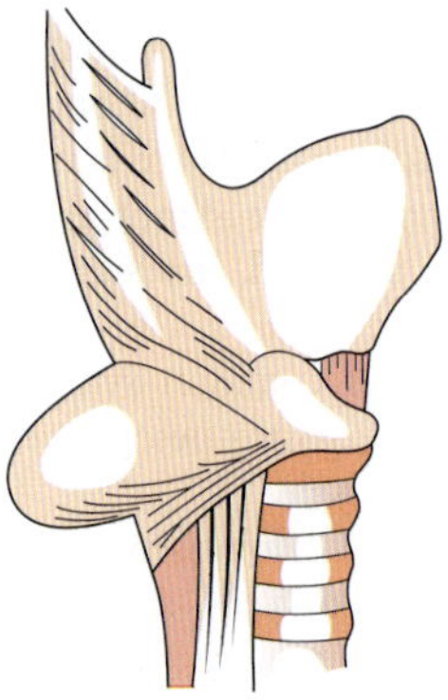

Figure 48.27 A pharyngeal pouch.

Radiological examination

A thin emulsion of barium is given to the patient as a barium swallow (Figure 48.28) or, ideally, as part of a videofluoroscopic swallowing study. Care should be exercised in patients who cough on swallowing, indicating they may have aspiration. A small volume of barium is sufficient to outline the pharynx, pouch and upper oesophagus. The videofluoroscopic study gives additional information about the pharyngeal contraction waves and the performance of the upper oesophageal sphincter.

Treatment

Surgery is indicated when the pouch is associated with progressive symptoms and particularly when a prominent cricopharyngeal bar of muscle associated with abnormality of the upper oesophageal sphincter mechanism causes considerable dysphagia. In elderly patients, a decision to operate may be influenced by their general condition. Preoperative chest physiotherapy and attention to the respiratory, cardiovascular and nutritional aspects of the patient are important. Perioperative antibiotics are recommended.

The preferred surgical technique is with endoscopic stapling of the diverticular wall. A double-bladed rigid endoscope is passed, with one blade in the diverticulum and one blade positioned in the oesophagus. An endoscopic linear stapler is then passed. One jaw of the stapler is placed in the oesophagus, the other in the pouch. The stapler is fired dividing the wall separating the two. The process should be repeated until the bottom of the pouch is reached. This has the effect of opening the pouch, incorporating it as part of the oesophageal wall and dividing the cricopharyngeus muscle. If the patient is symptom free after the procedure they may start graded peroral intake and early discharge.

In the classic external operation, the opening to the pouch is first identified using a pharyngoscope and a nasogastric tube placed into the oesophageal lumen for postoperative nutrition.

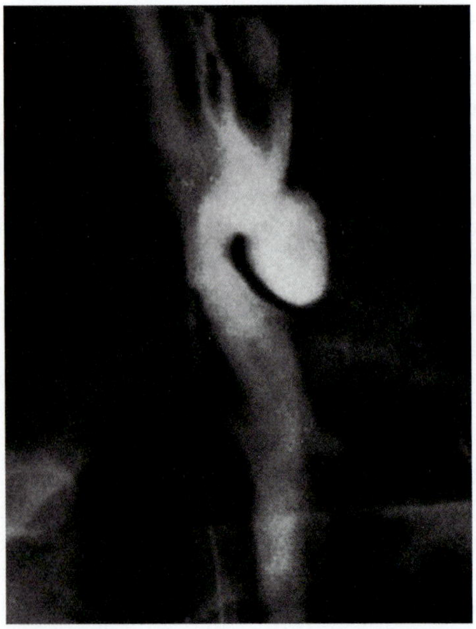

Figure 48.28 Barium swallow showing a pharyngeal pouch.

Gustav Killian, 1860–1921, Professor of Laryngology at Freiburg, and later at Berlin, Germany.

This initial endoscopy is often difficult because the normal oesophageal opening is small compared with the lumen of the pouch, but it may be better visualised using a Dohlmann's rigid endoscope. The pouch may be packed with ribbon gauze soaked in proflavin solution to further aid identification of its neck.

A lower neck incision along the anterior border of the left sternocleidomastoid muscle, or a transverse crease incision, is used and the muscle and carotid sheath are retracted laterally and the trachea and larynx medially. The pouch is found medially behind the lower pharynx and is carefully isolated and dissected back to its origin at Killian's dehiscence. It is then excised and the pharynx closed in two layers or, if it is small, the pouch may be invaginated into the pharyngeal lumen before closing the muscle layers. In all cases, a myotomy dividing the fibres of the cricopharyngeus muscle and the upper oesophageal circular muscle fibres must be performed. The wound is usually closed with drainage and the patient fed through a nasogastric tube for 3–7 days.

The average operating time with an endoscopic procedure is 20–30 minutes compared with 60–90 minutes with an external procedure. Inpatient stay is also decreased for patients undergoing an endoscopic procedure. The endoscopic technique is associated with a high symptomatic success rate and a low morbidity which is particularly important in the elderly.

Complications

The classic operation has been associated with wound infection, mediastinitis, pharyngeal fistula formation, recurrent laryngeal nerve palsy and stenosis of the upper oesophagus. Endoscopic division is associated with the same risks but at lower rates. The recurrence rates between the two procedures appear to be equal; longer-term follow up will establish this. Endoscopic stapling will also allow for safe reoperation if necessary.

Other approaches

Variations have been tried which include simply hitching up the pouch into a superior position without excising it, thus allowing the fundus and body to empty continuously into the oesophagus. This is unsatisfactory with larger pouches, and upper oesophageal myotomy is still required.

Carbon dioxide or argon laser division of the diverticular wall via a special pharyngoscope may also be used. These techniques are associated with a higher recurrence rate than both endoscopic and open repair.

Sideropenic dysphagia

Prolonged iron deficiency anaemia may lead to dysphagia, particularly in middle-aged women. In addition, they may have koilonychia, cheilosis, angular stomatitis together with lassitude and poor exercise tolerance. The dysphagia is caused by a postcricoid or upper oesophageal web and these patients have a higher incidence of postcricoid malignancy. The syndrome is associated with the names of Plummer and Vinson, Paterson and Brown Kelly.

TUMOURS OF THE OROPHARYNX

Benign

Benign tumours of the oropharynx are rare, papillomas being the most common. These are usually incidental findings and are rarely of any importance.

Malignant

The most important epithelial tumour is squamous cell carcinoma, which constitutes approximately 90 per cent of all epithelial tumours in the upper aerodigestive tract (Figures 48.29 and 48.30). In the oropharynx, the proportion is less (70 per cent) because of the higher incidence of lymphoma (25 per cent) and salivary gland tumours (5 per cent).

Aetiology

Squamous carcinomas of the oropharynx are strongly associated with cigarette smoking and consumption of alcohol. In countries where the consumption of tobacco and alcohol are associated with poor oral hygiene, these malignancies assume major importance. Because of the rich lymphatic drainage of the oropharynx, cervical node metastases are common. They may be the only presenting feature with an apparent occult primary

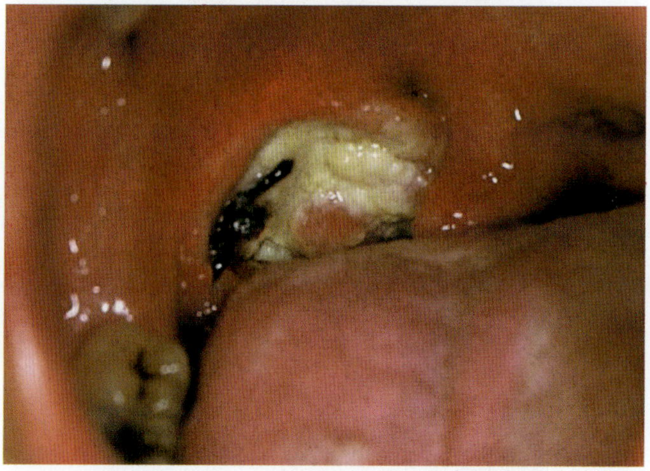

Figure 48.29 Squamous cell carcinoma of the right tonsil.

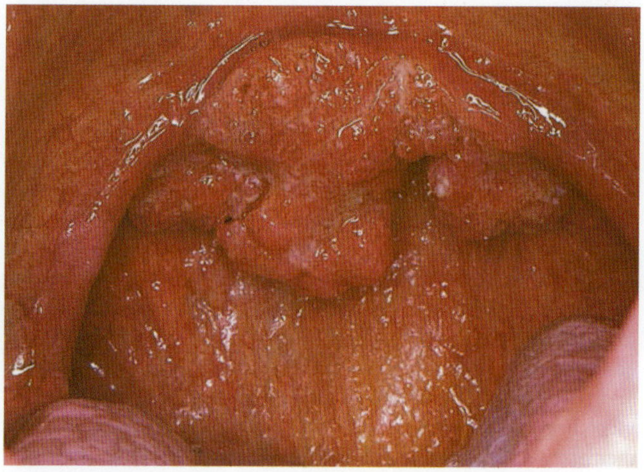

Figure 48.30 Squamous cell carcinoma of the soft palate.

Henry Stanley Plummer, 1874–1937, physician, The Mayo Clinic, Rochester, MN, USA, described this syndrome in 1912.
Porter Paisley Vinson, 1890–1959, physician, The Mayo Clinic, Rochester, MN, who later practised in Richmond, VA, USA.
Donald Rose Paterson, 1863–1939, surgeon, Ear, Nose and Throat Department, The Royal Infirmary, Cardiff, UK.
Adam Brown Kelly, 1865–1941, surgeon, Ear, Nose and Throat Department, The Royal Victoria Infirmary, Glasgow, UK.
Vinson, Paterson and Kelly all described this syndrome independently in 1919.

tumour often being unsuspected and missed in the tonsil or tongue base.

Treatment

Treatment varies with facilities around the world, but early tumours may be cured by chemoradiotherapy, laser excision or more conventional excision. Recurrent disease following radiotherapy is usually managed surgically and repair of the oropharynx may require regionally based myocutaneous flaps or free flaps with microvascular anastomosis. Neck dissection is required in a large proportion of cases of advanced disease. Postoperative dysphagia with aspiration as a result of interference in the complex neuromuscular control of the second phase of swallowing is a particular problem in these patients. This type of surgery is best carried out in a major centre undertaking this work on a regular basis.

Lymphoma of the head and neck

Lymphomas of the head and neck may arise in nodal or extranodal sites and both Hodgkin's disease and non-Hodgkin's lymphoma commonly present as lymph node enlargement in the neck. Hodgkin's disease is rare in the oropharynx, but non-Hodgkin's lymphoma accounts for 15–20 per cent of tumours at this site in some countries. Most are of the B-cell type and have features in common with other MALT tumours. Further evaluation with CT scanning of the thorax and abdomen, and bone marrow evaluation are essential. Fine-needle aspiration cytology of neck lymph nodes is now mandatory and flow cytometry of the aspirates have aided in diagnosis and classification of lymphomas.

Radiotherapy is the treatment of choice for localised non-Hodgkin's lymphoma and may give control rates as high as 75 per cent at five years. For disseminated non-Hodgkin's lymphoma, systemic chemotherapy is preferred.

TUMOURS OF THE HYPOPHARYNX

Benign

Benign tumours of the hypopharynx are very rare, the most common being the fibroma and the leiomyoma. They show a smooth, constant mass lying in the lumen of the hypopharynx or oesophagus.

Malignant

Malignant tumours of the hypopharynx are almost exclusively squamous cell carcinomas with a predominance of moderate and poor differentiation. The tumours are usually classified according to their probable anatomical site of origin from the pyriform fossa, post-cricoid region or posterior pharyngeal wall. Marked differences in the incidence of these tumours occur globally because of factors such as iron-deficiency anaemia (see above under Sideropenic dysphagia). They may be associated with marked submucosal spread of 10 mm or more, which further complicates evaluation. Tumours arising from the pyriform fossa and posterior pharyngeal wall may spread to upper or lower cervical nodes. Tumours arising in the post-cricoid area typically metastasise to paratracheal and paraoesophageal nodes, which may not be palpable. As with oropharyngeal tumours, alcohol and tobacco are two principal carcinogens. Post-cricoid carcinoma, though rare, is more common in women than men.

The diagnosis of hypopharyngeal carcinoma should be considered in all patients presenting with dysphagia, hoarseness or referred otalgia, particularly if they have a history of iron deficiency anaemia, smoking or significant alcohol consumption.

Fibreoptic endoscopic examination in clinic may show only subtle signs, such as oedema or pooling of saliva unilaterally in the pyriform fossa. Note should also be made that this region is not well seen on flexible gastroscopy. Preferred investigation is with direct rigid pharyngoscopy and oesophagoscopy with biopsy under a general anaesthetic. All regions of the neck must be assessed in a systematic manner. Fine-needle aspirate is advocated for suspicious nodes.

Radiological examination

A suspected primary requires a neck and staging CT and/or MRI of the neck.

Treatment

Squamous carcinoma of the hypopharynx commonly presents late and carries a poor prognosis. Early lesions may be treated with chemoradiotherapy or transoral endoscopic carbon dioxide laser resection. Major open excisional surgery is generally used for recurrence after radiotherapy or as primary excision in advanced disease. Total pharyngolaryngectomy is commonly required (Figure 48.31) and for lesions extending into the upper oesophagus, oesophagectomy with gastric pull-up or free flap reconstruction may be needed. Myocutaneous flaps, transposed jejunum or stomach are used to reconstruct the pharynx. Swallowing and voice rehabilitation are necessary to support patients after this major surgery if they are to adjust and maintain some quality of life (Summary box 48.7).

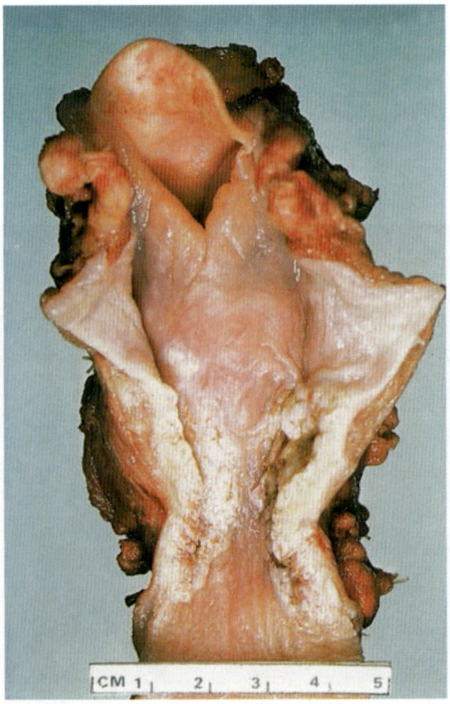

Figure 48.31 Total pharyngolaryngectomy specimen showing hypopharyngeal carcinoma (hypopharynx opened from posterior).

Thomas Hodgkin, 1798–1866, Curator of the Museum, and Demonstrator of Morbid Anatomy, Guy's Hospital, London, UK, described lymphadenoma in 1832.

Summary box 48.7

Tumours of the hypopharynx

- Variable symptoms – discomfort, pain, dysphagia, hoarseness
- Awareness increased by history of smoking and alcohol
- Expert examination with nasendoscopy
- Referral to expert for detailed assessment and treatment – radiotherapy, laser or extensive surgery

DISEASES OF THE LARYNX

Emergencies

Stridor

Stridor means noisy breathing. It may be inspiratory or expiratory, or occurring in both phases of respiration. Inspiratory stridor is usually due to an obstruction at or above the vocal folds and is most commonly the result of an inhaled foreign body or acute infections such as epiglottitis. Expiratory stridor is usually from the lower respiratory tract and gives rise to a prolonged expiratory wheeze. It is most commonly associated with acute asthma or acute infective tracheobronchitis. Biphasic stridor is usually due to obstruction or disease of the tracheobronchial airway and distal lungs (Summary box 48.8).

Summary box 48.8

Stridor

Inspiratory
- Foreign body or epiglottitis

Expiratory
- Acute asthma or infective tracheobronchitis

Biphasic
- Obstruction, disease of tracheobronchial airway or distal lungs

Stridor in children

Infants and children presenting with stridor need careful assessment with a full history and examination as appropriate. If, on presentation, a child is cyanosed and severely unwell, the airway must be secured as soon as possible, but a brief history with important pointers can often be obtained from the parents.

History

In infants in the first year of life, it is important to establish if the stridor is associated with particular activities such as swallowing, crying or movement. These may suggest congenital laryngomalacia or subglottic stenosis. If the stridor is exacerbated by feeding, particularly in the first 4 weeks of life, this suggests a vascular ring or tracheo-oesophageal fistula. If the cry is weak or abnormal, this suggests a vocal fold palsy. If the problem only occurs in association with an upper respiratory tract infection and, in particular, is biphasic, this would suggest congenital subglottic stenosis. In a young child, inspiratory stridor and drooling suggest acute epiglottitis, whereas biphasic stridor without drooling suggests laryngotracheobronchitis or croup (Summary box 48.9).

Summary box 48.9

Acute paediatric stridor

Congenital
- Laryngomalacia
- Laryngeal web
- Subglottic stenosis

Acquired
- Inflammatory
  - Angioneurotic oedema
- Traumatic
  - Impacted foreign body, laryngeal fracture
- Infective
  - Epiglottis, laryngotracheobronchitis
- Neurological
  - Vocal fold palsy
- Neoplasia
  - Benign laryngeal papillomatosis

Examination

It is important when possible to observe the child carefully at rest. Once a baby starts to cry, it may be impossible to study its resting respiratory pattern for some time. Ask the mother, not a nurse or a colleague, to move a baby or young child into different positions, such as face down and supine, and watch for changes in respiratory pattern and level of distress. Observe any drooling and, with neonates and infants, always try to watch the child being fed, listening to the trachea and chest with a stethoscope if possible. Always examine the whole child, looking for any evidence of congenital abnormalities before attempting any examination of the throat.

If a child is stridulous and drooling and sitting upright in its mother's arms or a chair, do not attempt to lie it down and do not attempt to look inside the mouth. These manoeuvres are potentially life-threatening as the child may aspirate a large quantity of thick saliva contained within the oral cavity. The child does not wish to attempt swallowing in the case of a retropharyngeal abscess, parapharyngeal abscess or acute epiglottitis as these conditions are so painful. It is particularly important in acute epiglottitis as the aspiration of thick saliva may be associated with further laryngeal spasm and a respiratory arrest. Restlessness, increasing tachycardia and cyanosis are important signs of hypoxia. If the child is not distressed and drooling, and not markedly stridulous, he/she may be cooperative enough that it is possible to look inside the mouth and check the palate, tongue and oropharynx. In stridulous children, particularly neonates and infants, a transcutaneous oximeter is invaluable. A resuscitation trolley with the necessary equipment for emergency intubation or tracheostomy should be close at hand if at all possible before commencing examination.

Investigation

Plain lateral radiographs of the neck and a chest radiograph can be obtained but only if the child's condition permits. If a child is severely stridulous, they should not be sent to a radiography department without access to medical staff or resuscitation equipment.

Examination under anaesthesia is essential in all children whose diagnosis remains in doubt. This requires a high level of skill and appropriate rigid laryngoscopes, bronchoscopes, endoscopic Hopkins' rods and an operating microscope should be made available if possible. Equipment should be available at all times to undertake an urgent tracheostomy to establish or maintain an airway.

Acute epiglottitis

In children, acute epiglottitis is of rapid onset. It tends to occur in children of two years of age and over. Stridor is usually associated with drooling of saliva. The condition is caused by *Haemophilus influenzae* infection, which initially causes a severe pharyngitis at the junction of the oro- and hypopharynx before producing inflammation and oedema of the laryngeal inlet. As it progresses, it involves the whole of the supraglottic larynx, with severe oedema of the aryepiglottic folds and epiglottis being the most notable component, hence the commonly used term 'acute epiglottitis'.

These children frequently require intensive management with emergency intubation or tracheostomy followed by oxygenation, humidification, continuous oximetry and antibiotics such as ampicillin or chloramphenicol. There may be associated septicaemia so blood cultures should be obtained. Attempted examination with a spatula into the mouth may precipitate a respiratory arrest and should be avoided. The incidence of acute epiglottitis has plummeted where *Haemophilus influenzae* vaccination programmes have occurred.

Laryngotracheobronchitis (croup)

Croup is usually of slower onset than acute epiglottitis and occurs most commonly in children under two years of age. It is usually viral in origin and the cases often occur in clusters. The children have biphasic stridor, and are often hoarse with a typical barking cough. Airway intervention is required less often, but admission to hospital with oxygenation and humidification, coupled with antibiotics, may be necessary if there are signs of secondary infection.

Foreign bodies

Both children and adults may inhale foreign bodies. Young children will attempt to swallow a wide variety of objects, but coins, beads and parts of toys are particularly common. In adults, the aspiration is usually food, particularly inadequately chewed bones and meat. This is more common in elderly edentulous adults. Occasionally, portions of dentures may be inhaled, particularly in association with road traffic accidents.

Clinical features

The history is paramount and a history of foreign body ingestion or inhalation in a child, even though the pain, dysphagia, coughing, etc. may have settled, should always be taken seriously.

Adults usually have a clear recall, which facilitates diagnosis. Fish bones may lodge in the tonsils or base of tongue with minimal symptoms, but small fish bones may give rise to para- and retropharyngeal abscess formation.

Examination

Examination may be prevented by trismus, pain and anxiety, but the presence of a foreign body may be suspected by a salivary pool within the pyriform fossa or adjacent oedema and erythema of the pharyngolaryngeal mucosa.

Radiology

Radiology may be helpful but is not critical. Fish bones are often invisible on plain radiographs and a normal plain radiograph does not exclude a foreign body within the pharynx, larynx, oesophagus or lungs.

Specialised studies may help in cases of doubt, using a CT scan or a gastrografin swallow in the case of a suspected oesophageal foreign body.

Treatment

In the case of an inhaled foreign body causing severe stridor in a neonate or infant, it may be removed either by hooking it from the pharynx with a finger or by inverting the child carefully by the ankles and slapping his/her back. In a larger child, it may be more appropriate to bend them over your knee with their head hanging down and again strike them firmly between the shoulders. In the case of adults, an impacted laryngeal foreign body may be coughed out using a Heimlich manoeuvre. This involves standing behind the patient, clasping the arms around the lower thorax, such that the knuckles of the clasped hands come into contact with the patient's xiphisternum, and then a brief, firm compression of the lower thorax may aid instant expiration of the foreign body. If none of these immediate emergency measures removes the foreign body and the patient is cyanosed and severely stridulous, an immediate cricothyroidotomy or tracheostomy may be necessary. In less urgent cases, and when a foreign body is strongly suspected, endoscopy under general anaesthesia may be indicated.

Other causes of acute pharyngolaryngeal oedema

Angioneurotic oedema, radiotherapy, laryngeal trauma associated with road traffic accidents, corrosives, scalds and smoke ingestion may all cause significant pharyngolaryngeal oedema, in addition to the acute infective conditions mentioned elsewhere. Hoarseness is the predominant symptom along with dysphagia prior to the increase in dyspnoea. If flexible laryngoscopic examination is possible, marked oedema of the supraglottis and pharynx can be seen. Humidified oxygen, adrenaline nebulisers, systemic antihistamines and steroids may be valuable. Morphine should not be given as it may cause respiratory depression and respiratory arrest. If the dyspnoea progresses, intubation or tracheostomy will be necessary.

TRACHEOSTOMY AND OTHER EMERGENCY AIRWAY MEASURES

This procedure relieves airway obstruction or protects the airway by fashioning a direct entrance into the trachea through the skin of the neck. Tracheostomy may be carried out as an emergency when the patient is *in extremis* and the larynx cannot be intubated, but it is not always an easy procedure, particularly in an obese patient. An easier alternative for the inexperienced is insertion of a large intravenous cannula or a small tube into the cricothyroid membrane, which lies in the midline immediately below the thyroid cartilage. Emergency intubation is a further option when the laryngotracheal airway is not obstructed and tracheostomy may be performed thereafter. **The time to do a tracheostomy is when you first think it may be necessary.**

Henry Judah Heimlich, born 1920, thoracic surgeon, Xavier University, Cincinnati, OH, USA.
in extremis is Latin for 'in the last things'.

If time allows, the following should be undertaken:

- inspection and palpation of the neck to assess the laryngotracheal anatomy in the individual patient;
- indirect or direct laryngoscopy;
- assessment of pulmonary function.

Whenever possible, the procedure should be adequately explained to the patient beforehand, with particular emphasis on the inability to speak immediately following the operation. Ample reassurance is required that they will not have 'lost' their voice permanently. The indications for tracheostomy are shown in Summary box 48.10.

Summary box 48.10

Indications for tracheostomy

Acute upper airway obstruction

- For example, an inhaled foreign body, a large pharyngolaryngeal tumour, or acute pharyngolaryngeal infections in children

Potential upper airway obstruction

- For example, after major surgery involving the oral cavity, pharynx, larynx or neck

Protection of the lower airway

- For example, protection against aspiration of saliva in unconscious patients as a consequence of head injuries, faciomaxillary injuries, comas, bulbar poliomyelitis or tetanus

Patients requiring prolonged artifical respiration

- Best performed within 10 days of ventilation

Emergency tracheostomy

If a skilled anaesthetist is unavailable, local anaesthesia is employed, but in desperate cases when the patient is unconscious, none is required. In patients who have suffered severe head and neck trauma and who may have an unstable cervical spine fracture, cricothyroidotomy may be more suitable. If it is possible, the patient should be laid supine with padding placed under the shoulders and the extended neck kept as steady as possible in the midline. This aids palpation of the thyroid and cricoid cartilage between the thumb and index finger of the free hand. The movements of the fingers of the free hand are important in this technique. The operation is more difficult in small children and thick-necked adults as the landmarks are difficult to palpate (Figures 48.32 and 48.33).

A vertical midline incision is made from the inferior aspect of the thyroid cartilage to the suprasternal notch and continued down between the infrahyoid muscles. There may be heavy bleeding from the wound at this point, particularly if the neck is congested as a result of the patient's efforts to breathe around an acute upper airway obstruction. No steps should be taken to control this haemorrhage, although an assistant and suction are valuable. The operator should feel carefully for the cricoid cartilage using the index finger of the free hand while retracting the skin edges by pressure applied by the thumb and middle finger. If the situation is one of extreme urgency, a further vertical incision straight into the trachea at the level of the second, third and fourth ring should be made immediately without regard to the presence of the thyroid isthmus. The knife blade is rotated through 90°, thus opening the trachea. At this point, the patient may cough violently as blood enters the airway. The operator should be aware of this possibility and avoid losing the position of the scalpel in the open trachea. Any form of available tube should be inserted into the trachea as soon as possible and blood and secretion sucked out. Once an airway has been established, haemostasis is then secured. With the emergency under control, the tracheostomy should be refashioned as soon as possible.

Should additional equipment and more time be available once the cricoid cartilage has been identified, blunt finger dissection inferiorly can be used to mobilise the thyroid isthmus, which should be divided between haemostats, clearing the trachea before making a vertical incision through the second to the fourth rings. A tracheal dilator is inserted through the tracheal incision and the edges of the tracheal wound are separated gently. In cases of suspected human immunodeficiency virus (HIV) infection or diphtheria, the surgeon places a swab over the wound so that the violent expiratory efforts which may follow do not contaminate the operator(s) with infected mucus and blood. When respiratory efforts have become less violent, a tracheostomy tube is inserted into the trachea and the dilator removed. It is important that the surgeon keeps a finger on the tube while the assistant ties the attached tapes around the patient's neck. Return the neck to a neutral position before tying the tapes firmly.

Elective tracheostomy

The advantage of an elective surgical procedure is that there is complete airway control at all times, unhurried dissection and careful placement of an appropriate tube. Close cooperation between the surgeon, anaesthetist and scrub nurse is essential,

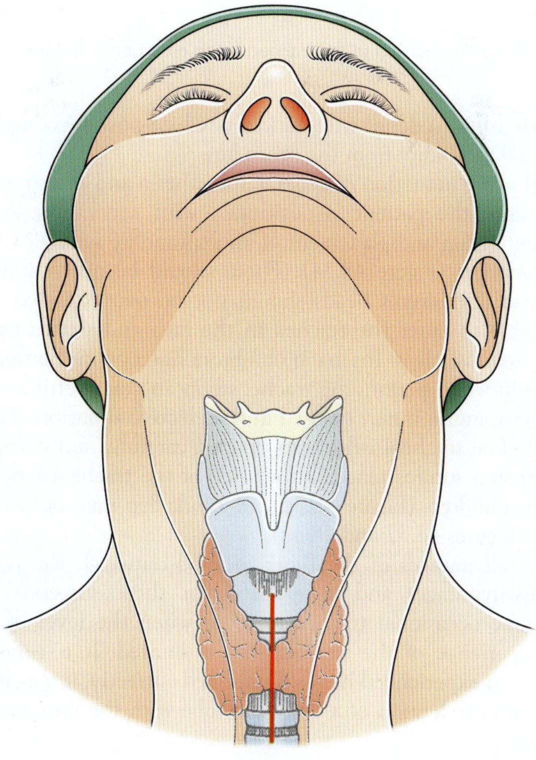

Figure 48.32 The position of skin incision in an emergency tracheostomy.

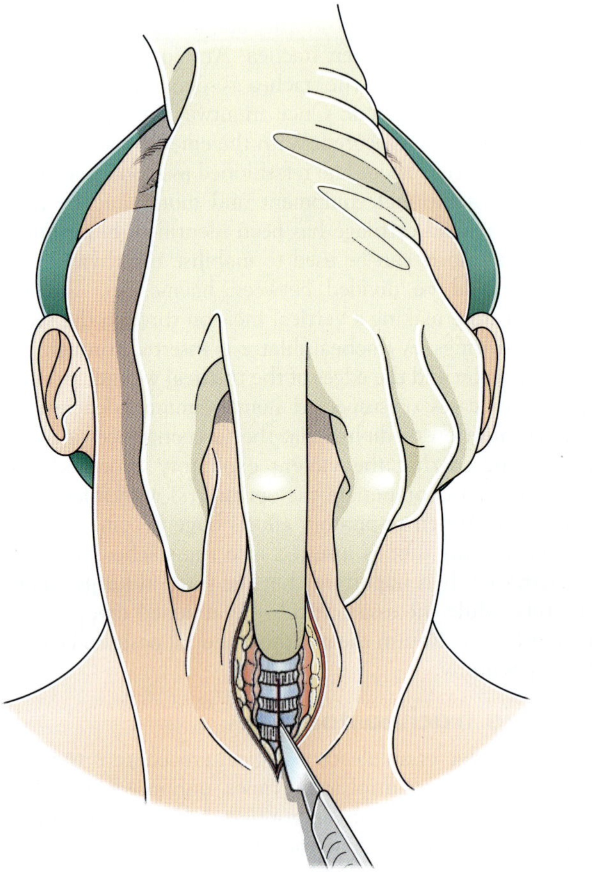

Figure 48.33 An incision in the trachea in an emergency tracheostomy.

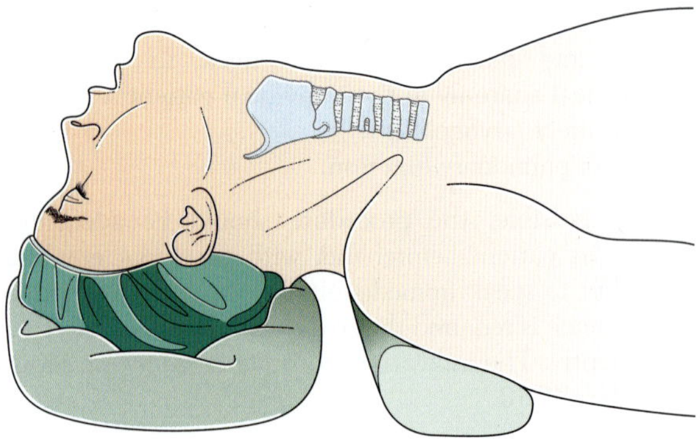

Figure 48.34 Position of the patient for elective tracheostomy.

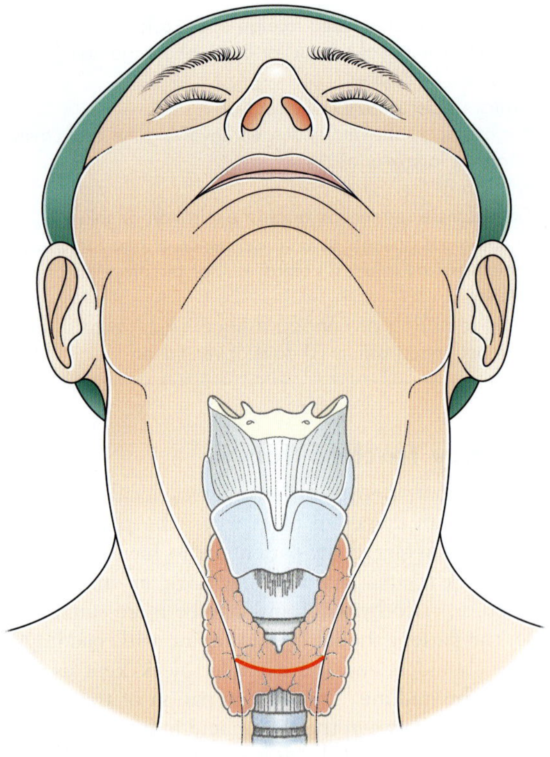

Figure 48.35 Position of a skin incision in an elective tracheostomy.

and attention to detail will markedly reduce possible complications and morbidity from the procedure.

Following induction of general anaesthesia and endotracheal intubation, the patient is positioned with a combination of head extension and placement of an appropriate sandbag under the shoulders (Figure 48.34). There should be no rotation of the head. Children's heads should not be overextended as it is possible to enter the trachea in the fifth and sixth rings in these circumstances. Insertion of a bronchoscope in the trachea may help when performing tracheostomy in young children. A transverse incision may be used in the elective situation (Figure 48.35). The tracheal isthmus is divided carefully and oversewn and tension sutures placed either side of the tracheal fenestration in children (Figure 48.36). A Bjork flap may be used in adults (Figures 48.37 and 48.38).

The advantages of the Bjork method outweigh the potential disadvantages and it is useful for those surgeons who undertake occasional tracheostomy or when the level of skill and experience of the nursing staff is limited. It is generally avoided in experienced hands. Performed correctly, it is safe and allows reintroduction of a displaced tube with the minimum of difficulty.

The inferiorly based flap is begun at its apex with an incision on the superior aspects of the second ring and extends down either side through the second and third rings. The tip of the flap should be stitched to the inferior edge of the transverse skin incision using horizontal mattress sutures through the structure of the second ring. These sutures should be generous enough so that they will not cut out. The first tracheal ring should not be violated in any circumstances.

In a paediatric patient who requires a tracheostomy, failure to remain in the midline may result in pneumothorax, as pleural spaces extend into the root of the neck laterally. Prior to incision of the trachea vertical stay sutures are placed lateral to the midline through the tracheal rings and left in place. A vertical incision is made between the second and third tracheal rings. No tracheal tissue is removed. These can provide traction for the trachea and allow for rapid tracheostomy tube reinsertion if accidental decannulation occurs prior to the establishment of

Viking Olaf Bjork, born 1918, formerly cardiac surgeon, Karolinska Sjukset, Stockholm, Sweden.

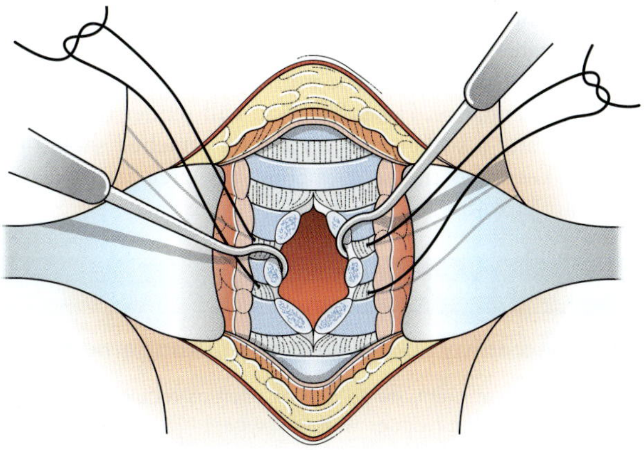

Figure 48.36 Tracheal fenestration in an elective tracheostomy.

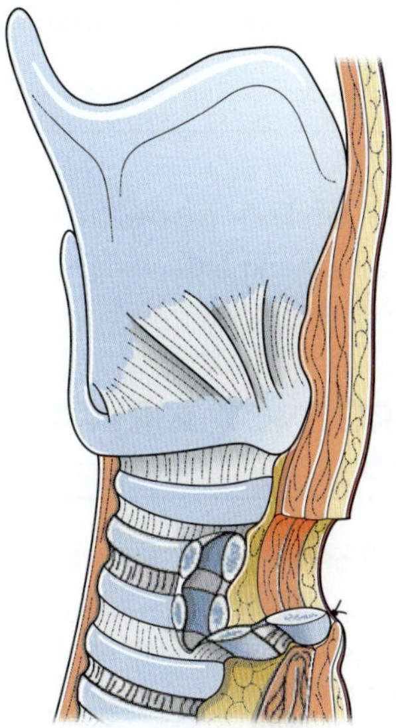

Figure 48.37 Bjork flap.

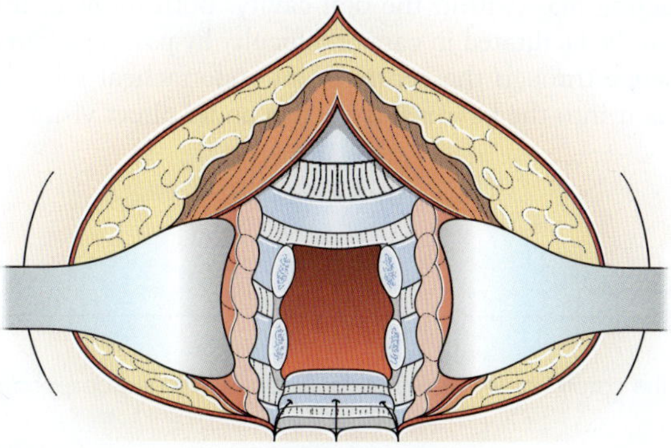

Figure 48.38 Fenestration in a Bjork flap.

the tract. Some surgeons will suture skin flaps to the trachea for additional safety.

Percutaneous tracheostomy

In many countries, tracheostomy may be performed percutaneously with bronchoscopic assistance. A transverse incision is made between the first and second tracheal rings, and blunt dissection of the midline is then performed. A 22-gauge needle is inserted between the second and third tracheal rings. When air is aspirated into the syringe, the guidewire is introduced. After the guidewire is protected, dilators are introduced. All dilators are inserted in a sequential manner from small to large diameter. The tracheotomy tube is then introduced along the dilator and guidewire. The guidewire and dilator are removed, the cuff of the tracheotomy tube is inflated, and the breathing circuit is connected. The endotracheal tube can then be removed.

Patients must have appropriate anatomy and no limitation of neck movement. If any doubt arises as to the suitability of a patient for percutaneous tracheostomy a surgical approach should be adopted. Percutaneous tracheostomy is rarely performed in children.

Tracheostomy tubes

These are basically made of two materials: silver or plastic. Both materials have been used to make tubes of various sizes with varying curves, angles, cuffs, inner tubes and speaking valves (Figures 48.39 and 48.40). A cuffed tube is used initially, which may be changed after 3–4 days to a non-cuffed plastic or silver tube. The pressure within the tube cuff should be carefully monitored and should be low enough so as not to occlude circulation in the mucosal capillaries. When in position, the tube should be retained by double tapes passed around the patient's neck with a reef knot on either side. It is important that the patient's head is flexed when the tapes are tied, otherwise they may become slack when the patient is moved from the position of extension, thereby resulting in a possible displacement of the tube if the patient coughs. Alternatively, the flanges of the plastic tube may be stitched directly to the underlying neck skin.

All forms of tracheostomy and cricothyroidotomy bypass the upper airway and have the following advantages:

- The anatomical dead space is reduced by approximately 50 per cent.
- The work of breathing is reduced.
- Alveolar ventilation is increased.
- The level of sedation needed for patient comfort is decreased and, unlike endotracheal intubation, the patient may be able to talk and eat with a tube in place.

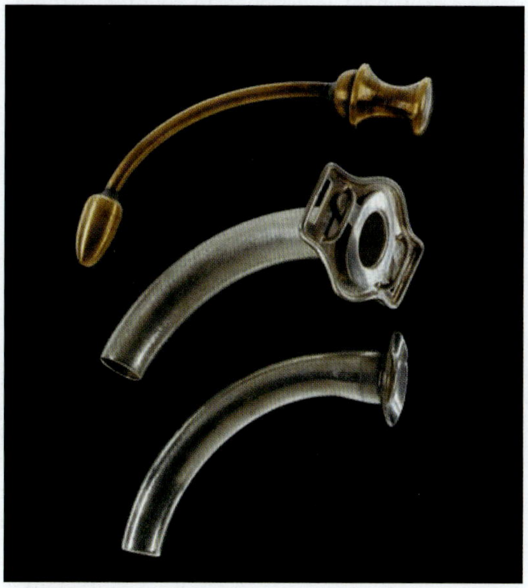

Figure 48.39 Silver tracheostomy tube. From above: introducer, outer tube and inner tube.

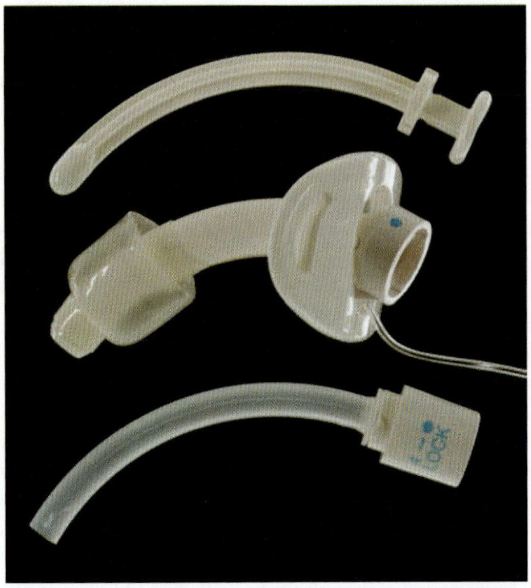

Figure 48.40 Modern plastic tracheostomy tube with introducer, low-pressure cuff and inner canula.

However, there are several disadvantages:

- Loss of heat and moisture exchange performed in the upper respiratory tract.
- Desiccation of tracheal epithelium, loss of ciliated cells and metaplasia.
- The presence of a foreign body in the trachea stimulates mucous production; where no cilia are present, this mucociliary stream is arrested.
- The increased mucus is more viscid and thick crusts may form and block the tube.
- Although many patients with a tracheostomy can feed satisfactorily, there is some splinting of the larynx, which may prevent normal swallowing and lead to aspiration; this aspiration may not be apparent.

Postoperative treatment is designed to counteract these effects and frequent suction and humidification are most important. A trolley must be placed by the bed containing a tracheal dilator, duplicate tubes and introducers, retractors and dressings. Oxygen is at hand and, in the initial period, a nurse must be in constant attendance. Humidification will render the secretions less viscid and a sucker with a catheter attached should be on hand to keep the tracheobronchial tree free from secretions (Summary box 48.11).

Summary box 48.11

Tracheostomy: postoperative management

- Suction – efficient, sterile and as often as required
- Humidification (with or without oxygen)
- A warm, well-ventilated room
- Position of the tube and patient
- Spare tube, introducer, tapes, tracheal dilator
- Change of tube, inner tube, possible speaking valve
- Physiotherapy
- Initiation of local decannulation protocols where indicated

Complications of tracheostomy

The intraoperative, early and late postoperative complications of tracheostomy are listed in Table 48.2.

OTHER EMERGENCY AIRWAY PROCEDURES

Fibreoptic endotracheal intubation

In most emergency situations, endotracheal intubation is the most direct and satisfactory method of securing the airway. Nasotracheal intubation in expert hands is also a well-established technique and is particularly useful if the patient has trismus, severe mandibular injuries, cervical spine rigidity or an obstructing mass within the oral cavity. Both forms of intubation can be facilitated in case of difficulty by passing a fibreoptic endoscope through the centre of an endotracheal tube, hence guiding it into the larynx and trachea under direct vision.

Table 48.2 Tracheostomy: complications.

Intraoperative complications	Haemorrhage Injury to paratracheal structures, particularly the carotid artery, recurrent laryngeal nerve and oesophagus Damage to the trachea
Early postoperative complications	Apnoea caused by a fall in the $P\text{CO}_2$ Haemorrhage Subcutaneous emphysema, pneumomediastinum and pneumothorax Accidental extubation, anterior displacement of the tube, obstruction of the tube lumen and tip occlusion against the tracheal wall Infection Swallowing dysfunction
Late postoperative complications	Difficult decannulation Tracheocutaneous fistula Tracheo-oesophageal fistula, tracheoinnominate artery fistula with severe haemorrhage Tracheal stenosis

Laryngeal mask airway

The laryngeal mask airway (LMA) is a wide-bore airway with an inflatable cuff at the distal end, which forms a seal in the pharynx around the laryngeal inlet. Provided the laryngotracheal airway is clear, the LMA provides a clear and secure airway. The technique can easily be learnt by non-anaesthetists and secures an airway in most cases. It comes in a range of sizes covering infants to large adults. It is particularly useful in cases of difficult intubation (Figure 48.41).

Transtracheal ventilation

This technique is simple and effective and allows ventilation for periods in excess of 1 hour providing time to allow for more elective intubation. The cricothyroid membrane is located by palpation of the neck with the index finger, and a 14- or 16-gauge plastic sheathed intravascular needle and a 10-mL syringe containing a few millilitres of lignocaine are introduced in the midline and directed downwards and backwards into the tracheal lumen. The needle is advanced steadily and negative pressure is placed on the syringe until bubbles of air are clearly seen (Figure 48.42). The tissues of the neck may be infiltrated with the anaesthetic if desired and the tracheal mucosa likewise partly anaesthetised by the introduction of 1–2 mL after gaining the lumen. The needle is removed and the plastic sheath cannula remains in the tracheal lumen and must be carefully held and fixed in place by the operator so that it does not come out of the lumen into the soft tissues of the neck. It is attached by means of a Luer connection to the high-pressure oxygen supply. Ventilation may be undertaken in a controlled manner with a jetting device with the chest being observed for appropriate movements.

If there is severe obstruction of the laryngopharynx by the foreign body or tumour, the exhaled outflow of gases can be aided by the placement of one or two further cannulae as exhalation ports. This procedure gains extremely rapid control of ventilation and requires a minimum of technical expertise. Its only notable complication is surgical emphysema of the neck tissues if the cannula dislodges from the tracheal lumen.

Cricothyroidotomy

Cricothyroidotomy has the advantages of speed and ease requiring little equipment and surgical expertise. However, its use for all but the briefest access to the airway remains controversial and there are conflicting reports with regard to the subsequent incidence of complications, particularly those of subglottic stenosis and long-term voice changes.

The patient's neck is extended and the area between the prominence of the thyroid cartilage and the cricoid cartilage below is palpated with the index finger of the free hand. In the emergency situation, a vertical skin incision is recommended with dissection rapidly carried down to the cricothyroid membrane. A 1-cm transverse incision is made through the membrane immediately above the cricoid cartilage and the scalpel twisted through a right angle to gain access to the airway. If available, artery forceps, dilator or tracheal hook will improve the aperture and insertion of an available tube (Figures 48.43 and 48.44).

Depending on the degree of emergency, it may be necessary for the surgeon to assess the results of the procedure by direct laryngoscopy and the authors recommend that careful consideration should be given to conversion of the cricothyroidotomy to a tracheostomy. Although there is debate about the frequency of subglottic stenosis following this procedure, there is general agreement that it is much increased if any long-term ventilation is undertaken via even a modestly sized tracheostomy tube through the cricothyroid membrane.

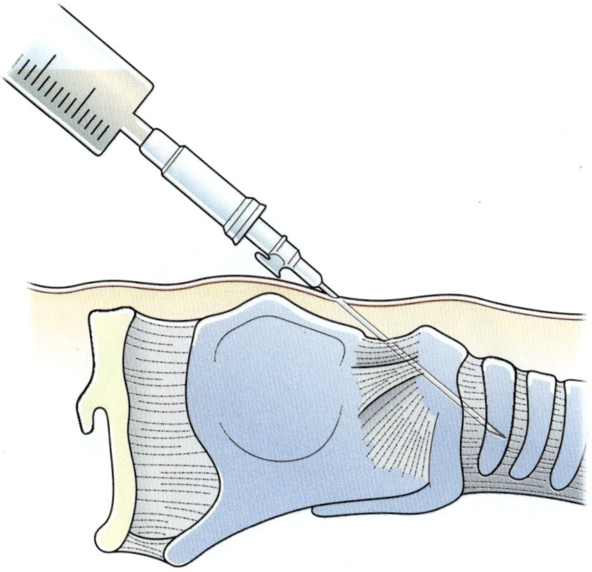

Figure 48.42 Transtracheal needle introduction.

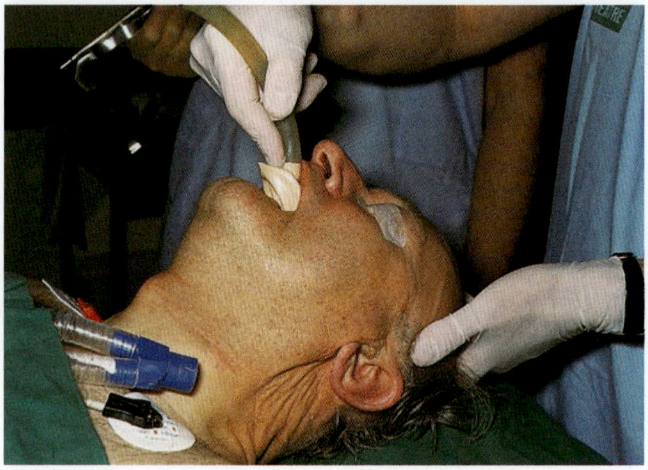

Figure 48.41 Laryngeal mask airway being inserted.

LARYNGEAL DISEASE CAUSING VOICE DISORDERS

Vocal nodules

These are fibrous thickenings of the vocal folds at the junction of the middle and anterior third (Figure 48.45), and are the result of vocal abuse; they are known as singers' nodules in adults and screamers' nodules in children. Speech therapy is

Luer was a German instrument maker who was working in Paris, France, at the end of the nineteenth century.

therefore the preferred treatment and the lesions will resolve spontaneously in most cases. Occasionally, the nodules will need to be surgically removed using modern microlaryngoscopic dissection or laser techniques, but speech therapy will still be required for postoperative voice rehabilitation (Summary box 48.12).

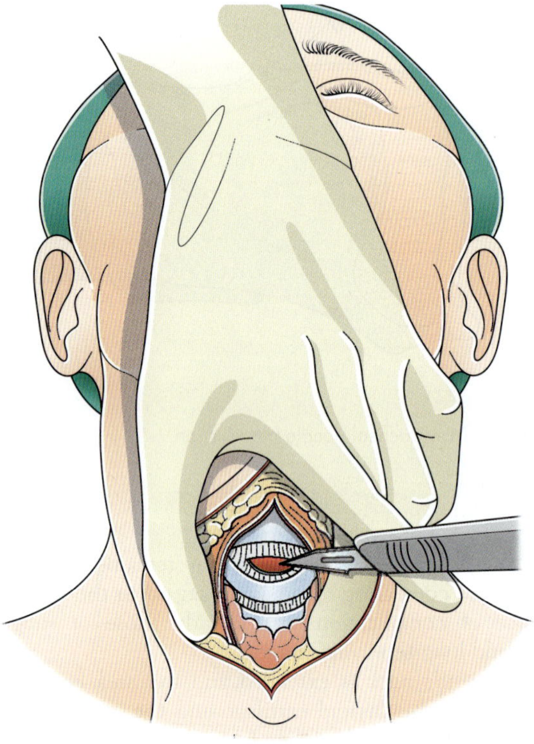

Figure 48.43 Incision in a cricothyroidotomy.

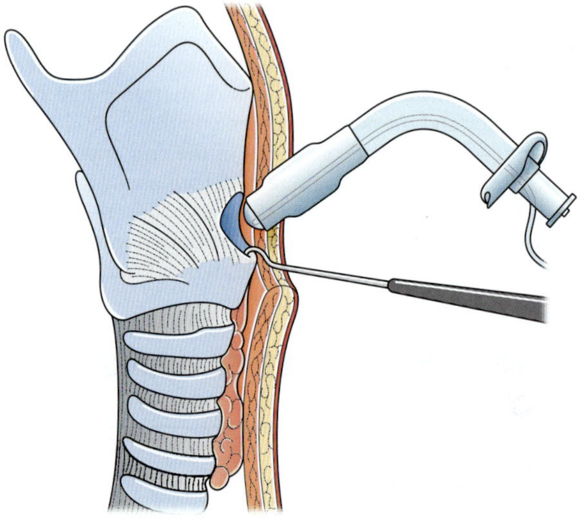

Figure 48.44 Insertion of a tube after cricothyroidotomy.

Summary box 48.12

Causes of hoarseness

- Mucosal disease, e.g. vocal nodule, polyps or laryngeal papillomatosis, acute or chronic laryngitis
- Neurological disease, e.g. vocal fold palsy
- Neoplasia, e.g. laryngeal tumours
- Non-specific voice disorders, functional dysphonia

Vocal fold polyps

These are usually unilateral and may be associated with an acute infective episode, cigarette smoking and vocal abuse (Figure 48.46). Speech therapy is again indicated, but they do usually require removal by microdissection or laser surgery.

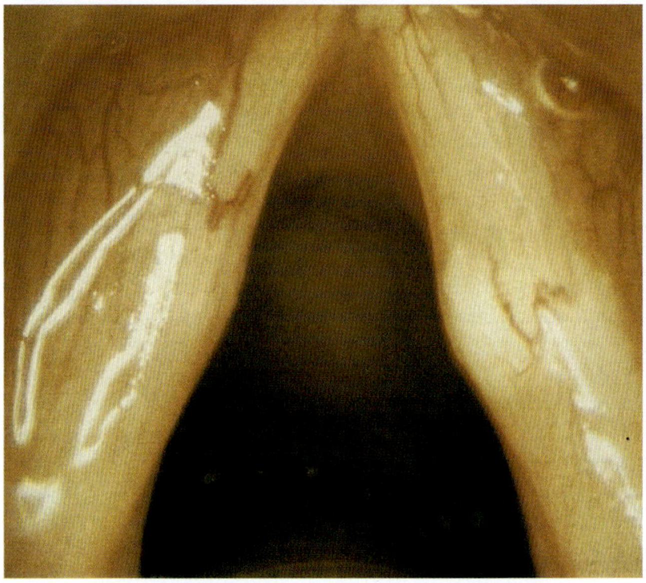

Figure 48.45 Vocal fold nodules.

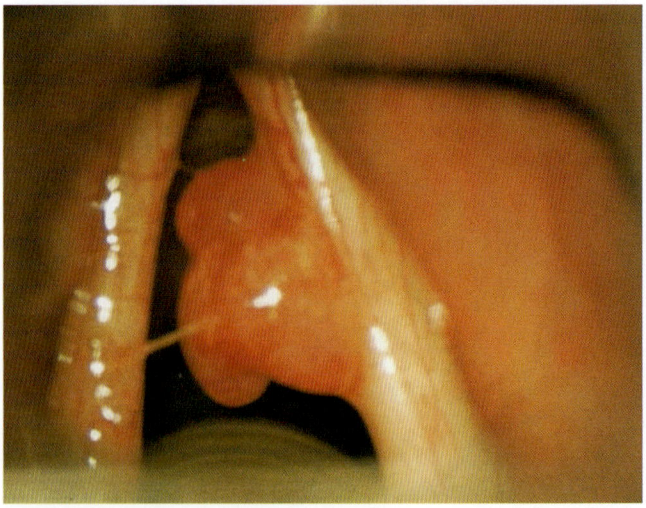

Figure 48.46 A vocal fold polyp.

Laryngeal papillomata

These are rare benign tumours occurring mainly in children, but can also present in adults. They are most commonly found on the vocal folds, but may spread throughout the larynx and tracheobronchial airway (Figure 48.47). They are caused by papillomaviruses and need removal by carbon dioxide laser or microsurgery to maintain a reasonable voice and airway. These patients are best managed in specialist centres, with the appropriate expertise. Antiviral treatment is of doubtful value at present. Papilloma vaccination is of unproven benefit.

Acute laryngitis

This often occurs in association with upper respiratory tract infections in association with a cough and pharyngitis. Usually viral, it may be localised to the larynx and it settles quickly if the voice is rested during the acute inflammation. Steam inhalations are soothing along with mild analgesia, but antibiotics are unnecessary (Summary box 48.13).

> **Summary box 48.13**
>
> **Warning**
>
> - Hoarseness lasting for 3–4 weeks should always be referred for an ENT opinion, particularly in smokers

Chronic laryngitis

Chronic laryngitis may be specific and can be caused by mycobacteria, syphilis and fungi. Treatment is directed towards the causative organism. Non-specific laryngitis is common, the main predisposing factors being smoking, chronic upper and lower respiratory sepsis and voice abuse. Gastro-oesophageal reflux has been implicated as a factor in laryngitis, vocal fold nodules and polyps, but the evidence is controversial. There is, however, a vogue for treatment with antireflux medication and proton pump inhibitors. Diagnosis of chronic laryngitis should not be made unless the larynx has been fully evaluated by a laryngologist.

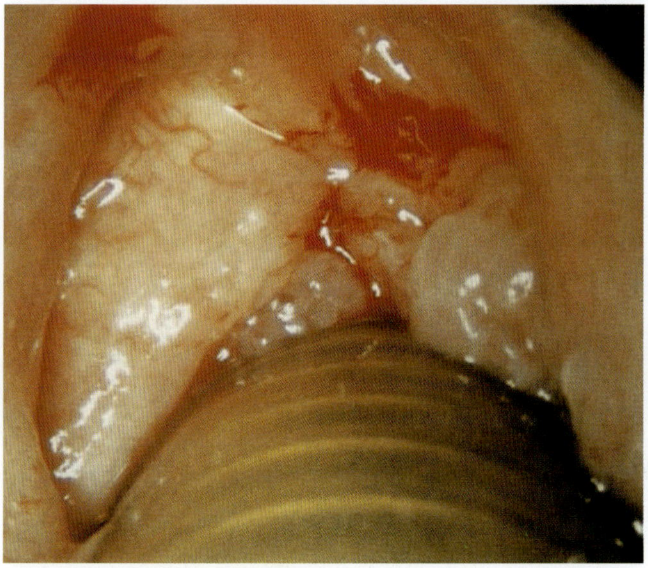

Figure 48.47 Laryngeal papillomata.

Vocal fold palsy

This may be unilateral or bilateral (Figure 48.48), but a unilateral left vocal fold palsy is the most common because of the long intrathoracic course of the left recurrent laryngeal nerve, which arches around the aorta and may be commonly involved in inflammatory and neoplastic conditions involving the left hilum. Lung cancer is the most common cancer in many parts of the world, and should be considered the cause of a left vocal palsy until proved otherwise.

Other malignant lesions can cause a similar effect and may arise in the nasopharynx, thyroid gland or oesophagus. Bilateral vocal fold paralysis is uncommon and tends to occur after thyroid surgery or head injuries (Summary box 48.14).

> **Summary box 48.14**
>
> **Causes of vocal fold palsy**
>
> Congenital (infants)
>
> Acquired
>
> - Traumatic
>   - Direct to neck
>   - Post-surgical, e.g. thyroidectomy
> - Infective
>   - Viral (rare)
> - Neoplastic
>   - Carcinoma of the lung involving the left hilum
>   - Carcinoma of the larynx
>   - Carcinoma of the thyroid
>   - Carcinoma of the oesophagus
> - Vascular
>   - Aortic aneurysm
> - Neurological
>   - Lower motor neurone disease

Clinical features

Unilateral recurrent laryngeal nerve palsy of sudden onset produces hoarseness, difficulty in swallowing liquids and a weakened cough. These symptoms may be short-lived and the voice may return to normal within a few weeks as the muscles in the opposite vocal fold compensate and move it across the midline to meet the paralysed vocal fold, which usually lies in the paramedian position. Bilateral recurrent laryngeal nerve palsy is an occasional and serious complication of thyroidectomy. Acute

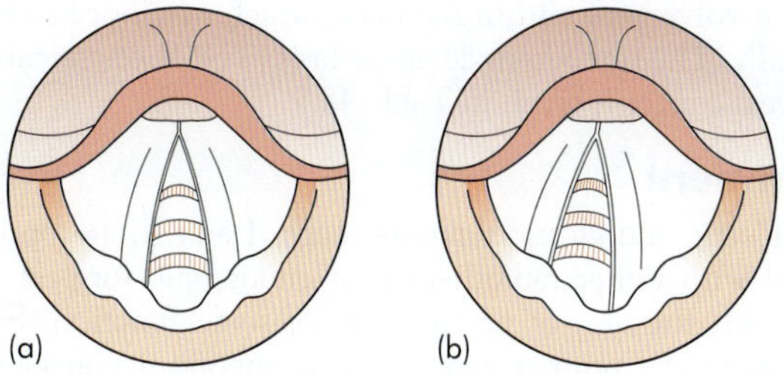

Figure 48.48 Vocal fold positions. (a) Normal; (b) unilateral vocal fold palsy.

dyspnoea occurs as a result of the paramedian position of both vocal folds, which reduce the airway to 2–3 mm and which tend to get sucked together on inspiration. In severe cases, tracheostomy or intubation is necessary immediately, otherwise death occurs from asphyxia.

Investigation of vocal fold paralysis is by a CT scan from skull base (including posterior fossa) to diaphragm. Approximately 20–25 per cent of vocal fold paralysis occurs without known pathology and spontaneous recovery may occur. When compensation does not occur, a unilateral paralysed fold may be medialised by a small external operation on the thyroid cartilage (thyroplasty).

In bilateral vocal fold palsy, surgery may be carried out to remove a small portion of the posterior aspect of one vocal fold or a portion of one arytenoid cartilage. These procedures are most easily performed endoscopically with a carbon dioxide laser. They increase the size of the posterior glottic airway, allowing the patient to be decannulated or even the avoidance of an initial tracheostomy.

TUMOURS OF THE LARYNX

Benign tumours of the larynx are extremely rare. Squamous carcinoma is the most common malignant tumour, being responsible for more than 90 per cent of tumours within the larynx. It is the most common head and neck cancer and previously almost always occurred in elderly male smokers. However, over the past two decades, the incidence among women is rising as a consequence of increased smoking habits. The incidence of laryngeal cancer in the three compartments, supraglottis, glottis and subglottis, varies around the world. The glottis is generally the most common site for cancer in patients in the UK, followed by the supraglottis (Figure 48.49).

Clinical features

Patients almost always present with voice change. If an early diagnosis can be made, i.e. confined to one vocal fold, treatment with radiotherapy or carbon dioxide laser excision is associated with a five-year disease-free survival of approximately 90 per cent. This rate drops dramatically once the lymphatically rich supraglottis or subglottis is involved because of spread to neck nodes. Tumour spread to just one neck gland halves the overall prognosis for the patient.

Investigations

Direct laryngoscopy, preferably a microlaryngoscopy, together with Hopkins' rod examination, allows precise determination of the extent of the tumour and biopsy confirms the histology. CT and MRI give further details of the extent of larger tumours, demonstrating spread outside the larynx and suspicious nodal involvement within the neck, which may not be obvious clinically. The tumour–node–metastasis (TNM) classification of laryngeal cancer is given in Table 48.3.

Treatment

Supraglottic and glottic tumours, stages I and II, are optimally treated with either radiotherapy or endoscopic surgical resection, with the aim of preservation of some function. Subsite location of the primary tumour is an important consideration when selecting the appropriate therapy. Transoral laser resection is a popular surgical treatment modality of stage I and II disease.

Table 48.3 Tumour–node–metastasis (TNM) classification of laryngeal carcinoma.

T – primary tumour

- TX Primary tumour cannot be assessed
- T0 No evidence of primary tumour
- Tis Carcinoma *in situ*
- Supraglottis
  - T1 Tumour limited to one subsite of supraglottis, with normal vocal fold mobility
  - T2 Tumour invades more than one subsite of supraglottis, with normal vocal fold mobility
  - T3 Tumour limited to larynx with vocal fold fixation and/or invades postcricoid area, medial wall of piriform sinus or pre-epiglottic tissues
  - T4 Tumour invades through cartilage and/or extends to other tissues beyond the larynx, e.g. to oropharynx, soft tissues of neck
- Glottis
  - T1 Tumour limited to vocal fold(s) (may involve anterior or posterior commissures) with normal mobility
  - T1a Tumour limited to one vocal fold
  - T1b Tumour involves both vocal folds
  - T2 Tumour extends to supraglottis and/or subglottis, and/or with impaired vocal fold mobility
  - T3 Tumour limited to the larynx with vocal fold fixation
  - T4 Tumour invades through thyroid cartilage and/or extends to other tissues beyond the larynx, e.g. to oropharynx, soft tissues of the neck
- Subglottis
  - T1 Tumour limited to the subglottis
  - T2 Tumour extends to vocal fold(s) with normal or impaired mobility
  - T3 Tumour limited to the larynx with vocal fixation
  - T4 Tumour invades through thyroid cartilage and/or extends to other tissues beyond the larynx, e.g. to oropharynx, soft tissues of the neck

N – regional lymph nodes

- N0 No regional lymph node metastases
- N1 Metastasis in a single ipsilateral lymph node 3 cm or less in greatest diameter
- N2 Metastasis in a single ipsilateral lymph node more than 3 cm or in multiple ipsilateral nodes or in bilateral or contralateral nodes

M – distant metastasis

Stage grouping

0	Tis	N0	M0
I	T1	N0	M0
II	T2	N0	M0
III	T1	N1	M0
	T2	N1	M0
	T3	N0, N1	M0
IV	T4	N0, N1	M0
	Any T	N2, N3	M0
	Any T	Any N	M1

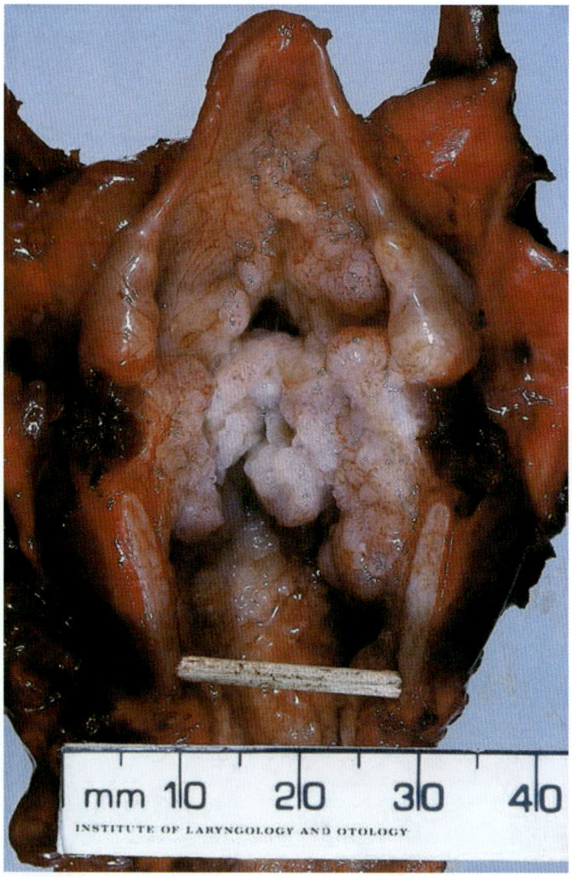

Figure 48.49 A total laryngectomy specimen with transglottic tumour.

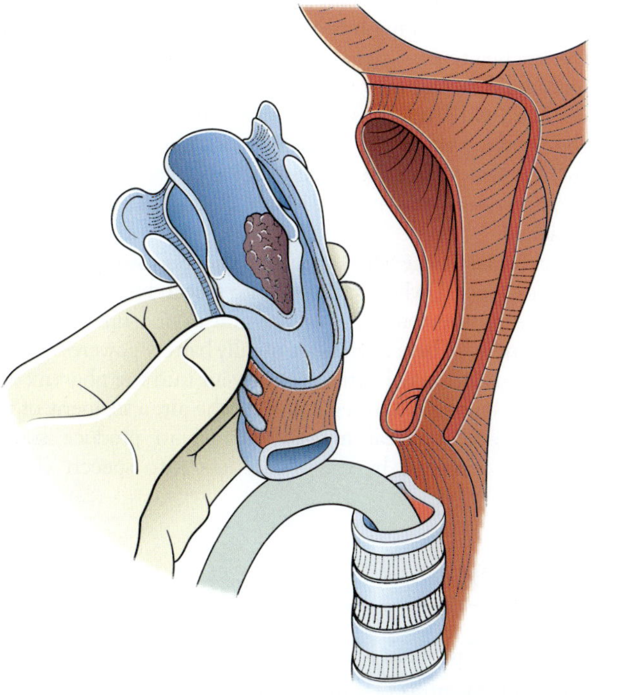

Figure 48.50 Larynx removal at laryngectomy with resultant pharyngeal defect.

A functional cricoarytenoid must be left intact. Both modalities are associated with similar survival rates. Chemotherapy is generally reserved for those patients with lymph node disease. Complications of organ-sparing treatment include aspiration, which if severe may require salvage laryngectomy.

Advanced laryngeal disease

Advanced stage laryngeal carcinomas (stage III) may be treated with radiotherapy for organ preservation or external partial laryngectomy. Stage IV disease is usually treated with total laryngectomy and adjuvant postoperative radiotherapy. In advanced stage disease chemotherapy is usually employed due to cervical lymph node spread.

After the larynx has been removed (Figure 48.50), the remaining trachea is brought out onto the lower neck as a permanent tracheal stoma and the hypopharynx, which is opened at the time of the operation, is closed to restore continuity for swallowing (Figure 48.51). Thus the upper aero- and digestive tracts are permanently disconnected. Part or all of the thyroid gland and associated parathyroid glands may also be removed, depending on the extent of the disease.

Vocal rehabilitation

The loss of the larynx as a generator of sound does not prevent patients speaking as long as an alternative source of vibration can be created in the pharynx. This can be achieved in one of three ways:

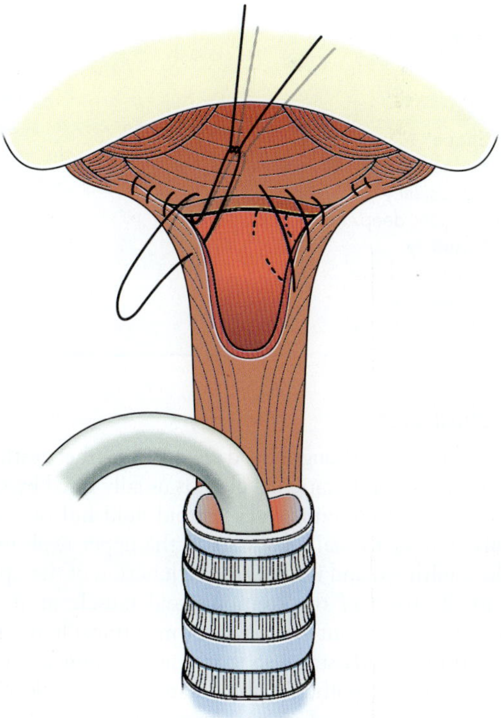

Figure 48.51 Transverse closure of the pharynx with an endotracheal tube in the end tracheostome.

1 A small one-way valve may be inserted through the back wall of the tracheal stoma into the pharynx. This allows air from the trachea to pass into the pharynx, but does not allow food and liquid to pass into the airway. These valves must not be confused with tracheostomy tubes. Like all foreign bodies, the speaking valves are associated with minor complications, such as the formation of granulations, bleeding or leakage of pharyngeal contents, and have continuing financial cost attached.
2 An external device when applied to the soft tissues of the neck produces sound, which is turned into speech by the vocal tract comprising the tongue, pharynx, oral cavity, lips, teeth and nasal sinuses. These devices are usually battery powered.
3 Some patients may learn to swallow air into the pharynx and upper oesophagus. On regurgitating the air, a segment of the pharyngo-oesophageal mucosa vibrates to produce sound, which is modified by the vocal tract into speech (Figure 48.52).

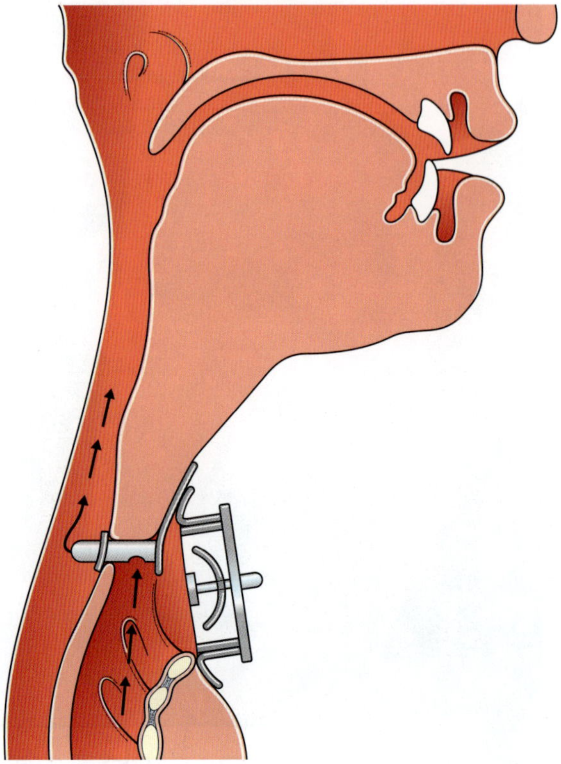

Figure 48.52 A Blom–Singer valve with a tracheo-oesophageal fistula.

THE NECK

Lump in the neck

The correct diagnosis of a lump in the neck can often be made with a careful history and examination. The clinical signs of size, site, shape, consistency, fixation to skin or deep structures, pulsation, compressibility, transillumination or the presence of a bruit still remain as important as ever (Summary box 48.15).

Summary box 48.15

Diagnosis of a lump in the neck

History
Physical signs
- Size
- Site
- Shape
- Surface
- Consistency
- Fixation: deep/superficial
- Pulsatility
- Compressibility
- Transillumination
- Bruit

Branchial cyst

A branchial cyst, thought to develop from the vestigial remnants of the second branchial cleft, is usually lined by squamous epithelium, and contains thick, turbid fluid full of cholesterol crystals. The cyst usually presents in the upper neck in early or middle adulthood and is found at the junction of the upper third and middle third of the sternomastoid muscle at its anterior border. It is a fluctuant swelling that may transilluminate and is often soft in its early stages so that it may be difficult to palpate. Other theories hypothesise that branchial cysts develop from cystic transformation of cervical lymph nodes.

If the cyst becomes infected, it becomes erythematous and tender and, on occasions, it may be difficult to differentiate from a tuberculous abscess. Ultrasound and fine-needle aspiration both aid diagnosis, and treatment is by complete excision, which is best undertaken when the lesion is quiescent. Although the anterior aspect of the cyst is easy to dissect, it may pass backwards and upwards through the bifurcation of the common carotid artery as far as the pharyngeal constrictors. It passes superficial to the hypoglossal and glossopharyngeal nerves, but deep to the posterior belly of the digastric. These structures and the spinal accessory nerve must be positively identified to avoid damage.

Branchial fistula

A branchial fistula may be unilateral or bilateral and is thought to represent a persistent second branchial cleft. The external orifice is nearly always situated in the lower third of the neck near the anterior border of the sternocleidomastoid, while the internal orifice is located on the anterior aspect of the posterior faucial pillar just behind the tonsil. However, the internal aspect of the tract may end blindly at or close to the lateral pharyngeal wall, constituting a sinus rather than a fistula. The tract is lined by ciliated columnar epithelium and, as such, there may be a small amount of recurrent mucous or mucopurulent discharge onto the neck. The tract follows the same path as a branchial cyst and requires complete excision, often by more than one transverse incision in the neck (Figure 48.53).

Cystic hygroma

Cystic hygromas usually present in the neonate or in early infancy, and occasionally may present at birth and be so large as to obstruct labour. The cysts are filled with clear lymph and lined by a single layer of epithelium with a mosaic appearance (Figure 48.54). Swelling usually occurs in the neck and may involve the parotid, submandibular, tongue and floor of mouth areas. The swelling may be bilateral and is soft and partially compressible, visibly increasing in size when the child coughs or cries. The characteristic that distinguishes it from all other neck swellings is that it is brilliantly translucent. The cheek, axilla, groin and mediastinum are other less frequent sites for a cystic hygroma.

The behaviour of cystic hygromas during infancy is unpredictable. Sometimes the cyst expands rapidly and occasionally respiratory difficulty ensues, requiring immediate aspiration and even, occasionally, a tracheostomy. The cyst may become infected.

Definitive treatment is complete excision of the cyst at an early stage. Injection of a sclerosing agent, for example picibanil (OK-432), may reduce the size of the cyst; however, they are commonly multicystic and if the injection is extracystic subsequent surgery may be more difficult.

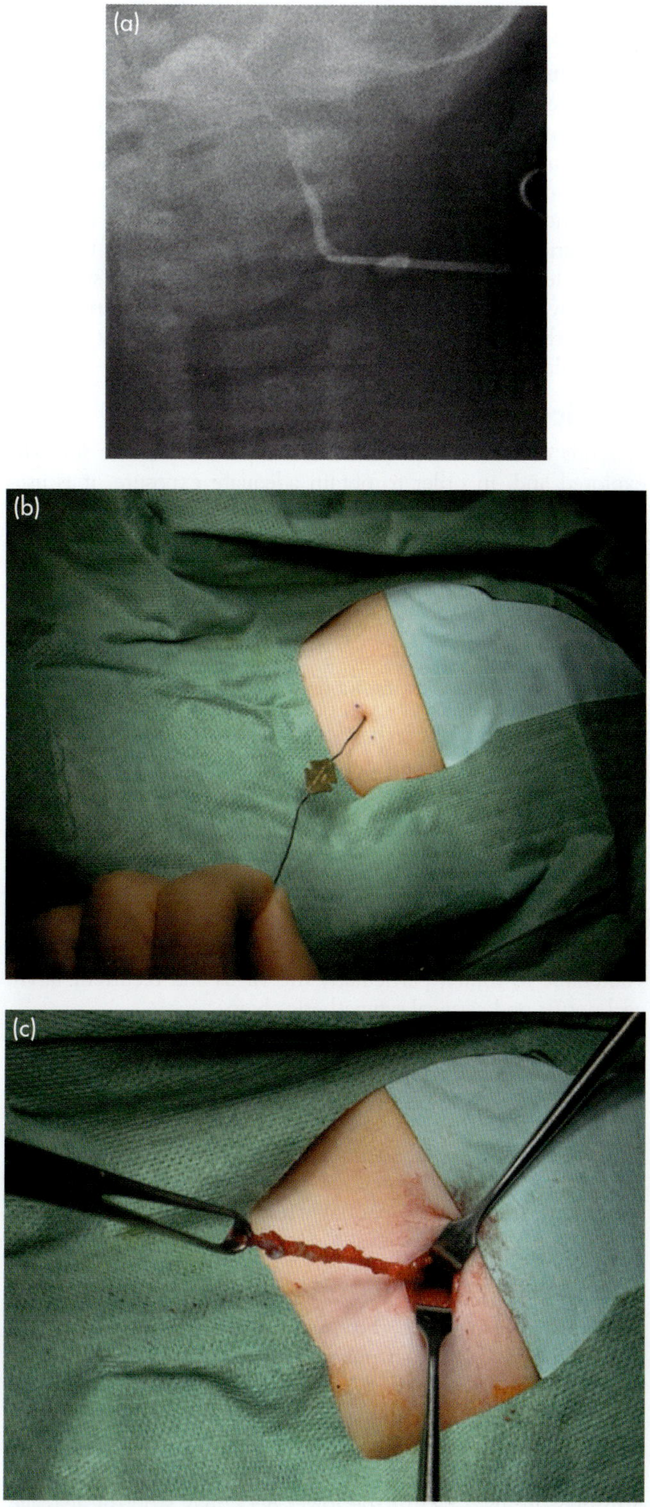

Figure 48.53 (a) Plain radiograph with radio-opaque dye in the fistula tract. (b) Probing of the fistula tract. (c) Excision of the fistula tract.

Thyroglossal duct cysts

Embryology

The thyroid gland descends early in fetal life from the base of the tongue towards its position in the lower neck with the isthmus lying over the second and third tracheal rings. At the time of its descent, the hyoid bone has not been formed and the track of the descent of the thyroid gland is variable, passing in front, through or behind the eventual position of the hyoid body. Thyroglossal duct cysts represent a persistence of this track and may therefore be found anywhere in or adjacent to the midline from the tongue base to the thyroid isthmus. Rarely, a thyroglossal cyst may contain the only functioning thyroid tissue in the body.

Clinical features

The cysts almost always arise in the midline but, when they are adjacent to the thyroid cartilage, they may lie slightly to one side of the midline. Classically, the cyst moves upwards on swallowing and with tongue protrusion, but this can also occur with other midline cysts such as dermoid cysts, as it merely indicates attachment to the hyoid bone.

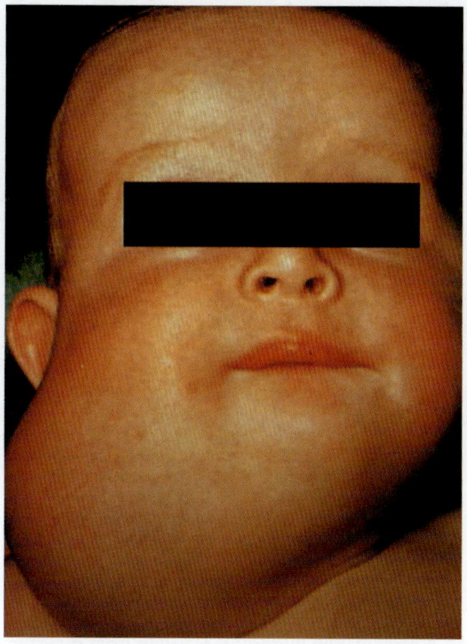

Figure 48.54 Cystic hygroma.

Thyroglossal cysts may become infected and rupture onto the skin of the neck presenting as a discharging sinus. Although they often occur in children, they may also present in adults, even as late as the sixth or seventh decade of life (Figure 48.55).

Treatment

Treatment must include excision of the whole thyroglossal tract, which involves removal of the body of the hyoid bone and the suprahyoid tract through the tongue base to the vallecula at the site of the primitive foramen caecum, together with a core of tissue on either side. This operation is known as Sistrunk's operation and prevents recurrence, most notably from small side branches of the thyroglossal tract.

TRAUMA TO THE NECK

Wounds above the hyoid bone

The cavity of the mouth or pharynx may have been entered and the epiglottis may be divided via the pre-epiglottic space. These wounds require repair with absorbable sutures on a formal basis under a general anaesthetic. If there is any degree of associated oedema or bleeding, particularly in relation to the tongue base or laryngeal inlet, it is advisable to perform a tracheostomy to avoid any subsequent respiratory distress.

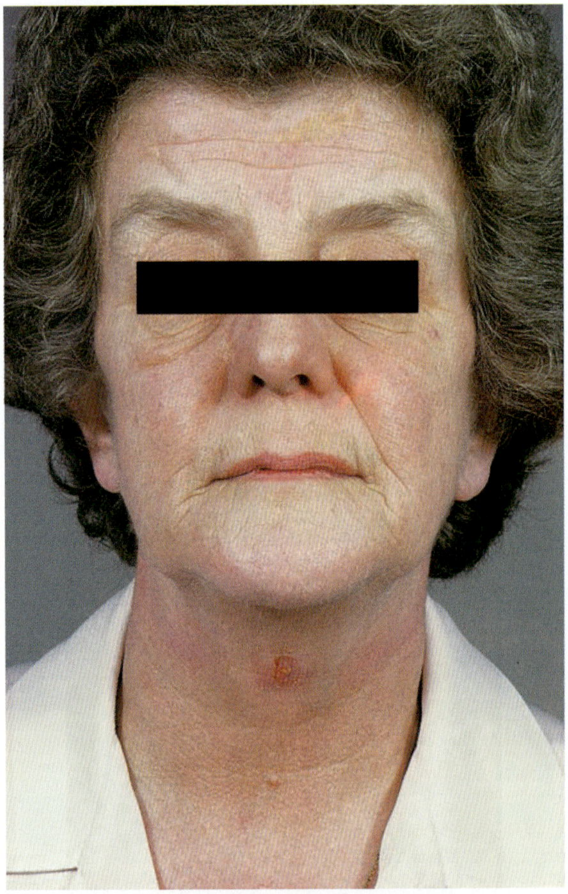

Figure 48.55 A patient with thyroglossal fistula from a cyst in the midline of the neck.

Wounds of the thyroid and cricoid cartilage

Blunt crushing injuries or severe laceration injuries to the laryngeal skeleton can cause marked haematoma formation and rapid loss of the airway. There may be significant disruption of the laryngeal skeleton. These patients should not have an endotracheal intubation for any length of time, even if this is the initial emergency way of protecting the airway. The larynx is a delicate three-tiered sphincter and the presence of a foreign body in its lumen after severe disruption gives rise to major fibrosis and loss of laryngeal function. These injuries are frequently an absolute indication for a low tracheostomy, following which the larynx can be carefully explored, damaged cartilages repositioned and sutured, and the paraglottic space drained.

An indwelling stent of soft sponge shaped to fit the laryngeal lumen and held by a nylon retaining suture through the neck may be left in place for approximately 5 days. This stent can be removed endoscopically after cutting the retaining suture and, as the laryngeal damage heals, the patient may then be decannulated.

Division of the trachea

Wounds of the trachea are rare. They should all be formally explored and, in order to obtain adequate exposure, it is usually necessary to divide and ligate the thyroid isthmus. A small tracheostomy below the wound followed by repair of the trachea with a limited number of submucosal sutures is appropriate. In self-inflicted wounds, the recurrent laryngeal nerves, which lie protected in the tracheo-oesophageal grooves, are rarely injured. Primary repair is rarely possible but may be undertaken at the time of formal exploration of a major neck wound.

Neurovascular injury

Penetrating wounds of the neck may involve the common carotid or the external or internal carotid arteries. Major haemorrhagic shock may occur. Venous air embolism may occur as a result of damage to one of the major veins, most commonly the internal jugular. Compression, resuscitation and exploration under general anaesthetic, with control of vessels above and below the injury, and primary repair should be undertaken. All cervical nerves are vulnerable to injury, particularly the vagus and recurrent laryngeal nerves and cervical sympathetic chain.

Thoracic duct injury

Wounds to the thoracic duct are rare and most often occur in association with dissection of lymph nodes in the left supraclavicular fossa. When damage to the duct is not recognised at the time of operation, chyle may subsequently leak from the wound in amounts up to 2 litres per day with profound effects on nutrition.

Treatment

Should the damage be recognised during an operation, the proximal end of the duct must be ligated. Ligation of the duct is not harmful because there are a number of anastomotic channels between the lymphatic and venous system in the lower neck. If undetected, chyle usually starts to discharge from the neck wound within 24 hours of the operation. On occasion, firm pressure by a pad to the lower neck may stop the leakage, but frequently this is unsuccessful and the wound should be re-explored and the damaged duct ligated.

Walter Ellis Sistrunk Jr, 1880–1933, Professor of Clinical Surgery, Baylor University College of Medicine, Dallas, TX, USA.

Inflammatory conditions of the neck

Ludwig's angina

Ludwig described a clinical entity characterised by a brawny swelling of the submandibular region combined with inflammatory oedema of the mouth. It is these combined cervical and intraoral signs that constitute the characteristic feature of the lesion, as well as the accompanying putrid halitosis.

The infection is often caused by a virulent streptococcal infection associated with anaerobic organisms and sometimes with other lesions of the floor of the mouth, such as carcinoma. The infection encompasses both sides of the mylohyoid muscle causing oedema and inflammation such that the tongue may be displaced upwards and backwards, giving rise to dysphagia and subsequently to painful obstruction of the airway. Unless treated, cellulitis may extend beneath the deep fascial layers of the neck to involve the larynx, causing glottic oedema and airway compromise.

Antibiotic therapy should be instituted as soon as possible using intravenous broad-spectrum antibiotics, with additional anaerobic cover.

In advanced cases when the swelling does not subside rapidly with such treatment, a curved submental incision may be used to drain both submandibular triangles. The mylohyoid muscle may be incised to decompress the floor of the mouth and corrugated drains placed in the wound, which is then lightly sutured. This operation may be conducted under local anaesthetic. Rarely, a tracheostomy may be necessary.

Cervical lymphadenitis

Cervical lymphadenitis is common due to infection or inflammation in the oral and nasal cavities, pharynx, larynx, ear, scalp and face.

Acute lymphadenitis

The affected lymph nodes are enlarged and tender, and there may be varying degrees of general constitutional disturbance such as pyrexia, anorexia and general malaise. The treatment in the first instance is directed to the primary focus of infection, for example tonsillitis or a dental abscess.

Chronic lymphadenitis

Chronic, painless lymphadenopathy may be caused by tuberculosis in young children or adults, or be secondary to malignant disease, most commonly from a squamous carcinoma in older individuals. Lymphoma and/or HIV infection may also present in the cervical nodes (Summary box 48.16).

Summary box 48.16

Causes of cervical lymphadenopathy

Inflammatory
- Reactive hyperplasia

Infective
- Viral
  - For example, infectious mononucleosis, HIV
- Bacterial
  - *Streptococcus, Staphylococcus*
  - Actinomycosis
  - Tuberculosis
  - Brucellosis
- Protozoan
  - Toxoplasmosis

Neoplastic
- Malignant
  - Primary, e.g. lymphoma
  - Secondary, e.g. squamous cell carcinoma
  - Known primary
  - Occult primary

Tuberculous adenitis

The condition most commonly affects children or young adults, but can occur at any age. The deep upper cervical nodes are most commonly affected, but there may be a widespread cervical lymphadenitis with many matting together. In most cases, the tubercular bacilli gain entrance through the tonsil of the corresponding side as the lymphadenopathy. Both bovine and human tuberculosis may be responsible. In approximately 80 per cent of patients, the tuberculous process is limited to the clinically affected group of lymph nodes, but a primary focus in the lungs must always be suspected.

As renal and pulmonary tuberculosis occasionally coexist, the urine should be examined carefully. Rarely, the patient may develop a natural resistance to the infection and the nodes may be detected at a later date as evidenced by calcification on radiography. This can also be seen after appropriate general treatment of tuberculosis adenitis. If treatment is not instituted, the caseated node may liquefy and break down with the formation of a cold abscess in the neck. The pus is initially confined by the deep cervical fascia, but after weeks or months, this may become eroded at one point and the pus flows through the small opening into the space beneath the superficial fascia. The process has now reached the well-known stage of a 'collar-stud' abscess. The superficial abscess enlarges steadily and, unless suitably treated, a discharging sinus results.

Investigation

Fine-needle aspirate taken from neck nodes with a suspicion of tuberculosis should be tested for the presence of acid-fast bacilli. Systemic investigation should not be neglected, with chest x-ray and Mantoux testing useful first-line investigations. Depending on the country of origin, where tuberculosis is diagnosed or suspected, the coexistence of other infectious diseases, such as HIV and malaria, should not be overlooked.

Treatment

The patient should be treated by appropriate chemotherapy, dependent on the sensitivities derived from the abscess contents. If an abscess fails to resolve despite appropriate chemotherapy and general measures, occasionally excision of the abscess and its surrounding fibrous capsule is necessary, together with the relevant lymph nodes. If there is active tuberculosis of another system, for example pulmonary tuberculosis, then removal of tuberculous lymph nodes in the neck is inappropriate. The nodes are commonly related to the internal jugular vein, common carotid and vagus nerve, and are usually associated with significant fibrosis making surgery difficult. A portion of the internal jugular vein may require excision, taking considerable care to avoid damage to the vagus or the cervical sympathetic trunk. To facilitate access, the sternocleidomastoid muscle

Wilhelm Friedrich von Ludwig, 1790–1865, Professor of Surgery and Midwifery, Tubingen, Germany.

For 600 years, the king's touch was believed to cure tuberculous adenitis. Charles II touched on an average 10 000 sufferers a year. In addition, he presented each with half a soverign.

should be divided, particularly if the disease is adjacent to the spinal accessory nerve or the hypoglossal nerve. The resected nodes should be sent for both histology and microbiology.

PRIMARY TUMOURS OF THE NECK

Neurogenic tumours

Chemodectoma (carotid body tumour)

This is a rare tumour that has a higher incidence in areas where people live at high altitudes because of chronic hypoxia leading to carotid body hyperplasia. The tumours most commonly present in the fifth decade and approximately 10 per cent of patients have a family history. There is an association with phaeochromocytoma. The tumours arise from the chemoreceptor cells on the medial side of the carotid bulb and, at this point, the tumour is adherent to the carotid wall. The cells of the chemodectoma are not hormonally active and the tumours are usually benign with only a small number of cases producing proven metastases.

Clinical features

There is often a long history of a slowly enlarging, painless lump at the carotid bifurcation. About one-third of patients present with a pharyngeal mass that pushes the tonsil medially and anteriorly. The mass is firm, rubbery, pulsatile, mobile from side to side but not up and down, and can sometimes be emptied by firm pressure, after which it slowly refills in a pulsatile manner. A bruit may also be present. Swellings in the parapharyngeal space, which often displace the tonsil medially, should not be biopsied from within the mouth.

Investigations

When a chemodectoma is suspected, a carotid angiogram can be carried out to demonstrate the carotid bifurcation, which is usually splayed, and a blush, which outlines the tumour vessels. MRI scanning also provides excellent detail in most cases. This tumour must not be biopsied and fine-needle aspiration is also contraindicated.

Treatment

Because these tumours rarely metastasise and their overall rate of growth is slow, the need for surgical removal must be considered carefully as complications of surgery are potentially serious. The operation is best avoided in elderly patients. Radiotherapy has no effect. In some cases, it may be possible to dissect the tumour away from the carotid bifurcation but, at times, when the tumour is large, it may not be separable from the vessels and resection will be necessary, such that all appropriate facilities should be available to establish a bypass while a vein graft is inserted to restore arterial continuity in the carotid system.

Vagal body tumours

Vagal paragangliomas arise from nests of paraganglionic tissue of the vagus nerve just below the base of the skull near the jugular foramen. They may also be found at various sites along the nerve down to the level of the carotid artery bifurcation (Figure 48.56).

They also present as slowly growing and painless masses in the anterolateral aspect of the neck, and may also have a long history, commonly of 2–3 years, before diagnosis. They may spread into the cranial cavity. Diagnosis is confirmed by CT and MRI scanning and additional MR angiogram or arteriography if necessary. Treatment is surgical excision.

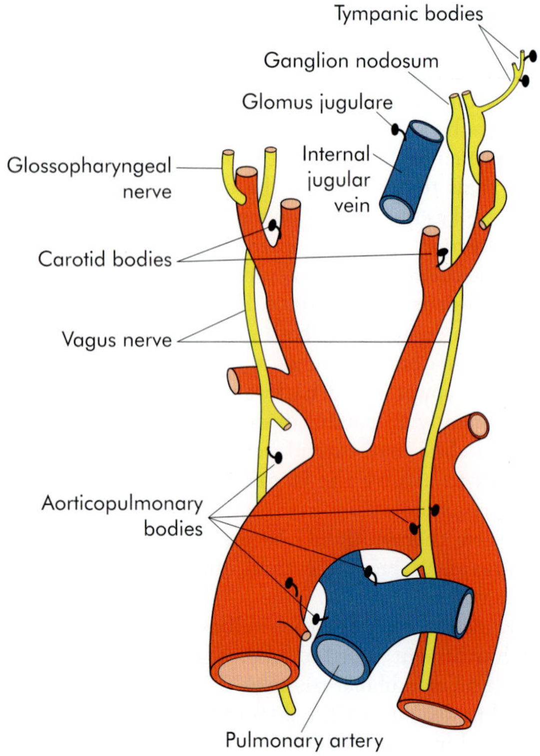

Figure 48.56 Sites for neurogenic tumours (paraganglionomas) in the neck.

Peripheral nerve tumours

Schwannomas are solitary and encapsulated tumours attached to or surrounded by nerve, although paralysis of the associated nerve is unusual. The vagus nerve is the most common site. Neurofibromas also arise from the Schwann cell and may be part of von Recklinghausen's syndrome of multiple neurofibromatosis. Multiple neurofibromatosis is an autosomal dominant, hereditary disease and the neurofibromata may be present at birth and often multiply.

Diagnosis requires CT or MRI scanning to differentiate them from other parapharyngeal tumours but, on occasions, the diagnosis must wait until excision.

Secondary carcinoma

Metastatic spread of squamous carcinoma to the cervical lymph nodes is a common occurrence from head and neck primary cancers. The nasopharynx, tonsil, tongue, pyriform fossa and supraglottic larynx must be carefully examined by panendoscopy for the primary growth before considering biopsy or any surgery on the neck. Investigation is further assisted by ultrasound and fine-needle aspirate of the neck node.

Management

The management of malignant cervical lymph nodes depends on the overall treatment regime:

Friedrich Daniel von Recklinghausen, 1833–1910, Professor of Pathology, Strasbourg, France, is credited with the description of generalized neurofibromatosis in 1882, although it was orgianally described by Robert Smith (1807–1873), Professor of Surgery, Trinity College Dublin in 1849.

- If surgery is being used to treat the primary disease and the cervical nodes are palpable and >3 cm, they may be excised with the primary lesion.
- If radiotherapy is used initially, as is always the case in carcinoma of the nasopharynx, then radiotherapy may also be given to the neck nodes, whatever their stage. In the case of the tongue, pharynx or larynx, however, if the node exceeds 3 cm in diameter, then surgery may be necessary for the neck nodes, even if the primary tumour is treated by chemoradiation.
- If radiotherapy is used initially with resolution of the primary tumour, but there is subsequent residual or recurrent nodal disease, then this situation will require cervical lymph node dissection.

Type of neck dissection

Classical radical neck dissection (Crile)

The classic operation involves resection of the cervical lymphatics and lymph nodes and those structures closely associated: the internal jugular vein, the accessory nerve, the submandibular gland and the sternocleidomastoid muscle. These structures are all removed *en bloc* and in continuity with the primary disease if possible. The main disability that follows the operation is weakness and drooping of the shoulder due to paralysis of the trapezius muscle as a consequence of excision of the accessory nerve.

Modified radical neck dissection

In selected cases, one or more of the three following structures are preserved: the accessory nerve, the sternocleidomastoid muscle or the internal jugular vein. Otherwise, all major lymph node groups and lymphatics are excised. Whichever structures are preserved should be clearly noted.

> **George Washington Crile**, 1864–1943, Professor of Surgery, Western Reserve University and one of the founders in 1921 of The Cleveland Clinic, Cleveland, OH, USA. He devised the small haemostatic forceps that goes by his name.

Selective neck dissection

In this type of dissection, one or more of the major lymph node groups is preserved along with the sternocleidomastoid muscle, accessory nerve and internal jugular vein. In these circumstances, the exact groups of nodes excised must be documented.

SUMMARY

The anatomical and physiological performance of the pharyngolarynx is involved in the important mechanisms of breathing, coughing, voice production and swallowing. A variety of congenital, traumatic, infectious and neoplastic conditions disturb these functions, giving rise to the common symptoms of pain, swelling, hoarseness, dyspnoea and dysphagia.

Squamous carcinomas are the most common malignancies, accounting for approximately 80 per cent of all head and neck tumours. Their incidence and anatomical site vary around the world, but they are mainly caused by the preventable aetiological agents of smoking and alcohol, although nasopharyngeal squamous carcinomas have additional genetic and environmental factors. These head and neck cancers have a high morbidity and mortality, and require expert treatment.

FURTHER READING

British Association of Otorhinolaryngology Head and Neck Surgery. *Head and neck cancer: Multidisciplinary management guidelines*, 4th edn. London: Royal College of Surgeons of England, 2011.

Bull P, Clarke R. *Diseases of the ear, nose and throat.* Oxford: Blackwell, 2007.

Dhillon R, East C. *Nose and throat, head and neck surgery*. Amsterdam: Elsevier, 2006.

Hibbert J (ed.). *Scott Brown's otolaryngology: Laryngology and head and neck surgery*, 6th edn. Oxford: Butterworth-Heinemann, 1997.

Lund VJ, Howard DJ. Ear, nose and throat emergencies, part II. In: Skinner DV, Swain A, Robertson C, Rodney Peyton JW (eds). *Cambridge textbook of accident and emergency medicine*. Cambridge: Cambridge University Press, 1997.

Probst R, Grevers G, Iro H. *Basic otorhinolaryngology*. Stuttgart: Georg Thieme, 2006.

Snow JB (ed.). *Ballenger's handbook of otorhinolaryngology, head and neck surgery*, 17th edn. Hamilton, ON: BC Decker, 2007.

Wei W, Sham J. *Cancer of the larynx and hypopharynx*. Oxford: Isis Medical Media, 2000.

CHAPTER

49 Oropharyngeal cancer

LEARNING OBJECTIVES

To understand:

- The relationship between oral cancers and the use of alcohol and tobacco
- The cardinal features of oropharyngeal cancer
- The investigation and treatment of patients with oropharyngeal cancer

INTRODUCTION AND EPIDEMIOLOGY

In the Western world, oral/oropharyngeal cancer is uncommon, accounting for only 2–4 per cent of all malignant tumours, although there is increasing evidence that the incidence is on the increase, particularly among young people. In the Indian subcontinent, however, oropharyngeal cancer remains the most common malignant tumour, accounting for 40 per cent of all cancers.

Epidemiology

The principal aetiological agents are tobacco and alcohol. In Europe and North America, this is mainly through cigarette smoking combined with alcohol abuse. Synergism between alcohol abuse and tobacco use in the development of squamous cell carcinoma (SCC) of the head and neck is well established, although evidence is gathering that the human papillomavirus (HPV16) is becoming increasingly responsible for tumours that arise particularly in the oropharynx of younger/middle-aged patients. Risk factors associated with cancer of the head and neck are outlined in Summary box 49.1.

Summary box 49.1

Risk factors associated with cancer of the head and neck

- Tobacco
- Alcohol
- Areca nut/pan masala
- Human papillomavirus
- Epstein–Barr virus
- Plummer–Vinson syndrome
- Poor nutrition

In the Indian subcontinent, the use of 'pan' (a combination of betel nut, areca nut, lime and tobacco) as well as reverse smoking (smoking a cheroot with the burning end inside the mouth) are responsible for the high incidence of oropharyngeal cancer. Betel quid appears to be the major carcinogen, although there is also a relationship between slaked lime and the areca nut and cancer.

INCIDENCE

The incidence is greater in men than in women and it is predominantly a disease of the elderly (those over 60 years of age). The incidence in women is increasing, particularly in younger patients, with oral tongue cancer being the cancer that is usually, but not exclusively, present.

ANATOMY

Lip and oral cavity

The oral cavity extends from the skin–vermilion border of the lips anteriorly to the junction of the soft palate superiorly and the line of the circumvallate papillae on the junction of the posterior one-third and anterior two-thirds of the tongue posteriorly. The anatomical sites that are frequently involved in mouth cancer include the floor of the mouth, the lateral border of the anterior tongue and the retromolar trigone (Figure 49.1). The retromolar trigone is defined as the attached mucosa overlying the ascending ramus of the mandible posterior to the last molar tooth and extending superiorly to the maxillary tuberosity.

Oropharynx

The oropharynx extends vertically from the oral surface of the soft palate to the superior surface of the hyoid bone (floor of vallecula). This includes the base of the tongue, the soft palate and the anterior and posterior tonsillar pillars, as well as the pharyngeal tonsils and the lateral and posterior pharyngeal walls. The

In India, habitual chewing of the rolled betel leaf with betel nut inside it with concentrated lime and storing the quid over long periods inside the cheek results in a high incidence of cancer of the cheek. Another routine habit among southern Indian rural dwellers is to roll the tobacco leaf and then smoke by putting the lighted end into the oral cavity; this almost always results in cancer of the palate or some other part of the oral cavity.

Henry Stanley Plummer, 1874–1937, physician, The Mayo Clinic, Rochester, MN, USA, described this syndrome in 1912.
Porter Paisley Vinson, 1890–1959, physician, The Mayo Clinic, Rochester, MN, who later practised in Richmond, VA, USA.

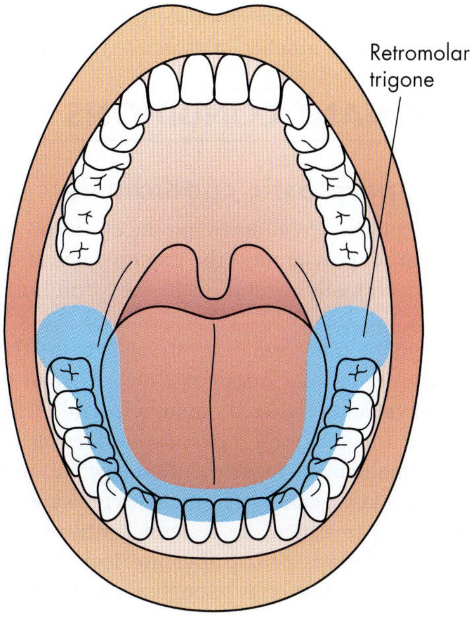

Figure 49.1 Common anatomical sites (blue) for oral squamous cell carcinoma.

lateral boundaries include the pharyngeal constrictor muscles and the medial aspect of the mandible.

PATHOLOGY

The anatomy of the oral cavity and the oropharynx is complex and the course of the nerves, blood vessels, lymphatic pathways and fascial planes influences the spread of disease. Fascial planes, including the periosteum, serve as barriers to the direct spread of tumours but contribute to the spread of tumours into the cervical lymph nodes. Perineural invasion acts as a conduit for the direct spread of tumours and profoundly impacts on prognosis and survival. Angioinvasion also carries a negative prognosis and correlates directly with distant metastases, particularly of oral tongue cancer.

Histology

Squamous cell carcinoma is the predominant histology for tumours arising in the oral cavity and oropharynx. Tumours mainly arise from the mucosal epithelium, although malignant salivary gland tumours from the minor salivary glands are a rare but important group of lesions. Lymphomas, particularly around Waldeyer's ring (tonsils, tongue base, lingual tonsil regions, posterior one-third of the tongue (see Figure 48.2, p. 674)), make up the last of the three principal pathological groups of oropharyngeal cancer.

Chronic exposure of the mucosal surface to carcinogenic substances, i.e. tobacco and alcohol, can produce multiple subclinical sites of carcinoma that can at any stage develop into malignant tumour. This pathological process supports the preventative measures of smoking cessation and alcohol rehabilitation in patients with head and neck cancer, thereby minimising the occurrence of synchronous and metachronous tumours (see below under Field changes and second primary tumours).

Premalignant lesions

The majority of oral carcinomas are not preceded by or associated with clinically obvious premalignant lesions. There is, however, a group of oral pathological conditions in which an association with malignant transformation exists (Summary box 49.2).

Summary box 49.2

Conditions associated with malignant transformation

High-risk lesions
- Erythroplakia
- Speckled erythroplakia
- Chronic hyperplastic candidiasis

Medium-risk lesions
- Oral submucous fibrosis
- Syphilitic glossitis
- Sideropenic dysphagia (Paterson–Kelly syndrome)

Low-risk/equivocal-risk lesions
- Oral lichen planus
- Discoid lupus erythematosus
- Discoid keratosis congenita

Clinical features

Premalignant lesions of the oral mucosa and oropharyngeal mucosa present as either:

- leukoplakia
- speckled leukoplakia
- erythroplakia/plasia.

Leukoplakia

Leukoplakia is defined as any white patch or plaque that cannot be characterised clinically or pathologically. It is purely a descriptive term with no histological correlation. Leukoplakia varies from a small, well-circumscribed, homogenous white plaque to an extensive lesion involving large surface areas of the oral mucosa. It may be smooth or wrinkled, fissured and vary in colour depending on the thickness of the lesion.

Speckled leukoplakia

This is a variation of leukoplakia arising on an erythematous base (Figure 49.2). It has the highest rate of malignant transformation.

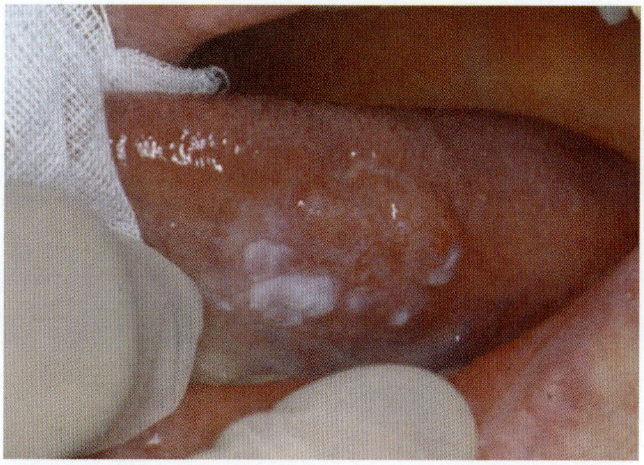

Figure 49.2 Speckled leukoplakia on the lateral border of the tongue. Histology confirms carcinoma *in situ*.

Heinrich Wilhelm Gottfried Waldeyer-Hartz, 1836–1921, Professor of Pathological Anatomy, Berlin, Germany.
Donald Rose Paterson, 1863–1939, surgeon, Ear, Nose and Throat Department, The Royal Infirmary, Cardiff, Wales.
Adam Brown Kelly, 1865–1941, surgeon, Ear, Nose and Throat Department, The Royal Victoria Infirmary, Glasgow, Scotland.

Erythroplakia

Erythroplakia is defined as any lesion of the oral mucosa that presents as a bright red plaque which cannot be characterised clinically or pathologically as any other recognisable condition. The lesions are irregular in outline and separated from adjacent normal mucosa (Figure 49.3). The surfaces may be nodular. These lesions occasionally coexist with leukoplakia.

FIELD CHANGE AND SECOND PRIMARY TUMOURS

The diffuse and chronic exposure of the mucosa of the upper aerodigestive tract to carcinogenic substances, e.g. tobacco and alcohol, causes widespread adverse changes in the mucosal epithelium. The consequence of the diffuse exposure is the development of separate tumours at different anatomical sites. These may present simultaneously, within six months (synchronous) or may be delayed (metachronous). Slaughter, in 1950, first proposed the concept of field change or 'cancerisation'. Separate primary tumours may not represent distinct genetic mutational events but rather the same clonal origin of cells, which migrate to separate sites in the upper aerodigestive tract. Nevertheless, minimising exposure of the oropharyngeal tissues to potential insults is the cornerstone of long-term management for patients with head and neck cancer.

Patients who develop a first tumour in the oral cavity and the oropharynx are more likely to develop a second primary tumour in the upper oesophagus. The overall rate of second primary tumour development is 15 per cent. In total, 80 per cent of these are metachronous tumours, of which 50 per cent develop within the first two years of initial presentation (Figure 49.4). The prevalence of synchronous second primary tumours is 4 per cent.

Potential for malignant change

The potential risk for malignant transformation:

- increases with increasing age of the patient;
- increases with increasing age of the lesion;
- is higher in smokers;
- increases with alcohol consumption;
- depends on the anatomical site of the premalignant lesion;
- is particularly high for leukoplakia on the floor of the mouth

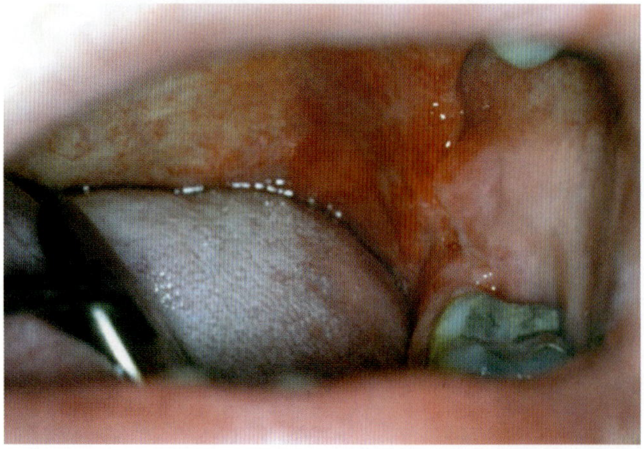

Figure 49.3 Erythroplakia of the left soft palate and lateral pharyngeal wall.

and ventral surface of the tongue, particularly in younger women, even in the absence of associated risk factors.

PREMALIGNANT CONDITIONS

Chronic hyperplastic candidiasis

Chronic hyperplastic candidiasis produces dense plaques of leukoplakia, particularly around the commissures of the mouth. The lesions occasionally extend on to the vermilion and even the facial skin (Figure 49.5). These lesions have a high incidence of malignant transformation, thought to be the result of invasion of the lesion by *Candida albicans*. A small percentage of patients have an associated immunological defect, which encourages the invasion of *C. albicans*, rendering the patient susceptible to malignant transformation. Specific management of chronic hyperplastic candidiasis includes prolonged (6 weeks) topical antifungal treatment or systemic antifungal treatment (2 weeks). If the lesions persist after medical therapy, surgical excision or laser vaporisation is strongly recommended.

Oral submucous fibrosis

Oral submucous fibrosis is a progressive disease in which fibrous bands form beneath the oral mucosa. Scarring produces con-

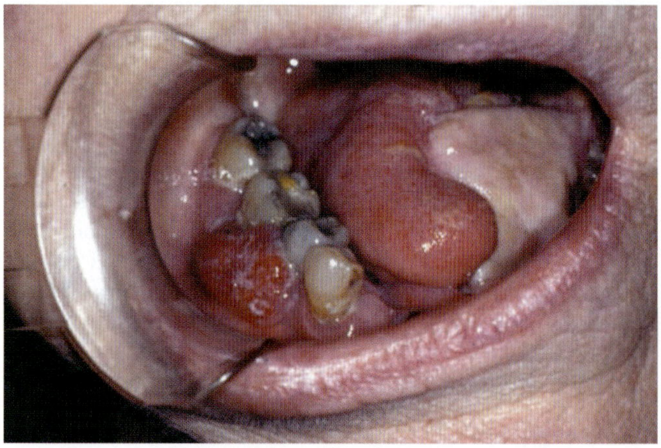

Figure 49.4 Metachronous tumour in the right mandibular alveolus after previous partial glossectomy and forearm flap reconstruction.

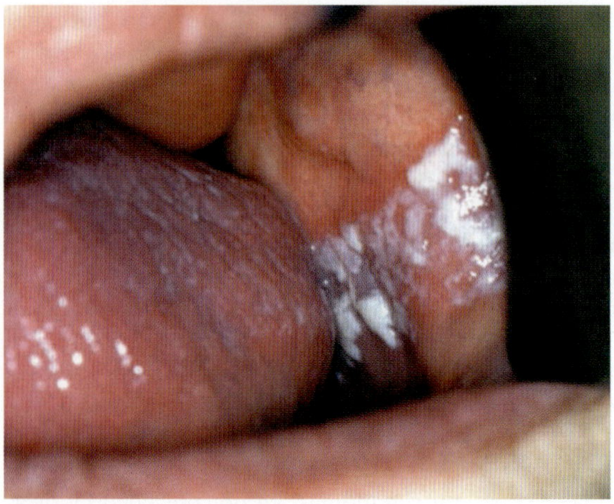

Figure 49.5 Chronic hyperplastic candidiasis of the left buccal mucosa.

tracture, resulting in limited mouth opening and restricted tongue movement. The condition is almost entirely confined to the Asian population and is characterised pathologically by epithelial fibrosis with associated atrophy and hyperplasia of the overlying epithelium (Figure 49.6). The epithelium also shows changes of epithelial dysplasia. Restricted mouth opening can be treated with either intralesional steroids or surgical excision and skin grafts.

Research strongly indicates that oral submucous fibrosis is significantly associated with the use of pan masala areca nut, with or without concurrent alcohol use. Tobacco smoking alone is not associated with oral submucous fibrosis.

Sideropenic dysphagia (Plummer–Vincent and Paterson–Kelly syndromes)

There is a well-known relationship between sideropenia (iron deficiency in the absence of anaemia) and the development of oral cancer. Sideropenia is common in Scandinavian women and leads to epithelial atrophy, which renders the oral mucosa vulnerable to irritation from topical carcinogens. Correction of the sideropenia with iron supplements reduces the epithelial atrophy and risk of malignant transformation.

CLASSIFICATION AND STAGING

TNM staging

Staging of head and neck cancer is defined by the American Joint Committee on Cancer (AJCC) and follows the TNM system. The system also takes into account the pretreatment computed tomography (CT) or magnetic resonance imaging (MRI) of the tumour. The T classification indicates the extent of the primary tumour and the N classification relates to the extent of regional neck metastases to the cervical lymph nodes; this is identical for all mucosal sites of the head and neck except for the nasopharynx. The M classification relates to distant metastasis. The risk of distant metastasis is dependent on nodal disease rather than the size of the primary tumour. Tumours close to the midline are at a greater risk of developing bilateral or contralateral cervical node metastasis.

The TNM staging system is outlined in Table 49.1.

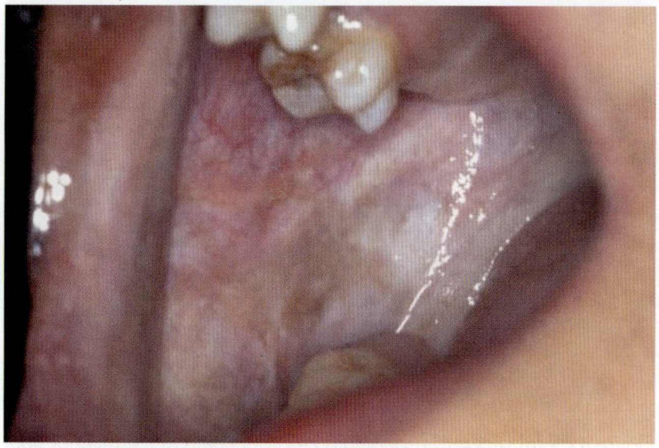

Figure 49.6 Oral submucous fibrosis of the right buccal mucosa and soft palate.

Table 49.1 The TNM staging system.

Primary tumour (T)

TX	Primary tumour cannot be assessed
T0	No evidence of primary tumour
Tis	Carcinoma *in situ*
T1	Tumour <2 cm in greatest dimension
T2	Tumour >2 but <4 cm
T3	Tumour >4 cm but <6 cm
T4	Tumour invades adjacent structures, e.g. mandible, skin

Regional lymph nodes (N)

NX	Regional lymph nodes cannot be assessed
N0	No regional lymph node metastasis
N1	Metastasis in a single ipsilateral lymph node <3 cm in greatest dimension
N2a	Metastasis in a single ipsilateral lymph node >3 cm but not more than 6 cm
N2b	Metastasis in multiple ipsilateral lymph nodes, none >6 cm in greatest dimension
N2c	Metastasis in bilateral or contralateral lymph nodes, none >6 cm in greatest dimension
N3	Metastasis in any lymph node >6 cm

Distant metastasis

M0	No evidence of distant metastasis
M1	Evidence of distant metastasis

Stage

0	Tis	N0	M0
I	T1	N0	M0
II	T2	N0	M0
III	T3	N0	M0
	T1, T2, T3	N1	M0
IV	T4	N0	M0
	Any T	N2	M0
	Any T	N3	M0
	Any T	Any N	M1

Patterns of lymph node metastasis

The cervical lymph nodes are divided into five principal levels as outlined in Figure 49.7.

The spread of tumour from the primary site has been well addressed. SCC in the oral cavity and lips tends to metastasise to lymph nodes at levels I, II and III. However, with SCC of the oral tongue there is a risk of skip metastasis directly to lymph node levels III or IV, without the involvement of higher-level lymph node groups. Tumours arising in the oropharynx commonly metastasise to lymph node levels II, III and IV, as well as retropharyngeal and contralateral nodal groups.

Distant metastases are relatively uncommon but sites involved include lung, brain, liver, bone and skin.

CLINICAL FEATURES

Between 25 and 50 per cent of patients with cancer of the oral cavity or oropharynx present late. Many of these patients are elderly and frail and delay visiting the doctor or the dentist partly because they wear dentures and are accustomed to the discomfort and associated ulceration. Occasionally, dental and medical practitioners fail to recognise that a lesion may be

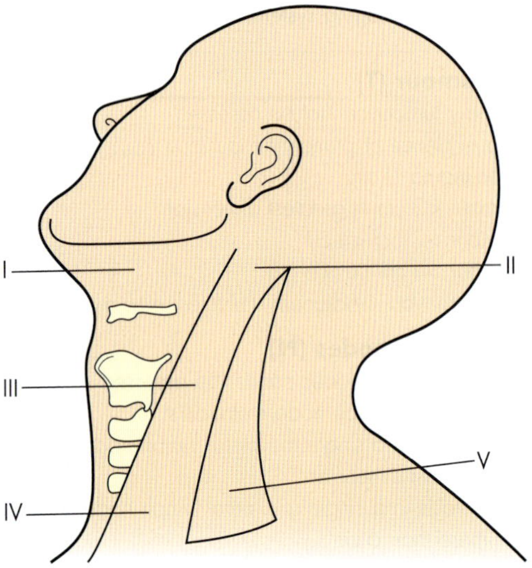

Figure 49.7 Cervical lymph nodes: (I) submandibular; (II) upper jugular; (III) middle jugular; (IV) lower jugular; (V) posterior triangle.

malignant and further delay referral. Moreover, early oral cancer is usually not painful until either the ulcer becomes infected or the tumour invades local sensory nerve fibres. Clinical presentation is markedly dependent on the anatomical site.

Lip cancer

Lip cancer presents early as it is readily visible to the patient. It usually arises as an ulcer on the vermilion border (Figure 49.8). In total, 95 per cent of carcinomas of the lip arise on the lower lip and 15 per cent arise in the central one-third and commissures. Tumours tend to spread laterally over the mucosal surface. Lymph node metastases, usually to the submental or submandibular nodes, occur late.

Oral cavity

Cancers of the oral cavity present in a variable way (Figure 49.9) but are often associated with persisting swelling or ulceration within the oral cavity (Summary box 49.3).

The duration of symptoms is highly variable, from several weeks to many months.

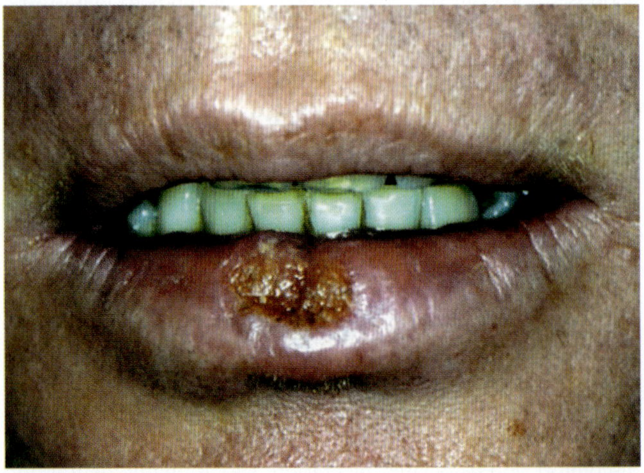

Figure 49.8 Squamous cell carcinoma of the lower lip.

Summary box 49.3

Clinical features of oral cancer

- Persistent oral swelling for >4 weeks
- Mouth ulceration for >4 weeks
- Sore tongue
- Difficulty swallowing
- Jaw or facial swelling
- Painless neck lump
- Unexplained tooth mobility
- Trismus

Oropharynx

Cancer of the oropharynx frequently presents much later than cancer of the lip and oral cavity. An ipsilateral or contralateral lump in the neck may be the single presenting complaint from a patient with a carcinoma arising from the tongue base, tonsil or soft palate. Palpable asymmetry, particularly in the tonsil, often represents submucosal infiltration of tumour. Deeper infiltration of the tongue base, pterygoid muscles or adherence of the tumour to the jaw results in poor mobility of the tongue or palate. Common clinical features of oropharyngeal cancer are outlined in Summary box 49.4.

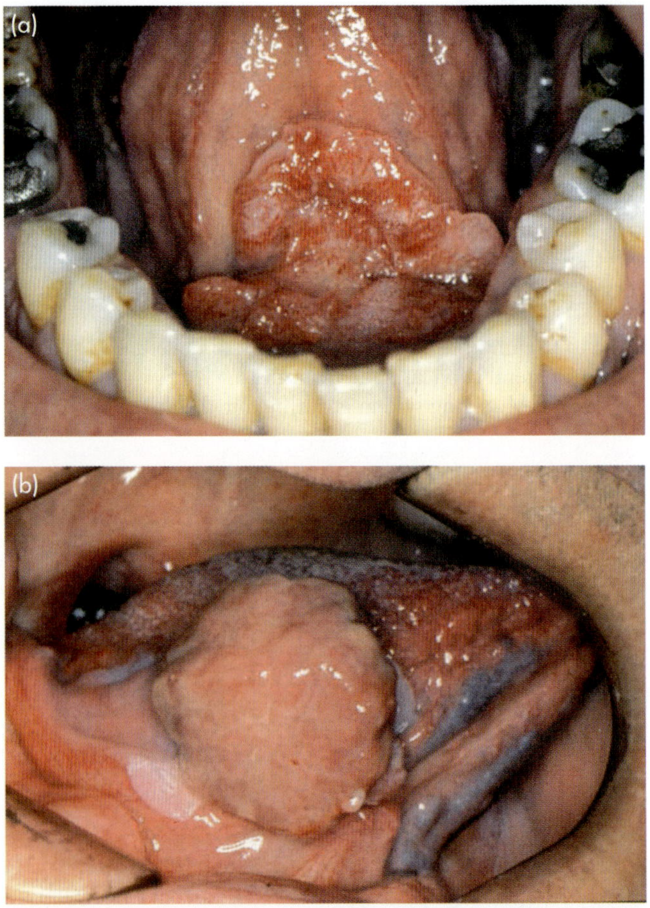

Figure 49.9 (a) Ulcerative squamous cell carcinoma of the anterior floor of the mouth. (b) Exophytic squamous cell carcinoma of the right lateral border of the tongue.

Summary box 49.4

Clinical features of oropharyngeal cancer

- Localised and persistent sore throat
- Difficulty and/or painful swallowing for >4 weeks
- Painless neck lump
- Unilateral tonsillar enlargement or ulceration
- Otalgia

INVESTIGATIONS

When a clinical diagnosis of oropharyngeal cancer is suspected, a comprehensive protocol of investigations should be instituted. An incisional biopsy should be carried out in all cases. Formal examination under anaesthetic is preferred in the vast majority of cases, not only to carry out the biopsy, but also to palpate and examine the extent of the tumour, which can be exquisitely tender in the conscious patient. Under the same anaesthetic, extraction of teeth with a dubious prognosis can be performed. Where available, and when the diagnosis is clear-cut, insertion of a percutaneous endoscopic gastrostomy (PEG) should be performed to facilitate feeding in the treatment phase. The biopsy should be generous and include the most suspicious area of the lesion, as well as normal adjacent tissue. Areas of necrosis or gross infection should be avoided.

Radiography

Plain radiography of the jaw is of limited value but does provide an opportunity for dental assessment. Before examination under anaesthesia, an orthopantomogram of the jaws is helpful to assess bony invasion, particularly from tumours arising on the alveolus and maxillary antrum.

Magnetic resonance imaging

MRI is the investigation of choice for cancer of the oral cavity and oropharynx, as it is not distorted by metallic dental restorations and provides excellent visualisation of soft-tissue infiltration of the tumour (Figure 49.10). Ideally, it should be performed before diagnostic biopsy as biopsy frequently distorts the image of the primary tumour. The specificity and sensitivity of MRI in diagnosing cervical node metastasis are similar to that of CT. Patients who suffer with claustrophobia may have difficulty in tolerating the investigation.

Computed tomography

CT is much more widely available than MRI but has limited value in oral cavity and oropharyngeal cancer. It is useful when bony invasion is suspected. CT of the thorax and abdomen is now indicated for all patients and not just those with proven cervical lymph node metastasis and large-volume disease.

Radionucleotide studies

A radioisotope bone scan of the facial skeleton adds little to the diagnosis and assessment of oropharyngeal cancer. The scan is not specific and tends to show increased uptake wherever there is increased metabolic activity in bone. A false-positive diagnosis is common and 'over-staging' of the disease frequent.

Fine-needle aspiration cytology

Fine-needle aspiration cytology (FNAC) is useful for the assessment and pathological diagnosis of enlarged cervical lymph nodes. It involves the use of a fine-needle puncture into the mass and immediate aspiration for cytological examination. It has few complications and does not spread tumour. It requires no specialist equipment other than a 21G or 23G needle and a 10-mL syringe. Aspiration should be carried out only when the needle enters the swelling. If the specimen can be assessed immediately by an expert cytologist, then it can be sent without fixation. If there is delay in microscopic examination, then the specimen, smeared on a microscope slide, should be fixed before transfer to the laboratory. The positive yield from FNAC is dependent not only on the quality of the aspirate, but also on the skill of the cytologist.

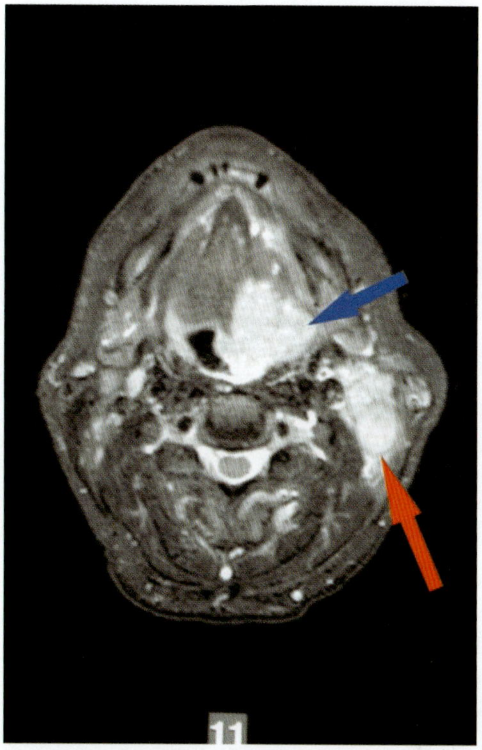

Figure 49.10 Magnetic resonance imaging of a primary tumour of the left tongue base (blue arrow) and neck node metastasis (red arrow).

Ultrasound

Ultrasound has limited use in the management of oropharyngeal cancer. It is useful as an adjunct in FNAC to ensure accurate aspiration of a deeply seated neck node swelling.

TREATMENT

General principles

The two principal treatment modalities of oropharyngeal cancer are surgery and radiotherapy. Small tumours can be managed either by primary radiotherapy or surgery. Large-volume disease, i.e. advanced tumour, usually requires a combination of surgery and radiotherapy. There is an increasing move to manage extensive disease of the oropharynx with chemoradiotherapy, provided that patients are medically fit to tolerate the toxicity. Factors that need to be taken into consideration include:

- the site of disease
- the stage

- histology
- concomitant medical disease
- social factors.

The management of head and neck cancer involves a team approach, whereby patients are assessed objectively by several specialists who agree on an optimum treatment strategy.

Cancer of the oral cavity is frequently managed with primary surgery whereas cancer of the oropharynx can be treated with either primary radiotherapy or primary surgery, or a combination, i.e. surgery for neck nodes and radiotherapy for the primary site.

When the tumour invades bone, e.g. the mandible, primary surgery is deemed appropriate as radiotherapy is less effective in controlling disease. Surgery is also more appropriate for bulky advanced disease, usually followed by postoperative radiotherapy. Tumours of intermediate size, e.g. T2 and T3 tumours, are more problematic and treatment regimes more controversial, hence the need for planning by a multidisciplinary team.

Cervical node involvement

When cervical lymph node involvement occurs, treatment should be geared towards a single modality to deal simultaneously with the lymph node disease and the primary tumour.

Histology

The degree of differentiation of SCC does not normally influence the management of the tumour alone. Management of verrucous carcinoma, a variant of SCC, is identical to that of any other SCC.

Malignant tumours of the minor salivary glands require primary surgery whereas lymphoma is managed by radiotherapy, or chemotherapy and radiotherapy, depending on the stage. Postoperative radiotherapy for minor salivary gland tumours is often indicated to reduce the risk of locoregional recurrence.

Age

Modern anaesthesia and postoperative critical care facilities have allowed major head and neck surgery to be carried out on patients with significant medical comorbidity. Advancing age is now not considered to be a contraindication to major head and neck cancer surgery. Conversely, young patients should not be denied radiotherapy for fear of inducing a second malignancy, e.g. sarcoma, in later life.

Previous radiotherapy

A second course of radiotherapy to a previously irradiated site is contraindicated as the tumour is likely to be radioresistant and reirradiation will invariably result in extensive tissue necrosis.

Field change

Surgery is preferred when multiple tumours are present or there is extensive premalignant change of the oropharyngeal mucosa. Radiotherapy is unsatisfactory as the entire oral cavity requires treatment, causing severe morbidity. In addition, subsequent postradiotherapy changes make the diagnosis of future premalignancy and malignancy more difficult.

Management of premalignant conditions

Elimination of associated aetiological factors is the basis of the management of premalignant oral mucosal lesions. Cessation of smoking, elimination of the areca nut/pan habit and reduction in alcohol consumption should be encouraged in all patients with premalignant lesions. A photographic record of the lesion is useful, particularly for long-term follow up. All erythroplakia and speckled leukoplakia should undergo urgent incisional biopsy. Biopsy from more than one site provides a better representation of histological changes within a lesion.

Severe epithelial dysplasia and carcinoma *in situ* should be ablated by surgical excision or laser vaporisation. Small lesions, particularly on the lateral border of the tongue or buccal mucosa, may be managed with surgical excision and primary closure by undermining the adjacent mucosa. Larger defects can be managed with laser vaporisation and allowed to epithelialise spontaneously (Figure 49.11). With mild-to-moderate epithelial dysplasia, treatment is facilitated by elimination of causative agents. Patients who continue to smoke should be managed as for severe dysplasia and carcinoma *in situ*. Patients who cease smoking and areca nut/pan habits may be followed up closely at three-monthly intervals.

LIP CANCER

Surgery and external beam radiotherapy are highly effective methods of treatment for lip cancer. The cure rate approaches 90 per cent for either modality.

Premalignant changes on the lower lip mucosa are frequently extensive and are best managed by a lower lip shave, in which

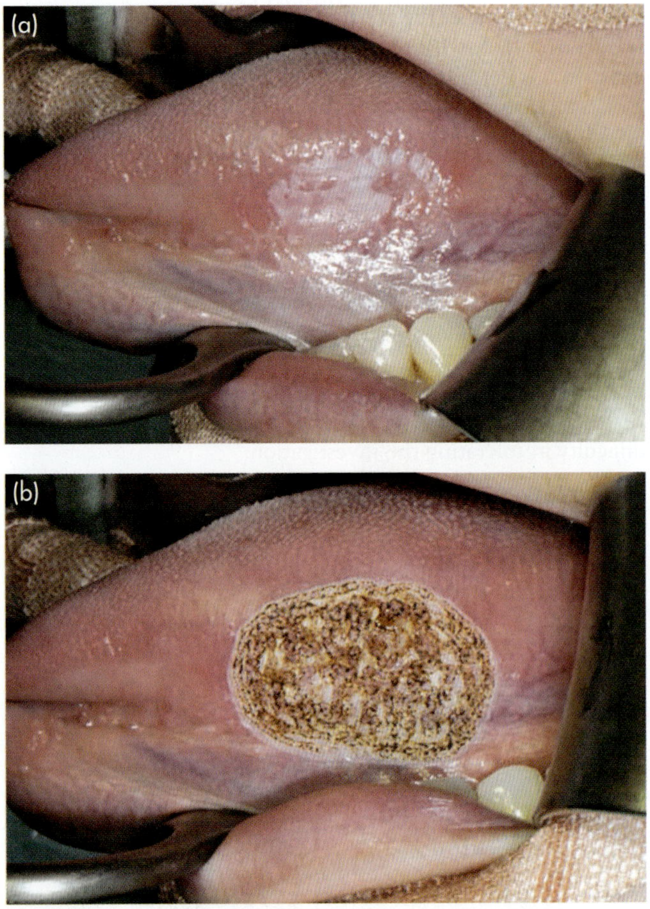

Figure 49.11 (a) Leukoplakia with severe dysplasia of the lateral border of the tongue. (b) Laser vaporisation.

the vermilion defect is closed by advancement of the lower labial mucosa.

Small tumours

Small tumours (<2 cm) of the lip can be managed with either a V- or W-shaped excision under local or general anaesthesia. The defect, which should be no larger than one-third of the total lip size, is closed in three layers – mucosa, muscle and skin – with particular attention paid to the correct alignment of the vermilion border (Figure 49.12).

Intermediate tumours

Larger tumours, which produce defects of between one-third and two-thirds the size of the lower lip, require local flaps for reconstruction. V or W excision will result in microstomia. Large central defects are best managed using the Johansen step technique (Figure 49.13). This allows closure of the defect by symmetrical advancement of soft-tissue flaps, utilising the excess skin in the labiomental grooves. Alternative techniques include the Bernard rotational flap.

Total lip reconstruction

Extensive tumours of the lower lip, which invade adjacent tissues (T4), have a high incidence of neck node metastasis. Patients with such advanced disease require surgery that may include unilateral or bilateral selective neck dissection and total excision of the lower lip and chin. The lower lip defect is best reconstructed with a forearm flap suspended with palmaris longus tendon (Figure 49.14).

TONGUE CANCER

Up to 30 per cent of patients with a T1 (<2 cm diameter) tumour (Figure 49.15) have occult metastasis at presentation and should undergo simultaneous treatment of the neck by either selective neck dissection or radiotherapy. When performing surgical excision of the primary tumour, a 2-cm margin in all planes should be achieved to ensure a wide, complete excision. Resection resulting in partial or hemiglossectomy can be performed with either a cutting diathermy or laser if available. Advanced tumours (T3 and T4) often encroach upon the floor of the mouth and, occasionally, the mandible. In these circumstances, a major resection of the tongue and floor of the mouth and mandible is required. T4 tumours of the oral tongue often cross the midline, for which total glossectomy is the only option to achieve adequate tumour clearance.

When a patient undergoes simultaneous neck dissection, the resection of the primary tumour should preferably be in continuity with the neck node specimen. This eliminates 'lingual' lymph nodes (lying between the primary tumour and submandibular (level I) nodes); these nodes may contain micro-deposits of tumour, which may lead to local recurrence.

Access

Access for oropharyngeal cancer is important to allow accurate assessment and clear visualisation to enable tumour clearance to be achieved. Access techniques include:

- transoral – small anterior oral tumours only;
- lip-split technique and paramedian or median mandibulotomy (Figure 49.16);
- visor incision (Figure 49.17).

Reconstruction

Small defects of the lateral tongue can be managed by primary closure or allowed to heal by secondary intention. Larger defects, e.g. T2, T3 and T4 resections, require formal reconstruction to encourage good speech and swallowing. A radial forearm flap either with skin (Figure 49.18) and/or fascia, utilising microvascular anastomosis, gives a good functional

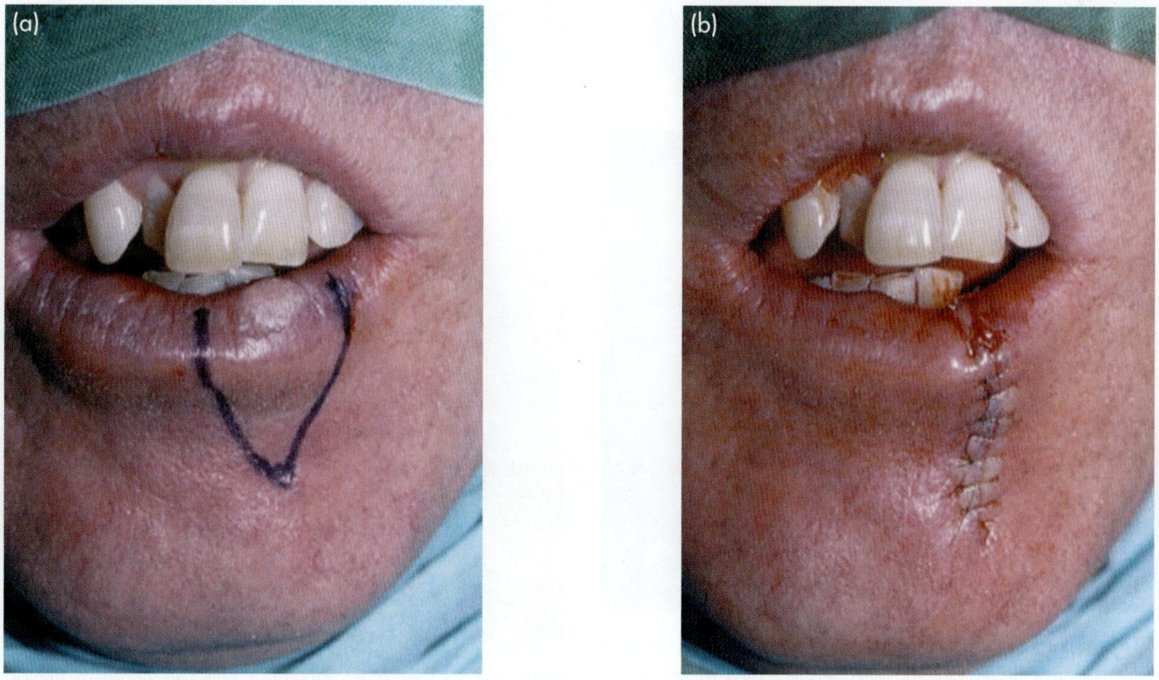

Figure 49.12 (a) Skin markings for wedge excision of the lower lip. (b) Primary closure.

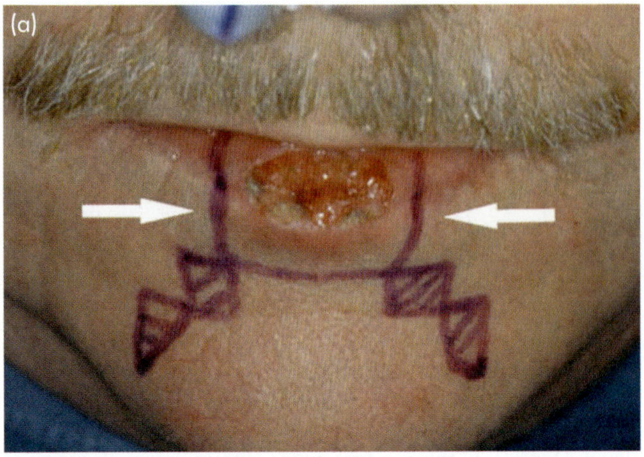

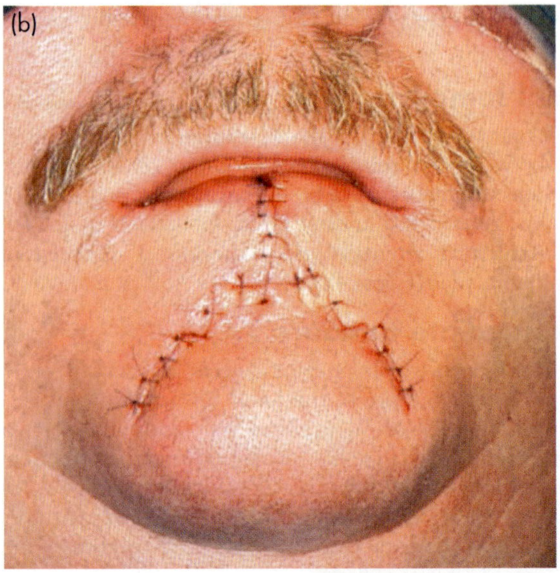

Figure 49.13 (a) Skin markings for Johansen step reconstruction. (b) Closure of lip and labiomental steps.

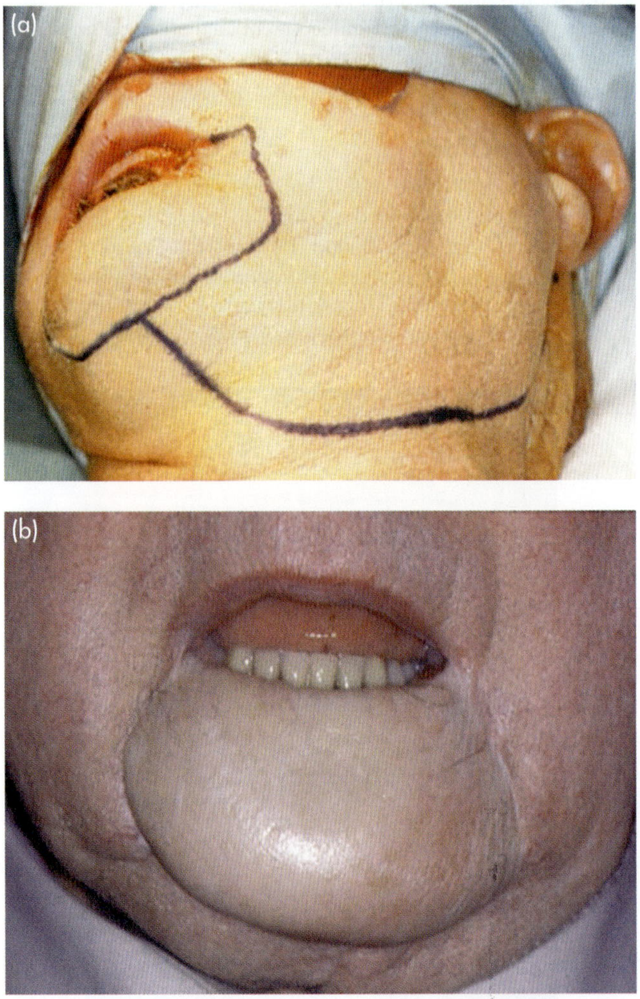

Figure 49.14 (a) Skin markings for total excision of the lower lip, chin and left selective neck dissection. (b) Postoperative view of the reconstructed lower lip using a radial artery forearm flap.

result. Large-volume defects, including total glossectomy, require more bulky flaps such as the rectus abdominus free flap. If feasible, the preservation of one or both hypoglossal nerves is useful to encourage floor of mouth function to help relearn swallowing.

FLOOR OF MOUTH

Carcinoma of the floor of the mouth can spread to the ventral surface of the anterior tongue or encroach upon the lower anterior alveolus (Figure 49.19). Surgical excision may include a partial anterior glossectomy and anterior mandibular resection. Only very small tumours of the floor of mouth can be managed by simple excision. The visor procedure provides excellent access (see Figure 49.17).

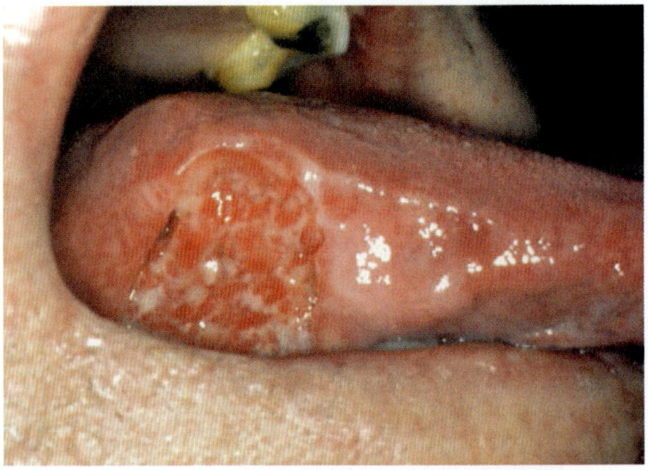

Figure 49.15 Ulcerative squamous cell carcinoma of the right lateral border of the tongue.

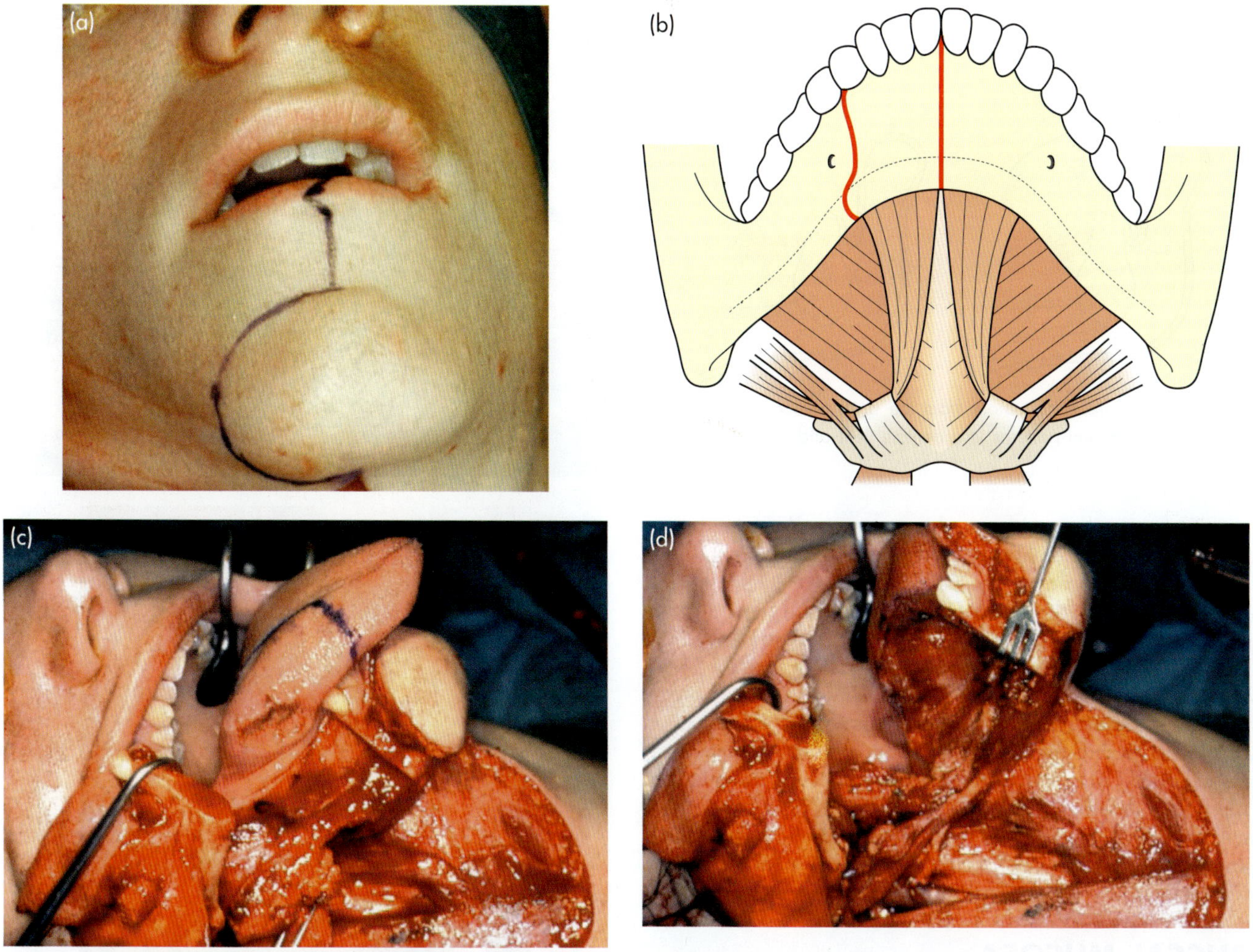

Figure 49.16 (a) Skin markings for lip split and mandibulotomy in continuity with neck dissection. (b) Paramedian and midline mandibulotomy. (c) Margins for primary tumour resection after mandibulotomy. (d) Tongue defect after right selective neck dissection, mandibulotomy and partial glossectomy.

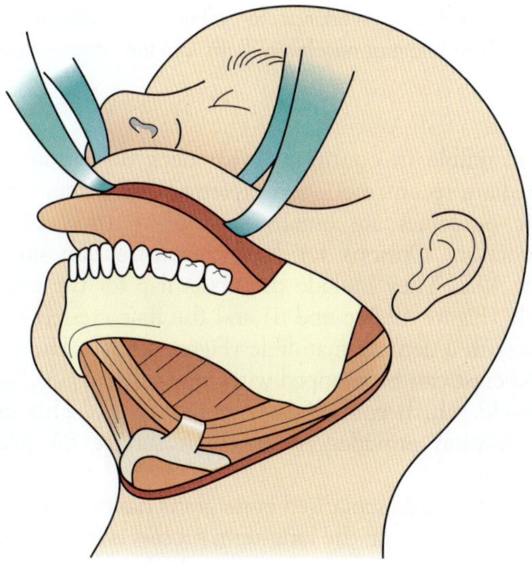

Figure 49.17 Visor approach to the anterior mandible/floor of the mouth and tongue.

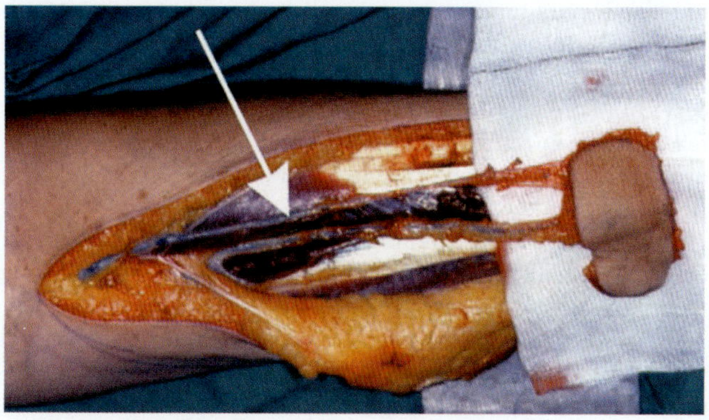

Figure 49.18 Radial artery forearm flap raised before division of vascular pedicle and cephalic vein (arrow).

Reconstruction

Small tumours of the floor of the mouth frequently require formal reconstruction. It is unacceptable to advance the cut surface of the ventral tongue to the labial mucosa as severe difficulties with speech, swallowing and mastication ensue. Simple soft-tissue defects of the anterior floor of mouth are best reconstructed with a radial artery forearm flap. If a patient

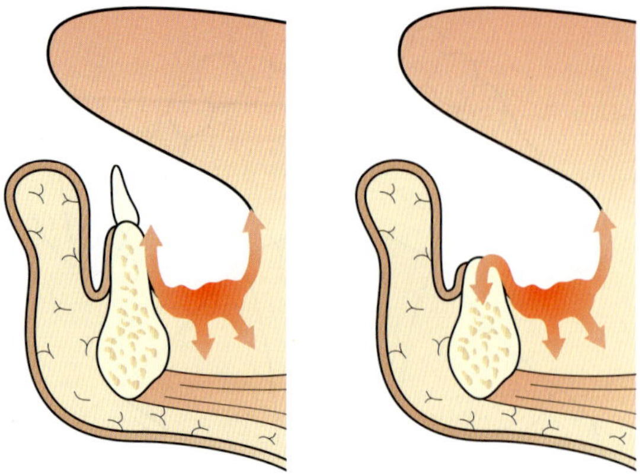

Figure 49.19 Spread of tumour from the anterior floor of the mouth showing the different patterns in a dentate (left) and edentulous (right) mandible.

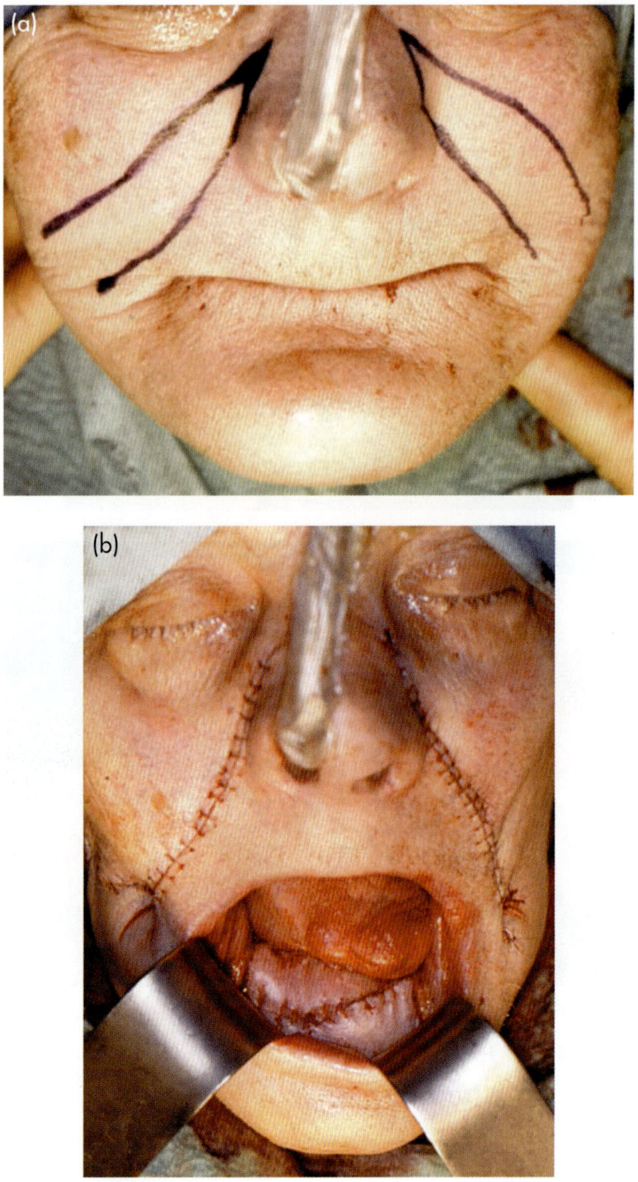

Figure 49.20 (a) Skin markings for bilateral nasolabial flaps. (b) Transposition of bilateral nasolabial flaps into the anterior floor of the mouth.

is unfit for microvascular free flap surgery or the facilities are limited, bilateral nasolabial flaps tunnelled into the mouth and interdigitated provide an acceptable alternative (Figure 49.20). Three weeks later their pedicles are divided and inset into the lateral floor of mouth defects. Large defects that involve rim resection of the anterior mandible may also be managed with soft tissue reconstruction only. Full-thickness resection of the anterior mandible, however, requires immediate reconstruction to prevent severe functional defects or a cosmetic deformity. Vascularised bone with a soft-tissue component provides the most up-to-date method of reconstruction. A fibula flap or a vascularised iliac crest graft (deep circumflex iliac artery (DCIA)) are two options in the management of anterior mandible defects with simultaneous floor of mouth defects.

BUCCAL MUCOSA

Squamous cell carcinoma of the buccal mucosa (Figure 49.21) should be excised widely, including the underlying buccinator muscle. Larger tumours occasionally extend onto the maxillary tuberosity, tonsillar fossa or mandibular alveolus. Facial skin involvement is rare but carries a poor prognosis. Although cervical node metastasis from buccal mucosa usually occurs less readily than in tongue and floor of mouth cancer, a simultaneous ipsilateral selective supraomohyoid neck dissection (levels I, II, III) is considered good practice.

Access for buccal carcinoma can be achieved either transorally for smaller lesions (T1, T2) or using the lip-splitting technique for larger lesions (T3, T4).

Reconstruction of the buccal mucosa prevents scarring and trismus. Options include the radial artery forearm flap or a temporalis muscle flap. Raw temporalis muscle inset into the buccal mucosal defect will epithelialise spontaneously over several weeks.

LOWER ALVEOLUS

Surgery is the treatment of choice for tumours that involve the mandibular alveolus (Figure 49.22a). Ipsilateral selective neck dissections should be performed for lateral tumours although the incidence of occult neck node metastasis is low. Bilateral selective neck dissection should be considered for anterior tumours. Bone invasion (Figure 49.22b) demands segmental resection of the mandible in continuity with neck dissection. Primary or immediate reconstruction is preferred as the functional and cosmetic outcomes are usually superior to those of delayed reconstruction. Options for bony reconstruction are shown in Table 49.2. They include the fibula flap for the edentulous mandible (Figure 49.22c and d) and the iliac crest (DCIA) for patients with a dentate mandible (Figure 49.23). The vascularised iliac crest can be wrapped with internal oblique abdominal wall muscle, which epithelialises spontaneously. This intraoral epithelialisation provides an excellent surface for prosthetic replacement.

Although non-vascularised bone grafts have a place in mandibular reconstruction, the long-term success is frequently low as many patients receive postoperative radiotherapy, which results in the loss of the bone and dehiscence of the titanium tray or reconstruction plate.

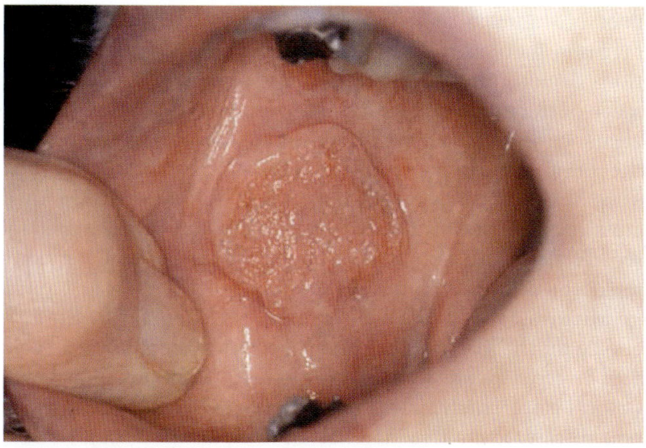

Figure 49.21 Exophytic squamous cell carcinoma of the right buccal mucosa.

Table 49.2 Mandibular reconstruction.

Method	Technique
No reconstruction	Primary closure
Soft tissue only	Pectoralis major myocutaneous flap
Alloplastic material	2.4 mm reconstruction plate alone
Combination alloplastic/soft tissue	2.4 mm reconstruction plate and pectoralis major flap
Non-vascularised bone grafts	Titanium tray and cancellous chips (iliac crest)
Vascularised bone grafts	Fibula (edentulous and dentate); iliac crest (dentate); scapula (concomitant large soft-tissue defect)

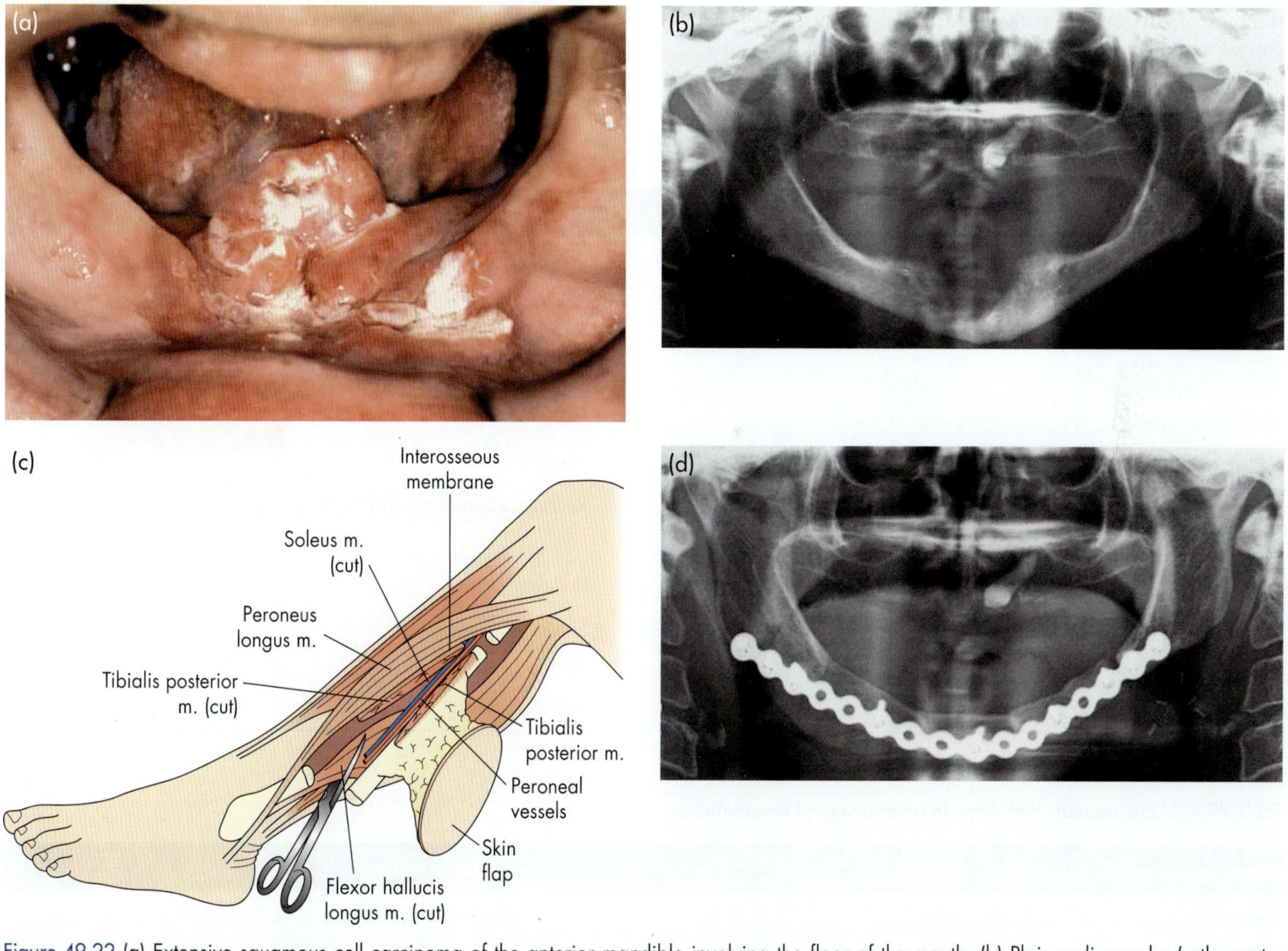

Figure 49.22 (a) Extensive squamous cell carcinoma of the anterior mandible involving the floor of the mouth. (b) Plain radiography (orthopantomogram) revealing bony destruction of the anterior mandible. (c) Osseocutaneous fibula flap. (d) Postoperative radiograph of the reconstructed mandible with fibula flap and reconstruction plate.

RETROMOLAR PAD

Tumours at this site frequently, but not always, invade the ascending ramus of the mandible. They also spread medially into the soft palate or even the tonsillar fossa. Access for excision is carried out via a lip split and mandibulotomy (see Figure 49.16). Small defects are managed either with a temporalis muscle flap or a radial artery forearm flap. Segmental mandibular resections require vascularised bone to achieve adequate reconstruction.

HARD PALATE AND MAXILLARY ALVEOLUS

The maxillary alveolus and hard palate are relatively uncommon sites for SCC. A tumour arising in these areas may arise either from the oral mucosa per se or from the maxillary antrum penetrating the oral cavity. In the Indian subcontinent, carcinoma of the hard palate is common and particularly associated with reverse smoking. Occasionally, malignant tumours of minor salivary glands present as swellings of the hard palate. Small tumours of the maxillary alveolus can be managed by transoral partial maxillectomy. More extensive tumours involving the floor of the maxillary sinus require wider access by a Weber–Ferguson incision (Figure 49.24). If the preoperative investigations demonstrate extension of the disease into the pterygoid space or the infratemporal fossa, the prognosis is poor as surgical clearance is difficult if not impossible. Tumour extending into the orbit requires simultaneous orbital exenteration or even a combined neurosurgical resection. The vascularised iliac crest graft is the method of choice for immediate maxillary reconstruction although the fibula provides adequate bony replacement to maintain facial contour.

Microvascular free tissue transfer remains the method of choice for the management of defects in the oropharynx (Table 49.3). Free flaps are superior reconstructive options to pedicled or local flaps, which may be used for salvage procedures or recurrent disease. Each 'free' flap has a principal blood supply and a concomitant venous drainage. The flaps can be tailored to the defect to include skin, fascia, bone and muscle. The techniques of free tissue transfer demand specialist training and a microscope to connect blood vessels in the neck after neck dissection, e.g. facial artery to the prepared artery attached to the flap. The vascular anatomy of microvascular free flaps is summarised in Table 49.4.

Table 49.3 Primary reconstructive options in oropharyngeal cancer.

Anatomical site	Microvascular free flap	Alternative flaps
Floor of mouth	Forearm	Nasolabial flaps (bilateral)
Lateral tongue	Forearm	Platysma skin flap
Total tongue/glossectomy	Rectus abdominus	Pectoralis major/lateral thigh
Buccal mucosa	Forearm	Temporalis muscle
Mandible		
Dentate	Iliac crest	Fibula
Edentulous	Fibula	Reconstruction plate and pectoralis major
Maxilla		
Low-level/hard palate	Temporalis muscle	Forearm
High	Iliac crest	Fibula
Soft palate/tonsil	Forearm	Temporalis muscle, galeal flap, pectoralis major
Tongue base	Forearm	Pectoralis major

Table 49.4 Microvascular 'free' flaps in oropharyngeal reconstruction.

Flap	Blood supply	Common variants
Forearm	Radial artery	Skin only; fascia only
Composite forearm	Radial artery	Skin and bone (radius)
Anterolateral thigh	Perforator vessels of the profunda femoris artery	Skin only; skin and muscle
Rectus abdominus	Deep inferior epigastric artery	Skin and muscle; muscle only
Fibula	Peroneal artery	Bone and skin; bone only; bone and fascia/fat
Ilium	Deep circumflex iliac artery	Bone only; bone and muscle; bone, muscle and skin
Scapula	Subscapular artery	Bone and skin; bone and muscle

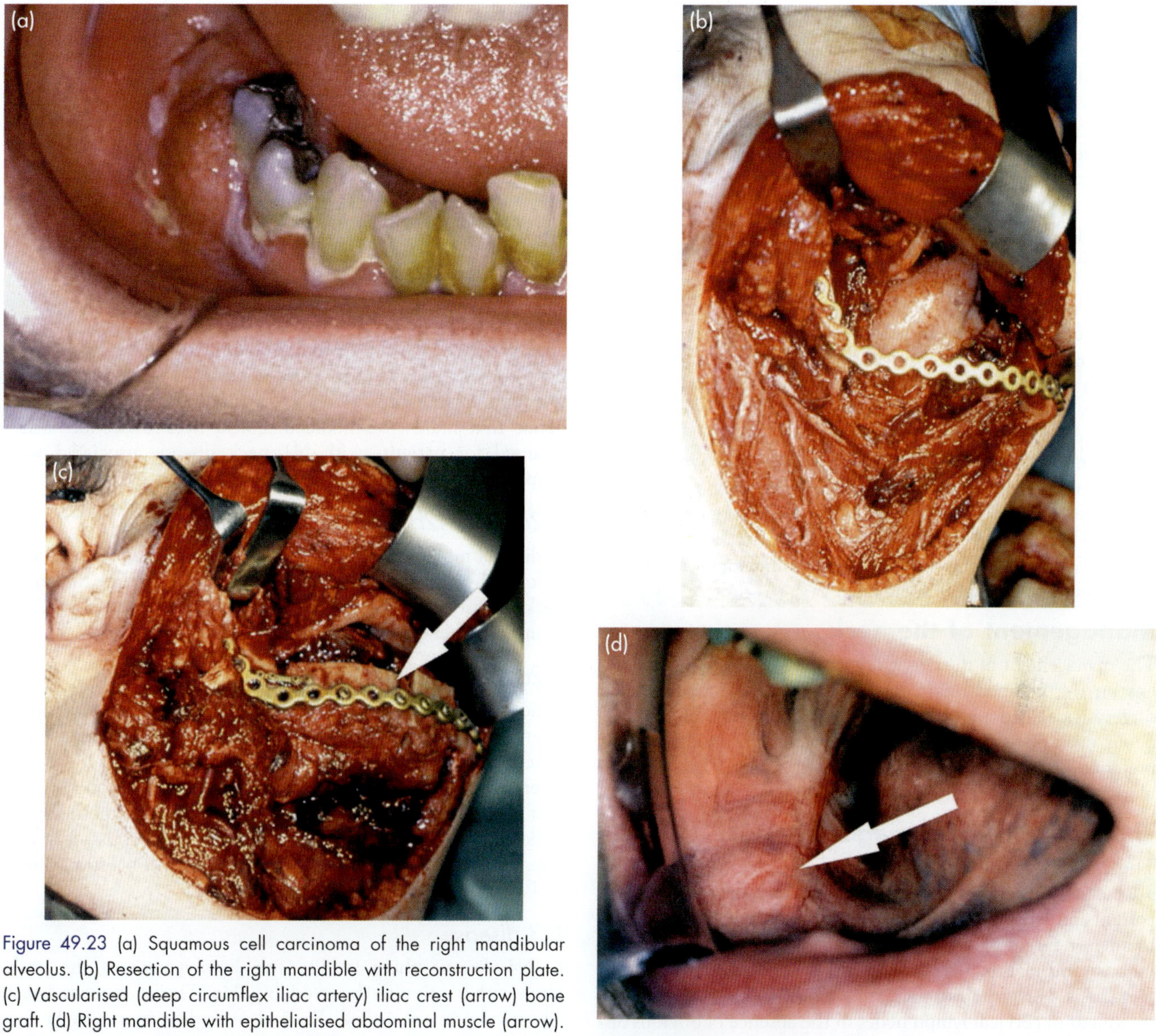

Figure 49.23 (a) Squamous cell carcinoma of the right mandibular alveolus. (b) Resection of the right mandible with reconstruction plate. (c) Vascularised (deep circumflex iliac artery) iliac crest (arrow) bone graft. (d) Right mandible with epithelialised abdominal muscle (arrow).

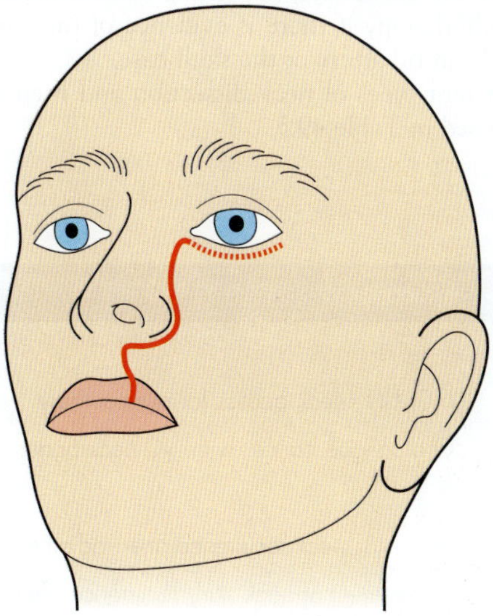

Figure 49.24 Weber–Ferguson incision for maxillectomy (lower eyelid extension is rarely required).

OROPHARYNX

Tumours of the oropharynx are frequently not amenable to surgery because of the morbid nature of the resection – small and intermediate (T1, T2) tongue base tumours may necessitate total glossectomy to achieve adequate clearance at the root of the tongue. Tumours of the soft palate and tonsil, however, can be managed with either primary surgery in continuity with neck dissection or primary radiotherapy. Subsequent defects of the tonsillar area can be managed with a forearm flap. Defects of the soft palate, including total soft palate reconstruction, are best managed with a combined reconstruction consisting of a superiorly based pharyngeal flap to line the nasal surface and a forearm flap for the oral surface of the new soft palate. Chemoradiotherapy is now increasingly used to manage tumours of the oropharynx in which organ preservation, but not necessarily function, is the goal. In patients with large-volume neck disease, e.g. N2 and N3, a combined modality of neck dissection followed by chemoradiotherapy to manage the tumour at the primary site and residual neck disease is gaining popularity.

Chemotherapy

The role of chemotherapy has evolved over the last 20–30 years. It was initially reserved for treatment of recurrent and incurable disease, often using single-agent therapy. Combination chemotherapy, particularly platinum agents and 5-fluorouracil, is now more effective in controlling recurrent and incurable disease. However, combination chemotherapy is associated with more severe side effects and a balance needs to be reached between efficacy, palliation and quality of life.

Chemotherapy also now has an important role in the treatment of locally advanced and previously untreated oropharyngeal carcinoma. There is compelling evidence that tumours of the tongue base may best be managed with primary chemoradiotherapy rather than radical surgery. The addition of chemotherapy with radiotherapy does, however, increase the morbidity and mortality rates. Patients who are frail or who have significant medical comorbidity may not tolerate the regime.

Chemoradiotherapy has been shown to improve survival in patients whose tumours are deemed unresectable, although organ preservation, i.e. swallowing and speech, is not always sustained. There is good evidence for the superiority of chemoradiotherapy over radiotherapy alone; however, chemoradiotherapy is rarely effective in large-volume disease.

Management of the neck

The management of the cervical lymph nodes is highly dependent on the planned treatment of the primary tumour. When surgery is deemed appropriate for the primary tumour, simultaneous neck dissection should be considered. If radiotherapy is preferred, treatment to the neck should be contemplated, particularly when there is a high risk of occult metastases, e.g. tongue.

The clinically node-negative neck

The cervical lymph nodes contain occult metastases in up to 30 per cent of patients. This is particularly significant with patients presenting with primary carcinomas of the tongue and, to a lesser extent, floor of mouth. Tumours arising in the buccal mucosa and mandibular alveolus are less likely to have occult metastasis. Nevertheless, increasing evidence exists that active treatment of cervical lymph nodes in the absence of obvious disease is considered good practice. Patients with carcinoma of the lateral tongue, floor of mouth and mandibular alveolus are best managed by supraomohyoid neck dissection (surgical removal of lymph node levels I, II and III in continuity with the primary tumour) (Figure 49.25).

Good evidence exists that carcinoma of the tongue can produce occult cervical metastasis directly to lymph node level IV. Consequently, the extended supraomohyoid neck dissection removing lymph node levels I, II, III and IV is indicated for patients with carcinoma of the tongue with N0 neck disease. Selective neck dissection is regarded as a staging as much as a therapeutic procedure. Patients who have two or more positive nodes or evidence of extracapsular spread should be managed with postoperative radiotherapy to the neck and the primary site.

Elective external beam radiotherapy is an alternative when radiotherapy is planned for the primary site.

The clinically node-positive neck

The presence of an isolated ipsilateral cytologically positive lymph node of <3 cm is now considered best managed by selective supraomohyoid neck dissection. There is good evidence that radical or modified radical neck dissection is not required for patients with N1 neck disease associated with oropharyngeal cancer.

N2a and N2b disease

Radical or modified radical neck dissection (Figure 49.26), often followed by postoperative radiotherapy, is appropriate to control neck disease. Patients unfit for surgery can be offered external beam radiotherapy palliation.

N2c disease

Patients with mouth cancer presenting with bilateral nodes often have a large, inoperable, primary tumour. Bilateral neck dissection can be undertaken, although morbidity is high. One internal jugular vein needs to be spared, usually on the side that is less involved with disease. Postoperative radiotherapy is indicated if there is multiple node involvement or extracapsular spread. Postoperative neck oedema and facial congestion occurs and may take months to resolve.

N3 disease

In N3 disease, there is extensive involvement of the neck, often with fixation to the overlying skin. This is associated with advanced primary disease. Radical neck dissection may be feasible in such circumstances, but strong consideration should be given to radiotherapy if there is evidence of tumour involving the internal carotid artery or the skull base.

The different types of neck dissection and their indications are summarised in Table 49.5.

Table 49.5 Neck dissection in oropharyngeal cancer.

Type of neck dissection	Lymph node levels removed	Indication
Selective		
Supraomohyoid	I–III	N0; N1; neck access for microsurgery
Extended supraomohyoid neck dissection	I–IV	Oral tongue cancer with N0 neck nodes; N1
Radical		
Full	I–V	N2; N3; neck recurrence after radiotherapy
Modified radical neck dissection	I–V, with preservation of internal jugular vein, accessory nerve and/or sternomastoid muscle	Involvement of neck skin; recurrence after selective neck dissection

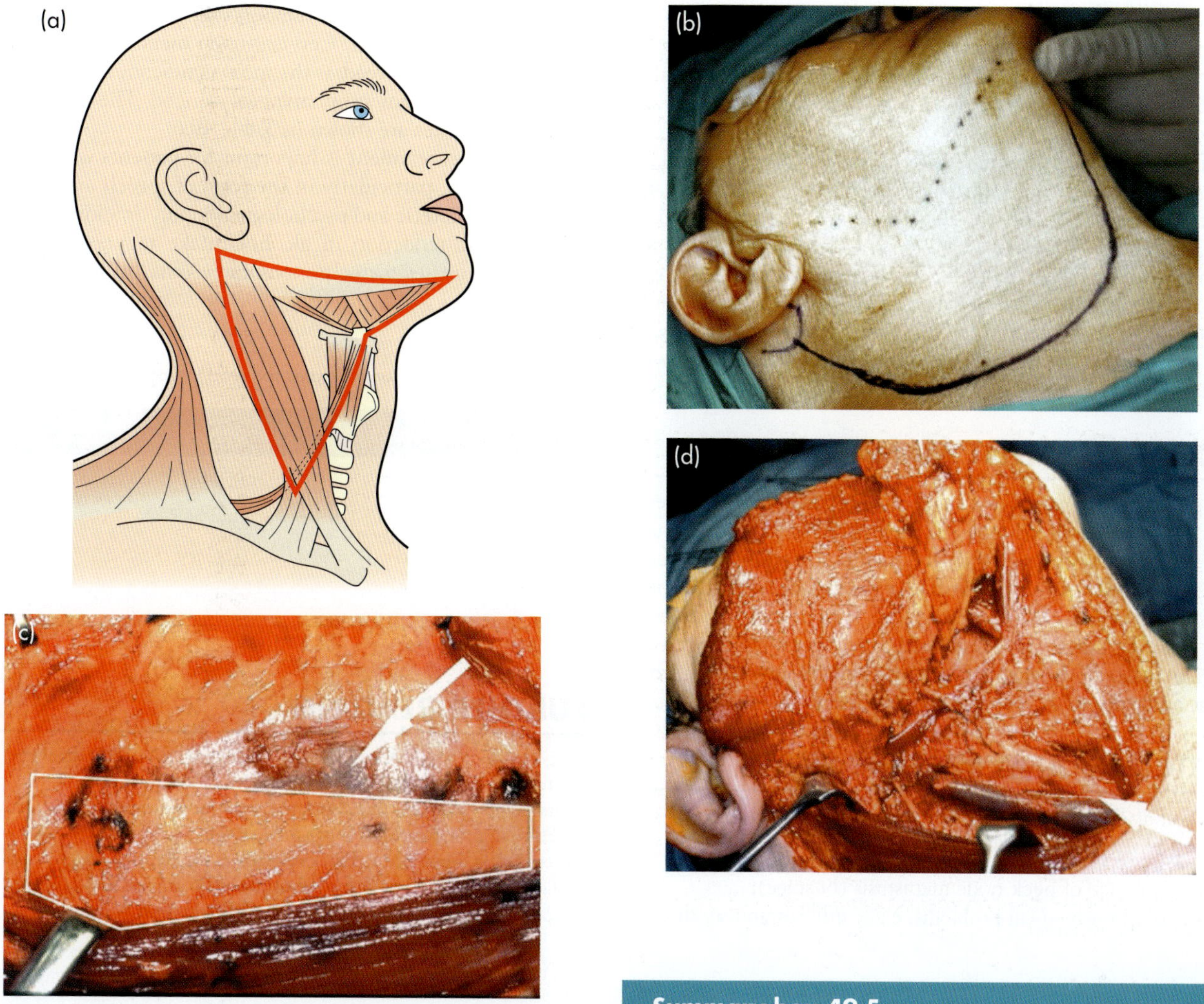

Figure 49.25 (a) Anatomical boundaries for supraomohyoid neck dissection (levels I, II, III). (b) Standard skin incision for neck dissection (solid line). (c) Deep cervical lymph nodes (box) posterolateral to the internal jugular vein (arrow). (d) Completed supraomohyoid neck dissection revealing great vessels of the neck (arrow).

COMPLICATIONS

Notwithstanding the general complications of major surgery, complications specifically associated with the treatment of oropharyngeal cancer are speech deficiencies, especially with resection of the anterior floor of the mouth and tongue; swallowing dysfunction and aspiration, especially after oropharyngeal resection; neurological injury, e.g. lingual nerve, hypoglossal nerve palsy; wound breakdown and cervical fistula formation; failure of internal fixation/reconstruction plates; failure of microvascular anastomosis; and flap failure. Other complications that may occur are listed in Summary box 49.5.

Patients undergoing treatment for oropharyngeal cancer frequently develop severe functional problems. The size and location of the tumour will dictate the extent of resection and the sacrifice of important structures.

Loss of tongue and floor of mouth musculature and the removal of bone and associated muscle attachments together

Summary box 49.5

Complications of treatment for oropharyngeal cancer

Surgical
- Accessory nerve palsy – shoulder dysfunction and pain
- Soft-tissue oedema, especially bilateral neck dissection
- Phrenic nerve injury
- Thoracic duct injury
- Cranial nerve injury
- Rupture of the carotid artery

Radiotherapy
- Osteoradionecrosis of the mandible
- Hypothyroidism
- Atherosclerosis of the carotid artery
- Neck and shoulder dysfunction
- Trismus
- Xerostomia
- Visual impairment
- Radiation neuritis

Chemotherapy
- Nausea and vomiting
- Diarrhoea
- Stomatitis
- Gastrointestinal upset
- Renal toxicity
- Leukopenia and thrombocytopenia

with the sacrifice of sensory and motor cranial nerves all greatly affect not only appearance but also speech, swallowing and nutritional status. Psychological disturbance is universal in patients undergoing major head and neck cancer surgery and radiotherapy.

The techniques of immediate reconstruction, particularly with microvascular flaps, minimise the complications and side effects but many patients are, nevertheless, radically changed for the remainder of their lives. Patients undergoing 'salvage' surgery following primary radiotherapy frequently undergo delayed wound healing, cervical fistula formation and, occasionally, carotid artery blowout/rupture. Skin anaesthesia associated with scar contracture creates additional problems, particularly with neck mobility and trismus.

POST-TREATMENT MANAGEMENT

Patients with oropharyngeal cancer need to be followed up regularly, not only to detect possible recurrence but also to manage the morbidity associated with treatment. In total, 70 per cent of recurrences occur in the first 12 months following treatment and 90 per cent in the first two years. Patients who survive for five years are cured and discharged. Recurrence after extensive surgery and radiotherapy is frequently beyond any further treatment and palliative care is a logical pathway.

OUTCOME AND PROGNOSIS

Survival after oropharyngeal cancer is directly related to:

- the size of the primary tumour (T stage);
- the evidence of neck node metastasis (N stage);
- concomitant medical problems, e.g. cardiorespiratory disease.

Patients with large primary tumours are more likely to develop cervical node metastasis. Cervical node metastasis, particularly with extracapsular spread, is the most significant factor in determining prognosis for oropharyngeal cancer. The overall five-year survival rates are shown in Table 49.6.

Supportive treatment is important for patients with oropharyngeal cancer, particularly in the form of speech and language support and dietetic and psychological input. Smoking cessation and a drastic reduction in alcohol intake reduces the risk of developing further metachronous carcinomas in the aerodigestive tract.

Table 49.6 Five-year survival rates for oropharyngeal cancer.

Stage at presentation	Survival rate (%)
I	80–90
II	65–75
III	40–50
IV	30

FURTHER READING

Langdon JF, Patel MA, Ord RA, Brennan PA. *Operative oral and maxillofacial surgery*, 2nd edn. London: Hodder Arnold, 2011.

Soutar DS, Tiwari R. *Excision and reconstruction head and neck cancer*. Edinburgh: Churchill Livingstone, 1994.

Urken ML, Cheney ML, Blackwell KE *et al. Atlas of regional and free flaps for head and neck reconstruction. Flap harvest and insetting*, 2nd edn. Philadelphia, PA: Lippincott Williams and Wilkins, 2012.

CHAPTER 50

Disorders of the salivary glands

LEARNING OBJECTIVES

To understand:
- The surgical anatomy of the salivary glands
- The presentation, pathology and investigation of salivary gland disease
- The medical and surgical treatment of stones, infections and tumours that affect salivary glands

INTRODUCTION

There are four main salivary glands, two submandibular glands and two parotid glands. In addition, there are multiple minor salivary glands.

MINOR SALIVARY GLANDS

Anatomy

The mucosa of the oral cavity contains approximately 450 minor salivary glands. They are distributed in the mucosa of the lips, cheeks, palate, floor of the mouth and retromolar area. These minor salivary glands also appear in other areas of the upper aerodigestive tract including the oropharynx, larynx and trachea as well as the sinuses. They have a histological structure similar to that of mucous-secreting major salivary glands. Overall, they contribute to 10 per cent of the total salivary volume (Summary box 50.1).

Summary box 50.1

Anatomy of salivary glands

- Two submandibular glands
- Two parotid glands
- Two sublingual glands
- Approximately 450 minor salivary glands

Common disorders of minor salivary glands

Cysts

Extravasation cysts are common and result from trauma to the overlying mucosa. They usually affect minor salivary glands within the lower lip, producing a variable swelling that is painless and usually, but not always, translucent (Figure 50.1). Some resolve spontaneously, but most require formal surgical excision that includes the overlying mucosa and the underlying minor salivary gland. Recurrence is rare.

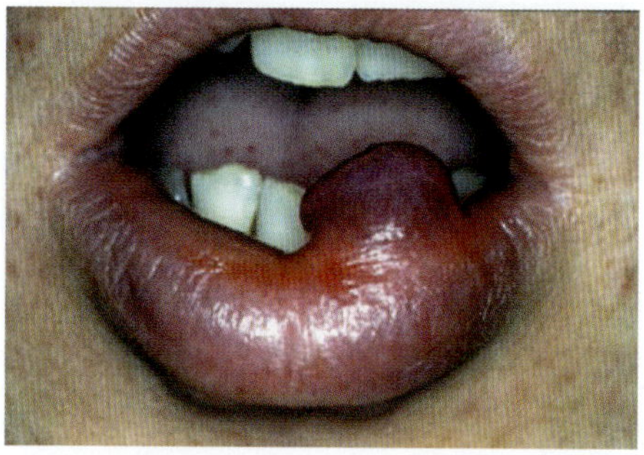

Figure 50.1 Mucous retention cyst. A translucent swelling on the lower lip is typical.

Tumours

Few tumours show more diversity in histological appearance and anatomical site than those that arise from mucous glands of the upper aerodigestive tract. Tumours of minor salivary glands are histologically similar to those of major glands; however, up to 90 per cent of minor salivary gland tumours are malignant. Although tumours of minor salivary gland origin occur anywhere in the upper aerodigestive tract, common sites for tumour formation include the upper lip, palate and retromolar regions. Less common sites for minor salivary gland tumours include the nasal and pharyngeal cavities. Minor salivary gland tumours have also been reported in the paranasal sinuses and throughout the pharynx. These tumours arise in submucosal seromucous glands that are found throughout the upper aerodigestive tract. Very rarely, a mucoepidermoid carcinoma can present as an intraosseous tumour of the mandible.

Benign minor salivary gland tumours present as painless, firm, slow-growing swellings. Overlying ulceration is extremely rare. Minor salivary gland tumours of the upper lip are managed by excision to include the overlying mucosa, with primary closure (Figure 50.2a–c).

Benign tumours of the palate, less than 1 cm in diameter, can be managed by excisional biopsy, and the defect is allowed to heal by secondary intention (Figure 50.3a–d). Where tumours of

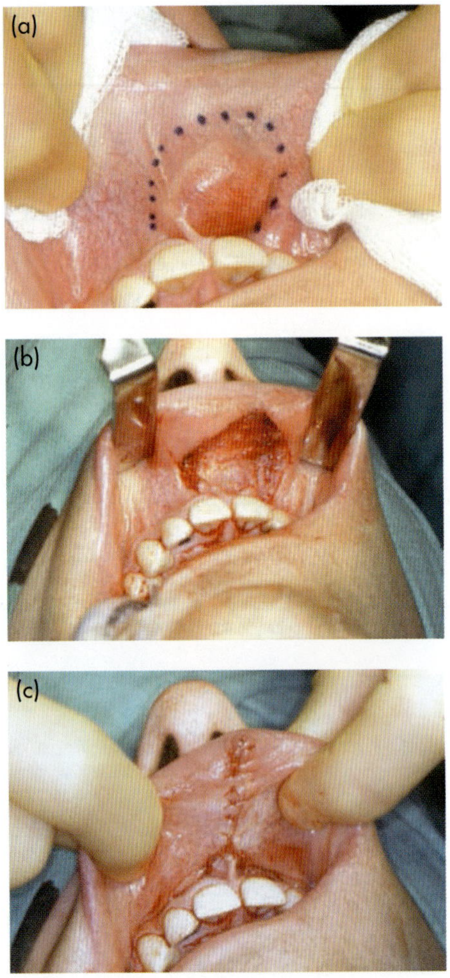

Figure 50.2 (a) Pleomorphic adenoma of the upper lip. (b) Tumour excised with overlying mucosa. (c) Primary closure of the defect.

the palate are greater than 1 cm in diameter, incisional biopsy is recommended to establish a diagnosis prior to formal excision.

Malignant minor salivary gland tumours are rare. They have a firm consistency, and the overlying mucosa may have a varied discolouration from pink to blue or black (Figure 50.4). The tumour may become necrotic with ulceration as a late presentation.

Malignant minor salivary gland tumours of the palate are managed by wide excision which may involve partial or total maxillectomy. The subsequent defect can be managed by either prosthetic obturation or immediate reconstruction. Various microvascular flaps have been designed to reconstruct maxillectomy defects, including radial forearm flap, fibular flap, rectus abdominus, latissimus dorsi and the vascularised iliac crest graft (Figure 50.5a and b).

THE SUBLINGUAL GLANDS

Anatomy

The sublingual glands are a paired set of minor salivary glands lying in the anterior part of the floor of mouth between the mucous membrane, the mylohyoid muscle and the body of the mandible close to the mental symphysis. Each gland has numerous excretory ducts that open either directly into the oral cavity

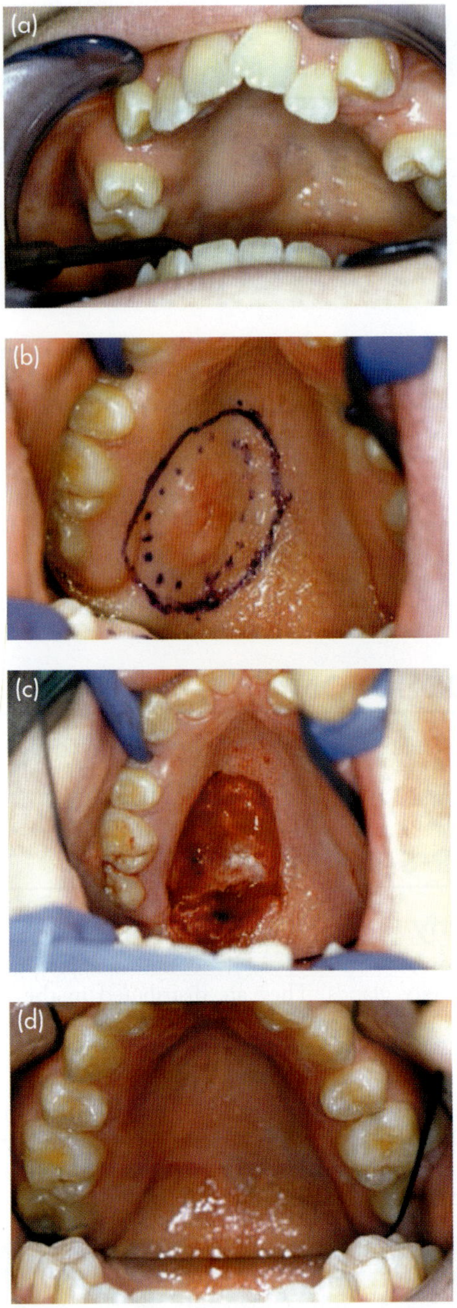

Figure 50.3 (a) Pleomorphic adenoma in the right palate in a 12-year-old girl. (b) Tumour marked out with adequate margins including the overlying mucosa. (c) The subsequent defect. (d) Healing by secondary intention three years after surgery.

or indirectly via ducts that drain into the submandibular duct (Summary box 50.2).

Summary box 50.2

Sublingual glands

- Problems are rare
- Minor mucous retention cysts may need surgery
- Plunging ranula is a retention cyst that tunnels deep
- Nearly all tumours are malignant

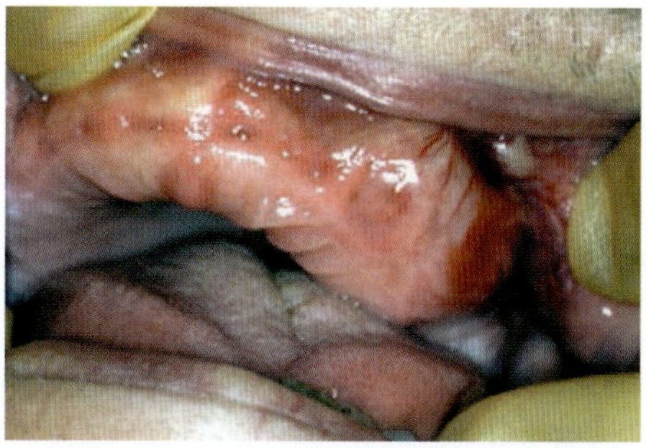

Figure 50.4 Adenoid cystic carcinoma of the left maxillary alveolus.

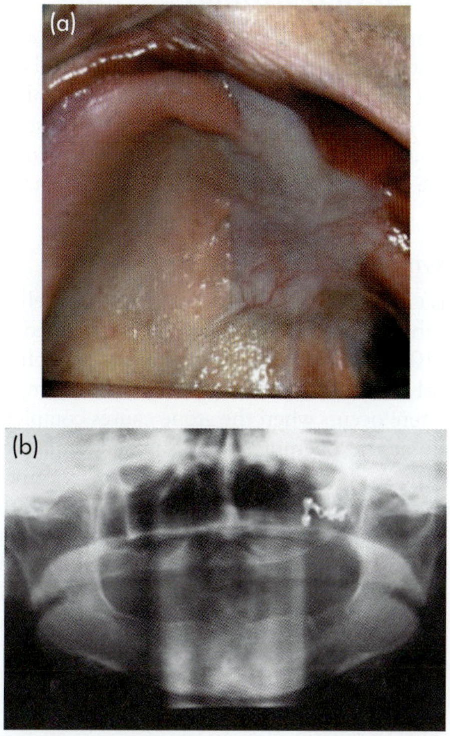

Figure 50.5 (a) Postoperative appearance following left maxillectomy and immediate reconstruction with a vascularised iliac crest graft and abdominal wall musculature (epithelialised). (b) Postoperative radiographic appearance of a reconstructed left maxilla with internal fixation.

Common disorders of the sublingual glands

Cysts

Minor mucous retention cysts develop in the floor of the mouth either from an obstructed minor salivary gland or from the sublingual salivary gland. The term 'ranula' should be applied only to a mucous extravasation cyst that arises from a sublingual gland. It produces a characteristic translucent swelling that takes on the appearance of a 'frog's belly' (ranula) (Figure 50.6). A ranula can resolve spontaneously, but many also require formal surgical excision of the cyst and the affected sublingual gland. Incision and drainage, however tempting, usually results in recurrence.

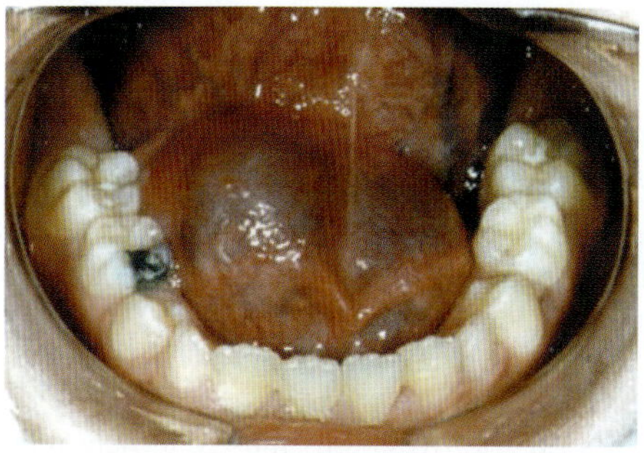

Figure 50.6 Large ranula affecting the floor of the mouth.

Plunging ranula

Plunging ranula is a rare form of mucous retention cyst that can arise from both sublingual and submandibular salivary glands. Mucus collects within the cyst, which perforates through the mylohyoid muscle diaphragm to enter the neck. Patients present with a dumb-bell-shaped swelling that is soft, fluctuant and painless in the submandibular or submental region of the neck (Figure 50.7a and b). Diagnosis is made on ultrasound or magnetic resonance imaging (MRI) examination. Excision is usually performed via a cervical approach removing the cyst and both the submandibular and sublingual glands. Smaller plunging ranulas can be treated successfully by transoral sublingual gland excision, with or without marsupialisation.

Tumours

Tumours involving the sublingual gland are extremely rare and are usually (85 per cent) malignant. They present as a hard or firm painless swelling in the floor of the mouth. Treatment requires wide excision involving the overlying mucosa and simultaneous neck dissection. Immediate reconstruction of the intraoral defect is recommended using, for example, a radial artery forearm flap.

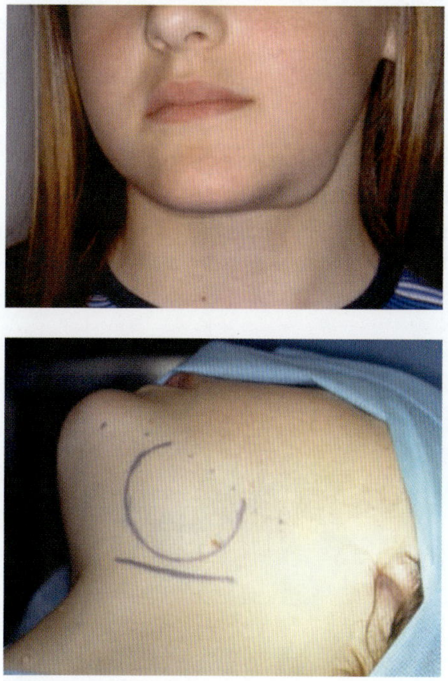

Figure 50.7 Plunging ranula in the left submandibular region.

Ranula is derived from 'rana', the Latin for frog.
Thomas Wharton, 1616–1673, physician, St Thomas's Hospital, London, UK, described the submandibular duct in 1656.

THE SUBMANDIBULAR GLANDS

Anatomy

The submandibular glands are paired salivary glands that lie below the mandible on either side. They consist of a larger superficial and a smaller deep lobe that are continuous around the posterior border of the mylohyoid muscle. Important anatomical relations include the anterior facial vein running over the surface of the gland and the facial artery. The deep part of the gland lies on the hyoglossus muscle closely related to the lingual nerve and inferior to the hypoglossal nerve. The gland is surrounded by a well-defined capsule that is derived from the deep cervical fascia which splits to enclose it. The gland is drained by a single submandibular duct (Wharton's duct) that emerges from its deep surface and runs in the space between the hyoglossus and mylohyoid muscles. It drains into the anterior floor of the mouth at the sublingual papilla. There are several lymph nodes immediately adjacent and sometimes within the superficial part of the gland (Summary box 50.3).

Summary box 50.3

Important anatomical relationships of the submandibular glands

- Lingual nerve
- Hypoglossal nerve
- Anterior facial vein
- Facial artery
- Marginal mandibular branch of the facial nerve

Ectopic/aberrant salivary gland tissue

The most common ectopic salivary tissue is the Stafne bone cyst. This presents as an asymptomatic, clearly demarcated radiolucency of the angle of the mandible, characteristically below the inferior dental neurovascular bundle (Figure 50.8). It is formed by invagination into the bone on the lingual aspect of the mandible of an ectopic lobe of the juxtaposed submandibular gland. No treatment is required.

Inflammatory disorders of the submandibular gland

Inflammation of the submandibular gland is termed sialadenitis. Submandibular sialadenitis may be acute, chronic or acute on chronic.

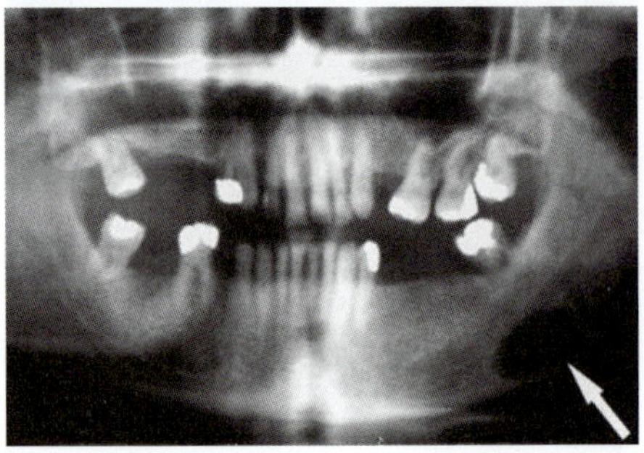

Figure 50.8 Plain radiographic appearance of a Stafne bone cyst.

Common causes are:

- Acute submandibular sialadenitis:
  - **Viral**. The paramyxovirus (mumps) is a viral illness of the salivary glands that usually produces parotitis. The submandibular glands are occasionally involved, causing painful tender swollen glands. Other viral infections of the submandibular gland are extremely rare.
  - **Bacterial**. Bacterial sialadenitis is more common than viral sialadenitis and occurs secondary to obstruction. Following infection and despite control of acute symptoms with antibiotics, the gland frequently becomes chronically inflamed and requires formal excision.
- Chronic submandibular sialadenitis.

Obstruction and trauma

The most common cause of obstruction within the submandibular gland is stone formation (sialothiasis) within the gland and its associated duct system. Eighty per cent of all salivary stones occur in the submandibular glands because their secretions are highly viscous. Eighty per cent of submandibular stones are radio-opaque and can be identified on plain radiography (Figure 50.9).

Clinical symptoms

Patients usually present with acute painful swelling in the region of the submandibular gland, precipitated by eating (Figure 50.10). The swelling occurs rapidly and often resolves spontaneously over 1–2 hours after the meal is completed. This classical picture occurs when the stone causes complete obstruction, usually at the opening of the submandibular duct. More frequently, the stone causes only partial obstruction when it lies within the hilum of the gland or within the duct in the floor of the mouth. In such circumstances, symptoms are more infrequent, producing minimal discomfort and swelling, not confined to mealtimes. Clinical examination reveals an enlarged firm submandibular gland, tender on bimanual examination. Pus may

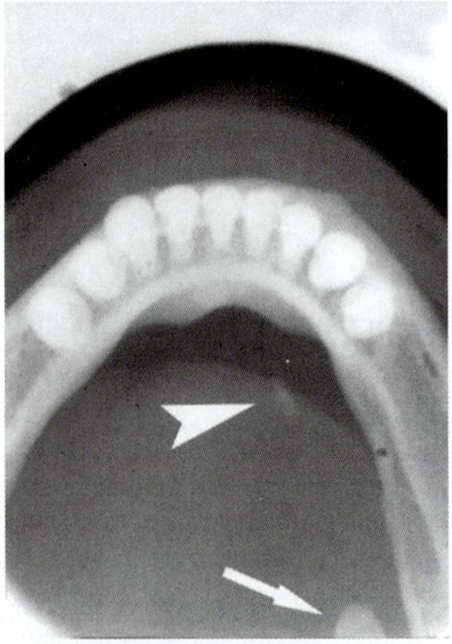

Figure 50.9 Lower occlusal x-ray highlighting a radio-opaque submandibular duct stone (arrowhead). Note the larger stone posteriorly located in the hilum of the gland (arrow).

Edward C Stafne, 1894–1981, dental surgeon, the Mayo Clinic, Rochester, MN, USA, described these cysts in 1942.

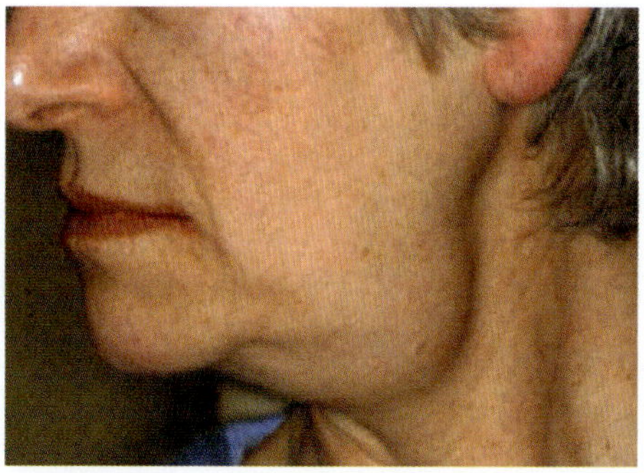

Figure 50.10 Acute left submandibular sialadenitis.

be visible, draining from the sublingual papilla (Figure 50.11), the consequence of chronic and non-specific bacterial infection.

Management

If the stone is lying within the submandibular duct in the floor of the mouth anterior to the point at which the duct crosses the lingual nerve (second molar region), the stone can be removed by incising longitudinally over the duct. Once the stone has been delivered, the wall of the duct should be left open to promote free drainage of saliva. Suturing the duct will lead to stricture formation and the recurrence of obstructive symptoms. Where the stone is proximal to the lingual nerve, i.e. at the hilum of the gland, stone retrieval via an intraoral approach should be avoided as there is a high risk of damage to the lingual nerve during exploration in the posterior lingual gutter. Treatment is by simultaneous submandibular gland excision and removal of the stone and ligation of the submandibular duct under direct vision. The retrieval of stone via an endoscopic approach, and/or removal by lithotripsy is gaining favour in some centres, but specialist equipment including a sialadenoscope is required.

Other causes of submandibular duct obstruction include external pressure, particularly trauma to the floor of the mouth from an overextended flange on a lower denture which impinges on the sublingual papilla causing inflammation and subsequent stricture.

Submandibular gland excision

Submandibular gland excision is indicated for:

- sialadenitis
- salivary tumours.

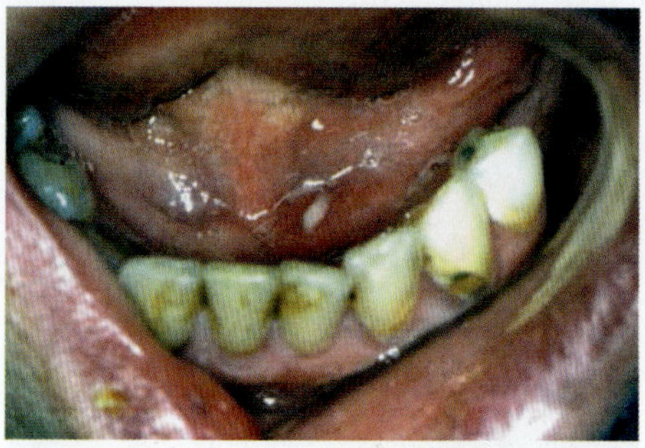

Figure 50.11 Acute suppurative submandibular sialadenitis. There is pus extruding from the left sublingual papilla.

Excision of the submandibular gland involves four distinct phases.

Incision and exposure of gland

Surgery is usually performed under endotracheal general anaesthesia with moderate neck extension and the chin rotated to the opposite side. The incision should be marked at least 3–4 cm below the lower border of the mandible to avoid damage to the marginal mandibular branch of the facial nerve (Figure 50.12a). The incision should be sited within the nearest skin crease and should be no more than 6 cm long. Infiltration with lidocaine with adrenaline is optional. Sharp dissection is performed down to the platysma muscle, which should be clearly identified to facilitate later closure (Figure 50.12b). The muscle is incised and then retracted. The underlying investing layer of deep cervical fascia is then divided, and the marginal mandibular branch of the facial nerve that normally runs on the deep surface of the platysma muscle is preserved. Posteriorly, the incision approaches the angular tract where the deep cervical fascia splits to form the investing layer around the sternomastoid muscle. Superficial veins, including the anterior facial vein, require ligation.

Gland mobilisation

Deepening the incision divides the submandibular gland capsule. In inflammatory conditions, the submandibular gland is excised by intracapsular dissection, mobilising the gland by sharp dissection. For tumours of the submandibular gland, extracapsular dissection by suprahyoid neck dissection is performed.

The superficial lobe of the submandibular gland is first mobilised by retracting superiorly with an Allis forceps. As dissection proceeds, the posterior belly and anterior belly of the digastric muscle are identified. Dissection posteriorly identifies the facial artery (Figure 50.13), which is divided to facilitate further mobilisation. The course of the facial artery is variable, sometimes penetrating the gland emerging on the upper border, and

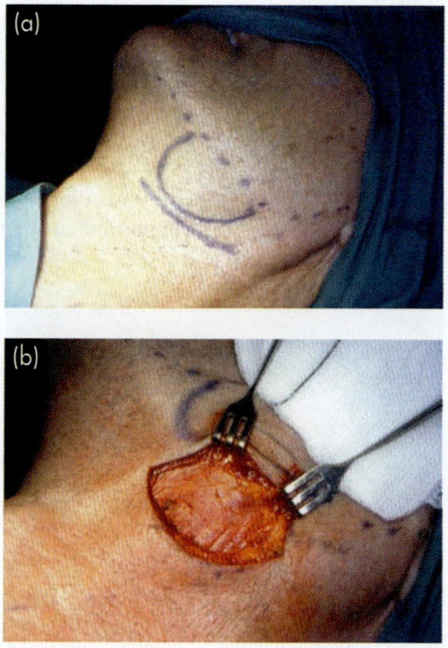

Figure 50.12 (a) Surface landmarks of submandibular gland excision. (b) Skin flaps elevated and platysma exposed.

Oscar Huntington Allis, 1836–1921, surgeon, The Presbyterian Hospital, Philadelphia, PA, USA.

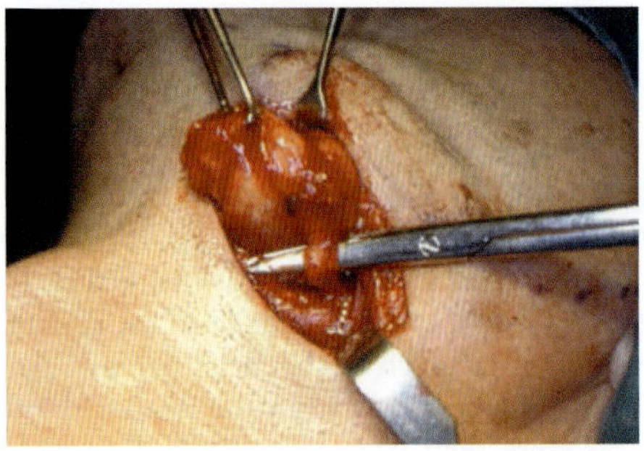

Figure 50.13 Submandibular gland mobilisation and exposure of the facial artery.

sometimes lying in a groove on the deeper aspect of the gland. The gland is further mobilised by blunt and sharp dissection. A number of small arteries and veins are encountered, which require control with bipolar diathermy.

Dissection of the deep lobe and identification of the lingual nerve

An important landmark in submandibular gland dissection is the posterior border of the mylohyoid muscle. Once identified, it can be retracted forwards to reveal the deep lobe of the gland. Several veins are usually encountered, which need to be controlled with diathermy. The gland is then retracted inferiorly, invariably attached to the lingual nerve through parasympathetic secretor motor fibres. In the presence of chronic infection and subsequent fibrosis, identification of the lingual nerve on the deep aspect of the gland is sometimes difficult. It is imperative that the lingual nerve is formally identified prior to division of the parasympathetic fibres. The gland is then pedicled entirely on the submandibular duct, which, once identified, is ligated. The gland is delivered and sent for histological examination. The hypoglossal nerves lie deep to the submandibular capsule and should not be damaged during intracapsular dissection (Figure 50.14).

Three cranial nerves are at risk during removal of the submandibular gland:

1. the marginal mandibular branch of the facial nerve
2. the lingual nerve
3. the hypoglossal nerve.

An adequate incision coupled with meticulous haemostasis allows the surgeon to identify these important structures during surgery.

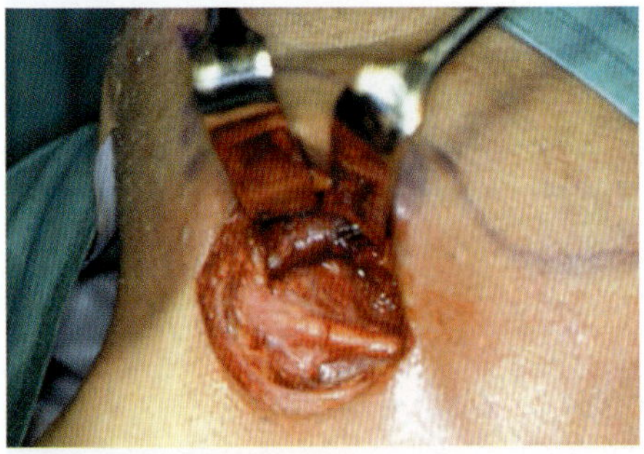

Figure 50.14 Bed of the submandibular triangle following submandibular gland removal, revealing the posterior edge of the mylohyoid muscle and the tendon of the digastric muscle.

Wound closure

Haemostasis is confirmed and a vacuum suction drain inserted. The wound is closed using a continuous resorbable suture to the platysma muscle, as the platysma muscle has a direct contribution to the depressor activity of the corner of the mouth. The skin may be closed with a subcuticular non-resorbable suture, removed 7 days after surgery. The drain remains for 24 hours.

Complications of submandibular gland excision

Complications are:

- haematoma
- wound infection
- marginal mandibular nerve injury
- lingual nerve injury
- hypoglossal nerve injury
- transection of the nerve to the mylohyoid muscle producing submental skin anaesthesia.

Tumours of the submandibular gland

Tumours of the submandibular gland are uncommon and usually present as a slow-growing, painless swelling within the submandibular triangle (Figure 50.15). Only 50 per cent of submandibular gland tumours are benign, in contrast to 80–90 per cent of parotid gland tumours (Table 50.1). In many circumstances, the swelling cannot, on clinical examination, be differentiated from submandibular lymphadenopathy. Most salivary neoplasms, even malignant tumours, are often slow-growing, painless swellings. Unfortunately, pain is not a reliable indication of malignancy as benign tumours often present with pain in the affected gland, presumably due to capsular distension or outflow obstruction.

Table 50.1 Salivary gland tumours – frequency and distribution.

Type	Location	Frequency	Malignant (%)
Major	Parotid	Common	10–20
	Submandibular	Uncommon	50
	Sublingual	Very rare	85
Minor	Upper aerodigestive tract	Rare	90

Clinical features of malignant salivary tumours

These include:

- facial nerve weakness
- rapid enlargement of the swelling
- induration and/or ulceration of the overlying skin
- cervical node enlargement.

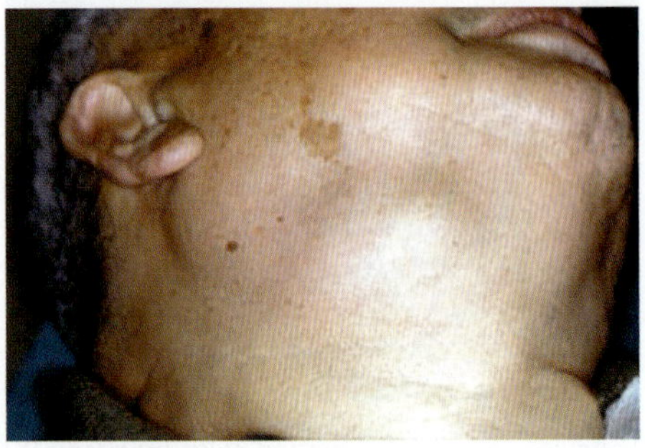

Figure 50.15 Benign tumour of the right submandibular gland.

Investigation

Computed tomography (CT) and MRI scanning are the most helpful techniques for imaging tumours arising in the major salivary glands. The tumour is intrinsic to the gland, and its border can be imaged to highlight whether it is circumscribed and probably benign, or diffuse, invasive and probably malignant. The scan will highlight the relationship of the tumour to other anatomical structures, which is helpful in planning surgery.

Open surgical biopsy is contraindicated as this may seed the tumour into surrounding tissues, making it impossible to eradicate microscopic deposits of tumour cells.

Fine-needle aspiration biopsy is a safe alternative to open biopsy. There is evidence to suggest that, provided the needle gauge does not exceed 18G, there is no risk of seeding viable tumour cells. The role of fine-needle aspiration biopsy is, however, controversial as it rarely alters surgical management.

Management of submandibular gland tumours

As with all salivary gland tumours, surgical excision with a cuff of normal tissue is the goal. When the tumour is small and entirely encased within the submandibular gland parenchyma, straightforward intracapsular submandibular gland excision is appropriate. However, benign tumours that are large and project beyond the submandibular gland are best served by suprahyoid neck dissection, preserving the marginal mandibular branch of the facial nerve, lingual nerve and hypoglossal nerves. This entails a full clearance of the submandibular triangle, involving the development of a subplatysmal skin flap (Figure 50.16a–e), dissection of periosteum along the lower border and inner aspect of the mandible, and delivery of the gland and tumour with a cuff of normal tissue. In cases of overt malignancy, modified neck dissection or radical neck dissection is appropriate. This may necessitate sacrifice of the lingual and hypoglossal nerves if the tumour is adherent to the deep bed of the gland (Figure 50.17a–d).

THE PAROTID GLAND

Anatomy

The parotid gland lies in a recess bounded by the ramus of the mandible, the base of the skull and the mastoid process. It lies on the carotid sheath and the XIth and XIIth cranial nerves and extends forward over the masseter muscle. The gland is enclosed in a sheath of dense deep cervical fascia. Its upper pole extends just below the zygoma and its lower pole into the neck.

Several important structures run through the parotid gland. These include:

- branches of the facial nerve;
- the terminal branch of the external carotid artery that divides into the maxillary artery and the superficial temporal artery;

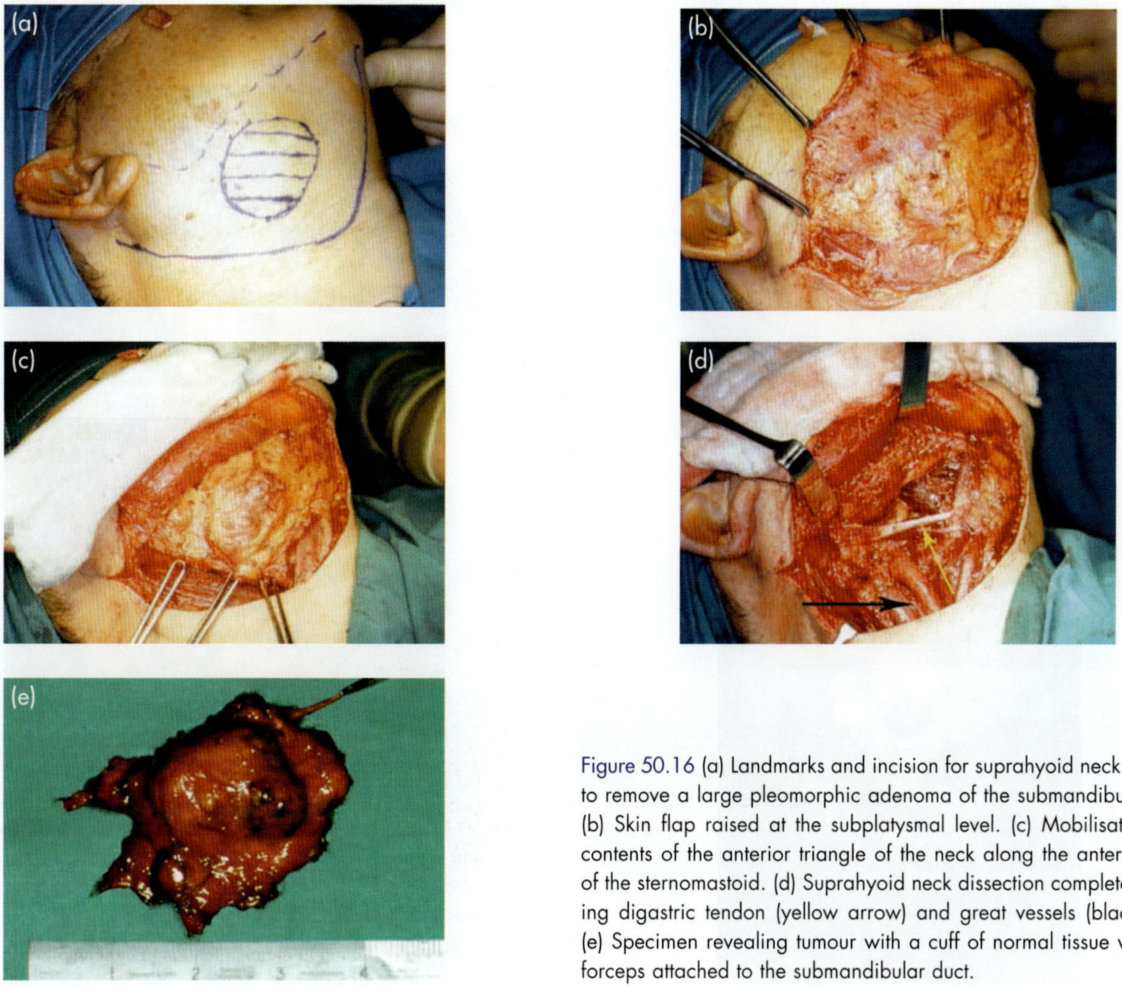

Figure 50.16 (a) Landmarks and incision for suprahyoid neck dissection to remove a large pleomorphic adenoma of the submandibular gland. (b) Skin flap raised at the subplatysmal level. (c) Mobilisation of the contents of the anterior triangle of the neck along the anterior border of the sternomastoid. (d) Suprahyoid neck dissection completed, revealing digastric tendon (yellow arrow) and great vessels (black arrow). (e) Specimen revealing tumour with a cuff of normal tissue with artery forceps attached to the submandibular duct.

- the retromandibular vein;
- intraparotid lymph nodes.

The gland is arbitrarily divided into deep and superficial lobes, separated by the facial nerve. Eighty per cent of the parotid gland lies superficial and 20 per cent deep to the nerve. An accessory lobe is occasionally present lying anterior to the superficial lobe on the masseter muscle.

Developmental disorders

Developmental disorders such as agenesis, duct atresia and congenital fistula are extremely rare.

Inflammatory disorders

Viral infections

Mumps is the most common cause of acute painful parotid swelling and predominantly affects children. It is spread via airborne droplets of infected saliva. The disease starts with a prodromal period of 1–2 days, during which the patient experiences fever, nausea and headache. This is followed by pain and swelling in one or both parotid glands. Parotid pain can be very severe and exacerbated by eating and drinking. Symptoms resolve within 5–10 days. The diagnosis is based on history and clinical examination; a recent contact with an infected patient with a painful parotid swelling is often sufficient to lead to a diagnosis. Atypical viral parotitis does occur and may present with predominantly unilateral swelling or even submandibular involvement. A single episode of infection confers lifelong immunity. Treatment of mumps is symptomatic with regular paracetamol and adequate oral fluid intake. Complications of orchitis, oophoritis, pancreatitis, sensorineural deafness and meningoencephalitis are rare, but are more likely to occur in adults.

Other viral agents that produce parotitis include Coxsackie A and B, parainfluenza 1 and 3, Echo and lymphocytic choriomeningitis.

Bacterial infections

Acute ascending bacterial sialadenitis is historically described in dehydrated elderly patients following major surgery. Reduced salivary flow secondary to dehydration results in ascending infection via the parotid duct into the parotid parenchyma. Acute bacterial parotitis is now more common with no obvious precipitating factors. The patient presents with a tender, painful parotid swelling that arises over several hours (Figure 50.18). There is generalised malaise, pyrexia and occasional cervical lymphadenopathy. The pain is exacerbated by eating or drinking. The parotid swelling may be diffuse, but often localises to the lower pole of the gland. Intraoral examination may reveal pus exuding from the parotid gland papilla. The infecting organism is usually *Staphylococcus aureus* or *Streptococcus viridans*, and treatment is with appropriate intravenous antibiotics. If the gland becomes fluctuant, ultrasound may identify abscess formation within the gland that may require aspiration with a large-bore needle or formal drainage under general anaesthesia. In the latter procedure, the skin incision should be made low to avoid

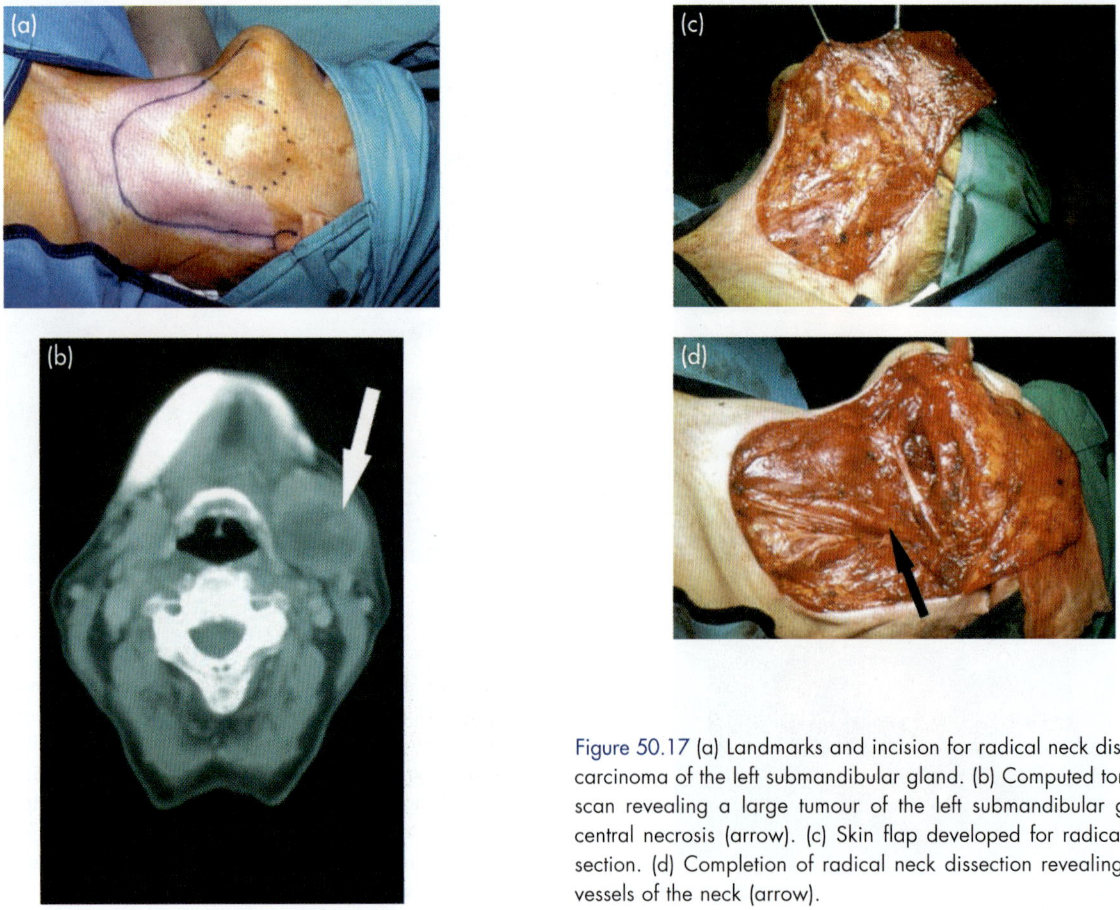

Figure 50.17 (a) Landmarks and incision for radical neck dissection for carcinoma of the left submandibular gland. (b) Computed tomographic scan revealing a large tumour of the left submandibular gland with central necrosis (arrow). (c) Skin flap developed for radical neck dissection. (d) Completion of radical neck dissection revealing the great vessels of the neck (arrow).

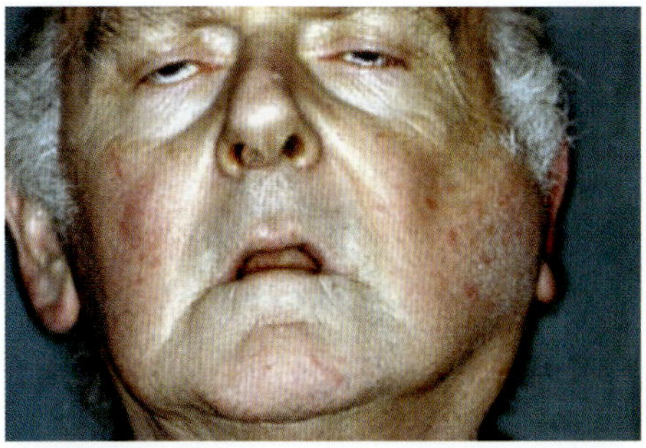

Figure 50.18 Acute left bacterial parotitis.

damage to the lower branch of the facial nerve. Blunt dissection using sinus forceps is preferred, and the cavity is opened to facilitate drainage. A drain is inserted and left *in situ* for 24–72 hours. Sialography is contraindicated during acute infection. Chronic bacterial sialadenitis is rare in the parotid gland.

Recurrent parotitis of childhood

Recurrent parotitis of childhood is a distinct clinical entity of unknown aetiology and variable prognosis. It is characterised by rapid swelling of one or both parotid glands, in which the symptoms are made worse by chewing and eating. Systemic upset with fever and malaise is variable. The symptoms usually last from 3 to 7 days, and are then followed by a quiescent period of weeks to several months. Children usually present between the ages of three and six years, although symptoms have been reported in infants as young as four months. The diagnosis is based on the characteristic history and can be confirmed by sialography. This shows a characteristic punctate sialectasis likened to a 'snowstorm' (Figure 50.19). The condition usually responds to short courses of antibiotics although, if recurrence is frequent, prophylactic low-dose antibiotics may be required for several months or even years. Few children require formal parotidectomy. However, if the onset of symptoms is late, e.g. adolescence/early adulthood, fewer patients respond to conservative measures and may require total conservative parotidectomy.

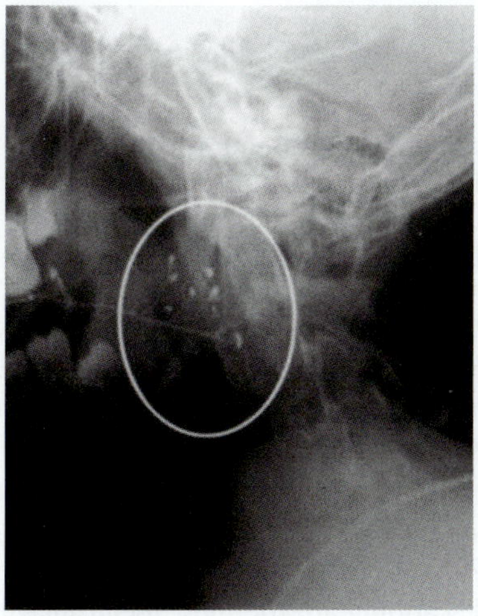

Figure 50.19 Characteristic 'snowstorm' appearance of recurrent parotitis of childhood (circled).

Human immunodeficiency virus-associated sialadenitis

Chronic parotitis in children is pathognomonic of human immunodeficiency virus (HIV) infection. The presentation of HIV-associated sialadenitis is very similar to classical Sjögren's syndrome in adulthood. Although HIV-associated sialadenitis and Sjögren's syndrome are histologically similar, the former condition is usually associated with a negative autoantibody screen. Other presentations of salivary gland disease in HIV-positive patients include multiple parotid cysts, which cause gross parotid swelling and facial disfigurement. CT and MRI demonstrate the characteristic 'Swiss cheese' appearance of multiple large cystic lesions (Figure 50.20). The swollen glands are usually painless and may regress on the institution of antiviral therapy. Parotidectomy, however, may be indicated to improve the appearance.

Obstructive parotitis

There are several causes of obstructive parotitis, which produces intermittent painful swelling of the parotid gland, particularly at mealtimes.

Papillary obstruction

Obstructive parotitis is less common than obstructive submandibular sialadenitis but, nevertheless, can be caused by trauma to the parotid papilla through either an overextended upper denture flange or a fractured upper molar tooth. The subsequent inflammation and oedema obstructs salivary flow, particularly at mealtimes. The patient usually experiences rapid onset pain and swelling at mealtimes. If left untreated, progressive scarring and fibrosis in and around the parotid duct papilla will produce a permanent stenosis. Symptoms are unlikely to resolve unless a papillotomy is performed. This is a simple procedure performed under either local or general anaesthesia. The parotid duct is

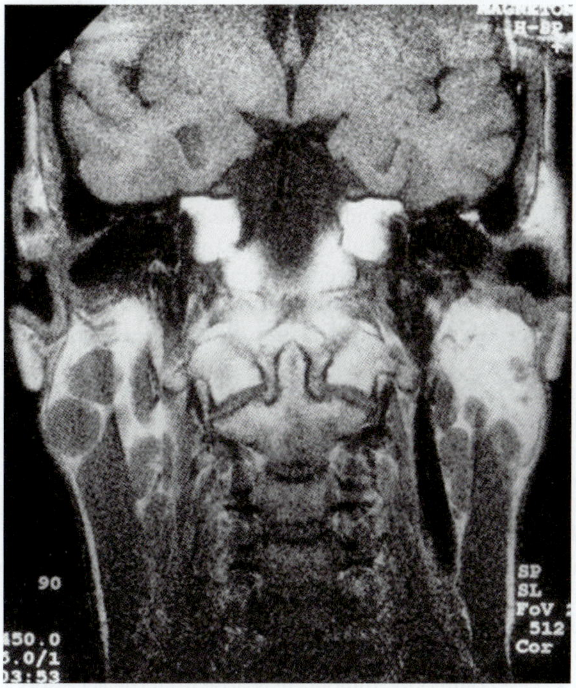

Figure 50.20 Magnetic resonance imaging scan. Giant bilateral parotid cysts in human immunodeficiency virus infection.

Henrik Samuel Conrad Sjögren, 1899–1986, Professor of Ophthalmology, Göthenburg, Sweden, described this condition in 1933.
A Swiss cheese is one with many holes in it.

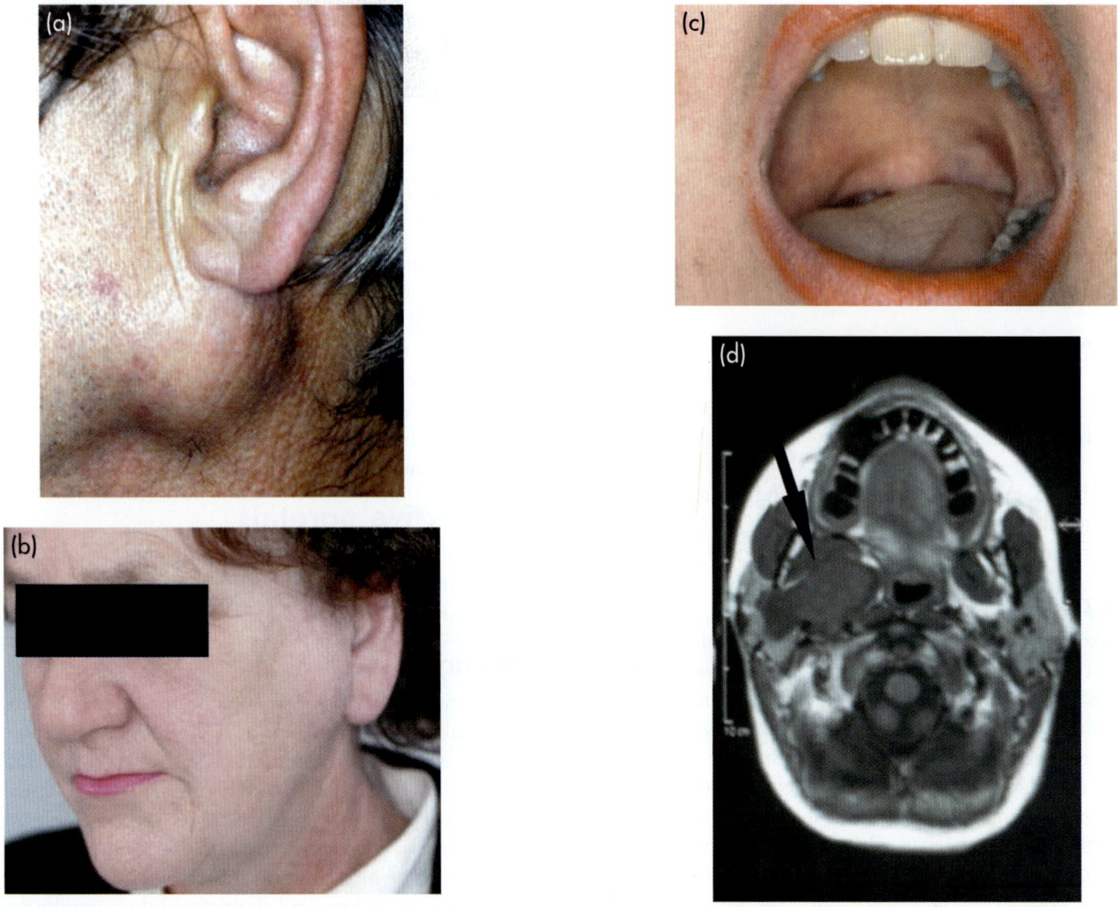

Figure 50.21 (a) Benign tumour of the left parotid gland producing characteristic deflection of the ear lobe. (b) Pleomorphic adenoma arising from the upper pole of the left parotid gland producing a pre-auricular swelling. (c) Deep lobe tumour of the right parotid presenting with a swelling of the right soft palate. (d) Magnetic resonance imaging scan revealing a large deep lobe tumour (arrow) of the right parotid gland, occupying the parapharyngeal space.

cannulated, and the distal parotid duct is laid open by incising longitudinally down onto the probe allowing free drainage of saliva.

Stone formation

Sialolithiasis is less common in the parotid gland (20 per cent) than in the submandibular gland (80 per cent). Parotid duct stones are usually radiolucent and rarely visible on plain radiography. They are frequently located at the confluence of the collecting ducts or located in the distal aspect of the parotid duct adjacent to the parotid papilla. Parotid gland sialography is usually required to identify the stone. A stone located in the collecting duct or within the gland may be managed by either endoscopic retrieval, lithotripsy or, least likely, surgical removal via a parotidectomy approach.

Tumours of the parotid gland

The parotid gland is the most common site for salivary tumours. Most tumours arise in the superficial lobe and present as slow-growing, painless swellings below the ear (Figure 50.21a), in front of the ear (Figure 50.21b) or in the upper aspect of the neck. Less commonly, tumours may arise from the accessory lobe and present as persistent swellings within the cheek. Rarely, tumours may arise from the deep lobe of the gland and present as parapharyngeal masses (Figure 50.21c and d). Symptoms include difficulty in swallowing and snoring. Clinical examination reveals a diffuse firm swelling in the soft palate and tonsil.

Some 80–90 per cent of tumours of the parotid gland are benign, the most common being pleomorphic adenoma (Table 50.2).

Malignant salivary gland tumours are divided into two distinct subgroups:

1 **Low-grade malignant tumours**, e.g. acinic cell carcinoma, are indistinguishable on clinical examination from benign neoplasms.
2 **High-grade malignant tumours** usually present as rapidly growing, often painless swellings in and around the parotid gland. The tumour presents as either a discrete mass with infiltration into the overlying skin (Figure 50.22) or a diffuse but hard swelling of the gland with no discrete mass. Presentation with advanced disease is common, and cervical lymph node metastases may be present.

Investigations

CT and MRI scanning are the most useful imaging techniques (Figure 50.23a and b). Fine-needle aspiration biopsy may aid in obtaining a preoperative diagnosis, but open surgical biopsy

Aldred Scott Warthin, 1866–1931, Professor of Pathology, University of Michigan, Ann Arbor, MI, USA.

Table 50.2 Classification of salivary gland tumours (simplified).

Type	Subgroup	Common examples
I Adenoma	Pleomorphic Monomorphic	Pleomorphic adenoma Adenolymphoma (Warthin's tumour)
II Carcinoma	Low grade	Acinic cell carcinoma Adenoid cystic carcinoma Low-grade mucoepidermoid carcinoma
	High grade	Adenocarcinoma Squamous cell carcinoma High-grade mucoepidermoid carcinoma
III Non-epithelial tumours		Haemangioma, lymphangioma
IV Lymphomas	Primary lymphomas Secondary lymphomas	Non-Hodgkin's lymphomas Lymphomas in Sjögren's syndrome
V Secondary tumours	Local Distant	Tumours of the head and neck especially Skin and bronchus
VI Unclassified tumours		
VII Tumour-like lesions	Solid lesions	Benign lymphoepithelial lesion Adenomatoid hyperplasia
	Cystic lesions	Salivary gland cysts

is contraindicated unless malignancy is suspected, and preoperative histological diagnosis is required as a prelude to radical parotidectomy.

All tumours of the superficial lobe of the parotid gland should be managed by superficial parotidectomy. There is no role for enucleation even if a benign lesion is suspected. The aim of superficial parotidectomy is to remove the tumour with a cuff of normal surrounding tissue. The term 'suprafacial parotidectomy' has been used as not all branches of the facial nerve need be formally dissected, particularly if a tumour lies in the lower pole of the parotid gland.

Parotidectomy

Superficial parotidectomy

Superficial parotidectomy is the most common procedure for parotid gland pathology. Surgery is performed under endotracheal general anaesthesia, which may or may not be accompanied by hypotensive anaesthesia to facilitate dissection, improve the visual surgical field and reduce blood loss. The operation has several distinct phases.

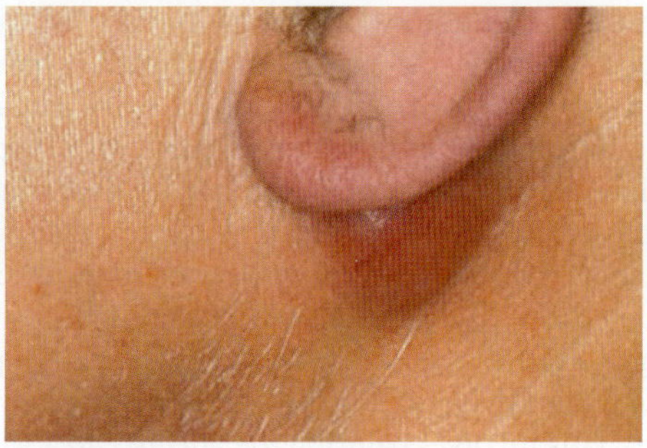

Figure 50.22 Malignant tumour of the left parotid gland with invasion of the overlying skin.

Incision and development of a skin flap

The most commonly used incision is the 'lazy S' pre-auricular–mastoid–cervical (Figure 50.24a). The incision is marked out and marked at three points along its length to facilitate closure. Infiltration with local anaesthetic and adrenaline is optional, but does aid in the development of the skin flap, improves visibility and reduces blood loss in the initial phase. The skin flap is developed in an anterior direction by either scalpel or scissors dissection. The plane of dissection is well below the hair follicles, just above the parotid fascia. The skin flap is developed forwards to the anterior border of the gland. Posterior undermining of the incision in the cervical region facilitates access to the anterior border of the sternomastoid muscle.

Mobilisation of the gland

This phase of the dissection aims to free the posterior margin of the gland, allowing identification of the facial nerve. Clips are applied along the fascia overlying the sternomastoid muscle, with the assistant applying traction anteriorly. By sharp dissection along the anterior border of the sternomastoid, an avascular plane is developed (Figure 50.24b), which requires elective transection of the great auricular nerve. At the lower end of the dissection, the external jugular vein is often encountered and ligated. The gland is gradually mobilised by sharp dissection up to and on to the anterior aspect of the mastoid process, identifying the posterior belly of the digastric muscle.

A second avascular plane is developed along the anterior border of the cartilaginous and bony external auditory meatus immediately anterior to the tragus. The two avascular planes are then connected by blunt and sharp dissection. By developing two broad avascular planes, identification of the facial nerve trunk is facilitated (Figure 50.24c). It is best achieved by scissors dissection in the line of the facial nerve trunk. Use of a facial nerve stimulator is optional. Landmarks commonly used to aid identification of the trunk of the facial nerve are:

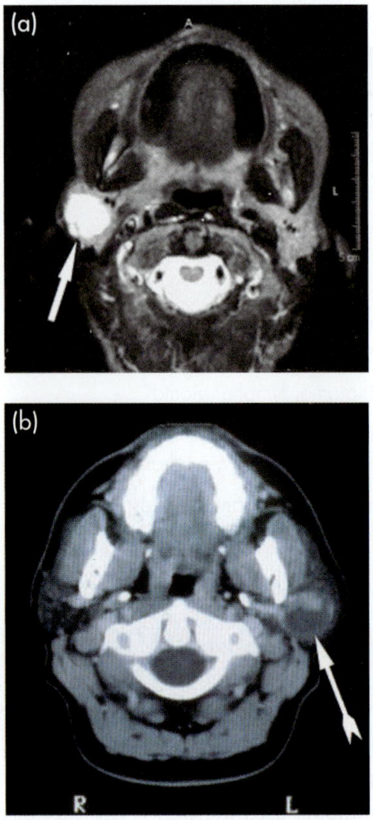

Figure 50.23 (a) Magnetic resonance imaging scan revealing a space-occupying lesion (arrow) in the right parotid gland; histology revealed pleomorphic adenoma. (b) Computed tomographic scan of the left parotid gland revealing a cystic lesion (arrow). Histology revealed acinic cell carcinoma.

- the inferior portion of the cartilaginous canal. This is termed Conley's pointer and indicates the position of the facial nerve, which lies 1 cm deep and inferior to its tip.
- the upper border of the posterior belly of the digastric muscle. Identification of this muscle not only mobilises the parotid gland, but also exposes an area immediately superior, in which the facial nerve is usually located.

Location of the facial nerve trunk

Once the facial nerve trunk is identified, gentle traction anteriorly facilitates further mobilisation. Control of haemorrhage at this stage is vital as bleeding, no matter how minor, significantly impedes visibility for the surgeon. Haemostasis can be achieved with bipolar diathermy, although caution is necessary, particularly when the facial nerve is approached. Damage to the stylomastoid artery, which lies immediately lateral to the nerve, can result in troublesome bleeding immediately prior to identification. Pledget swabs soaked in adrenaline are sometimes helpful in reducing the ooze associated with this phase of the dissection.

Dissection of the gland off the facial nerve

Once the facial nerve trunk is identified, further exposure of the branch of the facial nerve can be achieved by scissors dissection in the perineural plane immediately above the nerve. The tunnel thus created is then laid open, and divisions and branches of the facial nerve are followed to the periphery in a sequential manner, usually beginning with the upper division. The upper division divides into a temporal and a zygomatic branch, and the lower division into mandibular and cervical branches. In this way, the superficial lobe and its associated tumour are mobilised in a superior to inferior direction (Figure 50.24d). The upper division of the nerve is frequently tortuous in its course and can be damaged unless great care is taken during perineural dissection. It is often not necessary to dissect all branches of the facial nerve completely, as adequate tumour clearance can be achieved with a more conservative resection of the superficial lobe. When a branch of the facial nerve is adherent to the tumour or running through the tumour, it may require elective division. With the exception of the buccal branch, the transected nerve should be repaired immediately with a cable graft, harvested from the great auricular nerve.

Closure

The patient is placed into a Trendelenburg position to identify any residual bleeding vessels. A suction drain is applied for a period of 24–48 hours, and the wound closed in layers (Figure 50.24f).

Radical parotidectomy

Radical parotidectomy is performed for patients in whom there is clear histological evidence of a high-grade malignant tumour, e.g. squamous cell carcinoma. Low-grade malignant tumours can usually be managed by standard superficial parotidectomy. Radical parotidectomy involves removal of all parotid gland tissue and elective sectioning of the facial nerve, usually through the main trunk (Figure 50.25a–f). The surgery inevitably removes the ipsilateral masseter muscle and may also require simultaneous neck dissection, particularly where there is clinical, radiological and cytological evidence of lymph node metastases in the ipsilateral neck.

Complications of parotid gland surgery

Complications of parotid gland surgery include:

- haematoma formation;
- infection;
- temporary facial nerve weakness;
- transection of the facial nerve and permanent facial weakness;
- sialocoele;
- facial numbness;
- permanent numbness of the ear lobe associated with great auricular nerve transection;
- Frey's syndrome.

Frey's syndrome

Frey's syndrome (gustatory sweating) is now considered an inevitable consequence of parotidectomy, unless preventative measures are taken (see below). It results from damage to the autonomic innervation of the salivary gland with inappropriate regeneration of parasympathetic nerve fibres that stimulate the sweat glands of the overlying skin. The clinical features include sweating and erythema over the region of surgical excision of the parotid gland as a consequence of autonomic stimulation of salivation by the smell or taste of food. The symptoms are entirely variable and are clinically demonstrated by a starch iodine test. This involves painting the affected area with iodine, which is allowed to dry before applying dry starch, which turns blue on exposure to iodine in the presence of sweat. Sweating

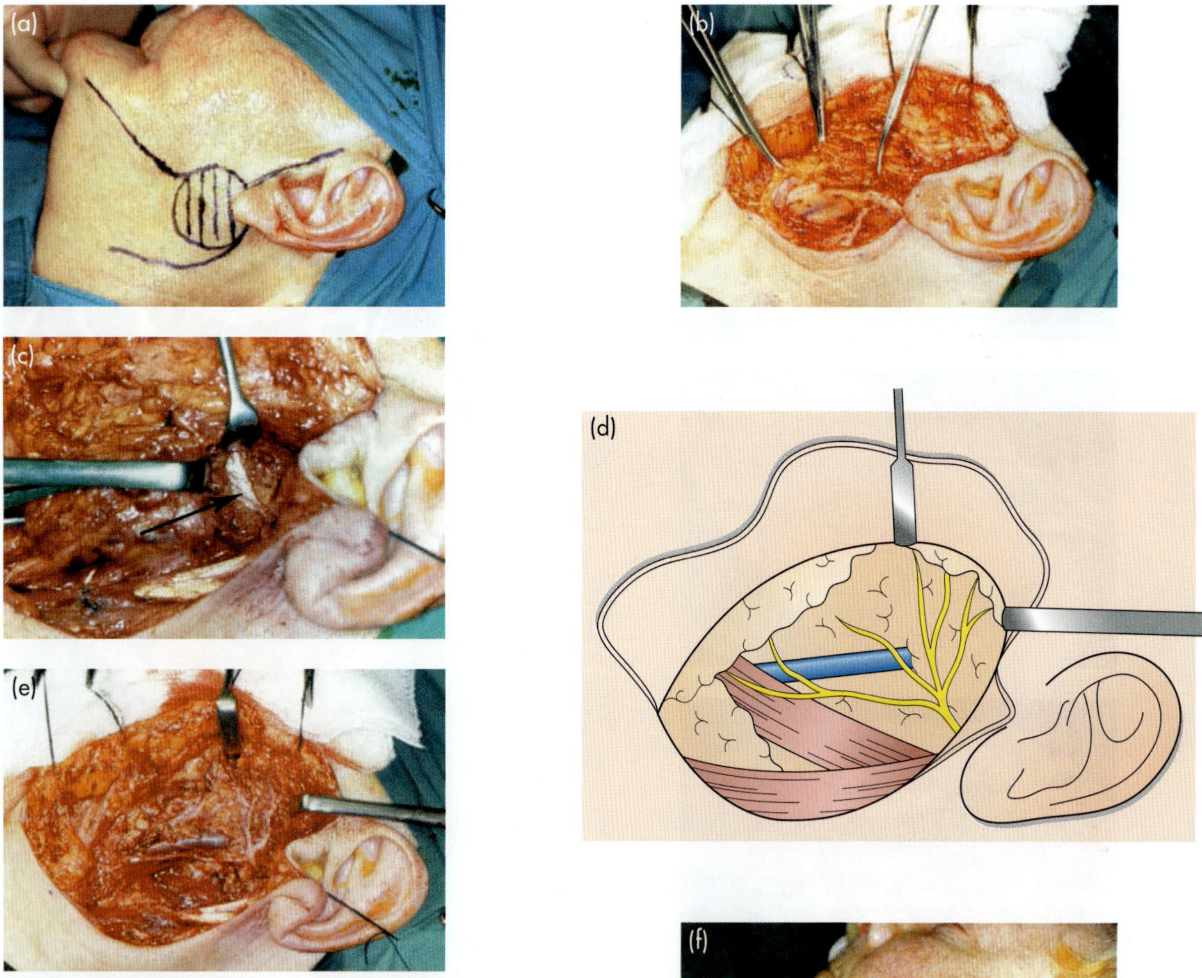

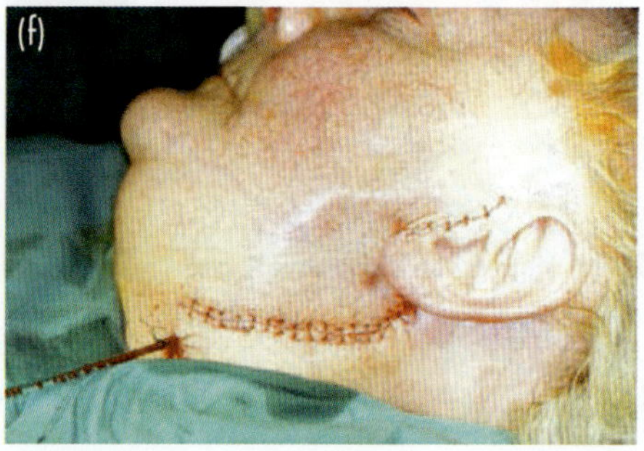

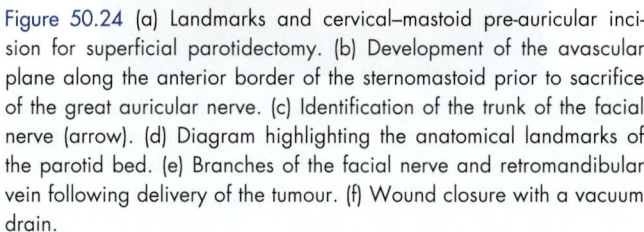

Figure 50.24 (a) Landmarks and cervical–mastoid pre-auricular incision for superficial parotidectomy. (b) Development of the avascular plane along the anterior border of the sternomastoid prior to sacrifice of the great auricular nerve. (c) Identification of the trunk of the facial nerve (arrow). (d) Diagram highlighting the anatomical landmarks of the parotid bed. (e) Branches of the facial nerve and retromandibular vein following delivery of the tumour. (f) Wound closure with a vacuum drain.

is stimulated by salivary stimulation.The management of Frey's syndrome involves the prevention as well as the management of established symptoms.

Prevention

There are a number of techniques described to prevent Frey's syndrome following parotidectomy. These include:

- sternomastoid muscle flap;
- temporalis fascial flap;
- insertion of artificial membranes between the skin and the parotid bed.

All these methods place a barrier between the skin and the parotid bed to minimise inappropriate regeneration of autonomic nerve fibres.

Management of established Frey's syndrome

Methods of managing Frey's syndrome include:

- antiperspirants, usually containing aluminium chloride;
- denervation by tympanic neurectomy;
- the injection of botulinum toxin into the affected skin.

The last is the most effective and can be performed as an outpatient.

Granulomatous sialadenitis

This is a group of rare conditions that affect the salivary glands producing a variety of signs and symptoms, particularly painless swellings of the parotid and/or submandibular glands. Systemic upset is variable. These include the following.

Mycobacterial infection

Tuberculosis and non-tuberculous sialadenitis typically present as a tumour-like swelling of the salivary gland. There is little pain and no fever. Preoperative investigations may be of some help, and the diagnosis is only confirmed when the swelling has

Lucie Frey, 1896–1944, physician, The Neurological Clinic, Warsaw, Poland.

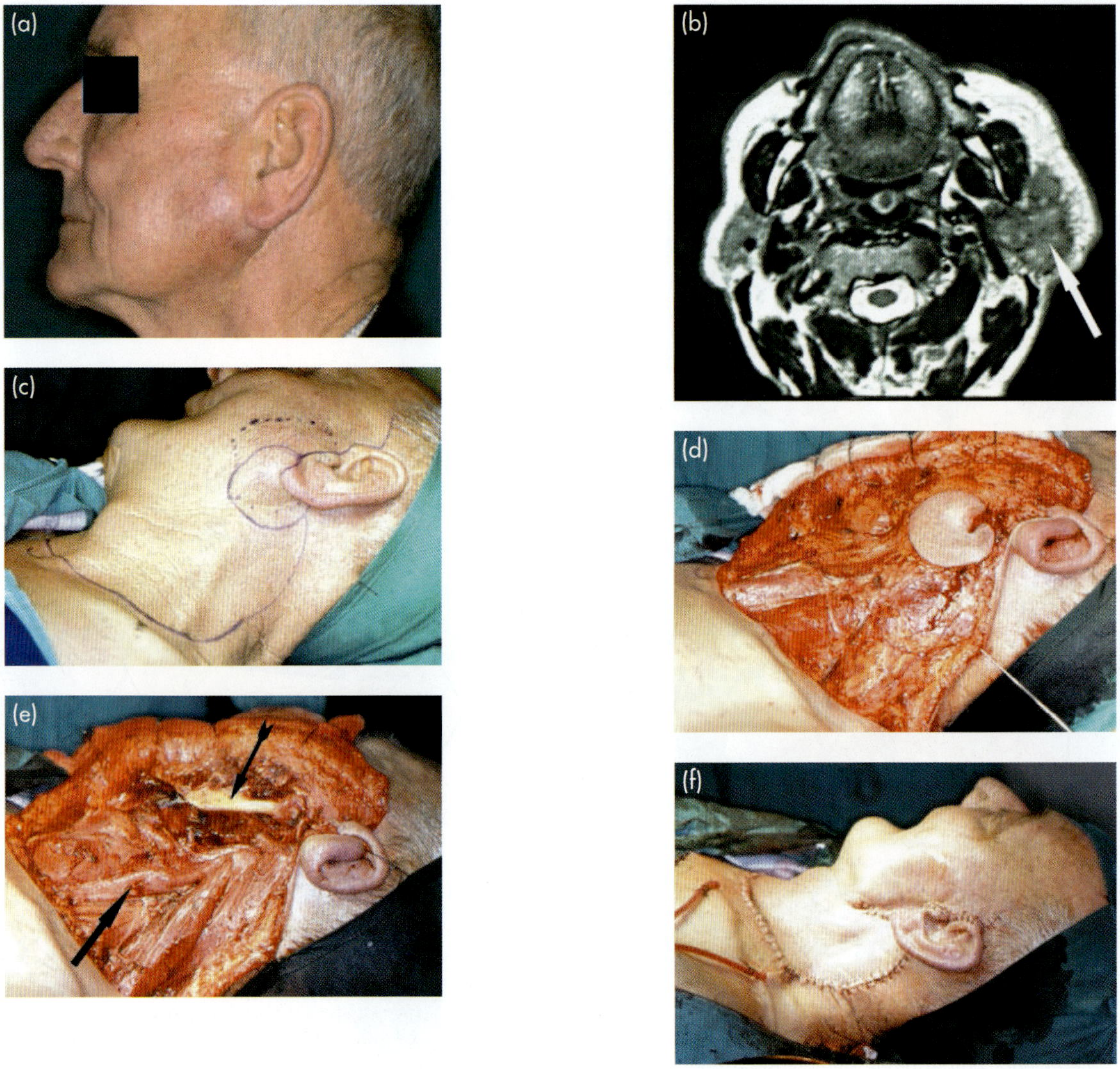

Figure 50.25 (a) High-grade malignant tumour in the left parotid gland. (b) Magnetic resonance imaging scan demonstrating a diffuse infiltrative malignant tumour of the left parotid gland (arrow). (c) Skin incision outlined for radical neck dissection and left radical parotidectomy including the removal of overlying skin. (d) Skin flap developed. (e) Appearance after left radical neck dissection and left radical parotidectomy. Posterior mandible (upper arrow) and great vessels of the neck (lower arrow) are visible. (f) Wound closure after left radical neck dissection.

been excised by either submandibular gland excision or formal parotidectomy.

Sarcoidosis

Sarcoidosis can affect the salivary tissue and presents with persistent salivary gland swelling that may be associated with xerostomia. Occasionally, the patient will present with a localised tumour-like swelling in one salivary gland, more commonly the parotid – the so-called sarcoid pseudotumour. In such circumstances, the diagnosis is only likely to be made following surgical excision for a presumed neoplasm.

Heerfordt's syndrome is sarcoidosis that involves parotid swelling, anterior uveitis, facial palsy and fever.

Other

These include cat scratch disease, toxoplasmosis, syphilis, deep mycoses and Wegener's granulomatosis, allergic sialadenitis and sialadenitis associated with radiotherapy of the head and neck.

Tumour-like lesions

There is a group of pathological conditions that affect the salivary glands which do not fall into any particular classification or category and are often difficult to diagnose. These include such conditions as sialadenosis, adenomatoid hyperplasia and multifocal monomorphic adenomatosis.

Sialadenosis

Sialadenosis (sialosis) is used to describe non-inflammatory swelling particularly affecting the parotid gland. It is usually occurs in association with a variety of conditions including diabetes mellitus, alcoholism, other endocrine diseases, pregnancy, drugs, bulimia and other eating disorders, and idiopathic diseases.

Most patients present between 40 and 70 years of age, and the salivary swellings are soft and often symmetrical (Figure 50.26). When the parotid glands are affected, patients may complain of

Christian Frederick Heerfordt, 1871–1953, a Danish ophthalmologist, described this syndrome in 1909.

a hamster-like appearance. Drug-induced sialosis is particularly common with sympathomimetic drugs. In many patients, no underlying disorder can be identified. Severe and prolonged malnutrition, as seen in eating disorders, produces sialadenosis by a process of glandular atrophy and fatty replacement. The pathological mechanism of sialadenosis can be associated with a process of neuropathy, which interferes with salivary gland function and subsequent acinar cell atrophy. This may be the case in diabetes mellitus, where autonomic neuropathy is a recognised complication as well as drug-induced sialosis.

The treatment of sialosis is unsatisfactory, but treatment is aimed at the correction of the underlying disorder. Drug-associated sialadenosis may regress when the drug responsible is withdrawn.

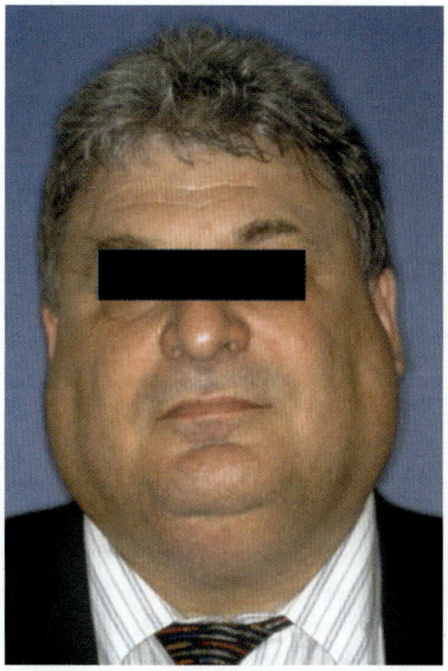

Figure 50.26 Sialosis of the parotid glands secondary to excess alcohol intake.

Degenerative conditions

Sjögren's syndrome

Sjögren's syndrome is an autoimmune condition causing progressive destruction of salivary and lacrimal glands. Primary Sjögren's syndrome differs from secondary Sjögren's syndrome in that xerostomia and keratoconjunctivitis sicca occur without the associated connective tissue disorder. However, the symptoms are often more severe, and the incidence of lymphomatous transformation (see below) in the primary group is higher than that in the secondary group (Table 50.3).

Table 50.3 Degenerative disorders.

Primary Sjögren's syndrome	More severe xerostomia
	Widespread exocrine gland dysfunction
	No connective tissue disorder
Secondary Sjögren's syndrome	M:F: 1:10
	Middle age
	Underlying connective tissue disorder
Benign lymphoepithelial lesion	20% develop lymphoma
	Diffuse parotid swelling 20% bilateral

Females are affected more than males in the ratio 10:1. Occasionally, there is enlargement of the salivary glands, more commonly the parotid rather than the submandibular glands. The glands are occasionally painful, and the patient sometimes develops a bacterial sialadenitis due to ascending infection from the associated xerostomia.

The characteristic pathological feature of Sjögren's syndrome is the progressive lymphocytic infiltration, acinar cell destruction and proliferation of duct epithelium in all salivary and lacrimal gland tissue. The diagnosis is based on the history as no single laboratory investigation is pathognomonic of either primary or secondary Sjögren's syndrome (Figure 50.27).

Management

Management of Sjögren's syndrome remains symptomatic. No known treatment modifies or improves the xerostomia or keratoconjunctivitis sicca. An ophthalmological assessment is important, and artificial tears are essential to preserve corneal function. For dry mouth, various artificial salivary substitutes are available, but patients often consume large volumes of water, carrying a bottle of water with them at all times. In the dentate patient, the use of salivary substitutes with fluoride is important to counter the risk of accelerating dental caries. Other oral complications include oral candidosis and accelerated periodontal disease.

Complications of Sjögren's syndrome

There is an increased incidence of developing lymphoma (most commonly monocytoid B-cell lymphoma) in patients with Sjögren's syndrome. The risk is highest within the primary group, and the onset of lymphoma is heralded by immunological change within the blood.

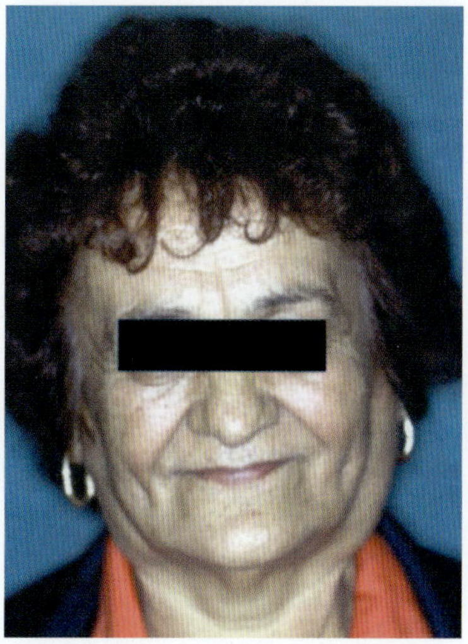

Figure 50.27 Clinical appearance of primary biliary cirrhosis associated with Sjögren's syndrome.

A **hamster** is a small nocturnal Eurasian rodent.

Benign lymphoepithelial lesion

The use of the word 'benign' to describe this lesion is misleading because 20 per cent of patients with benign lymphoepithelial lesion ultimately develop lymphoma. It is not possible to distinguish on histological grounds benign lymphoepithelial lesion from Sjögren's syndrome. Both are characterised by lymphocytic infiltration, acinar atrophy and ductal epithelial proliferation. Clinically, benign lymphoepithelial lesion presents as a diffuse swelling of the parotid gland. The swelling is firm, often painful and, in 20 per cent of patients, the presentation is bilateral. Most patients are female and over 50 years of age. Parotidectomy is often undertaken to establish a diagnosis. Prolonged follow up is essential.

Xerostomia

Xerostomia is a common symptom in many aspects of medical practice. Normal salivary flows decrease with age in both men and women, although many patients with xerostomia are post-menopausal women who also complain of a burning tongue or mouth. Common causes of xerostomia are:

- chronic anxiety states and depression;
- dehydration;
- anticholinergic drugs, especially antidepressants;
- salivary gland disorders – Sjögren's syndrome. Ascending parotitis is an occasional complication of xerostomia and is managed with antibiotics and increased fluid intake;
- radiotherapy to the head and neck.

Sialorrhoea

Certain drugs and oral infection produce a transient increase in salivary flow rates. In healthy individuals, excess salivation is rarely a symptom as excess saliva is swallowed spontaneously. Uncontrolled drooling is usually seen in the presence of normal salivary production. It is seen in children with mental and physical handicap, notably cerebral palsy.

Management

Uncontrollable drooling is managed surgically, and many operations are available. Surgical options include:

- bilateral submandibular duct repositioning and simultaneous sublingual gland excision;
- bilateral submandibular gland excision;
- transposition of the parotid ducts and simultaneous submandibular gland excision.

Most resting salivary gland flow arises from the submandibular glands, and surgery should be focused on this gland to control uncontrolled sialorrhoea.

FURTHER READING

Langdon J, Patel MF, Ord RA, Brennan P. *Operative oral and maxillofacial surgery*, 2nd edn. London: Hodder Arnold, 2011.

McGurk M, Renehan AE. *Controversies in the management of salivary gland disease*. Oxford: Oxford University Press, 2001.

PART

8 Breast and endocrine

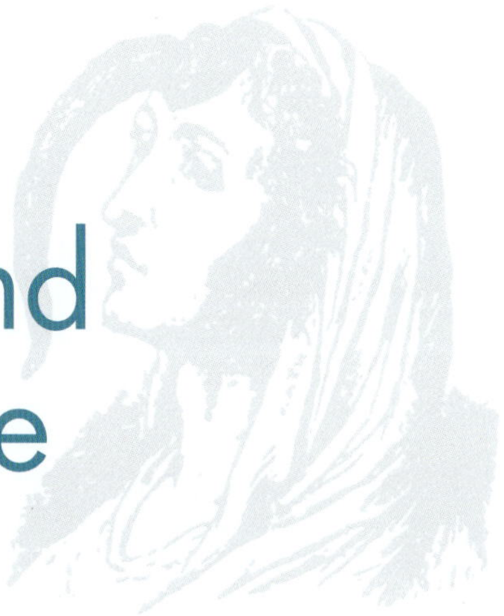

CHAPTER 51

The thyroid and parathyroid glands

LEARNING OBJECTIVES

- To understand the development and anatomy of the thyroid and parathyroid glands
- To know the physiology and investigation of thyroid and parathyroid function
- To be able to select appropriate investigations for thyroid swellings
- To know how to treat thyrotoxicosis and thyroid failure
- To know when to operate on a thyroid swelling
- To describe thyroid lobectomy
- To describe the investigation and management of hyperparathyroidism
- To know the risks and complications of thyroid and parathyroid surgery

EMBRYOLOGY

The thyroglossal duct develops from the median bud of the pharynx. The foramen caecum at the base of the tongue is the vestigial remnant of the duct. This initially hollow structure migrates caudally and passes in close continuity with, and sometimes through, the developing hyoid cartilage. The parathyroid glands develop from the third and fourth pharyngeal pouches (Figure 51.1). The thymus also develops from the third pouch. As it descends it takes the associated parathyroid gland with it which explains why the inferior parathyroid which arises from the third pharyngeal pouch normally lies inferior to the superior gland. However, the inferior parathyroid may be found anywhere along this line of descent. The developing thyroid lobes amalgamate with the structures that arise in the fourth pharyngeal pouch, i.e. the superior parathyroid gland and the ultimobranchial body. Parafollicular cells (C cells) from the neural crest reach the thyroid via the ultimobranchial body.

SURGICAL ANATOMY

The normal thyroid gland weighs 20–25 g. The functioning unit is the lobule supplied by a single arteriole and consists of 24–40 follicles lined with cuboidal epithelium. The follicle contains colloid in which thyroglobulin is stored (Figure 51.2). The arterial supply is rich, and extensive anastomoses occur between the main thyroid arteries and branches of the tracheal and oesophageal arteries (Figure 51.3). There is an extensive lymphatic network within the gland. Although some lymph channels pass directly to the deep cervical nodes, the subcapsular plexus drains principally to the central compartment juxtathyroid – 'Delphian' – and paratracheal nodes and nodes on the superior and inferior

Delphi, a sacred site near the Gulf of Corinth in Greece, is the place where Phythia, the snake-woman oracle, resided. She sat on a tripod clutching the ribbons of the monolithic 'omphalos' of the world and after inhaling sulphurous fumes, would utter meaningless jargon which was interpreted equivocally by the attendent priests for those who came to consult her. Formerly the purpose of these lymph nodes was uncertain, and they were therefore called 'Delphic'.

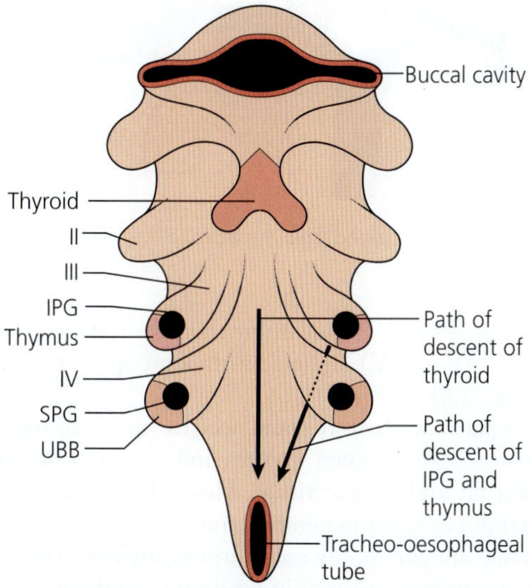

Figure 51.1 Embryology of thyroid and parathyroid. Diagram of an anterior view of the pharynx in a 4-week embryo showing the relationship of the third and fourth pharyngeal pouches to final position of the thyroid and parathyroid glands. IPG, inferior parathyroid; SPG, superior parathyroid; UBB, ultimobranchial body.

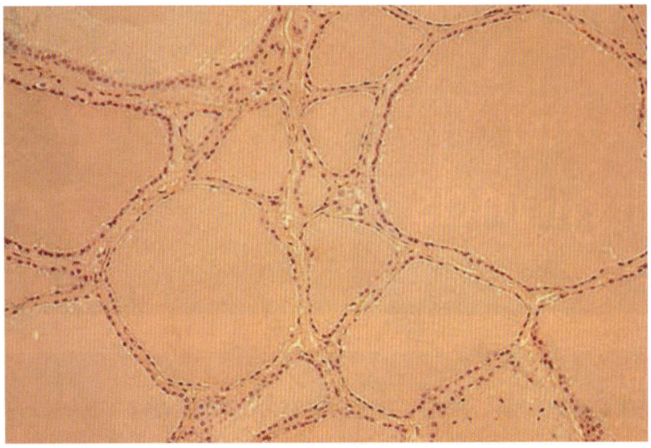

Figure 51.2 Histology of the normal thyroid.

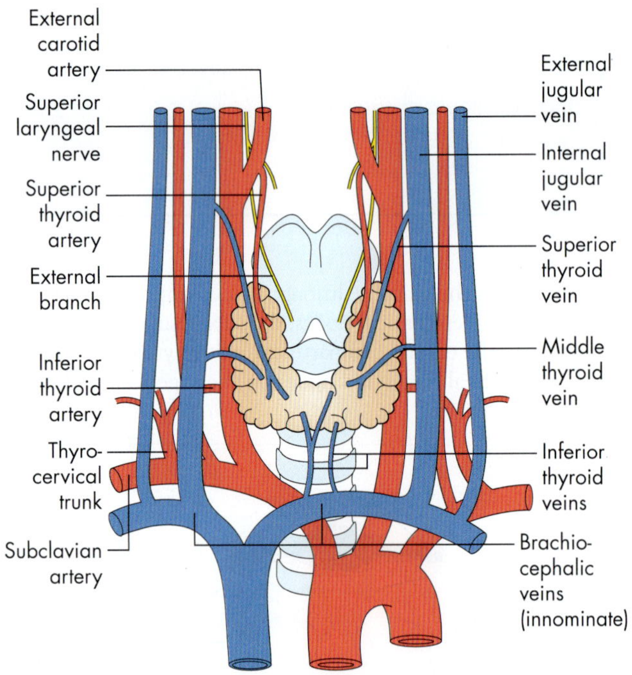

Figure 51.3 The thyroid gland from the front.

thyroid veins (level VI), and from there to the deep cervical (levels II, III, IV and V) and mediastinal groups of nodes (level VII) (Figure 51.4).

The normal parathyroid gland weighs up to 50 mg with a characteristic orange/brown colour and mobility within the surrounding fat and thymic tissue. Most adults have four parathyroid glands but supernumerary glands occur and nests of parathyroid tissue are commonly found in the thymus. The superior parathyroid is more consistent in position than the inferior. The superior gland is commonly found in fat above the inferior thyroid artery and close to the cricothyroid articulation. It should be noted that the anatomical and radiological site, usually described as above the artery and posterior to the recurrent laryngeal nerve (RLN), is different from the surgical anatomy when the thyroid lobe is mobilised and rotated anteriorly. When the superior gland enlarges it tends to pass behind the inferior thyroid artery and descend inferiorly behind the oesophagus. The inferior

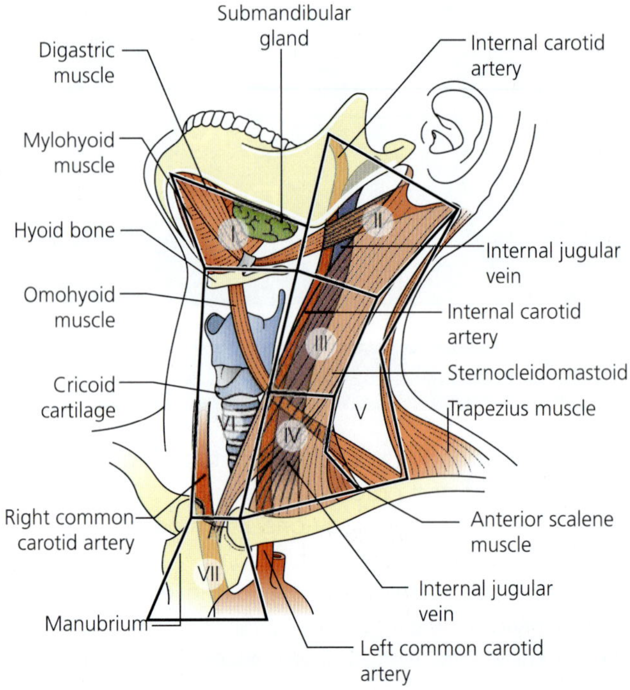

Figure 51.4 Cervical lymph node levels.

parathyroid gland is usually found under the capsule of the upper horn of the thymus or on the inferior pole of the thyroid lobe. A maldescended gland, however, can be found anywhere along the line of descent, virtually from the base of the skull to the aortopulmonary window (Figure 51.5) (Summary box 51.1).

Summary box 51.1

Embryology and anatomy

- Know the embryology of the thyroid and parathyroid glands
- Know the surgical and radiological anatomy of the thyroid

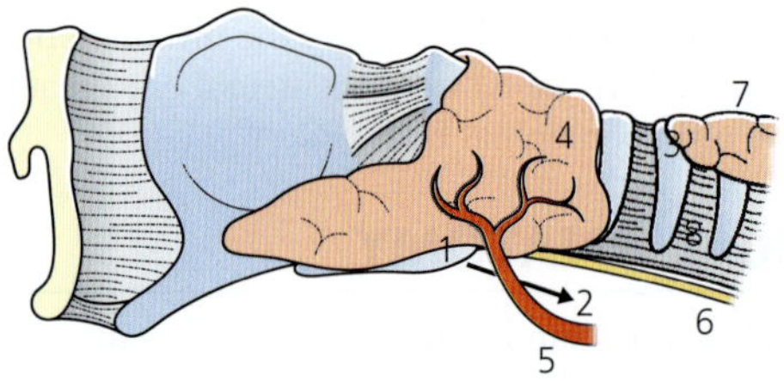

Figure 51.5 Surgical anatomy of the thyroid. The situation after mobilisation of the right lobe, and the relationships of the recurrent laryngeal nerve, inferior thyroid artery and the parathyroid glands as they are usually found. 1 and 2, common sites for superior parathyroid gland – the arrow shows the tendency for an enlarged gland to migrate from position 1 to position 2, i.e. in an inferior direction, to lie posterior to the inferior thyroid artery (5) and oesophagus (8); 3 and 4, common sites for inferior parathyroid gland (the upper horn of the thymus points like an index finger to the inferior parathyroid, which may lie under the fingernail); 5, recurrent laryngeal nerve; 6, thymus; 7, oesophagus. (see Figure 51.52).

PHYSIOLOGY

Thyroxine

The hormones tri-iodothyronine (T_3) and L-thyroxine (T_4) (extracted by EC Kendall in 1915) are bound to thyroglobulin within the colloid. Synthesis within the thyroglobulin complex is controlled by several enzymes, in distinct steps:

- trapping of inorganic iodide from the blood;
- oxidation of iodide to iodine;
- binding of iodine with tyrosine to form iodotyrosines;
- coupling of monoiodotyrosines and di-iodotyrosines to form T_3 and T_4.

When hormones are required, the complex is resorbed into the cell and thyroglobulin is broken down. T_3 and T_4 are liberated and enter the blood, where they are bound to serum proteins: albumin, thyroxine-binding globulin (TBG) and thyroxine-binding prealbumin (TBPA). The small amount of hormone that remains free in the serum is biologically active.

The metabolic effects of the thyroid hormones are due to unbound free T_4 and T_3 (0.03 and 0.3 per cent of the total circulating hormones, respectively). T_3 is the more important physiological hormone and is also produced in the periphery by conversion from T_4. T_3 is quick acting (within a few hours), whereas T_4 acts more slowly (4–14 days).

Parathormone

The parathyroid glands secrete the 84-amino acid peptide parathyroid hormone (PTH), which controls the level of serum calcium in extracellular fluid. PTH is released in response to a low serum calcium or high serum magnesium level. PTH activates osteoclasts to resorb bone, and increases calcium reabsorption from urine and renal activation of vitamin D with subsequent increased gut absorption of calcium. Renal excretion of phosphate is also increased.

Calcitonin

The parafollicular C cells of the thyroid are of neuroendocrine origin and arrive in the thyroid via the ultimobranchial body (Figure 51.1). They produce calcitonin which is a serum marker for recurrence of medullary thyroid cancer.

The pituitary–thyroid axis

Synthesis and liberation of thyroid hormones from the thyroid is controlled by thyroid-stimulating hormone (TSH) from the anterior pituitary. Secretion of TSH depends upon the level of circulating thyroid hormones and is modified in a classic negative feedback manner. In hyperthyroidism, when hormone levels in the blood are high, TSH production is suppressed whereas in hypothyroidism it is stimulated. Regulation of TSH secretion also results from the action of thyrotrophin-releasing hormone (TRH) produced in the hypothalamus.

Edward Calvin Kendall, 1886–1972, Professor of Physiological Chemistry, the Graduate Medical School, The Mayo Foundation, Rochester, MN, USA. He shared the 1950 Nobel Prize for Physiology or Medicine with Hench and Reichstein 'for their discoveries concerning the suprarenal hormones, their structure and biological effects'.

Thyroid-stimulating antibodies

A family of IgG immunoglobulins bind with TSH receptor sites (TRAbs) and activate TSH receptors on the follicular cell membrane. They have a more protracted action than TSH (16–24 versus 1.5–3 hours) and are responsible for virtually all cases of thyrotoxicosis not due to autonomous toxic nodules. Serum concentrations are very low but their measurement is not essential to make the diagnosis.

Therapeutic notes

T_4 is given once daily; an average replacement dose is 0.15 mg and a suppressive dose is 0.2 mg. T_3 is given three times daily, usually as a suppressive dose of 20 μg three times a day. Recombinant human TSH is now available and is used to maximise (radioactive) iodine uptake as an alternative to thyroid hormone withdrawal.

TESTS OF THYROID FUNCTION

There is a large variety of tests of thyroid function available to the endocrinologist; however, in a surgical setting investigations requested should be the minimum necessary to reach a diagnosis and formulate a management plan. Only a small number of parameters need to be measured as a routine, although this may require supplementation or to be repeated when inconclusive.

Serum thyroid hormones

Serum TSH

TSH levels can be measured accurately down to very low serum concentrations with an immunochemiluminometric assay. When the serum TSH level is in the normal range, it is redundant to measure the T_3 and T_4 levels. Interpretation of deranged TSH levels, however, depends on knowledge of the T_3 and T_4 values (Table 51.1). In the euthyroid state, T_3, T_4 and TSH levels will all be within the normal range. Florid thyroid failure results in depressed T_3 and T_4 levels, with gross elevation of the TSH. Incipient or developing thyroid failure is characterised by low normal values of the T_3 and T_4 and elevation of the TSH. In toxic states, the TSH level is suppressed and undetectable.

Table 51.1 Results of thyroid function tests in normal and pathological states.

Thyroid functional state	TSH (0.3–3.3 mU/L)	Free T_4 (10–30 nmol/L)	Free T_3 (3.5–7.5 μmol/L)
Euthyroid	Normal	Normal	Normal
Thyrotoxic	Undetectable	High	High
Myxoedema	High	Low	Low
Suppressive T_4 therapy	Undetectable	High	High (often normal)
T_3 toxicity	Low/undetectable	Normal	High

Thyroxine (T_4) and tri-iodothyronine (T_3)

These are transported in plasma bound to specific proteins (TBG). Only a small fraction of the total (0.03 per cent of T_4 and 0.3 per cent of T_3) is free and physiologically active. Assays of total hormone for both are now obsolete because of the confounding effect of circulating protein concentrations, influenced by the level of circulating oestrogen and nutritional state. Highly accurate radioimmunoassays of free T_3 and free T_4 are now routine. T_3 toxicity (with a normal T_4) is a distinct entity and may only be diagnosed by measuring the serum T_3, although a suppressed TSH level with a normal T_4 may suggest the diagnosis.

An appropriate combination to establish the functional thyroid status at initial assessment is serum TSH and assay of antithyroid antibodies supplemented by free T_4 and T_3 evaluation when TSH is abnormal.

Thyroid autoantibodies

Serum levels of antibodies against thyroid peroxidase (TPO) (previously referred to as thyroid microsomal antigen) and thyroglobulin are useful in determining the cause of thyroid dysfunction and swellings. Autoimmune thyroiditis may be associated with thyroid toxicity, failure or euthyroid goitre. Levels above 25 units/mL for TPO antibody and titres of greater than 1:100 for antithyroglobulin are considered significant, although a proportion of patients with histological evidence of lymphocytic (autoimmune) thyroiditis are seronegative. The presence of antithyroglobulin antibody interferes with assays of serum thyroglobulin with implications for follow up of thyroid cancers. TSH receptor antibodies (TSH-Rab or TRAB) are often present in Graves' disease. They are largely produced within the thyroid itself (Summary box 51.2).

Summary box 51.2

Thyroid investigations

Essential
- Serum: TSH (T_3 and T_4 if abnormal); thyroid autoantibodies
- FNAC of palpable discrete swellings; ultrasound guidance may reduce the 'Thy1' rate

Optional
- Corrected serum calcium
- Serum calcitonin (carcinoembryonic antigen may be used as an alternative screening test for medullary cancer)
- Imaging: chest radiograph and thoracic inlet if tracheal deviation/retrosternal goitre; ultrasound, CT and MRI scan for known cancer, some reoperations and some retrosternal goitres; isotope scan if discrete swelling and toxicity coexist

Thyroid imaging

Chest and thoracic inlet x-rays

Simple radiographs of the chest and thoracic inlet will rapidly and economically confirm the presence of significant retrosternal goitre and clinically important degrees of tracheal deviation and compression (Figure 51.6). Chest x-ray tends to underestimate the extent of retrosternal extensions. Pulmonary metastases may also be detected.

Ultrasound scanning

Ultrasound scanning gives good anatomical images of the thyroid and surrounding structures and while previously out of favour, high frequency ultrasound is now widely used (Figure 51.7). The drawback of ultrasound is that it may reveal thyroid swellings that are not clinically relevant and risks a cascade of unnecessary investigation, intervention and anxiety when used indiscriminately. However, in experienced hands, ultrasound can reduce the number of unsatisfactory aspiration cytology samples by permitting more targeted sampling, and is very reliable in the identification of nodes involved in thyroid cancer and the identification of larger parathyroid adenomas.

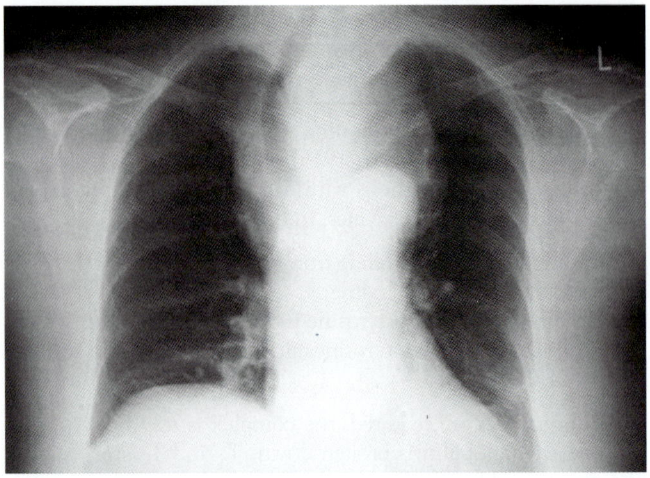

Figure 51.6 Chest radiograph showing retrosternal goitre with tracheal displacement.

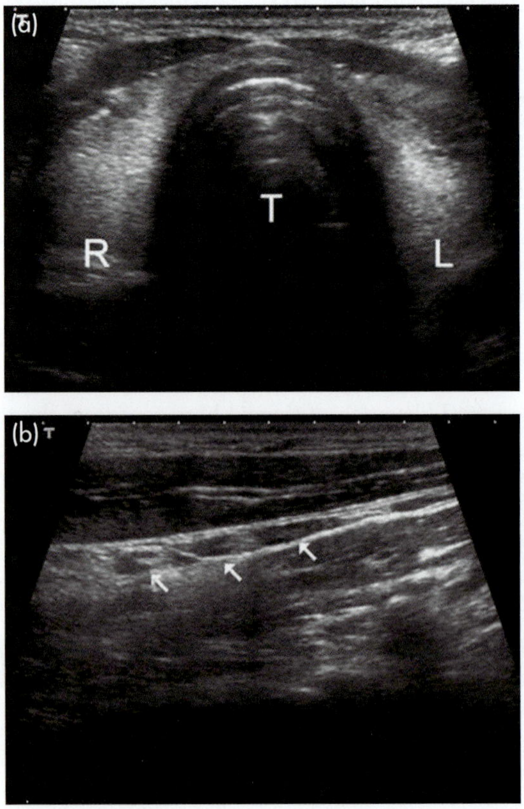

Figure 51.7 Ultrasound scanning. (a) Transverse scan of normal thyroid. R, right lobe; L, left lobe; T, trachea. (b) Longitudinal scan of normal jugular lymph nodes (white arrows).

Computed tomography, magnetic resonance imaging and positron emission tomography scanning

Routine computed tomography (CT) and magnetic resonance imaging (MRI) of unexceptional thyroid swellings is not indicated and is reserved for the assessment of known malignancy, to assess the extent of retrosternal and occasionally recurrent goitres (Figure 51.8). Iodine containing contrast agents may interfere with subsequent radioactive iodine uptake used for diagnostic scanning or therapy. The appearance and reporting of a retrosternal goitre on CT can give a misleading impression of the operative difficulty in delivery through a neck incision.

Positron emission tomography (PET)/CT scanning has an occasional role in the management of patients with obscure recurrent thyroid cancer but increasingly identifies incidental thyroid cancers in patients undergoing this investigation for other malignancies.

Isotope scanning

The uptake by the thyroid of a low dose of either radiolabelled iodine (^{123}I) or the cheaper technetium (^{99m}Tc) will demonstrate the distribution of activity in the whole gland (Figure 51.9). Routine isotope scanning is unnecessary and inappropriate for distinguishing benign from malignant lesions because the majority (80 per cent) of 'cold' swellings are benign and some (5 per cent) functioning or 'warm' swellings will be malignant. Its principal value is in the toxic patient with a nodule or nodularity of the thyroid. Localisation of overactivity in the gland will differentiate between a toxic nodule with suppression of the remainder of the gland, and toxic multinodular goitre with several areas of increased uptake with important implications for therapy.

Whole body scanning is used to demonstrate metastases, but the patient must have all normally functioning thyroid tissue ablated either by surgery or radioiodine before the scan is performed, because metastatic thyroid cancer tissue cannot compete with normal thyroid tissue in the uptake of iodine.

Fine-needle aspiration cytology

Fine-needle aspiration cytology (FNAC) is the investigation of choice in discrete thyroid swellings. FNAC has excellent patient compliance, is simple and quick to perform in the outpatient department and is readily repeated. This technique, developed in Scandinavia 40 years ago, is now routine throughout the world. FNAC results should be reported using standard terminology (Table 51.2). There is a trend to use ultrasound to guide the needle to achieve more accurate sampling and reduce the rate of unsatisfactory aspirates.

HYPOTHYROIDISM

A scheme for classifying hypothyroidism is given in Table 51.3.

Cretinism (fetal or infantile hypothyroidism)

Cretinism is the consequence of inadequate thyroid hormone production during fetal and neonatal development. 'Endemic

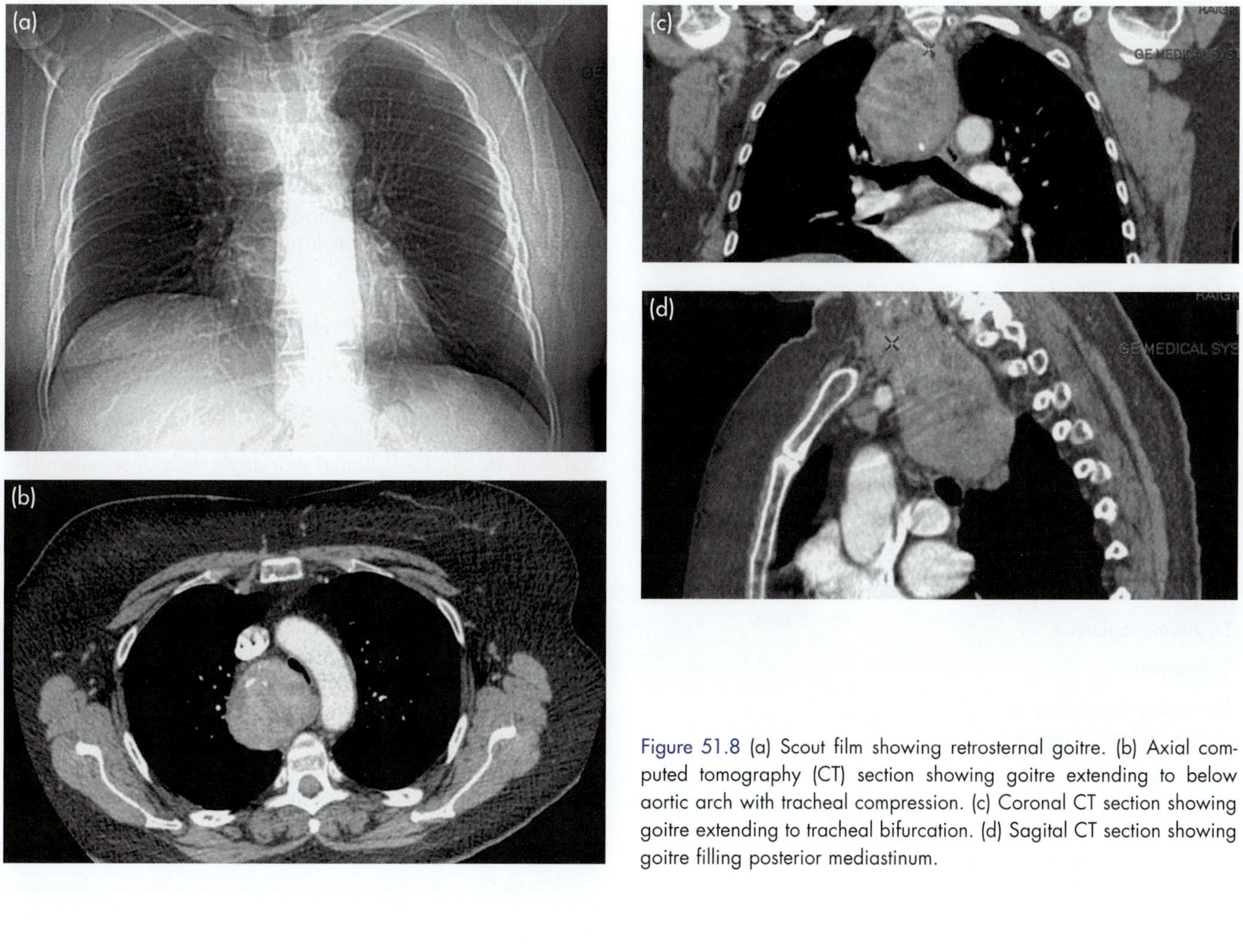

Figure 51.8 (a) Scout film showing retrosternal goitre. (b) Axial computed tomography (CT) section showing goitre extending to below aortic arch with tracheal compression. (c) Coronal CT section showing goitre extending to tracheal bifurcation. (d) Sagital CT section showing goitre filling posterior mediastinum.

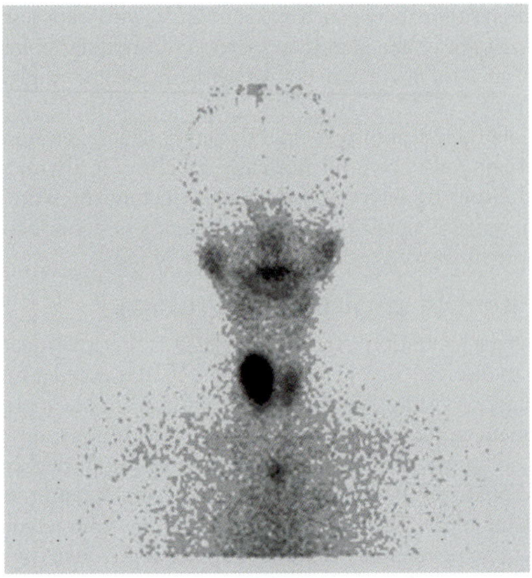

Figure 51.9 Technetium thyroid scan showing appearance of a 1-cm 'toxic' adenoma in the right thyroid lobe with suppression of uptake in the left lobe. The intense uptake gives a false impression of the size of the swelling.

Table 51.2 Classification of fine-needle aspiration cytology reports.

Thy1	Non-diagnostic
Thy1c	Non-diagnostic cystic
Thy2	Non-neoplastic
Thy3	Follicular
Thy4	Suspicious of malignancy
Thy5	Malignant

Table 51.3 Classification of hypothyroidism.

Autoimmune thyroiditis (chronic lymphocytic thyroiditis)	Non-goitrous: primary myxoedema
	Goitrous: Hashimoto's disease
Iatrogenic	After thyroidectomy
	After radioiodine therapy
	Drug induced (antithyroid drugs, para-aminosalicylic acid and iodides in excess)
Dyshormonogenesis	
Goitrogens	
Secondary to pituitary or hypothalamic disease	
Thyroid agenesis	
Endemic cretinism	Often goitrous and due to iodine deficiency

cretinism' is due to dietary iodine deficiency, whereas sporadic cases are due either to an inborn error of thyroid metabolism or complete or partial agenesis of the gland. A hoarse cry, macroglossia and umbilical hernia in a neonate with features of thyroid failure suggest the diagnosis. Immediate diagnosis and treatment with thyroxine within a few days of birth are essential to prevent *in utero* damage progressing and if physical and mental development is to be normal. In non-endemic areas and societies with iodised salt, sporadic hypothyroidism still occurs in 1 in 4000 live births, and biochemical screening of neonates for hypothyroidism using TSH and T_4 assays on a heel-prick blood sample is widespread. Women taking antithyroid drugs may give birth to a hypothyroid infant and radioactive iodine must never be given to pregnant women.

Adult hypothyroidism

The term myxoedema should be reserved for severe thyroid failure and not applied to the much more common mild thyroid deficiency. The signs of thyroid deficiency are:

- bradycardia
- cold extremities
- dry skin and hair
- periorbital puffiness
- hoarse voice
- bradykinesis, slow movements
- delayed relaxation phase of ankle jerks.

The symptoms are:

- tiredness
- mental lethargy
- cold intolerance
- weight gain
- constipation
- menstrual disturbance
- carpal tunnel syndrome.

Comparison of the facial appearance with a previous photograph may be helpful. Delayed relaxation of the ankle jerk reflex is the most useful clinical sign in making the diagnosis.

Thyroid function tests

These show low T_4 and T_3 levels with a high TSH (except in the rare event of pituitary failure) (Table 51.1). High serum levels of TPO antibodies are characteristic of autoimmune disease.

Treatment

Oral thyroxine (0.10–0.20 mg) as a single daily dose is curative. Caution is required in the elderly or those with cardiac disease and the replacement dose is then commenced at 0.05 mg daily and increased cautiously. If a rapid response is required, tri-iodothyronine (20 μg three times a day) may be used.

Myxoedema

The signs and symptoms of hypothyroidism are accentuated. The facial appearance is typical, and there is often supraclavicular puffiness, a malar flush and a yellow tinge to the skin (Figure 51.10). Myxoedema coma, characterised by altered mental state, hypothermia and a precipitating medical condition, for example cardiac failure or infection, carries a high mortality. Treatment comprises thyroid replacement, either a bolus of 0.50 mg of T_4 or 10 μg of T_3 either i.v. or orally every 4–6 hours. If the body

in utero is Latin for 'in the uterus'.
Myxoedema was first described in 1873 by Sir William Withey Gull, 1816–1890, physician, Guy's Hospital, London, UK.

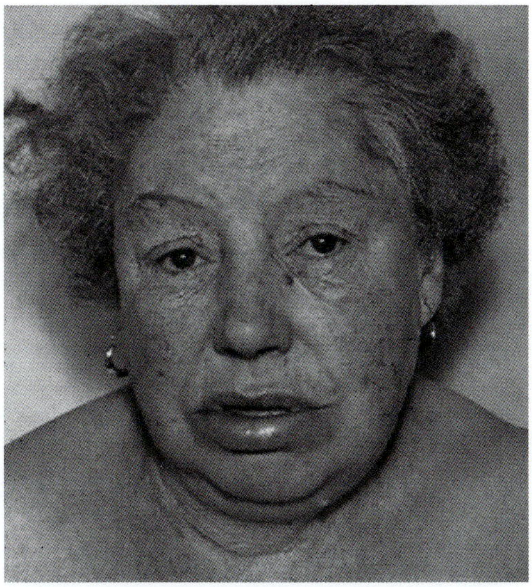

Figure 51.10 Myxoedema. Note the bloated look, pouting lips and dull expression (courtesy of Dr VK Summers, Liverpool, UK).

temperature is less than 30°C, the patient must be warmed slowly. Intravenous broad-spectrum antibiotics and hydrocortisone (in divided doses) are recommended.

Primary or atrophic myxoedema is considered to be an autoimmune disease similar to chronic lymphocytic (Hashimoto's) thyroiditis (see below) but without goitre formation. Delay in diagnosis is common and the degree of hypothyroidism is usually more severe than in goitrous autoimmune thyroiditis.

Dyshormonogenesis

Genetic deficiencies in the enzymes controlling the synthesis of thyroid hormones account for a minority of cases of neonatal hypothyroidism and goitre. These are usually inherited in an autosomal recessive pattern and a family history is common. If the biochemical effect is of moderate degree, thyroid enlargement may be the only manifestation and dyshormonogenesis should be considered in young patients presenting with euthyroid goitre. The most common abnormalities affect TPO activity and thyroglobulin synthesis. A classic example of dyshormonogenesis due to TPO deficiency is Pendred syndrome, in which goitre is associated with severe sensorineural hearing impairment and abnormality of the bony labyrinth observed on CT examination of the temporal bones.

THYROID ENLARGEMENT

The normal thyroid gland is impalpable. The term goitre (from the Latin guttur = the throat) is used to describe generalised enlargement of the thyroid gland. A discrete swelling (nodule) in one lobe with no palpable abnormality elsewhere is termed an isolated (or solitary) swelling. Discrete swellings with evidence of abnormality elsewhere in the gland are termed dominant (Summary box 51.3).

Hakaru Hashimoto, 1881–1934, Director of The Hashimoto Hospital, Mie, Japan, described chronic lymphocytic thyroiditis in 1912. The link to an autoimmune basis was defined by Roitt and his co-workers.

Summary box 51.3

Thyroid swellings

- Know how to describe thyroid swellings
- Use appropriate investigations
- Know the indications for surgery
- Select the appropriate procedure
- Describe and manage postoperative complications

A scheme for classifying thyroid enlargement is given in Table 51.4.

Table 51.4 Classification of thyroid swellings.

Simple goitre (euthyroid)	Diffuse hyperplastic	Physiological
		Pubertal
		Pregnancy
	Multinodular goitre	
Toxic	Diffuse (Graves' disease)	
	Multinodular	
	Toxic adenoma	
Neoplastic	Benign	
	Malignant	
Inflammatory	Autoimmune	Chronic lymphocytic thyroiditis
		Hashimoto's disease
	Granulomatous	De Quervain's thyroiditis
	Fibrosing	Riedel's thyroiditis
	Infective	Acute (bacterial thyroiditis, viral thyroiditis, 'subacute thyroiditis')
		Chronic (tuberculous, syphilitic)
	Other	Amyloid

Simple goitre

Aetiology

Simple goitre may develop as a result of stimulation of the thyroid gland by TSH, either as a result of inappropriate secretion from a microadenoma in the anterior pituitary (which is rare), or in response to a chronically low level of circulating thyroid hormones. The most important factor in endemic goitre is dietary deficiency of iodine (see below) but defective hormone synthesis probably accounts for many sporadic goitres (see below).

TSH is not the only stimulus to thyroid follicular cell proliferation and other growth factors, including immunoglobulins, exert an influence. The heterogeneous structural and functional response in the thyroid resulting in characteristic nodularity may

Ivan Maurice Roitt, born 1927, Emeritus Professor of Immunology, University College, London, UK. Elected Fellow of The Royal Society of London in 1983.
Vaughan Pendred, 1869–1946, a general practitioner of Durham, UK, described this syndrome in 1896. Exactly 100 years later the defect was mapped to chromosome 7q.

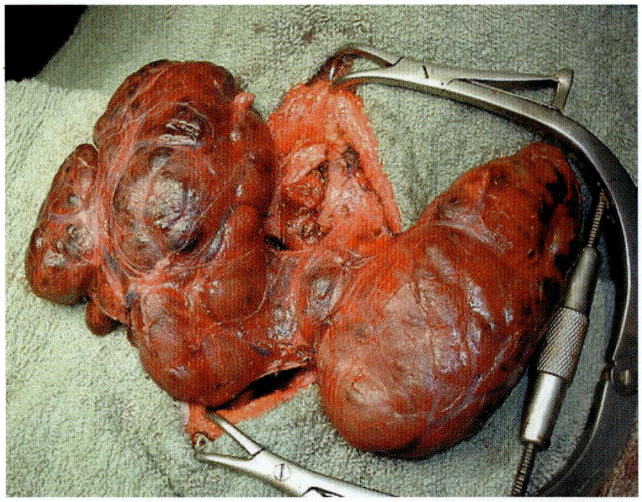

Figure 51.11 Total thyroidectomy for dyshormonogenetic goitre in a 14-year-old girl.

be due to the presence of clones of cells particularly sensitive to growth stimulation.

Iodine deficiency

The daily requirement of iodine is about 0.1–0.15 mg. In nearly all districts where simple goitre is endemic, there is a very low iodide content in the water and food. Endemic areas are in mountain ranges, such as the Rockies, Alps, Andes and Himalayas, and in the UK, areas of Derbyshire and Yorkshire. Endemic goitre is also found in lowland areas where the soil lacks iodide or the water supply comes from distant mountain ranges, e.g. the Great Lakes of North America, the plains of Lombardy, the Struma valley, the Nile valley and the Congo. Calcium is also goitrogenic and goitre is common in low iodine areas on chalk or limestone, for example Derbyshire and southern Ireland. Although iodides in food and water may be adequate, failure of intestinal absorption may produce iodine deficiency.

Dyshormonogenesis

Enzyme deficiencies of varying severity may be responsible for many sporadic goitres, i.e. in non-endemic areas (Figure 51.11). There is often a family history, suggesting a genetic defect. Environmental factors may compensate in areas of high iodine intake, e.g. goitre is almost unknown in Iceland where the fish diet is rich in iodine. Similarly, a low intake of iodine encourages goitre formation in those with a metabolic predisposition.

Goitrogens

Well-known goitrogens are the vegetables of the brassica family (cabbage, kale and rape), which contain thiocyanate, drugs such as para-aminosalicylic acid (PAS) and, of course, the antithyroid drugs. Thiocyanates and perchlorates interfere with iodide trapping; carbimazole and thiouracil compounds interfere with the oxidation of iodide and the binding of iodine to tyrosine.

Struma. The River Struma arises in the mountains of Bulgaria and flows into the Aegean Sea. Along its banks and those of its tributaries dwell peoples of several nationalities among whom endemic goitre has long been prevalent. Struma is a European continental term for goitre.

Surprisingly enough, iodides in large quantities are goitrogenic because they inhibit the organic binding of iodine and produce an iodide goitre. Excessive iodine intake may be associated with an increased incidence of autoimmune thyroid disease.

The natural history of simple goitre

Stages in goitre formation are:

- Persistent growth stimulation causes diffuse hyperplasia; all lobules are composed of active follicles and iodine uptake is uniform. This is a diffuse hyperplastic goitre, which may persist for a long time but is reversible if stimulation ceases.
- Later, as a result of fluctuating stimulation, a mixed pattern develops with areas of active lobules and areas of inactive lobules.
- Active lobules become more vascular and hyperplastic until haemorrhage occurs, causing central necrosis and leaving only a surrounding rind of active follicles.
- Necrotic lobules coalesce to form nodules filled either with iodine-free colloid or a mass of new but inactive follicles.
- Continual repetition of this process results in a nodular goitre. Most nodules are inactive, and active follicles are present only in the internodular tissue.

Diffuse hyperplastic goitre

Diffuse hyperplasia corresponds to the first stages of the natural history. The goitre appears in childhood in endemic areas but, in sporadic cases, it usually occurs at puberty when metabolic demands are high. If TSH stimulation ceases, the goitre may regress, but tends to recur later at times of stress, such as pregnancy. The goitre is soft, diffuse and may become large enough to cause discomfort. A colloid goitre is a late stage of diffuse hyperplasia when TSH stimulation has fallen off and when many follicles are inactive and full of colloid (Figure 51.12).

Nodular goitre

Nodules are usually multiple, forming a multinodular goitre (Figure 51.13). Occasionally, only one macroscopic nodule is found, but microscopic changes will be present throughout the gland; this is one form of a clinically solitary nodule. Nodules may be colloid or cellular, and cystic degeneration and haemorrhage are common, as is subsequent calcification. Nodules appear early in endemic goitre and later (between 20 and 30 years) in sporadic goitre, although the patient may be unaware of the goitre until his or her late 40s or 50s. All types of simple goitre are more common in the female than in the male owing to the presence of oestrogen receptors in thyroid tissue.

Diagnosis

Diagnosis is usually straightforward. The patient is euthyroid, the nodules are palpable and often visible; they are smooth, usually firm and not hard, and the goitre is painless and moves freely on swallowing. Hardness and irregularity, due to calcification, may simulate carcinoma. A painful nodule, sudden appearance, or rapid enlargement of a nodule raises suspicion of carcinoma but is usually due to haemorrhage into a simple nodule. Differential diagnosis from autoimmune thyroiditis may be difficult and the two conditions frequently coexist.

Investigations

Thyroid function should be assessed to exclude mild hyperthyroidism, and the presence of circulating thyroid antibodies tested

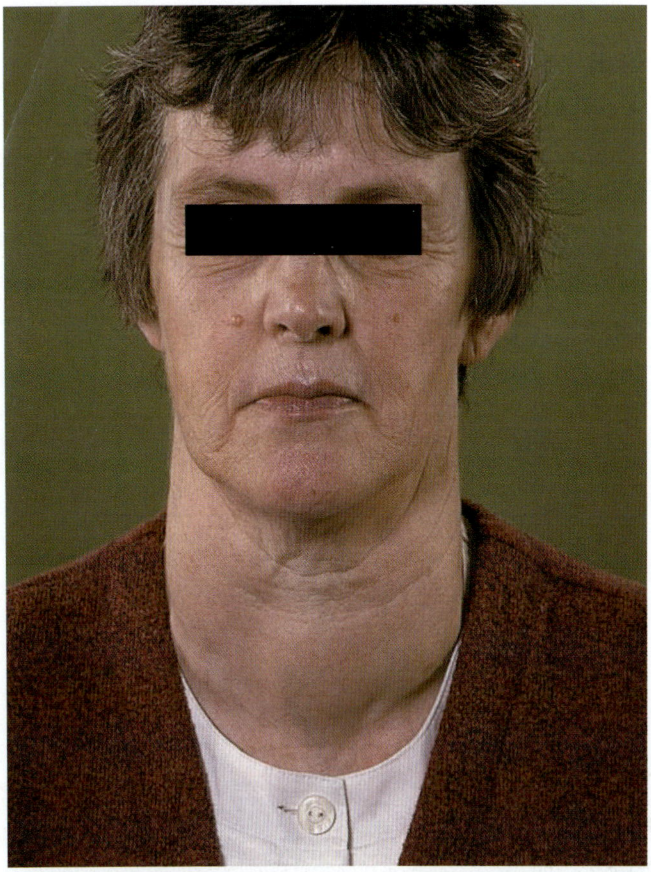

Figure 51.12 Colloid goitre.

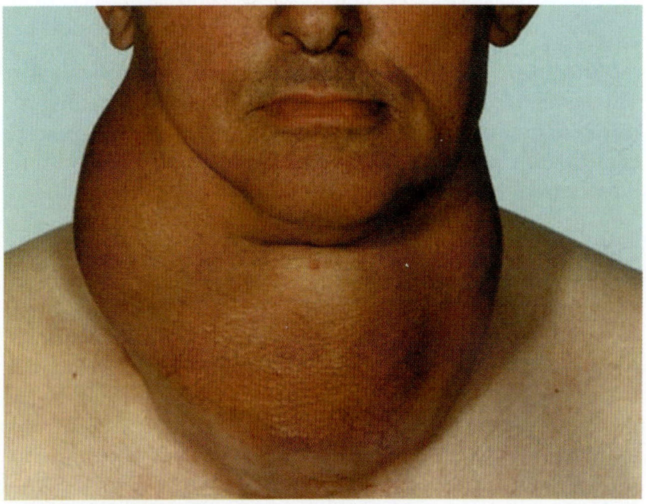

Figure 51.13 Large multinodular goitre.

to differentiate from autoimmune thyroiditis. Plain radiographs of the chest and thoracic inlet will rapidly demonstrate clinically significant tracheal deviation or compression. Ultrasound and CT give more detailed images but rarely influence clinical management. FNAC is only required for a dominant swelling in a generalised goitre.

Complications

Tracheal obstruction may be due to gross lateral displacement or compression in a lateral or anteroposterior plane by retrosternal extension of the goitre (Figures 51.6 and 51.8). Acute respiratory obstruction may follow haemorrhage into a nodule impacted in the thoracic inlet.

Secondary thyrotoxicosis

Transient episodes of mild hyperthyroidism are common, occurring in up to 30 per cent of patients.

Carcinoma

An increased incidence of cancer (usually follicular) has been reported from endemic areas. Dominant or rapidly growing nodules in long-standing goitres should always be subjected to aspiration cytology.

Prevention and treatment of simple goitre

In endemic areas, e.g. Switzerland, parts of the USA and Argentina, the incidence of goitre has been strikingly reduced by the introduction of iodised salt.

In the early stages, a hyperplastic goitre may regress if thyroxine is given in a dose of 0.15–0.2 mg daily for a few months.

Although the nodular stage of simple goitre is irreversible, more than half of benign nodules will regress in size over ten years. Most patients with multinodular goitre are asymptomatic and do not require operation. Operation may be indicated on cosmetic grounds, for pressure symptoms or in response to patient anxiety. Retrosternal extension with actual or incipient tracheal compression is also an indication for operation, as is the presence of a dominant area of enlargement that may be neoplastic.

There is a choice of surgical treatment in multinodular goitre: **total thyroidectomy** with immediate and lifelong replacement of thyroxine, or some form of partial resection, to conserve sufficient functioning thyroid tissue to subserve normal function while reducing the risk of hypoparathyroidism that accompanies total thyroidectomy. **Subtotal thyroidectomy** involves partial resection of each lobe, removing the bulk of the gland, leaving up to 8 g of relatively normal tissue in each remnant. The technique is essentially the same as described for toxic goitre, as are the postoperative complications. More often, however, the multinodular change is asymmetrically distributed, with one lobe more significantly involved than the other. In these circumstances, particularly in older patients, **total lobectomy** on the more affected side is the appropriate management with either subtotal resection (Dunhill procedure) or no intervention on the less affected side. In many cases, the causative factors persist and recurrence is likely. Reoperation for recurrent nodular goitre is more difficult and hazardous and, for this reason, an increasing number of thyroid surgeons favour **total thyroidectomy** in younger patients. However, when the first operation comprised unilateral lobectomy alone for asymmetric goitre, reoperation and completion total thyroidectomy is straightforward if required for progression of nodularity in the remaining lobe. Total lobectomy and total thyroidectomy have the additional advantage of being therapeutic for incidental carcinomas (see below).

After subtotal resection, it has been customary to give thyroxine to suppress TSH secretion, with the aim of preventing recurrence. Whether this is either necessary or effective is uncertain, although the evidence of benefit in endemic areas is better than elsewhere. There is some evidence that radioactive iodine may reduce the size of recurrent nodular goitre after previous

Sir Thomas Peel Dunhill, 1876–1957, surgeon, St Bartholomew's Hospital, London, UK.

subtotal resection and, in some circumstances, this may be a safer alternative than reoperation, particularly if there has been more than one previous thyroid procedure.

Clinically discrete swellings

Discrete thyroid swellings (thyroid nodules) are common and are present in 3–4 per cent of the adult population in the UK and USA. They are three to four times more frequent in women than men.

Diagnosis

A discrete swelling in an otherwise impalpable gland is termed **isolated** or **solitary**, whereas the preferred term is **dominant** for a similar swelling in a gland with clinical evidence of generalised abnormality in the form of a palpable contralateral lobe or generalised mild nodularity. About 70 per cent of discrete thyroid swellings are clinically isolated and about 30 per cent are dominant. The true incidence of isolated swellings is somewhat less than the clinical estimate. Clinical classification is inevitably subjective and overestimates the frequency of truly isolated swellings. When such a gland is exposed at operation or examined by ultrasonography, CT or MRI, clinically impalpable nodules are often detected. The true frequency of thyroid nodularity compared with the clinical detection rate by palpation is shown in Figure 51.14. Demonstrating the presence of impalpable nodules does not change the management of palpable discrete swellings and begs the question of the necessity of investigating incidentally found nodules. The importance of discrete swellings lies in the risk of neoplasia compared with other thyroid swellings. Some 15 per cent of isolated swellings prove to be malignant, and an additional 30–40 per cent are follicular adenomas. The remainder are non-neoplastic, largely consisting of areas of colloid degeneration, thyroiditis or cysts. Although the incidence of malignancy or follicular adenoma in clinically dominant swellings is approximately half of that of truly isolated swellings, it is substantial and cannot be ignored (Figure 51.15).

Investigation

Thyroid function

Serum TSH and thyroid hormone levels should be measured. If hyperthyroidism associated with a discrete swelling is confirmed biochemically, it indicates either a 'toxic adenoma' or a manifestation of toxic multinodular goitre. The combination of toxicity and nodularity is important and is an indication for isotope scanning to localise the area(s) of hyperfunction.

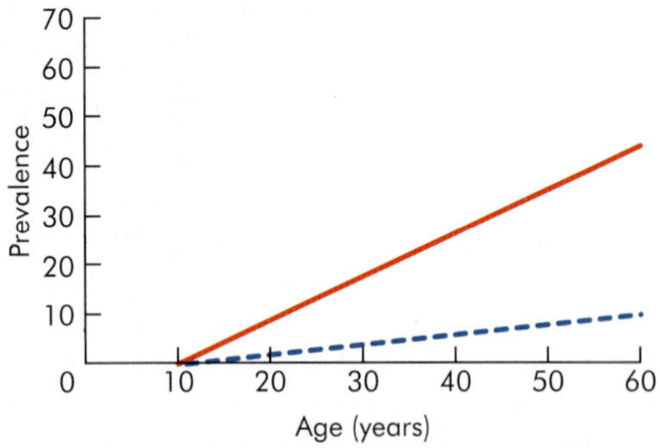

Figure 51.14 The prevalence of thyroid nodules detected on palpation (broken line) or by ultrasonography or post-mortem examination (solid line) (after Mazzaferri).

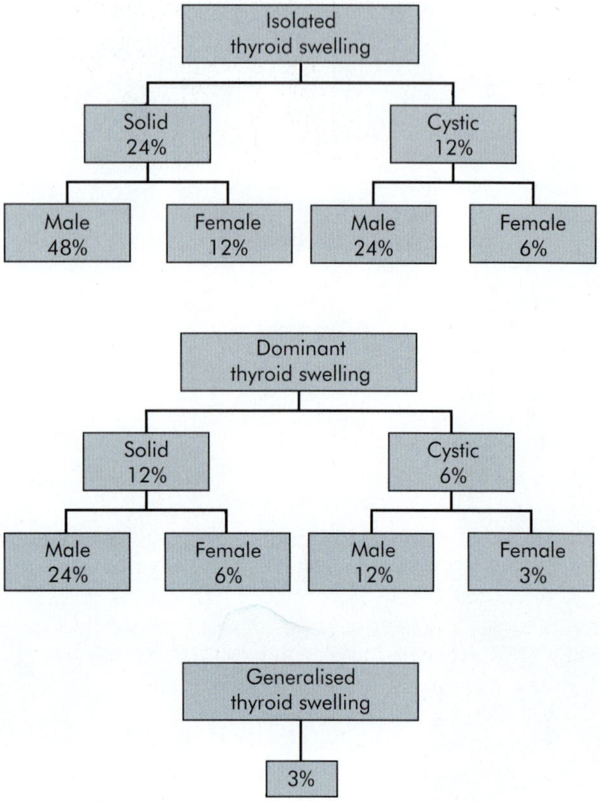

Figure 51.15 The risk of malignancy in thyroid swellings ('rule of twelve'). The risk of cancer in a thyroid swelling can be expressed as a factor of 12. The risk is greater in isolated versus dominant swellings, solid versus cystic swellings, and in men versus women.

Autoantibody titres

The autoantibody status may determine whether a swelling is a manifestation of chronic lymphocytic thyroiditis. The presence of circulating antibodies increases the risk of thyroid failure after lobectomy.

Isotope scan

Isotope scanning used to be the mainstay of investigation of discrete thyroid swellings to determine the functional activity relative to the surrounding gland according to isotope uptake.

On scanning, swellings are categorised as 'hot' (overactive), 'warm' (active) or 'cold' (underactive). A hot nodule is one that takes up isotope, while the surrounding thyroid tissue does not. Here the surrounding thyroid tissue is inactive because the nodule is producing such high levels of thyroid hormones that TSH secretion is suppressed (Figure 51.9). A warm nodule takes up isotope and so does normal thyroid tissue around it. A cold nodule takes up no isotope.

About 80 per cent of discrete swellings are cold, but only 15 per cent subsequently prove to be malignant and the use of this criterion as an indication for operation lacks discrimination. Routine isotope scanning has been abandoned except when toxicity is associated with nodularity.

Ultrasonography

This is widely used as a non-invasive supplement to clinical examination in determining the physical characteristics of thyroid swellings. It can demonstrate subclinical nodularity and cyst formation, the former is clinically irrelevant and the latter apparent at aspiration, which should be routine in all discrete swellings. There are a number of ultrasonic features in a thyroid swelling associated with thyroid neoplasia, including microcalcification and increased vascularity, but only macroscopic capsular breach and nodal involvement are diagnostic of malignancy. As an adjunct to FNAC it can reduce the rate of unsatisfactory specimens and is invaluable in the mapping of malignant lymphadenopathy.

Fine-needle aspiration cytology

Fine-needle aspiration cytology is the investigation of choice in discrete thyroid swellings. FNAC has excellent patient compliance, is simple and quick to perform in the outpatient department and is readily repeated.

Thyroid conditions that may be diagnosed by FNAC include colloid nodules (Figure 51.16), thyroiditis, papillary carcinoma (Figure 51.17), medullary carcinoma, anaplastic carcinoma and lymphoma. FNAC cannot distinguish between a benign follicular adenoma (Figure 51.18) and follicular carcinoma, as this distinction is dependent not on cytology but on histological criteria, which include capsular and vascular invasion.

Although FNAC was reported as highly accurate by Lowhagen and his colleagues (who were its pioneers) at the Karolinska Hospital, such high accuracy has not always been reproducible. There are very few false positives with respect to malignancy, but there is a definite false-negative rate with respect to both benign and malignant neoplasia. In addition, there can be a high rate of unsatisfactory aspirates, particularly in cystic or partly cystic swellings. These often yield only cyst fluid with macrophages and degenerate cells with few thyroid follicular cells upon which to report. After aspiration, a further sample for cytology should be taken from the cyst wall. There has been a recent trend to use ultrasound to guide the needle to achieve more accurate sampling and reduce the rate of unsatisfactory aspirates. Relatively few cysts are permanently abolished by one or more aspirations and, because of the risk of malignancy, recurrent cysts should be removed.

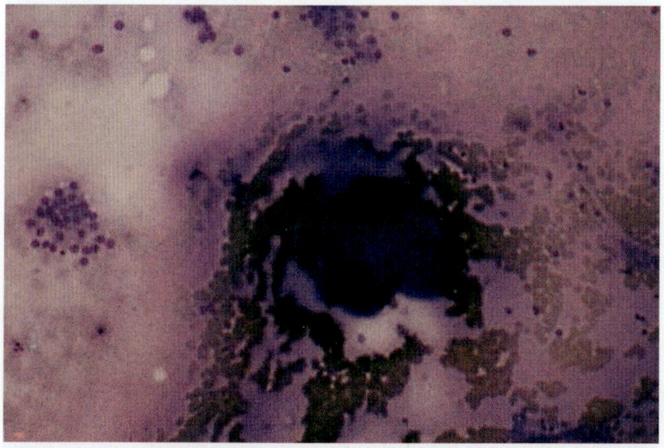

Figure 51.16 Thy2 aspiration cytology. Non-neoplastic appearances with scanty normal follicular cells together with colloid (= colloid nodule).

Torsten Lowhagen, cytologist, Department of Tumour Pathology, The Karolinska Hospital, Stockholm, Sweden. He was awarded the Papanicolaou Award in 1995.

Radiology

Chest and thoracic inlet radiographs may confirm tracheal deviation, compression or retrosternal extension and are required when either clinical suspicion or FNAC indicates malignancy.

Other scans

CT and MRI scans give excellent anatomical detail of thyroid swellings but have no role in the first line of investigation. They are most useful in assessing retrosternal (Figure 51.8) and recurrent swellings, particularly if initial surgery has been performed elsewhere. PET scan (Figure 51.19) may be useful, particularly in localising disease which does not take up radioiodine.

Laryngoscopy

Flexible laryngosopy has rendered indirect laryngosocpy obsolete and is widely used preoperatively to determine the mobility of the vocal cords, although usually for medicolegal rather than clinical reasons. Nevertheless, the presence of a unilateral cord palsy coexisting with a swelling suggestive of malignancy is usually diagnostic.

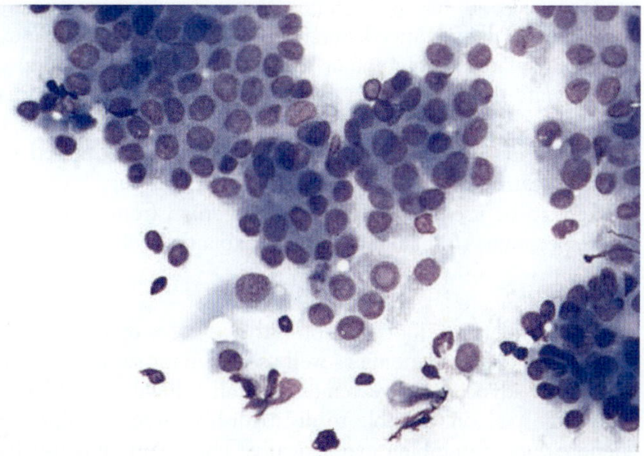

Figure 51.17 Thy5 aspiration cytology. Papillary carcinoma with typical cellular variability and nuclear inclusions.

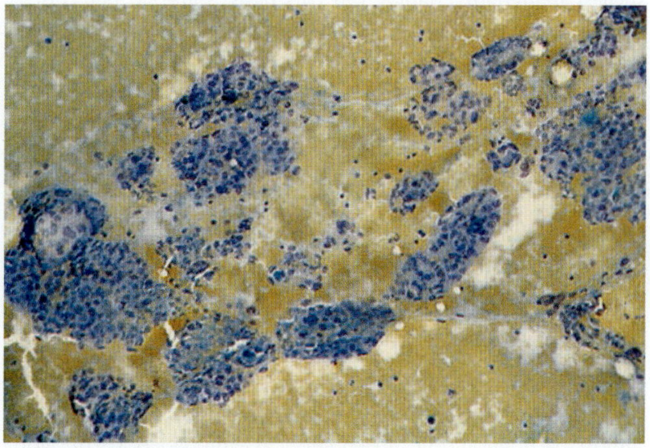

Figure 51.18 Thy3 aspiration cytology. Follicular neoplasm showing increased cellularity with a follicular pattern.

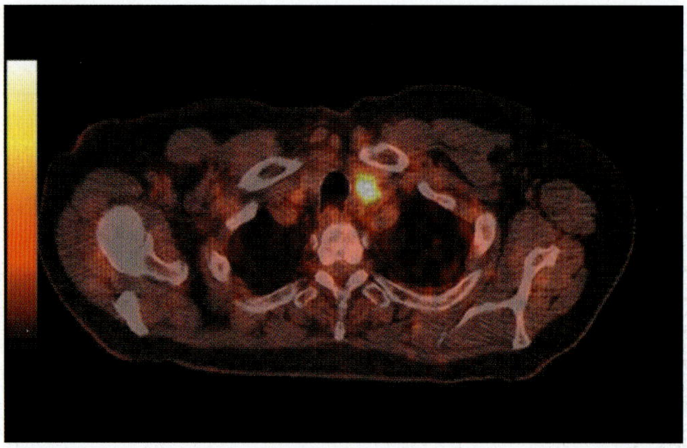

Figure 51.19 Fused computed tomography and positron emission tomography scans showing left-sided thyroid neoplasm (courtesy of Dr M Brooks, Aberdeen, UK).

Core biopsy

Core biopsy gives a strip of tissue for histological rather than cytological assessment. It has a high diagnostic accuracy but requires local anaesthesia, and may be associated with complications such as pain, bleeding, tracheal and recurrent laryngeal nerve damage. It has little application in routine assessment except in locally advanced, surgically unresectable malignancy (either anaplastic carcinoma or lymphoma) when a core biopsy may obviate the need for an operative biopsy. In some centres core biopsy is recommended following FNAC when a Thy1 FNAC (inadequate cytology) specimen has been obtained to avoid operating where the risk of malignancy is very low. It is unlikely to be useful in differentiating benign from malignant Thy3 specimens (follicular lesions) as explained below.

Treatment

The main indication for operation is the risk of neoplasia, which includes follicular adenoma as well as malignant swellings. The reason for advocating the removal of all follicular neoplasms is that it is seldom possible to distinguish between a follicular adenoma and carcinoma cytologically. The distinction usually depends on histological evidence of capsular or vascular invasion and FNAC cannot make this distinction although, on occasion, cellular nuclear features may be so abnormal as to suggest malignant change. On this basis, some 50 per cent of isolated swellings and 25 per cent of dominant swellings should be removed on the grounds of neoplasia. Even when the cytology is negative, the age and sex of the patient and the size of the swelling may be relative indications for surgery, especially when a large swelling is responsible for symptoms. Some patients are happier to have a swelling removed even when cytology is negative.

There are useful clinical criteria to assist in selection for operation according to the risk of neoplasia and malignancy. Hard texture alone is not reliable as tense cystic swellings may be suspiciously hard but a hard, irregular swelling with any apparent fixity, which is unusual, is highly suspicious. Evidence of recurrent laryngeal nerve paralysis, suggested by hoarseness and a non-occlusive cough and confirmed by laryngoscopy, is almost pathognomonic. Deep cervical lymphadenopathy along the internal jugular vein in association with a clinically suspicious swelling is almost diagnostic of papillary carcinoma. In most patients, however, such features are absent but there are risk factors associated with sex and age. The incidence of thyroid carcinoma in women is about three times that in men, but a discrete swelling in a male is much more likely to be malignant than in a female and it is seldom justifiable to avoid removing such a swelling in a man. The risk of carcinoma is increased at either end of the age range and a discrete swelling in a teenager of either sex must be provisionally diagnosed as carcinoma.

The risk increases as age advances beyond 50 years, more so in males.

Thyroid cysts

Routine FNAC (or ultrasonography) shows that over 30 per cent of clinically isolated swellings contain fluid and are cystic or partly cystic. Tense cysts may be hard and mimic carcinoma. Bleeding into a cyst often presents with a history of sudden painful swelling, which resolves to a variable extent over a period of weeks if untreated. Aspiration yields altered blood but reaccumulation is frequent. About 50 per cent of cystic swellings are the result of colloid degeneration, or of uncertain aetiology, because of an absence of epithelial cells in the lining. Although most of the remainder are the result of involution in follicular adenomas (Figure 51.20), some 10–15 per cent of cystic follicular swellings are histologically malignant (30 per cent in men and 10 per cent in women). Papillary carcinoma is often associated with cyst formation (Figure 51.21).

Most patients with discrete swellings, however, are women, aged 20–40 years, in whom the risk of malignancy, although significant, is low and the indications for operation are not clear-cut. FNAC is the most appropriate investigation to aid selection.

The indications for operation in isolated or dominant thyroid swellings are listed in Table 51.5.

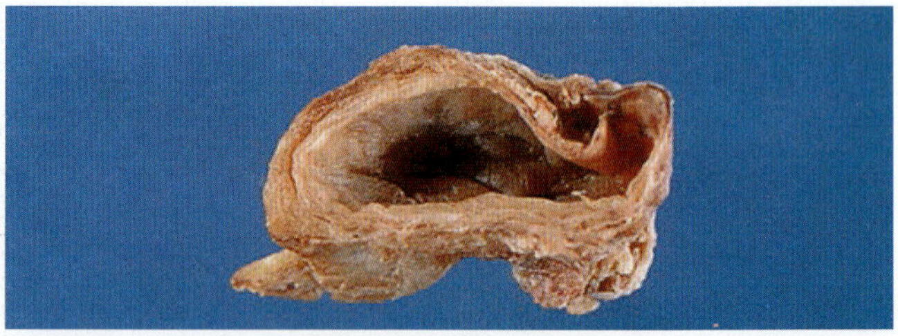

Figure 51.20 Apparently simple cystic thyroid swelling, the wall of which comprised follicular neoplastic tissue.

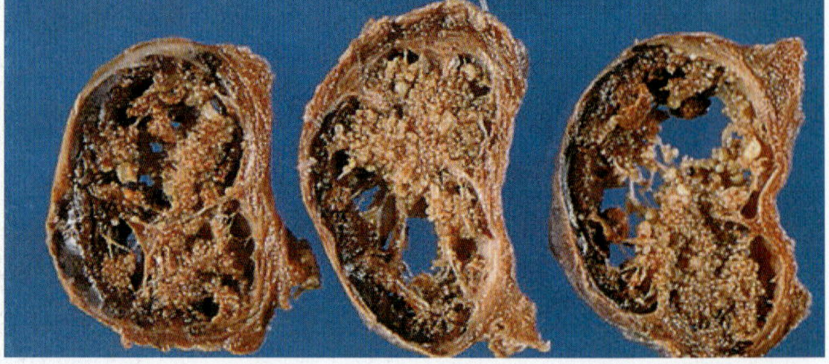

Figure 51.21 Cyst formation in a papillary carcinoma.

Table 51.5 Indications for operation in thyroid swellings.

Neoplasia	FNAC positive Thy3–5	
	Clinical suspicion	Age
		Male sex
		Hard texture
		Fixity
		Recurrent laryngeal nerve palsy
		Lymphadenopathy
		Recurrent cyst
Toxic adenoma		
Pressure symptoms		
Cosmesis		
Patient's wishes		

Selection of thyroid procedure

The choice of thyroid operation depends on:

- diagnosis (if known preoperatively);
- risk of thyroid failure;
- risk of recurrent laryngeal nerve injury;
- risk of recurrence;
- Graves' disease;
- multinodular goitre;
- differentiated thyroid cancer;
- risk of hypoparathyroidism.

Total and near-total thyroidectomy do not conserve sufficient thyroid tissue for normal thyroid function and thyroid replacement therapy is necessary. In most patients with negative antithyroid antibodies, one thyroid lobe will maintain normal function. In subtotal thyroidectomy, the volume of thyroid tissue preserved influences the risk of thyroid failure and larger remnants have a better chance of normal function but a higher risk of recurrence in Graves' disease.

Subtotal resections for colloid goitre run the risk of later growth of the remnant and, if a second operation is required years later, this greatly increases the risk to the RLN and parathyroids. In young patients, total thyroidectomy should be considered. It may be preferable to leave the least affected lobe untouched to permit a straightforward lobectomy in the future if required, rather than carry out subtotal resections.

In Graves' disease, preserving large remnants increases the risk of recurrence of the toxicity and, in these cases, it is better to err on the side of removing too much thyroid tissue rather than too little (Table 51.6). Thyroid failure need not be regarded as a failure of treatment but recurrent toxicity is.

The relative merits of routine total versus selective total thyroidectomy in differentiated thyroid cancer are discussed below (Summary box 51.4).

Summary box 51.4

Thyroid operations

All thyroid operations can be assembled from three basic elements:

1. Total lobectomy
2. Isthmusectomy
3. Subtotal lobectomy

Total thyroidectomy = 2 × total lobectomy + isthmusectomy

Subtotal thyroidectomy = 2 subtotal lobectomy + isthmusectomy

Near-total thyroidectomy = total lobectomy + isthmusectomy + subtotal lobectomy (Dunhill procedure)

Lobectomy = total lobectomy + isthmusectomy

Retrosternal goitre

Very few retrosternal goitres arise from ectopic thyroid tissue; most arise from the lower pole of a nodular goitre. If the neck is short and the pretracheal muscles are strong, as in men, the negative intrathoracic pressure tends to draw these nodules into the superior mediastinum.

Clinical features

A retrosternal goitre is often symptomless and discovered on a routine chest radiograph (Figure 51.6). There may, however, be severe symptoms:

Robert James Graves, 1796–1853, physician, Meath Hospital, Dublin, Ireland, published an account of exopthalmic goitre in 1835. He was President of the Royal College of Physicians of Ireland and elected Fellow of The Royal Society of London in 1849. There is a statue of him in the Royal College of Physicians in Ireland.

Table 51.6 Comparison of surgical options for Graves' disease.

	Total thyroidectomy	Subtotal thyroidectomy
Control of toxicity	Immediate	Immediate
Return to euthyroid state	Immediate	Variable – up to 12 months
Risk of recurrence	None	Lifelong – up to 5%[a]
Risk of thyroid failure	100%	Lifelong – up to 100% at 30 years[a]
Risk of permanent hypoparathyroidism	5%	1%
Need for follow up	Minimal	Lifelong

[a]The risk of recurrence and late failure are a function of the size of the remnant as a proportion of the total gland weight. Large remnants in small glands have a higher risk of recurrence and a low risk of failure, and small remnants in large glands have a higher risk of thyroid failure but a low risk of recurrence.

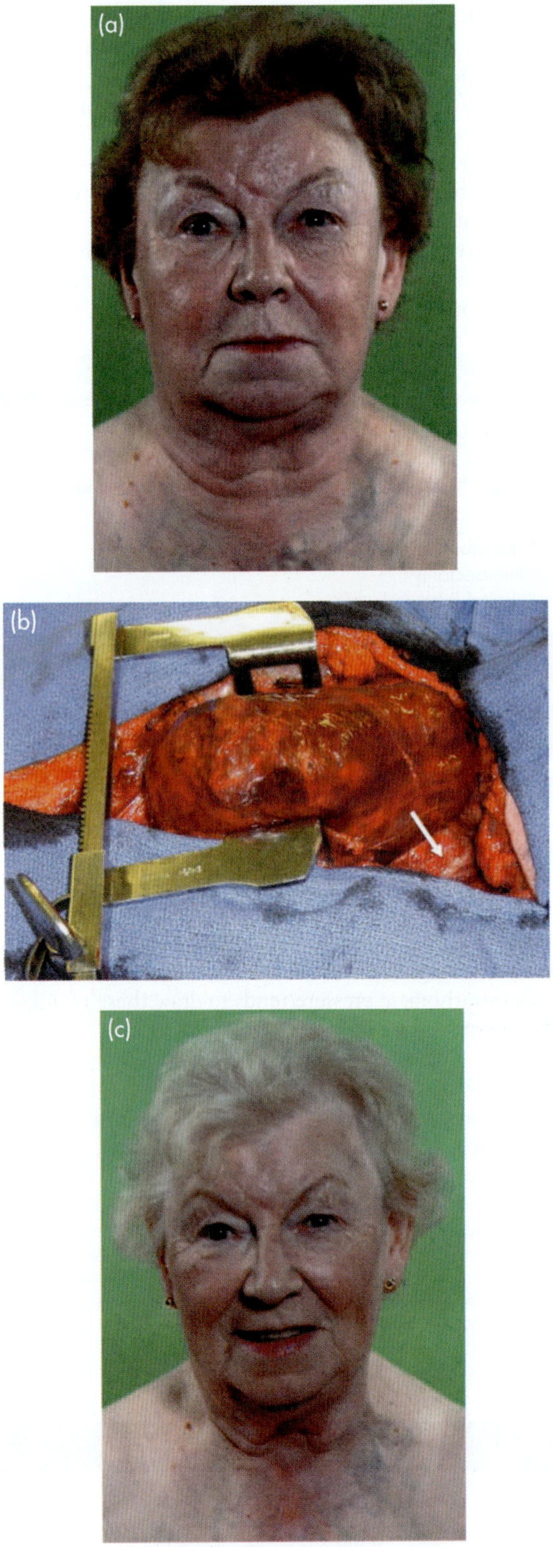

Figure 51.22 Retrosternal goitre with superior vena cava obstruction. (a) Preoperative appearance showing venous congestion. (b) Sternal split to deliver impacted left thyroid lobe. The recurrent laryngeal nerve is visible. (c) Postoperative appearance.

- Dyspnoea, particularly at night, cough and stridor (harsh sound on inspiration). Many patients attend a chest clinic with a diagnosis of asthma before the true nature of the problem is discovered.
- Dysphagia.
- Engorgement of facial, neck and superficial chest wall veins; in severe cases there may be obstruction of the superior vena cava (Figure 51.22).
- Recurrent nerve paralysis is rare; the goitre may also be malignant or toxic.

Chest and thoracic inlet radiographs show a soft-tissue shadow in the superior mediastinum, sometimes with calcification, and often causing deviation and compression of the trachea. CT scan gives the most accurate and, often dramatic, anatomical visualisation (Figure 51.8).

Significant tracheal compression and obstruction may be demonstrated objectively by a flow–volume loop pulmonary function test in which the rate of flow is plotted against the volume of air inspired and then expired. Deterioration in flow due to increase in tracheal compression, either acutely or in the long term, may be used to monitor progression of the disease and indicate the need for surgery. The changes are reversed by operation (Figure 51.23).

Treatment

If obstructive symptoms are present in association with thyrotoxicosis it is unwise to treat a retrosternal goitre with antithyroid drugs or radioiodine as these may enlarge the goitre. Resection can almost always be carried out from the neck, but median sternotomy is sometimes necessary (Figure 51.22b). The cervical part of the goitre should first be mobilised following division of the superior thyroid vessels and middle thyroid vein. Early division of the isthmus is often helpful. The retrosternal goitre can then be delivered by traction, which may be facilitated by inserting a series of sutures, finger or, traditionally, a spoon. Haemorrhage is rarely a problem because the goitre takes its blood supply with it from the neck. The recurrent laryngeal nerve should be identified before delivering the retrosternal goitre, as it may be abnormally displaced and is particularly vulnerable to injury from traction or tearing. If a large retrosternal goitre cannot be delivered intact, piecemeal delivery is possible but risks leaving a fragment of nodular goitre deep in the mediastinum resulting in

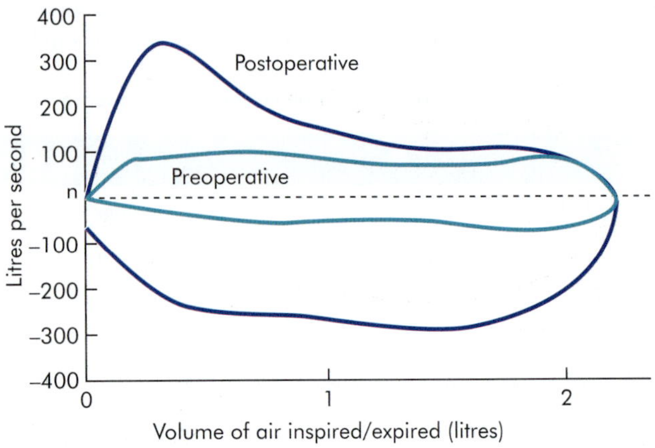

Figure 51.23 Flow–volume loops before and after operation on a goitre causing tracheal obstruction.

a very difficult reoperation many years later. Fragmentation must be avoided when malignancy is likely and all these problems are avoided with a timely median sternotomy.

Thyroid incidentaloma

The increased use of imaging modalities for non-thyroid head and neck pathology has created the clinical conundrum of the 'thyroid incidentaloma'. These are clinically unsuspected and impalpable thyroid swellings and, in some parts of the world, have reached 'epidemic' proportions. Injudicious reporting generates needless anxiety if the possibility of malignancy is raised inappropriately. The vast majority of impalpable thyroid swellings can be safely managed expectantly by a single annual review, with no intervention unless certain criteria are met or the swelling becomes palpable (Figure 51.24).

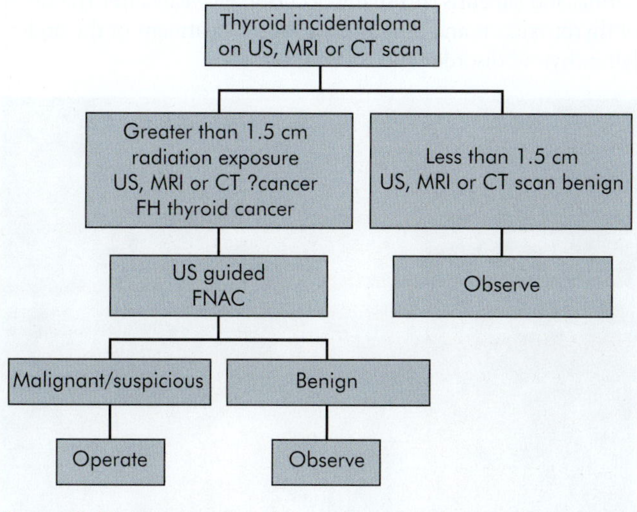

Figure 51.24 Management of thyroid incidentalomas. CT, computed tomography; FH, family history; FNAC, fine-needle aspiration cytology; MRI, magnetic resonance imaging; US, ultrasound.

HYPERTHYROIDISM

Thyrotoxicosis

The term thyrotoxicosis is retained because hyperthyroidism, i.e. symptoms due to a raised level of circulating thyroid hormones, is not responsible for all manifestations of the disease. Clinical types are:

- diffuse toxic goitre (Graves' disease);
- toxic nodular goitre;
- toxic nodule;
- hyperthyroidism due to rarer causes.

Diffuse toxic goitre

Graves' disease, a diffuse vascular goitre appearing at the same time as the hyperthyroidism, usually occurs in younger women and is frequently associated with eye signs. The syndrome is that of primary thyrotoxicosis (Figure 51.25); 50 per cent of patients have a family history of autoimmune endocrine diseases. The whole of the functioning thyroid tissue is involved, and the hypertrophy and hyperplasia are due to abnormal thyroid-stimulating antibodies (TSH-RAb) that bind to TSH receptor sites and produce a disproportionate and prolonged effect.

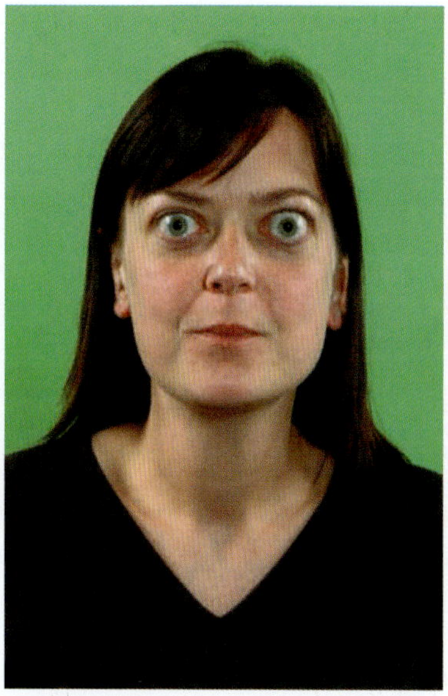

Figure 51.25 Graves' disease.

Toxic nodular goitre

A simple nodular goitre is present for a long time before the hyperthyroidism, usually in the middle-aged or elderly, and very infrequently is associated with eye signs. The syndrome is that of secondary thyrotoxicosis.

In many cases of toxic nodular goitre, the nodules are inactive, and it is the internodular thyroid tissue which is overactive. However, in some toxic nodular goitres, one or more nodules are overactive and here the hyperthyroidism is due to autonomous thyroid tissue as in a toxic adenoma.

Toxic nodule

A toxic nodule is a solitary overactive nodule, which may be part of a generalised nodularity or a true toxic adenoma. It is autonomous and its hypertrophy and hyperplasia are not due to TSH-RAb. TSH secretion is suppressed by the high level of circulating thyroid hormones and the normal thyroid tissue surrounding the nodule is itself suppressed and inactive.

Histology

The normal thyroid gland consists of acini lined with flattened cuboidal epithelium and filled with homogeneous colloid (Figure 51.3). In hyperthyroidism (Figure 51.26), there is hyperplasia of acini, which are lined by high columnar epithelium. Many of them are empty, and others contain vacuolated colloid with a characteristic 'scalloped' pattern adjacent to the thyrocytes.

Clinical features

The symptoms are:

- tiredness
- emotional lability
- heat intolerance
- weight loss
- excessive appetite
- palpitations.

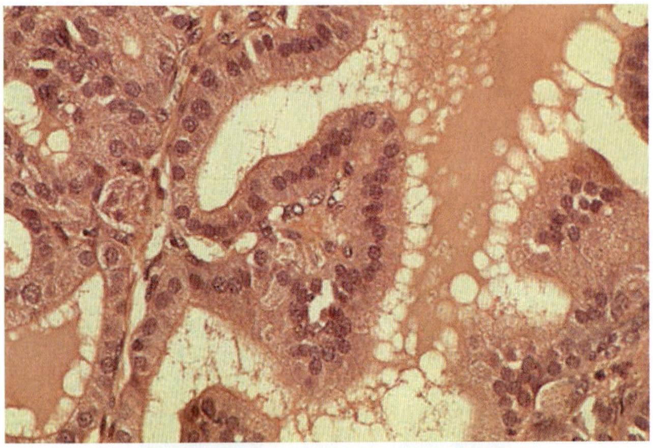

Figure 51.26 Histology of thyrotoxicosis.

The signs of thyrotoxicosis are:

- tachycardia
- hot, moist palms
- exophthalmos
- eyelid lag/retraction
- agitation
- thyroid goitre and bruit.

Symptomatology

Thyrotoxicosis is eight times more common in women than in men. It may occur at any age. The most significant symptoms are loss of weight despite a good appetite, a recent preference for cold, and palpitations. The most significant signs are the excitability of the patient, the presence of a goitre, exophthalmos and tachycardia or cardiac arrhythmia.

The goitre in primary thyrotoxicosis is diffuse and vascular; it may be large or small, firm or soft, and a thrill and a bruit may be present. The onset is abrupt, but remissions and exacerbations are not infrequent. Hyperthyroidism is usually more severe than in secondary thyrotoxicosis but cardiac failure is rare. Manifestations of thyrotoxicosis not due to hyperthyroidism per se, for example orbital proptosis, ophthalmoplegia and pretibial myxoedema, may occur in primary thyrotoxicosis.

In secondary thyrotoxicosis, the goitre is nodular. The onset is insidious and may present with cardiac failure or atrial fibrillation. It is characteristic that the hyperthyroidism is not severe. Eye signs other than lid lag and lid spasm (due to hyperthyroidism) are very rare.

Cardiac rhythm

A fast heart rate, which persists during sleep, is characteristic. Cardiac arrhythmias are superimposed on the sinus tachycardia as the disease progresses, and they are more common in older patients with thyrotoxicosis because of the prevalence of coincidental heart disease. Stages of development of thyrotoxic arrhythmias are:

1. multiple extrasystoles
2. paroxysmal atrial tachycardia
3. paroxysmal atrial fibrillation
4. persistent atrial fibrillation, not responsive to digoxin.

Myopathy

Weakness of the proximal limb muscles is commonly found if looked for. Severe muscular weakness (thyrotoxic myopathy), resembling myasthenia gravis, occurs occasionally. Recovery proceeds as hyperthyroidism is controlled.

Eye signs

Some degree of exophthalmos is common (Figure 51.25). It may be unilateral. True exophthalmos is a proptosis of the eye, caused by infiltration of the retrobulbar tissues with fluid and round cells, with a varying degree of retraction or spasm of the upper eyelid. (Lid spasm occurs because the levator palpebrae superioris muscle is partly innervated by sympathetic fibres.) This results in widening of the palpebral fissure so that the sclera may be seen clearly above the upper margin of the iris and cornea (above the 'limbus').

Spasm and retraction usually disappear when the hyperthyroidism is controlled. They may be improved by beta-adrenergic blocking drugs, for example guanethidine eye drops. Oedema of the eyelids, conjunctival injection and chemosis are aggravated by compression of the ophthalmic veins (Figure 51.27). Weakness of the extraocular muscles, particularly the elevators (inferior oblique), results in diplopia. In severe cases, papilloedema and corneal ulceration occur. When severe and progressive, it is known as malignant exophthalmos (Figure 51.28) and the eye may be destroyed. Graves' ophthalmopathy is an autoimmune disease in which there are antibody-mediated effects on the ocular muscles.

Exophthalmos tends to improve with time. Sleeping propped up and lateral tarsorrhaphy will help to protect the eye but will not prevent progression. Hypothyroidism increases proptosis by a few millimetres and should be avoided.

Improvement has been reported with massive doses of prednisone. Intraorbital injection of steroids is dangerous because of the venous congestion, and total thyroid ablation has not proved effective. When the eye is in danger, orbital decompression may be required (see Orbital swellings in Chapter 44).

Thyroid dermopathy ('pretibial myxoedema') (Figure 51.29) is a rare condition characterised by thickening of the skin, usually in areas of trauma, by deposition of hyaluronic acid in the dermis and subcutis. It usually occurs a few years after the onset of thyrotoxicosis and usually responds to treatment of the underlying thyroid disorder and topical steroids.

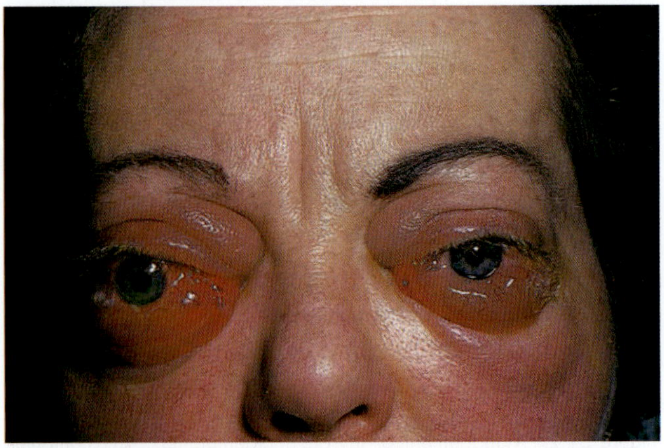

Figure 51.27 Severe Graves' ophthalmopathy (courtesy of Professor JS Bevan, Aberdeen, UK).

per se is Latin for 'through itself'.

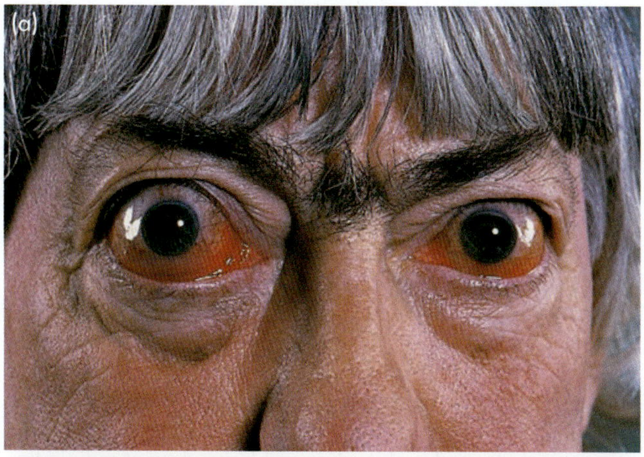

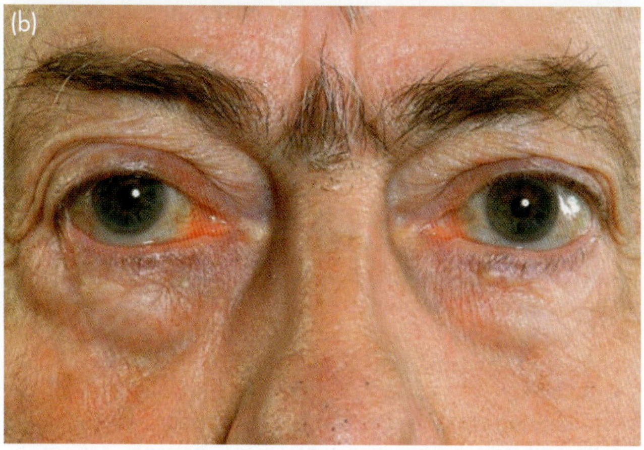

Figure 51.28 (a) Progressive (malignant) exophthalmos. (b) Following treatment with steroids, orbital radiotherapy and bilateral tarsorraphy (courtesy of Professor JS Bevan, Aberdeen, UK).

Diagnosis of thyrotoxicosis

Most cases are readily diagnosed clinically. Difficulty is most likely to arise in the differentiation of mild hyperthyroidism from an anxiety state when a goitre is present. In these cases, the thyroid status is determined by the diagnostic tests described earlier. A TRH test is rarely indicated.

T_3 thyrotoxicosis is diagnosed by estimating the free T_3. It should be suspected if the clinical picture is suggestive but routine tests of thyroid function reveal a normal T_4 but suppressed TSH. A thyroid scan is required to diagnose an autonomous toxic nodule (Figure 51.8) and differentiate it from a dominant swelling in a toxic multinodular goitre.

Thyrotoxicosis should always be considered in:

- children with a growth spurt, behaviour problems or myopathy;
- tachycardia or arrhythmia in the elderly;
- unexplained diarrhoea;
- loss of weight.

Principles of treatment of thyrotoxicosis

Non-specific measures are rest and sedation and in established thyrotoxicosis should be used only in conjunction with specific measures, i.e. the use of antithyroid drugs, surgery and radioiodine.

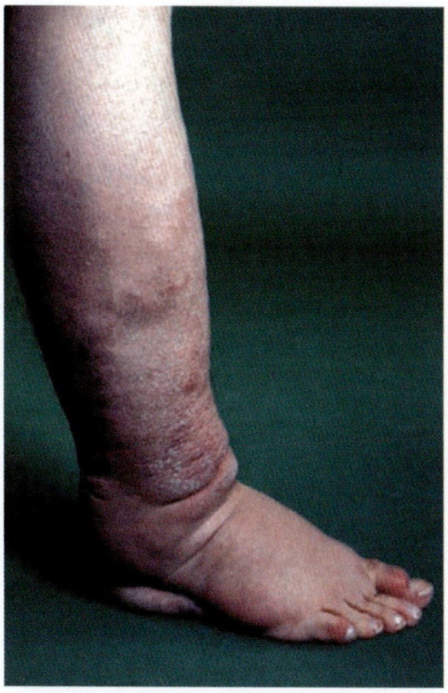

Figure 51.29 Thyroid dermopathy (pretibial myxoedema). It is usually symmetrical, and minor degrees are not uncommon but are easily missed. The earliest stage is a shiny red plaque of thickened skin with coarse hair, which may be cyanotic when cold. In severe cases, the skin of the whole leg below the knee is involved, together with that of the foot and the ankle, and there may be clubbing of the fingers and toes (thyroid acropachy).

Antithyroid drugs

Those in common use are carbimazole and propylthiouracil. β-Adrenergic blockers, such as propranolol and nadolol, are used to block the cardiovascular effects of the elevated T_4. Iodides, which may reduce the vascularity of the thyroid, should only be used as immediate preoperative preparation in the 10 days before surgery. Antithyroid drugs are used to restore the patient to a euthyroid state and to maintain this for a prolonged period in the hope that a permanent remission will occur, i.e. that production of thyroid-stimulating antibodies (TSH-RAb) will diminish or cease. Antithyroid drugs cannot cure a toxic nodule. The overactive thyroid tissue is autonomous and recurrence of the hyperthyroidism is certain when the drug is discontinued.

- **Advantages**. No surgery and no use of radioactive materials.
- **Disadvantages**. Treatment is prolonged and the failure rate is at least 50 per cent. The duration of treatment may be tailored to the severity of the toxicity with milder cases being treated for only six months and severe for two years before stopping therapy.

It is impossible to predict which patient is likely to go into permanent remission although large gland size, severity of disease and TSH-RAb levels are indicators of poor prognosis.

Some goitres enlarge and become very vascular during treatment, even if thyroxine is given at the same time. This is probably due to TSH-RAb stimulation during the prolonged course of treatment and not a direct effect of the drug.

Very rarely, there is a dangerous drug reaction, particularly agranulocytosis or aplastic anaemia. If a sore throat develops, the patient should be instructed to discontinue treatment, until the white cell count has been checked because of the risk of agranulocytosis.

Initially, 10 mg of carbimazole is given three or four times a day, with a latent interval of 7–14 days before clinical improvement is apparent. It is important to maintain a high concentration of the drug throughout the 24 hours by spacing the doses at 8- or 6-hourly intervals. When the patient becomes biochemically euthyroid, a maintenance dose of 5 mg two or three times a day is given for 6–24 months. An alternative technique is to continue with the high dose of carbimazole and inhibit all T_3 and T_4 production then giving a maintenance dose of 0.1–0.15 mg of thyroxine daily. There is no risk of producing iatrogenic thyroid insufficiency and follow up is less demanding ('block and replacement treatment').

The levels of TSH-RAb usually fall during treatment and this accounts for the permanent cure that occurs in 50 per cent of patients.

Surgery

In diffuse toxic goitre and toxic nodular goitre with overactive internodular tissue, surgery cures by reducing the mass of overactive tissue. Surgery achieves a cure by reducing the thyroid below a critical mass. After subtotal thyroidectomy the patient should return to a euthyroid state, albeit after a variable period of hypothyroidism. There are, however, the long-term risks of recurrence and eventual thyroid failure. In contrast, total/near total thyroidectomy accepts immediate thyroid failure and life-long thyroxine replacement to eliminate the risk of recurrence and simplify follow up. Operation may result in a reduction in TSH-RAb. In the autonomous toxic nodule, and in toxic nodular goitre with overactive autonomous toxic nodules, surgery cures by removing all the overactive thyroid tissue: this allows the suppressed normal tissue to function again.

- **Advantages**. The goitre is removed, the cure is rapid, and the cure rate is high if surgery has been adequate.
- **Disadvantages**. Recurrence of thyrotoxicosis occurs in approximately 5 per cent of cases when subtotal thyroidectomy is carried out. There is a risk of permanent hypoparathyroidism and nerve injury. Young women tend to have a poorer cosmetic result from the scar.

Every operation carries a risk, but with suitable preparation and an experienced surgeon the mortality is negligible and the morbidity low.

After subtotal resection thyroid failure is almost universal by 30 years although a few patients can develop recurrent toxicity many years after surgery. Long-term follow up is necessary to detect and treat both.

The incidence of permanent parathyroid insufficiency should be less than 5 per cent.

Radioiodine

Radioiodine destroys thyroid cells and, as in thyroidectomy, reduces the mass of functioning thyroid tissue to below a critical level.

- **Advantages**. No surgery and no prolonged drug therapy.
- **Disadvantages**. Isotope facilities must be available. The patient must be quarantined while radiation levels are high and avoid pregnancy and close physical contact, particularly with children. Eye signs may be aggravated.

The rate and timing of late thyroid failure are influenced by the dose selected (200–600 MBq). The higher dose is likely to result in thyroid failure in six months, whereas the lower dose may result in insufficiency which may reach a rate of 75–80 per cent after ten years. This is due to sublethal damage to those cells not actually destroyed by the initial treatment and this eventually causes failure of cellular reproduction. Indefinite follow up is essential.

There is no evidence that therapeutic radioiodine is carcinogenic or teratogenic. In some clinics, radioiodine is given to almost all patients including children. Response is slow, but a substantial improvement is to be expected in 8–12 weeks. Accurate dosage is difficult and, should there be no clinical improvement after 12 weeks, a further dose is given. Two or more doses are necessary in 20–30 per cent of cases. Follow-up requirements are reduced if a larger ablative dose of radioiodine is administered followed by routine replacement treatment with thyroxine.

Choice of therapy

Each case must be considered individually. Below are listed guiding principles on the most satisfactory treatment for a particular toxic goitre at a particular age; these must, however, be modified according to the facilities available and the personality, intelligence and wishes of the individual patient, business or family commitments and any other coexistent medical or surgical condition. Access to post-treatment care and availability of replacement thyroxine can be important considerations in the Third World.

In advising treatment, compliance, influenced by social and intellectual factors, is important; many patients cannot be trusted to take drugs regularly if they feel well, and indefinite follow up, which is essential after radioiodine or subtotal thyroidectomy, is a burden for all.

Diffuse toxic goitre

Most patients have an initial course of antithyroid drugs with radioiodine for relapse. Exceptions are those who refuse radiation, have large goitres, progressive eye signs or are pregnant.

Toxic nodular goitre

Toxic nodular goitre is often large and uncomfortable and enlarges still further with antithyroid drugs. A large goitre should be treated surgically because it does not respond as well or as rapidly to radioiodine or antithyroid drugs as does a diffuse toxic goitre.

Toxic nodule

Surgery or radioiodine treatment is appropriate. Resection is easy, certain and without morbidity. Radioiodine is a good alternative over the age of 45 years because the suppressed thyroid tissue does not take up iodine and there is thus no risk of delayed thyroid insufficiency.

Recurrent thyrotoxicosis after surgery

In general, radioiodine is the treatment of choice, but antithyroid drugs may be used in young women intending to have children. Further surgery has little place.

Failure of previous treatment with antithyroid drugs or radioiodine

In this case, surgery or thyroid ablation with ^{123}I is appropriate.

Special problems in treatment

Pregnancy

Radioiodine is absolutely contraindicated because of the risk to the fetus. The danger of surgery is miscarriage and the danger of antithyroid drugs is of inducing thyroid insufficiency in the mother and, because both TSH and antithyroid drugs cross the placenta, of the baby being born goitrous (Figure 51.30) and hypothyroid. The risk of either surgery in the second trimester, in competent hands, or careful administration of antithyroid drugs is very small and the choice is exactly as in the uncomplicated case.

Postpartum hyperthyroidism

Pregnancy may lead to an exacerbation of a variety of autoimmune diseases in the postpartum period. Postpartum hyperthyroidism may be a problem in a patient previously diagnosed with hyperthyroidism or may occur in a patient without any previous history of thyroid disease.

Children

Radioiodine is relatively contraindicated because of the theoretical risk of inducing thyroid carcinoma. There is an increased risk of recurrence after thyroidectomy because thyroid cells are highly active in the young. Children and adolescents should be treated with anti-thyroid drugs until the late teens, failing which total or near-total thyroidectomy by an expert surgeon should be undertaken.

The thyrocardiac

This is a patient with severe cardiac damage due wholly or partly to hyperthyroidism. The patient is usually middle aged or elderly with secondary thyrotoxicosis and the hyperthyroidism is not very severe: untreated Graves' disease sufficient to produce the level of emaciation and cardiomyopathy is rare in contemporary Western practice. The cardiac condition is far more significant than the hyperthyroidism, but this must be rapidly controlled to prevent further cardiac damage. Beta-blockade (propranolol or nadolol) can assist rapid control of cardiac effects.

Radioiodine is the treatment of choice together with antithyroid drugs started either before or after and continued until the radioiodine has had effect (usually 6 weeks).

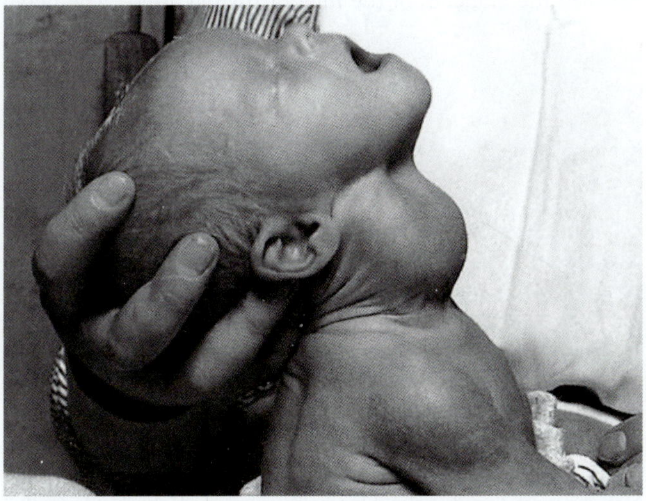

Figure 51.30 Transmitted thiouracil goitre. This does not occur if T_3 is given with antithyroid drugs, as it too crosses the placenta.

High titres of thyroid antibodies

Their presence indicates lymphatic infiltration of the goitre, i.e. a diffuse or focal thyroiditis, and a liability to spontaneous remission.

These patients are best treated with antithyroid drugs but if medical treatment fails, definitive treatment by operation or radioiodine is not contraindicated. Steroids may help to reduce pain and swelling.

Proptosis of recent onset

There is a conventional view that to terminate thyrotoxicosis abruptly by thyroidectomy or radioiodine when proptosis is recent may induce malignant exophthalmos. Although there is no real proof of this, it is reasonable to treat these patients with antithyroid drugs until the proptosis has been static for six months.

Hyperthyroidism due to other causes

Thyrotoxicosis factitia

Hyperthyroidism may be induced by taking thyroxine, but only if the dosage exceeds the normal requirements of 0.15–0.25 mg per day. Doses below the normal requirements simply suppress normal hormone production by the thyroid.

Jod–Basedow thyrotoxicosis

In European countries, diffuse toxic goitre is often called Basedow's disease or Jod–Basedow thyrotoxicosis (jod = German for iodine + Basedow). Large doses of iodide given to a patient with a hyperplastic endemic goitre that is iodine avid may produce temporary hyperthyroidism and, very occasionally, persistent hyperthyroidism.

Subacute/acute forms of autoimmune thyroiditis or of de Quervain's thyroiditis

In subacute or acute forms of autoimmune thyroiditis or of de Quervain's thyroiditis (see later), mild hyperthyroidism may occur in the early stages due to liberation of thyroid hormones from damaged tissue.

Secondary carcinoma

A large mass of secondary carcinoma will rarely produce sufficient hormone to induce mild hyperthyroidism.

Neonatal thyrotoxicosis

Neonatal thyrotoxicosis occurs in babies born to hyperthyroid mothers or to euthyroid mothers who have had thyrotoxicosis. High TSH-RAb titres are present in both mother and child because TSH-RAb can cross the placental barrier. The hyperthyroidism gradually subsides in 3–4 weeks time as the TSH-RAb titres fall in the baby's serum.

> The soil of New Zealand is heavily impregnated with **iodine**, but this does not prevent goitre in man, sheep and other animals (Sir Charles Hercus, former Professor of Public Health, University of Otago, New Zealand).

Karl Adolf Basedow, 1799–1854, a general practitioner of Merseburg, Germany, published his account of exopthalmic goitre in 1840.
Friedrich Joseph de Quervain, 1868–1940, Professor of Surgery, Berne, Switzerland, described this form of thyroiditis in 1902.

Surgery for thyrotoxicosis

Preoperative preparation

Traditional preparation aims to make the patient biochemically euthyroid at operation. The thyroid state is determined by clinical assessment, i.e. by improvement in previous symptoms and by objective signs such as weight gain and lowering of the pulse rate, and by serial estimations of the thyroid profile.

Preparation is as an outpatient and only rarely is admission to hospital necessary on account of severe symptoms at presentation, failure to control the hyperthyroidism or non-compliance with medication. Failure to control with antithyroid drugs is unusual but may be due to uneven dosage, i.e. not taking the drug at 6- or 8-hourly intervals.

Carbimazole 30–40 mg per day is the drug of choice for preparation. When euthyroid (after 8–12 weeks), the dose may be reduced to 5 mg 8-hourly or a 'block and replace' regime used (see above). The last dose of carbimazole may be given on the evening before surgery. Iodides are not used alone because, if the patient needs preoperative treatment, a more effective drug should be given.

An alternative method of preparation is to abolish the clinical manifestations of the toxic state, using β-adrenergic blocking drugs. These act on the target organs and not on the gland itself. Propranolol also inhibits the peripheral conversion of T_4 to T_3. The appropriate dosages are propranolol 40 mg three times a day or the longer-acting nadolol 160 mg once daily. Clinical response to beta-blockade is rapid and the patient may be rendered clinically euthyroid and operation arranged in a few days rather than weeks. The dose of β-adrenergic blocking drug is increased to achieve the required clinical response and quite often larger doses (propranolol 80 mg three times a day or nadololol 320 mg once daily) are necessary.

β-Adrenergic blocking drugs do not interfere with synthesis of thyroid hormones, and hormone levels remain high during treatment and for some days after thyroidectomy. It is, therefore, important to continue to give the drug for 7 days postoperatively.

Iodine may be given with carbimazole or a β-adrenergic blocking drug for the 10 days before operation. Iodide alone produces a transient remission and may reduce vascularity, thereby marginally improving safety. The use of iodine preparations is not universal because of more effective alternatives. Iodine gives an additional measure of safety in case the early morning dose of β-adrenergic blocking drug is mistakenly omitted on the day of operation.

Surgery

Preoperative investigations to be carried out and recorded are:

- **Thyroid function tests.**
- **Laryngoscopy.** Whether this is routine is a matter for local protocols. The outcome should have little impact on the operation because every recurrent laryngeal nerve must be routinely and obsessionally preserved.
- **Thyroid antibodies.**
- **Serum calcium estimation.**
- An **isotope scan** before preoperative preparation is necessary in patients with toxic nodular goitre if total thyroidectomy is not planned.

The extent of the resection depends on the size of the gland, the age of the patient, the experience of the surgeon, the need to minimise the risk of recurrent toxicity and the wish to avoid postoperative thyroid replacement (Table 51.6).

Technique

General anaesthesia with endotracheal intubation and muscle relaxation is routine. The patient is supine on the operating table with the table tilted up 15° at the head end to reduce venous engorgement (reverse Trendelenburg). A gel pad or sandbag is placed transversely under the shoulders and the neck is extended (with care particularly in the elderly) to make the thyroid gland more prominent and apply tension to skin, platysma and strap muscles, which makes dissection easier.

A gently curved skin crease incision is made midway between the notch of the thyroid cartilage and the suprasternal notch: a lower incision is easier to hide but is more likely to result in a hypertrophic scar. Flaps of skin, subcutaneous tissue and platysma are raised upwards to the superior thyroid notch and downwards to the suprasternal notch. The deep cervical fascia is divided in the midline between the sternothyroid muscles down to the plane of the thyroid capsule. The strap muscles are not divided as a routine but may be if greater exposure is required. The sternothyroid muscle is mobilised off the thyroid lobes, taking care to stay close to the muscle and outside the capsule.

In 30 per cent of patients, middle thyroid veins passing directly into the internal jugular vein require ligation and division. The plane between the medial aspect of the upper pole and the cricothyroid muscle is developed by keeping close to the thyroid to minimise the risk of trauma to the external branch of the superior laryngeal nerve. The branches of the superior thyroid artery splay out over the upper pole and the author's preference is to ligate these individually. This permits progressive downward delivery of even the highest upper pole. The lobe is then free to rotate medially out of its bed. The inferior thyroid arteries are not routinely ligated to preserve parathyroid blood supply.

The recurrent laryngeal nerve should be identified in its course in the operative field. It should first be sought below the level of the inferior thyroid artery as it passes obliquely upwards and forwards on the right (Figure 51.31) but parallel to the tracheo-oesophageal groove on the left. If not immediately seen, the nerve can usually be palpated as a taut strand crossing the tracheo-oesophageal groove. At a higher level, the nerve lies between the branches of the inferior thyroid artery. The nerve

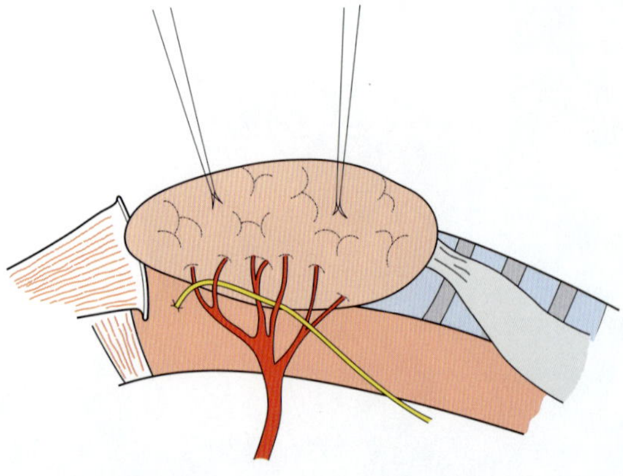

Figure 51.31 Identification of the recurrent laryngeal nerve (see text). Note how rotating the gland medially anteriorly kinks the nerve that is normally intimately related to the terminal branches of the inferior thyroid artery.

Carbimazole also has an immunosuppressive action on TSH-Rab production.

passes into the larynx under the inferior border of the inferior constrictor immediately behind the inferior cornu of the thyroid cartilage. If the right nerve cannot be found in its usual course, an anomalous (non-recurrent) nerve, present in 1 per cent of cases, should be suspected; this arises from the vagus trunk and usually passes from behind the carotid sheath, curving medially, forwards and upwards and may be mistaken for the inferior thyroid artery (Figure 51.32).

The parathyroid glands are identified by careful inspection in the common sites (Figure 51.4). The thymus is detached by serially dividing the inferior thyroid veins.

In subtotal thyroidectomy the isthmus is transected and the lobe resected obliquely from the medial and lateral aspects to produce a V-shaped surface (Figure 51.33). This facilitates subsequent suture of the divided surface for haemostasis. Care is required to avoid devascularisation of the parathyroids and damage to the recurrent laryngeal nerves particularly from the medial aspect. If a parathyroid gland is inadvertently or unavoidably excised or devascularised, it should be fragmented and autotransplanted immediately within the sternomastoid muscle.

Subtotal resection of each lobe is carried out, leaving a remnant of 4–5 g on each side. Absolute haemostasis is secured by ligation of individual vessels and by suture of the thyroid remnants to the tracheal fascia.

Total thyroidectomy (Figure 51.11) avoids transection of thyroid tissue by complete excision of the gland including the pyramidal lobe with preservation *in situ* or autotransplantation of as many parathyroids as can be identified.

The pretracheal muscles and cervical fascia are sutured and the wound closed. Randomised clinical trials have confirmed that routine drainage to the deep cervical space is not required.

New technology in thyroidectomy

The major immediate risk following thyroidectomy is haemorrhage and conventionally artery forceps, ligature and suture have been used to secure the meticulous haemostasis necessary to minimise the frequency. Ultrasonic shears and enhanced bipolar diathermy are increasingly used in thyroid surgery and may be advantageous in complex procedures. Identification of the RLN by electrical stimulation is popular in some centres but has no measurable impact on the incidence of RLN injury.

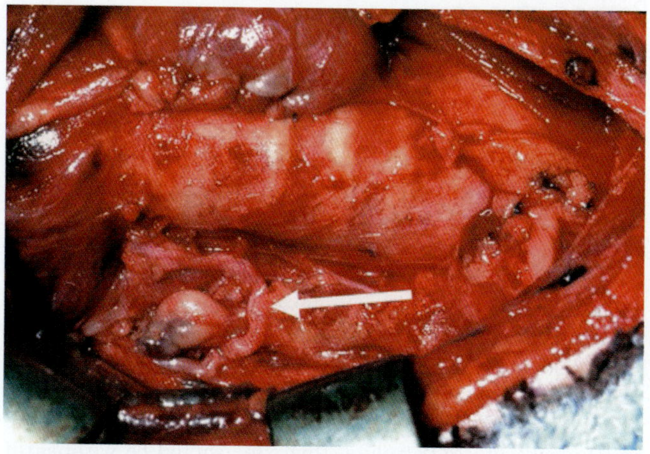

Figure 51.32 Operative photograph of non-recurrent laryngeal nerve (arrow). The inferior thyroid artery, as is often the case, is absent.

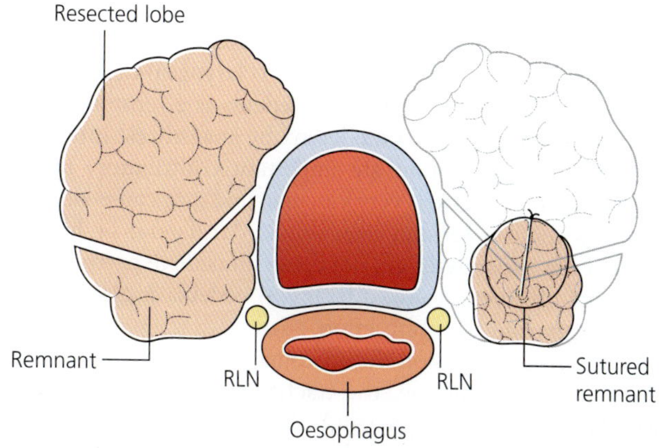

Figure 51.33 Technique of division of the mobilised thyroid lobe after division of the isthmus. The V-shaped resection margin facilitates subsequent suturing.

Postoperative complications

Haemorrhage

A tension haematoma deep to the cervical fascia is usually due to reactionary haemorrhage from one of the thyroid arteries; occasionally, haemorrhage from a thyroid remnant or a thyroid vein may be responsible. This is a rare but desperate emergency which requires urgent decompression by opening the layers of the wound, not simply the skin closure, to relieve tension before urgent transfer to theatre to secure the bleeding vessel (Figure 51.34).

A subcutaneous haematoma or collection of serum may form under the skin flaps and require evacuation in the following 48 hours. This should not be confused with the potentially life-threatening deep tension haematoma.

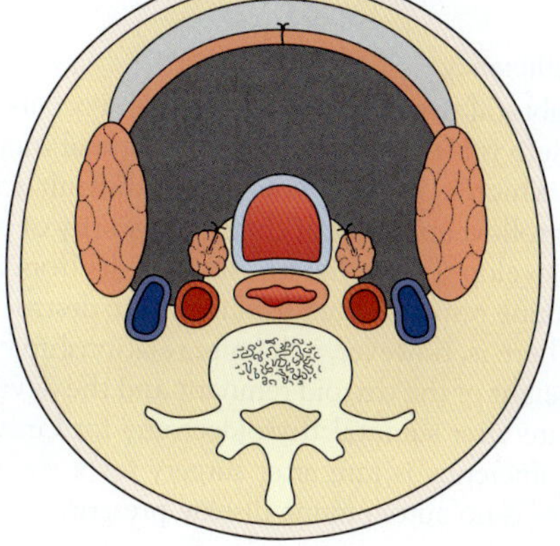

Figure 51.34 Postoperative haematoma. Subplatysmal haematoma may need evacuating (light grey) but tension haematoma (dark grey) deep to strap muscles requires urgent decompression and haemostasis.

Respiratory obstruction

This is very rarely due to collapse or kinking of the trachea (tracheomalacia). Most cases are due to laryngeal oedema. The most important cause of laryngeal oedema is a tension haematoma. However, trauma to the larynx by anaesthetic intubation and surgical manipulation are important contributory factors, particularly if the goitre is very vascular, and may cause laryngeal oedema without a tension haematoma. Unilateral or bilateral recurrent nerve paralysis will not cause immediate postoperative respiratory obstruction unless laryngeal oedema is also present, but will aggravate the obstruction.

If releasing a tension haematoma does not immediately relieve airway obstruction, the trachea should be intubated at once. An endotracheal tube can be left in place for several days; steroids are given to reduce oedema and a tracheostomy is rarely necessary. Intubation in the presence of laryngeal oedema may be very difficult and should be carried out by an experienced anaesthetist. Repeated unsuccessful attempts may aggravate the problem and, in a crisis, it is safer to perform a needle tracheostomy as a temporary measure; a large bore 12G intravenous cannula (diameter 2.3 mm) is satisfactory (see Emergency airway measures in Chapter 48).

Recurrent laryngeal nerve paralysis and voice change

Recurrent laryngeal nerve injury may be unilateral or bilateral, transient or permanent. Early routine postoperative laryngoscopy reveals a much higher incidence of transient cord paralysis than is detectable by simple assessment of the integrity of the voice and cough. Such temporary dysfunction is not clinically important however, but voice and cord function should be assessed at first follow up 4 weeks postoperatively. The British Association of Endocrine Surgeons audit revealed a RLN palsy rate of 1.8 per cent at one month declining to 0.5 per cent at three months for first-time operations. Permanent paralysis is rare if the nerve has been identified at operation. Injury to the external branch of the superior laryngeal nerve is more common because of its proximity to the superior thyroid artery. This leads to loss of tension in the vocal cord with diminished power and range in the voice. Patients, particularly those who use their voice professionally, must be advised that any thyroid operation will result in change to the voice even in the absence of nerve trauma. Fortunately, for most patients, the changes are subtle and only demonstrable on formal voice assessment.

Thyroid insufficiency

Following subtotal thyroidectomy this usually occurs within two years, but there is a small but progressive annual incidence over many years which is often insidious and difficult to recognise. With longer follow up it is clear that the majority of patients will eventually develop thyroid failure. This results from a change in the autoimmune response from stimulation to destruction of thyroid cells. There is, however, a definite relationship between the estimated weight of the thyroid remnant and the development of thyroid failure after subtotal thyroidectomy for Graves' disease. Thyroid insufficiency is rare after surgery for a toxic adenoma, because there is no autoimmune disease present.

Parathyroid insufficiency

This is due to removal of the parathyroid glands or infarction through damage to the parathyroid end artery; often, both factors occur together. Vascular injury is probably far more important than inadvertent removal. The incidence of permanent hypoparathyroidism should be less than 1 per cent and most cases present dramatically 2–5 days after operation but, very rarely, the onset is delayed for 2–3 weeks or if a patient with marked hypocalcaemia is asymptomatic.

Thyrotoxic crisis (storm)

This is an acute exacerbation of hyperthyroidism. It occurs if a thyrotoxic patient has been inadequately prepared for thyroidectomy and is now extremely rare. Very rarely, a thyrotoxic patient presents in a crisis and this may follow an unrelated operation. Symptomatic and supportive treatment is for dehydration, hyperpyrexia and restlessness. This requires the administration of intravenous fluids, cooling the patient with ice packs, administration of oxygen, diuretics for cardiac failure, digoxin for uncontrolled atrial fibrillation, sedation and intravenous hydrocortisone. Specific treatment is by carbimazole 10–20 mg 6-hourly, Lugol's iodine 10 drops 8-hourly by mouth or sodium iodide 1 g i.v. Propranolol intravenously (1–2 mg) or orally (40 mg 6-hourly) will block β-adrenergic effects.

Wound infection

Cellulitis requiring prescription of antibiotics, often by the general practitioner, is more common than most surgeons appreciate. A significant subcutaneous or deep cervical abscess is exceptionally rare and should be drained.

Hypertrophic or keloid scar

This is more likely to form if the incision overlies the sternum and in dark-skinned individuals. Intradermal injections of corticosteroid should be given at once and repeated monthly if necessary. Scar revision rarely results in significant long-term improvement.

Stitch granuloma

This may occur with or without sinus formation and is seen after the use of non-absorbable, particularly silk, suture material. Absorbable ligatures and sutures must be used throughout thyroid surgery. Some surgeons use a subcuticular absorbable skin suture rather than the traditional skin clips or staples. Skin staples, if used, can be removed safely in less than 48 hours because the skin closure is supported by the platysma stitch.

Postoperative care

About 25 per cent of patients develop transient hypocalcaemia and oral calcium may be necessary (1 g three to four times daily). If associated symptoms are severe, and serum calcium less than 1.90 mmol/L, 10 mL intravenous calcium gluconate 10 per cent (10 mL equivalent to 8.9 mg or 2.3 mmol calcium) should be given and alfacalcidol (1–2 μg oral daily) may be required to maintain normocalcaemia. To screen for parathyroid insufficiency, the serum calcium should be measured at the first review attendance 4–6 weeks after operation.

After subtotal resection, stability in terms of thyroid function takes time. It is important that biochemical (subclinical) thyroid failure should not be an indication for treatment during the first year, as the majority of patients with early subclinical failure, which is common, ultimately regain normality. Even when there are clinical features of failure, thyroxine should be withheld if possible during the first six months. Most patients who develop thyroid failure do so within the first two years, but there is a

Jean Guillaume Lugol, 1786–1851, physician, Hôpital St Louis, Paris, France.

continuing incidence thereafter. Recurrent thyrotoxicosis may occur at any time after operation. Follow up should therefore be for life.

Once a stable situation has been achieved, follow up after thyroid surgery should be carried out by an automated computerised system, which dramatically reduces the number of patient attendances at the thyroid clinic (Summary box 51.5).

Summary box 51.5

Hyperthyroidism

- Describe the causes
- Discuss the pros and cons of the three major treatment options
- Know how to prepare a patient for operation
- Describe appropriate surgical procedures
- Know about early and late postoperative management

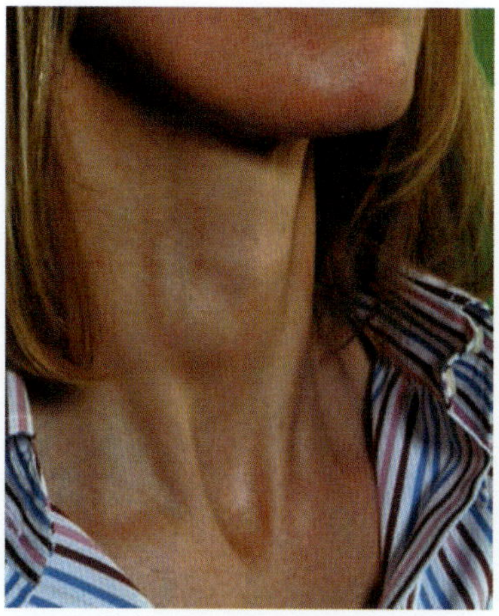

Figure 51.35 Isolated swelling in upper pole right thyroid lobe.

NEOPLASMS OF THE THYROID

Thyroid neoplasms are classified in Table 51.7 and the relative incidence of malignancies in Table 51.8.

Benign tumours

Follicular adenomas present as clinically solitary nodules (Figure 51.35) and the distinction between a follicular carcinoma and an adenoma can only be made by histological examination; in the adenoma there is no invasion of the capsule or of pericapsular blood vessels. Treatment is, therefore, by wide excision, i.e. lobectomy. The remaining thyroid tissue is normal so that prolonged follow up is unnecessary. It is doubtful if there is such an entity as a papillary adenoma and all papillary tumours should be considered as malignant even if encapsulated.

Table 51.7 Classification of thyroid neoplasms.

Benign	Follicular adenoma		
Malignant	Primary	Follicular epithelium – differentiated	Follicular Papillary
		Follicular epithelium – undifferentiated	Anaplastic
		Parafollicular cells	Medullary
		Lymphoid cells	Lymphoma
	Secondary	Metastatic	
		Local infiltration	

Table 51.8 Relative incidence of primary malignant tumour of the thyroid gland.

Relative incidence	(%)
Papillary carcinoma	60
Follicular carcinoma	20
Anaplastic carcinoma	10
Medullary carcinoma	5
Malignant lymphoma	5

Malignant tumours

The vast majority of primary malignancies are carcinomas derived from the follicular cells (Table 51.7). Dunhill classified them histologically as differentiated and undifferentiated: and the differentiated carcinomas are subdivided into follicular and papillary. Lymphoma and medullary cancers make up the remainder of primary malignancies. Metastases to the thyroid, most commonly from kidney and breast, are rare. Direct invasion by upper aerodigestive squamous cancer is a rare but lethal event. Lymph node and blood-borne metastases to bone and lung occur and may be the mode of presentation (Figure 51.36).

Aetiology of malignant thyroid tumours

The single most important aetiological factor in differentiated thyroid carcinoma, particularly papillary, is irradiation of the

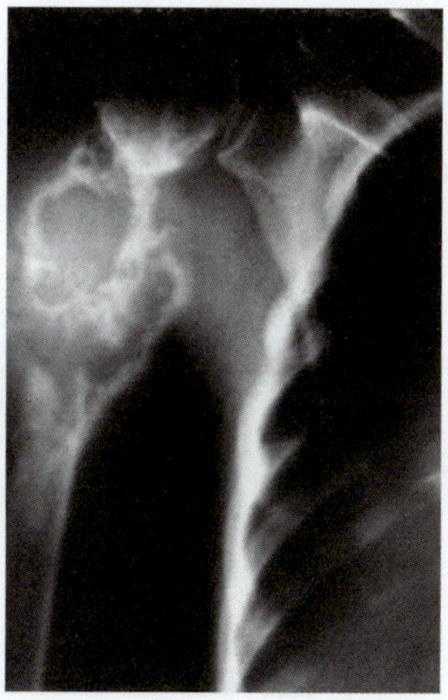

Figure 51.36 Metastasis in the humerus from thyroid carcinoma (courtesy of DS Devadatta, Vellore, India).

Circa 1600BC the Chinese used burnt sponge and seaweed to treat thyrotoxicosis.
In 1942, Saul Hertz from Boston, USA, and Arthur Roberts from Iowa, USA, first used radioactive iodine in the treatment of thyrotoxicosis.
In 1943, Edwin Bennett Astwood from Boston first treated thyrotoxicosis successfully with thiourea.

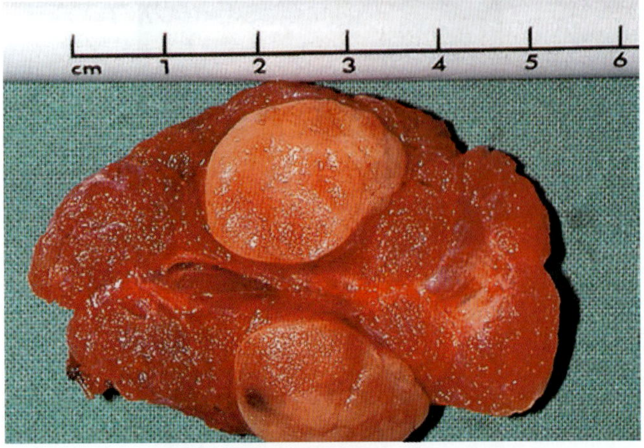

Figure 51.37 Follicular neoplasm of thyroid presenting as an isolated swelling.

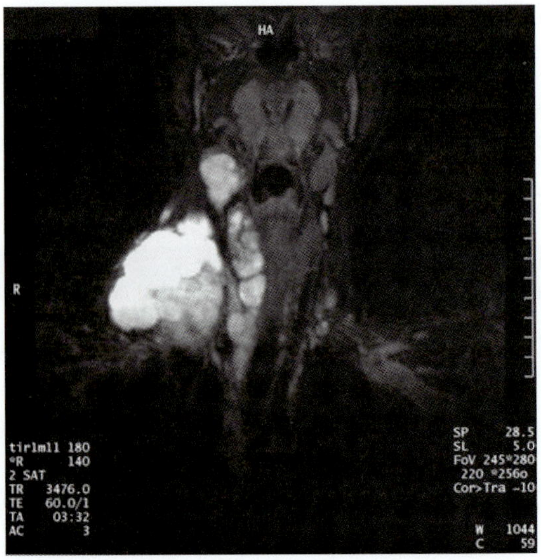

Figure 51.38 Magnetic resonance imaging scan of papillary cancer with multiple node metastases.

thyroid under five years of age. The incidence of childhood thyroid cancer in the Ukraine rose from 57 in the five years before the Chernobyl nuclear incident in 1986 to 577 in the subsequent ten years. In the town of Gomel, the incidence rose from <1 per million to 96 per million.

Short latency aggressive papillary cancer is associated with the *ret/PTC3* oncogene and later developing, possibly less aggressive, cancers with *ret/PTC1*. The incidence of follicular carcinoma is high in endemic goitrous areas, possibly due to TSH stimulation. Malignant lymphomas sometimes develop in autoimmune thyroiditis, and the lymphocytic infiltration in the autoimmune process may be an aetiological factor.

Clinical features of thyroid cancers

The annual incidence is about 3.7 per 100 000 of the population and the sex ratio is three females to one male. The overall mortality should be low because most patients are in a low-risk category but older patients have more aggressive disease with a worse prognosis. The most common presenting symptom is a thyroid swelling (Figures 51.35 and 51.37) and a five-year history is far from uncommon in differentiated growths. Enlarged cervical lymph nodes may be the presentation of papillary carcinoma. Recurrent laryngeal nerve paralysis is very suggestive of locally advanced disease.

Anaplastic growths are usually hard, irregular and infiltrating. A differentiated carcinoma may be suspiciously firm and irregular, but is often indistinguishable from a benign swelling. Small papillary tumours may be impalpable, even when lymphatic metastases are present. Pain, often referred to the ear, is frequent in infiltrating growths.

Diagnosis of thyroid neoplasms

Diagnosis is obvious on clinical examination in most cases of anaplastic carcinoma, although Riedel's thyroiditis (see later) is indistinguishable. The localised forms of granulomatous and lymphocytic thyroiditis may simulate carcinoma. It is not always easy to exclude a carcinoma in a multinodular goitre, and solitary nodules, particularly in the young male, are always suspect. Failure to take up radioiodine is characteristic of almost all thyroid carcinomas (only very rarely will differentiated carcinoma (primary or secondary) take up ^{123}I in the presence of normal thyroid tissue), but this also occurs in degenerating nodules and all forms of thyroiditis. TSH levels are often raised in carcinoma but this may be clouded by simultaneous elevation antithyroid antibodies. The key role of FNAC in preoperative diagnosis has already been discussed. There is a false-negative rate with all investigations, and lobectomy is appropriate when there is a strong clinical suspicion. Incisional biopsy may cause seeding of cells and local recurrence, and is not advised in a resectable carcinoma. In an anaplastic and obviously irremovable carcinoma, however, incisional or core needle biopsy is justified.

When a preoperative diagnosis is made, imaging with either ultrasound or MRI is required. CT, particularly with iodine containing contrast media, should be avoided. As well as additional information on the extent of the primary, this will give valuable information on nodal involvement (Figures 51.38 and 51.39) to permit preoperative planning for nodal dissection.

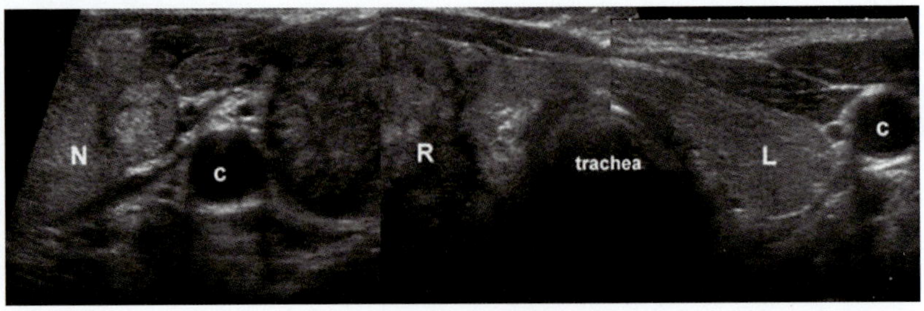

Figure 51.39 Composite ultrasound scan of papillary cancer of right thyroid lobe with extensive nodal metastases. N, enlarged nodes; C, carotid artery; R, primary carcinoma in right thyroid lobe; L, normal left thyroid lobe (courtesy Dr D McAteer, Aberdeen, UK).

Bernhard Moritz Carl Ludwig Riedel, 1846–1916, Professor of Surgery, Jena, Germany, described this form of thyroiditis in 1896.

Frozen section histology has a limited role in thyroid surgery. It cannot reliably differentiate encapsulated benign from malignant follicular neoplasms and is of more value in confirming whether nodes are involved with papillary cancer and thereby influencing the extent of nodal surgery.

Papillary carcinoma

Most papillary tumours contain a mixture of papillary and colloid-filled follicles and, in some, the follicular structure predominates. Nevertheless, if any papillary structure or characteristic cytology is present, the tumour will behave in a predictable fashion as a papillary carcinoma. Histologically the tumour shows papillary projections and characteristic pale, empty nuclei (Orphan Annie-eyed nuclei) (Figure 51.40). Papillary carcinomas are very seldom encapsulated.

Multiple foci may occur in the same lobe as the primary tumour or, less commonly, in both lobes. They may be due to lymphatic spread in the rich intrathyroidal lymph plexus, or to multicentric growth. Spread to the lymph nodes is common, but blood-borne metastases are unusual unless the tumour is extrathyroidal. The term extrathyroidal indicates that the primary tumour has infiltrated through the capsule of the thyroid gland although minimal invasion of the sternothyroid muscle is much less significant than infiltration into the oesophagus or trachea.

Microcarcinoma (occult carcinoma)

The reported prevalence of tiny foci of papillary carcinoma is related to the care with which the thyroid is examined histologically. In an autopsy study from Finland in which the thyroid was examined serially in 2-mm slices, an incidence of up to 36 per cent was reported. Clearly, the majority of such tumours never progress to become a clinically significant entity. A small percentage of cancers present with enlarged lymph nodes in the jugular chain or pulmonary metastases with no palpable abnormality of the thyroid. The primary tumour may be no more than a few millimetres in size and is often termed occult. Foci of papillary carcinoma may also be discovered in thyroid tissue resected for other reasons, for example Graves' disease. The term 'occult' was formally applied to all papillary carcinomas less than 1.5 cm in diameter but the preferred terminology now is microcarcinoma for cancers less than 1 cm. These have a uniformly excellent prognosis although those presenting with nodal or distant metastases justify more aggressive therapy.

Follicular carcinoma

These appear to be macroscopically encapsulated but, microscopically, there is invasion of the capsule and of the vascular spaces in the capsular region (Figure 51.41). Multiple foci are seldom seen and lymph node involvement is much less common than in papillary carcinoma. Blood-borne metastases are more common and the eventual mortality rate is twice that of papillary cancer (Figure 51.42).

Hürthle cell tumours are a variant of follicular neoplasm in which oxyphil (Hürthle, Askanazy) cells predominate histologically. Hurthle cell cancers are associated with a poorer prognosis and some hold that all Hurthle cell neoplasms are malignant.

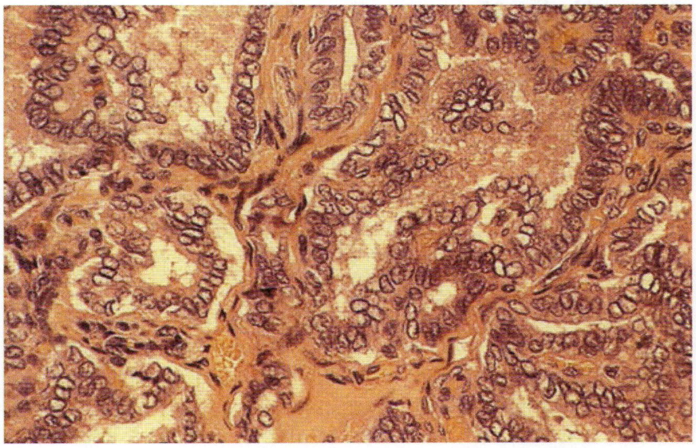

Figure 51.40 Histology of papillary thyroid carcinoma showing typical papillary projections and empty (Orphan Annie-eyed) nuclei (courtesy of Dr SWB Ewen, Aberdeen, UK).

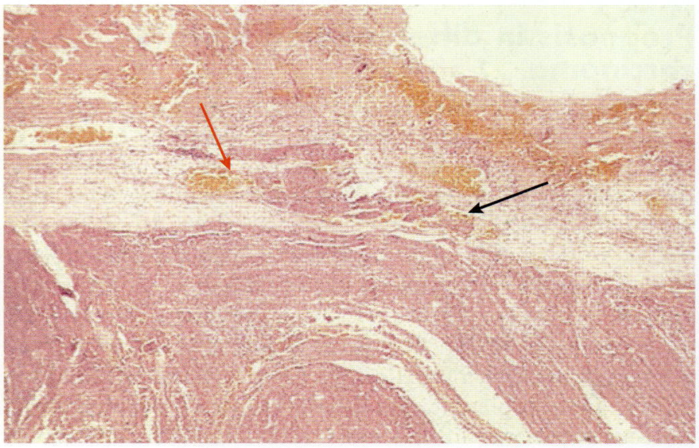

Figure 51.41 Histology of follicular thyroid carcinoma showing vascular (red arrow) and capsular (black arrow) invasion (courtesy of Dr SWB Ewen, Aberdeen, UK).

Table 51.9 Prognostic scoring in differentiated thyroid cancer.

	Age	Sex	Size	Metastases	Nodes	Extra-thyroid	Histological grade	Complete excision
AMES	+	+	+	+		+		
AGES	+		+	+		+	+	
MACIS	+		+	+		+		+
EORTC	+			+		+		
TNM	+	+	+	+	+	+		

AMES, age, metastases, extent, size; AGES, age, grade, extent, size; MACIS, metastases, age, completeness of excision, invasion, size; EORTC, European Organisation for Research and Treatment of Cancer; TNM, tumour, nodes, metastases – American Joint Committee on Cancer.

Orphan Annie is a character from a strip cartoon, who, along with others, such as Daddy Warbucks, is drawn with empty circles for eyes.

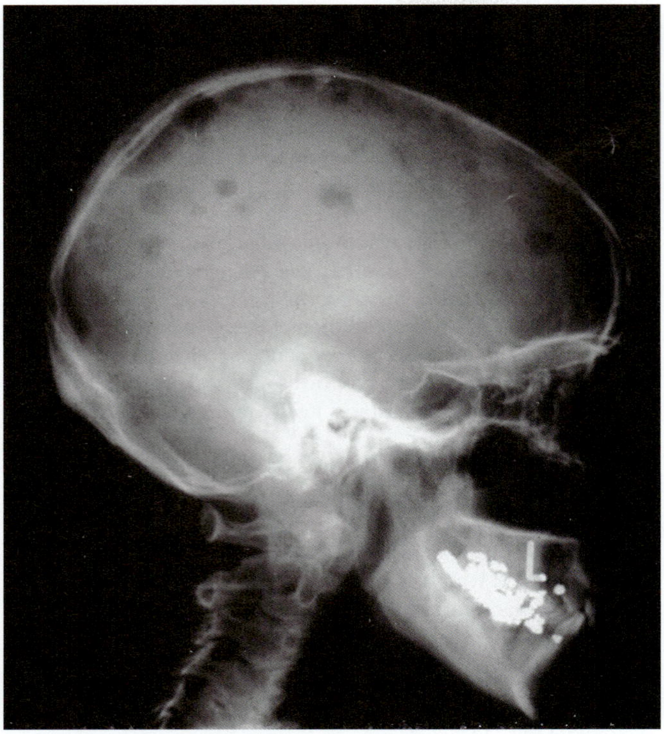

Figure 51.42 Follicular carcinoma of thyroid with skull secondaries.

Table 51.10 Tumour–node–metastasis (TNM) staging of thyroid cancer.

Tumour		
TX	Primary cannot be assessed	
T0	No evidence of primary	
T1	Tumour ≤2 cm	
	T1a: ≤1 cm	
	T1b: >1 cm ≤2 cm	
T2	Limited to thyroid, >2 cm but ≤4 cm	
T3	Limited to thyroid, >4 cm or any tumour with minimal extrathyroid extension	
T4	Any size with extensive extra thyroidal extension	
	T4a: moderately advanced	
	T4b: very advanced	
Nodes		
NX	Cannot be assessed	
N0	No regional node metastases	
N1	Regional node metastases	
	N1a: level VI	
	N1b: any/all other levels	
Metastases		
MX	Cannot be assessed	
M0	No metastases	
M1	Metastases present	
Stage	**Under 45 years**	**Over 45 years**
I	Any T, any N, M0	T1, N0, M0
II	Any T, any N, M1	T2, N0, M0
III		T3 or T1, T2 and N1a M0
IVA		T4 or T1,T2,T3, T4a and N1b M0
IVB		T4b Any N M0
IVC		Any T Any N M1

Prognosis in differentiated thyroid carcinoma

The prognosis in differentiated thyroid carcinoma compared to most cancers is excellent. Although influenced by histological type, prognosis is much more dependent on age at diagnosis, size of the tumour, metastatic disease and the presence of either extrathyroidal spread (in papillary cancer) or major capsular transgression (in follicular carcinoma). There are a multiplicity of scoring systems all of which identify the group of patients at high (40 per cent at 20 years) or low (1 per cent at 20 years) risk of death (Table 51.9). All patients should be TNM staged and this classification acknowledges the low risk of patients aged less than 45 years at presentation (Table 51.10). Approximately 80 per cent of patients are at a low risk of dying of thyroid cancer but suboptimal treatment, i.e. failure to eradicate all macroscopic disease at the first operation, may lead to increased recurrence and avoidable deaths many years after presentation. It is, however, important to avoid iatrogenic morbidity by overzealous treatment in those patients with a normal life expectancy.

Surgical treatment

Patients with large, locally aggressive or metastatic differentiated thyroid cancer (DTC) require total thyroidectomy, with excision of adjacent involved structures if necessary, and appropriate nodal surgery followed by radioiodine ablation with long-term TSH suppression. Such 'high risk' patients however are in the minority and there is continuing disagreement on the most appropriate operation for 'low risk' differentiated thyroid carcinoma, particularly with the increase in diagnosis of incidental microcarcinomas of less than 1 cm. Current guidelines advocate routine total thyroidectomy, often necessitating early reoperation and second lobectomy following a diagnostic first lobectomy with routine central compartment node dissection for all tumours greater than 1 cm. Total thyroidectomy facilitates the use of radioiodine for postoperative scanning to detect and subsequently ablate metastases results in lower thyroglobulin levels. An undetectable serum thyroglobulin is increasingly used as a proxy for cure. While this policy may reduce the rate of reoperation for recurrent disease it is unlikely to improve on existing 99 per cent survival in low risk patients and exposes patients to increased risk of RLN injury, hypoparathyroidism and later development of second cancers.

Local recurrence, in either the thyroid bed or contralateral lobe, should be exceptionally rare after total lobectomy, particularly in low risk cases. A randomised trial would have to recruit several thousand patients and take 50 years to resolve this debate. For the foreseeable future, many patients will be overtreated until a reliable method of identifying those who will benefit is established.

It is the author's current practice when a **preoperative diagnosis** of DTC has been made, usually on FNAC, to image the neck with ultrasound or MRI (Figures 51.36 and 51.37). The imaging will identify involved lymph node levels and permit

Karl Hürthle, 1866–1945, a German histopathologist who first drew attention to these cells.
Max Askanazy, 1865–1940, described these cells while working at the Pathological Anatomy Institute, Tübingen, Germany.

operative planning. Total thyroidectomy is recommended for tumours greater than 2 cm and those with nodal involvement or metastases and lobectomy for the remainder. Functional selective node dissection of involved node levels is performed as required. Lateral extension of the normal thyroidectomy incision generally gives adequate access to node levels 3–7. If access to level 2 is difficult an additional higher skin crease incision or alternatively a J-shaped utility incision may be made. Surgery should aim to remove all macroscopic disease (Figure 51.43).

There is a practical difference between a 'diagnostic' central compartment dissection in patients with no obvious nodal involvment and a 'therapeutic' clearance for macroscopic disease. A 'diagnostic' dissection can be limited to selective unilateral node dissection often with preservation of the thymus whereas a 'therapeutic' dissection requires clearance of all tissue to the level of the innominate vein. Very occasionally, it may be necessary to sacrifice the recurrent laryngeal nerve if it is completely encircled and, on even more rare occasions, extrathyroidal spread may require tracheal, oesophageal or laryngeal resection. Such procedures are not for the occasional surgeon. When the diagnosis of DTC is made **after diagnostic lobectomy** TSH suppression and review can be recommended with reoperation only for a clear indication. Indications for completion total thyroidectomy are the development of a new swelling or rising thyroglobulin. This is based on analysis of the outcome of thyroid lobectomy in the author's unit in both 'low' and 'high' risk patients since 1977.

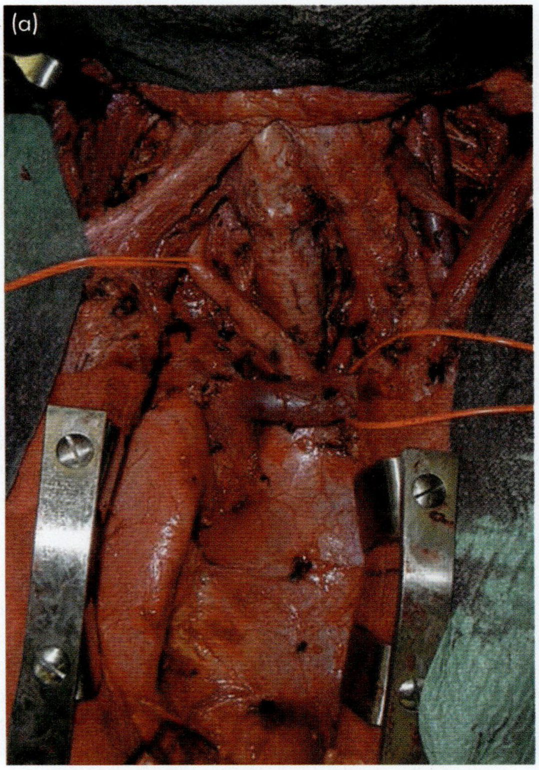

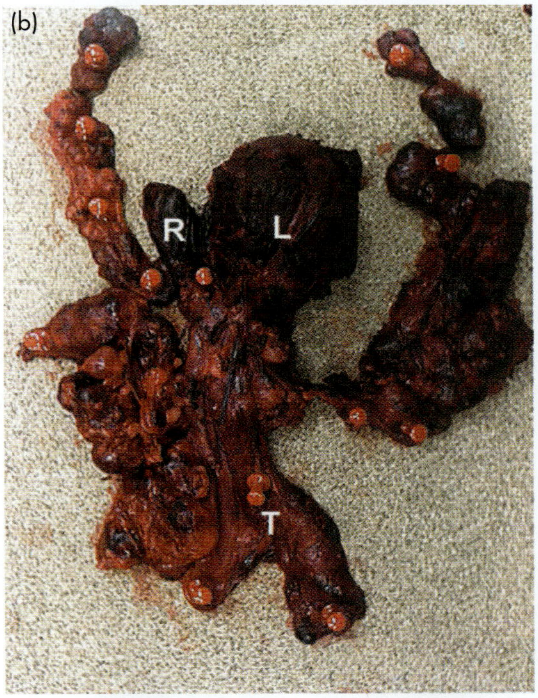

Figure 51.43 (a) Completed dissection for papillary cancer including median sternotomy with clearance of nodes from levels II–VII bilaterally and extensive mediastinal nodes. Vascular loops around innominate artery and vein. (b) Operative specimen. R, right thyroid lobe; L, enlarged left thyroid lobe with excised involved sternothyroid muscle; T, thymus. The remainder of the specimen comprises involved lymph nodes.

Additional measures

Thyroxine

It is standard practice to prescribe thyroxine in a dose of 0.1–0.2 mg daily, to suppress endogenous TSH production, for all patients after operation for differentiated thyroid carcinoma on the basis that most tumours are TSH dependent. Suppression of the TSH level should be confirmed by measurement. Failure of suppression to a level of <0.1 mU/L may indicate an inadequate dose of thyroxine or, more usually, that the patient is non-compliant. There is a trend to manage patients with undetectable thyroglobulin after radical treatment with a TSH level in the normal range because of some concern over the impact of long-term TSH suppression.

Thyroid hormone replacement is obviously necessary after total thyroidectomy and in the majority of patients after near-total thyroidectomy, and is usually given in the form of thyroxine. Patients with potential or actual distant metastases, who may require repeated radioiodine administration for scanning and therapy, should be given tri-iodothyronine (60–80 μg per day) because it is much shorter acting and, on stopping it, increased TSH secretion and thyroid avidity for iodine recovers quickly so that radioiodine may be given after 7 days. The patient is thereby spared the 4 weeks needed to develop thyroid insufficiency after stopping thyroxine before radioiodine may be given. An alternative to thyroxine withdrawal is to administer recombinant synthetic TSH over a 48-hour period to maximise iodine uptake. This is an equally effective but more expensive regime.

Radioiodine

If metastases take up radioiodine, they may be detected by scanning and treated with large doses of radioiodine. For effective

Leigh Walter Delbridge, formerly Professor of Surgery, University of Sydney, the Royal North Shore Hospital, NSW, Australia.
Radioactive iodine was first used in the treatment of thyrotoxicosis in 1942 by Herz and Roberts.
A Roberts, Isotope Department, The Massachusetts Institute of Technology, Boston, MA, USA.
John Carmel Watkinson, contemporary, otolaryngologist, Queen Elizabeth Hospital, Birmingham, UK.

scanning, all normal thyroid tissue must have been ablated either by surgery or preliminary radioiodine and the patient must be hypothyroid to improve uptake. Alternatively, synthetic recombinant TSH may be used to stimulate uptake. The indications for scanning after operations for differentiated carcinoma are also disputed, but radioiodine is indicated in patients with unresectable disease, local recurrence or metastatic disease, high-risk patients, and in those with a rising serum thyroglobulin level. A whole body scan can be carried out after empiric treatment with high-dose radioiodine 10 days later to allow decay of activity (Figure 51.44). Unfortunately, the more aggressive and de-differentiated the cancer the more likely it is not to take up radioiodine: those most in need of an effect are least likely to derive benefit.

If metastases have been treated, the serum thyroglobulin level and local protocols will determine when the scan should be repeated and further therapeutic doses of radioiodine given if necessary. Solitary distant metastases may be treated by external radiotherapy.

Thyroglobulin

The measurement of serum thyroglobulin is invaluable in the follow up and detection of metastatic disease in patients who have undergone surgery for differentiated thyroid cancer. It can be used after lobectomy, as after total thyroidectomy, provided that endogenous TSH production has been suppressed by T_4. This measurement reduces the need for serial radioactive iodine scanning but, when a rise occurs, imaging with neck ultrasound is appropriate. Surgery or therapeutic radioiodine is then indicated with a subsequent whole body scan once activity has decayed (Figure 51.45). This will confirm and locate metastatic disease which is iodine avid. The presence of circulating antithyroglobulin antibodies interferes with and invalidates thyroglobulin as a serum marker for recurrence, and occasionally, careful clinical palpation of the neck will be the first indication of local recurrence.

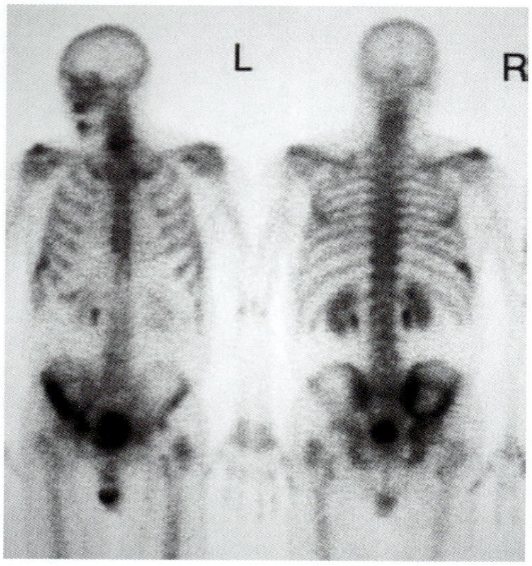

Figure 51.44 Whole body scan after total thyroidectomy and high-dose radioiodine for follicular carcinoma showing metastases in right shoulder, ribs and pelvis (courtesy of Dr M Brooks, Aberdeen, UK).

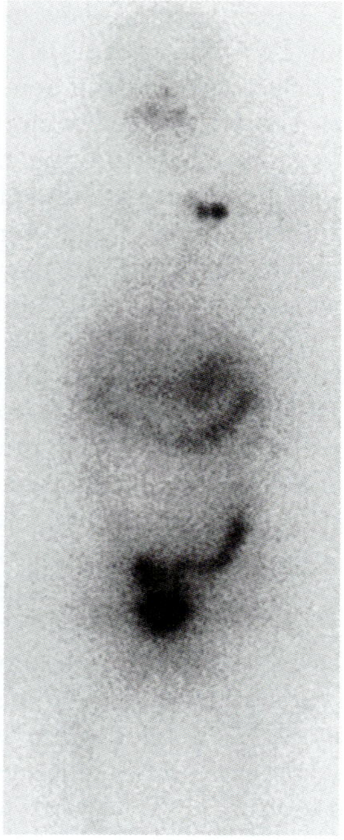

Figure 51.45 Whole body scan post-radioactive iodine ablation showing activity in recurrent lymph nodes in left level V.

Undifferentiated (anaplastic) carcinoma

This occurs mainly in elderly women and is much less often diagnosed now than in the past when many thyroid lymphomas were mistakenly classified histologically as anaplastic carcinomas. Local infiltration is an early feature of these tumours with spread by lymphatics and by the bloodstream. They are extremely lethal tumours and survival is calculated in months. Complete resection is justified if the disease appears confined to the thyroid and possibly the strap muscles and is only possible in a minority of patients. Even then the survival rarely exceeds six months and the median is around three months for the whole group. Some of these aggressive lesions present in an advanced stage with tracheal obstruction and they require urgent tracheal decompression. The trachea may be decompressed and tissue obtained for histology by isthmusectomy. Tracheostomy is best avoided. Radiotherapy should be given in all cases and may provide a worthwhile period of palliation, but there is little evidence to support the use of chemotherapy outwith clinical trials.

Medullary carcinoma

These are tumours of the parafollicular (C cells) derived from the neural crest and not from the cells of the thyroid follicle as are other primary thyroid carcinomas. The cells are not unlike those of a carcinoid tumour and there is a characteristic amyloid stroma (Figure 51.46). High levels of serum calcitonin and carcinoembryonic antigen are produced by many medullary tumours. Calcitonin levels fall after resection and rise again with recurrence making it a valuable tumour marker in the follow up of patients with this disease. Diarrhoea is a feature in 30 per cent of cases and this may be due to 5-hydroxytryptamine or prostaglandins produced by the tumour cells.

Some tumours are familial and account for 10–20 per cent of all cases. Medullary carcinoma may occur in combination with

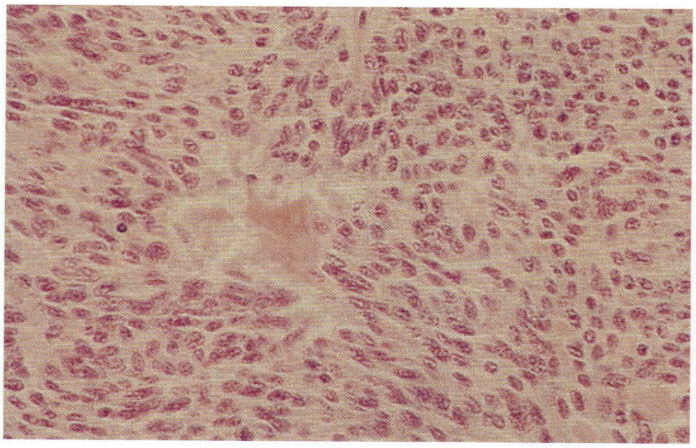

Figure 51.46 Histology of medullary carcinoma showing characteristic 'cell balls' and amyloid (courtesy of Dr SWB Ewen, Aberdeen, UK).

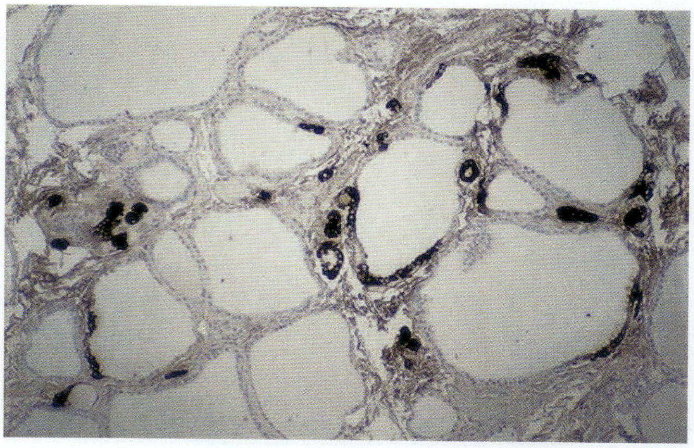

Figure 51.47 Hyperplasia of parafollicular C cells in a child from a family with medullary cancer (courtesy of Dr SWB Ewen, Aberdeen, UK).

adrenal phaeochromocytoma and hyperparathyroidism (usually due to hyperplasia) in the syndrome known as multiple endocrine neoplasia (MEN) type 2A (MEN-2A). The familial form of the disease frequently affects children and young adults, whereas the sporadic cases occur at any age with no sex predominance. When the familial form is associated with prominent mucosal neuromas involving the lips, tongue and inner aspect of the eyelids, with a Marfanoid habitus, the syndrome is referred to as MEN type 2B (see Chapter 52).

Involvement of lymph nodes occurs in 50–60 per cent of cases of medullary carcinoma and blood-borne metastases are common. As would be expected, tumours are not TSH dependent and do not take up radioactive iodine. The prognosis is variable and depends on the stage at diagnosis. Any nodal involvement virtually eliminates the prospect of cure and, unfortunately, even small tumours confined to the thyroid gland may have spread by the time of diagnosis, particularly in familial cancers. In common with many endocrine tumours the progression of disease may be very slow with a characteristically indolent course and long survival, even in the absence of cure.

Treatment

Treatment is by total thyroidectomy and either prophylactic or therapeutic resection of central and bilateral cervical lymph nodes.

Familial cases are now detected by genetic screening for the *RET* mutations, which identifies individuals who will develop medullary cancer later in life (Figure 51.47). The genetic tests are supplemented by estimating serum calcitonin levels in the basal state and after stimulation by either calcium or pentagastrin. A rise in calcitonin levels under these circumstances should lead to thyroidectomy, but even then the disease may be beyond the preinvasive C-cell hyperplasia stage (Figure 51.48). Prophylactic surgery is recommended for infants with the genetic trait. Detailed preoperative genetic and biochemical analyses permit a tailored approach to nodal surgery and may avoid unnecessarily radical surgery. A recent refinement as a result of preoperative genetic differentiation between sporadic and familial cancers suggests that lobectomy might be adequate treatment for sporadic cases.

In all cases, before embarking upon thyroid surgery, phaeochromocytoma must be excluded by measurement of urinary catecholamine levels.

Malignant lymphoma

In the past, many malignant lymphomas were diagnosed as small round-cell anaplastic carcinomas. Response to irradiation is dramatic (Figure 51.49) and radical surgery is unnecessary once the diagnosis is established by biopsy. Although the diagnosis may be made or suspected on FNAC, sufficient material is seldom available for immunocytochemical classification and core needle or open biopsy is usually necessary. In patients with tracheal compression, isthmusectomy is the most appropriate form of biopsy although the response to therapy is so rapid that this should rarely be necessary unless there has been difficulty in making a histological diagnosis. The prognosis is good if there is no involvement of cervical lymph nodes. Rarely, the tumour is part of widespread malignant lymphoma disease, and the prognosis in these cases is worse. Most lymphomas occur against a background of lymphocytic thyroiditis (Summary box 51.6).

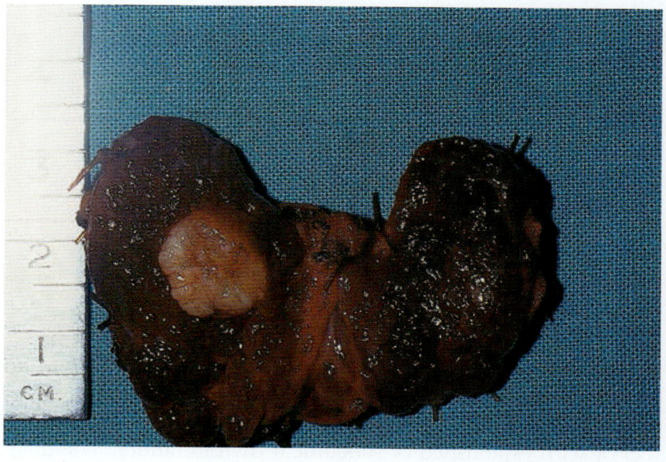

Figure 51.48 Total thyroidectomy specimen from a young girl undergoing surgery following genetic screening, showing a small medullary cancer in the right lobe.

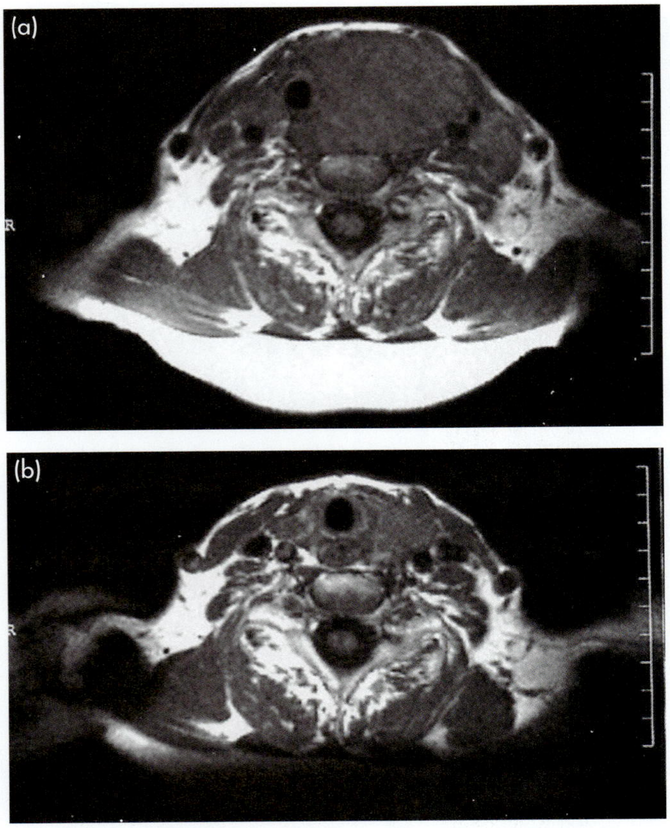

Figure 51.49 Magnetic resonance imaging scans of extensive malignant lymphoma (a) before and (b) after 7 days of external beam radiotherapy (courtesy of Dr FW Smith, Aberdeen, UK).

Summary box 51.6

Thyroid cancer

- Know the different pathological types and their behaviour
- Use appropriate investigations
- Be aware of the controversies in treatment
- Know about risk stratification and the possible effect on treatment
- Describe total thyroidectomy and node dissection
- Know how to manage the complications
- Understand the role of postoperative radioiodine therapy

THYROIDITIS

Chronic lymphocytic (autoimmune) thyroiditis

This common condition is usually associated with raised titres of thyroid antibodies. Not infrequently there is a family history of other autoimmune disease. It commonly presents as a goitre, which may be diffuse or nodular with a characteristic 'bosselated' feel or with established or subclinical thyroid failure. The diagnosis often follows investigation of a discrete swelling. Features of chronic lymphocytic (focal) thyroiditis are commonly present on histological examination in association with other thyroid disease, notably toxic goitre. Primary myxoedema without detectable thyroid enlargement represents the end stage of the pathological process.

Clinical features

The onset, thyroid status and the type of goitre vary profoundly from case to case. The onset may be insidious and asymptomatic, or so sudden and painful that it resembles the acute form of granulomatous thyroiditis. Mild hyperthyroidism may be present initially, but hypothyroidism is inevitable and may develop rapidly or extremely slowly. The goitre is usually lobulated, and may be diffuse or localised to one lobe. It may be large or small, and soft, rubbery or firm in consistency, depending upon the cellularity and the degree of fibrosis. The disease is most common in women at the menopause, but may occur at any age. Papillary carcinoma and malignant lymphoma are occasionally associated with autoimmune thyroiditis (Figure 51.50).

Diagnosis

Biochemical tests of thyroid function vary with the thyroid status and are of diagnostic value only if hypothyroidism is present. Significantly, raised serum levels of one or more thyroid antibodies are present in over 85 per cent of cases. Nevertheless, differential diagnosis from nodular goitre, carcinoma and malignant lymphoma of the thyroid is not always easy. FNAC is the most appropriate investigation although abundant lymphocytes may make the cytological distinction between autoimmune thyroiditis and lymphoma difficult. When there is doubt about neoplastic disease, which may coexist with thyroiditis, diagnostic lobectomy may be necessary.

Treatment

Full replacement dosage of thyroxine should be given for hypothyroidism and if the goitre is large or symptomatic, because some (under TSH stimulation) may subside with hormone therapy. More minor manifestations of the condition such as a small goitre with raised antibody titres, or histological evidence of thyroiditis in association with other thyroid disease, do not justify thyroxine replacement if thyroid function is biochemically normal; however, long-term surveillance is necessary because of

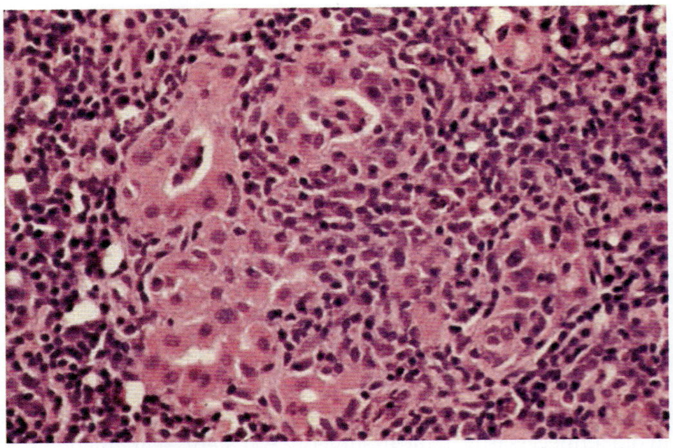

Figure 51.50 Autoimmune thyroiditis (Hashimoto's disease; struma lymphomatosa). Intense lymphocytic-plasma cell infiltration, acinar destruction and fibrosis. Compare with the normal histology shown in Figure 51.2.

the risk of late thyroid failure. Occasionally, the goitre increases despite hormone treatment and, in these circumstances, there may be a favourable response to steroid therapy. Thyroidectomy may be necessary if the goitre is large and causes discomfort. Increase in size of a long-standing lymphocytic goitre should be assessed urgently because of the possibility of the development of malignant lymphoma.

Granulomatous thyroiditis (subacute thyroiditis, de Quervain's thyroiditis)

This may follow a viral infection. In a typical subacute presentation, there is pain in the neck, fever, malaise and a firm, irregular enlargement of one or both thyroid lobes. There are raised inflammatory markers, absent thyroid antibodies, the serum T_4 is high normal or slightly raised, and the ^{123}I uptake of the gland is low. The condition is self-limiting and, in a few months, the goitre subsides and there may be a period of months of hypothyroidism before eventual recovery. In 10 per cent of cases the onset is acute, the goitre very painful and tender and there may be symptoms of hyperthyroidism. One-third of cases are asymptomatic but for the presence of the goitre. If diagnosis is in doubt, it may be confirmed by FNAC, radioactive iodine uptake and by a rapid symptomatic response to prednisone. The specific treatment for the acute case with severe pain is to give prednisone 10–20 mg daily for 7 days and the dose is then gradually reduced over the next month. If thyroid failure is prominent, treatment with thyroxine may be required until function recovers.

Riedel's thyroiditis

This is very rare, accounting for 0.5 per cent of goitres. Thyroid tissue is replaced by cellular fibrous tissue, which infiltrates through the capsule into muscles and adjacent structures, including parathyroids, recurrent nerves and carotid sheath. It may occur in association with retroperitoneal and mediastinal fibrosis and is most probably a collagen disease. The goitre may be unilateral or bilateral and is very hard and fixed. The differential diagnosis from anaplastic carcinoma can be made with certainty only by biopsy, when a wedge of the isthmus should also be removed to free the trachea. If unilateral, the other lobe is usually involved later and subsequent hypothyroidism is common. Treatment is with high-dose steroid, tamoxifen and thyroxine replacement. Reduction in size of the goitre and long-term improvement in symptoms are to be expected if treatment is commenced early (Summary box 51.7).

Summary box 51.7

Thyroiditis

- Be aware of the common and uncommon forms of thyroiditis
- Understand their effects on thyroid function

PARATHYROID HYPERPARATHYROIDISM

Primary hyperparathyroidism

Primary hyperparathyroidism is commonly a sporadic rather than familial condition associated with hypercalcaemia and inappropriately raised serum PTH levels due to enlargement of one or more glands and hypersecretion of PTH. The normal response to hypercalcaemia is PTH suppression.

Epidemiology

The prevalence of sporadic primary hyperparathyroidism increases with age and affects women more than men. Approximately 1 per cent of adults are hypercalcaemic on biochemical screening.

Familial hyperparathyroidism occurs as part of the following genetically determined conditions:

- MEN1 (multiple endocrine neoplasia type 1: Werner's syndrome);
- MEN2A (Sipple syndrome), rarely in MEN2B;
- Familial hyperparathyroidism.

Pathology

The majority (85 per cent) of patients with sporadic primary hyperparathyroidism have a single adenoma, approximately 13 per cent have hyperplasia affecting all four glands and about 1 per cent will have more than one adenoma or a carcinoma. In familial disease, multiple gland enlargement is usual.

There is a weak correlation between the size of an adenoma and the level of PTH (Figure 51.51). The histological differentiation between adenoma and hyperplasia can be difficult and the macroscopic findings are an important determinant in making the diagnosis. A single enlarged gland with three small normal glands is characteristic of a single adenoma regardless of the histology which may show considerable overlap between a hyperplastic and adenomatous gland. Multiple adenomas occur more frequently in older patients.

Parathyroid hyperplasia by definition affects all four glands (Figure 51.52).

Parathyroid carcinomas are large tumours and typically much more adherent or even frankly invasive than large adenomas. Histology demonstrates a florid desmoplastic reaction with dense fibrosis and capsular and vascular invasion.

Parathyroid cysts may be secondary to degeneration in nodules or adenomas, developmental and, while some present as a palpable neck swelling, small cysts are most often noted as

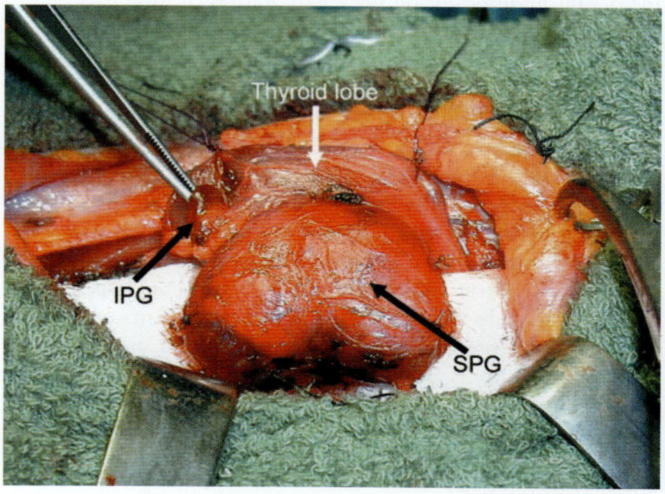

Figure 51.51 Parathyroid adenoma. Operative photograph showing normal left inferior parathyroid (IPG) and large left superior parathyroid adenoma (SPG).

Otto Werner, 1879–1936, a German physician who had a practice in a small town near the German–Danish border.
John Sipple, born 1930, Professor of Medicine, SUNY Medical Center, New York, NY, USA.

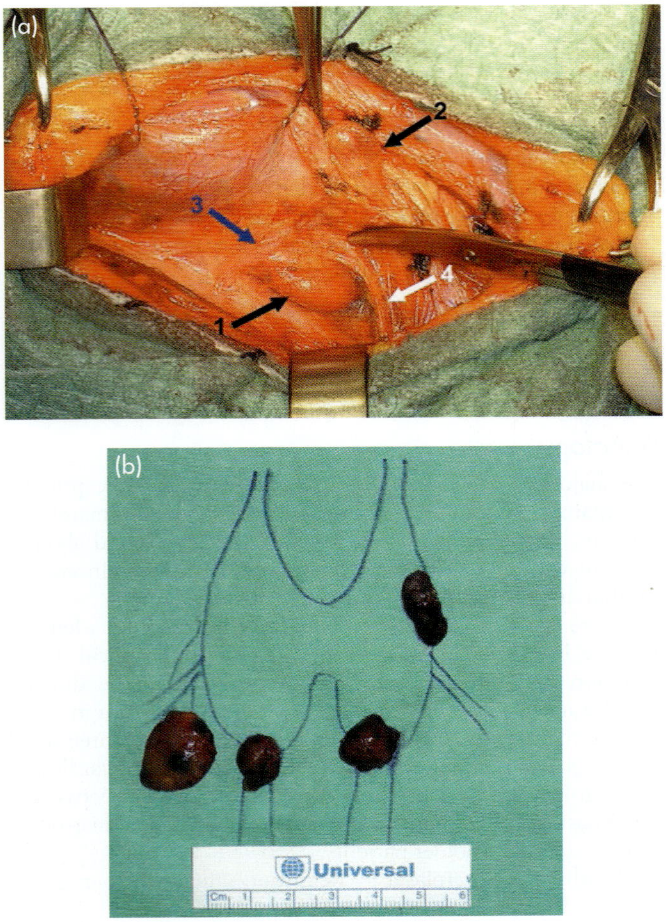

Figure 51.52 Parathyroid hyperplasia. (a) Mobilised right thyroid lobe showing enlarged superior and inferior parathyroid glands. Note how the superior gland has migrated posterior and inferior to the inferior thyroid artery. (b) Total parathyroidectomy specimens.

incidental findings during neck exploration. If aspirated preoperatively the diagnosis should be suspected from the watery clear fluid aspirated. The diagnosis is confirmed by a high PTH level.

Clinical presentation

The classic quartet of 'stones, bones, abdominal groans and psychic moans' is rarely observed in developed countries when the diagnosis is usually detected on serum calcium estimation well before the full picture of severe bone disease (von Recklinghausen's disease), renal calculi and calcinosis, pancreatitis and psychiatric disorder. Incidentally detected hypercalcaemia is rarely truly 'asymptomatic' and most patients experience an improved sense of well-being after surgery. Careful enquiry into family history is always appropriate and may reveal an index case for familial disease including familial primary HPT, MEN syndromes and familial hypocalciuric hypercalcaemia.

Diagnosis

Although ionised calcium is the physiologically active circulating element, total serum calcium is a satisfactory measure. The effect of binding to serum proteins must be corrected by upward or downward correction to a serum albumin level of 40 g/L. Inappropriate, i.e. elevated or normal PTH levels in the presence of high serum calcium is diagnostic of primary HPT. Hypophosphataemia and elevated urine calcium excretion are confirmatory.

Other causes of hypercalcaemia must be considered and excluded (Table 51.11). Advanced malignancy is the most common cause of hypercalcaemia in hospitalised patients, due to parathyroid hormone-related peptide (PTHrP) or bone metastases. The PTH level is suppressed.

Familial hypocalciuric hypercalcaemia is an autosomal dominant disorder characterised by mild elevation of calcium and PTH levels secondary to a missense mutation in the cell membrane calcium receptor. The low urinary excretion of calcium will discriminate this from HPT. Parathyroidectomy is not required. However, neonatal hyperparathyroidism is rare but is associated with severe hypercalcaemia in homozygous patients and urgent near-total parathyroidectomy is required.

Table 51.11 Causes of hypercalcaemia.

Endocrine	Primary hyperparathyroidism Thyrotoxicosis Phaeochromocytoma Adrenal crisis
Renal failure	Secondary hyperparathyroidism Tertiary hyperparathyroidism
Malignant disease	Skeletal secondaries Myeloma
Nutritional	Milk alkali syndrome Excess vitamin D intake
Granulomatous disease	Tuberculosis Sarcoidosis
Immobilisation	
Inherited disorders	Hypercalciuric hypercalcaemia

Treatment of primary hyperparathyroidism

At present surgery is the only curative option and should be offered to all patients with significant hypercalcaemia provided they are otherwise fit for the procedure. There are a number of medical strategies and therapies, particularly in mild hyperparathyroidism, which include simple expectant treatment until the calcium level or symptoms reach a level at which surgery becomes more attractive, low calcium diet, withdrawal of drugs (diuretics and lithium) which aggravate hypercalcaemia and, more recently, calcium reducing agents such as bisphosphanates and the calcium receptor agonist cinacalcet.

Occasionally, patients present with a parathyroid crisis and severe hypercalcaemia (serum calcium greater than 3.5 mmol/L). This results in confusion, nausea, abdominal pain, cardiac arrhythmias and hypotension with acute renal failure. Intravenous saline and bisphosphonate therapy (pamidronate) are required to correct the dehydration and hypercalcaemia. This is best done in a high-dependency unit or even intensive therapy unit setting to monitor the major physiological fluxes which result.

Indications for operation

Conventional indications for operation are shown in Table 51.12, but traditionally, endocrine surgeons have had a lower threshold for recommending operation than physicians. However, the widespread adoption of minimal access techniques for parathyroidectomy has changed many physicians' attitudes because of the perceived reduction in operative morbidity. There remains a cohort of patients with mild primary HPT and those with significant comorbidity where the decision for operation remains a matter of clinical judgement.

Table 51.12 Indications for parathyroidectomy in primary hyperparathyroidism.

Urinary tract calculi
Reduced bone density
High serum calcium[a]
? All in younger age group <50 years
Deteriorating renal function
Symptomatic hypercalcaemia

[a]Variously set between 2.85 and 3.00 mmol/L.

Preoperative localisation

There has been a paradigm shift in the use of preoperative imaging in primary hyperparathyroidism. Until a few years ago the maxim that the 'only localisation test necessary was to locate a good endocrine surgeon' (Doppman) was apposite when opinion favoured a conventional bilateral neck exploration. Skilled surgeons can achieve cure rates of the order of 98 per cent, with failure due to an ectopic adenoma not accessible through a cervical incision or, occasionally, failure to recognise multiple gland disease. While there should be minimal morbidity associated with a bilateral neck exploration, an image-guided targeted approach reduces this even further and has become routine in most major centres. Concerns that subtle abnormalities will be missed if all glands are not routinely visualised remain but have not translated into a significant clinical issue to date. There remains a cohort of patients in whom preoperative imaging does not localise an adenoma and the experience of the surgeon remains paramount in achieving a high cure rate.

High frequency neck ultrasound is non-invasive and should identify 75 per cent of enlarged glands. It gives better resolution but reduced penetration and cannot visualise the mediastinum (Figure 51.53). Nodular thyroid disease is a confounding factor.

Technetium-99m (99mTc)-labelled sestamibi (MIBI) isotope scans (Figure 51.54) also identify 75 per cent of abnormal parathyroid glands. The area scanned must include the mediastinum to detect ectopic glands. Single-photon emission computed tomography (SPECT) (Figure 51.55) gives a three-dimensional image which may influence the surgical approach. Concordance between ultrasound and sestamibi scan permits a targeted approach with confidence. However, the size of the adenoma is important and imaging and concordance decline with glands weighing less than 500 mg.

CT, PET and MRI imaging are not indicated prior to first-time neck exploration.

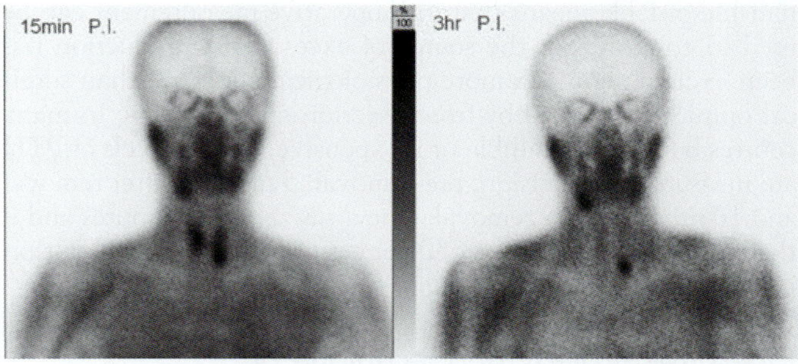

Figure 51.54 Technetium-sestamibi scans 15 minutes and 3 hours after injection showing retention of isotope in a left inferior parathyroid adenoma.

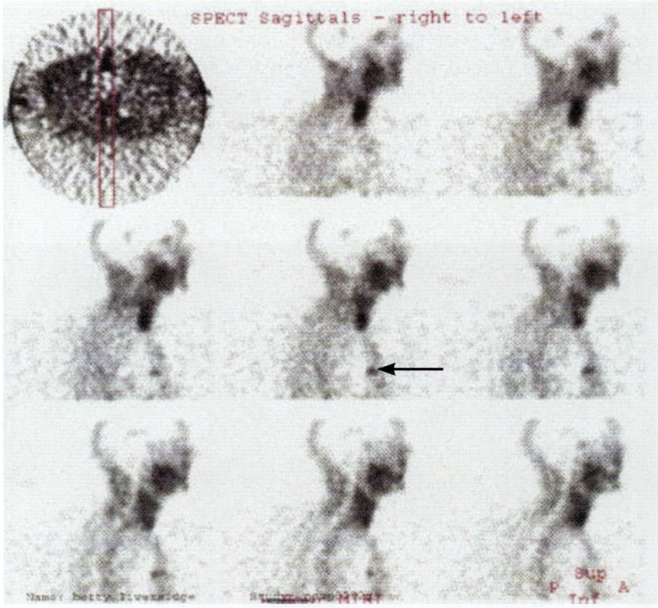

Figure 51.55 MIBI scan with single photon emission computed tomography showing hot spot in anterior mediastinum (arrow) (courtesy of Mr B Harrison, Sheffield, UK).

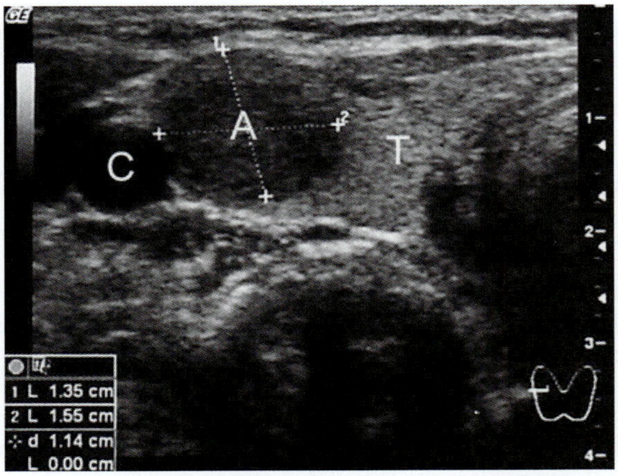

Figure 51.53 Ultrasound scan of parathyroid adenoma at upper pole right thyroid lobe. C, carotid artery; A, parathyroid adenoma; T, right thyroid lobe.

John L Doppman, contemporary, radiologist, Bethesda, MA, USA.
The noun isotope is derived from the Greek isos = equal and tops = place, meaning having an equal place on the periodic table.

Consent for surgery

Preoperative discussion must include the possibilities of:

- persistent hyperparathyroidism (5 per cent);
- recurrent laryngeal nerve injury (1 per cent);
- postoperative haemorrhage (1 per cent);
- permanent hypoparathyroidism;
- recurrent hyperparathyroidism.

Operation for primary hyperparathyroidism

There are a number of surgical options available, of which a targeted small incision approach and bilateral exploration using a conventional 'thyroidectomy' incision are the most frequently performed. Video-assisted (in which a video endoscope is used to reduce the size of incision and permit bilateral exploration) and totally endoscopic techniques with multiple punctures have not achieved much popularity. Methylene blue infusion to assist in gland identification has largely been abandoned. A gamma probe can be used to guide exploration following preoperative injection of technetium-labelled sestamibi. The short serum half-life of PTH means that intraoperative measurement can be used to confirm that the source of excess PTH production has been excised. This is a more physiological approach than surgical opinion supported by frozen section and is routine in many centres but is not infallible or inexpensive. Serum levels of PTH are measured pre-incision, pre-removal, 5 minutes after removal and 10 minutes after removal. The assay takes 30 minutes and if the percentage drop is not >50 per cent then further exploration is indicated.

Operative strategy and technique of parathyroidectomy

Targeted approach

General or local anaesthesia may be used. A head light and magnifying loupes or alternatively a 5-mm video laparoscope are useful. Confident preoperative localisation permits a 2–3 cm incision located over the site of the adenoma (Figure 51.56). This may be placed to permit extension to a formal bilateral exploration incision if the imaging is suboptimal. The subplatysmal plane is incised and either a midline or lateral approach to the strap muscles permits development of the plane between the thyroid capsule and carotid artery and jugular veins. The adenoma is easily identified in the anticipated site when imaging is concordant. It is carefully mobilised staying close to but avoiding rupture of the capsule. Identification of the recurrent laryngeal nerve is not routine and only bipolar diathermy should be used. Failure to immediately identify the gland may require an extended exploration which can be accomplished through a unilateral limited incision. Conversion to a formal neck incision and bilateral exploration should rarely be required if preoperative assessment has been rigorous.

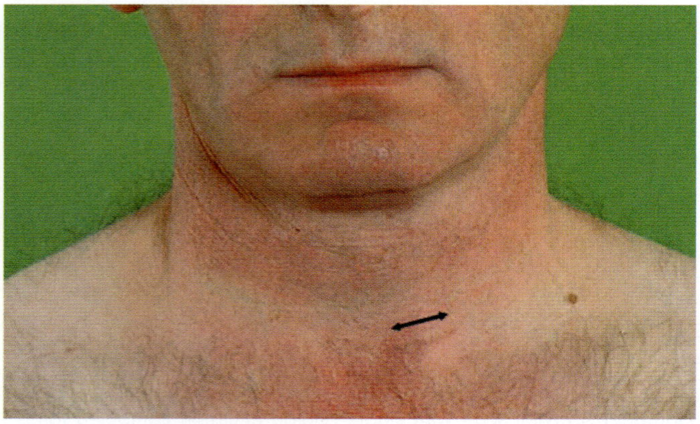

Figure 51.56 Targeted parathyroid surgery; a 2-cm incision over left inferior parathyroid adenoma.

Conventional approach

The patient is positioned in reverse Trendelenburg, with a silicone gel pad transversely under the shoulders to extend the neck with the head supported in a padded ring.

A transverse collar incision is made, the subplatysmal plane developed superiorly and inferiorly and the deep cervical fascia incised in the midline between the strap muscles. The thyroid lobes are mobilised with division of the middle thyroid vein when present. It is not normally necessary to divide the superior thyroid vessels unless the exploration proves difficult. Medial rotation of the thyroid lobe exposes the inferior thyroid artery and recurrent laryngeal nerve (Figures 51.5 and 51.52a). The glands are identified in a systematic manner commencing with the common sites and working sequentially through to the rare locations.

Superior gland:

1 in fat pad on surface of thyroid lobe above the inferior thyroid artery at level of cricothyroid articulation then

2 inferiorly behind the inferior thyroid artery and oesophagus then

3 divide superior thyroid vessels and rotate upper pole anteriorly.

Inferior gland:

1 along the thyrothymic axis then

2 on or under the capsule of the lower pole of the thyroid then

3 incise the fascia of the upper horn of thymus then

4 extend this down into the accessible mediastinal thymus then

5 within the carotid sheath (usually suggested by a tongue of ectopic thymus) then

6 transcervical thymectomy achieved by gentle upper retraction on the thymic lobe then

7 within the thyroid lobe which may require thyroid lobectomy.

All abnormal glands are excised and, in the event of sporadic four-gland disease, subtotal parathyroidectomy is carried out, preserving approximately 50 mg of one gland. This must be marked with a non-absorbable suture to facilitate any possible future re-exploration.

In patients with four-gland disease, transcervical thymectomy is recommended to reduce the risk of persistent or recurrent hyperparathyroidism. In patients with MEN-1, total parathyroidectomy reduces the risk of recurrence.

Preoperative imaging will identify the 1 per cent of patients with a mediastinal adenoma and allow a single curative operation (Figure 51.57a and b).

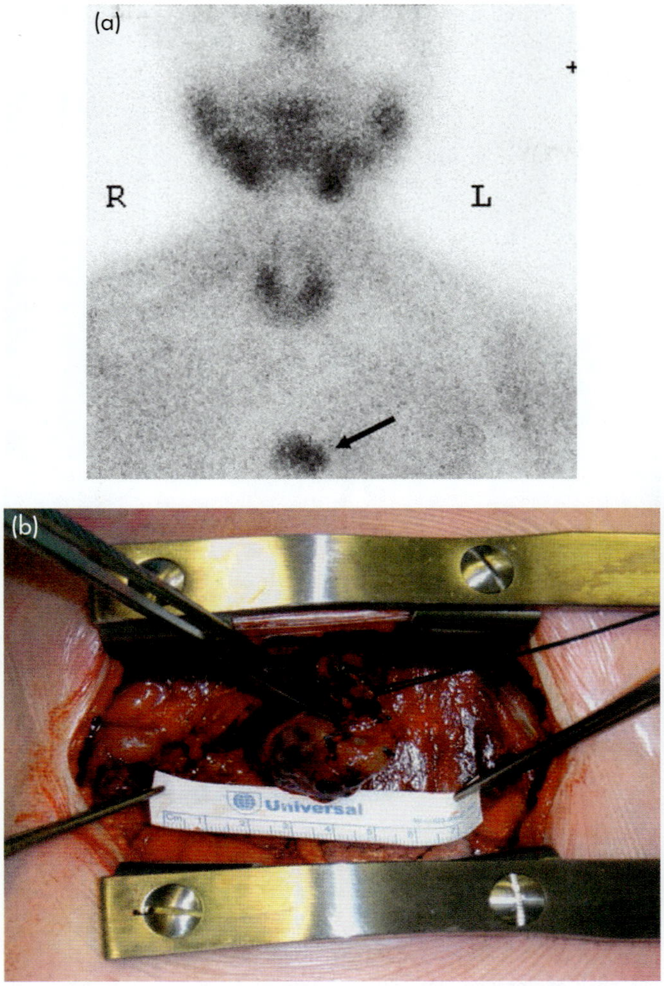

Figure 51.57 Mediastinal parathyroid adenoma. (a) Preoperative sestamibi scan with mediastinal adenoma (arrowed). (b) Operative photograph of median sternotomy showing a 4-cm parathyroid adenoma (courtesy Mr K Buchan, Aberdeen, UK).

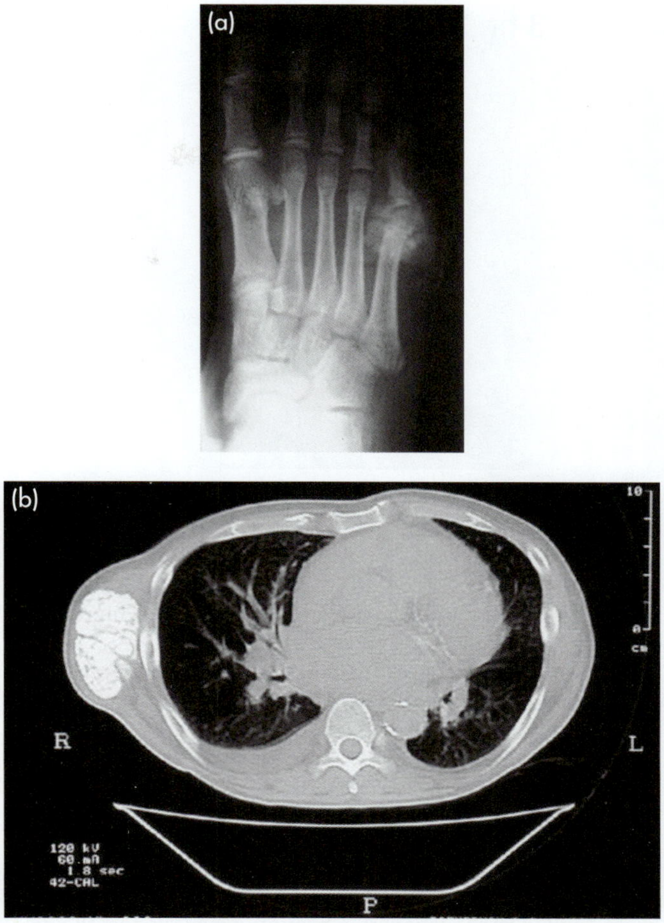

Figure 51.58 Secondary hyperparathyroidism. (a) Radiograph of ectopic calcification. (b) Computed tomography scan showing ectopic calcification in chest wall.

Secondary hyperparathyroidism

Chronic renal failure results in secondary hyperparathyroidism. The kidney cannot convert vitamin D into the physiologically active 1,25-cholecalciferol. Reduced intestinal absorption of calcium resulting in a low serum calcium and elevated phosphate due to renal failure to excrete phosphate increases secretion of parathyroid hormone. Prolonged stimulation results in parathyroid hyperplasia. Initially this is reversible following renal transplantation but when autonomous hyperfunction progresses after transplantation this is termed tertiary hyperparathyroidism.

Secondary hyperparathyroidism also occurs in vitamin D-deficient rickets, malabsorption and pseudohypoparathyroidism.

Clinical and biochemical features

These include bone pain, pruritus, muscle weakness, renal osteodystrophy and soft-tissue calcification (Figure 51.58a and b). Calciphylaxis (calcific uremic arteriolopathy) is the end stage of this condition with arteriolar occlusion resulting in cutaneous ulceration and gangrene. The systemic effects of these changes results in a high mortality and urgent parathyroidectomy may be required if the PTH is excessively high.

Treatment

Medical treatment of secondary hyperparathyroidism includes dietary phosphate restriction, calcium and vitamin D supplementation. Cinacalcet is not recommended except in patients unfit for surgery. Surgery is indicated when there is an excessive rise in the calcium/phosphate product and serum PTH. Patients are prepared with high-dose vitamin D (calcitriol) to reduce the severity of the profound hypocalcaemia which would otherwise follow parathyroidectomy. Preoperative dialysis is obligatory.

Operative strategy

Multiple-gland disease is usual although occasionally hyperparathyroidism secondary to single-gland disease is the cause rather than the consequence of renal failure. Options for management include total parathyroidectomy (Figure 51.52), total parathyoidectomy with autotransplantation of 50 mg parathyroid tissue into the brachioradilais or subtotal parathyroidectomy. The

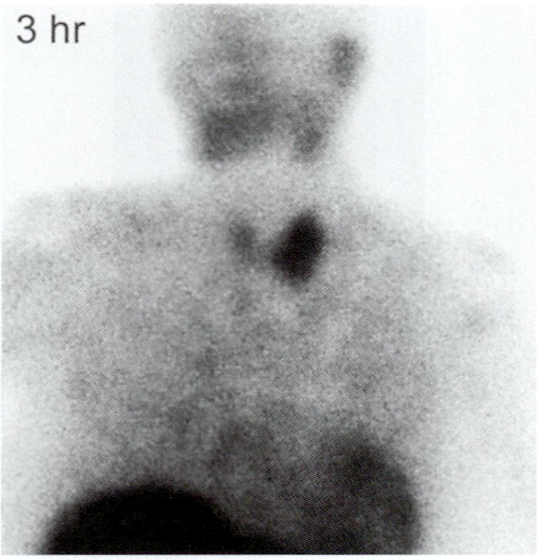

Figure 51.59 Technetium-sestamibi scan at 3 hours showing a left superior parathyroid carcinoma.

latter is preferred if renal transplantation is likely. Transcervical thymectomy is indicated.

Even after subtotal parathyroidectomy or autotransplantation postoperative hypocalcaemia is inevitable. Preoperative preparation and oral calcitriol and calcium are mandatory. Intravenous calcium and magnesium are often required.

Parathyroid carcinoma

Cancer of the parathyroid is rare accounting for 1 per cent of cases of hyperparathyroidism. Typical features are very high calcium and PTH levels often with a palpable neck swelling or occasionally lymphadenopathy. Scanning may support the diagnosis (Figure 51.59). The diagnosis is rarely known at the time of exploration but, if suspected, operation should include excision of the tumour mass with *en bloc* thyroid lobectomy and node dissection when indicated. The diagnosis is difficult to make histologically and may only become apparent when recurrent disease presents with hypercalcaemia, increased serum PTH and evidence of local recurrence. Adjuvant or palliative radiotherapy may be indicated and overall survival as in most endocrine cancers is reasonable with 85 per cent five-year survival.

Persistent hyperparathyroidism

The first operation is the best opportunity to cure hyperparathyroidism surgically and when competently performed should be successful in more than 95 per cent of procedures. If hypercalcaemia persists after a first neck exploration the diagnosis, preoperative investigations, operative findings and pathology must be reviewed carefully. Referral to a specialist centre is prudent. If reoperation is appropriate, further investigation is required to localise the abnormal parathyroid tissue, usually a missed adenoma. This may be readily apparent but can require a combination of ultrasound, sestamibi, CT, MRI, PET, selective angiography (Figure 51.60) and venous sampling for PTH. The latter may be difficult to interpret if normal venous drainage has been disrupted by previous operations.

When the site of an ectopic or missed adenoma is accurately identified, a second operation can be straightforward when performed through intact tissue planes. Re-exploration through previously explored tissues is more difficult and increases the

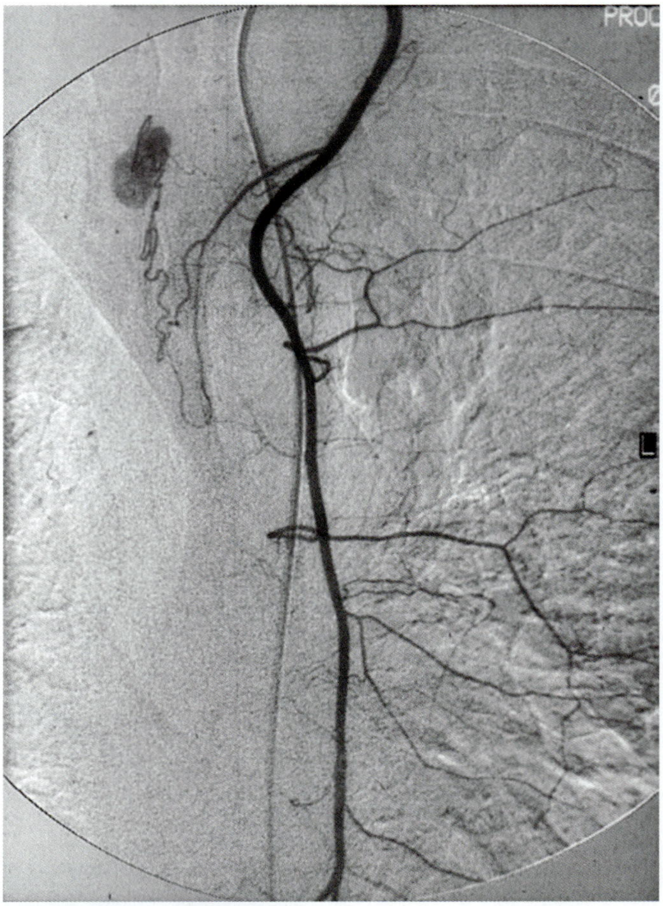

Figure 51.60 Selective arteriogram of internal mammary artery showing parathyroid tumour blush in a patient who had undergone three previous neck explorations for HPT (courtesy of Mr B Harrison, Sheffield, UK).

risks to the recurrent laryngeal nerves and of postoperative hypocalcaemia.

Recurrent hyperparathyroidism

Recurrent hyperparathyroidism is diagnosed when hypercalcaemia recurs more than 12 months after an initially curative operation. This may occur due to:

- missed pathology at the first operation;
- (rarely) development of a second adenoma;
- hyperplasia in autotransplanted tissue;
- parathyromatosis (disseminated nodules of parathyroid tissue within the soft tissues of the neck and superior mediastinum caused by rupture of abnormal parathyroid tissue at initial surgery).

Reoperative parathyroid surgery is associated with an increased risk of recurrent laryngeal nerve injury and postoperative hypocalcaemia.

HYPOPARATHYROIDISM

While there are rare congenital (DiGeorge) and medical (autoimmune polyglandular and Wilson) syndromes causing hypoparathyroidism, for practical purposes postoperative hypoparathyroidism is the dominant management issue in surgical practice. This results from removal, trauma or devascularisation of the parathyroid glands which may be deliberate but is more often inadvertent.

Symptoms and signs

The symptoms and signs of acute hypoparathyroidism are related to the level of serum calcium and range through mild circumoral and digital numbness and paraesthesia, to tetanic symptoms with carpopedal or laryngeal spasms, cardiac arrhythmia and fits. Chronic hypoparathyroidism can lead to abnormal bone demineralisation, cataracts, calcification in basal ganglia and consequent extrapyramidal disorders.

Percussion of the facial nerve just below the zygoma causes contraction of the ipsilateral facial muscles (Chvostek's sign). Carpopedal spasm can be induced by occlusion of the arm with a blood pressure cuff for 3 minutes (Trousseau's sign). Electrocardiogram changes include prolonged QT intervals and QRS complex changes.

Treatment

Acute symptomatic hypocalcaemia is a medical emergency and requires urgent correction by intravenous injection of calcium. Magnesium supplements may also be required. Oral calcium supplements (1 g three or four times daily) supplemented by 1–3 μg of 1-alpha-vitramin D if necessary should be given with a view to gradual withdrawal over the next 3–12 months. Lesser degrees of asymptomatic hypocalcaemia 1.90–2.10 mmol/L can be treated with oral calcium supplements of 3–4 g calcium per day in divided doses (Summary box 51.8).

Summary box 51.8

Management of postoperative hypocalcaemia

- Check serum calcium within 24 hours of total thyroidectomy or earlier if symptomatic
- Medical emergency if the level is <1.90 mmol/L: correct with 10 mL of 10 per cent calcium gluconate intravenously; 10 mL of 10 per cent magnesium sulphate intravenously may also be required
- Give 1 g of oral calcium three or four times daily
- Give 1–3 μg daily of oral 1-alpha-vitamin D if necessary

FURTHER READING

Machens A, Lorenz K, Dralle H. Individualization of lymph node dissection in RET (rearranged during transfection) carriers at risk for medullary thyroid cancer: value of pretherapeutic calcitonin levels. *Ann Surg* 2009; **250**: 305–10.

Monfared A, Gorti G, Kim D. Microsurgical anatomy of the laryngeal nerves as related to thyroid surgery. *Laryngoscope* 2002; **112**: 386–92.

Palazzo FF, Delbridge LW. Minimal access/minimally invasive parathyroidectomy for primary hyperparathyroidism. *Surg Clin N Am* 2004; **84**: 717–34.

Ravetto C, Colombo L, Dottorino ME. Usefulness of fine-needle aspiration in the diagnosis of thyroid carcinoma: a retrospective study of 37895 patients. *Cancer* 2000; **90**: 357–63.

Tan GH, Gahrib H. Thyroid incidentalomas: management approaches to nonpalpable nodules discovered incidentally on thyroid imaging. *Ann Intern Med* 1997; **126**: 226–31.

Tan CTK, Cheah WK, Delbridge LW. 'Scarless' (in the neck) endoscopic thyroidectomy (SET): an evidence-based review of published techniques. *World J Surg* 2008; **32**: 1349–57.

Wanebo H, Coburn M, Teates D, Cole B. Total thyroidectomy does not enhance disease control or survival even in high-risk patients with differentiated thyroid cancer. *Ann Surg* 1998; **227**: 912–21.

Angelo DiGeorge, born 1924, Professor of Paediatrics, Temple University, Philadelphia, PA, USA.
Samuel Alexander Kinnier Wilson, 1878–1956, Professor of Neurology, King's College Hospital, London, UK.
Frantisek Chvostek 1835–1884, physician, The Josefsacademie, Vienna, Austria.
Armand Trousseau, 1801–1867, physician, Hôtel Dieu, Paris, France.

CHAPTER 52

The adrenal glands and other abdominal endocrine disorders

LEARNING OBJECTIVES

To understand:
- The anatomy and function of the adrenal and other abdominal endocrine glands
- The diagnosis and management of these endocrine disorders
- The role of surgery in the management of these endocrine disorders

ADRENAL GLANDS

Anatomy

The weight of a normal adrenal gland is approximately 4 g. There are two distinct components to the gland: the inner adrenal medulla and the outer adrenal cortex (Figure 52.1). The adrenal glands are situated near the upper poles of the kidneys, in the retroperitoneum, within Gerota's capsule. The right adrenal gland is located between the right liver lobe and the diaphragm, close to and partly behind the inferior vena cava. The left adrenal gland lies close to the upper pole of the left kidney and the renal pedicle. It is covered by the pancreatic tail and the spleen (Figure 52.2). The adrenal glands are well supplied by blood vessels. The arterial blood supply branches from the aorta and the diaphragmatic and renal arteries and varies considerably. A large adrenal vein drains on the right side into the vena cava and on the left side into the renal vein.

Embryology

The two functional parts, the cortex and the medulla, arise from different blastodermic layers: mesodermal cells form the adrenal cortex and neuroectodermal cells migrate to the cortex from the neural crest during embryogenesis and form the adrenal medulla.

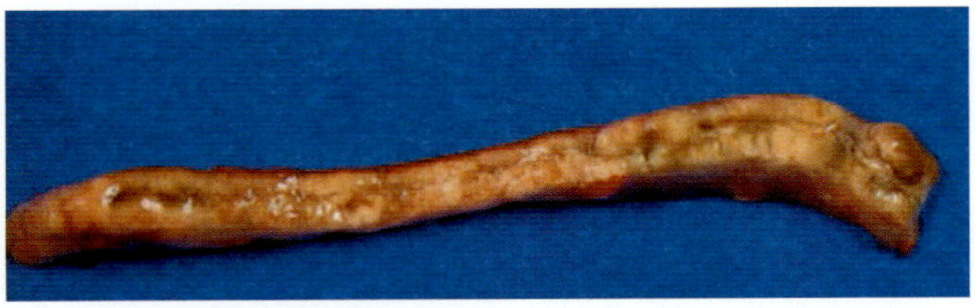

Figure 52.1 Cross-section of a normal adrenal gland. The inner, very thin layer between the two dark lines (zona reticularis) is the adrenal medulla.

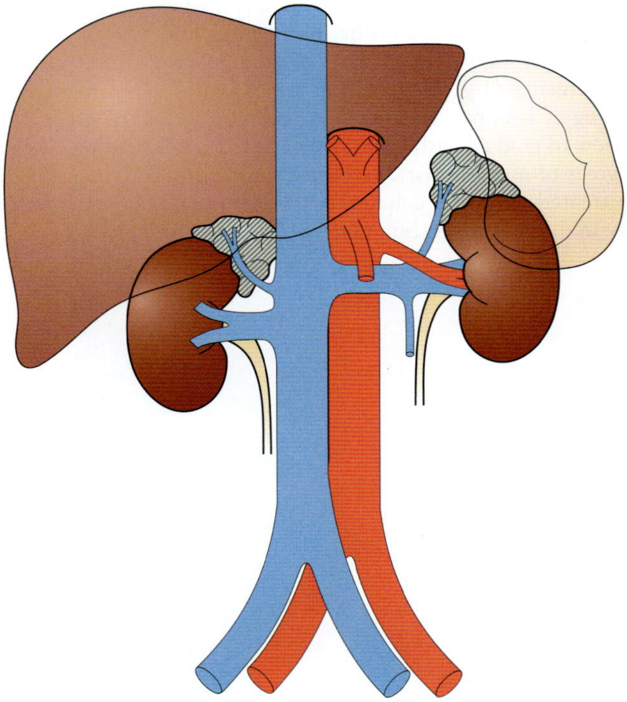

Figure 52.2 Position of the adrenal glands (hatched) in the retroperitoneum.

Histology

The adrenal cortex is arranged in a zonal configuration. The outer zona glomerulosa contains small, compact cells. The central zona fasciculata can be identified by larger, lipid-rich cells, which are arranged in radial columns. Compact and pigmented cells characterise the inner zona reticularis. The adrenal medulla consists of a thin layer of large chromaffin cells, which synthesise, store and secrete catecholamine.

Dumitru Gerota, 1867–1939, Professor of Surgery, Bucharest, Romania.

Function of the adrenal glands

The adrenal glands play a pivotal role in the response to stress. Catecholamines are secreted by the adrenal medulla and corticosteroids, aldosterone and cortisol are synthesised in the adrenal cortex. Cells of the adrenal medulla synthesise mainly adrenaline (epinephrine) but also noradrenaline (norepinephrine) and dopamine. These catecholamines act as hormones as they are secreted directly into the circulation. Their effects, which are mediated through α and β receptors on target organs, include the cardiovascular system, resulting in an increase in blood pressure and heart rate; vasoconstriction of vessels in the splanchnic system and vasodilatation of vessels in the muscles; bronchodilatation; and increased glycogenolysis in liver and muscles: all necessary for the flight/fight response. Cells of the zona glomerulosa produce aldosterone, which regulates sodium–potassium homeostasis. The target organs of aldosterone are the kidneys, the sweat and salivary glands and the intestinal mucosa. Aldosterone promotes sodium retention and potassium excretion. The most important regulators of aldosterone secretion are the renin–angiotensin system and the serum potassium concentration. Renin produced by the juxtaglomerular cells in the kidneys acts on its substrate angiotensinogen to generate angiotensin I. Angiotensin I is converted by angiotensin-converting enzyme (ACE) to the octapeptide angiotensin II, which is modified to angiotensin III. Both stimulate the secretion of aldosterone from the adrenal cortex. A decrease in renal blood flow (haemorrhage, dehydration, salt depletion, orthostasis, renal artery stenosis) or hyponatraemia increases renin secretion and leads to sodium retention, potassium excretion and an increase of plasma volume.

Cells of the zona fasciculata and zona reticularis synthesise cortisol and the adrenal androgens dehydroepiandrosterone (DHEA) and its sulphate (dehydroepiandrosterone sulphate (DHEAS)). DHEA and DHEAS are precursors of androgens and are converted in peripheral tissues such as fat. Cortisol secretion is regulated by adrenocorticotrophic hormone (ACTH), which is produced by the anterior pituitary gland. The hypothalamus controls ACTH secretion by secreting corticotropin-releasing hormone (CRH). The serum cortisol level inhibits the release of CRH and ACTH via a closed-loop system (negative feedback loop).

Cortisol has numerous metabolic and immunological effects. It increases gluconeogenesis and lipolysis, decreases peripheral glucose utilisation, immunological response and muscular mass. It affects fat distribution, wound healing and bone mineralisation; and alters mood (euphoria or, rarely, depression) and cortical alertness.

DISORDERS OF THE ADRENAL CORTEX

Incidentaloma

Definition

Incidentaloma is an adrenal mass, detected incidentally by imaging studies conducted for other reasons, not known previously to have been present or causing symptoms.

Incidence

The prevalence of adrenal masses in autopsy studies ranges from 1.4 to 8.7 per cent and increases with age. Incidentalomas may be detected on imaging studies in 1 per cent of patients. More than 75 per cent are non-functioning adenomas but Cushing's adenomas, phaeochromocytomas, metastases, adrenocortical carcinomas and Conn's tumours can all be found this way (Table 52.1).

Table 52.1 Prevalence of non-functioning and functioning tumours in patients with incidentalomas.

Tumour	Prevalence (%)
Non-functioning adenoma	78
Cushing's adenoma	7
Adrenocortical carcinoma	4
Phaeochromocytoma	4
Myelolipoma	2
Cyst	2
Metastases	2
Conn's adenoma	1

Diagnosis

When an incidentaloma is identified, a complete history and clinical examination are required. Occasionally, a previously occult endocrine disturbance will come to light. A biochemical work-up for hormone excess is needed and sometimes additional imaging studies are also required. The main goal is to exclude a functioning or malignant adrenal tumour.

Hormonal evaluation includes:

- morning and midnight plasma cortisol measurements;
- a 1-mg overnight dexamethasone suppression test;
- 24-hour urinary cortisol excretion;
- 12 or 24-hour urinary excretion of metanephrines or plasma-free metanephrines;
- serum potassium, plasma aldosterone and plasma renin activity;
- serum DHEAS, testosterone or 17-hydroxyestradiol (virilising or feminising tumour).

Computed tomography (CT) or magnetic resonance imaging (MRI) should be performed in all patients with adrenal masses. The likelihood of an adrenal mass being an adrenocortical carcinoma increases with the size of the mass (25 per cent >4 cm). Adrenal metastases are likely in patients with a history of cancer elsewhere and the sole indications for biopsy of an adrenal mass is to confirm a suspected metastasis from a distant primary site (Summary box 52.1).

Summary box 52.1

Adrenal gland biopsy

- Never biopsy an adrenal mass until phaeochromocytoma has been biochemically excluded
- The indication for adrenal gland biopsy is to confirm adrenal gland metastasis

Harvey Williams Cushing, 1869–1939, Professor of Surgery, Harvard University Medical School, Boston, MA, USA.

Treatment

The treatment of functional adrenal tumours is described below. Any non-functioning adrenal tumour greater than 4 cm in diameter and smaller tumours that increase in size over time should undergo surgical resection. Non-functioning tumours smaller than 4 cm should be followed-up after 6, 12 and 24 months by imaging (MRI) and hormonal evaluation.

Primary hyperaldosteronism – Conn's syndrome

Incidence

Primary hyperaldosteronism (PHA) is defined by hypertension, as a result of hypersecretion of aldosterone. In PHA, plasma renin activity is suppressed. Among patients with hypertension the incidence of PHA is approximately 2 per cent. Recent studies have revealed that up to 12 per cent of hypertensive patients have PHA with normal potassium levels, thus potassium levels are an inconsistent diagnostic feature of this disease, and cannot be relied on to confirm or exclude it.

Pathology

The most frequent cause of PHA with hypokalaemia is a unilateral adrenocortical adenoma (Figure 52.3). In 20–40 per cent of cases, bilateral micronodular hyperplasia is present. Rare causes of PHA are bilateral macronodular hyperplasia, glucocorticoid-suppressible hyperaldosteronism or adrenocortical carcinoma. In the subset of patients with normokalaemic PHA, 70 per cent have hyperplasia and 30 per cent unilateral adenoma.

Clinical features

Most patients are between 30 and 50 years of age with a female predominance. Apart from hypertension, patients complain of non-specific symptoms: headache, muscle weakness, cramps, intermittent paralysis, polyuria, polydypsia and nocturia.

Diagnosis

The key feature of the biochemical diagnosis is the assessment of potassium level and the aldosterone to plasma renin activity ratio. Antihypertensive and diuretic therapy, which cause hypokalaemia and influence the renin–angiotensin–aldosterone system, have to be discontinued. Once the biochemical diagnosis is confirmed, MRI or CT should be performed to distinguish unilateral from bilateral disease. Conn's adenomas usually measure between 1 and 2 cm and are detected by CT with a sensitivity of 80–90 per cent (Figure 52.4). Micronodular changes and small adenomas are often underdiagnosed. An apparent unilateral mass could be a non-functioning tumour in a patient with bilateral micronodular hyperplasia. Selective adrenal vein catheterisation can help before a decision on non-surgical or surgical treatment is made. During selective adrenal vein catheterisation, samples are obtained from the vena cava and from both adrenal veins and the aldosterone to cortisol ratio (ACR) is determined in each sample. A significant difference in the ACR ratio on one side indicates unilateral disease.

Treatment

The first-line therapy for PHA with bilateral hyperplasia is medical treatment with spironolactone. In most cases supplemental antihypertensive medication is necessary.

Unilateral laparoscopic adrenalectomy is an effective therapy in patients with clear evidence of unilateral or asymmetrical bilateral disease. A subtotal resection can be considered in the case of a typical single Conn's adenoma. In 10–30 per cent of patients who undergo an adrenalectomy, hypertension persists despite adequate diagnostic work-up and treatment, albeit at a lower level, requiring fewer medications to control it.

Cushing's syndrome

Definition

Hypersecretion of cortisol caused by endogenous production of corticosteroids is known as Cushing's syndrome. It can be either ACTH-dependent or ACTH-independent in origin. The most common cause (85 per cent) of ACTH-dependent Cushing's syndrome is Cushing's disease resulting from a pituitary adenoma that secretes an excessive amount of ACTH. Ectopic ACTH-producing tumours (small cell lung cancer,

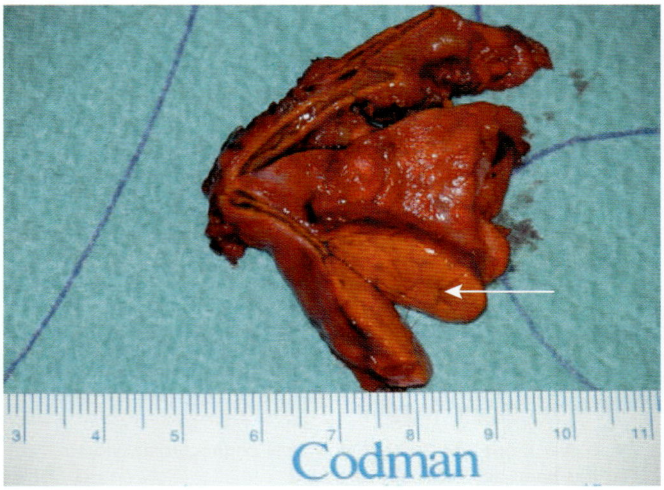

Figure 52.3 A Conn's adenoma (arrow) of the left adrenal gland; note the V-shaped normal adrenal tissue.

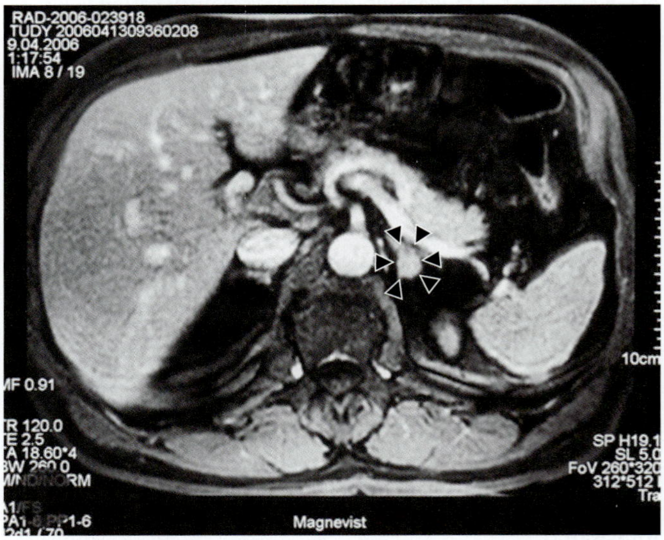

Figure 52.4 Computed tomography scan of a Conn's adenoma of the left adrenal gland (arrowheads).

Jerome William Conn, 1907–1981, Professor of Internal Medicine, The University of Michigan, Michigan, MI, USA.

foregut carcinoid) and CRH-producing tumours (medullary thyroid carcinoma, neuroendocrine pancreatic tumour) are more infrequent causes of ACTH-dependent Cushing's syndrome. Excessive or prolonged administration of cortisol-like drugs will produce the same clinical picture.

In about 15 per cent of patients, an ACTH-independent Cushing's syndrome (low ACTH levels) is caused by a unilateral adrenocortical adenoma. Adrenocortical carcinoma and bilateral macronodular or micronodular hyperplasia represent rare causes of hypercortisolism.

Clinical symptoms

The clinical features of Cushing's syndrome are shown in Summary box 52.2. The typical patient is characterised by a facial plethora, a buffalo hump and a moon face in combination with hypertension, diabetes and central obesity (Figures 52.5 and 52.6). However, clinical signs can be minimal or absent in patients with subclinical Cushing's syndrome.

Summary box 52.2

Clinical features of Cushing's syndrome

- Weight gain/central obesity
- Diabetes
- Hirsutism
- Hypertension
- Skin changes (abdominal striae, facial plethora, ecchymosis, acne)
- Muscle weakness
- Menstrual irregularity/impotence
- Depression/mania
- Osteoporosis
- Hypokalaemia

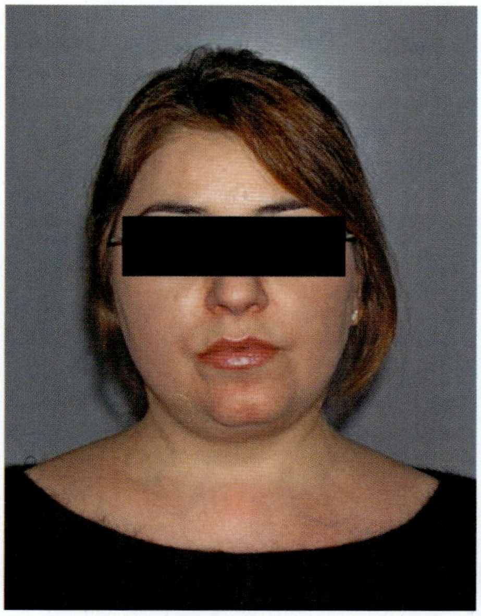

Figure 52.5 A 34-year-old patient with Cushing's syndrome whose symptoms included fullness of the face, weight gain and acne. Today, patients with Cushing's syndrome rarely have the full-blown appearance as shown in older textbooks.

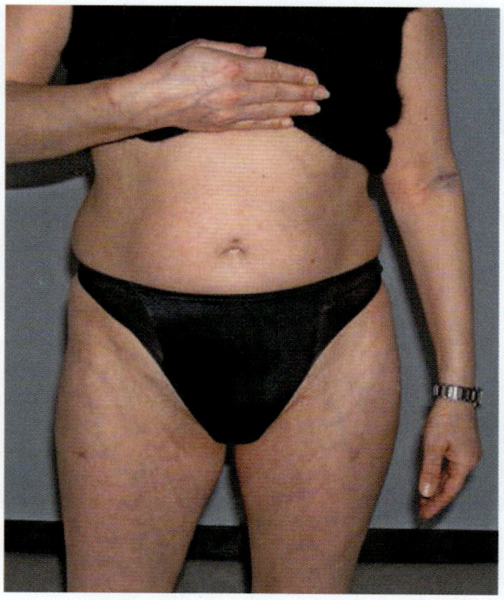

Figure 52.6 Discrete central obesity, ecchymosis and fragile skin in a patient with Cushing's syndrome.

Diagnosis

- Morning and midnight plasma cortisol levels are elevated, possibly with loss of diurnal rhythm.
- Dexamethasone fails to suppress 24-hour urinary cortisol excretion.
- Serum ACTH levels discriminate ACTH-dependent from ACTH-independent disease.

Elevated or normal ACTH levels provide evidence for an ACTH-producing pituitary tumour (85 per cent) or ectopic ACTH production. Therefore, in patients with elevated ACTH, MRI of the pituitary gland must be performed. If MRI is negative and additional venous sampling from the inferior petrosal sinus has excluded a pituitary microadenoma, a CT scan of the chest and abdomen is warranted to detect an ectopic ACTH-producing tumour. In patients with suppressed ACTH levels, a CT or MRI scan is performed to assess the adrenal glands.

Subclinical Cushing's syndrome is diagnosed if clinical symptoms are absent in the face of abnormal cortisol secretion.

Treatment

Medical therapy with metyrapone or ketoconazole reduces steroid synthesis and secretion and can be used to prepare patients with severe hypercortisolism preoperatively or if surgery is not possible. ACTH-producing pituitary tumours are treated by trans-sphenoidal resection or radiotherapy. If an ectopic ACTH source is localised, resection will correct hypercortisolism.

A unilateral adenoma is treated by adrenalectomy. In cases of bilateral ACTH-independent disease (Figure 52.7), bilateral adrenalectomy is the primary treatment. Patients with an ectopic ACTH-dependent Cushing's syndrome and an irresectable or unlocalised primary tumour should be considered for bilateral adrenalectomy as this controls hormone excess. Subclinical Cushing's syndrome caused by unilateral adenoma is treated by unilateral adrenalectomy.

Preoperative management

Patients with Cushing's syndrome are at an increased risk of hospital-acquired infection, thromboembolic and myocardial

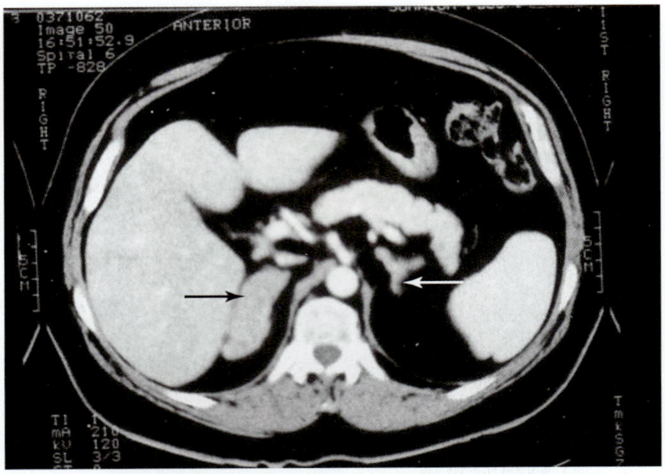

Figure 52.7 Bilateral asymmetrical hyperplasia of the adrenal glands (arrows) in a patient with Cushing's syndrome.

complications. Therefore, prophylactic anticoagulation and the use of prophylactic antibiotics are essential. Cushing-associated diseases (diabetes, hypertension) must be controlled by medical therapy preoperatively.

Postoperative management

After unilateral adrenalectomy supplemental cortisol should be given postoperatively because the contralateral gland will be suppressed. In total, 15 mg/hour is required parenterally for the first 12 hours followed by a daily dose of 100 mg for 3 days, which is gradually reduced thereafter. After unilateral adrenalectomy, the contralateral suppressed gland needs up to one year to recover adequate function. In 10 per cent of patients with Cushing's disease who undergo a bilateral adrenalectomy after failed pituitary surgery, the pituitary adenoma causes Nelson's syndrome due to continued ACTH secretion at high levels, causing hyperpigmentation as a result of chemical synergies between ACTH and melanocyte-stimulating hormone.

Adrenal metastases

Adrenal metastases are discovered at autopsy in one-third of patients with malignant disease (less frequently during life). In declining frequency, the most common primary tumours are breast, lung, renal, gastric, pancreatic, ovarian and colorectal cancer. In selected circumstances an adrenalectomy is appropriate, for example if it is the sole site of metastatic disease.

Adrenocortical carcinoma

Incidence

Adrenocortical carcinoma is a rare malignancy with an incidence of 1–2 cases per 1 000 000 population per year and a variable but generally poor prognosis. A slight female predominance is observed (1.5:1). The age distribution is bimodal with a first peak in childhood and a second between the fourth and fifth decades.

Pathology

The differentiation between benign and malignant adrenal tumours is challenging, even in the hands of an experienced pathologist. Criteria for malignancy are tumour size, the presence of necrosis or haemorrhage and microscopic features such as capsular or vascular invasion. These should be assessed in terms of a microscopic diagnostic score. Additional information is provided by immunohistochemistry. The macroscopic features are commonly multinodularity and heterogeneous structure (see Figure 52.8) with haemorrhage and necrosis.

Clinical presentation

Approximately 60 per cent of patients present with evidence of cortisol excess (Cushing's syndrome). Patients with non-functioning tumours frequently complain of abdominal discomfort or back pain caused by large tumours. However, with increasing use of abdominal imaging, a growing number of adrenocortical carcinomas are detected incidentally. Adrenal tumours secreting more than one hormone in excess, or feminising/masculanising steroids are likely to be malignant.

Diagnosis

The diagnostic work-up should include measurements of DHEAS, cortisol and catecholamines to exclude a phaeochromocytoma and a dexamethasone suppression test. MRI and CT are equally effective in imaging adrenocortical carcinoma (Figure 52.9). MRI angiography is useful to exclude tumour thrombus in the vena cava. As distant metastases are frequently present, a CT scan of the lungs is recommended. The World Health Organization classification of 2004 is based on the McFarlane classification and defines four stages: tumours <5 cm (stage I) or >5 cm (stage II), locally invasive tumours (III) or tumours with distant metastases (IV). Functioning tumours tend to do worse than non-functioning, but have the advantage of a serum marker which can be used for follow up and disease monitoring.

Treatment

Complete tumour resection (R0) is associated with favourable survival and should be attempted whenever possible. In order to prevent tumour spillage and implantation metastases, the capsule must not be damaged. *En bloc* resection with removal of locally involved organs is often required and in case of tumour thrombus in the vena cava thrombectomy is needed. Laparoscopic adrenalectomy is associated with a high incidence of local recurrence

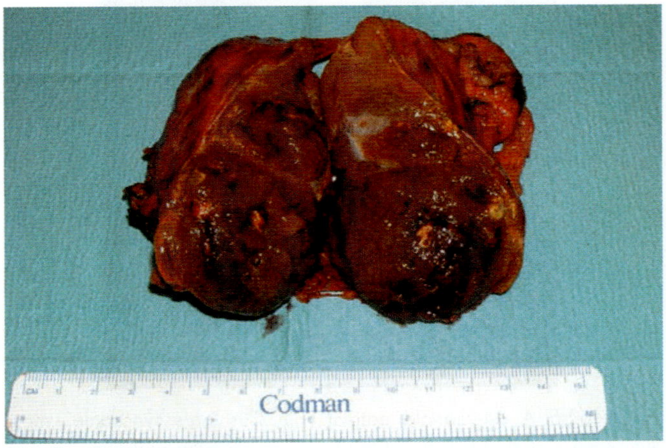

Figure 52.8 Adrenocortical carcinoma that caused Cushing's syndrome and virilisation in a female patient.

Don H Nelson, born 1925, Professor of Medicine, The University of Utah, Salt Lake City, UT, USA.

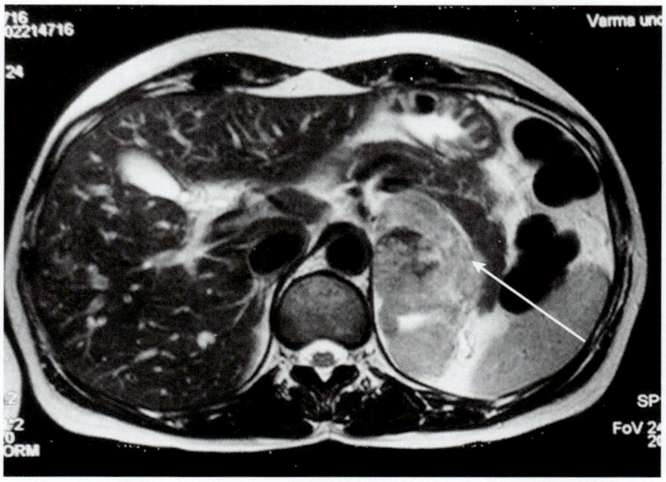

Figure 52.9 Magnetic resonance imaging of adrenocortical carcinoma (arrow) in a patient with cortisol and testosterone excess.

Summary box 52.3

Diseases associated with adrenal insufficiency

- Polyglandular autoimmune syndrome
- Tuberculosis
- After bilateral adrenalectomy
- Haemorrhage
- Metastases
- Systemic diseases (Boeck's disease, amyloidosis, Wilson's disease)
- Hereditary diseases (e.g. adrenoleukodystrophia, adrenogenital syndrome)
- HIV infection

and cannot be recommended. Tumour debulking plays a role in functioning tumours to control hormone excess.

Patients can be treated postoperatively with mitotane alone or in combination with etoposide, doxorubicin and cisplatin. Adjuvant radiotherapy may reduce the rate of local recurrence. After surgery, restaging every three months is required as the risk of tumour relapse is high. Prognosis depends on the stage of disease and complete removal of the tumour. Patients with stage I or II disease have a five-year survival rate of 25 per cent whereas patients with stage III and stage IV disease have five-year survival rates of 6 and 0 per cent, respectively.

Congenital adrenal hyperplasia (adrenogenital syndrome)

Virilisation and adrenal insufficiency in children are pathognomonic of congenital adrenal hyperplasia (CAH). This is an autosomal recessive disorder caused by a variety of enzymatic defects in the synthetic pathway of cortisol and other steroids from cholesterol. The most frequent defect (95 per cent) is the 21-hydroxylase deficiency, which has an incidence of 1 in 5000 live births. Excessive ACTH secretion is caused by the loss of cortisol and this leads to an increase in androgenic cortisol precursors and to CAH. CAH may present in girls at birth with ambiguous genitalia or as late-onset disease at puberty. Hypertension and short stature, caused by the premature epiphyseal plate closure, are common signs. Affected patients are treated by replacement of cortisol and with fludrocortisone. Large hypoplastic adrenals may need to be removed if symptomatic.

Adrenal insufficiency

Primary adrenal insufficiency is caused by the loss of function of the adrenal cortex (Summary box 52.3). It was first described by Thomas Addison in 1855. An early diagnosis is a clinical challenge, even today. Symptoms are only evident when about 90 per cent of the adrenal cortex is destroyed. Secondary adrenal insufficiency is defined as a deficiency of pituitary ACTH secretion. Tertiary adrenal deficiency is provoked by a loss of hypothalamic CRH secretion and is caused by therapeutic glucocorticoid administration, brain tumour or irradiation.

Acute adrenal insufficiency

Acute adrenal insufficiency usually presents as shock in combination with fever, nausea, vomiting, abdominal pain, hypoglycaemia and electrolyte imbalance. The Waterhouse–Friderichsen syndrome is a bilateral adrenal infarction associated with meningococcal sepsis and is rapidly fatal unless immediately treated. Because of intestinal symptoms and fever, the so-called Addisonian crisis is often misdiagnosed as an acute abdominal condition.

Chronic adrenal insufficiency

When symptoms develop over time, patients present with anorexia, weakness and nausea. As a result of negative feedback, ACTH and pro-opiomelanocortin (POMC) levels increase and cause hyperpigmentation of the skin and oral mucosa. Hypotension, hyponatraemia, hyperkalaemia and hypoglycaemia are commonly observed. The diagnosis of adrenal insufficiency is made using the ACTH stimulation test. Basal ACTH levels are found to be high with cortisol levels decreased. There is no rise in cortisol levels following the exogenous administration of ACTH (synacthen test).

Treatment

If a patient displays features of adrenal insufficiency, treatment must immediately be commenced, before awaiting the biochemical diagnosis. Initial blood samples can be used for later determinations of ACTH and cortisol levels. In addition to intravenous administration of hydrocortisone, 100 mg every 6 hours, 3 litres of saline is given in 6 hours under careful cardiovascular monitoring. Concomitant infections, which are frequently present, require treatment.

Chronic adrenal insufficiency is treated by replacement therapy with daily oral hydrocortisone (10 mg/m^2 body surface area) and fludrocortisone (0.1 mg). Patients must be advised about the need to take lifelong glucocorticoid and mineralocorticoid replacement therapy. To prevent an Addisonian crisis, patients must be aware of the need to increase the dose in case of illness or stress. If patients with adrenal insufficiency are scheduled for surgery, appropriate steroid cover must be administrated.

Thomas Addison, 1795–1860, physician, Guy's Hospital, London, UK, described the effects of disease of the suprarenal capsules in 1849.
Caesar Peter Moller Boeck, 1845–1917, Professor of Medicine, The University of Oslo, Norway.
Samuel Alexander Kinnier Wilson, 1878–1956, Professor of Neurology, King's College Hospital, London, UK, described this condition in 1912.
Rupert Waterhouse, 1875–1958, physician, The Royal United Hospital, Bath, UK, described the syndrome in 1911.
Carl Friderichsen, 1886–1979, Medical Superintendent, Sundby Hospital, Copenhagen, Denmark, gave his account of the syndrome in 1918.

DISORDERS OF THE ADRENAL MEDULLA AND NEURAL CREST-DERIVED TISSUE

Phaeochromocytoma and paraganglioma

Definition

These are tumours of the adrenal medulla and sympathetic ganglia which are derived from chromaffin cells and which produce catecholamines.

Aetiology

The prevalence of phaeochromocytoma in patients with hypertension is 0.1–0.6 per cent with an overall prevalence of 0.05 per cent in autopsy series. In total, 4 per cent of incidentalomas are phaeochromocytomas. Sporadic phaeochromocytomas occur around the fourth decade whereas patients with hereditary forms are diagnosed earlier. Phaeochromocytoma is known as the '10 per cent tumour' as 10 per cent of tumours are inherited, 10 per cent are extra-adrenal, 10 per cent are malignant, 10 per cent are bilateral and 10 per cent occur in children. With the recent advent of detailed genetic tests, however, the incidence of hereditary phaeochromocytomas has been shown to be higher.

Hereditary phaeochromocytomas occur in several tumour syndromes:

- **Multiple endocrine neoplasia type 2 (MEN 2)**: an autosomal dominant inherited disorder that is caused by activating germline mutations of the *RET* proto-oncogene.
- **Familial paraganglioma (PG) syndrome**: glomus tumours of the carotid body and extra-adrenal paraganglioma are characteristic in this hereditary tumour syndrome, which is caused by germline mutations within the succinate dehydrogenase complex subunit B (*SDHB*) *SDHD* and *SDHC* genes.
- **von Hippel–Lindau (VHL) syndrome**: those affected can develop early-onset bilateral kidney tumours, phaeochromocytomas, cerebellar and spinal haemangioblastomas and pancreatic tumours. Patients have a germline mutation in the *VHL* gene.
- **Neurofibromatosis (NF) type 1**: phaeochromocytomas in combination with fibromas on the skin and mucosae ('café-au-lait' skin spots) are indicative of a germline mutation in the *NF1* gene.

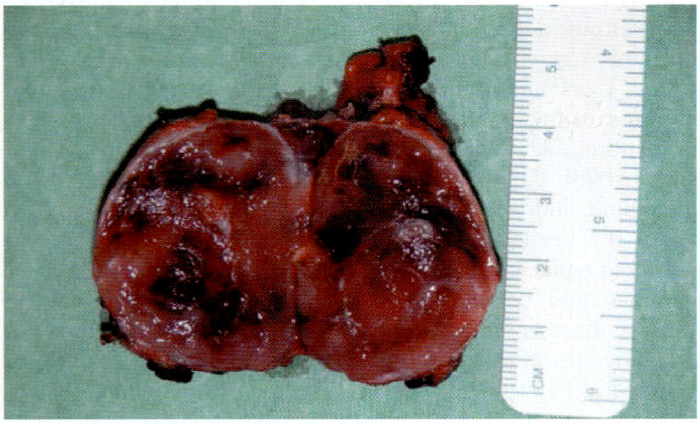

Figure 52.10 Gross appearance of a phaeochromocytoma.

Pathology

Phaeochromocytomas are greyish-pink on the cut surface and are usually highly vascularised. Areas of haemorrhage or necrosis are often observed (Figure 52.10). Microscopically, tumour cells are polygonal but the configuration varies considerably. The differentiation between malignant and benign tumours is difficult, except if metastases are present. An increased PASS (phaeochromocytoma of the adrenal gland scale score), a high number of Ki-67-positive cells, vascular invasion or a breached capsule all lean more towards malignant rather than benign.

Phaeochromocytomas may also produce calcitonin, ACTH, vasoactive intestinal polypeptide (VIP) and parathyroid hormone-related protein (PTHrP). In patients with MEN 2, the onset of phaeochromocytoma is preceded by adrenomedullary hyperplasia, sometimes bilateral. Phaeochromocytoma is rarely malignant in MEN 2.

Clinical features

Symptoms and signs are caused by catecholamine excess and are typically intermittent (Table 52.2). In total, 90 per cent of patients with the combination of headache, palpitations and sweating have a phaeochromocytoma. Paroxysms may be precipitated by physical training, induction of general anaesthesia and numerous drugs and agents (contrast media, tricyclic antidepressive drugs, metoclopramide and opiates). Hypertension may occur continuously, be intermittent or absent. A subset of patients are asymptomatic. More than 20 per cent of apparently sporadic phaeochromocytomas are caused by germline mutations in the *RET*, *SDHB*, *SDHC*, *SDHD* and *NF1* genes; genetic testing for these genes is therefore recommended, particularly in those aged under 50 years.

Table 52.2 Clinical signs of phaeochromocytoma.

Symptoms	Prevalence (%)
Hypertension	80–90
Paroxysmal	50–60
Continuous	30
Headache	60–90
Sweating	50–70
Palpitation	50–70
Pallor	40–45
Weight loss	20–40
Hyperglycaemia	40
Nausea	20–40
Psychological effects	20–40

Diagnosis

The first step in the diagnosis of a phaeochromocytoma is the determination of adrenaline and noradrenaline breakdown products, metanephrine and normetanephrine level, in a 12- or 24-hour urine collection. Levels that exceed the normal range by 2–40 times will be found in affected patients. Determination of plasma-free metanephrine and normetanephrine levels also

Eugen von Hippel, 1867–1939, Professor of Ophthalmology, Göttingen, Germany.
Arvid Lindau, 1892–1958, Professor of Pathology, Lund, Sweden.

has a high sensitivity. Biochemical tests should be performed at least twice. The biochemical diagnosis is followed by the localisation of the phaeochromocytoma. MRI is preferred because contrast media used for CT scans can provoke paroxysms. Classically, phaeochromocytomas show a 'Swiss cheese' configuration (Figure 52.11). ^{123}I-MIBG (metaiodobenzylguanidine) single-photon emission computed tomography (SPECT) will identify about 90 per cent of primary tumours and is essential for the detection of multiple extra-adrenal tumours and metastases (Figure 52.12). PET scanning using FDG PET or DOPA PET is yet more sensitive in detecting metastatic foci.

Treatment

Laparoscopic resection is now routine in the treatment of phaeochromocytoma. If the tumour is larger than 8–10 cm or radiological signs of malignancy are detected, an open approach should be considered.

Preoperative

Once a phaeochromocytoma has been diagnosed, an α-adrenoreceptor blocker (phenoxybenzamine) is used to block

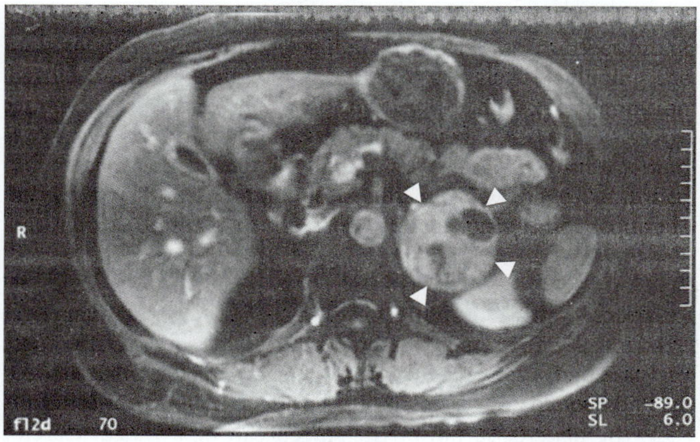

Figure 52.11 Magnetic resonance imaging of a sporadic phaeochromocytoma of the left adrenal gland (arrowheads).

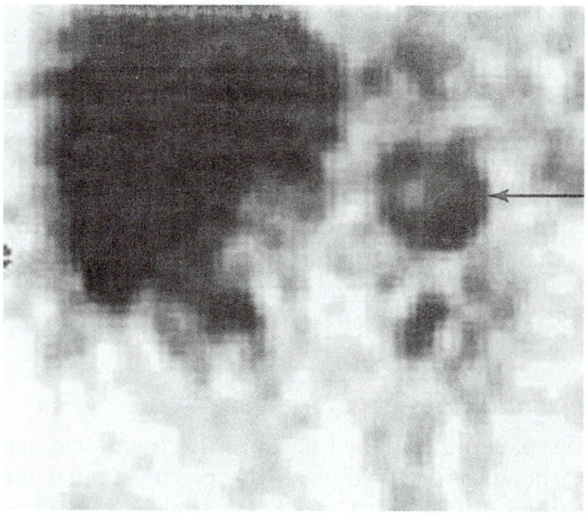

Figure 52.12 Meta-iodobenzylguanidine (MIBG) single-photon emission computed tomography scan of a phaeochromocytoma of the left adrenal gland (arrow) in the same patient as in Figure 52.11.

catecholamine excess and its consequences during surgery. With adequate medical pretreatment, the perioperative mortality rate has decreased from 20–45 per cent to less than 3 per cent. A dose of 20 mg of phenoxybenzamine initially should be increased daily by 10 mg until a daily dose of 100–160 mg is achieved and the patient reports symptomatic postural hypotension. Additional β-blockade is required if tachycardia or arrhythmias develop; this should not be introduced until the patient is α-blocked.

With adequate α-blockade preoperatively, anaesthesia should not be more hazardous than in patients with a non-functioning adrenal tumour; however, in some patients, dramatic changes in heart rate and blood pressure may occur and require sudden administration of pressor or vasodilator agents. A central venous catheter and invasive arterial monitoring are used. Special attention is required when the adrenal vein is ligated as a sudden drop in blood pressure may occur. The infusion of large volumes of fluid or administration of noradrenaline can be necessary to correct postoperative hypotension in the presence of unopposed α-blockade.

Postoperative

Patients should be observed for 24 hours in the intensive care or high dependency unit as hypovolaemia and hypoglycaemia may occur. Lifelong yearly biochemical tests should be performed to identify recurrent, metastatic or metachronous phaeochromocytoma (Summary box 52.4).

Summary box 52.4

Phaeochromocytoma

- Obtain a secure biochemical diagnosis
- Exclude family history
- Diagnosis confirmed, treat with α-blockers
- Plan surgical excision
- Yearly lifelong follow up

Malignant phaeochromocytoma

Definition

Approximately 10 per cent of phaeochromocytomas are malignant. This rate is higher in extra-adrenal tumours (paragangliomas). The diagnosis of malignancy implies metastases of chromaffin tissue, most commonly to lymph nodes, bone and liver.

Treatment

Surgical excision is the only chance for cure. Even in patients with metastatic disease, tumour debulking can be considered to reduce the tumour burden and to control the catecholamine excess. Symptomatic treatment can be obtained with α-blockers. Mitotane should be started as adjuvant or palliative treatment. Treatment with ^{131}I-MIBG or combination chemotherapy has resulted in a partial response in 30 per cent and an improvement of symptoms in 80 per cent of patients. The natural history is highly variable with a five-year survival rate of less than 50 per cent.

Phaeochromocytoma in pregnancy

Phaeochromocytomas in pregnancy may imitate an amnion infection syndrome or pre-eclampsia. Without adequate α-blockade, mother and unborn child are threatened by hypertensive crisis during delivery. In the first and second trimesters, the patient should be scheduled for laparoscopic adrenalectomy after adequate α-blockade; the risk of a miscarriage during surgery is high. In the third trimester, elective Caesarean with **consecutive** adrenalectomy should be performed. The maternal mortality rate is 50 per cent when a phaeochromocytoma remains undiagnosed.

Neuroblastoma

Definition

A neuroblastoma is a malignant tumour that is derived from the sympathetic nervous system in the adrenal medulla (38 per cent) or from any site along the sympathetic chain in the paravertebral sites of the abdomen (30 per cent), chest (20 per cent) and, rarely, the neck or pelvis.

Pathology

Neuroblastomas have a pale and grey surface, are encapsulated and show areas with calcification. With increased tumour size, necrosis and haemorrhage may be detected. They are characterised by the presence of immature cells derived from the neuroectoderm of the sympathetic nervous system. Mature cells are found only in ganglioneuroblastomas.

Clinical features

Predominantly, newborn infants and young children (<5 years of age) are affected. Symptoms are caused by tumour growth or by bone metastases. Patients present with a mass in the abdomen, neck or chest, proptosis, bone pain, painless bluish skin metastases, weakness or paralysis. Metastatic disease is present in 70 per cent of patients at presentation.

Diagnosis

Biochemical evaluation should include urinary excretion (24-hour urine) of vanillylmandelic acid (VMA), homovanillic acid (HVA), dopamine and noradenaline, as increased levels are present in about 80 per cent of patients. Accurate staging requires CT/MRI of the chest and abdomen, a bone scan, bone marrow aspiration and core biopsies as well as an MIBG scan. Staging is established according to the International Neuroblastoma Staging System (INSS).

Treatment

Prognosis can be predicted by the tumour stage and the age at diagnosis. Patients are classified as low, intermediate or high risk. Low-risk patients are treated by surgery alone (the addition of 6–12 weeks of chemotherapy is optional) whereas intermediate-risk patients are treated by surgery with adjuvant multiagent chemotherapy (carboplatin, cyclophosphamide, etoposide, doxorubicin). High-risk patients receive high-dose multiagent chemotherapy followed by surgical resection in responding tumours and myeloablative stem cell rescue. Patients assigned to the low-risk, intermediate-risk and high-risk groups have overall three-year survival rates of 90, 70–90 and 30 per cent, respectively.

Ganglioneuroma

Definition

A ganglioneuroma is a benign neoplasm that arises from neural crest tissue. Ganglioneuromas can occur in the adrenal medulla and are characterised by mature sympathetic ganglion cells and Schwann cells in a fibrous stroma.

Clinical features

Ganglioneuroma is found in all age groups but is more common before the age of 60. Ganglioneuromas occur anywhere along the paravertebral sympathetic plexus and in the adrenal medulla (30 per cent). Most often they are identified incidentally by CT or MRI performed for other indications.

Treatment

Treatment is by surgical excision, laparoscopic when adrenalectomy is indicated.

SURGERY OF THE ADRENAL GLANDS

Since its introduction in the 1990s, laparoscopic or retroperitoneoscopic adrenalectomy has become the 'gold standard' in the resection of adrenal tumours, except for tumours with signs of malignancy. The more popular approach is the laparoscopic transperitoneal approach, which offers a better view of the adrenal region than open surgery. The advantage of the retroperitoneoscopic approach is the minimal dissection required by this extra-abdominal procedure. In the case of small, bilateral tumours or in patients with hereditary tumour syndromes a subtotal resection is warranted, to avoid steroid dependence. The mortality rate ranges from 0 to 2 per cent in specialised centres.

An open approach should be considered if radiological signs, distant metastases, large tumours (>8–10 cm) or a distinct hormonal pattern suggest malignancy.

Laparoscopic adrenalectomy

Knowledge of the anatomy of the adrenal region is essential as anatomical landmarks guide the surgeon during operation. If these landmarks are respected, injury to the vena cava or renal vein, the pancreatic tail or the spleen can be avoided. Careful haemostasis is essential as small amounts of blood can impair the surgeon's view. To prevent tumour spillage, direct grasping of the adrenal tissue/tumour has to be avoided.

Right adrenalectomy

Position the patient right side up, with table brake. Use three ports to start. The dissection starts at the level of the periadrenal fat using careful coagulation and the peritoneum should be divided 2 cm below the edge of the liver from medial (inferior vena cava) to the lateral abdominal wall (Figure 52.13). This flap of peritoneum can then be used to retract the liver up and off the adrenal. A fourth port may be useful to hold the liver up. Identify the gland and mobilise gently, securing the vein with a clip or using one of the available energy devices, and remove the gland in a plastic catch bag.

Left adrenalectomy

With the patient positioned on his or her right side, mobilisation of the spleen will displace the pancreatic tail medially. The incision of Gerota's fascia is followed by identification of the adrenal vein, which runs into the renal vein in the space between the medial aspect of the kidney and the posterior aspect of the pancreatic tail. The resection is completed by mobilising

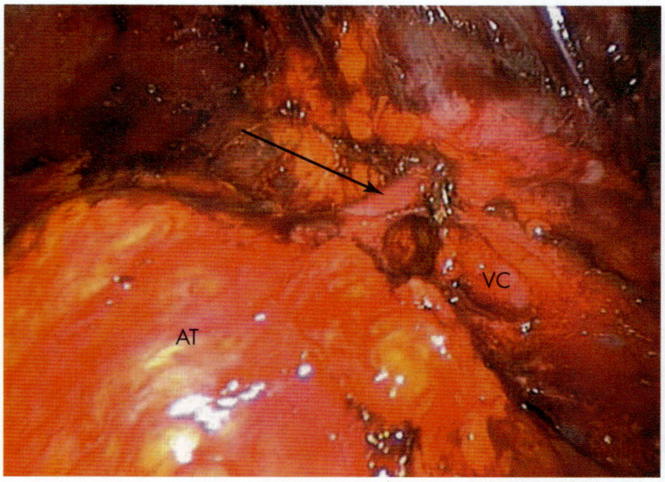

Figure 52.13 Laparoscopic view during a right adrenalectomy. Arrow indicates the adrenal vein. AT, adrenal tumour; VC, vena cava.

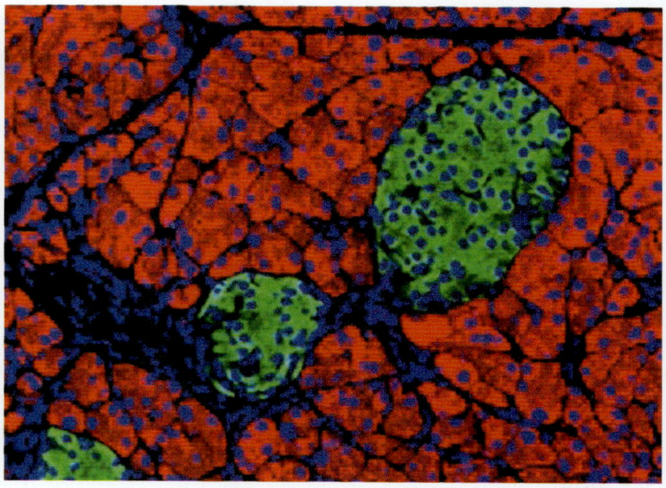

Figure 52.14 Immunofluorescent labelling of endocrine (insulin (green)) and exocrine (amylase (red)) pancreatic cells and the nuclear marker DAPI (blue) (courtesy of Dr Esni, Department of Surgery, University of Pittsburgh, USA).

the adrenal gland at the level of the periadrenal fat. Remove the gland in a bag and close the three port sites after infiltrating each with local anaesthesia.

Retroperitoneoscopic adrenalectomy

The first port is placed at the distal end of the 12th rib with the patient in the prone position. After a digital dissection into the retroperitoneum, Gerota's fascia is displaced ventrally. The right adrenal vein is covered by the retrocaval posterior aspect of the adrenal gland. The left adrenal vein is usually located at the medial inferior pole of the adrenal gland. High inflation pressures allow bloodless dissection effectively tamponading the veins. Being outside the abdominal cavity affords an excellent view.

Open adrenalectomy

An open adrenalectomy is almost exclusively performed when a malignant adrenal tumour is suspected. On the right side, the hepatic flexure of the colon is mobilised and the right liver lobe is cranially retracted to achieve an optimal exposure of the inferior vena cava and the adrenal gland. On the left side, the adrenal gland can be exposed after mobilisation of the splenic flexure of the colon, through the transverse mesocolon or through the gastrocolic ligament. The remaining dissection is the same as in laparoscopic adrenalectomy. A resection of regional lymph nodes is recommended in malignant adrenal tumours and should include resection of the tissue between the renal pedicle and the diaphragm.

PANCREATIC ENDOCRINE TUMOURS

Introduction

Pancreatic endocrine tumours (PET) represent an important subset of pancreatic neoplasms. They account for 5 per cent of all clinically detected pancreatic tumours. They consist of single or multiple, benign or malignant neoplasms and are associated in 10–20 per cent of cases with multiple endocrine neoplasia type 1 (MEN 1). They present as either functional tumours, causing specific hormonal syndromes, or non-functional tumours, with symptoms similar to those in patients with pancreatic adenocarcinoma. This section focuses on insulinomas, gastrinomas and non-functioning tumours because they represent 90 per cent of all PET (Table 52.3).

Function of the endocrine pancreas

The endocrine cells of the pancreas are grouped in the islets of Langerhans, which constitute approximately 1–2 per cent of the mass of the pancreas (Figure 52.14). There are about one million islets in a healthy adult human pancreas and their combined weight is 1–1.5 g. There are four main types of cell in the islets of Langerhans, which can be classified according to their secretions:

1. beta cells producing insulin (65–80 per cent of the islet cells);
2. alpha cells producing glucagon (15–20 per cent);
3. delta cells producing somatostatin (3–10 per cent);
4. pancreatic polypeptide (PP) cells containing polypeptide (1 per cent).

Insulinoma

Definition

This is an insulin-producing tumour of the pancreas causing the clinical scenario know as Whipple's triad, i.e. symptoms of hypoglycaemia after fasting or exercise, plasma glucose levels <2.8 mmol/L and relief of symptoms on intravenous administration of glucose.

George Hoyt Whipple, 1878–1976, Professor of Pathology, University of Rochester, Rochester, NY, USA, described this disease in 1907. He shared the 1934 Nobel Prize for Physiology or Medicine with George Richards Minot and William Parry Murphy 'for their discoveries concerning liver therapy against anaemias'.

Paul Langerhans, 1847–1888, Professor of Pathological Anatomy, Freiberg, Germany.

Table 52.3 Neuroendocrine tumours of the pancreas.

Tumour (syndrome)	Incidence (%)	Presentation	Malignancy (%)
Insulinoma	70–80	Weakness, sweating, tremor, tachycardia, anxiety, fatigue, dizziness, disorientation, seizures	<10
Gastrinoma	20–25	Intractable or recurrent peptic ulcer disease (haemorrhage, perforation), complications of peptic ulcer, diarrhoea	60–80
Non-functional tumours	30–50	Obstructive jaundice, pancreatitis, epigastric pain, duodenal obstruction, weight loss, fatigue	60–90
VIPoma	4	Profuse watery diarrhoea, hypotension, abdominal pain	80
Glucagonoma	4	Migratory necrolytic skin rash, glossitis, stomatitis, angular cheilitis, diabetes, severe weight loss, diarrhoea	80
Somatostatinoma	<5	Cholelithiasis, diarrhoea, neurofibromatosis	50
Carcinoid	<1	Flushing, sweating, diarrhoea, oedema	90
ACTHoma	<1	Cushing's syndrome	>90
GRFoma	<1	Acromegaly	30

ACTH, adrenocorticotrophic hormone; GRF, growth hormone-releasing factor; VIP, vasoactive intestinal polypeptide.

Incidence

Insulinomas are the most frequent of all the functioning PETs with a reported incidence of 2–4 cases per million population per year. Insulinomas have been diagnosed in all age groups with the highest incidence found in the fourth to the sixth decades. Women seem to be slightly more frequently affected.

Pathology

The aetiology and pathogenesis of insulinomas are unknown. No risk factors have been associated with these tumours. Virtually all insulinomas are located in the pancreas and tumours are equally distributed within the gland. Approximately 90 per cent are solitary and about 10 per cent are multiple and associated with MEN 1 syndrome.

Prognosis and predictive factors

No markers are available that reliably predict the biological behaviour of an insulinoma. Approximately 10 per cent are malignant. Insulinomas of <2 cm in diameter without signs of vascular invasion or metastases are considered benign.

Clinical features

Insulinomas are characterised by fasting hypoglycaemia and neuroglycopenic symptoms. The episodic nature of the hypoglycaemic attacks is caused by intermittent insulin secretion by the tumour. This leads to central nervous system symptoms such as diplopia, blurred vision, confusion, abnormal behaviour and amnesia. Some patients develop loss of consciousness and coma. The release of catecholamines produces symptoms such as sweating, weakness, hunger, tremor, nausea, anxiety and palpitations.

Biochemical diagnosis

A fasting test that may last for up to 72 hours is regarded as the most sensitive test. Usually, insulin, proinsulin, C-peptide and blood glucose are measured in 1- to 2-hour intervals to demonstrate inappropriately high secretion of insulin in relation to blood glucose. About 80 per cent of insulinomas are diagnosed by this test, most of them in the first 24 hours. Elevated C-peptide levels demonstrate the endogenous secretion of insulin and exclude factitious hypoglycaemia caused by insulin injection.

Differential diagnosis

The differential diagnosis of hypoglycaemia includes hormonal deficiencies, hepatic insufficiency, medication, drugs and enzyme defects. Occasionally, differentiating insulinoma from other causes of hypoglycaemia can be difficult. Nesidioblastosis is a rare disorder, mainly encountered in children, which is characterised by replacement of normal pancreatic islets by diffuse hyperplasia of islet cells.

Medical treatment of insulinoma

Medical management is reserved only for patients who are unable or unwilling to undergo surgical treatment or for unresectable metastatic disease. Diazoxide suppresses insulin secretion by direct action on the beta cells and offers reasonably good control of hypoglycaemia in approximately 50 per cent of patients. When surgical options to treat malignant insulinomas cannot be applied, chemotherapeutic options include doxorubicin and streptozotocin.

Surgical treatment of insulinoma

Indications for operation

After a positive fasting test and exclusion of diffuse abdominal metastases by ultrasound or CT scan, all patients should be advised to undergo surgical excision of insulinoma.

Preoperative localisation studies

Intraoperative exploration of the pancreas is the best method to use for localisation of insulinoma, yet the operating surgeon will need preoperative localisation! Insulinomas are detected in about 65 per cent of cases by endoscopic ultrasound (EUS), 33 per cent of cases by CT scan and abdominal ultrasound and 15 per cent of cases by magnetic resonance tomography. Intraoperative ultrasound (IOUS) of the pancreas is a vital tool

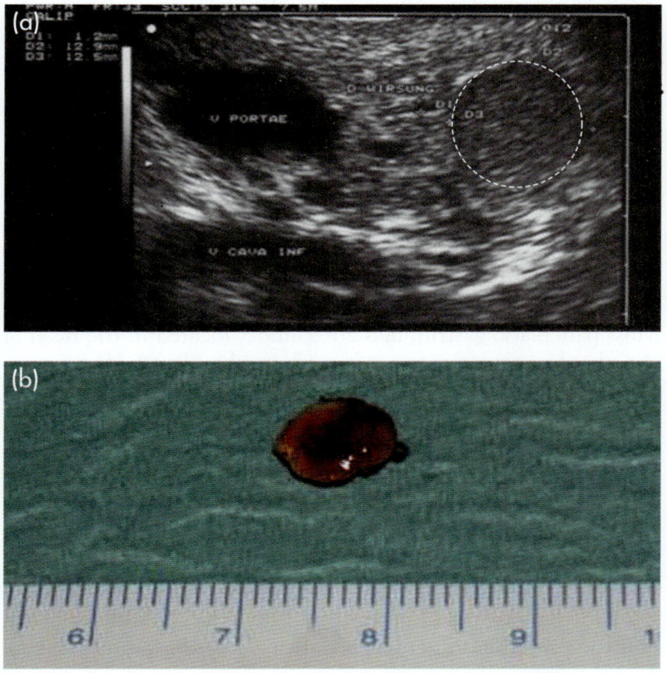

Figure 52.15 (a) Intraoperative ultrasound showing a typical insulinoma (dashed circle). v portae, portal vein; v cava inf, inferior vena cava; d wirsung, pancreatic duct. (b) Enucleated insulinoma.

after mobilisation of the gland. For preoperative localisation of an insulinoma, EUS has the highest sensitivity and should be used if laparoscopic resection is considered. If no lesion is identified and one can rely on the biochemical tests for diagnosis, laparotomy should follow, using IOUS.

Benign insulinoma

Surgical cure rates in patients with the biochemical diagnosis of insulinoma range from 90 to 100 per cent. At open surgery an extended Kocher manoeuvre and mobilisation of the head and then the distal pancreas is performed to explore the whole gland. IOUS should then be used to confirm the presence of a tumour, to find non-palpable lesions and also to identify the relation of the tumour to the pancreatic duct (Figure 52.15a). Tumour enucleation is the technique of choice (Figure 52.15b). For superficial tumours, laparoscopic enucleation is undertaken (Figure 52.16). Tumours located deep in the body or tail of the pancreas and those in close proximity to the pancreatic duct require distal pancreatectomy. Postoperatively, blood sugar levels begin to rise in most patients within the first few hours after removal of the tumour. To preserve pancreatic function and reduce the risk of iatrogenic diabetes mellitus, patients in whom tumour localisation is not successful at operation should not undergo blind resection.

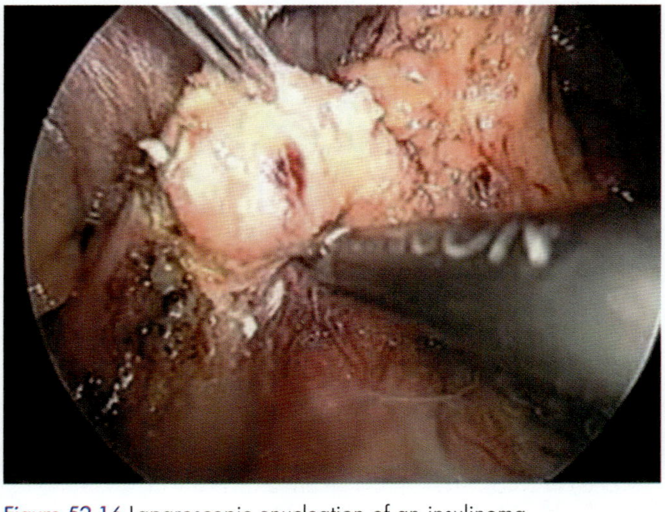

Figure 52.16 Laparoscopic enucleation of an insulinoma.

Malignant insulinoma

Aggressive attempts at resection are recommended as these tumours are much less virulent than adenocarcinomas.

Gastrinoma (Zollinger–Ellison syndrome)

Definition

Zollinger–Ellison syndrome (ZES) is a condition that includes: (1) fulminating ulcer diathesis in the stomach, duodenum or atypical sites; (2) recurrent ulceration despite 'adequate' therapy; and (3) non-beta islet cell tumours of the pancreas (gastrinoma).

Incidence

Gastrinomas account for about 20 per cent of PETs, second in frequency to insulinomas. Approximately 0.1 per cent of patients with duodenal ulcers have evidence of ZES. The reported incidence is between 0.5 and 4 cases per million population per year. ZES is more common in males than in females. The mean age at the onset of symptoms is 38 years, and the range is 7–83 years.

Pathology

The aetiology and pathogenesis of sporadic gastrinomas are unknown. At the time of diagnosis more than 60 per cent of tumours are malignant. Pancreatic gastrinomas are mainly found in sporadic disease; most are found in the head of the pancreas. More than 70 per cent of the gastrinomas in MEN 1 syndrome and most sporadic gastrinomas are located in the first and second part of the duodenum. Therefore, the anatomical area comprising the head of the pancreas, the superior and descending portion of the duodenum and the relevant lymph nodes has been called the 'gastrinoma triangle' because it harbours the vast majority of these tumours (Figure 52.17). All patients with gastrinomas should be tested for MEN 1 syndrome.

Prognosis and predictive factors

In general, the progression of gastrinomas is relatively slow with a five-year survival rate of 65 per cent and a ten-year survival rate of 51 per cent. Patients with complete tumour resection have excellent five- and ten-year survival rates (90–100 per cent). Patients with pancreatic tumours have a worse prognosis than those with primary tumours in the duodenum. There is no established marker to predict the biological behaviour of gastrinoma.

Clinical and biochemical features

Over 90 per cent of patients with gastrinomas have peptic ulcer disease, often multiple or in unusual sites. Diarrhoea is another

Emil Theodor Kocher, 1841–1917, Professor of Surgery, Berne, Switzerland. In 1909 he was awarded the Nobel Prize for Physiology or Medicine for his work on the thyroid.
Robert Milton Zollinger, 1903–1992, Professor of Surgery, Ohio State University, Columbus, OH, USA.
Edwin Homer Ellison, 1918–1970, Professor of Surgery, Marquette University, WI, USA.
Zollinger and Ellison described this condition in a joint paper in 1955 when they were both working at Ohio State University.

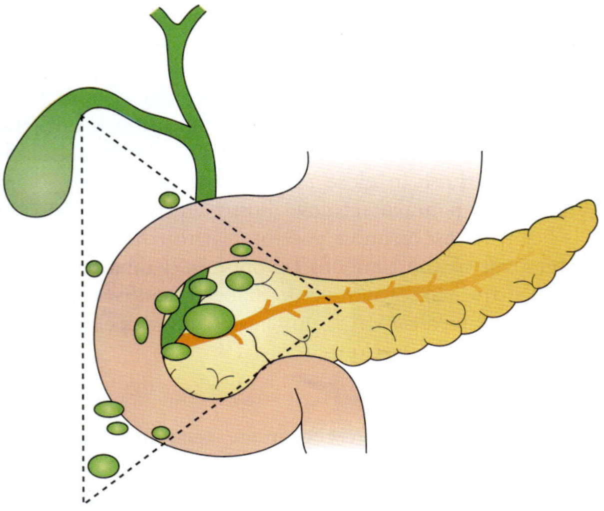

Figure 52.17 The gastrinoma triangle.

common symptom, caused by the large volume of gastric acid secretion. Abdominal pain from either peptic ulcer disease or gastro-oesophageal reflux disease (GORD) remains the most common symptom, occurring in more than 75 per cent of patients.

Biochemical diagnosis

If the patient presents with a gastric pH below 2.5 and a serum gastrin concentration above 1000 pg/mL (normal <100 pg/mL) then the diagnosis of ZES is confirmed. Unfortunately, the majority of patients have serum gastrin concentrations between 100 and 500 pg/mL and in these patients a secretin test should be performed. The secretin test is considered positive if an increase in serum gastrin of >200 pg/mL over the pretreatment value is obtained; this also rules out other causes of hypergastrinaemia (e.g. atrophic gastritis).

Differential diagnosis

The most common misdiagnoses are idiopathic peptic ulcer disease, chronic idiopathic diarrhoea and GORD. Other reasons for hypergastrinaemia are chronic atrophic gastritis, gastric outlet stenosis and retained antrum after gastric resection.

Medical treatment of gastrinoma

In most patients with ZES, gastric hypersecretion can be treated effectively with proton pump inhibitors. Octreotide can also help to control acid hypersecretion. Systemic chemotherapy is utilised in patients with diffuse metastatic gastrinomas. Streptozotocin in combination with 5-fluorouracil or doxorubicin is the first-line treatment.

Surgical treatment of gastrinoma

Indications for operation

Surgical exploration should be performed in all patients without diffuse metastases, to remove known malignant gastrinomas or benign ones.

Preoperative localisation studies

Pancreatic gastrinomas are often larger than 1 cm in diameter whereas gastrinomas of the duodenum are usually smaller. Therefore, it is nearly impossible to identify duodenal gastrinomas by preoperative imaging. Pancreatic gastrinomas are detected by EUS in about 80–90 per cent of cases, by CT in 39 per cent of cases and by MRI in 46 per cent of cases. In approximately one-third of patients, the results of conventional imaging studies are negative. On the basis of recent studies, either EUS or CT and somatostatin receptor scintigraphy (SRS) should be performed preoperatively for staging.

Pancreatic gastrinomas

Most pancreatic gastrinomas are solitary, located in the head of the gland or uncinate process, and can be identified at operation. Enucleation with peripancreatic lymph node dissection is the procedure of choice. Rarely, tumours are situated in the body or tail and should be treated by enucleation or distal resection. Even if a tumour is found in the pancreas, duodenotomy is recommended to detect additional tumours, if the patient has MEN 1.

Duodenal gastrinomas

The duodenum should be opened with a longitudinal incision and the posterior and anterior walls palpated separately (Figure 52.18). Duodenal tumours smaller than 5 mm can be enucleated with the overlying mucosa; larger tumours are excised with full-thickness excision of the duodenal wall.

Non-functional endocrine pancreatic tumours

Definition

PETs are clinically classified as non-functioning PETs (NF-PETs) when they do not cause a clinical syndrome.

Incidence

NF-PETs account for 30–50 per cent of all PETs. They are most often diagnosed in the fifth to sixth decades of life.

Pathology

NF-PETs cannot be differentiated from functional tumours by immunocytochemistry because they may also express hormones such as gastrin, insulin, etc. They usually stain positively for

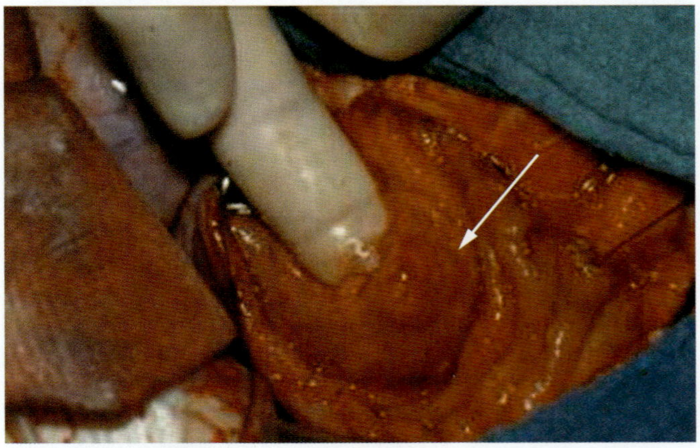

Figure 52.18 Palpation of a duodenal gastrinoma (arrow) after duodenotomy.

chromogranin A and synaptophysin. The tumours are usually large (>5 cm) and unifocal except in MEN 1 syndrome. They are distributed throughout the pancreas with a head to body to tail ratio of 7:1:1.5.

Prognosis and predictive factors

About 70 per cent of all NF-PETs are malignant. Overall five- and ten-year survival rates of 65 and 49 per cent, respectively, have been described. When comparing NF-PETs with functioning PETs, the NF-PETs have a worse prognosis.

Clinical features

Patients usually present late because of the lack of a clinical/hormonal marker of tumour activity. Therefore, in contrast to functioning PETs, patients with NF-PETs present with various non-specific symptoms, including jaundice, abdominal pain, weight loss and pancreatitis. In some cases liver metastases are the first presentation.

Biochemical diagnosis

Increased levels of chromogranin A have been reported in 50–80 per cent of NF-PETs; the level of chromogranin A sometimes correlates with the tumour burden. The combination of elevated chromogranin A and PP measurements increases the sensitivity of diagnosis from 84 to 96 per cent in NF-PETs.

Differential diagnosis

Differentiation from the more aggressive pancreatic adenocarcinoma is extremely important (Table 52.4). Recognition of NF-PETs is imperative because of their resectability and excellent long-term survival compared with their exocrine counterparts.

Table 52.4 Differences between pancreatic cancer and non-functioning endocrine pancreatic tumours (NF-PETs).

	Pancreatic cancer	NF-PETs
Tumour size	<5 cm	>5 cm
Computed tomography scan	Hypodensity	Hyperdensity
	No calcifications	Calcifications possible
Chromogranin A in blood	Negative	Positive
Somatostatin receptor scintigraphy	Negative	Positive

Medical treatment of non-functioning islet cell tumours

When surgical excision is not possible, chemotherapeutic options include streptozotocin, octreotide and interferon.

Surgical treatment of non-functioning islet cell tumours

Indications for operation

An aggressive surgical approach should be considered in malignant NF-PETs, even in the presence of distant metastases.

Preoperative localisation studies

Preoperative ultrasound or CT scan are the procedures of choice as these tumours are relatively large. Also, SRS should be performed to differentiate endocrine from non-endocrine pancreatic tumours.

Operative procedures

The major goal is a potentially curative resection. This may require partial pancreaticoduodenectomy as well as the synchronous or metachronous resection of liver metastases. Using an aggressive approach, curative resections are possible in up to 62 per cent of cases and overall five-year survival rates of around 65 per cent can be achieved. Repeated resections for resectable recurrences or metastases are justified to improve survival.

NEUROENDOCRINE TUMOURS OF THE STOMACH AND SMALL BOWEL

Definition and physiology

Neuroendocrine tumours (NET) of the gut and the pancreas arise from the diffuse neuroendocrine cell system, which can be found as single or clustered cells in the mucosa of the bronchi, stomach, gut, biliary tree, urogenital system and in the pancreas (see Chapters 71, 69 and 72 for NET of the appendix, colon and rectum, respectively). This cell system was first recognised as the 'clear cell system' by Feyrter in the 1930s and is identical to the APUD (amine precursor uptake and decarboxylation) system described by Pearse in 1970. All cells of the system secrete different neuroendocrine markers, such as synaptophysin, chromogranin A and neurone-specific enolase (NSE), and produce peptide hormones that are stored in granules, e.g. serotonin, somatostatin, PP or gastrin. In clinical practice chromogranin A is utilised as a tumour marker. The main functional test for NET of the jejunum and ileum (the NET that are most often encountered) is the measurement of the serotonin metabolite 5-hydroxyindoleacetic acid (5-HIAA) in urine.

Pathology

Neuroendocrine cells can form hyperplasias or tumours. In 1907, Oberndorfer coined the term 'carcinoids' for tumours arising from these cells. Although the term carcinoid continues to be used in clinical practice, these tumours do not always grow in a well-differentiated pattern reflecting the rather benign 'carcinoma-like', i.e. 'carcinoid', tumour. They can show different growth patterns, from benign tumours to high-grade undifferentiated carcinomas having a poor prognosis (neuroendocrine carcinomas). Therefore, they should always be addressed as NET, including a description of their histological pattern (benign, low- or high-grade malignant) and their anatomical site (e.g. stomach, ileum) according to the World Health Organization classification (2000). The relative distribution of NET in different organs is given in Table 52.5. Another classification based on embryological principles classifies NET as foregut (lung, stomach, pancreas), midgut (small bowel and appendix) and hindgut (colon and rectum) tumours.

Neuroendocrine tumours of the stomach

These tumours are rare. They comprise about 5 per cent of all NET of the gastrointestinal tract and have an incidence of

Anthony Guy Everson Pearse, 1916–2003, Professor of Histochemistry, The Royal Postgraduate Medical School, Hammersmith, London, UK.

Table 52.5 Relative distribution of neuroendocrine tumours in different organs.

Site	Distribution (%)
Lung	10
Stomach	5
Duodenum	2
Small bowel	25
Appendix	40
Colon	6
Rectum	15

approximately 0.2 cases per 100 000 population per year. There are four different types of gastric NET (Table 52.6). Types 1 and 2 are small benign tumours that arise from the enterochromaffin-like (ECL) cells in the gastric mucosa and grow in either a linear or a nodular pattern (Figure 52.19). Hypergastrinaemia may cause symptoms and the treatment of choice is endoscopic resection. Types 3 and 4 are almost always malignant and surgical resection should be undertaken if possible.

Pathogenesis, diagnosis and treatment

Type 1 tumours (ECLomas) are the most frequent NET of the stomach (approximately 80 per cent); they occur mostly in elderly women. Chronic hypergastrinaemia is the result of chronic atrophic gastritis and achlorhydria, the alkaline pH being the stimulus for hypersecretion of gastrin. They do not cause symptoms and are usually detected during gastroscopy for other reasons. Endoscopic resection is the treatment of choice. Antrectomy and resection of ECLomas should be undertaken only if there is recurrent disease and multiple (more than six) tumours, with at least one measuring >1 cm and infiltration of at least one into the submucosa.

The pathogenesis, diagnosis and treatment of type 2 tumours is similar to that of type 1. The only difference is the cause of the hypergastrinaemia, which in type 2 tumours is the result of MEN 1 syndrome, with multiple gastrinomas in the duodenum or, rarely, in the pancreas.

Type 3 tumours are rare, sporadic and solitary tumours of unknown origin. Serum gastrin is normal; upper gastrointestinal bleeding is the usual symptom that leads to endoscopy. Type 3 tumours are usually larger than 2 cm and often have lymph node and liver metastases at the time of diagnosis. Gastrectomy and lymph node dissection and resection of liver metastases is the treatment of choice. Liver metastases can also be treated by chemoembolisation.

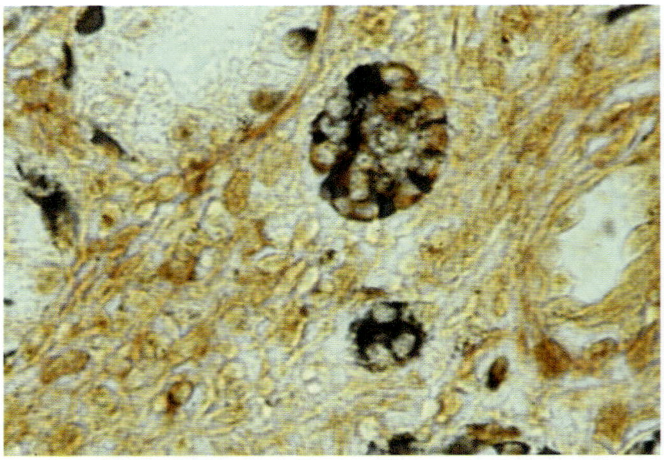

Figure 52.19 Immunostaining of chromogranin in micronodular hyperplasia of enterochromaffin-like (ECL) cells of the stomach associated with chronic atrophic gastritis.

Type 4 tumours present as large ulcerating malignancies similar to adenocarcinomas and should be treated accordingly. The prognosis of types 3 and 4 is poor (Table 52.6).

Neuroendocrine tumours of the small bowel

Introduction

These are the tumours that are most commonly referred to as 'carcinoid' tumours, as most NET of the gastrointestinal tract are found in the small bowel. They are also called 'midgut' tumours (together with NET of the appendix and the right colon). These tumours produce serotonin and cause the 'carcinoid' syndrome, but only in patients who have a large volume of liver metastases or if there is advanced local tumour growth draining into the

Table 52.6 Classification of gastric neuroendocrine tumours.

Type	Histological pattern	Size and location	Causative factor and prognosis
1	Benign, non-functional, well differentiated	Gastric corpus; <1 cm; mucosa/submucosa	ECLomas in chronic atrophic gastritis, hypergastrinaemia
2	Benign or low-grade malignant, differentiated	1–2 cm; angioinvasion; mucosa/submucosa	ECLomas with hypergastrinaemia as a result of gastrinoma in MEN 1
3	Low-grade malignant, differentiated	2 cm; invasion beyond submucosa	Sporadic ECLomas not related to hypergastrinaemia
4	Intermediate or small cell type, high-grade malignant (neuroendocrine carcinoma)	Different sizes	Causative factor unknown; prognosis poor

ECL, enterochromaffin-like; MEN, multiple endocrine neoplasia.

inferior vena cava and thereby bypassing the liver. NET of the duodenum (gastrinomas in MEN 1 syndrome, somatostatinomas and others) are very rare and are not discussed further.

Pathology

NET of the jejunum and ileum arise from a subgroup of cells of the diffuse neuroendocrine system, the enterochromaffin (EC) cells, which secrete serotonin and substance P. They are either solitary or more often multiple, are almost always malignant and metastasise early to the regional lymph nodes and the liver depending on the location of the primary tumour(s) (Figure 52.20).

Clinical symptoms

Symptoms that lead to the diagnosis are caused by either the primary tumour or its lymph node metastases. Acute or chronic, recurrent or persistent abdominal pain, ileus or, rarely, lower gastrointestinal bleeding may occur. Symptoms may be due to liver metastases, such as sudden painful reddening of the face and chest ('flushing'), diarrhoea or bronchospasm. These symptoms constitute 'carcinoid' syndrome. About 60 per cent of patients eventually develop cardiac symptoms because of stenosis and insufficiency of the pulmonary and, more rarely, the tricuspid valve, with enlargement and thickening of the wall of the right atrium. The aetiology is unknown but local effects of serotonin and kinins may contribute.

Abdominal symptoms are caused either by obstruction of the appendix by an appendiceal NET (leading to appendectomy) or by obstruction of the mesentery or the bowel lumen by growth of lymph node metastases in the mesentery near the bowel. Pain is caused by chronic ischaemia of the bowel (Figure 52.21), resulting not only from mesenteric lymph node metastases but also from constriction of mesenteric arteries and fibrosis of the mesentery by a so-called desmoplastic reaction.

Primary tumours in the jejunum and ileum rarely cause symptoms such as bleeding or intussusception as they usually only measure from a few millimetres up to 1 cm or at the most 2 cm in diameter (Figure 52.22). A polypoid NET of the terminal ileum may, however, cause ileocaecal intussusception.

Diagnosis

The diagnosis of NET of the small bowel is made by history, physical examination of the abdomen, imaging and an assessment of 5-HIAA in a 24-hour urine sample. It is positive in larger tumours only if metastases are present. Cross-sectional imaging, sonography, CT scan and MRI may show the primary tumour, mesenteric lymph node and liver metastases.

The best method for staging of NET is an octreotide (SRS) scan. This will show all tumour deposits provided that they are large enough and have a high somatostatin receptor density (Figure 52.23).

Surgical procedure

Surgery should be undertaken as soon as the diagnosis is made, even in the presence of liver metastases. The main goal is resection of the bowel primary tumour(s) and mesenteric lymph node metastases. This may entail resection of large amounts of bowel (100 cm or more), particularly if stage III or IV lymph node masses are found in the mesentery (Figure 52.24). In the presence of liver metastases, extrahepatic disease should be resected whenever possible. Metastatic disease in the mesenteric root will lead to long-term pain in the abdomen or back and to a poor quality of life, whereas liver metastases can be treated by chemotherapy or embolisation.

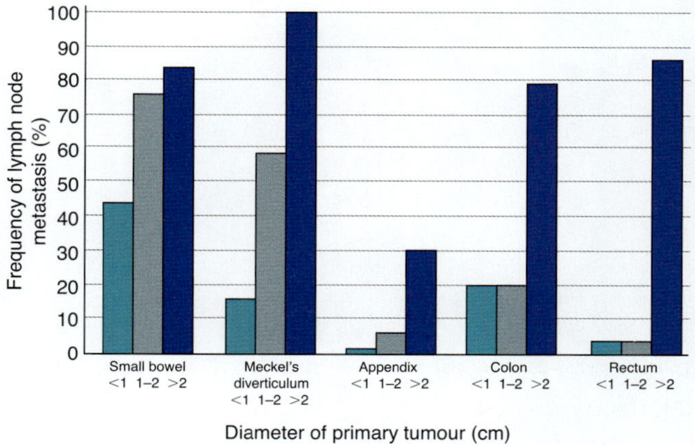

Figure 52.20 Relation of site and diameter of neuroendocrine tumours of the gut to frequency of lymph node metastasis.

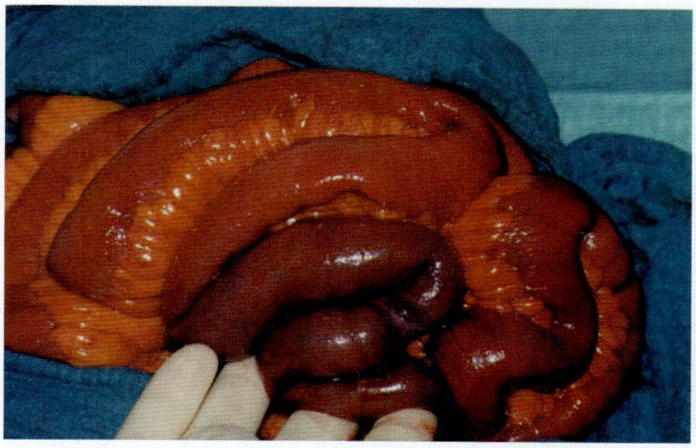

Figure 52.21 Chronic ischaemia of the small bowel caused by desmoplastic reaction and narrowing of vessels in the mesentery in a neuroendocrine tumour of the ileum.

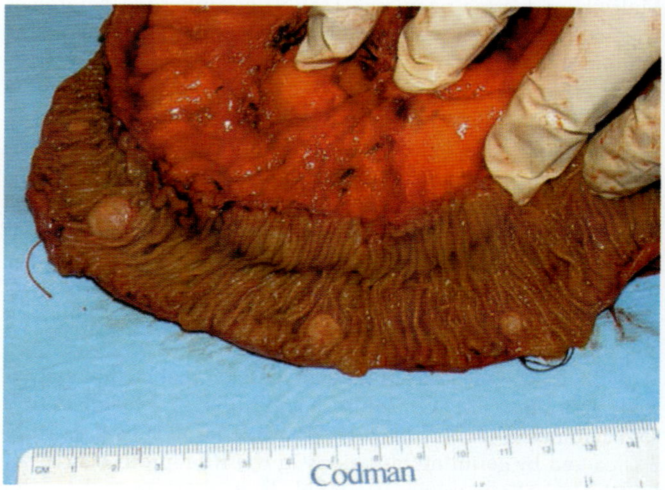

Figure 52.22 Multiple neuroendocrine tumours in the small bowel causing large lymph node metastases in the mesentery.

Johann Friedrich Meckel (the Younger), 1781–1833, Professor of Anatomy and Surgery, Halle, Germany.

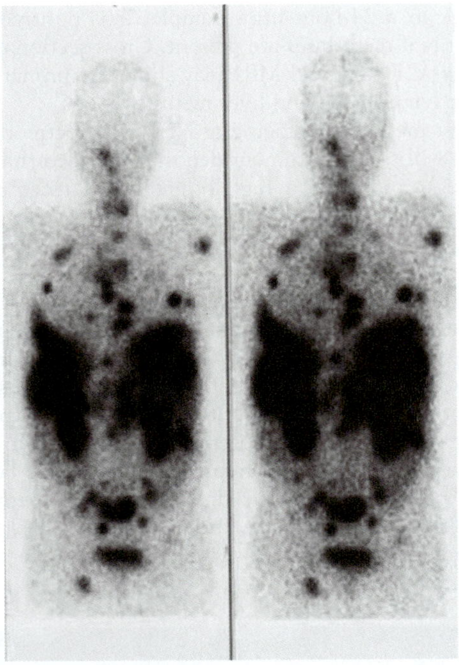

Figure 52.23 Octreotide scan of a patient with neuroendocrine tumour of the gut and diffuse metastases in different organs.

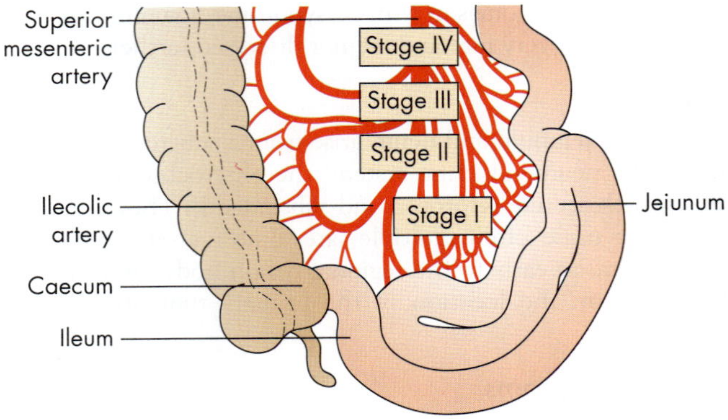

Figure 52.24 Bulky lymph node metastases can occur at different levels in the mesentery. To resect them completely, long segments of bowel must be resected, the closer to the mesenteric root the metastases are situated (adapted from Akerström, G., Hellman, P. and Öhrvall, U. (2001) Midgut and hindgut carcinoid tumours. In: Doherty, G.M. and Skogseid, B. (eds.). *Surgical Endocrinology*. Lippincott Williams & Wilkins, Philadelphia, PA, by kind permission).

Somatostatin and its analogues provide symptomatic treatment of the 'carcinoid' syndrome caused by a large volume of liver metastases. These drugs may also have an antiproliferative effect. Surgery to remove liver metastases is possible in approximately 10 per cent of patients. In others, embolisation, chemoembolisation, SRS using radioactively labelled octreotide, chemotherapy, biotherapy and also liver transplantation can be performed.

MULTIPLE ENDOCRINE NEOPLASIAS

Introduction

Multiple endocrine neoplasias (MEN) are inherited syndromes characterised by a combination of benign and malignant tumours in different endocrine glands. There are two main types, type 1 (MEN 1) and type 2 (MEN 2). The mode of inheritance is autosomal dominant in both.

MEN 1 is characterised by the triad of tumours in the anterior pituitary gland, mostly presenting as prolactinomas or non-functioning tumours, hyperplasia of the parathyroids causing primary hyperparathyroidism (pHPT) and pancreaticoduodenal endocrine tumours. The syndrome was first described by Wermer in 1954 and is therefore also called Wermer's syndrome. It is caused by germline mutations in the *menin* gene, located on chromosome 11.

MEN 2 is divided into three subtypes: familial medullary thyroid carcinoma (FMTC), MEN 2a and MEN 2b. Medullary thyroid carcinoma (MTC) plays the key role in all subtypes. MEN 2 is caused by germline mutations in the *RET* proto-oncogene, located on chromosome 10. MEN 2a is characterised by the combination of MTC, pHPT and mostly bilateral phaeochromocytomas. MTC combined with phaeochromocytoma alone is called Sipple's syndrome. FMTC is characterised by distinct mutations in *RET* and MTC alone as the clinical manifestation. MEN 2b comprises MTC, phaeochromocytoma and characteristic facial and oral mucosal neuromas and intestinal ganglioneuromatosis accompanied by a Marfanoid habitus (Figure 52.25).

The most important difference between MEN 1 and MEN 2, besides the different clinical pictures, is that MEN 2 is characterised by a well-understood genotype–phenotype correlation. This means that depending on the particular mutation in the *RET* proto-oncogene, the phenotypic appearance and the onset of endocrine tumours will be different and can be predicted from the type of mutation. This is not the case in MEN 1 syndrome.

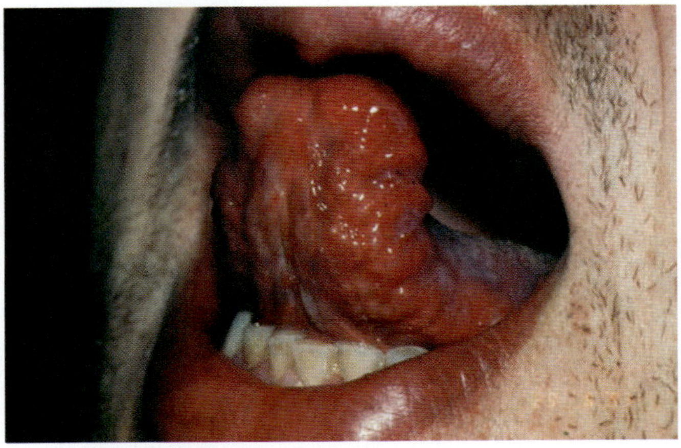

Figure 52.25 Neuromas of the tongue in a patient with multiple endocrine neoplasia type 2b.

Paul Wermer, 1898–1975, physician, The Presbyterian Hospital, New York, NY, USA, described this condition in 1954.

Table 52.7 Affected organs in multiple endocrine neoplasia type 1.

Endocrine gland affected	Frequency (%)	Hormone	Clinical syndrome
Parathyroids	90	PTH	pHPT
Pancreas, duodenum (mostly multiple)	50–80		
Gastrinoma		Gastrin	Zollinger–Ellison syndrome
Insulinoma		Insulin	Hypoglycaemia syndrome
Non-functioning tumours		PP	–
VIPoma		VIP	Verner–Morrison syndrome
Glucagonoma		Glucagon	Glucagonoma syndrome
Anterior pituitary gland:	30–60		
Prolactinoma		Prolactin	Galactorrhea
Non-functioning adenoma		–	Non-specific
Other manifestations			
Adrenals	40–50	Mostly non-functioning	
NET in lung, thymus, stomach	3–10	–	–
Lipoma	5–10	–	–

NET, neuroendocrine tumours; pHPT, primary hyperparathyroidism; PP, pancreatic polypeptide; PTH, parathormone; VIP, vasoactive intestinal polypeptide.

Multiple endocrine neoplasia type 1

Epidemiology

The prevalence of the syndrome is estimated to be around 0.04–0.2 cases per 1000 population per year. The penetrance is high with almost 100 per cent of mutation carriers developing the syndrome. The disease is equally distributed between men and women.

Clinical presentation

The clinical presentation depends on the affected organs. Tumours can occur synchronously (Table 52.7). Most of the mutation carriers identified in screening programmes are asymptomatic.

Parathyroids

In total, 90–100 per cent of patients suffering from MEN 1 develop pHPT and it is usually the first manifestation of the disease. MEN 1 pHPT is characterised by multiglandular disease so that all four parathyroids become hyperplastic in the course of the disease. The clinical presentation of MEN 1 pHPT is similar to that of the sporadic disease. Few patients have asymptomatic disease; most common in symptomatic disease is nephrolithiasis. Diagnosis is established by determination of parathyroid hormone (PTH) and calcium in serum and urine.

Endocrine pancreas

PETs occur in around 50–60 per cent of MEN 1 patients. In such patients taking part in screening programmes, 70–90 per cent are found to have non-functioning and functioning PETs. This high rate of detection of PETs is the result of the improvement in diagnostic procedures in the last decade, including EUS. MEN 1 PETs are the most common syndrome-associated cause of death. They are mostly multiple and often recur after surgery. Although most patients have multiple tumours, one hormone syndrome is usually dominant. The most common functional tumour is gastrinoma followed by insulinoma. VIPomas, glucagonomas and somatostatinomas are extremely rare. Non-functioning tumours can be asymptomatic for many years.

The diagnostic work-up is similar to that for sporadic PETs and includes hormone measurements, e.g. gastrin, insulin, PP, etc., and imaging.

Anterior pituitary gland

Tumours of the anterior pituitary gland are found in 30–60 per cent of patients with MEN 1. These are mostly microadenomas that present as prolactinomas or non-functioning tumours. Most prolactinomas can be treated with medication, thus avoiding operation.

Adrenal tumours and other organ manifestations

Adrenal involvement is common in MEN 1 patients and affects nearly 40–50 per cent of patients. Mostly non-functioning adenomas are found. Very rarely, adrenocortical carcinomas or phaeochromocytomas may develop.

Although very rare, manifestations of MEN 1 include NET of the lung, thymus, stomach, duodenum and small bowel. It is important to check for NETs of the thymus, as they are mostly malignant.

Genetic screening

Identification of the MEN 1 (*menin*) gene in 1997 formed the basis for direct mutational analysis of the gene and for family screening. After genetic counselling of the index patient, family members can be screened. Mutation carriers can then be included in screening programmes that make early detection of

John Sipple, born 1930, physician, The State University of New York, New York, NY, USA.
John V Verner, born 1927, an American physician.
AB Morrison, born 1921, an American physician.

endocrine tumours possible. Screening programmes should follow the consensus guidelines published by Brandi *et al.* in 2001. In cases of apparently sporadic endocrine tumours in patients younger than 40 years, genetic testing for MEN 1 is advised.

Operative therapy

Parathyroids

The indications for surgery in MEN 1 pHPT follow the same criteria as in sporadic disease but the choice of procedure is different. As multiglandular disease is present in all cases, resection follows the same rules as in secondary HPT. Therefore, the most common procedures are total parathyroidectomy, including cervical thymectomy or 3½-gland resection, leaving approximately 50 mg of parathyroid tissue behind, and cervical thymectomy. Selective resection of enlarged glands is obsolete because of the high rates of recurrence.

Endocrine pancreas

Indications for surgery and its extent are controversial. Most experts agree that MEN 1 gastrinoma and insulinoma have to be operated on to prevent liver metastases and to control hormonal excess, provided that diffuse liver metastases are not present. MEN 1 gastrinomas are more often located in the duodenum as multiple small tumours than in the pancreas. For gastrinomas located in the duodenum or pancreatic head (gastrinoma triangle, Figure 52.17), pylorus-preserving partial pancreaticoduodenectomy is recommended. In rare cases, the gastrinoma is located in the body or tail of the pancreas. In such cases, distal pancreatectomy with excision of tumours in the pancreatic head is the procedure of choice. In MEN 1 insulinoma the standard operative procedure is distal pancreatectomy with enucleation of tumours in the pancreatic head. Non-functioning PETs are operated on if they reach a size of 1 cm. Careful palpation and IOUS are essential in every pancreatic procedure for MEN 1 PETs.

Anterior pituitary gland

The indications for surgery in tumours of the anterior pituitary gland are the presence of symptomatic non-functional tumours or if medical therapy of prolactinoma fails. Most procedures can be performed through a trans-sphenoidal approach.

Adrenal tumours

Functional adrenal tumours in MEN 1 are rare and have to be operated on. Non-functioning tumours should be resected if they reach a size of 4 cm. Pre- and perioperative management follows the same rules as in sporadic adrenal tumours; therefore, phaeochromocytoma has to be ruled out in every patient. In most cases, a laparoscopic or retroperitoneoscopic approach can be used. If there is evidence for a malignant tumour, open surgery is preferred.

Multiple endocrine neoplasia type 2

In most patients with MEN 2a, the disease is caused by mutations of the *RET* proto-oncogene in codon 634. MTC is almost always the first manifestation of the syndrome. If phaeochromocytoma and pHPT do not occur, one must suspect the presence of the FMTC subtype. Patients with MEN 2b do not develop pHPT and in 95 per cent of cases mutations in codon 918 of the *RET* proto-oncogene are causative (Table 52.8).

Medullary thyroid carcinoma

MTC is characterised by multicentricity and is often accompanied by C-cell hyperplasia. These characteristics should lead to molecular diagnostic work-up (mutational analysis of the *RET* proto-oncogene) in patients with apparently 'sporadic' MTC. In contrast to sporadic MTC, the diagnosis in families with known mutation of the *RET* gene is mostly made much earlier, possibly as the result of mutational screening and calcitonin measurements. MTC is most aggressive in MEN 2b. It occurs in early childhood, much earlier than in MEN 2a, with lymph node metastases present in the early stages. Preventative surgery is advised around the age of one year.

Primary hyperparathyroidism

pHPT in MEN 2a is less common and has a milder clinical course than MEN 1 pHPT. It occurs in about 20–30 per cent of patients with MEN 2a. Most patients are asymptomatic but all parathyroid glands can become hyperplastic, mostly metachronously. The disease develops after the third decade of life typically.

Phaeochromocytoma

The frequency of phaeochromocytoma in MEN 2 is around 10–50 per cent and tumours can be bilateral. This can occur synchronously or metachronously. The tumours are almost always benign. Diagnostic work-up includes measurement of urinary catecholamines, abdominal CT or MRI, and 131I-MIBG scintigraphy (see above).

Operative therapy

Medullary thyroid carcinoma

Operative therapy for MEN 2 MTC in patients detected by genetic screening is a good example of efficient prophylactic surgery, as the likelihood of developing MTC is 100 per cent for most mutations. The mutation carriers can be operated on with no evidence of tumour in the thyroid, protecting them from MTC for the rest of their lives. Different *RET* mutations are associated with early or late onset of the disease. Risk groups have been defined to determine the appropriate age for thyroidectomy (Table 52.9).

Table 52.8 Frequency of diseases in multiple endocrine neoplasia type 2 related to mutation in different codons.

Syndrome	Frequently affected codons in *RET*	MTC (%)	pHPT (%)	PCC (%)
FMTC	533, 630, 768, 844	90–100	–	–
MEN 2a	609, 634, 790, 804	90–100	20–30	10–50
MEN 2b	883, 918	100	–	10–50

FMTC, familial medullary thyroid cancer; MEN 2a, multiple endocrine neoplasia type 2a; MEN 2b, multiple endocrine neoplasia type 2b; MTC, medullary thyroid cancer; PCC, phaeochromocytoma; pHPT, primary hyperparathyroidism; RET, RET proto-oncogene (RET = rearranged during transfection).

Table 52.9 Prophylactic thyroidectomy for medullary thyroid cancer depending on the site of mutation of the *RET* proto-oncogene in multiple endocrine neoplasia type 2 patients with normal calcitonin levels.

	Risk group		
	High	Medium	Low
Codon	883, 918, 922	609, 611, 618, 620, 634	768, 790, 791, 804, 891
Thyroidectomy at age (years)	< 1	6	<20

Phaeochromocytoma

The operative approach is laparoscopy or retroperitoneoscopy. Unilateral or bilateral subtotal resection may be feasible, which retains the healthy part of the gland and prevents postoperative dependence on cortisol and mineralocorticoid supplementation (see above) (Figure 52.26). Further phaeos can develop in the remnants that are left so continued surveillance is required.

Primary hyperparathyroidism

The clinical situation in MEN 2 pHPT is even more difficult than in MEN 1 pHPT because of the association with MTC in MEN 2. During neck surgery for MTC in a eucalcaemic patient, enlarged parathyroid glands should be removed. In cases in which neck surgery has already been performed for MTC, the surgical approach to MEN 2a pHPT should be more tailored to the individual patient. For example, in an older patient after thyroidectomy for MTC with mild asymptomatic hypercalcaemia, localisation procedures and a targeted approach may be appropriate.

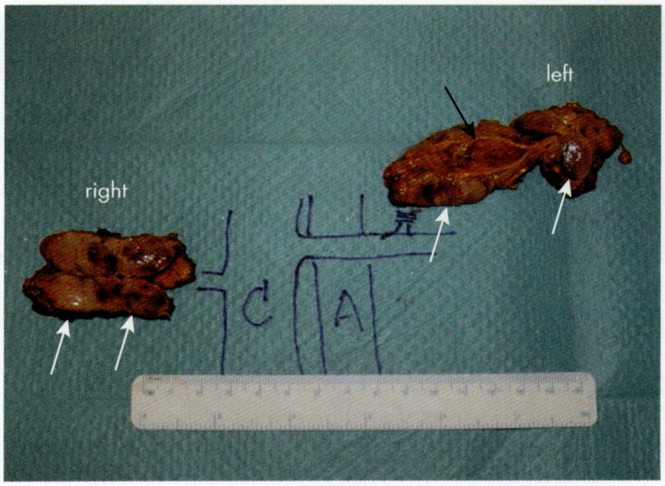

Figure 52.26 Bilateral multiple phaeochromocytomas in a patient with multiple endocrine neoplasia type 2a. A, aorta; C, vena cava; white arrows, tumours; black arrow, normal adrenal.

FURTHER READING

Allolio B, Fassnacht M. Clinical review: adrenocortical carcinoma: clinical update. *J Clin Endocrinol Metab* 2006; **91**: 2027–37.

Bartsch DK, Fendrich V, Langer P *et al.* Outcome of duodenopancreatic resections in patients with multiple endocrine neoplasia type 1. *Ann Surg* 2005; **242**: 757–64.

Brandi ML, Gagel RF, Angeli A *et al.* Guidelines for diagnosis and therapy of MEN type 1 and type 2. *J Clin Endocrinol Metab* 2001; **86**: 5658–71.

Hardy R, Lennard TWJ. Subtotal adrenalectomy. *Br J Surg* 2008; **95**: 1075–6.

Fendrich V, Langer P, Celik I *et al.* An aggressive surgical approach leads to long-term survival in patients with pancreatic endocrine tumors. *Ann Surg* 2006; **244**: 845–51.

Gaujoux S, Bonnet S, Leconte M *et al.* Risk factors for conversion and complications after unilateral laparoscopic adrenalectomy. *Br J Surg* 2011; **98**: 1392–9.

Ilias I, Pacak K. Diagnosis and management of tumors of the adrenal medulla. *Horm Metab Res* 2005; **37**: 717–21.

Madani R, Al-Hashmi M, Bliss R, Lennard TWJ. Ectopic phaeochromocytoma: does the rule of 10 apply? *World J Surg* 2007; **31**: 849–54.

Muth A, Hammarstedt L, Hellstrom M *et al.* Cohort study of patients with adrenal lesions discovered incidentally. *Br J Surg* 2011; **98**: 1383–91.

Norton JA, Fraker DL, Alexander HR *et al.* Surgery increases survival in patients with gastrinoma. *Ann Surg* 2006; **244**: 410–19.

Walz MK, Alesina PF, Wenger FA *et al.* Posterior retroperitoneoscopic adrenalectomy: results of 560 proceedures in 520 patients. *Surgery* 2006; **140**: 943–8.

Young WF Jr. Clinical practice: the incidentally discovered adrenal mass. *New Engl J Med* 2007; **356**: 601–10.

CHAPTER 53 The breast

LEARNING OBJECTIVES

To understand:
- Appropriate investigation of breast disease
- Breast anomalies and the complexity of benign breast disease
- The in-depth modern management of breast cancer

COMPARATIVE AND SURGICAL ANATOMY

The protuberant part of the human breast is generally described as overlying the second to the sixth ribs and extending from the lateral border of the sternum to the anterior axillary line. Actually, a thin layer of mammary tissue extends considerably further, from the clavicle above to the seventh or eighth ribs below and from the midline to the edge of the latissimus dorsi posteriorly. This fact is important when performing a mastectomy, the aim of which is to remove the whole breast. The anatomy of the breast is illustrated in Figure 53.1.

The **axillary tail** of the breast is of surgical importance. In some normal subjects it is palpable and, in a few, it can be seen premenstrually or during lactation. A well-developed axillary tail is sometimes mistaken for a mass of enlarged lymph nodes or a lipoma.

The **lobule** is the basic structural unit of the mammary gland. The number and size of the lobules vary enormously: they are most numerous in young women. From 10 to over 100 lobules empty via ductules into a lactiferous duct, of which there are 15–20. Each lactiferous duct is lined with a spiral arrangement of contractile myoepithelial cells and is provided with a terminal ampulla, a reservoir for milk or abnormal discharges.

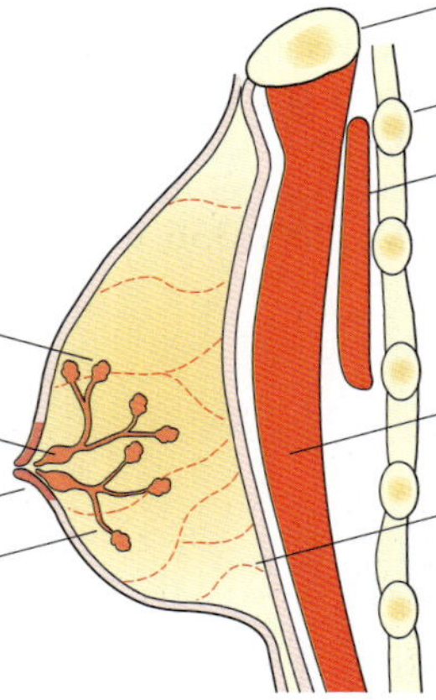

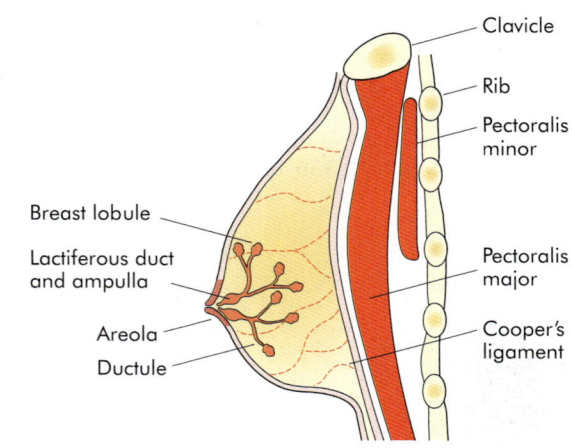

Figure 53.1 Cross-sectional anatomy of the breast.

The **ligaments of Cooper** are hollow conical projections of fibrous tissue filled with breast tissue; the apices of the cones are attached firmly to the superficial fascia and thereby to the skin overlying the breast. These ligaments account for the dimpling of the skin overlying a carcinoma.

The **areola** contains involuntary muscle arranged in concentric rings as well as radially in the subcutaneous tissue. The areolar epithelium contains numerous sweat glands and sebaceous glands, the latter of which enlarge during pregnancy and serve to lubricate the nipple during lactation (Montgomery's tubercles).

The **nipple** is covered by thick skin with corrugations. Near its apex lie the orifices of the lactiferous ducts. The nipple contains smooth muscle fibres arranged concentrically and longitudinally; thus, it is an erectile structure, which points outwards.

The **lymphatics** of the breast drain predominantly into the axillary and internal mammary lymph nodes. The axillary nodes receive approximately 85 per cent of the drainage and are arranged in the following groups:

- **lateral**, along the axillary vein;
- **anterior**, along the lateral thoracic vessels;
- **posterior**, along the subscapular vessels;
- **central**, embedded in fat in the centre of the axilla;
- **interpectoral**, a few nodes lying between the pectoralis major and minor muscles;
- **apical**, which lie above the level of the pectoralis minor tendon in continuity with the lateral nodes and which receive the efferents of all the other groups.

Sir Astley Paston Cooper, 1768–1841, surgeon, Guy's Hospital, London, UK, described these ligaments in 1845. He received a baronetcy and one thousand guineas for successfully removing an infected wen from the head of King George IV at Brighton in 1821. He described scrofulous swellings in the bosoms of young women, most of whom suffered from tuberculous cervical adenitis.

William Fetherston Montgomery, 1797–1859, obstetrician, Dublin, Ireland described these tubercles in 1837. He was instrumental in establishing the Chair of Obstetrics at the Irish College of Physicians.

The apical nodes are also in continuity with the supraclavicular nodes and drain into the subclavian lymph trunk, which enters the great veins directly or via the thoracic duct or jugular trunk. The **sentinel node** is defined as the first lymph node draining the tumour-bearing area of the breast. The importance of the sentinel node is described later.

The internal mammary nodes are fewer in number. They lie along the internal mammary vessels deep to the plane of the costal cartilages, drain the posterior third of the breast and are not routinely dissected although they were at one time biopsied for staging.

INVESTIGATION OF BREAST SYMPTOMS

Although an accurate history and clinical examination are important methods of detecting breast disease, there are a number of investigations that can assist in the diagnosis. Examination precedes palpation and requires careful observation of the patient both with the arms at rest and also elevated to lift the breast. Small lesions may betray their presence by dimpling or minor distortions when the patient moves.

Mammography

Soft tissue radiographs are taken by placing the breast in direct contact with ultrasensitive film and exposing it to low-voltage, high amperage x-rays (Figure 53.2). The dose of radiation is approximately 0.1 cGy and, therefore, mammography is a very safe investigation. The sensitivity of this investigation increases with age as the breast becomes less dense. In total, 5 per cent of breast cancers are missed by population-based mammographic screening programmes; even in retrospect, such carcinomas are not apparent. Thus, a normal mammogram does not exclude the presence of carcinoma. Digital mammography is being introduced, which allows manipulation of the images and computer-aided diagnosis. Tomo-mammography is also being assessed as a more sensitive diagnostic modality.

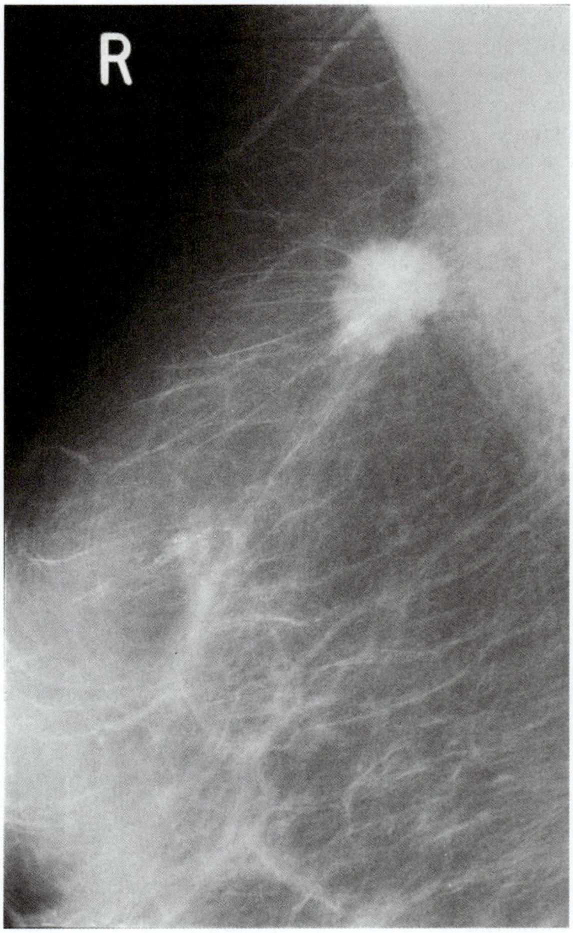

Figure 53.2 Mammogram showing a carcinoma.

Ultrasound

Ultrasound is particularly useful in young women with dense breasts in whom mammograms are difficult to interpret, and in distinguishing cysts from solid lesions (Figures 53.3 and 53.4). It can also be used to localise impalpable areas of breast pathology.

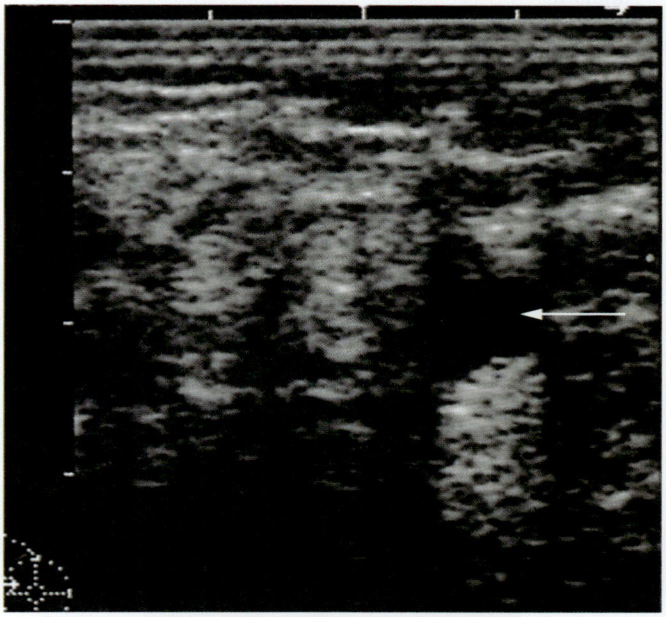

Figure 53.3 Ultrasound of the breast showing a cyst (arrow).

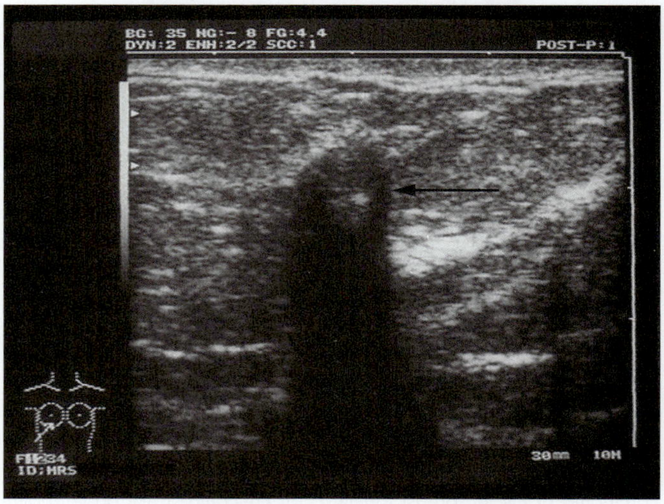

Figure 53.4 Ultrasound of the breast showing a carcinoma (arrow).

Gy is short for Gray, the SI unit for the absorbed dose of ionizing radiation.
Louis Harold Gray, 1905–1965, Director, The British Empire Cancer Campaign Research Unit in Radiobiology, Mount Vernon Hospital, Northwood, Middlesex, UK.

It is not useful as a screening tool and remains operator dependent. Increasingly, ultrasound of the axilla is performed when a cancer is diagnosed with guided percutaneous biopsy of any suspicious glands.

Magnetic resonance imaging

Magnetic resonance imaging (MRI) is of increasing interest to breast surgeons in a number of settings:

- It can be useful to distinguish scar from recurrence in women who have had previous breast conservation therapy for cancer (although it is less accurate within nine months of radiotherapy because of abnormal enhancement).
- It is becoming the standard of care when a lobular cancer is diagnosed to assess for multifocality and multicentricity and can be used to assess the extent of DCIS (ductal carcinoma *in situ*).
- It is the best imaging modality for the breasts of women with implants.
- It has proven to be useful as a screening tool in high-risk women (because of family history).
- It is less useful than ultrasound in the management of the axilla in both primary breast cancer and recurrent disease (Figure 53.5).

Although biopsies can be performed with MRI guidance this is complicated because of the configuration of the imaging system. With improved ultrasound equipment, an MRI-detected lesion can often be found on a second-look ultrasound and biopsied using this modality.

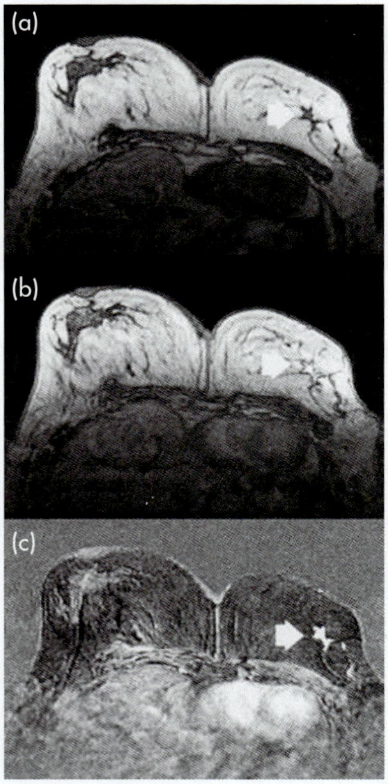

Figure 53.5 Magnetic resonance imaging scan of the breasts showing carcinoma of the left breast (arrows). (a) Pre-contrast; (b) post-gadolinium contrast; (c) subtraction image.

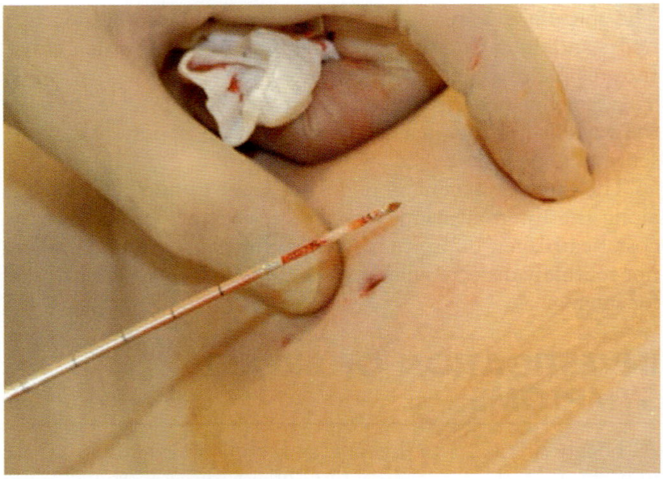
Figure 53.6 Corecut biopsy of breast.

Needle biopsy/cytology

Histology can be obtained under local anaesthesia using a spring-loaded core needle biopsy device (Figure 53.6). Cytology is obtained using a 21G or 23G needle and 10-mL syringe with multiple passes through the lump with negative pressure in the syringe. The aspirate is then smeared on to a slide, which is air dried or fixed (Figure 53.7). Fine-needle aspiration cytology (FNAC) is the least invasive technique of obtaining a cell diagnosis and is rapid and very accurate if both operator and cytologist are experienced. However, false negatives do occur, mainly through sampling error, and invasive cancer cannot be distinguished from *in situ* disease. A histological specimen taken by core biopsy allows a definitive preoperative diagnosis, differentiates between duct carcinoma *in situ* and invasive disease and also allows the tumour to be stained for receptor status. This is important before commencing neoadjuvant therapy.

Large-needle biopsy with vacuum systems

The sampling error decreases as the biopsy volume increases and using 8G or 11G needles allows more extensive biopsies to be

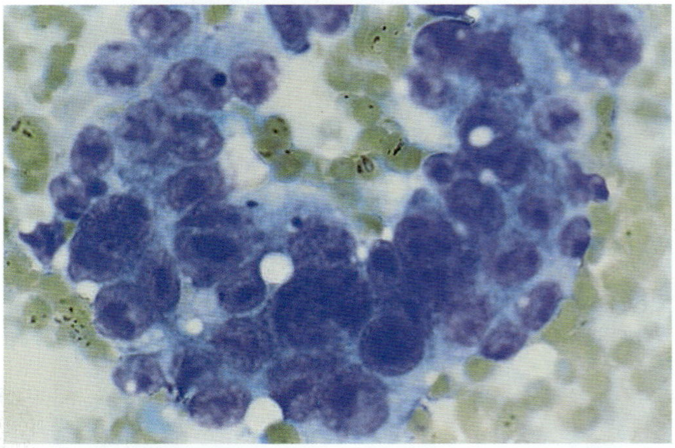
Figure 53.7 Fine-needle aspiration cytology (FNAC) showing grade III ductal carcinoma cells.

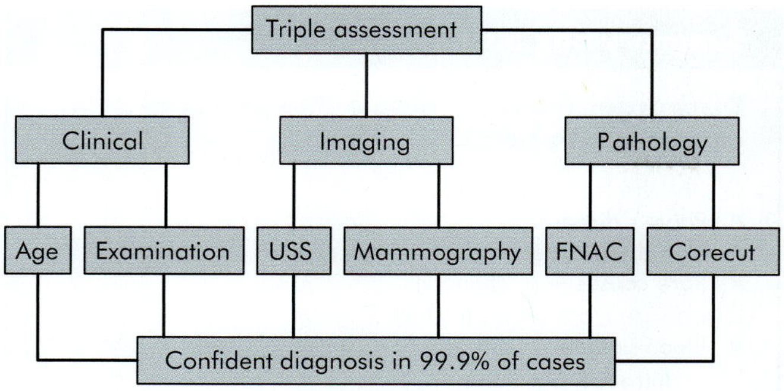

Figure 53.8 Triple assessment of breast symptoms. FNAC, fine-needle aspiration cytology; USS, ultrasound scan.

taken. This is useful in the management of microcalcifications or in the complete excision of benign lesions such as fibroadenomas.

Triple assessment

In any patient who presents with a breast lump or other symptoms suspicious of carcinoma, the diagnosis should be made by a combination of clinical assessment, radiological imaging and a tissue sample taken for either cytological or histological analysis (Figure 53.8), the so-called triple assessment. The positive predictive value (PPV) of this combination should exceed 99.9 per cent.

THE NIPPLE

Absence of the nipple is rare and is usually associated with amazia (congenital absence of the breast).

Supernumerary nipples not uncommonly occur along a line extending from the anterior fold of the axilla to the fold of the groin (Figure 53.9). This constitutes the milk line of lower mammals. Rarely, there is duplication of the nipple on a normal areola.

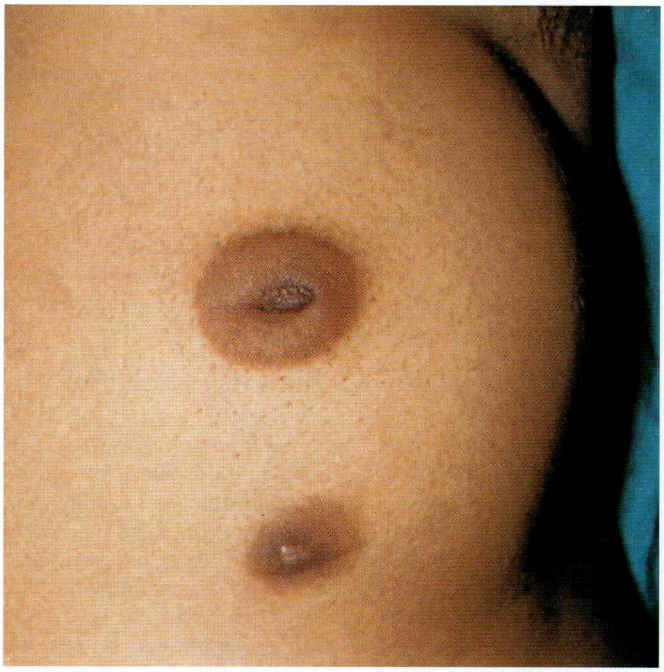

Figure 53.9 Accessory nipple with congenital retraction of the normal nipple.

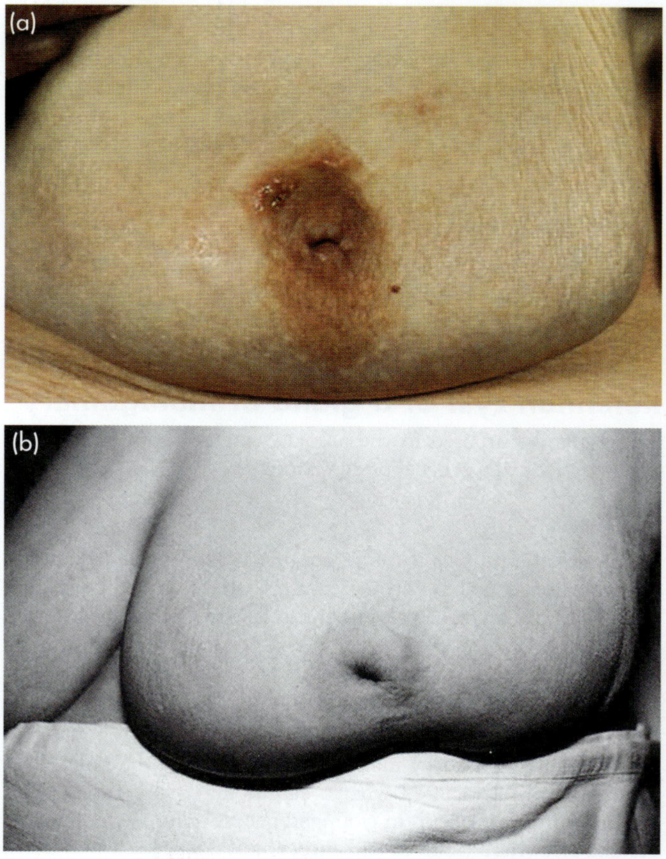

Figure 53.10 Recent nipple retraction. (a) Slit-like retraction of duct ectasia with mammary duct fistula. (b) Circumferential retraction with underlying carcinoma.

Nipple retraction

This may occur at puberty or later in life. Retraction occurring at puberty, also known as **simple nipple inversion**, is of unknown aetiology (benign horizontal inversion). In about 25 per cent of cases it is bilateral. It may cause problems with breastfeeding and infection can occur, especially during lactation, because of retention of secretions. Recent retraction of the nipple may be of considerable pathological significance. A slit-like retraction of the nipple may be caused by duct ectasia and chronic periductal mastitis (Figure 53.10a), but circumferential retraction, with or without an underlying lump, may well indicate an underlying carcinoma (Figure 53.10b).

Treatment

Treatment is usually unnecessary and the condition may spontaneously resolve during pregnancy or lactation.

Simple cosmetic surgery can produce an adequate correction but has the drawback of dividing the underlying ducts. Mechanical suction devices have been used to evert the nipple, with some effect.

Cracked nipple

This may occur during lactation and be the forerunner of acute infective mastitis. If the nipple becomes cracked during lactation, it should be rested for 24–48 hours and the breast should be emptied with a breast pump. Feeding should be resumed as soon as possible.

Papilloma of the nipple

Papilloma of the nipple has the same features as any cutaneous papilloma and should be excised with a tiny disc of skin. Alternatively, the base may be tied with a ligature and the papilloma will spontaneously fall off.

Retention cyst of a gland of Montgomery

These glands, situated in the areola, secrete sebum and if they become blocked a sebaceous cyst forms.

Eczema

Eczema of the nipples is a rare condition and is often bilateral; it is usually associated with eczema elsewhere on the body. It is treated with 0.5 per cent hydrocortisone (not a stronger steroid preparation).

Paget's disease

Paget's disease of the nipple must be distinguished from eczema. The former is caused by malignant cells in the subdermal layer and is usually associated with a carcinoma within the breast. Eczema tends to occur in younger people who have signs of eczema elsewhere (look at the antecubital fossae).

Summary box 53.1

Discharges from the nipple (the principal causes are in bold)

Discharge from the surface

- Paget's disease
- Skin diseases (eczema, psoriasis)
- Rare causes (e.g. chancre)

Discharge from a single duct

- Blood-stained
  - **Intraduct papilloma**
  - **Intraduct carcinoma**
  - Duct ectasia
- Serous (any colour)
  - **Fibrocystic disease**
  - **Duct ectasia**
  - Carcinoma

Discharge from more than one duct

- Blood-stained
  - **Carcinoma**
  - Ectasia
  - Fibrocystic disease
- Black or green
  - **Duct ectasia**
- Purulent
  - **Infection**
- Serous
  - **Fibrocystic disease**
  - Duct ectasia
  - Carcinoma
- Milk:
  - **Lactation**
  - Rare causes (hypothyroidism, pituitary tumour)

Discharges from the nipple

Discharge can occur from one or more lactiferous ducts. Management depends on the presence of a lump (which should always be given priority in diagnosis and treatment) and the presence of blood in the discharge or discharge from a single duct. Mammography is rarely useful except to exclude an underlying impalpable mass. Cytology may reveal malignant cells but a negative result does not exclude a carcinoma or *in situ* disease.

- A **clear, serous discharge** may be 'physiological' in a parous woman or may be associated with a duct papilloma or mammary dysplasia. Multiduct, multicoloured discharge is physiological and the patient may be reassured.
- A **blood-stained discharge** may be caused by duct ectasia, a duct papilloma or carcinoma. A duct papilloma is usually single and situated in one of the larger lactiferous ducts; it is sometimes associated with a cystic swelling beneath the areola.
- A **black or green discharge** is usually the result of duct ectasia and its complications (Summary box 53.1).

Treatment

Treatment must first be to exclude a carcinoma by occult blood test and cytology. Simple reassurance may then be sufficient but, if the discharge is proving intolerable, an operation to remove the affected duct or ducts can be performed (microdochectomy).

Microdochectomy

It is important not to express the blood before the operation as it may then be difficult to identify the duct in theatre. A lacrimal probe or length of stiff nylon suture is inserted into the duct from which the discharge is emerging. A tennis racquet incision can be made to encompass the entire duct or a periareolar incision used and the nipple flap dissected to reach the duct. The duct is then excised. A papilloma is nearly always situated within 4–5 cm of the nipple orifice.

Ductoscopy (inspection of the internal structure of the duct system) using microendoscopes is technically feasible but generally disappointing. The affected duct may not be visualised and biopsy systems are currently rudimentary.

Cone excision of the major ducts (after Hadfield) (subareolar resection)

When the duct of origin of nipple bleeding is uncertain or when there is bleeding or discharge from multiple ducts, the entire major duct system can be excised for histological examination without sacrifice of the breast form. A periareolar incision is made and a cone of tissue is removed with its apex just deep to the surface of the nipple and its base on the pectoral fascia. The resulting defect may be obliterated by a series of purse-string sutures although a temporary suction drain will reduce the chance of long-term deformity. It is vital to warn the patient that she will be unable to breastfeed after this and may experience altered nipple sensation.

Sir James Paget, 1874–1899, surgeon, St Bartholomew's Hospital, London, UK, described this disease of the nipple in 1874 and osteitis deformans in 1877.
Geoffrey John Hadfield, surgeon, Stoke Mandeville Hospital, Aylesbury, Buckinghamshire, UK.

BENIGN BREAST DISEASE

This is the most common cause of breast problems; up to 30 per cent of women will suffer from a benign breast disorder requiring treatment at some time in their lives. The most common symptoms are pain, lumpiness or a lump. The aim of treatment is to exclude cancer and, once this has been done, to treat any remaining symptoms.

Congenital abnormalities

Amazia

Congenital absence of the breast may occur on one (Figure 53.11) or both sides. It is sometimes associated with absence of the sternal portion of the pectoralis major (Poland's syndrome). It is more common in males.

Polymazia

Accessory breasts (Figure 53.12) have been recorded in the axilla (the most frequent site), groin, buttock and thigh. They have been known to function during lactation.

Mastitis of infants

Mastitis of infants is at least as common in boys as in girls. On the third or fourth day of life, if the breast of an infant is pressed lightly, a drop of colourless fluid can be expressed; a few days later, there is often a slight milky secretion, which disappears during the third week. This is popularly known as 'witch's milk' and is seen only in full-term infants. It is caused by stimulation of the fetal breast by prolactin in response to the drop in maternal oestrogens and is essentially physiological. True mastitis is uncommon and is predominately caused by *Staphylococcus aureus*.

Diffuse hypertrophy

Diffuse hypertrophy of the breasts occurs sporadically in otherwise healthy girls at puberty (benign virginal hypertrophy) and, much less often, during the first pregnancy. The breasts attain enormous dimensions and may reach the knees when the patient is sitting. The condition is rarely unilateral. This tremendous overgrowth is apparently caused by an alteration in the normal sensitivity of the breast to oestrogenic hormones and some success in treating it with anti-oestrogens has been reported. Treatment is otherwise by reduction mammoplasty.

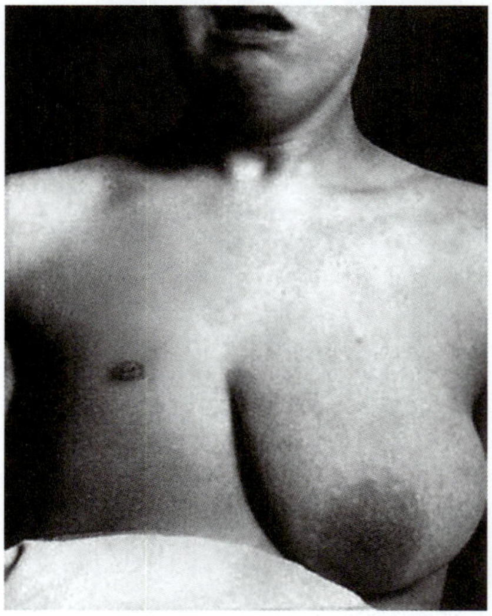

Figure 53.11 Congenital absence of the right breast.

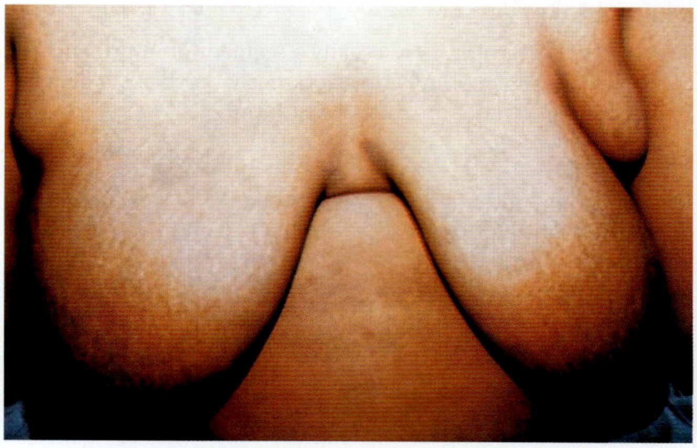

Figure 53.12 Bilateral accessory breasts.

Injuries of the breast

Haematoma

Haematoma, particularly a resolving haematoma, gives rise to a lump, which, in the absence of overlying bruising, is difficult to diagnose correctly unless it is biopsied.

Traumatic fat necrosis

Traumatic fat necrosis may be acute or chronic and usually occurs in stout, middle-aged women. Following a blow, or even indirect violence (e.g. contraction of the pectoralis major), a lump, often painless, appears. This may mimic a carcinoma, even displaying skin tethering and nipple retraction, and biopsy is required for diagnosis. A history of trauma is not diagnostic as this may merely have drawn the patient's attention to a pre-existing lump. A seatbelt may transect the breast with a sudden deceleration injury, as in a road traffic accident.

Acute and subacute inflammations of the breast

Bacterial mastitis

Bacterial mastitis is the most common variety of mastitis and is associated with lactation in the majority of cases.

Aetiology

Lactational mastitis is seen far less frequently than in former years. Most cases are caused by *S. aureus* and, if hospital acquired, are likely to be penicillin resistant. The intermediary is usually the infant; after the second day of life, 50 per cent of infants harbour staphylococci in the nasopharynx.

Although ascending infection from a sore and cracked nipple may initiate the mastitis, in many cases the lactiferous ducts will first become blocked by epithelial debris leading to stasis; this theory is supported by the relatively high incidence of mastitis in women with a retracted nipple. Once within the ampulla of the duct, staphylococci cause clotting of milk and, within this clot, organisms multiply.

Alfred Poland, 1822–1872, surgeon, Guy's Hospital, London, UK described this condition in 1841.

Clinical features

The affected breast, or more usually a segment of it, presents the classical signs of acute inflammation. Early on this is a generalised cellulitis but later an abscess will form.

Treatment

During the cellulitic stage the patient should be treated with an appropriate antibiotic, for example flucloxacillin or co-amoxiclav. Feeding from the affected side may continue if the patient can manage. Support of the breast, local heat and analgesia will help to relieve pain.

If an antibiotic is used in the presence of undrained pus, an 'antibioma' may form. This is a large, sterile, brawny oedematous swelling that takes many weeks to resolve.

It used to be recommended that the breast should be incised and drained if the infection did not resolve within 48 hours or if after being emptied of milk there was an area of tense induration or other evidence of an underlying abscess. This advice has been replaced with the recommendation that repeated aspirations under antibiotic cover (if necessary using ultrasound for localisation) be performed. This often allows resolution without the need for an incision scar and will also allow the patient to carry on breastfeeding.

The presence of pus can be confirmed with needle aspiration and the pus sent for bacteriological culture. In contrast to the majority of localised infections, fluctuation is a late sign. Usually, the area of induration is sector-shaped and, in early cases, about one-quarter of the breast is involved (Figure 53.13); in many late cases the area is more extensive (Figure 53.14). When in doubt, an ultrasound scan may clearly define an area suitable for drainage.

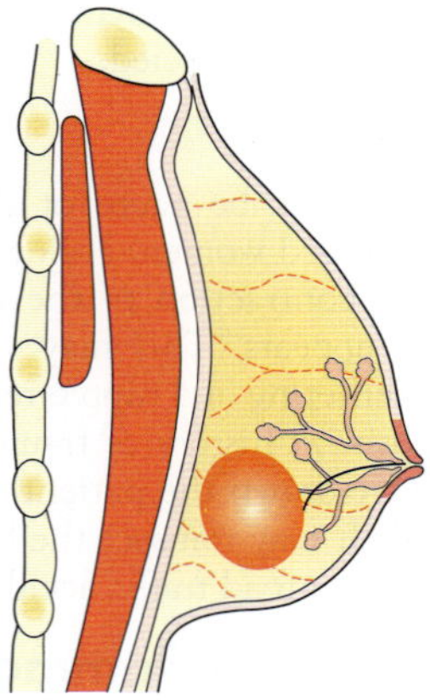

Figure 53.13 Intramammary breast abscess.

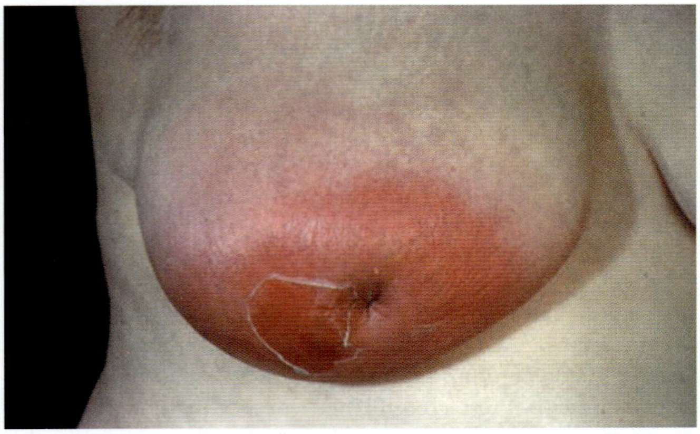

Figure 53.14 Large breast abscess.

Operative drainage of a breast abscess

This is less commonly needed as prompt commencement of antibiotics and repeated aspiration is usually successful. Incision of a lactational abscess is necessary if there is marked skin thinning and can usually be performed under local anaesthesia if an analgesic cream such as EMLA (lidocaine) is applied 30 minutes before surgery.

The usual incision is sited in a radial direction over the affected segment, although if a circumareolar incision will allow adequate access to the affected area this is preferred because it gives a better cosmetic result. The incision passes through the skin and the superficial fascia. A long artery forceps is then inserted into the abscess cavity. Every part of the abscess is palpated against the point of the artery forceps and its jaws are opened. All loculi that can be felt are entered.

Finally, the artery forceps having been withdrawn, a finger is introduced and any remaining septa are disrupted. The wound may then be lightly packed with ribbon gauze or a drain inserted to allow dependent drainage.

Chronic intramammary abscess

A chronic intramammary abscess, which may follow inadequate drainage or injudicious antibiotic treatment, is often a very difficult condition to diagnose. When encapsulated within a thick wall of fibrous tissue the condition cannot be distinguished from a carcinoma without the histological evidence from a biopsy.

Tuberculosis of the breast

Tuberculosis of the breast, which is comparatively rare, is usually associated with active pulmonary tuberculosis or tuberculous cervical adenitis.

Tuberculosis of the breast (Figure 53.15) occurs more often in parous women and usually presents with multiple chronic abscesses and sinuses and a typical bluish, attenuated appearance

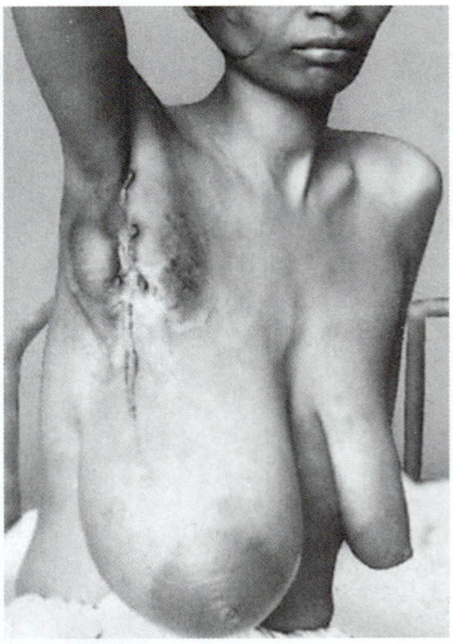

Figure 53.15 Tuberculosis of the breast with secondary suppurating axillary lymph nodes (courtesy of Professor AK Toufeeq, Lahore, Pakistan).

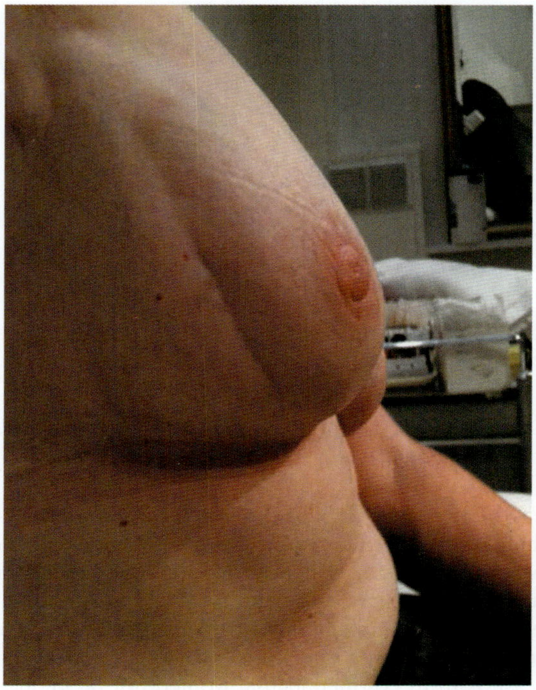

Figure 53.16 Mondor's disease of the right breast.

of the surrounding skin. The diagnosis rests on bacteriological and histological examination. Treatment is with anti-tuberculous chemotherapy. Healing is usual, although often delayed, and mastectomy should be restricted to patients with persistent residual infection.

Actinomycosis

Actinomycosis of the breast is rarer still. The lesions present the essential characteristics of faciocervical actinomycosis.

Mondor's disease

Mondor's disease is thrombophlebitis of the superficial veins of the breast and anterior chest wall (Figure 53.16), although it has also been encountered in the arm.

In the absence of injury or infection, the cause of thrombophlebitis (like that of spontaneous thrombophlebitis in other

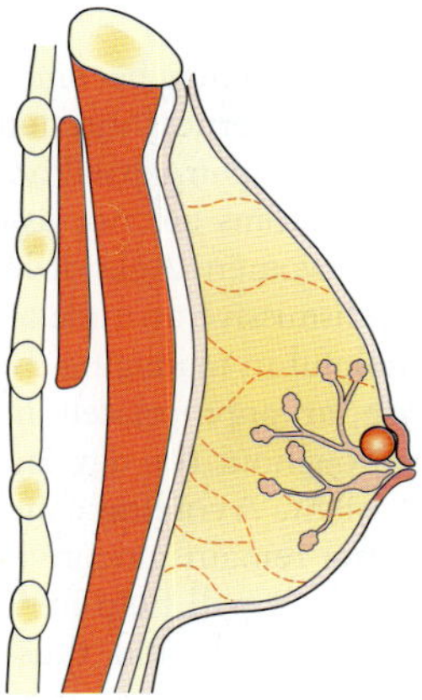

Figure 53.17 Subareolar abscess in duct ectasia.

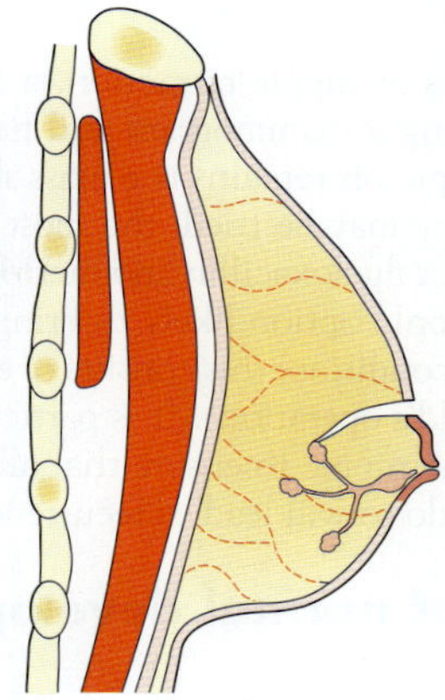

Figure 53.18 Mammary fistula originating in a chronic subareolar abscess.

sites) is obscure. The pathognomonic feature is a thrombosed subcutaneous cord, usually attached to the skin. When the skin over the breast is stretched by raising the arm, a narrow, shallow subcutaneous groove alongside the cord becomes apparent. The differential diagnosis is lymphatic permeation from an occult carcinoma of the breast. The only treatment required is restricted arm movements and, in any case, the condition subsides within a few months without recurrence, complications or deformity. There are case reports of Mondor's disease being associated with subsequent development of malignancy although this has been unsubstantiated by others and is thought to be coincidental.

Duct ectasia/periductal mastitis

Pathology

This is a dilatation of the breast ducts, which is often associated with periductal inflammation. The pathogenesis is obscure and almost certainly not uniform in all cases, although the disease is much more common in smokers.

The classical description of the pathogenesis of duct ectasia asserts that the first stage in the disorder is a dilatation in one or more of the larger lactiferous ducts, which fill with a stagnant brown or green secretion. This may discharge. These fluids then set up an irritant reaction in surrounding tissue leading to periductal mastitis or even abscess and fistula formation (Figures 53.17 and 53.18). In some cases, a chronic indurated mass forms beneath the areola, which mimics a carcinoma. Fibrosis eventually develops, which may cause slit-like nipple retraction.

An alternative theory suggests that periductal inflammation is the primary condition and, indeed, anaerobic bacterial infection is found in some cases. A marked association between recurrent periductal inflammation and smoking has been demonstrated. This was thought by some to indicate that arteriopathy is a contributing factor in its aetiology although others believe that smoking increases the virulence of the commensal bacteria. It is certainly clear that cessation of smoking increases the chance of a long-term cure.

Clinical features

Nipple discharge (of any colour), a subareolar mass, abscess, mammary duct fistula and/or nipple retraction are the most common symptoms.

Henri Mondor, 1885–1962, Professor of Surgery, Paris, France.

Treatment

In the case of a mass or nipple retraction, a carcinoma must be excluded by obtaining a mammogram and negative cytology or histology. If any suspicion remains the mass should be excised.

Antibiotic therapy may be tried, the most appropriate agents being co-amoxiclav or flucloxacillin and metronidazole. However, surgery is often the only option likely to bring about cure of this notoriously difficult condition; this consists of excision of all of the major ducts (Hadfield's operation). It is particularly important to shave the back of the nipple to ensure that all terminal ducts are removed. Failure to do so will lead to recurrence.

Aberrations of normal development and involution

Nomenclature

The nomenclature of benign breast disease is confusing. This is because over the last century a variety of clinicians and pathologists have chosen to describe a mixture of physiological changes and disease processes according to a variety of clinical, pathological and aetiological terminology. As well as leading to confusion, patients were often unduly alarmed or overtreated by ascribing a pathological name to a variant of physiological development. To address this confusion, a concept (aberrations of normal development and involution (ANDI)) has been developed and described by the Cardiff Breast Clinic.

Aetiology

The breast is a dynamic structure that undergoes changes throughout a woman's reproductive life and, superimposed upon this, cyclical changes throughout the menstrual cycle. This is illustrated in Figure 53.19. The pathogenesis of ANDI involves disturbances in the breast physiology extending from a perturbation of normality to well-defined disease processes. There is often little correlation between the histological appearance of the breast tissue and the symptoms.

Pathology

The disease consists essentially of four features that may vary in extent and degree in any one breast:

1 **Cyst formation**. Cysts are almost inevitable and very variable in size.

2 **Fibrosis**. Fat and elastic tissues disappear and are replaced with dense white fibrous trabeculae. The interstitial tissue is infiltrated with chronic inflammatory cells.

3 **Hyperplasia** of epithelium in the lining of the ducts and acini may occur, with or without atypia.

4 **Papillomatosis**. The epithelial hyperplasia may be so extensive that it results in papillomatous overgrowth within the ducts.

Clinical features

The symptoms of ANDI are many as the term is used to encompass a wide range of benign conditions, but often include an area of lumpiness (seldom discrete) and/or breast pain (mastalgia).

- A benign discrete lump in the breast is commonly a cyst or fibroadenoma. True lipomas occur rarely.
- Lumpiness may be bilateral, commonly in the upper outer quadrant or, less commonly, confined to one quadrant of one breast. The changes may be cyclical, with an increase in both lumpiness and often tenderness before a menstrual period.
- Non-cyclical mastalgia is more common in perimenopausal than postmenopausal women. It may be associated with ANDI or with periductal mastitis. It should be distinguished from referred pain, for example a musculoskeletal disorder. 'Breast' pain in postmenopausal women not taking hormone replacement therapy (HRT) is usually derived from the chest wall, back or neck.

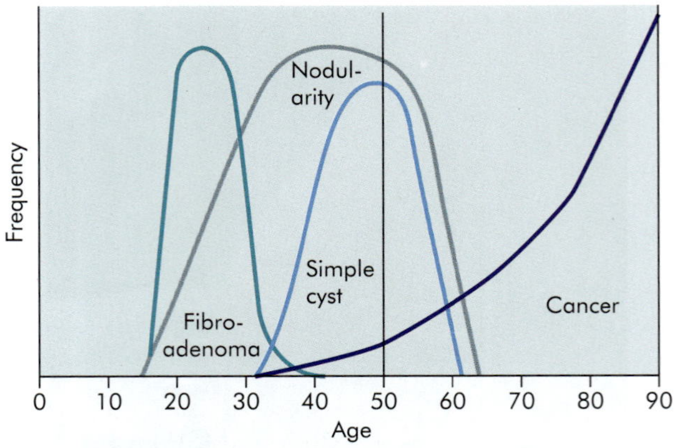

Figure 53.19 Normal breast changes throughout life. UK National Health Service Breast Screening Programme data.

About 5 per cent of breast cancers exhibit pain at presentation, but rarely as the sole presenting feature.

Treatment of lumpy breasts

If the clinician is confident that he or she is not dealing with a discrete abnormality (and clinical confidence is supported by mammography and/or ultrasound scanning if appropriate), then initially the woman can be offered firm reassurance. It is perhaps worthwhile reviewing the patient at a different point in the menstrual cycle, for example 6 weeks after the initial visit, and often the clinical signs will have resolved by that time. There is a tendency for women with lumpy breasts to be rendered unnecessarily anxious and to be submitted to multiple random biopsies because the clinician lacks the courage of his or her convictions. Rapid referral into the secondary health-care sytem often means patients are assessed without an intervening menstrual cycle and this may lead to additional concerns.

Treatment of mastalgia

Pronounced cyclical mastalgia may become a significant clinical problem if the pain and tenderness interfere with the woman's life, disturb her sleep and impair sexual activity. Initially, firm reassurance that the symptoms are not associated with cancer will help the majority of women. Acknowledgement that this is a real symptom, a non-dismissive attitude and an explanation of the aetiology are all helpful in managing this condition.

In the first instance, an appropriately fitting and supportive bra should be worn throughout the day and a soft bra (such as a sports bra) worn at night. Avoiding caffeine drinks is said to help, although the author remains unconvinced.

A patient symptom diary will help her to chart the pattern of pain throughout the month and thus determine whether this is cyclical mastalgia. This allows the majority of patients to adjust to the concept of a cyclical nature of their problem

Table 53.1 Treatment of breast pain.

Exclude cancer	
Reassure	Use pain chart if unsure if cyclical or non-cyclical. Also allows time for reassurance to become active!
Adequate support	Firm bra during the day and a softer bra at night
Exclude caffeine	Works for some although not very efficacious in author's practice
Consider medication	
Evening primrose oil (GLA)	Better effect in women over 40 years old than in younger women
Danazol, 100 mg three times a day	Start at 100 mg per day and increase (seldom used these days)
Tamoxifen	Not licensed for this indication but occasionally very helpful

but, if reassurance is inadequate, then a planned escalation of treatment (Table 53.1) could be advised. Oil of evening primrose, in adequate doses given over three months, will help more than half of these women. It appears to achieve higher response rates in those over 40 years of age rather than younger women. For those with intractable symptoms, an anti-gonadotrophin, such as danazol, or a prolactin inhibitor, such as bromocriptine, may be tried. Very rarely, it is necessary to prescribe an anti-oestrogen, for example tamoxifen, or a luteinising hormone-releasing hormone (LHRH) agonist to deprive the breast epithelium of oestrogenic drive. Ablative surgery should never be contemplated for breast pain and any patient seeking this treatment should be referred to a psychiatrist.

For non-cyclical mastalgia it is important to exclude extramammary causes such as chest wall pain. This is common in postmenopausal women who are not on HRT and the neck and shoulders are common sights of referred pain. It is seldom necessary these days to carry out a biopsy on a very localised tender area that might be harbouring a subclinical cancer as imaging is so much better. Treatment may be with non-steroidal analgesics or by injection with local anaesthetic on a 'trigger spot'.

Breast cysts

These occur most commonly in the last decade of reproductive life as a result of a non-integrated involution of stroma and epithelium. They are often multiple, may be bilateral and can mimic malignancy. Diagnosis can be confirmed by aspiration and/or ultrasound. They typically present suddenly and cause great alarm; prompt diagnosis and drainage provides immediate relief.

Treatment

A solitary cyst or small collection of cysts can be aspirated. If they resolve completely, and if the fluid is not blood-stained, no further treatment is required. However, 30 per cent will recur and require reaspiration. Cytological examination of cyst fluid is no longer practised routinely. If there is a residual lump or if the fluid is blood-stained, a core biopsy or local excision for histological diagnosis is advisable, which is also the case if the cyst reforms repeatedly. This will exclude cystadenocarcinoma, which is more common in elderly women.

Galactocoele

Galactocoele, which is rare, usually presents as a solitary, subareolar cyst and always dates from lactation. It contains milk and in long-standing cases its walls tend to calcify.

Fibroadenoma

These usually arise in the fully developed breast between the ages of 15 and 25 years, although occasionally they occur in much older women. They arise from hyperplasia of a single lobule and usually grow up to 2–3 cm in size. They are surrounded by a well-marked capsule and can thus be enucleated through a cosmetically appropriate incision. A fibroadenoma does not require excision unless associated with suspicious cytology, it becomes very large or the patient expressly desires the lump to be removed.

Giant fibroadenomas occasionally occur during puberty. They are over 5 cm in diameter and are often rapidly growing but, in other respects, are similar to smaller fibroadenomas and can be enucleated through a submammary incision. They are more common in the Afro-Caribbean population.

Phyllodes tumour

These benign tumours, previously sometimes known as serocystic disease of Brodie or cystosarcoma phyllodes, usually occur in women over the age of 40 years but can appear in younger women. They present as a large, sometimes massive, tumour with an unevenly bosselated surface. Occasionally, ulceration of overlying skin occurs because of pressure necrosis. Despite their size they remain mobile on the chest wall. Histologically, there is a wide variation in their appearance, with some of low malignant potential resembling a fibroadenoma and others having a higher mitotic index, which are histologically worrying. The latter may recur locally but, despite the name of cystosarcoma phyllodes, they are rarely cystic and only very rarely develop features of a sarcomatous tumour. These may metastasise via the bloodstream.

Treatment

Treatment for the benign type is enucleation in young women or wide local excision. Massive tumours, recurrent tumours and those of the malignant type will require mastectomy (Summary box 53.2).

When the diagnosis of carcinoma is in doubt

There will always be cases when the clinician cannot be sure whether a particular lump in the breast is an area of mammary dysplasia, a benign tumour or an early carcinoma.

If there is doubt on clinical, cytological or radiological examination, it is essential to obtain a tissue diagnosis. This is often

Sir Benjamin Collins Brodie, 1783–1862, surgeon, St George's Hospital, London, UK, described serocystic disease of the breast in 1840.
Phylloides – from the Greek = leaf-like.
Alexander Tietze, 1864–1927, Professor of Surgery, Breslau, Germany (now Wroclaw, Poland), described this condition in 1921.

Summary box 53.2

Benign breast disorder classification

Congenital disorders
- Inverted nipple
- Supernumerary breasts/nipples
- Non-breast disorders
- Tietze's disease (costochondritis)
- Sebaceous cysts and other skin conditions

Injury
Inflammation/infection
- *ANDI* (aberations of normal differentiation and involution)
  - Cyclical nodularity and mastalgia
  - Cysts
  - Fibroadenoma
- Duct ectasia/periductal mastitis
- Pregnancy-related
  - Galactocoele
  - Puerperal abscess

possible by needle biopsy. In the event of a negative result, open biopsy of the mass or large-gauge vacuum biopsy is necessary. Because of the possibility of reporting errors and because the histology is likely to be more difficult (if a diagnosis has not already been made), the author suggests that frozen-section reporting should be used rarely and certainly should not form the basis for a decision to undertake a mastectomy. Table 53.2 gives an algorithm for investigating any breast lump.

Risk of malignancy developing in association with benign breast pathology

The relative risks of malignancy developing according to different histological features found at biopsy are illustrated in Table 53.3.

These were elucidated 30 years ago but remain pertinent and a recent single-centre review reinforces the conclusion that the histological classification of the benign lesion in combination with a family history of breast cancer are important predictors of risk.

CARCINOMA OF THE BREAST

Breast cancer is the most common cause of death in middle-aged women in Western countries. In 2010, approximately one and three-quarter million new cases were diagnosed worldwide. In England and Wales, 1 in 12 women will develop the disease during their lifetime. The incidence is expected to continue rising as the population ages although more slowly than previously thought as the use of HRT has reduced in the USA and UK.

Aetiological factors

Geographical

Carcinoma of the breast occurs commonly in the Western world, accounting for 3–5 per cent of all deaths in women. In developing countries it accounts for 1–3 per cent of deaths.

Age

Carcinoma of the breast is extremely rare below the age of 20 years but, thereafter, the incidence steadily rises so that by the age of 90 years nearly 20 per cent of women are affected.

Gender

Less than 0.5 per cent of patients with breast cancer are male.

Genetic

It occurs more commonly in women with a family history of breast cancer than in the general population. Breast cancer related to a specific mutation accounts for about 5 per cent of breast cancers yet has far-reaching repercussions in terms of counselling and tumour prevention in these women. This will be discussed more fully in a subsequent section (see under Familial breast cancer).

Diet

Because breast cancer so commonly affects women in the 'developed' world, dietary factors may play a part in its causation. There is some evidence that there is a link with diets low in phyto-oestrogens. A high intake of alcohol is associated with an increased risk of developing breast cancer.

Endocrine

Breast cancer is more common in nulliparous women and breast-feeding in particular appears to be protective. Also protective is having a first child at an early age, especially if associated with late menarche and early menopause. It is known that in postmenopausal women, breast cancer is more common in the obese. This is thought to be because of an increased conversion of steroid hormones to oestradiol in the body fat. Recent studies have clarified the role of exogenous hormones, in particular the oral contraceptive pill and HRT, in the development of breast cancer. For most women the benefits of these treatments will far outweigh the small putative risk; however, long-term exposure to the combined preparation of HRT does significantly increase the risk of developing breast cancer. The recent fall in use of HRT in USA and UK has seen a reduction in the incidence of breast cancer in the 50- to 60-year-old cohort.

Previous radiation

This was considered to be of historical interest, as the majority of women exposed to the atomic bombs at Hiroshima and

Table 53.2 Investigation of a breast lump (after imaging performed) using fine-needle aspiration with cytology.

Cystic	Lump disappears; clear fluid (many colours)	Discharge patient
	Residual thickening; blood-stained fluid	Investigate – ?core biopsy
Solid	Benign	Offer excision or observe
	Atypical	Investigate – ?core biopsy
	Malignant	Treat for cancer

Table 53.3 Relative risk of invasive breast carcinoma based on pathological examination of benign breast tissue (American College of Pathologists Consensus Statement)[a].

No increased risk	Adenosis, sclerosing or florid
	Apocrine metaplasia
	Cysts, macro and/or micro
	Duct ectasia
	Fibroadenoma
	Fibrosis
	Hyperplasia
	Mastitis (inflammation)
	Periductal mastitis
	Squamous metaplasia
Slightly increased risk (1.5–2 times)	Hyperplasia, moderate or florid, solid or papillary
	Papilloma with a fibrovascular core
Moderately increased risk (5 times)	Atypical hyperplasia (ductal or lobular)
Insufficient data to assign a risk	Solitary papilloma of lactiferous sinus
	Radial scar lesion

[a]A combination with positive family history significantly increases the risks shown above.
After Page and Dupont (1978) by kind permission of the *Journal of the National Cancer Institute*, USA.

Nagasaki have now died. It is, however, a real problem in women who have been treated with mantle radiotherapy as part of the management of Hodgkin's disease, in which significant doses of radiation to the breast are received. The risk appears about a decade after treatment and is higher if radiotherapy occurred during breast development. A surveillance programme has been organised in the UK with MRI and mammographic screening.

Pathology

Breast cancer may arise from the epithelium of the duct system anywhere from the nipple end of the major lactiferous ducts to the terminal duct unit, which is in the breast lobule. The disease may be entirely *in situ*, an increasingly common finding with the advent of breast cancer screening, or may be invasive cancer. The degree of differentiation of the tumour is usually described using three grades: well differentiated, moderately differentiated or poorly differentiated. Commonly, a numerical grading system based on the scoring of three individual factors (nuclear pleomorphism, tubule formation and mitotic rate) is used, with grade III cancers roughly equating to the poorly differentiated group.

Previously, descriptive terms were used to classify breast cancer ('scirrhous', meaning woody, or 'medullary', meaning brain-like). More recently, histological descriptions have been used. These have been shown to have clinical correlations in the way that the tumour behaves and are likely to be used for the near future. However, with the increasing application of molecular markers there will be a change in the way that breast cancers are classified and it is likely that much more information about an individual tumour will be routinely reported, such as its likelihood of metastasis and to which therapeutic agents it will be susceptible. Gene array analysis of breast cancers has identified five subtypes. Some of these correlate with known markers such as oestrogen receptor status. There are specific gene signatures that are said to correlate with response to chemotherapy or poor prognosis; trials based upon these differences are planned. A commercial test is now available to patients with oestrogen-positive tumours to assess their risk of recurrence. This is based on analysis of 21 genes and may allow selection of patients in whom more aggressive therapy is indicated.

Current nomenclature

Ductal carcinoma is the most common variant with **lobular carcinoma** occurring in up to 15 per cent of cases. There are subtypes of lobular cancer including the classical type, which carries a better prognosis than the pleomorphic type. Occasionally, the picture may be mixed with both ductal and lobular features. There are different patterns of spread depending on histological type. If there is doubt whether a tumour is predominantly lobular in type, immunohistochemical analysis using the e-cadherin antibody, which reacts positively in lobular cancer, will help in diagnosis.

Rarer histological variants, usually carrying a better prognosis, include **colloid or mucinous carcinoma**, whose cells produce abundant mucin, **medullary carcinoma**, with solid sheets of large cells often associated with a marked lymphocytic reaction, and **tubular carcinoma**. Invasive lobular carcinoma is commonly multifocal and/or bilateral, hence the increasing use of MRI for assessment. Cases detected via the screening programme are often smaller and better differentiated than those presenting to the symptomatic service and are of a special type.

Inflammatory carcinoma is a fortunately rare, highly aggressive cancer that presents as a painful, swollen breast, which is warm with cutaneous oedema. This is the result of blockage of the subdermal lymphatics with carcinoma cells. Inflammatory cancer usually involves at least one-third of the breast and may mimic a breast abscess. A biopsy will confirm the diagnosis and show undifferentiated carcinoma cells. It used to be rapidly fatal but with aggressive chemotherapy and radiotherapy and with salvage surgery the prognosis has improved considerably.

In situ **carcinoma** is preinvasive cancer that has not breached the epithelial basement membrane. This was previously a rare, usually asymptomatic, finding in breast biopsy specimens but is becoming increasingly common because of the advent of mammographic screening; it now accounts for over 20 per cent of cancers detected by screening in the UK. *In situ* carcinoma may be ductal (DCIS) or lobular (LCIS), the latter often being multifocal and bilateral. Both are markers for the later development of invasive cancer, which will develop in at least 20 per cent of patients. Although mastectomy is curative, this constitutes overtreatment in many cases. The best treatment for *in situ* carcinoma is the subject of a number of ongoing clinical trials. DCIS may be classified using the Van Nuys system, which combines the patient's age, type of DCIS and presence of microcalcification, extent of resection margin and size of disease. Patients with a high score benefit from radiotherapy after excision, whereas those of low grade, whose tumour is completely excised, need no further treatment.

Staining for oestrogen and progesterone receptors is now considered routine, as their presence will indicate the use of adjuvant hormonal therapy with tamoxifen or an aromatase inhibitor (Figure 53.20). Tumours are also stained for c-erbB2 (also known as HER-2/neu) (a growth factor receptor) as patients who are positive can be treated with the monoclonal antibody trastuzumab (Herceptin®), either in the adjuvant or relapse setting.

The pathologist is an important member of the breast cancer team and will increasingly help decide which adjuvant therapies will be appropriate.

Paget's disease of the nipple

Paget's disease of the nipple (Figure 53.21a and b) is a superficial manifestation of an underlying breast carcinoma. It presents as an eczema-like condition of the nipple and areola, which persists despite local treatment. The nipple is eroded slowly and eventually disappears. If left, the underlying carcinoma will sooner or later become clinically evident. Nipple eczema should

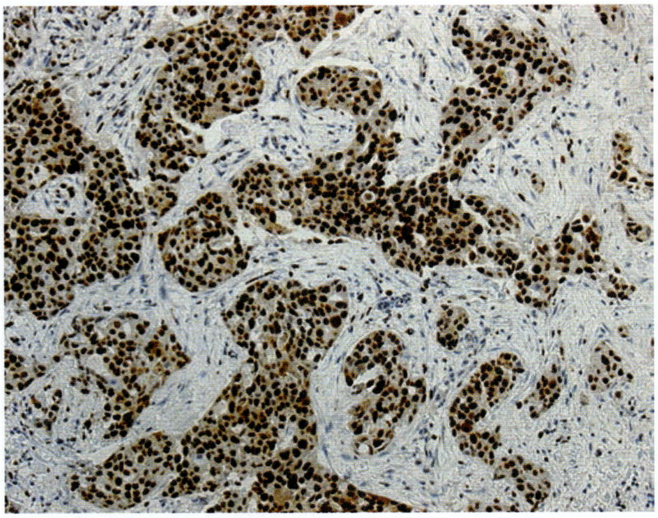

Figure 53.20 Immunohistochemical staining for oestrogen receptors.

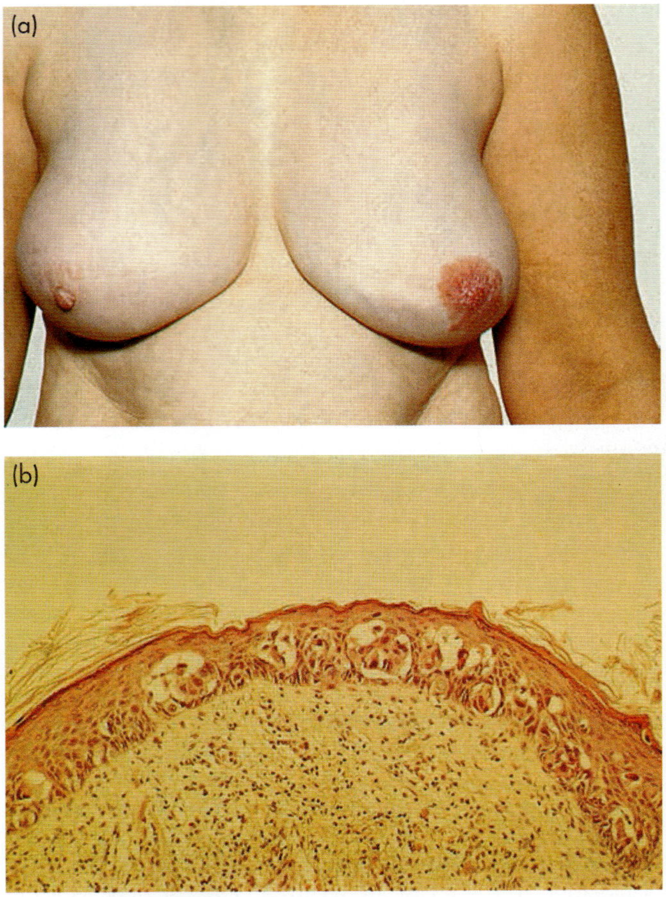

Figure 53.21 (a) Paget's disease of the nipple. (b) Histological appearance of Paget's disease.

be biopsied if there is any doubt about its cause. Microscopically, Paget's disease is characterised by the presence of large, ovoid cells with abundant, clear, pale-staining cytoplasm in the Malpighian layer of the epidermis.

The spread of breast cancer

Local spread

The tumour increases in size and invades other portions of the breast. It tends to involve the skin and to penetrate the pectoral muscles and even the chest wall if diagnosed late.

Lymphatic metastasis

Lymphatic metastasis occurs primarily to the axillary and the internal mammary lymph nodes. Tumours in the posterior one-third of the breast are more likely to drain to the internal mammary nodes. The involvement of lymph nodes has both biological and chronological significance. It represents not only an evolutional event in the spread of the carcinoma but is also a marker for the metastatic potential of that tumour. Involvement of supraclavicular nodes and of any contralateral lymph nodes represents advanced disease.

Spread by the bloodstream

It is by this route that skeletal metastases occur, although the initial spread may be via the lymphatic system. In order of

Marcello Malpighi, 1628–1694, Professor of Physic successively at Bologna, Pisa and Messina, and in 1691 physician to the Papal Court in Rome, Italy.

frequency, the lumbar vertebrae, femur, thoracic vertebrae, rib and skull are affected and these deposits are generally osteolytic. Metastases may also commonly occur in the liver, lungs and brain and, occasionally, the adrenal glands and ovaries; they have, in fact, been described in most body sites.

Clinical presentation

Although any portion of the breast, including the axillary tail, may be involved, breast cancer is found most frequently in the upper outer quadrant (Figures 53.22 and 53.23). Most breast cancers will present as a hard lump, which may be associated with indrawing of the nipple. As the disease advances locally there may be skin involvement with peau d'orange (Figure 53.24) or frank ulceration and fixation to the chest wall (Figure 53.25). This is described as cancer-en-cuirasse when the disease progresses around the chest wall. About 5 per cent of breast cancers in the UK will present with either locally advanced disease or symptoms of metastatic disease. This figure is much higher in the developing world. These patients must then undergo a staging evaluation so that the full extent of their disease can be ascertained. This will include a careful clinical examination, chest radiograph, computed tomography (CT) of the chest and abdomen and an isotope bone scan (Figure 53.26). This is important for both prognosis and treatment; a patient with widespread visceral metastases may obtain an increased length and quality of survival from systemic hormone therapy or chemotherapy but is unlikely to benefit from surgery as she will die from her metastases before local disease becomes a problem. In contrast, patients with relatively small tumours (<2 cm in diameter) confined to the breast and ipsilateral lymph nodes rarely need staging beyond a good clinical examination as the pick-up rate for distant metastases is so low. Currently, a chest radiograph, full blood count and liver function tests are all that are recommended for screening of patients with early-stage breast cancer.

Staging of breast cancer

Classical staging of breast cancer by means of the TNM (tumour–node–metastasis) or UICC (Union Internationale Contre le Cancer) criteria is used less often as we gain more knowledge of the biological variables that affect prognosis. It is becoming increasingly clear that it is these factors (discussed in more detail below) rather than anatomical mapping that influence outcome and treatment. Perhaps a more pragmatic approach would be to classify patients according to the treatment that they require (Table 53.4). Treatment recommendations are summarised in consensus statements such as those from the American Society of Clinical Oncology (ASCO) and the St Gallen Conference.

Prognosis of breast cancer

The best indicators of likely prognosis in breast cancer remain tumour size, grade and lymph node status; however, it is realised that some large tumours will remain confined to the breast

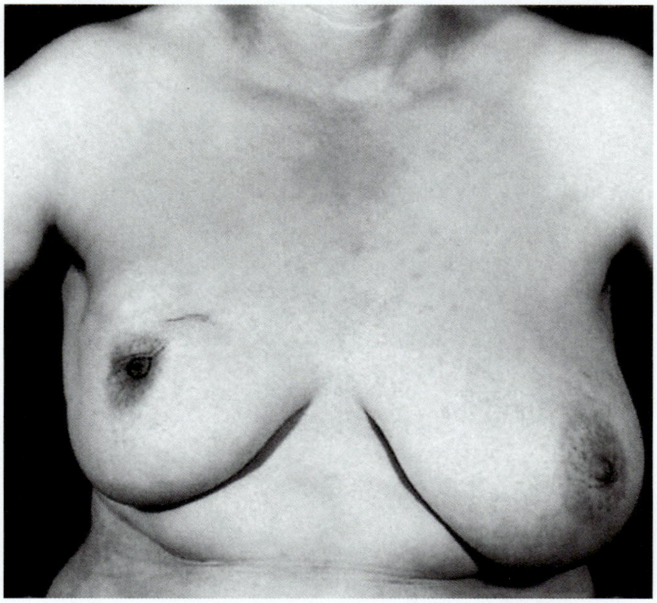

Figure 53.22 Invasive carcinoma of the right breast. Note the shrinking and elevation of the breast with nipple retraction.

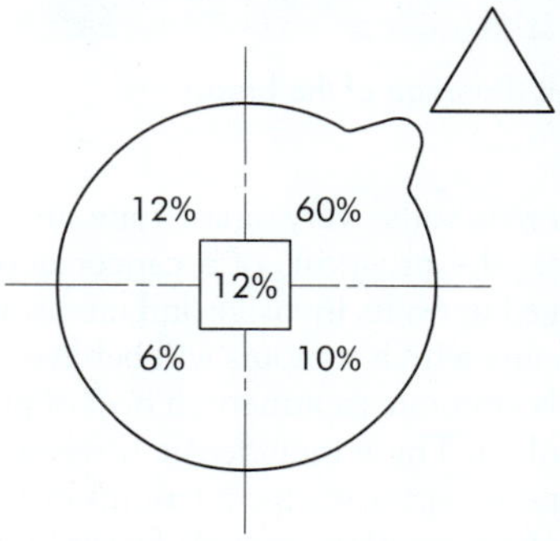

Figure 53.23 The relationship of carcinoma of the breast to the quadrants of the breast.

Table 53.4 A pragmatic classification of breast cancer.

Group	Approximate 5-year survival rate (%)	Example	Treatment
'Very low-risk' primary breast cancer	>90	Screen-detected DCIS, tubular or special types	Local
'Low-risk' primary breast cancer	70–90	Node negative with favourable histology	Locoregional with/without systemic
'High-risk' primary breast cancer	<70	Node positive or unfavourable histology	Locoregional with systemic
Locally advanced	<30	Large primary or inflammatory	Primary systemic
Metastatic	–	–	Primary systemic

DCIS, duct carcinoma *in situ*.

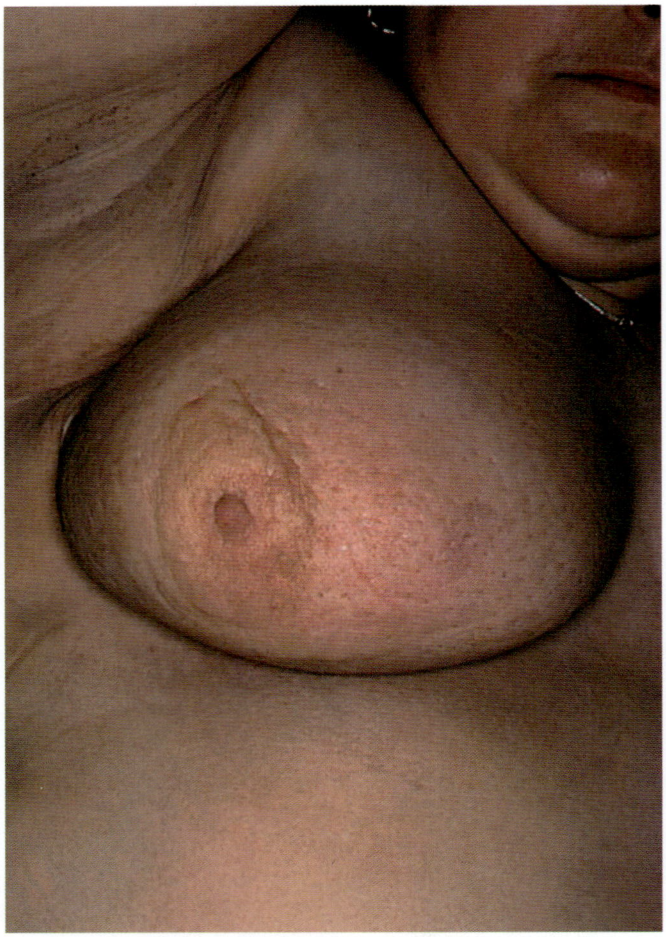

Figure 53.24 Peau d'orange of the breast.

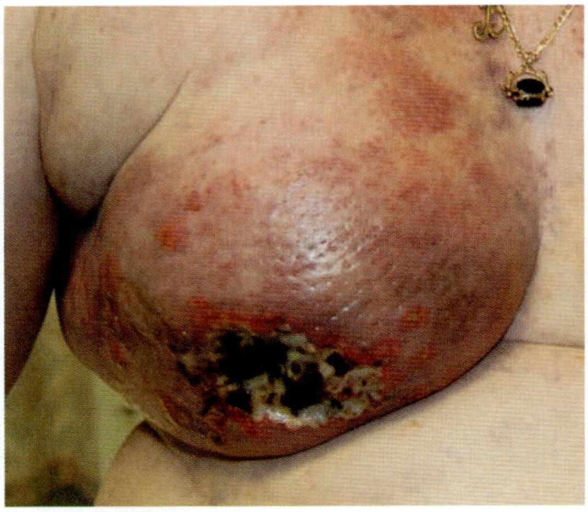

Figure 53.25 Ulcerated carcinoma of the right breast.

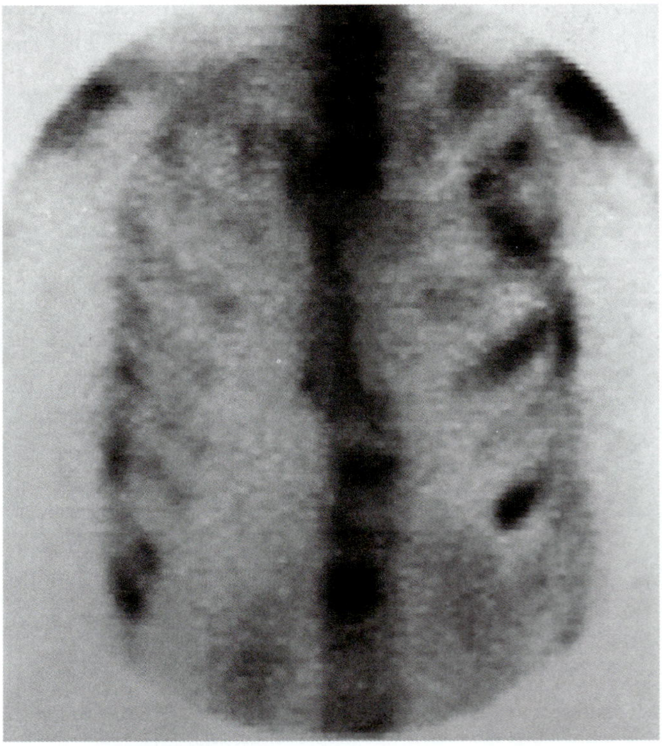

Figure 53.26 Skeletal isotope bone scan showing multiple 'hot-spots' due to metastases.

for decades whereas some very small tumours are incurable at diagnosis. Hence, the prognosis of a cancer depends not on its chronological age but on its invasive and metastatic potential. In an attempt to define which tumours will behave aggressively, and thus require early systemic treatment, a host of prognostic factors have been described. These include the histological grade of the tumour, hormone receptor status, measures of tumour proliferation such as S-phase fraction, growth factor analysis and oncogene or oncogene product measurements. Many others are under investigation but have proved of little practical value in patient management. Prognostic indices (such as the Nottingham prognostic index) have combined these factors to allow subdivision of patients into discrete prognostic groups. More recently, computer-aided programs (adjuvant online; www.adjuvantonline.com or in the UK Predict; www.predict.nhs.uk) have been developed, which incorporate the putative benefits of treatment allowing oncologist and patient to visualise the benefits of therapy.

Treatment of cancer of the breast

The two basic principles of treatment are to reduce the chance of local recurrence and the risk of metastatic spread. Treatment of early breast cancer will usually involve surgery with or without radiotherapy. Systemic therapy such as chemotherapy or hormone therapy is added if there are adverse prognostic factors such as lymph node involvement, indicating a high likelihood of metastatic relapse. At the other end of the spectrum, locally advanced or metastatic disease is usually treated by systemic therapy to palliate symptoms, with surgery playing a much smaller role. An algorithm for the management of breast cancer is shown in Summary box 53.3.

The multidisciplinary team approach

As in all branches of medicine, good doctor–patient communication plays a vital role in helping to alleviate patient anxiety. Participation of the patient in treatment decisions is of particular importance in breast cancer when there may be uncertainty as

Peau d'orange is French for 'orange skin'.

> **Summary box 53.3**
>
> **Algorithm for management of operable breast cancer**
>
> - Achieve local control
> - Appropriate surgery
>   - Wide local excision (clear margins) and radiotherapy, or
>   - Mastectomy ± radiotherapy (offer reconstruction – immediate or delayed)
>   - Combined with axillary procedure (see text)
>   - Await final pathology and receptor measurements
>   - Use risk assessment tool; stage if appropriate
> - Treat risk of systemic disease
>   - Offer chemotherapy if prognostic factors poor; include Herceptin if Her-2 positive
>   - Radiotherapy as decided above
>   - Hormone therapy if oestrogen receptor or progesterone receptor positive

to the best therapeutic option and the desire to treat the patient within the protocol of a controlled clinical trial. As part of the preoperative and postoperative management of the patient it is often useful to employ the skills of a trained breast counsellor and also to have available advice on breast prostheses, psychological support and physiotherapy, when appropriate.

In many specialist centres the care of breast cancer patients is undertaken as a joint venture between the surgeon, medical oncologist, radiotherapist and allied health professionals such as the clinical nurse specialist. This has been shown to be good for the patient, to lead to higher trial entry and to improve the mental health of the professionals in the breast team. There are published guidelines for the optimal management of patients with breast cancer, such as SIGN 84 (Scottish Intercollegiate Guidelines Network).

Local treatment of early breast cancer

Local control is achieved through surgery and/or radiotherapy (Summary box 53.4).

> **Summary box 53.4**
>
> **Treatment of early breast cancer**
>
> The aims of treatment are:
>
> - 'Cure': likely in some patients but late recurrence is possible
> - Control of local disease in the breast and axilla
> - Conservation of local form and function
> - Prevention or delay of the occurrence of distant metastases

Surgery

Surgery still has a central role to play in the management of breast cancer but there has been a gradual shift towards more conservative techniques, backed up by clinical trials that have shown equal efficacy between mastectomy and local excision followed by radiotherapy.

It was initially hoped that avoiding mastectomy would help to alleviate the considerable psychological morbidity associated with breast cancer, but recent studies have shown that over 30 per cent of women develop significant anxiety and depression following both radical and conservative surgery. After mastectomy women tend to worry about the effect of the operation on their appearance and relationships, whereas after conservative surgery they may remain fearful of a recurrence.

Mastectomy is indicated for large tumours (in relation to the size of the breast), central tumours beneath or involving the nipple, multifocal disease, local recurrence or patient preference. The radical Halsted mastectomy, which included excision of the breast, axillary lymph nodes and pectoralis major and minor muscles, is no longer indicated as it causes excessive morbidity with no survival benefit. The modified radical (Patey) mastectomy is more commonly performed and is thus described below. Simple mastectomy involves removal of only the breast with no dissection of the axilla, except for the region of the axillary tail of the breast, which usually has attached to it a few nodes low in the anterior group.

Patey mastectomy

The breast and associated structures are dissected *en bloc* (Figure 53.27) and the excised mass is composed of:

- the whole breast;
- a large portion of skin, the centre of which overlies the tumour but which always includes the nipple;
- all of the fat, fascia and lymph nodes of the axilla.

The pectoralis minor muscle is either divided or retracted to gain access to the upper two-thirds of the axilla. The axillary vein and nerves to the serratus anterior and latissimus dorsi (the thoracodorsal trunk) should be preserved. The intercostal brachial nerves are usually divided in this operation and the patient should be warned about sensation changes postoperatively.

The wound is drained using a wide-bore suction tube. Early mobilisation of the arm is encouraged and physiotherapy helps normal function to return very quickly; most patients are able to resume light work or housework within a few weeks.

Conservative breast cancer surgery

This is aimed at removing the tumour plus a rim of at least 1 cm of normal breast tissue. This is commonly referred to as a wide local excision. The term lumpectomy should be reserved for an operation in which a benign tumour is excised and in which a large amount of normal breast tissue is not resected. A quadrantectomy involves removing the entire segment of the breast that contains the tumour. Both of these operations are usually combined with axillary surgery, usually via a separate incision in the axilla. There are various options that can be used to deal with the axilla, including sentinel node biopsy, sampling, removal of the nodes behind and lateral to the pectoralis minor (level II) or a full axillary dissection (level III).

There is a somewhat higher rate of local recurrence following conservative surgery, even if combined with radiotherapy, but the long-term outlook in terms of survival is unchanged. Local recurrence is more common in younger women and in those with high-grade tumours and involved resection margins. Patients whose margins are involved should have a further local excision (or a mastectomy) before going on to radiotherapy. Excision of a breast cancer without radiotherapy leads to an unacceptable local recurrence rate.

The role of axillary surgery is to stage the patient and to treat

William Stewart Halsted, 1852–1922, Professor of Surgery, Johns Hopkins Medical School, Baltimore, MD, USA.
David Howard Patey, 1899–1976, surgeon, The Middlesex Hospital, London, UK.

the axilla. The presence of metastatic disease within the axillary lymph nodes remains the best single marker for prognosis; however, treatment of the axilla does not affect long-term survival, suggesting that the axillary nodes act not as a 'reservoir' for disease but as a marker for metastatic potential. It used to be accepted that only premenopausal women should have their axilla staged by operation as there was a good case for giving chemotherapy to lymph node-positive patients; however, it is now clear that postmenopausal women also benefit from chemotherapy and so all patients require axillary surgery. In postmenopausal patients, tamoxifen was once given regardless of axillary lymph node status, but it is now known that only hormone receptor-positive patients, irrespective of age, benefit from this. Axillary surgery should not be combined with radiotherapy to the axilla because of excess morbidity. Removal of the internal mammary lymph nodes is unnecessary.

Sentinel node biopsy

This technique has become the standard of care in the management of the axilla in patients with clinically node-negative disease. The sentinel node is localised peroperatively by the injection of patent blue dye (Figure 53.28) and radioisotope-labelled albumin in the breast. The recommended site of injection is in the subdermal plexus around the nipple although some still inject on the axillary side of the cancer. The marker passes to the primary node draining the area and is detected visually and with a hand-held gamma camera. Peropererative diagnosis allows completion axillary clearance if nodal disease is detected. This may be achieved with frozen-section analysis, touch imprint cytology (TIC) or by molecular methods. These involve homogenising the node and detection of a gene such as cytokeratin 19 or mammoglobin. In some cases there are only subcapsular micrometastases that are missed at frozen section. In patients in whom there is no tumour involvement of the sentinel node, further axillary dissection can be avoided. A nomogram outlining the chances of further axillary node positivity has been developed by the group at Memorial Sloan Kettering Hospital, New York, and is available on their website (www.mskcc.org/mskcc/html/15938.cfm). Recent trial results have called into question the utility of completion axillary clearance after a positive sentinel node has been detected but, at present, this remains controversial.

Radiotherapy

Radiotherapy to the chest wall after mastectomy is indicated in selected patients in whom the risks of local recurrence are high. This includes patients with large tumours and those with large numbers of positive nodes or extensive lymphovascular invasion. There is some evidence that postoperative chest wall radiotherapy improves survival in women with node-positive breast cancer.

It is conventional to combine conservative surgery with radiotherapy to the remaining breast tissue. Recurrence rates are too high for treatment by local excision alone except in special cases (small node-negative tumours of a special type). Trials are under way to investigate whether radiotherapy can be given intraoperatively at one sitting or as an accelerated postoperative course. This would have considerable advantages in making conservative surgery available in areas where radiotherapy is not currently used. It would also relieve the burden of the current demand for radiotherapy, which accounts for up to 40 per cent of activity in some departments.

Extrapolation from the Oxford overviews of systemic therapy

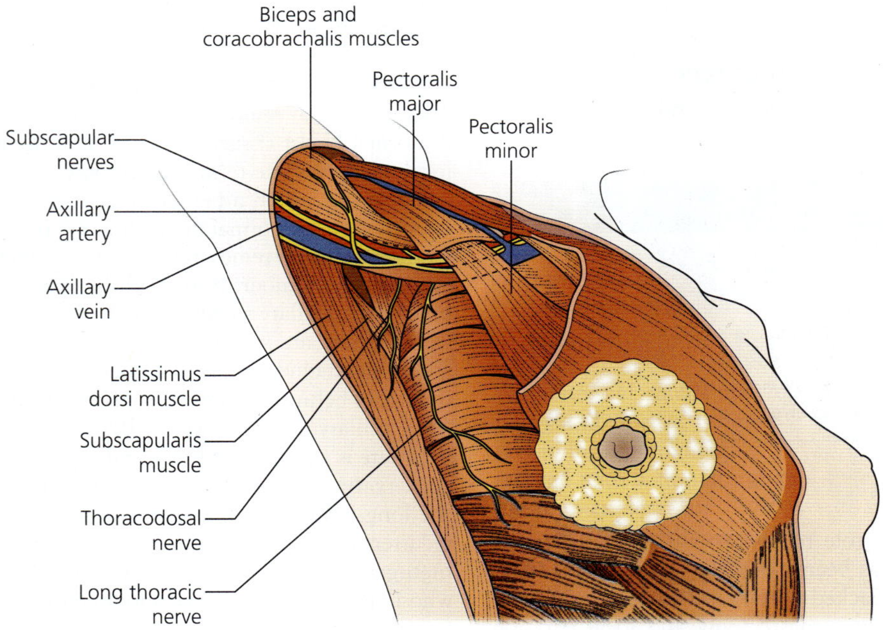

Figure 53.27 Radical mastectomy with pectoralis removed; the modified radical approach leaves the pectoralis major muscle intact.

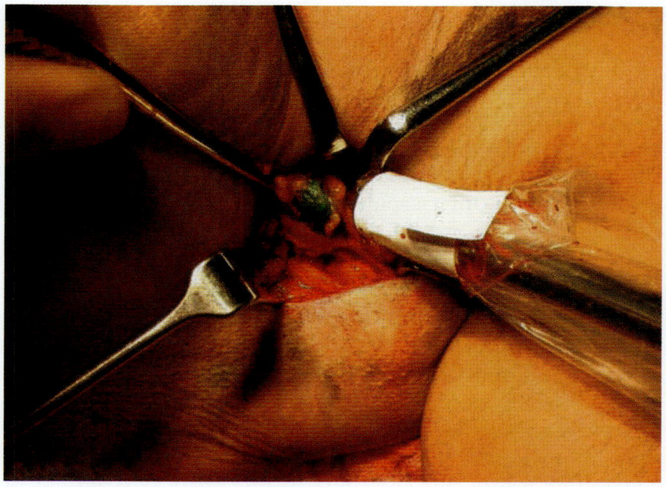

Figure 53.28 Sentinel node biopsy.

(carried out every five years) suggests that for every four local recurrences avoided, one additional life will be spared at 15 years. This means that it is important to get the first treatments right and avoid local recurrence.

Adjuvant systemic therapy

Over the last 25 years there has been a revolution in our understanding of the biological nature of carcinoma of the breast. It is now widely accepted that the outcomes of treatment are predetermined by the extent of micrometastatic disease at the time of diagnosis. Variations in the radical extent of local therapy might influence local relapse but probably do not alter long-term mortality from the disease. However, systemic therapy targeted at these putative micrometastases might be expected to delay relapse and prolong survival. As a result of many international clinical trials and recent world overview analyses, it can be stated with statistical confidence that the appropriate use of adjuvant chemotherapy or hormone therapy will improve relapse-free survival by approximately 30 per cent, which ultimately translates into an absolute improvement in survival of the order of 10 per cent at 15 years. Bearing in mind how common the disease is in northern Europe and the USA, these figures are of major public health importance.

Who to treat and with what are still questions for which absolute answers have yet to be found, but the data from the overviews of recent trials show that lymph node-positive and many higher risk node-negative women should be recommended adjuvant combined chemotherapy. Women with hormone receptor-positive tumours will obtain a worthwhile benefit from about five years of endocrine therapy, either 20 mg daily of tamoxifen if premenopausal or the newer aromatase inhibitors (anastrozole, letrozole and exemestane) if postmenopausal. It is no longer appropriate to give hormone therapy to women who do not have oestrogen or progesterone receptor-positive disease.

Hormone therapy

Tamoxifen has been the most widely used 'hormonal' treatment in breast cancer. Its efficacy as an adjuvant therapy was first reported in 1983 and it has now been shown to reduce the annual rate of recurrence by 25 per cent, with a 17 per cent reduction in the annual rate of death. The beneficial effects of tamoxifen in reducing the risk of tumours in the contralateral breast have also been observed, as has its role as a preventative agent (IBIS-I and NSABP-P1 trials). Trials studying the optimal duration of treatment suggest that five years of treatment is preferable to two years.

Other hormonal agents that are also beneficial as adjuvant therapy have been developed. These include the LHRH agonists, which induce a reversible ovarian suppression and thus have the same beneficial effects as surgical or radiation-induced ovarian ablation in premenopausal receptor-positive women, and the oral aromatase inhibitors (AIs) for postmenopausal women. The latter group of compounds are now licensed for treatment of recurrent disease, in which they have been shown to be superior to tamoxifen. A large trial comparing anastrazole to tamoxifen in the adjuvant setting has shown a beneficial effect for the aromatase inhibitor in terms of relapse-free survival, although no benefit for overall survival. There is an additional reduction in contralateral disease, which makes this drug suitable for a study of prevention, and the side-effect profile is different from that of tamoxifen. The AIs have been more expensive than tamoxifen but are all coming off patent protection and generic copies may allow more widespread use. There is an increase in bone density loss with patients on an AI and a bone density scan is advised prior to commencement with treatment of underlying osteopenia or osteoporosis.

Chemotherapy

Chemotherapy using a first-generation regimen such as a six-monthly cycle of cyclophosphamide, methotrexate and 5-fluorouracil (CMF) will achieve a 25 per cent reduction in the risk of relapse over a 10- to 15-year period. It is important to understand that this 25 per cent reduction refers to the likelihood of an event happening. For example, a woman with a 96 per cent chance of survival at, say, five years only has a 4 per cent chance of death over this time and the absolute benefit from chemotherapy would be an increase in survival rate of 1 per cent, to 97 per cent. This would not be a sufficient gain to offset the side effects of this potentially toxic therapy. However, for a woman with a 60 per cent chance of dying (40 per cent survival rate) a 25 per cent reduction in risk would increase her likelihood of survival to 55 per cent and thus treatment would be worthwhile. CMF is no longer considered adequate adjuvant chemotherapy and modern regimens include an anthracycline (doxorubicin or epirubicin) and the newer agents such as the taxanes.

Chemotherapy was once confined to premenopausal women with a poor prognosis (in whom its effects are likely to be the result, in part, of a chemical castration effect) but is being increasingly offered to postmenopausal women with poor prognosis disease as well. Chemotherapy may be considered in node-negative patients if other prognostic factors, such as tumour grade, imply a high risk of recurrence. The effect of combining hormone and chemotherapy is additive although hormone therapy is started after completion of chemotherapy to reduce side effects.

High-dose chemotherapy with stem cell rescue for patients with heavy lymph node involvement has now been shown in controlled trials to offer no advantage and has been abandoned.

Primary chemotherapy (neoadjuvant) is being used in many centres for large but operable tumours that would traditionally require a mastectomy (and almost certainly postoperative adjuvant chemotherapy). The aim of this treatment is to shrink the tumour to enable breast-conserving surgery to be performed. This approach is successful in up to 80 per cent of cases but is not associated with improvements in survival compared with conventionally timed chemotherapy. For older patients with breast cancers strongly positive for hormone receptors a similar effect can be seen with three months of endocrine treatment.

Newer 'biological' agents will be used more frequently as molecular targets are identified – the first of these, trastuzamab (Herceptin), is active against tumours containing the growth factor receptor c-erbB2. Other agents currently available include bevacizumab, a vascular growth factor receptor inhibitor, and lapitinab, an oral combined growth factor receptor inhibitor. It is unclear how and when these agents will be used, whether in combination or instead of standard chemotherapy agents.

Follow up of breast cancer

Patients with breast cancer used to be followed for life to detect recurrence and dissemination. This led to large clinics with little value for either patient or doctor. It is current practice to arrange yearly or two-yearly mammography of the treated and contralateral breast. There is a move to return the patient early to the care of the general practitioner with fast-track access back to the breast clinic if suspicious symptoms appear. There is currently no routine role for repeated measurements of tumour markers or imaging other than mammography.

Phenomena resulting from lymphatic obstruction in advanced breast cancer

Peau d'orange

Peau d'orange is caused by cutaneous lymphatic oedema. Where the infiltrated skin is tethered by the sweat ducts it cannot swell, leading to an appearance like orange skin. Occasionally, the same phenomenon is seen over a chronic abscess (Figure 53.24).

Late oedema of the arm is a troublesome complication of breast cancer treatment, fortunately seen less often now that radical axillary dissection and radiotherapy are rarely combined. However, it does still occur occasionally after either mode of treatment alone and appears at any time from months to years after treatment. There is usually no precipitating cause but recurrent tumour should be excluded because neoplastic infiltration of the axilla can cause arm swelling as a result of both lymphatic and venous blockage. This neoplastic infiltration is often painful because of brachial plexus nerve involvement.

An oedematous limb is susceptible to bacterial infections following quite minor trauma and these require vigorous antibiotic treatment. Antibiotics may need to be given for much longer than is normal and patients at risk of infection should have antibiotics readily available to enable treatment to be started promptly. Treatment of late oedema is difficult but limb elevation, elastic arm stockings and pneumatic compression devices can be useful.

Cancer-en-cuirasse

The skin of the chest is infiltrated with carcinoma and has been likened to a coat. It may be associated with a grossly swollen arm. This usually occurs in cases with local recurrence after mastectomy and is occasionally seen to follow the distribution of irradiation to the chest wall. The condition may respond to palliative systemic treatment but prognosis in terms of survival is poor.

Lymphangiosarcoma

Lymphangiosarcoma is a rare complication of lymphoedema with an onset many years after the original treatment. It takes the form of multiple subcutaneous nodules in the upper limb and must be distinguished from recurrent carcinoma of the breast. The prognosis is poor but some cases respond to cytotoxic therapy or irradiation. Interscapulothoracic (forequarter) amputation is rarely indicated.

Breast reconstruction

Despite an increasing trend towards conservative surgery, up to 50 per cent of women still require, or want, a mastectomy. These women can now be offered immediate or delayed reconstruction of the breast. Few contraindications to breast reconstruction exist. Even those with a limited life expectancy may benefit from the improved quality of life; however, patients do require counselling before this procedure so that their expectations of cosmetic outcome are not unrealistic.

The easiest type of reconstruction is using a silicone gel implant under the pectoralis major muscle. This may be combined with prior tissue expansion using an expandable saline prosthesis first (or a combined device), which creates some ptosis of the new breast. If the skin at the mastectomy site is poor (e.g. following radiotherapy) or if a larger volume of tissue is required, a musculocutaneous flap can be constructed either from the latissimus dorsi muscle (an LD flap) (Figure 53.29) or using the transversus abdominis muscle (a TRAM flap as shown in Figure 53.30). The latter gives an excellent cosmetic result in experienced hands but is a lengthy procedure and requires careful patient selection. It is now usually performed as a free transfer using microvascular anastomosis, although the pedicled TRAM from the contralateral side is still used. Variations on the TRAM flap requiring less muscle harvesting, such as the DIEP flap (based on deep inferior epigastric vessels), are increasingly being used.

The timing of reconstruction is difficult. Impediments to immediate reconstruction include insufficient theatre time and a lack of experienced reconstructive surgeons. In addition, if a patient is likely to need postoperative radiotherapy then a delayed reconstruction using a flap often gives a better result. Radiotherapy onto a prosthesis often leads to a high incidence of capsular contracture and unacceptable results.

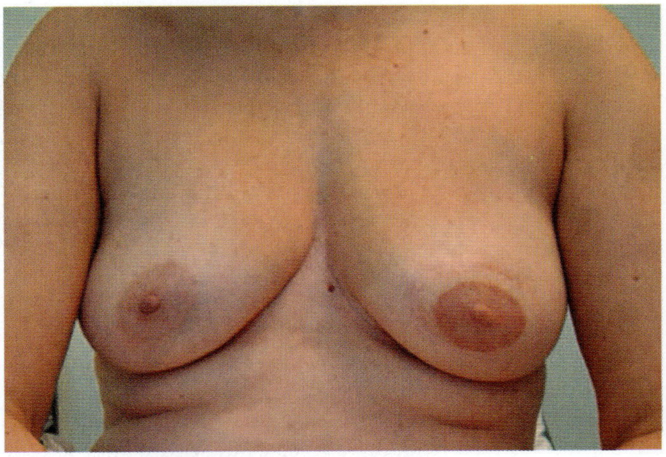

Figure 53.29 Reconstruction with latissimus dorsi flap.

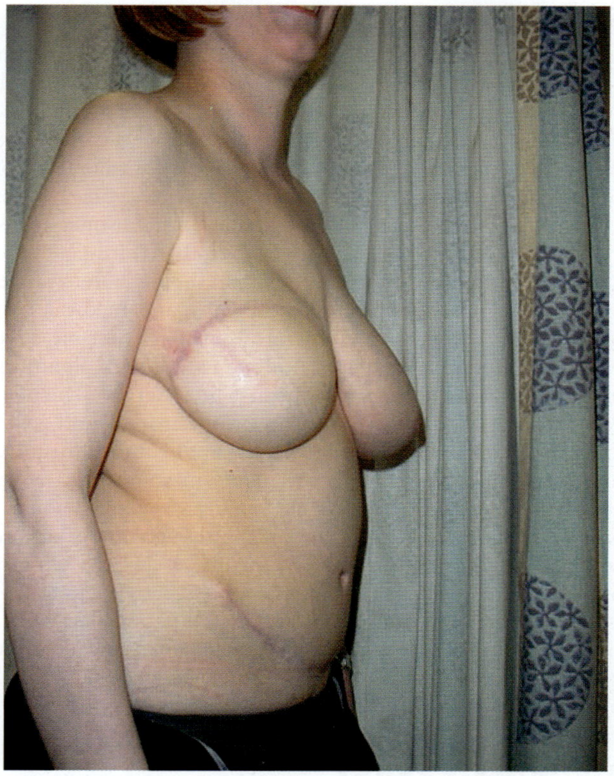

Figure 53.30 Transversus abdominus muscle flap.

Nipple reconstruction is a relatively simple procedure that can be performed under a local anaesthetic. Many different types of nipple reconstruction are described but the majority lose height with time. Tattooing of the reconstructed nipple is often required. Alternatively, the patient can be fitted with a prosthetic nipple. To achieve symmetry the opposite breast may require a cosmetic procedure such as reduction or augmentation mammoplasty, or mastopexy. A breast reconstructive service can be offered by a suitably trained breast surgeon, a plastic surgeon or, ideally, using a combined oncoplastic approach. The patient needs to be warned that breast reconstruction is seldom, if ever, one operation.

External breast prostheses that fit within the bra are the most common method of restoring volume fill and should be available for all women who do not have an immediate reconstruction.

Screening for breast cancer

Because the prognosis of breast cancer is closely related to stage at diagnosis it would seem reasonable to hope that a population screening programme that could detect tumours before they come to the patient's notice might reduce mortality from breast cancer. Indeed, a number of studies have shown that breast screening by mammography in women over the age of 50 years will reduce cause-specific mortality by up to 30 per cent. Following the publication in 1987 of the Forrest report, the National Health Service in the UK launched a programme of three-yearly mammographic screening for women between the ages of 50 and 64 years (now increased to 70 years). The introduction of this programme has undoubtedly improved the quality of breast cancer services but a number of questions remain unanswered, including the value of screening women under 50 years and the ideal interval between screenings. The psychological consequences of false alarms or false reassurances still need to be addressed and self-examination programmes that have failed to show any benefit for the population in terms of earlier detection of or decreased mortality from breast cancer remain controversial. The opponents of screening rightly point out that some women will have disease detected and treated that might never harm them in their lifetime. However, until we can identify this group and separate them from those in whom prompt diagnosis and treatment will be benficial, we will continue to treat everyone.

MRI is used to screen those at very high risk or where radiation might be hazardous (Li–Fraumeni syndrome). There is no place for thermography as a screening (or diagnostic) tool.

Familial breast cancer

Recent developments in molecular genetics and the identification of a number of breast cancer predisposition genes (*BRCA1*, *BRCA2* and *p53*) have done much to stimulate interest in this area. Yet women whose breast cancer is due to an inherited genetic change actually account for less than 5 per cent of all cases of breast cancer, that is about 1250 cases per year in the UK and 9000 cases in the USA. A much larger number of women will have a risk that is elevated above normal because of an as yet unspecified familial inheritance. These women have a risk of developing breast cancer that is 2–10 times above baseline. The risks associated with family history are summarised in Table 53.5.

Table 53.5 Likelihood of genetic mutation with family history.

No. of family cases <50 years old	*BRCA1* (%)[a]	*BRCA1* (%)[b]
2	4	3
3	17	13
4	41	33
5	55	44

[a] *BRCA1* is also associated with ovarian and, to a lesser extent, colorectal and prostate cancer.
[b] *BRCA2* is associated with familial male breast cancer.

The *BRCA1* gene has been associated with an increased incidence of breast (and ovarian) cancer and is located on the long arm of chromosome 17 (17q). The gene frequency in the population is approximately 0.0006. It does, however, occur with greater frequency in certain populations such as Ashkenazi Jews, in whom there is often a common (founder) mutation. *BRCA2* is located on chromosome 13q and there is an association with male breast cancer. Women who are thought to be gene carriers may be offered breast screening (and ovarian screening in the case of BRCA1, which is known to impart a 50 per cent lifetime risk of ovarian cancer), usually as part of a research programme, or genetic counselling and mutation analysis. Those who prove to be 'gene positive' have a 50–80 per cent risk of developing breast cancer, predominantly while premenopausal. Many will opt for prophylactic mastectomy. Although this does

Sir Andrew Patrick McEwen Forrest, Former Regius Professor of Clinical Surgery, The University of Edinburgh, Edinburgh, Scotland.
Ashkenazi Jews are Jews of Eastern or Central European descent.

not completely eliminate the risk, it does reduce it considerably. This work should be carried out in specialist centres.

For the great majority of women with a positive family history, who are unlikely to be carriers of a breast cancer gene, there are no currently proven breast cancer screening manoeuvres, although this is under investigation. Tamoxifen given for five years appears to reduce the risk of breast cancer by 30–50 per cent, and newer agents are currently under trial. Thus, these women are best served by being assessed and followed-up, preferably in a properly organised family history clinic.

Pregnancy

The effects of pregnancy on breast cancer are not well studied but it is thought that breast cancer presenting during pregnancy or lactation tends to be at a later stage, presumably because the symptoms are masked by the pregnancy; however, in other respects it behaves in a similar way to breast cancer in a non-pregnant young woman and should be treated accordingly. Thus, treatment is similar with some provisos: radiotherapy should be avoided during pregnancy, making mastectomy a more frequent option than breast conservation surgery; chemotherapy should be avoided during the first trimester but appears safe subsequently; most tumours are hormone receptor negative and so hormone treatment, which is potentially teratogenic, is not required. Becoming pregnant subsequent to a diagnosis of breast cancer appears not to alter the likely outcome, but women are usually advised to wait at least two years as it is within this time that recurrence most often occurs. The risk of developing breast cancer with oral contraceptive use is only slight, and disappears ten years after stopping the oral contraceptive pill.

Hormone replacement therapy

HRT does increase the risk of developing breast cancer if taken for prolonged periods and in certain high-risk groups. HRT may also prolong symptoms of benign breast disorders such as cysts and mastalgia and make mammographic appearances more difficult to interpret.

Patients who develop breast cancer while on HRT appear to have a more favourable prognosis. The consequences in terms of recurrence in women using HRT following breast cancer are unknown.

Treatment of advanced breast cancer

Breast cancer may occasionally present as metastatic disease without evidence of a primary tumour (that is with an occult primary). The diagnosis is made partly by exclusion of another site for the primary tumour and may be confirmed by histology with special immunohistological stains of the metastatic lesions. Management should be aimed at palliation of the symptoms and treatment of the breast cancer, usually by endocrine manipulation with or without radiotherapy.

Locally advanced inoperable breast cancer

Locally advanced inoperable breast cancer, including inflammatory breast cancer, is usually treated with systemic therapy, either chemotherapy or hormone therapy.

Occasionally, 'toilet mastectomy' or radiotherapy is required to control a fungating tumour but often incision through microscopically permeated tissues results in a worse outcome.

Metastatic carcinoma of the breast

Metastatic carcinoma of the breast will also require palliative systemic therapy to alleviate symptoms. Hormone manipulation is often the first-line treatment because of its minimal side effects. It is particularly useful for bony metastases. However, only about 30 per cent of these tumours will be hormone responsive and, unfortunately, in time, even these will become resistant to treatment. First-line hormone therapy for postmenopausal women is now anastrazole or one of the other third-generation aromatase inhibitors. Tamoxifen, ovarian suppression by surgery (for premenopausal women), radiotherapy and medical treatment are all in common use. When resistance to these has developed, other hormonal agents can prove useful, with about one-half of the response rate seen in the first-line therapy. The newer agents such as anti-progestins, pure anti-oestrogens and growth factor tyrosine kinase inhibitors are all candidates for this role.

Cytotoxic therapy is used particularly in younger women or those with visceral metastases and rapidly growing tumours. A variety of regimens is available and, although none prolongs survival, contrary to expectations, quality of life and symptom control is often better with more aggressive treatments, with responses being seen in up to 70 per cent of patients.

Local treatment may also prove useful for some metastatic disease, such as radiotherapy for painful bony deposits and internal fixation of pathological fractures.

THE MALE BREAST

Gynaecomastia

Idiopathic

Hypertrophy of the male breast may be unilateral or bilateral. The breasts enlarge at puberty and sometimes present the characteristics of female breasts.

Hormonal

Enlargement of the breasts often accompanied stilbestrol therapy for prostate cancer, now rarely used. It may also occur as a result of a teratoma of the testis, in anorchism and after castration. Rarely, it may be a feature of ectopic hormonal production in bronchial carcinoma and in adrenal and pituitary disease. Bodybuilders may use steroids to improve their physique, which may cause gynaecomastia. Some even go so far as to take tamoxifen to mask this symptom.

Associated with leprosy

Gynaecomastia is very common in men suffering from leprosy. This is possibly because of bilateral testicular atrophy, which is a frequent accompaniment of leprosy.

Associated with liver failure

Gynaecomastia sometimes occurs in patients with cirrhosis as a result of failure of the liver to metabolise oestrogens. It is associated with drugs that interfere with the hepatic metabolism of oestrogens. It is also seen with certain drugs such as cimetidine, digitalis and spironolactone.

Associated with Klinefelter syndrome

Gynaecomastia may occur in patients with Klinefelter's syndrome, a sex chromosome anomaly having 47XXY trisomy.

Harry Fitch Klinefelter Jr, born 1912, physician of Baltimore, MD, USA, described this syndrome in 1942.

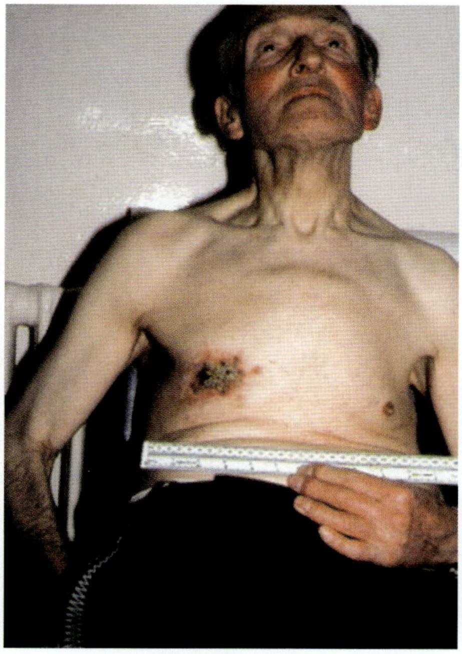

Figure 53.31 Carcinoma of the male breast.

Treatment

Provided that the patient is healthy and comparatively young, reassurance may be sufficient. If not, mastectomy with preservation of the areola and nipple can be performed. The patient must be warned about the side effects of this procedure, which are common and a cause of many medicolegal complaints in the UK.

Carcinoma of the male breast

Carcinoma of the male breast (Figure 53.31) accounts for less than 0.5 per cent of all cases of breast cancer. The known predisposing causes include gynaecomastia and excess endogenous or exogenous oestrogen. As in the female, it tends to present as a lump and is most commonly an infiltrating ductal carcinoma.

Treatment

Stage for stage the treatment is the same as for carcinoma in the female breast and prognosis depends upon stage at presentation. Adequate local excision, because of the small size of the breast, should always be with a 'mastectomy'.

OTHER TUMOURS OF THE BREAST

Lipoma

A true lipoma is very rare.

Sarcoma of the breast

Sarcoma of the breast is usually of the spindle-cell variety and accounts for 0.5 per cent of malignant tumours of the breast. Some of these growths arise in an intracanalicular fibroadenoma or may follow previous radiotherapy, e.g. for Hodgkin's lymphoma, many years previously. It may be impossible to distinguish clinically a sarcoma of the breast from a medullary carcinoma, but areas of cystic degeneration suggest a sarcoma and on incising the neoplasm it is pale and friable. Sarcoma tends to occur in younger women between the ages of 30 and 40 years. Treatment is by simple mastectomy followed by radiotherapy. The prognosis depends on the stage and histological type.

Metastases

On rare occasions cancer elsewhere may present with a metastasis in the breast. The breast is also occasionally infiltrated by Hodgkin's disease and other lymphomas.

FURTHER READING

Harris JR, Lippman M, Morrow M, Hellman S. *Diseases of the breast.* Philadelphia, PA: Lippincott, 2010.

Hughes LE, Mansel RE, Webster DJT. *Benign disorders and diseases of the breast*, 2nd edn. London: Baillière Tindall, 1989.

Sainsbury R. Breast operations. In: Kirk R (ed.). *General surgical operations*. Edinburgh: Churchill Livingstone, 2006.

SIGN 84. Management of breast cancer in women. A national clinical guideline. Available online at: www.sign.ac.uk/pdf/sign84.pdf.

PART

9 Cardiothoracic

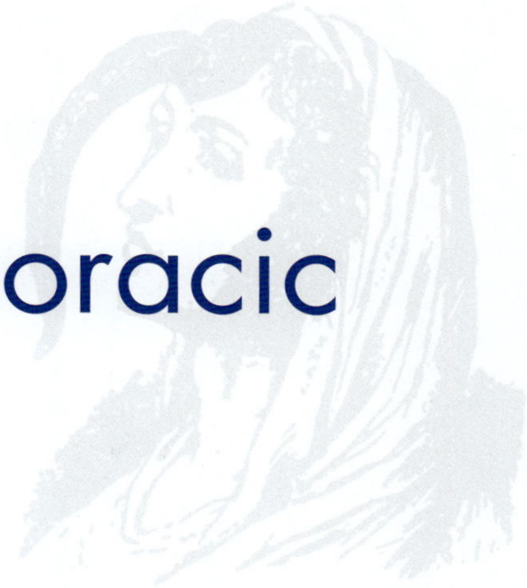

CHAPTER 54

Cardiac surgery

LEARNING OBJECTIVES

To understand:

- The important role of surgery in cardiac disease
- The role of investigation in planning surgery
- The management of coronary heart disease
- The role of surgery in valvular heart disease
- The special role of surgery in congenital heart disease
- The management of aortic vascular and pericardial disease

INTRODUCTION

In 1925, Sir Henry Souttar reported the first mitral commissurotomy in the *British Medical Journal*. He wrote that the heart should be as amenable to surgery as any other organ. He saw the main problem as being maintenance of blood flow, particularly to the brain, while surgery was being performed.

The first real advances occurred in the late 1940s and early 1950s, driven by surgeons who had gained confidence and experience under the pressures and opportunities provided by war, followed by the development of cardiopulmonary bypass in the mid-1950s. Recently, the well-being and lifespan of patients with congenital, valvular and degenerative heart disease has improved drastically due to the advances in the range, complexity, and technical expertise in cardiac surgery.

CARDIOPULMONARY BYPASS

Cardiopulmonary bypass (CPB) was first used successfully in 1953 by Gibbon and has since revolutionised cardiac surgery. It can be employed in any procedure in which the heart and lungs need to be stopped temporarily and their function replaced artificially. Before Gibbon's work, valve surgery under direct vision would not have been possible nor would the precise reconstructions needed to treat extensive coronary artery disease. Much of the success of modern CPB is attributable to the development of new biomaterials and sophisticated oxygenating devices, as well as a greater understanding of the pathophysiological consequences of CPB (Summary box 54.1).

Summary box 54.1

Alternative uses of CPB

- Rewarming from profound hypothermia
- Resuscitation in severe respiratory failure
- As an adjunct in pulmonary embolectomy
- In single- and double-lung transplantation
- In cardiopulmonary trauma
- In certain non-cardiac surgical procedures (e.g. resection of highly vascular tumours and tumours invading large blood vessels)

Surgical approach to the heart

The heart is approached mainly by a median sternotomy. An incision is made from the jugular or suprasternal notch to the lower end of the xiphisternum. The sternum is divided and retracted to expose the thymus superiorly and the pericardium inferiorly. The thymus, although atrophic in adults, often remains relatively vascular. The thymus and pleurae are dissected from the pericardium, and the pericardium is opened. Before cannulation for CPB, the patient is fully heparinised. Other incisions which can be used include left anterolateral thoracotomy.

Initiating cardiopulmonary bypass

Arterial cannulation

Conventionally, the great vessels are exposed and an aortic perfusion cannula is inserted into the ascending aorta, held in place by the purse-string suture. Air is excluded and the cannula connected to the bypass circuit. Alternatively, when it is inadvisable (aortic dissection), impractical (aortic root surgery) or impossible (severe adhesions) to cannulate the aorta, alternative arterial cannulation sites can be used, such as the femoral artery or the axillary artery.

Venous cannulation

A second purse-string suture is inserted into the right atrium by the appendage. A single 'two-stage' venous cannula placed in the right atrium establishes venous drainage. The venous pipe has end holes that sit in the inferior vena cava and side holes that sit in the right atrium (to take the drainage from the superior vena cava). Alternatively, the superior and inferior

Sir Henry Sessions Souttar, 1875–1974, surgeon, The London Hospital London, UK.
John Heysham Gibbon, 1903–1973, worked at Jefferson University, Philadelphia, PA, USA.

vena cavae may be cannulated separately to gain better control over the venous return and to facilitate surgery within the right atrium. Venous drainage from the femoral vein can offer an alternative, particularly during thoracic aortic procedures.

Cardiopulmonary bypass circuit

Once the circuit is connected (Figure 54.1), the CPB machine (the 'pump') gradually takes over the processes of circulation and ventilation. Once full flow is established (the required cardiac output depends on the body surface area of the patient), the ventilator is stopped and the heart can be isolated from the rest of the circulation. Blood is pumped from a venous reservoir and oxygenated using an oxygenator that allows gas exchange across its membrane.

The core systemic temperature can be lowered by passing the returning blood through a heat exchanger which can reduce the metabolic demands of the tissues. The degree of cooling is according to the severity and complexity of the surgical procedure, as well as the surgeon's preference.

The blood is also filtered to remove particulate emboli and returned to the systemic arterial circulation via a pump. Suction pumps can be employed to keep the area around the heart clear of blood, and to decompress the heart when used as vents.

Myocardial protection

Once CPB has been established, the ascending aorta is usually cross-clamped to obtain a bloodless operative field. The heart ceases to eject and becomes anoxic due to inhibition of coronary blood flow. Permanent myocardial damage can develop within 15–20 minutes, therefore most cardiac operations require some form of myocardial protection. Techniques of myocardial protection and the operative management of the myocardium have had a significant impact on the complexity of cardiac surgery. The methods of myocardial protection include intracoronary infusion of a cardioplegic solution, intermittent cross-clamp fibrillation and total circulatory arrest.

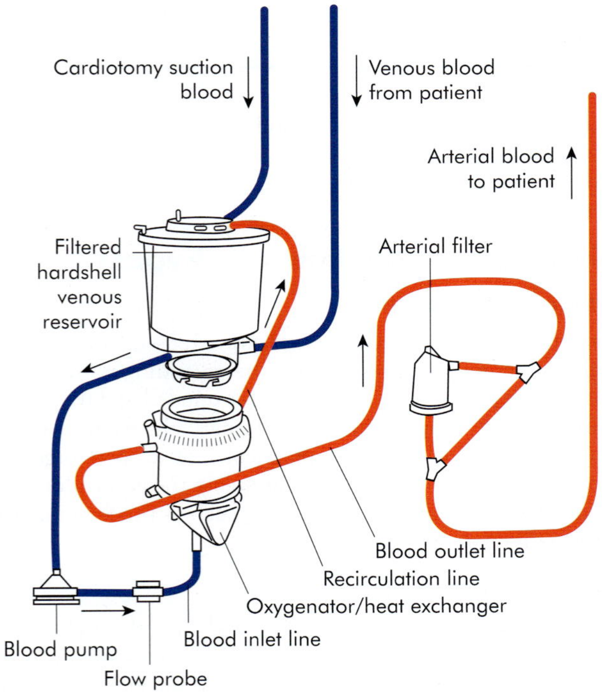

Figure 54.1 Components of the cardiopulmonary bypass (CPB) circuit. (Reproduced from Abraham JK. Cardiopulmonary bypass. Surgery 2000; **18**: 11, with permission from The Medical Publishing Company.)

Cardioplegic solutions vary in terms of temperature, pH, arresting agent, osmolality, and the presence of red cells and other factors. Most solutions contain potassium as the arresting agent. Potassium arrests the heart in diastole by depolarisation of the membrane. Cold (4–10°C) isotonic crystalloid or blood solutions aid myocardial protection by reducing metabolic requirements through local hypothermia. Warm cardioplegic solutions, on the other hand, may facilitate better myocardial repair recovery postoperatively by aiding intramyocardial enzyme activation.

Intermittent cross-clamp fibrillation is a technique in which intermittent ventricular fibrillation is induced by a small electrical charge. The heart does not eject and is relatively still, but not bloodless. The aorta is cross-clamped to render the heart ischaemic. The heart can tolerate short periods (10–20 minutes) of intermittent ischaemia, providing the heart is reperfused when the cross-clamp is released and allowed to beat following cardioversion for short periods during the operation.

Total circulatory arrest becomes necessary when visibility and clarity of the operative area is crucial, as in paediatric surgery or in surgery of the ascending aorta and arch of the aorta. CPB is instituted and the core body temperature reduced to 15–18°C (profound hypothermia). The metabolic rate of all organs of the body is reduced by 50 per cent with every 7°C drop in temperature. Using this technique, circulatory arrest can be tolerated for 20–30 minutes. Additional cerebral protection can be provided with ice packs placed around the head, pharmacological agents, and cerebral perfusion techniques.

Discontinuing cardiopulmonary bypass

At the end of the procedure, air must be meticulously excluded from the cardiac chambers. Once perfusion is restored to the coronary arteries (by removing the cross-clamp) the heart may beat spontaneously. If ventricular fibrillation is present, cardioversion may be required. Epicardial pacing wires may be placed to treat postoperative bradycardia or heart block. The patient is rewarmed, acidosis and hypokalaemia are corrected, and ventilation is restarted. The heart gradually takes over the circulation while the arterial flow from the CPB machine is reduced. When the blood pressure is acceptable and the surgeon is confident that the heart function is adequate, CPB is discontinued. The cannulae are removed and the anticoagulation is reversed by using protamine.

Complications of cardiopulmonary bypass

CPB is a complex technique and requires careful management between surgeon, anaesthetist and perfusionist to ensure that the patient remains safe. Difficulties can occur during cannulation (arterial tear), at the start of CPB (oxygenator failure) and at the end of CPB (coagulopathy). A summary is given in Summary box 54.2. Many complications can occur following blood exposure to the non-physiological surface of the CPB circuit. This leads to the activation of inflammatory cascades giving rise to a post-CPB systematic inflammatory response syndrome (SIRs) that can ultimately lead to multiorgan failure.

Recent developments include 'off-pump' surgery where the surgery is performed on the beating heart with the aid of stabilisers and minimal (mini) bypass, where all the elements of conventional bypass are made as compact as possible to eliminate the potential inflammatory effects.

Summary box 54.2

Potential complications of CPB

- Bleeding disorders
- Infection
- Air embolism
- Intestinal ischaemia/infarction
- Microembolisation
- Myocardial depression
- Neurological dysfunction
- Pancreatitis
- Post-cardiotomy syndrome
- Pulmonary injury
- Systemic organ dysfunction
- Vascular injury

CORONARY ARTERY BYPASS SURGERY

Introduction

Before the 1950s, surgical attempts to treat coronary artery disease (CAD) through augmentation of non-coronary flow to the myocardium via the creation of pericardial or omental adhesions had limited success. From the 1960s, the importance of aortocoronary saphenous vein grafts and the value of the internal mammary (internal thoracic artery) were increasingly recognised. The outcomes of coronary artery bypass graft (CABG) surgery were carefully monitored from the beginning and by the 1970s multiple large, prospectively randomised, multicentre trials were conducted. All showed that a subset of patients had improved survival after surgery. With the advent of percutaneous coronary intervention (PCI) in the 1980s, the patient population undergoing CABG has changed, becoming progressively sicker but often with the most to gain. Over the last decade, there have been major advances in PCI including the use of bare metal stents and the development of drug-eluting stents in an effort to reduce restenosis. The role of CABG in the treatment of ischaemic heart disease is continually questioned and less invasive therapies are being sought. A recent large multicentred trial compared CABG to PCI with drug-eluting stents and showed that CABG is still the 'gold standard' in certain groups of patients (Summary box 54.3).

Summary box 54.3

Coronary artery surgery

- Randomised controlled trials have confirmed improvement in survival following CABG for certain groups of patients

Coronary artery anatomy

The coronary arteries are branches of the ascending aorta, arising from ostia in the aortic sinuses above the aortic valve, the right from the anterior sinus and the left from the left posterior sinus (Figure 54.2).

Left coronary artery

The left main coronary artery, which arises from the aortic root, can be the site of significant stenosis ('left main stem disease') and carries the worst prognosis in terms of survival without surgery. The artery is inaccessible at its origin and therefore grafts are anastomosed to its branches, the left anterior

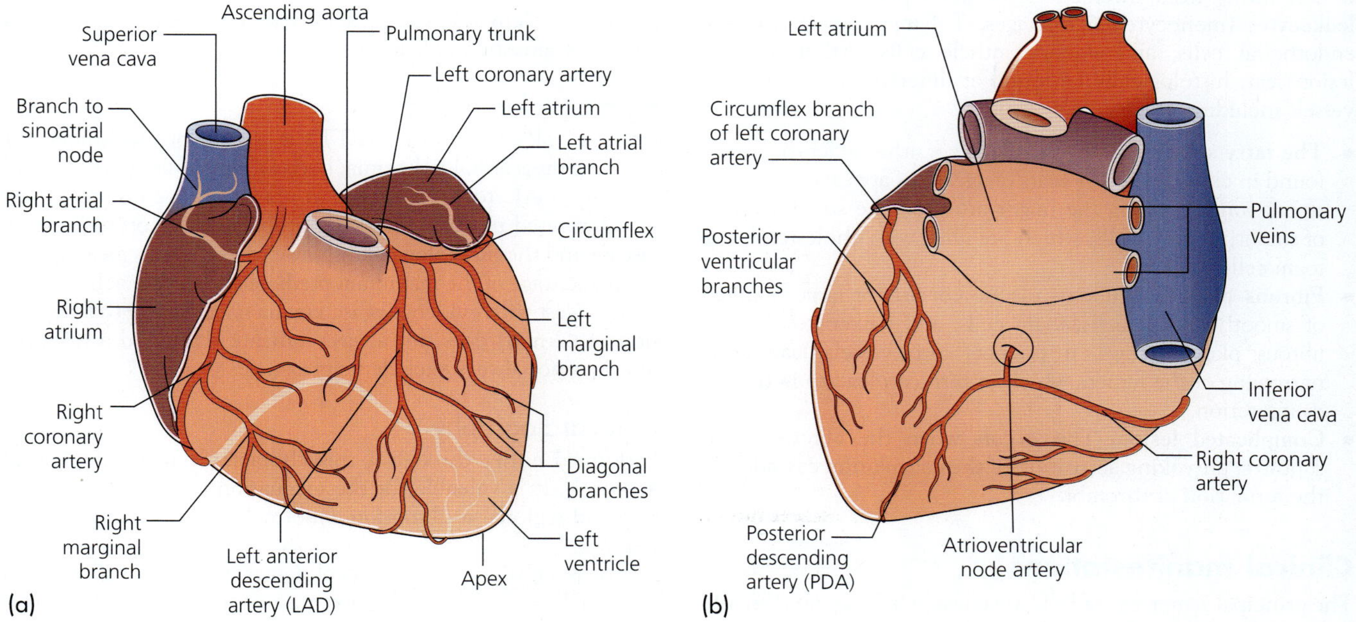

Figure 54.2 The heart, showing the distribution of the left and right coronary arteries. (a) Anterior surface of the heart and (b) base and diaphragmatic surface of the heart.

descending (LAD) artery or anterior interventricular artery and obtuse/marginal (OM) branches of the circumflex artery. The LAD is the most frequently diseased coronary artery and most often bypassed during CABG surgery.

Right coronary artery

The right coronary artery (RCA) passes from its origin anteriorly between the right atrial appendage and the pulmonary trunk and courses in the atrioventricular groove around the margin of the right ventricle. It continues as the posterior descending artery or interventricular artery. Common sites of stenosis of the RCA are in its proximal portion or at the bifurcation or crux. In the presence of disease at the bifurcation, a graft can be placed distally to the posterior descending artery.

The question of anatomical dominance is determined by the artery that supplies the posterior descending artery. In approximately 90 per cent of cases, the posterior descending artery arises from the RCA, a pattern referred to as 'right dominance'. The posterior descending artery can also arise from the circumflex artery, a pattern referred to as 'left dominance', which occurs in approximately 10 per cent of cases. A balanced pattern is one in which two posterior descending arteries, one arising from the right coronary artery and one from the circumflex artery, can exist (Figure 54.2).

Ischaemic heart disease

Ischaemic heart disease (IHD) is a major cause of morbidity and mortality in developed countries. The underlying pathology is mainly atherosclerosis of the coronary arteries.

Pathophysiology

Atherosclerosis is the process underlying the formation of focal obstructions or plaques in large- and medium-sized arteries. It is accepted that atherosclerosis is a chronic inflammatory process resulting from interactions between plasma lipoproteins, leukocytes (monocyte/macrophages, T lymphocytes), vascular endothelial cells, and smooth muscle cells. Atherosclerotic lesions can histologically be found at different stages in blood vessels including:

- **The fatty streak**. The first evidence of atherosclerosis can be found in children 10–14 years of age. This appears as a yellow streak running along the major arteries. The streak consists of smooth muscle cells, which are filled with cholesterol, and foam cells.
- **Fibrous plaque**. A fibrous plaque consists of large numbers of smooth muscle cells, foam cells, and leukocytes. As the fibrous plaque grows, it projects into vessels leading to narrowing of the lumen, which in turn can lead to ischaemia or infarction.
- **Complicated lesion**. This occurs when the fibrous plaque ruptures, provoking activation of the coagulation cascade and the formation of thrombi.

Clinical manifestations

The principal symptoms of IHD are chest pain or angina, breathlessness, fatigue, swelling, palpitations and syncope. Severity of symptoms and the extent to which the symptoms interfere with everyday activities form a significant part of the clinical history. An assessment of risk factors should be included (Summary box 54.4). Clinical examination follows and, although often normal, any evidence of myocardial ischaemia or stigmata of associated disease, such as diabetes or peripheral vascular disease, should be noted.

Summary box 54.4

Risk factors for IHD

- Advancing age
- Male gender
- Hyperlipidaemia
- Diabetes mellitus
- Hypertension
- Smoking
- Family history of IHD
- Obesity
- Reduced physical activity

Investigations

Non-invasive methods of diagnosis

Resting electrocardiography

As a baseline test, a 12-lead resting electrocardiogram (ECG) often provides the first indication of ischaemic cardiac disease and is essential in the acute clinical setting. However, it is not necessarily abnormal even in the presence of severe multivessel coronary heart disease. Evidence of previous myocardial infarction is seen commonly as Q waves and/or non-specific ST and T-wave changes.

Troponin and cardiac isoenzymes

These are useful in assessing patients with an acute coronary syndrome (ACS) when the diagnosis is in doubt. Standard enzyme measurement such as Troponin, creatine kinase MB (CKMB), and lactate dehydrogenase (LDH) can aid diagnosis, as well as having prognostic implications.

Exercise tolerance testing

Exercise tolerance testing (ETT) is a valuable technique for assessing myocardial ischaemia, both for diagnostic purposes and as a prognostic tool. However, an abnormal exercise test must be interpreted in the light of the probability of coronary artery disease and the physiological response to exercise as measured by the percentage of the maximum predicted heart rate achieved. A positive test with evidence of ischaemia on the ECG (ST depression of ≤2 mm) does not always indicate IHD, and a negative test does not always exclude its presence.

Echocardiography

Performed either through a transthoracic or transoesophageal approach, it is valuable for the evaluation of ventricular function and regional wall motion abnormalities, as well as valvular lesions.

Stress echocardiography can detect regional wall motion abnormalities brought on by exercise or the use of dobutamine or dipyridamole. It is a reliable method of identifying viable myocardium. Impaired but recoverable myocardium possesses a functional reserve that allows it to be temporarily recruited into action, whereas scar tissue does not. The development of real time three-dimensional ECHO (RT3DE) with the ability to carry out valve construction from different surfaces has recently revolutionised preoperative surgical planning in patients with complex valvular diseases.

Radionuclide studies and cardiac magnetic resonance imaging

The two main types of radionuclide study available are perfusion and blood pool studies. They allow an assessment of the perfusion and cellular integrity of viable myocardium. Cardiac magnetic resonance imaging (MRI) can be performed to evaluate the structure and function of the heart and blood vessels and offers an alternative to angiography.

Positron emission tomography

Positron emission tomography (PET) provides information on myocardial perfusion, metabolism and cell membrane function. Positron-emitting isotopes are used to label physiological substances, after which the regional distribution of these substances can be measured. PET is valuable in the diagnosis of coronary artery disease, particularly when the more widely available imaging modalities are inconclusive. It can identify injured but viable myocardium that is potentially salvageable by revascularisation.

Computed tomography

With the development of the latest computed tomography (CT) scanners, which have the ability to correct for respiratory and cardiac movements, multislice high-resolution CT scanning may become an alternative to coronary angiography. It allows for the assessment of coronary disease, particularly proximal coronary artery disease, and gives some information about the degree of coronary artery calcification.

Invasive methods of diagnosis

Coronary angiography

Selective coronary angiography provides the means of accurately diagnosing the presence and extent of coronary artery disease and remains the 'gold standard' diagnostic technique (Figure 54.3).

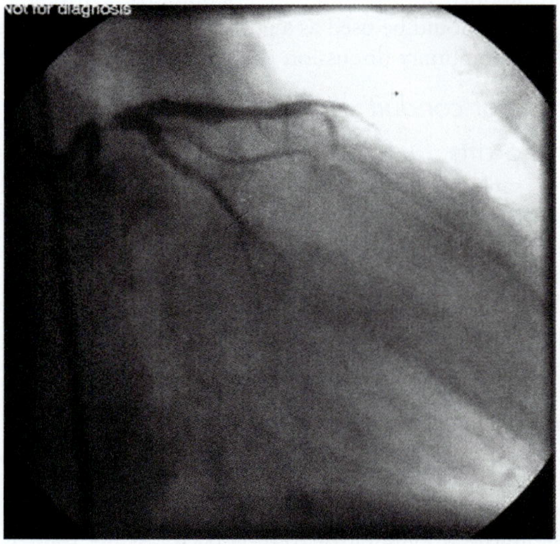

Figure 54.3 Coronary angiogram demonstrating severe stenosis in the left main stem prior to bifurcation of the left anterior descending and circumflex arteries.

In spite of the availability of newer imaging techniques, such as cardiac MRI, selective coronary angiography provides high image quality, demonstrating the extent, severity and location of coronary artery stenoses and the quality and size of the distal coronary arteries. Any stenosis in an artery of >70 per cent of the diameter (90 per cent reduction on cross-sectional area) is considered 'severe'. In addition, it allows assessment of ventricular function and provides the cardiac surgeon with information to determine operability, operative risk and probability of operative result. This test only outlines the coronary anatomy, does not demonstrate ischaemia and carries an overall complication rate of less than 1 per cent (Summary box 54.5).

Summary box 54.5

Coronary angiography

- 'Gold standard' for imaging of anatomy
- Demonstrates extent, severity and location of stenoses
- Reduction in diameter of >70 per cent is considered severe (90 per cent reduction in cross-sectional area)
- Demonstrates quality and size of distal arterial tree
- Aids diagnosis of ischaemia
- Evaluates suitability for surgery
- Aids in prognostic assessment

Indications for surgery

The decision to offer CABG is based on the balance between the expected benefit and the risks that the patient faces. The two issues to be addressed when deciding if a patient is suitable to have surgery are the appropriateness of revascularization, and the relative merits of CABG versus PCI.

Current best evidence shows that revascularization can be readily justified on symptomatic grounds in patients with persistent limiting symptoms (angina or angina equivalent) despite optimal medical therapy and/or on prognostic grounds in certain anatomical patterns of disease.

Recent guidelines on myocardial revascularization have been released by the Task Force on Myocardial Revascularization of the European Society of Cardiology (ESC) and the European Association for Cardio-Thoracic Surgery (EACTS) and identified patients with certain angiographic features who can benefit from surgery (Summary box 54.6).

Summary box 54.6

Indication for surgery

- >50 per cent stenosis of the left main stem ('critical left main stem disease')
- >50 per cent stenosis of the proximal left anterior interventricular artery
- Two or three main coronary arteries diseased ('triple-vessel disease')
- Poor ventricular function associated with multi-vessel disease

Chronic stable angina

Although PCI is increasingly being used for the treatment of stable angina, CABG is still indicated in the presence of certain angiographic features. Angina can be relieved by surgical revascularisation in most patients and symptomatic improvement can be expected for over ten years.

Acute coronary syndromes

A recently published meta-analysis showed substantial benefit with an early invasive strategy mainly in high risk patients. An invasive strategy always starts with angiography. After defining the anatomy and its associated risk features, a decision about the type of intervention can be made. The angiography in combination with ECG changes often identifies the culprit lesion and PCI, if desirable, can be recommended to treat the culprit lesion. Angiography should be performed urgently for diagnostic purposes in patients at high risk and in whom the differential diagnosis of other acute clinical situations is unclear. In stabilized patients after an episode of ACS, surgical indications are similar to those with stable chronic disease.

The optimal timing of revascularization is different for PCI and for CABG. While the benefit from PCI in patients with NSTE-ACS (non-ST-segment elevation acute coronary syndrome) is related to its early performance, the benefit from CABG is greatest when patients can undergo surgery after several days of medical stabilization.

Surgery for the complications of myocardial infarction

Myocardial infarction (MI) leads to myocyte necrosis, which may heal to form scar tissue or rupture if the ventricular wall gives way. Free rupture of the ventricle is usually fatal despite treatment. Ventricular septal rupture typically presents 3–7 days after infarction with pulmonary oedema, a pansystolic murmur and hypotension. The diagnosis is usually confirmed with echocardiography. Repair is with a pericardial or artificial Dacron patch. Papillary muscle necrosis causes acute mitral regurgitation, a pansystolic murmur and pulmonary oedema. Diagnosis is made by echocardiography and right heart catheterisation (showing large V waves). Mitral valve replacement is usually necessary, but the mortality rate is higher than in valve replacement for rheumatic heart disease as a result of the associated coronary artery disease. Ventricular aneurysm occurs following partial-thickness necrosis of the ventricular wall if the free wall is replaced with non-contractile fibrous tissue. Left ventricular function is affected because the fibrous wall balloons out during systole and reduces the actual stroke volume. Repair is undertaken using CPB, and CABG is undertaken at the same time if necessary combined with valve replacement

Patients undergoing valve replacement usually have coronary bypass surgery to any significant coronary lesions. However, several variables need to be carefully evaluated when considering the choice of a combined procedure and the overall operative risk: these include age >70 years, female sex and poor left ventricular function, as well as what the underlying valve pathology is and which valve is to be replaced.

Acute failure of percutaneous coronary angioplasty

Since the advent of intracoronary stents, the need for emergency CABG following complications of percutaneous transluminal coronary angioplasty (PTCA) is low at <1 per cent. The mortality rate in this group is significantly higher than for elective CABG.

Preparation for surgery

Clinical assessment

Before CABG, the severity and stability of the patient's IHD, the presence of significant valvular disease and the status of left ventricular function should be properly evaluated.

Any comorbid risk factors for IHD should be documented and, in particular, the state of coexisting diseases assessed. Attention is paid to the presence of carotid artery disease, peripheral vascular disease, respiratory status, preoperative diabetic control and presence of associated diabetic complications, significant renal dysfunction or coagulopathy. All medications taken by the patient are noted. Ideally, some should be stopped before surgery, in particular any anti-platelet agents, including aspirin and anticoagulants, as well as oral hypoglycaemics. Others drugs, such as diuretics and angiotensin-converting enzyme (ACE) inhibitors, are stopped on the discretion of the surgeon. However, apart from the exceptions noted, as a general rule all cardiac and antihypertensive medications should be taken preoperatively.

Risk assessment

Myocardial revascularization is appropriate when the expected benefits, in terms of survival or health outcomes exceed the expected negative consequences of the procedure. Therefore, risk assessment is an important aspect of contemporary clinical practice, being of value to clinicians and patients. Over the long term, it allows quality control and the assessment of health economics. Numerous different models have been developed for risk stratification in cardiac surgery including the EuroSCORE and STS (Society of Thoracic Surgeons).

The EuroSCORE validated to predict surgical mortality was recently shown to be an independent predictor of major adverse cardiac events (MACE). Therefore, it can be used to determine the risk of revascularization irrespective of, and even before, the selection of treatment strategy. However, it is important to acknowledge that no risk score can accurately predict events in an individual patient. Moreover, limitations exist with all databases used to build risk models, and differences in definitions and variable content can affect the performance of risk scores when they are applied across different populations. Ultimately, risk stratification should be used as a guide, while clinical judgement and multidisciplinary discussion (heart team) remain essential.

Selection of conduit

Venous grafts

The long saphenous vein is the most common vein used as a conduit as it is straightforward to harvest, provides good length and is easy to handle. The ten-year patency rate for long saphenous vein grafts is reported to be 50–60 per cent, with 10–15 per cent occluding in one year. However, recent studies suggest that the early use of lipid-lowering agents and anti-platelet agents, such as low-dose aspirin, can improve vein graft long term patency. In assessing the patient preoperatively, the legs should be checked for varicose veins. Alternative vein conduits include the short saphenous vein or upper limb veins, such as the cephalic vein.

Arterial grafts

The left internal mammary artery (LIMA) or internal thoracic artery has become the conduit of choice for the LAD. Since the mid-1980s, long patency rates of >98 per cent have been reported, with improved long-term survival and fewer reoperations. As

LIMA–LAD anastomosis avoids the late complication of vein graft atherosclerosis, particular interest has focused on the use of bilateral internal mammary artery (BIMA) grafts. However, there is still debate regarding the appropriateness in certain subgroups of patients, such as the obese diabetic in whom sternal wound complications appear higher.

The use of the radial artery as a second or alternative arterial bypass graft has enjoyed a revival. This has been driven to some extent by the developing concept of total arterial revascularisation and the belief that this will help improve long-term results of coronary surgery. Recent randomised controlled studies in the United States and UK have demonstrasted excellent patency rates at one and five years. In assessing a patient in whom a radial artery harvest is planned, an Allen's test is performed (Summary box 54.7). Alternative arterial bypass grafts include the gastroepiploic artery and the inferior epigastric artery.

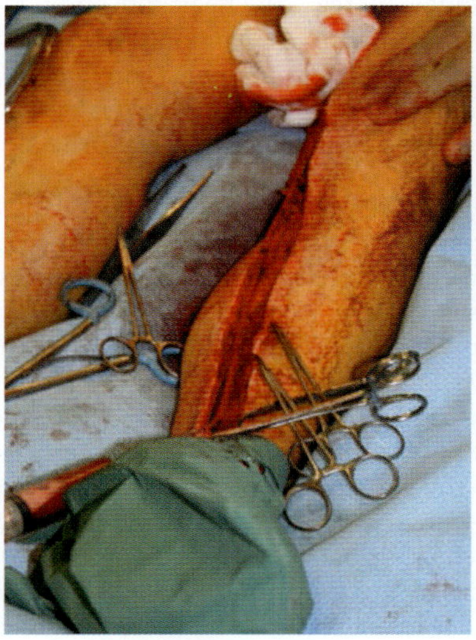

Figure 54.4 The long saphenous vein is exposed at the ankle, anterior to the medial malleolus, as far as the saphenofemoral junction (if required). The side branches are tied carefully and divided, and the vein is excised. Gentle distension of the vein through a cannula at its distal end allows inspection for leaks.

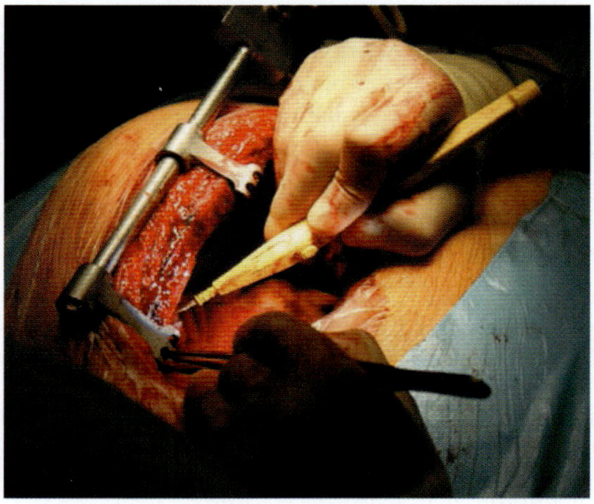

Figure 54.5 A pedicled left internal mammary artery is dissected off the chest wall and divided distally after systemic heparinisation. It is left attached to the subclavian artery proximally.

Summary box 54.7

Allen's test

- The patient makes a tight fist while the surgeon compresses both distal and ulnar arteries digitally; this squeezes blood from the hand
- The hand is then relaxed and compression of the ulnar artery is released; the speed of returning colour to the hand is assessed
- If colour returns in 5–7 seconds, patency and collateral flow from the ulnar artery is confirmed

The operation

Intraoperative monitoring includes monitoring of continuous central venous pressure and blood pressure (via a central line in the internal jugular or subclavian vein and radial artery line, respectively), urine output via a urinary catheter, temperature using a probe positioned at the nasal septum, and the ECG.

The operation commences with harvesting of the conduits (long saphenous vein from the leg (Figure 54.4) or/and radial artery), while the chest is opened via a median sternotomy and the LIMA is dissected from the chest wall (Figure 54.5). The patient is typically placed on CPB after heparinising, the aorta is cross-clamped and the heart arrested with cardioplegia. The grafts are anastomosed to coronary arteries distal to the stenosis (Figure 54.6).

The aortic cross-clamp is removed and the heart is reperfused with oxygenated blood. A side-biting clamp is applied to the ascending aorta and the proximal anastomoses are completed. Occasionally, the surgeon may opt to carry out the whole operation while the cross-clamp is applied to reduce the risks associated with aortic manipulation. The patient is warmed and weaned from CPB. The heparin is reversed and the patient is returned to the intensive care unit (ICU).

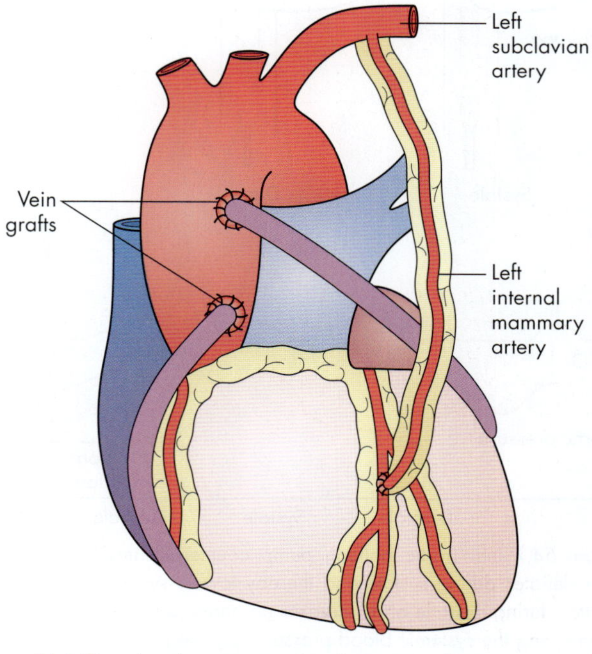

Figure 54.6 Completed coronary artery bypass grafts.

Edgar van Nuys Allen, 1900–1961, Professor of Medicine, The Mayo Clinic, Rochester, MN, USA.

Postoperative recovery

The majority of patients are extubated a few hours after returning from surgery and remain in the ICU for 24 hours or so. In some centres, 'fast tracking' appropriate patients allows for an earlier transfer to a recovery area or high-dependency unit (HDU). Discharge is routinely 4–8 days after surgery.

Postoperative complications

Bleeding

Significant bleeding occurs in approximately 2–3 per cent of patients. Rarely, acute cardiac tamponade or profound hypotension may occur in the early postoperative period and requires emergency resternotomy.

Arrhythmias

The most common postoperative arrhythmia is sinus tachycardia, closely followed by atrial fibrillation (AF). It occurs in around 30 per cent of patients undergoing CABG and often spontaneously reverts to sinus rhythm. Treatment includes correction of potassium (>4.5 mmol/L), the use of amiodarone or digoxin and, if necessary, cardioversion. Bradycardia is seldom seen, but temporary pacing via epicardial pacing wires inserted intraoperatively may be required in the postoperative period.

Poor cardiac output state

Myocardial function typically declines in the first few hours following cardiac surgery, presumably in response to an ischaemia/reperfusion-type injury. Often, inotropic agents are required at this time to support the heart and circulation. Occasionally, the patient develops a persistent low cardiac output state. The clinical manifestations of such a situation include poor peripheral perfusion, with poor urine output, a developing metabolic acidosis and low blood pressure.

There are several mechanisms that account for this complication in the early postoperative period, including depressed myocardial contractility, reduced preload, increased afterload and a disturbance in heart rate or rhythm.

Treatment is aimed at the underlying cause, but generally includes oxygenation, optimising preload, reducing afterload, managing any rhythm disturbances and improving contractility. If the low cardiac output state persists, the heart may require pharmacological or mechanical support.

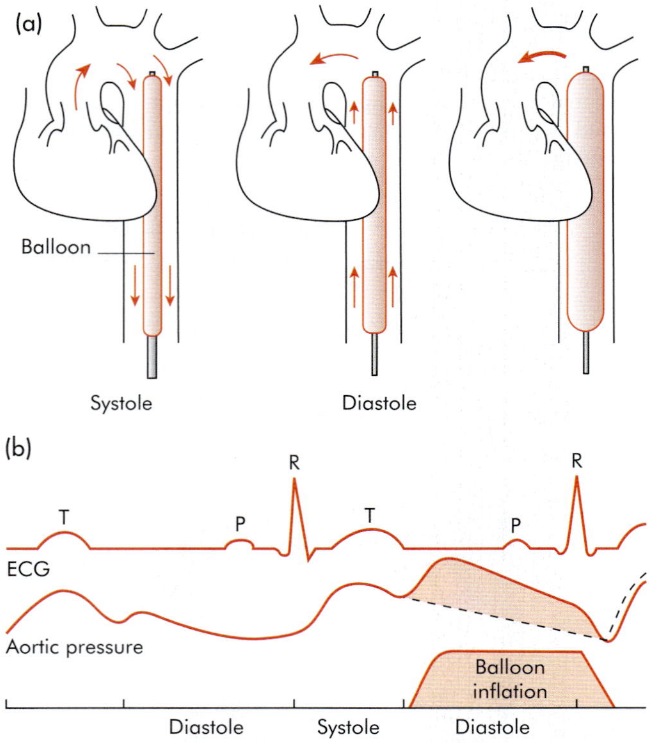

Figure 54.7 Intra-aortic balloon pump counterpulsation. (a) The balloon deflates during systole and thereby lowers systemic resistance. It inflates during diastole and increases coronary perfusion in addition to augmenting the systemic blood pressure. (b) The pressure changes and phases of the electrocardiogram (ECG) are shown.

Pharmacological support

Inotropic drugs act in a variety of ways to alter the systemic vascular resistance, increase the heart rate and increase the force of myocardial contractility. Commonly used inotropes include isoprenaline, dopamine, dobutamine, adrenaline (epinephrine) and noradrenaline (norepine); they are often used in conjunction with vasodilating agents that decrease the afterload.

Mechanical support

If low cardiac output persists despite inotropic support, the heart may require mechanical support while it recovers its function. Mechanical support can be achieved by using an intra-aortic balloon pump (IABP) counterpulsation, or a ventricular assist device (VAD).

IABP is a device that is inserted, either percutaneously or under direct vision, into the common femoral artery. It is threaded into the aorta until its tip lies just distal to the arch vessels (Figure 54.7). The balloon is triggered by the ECG, deflating during ventricular systole (thus reducing afterload) and inflating in diastole (displacing blood that perfuses the coronary arteries retrogradely). When the heart has recovered sufficiently, the balloon is removed.

VAD is a mechanical circulatory supporting device used to replace the function of a failing heart partially or completely. It can be used as a short-term measure typically for patients recovering from heart attacks or heart surgery, or as a long-term support for patients suffering from congestive heart failure. VAD pumps can be pulsatile which mimic the natural pulsing action of the heart, or continuous flow pumps. Blood is exposed in these devices to a non-biologic surface which can activate proinflammatory and coagulation cascades leading to strokes and bleeding. Another important complication associated with VAD is infection which can be caused Gram-positive bacteria, Gram-negative bacteria, and fungi.

Neurological dysfunction

Stroke leading to a focal neurological deficit occurs in approximately 2 per cent of patients following CABG. Embolisation, probably originating from the aortic arch or heart chambers, is the most common mechanism for territorial infarcts, with hypoperfusion leading to watershed infarcts. Diffuse neurological injury may occur leading to more subtle cognitive abnormalities in memory, concentration and attention.

Wound infection

Significant deep wound infection resulting in sternal dehiscence and mediastinitis occurs in around 0.5–2 per cent of patients.

This can be associated with significant morbidity with a prolonged hospital stay and further surgical interventions for debridement and/or rewiring of the sternum. It still has a significant mortality rate of as high as 40 per cent. Wound infections are more common in diabetics and the obese.

Mortality

In the UK, the overall mortality rate for patients undergoing CABG is 2–3 per cent. Multiple factors have been demonstrated to affect mortality after CABG, including age, gender, left ventricular function, use of LIMA and complete revascularisation.

Surgical outcome

Relief of symptoms

If revascularisation is complete, CABG alleviates or improves anginal symptoms in more than 90 per cent of patients at one year; this falls to 80 per cent at five years and 60 per cent at ten years. This symptomatic deterioration usually reflects progression of atherosclerotic disease in vein grafts and native coronary arteries.

Survival

Early surgical versus medical studies have reported survival rates to be 95 per cent at one year, 90 per cent at five years, 75 per cent at ten years and 60 per cent at 15 years. Through changes in surgical practice, such as an increased use of arterial conduits and the widespread use of dual antiplatelet therapy, B-blockers, and lipid-lowering agents, post-CABG survival may well improve in the future (Summary box 54.8).

Summary box 54.8

Coronary artery bypass surgery outcome

Mortality
- 2–3 per cent

Peroperative infarct
- 2–3 per cent

Angina
- Better in 90 per cent at one year
- 80 per cent at five years
- 60 per cent at ten years

Survival
- 95 per cent at one year
- 90 per cent at five years
- 75 per cent at ten years
- 60 per cent at 15 years

Off-pump coronary artery surgery

CABG without the use of CPB is a well-established and increasingly popular method that may be combined with a minimally invasive approach or carried out through a conventional sternotomy. It offers the advantages that it avoids the physiological stress associated with CPB and, to some extent, the aortic manipulation that can lead to neurological injury through atherosclerotic embolisation. Since the introduction of cardiac stabilising devices, such as the Octopus® (Figure 54.8), off-pump coronary artery bypass (OPCAB) grafting has become widespread. One of the concerns, however, associated with off-pump surgery is related to the quality of anastomosis as its carried out on a beating heart and bloody field which can limit the surgeon's vision.

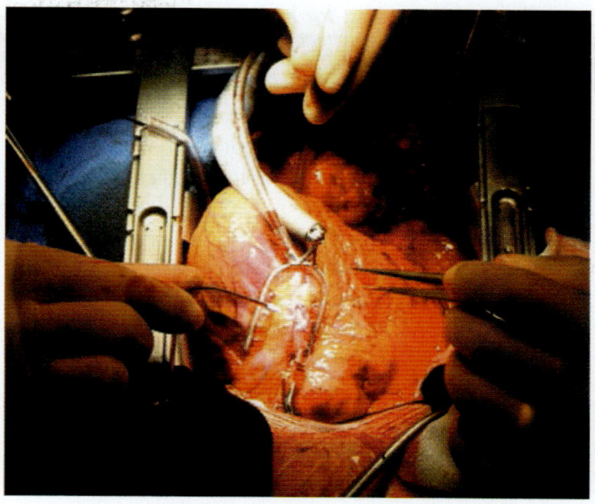

Figure 54.8 Off-pump coronary artery bypass using an Octopus stabiliser to perform the distal anastomosis.

The advantages of off-pump surgery over on-pump has recently been questioned especially with the development and use of the mini-bypass machines which offer a closed circuit and minimal unphysiological surface area, though reducing proinflammatory activation, but at the same time allow the surgeon to operate on a still heart in a bloodless field.

Minimal access surgery

Minimally invasive direct coronary artery bypass (MIDCAB) grafting is performed through a strategically placed minimal access incision and so avoids all invasive aspects of conventional CABG. Through an anterior submammary incision, the LIMA can be dissected down with the aid of a thoracoscope and grafted to the LAD. More lateral MIDCAB incisions allow access to other coronary vessels including branches of the circumflex artery. Patient selection remains, at least at present, a restriction to the ever-increasing minimally invasive methods being developed. Although not yet critically evaluated, one particular approach is to combine MIDCAB (typically LIMA to LAD) with PCI to other less accessible coronary arteries ('hybrid' coronary revascularisation).

VALVULAR HEART DISEASE

Introduction

Early surgical management of valvular heart disease concentrated on valvular repair. The heroic early procedures for valve stenosis were closed and therefore 'blind' commissurotomies. They were replaced by open procedures with full visualisation allowing precise repair and replacement. The first prosthetic valve replacement was performed by Harken in 1960 replacing the aortic valve, followed by a mitral valve replacement by Starr a

Dwight Emary Harken, 1910 – 1993, formerly Chief of Thoracic Surgery, The Peter Bent Brigham Hospital, Boston, MA, USA. Innovator in heart surgery, introduced the concept of intensive care unit and opened the first intensive care unit in 1951. Served as Chief of Thoracic Surgery at Harvard University for 22 years.
Albert Starr, born 1926, formerly Professor of Surgery, The University of Oregon, Portland, OR, USA. Medical Director, Providence Heart and Vascular Institute, Portland. Inventor of the world's first durable artificial mitral valve; winner of Lasker award in 2007 – an award given by the Lasker Foundation in the United States to a person (or persons) who has made major contributions to medical science or who has performed public service on behalf of medicine.

Table 54.1 Comparing options for heart valve surgery.

	Advantages	Disadvantages
Valve repair	Preservation of integral structures Improved haemodynamics Avoids long-term anticoagulation	Technical difficulties Variable failure rate
Valve replacement		
Mechanical	Readily available Extensive experience of use Used in any age group Durability, lifelong	Needs lifelong anticoagulation Susceptibility to infection
Biological		
Stented	Readily available Short period of anticoagulation	Limited lifespan
Stentless	Readily available Probably better haemodynamics with less outflow tract obstruction Short period of anticoagulation	Limited lifespan More difficult to insert
Homograft	No anticoagulation Improved haemodynamics Long-term outcome uncertain	Not readily available Technical difficulties

Table adapted from Sharpe DAC, Das SR. Heart valve surgery. *Surgery* 2000; **18**: 265–9.

year later. Continued improvements in perioperative care, myocardial protection and, in particular, the development of prosthetic heart valves have improved long-term haemodynamic effects, and provided symptom relief and prolonged survival. The majority of valvular operations involve surgery on the aortic or mitral valve; tricuspid and pulmonary valve surgery is rarely undertaken.

Surgical anatomy

Heart valves function to maintain pressure gradients between cardiac chambers and so ensure unidirectional flow of blood without reflux through the heart. The aortic valve is tricuspid with semilunar leaflets attached to the aortic wall at the annulus with the aortic sinuses being above the base of each leaflet, two of which form the origin or ostium of the coronary arteries. The intrinsic shape of the aortic semilunar valve allows blood to leave the ventricle during systole and prevents its regurgitation during diastole. If disease leads to disruption of the leaflets or the annulus, valve function will be affected.

The mitral valve is bileaflet; the anterior leaflet is larger in area. The leaflets, like those of the aortic valve, are attached to an annulus. The leaflets join at two commissures and are supported by a subvalvular apparatus consisting of chordae tendinae and papillary muscles. The papillary muscles contract in ventricular systole, pulling the cusps towards the atrioventricular orifice and holding blood within the ventricle. The proper functioning of the mitral valve depends on the integrity of the annulus, leaflets, chordae and papillary muscles. If surgical correction is required, emphasis is on the preservation of these structures when possible (Figure 54.9).

Surgical options for heart valve disease

The decision of whether to repair or replace the diseased valve depends on the underlying pathology, the severity of disease, and quality and/or involvement of the surrounding supporting structures. Generally, repair is increasingly favoured when possible in mitral valve disease, particularly in mitral regurgitation in which it has been shown to have good long-term outcomes. Repair is the operation of choice in tricuspid valve disease, but aortic valve surgery generally involves replacing the diseased valve (Table 54.1).

Important factors in selecting the type of procedure and prosthesis include the age of the patient and the need for anticoagulation. Because of uncertainties about its lifespan, there is debate about when a bioprosthetic valve should be used, with most accepting its use in those over 65 years. The need for anticoagulation may have an impact on choice of valve, particularly in women of child-bearing age, the elderly, the presence of congenital or acquired bleeding diathesis and when there is the need for further major surgery.

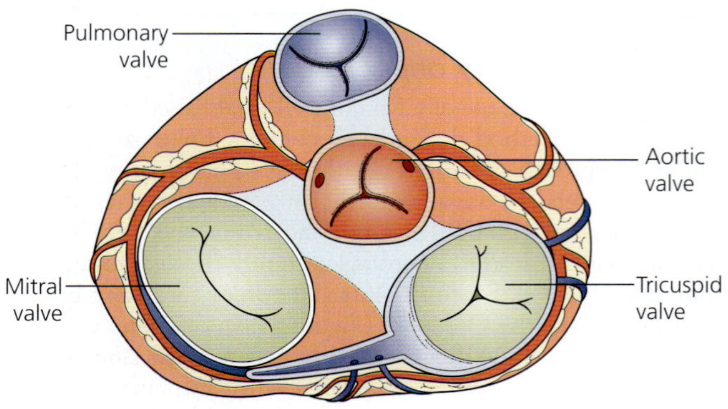

Figure 54.9 Four valves of the heart.

Types of prosthetic valves

Mechanical valves

Mechanical valves can be used in any age group to replace any valve (Figure 54.10). They are extremely durable, but the components of the valve are thrombogenic and therefore the patient requires systemic anticoagulation, usually with warfarin. This subjects the patients to a lifetime of blood tests, medication and the constant threat of haemorrhagic (intracerebral, epistaxis, gastrointestinal bleed) or thrombotic (cerebral infarction) complications.

Biological valves

Biological valves include **homograft** (or **allograft**) valves, removed from cadavers; **autografts**, a patient's own valve; and, most commonly, **heterografts** (or **xenografts**) prepared from animal tissues. All share the basic design of three semilunar leaflets with central flow, so decreasing pressure gradients and minimising turbulence (Figure 54.11). Heterograft 'tissue' valves are the most commonly used valves and can be stented with a limited durability of 10–15 years, whereas stentless (or frameless) valves are expected to have less late calcific degeneration, but are more technically difficult to insert.

Prosthetic valve dysfunction and complications

Structural valve failure

Bioprosthetic valves are vulnerable to degenerative changes. Structural failure rates for biological valves, although rare in those over 70 years of age, can reach 60 per cent after 15 years. However, newer biological valve have a reoperative rate of less than 10 per cent at 20 years. Structural failure of a mechanical valve is generally uncommon.

Paravalvular leak

Early-onset paravalvular leaks usually result from technical difficulties at insertion. Late-onset leaks can occur and may be related to an episode of endocarditis or, in the presence of bioprostheses, leaflet degeneration. The leak can cause haemolytic anaemia or haemodynamic compromise and the valve may need replacement.

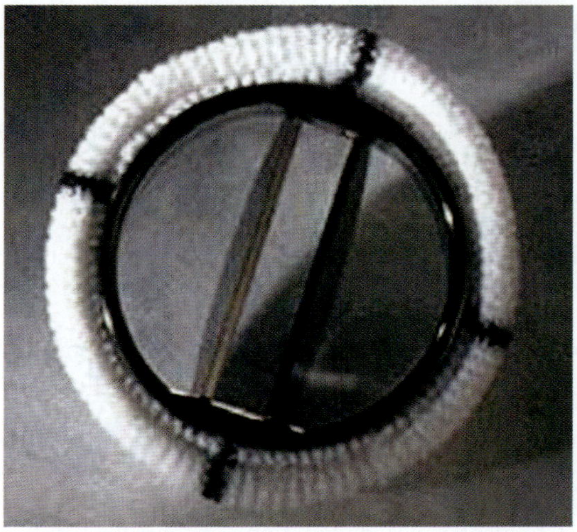

Figure 54.10 Bileaflet mechanical valve.

Thrombosis and thromboembolism

Thrombus formation on a prosthetic valve remains the most common complication of mechanical and biological valves (Figure 54.12). The risk of thromboembolism is greater with a valve in the mitral position (mechanical or biological) than with one in the aortic position. Improved haemodynamic function lowers the probability of thromboembolism. The incidence of thromboembolism in current mechanical valves is 0.5–3 per cent per patient-year.

Prosthetic valve endocarditis

The incidence of prosthetic valve endocarditis (PVE) is 2–4 per cent. The risk is lifelong and at its greatest in the first 15 weeks after surgery. The incidence of PVE is higher with mechanical and bioprosthetic valves and lowest with homograft and autograft valves. The diagnosis is suspected following symptoms of septicaemia, appearance of a new murmur or a septic embolus. It is confirmed with echocardiography, which may show vegetations and even abscess formation. A high index of suspicion is required and early multiple blood cultures are needed to confirm the diagnosis, identify the infective organism and choose appropriate antibiotic therapy. The most common organisms that can lead to PVE are the *Staphylococcus* species, particularly *Staphylococcus epidermidis* in early PVE and *Staphylococcus aureus* (at least 50 per cent of cases); the *Streptococcus* species, usually *Streptococcus viridans*, but also *Streptococcus pneumoniae*, and less commonly, Gram-negative bacilli, as well as fungal organisms.

The treatment of choice is early aggressive intravenous antibiotic therapy. Serial echocardiography to assess extent of infection into surrounding myocardial tissue, as well as functional assessment of the infected valve, may help in optimising decisions on timing of surgical intervention. The prognosis of PVE remains poor with an overall mortality rate of over 50 per cent.

Postoperative management

Antibiotic prophylaxis

Valve surgery, like all cardiac procedures, requires perioperative and immediate postoperative antibiotic prophylaxis. If prosthetic

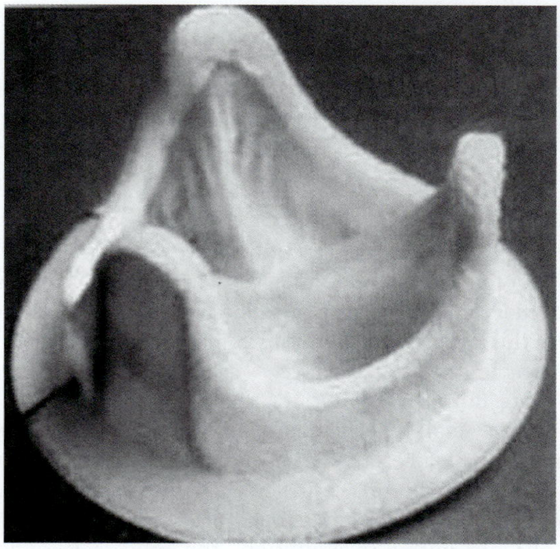

Figure 54.11 Porcine heterograft stented valve.

infective endocarditis is to be avoided, further prophylaxis with appropriate antibiotics is required during dental and minor surgical procedures in all patients with prosthetic heart valves.

Anti-thrombotic therapy

All patients with mechanical valves require warfarin, usually started on the second postoperative day. The use of anticoagulation or anti-platelet therapy with biological valves is variable and depends on the patient's underlying rhythm postoperatively.

Mitral valve disease

Approximately one-third of all valve surgery performed in the UK is for mitral valve disease, with increasing emphasis on valve repair as the importance of preserving the mitral valve apparatus has become apparent.

Mitral regurgitation

Any pathological process affecting the mitral valve apparatus may lead to mitral regurgitation. As such, there are many causes of regurgitation and they can be broadly classified into five headings (Summary box 54.9).

Summary box 54.9

Causes of mitral regurgitation and likely pathology

Degenerative
- Mitral valve prolapse
- Floppy valve: degeneration of the leaflets with/without chordal rupture
- Senile calcification: calcified annulus
- Connective tissue disorders (e.g. Marfan syndrome, Ehlers–Danlos syndrome): disruption of mitral valve apparatus

Ischaemic
- Papillary muscle rupture: following myocardial infarction
- Dynamic mitral regurgitation: as a result of transient ischaemia
- Poor left ventricular function: most common 'functional' cause secondary to myocardial ischaemia

Rheumatic
- Previous acute rheumatic fever: stiffened leaflets unable to coapt

Infective
- Endocarditis: leaflet destruction

Adapted from Hall R. Mitral valve disease. *Medicine* 1997; **25**: 27.

Pathophysiology

There is an important distinction between acute and chronic mitral regurgitation. The former is usually as a result of ischaemic papillary muscle rupture or following infective endocarditis, whereas the latter is a result of myxomatous degeneration of the leaflets leading to a floppy valve.

In acute mitral regurgitation, the left ventricle ejects blood back into a small poorly compliant left atrium, imposing a sudden volume load on the left atrium during ventricular systole. This leads to an abrupt rise in left atrial pressure followed by a rise in pulmonary venous pressure and pulmonary oedema.

In chronic mitral regurgitation, the process is sufficiently slow to allow compensatory left ventricular dilatation and hypertrophy, and dilatation of the left atrium without any significant increase in pressure, so protecting the pulmonary circulation. As the disease advances and left atrial dilatation can no longer cope, left atrial pressure begins to rise, leading to a rise in pulmonary venous pressure and progressive pulmonary congestion, and eventual congestive cardiac failure.

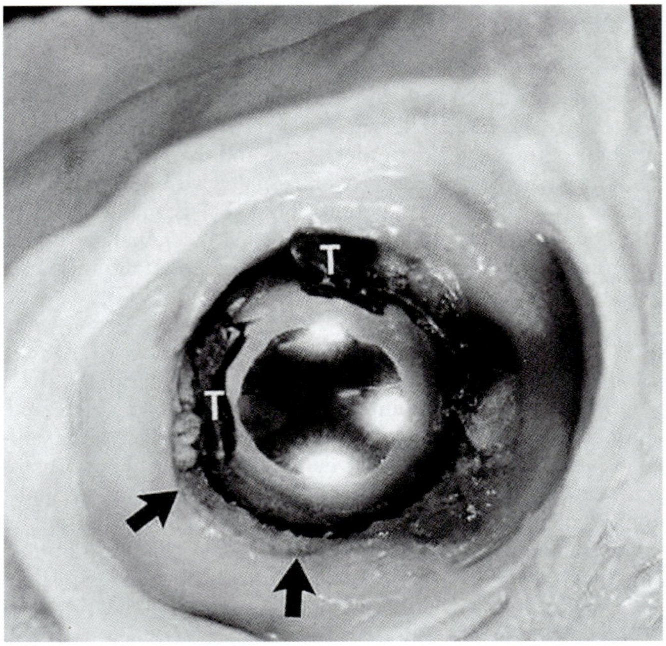

Figure 54.12 Thrombus (marked T and illustrated with the arrows) on the moving components of a ball-and-cage valve.

Clinical features

In acute mitral regurgitation, the patient is usually unwell, presenting with clinical and radiological evidence of acute pulmonary oedema and a loud apical pansystolic murmur. Patients with mild chronic mitral regurgitation are usually asymptomatic. With progressive pulmonary congestion and left ventricular failure, the patient develops fatigue, dyspnoea on exertion and orthopnoea. The development of atrial fibrillation with left atrial dilatation is common. The enlarged left ventricle leads to a heaving apical impulse and a pansystolic murmur.

Investigations

- **ECG** may show only left atrial hypertrophy (bifid P waves), left ventricular hypertrophy and atrial fibrillation.
- **Chest radiography**. There may be cardiomegaly with prominent pulmonary vasculature.
- **Echocardiography** is often combined with colour flow Doppler imaging, which shows the severity of the regurgitant jet of mitral regurgitation.
- **Coronary angiography**. To investigate the coronary arteries.

Indications for surgery

Indications for surgery include severe symptoms as assessed by the New York Heart Association (NYHA) functional classification system, a progressive increase in left ventricular volume leading to ventricular dysfunction, uncontrolled endocarditis and severe acute mitral regurgitation (Figure 54.13). Timing of

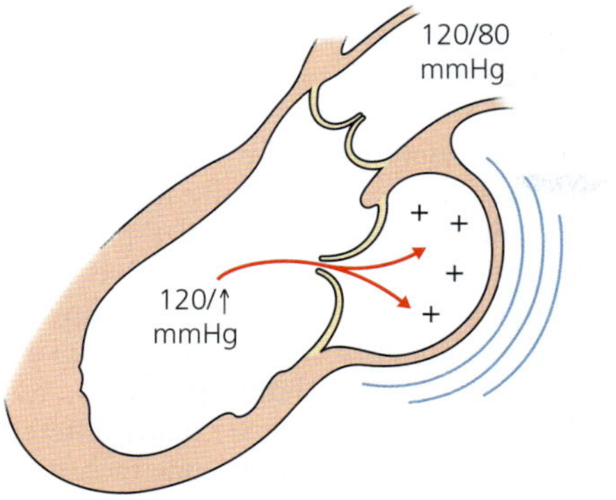

Figure 54.13 Features and pathophysiology of mitral regurgitation. There is a loud parasystolic murmur and the left atrium enlarges. The left ventricle enlarges as a consequence of volume overload.

surgery is crucial, as surgery performed too late in the natural history of the condition does not benefit the patient because of the damage already done.

Mitral stenosis

The most common cause of mitral stenosis remains rheumatic fever (Summary box 54.10), despite the fact that the incidence of overt rheumatic fever in the developed world has decreased. During the healing phase of acute rheumatic fever, the valve leaflets become adherent to each other at their free border so that the commissures become obliterated and the valve orifice narrows. Symptoms from mitral stenosis usually develop more than ten years after the acute attack.

Summary box 54.10

Causes of mitral valve disease

Stenosis
- Rheumatic heart disease (common)
- Calcification of valve or chordae
- Congenital (rare)

Regurgitation
- Rheumatic heart disease
- Valve prolapse
- Left ventricular dilatation or hypertrophy
- Ischaemia
- Bacterial endocarditis

Pathophysiology

Mitral stenosis slows ventricular filling during diastole and the pressure in the left atrium rises to maintain cardiac output. This leads to atrial hypertrophy and dilatation. Pulmonary congestion results from the rise in left atrial pressure but, with time, the lungs are protected against pulmonary oedema by constriction of the pulmonary vessels. However, this adaptive response, along with the passive 'back pressure' generated by the rise in left atrial pressure, leads to pulmonary hypertension. This leads to an increased demand on the right ventricle with eventual right heart failure and tricuspid regurgitation. The development of atrial fibrillation is common and can lead to a significant reduction in cardiac output. Atrial fibrillation predisposes to thrombi forming in the left atrium, which may embolise.

Clinical features

Patients may remain asymptomatic for years and then present with symptoms when the heart is stressed by an event such as pregnancy, fever or a chest infection, or with the onset of atrial fibrillation. The common symptoms are fatigue and dyspnoea on exertion, which result from the combination of reduced forward flow and increased back pressure. The resulting pulmonary congestion adds to the breathlessness and may produce a cough or haemoptysis. If mitral stenosis is advanced, there may also be a right ventricular heave due to right ventricular hypertrophy in response to pulmonary hypertension. Auscultation reveals an opening snap soon after the second heart sound, as the diseased valve is opened forcibly by the high pressure in the left atrium. The reverse happens when the valve closes and there is a loud 'tapping' first heart sound. In addition, a rumbling mid-diastolic murmur can be heard. The duration of the murmur is related to the severity of the mitral stenosis, increasing in length as the mitral stenosis becomes more severe.

Investigations

- **ECG** may show left atrial enlargement (P-mitrale) or AF. Right axis deviation and other ECG signs of right ventricular hypertrophy (tall QRS complexes in the right ventricular leads V1–3) may also be present.
- **Chest radiography**. There is a small aortic outline and a prominent pulmonary artery. The left atrium is enlarged (sometimes to an enormous degree) along with upper lobe diversion as a result of the raised pulmonary venous pressure. The right ventricle also appears enlarged (Figure 54.14).
- **Echocardiography**, in combination with colour flow Doppler imaging, allows assessment of the flow across the valve and, therefore, the degree of stenosis. Transoesophageal

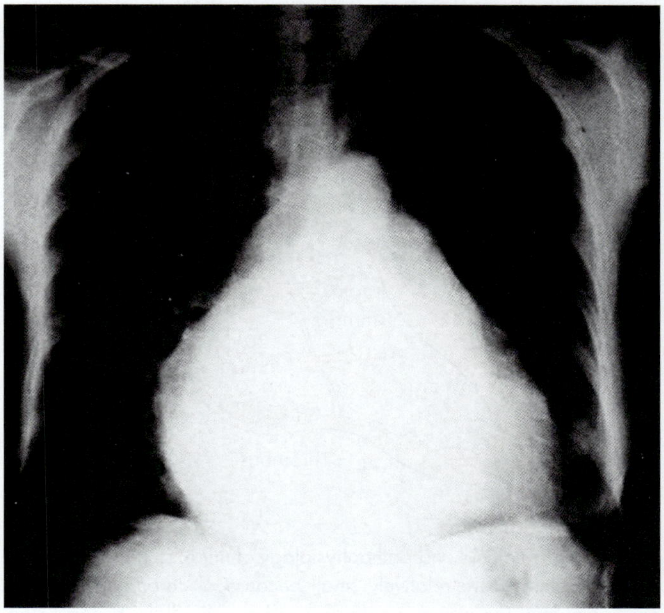

Figure 54.14 Chest radiograph of long-standing mitral stenosis, showing a massive left atrium.

echocardiography (TOE) may be better at assessing valve morphology in detail and excluding the presence of an atrial clot.

- **Coronary angiography**. To investigate the coronary arteries.

Indications for surgery

Medical management includes the use of anticoagulation in patients with AF or left atrial enlargement. Prophylactic antibiotics for endocarditis should be administered before invasive procedures. Tachyarrhythmias, including fast AF, which may lead to decompensation and cardiac failure, should be avoided. Digoxin is the mainstay of treatment, but other rate-controlling agents are increasingly used. Diuretics may provide some benefit. Surgery is indicated for severe symptoms (NYHA class III or IV), severe mitral stenosis (mitral valve area ≤1.5 cm^2), or signs of left ventricular dysfunction. These include an ejection fraction of less than 60 per cent and a left ventricular end systolic dimension (LVESD) of more than 45 mm, or systemic emboli. Prognosis is determined by the severity of the stenosis, the size of the atrium, the onset of AF, rising pulmonary artery pressure and the unpredictable risk of embolism from a large, fibrillating atrium (Figure 54.15). Surgical options include mitral valve repair or mitral valve replacement. Old surgical procedures, such as commissurotomy or valvotomy, are rarely currently performed.

Mitral valve operations

Depending on the type of procedure and approach to the mitral valve, a median sternotomy or, occasionally, a right thoracotomy is completed. The mitral valve can be approached directly through the left atrium in the interatrial groove, through the right atrium and then the interatrial septum, or through the left atrial appendage.

Mitral valve repair

The restoration of normal valve function and preservation of the mitral apparatus is preferable to replacement. The functional classification system developed by Carpentier serves as a guideline in valve reconstruction. It allows classification of any mitral insufficiency into one of three groups according to the amplitude of the leaflet motion and provides a useful framework for the mechanisms of failure of the mitral valve. As a rule, several valvular lesions or abnormalities are involved in a functional abnormality, with specific techniques developed to correct each lesion.

At surgery, the anatomy of the valvular apparatus and subvalvular structures has to be carefully inspected. In particular, the extent of annular dilatation, leaflet prolapse and chordal dysfunction are assessed. The mitral valve reconstruction is completed using various techniques, including insertion of a prosthetic ring annuloplasty (Figure 54.16), quadrangular resection of the leaflet, use of a sliding plasty, chordal shortening and chordal transposition. There are many different techniques which is an indication that so far, no one technique will address all the issues that can occur during mitral regurgitation. Valve repair, however, offers better preservation of ventricular function and avoids the need for prolonged anticoagulation as well as avoiding valve-related complications, such as PVE or structural dysfunction. Recent advances in surgical techniques and the development of various types of rings lead to increased use of mitral valve repair with excellent results making it the gold standard operation. The operative mortality is 1–3 per cent. Complication-free survival at five years ranges from 80 to 95 per cent.

Mitral valve replacement

When valve repair is not feasible mitral valve replacement is necessary. This usually involves a median sternotomy and access to the left atrium on CPB. The diseased valve is exposed, excised and a suitably sized mechanical or bioprosthetic valve is implanted. The atriotomy is closed following de-airing of the left heart. Intraoperative TOE can be used to assess adequate valve function.

The operative mortality rate for elective mitral valve replacement is approximately 5–6 per cent. This depends largely on the state of the myocardium and the general condition (including age) of the patient. Common serious in-hospital complications include stroke (<4 per cent) and renal failure (3 per cent), although any complication of heart surgery is possible. The longer-term prognosis for patients following mitral valve replacement is generally good in comparison with the natural history of mitral valve disease.

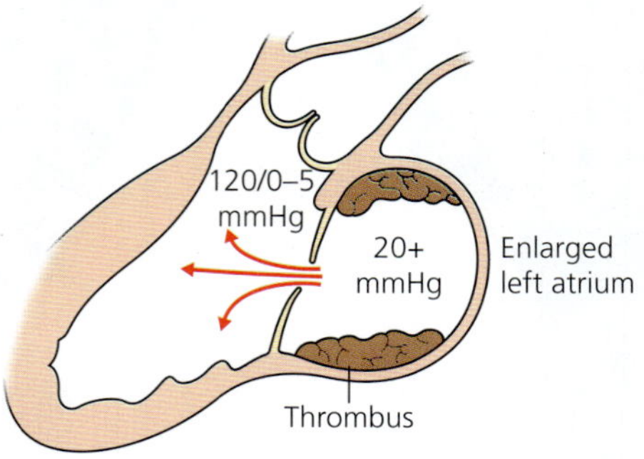

Figure 54.15 Features and pathophysiology of mitral stenosis. The aorta and left ventricle are relatively small because of chronically reduced cardiac output. The atrium is enlarged and may fibrillate, become stagnant and contain a thrombus. The ventricle fills with a turbulent jet that may be detected as a diastolic murmur or a thrill at the apex.

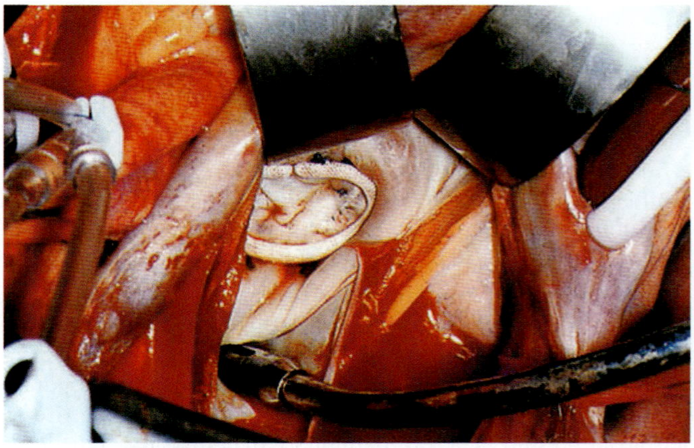

Figure 54.16 Operative view of the completed repair of a mitral valve using a Carpentier–Edwards annuloplasty ring (image courtesy of A Murday FRCS).

Alain Frédéric Carpentier, born 1933, cardiothoracic surgeon, Hôpital European Georges Pompidou, Paris, France, refered to as 'the father of modern mitral valve repair'.

Percutaneous mitral valve repair (MitraClip)

The MitraClip® is a device used to reduce mitral valve regurgitation. The method involves suturing of the leaflets of the mitral valve together so that regurgitation into the left atrium is prevented. The valve continues to open through the sides of the suture and therefore blood continues to flow into the left ventricle, although this method is less invasive, associated with rapid recovery, and reduced inhospital stay. However, it is technically demanding and long-term durability of the results of the device is unknown.

Recent data suggest that Mitraclip may be suitable for a small subset of high-risk or chronic heart failure patients, but not for the vast majority, who are better served by surgery, which leaves them with substantially less mitral regurgitation.

Aortic valve disease

Approximately two-thirds of all valve surgery performed in the UK is for aortic valve disease, which remains common despite a reduction in the incidence of rheumatic fever in the developed world.

Aortic stenosis

Aortic stenosis (AS), as opposed to aortic sclerosis, occurs when a pressure gradient can be demonstrated across the valve. Therefore, the difference is not absolute, as sclerosis can progress to stenosis. The common cause of aortic stenosis in adults is an acquired, degenerative, calcific process that results in immobile aortic valve cusps. Progressive fibrosis and calcification of a congenitally abnormal valve can mimic this degenerative process. The usual congenital abnormality is commissural fusion, leading to a bicuspid aortic valve, which occurs in approximately 1 per cent of the population (Figure 54.17).

Pathophysiology

A pressure gradient develops between the left ventricle and the aorta, with the left ventricle adapting to this systolic pressure overload by an increase in left ventricular wall thickness or hypertrophy. This adaptive response is an attempt to normalise left ventricular wall stress in the face of increased left ventricular systolic pressure, and may maintain a normal cardiac output, prevent left ventricular dilatation and avoid significant symptoms for a number of years. Eventually, myocardial function is affected and, together with insufficient left ventricular hypertrophy to normalise wall stress (load mismatch), ventricular contractility is reduced.

When aortic stenosis is severe and cardiac output is normal, a >50 mmHg gradient between peak systolic left ventricular and aortic pressure exists. As aortic stenosis worsens, cardiac output cannot increase with exertion and eventually becomes insufficient at rest. The reduction in ventricular contractility leads to an irreversible decline in left ventricular function, with dilatation and a rise in left ventricular end-diastolic pressure, to the point of overt left heart failure.

Clinical features

Patients are often asymptomatic until decompensation occurs, typically presenting with dyspnoea and angina, which is due to increased oxygen needs of the hypertrophied left ventricle, reduced coronary filling and inadequate cardiac output during exertion. Patients often describe a feeling of light-headedness or 'near' syncope on effort. Cardiac arrhythmias can also occur. Auscultation of the heart demonstrates a murmur that is typically harsh, ejection in nature and best heard over the aortic area with radiation to the carotids. With critical aortic stenosis and a fall in cardiac output, the murmur may become quieter. The apex beat may be displaced in late disease along with signs of cardiac congestion (Figure 54.18).

Investigations

- **ECG**. There is left ventricular hypertrophy with tall R waves in the lateral leads and sometimes a 'strain pattern' (S–T depression with inverted T waves in the lateral leads).
- **Chest radiography**. May be normal. Cardiomegaly and pulmonary congestion can be seen in the presence of left ventricular failure. Post-stenotic dilatation of the aorta is occasionally seen (Figure 54.19).

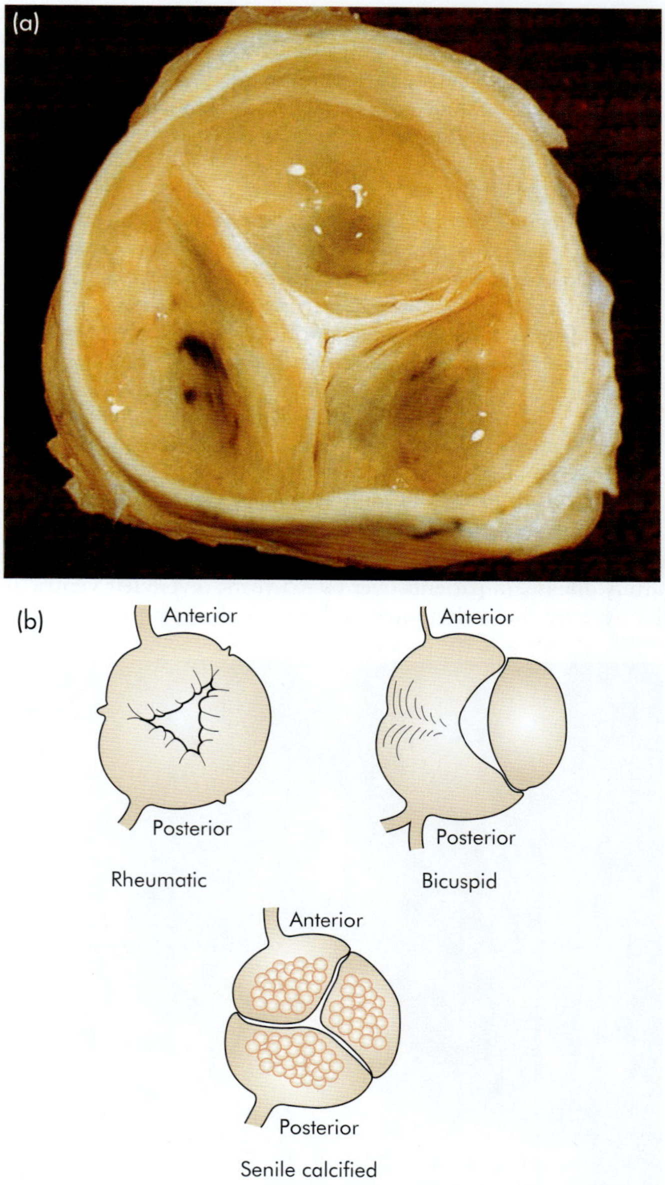

Figure 54.17 (a) Formaldehyde-treated aortic valve (normal tricuspid configuration). (b) Aortic stenosis, different pathologies.

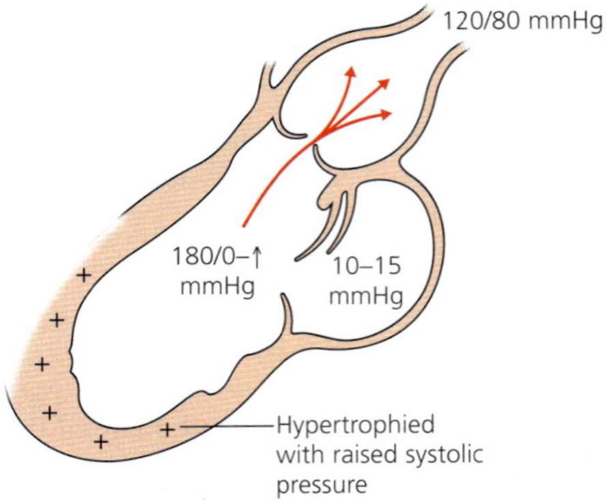

Figure 54.18 Features and pathophysiology of aortic stenosis. Haemodynamic changes in aortic stenosis. Aorta with post-stenotic dilatation.

- **Echocardiography** confirms the diagnosis and, together with colour flow Doppler imaging, allows assessment of the aortic valve gradient, calculation of valve area, and evaluation of left ventricular dimensions and wall thickness.
- **Coronary angiography**. To investigate the coronary arteries.

Indications for surgery

Medical management focuses on the avoidance of systemic hypotension and arterial vasodilatation, which may reduce myocardial perfusion pressure and therefore provoke ischaemia.

The natural history of symptomatic patients with aortic stenosis is dismal, with a ten-year mortality rate of 80–90 per cent. The patient is at risk of sudden death related to the severity of the stenosis. An estimated or actual peak systolic gradient of >6.7 kPa (50 mmHg) with impaired ventricular function on dynamic testing is sufficient indication for aortic valve replacement.

Indications for surgery in asymptomatic patients with severe aortic stenosis are controversial. Most would consider surgery in patients with left ventricular dysfunction, concomitant coronary artery disease, in patients over 60–65 years, severe left ventricular hypertrophy, arrhythmias and silent ischaemia.

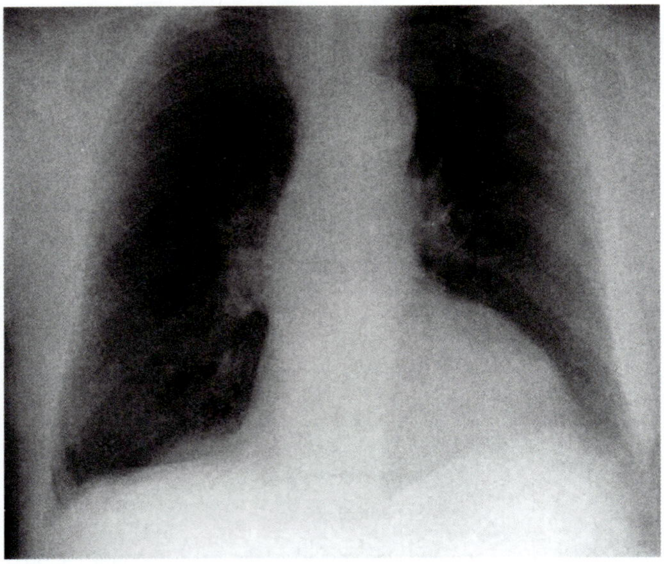

Figure 54.19 Chest radiograph in aortic stenosis.

Aortic regurgitation

The causes of aortic regurgitation can be classified according to the speed of development of the regurgitant jet (acute or chronic) or according to the anatomical location of pathology (valve leaflet or aortic wall). The causes of acute aortic regurgitation include infective endocarditis, aortic dissection and trauma. The common causes of chronic aortic regurgitation include degeneration leading to aortic root and/or annular dilatation, congenital bicuspid valve and previous rheumatic fever or endocarditis (Summary box 54.11).

Summary box 54.11

Causes of aortic regurgitation according to predominant anatomical location of pathology

Valve leaflet disease

- Congenital, e.g. bicuspid valve leading to degenerative changes, with ventricular septal defect
- Rheumatic heart disease
- Infective endocarditis

Aortic wall pathology

- Inflammatory, e.g. connective tissue disorders, such as ankylosing spondylitis, systemic lupus erythematosus, rheumatoid arthritis
- Systemic disease, e.g. tertiary syphilis
- Degenerative, e.g. Marfan syndrome, aortic root dissection, senile aortopathy, leading to aortic root/annular dilatation

Adapted from Petch M. Aortic valve disease. *Medicine* 1997; **25**: 31.

Pathophysiology

Acute aortic regurgitation imposes a volume load on the left ventricle because of backflow. It causes a sharp rise in left ventricular end-diastolic pressure, premature closure of the mitral valve and inadequate forward left ventricular filling. The result is sudden haemodynamic deterioration and acute respiratory compromise.

In chronic aortic regurgitation, volume load and left ventricular end-diastolic pressure increase gradually, leading to compensatory left ventricular dilatation and eccentric hypertrophy to maintain adequate cardiac output. Systolic and diastolic function is abnormal, and sudden deterioration can occur.

Clinical features

Long-standing aortic regurgitation is asymptomatic until the left ventricle begins to fail, when exertional dyspnoea may be the only symptom. Angina can also develop. A wide pulse pressure due to a reduction in diastolic pressure and collapsing pulse (waterhammer pulse) are commonly seen. Other manifestations of the wide pulse pressure include visible capillary pulsation of the nail bed (Quincke's sign), pulsatile head bobbing (de Musset's sign), visible arterial pulsation in the neck (Corrigan's sign), a 'pistol shot' sound on auscultating over the femoral artery (Traube's sign) and uvular pulsation (Müller's sign). The apex is displaced laterally, often visible and hyperdynamic or

Ludwig Traube, 1818–1876, physician, The Charité, Berlin, Germany. He worked alongside Rudolf Virchow (1821–1902) and was cofounder of the science of experimental pathology in Germany.

'thrusting' in nature because of the left ventricular hypertrophy. Auscultation reveals a high-pitched early diastolic murmur best heard at the left sternal edge (Figure 54.20).

Investigations

- **ECG**. There is left ventricular hypertrophy and sometimes a 'strain pattern'.
- **Chest radiography**. Cardiomegaly can be seen if the left ventricle is dilating; sometimes, the aortic shadow may also indicate dilatation.
- **Echocardiography**. This allows assessment of the underlying cause and severity of aortic regurgitation and enables the diameter of the aortic root, as well as left ventricular dimensions, to be determined. Colour flow Doppler imaging quantifies the size of the regurgitant jet.
- **Coronary angiography**. To investigate the coronary arteries.

Indications for surgery

Medical therapy with vasodilator drugs for the relief of dyspnoea or angina is designed to improve forward stroke volume and reduce regurgitant volume. However, symptomatic relief does not alter the need for valve surgery.

The indications for surgery are the onset of symptoms of NYHA class III or IV. Minor degrees of aortic regurgitation are well tolerated, but if the left ventricle deteriorates and dilates it may be too late for surgery. An end-diastolic pressure of >70 mmHg, an end-systolic pressure of >50 mmHg, an end systolic dimension of >50 mm and an end-diastolic dimension of >70 mm indicate severe pathology warranting surgical intervention, even in patients with mild symptoms (NYHA class II). Asymptomatic patients with left ventricular dysfunction during exercise should be followed up with regular echocardiography. Aortic valve replacement is recommended if there is progressive left ventricular dilatation or a fall in systolic function occurs (Summary box 54.12).

Aortic valve surgery

Unlike mitral valve surgery, there are few occasions when the aortic valve can be repaired and usually the valve requires replacement. However, in neonates and children, aortic valve repair or valvotomy is well established. Percutaneous aortic balloon valvotomy has a role in children, but appears to offer no benefits in adult aortic valve disease.

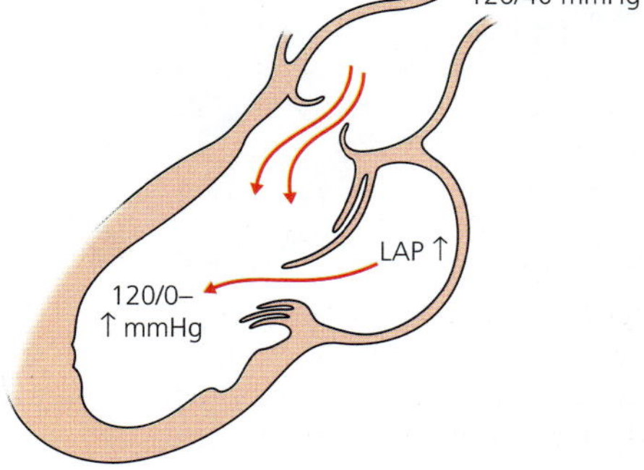

Figure 54.20 Haemodynamic consequences of aortic regurgitation. The left ventricle dilates and hypertrophies and there is a diastolic murmur. LAP, left atrial pressure.

Summary box 54.12

Causes of aortic valve disease

Stenosis
- Congenital
- Rheumatic heart disease
- Acquired calcification and fibrosis of valve or chordae tendineae with age

Regurgitation
- Rheumatic heart disease
- Infective endocarditis
- Congenital
- Inflammatory:
  - Systemic lupus erythematosus
  - Rheumatic ankylosing spondylitis
- Dilatation of aortic root:
  - Marfan syndrome
  - Dissection
- Systemic disease:
  - Syphilis
  - Ulcerative colitis

Aortic valve replacement

This is performed through a median sternotomy on CPB. The aorta is cross-clamped and opened proximally to reveal the diseased valve. Cardioplegic solution is infused into the coronary arteries to arrest the heart in diastole. The valve is then excised leaving the annulus *in situ*, but removing as much calcific debris as possible. The annulus is sized and the mechanical or biological valve is then sutured into position at the level of the native annulus and the aortotomy is closed.

The operative mortality rate for elective aortic valve surgery is <5 per cent, but is higher in emergency surgery, in surgery for endocarditis and in older patients.

Major complications include stroke (2 per cent), perioperative myocardial infarction (2 per cent) and heart block requiring a permanent pacemaker (<1 per cent). The major determinant of late survival after aortic valve surgery is preoperative left ventricular function. The five-year survival rate is approximately 75–85 per cent, with the majority of late deaths related to myocardial factors.

Transcatheter aortic-valve implantation

Although aortic valve replacement (AVR) is still the gold standard treatment, a significant number of patients affected by severe AS requiring AVR do not undergo surgery because they are considered too old or too frail for such an invasive procedure, or because they are affected by concomitant comorbidities that noticeably increase the operative risk. In such patients, transcatheter aortic valve implantation is an attractive alternative to standard AVR. Other indications include heavily calcified ascending aorta ('porcelain' aorta) and the presence of a severe congenital thoracic distortion.

There are different approaches for valve implantation; the most commonly used are transapical (antegrade) and transluminal (retrograde).

- **Transapical approach**. The main advantage of performing transapical procedures is that the feasibility does not rely on the absence of a concomitant peripheral vascular disease

Heinrich Irenaeus Quincke, 1842–1922, Professor of Medicine, Keil, Germany.
Louis Charles Alfred de Musset, 1810–1857, French poet and playwright in whom the sign traditionally was first noticed.
Sir Dominic John Corrigan, 1802–1880, physician, The Charitable Infirmary, Jervis Street, Dublin, Ireland.
Friedrich von Müller, 1858–1941, a physician of Munich, Germany.

or previous aortic surgery. This approach reduces the risk of calcium dislodgement due to the passage of a stiff transluminal device into a diseased aortic arch. In transapical transcatheter aortic-valve implantation (TAVI), the cardiac apex is prepared through a small left anterolateral mini-thoracotomy using a purse-string or a crossing suture reinforced by pledgets and, after the procedure, a chest tube is routinely inserted into the left pleura.

- **Transluminal approach**. This can be carried out via the femoral or subclavian artery. This is a useful technique for patients with previous cardiac surgery; however, the presence of peripheral vascular disease, small vessel diameters, tortuous vessels, aortic disease or previous aortic surgery contraindicates this approach.

Whichever approach is used, a balloon catheter is advanced into the left ventricle over a guidewire and positioned at the opening of the aortic valve. The existing aortic valve is dilated in order to make room for the prosthetic valve. Rapid right ventricular pacing is used to interrupt cardiac output through the existing aortic valve and to reduce movement during implantation. The new valve, mounted on a metal stent, is manipulated into position and is either self-expanding or deployed using balloon inflation. Deployment leads to obliteration of the existing aortic valve.

Complications associated with TAVI include mortality (5–18 per cent at 30 days), mild-to-moderate aortic regurgitation (30–50 per cent), stroke (3–9 per cent), perioperative open conversion (9–12 per cent), vascular complications (10–15 per cent) and atrioventricular block (4–8 per cent). A recent myocardial infarction (less than three months), severe pulmonary dysfunction, and the presence of an apical thrombus are contraindications for transapical TAVI, whereas a left ventricular ejection fraction (LVEF) below or equal to 20 per cent contraindicates all TAVI procedures.

CONGENITAL HEART DISEASE

Introduction

Congenital heart diseases are abnormalities of cardiac structure that are present from birth. Such abnormalities in the development of the heart typically arise in the third to eighth week of gestation. The first operation for congenital heart disease was the ligation of a patent ductus arteriosus (PDA) by Gross in 1938. With the development of neonatal CPB, improved methods of myocardial protection and microsurgical techniques, an increasing number of corrective and palliative operations is possible.

Development of the heart and fetal circulation and circulatory changes at birth

By 12 weeks of fetal life, the primitive vascular tube is fully developed. The fetal circulation differs from that of the adult in that the right and left ventricles pump blood in parallel rather than in series. Such an arrangement allows the heart and head to receive more highly oxygenated blood. In the fetus, this is possible because of the presence of three structural shunts: the ductus venosus, the foramen ovale and the ductus arteriosus (Figure 54.21).

Soon after birth, pulmonary vascular resistance falls because of the action of breathing and the resulting pulmonary vasodilatation. In addition, within 30 minutes of delivery, the ductus arteriosus constricts in response to an increase in blood oxygen levels. The result is a reversal of the pulmonary–systemic pressure gradient and termination of blood flow from the pulmonary artery into the aorta.

After birth, the act of cutting and tying the umbilical cord stops venous blood flow from the placenta. This lowers the pressure in the inferior vena cava and, with the fall in pulmonary vascular resistance, right atrial pressure falls. The result is closure of the foramen ovale. The abolition of venous return from the placenta also causes the ductus venosus to close.

The closure of the fetal circulatory shunts in the few hours following birth is functional, with complete structural closure typically taking several months. In 20 per cent of adults, the structural closure of the foramen ovale remains incomplete, but is of no cardiovascular significance.

Abnormalities of cardiac structure may arise from the persistence of normal fetal channels (PDA, patent foramen ovale), failure of septation (atrial septal defect, ventricular septal defect, tetralogy of Fallot), stenosis (intracardiac–supravalvular, valvular, infravalvular or extracardiac–coarctation of the aorta), atresia or abnormal connections (transposition of the great arteries, total anomalous venous drainage). Fetal echocardiography is now sufficiently sensitive to detect intracardiac lesions in the second trimester.

Incidence

Congenital heart disease is the most common congenital abnormality in the UK; the incidence of significant cardiac abnormalities is eight cases per 1000 live births. Many

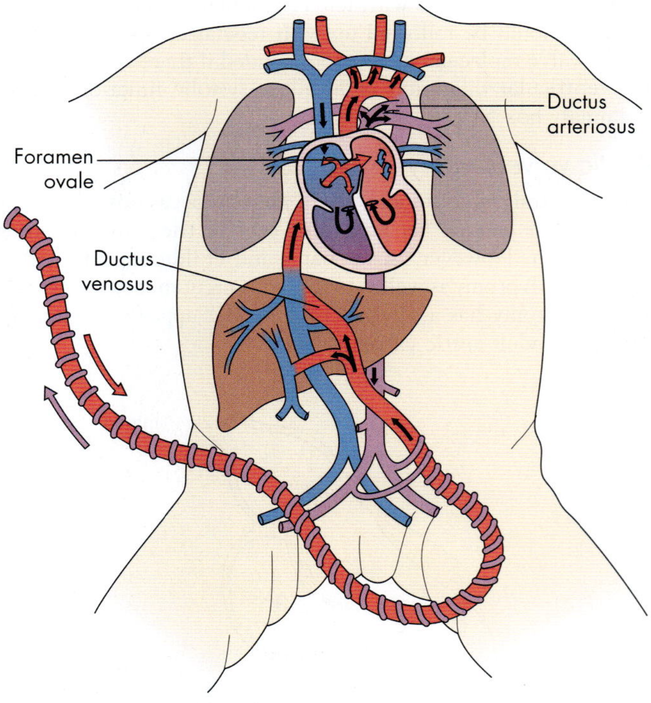

Figure 54.21 Fetal circulation.

Etienne Arthur Louis Fallot, 1850–1911, Professor of Medicine, Marseilles, France.
Jacqueline Ann Noonan, born 1921, paediatric cardiologist, The University of Kentucky College of Medicine, Lexington, KY, USA, described this condition in 1963.

PART 9 | CARDIOTHORACIC

spontaneous abortions or stillbirths have cardiac malformations or chromosomal abnormalities associated with structural heart defects. In neonates and children with congenital heart disease, 15 per cent will have more than one cardiac abnormality and 15 per cent will have another extracardiac abnormality.

Aetiology

There is often no obvious aetiology; most abnormalities appear to be multifactorial with both genetic and environmental influences. There are well-recognised associations (Summary box 54.13).

Summary box 54.13

Recognised associations with congenital heart disease

- Maternal (environmental) factors
  - Infection: rubella
  - Disease: systemic lupus erythematosus, diabetes mellitus
  - Drugs/medications: alcohol abuse, warfarin, phenytoin
- Genetic factors
  - Single gene defects: Marfan, Noonan and Holt–Oram syndromes
  - Chromosomal defects: trisomy 21 (Down syndrome), trisomy 18 (Edwards syndrome), trisomy 13 (Patau syndrome), Turner syndrome
  - Deletions: DiGeorge and Williams syndromes

Diagnosis

Occasionally, an antenatal diagnosis is possible, with severe congenital heart disease detected *in utero* at 16–18 weeks. If an infant is suspected of having a congenital heart disease, a diagnostic evaluation begins with an accurate history from the parents and specific questions about maternal health and drug intake during pregnancy. A detailed family history is important because some defects are familial. Clinical examination may reveal a murmur, evidence of heart failure, failure to thrive and cyanosis. In addition, congenital heart disease can present with hypertension, an arrhythmia, evidence of polycythaemia or a thromboembolic event. Investigation is much the same as for the adult patient and, with fetal echocardiography available, cardiac catheterisation is now avoided whenever possible.

Classification

Congenital heart disease can be broadly classified according to the presence or absence of cyanosis, although the distinction is not always clear-cut. The presence of central cyanosis, blueness of the trunk and mucous membranes, results from levels of deoxygenated haemoglobin of >3–5 g/dL in the arterial circulation.

Cyanotic congenital heart diseases make up one-third of cases and are usually more complex, although they do include simple defects. Cyanotic congenital cardiac lesions can involve:

- A right-to-left shunt resulting in decreased pulmonary blood flow. Many of these lesions consist of a septal defect in conjunction with a right-sided obstructive lesion, producing an obligatory right-to-left shunt. The most common cause of this is tetralogy of Fallot.
- Parallel systemic and pulmonary blood flow rather than in series. If there is no mixing, this is incompatible with life, so typically neonates have a patent foramen ovale that allows some mixing of the two circulations at this level. The most common example of this is transposition of the great vessels (TGV).
- Defects in the connections of the heart in which there is mixing of the systemic and pulmonary flows. An example of such a complex lesion is total anomalous pulmonary venous drainage.

Acyanotic congenital heart diseases represent the other two-thirds of cases and are usually less complex. Such defects result in an increase in the work imposed on the heart because of either:

- A left-to-right shunt with increased pulmonary blood flow, which causes an increase in volume work of the heart. Examples include PDA, atrial septal defect (ASD) and ventricular septal defect (VSD).
- Obstruction of the blood flow across a heart valve on the left side of the heart, such as aortic stenosis, or in the aorta itself, as occurs with coarctation of the aorta, leading to an increase in pressure and work of the heart.

Typically, acyanotic congenital heart disease presents as heart failure in infancy because of pulmonary congestion caused by increased pulmonary blood flow or increased pulmonary venous blood pressure resulting from an obstructive lesion. The common acyanotic cardiac defects can also present as a murmur in infancy or later.

Cyanotic congenital heart disease

Fallot's tetralogy

This is the most common cyanotic congenital heart disease found in children surviving to one year and accounts for about 4–6 per cent of all congenital heart diseases. The four intracardiac lesions originally described (Figure 54.22) were:

- VSD
- overriding aorta
- pulmonary (typically infundibular or subpulmonary) stenosis
- right ventricular hypertrophy.

Clinically, there may be no signs initially but, as pulmonary stenosis progresses, cyanosis typically develops within the first year of life. Squatting is an adaptation by the child to hypoxic spells. This increases systemic vascular resistance and the venous return to the heart and consequently blood is diverted into the pulmonary circulation with increased oxygenation. Lethargy and tiredness are also common. Classically the chest radiograph demonstrates a 'boot-shaped' heart with poorly developed lung vasculature. The diagnosis is confirmed with echocardiography. Surgery to correct the tetralogy can be performed early as a single complete primary repair or later following an initial palliative shunt, which diverts systemic blood into the pulmonary circulation and may be used to improve oxygenation. The results of surgery are good, with a late survival rate at five to ten years following correction of tetralogy of 95 per cent, an operative mortality rate for a repair of between 5 and 10 per cent, and an incidence of reoperation following tetralogy repair of 5–10 per cent.

Mary Clayton Holt, born 1924, cardiologist, The London Hospital for Women and Children, London, UK.
Samuel Oram, 1913–1991, cardiologist, King's College Hospital, London, UK.
Holt and Oram described this condition in a joint paper in 1960.
John Hilton Edwards, 1928–2007, Professor of Genetics, The University of Oxford, UK.

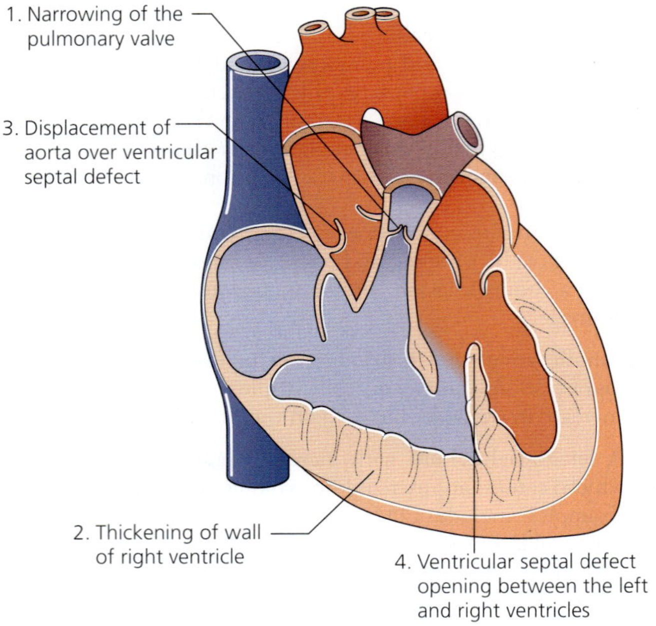

Figure 54.22 Fallot's tetralogy. Four abnormalities that result in insufficiently oxygenated blood being pumped to the body.

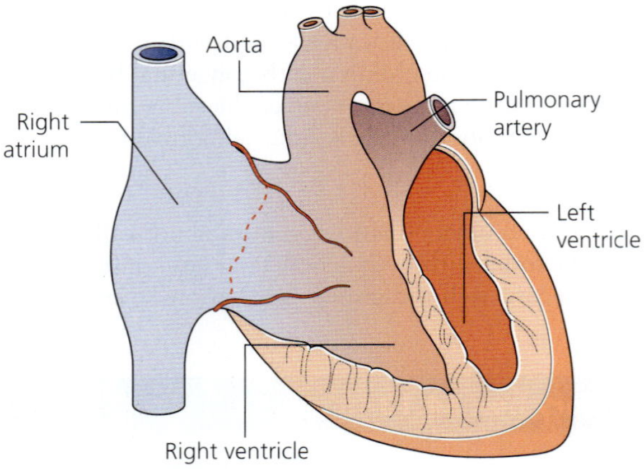

Figure 54.23 Transposition of the great vessels.

Transposition of the great vessels

The condition, first described by Morgagni, is the second most common cyanotic congenital heart disease and is the most common cause of cyanosis from a congenital cardiac defect discovered in the newborn period. TGV results from abnormal development and typically occurs when the aorta arises from the right ventricle and the pulmonary artery from the left ventricle (Figure 54.23). The resulting transposition causes the pulmonary and systemic circulations to run in parallel rather than in series, so that oxygenated pulmonary venous blood returns back to the lungs and desaturated systemic venous blood is pumped around the body. The situation is incompatible with life and mixing of the blood must occur through associated shunts such as a patent foramen ovale or associated VSD. The most obvious presentation is severe central cyanosis ocurring in the first 48 hours of life. However, if there is a large ASD or VSD, there may be minimal cyanosis initially. Typically, progress is poor and, as pulmonary vascular resistance declines in the neonatal period, high pulmonary flow develops, with cardiac enlargement and left ventricular failure.

The chest radiograph shows pulmonary plethora, with the heart having an 'egg on its side' appearance, with a small pedicle (aorta in front of pulmonary artery). Cardiac catheterisation and echocardiography confirm the diagnosis and delineate the anatomy. Initial palliation is by percutaneous (Rashkind) balloon atrial septostomy or, alternatively, intravenous prostaglandin to keep the ductus open. Definitive repair is usually by the arterial switch procedure, mostly carried out as a two-stage procedure, whereby the pulmonary artery is first banded to 'tone up' the left ventricle. However, the arterial switch procedure without prior pulmonary artery banding is increasingly being carried out in the newborn with TGV and an intact ventricular septum. The long-term results are impressive and it has replaced the atrial switch or baffle (Mustard or Senning) operations.

Total anomalous pulmonary venous drainage

Total anomalous pulmonary venous drainage (TAPVD) accounts for only 1–2 per cent of congenital heart disease. In this condition, the pulmonary venous drainage has become disconnected from the left atrium and drains into the systemic venous circulation at some other point (inferior vena cava, superior vena cava, coronary sinus or right atrium). Typically, TAPVD presents after the first week of life with cyanosis that is mild to moderate depending on pulmonary flow. Infants with high pulmonary flow develop cardiac failure, recurrent chest infections, failure to thrive and feeding difficulties. If high pulmonary flow is associated with a large ASD, cyanosis is often minimal and the lesion is tolerated well. If there is additional venous obstruction, cyanosis presents at birth with dyspnoea and pulmonary oedema. Echocardiography and cardiac (pulmonary) angiography are necessary to confirm the diagnosis and establish the location of the anomalous drainage.

The surgical principle is to re-establish the pulmonary venous drainage into the left atrium. The exact operative technique depends on the anatomy and type of TAPVD. The long-term results for survivors of the operation are generally good. Late death following repair is uncommon but, when it occurs, it is often caused by intimal fibroplasia of the pulmonary veins away from the anastomosis.

Eisenmenger's syndrome

Eisenmenger's syndrome is becoming less common as corrective surgery is undertaken increasingly early and fewer patients develop a fixed increase in their pulmonary vascular resistance. It occurs following the reversal of a left-to-right shunt across a previous left-to-right shunt, such as with an ASD, VSD or a patent ductus arteriosus. These congenital anomalies cause an increase in flow and higher right-sided pressures, which lead to compensatory right ventricular hypertrophy and a subsequent rise in pulmonary artery pressure. Increasing pulmonary hypertension leads to equalisation of pressures either side of the shunt but, at some point, the right-sided pressures will exceed those on the left side, resulting in shunt reversal and desaturated blood entering the left side of the circulation. Cyanosis and dyspnoea are the most common clinical features. Closure of the shunt is contraindicated if pulmonary hypertension is irreversible

William Jacobson Rashkind, born 1922, surgeon, The Childern's Hospital, Philadelphia, PA, USA.
William T Mustard, formerly Associate Professor of Surgey, The Hospital for Sick Children, Toronto, Ontario, Canada.
Ake Senning, 1915–2000, Professor of Surgery, The University Hospital, Zurich, Switzerland.

because the right-to-left shunt now serves to decompress the pulmonary circulation.

Acyanotic congenital heart disease

Patent ductus arteriosus

The ductus arteriosus, a normal fetal communication, facilitates the transfer of oxygenated blood from the pulmonary artery to the aorta, shunting blood away from the lungs. Normally, functional closure of the ductus occurs within a few hours of birth; it is abnormal if it persists beyond the neonatal period. The ductus closes in response to an increase in peripheral oxygen saturation and a drop in the resistance of the pulmonary circulation as the lungs expand; this causes the ductal tissue to contract through a prostaglandin inhibition mechanism. A cycloxygenase inhibitor (e.g. indomethacin) may be used therapeutically to close the ductus in the first few weeks of life. In premature babies, the ductus is more likely to remain patent for longer or permanently. In the isolated case of PDA, there is a left-to-right shunt of blood, resulting in a high pulmonary blood flow. Small shunts usually cause few symptoms and signs apart from the continuous machinery murmur in the left second intercostal space. Larger ducts cause cardiac failure and can uncommonly lead to shunt reversal with cyanosis and clubbing. The diagnosis is best confirmed by echocardiography with colour flow Doppler imaging. Cardiac catheterisation is performed only if additional lesions are suspected.

After six months of age, spontaneous closure of a PDA is rare. Most should be closed by preschool age, regardless of the absence of symptoms, if the risks of infective endocarditis, developing left ventricular failure or, rarely, Eisenmenger's syndrome are to be avoided. In the adult, surgical treatment is indicated if there is a persistent left-to-right shunt, even in the presence of pulmonary hypertension. In the premature infant, if medical treatment to close the ductus is unsuccessful, the lesion may be treated by interventional cardiology using an umbrella or coil duct occlusion device inserted percutaneously. If the lesion is very large or the patient very small, surgical closure via a left thoracotomy is preferred. This can be accomplished by either ligation or division of the PDA. The operative mortality rate is low and outcome generally very good.

Coarctation of the aorta

This accounts for 6–7 per cent of congenital heart disease and is defined as a haemodynamically significant narrowing of the aorta, usually in the descending aorta just distal to the left subclavian artery, around the area of the ductus arteriosus (Figure 54.24). The coarctation typically puts a pressure load on the left ventricle, which can ultimately fail. The upper body is well perfused but the lower body, including the kidneys, is poorly perfused, leading to fluid overload, excess renin secretion and acidosis. Coarctation usually affects boys and if it occurs in girls is suggestive of Turner's syndrome.

In the neonatal period, coarctation, often referred to as 'infantile' or preductal coarctation, presents with symptoms of heart failure. The child may appear well in the first few days of life because the coarctation is bypassed by the ductus arteriosus and oxygenated blood reaches the entire systemic circulation. As the ductus closes, the child becomes progressively more unwell. In adult-type coarctation, which is often juxtaductal or slightly postductal, obstruction is gradual with complications developing in adolescence or early adulthood. Hypertension is a common presenting problem in older children, often upper body hypertension only with development of enormous collateral vessels that may cause rib-notching and flow murmurs over the scapula. Other symptoms include prominent pulsation in the neck, tired legs or intermittent claudication on exercise. Clinical examination of the pulses may demonstrate a radio-femoral delay and a murmur that is continuous and heard best over the thoracic spine or below the left clavicle.

The chest radiograph classically demonstrates rib-notching from the age of six to eight years because of dilated posterior intercostal vessels. The heart is usually of normal size in the older child and shows a classical 'three sign' replacing the typical aortic knuckle. The upper part of the three sign is the dilated left subclavian, the middle part is the narrowing at the coarctation site, and the lower part is the post-stenotic dilatation of the descending aorta. Echocardiography is diagnostic, with cardiac catheterisation performed if other anomalies are present. Infant coarctation typically presents with cardiac failure, often requiring vigorous medical treatment, including the administration of prostoglandin to reopen the ductus and general resuscitation, before corrective surgery. Definitive treatment is usually surgical repair via a left thoracotomy. Coarctation presenting in the child or later typically requires surgical repair, as most patients die before the age of 40 years because of the associated complications. Percutaneous balloon dilatation is an alternative procedure in older children and adults and, in particular, for recoarctation. Without correction, the majority of deaths are caused by heart failure, infective endocarditis, rupture of the aorta or haemorrhagic stroke. The preoperative hypertension may not resolve despite surgical repair.

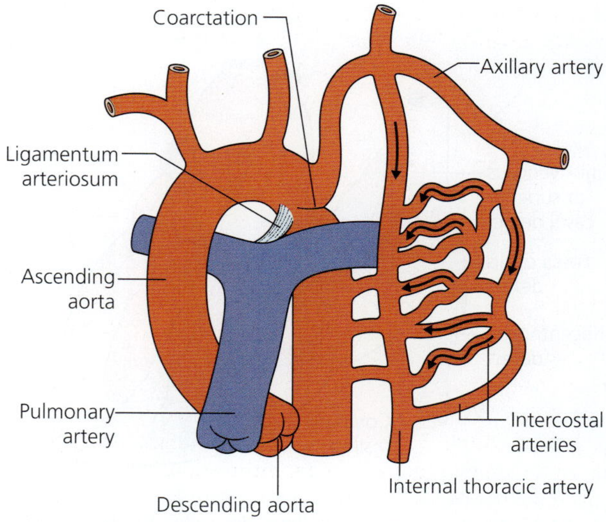

Figure 54.24 Coarctation of the aorta. Coarctation causes severe obstruction of blood flow in the descending thoracic aorta. The descending aorta and its branches are perfused by collateral channels from the axillary and internal thoracic arteries through the intercostal arteries (arrows).

Victor Eisenmenger, 1864–1932, Austrian physician who first described this condition in 1897, but the term 'Eisenmenger's syndrome' was first introduced in 1958 by Paul Hamilton Wood (1907–1962).

Henry Hubert Turner, 1892–1970, Professor of Medicine, The University of Oklahoma, Oklahoma City, OK, USA.

Atrial septal defects

An ASD is a defect in the septum between the left and right atria leading to a left-to-right shunt, the significance of which is determined by the size of the defect and the relative compliance of the ventricles. The development of the atrial septum is complex and abnormalities of development lead to three commonly recognised ASDs (Figure 54.25).

The most common type is an ostium secundum ASD. The anomaly is caused by a defect in the floor of the fossa ovalis, resulting in failure of the septum secundum to develop completely and cover the foramen ovale. Secundum defects are usually asymptomatic in childhood, with symptoms developing insidiously, typically presenting in middle age with congestive cardiac failure secondary to pulmonary hypertension or with atrial arrhythmias.

In ostium primum ASD, the anomaly is a form of partial atrioventricular canal defect or endocardial cushion defect. The abnormalities are confined to the atrial septum and are caused by the endocardial cushions failing to develop and so close the ostium primum part of the interatrial septum. The defect is associated with abnormalities of the mitral valve, leading to mitral regurgitation. There is a relatively high incidence of this abnormality in trisomy 21 (Down syndrome). Typically, the primum defect presents earlier than ostium secundum in childhood, with dyspnoea, recurrent chest infections and, if pulmonary hypertension develops, cyanosis.

A sinus venosus ASD is a rare defect and is the result of failure of partition of the pulmonary and systemic venous circulations. These defects are most commonly located high in the atrial septum at the junction of the superior vena cava and the right atrium. They are frequently associated with anomalous pulmonary venous drainage with right superior pulmonary veins draining into the superior vena cava or right atrium directly (Summary box 54.14).

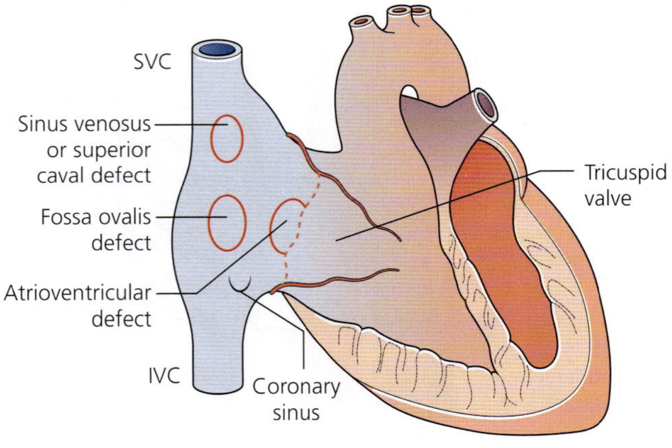

Figure 54.25 Atrial septum viewed from the right. The fossa ovalis is a useful reference point; the most common defect is in this area and is called a fossa ovalis (or ostium secundum) defect. A defect near the atrioventricular junction may be part of the spectrum of atrioventricular septal defects; if the defect is near the entry of the superior vena cava (SVC), it is commonly associated with anomalies of venous drainage into the atria. IVC, inferior vena cava.

Summary box 54.14

ASDs

- Common defects
  - Ostium secundum: fossa ovalis defect (approximately 70 per cent of ASDs)
  - Ostium primum: atrioventricular septal defect (approximately 20 per cent of ASDs)
  - Sinus venosus defect: often associated with anomalous pulmonary venous drainage (approximately 10 per cent of ASDs)
  - Patent foramen ovale: common in isolation, usually no left-to-right shunt (not strictly an ASD)
- Rarer defects
  - Inferior vena cava defects: a low sinus venosus defect and may allow shunting of blood into the left atrium
  - Coronary sinus septal defect: also known as unroofed coronary sinus with the left superior vena cava draining to the left atrium as part of a more complex lesion

Closure is performed during the first decade of life, even in the absence of symptoms, to avoid late-onset right ventricular failure, endocarditis and paradoxical emboli. In adults, closure is still appropriate for symptomatic improvement and avoidance of complications. The traditional method of closure involves open-heart surgery with CPB and closure of the defect either directly with sutures, as with most secundum defects, or, if the defect is large, using a pericardial or synthetic patch. Closure of small to moderate ASDs using percutaneous catheter-delivered devices in the cardiology catheter laboratory is increasingly common. Primum atrioventricular defect repairs may require additional mitral valve repair. The operative mortality rate for isolated atrioventricular defect repairs is <1 per cent, with an excellent prognosis. Surgical correction of complete atrioventricular canal defects, with closure of the ASD and ventricular septal components and mitral valve repair, is possible with a higher surgical mortality rate.

Ventricular septal defects

A VSD is a defect in the interventricular septum that allows a left-to-right shunting of blood. VSDs account for 20–30 per cent of congenital heart disease and affect approximately 2 in 1000 live births. They may occur in isolation or as part of a more complex set of cardiac abnormalities (e.g. tetralogy of Fallot, complete atrioventricular canal defect). Four major anatomical types of VSD are described, based on the anatomical subsections of the interventricular septum (Summary box 54.15 and Figure 54.26).

The VSD permits a left-to-right shunt at the ventricular level, with subsequent right ventricular volume overload and increased pulmonary blood flow. This may lead to progressive pulmonary oedema and congestive cardiac failure. Persistently elevated pulmonary blood flow and pulmonary vascular resistance also lead to irreversible pulmonary hypertension. They may eventually result in reversal of flow across the defect and Eisenmenger's syndrome. The clinical presentation reflects the magnitude of the left-to-right shunt, which in turn depends on the size of the VSD and the pulmonary and systemic vascular resistances. Small defects may close or cause little systemic disturbance (maladie de Roger); infants are asymptomatic with

Summary box 54.15

Types of VSD

- Perimembranous defect
  Also called conoventricular VSD; the most common defect (70–80 per cent), usually located within the membranous septum and may extend to the tricuspid valve annulus or base of the aortic valve
- Muscular defect
  Also called trabecular VSD; occurs in 10 per cent of cases and is located within the membranous septum and often multiple
- Atrioventricular defect
  Also called atrioventricular canal-type defect; occurs in 5 per cent of cases and is located in the atrioventricular canal beneath the tricuspid valve
- Subarterial defect
  Also called infundibular or subarterial VSD; occurs in 5–10 per cent of cases and lies within the conal septum immediately subaortic

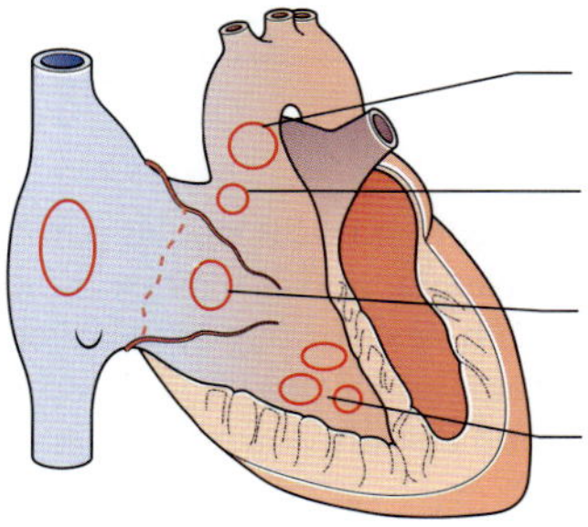

Figure 54.26 Ventricular septum viewed from the right, showing the characteristic sites of ventricular septal defects.

normal development. In the first five years, up to 30–50 per cent of VSDs close spontaneously. Clinically, a loud pansystolic murmur can be detected at the left sternal border because of high pressure flow between the ventricles. Large defects typically present with congestive cardiac failure in the first two months of life. Because of the size of the VSD, ventricular pressures are equalised and often only a soft systolic murmur is detected. If left untreated, pulmonary hypertensive changes start from about one year of age. Eisenmenger's syndrome, secondary to shunt reversal in such cases, may become evident in the second decade of life.

Echocardiography confirms the diagnosis and can estimate the degree of shunting across the defect. Cardiac catheterisation can quantify the various pressures within the cardiac chambers and so assess the degree of pulmonary hypertension, as well as demonstrating a step up in oxygen saturation between left and right ventricles. Generally, surgical closure is indicated for large defects, when there is failure to respond to medical therapy, for left-to-right shunts of >2:1, when there are signs of increasing pulmonary vascular resistance and in the presence of complications of VSD. These include: (1) aortic regurgitation, which occurs in about 5 per cent of defects; (2) infundibular stenosis, which tends to be progressive and leads to shunt reversal; and (3) infective endocarditis, often presenting with pneumonia or pleurisy as the infected 'emboli' in a VSD with a typical left-to-right shunt flows into the pulmonary circulation.

THE THORACIC AORTA

The most common pathology affecting the thoracic aorta is aneurysm formation or dissection.

Thoracic aortic aneurysms

A true aneurysm is a localised dilatation of a blood vessel involving all layers of the vessel, whereas a false aneurysm has compressed supporting tissue as its wall and is usually the result of a defect in the vessel intima (from trauma, dissection or previous surgery). Aneurysms are described as fusiform when the whole circumference is affected or saccular when only part of the circumference is involved.

Aortic aneurysms can develop anywhere along its length, but thoracic aortic aneurysms, including those that extend into the upper abdomen (thoracoabdominal aneurysms), account for 25 per cent, typically occurring in men in the fifth to seventh decade or younger in those with connective tissue disorders.

Aetiology

The most common aetiology is atherosclerosis, but connective tissue disorders account for many aneurysms in the aortic root and ascending aorta now that tertiary syphilis is rare. Marfan syndrome is associated with cystic medial degeneration involving the vessel wall and causes widening of the proximal aorta and aortic root, leading to aortic valve insufficiency. Other disorders associated with aneurysm formation and dissection include Ehlers–Danlos syndrome and osteogenesis imperfecta.

Trauma, typically following blunt chest injury, can lead to aneurysm formation, usually involving the descending aorta. However, these are usually false aneurysms containing haematoma from injury to the aortic vessel wall.

Clinical features

Many aneurysms are asymptomatic and are discovered incidentally on routine chest x-rays. Others present as a space-occupying lesion in the thorax with pain caused by pressure on adjacent structures (vertebra), hoarseness (left recurrent laryngeal nerve), dysphagia (oesophagus) and respiratory symptoms (left main bronchus). Aortic root aneurysms may lead to dilatation of the aortic root annulus and aortic regurgitation.

Rupture can lead to cardiac tamponade or haemorrhage into the left pleural space, leading to dyspnoea and, if the tracheobronchial airway or oesophagus is involved, haemoptysis or haematemesis, respectively.

Investigations

The diagnosis is confirmed by CT or MRI. Arteriography is not necessary for diagnosis but is often required to demonstrate the relation of the arch vessels to the aneurysm.

Indications for surgery

Without treatment, the aneurysm is likely to expand and ultimately rupture. Important factors to consider when planning treatment are age, comorbidity and coexisting coronary disease.

Edvard Ehlers, 1863–1937, Professor of Clinical Dermatology, Copenhagen Denmark.
Henri Alexandre Danlos, 1844–1912, dermatologist, Hôpital St Louis, Paris, France, gave his account of this condition in 1908.

Henri Louis Roger, 1809–1891, physician, Hôpital Saint-Eugene, Paris, France.
Benjamin Jean Antonin Marfan, 1858–1942, physician, L'hôpital des Enfantes-Malades, Paris, France, described Marfan syndrome in 1896.

In ascending aneurysms, the presence of progressive aortic valve insufficiency is an important indication for surgery. Other indications in this group, including Marfan-related aneurysms, are a diameter of 5–6 cm and the presence of symptoms. In descending aneurysms, indications for surgery include symptoms, acute enlargement and a diameter of approximately 6 cm.

Surgical options

The approach adopted for surgical treatment depends on the location of the aneurysm, but typically involves a median sternotomy, CPB and cooling the patient to 18°C before cross-clamping the aorta above the aneurysm (Figure 54.27). If the aortic root is involved, the aorta, together with its annulus and valve, is resected and a composite graft is sutured to the aortic root. The circulation is arrested and, after removal of the aortic cross-clamp, the distal anastomosis is completed. The coronary ostia require reimplantation into the graft (Bentall's operation). If the ascending aorta is involved, it is resected and replaced with a tube graft. For aortic arch aneurysms, surgery on this section of the aorta is a formidable undertaking because the cerebral and subclavian vessels have to be anastomosed to the graft, either separately or en bloc. Typically, it involves a period of circulatory arrest and some form of cerebral protection. Excision of a descending aortic aneurysm is with graft replacement under CPB with exposure via a left thoracotomy or with a heparin-bonded shunt. Increasingly, thoracic aneurysms at the aortic arch or more distal are repaired using a percutaneous approach via the femoral artery with insertion of an endovascular stent under radiological guidance.

Surgical outcome

The operative mortality rate is variable depending on the location and type of repair required but electively is between 5 and 15 per cent. An emergency repair has a considerably higher operative mortality rate. Long-term survival depends on underlying pathology but, for ascending aneurysm repairs, the five-year survival rate is approximately 65 per cent. The major complications of descending aneurysm repairs include paraplegia, renal failure and ventricular dysfunction.

Aortic dissection

This occurs when there is a defect or flap in the intima of the aorta, resulting in blood tracking into the aortic tissues splitting the medial layer and creating a false lumen. It most commonly occurs in the ascending aorta or less often just distal to the left subclavian artery. It is also more common in men, typically those aged 50–70 years, and in Afro-Caribbeans.

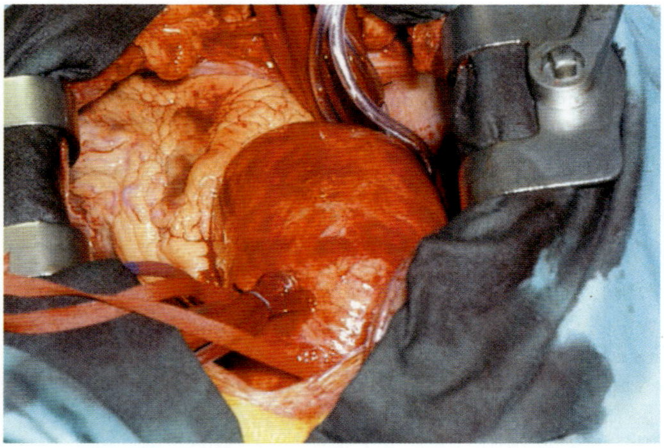

Figure 54.27 A large thoracic aortic aneurysm.

Aetiology

It usually occurs as a spontaneous or sporadic event, although very often a history of hypertension is noted. Other important associations include Marfan syndrome and pregnancy (Summary box 54.16).

Summary box 54.16

Predisposing factors for aortic dissection

- Age
- Hypertension
- Marfan syndrome
- Pregnancy
- Other connective tissue disorders, for example Ehlers–Danlos syndrome, giant cell arteritis, systemic lupus erythematosus
- Coarctation of the aorta
- Turner or Noonan syndromes
- Aortotomy site

Clinical features

The presentation is often a tearing intrascapular pain not unlike the pain of myocardial ischaemia, and it may be difficult to distinguish between the two. The extent of arterial dissection may produce widespread symptoms and signs.

The dissection can extend distally down the aorta to involve:

- the renal arteries (renal pain and renal failure);
- the mesenteric arteries (abdominal pain and bowel ischaemia);
- the spinal arteries (paraplegia);
- the iliac arteries (leg pain, pallor, loss or reduced pulses and limb ischaemia).

The dissection may track proximally to involve:

- the head and neck vessels (symptoms and signs of a stroke or transient ischaemic attack);
- the coronary vessels (myocardial infarction);
- the aortic root (aortic regurgitation).

The aneurysm may rupture back into the lumen or externally into the pericardium (cardiac tamponade) or mediastinum (left haemothorax).

Classification

There are two classifications, both of which are limited in their application but widely used. The DeBakey classification is based on the pattern of dissection, whereas the Stanford classification is based on whether the ascending aorta is involved (Figure 54.28).

Investigations

The diagnosis is suspected when chest radiography demonstrates a widened mediastinum, often associated with fluid in the left costophrenic angle. Diagnosis is confirmed by whatever method is most readily at hand and includes echocardiography, ideally TOE, CT of the thorax or MRI (Figure 54.29). Traditionally,

Hugh Henry Bentall, formerly Professor of Cardiac Surgery, The Royal Postgraduate Medical School, Hammersmith Hospital, London, UK.

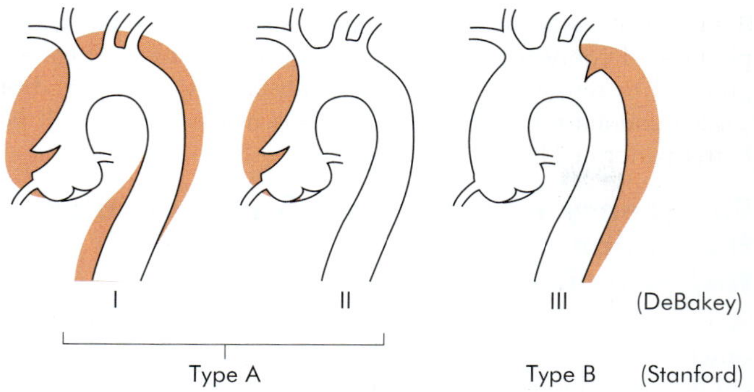

Figure 54.28 Stanford classification of aortic dissections according to whether the ascending aorta is involved (type A) or not (type B). This is simpler than the DeBakey classification (types I, II and III).

aortography was the 'gold standard' technique and it still provides excellent information before surgery but, increasingly, advanced three-dimensional CT angiography and MRI are used when available.

Management

In the emergency situation, before further imaging, blood pressure (which is usually high at presentation) should be brought under control to prevent extension of the dissection.

Surgical options

Type A (or type I and II) dissections

Those involving the ascending aorta usually require surgical intervention. The chest is opened through a median sternotomy and CPB is started with core cooling down to 18°C. The aorta is cross-clamped as high as possible and opened. Cardioplegia solution is infused into the coronary ostia to arrest the heart in diastole. If the intimal tear is present and localised, the ascending aorta is excised with the tear and replaced with a synthetic graft. The distal anastomosis is performed with circulatory arrest. Recently, there have been attempts to carry out endovascular stenting of type A dissection with variable degrees of success.

Type B (or type III) dissections

Initially, these are best managed medically with antihypertensive drugs. Surgery is indicated if the pain increases (signalling impending rupture), the aneurysm is expanding on serial chest radiographs or complications, such as organ, limb or neurological symptoms, develop. The operation may be performed with a heparin-bonded shunt or under CPB. There is a real risk of paraplegia from this operation, which should be mentioned specifically to the patient before operation. Use of percutaneously placed endovascular stents is likely to increase in the future, although currently its role in the acute setting remains to be established. There has been a shift in the surgical management of type B dissection towards endovascular stenting which can be a part of a hybrid operation including surgical replacement of parts of the aorta, such as the arch.

Outcomes

If dissection is untreated, the mortality rate is 50 per cent within 48 hours and 75 per cent within 1–2 weeks. Almost all patients with type A dissections will die if not operated on, whereas patients with type B dissections have a better prognosis. The

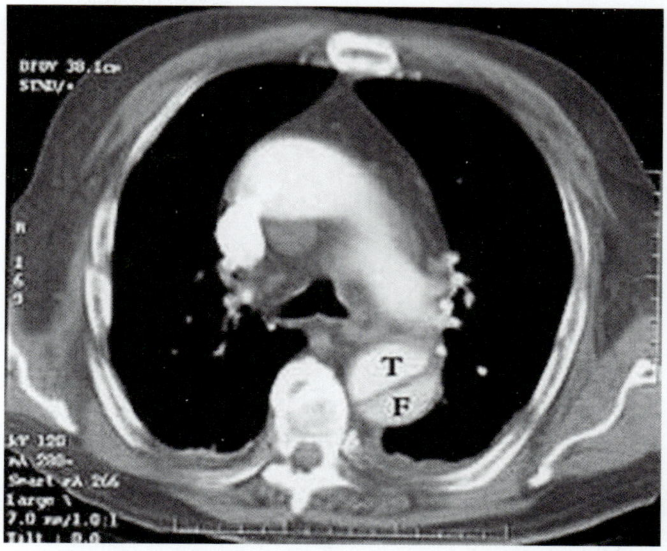

Figure 54.29 Computed tomography scan showing acute dissection of the descending thoracic aorta. F, false lumen; T, true lumen.

surgical mortality rate is variable but is around 15 per cent for proximal aortic dissection. The overall survival rate for patients leaving hospital, regardless of the type of dissection, is around 80 per cent at five years and 40 per cent at ten years.

PERICARDIAL DISEASE

There is a fibrous envelope covering the heart and separating it from the mediastinal structures. This fibrous structure includes a parietal layer and allows the heart to move with each beat. It is not essential for life because it can be left wide open after cardiac surgery without any ill-effects; however, there are a number of conditions affecting the pericardium that may present to the surgeon.

Pericardial effusion

There is a continuous production and resorption of pericardial fluid. If a disease process disturbs this balance, a pericardial effusion may develop. If the pressure exceeds the pressure in the atria, compression will occur, venous return will fall and the circulation will be compromised. This state of affairs is called 'tamponade'. A gradual build up of fluid (e.g. malignant infiltration) may be well tolerated for a long period before tamponade occurs, and the pericardial cavity may contain 2 litres of fluid. Acute tamponade (from penetrating trauma, during coronary angiography or postoperatively) may occur in minutes with small volumes of blood. The clinical features are low blood pressure with a raised jugular venous pressure and paradoxical pulse. Kussmaul's sign is a characteristic pattern that is seen when the jugular venous pressure rises with inspiration as a result of the impaired venous return to the heart.

Emergency treatment of pericardial tamponade is aspiration of the pericardial space. A wide-bore needle is inserted under local anaesthesia to the left of the xiphisternum, between the angle of the xiphisternum and the ribcage (Figure 54.30). The needle is advanced towards the tip of the scapula into the pericardial space. An ECG electrode attached to the needle will indicate when the heart has been touched. This will relieve

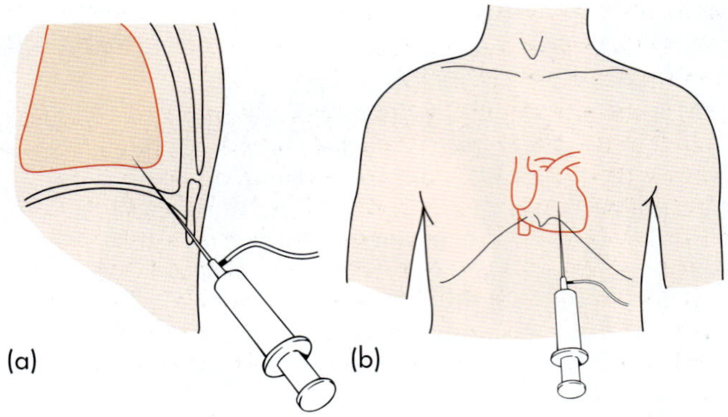

Figure 54.30 (a) Pericardial aspiration through the subxiphoid region. (b) Site of needle insertion for pericardial aspiration.

the situation temporarily until the cause of the tamponade is established. Penetrating wounds of the heart usually require exploration through a median sternotomy. Emergency room thoracotomy is rarely required. Chronic tamponade is usually a result of malignant infiltration of the pericardium (usually secondary carcinoma from breast or bronchus) or, very occasionally, uraemia or connective tissue disease. Treatment sometimes requires a pericardial window between the pericardial space and the pleural or peritoneal space.

Pericarditis

Infection and inflammation may also affect the pericardium. Acute pericarditis usually occurs following a viral illness. Treatment is with non-steroidal anti-inflammatory drugs and bed rest (in case there is an underlying myocarditis). Acute purulent pericarditis is uncommon, but requires urgent drainage and intravenous antibiotics with attention to the underlying cause.

Chronic pericarditis is an uncommon condition in which the pericardium becomes thickened and non-compliant. The heart cannot move freely and the stroke volume is reduced by the constrictive process. The central venous pressure is raised and the liver becomes congested. Peripheral oedema and ascites are also a feature. Treatment is aimed at relieving the constriction.

MANAGEMENT OF CARDIAC ARREST AFTER CARDIAC SURGERY

Introduction

The incidence of cardiac arrest after cardiac surgery is around 0.7–2.9 per cent with 17–79 per cent survival rates. Ventricular fibrillation (VF), tamponade and major bleeding account for most arrests. Multiple variables may dictate differences in the management of cardiac arrest after cardiac surgery when compared to other situations. Therefore, EACTS published guidelines for resuscitation of cardiac arrest post-cardiac surgery which are summarised below.

Cardiac arrest with 'non-shockable' rhythm

Cardiac surgical patients who have a non-VF/VT (ventricular tachycardia) arrest may have tamponade, tension pneumothorax, or severe hypovolaemia. Prompt treatment is associated with an excellent outcome. Resternotomy should be performed promptly if connecting the pacemaker and administrating atropine fail to resolve the arrest especially if prolonged period of cardiopulmonary resuscitation (CPR) is needed which will be better performed by internal massage.

Emergency resternotomy for ventricular fibrillation or pulseless ventricular tachycardia

A precordial thump may be performed if within 10 s of the onset of VF or pulseless VT, however, this should not delay cardioversion by defibrillation. In VF or pulseless VT, emergency resternotomy should be performed after three failed attempts at defibrillation.

Emergency resternotomy

After the identification of cardiac arrest, basic life support according to the ALS (advanced life support) guidelines should be initiated while preparing for emergency resternotomy. Emergency resternotomy may be required in 0.8–2.7 per cent of all patients undergoing cardiac surgery. Emergency resternotomy is a multipractitioner procedure, which should be rapidly performed with full aseptic technique.

Preperation for emergency resternotomy

- Don a gown and gloves in a sterile fashion.
- Apply the thoracic drape ensuring that the whole bed is covered. (If an all-in-one sterile drape is used, then there is no need to prepare the skin with antiseptic.)
- Use the scalpel to cut the sternotomy incision, including all sutures deeply down to the sternal wires.
- Cut all the sternal wires with the wire cutters. The sternal edges will separate a little which may relieve tamponade.
- Use suction to clear excessive blood or clot.
- Place the retractor between the sternal edges and open the sternum.
- If cardiac output is restored, wait for expert assistance. If there is no cardiac output, carefully identify the position of any grafts and then perform internal cardiac massage and internal defibrillation if required.

Internal cardiac massage

This is a potentially dangerous procedure. Risks include avulsion of a bypass graft, with the left internal mammary artery being at particular risk, and right ventricular rupture especially if it is thin or distended. Therefore, it is important to carefully remove any clot and identify structures at risk, such as grafts, before placing hands around the heart.

There are several methods of internal massage, however, the two-hand technique is the safest.

Two-hand technique

The heart should be inspected to locate the internal mammary and any other grafts if present followed by removing any blood clots. The right hand is passed over the apex of the heart and then advanced round the apex to the back of the heart, palm up and hand flat. The left hand is then placed flat onto the anterior surface of the heart and the two hands squeezed together at a rate of 100 per minute. Flat palms and straight fingers are important to avoid an unequal distribution of pressure onto the heart, thereby minimising the chance of trauma. If there is a mitral valve

Adolf Kussmaul, 1822–1902, successively Professor of Medicine at Heidelberg, Erlangen, Frieburg and Strasbourg, Germany.

replacement or repair, care should be taken not to lift the apex by the right hand, as this can cause a posterior ventricular rupture.

FURTHER READING

Bojar RM. *Manual of perioperative care in cardiac surgery*, 3rd edn. Oxford: Blackwell Science, 1999.

Bonow RO, Carabello BA, Chatterjee K *et al.* American College of Cardiology/American Heart Association Task Force on Practice Guidelines. *J Am Coll Cardiol* 2008; **52**: e1–142.

Dunning J, Fabbri A, Kolh PH *et al.* Guideline for resuscitation in cardiac arrest after cardiac surgery. *Eur J Cardiol Surg* **2009; 36**: 3–28.

Henry Edmunds L Jr. *Cardiac surgery in the adult*, 2nd edn, 2003. Available online from www.ctsnet.org/book/edmunds/.

Kirklin J, Barratt-Boyce B. *Cardiac surgery*, 3rd edn. Edinburgh: Churchill Livingstone, 2003.

Kolh P, Wijns W, Danchin N *et al.* Guidelines on myocardial revascularization. *Eur J Cardiothorac Surg* 2010; **38** (Suppl.): S1–S52.

Treasure T, Hunt I, Keogh B, Pagano D (eds). *The evidence for cardiothoracic surgery*. Shrewsbury: tfm, 2004.

CHAPTER 55

The thorax

LEARNING OBJECTIVES

To understand:
- The anatomy and physiology of the thorax
- Investigation of chest pathology
- The role of surgery in pleural disease
- The assessment of patients requiring lung surgery
- Surgical oncology as applied to chest surgery

INTRODUCTION

Anatomical development of the lungs

The lungs are derived from an outpouching of the primitive foregut during the fourth week of intrauterine life. This bud becomes a two-lobed structure, the ends of which ultimately become the lungs. The lobar arrangement is defined early and is fairly constant but anomalies of fissures and segments leading to anatomical variation in the adult are common.

The primitive lungs drain into the cardinal veins, which ultimately become the pulmonary veins draining into the left atrium. Variability in venous drainage is very common and is usually of little functional significance. At the most severe end of the spectrum is total anomalous drainage, which presents in early infant life because oxygenated blood is all directed back to the right heart.

Anatomy of the lungs

The left lung is divided by the oblique fissure, which lies nearer vertical than horizontal, so the upper and lower lobes could also be called anterior and posterior. On the right, the equivalent of the left upper lobe is further divided to give the middle lobe. Each lobe is composed of segments, with anatomically defined and named bronchial, pulmonary arterial and venous connections (Figure 55.1).

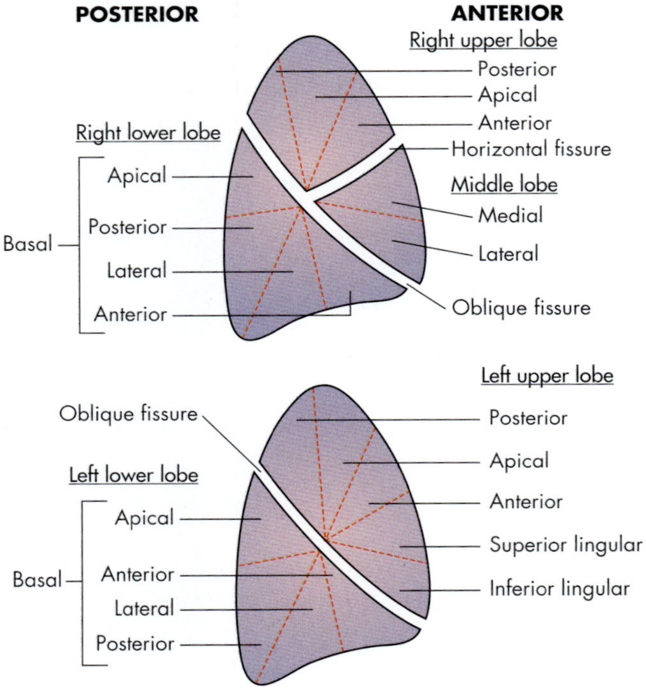

Figure 55.1 The lobar and segmental divisions of the lungs, right lung above and left lung below as if viewed from the side.

The right main bronchus (RMB) is shorter, wider and nearly vertical compared with the left main bronchus (LMB). As a consequence, inhaled foreign bodies are more likely to enter the right main bronchus than the left (Figure 55.2). The trachea and bronchi have a systemic arterial blood supply delivered by the bronchial arteries, which arise directly from the nearby thoracic aorta.

Lymphatic drainage tends to follow the bronchi. Lymph nodes are both named and identified by numbered 'stations', which are of importance in staging of lung cancer (Figure 55.3).

Mechanics of breathing

The intercostal muscles contract, causing the ribs to move upwards and outwards, thereby increasing the transverse and anteroposterior dimensions of the chest wall. The diaphragm contracts simultaneously and flattens, increasing the vertical dimension of the chest cavity. As the volume increases, the intrathoracic pressure falls and air flows in until the alveolar pressure is the same as the atmospheric pressure. The only force used in normal expiration is the elastic recoil of the lung.

Coughing to clear sputum is an essential part of recovery from surgery. In a vigorous cough, probably the only muscle in the body that is relaxed is the diaphragm; as the abdomen and chest wall muscles contract, the limbs are braced and the sphincters are tightened. When the intrathoracic and abdominal pressure is built up, the glottis is opened and the diaphragm is forced up

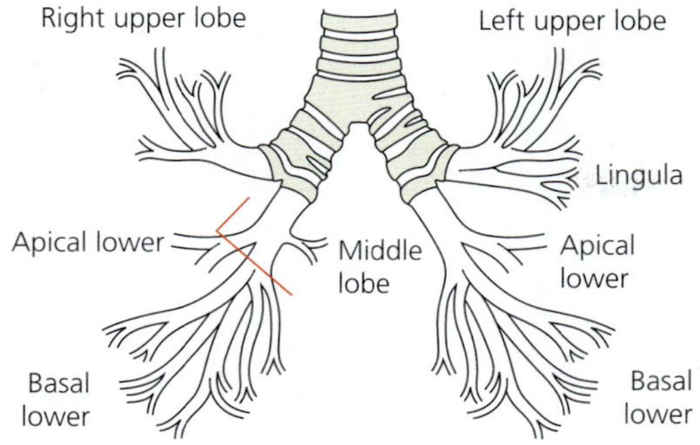

Figure 55.2 Surgical anatomy of the bronchial tree. To surgically remove the right lower lobe and conserve the middle lobe, the surgeon must be prepared to dissect and separately divide the apical bronchial segment (red line).

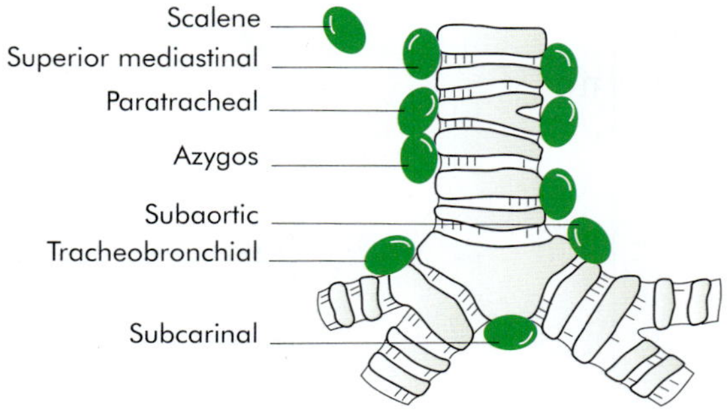

Figure 55.3 Lymph node stations related to the bronchial tree are particularly important in the staging of lung cancer, with N1 nodes (10–14) and N2 nodes (2–9) shown.

as a piston, or like the plunger of a syringe, to expel air at high velocity.

Investigation of the respiratory system

Any patient undergoing general anaesthesia requires some assessment of respiratory function. This may be a clinical appraisal of fitness but more detail is necessary for patients who are undergoing lung resection.

Pulmonary function tests

Pulmonary function tests (PFTs) are useful in determining the functional capacity of the patient and the severity of pulmonary disease, and in predicting the response to various treatments. The tests range from simple clinic or bedside measurements to those only available in specialist centres. Spirometry is the most commonly performed PFT and measures specifically the amount (volume) and/or speed (flow rate) of air that can be inhaled or exhaled. It is reported in both absolute values and as a predicted percentage of normal. Normal values vary, depending on gender, race, age and height. The most common parameters measured in spirometry are defined below and illustrated (Figure 55.4).

Peak expiratory flow rate

Peak expiratory flow rate (PEFR) is measured by a Wright peak flow meter or a peak flow gauge. This is the maximum airflow velocity achieved during an expiration delivered with maximal force from the total lung capacity. It is a reliable and reproducible test but has the disadvantage of being effort dependent, and it may therefore be affected by abdominal or thoracic wound pain. PEFR measurements are often used in managing asthma, but there are many other causes of low PEFR, such as a problem with large airway patency.

Forced expiratory volume in 1 second

The forced expiratory volume in 1 s (FEV_1) is the amount of air forcibly expired in 1 s. It is low in obstructive lung disease and may be normal in patients with poor gas exchange.

Forced vital capacity

The forced vital capacity (FVC) is the volume of air forcibly displaced following maximal inspiration to maximal expiration. The FEV_1 and the FVC can be measured using a Vitallograph and a ratio (FEV_1/FVC) can be calculated (Figure 55.4). A low ratio indicates obstruction and the test should be repeated after bronchodilators. A normal ratio (FVC and FEV_1 reduced to the same extent) indicates a restrictive pathology.

There are two physiological categories of lung disease: obstructive and restrictive (Table 55.1). In obstructive conditions, such as asthma or emphysema, the flow of air in and out of the lungs is impaired. In restrictive disease, such as lung fibrosis, the lungs have lost size or elasticity, becoming 'stiff' so that they do not fill or expand properly.

Table 55.1 Spirometry values in obstructive and restrictive lung diseases.

	Obstructive pattern	Restrictive pattern
PEFR	↓↓	Normal or ↓
FEV_1	↓↓	Normal or ↓
FVC	Normal or ↓	↓↓
FEV_1/FVC	<70	>80

FEV_1, forced expiratory volume in 1 s; FVC, forced vital capacity; PEFR, peak expiratory flow rate.

Diffusion capacity

The diffusion capacity (DLCO) is a measurement of the lung's ability to transfer gases and is often referred to as the 'transfer factor'. It cannot be performed at the bedside, requires the patient's current haemoglobin level and is a test of the integrity of the lung's alveolar-capillary surface area for gas exchange. In lung diseases that damage the alveolar walls, such as emphysema, or thicken the alveolar membrane, such as lung fibrosis, it may be reduced.

Oxygen saturation

Oxygen saturation (SpO_2) refers to the degree of oxygen molecules (O_2) carried in the blood attached to haemoglobin (Hb) molecules. It is a measure of how much oxygen the blood is carrying as a percentage of the maximum it could carry. The common method of monitoring the oxygenation of a patient's haemoglobin is through a pulse oximeter.

Basil Martin Wright, 1912–2001, member of the Scientific Staff of the Medical Research Council Research Centre, Northwick Park Hospital, Harrow, Middlesex, UK.

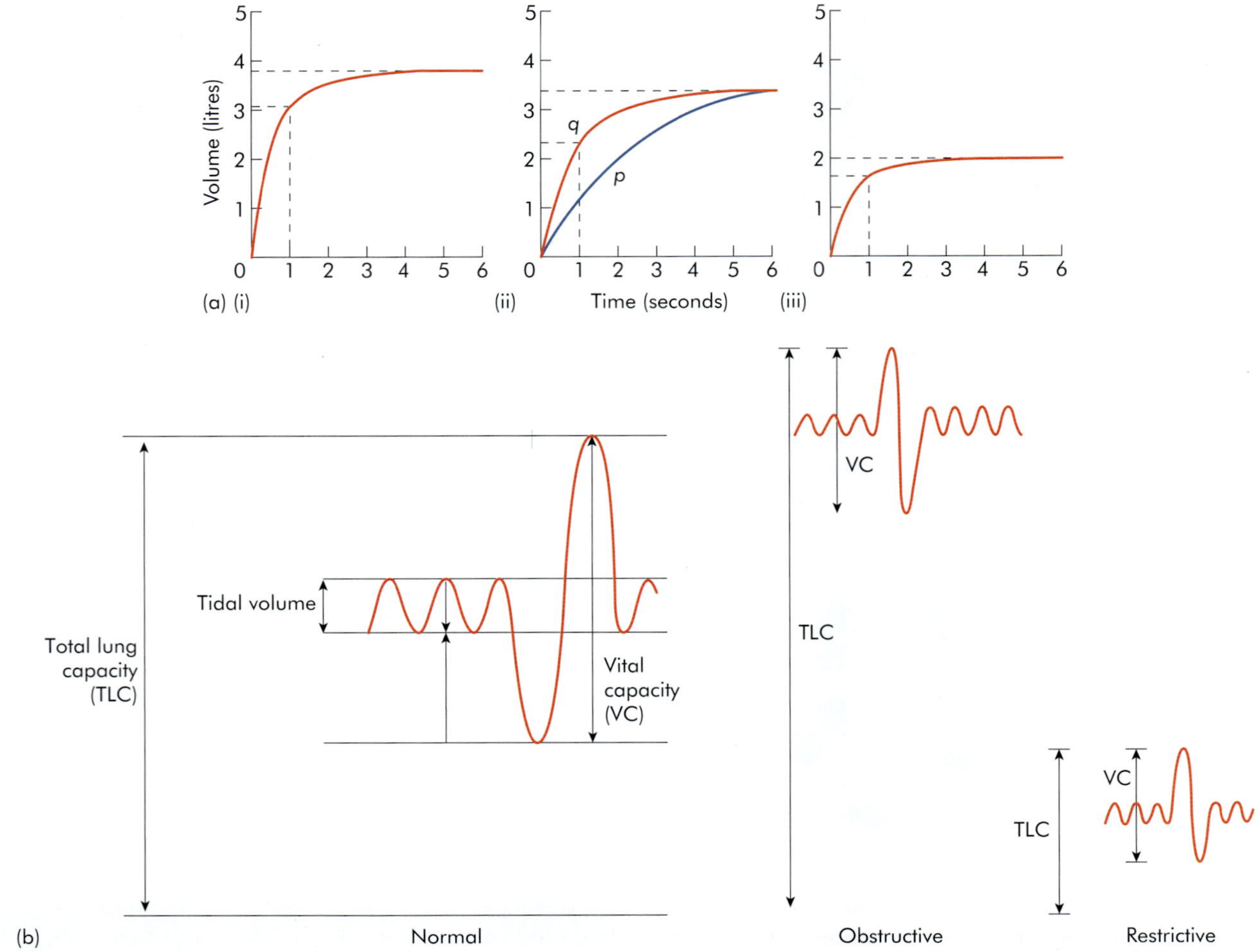

Figure 55.4 Spirometry. (a) Spirogram drawings obtained from a Vitallograph: (i) normal forced expiratory volume in 1 s (FEV_1) 31 litres, forced vital capacity (FVC) 3.8 litres, FEV_1/FVC 82 per cent; (ii) obstructive defect, reversible asthma, *p* before a bronchodilator, FEV_1 1.4 litres, FVC 3.5 litres, FEV_1/FVC 40 per cent; *q* after a bronchodilator, FEV_1 2.5 litres, FVC 3.5 litres, FEV_1/FVC 71 per cent; (iii) restrictive defect, fibrosing alveolitis, FEV_1 1.8 litres, FVC 2.0 litres, FEV_1/FVC 90 per cent. No change with bronchodilators. (b) Changes in lung volume in obstructive and restrictive lung disease. (Reproduced from Gray HH. Pulmonary embolism. *Medicine International* 1993; **21**: 477, by kind permission of the Medicine Group (Journals) Ltd.)

Blood gases

SpO_2 measured non-invasively with a pulse oximeter measures only oxygenation, not ventilation and provides no information regarding a patient's carbon dioxide or bicarbonate levels, blood pH, base deficit. This requires arterial blood sampling or 'blood gases' (Table 55.2).

Table 55.2 Arterial blood gases 'normal values'.

pH 7.35–7.45
$PaCO_2$ 4.5–6 kPa (35–50 mmHg)
PaO_2 11–14 kPa (83–105 mmHg)
Standard bicarbonate 22–28 mmol/L
Anion gap 10–16 mmol/L
Chloride 98–107 mmol/L

The pleura

The key to many aspects of practical chest surgery is an understanding of the pleura and of the mechanics of breathing. Management of the essentially healthy pleural space is logical and simple and needs minimal technology. On the other hand, when pleural disease is advanced, for example when there is gross pleural sepsis surrounding a leaking and trapped lung, management is difficult and the patient may require prolonged care with repeated interventions.

The physiology of pleural fluid

The turnover of fluid in the human pleural space is about 1–2 litres in 24 hours, with only 5–10 mL of fluid present at any one time as a film, about 20 μm thick, between the visceral and parietal pleura.

The mechanisms and equations given are simplifications, but serve to explain the clinical conditions encountered. The fluid is produced from the capillaries of the parietal pleura as a transudate, according to the Starling capillary loop pressures. However, there is a further negative force in the pleura. The elastic content of the lung causes it to recoil and collapse if not held open by the negative pressure in the pleura. This elastic recoil exerts about 4 mmHg negative pressure and favours accumulation of fluid. The secreting forces add up to about 11 mmHg in health. Pleural fluid is mainly reabsorbed (about 90 per cent) by the visceral pleura, whose capillaries are part of the pulmonary circulation. The principal force in absorption of pleural fluid is oncotic pressure (approximately 25 mmHg) less the difference in mean capillary hydrostatic pressure of the pulmonary capillary (8 mmHg). Thus, the overall absorbing pressure is 25 − 8 = 17 mmHg, producing a net drying effect (17 − 11) of about 6 mmHg (Figure 55.5).

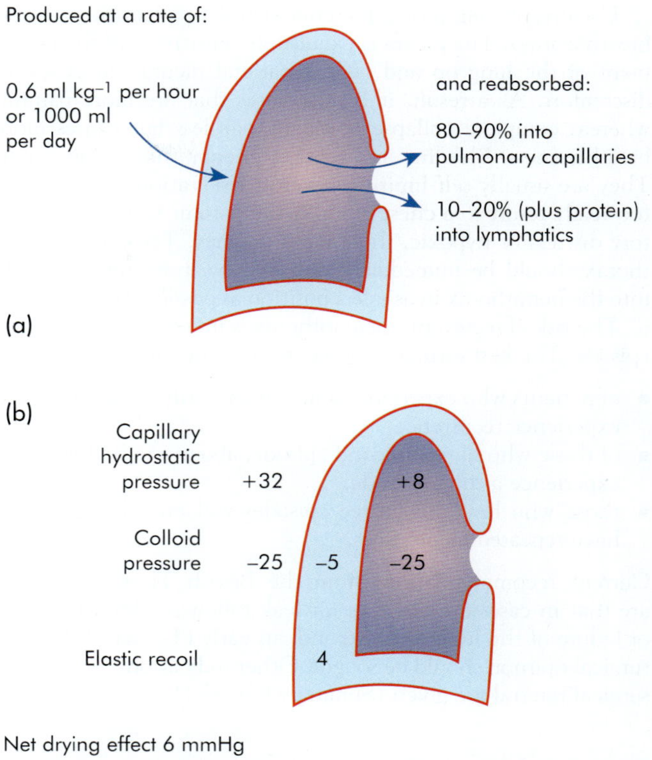

Figure 55.5 (a) Production and absorption of pleural fluid. (b) Normal pleural physiology. (See the text for an explanation of this simplistic physiological model.)

Gas in the pleural space

There is normally no free gas in the pleural space because the same physiological mechanism that absorbs air from a pneumothorax prevents any gas accumulating.

The partial pressures (water as saturated vapour pressure) of the gases in venous/end-capillary blood are:

PO_2	40 mmHg	5.3 kPa
PCO_2	46 mmHg	6.1 kPa
PN_2	573 mmHg	76.4 kPa
PH_2O	47 mmHg	6.3 kPa

These partial pressures add up to less than atmospheric pressure (760 mmHg). Free gas is therefore absorbed into the blood and lost to the atmosphere through the lungs, with the gases moving in relation to their solubility (carbon dioxide quickest and nitrogen slowest) and relative concentrations in the pleural space and the blood. This does not favour nitrogen, which constitutes about 80 per cent of atmospheric air. Breathing oxygen accelerates nitrogen removal by reducing the content of nitrogen in the blood and increasing the gradient for its absorption. Nitrous oxide anaesthesia is dangerous in the presence of a pneumothorax; nitrous oxide is very soluble and, although not normally present in the pleural space, it will be rapidly transported into the space if the patient is given nitrous oxide to breathe.

PLEURAL DISEASE

Pneumothorax

Pneumothorax is the presence of air outside the lung, within the pleural space. It must be distinguished from bullae or air cysts within the lung. Bullae can be the cause of an air leak from the lung and can therefore coexist with pneumothorax.

Spontaneous pneumothorax occurs when the visceral pleura ruptures without an external traumatic or iatrogenic cause. They are divided into primary spontaneous pneumothorax (PSP) and secondary spontaneous pneumothorax (SSP). Pneumothoraces can also cause occur following trauma or be caused by iatrogenic injury, such as insertion of a central line. Tension pneumothorax is when (independent of aetiology) there is a build up of positive pressure within the hemithorax, to the extent that the lung is completely collapsed, the diaphragm is flattened and the mediastinum is distorted and, eventually, the venous return to the heart is compromised. Any pleural breach is inherently valve-like because air will find its way out through the alveoli but cannot be drawn back in because the lung tissue collapses around the hole in the pleura. Patients being mechanically ventilated following trauma are at particular risk.

Surgical emphysema is the presence of air in the tissues. It requires a breach of an air-containing viscus in communication with soft tissues, and the generation of positive pressure to push the air along tissue planes. The most serious cause is a ruptured oesophagus. Mediastinal surgical emphysema can also occur with asthma or barotrauma from positive pressure ventilation. A poorly managed chest drain with intermittent build up of pressure allows air to track into the chest wall through the point where the drain breaches the parietal pleura.

Primary spontaneous pneumothorax

This is a common disease characteristically seen in young people from their mid-teens to late twenties. About 75 per cent of cases are in young men, who tend to be tall, and the condition runs in families. It is due to leaks from small blebs, vesicles or bullae, which may become pedunculated, typically at the apex of the upper lobe or on the upper border of the lower or middle lobes.

Secondary spontaneous pneumothorax

This occurs when the visceral pleura leaks as part of an underlying lung disease; any disease that involves the pleura may cause pneumothorax, including tuberculosis, any degenerative or cavitating lung disease and necrosing tumours. As such it tends to occur in older patients, often with a history of underlying lung disease, such as emphysema. The pneumothorax may be less well tolerated.

Ernest Henry Starling, 1866–1927, Professor of Physiology, University College, London, UK.

Usually, pneumothorax presents with sharp pleuritic pain and breathlessness. The pleura is exquisitely sensitive and the movement of the lung on and off the parietal pleura causes severe discomfort. As a result, it is mild cases that are more painful, whereas complete collapse is usually painless but causes more breathlessness. Bleeding and tension pneumothorax can occur. They are usually self-limiting; careful observation is wiser than too-ready resort to a chest drain. If the patient is not in respiratory distress or hypoxic, there is no urgency. Tension pneumothorax should be immediately relieved by inserting a cannula into the hemithorax in as safe a position as possible (Figure 55.6).

The risk of recurrent pneumothorax is increased after the first episode. The best estimates of recurrence rates are:

- of patients who experience a first event, only about one-third experience recurrence;
- of those who have a second episode, about one-half go on to experience a third episode;
- those who have had three episodes will probably go on to have repeated recurrences.

Current recommendations from the British Thoracic Society are that in cases of persistent air leak following drain insertion or failure of the lung to re-expand, an early (3–5 days) thoracic surgical opinion should be sought. Other indications for thoracic surgical referral are given (Summary box 55.1).

Summary box 55.1

Indications for surgical intervention for pneumothorax

- Second ipsilateral pneumothorax
- First contralateral pneumothorax
- Bilateral spontaneous pneumothorax
- Spontaneous haemothorax
- Professions at risk (e.g. pilots, divers)
- Pregnancy

Current recommendations focus on the use of small bore (10–14 Fr) chest drains, usually of a Seldinger-type inserted ideally under ultrasound guidance. However, knowledge of the role of the 'surgical' chest drain and how to safely insert it is still required.

Inserting and managing a chest drain

An intercostal tube connected to an underwater seal is central to the management of chest disease; however, the management of the pleura and of chest drains can be troublesome, even in experienced hands.

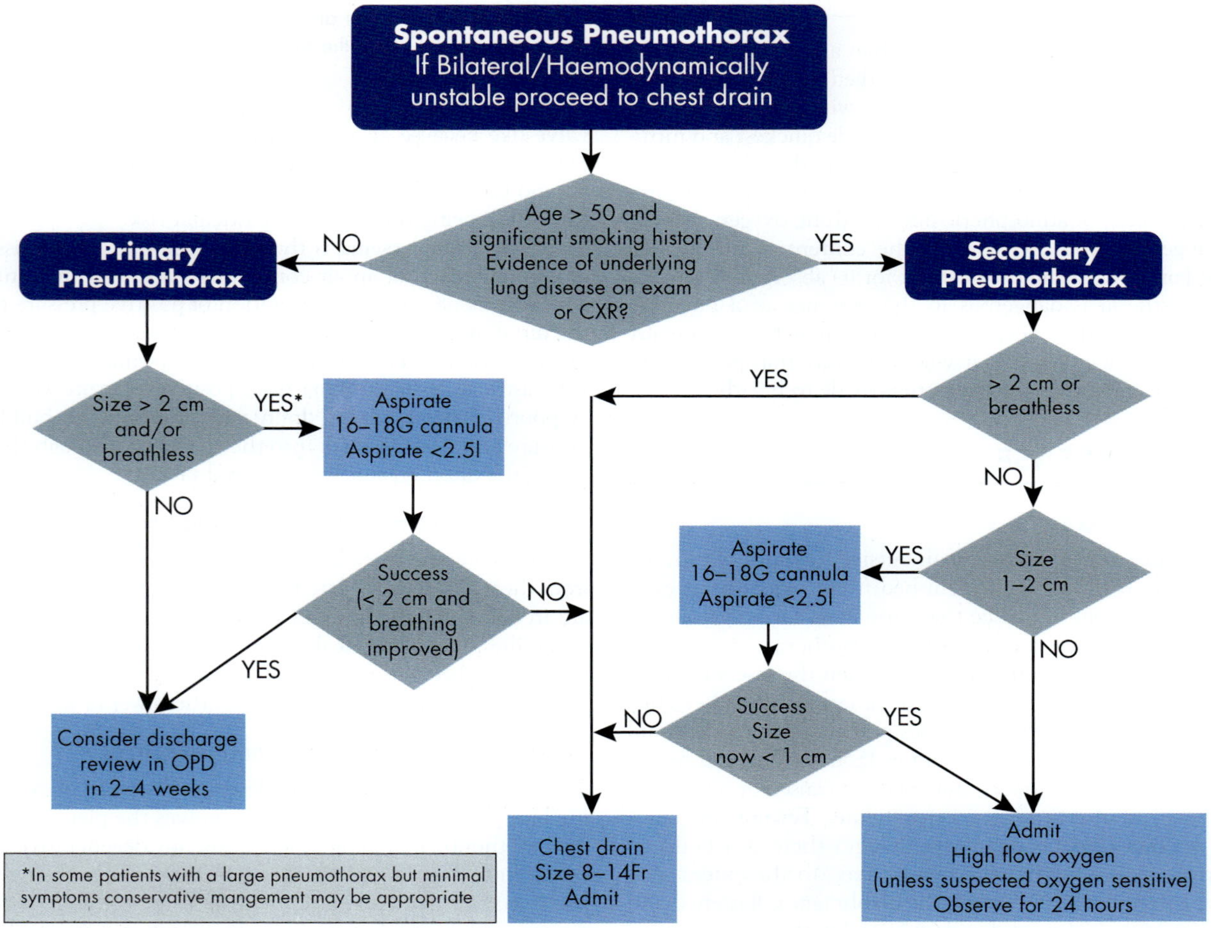

Figure 55.6 British Thoracic Society (BTS) guidelines on management of spontaneous pneumothorax (2010) (adapted from www.bts.org.uk).

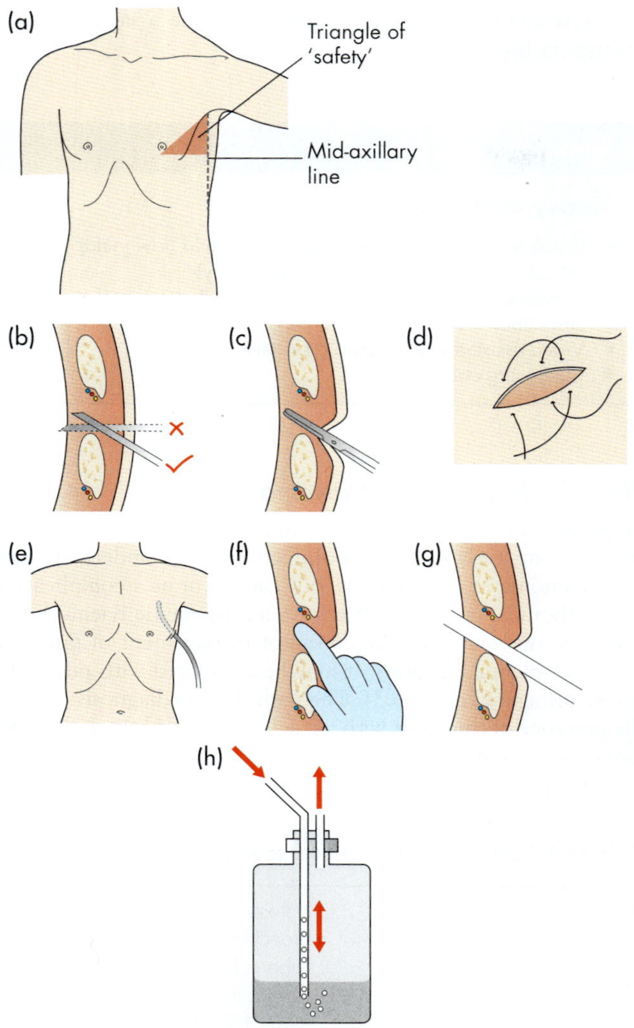

Figure 55.7 Insertion of chest drain: (a) triangle of safety; (b) penetration of the skin, muscle and pleura; (c) blunt dissection of the parietal pleura; (d) suture placement; (e) gauging the distance of insertion; (f) digital examination along the tract into the pleural space; (g) withdrawal of central trochar and positioning of drain; (h) underwater seal chest drain bottle.

The safest site for insertion of a drain (Figure 55.7) is in the triangle that lies:

- anterior to the mid-axillary line;
- above the level of the nipple;
- below and lateral to the pectoralis major muscle.

This will ideally find the fifth space. The technique includes the following:

- Meticulous attention to sterility throughout.
- Adequate local anaesthesia to include the pleura.
- Sharp dissection only to cut the skin.
- Blunt dissection with artery forceps down through the muscle layers; these should only be the serratus anterior and the intercostals.
- An oblique tract, so that the skin incision and the hole in the parietal pleura do not overlie each other and the drain is in a short tunnel, which reduces the chance of entraining air.
- A drain for pneumothorax and haemothorax should aim towards the apex of the lung. A drain for pleural effusion or empyema should be nearer the base. The drain should pass over the upper edge of the rib to avoid the neurovascular bundle that lies beneath the rib.
- The retaining stitch should be secure, but not obliterate the drain.
- A vertical mattress suture is inserted for later wound closure. This is vital for pneumothorax management, but should be omitted if the drain is for empyema (provided there is adherence of the pleura) because that tract should lie open.
- Connect the drain to an underwater seal device which functions as a one-way valve.
- After completion, check that the drain has achieved its objective by taking a chest x-ray.

It is preferable not to apply suction to the drain or to clamp it. The danger is that the clamp may be applied for transport and forgotten. Dangers of disconnection and siphoning are small or best averted in other ways apart from clamping. A bubbling drain should (almost) never be clamped. Remove the drain when it no longer has a function (Summary box 55.2).

Summary box 55.2

Suction on a pleural tube

- Beware! Inserting the drain, and not the suction, is the life-saving manoeuvre
- If the lung is reluctant to expand, the suction deviates the mediastinum
- If the lung is fragile, it may worsen an air leak

Definitive management of pneumothorax

Pleurectomy and pleurodesis

Surgery for pneumothorax can be performed by video-assisted thoracoscopic surgery (VATS) or as an open procedure (thoracotomy).

The object of the exercise is three-fold:

- to deal with any leaks from the lung;
- to search for and obliterate any blebs and bullae (**Bullectomy**);
- to make the visceral pleura adherent to the parietal pleura so that any subsequent leaks are contained and the lung cannot completely collapse.

Pleural adhesion is achieved in one of three ways:

- **Pleurectomy**: systematically strip the parietal pleura from the chest wall.
- **Pleural abrasion**: a scourer is used to scrape off the slick surface of the parietal pleura.
- **Chemical pleurodesis**: usually talc is used and is insufflated into the chest cavity.

Pleural effusion

Pleural effusion can be readily understood with reference to the physiological mechanisms governing the flux of pleural fluid given above. Pleural effusions are divided into exudates and transudates, depending on protein content (more (exudates) or less (transudates) than 30 g/L), and characterised further according to glucose content, pH and lactate dehydrogenase content. The following are the most common ways in which the pleural fluid balance is disturbed:

- **Elevated pulmonary capillary pressure.** If left atrial pressure rises, the pulmonary capillary pressure must rise with it, whether as a result of impaired cardiac performance or an overloaded circulation.
- **Reduced intravascular oncotic pressure.** If the plasma proteins fall because of renal or hepatic disease or malnutrition, the absorption mechanism fails.
- **Accumulation of pleural protein** due to obstruction of the mediastinal lymphatics secondary to lymphoma or cancers that invade the lymphatic system.
- **Excessive permeability of the capillaries to fluid and protein** as in inflammatory diseases, particularly the collagen vascular diseases. Of particular importance to the surgeon is the effusion associated with pleural infection (empyema) and malignant effusions.

Malignant pleural effusion

Pleural effusion is a common complication of cancer. This may be due to:

- lung cancer;
- pleural involvement with primary or secondary malignancy;
- mediastinal lymphatic involvement.

- **Lung cancer.** There may be direct involvement of the parietal and/or visceral pleura, collapse of the lung parenchyma and spread to the mediastinal lymphatics, or a combination of these, causing pleural fluid accumulation. It is usually regarded as a feature that puts lung cancer beyond surgical cure.
- **Pleural malignancy.** The only primary malignancy of the pleura seen with any regularity is malignant mesothelioma. This is a consequence of asbestos exposure with few exceptions. The peak of asbestos imports into the UK was from 1960 to 1975 and the incidence of mesothelioma is rising and is expected to peak in around 2015. Mesothelioma commonly presents with breathlessness because of pleural effusions, pain and systemic features of malignancy. Diffuse seeding of the parietal and visceral pleura is a common pattern of dissemination of cancers, particularly adenocarcinoma of any origin.
- **Mediastinal lymphatic involvement.** In many instances, particularly in breast cancer, there is no evident disease in the pleura. The disease is in the mediastinal lymphatics, which are obstructed, and this upsets the balance of physiological forces that control pleural fluid.

Surgery for patients with malignant pleural effusion

The surgeon has two roles:

- to make the diagnosis;
- to achieve effective palliation by draining the fluid and pleurodesis.

Diagnosis

Pleural biopsy can be obtained by a range of techniques with VATS being the most common. An unequivocally positive biopsy is useful but a negative biopsy may be a sampling error (Summary box 55.3).

Summary box 55.3

Biopsy of the pleura

- Cytological examination of the pleural fluid (low yield)
- Abrams' needle (low yield in malignancy)
- Computed tomography (CT)-guided needle biopsy of a suspicious area
- Video-assisted thoracoscopic surgery biopsy
- Open surgical biopsy

Pleural infection and empyema

Empyema is the end stage of pleural infection from any cause. It most commonly results from infection of the underlying lung by pneumonia or lung abscess, but can occur as a complication of any thoracic operation. It is seen if a traumatic haemothorax becomes infected or in the course of management of pneumothorax or pleural effusions. It may be associated with pus under the diaphragm (Table 55.3). The pathological diagnosis requires the presence of thick pus with a thick cortex of fibrin and coagulum over the lung.

Table 55.3 Conditions that predispose to empyema formation.

Pulmonary infection	Unresolved pneumonia Bronchiectasis Tuberculosis Fungal infections Lung abscess
Aspiration of pleural effusion	Any aetiology
Trauma	Penetrating injury Surgery Oesophageal perforation
Extrapulmonary sources	Subphrenic abscess
Bone infections	Osteomyelitis of ribs or vertebrae

When empyema presents *de novo* it usually follows pneumonia and three phases are described:

1. In the exudative phase, there is protein-rich (>30 g/L) effusion. If this becomes infected with the organisms from the lung (typically *Streptococcus milleri* and *Haemophilus influenzae* in children), the scene is set for empyema. At this stage, antibiotics may be all that is required. Aspiration or drainage to dryness in addition is preferred.
2. Over the next days, the fluid thickens to what is known as the fibrinopurulent phase. Drainage at this stage is prudent as antibiotics alone are unlikely to be curative.
3. The organising phase causes the lung to be trapped by a thick peel or 'cortex' for which surgical management may be required.

Leon David Abrams, formerly cardiothoracic surgeon, The United Birmingham Hospitals, Birmingham, UK.

Surgical management of pleural effusions and infections

Thoracoscopy or video-assisted thoracoscopic surgery

The direct-vision thoracoscope has been used for many years, but its use was limited mainly to performing biopsies. The instrument had a limited view and was uncomfortable to use for any length of time. All this has changed since the advent of video-assisted thoracoscopy (Figure 55.8) where the surgeon's hands are freed because the camera is attached to the thoracoscope, which can be operated by an assistant with the image displayed on a television screen. The surgeon is able to manipulate instruments with both hands to perform a variety of procedures. The number of ports required depends on the type and complexity of the surgery. The patient is usually positioned with the diseased side uppermost, having had a double lumen endotracheobronchial tube placed by the anaesthetist to allow for single-lung ventilation.

Pneumonectomy, lobectomy and empyema drainage are all possible. However, lung biopsy and the treatment of recurrent pneumothorax are the most frequent indications. The principal advantage is that a large incision is avoided resulting in less postoperative pain and a more rapid recovery.

VATS drainage, pleural biopsy and talc pleurodesis

VATS drainage, pleural biopsy and talc pleurodesis is an increasingly performed procedure for managing patients with an undiagnosed or malignant pleural effusion. It can be performed using a single or two ports and allows for direct visualisation of the pleural cavity for complete drainage, multiple pleural biopsies and excellent talc insufflation to achieve pleurodesis.

VATS debridement of empyema

Pleural infection, particularly early in its evolution, requires drainage but once the fluid component becomes fibrinopurulent and loculated it requires surgical debridement which can often be achieved through a VATS approach. The lung is isolated through the use of a double lumen tube, the patient is positioned disease side up, and the pleural cavity is entered. The fluid and debris are vigorously debrided, freeing the lung and allowing for re-expansion. At the end of the case, carefully positioned chest drains are placed to allow for dependent drainage. The drain/s must exit the skin anterior to the mid-axillary line otherwise the patient will have to lie on the drain(s), causing pain and possibly obstructing the tube. The drain should lie obliquely in its course through the skin and chest wall and into the pleura, or it will kink.

Following the procedure, the patient requires good analgesic control, typically patient controlled analgesia (PCA) and physiotherapy to help fully re-expand the lung prior to final removal of chest drains.

Decortication

If the lung fails to re-expand after drainage of the empyema, the more radical operation of decortication may be required (Figure 55.9). The fibrous cortex or peel from the entrapped underlying lung is removed so that the lung can expand to obliterate the pleural space. This is performed through a posterolateral thoracotomy and requires careful dissection to remove the parietal and visceral cortex, taking care not to damage the visceral pleura.

PRESENTATION OF LUNG DISEASE

Haemoptysis

Diseases causing repeated haemoptysis include carcinoma, bronchiectasis, carcinoid tumours and some infections. Severe mitral stenosis is now a rare cause. Patients with repeated haemoptysis should be investigated, at the very least by chest radiography and bronchoscopy. Haemoptysis following trauma may be from a lung contusion or injury to a major airway. Treatment depends on the underlying cause.

Common associated chest symptoms include cough with

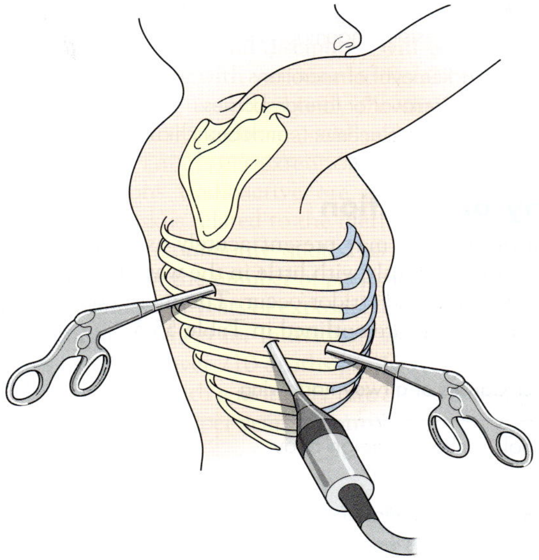

Figure 55.8 Video-assisted thoracoscopic surgery (VATS) utilises modern thoracoscopic instruments and digital technology and avoids large incisions.

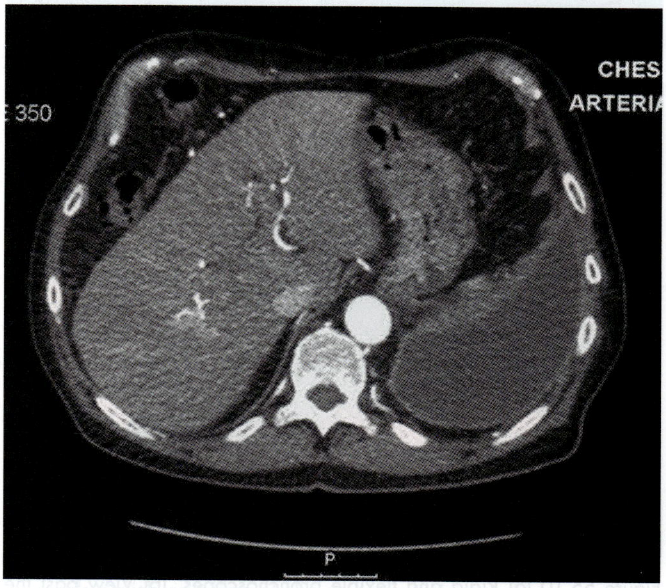

Figure 55.9 Chest computed tomography scan showing an empyema with a grossly thickened pleura.

(because of the involvement of, or extrinsic pressure on, the oesophagus) and superior vena caval obstruction.
- Small cell carcinoma is associated with the development of myopathies including the Eaton–Lambert syndrome, which is similar to myasthenia gravis (Summary box 55.5).

Summary box 55.5

Symptoms of lung cancer

- Haemoptysis <50% of patients
- Cough, new or changed pattern
- Pain
- Dyspnoea
- Clubbing
- Hoarseness
- Myopathies

Treatment of lung cancer

Careful investigation is required to determine which tumours are operable and will benefit from a major thoracic resection. The internationally agreed tumour–node–metastasis (TNM) staging system gives prognostic information on the natural history of the disease. Tumours graded up to T3, N1, M0 can be encompassed within an anatomical surgical resection and have a much improved prognosis when treated surgically, so the tumour must be staged accurately before resection (Table 55.6). A number of non-tumour factors, including the general fitness of the patient and the results of lung function tests, help to determine the appropriate treatment. In patients with incurable disease, treatment is palliative to maximise quality of life and disease-free survival.

Survival

Carcinoma of the bronchus generally has a low survival rate after diagnosis (Table 55.7). Important factors in determining

Table 55.6 The international tumour–node–metastasis (TNM) staging system.

Primary tumour (T)	
T0	No evidence of primary tumour
T1	Tumour ≤3 cm[a], surrounded by lung or visceral pleura, no bronchoscopic evidence of invasion, more proximal than the lobar bronchus T1a, Tumour ≤2 cm T1b, Tumour >2, but ≤3 cm
T2	Tumour >3, but ≤7 cm[a] or tumour with any of the following[b]: invades visceral pleura, involves main bronchus ≥2 cm distal to the carina, atelectasis/obstructive pneumonia extending to hilum, but not involving the entire lung T2a, Tumour >3, but ≤5 cm[a] T2b, Tumour >5, but ≤7 cm[a]
T3	Tumour >7 cm or directly invading chest wall, diaphragm, phrenic nerve, mediastinal pleura, or parietal pericardium; or tumour in the main bronchus <2 cm distal to the carina[c]; or atelectasis/obstructive pneumonitis of entire lung; or separate tumour nodules in the same lobe
T4	Tumour of any size with invasion of the mediastinum or involving the heart, great vessels, trachea, recurrent laryngeal nerve, oesophagus, vertebral body or carina, or separate tumour nodules in a different ipsilateral lobe
Nodal involvement (N)	
N0	No demonstrable metastasis or regional lymph node
N1	Metastasis to lymph nodes in the peribronchial or the ipsilateral hilar region, or both, including direct extension
N2	Metastasis to the ipsilateral, mediastinal and subcarinal lymph nodes
N3	Metastasis to the contralateral mediastinal lymph nodes, contralateral hilar lymph nodes, ipsilateral or contralateral scalene or supraclavicular lymph nodes
Distant metastasis (M)	
M0	No known distant metastasis
M1a	Separate tumour nodules in a contralateral lobe, or tumour with pleural nodules or malignant pleural dissemination[d]
M1b	Distant metastasis
Special situations	
T,N,M	T, N or M status not able to be assessed
Tis	Focus of *in situ* cancer
T1	Superficial spreading tumour of any size, but confined to the wall of the trachea or mainstream bronchus

[a]In the greatest dimension.
[b]T2 tumours with these features are classified as T2a if ≤5 cm.
[c]The uncommon superficial spreading tumour in central airways is classified as T1.
[d]Pleural effusions that are cytologically negative, non-bloody, transudative, and clinically judged not to be due to cancer are excluded.

Lee M Eaton, 1905–1958, a neurologist who was a Professor at The Mayo Clinic, Rochester, MN, USA.
Edward H Lambert, 1915–2003, Professor of Physiology, The University of Minnesota, MN, USA, regarded as an icon in neurology in the USA.
Eaton and Lambert described Eaton–Lambert syndrome in a joint paper in 1956.

prognosis are the histological type of the tumour, the spread (stage) and the general condition of the patient. Early detection and surgical resection offer the best hope for cure.

Diagnosis and staging

Increasing emphasis in recent years has been the early detection of lung cancer, with guidance on symptoms and signs of potential lung cancer that require urgent chest x-ray and referral to lung cancer team (Table 55.8).

Non-invasive investigations

Chest x-ray

A chest x-ray will detect most lung cancers but some, particularly early curable tumours, are hidden by other structures. Secondary effects such as pleural effusion, distal collapse and raised hemidiaphragm may be evident (Figure 55.12).

Computed tomography

This is the first investigation in suspected lung cancer. The surgeon needs to know if the primary is resectable (T stage) and which if any lymph nodes are involved (N stage). Lymph nodes of

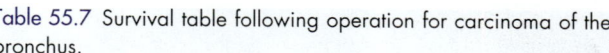

Table 55.7 Survival table following operation for carcinoma of the bronchus.

	(%)
Five-year survival according to presurgical staging	
Stage I	56–67
Stage II	39–55
Stage IIIa	23
Stage IIIb	<10
Five-year survival according to cell type	
Squamous cell carcinoma	35–50
Adenocarcinoma	25–45
Adenosquamous carcinoma	20–35
Undifferentiated carcinoma	15–25
Small cell carcinoma	0–5

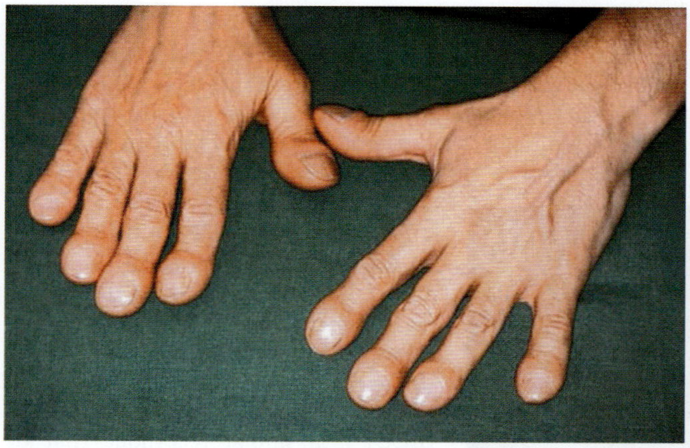

Figure 55.11 Example of finger clubbing in a patient with bronchogenic carcinoma.

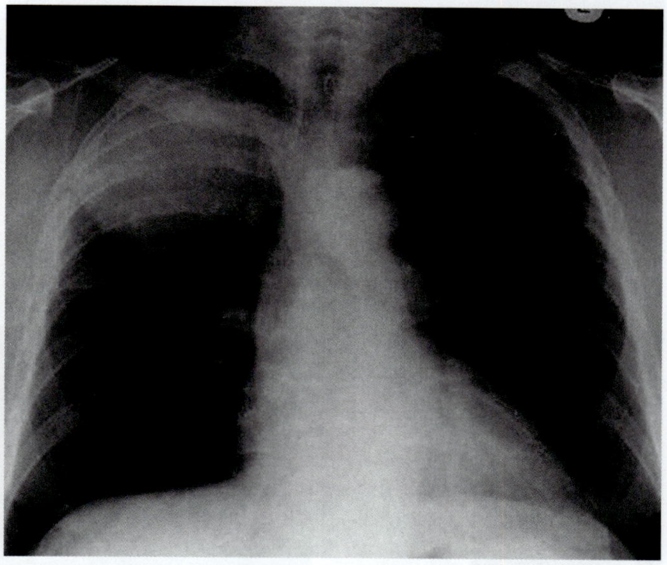

Figure 55.12 Chest x-ray of carcinoma of the lung. This patient has a large mass in the right upper lobe, causing Horner's syndrome.

Table 55.8 Recent National Institute for Health and Clinical Excellence (NICE) guidance on referral in patients with suspected lung cancer.

Symptoms and signs indicating urgent chest x-ray	Offer urgent chest x-ray to patients presenting with haemoptysis, or any of the following if unexplained or present for more than 3 weeks:	Cough Chest/shoulder pain Dyspnoea Finger clubbing Signs suggesting metastases (for example, in brain, bone, liver or skin) Weight loss Chest signs Hoarseness Cervical/supraclavicular lymphadenopathy
Symptoms and signs indicating urgent referral	Offer urgent referral to lung cancer multidisciplinary team (MDT) (usually the chest physician) while waiting for chest x-ray results if any of the following are present:	Persistent haemoptysis in a smoker or ex-smoker older than 40 years Signs of superior vena cava obstruction (swelling of the face and/or neck with fixed elevation of jugular venous pressure) Stridor
	Offer urgent referral to lung cancer MDT (usually the chest physician) if:	A chest x-ray or CT scan suggests lung cancer (including pleural effusion and slowly resolving consolidation) or Chest x-ray is normal, but there is a high suspicion of lung cancer

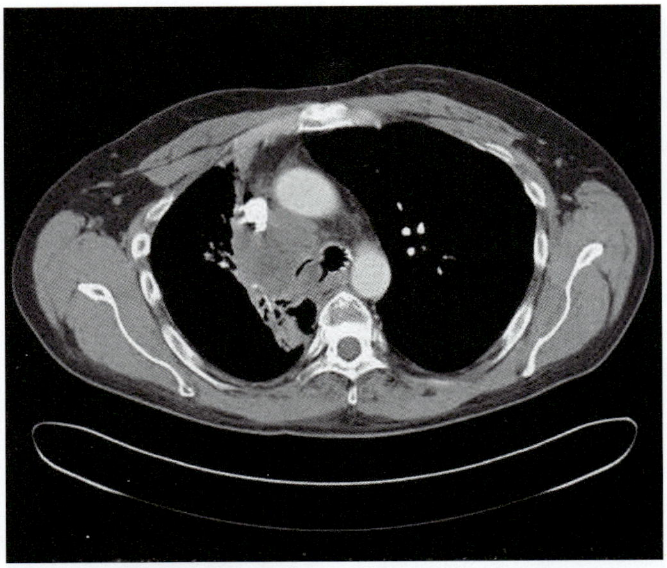

Figure 55.13 Paratracheal lymphadenopathy shown on a computed tomography scan.

more than 2 cm in diameter are likely to be involved in the disease (70 per cent) (Figure 55.13) and those less than 10 mm in the shorter axis are unlikely to be involved. If the presence of cancer in the nodes is critical to management, further evidence from positron emission tomography with radiolabelled fluorodeoxyglucose (FDG-PET) or biopsy (see below) is essential. Remote metastases to the liver, adrenals or elsewhere may be detected.

Positron emission tomography

The patient is given radiolabelled FDG, which is taken up by all metabolising cells but more avidly by cancer cells. The FDG enters the Kreb's cycle but cannot complete it and accumulates in proportion to the glucose avidity of the cells. High accumulation is associated with lung cancers and secondaries. Infection or other inflammation, and lymphadenopathy secondary to it, are also FDG avid (Figure 55.14).

Sputum cytology

Sputum cytology may reveal malignant cells, but the false-negative rate is high.

Invasive investigations

Once lung cancer is suspected, diagnosis and further staging are sought. The choice of investigation depends on the position of the primary tumour in the lung (peripheral or central) and the clinical stage of the cancer (presence of enlarged lymph nodes or metastasis).

Bronchoscopy

A flexible bronchoscopy is usually performed under sedation particularly in more centrally placed lung cancers. It allows assessment of the segmental airway, cytological testing through bushing and washing of the concerned segmental bronchi and transbronchial needle aspiration (TBNA).

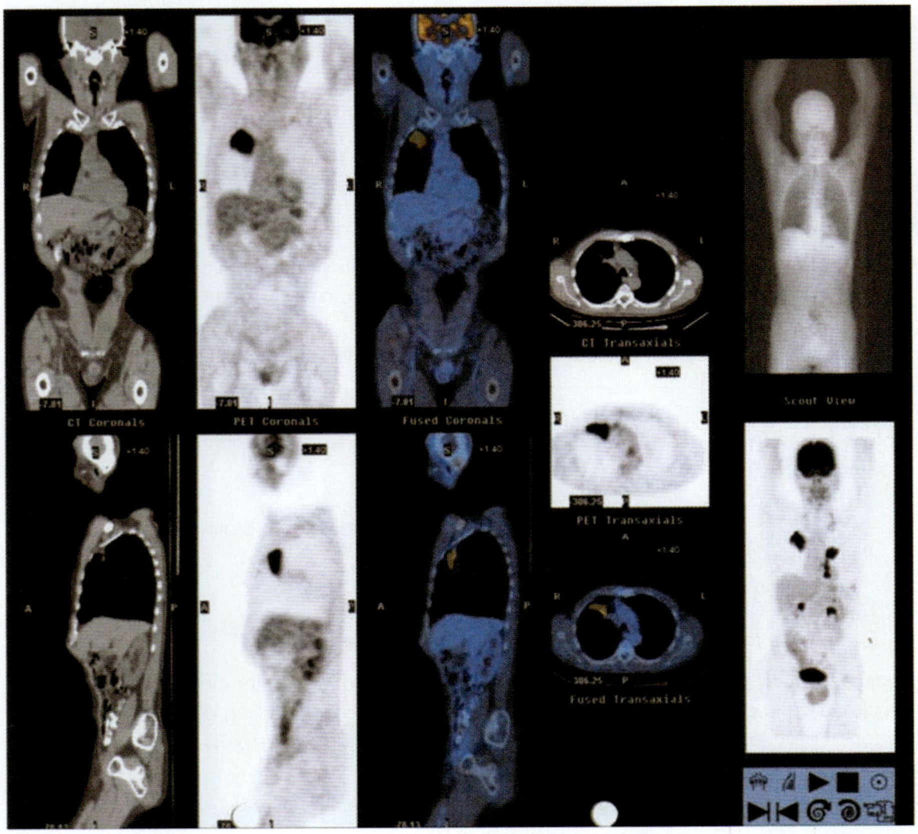

Figure 55.14 Multiple FDG-avid mediastinal lymph nodes shown on a positron emission tomography/computed tomography scan (courtesy of Dr Sally Barrington).

Endobronchial ultrasound

Endobronchial ultrasound (EBUS) allows bronchoscopic assessment of suspicious mediastinal lymph nodes with an ultrasound probe incorporated into the tip of the bronchoscope to aid TBNA (Figure 55.15). Endoscopic ultrasound (EUS) is a similar technique that by passing down the oesophagus allows fine needle aspiration (FNA) of less approachable mediastinal lymph nodes.

Computed tomography-guided biopsy

Percutaneous CT-guided FNA may give a good yield of cells for cytological examination. Alternatively, a core of tissue can be obtained for formal histology. These techniques are best for larger and more peripheral lesions. Pneumothorax is common (30 per cent), but rarely requires intercostal tube drainage. The contraindications include poor respiratory reserve when even a small pneumothorax would be hazardous.

Surgical diagnosis and staging

Mediastinoscopy, mediastinotomy, VATS or thoracotomy lymph node/lung biopsy are aimed at establishing a tissue

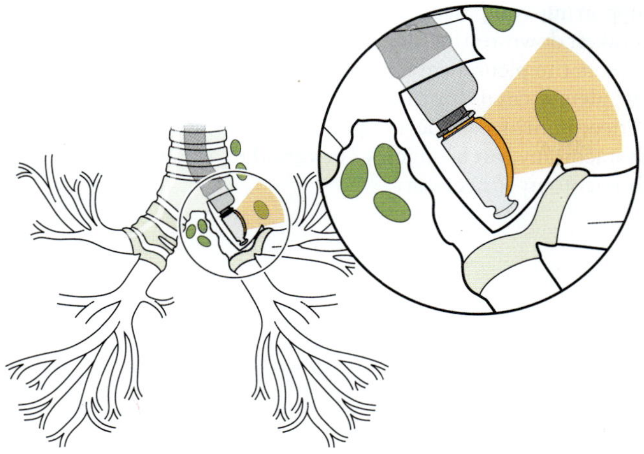

Figure 55.15 Endobronchial ultrasound (EBUS) allows accurate diagnosis of enlarged mediastinal lymph nodes for diagnosis and staging of lung cancer.

diagnosis and assessing the degree of spread (staging), which determines resectability. Histological proof of the status of mediastinal nodes may be important to avoid unnecessary thoracotomy for incurable cancers and, conversely, to not deny surgery to patients whose lymph nodes are enlarged but benign.

Mediastinoscopy

This procedure is performed under general anaesthesia with the patient supine and his or her neck extended (Figure 55.16). A transverse incision is made 2 cm above the sternal notch and deepened until the strap muscles are reached. These are retracted laterally and the thyroid isthmus is retracted superiorly to reveal the pretracheal fascia. Careful blunt dissection in this plane allows access to the paratracheal and subcarinal nodes. A mediastinoscope is introduced for direct visualisation and biopsy. Great caution should be used in the presence of superior vena caval obstruction. Complications include pneumothorax and haemorrhage.

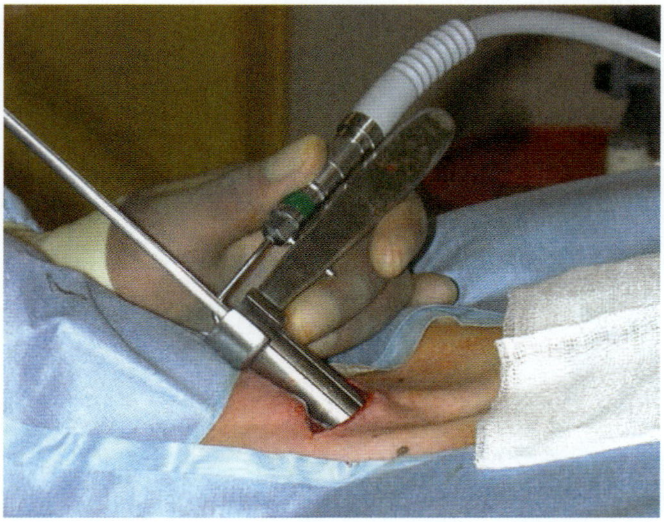

Figure 55.16 Mediastinoscopy. The mediastinoscope slides down immediately in front of the trachea, behind the aortic arch, and behind and between the great vessels of the head and neck.

Sir Hans Adolf Krebs, 1900–1981, Professor of Biochemistry, The University of Oxford, Oxford, UK. Was elected as a Fellow of the Royal Society of London in 1947; he is known best for identification of the urea cycle and the citric acid cycle. The latter known as the Kreb's cycle, earned him a share of the Nobel Prize in Physiology or Medicine in 1953.

Mediastinotomy

An incision is made through the second intercostal space to gain access to some of the mediastinal lymph nodes on the affected side. On the left, this includes lymph nodes in the para-aortic or sub-aortic fossa. Damage to the internal mammary artery and the phrenic nerve must be avoided. Mediastinal extension of tumour can also be assessed, for example left upper lobe tumours which invade the mediastinum around the aortic arch.

These techniques may also be used in the diagnosis of other mediastinal conditions, including:

- lymphoma;
- anterior mediastinal tumours;
- thymoma;
- sarcoid, tuberculosis or any other cause of lymphadenopathy.

VATS mediastinal lymph node and lung biopsy

For inaccessible mediastinal lymph nodes, or when diagnosis of the lung tumour has not been possible through radiological or bronchoscopic techniques, VATS performed through two or three ports allows diagnosis of the tumour, staging of the mediastinum and gives the opportunity to assess the likely operability of the lung cancer.

Surgical approach to lung cancer resection

Thoracotomy

Although the most frequent reason for thoracotomy is lung cancer, all surgeons dealing with trauma should be able to perform a thoracotomy, if required. The standard route into the thoracic cavity is through a posterolateral thoracotomy. The incision is used for access to the:

- lung and major bronchi;
- pleura;
- thoracic aorta;
- oesophagus;
- posterior mediastinum.

A double-lumen endotracheal tube is used to allow ventilation of one lung while the other is collapsed, to facilitate surgery and to protect the non-operated lung and retain control of ventilation (Figure 55.17).

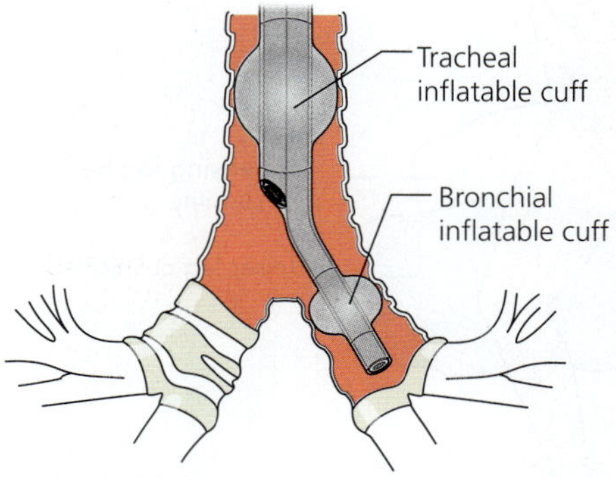

Figure 55.17 The double-lumen tube permits separate ventilation of the right and left lungs.

The patient is turned to the lateral position with the affected side up (Figure 55.18). The lower leg is flexed at the hip and the knee, with a pillow between the legs. Table supports are used to maintain the position and additional strapping is used at the hips for stability. The patient's hips are placed below the break point of the operating table to allow opening of the intercostal spaces as the table is angulated. The upper arm may be supported by a bracket in a position of 90° flexion. The lower arm is flexed and positioned by the head. It is important for both the surgeon and the anaesthetist to be completely satisfied with the position of the patient and the tube and lines at this stage.

- The incision passes 1–2 cm below the tip of the scapula, and extends posteriorly and superiorly between the medial border of the scapula and the spine.
- The incision is deepened through the subcutaneous tissues to the latissimus dorsi. This muscle is divided with coagulating diathermy, taking care over haemostasis.
- A plane of dissection is developed by hand deep to the scapula and serratus anterior. The ribs can be counted down from the highest palpable rib (which is usually the second) and the sixth rib periosteum is scored with the diathermy near its upper border. A periosteal elevator is used to lift the periosteum off the superior border of the rib or alternatively the intercostal muscle is cut with diathermy just above the rib (Figure 55.19).
- This reveals the pleura, which may be entered by blunt dissection. A rib spreader is inserted between the ribs and opened gently to prevent fracture.
- Exposure may be facilitated by dividing the rib at the costal angle or by dividing the costotransverse ligament. Resection of a rib is not usually required.
- The anaesthetist is now able to deflate the affected lung to allow a better view of the intrathoracic structures.

In an emergency thoracotomy for penetrating wounds of the heart, a more anterior approach is used and no specialised supporting equipment is required (Figure 55.20). The incision is taken down to the fourth or fifth rib with a scalpel, and using scissors the pleural cavity opened. This gives rapid access to the left pleural cavity in cases of massive left haemothorax and the pericardium if cardiac tamponade is supected. A left anterior thoracotomy can be quickly converted to a clamshell or bilateral thoracotomy if necessary.

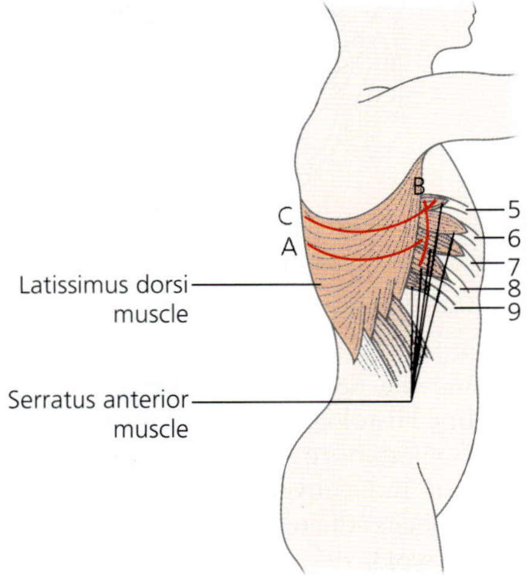

Figure 55.19 Incision and layers encountered during anterolateral thoracotomy. A The latissimus dorsi is divided in line with the skin incision. B If the serratus anterior is divided, it should be close to its attachment to ribs 6, 7 and 8. It can be left intact and mobilised along its inferior border. C The intercostal muscles are stripped off the upper border of the rib.

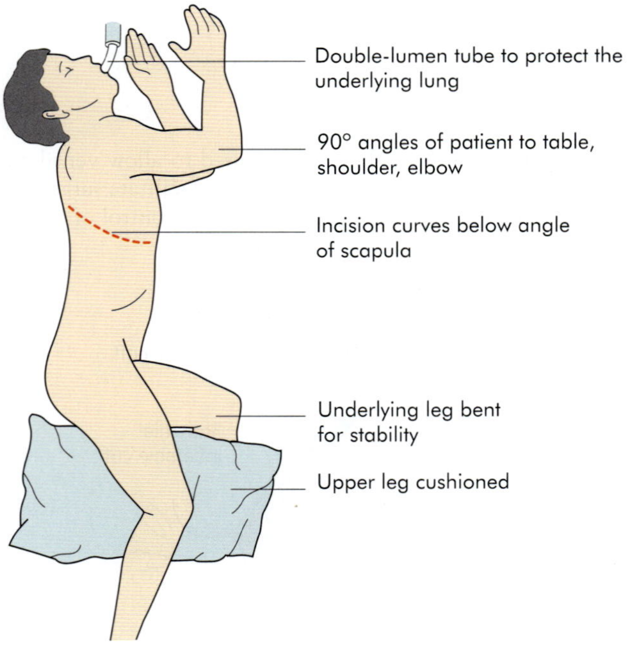

Figure 55.18 Correct positioning for thoracotomy.

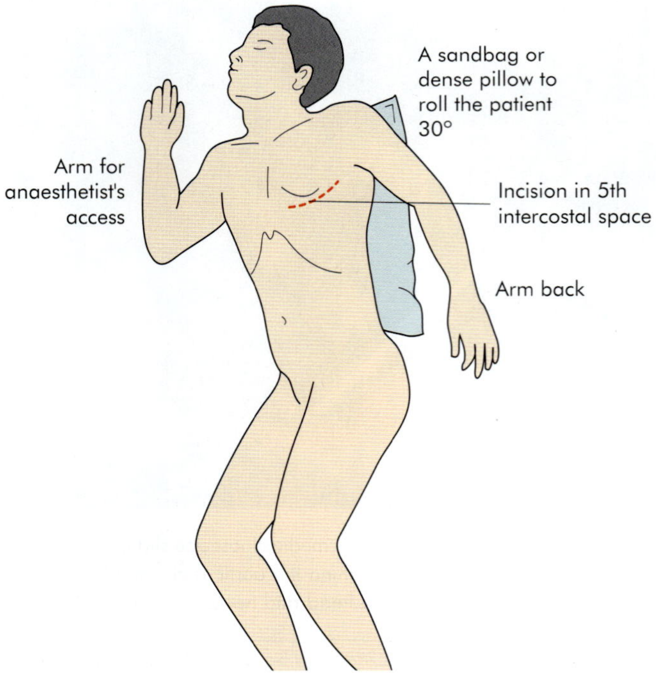

Figure 55.20 Emergency left anterior thoracotomy for access to the heart. Requires no special supports or devices.

Following the operation, 24–28 Fr chest drain/s are placed, typically through the seventh or eighth intercostal space, anterior to the mid-axillary line, so that the patient does not lie on them. Even if the site to be drained is posterior, as in empyema, the drains are tunnelled to come out more anteriorly for easier management. The thoracotomy is closed using paracostal sutures placed around the rib above and below to reapproximate the ribs or alternatively intercostal muscle is sutured to the intercostal muscle below the stripped rib with a continuous absorbable suture. The fascia and muscle layer are closed in layers using an absorbable suture. Skin closure is a matter of personal preference.

Analgesia is an important aspect of postoperative care and the process may be started prior to thoracotomy with an epidural catheter placed by the anaesthetist, or intraoperatively by infiltrating the intercostal nerves in the region of the incision with a long-acting local anaesthetic via a surgically sited paravertebral catheter. Various strategies have been developed to deliver analgesics postoperatively to facilitate a normal breathing pattern.

Video-assisted thoracoscopic surgery

Various approaches utilising thoracoscopic techniques can be used to gain access to the chest cavity and facilitate lung resection. A combination of a smaller thoracotomy incision and VATS has been described, but increasingly lung resections can be performed through three or four port incisions and the dissection of hilar structures completed entirely through VATS. The technique avoids rib-spreading and appears to reduce postoperative pain, length of stay and aids a speedier recovery.

Surgical management of lung cancer

The principle of surgery is to remove all cancer (the primary and the regional lymph nodes), but to conserve as much lung as possible. The selection of patients in terms of the stage of the lung cancer and fitness to undergo such surgery is paramount. Surgery with curative intent is offered to patients with early stage lung cancer (T1–3, N0–1) (Table 55.9). Assessment of a patient's fitness to undergo lung cancer resection involves considering premorbid conditions which can be aided using risk scores such as Thorascore, cardiovascular function and lung function (Table 55.10). Lung function particularly will aid the surgeon in selecting the type of procedure offered and likely breathlessness or dyspnoea following lung resection.

Table 55.9 National Institute for Health and Clinical Excellence (NICE) recommendations for surgery for non-small cell lung cancer.

Surgery with curative intent for non-small cell lung cancer (NSCLC)
Offer patients with NSCLC who are fit for surgery, open or thoracoscopic lobectomy as the treatment of first choice. If complete resection is possible, consider segmentectomy or wedge resection for patients with smaller tumours (T1a–b, N0, M0) and borderline fitness
Offer more extensive surgery (bronchoangioplastic surgery, bilobectomy, pneumonectomy) only when needed to obtain clear margins
Perform hilar and mediastinal lymph node sampling or en bloc resection for all patients undergoing surgery with curative intent
For T3 NSCLC with chest wall involvement, aim for complete resection by extrapleural or en bloc chest wall resection

Table 55.10 National Institute for Health and Clinical Excellence (NICE) recommendations for assessing fitness for treatment with curative intent (including surgery).

Perioperative mortality	Consider global risk score, such as Thoracoscore	Ensure patient is aware of risk before consenting
Cardiovascular function	Assess risk factors and cardiac functional capacity	Avoid surgery within 30 days of myocardial infarction (MI)
		Optimise primary cardiac treatment and begin secondary cardiac prophylaxis as soon as possible
		Offer surgery if two or fewer risk factors and good cardiac functional capacity
		Seek cardiology review if active cardiac condition, three or more risk factors or poor cardiac functional capacity
		Consider revascularisation before surgery in stable angina
		Continue anti-ischaemic treatment in perioperative period. Discuss perioperative platelet treatment if patient has a coronary stent
Lung function	Perform spirometry, measure T_LCO if disproportionate breathlessness or other lung pathology, perform segment count and assess exercise tolerance,	Offer surgery if normal FEV_1 and good exercise tolerance or FEV_1 or T_LCO below 30% and patient accepts the risks of dyspnoea
	and consider shuttle walk testing (cut-off 400 m) and cardiopulmonary exercise testing (cut-off 15 mL/kg/minute) if moderate to high risk of postoperative dyspnoea	Offer radiotherapy with curative intent if lung function poor but patient is otherwise suitable for radiotherapy with curative intent and volume of irradiated lung is small

From NICE clinical guideline 21, available from: www.nice.org.uk/nicemedia/live/13465/54208/54208.pdf

Choice of lung resection

Segmentectomy and wedge resection

Segmentectomy and wedge resections are performed in patients with small tumours and with borderline fitness through thoracotomy or VATS. Each lobe of the lung has segments which allows anatomical dissection and ligation of the segmental pulmonary artery, vein and bronchus (segmentectomy) (Figure 55.2) or non-anatomical excision can be performed (wedge resection) combined with removal of regional lymph nodes.

Lobectomy

Lobectomy remains the treatment of choice in patients with early stage lung cancer. The surgery can be performed via thoracotomy or VATS. Following dissection of the fissure and hilar structures, the branches of the pulmonary artery and veins to the lobe are isolated and ligated. The bronchus is usually stapled but can be sewn.

At the completion of the operation, the remaining lung is reinflated. Some air leak is common and usually settles within a few days. One or two intercostal drains are inserted. The patient does not routinely need intensive care and postoperative ventilation is best avoided. The 30-day mortality rate is 2–3 per cent, with morbidity such as chest infection or cardiac arrhythmia of around 10 per cent. The average length of stay is around 5–7 days.

Pneumonectomy

Pneumonectomy is removal of a whole lung and has a higher mortality rate (5–8 per cent). The surgeon must be satisfied that the patient is fit to tolerate this procedure from the preoperative work up. This procedure is reserved for either centrally placed tumours involving the main bronchus or those that straddle the fissure. At thoracotomy, an inspection of the lung and direct palpation of the mass will determine resectability and lymph node spread. Fixation of the tumour to the aorta, heart or oesophagus implies irresectability. Involvement of the mediastinal lymph node chain is associated with a poor prognosis. With modern preoperative imaging, resection is abandoned in only about 3 per cent of cases.

Pneumonectomy is anatomically more straightforward than lobectomy and involves dissecting and ligating the main pulmonary artery, the superior and inferior pulmonary veins and the main bronchus which is divided so that no blind stump remains (Figure 55.21). The technique of stump closure is important if a bronchopleural fistula is to be avoided. The tissues are carefully handled and the stump is usually stapled and sometimes covered using pleural, pericardium or a vascular pedicle such as an intercostal muscle. Drainage of the space is a matter of debate. Most use an underwater-seal drain and either leave it unclamped or unclamp it for 1 minute every hour until the drainage ceases; others prefer not to drain. The critical point is that no suction should be applied as there is now a sealed space with the mobile mediastinum on one side of it. The air in the pneumonectomy space is gradually absorbed and the fluid level within the space rises (Figure 55.22).

Complications of lung resection

- **Bleeding**. Bleeding should be avoidable by the use of a careful surgical technique, but may be severe in the presence of dense adhesions.
- **Respiratory infection**. Many of these patients are ex-smokers and so basal collapse and hypoxaemia are common postoperatively.
- **Persistent air leak**. Chest drains are placed at the time of surgery to deal with the air leak. Rarely, the air leak persists and the remaining lung does not expand. Repeat thoracotomy may then be necessary to seal the leak.
- **Bronchopleural fistula**. Bronchopleural fistula is a serious complication. Following pneumonectomy, the space left behind is initially filled with air. This is slowly reabsorbed and the space fills with tissue fluid. The fluid level rises until the air is finally reabsorbed. Dehiscence of the bronchial stump leads to the development of a bronchopleural fistula and the fluid in the space (which is almost inevitably infected) is expectorated in large quantities. This complication has a high morbidity and mortality rate.

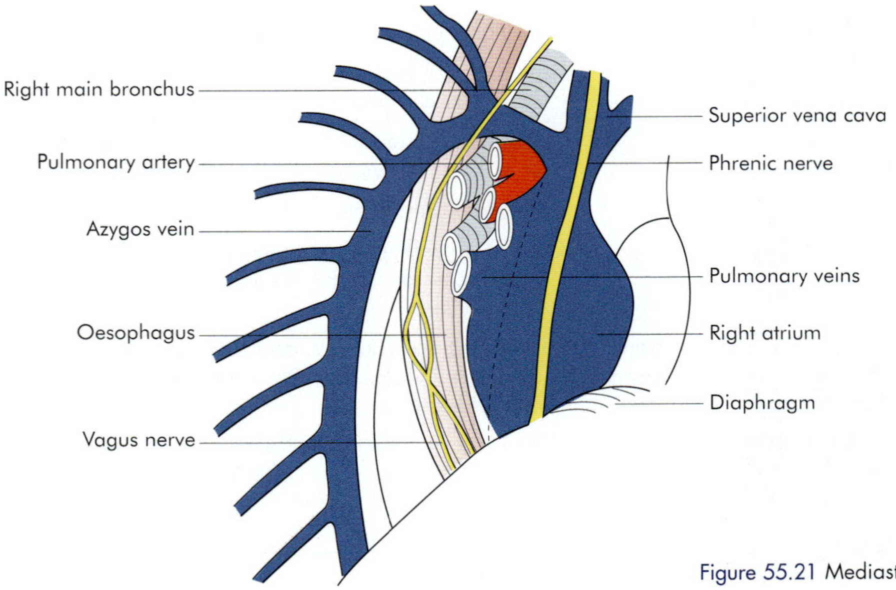

Figure 55.21 Mediastinal structures after removal of right lung.

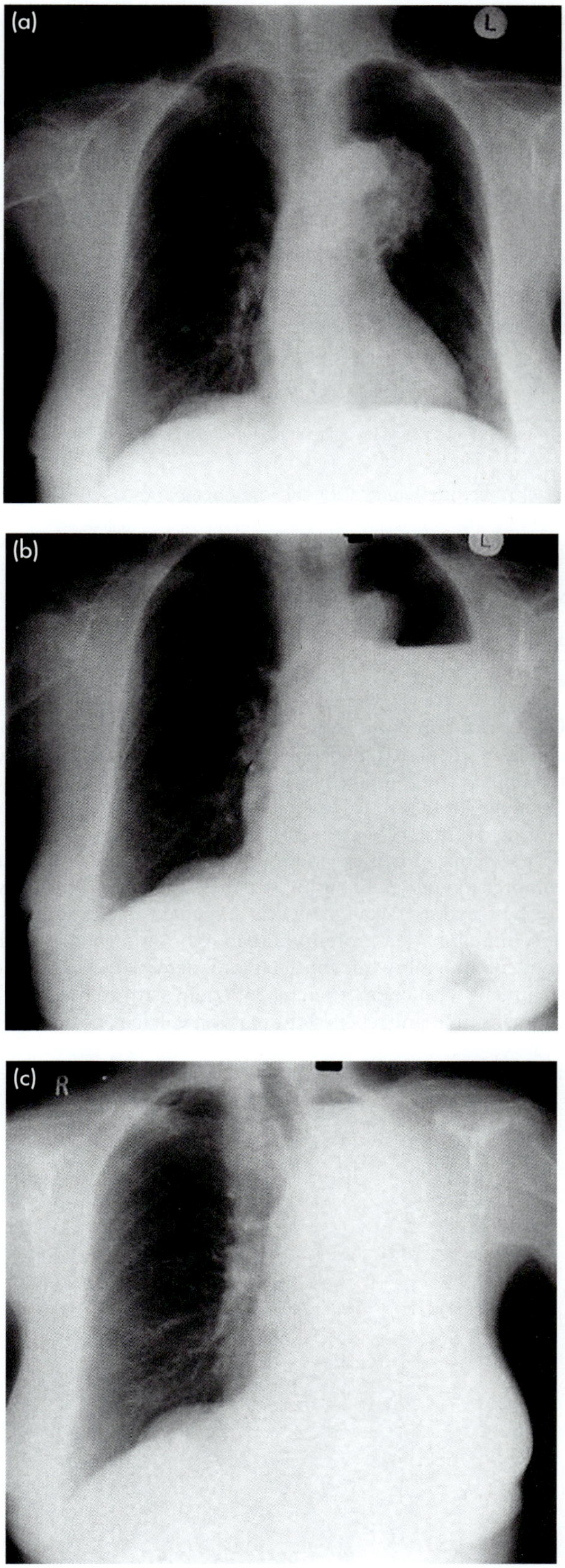

Figure 55.22 Chest radiographs (a) pre- and (b) post-pneumonectomy, with rising fluid level (c) in the left haemothorax.

The patient is nursed sitting up and turned so that the affected space is dependent, to prevent infected fluid from entering the remaining lung while arrangements are made to site a pleural drain. This should be connected to an underwater seal, but not suction. Bronchopleural fistulas are unlikely to resolve spontaneously and management is highly specialised.

Postoperative care

Patients have limited respiratory reserve following lung resection, so infection and fluid overload are to be avoided. Once air leaks have settled, the drains are removed. Mobilisation, breathing exercises and regular physiotherapy are begun as soon as the patient's condition permits.

Postoperative pain

It is important to deal with post-thoracotomy pain effectively so that a normal breathing pattern and gas exchange are achieved in the early postoperative period. Three strategies are routinely used in combination:

- patient-controlled analgesia (PCA) with intravenous boluses of opiates;
- paravertebral/extrapleural or epidural catheter-delivered local anaesthetic;
- background oral analgesia with paracetamol.

Long-term post-thoracotomy pain can be reduced by careful attention to detail during the operation. Sources of avoidable chronic pain include rib fracture and the entrapment of intercostal nerves during wound closure.

BENIGN LUNG TUMOURS

Benign tumours of the lung are uncommon and account for fewer than 15 per cent of solitary lesions seen on chest x-rays. A peripheral tumour usually causes no symptoms until it is large; a central tumour may present with haemoptysis and signs of bronchial obstruction while small. A tumour is likely to be benign if it has not increased in size on chest x-rays for more than two years or it has some degree of calcification; however, a tissue diagnosis is usually pursued.

Most benign nodules are granulomas (tuberculosis or histoplasmosis). The most common benign tumour is a hamartoma, a developmental abnormality containing mesothelial and endothelial elements. Diagnosis (and definitive treatment) is achieved by excision of the lesion. Any of the mesodermal elements of the lung may form a mesodermal tumour (chondroma, lipoma, leiomyoma). Deposits of amyloid may give similar radiographic appearances of a nodule (pseudotumour).

Bronchopulmonary carcinoid tumours

These carcinoid tumours are derived from the neuroendocrine cells of bronchial glands. Most (80 per cent) are found in the major bronchi and are characteristically slow growing and highly vascular. They are currently classified within a spectrum of neuroendocrine tumours. Most behave in a benign way; however, approximately 15 per cent metastasise. The patient often presents with a history of recurrent pneumonia or haemoptysis, but carcinoid syndrome is rare unless there is extensive pulmonary or hepatic metastases. Surgical excision is preferred as prognosis following complete resection is excellent (>90 per cent ten-year survival). Segmental or wedge resection may be sufficient for a small peripheral tumour, while lobectomy or pneumonectomy may be necessary for central tumours. Where possible, a lung-sparing bronchoplastic or sleeve resection should be considered. This allows resection of proximal endobronchial lesions in an effort to preserve more distal, uninvolved lung parenchyma.

THE MEDIASTINUM

The mediastinum refers to the central area in the chest between the thoracic inlet and the diaphragm, between the right and left pleural surfaces and which extends from the inner aspect of the sternum to the vertebral column. It contains the heart, great vessels, trachea and the oesophagus, and is arbitrarily subdivided into compartments (superior, inferior, anterior, middle and posterior). Much of the regional lymph node chains draining the chest and its organs are also found in the mediastinum. Various surgical procedures to approach structures and particularly lymph nodes in the mediastinum have been described earlier under Surgical diagnosis and staging, and are performed usually as diagnostic procedures. The surgical approach when mediastinal tumours require resection depends on the antomical location of the tumour (Figure 55.23) and includes median sternotomy for anterior mediastinal pathology, thoracotomy or VATS for posterior mediastinal pathology and transcervical (neck incisions) for superior mediastinal pathology. The middle mediastinum can usually be approached through thoracotomy or VATS.

Primary tumours of the mediastinum

Thymoma, neurogenic tumours, germ cell tumours and lymphoma are the usual primary tumours of the mediastinum.

- **Thymoma**. This is the most common mediastinal tumour, accounting for 25 per cent of the total and is derived from the thymus gland (Figure 55.24). Thymomas vary in behaviour from benign to aggressively invasive as reflected in the Masaoka classification system used to stage thymomas (Table 55.11). They are often related to myaesthenia gravis (MG), a neuromuscular condition which can have a high associated incidence of thymomas, and interestingly may respond to excision of the thymus gland even when the gland has no associated thymoma present. The only reliable indicator of malignancy is capsular invasion. Diagnosis and treatment are best achieved by complete thymectomy, which is usually performed as a median sternotomy. However, if the thymoma is small or when the patient has MG and the thymus is being excised as a treatment, a transcervical approach with or without an additional VATS procedure can be performed.

Table 55.11 Masaoka thymoma staging system.

Stage	Description
I	Macroscopically completely encapsulated Microscopically no capsular invasion
II	Macroscopic invasion into surrounding fatty tissue or mediastinal pleura Microscopic invasion into the capsule
III	Macroscopic invasion into neighbouring organs (pericardium, great vessels, lungs)
IVA	Pleural or pericardial dissemination
IVB	Lymphogenous or hematogenous metastasis

After Masaoka A *et al.*, *Cancer* 1981; **48**: 2485.

- **Germ cell tumour**. The anterior mediastinum is the most common site of extragonadal germ cell tumours. They account for 13 per cent of all mediastinal masses and cysts and contain elements from all three cell types (mesoderm, endoderm and ectoderm). They tend to present in young adults and 75 per cent are benign and cystic, although they may cause compression of neighbouring structures; hence, dermoid cysts are best excised. Malignancy is suspected if elevated levels of serum alpha-fetoprotein, human chorionic gonadotrophin and carcinoembryonic antigen are detected. After initial treatment with chemotherapy, a patient with tumour marker normalisation and a persistent mass on CT may be considered

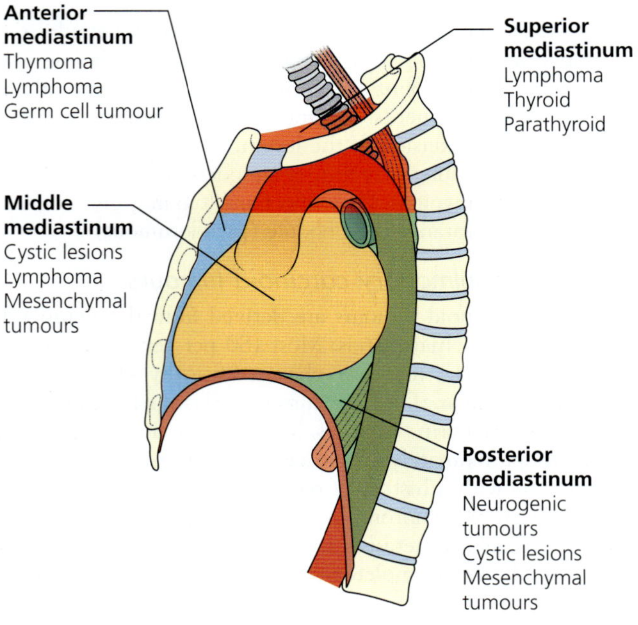

Figure 55.23 Mediastinal pathology. Subdivisions of the mediastinum with the most common mediastinal masses.

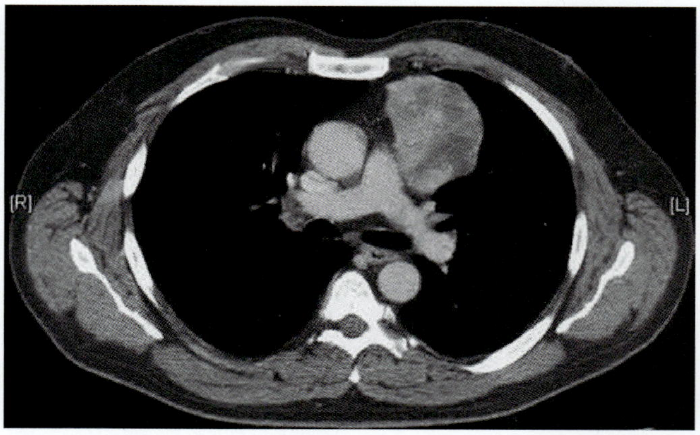

Figure 55.24 Computed tomography scan showing a thymoma presenting as a mediastinal mass.

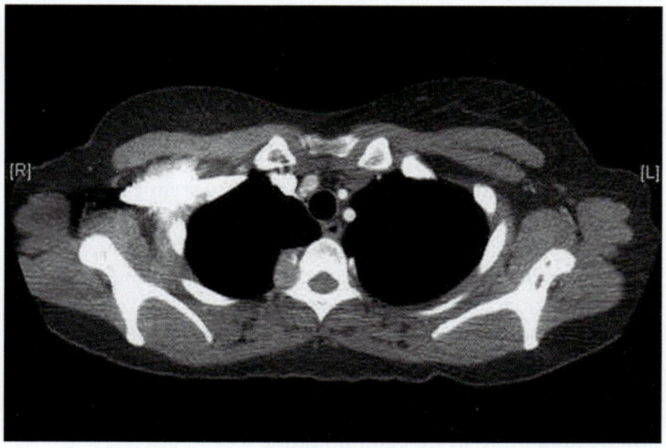

Figure 55.25 Computed tomography scan showing a right-sided paravertebral neurogenic tumour.

for surgical resection. If tumour markers fail to normalise, further chemotherapy is usually offered.

- **Lymphoma**. Lymphoma is a common cause of a mediastinal mass lesion, particularly the anterior mediastinum, and can lead to superior vena cava obstruction or other symptoms of local compression. The main treatment is chemotherapy, and surgery is rarely required apart from obtaining tissue for diagnosis.
- **Mesenchymal tumours**. Lipomas are common in the anterior mediastinum. Other mesenchymal tumours are very rare.
- **Thyroid**. Ectopic thyroid tissue (and parathyroid) may be found in the anterior mediastinum, but usually the mass is an extension of a thyroid lesion (retrosternal goitre). Excision of retrosternal thyroids may be required if there is local airway compression and stridor and can be performed via a transcervical incision, but occasionally median sternotomy may be required.
- **Neurogenic tumours**. These may derive from the sympathetic nervous system or the peripheral nerves and are more prevalent in the posterior mediastinum. They may be painful but are more often discovered accidentally on routine chest radiography and can be quite large (Figure 55.25). They include neuroblastoma in childhood, and schwannomas

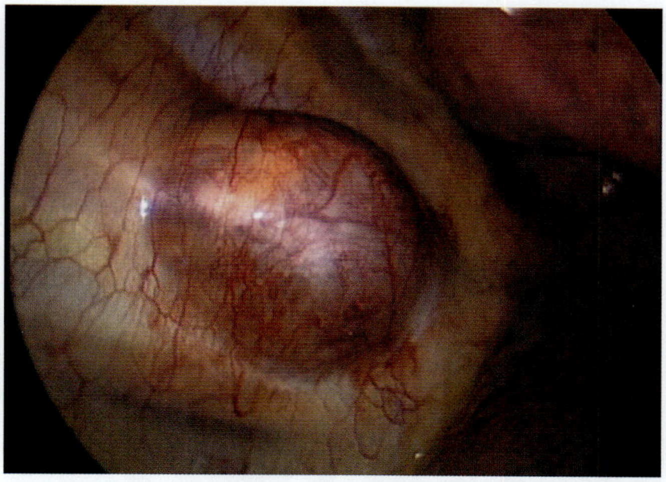

Figure 55.26 Video-assisted thoracoscopic surgery (VATS) image of a neurogenic tumour attached to the posterolateral chest wall prior to excision.

and neurofibromas in adults, which are usually benign. Phaeochromocytoma arises from the sympathetic chain and produces the characteristic endocrine syndrome. Excision of neurogenic tumours is generally recommended particularly if the patient is developing symptoms. This can be performed through a thoracotomy, though for smaller tumours a VATS approach can be used (Figure 55.26).
- **Enlarged mediastinal lymph nodes** are commonly involved by metastatic tumour mimicking a primary mediastinal lesion. Symptoms are generally secondary to compression or invasion of a structure within the mediastinum. Surgery, such as mediastinoscopy, is reserved for diagnosis only.

Other conditions of the mediastinum

Many of the primary tumours, such as neurogenic tumours and germ cell tumours, can present as cysts or have a cystic quality. In addition, the mediastinum can contain other cysts often with an embryological aetiology. Thymic cysts, pericardial cysts, bronchogenic and foregut cysts can all present asymptomatically or with local compression (Figure 55.27). Surgical excision is recommended if diagnosis is unclear or the patient has symptoms.

MEDICAL CONDITIONS FOR WHICH SURGERY MAY BE REQUIRED

Bronchiectasis

Bronchiectasis is chronic irreversible dilatation of the medium-sized bronchi, which may occur following a suppurative pneumonia or bronchial obstruction. It is the pathological end-stage of a range of conditions. If generalised, it is almost never considered for surgical resection. Cases caused by whooping cough and measles are decreasing in frequency in developed countries.

Treatment

Removal of the bronchiectatic part of the lung for symptoms of bleeding, recurrent infection or copious symptoms can be very effective when the disease is localised.

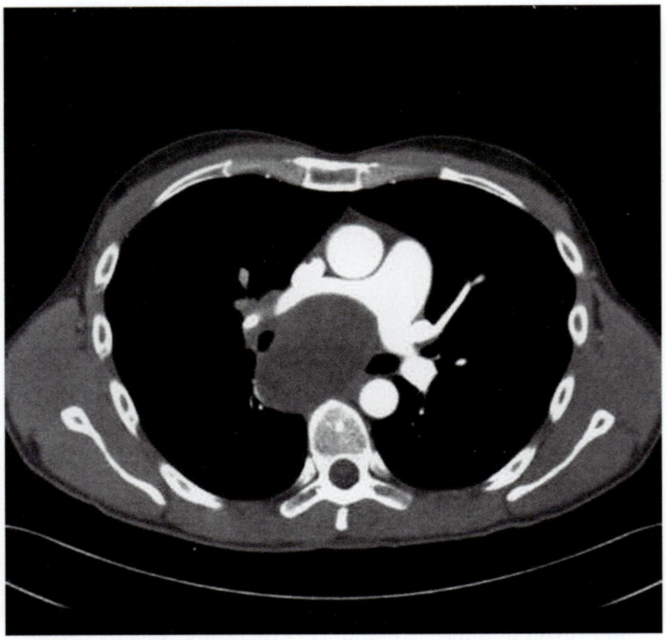

Figure 55.27 Computed tomography scan of the chest showing a bronchiogenic cyst splaying the carina.

Table 55.12 Causes of lung abscess.

Specific pneumonia	Streptococcal Staphylococcal Pneumococcal *Klebsiella* spp. Anaerobic
Bronchial obstruction	Carcinoma Carcinoid Foreign body Postoperative atelectasis
Chronic respiratory sepsis	Sinusitis Tonsillitis Dental infection
Septicaemia	
Penetrating lung injury	

Lung abscess

The causes of lung abscess are shown in Table 55.12. The chest radiograph shows a cavity with a fluid level or, in mycetoma, a fungal ball. Most acute abscesses resolve with appropriate antibiotic therapy and postural drainage. Surgery is avoided. Small radiologically sited drains are sometimes used in the intensive care unit.

Tuberculosis

Surgery is rarely indicated for tuberculosis in developed countries but, when it is, it must be combined with adequate antitubercular chemotherapy or the benefit of surgery will be lost (Summary box 55.6).

Summary box 55.6

Tuberculosis: indications for surgery

- Suspicious lesion on chest radiograph in which neoplasia cannot be excluded
- Chronic tuberculous abscess, resistant to chemotherapy
- Aspergilloma within a tuberculous cavity
- Life-threatening haemoptysis

Diagnosis

Surgical procedures may be necessary to establish the diagnosis if suspected clinically, but sputum or pus cultures are persistently negative.

Complications, such as an aspergilloma in a chronic cavity causing life-threatening haemoptysis, may require lobectomy.

Pulmonary sequestration

This describes a section of non-functional lung separated from the normal bronchial connection with other abnormalities of development, which often include a direct systemic arterial supply from the aorta. Venous return is to the pulmomary veins in the majority of cases. The segment becomes cystic and infected, resulting in the common appearance of a solid lung mass that may be homogenous or heterogenous, occasionally with cystic changes on CT scan. Interlobar sequestration occurs within the lung substance. It may present with recurrent chest infections and/or haemoptysis. Patients with extralobar sequestration are usually asymptomatic as air spaces are not present, and therefore usually present as an incidental finding.

Lung cysts

Developmental lung cysts have a tendency to become infected. Acquired lung cysts may contain air or fluid and may be single or multiple. Pulmonary hydatid disease is a cause in endemic areas. Air cysts (bullae) may be spontaneous, but may be secondary to emphysematous degeneration (Figure 55.28).

LUNG TRANSPLANTATION

Lung transplantation is an established therapy for those with end-stage parenchymal or pulmonary vascular disease, which is limited by the number of donor lungs available.

CHEST TRAUMA

The approach to trauma must be methodical and exact, because the signs, particularly in the presence of other injury, may easily be missed. The general principles of resuscitation and ATLS (advanced trauma and life support) must be followed.

Thoracic trauma is responsible for over 70 per cent of all deaths following road traffic accidents. Blunt trauma to the chest in isolation is fatal in 10 per cent of cases, rising to 30 per cent if other injuries are present. The indications for emergency room thoractomy in blunt chest trauma include massive haemothorax,

Theodor Albrecht Edwin Klebs, 1834–1913, Professor of Bacteriology successively in Prague, The Czech Republic; in Zurich, Switzerland; and at The Rush Medical College, Chicago, IL, USA.

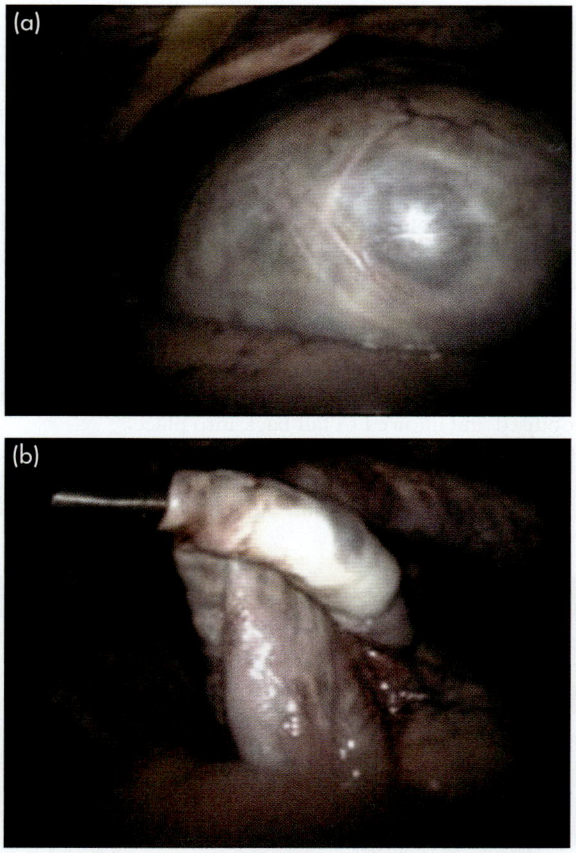

Figure 55.28 (a) A large solitary bulla seen on videothoracoscopy. (b) The bulla deflated and rolled in preparation for staple resection.

suspected cardiac tamponade and witnessed cardiac arrest in the resuscitation area. Success rates are low. Penetrating thoracic wounds vary according to the prevalence of civil violence, with a mortality rate of 3 per cent for simple stabbing to 15 per cent for gunshot wounds. The indications for emergency room thoracotomy are similar to blunt chest trauma. The standard approach is a left anterior thoracotomy, unless the penetrating injury is in the right chest, however it may be necessary to extend the incision to bilateral thoracotomies or a clam-shell incision.

Early deaths after thoracic trauma are caused by hypoxaemia, hypovolaemia and tamponade. The first steps in treating such patients should be to diagnose and treat these problems as early as possible because they may be readily corrected. Young patients have a large physiological reserve, and serious injury may be overlooked until this reserve is used up, by which time the situation is critical and may be irretrievable. The best approach is to remain highly suspicious if life-threatening conditions are to be anticipated and treated. Early consultation with a regional thoracic centre is advised in cases of doubt. In an emergency, it is essential that experienced help is summoned.

Management of chest trauma is covered in detail in Chapter 28.

THE DIAPHRAGM

The diaphragm is the fibromuscular structure separating the thorax from the abdomen (Figure 55.29).

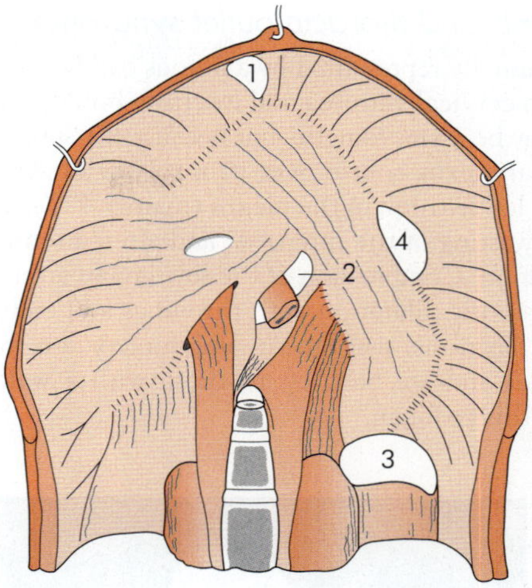

Figure 55.29 Diagram of sites of hernias. The usual sites of congenital diaphragmatic hernia: 1, foramen of Morgagni; 2, oesophageal hiatus; 3, foramen of Bochdalek (pleuroperitoneal hernia); and 4, dome.

Diaphragmatic disorders

Disorders of the diaphragm can be broadly classified as disorders of innervation, leading to paralysis of the diaphragm, with elevation and reduction of thoracic volume leading to breathlessness; or disorders of anatomy, which are further categorised into congenital diaphragmatic hernias or acquired hernias usually secondary to trauma. There are two well-recognised congenital sites where abdominal viscera can herniate into the chest (Figure 55.30):

- **The foramen of Morgagni**. A hernia in the anterior part of the diaphragm with a defect between the sternal and costal attachments. The most commonly involved viscus is the transverse colon.
- **The foramen of Bochdalek**. Through the dome of the diaphragm posteriorly.

Traumatic rupture of the diaphragm may occur with blunt trauma. Unless there is severe bleeding or strangulation of the viscera it is best managed at an interval. In a severely injured patient being ventilated, it can wait until other injuries are dealt with and weaning from the ventilator is being considered.

When the diaphragm is breached as in anatomical disorders, repair with either primary closure or with a mesh is usually possible via a thoracotomy. Diaphragmatic paralysis, particularly idiopathic unilateral paralysis can be plicated returning the diaphragm to a lower position and improving thoracic volume.

THE CHEST WALL

Tumours of the chest wall

These can be tumours of any component of the chest wall, i.e. bone, cartilage and soft tissue. They are treated similarly to those that occur in other sites and require specialist surgical input only if major resection and chest wall reconstruction are contemplated.

Other diseases of the chest wall

Congenital abnormalities are often incidental findings on chest x-ray (bifid rib), but there are some important exceptions.

Giovanni Batista Morgagni, 1682–1771, Professor of Anatomy, Padua, Italy for 59 years. He is regarded as the 'Founder of Morbid Anatomy'.
Victor Alexander Bochdalek, 1801–1883, Professor of Anatomy, Prague, The Czech Republic.

Cervical rib and thoracic outlet syndrome

This rib is usually represented by a fibrous band originating from the seventh cervical vertebra and inserting onto the first thoracic rib. It may be asymptomatic, but because the subclavian artery and brachial plexus course over it, a variety of symptoms may occur. The lower trunk of the plexus (mainly T1) is compressed, leading to wasting of the interossei and altered sensation in the T1 distribution. Compression of the subclavian artery may result in a post-stenotic dilatation with thrombus and embolus formation. The diagnosis, assessment and surgery are fraught with uncertainties and are best left to those with a well-developed interest in this problem.

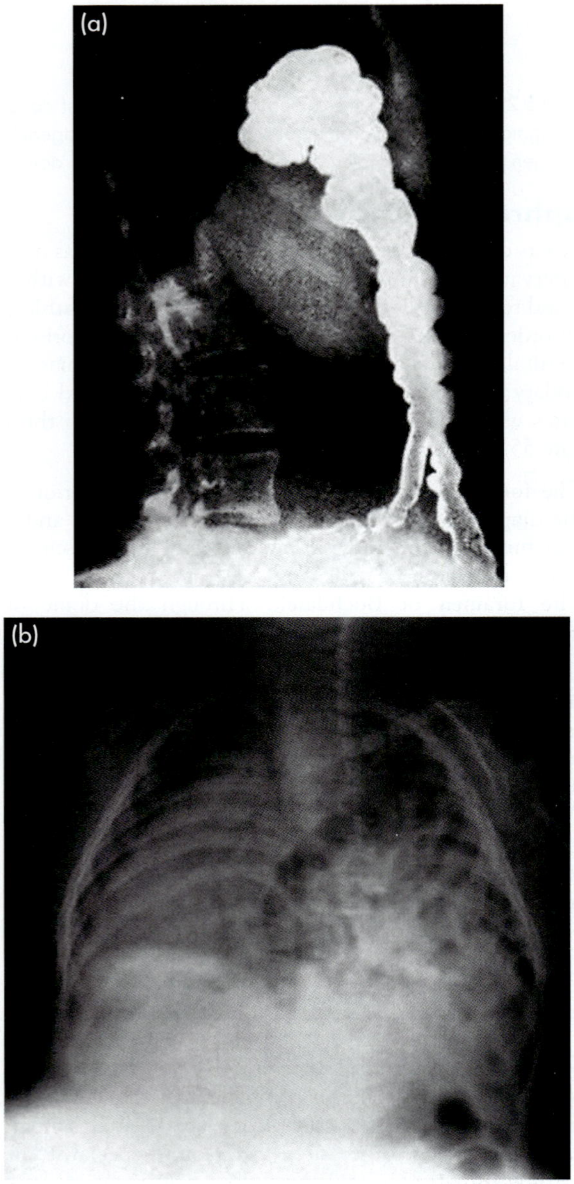

Figure 55.30 Chest x-ray of congenital diaphragmatic hernia. (a) Colon occupying a Morgagni hernia (courtesy of Dr Oliver Smith, Birmingham, UK). (b) Foramen of Bochdalek hernia on the left side in an infant. The left pleural cavity is occupied by intestine, the mediastinum is displaced to the right and the right lung is aerated very little.

Pectus excavatum

The sternum is depressed, with a dish-shaped deformity of the anterior portions of the ribs on one or both sides. It is never a cause of respiratory problems. It can be repaired to improve its cosmetic appearance either as an open procedure (the Ravitch procedure) which involves resecting the affected costal cartilages and mobilising the sternum, or as a minimally invasive technique, the Nuss procedure. A metal bar is paced behind the sternum to hold this central panel in its new position and has to be removed after a period of time (Figure 55.31a,b).

Pectus carinatum (pigeon chest)

In this condition, the sternum is elevated above the level of the ribs and treatment is offered for cosmetic reasons. The sternum is mobilised and allowed to fall back into place.

It often comes to light during the growth spurt at adolescence when, of course, the teenager is particularly sensitive about appearance. Most patients are asymptomatic and the only

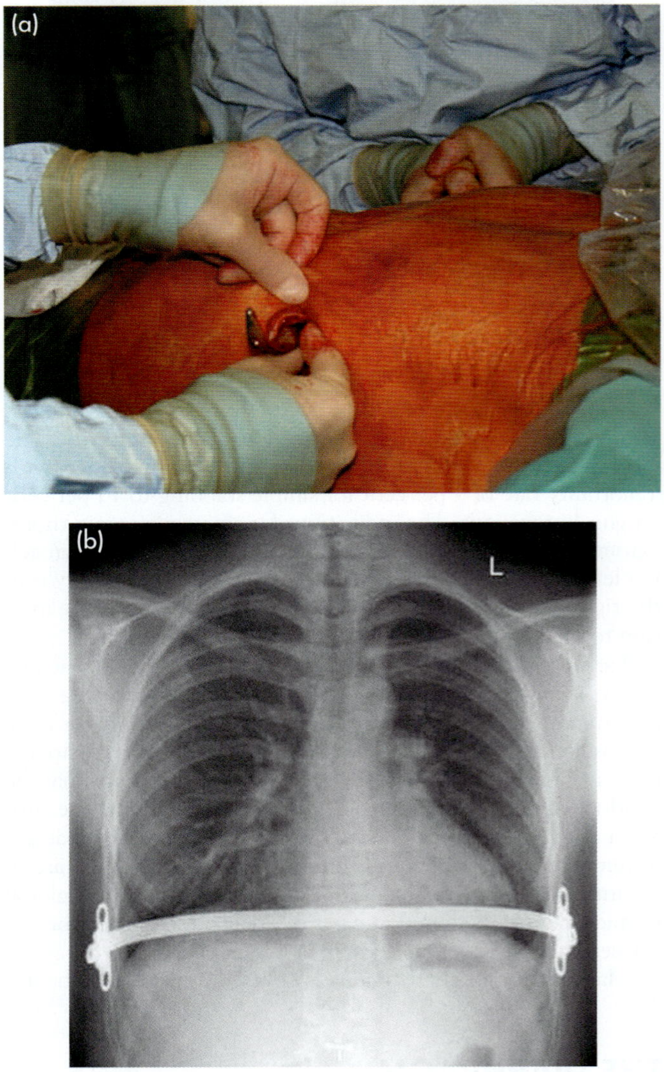

Figure 55.31 (a) Insertion of preformed bar placed thoracoscopically beneath the pectus excavatum. (b) Chest x-ray following insertion of a metal bar bracing the sternum forward (the Nuss procedure).

cojustification for treatment is on cosmetic grounds. Some surgeons make a very good case for this, but the risk of morbidity and of a less than perfect result must be clearly spelt out to the patients and their parents. Surgery involves mobilising the sternum with the costal cartilages so that the sternum can be flattened to a more anatomical position. Surgery is best left until the late teens, when further growth of the chest wall is unlikely.

FURTHER READING

British Thoracic Society Pleural Disease Guideline 2010. *Thorax 2010*; **65** (Suppl. 2): 1–76.

Guidelines on the radical management of patients with lung cancer. *Thorax* 2010; **65** (Suppl. 3): 1–27.

PART

10 Vascular

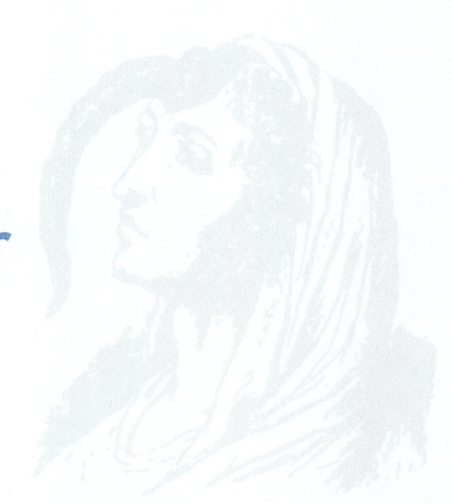

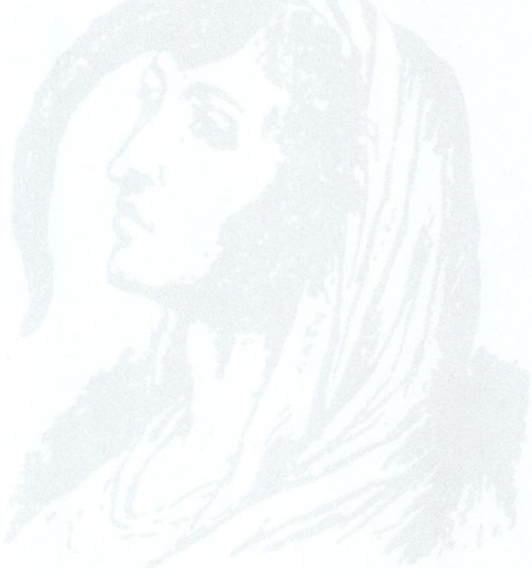

CHAPTER

56 Arterial disorders

LEARNING OBJECTIVES

To understand:

- The nature and associated features of occlusive arterial disease
- The investigation and treatment options for occlusive arterial disease
- The principles of management of the severely ischaemic limb
- The nature and presentation of aneurysmal disease, particularly of the abdominal aorta
- The investigation and treatment options for aneurysmal disease
- The arteritides and vasospastic disorders

INTRODUCTION

Arterial disorders represent the most common cause of morbidity and death in Western societies. Much of this is due to the effects of atheroma on the arteries supplying the heart muscle (coronary thrombosis and myocardial infarction) and brain (stroke), although atheroma is also common at other sites. This chapter addresses diseases that are typically the province of the vascular surgeon, namely those affecting the arteries of the body, excluding those of the heart and those within the cranium.

ARTERIAL STENOSIS AND OCCLUSION

Cause and effect

Arterial stenosis or occlusion is commonly caused by atheroma, but can occur acutely as a result of emboli or trauma. Stenosis or occlusion produces symptoms and signs that are related to the organ supplied by the artery: e.g. lower limb (claudication, rest pain and gangrene); brain (transient ischaemic attacks and stroke); myocardium (angina and myocardial infarction); kidney (hypertension and renal failure) (Figure 56.1); intestine (abdominal pain and infarction). The severity of the symptoms is related to the size of the vessel occluded and whether the stenosis or occlusion occurs suddenly (acute) in a previously normal artery or gradually (chronic) with progressive narrowing of the artery over time. In chronic arterial narrowing, a collateral circulation may develop and provide an alternative route for blood flow which reduces symptoms until a critical stenosis or occlusion has developed (Figure 56.2).

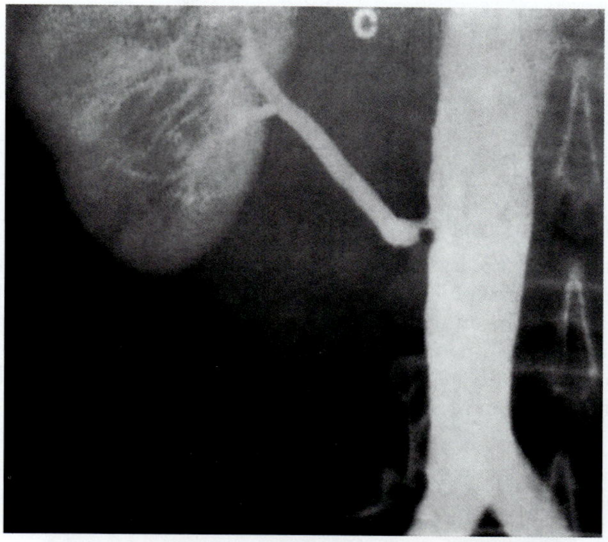

Figure 56.1 Renal artery stenosis. Angiogram by retrograde femoral catheterisation. Note the post-stenotic dilatation.

Features of chronic arterial stenosis or occlusion in the leg

Intermittent claudication

Intermittent claudication is a cramp-like pain felt in the muscles that is:

- brought on by walking;
- not present on taking the first step (unlike osteoarthritis);
- relieved by standing still (unlike nerve compression from a lumbar intervertebral disc prolapse or osteoarthritis of the spine or spinal stenosis).

The distance that a patient is able to walk without stopping varies only slightly from day to day. It is altered by walking up hill, the speed of walking, carrying heavy weights and changes in general health, such as anaemia or heart failure.

The pain of claudication is usually felt in the calf because the superficial femoral artery is the most commonly affected (70 per cent of cases). Aortoiliac disease (30 per cent of cases) may cause

Claudication from the Latin *claudicare*, to limp. The Roman emperor Claudius (10BC to 54AD) walked with a limp, which was possibly due to poliomyelitis.

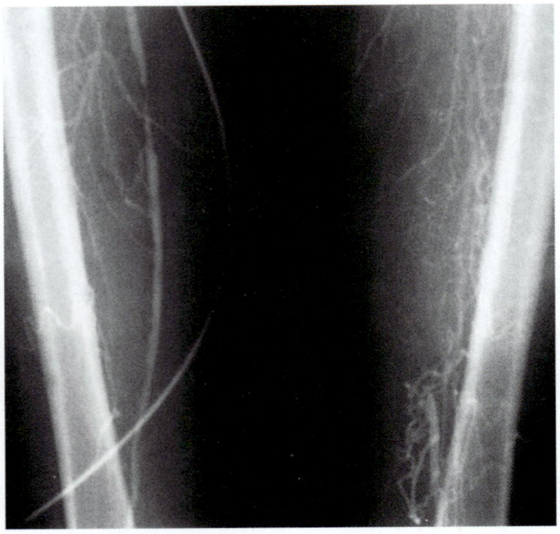

Figure 56.2 Right superficial femoral stenosis. Left superficial femoral occlusion with collateral vessels present, causing claudication.

thigh or buttock claudication. Buttock claudication in association with sexual impotence resulting from arterial insufficiency is eponymously called Leriche's syndrome. It is very rare.

Rest pain

Rest pain occurs with the limb at rest and is felt in the foot; it is exacerbated by lying down or elevation of the foot. Characteristically, the pain is worse at night and it may be lessened by hanging the foot out of bed or by sleeping in a chair. The pressure of bed clothes on the foot usually makes the pain worse.

Ulceration and gangrene

Ulceration occurs with severe arterial insufficiency and may present as a painful erosion between the toes or as shallow, nonhealing ulcers on the dorsum of the feet, on the shins and especially around the malleoli. The blackened mummified tissues of frank gangrene are unmistakable (Figure 56.3), and superadded infection often makes the gangrene wet.

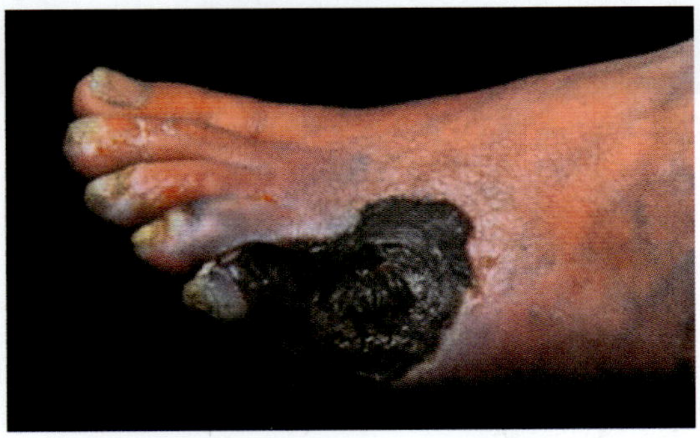

Figure 56.3 Severe chronic ischaemia with dry gangrene.

Rene Leriche, 1879–1955, Professor of Surgery, Strasbourg, France, described this syndrome (although the syndrome is credited to Leriche, the condition was first described by Robert Graham (1786–1845), physician at the Royal Infirmary in Glasgow, UK).

Colour, temperature, sensation and movement

An acutely ischaemic foot is often cold, white, paralysed and insensate. However, a chronically ischaemic limb tends to equilibrate with the temperature of its surroundings and may feel quite warm under the bedclothes. Chronic ischaemia does not produce paralysis and sensation is usually intact. Elevation of the limb produces pallor which changes to a red/purple colour when the limb is allowed to hang down (dependent rubor or the sunset foot sign). The capillary refill time may be elicited by pressing the skin of the heel or toe causing blanching and then releasing to allow colour to return (normally this takes 2–3 seconds, but may be prolonged to 10 seconds in severe ischaemia (Figure 56.4)).

Arterial pulses

It is standard practice to examine the femoral, popliteal, posterior tibial and dorsalis pedis arteries, together with the abdomen for an aneurysm which may coexist with occlusive disease. Diminution of a pulse can often be appreciated by comparing it with its opposite number. Popliteal pulses are difficult to feel and, if prominent, may suggest popliteal aneurysm. Pulsation distal to an arterial occlusion is usually absent although the presence of a highly developed collateral circulation may allow distal pulses to be normal – this is most likely to occur with an iliac stenosis. In this case, exercise (walking until claudication develops) usually causes the pulse to disappear as vasodilation occurs below the obstruction causing the pulse pressure to reduce. An arterial bruit, heard on auscultation over the pulse, indicates turbulent flow and suggests a stenosis. It is an unreliable clinical sign as tight stenoses often do not have bruits. A continuous 'machinery' murmur over an artery usually indicates an arteriovenous fistula (Summary box 56.1).

Summary box 56.1

Features of chronic lower limb arterial stenosis or occlusion

- Intermittent claudication
- Rest pain
- Dependent rubor or sunset foot
- Ulceration
- Gangrene
- Arterial pulsation diminished or absent
- Arterial bruit
- Slow capillary refilling

Relationship of clinical findings to site of disease

In most cases, the site of arterial obstruction can be determined from the symptoms and signs (Table 56.1). Severe ischaemia (rest pain, ulceration, gangrene) is usually caused by multilevel disease, e.g. iliac and femoropopliteal disease.

Risk factors and natural history

The common modifiable risk factors for occlusive arterial disease are smoking, hypertension, diabetes mellitus and hyperlipidaemia.The natural history of claudication is often to improve if the patient stops smoking and exercises. This encourages development of collaterals and the risk of limb loss is very low. For patients with rest pain or worse, intervention is usually required to prevent major amputation.

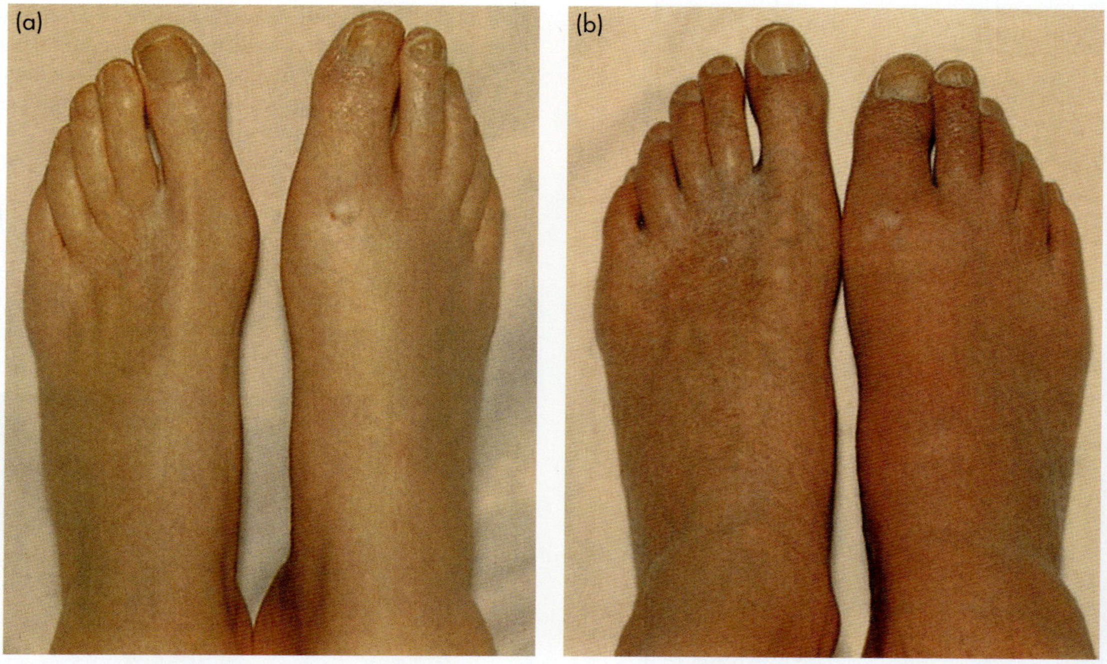

Figure 56.4 Colour changes with elevation (a) and dependency (b).

Table 56.1 Relationship of clinical findings to site of disease.

Aortoiliac obstruction	Claudication in both buttocks, thighs and calves
	Femoral and distal pulses absent in both limbs
	Bruit over aortoiliac region
	Impotence (Leriche)
Iliac obstruction	Unilateral claudication in the thigh and calf and sometimes the buttock
	Bruit over the iliac region
	Unilateral absence of femoral and distal pulses
Femoropopliteal obstruction	Unilateral claudication in the calf
	Femoral pulse palpable with absent unilateral distal pulses
Distal obstruction	Femoral and popliteal pulses palpable
	Ankle pulses absent
	Claudication in calf and foot

The best results from surgery are obtained by operation on the larger vessels, which allows a high volume of blood flow through bypass grafts. For instance, aortoiliac bypass is longer lasting than femorotibial bypass.

Investigation of arterial occlusive disease

Most patients with symptoms of arterial disease do not need invasive treatment, such as angioplasty or surgical reconstruction, and the decision whether or not to intervene can often be made without recourse to special investigations.

General investigation

Patients with arterial disease tend to be elderly and atherosclerosis is a generalised disease; if active intervention is contemplated, full assessment is essential. Many patients have age-related diseases, such as cardiac ischaemia, chronic obstructive pulmonary disease and malignancy. Blood tests to exclude anaemia, diabetes, renal disease and lipid abormalities should include a full blood count, blood glucose, lipid profile and serum urea and electrolytes. High blood viscosity (polycythaemia and thrombocythaemia) may be caused by smoking, but may also be associated with cancer; renal impairment (raised serum creatinine and low glomerular filtration rate (GFR)) may be caused by drugs and may be exacerbated by intravenous contrast agents used during angiography.

An electrocardiogram (ECG) may show coronary ischaemia, left ventricular hypertrophy or rhythm abnormalities, although a normal ECG does not rule out these conditions. More information may be gained by a cardiac echo or exercise testing. Arterial blood gases and pulmonary function test may be appropriate in patients with severe lung disease.

Doppler ultrasound blood flow detection

A hand-held Doppler ultrasound probe is very useful in the assessment of occlusive arterial disease (Figures 56.5 and 56.6). A continuous-wave ultrasound signal is transmitted from the probe at an artery and the reflected beam is picked up by a receiver within the probe itself. The change in frequency in the reflected beam compared with that of the transmitted beam is due to the Doppler shift, resulting from the reflection of the beam by moving blood cells. The frequency change may be converted into an audio signal that is typically pulsatile. Doppler ultrasound equipment can be used in conjunction with a sphygmomanometer to assess systolic pressure in small vessels. This is possible even when the arterial pulse cannot be palpated. Both the pressure and signal quality are important; a normal artery has a triphasic signal that can be detected by a trained observer. However, although the presence of a Doppler signal indicates moving blood, it does not necessarily indicate that the blood flow is sufficient to maintain limb viability and prevent limb loss.

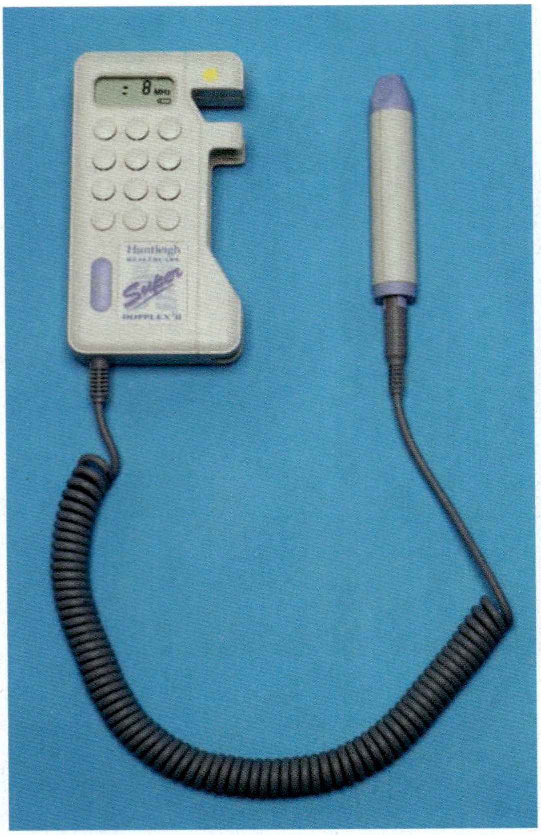

Figure 56.5 Simple hand-held Doppler ultrasound probe.

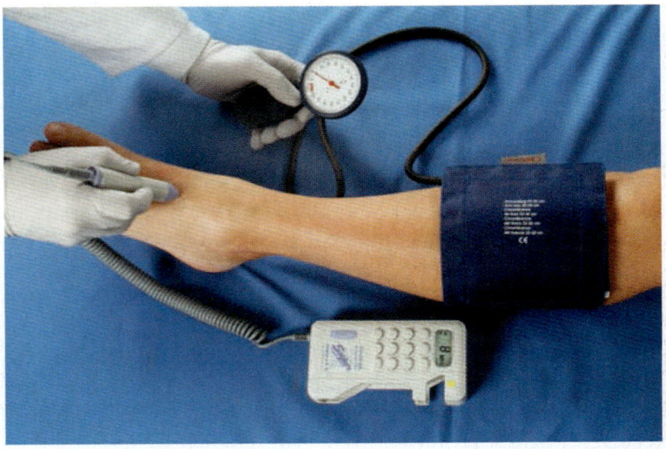

Figure 56.6 Hand-held Doppler probe and sphygmomanometer used to determine systolic pressure in the dorsalis pedis artery, as part of assessing the ankle–brachial pressure index.

The ankle–brachial pressure index (ABPI) is the ratio of systolic pressure at the ankle to that in the arm. The highest pressure in the dorsalis pedis, posterior tibial or peroneal artery serves as the numerator, with the highest brachial systolic pressure being the denominator. Resting ABPI is normally about 1.0; values below 0.9 indicate some degree of arterial obstruction (claudication), less than 0.5 suggests rest pain and less than 0.3 indicates imminent necrosis. However, the values are merely a guide and normal values may be present with intermittent claudication. Retesting after exercise can be useful; a normal ABPI may subsequently fall in patients with ischaemia. Artificially high readings can be caused by calcified, incompressible arteries which are often found in diabetics.

Duplex scanning

This major non-invasive technique uses B-mode ultrasound to provide an image of vessels (Figures 56.7 and 56.8). The image is created because of the varying ability of different tissues to reflect the ultrasound beam. A second ultrasound beam is then used to insonate the imaged vessel and the Doppler shift

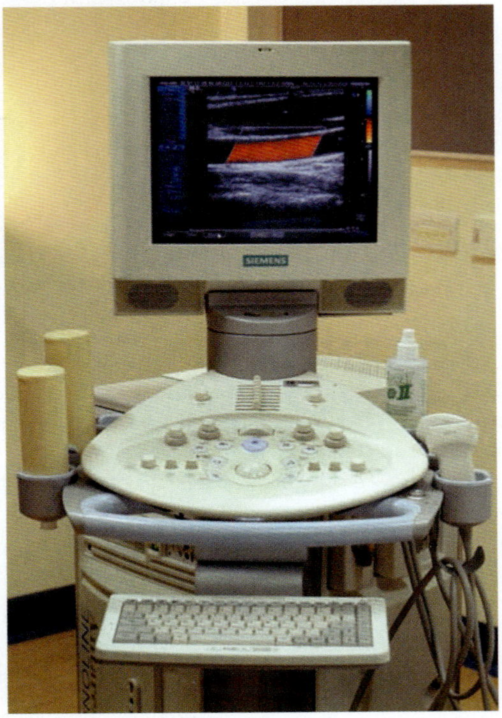

Figure 56.7 Colour duplex scanner.

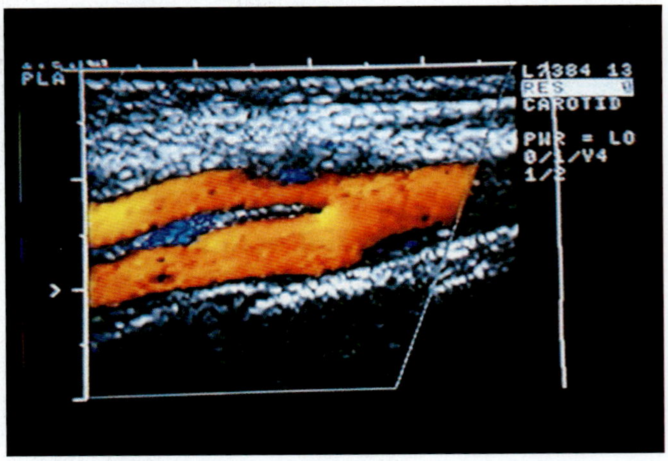

Figure 56.8 Colour duplex scan of carotid vessels in neck showing stenosis at common carotid bifurcation (courtesy of Dr Paul Allan, Royal Infirmary, Edinburgh, UK).

obtained is analysed by a computer. Most scanners now have colour coding which allows detailed visualisation of blood flow, turbulence, etc. Different colours indicate changes in direction and velocity of flow with areas of high flow usually indicating a stenosis. In experienced hands, Duplex scanning is as accurate as angiography and has the advantages of cost-effectiveness and safety. However, the aortoiliac segment can be difficult to visualise particularly in obese patients. A computed tomography (CT) angiogram can provide better imaging of this segment in these cases (see below).

Angiography

Angiography is invasive and only appropriate if intervention is being contemplated. It involves injection of a radio-opaque dye into the arterial tree by a percutaneous catheter method (Seldinger technique) usually involving the femoral artery (Figures 56.9 and 56.10). Hazards include bleeding, haematoma, false aneurysm formation, thrombosis, arterial dissection, distal embolisation, renal dysfunction and allergic reaction. Digital subtraction angiography (DSA) is now the standard technique whereby the images obtained are digitised by computer and the extraneous background (bone, soft tissues, etc.) is removed to provide clearer images. CT angiography and magnetic resonance (MR) angiography (Figure 56.11) are new techniques gaining in popularity although the image quality is not as good as DSA. They can be useful where duplex scanning is not possible (intrathoracic arteries) or produces poor images (aortoiliac segment). MR has the added advantage of avoiding the need for ionising radiation.

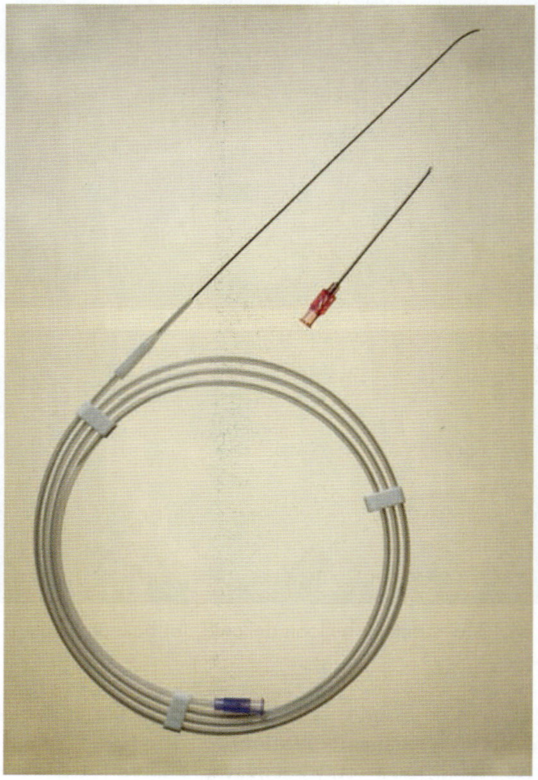

Figure 56.9 Seldinger needle and guidewire for introducing an arterial catheter.

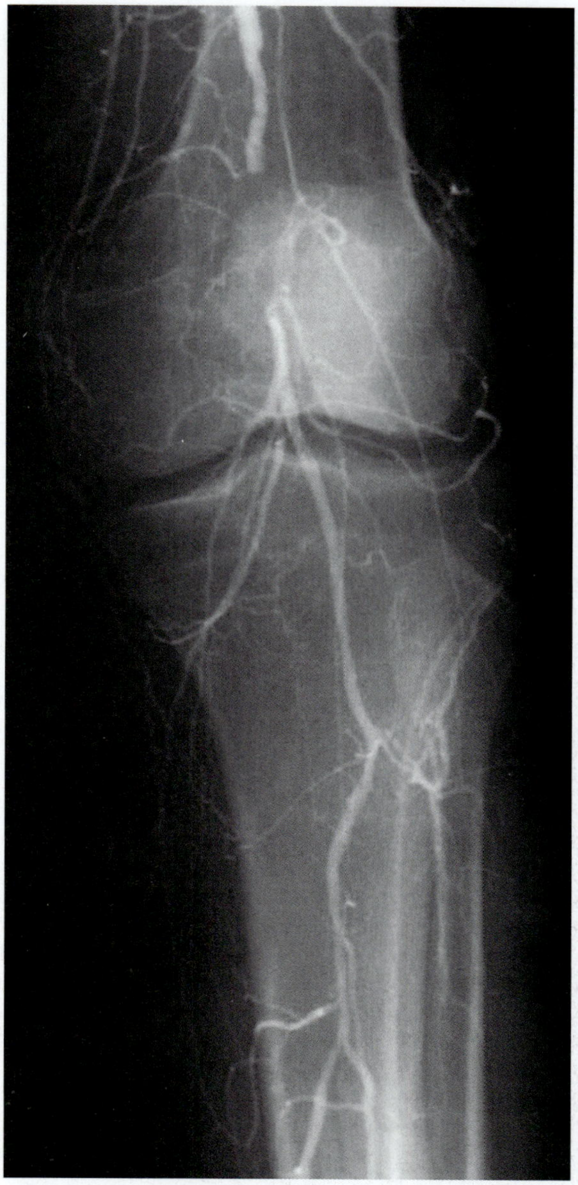

Figure 56.10 Arterial occlusion just above the knee causing claudication of the calf; good collateral circulation (arteriogram by the Seldinger technique).

Non-surgical management of arterial stenosis or occlusion

General

For many patients with claudication, stopping smoking and regular exercise (walking) will lead to improvement of symptoms over the first six months as collaterals develop. Walking regularly within the limits of the disability is ideal; there is nothing to be gained from walking in pain. Supervised exercise programmes, dietary advice, and weight loss in obese patients, will help. If this advice is followed, the risk of progression to critical leg ischaemia and amputation is very small. Unfortunately, claudication is often a marker of silent coronary and cerebral arterial disease and 50 per cent of claudicants will

Sven Ivar Seldinger, 1921–1998, radiologist, Karolinska Institute, Stockholm, Sweden, introduced percutaneous arterial catheterisation in 1953.

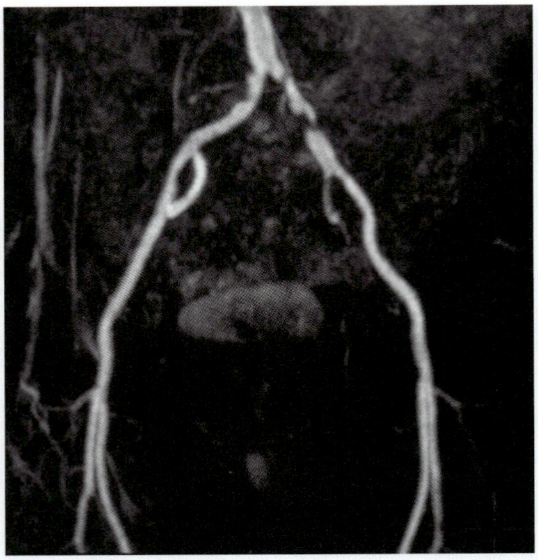

Figure 56.11 Magnetic resonance angiogram showing a tight stenosis at the midpoint of the left common iliac artery.

die within ten years from myocardial infarction or stroke. Patients with rest pain or tissue necrosis require urgent revascularisation to prevent limb loss.

Drugs

Medication may be required for diseases associated with arterial disorders, such as hypertension and diabetes; some antihypertensives (particularly β-blockers) may exacerbate claudication. Raised blood lipids require active drug treatment, but even when the lipid profile is normal, a statin should be prescribed as they may stabilise atherosclerotic plaques and protect against cardiac death. An antiplatelet agent is also necessary, usually 75 mg/day of aspirin, with 75 mg/day of clopidogrel as an alternative for those who are aspirin intolerant. Other agents, such as vasodilators, are unlikely to prove beneficial. Drugs are now available to help with smoking cessation.

Transluminal angioplasty and stenting

Arterial occlusive disease may be treated by inserting a balloon catheter into an artery and inflating it within a narrowed or blocked area (Figures 56.12 and 56.13). This technique is suitable for patients with claudication, rest pain or tissue necrosis, and is usually done in the radiology department (Figures 56.14 and 56.15). The basic method involves percutaneous femoral artery puncture under local anaesthetic followed by insertion of a guidewire which is negotiated through the stenosis or occlusion under fluoroscopic control. A balloon catheter is then inserted over the guidewire and positioned within the lesion. The balloon is then inflated at high pressure for approximately 1 minute and deflated. Satisfactory dilation of the lesion is confirmed by performing an angiogram. Percutaneous transluminal angioplasty (PTA) has proved very successful in dilating the iliac and femoropopliteal segments; the results below the knee are less successful. Long occlusions may be treated by the technique of subintimal angioplasty where the guidewire crosses the lesion in the subintimal space (in the arterial wall) and a new lumen is created by inflation of the balloon. Complications occur in about 5 per cent of cases and include failure, haematoma, bleeding, thrombosis and distal embolisation.

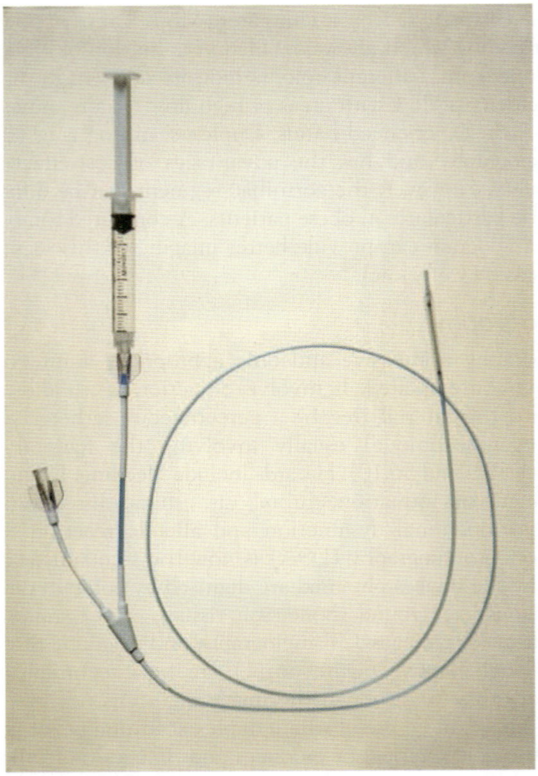

Figure 56.12 Balloon catheter for percutaneous transluminal angioplasty.

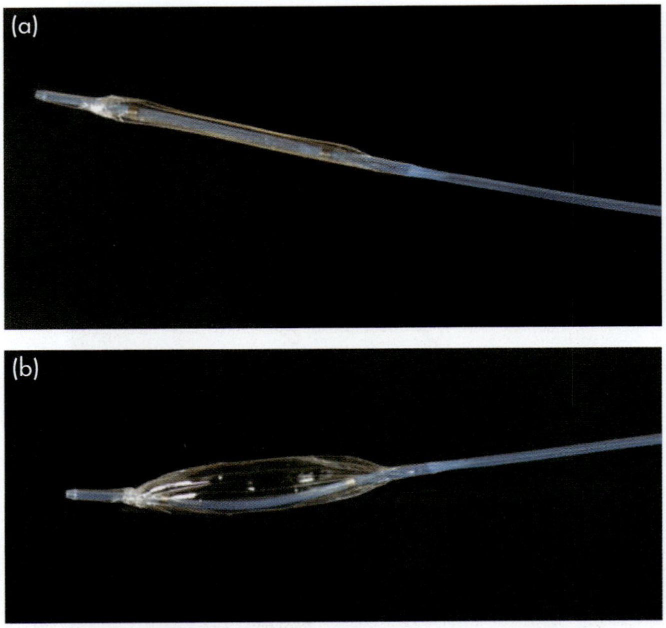

Figure 56.13 (a) Catheter balloon deflated; (b) balloon inflated.

If the vessels fail to stay adequately dilated (often caused by elastic recoil of the artery), it may be possible to hold the lumen open using a metal stent (Figures 56.16 and 56.17). This may be

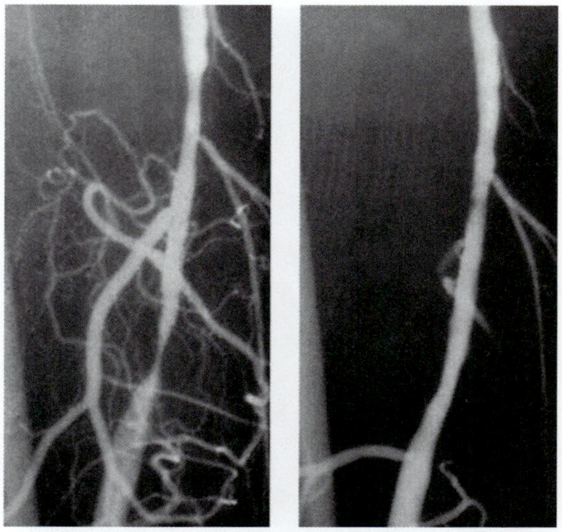

Figure 56.14 Narrowed superficial femoral artery before and after transluminal angioplasty (courtesy of J McIvor, FRCR, London, UK). The advantage of this technique is that it can be carried out under local anaesthesia using the Seldinger technique of percutaneous arterial puncture, and is therefore especially useful in the treatment of patients who are medically unfit for major surgery.

introduced on a balloon catheter and expanded by balloon inflation; or alternatively a self-expanding stent may be used which is contained inside a plastic sheath and deployed by withdrawal of the sheath.

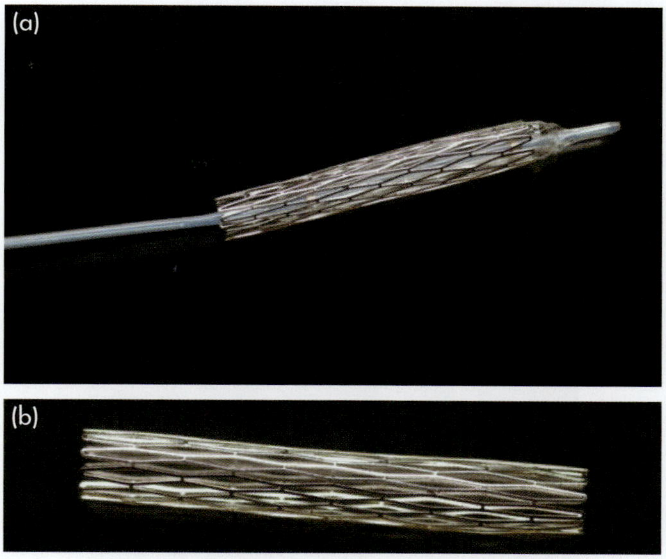

Figure 56.16 (a) Balloon catheter carrying stent; (b) expanded stent.

Operations for arterial stenosis or occlusion

Site of disease and type of operation

Surgical operations are usually reserved for patients with severe symptoms where angioplasty has failed or is not possible. Aortoiliac occlusion responds well to aortofemoral bypass

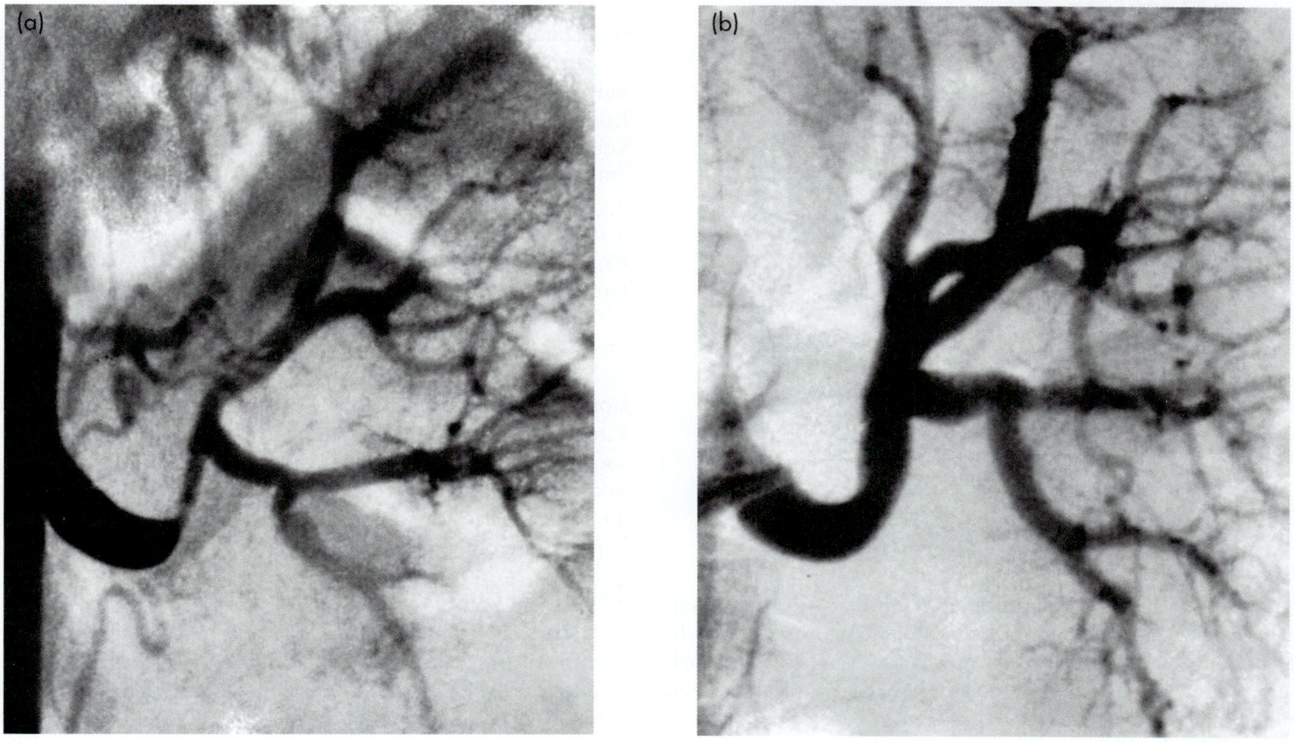

Figure 56.15 Before (a) and after (b) balloon dilatation of a severely stenosed left renal artery in a 20-year-old woman with uncontrollable hypertension. The blood pressure fell to normal after the procedure. The stenosis was probably due to fibromuscular hyperplasia, but no tissue was available for histological diagnosis.

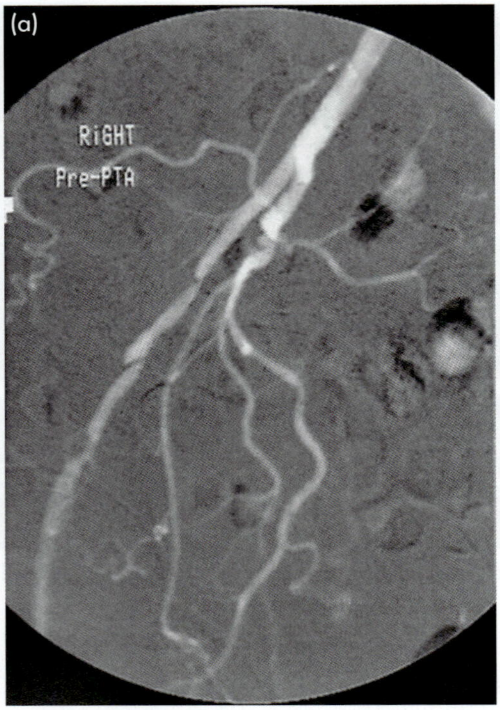

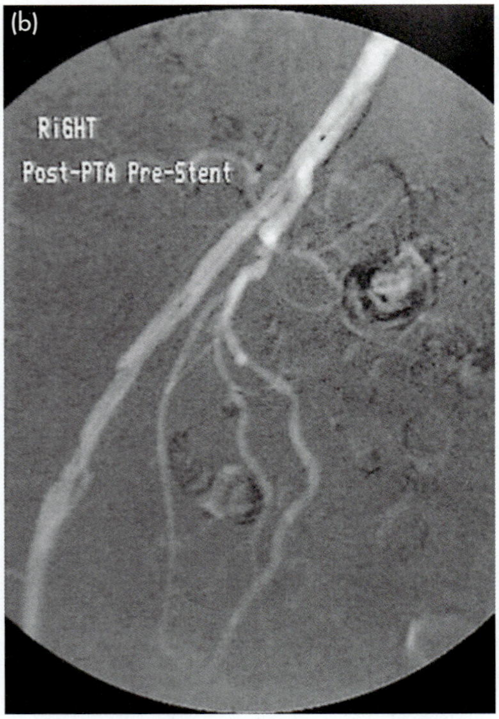

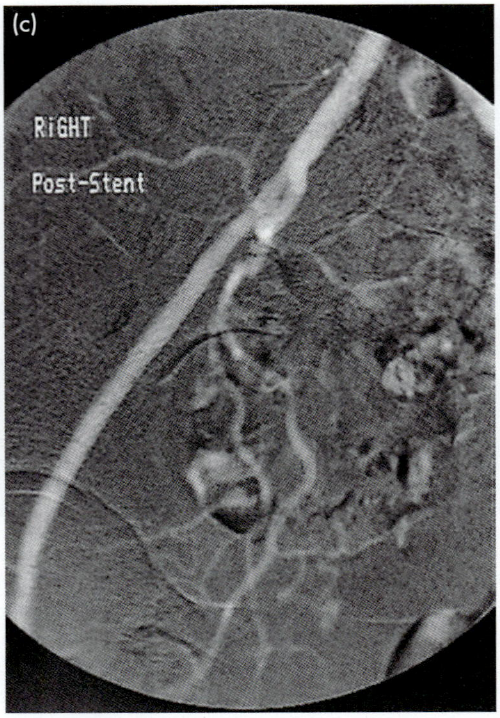

Figure 56.17 (a) External iliac artery stenosis before dilatation; (b) after dilatation by percutaneous transluminal angioplasty; and (c) dilated artery patency assured by stent (courtesy of Johnson and Johnson Interventional Systems, Bracknell, UK, and Dr W Shaw, Ninewells Hospital, Dundee, UK).

(Figure 56.18a) using a Dacron graft (Figure 56.19a); although the operation carries a mortality rate of about 5 per cent. In unfit patients, an axillofemoral bypass is an alternative although patency rates are less. If only one iliac system is occluded, an iliofemoral or femorofemoral crossover graft may be performed.

Superficial femoral artery disease can be treated by femoropopliteal bypass (Figure 56.18b); long-term graft patency is determined by the quality of inflow and outflow, graft length (whether the distal anastomosis is above or below the knee) and the conduit used for the bypass. Autogenous saphenous vein gives the best results and can be used reversed or *in situ* after valve disruption. If the long saphenous vein is not available from either leg, short saphenous or arm veins may be used. If no vein is available, a prosthetic polytetrafluoroethylene (PTFE) graft may be employed (Figure 56.19b), although patency rates are less; many surgeons construct the lower anastomosis using a small collar of vein (Miller cuff) between the PTFE and the recipient artery, which may improve patency. Isolated common femoral artery or profunda disease can be treated with endarterectomy and patch (vein or prosthetic) or a short bypass in the groin.

Sometimes, in patients with critical leg ischaemia, the occlusion extends beyond the popliteal artery into the tibial vessels. Limb salvage can be attempted with a femorodistal bypass with success even more dependent on the state of the run-off vessel and the quality of the vein conduit (minimum diameter 3 mm). The risk of early graft failure with limb loss is high and these long bypasses are only appropriate for limb salvage.

Technical details

For aortofemoral bypass, the aorta is approached through a midline or transverse abdominal incision. The common femoral arteries and their branches are exposed through vertical groin incisions. The small bowel is retracted to the right and the posterior peritoneum opened. Retroperitoneal tunnels are made from the aorta to the groins. Heparin (5000 U) is given intravenously and the vessels clamped. A vertical incision is made in the anterior aspect of the aorta to which an obliquely cut, bifurcated

Justin H Miller, vascular surgeon, Royal Adelaide Hospital, Adelaide, SA, Australia.

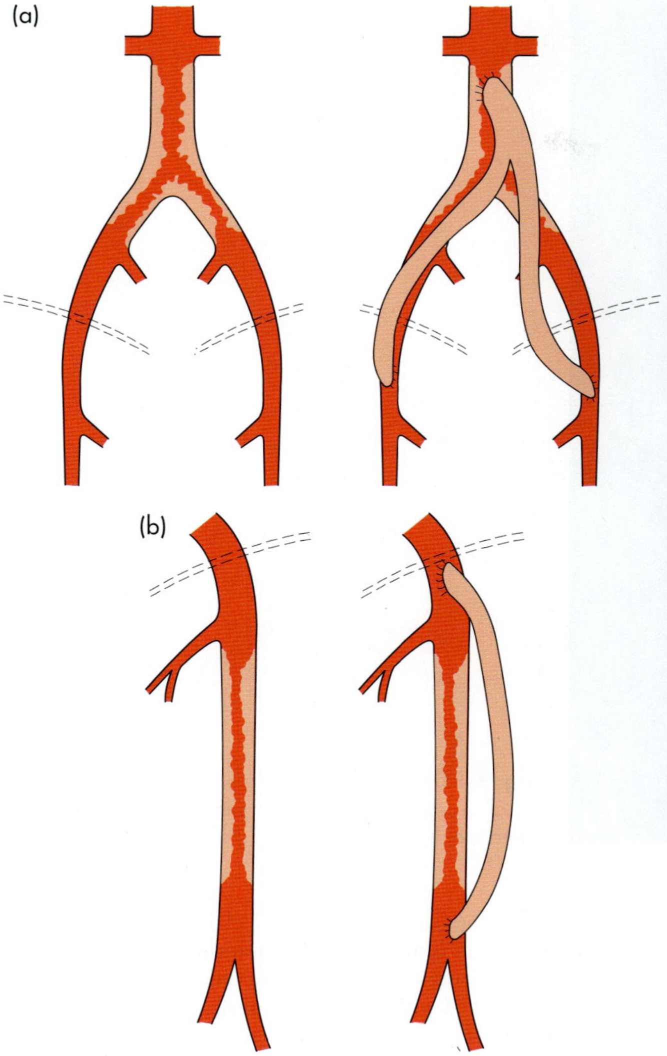

Figure 56.18 (a) Atherosclerotic narrowing of the aortic bifurcation. Aortobifemoral graft to bypass stenosis. (b) Superficial femoral artery occlusion. Femoropopliteal graft used to bypass the occluded area into good 'run off' below.

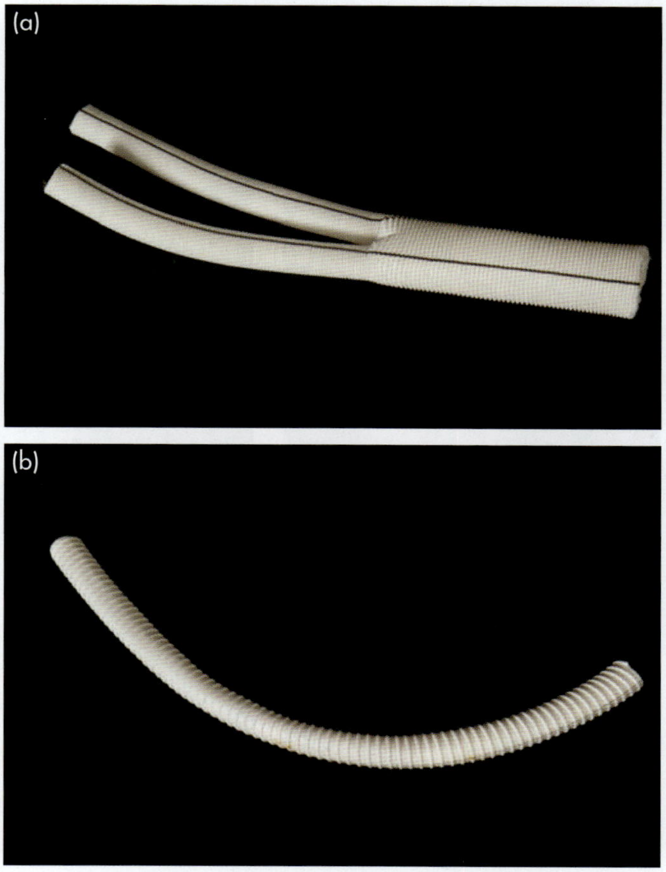

Figure 56.19 (a) Dacron bifurcation graft; (b) polytetrafluoroethylene graft.

Dacron graft is sutured end-to-side. The graft limbs are then fed down to the groins where they are anastomosed end-to-side to the common femoral arteries or, if there is evidence of profunda stenosis, to an arteriotomy running from the common femoral vessel down into the profunda. The posterior peritoneum is closed over the Dacron to prevent adhesion of the graft to bowel, and the abdomen and groin wounds are closed.

For femoropopliteal bypass, the popliteal artery above or below the knee is exposed through a medial incision. The common femoral artery is exposed at groin level. The long saphenous vein may be used in two different ways. First, it may be excised, its tributaries tied, and the vein used in a reversed fashion so the valves do not obstruct the flow of blood. Alternatively, it may be left in place (*in situ*) and the valves disrupted with a valvulotome. The graft is sutured to the femoral artery proximally and to the popliteal artery distally. Femorodistal bypass involves fashioning the distal anastomosis to a tibial vessel. If no suitable vein is available, prosthetic material (usually PTFE) may be used, with or without a small vein collar (Miller cuff) at its distal end (Figure 56.20a,b).

A femorofemoral crossover graft involves tunnelling a prosthetic graft subcutaneously above the pubis between the groins. An axillofemoral graft is tunnelled subcutaneously between the axillary artery proximally, to reach one or both of the femoral arteries; the patency rates of an axillobifemoral bypass is better than an axillo(uni)femoral bypass.

Results of operation

Long-term results of aortoiliac reconstructive surgery are good, usually marred only by progressive infrainguinal disease. Femoropopliteal surgery is less successful. Immediate postoperative success for vein bypass exceeds 90 per cent, but the five-year patency is around 60 per cent. PTFE bypass yields poorer results than vein bypass, with five-year success rates of less than 50 per cent. Although the results of femorodistal bypass are even less satisfactory, such surgery can ensure limb salvage in patients who are generally debilitated and whose expected lifespan is limited; long-term patency is less important.

Other sites of atheromatous occlusive disease

The principles of arterial surgery outlined above can be applied at other arterial sites. Carotid stenosis (at the carotid bifurca-

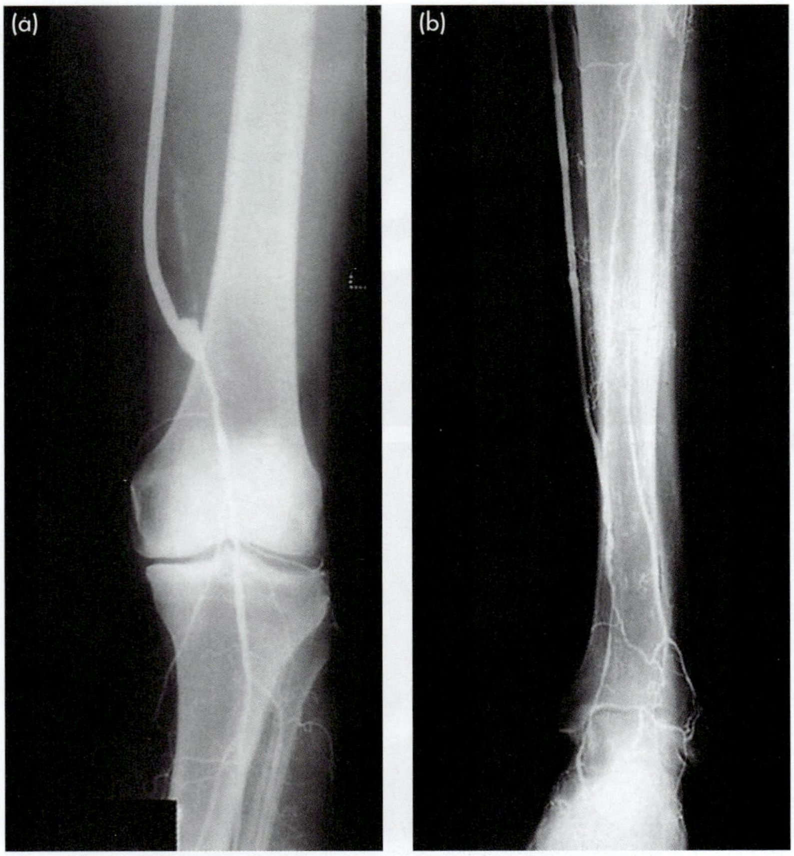

Figure 56.20 (a) Completion angiogram of femoropopliteal bypass graft (with Miller cuff). (b) Completion angiogram of femorodistal bypass graft *in situ*.

tion in the neck) may cause transient ischaemic attacks (TIA). These short-lived mini-strokes are often recurrent and cause unilateral motor or sensory loss in the arm, leg or face, transient blindness (amaurosis fugax) or speech impairment. They are caused by distal embolisation of platelet thrombi that form on the atheromatous plaque into the cerebral circulation. They are a warning of impending major stroke. Patients should be assessed with a duplex scan. If a tight stenosis (>70 per cent) is detected, carotid endarterectomy should be offered (Figure 56.21). Current guidelines for carotid endarterectomy are listed in Summary box 56.2. This involves clamping the vessels, an arteriotomy in the common carotid artery continued up into the internal carotid artery through the diseased segment, removal of the occlusive disease (endarterectomy) and closure of the arteriotomy, often with a patch. Many surgeons also use a temporary shunt to maintain cerebral blood flow while the carotid system is clamped.

Summary box 56.2

Indications for carotid endarterectomy in symptomatic patients

70% or greater carotid stenosis and:

- Ipsilateral amaurosis fugax or monocular blindness
- Contralateral facial paralysis or paraesthesia
- Arm/leg paralysis or paraesthesia
- Hemianopia
- Dysphasia (if dominant hemisphere)
- Sensory or visual inattention/neglect

Subclavian artery stenosis may cause claudication in the arm or digital ischaemia from distal embolisation. It may be treated by angioplasty or surgical bypass. Sometimes subclavian artery lesions are associated with neck pathology, such as a cervical rib which should be removed during arterial repair (see Chapter 57, Figure 57.37). Subclavian steal syndrome may occur if the first part of the subclavian artery is occluded. Arm exercise causes syncope because of reversed flow in the vertebral artery leading to cerebral ischaemia. It can be treated by angioplasty or surgery and is rare.

Mesenteric artery occlusive disease may cause pain after eating (intestinal angina) and weight loss. In general, two of the three enteric vessels (coeliac axis, superior mesenteric artery, inferior mesenteric artery) must be occluded to produce symptoms and other intestinal disorders must be excluded before treatment with PTA, endarterectomy or bypass.

Renal artery stenosis may cause hypertension and eventual renal failure. Although it is possible to improve renal blood flow with PTA or surgery, the mainstay of treatment is drugs to control hypertension, diabetes, etc.

GANGRENE

Gangrene refers to death of macroscopic portions of tissue which turn black because of the breakdown of haemoglobin and the formation of iron sulphide. It usually affects the most distal part of a limb because of arterial obstruction (from thrombosis, embolus or arteritis). Dry gangrene occurs when the tissues are desiccated by gradual slowing of the bloodstream; it is typically

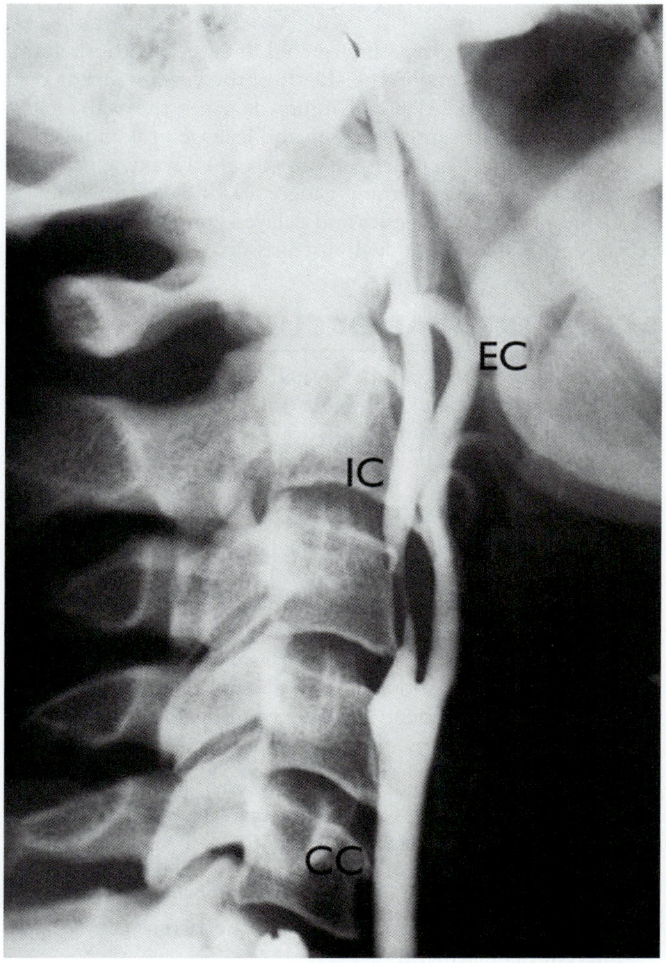

Figure 56.21 Carotid stenosis. A unilateral localised stenosis suitable for operation. CC, common carotid; EC, external carotid; IC, internal carotid.

the result of atheromatous occlusion of arteries. Wet gangrene occurs when superadded infection and putrefaction are present. Crepitus may be palpated as a result of infection by gas-forming organisms commonly in diabetic foot problems.

Separation of gangrene

A zone of demarcation between the truly viable and the dead or dying tissue will eventually appear. Separation is achieved by the development of a layer of granulation tissue, which forms between the dead and the living parts. In dry gangrene, if the blood supply of the proximal tissues is adequate, the final line of demarcation appears in a matter of days and separation occurs neatly and with the minimum of infection. If bone is involved, complete separation takes longer than when soft tissues alone are affected, and the stump tends to be conical as the bone has a better blood supply than its coverings. In moist gangrene, the infection and suppuration extends into the neighbouring living tissue, causing the final line of demarcation to be more proximal than in dry gangrene.

If the arterial supply to the proximal living tissue is poor, the line of final demarcation is very slow to form or does not develop at all. Unless the arterial supply can be improved, the gangrene will spread to adjacent tissues or will suddenly appear as 'skip' areas further up the limb. These skip lesions may occur on the other side of the foot, on the heel, on the dorsum of the foot or even in the calf. Infection may also cause gangrene to spread proximally into areas of extensive inflammation. To attempt local amputation in the presence of poor circulation will fail and gangrene will reappear in the wound or skin edges.

Treatment of gangrene

How much of a limb or digit can be salvaged depends on the blood supply proximal to the gangrene. Poor circulation can sometimes be improved by radiological or surgical intervention and this may allow a more conservative debridement or distal amputation. However, major limb amputation may be required in the presence of life-threatening sepsis, when the blood supply cannot be improved or in patients whose limb is useless because of contractures, stroke, etc.

Specific varieties of gangrene

Diabetic gangrene

Diabetic gangrene is usually caused by a combination of three factors – ischaemia secondary to atheroma, peripheral neuropathy which leads to trophic skin changes and immunosuppression caused by excess of sugar in the tissues which predisposes to infection (Figure 56.22). The neuropathy is usually sensory which favours the neglect of minor injuries and infections. Motor involvement is frequently accompanied by loss of reflexes and deformities (neuropathic joints). Thick callosities develop on the sole of the foot which together with poor chiropody may allow the entry of infection that can spread rapidly and proximally in subfascial planes. Treatment depends on the degree of arterial involvement which should be investigated and treated rapidly with angioplasty or surgery. The gangrene is treated by drainage of pus, debridement of dead tissue with local amputation of necrotic digits and antibiotics.

Bedsores

A bedsore is gangrene caused by local pressure (Figure 56.23). Bedsores are predisposed to by five factors: pressure, injury, anaemia, malnutrition and moisture. They can appear and extend rapidly in immobile patients and in those with debili-

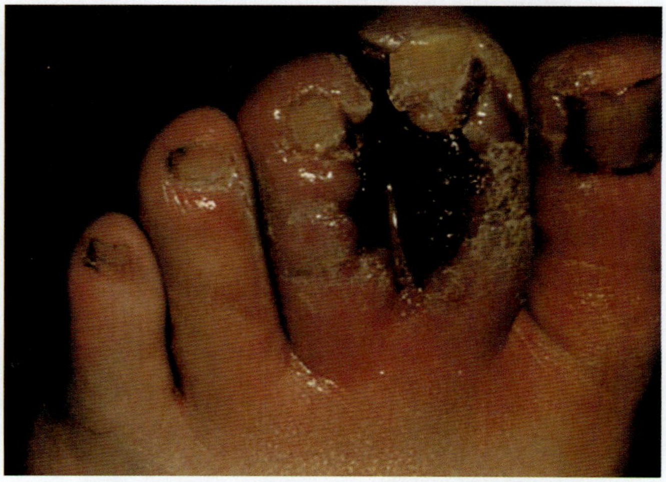

Figure 56.22 Diabetic gangrene.

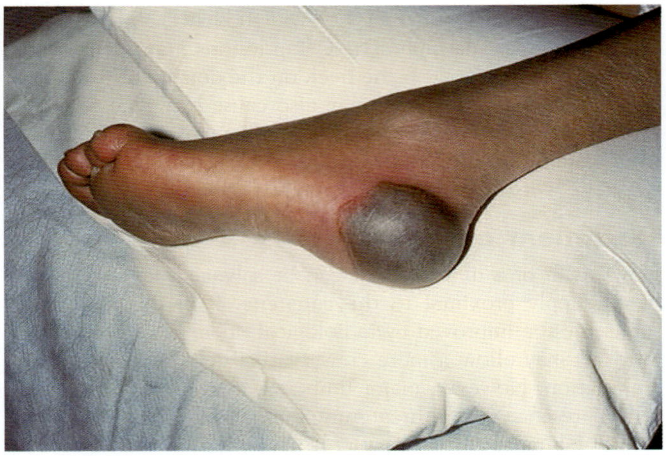

Figure 56.23 Bedsores typically appear over areas exposed to pressure, such as the sacrum and (as in this case) the heel.

tating illness. Prophylactic measures must be taken, including the avoidance of pressure over bony prominences by the use of foam blocks or similar, regular turning, and nursing on specially designed beds that reduce the pressure to the skin. A water bed or a ripple bed is sometimes desirable. Injury from wrinkled sheets and maceration of the skin by sweat, urine, faeces or pus must be prevented by skilled nursing and the use of appropriate dressings.

A bedsore can be expected if erythema appears that does not change colour on pressure. Once pressure sores develop, they are difficult to heal. They should be kept clean and debrided if necessary. Advice from a plastic surgeon should be sought for major lesions; vacuum dressings and rotation flaps can be effective.

Frostbite

Frostbite is caused by exposure to cold. It is seen both in climbers at high altitudes and in the elderly or the vagrant during cold weather (Figure 56.24). Cold injury damages the wall of the blood vessel which causes swelling and leakage of fluid together with severe pain. When the pain disappears, a waxy appearance remains; blistering and then gangrene follow. Treatment is gradual rewarming, analgesics and delayed conservative amputation after demarcation of devitalised tissue.

ACUTE ARTERIAL OCCLUSION

Sudden occlusion of an artery is usually caused by an embolus. It may also happen when thrombosis occurs on an atherosclerotic plaque, although the outcome is usually less dramatic because collaterals are likely to have developed in chronic arterial stenosis.

Embolic occlusion

An embolus is a body that is foreign to the bloodstream and which may become lodged in a vessel and cause obstruction. It is often a thrombus that has become detached from the heart or a more proximal vessel. Sources include the left atrium in atrial fibrillation, a left ventricular mural thrombus following myocardial infarction; vegetations on heart valves in infective endocarditis, thrombi in aneurysms and on atheroscerotic plaques. Emboli may lodge in any organ and cause ischaemic symptoms.

- **Arm and leg.** Pain, pallor, paralysis, pulselessness and paraesthesia (Figure 56.25). Acute arterial occlusion due to an embolus differs from occlusion due to thrombosis on pre-existing atheroma; in the latter case, a collateral circulation has often built up over time (Figures 56.26 and 56.27). It is essential to differentiate between the two as they require different management.

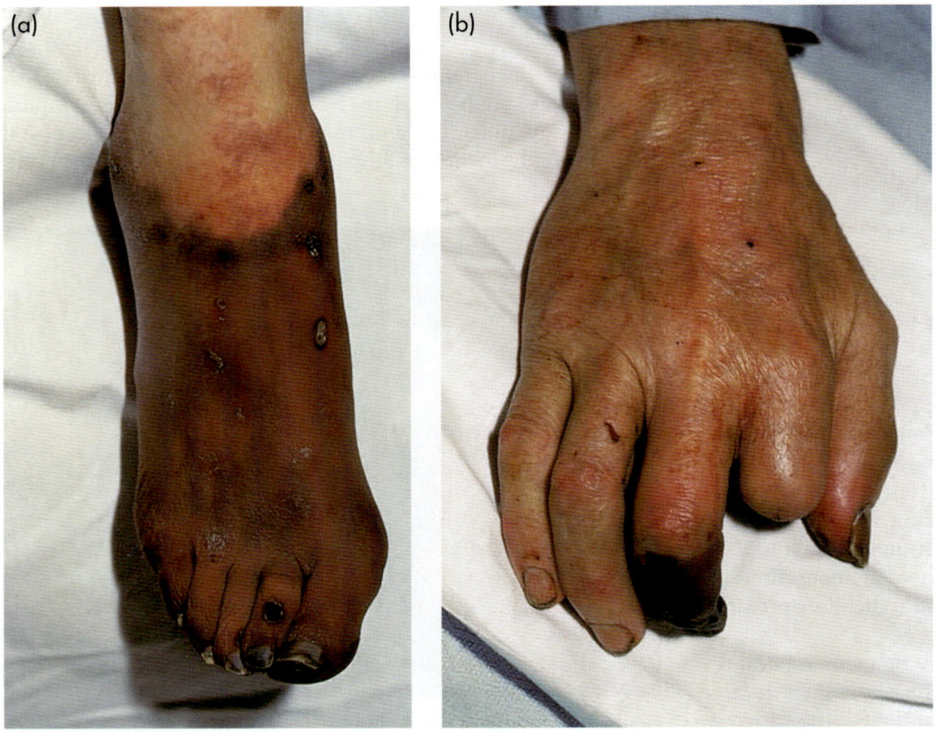

Figure 56.24 (a) Frostbite of the foot. Note the clear demarcation. (b) Frostbite of the middle finger in the same patient. The index finger was lost two years before, also from frostbite.

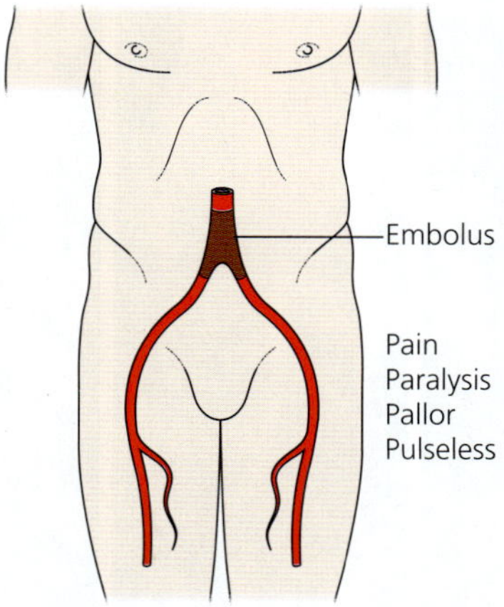

Figure 56.25 The symptoms and signs of embolism (four Ps). The fifth feature, anaesthesia, is often stated to be paraesthesia (the fifth P) but, in truth, complete loss of sensation in the toes and feet is characteristic.

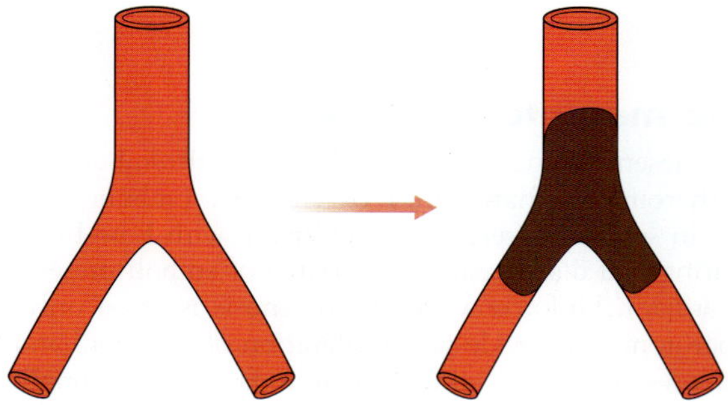

Figure 56.26 Aortic bifurcation embolus. Source of embolus is a recent myocardial infarct or atrial fibrillation. This causes severe, dramatic symptoms.

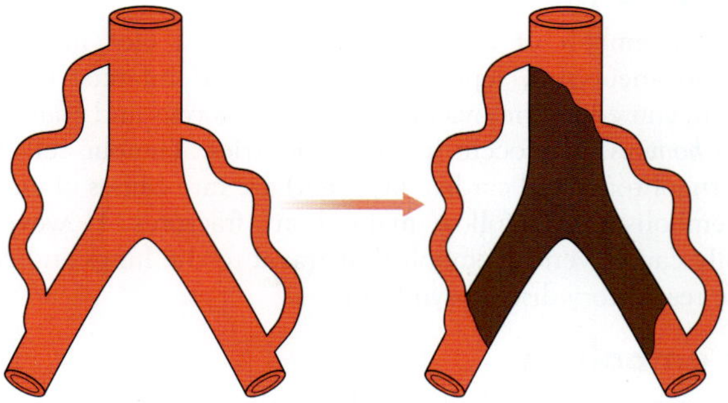

Figure 56.27 Aortic bifurcation thrombosis. No source of embolus but previous claudication. Claudication worse but no dramatic event.

- **Brain**. The middle cerebral artery (or its branches) is most commonly affected, resulting in major or minor (TIA) stroke.
- **Retina.** Amaurosis fugax is fleeting blindness caused by a minute thrombus emanating from an atheromatous plaque in the carotid artery passing into the central retinal artery. Lasting obstruction causes permanent blindness.
- **Mesenteric vessels**. Possible gangrene of the corresponding loop of intestine.

Acute limb ischaemia

Clinical features

Embolic arterial occlusion is an emergency that requires immediate treatment. Ischaemia beyond 6 hours is usually irreversible and results in limb loss. The leg is often affected, with pain, pallor, paralysis, loss of pulsation and paraesthesia (or anaesthesia) (Figure 56.25). The limb is cold and the toes cannot be moved, which contrasts with venous occlusion when muscle function is not affected. The diagnosis can be made clinically in a patient who has no history of claudication and has a source of emboli, who suddenly develops severe pain or numbness of the limb, which becomes cold and mottled. Movement becomes progressively more difficult and sensation is lost. Pulses are absent distally, but the femoral pulse may be palpable, even thrusting, as distal occlusion results in forceful expansion of the artery with each pressure wave despite the lack of flow. A similar picture will occur in the arm with a brachial embolus.

Treatment

Because of the ensuing stasis, a thrombus can extend distally and proximally to the embolus. The immediate administration of 5000 U of heparin intravenously can reduce this extension and maintain patency of the surrounding (particularly the distal) vessels until the embolus can be treated. The relief of pain is essential because it is severe and constant. Embolectomy and thrombolysis are the treatments available for patients with limb emboli.

Embolectomy

Local or general anaesthesia may be used. The artery (usually the femoral), bulging with clot, is exposed and held in slings. Through a longitudinal or transverse incision, the clot begins to extrude and is removed, together with the embolus (Figure 56.28), with the help of a Fogarty balloon catheter. The catheter, with its balloon tip, is introduced both proximally and distally until it is deemed to have passed the limit of the clot. The

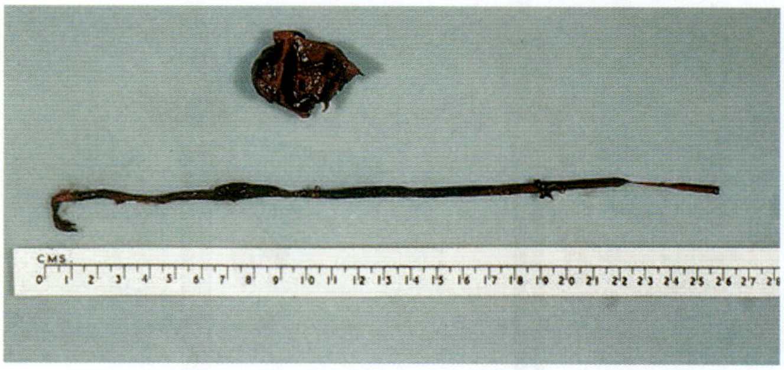

Figure 56.28 Embolic material removed from the common femoral artery, along with a long distal extension thrombus.

Thomas J Fogarty, born 1934, surgeon, University of Oregon Medical School, Portland, OR, USA. Since 1993, Professor of Surgery, Stanford University, CA, USA; patented his catheter in 1969; first balloon angioplasty performed with a Fogarty catheter in 1965; recipient of Inventor of the Year Award given by San Francisco Patent and Trademark Association. He became very interested in wine and established the Thomas Fogarty Winery and Vineyards in California in 1981.

balloon is inflated and the catheter withdrawn slowly, together with any obstructing material (Figure 56.29). The procedure is repeated until back bleeding occurs. An angiogram may be performed in the operating theatre at the end of the procedure to ensure that flow to the distal leg has been restored. Postoperatively, heparin therapy is continued until long-term anticoagulation with warfarin is established to reduce the chance of further embolism.

Compartment syndrome

In limbs that have been subject to sudden ischaemia followed by revascularisation, oedema is likely. Muscles swell within fixed fascial compartments and this can itself be a cause of ischaemia, with both local muscle necrosis and nerve damage due to pressure, and distal effects such as renal failure secondary to the liberation of muscle breakdown products. The treatment is urgent fasciotomy to release the compression. The usual site for fasciotomy is the calf (especially the anterior tibial compartment), but compartment syndrome may occasionally affect the thigh and the arm.

Intra-arterial thrombolysis

If ischaemia is not so severe that immediate operation is essential, it may be possible to treat either embolus or thrombosis by intra-arterial thrombolysis (Figure 56.30). At arteriography of the ischaemic limb (usually via the common femoral artery), a narrow catheter is passed into the occluded vessel and left embedded within the clot. Tissue plasminogen activator (TPA) is infused through the catheter and regular arteriograms are carried out to check on the extent of lysis, which, in successful cases, is achieved within 24 hours. The method should be abandoned if there is no progression of dissolution of clot with time. There are several contraindications to thrombolysis, the most important of which are recent stroke, bleeding diathesis and pregnancy, and results in those over 80 years old are poor.

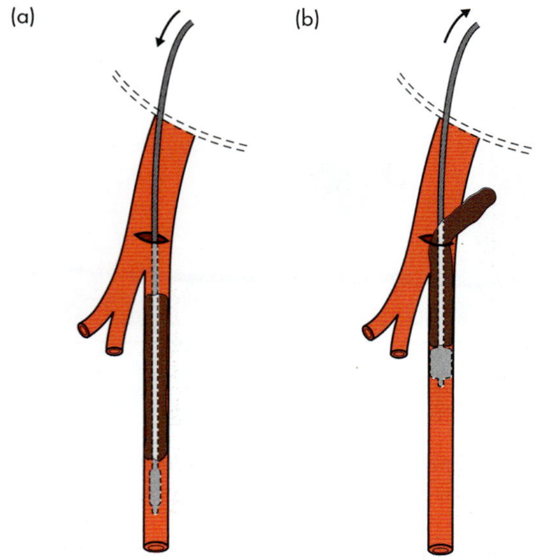

Figure 56.29 (a) A Fogarty catheter is inserted through an arteriotomy in the common femoral artery and fed distally down the superficial femoral artery and through the embolus. (b) The balloon is inflated and the catheter withdrawn, removing the embolus; the deep femoral and iliac arteries are similarly treated.

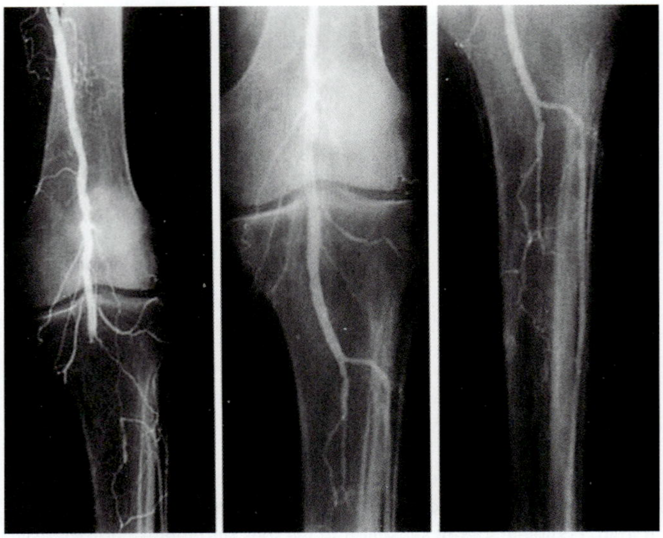

Figure 56.30 Angiogram of an occluded popliteal artery before thrombolysis (left), during successful lysis (middle) and after completion of lysis (right).

Acute mesenteric ischaemia

Acute mesenteric occlusion may be either thrombotic (following atheromatous narrowing) or embolic. Embolic occlusion results in sudden, severe abdominal pain, with bowel emptying (vomiting and diarrhoea) and a source of emboli present (usually cardiac). Unfortunately, the diagnosis is often only made at laparotomy with widespread infarction of the small and large bowel present; in this situation, it is fatal. Occasionally, the degree of bowel infarction is more limited; resection of the dead bowel and embolectomy of the superior mesenteric artery, or bypass surgery can reduce the otherwise high mortality rate in these patients. A 'second look' laparotomy 24 hours later to check the viability of the bowel is often indicated.

Other forms of emboli

Infective emboli of bacteria or an infected clot may cause mycotic aneurysms, septicaemia or infected infarcts. Parasitic emboli, caused by the ova of *Taenia echinococcus* and *Filaria sanguinis hominis*, may occur in some countries. Tumour cells (e.g. hypernephroma and cardiac myxoma) are rare causes of emboli. Fat embolism may follow major bony fractures. However, it usually causes venous emboli that travel to the lungs and cause acute respiratory distress syndrome.

Air embolism

Air may be accidentally injected into the venous circulation or sucked into an open vein during head and neck surgery or a cut throat. It may also occur following Fallopian tube insufflation or illegal abortion. If a large volume of air reaches the right side of the heart it may form an air lock within the pulmonary artery and cause acute right heart failure.

The treatment of air embolism is to put the patient in a head-down (Trendelenburg) position to encourage the air to enter the veins in the lower part of the body. The patient should also be placed on the left side to help the air to float to the ventricular apex, away from the ostium of the pulmonary artery. In extreme

Gabrielle Falloppio (Fallopius), 1523–1563, Professor of Anatomy, Surgery and Botany, Padua, Italy.

cases, air may be aspirated from the heart through a needle introduced below the left costal margin.

Therapeutic embolisation

This is used to arrest haemorrhage from the gastrointestinal, urinary (Figure 56.31), gynaecological and respiratory tracts, to treat arteriovenous malformations by blocking their arterial supply and to control the growth of unresectable tumours. Arterial embolisation requires accurate selective catheterisation using the Seldinger technique. A variety of materials may be used, including gelfoam sponge, plastic microspheres, balloons, ethyl alcohol, quick-setting plastics and metal coils.

AMPUTATION

General

Amputation should be considered when part of a limb is dead, deadly or a dead loss. A limb is dead when arterial occlusive disease is severe enough to cause infarction of macroscopic portions of tissue, i.e. gangrene. The occlusion may be in major vessels (atherosclerotic or embolic occlusions) or in small peripheral vessels (diabetes, Buerger's disease, Raynaud's disease, inadvertent intra-arterial injection). If the obstruction cannot be reversed and the symptoms are severe, amputation is required.

A limb is deadly when the putrefaction and infection of moist gangrene spreads to surrounding viable tissues. Cellulitis and severe toxaemia are the result. Amputation is required as a life-saving operation. Antibiotic cover should be broad and massive. Other life-threatening situations for which amputation may be required include gas gangrene (as opposed to simple infection), neoplasm (such as osteogenic sarcoma) and arteriovenous fistula.

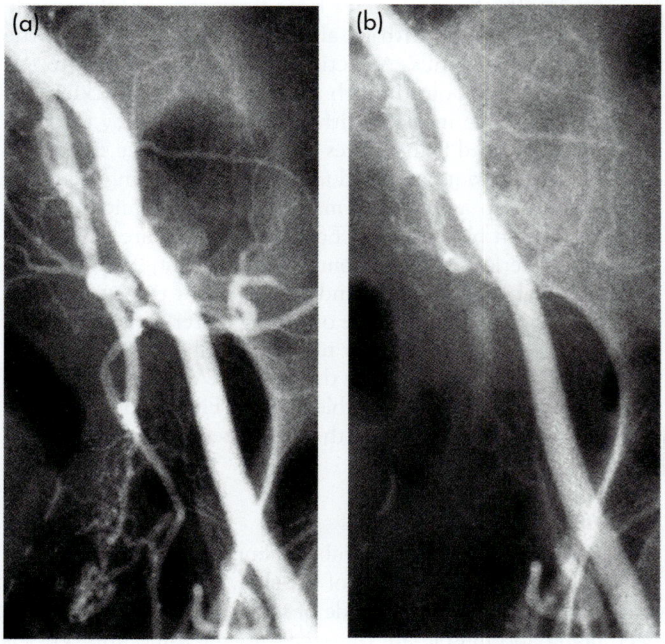

Figure 56.31 Before (a) and after (b) therapeutic embolisation of the internal iliac artery in a patient with gross haematuria from an ulcerating bladder carcinoma (courtesy of F McIvor, FRCR, London, UK).

A limb may be deemed a dead loss in the following circumstances: first, when there is relentless severe rest pain without gangrene and reconstruction is not possible – amputation will improve quality of life; second, when a contracture or paralysis makes the limb impossible to use and renders it a hindrance; and third, when there is major unrecoverable traumatic damage (Summary box 56.3).

Summary box 56.3

Indications for amputation

- Dead limb
  - Gangrene
- Deadly limb
  - Wet gangrene
  - Spreading cellulitis
  - Arteriovenous fistula
  - Other (e.g. malignancy)
- 'Dead loss' limb
  - Severe rest pain with unreconstructable critical leg ischaemia
  - Paralysis
  - Other (e.g. contracture, trauma)

Distal and transmetatarsal amputation

In patients with small-vessel disease, typically caused by diabetes, gangrene of the toes may occur with relatively good blood supply to the surrounding tissues. In such circumstances, local amputation of the digits can result in healing. However, if the metatarsophalangeal joint region is involved, a ray excision is required, taking part of the metatarsal and cutting tendons back. Most surgeons leave the wound open. Early mobility aids drainage provided that cellulitis is not present. For less extensive gangrene, if amputation is taken through a joint, healing is improved by removing the cartilage from the joint surface. A transmetatarsal amputation may be required when several toes are affected, but the proximal circulation is adequate. The wound may be closed with a viable long plantar flap (Figure 56.32) or left open.

Major amputation

Choice of operation

The major choice is between an above- or below-knee operation. A below-knee amputation preserves the knee joint and gives the best chance of walking again with a prosthesis. However, an above-knee amputation is more likely to heal and may be appropriate if the patient has no prospect of walking again. If the femoral pulse is absent, the amputation should be above the knee. Unfortunately, the presence of a femoral pulse does not guarantee healing of a below-knee amputation and sometimes a

Sir William Ferguson (1808–1877), surgeon, Royal Infirmary, Edinburgh, later Professor of Surgery, King's College Hospital, London, said that amputation is 'one of the meanest, and yet one of the greatest operations in surgery: mean, when resorted to where better may be done – great, as the only step to give comfort and prolong life'.

Sir Edward 'Weary' Dunlop, a great Australian surgeon. During the Second World War, as a prisoner of war (POW) held by the Japanese while looking after other POWs working on the Burma–Siam Railway, he made prosthetic lower limbs for amputees out of bamboo.

Leo Buerger, 1879–1943, Professor of Urologic Surgery, New York Polyclinic Medical School, New York, NY, USA, described thromboangitis obliterans in 1908.
Maurice Raynaud, 1834–1881, physician, Hospital Lariboisiere, Paris, France, described this condition in 1862.

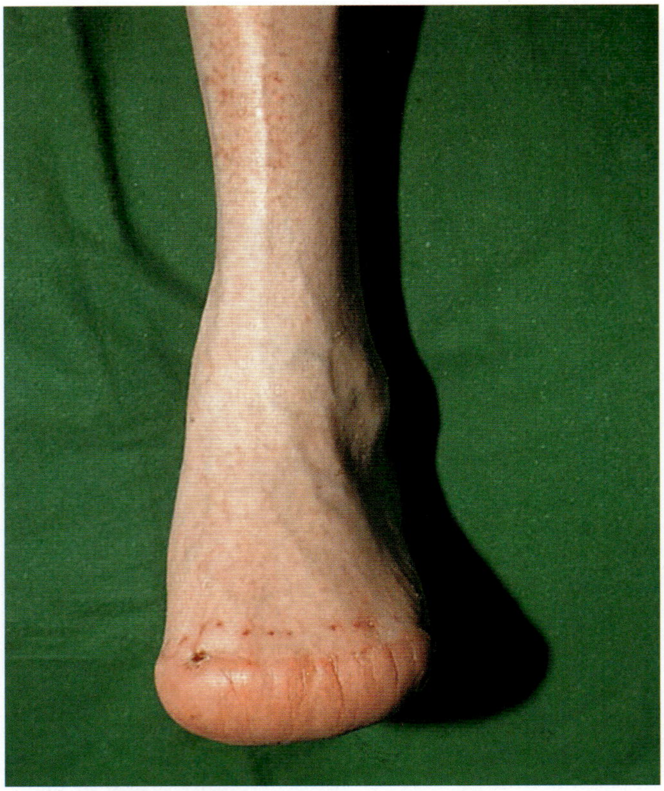

Figure 56.32 Transmetatarsal amputation for diabetic gangrene of the toes.

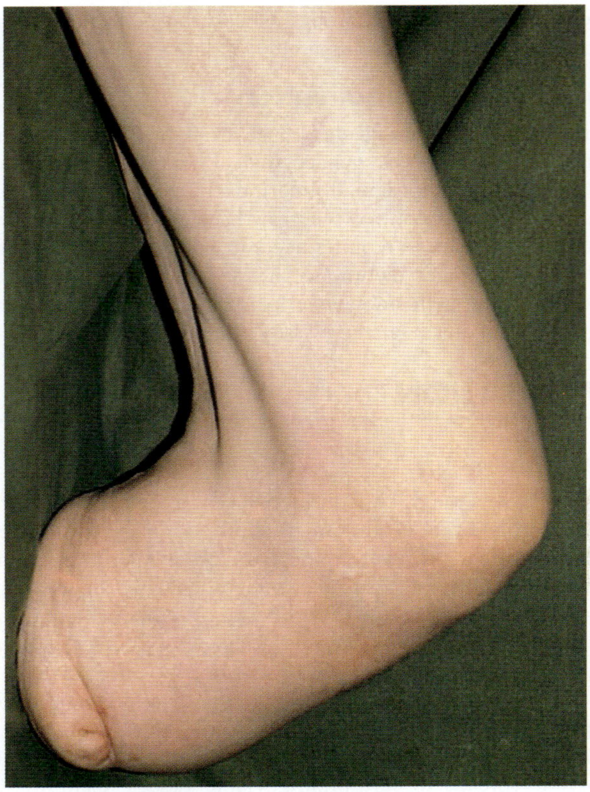

Figure 56.33 Classic long posterior flap type of below-knee amputation.

failed below-knee amputation may require revision to an above-knee procedure.

For above- or below-knee amputations with a good stump shape, it is possible to hold a prosthesis in place simply by suction, without any cumbersome and unsightly straps. The stump should be of sufficient length to give the required leverage, i.e. not less than 8 cm below the knee (preferably 10–12 cm) and not less than 20 cm above the knee.

Below-knee amputations

Two types of skin flap are commonly used: long posterior flap and skew flap (described by KP Robinson). For both methods, the total length of flap must be at least one and a half times the diameter of the leg at the point of bone section.

The long posterior flap technique is the older method and remains the more popular probably because of its relative simplicity (Figure 56.33). Anteriorly, the incision is deepened to bone and the lateral and posterior incisions are fashioned to leave the bulk of the gastrocnemius muscle attached to the flap, muscle and skin being transected together at the same level. If bleeding is inadequate, the amputation is refashioned at a higher level. Blood vessels are identified and ligated. Nerves are not clamped, but pulled down gently and transected as high as possible. Vessels in nerves are ligated. The fibula is divided 2 cm proximal to the level of tibial division using bone cutters. The tibia is cleared and transected at the desired level, the anterior aspect of the bone being sawn obliquely before the cross-cut is made. This, with filing, gives a smooth anterior bevel, which prevents pressure necrosis of the flap. The long muscle/skin flap is tapered after removing the bulk of the soleus muscle (much of the gastrocnemius may be left, unless it is very bulky). The area is washed with saline to remove bone fragments and the muscle and fascia are sutured with an absorbable material to bring the flap over the bone ends. A suction drain is placed deep to the muscle and brought out through a stab incision in the skin. The skin flap should lie in place with all tension taken by the deep sutures. Interrupted skin sutures are inserted. Gauze, wool and crepe bandages are usually used for the stump dressing.

The skew flap amputation makes use of anatomical knowledge of the skin blood supply. Equally long flaps are developed; they join anteriorly 2.5 cm from the tibial crest, overlying the anterior tibial compartment, and posteriorly at the exact opposite point on the circumference of the leg. After division of bone and muscle in a fashion similar to that described above, the gastrocnemius flap is sutured over the cut bone end to the anterior tibial periosteum with absorbable sutures. Finally, drainage and skin sutures are inserted and the limb dressed as for the long posterior flap operation.

Above-knee amputation

The site is chosen as indicated above, but may need to be higher if bleeding is poor on incision of the skin. Equal curved anterior and posterior skin flaps are made of sufficient total length. Skin, deep fascia and muscle are transected in the same line. Vessels are ligated. The sciatic nerve is pulled down and transected cleanly as high as possible and the accompanying artery ligated.

James Syme, 1799–1871, Regius Professor of Clinical Surgery, University of Edinburgh, Edinburgh, UK.
Rocco Gritti, 1828–1920, surgeon, Milan, Italy, described this operation in 1857.
Sir William Stokes, 1839–1900, surgeon, Dublin, Ireland described his modification of Gritti's operation in 1870.
Kingsley Peter Robinson, formerly surgeon, The Westminister Hospital, London, UK

Muscle and skin are retracted and the bone cleared and sawn at the point chosen. Haemostasis is achieved. The muscle ends are united over the bone by absorbable sutures incorporating the fascia. A suction drain deep to the muscle is brought out through the skin clear of the wound. The fascia and subcutanous tissues are further brought together so that the skin can be apposed by interrupted sutures. Gauze, wool and crepe bandages form the stump dressing.

Postoperative care of an amputee

Opiate pain relief should be given regularly. Care of the good limb must not be forgotten as a pressure ulcer on the remaining foot will delay mobilisation, despite satisfactory healing of the stump. Exercise and mobilisation are of the greatest importance. After surgery, flexion deformity must be prevented and exercises started to build up muscle power and coordination. Mobility is progressively increased with walking between bars and the use of an inflatable artificial limb, which allows weight-bearing to be started before a pylon or temporary artificial limb is ready (Figure 56.34). Early assessment of the home is part of the programme; it allows time for minor alterations, such as the addition of stair rails, movement of furniture to give support near doors and provision of clearance in confined passages.

Complications

Early complications include haemorrhage (which requires return to the operating theatre for haemostasis), haematoma (which requires evacuation) and infection (usually in association with a haematoma). Any abscess must be drained and appropriate antibiotics given. Gas gangrene can occur in a mid-thigh stump from faecal contamination. Wound dehiscence and gangrene of the flaps are caused by ischaemia; a higher amputation may be necessary. Amputees are at risk of deep vein thrombosis and pulmonary embolism in the early postoperative period and prophylaxis with subcutaneous heparin is essential.

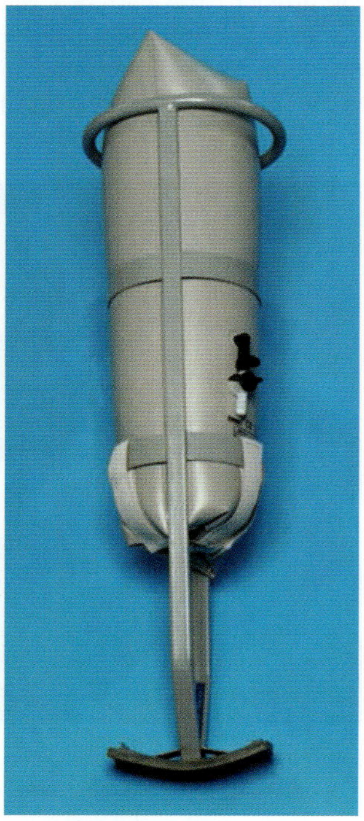

Figure 56.34 Inflatable artificial limb.

Later complications include pain resulting from unresolved infection (sinus, osteitis, sequestrum), a bone spur, a scar adherent to bone and an amputation neuroma. Patients frequently remark that they can feel the amputated limb (phantom limb) and sometimes remark that it is painful (phantom pain). The surgeon's attitude should be one of firm reassurance that this sensation will almost certainly disappear with time; amitriptyline or gabapentin may help. Other late complications include ulceration of the stump because of pressure effects of the prosthesis or increased ischaemia.

ANEURYSM

General

Dilatations of localised segments of the arterial system are called 'aneurysms'. They can either be true aneurysms, containing the three layers of the arterial wall (intima, media, adventitia) in the aneurysm sac, or false aneurysms, having a single layer of fibrous tissue as the wall of the sac, e.g. aneurysm following trauma. Aneurysms can also be grouped according to their shape (fusiform, saccular) or their aetiology (atheromatous, traumatic, mycotic, etc.). The term 'mycotic' is a misnomer because, although it indicates infection as the cause of the aneurysm, it is due to bacteria, not fungi. Aneurysms may occur in the aorta, iliac, femoral, popliteal, subclavian, axillary, carotid, cerebral, mesenteric, splenic and renal arteries and their branches. The majority are true fusiform atherosclerotic aneurysms (Summary box 56.4).

Summary box 56.4

Classification of aneurysms

- Wall
  - True (three layers: intima, media, adventitia)
  - False (single layer of fibrous tissue)
- Morphology
  - Fusiform
  - Saccular
- Aetiology
  - Atheromatous
  - Mycotic (bacterial rather than fungal)
  - Collagen disease
  - Traumatic

Clinical features

All aneurysms can cause symptoms, as a result of compression of surrounding structures, thrombosis, rupture or the release of emboli. The symptoms relate to the vessel affected and the tissues it supplies. Many aneurysms of clinical significance can be palpated and, typically, an expansile pulsation is felt. Transmitted pulsation through a mass lesion, cyst or abscess lying adjacent to a large artery may be mistaken for aneurysmal pulsation. Before incising a swelling believed to be an abscess, it is essential to make sure that it does not pulsate. Finally, a tortuous (and often ectatic) artery, usually the innominate or carotid, may seem like an aneurysm to the inexperienced clinician.

Abdominal aortic aneurysm

Abdominal aortic aneurysm is by far the most common type of large vessel aneurysm and is found in 2 per cent of the population at autopsy; 95 per cent have associated atheromatous degeneration and 95 per cent occur below the renal arteries. Most remain asymptomatic until rupture occurs; the risk of rupture increases with increasing size (diameter) of the aneurysm. Asymptomatic aneurysms are found incidentally on physical examination, radiography or ultrasound investigation. It may be appropriate to screen for abdominal aortic aneurysms with ultrasound; a national screening programme has recently started in England and offers an ultrasound scan to men in their 65th year. Symptomatic aneurysms may cause minor symptoms, such as back and abdominal discomfort, before sudden, severe back and/or abdominal pain develops from expansion and rupture.

Asymptomatic abdominal aortic aneurysm

An asymptomatic abdominal aortic aneurysm (Figure 56.35) in an otherwise fit patient should be considered for repair if >55 mm in diameter (measured by ultrasonography). The annual incidence of rupture rises from 1 per cent or less in aneurysms that are <55 mm in diameter to a significant level, perhaps as high as 20 per cent, in those that are 70 mm in diameter. Assuming open elective surgery (transabdominal) carries a 5 per cent mortality rate, the balance is in favour of elective operation once the diameter is >55 mm, provided there is no major comorbidity. Regular ultrasonographic assessment is indicated for asymptomatic aneurysms <55 mm in diameter.

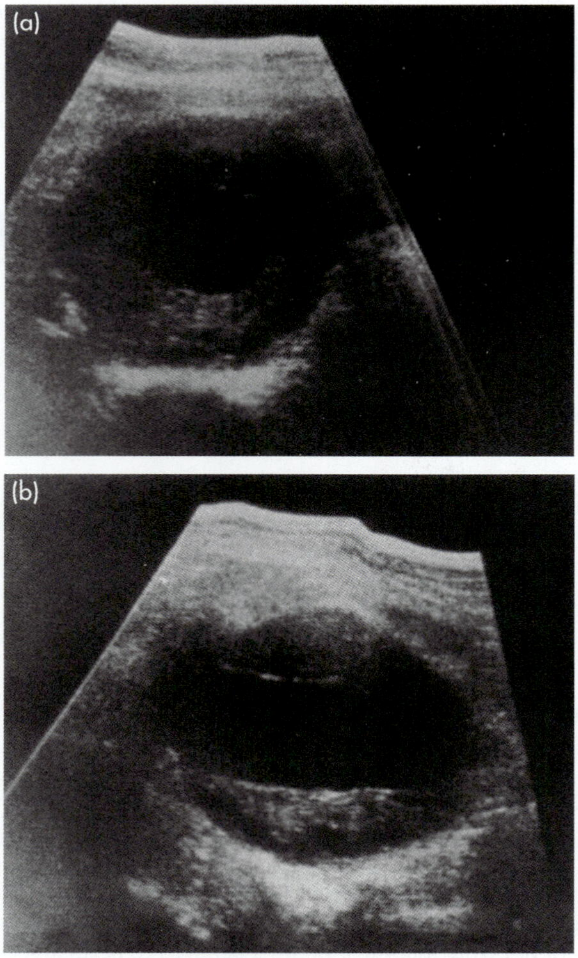

Figure 56.35 Ultrasonogram of an aortic aneurysm showing the large clot-filled sac with a small central lumen (a) transverse and (b) longitudinal scans.

Investigations

Full blood count, electrolytes, liver function tests, coagulation tests and blood lipid estimation should be performed. Blood should be crossmatched a few days prior to surgery. Many patients now have an anaesthetic assessment and the need for cardiac and respiratory function tests are decided at this time. An electrocardiogram and chest radiograph are essential; further assessment may include echocardiography or isotope ventriculography, cardiopulmonary exercise testing and spirometry.

The morphology of the aneurysm is best assessed by CT scan (Figures 56.36 and 56.37). Fifty per cent of aneurysms are suitable for endovascular (minimally invasive) repair usually via the femoral arteries in the groin. If lower limb pulse is absent, there may be associated arterial occlusive disease which should be assessed by duplex scanning initially. Further assessment with CT, MR or digital subtraction angiography may be required and angioplasty may be appropriate. The aneurysm is often filled with circumferential clot (Figure 56.38a), which produces a falsely narrowed appearance on digitial subtraction angiography (Figure 56.38b); this method should not therefore be used to assess aneurysm size.

Choice of operation – open or endovascular repair

Open surgical procedure

Under general anaesthesia, with the patient lying supine, a full-length midline or supraumbilical transverse incision is made. The small bowel is lifted to the patient's right and the aorta identified. The posterior peritoneum overlying the aorta is opened and the upper limit of the aneurysm identified. The aorta immediately above the dilatation is exposed; this is generally just inferior to the left renal vein and renal arteries (Figure 56.39).

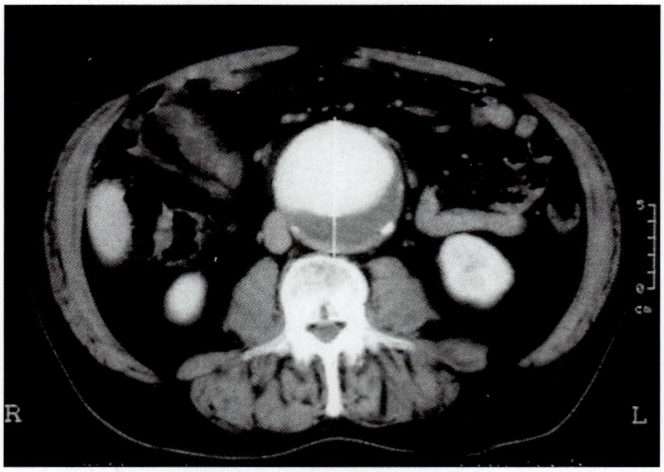

Figure 56.36 Computed tomogram of the abdomen showing an aortic aneurysm. Blood flowing through the thrombus-containing sac is enhanced by intravascular contrast and therefore appears white while the thrombus remains unenhanced.

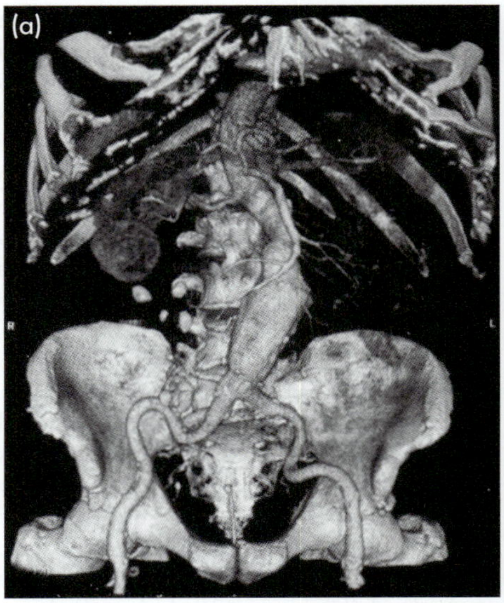

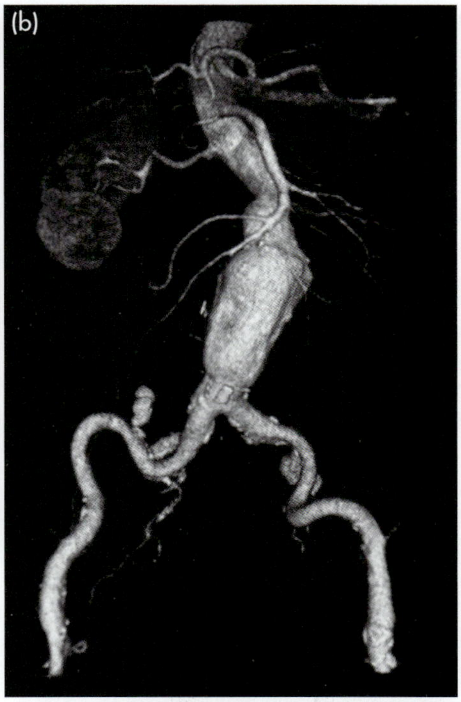

Figure 56.37 (a) Spiral computed tomogram showing an infrarenal abdominal aortic aneurysm; (b) with the bony elements subtracted.

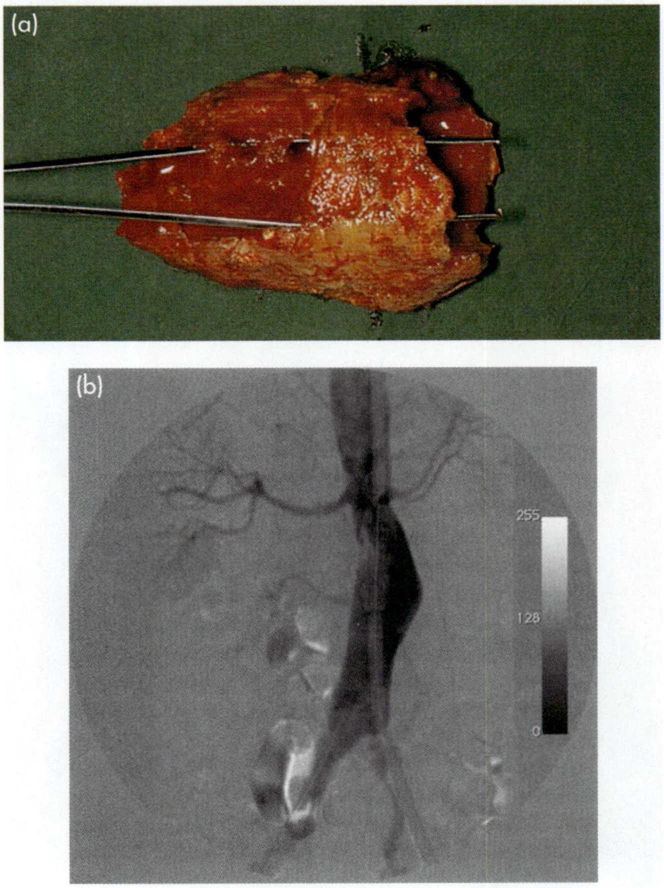

Figure 56.38 (a) Thrombus removed from an abdominal aortic aneurysm; this thrombus is the reason an angiogram may give a false impression of aneurysm diameter on digital subtraction angiography (b).

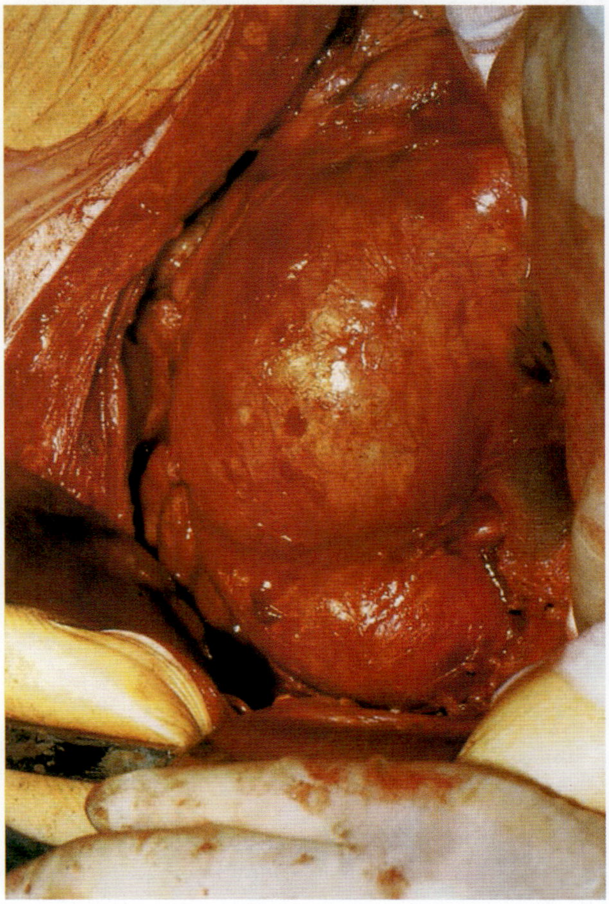

Figure 56.39 Operative appearance of a huge, non-ruptured infrarenal abdominal aortic aneurysm.

The common iliac arteries are then exposed and clamps applied above and below the lesion. Many surgeons give systemic heparin before clamping. The aneurysm is opened longitudinally and back-bleeding from lumbar and mesenteric vessels controlled by sutures placed from within the sac. Upper and lower aortic necks are prepared to which an aortic prosthesis is then sutured end to end inside the sac with a monofilament non-absorbable suture (Figure 56.40). Clamps are released slowly to prevent sudden hypotension. If haemostasis is satisfactory at this point, the aneurysm sac is closed around the prosthesis to exclude both it and the suture lines from the bowel to reduce the risk of adherence and potential fistula formation. The abdomen is then closed. Occasionally, when the iliac vessels are also involved with dilatation or severe atheroma, it is necessary to construct an aortobi-iliac or aortobifemoral bypass, rather than use a simple aorto-aortic tube.

Endovascular aneurysm repair

Endovascular aneurysm repair (EVAR) is now established in clinical practice and has been shown to have reduced mortality compared to open repair over the first six years. Currently, about 50 per cent of infrarenal aneurysms are suitable for EVAR which is dependent on the morphology of the aneurysm when assessed by CT scan. Common causes of unsuitability include a short, flared or angulated neck and difficult iliac artery access because of narrowing or tortuosity. The usual technique is to expose both femoral arteries (under general or local anaesthetic) which allows access to the aorta. Then, under radiological control, guidewires and catheters are used to cross the aneurysm and an angiogram performed to mark the level of the renal arteries.

The endovascular prosthesis (often termed a 'stent graft') is usually made up of three separate parts – a main body (Figure 56.41a) and two limbs which are enclosed in separate delivery catheters (Figure 56.41b). Some types have only two pieces – a main body with ipsilateral limb attached and a separate contralateral limb. The prosthesis is made from Dacron or PTFE with integral metallic stents for support. The delivery catheter is inserted in the aneurysm sac and the stent graft deployed by withdrawal of the delivery system. Most systems now have hooks or barbs to anchor the prosthesis in the aortic wall and some surgeons inflate a moulding balloon catheter in the stent graft to ensure the hooks and barbs are engaged and a good seal is obtained (Figure 56.42). Although the top edge of the fabric of the stent graft has to be deployed below the renal arteries (infrarenal fixation), some systems have additional bare metal stents at the proximal end of the main body which lie across

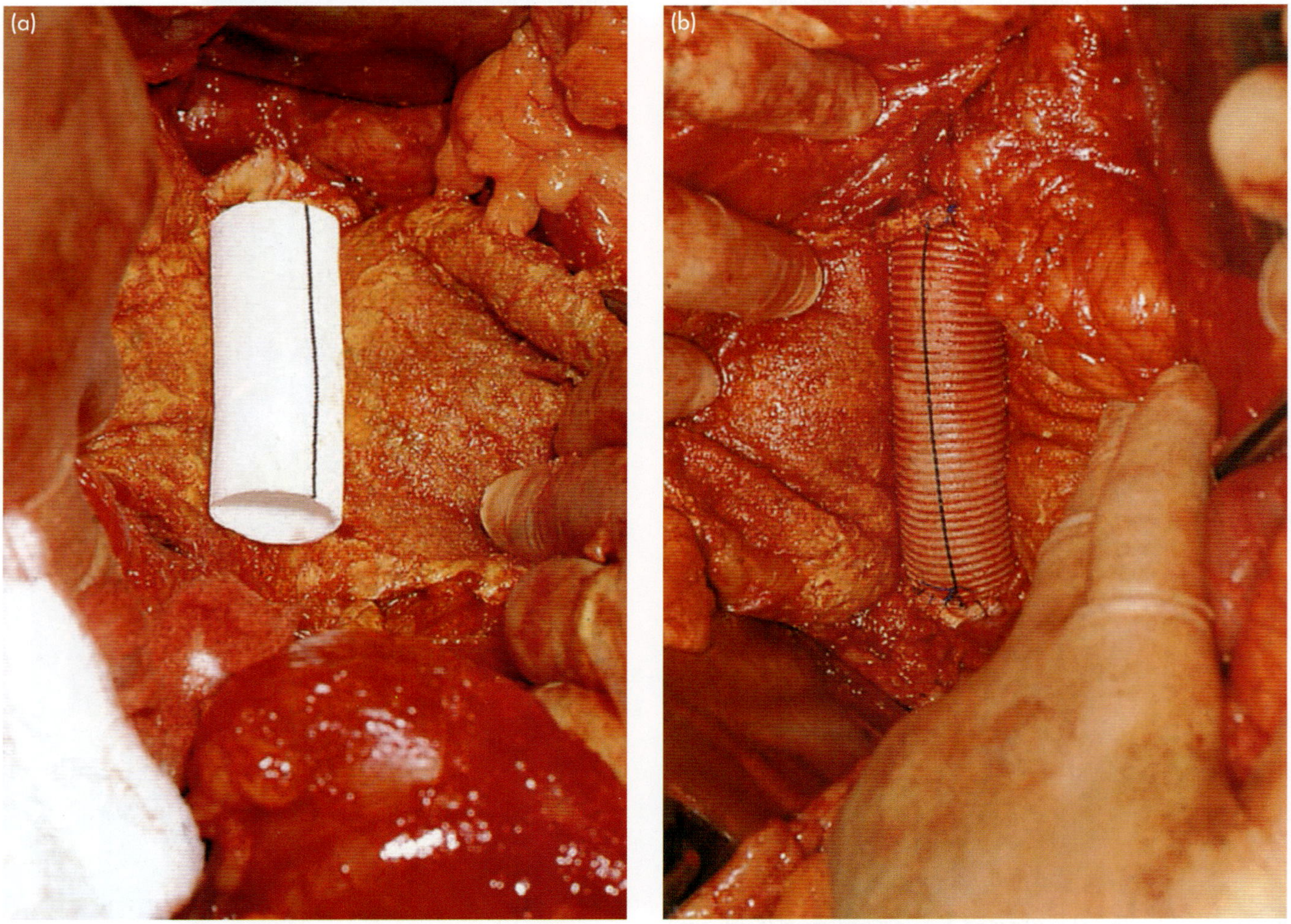

Figure 56.40 (a) Aneurysm sac opened. Note that the posterior wall of the aorta immediately above and below the sac is not divided. A Dacron tube graft is laid in place within the sac ready for suture. (b) Graft sutured in place and vascular clamps removed.

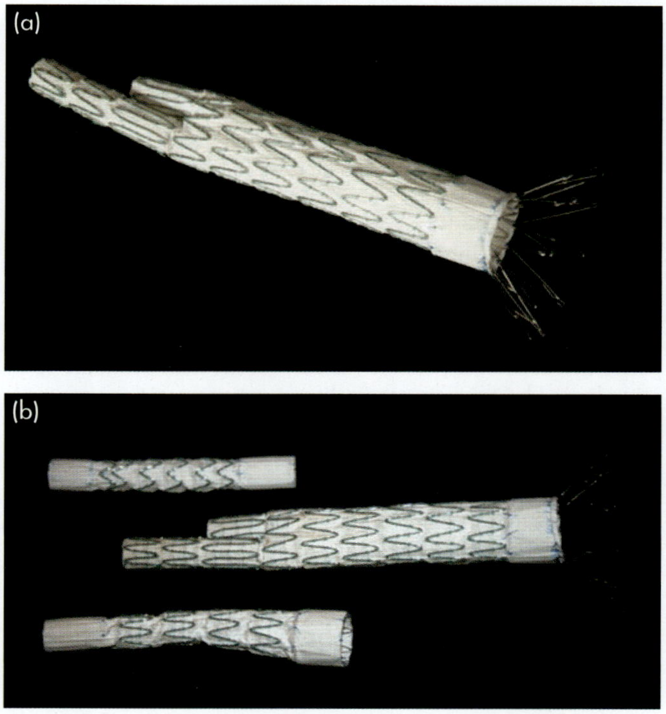

Figure 56.41 (a) Endovascular prosthesis main body (b) with separate limbs.

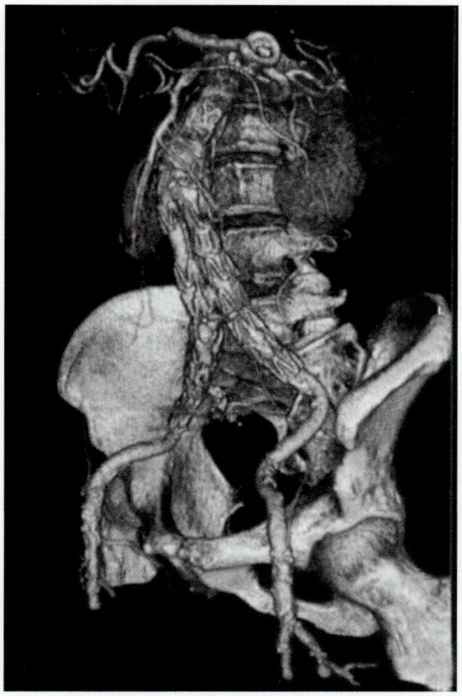

Figure 56.42 Spiral computed tomogram showing an endoluminal aortoiliac 'stent graft'. The metallic stent structure is clearly observed.

the renal arteries to give better support and fixation (suprarenal fixation). Blood flows between the metal struts of the stent into the renal arteries. Success is dependent on a good seal between the stent graft and the proximal and distal 'landing zones' in the aorta and iliac arteries. Failure to achieve a good seal results in an endoleak which means that the aneurysm is not excluded from the circulation and may still expand and rupture. Patients who undergo EVAR require life-long follow up and surveillance with duplex or CT scans to detect endoleak, disconnection of the components and migration of the stent graft, all of which predispose to late rupture (Figure 56.43).

Ruptured abdominal aortic aneurysm

Abdominal aortic aneurysms can rupture anteriorly into the peritoneal cavity (20 per cent) or posterolaterally into the retroperitoneal space (80 per cent). Less than 50 per cent of patients with rupture survive to reach hospital. Anterior rupture results in free bleeding into the peritoneal cavity; very few patients reach hospital alive. Posterior rupture on the other hand produces a retroperitoneal haematoma (Figure 56.44). Often a brief period ensues when a combination of moderate hypotension and the resistance of the retroperitoneal tissues arrests further haemorrhage and may allow transport to hospital. The patient may remain conscious, but in severe pain. If no operation is performed, death is virtually inevitable. Operative mortality is around 50 per cent and the overall combined mortality (community and hospital) is around 80–90 per cent.

Ruptured abdominal aortic aneurysm is a surgical emergency; it should be suspected in a patient with the triad of severe abdominal and/or back pain, hypotension and a pulsatile abdominal mass. If there is doubt about the presence of an aneurysm an ultrasound scan may help, but this cannot diagnose rupture. CT scanning is performed in an increasing number of patients to establish the diagnosis and to determine whether an endovascular repair is possible.

Good venous access is needed for infusion of saline or volume expanding fluids, but the systolic blood pressure should not be raised any more than is necessary to maintain consciousness and permit cardiac perfusion (<100 mmHg). Many surgeons now adopt a policy of permissive hypotension where fluids are withheld if the patients is conscious (and cerebral perfusion is therefore adequate), in order to avoid provoking further uncontrolled haemorrhage. After CT scanning, the patient should be transferred immediately to an operating theatre where a urinary

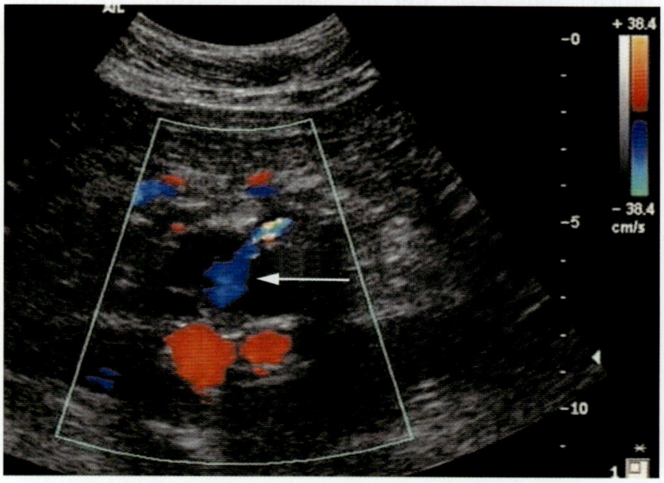

Figure 56.43 Duplex ultrasound scan post-endovascular aneurysm repair (EVAR) showing aortic sac in cross-section and two limbs of EVAR (red ovals). There is a type II endoleak from the inferior mesenteric artery with blood flowing retrogradely into the aneurysm sac (arrow).

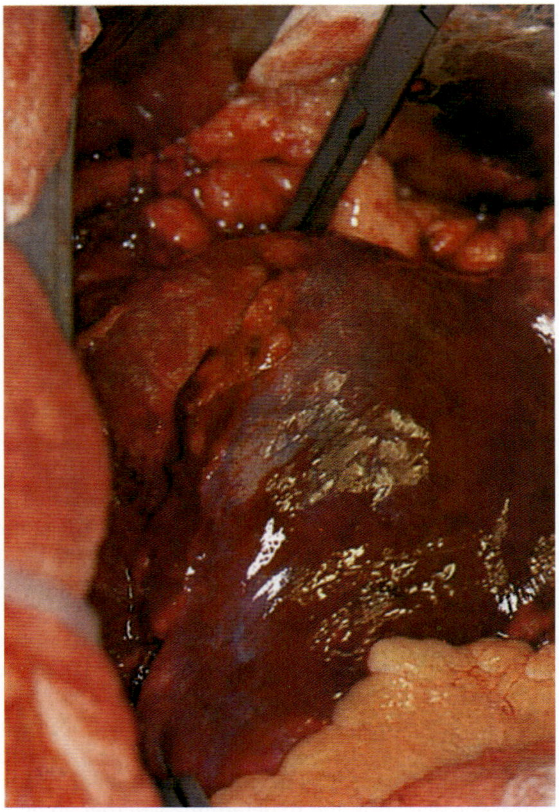

Figure 56.44 The retroperitoneal haematoma of a ruptured aortic aneurysm. The aortic pulsation is palpated through the haematoma at its upper limit and fingers are insinuated on each side of the aorta. With finger control, the upper clamp is positioned and closed on the aorta. The procedure is then as for a planned case. In this illustration, the clamp is at the proximal end of the aneurysm; the haematoma has spread from the left paracolic gutter to encircle the aneurysm and the aortic bifurcation.

catheter and arterial line are usually inserted. If the patient appears stable, surgery may be delayed until cross-matched blood is available, but surgery should commence immediately if haemodynamic instability develops and the patient collapses. The abdomen is usually prepared and draped with the patient awake. It should always be remembered that the treatment of ruptured aneurysm is operation, not monitoring and resuscitation (Summary box 56.5).

Summary box 56.5

Management of ruptured abdominal aortic aneurysm

- Early diagnosis (abdominal/back pain, pulsatile mass, shock)
- Immediate resuscitation (oxygen, intravenous replacement therapy, central line)
- Maintain systolic pressure, but not >100 mmHg, consider permissive hypotension
- Urinary catheter
- Cross-match six units of blood
- Rapid transfer to the operating theatre

Symptomatic abdominal aortic aneurysm

These patients most commonly present with abdominal and/or back pain, but the aneurysm is not ruptured on CT scan. Pain may also occur in the thigh and groin because of nerve compression. Gastrointestinal, urinary and venous symptoms can also be caused by pressure from an abdominal aneurysm. About 3 per cent of all aneurysms cause pain as a result of inflammation of the aneurysm itself (Figure 56.45). Finally, a few cause symptoms from distal embolisation of fragments of their intraluminal thrombus. An operation is usually indicated in patients who are otherwise reasonably fit. Pain may be a warning sign of stretching of the aneurysm sac and imminent rupture; surgery should be performed as soon as possible (usually on the next available operating list). The operative mortality of symptomatic aneurysms is usually higher than elective cases.

Postoperative complications

The most common complications after open repair are cardiac (ischaemia and infarction) and respiratory (atelectasis and lower lobe consolidation). A degree of colonic ischaemia because of a lack of a collateral blood supply occurs in about 10 per cent of patients, but fortunately this usually resolves spontaneously. Renal failure is an uncommon event after elective procedures but may complicate procedures undertaken for rupture. Renal

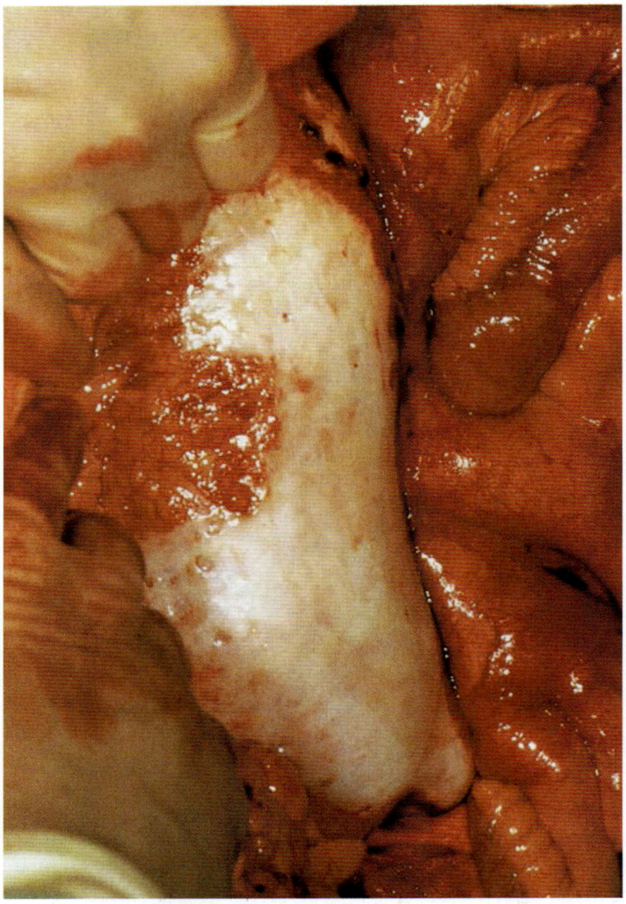

Figure 56.45 An inflammatory abdominal aortic aneurysm. Note the white 'icing' effect. Such lesions can be technically difficult to manage.

failure is more likely if there is preoperative renal impairment or considerable intraoperative blood loss. Neurological complications include sexual dysfunction and spinal cord ischaemia. An aortoduodenal fistula is an uncommon but treatable complication of abdominal aortic replacement surgery. It should be suspected whenever haematemesis or melaena occurs in the months or years after operation. Prosthetic graft infection is also uncommon; it may require removal of the graft and limb revascularisation by insertion of an axillobifemoral bypass.

Cardiac, respiratory, renal and neurological complications are less common after endovascular repair. However, there are complications that are unique to EVAR such as endoleak, graft migration, metal strut fracture and graft limb occlusion. Life-long surveillance with duplex or CT (together with plain abdominal x-ray for strut fracture) is required to detect endoleak and migration. High pressure endoleaks may require repeat ballooning or a proximal cuff or distal limb extension to reseal the endograft. Migration may also require extension of the graft. Overall, 10–20 per cent of patients with EVAR will require secondary interventions to treat complications at some future date, although many of the interventions can be performed via a percutaneous approach via the femoral artery in the angiography suite.

Peripheral aneurysm

Popliteal aneurysm

Popliteal artery aneurysm accounts for 70 per cent of all peripheral aneurysms; two-thirds are bilateral. Examination of the abdominal aorta is indicated if a popliteal aneurysm is found because one-third are accompanied by aortic dilatation. Popliteal aneurysms present as a swelling behind the knee or with symptoms caused by complications, such as severe ischaemia following thrombosis or distal ischaemia as a result of emboli. The diagnosis is usually confirmed with duplex scanning, but assessment of the distal vessels (with CT, MR or DSA) is important prior to repair if the foot pulses are diminished or absent. An asymptomatic aneurysm should be considered for elective repair to prevent future complications, especially if it exceeds 25 mm in diameter. Some surgeons would also offer elective repair if the sac contained thrombus because this may predispose to distal emboli. Surgery usually involves a medial approach to the above and below knee popliteal arteries, ligation of the aneurysm and restoration of flow to the foot with a bypass graft using saphenous vein. An alternative is a posterior approach and an inlay graft.

In the acute situation, the presentation is usually with a thrombosed aneurysm and an ischaemic foot. Surgery is often unsuccessful because the distal vessels are thrombosed and difficult to clear. Attempts should be made with a Fogarty catheter and intra-arterial thrombolysis. The limb loss rate is high (50 per cent).

Femoral aneurysm

True aneurysm of the femoral artery is uncommon. Complications occur in less than 3 per cent so conservative treatment is generally indicated, but it is important to look for aneurysms elsewhere as over half are associated with abdominal or popliteal aneurysms. Large aneurysms should be repaired. False aneurysm of the femoral artery occurs in 2 per cent of patients after arterial surgery at this site. Local repair may involve reanastomosis of the bypass in the groin under suitable antibiotic cover. However, if infection is the cause, the treatment may involve excision of the infected graft and insertion of a further bypass routed around the infected area. In the latter case, the failure rate is high, and limb loss may be unavoidable. For false aneurysms caused by femoral artery puncture, thrombin injection under ultrasound guidance may be successful and avoids surgery; the alternative is arterial repair and suturing the puncture site in the artery.

Iliac aneurysm

This usually occurs in conjunction with aortic aneurysm and only rarely on its own. On its own, it is difficult to diagnose clinically so about half present already ruptured. Open surgery usually involves an inlay graft, but some iliac aneurysms may be suitable for endovascular repair.

Arteriovenous fistula

Communication between an artery and a vein (or veins) may be either a congenital malformation or the result of trauma. Arteriovenous fistulae for haemodialysis access are also created surgically. All arteriovenous communications have a structural and a physiological effect. The structural effect of arterial blood flow on the veins is characteristic; they become dilated, tortuous and thick walled (arterialised). The physiological effect, if the fistula is big enough, is an increase in cardiac output. In extreme circumstances, this can cause left ventricular enlargement and even cardiac failure.

A pulsatile swelling may be present if the lesion is superficial. A thrill is detected on palpation and auscultation reveals a buzzing continuous bruit ('machinery murmur'). Dilated veins may be seen, in which there is rapid blood flow. Pressure on the artery proximal to the fistula reduces the swelling and the thrill and bruit cease.

Duplex scan and/or angiography confirms the lesion, which is noteworthy for the speed with which venous filling occurs.

Management

Treatment is by embolisation. Excisional surgery can be advocated only rarely, perhaps for severe deformity or recurrent haemorrhage; the assistance of a plastic surgeon is wise. It is important to realise that ligation of a 'feeding' artery on its own is of no lasting value and is actually detrimental as it may preclude treatment by embolisation.

ARTERITIS AND VASOSPASTIC CONDITIONS

Thromboangiitis obliterans (Buerger's disease)

This is characterised by occlusive disease of small- and medium-sized arteries (plantar, tibial, radial, etc.), thrombophlebitis of the superficial or deep veins, and Raynaud's syndrome; it occurs in male smokers, usually under the age of 30 years. Often, only one or two of the three manifestations are present. Histologically, there are inflammatory changes in the walls of arteries and veins, leading to thrombosis. Treatment is total abstinence from smoking, which arrests, but does not reverse, the disease. Established arterial occlusions are treated as for atheromatous disease, but amputations may eventually be required.

Other types of arteritis

Arteritis occurs in association with many connective tissue disorders, e.g. rheumatoid arthritis, systemic lupus erythematosus and polyarteritis nodosa. This is usually the province of the specialist physician, but the surgeon may be called on to carry out minor amputations. Sympathectomy has previously been used, but is usually ineffective.

Temporal arteritis is a disease in which localised infiltration with inflammatory and giant cells leads to arterial occlusion, ischaemic headache and tender, palpable, pulseless (thrombosed) arteries in the scalp. Irreversible blindness occurs if the ophthalmic artery becomes occluded. The surgeon may be required to perform a temporal artery biopsy, but this should not delay immediate steroid therapy to arrest and reverse the process before the ophthalmic artery is involved. The length of the biposy should be at least 1 cm.

Takayasu's disease is an arteritis that obstructs major arteries, particularly the large vessels coming off the aortic arch. It usually pursues a relentless course.

Cystic myxomatous degeneration

This is typified by an accumulation of clear jelly (like a synovial ganglion) in the outer layers of a main artery, especially the popliteal artery. The lesion may narrow the vessel causing claudication. Duplex scan is the investigation of choice. Decompression, by removal of the myxomatous material, is often all that is required, but the 'ganglion' may recur, necessitating excision of part of the artery with interposition vein graft repair.

Raynaud's disease

This idiopathic condition usually occurs in young women and affects the hands more than the feet. There is abnormal sensitivity in the arteriolar response to cold. These vessels constrict and the digits (usually the fingers) turn white and become incapable of fine movements. The capillaries then dilate and fill with slowly flowing deoxygenated blood, resulting in the digits becoming swollen and dusky. As the attack passes off, the arterioles relax, oxygenated blood returns into the dilated capillaries and the digits become red. Thus, the condition is recognised by the characteristic sequence of blanching, dusky cyanosis and red engorgement, often accompanied by pain. Superficial necrosis is very uncommon. This condition must be distinguished from Raynaud's syndrome, which has similar features (see below). Treatment of Raynaud's disease consists of protection from cold and avoidance of pulp and nailbed infection. Calcium antagonists, such as nifedipine, may also have a role to play and electrically heated gloves can be useful in winter. Sympathectomy has been used in the past, but it is either ineffective or its effects are short-lived.

Raynaud's syndrome

Although peripheral vasospasm may be noted in atherosclerosis, thoracic outlet syndrome, carpal tunnel syndrome, etc., the term 'Raynaud's syndrome' is most often used for a peripheral arterial manifestation of a collagen disease, such as systemic lupus erythematosus or rheumatoid arthritis. The clinical features are as for Raynaud's disease, but they may be much more aggressive. Raynaud's syndrome may also follow the use of vibrating tools. In this context, it is a recognised industrial disease and is known as 'vibration white finger'.

Treatment is directed primarily at the underlying condition, although the conservative measures outlined above are often helpful. The syndrome when secondary to collagen disease leads frequently to necrosis of digits and multiple amputations. Sympathectomy yields disappointing results and is not recommended. Nifedipine, steroids and vasospastic antagonists may all have a role in treatment. Patients with vibration white finger should avoid vibrating tools.

Acrocyanosis

Acrocyanosis may be confused with Raynaud's disease, but it is painless and not episodic. It tends to affect young women and the mottled cyanosis of the fingers and/or toes may be accompanied by paraesthesia and chilblains.

Cervical sympathectomy

Open cervical sympathectomy was previously performed for vasospastic conditions affecting the hands and to treat palmar (sometimes axillary) hyperhidrosis. The operation is now obsolete, having been replaced by endoscopic transthoracic sympathectomy. Furthermore, it has been increasingly recognised that the vasospastic conditions do not respond to this form of treatment, rendering the endoscopic intervention a therapy that is suitable solely for hyperhidrosis.

An endoscope, often a rigid cystoscope, is used. The ipsilateral lung may be deflated by the anaesthetist and a cannula inserted into the chest wall to permit easy access for the scope. The sympathetic chain is visualised and a coagulating electrode used to ablate the ganglia below the stellate. The scope and cannula are then removed, the lung inflated and the small chest wound closed.

Lumbar sympathectomy

Lumbar sympathectomy has been used to treat chronic lower limb ischaemia in the past. Lumbar sympathectomy by open operation has, however, been obsolete for several years and even chemical sympathectomy, its minimally invasive equivalent, can now be regarded as outdated. Chemical sympathectomy requires the injection of small quantities of a sclerosant into the lumbar sympathetic chain under radiographic control.

FURTHER READING

Ascher E, Haimovici H (eds). *Haimovici's vascular surgery*, 5th edn. Oxford: Blackwell Publishing, 2003.

Cronenwett J, Johnstone W (eds). *Rutherford's vascular surgery*, 7th edn. Philadelphia, PA: WB Saunders, 2010.

Davies AH, Brophy CM, Lumley J (eds). *Vascular surgery*. Philadelphia, PA: Springer, 2005.

Donnelly R, London NJM (eds). *The ABC of arterial and venous disease*, 2nd edn. Oxford: Wiley-Blackwell, 2009.

Moore WS (ed.). *Vascular and endovascular surgery: a comprehensive review*, 7th edn. Philadelphia, PA: WB Saunders, 2005.

Mikito Takayasu, 1860–1938, Japanese ophthalmologist described this disease in 1908.

CHAPTER

57 Venous disorders

LEARNING OBJECTIVES

To understand:
- Venous anatomy and the physiology of venous return
- The pathophysiology of venous disease
- The clinical significance and management of varicose veins
- Deep venous thrombosis
- Venous insufficiency and venous ulceration

THE ANATOMY OF THE VENOUS SYSTEM OF THE LIMBS

Arterial blood flows through the main axial arteries of the upper and lower limbs before returning via the deep and superficial veins. All of the veins of the upper and lower limbs contain valves, which ensure that blood flows towards the heart.

The superficial venous trunks in the leg are the greater (long) and lesser (short or small) saphenous veins (Figure 57.1a and b), which lie above the muscle fascia of the limb. The cephalic and basilic veins are the superficial venous trunks of the arm (Figure 57.1c and d). Although the long saphenous vein is classically said to join the femoral vein at the saphenofemoral junction, a fixed point in the groin 2.5 cm below and lateral to the pubic tubercle, it is usually encountered somewhat higher. The lesser saphenous vein joins the popliteal vein at the saphenopopliteal junction at a variable site in the popliteal fossa but generally proximally to the knee joint crease. Blood passing up the superficial veins enters the deep veins at the saphenopopliteal and saphenofemoral junctions.

In the calf and thigh there are a number of valved perforating (communicating) veins that join the superficial to the deep veins at inconstant sites and which allow blood to flow from the superficial to the deep venous system. The most important of these are the direct perforating veins of the medial and lateral calf and the communicating veins around the knee and in the mid-thigh.

The deep veins of the lower limb include three pairs of venae commitantes, which accompany the three crural arteries (anterior and posterior tibial and peroneal arteries). These six veins intercommunicate and join in the popliteal fossa to form the popliteal vein, which also receives the soleal and gastrocnemius veins.

The popliteal vein passes up through the adductor hiatus to enter the subsartorial canal as the superficial femoral vein, which receives the deep (profunda) femoral vein (or veins) in the femoral triangle to become the common femoral vein, which then changes its name to the external iliac vein as it passes behind the inguinal ligament. The internal iliac vein joins with the external iliac vein in the pelvis to form the common iliac vein. The left common iliac vein passes behind the right common iliac artery to join the right common iliac vein on the right side of the abdominal aorta to form the inferior vena cava.

VENOUS PATHOPHYSIOLOGY

Blood enters the lower limb through the femoral arteries before passing through arterioles into the capillaries, which have a pressure of about 32 mmHg at their arterial ends. This pressure is reduced along the course of the capillaries and is approximately 12 mmHg at the venular end of the capillary. The pressure continues to fall in the main veins and is as low as −5 mmHg at the upper end of the vena cava where it enters the right atrium.

The venous pressure in a foot vein on standing is equivalent to the height of a column of blood extending from the heart to the foot, e.g. approximately 100 mmHg (Figure 57.2). To enable blood to be returned against gravity in the standing position, an auxiliary pump is required in the lower limb. This is the calf muscle pump, which is augmented to a lesser extent by the thigh and foot pumps. The deep veins of the calf are capacious and are joined by blind-ending sacks called the soleal sinusoids, which force blood into the popliteal and crural veins during calf muscle pump contraction, e.g. walking. The foot pump also ejects blood from the plantar veins during walking. As the calf muscles contract, the veins are compressed and the valves only allow blood to pass in the direction of the heart. The pressure within the calf compartment rises to 200–300 mmHg during muscle contraction. During muscle relaxation the pressure falls and blood from the superficial veins enters the deep veins through the saphenous junctions and the perforating veins. Each time this occurs the pressure falls in the superficial venous compartment until a threshold is reached, when the venous inflow keeps pace with ejection from the deep veins. This is normally around 30 mmHg, a fall of approximately two-thirds of the resting venous pressure. The net reduction in the pressure of the superficial system is dependent on the presence of patent deep veins, perforating veins and superficial veins, which must contain competent valves. Ambulatory venous hypertension is a consequence of

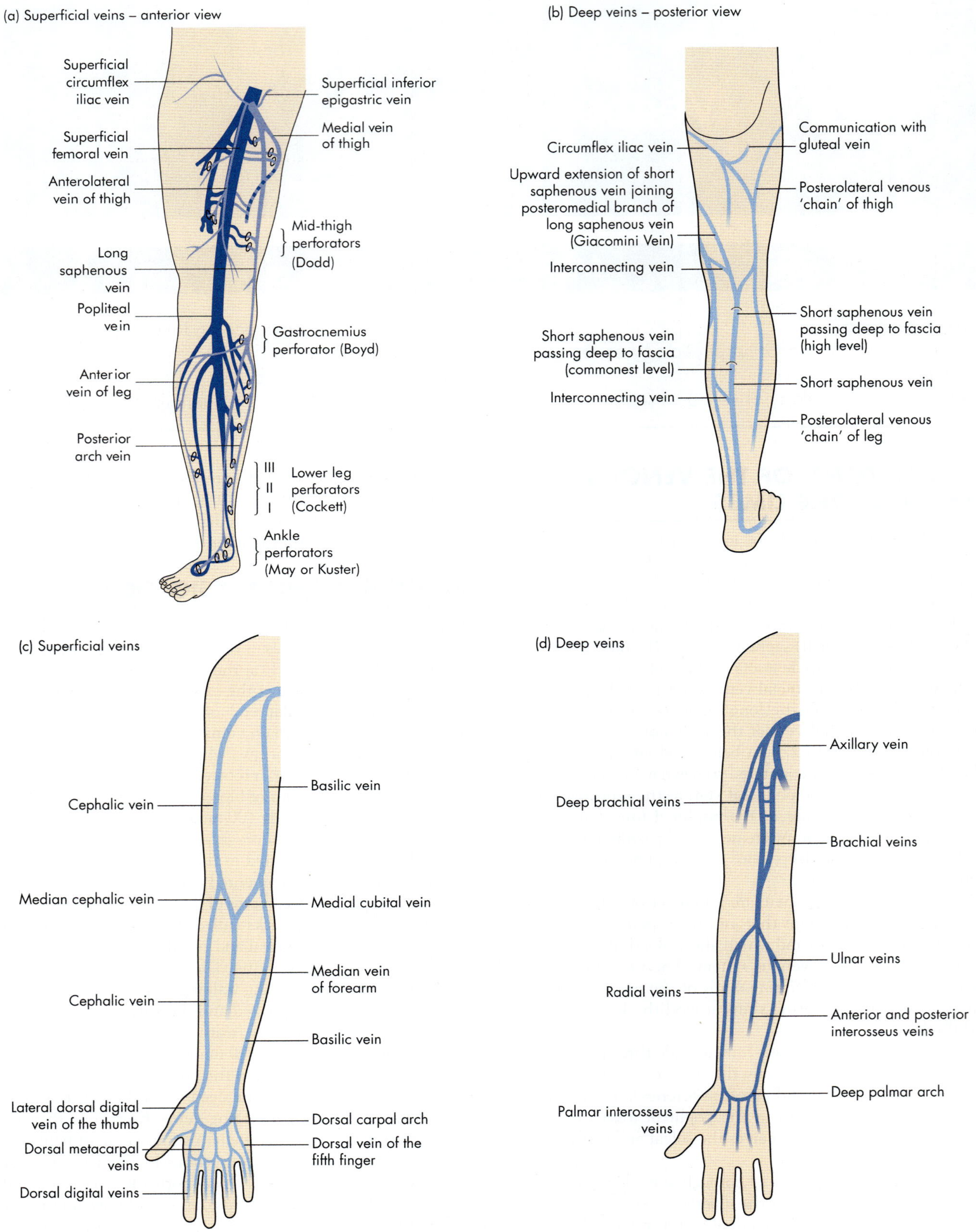

Figure 57.1 (a and b) Anatomy of the superficial and deep veins of the lower limb. (c and d) Anatomy of the superficial and deep veins of the upper limb. The innumerable branch veins and those lying within muscle are omitted. The tibial and peroneal veins of the leg are usually paired veins uniting in their upper parts.

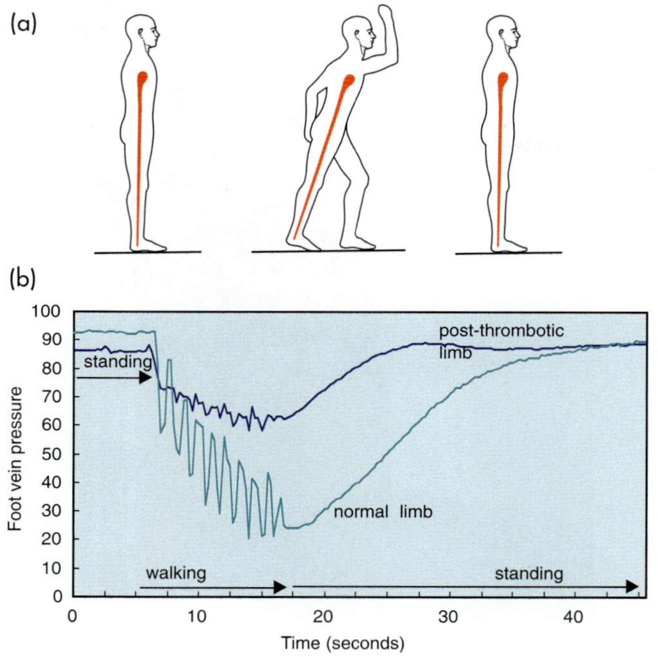

Figure 57.2 (a) Effect of exercise on the superficial venous pressure in health and disease; (b) physiology of the calf muscle pump; pressure traces.

valve failure (reflux) or obstruction in the venous system and may eventually lead to lipodermatosclerosis and ulceration.

The pathophysiology of varicose vein development is probably related to changes in the vein wall (dysfunctional smooth muscle cell proliferation, collagen deposition, decreased elastin content and increased matrix metalloproteinases) leading to venous dilatation and secondary valvular incompetence rather than to a primary valvular defect, which occurs in a small group of patients who have total lack of venous valves. Secondary varicose veins may develop in patients with post-thrombotic limbs and in patients with congenital abnormalities such as the Klippel–Trenaunay syndrome or multiple arteriovenous fistulae.

Simplistically, venous disease can be divided into superficial venous incompetence and deep venous incompetence or a combination of these along with their clinical presentations.

VARICOSE VEINS

Varicose veins are defined as dilated, usually tortuous, subcutaneous veins ≥3 mm in diameter measured in the upright position with demonstrable reflux.

Epidemiology

The adult prevalence of visible varicose veins is 25–30 per cent in women and 15 per cent in men. Factors affecting prevalence include:

- gender: the vast majority of studies report a higher prevalence in women than men, the Edinburgh Vein Study being the main exception;
- age: the prevalence of varicose veins increases with age. In the Edinburgh Vein Study, the prevalence of trunk varicosities in the age groups 18–24 years, 25–34 years, 35–44 years, 45–57 years and 55–64 years was 11.5, 14.6, 28.8, 41.9 and 55.7 per cent, respectively;
- ethnicity: does seem to influence the prevalence of varicose veins;
- body mass and height: increasing body mass index and height may be associated with a higher prevalence of varicose veins;
- pregnancy: appears to increase the risk of varicose veins;
- family history: evidence supports familial susceptibility to varicose veins;
- occupation and lifestyle factors: there is inconclusive evidence regarding increased prevalence of varicose veins in smokers, patients who suffer constipation and occupations which involve prolonged standing.

Klippel and Trenaunay described the condition in 1900. Seven years later, Frederick Parkes-Weber, 1863–1962, an English physician, also described the condition, hence also called Klippel–Trenaunay–Weber syndrome.

Classification

The CEAP (clinical – etiology – anatomy – pathophysiology) classification for chronic venous disorders is widely utilised.

Clinical classification

- C0: no signs of venous disease
- C1: telangectasia or reticular veins
- C2: varicose veins
- C3: oedema
- C4a: pigmentation or eczema
- C4b: lipodermatosclerosis or atrophie blanche
- C5: healed venous ulcer
- C6: active venous ulcer

Each clinical class is further characterised by a subscript depending upon whether the patient is symptomatic (S) or asymptomatic (A) e.g. C2S.

Etiologic classification

- Ec: congenital
- Ep: primary
- Es: secondary (post-thrombotic)
- En: no venous cause identified

Anatomical classification

- As: superficial veins
- Ap: perforator veins
- Ad: deep veins
- An: no venous location identified

Pathophysiological classification

- Pr: reflux
- Po: obstruction
- Pr,o: reflux and obstruction
- Pn: no venous pathophysiology identifiable

Clinical features

Symptoms

Varicose veins frequently cause symptoms, the most common being aching or heaviness, which typically increases throughout the day or with prolonged standing and is relieved by elevation or compression hosiery. Other less common symptoms include ankle swelling and itching while complications (bleeding, superficial thrombophlebitis, eczema,

Maurice Klippel, 1858–1942, neurologist, La Salpêtrière, Paris, France.
Paul Trenaunay, born 1875, a French neurologist.

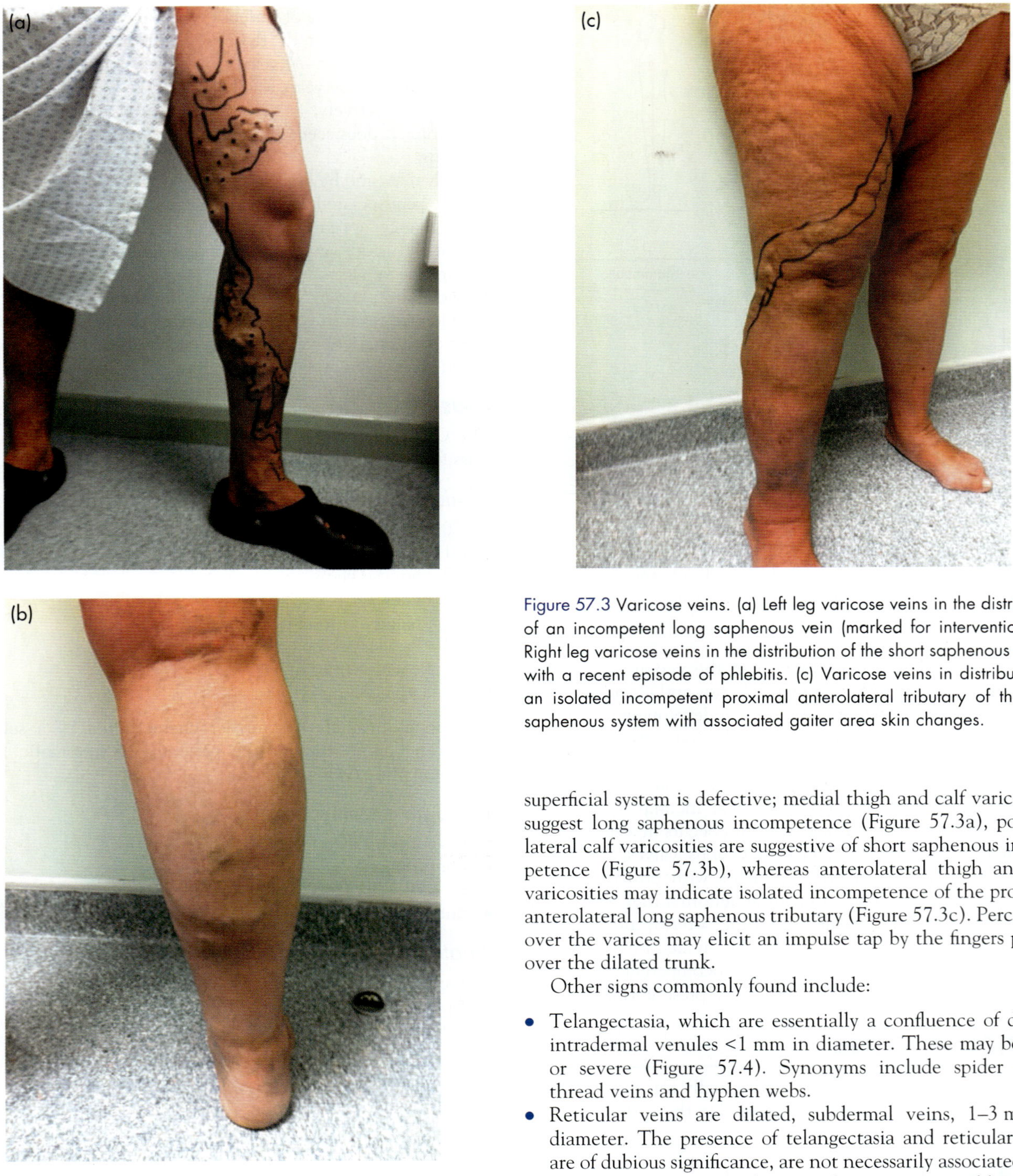

Figure 57.3 Varicose veins. (a) Left leg varicose veins in the distribution of an incompetent long saphenous vein (marked for intervention). (b) Right leg varicose veins in the distribution of the short saphenous system with a recent episode of phlebitis. (c) Varicose veins in distribution of an isolated incompetent proximal anterolateral tributary of the long saphenous system with associated gaiter area skin changes.

lipodermatosclerosis and ulceration) represent important indications for investigation and intervention. The Edinburgh Vein Study failed to show any evidence that the extent of valvular incompetence was related to the severity of symptoms.

Signs

The presence of tortuous dilated subcutaneous veins are usually clinically obvious. These are confined to the long and lesser saphenous systems in approximately 60 and 20 per cent of cases, respectively. The distribution of varicosities may indicate which superficial system is defective; medial thigh and calf varicosities suggest long saphenous incompetence (Figure 57.3a), posterolateral calf varicosities are suggestive of short saphenous incompetence (Figure 57.3b), whereas anterolateral thigh and calf varicosities may indicate isolated incompetence of the proximal anterolateral long saphenous tributary (Figure 57.3c). Percussion over the varices may elicit an impulse tap by the fingers placed over the dilated trunk.

Other signs commonly found include:

- Telangectasia, which are essentially a confluence of dilated intradermal venules <1 mm in diameter. These may be mild or severe (Figure 57.4). Synonyms include spider veins, thread veins and hyphen webs.
- Reticular veins are dilated, subdermal veins, 1–3 mm in diameter. The presence of telangectasia and reticular veins are of dubious significance, are not necessarily associated with major varicose veins and are purely a cosmetic problem.
- In saphena varix (Figure 57.5), there is a large groin varicosity which presents as a (usually painless) lump, emergent when standing and disappearing when recumbent. Gentle palpation over the varix during coughing may elicit a thrill.
- Atrophie blanche (Figure 57.6) is localised white atrophic skin frequently surrounded by dilated capillaries and hyperpigmentation, usually seen around the ankle.
- Corona phlebectasia are fan-shaped patterns of small intradermal veins on the medial or lateral aspects of the ankle or foot. Synonyms include malleolar or ankle flares.

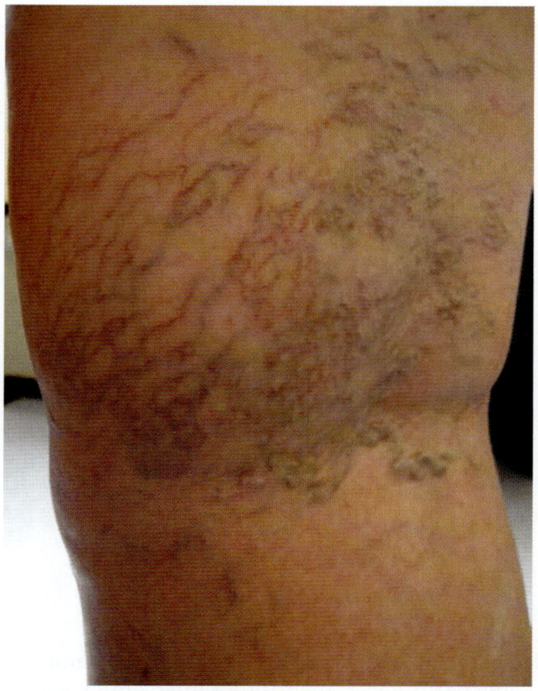
Figure 57.4 Severe telengectasia.

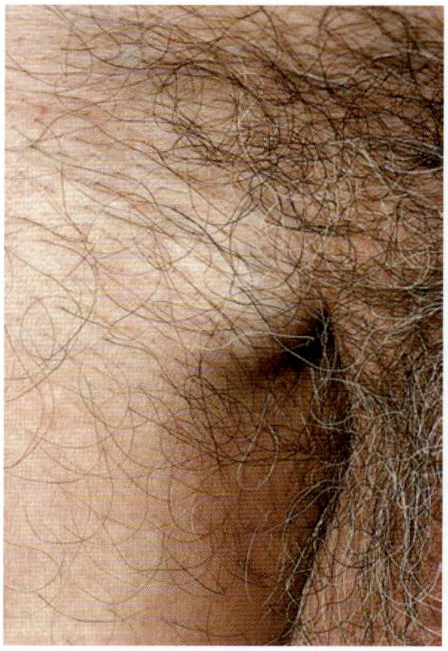
Figure 57.5 A saphena varix.

- Pigmentation (Figure 57.7) is usually a brown discolouration (because of haemosiderin deposition) of the skin, most frequently affecting the gaiter area, and may be associated with phlebitis and ulceration.
- Eczema (Figure 57.8a); this is an erythematous dermatitis which may progress to blistering, weeping or scaling eruption of the skin, not to be confused with contact dermatitis (Figure 57.8b).
- Dependent pitting oedema as a result of increase in volume of fluid in skin and subcutaneous tissue characteristically increases throughout the day, and is relieved by elevation and compression hosiery/bandaging. The oedema is usually confined to the ankle area but may extend to the foot and rest of the leg.

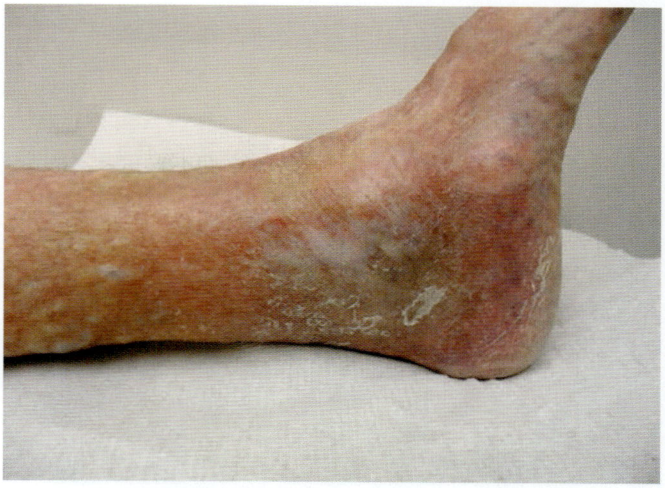
Figure 57.6 Atrophie blanche.

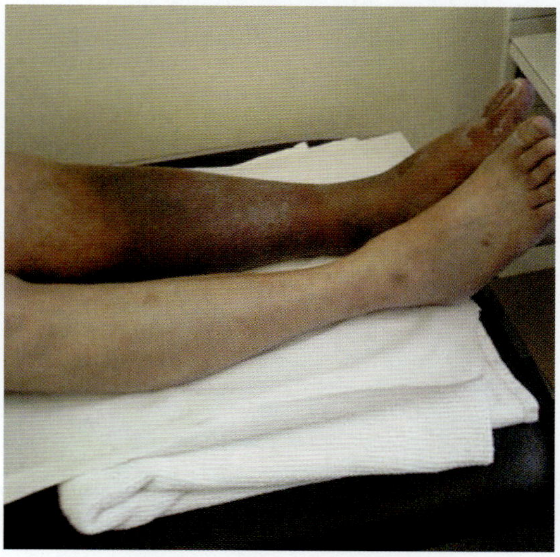
Figure 57.7 Pigmentation: brown discoloration of the skin, most frequently affecting the gaiter area associated with chronic venous insufficiency.

- Lipodermatosclerosis (Figure 57.9) is a localised chronic inflammation and fibrosis of the skin and subcutaneous tissues of the leg, a sign of severe chronic venous disease.
- Ulceration (Figure 57.10) is a full thickness epidermal defect, most frequently affecting the gaiter area.

Investigation

Tourniquet tests have now largely been abandoned. There is good evidence to support the policy of duplex ultrasound scanning for all patients with varicose veins prior to any intervention. This policy facilitates a more accurate surgical approach, reduces the incidence of varicose vein recurrence, and allows assessment regarding suitability for endovenous intervention. Clinical acumen combined with continuous wave hand-held Doppler examination will miss up to 30 per cent of important connections between superficial and deep veins and information

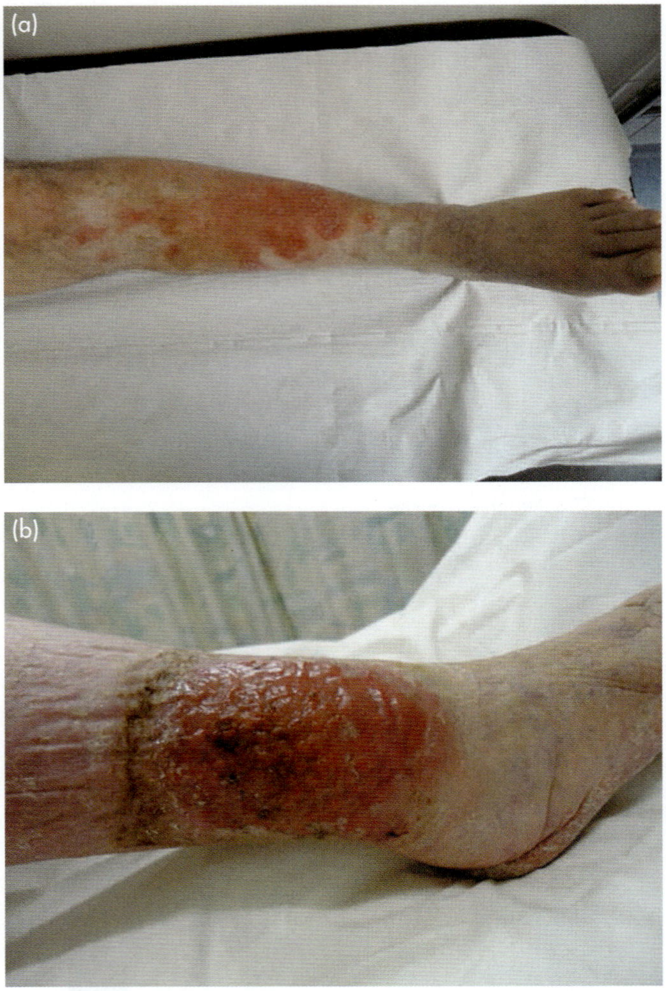

Figure 57.8 Excema. (a) Erythematous dermatitis; (b) contact dermatitis.

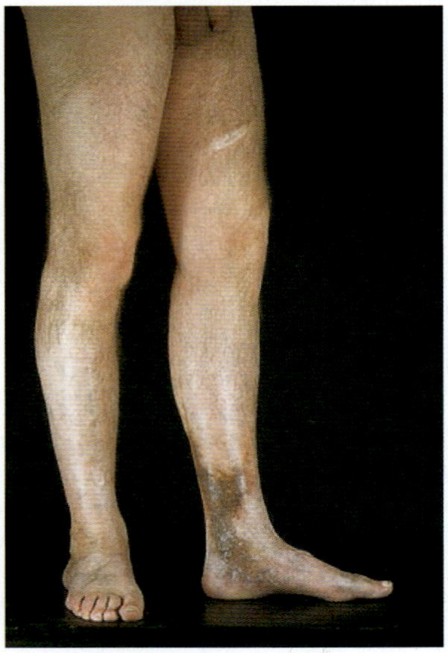

Figure 57.9 Lipodermatosclerosis of the calf skin.

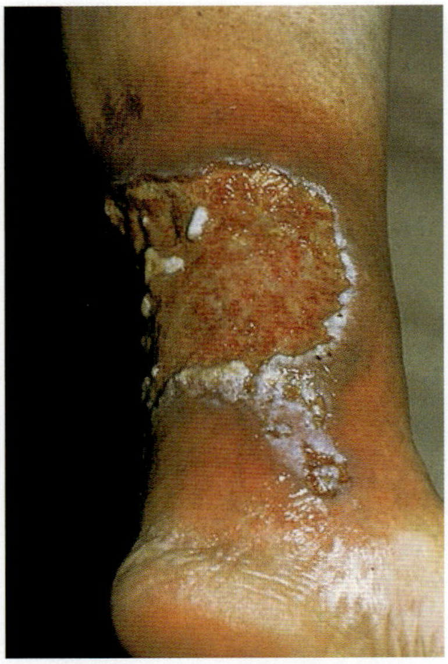

Figure 57.10 A venous ulcer.

on affected veins when compared to duplex scanning; thus, it should only be utilised as the basis for intervention when duplex scanning is not available.

Hand-held continuous wave Doppler emits a sound when blood flows past the transmitting and receiving crystals. A uniphasic signal indicates flow in one direction. Forward and reverse flow produces a biphasic signal which is indicative of blood refluxing through incompetent valves. A biphasic signal following a calf squeeze performed with the Doppler probe over the saphenofemoral junction suggests the presence of junctional incompetence. A biphasic signal over the saphenopopliteal junction or lesser saphenous vein is not an accurate method of establishing incompetence of the lesser saphenous vein as its termination is variable and it is difficult to separate lesser saphenous incompetence from popliteal valvular incompetence. In all cases of biphasic lesser saphenous signal a duplex scan should be performed.

Duplex ultrasound imaging

Duplex ultrasound imaging has become the main stay of investigation for varicose veins. A high-frequency linear array transducer of 7.5–13 MHz is appropriate for the majority of lower limbs in order to obtain good quality images. The B mode settings (depth, focal zone, overall gain and dynamic gain) should be optimised to ensure the area of interest is in the centre and occupies the majority of the image, and that the lumen of the vein appears as a dark void in the subcutaneous and deep tissues. The pulsed wave spectral or colour Doppler settings should be optimised for the low flow velocities encountered within veins. It is conventional to use blue to represent antegrade venous flow towards the heart and red for the reverse. Visible venous flow can be augmented by a calf squeeze.

The aim of the duplex scan in patients with varicose veins is to establish:

- which saphenous junctions are incompetent and their locations;
- the extent of reflux in the saphenous veins and their diameters;
- the number, location and diameter of incompetent perforating veins;

- other relevant veins that demonstrate reflux;
- the source of all superficial varices if not from the veins already described;
- the competence and evidence of previous venous thrombosis in the deep venous system.

In order to standardise measurements of venous diameter and reflux, it is recommended that examination of the superficial veins is performed with the patient standing. Venous reflux is defined as retrograde flow in the reverse direction to physiological flow lasting for more than 0.5 seconds. Reflux may be elicited by release of a calf or foot squeeze for proximal or calf varicosities respectively, manual compression over varicosity clusters, pneumatic calf cuff deflation, active foot dorsiflexion and relaxation or the Vasalva manoeuvre.

The patient should stand facing towards the examiner with the leg rotated outwards, heel on the ground and weight on the opposite limb (Figure 57.11). The scan should begin in the groin, using a transverse view to identify the long saphenous vein and common femoral vein lying medial to the common femoral artery (the 'Micky Mouse' sign – Figure 57.12). Saphenofemoral junction (SFJ) competence is assessed in the transverse view and potential destinations for reflux including the greater or long saphenous vein (LSV), the accessory anterior saphenous vein and other major thigh tributaries superficial to the saphenous fascia are noted. The full length of the LSV within its fascial compartment, known as the 'saphenous eye', should be examined (Figure 57.13), and its diameter measured just below the SFJ, mid-thigh, above and below the knee joint, mid-calf and ankle. The groin is next examined for reflux in the longitudinal plane in the common femoral vein, superficial femoral vein and SFJ using spectral and/or colour Doppler (Figure 57.14). The presence and competence of thigh and calf perforators should be noted. For examination of the lesser or short saphenous vein (SSV) and posterior thigh extension of the SSV (Giacomini vein), the patient is positioned facing away, knee slightly flexed, heel on the ground and the weight taken on the opposite leg. If the saphenopopliteal junction (SPJ) is incompetent, the level of the SPJ in relation to the knee crease and whether the SSV joins the popliteal vein posteriorly, medially or laterally is noted. In the transverse view, the SSV vein is followed distally, checking its competence and diameter in the proximal, mid and distal

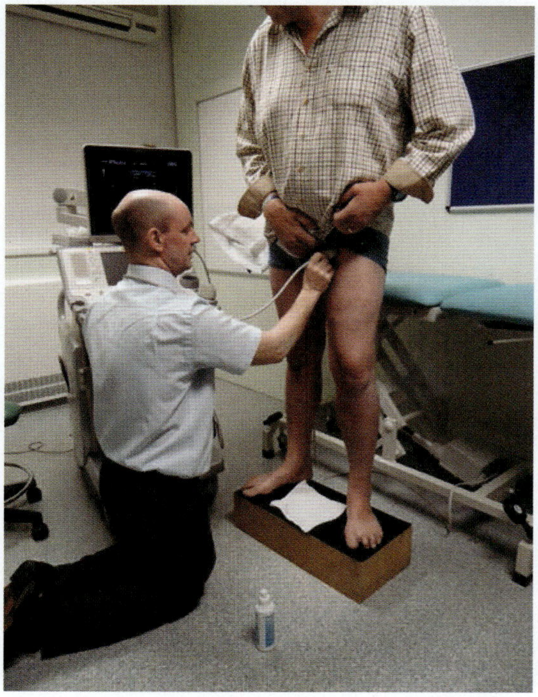

Figure 57.11 Patient position for venous duplex examination of the long saphenous system.

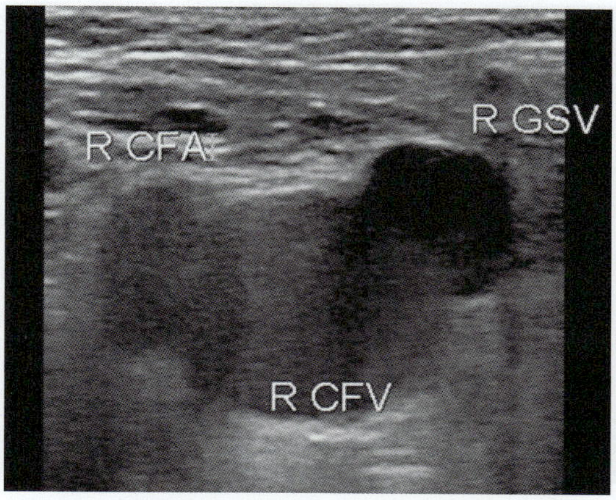

Figure 57.12 'Micky Mouse' transverse B mode image of right common femoral vein (R CFV) and right common femoral artery (R CFA) and greater saphenous vein (GSV) at the saphenofemoral junction (SFJ).

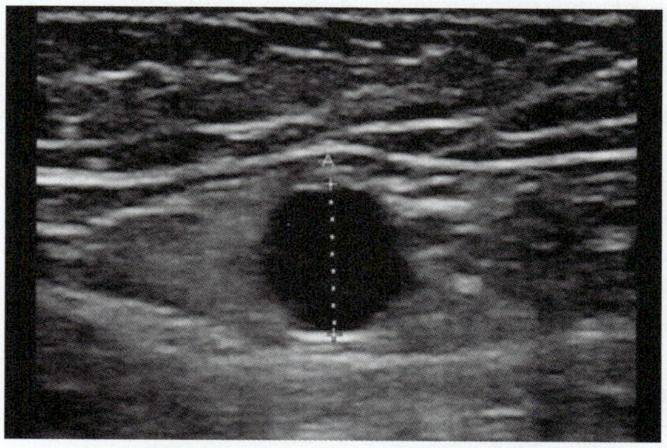

Figure 57.13 'Saphenous eye' transverse B mode view of long saphenous vein in fascial compartments of the thigh.

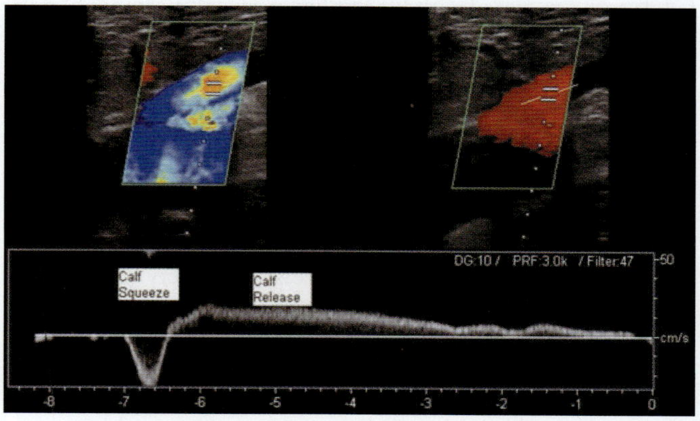

Figure 57.14 Duplex scan of the saphenofemoral junction showing antegrade and retrograde flow.

Antonio Maria Valsalva, 1666–1723, Professor of Anatomy, Bologna, Italy.

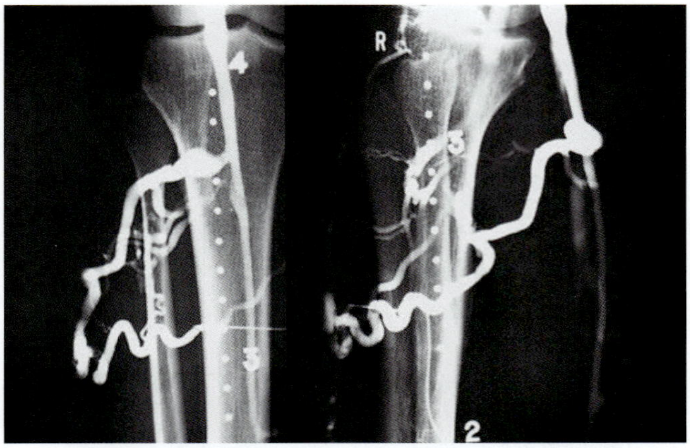

Figure 57.15 Varicogram.

calf. Finally, the patency and competence of the popliteal vein is assessed.

Very occasionally, investigations other than duplex are required, usually when duplex demonstrates reflux in superficial varicosities but fails to identify any site of junctional incompetence. Varicography involves injection of contrast directly into superficial varices which allows detailed mapping of the varices to their termination. This can be useful in patients with recurrent varicose veins or with complex anatomy (Figure 57.15). Descending intravenous venography where contrast is injected via the deep veins or magnetic resonance venography is useful when lower limb varicosities appear to arise from pelvic vein incompetence.

Management

Patients who have asymptomatic varicose veins can simply be reassured. Indications for referral to a vascular surgeon include C2 disease associated with bleeding, superficial thrombophlebitis or symptoms which are impairing quality of life, or C3–6 disease.

Compression hosiery

Compression hosiery relies on graduated external pressure to improve deep venous return. Compression hosiery can be knee length or thigh length; there is no evidence which length of stocking is more effective and hence below-knee stockings are usually prescribed as they are easier to don and have much better patient acceptance. Compression hosiery is classified according to the pressure exerted, and the British classification class 1 stockings exert pressure of 14–17 mmHg, class 2 exert 18–24 mmHg and class 3 exert 25–35 mmHg. Compression hosiery significantly improves varicose vein symptoms but is not popular with patients with compliance rates and long-term tolerance being universally poor. There is no evidence to suggest that compression hosiery prevents the occurrence or progression of varicose veins. Finally, the incorrect application of compression hosiery can have serious consequences (pressure necrosis, tourniquet effects); thus assessment, prescription and application of compression hosiery should be limited to those with the appropriate skills and training.

Ultrasound-guided foam sclerotherapy

Ultrasound-guided foam sclerotherapy involves the injection of detergent directly into the superficial veins. The most commonly used (and only sclerosant recognised for treatment in the UK) is sodium tetradecyl sulphate although others are available on a named patient basis. The detergent destroys the lipid membranes of endothelial cells causing them to shed, leading to thrombosis, fibrosis and obliteration (sclerosis). The procedure commences with the patient standing, and the sites of venous cannulation are selected and marked using ultrasound. Then, with the patient supine, the major venous trunks and superficial varicosities to be treated are all cannulated using ultrasound guidence (Figure 57.16). This is performed before injection as the injection quickly spreads through the superficial varicosities making further cannulation difficult. Once all injection sites are cannulated the injection can be prepared. The most widely used method is that of Tessari, which utilises two syringes connected using a three-way tap. A 1:3 or 1:4 ratio mixture of sclerosant and air is drawn into one syringe, and is then oscillated vigorously between the two syringes about 10 or 20 times (Figure 57.17). The foam produced in this way is stable for about 2 minutes so it

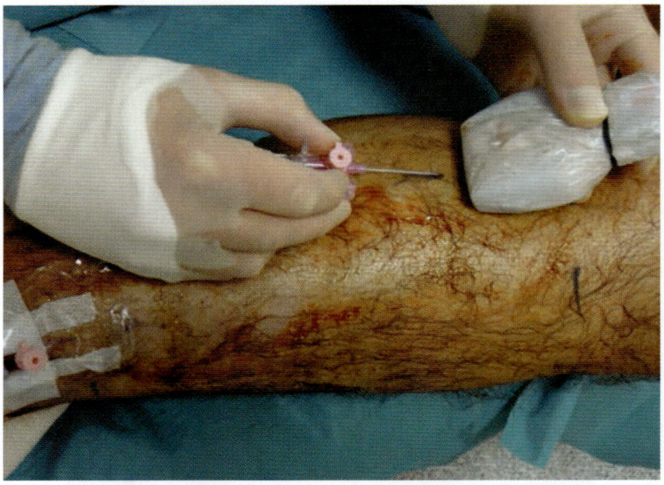

Figure 57.16 Foam sclerotherapy; cannulation of varicosities for ultrasound-guided foam sclerotherapy.

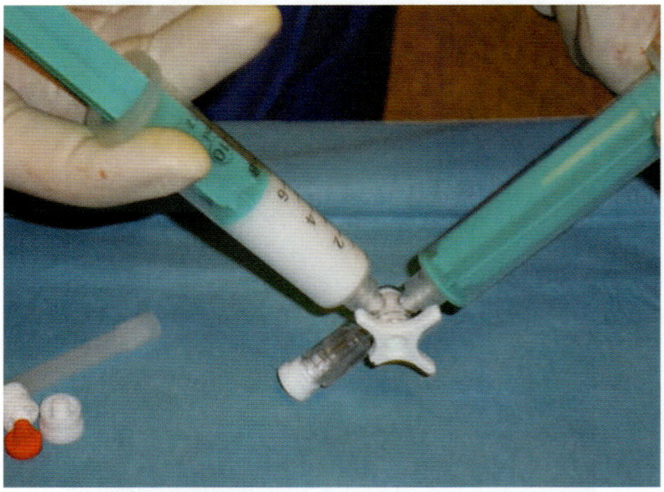

Figure 57.17 Foam sclerotherapy; Tessari method of foam sclerosant preparation.

Carlo Giacomini, 1840–1898, anatomist, Turin, Italy, on his death left his skeleton to the Anatomical Museum in Turin.
Lorenzo Tessari, born 1949, an Italian physician.
William George Fegan, 1921–2007, Emeritus Profesor of Surgery, Trinity College, Dublin, Ireland.

should be injected as soon as it has been made. The leg is then elevated to empty the veins of blood, and injection of foam commences first with superficial varicosities and ends with injection of the LSV or SSV. Only 1 or 2 mL of foam should be injected at a time and the distribution of the foam should be monitored and massaged with the ultrasound probe. When the foam is visualised at the site of junctional incompetence no further foam should be injected. The maximum volume of foam which should be injected at a single session should not exceed 10–12 mL as the incidence of complications are directly related to the volume of foam injected. Compression bandaging or hosiery is then applied and left *in situ* for 7–10 days. Sclerotherapy improves varicose vein-related symptoms, but recurrence rates and the need for reintervention are relatively high. Foam is superior to liquid sclerotherapy, as popularised by George Fegan, in achieving LSV obliteration at two years. Some complications (phlebitis, pigmentation, headache, visual disturbance, chest tightness, cough) are relatively common. There is no robust randomised controlled trial data to influence choice of sclerosant, local pressure dressings, or duration of postsclerotherapy compression. Short-term bandaging is better tolerated than more prolonged bandaging.

Endovenous laser ablation

Endovenous laser ablation (EVLA) as a treatment for varicose veins was first described in 2001, and involves the insertion of a laser fibre into the lumen of an incompetent truncal vein, with subsequent thermal ablation of the vein. The vast majority of patients with primary and recurrent varicose veins are suitable for EVLA, with success reported in treating the long, short and anterior saphenous veins, perforators and varicosities themselves. The factors which may preclude EVLA pertain to either the patient (unsuitable for local anaesthesia, e.g. needle phobia) or the vein (excess tortuosity, thrombophlebitis).

The procedure begins with ultrasound-guided marking of the truncal vein to be treated and the site of proposed cannulation. The varicosities are also marked at this stage if concomitant treatment (phlebectomy, foam sclerotherpy) is to be undertaken. The patient is then positioned on the procedure couch in the reverse Trendelenburg position. For the LSV, the patient is supine with the hip of the leg to be treated externally rotated and slightly flexed. A pillow under the contralateral hip/lower back may improve patient comfort. For the SSV, the patient is positioned in the prone position. The vein is then cannulated percutaneously under ultrasound guidance, at the lowest point of reflux. A wire is then passed through the needle into the superficial vein through the site of junctional incompetence into the deep vein. The catheter is then passed over the wire and positioned within 1 cm of the site of junctional incompetence. Accurate positioning of the catheter tip (and thus the laser fibre tip) with ultrasound is crucial (Figure 57.18). Following the administration of perivenous tumescent anaesthesia (Figure 57.19a and b), the laser fibre is introduced into the catheter (Figure 57.20), passed to the catheter tip and laser energy is used to ablate the vein.

The tumescent anaesthesia during EVLA provides analgesia and compresses the vein, increasing the contact area between the vein wall and laser fibre. It also protects adjacent structures (skin, nerves) by causing hydrodissection and acting as a heat sink. Dilute lidocaine with adrenaline and bicarbonate warmed to body temperature is recommended. It is important not to exceed the recommended dose.

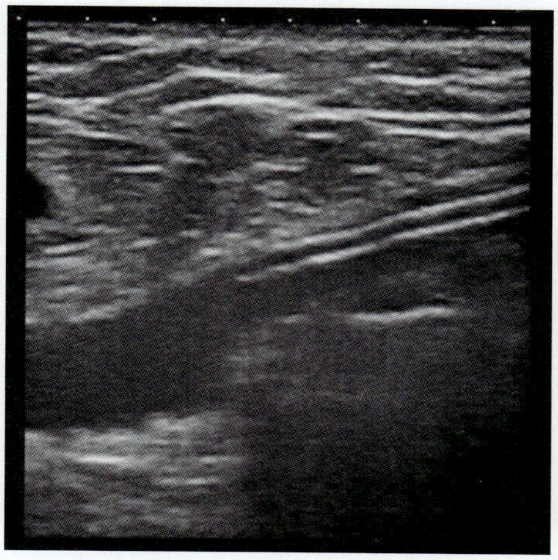

Figure 57.18 Endovenous laser ablation. B mode image of catheter tip positioning at saphenofemoral junction.

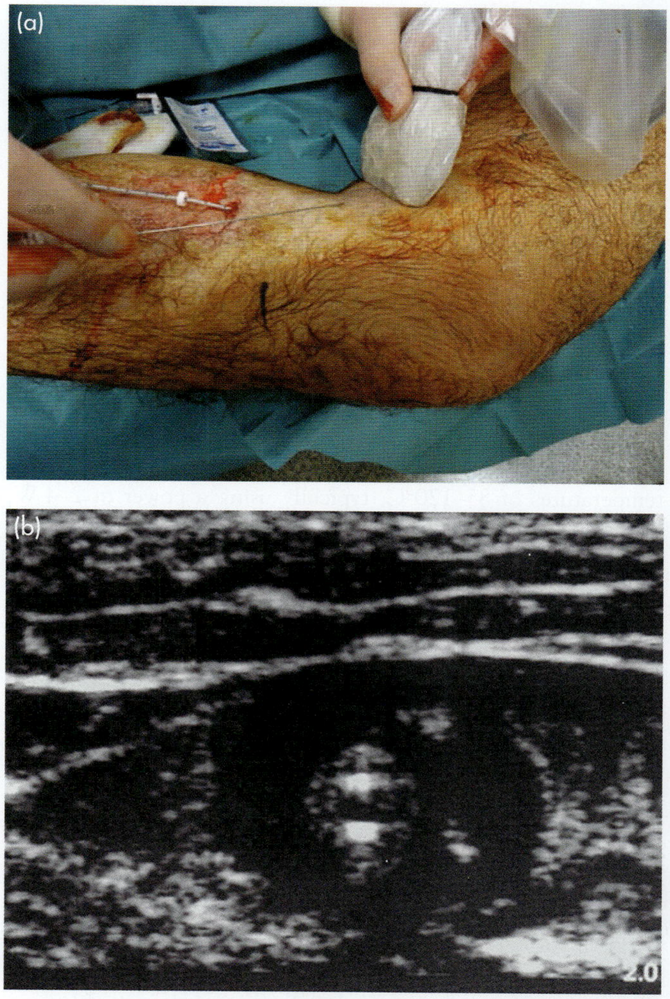

Figure 57.19 Endovenous laser ablation. (a) Ultrasound-guided infiltration of perivenous tumescent anaesthetic. (b) Ultrasound image of perivenous halo of anaesthetic infiltration.

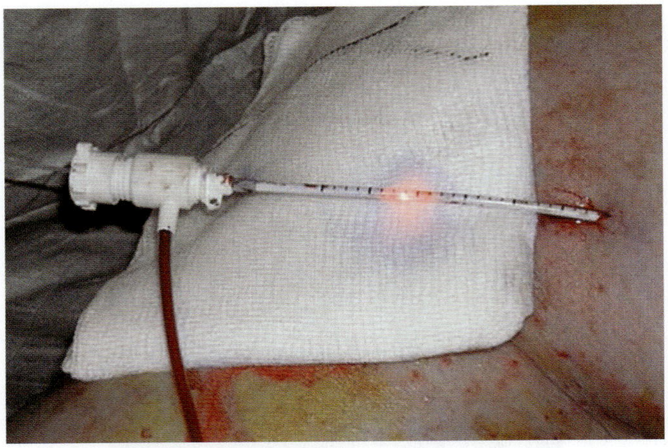

Figure 57.20 Endovenous laser ablation fibre introduced through catheter.

As EVLA treats only junctional and truncal incompetence, debate exists regarding the management of varicosities. These can be managed concomitantly or sequentially by either phlebectomy or sclerotherapy. Concomitant phlebectomies (Figure 57.21) result in a more rapid improvement in disease-specific quality of life, and allow the vast majority of patients to complete treatment in a single visit. Compression and analgesia are usually recommended in the early postoperative period.

Radiofrequency ablation

Radiofrequency ablation (RFA) is a minimally invasive endovascular therapy that uses a bipolar catheter to generate thermal energy to ablate the vein. Preoperative planning and consent, patient positioning, tumescent anaesthesia administration and postoperative management are identical to EVLA. The main differences include vein cannulation and method of ablation. The vein to be treated is cannulated with a 7FG sheath using ultrasound guidance and the catheter is introduced through the sheath and the catheter tip positioned not within 2 cm of the incompetent junction (Figure 57.22). The catheter generates temperatures of 85–120°C, typically using a power of 2–4 W,

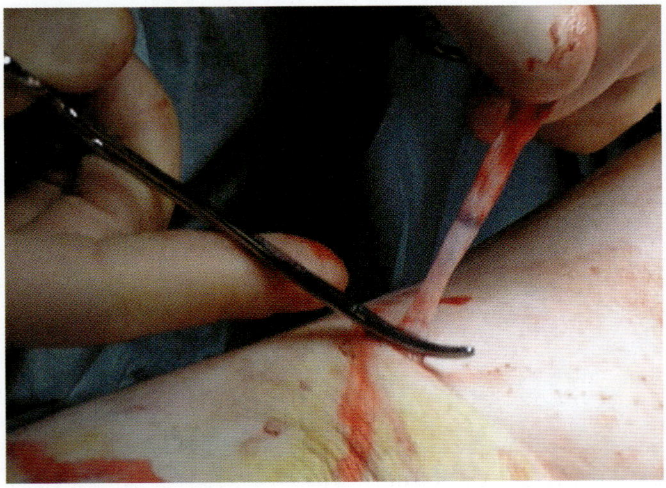

Figure 57.21 Phlebectomies performed under tumescent anaesthesia following endovenous thermal ablation.

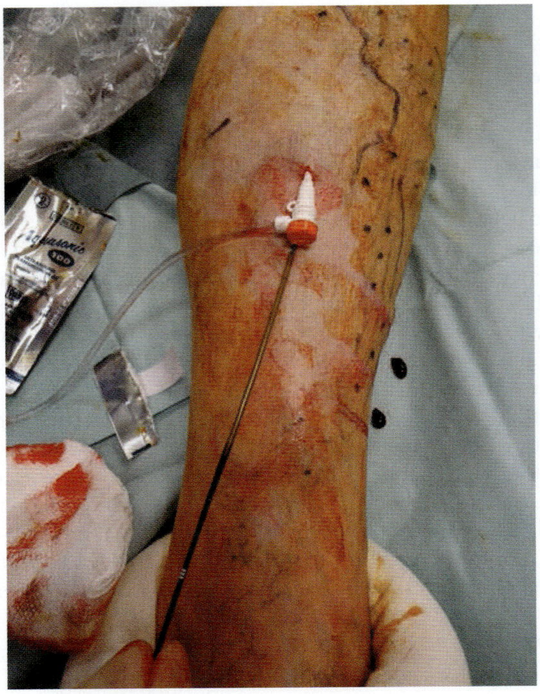

Figure 57.22 Radiofrequency ablation – introducing catheter through sheath.

to ablate the vein. The thermal energy can be applied continuously using a continuous pull-back technique or sequentially over 7-cm segments depending on the RFA catheter of choice. Recent trials comparing RFA and EVLA suggest the former may be associated with less pain and bruising.

The incidence of complications following endovenous interventions are low but include thromboembolic complications (<1 per cent), phlebitis (<5 per cent – reduced with non-steroidal anti-inflammatory drugs (NSAIDs) and skin burns (<2 per cent – the majority occurring in patients not given tumescence).

Surgery

The principles of the operation are to ligate the point of junctional incompetence and to remove the refluxing trunk and dilated tributaries. Preoperatively, a careful consent is taken, explaining the risks of infection, minor nerve injury and recurrence, and the varicose veins must be tramlined using an indelible marker pen to enable accurate identification varicosities during surgery. The operation is usually performed under general anaesthesia but locoregional anaesthesia is possible.

Saphenofemoral ligation and long saphenous stripping

An oblique groin incision is made at the level of and lateral to the pubic tubercle. The long saphenous vein is identified and dissected to the SFJ, which should be clearly established before the vein is divided to avoid disasters (Figure 57.23). Six LSV tributaries are normally encountered close to the SFJ, the superficial inferior epigastric vein and superficial circumflex iliac vein laterally, the deep and superficial external pudendal veins medially, and usually more distally the anterolateral and posteriomedial thigh veins, which should be ligated and divided. A flush SFJ ligation is then peformed and the LSV retrogradely

William Wayne Babcock, 1872–1963, Professor of Surgery, Temple University Medical College, Philadelphia, PA, USA.
Karl Ritter von Edenberg Langer, 1819–1887, Professor of Anatomy, Vienna, Austria described these lines in 1862.

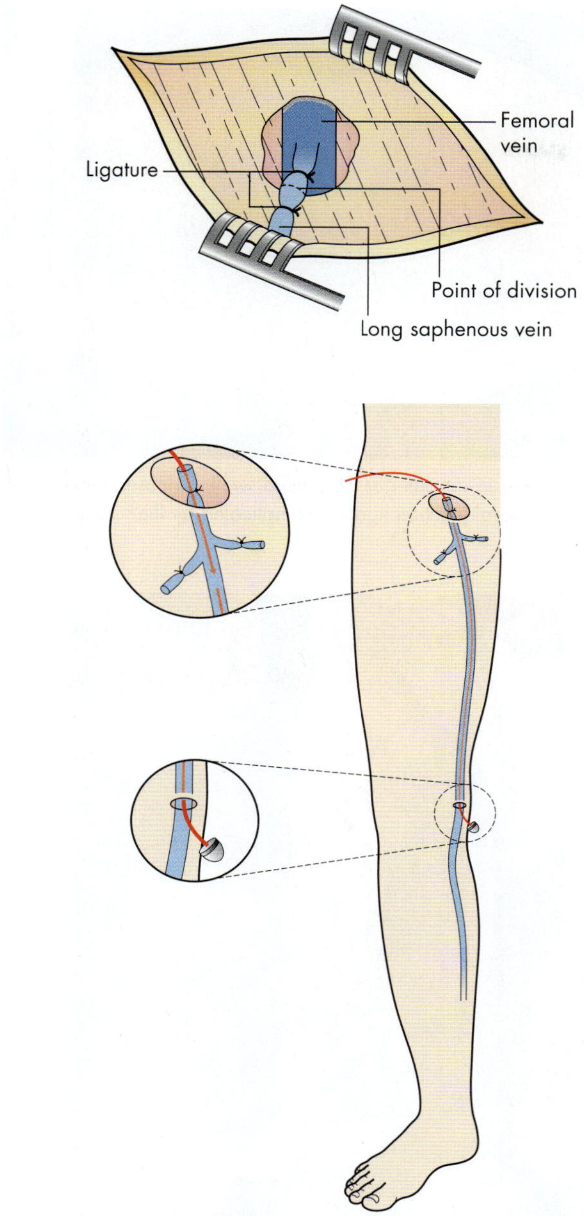

Figure 57.23 Saphenofemoral junction ligation and stripping.

stripped to the knee. The tributary varicosities should then be avulsed through small incision along Langer's lines, using small hooks or mosquito forceps. Closure of the cribriform fascia, with sutures or synthetic patches, over the ligated SFJ, has not been demonstrated to reduce groin recurrence. Stripping the LSV reduces the rate of reintervention for recurrent varicose veins, but it should only be stripped to knee level, as stripping to the ankle does not improve symptomatic relief, but significantly increases the risk of saphenous nerve injury.

Saphenopopliteal junction ligation and lesser saphenous stripping

Preoperative duplex to mark the position of the SPJ is highly recommended (Figure 57.24). The patient is positioned in the prone position, a transverse incision is made over the premarked

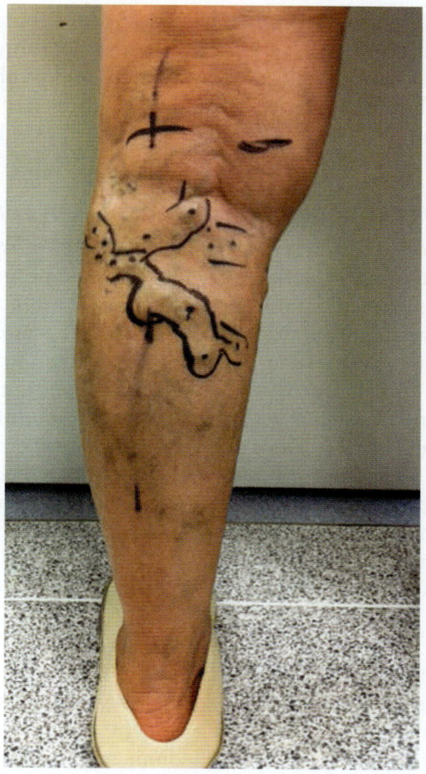

Figure 57.24 Preoperative marking of saphenopopliteal junction and short saphenous vein mapped using duplex scanning.

SPJ, the fascia is divided and the SSV is exposed. The SPJ can then be formally dissected with a flush ligation or the SSV can be gently retracted and ligated as proximally as possible. No good evidence exists to favour one technique over the other, but proponents of the flush ligation would argue that it avoids leaving a stump of SSV, a common source of recurrence, while proponents of the simple SSV ligation technique argue it reduces the incidence of the most common serious complications, nerve injury and popliteal vein injury. The SSV can then either be stripped or the proximal section of the vein can be resected. Those who strip argue it reduces the incidence of recurrence while opponents feel it increases the incidence of sural nerve injury. There are no randomised trials comparing these techniques.

Perforator ligation

The majority of studies assessing the role of perforator ligation have been in patients with venous ulcers analysing the effects on ulcer healing, and even in this situation randomised controlled data are lacking. The role of perforator ligation in patients with uncomplicated varicose veins is even less clear. The traditional procedure described by Linton and Cockett has fallen out of favour due to the associated high incidence of wound complications. In uncomplicated varicose veins, perforators may be ligated through a small, duplex-guided incision, while in patients with skin changes, subfascial endoscopic perforator ligation may be preferred, although the benefits are unproven.

Phlebectomies

These may be performed following treatment of junctional incompetence and axial vein reflux or as sole treatment under local anaesthetic in patients with isolated tributary incompetence. Phlebectomies are usually performed through small stab incisions using small mosquito forceps and/or phlebectomy hooks which have been demonstrated to be superior in terms of bruising, pain and generic quality of life than transilluminated-powered phlebectomy (TIPP).

Complications of standard varicose vein surgery

Complications (minor and major) are reported in up to 20 per cent of patients who undergo traditional varicose vein surgery. Wound infections, the most common complication, are reduced by prophylactic antibiotics. Nerve injury is the most common serious complication. The incidence of saphenous nerve neuralgia is up to 7 per cent following LSV stripping to the knee (the incidence is higher with stripping to the ankle). The incidence of sural nerve neuropraxia and common peroneal nerve injury may be as high as 20 and 4 per cent, respectively, following SSV surgery. The incidence of venous thromboembolic complications is approximately 0.5 per cent following varicose vein surgery, however patient risk factors must be individually assessed and appropriate prophylaxis administered according to guidelines.

Comparison of interventions

Endovenous and traditional surgery for varicose veins appear equally beneficial in improving generic and disease-specific quality of life in the short to medium term. However in the early postoperative period, traditional surgery is associated with higher pain scores and analgesic requirement, and more severe disability in terms of physical, social and psychological quality of life although the clinical significance of this is unclear. Thus endovenous interventions, by minimising the immediate postoperative quality of life impairment, result in a more rapid return to work and normal activities. Adequately powered, long-term comparisons of recurrence rates following surgery and endovenous interventions are awaited.

Recurrent varicose veins

Approximately 10–20 per cent of patients who present to hospital with varicose veins have had previous intervention. Prospective data on long-term results following intervention for recurrent varicose veins are sparse and the criteria for defining recurrence are variable.

Significant clinical recurrence five to ten years following varicose vein surgery occurs in 10–35 per cent of patients, but minor/duplex detected recurrence is much more common being in the order of 70 per cent. Causes of recurrence are controversial but include: neo-revascularisation; reflux in residual axial vein; inadequate initial surgery; and new junctional reflux. Recurrence is more common following short than long saphenous vein surgery and in patients with high BMI (body mass index), while stripping of the incompetent axial vein reduces recurrence rates. Limited data suggest recurrence rates following endovenous thermal ablation may be lower and of different aetiology (axial vein recannalisation) than following surgery. Recurrent varicose veins often have an atypical distribution and duplex assessment is mandatory (Figures 57.25 and 57.26). Surgery for recurrent varicose veins is associated with a high (40 per cent) complication rate, the most common being lymph leak and wound infection, thus endovenous interventions would seem to offer an attractive alternative, where feasible.

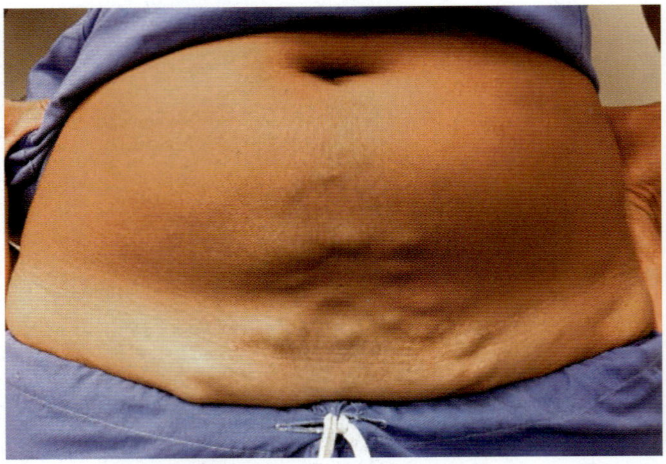

Figure 57.25 Recurrent anterior abdominal wall varicose veins following saphenofemoral junction ligation complicated by iliac deep venous thrombosis.

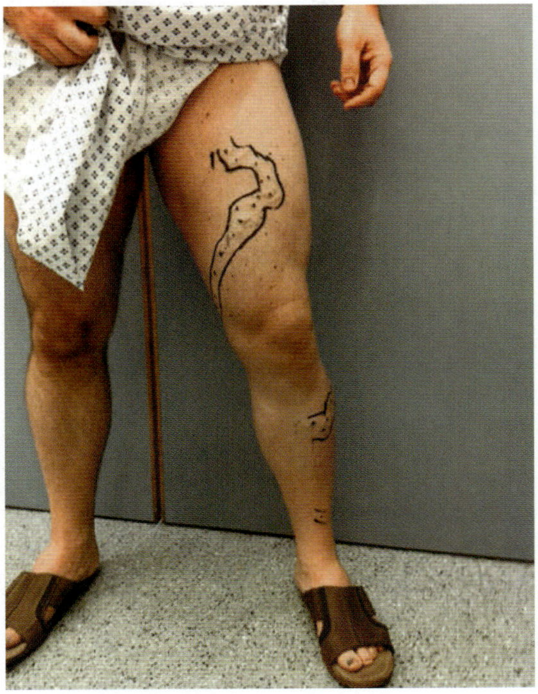

Figure 57.26 Recurrent varicose veins secondary to an incompetent thigh perforator.

Pelvic congestion syndrome

Pelvic congestion syndrome (PCS) is among the differential diagnoses to be considered in female patients presenting with chronic pelvic pain. PCS sufferers are typically premenopausal, multiparous women aged 20–45 years, who present with severe dull aching pelvic pain thought to be the direct result of ovarian and pelvic varicosities. The pain is usually non-cyclical, and may be precipitated by prolonged standing. Other symptoms include dysmenorrhoea, menorrhagia, rectal discomfort or urinary frequency. Signs may include tenderness over the uterus/ovaries, vulval varicosities and haemorrhoids. There may be vulval and

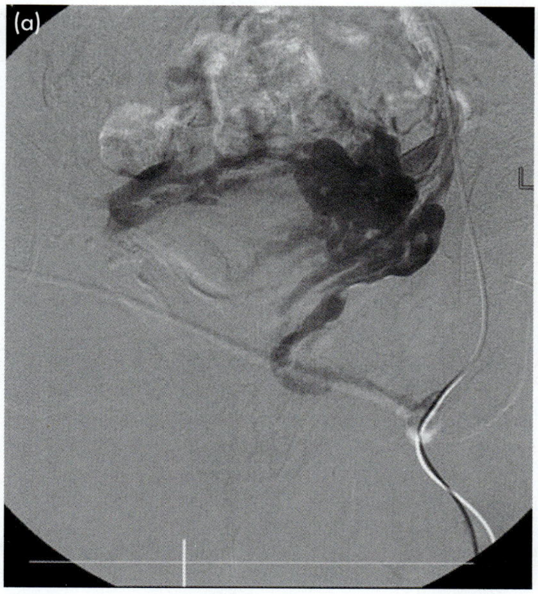

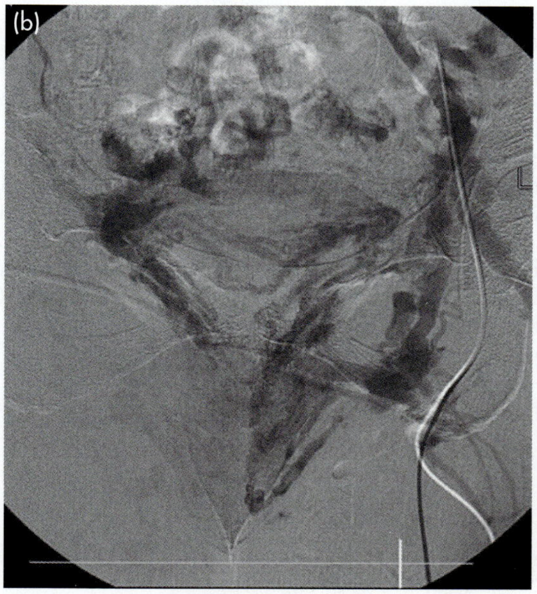

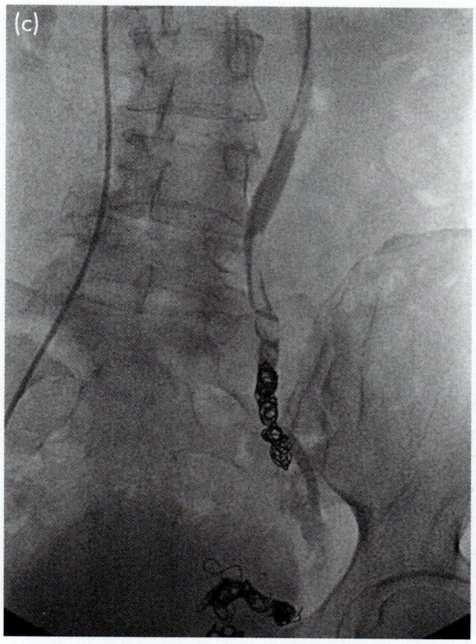

Figure 57.27 (a–c) Left ovarian vein incompetence supplying pelvic and pudendal varicosities (diagnostic venogram and therapeutic embolisation).

atypically distributed thigh varicosities. The road to a diagnosis of PCS is often a long and laborious one, usually only made following extensive investigations to exclude other more common causes of pelvic pain. Abdominal, pelvic and transvaginal duplex examinations allow dynamic visualisation of pelvic blood flow and should be the initial investigations of choice, as they are rapid, readily accessible outpatient procedures which are also valuable in excluding other pathologies. However, the sensitivity for PCS of magnetic resonance venography or diagnostic venography is superior.

Medical treatments for PCS include psychotherapy, progestins, danazol, gonadotrophin receptor agonists (GnRH) with hormone replacement therapy, and NSAIDs. Historical open surgical procedures (extraperitoneal resection of ovarian veins) have now largely been superceded by percutaneous pelvic vein embolisation (Figure 57.27c), reducing peri- and postprocedural morbidity while maintaining high success rates.

VENOUS THROMBOSIS

Venous thrombosis is the formation of a semi-solid coagulum within the venous system and may occur in the superficial system (usually described as superficial thrombophlebitis) or the deep system (deep venous thrombosis or DVT). Venous thrombosis of the deep veins of the leg may be complicated by the immediate risk of pulmonary embolus and sudden death. Subsequently, patients are at risk of developing a post-thrombotic limb (Figure 57.28) and venous ulceration. While DVT may occur in the upper limb, it is the leg that gives rise to the vast majority of the morbidity and subsequent complications of this condition.

Aetiology

The three factors described by Virchow over a century ago are still relevant in the development of venous thrombosis. These are:

- changes in the vessel wall (endothelial damage);
- stasis, which is diminished blood flow through the veins;
- coagulability of blood (thrombophilia).

There are many predisposing causes for venous thrombosis. These are listed in Table 57.1. The most important factor is a hospital admission for the treatment of a medical or surgical condition. Injury, especially fractures of the lower limb and pelvis, pregnancy and the oral contraceptive pill are other well-recognised predisposing factors. Endothelial damage is now known to be critically important. The interaction of the endothelium with inflammatory cells, or previous deep vein damage, renders the endothelial surface hypercoagulable and less fibrinolytic.

Stasis is a predisposing factor seen in many of the conditions described in Table 57.1, especially in the postoperative period, in patients with heart failure and in those with arterial ischaemia.

Rudolf Ludwig Carl Virchow, 1821–1902, Professor of Pathology, Berlin, Germany.

Table 57.1 Risk factors for venous thromboembolism.

Patient factors	Age
	Obesity
	Varicose veins
	Immobility
	Pregnancy
	Puerperium
	High-dose oestrogen therapy
	Previous deep vein thrombosis or pulmonary embolism
	Thrombophilia (see *Table 57.2*)
Disease or surgical procedure	Trauma or surgery, especially of pelvis, hip and lower limb
	Malignancy, especially pelvic, and abdominal metastatic
	Heart failure
	Recent myocardial infarction
	Paralysis of lower limb(s) infection
	Inflammatory bowel disease
	Nephrotic syndrome
	Polycythaemia
	Paraproteinaemia
	Paroxysmal nocturnal haemoglobinuria antibody or lupus anticoagulant
	Behçet's disease
	Homocystinaemia

A number of conditions are associated with increased coagulability of the blood (thrombophilia) (Table 57.2). Deficiencies of antithrombin, activated protein C and protein S have all been shown to predispose to venous thrombosis in young patients. Activated protein C deficiency is associated with inheritance of the factor V Leiden gene and may account for the higher incidence of venous thrombosis in Caucasian populations (being present in 6–7 per cent). It results in a small increase in the risk of venous thrombosis, although it may act in concert with some of the other predisposing factors. A thrombophilic cause should be sought in any patient presenting with an episode of venous thrombosis who gives a family history of deep vein thrombosis or in whom there is no other predisposing factor.

Although the development of deep vein thrombosis is probably multifactorial, immobility (and hence stasis) remains one of the most important factors. Deep vein thrombosis is recognised as a complication of long-haul flights and other forms of travel.

Table 57.2 Abnormalities of thrombosis and fibrinolysis (thrombophylia) that lead to an increased risk of venous thrombosis.

Congenital	Deficiency of antithrombin III, protein C or protein S
	Antiphospholipid antibody or lupus anticoagulant
	Factor V Leiden gene defect or activated protein C resistance
	Dysfibrinogenaemias
Acquired	Antiphospholipid antibody or lupus anticoagulant

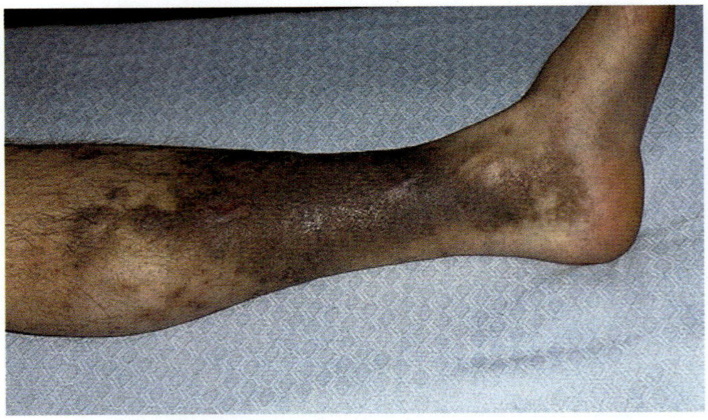

Figure 57.28 Post-thrombotic leg.

Pathology

A thrombus often develops in the soleal veins of the calf, initially as a platelet aggregate. Subsequently, fibrin and red cells form a mesh until the lumen of the vein wall occludes. The coralline thrombus then progresses as a propagated loose red fibrin clot containing many red cells (Figure 57.29). This is likely to extend up to the next large venous branch and it is possible for the clot to break off and embolise to the lung as a pulmonary embolism. In this situation the embolus arising from the lower leg veins becomes detached, passes through the large veins of the limb and vena cava, through the right heart and lodges in the pulmonary arteries. This may totally occlude perfusion to all or part of one or both lungs (pulmonary embolism). Acute right heart obstruction may lead to sudden collapse and death. Lung infarction is rare as the lung has a dual blood supply (bronchial and pulmonary arteries). Moderate-sized emboli can cause pyramidal-shaped infarcts.

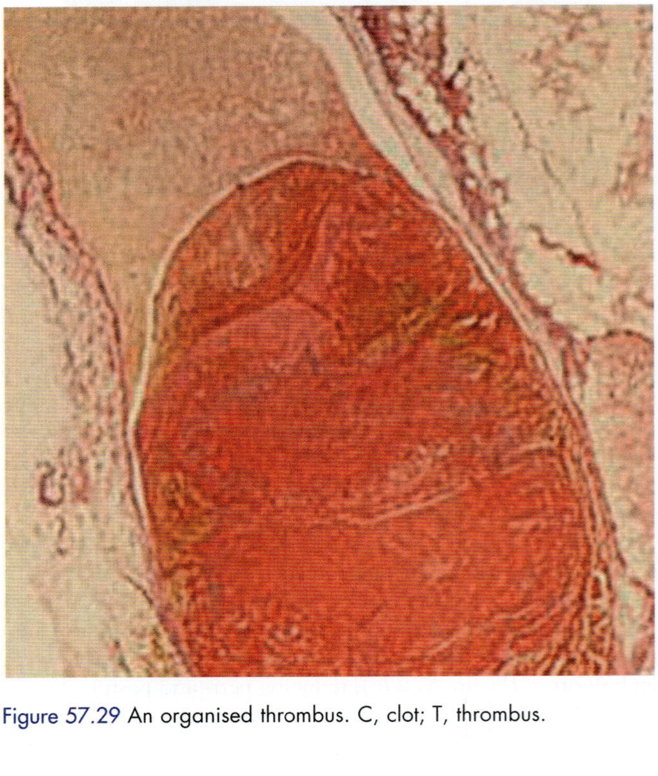

Figure 57.29 An organised thrombus. C, clot; T, thrombus.

Diagnosis

The most common presentation of a deep vein thrombosis is pain and swelling, especially in the calf – usually in one lower limb; however, bilateral deep vein thromboses are common, occurring in up to 30 per cent. When the swelling is bilateral, deep vein thromboses must be differentiated from other causes of systemic oedema, such as hypoproteinaemia, renal failure and heart failure. Some patients have no symptoms of thrombosis and may first present with signs of a pulmonary embolism, e.g. pleuritic chest pain, haemoptysis and shortness of breath. Patients may also develop shortness of breath from chronic pulmonary hypertension. Sometimes the leg appears cellulitic and, very occasionally, it may be white or cyanosed: phlegmasia alba dolens and phlegmasia cerulia dolens (Figure 57.30). Patients who present with venous gangrene (Figure 57.31) often have an underlying neoplasm.

Clinical examination for DVT is unreliable. Physical signs may also be absent. Mild pitting oedema of the ankle, dilated surface veins, a stiff calf and tenderness over the course of the deep veins should be sought. Leg pain occurs in about 50 per cent of patients with DVT but is non-specific. Homans' sign – resistance (not pain) of the calf muscles to forcible dorsiflexion – is not specific and should not be elicited. Tenderness occurs in 75 per cent of patients but is also found in 50 per cent of patients without objectively confirmed DVT. The pain and tenderness associated with DVT does not usually correlate with the size, location or extent of the thrombus. Clinical signs and symptoms of pulmonary embolism occur in about 10 per cent of patients with confirmed DVT.

A low-grade pyrexia may be present, especially in a patient who is having repeated pulmonary emboli. Patients may have signs of cyanosis, dyspnoea, raised neck veins, a fixed split second heart sound and a pleural rub if they are having pulmonary emboli causing right heart strain, although these signs may be subtle or lacking.

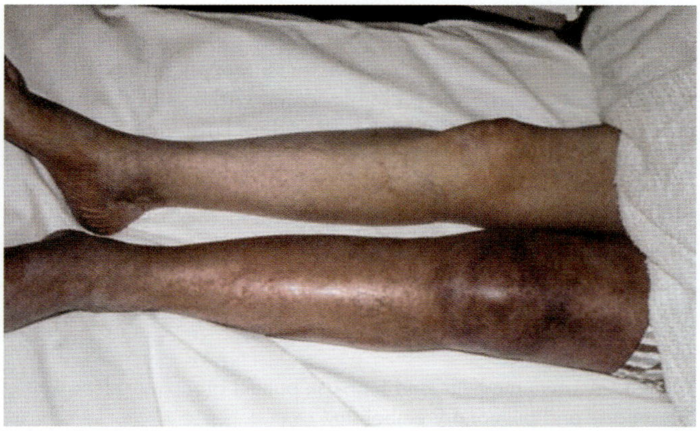

Figure 54.30 Phlegmasia cerulia dolens.

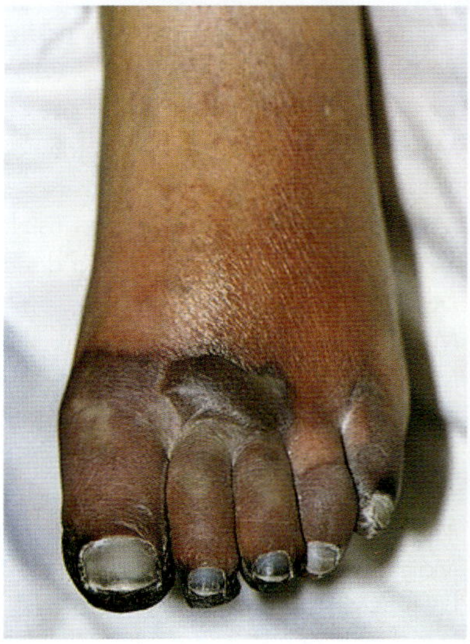

Figure 57.31 A foot with venous gangrene. The gangrene is symmetrical involving all of the toes. There is no clear-cut edge and there is marked oedema of the foot.

Investigation

The diagnosis of deep vein thrombosis and pulmonary embolism should be established by special investigations as the symptoms and signs are non-specific and may be entirely lacking. In addition, treatment with anticoagulation is not without risk and the diagnosis must be made with reasonable certainty.

Patients who present to an Accident and Emergency department with an idiopathic thrombosis usually have a d-dimer measurement where the modified Wells score is long than 4 or there is clinical suspicion (Table 57.3). If this is greater than the normal range there is no indication for further investigation but, if raised, a duplex compression ultrasound examination of the deep veins should be performed. The deep veins of the lower limb are located and compressed. Filling defects in flow and a lack of compressibility indicate the presence of a thrombosis (Figure 57.32). This is accurate and reliable for femoral and popliteal clots but less certain in tibial vein clots.

Ascending venography, which shows a thrombus as a filling defect, is now rarely required unless other measures are being considered (Figure 57.33). Magnetic resonance imaging

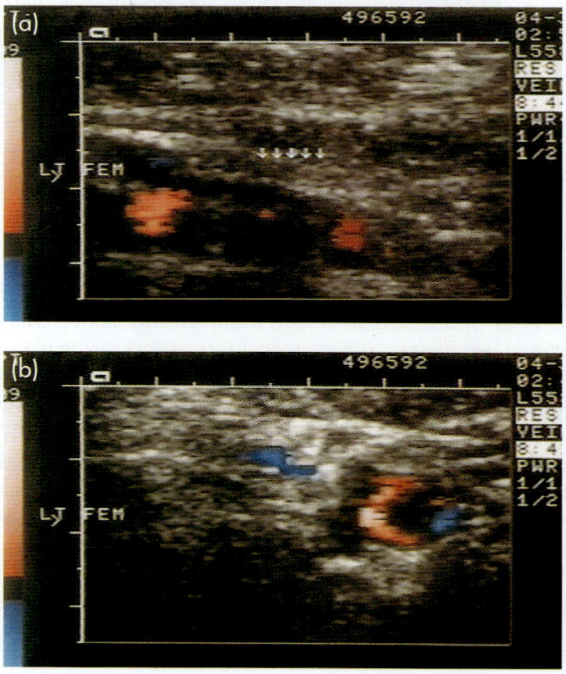

Figure 57.32 A longitudinal (a) and transverse (b) section of a duplex scan of a vein containing a thrombus.

John Homans, 1877–1957, Professor of Clinical Surgery, Harvard University Medical School, Boston, MA, USA.

Table 57.3 Modified Wells criteria for predicting pulmonary embolism.

Variable	Points
Clinical signs and symptoms of DVT (minimum of leg swelling and pain on palpation of deep veins)	3.0
Alternative diagnosis less likely than PE	3.0
Heart rate >100	1.5
Immobilisation >3 days or surgery within past 4 weeks	1.5
Previous DVT or PE	1.5
Haemoptysis	1.0
Malignancy (treatment or palliation within past 6 months)	1.0

DVT, deep venous thrombosis; PE, pulmonary embolism.
A score of <4 means PE is unlikely; >4 is suggestive of PE.

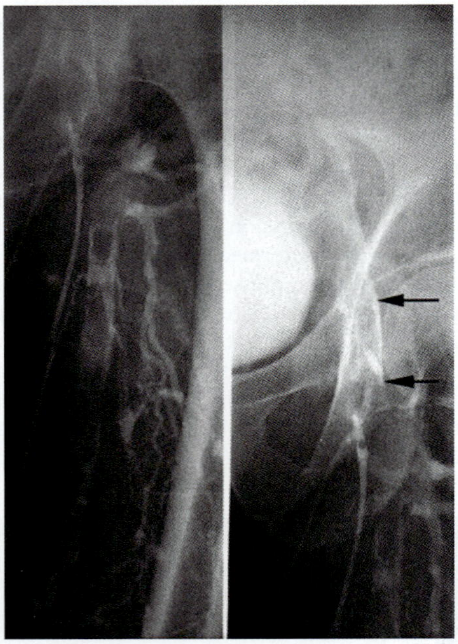

Figure 57.33 An ascending venogram of a deep vein thrombosis seen as filling defects (arrows) with contrast passing around the thrombus.

(MRI) uses a magnet to produce detailed pictures of the inside of the body by aligning hydrogen atoms in the tissues. Magnetic resonance venography is now as accurate as contrast venography.

Pulmonary embolism is diagnosed definitively by computed tomography (CT) scanning of the pulmonary arteries, which can show filling defects in the pulmonary arteries (Figure 57.34). Pulmonary angiography is rarely required unless interventional treatment is being considered. Radionucleotide imaging has now been superceded by CT pulmonary angiography and should not normally be used.

The differential diagnosis of a deep vein thrombosis includes a ruptured Baker's cyst, a calf muscle haematoma, a ruptured plantaris muscle, a thrombosed popliteal aneurysm and arterial ischaemia. Duplex scanning will detect many of these conditions but often patients present with non-specific pain in the calf that resolves with no firm diagnosis being made. The differential

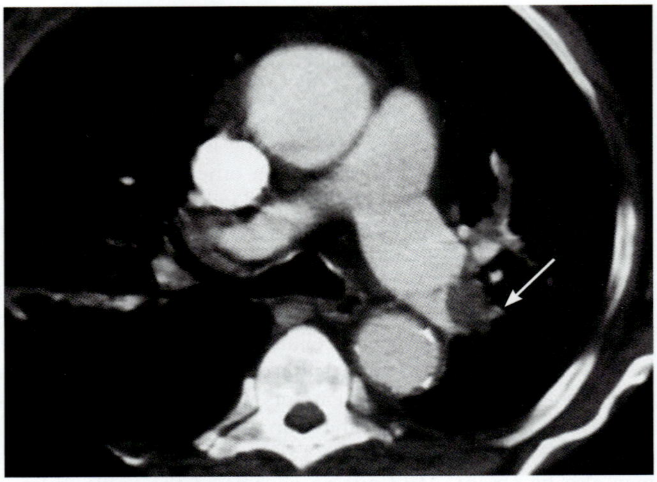

Figure 57.34 A computed tomography scan showing pulmonary emboli as filling defects (arrow) in the pulmonary artery.

diagnosis of a pulmonary embolism includes myocardial infarction, pleurisy and pneumonia.

Prophylaxis

Patients who are being admitted for surgery can be graded as low, moderate or high risk (Table 57.4). Patients in the medium or high risk groups should be considered for anticoagulation prophylaxis.

Prophylactic methods can be divided into mechanical and pharmacological. A variety of mechanical methods have been tried but only the use of graduated elastic compression stockings and external pneumatic compression have been shown to be worthwhile by reducing the incidence of thrombosis.

Table 57.4 Low-, medium- and high-risk patient groups for deep vein thrombosis and pulmonary embolism.

Risk groups	
Low	Minor surgery <30 minutes. Any age. No risk factors
	Major surgery >30 minutes. Age <40. No other risk factors
	Minor trauma or medical illness, any age. No risk factors
Moderate	Major surgery. Age 40+ or other risk factors
	Major medical illness: heart/lung disease, cancer, inflammatory bowel disease
	Major trauma/burns
	Minor surgery, trauma, medical illness in patient with previous DVT, PE or thrombophilia
High	Major orthopaedic surgery or fracture pelvis, hip, lower limb
	Major abdominal/pelvic surgery for cancer
	Major surgery, trauma, medical illness in patient with DVT, PE or thrombophilia
	Lower limb paralysis (e.g. stroke, paraplegia)
	Major lower limb amputation

DVT, deep venous thrombosis; PE, pulmonary embolism.

William Morrant Baker, 1839–1896, surgeon, St Bartholomew's Hospital, London, UK, described these cysts in 1877.

Pharmacological methods are more effective than mechanical methods at risk reduction although they carry an increased risk of bleeding. In the past, low-dose unfractionated heparin was used both intravenously and subcutaneously. Most patients now start on low molecular weight heparin given subcutaneously, with the dose based on the patient's weight. This does not require monitoring and has a reduced risk of heparin-induced thrombocytopenia. It can be given once a day and has a lower risk of bleeding complications. Unfractionated heparin and warfarin are now rarely used in the prophylaxis of deep vein thrombosis. A combination of mechanical and pharmacological treatment with heparin can be used in patients considered at high risk.

Treatment of a deep vein thrombosis

Patients who are confirmed to have a deep vein thrombosis on duplex imaging should be started on subcutaneous low molecular weight heparin and rapidly anticoagulated with warfarin unless there is a specific contraindication. Warfarin is usually started at a dose of 10 mg on day 1, 10 mg on day 2 and 5 mg on day 3. A prothrombin time taken on days 2 and 3 along with a warfarin dose algorithm guides the maintenance dose of warfarin.

The great majority of patients are treated with heparin and warfarin in this way. Thrombolysis should be considered, however, in patients with an iliac vein thrombosis, especially if they are seen early and the limb is extremely swollen. Very few surgeons now carry out surgical venous thrombectomy, although it may still be attempted in patients with threatened venous gangrene and phlegmasia cerulia dolens. If performed, a venous thrombectomy should be accompanied by an arteriovenous fistula to increase venous flow through the vein that has had the thrombus removed, however the results are, at best, modest.

During thrombolysis, tissue plasminogen activator (or more usually urokinase in the United States) is administered directly into the thrombus, either via the popliteal vein or by direct puncture in the groin. New devices are being marketed that physically disrupt the thrombus at the same time as local lysis is carried out. Some thrombi can be compressed by stent grafting, allowing the venous lumen to be opened, especially in the iliac region. This technique is most useful in patients who have a malignant cause for their venous obstruction.

Treatment of pulmonary embolus

Most pulmonary emboli can be treated by anticoagulation and observation but severe right heart strain and shortness of breath indicate the need for fibrinolytic treatment or radiologically guided catheter embolectomy. Rarely, patients who are on the point of cardiac arrest should undergo surgical pulmonary embolectomy.

Prophylaxis against pulmonary embolism

In patients who are considered at high risk of embolism or when anticoagulants are contraindicated, an inferior vena cava filter may be inserted to prevent the onward passage of any emboli. Filters can also be placed in patients who continue to have pulmonary emboli despite adequate anticoagulation. A large number of different types of filter are now available, some of which are removable (temporary filters). There are no good randomised trials to determine which filter is best.

Superficial thrombophlebitis

This is a superficial venous thrombosis. The term 'thrombophlebitis' implies a major inflammatory component; however, this is rarely seen. Common causes include external trauma (especially to varicose veins), venepunctures and infusions of hyperosmolar solutions and drugs. The presence of an intravenous cannula for longer than 24–48 hours often leads to local thrombosis. Some systemic diseases, such as thromboangiitis obliterans (Buerger's disease) and malignancy, especially of the pancreas, can lead to a flitting thrombophlebitis (thrombophlebitis migrans), affecting different veins at different times. Finally, coagulation disorders, such as polycythaemia, thrombocytosis and sickle cell disease are often associated, as is a concomitant thrombosis within the deep veins.

The surface vein feels solid and is tender on palpation. The overlying skin may be attached to the vein and in the early stages may be erythematous before gradually turning brown. A linear segment of vein of variable length can be easily palpated once the inflammation has died down.

A full blood count, coagulation screen and duplex scan of the deep veins should usually be obtained. Any suggestion of an associated malignancy should be investigated using appropriate endoscopy and imaging studies, such as an abdominal CT scan.

Most patients are treated with NSAIDs and the condition resolves spontaneously. Rarely, infected thrombi require incision or excision. Ligation to prevent propagation into the deep veins is almost never required, although some authors advocate saphenofemoral ligation when the thrombus is seen on ultrasound to be at the saphenofemoral junction. Associated deep vein thrombosis or thrombophilias are treated by anticoagulation.

LEG ULCERATION

Venous disease is responsible for between 60 and 70 per cent of all ulcers in the lower leg. There are many other causes of leg ulcers and these must be excluded in any patient presenting with ulceration:

- venous disease: superficial incompetence; deep venous damage (post-thrombotic);
- arterial ischaemic ulcers;
- rheumatoid ulcers;
- traumatic ulcers;
- neuropathic ulcers (diabetes);
- neoplastic ulcers (squamous cell carcinoma and basal cell carcinoma);
- infections, especially in Third World countries.

Up to 20 per cent of patients have evidence of arterial disease, which may be the sole cause of ulceration or may be a mixed factor in the development of an ulcer in association with venous disease.

Aetiology of ulceration

The exact pathophysiology of ulcer development has not been established. Originally, it was thought that static blood within the superficial veins led to hypoxia, which caused tissue death (stasis ulcers). This was not confirmed by investigation of venous oxygen saturation, which was found to be higher in ulcerated limbs. This led to the concept of arteriovenous fistulae, which were thought to develop in response to the high venous pressure; however, this could not be confirmed. High venous pressure was found to be associated with a pericapillary infiltrate. This includes fibrin and other proteins, which are known to lead to fibrosis. It was hypothesised that these 'cuffs' could act as a diffusion block.

Leukocytes were found to decrease in the venous effluent coming out of dependent limbs. This decrease in leukocyte passage was shown to increase if short-term venous hypertension was induced by application of a tourniquet. This led to the concept of white cell 'trapping', which, however, has not been confirmed by further investigation. Polymorphonuclear leukocytes were not found within the tissues but increased numbers of mast cells, monocytes and lymphocytes have been found in periulcer tissues.

Reactive oxygen species are increased in the ulcer environment and these may generate free radicals, leading to tissue damage. Proteolytic enzymes are also increased in ulcers and the fibroblasts in the ulcer surrounds are also abnormal, being in a 'senescent' state. Growth factors may be inhibited, leading to poor repair, and their absence may also lead to ulceration. It is proving difficult to show whether any of these factors is the cause of or the result of an ulcer.

At present, ambulatory venous hypertension is the only accepted underlying cause of ulceration. This also explains why venous ulcers are never seen in the upper limb. It is important to try and define the exact mechanism of ulcer development. Venous hypertension may be the result of primary valve incompetence of the saphenous veins, incompetence of the perforating veins or incompetence or obstruction of the deep veins.

Clinical features

The ulcer must be carefully examined. A venous ulcer usually has a gently sloping edge and the floor contains granulation tissue covered by a variable amount of slough and exudate. Any significant elevation of the ulcer edge should indicate the need for a biopsy to exclude a carcinoma (usually a squamous cell).

The venous ulcer of the leg characteristically develops in the skin of the gaiter region, the area between the muscles of the calf and the ankle. This is the region where many of the Cockett perforators join the posterior tibial vein to the surface vein, known as the posterior arch vein. The majority of ulcers develop on the medial side of the calf but ulcers associated with lesser saphenous incompetence may develop on the lateral side of the leg. Ulcers can develop on any part of the calf skin in patients with post-thrombotic legs; however, venous ulcers rarely extend onto the foot or into the upper calf and, if there is ulceration at these sites, other diagnoses should be seriously considered. Ulcers often develop in response to minor trauma; many patients notice some itching, perhaps associated with mast cell degranulation, before the ulcers develop. Almost all venous ulcers have surrounding haemasiderosis (seen as pigmentation) and the more chronic ulcers develop lipodermatosclerosis with associated fibrosis of the subcutaneous tissue (Figure 57.10). This is manifest as thickening, pigmentation, inflammation and induration of the calf skin. The pigmentation comes from haemosiderin and melanin and the haemosiderin itself may be an important factor in the ulcer development.

A full examination of the front and back of the limbs with the patient standing should be carried out to assess the presence of varicosities and truncal incompetence of the saphenous systems (note that venous ulcers are not always accompanied by varicose veins).

All patients should have their pulses palpated and, if there is any doubt, their Doppler pressures should be measured. Sensation and proprioception should be assessed to exclude neuropathy, especially in diabetic patients. A careful examination of the hand and other joints may confirm the presence of rheumatoid arthritis or osteoarthritis.

Investigation

Most vascular surgeons will carry out a duplex scan when the patient with an ulcer is first seen to assess the state of the deep and superficial veins. The presence of reflux in these veins does not confirm a venous ulcer but supports the diagnosis in the absence of another cause and helps direct treatment.

All patients presenting for the first time with a new leg ulcer should have a full blood count, blood glucose, erythrocyte sedimentation rate (ESR) or C-reactive protein (CRP) and sickle cell test if they have an appropriate racial background. Anaemia can both cause ulcers (e.g. sickle cell disease and pernicious anaemia) and be a result of ulceration (e.g. iron deficiency anaemia and the anaemia of chronic disease). Polycythaemia is a rare cause of ulceration. An antibody screen should be obtained if the ulcer appears 'atypical' or there is any suggestion of joint disease (e.g. rheumatoid arthritis). All patients presenting with a new ulcer should have their Doppler pressures measured, unless the foot pulses are easily palpable and have been confirmed as such by a vascular specialist.

Management

When the diagnosis of a 'probable venous ulcer' has been made, patients are initially treated by a compression bandaging regimen, which can be applied in a specialised clinic or by a trained district or practice nurse. Patients with new ulcers should ideally be assessed in a specialised ulcer clinic to confirm the diagnosis and agree the correct treatment regimen.

Many bandaging regimens have been described but three types usually suffice. A multilayered elastic compression bandaging system has been shown to be effective (Charing Cross four-layer bandage), as has a rigid multilayered system (Steripaste™ three-layer bandage). A low-compression regimen is desirable for mixed venous/arterial ulcers. The alternative to these bandaging regimens is to apply a bland absorbent leak-proof dressing beneath a graduated elastic compression stocking (class II). Recent data suggest that this regimen may be equally effective in attaining ulcer healing.

These compression regimens are ideally applied by trained staff on a bi-weekly or weekly basis until the ulcer is starting to heal and the amount of exudate is reduced. Longer periods between dressing changes can then be instituted. At each attendance ulcer size must be measured to monitor improvement. Antibiotics do not speed ulcer healing in the absence of cellulitis and all other specific ulcer-healing drugs are of dubious validity. Failure to heal an ulcer may indicate that it has another or coexisting cause (e.g. malignancy, rheumatoid arthritis or arterial ischaemia). Biopsies are indicated if malignancy is suspected and it is important to remember that a Marjolin's type of ulcer (a squamous cell or basal cell carcinoma) can develop in a chronic long-standing venous ulcer (Figure 57.35).

Once these factors have been excluded, consideration may be given to healing the ulcer by excision and grafting in appropriate cases. A number of biological dressings have been developed, including fetal keratinocytes and collagen meshes, which have been shown to improve healing; however, they are not cost-effective for the majority of ulcers. Pinch grafts and

A gaiter is a leather or cloth covering for the lower leg and ankle. The name is derived from the French 'guetre' for the same piece of clothing.
Frank Bernard Cockett, formerly surgeon, St Thomas's Hospital, London, UK.
Jean-Nicholas Marjolin, 1780–1850, surgeon, Paris, France, described the development of carcinomatous ulcers in scars in 1828.
Charing Cross. This method of treating venous ulcers was introduced at Charing Cross Hospital, London, UK.

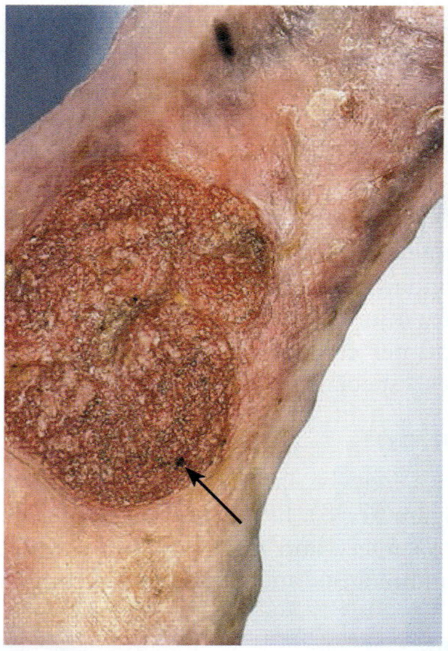

Figure 57.35 A Marjolin's ulcer (a squamous cell cancer arising in a chronic venous ulcer; arrow).

ulcer excision with mesh grafting have been shown to provide good early healing with moderate long-term results (50 per cent healed at five years).

The Eschar trial has confirmed that surgery to sites of superficial venous incompetence does not speed ulcer healing and this practice should be abandoned unless new evidence is provided of its efficacy.

Prevention of recurrence

Once an ulcer has healed the patient must be re-evaluated in an attempt to prevent recurrence. Patients with normal deep veins should be offered treatment to obliterate any sites of saphenous or perforator reflux. The Eschar study has confirmed the results of other studies showing that this treatment is effective in reducing the incidence of ulcer recurrence in patients with **normal** deep veins. Some patients will decline treatment and others will be considered unsuitable for major interventions on their veins.

Elastic stockings (normally class II) should be prescribed for all patients with evidence of post-thrombotic deep vein damage and these remain an alternative treatment for patients with superficial venous disease who decline intervention. Although ideally these should be above-knee stockings in many cases, the pragmatist will prescribe below-knee stockings as most patients will otherwise not comply. Stockings need to be worn during the day and are a lifelong prescription. Used effectively, they will reduce the incidence of any further DVTs and reduce although not eliminate the chance of further ulceration. Studies are required to determine whether laser ablation and foam sclerotherapy are as satisfactory as surgery in achieving prolonged ulcer-free periods.

Prognosis

Nearly all venous ulcers can be healed but, even in those who have successful surgery or wear their stockings religiously, there is a 20–30 per cent incidence of reulceration by five years. The greatest risk of reulceration is in the post-thrombotic leg.

CONGENITAL VENOUS ANOMALIES

There are four main types of anomaly:

1 aplasia;
2 hypoplasia;
3 duplication;
4 persistence of vestigial vessels.

Aplasia is most commonly seen in the inferior vena cava and has a similar presentation to the post-thrombotic limb. Membranous occlusion of the left common iliac vein (May–Thurner–Cockett syndrome) often develops where the vein passes behind the right common iliac artery (iliac vein compression syndrome) This leads to an iliac vein thrombosis, which most commonly affects the left common and external iliac veins. Membranes may also narrow the hepatic veins, which can become totally occluded, leading to a Budd–Chiari syndrome.

Hypoplasia results in a narrow vein.

Duplications are quite common, with double vena cava, femoral and renal veins; they often present as an incidental finding.

Klippel–Trenaunay syndrome

This is a combined anomaly of a cutaneous naevus, persistent vestigial veins with varicose veins, and soft tissue and bone hypertrophy. The condition is a mesodermal abnormality that is not familial (Figure 57.36).

Segments of the deep veins are hypoplastic or aplastic and there may be an associated obstruction of the lymphatics. The condition must be distinguished from the Parkes Weber syndrome, in which there are multiple arteriovenous fistulae causing venous hypertension, ulceration and high-output cardiac failure.

Virtually all patients with Klippel–Trenaunay syndrome should be treated conservatively with elastic compression hosiery; however, some will benefit from laser ablation of the naevus, stapling of the bones to avoid leg length discrepancy and occasional removal of large superficial varicose veins, provided the deep veins are normal. Low molecular weight heparin should be given to all patients having surgery as this syndrome is associated with an increased risk of deep vein thrombosis.

ENTRAPMENT OF VEINS

The axillary vein and the popliteal vein are the two veins that are most commonly compressed. The former is compressed at the thoracic outlet between the first rib and the clavicle, where it usually presents as an axillary vein thrombosis (see below) (Figure 57.37a). The latter is compressed by an abnormal insertion of the gastrocnemius muscles. Entrapment may cause discomfort and swelling of the limb during exercise before thrombosis develops. Treatment is by surgical decompression, excising the first rib or dividing the abnormal musculature of the gastrocnemius insertion.

AXILLARY VEIN THROMBOSIS

Thrombosis of the axillary vein may occur following excessive exercise in a patient with an anatomically abnormal thoracic outlet but is also associated with excessive muscle bulk as found

Hans Chiari, 1851–1916, Professor of Pathological Anatomy, Strasbourg, Germany (Strasbourg was returned to France after the end of World War I, in 1918), gave his account of this condition in 1898.

George Budd, 1808–1882, Professor of Medicine, King's College Hospital, London, UK, described this syndrome in 1845.
Frederick Parkes Weber, 1863–1962, physician, The German Hospital, Dalston, London, UK.

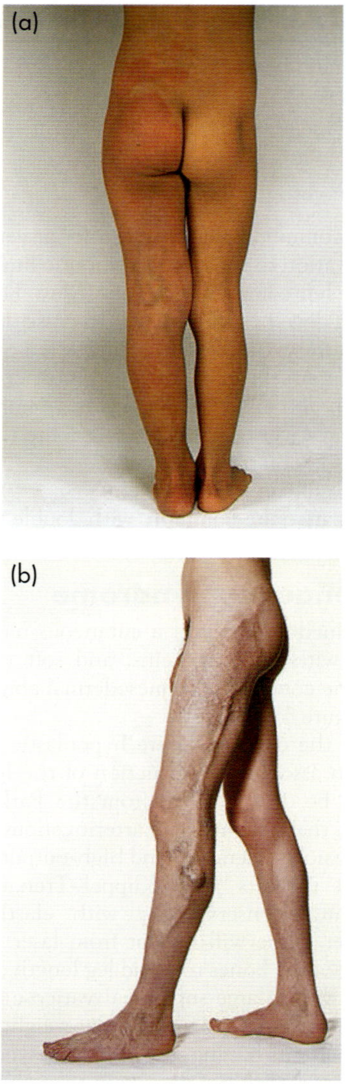

Figure 57.36 Two patients with Klippel–Trenaunay syndrome. (a) This patient has a longer leg and a capillary naevus. (b) This patient has a large lateral anomalous axial vein.

in weightlifters. The vein may be compressed by a cervical rib if this is present (Figure 57.37b). The arm is swollen and painful and, at an early stage, the thrombus can be removed by thrombolysis delivered through one of the arm veins. The vein must then be imaged to see if there is any compression on elevation of the arm. Thoracic outlet decompression can be carried out by resecting the cervical rib or first rib if this is confirmed.

VENOUS INJURY

Blunt or penetrating trauma almost always damages some small and medium-sized veins, which can be safely ignored or ligated without causing any problems. Larger axial venous channels have, in the past, been ligated when injured, but it is now recognised that these axial veins should be repaired whenever possible to reduce subsequent morbidity (pain and swelling in the tissues being drained) and limb loss when associated with a concomitant arterial injury. Many venous injuries remain undiagnosed at the time of injury (e.g. crural vein damage associated with a fractured tibia) and only present many years later when post-thrombotic changes become apparent. Venous injuries occur from both civilian and military trauma but the incidence of venous military injuries has been particularly well documented. In total, 40–50 per cent of arterial injuries have concomitant venous injuries, especially in the popliteal fossa.

> Henry IV of Navarre, 1553–1610, led his army into the Battle of Ivry, shouting 'rally round the white plume of Navarre'. He used his sword to such good effect that he could not use his arm for 6 weeks probably from an axillary vein thrombosis.

Classification

Venous injuries may be lacerated, contused or torn apart by stretching (Figure 57.38). Iatrogenic injuries result from damage at the time of surgery and from punctures caused by catheter insertion by radiologists and physicians. Thrombosis, haemor-

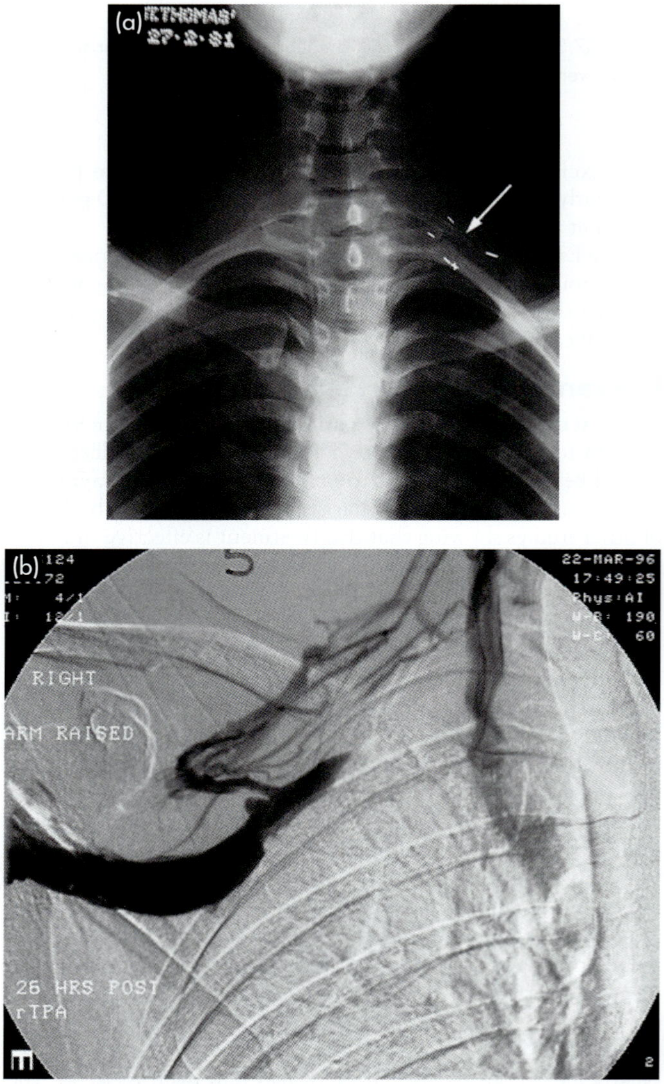

Figure 57.37 Thoracic outlet syndrome. (a) Cervical ribs; (b) elevation of the arm causing occlusion of the axillary vein with collateral fillings. The patient has had previous surgery on the left side.

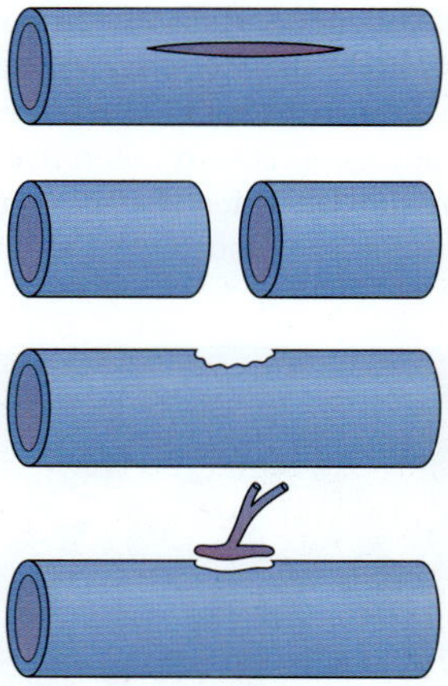

Figure 57.38 Types of venous damage. (a) Incision; (b) transection; (c) irregular laceration; (d) avulsion of a tributary.

rhage and embolisation are all common complications and arteriovenous fistulae may develop when a penetrating needle transfixes the vein and artery.

Associated injuries to soft tissue, arteries and bones often overshadow the venous injury. Massive haemorrhage from the pelvic bones or the inferior vena cava can rapidly lead to hypovolaemic shock and death if left untreated. Haematomas are common and engorgement, cyanosis and swelling are also indicative of a major venous injury.

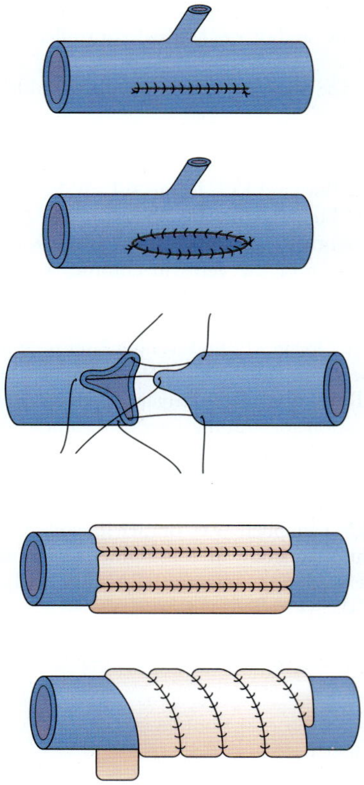

Figure 57.39 Types of venous repair. (a) Lateral suture; (b) patch graft; (c) Carrel triangulation technique of venous anastomosis; (d) panel graft; (e) spiral graft.

Investigations are rarely helpful and rapid exploration is usually required except in the case of unstable pelvic fractures where external fixation has dramatically improved the outcome of these injuries by stabilising the injury. Embolisation and stent grafting can have a limited role, especially if the venous injury is relatively inaccessible or an arteriovenous fistula has developed.

The patient must be adequately resuscitated, have blood cross-matched and have good intravenous access obtained via a central venous pressure line if possible, provided that there are no injuries around the neck or thorax. Gentle wound exploration, under tourniquet control when possible, should assess the extent of the injuries before the vessels are dissected out and clamped. Different types of repair are shown in Figure 57.39; the type of repair carried out depends on the extent of the venous injury, including how much venous wall has been lost or damaged. Lateral sutures and vein patches are ideal methods of repair and end-to-end anastomosis is satisfactory provided that it is not carried out under tension.

Vein replacement should be by autogenous tissue whenever possible, using vein harvested from another site, e.g. the internal jugular vein or the long saphenous vein from an undamaged limb. Artificial grafts, such as polytetrafluoroethylene (PTFE) grafts, are likely to get infected in contaminated wounds and have given poor results in recent conflicts. The use of anticoagulants and an arteriovenous fistula to reduce the risk of thrombosis in the vein graft are controversial and depend on the associated injuries that are present. In contaminated wounds, tetanus, toxoid and antibiotics should be given. A fasciotomy should always be considered if there is a concomitant arterial and venous injury.

Prognosis

It is now recognised that repair of a major axial vein can be carried out with a 70–80 per cent success rate, reducing the morbidity of a combined arterial and venous injury considerably (especially limb loss). Complex repairs should not, however, be carried out if a patient's life is at risk, when ligation may have to suffice in the short term.

VENOUS TUMOURS

Cystic degeneration of the vein wall is an uncommon cause of venous occlusion. It may be detected by ultrasound. The cyst may be deroofed or the venous segment excised.

Venous malformation cavernous angioma/haemangioma

These malformations are common, representing one end of a spectrum of arteriovenous malformations. They often affect the skin but also extend into the deep tissues, including bones and joints. They usually present with variable swelling and dilated veins beneath the skin. Occasionally, there is no visible mass and the complaint is one of pain. Haemorrhage and thrombophlebitis may exacerbate the pain. A soft compressible mass, which is venous in colour especially if it is under the skin, is usually present (Figure 57.40a). A dark blue tinge is often apparent even if the malformation is deeply situated. Nodules within the mass usually represent previous episodes of thrombosis. The size and extent of the haemangioma are best visualised by nuclear magnetic resonance with a short tau inversion recovery (STIR) sequence (Figure 57.40b) or CT scanning with contrast

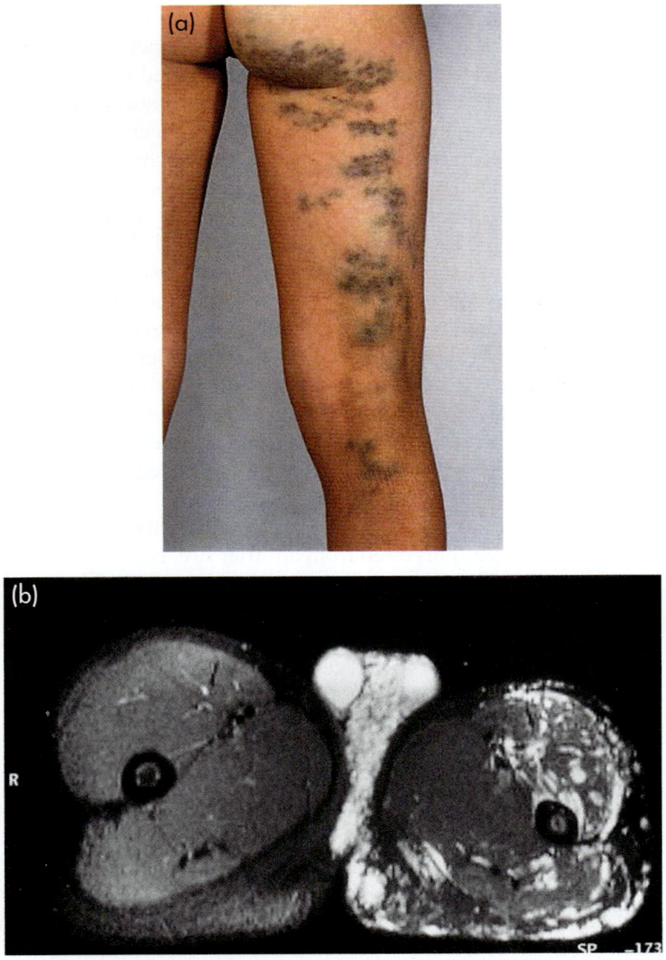

Figure 57.40 (a) Venous angioma of the leg. (b) Magnetic resonance with a short tau inversion recovery sequence showing angioma in white throughout the limb.

enhancement. Venography rarely shows an abnormality, but direct puncture with contrast injection shows the connections of the malformation.

Treatment is a highly specialised area. Treatment options nowadays rarely initially involve surgical excision as once this is done future embolisation and sclerotherapy is very difficult. No treatment is entirely curative because it is difficult to remove all of the angiomatous tissue or sclerose the angioma completely. Sclerosis can be dangerous when the veins connect to the deep system, particularly near the central nervous system.

Leiomyomas and leiomyosarcomas of the vein wall

These are extremely rare tumours that are usually slow growing. They present with pain and a mass with signs of venous obstruction, e.g. oedema and distended veins. Duplex scanning, CT (Figure 57.41) and magnetic resonance imaging show a filling defect within the vein wall. Treatment is by resection with replacement by autogenous vein taken from another site. Rarely, a PTFE graft is required. When the tumour affects the vena cava it must be resected and replaced with a prosthetic graft.

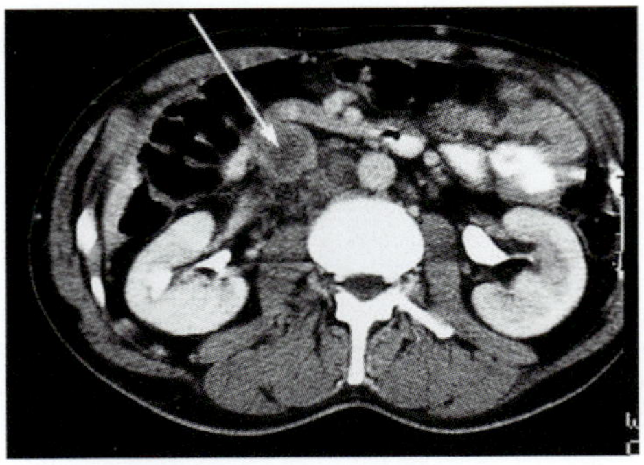

Figure 57.41 Inferior vena cava containing a filling defect from a leiomyosarcoma.

FURTHER READING

Barwell JR, Davies CE, Deacon J *et al.* Comparison of surgery and compression with compression alone in chronic venous ulceration (ESCHAR study): randomised controlled trial. *Lancet* 2004; **363**: 1857–9.

Bergan JJ. *The vein book.* Burlington, MA: Elsevier Academic Press, 2006.

Brar R, Nordon IM, Hinchliffe RJ *et al.* Surgical management of varicose veins; meta-analysis. *Vascular* 2010; **18**: 205–10.

Browse NL, Burnand KG, Irvine AT, Wilson N. *Diseases of the veins*, 2nd edn. London: Arnold, 1999.

Coleridge-Smith P, Labropoulos N, Partsch K *et al.* Duplex ultrasound investigation of the veins in chronic venous disease of the lower limbs – UIP consensus statement. *Eur J Vasc Endovasc Surg* 2006; **31**: 83–92.

Darwood RJ, Gough MJ. Endovenous laser treatment for uncomplicated varicose veins. *Phlebology* 2009; **24**(Suppl. 1): 50–61.

Eklof B, Rutherford RB, Bergan JJ *et al.* Revision of the CEAP classification for chronic venous disorders: consensus statement. *J Vasc Surg* 2004; **40**: 1248–52.

Gohel MS, Davies AH. Radiofrequency ablation for uncomplicated varicose veins. *Phlebology* 2009; **24**(Suppl. 1): 42–9.

Michaels JA, Campbell WB, Brazier JE *et al.* Randomised clinical trial, observational study and assessment of cost-effectiveness of the treatment of varicose veins (REACTIV trial). *Health Technol Assess* 2006; **10**: 1–196.

Tisi PV, Beverley C, Rees A. Injection sclerotherapy for varicose veins. *Cochrane Database Syst Rev* 2006; (**4**): CD001732.

CHAPTER

58 Lymphatic disorders

LEARNING OBJECTIVES

To understand:

- The main functions of the lymphatic system
- The development of the lymphatic system
- The various causes of limb swelling
- The aetiology, clinical features, investigations and treatment of lymphoedema

INTRODUCTION

The lymphatic system was first described by Erasistratus in Alexandria more than 2000 years ago. William Hunter, in the late eighteenth century, was the first to describe the function of the lymphatic system. Starling's pioneering work on the hydrostatic and haemodynamic forces controlling the movement of fluid across the capillary provided further insights into the function of the lymphatics. However, there is much about the lymphatic system that is not understood and debate continues over the precise aetiology of the most common abnormality of the system, namely lymphoedema.

ANATOMY AND PHYSIOLOGY OF THE LYMPHATIC SYSTEM

Functions

The principal function of the lymphatics is the return of protein-rich fluid to the circulation through the lymphaticovenous junctions in the jugular area. Thus, water, electrolytes, low molecular weight moieties (polypeptides, cytokines, growth factors) and macromolecules (fibrinogen, albumin, globulins, coagulation and fibrinolytic factors) from the interstitial fluid (ISF) return to the circulation via the lymphatics. Intestinal lymph (chyle) transports cholesterol, long-chain fatty acids, triglycerides and the fat-soluble vitamins (A, D, E and K) directly to the circulation, bypassing the liver. Lymphocytes and other immune cells also circulate within the lymphatic system.

Development and macroanatomy

In the human embryo lymph sacs develop at 6–7 weeks' gestation as four cystic spaces, one on either side of the neck and one in each groin. These cisterns enlarge and develop communications that permit lymph from the lower limbs and abdomen to drain via the cisterna chyli into the thoracic duct, which in turn drains into the left internal jugular vein at its confluence with the left subclavian vein. Lymph from the head and right arm drains via a separate lymphatic trunk, the right lymphatic duct, into the right internal jugular vein. Lymphatics accompany veins everywhere except in the cortical bony skeleton and central nervous system, although the brain and retina possess cerebrospinal fluid and aqueous humour, respectively.

The lymphatic system comprises lymphatic channels, lymphoid organs (lymph nodes, spleen, Peyer's patches, thymus, tonsils) and circulating elements (lymphocytes and other mononuclear immune cells). Lymphatic endothelial cells are derived from embryonic veins in the jugular and perimesonephric areas from where they migrate to form the primary lymph sacs and plexus. Both transcription (e.g. Prox1) and growth (e.g. VEGF-C) factors are essential for these developmental events.

William Hunter, 1718–1783, anatomist and obstetrician who became the first Professor of Anatomy at the Royal Academy of Arts, London, UK. He was the elder brother of John Hunter, the anatomist and surgeon.

Microanatomy and physiology

Lymphatic capillaries

Lymphatics originate within the ISF space from specialised endothelialised capillaries (initial lymphatics) or non-endothelialised channels such as the spaces of Disse in the liver. Initial lymphatics are unlike arteriovenous capillaries in that:

- they are blind-ended;
- they are much larger (50 μm);
- they allow the entry of molecules of up to 1000 kDa in size because the basement membrane is fenestrated, tenuous or even absent and the endothelium itself possesses intra- and intercellular pores;
- they are anchored to interstitial matrix by filaments. In the resting state, initial lymphatics are collapsed. When ISF volume and pressure increases, initial lymphatics and their pores are held open by these filaments to facilitate increased drainage.

Terminal lymphatics

Initial lymphatics drain into terminal (collecting) lymphatics

Erasistratus of Chios, c.300–250 BC, of the Medical School at Alexandria in Egypt is regarded by many as the first physiologist.
Ernest Henry Starling, 1866–1927, Professor of Physiology, University College, London, UK.
Josef Disse, 1852–1912, a German anatomist.

that possess bicuspid valves and endothelial cells rich in the contractile protein actin. Larger collecting lymphatics are surrounded by smooth muscle. Valves partition the lymphatics into segments (lymphangions) that contract sequentially to propel lymph into the lymph trunks.

Lymph trunks

Terminal lymphatics lead to lymph trunks, which have a structure similar to that of veins, namely a single layer of endothelial cells, lying on a basement membrane overlying a media comprising smooth muscle cells that are innervated with sympathetic, parasympathetic and sensory nerve endings. About 10 per cent of lymph arising from a limb is transported in deep lymphatic trunks that accompany the main neurovascular bundles. The majority, however, is conducted against venous flow from deep to superficial in epifascial lymph trunks. Superficial trunks form lymph bundles of various sizes, which are located within strips of adipose tissue, and tend to follow the course of the major superficial veins.

Starling's forces

The distribution of fluid and protein between the vascular system and ISF depends on the balance of hydrostatic and oncotic pressures between the two compartments (Starling's forces), together with the relative impermeability of the blood capillary membrane to molecules over 70 kDa. In health there is net capillary filtration, which is removed by the lymphatic system.

Transport of particles

Particles enter the initial lymphatics through interendothelial openings and vesicular transport through intraendothelial pores. Large particles are actively phagocytosed by macrophages and transported through the lymphatic system intracellularly.

Mechanisms of lymph transport

Resting ISF is negative (−2 to −6 mmH2O), whereas lymphatic pressures are positive, indicating that lymph flows against a small pressure gradient. It is believed that prograde lymphatic flow depends upon three mechanisms:

1. transient increases in interstitial pressure secondary to muscular contraction and external compression;
2. the sequential contraction and relaxation of lymphangions;
3. the prevention of reflux because of valves.

Lymphangions are believed to respond to increased lymph flow in much the same way as the heart responds to increased venous return in that they increase their contractility and stroke volume. Contractility is also enhanced by noradrenaline, serotonin, certain prostaglandins and thromboxanes, and endothelin-1. Pressures of up to 30–50 mmHg have been recorded in normal lymph trunks and up to 200 mmHg in severe lymphoedema. Lymphatics may also modulate their own contractility through the production of nitric oxide and other local mediators. Transport in the thoracic and right lymph ducts also depends upon intrathoracic (respiration) and central venous (cardiac cycle) pressures. Therefore, cardiorespiratory disease may have an adverse effect on lymphatic function.

In summary, in the healthy limb, lymph flow is largely due to intrinsic lymphatic contractility, although this is augmented by exercise, limb movement and external compression. However, in lymphoedema, when the lymphatics are constantly distended with lymph, these external forces assume a much more important functional role.

ACUTE INFLAMMATION OF THE LYMPHATICS

Acute lymphangitis is an infection, often caused by *Streptococcus pyogenes* or *Staphylococcus aureus*, which spreads to the draining lymphatics and lymph nodes (lymphadenitis) where an abscess may form. Eventually this may progress to bacteraemia or septicaemia. The normal signs of infection (rubor, calor, dolor) are present and a red streak is seen in the skin along the line of the inflamed lymphatic (Figure 58.1). The part should be rested to reduce lymphatic drainage and elevated to reduce swelling, and the patient should be treated with intravenous antibiotics based upon actual or suspected sensitivities. Failure to improve within 48 hours suggests inappropriate antibiotic therapy, the presence of undrained pus or the presence of an underlying systemic disorder (malignancy, immunodeficiency). The lymphatic damage caused by acute lymphangitis may lead to recurrent attacks of infection and lymphoedema; patients with lymphoedema are prone to so-called acute inflammatory episodes (see below).

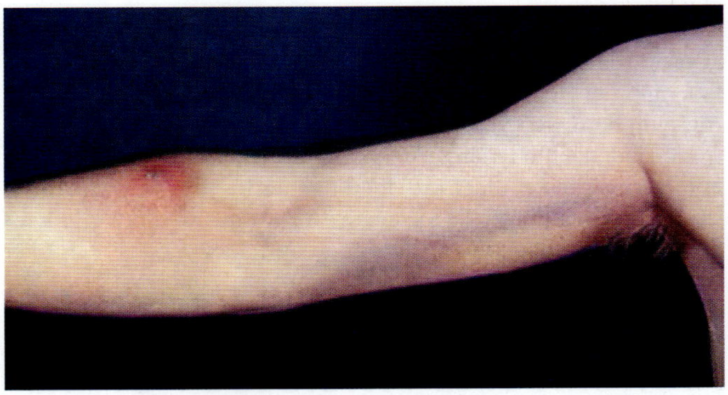

Figure 58.1 Acute lymphangitis of the arm. Erythematous streaks extend from the site of primary infection on the volar aspect of the forearm to epicondylar nodes at the elbow and from there to enlarged and tender axillary lymph nodes.

LYMPHOEDEMA

Definition

Lymphoedema may be defined as abnormal limb swelling caused by the accumulation of increased amounts of high protein ISF secondary to defective lymphatic drainage in the presence of (near) normal net capillary filtration.

The scope of the clinical problem

At birth, 1 in 6000 people will develop lymphoedema with an overall prevalence of 0.13–2 per cent. The condition is not only associated with significant physical symptoms and complications but is also a frequent cause of emotional and psychological distress, which can lead to difficulties with relationships, education and work (Summary box 58.1).

Despite this significant impact on quality of life, many sufferers choose not to seek medical advice because of embarrassment and a belief that nothing can be done. Patients who do come

Summary box 58.1

Symptoms frequently experienced by patients with lymphoedema

- Swelling, clothing or jewellery becoming tighter
- Constant dull ache, even severe pain
- Burning and bursting sensations
- General tiredness and debility
- Sensitivity to heat
- 'Pins and needles'
- Cramp
- Skin problems, including flakiness, weeping, excoriation and breakdown
- Immobility, leading to obesity and muscle wasting
- Backache and joint problems
- Athlete's foot
- Acute infective episodes

forward for help, especially those with non-cancer-related lymphoedema, often find they have limited access to appropriate expertise and treatment. Lymphoedema is often misdiagnosed and mistreated by doctors, who frequently have a poor understanding of the importance of the condition, believing it to be primarily a cosmetic problem in the early stages. However, making an early diagnosis is important because relatively simple measures can be highly effective at this stage and can prevent the development of disabling late disease, which is often very difficult to treat. It is also an opportunity for patients to make contact with patient support groups (Summary box 58.2).

Summary box 58.2

What every patient with lymphoedema should receive

- An explanation of why the limb is swollen and the underlying cause
- Guidance on skin hygiene and care and the avoidance of acute infective episodes
- Antifungal prophylactic therapy to prevent athlete's foot
- Rapid access to antibiotic therapy if necessary, hospital admission for acute infective episodes
- Appropriate instructions regarding exercise therapy
- Manual lymphatic drainage (MLD)
- Multilayer lymphoedema bandaging (MLLB)
- Compression garments and, if appropriate, specialised footwear
- Advice on diet
- Access to support services and networks

The severity of unilateral limb lymphoedema can be classified as:

- mild: <20 per cent excess limb volume;
- moderate: 20–40 per cent excess limb volume;
- severe: >40 per cent excess limb volume.

Pathophysiology

The ISF compartment (10–12 litres in a 70-kg man) constitutes 50 per cent of the wet weight of the skin and subcutaneous tissues and, in order for oedema to be clinically detectable, its volume has to double. About 8 litres (protein concentration approximately 20–30 g/L, similar to ISF) of lymph is produced each day and travels in afferent lymphatics to lymph nodes. There, the volume is halved and the protein concentration doubled, resulting in 4 litres of lymph re-entering the venous circulation each day via efferent lymphatics. In one sense, all oedema is lymphoedema in that it results from an inability of the lymphatic system to clear the ISF compartment. However, in most types of oedema this is because the capillary filtration rate is pathologically high and overwhelms a normal lymphatic system, resulting in the accumulation of low-protein oedema fluid. In contrast, in true lymphoedema, when the primary problem is in the lymphatics, capillary filtration is normal and the oedema fluid is relatively high in protein. Of course, in a significant number of patients with oedema there is both abnormal capillary filtration and abnormal lymphatic drainage, as in chronic venous insufficiency (CVI) for example.

Lymphoedema results from lymphatic aplasia, hypoplasia, dysmotility (reduced contractility with or without valvular insufficiency), obliteration by inflammatory, infective or neoplastic processes, or surgical extirpation. Whatever the primary abnormality, the resultant physical and/or functional obstruction leads to lymphatic hypertension and distension, with further secondary impairment of contractility and valvular competence. Lymphostasis and lymphotension lead to the accumulation in the ISF of fluid, proteins, growth factors and other active peptide moieties, glycosaminoglycans and particulate matter, including bacteria. As a consequence, there is increased collagen production by fibroblasts, an accumulation of inflammatory cells (predominantly macrophages and lymphocytes) and activation of keratinocytes. The end result is protein-rich oedema fluid, increased deposition of ground substance, subdermal fibrosis and dermal thickening and proliferation. Lymphoedema, unlike all other types of oedema, is confined to the epifascial space. Although muscle compartments may be hypertrophied because of the increased work involved in limb movement, they are characteristically free of oedema.

Classification

Two main types of lymphoedema are recognised:

1. **Primary lymphoedema**, in which the cause is unknown (or at least uncertain and unproven); it is thought to be caused by 'congenital lymphatic dysplasia'.
2. **Secondary or acquired lymphoedema**, in which there is a clear underlying cause.

Primary lymphoedema is usually further subdivided on the basis of the presence of family history, age of onset and lymphangiographic findings (Tables 58.1 and 58.2) (see below).

Risk factors for lymphoedema

Although the true risk factor profile for lymphoedema is not currently known, a number of factors are thought to predispose an individual to its development and predict progression, severity and outcome of the condition (Table 58.3).

Symptoms and signs

In most cases, the diagnosis of primary or secondary lymphoedema can be made and the condition can be differentiated from other causes of a swollen limb on the basis of history and exami-

Table 58.1 Aetiological classification of lymphoedema.

Primary lymphoedema	Congenital (onset <2 years old): sporadic; familial (Nonne–Milroy's disease)
	Praecox (onset 2–35 years old): sporadic; familial (Letessier–Meige's disease)
	Tarda (onset after 35 years old)
Secondary lymphoedema	Parasitic infection (filariasis)
	Fungal infection (tinea pedis)
	Exposure to foreign body material (silica particles)
	Primary lymphatic malignancy
	Metastatic spread to lymph nodes
	Radiotherapy to lymph nodes
	Surgical excision of lymph nodes
	Trauma (particularly degloving injuries)
	Superficial thrombophlebitis
	Deep venous thrombosis

Table 58.2 Clinical classification of lymphoedema.

Grade (Brunner)	Clinical features
Subclinical (latent)	There is excess interstitial fluid and histological abnormalities in lymphatics and lymph nodes, but no clinically apparent lymphoedema
I	Oedema pits on pressure and swelling largely or completely disappears on elevation and bed rest
II	Oedema does not pit and does not significantly reduce upon elevation, positive Stemmer's sign
III	Oedema is associated with irreversible skin changes, i.e. fibrosis, papillae

nation without recourse to complex investigation (Table 58.4). Unlike other types of oedema, lymphoedema characteristically involves the foot (Figure 58.2). The contour of the ankle is lost through infilling of the submalleolar depressions, a 'buffalo hump' forms on the dorsum of the foot, the toes appear 'square' because of confinement of footwear and the skin on the dorsum of the toes cannot be pinched because of subcutaneous fibrosis (Stemmer's sign). Lymphoedema usually spreads proximally to knee level and less commonly affects the whole leg (Figure 58.3). In the early stages, lymphoedema will 'pit' and the patient will report that the swelling is down in the morning. This represents a reversible component to the swelling, which can be controlled. Failure to do so allows fibrosis, dermal thickening and hyperkeratosis to occur. In general, primary lymphoedema progresses more slowly than secondary lymphoedema. Chronic eczema fungal infection of the skin (dermatophytosis) and nails (onychomycosis), fissuring, verrucae and papillae (warts) are frequently seen in advanced disease. Ulceration is unusual, except in the presence of chronic venous insufficiency.

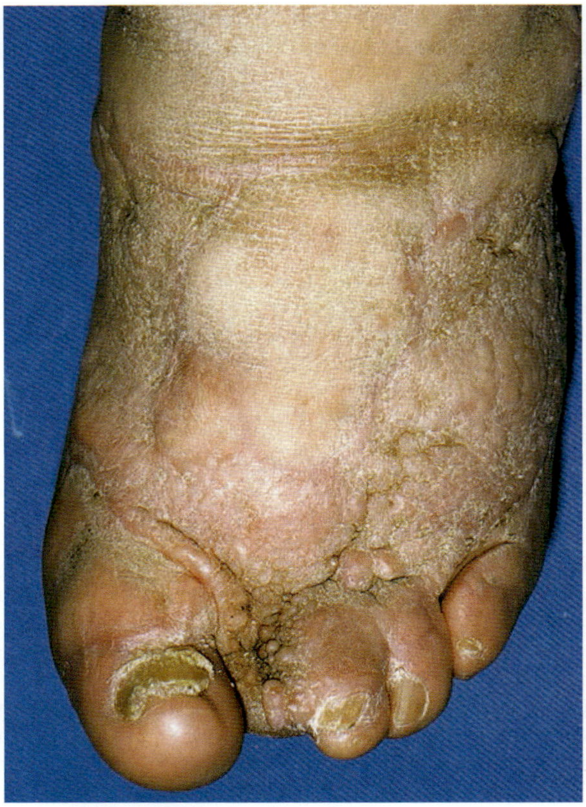

Figure 58.2 The foot of a patient with typical lymphoedema.

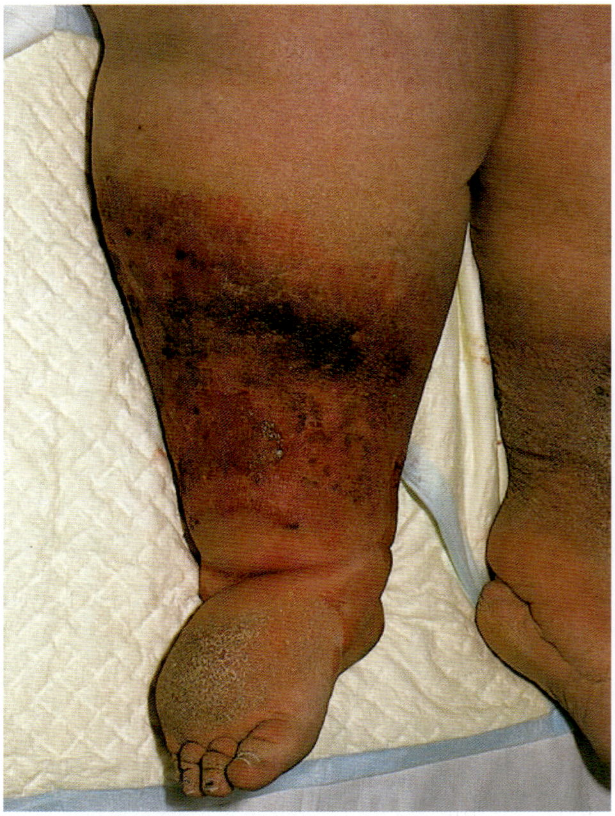

Figure 58.3 The lower leg of a patient with typical lymphoedema.

Table 58.3 Risk factors for lymphoedema.

Upper limb/trunk lymphoedema	Lower limb lymphoedema
Surgery with axillary lymph node dissection, particularly if extensive breast or lymph node surgery	Surgery with inguinal lymph node dissection
Scar formation, fibrosis and radiodermatitis from postoperative axillary radiotherapy	Postoperative pelvic radiotherapy
Radiotherapy to the breast or to the axillary, internal mammary or subclavicular lymph nodes	Recurrent soft tissue infection at the same site
Drain/wound complications or infection	Obesity
Cording (axillary web syndrome)	Varicose vein stripping and vein harvesting
Seroma formation	Genetic predisposition/family history of chronic oedema
Advanced cancer	Advanced cancer
Obesity	Intrapelvic or intra-abdominal tumours that involve or directly compress lymphatic vessels
Congenital predisposition	Orthopaedic surgery
Trauma in an 'at-risk' arm (venepuncture, blood pressure measurement, injection)	Poor nutritional status
Chronic skin disorders and inflammation	Thrombophlebitis and chronic venous insufficiency, particularly post-thrombotic syndrome
Hypertension	Any unresolved asymmetrical oedema
Taxane chemotherapy	Chronic skin disorders and inflammation
Insertion of pacemaker	Concurrent illnesses such as phlebitis, hyperthyroidism, kidney or cardiac disease
Arteriovenous shunt for dialysis	Immobilisation and prolonged limb dependency
Air travel	Air travel
Living in or visiting an area for endemic lymphatic filariasis	Living in or visiting an area for endemic lymphatic filariasis

Reproduced with permission from: Lymphoedema Framework. *Best practice management of lymphoedema*. International Consensus. London: MEP Ltd, 2006. © MEP Ltd 2006.

Lymphangiomas are dilated dermal lymphatics that 'blister' onto the skin surface. The fluid is usually clear but may be blood-stained. In the long term, lymphangiomas thrombose and fibrose, forming hard nodules that may raise concerns about malignancy. If lymphangiomas are <5 cm across, they are termed lymphangioma circumscriptum, and if they are more widespread, they are termed lymphangioma diffusum. If they form a reticulate pattern of ridges then it has been termed lymphoedema *ab igne*. Lymphangiomas frequently weep (lymphorrhoea, chylorrhoea), causing skin maceration, and they act as a portal for infection. Protein-losing diarrhoea, chylous ascites, chylothorax, chyluria and discharge from lymphangiomas suggest lymphangectasia (megalymphatics) and chylous reflux.

Ulceration, non-healing bruises and raised purple-red nodules should lead to suspicion of malignancy. Lymphangiosarcoma was originally described in postmastectomy oedema (Stewart–Treves' syndrome) and affects around 0.5 per cent of patients at a mean onset of ten years. However, lymphangiosarcoma can develop in any long-standing lymphoedema, but usually takes longer to manifest (20 years). It presents as single or multiple bluish/red skin and subcutaneous nodules that spread to form satellite lesions, which may then become confluent. The diagnosis is usually made late and confirmed by skin biopsy. Amputation offers the best chance of survival but, even then, most patients live for less than three years. It has been suggested that lymphoedema leads to an impairment of immune surveillance and so predisposes to other malignancies, although the causal association is not as definite as it is for lymphangiosarcoma (Summary box 58.3).

Fred Waldorf Stewart, 1894–1991, Chairman of Pathology, Memorial Sloan-Kettering Hospital, New York, NY, USA. An annual award was instituted in his name by the Department of Pathology called the Fred Waldorf Stewart Award.

Summary box 58.3

Malignancies associated with lymphoedema

- Lymphangiosarcoma (Stewart–Treves' syndrome)
- Kaposi's sarcoma (HIV)
- Squamous cell carcinoma
- Liposarcoma
- Malignant melanoma
- Malignant fibrous histiocytoma
- Basal cell carcinoma
- Lymphoma

Ab igne is Latin for 'from fire'.
William Morrant Baker, 1839–1896, surgeon, St Bartholomew's Hospital, London, UK, described these cysts in 1877.
Norman Treves, 1894–1964, an American surgeon. He had a special interest in male breast cancer.
Stewart and Treves reported this condition in a joint paper in 1948.

Table 58.4 Differential diagnosis of the swollen limb.

Non-vascular or lymphatic	General disease states	Cardiac failure from any cause
		Liver failure
		Hypoproteinaemia due to nephrotic syndrome, malabsorption, protein-losing enteropathy
		Hypothyroidism (myxoedema)
		Allergic disorders, including angioedema and idiopathic cyclic oedema
		Prolonged immobility and lower limb dependency
	Local disease processes	Ruptured Baker's cyst
		Myositis ossificans
		Bony or soft-tissue tumours
		Arthritis
		Haemarthrosis
		Calf muscle haematoma
		Achilles tendon rupture
	Retroperitoneal fibrosis	May lead to arterial, venous and lymphatic abnormalities
	Gigantism	Rare
		All tissues are uniformly enlarged
	Drugs	Corticosteroids, oestrogens, progestagens
		Monoamine oxidase inhibitors, phenylbutazone, methyldopa, hydralazine, nifedipine
	Trauma	Painful swelling due to reflex sympathetic dystrophy
	Obesity	Lipodystrophy
		Lipoidosis
Venous	Deep venous thrombosis	There may be an obvious predisposing factor, such as recent surgery
		The classical signs of pain and redness may be absent
	Post-thrombotic syndrome	Swelling, usually of the whole leg, due to iliofemoral venous obstruction
		Venous skin changes, secondary varicose veins on the leg and collateral veins on the lower abdominal wall
		Venous claudication may be present
	Varicose veins	Simple primary varicose veins are rarely the cause of significant leg swelling
	Klippel–Trenaunay's syndrome and other malformations	Rare
		Present at birth or develops in early childhood
		Comprises an abnormal lateral venous complex, capillary naevus, bony abnormalities, hypo(a)plasia of deep veins and limb lengthening
		Lymphatic abnormalities often coexist
	External venous compression	Pelvic or abdominal tumour including the gravid uterus
		Retroperitoneal fibrosis
	Ischaemia–reperfusion	Following lower limb revascularisation for chronic and particularly chronic ischaemia
Arterial	Arteriovenous malformation	May be associated with local or generalised swelling
	Aneurysm	Popliteal
		Femoral
		False aneurysm following (iatrogenic) trauma

PRIMARY LYMPHOEDEMA

Aetiology

It has been proposed that all cases of primary lymphoedema are due to an inherited abnormality of the lymphatic system, sometimes termed 'congenital lymphatic dysplasia'. However, it is possible that many sporadic cases of primary lymphoedema occur in the presence of a (near-)normal lymphatic system and are actually examples of secondary lymphoedema for which the triggering events have gone unrecognised. These might include seemingly trivial (but repeated) bacterial and/or fungal infections, insect bites, barefoot walking (silica), deep venous thrombosis (DVT) or episodes of superficial thrombophlebitis. In animal models, simple excision of lymph nodes and/or trunks leads to acute lymphoedema, which resolves within a few weeks, presumably because of the development of collaterals. The human condition can only be mimicked by inducing extensive lymphatic obliteration and fibrosis. Even then, there may be considerable delay between the injury and the onset of oedema. Primary lymphoedema is much more common in the legs than the arms. This may be because of gravity and a bipedal posture, the fact that the lymphatic system of the leg is less well developed, or the increased susceptibility of the leg to trauma and/or infection. Furthermore, loss of the venoarteriolar reflex (VAR), which protects lower limb capillaries from excessive hydrostatic forces in the erect posture, with age and disease (CVI, diabetes), may be important.

Classification

Primary lymphoedema is usually classified on the basis of apparent genetic susceptibility, age of onset or lymphangiographic findings. None of these is ideal and the various classification systems in existence can appear confusing and conflicting as various terms and eponyms are used loosely and interchangeably. This has hampered research and efforts to gain a better understanding of underlying mechanisms, the effectiveness of therapy and prognosis.

Genetic susceptibility

Primary lymphoedema is often subdivided into those cases in which there appears to be a genetic susceptibility or element to the disease, and those in which there is not. The former may be further divided into those cases that are familial (hereditary), when typically the only abnormality is lymphoedema and there is a family history, and those cases that are syndromic, when the lymphoedema is only one of several congenital abnormalities and is either inherited or sporadic. Syndromic lymphoedema may be sporadic and chromosomal (Turner's (XO karyotype), Klinefelter's (XXY), Down's (trisomy 21) syndrome) or clearly inherited and related to an identified or presumed single-gene defect (lymphoedema–distichiasis (autosomal dominant defect in *FOXC2* gene)), or of uncertain genetic aetiology (yellow-nail and Klippel–Trenaunay–Weber's syndromes). Familial (hereditary) lymphoedema can be difficult to distinguish from non-familial lymphoedema because a reliable family history may be unobtainable, the nature of the genetic predisposition is unknown and the genetic susceptibility may only translate into clinical disease in the presence of certain environmental factors. Although the distinction may not directly affect treatment, the patients are often concerned lest they be 'passing on' the disease to their children.

Two main forms of familial (hereditary) lymphoedema are recognised – Nonne–Milroy (type I) and Letessier–Meige (type II) – although it is likely that both eponymous diseases overlap and represent more than a single disease entity and genetic abnormality. Milroy's disease is estimated to be present in 1 in 6000 live births and is probably inherited in an autosomal dominant manner with incomplete (about 50 per cent) penetrance. In some families, the condition may be related to abnormalities in the gene coding for a vascular endothelial growth factor receptor 3 (VEGFR3) on chromosome 5. The disease is characterised by brawny lymphoedema of both legs (and sometimes the genitalia, arms and face), which develops from birth or before puberty. The disease has been associated with a wide range of lymphatic abnormalities on lymphangiography. Meige's disease is similar to Milroy's disease, except that the lymphoedema generally develops between puberty and middle age (50 years). It usually affects one or both legs but may involve the arms. Some, but not all, cases appear to be inherited in an autosomal dominant manner. Lymphangiography generally shows aplasia or hypoplasia.

Age of onset

Lymphoedema congenita (onset at or within two years of birth) is more common in males and is more likely to be bilateral and involve the whole leg. Lymphoedema praecox (onset from 2 to 35 years) is three times more common in females, has a peak incidence shortly after menarche, is three times more likely to be unilateral than bilateral and usually only extends to the knee. Lymphoedema tarda develops, by definition, after the age of 35 years and is often associated with obesity, with lymph nodes being replaced with fibrofatty tissue. The cause is unknown. Lymphoedema developing for the first time after 50 years should prompt a thorough search for underlying (pelvic, genitalia) malignancy. It is worth noting that, in such patients, lymphoedema often commences proximally in the thigh rather than distally (Figure 58.4).

Lymphangiographic classification

Browse has classified primary lymphoedema on the basis of lymphangiographic findings (Table 58.5 and Figures 58.5 and 58.6). These findings may be related to the clinical presentations described above. Some patients with lymphatic hyperplasia possess megalymphatics in which lymph or chyle refluxes freely under the effects of gravity against the physiological direction of flow. The megalymphatics usually end in thin-walled vesicles on the skin, serous surfaces (chylous ascites, chylothorax), intestine (protein-losing enteropathy), kidney or bladder (chyluria) (Figure 58.7).

SECONDARY LYMPHOEDEMA

This is the most common form of lymphoedema. There are several well-recognised causes including infection, inflammation, neoplasia and trauma (Table 58.6).

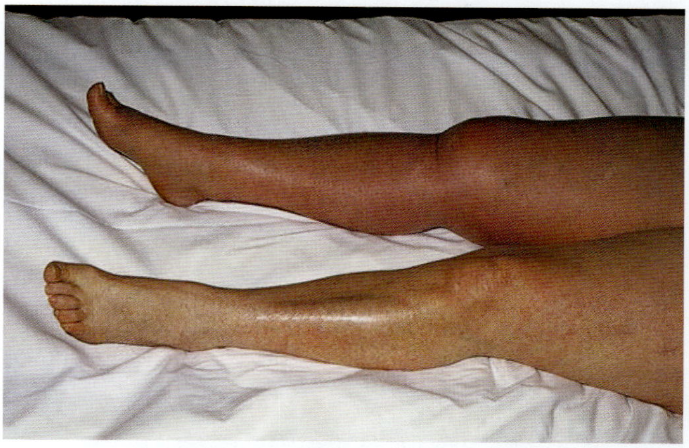

Figure 58.4 This patient, in her sixth decade, presented with rapid onset of lymphoedema of the right leg. On further investigation she was found to have locally advanced bladder carcinoma. Note that unlike most cases of lymphoedema the swelling is greater proximally than distally.

Sir Norman Leslie Browse, formerly Professor of Surgery, the United Medical and Dental Schools of Guy's and St Thomas's Hospitals, London, UK; former President of the Royal College of Surgeons of England.

Henry Hubert Turner, 1892–1970, Professor of Medicine, The University of Oklahoma, OK, USA.
Harry Fitch Klinefelter, Jr, born 1912, Associate Professor of Medicine, The Johns Hopkins University Medical School, Baltimore MD, USA, described this syndrome in 1942.
John Langdon Haydon Down (sometimes given as Langdon-Down), 1828–1896, physician, The London Hospital, London, UK.
Max Nonne, 1861–1959, a neurologist of Hamburg, Germany, described this disease in 1891.
William Forsyth Milroy, 1855–1942, Professor of Clinical Medicine, Columbia University, New York, NY, USA, described the condition in 1892.
Henri Meige, 1866–1940, physician, La Salpêtrière, Paris, France, gave his description of the disease in 1899.

Table 58.5 Lymphangiographic classification of primary lymphoedema.

	Congenital hyperplasia (10%)	Distal obliteration (80%)	Proximal obliteration (10%)
Age of onset	Congenital	Puberty (praecox)	Any age
Sex distribution	Male > female	Female > male	Male = female
Extent	Whole leg	Ankle, calf	Whole leg, thigh only
Laterality	Unilateral = bilateral	Often bilateral	Usually unilateral
Family history	Often positive	Often positive	No
Progression	Progressive	Slow	Rapid
Response to compression therapy	Variable	Good	Poor
Comments	Lymphatics are increased in number; although functionally defective, there is usually an increased number of lymph nodes. May have chylous ascites, chylothorax and protein-losing enteropathy	Absent or reduced distal superficial lymphatics. Also termed aplasia or hypoplasia	There is obstruction at the level of the aortoiliac or inguinal nodes. If associated with distal dilatation, the patient may benefit from lymphatic bypass operation. Other patients have distal obliteration as well

Filariasis

This is the most common cause of lymphoedema worldwide, affecting up to 100 million individuals. It is particularly prevalent in Africa, India and South America where 5–10 per cent of the population may be affected. The viviparous nematode *Wucheria bancrofti*, whose only host is man, is responsible for 90 per cent of cases and is spread by the mosquito. The disease is associated with poor sanitation. The parasite enters lymphatics from the blood and lodges in lymph nodes, where it causes fibrosis and obstruction, due partly to direct physical damage and partly to the immune response of the host. Proximal lymphatics become grossly dilated with adult parasites. The degree of oedema is often massive, in which case it is termed elephantiasis (Figure 58.8). Immature parasites (microfilariae) enter the blood at night and can be identified on a blood smear, in a centrifuged specimen of urine or in lymph itself. A complement fixation test is also available and is positive in present or past infection. Eosinophilia is usually present. Diethylcarbamazine destroys the parasites but does not reverse the lymphatic changes, although there may be some regression over time. Once the infection has been cleared, treatment is as for primary lymphoedema. Public health measures to reduce mosquito breeding, protective clothing and mosquito netting may be usefully employed to combat the condition (Summary box 58.4).

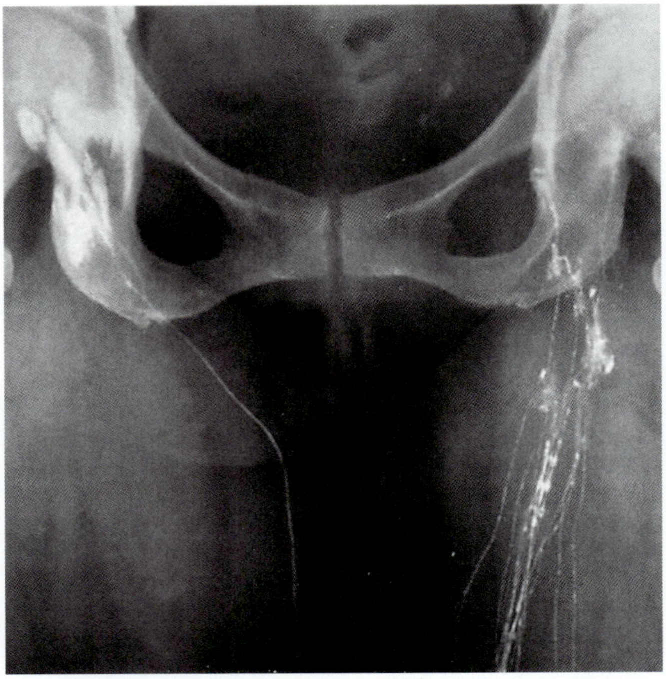

Figure 58.5 This patient presented with congenital lymphoedema of the right leg. The lymphangiogram shows lymphatic hypoplasia.

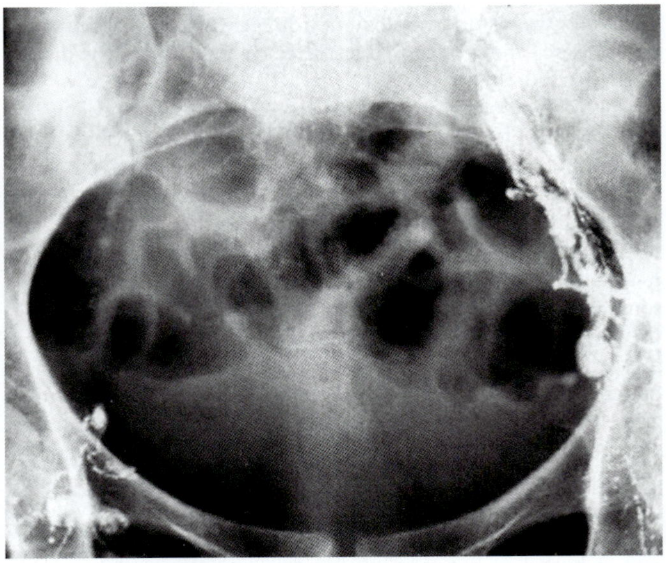

Figure 58.6 This patient presented with lymphoedema of the right leg. A bipedal lymphangiogram demonstrated normal lymphatics in the right leg up to the inguinal nodes, but no progression of contrast above the inguinal ligament – a case of proximal obstruction.

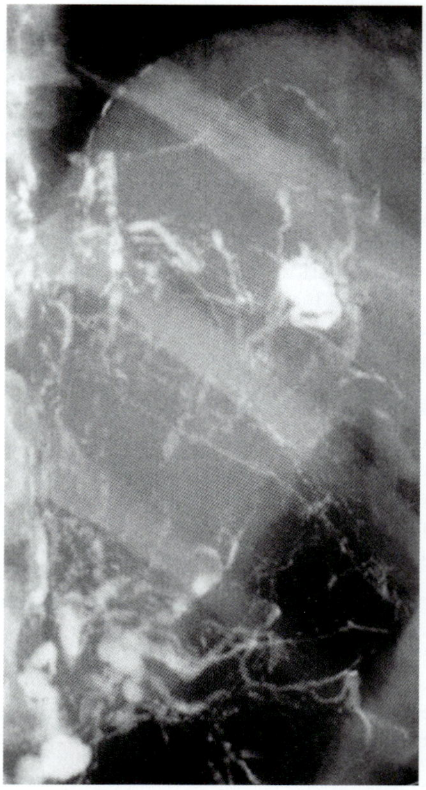

Figure 58.7 Lymphangiogram demonstrating reflux from dilated para-aortic vessels into the left kidney in a patient with filariasis who presented with chyluria.

Summary box 58.4

Features of filariasis

Acute
- Fever
- Headache
- Malaise
- Inguinal and axillary lymphadenitis
- Lymphangitis
- Cellulitis, abscess formation and ulceration
- Funiculo-epididymo-orchitis

Chronic
- Lymphoedema of legs (arm, breast)
- Hydrocoele
- Abdominal lymphatic varices
  - Chyluria
  - Lymphuria

Endemic elephantiasis (podoconiosis)

This is common in the tropics and affects more than 500 000 people in Africa. The barefoot cultivation of soil composed of alkaline volcanic rocks leads to destruction of the peripheral lymphatics by particles of silica, which can be seen in macrophages in draining lymph nodes. Plantar oedema develops in childhood and rapidly spreads proximally. The condition is prevented and its progression is slowed by the wearing of shoes.

Table 58.6 Classification of causes of secondary lymphoedema.

Classification	Example(s)
Trauma and tissue damage	Lymph node excision
	Radiotherapy
	Burns
	Variscose vein surgery/harvesting
	Large/circumferential wounds
	Scarring
Malignant disease	Lymph node metastases
	Infiltrative carcinoma
	Lymphoma
	Pressure from large tumours
Venous disease	Chronic venous insufficiency
	Venous ulceration
	Post-thrombotic syndrome
	Intravenous drug use
Infection	Cellulitis/erysipelas
	Lymphadenitis
	Tuberculosis
	Filariasis
Inflammation	Rheumatoid arthritis
	Dermatitis
	Psoriasis
	Sarcoidosis
	Dermatosis with epidermal involvement
Endocrine disease	Pretibial myxoedema
Immobility and dependency	Dependency oedema
	Paralysis
Factitious	Self-harm

Reproduced with permission from: Lymphoedema Framework. *Best practice management of lymphoedema*. International Consensus. London: MEP Ltd, 2006. © MEP Ltd 2006.

Bacterial infection

Lymphangitis and lymphadenitis can cause lymphatic destruction that predisposes to lymphoedema complicated by further acute inflammatory episodes. Interestingly, in such patients, lymphangiography has revealed abnormalities in the contralateral, unaffected limb, suggesting an underlying, possibly inherited, susceptibility. Lymphatic and lymph node destruction by tuberculosis is also a well-recognised cause of lymphoedema, especially in developing countries.

Malignancy and its treatment

Treatment (surgery, radiotherapy) for breast carcinoma is the most common cause of lymphoedema in developed countries, but is decreasing in incidence as surgery becomes more conservative (see Chapter 53). Lymphoma may present with lymphoedema, as may malignancy of the pelvic organs and external genitalia. Kaposi's sarcoma developing in the course of human immunodeficiency virus (HIV)-related illness may cause lymphatic obstruction and is a growing cause of lymphoedema in certain parts of the world.

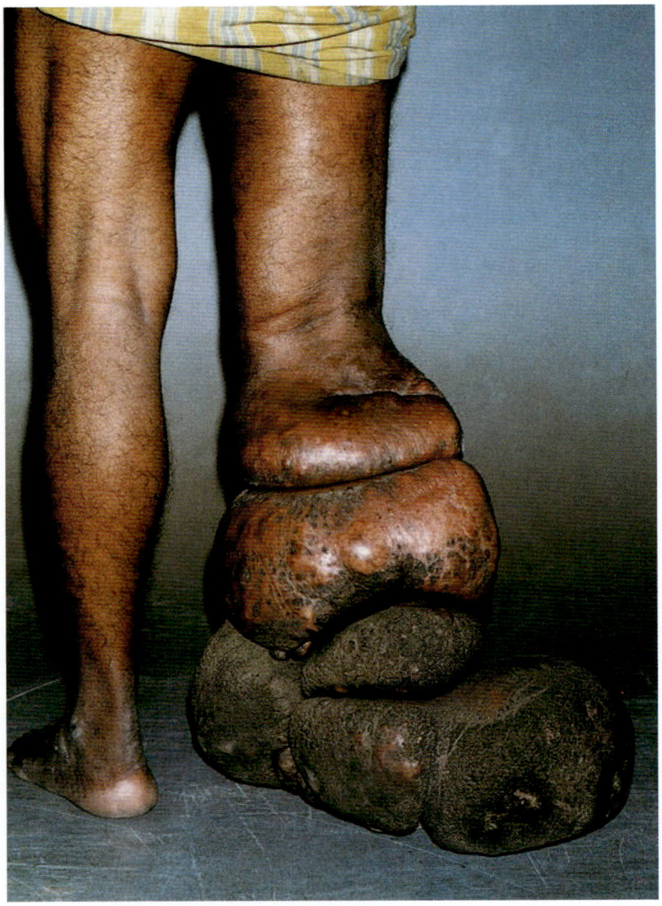

Figure 58.8 Elephantiasis due to filariasis.

Trauma

It is not unusual for patients to develop chronic localised or generalised swelling following trauma. The aetiology is often multifactorial and includes disuse, venous thrombosis and lymphatic injury or destruction. Degloving injuries and burns are particularly likely to disrupt dermal lymphatics. Tenosynovitis can also be associated with localised subcutaneous lymphoedema, which can be a cause of troublesome persistent swelling following ankle and wrist 'sprains' and repetitive strain injury.

Lymphoedema and chronic venous insufficiency

It is important to appreciate the relationship between lymphoedema and CVI as both conditions are relatively common and so often coexist in the same patient, and it can be difficult to unravel which components of the patient's symptom complex are caused by each. There is no doubt that superficial venous thrombophlebitis (SVT) and DVT can both lead to lymphatic destruction and secondary lymphoedema, especially if recurrent. Lymphoedema is an important contributor to the swelling of the postphlebitic syndrome. It has also been suggested that lymphoedema can predispose to DVT, and possible SVT, through immobility and acute inflammatory episodes. Certainly, tests of venous function (duplex ultrasonography, plethysmography) are frequently abnormal in patients with lymphoedema.

It is not uncommon to see patients (usually women) with lymphoedema in whom a duplex ultrasound scan has revealed superficial reflux (such reflux is present subclinically in up to one-third of the adult population). Although isolated, superficial venous reflux rarely, if ever, leads to limb swelling; such patients are frequently misdiagnosed as having venous disease rather than lymphoedema, and are subjected mistakenly to varicose vein surgery. Not only will such surgery invariably fail to relieve the swelling, it will usually make it worse as saphenofemoral and saphenopopliteal ligation, together with saphenous stripping, will compromise still further drainage through the subcutaneous lymph bundles (which follow the major superficial veins) and draining inguinal and popliteal lymph nodes.

Miscellaneous conditions

Rheumatoid and psoriatic arthritis (chronic inflammation and lymph node fibrosis), contact dermatitis, snake and insect bites, and retroperitoneal fibrosis are all rare but well-documented causes of lymphoedema. Pretibial myxoedema is due to the obliteration of initial lymphatics by mucin.

Conditions mimicking lymphoedema

Factitious lymphoedema

This is caused by application of a tourniquet (a 'rut' and sharp cut-off is seen on examination) or 'hysterical' disuse in patients with psychological and psychiatric problems.

Immobility

Generalised or localised immobility of any cause leads to chronic limb swelling that can be misdiagnosed as lymphoedema, for example the elderly person who spends all day (and sometimes all night) sitting in a chair (armchair legs), the hemiplegic stroke patient and the young patient with multiple sclerosis.

Lipoedema

This presents almost exclusively in women and comprises bilateral, usually symmetrical, enlargement of the legs and, sometimes, the lower half of the body because of the abnormal deposition of fat. It may or may not be associated with generalised obesity. There are a number of features that help to differentiate the condition from lymphoedema but, of course, lipoedema may coexist with other causes of limb swelling. It has been proposed that lipoedema results from, or at least is associated with, fatty obliteration of lymphatics and lymph nodes (Summary box 58.5).

INVESTIGATION OF LYMPHOEDEMA

Are investigations necessary?

It is usually possible to diagnose and manage lymphoedema purely on the basis of history and examination, especially when the swelling is mild and there are no apparent complicating features. In patients with severe, atypical and multifactorial swelling, investigations may help confirm the diagnosis, inform management and provide prognostic information.

'Routine' tests

These include a full blood count, urea and electrolytes, creati-

Summary box 58.5

Features of lipoedema that help differentiate it from lymphoedema

- Occurs almost exclusively in women
- Onset nearly always coincides with puberty
- Nearly always bilateral and symmetrical
- Involvement of trunk
- The feet are not involved, leading to an inverse shouldering effect at the malleoli
- No pitting
- No response to elevation or compression
- No skin changes of lymphoedema (negative Stemmer's sign)
- MRI shows subcutanteous fat but no fluid accumulation

nine, liver function tests, thyroid function tests, plasma total protein and albumin, fasting glucose, C-reactive protein, urine dipstick including observation for chyluria, blood smear for microfilariae, chest radiograph and ultrasound.

Lymphangiography

Direct lymphangiography involves the injection of contrast medium into a peripheral lymphatic vessel and subsequent radiographic visualisation of the vessels and nodes. It remains the 'gold standard' for showing structural abnormalities of larger lymphatics and nodes (Figure 58.9). However, it can be technically difficult, it is unpleasant for the patient, it may cause further lymphatic injury and, largely, it has become obsolete as a routine method of investigation. Few centres now perform this technique and those that do generally reserve it for preoperative evaluation of the rare patient with megalymphatics who is being considered for bypass or fistula ligation. Indirect lymphangiography involves the intradermal injection of water-soluble, non-ionic contrast into a web space, from where it is taken up by lymphatics and then followed radiographically. It will show distal lymphatics but not normally proximal lymphatics and nodes.

Isotope lymphoscintigraphy

This has largely replaced lymphangiography as the primary diagnostic technique in cases of clinical uncertainty. Radioactive technetium-labelled protein or colloid particles are injected into an interdigital web space and specifically taken up by lymphatics, and serial radiographs are taken with a gamma camera. The technique provides a qualitative measure of lymphatic function rather than quantitative function or anatomical detail. Quantitative lymphoscintigraphy is performed using a dynamic (exercise) component in addition to the static test and provides information on lymphatic transport.

Computed tomography

A single, axial computed tomography (CT) slice through the midcalf has been proposed as a useful diagnostic test for lymphoedema (coarse, non-enhancing, reticular 'honeycomb' pattern in an enlarged subcutaneous compartment), venous oedema (increased volume of the muscular compartment) and lipoedema (increased subcutaneous fat). CT can also be used to exclude pelvic or abdominal mass lesions.

Magnetic resonance imaging

Magnetic resonance imaging (MRI) can provide clear images of lymphatic channels and lymph nodes, and can be useful in the assessment of patients with lymphatic hyperplasia. MRI can also distinguish venous and lymphatic causes of a swollen limb, and detect tumours that may be causing lymphatic obstruction.

Ultrasound

Ultrasound can provide useful information about venous function including DVT and venous abnormalities.

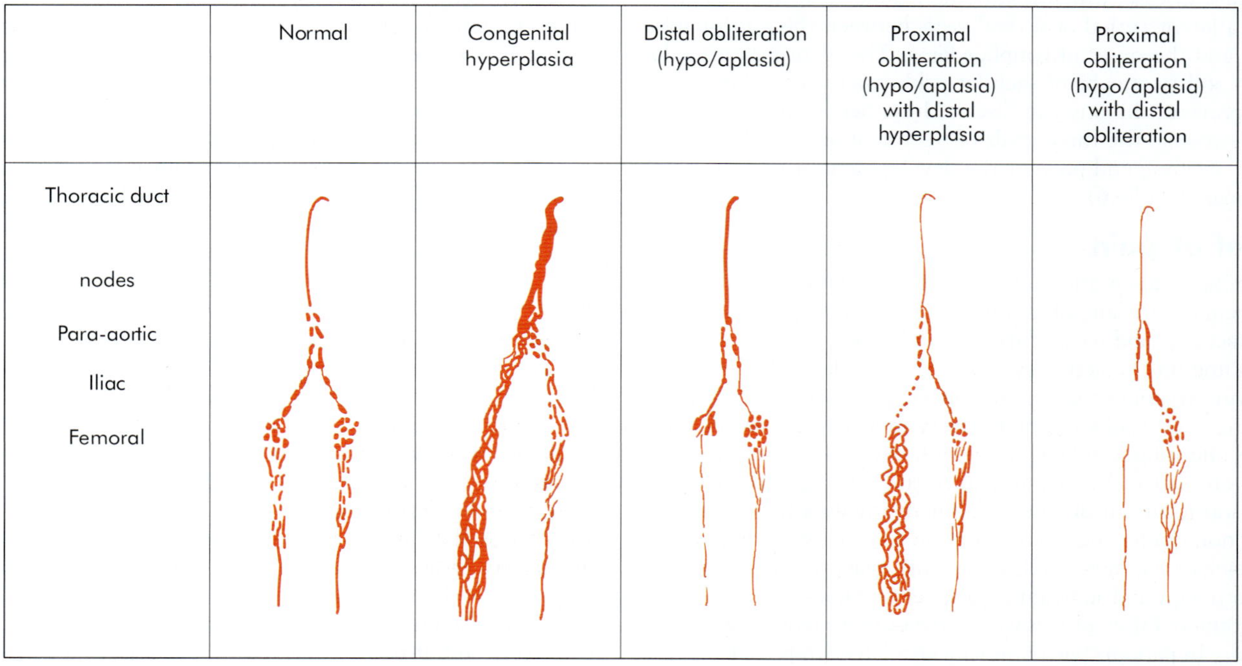

Figure 58.9 Lymphangiographic patterns of primary lymphoedema.

Pathological examination

In cases in which malignancy is suspected, samples of lymph nodes may be obtained by fine-needle aspiration, needle core biopsy or surgical excision. Skin biopsy will confirm the diagnosis of lymphangiosarcoma.

Limb volume measurement

While not helpful in the diagnosis of lymphoedema, limb volume measurement is a useful tool to determine severity of lymphoedema, guide management and assess response to treatment. Limb volume is typically measured at diagnosis, following intensive treatment and at follow up. In unilateral limb swelling the affected side can be compared to the contralateral unaffected limb. In bilateral swelling the volume of both limbs is tracked with time. Measurements are recorded in millilitres or expressed as a percentage of the normal limb. Water plethysmography (water displacement) is the 'gold standard' method but is limited by practicalities of measurement and hygiene issues. Other options include circumferential limb measurements and perometry (infrared light beams measure the outline of the limb to calculate volume).

MANAGEMENT OF LYMPHOEDEMA

Overview

The evaluation of the lymphoedema patient needs to be 'holistic' and their care delivered by a multiprofessional team comprising physical therapists, nurses, orthotists, physicians (dermatologists, oncologists, palliative care specialists), surgeons and social service professionals. Although surgery itself has a very small role, surgeons (especially those with breast and vascular interests) are frequently asked to oversee the management of these patients. Early diagnosis and institution of management are essential because at that stage relatively simple measures can be highly effective and will prevent the development of disabling late-stage disease, which is extremely difficult to treat. There is often a latent period of several years between the precipitating event and the onset of lymphoedema. The identification, education and treatment of such 'at-risk' patients can slow down, even prevent, the onset of disease. In patients with established lymphoedema, the three goals of treatment are to relieve pain, reduce swelling and prevent the development of complications (Summary box 58.6).

Relief of pain

On initial presentation, 50 per cent of patients with lymphoedema complain of significant pain. The pain is usually multifactorial and its severity and underlying cause(s) will vary depending on the aetiology of the lymphoedema. For example, following treatment for breast cancer, pain may arise from the swelling itself (radiation and surgery induced); nerve (brachial plexus and intercostobrachial nerve), bone (secondary deposits, radiation necrosis) and joint (arthritis, bursitis, capsulitis) disease; and recurrent disease. Treatment involves the considered use of non-opioid and opioid analgesics, corticosteroids, tricyclic antidepressants, muscle relaxants, anti-epileptics, nerve blocks, physiotherapy and adjuvant anticancer therapies (chemo-, radio- and hormonal therapy), as well as measures to reduce swelling if possible. In patients with non-cancer-related lymphoedema, the best way to reduce pain is to control swelling and prevent the development of complications. Whatever the cause, pain is a somatopsychic experience that is affected by mood and morale. These issues are important in patients with both cancer-related lymphoedema, who are concerned about recurrent disease, and non-cancer-related disease, who often have poor self-esteem and problems with body image and perception.

Summary box 58.6

Initial evaluation of the patient with lymphoedema

- History (age of onset, location, progression, exacerbating and relieving features)
- Past medical history including cancer history
- Family history
- Obesity (diet, height and weight, body mass index)
- Complications (venous, arterial, skin, joint, neurological, malignant)
- Assessment of physical, emotional and psychosocial symptoms
- Social circumstances (mobility, housing, education, work)
- Special needs (footwear, clothing, compression garments, pneumatic devices, mobility aids)
- Previous and current treatment
- Pain control
- Compliance with therapy and ability to self-care

Control of swelling

Physical therapy for lymphoedema comprising bed rest, elevation, bandaging, compression garments, massage and exercises was first described at the end of the nineteenth century, and through the twentieth century various eponymous schools developed. Although there is little doubt that physical therapy can be highly effective in reducing swelling, its general acceptance and practice has been hampered by a lack of proper research and confusing terminology. The current preferred term is decongestive lymphoedema therapy (DLT), which comprises two phases. The first is a short intensive period of therapist-led care and the second is a maintenance phase in which the patient uses a self-care regimen with occasional professional intervention. The intensive phase comprises skin care, manual lymphatic drainage (MLD) and multi-layer lymphoedema bandaging (MLLB), and exercises. The length of intensive treatment will depend upon the disease severity, the degree of patient compliance and the willingness and ability of the patient to take more responsibility for the maintenance phase. However, weeks rather than months should be the goal.

Skin care

The patient must be carefully educated in the principles and practice of skin care. The patient should inspect the affected skin daily, with special attention paid to skinfolds, where maceration may occur. The limb should be washed daily; the use of bath oil, e.g. Balneum, is recommended as a moisturiser and the limb must be carefully dried afterwards. A hair drier on low heat is more effective and hygienic, and less traumatic, than a towel. If the skin is in good condition daily application of a bland emollient, e.g. aqueous cream, is recommended to keep the skin hydrated. If the skin is dry and flaky then a bland ointment, e.g. 50:50 white soft paraffin/liquid paraffin (WSP/LP), should be used twice daily and, if there is marked hyperkeratosis, a keratolytic agent, such as 5 per cent salicylic acid, should be added. Many commercially available soaps, creams and lotions contain sensitisers, e.g. lanolin in E45 cream, and are best avoided as patients with lymphoedema are highly susceptible to contact dermatitis (eczema). Apart from causing intense discomfort, eczema acts as an entry point for infection. Management comprises avoidance of the allergen (patch testing may be required) and topical corticosteroids. Fungal infections are common, difficult to eradicate and predispose to acute inflammatory episodes. Chronic application of antifungal creams leads to maceration and it is better to use powders in shoes and socks. Ointment containing 3 per cent benzoic acid helps prevent athlete's foot and can be used safely over long periods. Painting at-risk areas with an antiseptic agent such as eosin may be helpful. Lymphorrhoea is uncommon but extremely troublesome. Management comprises emollients, elevation, compression and sometimes cautery under anaesthetic (Summary box 58.7).

Summary box 58.7

Skin care

- Protect hands when washing up or gardening; wear a thimble when sewing
- Never walk barefoot and wear protective footwear outside
- Use an electric razor to depilate
- Never let the skin become macerated
- Treat cuts and grazes promptly (wash, dry, apply antiseptic and a plaster)
- Use insect repellent sprays and treat bites promptly with antiseptics and antihistamines
- Seek medical attention as soon as the limb becomes hot, painful or more swollen
- Do not allow blood to be taken from, or injections to be given into, an affected arm (and avoid blood pressure measurement)
- Protect the affected skin from sun (shade, high-factor sun block)
- Consider taking antibiotics if going on holiday

Apart from lymphangiosarcoma, acute inflammatory episodes are probably the most serious complications of lymphoedema and frequently lead to emergency hospital admission. About 25 per cent of primary and 5 per cent of secondary lymphoedema patients are affected. Acute inflammatory episodes start rapidly, often without warning or a precipitating event, with tingling, pain and redness of the limb. Patients feel 'viral' and severe attacks can lead to the rapid onset of fever, rigors, headache, vomiting and delirium. Patients who have suffered previous attacks can usually predict the onset and many learn to carry antibiotics with them and self-medicate at the first hint of trouble. This may stave off a full-blown attack and prevent the further lymphatic injury that each acute inflammatory episode causes. It is rarely possible to isolate a responsible bacterium but the majority are presumed to be caused by group A β-haemolytic streptococci and/or staphylococci. The diagnosis is usually obvious but dermatitis, thrombophlebitis and DVT are in the differential diagnosis. Oral amoxycillin is the treatment of choice with erythromycin or clarithromycin in those with penicillin allergy. Flucloxacillin should be added for those with evidence of *S. aureus* infection (folliculitis, crusted dermatitis). Oral clindamycin is a second line agent for those with failure to respond to initial therapy. Hospital admission is required for patients with: signs of septicaemia; continuing or deteriorating systemic signs after 48 hours of antibiotic treament; unresolving or deteriorating local signs despite trials of first- and second-line antibiotics. Intravenous amoxycillin or benzyl penicillin with clindamycin in penicillin-allergic patients or as second-line therapy is most commonly recommended. Bed rest will reduce lymphatic drainage and the spread of infection, elevation will reduce the oedema and heparin prophylaxis will reduce the risk of DVT. Analgesia is often required but non-steroidal anti-inflammatories (NSAIDs) should be avoided as they have been associated with increased complications including necrotising fasciitis. Any lymphatic massage should be ceased in the presence of active infection. Amoxycillin can be taken by patients who self-medicate. The use of long-term prophylactic antibiotics is not evidence based, but penicillin V 500 mg daily is probably reasonable in patients who suffer two or more attacks per year. However, the benefits of scrupulous compliance with physical therapy and skin care cannot be underestimated.

Manual lymphatic drainage

Several different techniques of MLD have been described and the details are beyond the scope of this chapter. However, they all aim to evacuate fluid and protein from the interstitial space and stimulate lymphangion contraction with decongestion of impaired lymphatic pathways and development of collateral routes. The therapist should perform MLD daily; they should also train the patient (and/or carer) to perform a simpler, modified form of massage termed simple lymphatic drainage (SLD). In the intensive phase, SLD supplements MLD and, once the maintenance phase is entered, SLD will carry on as daily massage.

Multilayer lymphoedema bandaging and compression garments

Elastic bandages provide compression, produce a sustained high resting pressure and 'follow in' as limb swelling reduces. However, the sub-bandage pressure does not alter greatly in response to changes in limb circumference consequent upon muscular activity and posture. By contrast, short-stretch bandages exert support through the production of a semi-rigid casing where the resting pressure is low but changes quite markedly in response to movement and posture. This pressure variation produces a massaging effect within the limb and stimulates lymph flow. Whether the aim is to provide support or compression, the pressure exerted must be graduated (100 per cent ankle/foot, 70 per cent knee, 50 per cent mid-thigh, 40 per cent groin).

Non-invasive assessment of the ankle–brachial pressure index (ABPI) using a hand-held Doppler ultrasound device is usually necessary prior to commencing any form of compression therapy, as it is rarely possible to feel pulses in the lymphoedematous limb. Standard MLLB and compression is used in patients with ABPI ≥0.8 and modified techniques with lower pressures in those with moderate arterial disease (ABPI 0.5–0.8). MLLB is contraindicated in severe arterial insufficiency (ABPI <0.5), uncontrolled heart failure and severe peripheral neuropathy.

It is generally believed that non-elastic MLLB is preferable (and arguably safer) in patients with severe swelling during the intensive phase of DLT (Summary box 58.8), whereas compression (hosiery, sleeves) is preferable in milder cases and during the maintenance phase. MLLB is highly skilled and to be effective and safe it needs to be applied by a specially trained therapist. It is also extremely labour intensive, needing to be changed daily.

Summary box 58.8

Effects of MLLB

- Reduces oedema
- Restores shape to the affected area
- Reduces skin changes (hyperkeratosis, papillomatosis)
- Eliminates lymphorrhoea
- Supports inelastic skin
- Softens subcutaneous tissues

Compression garments form the mainstay of management in most clinics. The control of lymphoedema requires higher pressures (30–40 mmHg arm, 40–60 mmHg leg) than are typically used to treat CVI. These may be reduced to 15–25 mmHg in those with moderate arterial insufficiency (Figure 58.10). Confusingly, the British (classes I: 14–17 mmHg; II: 18–24 mmHg; III: 25–35 mmHg) and international (USA) (classes I: 20–30 mmHg; II: 30–40 mmHg; III: 40–50 mmHg; IV: 50–60 mmHg) standards are different. The patient should put the stocking on first thing in the morning before rising. It can be difficult to persuade patients to comply. Putting lymphoedema-grade stockings on and off is difficult and many patients find them intolerably uncomfortable, especially in warm climates. Furthermore, although intellectually they understand the benefits, emotionally they may find wearing them presents a greater body image problem than the swelling itself.

Enthusiasm for pneumatic compression devices has waxed and waned. Unless the device being used allows the sequential inflation of multiple chambers up to >50 mmHg, it will probably be ineffective for lymphoedema. The benefits to the patient are maximised and complications are minimised if these devices are used under the direction of a physical therapist as part of an overall package of care.

Exercise

Lymph formation is directly proportional to arterial inflow and 40 per cent of lymph is formed within skeletal muscle. Vigorous exercise, especially if it is anaerobic and isometric, will tend to exacerbate lymphoedema and patients should be advised to avoid prolonged static activities, for example carrying heavy shopping bags or prolonged standing. In contrast, slow, rhythmic isotonic movements (e.g. swimming) and massage will increase venous and lymphatic return through the production of movement between skin and underlying tissues (essential to the filling of initial lymphatics) and augmentation of the muscle pumps. Exercise also helps to maintain joint mobility. Patients who are unable to move their limbs benefit from passive exercises. When at rest, the lymphoedematous limb should be positioned with the foot/hand above the level of the heart. A pillow under the mattress or blocks under the bottom of the bed will encourage the swelling to go down overnight.

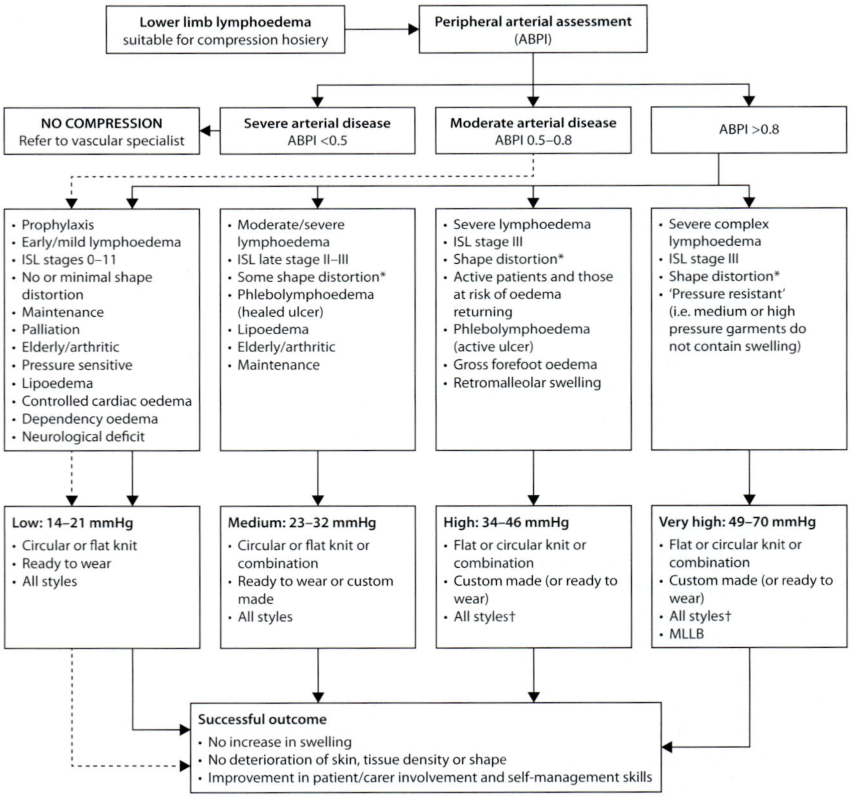

*For patients with shape distortion, flat knit hosiery is often preferable.
†Including inelastic adjustable compression device.

Figure 58.10 Compression garments for lower limb oedema and lymphovenous oedema. Reproduced with permission from: Lymphoedema Framework. *Best Practice Management of Lymphoedema*. International Consensus. London: MEP Ltd, 2006. © MEP Ltd 2006.

Drugs

There are considerable, and scientifically inexplicable, differences in the use of specific drugs for venous disease and lymphoedema between different countries. The benzpyrones are a group of several thousand naturally occurring substances, of which the flavonoids have received the most attention. Enthusiasts will argue that a number of clinical trials have shown benefit from these compounds, which are purported to reduce capillary permeability, improve microcirculatory perfusion, stimulate interstitial macrophage proteolysis, reduce erythrocyte and platelet aggregation, scavenge free radicals and exert an anti-inflammatory effect. Detractors will argue that the trials are small and poorly controlled with short follow up and 'soft' end points, and that any benefits observed can be explained by a placebo effect. In the UK, oxerutins (Paroven®) are the only such drugs licensed for venous disease and none has a license for lymphoedema. Diuretics are of no value in pure lymphoedema. Their chronic use is associated with side effects, including electrolyte disturbance, and should be avoided.

With increasing understanding of lymphangiogenesis pathways there is hope that specific pharmacological targets or gene therapy may become available in the future but this remains in the very early stages at present.

Surgery

Only a small minority of patients with lymphoedema benefit from surgery. Operations fall into three categories: bypass procedures, liposuction and reduction procedures.

Bypass procedures

The rare patient with proximal ilioinguinal lymphatic obstruction and normal distal lymphatic channels might benefit, at least in theory, from lymphatic bypass. A number of methods have been described including the omental pedicle, the skin bridge (Gillies), anastomosing lymph nodes to veins (Neibulowitz) and the ileal mucosal patch (Kinmonth). More recently, direct lymphaticovenular anastomosis (LVA) has been carried out on vessels of 0.3–0.8 mm diameter using supermicrosurgical techniques. The procedures are technically demanding and not without morbidity. They are more ofen attempted in the upper limb following lymph node resection or radiotherapy for breast cancer. The outcomes are best in patients with earlier stages of lymphoedema for whom the majority can be controlled with best medical therapy alone. In those with later stage disease who have failed conservative management, the outcomes of LVA have generally been disappointing.

Liposuction

Liposuction has been used in the treament of chronic lymphoedema. It is usually reserved for patients who have progressed to non-pitting oedema. Case series reported thus far have shown promising results with more than 100 per cent reduction in limb oedema volume which can be maintained by ongoing use of compression hosiery for at least one year. While liposuction appears to be safe, results of long-term efficacy and effects on the incidence of future lymphoedema complications (e.g. infection) are awaited.

Sir Harold Delf Gilles, 1882–1960, plastic surgeon, St Bartholomew's Hospital, London, UK. Born in New Zealand, widely considered the 'Father of Plastic Surgery', started his craft to better the lives of the victims of the First World War. Later he became a pioneer in 'gender reassignment (sex-change) surgery'. He was joined in private practice by his cousin, the other world famous plastic surgeon, Sir Archibald McIndoe. He excelled in most sports – cricket, rowing, golf, and was an accomplished painter.

Limb reduction procedures

These are indicated when a limb is so swollen that it interferes with mobility and livelihood. These operations are not 'cosmetic' in the sense that they do not create a normally shaped leg and are usually associated with significant scarring. Four operations have been described.

Sistrunk

A wedge of skin and subcutaneous tissue is excised and the wound closed primarily. This is most commonly carried out to reduce the girth of the thigh.

Homans

First, skin flaps are elevated, and then subcutaneous tissue is excised from beneath the flaps, which are then trimmed to size to accommodate the reduced girth of the limb and closed primarily. This is the most satisfactory operation for the calf (Figure 58.11). The main complication is skin flap necrosis. There must be at least six months between operations on the medial and lateral sides of the limb and the flaps must not pass the midline. This procedure has also been used on the upper limb, but is contraindicated in the presence of venous obstruction or active malignancy.

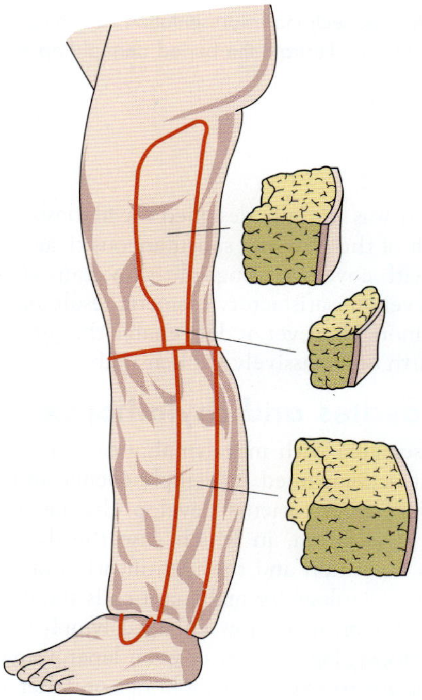

Figure 58.11 Homans' procedure involves raising skin flaps to allow the excision of a wedge of skin and a larger volume of subcutaneous tissue down to the deep fascia. Surgery to the medial and lateral aspects of the leg must be separated by at least six months to avoid skin flap necrosis.

John Bernard Kinmonth, 1916–1982, surgeon, St Thomas's Hospital, London, UK.
Walter Ellis Sistrunk, 1880–1933, Professor of Clinical Surgery, Baylor University College of Medicine, Dalls, TX, USA.
Frederick Thompson, 1910–1975, plastic surgeon, The Middlesex Hospital, London, UK.
Major-General Sir Richard Havelock Charles, 1887–1934, a surgeon in The Indian Medical Service.

Thompson

This is a modification of the Homans' procedure aimed to create new lymphatic connections between the superficial and deep systems. One skin flap is denuded (shaved of epidermis), sutured to the deep fascia and buried beneath the second skin flap (the so-called 'buried dermal flap') (Figure 58.12). This procedure has become less popular as pilonidal sinus formation is common. The cosmetic result is no better than that obtained with the Homans' procedure and there is no evidence that the buried flap establishes any new lymphatic connections.

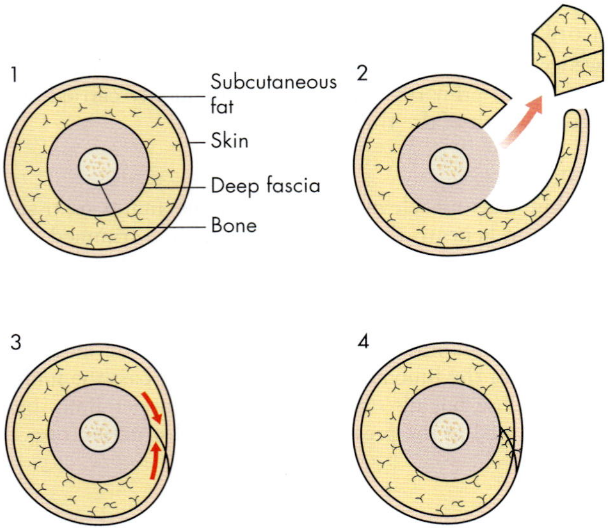

Figure 58.12 A cross-sectional representation of Thompson's reduction operation; red arrows illustrate the buried dermal flap sutured to deep fascia.

Charles

This operation was initially designed for filariasis and involved excision of all of the skin and subcutaneous tissues down to the deep fascia, with coverage using split-skin grafts (Figure 58.13). This leaves a very unsatisfactory cosmetic result and graft failure is not uncommon. However, it does enable the surgeon to reduce greatly the girth of a massively swollen limb.

Chylous ascites and chylothorax

These are associated with megalymphatics. The diagnosis may be obvious if accompanied by lymphoedema and lymphangioma. However, some patients develop chylous ascites and/or chylothorax in isolation, in which case the diagnosis can be confirmed by aspiration and the identification of chylomicrons in the aspirate. Cytology for malignant cells should also be carried out. A CT scan may show enlarged lymph nodes and CT with guided biopsy, laparoscopy or even laparotomy and biopsy may be necessary to exclude lymphoma or other malignancy. Lymphangiography may indicate the site of a lymphatic fistula that can be surgically ligated. Even if no localised lesion is identified, it may be possible to control leakage at laparotomy or even remove a segment of affected bowel. If the problem is

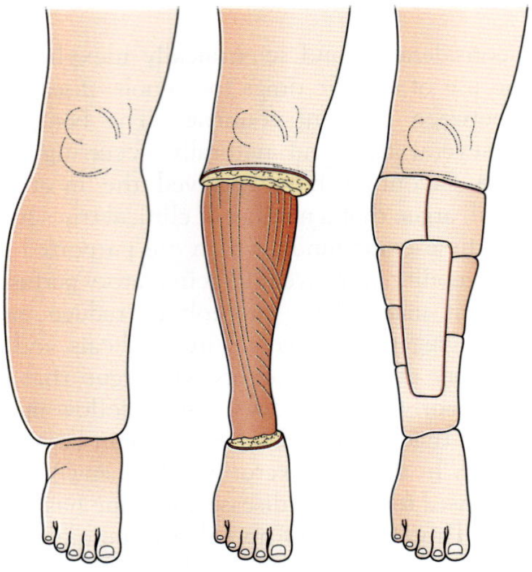

Figure 58.13 The Charles procedure involves circumferential excision of lymphoedematous tissue down to and including the deep fascia followed by split-skin grafting. This procedure gives a very poor cosmetic result but does allow the surgeon to remove very large amounts of tissue and is particularly useful in patients with severe skin changes.

too diffuse to be corrected surgically, a peritoneal venous shunt may be inserted, although occlusion and infection are important complications. Medical treatment comprising the avoidance of fat in the diet and the prescription of medium-chain triglycerides (which are absorbed directly into the blood rather than via the lymphatics) may reduce swelling. Chylothorax is best treated by pleurodesis, but this may lead to death from lymph-logged lungs as the excess lymph has nowhere to drain.

Chyluria

Filariasis is the most common cause, with chyluria occurring in 1–2 per cent of cases 10–20 years after initial infestation. It usually presents as painless passage of milky white urine, particularly after a fatty meal. The chyle may clot, leading to renal colic, and hypoproteinaemia may result. Chyluria may also be caused by ascariasis, malaria, tumour and tuberculosis. Intravenous urography and/or lymphangiography will often demonstrate the lymphourinary fistula. Treatment includes a low-fat and high-protein diet, increased oral fluids to prevent clot colic, and laparotomy and ligation of the dilated lymphatics. Attempts have also been made to sclerose the lymphatics either directly or via instrumentation of the bladder, ureter and renal pelvis.

FURTHER READING

Lee B-B, Bergan J, Rockson SG. *Lymphedema: a concise compendium of theory and practice*. New York: Springer, 2011.

Lymphoedema Framework. *Best practice for the management of lymphoedema. International consensus*. London: MEP Ltd, 2006.

Szuba A, Rockson SG. Lymphedema: anatomy, physiology and pathogenesis. *Vasc Med* 1997; **2**: 321–6.

Twycross R, Jenns K, Todd J. *Lymphoedema*. Oxford: Radcliffe Medical Press, 2000.

PART

11 Abdominal

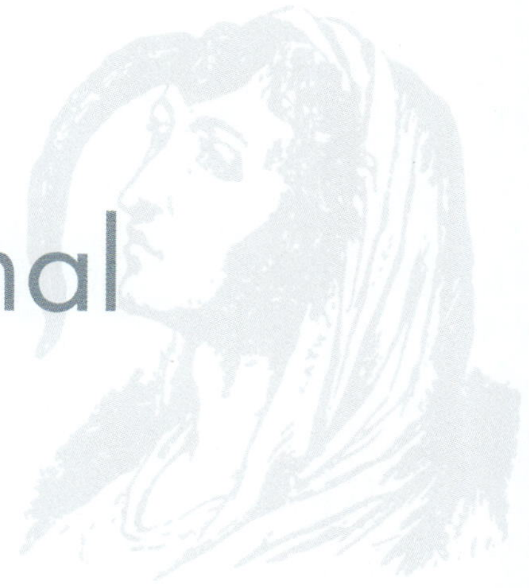

CHAPTER

59 History and examination of the abdomen

LEARNING OBJECTIVES

To understand:

- The pathway for clinical diagnosis of a patient presenting with an abdominal complaint
- The importance of recognising the organ or system responsible for the clinical features
- The pathophysiological basis of common abdominal symptoms and signs

To identify:

- Leading questions based on the organ or system affected and reach the most likely differential diagnosis
- The relevant physical signs and come to an appropriate clinical diagnosis

INTRODUCTION

Abdominal symptoms are possibly the most frequent of all symptoms encountered in surgical practice. Most symptoms arise from intra-abdominal organs or systems while some may originate extraabdominally and are then referred to the abdomen.

GATHERING INFORMATION

The first step is to obtain a history from the patient. But even before that, initial observations provide clues to the direction which the history should take; general appearance, gait, position in bed, facial expression, tone of the speech, all provide useful hints. The patient will be frightened and may well be in severe pain; therefore, the clinician should try to comfort the patient and gain their confidence, especially in cases of abdominal pain presenting as an emergency.

Obtaining a history

During the initial part of the interview with the patient, it is best to encourage the patient to explain their problem without interruption. After that, leading questions are used to fill any gaps left in the patient's history.

Presenting complaint

One should start with an open question inviting the patient to explain their reason for seeking medical advice.

Duration of the presenting complaint

The duration of symptoms will profoundly affect the differential diagnosis. For example, abdominal pain, which lasts for a few hours, may be ureteric colic whereas long-standing abdominal pain may be more suggestive of peptic ulceration.

History of the presenting complaint

Once the patient has finished explaining their problem, leading questions should be used to support or exclude the likely diagnoses. One way to do this is to enquire exactly when the patient last felt well and then ask about all that has happened since. At this stage it should be possible to identify a likely organ or system responsible for the patient's symptoms and come to a differential diagnosis. For example, a patient who presents with episodic loose stools, left-sided abdominal pain and sense of incomplete evacuation of bowel is likely to have pathology in the colon or rectum. In this case the relevant questions would be whether there was blood and mucus in the stools, and if there were constitutional symptoms suggestive of anaemia, malignancy and a family history of colon cancer.

Some patients may volunteer information that at first may not sound relevant but must be heeded. This is particularly important in the Asian subcontinent where people do resort to alternative medicines, which may have their own side effects.

Past history

The past history is important as it may have a bearing on the diagnosis and management. For example, control of diabetes will be difficult in the presence of intra-abdominal suppuration until the pus is drained. Some symptoms and signs may be due to comorbid conditions. A patient with abdominal pain due to gallstones may also have bilateral ankle oedema due to congestive cardiac failure. A tendency towards depression and anxiety may have an effect on the outcome of surgery.

Drug history and allergies

Some drugs will have an effect on the symptoms and signs or will have to be discontinued prior to surgery if they are not to cause complications. For example, a patient on a beta-blocker with abdominal bleeding will not have tachycardia proportionate to the blood loss. A patient on long-term steroids will need intravenous steroids to prevent an adrenal crisis in the perioperative period.

Social history

The use of alcohol and illicit drugs, smoking and occupation are important. Family background will give an idea as to the possible family support that can be expected after discharge from hospital.

Family history

Genetic disorders including adverse reactions to anaesthetics and medications need to be recorded. Any family history of cancer, particularly in a first-degree relative, is especially important.

Review of the systems

A system review should highlight any comorbid disease, such as cardiac, vascular, respiratory or endocrine problems (Summary box 59.1).

Summary box 59.1

Principles of history-taking

- Identify the reason for consultation
- Identify the duration and evolution of the problem
- Recognise the most likely organ or system affected
- Recall the relevant leading questions
- Select the most likely pathology from a list of differential diagnoses

CLINICAL PRESENTATION OF ABDOMINAL PROBLEMS

Pain, dyspepsia and alteration of bowel habit are the three common clinical presentations of pathology in the abdomen. However, it is important to be vigilant about insidious presentations of malignancies. Classic examples are right colon cancers presenting with symptoms of anaemia, malignant infiltrations of the liver with weight loss, gastric cancers with loss of appetite, abdominal lymphomas with weight loss and fever, ovarian cancers with abdominal distension, adrenal cancers with weight gain, and malignant obstructions of the extrahepatic biliary tree presenting with jaundice (Summary box 59.2).

Summary box 59.2

Sources of abdominal symptoms

- Abdominal pain, dyspepsia and alteration of bowel habit are the three common clinical presentations of abdominal pathology
- Occult malignancies may have atypical presentations

Abdominal pain

Pain is the most common of all abdominal symptoms. This may be due to inflammatory, infective or obstructive pathology. These can arise from abdominal viscera or be referred from a site outside the abdomen, such as the lungs as in pneumonia or the heart as in angina. Sometimes there may be abdominal pain for which no organic cause can be found, a situation labelled 'functional abdominal pain' for want of a better term. Common examples are dyspepsia or irritable bowel syndrome (IBS).

Acute medical conditions

Acute abdominal pain from medical conditions such as diabetic ketoacidosis and porphyrias may present as apparent surgical emergencies. It is also important to be vigilant about the atypical presentations of life-threatening abdominal problems and hidden malignancies. For example, an elderly man presenting with vague abdominal pain combined with an episode of fainting may have a leaking abdominal aortic aneurysm. Young alcoholics presenting to the Accident and Emergency department with abdominal pain and a recent history of trauma may be developing traumatic acute pancreatitis or a traumatic subcapsular haematoma of the spleen. The elderly patient presenting with a clinical picture of acute appendicitis and anaemia should arouse suspicion of a concomitant caecal cancer as a cause of obstructive appendicitis.

Abdominal pain and dyspepsia

The word dyspepsia is used to describe a multitude of symptoms, such as upper abdominal pain, abdominal distension, discomfort, early satiety, nausea, vomiting, heartburn, acid regurgitation and water brash; all these symptoms are referable to the upper gastrointestinal tract. They are called 'organic dyspepsias', the most common cause of which is gastro-oesophageal reflux disease. Other causes are peptic ulcer, gallstones, chronic pancreatitis and oesophagogastric cancer. However, in approximately 50 per cent of patients a definitive diagnosis cannot be made. In these cases the term 'functional dyspepsia' is used.

Abdominal pain and change of bowel habits

Alteration in bowel habit makes the colon the likely source of pathology. The onset, nature, duration, type of alteration (constipation or diarrhoea) and its relationship to abdominal pain will help to differentiate organic pathology causing obstruction or inflammation (colon cancer and inflammatory bowel disease) from functional conditions such as IBS. When patients complain of diarrhoea, they may imply different meanings – some use the term for loose stools, while others may mean frequent but normal stools. A long-standing increase in frequency of stools, with left-sided abdominal pain prior to defecation which eases after defecation, all points to IBS. However, if such symptoms are of short duration in an adult and are associated with blood and mucus in the stools with weight loss, a left colonic carcinoma is more likely. If a patient with such symptoms presents as an emergency with worsening abdominal pain and absolute constipation, then the most likely diagnosis is one of acute-on-chronic intestinal obstruction, from a stenotic left colon cancer. If the patient also has a distended abdomen and tenderness over the caecal area, then closed-loop obstruction with impending caecal rupture must be suspected and urgent surgery will be needed. However, a history of previous abdominal surgery changes the situation again; now, adhesions entrapping the small bowel is the most likely source of the symptoms. However, a small incarcerated femoral hernia could also be the cause. This can easily be missed, especially in an obese patient (Summary box 59.3).

Summary box 59.3

Classic presentations of abdominal pathology

- Obstructive and inflammatory pathology must be excluded in patients with abdominal pain and altered bowel habit
- Closed-loop obstruction with tenderness in the right iliac fossa is indicative of imminent caecal rupture
- Caecal cancer classically presents with anaemia
- Patients who have had previous abdominal surgery may have adhesions
- Check carefully for small incarcerated hernias, particularly femoral, in obese patients

Summary box 59.4

Nerves responsible for abdominal pain

- Abdominal wall and parietal peritoneum are supplied by the somatic nerves
- Abdominal organs and the visceral peritoneum are supplied by the autonomic nervous system
- Skin, muscles and parietal peritoneum are supplied by the iliohypogastric and ilioinguinal nerve and the lower six intercostal nerves
- Afferent pain fibres from the abdominal organs and visceral peritoneum travel with sympathetic nerves

PATHOPHYSIOLOGICAL BASIS OF COMMON ABDOMINAL SYMPTOMS AND SIGNS

The abdominal wall and parietal peritoneum are supplied by the somatic nervous system, while the abdominal organs and visceral peritoneum are innervated by the autonomic nervous system. Therefore pain will appear to change in position and nature as the underlying pathology spreads from a local intraperitoneal structure to the parietal peritoneum.

The skin and the muscles of the abdominal wall are supplied by the lateral and anterior cutaneous branches of the lower six intercostal nerves and the iliohypogastric and ilioinguinal nerve (Figure 59.1). The dermatome levels of the xiphoid process, umbilicus and pubis are T7, T10 and T12, respectively. The parietal peritoneum is supplied segmentally by the same nerves that innervate the overlying muscles. The central part of the diaphragmatic peritoneum is supplied by the phrenic nerve (C4); therefore, pain arising in this region is referred to the tip of the shoulder as it has the same segmental supply. The peripheral rim of the diaphragmatic peritoneum is supplied by the intercostal nerves. The obturator nerve is the chief nerve supply of the pelvic parietal peritoneum (Summary box 59.4).

Pain from the viscera is principally due to ischaemia, muscle spasm and stretching of the visceral peritoneum. Unlike somatic pain, autonomic pain is deep and poorly localised. This pain is transmitted via sympathetic fibres and so is referred to the appropriate somatic distribution of that nerve root from T1 to L2 (Figure 59.2). However, when an inflamed organ touches the parietal peritoneum, the pain becomes sharp and localises to the appropriate segmental dermatome of the abdominal wall. Pain arising from the parietal peritoneum may radiate to the back or the front along the appropriate dermatome. This referral pattern is classically seen in acute cholecystitis when an inflamed gall bladder touches the parietal peritoneum. Pain then radiates round to the back along the involved dermatome. The overlying muscle and the skin is supplied by the same nerve root, so when the patient takes a deep breath the tenderness in the right subcostal region is markedly increased, causing the patient to stop breathing; this is Murphy's sign. In children with abdominal pain, who hold their right hip in a flexed position to obtain relief from the pain, one should suspect retrocaecal appendicitis causing irritation of the psoas muscle.

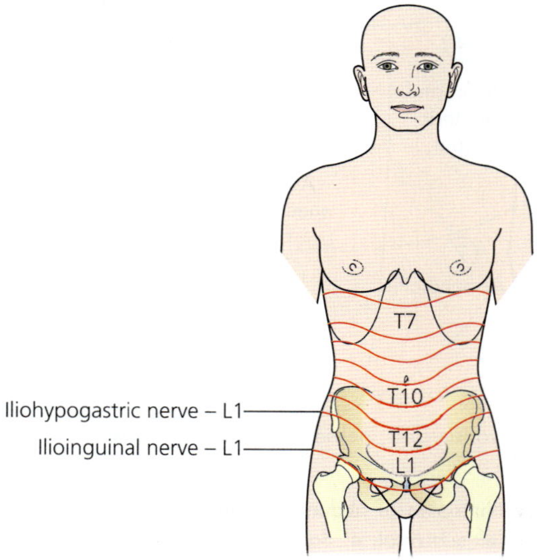

Figure 59.1 Distribution of the anterior abdominal wall dermatomes and nerves.

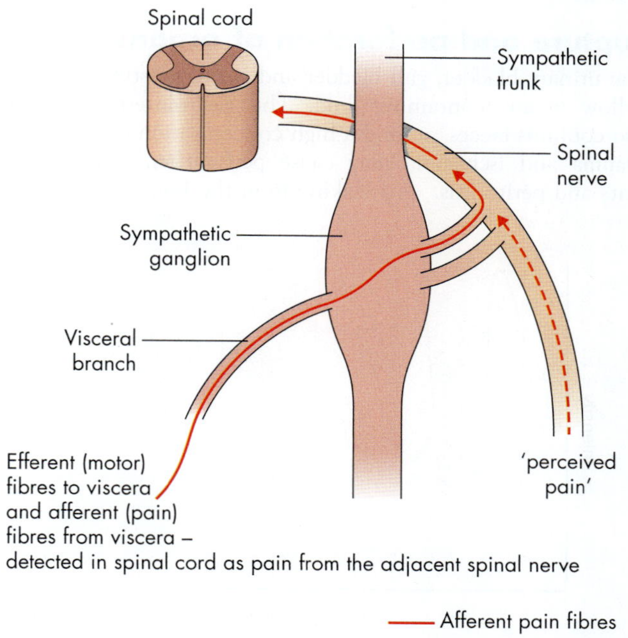

Figure 59.2 Pathways for parietal and visceral pain. (From 25th Edition of Bailey and Love, courtesy of Mr Simon Paterson-Brown, Consultant Surgeon, Royal Infirmary of Edinburgh.)

John Apley, 1909–1980, consultant paediatrician, Bristol, UK. The further away the chronic abdominal pain in a child is from the umbilicus, the more likely an organic cause.

The pattern of pain distribution from the various regions of the gut is most easily understood by appreciating that the gut develops with its own nerve supply. Pain arising from the foregut is felt in the epigastric region while pain from the mid-gut, which includes the small bowel, appendix and ascending colon, is referred to the periumbilical region (Summary box 59.5).

Summary box 59.5

Specific characteristics of abdominal pain

- Visceral pain arises from ischaemia, muscle spasm and stretching of the visceral peritoneum
- Autonomic pain, deep and poorly localised, is referred to the equivalent somatic distribution of that nerve root from T1 to L2
- When an inflamed organ touches the parietal peritoneum, pain is then localised to the segmental dermatome of the abdominal wall
- The pain in the parietal peritoneum may radiate to back or front along the dermatome

Obstruction

Central colicky abdominal pain is a classical presentation of small bowel obstruction. The central distribution is because of the segmental nerve supply of the mid-gut. When the peristaltic waves hit an obstruction, the contractions increase to overcome the resistance producing the colic. The pain reaches a crescendo and then disappears in minutes when the peristaltic wave passes (Figure 59.3). This is different from that of biliary colic. When the gall bladder contracts against a stone, pain is relatively insidious in onset and reaches its peak in about half an hour and then eases off. A basal pain persists between the bouts of colic (Summary box 59.6).

Rupture and perforation of organs

The urinary bladder, gall bladder and gastrointestinal tract are hollow organs containing fluid. The gastrointestinal system also contains faeces, air and a high concentration of organisms. Trauma and ischaemia may cause perforation, leak of contents and peritonitis. Air leaking from the bowel gets trapped between the liver and abdominal wall; hence the loss of hepatic dullness, a physical sign that supports the diagnosis of perforation of a hollow viscus. Rupture of the bowel causes sudden pain. The initial site of onset of the pain may give a clue as to the organ involved and so help with the differential diagnosis. For example, the diagnosis of a perforated peptic ulcer is supported by a past history of ulcer-type pain followed by sudden onset of upper abdominal pain. In such a patient who has peritonitis the abdominal wall will not move with respiration. The patient will have thoracic respiration with shallow breathing.

Summary box 59.6

Colicky abdominal pain

- The pain of 'small bowel colic' comes in waves and disappears completely in minutes when the peristaltic wave ceases
- Pain of biliary colic is insidious in onset, reaches the peak in half an hour or so and does not ease off completely between spasms

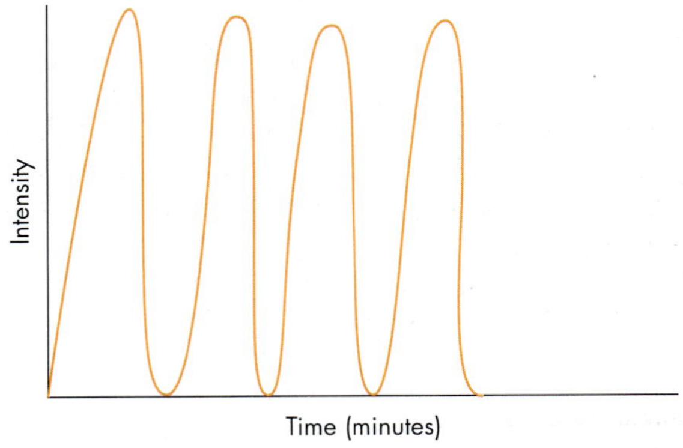

Figure 59.3 Time/intensity graph for the pain of obstruction. (From 25th Edition of Bailey and Love, courtesy of Mr Simon Paterson-Brown, Consultant Surgeon, Royal Infirmary of Edinburgh.)

The abdomen is divided into nine areas for ease of description (Figure 59.4). These regions are demarcated by the midclavicular lines in the vertical axis and by the transpyloric and transtubercular lines in the horizontal axis. Figure 59.4 also indicates some of the common organs and pathological processes that commonly cause pain experienced in these regions.

EXAMINATION OF THE ABDOMEN

Abdominal examination must be preceded by a detailed general examination of the patient as a whole. Physical examination

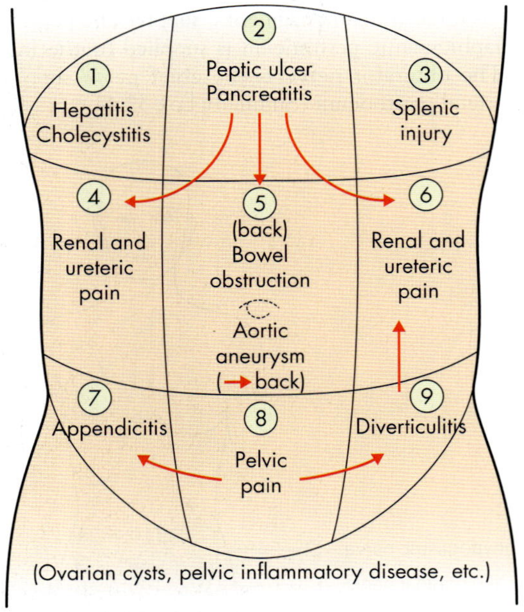

Figure 59.4 Nine sites of abdominal pain: 1, right subcostal; 2, epigastrium; 3, left subcostal; 4, right flank; 5, periumbilical; 6, left flank loin; 7, right iliac fossa; 8, suprapubic/hypogastrium; 9, left iliac fossa. (From 25th Edition of Bailey and Love, courtesy of Mr Simon Paterson-Brown, Consultant Surgeon, Royal Infirmary of Edinburgh.)

John Benjamin Murphy, 1857–1916, Professor of Surgery, Northwestern University, Chicago, IL, USA. He described his sign in 1903. He was the son of Irish immigrants fleeing the potato famine in Ireland, and was known as the 'Stormy Petrel' of American surgery, demonstrating the benefit of appendicectomy over conservative treatment amongst many things.

should be systematic using the following sequence: inspection, palpation, percussion and auscultation (Summary box 59.7).

Summary box 59.7

Inspection of abdomen

- Kneel beside the bed with eyes level with patient's anterior abdominal wall
- Look for skin colour changes (Grey Turner and Cullen's signs)
- Look for surgical scars
- Check for lumps and distended veins and pulsation
- Watch the abdomen move with respiration
- Intra-abdominal lumps vanish or become less prominent when the patient tenses the abdominal wall by lifting the head from the bed

General examination

Observation of the patient's general condition is useful even before starting to take the history, especially in the emergency situation. If a patient resorts to the knee–elbow position to get relief from pain, it indicates that the pain is of pancreatic origin (Figure 59.5). In the outpatient clinic, a patient with loose clothing (most likely caused by significant weight loss) may well have an underlying malignant process. The differential diagnosis will include tuberculosis, Crohn's disease or chronic pancreatitis. In a patient with anaemia, a clinician should check for nodes in the supraclavicular region from gastric cancer, other nodal masses from lymphoma, as well as a caecal mass and malignant hepatomegaly when the liver will be large with hard nodules. Bilateral lower limb oedema is a significant finding, which may point to heart, liver or renal failure as well as obstruction of the veins in the pelvis (Summary box 59.8).

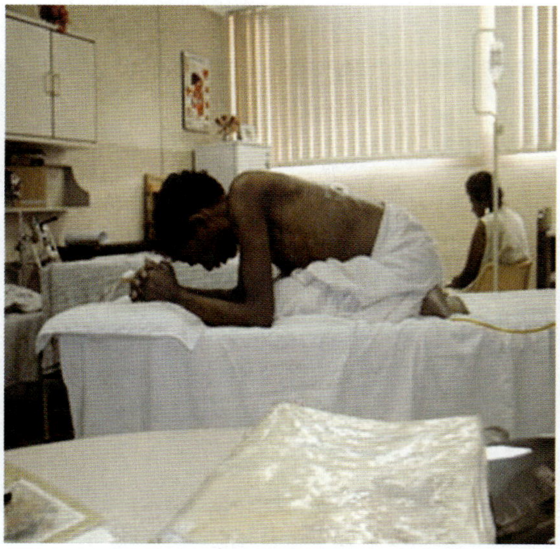

Figure 59.5 Classical position adopted to ease pancreatic pain (patient with chronic pancreatitis).

Summary box 59.8

Sources of physical signs in abdominal examination

- Malignancy, tuberculosis, Crohn's disease and chronic pancreatitis should be suspected in a patient who appears to have lost weight
- Occult gastrointestinal bleeding from chronic peptic ulceration and right colon cancers should be excluded in patients with anaemia
- The cause of bilateral lower limb oedema may be in the heart, liver, kidneys or in venous obstruction in the pelvis

Inspection

Scars, distension, peristalsis, masses, dilated veins, pulsations and abdominal wall swellings suggestive of hernia should all be carefully sought. In an abdominal emergency look for Grey Turner's sign – skin discoloration of flanks due to retroperitoneal haemorrhage in severe acute pancreatitis and leaking abdominal aortic aneurysm. The other cause of skin colour change is Cullen's sign – discoloration around the umbilicus from severe acute pancreatitis, ruptured ectopic pregnancy or trauma to the liver. In these situations blood tracks to the umbilicus along the ligamentum teres (Figure 59.6).

In a patient with acute abdominal pain, always check to see if the abdominal wall moves with respiration. If only the thorax moves then peritonitis should be suspected. Visible abdominal masses, mobility on respiration and peristalsis are all best observed by the clinician kneeling by the patient's bed so that the observer's eye is at the level of the patient's anterior abdominal wall. The same position is useful during palpation for abdominal masses (Figure 59.7).

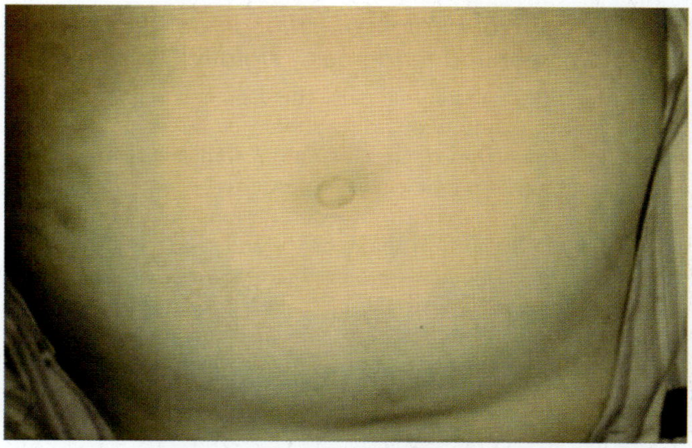

Figure 59.6 Cullen's and Grey Turner's sign of skin discolouration of flanks and around umbilicus (courtesy of Mr Pradip Datta, Honorary Consultant Surgeon, Wick, Scotland).

George Grey Turner, 1877–1951, Professor of Surgery, the University of Durham (1927–1934) and at the Royal Postgraduate Medical School, Hammersmith Hospital, London, UK (1935–1946). He had the surgical club, Grey Turner Surgical Club, named after him. It is said that he dressed shabbily so that when his friends met him they used to ask him to 'mend the clock'. He had a habit of keeping his cup of tea warm by covering it with his bowler hat!

Thomas Stephen Cullen, 1868–1953, Professor of Gynaecology, the Johns Hopkins University, Baltimore, MD, USA, described the sign in ruptured ectopic pregnancy in 1916.

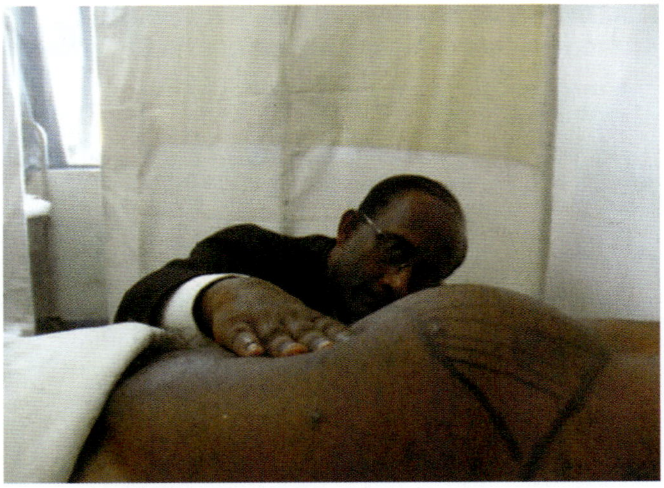

Figure 59.7 Eye at the level of patient's abdominal wall.

Palpation

Palpation should be performed in a systematic manner checking all nine regions of the abdomen (Figure 59.4). Palpation is started in the region furthest away from the site of pain. The examiner should observe the patient's facial expression throughout. It may help to divert the patient's attention by having a conversation. Watch their face so that you spot discomfort immediately. A relaxed patient with a pillow under the flexed knees makes the procedure easier. A gentle approach and warm hands will allay the patient's fears. Palpate superficially to identify tender areas then follow this with deep palpation. Take special care wherever tenderness is found in superficial palpation. Finally, palpation during respiration is performed to identify those structures like the liver and spleen which move with respiration.

Signs of parietal peritoneal irritation (tenderness, guarding, rebound tenderness, rigidity)

In the presence of abdominal pain, the degree of abdominal wall rigidity and involuntary guarding should be assessed. Guarding represents contraction of the abdominal wall muscles over the area of pain. This might occur 'voluntarily' when the patient wishes to avoid the pain from examination, or 'involuntarily' when the muscles go into spasm as the inflamed viscus touches the parietal peritoneum. This produces a reflex spasm of the overlying abdominal wall muscles. The presence of rebound tenderness indicates underlying peritoneal inflammation and is best examined using gentle percussion, although pain on coughing is also found when there is rebound tenderness. When the underlying peritoneal inflammation becomes generalised, the abdomen is 'board-like rigid' to palpation, and selective tenderness can no longer be elicited. This sign represents widespread involuntary guarding. The progression from tenderness, guarding, rebound tenderness are all stages in the evolution of generalised peritonitis.

Abdominal masses

A mass arising from the anterior abdominal wall will usually be mobile when the patient is relaxed. On contracting the abdominal wall muscles (ask the patient to lift their legs with the knees extended, or by a Valsalva manoeuvre for laterally placed swellings), lumps superficial to the abdominal wall muscles will become more obvious, and those attached to the deep fascia will become less mobile. Those arising within the muscle layer will become fixed and remain unchanged in size. Lumps arising deep to the abdominal wall (i.e. within the peritoneal cavity or behind the peritoneum) will become impalpable or less prominent on tensing the anterior abdominal wall muscles.

Intraperitoneal lumps in contact with the diaphragm will move on respiration (i.e. swellings arising from liver, gall bladder, spleen, stomach, kidneys and suprarenals). Retroperitoneal masses are usually fixed and certainly do not move with respiration; an enlarged kidney is 'ballotable' and bimanually palpable. Normal aortic pulsations can be both seen and felt in a thin abdomen, but expansile pulsation is characteristic of an abdominal aortic aneurysm. This should be differentiated from transmitted pulsation of a mass sitting on the aorta (e.g. pseudocyst of the pancreas).

When 'palpating during inspiration', the examining hand is placed distal to the normal site of the organ, and is held there until the edge of the organ descends and touches the examiner's fingers (Figure 59.8). Liver, spleen, gall bladder and kidneys are best palpated during inspiration.

In the female an abdominal mass, whose lower limit cannot be made out, must be arising from the pelvis. If the mass can be moved in a transverse direction, then it is likely to be an uterine or ovarian mass (Figure 59.9). If the lower limit of an abdominal mass is palpable and it is mobile, then it will be an intra-abdominal mass; the origin of this mass will be dependent upon the site (Figure 59.10) and the pathology dependent upon the clinical features as a whole. If a mass is of recent origin overlying a laparoscopic scar, without any signs of inflammation, consider a secondary metastasis of an intra-abdominal malignancy (Figure 59.11).

Spleen

In a healthy patient the spleen is not palpable. The enlarged spleen descends downwards, forwards and medially. Palpation

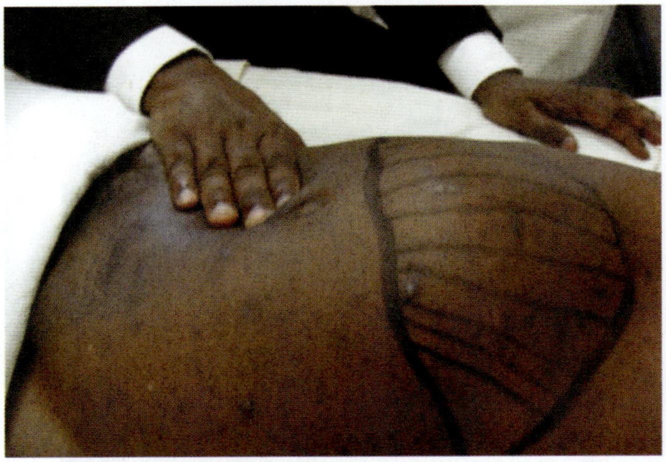

Figure 59.8 Palpation during inspiration. Examining hand is placed distal to the intended site of the organ until the edge of the organ descends and hits the hand.

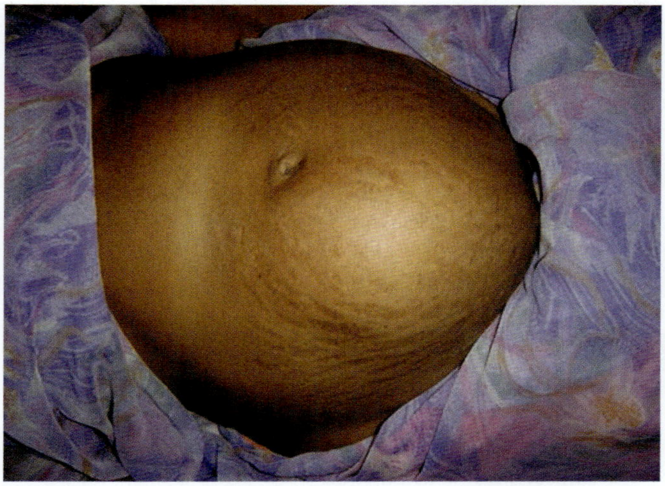

Figure 59.9 Large suprapubic mass. Patient referred with diagnosis of ovarian tumour with liver metastasis; investigations showed fibroid uterus with multiple haemangiomas in the liver.

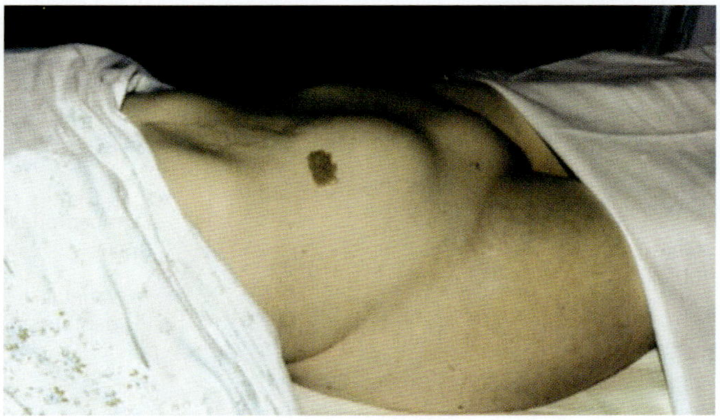

Figure 59.10 Mass in the right iliac fossa: carcinoma caecum (courtesy of Mr Pradip Datta, Honorary Consultant Surgeon, Wick, Scotland).

for an enlarged spleen is best performed in a supine patient. The examining hand should start in the right lower abdomen, with the tips of the fingers pointing upwards and pressed inwards. The patient is then asked to take a deep breath, and if the spleen is enlarged the lower edge with the characteristic notch will touch the fingers. If it is not palpable, then the hand is gradually moved upwards in the direction of the position of the edge of the normal-sized spleen with each breath. If the spleen is still not palpable, the patient is moved to the right lateral position and the examination repeated.

Liver

In a supine patient, the hand is placed in line with the potential enlarged liver edge lateral to the rectus muscle (Figure 59.8). The patient is then asked to take a deep breath. If the liver is enlarged sufficiently below the costal margin, then surface irregularities can also be felt.

Percussion

Percussion helps to distinguish distension due to bowel gas from free fluid in the abdomen and solid masses. Percussion is most sensitive when the examiner moves from resonant parts of the abdomen to dull ones. In patients with free fluid in the peritoneal cavity, percussion from the centre to the periphery reveals dullness of flanks. Shifting dullness is elicited if the patient is re-examined lying on their side. The margin of dullness is then found to shift when the patient has moved.

Percussion is a very sensitive and refined method of testing for rebound tenderness. If the patient winces with pain on abdominal percussion it denotes underlying peritonitis.

Auscultation

High-pitched bowel sounds are heard during early stages of mechanical intestinal obstruction. Aortic and iliac bruits are heard when blood flows through a stenosis. A succession splash is a sound like 'shaking a half-filled bottle with water' and is found most often in patients with gastric stasis due to gastric outlet obstruction. In generalised peritonitis, bowel sounds will not be heard or be very few and far between.

Inspection of hernial sites, examination of genitalia, inspection of anal region and digital rectal examination

Abdominal examination is not complete until all external hernial sites and the anal area have been carefully inspected, the genitalia examined and a digital rectal examination performed. A vaginal examination will also be needed in females. The spine and renal angles should be examined.

VALUE OF OBSERVATION AND REVIEW

In the case of acute abdominal pain, there will be a group of patients in whom, after full clinical assessment, the surgeon is still uncertain about the need for an urgent operation. This is probably the most difficult group to deal with compared with those in whom an urgent operation is either clearly required, or clearly not required, and undoubtedly the one in which the majority of errors occur. Further urgent investigations are obviously important in this group and these are discussed in some detail elsewhere in this book. However, while these are taking place, a period of observation with regular review is essential. This period of observation has now become an integral part of the early management of patients with acute abdominal pain.

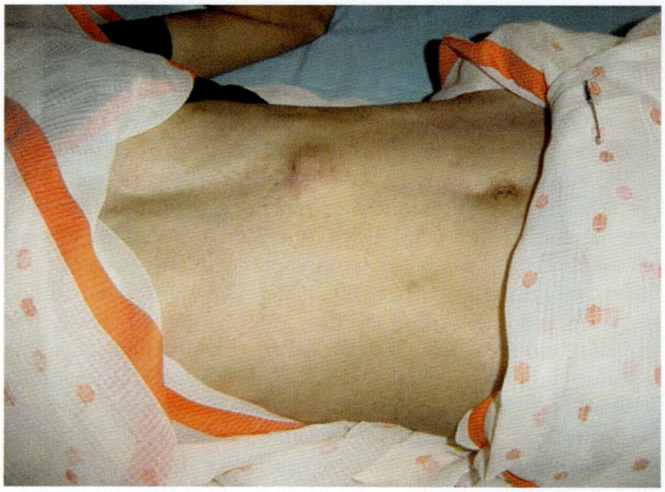

Figure 59.11 Port site metastasis after laparoscopic cholecystectomy in a patient with carcinoma gall bladder.

CHAPTER 60

Abdominal wall, hernia and umbilicus

LEARNING OBJECTIVES

To know and understand:

- Basic anatomy of the abdominal wall and its weaknesses
- Causes of abdominal hernia
- Types of hernia and classifications
- Clinical history and examination findings in hernia
- Complications of abdominal hernia
- Non-surgical and surgical management of hernia – including mesh
- Complications of hernia surgery
- Other abdominal wall conditions

THE ABDOMINAL WALL

Basic anatomy and function related to pathology

The abdominal wall is a complex structure composed primarily of muscle, bone and fascia. Its major function is to protect the enclosed organs of the gastrointestinal and urogenital tracts but a secondary role is mobility, being able to flex, extend, rotate and vary its capacity. Flexibility requires elasticity and stretch which compromise abdominal wall strength.

The roof of the abdomen is formed by the diaphragm separating the thoracic cavity above with negative pressure from the abdomen below with positive pressure. Weakness of the diaphragm can lead to much of the bowel being drawn into the chest down this pressure gradient. The bony pelvis forms the floor of the cavity but a muscular central portion, the perineum, may also weaken and allow rectum, bladder and gynaecological organs to bulge downwards, a condition called prolapse.

The overall design of the abdominal muscles is best seen on a transverse computed tomography (CT) scan through the midabdomen. Posteriorly the muscles are strong, further supported by the vertebral column, ribs and pelvis. Two regions called the posterior triangles represent areas of weakness which can lead to rare lumbar hernias. Laterally there are three thin muscle layers whose fibres criss-cross for strength and flexibility. Surgeons can make use of these layers, by making releasing incisions, separating the layers and then sliding one layer on another to increase girth and allow closure of defects in the centre of the abdomen, e.g. the 'Ramirez slide' used in large incisional hernia repair (Figure 60.1).

Anteriorly the two powerful rectus abdominus muscles extend vertically from ribs to pelvis. Herniation through these strong muscles does not occur naturally but their central join, the linea alba, is an area of weakness resulting in epigastric and paraumbilical herniation. Divarification of the recti is the condition where the linea alba stretches laterally as the two rectus muscles separate. It occurs in the upper abdomen in middle-aged, overweight men (Figure 60.2) but also as a result of birth trauma in the female when it occurs below the umbilicus.

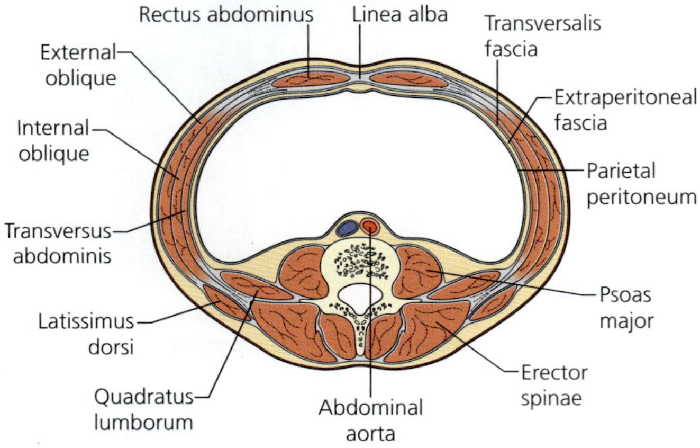

Figure 60.1 A cross section of the midabdomen showing the muscular layout.

Abdominal pressure

The positive pressure within the abdomen is used by a surgeon when drains are placed to allow blood, pus, bile, bowel content and urine to flow outwards down the pressure gradient. However, this constant pressure from within can also lead to the condition of abdominal hernia where tissue, meant to be within the abdominal cavity, is forced outwards through defects in the muscular wall.

ABDOMINAL HERNIA

A hernia is the bulging of part of the contents of the abdominal cavity through a weakness in the abdominal wall.

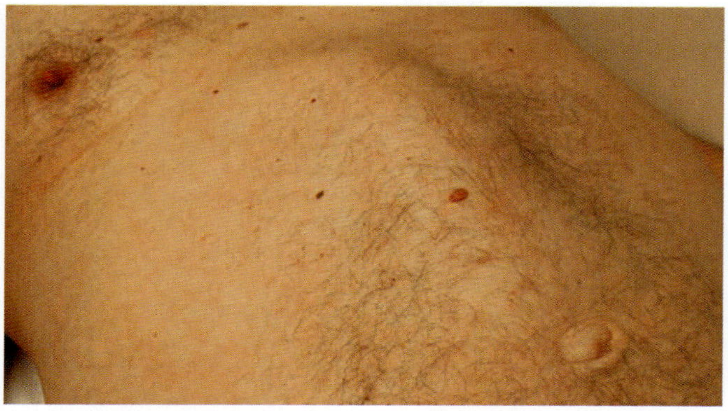

Figure 60.2 Divarification.

Anatomical causes of abdominal wall herniation

Despite the complex design of the abdominal wall, the only natural weaknesses caused by inadequate muscular strength are the lumbar triangles and the posterior wall of the inguinal canal (Figure 60.3).

Many structures pass into and out of the abdominal cavity creating weakness which can lead to hernia formation. The most common example is the inguinal canal in the male along which the testis descends from abdomen to scrotum at the time of birth. The testicular artery, veins and vas pass though this canal (the round ligament in the female). The resultant weakness leads to an indirect or lateral-type inguinal hernia. In adult surgery, 80 per cent of all hernia repairs are for inguinal hernia. The evolutionary advantage of testicular descent must outweigh the disadvantage of a high risk of herniation. Other examples are: oesophagus → hiatus hernia, femoral vessels → femoral hernia, obturator nerve → obturator hernia, sciatic nerve → sciatic hernia.

An inguinal hernia (indirect) also occurs through the developmental failure of the processus vaginalis to close. As the testis descends, it pulls a tube of peritoneum along with it. This tube should naturally fibrose and become obliterated but often it fails to fibrose and allows a hernia to form. Recent studies have shown that calcitonin gene-related peptide and hepatocyte growth factor influence the closure of the processus raising the possibility of a hormonal cause of hernia development.

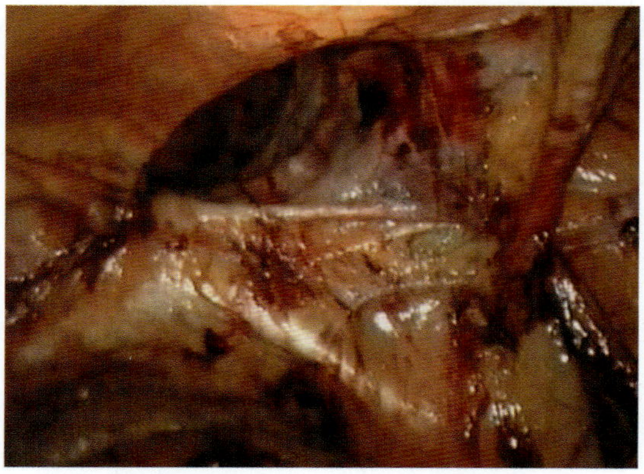

Figure 60.3 Posterior wall defect.

Failure of normal development may lead to weakness of the abdominal wall. Examples are diaphragmatic, umbilical and epigastric hernias. Muscles which should unite during development fail to form strong unions with hernia development at birth or in later life.

Herniation at the umbilicus has both components, i.e. weakness due to structures passing through the abdominal wall in fetal life and developmental failure of closure.

The risk of inguinal hernia is related to the anatomical shape of the pelvis and is higher in patients having a wider and shorter pelvis.

Weakness of abdominal muscles may be the result of sharp trauma. Most commonly, this results from abdominal surgery but also occurs after stabbing. A surgical scar, even with perfect wound healing, has only 70 per cent of the initial muscle strength. This loss of strength can result in herniation in at least 10 per cent of surgical incisions. Smaller laparoscopic port-site incisions have a hernia rate of 1 per cent. Increasing use of this surgical approach should lead to a fall in the incidence of incisional hernia.

Muscle damage by blunt trauma or tearing of the abdominal muscles requires exceptional force and is rare.

The sudden presence of a mass in the rectus muscle may be a rectus sheath haematoma, occasionally due to trauma but nowadays more often due to excessive anticoagulation therapy.

Primary muscle pathology and neurological conditions can lead to muscle weakness and occasionally present to the surgeon as a 'hernia' (Summary box 60.1).

Summary box 60.1

Causes of hernia

- Basic design weakness
- Weakness due to structures entering and leaving the abdomen
- Developmental failures
- Genetic weakness of collagen
- Sharp and blunt trauma
- Weakness due to ageing and pregnancy
- Primary neurological and muscle diseases
- ? Excessive intra-abdominal pressure

Pathophysiology of hernia formation

A normal abdominal wall has sufficient strength to resist high abdominal pressure and prevent herniation of content. Herniation has been attributed to high pressures from constipation, prostatic symptoms, excessive coughing in respiratory disease and obesity. However, it has been shown that hernia is no more common in Olympic weight lifters than the general population, suggesting that high pressure is not a major factor in causing a hernia. Many patients will first notice a hernia after excessive straining.

There is good evidence that hernia is a 'collagen disease' and due to an inherited imbalance in the types of collagen. This is supported by histological evidence and relationships between hernia and other diseases related to collagen, such as aortic aneurysm.

Hernia development is more common in pregnancy due to hormonally induced laxity of pelvic ligaments. It is also more common in the elderly due to degenerative weakness of muscles and fibrous tissue. A recent Swedish report has shown that inguinal hernia is less common in obese patients with hernia risk being negatively related to body mass index (BMI) contrary to widespread belief. Hernia is more common in smokers.

Common principles in abdominal hernia

An abdominal wall hernia has two essential components, a defect in the wall and content, that is tissue which has been forced outwards through the defect. The weakness may be entirely in muscle, such as an incisional hernia. It may also be in fascia, like an epigastric hernia through the linea alba. It may have a bony component, such as a femoral hernia. The weakness in the wall is usually the narrowest part of the hernia which expands into the subcutaneous fat outside of the muscle. The defect varies in size and may be very small or indeed very large. The nature of the defect is important to understanding the risk of hernia complications. A small defect with rigid walls traps the content and prevents it from freely moving in and out of the defect, increasing the risk of complications.

The content of the hernia may be tissue from the extraperitoneal space alone, such as fat within an epigastric hernia or urinary bladder in a direct inguinal hernia. However, if such a hernia enlarges then peritoneum may also be pulled into the hernia secondarily along with intraperitoneal structures such as bowel or omentum; a good example is a 'sliding type' of inguinal hernia.

More commonly, when peritoneum is lying immediately deep to the abdominal wall weakness, pressure forces the peritoneum through the defect and into the subcutaneous tissues. This 'sac' of peritoneum allows bowel and omentum to pass through the defect. In most cases, the intraperitoneal organs can move freely in and out of the hernia, a 'reducible' hernia, but if adhesions form or the defect is small, bowel can become trapped and unable to return to the main peritoneal cavity, an 'irreducible' hernia, with high risk of further complications. The narrowest part of the sac, at the abdominal wall defect, is called the 'neck of the sac'.

When tissue is trapped inside a hernia it is in a confined space. The narrow neck acts as a constriction ring impeding venous return and increasing pressure within the hernia. Resulting tension leads to pain and tenderness. If the hernia contains bowel then it may become 'obstructed', partially or totally. If the pressure rises sufficiently, arterial blood is not able to enter the hernia and the contents become ischaemic and may infarct. The hernia is then said to have 'strangulated'. The wall of the bowel perforates, releasing infected, toxic bowel content into the tissues and ultimately back into the peritoneal cavity. The risk of strangulation is highest in hernias which have a small neck of rigid tissue leading first to irreducibility and on to strangulation. The term 'incarcerated' is not clearly defined and used to imply a hernia which is irreducible and developing towards strangulation (Summary box 60.2).

In a special circumstance (Richter's hernia) only part of the bowel wall enters the hernia. It may be small and difficult or even impossible to detect clinically. Bowel obstruction may not be present but the bowel wall may still become necrotic and perforate with life-threatening consequences. Femoral hernia may present in this way often with diagnostic delay and high risk to the patient (Figure 60.4).

Summary box 60.2

Types of hernia by complexity

- Occult – not detectable clinically; may cause severe pain
- Reducible – a swelling which appears and disappears
- Irreducible – a swelling which cannot be replaced in the abdomen, high risk of complications
- Strangulated – painful swelling with vascular compromise, requires urgent surgery
- Infarcted – when contents of the hernia have become gangrenous, high mortality

An interstitial hernia occurs when the hernia extends between the layers of muscle and not directly through them. This is typical of a Spigelian hernia (see below under Spigelian hernia).

An internal hernia is a termed used when adhesions form within the peritoneal cavity leading to abnormal pockets into which bowel can enter and become trapped. As there is no defect within the abdominal wall, the term 'hernia' is confusing.

Clinical history and diagnosis in hernia cases

Patients are usually aware of a lump on the abdominal wall under the skin. Self-diagnosis is common. The hernia is usually painless but patients may complain of an aching or heavy feeling. Sharp, intermittent pains suggest pinching of tissue. Severe pain should alert the surgeon to a high risk of strangulation. One should determine whether the hernia reduces spontaneously or needs to be helped. The patient should be asked about symptoms which might suggest bowel obstruction.

It is important to know if this is a primary hernia or whether it is a recurrence after previous surgery. Recurrent hernia is more difficult to treat and may require a different surgical approach.

General questions regarding the cardiac and respiratory systems are necessary to assess a patient's anaesthetic risk.

In a male with a groin hernia, history of prostatic symptoms indicates a high risk of postoperative urinary retention.

Intake of anticoagulants such as warfarin is important as this impacts on future surgery. Many hernia operations can be performed as a day case or single overnight stay, so that suitability for such treatment needs to be assessed, including home support, distance from the hospital, mobility levels, etc.

Examination for hernia

The patient should be examined lying down initially and then standing as this will usually increase hernia size. In some

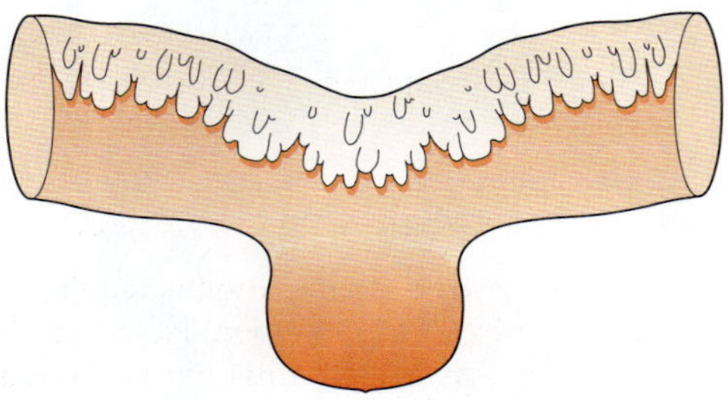

Figure 60.4 Diagrammatic representation of gangrenous Richter's hernia from a case of strangulated femoral hernia.

August Gottlieb Richter, 1742–1812, lecturer in Surgery, Göttingen, Germany described this form of hernia in 1777.

cases no hernia will be apparent with the patient lying. The patient is asked to cough, when an occult hernia may appear. Divarification is best seen by asking a supine patient to simply lift his head off the pillow.

The overlying skin is usually of normal colour. If bruising is present this may suggest venous engorgement of the content. If there is overlying cellulitis then hernia content is strangulating and the case should be treated as an emergency.

In most cases a cough impulse is felt. Gentle pressure is applied to the lump and the patient is asked to cough. If an impulse is felt this is due to increased abdominal pressure being transmitted into the hernia. In cases where the neck is tight and the hernia irreducible there may be no cough impulse. This can lead to failure of diagnosis and is typical of femoral hernia where lack of an impulse leads the clinician to misdiagnose a lymph node. Cough impulse can also occur in a saphena varix (see Chapter 57) which may be referred to a surgeon as a suspected inguinal hernia. It is not unusual for a patient to describe an intermittent swelling but the surgeon finds nothing on examination. This is due to muscle tightening in an anxious patient (Summary boxes 60.3 and 60.4).

Summary box 60.3

Checks

- Reducibility
- Cough impulse
- Tenderness
- Overlying skin colour changes
- Multiple defects/contralateral side
- Signs of previous repair
- Scrotal content for groin hernia
- Associated pathology

Summary box 60.4

Examination

- A swelling with a cough impulse is not necessarily a hernia
- A swelling with no cough impulse may still be a hernia

If, on lying, the hernia does not reduce spontaneously, the surgeon asks the patient to attempt reduction as he may be well practised in this task while the surgeon might cause unnecessary discomfort. If neither the patient nor surgeon can reduce the hernia then treatment is more urgent. An irreducible hernia may influence the decision between open and laparoscopic surgery. With the hernia reduced, the surgeon assesses the size, rigidity and number of defects. Multiple defects may be present in incisional hernia.

Investigations for hernia

For most hernias, no specific investigation is required, the diagnosis being made on clinical examination. However, the patient may have symptoms suggesting a hernia but no hernia is found or have a swelling suggestive of hernia but with clinical uncertainty. It is important to be certain that any symptoms described are due to a hernia and not to coexisting pathology. There may also be a requirement for more detailed information than can be found by examination alone. Plain x-ray of the abdomen is of little value (Figure 60.5) although a hiatus hernia and diaphragmatic hernia may be seen on chest x-ray. Ultrasound scan may be helpful in cases of irreducible hernia, where the differential diagnosis includes a mass or fluid collection, or when the nature of the hernia content is in doubt. Ultrasound is very useful in the early postoperative period when a haematoma or seroma may develop and be difficult to distinguish from an early recurrence. Ultrasound is non-invasive and low cost but operator dependent.

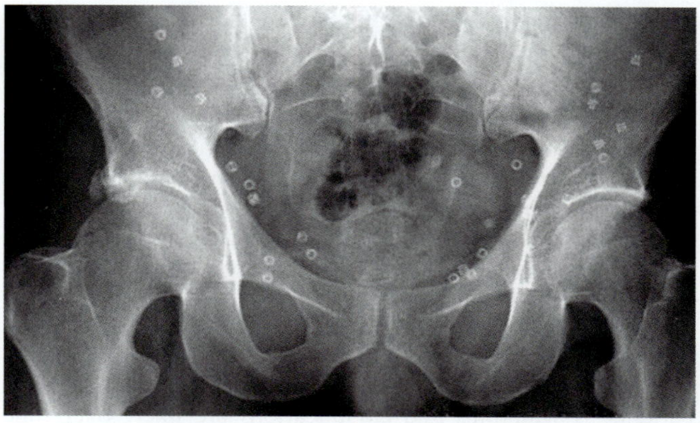

Figure 60.5 X-ray showing staples causing chronic pain after transabdominal preperitoneal repair.

Computed tomography scanning is helpful in complex incisional hernia, determining the number and size of muscle defects, identifying the content, giving some indication of presence of adhesions and excluding other intra-abdominal pathology such as ascites, occult malignancy, portal hypertension, etc.

Contrast barium radiology is occasionally useful in the absence of CT. Contrast may also be injected directly into the peritoneum, a herniagram, to identify an occult sac, especially in occult inguinal hernia. Magnetic resonance imaging (MRI) can help in the diagnosis of sportsman's groin where pain is the presenting feature and the surgeon needs to distinguish an occult hernia from an orthopaedic injury.

Laparoscopy itself may be used. In incisional hernia, initial laparoscopy may determine that a laparoscopic approach is feasible or not depending on the extent of adhesions. In inguinal hernia repair by the transabdominal route, initial laparoscopy can determine the presence of an occult contralateral hernia which has been described in up to 20 per cent of patients (Summary box 60.5).

Summary box 60.5

Investigations

- Plain x-ray – of little value
- Ultrasound scan – low cost, operator dependent
- CT scan – incisional hernia
- MRI scan – good in sportsman's groin with pain
- Contrast radiology – especially for inguinal hernia
- Laparoscopy – useful to identify occult contra lateral inguinal hernia

Management principles

An abdominal wall hernia does not necessarily require repair. A patient may request surgery for relief of symptoms of discomfort, cosmesis or to establish the diagnosis when in doubt. The surgeon should recommend repair when complications are likely, the most worrying being strangulation with bowel obstruction and bowel infarction. All cases of femoral hernia, with high risk of strangulation, should be repaired surgically. Any case of irreducible hernia, especially where there is pain and tenderness, should be offered repair unless coexisting medical factors place the patient at very high risk from surgery or anaesthesia. Increasing difficulty in reduction and increasing size are indications for surgery. Surgery should be offered to younger adult patients as symptoms and complications are likely over time (Summary box 60.6).

Summary box 60.6

Management

- Not all hernias require surgical repair
- Small hernias can be more dangerous than large
- Pain, tenderness and skin colour changes imply high risk of strangulation
- Femoral hernia should always be repaired

In reality, most patients with a hernia should be offered repair. In the elderly, if the hernia is asymptomatic, small in size, can be reduced easily and is not causing anxiety then observation alone should be sufficient. This policy, called 'watchful waiting' has been studied in asymptomatic inguinal hernia. One study reported such a policy to be safe but a second study was abandoned when a small number of patients developed strangulation. A truss can be used to control a hernia but few surgeons would recommend this approach. Small paraumbilical hernias are often seen. They cause few symptoms and usually contain fat or omentum with a very low risk of complications.

Large incisional hernias, particularly recurrent, present a major problem. Surgical repair is a complex procedure with significant risk of complications and later recurrence. When the neck is wide, the risk of strangulation is low. In the obese and elderly patient, these risks may outweigh the benefits of surgery and it is common for surgeons to adopt a conservative approach.

Any patient who presents with acute pain in a hernia, particularly if irreducible, should be offered surgery. Often, in a patient with an irreducible hernia, after admission to hospital and adequate analgesia, the hernia will reduce due to muscle relaxation. The likelihood of similar episodes is very high and surgery should be recommended at this admission or soon after.

Operative approaches to hernia

All surgical repairs follow the same basic principles:

1. reduction of the hernia content into the abdominal cavity with removal of any non-viable tissue and bowel repair if necessary;
2. excision and closure of a peritoneal sac if present or replacing it deep to the muscles;
3. reapproximation of the walls of the neck of the hernia if possible;
4. permanent reinforcement of the abdominal wall defect with sutures or mesh.

Reduction of hernia content is essential for a successful repair. It is rare that a surgeon fails to reduce the hernia but extensive dissection can lead to bowel injury sometimes requiring bowel resection with subsequent risks of infection and bowel anastomotic complications.

Excision and closure of the peritoneal sac is ideal but not essential. During laparoscopic repair of incisional hernia, surgeons will often leave the sac *in situ* after reducing hernia contents and simply fix a mesh over the neck to prevent recurrence. There is risk of fluid formation within the sac (seroma). This is a common complication in all forms of hernia repair. In lateral (indirect) inguinal hernia, most surgeons excise the peritoneal sac but some leading experts recommend that it be dissected from surrounding tissue and simply pushed back through the deep inguinal ring. In laparoscopic repair of inguinal hernias, surgeons simply pull the sac back into the abdominal cavity from within and do not excise it.

Closure of the abdominal wall defect is ideal but may not be possible when the defect is large or when tissues are rigid. Plastic surgical techniques have been developed to 'borrow' tissue from elsewhere in order to cover large muscle defects but usually at the cost of leaving a weak area elsewhere. Over the past 20 to 30 years, surgeons have realised that simple closure of a hernia defect by sutures alone leads to a high recurrence rate.

Additional reinforcement of the defect with a non-absorbable mesh is now widely practised in most hernia repairs and evidence has shown that recurrence rates have improved but recurrence still remains a problem. A recent large-scale study reported that mesh repair delays but does not prevent recurrence. With improved surgical techniques and new meshes it is hoped that recurrence after surgery will fall further. Mesh repair has become so important in hernia surgery that some understanding of mesh technology is essential for the modern surgeon.

Mesh in hernia repair

The term 'mesh' refers to prosthetic material, either a net or a flat sheet which is used to strengthen a hernia repair. Mesh can be used:

- to bridge a defect: the mesh is simply fixed over the defect as a tension-free patch;
- to plug a defect: a plug of mesh is pushed into the defect;
- to augment a repair: the defect is closed with sutures and the mesh added for reinforcement.

A well-placed mesh should have good overlap around all margins of the defect, at least 2 cm but up to 5 cm if possible. Suturing a mesh edge-to-edge into the defect (inlay), with no overlap, is not recommended. Mesh plug repairs have gained some popularity in small defects especially where overlap is hard to achieve. Plug operations are fast but plugs can form a dense 'meshoma' of plug and collagen. Other complications include migration, erosion into adjacent organs, fistula formation and chronic pain.

Mesh types

The wide array of meshes available can be classified as follows.

Gross structure

Net meshes are woven or knitted. Flat sheets are not porous but can be perforated with multiple holes. Net meshes allow fibrous tissue in growth between the strands and becoming adherent and integrated into host tissues within a few months. Initial fixation of the mesh is by glue, sutures or staples which may be absorbable. In laparoscopic inguinal hernia, no fixation is required at all as friction is sufficient to hold the mesh. 'Sheet' meshes do not allow host tissue in growth but become encapsulated by fibrous tissue. They always require strong, non-absorbable fixation to prevent mesh migration.

Synthetic mesh

The majority of meshes used today are synthetic polymers of polypropylene, polyester or polytetrafluoroethylene (PTFE) (Figure 60.6a,b). They are non-absorbable and provoke little tissue reaction. Polypropylene makes a strong monofilament mesh. It does not have any antibacterial properties but its hydrophobic nature and monofilament microstructure impede bacterial in-growth. Polyester is a braided filament mesh. This structure may allow infection to take hold, aided by its hydrophilic property. However this property also allows rapid vascular and cellular infiltration within the fibrils aiding host immune responses to infection and providing a stronger host–tissue interface. PTFE meshes are flat sheets and as a result do not allow any tissue in-growth. They are used as a non-adhesive barrier between tissue layers.

Weight and porosity

Synthetic meshes are very strong and early meshes were much stronger than a human abdominal wall so are considered as 'over-engineered'. All meshes provoke a fibrous reaction. More dense or heavyweight meshes provoke a greater reaction leading to collagen contraction and stiffening. The term 'mesh shrinkage' is often used to describe a progressive decrease in size of a mesh over time. It is due to natural contraction of fibrous tissue embedded in the mesh, reducing the area of mesh itself. This can lead to tissue tension and pain, a common complication of mesh repair. It can also lead to hernia recurrence if the mesh no longer covers the defect. Meshes can shrink by up to 50 per cent and, in occasional cases, even more. Meshes with thinner strands and larger spaces between them, 'lightweight, large-pore meshes', are preferred as they have better tissue integration, less shrinkage, more flexibility and improved comfort.

The terms 'light, medium and heavy' are not precisely defined but meshes less than 40 g/m^2 are generally referred to as light and meshes more than 80 g/m^2 are heavy.

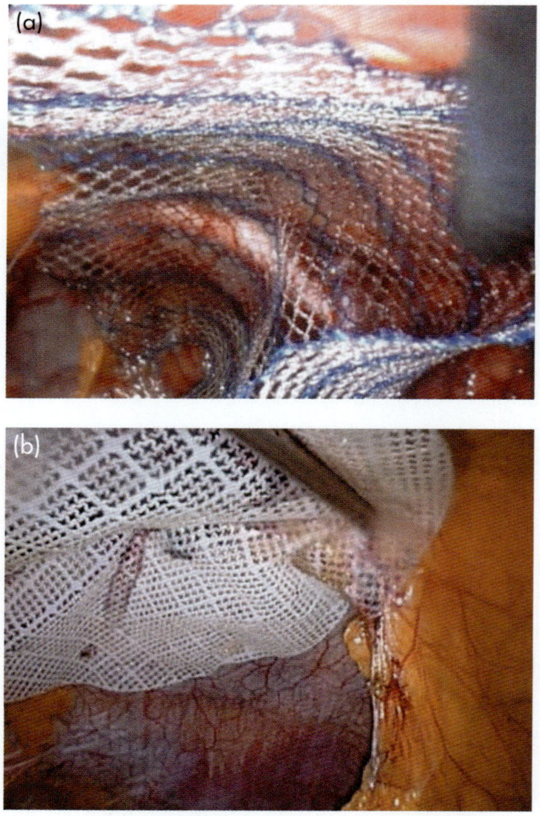

Figure 60.6 (a) Polypropylene mesh in totally extraperitonal (TEP) inguinal hernia repair and (b) polytetrafluoroethylene (PTFE) mesh in paraumbilical hernia repair.

Biological mesh

There are 'biological meshes' which are sheets of sterilised, decellularised, non-immunogenic connective tissue. They derive from human or animal dermis, bovine pericardium or porcine intestinal submucosa. They provide a 'scaffold' to encourage neovascular in-growth and new collagen deposition. Host enzymes eventually break down the biological implant which is replaced and remodelled with 'normal' host fibrous tissue. The rates of enzymatic degradation and collagen deposition vary between products and also depend on the local environment of the mesh. In the presence of infection, some biological meshes rapidly break down and weaken before remodelling can occur. Others remain strong, their labyrinthine microstructure allowing vascular in-growth to aid infection resistance. The choice of biological mesh depends on the clinical situation for which it is to be used. They are expensive.

Absorbable meshes

There are also synthetic absorbable meshes, such as those made from polyglycolic acid fibre. They are used in temporary abdominal wall closure and to buttress sutured repairs. They have no current role in hernia repair as they absorb and induce minimal collagen deposition.

Tissue-separating meshes

Most meshes induce fibrosis and, if placed within the peritoneal cavity, promote unwanted adhesions. New meshes have been designed for intraperitoneal use. Most of these have very different surfaces, one being sticky and one being slippery. Good adherence and host–tissue in-growth is required on the parietal (muscle) side of the mesh but the opposite (bowel) side needs to prevent adhesions to bowel. Usually one side of the mesh is coated by material which prevents adhesions (Figure 60.7), such as polycellulose, collagen, PTFE, etc. A recent mesh made entirely of a sheet of condensed PTFE with multiple perforations can be used intraperitoneally as the peritoneum will grow in through its perforations while bowel will not adhere to its inside (Summary box 60.7).

Positioning the mesh

The strength of a mesh repair depends on host–tissue in-growth. Meshes should be placed on a firm, well-vascularised tissue bed with generous overlap of the defect. The mesh can be placed:

- just outside of the muscle in the subcutaneous space (onlay);
- within the defect (inlay) – only applies to mesh plugs in small defects;

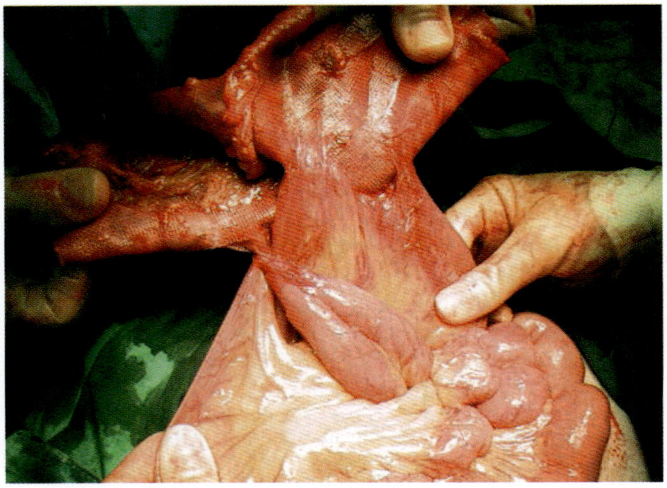

Figure 60.7 Adhesions to mesh.

Summary box 60.7

Mesh characteristics

- Woven, knitted or sheet
- Synthetic or biological – mainly synthetic
- Light, medium or heavyweight – lightweight becoming more popular
- Large pore, small pore – large pore causes less fibrosis and pain
- Intraperitoneal use or not – non-adhesive mesh on one side
- Non-absorbable or absorbable – mainly non-absorbable

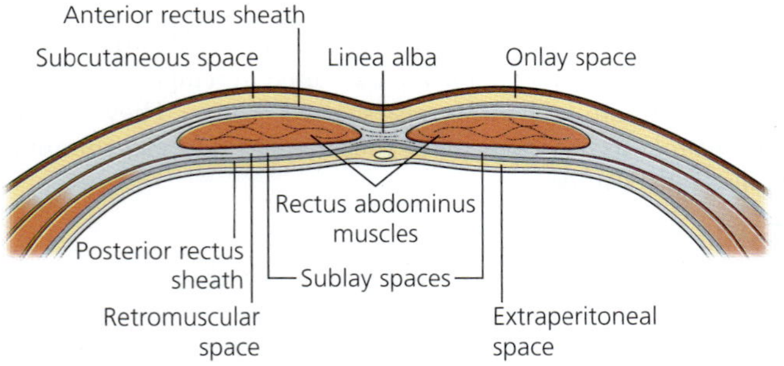

Figure 60.8 Diagrammatic representation of the various layers into which meshes are placed in ventral hernia repair.

- between fascial layers in the abdominal wall (intraparietal or sublay);
- immediately extraperitoneally, against muscle or fascia (also sublay);
- intraperitoneally.

At open surgery all of these planes are used but laparoscopic surgeons currently only use intraperitoneal or extraperitoneal planes (Figure 60.8).

Limitations to the use of mesh

The presence of infection limits the use of mesh, particularly heavyweight types. If a mesh becomes infected then it often needs to be removed. Some infected meshes can be salvaged using a combination of debridement of non-incorporated mesh, appropriate antibiotics and modern vacuum-assisted dressings.

Meshes are expensive, especially those for intraperitoneal use, but prices are falling and there are reports of low-cost solutions such as mosquito netting!

SPECIFIC HERNIA TYPES

Hernia sites are shown in Figure 60.9.

Inguinal hernia

The inguinal hernia, often referred to as a 'rupture' by patients, is the most common hernia in men and women but much more common in men. There are two basic types which are fundamentally different in anatomy, causation and complications. However, they are anatomically very close to one another, surgical repair techniques are very similar and ultimate reinforcement of the weakened anatomy is identical so they are often referred to together as inguinal hernia (Summary box 60.8).

Summary box 60.8

Inguinal hernia

- Types – lateral (oblique, indirect); medial (direct), sliding
- Origin – congenital or acquired
- Anatomy – inguinal canal
- Classification – latest European Hernia Society
- Diagnosis – usually clinical but radiological in special circumstances
- Surgery – open and laparoscopic

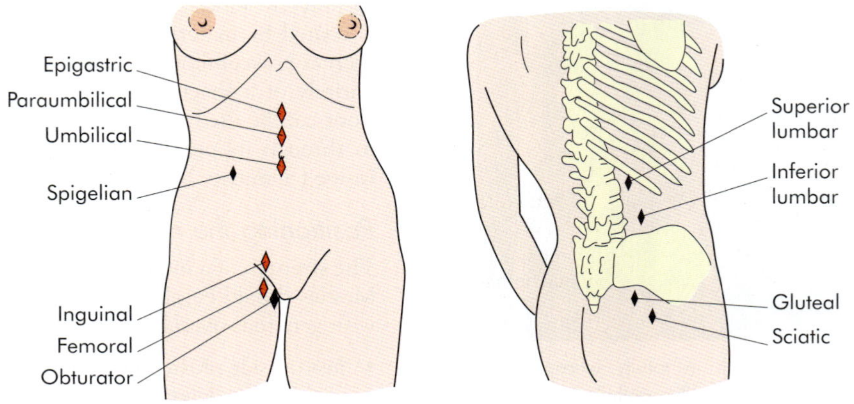

Figure 60.9 Diagram to show the sites of abdominal wall hernias, common in red and rare in black. Incisional and parastomal hernias can be found at various sites.

PART 11 | ABDOMINAL

The congenital inguinal hernia is known as indirect, oblique or lateral while the acquired hernia is called direct or medial. There is a third 'sliding' hernia which is acquired but is lateral in position (see below).

Basic anatomy of the inguinal canal

As the testis descends from the abdominal cavity to the scrotum in the male it firsts passes through a defect called the deep inguinal ring in the transversalis fascia, just deep to the abdominal muscles. This ring lies midway between the anterior superior iliac spine and the pubic tubercle, approximately 2–3 cm above the femoral artery pulse in the groin. The inferior epigastric vessels lie just medial to the deep inguinal ring passing from the iliac vessels to the rectus abdominus muscle. Muscle fibres of the innermost two layers of the lateral abdominal wall, the transversus muscle and the internal oblique muscle, arch over the deep inguinal ring from lateral to medial before descending to become attached to the pubic tubercle. These two muscles fuse and become tendinous, hence this arch is referred to as the conjoint tendon. Below this arch there is no muscle but only transversalis fascia and external oblique aponeurosis resulting in weakness (Figure 60.10).

The testis proceeds medially and downwards along the inguinal canal. Anterior to the canal is the aponeurosis of the external oblique muscle whose fibres run downwards and medially. The testis finally emerges through a v-shaped defect in the aponeurosis, the superficial inguinal ring, and descends into the scrotum. The inguinal canal is roofed by the conjoint tendon, its posterior wall is transversalis fascia, an anterior wall is the external oblique aponeurosis and a floor which is also external oblique which rolls inwards at its lower margin and thickens to become the inguinal ligament (Poupart's). The inguinal canal in the male contains the testicular artery, veins, lymphatics and the vas deferens. In the female, the round ligament descends through the canal to end in the vulva. Three important nerves, the ilioinguinal, the iliohypogastric and the genital branch of the genitofemoral nerve also pass through the canal.

As the testis descends, a tube of peritoneum is pulled with the testis and wraps around it ultimately to form the tunica vaginalis. This peritoneal tube should obliterate, possibly under hormonal control, but it commonly fails to fuse either in part or totally. As a result, bowel within the peritoneal cavity is able to pass inside the tube down towards the scrotum. Inguinal hernia in neonates and young children is always of this congenital type. However, in other patients, the muscles around the deep inguinal ring are able to prevent a hernia from developing until later in life, when under the constant positive abdominal pressure, the deep inguinal ring and muscles are stretched and a hernia becomes apparent. As the hernia increases in size, the contents are directed down into the scrotum. These hernias can become massive and may be referred to as a scrotal hernia (Figure 60.11).

An indirect hernia is lateral as its origin is lateral to the inferior epigastric vessels. It is also oblique as the hernia passes obliquely from lateral to medial through the abdominal muscle layers.

The second type of inguinal hernia, referred to as direct or medial, is acquired. It is a result of stretching and weakening of the abdominal wall just medial to the inferior epigastric (IE) vessels. Looked at from within the abdominal cavity, there is a triangle referred to as Hasselbach's triangle, whose three sides are the IE vessels laterally, the lateral edge of the rectus abdominus muscle medially and the pubic bone below (the iliopubic tract) (Figure 60.12). This area is weak as the abdominal wall here only consists of transversalis fascia covered by the external oblique aponeurosis. A direct, medial hernia is more likely in elderly

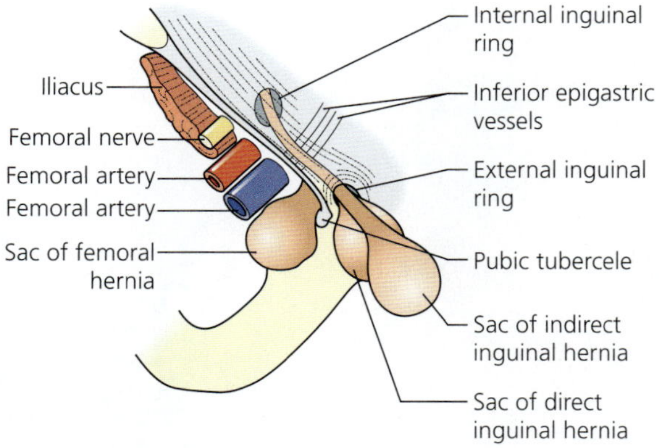

Figure 60.10 The close relationships of direct inguinal, indirect inguinal and femoral hernias.

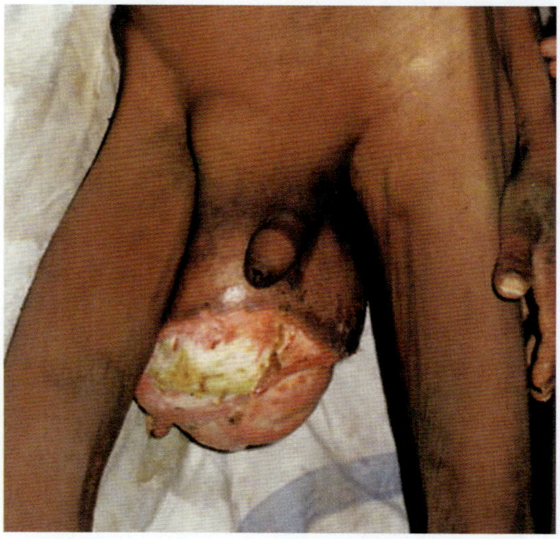

Figure 60.11 A huge scrotal hernia that has descended into the scrotum. The overlying skin has become gangrenous and sloughed away (courtesy of Dr Anupam Rai, Jabalpur, India).

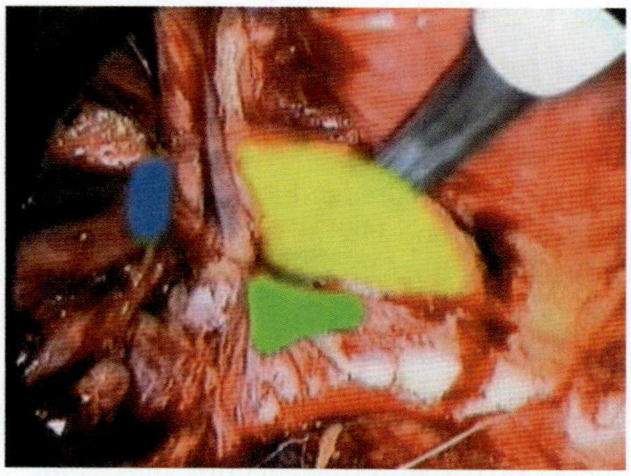

Figure 60.12 Laparoscopic view of posterior inguinal region with hernia defects highlighted: yellow – medial inguinal; blue – lateral inguinal; green – femoral.

patients. It is broadly based and therefore unlikely to strangulate. The medially placed bladder can be pulled into a direct hernia (Figure 60.13).

The third type of inguinal hernia is referred to as a sliding hernia. This is also an acquired hernia due to weakening of the abdominal wall but this occurs at the deep inguinal ring lateral to the IE vessels. Retroperitoneal fatty tissue is pushed downwards along the inguinal canal. As more tissue enters the hernia, peritoneum is pulled with it, thus creating a sac. However the sac has formed secondarily, distinguishing it from a classic indirect hernia. On the left side, sigmoid colon may be pulled into a sliding hernia and on the right side the caecum. Surgeons need extra caution during repair as the wall of the large bowel may not be covered by peritoneum and can be damaged.

Occasionally, both lateral and medial hernias are present in the same patient (pantaloon hernia).

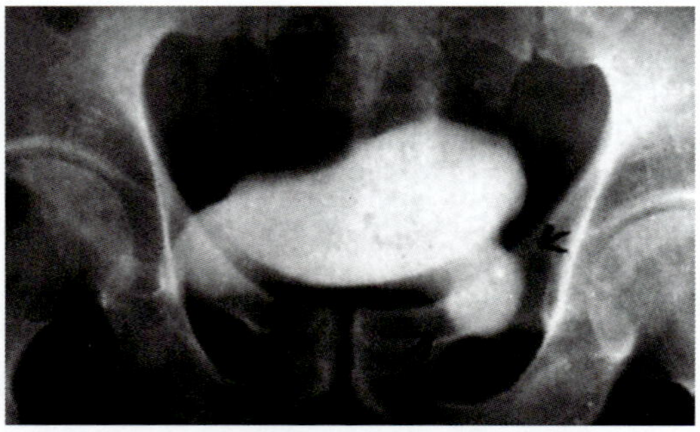

Figure 60.13 This cystogram shows the urinary bladder, part of which has descended into a left direct inguinal hernia.

Classification

Many surgeons over the past hundred years have attempted to classify inguinal (and femoral) hernias, including Casten, Halverson and McVay, Zollinger, Ponka, Gilbert and Nyhus. The European Hernia Society has recently suggested a simplified system of:

- primary or recurrent (P or R);
- lateral, medial or femoral (L, M or F);
- defect size in finger breadths assumed to be 1.5 cm.

A primary, indirect, inguinal hernia with a 3-cm defect size would be PL2.

Diagnosis of an inguinal hernia

In most cases, the diagnosis of an inguinal hernia is simple and patients often know their diagnosis as they are so common. Usually these hernias are reducible presenting as intermittent swellings, lying above and lateral to the pubic tubercle with an associated cough impulse. Often the hernia will reduce on lying and reappear on standing. With the patient lying down, the patient is asked to reduce the hernia if it has not spontaneously reduced. If the patient cannot then the surgeon gently attempts to reduce the hernia. Once reduced, the surgeon identifies the bony landmarks of the anterior superior iliac spine and pubic tubercle to landmark the deep inguinal ring at the mid-inguinal point. Gentle pressure is applied at this point and the patient asked to cough. If the hernia is controlled with pressure on the deep inguinal ring then it is likely to be indirect/lateral and if the hernia appears medial to this point then it is direct/medial. Other examination techniques have been suggested but even experienced surgeons find it difficult to distinguish lateral and medial hernias with certainty (Figure 60.14).

Diagnostic difficulties

Confirmation of the diagnosis may not be possible when the patient describes an intermittent swelling but nothing is found on examination. Surgeons will often accept the diagnosis on history alone but re-examination at a later date or investigation by ultrasound scan may be requested.

If an inguinal hernia becomes irreducible and tense there may be no cough impulse. Differential diagnosis would include a lymph node groin mass or an abdominal mass. Such cases require urgent investigation by either ultrasound or CT scan (Figure 60.15).

Large scrotal hernias may be misdiagnosed as a hydrocoele or other testicular swelling. The surgeon should be able to identify the upper limit of a scrotal swelling but a large scrotal hernia has no upper limit as it extends back along the inguinal canal to the

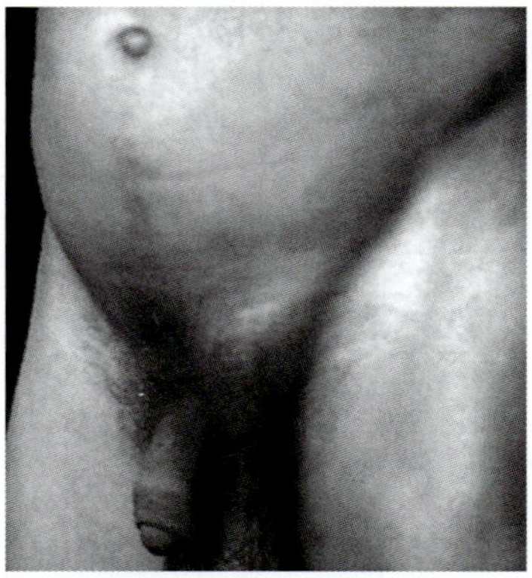

Figure 60.14 Oblique left inguinal hernia that became apparent when the patient coughed and persisted until it was reduced when he lay down.

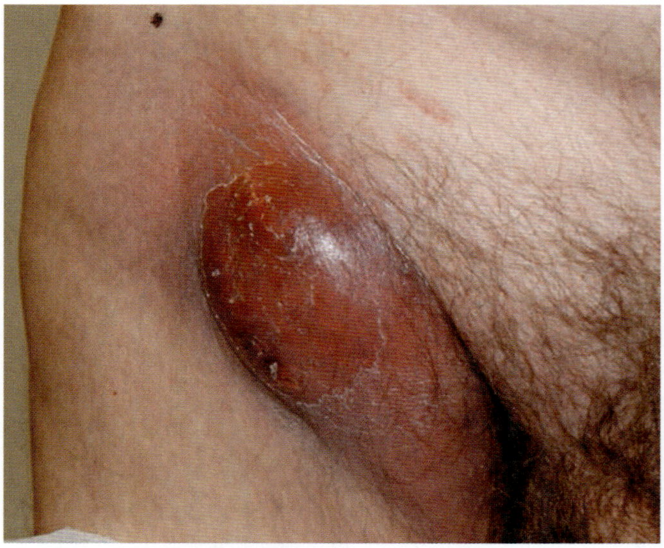

Figure 60.15 Malignant mass of nodes.

peritoneal cavity. In cases of doubt, ultrasound scanning should establish the diagnosis.

As inguinal hernia is so common, less-experienced clinicians might suggest this diagnosis when referring cases of femoral hernia or spigelian hernia. Also patients with a saphena varix may present with a swelling which increases in size on standing and with a definite cough impulse and be misdiagnosed as a hernia. The same can be true for a varicocoele.

It is essential to examine the scrotal contents to exclude other pathologies and to check that the patient has two testes. It is important to examine the opposite side as contralateral hernia is common. Even if the contralateral side is weak, then bilateral repair should be recommended as the risk of contralateral recurrence is high. Ten per cent of all patients will present with bilateral inguinal hernias and up to 20 per cent more will have an occult contralateral hernia on laparoscopic evaluation. A patient with a single hernia has a lifetime 33 per cent risk of developing a hernia on the other side. Some surgeons have suggested that all patients should be offered bilateral repair especially if laparoscopic surgery is planned, but this is not widespread practice at present.

Investigations for inguinal hernia

Most cases require no diagnostic tests but ultrasound scanning, CT scan and MRI scan are occasionally used. A herniogram involves the injection of contrast into the peritoneal cavity followed by screening which shows the presence of a sac or asymmetric bulging of the inguinal anatomy.

Management of inguinal hernia

It is safe to recommend no active treatment in cases of early, asymptomatic, direct hernia, particularly in elderly patients who do not wish surgical intervention. These patients should be warned to seek early advice if the hernia increases in size or becomes symptomatic. Surgical trusses are not recommended but may be required for occasional patients who refuse any form of surgical intervention.

Elective surgery for inguinal hernia is a common and simple operation. It can be undertaken under local, regional or general anaesthesia with minimal risk even in high-risk patients.

Herniotomy

In children who have lateral hernias with a persistent processus, it is sufficient only to remove and close the sac. This is called a herniotomy. In adult surgery, herniotomy alone has a high recurrence rate and some form of muscle strengthening is added (herniorrhaphy).

Open suture repair

In 1890, Eduardo Bassini described suture repair for inguinal hernia (Figure 60.16). This was a massive leap forward and has been the basis of open repair for over 100 years. The surgeon enters the inguinal canal by opening its anterior wall, the external oblique aponeurosis. The spermatic cord is dissected free and the presence of a lateral or a medial hernia is confirmed. The sac of a lateral hernia is separated from the cord, opened and any contents reduced. The sac is then sutured closed at its neck and excess sac removed. If there is a medial hernia then it is inverted and the transversalis fascia is suture plicated. Sutures are now placed between the conjoint tendon above and the inguinal ligament below, extending from the pubic tubercle to the deep

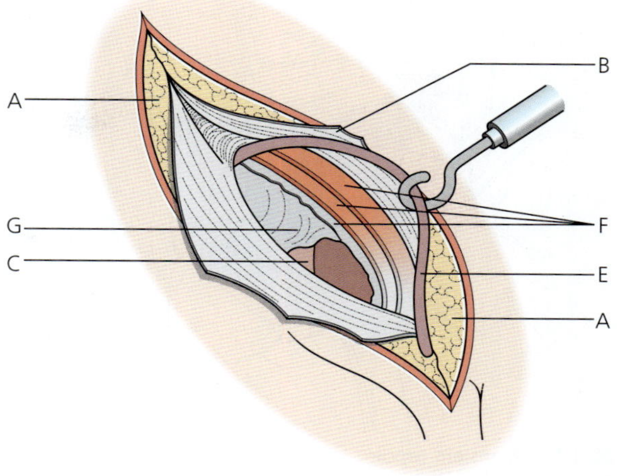

Figure 60.16 Bassini's original diagram. A, subcutaneous fat; B, external oblique; C, iliac vein; E, spermatic cord; F, nerves in inguinal canal; G, transversalis fascia.

inguinal ring. The posterior wall of the inguinal canal is thus strengthened.

Over 150 modifications to the Bassini operation have been described with little or no benefit except for the Shouldice modification. In this operation, the transversalis fascia is opened by a central incision from the deep inguinal ring to the pubic tubercle and then closed to create a double-thick, two-layered posterior wall (double breasting). The external oblique is closed in similar fashion. Expert centres have reported lifetime failure rates of less than 2 per cent after Shouldice repair but it is a technically demanding operation which, in general hands, gives results identical to the Bassini repair.

Today, when a Bassini-type operation is done, most surgeons use a continuous, non-absorbable nylon or polypropylene suture which is darned between the conjoint tendon and inguinal ligament. This operation was described by Maloney, and recently published large randomised trials have reported excellent results when compared to mesh techniques. It is the most common operation performed in countries where mesh is too expensive.

Suture repair is still under development, and recently, Desarda has described an operation where a 1–2-cm strip of external oblique aponeurosis lying over the inguinal canal is isolated from the main muscle but left attached both medially and laterally. It is then sutured to the conjoint tendon and inguinal ligament, reinforcing the posterior wall of the inguinal canal. As the abdominal muscles contract, this strip of aponeurosis tightens to add further physiological support to the posterior wall. This operation is currently being evaluated.

Open flat mesh repair

Synthetic mesh has been used since the 1950s to reinforce hernia repair, and in the 1980s Lichtenstein described a tension-free, simple, flat, polypropylene mesh repair for inguinal hernia (Figure 60.17). The initial part of the operation is identical to Bassini. Once the hernia sac has been removed and any medial defect closed, a piece of mesh, measuring 8 × 15 cm, is placed over the posterior wall, behind the spermatic cord, and is split to wrap around the spermatic cord at the deep inguinal ring. Loose sutures hold the mesh to the inguinal ligament and conjoint tendon. Two major advantages are claimed: lowered

Eduardo Bassini, 1844–1924, Professor of Surgery, Padua, Italy, described this method of herniorraphy in 1889.

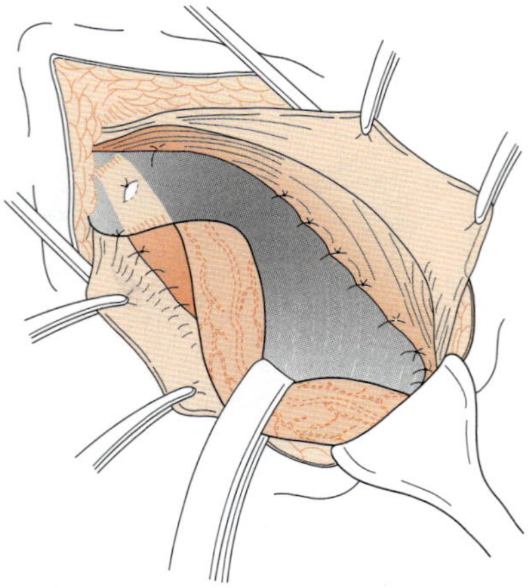

Figure 60.17 Lichtenstein repair.

hernia recurrence rates and accelerated postoperative recovery. Randomised trials show that hernia recurrence within the first two years is lowered but acute pain scores are similar. Recent research comparing the Lichtenstein repair with laparoscopic surgery has identified chronic pain as the most common complication of open flat mesh repair with rates reported as high as 20 per cent. Nonetheless, today, the Lichtenstein repair is the most common operation for inguinal hernia in the developed world.

Open plug/device/complex mesh repair

Surgeons and industry have been highly creative, attempting to improve on simple flat mesh repair. A surgeon in Europe has over 200 different products and techniques from which to choose. Shaped mesh plugs have gained much attention being simple to insert into the defect and requiring little if any fixation. However, they can become solid (meshoma) and also migrate. Meshes have been designed to be placed beneath the transversalis fascia. The surgeon introduces a finger through the deep inguinal ring and bluntly (and blindly) opens the preperitoneal space deep to the inguinal canal into which a mesh is inserted. A two-layered mesh ('hernia system'), in which the inner layer is placed deep to transversalis fascia and the outer layer superficial to it, is also gaining popularity. To date, there is little evidence to show any of these techniques is superior to the Lichtenstein operation.

Open preperitoneal repair

This approach was first described by Annandale in 1880, but was largely discarded until the 1950s when Stoppa, a French surgeon, described it with mesh reconstruction. It is useful when multiple attempts at open standard surgery have failed and the hernia(s) keeps recurring. It may now be superseded by the totally extraperitoneal laparoscopic approach which is modelled on the Stoppa operation and first described by Ger, also French.

Laparoscopic inguinal hernia repair

Two techniques are described and have been extensively studied in randomised trials. The totally extraperitoneal (TEP) approach is more widely used than the transabdominal preperitoneal (TAPP) approach. In both, the aim of surgery is to reduce the hernia and hernia sac within the abdomen and then place a 10 × 15 cm mesh just deep to the abdominal wall, extending across the midline into the retropubic space and 5 cm lateral to the deep inguinal ring. The mesh covers Hasselbach's triangle, the deep inguinal ring and the femoral canal. In TEP, the surgeon is able to create a space just deep to the abdominal muscles without entering the peritoneal cavity whereas, in TAPP, the surgeon enters the peritoneal cavity then incises the peritoneum above the hernia defects and reflects it away from the muscles, essentially entering the same space as in TEP. Once the hernia is reduced, an identical mesh is inserted and the peritoneum closed over the mesh (Figures 60.18 and 60.19).

Over 60 randomised trials have compared laparoscopic surgery with the Lichtenstein repair. They show that, although the laparoscopic operation takes longer to perform, proven advantages are reduced pain both following surgery and up to five years later, more rapid return to full activity and reduced incidence of the wound complications of infection, bleeding and seroma. Laparoscopic surgery is of particular benefit in bilateral cases and in patients with hernia recurrence after open surgery. National statistics show that the proportion of cases performed laparoscopically is slowly rising but all agree that there is a slow learning curve associated with these technically demanding operations (Summary box 60.9).

Summary box 60.9

Operations for inguinal hernia

- Herniotomy
- Open suture repair
  - Bassini
  - Shouldice
  - Desarda
- Open flat mesh repair
  - Lichtenstein
- Open complex mesh repair
  - Plugs
  - Hernia systems
- Open preperitoneal repair
  - Stoppa
- Laparoscopic repair
  - TEP
  - TAPP

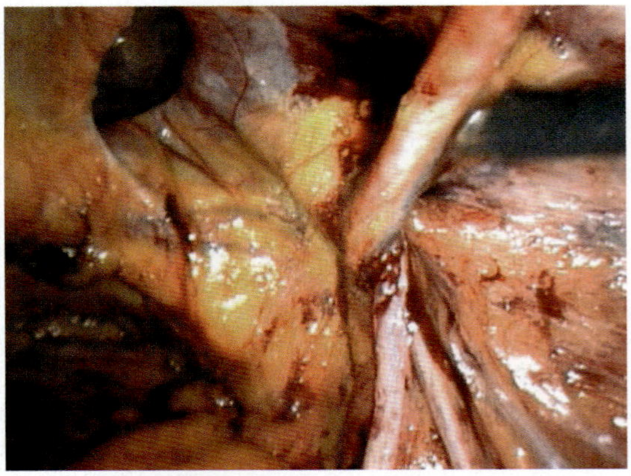

Figure 60.18 Right/medial direct hernia – laparascopic view. Note the medial (direct) defect upper left, the inferior epigastric vessels upper right and the structures of the spermatic cord lower right.

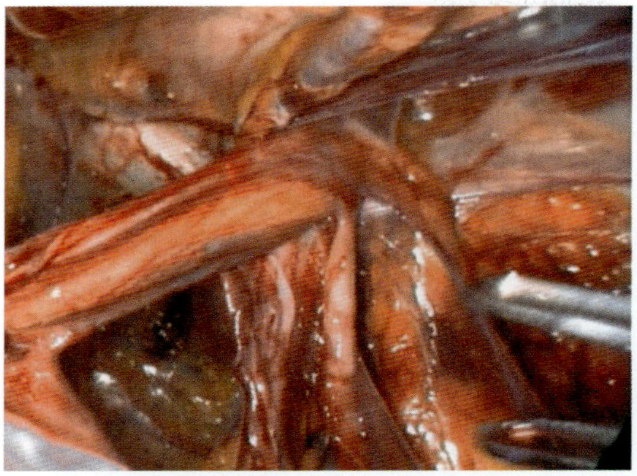

Figure 60.19 Right/lateral indirect hernia – laparoscopic view.

Emergency inguinal hernia surgery

Ninety-five per cent of inguinal hernia patients present at clinics and only 5 per cent present as an emergency with a painful irreducible hernia which may progress to strangulation and possible bowel infarction. The morbidity and mortality of emergency inguinal hernia surgery is high and surgery needs to be performed rapidly in a well-resuscitated patient with adequate postoperative high dependency or intensive care if necessary. The principles of surgery are the same as in an elective setting. Open surgery is preferred when a hernia is irreducible or if there is any risk of bowel resection. Infection may complicate these cases but most surgeons would still use a lightweight, synthetic mesh repair covered by appropriate antibiotics.

Complications of inguinal hernia surgery

Despite this being a common procedure and technically straightforward, postoperative complications are common. Immediate complications include bleeding (which may be due to accidental damage to the inferior epigastric or iliac vessels) and urinary retention which may require catheterisation. Occasional overenthusiastic infusion of local anaesthetic may lead to femoral nerve blockade, the patient being unable to move a leg. This usually resolves over 12 hours but is alarming.

Over the next week, seroma formation and wound infection may occur. Seroma is due to an excessive inflammatory response to sutures or mesh and cannot be prevented. In most cases the fluid resolves spontaneously but may require aspiration. After laparoscopic surgery, a seroma may be misdiagnosed as an early recurrence. Wound infection is not uncommon. Many surgeons use routine prophylactic antibiotics but recent studies suggest little benefit even when mesh is used.

In the longer term, hernia recurrence and chronic pain are the main concerns. No operation can guarantee to be recurrence free. Evidence shows that mesh repairs have lower recurrence rates than suture repairs but there is no difference between the various mesh repairs and no difference between open and laparoscopic surgery. There is very strong evidence that specialist hernia surgeons will have lower recurrence rates whatever technique they use.

Chronic pain, defined as pain present three months after surgery, is common after all forms of surgery. It is less common and less severe after laparoscopic surgery. Different types of pain have been described but the most severe is neuralgic pain due to nerve irritation. This may be the result of nerve injury at the time of operation or chronic irritation of nerves by suture material or mesh. Careful identification and protection of all three nerves passing along the inguinal canal reduces the incidence of neuralgic pain. This type of pain is also very uncommon after laparoscopic surgery which is performed at a deeper level away from the nerves. Some contribution to chronic pain may be due to the mesh which can become embedded in a dense collagenous reaction with shrinkage. This causes tissue tension and rigidity.

Rarely, damage to the testicular artery can lead to testicular infarction, perhaps the most serious complication of inguinal hernia surgery. There is no good evidence that hernia surgery has an effect on male fertility despite extensive study in this area (Summary box 60.10).

Summary box 60.10

Complications

- Early – pain, bleeding, urinary retention, anaesthetic related
- Medium – seroma, wound infection
- Late – chronic pain, testicular atrophy

Sportsman's hernia

This specific entity is well described and presents as severe pain in the groin area, extending into the scrotum and upper thigh. It is almost entirely restricted to young men who play contact sports such as football and rugby. The pain can be debilitating and prevent the patient from exercising. On examination there may be some tenderness in the region of the inguinal canal, over the pubic tubercle and over the insertion of the thigh adductor muscles. Usually no hernia can be felt and only occasionally can a true inguinal hernia be found.

In most cases, the pain is due to an orthopaedic injury, such as adductor strain or pubic symphasis diastasis. However, some believe that it can be due to muscle tearing (Gilmore's groin) or stretching of the posterior wall of the inguinal canal. Other causes of pain should be excluded, such as hip, pelvic or lumbar spinal disease and bladder/prostate problems. MRI scanning is most likely to detect an orthopaedic problem but ultrasound, herniography or even laparoscopy may be used.

There are many anecdotal reports of successful treatment using all types of inguinal hernia surgery, suture and mesh, open and laparoscopic, but no randomised trials. Hernia surgery should be a last resort and the patient warned of a significant risk of failure to cure the pain.

Femoral hernia

Basic anatomy

The iliac artery and vein pass below the inguinal ligament to become the femoral vessels in the leg. The vein lies medially and the artery just lateral to the artery with the femoral nerve lateral to the artery. They are enclosed in a fibrous sheath. Just medial to the vein is a small space containing fat and some lymphatic tissue (node of Cloquet). It is this space which is exploited by a femoral hernia. The walls of a femoral hernia are the femoral vein laterally, the inguinal ligament anteriorly, the pelvic bone covered by the

Sir Astley Paston Cooper, 1768–1841, surgeon, Guy's Hospital, London, UK. He received a baronetcy and one thousand guineas for successfully removing an infected wen from the head of King George IV at Brighton in 1821.

Jules Germain Cloquet, 1790–1883, Professor of Anatomy and Surgery, Paris, France.
Manoel Louise Antonio don Gimbernat, 1734–1816, Professor of Anatomy, Barcelona, Spain and later Director of the Royal College of Surgeons in Spain.

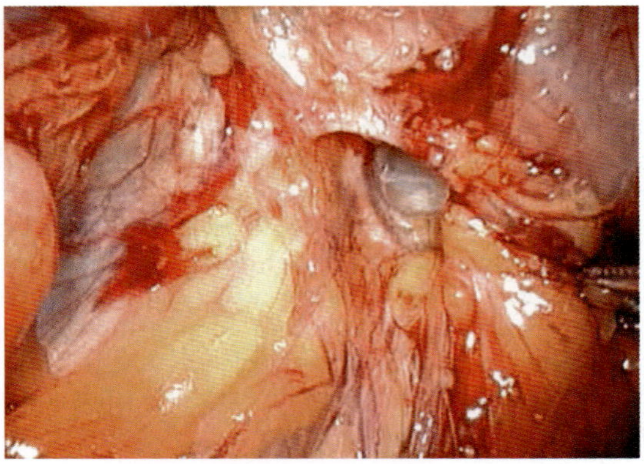

Figure 60.20 Left femoral hernia – laparoscopic view. Note the iliac vein left and lateral to the femoral hernia defect.

ileopectineal ligament (Astley Cooper's) posteriorly and the lacunar ligament (Gimbernat's) medially. This is a strong curved ligament with a sharp unyielding edge which impedes reduction of a femoral hernia (Figure 60.20).

The female pelvis has a different shape to the male, increasing the size of the femoral canal and the risk of hernia. In old age, the femoral defect increases and femoral hernia is commonly seen in low-weight, elderly females. There is a substantial risk of developing a femoral hernia after a sutured inguinal hernia repair (Denmark Hernia Registry) (Summary box 60.11).

Summary box 60.11

Femoral hernia

- Less common than inguinal hernia
- It is more common in females than in males
- Easily missed on examination
- Fifty per cent of cases present as an emergency with very high risk of strangulation

Diagnosis of femoral hernia

Diagnostic error is common and often leads to delay in diagnosis and treatment. The hernia appears below and lateral to the pubic tubercle and lies in the upper leg rather than in the lower abdomen. Inadequate exposure of this area during routine examination leads to failure to detect the hernia. The hernia often rapidly becomes irreducible and loses any cough impulse due to the tightness of the neck. It may only be 1–2 cm in size and can easily be mistaken for a lymph node. As it increases in size, it is reflected superiorly and becomes difficult to distinguish from a medial direct hernia which arises only a few centimetres above the femoral canal. A direct inguinal hernia leaves the

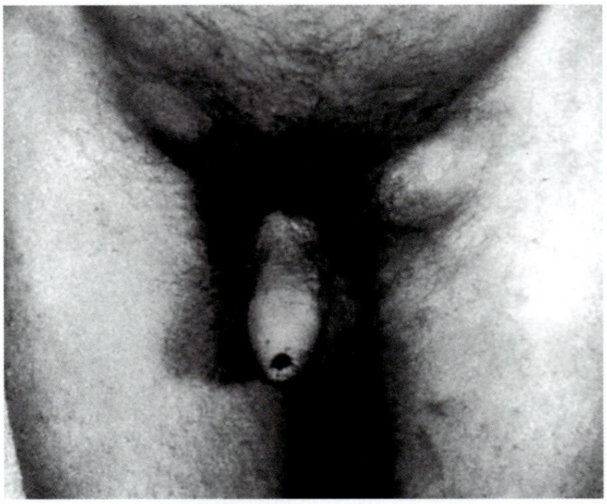

Figure 60.21 The patient has a left femoral and a right inguinal hernia.

abdominal cavity just above the inguinal ligament and a femoral hernia just below (Figure 60.21) (Summary box 60.12).

Summary box 60.12

Differential diagnosis

- Direct inguinal hernia
- Lymph node
- Saphena varix
- Femoral artery aneurysm
- Psoas abscess
- Rupture of adductor longus with haematoma

Investigations

In routine cases, no specific investigations are required. However, if there is uncertainly then ultrasound or CT should be requested. In the emergency patient, bowel obstruction usually occurs and a plain x-ray is likely to show small bowel obstruction. All patients with unexplained small bowel obstruction should undergo careful examination for a femoral hernia. It is now common to perform CT scanning in cases of bowel obstruction primarily to exclude malignancy, but it can identify an obstructing femoral hernia missed by clinicians.

Surgery for femoral hernia

There is no alternative to surgery for femoral hernia and it is wise to treat such cases with some urgency. There are three open approaches and appropriate cases can be managed laparoscopically.

Low approach (Lockwood)

This is the simplest operation for femoral hernia but only suitable when there is no risk of bowel resection. It can easily be performed under local anaesthesia. A transverse incision is made over the hernia. The sac of the hernia is opened and its contents reduced. The sac is also reduced and non-absorbable sutures placed between the inguinal ligament above and the fascia overlying the bone below. A small incision can be made in the medial lacunar ligament to aid reduction but there may be an abnormal branch of the obturator artery just deep to it which can bleed. The femoral vein, lateral to the hernia, needs to be protected. Some surgeons place a mesh plug into the hernia defect for further re-enforcement.

The inguinal approach (Lotheissen)

The initial incision is identical to that of a Bassini or Lichtenstein operation into the inguinal canal. The spermatic cord (or round ligament) is mobilised and the transversalis fascia opened from deep inguinal ring to pubic tubercle. A femoral hernia lies immediately below this incision and can be reduced by a combination of pulling from above and pushing from

Charles Barrett Lockwood, 1856–1914, surgeon, St Bartholomew's Hospital, London, UK.

below. If necessary, the peritoneum can be opened to help with reduction. Once reduced, the neck of the hernia is closed with sutures or a mesh plug, protecting the iliac vein throughout. The layers are closed as for inguinal hernia and the surgeon may place a mesh into the inguinal canal to protect against development of an inguinal hernia.

Some surgeons believe that exploration of the femoral canal to exclude a hernia should be a routine part of inguinal hernia surgery but most surgeons do not do this.

High approach (McEvedy)

This more complex operation is ideal in the emergency situation where the risk of bowel strangulation is high. It requires regional or general anaesthesia. A horizontal incision (classically vertical) is made in the lower abdomen centred at the lateral edge of the rectus muscle. The anterior rectus sheath is incised and the rectus muscle displaced medially. The surgeon proceeds deep to the muscle in the preperitoneal space. The femoral hernia is reduced and the sac opened to allow careful inspection of the bowel, and a decision made regarding the need for bowel resection. This is performed if necessary. In dubious cases, the bowel is replaced into the peritoneal cavity for 5 minutes and then re-examined. The femoral defect is then closed with sutures, mesh or plug. This approach allows a generous incision to be made in the peritoneum which aids inspection of the bowel and facilitates bowel resection.

Laparoscopic approach

Both the TEP and TAPP approaches can be used for femoral hernia and a standard mesh inserted. This is ideal for reducible femoral hernias presenting electively but not in emergency cases nor for irreducible hernia.

VENTRAL HERNIA

This term refers to hernias of the anterior abdominal wall. Inguinal and femoral hernias are not included even though they are ventral. Lumbar hernia is included despite being dorsolateral. The European Hernia Society classification (2009) distinguished primary ventral from incisional hernia but did not include parastomal hernia. We have included parastomal hernia and traumatic hernia (Summary box 60.13).

Summary box 60.13

Ventral hernias

- Umbilical – paraumbilical
- Epigastric
- Incisional
- Parastomal
- Spigelian
- Lumbar
- Traumatic

Umbilical hernia

The umbilical defect is present at birth but closes as the stump of the umbilical cord heals, usually within a week of birth. This process may be delayed, leading to the development of herniation in the neonatal period. The umbilical ring may also stretch and reopen in adult life.

Umbilical hernia in children

This common condition occurs in up to 10 per cent of infants, with a higher incidence in premature babies. The hernia appears within a few weeks of birth and is often symptomless but increases in size on crying and assumes a classical conical shape. Sexes are equally affected but the incidence in black infants is up to eight times higher than in white. Obstruction and/or strangulation are extremely uncommon below the age of three years.

Treatment

Conservative treatment is indicated under the age of two years when the hernia is symptomless. Parental reassurance is all that is necessary. Ninety-five per cent of hernias will resolve spontaneously. If the hernia persists beyond the age of two years it is unlikely to resolve and surgical repair is indicated.

Operation

A small curved incision is made immediately below the umbilicus. The neck of the sac is defined, opened and any contents are returned to the peritoneal cavity. The sac is closed and redundant sac is excised. The defect in the linea alba is closed with interrupted sutures (Summary box 60.14).

Summary box 60.14

Umbilical hernia in children

- Common in infants and most resolve spontaneously
- Rarely strangulate

Umbilical hernia in adults

Conditions which cause stretching and thinning of the midline raphe (linea alba), such as pregnancy, obesity and liver disease with cirrhosis, predispose to reopening of the umbilical defect. In adults, the defect in the median raphe is immediately adjacent to (most often above) the true umbilicus, although at operation this is indistinguishable. The term paraumbilical hernia is commonly used (Figure 60.22). The defect is rounded with a well-defined fibrous margin. Small umbilical hernias often contain extraperitoneal fat or omentum. Larger hernias can contain small or large bowel but, even when very large, the neck of the sac is narrow compared with the volume of its contents. As a result, in adults, umbilical hernias which include

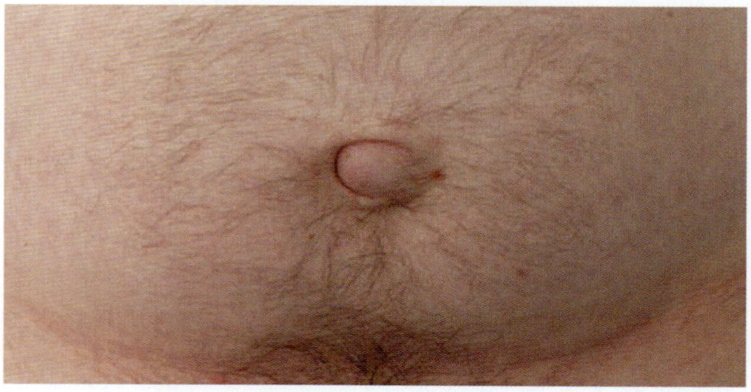

Figure 60.22 A small paraumbilical hernia.

George Lotheissen, 1868–1941, surgeon, the Kaiser Franz Joseph Hospital, Vienna, Austria, described this operation in 1898.
Peter George McEvedy, 1890–1951, surgeon, Ancoats Hospital, Manchester, UK.

bowel are prone to become irreducible, obstructed and strangulated.

Clinical features

Patients are commonly overweight with a thinned and attenuated midline raphe. The bulge is typically slightly to one side of the umbilical depression, creating a crescent-shaped appearance to the umbilicus (Figure 60.23). Women are affected more than men. Most patients complain of pain due to tissue tension or symptoms of intermittent bowel obstruction. In large hernias, the overlying skin may become thinned, stretched and develop dermatitis.

Treatment

Because of the high risk of strangulation, operation should be advised in cases where the hernia contains bowel. Small hernias may be left alone if they are asymptomatic, but they may enlarge and require surgery at a later date. Surgery may be performed open or laparoscopically.

Open umbilical hernia repair

Very small defects less than 1 cm in size may be closed with a simple figure-of-eight suture, or repaired by a darn technique where a non-absorbable, monofilament suture is criss-crossed across the defect and anchored firmly to the fascia all around.

Defects up to 2 cm in diameter may be sutured primarily with minimal tension, although the larger the defect, the more tension and the more likely it is that mesh reinforcement will be beneficial. The classical repair was described by Mayo. A transverse incision is made and the hernia sac dissected, opened and its content reduced. Any non-viable tissue is removed, sometimes involving bowel resection. The peritoneum is closed. The defect in the anterior rectus sheath is extended laterally on both sides and elevated to create an upper and lower flap. The lower flap is then inserted beneath the upper flap and sutured to it, with the upper flap being brought downwards over it so that the tissue is two-layered (double breasted). Non-absorbable sutures are used. There is often a large subcutaneous space. A suction drain is placed to reduce the risk of seroma and haematoma. The skin is closed but stretched or redundant skin may need to be excised (apronectomy) to achieve a better cosmetic result. Today, with modern suture materials, surgeons simply close the anterior sheath in a single layer.

For defects larger than 2 cm in diameter, mesh repair is recommended (Figure 60.24). The mesh may be placed in one of several anatomical planes:

- Within the peritoneal cavity – a tissue separating mesh is placed through the defect and spread out on the underside of the abdominal wall and fixed to it, ideally, with an overlap of 5 cm in each direction. This is a quick repair but requires the use of expensive mesh.
- In the retromuscular space – the linea alba is opened both vertically and both left and right posterior rectus sheaths are incised 1 cm to the side of the midline exposing the rectus muscle. The posterior sheaths are sutured together and the muscles elevated away from the sheath to develop the retromuscular space into which a sheet of mesh is placed and fixed by sutures. The mesh should overlap the midline by 5 cm laterally and the umbilicus vertically. It should therefore be a minimum diameter of 10 cm. A drain may be placed deep to the linea alba. This is a very secure repair but requires extensive dissection.
- In the extraperitoneal space – it is difficult, but possible, to develop the plane below the posterior rectus sheath, just outside the peritoneum. Care must be taken to avoid 'button-holing' the peritoneum as it is thin and fragile. Mesh can then be tucked into in this space, ensuring a good overlap as before. Ideally, the linea alba is closed over the mesh but if this is not possible, a flap of peritoneal sac can be used to cover the mesh. This is a good repair, but if the peritoneum is extensively damaged during the dissection, it will have to be abandoned in favour of an alternative technique.
- In the subcutaneous plane – this is the simplest technique, called an onlay mesh. The peritoneal sac and contents are dealt with as above. An attempt is made to close linea alba vertically with sutures and a disc of mesh is placed on the anterior rectus sheath and sutured to it. The mesh is lying in the subcutaneous space and is prone to infection.

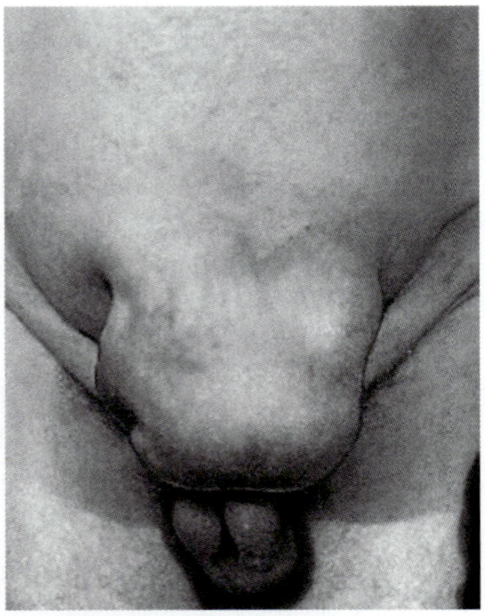

Figure 60.23 A large paraumbilical hernia.

William James Mayo, 1861–1939, surgeon, the Mayo Clinic, Rochester, MN, USA, described this operation in 1901. He and his brother Charles Horace Mayo (1865–1939) joined their father's private practice in Rochester. This practice became the Mayo Clinic. Their father William Worrall Mayo was born in Manchester, UK in 1919.

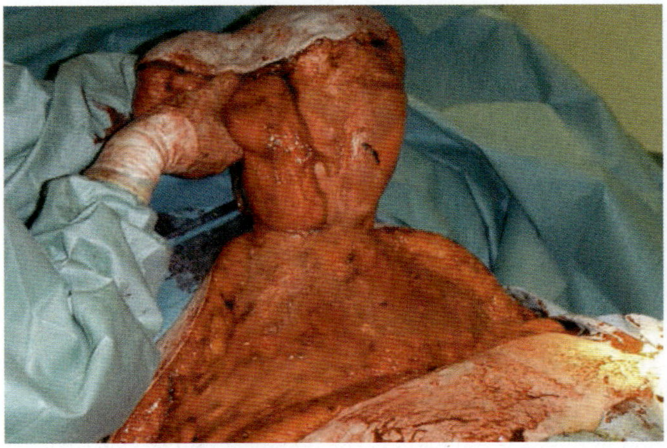

Figure 60.24 A massive paraumbilical hernia – operative view.

Laparoscopic umbilical hernia repair

Three ports are placed laterally on the abdominal wall, usually on the left side unless adhesions from previous surgery are likely. The contents of the hernia are reduced by traction and external pressure. The falciform ligament above and the median umbilical fold below may need to be taken down if they interfere with mesh placement. A disc of non-adherent mesh, designed for intraperitoneal use, is introduced and positioned on the under surface of the abdominal wall, centred on the defect. It is then fixed to the peritoneum and posterior rectus sheaths using staples, tacks or sutures. This is a simple and secure repair which achieves generous overlap without surgical damage to umbilicus and surrounding fascia (Figure 60.25). However, it requires specialised equipment and expensive tissue-separating mesh. Intraperitoneal meshes can cause severe pain lasting for 24–48 hours after surgery which can mimic peritonitis.

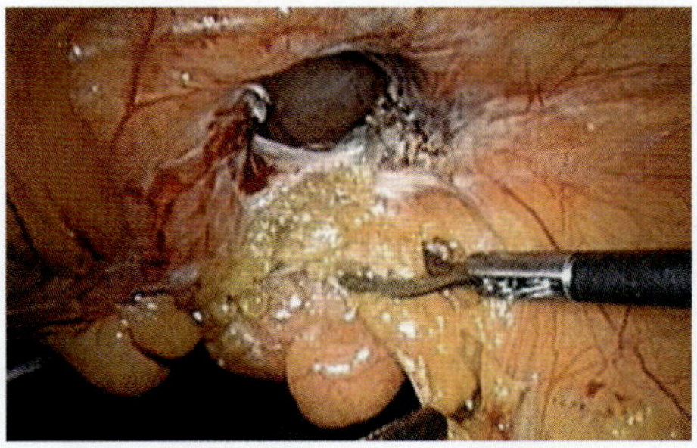

Figure 60.25 Paraumbilical defect – laparoscopic view.

Emergency repair of umbilical hernia

Incarceration, bowel obstruction and strangulation are frequent because of the narrow neck and the fibrous edge of the defect in the midline raphe. Delay to surgery can lead to gangrene of omentum or bowel. Large hernias are often multiloculated and there may be strangulated bowel in one component when other areas are clinically soft and non-tender hernia.

Operation

In cases of simple incarceration without clinical evidence of strangulation, repair may be attempted laparoscopically but reduction of the contents can be very difficult if the hernia contains bowel. The majority of emergency repairs are performed by open surgery. In the presence of established strangulation it is unwise to place mesh at all because of the risk of infection, so an open sutured repair should be performed, accepting a high risk of later recurrence. Alternatively, a two-stage repair could be planned: the hernia contents being dealt with initially with little attempt made to close the defect and then subsequent definitive mesh repair once sepsis has been controlled (Summary box 60.15).

Summary box 60.15

Umbilical hernia in adults

- Common in overweight men or multiparous women
- Progressively increase in size and may get very large indeed
- Round defect with rigid fibrous margins
- Surgery advised because of risk of obstruction and strangulation

Epigastric hernia

These arise through the midline raphe (linea alba) anywhere between the xiphoid process and the umbilicus, usually midway. When close to the umbilicus they are called supraumbilical hernias. Epigastric hernias begin with a transverse split in the midline raphe so, in contrast to umbilical hernias, the defect is elliptical. It has been hypothesised that the defect occurs at the site where small blood vessels pierce the linea alba or, more likely, that it arises at weaknesses due to abnormal decussation of aponeurotic fibres related to heavy physical activity (Figure 60.26).

Epigastric hernia defects are usually less than 1 cm in maximum diameter and commonly contain only extraperitoneal fat which gradually enlarges, spreading in the subcutaneous plane to resemble the shape of a mushroom. When very large they may contain a peritoneal sac but rarely any bowel. More than one hernia may be present. The most common cause of 'recurrence' is failure to identify a second defect at the time of original repair.

Clinical features

The patients are often fit, healthy males between 25 and 40 years of age. These hernias can be very painful even when the swelling is the size of a pea due to the fatty contents becoming nipped sufficiently to produce partial strangulation. The pain may mimic that of a peptic ulcer but symptoms should not be ascribed to the hernia until gastrointestinal pathology has been excluded. A soft midline swelling can often be felt more easily than it can be seen. It may be locally tender. It is unlikely to be reducible because of the narrow neck. It may resemble a lipoma. A cough impulse may or may not be felt.

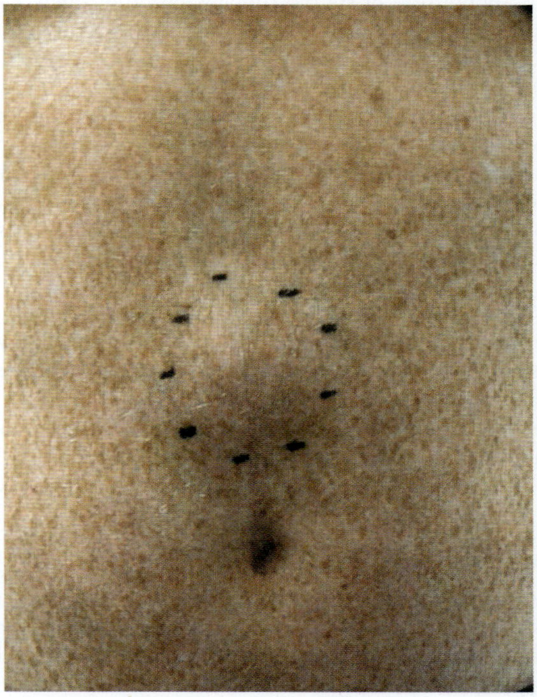

Figure 60.26 Epigastric hernia – external view.

Treatment

Very small epigastric hernias have been known to disappear spontaneously, probably due to infarction of the fat. Small to moderate-sized hernias without a peritoneal sac are not inherently dangerous and surgery should only be offered if the hernia is sufficiently symptomatic.

Operation

This may be done by open or laparoscopic surgery. At open surgery, a vertical or transverse incision is made over the swelling and down to the linea alba. Protruding extraperitoneal fat can simply be pushed back through the defect or excised. Often a small vessel is present in the hernia content which can cause troublesome bleeding. The defect in the linea alba is closed with non-absorbable sutures in adults and absorbable sutures in children. In larger hernias and when a peritoneal sac is present, the surgical approach is similar to an umbilical mesh repair.

Laparoscopic repair is very similar to that for umbilical hernia except that the defect is hidden behind the falciform ligament which must be taken down from the undersurface of the abdominal wall. The margins of the defect must be clearly exposed and the fatty contents reduced before the mesh is placed. Simply placing a mesh under the linea midline may not in fact remove the hernia when its contents are extraperitoneal fat.

Incisional hernia

These arise through a defect in the musculofascial layers of the abdominal wall in the region of a postoperative scar. Thus they may appear anywhere on the abdominal surface.

Incidence and aetiology

Incisional hernias have been reported in 10–50 per cent of laparotomy incisions and 1–5 per cent of laparoscopic port-site incisions. Factors predisposing to their development are patient factors (obesity, general poor healing due to malnutrition, immunosuppression or steroid therapy, chronic cough, cancer), wound factors (poor quality tissues, wound infection) and surgical factors (inappropriate suture material, incorrect suture placement).

An incisional hernia usually starts as disruption of the musculofascial layers of a wound in the early postoperative period. Often the event passes unnoticed if the overlying skin wound has healed securely. Many incisional hernias may be preventable with the use of good surgical technique. The classic sign of wound disruption is a serosanguinous discharge.

Clinical features

These hernias commonly appear as a localised swelling involving a small portion of the scar but may present as a diffuse bulging of the whole length of the incision (Figure 60.27). There may be several discrete hernias along the length of the incision and unsuspected defects are often found at operation (Figure 60.28). Incisional hernias tend to increase steadily in size with time. The skin overlying large hernias may become thin and atrophic so that peristalsis may be seen in the underlying intestine. Vascular damage to skin may lead to dermatitis. Attacks of partial intestinal obstruction are common as there are usually coexisting internal adhesions. Strangulation is less frequent and most likely to occur when the fibrous defect is small and the sac is large. Most incisional hernias are broad-necked and carry a low risk of strangulation (Summary box 60.16).

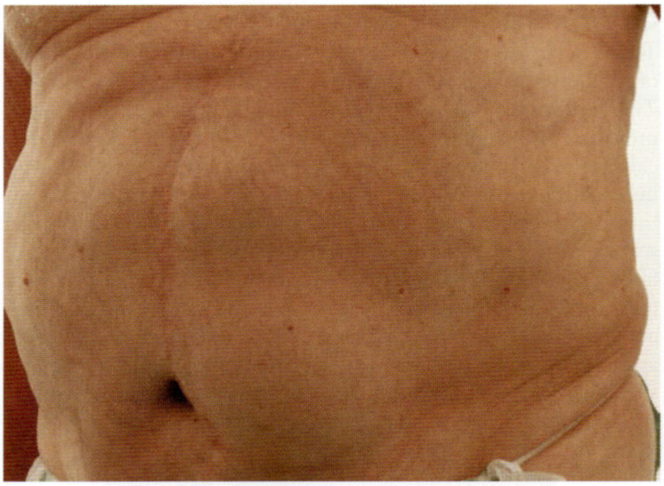

Figure 60.27 A large multilocular incisional hernia.

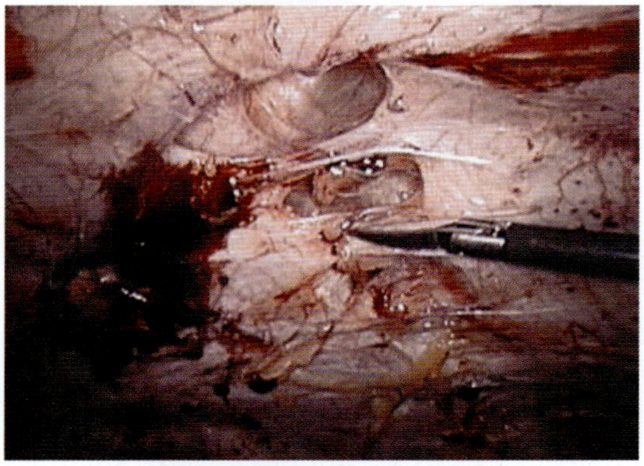

Figure 60.28 Multiple defects seen during laparoscopic operation.

Summary box 60.16

Incisional hernia

- Incidence 10–50 per cent after surgery
- Causation due to patient, wound and surgeon factors
- Wide variation in size
- Often multiple defects within the same scar
- Obstruction is common but strangulation is rare
- Open and laparoscopic repairs possible

Treatment

Asymptomatic incisional hernias may not require treatment at all. The wearing of an abdominal binder or belt may prevent the hernia from increasing in size.

Principles of surgery

For the majority of incisional hernias, surgery is relatively straightforward and both open and laparoscopic options are available. A number of principles apply, irrespective of the technique used.

The repair should cover the whole length of the previous incision. Approximation of the musculofascial layers should be done with minimal tension and prosthetic mesh should be used to reduce the risk of recurrence. Mesh may be contraindicated in a contaminated field, e.g. bowel injury during the dissection but, in a clean-contaminated field, such as after an elective bowel resection, mesh may be used if placed in a different anatomical plane to the contamination, such as in the extraperitoneal/retromuscular space. Appropriate systemic antibiotics should be used.

Open repair

Simple suture techniques without the use of prosthetic mesh for reinforcement, even with layered closure such as in Mayo, 'keel' or da Silva repairs, are not recommended today because of the high risk of recurrence. However, they may be the only option in the presence of gross contamination such as peritonitis.

The previous incision is opened along its full length to reveal any clinically unsuspected defects. The hernial sac, its neck and the margins of the defect are fully exposed. The sac can be opened, contents reduced, local adhesions divided and any redundant sac excised to allow safe reclosure of the peritoneum.

Mesh can be placed in one of several planes as for umbilical hernia repair. The simplest approach is an onlay mesh but increasingly the retromuscular sublay repair is preferred by expert surgeons and is described below.

Retromuscular sublay mesh repair

Vertical incisons are made through the fascia surrounding the rectus abdominus muscles so that the muscle can be separated and elevated from the posterior rectus sheath below. If possible, the medial edges of the posterior rectus sheath edges are sutured together with a continuous suture. In very large defects this may not be possible and below the arcuate line, the posterior sheath is deficient, being peritoneum and transversalis fascia only. In the case of transverse incision, where the defect extends lateral to the rectus sheath, internal oblique and transversus abdominis muscles form the posterior layer. A sheet of lightweight, large-pore prosthetic, elastic mesh is then laid between this posterior rectus sheath and belly(s) of the rectus muscle. It is fixed to the sheath by interrupted sutures. The mesh must be large enough to ensure 5 cm overlap of the underlying fascial defect in all directions. Careful haemostasis and meticulous asepsis are essential during this operation. The anterior rectus sheaths are then sutured together over the mesh so that, ideally, the mesh is completely covered by muscle and fascia and is not lying in the subcutaneous plane. Redundant skin may need to be excised. The risk of postoperative serous fluid collections is reduced by suction drainage.

Laparoscopic repair

Incisional hernias are increasingly being repaired by laparascopic mesh techniques. Laparoscopy and division of adhesions is initially performed. Hernia contents are reduced and the fibrous margins of the hernia defect(s) are exposed. Often the falciform ligament and median umbilical fold need to be taken down. Some surgeons prefer to suture close the muscle defects first and then reinforce with mesh. Others simply fix the mesh under the defect with adequate overlap. The use of a tissue-separating mesh is essential. Various techniques have been described to size and then position the mesh accurately. The mesh is fixed to the abdominal wall by staples or transfascial sutures which pass through all muscle layers to hold the mesh.

In the presence of dense peritoneal adhesions, the laparoscopic surgeon needs to take great care as injury to bowel is possible and may not be recognised. Diathermy is not used. If occult bowel injury does occur it can lead to postoperative peritonitis which is an extremely dangerous complication.

Management of the very large incisional hernia

Very large incisional hernias often require careful thought before treatment begins. If the volume of the sac is more than 25 per cent of the volume of the abdominal cavity (and this can be calculated from CT scan images) then there are likely to be issues of loss of abdominal domain when the hernia is repaired. The contents of the hernia, which have been outside the abdominal cavity for a long time, will not fit back inside, or if they do, it will result in high tension. High intra-abdominal pressure can lead to visceral compression and pulmonary complications due to impaired diaphragmatic movement. A tight abdomen can lead to wound breakdown and failure of the repair.

Techniques to overcome the potential loss of abdominal domain include preoperative abdominal expansion with progressive preoperative pneumoperitoneum over several weeks, resection of the omentum and/or colon at the time of repair, the use of prosthetic mesh to span the uncloseable gap in the musculofascial layer, or the use of musculofascial advancement or transposition flaps to achieve closure.

Even if loss of domain is not a concern, large defects can still be very difficult to close and the same special techniqes may need to be used to avoid producing excessive tension in the repair. The Ramirez component separation technique, which incorporates relaxing incisions in the external oblique aponeurosis and/or the posterior sheath, is very useful as this enables either the anterior or posterior component of the rectus sheath to be drawn together. It may then be reinforced with a mesh.

Patients with poor quality or redundant skin may benefit from a wedge excision of skin and fat (lipectomy) to improve the abdominal contour postoperatively. Repair of these very large hernias is highly specialised surgery and is best done in specialist centres.

Reducing the risk of incisional hernia

The incidence of incisional hernia may be reduced by improving the patients's general conditon preoperatively where possible – e.g. weight loss for obesity, or improving nutritonal state for malnutrition. Closing the fascial layers with non-absorbable, or very slowly absorbable, sutures of adequate gauge is important. Traditional teaching was that sutures should be 1 cm deep and 1 cm apart. Recent work has shown that lower incisional hernia rates and reduced infection rates are gained when smaller and closer bites are used with a 2/0 suture rather than traditional heavier materials.

There is no evidence that interrupted sutures are better or worse than continuous. However, if continuous suturing is used, the tissue bites must not be too near the fascial edge nor pulled too tight or they may cut out. It has also been confirmed that the optimal ratio of suture length to wound length is 4:1 (Jenkins' rule). If less length than this is used, the suture bites are too far apart or too tight and the converse applies if more length than this is used.

Drains should be brought out through separate incisions and not through the wound itself as this leads to hernia formation.

Recent reports have suggested that placement of a prophylactic mesh in patients at high risk of hernia formation will substantially reduce that risk. This has been reported in obese patients undergoing bariatric surgery and also to prevent parastomal herniation which occurs in up to 50 per cent of patients.

Spigelian hernia

These hernias are uncommon although are probably underdiagnosed. They affect men and women equally and can occur at any age, but are most common in the elderly. They arise through a defect in the Spigelian fascia which is the aponeurosis of the transversus abdominis muscle. Often these hernias advance through the internal oblique as well and spread out deep to the external oblique aponeurosis. The Spigelian fascia extends between the transversus muscle and the lateral border of the rectus sheath from the costal margin to the groin where it blends into the conjoint tendon. Most Spigelian hernias appear below the level of the umbilicus near the edge of the rectus sheath but they can be found anywhere along the 'Spigelian line' (Figure 60.29). There is a common misconception that they protrude below the arcuate line owing to deficiency of the posterior rectus sheath at that level, but in fact the defect is almost always above the arcuate line. In young patients they usually contain extraperitoneal fat only but in older patients there is often a peritoneal sac and they can become very large indeed.

They have also been described in infants and may be congenital, reflecting incomplete differentiation of the mesenchymal layers within the abdominal wall.

Clinical features

Young patients usually present with intermittent pain, due to pinching of the fat, similar to an epigastric hernia. A lump may or may not be palpable as the fatty hernia is small and the overlying external oblique is intact. Older patients generally present with a reducible swelling at the edge of the rectus sheath and may have symptoms of intermittent obstruction. The diagnosis should be suspected because of the location of the symptoms and is confirmed by CT. Ultrasound scanning has the advantage that it can be performed in the upright patient as no defect may be visible with the patient lying down.

Treatment

Surgery is recommended as the narrow and fibrous neck predisposes to strangulation. Surgery can be open or laparoscopic.

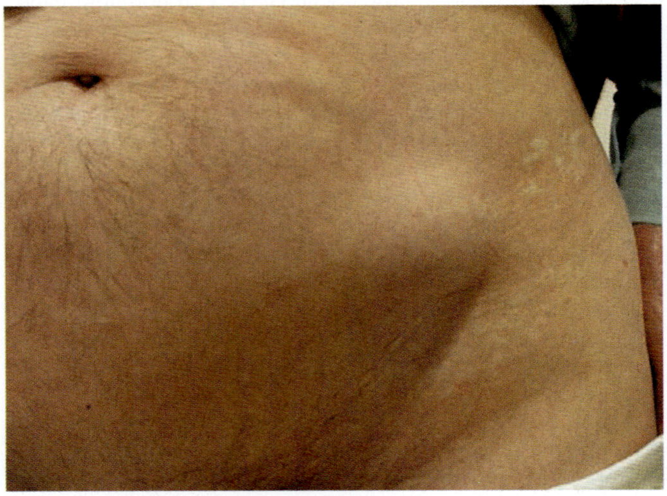

Figure 60.29 Spigelian hernia.

At open surgery a skin crease is made over the hernia, but no abnormality will be seen until the external oblique is opened. The sac and contents are dealt with and the small defect in the Spigelian fascia is repaired by suture or mesh laid deep to external oblique aponeurosis. The plane of the mesh can be extended medially into the posterior rectus sheath if required. The external oblique aponeurosis is closed over the mesh.

Laparoscopy is useful if no sac is palpable, but in young patients with a hernia only containing extraperitoneal fat, no hernia will be seen from within the peritoneum. In such cases, the peritoneum can be incised and the extraperitoneal plane explored for the small defect, which can then be closed either by suture or mesh. When an intraperitoneal sac is present, laparoscopic repair can be performed using either the intraperitoneal onlay of mesh (IPOM) or TAPP technique (Summary box 60.17).

Summary box 60.17

Spigelian hernia

- Rare
- Often misdiagnosed
- High risk of complications

Lumbar hernia

Most primary lumbar hernias occur through the inferior lumbar triangle of Petit bounded below by the crest of the ilium, laterally by the external oblique muscle and medially by the latissimus dorsi (Figure 60.30). Less commonly, the sac comes through the superior lumbar triangle, which is bounded by the 12th rib above, medially by the sacrospinalis and laterally by the posterior border of the internal oblique muscle. Primary lumbar hernias are rare, but may be mimicked by incisional hernias arising through flank incisions for renal operations or through incisions for bone grafts harvested from the iliac crest.

Differential diagnosis

A lumbar hernia must be distinguished from:

- a lipoma;
- a cold (tuberculous) abscess pointing to this position;
- pseudo-hernia due to local muscular paralysis. Lumbar pseudo-hernia can result from any interference with the nerve supply of the affected muscles, the most common cause being injury to the subcostal nerve during a renal operation.

Treatment

The natural history is for these hernias to increase in size and surgery is recommended. Lumbar hernias can be approached by open or laparoscopic surgery. The defects can be difficult to close with sutures and mesh is recommended.

The TAPP laparoscopic approach is gaining popularity. With the patient in a semilateral position ports are inserted well away from the defect. The peritoneum is incised above the hernia and dissected back to expose the muscle defect. The content, often extraperitoneal fat, is reduced and a mesh fixed with ample overlap. The peritoneum can then be resutured or tacked back to cover the mesh.

Lumbar incisional hernias can be approached in the same way but large ones, especially if there is a component of neuropathic

Adrian Van der Spieghel (Spigelius), 1578–1625, Professor of Anatomy, Padua, Italy.
Jean Louis Petit, 1674–1750, Director of the Academie de Chirurgie, Paris, France.

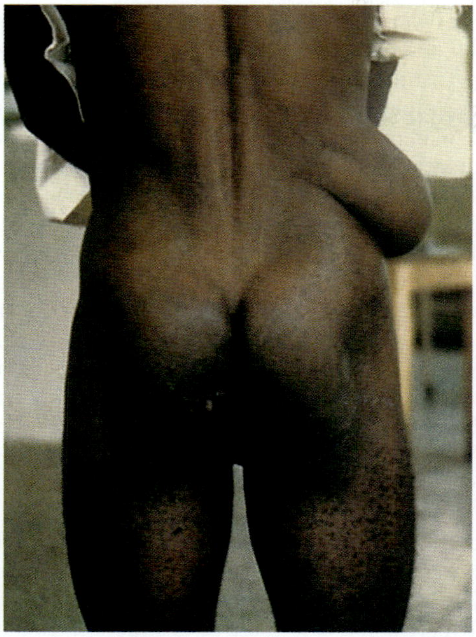

Figure 60.30 Inferior lumbar hernia, which contained caecum, appendix and small bowel. Note the filarial skin rash on the buttocks (courtesy of VJ Hartfield, formerly of SE Nigeria).

muscle atrophy causing a diffuse bulge (pseudo-hernia), can be very difficult and muscle-flap double-breasting with mesh reinforcement may be required.

Parastomal hernia

When surgeons create a stoma, such as a colostomy or ileostomy, they are effectively creating a hernia by bringing bowel out through the abdominal wall. The muscle defect created tends to increase in size over time and can ultimately lead to massive herniation around the stoma. The rate of parastomal hernia is over 50 per cent. For patients, it is very difficult to manage a stoma which is lying adjacent to or atop of a large hernia. Stoma appliance bags fit poorly leading to leakage.

The ideal surgical solution for the patient is to rejoin the bowel and remove the stoma altogether but this is not always possible. The stoma may be resited but further recurrence is likely. Various open suture and mesh techniques have been described to repair parastomal hernia but failure rates are high. Meshes are best placed in the retromuscular space. Laparoscopic repair is also possible using a large mesh with a central hole. It can be positioned around the bowel onto the parietal peritoneum.

Recent reports (Israelson) have described the use of prophylactic mesh insertion at the time of formation of the stoma. A lightweight, polypropylene mesh is inserted in the retromuscular space so that the bowel passes through a hole in the mesh centre. Using this technique, parastomal hernia rates have been reduced significantly.

Traumatic hernia

These hernias arise through non-anatomic defects caused by injury. They can be classified into three types:

1. Hernias through abdominal stab wound sites. These are effectively incisional hernias.
2. Hernias protruding through splits or tears in the abdominal muscles following blunt trauma.
3. Abdominal bulging secondary to muscle atrophy which occurs as a result of nerve injury or other traumatic denervation. Akin to the lumbar pseudo-hernia seen after open nephrectomy, these can arise following chest injury with damage to the intercostal nerves.

Clinical features

Traumatic hernias present as any other hernia. The key to the aetiology is in the history and the non-anatomic location of the hernia.

Treatment

Surgery may be justified if the hernia is sufficiently symptomatic, or if investigations suggest a narrow neck and hence a risk of obstruction or strangulation. Stab wound traumatic hernias are straightforward to repair using open or laparoscopic techiques as for other ventral hernias. Diffuse abdominal bulges are more difficult to correct and require some form of plication of the stretched musculofascial layer with mesh reinforcement to prevent further bulging in the future. Some bulging may persist however.

Rare external hernias

Perineal hernia

This type of hernia is very rare and includes:

- postoperative hernia through a perineal scar, which may occur after excision of the rectum;
- median sliding perineal hernia, which is a complete prolapse of the rectum;
- anterolateral perineal hernia, which occurs in women and presents as a swelling of the labium majus;
- posterolateral perineal hernia, which passes through the levator ani to enter the ischiorectal fossa.

Treatment

A combined abdominoperineal operation is generally the most satisfactory for the last two types of hernia. The hernia is exposed by an incision directly over it. The sac is opened and its contents are reduced. The sac is cleared from surrounding structures and the wound closed. With the patient in semi-Trendelenburg position, either laparoscopically or at open surgery, the abdomen is opened and the mouth of the sac is exposed. The sac is inverted, ligated and excised and the pelvic floor repaired by muscle apposition and, if indicated, buttressing of the repair with prosthetic mesh.

Obturator hernia

Obturator hernia, which passes through the obturator canal, occurs six times more frequently in women than in men. Most patients are over 60 years of age. The swelling is liable to be overlooked because it is covered by the pectineus. It seldom causes a definite swelling in Scarpa's triangle, but if the limb is flexed, abducted and rotated outwards, the hernia sometimes becomes apparent. The leg is usually kept in a semiflexed position and movement increases the pain. In more than 50 per cent of cases of strangulated obturator hernia, pain is referred along the obturator nerve by its geniculate branch to the knee. On vaginal or rectal examination the hernia can sometimes be felt as a tender swelling in the region of the obturator foramen.

These hernias have often undergone strangulation, frequently of the Richter type, by the time of presentation.

Treatment

Operation is indicated. The diagnosis is rarely made preoperatively and so it is often approached through a laparotomy incision. Full Trendelenburg position is adopted. The constricting agent is the obturator fascia which can be stretched by inserting the operator's index finger, or suitable forceps, through the gap in the fascia. Content is reduced. If incision of the fascia is required, it is made parallel to the obturator vessels and nerve. The contents of the sac are dealt with in standard manner. The defect cannot be simply closed as one margin is bone and the obturator nerve and vessels run through it. It is best closed using a mesh plug. In the absence of mesh or in an infected field, the broad ligament can be used as a plug.

Laparoscopic TAPP repair may also be performed again using a mesh. To avoid nerve injury, glue can be used to fix a mesh over the defect.

Gluteal and sciatic hernias

Both of these hernias are very rare. A gluteal hernia passes through the greater sciatic foramen, either above or below the piriformis. A sciatic hernia passes through the lesser sciatic foramen. Differential diagnosis must be made between these conditions and:

- a lipoma or other soft tissue tumour beneath the gluteus maximus;
- a tuberculous abscess;
- a gluteal aneurysm.

All doubtful swellings in this situation can be characterised with CT scanning but, if in doubt, they should be explored by operation.

UMBILICAL CONDITIONS IN THE ADULT

Chronic infection

Chronic infection occurs in the umbilical area, particularly in patients with poor hygiene. It may also occur in the obese and when a paraumbilical hernia is present. It can be due to a plug of keratin causing chronic irritation. It is often encountered during elective surgery and may complicate the insertion of a laparoscope port at the umbilicus. A range of bacteria and fungi can be involved. Occasionally, a rapid onset, superficial cellulitis occurs even after minor surgery in this region. It is normally a streptococcus and treated with penicillin or other appropriate antibiotic. Pre-existing infection should be treated prior to surgery where possible.

Chronic fistula

Patients may present with a persistent discharge from the umbilical area. This may be due to simple, superficial infection or possibly an infected epidermoid cyst within the umbilicus. However, it may also be due to a fistulous connection to deeper structures.

In normal patients, the umbilicus is connected to the liver, bladder and gynaecological organs by various ligaments. Diseases of these organs, such as infection or malignancy, can extend along these ligaments to appear at the umbilicus as a mass or fistulous discharge.

Chronic fistula may be a complication of umbilical hernia repair due to chronic infection of a mesh or around non-absorbable suture material. In most cases this problem arises soon after surgery but occasionally a chronic infection can occur months or even years after an operation. Antibiotics may help but most commonly the synthetic suture or mesh will need to be removed with a risk of recurrence of the hernia.

In fetal life the umbilicus was also connected to the gut by the vitellointestinal duct. In most patients this duct becomes totally obliterated and vanishes. The bowel end of the duct may persist as a Meckel's diverticulum. More rarely, the umbilical end persists leading to chronic discharge. If an abnormal connection between bowel and umbilicus persists then this band can act as a cause of adhesional intestinal obstruction.

Patent urachus

A connection between the urinary bladder and umbilicus usually presents in later life. This is due to increased pressure in the bladder as a result of obstruction from conditions such as prostatic hypertrophy. The cause of obstruction should be dealt with initially but if the problem persists then surgical excision of the patent urachus might be considered.

Malignancy at the umbilicus

Primary squamous carcinoma may occur. If tumour presents at the umbilicus it is most likely due to spread from internal organs along internal ligaments, for example from the liver along the falciform ligament. A malignant mass at the umbilicus is called a Sister Joseph's nodule. It usually indicates very advanced malignant disease and surgery probably has little to offer (Figure 60.31).

GENERAL INFECTION OF THE ABDOMINAL WALL

The skin of the abdominal wall, like all skin, is prone to develop superficial infection which may be spontaneous, due to minor trauma or to infection of skin lesions such as an epidermoid cyst. While antibiotics will suffice in most patients, if an abscess develops then surgical drainage may be required.

The close proximity of bowel and bowel organisms opens the abdominal wall to attack from a wide range of highly virulent bacteria. Most commonly, these are released during abdominal surgery such as appendicectomy and hence the need for appropriate antibiotic prophylactic cover.

Synergistic gangrene

This rare condition is due to the synergistic action of non-haemolytic streptococcus and staphylococcus causing rapid tissue necrosis and overwhelming systemic infection (Figure 60.32). It requires immediate administration of high-dose,

> The neoplastic nodule sited at the umbilicus is known as **Sister Joseph's nodule**. Sister Mary Joseph made the observation that her patients with terminal cancer sometimes developed a red papular lesion in the umbilicus. She and William Mayo published this observation in 1928. However, it was Hamilton Bailey who coined the term 'Sister Mary Joseph's nodule' in 1949.
> **Sister Mary Joseph (nee Julia Dempsey)**, Nursing Superintendent, St Mary's Hospital, which became the Mayo Clinic, Rochester, MN, USA. The Mayo Clinic in Rochester, MN, USA, was founded in 1889 as the St Mary's Hospital by William Worrall Mayo and his two sons, William James Mayo and Charles Horace Mayo, both of whom became surgeons to the hospital.

Antonio Scarpa, 1747–1832, Professor of Anatomy, Pavia, Italy.
Johann Frederick Meckel (the Younger), 1781–1833, Professor of Anatomy and Surgery, Halle, Germany, described his diverticulum in 1809.
Alexis Littre, 1658–1726, surgeon and lecturer in Anatomy, Paris, France, described Meckel's diverticulum in a hernial sac in 1700, 81 years before Meckel was born.

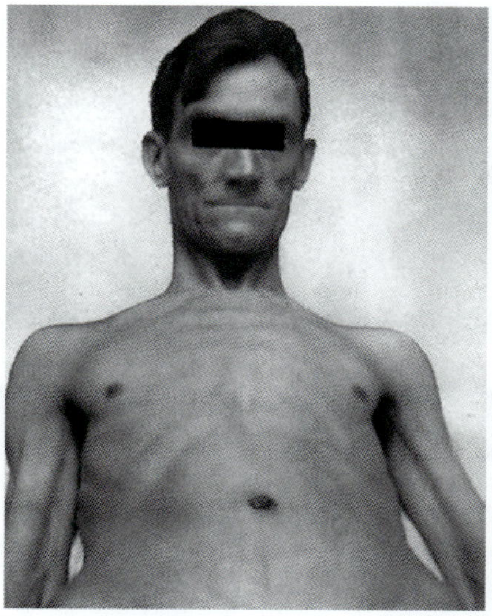

Figure 60.31 Secondary nodule at the umbilicus – Sister Joseph's nodule.

broad-spectrum, powerful antibiotics in combination with early debridement of any non-viable tissue. Hyperbaric oxygen therapy has been advocated.

Other forms of severe abdominal wall infections occur, generally known as necrotising fasciitis (e.g. Fournier's gangrene). All of these conditions have a high associated morbidity and mortality. They occur in debilitated and immune-compromised patients but can occasionally occur in healthy patients. Rapid diagnosis and aggressive surgical debridement treatment is the key to success.

Cutaneous fistula

Due to the thickness of the abdominal wall, it is rare for abdominal inflammatory conditions to discharge spontaneously through the wall to the skin. Chronic intraperitoneal abscesses arising after occult bowel perforation, appendicitis, diverticulitis and cholecystitis are the most likely sources. CT scanning will locate the internal abscess and suggest the likely origin. Treatment today is usually by CT or ultrasound-guided drainage but the surgeon may be called on to remove the source organ, e.g. gall bladder.

Malignancy in its later stages can occasionally erode through the abdominal wall.

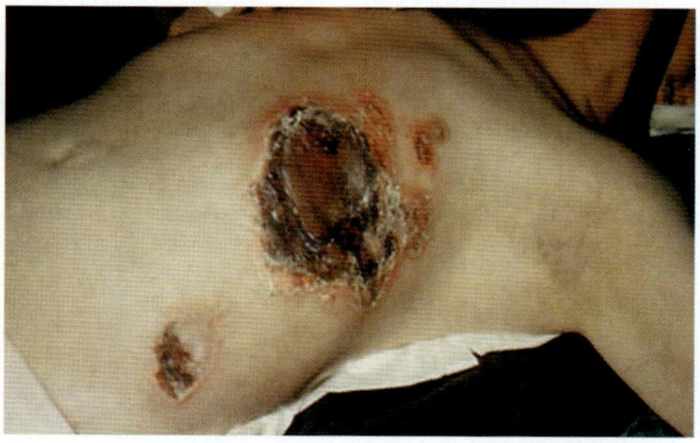

Figure 60.32 Bacterial synergistic gangrene of the chest and abdominal wall. The area has become gangrenous and looks like suede leather. Beware of amoebiasis cutis.

Crohn's disease also has a tendency to fistulate into adjacent organs and may develop an enterocutaneous fistula.

Abdominal compartment syndrome

Surgeons are increasingly aware of the harmful effect of high intra-abdominal pressures which can occur in severe intra-abdominal sepsis, such as pancreatitis and also aortic aneurysm rupture. High pressure leads to reduced blood flow and tissue ischaemia which contributes to multiorgan failure. While the abdominal wall has elasticity, if intra-abdominal volume increases due to fluid, gas, pus, tissue oedema, etc., then maximal capacity may be reached and pressure rises to a critical level. Tension releasing incisions, equivalent to a fasciotomy, have been suggested although this is not widely practised.

In some cases, after surgery for severe intraperitoneal sepsis, the surgeon cannot close the abdomen and may leave the incision wide open, covering abdominal contents with mesh or a saline-soaked dressing, planning to return at a future date to close the defect. This is called a laparostomy.

Neoplasms of the abdominal wall

As the abdominal wall is composed of muscle, fascia and bone, benign and malignant tumours can arise from each although these are rare.

Desmoid tumour

This is usually considered by pathologists to be a hamartoma and is more common in women. Some however believe it to be a fibroma and possibly the result of repeated trauma. Desmoids have been reported in familial adenomatous polyposis (FAP). Histologically they contain plasmoidal cell masses resembling giant cells. They undergo central myxomatous change. Surgical excision with a wide margin is required to prevent recurrence which is a frequent problem.

Fibrosarcoma

These tumours can occur anywhere in the body. They are generally highly malignant and respond poorly to both radio- and chemotherapy. Wide excision will often require plastic surgical reconstruction.

FURTHER READING

Kingsnorth AN, LeBlanc KA. *Management of abdominal hernias*, 3rd edn. London: Edward Arnold, 2003.

Millbourn D, Cengiz Y, Israelsson LA. Effect of stitch length on wound complications after closure of midline incisions. *Arch Surg* 2009; **144**(11): 1056–9.

WEBSITE ADDRESSES

Classification of groin hernia: www.herniaweb.org/documents/EHS_groin_hernia_classification.pdf

Guidelines for management of groin hernia:www.herniaweb.org/documents/EHS_Guidelines.pdf

European classification of primary and incisional abdominal wall hernias: www.ncbi.nlm.nih.gov/pmc/articles/PMC2719726/

NICE guidelines for laparoscopic inguinal hernia repair: guidance.nice.org.uk/TA83

SIGN guidelines for antibiotics in surgery (including hernia): www.sign.ac.uk/pdf/sign104.pdf

CHAPTER 61

The peritoneum, omentum, mesentery and retroperitoneal space

LEARNING OBJECTIVES

To recognise and understand:

- The causes and complications of localised and generalised peritonitis
- The clinical features of peritonitis and intraperitoneal abscess
- The principles of surgical management in patients with peritonitis and intraperitoneal abscess
- The causes and pathophysiology of ascites
- The pathophysiology and complications of adhesion formation
- The spectrum of mesenteric and retroperitoneal conditions

ANATOMY AND PHYSIOLOGY

Embryology

The peritoneal cavity, mesenteries and omentum have an anatomical complexity which can perhaps only be truly understood with surgical experience. Nevertheless, an understanding of the geometric alterations occurring during early gastrointestinal (GI) morphogenesis (regionalisation, elongation and coiling) of the derivatives of the endoderm (E = epithelium) and the visceral mesoderm (M = muscle and most of the rest) along with the later fusion of adjacent layers of peritoneum will give an appreciation of how the adult disposition is as it is.

Adult arrangement and functions

The peritoneal cavity is the largest cavity in the body, the surface area of its lining membrane (2 m^2 in an adult) being nearly equal to that of the skin. The peritoneal membrane is composed of flattened polyhedral cells (mesothelium), one layer thick, resting upon a thin layer of fibroelastic tissue. This membrane is conveniently divided into two parts – the visceral peritoneum surrounding the viscera and the parietal peritoneum lining the other surfaces of the cavity. Beneath the peritoneum, supported by a small amount of areolar tissue, lies a network of lymphatic vessels and rich plexuses of capillary blood vessels from which all absorption and exudation must occur. In health, only a few millilitres of peritoneal fluid is found in the peritoneal cavity. The fluid is pale yellow, somewhat viscid and contains lymphocytes and other leukocytes; it lubricates the viscera, allowing easy movement and peristalsis. The parietal portion is richly supplied with nerves and, when irritated, causes severe pain that is accurately localised to the affected area. The visceral peritoneum, in contrast, is poorly supplied with nerves (these being situated around blood vessels) and its irritation causes pain that is usually poorly localised to the midline.

The peritoneum has a number of functions (Summary box 61.1).

The peritoneum has the capacity to absorb large volumes of fluid: this ability is used during peritoneal dialysis in the treatment of renal failure. However, the peritoneum can also produce large volumes of fluid (ascites) and an inflammatory exudate when injured (peritonitis). During expiration, intra-abdominal pressure is reduced and peritoneal fluid, aided by capillary attraction, travels in an upward direction towards the diaphragm. Experimental evidence shows that particulate matter and bacteria are absorbed within a few minutes into the lymphatic network through a number of 'pores' within the diaphragmatic peritoneum. The circulation of peritoneal fluids may be responsible for the occurrence of abscesses distant from primary disease. When parietal peritoneal defects are created, healing occurs not from the edges but by the development of new mesothelial cells throughout the surface of the defect. In this way, large defects heal as rapidly as small defects.

Summary box 61.1

Functions of the peritoneum

- In health
  - Visceral lubrication
  - Fluid and particulate absorption
- In disease
  - Pain perception (mainly parietal)
  - Inflammatory and immune responses
  - Fibrinolytic activity

SCOPE OF DISEASE

The peritoneum, mesentery and omentum may be the site of a variety of conditions that reflect their relationship to other anatomical structures or in some instances their primary functions (Summary box 61.2).

Summary box 61.2

Scope of disease

Intraperitoneal disease
- Peritonitis
  - Primary
  - Secondary
- Abscess
- Ascites
  - Transudate
  - Exudate
- Tumours
  - Primary
  - Secondary
- Adhesions

Omental disease
- Hernia
- Adhesions
- Torsion
- Neoplasia

Mesenteric disease
- Trauma
- Ischaemia
- Inflammation
- Cysts
- Neoplasia

Retroperitoneal disease
- Chronic inflammation/fibrosis
- Abscess
- Tumours

PERITONITIS

Peritonitis is simply defined as inflammation of the peritoneum and may be localized or generalised. Most cases of peritonitis are caused by an invasion of the peritoneal cavity by bacteria, so that when the term 'peritonitis' is used without qualification, acute bacterial peritonitis is often implied. In this instance, free fluid spills into the peritoneal cavity and circulates largely directed by the normal peritoneal attachments and gravity. For example, spillage from a perforated peptic ulcer may run down the right paracolic gutter leading to presentation with pain in the right iliac fossa (Valentino's syndrome). Even in patients with non-bacterial peritonitis (e.g. acute pancreatitis, intraperitoneal rupture of the bladder or haemoperitoneum), the peritoneum often becomes infected by transmural spread of organisms from the bowel. Such translocation is a feature of the systemic inflammatory response on the bowel and it is not long (often a matter of hours) before a bacterial peritonitis develops. Most duodenal and gastric perforations are initially sterile for up to several hours before becoming secondarily infected. Other causes of peritoneal inflammation are shown in Summary box 61.3.

Summary box 61.3

Causes of peritoneal inflammation

- Bacterial, gastrointestinal and non-gastrointestinal
- Chemical, e.g. bile, barium
- Allergic, e.g. starch peritonitis
- Traumatic, e.g. operative handling
- Ischaemia, e.g. strangulated bowel, vascular occlusion
- Miscellaneous, e.g. familial Mediterranean fever

Although acute bacterial peritonitis most commonly arises from a perforation of a viscus of the alimentary tract, other routes of infection can include the female genital tract and exogenous contamination. There are also less common forms in which the aetiology is a primary 'spontaneous' peritonitis, in which a pure infection with streptococcal, pneumococcal or haemophilus bacteria occurs. Summary box 61.4 outlines the main causes of bacterial peritonitis.

Summary box 61.4

Paths to peritoneal infection

- Gastrointestinal perforation, e.g. perforated ulcer, appendix, diverticulum
- Transmural translocation (no perforation), e.g. pancreatitis, ischaemic bowel
- Exogenous contamination, e.g. drains, open surgery, trauma
- Female genital tract infection, e.g. pelvic inflammatory disease
- Haematogenous spread (rare), e.g. septicaemia

Microbiology

Bacteria from the gastrointestinal tract

The number of bacteria within the lumen of the gastrointestinal tract is normally low until the distal small bowel is reached. However, disease leading to stasis and overgrowth (e.g. obstruction, chronic and acute motility disturbances) may increase proximal colonisation. The biliary and pancreatic tracts are also normally free from bacteria, although they may be infected in disease, e.g. gallstones. Peritoneal infection is usually caused by two or more bacterial strains. Gram-negative bacteria contain endotoxins (lipopolysaccharides) in their cell walls that have multiple toxic effects on the host, primarily by causing the release of tumour necrosis factor (TNF) from host leukocytes. Systemic absorption of endotoxin may produce endotoxic shock with hypotension and impaired tissue perfusion. Other bacteria such as *Clostridium welchii* produce harmful exotoxins. Bacteroides are commonly found in peritonitis. These Gram-negative, non-sporing organisms, although predominant in the lower intestine, often escape detection because they are strictly anaerobic and slow to grow on culture media unless there is an adequate carbon dioxide tension in the anaerobic apparatus. In many laboratories, the culture is discarded if there is no growth in 48 hours. These organisms are resistant to penicillin and streptomycin but sensitive to metronidazole, clindamycin,

Rudolph Valentino, Italian actor died during surgery for this in New York in 1926, aged 31 years.
William Henry Welch, 1850–1934, Professor of Pathology, Johns Hopkins University, Baltimore, MD, USA, discovered the causative organism of gas gangrene in 1892.
William Alexander Gillespie, formerly Professor of Clinical Bacteriology, the University of Bristol, Bristol, UK.

lincomycin and cephalosporin compounds. Since the widespread use of metronidazole (Flagyl), Bacteroides infections have greatly diminished.

Non-gastrointestinal causes of peritonitis

Pelvic infection via the Fallopian tubes is responsible for a high proportion of 'non-gastrointestinal' infections. The most common offending organisms are chlamydia and gonococcus. These organisms lead to a thinning of cervical mucus and allow bacteria from the vagina into the uterus and oviducts, causing infection and inflammation. A variant of transperitoneal spread of such organisms is perihepatitis which can cause scar tissue to form on Glisson's capsule, a thin layer of connective tissue surrounding the liver (Fitz-Hugh–Curtis syndrome). Other bacterial variants that are discussed separately include tuberculosis and other mycobacterial strains and those causing primary peritonitis (pneumococcus, staphylococcus and streptococcus spp). Fungal peritonitis is uncommon but may complicate severely ill patients (Summary box 61.5).

Summary box 61.5

Microorganisms in peritonitis

Gastrointestinal source
- *Escherichia coli*
- *Streptococci*
- *Bacteroides*
- *Clostridium*
- *Klebsiella pneumoniae*

Other sources
- *Chlamydia trachomatis*
- *Neisseria gonorrhoeae*
- *Haemolytic streptococci*
- *Staphylococcus*
- *Streptococcus pneumoniae*
- *Mycobacterium tuberculosis* and other spp.
- Fungal infections

Localised peritonitis

Anatomical and pathological factors may favour the localisation of peritonitis.

Anatomical

The greater sac of the peritoneum is divided into (1) the subphrenic spaces, (2) the pelvis and (3) the peritoneal cavity proper. The last is divided into a supracolic and an infracolic compartment by the transverse colon and transverse mesocolon, which deters the spread of infection from one to the other. When the supracolic compartment overflows, as is often the case when a peptic ulcer perforates, it does so over the colon into the infracolic compartment or by way of the right paracolic gutter to the right iliac fossa and hence to the pelvis.

Pathological

The clinical course is determined in part by the manner in which adhesions form around the affected organ. Inflamed peritoneum loses its glistening appearance and becomes reddened and velvety. Flakes of fibrin appear and cause loops of intestine to become adherent to one another and to the parietes. There is an outpouring of serous inflammatory exudate rich in leukocytes and plasma proteins that soon becomes turbid; if localisation occurs, the turbid fluid becomes frank pus. Peristalsis is retarded in affected bowel and this helps to prevent distribution of the infection. The greater omentum, by enveloping and becoming adherent to inflamed structures, often forms a substantial barrier to the spread of infection (see below).

Theodor Albrecht Edwin Klebs, 1834–1913, Professor of Bacteriology successively at Prague, The Czech Republic; Zurich, Switzerland; and The Rush Medical College, Chicago, IL, USA.

Diffuse (generalised) peritonitis

A number of factors may favour the development of diffuse peritonitis:

- Speed of peritoneal contamination is a prime factor. If an inflamed appendix or other hollow viscus perforates before localisation has taken place, there will be an efflux of contents into the peritoneal cavity, which may spread over a large area almost instantaneously. Perforation proximal to an obstruction or from sudden anastomotic separation is associated with severe generalised peritonitis and a high mortality rate.
- Stimulation of peristalsis by the ingestion of food or even water hinders localisation. Violent peristalsis occasioned by the administration of a purgative or an enema may cause the widespread distribution of an infection that would otherwise have remained localised.
- The virulence of the infecting organism may be so great as to render the localisation of infection difficult or impossible.
- Young children have a small omentum, which is less effective in localising infection.
- Disruption of localised collections may occur with injudicious handling, e.g. appendix mass or pericolic abscess.
- Deficient natural resistance ('immune deficiency') may result from use of drugs (e.g. steroids), disease (e.g. acquired immune deficiency syndrome (AIDS)) or old age.

With appropriate treatment, localised peritonitis usually resolves; in about 20 per cent of cases, an abscess follows. Infrequently, localised peritonitis becomes diffuse. Conversely, in favourable circumstances, diffuse peritonitis can become localised, most frequently in the pelvis or at multiple sites within the abdominal cavity.

Clinical features

Localised peritonitis

The initial symptoms and signs of localised peritonitis are those of the underlying condition – usually visceral inflammation (hence abdominal pain, specific GI symptoms + malaise, anorexia and nausea). When the peritoneum becomes inflamed, abdominal pain will worsen and, in general, temperature and pulse rate will rise. The pathognomonic signs are localised guarding (involuntary abdominal wall contraction to protect the viscus from the examining hand), a positive 'release' sign (rebound tenderness) and, sometimes, rigidity (involuntary constant contraction of the abdominal wall over the inflamed parietes). If inflammation arises under the diaphragm, shoulder tip ('phrenic') pain may be felt as the pain is referred to the C5 dermatome. In cases of pelvic peritonitis arising from an inflamed

Named after the two physicians, Thomas Fitz-Hugh, Jr and Arthur Hale Curtis who first reported this condition in 1934 and 1930, respectively.
Theodor Escherich, 1857–1911, Professor of Paediatrics, Vienna, Austria discovered the *Bacterium Coli Commune* in 1886.

appendix in the pelvic position or from salpingitis, the abdominal signs are often slight; there may be deep tenderness of one or both lower quadrants alone, but a rectal or vaginal examination reveals marked tenderness of the pelvic peritoneum.

Diffuse (generalised) peritonitis

Early

Abdominal pain is severe and made worse by moving or breathing. It is first experienced at the site of the original lesion and spreads outwards from this point. The patient usually lies still. Tenderness and generalised guarding are found on palpation when the peritonitis affects the anterior abdominal wall. Infrequent bowel sounds may still be heard for a few hours but they cease with the onset of paralytic ileus. Pulse and temperature rise in accord with degree of inflammation and infection.

Late

If resolution or localisation of generalised peritonitis does not occur, the abdomen will become rigid (generalised rigidity). Distension is common and bowel sounds are absent. Circulatory failure ensues, with cold, clammy extremities, sunken eyes, dry tongue, thready (irregular) pulse and drawn and anxious face (Hippocratic facies; Figure 61.1). The patient finally lapses into unconsciousness. With early diagnosis and adequate treatment, this condition is rarely seen in modern surgical practice (Summary box 61.6).

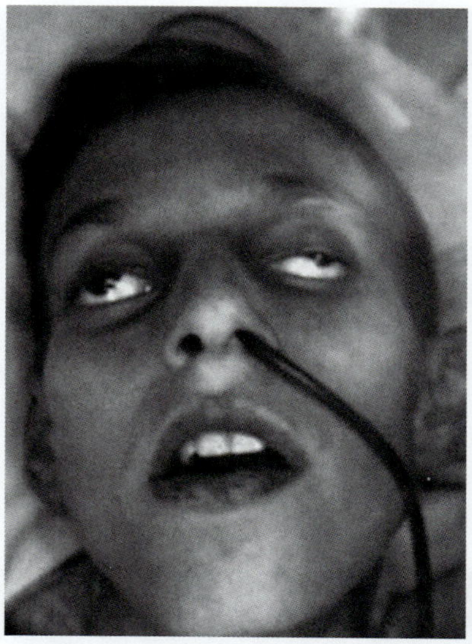

Figure 61.1 The Hippocratic facies in terminal diffuse peritonitis.

Summary box 61.6

Clinical features of peritonitis

- Abdominal pain, worse on movement, coughing and deep respiration
- Constitutional upset: anorexia, malaise, fever, lassitude
- GI upset: nausea ± vomiting
- Pyrexia (may be absent)
- Raised pulse rate
- Tenderness ± guarding/rigidity/rebound of abdominal wall
- Pain/tenderness on rectal/vaginal examination (pelvic peritonitis)
- Absent or reduced bowel sounds
- 'Septic shock' (systemic inflammatory response syndrome (SIRS) and multiorgan dysfunction syndrome (MODS)) in later stages

Diagnostic aids

Investigations may elucidate a doubtful diagnosis, but the importance of a careful history and repeated examination must not be forgotten.

Bedside

- Urine dipstix for urinary tract infection
- ECG if diagnostic doubt (as to cause of abdominal pain) or cardiac history.

Bloods

- Baseline U&E for treatment
- Full blood count for white cell count (WCC)
- Serum amylase estimation may establish the diagnosis of acute pancreatitis provided that it is remembered that moderately raised values are frequently found following other abdominal catastrophes and operations, e.g. perforated duodenal ulcer
- Group and save serum may be taken as an adjunct to impending surgery.

Imaging

- Erect chest radiograph to demonstrate free subdiaphramatic gas (Figure 61.2a).
- A supine radiograph of the abdomen may confirm the presence of dilated gas-filled loops of bowel (consistent with a paralytic ileus), occasionally show other gas-filled structures that may aid diagnosis, e.g. biliary tree; the faecal pattern may act as a guide to colonic disease (absent in sites of significant inflammation, e.g. diverticulitis). In the patient who is too ill for an 'erect' film, a lateral decubitus film can show gas beneath the abdominal wall (if CT unavailable).
- Multiplanar computed tomography (CT) is increasingly used to identify the cause of peritonitis (Figures 61.2b and 61.3) and may also influence management decisions, e.g. surgical strategy. There is an abundance of recent published evidence to support its use in managing acute abdominal pain.
- Ultrasound scanning has undoubted value in certain situations such as pelvic peritonitis in females and localised right upper quadrant peritonism.

Invasive

- In the era of access to high quality CT scanning, peritoneal diagnostic aspiration has little residual value.

Management

General care of the patient

The care of critically ill surgical patients is described in detail in Chapters 14, 17 and 21. Nutritional support is covered in Chapter 18 and anaesthesia and pain relief in Chapter 15. Depending on degree (localised/generalised), duration and severity, patients will require some or all of the following.

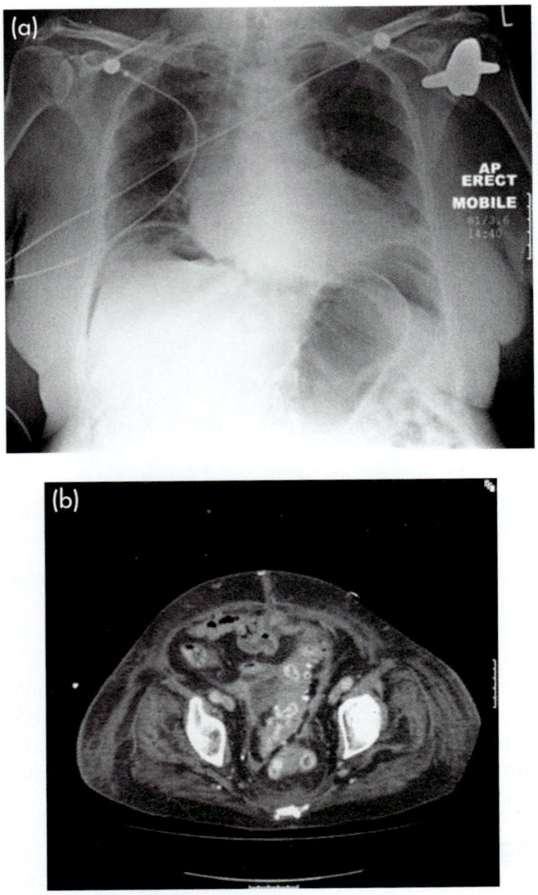

Figure 61.2 (a) Gas under the diaphragm in a patient with free perforation and peritonitis; (b) representative computed tomography axial image through the pelvis of the same patient showing perforated sigmoid diverticular disease.

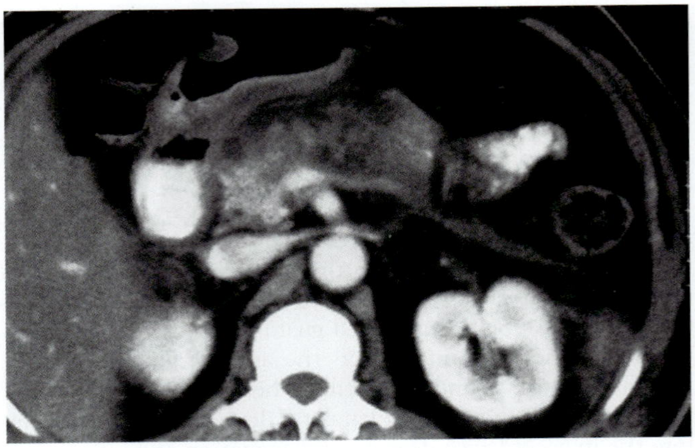

Figure 61.3 Acute pancreatitis seen on computed tomography scanning with swelling of the gland and surrounding inflammatory changes (courtesy of Dr J Healy, Chelsea and Westminster Hospital, London, UK).

Correction of fluid loss and circulating volume

Patients are frequently hypovolaemic with electrolyte disturbances. The plasma volume must be restored and electrolyte concentrations corrected. Fluid balance should be monitored and pre-existent and ongoing losses corrected. Special measures may be needed for cardiac, pulmonary and renal support, especially if septic shock is present (see Chapter 2), including central venous pressure monitoring in patients with concurrent disease.

Urinary catheterisation ± gastrointestinal decompression

A urinary catheter will give a guide to central perfusion and will be required if abdominal surgery is to proceed. A nasogastric tube is commonly passed to allow drainage ± aspiration until paralytic ileus has resolved.

Antibiotic therapy

Administration of parenteral broad-spectrum (aerobic and anaerobic) antibiotics prevents the multiplication of bacteria and the release of endotoxins.

Analgesia

The patient should be nursed in the sitting-up position and must be relieved of pain before and after operation. If appropriate expertise is available, epidural infusion may provide excellent analgesia. Freedom from pain allows early mobilisation and adequate physiotherapy in the postoperative period, which helps to prevent basal pulmonary collapse, deep-vein thrombosis and pulmonary embolism.

Specific treatment of the cause

While difficult to generalise, in patients where specific treatment has not been guided by CT scanning, early surgical intervention is to be preferred to a 'wait and see' policy assuming that the patient is fit for anaesthesia and that resuscitation has resulted in a satisfactory restitution of normal body physiology. This rule is particularly true for previously healthy patients and those with postoperative peritonitis. More caution is, of course, required in patients at high operative risk because of comorbidity or advanced age.

In those patients with a preoperative diagnosis, if the cause of peritonitis is amenable to surgery, operation must be carried out as soon as the patient is fit. This is usually within a few hours. In peritonitis caused by pancreatitis or salpingitis, or in cases of primary peritonitis of streptococcal or pneumococcal origin, non-operative treatment is preferred provided the diagnosis can be made with confidence. It is beyond the remit of this chapter to cover specific causes of peritonitis and their treatment, be it by open or laparoscopic approach. However, in general, surgery is directed to removing (or diverting) the cause and subsequent adequate peritoneal lavage ± drainage. In operations for generalised peritonitis it is essential that, after the cause has been dealt with, the whole peritoneal cavity is explored with the sucker and, if necessary, mopped dry until all seropurulent exudate is removed. The use of a large volume of saline (typically 3 litres) containing dissolved antiseptic or antibiotic has been shown to be effective (Summary box 61.7).

Prognosis and complications

With modern treatment, diffuse peritonitis carries a mortality rate of about 10 per cent reflecting the degree and duration of peritoneal contamination, age and fitness of the patient and the

> **Summary box 61.7**
>
> **Management of peritonitis**
>
> General care of patient
> - Correction of fluid and electrolyte imbalance
> - Insertion of nasogastric drainage tube and urinary catheter
> - Broad-spectrum antibiotic therapy
> - Analgesia
> - Vital system support
>
> Operative treatment of cause when appropriate
> - Remove or divert cause
> - Peritoneal lavage ± drainage

nature of the underlying cause. The systemic and local complications are shown in Summary box 61.8. Paralytic ileus is covered in detail in Chapter 69; abscess formation and adhesions are covered below.

> **Summary box 61.8**
>
> **Complications of peritonitis**
>
> - Systemic complications
>   - Bacteraemic/endotoxic shock
>   - Systemic inflammatory response syndrome
>   - Multiorgan dysfunction syndrome
>   - Death
> - Abdominal complications
>   - Paralytic ileus
>   - Residual or recurrent abscess/inflammatory mass
>   - Portal pyaemia/liver abscess
>   - Adhesional small bowel obstruction

SPECIAL FORMS OF PERITONITIS

Bile peritonitis

Unless there is reason to suspect that the biliary tract was damaged during operation or the patient has proven acute cholecystitis, it is improbable that bile as a cause of peritonitis will be thought of until the abdomen has been opened. The common causes of bile peritonitis are shown in Summary box 61.9.

Unless the bile has extravasated slowly and the collection becomes shut off from the general peritoneal cavity, there are symptoms (often severe pain) and signs of diffuse peritonitis. After a few hours a tinge of jaundice is not unusual. Laparotomy (or laparoscopy) should be undertaken with evacuation of the bile and peritoneal lavage. The source of bile leakage should be identified and treated accordingly. Infected bile is more lethal than sterile bile. A 'blown' duodenal stump should be drained as it is too oedematous to repair, but sometimes it can be covered by a jejunal patch. The patient is often jaundiced from absorption of peritoneal bile, but the surgeon must ensure that the abdomen is not closed until any obstruction to a major bile duct has been either excluded or relieved. Bile leaks after cholecystectomy or liver trauma may be dealt with by percutaneous (ultrasound-guided) drainage and endoscopic biliary stenting to reduce bile duct pressure. The drain is removed when dry and the stent at 4–6 weeks.

> **Summary box 61.9**
>
> **Causes of bile peritonitis**
>
> - Perforated cholecystitis
> - Postcholecystectomy
>   - Cystic duct stump leakage
>   - Leakage from an accessory duct in the gall bladder bed
>   - Bile duct injury
>   - T-tube drain dislodgement (or tract rupture on removal)
> - Following other operations/procedures
>   - Leaking duodenal stump postgastrectomy
>   - Leaking biliary–enteric anastomosis
>   - Leakage around percutaneous placed biliary drains
> - Following liver trauma

Primary peritonitis

Primary pneumococcal peritonitis may complicate nephrotic syndrome or cirrhosis in children. Otherwise healthy children, particularly girls between three and nine years of age, may also be affected, and it is likely that the route of infection is sometimes via the vagina and Fallopian tubes. At other times, and always in males, the infection is blood-borne and secondary to respiratory tract or middle ear disease. The prevalence of pneumococcal peritonitis has declined greatly and the condition is now rare.

Clinical features

The onset is sudden and the earliest symptom is pain localised to the lower half of the abdomen. The temperature is raised to 39°C or more and there is usually frequent vomiting. After 24–48 hours, profuse diarrhoea is characteristic. There is usually increased frequency of micturition. The last two symptoms are caused by severe pelvic peritonitis. On examination, peritonism is usually diffuse but less prominent than in most cases of a perforated viscus leading to peritonitis.

Investigation and treatment

A leukocytosis ≥30 000 μL with approximately 90 per cent polymorphs suggests pneumococcal peritonitis rather than another cause, e.g. appendicitis. After starting antibiotic therapy and correcting dehydration and electrolyte imbalance, early surgery is required unless spontaneous infection of pre-existing ascites is strongly suspected, in which case a diagnostic peritoneal tap is useful. Laparotomy or laparoscopy may be used. Should the exudate be odourless and sticky, the diagnosis of pneumococcal peritonitis is practically certain, but it is essential to perform a careful exploration to exclude other pathology. Assuming that no other cause for the peritonitis is discovered, some of the exudate is aspirated and sent to the laboratory for microscopy, culture and sensitivity tests. Thorough peritoneal lavage is carried out and the incision closed. Antibiotic and fluid replacement therapy are continued and recovery is usual.

Other organisms are now known to cause some cases of primary peritonitis in children, including *Haemophilus*, other streptococci and a few Gram-negative bacteria. Underlying pathology (including an intravaginal foreign body in girls) must always be excluded before primary peritonitis can be diagnosed with certainty. Idiopathic streptococcal and staphylococcal peritonitis can also occur in adults.

Tuberculous peritonitis

Intra-abdominal tuberculosis is very common in the developing world where all general surgeons are familiar with its presentation and management. The incidence is however also rising in areas of the developed world as a consequence of migration and immunosuppression where *Mycobacterium avium-intracellulare* is becoming increasingly prevalent with the widespread increase in human immunodeficiency virus (HIV) coinfection. Abdominal tuberculosis (TB) includes intraperitoneal, GI tract and solid organ disease forms with TB peritonitis being a common site-specific variant. Although still uncommon, TB peritonitis requires some specific mention since it is often diagnosed late in the course of the disease, resulting in undue patient morbidity and mortality.

Tuberculosis can spread to the peritoneum through the GI tract (typically ileocaecal region) via mesenteric lymph nodes or directly from the blood, usually from the 'miliary' (Figure 61.4a) but occasionally the 'cavitating' form of pulmonary TB, lymph and the Fallopian tubes; 50–83 per cent of patients with abdominal TB can be expected to have peritoneal involvement. Clinical or subclinical ascites is reported in virtually all patients with TB peritonitis and is frequently a presenting feature. In the most common form of the disease, wet-type peritonitis, ascites may be localised or generalised throughout the peritoneal cavity. Multiple tubercle deposits appear on both layers of the peritoneum. Diagnosis is via abdominal ultrasound or CT to detect ascites and lymphadenopathy ± diffuse thickening of the peritoneum, mesentery and/or omentum (Figure 61.4b). Ascitic fluid is typically a straw-coloured exudate (protein >25–30 g/L) with white cells >500 mm^3 and lymphocytes >40 per cent. Unfortunately, diagnostic smears for acid-fast bacilli are diagnostic in <3 per cent of patients and culture may take up to 4–8 weeks with no guarantee of a positive result. Laparoscopy and peritoneal biopsy may thus be helpful to couple typical appearances with histology. Management is principally supportive (nutrition and hydration) and medical (systemic antituberculous therapy) although surgery may be required for specific complications such as intestinal obstruction.

The main features are summarized in Summary box 61.10.

Summary box 61.10

Tuberculous peritonitis

- Acute (may be clinically indistinguishable from acute bacterial peritonitis) and chronic forms
- Abdominal pain, sweats, malaise and weight loss are frequent
- Ascites common, may be loculated
- Caseating peritoneal nodules are common – distinguish from metastatic carcinoma and fat necrosis of pancreatitis
- Intestinal obstruction may respond to antituberculous treatment without surgery

Familial Mediterranean fever (periodic peritonitis)

Familial Mediterranean fever (periodic peritonitis) is characterised by abdominal pain and tenderness, mild pyrexia, polymorphonuclear leukocytosis and, occasionally, pain in the

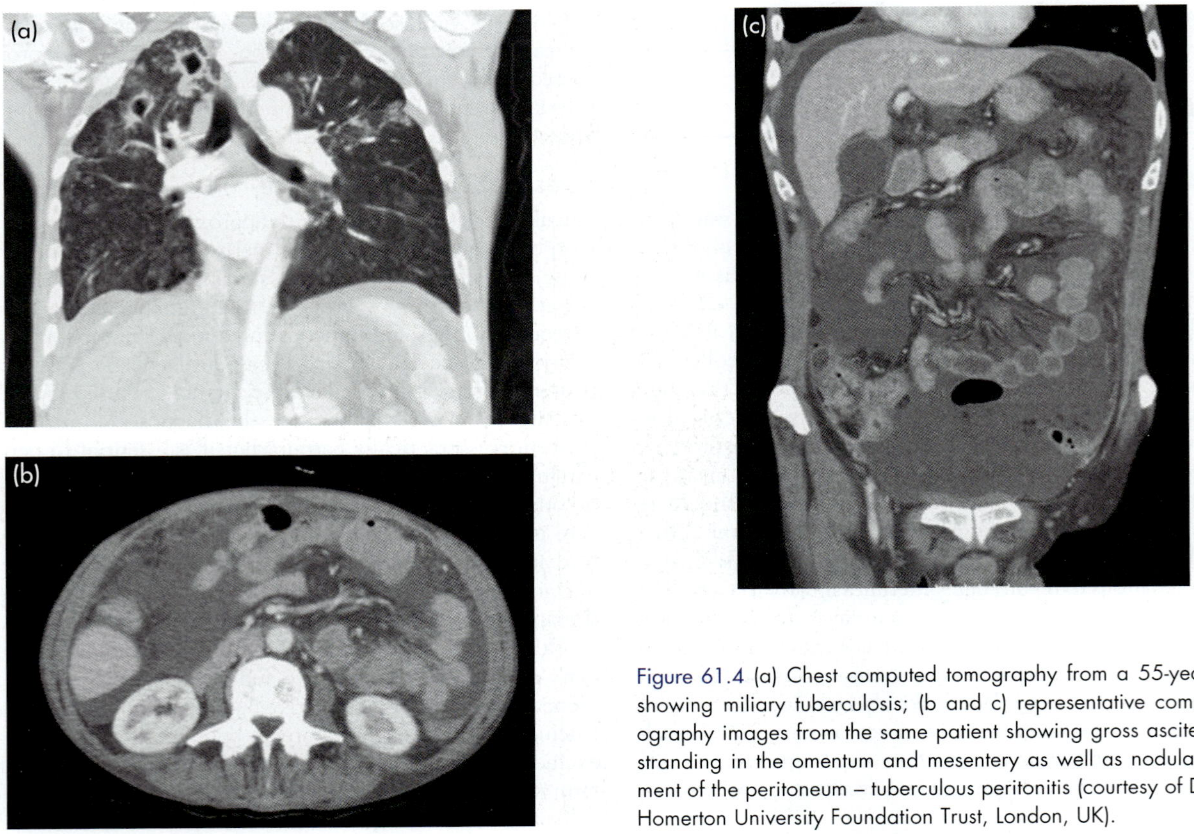

Figure 61.4 (a) Chest computed tomography from a 55-year-old man showing miliary tuberculosis; (b and c) representative computed tomography images from the same patient showing gross ascites, nodular stranding in the omentum and mesentery as well as nodular enhancement of the peritoneum – tuberculous peritonitis (courtesy of Dr S Burke, Homerton University Foundation Trust, London, UK).

thorax and joints. The duration of an attack is 24–72 hours, when it is followed by complete remission, but exacerbations recur at regular intervals. Most of the patients have undergone appendicectomy in childhood. This disease, often familial, is limited principally to Arab, Armenian and Jewish populations; other races are occasionally affected. Mutations in the *MEFV* (Mediterranean fever) gene appear to cause the disease. This gene produces a protein called pyrin, which is expressed mostly in neutrophils but whose exact function is not known.

Usually, children are affected but it is not rare for the disease to make its first appearance in early adult life, with cases in women outnumbering those in men by two to one. Exceptionally, the disease becomes manifest in patients over 40 years of age. At operation, which may be necessary to exclude other causes (but should be avoided if possible), the peritoneum is inflamed, particularly in the vicinity of the spleen and the gall bladder. There is no evidence that the interior of these organs is abnormal. Colchicine therapy is used during attacks and to prevent recurrent attacks.

INTRAPERITONEAL ABSCESS

Following intraperitoneal sepsis (usually manifest first as local or diffuse peritonitis), the anatomy of the peritoneal cavity is such that with the influence of gravity (depending on patient position – sitting or supine), abscess development usually occupies one of a number of specific abdominal or pelvic sites (Figure 61.5).

In general, the symptoms and signs of a purulent collection may be vague and consist of nothing more than lassitude, anorexia and malaise; pyrexia (often low-grade), mild tachycardia and localised tenderness. Certain sites have more specific clinical features (Summary box 61.11). Larger abscesses will give rise to the picture of swinging pyrexia and pulse and a palpable mass. Blood tests will reveal elevated inflammatory markers.

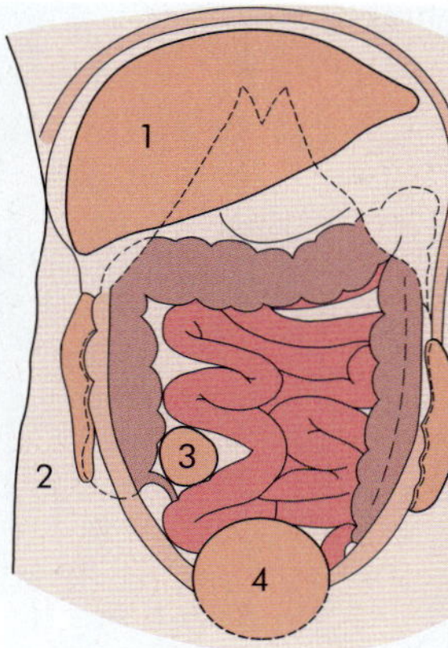

Figure 61.5 Common situations for residual abscesses: (1) subphrenic; (2) paracolic; (3) right iliac fossa; (4) pelvic.

Summary box 61.11

Clinical features of an abdominal/pelvic abscess

Symptoms
- Malaise, lethargy – failure to recover from surgery as expected
- Anorexia and weight loss
- Sweats ± rigors
- Abdominal/pelvic pain
- Symptoms from local irritation, e.g. shoulder tip/hiccoughs (subphrenic), diarrhoea and mucus (pelvic), nausea and vomiting (any upper abdominal)

Signs
- Increased temperature and pulse ± swinging pyrexia
- Localised abdominal tenderness ± mass (including on pelvic exam)

Pelvic abscess

The pelvis is the most common site of abscess formation because the vermiform appendix is often pelvic in position and the Fallopian tubes are also frequent sites of infection. A pelvic abscess can also occur as a sequel to any case of diffuse peritonitis and is common after anastomotic leakage following colorectal surgery.

Clinical features

The most characteristic symptoms are of pelvic pain, diarrhoea and the passage of mucus in the stools. Rectal examination reveals a bulging of the anterior rectal wall, which, when the abscess is ripe, becomes softly cystic.

Investigation and management

Left to nature, a proportion of these abscesses burst into the rectum, after which the patient nearly always recovers rapidly. If this does not occur, the abscess should be drained deliberately. In women, vaginal drainage through the posterior fornix is often chosen. In other cases, when the abscess is definitely pointing into the rectum, rectal drainage (Figure 61.6) is employed. If any uncertainty exists, the presence of pus should be confirmed by ultrasound or CT scanning (Figure 61.7). Laparotomy is almost never necessary and rectal drainage of a pelvic abscess is far preferable to suprapubic drainage, which risks exposing the general peritoneal cavity to infection. Drainage tubes can also be inserted percutaneously or via the vagina or rectum under ultrasound or CT guidance.

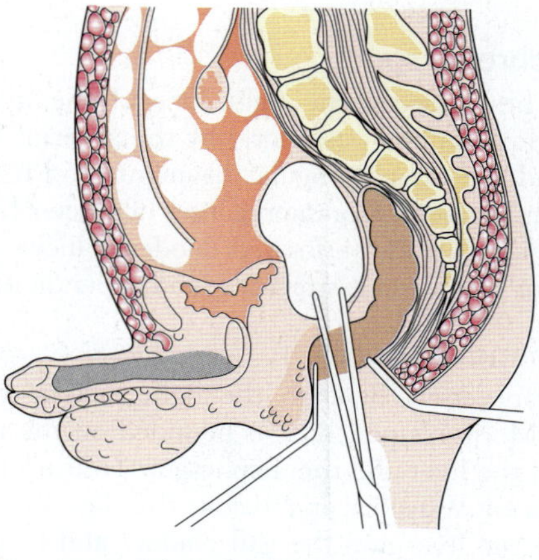
Figure 61.6 Opening a pelvic abscess into the rectum.

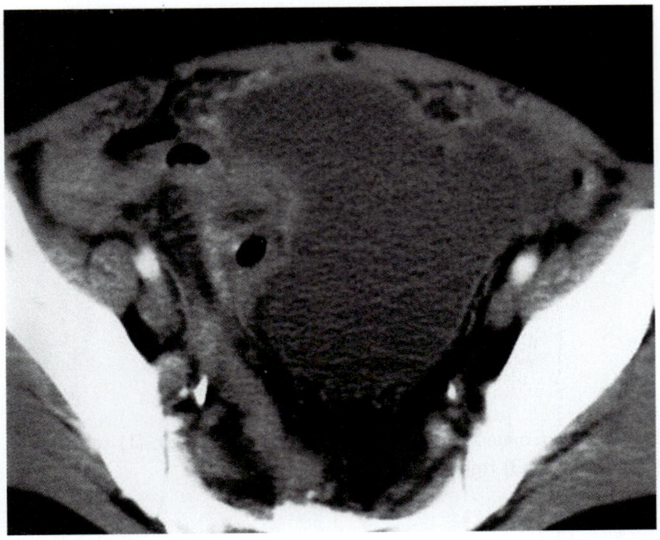

Figure 61.7 A pelvic abscess seen on computed tomography scanning (courtesy of Dr J Healy, Chelsea and Westminster Hospital, London, UK).

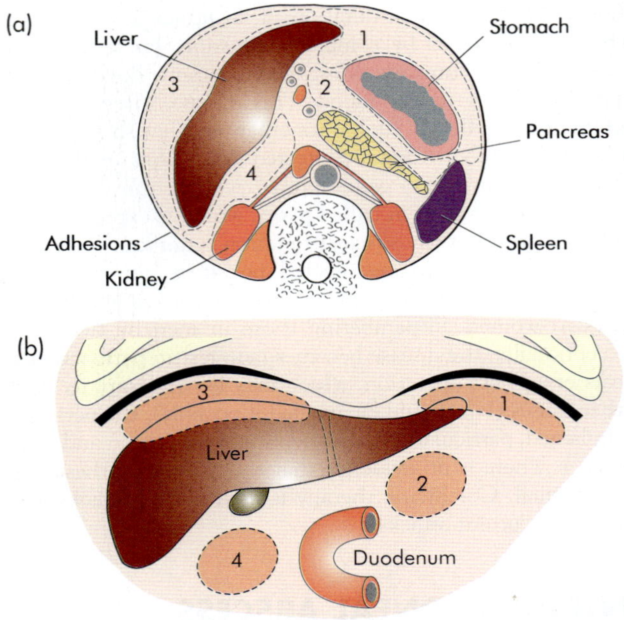

Figure 61.8 (a) Intraperitoneal abscesses on transverse section: (1) the left subphrenic space, (2) left subhepatic space/lesser sac, (3) right subphrenic space, (4) right subhepatic space. (b) Intraperitoneal abscesses on sagittal section: (1) left subphrenic, (2) left subhepatic/lesser sac, (3) right subphrenic, (4) right subhepatic.

Intraperitoneal abscess

Anatomy

The complicated arrangement of the peritoneum results in the formation of four intraperitoneal spaces in which pus may commonly collect (Figure 61.8).

Left subphrenic space

This is bounded above by the diaphragm and behind by the left triangular ligament and the left lobe of the liver, the gastrohepatic omentum and the anterior surface of the stomach. To the right is the falciform ligament and to the left the spleen, gastrosplenic omentum and diaphragm. The common cause of an abscess here is an operation on the stomach, the tail of the pancreas, the spleen or the splenic flexure of the colon.

Left subhepatic space/lesser sac

The most common cause of infection here is complicated acute pancreatitis. In practice, a perforated gastric ulcer rarely causes a collection here because the potential space is obliterated by adhesions.

Right subphrenic space

This space lies between the right lobe of the liver and the diaphragm. It is limited posteriorly by the anterior layer of the coronary and the right triangular ligaments and to the left by the falciform ligament. Common causes of abscess here are perforating cholecystitis, a perforated duodenal ulcer, a duodenal cap 'blow-out' following gastrectomy and appendicitis.

Right subhepatic space

This lies transversely beneath the right lobe of the liver in Rutherford Morison's pouch. It is bounded on the right by the right lobe of the liver and the diaphragm. To the left is situated the foramen of Winslow and below this lies the duodenum. In front are the liver and the gall bladder and behind are the upper part of the right kidney and the diaphragm. The space is bounded above by the liver and below by the transverse colon and hepatic flexure. It is the deepest space of the four and the most common site of a subphrenic abscess, which usually arises from appendicitis, cholecystitis, a perforated duodenal ulcer or following upper abdominal surgery.

Clinical features

The symptoms and signs of subphrenic infection are frequently non-specific and it is well to remember the aphorism, 'pus somewhere, pus nowhere, pus under the diaphragm'. A common history is that, when some infective focus in the abdominal cavity has been dealt with, the condition of the patient improves temporarily but, after an interval of a few days or weeks, symptoms of toxaemia reappear. The condition of the patient steadily, and often rapidly, deteriorates. Sweating, wasting and anorexia are present. There is sometimes epigastric fullness and pain, or pain in the shoulder on the affected side due to irritation of sensory fibres in the phrenic nerve, this being referred along the descending branches of the cervical plexus. Persistent hiccoughs may be a presenting symptom. A swinging pyrexia is usually present. If the abscess is anterior, abdominal examination will reveal some tenderness, rigidity or even a palpable swelling. Sometimes the liver is displaced downwards but more often it is fixed by adhesions.

Investigation and management

Examination of the chest and plain radiograph are important, as in the majority of cases, collapse of the lung or evidence of basal effusion or even an empyema are evident. The modern management of an abscess is by radiological diagnosis using ultrasound or CT guidance (Figure 61.9) followed by drainage. The same tube can be used to instill antibiotic solutions or irrigate the

James Rutherford Morison, 1853–1939, Professor of Surgery, The University of Durham, Durham, UK.
Jacob Benignus Winslow, 1669–1760, Professor of Anatomy, Physic and Surgery, Paris, France.

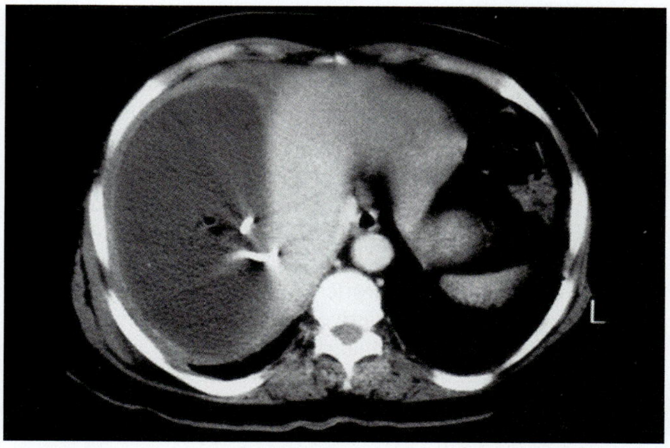

Figure 61.9 A subphrenic abscess drained under computed tomography guidance (courtesy of Dr J Healy, Chelsea and Westminster Hospital, London, UK).

abscess cavity if necessary. In some instances, monitoring may be appropriate by either clinically marking out limits on the abdominal wall (if palpable) with daily examination. However, more commonly, repeat ultrasound or CT scanning will be required. Radiolabelled white cell scanning may occasionally prove helpful when other imaging techniques have failed. In most cases, with the aid of percutaneous drainage and antibiotic treatment, the abscess or mass gradually reduces in size until, finally, it is undetectable. Open drainage of an intraperitoneal collection is thus now uncommon but may be necessary. If a swelling can be detected in the subcostal region or in the loin, an incision is made over the site of maximum tenderness or over any area where oedema or redness is discovered. Cautious blunt finger exploration can then be used to avoid dissemination of pus into the peritoneal or pleural cavities and minimise the risk of an intestinal fistula. When the cavity is reached, all of the fibrinous loculi must be broken down with the finger and one or two drainage tubes fully inserted. These drains are withdrawn gradually during the next 10 days and the closure of the cavity can be checked by sinograms or scanning. Appropriate antibiotics are also given.

ASCITES

Ascites is defined as an accumulation of excess serous fluid within the peritoneal cavity.

Pathophysiology

The balanced effects of plasma and peritoneal colloid osmotic and hydrostatic pressures determine the exchange of fluid between the capillaries and the peritoneal fluid. Protein-rich fluid enters the peritoneal cavity when capillary permeability is increased, as in peritonitis and carcinomatosis peritonei. Capillary pressure may be increased because of generalised water retention, cardiac failure, constrictive pericarditis or vena cava obstruction. Capillary pressure is raised selectively in the portal venous system in the Budd–Chiari syndrome, cirrhosis of the liver or extrahepatic portal venous obstruction. Plasma colloid osmotic pressure may be lowered in patients with reduced nutritional intake, diminished intestinal absorption, abnormal protein losses or defective protein synthesis such as occurs in cirrhosis. Peritoneal lymphatic drainage may be impaired, resulting in the accumulation of protein-rich fluid. A list of causes of ascites is given in Summary box 61.12.

Summary box 61.12

Causes of ascites

Transudates (protein <25 g/L)
- Low plasma protein concentrations
  - Malnutrition
  - Nephrotic syndrome
  - Protein-losing enteropathy
- High central venous pressure
  - Congestive cardiac failure
- Portal hypertension
  - Portal vein thrombosis
  - Cirrhosis

Exudates (protein >25 g/L)
- Tuberculous peritonitis
- Peritoneal malignancy
- Budd–Chiari syndrome (hepatic vein occlusion or thrombosis)
- Pancreatic ascites
- Chylous ascites
- Meigs' syndrome

Clinical features

Ascites can usually only be recognised clinically when the amount of fluid present exceeds 1.5 L depending on body habitus: in the obese a greater quantity than this is necessary before there is clear evidence. The abdomen is distended evenly with fullness of the flanks, which are dull to percussion. Usually, shifting dullness is present but when there is a very large accumulation of fluid this sign is absent. In such cases, on flicking the abdominal wall, a characteristic fluid thrill is transmitted from one side to the other. In women, ascites must be differentiated from an enormous ovarian cyst.

Congestive heart failure, the most common cause of ascites, results in increased venous pressure in the vena cava and consequent obstruction to the venous outflow from the liver. The ascitic fluid is light yellow and of low specific gravity, about 1.010, with a low protein concentration (<25 g/L). Patients with constrictive pericarditis (Pick's disease) have both peritoneal and pleural effusions because of engorgement of the venae cavae consequent upon the diminished capacity of the right side of the heart. Ascites occurs with low plasma albumin concentrations, for example in patients with albuminuria or starvation. The ascites in this instance is caused by alterations in the osmotic pressure of the capillary blood and has a low specific gravity.

In cirrhosis, there is obstruction to the portal venous system, which is caused by obliterative fibrosis of the intrahepatic venous bed. In the Budd–Chiari syndrome (see Chapter 65), thrombosis or obstruction of the hepatic veins is responsible for obstruction to venous outflow from the liver. The ascites seen in patients with peritoneal metastases is caused by excessive exudation of fluid and lymphatic blockage. The fluid is dark yellow and frequently blood-stained. The specific gravity, 1.020 or over, and the protein content (>25 g/L) are high. Microscopic

Harrith M Hasson, Clinical Professor of Obstetrics and Gynaecology, University of Chicago.
George Budd, 1808–1882, Professor of Medicine, King's College Hospital, London, UK, described this syndrome in 1845.

examination often reveals cancer cells, especially if large quantities of fluid are 'spun down' to produce a concentrated deposit for sampling. Rarely, ascites and pleural effusion are associated with solid fibromas of the ovary (Meigs' syndrome). The effusions disappear when the tumour is excised.

Investigation

In addition to relevant investigations that may determine the underlying cause, e.g. liver and cardiac function tests, ultrasound and/or CT imaging (Figure 61.10) will determine much smaller quantities of ascites than possible clinically. These will often also diagnose aetiology, e.g. carcinomatosis, liver disease. Ascitic aspiration or tap (below) is now most commonly performed under imaging guidance to minimise the risk of visceral injury. The bladder having been emptied, puncture of the peritoneum is carried out under local anaesthetic using a moderately sized trocar and cannula. Alternatively, a peritoneal drain may be inserted. In cases where the effusion is caused by cardiac failure, the fluid must be evacuated slowly. Fluid is sent for microscopy/cytology, culture, including mycobacteria, and analysis of protein content and amylase. Unless other measures are taken the fluid soon reaccumulates, and repeated tappings remove valuable protein.

Treatment

Treatment of the specific cause is undertaken whenever possible; for example, if portal venous pressure is raised, it may be possible to lower it by treatment of the primary condition. Dietary sodium restriction to 200 mg/day may be helpful, but diuretics are usually required. In rare cases in which ascites accumulates rapidly after paracentesis and the patient is otherwise fit, permanent drainage of the ascitic fluid via a peritoneovenous shunt (e.g. LeVeen, Denver) may render the patient more comfortable. Similar in concept to shunts for hydrocephalus (see Chapter 43), a catheter (e.g. of silicone) is constructed with a valve so as to allow one-way flow from the peritoneum to a central vein (e.g. internal jugular). A chamber placed subcutaneously over the chest wall may be included for manual compression. Insertion is relatively simple. The complications include overloading the venous system, cardiac failure and disseminated intravascular coagulopathy. The frequency of these complications may be reduced by evacuating ascitic fluid and partially replacing it with normal saline at the time of shunt insertion.

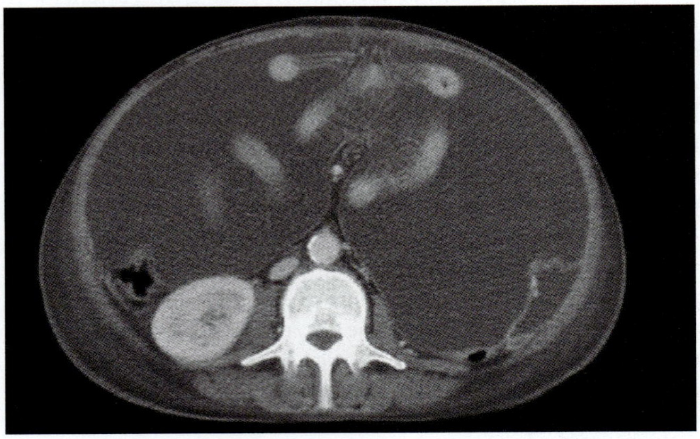

Figure 61.10 Computed tomography scan showing gross ascites.

The procedure may also be used for patients with terminal malignant ascites, giving improved quality of life despite the risk of further dissemination of malignant cells.

Special cases

Chylous ascites

In some patients the ascitic fluid appears milky because of an excess of chylomicrons (triglycerides). Most cases are associated with malignancy, usually lymphomas; other causes are cirrhosis, tuberculosis, filariasis, nephrotic syndrome, abdominal trauma (including surgery), constrictive pericarditis, sarcoidosis and congenital lymphatic abnormality. The prognosis is poor unless the underlying condition can be cured. In addition to other measures used to treat ascites, patients should be placed on a fat-free diet with medium-chain triglyceride supplements.

TUMOURS OF THE PERITONEUM

Primary tumours

Primary tumours of the peritoneum are rare and in most cases take their origin not from the serous layer but from some adjacent structure, e.g. lipoma from appendices epiploicae, fibroma from connective tissue. Mesothelioma of the peritoneum is less frequent than in the pleural cavity but equally lethal. Asbestos is a recognised cause. It has a predilection for the pelvic peritoneum. Chemocytotoxic agents are the mainstay of treatment. Desmoid tumours which have a relationship to the peritoneum are considered under familial adenomatous polyposis (Chapter 69).

Secondary tumours

Carcinomatosis peritonei

This is a common terminal event in many cases of carcinoma of the stomach, colon, ovary or other abdominal organs and also of the breast and bronchus. The peritoneum, both parietal and visceral, is studded with secondary growths and the peritoneal cavity becomes filled with clear, straw-coloured or blood-stained ascitic fluid.

The main forms of peritoneal metastases are:

- discrete nodules – by far the most common variety;
- plaques varying in size and colour;
- diffuse adhesions – this form occurs at a late stage of the disease and gives rise, sometimes, to a 'frozen pelvis'.

Gravity probably determines the distribution of free malignant cells within the peritoneal cavity. Cells not caught in peritoneal folds gravitate into the pelvic pouches or into a hernial sac, the enlargement of which is occasionally the first indication of the condition. Implantation occurs also on the greater omentum, the appendices epiploicae and the inferior surface of the diaphragm. The main differential diagnosis is from tuberculous peritonitis (tubercles are greyish and translucent and closely resemble the discrete nodules of peritoneal carcinomatosis). Investigation and treatment are as for underlying malignancy.

Pseudomyxoma peritonei

This rare condition occurs more frequently in women. The abdomen is filled with a yellow jelly, large quantities of which are often encysted. The condition is associated with mucinous

Friedel Pick, 1867–1926, physician, Prague, The Czech Republic, described this disease in 1896.
Joe Vincent Meigs, 1892–1963, Professor of Gynaecology, Harvard University Medical School, Boston, MA, USA.
Harry LeVeen, Professor of Surgery, the University of South Carolina, SC, USA.

cystic tumours of the ovary and appendix. Recent studies suggest that most cases arise from a primary appendiceal tumour with secondary implantation on to one or both ovaries. It is often painless and there is frequently no impairment of general health. Pseudomyxoma peritonei does not give rise to extraperitoneal metastases. Although an abdomen distended with what seems to be fluid that cannot be made to shift should raise the possibility, the diagnosis is more often suggested by ultrasound and CT scanning or made at operation. At laparotomy, masses of jelly are scooped out. The appendix, if present, should be excised together with any ovarian tumour. Unfortunately, recurrence is inevitable, but patients may gain symptomatic benefit from repeated 'debulking' surgery. Occasionally, the condition responds to radioactive isotopes or intraperitoneal chemotherapy. The role of early radical peritoneal excision is uncertain.

Peritoneal loose bodies (peritoneal mice)

Peritoneal loose bodies (peritoneal mice) may be confused with a small tumour but almost never cause symptoms. One or more may be found in a hernial sac or in the pouch of Douglas. The loose body may come from an appendix epiploica that has undergone axial rotation followed by necrosis of its pedicle and detachment but they are also found in those who suffer from subacute attacks of pancreatitis. These hyaline bodies attain the size of a pea or bean and contain saponified fat surrounded by fibrin.

ADHESIONS

Pathophysiology

Adhesions are strands of fibrous tissue that form, usually as a result of surgery, between surgically injured tissues. After injury, there is bleeding and an increase in vascular permeability with extravasation of fibrinogen-rich fluid from the injured surfaces forming a temporary fibrin matrix. An inflammatory response ensues with cell migration, release of cytokines, and activation of the coagulation cascade. The activation of the coagulation system results in thrombin formation, which is necessary for the conversion of fibrinogen to fibrin. In the absence of fibrinolysis, adhesions will form within 5–7 days as the matrix gradually becomes more organised with collagen secretion by fibroblasts. Fibrinolysis is therefore the key factor in determining whether an adhesion persists. This is governed by several cascades and activators that may account for interindividual differences (Chapter 59). Of great importance however to the surgeon is the fact that ischaemic tissue loses its ability to break down fibrin and inhibits fibrinolysis in adjacent tissues.

Complications

The most common adhesion-related problem is small bowel obstruction (SBO). Adhesions are the most frequent cause of SBO in the developed world and are responsible for 60–70 per cent of SBO (see Chapter 69). Adhesions are implicated as a major cause of secondary infertility (beyond the remit of this text). The relationship of adhesions to chronic abdominal and pelvic pain is contentious. Unguided division of adhesions has not been shown to reduce chronic abdominal pain in definitive randomised controlled trials although conscious pain mapping (laparoscopy under local anaesthesia) to direct lysis may improve success rates.

Prevention

Because of the scale of the problem there has been significant research into ways of preventing postoperative adhesion formation. Minimising the production of ischaemic tissue by careful operative technique, including meticulous control of bleeding, remain however the most critical concepts. The evolution of laparoscopic bowel surgery has been shown by collective review data to result in reduced adhesion-related readmissions for a number of abdominal and pelvic procedures, e.g. cholecystectomy, hysterectomy and colectomy. It should be noted however that only one randomised controlled trial (after Crohn's resection) has ever shown a definitive effect and this was not confirmed by evidence synthesis at Cochrane review.

The effect of a number of drugs including anti-inflammatory drugs like aspirin and steroids, some hormones, anticlotting agents, antibiotics, vitamin E and even methylene blue have been investigated in adhesion prevention but have not achieved widespread use either because of side effects or lack of consistent evidence of effectiveness. Many barrier methods of reducing adhesions have also been trialled. Adept® (4 per cent icodextrin solution) is a solution applied inside the abdomen at the time of surgery and has been shown to reduce the extent and severity of adhesion formation in animal models. It has also been used widely as a peritoneal dialysis solution for many years. Interceed TC7® is a mesh-like product (oxidised regenerated cellulose) which quickly forms a soft gelatinous mass around healing tissues and is absorbed within 2 weeks. It has been shown to significantly reduce the number of adhesions at the site where it is used. However, it is worth noting that a reduction in the number of adhesions in such studies does not necessarily equate to a reduction in adhesion-related problems in the future. In a review of seven randomised trials looking at a similar barrier-type product (hyaluronic acid/carboxymethyl membrane), there was a significant reduction in the incidence, extent and severity of adhesions but no reduction in the incidence of intestinal obstruction or operative intervention. Such barriers when placed around bowel anastomosis also led to a significant increase in the anastomotic leaks. For these reasons barrier approaches have not gained popularity.

Special forms of intraperitoneal fibrosis

Sclerosing encapsulating peritonitis

Also known as abdominal cocoon syndrome, sclerosing encapsulating peritonitis (SEP) is described in patients as a complication of long-term peritoneal dialysis or portovenous shunting. The peritoneal cavity becomes obliterated as a result of gross subserosal thickening by fibrosis leading to bowel obstruction and other sequelae. Surgery should be undertaken with trepidation and avoided if possible.

Diffuse fibromatosis

This is a variant of intra-abdominal fibromatosis (IAF) and is actually a rare tumour characterised by an abnormal proliferation of myofibroblasts. Although non-metastasising, and said to be benign, it can nevertheless prove widely invasive, compressing and infiltrating surrounding tissues such as the bowel and mesentery with complications thereof. IAF is very rare within the general population but has a recognised association with familial adenomatous polyposis (FAP).

James Douglas, 1675–1742, anatomist and male midwife, London, UK.

THE OMENTUM

Rutherford Morison called the greater omentum 'the abdominal policeman'. The greater omentum attempts, often successfully, to limit intraperitoneal infective and other noxious processes (Figure 61.11). For instance, an acutely inflamed appendix is often found wrapped in omentum, and this saves many patients from developing diffuse peritonitis. Some sufferers of herniae are also greatly indebted to this structure, for it often plugs the neck of a hernial sac and prevents a coil of intestine from entering and becoming strangulated. It can, of course, also be a cause of obstruction (acting as a large adhesion). The omentum is usually involved in tuberculous peritonitis and carcinomatosis of the peritoneum.

Torsion of the omentum

Torsion of the omentum is a rare emergency and consequently is seldom diagnosed correctly. It is usually mistaken for appendicitis with somewhat abnormal signs. It may be primary, or secondary to adhesion of the omentum to an old focus of infection or hernia. The patient is most frequently a middle-aged, obese man. A tender lump may be present in the abdomen. The blood supply having been jeopardised, the twisted mass sometimes becomes gangrenous, in which case bacterial peritonitis may follow. Treatment is surgical; the pedicle above the twist is ligated securely and the mass removed.

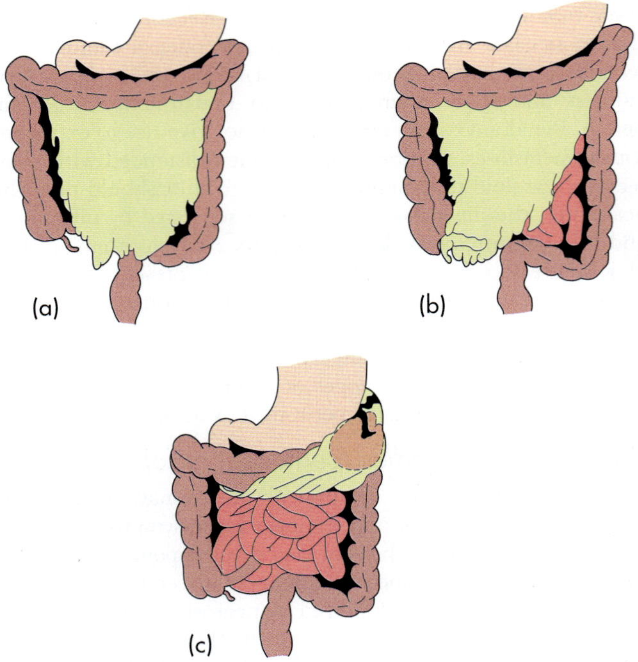

Figure 61.11 The greater omentum. (a) Normal; (b) in appendicitis; (c) in a (comparatively small) laceration of the spleen.

THE MESENTERY

Mesenteric injury

A wound of the mesentery can follow severe abdominal contusion and is a cause of haemoperitoneum. More commonly, it is injured by a torsional force, so-called seatbelt syndrome. This occurs during a vehicular collision when a seatbelt is being worn with sudden deceleration resulting in a torn mesentery. This possibility should be borne in mind, particularly as multiple injuries may distract attention from this injury (the management of abdominal trauma is covered in Chapter 23). Aside from control of any ongoing haemorrhage, associated ischaemic or ruptured gut will require resection.

Ischaemia

Torsion of the mesentery is covered under midgut volvulus and volvulus of the small intestine (see Chapter 70). Embolism and thrombosis of mesenteric vessels leading to intestinal ischaemia are also covered in Chapter 70.

Inflammation

A number of somewhat miscellaneous conditions are best described under this umbrella term.

Acute non-specific ileocaecal mesenteric adenitis

Non-specific mesenteric adenitis was so named to distinguish it from specific (tuberculous) mesenteric adenitis. It is now much more common than the tuberculous variety. The aetiology often remains unknown, although some cases are associated with *Yersinia* infection of the ileum. In other cases, an unidentified virus is blamed. In about 25 per cent of cases, a respiratory infection precedes an attack of non-specific mesenteric adenitis. This self-limiting disease is never fatal but may be recurrent. Its significance thus mainly lies in its differential diagnosis with appendicitis in children.

Diagnosis

During childhood, acute non-specific mesenteric adenitis is a common condition. The typical history is one of short attacks of central abdominal pain lasting from 10 to 30 minutes, commonly associated with vomiting. The patient seldom looks ill. In more than half of the cases the temperature is elevated. Abdominal tenderness is poorly localised, and when present, shifting tenderness is a valuable sign for differentiating the condition from appendicitis. The neck, axillae and groins should be palpated for enlarged lymph nodes. There is often a leukocytosis of 10 000–12 000 μL (10–12 × 109 L) or more on the first day of the attack, but this falls on the second day.

Treatment

When the diagnosis can be made with assurance, bed rest and simple analgesia is the only treatment necessary. If at a second examination a few hours later, acute appendicitis cannot be excluded, it is safer to perform either appendicectomy or diagnostic laparoscopy. If surgery is mistakenly undertaken, there is a small increase in the amount of peritoneal fluid. The ileocaecal mesenteric lymph nodes are enlarged and can be seen and felt between the leaves of the mesentery. In very acute cases they are distinctly red, and many of them are the size of a walnut. The nodes nearest the attachment of the mesentery are the largest. They are not adherent to their peritoneal coats and, if a small incision is made through the overlying peritoneum, a node is extruded easily.

Alexander Emile Jean Yersin, 1863–1943, bacteriologist, The Institute Pasteur, Paris, France.

Tuberculosis of the mesenteric lymph nodes

Tuberculous mesenteric lymphadenitis is considerably less common than acute non-specific lymphadenitis. Tubercle bacilli, usually, but not necessarily, bovine, are ingested and enter the mesenteric lymph nodes by way of Peyer's patches. Sometimes only one lymph node is infected; usually there are several; occasionally massive involvement occurs. The presentation may be with abdominal pain (a rare differential for appendicitis) or with general constitutional symptoms (pyrexia, weight loss, etc.). Calcified lymph nodes may be demonstrated on a plain radiograph of the abdomen where they must be distinguished from other calcified lesions, e.g. renal or ureteric stones.

Misty mesentery

The term 'misty mesentery' indicates a pathological increase in mesenteric fat attenuation at CT (Figure 61.12). It is frequently observed on multidetector CT (MDCT) scans performed during daily clinical practice and may be caused by various pathological conditions, including oedema, inflammation (especially in association with pancreatitis), haemorrhage, neoplastic infiltration (especially otherwise occult lymphoma) or sclerosing mesenteritis. In patients suffering from acute abdominal disease, misty mesentery may be considered a feature of the underlying disease. Otherwise, it may represent an incidental finding on MDCT performed for other reasons. Follow-up scans may be required to dictate whether further investigation is required depending on progression or resolution. It should be noted that the term 'mesenteric panniculitis' is frequently used synonymously with 'misty mesentery'. Correctly this term should be reserved for the mesenteric manifestation of Weber–Christian disease; isolated lipodystrophy and mesenteric lipogranuloma. It is a very rare (2–300 cases reported worldwide) benign inflammatory or fibrotic change in the mesentery of the bowel.

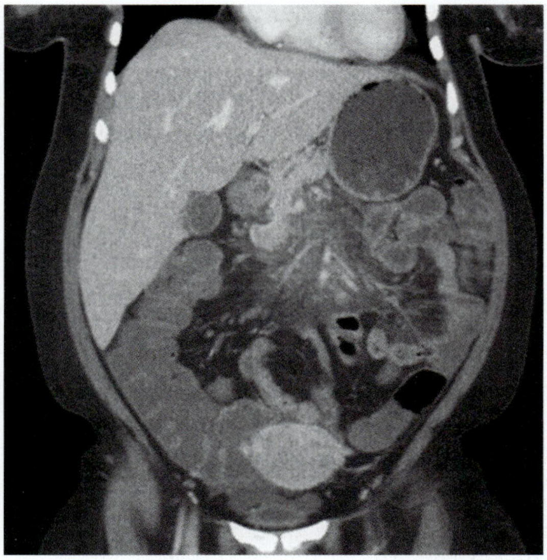

Figure 61.12 Computed tomography scan showing 'misty mesentery' in a patient with probable peritoneal inflammation secondary to acute pancreatitis (courtesy of Dr K Patel, Homerton University Foundation Trust, London, UK).

Mesenteric cysts

Cysts may occur in the mesentery of either the small intestine (60 per cent) or the colon (40 per cent) and can be classified as:

- chylolymphatic;
- enterogenous;
- urogenital remnant (actually retroperitoneal but project into peritoneum);
- dermoid.

Pathology

Chylolymphatic cyst

This is the most common variety, probably arising in congenitally misplaced lymphatic tissue that has no efferent communication with the lymphatic system (most frequently in the mesentery of the ileum). The thin wall of the cyst, which is composed of connective tissue lined by flat endothelium, is filled with clear lymph or, less frequently, with chyle varying in consistency from watered milk to cream. Occasionally, the cyst attains a great size. More often unilocular than multilocular, a chylolymphatic cyst is almost invariably solitary, although there is an extremely rare variety in which myriads of cysts are found in the various mesenteries of the abdomen. A chylolymphatic cyst has a blood supply that is independent from that of the adjacent intestine and, thus, enucleation is possible without the need for resection of gut.

Enterogenous cysts

These are believed to be derived either from a diverticulum of the mesenteric border of the intestine that has become sequestrated from the intestinal canal during embryonic life or from a duplication of the intestine (see Chapter 8). An enterogenous cyst has a thicker wall than a chylolymphatic cyst and it is lined by mucous membrane, sometimes ciliated. The content is mucinous and is either colourless or yellowish brown as a result of past haemorrhage. The muscle in the wall of an enteric duplication cyst and the bowel with which it is in contact have a common blood supply; consequently, removal of the cyst always entails resection of the related portion of intestine.

Urogenital remnant

A cyst developing in the retroperitoneal space (see below) often attains very large dimensions and has first to be distinguished from a large hydronephrosis. Even after the latter condition has been eliminated by scanning or urography, a retroperitoneal cyst can seldom be distinguished with certainty from a retroperitoneal tumour until displayed at operation. The cyst may be unilocular or multilocular. Many of these cysts are believed to be derived from a remnant of the Wolffian duct, in which case they are filled with clear fluid.

Clinical features

These are shown for mesenteric cysts in general in Summary box 61.13.

Investigation and treatment

Ultrasound and CT scanning will demonstrate the lesion and may allow diagnosis of cyst type (Figure 61.14a,b). There are no suitable medical therapies. The goal of surgical therapy is complete excision of the mass. The preferred treatment of

Kaspar Friedrich Wolff, 1733–1794, Professor of Anatomy and Physiology, St Petersburg, Russia, described the mesonephric duct and body in 1759.

Summary box 61.13

Mesenteric cysts: clinical features

- Cysts occur most commonly in adults with a mean age of 45 years
- Twice as common in women as in men
- Rare – incidence around 1 per 140 000
- Approximately one-third of cases occur in children younger than 15 years
- The mean age of children affected is 4.9 years
- The most common presentation is of a painless abdominal swelling with characteristic physical signs
    - there is a fluctuant swelling near the umbilicus
    - the swelling moves freely in a plane at right angles to the attachment of the mesentery (Tillaux's sign) (Figure 61.13)
    - there is a zone of resonance around the cyst
- Other presentations are with recurrent attacks of abdominal pain with or without vomiting (pain resulting from recurring temporary impaction of a food bolus in a segment of bowel narrowed by the cyst or possibly from torsion of the mesentery) and acute abdominal catastrophe, due to
    - torsion of that portion of the mesentery containing the cyst
    - rupture of the cyst, often as a result of a comparatively trivial accident
    - haemorrhage into the cyst
    - infection

mesenteric cysts is enucleation, although bowel resection is frequently required to ensure that the remaining bowel is viable. Bowel resection may be required in 50–60 per cent of children with mesenteric cysts, whereas resection is necessary in about one-third of adults (Figure 61.14c). If enucleation or resection is not possible because of the size of the cyst or because of its location deep within the root of the mesentery, the third option is partial excision with marsupialisation of the remaining cyst into the abdominal cavity. Approximately 10 per cent of patients require this form of therapy; If marsupialisation is performed, the cyst lining should be sclerosed with 10 per cent glucose solution, diathermy, or tincture of iodine to minimise recurrence. Recurrence rates vary from 0 to 13 per cent.

Differential diagnosis

The following, although not being mesenteric cysts in the true meaning of the term, give rise to the same physical signs:

- serosanguinous cyst, probably traumatic in origin although a history of an accident is seldom obtained;
- tuberculous abscess of the mesentery;
- hydatid cyst of the mesentery.

Neoplasms of the mesentery

The mesentery is necessarily affected by local lymphatic spread of carcinoma arising from the peritoneal viscera. Other benign and malignant tumours are less common (Summary box 61.14).

Tumours situated in the mesentery give rise to physical signs that are similar to those of a mesenteric cyst, the sole exception being that they sometimes feel solid. If indicated, a benign tumour of the mesentery is excised in the same way as an enterogenous mesenteric cyst, i.e. with resection of the adjacent intestine. A malignant tumour of the mesentery requires biopsy confirmation and specific, usually non-surgical, treatment, e.g. chemotherapy for lymphoma.

Summary box 61.14

Mesenteric tumours

Benign
- Lipoma
- Fibroma
- Fibromyxoma

Malignant
- Lymphoma
- Secondary carcinoma

THE RETROPERITONEAL SPACE

Retroperitoneal chronic inflammation/fibrosis

This is a relatively rare diagnosis characterised by the development of a flat grey/white plaque of tissue which is found first in the low lumbar region but then spreads laterally and upwards to encase the common iliac vessels, ureters and aorta. Histological appearances vary from active inflammation with a high cellular content interspersed with bundles of collagen through to one of acellularity and mature fibrosis/calcification. Its aetiology is obscure in most cases (idiopathic) being allied to other fibromatoses (others being Dupuytren's contracture and Peyronie's disease). In other patients the cause is known (Summary box 61.15).

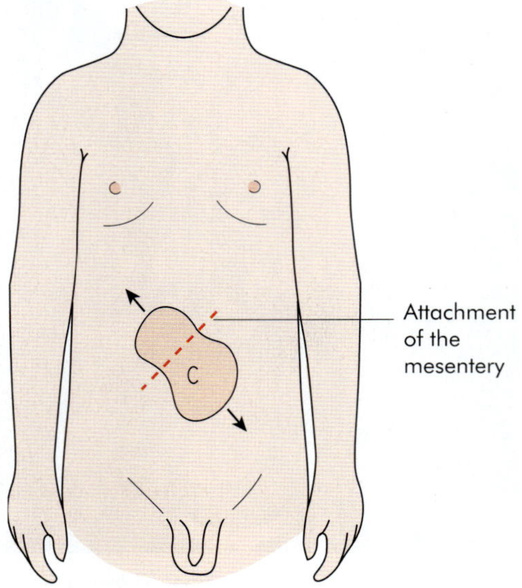

Figure 61.13 A mesenteric cyst moves freely in the direction of the arrows, i.e. at right angles to the attachment of the mesentery (Tillaux's sign).

PART 11 | ABDOMINAL

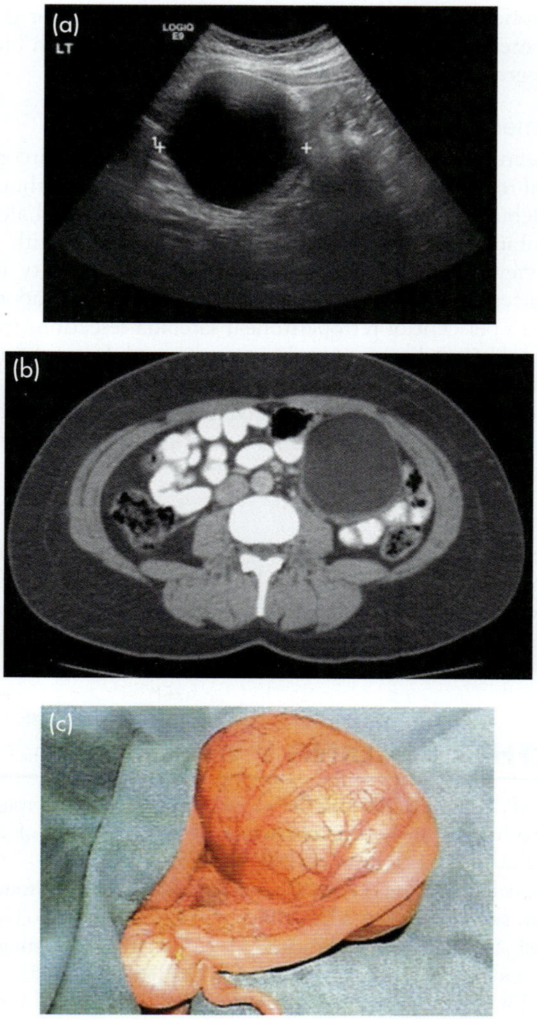

Figure 61.14 A mesenteric enterogenous cyst in a 37-year-old female presenting with an asymptomatic palpable abdominal mass: (a) ultrasound findings; (b) computed tomography findings; (c) intraoperative findings requiring en masse small bowel resection (courtesy of Mr F Olagbaiye, Homerton University Foundation Trust, London, UK).

Summary box 61.15

Causes of retroperitoneal fibrosis

Benign
- Idiopathic (Ormond's disease)
- Chronic inflammation
- Extravasation of urine
- Retroperitoneal irritation by leakage of blood or intestinal content
- Aortic aneurysm (inflammatory type)
- Trauma
- Drugs (chemotherapeutic agents and previously methysergide)

Malignant
- Lymphoma
- Carcinoid tumours
- Secondary deposits (especially from carcinoma of stomach, colon, breast and prostate)

The clinical presentation may be one of ill-defined chronic backache or may occur as a result of compromise to involved structures, e.g. lower limb or scrotal oedema secondary to venous occlusion, or chronic renal failure secondary to ureteric obstruction. Treatment will be directed to the cause, to the modification of disease activity when appropriate, e.g. immune suppression with steroids and restoration of flow in affected structures, e.g. ureteric stenting.

Retroperitoneal (psoas) abscess

The retroperitoneal space can also be a site for abscess formation which for practical purposes is almost synonymous with psoas abscess. Psoas abscess is a relatively uncommon diagnosis whose true incidence is not well described. At the beginning of the twentieth century, psoas abscess was mainly caused by tuberculosis of the spine (Pott's disease). With the decline of *Mycobacterium tuberculosis* as a major pathogen in developed countries a psoas abscess was mostly found secondary to direct spread of infection from the inflamed ± perforated digestive or urinary tract. In recent years, a primary psoas abscess due to haematogenous spread from an occult source is more common, especially in immunocompromised and older patients as well as in association with intravenous drug misuse.

Clinical presentation is with back pain, lassitude and fever. A swelling may point to the groin as it tracks along ileopsoas (see Chapter 73). Pain may be elicited by passive extension of the hip or a fixed flexion of the hip evident on inspection.

Radiological investigation is via CT scanning (Figure 61.15) and treatment usually by percutaneous CT-guided drainage and appropriate antibiotic therapy.

Retroperitoneal tumours

Although swellings in the retroperitoneum may include abscess, haematoma, cysts (see above) and spread of malignancy from retroperitoneal organs (kidney, ureter, adrenal), the term retroperitoneal tumour is usually confined to primary tumours arising in other tissues in this region, e.g. muscles, fat, lymph nodes and nerves. The management of such tumours is now frequently by referral to a specialist centre and this should be done before biopsy which may compromise subsequent surgical cure. The two most common are briefly described.

Retroperitoneal lipoma

The patient may seek advice on account of a swelling or because of indefinite abdominal pain. Women are more often affected. These swellings sometimes reach an immense size. Diagnosis is usually by ultrasound and CT scanning. A retroperitoneal lipoma sometimes undergoes myxomatous degeneration, a complication that does not occur in a lipoma in any other part of the body. Moreover, a retroperitoneal lipoma is often malignant (liposarcoma) (see below) and may increase rapidly in size.

Retroperitoneal sarcoma

Retroperitoneal sarcomas are rare tumours accounting for only 1–2 per cent of all solid malignancies (10–20 per cent of all sarcomas are retroperitoneal). The peak incidence is in the fifth decade of life, although they can occur at almost any age. The most common types of retroperitoneal soft tissue sarcomas in adults vary from study to study. However, in most studies, the most frequently encountered cell types are:

Baron Guillaume Dupuytren, 1777–1835, Surgeon in Chief, Hôtel Dieu, Paris, France, described this condition in 1831.
Francois de la Peyronie, 1678–1747, surgeon to King Louis XIV of France and founder of the Royal Academy of Surgery, Paris, France.
JK Ormond, an American urologist.

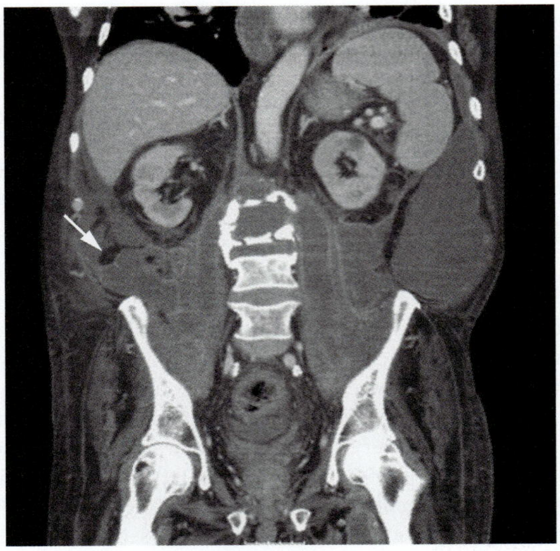

Figure 61.15 Representative sagittal computed tomography reconstruction of a right-sided psoas abscess (courtesy of Dr K Patel, Homerton University Foundation Trust, London, UK).

- liposarcoma;
- leiomyosarcoma;
- malignant fibrous histiocytoma (MFH).

Clinical features

Patients with sarcomas present late, because these tumours arise in the large potential spaces of the retroperitoneum and can grow very large without producing symptoms. Moreover, when symptoms do occur, they are non-specific, such as abdominal pain and fullness, and are easily dismissed as being caused by other less serious processes. Retroperitoneal sarcomas, therefore, are usually very large at the time of presentation.

Investigation

Detailed multiplanar imaging (CT + magentic resonance imaging) with reconstructions are required not only for tumour detection, staging and operative planning, but also for guiding percutaneous or surgical biopsy of these tumours. Such biopsies have a greater role than for other sarcomas.

Treatment

The definitive treatment of primary retroperitoneal sarcomas is surgical resection. Chemotherapy and radiotherapy without surgical debulking have rarely been beneficial, when used alone or in combination A multidisciplinary team approach with imaging review will be required when assessing operability (based on adjacency or involvement of vital structures) and approach. Up to 75 per cent of retroperitoneal sarcoma resections involve resection of at least one adjoining intra-abdominal visceral organ (commonly large or small bowel or kidney). The most common types of vascular involvement precluding resection are involvement of the proximal superior mesenteric vessels or involvement of bilateral renal vessels.

Prognosis

In the vast majority of sarcomas, cell type has no impact on treatment and long-term survival. Survival rates are, in general, poor, even after complete resection, these being in the order of 35–50 per cent (excluding low grade liposarcomas, which may frequently be cured by resection).

FURTHER READING

Burke AP, Sobin LH, Shekitka KM *et al.* Intra-abdominal fibromatosis. A pathologic analysis of 130 tumors with comparison of clinical subgroups. *Am J Surg Pathol* 1990; **14**: 335–41.

Mendenhall WM, Zlotecki RA, Hochwald SN *et al.* Retroperitoneal soft tissue sarcoma. *Cancer* 2005; **104**: 669–75.

Rasheed S, Zinicola R, Watson D *et al.* Intra-abdominal and gastrointestinal tuberculosis. *Colorectal Dis* 2007; **9**: 773–83.

Sadler TW. *Langman's medical embryology* (with CD-ROM), 11th edn. Baltimore, MD: Lippincott Williams and Wilkins, 2010.

Schnüriger B, Barmparas G, Branco BC *et al.* Prevention of postoperative peritoneal adhesions: a review of the literature. *Am J Surg* 2011; **201**: 111–21.

CHAPTER

62 The oesophagus

LEARNING OBJECTIVES

To understand:

- The anatomy and physiology of the oesophagus and their relationship to disease
- The clinical features, investigations and treatment of benign and malignant disease with particular reference to the common adult disorders

BACKGROUND

Surgical anatomy

The oesophagus is a muscular tube, approximately 25 cm long, mainly occupying the posterior mediastinum and extending from the upper oesophageal sphincter (the cricopharyngeus muscle) in the neck to the junction with the cardia of the stomach. The musculature of the upper oesophagus, including the upper sphincter, is striated. This is followed by a transitional zone of both striated and smooth muscle with the proportion of the latter progressively increasing so that, in the lower half of the oesophagus, there is only smooth muscle. It is lined throughout with squamous epithelium. The parasympathetic nerve supply is mediated by branches of the vagus nerve that has synaptic connections to the myenteric (Auerbach's) plexus. Meissner's submucosal plexus is sparse in the oesophagus.

The upper sphincter consists of powerful striated muscle. The lower sphincter is more subtle, and is created by the asymmetrical arrangement of muscle fibres in the distal oesophageal wall just above the oesophagogastric junction. It is helpful to remember the distances 15, 25 and 40 cm for anatomical location during endoscopy (Figure 62.1).

Physiology

The main function of the oesophagus is to transfer food from the mouth to the stomach in a coordinated fashion. The initial movement from the mouth is voluntary. The pharyngeal phase of swallowing involves sequential contraction of the oropharyngeal musculature, closure of the nasal and respiratory passages, cessation of breathing and opening of the upper oesophageal sphincter. Beyond this level, swallowing is involuntary. The body of the oesophagus propels the bolus through a relaxed lower oesophageal sphincter (LOS) into the stomach, taking air with it (Figure 62.2). This coordinated oesophageal wave that follows a conscious swallow is called primary peristalsis. It is under vagal control, although there are specific neurotransmitters that control the LOS.

The upper oesophageal sphincter is normally closed at rest and serves as a protective mechanism against regurgitation of oesophageal contents into the respiratory passages. It also serves to stop air entering the oesophagus other than the small amount that enters during swallowing.

The LOS is a zone of relatively high pressure that prevents gastric contents from refluxing into the lower oesophagus (Figure 62.3). In addition to opening in response to a primary peristaltic wave, the sphincter also relaxes to allow air to escape from the stomach and at the time of vomiting. A variety of factors influence sphincter tone, notably food, gastric distension, gastrointestinal hormones, drugs and smoking. The arrangement of muscle fibres, their differential responses to specific neurotransmitters and the relationship to diaphragmatic contraction all contribute to the action of the LOS. The presence of the physiological sphincter was first demonstrated by Code using manometry with small balloons. Nowadays, LOS pressure is measured by perfused tubes or microtransducers. The normal LOS is 3–4 cm long

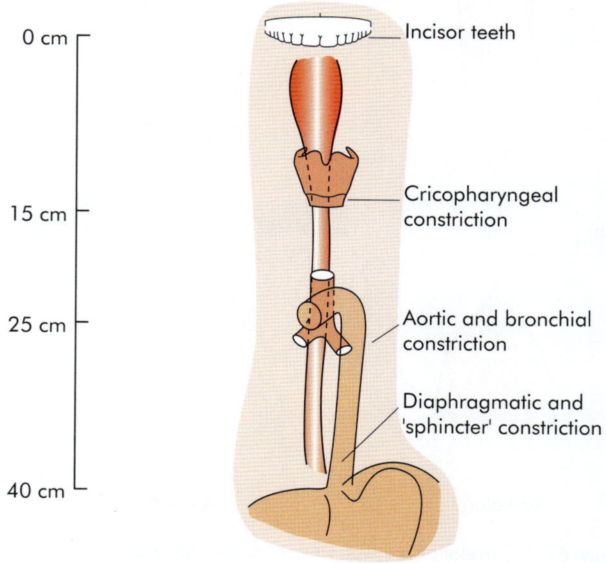

Figure 62.1 Endoscopic landmarks. Distances are given from the incisor teeth. They vary slightly with the build of the individual.

Leopold Auerbach, 1828–1897, Professor of Neuropathology, Breslau, Germany (now Wroclaw, Poland), described the myenteric plexus in 1862.
George Meissner, 1829–1905, Professor of Physiology, Göttingen, Germany, described the submucosal plexus in 1852.

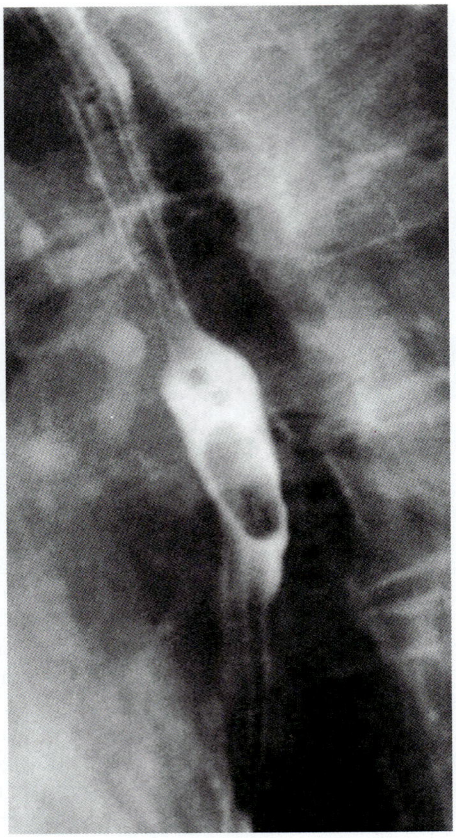

Figure 62.2 A bolus of barium or food usually takes air with it into the stomach.

and has a pressure of 10–25 mmHg. Accurate measurement of sphincter relaxation is achieved using a device (Dent sleeve) that straddles the high-pressure zone.

Manometry is also used to assess the speed and amplitude of oesophageal body contractions and ensure that peristalsis is propagated down the entire length of the oesophagus (Figure 62.4). Secondary peristalsis is the normal reflex response to a stubborn food bolus or refluxed material designed to clear the oesophagus by a contraction that is not preceded by a conscious swallow. It is worth remembering that the majority of clearance swallows to neutralise refluxed gastric acid are, however, achieved by primary peristalsis, which carries saliva with its high bicarbonate content down to the lower oesophagus. Tertiary contractions are non-peristaltic waves that are infrequent (<10 per cent) during laboratory-based manometry, although readily detected if manometry is undertaken while the patient eats a meal (Figure 62.5).

Symptoms

Dysphagia

Dysphagia is used to describe difficulty with swallowing. When there is a problem with swallowing in the voluntary (oral or pharyngeal) phases, patients will usually say that they cannot swallow properly, but they do not characteristically describe 'food sticking'. Instead, when they try to initiate a conscious swallow, food fails to enter the oesophagus, stays in the mouth or enters the airway causing coughing or spluttering. Virtually all causes of this type of dysphagia are chronic neurological or muscular diseases. Oesophageal dysphagia occurs in the involuntary phase and is characterised by a sensation of food sticking. The nature of this type of dysphagia is often informative regarding a likely diagnosis. Dysphagia may occur acutely or in a chronic fashion, can affect solids and/or fluids and be intermittent or progressive. While many patients point to a site of impaction, this is unreliable.

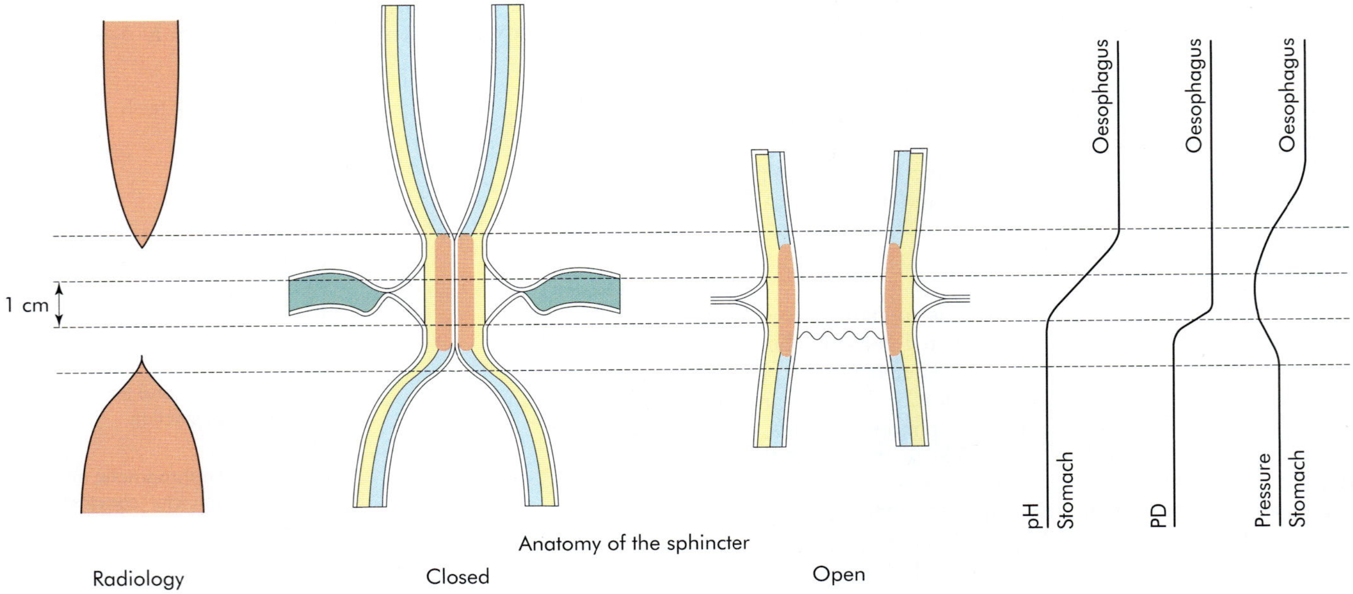

Figure 62.3 Correlation between the radiological appearances of a barium column and the lower oesophageal sphincter open and closed. The three curves on the right, set up vertically, show the pH gradient, the mucosal potential difference (PD) marking the junction of squamous and columnar epithelium and the high-pressure zone of the sphincter.

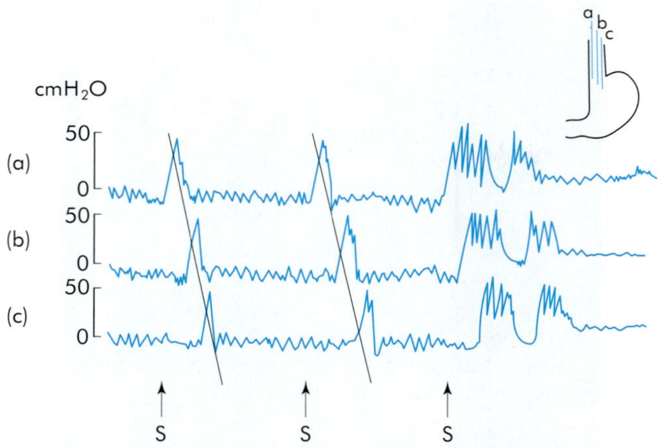

Figure 62.4 Manometric recording from the body of a normal oesophagus. Peristalsis is seen in the first and last panels, but other waves are simultaneous. Non-peristaltic simultaneous contractions are called 'tertiary contractions'.

Odynophagia

Odynophagia refers to pain on swallowing. Patients with reflux oesophagitis often feel retrosternal discomfort within a few seconds of swallowing hot beverages, citrus drinks or alcohol. Odynophagia is also a feature of infective oesophagitis and may be particularly severe in chemical injury.

Regurgitation and reflux

Regurgitation and reflux are often used synonymously. It is helpful to differentiate between them, although it is not always possible. Regurgitation should strictly refer to the return of oesophageal contents from above a functional or mechanical obstruction. Reflux is the passive return of gastroduodenal contents to the mouth as part of the symptomatology of gastro-oesophageal reflux disease (GORD). Loss of weight, anaemia, cachexia, change of voice due to refluxed material irritating the vocal cords and cough or dyspnoea due to tracheal aspiration may all accompany regurgitation and/or reflux.

Chest pain

Chest pain similar in character to angina pectoris may arise from an oesophageal cause, especially gastro-oesophageal reflux and motility disorders. Exercise-induced chest pain can be due to reflux (Summary box 62.1).

Summary box 62.1

Symptoms of oesophageal disease

- Difficulty in swallowing described as food or fluid sticking (oesophageal dysphagia) must rule out malignancy
- Pain on swallowing (odynophagia) suggests inflammation and ulceration
- Regurgitation or reflux (heartburn) common in gastro-oesophageal reflux disease
- Chest pain is difficult to distinguish from cardiac pain

Investigations

Radiography

Contrast radiography has been somewhat overshadowed by endoscopy but remains a useful investigation for demonstrating narrowing, space-occupying lesions, anatomical distortion or abnormal motility. An adequate barium swallow should be tailored to the problem under investigation. It may be helpful to give a solid bolus (bread or marshmallow) if a motility disorder is suspected. Video recording is useful to allow subsequent replay and detailed analysis. Barium radiology is, however, inaccurate in the diagnosis of gastro-oesophageal reflux, unless reflux is gross, and should not be used for this purpose. Plain radiographs will show some foreign bodies.

Cross-sectional imaging by computed tomography (CT) scanning is now an essential investigation in the assessment of neoplasms of the oesophagus and can be used in place of a contrast swallow to demonstrate perforation. The role of CT and other cancer-specific tests is described later.

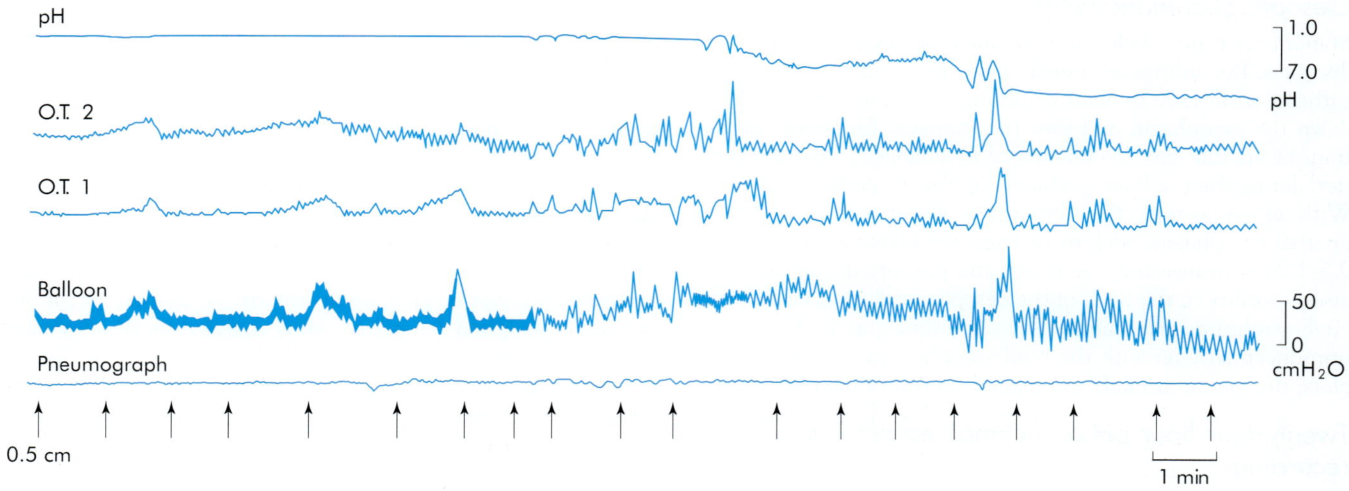

Figure 62.5 Triple water-perfused tube study of normal lower oesophagus and lower oesophageal sphincter. Note that the swallowing contractions (S) in the body of the oesophagus are sequential, i.e. peristaltic.

Endoscopy

Endoscopy is necessary for the investigation of most oesophageal conditions. It is required to view the inside of the oesophagus and the oesophagogastric junction, to obtain a biopsy or cytology specimen, for the removal of foreign bodies and to dilate strictures. Traditionally, there are two types of instrument available, the rigid oesophagoscope and the flexible video endoscope, but the rigid instrument is now virtually obsolete.

For flexible video gastroduodenoscope, general anaesthesia is not required; most examinations can be done on an outpatient basis, and the quality of the magnified image is superb. The technology associated with video endoscopy continues to improve. Novel techniques that rely on fluorescence and narrow band imaging to enhance visual contrast are becoming increasingly used for the identification of mucosal abnormalities that are not easily seen with white light, for instance in patients with Barrett's oesophagus undergoing endoscopic surveillance.

As a matter of routine, the stomach and duodenum are examined as well as the oesophagus. If a stricture is encountered, it may be helpful to dilate it to allow a complete inspection of the upper gastrointestinal tract, but this decision should be dictated by clinical circumstances and an appreciation of the perforation risk.

Endosonography

Endoscopic ultrasonography relies on a high-frequency (5–30 MHz) transducer located at the tip of the endoscope to provide highly detailed images of the layers of the oesophageal wall and mediastinal structures close to the oesophagus. Radial echoendoscopes have a rotating transducer that creates a circular image with the endoscope in the centre, and this type of scanner is widely used to create diagnostic transverse sectional images at right angles to the long axis of the oesophagus (Figure 62.6). Linear echoendoscopes produce a sectoral image in the line of the endoscope and are used to biopsy submucosal oesophageal lesions or mediastinal masses such as lymph nodes (Figure 62.7). Radial scanners without optical components are available for passage through narrow strictures over a guidewire, and there are even catheter probes that can be passed down the endoscope biopsy channel.

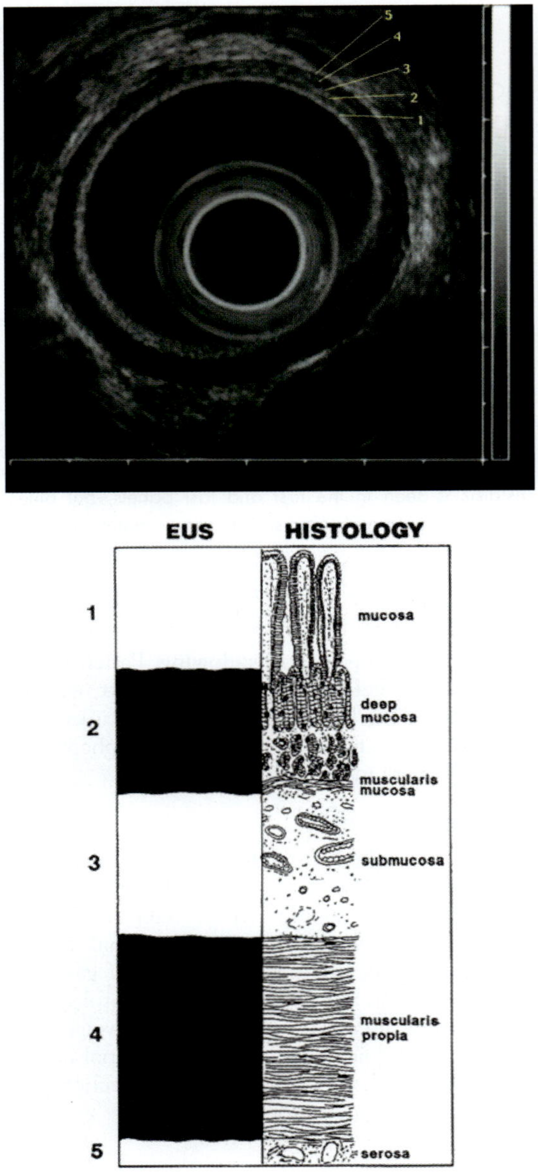

Figure 62.6 Radial endosonography indicating wall layers as alternating hyper- and hypoechoic bands.

Oesophageal manometry

Manometry is now widely used to diagnose oesophageal motility disorders. Recordings are usually made by passing a multilumen catheter with three to eight recording orifices at different levels down the oesophagus and into the stomach. Electronic microtransducers that are not influenced by changes in patient position during the test have gradually supplanted perfusion systems. With either system, the catheter is withdrawn progressively up the oesophagus, and recordings are taken at intervals of 0.5–1.0 cm to measure the length and pressure of the LOS and assess motility in the body of the oesophagus during swallowing. High-resolution manometry uses a multiple (up to 30) microtransducer catheter with the results displayed as spaciotemporal plots; this system is likely to supplant conventional manometry.

Twenty-four hour pH and combined pH-impedance recording

Prolonged measurement of pH is now accepted as the most accurate method for the diagnosis of gastro-oesophageal reflux. It is particularly useful in patients with atypical reflux symptoms, those without endoscopic oesophagitis and when patients respond poorly to intensive medical therapy. A small pH probe is passed into the distal oesophagus and positioned 5 cm above the upper margin of the LOS, as defined by manometry. The probe is connected to a miniature digital recorder that is worn on a belt and allows most normal activities. Patients mark symptomatic events such as heartburn. A 24-hour recording period is usual, and the pH record is analysed by an automated computer program. An oesophageal pH < 4 at the level of the pH electrode is conventionally considered the cut-off value and, in most oesophageal laboratories, the total time when pH is < 4 in a 24-hour period does not exceed 4 per cent in a healthy adult. Patterns of reflux and the correlation between symptoms and oesophageal pH < 4 can be calculated. Most laboratories use a scoring system (Johnson–DeMeester) to create a numerical value, above which reflux is considered pathological.

aspiration pneumonitis may allow the problem to be recognised at a time when intervention may be appropriate and feasible. Covering the communication with a self-expanding metal stent is the usual solution. Erosion into a major vascular structure is invariably fatal.

Penetrating injury

Perforation by knives and bullets is uncommon, even in war, as the oesophagus is a relatively small target surrounded by other vital organs.

Foreign bodies

The oesophagus may be perforated during removal of a foreign body but, occasionally, an object that has been left in the oesophagus for several days will erode through the wall.

Instrumental perforation

Instrumentation is by far the most common cause of perforation. Modern instrumentation is remarkably safe, but perforation remains a risk that should never be forgotten (Summary box 62.4).

Summary box 62.4

Instrumental perforation

- Prevention of perforation is better than cure

Perforation related to diagnostic upper gastrointestinal endoscopy is unusual with an estimated frequency of about 1:4000 examinations. Perforation can occur in the pharynx or oesophagus, usually at sites of pathology or when the endoscope is passed blindly. A number of patient-related factors are associated with increased risk, including large anterior cervical osteophytes, the presence of a pharyngeal pouch and mechanical causes of obstruction. Perforation may follow biopsy of a malignant tumour.

Patients undergoing therapeutic endoscopy have a perforation risk that is at least ten times greater than those undergoing diagnostic endoscopy. The oesophagus may be perforated by guidewires, graduated dilators or balloons, or during the placement of self-expanding stents. The risk is considerably higher in patients with malignancy.

Diagnosis of instrumental perforation

In most cases, a combination of technical difficulties and an interventional procedure should lead to a high index of suspicion. History and physical signs may be useful pointers to the site of perforation.

Cervical perforation may result in pain localised to the neck, hoarseness, painful neck movements and subcutaneous emphysema. Intrathoracic and intra-abdominal perforations, which are more common, can give rise to immediate symptoms and signs either during or at the end of the procedure, including chest pain, haemodynamic instability, oxygen desaturation or visual evidence of perforation. Within the first 24 hours, patients may additionally complain of abdominal pain or respiratory difficulties. There may be evidence of subcutaneous emphysema, pneumothorax or hydropneumothorax. In some patients, the diagnosis may be missed and recognised only at a late stage beyond 24 hours, as unexplained pyrexia, systemic sepsis or the development of a clinical fistula.

Prompt and thorough investigation is the key to management. Careful endoscopic assessment at the end of any procedure combined with a chest x-ray will identify many cases of perforation immediately. If not recognised immediately, then early and late suspected perforations should be assessed by a water-soluble contrast swallow. If this is negative, a dilute barium swallow should be considered. A CT scan can be used to replace a contrast swallow or as an adjunct to accurately delineate specific fluid collections.

Treatment of oesophageal perforations

Perforation of the oesophagus usually leads to mediastinitis. The loose areolar tissues of the posterior mediastinum allow a rapid spread of gastrointestinal contents. The aim of treatment is to limit mediastinal contamination and prevent or deal with infection. Operative repair deals with the injury directly, but imposes risks of its own; non-operative treatment aims to limit the effects of mediastinitis and provide an environment in which healing can take place.

The decision between operative and non-operative management rests on four factors. These are:

1. the site of the perforation (cervical versus thoracoabdominal oesophagus);
2. the event causing the perforation (spontaneous versus instrumental);
3. underlying pathology (benign or malignant);
4. the status of the oesophagus before the perforation (fasted and empty versus obstructed with a stagnant residue).

It follows that most perforations that can be managed non-operatively occur in the context of small instrumental perforations of a clean oesophagus without obstruction, where leakage is likely to be confined to the nearby mediastinum at worst (Table 62.1).

Table 62.1 Management options in perforation of the oesophagus.

Factors that favour non-operative management	Factors that favour operative repair
Small septic load	Large septic load
Minimal cardiovascular upset	Septic shock
Perforation confined to mediastinum	Pleura breached
Perforation by flexible endoscope	Boerhaave's syndrome
Perforation of cervical oesophagus	Perforation of abdominal oesophagus

Instrumental perforations in the cervical oesophagus are usually small and can nearly always be managed conservatively. The development of a local abscess is an indication for cervical drainage preventing the extension of sepsis into the mediastinum.

The conservative management of an instrumental perforation in the thoracoabdominal parts of the oesophagus can be undertaken when the perforation is detected early and prior to oral alimentation. General guidelines for non-operative management include:

- pain that is readily controlled with opiates;
- absence of crepitus, diffuse mediastinal gas, hydropneumothorax or pneumoperitoneum;
- mediastinal containment of the perforation with no evidence of widespread extravasation of contrast material;
- no evidence of ongoing luminal obstruction or a retained foreign body.

In addition, conservative management might be appropriate in patients who have remained clinically stable despite diagnostic delay. The principles of non-interventional management involve hyperalimentation, preferably by an enteral route, nasogastric suction and broad-spectrum intravenous antibiotics.

Surgical management is required whenever patients:

- are unstable with sepsis or shock;
- have evidence of a heavily contaminated mediastinum, pleural space or peritoneum;
- have widespread intrapleural or intraperitoneal extravasation of contrast material.

Ongoing luminal obstruction (often related to malignancy) in a frail patient considered unfit for major surgery can be dealt with by placement of a covered self-expanding stent. Expanding metal stents should be used with caution in patients with benign disease as they cause significant tissue reaction and some designs are impossible to remove at a later date. Biodegradable and removable stents are being developed and may be used alone or as a bridge to later definitive treatment where perforation accompanies obstruction.

For patients requiring surgery, the choice rests between direct repair, the deliberate creation of an external fistula or, rarely, oesophageal resection with a view to delayed reconstruction. Direct repair is preferred by many surgeons if the perforation is recognised early (within the first 4–6 hours) and the extent of mediastinal and pleural contamination is small. After 12 hours, the tissues become swollen and friable and less suitable for direct suture. The hole in the mucosa is always bigger than the hole in the muscle, and the muscle should be incised to see the mucosal edges clearly. It is essential that there should be no obstruction distal to the repair. A variety of local tissues (gastric fundus, pericardium, intercostal muscle) have been used to buttress such repairs.

Primary repair is inadvisable with late presentation and in the presence of widespread mediastinal and pleural contamination. These patients tend to be more ill as a result of the delay, and the aim of treatment should be to achieve wide drainage with the creation of a controlled fistula and distal enteral feeding. This can usually be achieved by placing a T-tube into the oesophagus along with appropriately located drains and a feeding jejunostomy. In unusual circumstances, for instance with extensive necrosis following corrosive ingestion, emergency oesophagectomy may be necessary. Oesophagostomy and gastrostomy should be performed with a view to delayed reconstruction.

MALLORY–WEISS SYNDROME

Forceful vomiting may produce a mucosal tear at the cardia rather than a full perforation. The mechanism of injury is different. In Boerhaave's syndrome, vomiting occurs against a closed glottis, and pressure builds up in the oesophagus. In Mallory–Weiss syndrome, vigorous vomiting produces a vertical split in the gastric mucosa, immediately below the squamocolumnar junction at the cardia in 90 per cent of cases. In only 10 per cent is the tear in the oesophagus (Figure 62.11). The condition presents with haematemesis. Usually, the bleeding is not severe, but endoscopic injection therapy may be required for the occasional, severe case. Surgery is rarely required. There are two other injuries to the oesophagus that lie within the spectrum of the mucosal tear of Mallory–Weiss and the full-thickness tear of Boerhaave. Intramural rupture produces a dissection within the oesophageal wall that causes severe chest pain, often with odynophagia. It is best diagnosed by contrast radiology. Intramural haematoma is seen most often in elderly patients on anticoagulants or patients with coagulation disorders, and usually follows an episode of vomiting. Large haematomas causing dysphagia can occur extending from the cardia up to the carina. The diagnosis is readily made on endoscopy. Both intramural rupture and intramural haematoma can be managed conservatively. Symptoms usually resolve in 7–14 days, and oral intake can be reinstituted as soon as symptoms allow.

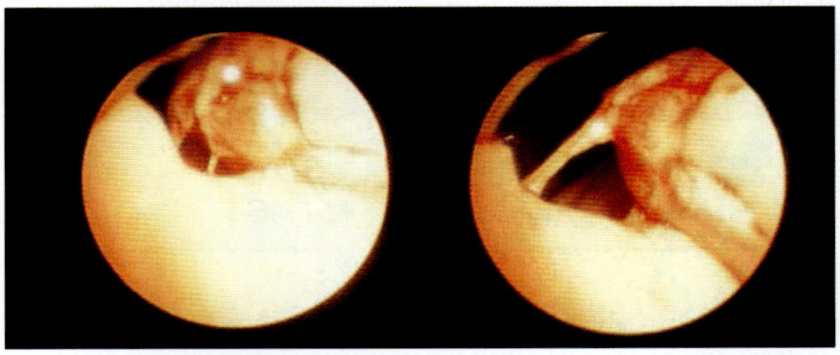

Figure 62.11 The endoscopic appearance of a mucosal tear at the cardia (Mallory–Weiss).

CORROSIVE INJURY

Corrosives such as sodium hydroxide (lye, caustic soda) or sulphuric acid may be taken in attempted suicide. Accidental ingestion occurs in children and when corrosives are stored in bottles labelled as beverages. All can cause severe damage to the mouth, pharynx, larynx, oesophagus and stomach. The type of agent, its concentration and the volume ingested largely determine the extent of damage. In general, alkalis are relatively odourless and tasteless, making them more likely to be ingested in large volume. Alkalis cause liquefaction, saponification of fats, dehydration and thrombosis of blood vessels that usually leads to fibrous scarring. Acids cause coagulative necrosis with eschar formation, and this coagulant may limit penetration to deeper layers of the oesophageal wall. Acids also cause more gastric damage than alkalis because of the induction of intense pylorospasm with pooling in the antrum.

Symptoms and signs are notoriously unreliable in predicting the severity of injury. The key to management is early endoscopy by an experienced endoscopist to inspect the whole of the oesophagus and stomach (Figure 62.12). Deep ulcers and the recognition of a grey or black eschar signify the most severe lesions with the greatest risk of perforation. Minor injuries with only oedema of the mucosa resolve rapidly with no late sequelae. These patients can safely be fed. With more severe injuries, a feeding jejunostomy may be appropriate until the patient

George Kenneth Mallory, born 1926, Professor of Pathology, Boston University, Boston, MA, USA.
Soma Weiss, 1898–1942, Professor of Medicine, Harvard University Medical School, Boston, MA, USA.

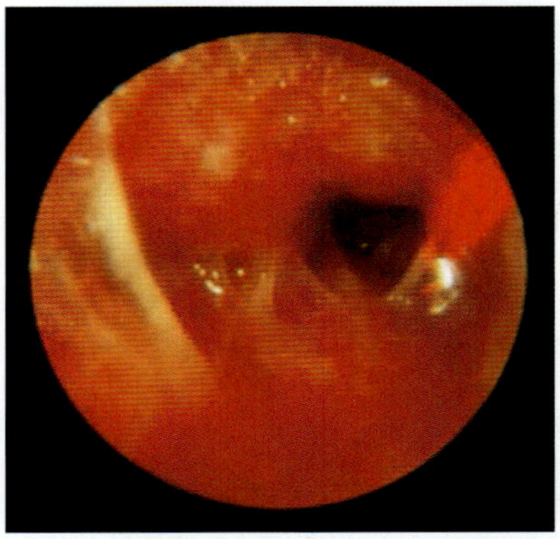

Figure 62.12 Acute caustic burn in the haemorrhagic phase.

can swallow saliva satisfactorily. The widespread use of broad-spectrum antibiotics and steroids is not supported by evidence.

Regular endoscopic examinations are the best way to assess stricture development (Figure 62.13). Significant stricture formation occurs in about 50 per cent of patients with extensive mucosal damage (Figure 62.14). The role and timing of repeat endoscopies with or without dilatation in such patients remains controversial. Other than the need for emergency surgery for bleeding or perforation, elective oesophageal resection should be deferred for at least three months until the fibrotic phase is established. Oesophageal replacement is usually required for very long or multiple strictures. Resection can be difficult because of perioesophageal inflammation in these patients. Because of associated gastric damage, colon may have to be used as the replacement conduit.

There is also controversy regarding the risk of developing carcinoma in the damaged oesophagus and stomach and how this might influence management. The lifetime risk is certainly less than 5 per cent. Some surgeons advocate resection and replacement, while others believe that oesophageal bypass and endoscopic surveillance is preferable, as removal of the badly damaged oesophagus from a scarred mediastinum can be hazardous (Summary box 62.5).

Summary box 62.5

Corrosive injury

- Skilled early endoscopy is mandatory

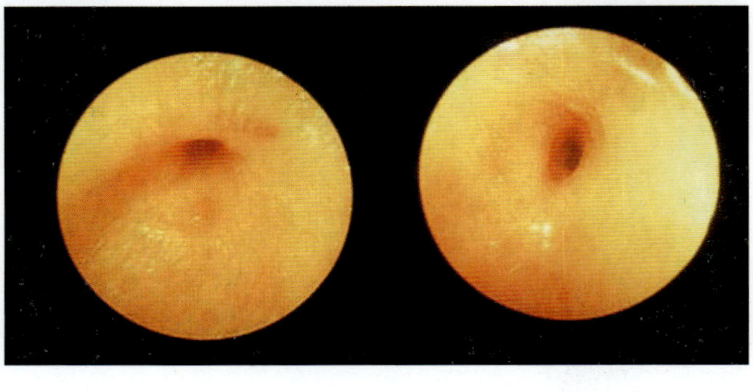

Figure 62.13 The late result of a caustic alkali burn with a high oesophageal stricture.

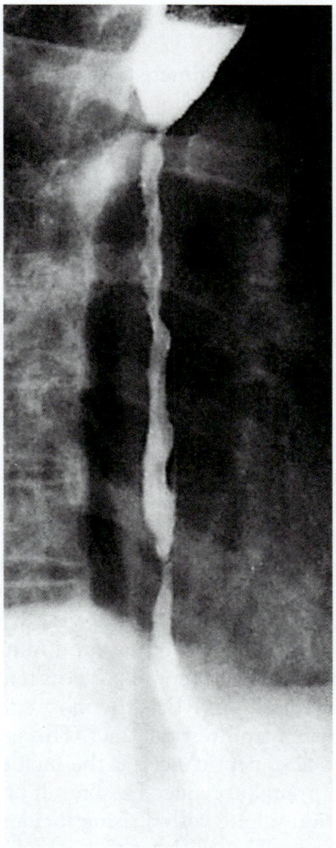

Figure 62.14 Caustic or lye stricture with marked stenosis high in the body of the oesophagus. The strictures are frequently multiple and difficult to dilate unless treated energetically at an early stage.

DRUG-INDUCED INJURY

Many medications, such as antibiotics and potassium preparations, are potentially damaging to the oesophagus, as tablets may remain for a long time, especially if taken without an adequate drink. Acute injury presents with dysphagia and odynophagia, which may be severe. The inflammation usually resolves within 2–3 weeks, and no specific treatment is required apart from appropriate nutritional support. A stricture may follow.

GASTRO-OESOPHAGEAL REFLUX DISEASE

Aetiology

Normal competence of the gastro-oesophageal junction is maintained by the LOS. This is influenced by both its physiological function and its anatomical location relative to the diaphragm and the oesophageal hiatus. In normal circumstances, the LOS transiently relaxes as a coordinated part of swallowing, as a means of allowing vomiting to occur and in response to stretching of the gastric fundus, particularly after a meal to allow swallowed air to be vented. Most episodes of physiological reflux occur during postprandial transient lower oesophageal sphincter relaxations (TLOSRs). In the early stages of GORD, most pathological reflux occurs as a result of an increased number of

TLOSRs rather than a persistent fall in overall sphincter pressure. In more severe GORD, LOS pressure tends to be generally low, and this loss of sphincter function seems to be made worse if there is loss of an adequate length of intra-abdominal oesophagus.

The absence of an intra-abdominal length of oesophagus results in a sliding hiatus hernia. The normal condensation of peritoneal fascia over the lower oesophagus (the phreno-oesophageal ligament) is weak, and the crural opening widens allowing the upper stomach to slide up through the hiatus. The loss of the normal anatomical configuration exacerbates reflux, although sliding hiatus hernia alone should not be viewed as the cause of reflux. Sliding hiatus hernia is associated with GORD and may make it worse but, as long as the LOS remains competent, pathological GORD does not occur. Many GORD sufferers do not have a hernia, and many of those with a hernia do not have GORD. It should be noted that rolling or paraoesophageal hiatus hernia is a quite different and potentially dangerous condition (see under Paraoesophageal ('rolling') hiatus hernia below). A proportion of patients have a rolling hernia and symptomatic GORD or a mixed hernia with both sliding and rolling components. Reflux oesophagitis that is visible endoscopically is a complication of GORD and occurs in a minority of sufferers overall, but in around 40 per cent of patients referred to hospital.

In Western societies, GORD is the most common condition affecting the upper gastrointestinal tract. This is partly due to the declining incidence of peptic ulcer as the incidence of infection with *Helicobacter pylori* has reduced as a result of improved socioeconomic conditions along with a rising incidence of GORD in the last 20–30 years. The cause of the increase is unclear, but may be due in part to increasing obesity. The strong association between GORD, obesity and the parallel rise in the incidence of adenocarcinoma of the oesophagus represents a major health challenge for most Western countries.

Clinical features

The classical triad of symptoms is retrosternal burning pain (heartburn), epigastric pain (sometimes radiating through to the back) and regurgitation. Most patients do not experience all three. Symptoms are often provoked by food, particularly those that delay gastric emptying (e.g. fats, spicy foods). As the condition becomes more severe, gastric juice may reflux to the mouth and produce an unpleasant taste often described as 'acid' or 'bitter'. Heartburn and regurgitation can be brought on by stooping or exercise. A proportion of patients have odynophagia with hot beverages, citrus drinks or alcohol. Patients with nocturnal reflux and those who reflux food to the mouth nearly always have severe GORD. Some patients present with less typical symptoms such as angina-like chest pain, pulmonary or laryngeal symptoms. Dysphagia is usually a sign that a stricture has occurred, but may be caused by an associated motility disorder.

Because GORD is such a common disorder, it should always be the first thought when a patient presents with oesophageal symptoms that are unusual or that defy diagnosis after a series of investigations.

Diagnosis

In most cases, the diagnosis is assumed rather than proven, and treatment is empirical. Investigation is only required when the diagnosis is in doubt, when the patient does not respond to a proton pump inhibitor (PPI) or if dysphagia is present. The most appropriate examination is endoscopy with biopsy. If the typical appearance of reflux oesophagitis, peptic stricture or Barrett's oesophagus is seen, the diagnosis is clinched, but visible oesophagitis is not always present, even in patients selected as above. This is compounded in clinical practice by the widespread use of PPIs, which cause rapid healing of early mucosal lesions. Many patients will have received such treatment before referral. The endoscopic appearances of the normal oesophagus, hiatus hernia, oesophagitis and stricture are shown in Figures 62.15, 62.16, 62.17, 62.18, 62.19, 62.20 and 62.21. It is worth remembering that the correlation between symptoms and endoscopic appearances is poor. On the other hand, there is a strong correlation between worsening endoscopic appearances and the duration of oesophageal acidification on pH testing.

In patients with atypical or persistent symptoms despite therapy, oesophageal manometry and 24-hour oesophageal pH recording (ideally with impedance measurement) may be justified to establish the diagnosis and guide management (Summary box 62.6).

Summary box 62.6

Diagnostic measurement in GORD

- 24-hour pH recording is the 'gold standard' for diagnosis of GORD
- TLOSRs are the most important manometric findings in GORD
- The length and pressure of the LOS are also important

As a matter of routine, PPIs are stopped 1 week before oesophageal pH recording, but acid secretion is sometimes reduced for 2 weeks or more, and this can necessitate repeat examination after a prolonged interval without a PPI. Manometry and pH recording are essential in patients being considered for antireflux surgery. While the main purpose of the test is objectively to quantify the extent of reflux disease, it is also used to rule out a diagnosis of achalasia. In the early stages of achalasia, chest pain can dominate the clinical picture and, when associated with

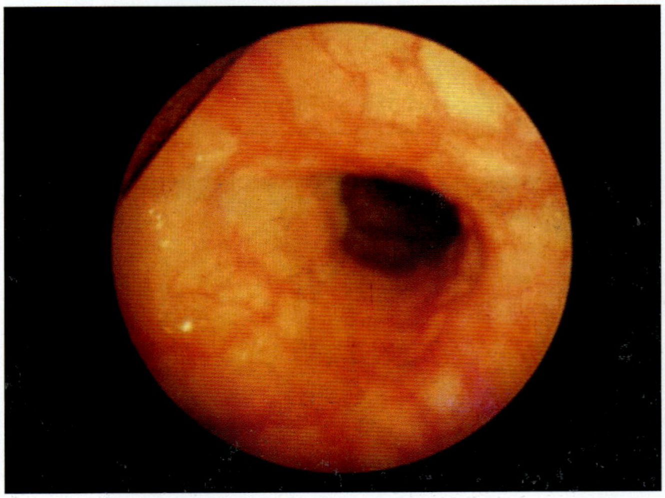

Figure 62.15 The endoscopic appearance of the normal squamous mucosa in the body of the oesophagus.

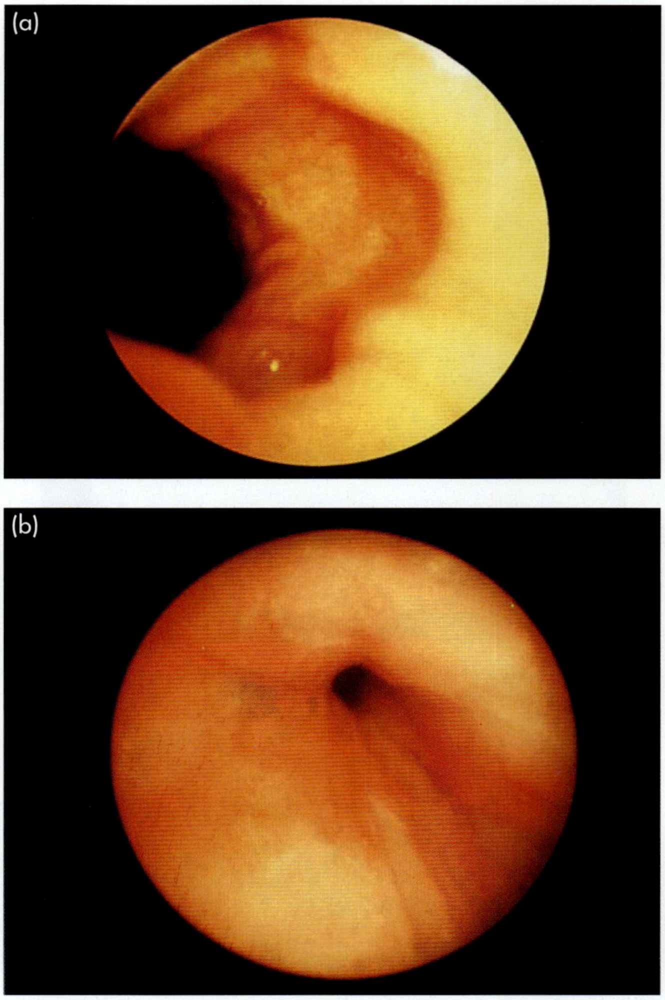

Figure 62.16 The normal lower oesophageal sphincter: (a) open; (b) closed.

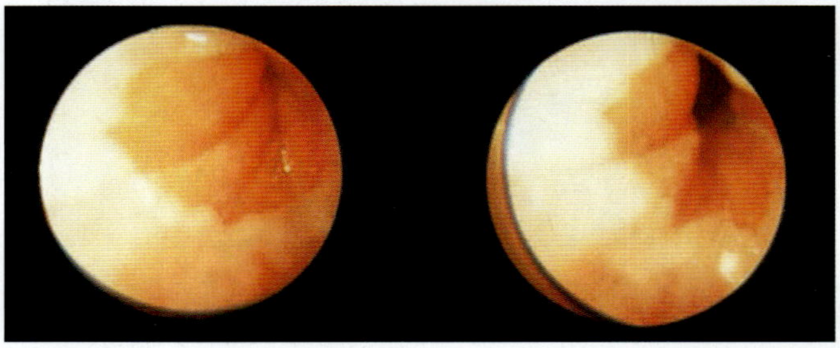

Figure 62.17 The squamocolumnar junction is clearly seen in the lower oesophagus with a normal sharp demarcation.

intermittent swallowing problems and non-specific symptoms, it is easy to see how a clinical diagnosis of GORD might be made. Patients with achalasia can also have an abnormal pH study as a result of fermentation of food residue in a dilated oesophagus. Usually, the form of the pH trace is different from that of GORD, with slow undulations of pH rather than rapid bursts of reflux, but the complete absence of peristalsis on manometry is pathognomonic of achalasia.

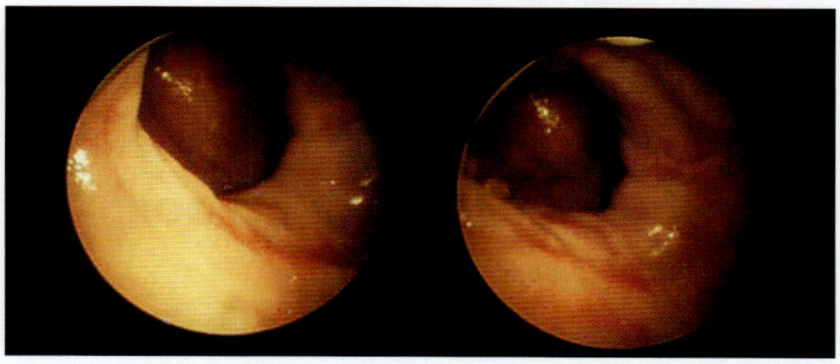

Figure 62.18 Sliding hiatus hernia. The diaphragm can be seen constricting the upper stomach.

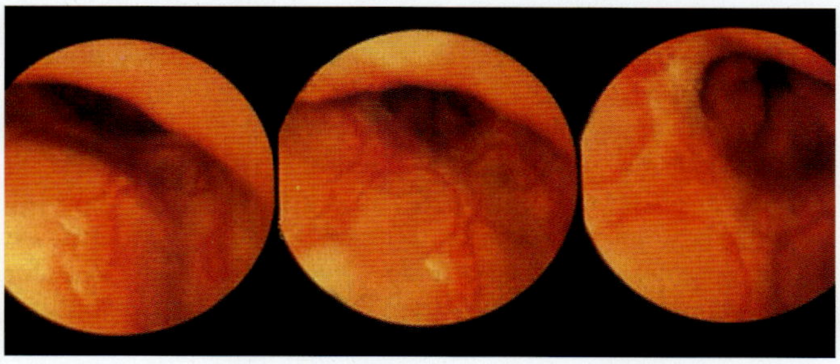

Figure 62.19 Reflux oesophagitis.

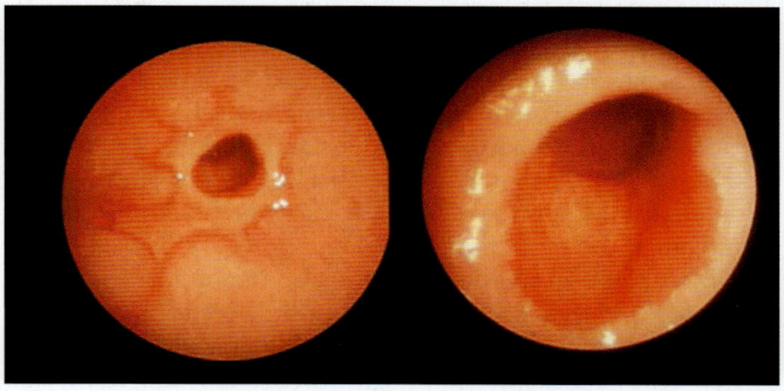

Figure 62.20 Benign stricture with active oesophagitis (left) and healed with columnar epithelium (right).

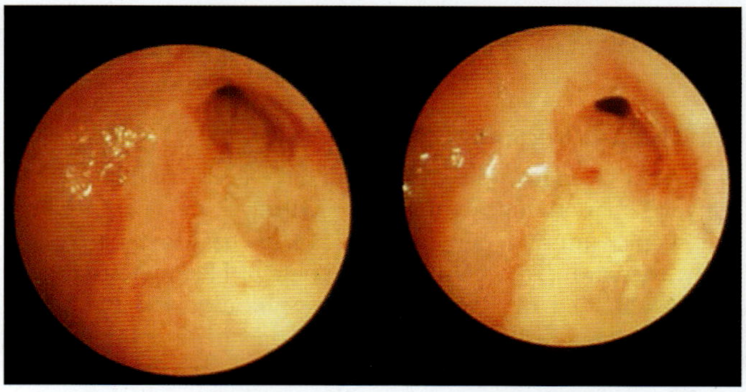

Figure 62.21 Ulceration associated with a benign peptic stricture.

Barium swallow and meal examination gives the best appreciation of gastro-oesophageal anatomy (Figure 62.22). This may be important in the context of surgery for rolling or mixed hiatus hernias, but it is unimportant in most patients with GORD.

Management of uncomplicated GORD

Medical management

Most sufferers from GORD do not consult a doctor and do not need to do so. They self-medicate with over-the-counter medicines such as simple antacids, antacid–alginate preparations and H2-receptor antagonists. Consultation is more likely when symptoms are severe, prolonged and unresponsive to the above treatments. Simple measures that are often neglected include advice about weight loss, smoking, excessive consumption of alcohol, tea or coffee, the avoidance of large meals late at night and a modest degree of head-up tilt of the bed. Tilting the bed has been shown to have an effect that is similar to taking an H2-receptor antagonist. The common practice of using additional pillows has no significant effect.

PPIs are the most effective drug treatment for GORD. Indeed, they are so effective that, once started, patients are very reluctant to stop taking them. Given an adequate dose for 8 weeks, most patients have a rapid improvement in symptoms (within a few days), and more than 90 per cent can expect full mucosal healing at the end of this time. For this reason, a policy of 'step-down' medical treatment is advocated based on the general advice outlined above and a standard dose of a PPI given for 8 weeks. At the end of that time, the dose of PPI is reduced to that which keeps the patient free of symptoms, and this might even mean the cessation of PPI treatment. Because most patients do not make major lifestyle changes and because PPIs are so effective, many remain on long-term treatment. For the minority who do not respond adequately to a standard dose, a trial at an increased dose or the addition of an H2-receptor antagonist is recommended. If unsuccessful, these patients should be formally investigated.

Proton pump inhibitor therapy is also important in patients with reflux-induced strictures, resulting in significant prolongation of the intervals between endoscopic dilatation. As yet, fears that chronic acid suppression might have serious long-term side effects including the risk of gastric cancer seem unwarranted.

Surgery

Strictly speaking, the need for surgery should have been reduced as medication has improved so much. Paradoxically, the number of antireflux operations has remained relatively constant and may even be increasing. This is probably due partly to increased patient expectations and partly to the advent of minimal access surgery, which has improved the acceptability of procedures.

Endoscopic treatments

A number of endoscopic treatments have been tried in the last ten years that attempt to augment a failing LOS. These involve endoscopic suturing devices that plicate gastric mucosa just below the cardia to accentuate the angle of His, radiofrequency ablation applied to the level of the sphincter and the injection of submucosal polymers into the lower oesophagus. The procedures have generally been applied to patients with only small hiatus hernias or none at all, so only a small proportion of patients who present to hospitals are suitable. While all methods produce some temporary improvement in symptoms and objective assessments of reflux, failure rates at one year are over 50 per cent, and there are no large case series that have reported long-term outcomes.

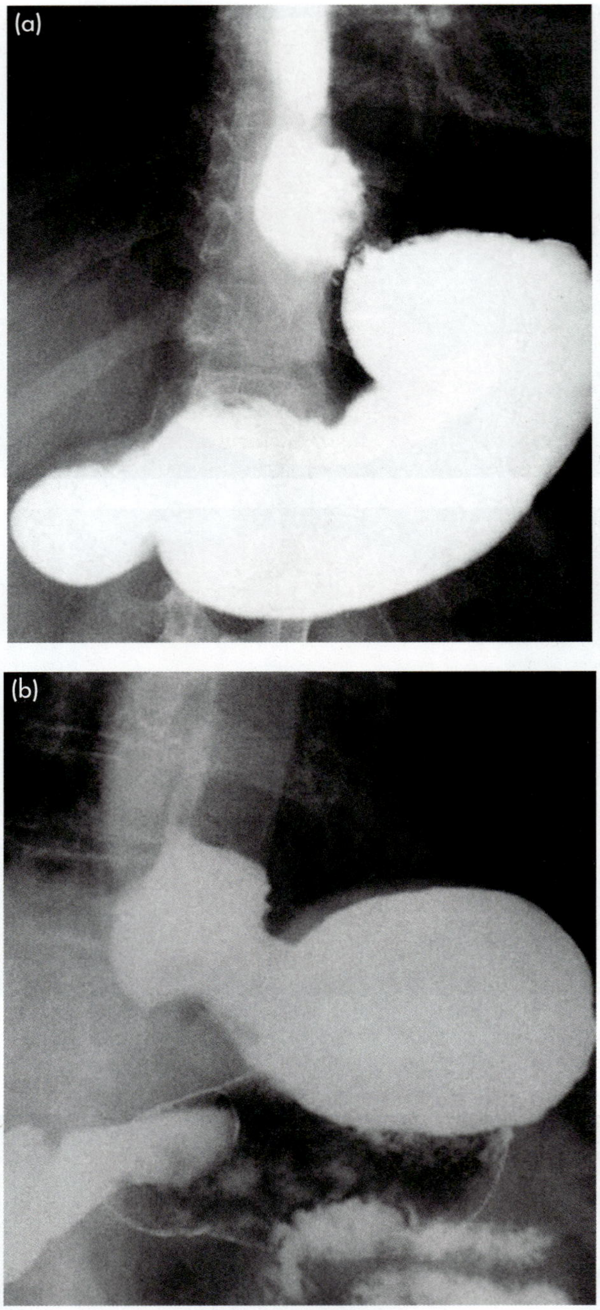

Figure 62.22 (a) Sliding hiatus hernia with a sphincter and diaphragmatic crural narrowing clearly shown. (b) Another sliding hernia in which the sphincter is lax, and the diaphragm is wide open. The patient is in the Trendelenburg position to demonstrate barium in the fundus. This unphysiological position may stimulate 'reflux' in those who do not have gastro-oesophageal reflux disease (GORD).

Surgical treatments

The indication for surgery in uncomplicated GORD is

essentially patient choice. The risks and possible benefits need to be discussed in detail. Risks include a small mortality rate (0.1–0.5 per cent, depending on patient selection), failed operation (5–10 per cent) and side effects such as dysphagia, gas bloat or abdominal discomfort (10 per cent). With current operative techniques, 85–90 per cent of patients should be satisfied with the result of an antireflux operation. Patients who are asymptomatic on a PPI need a careful discussion of the risk side of the equation. Those who are symptomatic on a PPI need a careful clinical review to make sure that they will benefit from an operation. Reasons for failure on a PPI include 'volume' reflux (a good indication for surgery), a 'hermit' lifestyle in which the least deviation from lifestyle rules leads to symptoms (a good indication), psychological distress with intolerance of minor symptoms (a poor indication; these patients are likely to be dissatisfied with surgery), poor compliance (a good indication if the reason for poor compliance is the side effects of treatment, otherwise a bad indication) and misdiagnosis of GORD.

Which operation?

There are many operations for GORD, but they are virtually all based on the creation of an intra-abdominal segment of oesophagus, crural repair and some form of wrap of the upper stomach (fundoplication) around the intra-abdominal oesophagus. The contribution of each component to operative success is widely debated, but it is clear that operations that fail to address all three components have inferior success rates. The major types of antireflux operation were all developed in the 1950s (Figure 62.23). When performed correctly, these are all effective operations. Randomised clinical trials do not show a clear advantage for any one operation over the others. One meta-analysis, however, has come down in favour of the Toupet posterior partial fundoplication over the Nissen total fundoplication when performed laparoscopically.

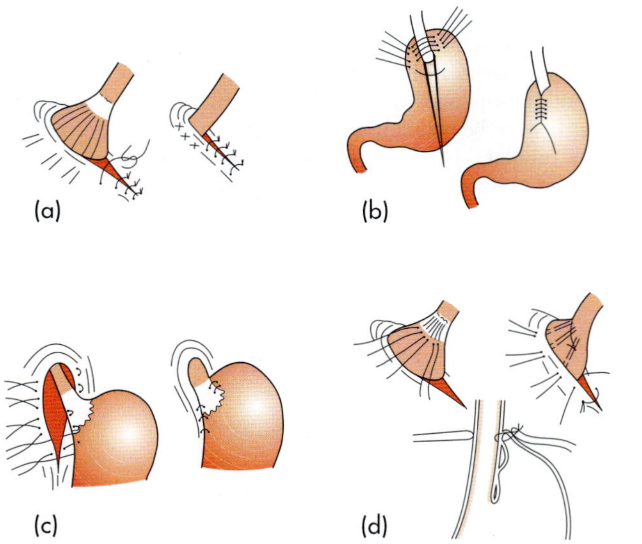

Figure 62.23 Various operations for the surgical correction of gastro-oesophageal reflux disease. (a) The original Allison repair of hiatus hernia (this is ineffective and is no longer done); (b) Nissen fundoplication; (c) Hill procedure; (d) Belsey mark IV operation.

Total fundoplication (Nissen) tends to be associated with slightly more short-term dysphagia but is the most durable repair in terms of long-term reflux control. Partial fundoplication, whether performed posteriorly (Toupet) or anteriorly (Dor, Watson), has fewer short-term side effects, although this is sometimes at the expense of a slightly higher long-term failure rate. One disadvantage of total fundoplication is the creation of an overcompetent cardia, resulting in the 'gas bloat' syndrome in which belching is impossible. The stomach fills with air, the patient feels very full after small meals and passes excessive flatus. This does not seem to occur with partial fundoplication. The problem has been largely overcome by the 'floppy' Nissen technique in which the fundoplication is loose around the oesophagus and is kept short in length. While the other short-term side effects of fundoplication usually resolve within three months of surgery, this is rarely the case for gas bloat. The problem is best remedied by conversion to a partial fundoplication.

As with primary surgery, a variety of revisional procedures have been described. For most patients, recurrent reflux relates to anatomical failure, so the solution is a revisional fundoplication. A very small proportion of patients may undergo more than two operations to correct recurrent reflux or unacceptable side effects. Revisional surgery carries a lower chance of success and, in some patients, local revision is technically impossible. The final resort is partial gastrectomy with a Roux-en-Y reconstruction. This reduces gastric acid secretion and diverts bile and pancreatic secretions away from the stomach. Thus, the volume of potential refluxate in the stomach is reduced and, because of its changed composition, it is less damaging to the oesophagus.

For many years, the relative merits of thoracic and abdominal approaches were hotly debated. The introduction of minimal access surgery has made this debate practically obsolete, and most antireflux operations are now done with a laparoscopic approach.

Laparoscopic fundoplication

Five cannulae are inserted in the upper abdomen (Figure 62.24). The cardia and lower oesophagus are separated from the diaphragmatic hiatus. An appropriate length of oesophagus is mobilised in the mediastinum. The fundus may be mobilised by dividing the short gastric vessels that tether the fundus to the spleen. The hiatus is narrowed by sutures placed behind the oesophagus. In total (Nissen) fundoplication, the fundus is drawn behind the oesophagus and then sutured to itself in front of the oesophagus (Figure 62.25a). In partial fundoplication, the fundus is drawn either behind or in front of the oesophagus and sutured to it on each side, leaving a strip of exposed oesophagus either at the front (Figure 62.25b) or at the back.

Complications of gastro-oesophageal reflux disease

Stricture

Reflux-induced strictures (see Figure 62.21) occur mainly in the late middle-aged and the elderly, but they may present in children. It is important to distinguish a benign reflux-induced stricture from a carcinoma. This is not usually difficult on the basis of location (immediately above the oesophagogastric junction), length (only about 1–2 cm) and smooth mucosa, but sometimes

Rudolph Nissen, 1896–1981, Professor of Surgery, Istanbul, Turkey, and later at Basle, Switzerland.
André M Toupet, born 1915, surgeon, St Cloud Hospital, Senior Consultant, University of Paris, France, proposed his technique in 1963.
Philip Rowland Allison, 1907–1974, Professor of Surgery, Oxford University, Oxford, UK.
Lucius David Hill, surgeon, The Mason Clinic, Seattle, MN, USA.
Ronald Herbert Robert Belsey, 1910–2007, thoracic surgeon, The Frenchay Hospital, Bristol, UK, came to be known by his colleagues as 'the B'.

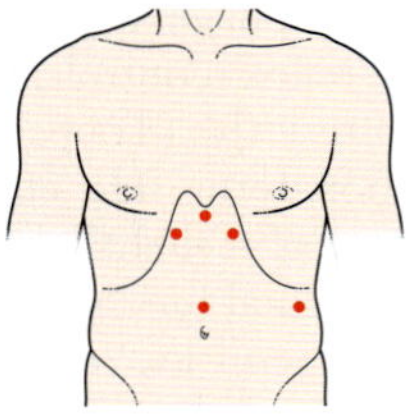

Figure 62.24 Laparoscope cannula sites for laparoscopic fundoplication.

a cancer spreads under the oesophageal mucosa at its upper margin, producing a benign-looking stricture.

Peptic strictures generally respond well to dilatation and long-term treatment with a PPI. As most patients are elderly, antireflux surgery is not usually considered. However, it is an alternative to long-term PPI treatment, just as in uncomplicated GORD in younger and fitter patients. Most patients do not require anything other than a standard operation (Summary box 62.7).

Summary box 62.7

Peptic stricture

- Day-case dilatation and PPI for peptic stricture

Oesophageal shortening

The issue of oesophageal shortening continues to provoke debate. There can be no doubt that, in the presence of a large sliding hiatus hernia, the oesophagus is short, but this does not necessarily mean that, with mobilisation from the mediastinum, it cannot easily be restored to its normal length. The extent to which severe inflammation in the wall of the oesophagus causes fibrosis and real shortening is less clear. If a good segment of intra-abdominal oesophagus cannot be restored without tension, a Collis gastroplasty should be performed (Figure 62.26). This produces a neo-oesophagus around which a fundoplication can be done (Collis–Nissen operation) (Summary box 62.8).

Summary box 62.8

GORD

- Is due to loss of competence of the LOS and is extremely common
- May be associated with a hiatus hernia, which may be sliding or, less commonly, rolling (paraoesophageal)
- The most common symptoms are heartburn, epigastric discomfort and regurgitation, often made worse by stooping and lying
- Achalasia and GORD are diagnostically easily confused

  Dysphagia may occur, but a neoplasm must be excluded

  Diagnosis and treatment can be instituted on clinical grounds
- Endoscopy may be required and 24-hour pH is the 'gold standard'

  Management is primarily medical (PPIs being the most effective), but surgery may be required; laparoscopic fundoplication is the most popular technique

  Stricture may develop in time

Barrett's oesophagus (columnar-lined lower oesophagus)

Barrett's oesophagus is a metaplastic change in the lining mucosa of the oesophagus in response to chronic gastro-oesophageal reflux (Figure 62.27). Many of these patients do not have particularly severe symptoms, although they do have the most abnormal pH profiles. This adaptive response involves a mosaic of cell types, probably beginning as a simple columnar epithelium that becomes 'specialised' with time. The hallmark of 'specialised' Barrett's epithelium is the presence of mucus-secreting goblet cells (intestinal metaplasia). One of the great mysteries of GORD is why some people develop oesophagitis and others develop Barrett's oesophagus, often without significant oesophagitis. In Barrett's oesophagus, the junction between squamous oesophageal mucosa and gastric mucosa moves proximally. It may be difficult to distinguish a Barrett's oesophagus from a tubular, sliding hiatus hernia during endoscopy, as the two often coexist (Figure 62.28) or where the visible Barrett's segment is very short. The key is where the gastric mucosal folds end. The mucosa in the body of the stomach has longitudinal

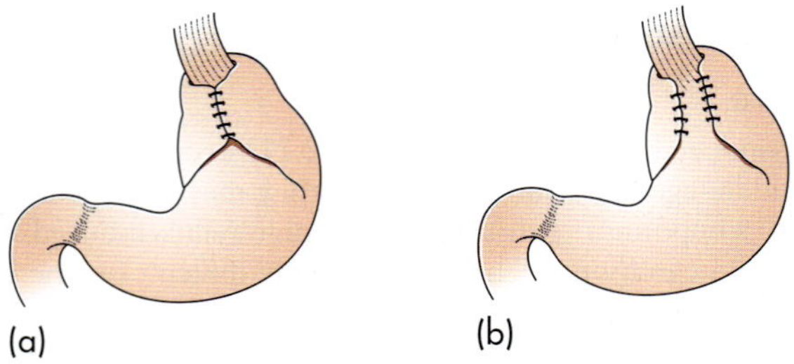

Figure 62.25 (a) Total (Nissen) fundoplication; (b) partial fundoplication (Toupet).

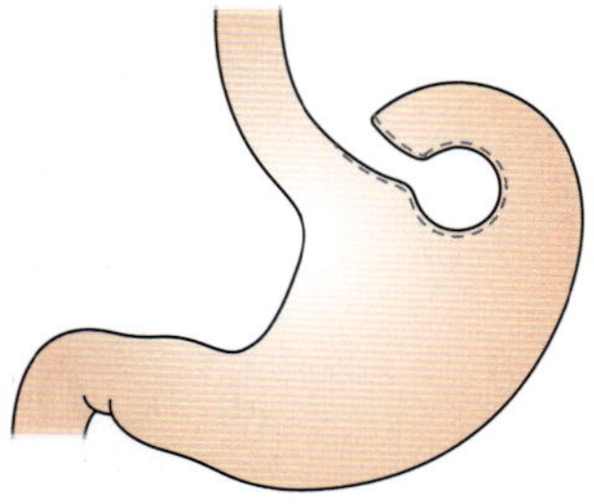

Figure 62.26 Collis gastroplasty to produce a neo-oesophagus around which a Nissen fundoplication is done. The operation may be performed by a laparoscopic as well as an open approach using circular and linear staplers.

John Leigh Collis, 1911–2003, Professor of Thoracic Surgery, the University of Birmingham, Birmingham, UK.

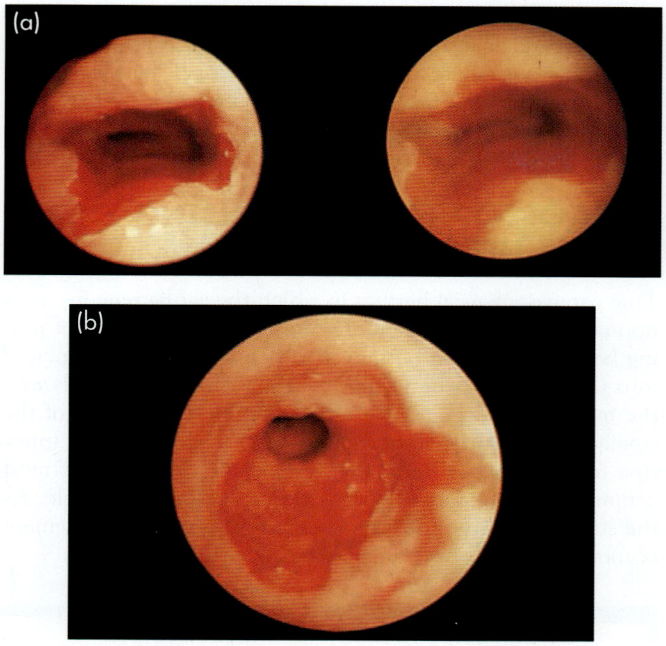

Figure 62.27 Barrett's oesophagus with proximal migration of the squamocolumnar junction (a) and with a view of the distal oesophagus (b).

folds; the columnar lining of Barrett's oesophagus is smooth. Strictures can occur in Barrett's oesophagus and nearly always appear at the new squamocolumnar junction (Figure 62.29). Rarely, a stricture may occur in the columnar segment after healing of a Barrett's ulcer (Figure 62.30). When intestinal metaplasia occurs, there is an increased risk of adenocarcinoma of the oesophagus (Summary box 62.9), which is about 25 times that of the general population (Figures 62.30, 62.31 and 62.32).

Patients who are found to have Barrett's oesophagus may be submitted to regular surveillance endoscopy with multiple biopsies in the hope of finding dysplasia or *in situ* cancer rather than allowing invasive cancer to develop and cause symptoms. There

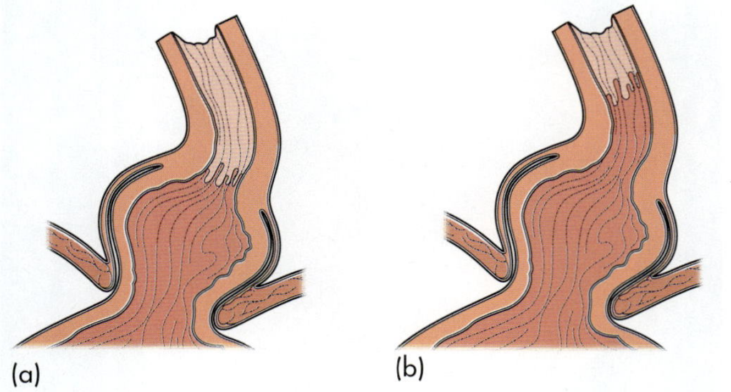

Figure 62.28 (a) The relationship between the lower oesophageal sphincter, the squamocolumnar junction and the diaphragm in sliding hiatus hernia. (b) Barrett's oesophagus and sliding hernia.

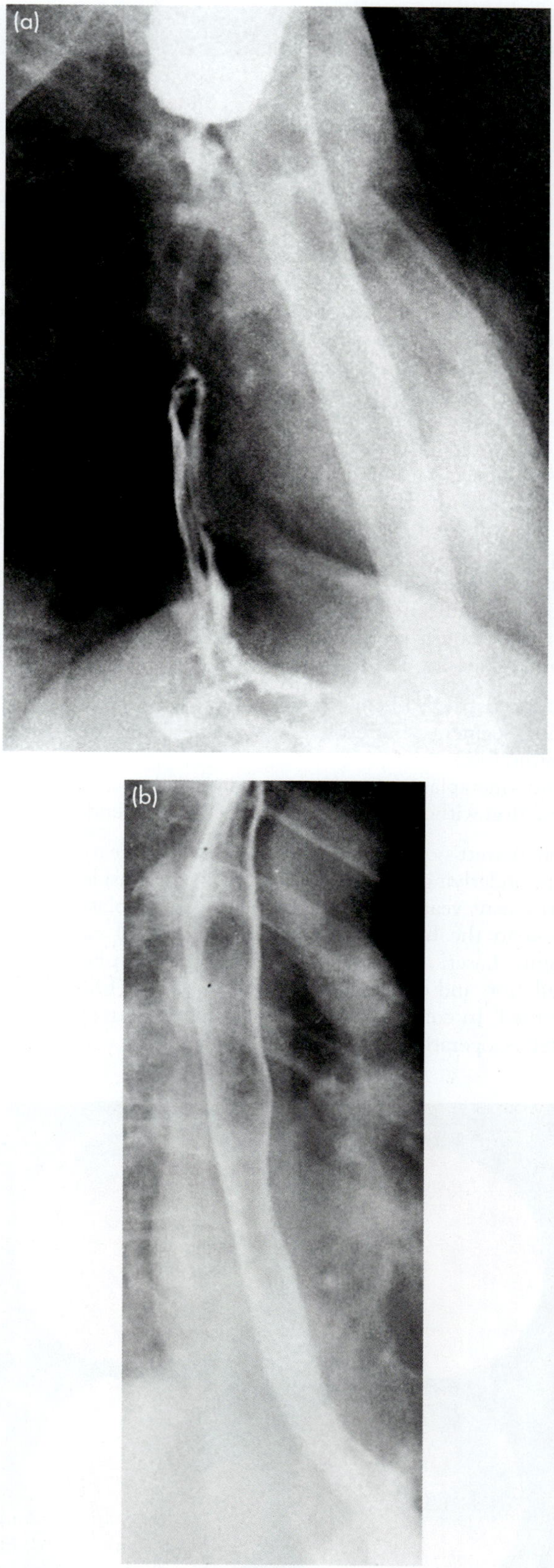

Figure 62.29 The radiological appearance of a mid-oesophageal stricture in a patient with Barrett's oesophagus (a) and in a patient with a normal lumen following dilatation (b).

Summary box 62.9

Barrett's oesophagus

- Intestinal metaplasia is an important risk factor for the development of adenocarcinoma
- Do not confuse Barrett's ulcer with oesophagitis

is as yet no general agreement about the benefits of surveillance endoscopy, nor about its ideal frequency. Annual endoscopy has been widely practised, but two-year intervals are probably adequate, provided no dysplasia has been detected. A significant problem is that the incidence of Barrett's oesophagus in the community is estimated to be at least ten times the incidence discovered in dyspeptic patients referred for endoscopy. Thus, adenocarcinoma in Barrett's oesophagus often presents with invasive cancer without any preceding reflux symptoms.

Until recently, Barrett's oesophagus was not diagnosed until there was at least 3 cm of columnar epithelium in the distal oesophagus. With the better appreciation of the importance of intestinal metaplasia, Barrett's oesophagus may be diagnosed if there is any intestinal metaplasia in the oesophagus. The relative risk of cancer probably increases with increasing length of abnormal mucosa. The following terms are widely used:

- classic Barrett's (3 cm or more columnar epithelium);
- short-segment Barrett's (less than 3 cm of columnar epithelium);
- cardia metaplasia (intestinal metaplasia at the oesophagogastric junction without any macroscopic change at endoscopy).

When Barrett's oesophagus is discovered, the treatment is that of the underlying GORD. There has been considerable interest in recent years in endoscopic methods of ablating Barrett's mucosa in the hope of eliminating the risk of cancer development. Laser, photodynamic therapy, argon-beam plasma coagulation and endoscopic mucosal resection (EMR) have all been used. In conjunction with high-dose PPI treatment or an antireflux operation, these endoscopic methods can result in a neosquamous lining. There is no evidence yet that any of these methods is reliable in eliminating cancer risk. Residual islands of Barrett's epithelium can persist, glands may be buried beneath the new lining, and damage to the oesophageal wall may cause stricturing.

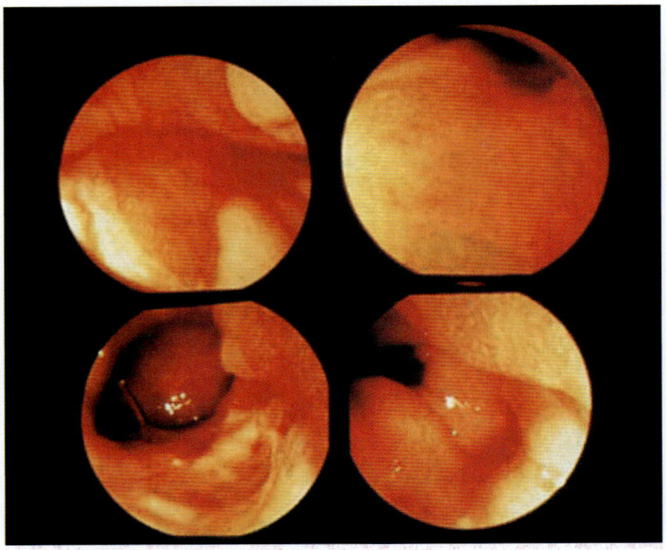

Figure 62.30 Barrett's ulcer in the columnar cell-lined oesophagus.

PARAOESOPHAGEAL ('ROLLING') HIATUS HERNIA

True paraoesophageal hernias in which the cardia remains in its normal anatomical position are rare. The vast majority of rolling hernias are mixed hernias in which the cardia is displaced into the chest and the greater curve of the stomach rolls into the mediastinum (Figure 62.33). Sometimes, the whole of the stomach lies in the chest (Figure 62.34). Colon or small intestine may sometimes lie in the hernia sac. The hernia is most common in the elderly, but may occur in young fit people. As the stomach rolls up into the chest, there is always an element of rotation (volvulus) (Summary box 62.10).

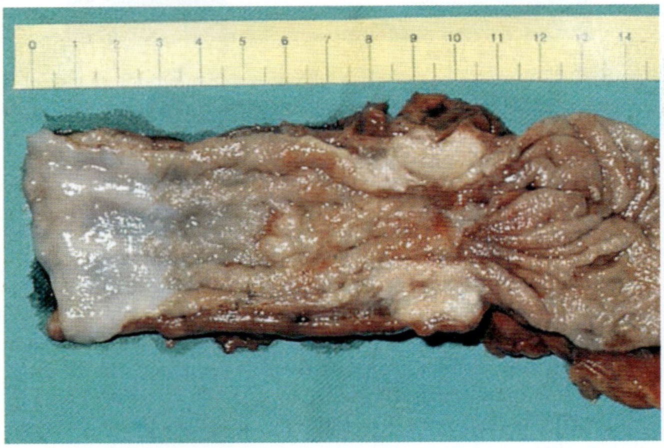

Figure 62.31 The macroscopic appearances of an adenocarcinoma in Barrett's oesophagus.

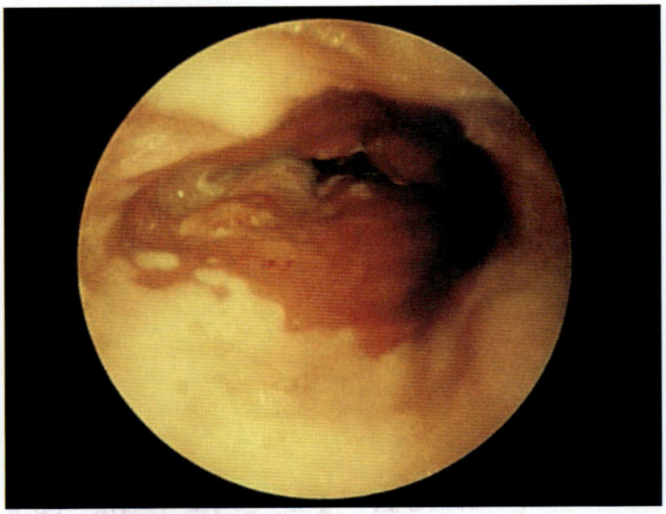

Figure 62.32 Endoscopic view of carcinoma in Barrett's oesophagus.

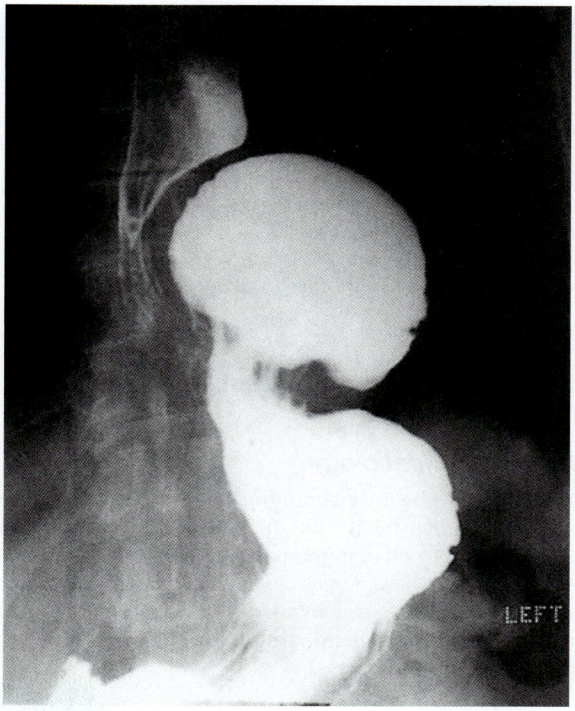

Figure 62.33 A paraoesophageal hernia showing the gastro-oesophageal junction just above the diaphragm and the fundus alongside the oesophagus, compressing the lumen.

Summary box 62.10

'Rolling' hiatus hernia

- Potentially dangerous, because of volvulus

The symptoms of rolling hernia are mostly due to twisting and distortion of the oesophagus and stomach. Dysphagia is common. Chest pain may occur from distension of an obstructed stomach. Classically, the pain is relieved by a loud belch. Symptoms of GORD are variable. Strangulation, gastric perforation and gangrene can occur. Emergency presentation with any of these complications carries high mortality on account of a combination of late diagnosis, generally elderly patients with comorbid diseases and the complexity of surgery involved.

The hernia may be visible on a plain radiograph of the chest as a gas bubble, often with a fluid level behind the heart (Figure 62.35). A barium meal is the best method of diagnosis. The endoscopic appearances may be confusing, especially in large hernias when it is easy to become disorientated.

Symptomatic rolling hernias nearly always require surgical repair as they are potentially dangerous. The risk of an asymptomatic patient developing a significant problem when a rolling hiatus hernia is discovered incidentally has probably been overestimated in the past. The annual risk is probably no more than 1 per cent. Patients who present as an emergency with acute chest pain may be treated initially by nasogastric tube to relieve the distension that causes the pain, followed by operative repair. If the pain is not relieved or perforation is suspected, immediate operation is mandatory.

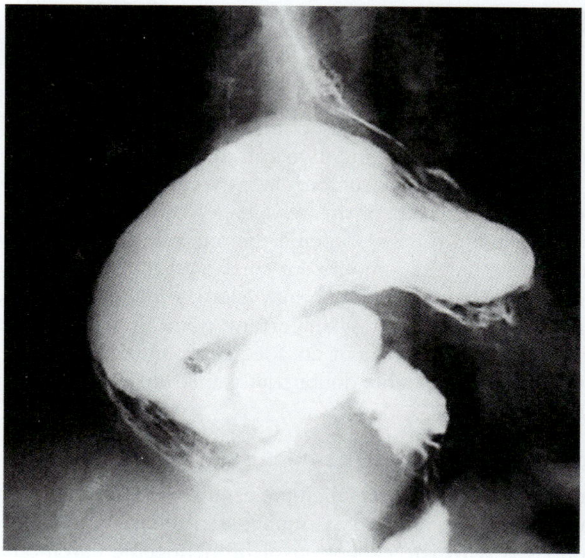

Figure 62.34 A huge paraoesophageal hernia with an upside-down stomach and the pylorus just below the hiatus.

Emergency surgery needs to be tailored to the problem encountered and the fitness of the patient. Elective surgery involves reduction of the hernia, excision of the sac, reducing the crural defect and some form of retention of the stomach in the abdomen. Some surgeons perform a fundoplication, arguing that this is a very effective means of maintaining reduction and that it deals with the associated GORD. Others argue that fundoplication should only be done if reflux can be conclusively demonstrated beforehand. Surprisingly, both philosophies achieve good results. Laparoscopic repair has recently become popular. Full anatomical repair of a large rolling hernia can be difficult by this approach and requires considerable expertise. Secure closure of the hiatal defect can be a problem, and some surgeons advocate mesh to reinforce the repair.

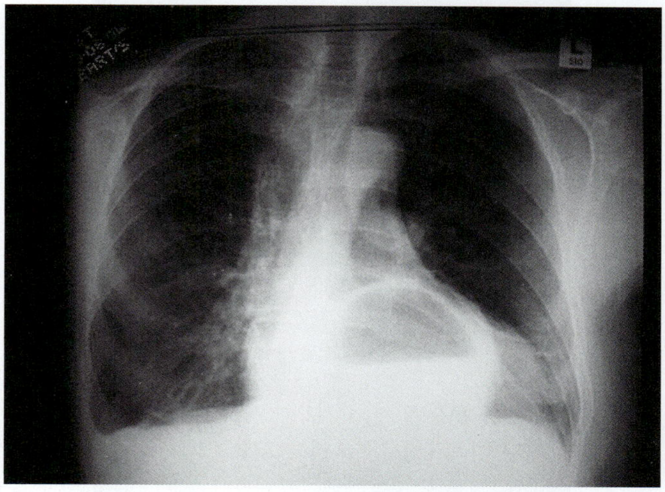

Figure 62.35 A gas bubble seen on a plain chest radiograph, showing the fundus of the stomach in the chest. Courtesy of Dr Stephen Ellis, Barts and the London NHS Trust.

NEOPLASMS OF THE OESOPHAGUS

Benign tumours

Benign tumours of the oesophagus are relatively rare. True papillomas, adenomas and hyperplastic polyps do occur, but the majority of 'benign' tumours are not epithelial in origin and arise from other layers of the oesophageal wall (gastrointestinal stromal tumour (GIST), lipoma, granular cell tumour). Most benign oesophageal tumours are small and asymptomatic, and even a large benign tumour may cause only mild symptoms (Figure 62.36). The most important point in their management is usually to carry out an adequate number of biopsies to prove beyond reasonable doubt that the lesion is not malignant (Figure 62.37).

Malignant tumours

Non-epithelial primary malignancies are also rare, as is malignant melanoma. Secondary malignancies rarely involve the oesophagus with the exception of bronchogenic carcinoma by direct invasion of either the primary and/or contiguous lymph nodes.

Carcinoma of the oesophagus

Cancer of the oesophagus is the sixth most common cancer in the world. In general, it is a disease of mid to late adulthood, with a poor survival rate. Only 5–10 per cent of those diagnosed will survive for five years (Summary box 62.11).

Summary box 62.11

Carcinoma of the oesophagus

- Squamous cell usually affects the upper two-thirds; adenocarcinoma usually affects the lower-third
- Common aetiological factors are tobacco and alcohol (squamous cell) and GORD (adenocarcinoma)
- The incidence of adenocarcinoma is increasing
- Lymph node involvement is a bad prognostic factor
- Dysphagia is the most common presenting symptom, but is a late feature
- Accurate pretreatment staging is essential in patients thought to be fit to undergo 'curative' treatment

Pathology and aetiology

Squamous cell cancer (Figures 62.38 and 62.39) and adenocarcinoma (Figures 62.40 and 62.41) are the most common types. Squamous cell carcinoma generally affects the upper two-thirds of the oesophagus and adenocarcinoma the lower one-third. Worldwide, squamous cell cancer is most common, but adenocarcinoma predominates in the West and is increasing in incidence.

Geographical variation in oesophageal cancer

The incidence of oesophageal cancer varies more than that of any other cancer. Squamous cell cancer is endemic in the

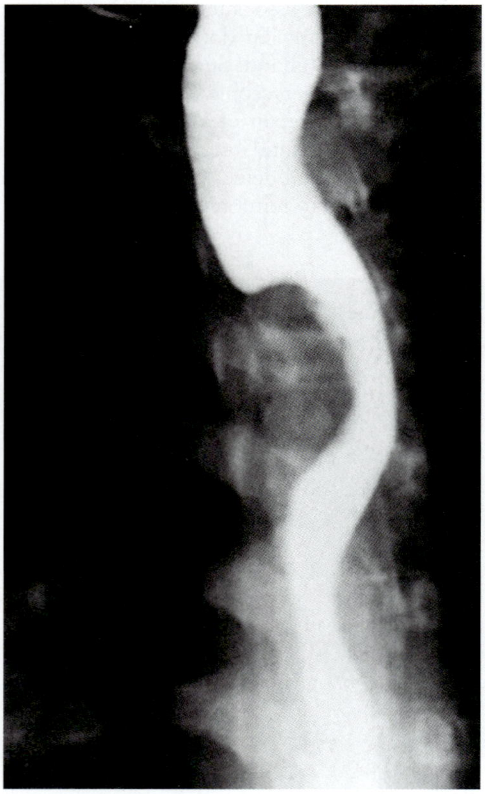

Figure 62.36 Classic appearance of a large oesophageal gastrointestinal stromal tumour on barium swallow.

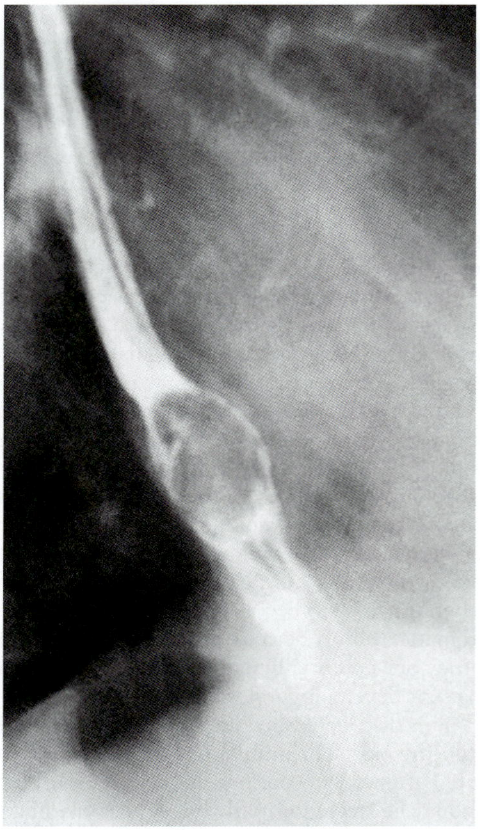

Figure 62.37 An intraluminal polyp that proved to be a leiomyosarcoma.

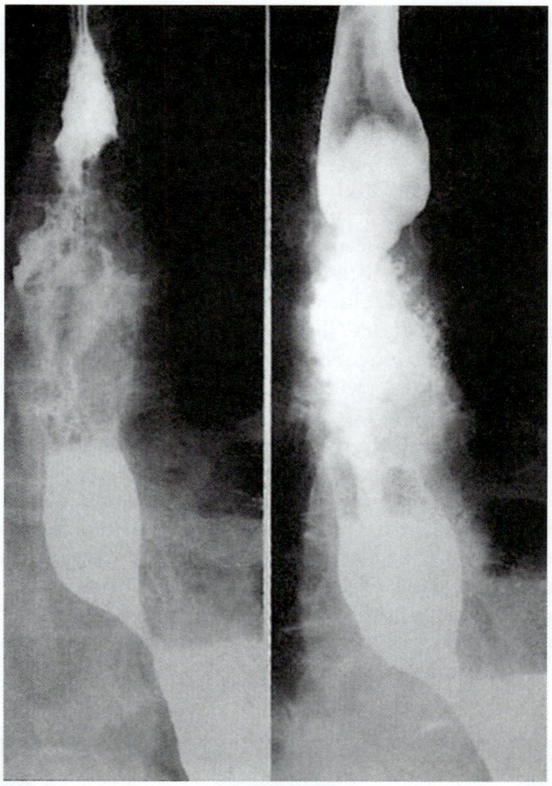

Figure 62.38 The classic appearances of a mid-oesophageal proliferative squamous cell carcinoma.

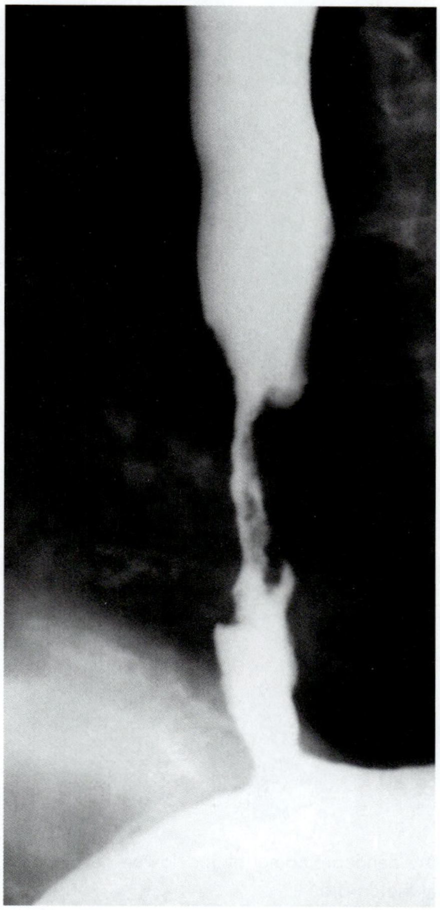

Figure 62.39 Squamous cell carcinoma of the oesophagus producing an irregular stricture with shouldered margins.

Transkei region of South Africa and in the Asian 'cancer belt' that extends across the middle of Asia from the shores of the Caspian Sea (in northern Iran) to China. The highest incidence in the world is in Linxian in Henan province in China, where it is the most common single cause of death, with more than 100 cases per 100 000 population per annum. The cause of the disease in the endemic areas is not known, but it is probably due to a combination of fungal contamination of food and nutritional deficiencies. In Linxian, supplementation of the diet with beta-carotene, vitamin E and selenium has been shown to reduce the incidence.

Away from the endemic areas, tobacco and alcohol are major factors in the occurrence of squamous cancer. Incidence rates vary from less than 5:100 000 in white people in the US to 26.5:100 000 in some regions of France.

In many Western countries, the incidence of squamous cell cancer has fallen or remained static, but the incidence of adenocarcinoma of the oesophagus has increased dramatically since the mid-1970s at a rate of 5–10 per cent per annum. The change is greater than that of any other neoplasm in this time. Adenocarcinoma now accounts for 60–75 per cent of all oesophageal cancers in several countries. The reason for this change is not understood. A similar rate of increase in GORD over the same period, which mirrors an increase in obesity in the West, is likely to be an important factor, particularly through the link to Barrett's oesophagus. There has been a similar increase in the incidence of carcinoma of the cardia of the stomach, which suggests that cancer of the cardia and adenocarcinoma of the oesophagus may share common aetiological factors. With a falling incidence of cancer in the rest of the stomach, more than 60 per cent of all upper gastrointestinal cancers in the West involve the cardia or distal oesophagus.

Both adenocarcinomas and squamous cell carcinomas tend to disseminate early. Sadly, the classical presenting symptoms of dysphagia, regurgitation and weight loss are often absent until the primary tumour has become advanced, and so the tumour is often well established before the diagnosis is made. Tumours can spread in three ways: invasion directly through the oesophageal wall, via lymphatics or in the bloodstream. Direct spread occurs both laterally, through the component layers of the oesophageal wall, and longitudinally within the oesophageal wall. Longitudinal spread is mainly via the submucosal lymphatic channels of the oesophagus. The pattern of lymphatic drainage is therefore not segmental, as in other parts of the gastrointestinal tract. Consequently, the length of oesophagus involved by tumour is frequently much longer than the macroscopic length of the malignancy at the epithelial surface. Lymph node spread occurs commonly. Although the direction of spread to regional lymphatics is predominantly caudal, the involvement of lymph nodes is potentially widespread and can also occur in a cranial direction. Any regional lymph node from the superior mediastinum to the coeliac axis and lesser curve of the stomach may be involved regardless of the location of the primary lesion within the oesophagus. Haematogenous spread may involve a

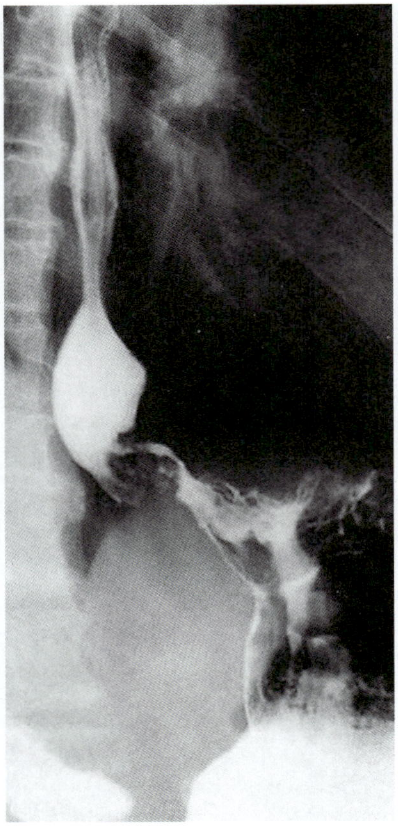

Figure 62.40 Adenocarcinoma of the lower oesophagus, spreading upwards from the cardia.

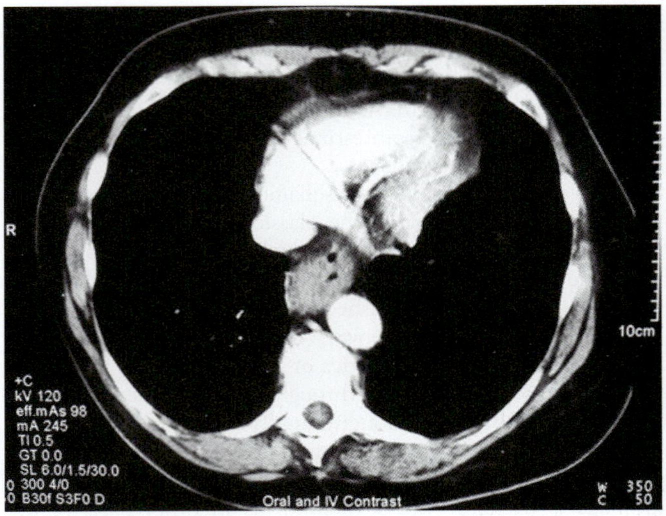

Figure 62.41 Computed tomography scan showing a primary tumour of the lower oesophagus.

variety of different organs including the liver, lungs, brain and bones. Tumours arising from the intra-abdominal portion of the oesophagus may also disseminate transperitoneally.

Clinical features

Most oesophageal neoplasms present with mechanical symptoms, principally dysphagia, but sometimes also regurgitation, vomiting, odynophagia and weight loss. Clinical findings suggestive of advanced malignancy include recurrent laryngeal nerve palsy, Horner's syndrome, chronic spinal pain and diaphragmatic paralysis. Other factors making surgical cure unlikely include weight loss of more than 20 per cent and loss of appetite. Cutaneous tumour metastases or enlarged supraclavicular lymph nodes may be seen on clinical examination and indicate disseminated disease. Hoarseness due to recurrent laryngeal nerve palsy is a sign of advanced and incurable disease. Palpable lymphadenopathy in the neck is likewise a sign of advanced disease.

Patients with early disease may have non-specific dyspeptic symptoms or a vague feeling of 'something that is not quite right' during swallowing. Some are diagnosed during endoscopic surveillance of patients with Barrett's oesophagus and, while this does identify patients with the earliest stages of disease, such programmes have little overall impact, as most patients with Barrett's oesophagus are unknown to the medical profession and make their first presentation with a symptomatic and therefore usually locally advanced oesophageal cancer. The widespread use of endoscopy as a diagnostic tool does, nevertheless, provide an opportunity for early diagnosis (Figure 62.42). Biopsies should be taken of all lesions in the oesophagus (Figures 62.43 and 62.44), no matter how trivial they appear and irrespective of the indication for the examination.

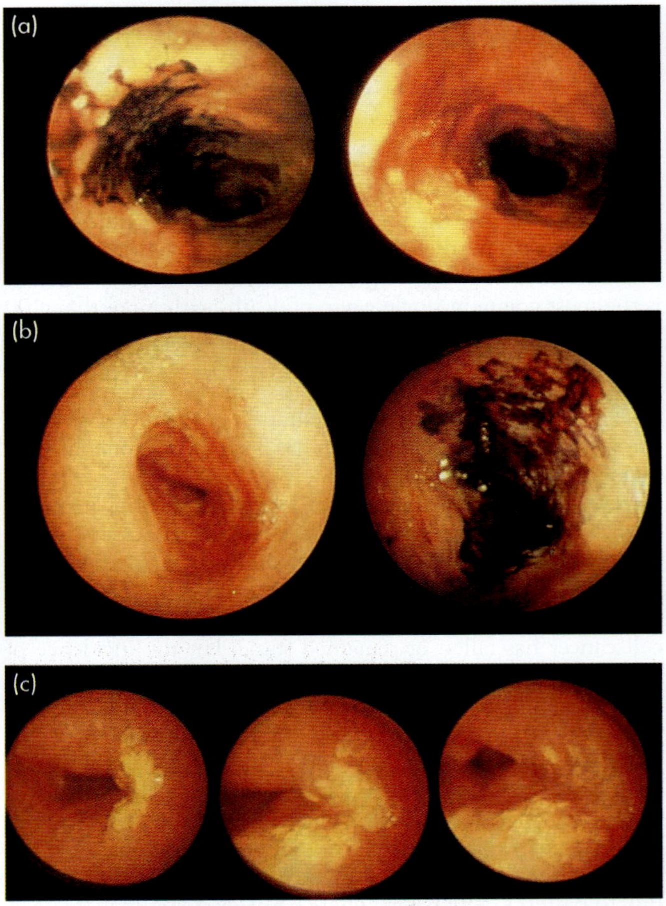

Figure 62.42 Carcinoma *in situ* showing the varied presentations: (a) occult form; (b) erythroplakia; (c) leukoplakia. The right-hand pictures in (a) and (b) demonstrate the use of vital staining with methylene blue.

Johann Friefrich Horner, 1831–1886, Professor of Ophthalmology, Zurich, Switzerland, described this syndrome in 1869.

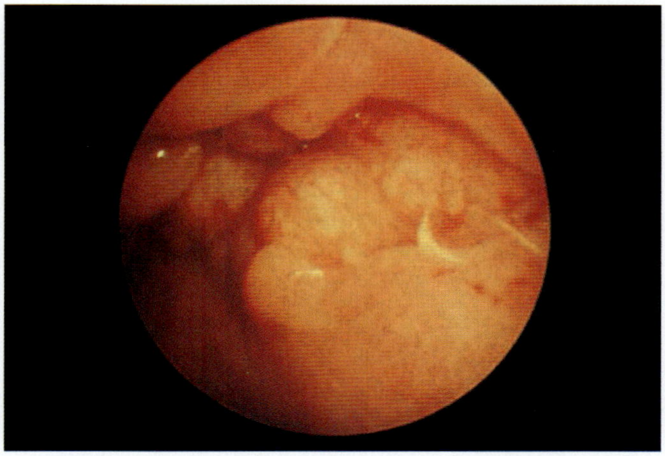

Figure 62.43 Endoscopic appearances of a mid-oesophageal squamous cell carcinoma.

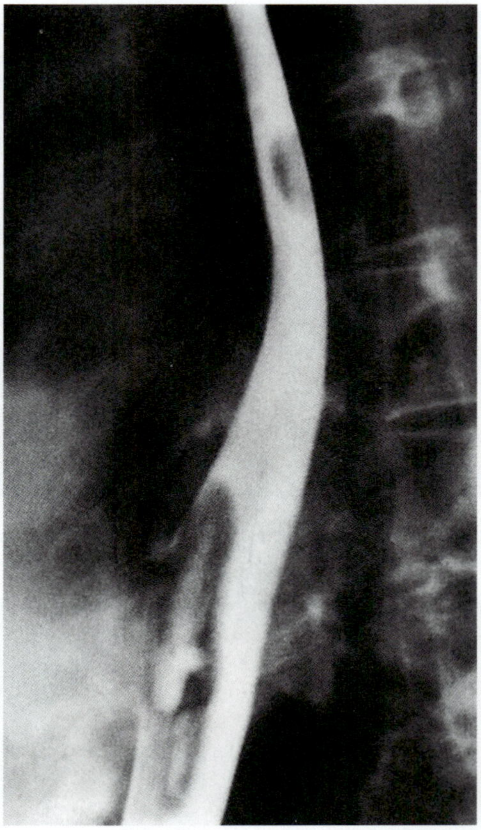

Figure 62.44 Beware the differential diagnosis of infection, for what appears to be a tumour. This mid-oesophageal mass was actually tuberculosis.

Investigation

Endoscopy is the first-line investigation for most patients. It provides an unrivalled direct view of the oesophageal mucosa and any lesion allowing its site and size to be documented. Cytology and/or histology specimens taken via the endoscope are crucial for accurate diagnosis. The combination of histology and cytology increases the diagnostic accuracy to more than 95 per cent. The chief limitation of conventional endoscopy is that only the mucosal surface can be studied and biopsied. Other investigations are therefore usually required to define the extent of local or distant spread. The improved image resolution of modern endoscopes and novel techniques involving magnification and the use of dyes to enhance surface detail may lead to more early lesions being recognised (see Figure 62.42).

General assessment and staging

Once the initial diagnosis of a malignant oesophageal neoplasm has been made, patients should be assessed first in terms of their general health and fitness for potential therapies. Their preferences should also be considered. Most potentially curative therapies include radical surgery, although chemoradiotherapy is an alternative in squamous cell carcinoma. Patients who are unfit for, or who do not wish to contemplate, radical treatments should not be investigated further, but should be diverted to appropriate palliative therapies, depending on symptoms and current quality of life. Only those patients suitable for potentially curative therapies should proceed to staging investigations to rule out haematogenous spread and then to assess locoregional stage (endoscopic ultrasound (EUS) ± laparoscopy). This will distinguish between early (T1/T2, N0) and advanced lesions (T3/T4, N1) and indicate whether surgery alone or multimodal therapy is most appropriate. Where attempted cure is deemed possible, the aim should be to provide the best chance of cure while minimising perioperative risks. In general, surgery alone should be reserved for patients with early disease, and multimodal therapy should be used in patients with locally advanced disease, in whom the chance of cure by surgery alone is small (generally less than 20 per cent).

The most widely used pathological staging system is the World Health Organization (tumour–nodes–metastasis TNM) classification.

Table 62.2 shows the TNM system for oesophageal cancer in its most updated form. Like all pathological systems, it is reliant on the nature and extent of the surgery performed. For example, performing more extensive radical surgical lymphadenectomy provides a more accurate assessment of the 'N' stage. There is evidence that many patients described as N0 in the past were probably N1, a phenomenon described as stage migration.

Staging information may be gathered before the commencement of therapy, during therapy (e.g. at open operation) or following treatment (histology or post-mortem). The techniques commonly used to provide preoperative staging data are described in Figure 62.45, along with a suggested algorithm.

Blood tests

These are of limited value. Blood tests reveal nothing about local invasion or regional lymph node spread and, to date, no reliable tumour marker for oesophageal cancer has been isolated from peripheral blood. The presence of abnormal liver function tests (LFTs) may suggest the presence of liver metastases, but this is generally too insensitive to be diagnostic. Many patients with known liver metastases have normal LFTs. At best, abnormal LFTs only reinforce the clinical suspicion of spread to the liver, and further imaging is usually required to confirm the diagnosis.

Transcutaneous ultrasound

It is difficult to visualise mediastinal structures with transcutaneous ultrasound. With the relatively low-frequency sound waves

Table 62.2 TNM staging scheme for oesophageal cancer.

Tis	High-grade dysplasia
T1	Tumour invading lamina propria or submucosa
T2	Tumour invading muscularis propria
T3	Tumour invading beyond muscularis propria
T4a	Tumour invading adjacent structures (pleura, pericardium, diaphragm)
T4b	Tumour invading adjacent structures (trachea, bone, aorta)
N0	No lymph node metastases
N1	Lymph node metastases in 1–2 nodes
N2	Lymph nodes metastases in 3–6 nodes
N3	Lymph node metastases in 7 or more lymph nodes
M0	No distant metastases
M1	All other distant metastases
Stage	1A: T1N0M0; 1B: T2N0M0; 2A: T3N0M0; 2B: T1/2N0M0; 3A: T4aN0M0, T3N1M0, T1/2N2M0; 3B: T3N2M0; 3C: T4aN1/2M0, T4bN0-3M0, T1-4N3M0; 4: T1-4N1-3M1

used, good depth of tissue penetration is achieved at the expense of poor image resolution. In addition, the mediastinal organs are surrounded by bone and air, which renders them largely inaccessible to external ultrasound. The technique is therefore used mainly to assess spread to the liver, the whole of which can be clearly visualised by standard transcutaneous ultrasound. Haematogenous spread can be more fully assessed by combining ultrasound with chest radiography, although this combination is less accurate than CT scanning.

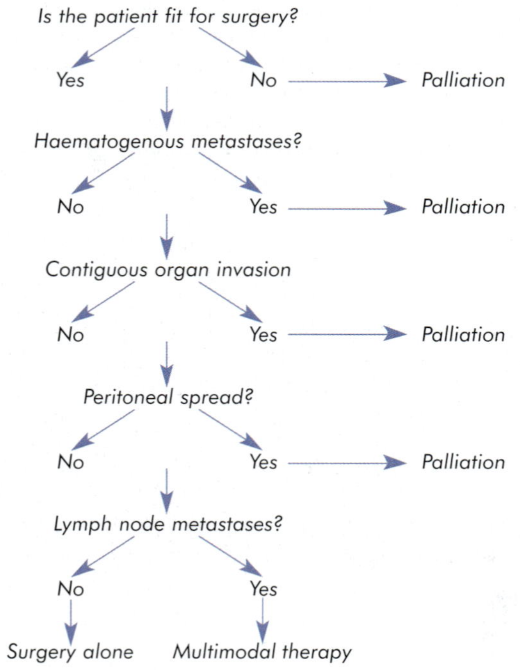

Figure 62.45 Algorithm for the management of oesophageal cancer.

Bronchoscopy

Many middle- and upper-third oesophageal carcinomas (and therefore usually squamous carcinomas) are sufficiently advanced at the time of diagnosis that the trachea or bronchi are already involved (Figure 62.46). Bronchoscopy may reveal either impingement or invasion of the main airways in over 30 per cent of new patients with cancers in the upper third of the oesophagus. In some cases, therefore, bronchoscopy alone can confirm that the tumour is locally unresectable.

Laparoscopy

This is a useful technique for the diagnosis of intra-abdominal and hepatic metastases. It has the advantage of enabling tissue samples or peritoneal cytology to be obtained and is the only modality reliably able to detect peritoneal tumour seedlings (Figure 62.47). This is particularly important for tumours arising from the intra-abdominal portion of the oesophagus, cardia and where there is a potential communication between a full-thickness tumour and the peritoneal cavity, for instance where there is a hiatus hernia.

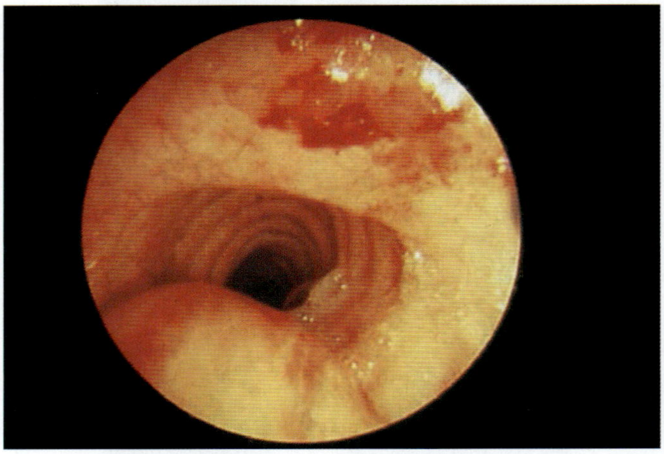

Figure 62.46 Invasion into the posterior wall of the trachea from an oesophageal carcinoma.

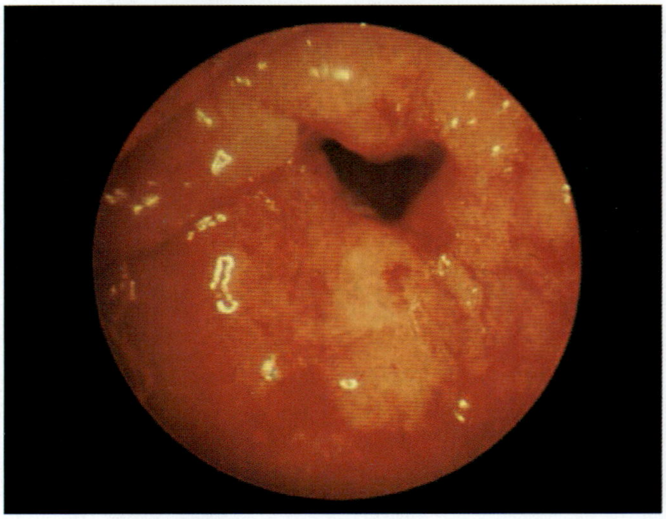

Figure 62.47 Adenocarcinoma of the cardia. Transcoelomic spread may occur with this type of lesion.

Computed tomography

Computed tomography scanning is the modality most used to identify haematogenous metastases (Figure 62.48). Distant organs are easily seen and metastases within them visualised with high accuracy (94–100 per cent). The normal thoracic oesophagus is easily demonstrated by CT scanning. The mediastinal fat planes are usually clearly imaged in healthy individuals, and any blurring or distortion of these images is a fairly reliable indicator of abnormality. In cachectic patients with dysphagia and malnutrition, the mediastinal fat plane may be virtually absent, making local invasion difficult to assess. Spiral and thin-slice CT permit structures such as lymph nodes to be adequately imaged, down to a minimum diameter of about 5 mm. Smaller nodes cannot be reliably visualised, and it is not possible to distinguish between enlarged lymph nodes that have reactive changes only and metastatic nodes. Similarly, micrometastases within normal-sized nodes cannot be detected.

Magnetic resonance imaging

Magnetic resonance imaging (MRI) does not expose the patient to ionising radiation and needs no intravascular contrast medium, although intraoesophageal air or contrast media may help to assess wall thickness. Distant metastases to organs such as the liver are usually reliably identified by MRI but, at the present time, there do not seem to be additional benefits over CT.

Endoscopic ultrasound

After haematogenous spread, the two principal prognostic factors for oesophageal cancer are the depth of tumour penetration through the oesophageal wall and regional lymph node spread. Although CT will detect distant metastasis, its limited axial resolution precludes a reliable assessment of both the depth of wall penetration and lymph node involvement. Endoscopic ultrasound can determine the depth of spread of a malignant tumour through the oesophageal wall (T1–3), the invasion of adjacent organs (T4) and metastasis to lymph nodes (N0 or N1) (Figures 62.49, 62.50 and 62.51). It can also detect contiguous spread downward into the cardia and more distant metastases to the left lobe of the liver.

Endoscopic ultrasound visualises the oesophageal wall as a multilayered structure. The layers represent ultrasound interfaces rather than true anatomical layers, but there is close enough

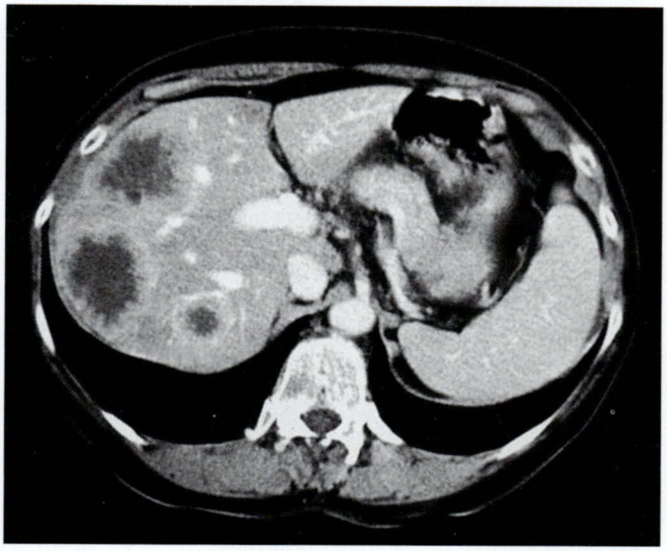

Figure 62.48 Computed tomography scan demonstrating liver metastases.

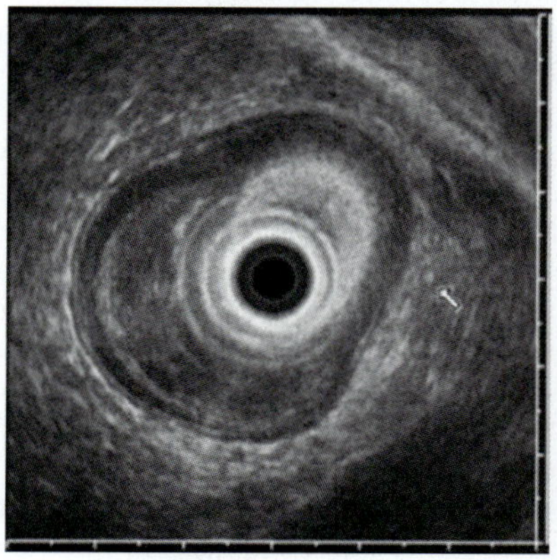

Figure 62.49 Endosonography demonstrating an 'early' tumour. Note the preservation of the outer dark wall layer that represents the muscle coat.

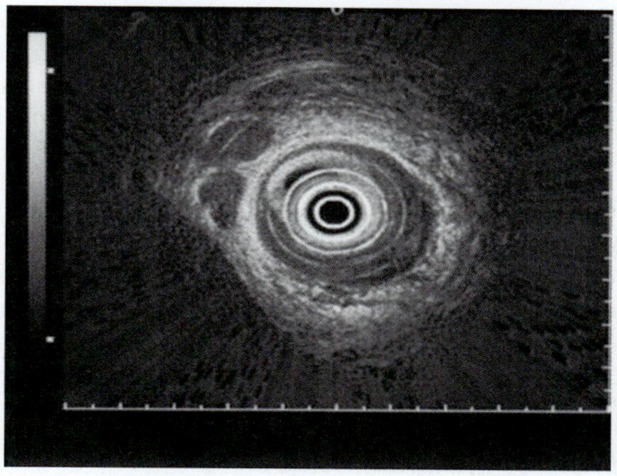

Figure 62.50 Endosonography demonstrating an 'advanced' local tumour. Note the breach of the outer white line that represents the interface between the oesophageal wall and the mediastinum.

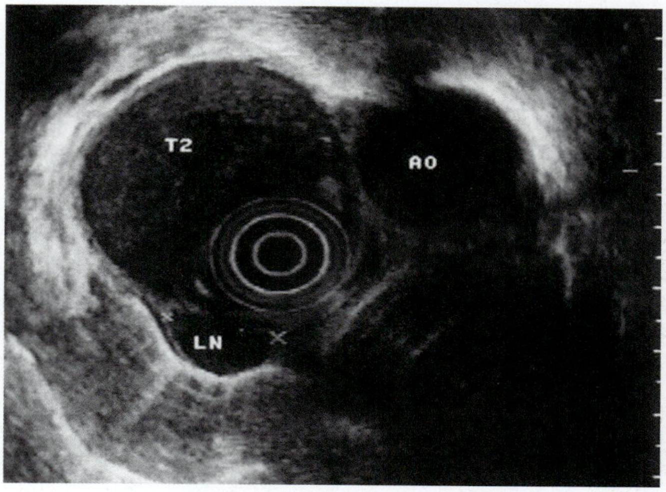

Figure 62.51 Endosonography demonstrating malignant nodes. These are usually large, hypoechoic and round compared with normal nodes.

correlation to allow accurate assessment of the depth of invasion through the oesophageal wall. Structures smaller than 5 mm can be clearly seen enabling very small nodes to be imaged. The EUS image morphology of such structures provides an additional means of distinguishing malignant from reactive or benign lymph nodes. For submucosal lesions, EUS can demonstrate the wall layer of origin of a lesion, suggesting the likely histological type.

Narrow EUS instruments are available for insertion over a guidewire to minimise the risk of technical failure, and linear array echoendoscopes can be used to biopsy lesions that might signify incurability outside the wall of the gastrointestinal tract (e.g. coeliac lymph nodes).

Positron emission tomography/computed tomography scanning

Positron emission tomography (PET) in the context of cancer staging relies on the generally high metabolic activity (particularly in the glycolytic pathway) of tumours compared with normal tissues. The patient is given a small dose of the radiopharmaceutical agent 18F-fluorodeoxyglucose (FDG). This enters cells and is phosphorylated. FDG-6-phosphate cannot be metabolised further and, because it is a highly polar molecule, it cannot easily diffuse back out of the cell. After intravenous injection of FDG, it continuously accumulates in metabolically active cells. Primary oesophageal cancers are usually sufficiently active to be easily visible, and spatial resolution of positive PET areas occurs down to about 5–8 mm. When used in isolation, there are problems with the anatomical location of these areas. This has been significantly improved by combining PET with CT (Figure 62.52). Although there are wide variations between centres, a change in stage is frequently reported in around 15 per cent of patients. It has also been suggested that a reduction in PET activity following chemotherapy might be a way of predicting 'responders' to this approach.

Treatment of malignant tumours

Principles

At the time of diagnosis, around two-thirds of all patients with oesophageal cancer will already have incurable disease. The aim of palliative treatment is to overcome debilitating or distressing symptoms while maintaining the best quality of life possible for the patient. Some patients do not require specific therapeutic interventions, but do need supportive care and appropriate liaison with community nursing and hospice care services.

As dysphagia is the predominant symptom in advanced oesophageal cancer, the principal aim of palliation is to restore adequate swallowing. A variety of methods are available and, given the short life expectancy of most patients, it is important that the choice of treatment should be tailored to each individual. Tumour location and endoscopic appearance are important in this regard, as is the general condition of the patient.

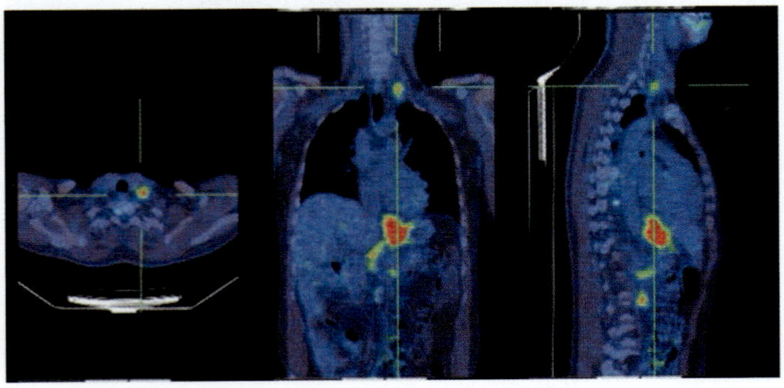

Figure 62.52 Positron emission tomography/computed tomography demonstrating a primary tumour and a distant metastatic node.

Once oesophageal neoplasms reach the submucosal layer of the oesophagus, the tumour has access to the lymphatic system, meaning that, even at this early local stage, there is an incidence of nodal positivity for both squamous cell carcinoma and adenocarcinomas of between 10 and 50 per cent. The principle of oesophagectomy is to deal adequately with the local tumour in order to minimise the risk of local recurrence and achieve an adequate lymphadenectomy to reduce the risk of staging error. Although studies in Japan would indicate that more extensive lymphadenectomy is associated with better survival, this may simply reflect more accurate staging. A number of studies support the view that the proximal extent of resection should ideally be 10 cm above the macroscopic tumour and 5 cm distal. When such a margin cannot be achieved proximally, particularly with squamous cell carcinoma, there is evidence that postoperative radiotherapy can minimise local recurrence, although not improve survival.

Adenocarcinoma commonly involves the gastric cardia and may therefore extend into the fundus or down the lesser curve. Some degree of gastric excision is essential in order to achieve adequate local clearance and accomplish an appropriate lymphadenectomy. Excision of contiguous structures, such as crura, diaphragm and mediastinal pleura, needs to be considered as a method of creating negative resection margins.

The rarity of intramucosal cancer in symptomatic patients means that there are no randomised studies to compare different approaches to this type of very early disease. Even in Barrett's oesophagus, where high-grade dysplasia and early cancer coexist, many centres favour oesophagectomy in fit patients. Endoscopic mucosal resection for these apparently early lesions has become increasingly popular, providing either a cure or at least sufficient histological information upon which to base a further management strategy. Photodynamic therapy (PDT) is an alternative approach that has largely been used in patients who were either unfit or unwilling to undergo surgery. This endoscopic technique relies on the administration of a photosensitiser that is taken up preferentially by dysplastic and malignant cells followed by exposure of an appropriate segment of the oesophagus to laser light. The main drawback is skin photosensitisation, so patients must avoid sunlight exposure in the short term. PDT is also associated with a risk of stricture formation although, as the technique and photosensitising agents improve, these problems are reducing.

Surgery alone is best suited to patients with disease confined to the oesophagus (T1, T2) without nodal metastasis (N0). As a result of careful preoperative investigation, most of these patients are now identifiable and can be offered surgery alone, with a prospect of cure between 50 and 80 per cent. Patients with more advanced stages of disease require either multimodal approaches or entry into appropriate trials.

It is essential that oesophagectomy should be performed with a low hospital mortality and complication rate. Case selection, volume and experience of the surgical team are all important. Preoperative risk analysis has shown that this can play a major part in reducing hospital mortality. There are really no circumstances in the Western world in which surgery should be undertaken if it is not part of an overall treatment plan aimed at cure (Summary box 62.12).

Summary box 62.12

Treatment of carcinoma of the oesophagus

- Radical oesophagectomy is the most important aspect of curative treatment
- Neoadjuvant treatments before surgery may improve survival in a proportion of patients
- Chemoradiotherapy alone may cure selected patients, particularly those with squamous cell cancers
- Useful palliation may be achieved by chemo/radiotherapy or endoscopic treatments

Treatments with curative intent

Surgery

Histological tumour type, location and the extent of the proposed lymphadenectomy all influence the operative approach. This is largely an issue of surgical preference, although it should be recognised that a left thoracoabdominal approach is limited proximally by the aortic arch and should be avoided when the primary tumour is at or above this level. Similarly, transhiatal oesophagectomy is unsuitable for most patients with squamous cell carcinoma because a complete mediastinal lymphadenectomy is not easily achieved by this approach. The most widely practised approach in the West is the two-phase Ivor Lewis (sometimes called Lewis–Tanner) operation (Figure 62.53), with an initial laparotomy and construction of a gastric tube, followed by a right thoracotomy to excise the tumour and create an oesophagogastric anastomosis. The closer this is placed to the apex of the thoracic cavity, the fewer problems there are

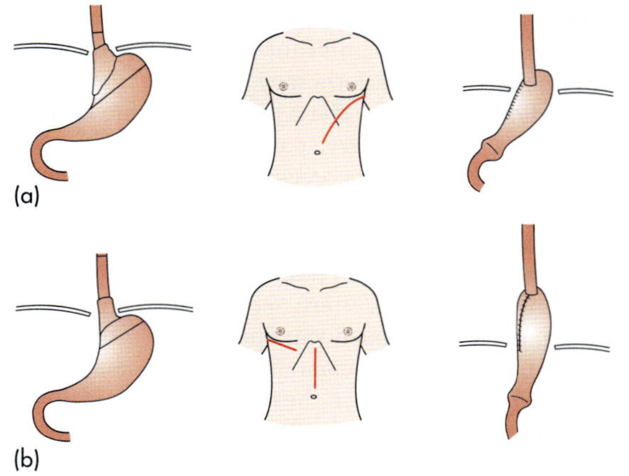

Figure 62.53 The two usual approaches for surgery of the oesophagus are the thoracoabdominal (a), which opens the abdominal and thoracic cavities together, and the two-stage Ivor Lewis approach (b), in which the abdomen is opened first, closed and then the thoracotomy is performed. In the McKeown operation, a third incision in the neck is made to complete the cervical anastomosis.

with reflux disease. Three-phase oesophagectomy (McKeown) may be more appropriate for more proximal tumours in order to achieve better longitudinal clearance, although the additional distance gained is less than many surgeons believe. A third cervical incision also permits lymphadenectomy in this region.

The extent of lymphadenectomy is highly controversial. For squamous cell carcinoma, because a higher proportion of patients will have middle- and upper-third tumours in the thoracic oesophagus, the rationale behind a three-phase operation with three-field lymphadenectomy is more understandable, even though this approach has not been widely adopted in the West. For adenocarcinoma, the incidence of metastases in the neck is relatively low in the context of patients who would otherwise be curable. For this reason, two-phase operations with two-field lymphadenectomy seem the most logical operations. While two-field lymphadenectomy does not substantially increase operative morbidity or mortality, the same cannot be said for more extended operations.

The introduction of minimal access techniques has been pioneered in Australia by Gotley and Smithers and in North America by Luketich. In experienced hands, the open operation can be reproduced without significant compromise. As yet, benefits seem to be confined to reduced wound pain and the absence of specific complications associated with long incisions.

While many centres have reduced hospital mortality to single figures following oesophagectomy, the complication rate remains high. At least one-third of all patients will develop some significant complication after surgery. The most common of these is respiratory, followed by anastomotic leakage, chylothorax and injury to the recurrent laryngeal nerves. The most common late problem is benign anastomotic stricture, which seems to be higher with cervical rather than with intrathoracic anastomoses, although the problem is usually easily dealt with by endoscopic dilatation.

Lesions of the cardia that do not involve the oesophagus to any significant extent may be dealt with by extended total gastrectomy to include the distal oesophagus, or by proximal gastrectomy and distal oesophagectomy (Summary box 62.13).

Summary box 62.13

Oesophagogastric surgery

- Beware of satellite nodules proximal to the primary lesion
- Carefully preserve the blood supply of the stomach, both venous and arterial
- Right thoracic approach gives easy access to the oesophagus

Two-phase oesophagectomy (abdomen and right chest, Ivor Lewis)

Mobilisation of the stomach must be done with care as it is essential to have a tension-free, well-vascularised stomach for transposition. The left gastric, short gastric and left gastroepiploic arteries are all divided. The viability of the transposed stomach mainly depends on the right gastroepiploic and, to a lesser extent, the right gastric vessels. It should be noted that venous drainage is as important as arterial supply, and it is essential to perform an accurate anatomical dissection that preserves the

Ivor Lewis, 1895–1982, surgeon, the North Middlesex Hospital, London, UK, and later at Rhyl, North Wales, UK.
Norman Cecil Tanner, 1906–1982, surgeon, Charing Cross Hospital, London, UK.
Kenneth Charles McKeown, 1912–1995, surgeon, Darlington Memorial Hospital, Darlington, County Durham, UK.

right gastroepiploic vein as well as the artery. The stomach is divided to remove the cardia and the upper part of the lesser curve, including the whole of the left gastric artery and its associated lymph nodes.

The approach to the oesophagus through the right chest is straightforward. A thoracotomy with entry above the fifth rib gives excellent access to the mediastinum and the thoracic inlet. The azygos vein is divided, and the whole of the intrathoracic oesophagus can be mobilised along with the thoracic duct (which is ligated by most surgeons) and the mediastinal lymph nodes. The oesophagus is divided just below the thoracic inlet. As most lesions are in the lower or middle thirds, this usually gives adequate proximal clearance of at least 5 cm. Carcinomas of the upper thoracic oesophagus are almost always incurable at the time of diagnosis, and invasion of the trachea is common. If one of these lesions is resectable, it is essential to use an incision in the neck (McKeown or three-phase operation) and to resect more of the oesophagus than is customary in the operation of subtotal oesophagectomy.

Oesophagogastric anastomosis may be performed equally well by hand or by stapler. Both methods require attention to detail. In experienced hands, clinical anastomotic leakage should be less than 5 per cent. Most surgeons still prefer to keep the patient nil-by-mouth for 5–7 days. Most centres have abandoned the use of routine contrast swallows in patients who are clinically well. Conversely, aggressive investigation of a suspected leak is mandatory for any unexplained fever or clinical event. This may involve contrast radiology, CT scan or endoscopy to resolve the situation adequately.

Postoperative nutritional support remains controversial. There is general agreement that parenteral feeding is associated with more nosocomial infection, including pneumonia, than enteral feeding. It is also expensive. If nutritional support is given, a feeding jejunostomy is probably the best method.

Transhiatal oesophagectomy (without thoracotomy)

This approach was popularised for cancer by Orringer, adapting a technique developed in Brazil by Pinotti for the removal of Chagasic megaoesophagus (see below under Achalasia). The stomach is mobilised through a midline abdominal incision, and the cervical oesophagus is mobilised through an incision in the neck. The diaphragm is then opened from the abdomen, and the posterior mediastinum is entered. The lower oesophagus and the tumour are mobilised under direct vision, and the upper oesophagus is mobilised by blunt dissection. This approach can provide an adequate removal of the tumour and lymph nodes in the lower mediastinum, but it is not possible to remove the nodes in the middle or upper mediastinum. It may be a useful procedure for lesions of the lower oesophagus, but is hazardous for a middle-third lesion that may be adherent to the bronchus or to the azygos vein.

Neoadjuvant treatments with surgery

Apart from the earliest stages of disease, surgery alone produces relatively few cures in either squamous cell carcinoma or adenocarcinoma patients. This led to a number of trials throughout the 1980s and 1990s to investigate the value of chemotherapy and surgery or chemoradiotherapy and surgery compared with surgery alone. Some studies relate only to squamous cell cancer, and many are open to criticism on the grounds of trial design or patient numbers. Nevertheless, positive results in favour of neoadjuvant therapy for adenocarcinoma in two studies as well as a limited meta-analysis indicate that it is no longer appropriate to consider surgery alone as the 'gold standard' treatment for most patients who are surgical candidates with adenocarcinoma. The exact role of surgery in a multimodal approach to squamous cell carcinoma is an unresolved issue.

Gastro-oesophageal reflux following oesophagogastric resection

Gastro-oesophageal reflux may be a major problem following any operation that involves resecting the cardia. Reflux may present with the typical symptoms of GORD or with a peptic stricture at the site of the anastomosis. However, the presentation may be different with a miserable patient who fails to thrive following the operation and who is then suspected of having recurrent cancer. This atypical presentation is particularly common following total gastrectomy with an inadequate reconstruction that allows bile reflux (Summary box 62.14).

Summary box 62.14

Postoesophagectomy

- Reflux may be a problem following resection
- Symptoms may be atypical
- Reflux may be limited or avoided by subtotal oesophagectomy and gastric transposition high in the chest

Non-surgical treatments

Radiotherapy alone was widely used as a single-modality treatment for squamous cell carcinoma of the oesophagus until the late 1970s. The five-year survival rate overall was 6 per cent. As a result, multimodal approaches were adopted throughout the 1980s, initial trials indicating that similar long-term survival rates could be obtained with surgery. Subsequent randomised studies essentially confined to patients with squamous cell carcinoma have indicated significant survival advantages with chemoradiotherapy over radiotherapy alone. While it is clear that chemoradiotherapy does offer a prospect of cure for patients who may not be fit for surgery, particularly in squamous cell carcinoma, the high rate of locoregional failure has meant that surgery remains the mainstay of attempted curative treatments for both adenocarcinoma and squamous cell carcinoma in patients who have potentially resectable disease and are fit for oesophagectomy. In most Western series, this represents about one-third of patients with adenocarcinoma and a slightly lower percentage of patients with squamous cell carcinoma. There has been no formal comparison of the results of definitive radiotherapy or chemoradiotherapy and surgical resection, and it is therefore impossible to make dogmatic statements about the relative merits of each form of treatment (Summary box 62.15).

Summary box 62.15

Alternative therapeutic approaches

- Chemoradiotherapy may be a useful alternative to surgery, especially in unfit patients

Mark Burton Orringer, surgeon, Ann Arbor, MI, USA.
Walter Pinotti, Professor of Surgery, Sao Paulo, Brazil.
Carlos Justiniano Ribeiro Chagas, 1879–1934, Director, the Oswaldo Cruz Institute, and Professor of Tropical Medicine, the University of Rio de Janiero, Brazil.

Palliative treatment

Surgical resection and external beam radiotherapy may be used for palliation, but are not suitable when the expected survival is short, as most of the remainder of life will be spent recovering from the 'treatment'. Surgical bypass is likewise too major a procedure for use in a patient with limited life expectancy. A variety of relatively simple methods of palliation are now available that will produce worthwhile relief of dysphagia with minimal disturbance to the patient (Summary box 62.16).

Summary box 62.16

Palliation

- Palliation should be simple and effective

Intubation has been used for many years following the invention of the Souttar tube, which was made of coiled silver wire. A variety of rigid plastic or rubber tubes were developed for placement under endoscopic and/or radiological control. The technology of intubation has now moved on with the development of various types of expanding metal stent (Figure 62.54). These are also inserted under radiographic or endoscopic control. The stent is collapsed during insertion and released when it is in the correct position. Expanding stents produce a wider lumen for swallowing than rigid tubes. More importantly, it is not necessary to dilate the oesophagus to beyond 8 mm to insert the unexpanded stent through the tumour, so there is a lower risk of injury to the oesophagus.

Endoscopic laser treatment may be used to core a channel through the tumour. It is based on thermal tumour destruction. It produces a worthwhile improvement in swallowing, but has the disadvantage that it has to be repeated every few weeks. Lasers may also be used to unblock a stent that has become occluded by tumour overgrowth. **Other endoscopic methods** include bipolar diathermy, argon-beam plasma coagulation and alcohol injection.

Brachytherapy is a method of delivering intraluminal radiation with a short penetration distance (hence the term brachy) to a tumour. An introduction system is inserted through the tumour, and the treatment is then delivered in a single session lasting approximately 20 minutes. The equipment is expensive to purchase, but running costs are low.

While the above methods are suitable for patients with very advanced disease, the elderly and those with significant comorbidities that would make more aggressive strategies inappropriate, an increasing proportion of patients (particularly with adenocarcinoma) are being treated by platinum-based chemotherapy. In general, this leads to only a modest prolongation of survival but a better quality of life than in those receiving an endoscopic treatment alone.

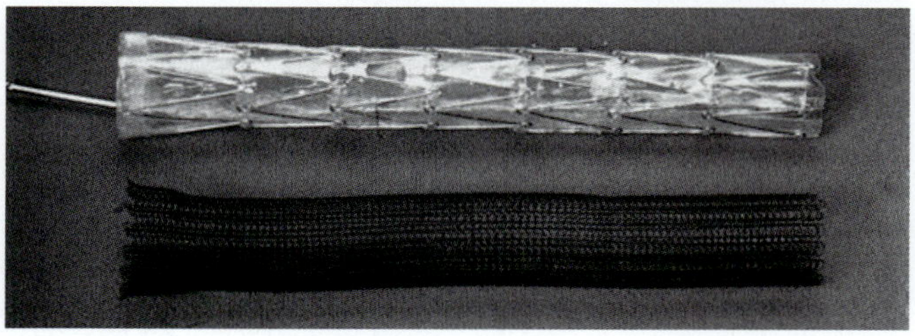

Figure 62.54 Expanding metal stents, covered and uncovered.

Malignant tracheo-oesophageal fistula

Malignant tracheo-oesophageal fistula is a sign of incurable disease. Some have advocated surgical bypass and oesophageal exclusion, but this is a major procedure. An expanding metal stent is probably the best treatment.

Post-cricoid carcinoma

Post-cricoid carcinoma is considered in Chapter 48 in neoplasms of the pharynx.

MOTILITY DISORDERS AND DIVERTICULA

Oesophageal motility disorders

A motility disorder can be readily understood when a patient has dysphagia in the absence of a stricture, and a barium-impregnated food bolus is seen to stick in the oesophagus. If this can be correlated with a specific abnormality on oesophageal manometry, accepting that this is the cause of the patient's symptoms may be straightforward. Unfortunately, this is often not the case. Pain, with or without a swallowing problem, is frequently the dominant symptom, and patients often undergo extensive hospital investigation before the oesophagus is considered as a source of symptoms. Symptoms are often intermittent, and the correlation between symptoms and test 'abnormalities' is poor. Much harm may be done by inappropriate enthusiastic surgery for ill-defined conditions. It should also be remembered that oesophageal dysmotility may be only a feature of a general disturbance in gastrointestinal function (Summary box 62.17).

Summary box 62.17

Oesophageal motility disorders

- May be part of a more diffuse gastrointestinal motility problem
- May be associated with GORD

It is convenient to classify oesophageal motility disorders as in Table 62.3.

Functional pain and the oesophagus

Pain that is assumed to arise from dysfunction of the gastrointestinal tract may reflect abnormal motor activity, abnormal perception or a combination of the two. There is evidence that all three exist. Very high-pressure uncoordinated contractions ('spasm') have been shown to correlate with pain. Distension of a balloon in the oesophagus indicates that some patients have a low threshold for the sensation of pain (visceral hypersensitivity), and this itself may reflect local or central neuronal dysfunction. In practice, the difficulty is in understanding the relative contributions of these elements, so that a logical treatment might follow.

Sir Henry Sessions Souttar, 1875–1964, surgeon, the London Hospital, London, UK.

Table 62.3 Classification of oesophageal motility disorders

Disorders of the pharyngo-oesophageal junction	Neurological – stroke, motor neurone disease, multiple sclerosis, Parkinson's disease
	Myogenic – myasthenia, muscular dystrophy
	Pharyngo-oesophageal (Zenker's) diverticulum
Disorders of the body of the oesophagus	Diffuse oesophageal spasm
	Nutcracker oesophagus
	Autoimmune disorders – especially systemic sclerosis (CREST)
	Reflux associated
	Idiopathic
	Allergic
	Eosinophilic oesophagitis
	Non-specific oesophageal dysmotility
Disorders of the lower oesophageal sphincter	Achalasia
	Incompetent lower sphincter (i.e. GORD)

CREST, calcinosis, Raynaud's syndrome, (o)esophageal motility disorders, sclerodactyly and telangiectasia; GORD, gastro-oesophageal reflux disease.

Achalasia

Pathology and aetiology

Achalasia (Greek 'failure to relax') is uncommon, but merits prominence because it is reasonably understood and responds to treatment. It is due to loss of the ganglion cells in the myenteric (Auerbach's) plexus, the cause of which is unknown. In South America, chronic infection with the parasite *Trypanosoma cruzi* causes Chagas' disease, which has marked clinical similarities to achalasia. Achalasia differs from Hirschsprung's disease of the colon because the dilated oesophagus usually contains few ganglion cells, whereas the dilated colon contains normal ganglion cells proximal to a constricted, aganglionic segment. Histology of muscle specimens generally shows a reduction in the number of ganglion cells (and mainly inhibitory neurones) with a variable degree of chronic inflammation. In so-called 'vigorous achalasia', which may be an early stage of the disease, there is inflammation and neural fibrosis, but normal numbers of ganglion cells (Summary box 62.18).

The classic physiological abnormalities are a non-relaxing LOS and absent peristalsis in the body of the oesophagus. While most patients have almost no recognisable contractions, 'vigorous' achalsia has been recognised for many years as a condition where, in its earliest stages, the oesophagus is of normal calibre and still exhibits contractile (although non-peristaltic) activity. In some patients, these uncoordinated contractions result in pain as much as a sense of food sticking. High-resolution manometry indicates that there are a number of contraction patterns and these may be important in predicting the outcome of treatment. With time, the oesophagus dilates and contractions disappear, so that the oesophagus empties mainly by the hydrostatic pressure of its contents. This is nearly always incomplete, leaving residual food and fluid. The gas bubble in the stomach is frequently absent, as no bolus with its accompanying normal gas passes through the sphincter. The 'megaoesophagus' becomes tortuous with a persistent retention oesophagitis due to fermentation of food residues (Figure 62.55), and this may account for the increased incidence of carcinoma of the oesophagus (Summary box 62.19).

Harald Hirschsprung, 1831–1916, physician, the Queen Louise Hospital for Children, and Professor of Paediatrics, Copenhagen, Denmark, described congenital megacolon in 1888.

Summary box 62.18

Achalasia

- Is uncommon
- Is due to selective loss of inhibitory neurones in the lower oesophagus
- The causes dysphagia and carcinoma must be excluded
- Treatment is by either endoscopic dilatation or surgical myotomy

Summary box 62.19

Lower oesophageal stricture

- Beware pseudoachalasia; look for tumour

Pseudoachalasia is an achalasia-like disorder that is usually produced by adenocarcinoma of the cardia (Figure 62.56), but has also been described in relation to benign tumours at this level. It has been presumed that the inability of the sphincter to relax is linked to the loss of body peristalsis, but other cancers outside the oesophagus (bronchus, pancreas) have also been associated with pseudoachalasia.

Clinical features

The disease is most common in middle life, but can occur at any age. It typically presents with dysphagia, although pain (often mistaken for reflux) is common in the early stages. Patients often present late and, having had relatively mild symptoms, remain untreated for many years. Regurgitation is frequent, and there may be overspill into the trachea, especially at night.

Diagnosis

Achalasia may be suspected at endoscopy by finding a tight cardia and food residue in the oesophagus. Barium radiology may show hold-up in the distal oesophagus, abnormal contractions in the oesophageal body and a tapering stricture in the distal oesophagus, often described as a 'bird's beak' (see Figure 62.55). The gastric gas bubble is usually absent. These typical features of well-developed achalasia are often absent, and endoscopy and radiology can be normal. A firm diagnosis is established by oesophageal manometry. Classically, the LOS does not relax completely on swallowing, there is no peristalsis and there is a raised resting pressure in the oesophagus (Figure 62.57). The LOS pressure may be elevated, but is often normal.

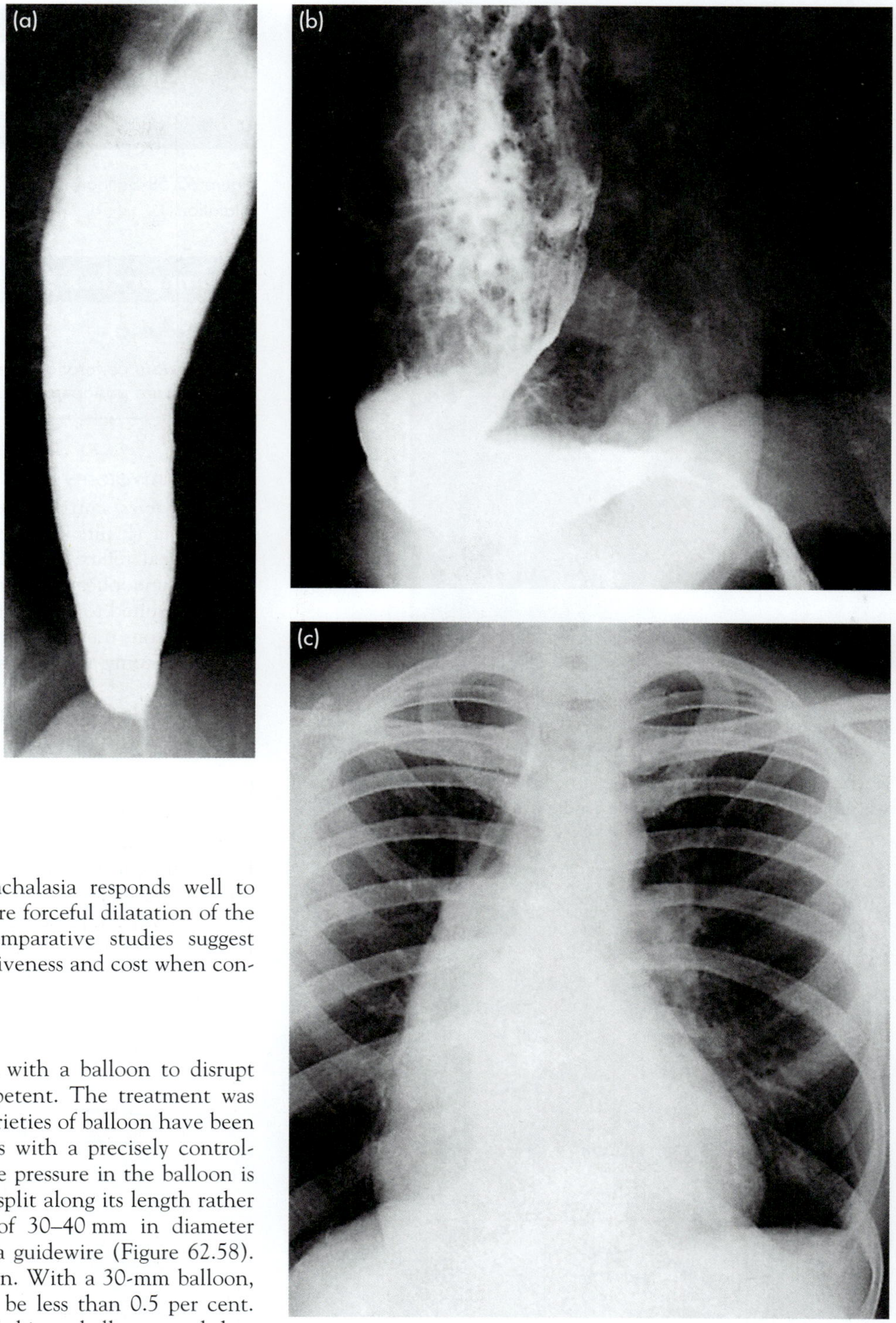

Figure 62.55 Achalasia of the oesophagus. (a) Barium swallow showing the smooth outline of the stricture, which narrows to a point at its lower end. (b) Tortuosity and sigmoid appearance of the lower oesophagus. (c) Mediastinal shadow due to a large, fluid-filled oesophagus.

Treatment

Alone among motility disorders, achalasia responds well to treatment. The two main methods are forceful dilatation of the cardia and Heller's myotomy. Comparative studies suggest equivalence in terms of safety, effectiveness and cost when considered over a number of years.

Pneumatic dilatation

This involves stretching the cardia with a balloon to disrupt the muscle and render it less competent. The treatment was first described by Plummer. Many varieties of balloon have been used but, nowadays, plastic balloons with a precisely controlled external diameter are used. If the pressure in the balloon is too high, the balloon is designed to split along its length rather than expanding further. Balloons of 30–40 mm in diameter are available and are inserted over a guidewire (Figure 62.58). Perforation is the major complication. With a 30-mm balloon, the incidence of perforation should be less than 0.5 per cent. The risk of perforation increases with bigger balloons, and they should be used cautiously for progressive dilatation over a period of weeks. Forceful dilatation is curative in 75–85 per cent of cases. The results are best in patients aged more than 45 years (Summary box 62.20).

Ernst Heller, 1877–1964, surgeon, St George's Krankenhaus, Leipzig, Germany, described his operation in 1914 when he performed a double myotomy. In 1923, JH Zaaijer from Leiden in The Netherlands reported that a single anterior mytomy is as good which is performed today.

Henry Stanley Plummer, 1874–1937, physician, the Mayo Clinic, Rochester, MN, USA.

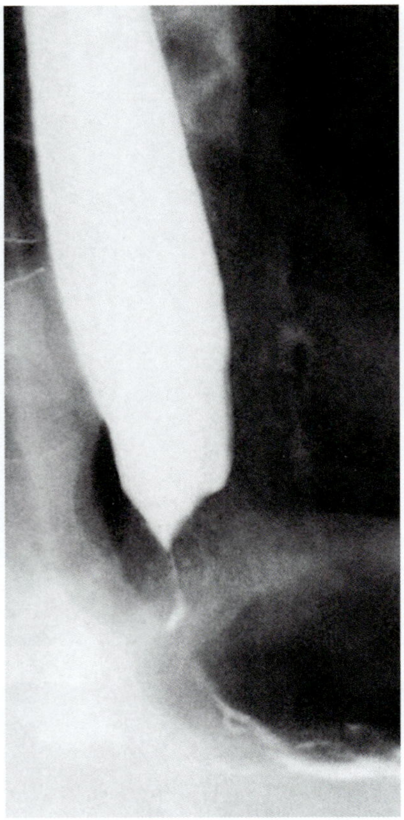

Figure 62.56 Almost achalasia, but note the irregularity of the taper, which indicates carcinoma of the cardia.

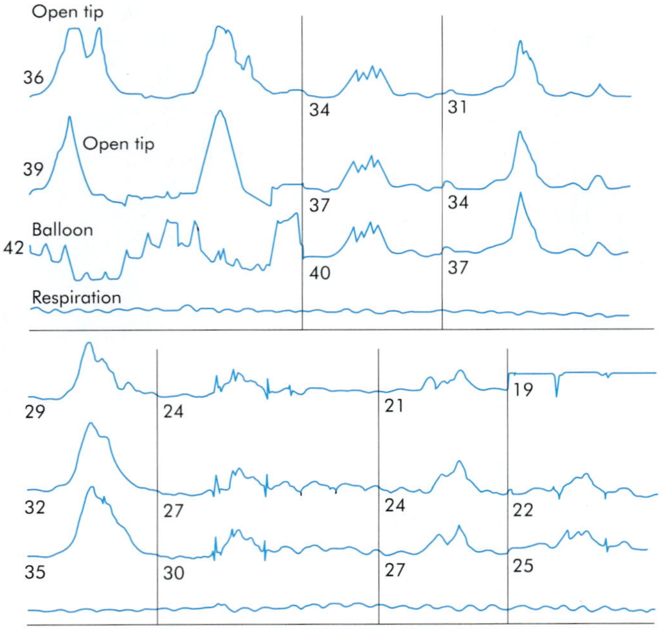

Figure 62.57 Manometry in achalasia, showing simultaneous contractions in the body of the oesophagus and incomplete relaxation of the lower oesophageal sphincter (LOS) in response to swallowing.

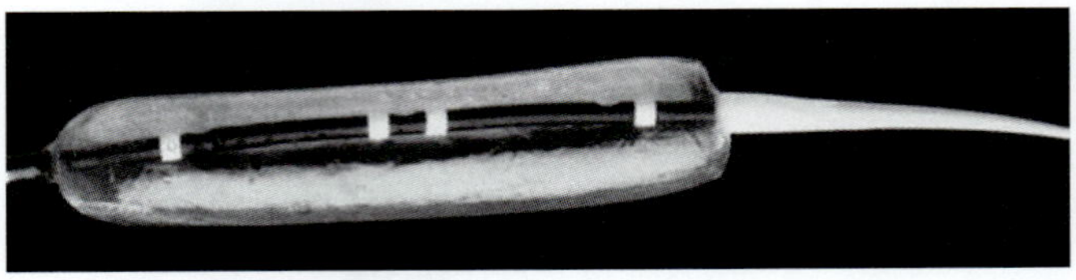

Figure 62.58 Balloon dilator for the treatment of achalasia by forceful dilatation.

Summary box 62.20

Achalasia

- Beware perforation due to dilatation of achalasia
- Beware postoperative reflux

Heller's myotomy

This involves cutting the muscle of the lower oesophagus and cardia (Figure 62.59). The major complication is gastro-oesophageal reflux, and most surgeons therefore add a partial anterior fundoplication (Heller-Dor's operation). The procedure is ideally suited to a minimal access laparoscopic approach, and most surgeons use intraoperative endoscopy to judge the extent of the myotomy and to ensure that the narrow segment is abolished.

It is successful in more than 90 per cent of cases and may be used after failed dilatation.

Botulinum toxin

This is done by endoscopic injection into the LOS. It acts by interfering with cholinergic excitatory neural activity at the LOS. The effect is not permanent, and the injection usually

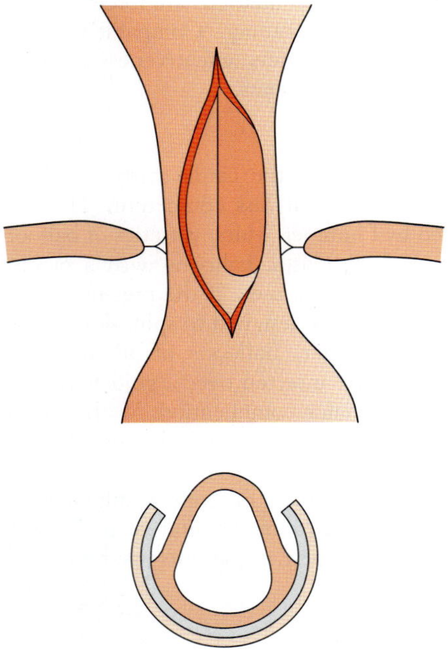

Figure 62.59 Heller's myotomy. The incision should not go too far on to the stomach. The lateral extent must enable the mucosa to pout out, to prevent the edges healing together.

has to be repeated after a few months. For this reason, its use is restricted to elderly patients with other comorbidities.

Drugs

Drugs such as calcium channel antagonists have been used but are ineffective for long-term use. However, sublingual nifedipine may be useful for transient relief of symptoms if definitive treatment is postponed.

Other oesophageal motility disorders

Disorders of the pharyngo-oesophageal junction

With the exception of Zenker's diverticulum (see below), most patients with oropharyngeal dysphagia have generalised neurological or muscular disorders with pharyngeal involvement. A small number of patients who have sustained a cerebrovascular accident benefit from myotomy of the cricopharyngeus to alleviate pooling of saliva and nocturnal aspiration, but they should have good deglutition and phonation before this is performed. The operation is also effective in patients with oculopharyngeal muscular dystrophy.

Disorders of the body of the oesophagus

Diffuse oesophageal spasm and nutcracker oesophagus

Diffuse oesophageal spasm is a condition in which there are incoordinate contractions of the oesophagus, causing dysphagia and/or chest pain. The condition may be dramatic, with spastic pressures on manometry of 400–500 mmHg, marked hypertrophy of the circular muscle and a corkscrew oesophagus on barium swallow (Figure 62.60). These abnormal contractions are more common in the distal two-thirds of the oesophageal body, and this may have some relevance to treatment. Making the diagnosis when chest pain is the only symptom may be difficult. Prolonged ambulatory oesophageal manometry that correlates episodes of chest pain with manometric abnormalities may establish the diagnosis.

There is no proven pharmacological or endoscopic treatment. Calcium channel antagonists, vasodilators and endoscopic dilatation have only transient effects. While the severity and frequency of symptoms may be tolerated by most patients, sometimes the combination of chest pain and dysphagia is sufficiently severe that malnutrition begins. In these patients, extended oesophageal myotomy up to the aortic arch may be required. Surgical treatment of diffuse spasm is more successful in improving dysphagia than chest pain, and caution should be exercised in patients in whom chest pain is the only symptom.

Nutcracker oesophagus is a condition in which peristaltic pressures of more than 180 mmHg develop. It is said to cause chest pain, but there is still some debate as to whether it is a real disorder.

Oesophageal involvement in autoimmune disease

Oesophageal involvement is mainly seen in systemic sclerosis, but may be a feature of polymyositis, dermatomyositis, systemic lupus erythematosus, polyarteritis nodosa or rheumatoid disease. While most involve weak peristalsis, swallowing difficulties may be compounded by pharyngeal problems in the disorders that primarily affect skeletal muscle (e.g. polymyositis) or extraoesophageal problems such as involvement of the cricoarytenoid joint in rheumatoid disease or dry mouth in Sjögren's syndrome. In systemic sclerosis, smooth muscle atrophy causes hypoperistalsis (Figure 62.61). The LOS is involved, leading to a loss of the antireflux barrier. A wide range of symptoms can follow from mild to severe dysphagia accompanied by regurgitation and aspiration. Reflux can be severe and is exacerbated by weak acid clearance so that strictures can occur. There are no drugs that specifically correct the motor disorder, and medical treatment is mainly directed at minimising reflux-induced damage with PPIs. A small number of patients may require antireflux surgery.

Eosinophilic oesophagitis is a disorder that occurs in children and adults either alone or as a manifestation of eosinophilic gastroenteritis. It is characterised by eosinophilic infiltration of the oesophageal wall, presumably of allergic or idiopathic origin. The most common presenting symptom is dysphagia,

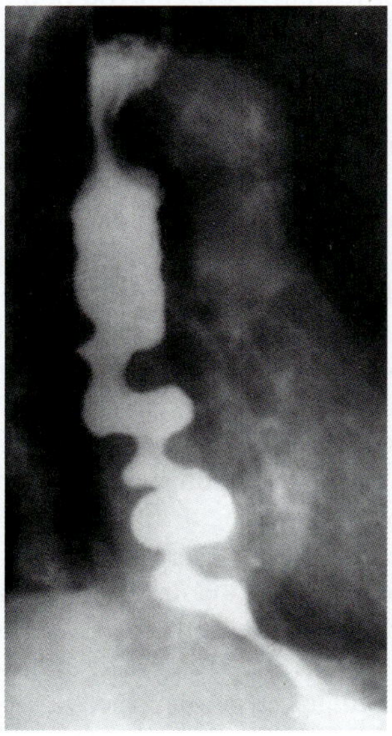

Figure 62.60 Corkscrew oesophagus in diffuse oesophageal spasm.

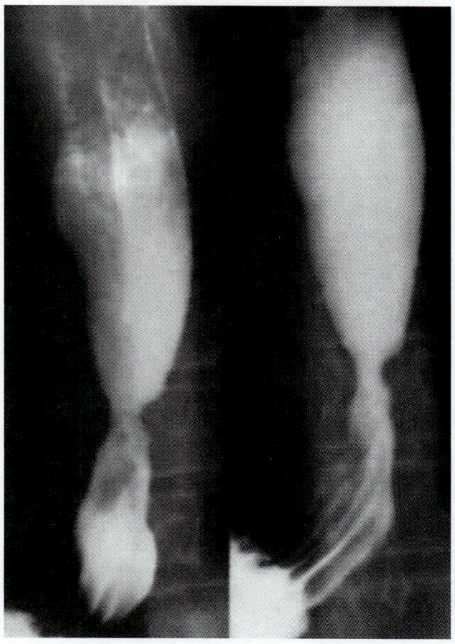

Figure 62.61 Advanced scleroderma of the oesophagus. The oesophagus dilates, and the lower oesophageal sphincter is widely incompetent.

Friedrich Albert Zenker, 1825–1898, Professor of Pathology, Dresden, Germany.

and more than half have some history of atopy. The oesophagus often seems narrow and friable on endoscopy and may include mucosal rings. The most important feature is the development of deep ulcers leading to stricture development, especially in the proximal oesophagus. The diagnosis is established by endoscopic biopsy.

Elimination diets, topical and systemic steroids all seem to be helpful in the short term, but there is scant information on the long-term impact of any particular approach. Immunotherapy directed against interleukin (IL)-5, which has a major role in eosinophil recruitment, seems to be a promising innovative approach. Although endoscopic dilatation has been recommended, this can create deep ulcers and further scarring, so should be used with caution and only when the above therapies fail.

Pharyngeal and oesophageal diverticula

Most oesophageal diverticula are **pulsion** diverticula that develop at a site of weakness as a result of chronic pressure against an obstruction. Symptoms are mostly caused by the underlying disorder unless the diverticulum is particularly large. **Traction** diverticula (Figure 62.62) are much less common. They are mostly a consequence of chronic granulomatous disease affecting the tracheobronchial lymph nodes due to tuberculosis, atypical mycobacteria or histoplasmosis. Fibrotic healing of the lymph nodes exerts traction on the oesophageal wall and produces a focal outpouching that is usually small and has a conical shape. There may be associated broncholithiasis, and additional complications may occur, such as aerodigestive fistulation (Figure 62.63) and bleeding.

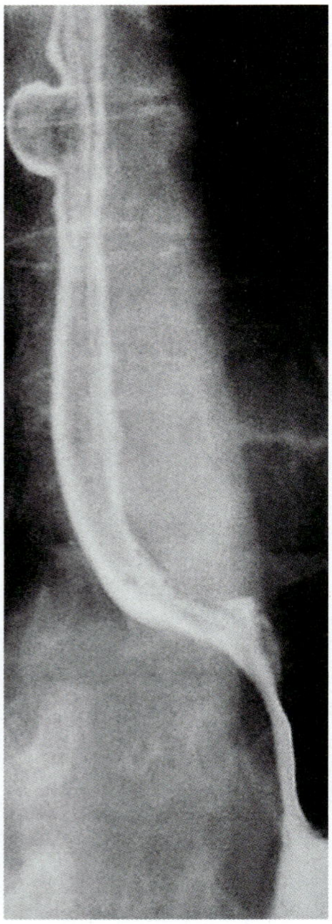

Figure 62.62 Mid-oesophageal traction diverticulum with the mouth facing downwards.

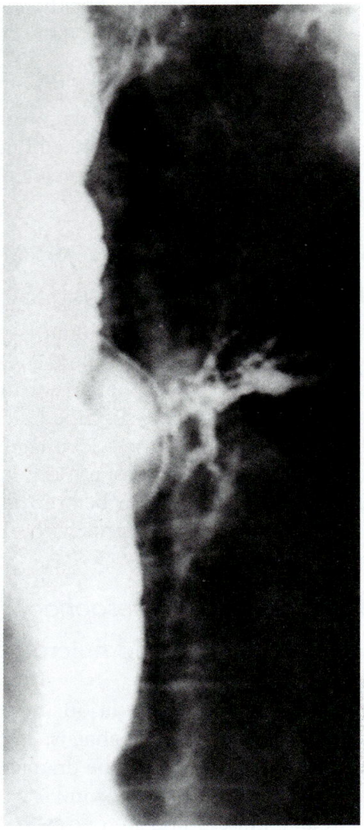

Figure 62.63 Mid-oesophageal diverticulum with a tracheo-oesophageal fistula.

Zenker's diverticulum (pharyngeal pouch) is not really an oesophageal diverticulum as it protrudes posteriorly above the cricopharyngeal sphincter through the natural weak point (the dehiscence of Killian) between the oblique and horizontal (cricopharyngeus) fibres of the inferior pharyngeal constrictor (Figures 62.64 and 62.65). The exact mechanism that leads to its formation is unknown, but it involves loss of the coordination between pharyngeal contraction and opening of the upper sphincter. When the diverticulum is small, symptoms largely reflect this incoordination with predominantly pharyngeal dysphagia. As the pouch enlarges, it tends to fill with food on eating, and the fundus descends into the mediastinum. This leads to halitosis and oesophageal dysphagia. Treatment can be undertaken endoscopically with a linear cutting stapler to divide the septum between the diverticulum and the upper oesophagus, producing a diverticulo-oesophagostomy, or can be done by open surgery involving pouch excision, pouch suspension (diverticulopexy) and/or myotomy of the cricopharyngeus. All techniques have good results.

Mid-oesophageal diverticula are usually small pulsion diverticula of no particular consequence. The underlying motility disorder does not usually require treatment. Some pulsion diverticula may fistulate into the trachea (Figure 62.63), but this is more common with traction diverticula in granulomatous disease.

Henrik Samuel Conrad Sjögren, 1899–1986, Professor of Ophthalmology, Gothenburg, Sweden.
Gustav Killian, 1860–1921, Professor of Laryngology at Freiburg, and later at Berlin, Germany.

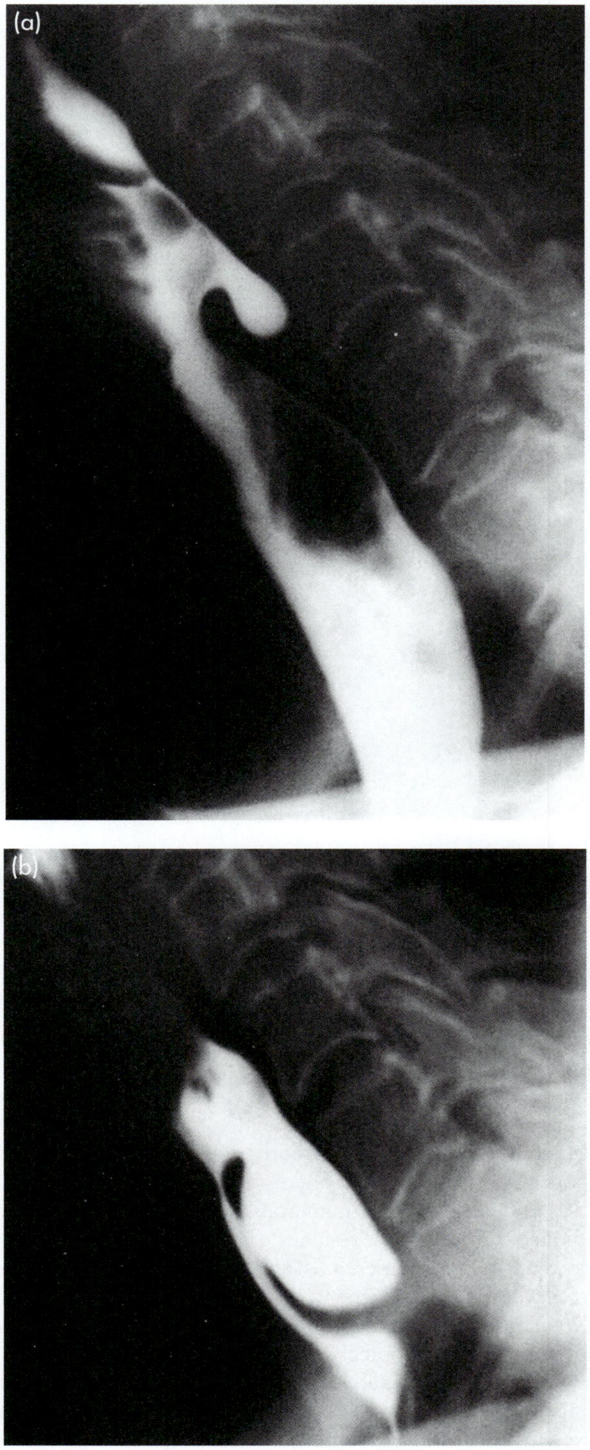

Figure 62.64 The typical appearances of: (a) a small pharyngeal pouch with a prominent cricopharyngeal impression and 'streaming' of barium, indicating partial obstruction; and (b) a large pouch extending behind the oesophagus towards the thoracic inlet.

Epiphrenic diverticula are pulsion diverticula situated in the lower oesophagus above the diaphragm (Figure 62.66). They may be quite large, but cause surprisingly few symptoms. They again probably reflect some loss of coordination between an

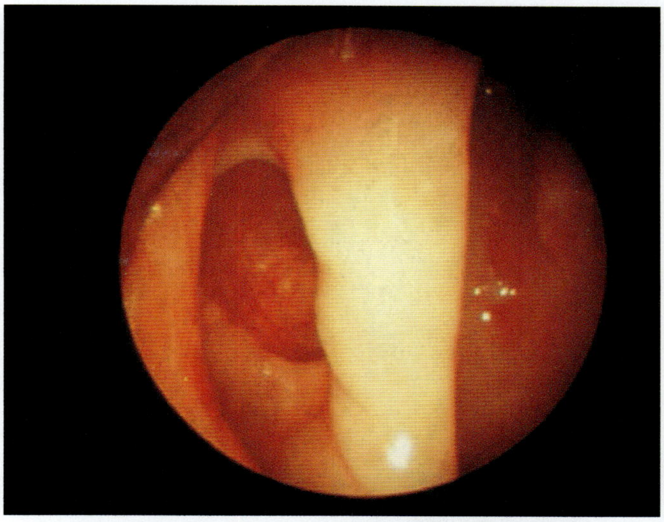

Figure 62.65 The endoscopic appearance of the mouth of a pharyngeal pouch posterior to the normal opening (left) of the oesophagus.

incoming pressure wave and appropriate relaxation of the LOS. This needs to be acknowledged in the surgical management of the patient. The diverticulum, in isolation, should not be assumed to account for a patient's illness just because it looks dramatic on a radiograph. Large diverticula may be excised, and this should be combined with a myotomy from the site of the diverticulum down to the cardia to relieve functional obstruction (Summary box 62.21).

Summary box 62.21

Oesophageal diverticula

- Diverticula are indicators of a motor disorder and not necessarily the cause of symptoms

Diffuse intramural pseudodiverticulosis is a rare condition in which there are multiple tiny outpouchings from the lumen of the oesophagus. The pseudodiverticula are dilated excretory ducts of oesophageal sebaceous glands. It is questionable whether the condition produces any symptoms in its own right.

OTHER NON-NEOPLASTIC CONDITIONS

Schatzki's ring

Schatzki's ring is a circular ring in the distal oesophagus (Figure 62.67), usually at the squamocolumnar junction. The cause is obscure, but there is a strong association with reflux disease. The core of the ring consists of variable amounts of fibrous tissue and cellular infiltrate. Most rings are incidental findings. Some are associated with dysphagia and respond to dilatation in conjunction with medical antireflux therapy.

Richard Schatski, 1901–1992, American radiologist, a German by birth and medical training, he became Chief of Radiology Department, Mount Auburn Hospital, Cambridge. MA, USA.

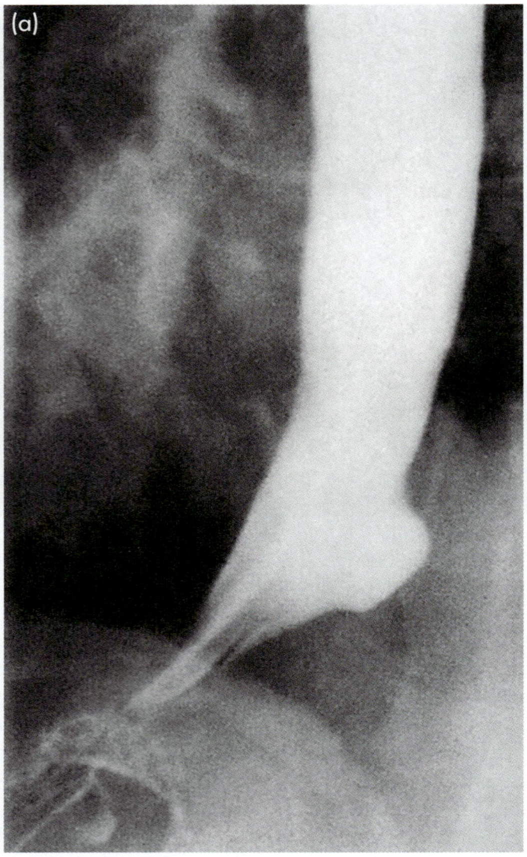

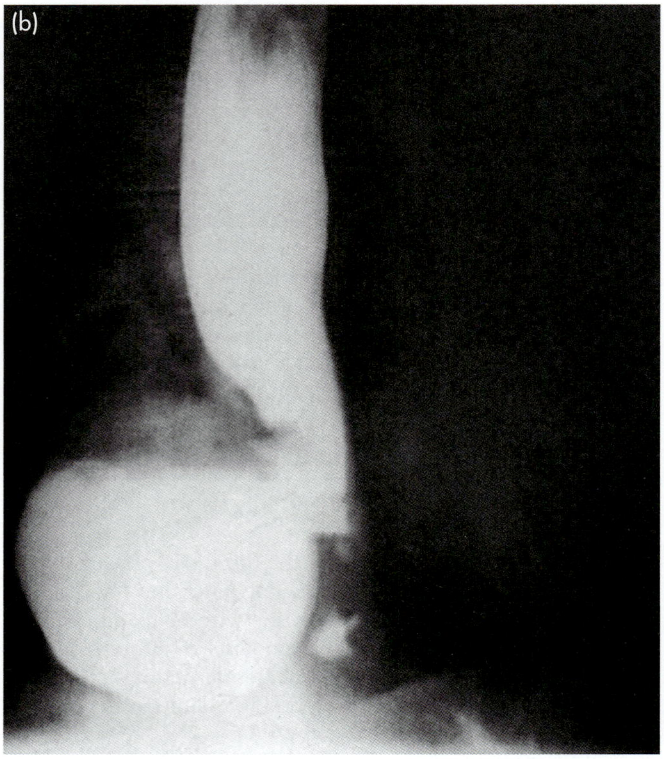

Figure 62.66 Epiphrenic diverticulum proximal to the gastro-oesophageal sphincter. (a) Small and asymptomatic; (b) large, symptomatic and appearing as a gas-filled bubble on the chest radiograph.

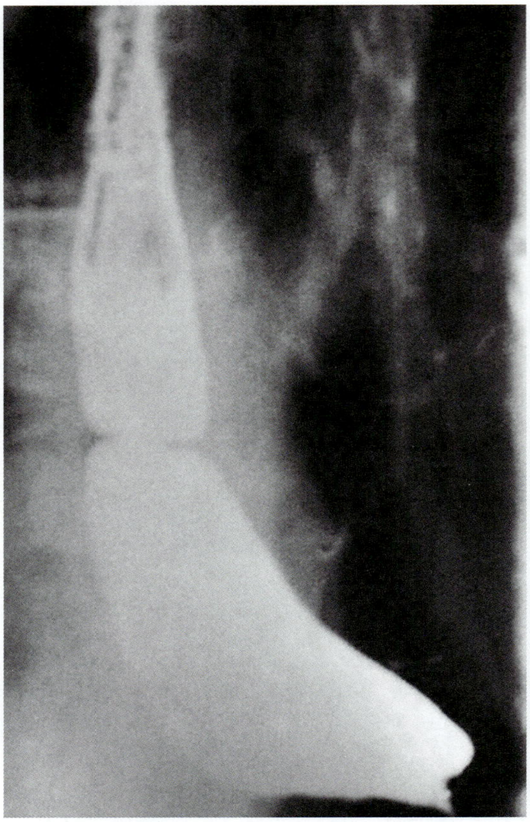

Figure 62.67 Schatzki's ring, a thin submucosal web completely encircling the whole of the lumen, usually situated at the squamocolumnar junction.

Oesophageal infections

Bacterial infection of the oesophagus is rare, but fungal and viral infections do occur. They are particularly important in immunocompromised patients.

Oesophagitis due to *Candida albicans* is relatively common in patients taking steroids (especially transplant patients) or those undergoing cancer chemotherapy. It may present with dysphagia or odynophagia. There may be visible thrush in the throat. Endoscopy shows numerous white plaques that cannot be moved, unlike food residues (Figure 62.68). Biopsies are diagnostic. In severe cases, a barium swallow may show dramatic mucosal ulceration and irregularity that is surprisingly similar to the appearance of oesophageal varices (Figures 62.69 and 62.70). Treatment is with a topical antifungal agent.

Dysphagia and odynophagia can also be caused by herpes simplex virus and cytomegalovirus (CMV). With the former, there may be a history of a herpetic lesion on the lip some days earlier, and endoscopy may reveal vesicles or small ulcers with raised margins, usually in the upper half of the oesophagus. CMV infection may be apparent in graft-versus-host disease following bone marrow transplantation. It has a characteristic endoscopic appearance with a geographical, serpiginous border. In both cases, endoscopic biopsy is diagnostic.

Chagas' disease

This condition is confined to South American countries, but is of interest because oesophageal symptoms occur that are similar

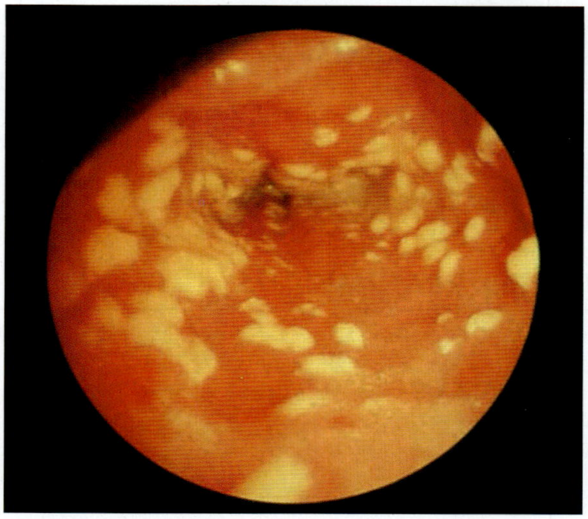

Figure 62.68 Endoscopic appearance of oesophageal candidiasis.

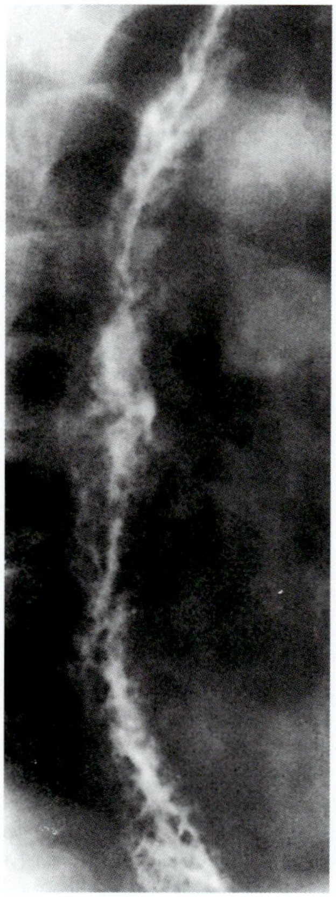

Figure 62.69 Oesophageal candidiasis with shaggy appearance of mucosal defects.

to severe achalasia. It is caused by a protozoan, *Trypanosoma cruzi*, transmitted by an insect vector. Parasites reach the bloodstream and, after a long latent period, there is damage particularly to cardiac and smooth muscle. Destruction of both Auerbach's and Meissner's plexuses leads to acquired megaoesophagus.

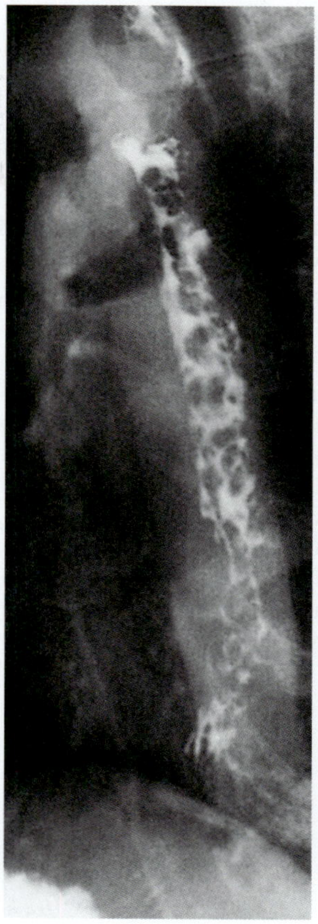

Figure 62.70 Oesophageal varices with smooth outline of the filling defects.

Crohn's disease

The oesophagus is not commonly affected by symptomatic Crohn's disease. However, pathological studies indicate that it may be present in 20 per cent of patients without symptoms. Symptoms are often severe, and a diagnosis of reflux oesophagitis is usually made on the basis of retrosternal pain and dysphagia. Endoscopy shows extensive oesophagitis that extends much further proximally than reflux oesophagitis. Biopsies may be diagnostic, but may show only non-specific inflammation. In severe cases, deep sinuses occur, and fistulation has been described. Crohn's oesophagitis is said to respond poorly to medical treatment and, although balloon dilatation of strictures and surgical resection for multiple internal fistulae have both been described, these interventions should be used with great caution.

Plummer–Vinson syndrome

This is also called the Paterson–Kelly syndrome or **sideropenic dysphagia**. The original descriptions are vague and poorly supported by evidence of a coherent syndrome. Dysphagia is said to occur because of the presence of a postcricoid web that is associated with iron deficiency anaemia, glossitis and koilonychia. The classical syndrome is rarely complete. Some patients may have oropharyngeal leukoplakia, and this may account for an alleged increased risk of developing hypopharyngeal cancer.

Porter Paisley Vinson, 1890–1959, physician, the Mayo Clinic, Rochester, MN, who later practised in Richmond, VA, USA.
Adam Brown Kelly, 1865–1941, surgeon, the Ear, Nose and Throat Department, the Royal Victoria Infirmary, Glasgow, UK.
Donald Rose Paterson, 1863–1939, surgeon, the Ear, Nose and Throat Department, the Royal Infirmary, Cardiff, Wales, UK.
Vinson, Kelly and Paterson, all described this syndrome independently in 1919.

Webs certainly occur in the upper and middle oesophagus, usually without any kind of associated syndrome. They are nearly always thin diaphanous membranes identified coincidentally by contrast radiology. Even symptomatic webs that cause a degree of obstruction may be inadvertently ruptured at endoscopy. Few require formal endoscopic dilatation.

Vascular abnormalities affecting the oesophagus

Several congenital vascular anomalies may produce dysphagia by compression of the oesophagus. Classically, this results from an aberrant right subclavian artery (arteria lusoria). However, the oesophagus is more commonly compressed by vascular rings, such as a double aortic arch. Dysphagia occurs in only a minority of cases and usually presents early in childhood, although it can occur in the late teens. Treatment is usually by division of the non-dominant component of the ring.

In adults, acquired causes include aneurysm of the aorta, diffuse cardiac enlargement and pressure from the left common carotid or vertebral arteries. It is rare that symptom severity justifies surgical intervention.

Mediastinal fibrosis

This rare condition can occur alone or in conjunction with retroperitoneal fibrosis. The cause is unknown and, while the major consequences are usually cardiovascular as a result of caval compression, dysphagia can occur. The existence of irreparable cardiovascular problems usually precludes surgical intervention on the oesophagus.

FURTHER READING

Castell DO, Richter JE. *The esophagus*, 4th edn. Baltimore, MD: Lippincott, Williams & Wilkins, 2003.

Griffin SM, Raimes SA. *Oesophago-gastric surgery*, 4th edn. London: WB Saunders, 2009.

Jamieson GG. *Surgery of the oesophagus*. Edinburgh: Churchill Livingstone, 1988.

Pearson FG, Cooper JD, Deslauriers J *et al*. *The esophagus*, 2nd edn. Edinburgh: Churchill Livingstone, 2002.

Sharma P, Sampliner RE. *Barrett's oesophagus and esophageal adenocarcinomas*, 2nd edn. Oxford: Blackwell, 2006.

CHAPTER 63

Stomach and duodenum

LEARNING OBJECTIVES

- To understand the gross and microscopic anatomy and pathophysiology of the stomach in relation to disease
- To be able to decide on the most appropriate techniques to use in the investigation of patients with complaints relating to the stomach and duodenum
- To understand the critical importance of gastritis and *Helicobacter pylori* in upper gastrointestinal disease
- To be able to investigate and treat peptic ulcer disease and its complications
- To be able to recognise the presentation of gastric cancer and understand the principles involved in its treatment
- To know about the causes of duodenal obstruction and the presentation of duodenal tumours

INTRODUCTION

The function of the stomach is to act as a reservoir for ingested food. It also serves to break down foodstuffs mechanically and commence the processes of digestion before these products are passed on into the duodenum.

GROSS ANATOMY OF THE STOMACH AND DUODENUM

Blood supply

Arteries

The stomach has an arterial supply on both lesser and greater curves (Figure 63.1). On the lesser curve, the left gastric artery, a branch of the coeliac axis, forms an anastomotic arcade with the right gastric artery, which arises from the common hepatic artery. Branches of the left gastric artery pass up towards the cardia. The gastroduodenal artery, which is also a branch of the hepatic artery, passes behind the first part of the duodenum, highly relevant with respect to the bleeding duodenal ulcer. Here it divides into the superior pancreaticoduodenal artery and the right gastroepiploic artery. The superior pancreaticoduodenal artery supplies the duodenum and pancreatic head, and forms an anastomosis with the inferior pancreaticoduodenal artery, a branch of the superior mesenteric artery. The right gastroepiploic artery runs along the greater curvature of the stomach, eventually forming an anastomosis with the left gastroepiploic artery, a branch of the splenic artery. This vascular arcade, important for the construction of the gastric conduit in oesophageal resection, is often variably incomplete. The fundus of the stomach is supplied by the vasa brevia (or short gastric arteries), which arise from near the termination of the splenic artery.

Veins

In general, the veins are equivalent to the arteries, those along the lesser curve ending in the portal vein and those on the greater curve joining via the splenic vein. On the lesser curve, the coronary vein is particularly important. It runs up the lesser

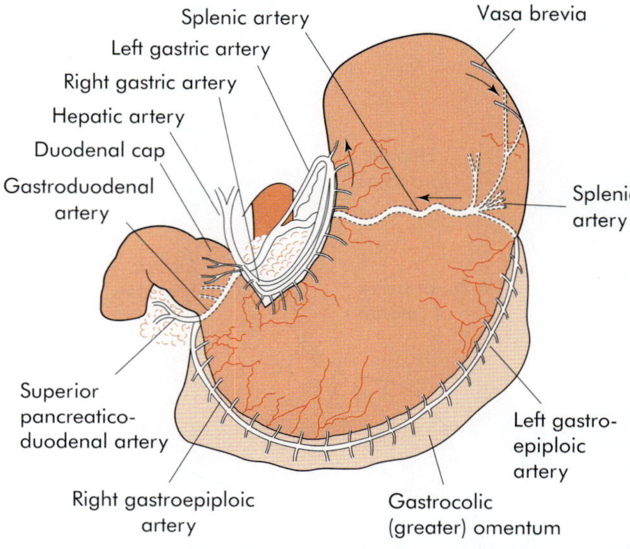

Figure 63.1 The arterial blood supply of the stomach.

curve towards the oesophagus and then passes left to right to join the portal vein. This vein becomes markedly dilated in portal hypertension.

Lymphatics

The lymphatics of the stomach are of considerable importance in the surgery of gastric cancer and are therefore described in detail in the section Spread of carcinoma of the stomach.

Nerves

As with the entire gastrointestinal tract, the stomach and duodenum possess both intrinsic and extrinsic nerve supplies. The intrinsic nerves exist principally in two plexuses, the myenteric plexus of Auerbach and the submucosal plexus of Meissner. Compared with the rest of the gut, the submucosal plexus of the stomach contains relatively few ganglionic cells, as does the myenteric plexus in the fundus. However, in the antrum the ganglia of the myenteric plexus are well developed. The extrinsic supply is derived mainly from the vagus nerves (CN XI), fibres of which originate in the brainstem. The vagal plexus around the oesophagus condenses into bundles that pass through the oesophageal hiatus (Figure 63.2), the posterior bundle being usually identifiable as a large nerve trunk. Vagal fibres are both afferent (sensory) and efferent. The efferent fibres are involved in the receptive relaxation of the stomach and the stimulation of gastric motility, as well as having the well-known secretory function. The sympathetic supply is derived mainly from the coeliac ganglia.

MICROSCOPIC ANATOMY OF THE STOMACH AND DUODENUM

The gastric epithelial cells are mucus producing and are turned over rapidly. In the pyloric part of the stomach, and also the duodenum, mucus-secreting glands are found. Most of the specialised cells of the stomach (parietal and chief cells) are found in the gastric crypts (Figure 63.3). The stomach also has numerous endocrine cells.

Parietal cells

These are in the body (acid-secreting portion) of the stomach and line the gastric crypts, being more abundant distally. They are responsible for the production of hydrogen ions to form hydrochloric acid. The hydrogen ions are actively secreted by the proton pump, a hydrogen–potassium-ATPase (Sachs), which exchanges intraluminal potassium for hydrogen ions. The potassium ions enter the lumen of the crypts passively, but the hydrogen ions are pumped against an immense concentration gradient (1 000 000:1).

Chief cells

These lie principally proximally in the gastric crypts and produce pepsinogen. Two forms of pepsinogen are described: pepsinogen I and pepsinogen II. Both are produced by the chief cell, but pepsinogen I is produced only in the stomach. The ratio between pepsinogens I and II in the serum decreases with gastric atrophy. Pepsinogen is activated in the stomach to produce the digestive protease, pepsin.

Endocrine cells

The stomach has numerous endocrine cells, which are critical to its function. In the gastric antrum, the mucosa contains G cells, which produce gastrin. Throughout the body of the stomach, enterochromaffin-like (ECL) cells are abundant and produce histamine, a key factor in driving gastric acid secretion. In addition, there are large numbers of somatostatin-producing D cells throughout the stomach, and somatostatin has a negative regulatory role. The peptides and neuropeptides produced in the stomach are discussed later.

Duodenum

The duodenum is lined by a mucus-secreting columnar epithelium. In addition, Brunner's glands lie beneath the mucosa and are similar to the pyloric glands in the pyloric part of the stomach. Endocrine cells in the duodenum produce cholecystokinin and secretin.

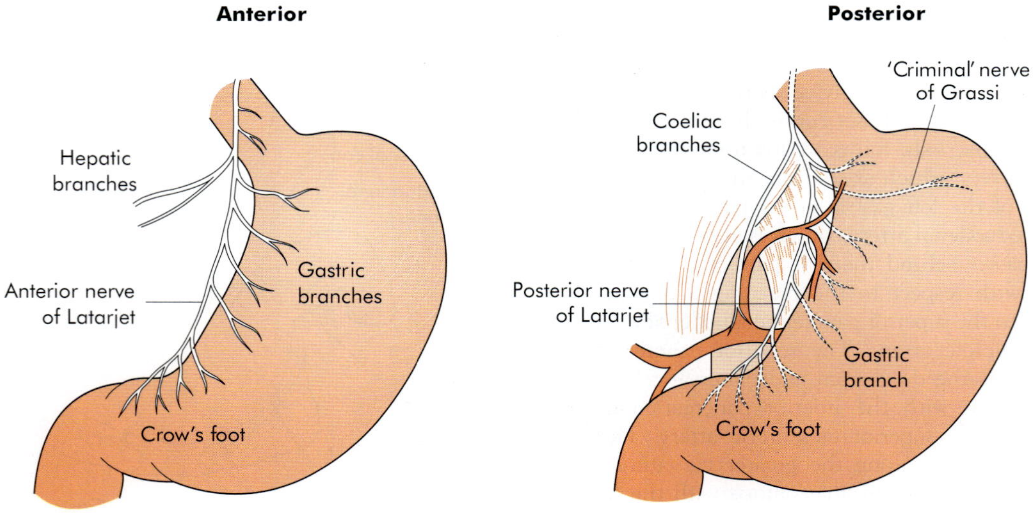

Figure 63.2 The anatomy of the anterior and posterior vagus nerves in relation to the stomach.

Leopold Auerbach, 1828–1897, Professor of Neuropathology, Breslau, Germany (now Wroclaw, Poland), described the myenteric plexus in 1862.
George Meissner, 1829–1905, Professor of Physiology, Göttingen, Germany, described the submucosal plexus in 1852.
George Sachs, Professor of Medicine, CURE, Los Angeles, CA, USA.
Johann Conrad Brunner, 1653–1729, Professor of Anatomy at Heidelberg, Germany and later at Strasbourg, France, described these glands in 1687.

PHYSIOLOGY OF THE STOMACH AND DUODENUM

The stomach mechanically breaks up ingested food and, together with the actions of acid and pepsin, forms chyme that passes into the duodenum. In contrast with the acidic environment of the stomach, the environment of the duodenum is alkaline, due to the secretion of bicarbonate ions from both the pancreas and the duodenum. This neutralises the acid chyme and adjusts the luminal osmolarity to approximately that of plasma. Endocrine cells in the duodenum produce cholecystokinin, which stimulates the pancreas to produce trypsin and the gall bladder to contract. Secretin is also produced by the endocrine cells of the duodenum. This hormone inhibits gastric acid secretion and promotes production of bicarbonate by the pancreas (Summary box 63.1).

Summary box 63.1

The anatomy and physiology of the stomach

- The stomach acts as a reservoir for food and commences the process of digestion
- Gastric acid is produced by a proton pump in the parietal cells, which in turn is controlled by histamine acting on the H_2-receptors
- The histamine is produced by the endocrine gastric ECL cells in response to a number of factors, particularly gastrin and the vagus
- Proton pump inhibitors abolish gastric acid production, whereas H_2-receptor antagonists only markedly reduce it
- The gastric mucous layer is essential to the integrity of the gastric mucosa

Gastric acid secretion

The secretion of gastric acid and pepsin tends to run in parallel, although the understanding of the mechanisms of gastric acid secretion is considerably greater than that of pepsin. Numerous factors are involved to some degree in the production of the gastric acid. These include neurotransmitters, neuropeptides and peptide hormones. This complexity need not detract from the fact that there are basic principles that are relatively easily understood (Figure 63.4). Hydrogen ions are produced by the parietal cell by the proton pump. Although numerous factors can act on the parietal cell, the most important of these is histamine, which acts via the H_2-receptor. Histamine is produced, in turn, by the ECL cells of the stomach and acts in a paracrine (local) fashion on the parietal cells. These relationships explain why proton pump inhibitors can abolish gastric acid secretion, as they act on the final common pathway – hydrogen ion secretion. H_2-receptor antagonists have profound effects on gastric acid secretion, but this is not insurmountable (Figure 63.4). The ECL cell produces histamine in response to a number of stimuli that include the vagus nerve and gastrin. Gastrin is released by the G cells in response to the presence of the food in the stomach. The production of gastrin is inhibited by acid, hence creating a negative feedback loop. Various other peptides, including secretin, inhibit gastric acid secretion.

Classically, three phases of gastric secretion are described. The cephalic phase is mediated by vagal activity, secondary

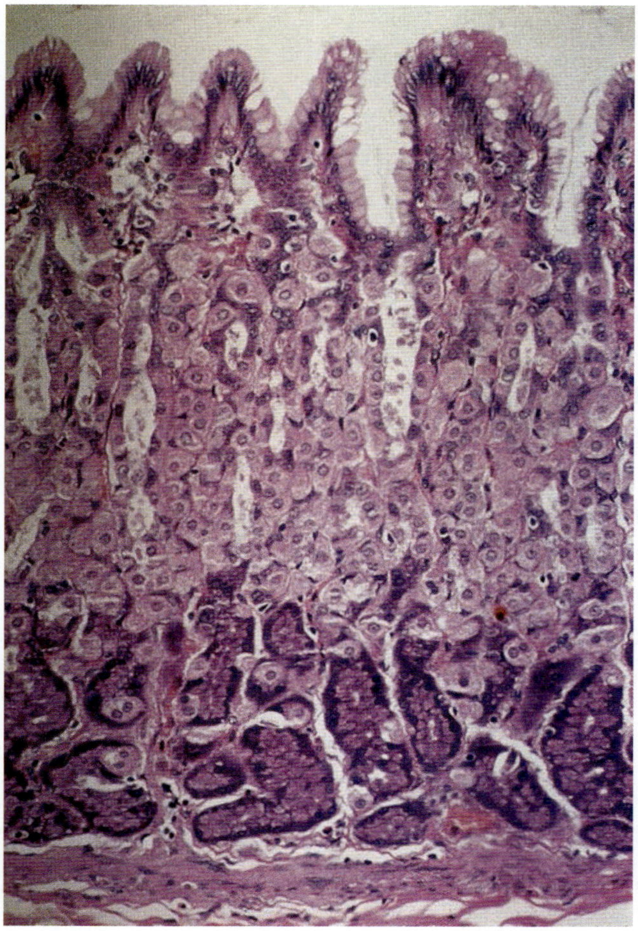

Figure 63.3 The histological appearance of a gastric gland. The mucus-secreting cells are seen at the mucosal surface, the eosinophilic parietal cells superficially in the glands, and the basophilic chief cells in the deepest layer.

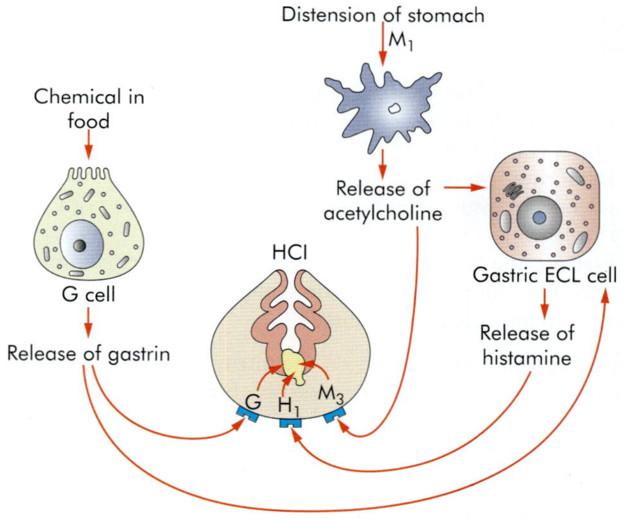

Figure 63.4 The parietal cell in relation to the mechanism of gastric acid secretion. G, gastrin receptor; H, histamine receptor; M, muscarinic receptor.

to sensory arousal as first demonstrated by Pavlov. The gastric phase is a response to food within the stomach, which is mediated principally, but not exclusively, by gastrin. In the intestinal phase, the presence of chyme in the duodenum and small bowel inhibits gastric emptying and, the acidification of the duodenum leads to the production of secretin, which inhibits gastric acid secretion, along with numerous other peptides originating from the gut. The stomach also possesses somatostatin-containing D cells. Somatostatin is released in response to a number of factors including acidification. This peptide acts probably on the G cell, the ECL cell and the parietal cell itself to inhibit the production of acid.

Gastric mucus and the gastric mucosal barrier

The gastric mucous layer is essential to the integrity of the gastric mucosa. It is a viscid layer of mucopolysaccharides produced by the mucus-producing cells of the stomach and the pyloric glands. Gastric mucus is an important physiological barrier to protect the gastric mucosa from mechanical damage, and also the effects of acid and pepsin. Its considerable buffering capacity is enhanced by the presence of bicarbonate ions within the mucus. Many factors can lead to the breakdown of this gastric mucous barrier. These include bile, non-steroidal anti-inflammatory drugs (NSAIDs), alcohol, trauma and shock. Tonometry studies have shown that, of all the gastrointestinal tract, the stomach is the most sensitive to ischaemia following a hypovolaemic insult and also the slowest to recover. This may explain the high incidence of stress ulceration in the stomach.

Peptides and neuropeptides in the stomach and duodenum

As with most of the gastrointestinal tract, the endocrine cells of the stomach produce peptide hormones and neurotransmitters. Previously, nerves and endocrine cells were considered distinct in terms of their products. However, it is increasingly realised that there is enormous overlap within these systems. Many peptides recognised as hormones may also be produced by neurones, hence the term neuropeptides. The term 'messenger' can be used to describe all such products. There are three conventional modes of action that overlap.

1 **Endocrine**. The messenger is secreted into the circulation, where it affects tissues that may be remote from the site of origin (Bayliss and Starling).
2 **Paracrine**. Messengers are produced locally and have local effects on tissues. Neurones and endocrine cells both act in this way.
3 **Neurocrine** (classical neurotransmitter). Messengers are produced by the neurone via the synaptic knob and pass across the synaptic cleft to the target.

Many peptide hormones act on the intrinsic nerve plexus of the gut (see later) and influence motility. Similarly, neuropeptides may influence the structure and function of the mucosa. Some of these peptides, neuropeptides and neurotransmitters are shown in Table 63.1.

Table 63.1 Function and source of peptides and neuropeptides in the stomach.

Function	Source
Stimulate secretion	
Gastrin	G cells
Histamine	ECL cells
Acetylcholine	Neurones
Gastrin-releasing peptide	Neurones and mucosa
Cholecystokinin (CCK)	Duodenal endocrine cells
Inhibit secretion	
Somatostatin	D cells and neurones
Secretin	Duodenal endocrine cells
Enteroglucagon	Small intestinal endocrine cells
Prostaglandins	Mucosa
Neurotensin	Neurones
GIP	Duodenal and jejunal endocrine cells
PYY	Small intestinal endocrine cells
Stimulate motility	
Acetylcholine	Neurones
5-HT	Neurones
Histamine	ECL cell
Substance P	Neurones
Substance K	Neurones
Motilin	Neurones
Gastrin	G cells
Angiotensin	
Inhibit motility	
Somatostatin	D cells and neurones
VIP	Neurones
Nitric oxide	Neurones and smooth muscle
Noradrenaline	Neurones
Encephalin	Neurones
Dopamine	Neurones

ECL, entrochromaffin-like cells; GIP, gastric inhibitory polypeptide; PYY, peptide YY; VIP, vasoactive intestinal peptide.

Gastroduodenal motor activity

The motility of the entire gastrointestinal tract is modulated to a large degree by its intrinsic nervous system. Critical in this process is the migrating motor complex (MMC). In the fasted state, and after food has cleared, in the small bowel there is a period of quiescence lasting in the region of 40 minutes (phase I). There follows a series of waves of electrical and motor activity, also lasting for about 40 minutes, propagated from the fundus of the stomach in a caudal direction at a rate of about 3 per minute (phase II). These pass as far the pylorus, but not beyond. Duodenal slow waves are generated in the duodenum at a rate of about 10 per minute, which carry down the small bowel. The amplitude of these contractions increases to a maximum in phase III, which lasts for about 10 minutes. This 90-minute

Ivan Petrovich Pavlov, 1849–1936, Professor of Physiology, The Medico-Chirurgical Academy, St Petersburg, Russia.
Sir William Maddock Baylis, 1860–1924, Professor of Physiology, University College, London, UK.
Ernst Henry Starling, 1866–1927, Professor of Physiology, University College, London, UK.

cycle of activity is then repeated. From the duodenum, the MMC moves distally at 5–10 cm/min, reaching the terminal ileum after 1.5 hours.

Following a meal, the stomach exhibits receptive relaxation, which lasts for a few seconds. Following this, adaptive relaxation occurs, which allows the proximal stomach to act as a reservoir. Most of the peristaltic activity is found in the distal stomach (the antral mill) and the proximal stomach demonstrates only tonic activity. The pylorus, which is most commonly open, contracts with the peristaltic wave and allows only a few millilitres of chyme through at a time. The antral contraction against the closed sphincter is important in the milling activity of the stomach. Although the duodenum is capable of generating ten waves per minute, after a meal it only contracts after an antral wave reaches the pylorus. The coordination of the motility of the antrum, pylorus and duodenum means that only small quantities of food reach the small bowel at a time. Motility is influenced by numerous factors, including mechanical stimulation and neuronal and endocrine influences (Table 63.1).

INVESTIGATION OF THE STOMACH AND DUODENUM

Flexible endoscopy

Flexible endoscopy is the 'gold standard' investigation of the upper gastrointestinal tract. The original flexible endoscopes were fibreoptic (Hirschowitz), but now most use a solid-state camera mounted at the instrument's tip (Figures 63.5 and 63.6). Other members of the endoscopy team see the image and this is useful when taking biopsies or performing interventional techniques, and also facilitates teaching and training (Summary box 63.2).

Summary box 63.2

The investigation of gastric disorders

- Flexible endoscopy is the most commonly used and sensitive technique for investigating the stomach and duodenum
- Great care needs to be exercised in performing endoscopy to avoid complications and missing important pathology
- Axial imaging, particularly multislice CT, is useful in the staging of gastric cancer, although it may be less sensitive in the detection of liver metastases than other modalities
- CT/PET is useful in staging gastric cancer
- Endoscopic ultrasound is the most sensitive technique in the evaluation of the 'T' stage of gastric cancer and in the assessment of duodenal tumours
- Laparoscopy is very sensitive in detecting peritoneal metastases, and laparoscopic ultrasound provides an accurate evaluation of lymph node and liver metastases

Flexible endoscopy is more sensitive than conventional radiology in the assessment of the majority of gastroduodenal conditions. This is particularly the case for peptic ulceration, gastritis and duodenitis. In upper gastrointestinal bleeding, endoscopy is far superior to any other investigation and offers the possibility of endoscopic therapy. In most circumstances it is the only investigation required.

Basil I Hirschowitz, born 1925 in South Africa, Professor Emeritus of Medicine, Physiology and Biophysics, University of Alabama, Birmingham, AL, USA and given Lifetime Achievement Award as Physician of the Year.

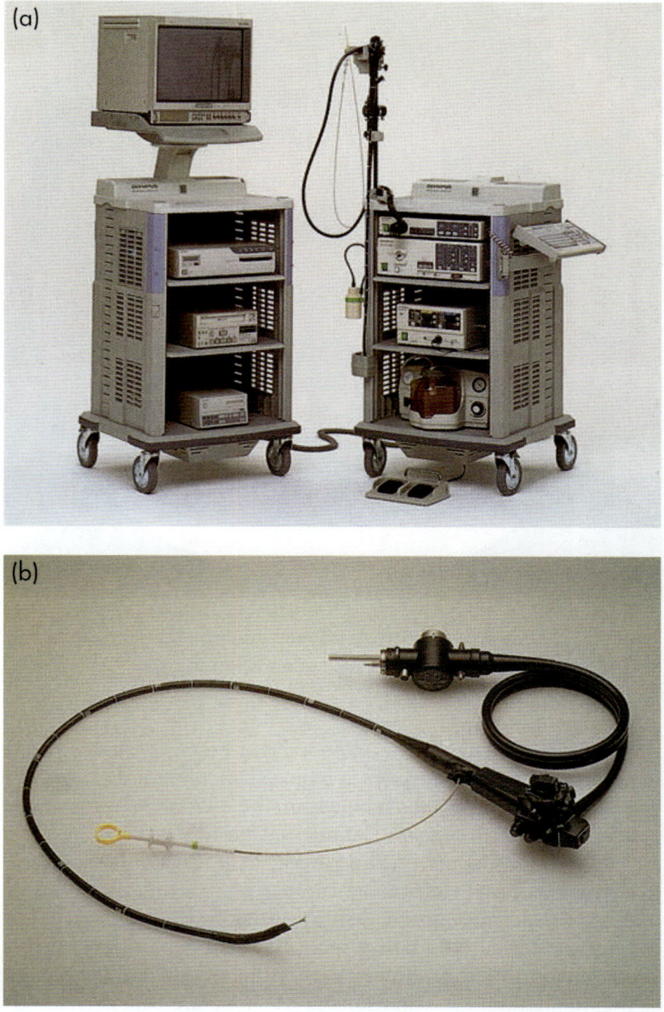

Figure 63.5 A video-gastroscope (courtesy of Keymed (Medical and Industrial Equipment Ltd)). (a) The camera stack. (b) The gastroscope, and biopsy forceps, in the working channel.

Fibreoptic endoscopy is generally a safe investigation, but it is important that all personnel undertaking these procedures are adequately trained and that resuscitation facilities are always available. Careless and rough handling of the endoscope during intubation of a patient may result in perforations of the pharynx and oesophagus. Any other part of the upper gastrointestinal tract may also be perforated. An inadequately performed endoscopy is also dangerous as a serious condition may be overlooked. This is particularly the case in respect of early and curable gastric cancer, the appearances of which may often be extremely subtle and may be missed by inexperienced endoscopists. A more experienced endoscopist will have a higher index of suspicion for any mucosal abnormalities and will take more biopsies. Spraying the mucosa with dye endoscopically may allow better discrimination between normal and abnormal mucosa, so allowing a small cancer to be more easily seen. In the future, advances in technology may allow 'optical biopsy' to determine the nature of mucosal abnormalities in real time.

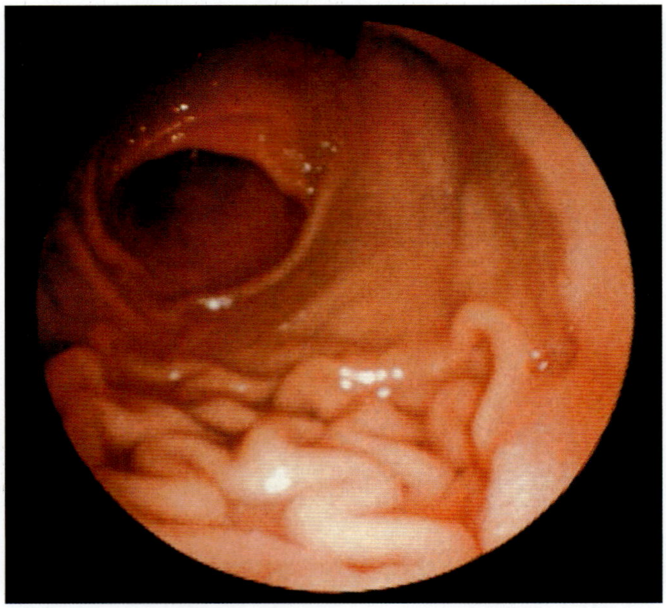

Figure 63.6 A view of the normal stomach during endoscopy (courtesy of GNJ Tytgat, Amsterdam, The Netherlands).

Upper gastrointestinal endoscopy can be performed without sedation, but when sedation is required incremental doses of a benzodiazepine are usually administered. Sedation is of particular concern in the case of gastrointestinal bleeding as it may have a more profound effect on the patient's cardiovascular stability. It has now become the standard to use pulse oximetry to monitor patients during upper gastrointestinal endoscopy, and nasal oxygen is often also administered. Buscopan is useful to abolish duodenal motility for examinations of the second and third parts of the duodenum. Examinations of this type are best carried out using a side-viewing endoscope such as is used for endoscopic retrograde cholangiopancreatography (ERCP).

Some patients are relatively resistant to sedation with benzodiazepenes, particularly those who are accustomed to drinking alcohol. Increasing the dose of benzodiazepines in these patients may not result in any useful sedation, but merely make the patient more restless and confused. Such patients are sometimes better endoscoped fully awake using a local anaesthetic throat spray and a narrow-gauge endoscope. Whatever the circumstances, it is important that resuscitation facilities are available, including agents that reverse the effects of benzodiazepines, such as flumazenil.

The technology associated with upper gastrointestinal endoscopy is continuing to advance. Instruments which allow both endoscopy and endoluminal ultrasound to be performed simultaneously (see below) are used routinely. Bleeding from the stomach and duodenum can be treated with a number of haemostatic measures. These include injection with various substances, diathermy, heater probes and lasers. These approaches appear to be useful in the treatment of bleeding ulcers, although there are few good controlled trials in this area. There is no good evidence that such interventional procedures at the moment work in patients who are bleeding from very large vessels, such as the gastroduodenal artery or splenic artery, although technology may overcome this problem in the future.

Contrast radiology

Upper gastrointestinal radiology is not used as much as in previous years, as endoscopy is a more sensitive investigation for most gastric problems. Computed tomography (CT) imaging with oral contrast has also replaced contrast radiology in many of the areas where anatomical information is sought, e.g. large hiatus hernias of the rolling type and chronic gastric volvulus. In these conditions it may be difficult for the endoscopist to determine exactly the anatomy or, indeed, negotiate the deformity to see the distal stomach.

Ultrasonography

Standard ultrasound imaging can be used to investigate the stomach, but used conventionally it is less sensitive than other modalities. In contrast, endoluminal ultrasound and laparoscopic ultrasound are probably the most sensitive techniques available in the preoperative staging of gastric cancer. In endoluminal ultrasound, the transducer is usually attached to the distal tip of the instrument. However, devices have been developed which may be passed down the biopsy channel, albeit with poorer image quality. Five layers (Figure 63.7) of the gastric wall may be identified on endoluminal ultrasound and the depth of invasion of a tumour can be assessed with exquisite accuracy (90 per cent accuracy for the 'T' component of the staging). Enlarged lymph nodes can also be identified and the technique's accuracy in this situation is about 80 per cent. Finally, it may be possible to identify liver metastases not seen on axial imaging. Laparoscopic ultrasound is also a very sensitive imaging modality to a large measure because of the laparoscopy itself (see below). It is one of the most sensitive methods of detecting liver metastases from gastric cancer.

An additional use of ultrasound is in the assessment of gastric emptying. Swallowed contrast is utilised, which is designed to be easily seen using an ultrasound transducer. The emptying of this contrast is then followed directly. The accuracy of the technique is similar to that of radioisotope gastric emptying studies (see below).

CT scanning and magnetic resonance imaging

The resolution of CT scanners is continuing to improve, and multislice CT is of increasing value in the investigation of the stomach, especially gastric malignancies (Figure 63.8). The presence of gastric wall thickening associated with a carcinoma

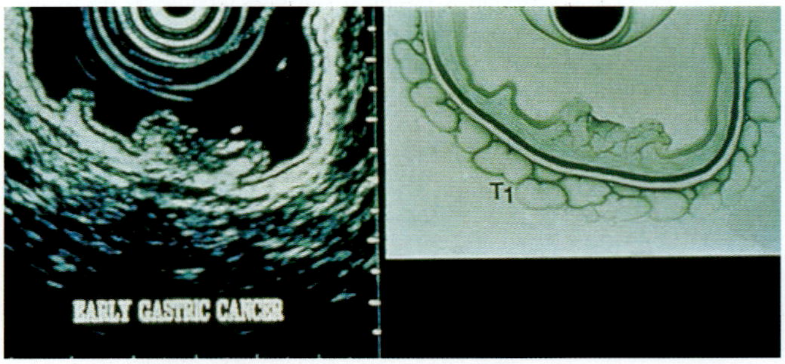

Figure 63.7 Endoscopic ultrasound of the stomach. Five layers can be identified in the normal stomach. A gastric cancer is shown invading the muscle of the gastric wall (courtesy of KeyMed (Medical and Industrial Equipment Ltd)).

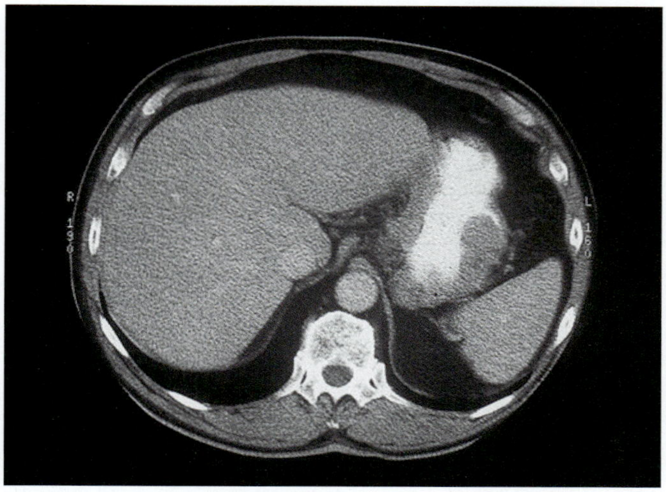

Figure 63.8 A computed tomography scan of the abdomen, showing a gastric cancer arising in the body of the stomach.

of any reasonable size can be easily detected by CT, but the investigation lacks sensitivity in detecting smaller and curable lesions. It is much less accurate in 'T' staging than endoluminal ultrasound. Lymph node enlargement can be detected and, based on the size and shape of the nodes, it is possible to be reasonably accurate in detecting nodal involvement with tumour. However, as with all imaging techniques, it is limited. Microscopic tumour deposits in lymph nodes cannot be detected when the node is not enlarged and, in contrast, lymph nodes may undergo reactive enlargement but not contain tumour. These problems apply to all imaging techniques.

The detection of small liver metastases is improving, although in general terms metastases from gastric cancer are less easy to detect using CT than those, for instance, from colorectal cancer. This is because metastases from gastric cancer may be of the same density as liver and may not handle the intravenous contrast any differently. At present, magnetic resonance imaging (MRI) scanning does not offer any specific advantage in assessing the stomach, although it has a higher sensitivity for the detection of gastric cancer liver metastases than conventional CT imaging.

CT/positron emission tomography

Positron emission tomography (PET) is a functional imaging technique which relies on the uptake of a tracer in most cases by metabolically active tumour tissue. Fluorodeoxyglucose (FDG) is the most commonly used tracer. This tracer has a short half-life hence manufacture and use have to be carefully coordinated. To be of value, anatomical and functional informations need to be linked hence PET/CT is now used universally. It is increasingly being used in the preoperative staging of gastro-oesophageal cancer as it will demonstrate occult spread which renders the patient surgically incurable in up to 10 per cent of patients who would otherwise have undergone major resections (Figure 63.9). PET/CT may also be used to determine the response to neoadjuvant chemotherapy in oesophagogastric malignancies although this is the subject of ongoing studies.

Laparoscopy

This technique is now well used in the assessment of patients with gastric cancer. Its particular value is in the detection of peritoneal disease, which is difficult by any other technique, unless the patient has ascites or bulky intraperitoneal disease. Its main limitation is in the evaluation of posterior extension but other techniques are available to evaluate posterior invasion, especially CT and endoluminal ultrasound. Usually laparoscopy is combined with peritoneal cytology unless laparotomy follows immediately.

Gastric emptying studies

These are useful in the study of gastric dysmotility problems, particularly those that follow gastric surgery. The principle of the examination is that a radioisotope-labelled liquid and solid meal are ingested by the patient and the emptying of the stomach is followed on a gamma camera. This allows the proportion of activity in the remaining stomach to be assessed numerically, and it is possible to follow liquid and solid gastric emptying independently (Figure 63.10).

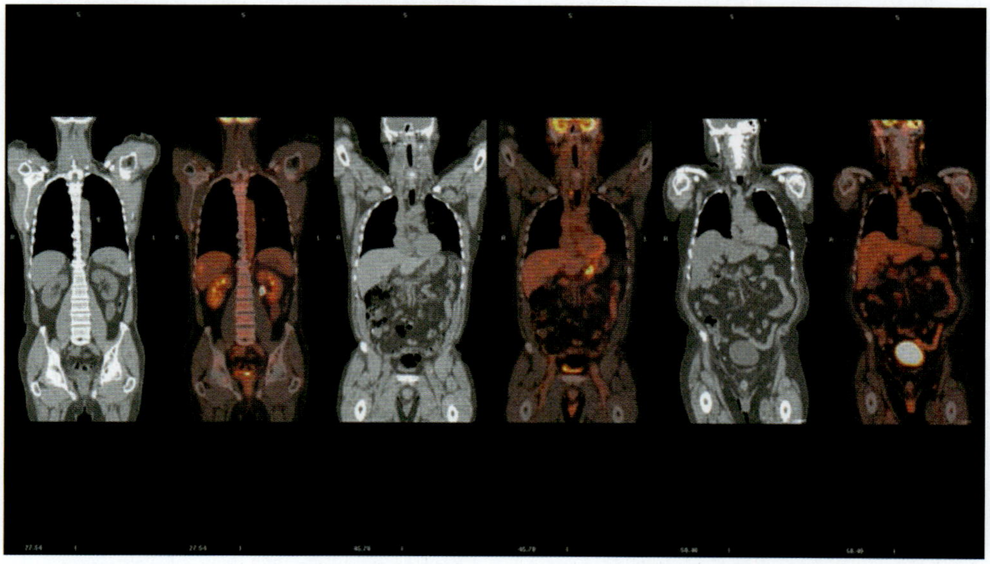

Figure 63.9 Computed tomography/positron emission tomography of a patient with gastric cancer. The middle pair of images shows the primary tumour. The two images on the left show unsuspected liver metastases, whereas the two on the right show a left cervical node positive for metastases.

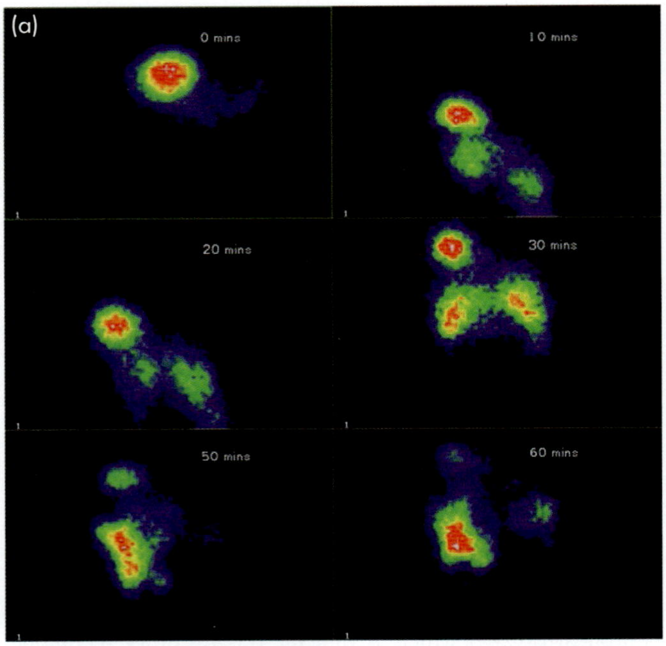

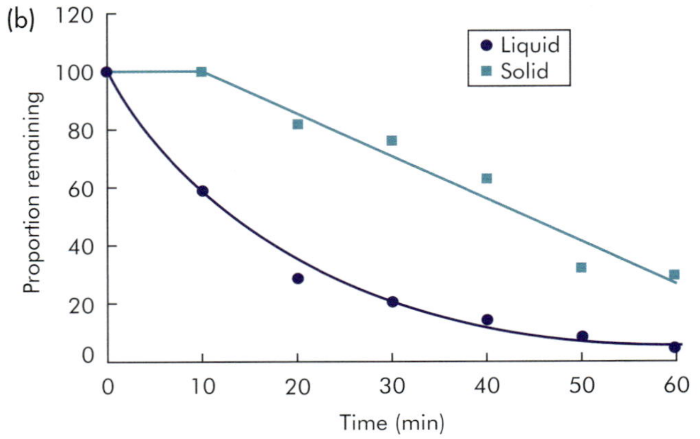

Figure 63.10 Dual-phase solid and liquid gastric emptying. The use of two isotopic labels allows the liquid and solid phases of the emptying to be followed separately. (a) Image acquisition. (b) Gastric emptying curves in a normal individual showing typical lag period in solid phase before linear emptying (courtesy of Dr V Lewington, Southampton, UK).

Angiography

Angiography is used most commonly in the investigation of upper gastrointestinal bleeding that is not identified using endoscopy. Therapeutic embolisation may also be of value in the treatment of bleeding in patients in whom surgery is difficult or inadvisable.

HELICOBACTER PYLORI

Over the last 30 years, this organism has proved to be of overwhelming importance in the aetiology of a number of common gastroduodenal diseases such as chronic gastritis, peptic ulceration and gastric cancer. The organism had unquestionably been observed by a number of workers since Bircher's first description in 1874, but it was not until 1980 that Warren and Marshall, with enthusiasm but perhaps a lack of caution, ingested the organism to confirm that Koch's postulates could be fulfilled with respect to the gastritis that they succeeded in causing in themselves. Eradication therapy was then employed with mixed success, but both received the Nobel Prize for Medicine and Physiology in 2005. The organism is spiral shaped and is fastidious in its requirements, being difficult to culture outside the mucous layer of the stomach.

One of the characteristics of the organism is its ability to hydrolyse urea, resulting in the production of ammonia, a strong alkali. The effect of ammonia on the antral G cells is to cause the release of gastrin via the previously described negative-feedback loop. This is probably responsible for the modest, but inappropriate, hypergastrinaemia in patients with peptic ulcer disease, which, in turn, may result in gastric acid hypersecretion. The organism's obligate urease activity is utilised by various tests used to detect the presence of the organism, including the 13C and 14C breath tests and the CLO test (a commercially available urease test kit), which is performed on gastric biopsies. The organism can also be detected histologically (Figure 63.11), using the Giemsa or the Ethin–Starey silver stains, and cultured using appropriate media. Previous or current infection with the organism may also be detected serologically. Breath tests or faecal antigen tests are recommended for the pretreatment diagnosis of *H. pylori* infection in the community. Less accurate, hospital-based serology tests have a place within the non-invasive test and treat strategy.

Infection with *H. pylori* leads to the disruption of the gastric mucous barrier by the enzymes produced by the organism, and the inflammation induced in the gastric epithelium is the basis of many of the associated disease processes. The association of

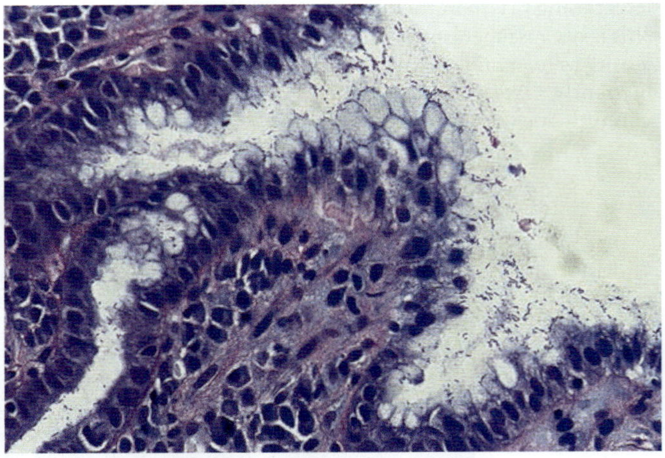

Figure 63.11 Antral mucosa showing colonisation with *Helicobacter pylori* (modified Giemsa stain).

Warren and Marshall were awarded (among many other awards) the Nobel Prize for Physiology or Medicine in 2005 'for their discovery of the bacterium *Helicobacter pylori* and its role in gastritis and peptic ulcer disease'. Marshall ingested the bacteria to prove that *H. pylori* was indeed the causative organism.
Robert Koch, 1843–1910, Professor of Hygiene and Bacteriology, Berlin, Germany, started his postulates in 1882. These define the conditions which must be met before an organism can be shown to be the causal agent for a particular disease.

John Robin Warren, born 1937, pathologist, the Royal Perth Hospital, Perth, WA, Australia.
Barry James Marshall, born 1951, physician, the Royal Perth Hospital, Perth, WA, Australia; later became Professor of Medicine at the University of Virginia, VA, USA.
Gustav Giemsa, 1867–1948, a bacteriologist who became Privatdozent in Chemotherapy at the University of Hamburg, Hamburg, Germany.

the organism with chronic (type B) gastritis is not in doubt. Some strains of *H. pylori* produce cytotoxins, notably the *Cag A* and *Vac A* products, and the production of cytotoxins seem to be associated with the ability of the organism to cause gastritis, peptic ulceration and cancer. The effect of the organism on the gastric epithelium is to incite a classical inflammatory response that involves the migration and degranulation of acute inflammatory cells, such as neutrophils, and also the accumulation of chronic inflammatory cells, such as macrophages and lymphocytes.

It is evident how *H. pylori* infection results in chronic gastritis and also how this may progress to gastric ulceration, but for a while it remained an enigma as to how the organism could be involved in duodenal ulceration, as the normal duodenum is not colonised. As mentioned above, the production of ammonia does increase the level of circulating gastrin and it has been shown subsequently that eradication of the organism in patients with duodenal ulcer disease will reduce the acid levels to normal. However, the overlap in gastric acid secretion between normal subjects and those with duodenal ulcers is considerable and the modestly increased acid levels in patients with *Helicobacter*-associated antral gastritis are insufficient to explain the aetiology of duodenal ulceration.

The explanation can probably be found in the phenomenon of duodenal gastric metaplasia. Gastric metaplasia is the normal response of the duodenal mucosa to excess acidity. It can be thought of in the same way as any other metaplasia in the gastrointestinal tract: an attempt by the mucosa to resist an injurious stimulus. Although normal duodenal mucosa cannot be infected with *H. pylori*, gastric metaplasia in the duodenum is commonly infected and this infection results in the same inflammatory process that is observed in the gastric mucosa. The result is duodenitis, which is almost certainly the precursor of duodenal ulceration.

Infection with *H. pylori* may be the most common human infection. The incidence of infection within a population increases with age, and in many populations infection rates of 80–90 per cent are not unusual. Up to 50 per cent of the world's population may be infected with helicobacter. It appears that most infection is acquired in childhood and the possibility of infection is inversely related to socioeconomic group. The means of spread has not been identified, but the organism can occur in the faeces and faecal–oral spread seems most likely. The organism is not normally found in saliva or dental plaque. There is evidence in different environments and in different population groups that the manifestations of the infection may be different. Predominantly antral gastritis, which is commonly seen in the West, results initially in increased levels of acid production and peptic ulcer disease, whereas gastritis affecting the body, common in the developing world, may lead to hypochlorhydria and gastric neoplasia.

It has been known since 1984 that *Helicobacter* infection is amenable to treatment with antibiotics. The profound hypochlorhydria produced by proton pump inhibitors combined with antibiotics is also effective in eradicating the organism. Commonly used eradication regimes include a proton pump inhibitor and two antibiotics, such as metronidazole and amoxycillin. Very high eradication rates, in the region of 90 per cent, can be achieved with combinations that include the antibiotic clarithromycin, although it may be that in the future antibiotic resistance will become a problem. Reinfection following successful eradication appears rare (<0.5 per cent) but incomplete eradication is a more important clinical problem.

At present, eradication therapy is recommended for patients with duodenal ulcer disease, but not for patients with non-ulcer dyspepsia or in asymptomatic patients who are infected. However, recent data show that a proportion of patients with non-ulcer dyspepsia do respond to treatment. *H. pylori* is now classed by the World Health Organisation as a class 1 carcinogen and it may be that further epidemiological studies on the risk of gastric cancer change the current advice on treatment.

GASTRITIS

The understanding of gastritis has increased markedly following elucidation of the role of *H. pylori* in chronic gastritis (Summary box 63.3).

Summary box 63.3

Gastritis

- The spiral bacterium *H. pylori* is critical in the development of type B gastritis, peptic ulceration and gastric cancer
- Infection appears to be acquired mainly in childhood and the infection rate is inversely associated with socioeconomic status
- Eradication, recommended specifically in patients with peptic ulcer disease, can be achieved in up to 90 per cent of patients with a combination of a proton pump inhibitor and antibiotics, and reinfection is uncommon (<0.5 per cent)
- Erosive gastritis is usually related to the use of NSAIDs
- Type A gastritis is an autoimmune process and is associated with the development of pernicious anaemia and gastric cancer

Type A gastritis

This is an autoimmune condition in which there are circulating antibodies to the parietal cell. This results in the atrophy of the parietal cell mass, hence hypochlorhydria and ultimately achlorhydria. As intrinsic factor is also produced by the parietal cell there is malabsorption of vitamin B12, which, if untreated, may result in pernicious anaemia. In type A gastritis, the antrum is not affected and the hypochlorhydria leads to the production of high levels of gastrin from the antral G cells. This results in chronic hypergastrinaemia. This, in turn, results in hypertrophy of the ECL cells in the body of the stomach, which are not affected by the autoimmune damage. Over time it is apparent that microadenomas develop in the ECL cells of the stomach, sometimes becoming identifiable tumour nodules. Very rarely, these tumours can become malignant. Patients with type A gastritis are predisposed to the development of gastric cancer, and screening such patients endoscopically may be appropriate.

Type B gastritis

There are abundant epidemiological data to support the association of this type of gastritis with *H. pylori*. Most commonly, type B gastritis affects the antrum, and it is these patients who are prone to peptic ulcer disease. *Helicobacter*-associated pangastritis is also a very common manifestation of infection, but gastritis affecting the corpus alone does not seem to be associated. However, there are some data to suggest that *Helicobacter* may be involved in the initiation of the process. Patients with pangastritis seem to be most prone to the development of gastric cancer.

Intestinal metaplasia is associated with chronic pangastritis with atrophy. Although intestinal metaplasia per se is common, intestinal metaplasia associated with dysplasia has significant malignant potential and, if this condition is identified, endoscopic screening may be appropriate.

Reflux gastritis

This is caused by enterogastric reflux and is particularly common after gastric surgery. Its histological features are distinct from other types of gastritis. Although commonly seen after gastric surgery, it is occasionally found in patients with no previous surgical intervention or who have had a cholecystectomy. Bile chelating or prokinetic agents may be useful in treatment and as a temporising measure to avoid consideration of revisional surgery. Operation for the condition should be reserved for the most severe cases.

Erosive gastritis

This is caused by agents that disturb the gastric mucosal barrier; NSAIDs and alcohol are common causes. The NSAID-induced gastric lesion is associated with inhibition of the cyclo-oxygenase type 1 (COX-1) receptor enzyme, hence reducing the production of cytoprotective prostaglandins in the stomach. Many of the beneficial anti-inflammatory activities of NSAIDs are mediated by COX-2, and the use of specific COX-2 inhibitors reduces the incidence of these side effects. However, taken long term, COX-2 inhibitors are associated with cardiovascular complications in common with many NSAIDs.

Stress gastritis

This is a common sequel of serious illness or injury and is characterised by a reduction in the blood supply to superficial mucosa of the stomach. Although common, this is not usually recognised unless stress ulceration and bleeding supervene, in which case treatment can be extremely difficult. The condition also sometimes follows cardiopulmonary bypass. Prevention of the stress bleeding from the stomach is much easier than treating it, and hence the routine use of H_2-antagonists with or without barrier agents, such as sucralfate, in patients who are on intensive care. These measures have been shown to reduce the incidence of bleeding from stress ulceration.

Ménétrier's disease

This is an unusual condition characterised by gross hypertrophy of the gastric mucosal folds, mucus production and hypochlorhydria. The condition is premalignant and may present with hypoproteinaemia and anaemia. There is no treatment other than a gastrectomy. The disease seems to be caused by overexpression of transforming growth factor alpha (TGF-α). Like epidermal growth factor (EGF), this peptide also binds to the EGF receptor. The histological features of Ménétrier's disease may be reproduced in transgenic mice overexpressing TGF-α.

Lymphocytic gastritis

This type of gastritis is seen rarely. It is characterised by the infiltration of the gastric mucosa by T cells and is probably associated with *H. pylori* infection. The pattern of inflammation resembles that seen in coeliac disease or lymphocytic colitis.

Other forms of gastritis

Eosinophilic gastritis appears to have an allergic basis, and is treated with steroids and cromoglycate. Granulomatous gastritis is seen rarely in Crohn's disease and also may be associated with tuberculosis. Acquired immunodeficiency syndrome (AIDS) gastritis is secondary to infection with cryptospiridiosis. Phlegmonous gastritis is a rare bacterial infection of the stomach found in patients with severe intercurrent illness. It is usually an agonal event.

PEPTIC ULCER

Although the name 'peptic' ulcer suggests an association with pepsin, this is essentially unimportant as in the absence of acid, for instance in type A gastritis with atrophy, peptic ulcers do not occur. All peptic ulcers can be healed by using proton pump inhibitors, which can render a patient virtually achlorhydric (Summary box 63.4).

Summary box 63.4

Peptic ulceration

- Most peptic ulcers are caused by *H. pylori* or NSAIDs and changes in epidemiology mirror changes in these principal aetiological factors
- Duodenal ulcers are more common than gastric ulcers, but the symptoms are indistinguishable
- Gastric ulcers may become malignant and an ulcerated gastric cancer may mimic a benign ulcer
- Gastric antisecretory agents and *H. pylori* eradication therapy are the mainstay of treatment, and elective surgery is very rarely performed
- The long-term complications of peptic ulcer surgery may be difficult to treat
- The common complications of peptic ulcers are perforation, bleeding and stenosis
- The treatment of the perforated peptic ulcer is primarily surgical, although some patients may be managed conservatively

Common sites for peptic ulcers are the first part of the duodenum and the lesser curve of the stomach, but they also occur on the stoma following gastric surgery, the oesophagus and even in a Meckel's diverticulum, which contains ectopic gastric epithelium. In general, the ulcer occurs at a junction between different types of epithelia, the ulcer occurring in the epithelium least resistant to acid damage.

In the past, much distinction has been made between acute and chronic peptic ulcers, but this difference can sometimes be difficult to determine clinically. It is probably best to consider that there is a spectrum of disease from the superficial gastric and duodenal ulceration, frequently seen at endoscopy, to deep chronic penetrating ulcers. This does not minimise the importance of acute stress ulceration. These ulcers can both perforate and bleed.

For many years, the cause of peptic ulceration remained an

Pierre Eugene Meneterier, 1859–1935, a French histopathologist who later became Professor of Medical History in the Faculty of Medicine, Paris, France.
Johann Frederick Meckel (the Younger), 1781–1833, Professor of Anatomy and Surgery, Halle, Germany, described his diverticulum in 1809.

enigma. When comparing groups of patients with duodenal and prepyloric peptic ulcers with normal subjects, gastric acid levels are higher, but the overlap is very considerable. Patients with gastric ulceration have relatively normal levels of gastric acid secretion. As peptic ulceration will occur in the presence of very high acid levels, such as those found in patients with a gastrinoma (Zollinger–Ellison syndrome), and as all ulcers can be healed in the absence of acid, it is clear that acid is important. In patients with a gastrinoma it may be the only aetiological factor, but this is not the case in the majority of patients. As with many diseases, genetic factors may be involved to a limited degree and social stress has also been falsely implicated (Asher).

It is now widely accepted that infection with *H. pylori* and the consumption of NSAIDs are the most important factors in the development of peptic ulceration. In combination, *H. pylori* and NSAIDs act synergistically to promote ulcer development and ulcer bleeding. Cigarette smoking predisposes to peptic ulceration and increases the relapse rate after treatment, with either gastric antisecretory agents or, in the past, elective surgery. Multiple other factors may be involved in transition between the superficial and the deep penetrating chronic ulcer, but they are of lesser importance.

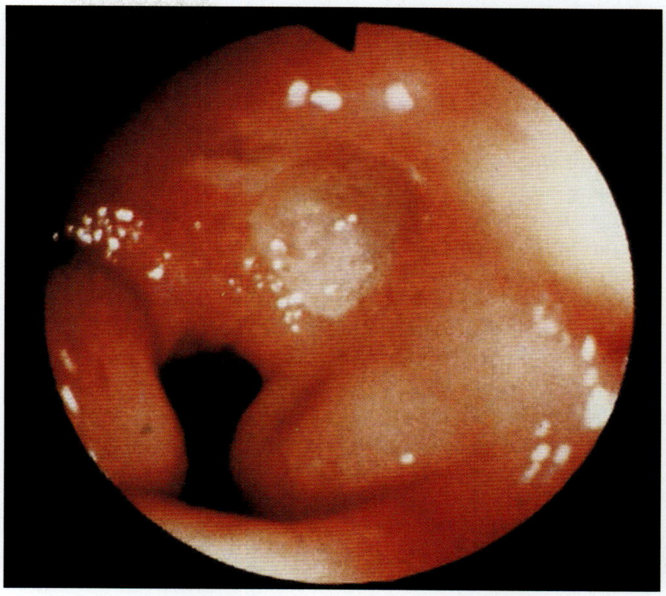

Figure 63.12 Duodenal ulcer at gastroduodenoscopy (courtesy of Dr GNJ Tytgat, Amsterdam, The Netherlands).

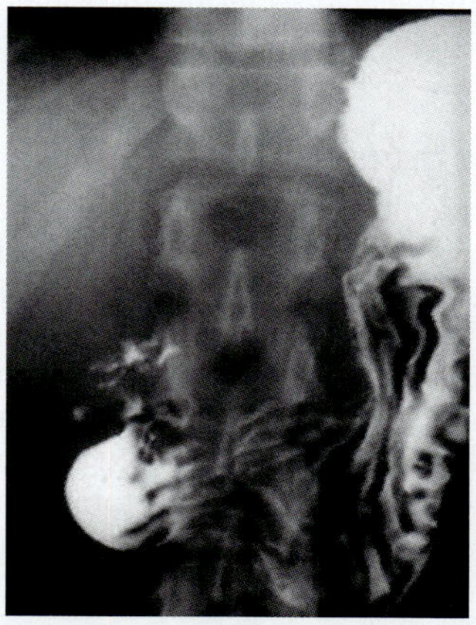

Figure 63.13 Duodenal ulcer shown by barium meal.

Duodenal ulceration

Incidence

There have been marked changes in the last two decades in the demography of patients presenting with duodenal ulceration in the West. First, even before the introduction of H_2-receptor antagonists, the incidence of duodenal ulceration and the frequency of elective surgery for the condition were falling. This trend has continued and now, in the West, dyspeptic patients presenting with a duodenal ulcer at gastroscopy are uncommon. In part, this may relate to the widespread use of gastric antisecretory agents and *H. pylori* eradication therapy for patients with dyspepsia. Second, the peak incidence is now in a much older age group than previously and, although it is still more common in men, the difference is less marked. These changes mirror the changes, at least in part, in the epidemiology of *H. pylori* infection. In Eastern Europe, the disease remains common and, from having been uncommon in some developing nations, it is now observed more frequently. Again, the relationship with *H. pylori* appears convincing.

Pathology

Most occur in the first part of the duodenum (Figures 63.12 and 63.13). A chronic ulcer penetrates the mucosa and into the muscle coat, leading to fibrosis. The fibrosis causes deformities such as pyloric stenosis. When an ulcer heals, a scar can be observed in the mucosa. Sometimes there may be more than one duodenal ulcer. The situation in which there is both a posterior and an anterior duodenal ulcer is referred to as 'kissing ulcers'. Anteriorly placed ulcers tend to perforate and, in contrast, posterior duodenal ulcers tend to bleed, sometimes by eroding into the gastroduodenal artery. Occasionally, the ulceration may be so extensive that the entire duodenal cap is ulcerated and devoid of mucosa. With respect to the giant duodenal ulcer, malignancy in this region is so uncommon that under normal circumstances surgeons can be confident that they are dealing with benign disease, even though from external palpation it may not appear so. In the stomach the situation is different.

> Richard Asher, 1912–1969, physician, the Central Middlesex Hospital, London, UK. Ridiculed the concept that the stress of modern living caused peptic ulceration by pointing out that the same claim was made for syphilis! It is an interesting coincidence that both diseases have strong aetiological associations with spiral organisms.

Histopathology

Microscopically, destruction of the muscular coat is observed and the base of the ulcer is covered with granulation tissue, the arteries in this region showing the typical changes of endarteritis obliterans. Sometimes the terminations of nerves can be seen among the fibrosis. The pathological appearances of the healing ulcer must be carefully interpreted as some of the epithelial downgrowths can be misinterpreted as invasion. This is unlikely to be important in duodenal ulcers when malignancy rarely, if ever, occurs, but it is much more important with gastric ulcers.

Robert Milton Zollinger, 1903–1992, Professor of Surgery, the Ohio State University, Columbus, OH, USA.
Edwin Homer Ellison, 1918–1970, Professor of Surgery, Marquette University, WI, USA.
Zollinger and Ellison described this condition in a joint paper in 1955 when they were both working at the Ohio State University.

Gastric ulcers

Incidence

As with duodenal ulceration, *H. pylori* and NSAIDs are the important aetiological factors. Gastric ulceration is also associated with smoking; other factors are of lesser importance.

There are marked differences between the populations afflicted by chronic gastric ulceration compared with duodenal ulceration. First, gastric ulceration is substantially less common than duodenal ulceration. The sex incidence is equal and the population with gastric ulcers tends to be older. It is more prevalent in low socioeconomic groups and is considerably more common in the developing world than in the West.

Pathology

This is essentially similar to that of a duodenal ulcer, except that gastric ulcers tend to be larger. Fibrosis, when it occurs, may result in the now rarely seen hourglass contraction of the stomach. Large chronic ulcers may erode posteriorly into the pancreas and, on other occasions, into major vessels such as the splenic artery. Less commonly, they may erode into other organs such as the transverse colon. Chronic gastric ulcers are much more common on the lesser curve (especially at the incisura angularis; Figures 63.14 and 63.15) than on the greater curve and, even when high on the lesser curve, they tend to be at the boundary between the acid-secreting and the non-acid-secreting epithelia. With atrophy of parietal cell mass, non-acid-secreting epithelium migrates up the lesser curvature.

Malignancy in gastric ulcers

Chronic duodenal ulcers are not associated with malignancy and, in contrast, gastric ulcers are. Widely varying estimates are made of the incidence of gastric malignancy in gastric ulcers. The reason for this is that the authors reporting such diverse incidences are describing different clinical situations. Two clinical extremes must be distinguished to understand this problem properly. First, there is the situation in which a benign chronic gastric ulcer undergoes malignant transformation. This is known to happen, albeit rarely. The contrasting clinical extreme is

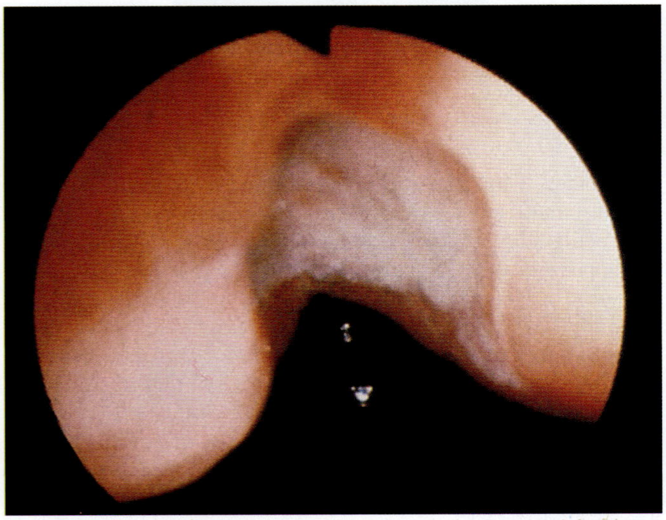

Figure 63.14 Benign incisural gastric ulcer shown at gastroscopy (courtesy of Dr GNJ Tytgat, Amsterdam, The Netherlands).

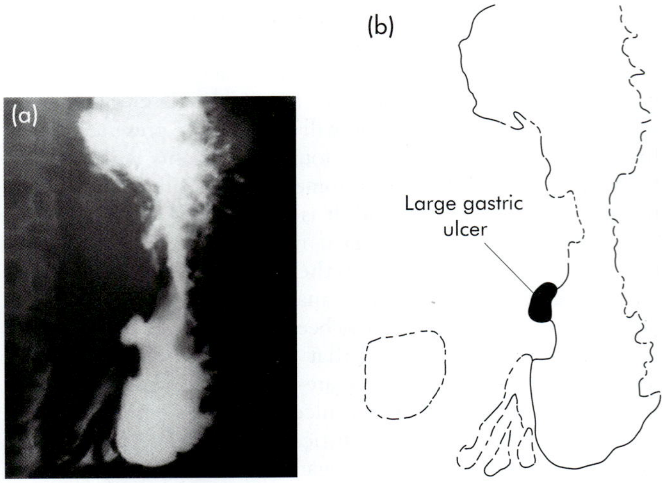

Figure 63.15 Benign gastric ulcer shown on barium meal. (a) Radiograph. (b) Diagrammatic outline.

the patient identified as having an ulcer in the stomach, either endoscopically or on contrast radiology, which is assessed as benign but biopsies reveal malignancy. In this situation the patient does not have, and probably never has had, chronic peptic ulceration in the stomach but has presented with an ulcerated cancer. This situation is common, although whether a lesion found in the stomach is described as being benign or malignant on clinical grounds depends very much on the skill and experience of the endoscopist or radiologist.

It is fundamental that any gastric ulcer should be regarded as being malignant, no matter how classic the features of a benign gastric ulcer. Multiple biopsies should always be taken, perhaps as many as ten well-targeted biopsies, before an ulcer can be tentatively accepted as being benign. Even then it is important that further biopsies are taken while the ulcer is healing and when healed. Modern antisecretory agents can frequently heal the ulceration associated with gastric cancer but, clearly, are ineffective in treating the malignancy itself. At operation, even experienced surgeons may have difficulty distinguishing between the gastric cancer and a benign ulcer. Operative strategies differ so radically that it is essential, if at all possible, that a confident diagnosis is made before operation. If, at operation, it is determined that the ulcer is probably benign it should, nonetheless, be excised, in totality if possible, and submitted for histological examination. It is not known whether a patient's survival is compromised by this approach if the ulcer turns out to be malignant on biopsy, as convincing data are not available.

Other peptic ulcers

The prepyloric gastric ulcer was in the past difficult to treat, a problem overcome with the introduction of proton pump inhibitors. Pyloric channel ulcers are similar to duodenal ulcers. Both prepyloric and pyloric ulcers may be malignant, and biopsy is essential. Stomal ulcers occur after a gastroenterostomy or a gastrectomy of the Billroth II type. The ulcer is usually found on the jejunal side of the stoma.

Clinical features of peptic ulcers

Although many textbooks try to create differences in the clinical features of gastric and duodenal ulceration, detailed analysis has shown that they cannot be differentiated on the basis of symptoms. The demographic characteristics of groups of patients with gastric and duodenal ulceration do differ but this does not allow discrimination.

Pain

The pain is epigastric, often described as gnawing and may radiate to the back. Eating may sometimes relieve the discomfort. The pain is normally intermittent rather than intractable.

Periodicity

One of the classic features of untreated peptic ulceration is periodicity. Symptoms may disappear for weeks or months to return again. This periodicity may be related to the spontaneous healing of the ulcer.

Vomiting

While this occurs, it is not a notable feature unless stenosis has occurred.

Alteration in weight

Weight loss or, sometimes, weight gain may occur. Patients with gastric ulceration are often underweight but this may precede the occurrence of the ulcer.

Bleeding

All peptic ulcers may bleed. The bleeding may be chronic and presentation with microcytic anaemia is not uncommon. All such patients should be investigated with endoscopy. Acute presentation with haematemesis and melaena is discussed below under Haematemesis and melaena.

Clinical examination

Examination of the patient may reveal epigastric tenderness but, except in extreme cases (for instance gastric outlet obstruction), there is unlikely to be much else to find.

Investigation of the patient with suspected peptic ulcer

Gastroduodenoscopy

This is the investigation of choice in the management of suspected peptic ulceration and in the hands of a well-trained operator is highly sensitive and specific.

In the stomach, any abnormal lesion should be multiple biopsied, and in the case of a suspected benign gastric ulcer numerous biopsies must be taken in order to exclude, as far as possible, the presence of a malignancy. Commonly, biopsies of the antrum will be taken to see whether there is histological evidence of gastritis and a CLO test performed to determine the presence of *H. pylori*. A 'U' manoeuvre should be performed to exclude ulcers around the gastro-oesophageal junction. This is important as the increasing incidence of cancer at the gastro-oesophageal junction requires that all mucosal abnormalities in this region should undergo multiple biopsy. Similarly, if a stoma is present, for instance after gastroenterostomy or Billroth II gastrectomy, it is important to enter both afferent and efferent loops. Almost all stomal ulcers will be very close to the junction between the jejunal and gastric mucosa. Attention should be given to the pylorus to note whether there is any prepyloric or pyloric channel ulceration, and also whether it is deformed, which is often the case with chronic duodenal ulceration. In the duodenum, care must be taken to view all of the first part. It is not infrequent for an ulcer to be just beyond the pylorus and easily overlooked.

Treatment of peptic ulceration

The vast majority of uncomplicated peptic ulcers are treated medically. Surgical treatment of uncomplicated peptic ulceration has decreased markedly since the 1960s and is now seldom performed in the West. Surgical treatment was aimed principally at reducing gastric acid secretion and, in the case of gastric ulceration, removing the diseased mucosa. When originally devised, medical treatment also aimed to reduce gastric acid secretion, initially using the highly successful H_2-receptor antagonist and, subsequently, proton pump inhibitors. This has now largely given way to eradication therapy.

Medical treatment

It is reasonable that a doctor managing a patient with an uncomplicated peptic ulcer should suggest modifications to the patient's lifestyle, particularly the cessation of cigarette smoking. This advice is rarely followed and pharmacological measures form the mainstay of treatment.

H_2-receptor antagonists and proton pump inhibitors

H_2-antagonists (Black) revolutionised the management of peptic ulceration. Most duodenal ulcers and gastric ulcers can be healed by a few weeks of treatment with these drugs provided that they are taken and absorbed. There remained, however, a group of patients who were relatively refractory to conventional doses of H_2-receptor antagonists. This is largely now irrelevant as proton pump inhibitors can effectively render a patient achlorhydric and all benign ulcers will heal using these drugs, the majority within 2 weeks. Symptom relief is impressively rapid, most patients being asymptomatic within a few days. Like H_2-antagonists, proton pump inhibitors are safe and relatively devoid of serious side effects. The problem with all gastric antisecretory agents is that following cessation of therapy relapse is almost universal.

Eradication therapy

Eradication therapy is now routinely given to patients with peptic ulceration, and this is described earlier in this chapter. Evidence suggests that if a patient has a peptic ulcer and *H. pylori* is the principal aetiological factor (essentially the patient not taking NSAIDs), then complete eradication of the organism will cure the disease and reinfection as an adult is uncommon. Eradication therapy is therefore the mainstay of treatment for peptic ulceration. It is extremely economical by comparison with prolonged courses of antisecretory agents or surgery. It is also considerably safer than surgical treatment.

There are some patients with peptic ulcers in whom eradication therapy may not be appropriate and this includes patients with NSAID-associated ulcers. Such patients should avoid these drugs if possible and, if not, they should be co-prescribed with a potent antisecretory agent. Similarly, patients with stomal ulceration are not effectively treated with eradication therapy and

Sir James Whyte Black, 1924–2002, Professor of Analytical Pharmacology, King's College Hospital Medical School, London, UK, introduced beta-blockers and H receptor antagonists. For this work he shared the 1988 Nobel Prize for Physiology or Medicine with Gertrude Bion and George Hitchings.

require prolonged prescription of antisecretory agents. Patients with Zollinger–Ellison syndrome should be treated in the long term with proton pump inhibitors unless the tumour can be adequately managed by surgery.

Ulcers that fail to heal

The introduction of antisecretory agents and effective treatments for *H. pylori* have revolutionized the management of peptic ulcers. Despite these advances, peptic ulceration fails to heal in a small minority of patients. Endoscopic re-evaluation should be regarded as mandatory to confirm healing of gastric ulcers. Furthermore, endoscopy permits the differentiation between a refractory ulcer and persistent symptoms despite ulcer healing. The most common cause of failed healing is persistent *H. pylori* infection. Biopsies should be repeated at the time of endoscopy as false-negative results with breath tests may be expected soon after eradication therapy and serum antibody titres may not fall for six months after successful eradication. Failure of eradication is usually due to poor compliance or bacterial resistance and bacteriological culture will guide further attempts at *H. pylori* eradication. The ingestion of NSAIDs should once again be addressed. A diagnosis of Zollinger–Ellison syndrome (described in detail below under Zollinger–Ellison syndrome) should be suspected in *H. pylori* negative, non-NSAID-related peptic ulceration and serum gastrin levels should be measured.

Surgical treatment of uncomplicated peptic ulceration

From its peak in the 1960s, the incidence of surgery for uncomplicated peptic ulceration has fallen markedly, to the extent that peptic ulcer surgery is now of little more than historical interest. A description of operations used in the treatment of peptic ulcers is still necessary because surgery is occasionally employed for the complicated ulcer and, in addition, many patients are left suffering from the consequences of the more destructive operations.

Operations for duodenal ulceration

Duodenal ulcer surgery (rationale)

Procedures devised for the treatment of duodenal ulcers have the common aim of excluding the damaging effects of acid from the duodenum. This has been achieved by diversion of the acid away from the duodenum, reducing the secretory potential of the stomach, or both. All of the operations devised achieved their aim to some extent, but with varying degrees of morbidity, mortality and postoperative side effects. There is now no role for acid-reducing operations in the routine management of peptic ulcer disease but, occasionally, operations which involve gastrectomy have to be performed in the emergency situation. In addition, many patients have had such operations performed and suffer from the sequelae. Hence it is important for the clinician to understand the anatomical and physiological consequences of surgery. The operations are described in historical sequence.

Billroth II gastrectomy

The first successful gastrectomy was performed by Billroth in January 1881, and Wolfler performed the first gastroenterostomy in the same year. The original Billroth operations consisted of a gastric resection with gastroduodenal anastomosis (Billroth I technique) (Figure 63.16). The Billroth II operation was devised more by accident than design (Figure 63.17). A gastroenterostomy (Figure 63.18) was performed on a gravely ill patient with a pyloric cancer, who was not expected to survive. Contrary to expectations, the patient improved and the stomach distal to the anastomosis was resected. It soon became evident that the use of a gastrojejunal anastomosis after gastric resection could be safer and easier than the Billroth I procedure, and it became popular and effective in the surgical treatment of duodenal ulcer. Because of its disadvantages, such as higher operative mortality and morbidity, it has not been used for many years in the patient with an uncomplicated ulcer, but it is still used occasionally in the treatment of a complicated ulcer with a 'difficult' duodenum. In Billroth II gastrectomy, or its close relation Polya gastrectomy, the antrum and distal body of the stomach are

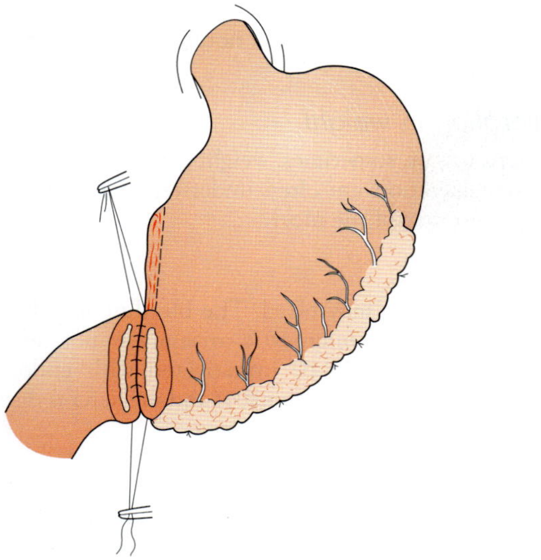

Figure 63.16 Billroth I gastrectomy. The lower half of the stomach is removed and the cut stomach anastomosed to the first part of the duodenum.

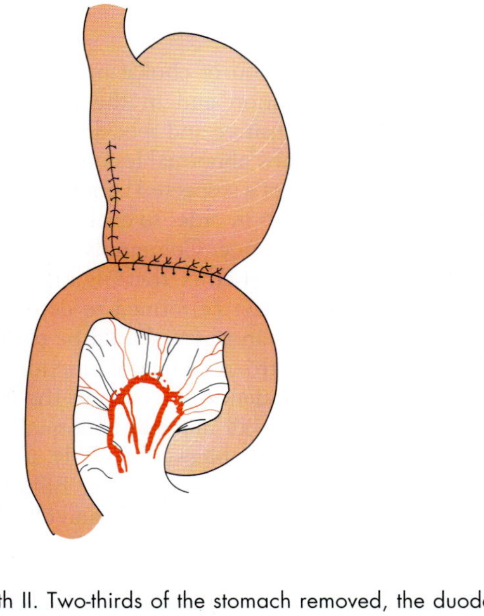

Figure 63.17 Billroth II. Two-thirds of the stomach removed, the duodenal stump is closed and the stomach anastomosed to the jejunum.

Christian Albert Theodor Billroth, 1829–1894, Professor of Surgery, Vienna, Austria.
Anton Wolfler, 1850–1917, Professor of Surgery, Prague, The Czech Republic.
Eugen (Janö) Alexander Pólya, 1876–1944, surgeon, St Stephen's Hospital,Budapest, Hungary.

Table 63.2 Operative mortality, side effects and incidence of recurrence following duodenal ulcer operations.

Operation	Operative mortality (%)	Significant side effects (%)	Recurrent ulceration (%)
Gastrectomy	1–2	20–40	1–4
Gastroenterostomy alone	<1	10–20	50
Truncal vagotomy and drainage	<1	10–20	2–7
Selective vagotomy and drainage	<1	10–20	5–10
Highly selective vagotomy	<0.2	<5	2–10
Truncal vagotomy and antrectomy	1	10–20	1

mobilised by opening the greater and lesser omentum and dividing the gastroepiploic arteries, right gastric artery and the left gastric artery arcade at the limit of the resection. The duodenum is closed off either by suture or using staples, sometimes with difficulty in patients with a very deformed duodenum. Various techniques are available to close the difficult duodenum and, *in extremis*, a catheter may be placed in the duodenal stump, the duodenum closed around it and a catheter brought out through the abdominal wall. Following resection, the distal end of the stomach is narrowed by the closure of the lesser curve aspect of the remnant. The greater curve aspect is then anastomosed, usually in a retrocolic fashion, to the jejunum leaving as short an afferent loop as feasible (Figure 63.17). Even when well performed, this procedure has an operative mortality rate of a few per cent and morbidity is not unusual. A common cause of morbidity is leakage from the duodenal stump, which is particularly associated with kinking of the afferent loop. Leakage from the gastrojejunal anastomosis is unusual unless it is under tension or the stomach has been devascularised during the mobilisation. The incidence of side effects following gastrectomy is considerable, as shown in Table 63.2. Recurrence of the ulcer at the stoma is uncommon but can occur, especially as this procedure is traditionally not combined with the vagotomy.

Gastrojejunostomy

Because of the potential for mortality after gastrectomy, the use of gastrojejunostomy alone in the treatment of duodenal ulceration was developed (Figure 63.18). Reflux of alkali from the small bowel into the stomach reduced duodenal acid exposure and was often successful in healing the ulcer. However, because the jejunal loop was exposed directly to gastric acid, stomal ulceration was extremely common, hence the procedure in isolation was ineffective.

Truncal vagotomy and drainage

Truncal vagotomy was first introduced in 1943 by Dragstedt and, for many years, combined with drainage, was the mainstay of treatment of duodenal ulceration (Figure 63.19). The principle of the operation is that section of the vagus nerves, which are critically involved in the secretion of gastric acid, reduces the maximal acid output by approximately 50 per cent. Because the vagal nerves are motor to the stomach, denervation of the antropyloroduodenal segment results in gastric stasis in a substantial proportion of patients on whom truncal vagotomy alone is performed. This was first noted by Dragstedt, who did not perform a drainage procedure when he first introduced the operation. The most popular drainage procedure is the Heineke–Mikulicz pyloroplasty (Figure 63.20). It is simple to perform and involves the longitudinal section of the pyloric ring. The incision is closed transversely. Gastrojejunostomy (Figure 63.18) was the alternative drainage procedure to pyloroplasty. This is performed through opening the lesser sac and performing an anastomosis between the most dependent part of the antrum and the first jejunal loop. An isoperistaltic anastomosis was most commonly performed. The operation of truncal vagotomy and drainage is substantially safer than gastrectomy (Table 63.2). However, the side effects of surgery are, in fact, little different from those that follow gastrectomy.

Lester Reynolds Dragstedt, 1893–1975, Professor of Surgery, Chicago, IL, USA. He was a physiologist to start with and later became a surgeon. His physiological mind made him consider that vagotomy would be a treatment for peptic ulcer. Accordingly, he performed the first vagotomy in 1943.

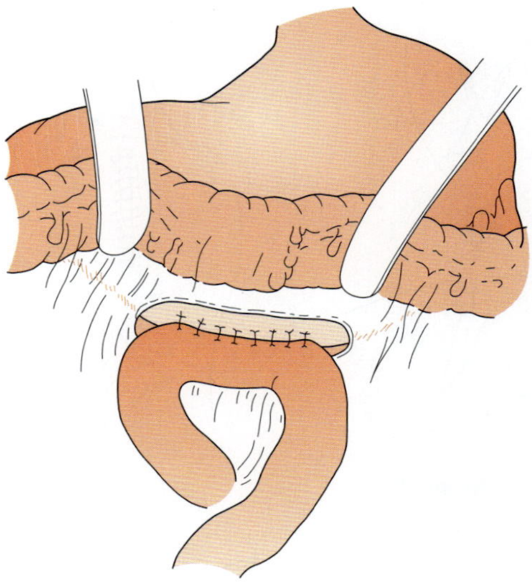

Figure 63.18 Gastroenterostomy. The jejunum is anastomosed to the posterior, dependent, wall of the stomach.

Highly selective vagotomy

In 1968, Johnston and Amdrup independently devised the operation of highly selective vagotomy in which only the parietal cell mass of the stomach was denervated (Figure 63.21). This proved to be the most satisfactory operation for duodenal ulceration, with a low incidence of side effects and acceptable recurrence rates when performed to a high technical standard. This operation became the 'gold standard' for operations on duodenal ulceration in the 1970s. The operative mortality was

Walther Hermann Heineke, 1834–1901, surgeon of Erlangen, Germany.
Johann von Mikulicz-Radecki, 1850–1905, Professor of Surgey, Breslau, Germany (now Wroclaw, Poland).

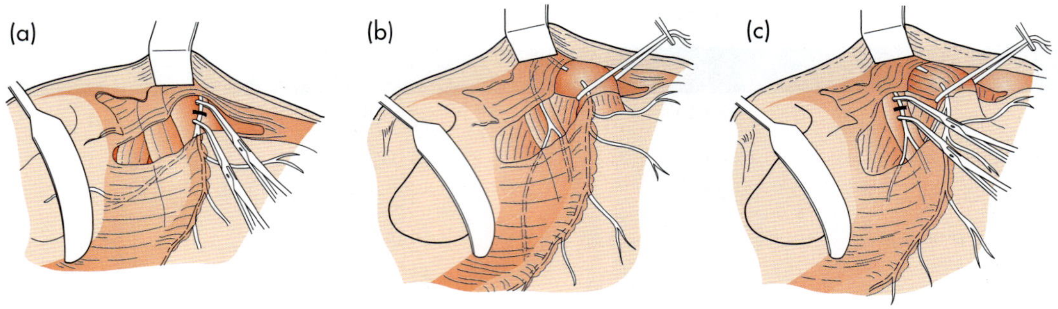

Figure 63.19 Truncal vagotomy. (a) Division of the anterior vagus. (b) Mobilisation of the oesophagus. (c) Division of the posterior vagus.

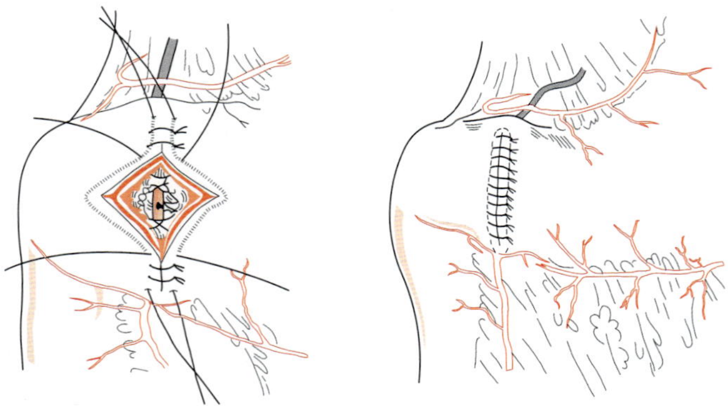

Figure 63.20 Pyroplasty.

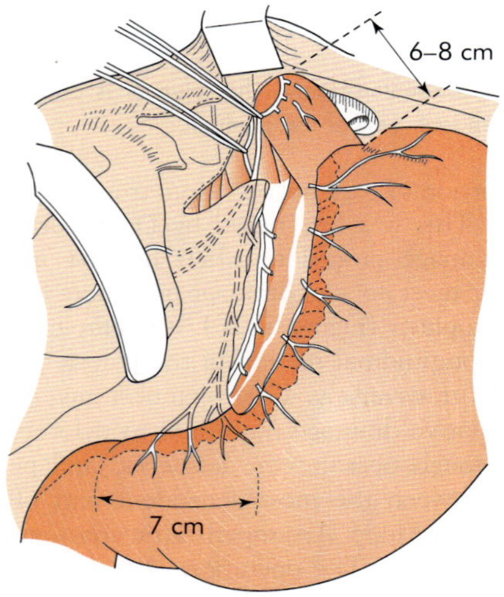

Figure 63.21 Highly selective vagotomy. The anterior and posterior vagus nerves are preserved but all branches to the fundus and body of the stomach are divided.

lower than any other definitive operation for duodenal ulceration, in all probability because the gastrointestinal tract was not opened during this procedure. The unpleasant effects of peptic ulcer surgery were largely avoided, although loss of receptive relaxation of the stomach did occur, leading to epigastric fullness and sometimes mild dumping. However, the severe symptoms that occur after other more destructive gastric operations did not occur. It is often said that recurrent ulceration is the Achilles heel of this operation although, when performed well, recurrence was no more common than after truncal vagotomy. The operation disappeared from routine use with the advent of antisecretory agents and eradication therapy.

Truncal vagotomy and antrectomy

For completeness, this operation should be mentioned as at one stage it was popular in the USA. In addition to a truncal vagotomy, the antrum of the stomach is removed, thus removing the source of gastrin, and the gastric remnant is joined to the duodenum. The recurrence rates after this procedure are exceedingly low. However, the operative mortality is higher than after vagotomy and drainage (Table 63.2) and the incidence of unpleasant side effects is similar.

Operations for gastric ulcer

In contrast with duodenal ulcer surgery, when the principal objective was to reduce duodenal acid exposure, in gastric ulceration the diseased tissue is usually removed as well. This has the advantage that malignancy can then be confidently excluded. As with duodenal ulceration, such surgery is not now performed except for complications of gastric ulcer.

Billroth I gastrectomy

This was the standard operation (Figure 63.16) for gastric ulceration until medical treatments became prevalent. The distal stomach is mobilised and resected in the same way as in the Billroth II gastrectomy. This resection should include the ulcer that is usually situated on the lesser curve. The cut edge of the remnant is then partially closed from the lesser curve aspect, leaving a stoma at the greater curve aspect, which should be similar in size to the duodenum. Reconstruction may be facilitated by mobilising the duodenum using Kocher's manoeuvre. The incidence of recurrent ulceration after this operation is low, but it carries with it the morbidity and mortality associated with any gastric resection.

Sequelae of peptic ulcer surgery

There are a number of sequelae of peptic ulcer surgery, which include recurrent ulceration, small stomach syndrome, bilious vomiting, early and late dumping, diarrhoea and malignant transformation. These sequelae principally follow from the more destructive operations that are now seldom performed. However, a substantial number of patients suffer from side effects from operations undertaken in the past. Approximately 30 per cent of patients can expect to suffer a degree of dysfunc-

David Johnston, Professor of Surgery, the University of Leeds, Leeds, UK.
Eric Amdrup, 1923–1998, Professor of Surgery, Aarhus, Denmark.
Emil Theodor Kocher, 1841–1917, Professor of Surgery, Berne, Switzerland. In 1909 he was awarded the Nobel Prize for Physiology or Medicine for his work on the thyroid.

tion following peptic ulcer surgery (Table 63.2) and, in about 5 per cent of such patients, the symptoms will be intractable.

Recurrent ulceration

Although mentioned first, this is by far the easiest problem to treat. Just as all peptic ulcers will heal with potent antisecretory agents, so will ulcers that are recurrent after ulcer surgery.

As with other peptic ulcers, recurrent ulcers may present with complications, particularly bleeding and perforation. In this respect, the complication of gastrojejuno-colic fistula requires a particular mention. In this rare condition, the anastomotic ulcer penetrates into the transverse colon. Patients suffer from diarrhoea that is severe and follows every meal. They have foul breath and may vomit formed faeces. Severe weight loss and dehydration are rapid in onset, and for this reason the condition may be mistaken for malignancy. The major factor producing the nutritional disturbance is the severe contamination of the jejunum with colonic bacteria. A number of imaging techniques can be used to detect the fistula, most commonly CT with oral contrast or indeed a barium enema. Endoscopy may not convincingly demonstrate the fistula and, in about one-half of such cases, the barium meal will not reveal the problem. The treatment of gastrocolic fistula consists of first correcting the dehydration and malnutrition and then performing revisional surgery.

Small stomach syndrome

Early satiety follows most ulcer operations to some degree, including highly selective vagotomy. In this latter circumstance, although there is no anatomical disturbance of the stomach there is loss of receptive relaxation. Fortunately, this problem does tend to get better with time and revisional surgery is not necessary.

Bile vomiting

Bile vomiting can occur after any form of vagotomy with drainage or gastrectomy. Commonly, the patient presents with vomiting a mixture of food and bile or sometimes some bile alone after a meal. Often, eating will precipitate abdominal pain and reflux symptoms are common. Bile chelating agents can be tried but are usually ineffective. In intractable cases, revisional surgery may be indicated. The nature of that revisional surgery depends very much on the original operation. Following gastrectomy, Roux-en-Y diversion is probably the best treatment. In patients with a gastroenterostomy, this can be taken down and, in most circumstances a small pyloroplasty can be performed. In patients with a pyloroplasty, reconstruction of the pylorus has been attempted but, in general terms, the results of this operation have been rather poor. Antrectomy and Roux-en-Y reconstruction may be the better option.

Early and late dumping

Although considered together because the symptoms are similar, early and late dumping have different aetiologies. A common feature, however, is early rapid gastric emptying. Many patients have both early and late dumping.

Early dumping

Early dumping consists of abdominal and vasomotor symptoms that are found in about 10 per cent of patients following gastrectomy or vagotomy and drainage. It also affects a small percentage of patients following highly selective vagotomy due to the loss of receptive relaxation of the stomach. The small bowel is filled with foodstuffs from the stomach, which have a high osmotic load, and this leads to the sequestration of fluid from the circulation into the gastrointestinal tract. This can be observed by the rise in the packed cell volume while the symptoms are present. All of the symptoms shown in Table 63.3 can be related to this effect on the gut and the circulation.

The principal treatment is dietary manipulation. Small, dry meals are best, and avoiding fluids with a high carbohydrate content also helps. Fortunately, following operation, the syndrome tends to improve with time. For some reason, however, there is a group of patients who suffer intractable dumping regardless of any of these measures. The somatostatin analogue octreotide given before meals has been shown to be useful in some individuals and the long-acting preparation may also be useful. However, this treatment can lead to the development of gallstones and it does not help the diarrhoea from which many patients with dumping also suffer.

Revisional surgery may be occasionally required. In patients with a gastroenterostomy, the drainage may be taken down or, in the case of a pyloroplasty, repaired. Alternatively, antrectomy with Roux-en-Y reconstruction is often effective, although the procedure is of greater magnitude; following gastrectomy, it is the revisional procedure of choice.

Table 63.3 Features of early and late dumping.

	Early	Late
Incidence	5–10%	5%
Relation to meals	Almost immediate	Second hour after meal
Durations of attack	30–40 minutes	30–40 minutes
Relief	Lying down	Food
Aggravated by	More food	Exercise
Precipitating factor	Food, especially carbohydrate-rich and wet	As early dumping
Major symptoms	Epigastric fullness, sweating, light-headedness, tachycardia, colic, sometimes diarrhoea	Tremor, faintness, prostration

Late dumping

This is reactive hypoglycaemia. The carbohydrate load in the small bowel causes a rise in the plasma glucose, which, in turn, causes insulin levels to rise, causing a secondary hypoglycaemia. This can be easily demonstrated by serial measurements of blood glucose in a patient following a test meal. The treatment is essentially the same as for early dumping. Octreotide is very effective in dealing with this problem.

Postvagotomy diarrhoea

This can be the most devastating symptom to afflict patients having peptic ulcer surgery. Most patients will suffer some looseness of bowel action to some degree (with the exception of highly selective vagotomy) but, in about 5 per cent, it may be intractable. Despite much investigation, the precise aetiology of the problem is uncertain. It is related, to some degree, to rapid gastric emptying. In all probability, the denervation of the upper gastrointestinal tract as a result of the vagotomy is also important. Exaggerated gastrointestinal peptide responses may also aggravate the condition.

The diarrhoea in postvagotomy patients may take several forms. It may be severe and explosive, the patient experiencing a considerable degree of urgency. The patients sometimes describe the diarrhoea as feeling like passing boiling water. At the other extreme, some patients only have minor episodes of diarrhoea, which are not as directly related to food.

Many authors regard diarrhoea and dumping as being essentially the same problem. However, many patients with severe diarrhoea do not have any of the other symptoms of dumping and likewise some patients with dumping do not experience any significant diarrhoea.

The condition is difficult to treat. The patient should be managed as for early dumping and antidiarrhoeal preparations may be of some value. Octreotide is not effective in this condition and the results of revisional surgery are too unpredictable to make this an attractive treatment option.

Malignant transformation

Many large studies now confirm that operations such as gastrectomy or vagotomy and drainage are independent risk factors for the development of gastric cancer. The increased risk appears to be approximately four times that of the control population.

It is not difficult to understand the increased incidence of gastric cancer, as bile reflux gastritis, intestinal metaplasia and gastric cancer are linked. The lag phase between operation and the development of malignancy is at least ten years. Highly selective vagotomy does not seem to be associated with an increased incidence of gastric cancer in the long term.

Nutritional consequences

Nutritional disorders are more common after gastrectomy than after vagotomy and drainage. Weight loss is common after gastrectomy and the patient may, in fact, never return to their original weight. Nutritional advice advising the taking of small meals is often more useful. Anaemia may be due to either iron or vitamin B12 deficiency.

Iron-deficiency anaemia occurs after both gastrectomy and vagotomy and drainage and is probably multifactorial in origin. Reduced iron absorption is probably the most important factor, although the loss of blood from the gastric mucosa may also be important. Vitamin B12 deficiency is prone to occur after total gastrectomy. However, because of the very large vitamin B12 stores that most patients have, this may be very late in occurring. Vitamin B12 supplementation after total gastrectomy is essential. Rarely, vitamin B12 deficiency may occur after lesser forms of gastrectomy. In such patients the cause is probably a combination of reduced intrinsic factor production and also the fact that some patients have bacterial colonisation, which results in the destruction of the vitamin B12 in the gut.

Bone disease is seen principally after gastrectomy, and mainly in women. The condition is essentially indistinguishable from the osteoporosis commonly seen in postmenopausal women. It is only the frequency and magnitude of the disorder that distinguish it. Treatment is with dietary supplementation, calcium and vitamin D, and exercise.

Gallstones

The development of gallstones is strongly associated with truncal vagotomy. Following truncal vagotomy, the biliary tree, as well as the stomach, is denervated, leading to stasis and hence stone formation. Patients developing symptomatic gallstones will require cholecystectomy. However, this may induce or worsen other postpeptic ulcer surgery syndromes such as bilious vomiting and postvagotomy diarrhoea.

The complications of peptic ulceration

The common complications of peptic ulcer are perforation, bleeding and stenosis. Bleeding and stenosis are considered below in the relevant sections.

Perforated peptic ulcer

Epidemiology

Despite the widespread use of gastric antisecretory agents and eradication therapy, the incidence of perforated peptic ulcer has changed little. However, there has been a considerable change in the epidemiology of perforated peptic ulcer in the West over the last two decades. Previously, most patients were middle aged, with a ratio of 2:1 of male:female. With time, there has been a steady increase in the age of the patients suffering this complication and an increase in the numbers of females, such that perforations now occur most commonly in elderly female patients. NSAIDs appear to be responsible for most of these perforations.

Clinical features

The classic presentation of perforated duodenal ulcer is instantly recognisable (Figure 63.22). The patient, who may have a history of peptic ulceration, develops sudden onset severe generalised abdominal pain due to the irritant effect of gastric acid on the peritoneum. Although the contents of an acid-producing stomach are relatively low in bacterial load, bacterial peritonitis supervenes over a few hours, usually accompanied by a deterioration in the patient's condition. Initially, the patient may be shocked with a tachycardia but a pyrexia is not usually observed until some hours after the event. The abdomen exhibits a board-like rigidity and the patient is disinclined to move because of the pain. The abdomen does not move with respiration. Patients with this form of presentation need an operation, without which the patient will deteriorate with a septic peritonitis.

This classic presentation of the perforated peptic ulcer is observed less commonly than in the past. Very frequently, the

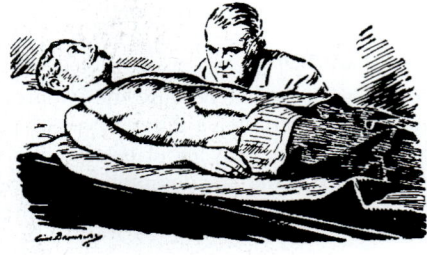

Figure 63.22 A sketch of Mr Hamilton Bailey watching for abdominal movement on respiration. In the case of a classically presenting perforated ulcer, the abdominal movement is restricted or absent.

elderly patient who is taking NSAIDs will have a less dramatic presentation, perhaps because of the use of potent anti-inflammatory drugs (steroids). The board-like rigidity seen in the abdomen of younger patients may also not be observed and a higher index of suspicion is necessary to make the correct diagnosis. In other patients, the leak from the ulcer may not be massive. They may present only with pain in the epigastrium and right iliac fossa as the fluid may track down the right paracolic gutter. Sometimes perforations will seal owing to the inflammatory response and adhesion within the abdominal cavity, and so the perforation may be self-limiting. All of these factors may combine to make the diagnosis of perforated peptic ulcer difficult.

By far the most common site of perforation is the anterior aspect of the duodenum. However, the anterior or incisural gastric ulcer may perforate and, in addition, gastric ulcers may perforate into the lesser sac, which can be particularly difficult to diagnose. These patients may not have obvious peritonitis.

Investigations

An erect plain chest radiograph will reveal free gas under the diaphragm in an excess of 50 per cent of cases with perforated peptic ulcer (Figure 63.23) but CT imaging is more accurate (see below). All patients should have serum amylase performed, as distinguishing between peptic ulcer, perforation and pancreatitis can be difficult. Measuring the serum amylase, however, may not remove the diagnostic difficulty. It can be elevated following perforation of a peptic ulcer although, fortunately, the levels are not usually as high as the levels commonly seen in acute pancreatitis. Several other investigations are useful if doubt remains. A CT scan will normally be diagnostic in both conditions.

Treatment

The initial priorities are resuscitation and analgesia. Analgesia should not be withheld for fear of removing the signs of an intra-abdominal catastrophe. In fact, adequate analgesia makes the clinical signs more obvious. It is important, however, to titrate the analgesic dose. Following resuscitation, the treatment is principally surgical. Laparotomy is performed, usually through an upper midline incision if the diagnosis of perforated peptic ulcer can be made with confidence. This is not always possible and hence it may be better to place a small incision around the umbilicus to localise the perforation with more certainty. Alternatively, laparoscopy may be used. The most important component of the operation is a thorough peritoneal toilet to remove all of the fluid and food debris. If the perforation is in the duodenum it can usually be closed by several well-placed sutures, closing the ulcer in a transverse direction as with a pyloroplasty. It is important that sufficient tissue is taken in the suture to allow the edges to be approximated, and the sutures should not be tied so tight that they tear out. It is common to place an omental patch over the perforation in the hope of enhancing the chances of the leak sealing. If the perforation is difficult to close primarily, it is frequently possible to seal the leak with an omental patch alone, and many surgeons now employ this strategy for all perforations. When securing the omental patch it is important not to tie the sutures too tight so as to obliterate the omental blood supply. Gastric ulcers should, if possible, be excised and closed, so that malignancy can be excluded. Occasionally, a patient is seen who has a massive duodenal or gastric perforation such that simple closure is impossible; in these patients a Billroth II gastrectomy or subtotal gastrectomy with Roux-en-Y reconstruction are useful operations.

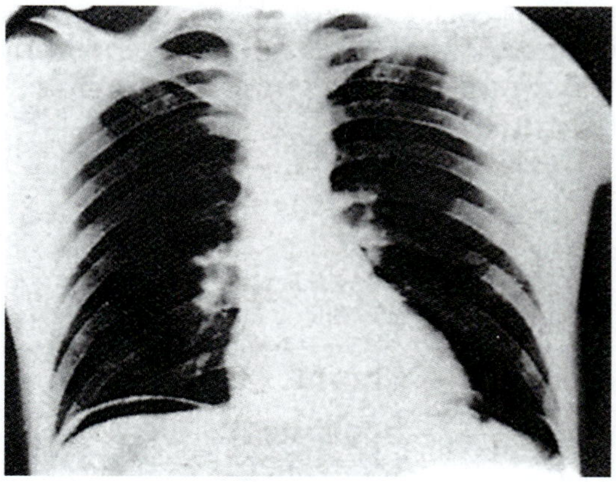

Figure 63.23 Plain abdominal radiograph of a perforated ulcer, showing air under the diaphragm.

All patients should be treated with systemic antibiotics in addition to a thorough peritoneal lavage. In the past, many surgeons performed definitive procedures such as either truncal vagotomy and pyloroplasty or, more recently and probably more successfully, highly selective vagotomy during the course of an operation for a perforation. Studies show that in well-selected patients and in expert hands this is a very safe strategy. However, nowadays, surgery is confined to first-aid measures most commonly, and the peptic ulcer is treated medically as described earlier in this chapter. Following operation, gastric antisecretory agents should be started immediately.

Perforated peptic ulcers can often be managed by minimally invasive techniques if the expertise is available. The principles of operation are, however, the same; thorough peritoneal toilet is performed and the perforation is closed by intracorporeal suturing. Whatever technique is used, it is important that the stomach is kept empty postoperatively by nasogastric suction, and that gastric antisecretory agents are commenced to promote healing of the residual ulcer.

A great deal has been written about the conservative management of perforated ulcer. Some writers say that virtually all patients can be managed conservatively, whereas most surgeons have difficulty in understanding how a patient who is ill with widespread peritonitis and who has food debris widely distributed through the abdominal cavity will improve without an operation. However, undoubtedly, there are patients who have small leaks from a perforated peptic ulcer and relatively mild peritoneal contamination, who may be managed with intravenous fluids, nasogastric suction and antibiotics. These patients are in the minority. A number of factors have been associated with poor outcome after perforated peptic ulcer, including:

- delay in diagnosis (>24 hours)
- medical comorbidities
- shock
- increasing age (>75).

There is little evidence to advocate the conservative management of patients who exhibit any of these characteristics.

Patients who have suffered one perforation may suffer another one. Therefore, they should be managed aggressively to ensure that this does not happen. In patients with *Helicobacter*-associated ulcers, eradication therapy is appropriate. Life-long treatment with proton pump inhibitors is a reasonable option, especially in those who have to continue with NSAID treatment (Summary box 63.4).

HAEMATEMESIS AND MELAENA

Upper gastrointestinal haemorrhage remains a major medical problem with an incidence of over 100/100 000 per year in Western practice that increases with increasing age. Haemorrhage is strongly associated with NSAID use. Despite improvements in diagnosis and the proliferation in treatment modalities over the last few decades, an in-hospital mortality of 5–10 per cent can be expected. This rises to 33 per cent when bleeding is first observed in patients who are hospitalised for other reasons. In patients in whom the cause of bleeding can be found, the most common causes are peptic ulcer, erosions, Mallory–Weiss tear and bleeding oesophageal varices (Table 63.4).

Table 63.4 Causes of upper gastrointestinal bleeding.

Condition	%
Ulcers	60
Oesophageal	6
Gastric	21
Duodenal	33
Erosions	26
Oesophageal	13
Gastric	9
Duodenal	4
Mallory–Weiss tear	4
Oesophageal varices	4
Tumour	0.5
Vascular lesions, e.g. Dieulafoy's disease	0.5
Others	5

Whatever the cause, the principles of management are identical. First, the patient should be adequately resuscitated and, following this, the patient should be investigated urgently to determine the cause of the bleeding. Only then should treatment of a definitive nature be instituted. For any significant gastrointestinal bleed, intravenous access should be established and, for those with severe bleeding, central venous pressure monitoring should be set up and bladder catheterisation performed. Blood should be cross-matched and the patient transfused as clinically indicated, usually when >30 per cent of blood volume has been lost. There is no evidence for the use of intravenous proton pump inhibitors prior to endoscopy. As a general rule, most gastrointestinal bleeding will stop, albeit temporarily, but there are sometimes instances when this is not the case. In these circumstances, resuscitation, diagnosis and treatment should be carried out simultaneously. There are occasions when life-saving manoeuvres have to be undertaken without the benefit of an absolute diagnosis. For instance, in patients with known oesophageal varices and uncontrollable bleeding, a Sengstaken–Blakemore tube may be inserted before an endoscopy has been carried out. This practice is not to be encouraged, except *in extremis*. In some patients, bleeding is secondary to a coagulopathy. The most important current causes of this are liver disease and inadequately controlled warfarin therapy. In these circumstances the coagulopathy should be corrected, if possible, with fresh-frozen plasma or concentrated clotting factors.

Upper gastrointestinal endoscopy should be carried out by an experienced operator as soon as practicable after the patient has been stabilised. In patients in whom the bleeding is relatively mild, endoscopy may be carried out on the morning after admission. In all cases of severe bleeding it should be carried out immediately. A number of scoring systems have been advocated for the assessment of rebleeding and death after upper gastrointestinal haemorrhage. Perhaps the most useful of these is the Rockall score. This can be used in a pre-endoscopy format to stratify patients to safe early discharge and postendoscopy it can relatively accurately predict rebleeding and death.

Bleeding peptic ulcers

The epidemiology of bleeding peptic ulcers exactly mirrors that of perforated ulcers. In recent years, the population affected has become much older and the bleeding is commonly associated with the ingestion of NSAIDs. Diagnosis can normally be made endoscopically, although occasionally the nature of the blood loss precludes accurately identifying the lesion. However, the more experienced the endoscopist, the less likely this is to be a problem.

Medical and minimally interventional treatments

Medical treatment has limited efficacy. All patients are commonly started on either an H_2-antagonist or a proton pump antagonist, and recent evidence confirms the benefit of proton pump inhibitor administration to prevent rebleeding after endoscopy. Furthermore, meta-analysis of studies suggests that tranexamic acid, an inhibitor of fibrinolysis, may reduce overall mortality.

Therapeutic endoscopy can achieve haemostasis in approximately 70 per cent of cases, with the best evidence supporting a combination of adrenaline injection with heater probe and/or clips. Therapeutic endoscopy will probably never be effective in patients who are bleeding from large vessels and with which the majority of the mortality is associated.

In patients where the source of bleeding cannot be identified or in those who rebleed after endoscopy, angiography with transcatheter embolisation may offer a valuable alternative to surgery in expert centres. The risk of significant ischaemia following embolisation is low because of the rich collateral blood supply of the stomach and duodenum. The surgeon should be mindful that rescue surgery after failed embolisation is associated with poor outcome and it may be advantageous to proceed directly to surgery.

Surgical treatment

Criteria for surgery are well worked out. A patient who continues to bleed requires surgical treatment. The same applies to a

George Kenneth Mallory, born 1926, Professor of Pathology, Boston University, Boston, MA,USA.
Soma Weiss, 1898–1942, Professor of Medicine, Harvard University Medical School, Boston, MA, USA.
Robert William Sengstaken, born 1923, surgeon, Garden City, New York, NY, USA.
Arthur Hendley Blakemore, Associate Professor of Surgery, the Columbia College of Physicians and Surgeons, New York, NY, USA.
Sengstaken and Blakemore originally described the tube in 1950.

significant rebleed. Patients with a visible vessel in the ulcer base, a spurting vessel or an ulcer with a clot in the base are statistically likely to require surgical treatment to stop the bleeding. Elderly and unfit patients are more likely to die as a result of bleeding than younger patients. Ironically, they should have early surgery. A patient who has required more than six units of blood in general needs surgical treatment.

The aim of the operation is to stop the bleeding. The advent of endoscopy has greatly helped in the management of upper gastrointestinal bleeding as a surgeon can usually be confident about the site of bleeding prior to operation. The most common site of bleeding from a peptic ulcer is the duodenum. In tackling this, it is essential that the duodenum is fully mobilised. This should be done before the duodenum is opened as it makes the ulcer much more accessible and also allows the surgeon's hand to be placed behind the gastroduodenal artery, which is commonly the source of major bleeding. Following mobilisation, the duodenum, and usually the pylorus, is opened longitudinally as in a pyloroplasty (Figure 63.20). This allows good access to the ulcer, which is usually found posteriorly or superiorly. Accurate haemostasis is important and can be achieved initially by direct pressure. It is the vessel within the ulcer that is bleeding and this should be controlled using well-placed sutures on a small round-bodied needle that under-run the vessel. The placing of more and more inaccurately positioned sutures is counterproductive. Following under-running, it is often possible to close the mucosa over the ulcer. The pyloroplasty is then closed with interrupted sutures in a transverse direction as in the usual fashion. In a giant ulcer the first part of the duodenum may be destroyed making primary closure impossible. In this circumstance one should proceed to subtotal gastrectomy with Roux-en-Y reconstruction. The duodenal stump may then be closed using the Nissen technique with T-tube drainage.

The principles of management of bleeding gastric ulcers are essentially the same. The stomach is opened at an appropriate position anteriorly and the vessel in the ulcer under-run. If the ulcer is not excised then a biopsy of the edge needs to be taken to exclude malignant transformation. Sometimes the bleeding is from the splenic artery and if there is a lot of fibrosis present then the operation may be challenging. However, most patients can be managed by conservative surgery. Gastrectomy for bleeding has been widely practised in the past, but is associated with a high perioperative mortality even if the incidence of recurrent bleeding is less.

Bearing in mind that most patients nowadays are elderly and unfit, the minimum surgery that stops the bleeding is probably optimal. Acid can be inhibited by pharmacological means and appropriate eradication therapy will prevent ulcer recurrence. Definitive acid-lowering surgery is not now required. Patients on long-term NSAIDs can be managed as outlined earlier.

Stress ulceration

This commonly occurs in patients with major injury or illness, who have undergone major surgery or who have major comorbidity. Many such patients are found in intensive care units. There seems little doubt that the incidence of this problem has reduced in recent years due to the widespread use of prophylaxis. Acid inhibition and the nasogastric or oral administration of sucralfate has been shown to reduce the incidence of stress ulceration. There is no doubt that it is far better to prevent this condition than to try to treat it once it occurs. Endoscopic means of treating stress ulceration may be ineffective and operation may be required. The principles of management are the same as for the chronic ulcer.

Gastric erosions

Erosive gastritis has a variety of causes, especially NSAIDs. Fortunately, most such bleeding settles spontaneously, but when it does not it can be a major problem to treat. In general terms, although there is a diffuse erosive gastritis, there is one (or more) specific lesion that has a significant-sized vessel within it. This should be dealt with appropriately, preferably endoscopically, but sometimes surgery is necessary.

Mallory–Weiss tear

This is a longitudinal tear at the gastro-oesophageal junction, which is induced by repetitive and strenuous vomiting. Doubtless, many such lesions occur and do not cause bleeding. When it is a cause of haematemesis, the lesion may often be missed as it can be difficult to see as it is just below the gastro-oesophageal junction, a position that can be difficult for the inexperienced endoscopist. Occasionally, these lesions continue to bleed and require surgical treatment. Often the situation arises in which the surgeon does not have guidance from the endoscopists as regards the site of bleeding, and a high index of suspicion in such circumstances is important. The experienced surgeon will perform on-table endoscopy prior to embarking on surgery. The stomach is opened by longitudinal gastrotomy and the upper section is carefully inspected. It is normally possible to palpate the longitudinal mucosal tear with a little induration at the edges, which gives a clue to the lesion's location. Under-running is all that is required.

Dieulafoy's disease

This is essentially a gastric arterial venous malformation that has a characteristic histological appearance. Bleeding due to this malformation is one of the most difficult causes of upper gastrointestinal bleeding to treat. The lesion itself is covered by normal mucosa and, when not bleeding, it may be invisible. If it can be seen while bleeding, all that may be visible is profuse bleeding coming from an area of apparently normal mucosa. If this occurs, the cause is instantly recognisable. If the lesion can be identified endoscopically there are various means of dealing with it, including injection of sclerosant and endoscopic clips. If it is identified at operation then only a local excision is necessary. Occasionally, a lesion is only recognised after gastrectomy and sometimes not even then. The pathologist, as well as the endoscopist, may have difficulty in finding it.

Tumours

All of the gastric tumours described below may present with chronic or acute upper gastrointestinal bleeding. Bleeding is not normally torrential but can be unremitting. Gastric stromal tumours commonly present with bleeding and have a characteristic appearance, as the mucosa breaks down over the tumour in the gastric wall (Figure 63.24). Whatever the nature, the tumours should be dealt with as appropriate.

Portal hypertension and portal gastropathy

The management of bleeding gastric varices is very challenging. Fortunately, most bleeding from varices is oesophageal and this

Paul Georges Dieulafoy, 1839–1911, Professor of Medicine and Chief of Medical Services at the Hôtel Dieu, Paris, France.

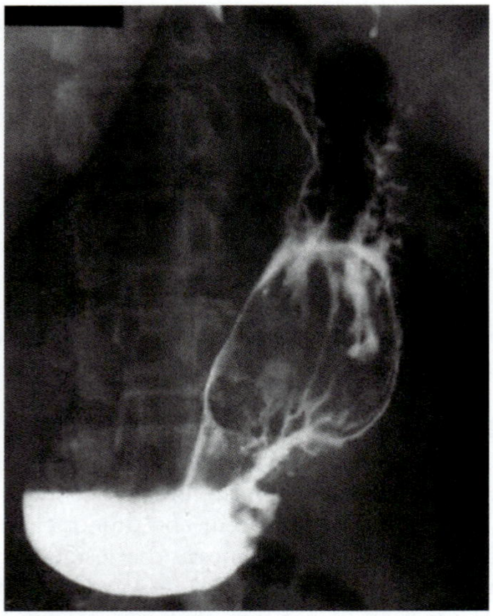

Figure 63.24 Smooth muscle tumour of the stomach, with ulceration.

is much more amenable to sclerotherapy, banding and balloon tamponade. Gastric varices may also be injected, although this is technically more difficult. Banding can also be used, again with difficulty. The gastric balloon of the Sengastaken–Blakemore tube can be used to arrest the haemorrhage if it is occurring from the fundus of the stomach or gastro-oesophageal junction. Octreotide is a somatostatin analogue that reduces portal pressure in patients with varices, and trials suggest that it is of value in arresting haemorrhage in these patients, although its overall effect on mortality remains in doubt. Glypressin is also said to be of use.

Most surgeons prefer to avoid acute surgery on bleeding varices as, in contrast with elective operations for portal hypertension, acute shunts are attended by considerable operative mortality. For this reason the acute TIPSS procedure (transjugular intrahepatic portosystemic shunt), which is described in Chapter 65, can be an extremely useful, although technically demanding, procedure.

Portal gastropathy

Portal gastropathy is essentially the same disease process as described above. The mucosa is affected by the increased portal pressure and may exude blood, even in the absence of well-developed visible varices. The treatment is as above.

Aortic enteric fistula

This diagnosis should be considered in any patient with haematemesis and melaena that cannot be otherwise explained. Contrary to expectation, the bleeding from such patients is not always massive, although it can be. Very often there is nothing much to distinguish between the bleeding from the aortic enteric fistula and any other recurrent upper gastrointestinal bleeding. The vast majority of patients will have had an aortic graft and, in the absence of this, the diagnosis is unlikely. However, it is occasionally seen in patients with an untreated aortic aneurysm. A well-performed CT scan will commonly allow the diagnosis to be made with certainty. The condition should be managed by an expert vascular surgeon as, whether secondary or primary, the morbidity and mortality are high.

GASTRIC OUTLET OBSTRUCTION

The two common causes of gastric outlet obstruction are gastric cancer (see below) and pyloric stenosis secondary to peptic ulceration. Previously, the latter was more common. Now, with the decrease in the incidence of peptic ulceration and the advent of potent medical treatments, gastric outlet obstruction should be considered malignant until proven otherwise, at least in the West.

The term 'pyloric stenosis' is normally a misnomer. The stenosis is seldom at the pylorus. Commonly, when the condition is due to underlying peptic ulcer disease, the stenosis is found in the first part of the duodenum, the most common site for a peptic ulcer. True pyloric stenosis can occur due to fibrosis around a pyloric channel ulcer. However, in recent years, the most common cause of gastric outlet obstruction has been gastric cancer. In this circumstance the metabolic consequences may be somewhat different from those of benign pyloric stenosis because of the relative hypochlorhydria found in patients with gastric cancer (Summary box 63.5).

Summary box 63.5

Gastric outlet obstruction

- Gastric outlet obstruction is most commonly associated with long-standing peptic ulcer disease and gastric cancer
- The metabolic abnormality of hypochloraemic alkalosis is usually only seen with peptic ulcer disease and should be treated with isotonic saline with potassium
- Endoscopic biopsy is essential to determine whether the cause of the problem is malignancy
- Aggressive medical therapy for peptic ulcer disease often leads to resolution
- Endoscopic dilatation of the gastric outlet may be effective in the less severe cases of benign stenosis
- Operation is frequently required, with a drainage procedure being performed for benign disease and appropriate resectional surgery if malignant

Clinical features

In benign gastric outlet obstruction there is usually a long history of peptic ulcer disease. Nowadays, as most patients with peptic ulcer symptoms are treated medically, it is easy to understand why the condition is becoming much less common. In some patients the pain may become unremitting and in other cases it may largely disappear. The vomitus is characteristically unpleasant in nature and is totally lacking in bile. Very often it is possible to recognise foodstuff taken several days previously. The patient commonly complains of losing weight, and appears unwell and dehydrated. When examining the patient, it may be possible to see the distended stomach and a succussion splash may be audible on shaking the patient's abdomen.

Metabolic effects

These are most interesting as the metabolic consequences of benign pyloric stenosis are unique. The vomiting of hydrochloric acid results in hypochloraemic alkalosis. Initially, the sodium and potassium may be relatively normal. However, as dehydration progresses, more profound metabolic abnormalities arise, partly related to renal dysfunction. Initially, the urine has a low chloride and high bicarbonate content, reflecting the primary metabolic abnormality. This bicarbonate is excreted along with sodium, and so with time the patient becomes progressively hyponatraemic and more profoundly dehydrated. Because of the dehydration, a phase of sodium retention follows and potassium and hydrogen are excreted in preference. This results in the urine becoming paradoxically acidic and hypokalaemia ensues. Alkalosis leads to a lowering in the circulating ionised calcium, and tetany can occur.

Management

Treating the patient involves correcting the metabolic abnormality and dealing with the mechanical problem. The patient should be rehydrated with intravenous isotonic saline with potassium supplementation. Replacing the sodium chloride and water allows the kidney to correct the acid–base abnormality. Following rehydration, it may become obvious that the patient is also anaemic, the haemoglobin being spuriously high on presentation.

It is notable that the metabolic abnormalities may be less if the obstruction is due to malignancy, as the acid–base disturbance is less pronounced.

The stomach should be emptied using a wide-bore gastric tube. A large nasogastric tube may not be sufficiently large to deal with the contents of the stomach, and it may be necessary to pass an orogastric tube and lavage the stomach until it is completely emptied. This then allows investigation of the patient with endoscopy and contrast radiology. Biopsy of the area around the pylorus is essential to exclude malignancy. The patient should also have a gastric antisecretory agent, initially given intravenously to ensure absorption.

Early cases may settle with conservative treatment, presumably as the oedema around the ulcer diminishes as the ulcer is healed. Traditionally, severe cases are treated surgically, usually with a gastroenterostomy rather than a pyloroplasty. Endoscopic treatment with balloon dilatation has been practised and may be most useful in early cases. However, this treatment is not devoid of problems. Dilating the duodenal stenosis may result in perforation. The dilatation may have to be performed several times and may not be successful in the long term. Occasionally, duodenal stent insertion will be considered in specialist centres.

Other causes of gastric outlet obstruction

Adult pyloric stenosis

This is a rare condition and its relationship to the childhood condition is unclear, although some patients have a long history of problems with gastric emptying. It is commonly treated by pyloroplasty rather than pyloromyotomy.

Pyloric mucosal diaphragm

The origin of this rare condition is unknown. It usually does not become apparent until middle age. When found, simple excision of the mucosal diaphragm is all that is required.

GASTRIC POLYPS

A number of conditions manifest as gastric polyps. Their main importance is that they may actually represent early gastric cancer. Biopsy is essential.

The most common type of gastric polyp is metaplastic. These are associated with *H. pylori* infection and regress following eradication therapy. Inflammatory polyps are also common. Fundic gland polyps deserve particular attention. They seem to be associated with the use of proton pump inhibitors and are also found in patients with familial polyposis. None of the above polypoid lesions has proven malignant potential. True adenomas have malignant potential and should be removed, but they account for only 10 per cent of polypoid lesions. Gastric carcinoids arising from the ECL cells are seen in patients with pernicious anaemia and usually appear as small polyps.

GASTRIC CANCER

Carcinoma of the stomach is a major cause of cancer mortality worldwide. Its prognosis tends to be poor, with cure rates little better than 5–10 per cent, although better results are obtained in Japan, where the disease is common. Gastric cancer is actually an eminently curable disease provided that it is detected at an appropriate stage and treated adequately. It rarely disseminates widely before it has involved the lymph nodes and, therefore, there is an opportunity to cure the disease prior to dissemination. Early diagnosis is therefore the key to success with this disease. Unfortunately, the late presentation of many cases is the cause of the poor overall survival figures. The only treatment modality able to cure the disease is resectional surgery (Summary box 63.6).

Summary box 63.6

Gastric cancer

- Gastric cancer is one of the most common causes of cancer death in the world
- The outlook is generally poor, owing to the advanced stage of the tumour at presentation
- Better results are obtained in Japan, which has a high population incidence, screening programmes and a high-quality surgical treatment
- The aetiology of gastric cancer is multifactorial, but *H. pylori* is an important factor for distal but not proximal gastric cancer
- Early gastric cancer is associated with very high cure rates
- Gastric cancer can be classified into intestinal and diffuse types, the latter having a worse prognosis
- In the West, proximal gastric cancer is now more common than distal cancer and is usually of the diffuse type
- Spread may be by lymphatics, blood, transcoelomic or direct, but distant metastases are uncommon in the absence of lymph node involvement
- The treatment of curable cases is by radical surgery and removal of the second tier of nodes (around the principal arterial trunks) may be advantageous
- Gastric cancer is chemosensitive and chemotherapy improves survival in patients having surgery for the condition and in advanced disease

Incidence

There are marked variations in the incidence of gastric cancer worldwide. In the UK, it is approximately 15/100 000 per year, in the USA 10/100 000 per year and in Eastern Europe 40/100 000 per year. In Japan, the disease is much more common, with an incidence of approximately 70/100 000 per year, and there are small geographical areas in China where the incidence is double that in Japan. These underlying epidemiological data make it clear that this is an environmental disease. In general, men are more affected by the disease than women and, as with most solid-organ malignancies, the incidence increases with age.

At present, marked changes are being observed in the West in terms of the incidence and site of gastric cancer and the population affected, changes that to date have not been observed in Japan. First, the incidence of gastric cancer is continuing to fall at about 1 per cent per year. This reduction exclusively affects carcinoma arising in the body and distal stomach. In contrast, there appears to be an increase in the incidence of carcinoma in the proximal stomach, particularly the oesophagogastric junction. Carcinoma of the distal stomach and body of the stomach is most common in low socioeconomic groups, whereas the increase in proximal gastric cancer seems to affect principally higher socioeconomic groups. Proximal gastric cancer does not seem to be associated with *H. pylori* infection, in contrast with carcinoma of the body and distal stomach.

Aetiology

Gastric cancer is a multifactorial disease (Correa). Epidemiological studies point to a role for *H. pylori*, although there is argument about how important this factor is. Studies reveal a correlation between the incidence of gastric cancer in various populations and the prevalence of *H. pylori* infection, but other factors are also important. There is insufficient evidence at the moment to support eradication programmes in asymptomatic patients who are infected with *Helicobacter*, with a view to reducing the population incidence of gastric cancer. However, clinical trials may subsequently change this view. As mentioned above, *Helicobacter* seems to be principally associated with carcinoma of the body and distal stomach rather than the proximal stomach. As *Helicobacter* is associated with gastritis, gastric atrophy and intestinal metaplasia, the association with malignancy is perhaps not surprising.

Several other risk factors have been identified as being important in the aetiology of gastric cancer. Patients with pernicious anaemia and gastric atrophy are at increased risk, as are those with gastric polyps. Patients who have had peptic ulcer surgery, particularly those who have had drainage procedures such as Billroth II or Polya gastrectomy, gastroenterostomy or pyloroplasty, are at approximately four times the average risk. Presumably, duodenogastric reflux and reflux gastritis are related to the increased risk of malignancy in these patients. Intestinal metaplasia is a risk factor. Carcinoma is associated with cigarette smoking and dust ingestion from a variety of industrial processes. Diet appears to be important, as illustrated by the often quoted example of the change in the incidence of gastric cancer in Japanese families living in the USA. The high incidence of gastric cancer in some pockets in China is probably environmental and probably diet related. The ingestion of substances such as spirits may induce gastritis and, in the long term, cancer. Excessive salt intake, deficiency of antioxidants and exposure to *N*-nitroso compounds are also related. The aetiology of proximal gastric cancer remains an enigma. It is not associated with *Helicobacter* but is associated with obesity and higher socioeconomic status. Genetic factors are also important but imperfectly elucidated (see below).

Clinical features

The features of advanced gastric cancer are usually obvious. However, curable gastric cancer has no specific features to distinguish it symptomatically from benign dyspepsia. The key to improving the outcome of gastric cancer is early diagnosis and, although in Japan there is a screening programme, most curable cases are picked up by the liberal use of gastroscopy in patients with dyspepsia. In the West it is much more difficult as the population incidence is much lower. Hence the cost-effectiveness of performing gastroscopy for mild dyspeptic symptoms is low. However, a high index of suspicion is necessary as only endoscoping patients with symptoms of advanced cancer is unlikely to be beneficial as such patients are not surgically curable. It is important to note that gastric antisecretory agents will improve the symptoms of gastric cancer so the disease should be excluded preferably before therapy is started.

In advanced cancer, early satiety, bloating, distension and vomiting may occur. The tumour frequently bleeds, resulting in iron deficiency anaemia. Obstruction leads to dysphagia, epigastric fullness or vomiting. With pyloric involvement the presentation may be of gastric outlet obstruction, although the alkalosis is usually less pronounced or absent compared with when duodenal ulceration leads to obstruction. In recent years, gastric outlet obstruction is more commonly associated with malignancy than benign disease. Non-metastatic effects of malignancy are seen, particularly thrombophlebitis (Trousseau's sign) and deep venous thrombosis. These features result from the effects of the tumour on thrombotic and haemostatic mechanisms.

Site

The proximal stomach is now the most common site for gastric cancer in the West. Because so many malignancies occur at the oesophagogastric junction, and because the lower oesophagus is also a very common site of adenocarcinoma, it is artificial to separate the stomach from the oesophagus. Therefore, it is best to consider the whole of the upper gastrointestinal tract from the cricopharyngeus to the pylorus. The incidence of cancer at these various sites is shown in Figure 63.25. It can be seen that just under 60 per cent of all of the malignancies occurring in the oesophagus and stomach occur in proximity to the oesophagogastric junction. Adenocarcinoma at this site has doubled in incidence in the UK over the last 30 years. This high prevalence of proximal gastric cancer is not seen in Japan, where distal cancer still predominates, as it does in most of the rest of the world.

Pathology

The most useful classification of gastric cancer is the Lauren classification. In this system there are principally two forms of gastric cancer: intestinal gastric cancer and diffuse gastric cancer. In intestinal gastric cancer, the tumour resembles a carcinoma elsewhere in the tubular gastrointestinal tract and forms polypoid tumours or ulcers. It probably arises in areas of intestinal metaplasia. In contrast, diffuse gastric cancer infiltrates deeply into the stomach without forming obvious mass lesions, but spreads widely in the gastric wall. Not surprisingly, this has a much worse prognosis. A small proportion of gastric cancers are of mixed morphology.

Armand Trousseau, 1801–1867, physician, Hôtel Dieu, Paris. The sign led him to suspect that he had gastric cancer himself. He actually had pancreatic cancer which was diagnosed at postmortem.

P Correa, a pathologist of New Orleans, LA, USA, produced a cogent hypothesis to explain the development of the intestinal type of gastric cancer.

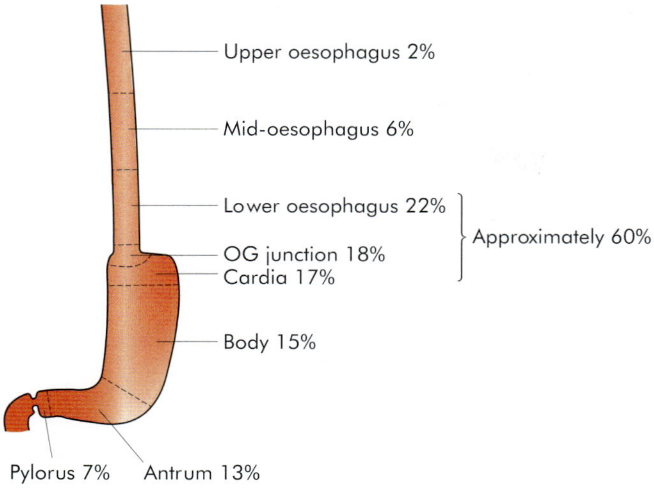

Figure 63.25 The incidence of cancer in the various parts of the upper gastrointestinal tract in the UK. OG, oesophagogastric.

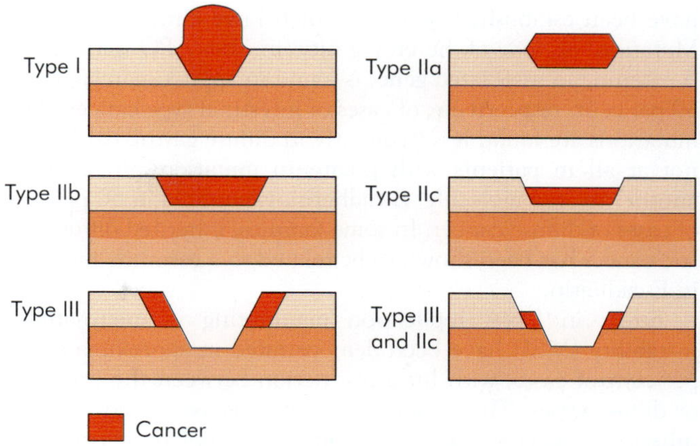

Figure 63.26 Early gastric cancer, Japanese classification.

Gastric cancer can be divided into early gastric cancer and advanced gastric cancer. Early gastric cancer is defined as cancer limited to the mucosa and submucosa with or without lymph node involvement (T1, any N). The classification is shown in Figures 63.26 and 63.27. This can be either protruding, superficial or excavated in the Japanese classification. This type of cancer is eminently curable, and even early gastric cancers associated with lymph node involvement have five-year survival rates in the region of 90 per cent. In Japan, approximately one-third of gastric cancers diagnosed are in this stage. However, in the UK it is uncommon to detect gastric cancers at this stage. A number of reasons probably still account for this. First, because gastric cancer is less common in the UK, dyspeptic patients are not always referred for endoscopy at an appropriate stage. Second, endoscopists are unfamiliar with the appearances of early gastric cancer and in all probability many such cases are missed.

Advanced gastric cancer involves the muscularis. Its macroscopic appearances have been classified by Bormann into four types (Figures 63.28 and 63.29). Types III and IV are commonly incurable.

The molecular pathology of gastric cancer

Although the molecular pathology of gastric cancer is less well worked out than colorectal cancer, several genetic events

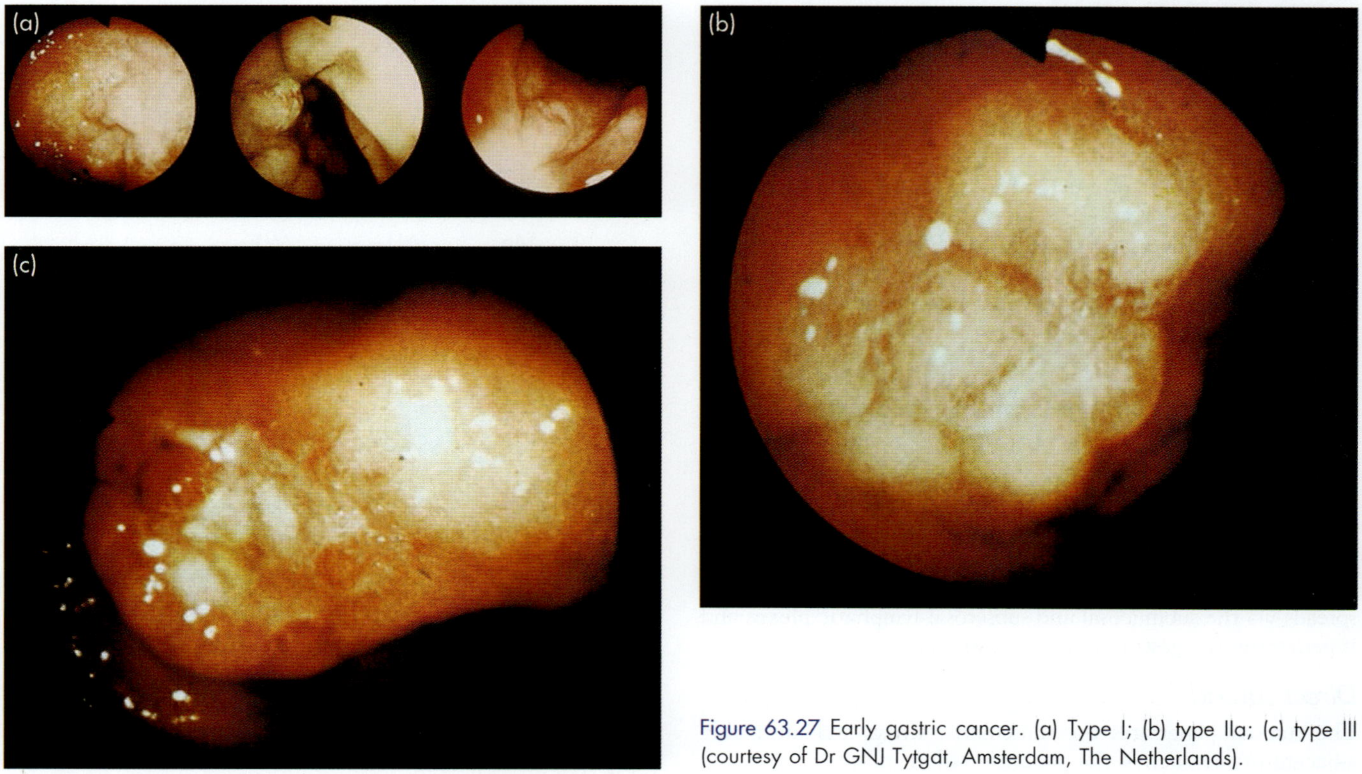

Figure 63.27 Early gastric cancer. (a) Type I; (b) type IIa; (c) type III (courtesy of Dr GNJ Tytgat, Amsterdam, The Netherlands).

have been established, some of which have clinical relevance. Mutation or loss of heterozygosity in the *APC* gene or in β-catenin, an associated gene, is found in approximately 50 and 30 per cent, respectively, of cases of intestinal type cancer. *APC* mutations are found less frequently in diffuse gastric cancer and not at all in patients with β-catenin mutations. In contrast, another related molecule, E-cadherin, is mutated in 50 per cent of cases of diffuse cancer. In some families, inherited diffuse gastric cancer has been shown to be related to a germline mutation in E-cadherin.

Errors in DNA replication manifesting as microsatellite instability (MSI) have been demonstrated in approximately 15 per cent of cases, with little distinction between the intestinal or diffuse types. This genetic phenotype is associated with the inherited cancer syndrome hereditary non-polyposis colorectal cancer syndrome (HNPCC) or the Lynch syndrome. However, most cases of MSI are a result of an acquired mutation in the tumour itself. These findings serve to illustrate that there are important differences between the two types of cancer at a molecular level.

Inactivation of *p53*, a tumour-suppressor gene, is found in around 30 per cent of both intestinal and diffuse gastric cancer.

Several growth factor receptors are overexpressed/amplified in gastric cancer; these include c-Met, k-Sam and c-ErbB2. Similarly, several growth factors may be overexpressed, including transforming growth factor α, the epidermal growth factor and vascular endothelial growth factor (VGEF).

Lastly, loss of heterozygosity at the *bcl-2* gene, an inhibitor of apoptosis, is associated with intestinal-type cancer.

These genetic changes may be involved in the familial predisposition to gastric cancer. Well-known syndromes such as HNPCC have gastric cancer as part of their spectrum.

Staging

The International Union Against Cancer (UICC) staging system is shown in Table 63.5. Important changes have been made in the seventh edition of the TNM staging system that are worthy of discussion. In an attempt to reflect the current evidence base and to improve outcome prediction for individual patients all gastric tumours whose epicentre is within 5 cm of the gastro-oesophageal junction and extend into the oesophagus are now classified according to the oesophageal system. Tumours whose epicentre is within 5 cm of the gastro-oesophageal junction but do not extend into the oesophagus, and all other gastric cancers are staged using the revised gastric staging system. In addition, any tumour that perforates the serosa is now classified as T4 disease.

Table 63.5 International Union Against Cancer (UICC) staging of gastric cancer.

T1	Tumour involves lamina propria, submucosa		
	T1a lamina propria		
	T1b submucosa		
T2	Tumour invades muscularis propria		
T3	Tumour involves subserosa		
T4a	Tumour perforates serosa		
T4b	Tumour invades adjacent organs		
N0	No lymph nodes		
N1	Metastasis in 1–2 regional nodes		
N2	Metastasis in 3–6 regional nodes		
N3a	Metastasis in 7–15 regional nodes		
N3b	Metastasis in more than 15 regional nodes		
M0	No distant metastasis		
M1	Distant metastasis (this includes peritoneum and distant lymph nodes)		
Staging			
IA	T1	N0	M0
IB	T1	N1	M0
	T2	N0	M0
IIA	T1	N2	M0
	T2	N1	M0
	T3	N0	M0
IIB	T1	N3	M0
	T2	N2	M0
	T3	N1	M0
	T4a	N0	M0
IIIA	T2	N3	M0
	T3	N2	M0
	T4a	N1	M0
IIIB	T3	N3	M0
	T4a	N2	M0
	T4b	N0–1	M0
IIIC	T4a	N3	M0
	T4b	N2–3	M0
IV	Any T	Any N	M1

Spread of carcinoma of the stomach

No better example of the various modes by which carcinoma spreads can be given than the case of stomach cancer. It is important to note that distant spread is unusual before the disease spreads locally, and distant metastases are uncommon in the absence of lymph node metastases. The intestinal and diffuse types of gastric cancer spread differently. The diffuse type spreads via the submucosal and subserosal lymphatic plexus and it penetrates the gastric wall at an early stage.

Direct spread

The tumour penetrates the muscularis, serosa and ultimately adjacent organs such as the pancreas, colon and liver.

Lymphatic spread

This is by both permeation and emboli to the affected tiers (see below) of nodes. This may be extensive, the tumour even appearing in the supraclavicular nodes (Troisier's sign). Unlike malignancies such as breast cancer, nodal involvement does not imply systemic dissemination.

Charles Emil Troisier, 1844–1919, Professor of Pathology, Paris, France.

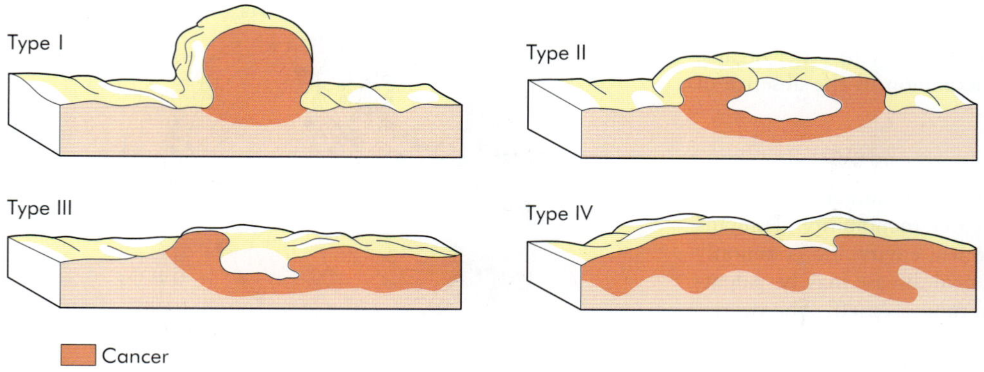

Figure 63.28 Borrmann classification of advanced gastric cancer.

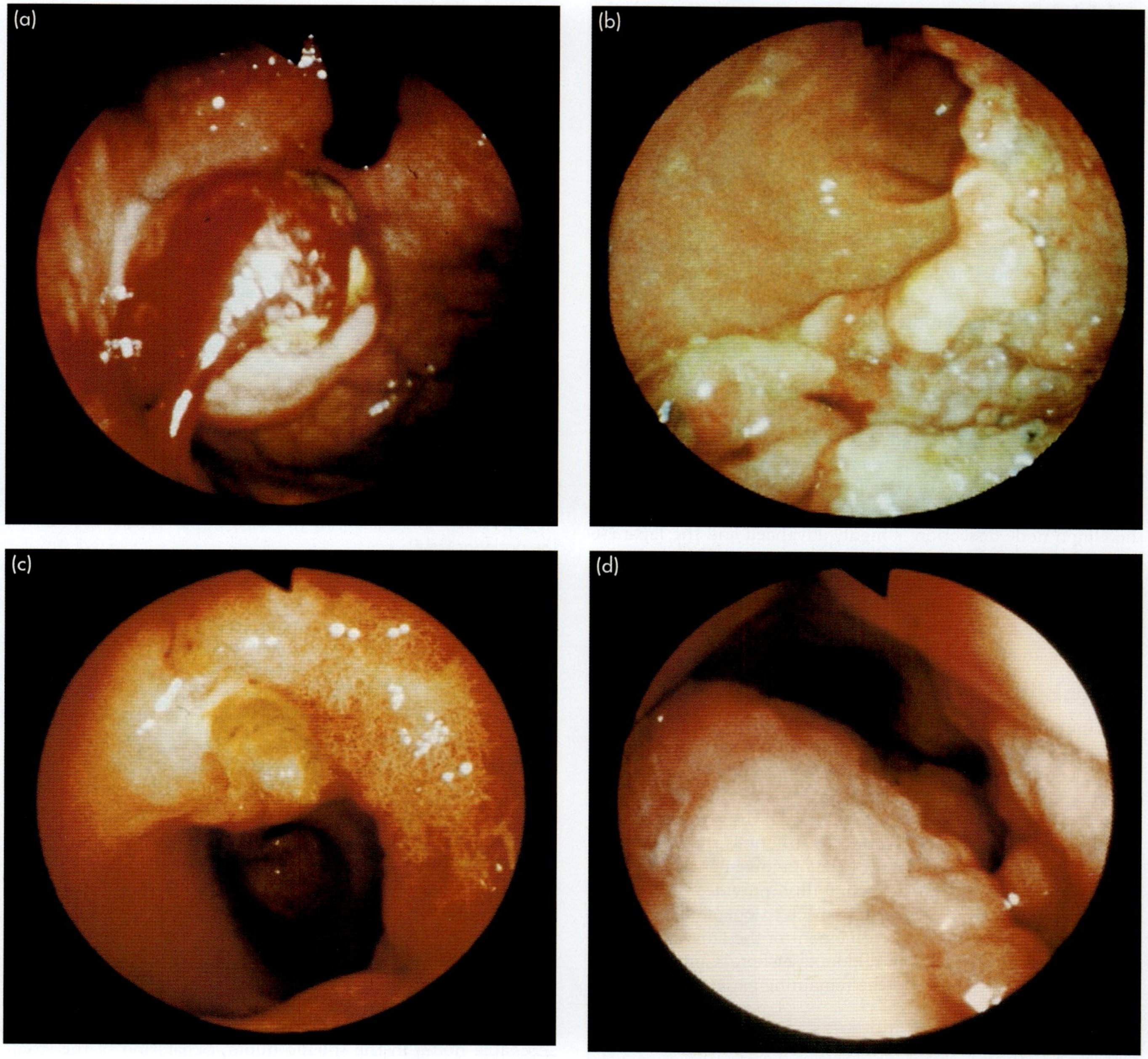

Figure 63.29 Advanced gastric cancer. (a) Type I; (b) type II; (c) type III; (d) type IV (linitus plastica) (courtesy of Dr GNJ Tytgat, Amsterdam, The Netherlands).

Blood-borne metastases

These occur first to the liver and subsequently to other organs, including lung and bone. This is uncommon in the absence of nodal disease.

Transperitoneal spread

This is a common mode of spread once the tumour has reached the serosa of the stomach and indicates incurability. Tumours can manifest anywhere in the peritoneal cavity and commonly give rise to ascites. Advanced peritoneal disease may be palpated either abdominally or rectally as a tumour 'shelf'. The ovaries may sometimes be the sole site of transcoelomic spread (Krukenberg's tumours). Tumour may spread via the abdominal cavity to the umbilicus (Sister Joseph's nodule). Transperitoneal spread of gastric cancer can be detected most effectively by laparoscopy and cytology.

Lymphatic drainage of the stomach

Understanding the lymphatic drainage of the stomach is the key to comprehending the radical surgery of gastric cancer. The lymphatics of the antrum drain into the right gastric lymph node superiorly, and right gastroepiploic and subpyloric lymph nodes inferiorly. The lymphatics of the pylorus drain into the right gastric suprapyloric nodes superiorly and the subpyloric lymph nodes situated around the gastroduodenal artery inferiorly. The efferent lymphatics from suprapyloric lymph nodes converge on the para-aortic nodes around the coeliac axis, whereas the efferent lymphatics from the subpyloric lymph nodes pass up to the main superior mesenteric lymph nodes situated around the origin of the superior mesenteric artery. The lymphatic vessels related to the cardiac orifice of the stomach communicate freely with those of the oesophagus.

The prognosis of operable cases of carcinoma of the stomach depends on whether or not there is histological evidence of regional lymph node involvement. Retrograde (downwards) spread may occur if the upper lymphatics are blocked. In Japan, the lymph node dissection is highly advanced and the Japanese Research Society for Gastric Cancer has assigned a number to each lymph node station to aid the pathological staging (Figure 63.30). Many centres in the West now perform surgery that involves a radical lymphadenectomy but, in other centres, both the staging and surgery are less developed.

Operability

It is important that patients with incurable disease are not subjected to radical surgery that cannot help them, hence the value of CT/PET and preoperative laparoscopy. Unequivocal evidence of incurability is haematogenous metastases, involvement of the distant peritoneum, N4 nodal disease and disease beyond the N4 nodes, and fixation to structures that cannot be removed. It is important to note that involvement of another organ per se does not imply incurability, provided that it can be removed. Controversies with respect to operability include N3 nodal involvement and involvement of the adjacent peritoneum, performed in Japan but seldom elsewhere. Curative resection should be considered on the remaining patients.

Friedrich Ernst Krukenberg, 1870–1946, ophthalmologist of Halle, Germany. In 1896 while studying pathology, he published his description of a fibrosarcoma of the ovary which became known as Krukenberg tumour of the ovary. He became an ophthalmologist who practised privately.

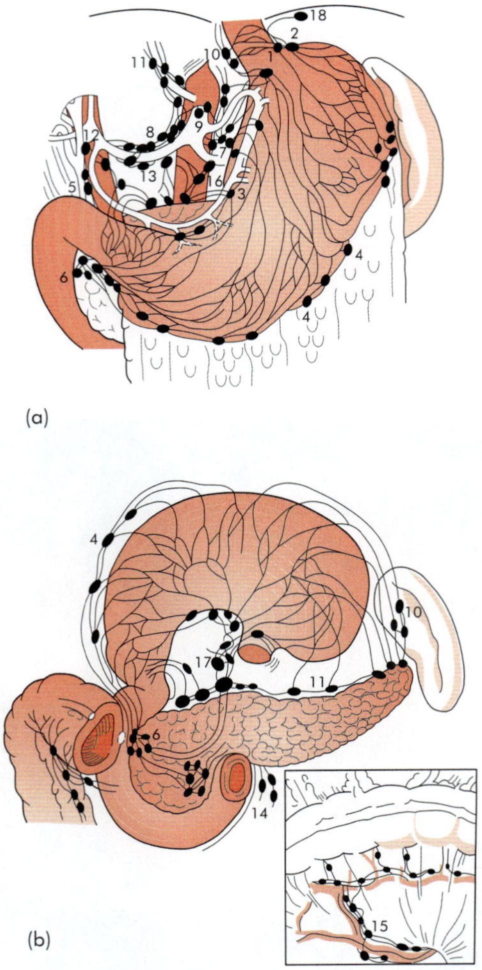

Figure 63.30 Lymphatic drainage of the stomach and nodal stations by the Japanese classification. (a) The anterior view of the stomach. (b) The posterior view.

Most operable patients should have neoadjuvant chemotherapy as described below as this improves survival.

Total gastrectomy

This is best performed through a long upper midline incision. The stomach is removed en bloc, including the tissues of the entire greater omentum and lesser omentum (Figure 63.31). In commencing the operation, the transverse colon is completely separated from the greater omentum. The dissection may then be commenced proximally or, more usually, distally. The subpyloric nodes are dissected and the first part of the duodenum is divided, usually with a surgical stapler. The hepatic nodes are dissected down to clear the hepatic artery; this dissection also includes the suprapyloric nodes. The right gastric artery is taken on the hepatic artery. The lymph node dissection is continued to the origin of the left gastric artery, which is divided flush with its origin. The dissection is continued along the splenic artery, taking all of the nodes at the superior aspect of the pancreas and accessible nodes in the splenic hilum. Separation of the stomach from the spleen, if this organ is not going to be removed, is carried out and this then allows access to the nodal tissues

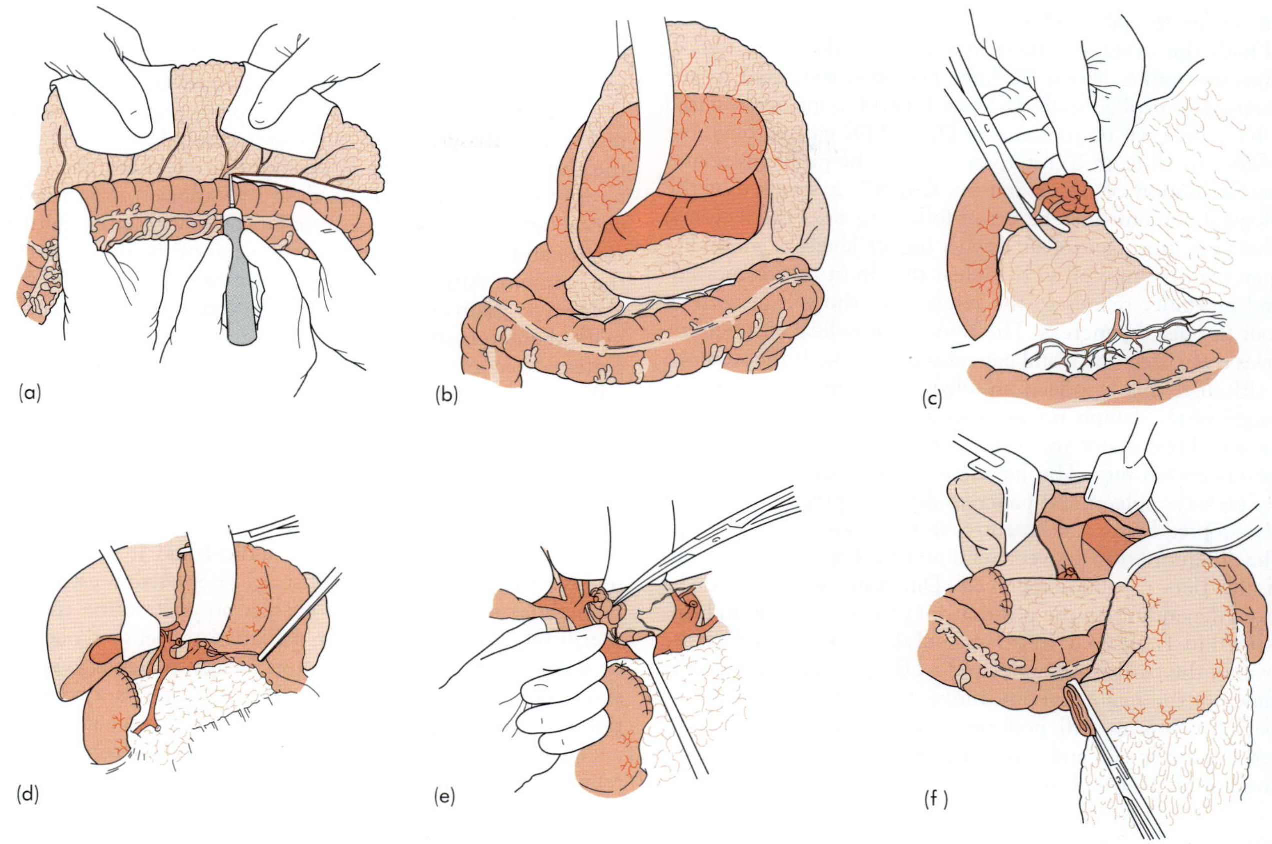

Figure 63.31 Radical total gastrectomy. (a) Dissection of omentum off the transverse colon. (b) Exposure of the lesser sac. (c) Splenectomy. (d) Division and oversewing of the duodenum. (e) Dissection of the left gastric artery nodes (group 17). (f) Mobilisation of the oesophagus.

around the upper stomach and oesophagogastric junction. The oesophagus can then be divided at an appropriate point using a combination of stay sutures and a soft non-crushing clamp, usually of the right-angled variety. It is important that the resection margins are well clear of the tumour (>5 cm). Involvement of either proximal or distal resection margin carries an appalling prognosis and, if in doubt, frozen section should be performed. There is some controversy regarding the management of the spleen and distal pancreas in this procedure and this is discussed below.

Gastrointestinal continuity is reconstituted by means of a Roux loop. Other methods of reconstruction should be discouraged because of poor functional results. The alimentary limb of the Roux loop should be at least 50 cm long to avoid bile reflux oesophagitis. The simplest means of effecting the oesophagojejunostomy is to place a purse string in the cut end of the oesophagus and, using a circular stapler introduced through the blind end of the Roux loop, staple the end of the oesophagus onto the side of the Roux loop. The blind open end of the Roux loop may then be closed either with sutures or, alternatively, with a linear stapler. The anastomosis can also be fashioned end to end. The Roux loop may be placed in either an anticolic or retrocolic position. The jejunojejunostomy is undertaken at a convenient point in the usual fashion (end to side, Figure 63.32).

There remains some controversy about the extent of the lymphadenectomy required for the optimal treatment of curable gastric cancer. In Japan, at least a D2 gastrectomy (removal of the second-tier of nodes) is performed on all operable gastric cancer and some centres are practising more radical surgery (D3 and even D4 resections). Certainly, the results of surgical treatment stage for stage in Japan are much better than commonly reported in the West, and the Japanese contention is that the difference is principally related to the staging and the quality of the surgery. It is observed that the physical proportions of the average Japanese

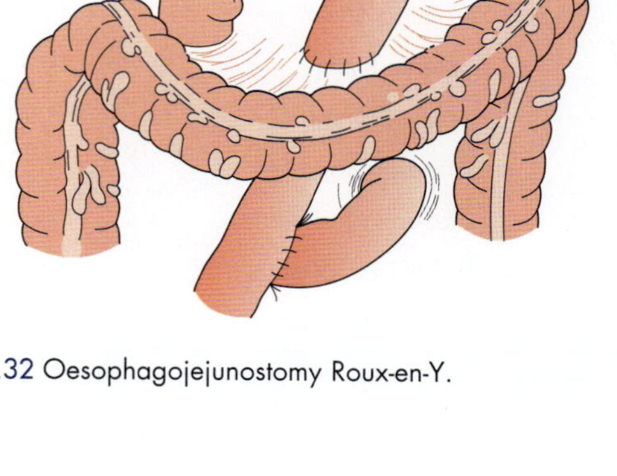

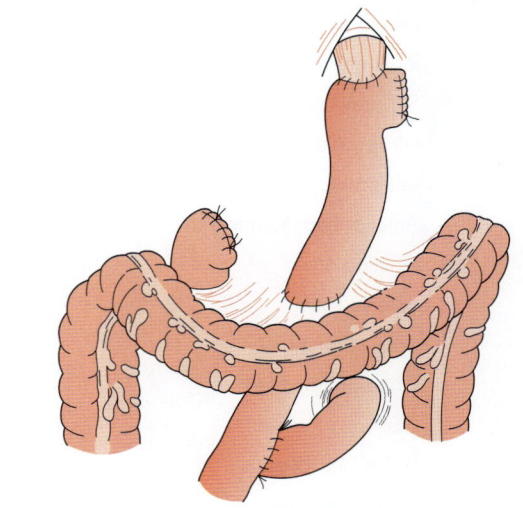

Figure 63.32 Oesophagojejunostomy Roux-en-Y.

patient favour the performance of more radical procedures compared with the average patient in the West. However, radical lymphadenectomies above D2 have not been subjected to any randomised controlled trials. In the UK and Europe, randomised trials have been set up to compare D1 and D2 gastrectomy, but the results are difficult to interpret. One of the problems relates to standardisation of the operation. Overall, it seems that the oncological outcome may be better following a D2 gastrectomy, but this operation is associated with higher levels of morbidity and peroperative mortality. It is clear that most of this morbidity and mortality relates to the removal of the spleen with or without the distal pancreas. The traditional radical gastrectomy removes the spleen and distal pancreas en bloc with the stomach and, although this is indeed an adequate means of performing clearance of the lymph nodes around the splenic artery, there now seems little doubt that adding this substantially increases the complication rate. The Japanese D2 gastrectomy will commonly preserve spleen and pancreas and this practice has been widely adopted by specialist centres in the West.

The differentiation between a D1 and a D2 operation depends upon the tiers of nodes removed. Different tiers need to be removed depending on the positions of primary tumour and this is outlined in Table 63.6. In general, a D1 resection involves the removal of the perigastric nodes and a D2 resection involves the clearance of the major arterial trunks. In practice, the majority of specialist centres will perform a radical total gastrectomy, conserving the spleen and pancreas, with D2 lymphadenectomy sparing station 10 lymph nodes.

Subtotal gastrectomy

For tumours distally placed in the stomach, it appears unnecessary to remove the whole stomach. However, the operation is very similar to that of a total gastrectomy except that the proximal stomach is preserved, the blood supply being derived from the short gastric arteries. Following the resection, the simplest form of reconstruction is to close the stomach from the lesser curve, near the oesophagogastric junction, with either sutures or staples and then perform an anastomosis of the greater curve to the jejunum. Although this can be performed as in a Billroth II/Polya-type gastrectomy, this reconstruction may result in quite marked enterogastric reflux and bile reflux oesophagitis, and the preferred reconstruction is to perform the reconstruction using a Roux loop.

Palliative surgery

In patients suffering from significant symptoms of either obstruction or bleeding, palliative resection is appropriate. A palliative gastrectomy need not be radical and it is sufficient to remove the tumour and reconstruct the gastrointestinal tract. Sometimes it is impossible to resect an obstructing tumour in the distal stomach and other palliative procedures need to be considered, although the prognosis in such patients, even in the short term, is poor. A high gastroenterostomy is a poor operation that very frequently does not allow the stomach to empty adequately, but may produce the additional problem of bile reflux. A Roux loop with a wide anastomosis between the stom-

Table 63.6 The lymph node stations (see Figure 63.30) that need to be removed in a D1 (N1 nodes removed) or a D2 (N2 nodes removed) resection.

LN number		Site of cancer			
		Antrum	Middle	Cardia	Cardia and oesophagus
1	Right cardia	N2	N1	N1	N1
2	Left cardial		N1	N1	N1
3	Lesser curve	N1	N1	N1	N1
4sa	Short gastric	N1	N1	N1	N1
4sb	Left gastroepiploic	N1	N1	N1	N1
4d	Right gastroepiploic	N1	N1	N2	N2
5	Suprapyloric	N1	N1	N2	N2
6	Infrapyloric	N1	N1	N2	N2
7	Left gastric artery	N2	N2	N2	N2
8a	Anterior hepatic artery	N2	N2	N2	N2
9	Coeliac artery	N2	N2	N2	N2
10	Splenic hilum		N2	N2	N2
11	Splenic artery		N2	N2	N2
19	Infradiaphragmatic				N2
20	Oesophageal hiatus			N2	N1
110	Lower oesophagus				N2
111	Supradiaphragmatic				N2

The nodes in stations 12–18 are not routinely removed in a D1 or D2 gastrectomy.

ach and jejunum may be a better option, although even this may not allow the stomach to empty particularly well. Gastric exclusion and oesophagojejunostomy is practised by some surgeons. For inoperable tumours situated in the cardia, either palliative intubation, stenting or another form of recanalisation can be used (Chapter 62). Recanalisation appears to offer better functional results.

Postoperative complications of gastrectomy

Radical gastrectomy is complex major surgery and predictably there is a large number of potential complications of the operation. Leakage of the oesophagojejunostomy should be uncommon in experienced hands. When it occurs it can often be managed conservatively as the Roux-en-Y reconstruction means that it is mainly saliva and ingested food that leaks. Some patients may establish a fistula from the wound or drain site and others may need radiological or surgically placed drains. It is unclear whether a nasoenteric tube should be used routinely. Many surgeons use such tubes routinely, but this is not supported by any evidence base. It is common practice to perform a water-soluble contrast swallow at 5–7 days after the operation to determine whether the anastomosis is intact, and finding a small radiological leak is not uncommon. It is unusual to detect a major leak in the absence of clinical signs. Physiological scoring systems to predict those patients likely to experience significant complications offer potential in this area.

As with any gastrectomy, leakage from the duodenal stump can occur. This is usually due to a degree of distal obstruction and care must be taken when performing the Roux-en-Y anastomosis that there is no kinking. Paraduodenal collections can be drained radiologically, which will often convert the collection into an external fistula. Biliary peritonitis requires a laparotomy and peritoneal toilet, and in this circumstance it is best to leave a Foley catheter in the duodenum to establish a controlled duodenal fistula. If it is established that there is no distal obstruction, or if any such obstruction is managed, then with time the fistula will close.

The presence of septic collections along with a very radical vascular dissection may lead to catastrophic secondary haemorrhage from the exposed or divided blood vessels. This situation may be very difficult to manage, whether or not reoperation or interventional radiology is employed.

Long-term complications of surgery

It is surprising that, considering the radical nature of the total gastrectomy, many patients, particularly the younger ones, have good functional results. However, most patients will have a reduced capacity, particularly in the short term. They need to be given detailed nutritional advice, the substance of which is to eat small meals and often, while the jejunum or small gastric remnant adapts. In fact, there is very little functional difference between patients who have a total gastrectomy and those who have a subtotal gastrectomy. Various attempts have been made to try and improve the short-term functional results by forming a jejunal pouch and attaching this to the oesophagus. Most surgeons do not perform this as in the long term there seems little functional advantage. It is surprising that these patients only infrequently suffer from the complications of gastric surgery, such as dumping and diarrhoea. Nutritional deficiencies may occur and the patient should be monitored with this in mind. The loss of the parietal mass leads to vitamin B12 deficiency and replacement should be given routinely.

Outlook after surgical treatment

The outlook after surgical treatment varies considerably between the West and Japan. In Japan, approximately 75 per cent of patients will have a curative resection and, of these, the overall five-year survival rate will be in the region of 50–70 per cent. In contrast, in the West most series show that only 25–50 per cent of patients undergoing surgery will have a curative operation and the five-year survival rate in such patients is only about 25–30 per cent, although in some series it approaches Japanese levels. A combination of differences in staging and a higher standard of surgery in Japan probably accounts for the differences. Staging is clearly crucial when survival figures are being compared. The more thorough the staging, the higher the stage is likely to be and, therefore, stage for stage the outcome seems better in patients who are adequately staged pathologically. This phenomenon is termed 'stage migration'.

Other treatment modalities

Because of the failure of radical surgery to cure advanced gastric cancer, there has been an interest in the use of radiotherapy and chemotherapy.

Radiotherapy

The routine use of radiotherapy is controversial as the results of clinical trials are inconclusive. There are a number of radiosensitive tissues in the region of the gastric bed, which limits the dose that can be given. Radiotherapy has a role in the palliative treatment of painful bony metastases.

Chemotherapy

Gastric cancer may respond well to combination cytotoxic chemotherapy and neoadjuvant chemotherapy improves the outcome following surgery. Most patients therefore should have prior chemotherapy. There are a number of well-investigated regimes, but the best results are currently obtained using a combination of epirubacin, *cis*-platinum and infusional 5-FU or an oral analogue such as capecitabine. The same regimen is used as first line for patients with inoperable disease although oxaliplatin is being substituted for *cis*-platinum as it has fewer side effects. Second-line treatment using combinations which include taxotere are increasingly being used. Chemotherapy for advanced disease is palliative. Newer biological agents such as trastuzumab (Herceptin®) offer potential advantages to survival in the minority of patients (<20 per cent) with *HER2*-positive gastric cancer. However, the absolute survival advantages are small (approximately four months) and the cost of treatment is high. Nevertheless, trastuzumab has been approved for use in metastatic *HER2*-positive gastric cancer in the UK and European Union.

Pattern of relapse following surgical treatment

As might be expected, the most common site of relapse following radical gastrectomy is the gastric bed, representing inadequate extirpation of the primary tumour. Widespread nodal intraperitoneal metastases, distant nodal metastases and liver metastases are all common. Dissemination to the lung and bones usually only occurs after liver metastases are already established.

Frederic Eugene Basil Foley, 1891–1966, urologist, Anker Hospital, St Paul, MN, USA.

GASTROINTESTINAL STROMAL TUMOURS

Gastrointestinal stromal tumours (GIST) may arise in any part of the gastrointestinal tract but 50 per cent will be found in the stomach. Previously named leiomyoma and leiomyosarcoma, the term GIST is now used, recognising their particular distinct phenotype. They are tumours of mesenchymal origin and are observed equally commonly in males and females. The tumours are universally associated with a mutation in the tyrosine kinase *c-kit* oncogene. These tumours are sensitive to the tyrosine kinase antagonist imatinib, and an 80 per cent objective response rate can be observed. Tumours with mutations in exon 11 of *c-kit* are particularly sensitive to this drug. The biological behaviour of these tumours is unpredictable but size and mitotic index are the best predictors of metastasis. Peritoneal and liver metastases are most common but spread to lymph nodes extremely rare.

The incidence of the condition is unclear as small stromal tumours of the stomach are probably quite common and remain unnoticed. Clinically obvious tumours are considerably less common than gastric cancer. GIST comprise 1–3 per cent of all gastrointestinal neoplasia.

The only ways that many stromal tumours are recognised are either that the mucosa overlying the tumour ulcerates (see Figure 63.24), leading to bleeding, or that they are noticed incidentally at endoscopy. Because the mucosa overlying the tumour is normal, endoscopic biopsy can be uninformative unless the tumour has ulcerated. Targeted biopsy by endoscopic ultrasound is more helpful. Larger tumours present with non-specific gastric symptoms and, in many instances, they may be thought to be gastric cancer initially (Figure 63.33).

As the biological behaviour is difficult to predict, the best guide is to consider the size of the tumour. Tumours over 5 cm in diameter should be considered to have metastatic potential. If easily resectable, surgery is the primary mode of treatment. Smaller tumours can be treated by wedge excision although the appropriate management of asymptomatic diminutive tumours found incidentally at endoscopy is unclear. Larger tumours may require a gastrectomy or duodenectomy (see Chapter 68) but lymphadenectomy is not required. Larger tumours which require multivisceral resection may be better treated with three to six months of imatinib prior to operation as this will usually radically reduce the size and vascularity of the tumours. Adjuvant imatinib for large resected tumours of high malignant potential should probably be continued indefinitely.

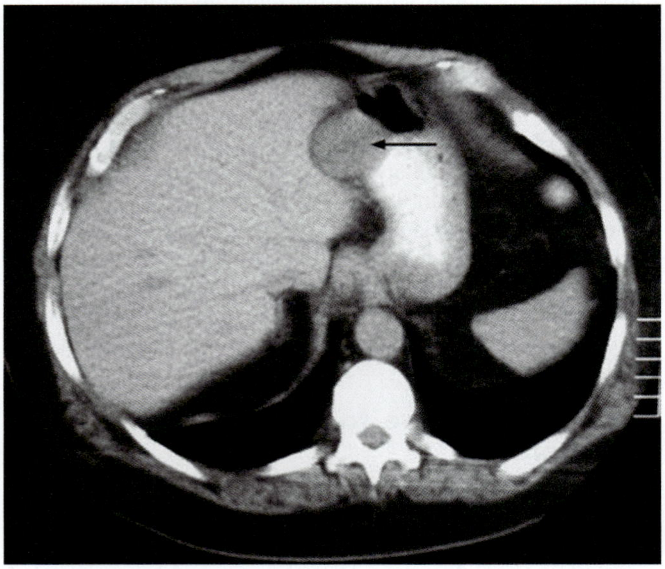

Figure 63.33 Computed tomography of the upper abdomen showing a 3.5 cm gastrointestinal stromal tumour arising from the gastric wall.

The prognosis of advanced metastatic GIST has been dramatically improved with imatinib chemotherapy but resection of metastases, especially from the liver, still has an important role.

GASTRIC LYMPHOMA

Gastric lymphoma is an interesting disease and some aspects of the management are controversial. It is first important to distinguish primary gastric lymphoma from involvement of the stomach in a generalised lymphomatous process. This latter situation is more common than the former. Unlike gastric carcinoma, the incidence of lymphoma seems to be increasing. Primary gastric lymphoma accounts for approximately 5 per cent of all gastric neoplasms.

Gastric lymphoma is the most common in the sixth decade and the presentation is no different from gastric cancer, the common symptoms being pain, weight loss and bleeding. Acute presentations of gastric lymphoma, such as haematemesis, perforation or obstruction, are not common. Primary gastric lymphomas are B cell derived, the tumour arising from the mucosa-associated lymphoid tissue (MALT). Primary gastric lymphoma remains in the stomach for a prolonged period before involving the lymph nodes. At an early stage, the disease takes the form of a diffuse mucosal thickening, which may ulcerate. Diagnosis is made as a result of the endoscopic biopsy and seldom on the basis of the endoscopic features alone, which are not specific.

Following diagnosis, adequate staging is necessary, primarily to establish whether the lesion is a primary gastric lymphoma or part of a more generalised process. CT scans of the chest and abdomen and bone marrow aspirate are required, as well as a full blood count.

Although the treatment of primary gastric lymphoma is somewhat controversial, it seems most appropriate to use surgery alone for the localised disease process. No benefit has been shown from adjuvant chemotherapy, although some oncologists contend that primary gastric lymphoma can be treated by chemotherapy alone. Chemotherapy alone is appropriate for patients with systemic disease.

Some of the more controversial aspects of gastric lymphoma concern the role of *H. pylori*. Lymphocytes are not found to any degree in normal gastric mucosa, but are found in association with *Helicobacter* infection. It has also been shown that early gastric lymphomas may regress and disappear when the *Helicobacter* infection is treated.

Gastric involvement with the diffuse lymphoma

These patients are treated with chemotherapy, sometimes with dramatic and rapid responses. Surgeons are frequently asked to deal with the complications of gastric involvement. The two common complications are bleeding and perforation. Both may occur at presentation, but more usually may follow the

Peter Gersohn Isaacson, Emeritus Professor of Pathology and Consultant Histopathologist, University College, London, UK.

chemotherapy when there is rapid regression and necrosis of the tumour. These operations can be technically very challenging and normally require gastrectomy.

DUODENAL TUMOURS

Benign duodenal tumours

Duodenal villous adenomas occur principally in the periampullary region. Although generally uncommon, they are often found in patients with familial adenomatous polyposis. The appearances are similar to those adenomas arising in the colon and, as they have malignant potential, they should be locally excised with histologically clear margins (Summary 63.7).

Summary box 63.7

Duodenal tumours

- Duodenal villous adenomas are commonly found around the ampulla of Vater and are premalignant
- Duodenal carcinoma is uncommon, but the most common site for adenocarcinoma is in the small intestine
- Both adenoma and carcinoma occur commonly in patients with familial polyposis and screening these patients is advised
- Pancreatic cancer is the most common cause of duodenal obstruction

Duodenal adenocarcinoma

Although uncommon, this is the most common site for adenocarcinoma arising in the small bowel. Most tumours originate in the periampullary region and commonly arise in pre-existing villous adenomas. Patients present with anaemia due to ulceration of the tumour or obstruction as the polypoid neoplasm begins to obstruct the duodenum. Direct involvement in the ampulla leads to obstructive jaundice. Histologically, the lesion is a typical adenocarcinoma and the metastases are commonly to regional lymph nodes and the liver. At presentation, about 70 per cent of the patients have resectable disease and for those who survive operation the five-year survival rate is in the region of 20 per cent, this approximately equating to cure. Poor prognostic features in the resected specimen include regional lymph node metastases, transmural involvement and perineural invasion. Curative surgical treatment will normally involve a pancreaticoduodenectomy (Whipple's procedure). Patients with familial polyposis, which is due to a mutation in the *APC* gene on chromosome 5, are predisposed to periampullary cancer, which is one of the most common causes of death in patients who have had their colon removed. Other duodenal malignancies include GISTs (see above) and neuroendocrine tumours.

Neuroendocrine tumours

A number of neuroendocrine neoplasms occurs in the duodenum. It is a common site for primary gastrinoma (Zollinger–Ellison syndrome). Non-functioning neuroendocrine tumours (usually called carcinoid tumours) also occur but uncommonly in comparison to the ileum.

Zollinger–Ellison syndrome

This syndrome is mentioned here because the gastrin-producing endocrine tumour is often found in the duodenal loop, although it also occurs in the pancreas, especially the head. It is a cause of persistent peptic ulceration. Before the development of potent gastric antisecretory agents, the condition was recognised by the sometimes fulminant peptic ulceration which did not respond to gastric surgery short of total gastrectomy. It was also recognisable from gastric secretory studies in which the patient had a very high basal acid output but no marked response to pentagastrin, as the parietal cell mass was already nearly maximally stimulated by pathological levels of gastrin. The advent of proton pump inhibitors such as omeprazole has rendered this extreme endocrine condition fully controllable, but also less easily recognised.

Gastrinomas may be either sporadic or associated with the autosomal dominantly inherited multiple endocrine neoplasia (MEN) type I (in which a parathyroid adenoma is almost invariable). The tumours are most commonly found in the 'gastrinoma triangle' (Passaro) defined by the junction of the cystic duct and common bile duct superiorly, the junction of the second and third parts of the duodenum inferiorly, and the junction of the neck and body of the pancreas medially (essentially the superior mesenteric artery). Many are found in the duodenal loop, presumably arising in the G cells found in Brunner's glands. It is extremely important that the duodenal wall is very carefully inspected endoscopically and also at operation. Very often all that can be detected is a small nodule that projects into the medial wall of the duodenum.

Even malignant sporadic gastrinomas may have a very indolent course. The palliative resection of liver metastases may be beneficial and liver transplantation is practised in some centres, as for other gut endocrine tumours, with reasonable long-term results. However, the minority of tumours found to the left of the superior mesenteric artery (outside the 'triangle') seems to have a worse prognosis, more having liver metastases at presentation. In MEN type I, the tumours may be multiple and the condition is incurable. Even in this situation, as with sporadic gastrinoma, surgical treatment should be employed to remove any obvious tumours and associated lymphatic metastases, as the palliation achieved may be good.

DUODENAL OBSTRUCTION

Duodenal obstruction in the adult is usually due to malignancy, and cancer of the pancreas is the most common cause. About one-fifth of patients with pancreatic cancer treated with endoscopic stenting will develop obstruction. Treatment is usually by gastroenterostomy but duodenal stenting is increasingly being used. In patients having a surgical biliary bypass for pancreatic cancer, gastric drainage may be necessary.

A variety of other malignancies can cause duodenal obstruction, including metastases from colorectal and gastric cancer. Primary duodenal cancer is much less common as a cause of obstruction than these other malignancies.

Annular pancreas may rarely cause duodenal obstruction. Obstruction usually follows an attack of pancreatitis and, on occasions, the obstruction may be mistaken for malignancy.

Arteriomesenteric compression is an ill-defined condition

Allen Oldfather Whipple, 1881–1963, Director of Surgical Services, The Presbyterian Hospital, and Professor of Surgery, the College of Physicians and Surgeons, New York, NY, USA.

Edward Passaro, Professor of Surgery, Los Angeles, CA, USA.

in which it is proposed that the fourth part of the duodenum is compressed between the superior mesenteric artery and the vertebral column; when it is convincingly demonstrated and causing weight loss, duodenojejunostomy may be performed.

OTHER GASTRIC CONDITIONS

Acute gastric dilatation

This condition usually occurs in association with pyloroduodenal disorders or postsurgery without nasogastric suction. The stomach, which may also be atonic, dilates enormously. Often the patient is also dehydrated and has electrolyte disturbances. Failure to treat this condition can result in a sudden massive vomit with aspiration into the lungs. The treatment is nasogastric suction, with a large-bore tube, fluid replacement and treatment of the underlying condition.

Trichobezoar and phytobezoar

Trichobezoar (hair balls) (Figure 63.34) are unusual and are virtually exclusively found in female psychiatric patients, often young. It is caused by the pathological ingestion of hair, which remains undigested in the stomach. The hair ball can lead to ulceration and gastrointestinal bleeding, perforation or obstruction. The diagnosis is made easily at endoscopy or, indeed, from a plain radiograph. Treatment consists of removal of the bezoar, which may require open surgical treatment. Phytobezoars are made of vegetable matter and found principally in patients who have gastric stasis. Often this follows gastric surgery.

Foreign bodies in the stomach

A variety of ingested foreign bodies reach the stomach, and very often these can be seen on a plain radiograph. If possible, they should be removed endoscopically but, if not, most can be left to pass normally. Even objects such as needles, with which there is understandable anxiety, will seldom cause harm. In general, an object which leaves the stomach will pass spontaneously. In contrast, attempted removal at laparotomy can be very difficult as the object may be much more difficult to find than might be expected. Most adults who swallow foreign bodies have ill-defined psychiatric problems and may appear to relish the attention associated with serial laparotomies. The treatment should therefore be expectant and intervention reserved for patients with symptoms in whom the foreign body is failing to progress.

Volvulus of the stomach

Rotation of the stomach usually occurs around the axis and between its two fixed points, i.e. the cardia and the pylorus. In theory, rotation can occur in the horizontal (organoaxial) or vertical (mesenteroaxial) direction but, commonly, it is the former which occurs. This condition is usually associated with a large diaphragmatic defect around the oesophagus (paraoesophageal herniation) (Figure 63.35). What commonly happens is that the transverse colon moves upwards to lie under the left diaphragm, thus taking the stomach with it, and the stomach and colon may both enter the chest through the eventration of the diaphragm. The condition is commonly chronic, the patient presenting with difficulty in eating. An acute presentation with ischaemia may occur. Endoscopically, it can be

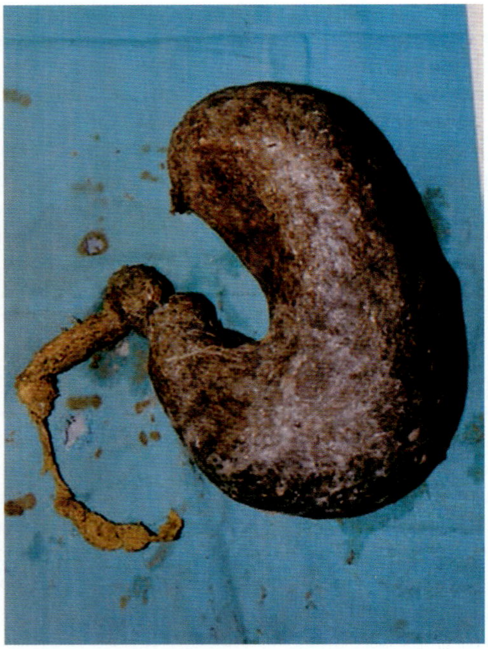

Figure 63.34 Trichobezoar of the stomach in a girl aged 15 years.

Bezoars are masses of foreign material in the stomach or intestines of animals, and are relatively common. In some primitive communities a gastric bezoar from a goat is accredited with magical healing properties.

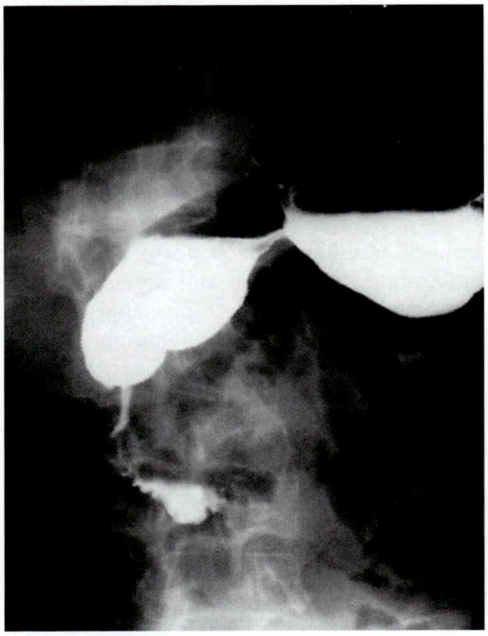

Figure 63.35 Barium meal showing organoaxial volvulus of the stomach associated with eventration of the diaphragm.

extremely difficult to sort out the anatomy, and this is one situation in which the contrast radiograph is superior.

Treatment

If the problem is causing symptoms then surgical treatment is the only satisfactory approach. Traditionally, open surgery has been employed but this problem is suitable for laparoscopic treatment if appropriate skill is available. If there is a hernia, the sac and its contents (usually the stomach) should be reduced. The defect in the diaphragm should be closed, if necessary, with a mesh. It is advisable to separate the stomach from the transverse colon and then perform an anterior gastropexy to fix the stomach to the anterior abdominal wall. The results from this treatment are good.

FURTHER READING

McCulloch P, Nita ME, Kazi H, Gama-Rodrigues J. Extended versus limited lymph nodes dissection technique for adenocarcinoma of the stomach. *Cochrane Database Syst Rev* 2003; (**4**): CD001964.

Paterson-Brown S, Garden OJ. *Companion to specialist surgical practice*. Philadelphia, PA: WB Saunders, 2009.

Sano T, Aiko T. New Japanese classifications and treatment guidelines for gastric cancer: revision concepts and major revised points. *Gastric Cancer* 2011; **14**: 97–100.

Sobin LH, Gospodarowicz MK, Wittekind C (eds). *UICC TNM classification of malignant tumours*, 7th edn. New York: Wiley, 2009.

Wagner AD, Unverzagt S, Grothe W *et al*. Chemotherapy for advanced gastric cancer. *Cochrane Database Syst Rev* 2010; (**3**): CD004064.

CHAPTER

64 Bariatric surgery

LEARNING OBJECTIVES

To know and understand:

- What morbid obesity is
- Who is eligible for bariatric surgery
- What surgical procedures are currently available
- Outcomes and complications
- What the future holds for bariatric surgery

INTRODUCTION

Surgical management for obesity has been available for decades. The first recorded proper bariatric operation, the jejunoileal bypass (JIB), was described in 1954. The JIB was the most popular procedure in the 1960s but fell into disrepute because of various complications, some of which were lethal. To avoid these complications Edward Mason devised the vertical banded gastroplasty which after various iterations stood the test of time until he devised the gastric bypass which then became the gold standard in the United States. To improve on the older JIB operation, Nicola Scopinaro from Italy modified the procedure as a biliopancreatic diversion (BPD) which was further modified by Marceau with a duodenal switch. In the 1980s, gastric bands were introduced to the market, at first as non-adjustable then as adjustable bands.

The laparoscopic era heralded a paradigm shift in bariatric surgery such that all procedures are now able to be carried out laparoscopically. Open surgery has all but disappeared except for some complex revisional procedures. Furthermore, the growth in recent decades of obesity surgery has led to a much more professional approach to the subject with the establishment of a multidisciplinary team (MDT) for patient selection and follow up, emphasis on quality improvement and accreditation of surgeons and units as well as a constant search for more effective and safer surgical methods of treatment. There is now universal agreement that obesity surgery is better termed metabolic surgery because of its profound effects on the various hormones which affect insulin sensitivity.

CAUSES OF OBESITY AND EPIDEMIOLOGY

Obesity is a multifactorial metabolic disorder which essentially manifests itself as a surplus of unexpended energy stored as fat. The contributing factors include genetic predisposition, eating disorders, psychological issues, poor diet, lack of exercise and comorbid conditions predisposing to obesity. The outcome of excess fat storage is often the development of a metabolic syndrome which drives the excess incidence of associated comorbidities. Table 64.1 shows the comorbidities associated with morbid obesity all of which can be improved by weight loss.

Morbid obesity is defined as a body mass index (BMI) equal to or greater than 40 kg/m^2 (Table 64.2). A patient with a BMI of 40 kg/m^2 is around 80 per cent above their ideal body weight. A 40-year-old women with a BMI of 40 kg/m^2 has an excess mortality of 8–12 years and will die younger than her peer group with a normal BMI. As BMI increases further so does the incidence

Nicola Scopinaro, born 1945. Professor of Surgery, University of Genoa, Italy. A charismatic figure and one of the most influential figures in the development of bariatric surgery.

Table 64.1 List of comorbidities associated with obesity which can be alleviated by surgical induced weight loss.

Comorbidity	
Metabolic syndrome	Type II diabetes mellitus
	High blood pressure
	Dyslipidaemia
Obstructive sleep apnoea	
Venous and lymphatic stasis	
Osteoarthritis	
Decreased mobility	
Chronic respiratory hypoventilation (Pickwickian syndrome)	
Hypertrophic cardiomyopathy	
Pseudotumour cerebri (idiopathic intracranial hypertension)	
Poor quality of life	
Urinary stress incontinence	
Gastro-oesophageal reflux disease	

Edward Mason, born 1920 (in the back seat of a taxi). Emeritus Professor of Surgery, University of Iowa, IA, USA. Best known as the 'father of obesity surgery'.

Table 64.2 Definition of body mass index (BMI).

Normal	BMI = 20–25 kg/m^2
Morbid obesity	BMI >40 kg/m^2
	BMI >35 kg/m^2 with comorbidity

BMI = weight (kg)/height (m)^2.

of associated comorbidities and the chance of premature death. The cause of death usually results from advanced metabolic syndrome causing premature atherosclerosis and diabetes.

In the UK, 2 per cent of females and 0.8 per cent of males have a BMI >40 kg/m^2 while in the US these figures are much higher. The international trend is for obesity incidence to increase such that the definition of a normal BMI of 20–25 kg/m^2 has been called into question. The comorbidities caused by obesity have become one of the world's greatest health-care problems as we do not seem to be able to stop the increase in obesity levels despite educating the public.

Non-surgical treatment for morbid obesity usually involves the patient trying various diets and attempts at exercising more regularly as well as other lifestyle changes. This can be aided by slimming clubs, professional dietician advice, personal exercise trainers and some pharmacological agents. Sadly, for morbidly obese patients, these have a 97 per cent long-term failure rate which is the main driver for surgical means to deal with the disorder. Even after initially successful bariatric surgery there is always a trend for gradual weight regain over the long term. This requires the bariatric patient to continue to address diet and exercise requirements. It must always be emphasised to patients that bariatric surgery does not cure the obesity problem but is an adjunct to help them to manage the problem more readily.

RELEVANT ANATOMY AND PHYSIOLOGY

Most bariatric procedures are aimed at the stomach in an attempt to restrict the amount the patient can eat. Some of these procedures also add an element of gastric and small intestinal bypass to produce a degree of malabsorption. Experimentally there are also approaches trying neuromodulation of the vagus or gastric muscle in order to create increased satiety.

The stomach receives food and starts the digestive process by adding acid and pepsin during the tituration process. The fundic area of the stomach also produces grehlin which is the only known hormone that stimulates appetite. During a meal levels of grehlin drop while between meals grehlin levels rise to stimulate the need to eat again. In addition, the stomach during filling undergoes adaptive relaxation mediated by the vagus so that it will accommodate food at a constant pressure. The jejunum and ileum also produce peptide hormones such as glucagon-like peptide-1 (GLP-1), peptide-YY (PYY) and cholecystokinin (CCK) which also have a role in stimulating the release of insulin and reducing appetite.

RATIONALE FOR OBESITY SURGERY

Obesity is dangerous to health due to the excess incidence of comorbidities that obese patients often develop, especially the metabolic syndrome. Many studies have suggested that if weight loss is induced surgically this leads to improvement in various comorbidities which translates into increased life expectancy. The best study so far is the well-known Swedish Obese Subjects study, which started in 1987, where the investigators matched over 2000 surgically treated patients with 2000 medically treated patients and followed these cohorts up for 15 years. Essentially this research has demonstrated that surgically induced weight loss increases life expectancy, and ameliorates diabetes, hypertension, hyperlipidaemia, obstructive sleep apnoea and atherosclerosis rates. In addition, these workers also have demonstrated that bariatric surgery leads to an improved quality of life and the patient being more likely to be employed as well as costing the health service less money. There is also some evidence from these workers as well as others that bariatric surgery reduces the incidence of some cancers. All published expert reports have supported bariatric surgery as being justifiable, namely the National Institute for Health in the US and the National Institute for Clinical Excellence in the UK. It should also be emphasized to potential patients that obesity surgery is not cosmetic surgery – it is designed to prevent the comorbidities that obesity causes with the long-term aim to increase life expectancy and quality of life (Summary box 64.1).

Summary box 64.1

Rationale for surgery

- Increase life expectancy
- Decrease comorbidities
- Decrease health-care costs to society

One of the biggest issues with bariatric surgery is who will pay for it. Rationing is inevitable in countries with a socialised health-care system, which nowadays is our biggest challenge. Who takes priority – a 55-year-old man with multiple comorbidities who is costing the health service a considerable amount of money or a 25-year-old man who is morbidly obese but as yet has not developed any comorbidities? No one has a clear answer to this ethical dilemma although ideally they should both be offered surgery.

PATIENT SELECTION AND PREPARATION FOR SURGERY

The criteria for patient selection are universally agreed (Table 64.3) although the evidence base for them has never been clearly delineated. Indeed, many bariatric surgeons think they are too conservative and need to be revised in light of new knowledge. There will always be some exceptions to the guidelines but for most part they should be followed. There is also an increasing trend for bariatric surgery to be carried out in younger patients, especially those in the paediatric age group where it is becoming clear that delaying surgery to adulthood is detrimental to their health.

All surgical candidates should been seen by the bariatric MDT (Table 64.4). All patients need some dietetic assessment which may help to choose the correct operation for them. In addition, they must be seen by a physician with an interest in obesity to screen for endocrine disorders and to establish the degree of metabolic syndrome present. All patients should also

Table 64.3 Selection criteria for obesity surgery (based on the International Federation for Surgery of Obesity and the National Institute for Clinical Excellence).

Body mass index (BMI) >40 kg/m^2 or BMI 35–39 kg/m^2 with serious comorbid disease treatable by weight loss
Minimum of 5 years obesity
Failure of conservative treatment
No alcoholism or major untreated psychiatric illness
Avoid if likely to get pregnant within 2 years
Age limits 18–55 (relative)
Acceptable operative risk on preoperative assessment

Table 64.4 Obesity multidisciplinary team (MDT) – all with required bariatric training.

Surgeon with a bariatric training
Physician with a special interest in obesity
Dietician
Specialist bariatric nurse
Anaesthetist
Skilled theatre staff
Psychiatrist/psychologist with interest in eating disorders

have a psychological screen to determine whether there are unresolved issues to be dealt with either pre- or postoperatively.

The risks of bariatric surgery need particular attention when counselling patients as the global risk of perioperative death is around 1 per cent although it is much lower than this for some procedures, especially in fitter patients. Involvement of the family or carers in decision-making is also crucial (Summary box 64.2).

Summary box 64.2

Patient selection

- Follow national guidelines
- Need MDT assessment
- Patient must understand risk/complications

Preoperatively patients are generally put on a low carbohydrate diet for a minimum of 2 weeks to shrink the liver to allow for adequate working space to carry out the surgery. A preoperative baseline metabolic screen (Table 64.5) is also desirable to determine the levels of vitamins, minerals and micronutrients which are essential for health. It is well recognised that many bariatric patients preoperatively suffer from vitamin and micronutrient deficiencies, usually due to their poor diet.

SURGICAL TREATMENT

The choosing of the best surgical procedure for an individual patient is not an exact science. What is clear is that there is no perfect operation free of side effects or complications. Some procedures are more effective than others albeit at the cost of higher perioperative rates of morbidity and mortality. It is unclear what the end point of bariatric surgery should be: is it maximum weight loss regardless of risk or just enough weight loss to alleviate comorbidities at minimum risk? Intuitively, it should be maximum weight loss with least risk and side effects, which requires a very detailed discussion of the options available with each individual patient.

As with other high-risk surgical procedures there is a volume–outcome effect thus it behoves any commissioner of bariatric services to fund only established high-volume centres in order to reduce complications and improve outcomes.

Table 64.5 Preoperative nutrition screen.

All patients	Full blood count, urea and electrolytes, liver function tests
	Fasting lipid profile
	Fasting glucose, HbA1C (if diabetic)
	Vitamins A, D and E
	Parathyroid hormone
Bypass patients	Magnesium, calcium and phosphate
	Ferritin, vitamin B12, folate and coagulation screen
	Zinc, selenium, copper and C-reactive protein

CURRENT SURGICAL OPTIONS

The surgical options have varying degrees of gastric restriction from pure (banding) to least (standard biliopancreatic diversion (BPD)). Varying degrees of malabsorption also pertain from none (banding) to severe (BPD). All procedures are usually carried out laparoscopically and increasingly through fewer access ports as instrumentation and techniques improve. With appropriate training some procedures can be carried out through a single umbilical incision although the future role of this approach is as yet unclear. Furthermore, some surgeons are now experienced at carrying out some procedures transvaginally leaving no abdominal scars at all!

Gastric banding

Around half of all surgical procedures in many countries are gastric bands which involves putting an adjustable band around the upper stomach leaving a small pouch just below the cardia (Figure 64.1). The degree of restriction can be controlled by the amount of fluid injected into the subcutaneous port. This operation is especially popular in Australia where excellent results are obtained. The perception that the band is reversible is important to some patients (although in reality it is a disadvantage). Gastric banding is certainly the least risky procedure (0.1 per cent perioperative mortality) as it does not involve cutting any stomach or bowel and is a relatively easy operation to perform in most patients who have a BMI <50 kg/m^2.

Most patients can expect to lose around 45–50 per cent of their excess weight, especially if the quality of follow up is intensive. However, there is a wide variation in results with

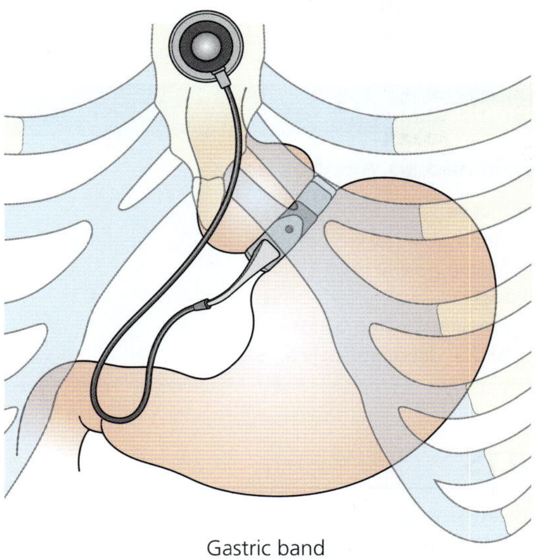

Figure 64.1 Gastric band.

some patients obtaining poor weight loss eventually requiring a revisional procedure. Furthermore, bands can fail due to prolapse of the stomach through the band or the band can slip up or down from its initial position. Bands can also erode into the stomach. Although the incidence of these complications is relatively low (<5 per cent) up to 30 per cent of patients are deemed long-term failures due to insufficient weight loss. It may be that these patients have been poorly selected in the first place or the quality of their follow up has not been very good.

One disadvantage of the gastric band is the need for continual band adjustments in the early postoperative period and occasional long-term adjustments. It is generally considered a labour-intensive procedure which requires a lot of patient compliance to get good results. Another disadvantage of the gastric band is that when a revisional procedure is indicated it is a much higher-risk procedure due to adhesions and gastric wall thickening.

However, gastric banding has a place in properly selected patients who have the correct attitude and understanding of the postoperative requirements. In selected patients a band can even be inserted as a day-case procedure. It should generally be avoided in binge eating patients and those whose eating habits involve excessive sweets and chocolate.

Sleeve gastrectomy

This relatively new operation requires less postoperative monitoring as it does not require any adjustments although it is a riskier procedure than gastric banding (0.2 per cent operative mortality). The long staple line can leak despite various manoeuvres to avoid leakage, such as applying reinforcing material and/or gluing. Another attraction of this procedure is that as it removes most of the grehlin-secreting area of the stomach it may have a beneficial effect on reducing appetite (Figure 64.2).

Around 65 per cent excess weight loss can be expected at two years which is as good as gastric bypass without any malabsorption issues. However, there is a tendency for the sleeve to expand over time. A resleeving procedure is well described or alternatively it is relatively straightforward to convert the procedure to a gastric bypass or a BPD with a duodenal switch. Indeed, many bariatric surgeons believe that in patients with a BMI >50 kg/m^2 who want a gastric bypass, it is safer to do a sleeve gastrectomy first and convert only those patients who regain weight to a gastric bypass. The exact percentage of how many patients might require a second procedure is not yet clear but is probably around 10–20 per cent depending on patient selection. Thus, the concept of bariatric surgery as a staged procedure has been mooted with the first stage being a sleeve gastrectomy and the second a gastric bypass or BPD with a duodenal switch. The second stage in most cases will not be needed.

The true place for sleeve gastrectomy as a primary bariatric procedure is still unclear and more long-term data are needed. Despite this, the frequency of this procedure is accelerating at a remarkable rate largely because of the relative technical ease of doing the procedure, the lack of potential malabsorption problems and the option of doing a relatively safe second-stage procedure if needed.

Roux-en-Y gastric bypass

The gastric bypass is a very effective weight loss procedure but is performed with a myriad of technical variations making comparisons difficult. However, overall it produces 65–75 per cent excess weight loss albeit at a higher risk of around 0.5 per cent perioperative mortality.

Gastric bypass is a very effective operation for alleviating and even curing type II diabetes – the result being almost immediate and independent of weight loss. There are two major theories as to how this happens (Table 64.6), given that other bariatric procedures such as banding and sleeve gastrectomy are dependent on weight loss to resolve the diabetes. Over 80 per cent of patients will have their diabetes permanently resolved (Table 64.7).

There are many variations in the actual gastric bypass technique, e.g. antecolic versus retrocolic Roux limb placement, varying alimentary and biliary limb lengths, additional banding of the gastrojejunal anastomosis to prevent dilatation, varying methods of doing the gastrojejunal anastomosis and varying methods of closing potential hernia spaces (Figure 64.3). There is a need to consolidate knowledge about the outcomes of these variations in order to standardise the procedure.

Although weight loss is generally very good the downside of this procedure is the need for careful postoperative metabolic

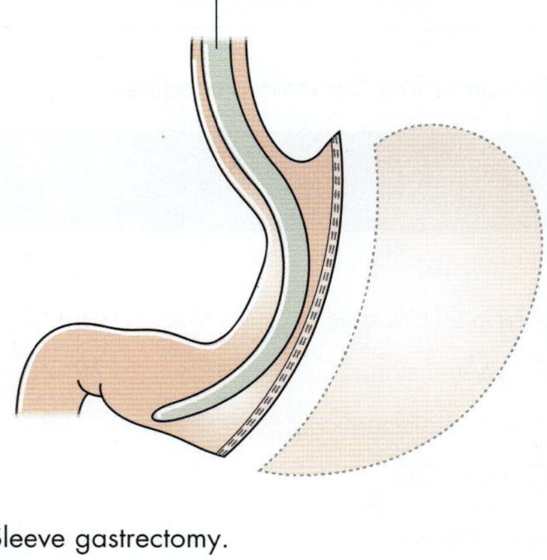

Figure 64.2 Sleeve gastrectomy.

follow up to avoid deficiency syndromes. Additional multivitamins, iron and calcium are needed for all patients as well as vitamin B12 administration. Some surgeons also recommend periodic bone densitometry measurements to avoid premature osteoporosis.

Biliopancreatic diversion – with or without a duodenal switch

This procedure, which produces the most malabsorption of all operations, is the most effective with 75–85 per cent excess weight loss but at the expense of the highest perioperative mortality of 1–2 per cent. Additionally as time goes by, if the patient does not adhere to their vitamin and micronutrient supplementation regime they are at severe risk of many deficiency syndromes. Furthermore, due to the extreme malabsorption these operations produce there is a need for a high protein intake of around 90 g/day which many patients find difficult. If this is not achieved then protein calorie malnutrition can be a problem. In correctly selected patients however, the BPD can be very effective, especially in those patients with a very high BMI. A BPD also has the same rapid effect as a gastric bypass for alleviating diabetes independent of weight loss (Tables 64.6 and 64.7).

The duodenal switch variation of the BPD was designed to reduce the need for taking vitamin B12 and reduce the incidence of anastomotic strictures at the gastrojejunal anastomosis. In the standard BPD, approximately two-thirds of the distal stomach is removed while in the duodenal switch variation there is a vertical sleeve gastrectomy. In the duodenal switch variation, the anastomosis is made to the first part of the duodenum rather than the stomach as in the standard BPD. The limb lengths also vary, as shown in Figure 64.4. In reality, there is very little difference between these two procedures in terms of weight loss and long-term complications despite some assertions to the contrary (Summary box 64.3).

Table 64.6 Theories on mechanisms of how a gastric bypass/biliopancreatic diversion ameliorates diabetes.

Foregut hypothesis	Bypass of proximal duodenum and jejunum reduces stimulated secretion of anti-incretin factors which normally inhibit insulin secretion thus allowing the unopposed effects of incretins to stimulate insulin secretion
Hindgut hypothesis	Rapid delivery of small bowel content into the distal jejunum and ileum exaggerates stimulated incretin (glucagon-like peptide-1 and peptide-YY) release which stimulates insulin secretion

Summary box 64.3

Established surgical options

- Restrictive
  - Adjustable gastric banding
  - Sleeve gastrectomy
- Bypass
  - Proximal gastric bypass
  - BPD ± duodenal switch

RESULTS

When discussing results of bariatric surgery there is an immediate problem in defining success. Traditionally it has been considered as losing at least 50 per cent of the excess weight in the first 12–24 months. The excess weight of a patient is their current weight minus their ideal body weight (at BMI 25 kg/m^2). For a given procedure that removes say 50 per cent of excess weight, the higher the initial BMI of the patient the more weight is removed but the patient may still be considerably overweight after surgery compared to a lower BMI patient. Furthermore, many comorbidities are improved with only 10–20 per cent of excess weight loss thus the end point of removing as much weight as possible may not always be necessary from a health and longevity point of view. Other outcomes such as improved quality of life may also be as important. In general terms, however, most surgeons strive for an effective operation which is usually perceived as reducing as much weight as possible for the given risk of the procedure. In addition, it should also resolve or ameliorate any of the comorbidities which are linked to obesity (Table 64.1). Table 64.7 shows the usual outcomes for bariatric procedures.

While there is a spectrum of weight loss results between the various procedures there is also a variation in weight loss for each individual procedure which is usually a function of patient selection and postoperative follow up. For example, restrictive procedures are notorious for good early results but as time goes by the patient learns to cheat more effectively, eats more soft calories and becomes complacent about exercise. This results in weight regain which is always difficult to manage and in some cases will result in revisional surgery which is always more risky than a primary procedure. In addition, patients will often 'move

Table 64.7 Outcomes from bariatric procedures.

	Restrictive (bands, sleeve gastrectomy)	Combined gastric bypass	Malabsorptive BPD with or without a duodenal switch
Excess weight loss (%)	48–68	62	72
Resolution of type 2 diabetes (%)	48–72	84	98
Resolution of hypertension, (%)	28–73	75	81
Improvement in dyslipidaemia (%)	71–81	94	100
Operative mortality (%)	0.1	0.5	1.10

BPD, biliopancreatic diversion.

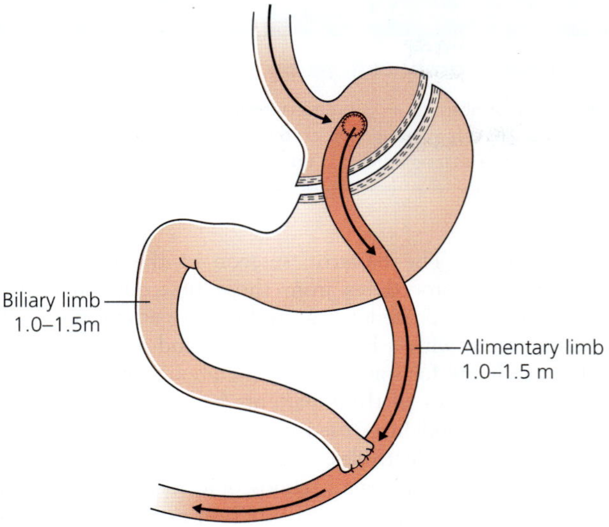

Figure 64.3 Gastric bypass.

the goal posts' wanting a better result than the surgery promises. Thus, a clear understanding of the end point of surgery must be agreed before embarking on any procedure, i.e. amount of weight loss or resolution of comorbidities or, usually, a combination of both. If this is written down and agreed preoperatively this avoids misunderstandings postoperatively.

It behoves the surgeon to get the operation right the first time for an individual patient after a thorough understanding of what risks they are prepared to take for a particular outcome. This will vary from patient to patient. Those patients who are very risk averse, often young with young children, will understandably often want an operation with the least postoperative mortality even though it may not result in as much weight loss as another more risky procedure. Conversely, a patient without children who is older and much heavier may be keen to undergo a more risky procedure to maximise their weight loss. It is a matter of considerable judgement on both the patient and surgeon's part to decide what is the most suitable procedure for a given patient. Discussion at a bariatric MDT is always desirable in order that every member of the bariatric team has a chance to express their views about the suitability of any particular procedure for the patient in question.

COMPLICATIONS

Carrying out surgery in obese patients generally is more risky than surgery in lean patients no matter what type of surgery is contemplated. Obese patients are more likely to suffer from cardiorespiratory comorbidities which increase surgical complications. Furthermore, they are often hypercoagulable with an increased risk of deep-vein thrombosis and pulmonary embolism. Most of the general risks of surgery, such as bleeding and infection, are also more likely to occur. The specific risks in relation to the actual surgical procedure will vary from procedure to procedure and are listed in Table 64.8.

Perioperative mortality should be minimal but is higher in those patients with the most severe comorbidities. Severe unstable cardiovascular disease is an absolute contraindication to bariatric surgery. Super-obese (BMI >50 kg/m^2) males also have a higher risk of perioperative mortality as well as patients with a past history of pulmonary embolism. For the latter a prophylactic

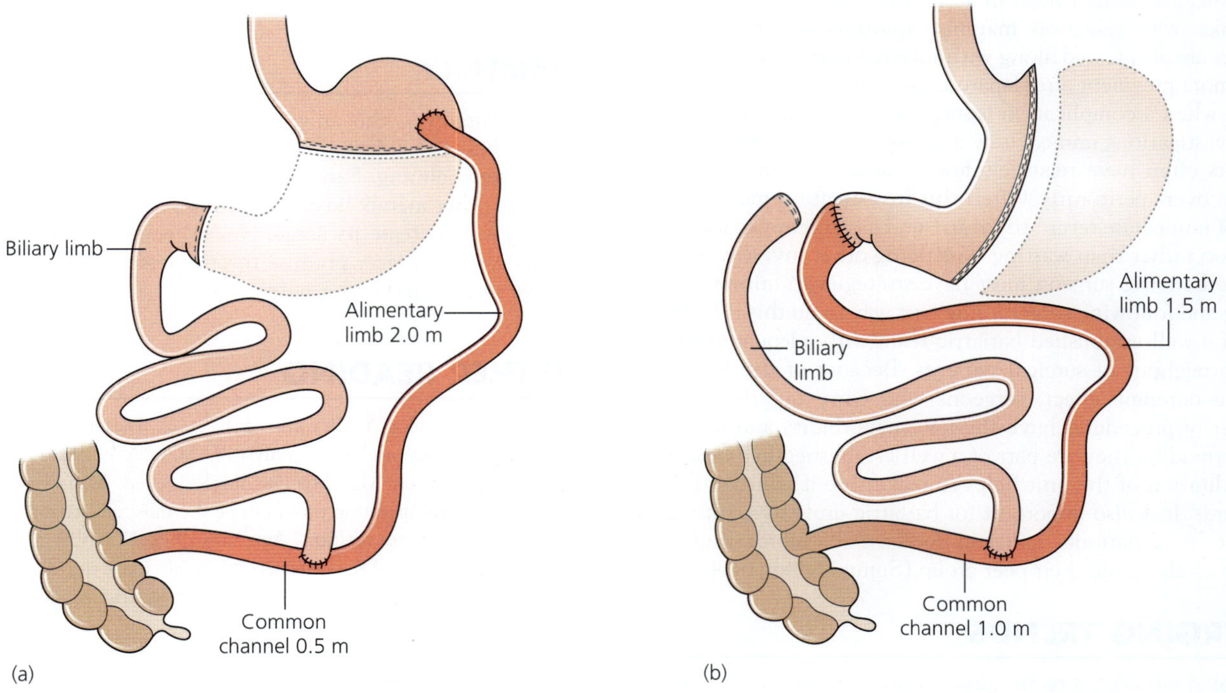

Figure 64.4 (a) Standard biliopancreatic diversion (BPD); (b) BPD with duodenal switch variation.

Table 64.8 Risks of bariatric procedures.

Risk	
General risks of bariatric surgery	Bleeding
	Infection
	Deep vein thrombosis (± pulmonary embolism)
	Accidental bowel perforation
	Perioperative mortality (see Table 64.6)
Risks of specific bariatric procedures	Internal herniation (gastric bypass and BPD)
	Staple line/anastomotic leak (gastric bypass, sleeve gastrectomy, BPD)
	Band slippage/erosion
	Pouch dilatation (gastric band, gastric bypass, sleeve gastrectomy)
Long-term risks of all bariatric surgery	Protein calorie malnutrition
	Vitamin and micronutrient depletion syndromes
	Weight regain

BPD, biliopancreatic diversion.

preoperative caval filter should be considered. Even if there is no history of deep-vein thrombosis, a pulmonary embolism is still a leading cause of perioperative mortality despite the usual prophylactic precautions of graded calf compression stockings, intraoperative calf compression, intraoperative low molecular weight heparin, early mobilisation and extended postoperative low molecular weight heparin administration.

Leaks from resection margins, anastomoses or off-camera injuries are also feared along with internal hernias which appear to be more prevalent after laparoscopic surgery. The key message is that when a complication is suspected it is important to carry out investigations immediately and not delay as morbidly obese patients often have relatively few clinical signs and symptoms despite overt peritonitis. Often this investigation may take the form of immediate return to theatre and laparoscopy to assess the situation rather than wasting time doing other investigations.

The bariatric surgeon must have strategies to minimise risks during and following surgery. The best way to do this is by being part of a well-established bariatric team with adequate training and throughput of surgical patients. Because of the beneficial volume–outcome effect, surgeons who carry out the greatest number of procedures have the lowest morbidity and mortality rates providing they are part of a well-established bariatric unit. Accreditation of the unit helps to make sure it adheres to high standards. It is also important for bariatric units to submit their patients to a national bariatric database for monitoring their outcomes alongside their peer group (Summary box 64.4).

Summary box 64.4

Minimise complications by

- Subspecialisation in bariatric surgery
- Work in a high volume accredited unit
- Compare outcomes with a national database

EMERGING TRENDS

Typical of all surgical techniques bariatric procedures are rapidly evolving along with improvements in technology and evidence of effectiveness. The bariatric surgeon of the future will be doing different procedures from those of today, more likely with an array of procedures according to patient needs. The diabetic patient with a BMI between 30 and 34 kg/m^2 is likely to be a candidate for some form of metabolic surgery when the results from studies in these patients become available. Some of the surgical modalities used may be neuromodulation using gastric-implanted electrodes, vagal blocking using electrodes around the abdominal vagus, endoscopically placed intraluminal sleeves, endoscopic gastric restriction procedures as well as improvements in the current operations, especially involving less abdominal wall trauma by using single incision and transvaginal approaches. Careful evaluation will determine their place in the armamentarium for managing obesity and related metabolic conditions (Summary box 64.5).

Summary box 64.5

Experimental options

- Vagal stimulation
- Endoluminal sleeve
- Natural orifice endoscopic surgery

SUMMARY

Bariatric surgery is the only effective long-term treatment for morbid obesity. Evidence for its initial and medium-term success is overwhelming. Extension of the principles of surgery for obesity to other metabolic conditions, especially type II diabetes mellitus, will increase its usage. Newer techniques for performing this type of surgery promise to offer less complications, less invasive surgery and better outcomes.

FURTHER READING

Buchwald H, Avidor Y, Braunwald E *et al.* Bariatric surgery – a systematic review and meta-analysis. *JAMA* 2004; **292**: 1724–37.

Poiries WJ, Swanson MS, MacDonald KG *et al.* Who would have thought it? An operation proves to be the most effective therapy for adult-onset diabetes mellitus. *Ann Surg* 1995; **222**: 339–52.

Sjostrum L, Lindross AK, Peltonen M *et al.* Lifestyle, diabetes and cardiovascular risk factors 10 years after bariatric surgery. *N Engl J Med* 2004; **351**: 2683–93.

Sjostrum L, Narbro K, Sjostrum D *et al.* Effects of bariatric surgery on mortality in Swedish obese subjects. *N Engl J Med* 2007; **357**: 741–52.

CHAPTER

65 The liver

LEARNING OBJECTIVES

To understand:

- The anatomy of the liver
- The signs of acute and chronic liver disease
- The investigation of liver disease
- The management of liver trauma, infections, cirrhosis and tumours

INTRODUCTION

The liver is the largest organ in the body, weighing 1.5 kg in the average 70-kg man. The liver parenchyma is entirely covered by a thin capsule and by visceral peritoneum on all but the posterior surface of the liver, termed the 'bare area'. The liver is divided into a large right lobe, which constitutes three-quarters of the liver parenchyma, and a smaller left lobe.

ANATOMY OF THE LIVER

Ligaments and peritoneal reflections

The liver is fixed in the right upper quadrant by peritoneal reflections that form ligaments. On the superior surface of the left lobe is the left triangular ligament. Dividing the anterior and posterior folds of this ligament allows the left lobe to be mobilised from the diaphragm and the left lateral wall of the inferior vena cava (IVC) to be exposed. The right triangular ligament fixes the entire right lobe of the liver to the undersurface of the right hemidiaphragm. Division of this ligament allows the liver to be mobilised from under the diaphragm and rotated to the left. Another major supporting structure is the falciform ligament (remnant of the umbilical vein), which runs from the umbilicus to the liver between the right and left lobes, passing into the interlobar fissure. From the fissure, it passes anteriorly on the surface of the liver, attaching it to the posterior aspect of the anterior abdominal wall. Division of the superior leaves of the falciform ligament allows exposure of the suprahepatic IVC, lying within a thin sheath of fibrous tissue. The final peritoneal reflection is between the stomach and the liver. This lesser omentum is often thin and fragile, but contains the hilar structures in its free edge.

Liver blood supply

The blood supply to the liver is unique, 80 per cent being derived from the portal vein and 20 per cent from the hepatic artery. The arterial blood supply in most individuals is derived from the coeliac trunk of the aorta, where the hepatic artery arises along with the splenic artery. After supplying the gastroduodenal artery, it branches at a very variable level to produce the right and left hepatic arteries. The right artery supplies the majority of the liver parenchyma and is therefore the larger of the two arteries. There are many anatomical variations, knowledge of which is essential for safe surgery on the liver. The blood supply to the right lobe of the liver may be partly or completely supplied by a right hepatic artery arising from the superior mesenteric artery. This vessel passes posterior to the uncinate process and head of the pancreas, and runs to the liver on the posterior wall of the bile duct. Similarly, the arterial blood supply to the left lobe of the liver may be derived from the coeliac trunk via its left gastric branch. This vessel runs between the lesser curve of the stomach and the left lobe of the liver in the lesser omentum (Figure 65.1).

Structures in the hilum of the liver

The porta hepatis, a transverse fissure on the visceral surface of the liver, is the hilum of the liver. The hepatic artery, portal vein and bile duct are present within the free edge of the lesser omentum or the 'hepatoduodenal ligament' and together with nerves and lymphatics enter the liver at the porta hepatis. To expose these structures requires division of the overlying peritoneum followed by the division of small vessels and the lymphatic plexus. The usual anatomical relationship of these structures is for the bile duct to be within the free edge, the hepatic artery to be above and medial, and the portal vein to lie posteriorly. Within this ligament, the common hepatic duct is joined by the cystic duct at a varying level to form the common bile duct. The common hepatic artery branches at a variable level within the ligament to form two, or often three, main arterial branches to the liver. The right hepatic artery crosses the bile duct either anteriorly or posteriorly before giving rise to the cystic artery (see Figure 67.1 in Chapter 67). Multiple small hepatic arterial branches provide blood to the bile duct, principally from the right hepatic artery. The portal vein arises from the confluence of the splenic vein and the superior mesenteric vein behind the neck of the pancreas. It has some important tributaries, including the left gastric vein which joins just above the pancreas.

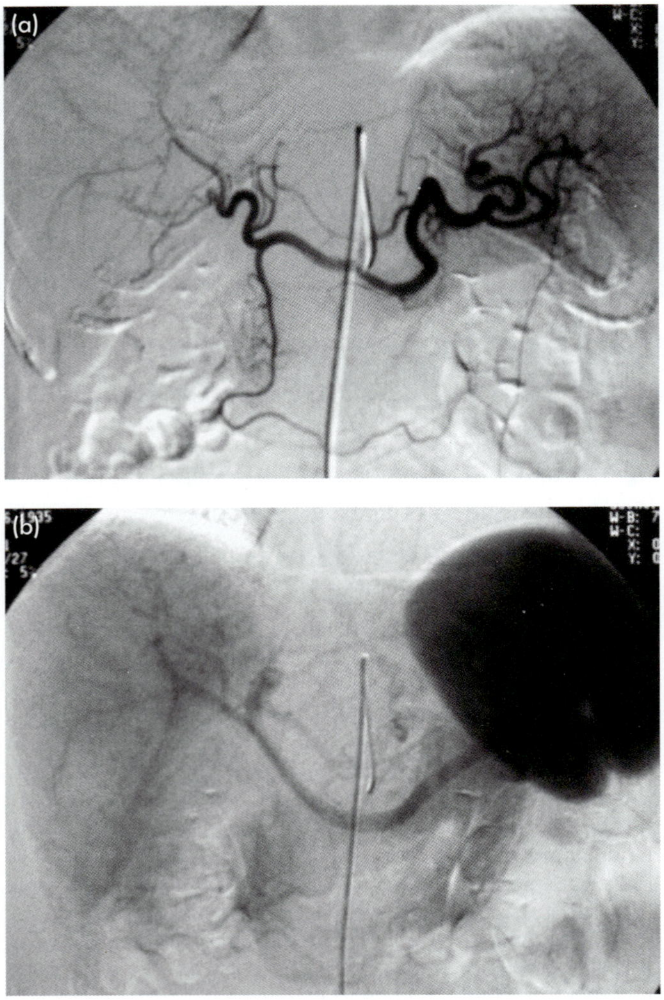

Figure 65.1 Hepatic angiography/conventional arterial anatomy. Arterial (a) and venous (b) phase of a selective hepatic angiogram. The hepatic artery usually arises from the coeliac trunk, along with the splenic artery, and gives rise to the gastroduodenal artery before dividing into the right and left hepatic arteries. The portal vein forms from the superior mesenteric and splenic veins, and divides into right and left branches in the hilum of the liver.

Division of structures at the hilum

At the hilum, the major structures are divided into right and left branches. The right and left hepatic ducts arise from the hepatic parenchyma and join to form the common hepatic duct. The left duct has a longer extrahepatic course of approximately 2 cm. Once within the liver parenchyma, the duct accompanies the branches of the hepatic artery and portal vein within a fibrous sheath. The portal vein often gives off two large branches to the right lobe, which are usually outside the liver for a short length, before giving a left portal vein branch that runs behind the left hepatic duct.

Venous drainage of the liver

The venous drainage of the liver is via the hepatic veins into the IVC. The vena cava lies within a groove in the posterior wall of the liver. Above the liver, it immediately penetrates the diaphragm to join the right atrium, whereas below the liver parenchyma, there is a short length of vessel before the insertion of the renal veins. The inferior hepatic veins are short vessels that pass directly between the liver parenchyma and the anterior wall of the IVC. The major venous drainage is through three large veins that join the IVC immediately below the diaphragm. Outside the liver, these vessels are surrounded by a thin fibrous layer. The right hepatic vein can be exposed fully outside the liver, but the middle and left veins usually join within the liver parenchyma. The right kidney and adrenal gland lie immediately adjacent to the retrohepatic IVC. The right adrenal vein drains into the IVC at this level, usually via one main branch. The IVC can be mobilised fully from the retroperitoneal tissues and, in the healthy state, there are no large vessels in this tissue plane.

SEGMENTAL ANATOMY OF THE LIVER

Understanding the internal anatomy of the liver has greatly facilitated safe liver surgery. Couinaud, a French anatomist, described the liver as being divided into eight segments (Figure 65.2). Each of these segments can be considered as a functional

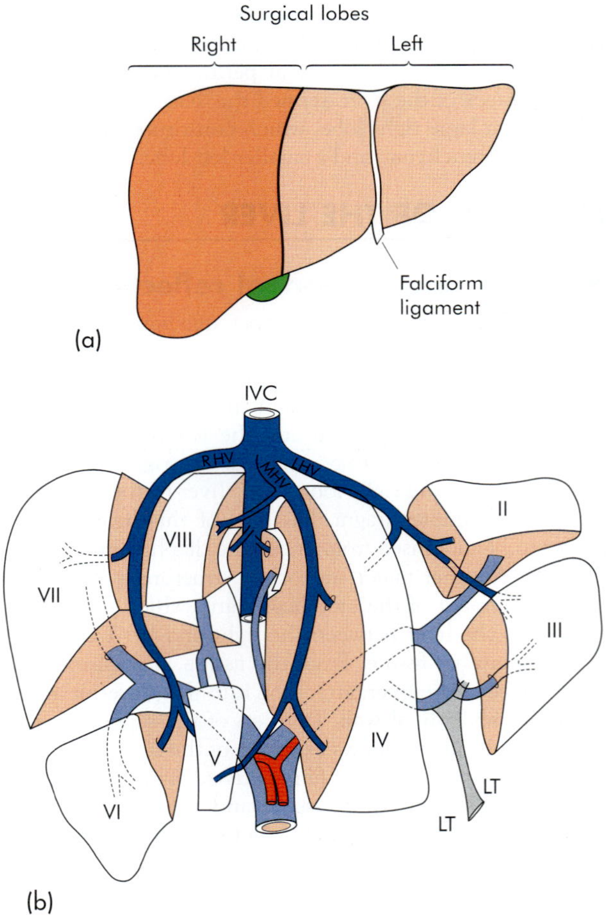

Figure 65.2 (a) The 'surgical' labels of the liver compared with the usual anatomical division into right and left lobes by the falciform ligament. (b) Segments of the liver (after Couinaud). IVC, inferior vena cava; LHV, left hepatic vein; LT, ligamentum teres; MHV, middle hepatic vein; RHV, right hepatic vein.

unit, with a branch of the hepatic artery, portal vein and bile duct, and drained by a branch of the hepatic vein. The overall anatomy of the liver is divided into a functional right and left 'unit' along the line between the gall bladder fossa and the middle hepatic vein (Cantlie's line). Liver segments (V–VIII), to the right of this line, are supplied by the right hepatic artery and the right branch of the portal vein, and drain bile via the right hepatic duct. To the left of this line (segments I–IV), functionally, is the left liver, which is supplied by the left branch of the hepatic artery and the left portal vein branch, and drains bile via the left hepatic duct (Summary box 65.1).

Summary box 65.1

Liver anatomy

- There are two anatomical lobes with separate blood supply, bile duct and venous drainage
- Dual blood supply (20 per cent hepatic artery and 80 per cent portal vein)
- The liver regenerates fully after partial resection
- Resection is based on anatomical lines to preserve maximal functioning liver

The hepatic lobules

The functional units within the liver segments are the liver lobules. These comprise plates of liver cells separated by the hepatic sinusoids, large, thin-walled venous channels that carry blood to the central vein, a tributary of the hepatic vein, from the portal tracts, which contain branches of the hepatic artery and portal vein. During passage through the sinusoids, the many functions of the liver take place, including bile formation, which is channelled in an opposite direction to the blood flow to drain via the bile duct tributaries within the portal tracts.

Embryology

The liver is a foregut structure and forms as a small endodermal bud early in gestation. The cell population is bipotential, and cells may develop into hepatocytes or intrahepatic ductal cells. The liver endothelium is derived from the vitelline and umbilical veins, which merge with the endodermal bud to form the liver sinusoids. The supporting connective tissue, haemopoietic cells, and Kupffer cells are derived from the mesoderm of the septum transversum which is a mass of mesenchymal connective tissue.

ACUTE AND CHRONIC LIVER DISEASE

Liver function and tests

Adequate liver function is essential to survival; humans will survive for only 24–48 hours in the anhepatic state despite full supportive therapy. The liver is central to many key metabolic pathways (Summary box 65.2).

An awareness of the currently available liver function tests and their significance is essential (Table 65.1).

Bilirubin is synthesised in the liver and excreted in bile. Increased levels may be associated with increased haemoglobin breakdown, hepatocellular dysfunction resulting in impaired bilirubin transport and excretion, or biliary obstruction. In patients with known parenchymal liver disease, progressive elevation of bilirubin in the absence of a secondary complication suggests deterioration in liver function. The serum alkaline phosphatase is particularly elevated with cholestatic liver disease or biliary obstruction. The transaminase levels (aspartate transaminase (AST) and alanine transaminase (ALT)) reflect acute hepatocellular damage, as does the gamma-glutamyl transpeptidase (GGT) level, which may be used to detect the liver injury associated with acute alcohol ingestion. The synthetic functions of the liver are reflected in the ability to synthesise proteins (albumin level) and clotting factors (prothrombin time). The standard method of monitoring liver function in patients with chronic liver disease is serial measurement of bilirubin, albumin and prothrombin time.

Summary box 65.2

Main functions of the liver

- Maintaining core body temperature
- pH balance and correction of lactic acidosis
- Synthesis of clotting factors
- Glucose metabolism, glycolysis and gluconeogenesis
- Urea formation from protein catabolism
- Bilirubin formation from haemoglobin degradation
- Drug and hormone metabolism and excretion
- Removal of gut endotoxins and foreign antigens

Table 65.1 Routinely available tests of liver function.

Test	Normal range
Bilirubin	5–17 μmol/L
Alkaline phosphatase (ALP)	35–130 IU/L
Aspartate transaminase (AST)	5–40 IU/L
Alanine transaminase (ALT)	5–40 IU/L
Gamma-glutamyl transpeptidase (GGT)	10–48 IU/L
Albumin	35–50 g/L
Prothrombin time (PT)	12–16 s

Clinical signs of impaired liver function

These signs depend on the severity of dysfunction and whether it is acute or chronic.

Acute liver failure

Causes of acute liver failure

In the early stages, there may be no objective signs, but with severe dysfunction the onset of clinical jaundice may be associated with neurological signs of liver failure (hepatic encephalopathy), consisting of a liver flap, drowsiness, confusion and, eventually, coma (Summary box 65.3).

Treatment of acute liver failure

The overall mortality from acute liver failure is approximately 50 per cent, even with the best supportive therapy (Summary box 65.4).

Karl Wilhelm von Kupffer, 1829–1902, Professor of Anatomy at Kiel (1867), Königsberg (1875), and Munich, Germany (1880), described these 'stellate cells' in 1880.
King's College Hospital, London, UK, a pioneering centre for liver transplantation.

Summary box 65.3

Causes of acute liver failure

- Viral hepatitis (hepatitis A, B, C, D, E)
- Drug reactions (halothane, isoniazid–rifampicin, antidepressants, non-steroidal anti-inflammatory drugs, valproic acid)
- Paracetamol overdose
- Mushroom poisoning
- Shock and multiorgan failure
- Acute Budd–Chiari syndrome
- Wilson's disease
- Fatty liver of pregnancy

Summary box 65.4

Supportive therapy for acute liver failure

- Fluid balance and electrolytes
- Acid–base balance and blood glucose monitoring
- Nutrition
- Renal function (haemofiltration)
- Respiratory support (ventilation)
- Monitoring and treatment of cerebral oedema
- Treat bacterial and fungal infection

Liver transplantation is appropriate for some patients with acute liver failure (Summary box 65.5), although the short-term results are poor in comparison with liver transplantation for chronic liver disease.

Summary box 65.5

Criteria for orthotopic liver transplantation in acute liver failure

- Paracetamol induced
  pH <7.30 (irrespective of grade of encephalopathy)
  or prothrombin time (PT) >100 s + serum creatinine >300 μmol/L + grade 3 or 4 encephalopathy.
- Non-paracetamol induced (irrespective of encephalopathy)
  PT >100 s

or any three of the following:

Age <10 years or >40 years
Aetiology non-A, non-B, halothane or idiosyncratic drug reaction
More than 7 days' jaundice before encephalopathy
PT >50 s
Bilirubin >300 μmol/L

O'Grady *et al.* *Gastroenterology* 1989; **97**: 439–45.

Chronic liver disease

Lethargy and weakness are common features irrespective of the underlying cause. This often precedes clinical jaundice, which indicates the liver's inability to metabolise bilirubin. The serum bilirubin level reflects the severity of the underlying liver disease. Progressive deterioration in liver function is associated with a hyperdynamic circulation involving a high cardiac output, large pulse volume, low blood pressure and flushed warm extremities. Fever is a common feature, which may be related to underlying inflammation and cytokine release from the diseased liver or may be due to bacterial infection, to which patients with chronic liver disease are predisposed. Skin changes may be evident, including spider naevi*, cutaneous vascular abnormalities that blanch on pressure, palmar erythema and white nails (leuconychia). Endocrine abnormalities are responsible for hypogonadism and gynaecomastia. The mental derangement associated with chronic liver disease is termed 'hepatic encephalopathy'. This is associated with memory impairment, confusion, personality changes, altered sleep patterns and slow, slurred speech. The most useful clinical sign is the flapping tremor demonstrated by asking the patient to extend his or her arms and hyperextend the wrist joint. Abdominal distension due to ascites is a common late feature. This may be suggested clinically by the demonstration of a fluid thrill or shifting dullness. Protein catabolism produces loss of muscle bulk and wasting, and a coagulation defect is suggested by the presence of skin bruising. A patient with the typical features of end-stage chronic liver disease is shown in Figure 65.3 (Summary box 65.6).

Classifying the severity of chronic liver disease

Two prognostic models commonly used to assess the severity of chronic liver disease and perioperative risk are the Child–Turcotte–Pugh (CTP) Classification and the Model for End-Stage Liver Disease (MELD) score. The CTP classification has been modified from the original Child classification which was developed to predict mortality following shunt surgery in cirrhotic patients. The CTP classification is shown in Table 65.2. The MELD score was originally developed to predict short-term

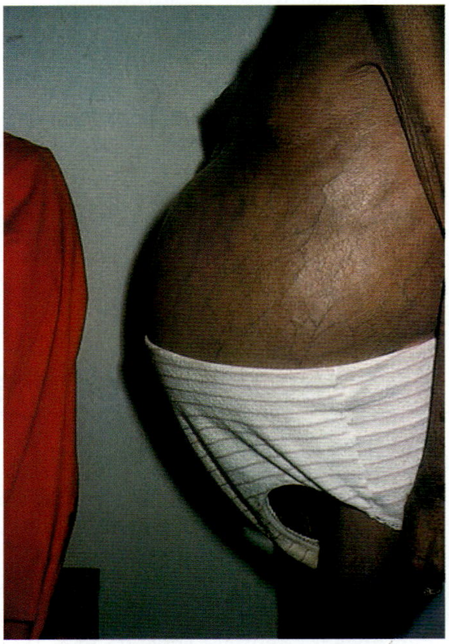

Figure 65.3 A patient with end-stage liver cirrhosis disease, demonstrating muscle wasting and gross abdominal distension due to ascites.

*An older Miss Muffet
Decided to rough it
And lived upon whisky and gin.
Red hands and a spider
Developed outside her
Such are the wages of sin. William Bennet Bean, 1909–89, Professor of Internal Medicine, University of Iowa, USA.

Summary box 65.6

Features of chronic liver disease

- Lethargy
- Fever
- Jaundice
- Protein catabolism (wasting)
- Coagulopathy (bruising)
- Cardiac (hyperdynamic circulation)
- Neurological (hepatic encephalopathy)
- Portal hypertension
  - Ascites
  - Oesophageal varices
  - Splenomegaly
- Cutaneous
  - Spider naevi
  - Palmar erythema

prognosis in patients undergoing transjugular intrahepatic portosystemic shunt insertion, but has now been adopted to prioritise patients awaiting liver transplantation. In the MELD model, the survival probability of patients with end-stage liver disease is computed based on the patient's international normalised ratio (INR), serum bilirubin and serum creatinine.

Table 65.2 Child–Turcotte–Pugh (CTP) classification of hepatocellular function in cirrhosis.

Points	1 point each	2 points each	3 points each
Bilirubin (μmol/L)	<34	34–50	>50
Albumin (g/L)	>35	25–35	<25
Ascites	None	Easily controlled	Poorly controlled
Encephalopathy	None	Grade I–II	Grade III–IV
INR	<1.7	1.7–2.2	>2.2

CTP A = 5–6 points; CTP B = 7–9 points; CTP C = 10–15 points.
INR, international normalised ratio.

IMAGING THE LIVER

The major advances that have taken place over recent years in surgical approaches to the liver and the enormous improvement in the safety of liver surgery are a result of the careful individualised planning of surgery achieved through improvements in preoperative imaging. The ideal choice of imaging modality is determined by the likely liver pathology and the locally available equipment and radiological expertise (Table 65.3).

Ultrasound

This is the first-line test owing to its safety and wide availability. It is entirely operator dependent. It is useful for determining bile duct dilatation, the presence of gallstones (Figure 65.4) and the presence of liver tumours. Ultrasound can reliably differentiate between cystic and solid masses. Doppler ultrasound allows flow in the hepatic artery, portal vein and hepatic veins to be assessed. In some countries, it is used as a screening test for the development of primary liver cancers in a high-risk population. Ultrasound is useful in guiding the percutaneous biopsy of a liver lesion, and aspiration of liver abscesses.

Table 65.3 Imaging the liver.

Imaging modality	Principal indication
Ultrasound	Standard first-line investigation
Spiral CT	Anatomical planning for liver surgery
MRI	Alternative to spiral CT
MRCP	First-line, non-invasive cholangiography
ERCP	Imaging the biliary tract when endoscopic intervention is anticipated (e.g. ductal stones)
PTC	Biliary tract imaging when ERCP impossible or failed
Angiography	To detect vascular involvement by tumour
Nuclear medicine	To quantify biliary excretion and tumour spread
Laparoscopy/ laparoscopic ultrasound	To detect peritoneal tumour spread and superficial liver metastases

CT, computed tomography; ERCP, endoscopic retrograde cholangiopancreatography; MRCP, magnetic resonance cholangiopancreatography; MRI, magnetic resonance imaging; PTC, percutaneous transhepatic cholangiography.

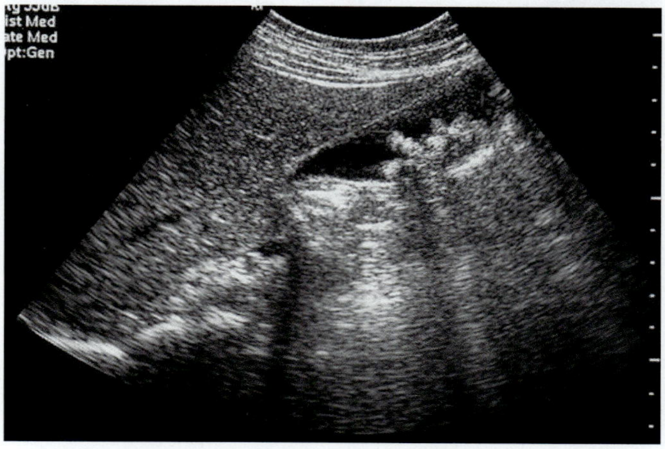

Figure 65.4 Ultrasound scan of the upper abdomen, showing the liver on the left and a gall bladder containing multiple gallstones centrally. The stones can be seen to cast an acoustic shadow.

Computed tomography

Modern computed tomography (CT) technology has inceased the accuracy of diagnosis and staging of liver lesions, and contrast-enhanced computed tomography is currently the most widely used and best validated modality for liver imaging. This provides fine detail of liver lesions down to less than 1 cm in diameter and gives information on their nature (Figure 65.5). Oral contrast enhancement allows visualisation of the stomach and duodenum in relation to the liver hilum. The early arterial phase of the intravenous contrast vascular enhancement is particularly useful for detecting small primary liver cancers, owing to their preferential arterial blood supply. The venous phase

CG Child, surgeon, Michigan, USA. Child and JG Turcotte first proposed the scoring system in 1964. In 1972, Pugh modified the scoring system by replacing nutritional status by prothrombin time or international normalised ratio.

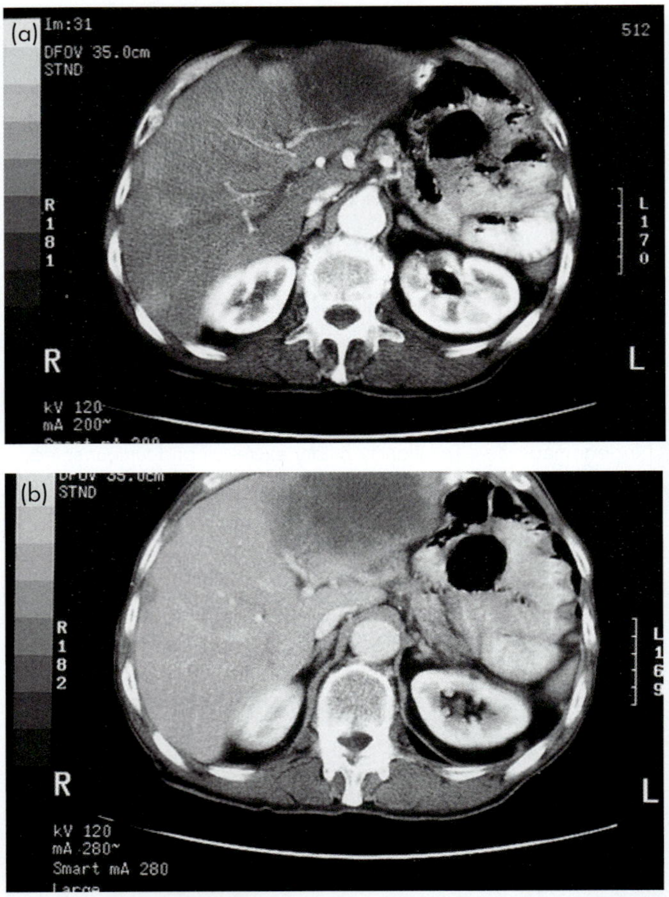

Figure 65.5 Computed tomography (CT) scan of a patient with a liver tumour in the left lobe of the liver, using intravenous contrast enhancement. The vascularity of the lesion and, hence, its possible nature can be determined from the arterial (a) and venous (b) phases of the scan.

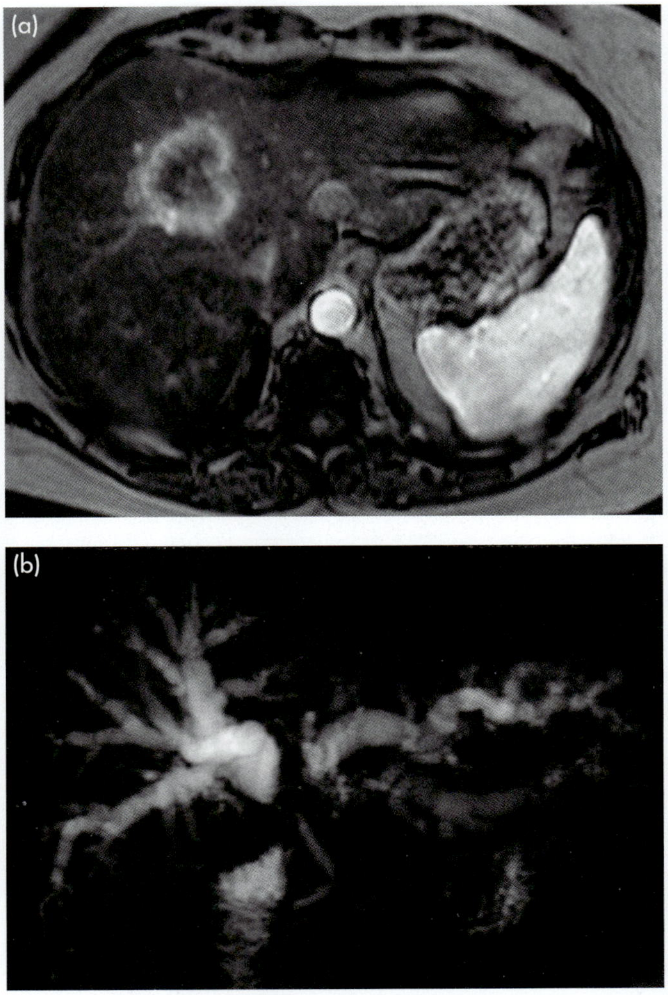

Figure 65.6 The role of magnetic resonance imaging (MRI) in liver disease. MRI is increasingly used for imaging the liver. It may be used for cross-sectional imaging for staging liver cancers (MRI) (a), for non-invasive cholangiography to demonstrate a hilar stricture (magnetic resonance cholangiopancreatography, MRCP) (b), or for the non-invasive assessment of blood vessels (magnetic resonance angiography, MRA).

maps the branches of the portal vein within the liver and the drainage via the hepatic veins. Inflammatory liver lesions often exhibit rim enhancement with intravenous contrast, whereas the common haemangioma characteristically shows late venous enhancement. The density of any liver lesion can be measured, which can be useful in establishing the presence of a cystic lesion. CT has high accuracy in determining the stage, and high sensitivity and specificity in determining resectability of liver tumours. Local and distant metastases can also be detected, although peritoneal metastases are often missed on CT.

Magnetic resonance imaging

Magnetic resonance imaging (MRI) (Figure 65.6) would appear to be as effective an imaging modality as CT in the majority of patients with liver disease. It does, however, offer several advantages. First, the use of iodine-containing intravenous contrast agents is precluded in many patients because of a history of allergy. These patients should be offered MRI rather than contrast CT. Second, magnetic resonance cholangiopancreatography (MRCP) provides excellent quality, non-invasive imaging of the biliary tract, the accuracy of which is comparable to direct cholangiography by endoscopic retrograde cholangiopancreatography (ERCP) or percutaneous transhepatic cholangiography (PTC). Complementary to CT, MRI and MRCP are the best imaging modalities for suspected hilar cholangiocarcinoma. It is useful for diagnostic questions when ERCP has failed or is impossible due to previous surgery. Magnetic resonance angiography (MRA) similarly provides high-quality images of the hepatic artery and portal vein, without the need for arterial cannulation. It is used as an alternative to selective hepatic angiography for diagnosis. It is particularly useful in patients with chronic liver disease and coagulopathy in whom the patency of the portal vein and its branches is in question.

Endoscopic retrograde cholangiopancreatography

ERCP (Figure 65.7a) is performed in patients with obstructive jaundice when an endoscopic intervention is anticipated based on imaging (endoscopic removal of common bile duct

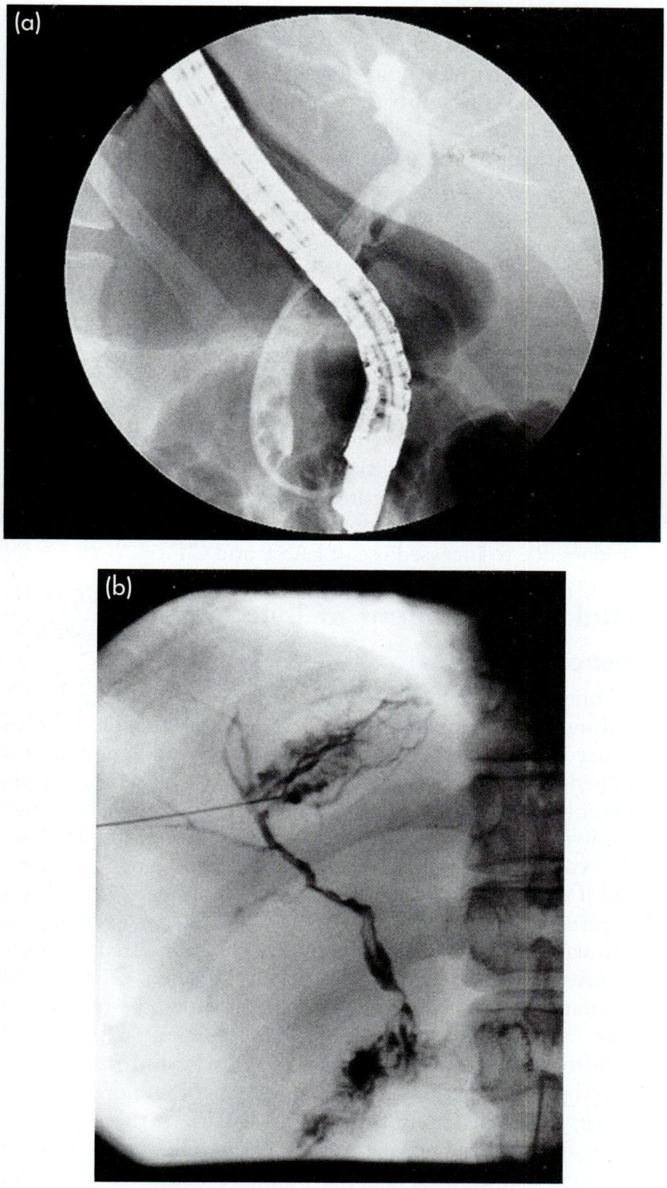

Figure 65.7 (a) Endoscopic retrograde cholangiopancreatography demonstrating the biliary tract with multiple stones in the distal common bile duct. (b) Percutaneous transhepatic cholangiography. Some contrast has extravasated at the site of hepatic puncture of the percutaneously placed needle, but the biliary tract is clearly demonstrated and shows the multiple strictures typical of primary sclerosing cholangitis.

(CBD) stones, biliary drainage in a septic patient or insertion of a biliary tract stent). A preoperative check of coagulation is essential, along with prophylactic antibiotics and an explanation of the main complications, which include pancreatitis, cholangitis and bleeding or perforation of the duodenum related to sphincterotomy.

Percutaneous transhepatic cholangiography

PTC is indicated where endoscopic cholangiography has failed or is impossible, e.g. in patients with previous pancreatoduodenectomy or Pólya gastrectomy. It is often required in patients with hilar bile duct tumours to guide external drainage of the obstructed bile ducts to relieve jaundice, evaluate resectability and to direct stent insertion (Figure 65.7b).

Angiography

Selective visceral angiography (see Figure 65.1) can provide accurate assessment of vascular involvement by tumour, but the technique is invasive. CT and MRA have evolved and their diagnostic accuracy is comparable to conventional angiography which is nowadays mostly employed for therapeutic intervention only. Therapeutic interventions include the occlusion of arteriovenous malformations, the embolisation of bleeding sites in the liver and the treatment of liver tumours (transarterial embolisation, TAE).

Nuclear medicine scanning

Radioisotope scanning can provide important diagnostic information. HIDA is a technetium-99m (^{99m}Tc)-labelled radionuclide that is administered intravenously, removed from the circulation by the liver, processed by hepatocytes and excreted in the bile. Imaging under a gamma camera allows its uptake and excretion to be monitored in real time. This is a useful non-invasive test when there is suspicion of bile leak.

18F-2-fluoro-2-deoxy-D-glucose positron emission tomography (FDG–PET) depends on the avid uptake of glucose by cancerous tissue in comparison with benign or inflammatory tissue. Deoxyglucose is labelled with the positron emitter fluorine-18 (18FDG), and this is administered to the patient prior to imaging by positron emission tomography (PET). A three-dimensional image of the whole body is obtained, highlighting areas of increased glucose metabolism (Figure 65.8). PET or

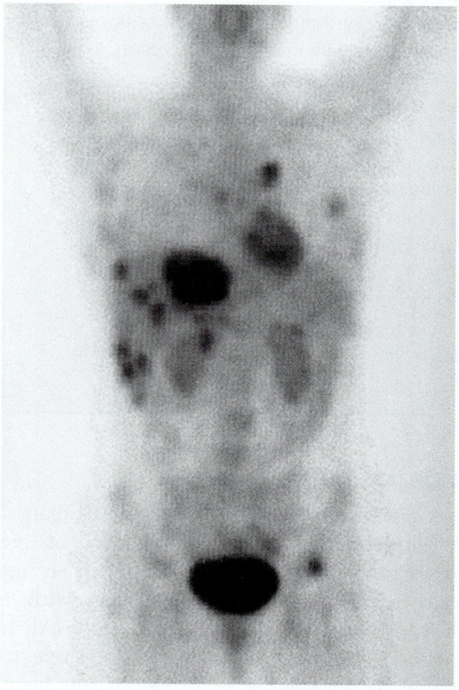

Figure 65.8 Whole-body positron emission tomography in a patient with colorectal metastases showing widespread areas of 18F-2-fluoro-2-deoxy-D-glucose uptake, indicating the sites of metastatic disease.

Eugen (Janö) Alexander Pólya, 1876–1944, surgeon, St Stephen's Hospital, Budapest, Hungary.

integrated PET-CT can be useful in the diagnosis of regional lymph node metastases and distant metastases particularly when CT and MRI findings are equivocal.

Laparoscopy

Laparoscopy is useful for the staging of hepatopancreatobiliary cancers particularly primary liver and biliary tract cancers. Lesions overlooked by conventional imaging are mainly peritoneal metastases and superficial liver tumours. These lesions can be detected at laparoscopy, thus avoiding an unnecessary laparotomy. A liver biopsy to confirm or exclude chronic liver disease can also be performed during laparoscopy.

LIVER TRAUMA

General

The liver is the second most common organ injured in abdominal trauma.

Liver trauma can be divided into blunt and penetrating injuries. Blunt injury produces contusion, laceration and avulsion injuries to the liver, often in association with splenic, mesenteric or renal injury. Penetrating injuries, such as stab and gunshot wounds, are often associated with chest or pericardial involvement (Summary box 65.7). Blunt injuries are more common and have a higher mortality than penetrating injuries.

Summary box 65.7

Management of liver trauma

- Remember associated injuries
- At-risk groups
  - Stabbing/gunshot in lower chest or upper abdomen
  - Crush injury with multiple rib fractures
- Resuscitate
  - Airway
  - Breathing
  - Circulation
- Assessment of injury
  - CT chest and abdomen with contrast
  - Laparotomy if haemodynamically unstable
- Treatment
  - Correct coagulopathy
  - Suture lacerations
  - Resect if major vascular injury
  - Packing if diffuse parenchymal injury

Diagnosis of liver injury

The liver is an extremely well-vascularised organ, and blood loss is therefore the major early complication of liver injuries. Clinical suspicion of a possible liver injury is essential, as a laparotomy by an inexperienced surgeon with inadequate preparation preoperatively is doomed to failure. All lower chest and upper abdominal stab wounds should be suspect, especially if considerable blood volume replacement has been required. Similarly, severe crushing injuries to the lower chest or upper abdomen often combine rib fractures, haemothorax and damage to the spleen and/or liver. Focused assessment sonography in trauma (FAST) performed in the emergency room by an experienced operator can reliably diagnose free intraperitoneal fluid. Patients with free intraperitoneal fluid on FAST and haemodynamic instability, and patients with a penetrating wound will require a laparotomy and/or thoracotomy once active resuscitation is under way. Owing to the opportunity for massive ongoing blood loss and the rapid development of a coagulopathy, the patient should be directly transferred to the operating theatre while blood products are obtained and volume replacement is taking place. Patients who are haemodynamically stable should have a contrast-enhanced CT scan of the chest and abdomen as the next step. This will demonstrate evidence of parenchymal damage to the liver or spleen, as well as associated traumatic injuries to their feeding vessels. Free fluid can also be clearly established. The chest scan will help to exclude injuries to the great vessels and demonstrate damage to the lung parenchyma. Additional investigations that may be of value include diagnostic peritoneal lavage, which can confirm the presence of haemoperitoneum, but this is rarely performed nowadays due to inceased use of FAST and CT.

Initial management of liver injuries

Penetrating

The initial management is maintenance of airway patency, breathing and circulation (ABC) following the principles of advanced trauma life support (ATLS). Peripheral venous access is gained with two large-bore cannulae and blood sent for crossmatch of ten units of blood, full blood count, urea and electrolytes, liver function tests, clotting screen, glucose and amylase. Initial volume replacement should be with colloid or O-negative blood if necessary. Arterial blood gases should be obtained and the patient intubated and ventilated if the gas exchange is inadequate. Intercostal chest drains should be inserted if associated pneumothorax or haemothorax is suspected. Once initial resuscitation has commenced, the patient should be transferred to the operating theatre, with further resuscitation performed on the operating table. The necessity for fresh-frozen plasma and cryoprecipitate should be discussed with the blood transfusion service immediately the patient arrives, as these patients rapidly develop irreversible coagulopathies due to a lack of fibrinogen and clotting factors. Standard coagulation profiles are inadequate to evaluate this acute loss of clotting factors, and factors should be given empirically, aided by the results of thromboelastography (TEG), if available (Figure 65.9). A contrast CT prior to laparotomy should be considered if the patient is haemodynamically stable.

Blunt trauma

With blunt injuries, the initial plan for resuscitation and management is as outlined above for penetrating injuries. Patients who are haemodynamically unstable will require an immediate laparotomy. For the patient who is haemodynamically stable, imaging by CT should be performed to further evaluate the nature of the injury. Most patients with blunt liver injury who are haemodynamically stable can be managed conservatively. The indication for discontinuing conservative treatment for blunt liver trauma would be development of haemodynamic instability, evidence of ongoing blood loss despite correction of any underlying coagulopathy and the development of signs of generalised peritonitis. Interventional radiology has an

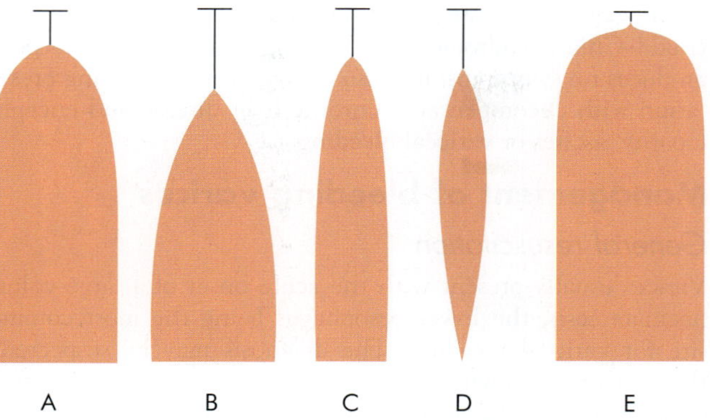

Figure 65.9 Thromboelastography (TEG). This dynamic form of assessing the coagulation status is being used increasingly for intraoperative monitoring. The shape of the TEG trace defines the nature of the underlying coagulation deficiency as shown. A, normal; B, delayed clot formation; C, reduced clot strength; D, clot lysis; E, hypercoagulable.

important role in management of liver trauma and embolisation to control hepatic artery bleeding is safe and effective in a stable patient with no evidence of hollow viscus perforation.

The surgical approach to liver trauma

Good access is vital. A 'rooftop' incision with midline extension to the xiphisternum and retraction of the costal margins gives excellent access to the liver and spleen. If the laparotomy has been started through a midline incision, a transverse lateral extension to the right can be added to improve access to the liver. Compression of the liver with packs and correction of coagulopathy, if present, will control most of the active bleeding. If bleeding persists, further control can be achieved by vascular inflow occlusion by placing an atraumatic clamp across the foramen of Winslow (the Pringle manoeuvre). A stab incision in the liver can be sutured with a fine absorbable monofilament suture. Lacerations to the hepatic artery should be identified and repaired with 6/0 Prolene suture. If unavoidable, the hepatic artery may be ligated, although parenchymal necrosis and abscess formation will result in some individuals. Portal vein injuries should be repaired with 5/0 Prolene. Inflow occlusion facilitates suturing of lacerations and vessels.

If bleeding persists despite inflow occlusion, consider major hepatic vein or IVC injuries, and also look for abberant arteries to the liver. Deceleration injuries often produce lacerations of the liver parenchyma adjacent to the anchoring ligaments of the liver. These may be amenable to suture with an absorbable monofilament suture. Again, inflow occlusion may facilitate this suturing and, if necessary, the sutures can be buttressed to prevent them cutting through the liver parenchyma. With more severe deceleration injuries, a portion of the liver may be avulsed. These injuries are more complex as they are associated with a devitalised portion of the liver and, often, major injuries to the hepatic veins and IVC. Diffuse parenchymal injuries should be treated by packing the liver to produce haemostasis. This is effective for the majority of liver injuries if the liver is packed against the natural contour of the diaphragm by packing from below. Large abdominal packs should be used to ease their removal, and the abdomen closed to facilitate compression of the parenchyma. Care should be taken to avoid overzealous packing, as this may produce pressure necrosis of the liver parenchyma or abdominal compartment syndrome.

James Hogarth Pringle, 1863–1941, surgeon, The Royal Infirmary, Glasgow, UK. Born in Australia and trained in Edinburgh, he was a strong supporter of women in medicine; he performed the first successful autologous vein graft in the UK and the first excision and block dissection for malignant melanoma. He and his father, George Hogarth Pringle (1830 –1872, who practised in Australia), formed a famous team of surgical innovators.

Crush injuries to the liver often result in large parenchymal haematomas and diffuse capsular lacerations. Suturing is usually ineffective, and perihepatic packing which involves placing packs above, behind and below the liver, is the most useful method of providing haemostasis. Necrotic tissue should be removed, but poorly perfused, though viable, liver left *in situ*. If packing is necessary, the patient should have the packs removed after 48 hours, and usually no further surgical intervention is required. Antibiotic cover is advisable, and full reversal of any coagulopathy is essential. If a major liver vascular injury is suspected at the time of the initial laparotomy, then referral to a specialist centre should be considered. A common surgical approach in these circumstances would be to place the patient on venovenous bypass using cannulae in the femoral vein via a long saphenous cut-down with the blood returned, using a roller pump, to the superior vena cava (SVC) via an internal jugular line. Venovenous bypass allows the IVC to be safely clamped to facilitate caval or hepatic vein repair. A rapid infuser blood transfusion machine facilitates the delivery of large volumes of blood instantaneously. Once prepared, the patient is relaparotomised via the rooftop incision with a midline extension to the xiphisternum. The liver is mobilised by division of the supporting ligaments, and complete vascular isolation of the liver is achieved by occluding the hilar inflow and the IVC above the renal veins and at the level of the diaphragm with atraumatic vascular clamps. Venous return is provided by the venovenous bypass. Warm ischaemia of the liver is tolerated for up to 45 minutes, allowing sufficient time in a blood-free field for repair of injuries to the IVC or hepatic veins.

Other complications of liver trauma

A subcapsular or intrahepatic haematoma requires no specific intervention and should be allowed to resolve spontaneously. Abscesses may form as a result of secondary infection of an area of parenchymal ischaemia, especially after penetrating trauma. Treatment is with systemic antibiotics and aspiration under ultrasound guidance once the necrotic tissue has liquefied. Bile collections require aspiration under ultrasound guidance or percutaneous insertion of a pigtail drain. The site of origin of a biliary fistula should be determined by endoscopic or percutaneous cholangiography, and biliary decompression achieved by nasobiliary or percutaneous transhepatic drainage or endoprosthesis insertion. If this fails to control the fistula, the affected portion of the liver may require resection. Late vascular complications include hepatic artery aneurysm and arteriovenous or arteriobiliary fistulae (Figure 65.10). These are best treated nonsurgically by a specialist hepatobiliary interventional radiologist. The feeding vessel can be embolised transarterially.

Hepatic failure may occur following extensive liver trauma. This will usually reverse with conservative supportive treatment if the blood supply and biliary drainage of the liver are intact (Summary box 65.8).

Jacob Benignus Winslow, 1669–1760, Professor of Anatomy, Physic and Surgery, Paris, France.

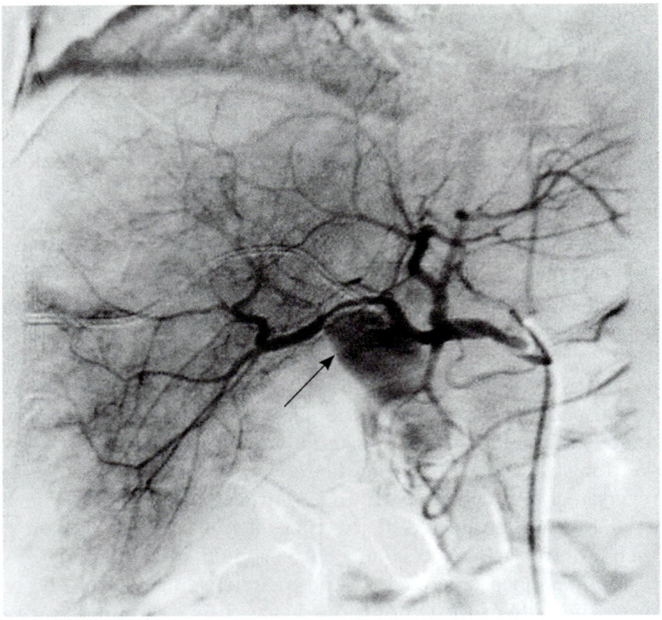

Figure 65.10 Hepatic aneurysm following liver trauma. An aneurysm arising from the right hepatic artery (arrow), which can be optimally treated by the interventional radiologist using transarterial embolisation.

Summary box 65.8

Other complications of liver trauma

- Intrahepatic haematoma
- Liver abscess
- Bile collection
- Biliary fistula
- Hepatic artery aneurysm
- Arteriovenous fistula
- Arteriobiliary fistula
- Liver failure

Long-term outcome of liver trauma

The capacity of the liver to recover from extensive trauma is remarkable, and parenchymal regeneration occurs rapidly. Late complications are rare, but the development of biliary tract strictures many years after recovery from liver trauma has been reported. The treatment depends on the mode of presentation and the extent and site of stricturing. A segmental or lobar stricture, associated with atrophy of the corresponding area of liver parenchyma and compensatory hypertrophy of the other liver lobe, may be treated expectantly. A dominant extrahepatic bile duct stricture associated with obstructive jaundice may be treated initially with endobiliary balloon dilatation or stenting, but will usually require surgical correction using a Roux-en-Y hepatodochojejunostomy.

PORTAL HYPERTENSION

An elevation in portal pressure is most commonly found in the presence of liver cirrhosis, although it may be present in patients with extrahepatic portal vein occlusion, intrahepatic veno-occlusive disease or occlusion of the main hepatic veins (Budd–Chiari syndrome (BCS)). As portal hypertension per se produces no symptoms, it is usually diagnosed following presentation with decompensated chronic liver disease and encephalopathy, ascites or variceal bleeding.

Management of bleeding varices

General resuscitation

Varices usually present with the acute onset of a large-volume haematemesis, the lower oesophagus being the most common site for variceal bleeding. The diagnosis may be suspected if the patient is known to have liver cirrhosis, but it needs to be confirmed following initial resuscitation of the patient. Variceal haemorrhage is a medical emergency. Patients with massive haemorrhage should be admitted to the intensive treatment unit (ITU). Venous access should be obtained through two large bore peripheral cannulae. Colloids should be administered while adequate blood is obtained (initially ten units). Liver function tests will reveal underlying liver disease, and a coagulation profile will reveal any underlying coagulopathy. Blood volume should be replaced with colloids, plasma expanders and blood transfusions. Hypervolaemia should be avoided since this may increase portal pressure and exacerbate the bleeding. Vitamin K is administered (10 mg intravenously (i.v.)), but correction of a coagulopathy will require the administration of fresh-frozen plasma (FFP). An associated thrombocytopenia is usually secondary to hypersplenism due to cirrhosis and is treated if the platelet count falls below 50×10^9/L. Treatment with a splanchnic vasoconstrictor should be started. Administration of a prophylactic antibiotic is recommended to prevent or treat associated bacterial infection. As soon as the patient is haemodynamically stabilised an upper gastrointestinal endoscopy should be performed to establish the diagnosis because 50 per cent of patients with portal hypertension will have a non-variceal source of bleeding. Variceal bleeding is often associated with hepatic encephalopathy and, in these circumstances and when bleeding is severe, endotracheal intubation will be required for endoscopy. Bronchial aspiration is a frequent complication of variceal bleeding (Summary box 65.9).

Summary box 65.9

Management of bleeding oesophageal varices

- Blood transfusion
- Correct coagulopathy
- Oesophageal balloon tamponade (Sengstaken–Blakemore tube)
- Drug therapy (vasopressin/octreotide)
- Endoscopic sclerotherapy or banding
- Assess portal vein patency (Doppler ultrasound or CT)
- Transjugular intrahepatic portosystemic stent shunts (TIPSS)
- Surgery
    - Portosystemic shunts
    - Oesophageal transection
    - Splenectomy and gastric devascularisation

If the rate of blood loss prohibits endoscopic evaluation, a Sengstaken–Blakemore tube may be inserted to provide temporary haemostasis. This is shown diagrammatically in Figure 65.11. Once inserted, the gastric balloon is inflated with 300 mL

Robert William Sengstaken, born 1923, surgeon, Garden City, New York, NY, USA.
Arthur Hendley Blakemore, Associate Professor of Surgery, The Columbia College of Physicians and Surgeons, New York, NY, USA.

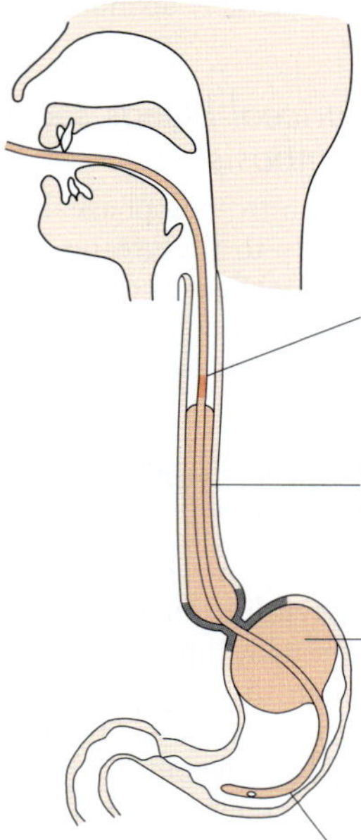

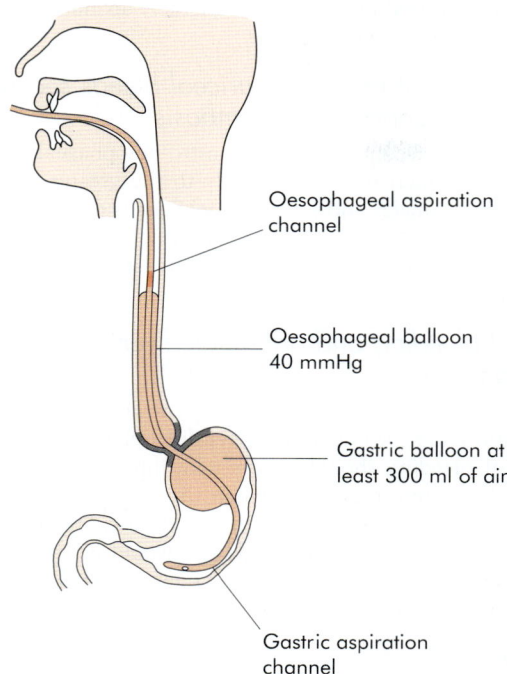

Figure 65.11 Oesophageal balloon tamponade.

of air and retracted to the gastric fundus, where the varices at the oesophagogastric junction are tamponaded by the subsequent inflation of the oesophageal balloon to a pressure of 40 mmHg. The two remaining channels allow gastric and oesophageal aspiration. An x-ray is used to confirm the position of the tube. The balloons should be temporarily deflated after 12 hours to prevent pressure necrosis of the oesophagus. Aspiration pneumonia and oesophageal ulceration are other complications. Balloon tamponade is very effective in stopping bleeding and once the patient is stabilised, a more definitive treatment can be carried out.

Drug treatment for variceal bleeding

Splanchnic vasoconstrictors reduce portal flow and pressure and should be started early in the treatment of variceal haemorrhage. Vasopressin is a potent vasocontrictor and has been the most extensively used drug for the initial control of variceal haemorrhage, but it can cause myocardial ischaemia, arrhythmias, mesenteric and limb ischaemia. Terlipressin, somatostatin and octreotide are safer than vasopressin and equally effective.

Endoscopic treatment of varices

Treatment with a vasoconstrictor (see above) combined with endoscopic therapy is the standard medical treatment for acute variceal bleeding. The two most commonly used endoscopic techniques are endoscopic band ligation which involves placing a constricting rubber band at the base of the varix, and endoscopic sclerotherapy which involves injection of a sclerosant, such as polidocanol (1–3 per cent) or ethanolamine (5 per cent), into or around the varix. Although both are effective in controlling the bleed, banding is significantly better in preventing rebleeding and is the preferred option. The majority of variceal bleeds will respond to a single course.

Transjugular intrahepatic portosystemic stent shunts

The emergency management of variceal haemorrhage has been revolutionised by the introduction of transjugular intrahepatic portosystemic stent shunts (TIPSS) in 1988. Over a short period, it has become the main treatment of variceal haemorrhage that has not responded to drug treatment and endoscopic therapy. The shunts are inserted under local anaesthetic, analgesia and sedation using fluoroscopic guidance and ultrasonography. Via the internal jugular vein and SVC, a guidewire is inserted into a hepatic vein and through the hepatic parenchyma into a branch of the portal vein. The track through the parenchyma is then dilated with a balloon catheter to allow insertion of a metallic stent, which is expanded once a satisfactory position is achieved (Figure 65.12) to form a channel between systemic and portal venous systems. A satisfactory drop in portal venous pressure is usually associated with good control of the variceal haemorrhage. The main early complication of this technique is perforation of the liver capsule, which can be associated with fatal intraperitoneal haemorrhage. TIPSS occlusion may result in further variceal haemorrhage and occurs more commonly in patients with well-compensated liver disease and good synthetic function. Post-shunt encephalopathy is the confusional state caused by the portal blood bypassing the detoxification of the liver. It occurs in about 40 per cent of patients, a similar incidence to that found after surgical shunts. If severe, the lumen of the TIPSS can be reduced by insertion of a smaller stent. The

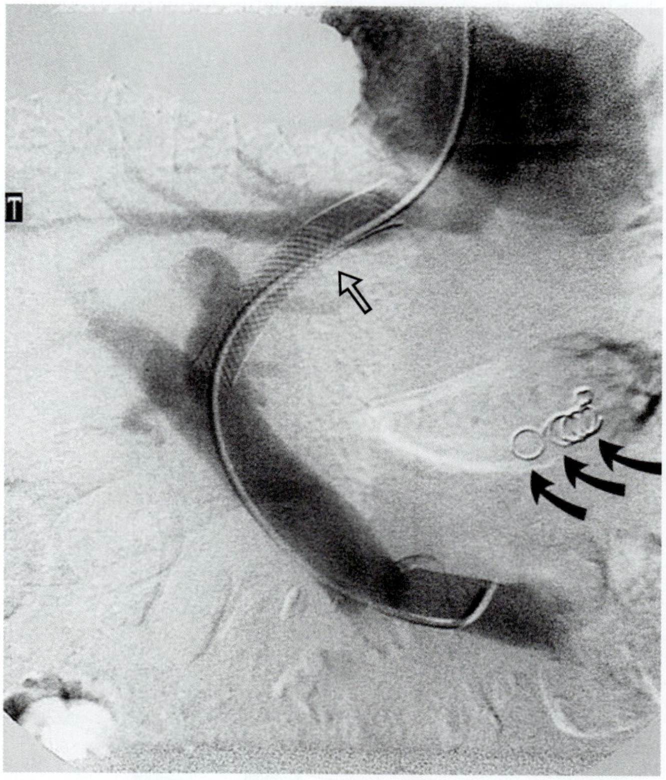

Figure 65.12 A check angiogram following insertion of a transjugular intrahepatic portosystemic stent shunt (open arrow). Injection of contrast into the portal vein flows through the metallic stent and outlines the right hepatic vein. Pressure measurements are taken from within the portal vein before and after insertion. Solid arrows indicate coils placed at the site of previous embolisation.

main contraindication to TIPSS is portal vein occlusion. The main long-term complication of TIPSS is stenosis of the shunt, which is common (approximately 50 per cent at one year) and may present as further variceal haemorrhage.

Surgical shunts for variceal haemorrhage

The increasing availability of liver transplantation and TIPSS has greatly reduced the indications for surgical shunts. It is rarely considered for the acute management of variceal haemorrhage, as the morbidity and mortality in these circumstances are high. The main current indication for a surgical shunt is a patient with Child's grade A cirrhosis, in whom the initial bleed has been controlled by sclerotherapy. Long-term β-blocker therapy and chronic sclerotherapy or banding are the main alternatives.

Surgical shunts are an effective method of preventing rebleeding from oesophageal or gastric varices, as they reduce the pressure in the portal circulation by diverting the blood into the low-pressure systemic circulation. Shunts may be divided into selective (e.g. splenorenal) and non-selective (e.g. portocaval), the former attempting to preserve blood flow to the liver while decompressing the left side of the portal circulation responsible for giving rise to the oesophageal and gastric varices. Selective shunts may be associated with a lower incidence of portal systemic encephalopathy (PSE), a confusional state commonly found in patients with chronic liver disease who have undergone radiological or surgical portosystemic shunts. The different types of surgical shunt are shown in Figure 65.13. There is no evidence that prophylactic shunting is beneficial in patients with varices that have not bled.

Oesophageal stapled transection

This technique for the management of bleeding oesophageal varices uses the circular stapling device for stapling and resecting a doughnut ring of the lower oesophagus. As with surgical shunts in the acute situation, it was associated with a high perioperative mortality and has been largely abandoned in centres where TIPSS is available.

Management of recurrent variceal bleeds secondary to splenic or portal vein thrombosis

Treatment is by splenectomy and gastro-oesophageal devascularisation, in which the blood supply to the greater and lesser curve of the stomach and lower oesophagus is divided. Splenic vein thrombosis may be seen secondary to chronic pancreatitis, and portal vein thrombosis is a common late complication of liver cirrhosis.

Variceal bleeding and orthotopic liver transplantation

Liver transplantation is the only therapy which will treat portal hypertension and the underlying liver disease. The management of variceal bleeding should always take into account the possibility of liver transplantation when this is available. Previous surgical shunts greatly increase the morbidity associated with orthotopic liver transplantation. TIPSS would be the preferred management for bleeds resistant to sclerotherapy, as long as placement is optimal.

Ascites

The accumulation of free peritoneal fluid is a common feature of advanced liver disease independent of the aetiology. The fluid accumulation is usually associated with abdominal discomfort and a dragging sensation. Development is usually insidious. The aetiology of the ascites must be established (Summary box 65.10).

Imaging by CT will confirm the ascites and demonstrate the irregular and shrunken nature of a cirrhotic liver and associated splenomegaly. Intravenous contrast enhancement will allow abdominal varices to be demonstrated and assess patency of the portal vein, as portal vein thrombosis is a common predisposing

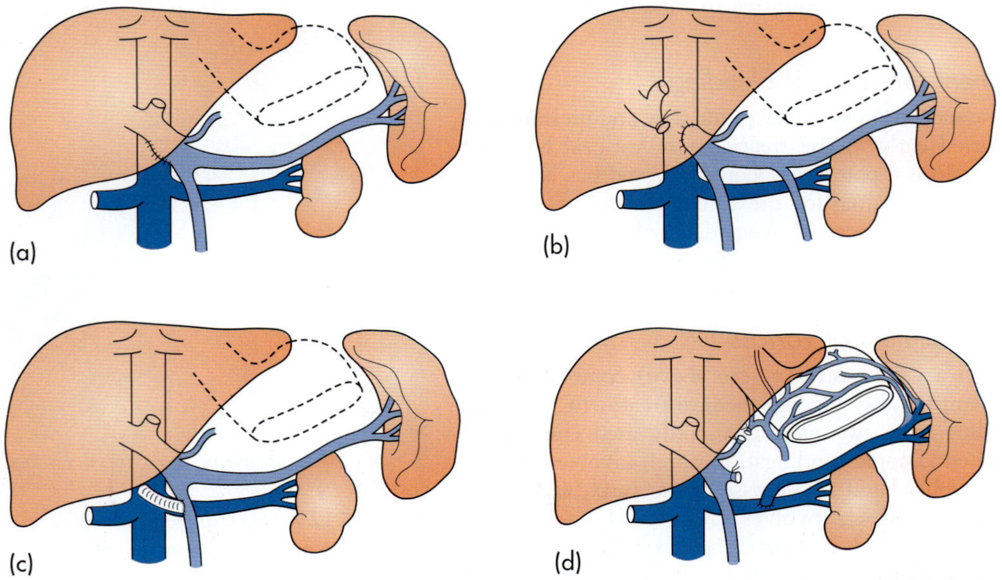

Figure 65.13 (a–d) Surgical shunts. Surgical shunts for portal hypertension involve shunting portal blood into the systemic veins. This commonly involves a side-to-side portocaval anastomosis (a) or end-to-side portocaval (b), mesocaval (c) or splenorenal (d) anastomoses.

Summary box 65.10

Determining the cause of ascites

- Imaging (ultrasound or CT)
  - Irregular cirrhotic liver
  - Portal vein patency
  - Splenomegaly of cirrhosis
- Aspiration
  - Culture and microscopy
  - Protein content
  - Cytology
  - Amylase level

factor to the development of ascites in chronic liver disease. In patients without evidence of liver disease, malignancy is a common cause, and the primary site may also be established on CT. Aspiration of the peritoneal fluid allows the measurement of protein content to determine whether the fluid is an exudate or transudate, and an amylase estimation to exclude pancreatic ascites. Cytology will determine the presence of cancerous cells, and both microscopy and culture will exclude primary bacterial peritonitis and tuberculous peritonitis.

Treatment of ascites in chronic liver disease

The initial treatment is to restrict additional salt intake and commence diuretics using either spironolactone or furosemide. This should be combined with advice on avoiding any precipitating factors for impaired liver function, such as alcohol intake in patients with alcoholic cirrhosis. Patients on diuretics should be monitored for the development of hyponatraemia and hypokalaemia (Summary box 65.11).

Summary box 65.11

Treatment of ascites in chronic liver disease

- Salt restriction
- Diuretics
- Abdominal paracentesis
- Peritoneovenous shunting
- Transjugular intrahepatic portosystemic stent shunts (TIPSS)
- Liver transplantation

Abdominal paracentesis

Patients who fail to respond to diuretic treatment may require repeated percutaneous aspiration of large volume of the ascites (abdominal paracentesis), combined with volume replacement using salt-poor or standard human albumin solution, dependent on the serum sodium level. Paracentesis provides only short-term symptomatic relief.

Peritoneovenous shunting

The LeVeen shunt is designed for the relief of ascites due to chronic liver disease. One end of the silastic tube is inserted into the ascites within the peritoneal cavity and the other end is tunnelled subcutaneously to the neck, where it is inserted under direct vision into the internal jugular vein and fed into the SVC. Owing to a one-way valve within the tubing, peritoneal fluid is drawn from the abdomen and drained to the circulation due to the lower pressure in the SVC in comparison with the abdomen during the respiratory cycle. Complications include occlusion, displacement, infection and disseminated intravascular coagulation. In an attempt to prevent the high occlusion rate, a further development was the insertion of a chamber placed over the costal margin to allow digital pressure and evacuation of any debris within the peritoneovenous shunt (Denver shunt). Peritovenous shunts are rarely performed nowadays.

TIPSS for ascites

The use of TIPSS for ascites is for symptomatic relief. In patients with intractable ascites, TIPSS is a good alternative to repeated paracentesis, but post-stent encephalopathy is common (about 40 per cent), and the majority of stents will stenose on follow up (approximately 50 per cent by one year).

Liver transplantation for ascites

Diuretic-resistant ascites is an indication for liver transplantation if associated with deterioration in liver function (rising bilirubin, dropping albumin, prolonged prothrombin time). The patient's age, underlying aetiology of liver disease and associated medical problems will be the major factors determining suitability for liver transplantation. In those considered inappropriate for liver transplantation, management is aimed at symptomatic control of ascites.

CHRONIC LIVER CONDITIONS

There are several chronic liver conditions, which, although rare, are important to recognise because they require a specific plan for investigation and treatment, and may present mimicking a more common clinical condition (Table 65.4).

Table 65.4 Important chronic liver conditions.

Condition	Common presentations
Budd–Chiari syndrome	Ascites
Primary sclerosing cholangitis (PSC)	Abnormal LFTs or jaundice
Primary biliary cirrhosis (PBC)	Malaise, lethargy, itching, abnormal LFTs
Caroli's disease	Abdominal pain, sepsis
Simple liver cysts	Coincidental finding, pain
Polycystic liver disease	Hepatomegaly, pain

LFTs, liver function tests.

Budd–Chiari syndrome

This is a condition principally affecting young females, in which the venous drainage of the liver is occluded by hepatic venous thrombosis or obstruction from a venous web. As a result of venous outflow obstruction, the liver becomes acutely congested, with the development of impaired liver function and, subsequently, portal hypertension, ascites and oesophageal varices. In an acute thrombosis, the patient may rapidly progress

Harry H LeVeen, 1914–1996, Professor of Surgery, The University of South Carolina, SC, USA, devised his shunt in the 1970s.

to fulminant liver failure but, in the majority of cases, abdominal discomfort and ascites are the main presenting features. If chronic, the liver progresses to established cirrhosis. The cause of the venous thrombosis needs to be established, and an underlying myeloproliferative disorder or procoagulant state is commonly found, such as anti-thrombin 3, protein C or protein S deficiency. The diagnosis is commonly suspected in a patient presenting with ascites, in whom a CT scan shows a large congested liver (early stage, Figure 65.14) or a small cirrhotic liver in which there is gross enlargement of segment I (the caudate lobe). This feature results from preservation and hypertrophy of the segment with direct venous drainage to the IVC in the face of atrophy of the rest of the liver due to venous obstruction (Figure 65.15). IVC compression or occlusion from the segment I hypertrophy is also a common feature, as is thrombosis of the portal vein. Confirmation of the suspected diagnosis is by hepatic venography via a transjugular approach, which demonstrates occlusion of the hepatic veins and may allow a transjugular biopsy.

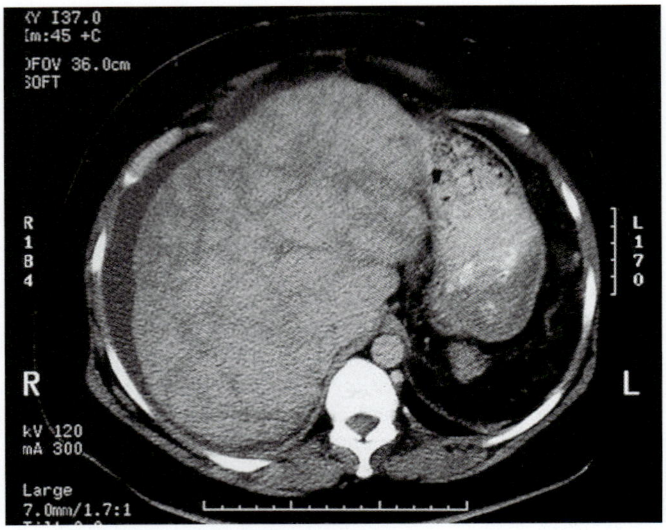

Figure 65.14 Computed tomography scan in early Budd–Chiari syndrome.

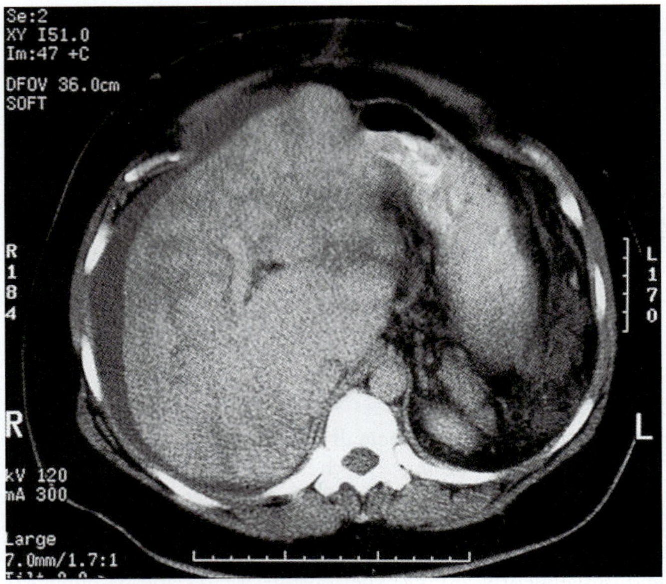

Figure 65.15 Segment I hypertrophy with Budd–Chiari syndrome.

Treatment of BCS must be tailored to the individual patient and, in particular, to the stage of disease at presentation. Patients presenting in fulminant liver failure should be considered for liver transplantation, as should those with established cirrhosis and the complications of portal hypertension. Those in whom cirrhosis is not established may be considered for portosystemic shunting by TIPSS, portocaval shunt or mesoatrial shunting. IVC compression may be relieved by the insertion of a retrohepatic expandable metallic stent. If the BCS is treated satisfactorily, the prognosis of this patient group is largely dependent on the underlying aetiology and whether this is amenable to treatment. Patients are usually left on lifelong anticoagulation with warfarin.

Primary sclerosing cholangitis

This condition often presents in young adults with mild nonspecific symptoms, and biliary disease is suggested by the finding of abnormal liver function tests. Rarely, the first presentation is with jaundice due to biliary obstruction. The disease process results in progressive fibrous stricturing and obliteration of both the intrahepatic and the extrahepatic bile ducts. Although the aetiology is unknown, a genetic predisposition is likely owing to its association with ulcerative colitis (UC). In patients with primary sclerosing cholangitis (PSC) and UC, the condition usually progresses even if the diseased colon is removed. The diagnosis is principally based on the findings at cholangiography, in which irregular, narrowed bile ducts are demonstrated in both the intrahepatic and the extrahepatic biliary tree (Figure 65.16). If the radiological appearances are equivocal, a liver biopsy is required to demonstrate the fibrous obliteration of the biliary tracts. There is no specific treatment that can reverse the ductal changes, and the patients usually slowly progress to progressive cholestasis and death from liver failure. There is a strong predisposition to cholangiocarcinoma (CCA), and this should be considered in any patient with PSC in whom a new or dominant stricture is demonstrated on cholangiography.

Diagnosis of CCA in PSC is greatly facilitated by biliary brush cytology, as imaging rarely shows evidence of a mass lesion even in patients with advanced CCA. Further, imaging cannot reliably differentiate between inflammatory and malignant biliary strictures. Serum CA 19-9 level may be increased but the sensitivity of CA 19-9 in detecting CCA in PSC is approximately 60 per cent. Patients with good liver function, no dominant strictures and negative biliary cytology may simply be monitored for disease progression. The only useful treatment modality is liver transplantation, which is associated with excellent results if carried out before bile duct cancer has developed. Temporary relief of obstructive jaundice due to a dominant bile duct stricture can be achieved by biliary stenting, although there is considerable risk of cholangitis from the introduction of bacteria to the biliary tract.

Primary biliary cirrhosis

As with PSC, the presentation of patients with primary biliary cirrhosis (PBC) is often hidden, with general malaise, lethargy and pruritus prior to the development of clinical jaundice or the finding of abnormal liver function tests. The condition is largely confined to females. Diagnosis is suggested by the finding

George Budd, 1808–1882, Professor of Medicine, King's College Hospital, London, UK, described this syndrome in 1845.
Hans Chiari, 1851–1916, Professor of Pathological Anatomy, Strasbourg, Germany (Strasbourg was returned to France after the end of the First World War in 1918) gave his account of this condition in 1898.

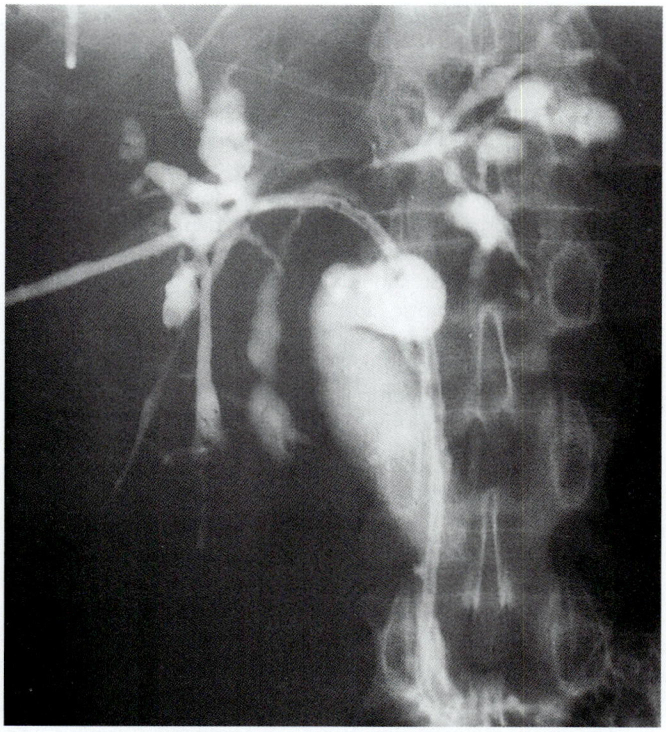

Figure 65.16 Primary sclerosing cholangitis (PSC). Percutaneous cholangiography showing the characteristic extensive bile duct strictures and dilatations associated with PSC.

of circulating anti-smooth muscle antibodies and, if necessary, is confirmed by liver biopsy. The condition is slowly progressive, with deterioration in liver function resulting in lethargy and malaise. It may be complicated by the development of portal hypertension and the secondary complications of ascites and variceal bleeding. The mainstay of treatment is liver transplantation, which should be considered when the patient's general condition starts to deteriorate with inability to lead a normal lifestyle.

Caroli's disease

This is congenital dilatation of the intrahepatic biliary tree, which is often complicated by the presence of intrahepatic stone formation. Presentation may be with abdominal pain or sepsis. Imaging is usually diagnostic, with the finding on ultrasound or CT of intrahepatic biliary lakes containing stones. Biliary stasis and stone formation combine to predispose to biliary sepsis, which may be life-threatening. Another well-recognised complication is the development of carcinoma. No specific treatment is available. Acute infective episodes are treated with antibiotics. Obstructed and septic bile ducts may be drained either radiologically or surgically. Malignant change within the ductal system results in cholangiocarcinoma, which may be amenable to resection. Segmental involvement of the liver by Caroli's disease may be treated by resection of the affected part, although the ductal dilatation is usually diffuse. Liver transplantation is a radical but definitive treatment.

Simple cystic disease

Liver cysts are a common coincidental finding in patients undergoing abdominal ultrasound. Radiological findings to suggest that a cyst is simple are that it is regular, thin walled and unilocular, with no surrounding tissue response and no variation in density within the cyst cavity. If these criteria are confirmed and the cyst is asymptomatic, no further tests or treatment are required. Large cysts may be associated with symptoms of abdominal discomfort possibly related to stretching of the overlying liver capsule, acute pain associated with haemorrhage in the cyst, or may present as right upper quadrant abdominal mass. Aspiration of the cyst contents under radiological guidance provides a sample for culture, microscopy and cytology, and allows the symptomatic response to cyst drainage to be assessed. Aspiration alone is usually associated with cyst and symptom recurrence, in which case more definitive treatment is required. Laparoscopic deroofing is the treatment of choice for large symptomatic cysts and is associated with good long-term symptomatic relief.

Polycystic liver disease

This is a congenital abnormality associated with cyst formation within the liver and often other abdominal organs, principally the pancreas and kidney. Those associated with renal cysts may have autosomal dominant inheritance. The cysts are often asymptomatic and incidental findings on ultrasound. They usually have no effect on organ function and require no specific treatment. Massive polycystic disease of the liver is rare, but can give rise to discomfort or pain. This often responds to treatment with simple analgesics. Severe pain often indicates haemorrhage into a cyst, which may be confirmed by ultrasound or CT scan. Cyst discomfort that is not adequately controlled by oral analgesics may be treated by open or laparoscopic fenestration of the liver cysts, although the results are less favourable than with simple cysts. Ultimately, massive polycystic liver disease may require liver transplantation.

LIVER INFECTIONS

Viral hepatitis

Viral hepatitis is a major world health problem. In addition to the well-recognised acute and chronic liver diseases produced by hepatitis A, B and C, other hepatitis viruses have been isolated, including hepatitis D, which is usually detected only in patients with hepatitis B virus (HBV) infection, and hepatitis E, which produces a self-limiting hepatitis due to faeco-oral spread similar to hepatitis A (Table 65.5).

Hepatitis A presents with anorexia, weakness and general malaise for several weeks prior to the development of clinical jaundice, often accompanied by tenderness on palpation of an enlarged liver. The condition is spread by the faeco-oral route and often spreads rapidly in closed communities. Liver function tests will be compatible with an acute hepatitis, with elevation of bilirubin and transaminases. Diagnosis is confirmed by the antibody titre to hepatitis A. The condition is virtually always self-resolving, although rarely the viral hepatitis can lead to fulminant liver failure. Once the clinical condition resolves, the liver tends to recover fully, with no functional deficit and no long-term sequelae.

Hepatitis B is a more serious condition in most respects than hepatitis A. Although it can also produce an acute self-resolving hepatitis, the virus is often not cleared and produces chronic hepatitis B causing long-term liver damage, with the

Jacques Caroli, 1902–1979, Professor of Medicine, St Antoine Hospital, Paris, France, described the disease in 1958.

Table 65.5 Liver infections and their treatment.

Condition	Causative agent	Treatment
Viral hepatitis	Hepatitis A, B, C	Supportive, anti-viral agents (lamivudine, interferon, ribavirin)
		Liver transplant for cirrhosis
Ascending cholangitis	Enteric bacteria	Antibiotics (cephalosporin)
	Relieve obstruction	
Pyogenic liver abscess	*Streptococcus milleri*	Antibiotics
	Escherichia coli	Aspiration
	Streptococcus faecalis	Drainage
Amoebic liver abscess	Entamoeba	Metronidazole
Hydatid liver disease	Echinococcus	Mebendazole
		Resection/omentoplasty

development of liver cirrhosis and hepatocellular carcinoma. Therefore, patients may present acutely with malaise, anorexia, abdominal pain and clinical jaundice due to active hepatitis, or at a late stage owing to the complications of cirrhosis, most commonly ascites or variceal bleeding. Treatment for acute hepatitis is antivirals and supportive. In patients with cirrhosis, treatment is initially dictated by the specific complication at presentation (see above under Treatment of ascites in chronic liver disease). In established cirrhosis, liver transplantation may be considered if viral eradication or suppression can be achieved with anti-viral agents (e.g. lamivudine). Without viral suppression, death from reinfection of the transplanted liver is common. The hepatitis virus greatly increases the risk of primary liver cancer, which usually appears at the stage when the liver parenchyma has become cirrhotic. The assessment and management of HBV cirrhosis with hepatocellular carcinoma (HCC) is discussed below under Liver tumours.

Hepatitis C has become one of the most common causes of chronic liver disease worldwide and, in many countries, a large percentage of the population has been exposed; 1 per cent of potential blood donors worldwide are hepatitis C virus (HCV) positive. Transmission is often related back to blood transfusion, and routine screening of blood for HCV has only recently been introduced in many countries. Chronic HCV infection is an important health problem because currently there is no vaccine available to prevent the disease and current anti-viral treatment has limitations. As with hepatitis B, it may present as an acute hepatitis or progress to chronic hepatitis which may lead to development of liver cirrhosis and hepatocellular carcinoma. Chronic hepatitis C infection can remain hidden until the development of cirrhosis and the complications of portal hypertension or until development of hepatocellular carcinoma. Acute hepatitis C progresses to chronic infection and cirrhosis in about 20 per cent of cases. Decompensation of cirrhosis suggested by deterioration in liver function, encephalopathy, ascites or bleeding in a patient with known HCV cirrhosis necessitates an urgent assessment for liver transplantation, if available. Reinfection of the graft with HCV after liver transplantation occurs in almost all patients.

Ascending cholangitis

Ascending bacterial infection of the biliary tract is usually associated with obstruction and presents with clinical jaundice, rigors and a tender hepatomegaly. The diagnosis is confirmed by the finding of dilated bile ducts on ultrasound, an obstructive picture of liver function tests and the isolation of an organism from the blood on culture. The condition is a medical emergency, and delay in appropriate treatment results in organ failure secondary to septicaemia. Once the diagnosis has been confirmed, the patient should be commenced on a first-line broad-spectrum antibiotic and rehydrated, and arrangements should be made for urgent endoscopic or percutaneous transhepatic drainage of the biliary tree. Biliary stone disease is a common predisposing factor, and the causative ductal stones may be removed at the time of endoscopic cholangiography by endoscopic sphincterotomy.

Pyogenic liver abscess

The aetiology of a pyogenic liver abscess is unexplained in the majority of patients. It has an increased incidence in the elderly, diabetics and the immunosuppressed, who usually present with anorexia, fevers and malaise, accompanied by right upper quadrant discomfort. The diagnosis is suggested by the finding of a multiloculated cystic mass on ultrasound or CT scan (Figure 65.17) and is confirmed by aspiration for culture and sensitivity. The most common organisms are *Streptococcus milleri* and *Escherichia coli*, but other enteric organisms such as *S. faecalis*, *Klebsiella* and *Proteus vulgaris* also occur, and mixed growths are common. Opportunistic pathogens include staphylococci. Treatment is with antibiotics and ultrasound-guided aspiration. First-line antibiotics to be used are a penicillin, aminoglycoside and metronidazole or a cephalosporin and metronidazole. Often, repeated aspirations may be necessary. Percutaneous drainage without ultrasound guidance should be avoided as an empyema may follow drainage through the pleural space. A source for the liver abscess should be sought, particularly from the colon. Atypical clinical or radiological findings should raise the possibility of a necrotic neoplasm.

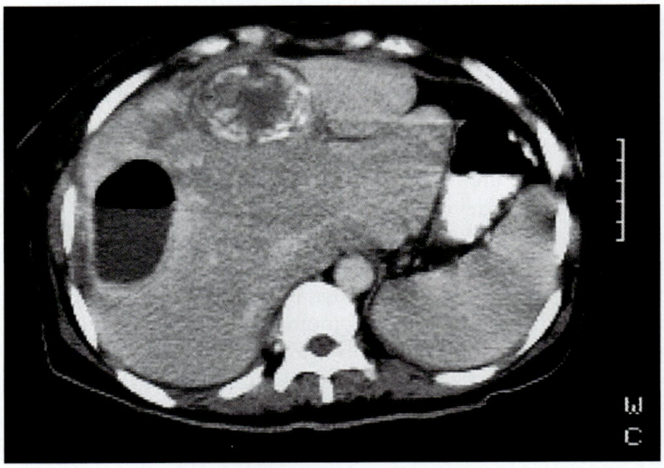

Figure 65.17 Liver abscess. Computed tomography scan showing an air–fluid level and rim enhancement with intravenous contrast typical of a liver abscess. In the adjacent liver is a calcified hydatid cyst.

Amoebic liver abscess

Entamoeba histolytica is endemic in many parts of the world. It exists in vegetative form outside the body and is spread by the faeco-oral route. The most common presentation is with dysentery, but it may also present with an amoebic abscess, the common sites being paracaecal and in the liver. The amoebic cyst is ingested and develops into the trophozoite form in the colon, and then passes through the bowel wall and to the liver via the portal blood. Diagnosis is by isolation of the parasite from the liver lesion or the stool and confirming its nature by microscopy. Often patients with clinical signs of an amoebic abscess will be treated empirically with metronidazole (400–800 mg, three times a day, for 7–10 days) and investigated further only if they do not respond. Resolution of the abscess can be monitored using ultrasound.

Hydatid liver disease

This is a very common condition in countries around the Mediterranean. The causative tapeworm, *Echinococcus granulosus*, is present in the dog intestine, and ova are ingested by humans and pass in the portal blood to the liver. Liver abscesses are often large by the time of presentation with upper abdominal discomfort or may present after minor abdominal trauma as an acute abdomen due to rupture of the cyst into the peritoneal cavity. Diagnosis is suggested by the finding of a multiloculated cyst on ultrasound and is further supported by the finding of a floating membrane within the cysts on CT scan (Figure 65.18). Active cysts contain a large number of smaller daughter cysts (Figure 65.19), and rupture can result in these implanting and growing within the peritoneal cavity. Liver cysts can also rupture through the diaphragm producing an empyema, into the biliary tract producing obstructive jaundice, or into the stomach. Clinical and radiological diagnosis can be supported by serology for antibodies to hydatid antigen in the form of an enzyme-linked immunosorbent assay (ELISA). Treatment is indicated to prevent progressive enlargement and rupture of the cysts. In the first instance, a course of albendazole or mebendazole may be tried. There are many reports that percutaneous treatment of hydatid cysts is safe and effective. Percutaneous treatment constitutes an intial course of albendazole followed by **p**uncture of the cyst under image guidance, **a**spiration of the cysts contents, **i**nstillation of hypertonic saline in the cyst cavity and **r**easpiration (PAIR). PAIR should only be attempted if there is no communication with the biliary tree. Failure to respond to medical treatment or percutaneous treatment usually requires surgical intervention. The surgical options range from liver resection or local excision of the cysts to deroofing with evacuation of the contents. Contamination of the peritoneal cavity at the time of surgery with active hydatid daughters should be avoided by continuing drug therapy with albendazole and adding peroperative praziquantel. This should be combined with packing of the peritoneal cavity with 20 per cent hypertonic saline-soaked packs and instilling 20 per cent hypertonic saline into the cyst before it is opened. A biliary communication should be actively sought and sutured. The residual cavity may become infected, and this may be reduced, as may bile leakage, by packing the space with pedicled greater omentum (an omentoplasty). Calcified cysts may well be dead. If doubt exists as to whether a suspected cyst is active, it can be followed on ultrasound, as active cysts gradually become larger and more superficial in the liver. Rupture of daughter hydatids into the biliary tract may result in obstructive jaundice or acute cholangitis. This may be treated by endoscopic clearance of the daughter cysts prior to cyst removal from the liver.

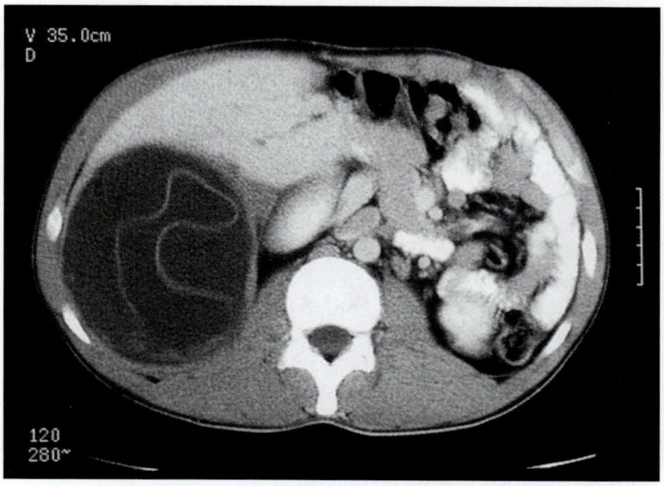

Figure 65.18 Hydatid liver cyst. Active hydatid disease usually produces a non-calcified liver cyst and, within the cyst, floating layers of the germinal membrane can be seen.

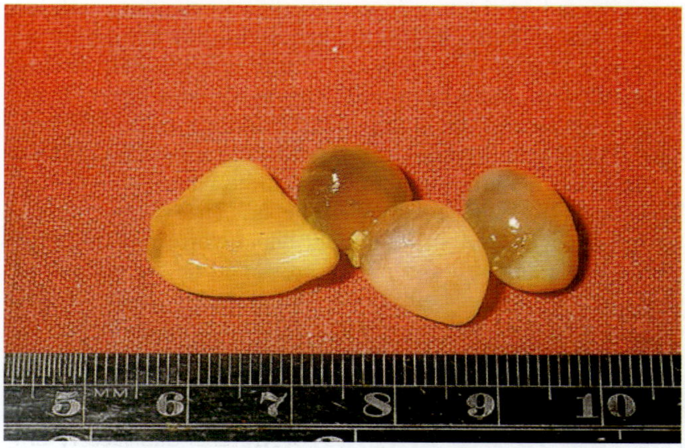

Figure 65.19 Hydatid 'daughter' cysts. These were removed from the bile duct of a patient presenting with obstructive jaundice due to a hydatid liver cyst communicating with the bile duct. Endoscopic removal should also be considered.

LIVER TUMOURS

Surgical approaches to resection of liver tumours

Adequate exposure of the liver is an absolute prerequisite to safe liver surgery. A transverse abdominal incision in the right upper quadrant with a vertical midline extension to the xiphoid provides excellent access to the liver if adequate retraction of the costal margin is employed using a costal margin retractor. If necessary, the incision can be extended across the midline transversely in the left upper quadrant. Thoracoabdominal incisions are no longer required. The procedure for complete mobilisation of the liver is described, although this will not be necessary in all cases. There are many variations in surgical technique.

Mobilisation of the liver

The falciform ligament is first divided and followed along the anterior surface of the liver towards the suprahepatic IVC. The left triangular ligament is divided, facilitated by placing an abdominal pack in front of the oesophagogastric junction. The right triangular ligament is then divided by retraction of the diaphragm away from the right lobe parenchyma. On exposure of the bare area of the liver, the IVC can be seen as it passes behind the liver, and this can be slung above the renal veins below the liver and at the level of the main hepatic veins. Mobilisation of the liver is completed by division of the lesser omentum. Removing the liver from the IVC is achieved by lifting the liver anteriorly to expose the multiple small veins (inferior hepatic veins) passing between the liver parenchyma and the IVC. These should be suture ligated to ensure haemostasis. This proceeds from above the renal veins until the main hepatic veins are reached below the diaphragm.

Dissection of the hilum

The peritoneum overlying the hilar triad is divided. The CBD is then exposed on the free edge of the lesser omentum, mobilisation being facilitated by ligation and division of the cystic duct and artery followed by removal of the gall bladder. Slinging the CBD with an elastic sling allows exposure of the common hepatic artery and dissection of the main right and left branches. These again may be slung to allow the remaining lymphatic tissue surrounding the portal vein to be ligated and divided. The possibility of an aberrant right hepatic artery lying posterior to the bile duct or an accessory left hepatic artery from the left gastric artery in the lesser omentum should be considered and carefully excluded. Dissection of the hilar bile ducts requires careful retraction on segment IV of the liver, and division of the small vessels and bile duct branches passing between segment IV and the confluence of the right and left hepatic ducts.

Division of the parenchyma

Once the liver has been adequately mobilised and the hilar vessels have been exposed, the main inflow vessels and bile duct to the liver lobe to be resected can be divided. The arterial branch should be transfixed with 4/0 Prolene, the bile duct transfixed with 4/0 PDS and the portal vein branch with a 4/0 Prolene suture. Division of the inflow vessels produces a line of demarcation between the right and left liver, passing to the right of and parallel with the falciform ligament. The parenchyma is divided along this plane of demarcation commencing by diathermy of the liver capsule. The ultrasound dissector (Cavitron ultrasonic surgical aspirator (CUSA)) is the most common method used for division of the parenchyma. This allows the parenchyma to be divided, leaving the vessels and bile duct branches to be diathermied or ligated depending on their size. Dissection continues on an even plane until the hepatic vein branches are approached from within the liver parenchyma, when they are ligated or stapled, and then divided (Figure 65.20).

Segmental and local resections

These are considered in patients whose liver tumours can be excised with an adequate margin (generally considered to be 1 cm) without a formal right or left lobe liver resection. The segments that can be removed individually are those shown in Figure 65.2. Each carries its own blood supply, venous drainage and bile drainage. The extent of mobilisation of the liver required (described above under Mobilisation of the liver) depends on the segment to be resected. Hilar dissection may not be necessary. Segmental resections are used particularly in patients with HCC and underlying liver disease (e.g. HBV or HCV) to minimise the risk of postoperative liver failure (Figure 65.21). Local resections are principally used for patients with multiple liver metastases when removal of the tumour mass with a minimum margin of 1 cm of normal liver parenchyma is required.

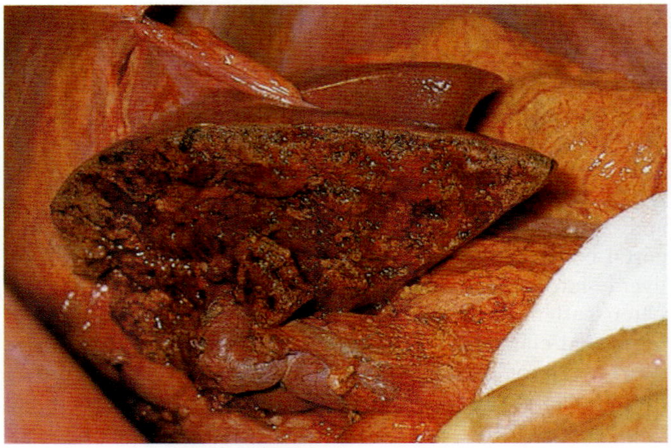

Figure 65.20 Hepatectomy post-resection. Cut surface of the residual liver following a right hepatectomy in which segments V–VIII have been removed. On the lower edge, the portal vein and bile duct can be visualised.

Laparoscopic liver resections

With advances in minimal access surgery, the application of laparoscopic surgery in performing liver resections has evolved considerably. However, success in laparoscopic liver resections requires expertise both in advanced laparoscopic techniques and in liver surgery. Wedge resections of superficial and peripherally located tumours, and left lateral liver resections are commonly performed in most centres. Major right and left hepatectomies are also being performed in selected centres.

Blood loss and transfusion

The reduction of blood loss during liver surgery has been one of the major achievements in the last decade, and resection without blood transfusion is often possible. Better understanding of the segmental anatomy of the liver, better patient selection for surgery, reducing central venous pressure (<10 mmHg) during parenchymal transection have all helped to reduce the need for blood transfusions. Intraoperative cell saver, used in non-cancer cases and during liver transplantation, has reduced the need for autologous blood transfusions. Devices such as the ultrasound dissector have helped, but clamp crushing (Kelly clysis) is equally effective in achieving parenchymal transection with minimal blood loss. Better control of the coagulation cascade has been achieved using TEG (see Figure 65.9), and the antifibrinolytic drug aprotinin has significantly reduced bleeding in patients with liver disease and an underlying coagulopathy. Oozing from the resected surface can be reduced by the topical application of fibrin glue or fibrin-impregnated collagen fleece.

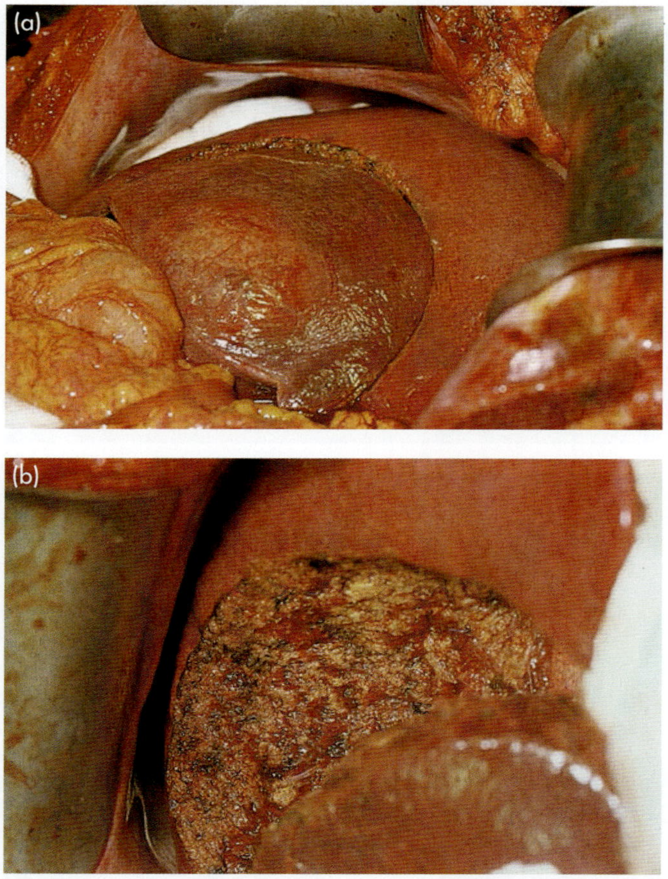

Figure 65.21 Segmental resection. Removal of a primary liver tumour by resection of liver segment VI (a and b) in a patient with well-compensated liver cirrhosis.

The main alternative is use of the argon-beam coagulator. Temporary clamping of the portal vein and hepatic artery in the hepatoduodenal ligament (Pringle manoeuvre) can prevent excessive blood loss during parenchymal transection. The optimal duration of the Pringle manoeuvre is unknown, but it can be applied intermittently, e.g. cycles of 15 minutes inflow occlusion followed by 5 minutes of reperfusion, until parenchymal transection is complete.

Benign liver tumours

Haemangiomas

These are the most common liver lesions, and the reported incidence has increased with the widespread availability of diagnostic ultrasound. They consist of an abnormal plexus of vessels, and their nature is usually apparent on ultrasound. If diagnostic uncertainty exists, CT scanning with delayed contrast enhancement shows the characteristic appearance of slow contrast enhancement due to small vessel uptake in the haemangioma. Often, haemangiomas are multiple. Lesions found incidentally require confirmation of their nature and no further treatment. The management of 'giant' haemangiomas is more controversial. Occasional reports of rupture of haemangiomas have led some to consider resection for the large lesions, especially if they appear to be symptomatic. They have little if any malignant potential, and this is no indication for surgery. Percutaneous biopsy of these lesions should be avoided as they are vascular lesions and may bleed profusely into the peritoneal cavity.

Hepatic adenoma

Hepatic adenomas (Figure 65.22) are rare benign liver tumours. They occur mostly in women of child-bearing age. Imaging by CT or MRI demonstrates a well-circumscribed and vascular solid tumour. They usually develop in an otherwise normal liver. Unfortunately, there are no characteristic radiological features to differentiate these lesions from HCC. Arterial phase CT demonstrates a well-developed peripheral arterialisation of the tumour. Biopsy may be necessary for confirmation and characterisation of the nature of these lesions. These tumours may bleed and are thought to have malignant potential, and resection is therefore the treatment of choice. An association with sex hormones (including the oral contraceptive pill) is well recognised, and regression of symptomatic adenomas on withdrawal of hormone stimulation is well documented.

Focal nodular hyperplasia

This is an unusual benign condition of unknown aetiology in which there is a focal overgrowth of functioning liver tissue supported by fibrous stroma. Patients are usually middle-aged

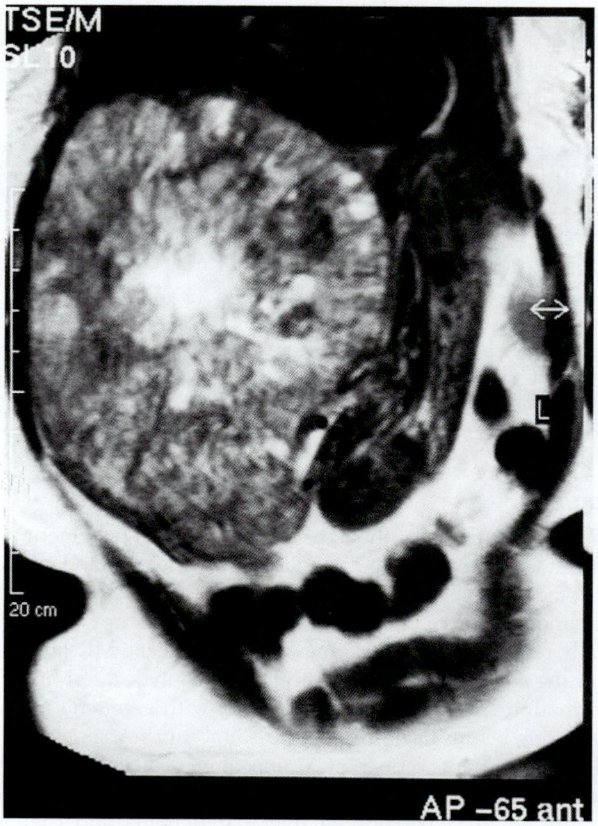

Figure 65.22 Hepatic adenoma. Magnetic resonance imaging scan of a giant hepatic adenoma. These lesions are thought to be premalignant, they may haemorrhage and, in some cases, their growth is sex hormone sensitive. Withdrawal of hormone preparations may allow spontaneous regression.

females, and there is no association with underlying liver disease. Ultrasound shows a solid tumour mass but does not help in discrimination. Contrast CT or/and MRI may show central scarring and evidence of a well-vascularised lesion. Again, these appearances are not specific for focal nodular hyperplasia (FNH). FNH contain both hepatocytes and Kupffer cells. MRI using liver-specific contrast agents, such as gadoxetic acid, which is taken up by hepatocytes and excreted in bile or superparamagnetic iron oxide which is taken up by Kupffer cells, may be useful in determining the hepatocellular origin of FNH and allowing differentiation of FNH from metastatic cancer. Similarly, a sulphur colloid liver scan may be useful, since Kupffer cells take up the colloid. FNH do not have any malignant potential and, once the diagnosis is confirmed, they do not require any treatment.

Surgery for liver metastases

Outcome

The role of surgery in the treatment of colorectal liver metastases is now well established, based on prospective data on resected patients compared with unresected patients with a similar stage of disease. The role of resection of liver metastases from other primary sites has not been well defined. The resectability rate for liver metastases from colorectal cancer is 20–30 per cent. The expected patient survival rate for resection of colorectal metastases is approximately 35 per cent at five years, with few cancer-related deaths beyond this period. Solitary, multiple unilobar and multiple bilobar liver metastases are all considered for resection, although cure rates will vary significantly (Summary box 65.12).

Summary box 65.12

Prognostic factors in patients undergoing resection of colorectal liver metastases

- Stage of primary
- Time from primary resection
- Carcinoembryonic antigen (CEA) level
- Size of largest lesion
- Number of lesions

Staging

This involves defining the extent of the liver involvement with metastases and excluding extrahepatic disease. A standard work up would involve oral and intravenous contrast CT scans of the liver and abdomen, chest CT scan and colonoscopy to look for locally recurrent or synchronous colonic cancers. MRI and PET scanning are useful in the clarification of equivocal lesions. This information should be taken in parallel with a general medical evaluation before deciding on the suitability for surgery of an individual patient. The typical appearance of colorectal liver metastases on contrast CT is shown in Figure 65.23. These patients usually have normal liver parenchyma and therefore tolerate a 60–70 per cent resection of liver parenchyma without risk of postoperative liver failure (Summary box 65.13). Tumour markers are useful but have low specificity. Histological confirmation prior to undertaking surgery is not necessary and percutaneous biopsy of resectable lesions should be avoided as

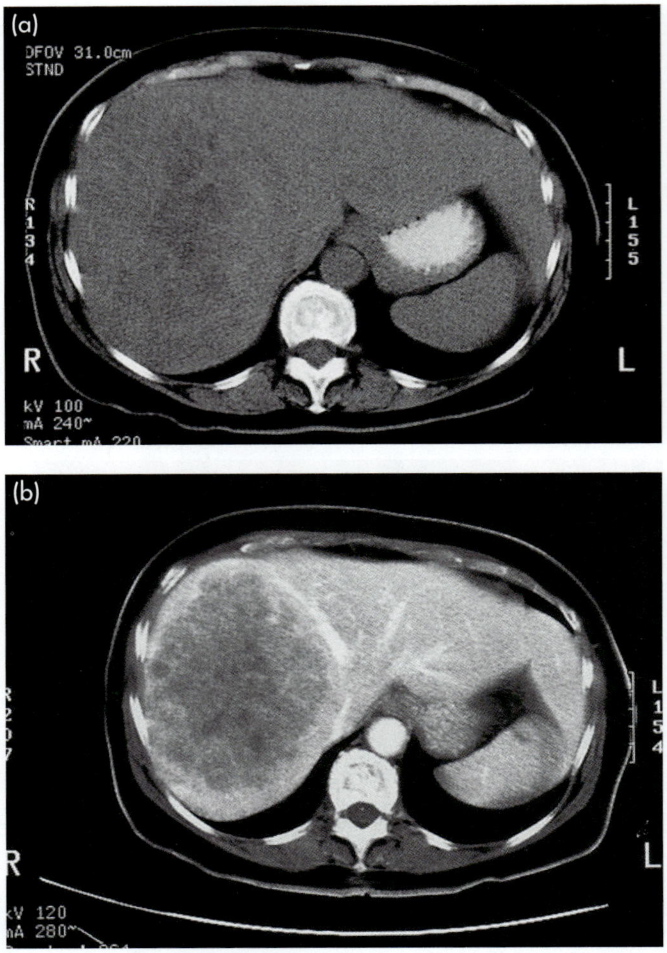

Figure 65.23 Colorectal liver metastases on computed tomography (CT) scan: (a) after oral contrast CT; (b) after intravenous contrast. The colorectal liver metastasis occupying the entire right lobe of the liver is difficult to visualise on oral contrast CT. The addition of intravenous contrast shows its lack of enhancement and its relationship to the hepatic veins.

there is good evidence that malignant cells can seed along the biopsy track.

Summary box 65.13

Staging and assessment with colorectal liver metastases

- General medical assessment
- CT, PET-CT or MRI of the abdomen/pelvis with contrast (? resectability)
- Chest CT
- Review histology of primary (? risk of local recurrence)
- Colonoscopy
- Liver function tests and tumour markers

Surgical approach

The basic surgical approach to liver resection is outlined above. A search for local recurrent disease, peritoneal deposits and regional lymph node involvement should be made at the start of the laparotomy. Planar imaging often overlooks peritoneal or superficial liver metastatic deposits. Coeliac node involvement in patients with liver metastases considerably reduces the overall survival whether or not the liver and nodal disease is resected. Intraoperative ultrasound with bimanual palpation of the liver is valuable in assessing the number of lesions and resectability.

Downstaging therapies

There have been major advances in the management of patients with colorectal liver metastases who, until recently, would have been considered 'unresectable' due to the size or distribution of their metastases. Chemotherapy with 5-fluorouracil (5FU) and folinic acid produces a response rate of approximately 30 per cent but, when combined with oxaliplatin, the response rate increases to 50–60 per cent, often with a dramatic size reduction of the lesions. The combination of chemotherapy with monoclonal antibodies (mAbs) that recognise vascular endothelial growth factor (VEGF) receptor or the epidermal growth factor receptor (EGFR) may provide additional benefit. Long-term follow up of patients downstaged with chemotherapy, who have proceeded to resection of their cancers, have shown five-year survival rates of 30–40 per cent.

Patients with bilobar metastases with a lesion centrally within the right lobe and a second lesion peripherally in the left lobe may have resection of their metastases in two stages to allow for regeneration of the liver parenchyma between the procedures. Good long-term survival has been reported for this group of patients.

Portal vein embolisation is a third development to affect patients previously deemed unresectable. Patients who require a right or extended right hepatectomy and in whom the left lobe volumes are congenitally small (<30 per cent of functioning parenchyma) have an increased risk of post-resection liver failure. This can be reduced by preoperative (3–6 weeks) percutaneous embolisation of the right portal vein branch, which produces atrophy of the affected lobe and hypertrophy of the contralateral lobe.

In patients who cannot be rendered resectable, systemic chemotherapy has been shown to produce survival and quality of life benefit. Many techniques are now available that produce local ablation of the tumours, including cryotherapy, interstitial laser hyperthermia, radiofrequency ablation (RFA), microwave therapy, focused ultrasound and electrolytic therapy. These techniques may produce survival benefit along with chemotherapy in the palliative setting, but there is little objective evidence of long-term survival, and they should therefore be restricted to patients who cannot be offered surgical resection (Summary box 65.14).

Summary box 65.14

Strategies for 'unresectable' colorectal liver metastases

- Neoadjuvant chemotherapy
- Anti-VEGF or EGFR monoclonal antibody therapy
- Two-stage liver resection
- Portal vein embolisation
- Ablation techniques

Approximately 15–20 per cent of patients with colorectal cancer present with synchronous liver metastases. However, the timing of resection of the liver metastases in these patients is controversial. For most patients, a staged approach consisting of resection of the colorectal primary first followed by liver resection at a later date is the standard treatment. In selected patients in whom the colorectal primary is small and asymptomatic, the liver resection may be performed first to prevent progression of the liver metastases. In patients requiring minor liver resection for small metastases, simultaneous liver and colorectal resections is safe and effective. Similarly, a right-sided colonic resection which is usually straightforward can be combined with liver resection safely. Combining major liver resection with major colorectal resection is controversial.

Hepatocellular carcinoma

Primary liver cancer (HCC) is one of the world's most common cancers, and its incidence is expected to rise rapidly over the next decade due to the association with chronic liver disease, particularly HBV and HCV. Many patients known to have chronic liver disease are now being screened for the development of HCC by serial ultrasound scans of the liver or serum measurements of alpha-fetoprotein (AFP). Patients often present in middle age, either because of the symptoms of chronic liver disease (malaise, weakness, jaundice, ascites, variceal bleed, encephalopathy) or with the anorexia and weight loss of an advanced cancer. The surgical treatment options include resection of the tumour and liver transplantation. Which option is most appropriate for an individual patient depends on the stage of the underlying liver disease, the size and site of the tumour, the availability of organ transplantation and the management of the immunosuppressed patient.

Staging and clinical assessment of HCC

In addition to a general assessment of the patient's fitness for surgery, crucial information is the severity of the underlying liver disease, based on CTP classification (see Table 65.2) or MELD score, and the size, number and site of the tumour. As chronic liver disease predisposes to these tumours, they are often multifocal by the time of diagnosis. Extensive liver resections in patients with advanced cirrhosis are associated with a high mortality due to liver failure and sepsis. In contrast, extensive resections for HCC in a non-cirrhotic liver are associated with a low risk of liver failure, and resection rather than transplantation would be the treatment option of choice. Tumours often metastasise to the lung and bone and, therefore, a chest CT scan and a bone scan are useful staging investigations. Evidence of intraperitoneal disease is difficult to determine by CT scan, and laparoscopy may be useful for this purpose. The intrahepatic distribution of HCC is equally difficult to determine within the cirrhotic liver. Ultrasound, early arterial phase-enhanced spiral CT scan and contrast MRI are the most useful investigations that are currently available. Wedged hepatic venous pressure (WHVP) measurements are useful in cirrhotic patients. An elevated WHVP suggests portal hypertension and is an independent predictor of poor outcome after liver resection in cirrhotic patients. Indocyanine green (ICG) clearance test is useful to assess liver function preoperatively in cirrhotic patients. Intravenously injected ICG is exclusively eliminated by hepatocytes and excreted into bile and does not enter enterohepatic circulation. The plasma clearance of ICG has been used as an indicator of hepatic blood flow and hepatic function. Generally, cirrhotic patients who are CTP class A and have a high ICG clearance are suitable for major liver resections.

Surgical approach to HCC

The surgical approach should remove the known cancer with a 1- to 2-cm margin of unaffected liver tissue. In patients with associated chronic liver disease, the volume of liver resected should be minimised to reduce the incidence of postoperative liver failure. Local or segmental resections are preferred to major resections (see Figure 65.21). In carefully selected patients, liver transplantation is an effective treatment. Patients with cirrhosis who have a single HCC less than 5 cm in diameter or multiple HCCs each less than 3 cm, and with no evidence of vascular invasion or extrahepatic spread are ideal candidates for liver transplantation.

Non-surgical therapy for hepatocellular carcinoma

The majority of patients diagnosed with HCC will not be amenable to surgical resection because of the advanced stage of the cancer or the severity of the underlying liver disease. Those patients awaiting liver transplantation may develop progressive disease before a suitable donor liver is found, because of the long waiting list for transplantation. Patients with unresectable disease can be offered local ablative treatments, such as transarterial embolisation (TAE), transarterial chemoembolisation (TACE), percutaneous ethanol ablation (PEA) or RFA (Figure 65.24). These local ablative treatments may also be used as bridging procedures to liver transplantation.

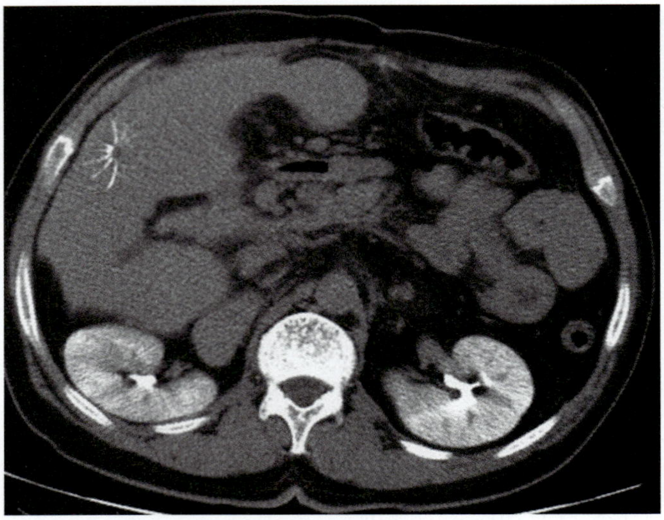

Figure 65.24 Computed tomography scan after radiofrequency ablation for hepatocellular carcinoma.

Follow up and adjuvant treatment

There is little evidence that adjuvant chemotherapy will improve the prognosis of patients following resection of HCC, but trials with the multikinase inhibitor Sorafenib are ongoing. Chemotherapy may damage the function of the liver in those with underlying chronic liver disease. AFP is a clinically useful tumour marker for follow up, although its low sensitivity would suggest that imaging should also be used.

Cholangiocarcinoma

Presentation, pathology and natural history

Bile duct cancers typically present with painless obstructive jaundice. Elderly patients are frequently affected, but patients with PSC may develop these tumours at a much earlier age. These tumours are typically slow growing and often arise at the confluence of the right and left hepatic ducts (Klatskin tumours), eventually invading the liver parenchyma. Cancers at this site are usually fibrous and produce tight duct strictures. Distal bile duct cholangiocarcinomas are more frequently polypoidal and obstruct the lumen of the duct. Investigation, staging and management of bile duct and gall bladder malignancies are discussed in Chapter 67.

FURTHER READING

Blumgart LH. *Surgery of the liver, biliary tract and pancreas*, 4th edn. Philadelphia, PA: WB Saunders, 2007.

Dooley JS, Lok ASF, Burroughs AK, Heathcote EJ (eds). *Sherlock's diseases of the liver and biliary system*, 12th edn. Oxford: Wiley-Blackwell, 2011.

Townsend CM. *Sabiston textbook of surgery*, 18th edn. London: Elsevier Health Sciences, 2007.

CHAPTER 66

The spleen

LEARNING OBJECTIVES

To understand:
- The function of the spleen
- The common pathologies involving the spleen
- The principles and potential complications of splenectomy
- The potential advantages of laparoscopic splenectomy
- The benefits of splenic conservation
- The importance of prophylaxis against infection following splenectomy

EMBRYOLOGY, ANATOMY AND PHYSIOLOGY

Embryology

Fetal splenic tissue develops from condensations of mesoderm in the dorsal mesogastrium. This peritoneal fold attaches the dorsal body wall to the fusiform swelling in the foregut that develops into the stomach. This condensation divides the mesogastrium into two parts, one between the fetal splenic tissue and the stomach to form the gastrosplenic ligament and the other between it and the left kidney to form the lienorenal ligament.

Anatomy

The weight of the normal adult spleen is 75–250 g. It lies in the left hypochondrium between the gastric fundus and the left hemidiaphragm, with its long axis lying along the tenth rib. The hilum sits in the angle between the stomach and the kidney and is in contact with the tail of the pancreas. The concave visceral surface lies in contact with these structures, and the lower pole extends no further than the mid-axillary line. There is a notch on the inferolateral border, and this may be palpated when the spleen is enlarged. The tortuous splenic artery arises from the coeliac axis and runs along the upper border of the body and tail of the pancreas, to which it gives small branches. The short gastric and left gastroepiploic branches pass between the layers of the gastrosplenic ligament. The main splenic artery generally divides into superior and inferior branches, which, in turn, subdivide into several segmental branches.

The splenic vein is formed from several tributaries that drain the hilum. The vein runs behind the pancreas, receiving several small tributaries from the pancreas before joining the superior mesenteric vein at the neck of the pancreas to form the portal vein.

The splenic pulp is invested by an external serous and internal fibroelastic coat which is reflected inwards at the hilum onto the vessels to form vascular sheaths. The lymphatic drainage comprises efferent vessels in the white pulp that run with the arterioles and emerge from nodes at the hilum. These nodes and lymphatics drain via retropancreatic nodes to the coeliac nodes.

Sympathetic nerve fibres run from the coeliac plexus and innervate splenic arterial branches.

Physiology

The splenic parenchyma consists of white and red pulp that is surrounded by serosa and a collagenous capsule with smooth muscle fibres. These penetrate the parenchyma as trabeculae of dense connective tissue fibres rich in collagen and elastic tissue. These, with the reticular framework, support the cells of the spleen and surround the vessels in the splenic pulp. The white pulp comprises a central trabecular artery surrounded by nodules with germinal centres and periarterial lymphatic sheaths that provide a framework filled with lymphocytes and macrophages. Arteries from the central artery and the peripheral 'penicillar' arteries pass into the marginal zone that lies at the edge of the white pulp. Plasma-rich blood that has passed through the central lymphatic nodules is filtered as it passes through the sinuses within the marginal zone, and particles are phagocytosed. Immunoglobulins produced in the lymphatic nodules enter the circulation through the sinuses in the marginal zone, beyond which lies the red pulp, which consists of cords and sinuses. Cell-concentrated blood passes in the trabecular artery through the centre of the white pulp to the red pulp cords. Red cells must elongate and become thinner to pass from the cords to the sinuses, a process that removes abnormally shaped cells from the circulation (Figure 66.1). As 90 per cent of the blood passing through the spleen moves through an open circulation in which blood flows from arteries to cords, and thence sinuses, splenic pulp pressure reflects the pressure throughout the portal system. The remaining 10 per cent of the blood flow through the spleen bypasses the cords and sinuses by direct arteriovenous communications. The overall flow rate of blood is about 300 mL/min.

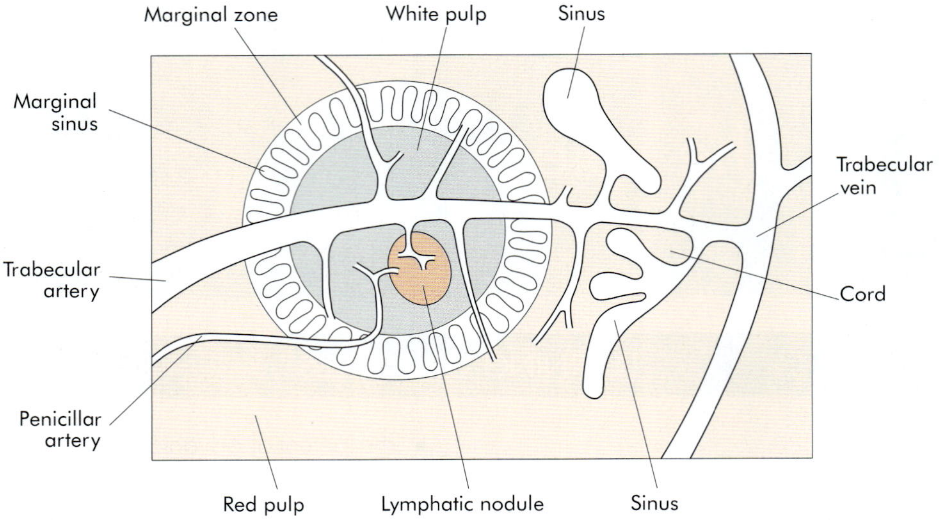

Figure 66.1 A central trabecular artery passing through the white pulp into the surrounding red pulp. A blood flow skimming effect results in most of the plasma passing down the branches of the artery while the cells pass in the central trabecular artery directly into the red pulp (courtesy of Professor TG Allen-Mersh, Westminster and Charing Cross Hospitals, London, UK).

FUNCTIONS OF THE SPLEEN

Although the spleen was previously thought to be dispensable, increasing knowledge of its function has led to a conservative approach in the management of conditions involving the spleen. It is now recognised that an incidental splenectomy during the course of another operative procedure increases the risk of complication and death. The surgeon should therefore normally endeavour to preserve the spleen to maintain the following functions:

- **Immune function**. The spleen processes foreign antigens and is the major site of specific immunoglobulin M (IgM) production. The non-specific opsonins, properdin and tuftsin, are synthesised. These antibodies are of B- and T-cell origin and bind to the specific receptors on the surface of macrophages and leukocytes, stimulating their phagocytic, bactericidal and tumoricidal activity.
- **Filter function**. Macrophages in the reticulum capture cellular and non-cellular material from the blood and plasma. This will include the removal of effete platelets and red blood cells. This process takes place in the sinuses and the splenic cords by the action of the endothelial macrophages. Iron is removed from the degraded haemoglobin during red cell breakdown and is returned to the plasma. Removed non-cellular material may include bacteria and, in particular, pneumococci.
- **Pitting**. Particulate inclusions from red cells are removed, and the repaired red cells are returned to the circulation. These include Howell–Jolly and Heinz bodies, which represent nuclear remnants and precipitated haemoglobin or globin subunits, respectively.
- **Reservoir function**. This function in humans is less marked than in other species, but the spleen does contain approximately 8 per cent of the red cell mass. An enlarged spleen may contain a much larger proportion of the blood volume.
- **Cytopoiesis**. From the fourth month of intrauterine life, some degree of haemopoiesis occurs in the fetal spleen. Stimulation of the white pulp may occur following antigenic challenge, resulting in the proliferation of T and B cells and macrophages. This may also occur in myeloproliferative disorders, thalassaemias and chronic haemolytic anaemias (Summary box 66.1).

Summary box 66.1

Functions of the spleen

- Immune
- Filter function
- Pitting
- Reservoir
- Cytopoiesis

INVESTIGATION OF THE SPLEEN

Conditions that result in splenomegaly can be diagnosed on the basis of the history and examination findings and from laboratory examination. In haemolytic anaemia, a full blood count, reticulocyte count and tests for haemolysis will determine the cause of the anaemia. Splenomegaly associated with portal hypertension caused by cirrhosis is diagnosed on the history, physical signs of liver dysfunction, abnormal tests of liver function and endoscopic evidence of oesophageal varices. Sinistral or segmental portal hypertension may result from isolated occlusion of the splenic vein by pancreatic inflammation or tumour. As many conditions that cause splenomegaly are associated with lymphadenopathy, investigation should be directed at those disease processes known to be associated with both physical signs. Lymph node biopsy may be required.

William Henry Howell, 1860–1945, Professor of Physiology, Johns Hopkins University, Baltimore, MD, USA
Justin Marie Jules Jolly, 1870–1953, Professor of Histopathology, College de France, Paris, France.
Robert Heinz, 1865–1924, Professor of Pharmacology and Toxicology, Erlangen, Germany.

often pale and jaundiced at presentation and, in established cases, lassitude and undue fatigue are present.

In some families, the disease is characterised by a severe crisis of red blood cell destruction, during which the erythrocyte count may fall from 4.5×10^6 to 1.5×10^6/mL within a week. Such crises are characterised by the onset of pyrexia, abdominal pain, nausea, vomiting and extreme pallor followed by increased jaundice. These episodes may be precipitated by acute infection. Any child with gallstone disease should be investigated for hereditary spherocytosis and a family history sought.

Examination reveals splenomegaly, and the liver may also be palpable. Chronic leg ulcers may arise in adults with the disease.

Haematological investigations include the fragility test. Erythrocytes begin to haemolyse in 0.47 per cent saline solution but, in this condition, haemolysis may occur in 0.6 per cent or even stronger solutions. Immature red blood cells (reticulocytes), which differ from adult cells by possessing a reticulum, are discharged into the circulation by the bone marrow to compensate for the loss of erythrocytes by haemolysis.

Faecal urobilinogen is increased as this route excretes most of the urinobilinogen.

Radioactive chromium (^{51}Cr) labelling of the patient's own red cells will demonstrate the severity of red cell destruction. Daily scanning over the spleen will show the degree of red cell sequestration by the spleen. The presence of high levels of splenic radioactivity generally predicts a good response to splenectomy, but this test is used less commonly.

All patients with hereditary spherocytosis should be treated by splenectomy but, in juvenile cases, this is generally delayed until six years of age to minimise the risk of post-splenectomy infection, but before gallstones have had time to form. Ultrasonography should be performed preoperatively to determine the presence or absence of gallstones.

Acquired autoimmune haemolytic anaemia

This condition is divided into immune and non-immune-mediated forms. It may arise following exposure to agents such as chemicals, infection or drugs, e.g. alpha-methyldopa, or be associated with another disease (e.g. systemic lupus erythematosus). In most instances, the cause is unknown, and red cell survival is reduced because of an immune reaction triggered by immunoglobulin or complement on the red cell surface. This condition is more common in women after the age of 50 years. In half the patients, the spleen is enlarged and, in 20 per cent of cases, pigment gallstones are present.

Anaemia is invariably present and may be associated with spherocytosis because of red cell membrane damage. In the immune type, antibody, which coats the red cells, can be detected by agglutination when anti-human globulin is added to a suspension of the patient's erythrocytes (Coombs' test positive). The disease runs an acute self-limiting course, and no treatment is necessary. Splenectomy should, however, be considered if corticosteroids are ineffective, when the patient is developing complications from long-term steroid treatment or if corticosteroids are contraindicated. Eighty per cent of patients respond to splenectomy.

Thalassaemia (synonyms: Cooley's anaemia, Mediterranean anaemia)

Thalassaemia (Greek, *Thalassa* meaning sea (because the disease occurs in people of Mediterranean origin)) results from a defect in haemoglobin peptide chain synthesis and is transmitted most commonly as a recessive trait. The disease is really a group of related diseases, alpha, beta and gamma, depending upon which haemoglobin peptide chain's rate of synthesis is reduced. Most patients suffer from betathalassaemia, in which a reduction in the rate of beta-chain synthesis results in a decrease in haemoglobin A. Intracellular precipitates (Heinz bodies) contribute to premature red cell destruction.

Graduations of the disease range from heterozygous thalassaemia minor to homozygous thalassaemia major, which is associated with chronic anaemia, jaundice and splenomegaly. Patients with homozygous thalassaemia major frequently develop clinical signs in the first year of life, and these include retarded growth, enlarged head with slanting eyes and depressed nose, leg ulcers, jaundice and abdominal distension secondary to splenomegaly.

Red cells are small, thin and misshapen and have a characteristic resistance to osmotic lysis. In the more severe forms, nucleated red cells and other immature blood cells are seen. The final diagnosis is by haemoglobin electrophoresis.

Blood transfusion may be required to correct profound anaemia, but the patient may become transfusion dependent because of the development of hypersplenism. Splenectomy is therefore of benefit in patients who require frequent blood transfusion and if haemolytic antibodies have developed as a result.

Sickle cell disease

Sickle cell disease is a hereditary, autosomal recessive haemolytic anaemia occurring mainly among those of African origin in whom the normal haemoglobin A is replaced by haemoglobin S (HbS). The HbS molecule crystallises when the blood oxygen tension is reduced, thus distorting and elongating the red cell. The resulting increased blood viscosity may obstruct the flow of blood in the spleen. Splenic microinfarcts are therefore common.

The sickle cell trait can be detected in 9 per cent of those of African origin, but most are asymptomatic; sickle cell disease occurs in about 1 per cent of Africans. Depending upon the vessels affected by vascular occlusion, patients may complain of bone or joint pain, priapism, neurological abnormalities, skin ulcers or abdominal pain due to visceral blood stasis. The diagnosis is made by the finding of characteristic sickle-shaped cells on blood film, although this investigation has largely been replaced by haemoglobin electrophoresis.

Hypoxia that provokes a sickling crisis should be avoided and is particularly relevant in patients undergoing general anaesthesia. Adequate hydration and partial exchange transfusion may help in a crisis. Splenectomy is of benefit in a few patients in whom excessive splenic sequestration of red cells aggravates the anaemia. Chronic hypersplenism usually occurs in late childhood or adolescence, although *Streptococcus pneumoniae* infection may precipitate an acute form in the first five years of life.

Porphyria

Porphyria is a hereditary error of haemoglobin catabolism in which porphyrinuria occurs. Abdominal crises, characterised by severe intestinal colic and constipation, can be precipitated by the administration of barbiturates. The patient is anaemic and may suffer from photosensitivity; in advanced forms of the disease, neurological and mental symptoms are present. The splenomegaly associated with this condition may be overlooked. The urine may be orange and develops a port-wine colour after

Ronin Royston Amos Coombs, 1921–2006, Qucik Professor of Immunology, University of Cambridge, Cambridge, UK described this test in 1945.
Thomas Benton Cooley, 1871–1945, Professor of Pediatrics, Wayne University, Detroit, MI, USA, described this type of anaemia in 1927.

a few hours of exposure to the air. Splenectomy has little role to play in the management of this condition.

Gaucher's disease

This lipid storage disease is characterised by storage of glucocerebroside in the reticuloendothelial system and in the spleen. Enormous splenic enlargement may be associated with yellowish-brown discolouration of the skin on the hands and face, anaemia and conjunctival thickening (pinguecula). Slavonic and Jewish races are more prone to the disease, and the detection of Gaucher cells in the bone marrow confirms the diagnosis. Splenectomy is indicated only for severe symptoms related to the splenomegaly.

Hypersplenism due to portal hypertension

Splenomegaly is an invariable feature of portal hypertension (Figure 66.7) and results in the thrombocytopenia and granulocytopenia observed in these patients. These may be improved if the portal hypertension is relieved by shunt surgery or liver transplantation. Splenectomy would normally be required only in those patients whose segmental portal hypertension has resulted in symptomatic oesophagogastric varices.

Felty's syndrome

Patients with rheumatoid arthritis may develop leukopenia. This is referred to as Felty syndrome if it is extreme and associated with splenomegaly. There is no definite relationship between the severity of the arthritic changes and the leukopenia and splenomegaly. Splenectomy produces only a transient improvement in the blood picture, but rheumatoid arthritis may respond to steroid therapy to which it had previously become resistant.

NEOPLASMS

Haemangioma is the most common benign tumour of the spleen and may rarely develop into a haemangiosarcoma that is managed by splenectomy. The spleen is rarely the site of metastatic disease. Lymphoma is the most common cause of neoplastic enlargement, and splenectomy may play a part in its management. Splenectomy may be required to achieve a diagnosis in the absence of palpable lymph nodes or to relieve the symptoms of gross splenomegaly. However, the need for staging laparoscopy has largely receded with the advent of CT scanning. Its use has been restricted to those patients in whom a definite histological diagnosis of intra-abdominal disease will affect management. Thus, selected patients with stage IA or IIA Hodgkin's disease may be candidates for staging laparotomy or laparoscopy. In the absence of obvious liver or intra-abdominal nodal disease, splenectomy is an integral part of the staging procedure to exclude splenic involvement, which would alter the method of treatment.

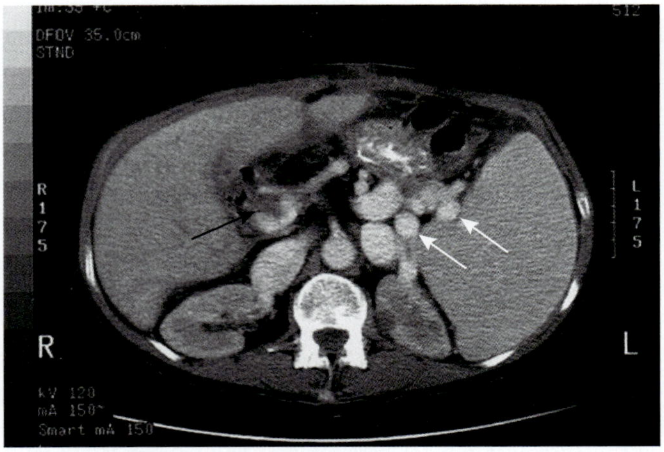

Figure 66.7 Computed tomographic scan showing an enlarged spleen in a patient with portal hypertension secondary to portal vein thrombosis. Clot is evident within the lumen of the portal vein (black arrow), and large varices (white arrows) are present at the splenic hilus.

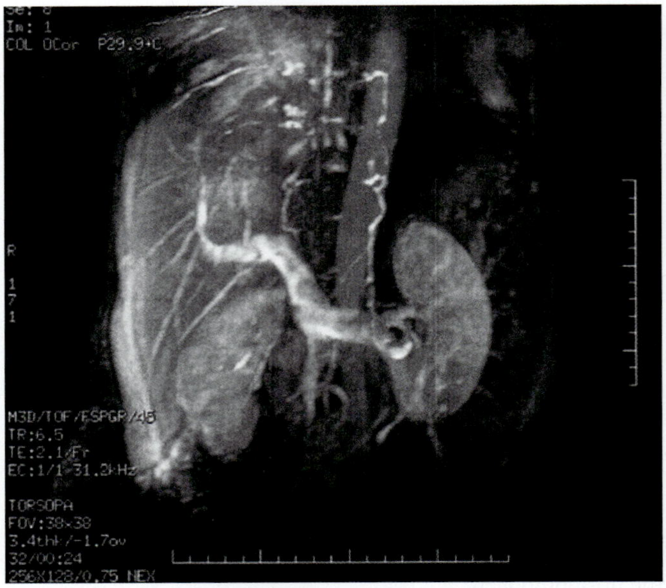

Figure 66.8 Magnetic resonance imaging (MRI) scan showing massive hepatosplenomegaly secondary to myelofibrosis. Note the prominent portal system and the left kidney, which is superimposed over the grossly enlarged spleen.

Myelofibrosis results from an abnormal proliferation of mesenchymal elements in the bone marrow, spleen, liver and lymph nodes. Most patients present over the age of 50 years, and the spleen may produce pain owing to its gross enlargement (Figure 66.8) or from splenic infarcts. Splenectomy reduces the need for transfusion and may relieve the discomfort resulting from the splenomegaly.

SPLENECTOMY

The common indications for splenectomy are:

- trauma resulting from an accident or during a surgical procedure, as for example during mobilisation of the oesophagus, stomach, distal pancreas or splenic flexure of the colon;
- removal en bloc with the stomach as part of a radical gastrectomy or with the pancreas as part of a distal or total pancreatectomy;
- to reduce anaemia or thrombocytopenia in spherocytosis, idiopathic thrombocytopenic purpura or hypersplenism;
- in association with shunt or variceal surgery for portal hypertension (Summary box 66.2).

Philippe Charles Ernest Gaucher, 1854–1918, physician, Hôpital St Louis, Paris, France, described familial splenic anaemia in 1882.
Augustus Roi Felty, 1895–1964, physician, Hartford Hospital, CT, USA, described this disease in 1924.

Summary box 66.2

Indications for splenectomy

- Trauma
  - Accidental
  - Operative
- Oncological
  - Part of en bloc resection
  - Diagnostic
  - Therapeutic
- Haematological
  - Spherocytosis
  - Purpura (ITP)
  - Hypersplenism
- Portal hypertension
  - Variceal surgery

Preoperative preparation

In the presence of a bleeding tendency, transfusion of blood, fresh-frozen plasma, cryoprecipitate or platelets may be required. Coagulation profiles should be as near normal as possible at operation, and platelets should be available for patients with thrombocytopenia at operation and in the early postoperative period.

Antibiotic prophylaxis appropriate to the operative procedure should be given and consideration should be given to the risk of post-splenectomy sepsis (see below under Postoperative complications).

Technique of open splenectomy

Most surgeons use a midline or transverse left subcostal incision for open splenectomy. Rarely, a thoracoabdominal incision may be necessary for a massive spleen that is adherent to the diaphragm. Passage of a nasogastric tube following induction of the anaesthetic enables the stomach to be emptied.

In elective splenectomy, the gastrosplenic ligament is opened up, and the short gastric vessels are divided. The splenic vessels at the superior border of the pancreas are suture-ligated. The posterior surface of the spleen is exposed, the posterior leaf of the lienorenal ligament divided with long curved scissors, and the spleen rotated medially along with the tail and body of the pancreas (Figure 66.9). The pancreas is separated from the hilar vessels, which are ligated and divided. Accessory splenic tissue in the splenic hilum or omentum should be excluded by a careful search at operation. There is no need to drain the wound if haemostasis is secured adequately.

The segmental vasculature of the spleen does make it possible to undertake limited resection of the parenchyma. Haemostasis can be achieved by ligation of, or application of, metal clips to intrasplenic vessels, and by careful application of topical haemostatic agents or mesh. Conservative splenic surgery is therefore possible in some cases of splenic trauma and other pathology, such as splenic cysts.

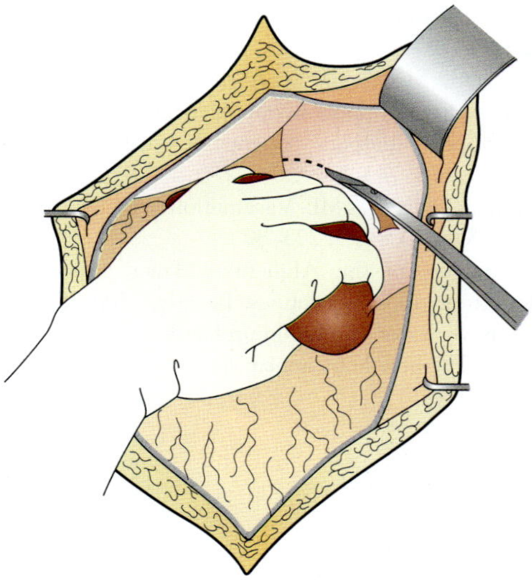

Figure 66.9 Diagrammatic view of the approach required to divide the short gastric vessels anteriorly and the lienorenal ligament posteriorly.

Technique of laparoscopic splenectomy

The patient is placed on the right side with the space between the left ilium and costal margin exposed. Placement of access ports is often determined by the size of the patient and the spleen. Insufflation of the abdomen can be performed once access is obtained through an incision 1 cm from the costal margin at the left mid-clavicular line. A further trocar is inserted close to the costal margin below the xiphoid. A 12-mm trocar is inserted at a similar distance from the costal margin at the posterior axillary line. The splenocolic ligament is divided to give access to the lower splenic pole. The spleen is separated from the kidney and diaphragm before the gap between the splenic hilum and the tail of the pancreas is enlarged. The spleen is elevated to expose the splenic hilum, which is secured and divided with an endoscopic vascular stapler (Figure 66.10). Two or three applications of the instrument may be required to secure the hilum and the short gastric vessels. Any remaining attachments to the diaphragm are divided before a self-retaining opening bag is introduced through the incision of the open laparoscopy after removal of the 12-mm port. The spleen is placed in the bag, the mouth of which is pulled out of the abdominal opening before the spleen is crushed and retrieved with an instrument. The operation may be undertaken as a hand-assisted procedure particularly when the spleen is grossly enlarged.

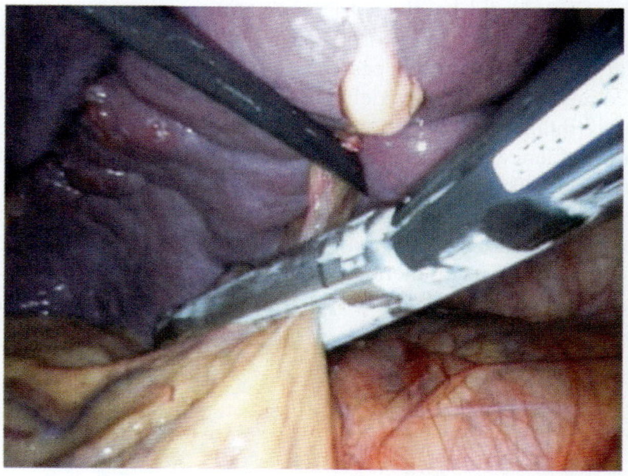

Figure 66.10 Photograph showing a stapling gun across the hilus of spleen for division of the splenic vessels during laparoscopic splenectomy.

Postoperative complications

Immediate complications specific to splenectomy include haemorrhage resulting from a slipped ligature. Haematemesis from gastric mucosal damage and gastric dilatation is uncommon. Left basal atelectasis is common, and a pleural effusion may be present. Adjacent structures at risk during the procedure include the stomach and pancreas. A fistula may result from damage to the greater curvature of the stomach during ligation of the short gastric vessels. Damage to the tail of the pancreas may result in pancreatitis, a localised abscess or a pancreatic fistula. Postoperative thrombocytosis may arise and, if the blood platelet count exceeds 1×10^6/mL, prophylactic aspirin is recommended to prevent axillary or other venous thrombosis.

Post-splenectomy septicaemia may result from *Streptococcus pneumoniae*, *Neisseria meningitides*, *Haemophilus influenzae* and *Escherichia coli*. The risk is greater in the young patient, in splenectomised patients treated with chemoradiotherapy and in patients who have undergone splenectomy for thalassaemia, sickle cell disease and autoimmune anaemia or thrombocytopenia.

Opportunist post-splenectomy infection (OPSI) is a major concern. Published guidelines emphasise that most infections after splenectomy could be avoided through measures that include offering patients appropriate and timely immunisation, antibiotic prophylaxis, education and prompt treatment of infection. The benefit of prophylactic antibiotics in this setting remains controversial. It is thought that children who have undergone splenectomy before the age of five years should be treated with a daily dose of penicillin until the age of ten years. Prophylaxis in older children should be continued at least until the age of 16 years, but its use is less well defined in adults. Furthermore, compliance is problematic in the long term but, as the risk of overwhelming sepsis is greatest within the first 2–3 years after splenectomy, it seems reasonable to give prophylaxis during this time. However, all patients with compromised immune function should receive prophylaxis. Satisfactory oral prophylaxis can be obtained with penicillin, erythromycin or amoxicillin, or co-amoxiclav. Suspected infection can be treated intravenously with these same antibiotics and cefotaxime, ceftriaxone or chloramphenicol in patients allergic to penicillin and cephalosporins. If elective splenectomy is planned, consideration should be given to vaccinating against pneumococcus, meningococcus C (both repeated every five years) and *H. influenza* type B (Hib) (repeated every ten years). The latter two vaccines are commonly delivered as a combined preparation. Yearly influenza vaccination has been recommended as there is some evidence that it may reduce the risk of secondary bacterial infection. Such vaccinations should be administered at least 2 weeks before elective surgery or as soon as possible after recovery from surgery but before discharge from hospital. Pneumococcal vaccination is recommended in those patients aged over two years. *Haemophilus influenzae* type b vaccination is recommended irrespective of age. Asplenic patients should carry a medical alert and an up-to-date vaccination card. They require specific advice regarding travel and animal handling. Patients who have undergone splenectomy and are travelling to countries where malaria is present are strongly advised to use all physical anti-mosquito barriers, as well as anti-malarial therapy, since they are at increased risk of severe malaria. Overwhelming post-splectomy sepsis due to *Capnocytophaga canimorsus* may result from dog, cat or other animal bites.

In the trauma victim, vaccination can be given in the postoperative period, and the resulting antibody levels will be protective in the majority of cases. Antibody levels are, however, less than 50 per cent of those achieved if vaccination is given in the presence of an intact spleen. Protection following vaccination is not always guaranteed (Summary box 66.3).

Summary box 66.3

Splenectomy

- Remember preoperative immunisation
- Prophylactic antibiotics in the long term
- OPSI is a real clinical danger
- Splenic conservation should be considered

The spleen dislikes, distrusts and devours spheroidal red cells.
Arthur Rendle Short 1880–1953

Professor of Surgery, University of Bristol, UK

FURTHER READING

Bisharat N, Omari H, Lavi I, Raz R. Risk of infection and death among post-splenectomy patients. *J Infect* 2001; **43**: 182–6.

Davies JM, Barnes R, Milligan D. Update of guidelines for the prevention and treatment of infection in patients with an absent or dysfunctional spleen. *Clin Med* 2002; **2**: 440–3.

Di Sabatino A, Carsetti R, Corazza GR. Post-splenectomy and hyposplenic states. *Lancet* 2011; **378**: 86–97.

Glasgow RE, Mulvihill SJ. Laparoscopic splenectomy. *World J Surg* 1999; **23**: 384–8.

Mourtzoukou EG, Mikhael J, Northridge K *et al.* Short-term and long-term failure of laparoscopicsplenectomy in adult immune thrombocytopenic purpura patients: a systematic review. *Am J Hematol* 2009; **84**: 743–8.

Pappas G, Peppas G, Falagas ME. Vaccination of asplenic or hyposplenic adults. *Br J Surg* 2008; **95**: 273–80.

Society for Surgery of the Alimentary Tract. Prophylaxis against postsplenectomy sepsis guidelines. Beverly, MA: SSAT. Available online from www.ssat.com/cgi-bin/spleen7.cgi.

Weatherall DJ. The hereditary anaemias. *Br Med J* 1997; **314**: 492–6

Albert Ludwig Siegmund Neisser, 1855–1916, Director of the Dermatological Institute, Breslau, Germany (now Wroclaw, Poland).
Theodor Escherich, 1857–1911, Professor of Paediatrics, Austria, Vienna.

CHAPTER 67

The gall bladder and bile ducts

LEARNING OBJECTIVES

- To understand the anatomy and physiology of the gall bladder and bile ducts
- To be familiar with the pathophysiology and management of gallstones
- To be aware of unusual disorders of the biliary tree
- To be aware of malignant disease of the gall bladder and bile ducts

SURGICAL ANATOMY AND PHYSIOLOGY

The gall bladder lies on the underside of the liver in the main liver scissura at the junction of the right and left lobes of the liver. The relationship of the gall bladder to the liver varies between being embedded within the liver substance to being suspended by a mesentry. It is a pear-shaped structure, 7.5–12 cm long, with a normal capacity of about 25–30 mL. The anatomical divisions are a fundus, a body and a neck that terminates in a narrow infundibulum. The muscle fibres in the wall of the gall bladder are arranged in a criss-cross manner, being particularly well developed in its neck. The mucous membrane contains indentations of the mucosa that sink into the muscle coat; these are the crypts of Luschka.

The cystic duct is about 3 cm in length, but the length is variable. The lumen is usually 1–3 mm in diameter. The mucosa of the cystic duct is arranged in spiral folds known as the 'valves of Heister' and the wall is surrounded by a sphincteric structure called the 'sphincter of Lütkens'. The cystic duct joins the supraduodenal segment of the common hepatic duct in 80 per cent of cases; however, the anatomy may vary and the junction may be much lower in the retroduodenal or even retropancreatic part of the bile duct. Occasionally, the cystic duct may join the right hepatic duct or even a right hepatic sectorial duct (see below).

The common hepatic duct is usually less than 2.5 cm long and is formed by the union of the right and left hepatic ducts. The common bile duct is about 7.5 cm long and formed by the junction of the cystic and common hepatic ducts. It is divided into four parts:

- **Supraduodenal portion**. About 2.5 cm long, running in the free edge of the lesser omentum.
- **Retroduodenal portion**.
- **Infraduodenal portion** lies in a groove, but at times in a tunnel, on the posterior surface of the pancreas.
- **Intraduodenal portion** passes obliquely through the wall of the second part of the duodenum, where it is surrounded by the sphincter of Oddi, and terminates by opening on the summit of the ampulla of Vater.

The cystic artery, a branch of the right hepatic artery, usually arises behind the common hepatic duct (Figure 67.1).

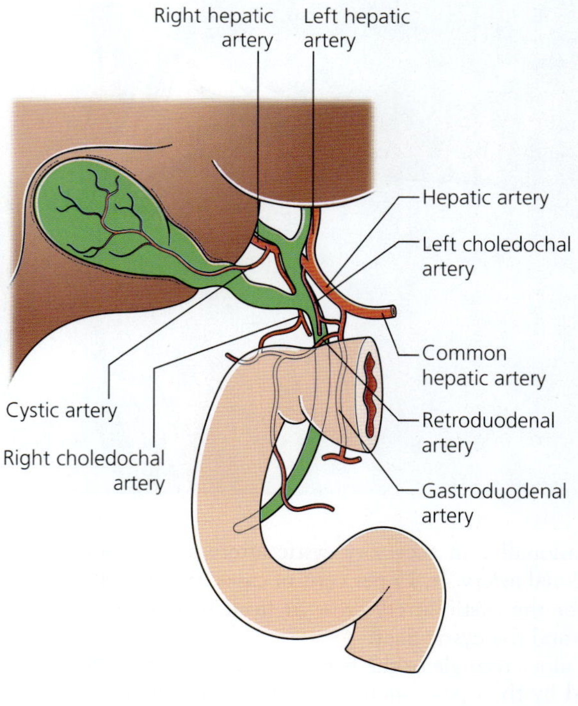

Figure 67.1 The anatomy of the gall bladder and bile ducts. Note the arrangement of the arterial tree.

Hubert Luschka, 1820–1875, Professor of Anatomy, Tübingen, Germany.
Lorenz Heister, 1683–1758, Professor of Surgery and Botany, Helmstädt, Germany.
Ruggero Oddi, 1864–1913, physiologist, Perugia, Italy.
Abraham Vater, 1684–1751, Professor of Anatomy and Botany, Wittenberg, Germany.

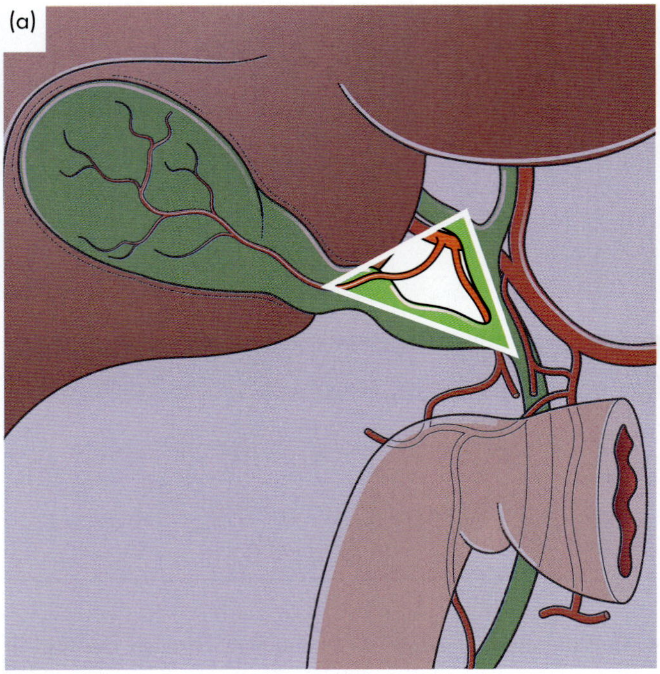

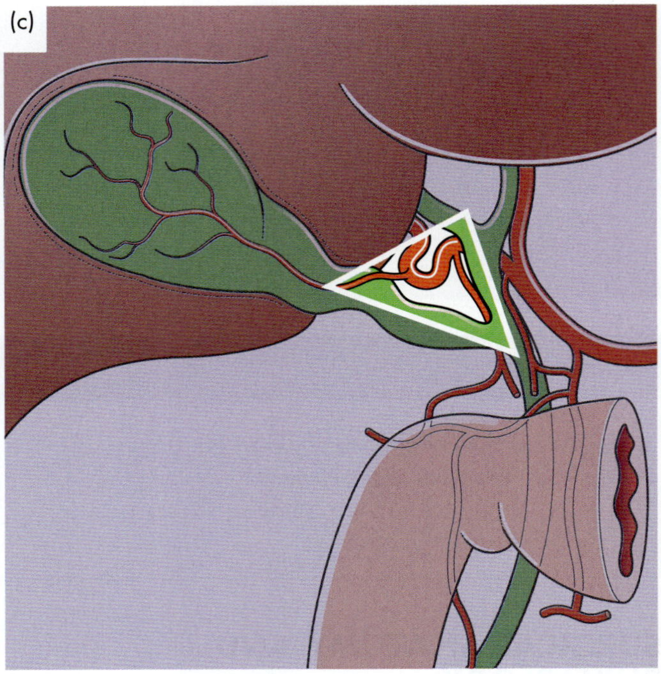

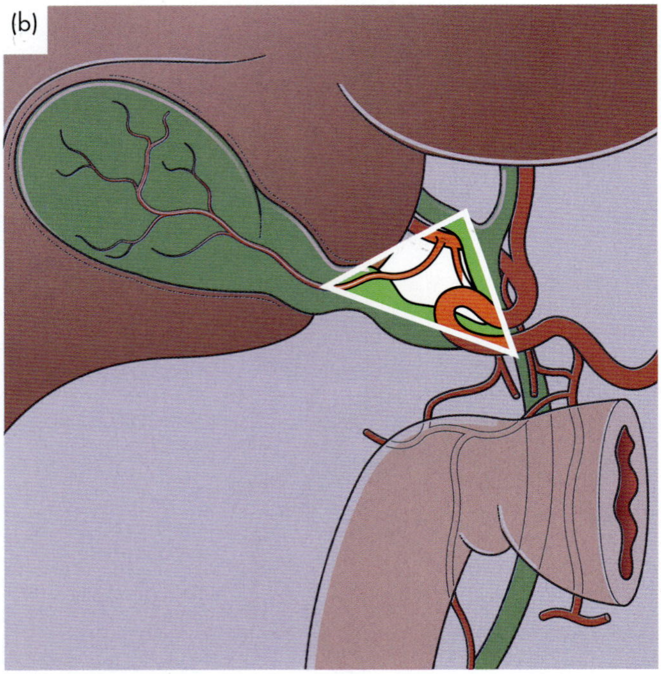

Figure 67.2 (a) Usual anatomy of Calot's triangle; (b) tortuous common hepatic artery; (c) tortuous right hepatic artery with short cystic aterery; (b) and (c) are examples of so-called 'caterpillar turn' or 'Moynihan's hump' which if not recognised can lead to inadvertent arterial injury or bleeding during cholecystectomy.

Occasionally, an accessory cystic artery arises from the gastroduodenal artery. In 15 per cent of cases, the right hepatic artery and/or the cystic artery cross in front of the common hepatic duct and the cystic duct.

Calot's triangle or the hepatobiliary triangle is the space bordered by the cystic duct inferiorly, the common hepatic artery medially and the superior border of the cystic artery. This was described in 1891 by Jean-François Calot. It is an important surgical landmark and should be identified by surgeons performing a cholecystectomy to avoid damage to the extrahepatic biliary system (Figure 67.2a).

The most dangerous anomalies are where the hepatic artery takes a tortuous course on the front of the origin of the cystic duct (Figure 67.2b), or the right hepatic artery is tortuous and the cystic artery short (Figure 67.2c). The tortuosity is known as the 'caterpillar turn' or 'Moynihan's hump'. This variation is the cause of many problems during a difficult cholecystectomy with inflammation in the region of the cystic duct.

Lymphatics

The lymphatic vessels of the gall bladder (subserosal and submucosal) drain into the cystic lymph node of Lund (the sentinel lymph node), which lies in the fork created by the junction of the cystic and common hepatic ducts. Efferent vessels from this lymph node go to the hilum of the liver, and to the coeliac lymph nodes. The subserosal lymphatic vessels of the gall bladder also connect with the subcapsular lymph channels of the liver, and this accounts for the frequent spread of carcinoma of the gall bladder to the liver.

Surgical physiology

Bile is produced by the liver and stored in the gall bladder from which it is released into the duodenum. As it leaves the liver, it is composed of 97 per cent water, bile salts (cholic and cheno-

Berkeley George Andre Moynihan, (Lord Moynihan of Leeds), 1865–1936, Professor of Clinical Surgery, University of Leeds, UK. Moynihan felt that English surgeons knew little about the work of their colleagues both at home and abroad. Therefore, in 1909, he established a small travelling club which, in 1929, became the Moynihan Chirurgical Club. It still exists. He took a leading part in founding the British Journal of Surgery in 1913 and became the first chairman of the editorial committee until his death.

Jean-François Calot, 1861–1944, surgeon, Paris, France.
Fred Bates Lund, 1865–1950, surgeon, Boston City Hospital, Boston, MA, USA.

deoxycholic acids, deoxycholic and lithocholic acids), phospholipids, cholesterol and bilirubin. The liver excretes bile at a rate estimated to be approximately 40 mL/hour. About 95 per cent of bile salts are reabsorbed in the terminal ileum (enterohepatic circulation).

FUNCTIONS OF THE GALL BLADDER

The gall bladder is a reservoir for bile. During fasting, resistance to flow through the sphincter of Oddi is high, and bile excreted by the liver is diverted to the gall bladder. After feeding, the resistance to flow through the sphincter is reduced, the gall bladder contracts and the bile enters the duodenum. These motor responses of the biliary tract are in part effected by the hormone cholecystokinin.

The second function of the gall bladder is concentration of bile by active absorption of water, sodium chloride and bicarbonate by the mucous membrane of the gall bladder. The hepatic bile which enters the gall bladder becomes concentrated 5–10 times, with a corresponding increase in the proportion of bile salts, bile pigments, cholesterol and calcium.

The third function of the gall bladder is the secretion of mucus – approximately 20 mL is produced per day. With complete obstruction of the cystic duct in an otherwise healthy gall bladder, a mucocoele may develop as a result of ongoing mucus secretion by the gall bladder mucosa.

RADIOLOGICAL INVESTIGATION OF THE BILIARY TRACT

Plain x-rays

The skillfully taken plain x-ray of the gall bladder will show radiopaque gallstones in 10 per cent of patients (Figure 67.3). Rarely, the centre of a stone may contain radiolucent gas in a

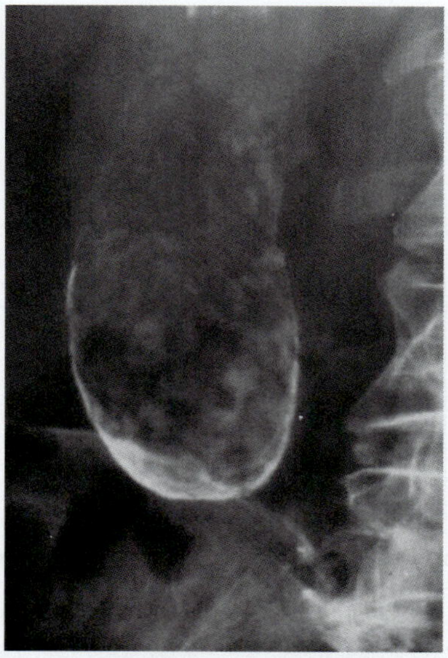

Figure 67.4 Porcelain gall bladder.

triradiate or biradiate fissure and this gives rise to characteristic dark shapes on a radiograph – the 'Mercedes–Benz' or 'seagull' sign.

A plain x-ray may also show the rare cases of calcification of the gall bladder, a so-called 'porcelain' gall bladder (Figure 67.4). Today, this is more commonly seen on computed tomography (CT) scan (Figure 67.5). The importance of this appearance is that it is associated with carcinoma in up to 25 per cent of cases and is an indication for cholecystectomy. Gas may be seen in the wall of the gall bladder (emphysematous cholecystitis) (Figure 67.6). Gas in the biliary tree may be seen after endoscopic sphincterotomy or surgical anastomosis.

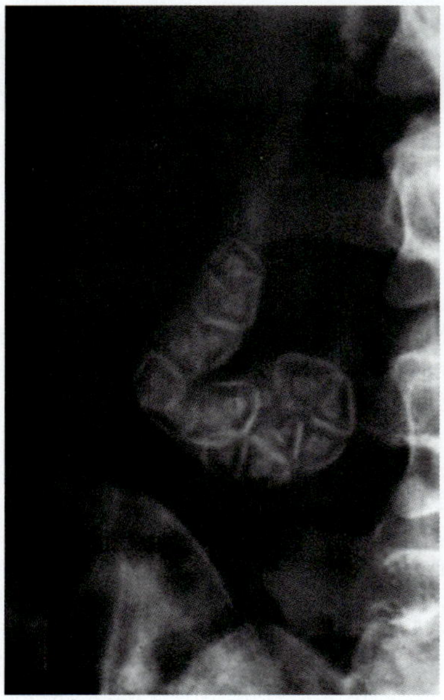

Figure 67.3 Plain radiograph showing radiopaque stones in the gall bladder. Radiopaque stones are rare (10 per cent).

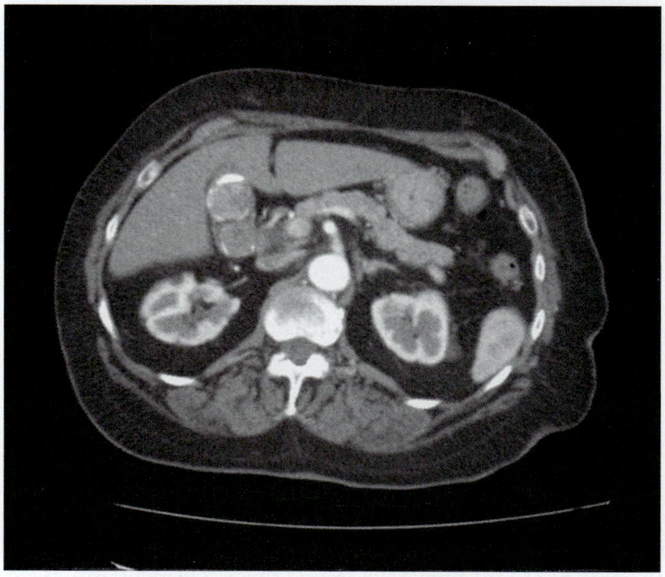

Figure 67.5 Computed tomography scan demonstrating calcification in the gall bladder wall ('porcelain gall bladder').

Mercedes–Benz sign, takes its name from the insignia displayed on the bonnet of a Mercedes–Benz car.

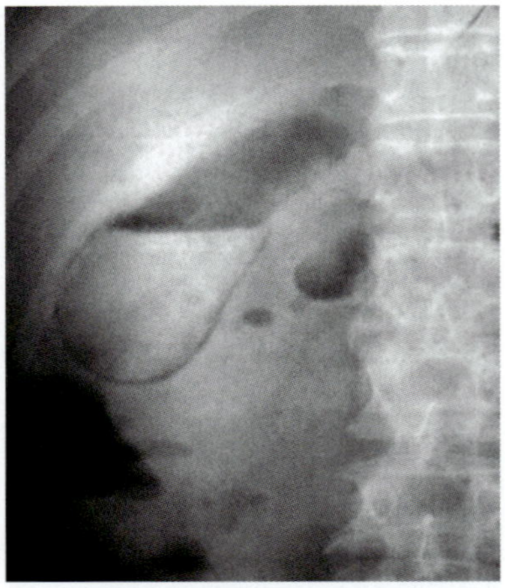

Figure 67.6 Gas in the gall bladder and gall bladder wall (*Clostridium perfringens*). Emergency surgery is indicated.

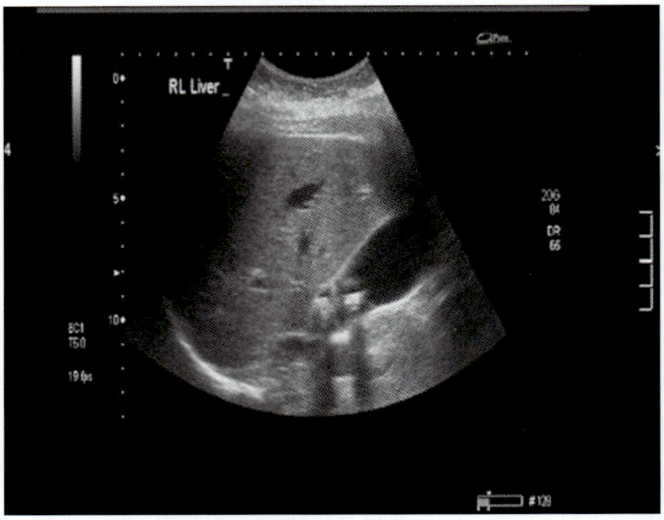

Figure 67.8 Ultrasound examination. Gallstones noted at the neck of the gall bladder with associated acoustic shadowing.

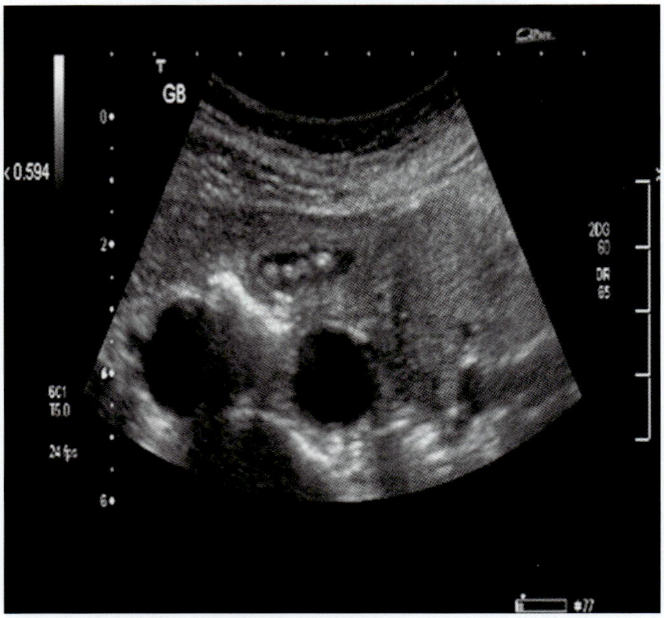

Figure 67.7 Ultrasound examination. Multiple gallstones noted within the gall bladder.

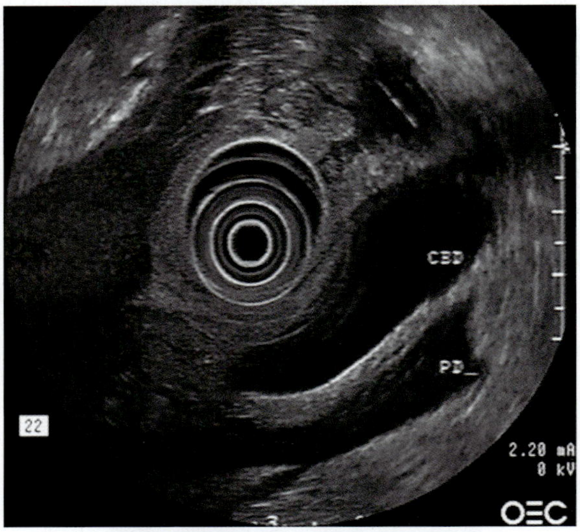

Figure 67.9 Endoscopic ultrasonography. CBD, common bile duct; PD, pancreatic duct.

Oral cholecystography and intravenous cholangiography

Oral and intravenous cholecystography are of interest for historical purposes only, as they were relatively inaccurate and have been replaced by more accurate imaging modalities.

Ultrasonography

Transabdominal ultrasonography (Figures 67.7 and 67.8) is the initial imaging modality of choice as it is accurate, readily available, inexpensive and quick to perform. However, it is operator dependent and may be suboptimal due to excessive body fat and intraluminal bowel gas. It can demonstrate biliary calculi, the size of the gall bladder, the thickness of the gall bladder wall, the presence of inflammation around the gall bladder, the size of the common bile duct and, occasionally, the presence of stones within the biliary tree.

In the patient who presents with obstructive jaundice, ultrasonography is particularly helpful as it can identify intra- and extrahepatic biliary dilation and often the level of obstruction. In addition, the cause of the obstruction may also be identified, such as gallstones in the gall bladder, common hepatic or common bile duct stones or lesions in the wall of the common bile duct suggestive of a cholangiocarcinoma or enlargement of the pancreatic head indicative of a pancreatic carcinoma.

Endoscopic ultrasonography utilises a specially designed endoscope with an ultrasound transducer at its tip which allows the gastroenterologist to visualise the liver and biliary tree from within the stomach and duodenum (Figure 67.9). It is an accurate technique to determine the presence of stones in the common bile duct. In addition, it has been shown to be highly accurate in diagnosing and staging both pancreatic and periampullary cancers.

Radioisotope scanning

Technetium-99m (^{99m}Tc)-labelled derivatives of iminodiacetic acid (HIDA, IODIDA) when injected intravenously are selectively taken up by the retroendothelial cells of the liver and excreted into the bile. This allows for visualisation of the biliary tree and gall bladder. In 90 per cent of normal individuals the gall bladder is visualised within 30 minutes following injection with 100 per cent being seen within 1 hour (Figure 67.10). The bowel is seen usually within 1 hour in the majority of patients. Non-visualisation of the gall bladder is suggestive of acute cholecystitis. If the patient has a contracted gall bladder as often seen in chronic cholecystitis, the gall bladder visualisation may be reduced or delayed.

Biliary scintigraphy may also be helpful in diagnosing bile leaks and iatrogenic biliary obstruction. When there is a suspicion of a bile leak following a cholecystectomy, radioisotope imaging should be one of the initial investigations performed. It can identify and quantitate the leak thus helping the surgeon determine whether or not an operative or conservative approach is warranted. If available, endoscopic retrograde cholangiopancreatography (ERCP) should be considered as this is both diagnostic and potentially therapeutic. The most common bile leak following cholecystectomy is from the cystic duct. This can be treated by the gastroenterologist placing a biliary endoprosthesis (stent) in the common bile duct across the origin of the cystic duct.

Computed tomography

Unlike ultrasonography, CT is less affected by body habitus and is not operator dependent. It allows visualisation of the liver, bile ducts, gall bladder and pancreas (Figure 67.11) and is particularly useful in detecting hepatic and pancreatic lesions and is the modality of choice in the staging of cancers of the liver, gall bladder, bile ducts and pancreas. It can identify the extent of the primary tumour and defines its relationship to other organs and blood vessels (Figure 67.12). In addition, the presence of enlarged lymph nodes or metastatic disease can be seen.

Improvements in CT technology, such as multidetector scanners, which allow for three-dimensional reconstruction of the biliary tree have led to greater diagnostic accuracy and have increased the accuracy of CT in assessing benign disease.

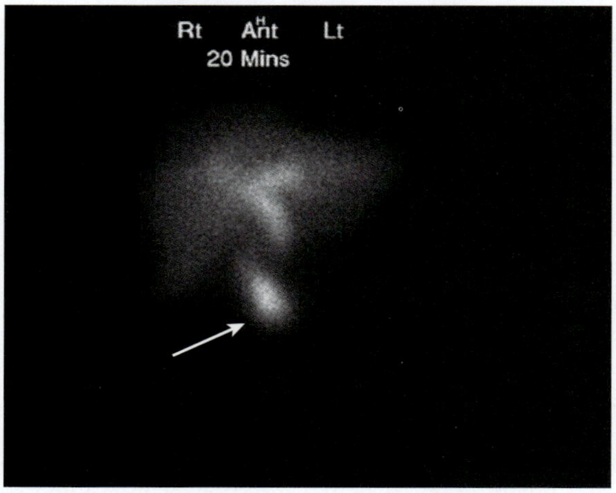

Figure 67.10 Dimethyl iminodiacetic acid (HIDA) scan.

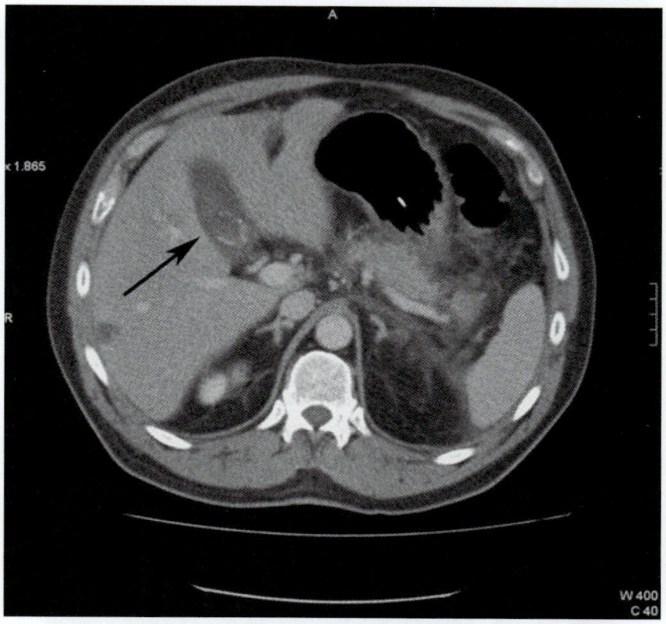

Figure 67.11 Computed tomography scan demonstrating a gallstone within the gall bladder (arrowed).

Magnetic resonance cholangiopancreatography

Magnetic resonance cholangiopancreatography (MRCP) is an imaging technique based on the principles of nuclear magnetic resonance used to image the gall bladder and biliary system. It is non-invasive and can provide either cross-sectional or projection images (Figures 67.13 and 67.14). Excellent images can be obtained of the biliary tree demonstrating ductal obstruction, strictures or other intraductal abnormalities. Images comparable to those obtained at ERCP or percutaneous transhepatic cholangiography (PTC) can be achieved non-invasively without the potential complications of either technique.

Endoscopic retrograde cholangiopancreatography

This technique remains widely used as both a diagnostic and therapeutic modality. Using a side-viewing endoscope the ampulla of Vater can be identified and cannulated. Injection

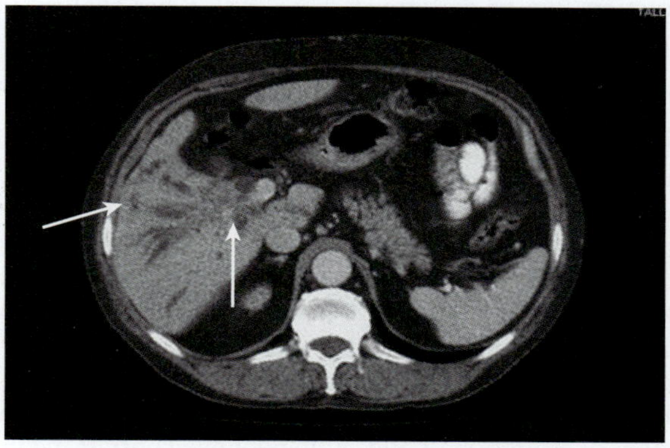

Figure 67.12 Computed tomography scan demonstrating a hilar mass.

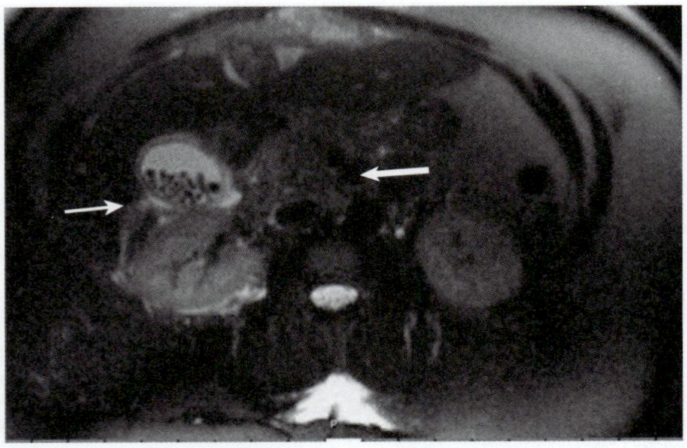

Figure 67.13 Magnetic resonance cholangiopancreatography cross-sectional image demonstrating a hilar mass (thick arrow) and gallstones (thin arrow).

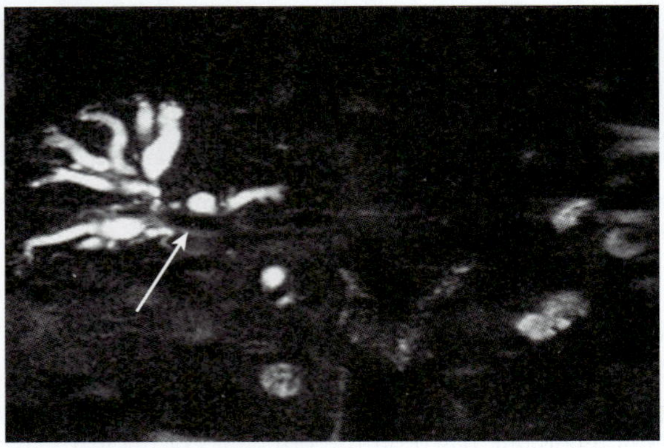

Figure 67.14 Magnetic resonance cholangiopancreatography demonstrating hilar obstruction (arrow). Same case as seen in Figure 67.12.

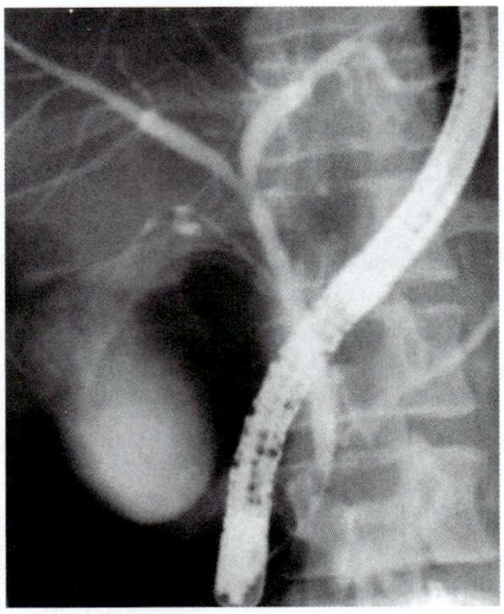

Figure 67.15 Endoscopic retrograde cholangiopancreatography: normal cholangiogram.

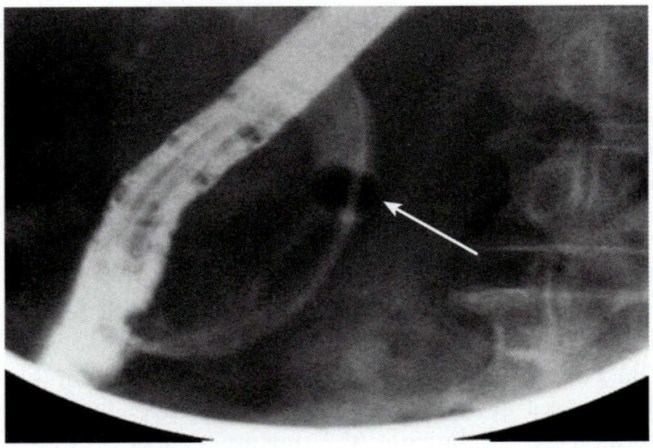

Figure 67.16 Endoscopic retrograde cholangiopancreatography showing common duct obstruction due to a stone (arrow).

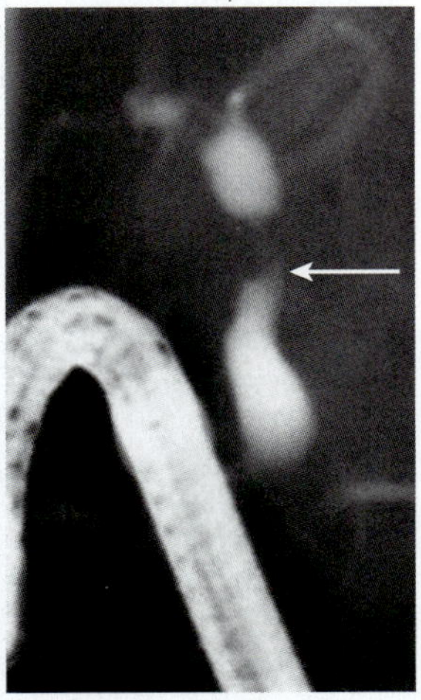

Figure 67.17 Endoscopic retrograde cholangiopancreatography: partial occlusion of the bile duct by a malignant stricture (arrow).

of water-soluble contrast directly into the bile duct provides excellent images of the ductal anatomy (Figure 67.15) and can identify causes of obstruction, such as calculi (Figure 67.16) or malignant strictures (Figure 67. 17). While the widespread availability of ultrasound and MRCP has reduced its diagnostic use, ERCP still has a real role in the assessment of the patient with obstructive jaundice. In this group of patients, it is especially useful in determining the cause and level of obstruction.

During ERCP, bile aspirates can be sent for cytological and microbiological examination, and endoluminal brushings can be taken from strictures for cytological studies. Therapeutic interventions, such as stone removal or stent placement to relieve the obstruction, can be performed. Thus, ERCP has evolved into a mainly therapeutic rather than a diagnostic technique.

Percutaneous transhepatic cholangiography

This is an invasive technique in which the bile ducts are cannulated directly. It is only undertaken once a bleeding tendency has been excluded and the patient's prothrombin time is normal. Antibiotics should be given prior to the procedure. Usually, under fluoroscopic control, a needle (the Chiba or Okuda needle) is introduced percutaneously into the liver substance. Under radiological control (either ultrasound or CT), a bile duct is cannulated. Successful entry is confirmed by contrast injection or aspiration of bile. Water-soluble contrast medium is injected to demonstrate the biliary system. Multiple images can be taken demonstrating areas of strictures or obstruction (Figure 67.18). Bile can be sent for cytology. In addition, this technique enables placement of a catheter into the bile ducts to provide external biliary drainage or the insertion of indwelling stents. The scope of this procedure can be further extended by leaving

Evarts Ambrose Graham, 1883–1957, Bixby Professor of Surgery, Washington University, St Louis, MO, USA.
Warren Henry Cole, 1898–1990, Emeritus Professor of Surgery, University of Illinois, Chicago, IL, USA. Introduced cholecystography in 1924.
Kunio Okuda, 1921–2003, Professor of Medicine, Chiba University, Japan.

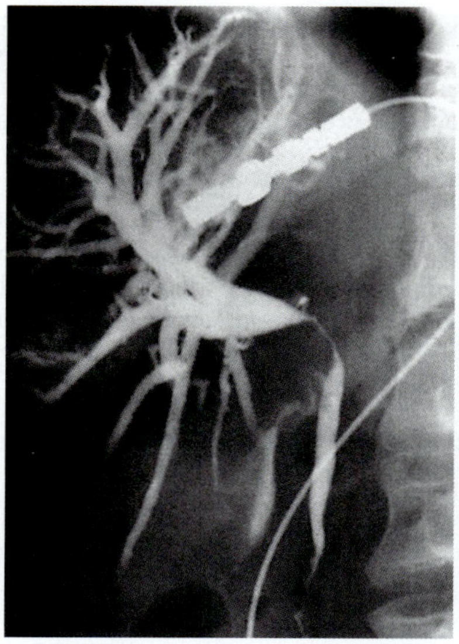

Figure 67.18 Transhepatic cholangiogram showing a stricture of the common hepatic duct (courtesy of Miss Phyllis George, FRCS, London, UK).

the drainage catheter *in situ* for a number of days and then dilating the track sufficiently for a fine flexible choledochoscope to be passed into the intrahepatic biliary tree in order to diagnose strictures, take biopsies and remove stones.

In general, if a malignant stricture at the level of the confluence of the right and left hepatic ducts or higher is suspected in a jaundiced patient, a PTC is preferred to ERCP as successful drainage is more likely (Summary box 67.1).

Summary box 67.1

Investigation of the biliary tree

- Ultrasound: stones and biliary dilation
- Plain radiograph: calcification
- MRCP: anatomy and stones
- MDR-CT scan: anatomy liver, gall bladder and pancreas cancer
- Radioisotope scanning (HIDA scan): function
- ERCP: anatomy, stones and biliary strictures
- PTC: anatomy and biliary strictures
- Endoscopic ultrasound (EUS): anatomy, stones

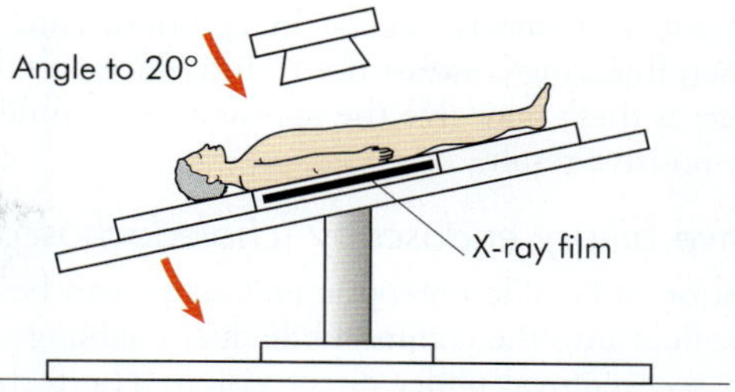

Figure 67.19 Preoperative cholangiography using a radiolucent table-top.

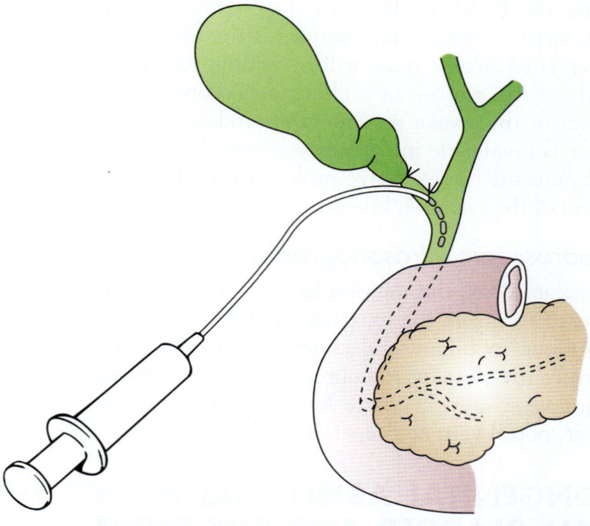

Figure 67.20 Peroperative cholangiography. Technique of introducing contrast.

Intraoperative imaging techniques

Peroperative cholangiography

During open or laparoscopic cholecystectomy, a catheter can be placed in the cystic duct and contrast injected directly into the biliary tree. The technique defines the anatomy and in the main is used to exclude the presence of stones within the bile ducts (Figures 67.19, 67.20 and 67.21). A single x-ray plate or image intensifier can be used to obtain and review the images intraoperatively. Irrespective of the technique used, the operating table should be tilted head down approximately 20° to facilitate

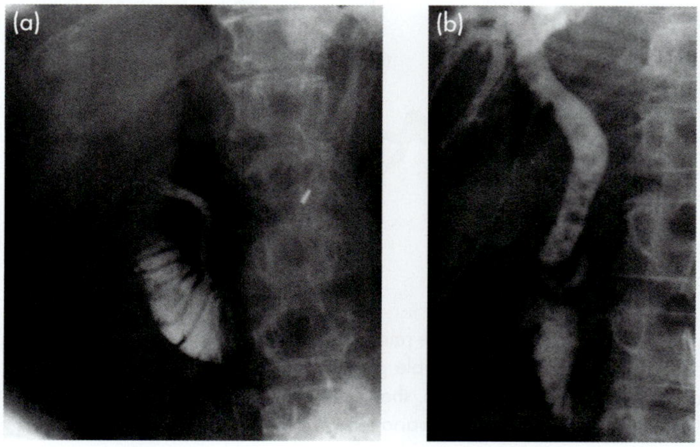

Figure 67.21 Peroperative cholangiography. (a) Normal common bile duct: gentle infusion of contrast which passes without hindrance into the duodenum. (b) The common bile duct is dilated with multiple stones. Contrast is seen to reflux into the pancreatic duct. A sphincterotomy was performed.

filling of the intrahepatic ducts. In addition, care should be taken when injecting contrast not to introduce air bubbles into the system as these may give the appearance of stones and lead to a false-positive result.

Operative biliary endoscopy (choledochoscopy)

At operation, a flexible fibreoptic endoscope can be passed via the cystic duct into the common bile duct enabling stone identification and removal under direct vision. The technique can be combined with an x-ray image intensifier to ensure complete clearance of the biliary tree. After exploration of the bile duct, a tube can be left in the cystic duct remnant or in the common bile duct (a T-tube) and drainage of the biliary tree established. After 7–10 days, a track will be established. This track can be used for the passage of a choledochoscope to remove residual stones in the awake patient in an endoscopy suite. This technique is invaluable in the management of difficult stone disease and prevents the excessive prolongation of an operative exploration of the common bile duct.

Laparoscopic ultrasonography

At laparoscopy, the use of a laparoscopic ultrasound probe can be used to image the extrahepatic biliary system. It is a useful technique in biliary and pancreatic tumour staging as it can identify the primary tumour and determine its relationship to major vessels, such as the hepatic artery, superior mesenteric artery, portal vein and superior mesenteric vein.

CONGENITAL ABNORMALITIES OF THE GALL BLADDER AND BILE DUCTS

Embryology

The hepatic diverticulum arises from the ventral wall of the foregut and elongates into a stalk to form the choledochus. A lateral bud is given off, which is destined to become the gall bladder and cystic duct. The embryonic hepatic duct sends out many branches which join up the canaliculi between the liver cells. As is usual with embryonic tubular structures, hyperplasia obliterates the lumina of this ductal system; normally, recanalisation subsequently occurs and bile begins to flow. During early fetal life, the gall bladder is entirely intrahepatic.

Absence of the gall bladder

Occasionally, the gall bladder is absent. Failure to visualise the gall bladder is not necessarily a pathological problem.

The Phrygian cap

The Phrygian cap (Figure 67.22) is present in 2–6 per cent of cholecystograms and may be mistaken for a pathological deformity of the organ. 'Phrygian cap' refers to hats worn by the people of Phrygia, an ancient country of Asia Minor; it was rather like a liberté cap of the French Revolution.

Floating gall bladder

The gall bladder may hang on a mesentery, which makes it liable to undergo torsion.

Absence of the cystic duct

This is usually a pathological, as opposed to an anatomical, anomaly and indicates the recent passage of a stone or the presence of a stone at the lower end of the cystic duct, which is ulcerating into the common bile duct. The main danger at surgery is damage to the bile duct, and particular care to identify the correct anatomy is essential before division of any duct.

Low insertion of the cystic duct

The cystic duct opens into the common bile duct near the ampulla. All variations of this anomaly can occur (Figure 67.23). At operation, they are not important. Dissection of a cystic duct which is inserted low in the bile duct should be avoided, as removal will damage the blood supply to the common bile duct and can lead to stricture formation.

An accessory cholecystohepatic duct

Ducts passing directly into the gall bladder from the liver are not uncommon. Larger ducts should be closed, but before doing so the precise anatomy should be carefully ascertained to ensure a right hepatic duct is not being ligated (Figure 67.23).

EXTRAHEPATIC BILIARY ATRESIA

Aetiology and physiology

Atresia is present in approximately 1 per 12 000 live births, and affects males and females equally. The extrahepatic bile

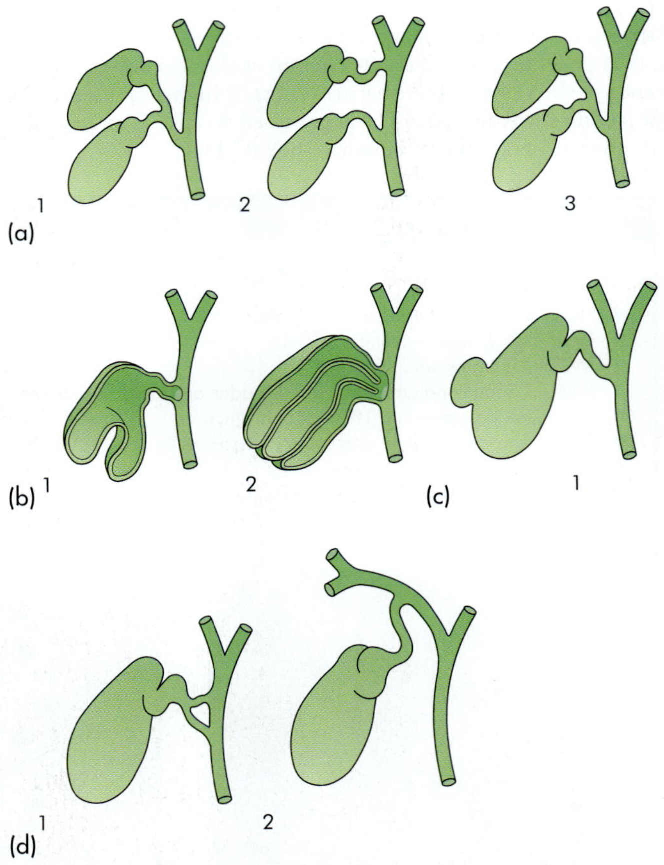

Figure 67.22 The main variations in gall bladder and cystic duct anatomy. (a) Double gall bladder; (b) septum of the gall bladder; 1 is the most common, the so-called 'Phrygian cap'; (c) diverticulum of the gall bladder; (d) variations in cystic duct insertion.

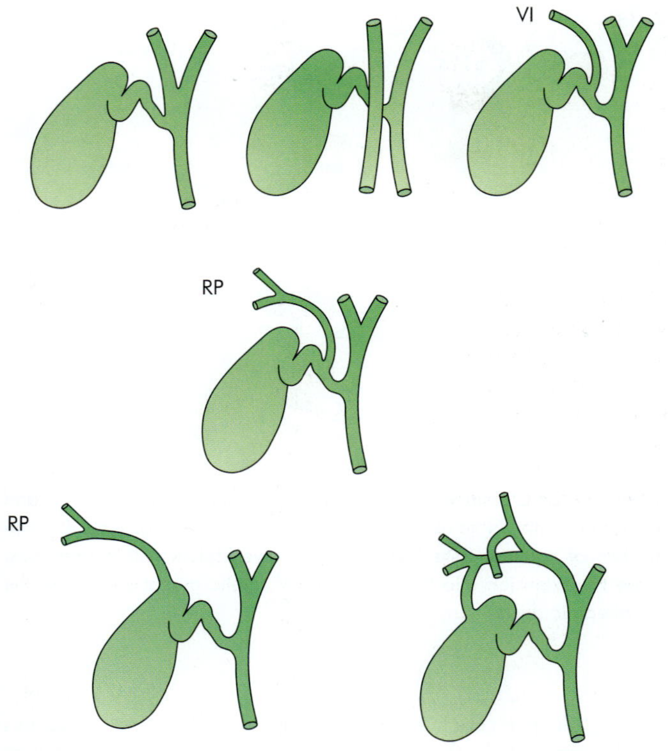

Figure 67.23 Patterns of cystic duct anatomy – note segment VI drainage into the cystic duct and the drainage of the right posterior (RP) sectorial duct into the neck of the gall bladder, or an accessory duct, the so-called duct of Luschka.

ducts are progressively destroyed by an inflammatory process which starts around the time of birth. The aetiology is unclear. Intrahepatic changes also occur and eventually result in biliary cirrhosis and portal hypertension. Untreated, death from the consequences of liver failure occurs before the age of three years.

The inflammatory destruction of the bile ducts has been classified into three main types (Figure 67.24):

- type I: atresia restricted to the common bile duct;
- type II: atresia of the common hepatic duct;
- type III: atresia of the right and left hepatic ducts.

In about 20 per cent of cases, associated anomalies include cardiac lesions, polysplenia, situs inversus, absent vena cava and a preduodenal portal vein.

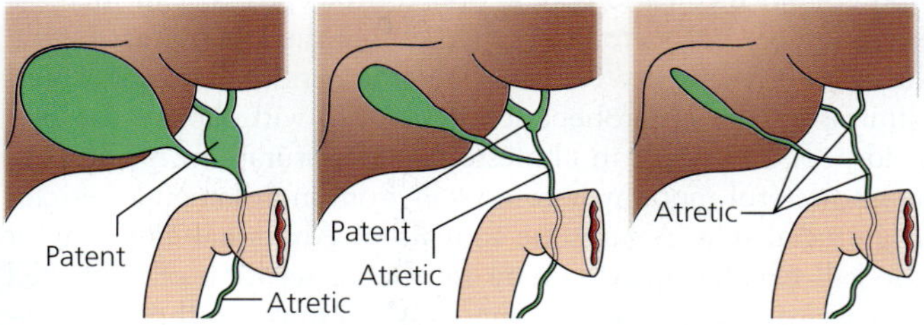

Figure 67.24 Classification of biliary atresia. Gall bladder filling provides a clue to the type of atresia.

Clinical features

About one-third of patients are jaundiced at birth. In all, however, jaundice is present by the end of the first week and deepens progressively. Liver function tests show an obstructive pattern with elevated bilirubin and alkaline phosphatase. The meconium may be a little bile stained, but later the stools are pale and the urine is dark. Prolonged steatorrhoea gives rise to osteomalacia (biliary rickets). Pruritus is severe. Clubbing and skin xanthomas, probably related to a raised serum cholesterol, may be present.

Differential diagnosis

This includes any form of jaundice in a neonate giving a cholestatic picture. Examples are alpha$_1$-antitrypsin deficiency, cholestasis associated with intravenous feeding, choledochal cyst and inspissated bile syndrome. Neonatal hepatitis is the most difficult to differentiate. Both extrahepatic biliary atresia and neonatal hepatitis are associated with giant cell transformation of the hepatocytes. Liver biopsy and radionuclide excretion scans are essential.

Treatment

Patent segments of proximal bile duct are found in 10 per cent of type I lesions. A direct Roux-en-Y hepaticojejunostomy will achieve bile flow in 75 per cent, but progressive fibrosis results in disappointing long-term results. A simple biliary-enteric anatomosis is not possible in the majority of cases in which the proximal hepatic ducts are either very small (type II) or atretic (type III). These are treated by the Kasai procedure, in which radical excision of all bile duct tissue up to the liver capsule is performed. A Roux-en-Y loop of jejunum is anastomosed to the exposed area of liver capsule above the bifurcation of the portal vein creating a portoenterostomy. The chances of achieving effective bile drainage after portoenterostomy are maximal when the operation is performed before the age of 8 weeks, and approximately 90 per cent of children whose bilirubin falls to within the normal range can be expected to survive for ten years or more. Early referral for surgery is critical.

Postoperative complications include bacterial cholangitis, which occurs in 40 per cent of patients. Repeated attacks lead to hepatic fibrosis and 50 per cent of long-term survivors develop portal hypertension, with one-third having variceal bleeding.

Liver transplantation should be considered in children in whom a portoenterostomy is unsuccessful. Results are improving with 70–80 per cent alive two to five years following transplant.

CONGENITAL DILATATION OF THE INTRAHEPATIC DUCTS (CAROLI'S DISEASE)

This rare condition is characterised by multiple irregular saccular dilatations of the intrahepatic ducts separated by segments of normal or stenotic ducts with a normal extrahepatic biliary system. The aetiology is unknown, but it is considered to be hereditary. It can be divided into a simple and periportal fibrotic type. The periportal fibrotic type presents in childhood and is associated with biliary stasis, stone formation and cholangitis, whereas the simple type presents later with episodes of

Morio Kasai, 1922–2008, Professor of Surgery, Tokyo University, Japan, described his operation in 1955.

abdominal pain and biliary sepsis. Associated conditions include congenital hepatic fibrosis, polycystic liver and, rarely, cholangiocarcinoma. The mainstays of treatment are antibiotics for the cholangitis and the removal of calculi. As the condition can be limited to one lobe of the liver, lobectomy may be indicated.

Choledochal cyst

Cystic disease of the biliary system is rare. Choledochal cysts are congenital dilations of the intra- and/or extrahepatic biliary system. The pathogenesis is unclear. Anomalous junctions of the biliary pancreatic junction are frequently observed, but whether or not these play a role in the pathogenesis of the condition is unclear. Todani and colleagues proposed a classification of cystic disease of the biliary tract (Figure 67.25). Type I cysts are the most common and account for approximately 75 per cent of patients.

Patients may present at any age with jaundice, fever, abdominal pain and a right upper quadrant mass on examination, however, 60 per cent of cases are diagnosed before the age of ten years. Pancreatitis is not an infrequent presentation in adults. Patients with choledochal cysts have an increased risk of developing cholangiocarcinoma with the risk varying directly with the age at diagnosis.

Ultrasonography will confirm the presence of an abnormal cyst and magnetic resonance imaging (MRI/MRCP) will reveal the anatomy, in particular the relationship between the lower end of the bile duct and the pancreatic duct. CT is also useful for delineating the extent of the intra- or extrahepatic dilation.

Radical excision of the cyst is the treatment of choice with reconstruction of the biliary tract using a Roux-en-Y loop of jejunum. Complete resection of the cyst is important because of the association with the development of cholangiocarcinoma. Resection and Roux-en-Y reconstruction is also associated with a reduced incidence of stricture formation and recurrent cholangitis.

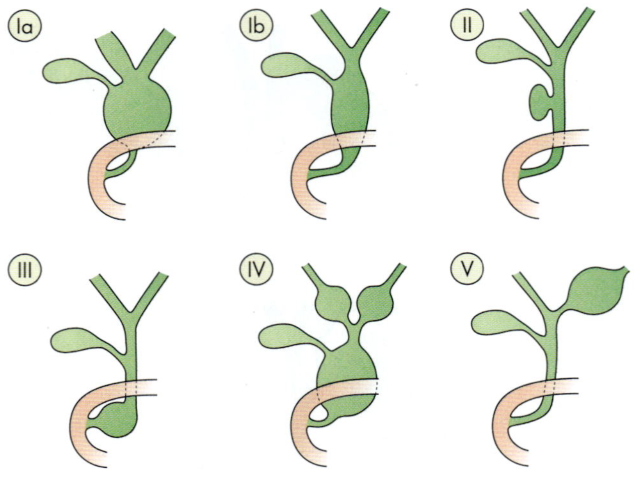

Figure 67.25 Classification of types of choledochal cyst. Type Ia and b: diffuse cystic. Note extension into pancreas of type Ib. Type II: diverticulum of common bile duct. Type III: diverticulum within pancreas. Type IV: extension into the liver. Type V: cystic dilatation only of the intrahepatic ducts.

TRAUMA

Injuries to the gall bladder and extrahepatic biliary tree are rare. They occur as a result of blunt or penetrating abdominal trauma. Operative trauma is perhaps more frequent than external trauma. The physical signs are those of an acute abdomen. Management depends on the location and extent of the biliary and associated injury. In the stable patient, a transected bile duct is best repaired by a Roux-en-Y choledochojejunostomy. Injuries to the gall bladder can be dealt with by cholecystectomy.

TORSION OF THE GALL BLADDER

This is very rare and requires a long mesentery, which often occurs in an older patient with a large mucocoele of the gall bladder. The patient presents with extreme pain and an acute abdomen. Immediate exploration is indicated, with cholecystectomy as the only treatment.

GALLSTONES (CHOLELITHIASIS)

Gallstones are the most common biliary pathology. It is estimated that gallstones affect 10–15 per cent of the population in western societies. They are asymptomatic in the majority of cases (>80 per cent). In the UK, the prevalence of gallstones at the time of death is estimated to be 17 per cent and may be increasing. Approximately, 1–2 per cent of asymptomatic patients will develop symptoms requiring surgery per year, making cholecystectomy one of the most common operations performed by general surgeons.

Causal factors in gallstone formation

Gallstones can be divided into three main types: cholesterol, pigment (brown/black) or mixed stones. In the United States and Europe, 80 per cent are cholesterol or mixed stones, whereas in Asia, 80 per cent are pigment stones. Cholesterol or mixed stones contain 51–99 per cent pure cholesterol plus an admixture of calcium salts, bile acids, bile pigments and phospholipids.

Cholesterol, which is insoluble in water, is secreted from the canalicular membrane in phospholipid vesicles. Whether cholesterol remains in solution depends on the concentration of phospholipids and bile acids in bile, and the type of phospholipid and bile acid. Micelles formed by the phospholipid hold cholesterol in a stable thermodynamic state. When bile is supersaturated with cholesterol or bile acid concentrations are low, unstable unilamellar phospholipid vesicles form, from which cholesterol crystals may nucleate, and stones may form. The process of gallstone formation is complex (Figure 67.26), and many areas remain unclear. Obesity, high-caloric diets and certain medications (e.g. oral contraceptives) can increase secretion of cholesterol and supersaturate the bile increasing the lithogenicity of bile. Resection of the terminal ileum, which diminishes the enterohepatic circulation, will deplete the bile acid pool and result in cholesterol supersaturation. Nucleation of cholesterol monohydrate crystals from multilamellar vesicles is a crucial step in gallstone formation. Abnormal emptying of the gall bladder function may aid the aggregation of nucleated cholesterol crystals; hence, removing gallstones without removing the gall bladder inevitability leads to gallstone recurrence.

Pigment stone is the name used for stones containing less

Takuji Todani, contemporary, Department of Surgery, Okayama University Medical School, Japan, in 1977 modified Alonso-Lej's classification of choledochal cysts.

than 30 per cent cholesterol. There are two types – black and brown. Black stones are largely composed of an insoluble bilirubin pigment polymer mixed with calcium phosphate and calcium bicarbonate. Overall, 20–30 per cent of stones are black. The incidence rises with age. Black stones are associated with haemolysis, usually hereditary, spherocytosis or sickle cell disease. For reasons that are unclear, patients with cirrhosis have a higher instance of pigmented stones.

Brown pigment stones contain calcium bilirubinate, calcium palmitate and calcium stearate, as well as cholesterol. Brown stones are rare in the gall bladder. They form in the bile duct and are related to bile stasis and infected bile. Stone formation is related to the deconjugation of bilirubin deglucuronide by bacterial β-glucuronidase. Insoluble unconjugated bilirubinate precipitates. Brown pigment stones are also associated with the presence of foreign bodies within the bile ducts, such as endoprosthesis (stents), or parasites, such as *Clonorchis sinensis* and *Ascaris lumbricoides*.

Clinical presentation

Gallstones may remain symptomatic, being detected incidentally as imaging is performed for other symptoms. If symptoms occur, patients typically complain of right upper quadrant or epigastric pain, which may radiate to the back. This may be described as colicky, but more often is dull and constant. Other symptoms include dyspepsia, flatulence, food intolerance, particularly to fats, and some alteration in bowel frequency. Biliary colic is typically present in 10–25 per cent of patients. This is described as a severe right upper quadrant pain which ebbs and flows associated with nausea and vomiting. Pain may radiate to the chest. The pain is usually severe and may last for minutes or even several hours. Frequently, the pain starts during the night and wakes the patient. Minor episodes of the same discomfort may occur intermittently during the day. Dyspeptic symptoms may coexist and be worse after such an attack. As the pain resolves, the patient improves and is able to eat and drink again, often only to suffer further episodes. It is of interest that a patient may have several episodes of this nature over a period of a few weeks and then no more trouble for some months. Jaundice may result if the stone migrates from the gall bladder and obstructs the common bile duct. Rarely, a gallstone can lead to bowel obstruction (gallstone ileus) (Summary box 67.2).

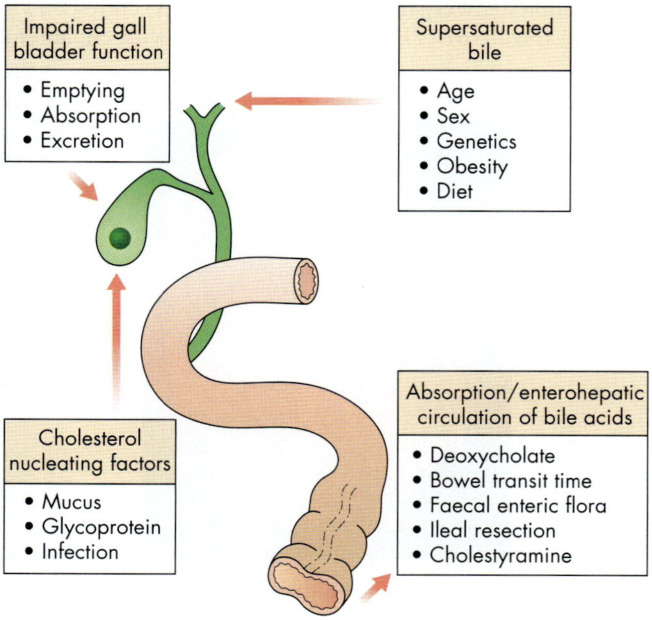

Figure 67.26 Factors associated with gallstone formation.

Summary box 67.2

Effects and complications of gallstones

- Biliary colic
- Acute cholecystitis
- Chronic cholecystitis
- Empyema of the gall bladder
- Mucocoele
- Perforation
- Biliary obstruction
- Acute cholangitis
- Acute pancreatitis
- Intestinal obstruction (gallstone ileus)

When the symptoms do not resolve, but progress to continued pain with fever and leukocytosis, the diagnosis of acute cholecystitis should be considered. The differential diagnosis is given in Summary box 67.3.

Summary box 67.3

Differential diagnosis of acute cholecystitis

- Common
  - Appendicitis
  - Perforated peptic ulcer
  - Acute pancreatitis
- Rare
  - Acute pyelonephritis
  - Myocardial infarction
  - Pneumonia – right lower lobe

Diagnosis

A diagnosis of gallstone disease is based on the history and physical examination with confirmatory radiological studies, such as transabdominal ultrasonography and radionuclide scans (see above under Radiological investigation of the biliary tract). In the acute phase, the patient may have right upper quadrant tenderness that is exacerbated during inspiration by the examiner's right subcostal palpation (Murphy's sign). A positive Murphy's sign suggests acute inflammation and may be associated with a leukocytosis and moderately elevated liver function tests. A mass may be palpable as the omentum walls off an inflamed gall bladder. Fortunately in the majority of cases, the process is limited by the stone slipping back into the body of the gall bladder and the contents of the gall bladder escaping by way of the cystic duct. This achieves adequate drainage of the gall bladder and enables the inflammation to resolve.

If resolution does not occur, an empyema of the gall bladder may result. The wall may become necrotic and perforate, with development of localised peritonitis. The abscess may then perforate into the peritoneal cavity with a septic peritonitis –

however, this is uncommon, because the inflamed gall bladder is usually localised by omentum which contains the perforation.

A palpable, non-tender gall bladder (Courvoisier's sign) portends a more sinister diagnosis. This usually results from a distal common duct obstruction secondary to a peripancreatic malignancy. Rarely, a non-tender, palpable gall bladder results from complete obstruction of the cystic duct with reabsorption of the intraluminal bile salts and secretion of uninfected mucus secreted by the gall bladder epithelium leading to a mucocoele of the gall bladder.

Treatment

Most consider that it is safe to observe patients with asymptomatic gallstones, with cholecystectomy reserved for patients who develop symptoms or complications. However, prophylactic cholecystectomy may be considered for diabetic patients, those with congenital haemolytic anaemia and those patients who are undergoing bariatric surgery for morbid obesity as it has been found in these groups that the risk of developing symptoms is increased. For patients with biliary colic or cholecystitis, cholecystectomy is the treatment of choice if there are no medical contraindications.

Experience shows that in more than 90 per cent of cases, the symptoms of acute cholecystitis subside with conservative measures. Non-operative treatment is based on four principles:

- Nil per mouth (NPO) and intravenous fluid administration until the pain resolves.
- Administration of analgesics.
- Administration of antibiotics. As the cystic duct is blocked in most instances, the concentration of antibiotic in the serum is more important than its concentration in bile. A broad-spectrum antibiotic effective against Gram-negative aerobes is most appropriate (e.g. cefazolin, cefuroxime or gentamicin).
- Subsequent management. When the temperature, pulse and other physical signs show that the inflammation is subsiding, oral fluids are reinstated followed by regular diet. Ultrasonography is performed to confirm the diagnosis. If jaundice is present, an MRCP is performed to exclude choledocholithiasis. If there is any concern regarding the diagnosis or presence of complications, such as perforation, a CT should be performed. Cholecystectomy may be performed on the next available list, or the patient may be allowed home to return later when the inflammation has completely resolved.

Conservative treatment must be abandoned if the pain and tenderness increase; depending on the status of the patient, either operative intervention and cholecystectomy should be performed or if the patient has comorbid conditions, a percutaneous cholecystostomy can be performed by a radiologist under ultrasound control. This will usually rapidly relieve symptoms, however an interval cholecystectomy will be required once the patient's condition has stabilised.

The timing of surgery in acute cholecystitis remains controversial with many units favouring an early intervention within the first week, whereas others suggest that a delayed approach is preferable. Early cholecystectomy during acute cholecystitis appears to be safe and shortens the total hospital stay.

Provided that the operation is undertaken within 5–7 days of the onset of the attack, the surgeon is experienced and excellent operating facilities are available, good results are achieved. Nevertheless, the conversion rate in laparoscopic cholecystectomy is higher in acute than in elective surgery. If an early operation is not indicated, one should wait approximately 6 weeks for the inflammation to subside before operating.

EMPYEMA OF THE GALL BLADDER

Empyema may be a sequel of acute cholecystitis or the result of a mucocoele becoming infected. The gall bladder is distended with pus. The optimal treatment is drainage (cholecystostomy, see above under Gallstones (cholelithiasis)) and, later, cholecystectomy.

Acalculous cholecystitis

Acute and chronic inflammation of the gall bladder can occur in the absence of stones and give rise to a clinical picture similar to calculous cholecystitis. Some patients have non-specific inflammation of the gall bladder, whereas others have one of the cholecystoses (see below). Acute acalculous cholecystitis is particularly seen in critically ill patients and those recovering from major surgery, trauma and burns. The diagnosis is often missed and the mortality rate is high.

THE CHOLECYSTOSES (CHOLESTEROSIS, POLYPOSIS, ADENOMYOMATOSIS AND CHOLECYSTITIS GLANDULARIS PROLIFERANS)

This is a relatively uncommon group of conditions affecting the gall bladder, in which there are chronic inflammatory changes with hyperplasia of all tissue elements.

Cholesterosis ('strawberry gall bladder')

In the fresh state, the interior of the gall bladder looks something like a strawberry; the yellow specks (submucous aggregations of cholesterol crystals and cholesterol esters) correspond to the seeds (Figure 67.27). It may be associated with cholesterol stones.

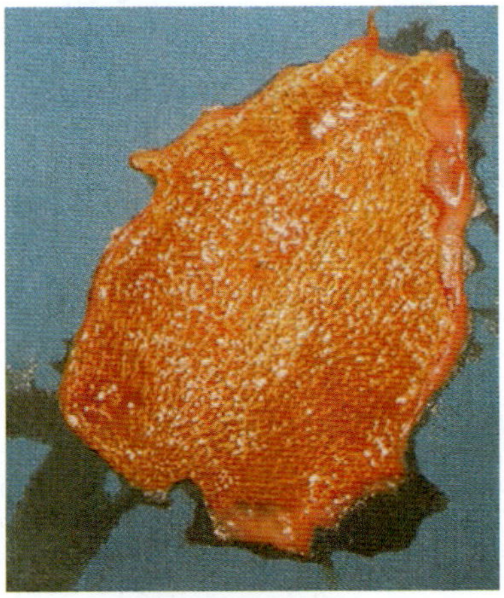

Figure 67.27 The interior of a strawberry gall bladder (cholesterosis) (courtesy of Dr Sanjay P Thakur, Patna, India).

Ludwig Courvoisier, 1843–1918, Professor of Surgery, Basle, Switzerland, described his sign (also referred to as a law) in 1890.
Charles Frederick Morris Saint, 1886–1973, Emeritus Professor of Surgery, Cape Town, South Africa.

Cholesterol polyposis of the gall bladder

Cholecystography shows negative shadows in a functioning gall bladder, or on ultrasound there is a well-defined polyp present. These are due either to cholesterol polyposis or adenomatous change. With high resolution ultrasonography, they are seen more frequently, and surgery is advised only if there is a change in size over time or are larger than 1 cm.

Cholecystitis glandularis proliferans (polyp, adenomyomatosis and intramural diverticulosis)

Figure 67.28 summarises the varieties of this condition. A polyp of the mucous membrane is fleshy and granulomatous. All layers of the gall bladder wall may be thickened, but sometimes an incomplete septum forms that separates the hyperplastic from the normal. Intraparietal 'mixed' calculi may be present. These can be complicated by an intramural, and later extramural, abscess and potentially fistula formation. If symptomatic, the patient is treated by cholecystectomy.

Diverticulosis of the gall bladder

Diverticulosis of the gall bladder is usually manifest as black pigment stones impacted in the outpouchings of the lacunae of Luschka. Diverticulosis of the gall bladder may be demonstrated by cholecystography, especially when the gall bladder contracts after a fatty meal. There are small dots of contrast medium just within and outside the gall bladder (Figure 67.29). A septum may also be present to be distinguished from the Phrygian cap. The treatment is cholecystectomy.

Typhoid infection of the gall bladder

Salmonella typhi or *S. typhimurium* can infect the gall bladder. Acute cholecystitis can occur. More frequently, chronic cholecystitis occurs, the patient being a typhoid carrier excreting the bacteria in the bile. Gallstones may be present (surgeons should not give patients their stones after their operation if there is any suspicion of typhoid!). It is debatable whether the stones are secondary to the *Salmonella* cholecystitis or whether pre-existing stones predispose the gall bladder to chronic infection. Salmonellae can, however, frequently be cultured from these stones. Treatment with ampicillin and cholecystectomy are indicated. In cases of penicillin allergy, a quinolone antibiotic can be used.

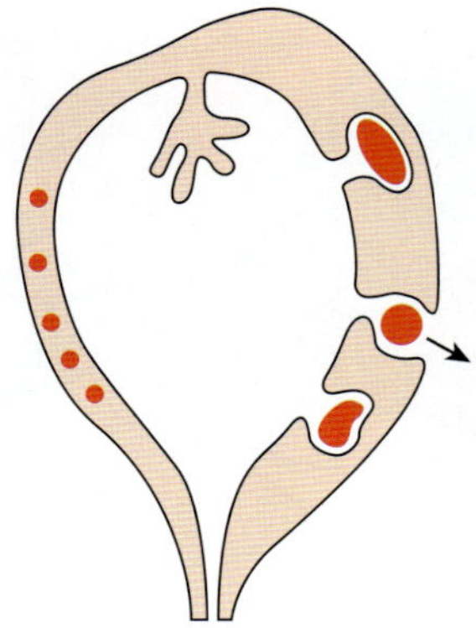

Figure 67.28 Types of cholecystitis glandularis proliferans (polypus, intramural or diverticular stones and fistula).

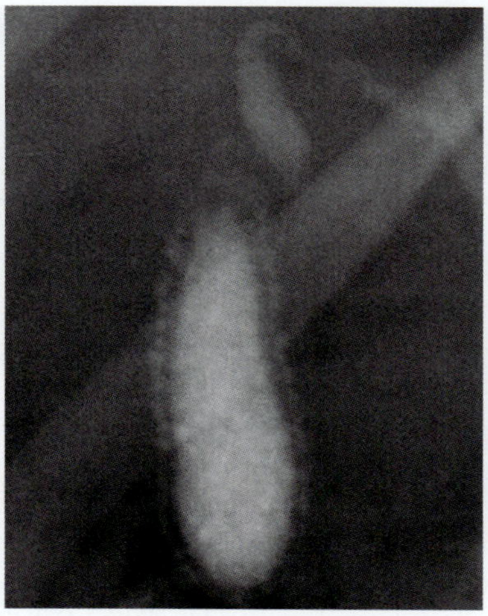

Figure 67.29 Cholecystogram showing diverticulosis with dots of contrast medium in the gall bladder wall.

CHOLECYSTECTOMY

Preparation for operation

After appropriate history taking and assessment of the patient's fitness for the procedure, a full blood count and biochemical profile should be performed to exclude anaemia and to identify abnormal liver function. A blood coagulation screen should be checked if there is a history of jaundice or liver function is abnormal. Prophylactic antibiotics should be administered either with the premedication or at the time of induction of anaesthesia. A second-generation cephalosporin is appropriate. Subcutaneous heparin or anti-embolic stockings should be prescribed. The patient must sign a consent form to indicate that he or she is fully aware of the procedure being undertaken, alternative options and the risks involved and complications that may occur (Summary box 67.4).

Summary box 67.4

Preparation for operation

- Full blood count
- Renal profile and liver function tests
- Prothrombin time
- Chest x-ray and electrocardiogram (if over 45 years or medically indicated)
- Antibiotic prophylaxis
- Deep vein thrombosis prophylaxis
- Informed consent

Laparoscopic cholecystectomy

The preparation and indications for cholecystectomy are the same whether it is performed by laparoscopy or by open techniques. Laparoscopic cholecystectomy is the procedure of choice for the majority of patients with gall bladder disease. The key, as in open surgery, is the identification and safe dissection of Calot's triangle (Figure 67.30).

Daniel Elmer Salmon, 1850–1914, veterinary pathologist, Chief of the Bureau of Animal Industry, Washington, DC, USA.

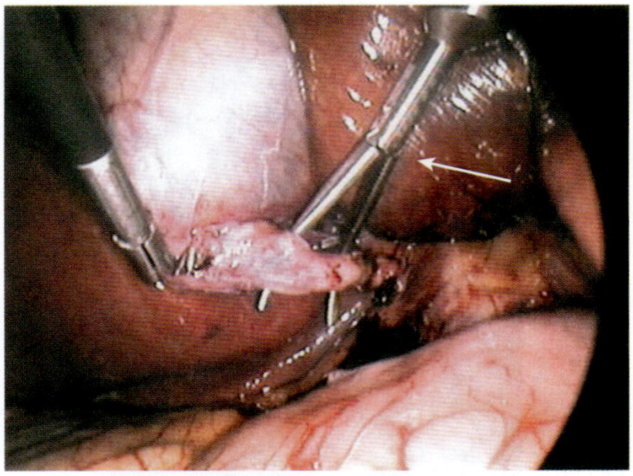

Figure 67.30 Operative image of a laparoscopic cholecystectomy. Laparoscopic forceps (arrow) are used to dissect Calot's triangle.

The patient is placed supine on the operating table. Following induction and maintenance of general anaesthetic, the abdomen is prepared in a standard fashion. Pneumoperitoneum is established. A number of techniques are described. The author's preference is to use an open subumbilical cutdown with direct visualisation of the peritoneum to place the initial port. This port will function as the camera port. An angled telescope (30°) is preferred. Many surgeons use a 'closed' technique using a Verres needle to establish pneumoperitoneum prior to placing the initial trocar.

Additional operating ports are inserted in the subxiphoid area and in the right subcostal area. The patient is placed in a reverse Trendelburg position slightly rotated to the left. This exposes the fundus of the gall bladder which is retracted towards the diaphragm. The neck of the gall bladder is then retracted towards the right iliac fossa exposing Calot's triangle. This area is laid widely open by dividing the peritoneum on the posterior and on the anterior aspect. The cystic duct is carefully defined, as is the cystic artery. The gall bladder is separated from the liver bed for about 2 cm to allow for confirmation of the anatomy. Unless there are specific indications (see below), a routine cholangiogram is not performed. However, if doubt exists regarding the anatomy, a cholangiogram is warranted. Once the anatomy is clearly defined and the triangle of Calot has been laid widely open, the cystic duct and artery are clipped and divided. The gall bladder is then removed from the gall bladder bed by sharp or cautery dissection and once free removed via the umbilicus.

Open cholecystectomy

For patients in whom a laparoscopic approach is not indicated or in whom conversion from a laparoscopic approach is required an open cholecystectomy is performed.

Either an upper midline or a short right upper transverse incision is made centred over the lateral border of the rectus muscle. The gall bladder is appropriately exposed and packs are placed on the hepatic flexure of the colon, the duodenum and the lesser omentum to ensure a clear view of the anatomy of the porta hepatis. These packs may be retracted using the hand of the assistant ('It is the left hand of the assistant that does all the work' – Moynihan), or, alternatively, a stabilised ring retractor can be used to keep the packs in position.

An artery or Duval forceps is placed on the infundibulum of the gall bladder and the peritoneum overlying Calot's triangle is placed on a stretch. The peritoneum is then divided close to the wall of the gall bladder and the fat in the triangle of Calot carefully dissected away to expose the cystic artery and the cystic duct. The cystic duct is cleaned down to the common bile duct, whose position is clearly ascertained. The cystic artery is tied and divided. The whole of the triangle of Calot is displayed to ensure that the anatomy of the ducts is clear and the cystic duct is then divided between ligatures (Figure 67.31). The gall bladder is then dissected away from the gall bladder bed.

Some golden rules to observe in case of difficulty:

- When the anatomy of the triangle of Calot is unclear, blind dissection should stop.
- Bleeding adjacent to the triangle of Calot should be controlled by pressure and not by blind clipping or clamping.
- When there is doubt about the anatomy, a retrograde or 'fundus-first' cholecystectomy dissecting on the gall bladder wall down from the fundus to the cystic duct can be helpful.
- If the cystic duct is densely adherent to the common bile duct and there is the possibility of a Mirizzi syndrome (a stone ulcerating through the neck of the gall bladder into the common hepatic duct), the infundibulum of the gall bladder should be opened, the stone removed and the infundibulum oversewn. Attempts to completely dissect out the cystic duct will only lead to common hepatic or common bile duct injury.
- A cholecystostomy is rarely indicated, but, if it has to be done, as many stones as possible should be extracted and a large Foley catheter (14 F) placed in the fundus of the gall bladder with a direct track externally. By so doing, should stones be left behind in the gall bladder, these can be subsequently extracted with a choledochoscope.

Indications for choledochotomy

In an environment in which neither the modern diagnostic armamentarium described at the beginning of this chapter nor peroperative cholangiography is available, it is well to remember the traditional indications for choledochotomy, which are:

- palpable duct stones;
- jaundice or a history of jaundice or cholangitis;
- a dilated common bile duct;
- abnormal liver function tests, in particular a raised alkaline phosphatase.

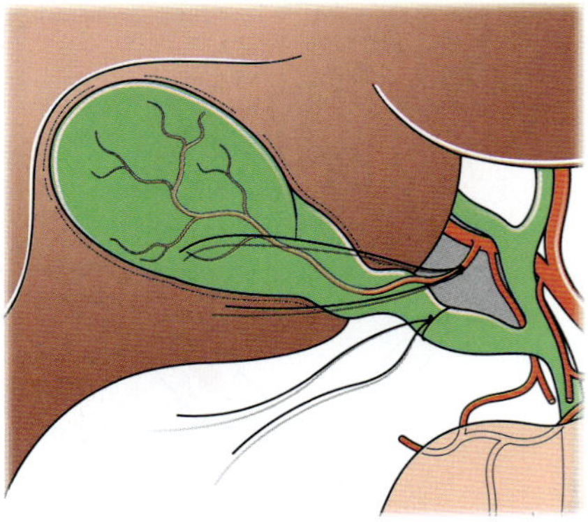

Figure 67.31 Ligatures are passed and tied around the cystic artery and cystic duct. The grey shaded area represents Calot's triangle.

Pierre Alfred Duval, 1874–1941, French surgeon.
Pablo Luis Mirizzi, 1893–1964, surgeon Cordoba, Argentina. Described this condition in 1932. First to introduce interoperative cholangiogram in 1931.
Frederic Eugene Basil Foley, 1891–1965, urologist, The Miller and Anker Hospitals, St Paul, MN, USA.

Unless the expertise is available, it is probably inadvisable to perform a choledochotomy laparoscopically; rather one should rely on endoscopic techniques or convert to an open operation. The incidence of symptomatic stones in the bile duct varies from 5 to 8 per cent. These can, in the main, be dealt with endoscopically without resort to opening the duct. However, current trials suggest that in experienced hands the morbidity of the two techniques is identical.

Complications of cholecystectomy

Recovery after laparoscopic cholecystectomy is associated with less pain, enhanced recovery and faster return to normal activity. The majority of patients undergoing an elective procedure can have this procedure performed as a day case, avoiding hospital admission. Any untoward symptoms in the postoperative period, such as fevers, chills or abdominal pain require immediate investigation.

The operative mortality for cholecystectomy is less than 1 per cent. Factors increasing the risk for postoperative mortality include advanced age, comorbid conditions and acute presentation. Complications can occur in 10–15 per cent of cases. Serious complications of laparoscopic cholecystectomy fall into two major areas: access complications or bile duct injuries. The latter are rare occurring in approximately 0.5 per cent of cases. In the main, biliary injury results from poor dissection and failure to adequately define the surgical anatomy. Controversy exists as to whether or not the use of operative cholangiography reduces the incidence of bile duct injury. The majority of surgeons use cholangiography only in selected cases.

Patients who develop jaundice in the postoperative period require urgent investigation. This is especially true if the jaundice is associated with infection, a condition called cholangitis.

The first step in management is to undertake an immediate ultrasound scan. This will demonstrate whether there is intra- or extrahepatic ductal dilation. The anatomy needs to be defined by either an ERCP or a MRCP. The former will also allow therapeutic maneouvres such as removal of an obstructing stone or insertion of a stent across a biliary leak. If a fluid collection is present in the subhepatic space drainage catheters may be required. These can be inserted under radiological control or if this expertise is not available at open operation. Small biliary leaks will usually resolve spontaneously, especially if there is no distal obstruction. Should the common bile duct be damaged, the patient should be referred to an appropriate expert for reconstruction of the duct.

About 15 per cent of injuries to the bile ducts are recognised at the time of operation, in the remaining 85 per cent of cases, the injury declares itself postoperatively by: (1) a profuse and persistent leakage of bile if drainage has been provided, or bile peritonitis if such drainage has not been provided; and (2) deepening obstructive jaundice. When the obstruction is incomplete, jaundice is delayed until subsequent fibrosis renders the lumen of the duct inadequate.

Any postoperative elevation in serum bilirubin or suggestion of duct damage requires investigation and the nature of the bile duct injury clarified. The surgical repair and subsequent outcome is related to the level of injury, which is determined using the Bismuth classification.

In a debilitated patient, temporary external biliary drainage may be achieved by passing a catheter percutaneously into an intrahepatic duct. Also, stents may be passed through strictures at the time of ERCP and left to drain into the duodenum. When the general condition of the patient has improved, definitive surgery can be undertaken. The principles of surgical repair are maintenance of duct length and restoration of biliary drainage. For benign stricture or duct transection, the preferred treatment is immediate Roux-en-Y choledochojejunostomy performed by an experienced surgeon. For a stricture of recent onset through which a guidewire can be passed, balloon dilatation with insertion of a stent is an acceptable alternative provided that the services of an experienced endoscopist are available. The outcome of such surgery is good, with 90 per cent patients having no further cholangitis or stricture formation.

Late symptoms after cholecystectomy

In up to 15 per cent of patients, cholecystectomy fails to relieve the symptoms for which the operation was performed. Such patients may be considered to have a 'post-cholecystectomy' syndrome. However, such problems are usually related to the preoperative symptoms and are merely a continuation of those symptoms. Full investigation should be undertaken to confirm the diagnosis and exclude the presence of a stone in the bile duct, a stone in the cystic duct stump or operative damage to the biliary tree. This is best performed by MRCP or ERCP, the latter which has the added advantage that if a stone is in the common bile duct it can be removed.

Post-cholecystectomy choledocholithiasis

Duct stones may occur many years after a cholecystectomy or be related to the development of new pathology, such as infection of the biliary tree or infestation by *Ascaris lumbricoides* or *Clinorchis sinensis*. Any obstruction to the flow of bile can give rise to stasis with the formation of stones within the duct. The consequences of duct stones are either obstruction to bile flow or infection. Stones in the bile ducts are more often associated with infected bile (80 per cent) than are stones in the gall bladder.

Symptoms

The patient may be asymptomatic but usually has bouts of pain, jaundice and fever. The patient is often ill and feels unwell. The term 'cholangitis' is given to the triad of pain, jaundice and fevers sometimes known as 'Charcot's triad'.

Signs

Tenderness may be elicited in the epigastrium and the right hypochondrium. In the jaundiced patient, it is useful to remember Courvoisier's law – 'in obstruction of the common bile duct due to a stone, distension of the gall bladder seldom occurs; the organ usually is already shrivelled'. In obstruction from other causes, distension is common by comparison. However, if there is no disease in the gall bladder and the obstruction is due to a cancer of the ampulla, pancreas or bile duct, then the gall bladder may well be distended.

Management

It is essential to determine whether the jaundice is due to liver disease, disease within the duct, such as sclerosing cholangitis, or obstruction. Ultrasound scanning, liver function tests, liver biopsy if the ducts are not dilated, and MRI or ERCP will identify the nature of the obstruction.

Jean-Martin Charcot, 1825–1893, physician, neurologist and professor of anatomical pathology, La Salpêtrière, Paris, France. His name is associated with a host of medical eponyms.

The patient may be ill. Pus may be present within the biliary tree and liver abscesses may be developing. Full supportive measures are required with rehydration, attention to clotting, exclusion of diabetes and starting the appropriate broad-spectrum antibiotics. As soon as resuscitation has taken place, relief of the obstruction is essential. Endoscopic papillotomy is the preferred first technique with a sphincterotomy, removal of the stones using a Dormia basket or the placement of a stent if stone removal is not possible (Figure 67.32 and 67.33). If this technique fails, percutaneous transhepatic cholangiography can be performed to provide drainage and subsequent percutaneous choledochoscopy. Surgery, in the form of choledochotomy, is now rarely used for this situation as most patients can be managed by minimally invasive techniques (Figure 67.34).

Choledochotomy

When faced with a sick patient whose investigations show that the cause of the cholangitis is stones in the common bile duct and minimally invasive techniques for stone extraction are not available, the surgeon has no alternative but to undertake a laparotomy. The aim of this surgery is to drain the common bile duct and remove the stones through a longitudinal incision in the duct. When the duct is clear of stones, a T-tube is inserted and the duct closed around it; the long limb is brought out on the right side and the bile allowed to drain externally. When the bile has become clear and the patient recovered, a cholangiogram is performed by the radiologist. If residual stones are found, the tube is left in place for 6 weeks so that the track is 'mature'. The radiologist can then use the track for percutaneous removal of the stones (Figure 67.34). Once the radiologist has removed the tube, the track will close and the patient make a rapid recovery.

Stricture of the bile duct

The causes of benign biliary stricture are given in Summary box 67.5. Bile duct strictures may be investigated radiologically (Summary box 67.6).

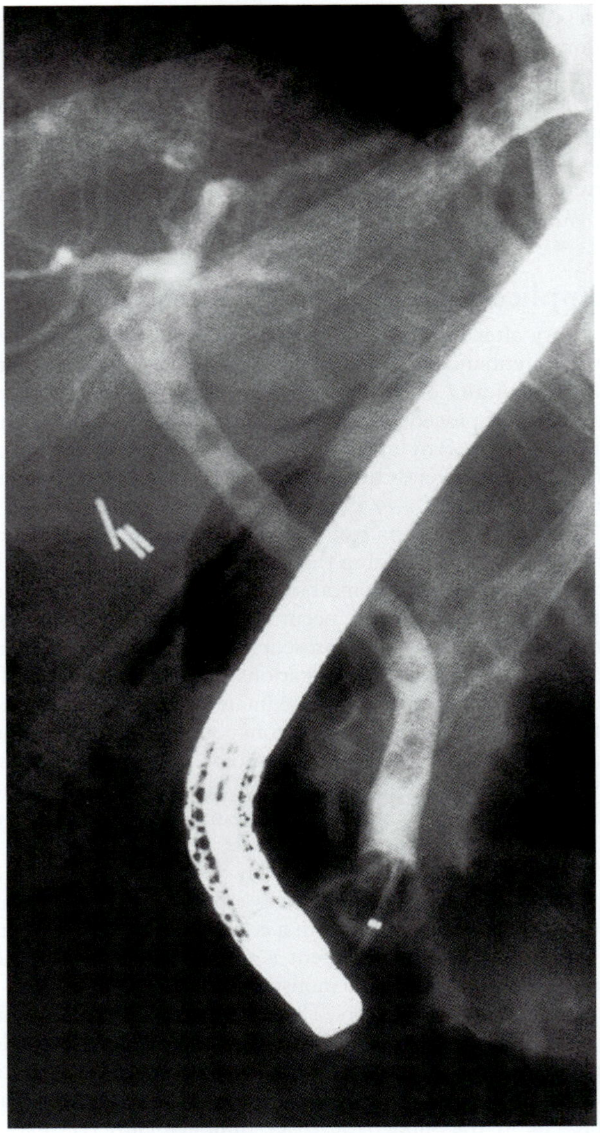

Figure 67.32 Endoscopic retrograde cholangiopancreatography showing multiple stones in the common bile duct in a patient who presented with jaundice 4 days following laparoscopic cholecystectomy.

Summary box 67.5

Causes of benign biliary stricture

- Congenital
  - Biliary atresia
- Bile duct injury at surgery
  - Cholecystectomy
  - Choledochotomy
  - Gastrectomy
  - Hepatic resection
  - Transplantation
- Inflammatory
  - Stones
  - Cholangitis
  - Parasitic
  - Pancreatitis
  - Sclerosing cholangitis
  - Radiotherapy
- Trauma
- Idiopathic

Summary box 67.6

Radiological investigation of biliary strictures

- Ultrasonography
- Cholangiography via T-tube, if present
- ERCP
- MRCP
- Percutaneous transhepatic cholangiography (Figure 67.18)
- CT scan

PRIMARY SCLEROSING CHOLANGITIS

Primary sclerosing cholangitis is an idiopathic fibrosing inflammatory condition of the biliary tree which affects both

H Joachim Burhenne, 1925–1996, born in Germany, Professor and Head of the Department of Radiology, University of British Columbia, Vancouver, Canada. He developed his technique in 1974. He was an award-winning photographer, an accomplished violinist and published a book on ski touring.

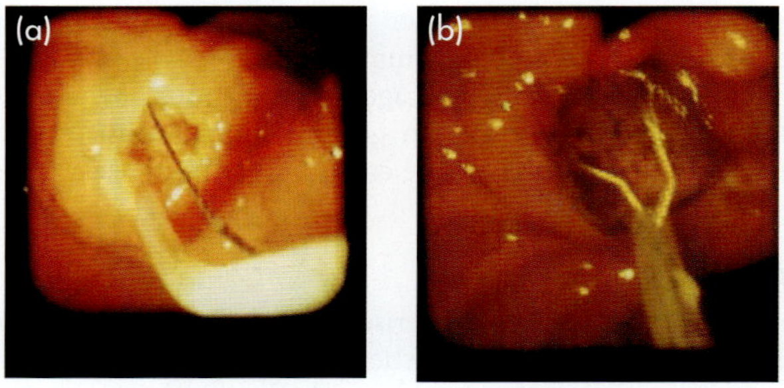

Figure 67.33 (a) Endoscopic sphincterotomy; (b) extraction of a stone from the bile duct through the ampulla.

intrahepatic and extrahepatic ducts. It is of unknown origin, but the association of hypergammaglobulinaemia and elevated markers such as smooth muscle antibodies and antinuclear factor suggest an immunological basis. The majority of patients are between 30 and 60 years. There appears to be a male predominance and a strong association with inflammatory bowel disease especially ulcerative colitis.

Common symptoms include right upper quadrant discomfort, jaundice, pruritus, fever, fatigue and weight loss. Investigation reveals a cholestatic pattern to the liver function tests with elevation of the serum alkaline phosphatase and gamma glutamyl transferase and smaller rises in the aminotransferases. Bilirubin values can be variable and may fluctuate. Imaging studies such as MRCP or ERCP may demonstrate stricturing and beading of the bile ducts (Figure 67.35). A liver biopsy is helpful in confirming the diagnosis and may help guide therapy by excluding cirrhosis. The important differential diagnoses are secondary sclerosing cholangitis and cholangiocarcinoma. The latter condition may be very difficult to diagnose and a high index of suspicion is required especially in the setting of an unexplained deterioration.

Medical management with antibiotics, vitamin K, cholestyramine, steroids and immunosuppressant drugs, such as azathioprine, is generally unsuccessful. Endoscopic stenting of dominant strictures and, in selected patients with predominantly extrahepatic disease, operative resection may be worthwhile. For patients with cirrhosis, liver transplantation is the best option. Five-year survival following transplantation in high-volume centres is in excess of 80 per cent.

PARASITIC INFESTATION OF THE BILIARY TRACT

Biliary ascariasis

The round worm, *Ascaris lumbricoides*, commonly infests the intestine of inhabitants of Asia, Africa and Central America. It may enter the biliary tree through the ampulla of Vater and cause biliary pain. Complications include strictures, suppurative cholangitis, liver abscesses and empyema of the gall bladder. In the uncomplicated case, antispasmodics can be given to relax the sphincter of Oddi and the worm will return to the small intestine to be dealt with by antihelminthic drugs. Operation may be necessary to remove the worm or deal with complications. Worms can be extracted via the ampulla of Vater by ERCP.

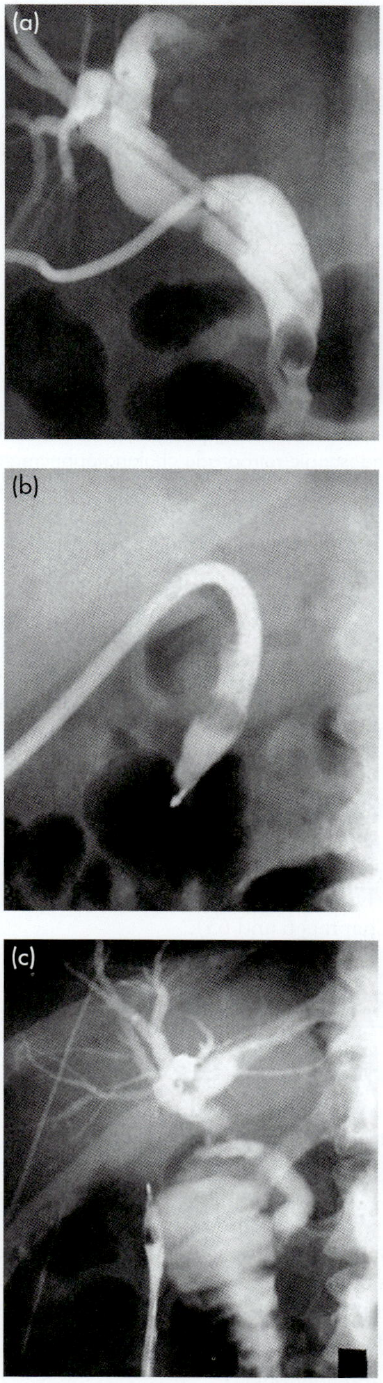

Figure 67.34 Extraction of a stone from the common bile duct by the Burhenne technique. (a) A T-tube *in situ* with a stone in the duct. (b) A steerable catheter has been manipulated into the duct and a basket placed around the stone. (c) The stone being extracted from the bile duct along the T-tube track.

Clonorchiasis (Asiatic cholangiohepatitis)

The disease is endemic in the Far East. The fluke, up to 25 mm long and 5 mm wide, inhabits the bile ducts, including the intrahepatic ducts. Fibrous thickening of the duct walls occur. Many cases are asymptomatic. Complications include biliary

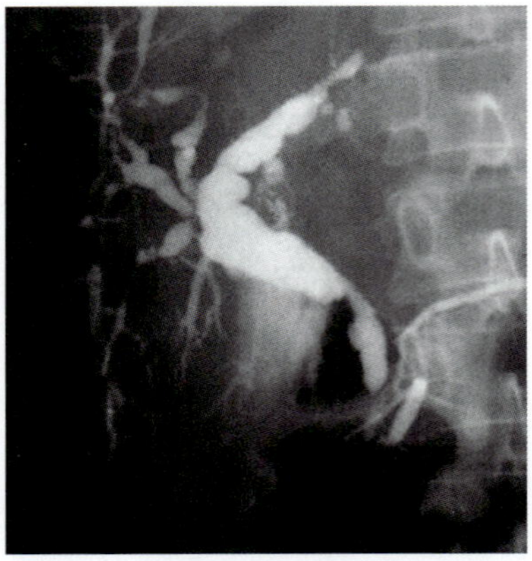

Figure 67.35 Sclerosing cholangitis in a patient with ulcerative colitis visualised by endoscopic retrograde cholangiopancreatography.

pain, stones, cholangitis, cirrhosis and bile duct carcinoma. Choledochotomy and T-tube drainage and, in some cases, choledochoduodenostomy are required. Because a process of recurrent stone formation is set up, a choledochojejunostomy with a Roux loop fixed to the adjacent abdominal wall is performed in some centres to allow easy subsequent access to the duct system.

Hydatid disease

A large hydatid cyst may obstruct the hepatic ducts. Sometimes, a cyst will rupture into the biliary tree and its contents cause obstructive jaundice or cholangitis, requiring appropriate surgery (see Chapters 6 and 65).

TUMOURS OF THE BILE DUCT

Benign tumours of the bile duct

These are uncommon and need to be distinguished from other benign conditions.

They may be an incidental finding on imaging. For symptomatic patients, the duration of symptoms may vary from a few days to months and their clinical presentation may in fact mimic the more common conditions, such as cholecystitis, choledocholithiasis, cholangiocarcinoma or pancreatic cancer.

Benign neoplasms causing biliary obstruction may be classified as follows:

- papilloma and adenoma
- multiple biliary papillomatosis
- granular cell myoblastoma
- neural tumours
- leiomyoma
- endocrine tumours.

Papilloma and adenoma

The most common benign neoplasms arise from the glandular epithelium lining the bile ducts. They can occur throughout the biliary system, but are more frequent in the periampullary area. Lesions in this area may protrude through the ampulla of Vater and be visible at endoscopy. Jaundice is the most common symptom occurring in greater than 90 per cent of cases. Coexisting gallstones are uncommon.

Treatment depends on the age, general status of the patient and site of the disease, but in general should consist of total resection of the lesion. In some cases, a wide local resection can be performed.

Papillomatosis

This rare condition is characterised by the presence of multiple mucus-secreting tumours of the biliary epithelium. Patients present with obstructive jaundice which may be intermittent often complicated by cholangitis. These tumours have a malignant potential and should be resected. This may involve liver resection if the disease is confined to a hepatic lobe. If both lobes are affected, then liver transplantation may be required.

Granular cell myoblastoma, neural tumours, leiomyomata and endocrine tumours are extremely uncommon. In general, if biliary obstruction occurs it should be relieved by either biliary resection, bypass or endoscopic stenting.

Malignant tumours of the biliary tract

Malignant tumours of the gall bladder and extrahepatic biliary tree are uncommon. Gall bladder cancer is the predominant type accounting for 60–70 per cent of cases with the remainder distributed between the intra- and extrahepatic biliary tree (Summary box 67.7).

Summary box 67.7

Bile duct cancer (cholangiocarcinoma)

- Rare, but incidence increasing
- Most patients present with abnormal liver function tests or frank jaundice
- Diagnosis by ultrasound, MDR-CT or MRCP scanning
- Majority of patients receive palliative care only
- Complete surgical excision possible in less than 10 per cent
- Prognosis poor – 90 per cent dead in one year from liver failure or biliary sepsis
- Adjuvant chemoradiation therapy has limited role

Unfortunately, due to advanced stage at presentation, surgical resection, which offers the best survival, is only possible in a minority of patients. Thus for most patients treatment is generally palliative in nature and survival limited.

Incidence

Cholangiocarcinoma is a rare malignancy accounting for 1–2 per cent of new cancers in a western practice. The overall annual incidence is 1–1.5 per 100 000 with two-thirds of patients being older than 65 years. It appears to be more common in males with a male:female ratio of approximately 1.5:1.

Anatomically, tumours involving the biliary confluence (hilar cholangiocarcinoma or Klatskin tumours) account for 60 per cent of cases with the remainder in the distal bile duct (20–30 per cent) or intrahepatic (10–20 per cent).

Risk factors

A minority of patients presenting with cholangiocarcinoma are noted to have a known risk factor (Summary box 67.8). The major risk factor in western practice is primary sclerosing cholangitis (PSC). It is estimated that a long-standing history of PSC increases the risk of developing biliary tract cancer by 20-fold compared to the normal population. It appears that patients with PSC and concomitant inflammatory bowel disease are at significantly higher risk of developing cancer compared to those without the disease. Cholangiocarcinoma appears to occur at an earlier age in patients with PSC (30–50 years of age) compared to the general population. In addition, disease is usually multifocal and detected at advanced stage with resultant poor prognosis.

Summary box 67.8

Risk factors for cholangiocarcinoma

- Chronic inflammatory conditions
  - Primary sclerosing cholangitis
  - Oriental cholangiohepatitis
  - Hepatitis C infection
- Parasitic infections
  - *Opisthorchis viverrini*
  - *Clonorchis sinensis*
- Congenital
  - Choledochal cysts
  - Caroli's disease
- Chemical agents
  - Thorium dioxide (Thorotrast®)
  - Vinyl chloride
  - Dioxin
  - Asbestos
- Postsurgical
  - Biliary-enteric anastomosis

Congenital cystic disease (Caroli's disease, choledochal cysts), hepatolithiasis, oriental cholangiohepatitis, hepatitis C viral infection and infestation with liver flukes have also been associated with an increased risk of cholangiocarcinoma. Liver fluke infestations are particularly important in South-East Asia. *Opisthorchis viverrini* and *Clonorchis sinensis* infestation is important in Thailand, Laos and western Malaysia. While the pathophysiology is unclear, it is hypothesised that these parasites cause chronic inflammination which leads to DNA changes and mutations through production of carcinogens and free radicals, which stimulate cellular proliferation in the intrahepatic bile ducts and ultimately can lead to invasive cancer.

Other risk factors suggested include chemical carcinogens, such as thorium dioxide, vinyl chloride, dioxin and asbestos.

Clinical features

Early symptoms of cholangiocarcinoma are often non-specific with abdominal pain, early satiety, anorexia and weight loss commonly seen. Symptoms associated with biliary obstruction (puritus and jaundice) may be present in a minority of patients. In these patients, examination often demonstrates clinical signs of jaundice, cachexia is often noticeable and a palpable gall bladder is present if the obstruction is in the distal common bile duct (Courvoisier's sign).

Investigations

Biochemical investigations will confirm the presence of obstructive jaundice (elevated bilirubin, alkaline phosphatase and γ-glutamyltransferase). The tumour marker CA 19-9 may also be elevated. Imaging studies, such as ultrasound, multidetector row computed tomography (MDR-CT) and MRI/MRCP, are essential for diagnosis and staging. These studies allow the level of biliary obstruction to be defined and determine the locoregional extent of disease and the presence of metastases (Figure 67.36).

Direct cholangiography using ERCP or PTC are also used following non-invasive studies. Both can define the level of obstruction and allow access to the biliary system for biopsy and placement of endobiliary stents for biliary drainage. The choice between either modality depends on local availability and the anatomical site of the tumour with PTC preferred for more proximal lesions and ERCP favoured for distal tumours. Cytology can be obtained from either procedure, but it is often non-diagnostic.

Recent work has suggested that combined positron emission tomography (PET) and MDR-CT scanning may be useful in staging cholangiocarcinoma, but further work is required to determine the true value of this modality.

Treatment

A multidisciplinary approach is required in all cases. The choice of treatment depends on the site of the disease and its extent. Unfortunately, the majority of patients present with advanced disease. However, 10–15 per cent are suitable for surgical resection which offers the only hope for long-term survival. The aim of surgical resection is to achieve a complete resection with negative pathological margins and safely restore biliary–enteric continuity. Depending on the site of disease, resections may involve excision of a lobe of the liver and reconstruction of the biliary tree. With the improved techniques associated with hepatic resection, the perioperative mortality rate is now less than 5 per cent. Distal common duct tumours may require a pancreaticoduodenectomy (Whipple procedure).

Liver transplantation has been suggested by some authors for selected patients who have locally unresectable disease

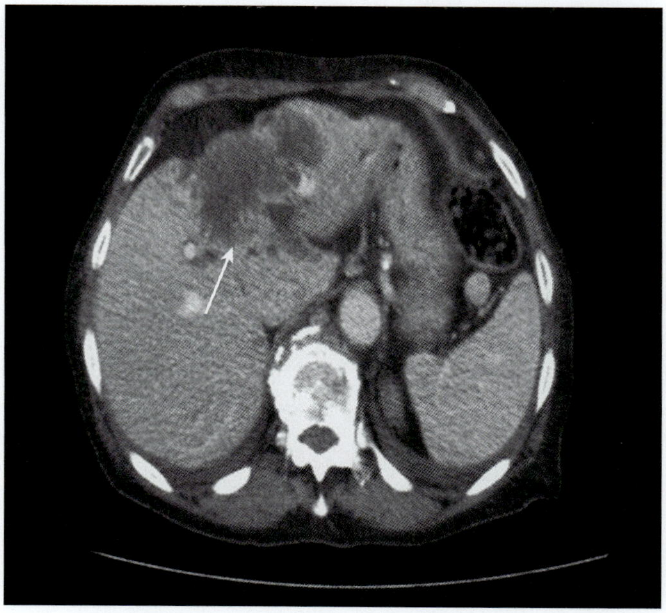

Figure 67.36 A computed tomography scan demonstrating a hilar cholangiocarcinoma (arrowed).

without evidence of distant metastases. Transplantation is often combined with neoadjuvant chemoradiation therapy. While emerging data are encouraging, this aggressive approach remains unproven and is reserved for selected patients in specialised centres.

Following resection, the median survival is approximately 18 months, with 20 per cent of patients surviving five years post-resection. Survival appears better for distal tumours compared to those involving the upper third of the biliary tree. Adjuvant chemotherapy or radiotherapy has a limited role to play and has not been demonstrated to add survival benefit following surgical resection. However, patients at high risk for recurrence (positive surgical margins or node positive) may benefit from adjuvant therapy and should be referred for a medical or radiation oncology opinion.

The majority of patients who present with unresectable disease are candidates for palliative therapy. The aim is to maintain or improve quality of life by relieving symptoms and preventing cholestatic liver failure. Biliary obstruction can be relieved by either endoscopic (ERCP) or percutaneous (PTC) methods. Surgical bypass rarely has a role apart from patients who present with a distal bile duct lesion and are found to have unresectable disease at operation.

Carcinoma of the gall bladder

Incidence

This is a rare disease, but extremely variable by geographical region and racial–ethnic groups. The highest incidence is among Chileans, American Indians and residents in parts of northern India, where it accounts for as much as 9 per cent of all biliary tract disease. Women appear to have a higher incidence across all geographic areas. In western practice, gall bladder cancer accounts for less than 1 per cent of new cancer diagnoses. The disease usually presents in the seventh or eighth decade. The aetiology is unclear, but there appears to be an association with pre-existing gallstone disease suggesting that chronic inflammation may play a role in a manner similar to tumours of the common bile duct. Calcification of the gall bladder wall, presumably due to chronic inflammation (porcelain gall bladder), is also associated with an increased risk of cancer (Figure 67.5). Chronic infection may also promote development of gall bladder cancer and the risk in typhoid carriers is significantly increased over the general population.

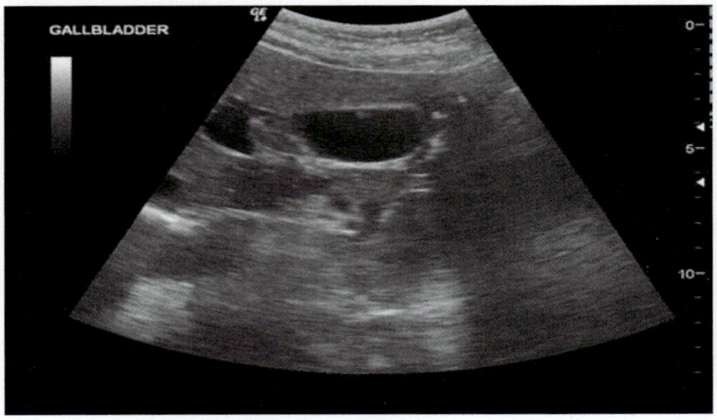

Figure 67.37 Ultrasound demonstrating gall bladder polyp. Note lack of acoustic shadow.

Gall bladder polyps may be found in approximately 5 per cent of patients who undergo ultrasonography (Figure 67.37). The majority are either adenomyomatosis or cholesterol polyps and have no malignant potential. True adenomatous polyps do occur and have malignant potential (Summary box 67.9).

Summary box 67.9

Gall bladder cancer

- Very rare
- Similar presentation to benign biliary disease, i.e. gallstones
- Diagnosis by ultrasound, CT scan, MRI/MRCP
- Most patients present with advanced disease
- Surgical resection in less than 10 per cent – remainder receive palliative treatment
- Prognosis is poor – median survival approximately six months

Pathology

The majority (90 per cent) of cases are adenocarcinoma. Squamous carcinomas also occur and are believed to arise from areas of mucosal squamous metaplasia.

At operation, localised carcinomas are difficult to differentiate from chronic cholecystitis; the most commonly presenting tumour is nodular and infiltrative, with thickening of the gall bladder wall, often extending to the whole gall bladder. The tumour spreads by direct extension into the liver, seeding of the peritoneal cavity and involvement of the perihilar lymphatics and neural plexuses. At the time of presentation, the majority of tumours are advanced (Figure 67.38).

Clinical features

Patients may be asymptomatic at the time of diagnosis. Symptoms, if present, are usually indistinguishable from those of benign gall bladder disease, such as biliary colic or cholecystitis, particularly in older patients. Jaundice and anorexia are late features. A palpable mass is a late sign.

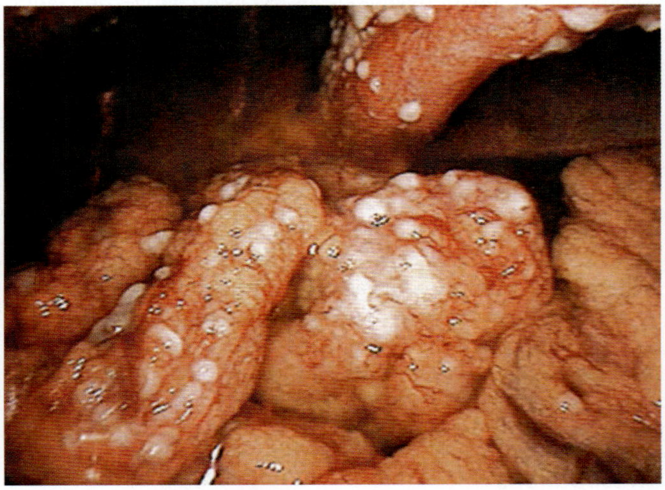

Figure 67.38 Laparoscopic staging in a patient with gall bladder carcinoma demonstrating gross peritoneal metastases.

Investigation

Laboratory findings are generally non-specific, but may be consistent with biliary obstruction. Non-specific findings, such as anaemia, leukocytosis, mild elevation in transaminases and increased inflammatory markers, such as ESR or C-reactive protein, may be present. Serum CA19-9 is elevated in approximately 80 per cent of patients.

The preoperative diagnosis is often made on ultrasonography, and confirmed by a MDR-CT scan or MRI/MRCP. Preoperative staging should be aimed at determining the local extent of diseases and excluding the presence of distant metastases (Summary box 67.10). A percutaneous biopsy under radiological guidance is often done to obtain tissue for pathological examination. In selected cases, a laparoscopic examination is useful in staging the disease. Laparoscopy can detect peritoneal or liver metastases which would preclude further surgical resection (Figure 67.38).

Summary box 67.10

Aim of staging gall bladder cancer

- Assessment of local disease
- Detection of metastatic disease
  - Liver
  - Peritoneal
  - Lymphatic
  - Extra-abdominal disease

Treatment and prognosis

The majority of patients have advanced disease at presentation, and are not candidates for surgical therapy. Surgery is indicated in only very selected cases.

Cholecystectomy should be performed for all gall bladder polyps greater than 1 cm. Polyps less than 1 cm can be followed with serial ultrasonography to detect any change in size or character as the incidence of malignancy in polyps less than 1 cm is extremely low.

Radical en-bloc resections which may include segmental or extended hepatectomy, bile duct resection and regional lymphadenectomy should be considered in selected patients. The aim is to remove the tumour entirely and achieve negative histopathological margins.

Patients can have the disease diagnosed following histopathological examination of the gall bladder removed for presumed benign disease. In these cases, the need for further surgery is determined by the stage of disease. For early stage disease confined to the mucosa or muscle of the gall bladder, no further treatment is indicated. However, for transmural disease, a radical en-bloc resection of the gall bladder fossa and surrounding liver along with the regional lymph nodes should be performed. If the initial procedure was performed laparoscopically, the surgeon should examine the laparoscopic port sites. Routine resection of port sites is no longer recommended. However, it is recognised that the finding of disease at the port sites is a sign of generalised peritoneal disease and portends a very poor prognosis.

For the majority of patients, a non-operative approach to palliation is best. Obstructive jaundice can be relieved by endoscopic and/or percutaneous methods. The value of adjuvant therapy is unproven.

Gall bladder cancer for most patients is a lethal disease with a grim prognosis. The median survival is less than six months and a five-year survival figure of 5 per cent reported.

FURTHER READING

Bland KI, Sarr MG, Buchler MW *et al.* (eds). *Liver and biliary surgery: handbooks in general surgery*. New York: Springer, 2010.

Blumgart LH (ed.). *Surgery of the liver and biliary tract*, 4th edn. London: WB Saunders, 2006.

Carter DC, Russell RCG, Pitt HA, Bismuth H (eds). *Rob and Smith's operative surgery: hepatobiliary and pancreatic surgery*. London: Chapman & Hall, 1996.

Dooley JS, Lok A, Burroughs A, Heathcoate J (eds). *Sherlock's diseases of the liver and biliary system*, 12th edn. Oxford: Wiley-Blackwell, 2011.

Jarnagin W. *Blumgart's surgery of the liver, pancreas and biliary tract*, 5 edn. Philadelphia, PA: WB Saunders, 2012.

Sherlock S, Dooley J (eds). *Diseases of the liver and biliary system*, 11th edn. Oxford: Blackwell Publishing, 2001.

CHAPTER 68

The pancreas

LEARNING OBJECTIVES

To understand:

- The anatomy and physiology of the pancreas
- Investigations of the pancreas
- Congenital abnormalities of the pancreas
- Assessment and management of pancreatitis
- Diagnosis and treatment of pancreatic cancer

ANATOMY AND PHYSIOLOGY

Anatomy

The name 'pancreas' is derived from the Greek '*pan*' (all) and '*kreas*' (flesh). For a long time, its glandular function was not understood, and it was thought to act as a cushion for the stomach. The pancreas is situated in the retroperitoneum. It is divided into a head, which occupies 30 per cent of the gland by mass, and a body and tail, which together constitute 70 per cent. The head lies within the curve of the duodenum, overlying the body of the second lumbar vertebra and the vena cava. The aorta and the superior mesenteric vessels lie behind the neck of the gland. Coming off the side of the pancreatic head and passing to the left and behind the superior mesenteric vein is the uncinate process of the pancreas. Behind the neck of the pancreas, near its upper border, the superior mesenteric vein joins the splenic vein to form the portal vein (Figures 68.1 and 68.2). The tip of the pancreatic tail extends up to the splenic hilum.

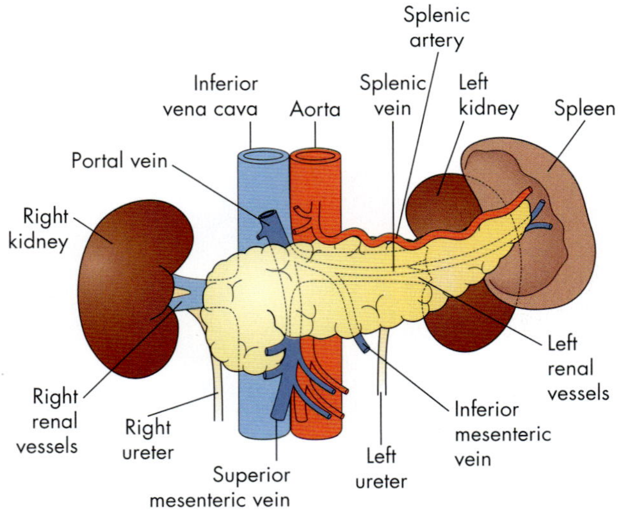

Figure 68.1 The posterior relations of the pancreas.

The pancreas weighs approximately 80 g. Of this, 80–90 per cent is composed of exocrine acinar tissue, which is organised into lobules. The main pancreatic duct branches into interlobular and intralobular ducts, ductules and, finally, acini. The main duct is lined by columnar epithelium, which becomes cuboidal in the ductules. Acinar cells are clumped around a central lumen, which communicates with the duct system. Clusters of endocrine cells, known as islets of Langerhans, are distributed throughout the pancreas. Islets consist of different cell types: 75 per cent are B cells (producing insulin); 20 per cent are A cells (producing glucagon); and the remainder are D cells (producing somatostatin) and a small number of pancreatic polypeptide cells. Within an islet, the B cells form an inner core surrounded by the other cells. Capillaries draining the islet cells drain into the portal vein, forming a pancreatic portal system.

There are nine key processes that occur during pancreatic embryogenesis (Table 68.1). Malrotation of the ventral bud in the fifth week results in an annular pancreas, while the mode of ductule fusion in the seventh week produces the various possible ductular patterns. Between the 12th and 40th weeks of fetal life, the pancreas differentiates into exocrine and endocrine

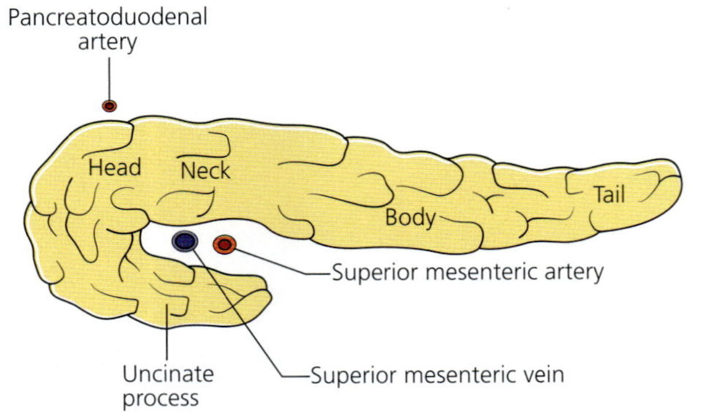

Figure 68.2 Transverse section of the pancreas. Note the position of the uncinate process behind the vessels.

Paul Langerhans, 1847–1888, Professor of Pathological Anatomy, Freiberg, Germany, described the islets in 1869, in his doctoral thesis. He later contracted tuberculosis, resigned and moved to warmer climes in Madeira, where he also studied marine worms.

Johann Georg Wirsung, 1589–1643, Professor of Anatomy, Padua, Italy, described the pancreatic duct in 1642, when dissecting the cadaver of a man hanged for murder. He died a year later from an assassin's bullet, on his doorstep.

elements. The primitive ducts and their ductules are responsible for the lobular arrangement of the pancreas. Congenital anomalies of the pancreas are varied and arise during the early phase of development (Summary box 68.1). The anatomy of the pancreatic duct is variable as a result of the primordial bud development. The dorsal duct is expressed in a variable manner in the adult, as outlined in Figure 68.3. Approximately 10 per cent of patients will have a significant flow from the main duct through the accessory papilla. The anatomy of the main duodenal papilla, also known as the ampulla of Vater, is also variable (Figure 68.4). The outlet of each duct is protected by a complex sphincter mechanism (sphincter of Oddi) (Figure 68.5).

Summary box 68.1

Anomalies of the pancreas

- Aplasia
- Hypoplasia
- Hyperplasia
- Hypertrophy
- Dysplasia
- Variations and anomalies of the ducts[a]
  - Pancreas divisum
  - Rotational anomalies
- Annular pancreas[a]
- Pancreatic gall bladder
- Polycystic disease[a]
- Congenital pancreatic cysts
  - Cystic fibrosis[a]
  - von Hippel–Lindau syndrome
- Ectopic pancreatic tissue, accessory pancreas[a]
- Vascular anomalies
- Choledochal cysts[a]
- Horseshoe pancreas

[a]The more frequent anomalies encountered in surgical practice.

Table 68.1 Steps in the development of the pancreas.

1	Day 26	Dorsal pancreatic duct arises from the dorsal side of the duodenum
2	Day 32	Ventral bud arises from the base of the hepatic diverticulum
3	Day 37	Contact occurs between the two buds. Fusion by the end of week 6
4	Week 6	Ventral bud produces the head and uncinate process
5	Week 6	Ducts fuse
6	Week 6	Ventral duct and distal portion of the dorsal duct form the main duct (duct of Wirsung)
7	Week 6	Proximal dorsal duct forms the duct of Santorini
8	Month 3	Acini appear
9	Months 3–4	Islets of Langerhans appear and become biologically active

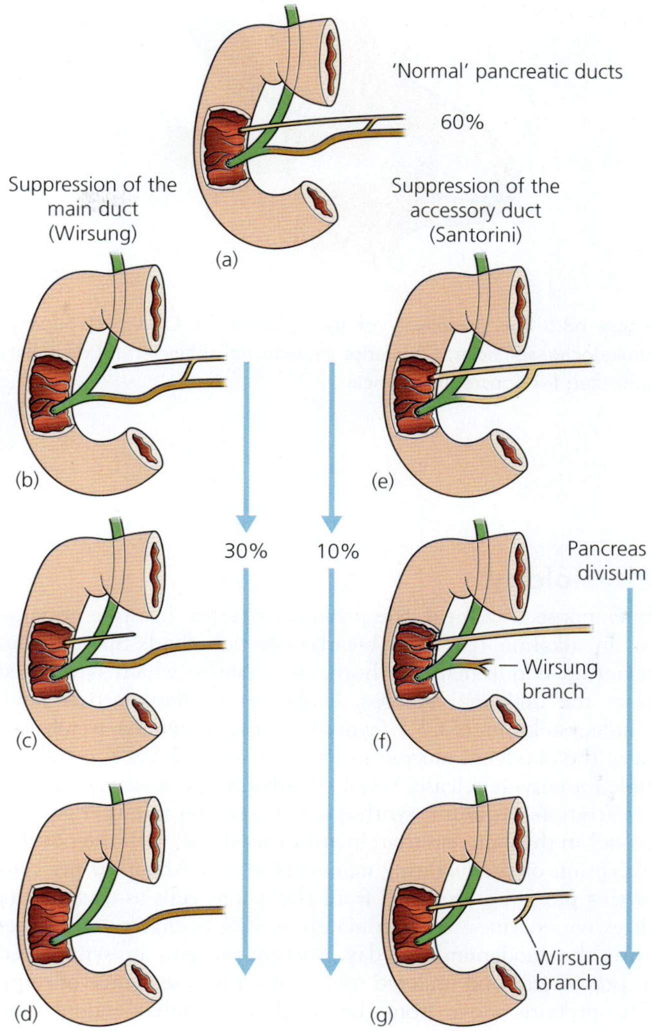

Figure 68.3 Variations in the pancreatic ducts. (a) Normal. (b–d) Progressive suppression of the accessory duct (30 per cent). (e–g) Progressive suppression of the main duct (10 per cent). (f) Pancreas divisum – the ventral duct drains only the uncinate process.

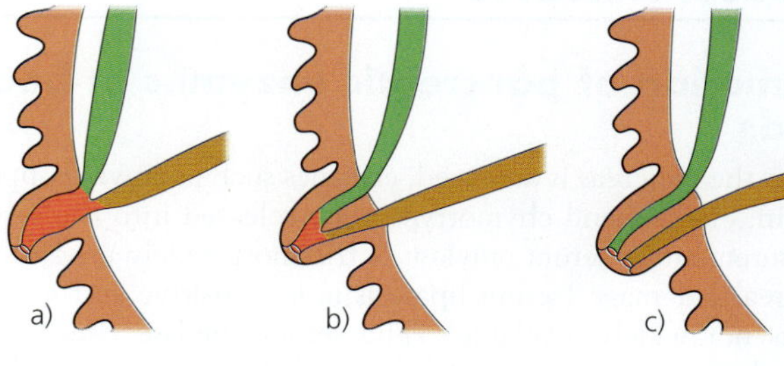

Figure 68.4 Variations in the relation of the common bile duct and main pancreatic duct at the main duodenal papilla. In (a), there is a common channel with no sphincter mechanism protecting flow between the ducts. In (b), there is a partial common channel, while in (c), there is separation of the two channels. Gallstone pancreatitis is more likely with (a) and (b).

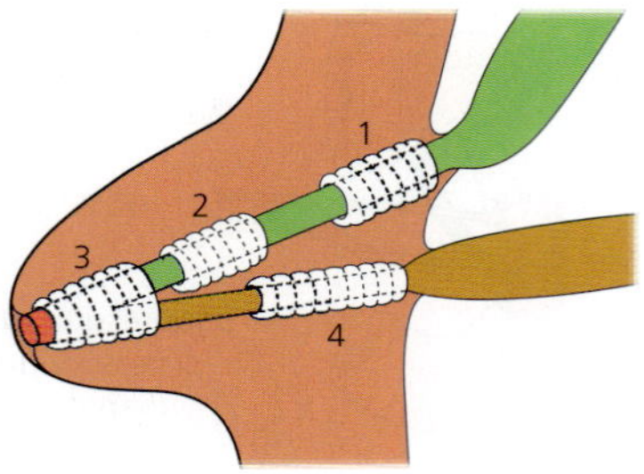

Figure 68.5 The complexity of the sphincter of Oddi. (1) Superior choledochal sphincter; (2) inferior choledochal sphincter; (3) ampullary sphincter; (4) pancreatic sphincter.

Physiology

In response to a meal, the pancreas secretes digestive enzymes in an alkaline (pH 8.4) bicarbonate-rich fluid. Spontaneous secretion is minimal; the hormone secretin, which is released from the duodenal mucosa, evokes a bicarbonate-rich fluid. Cholecystokinin (CCK) (synonym: pancreozymin) is released from the duodenal mucosa in response to food. CCK is responsible for enzyme release. Vagal stimulation increases the volume of secretion. Protein is synthesised at a greater rate (per gram of tissue) in the pancreas than in any other tissue, with the possible exception of the lactating mammary gland. About 90 per cent of this protein is exported from the acinar cells as a variety of digestive enzymes. Approximately 6–20 g of digestive enzymes enter the duodenum each day. Nascent proteins are synthesised as preproteins and undergo modification in a sequence of steps. The proteins move from the rough endothelial endoplasmic reticulum to the Golgi complex, where lysosomes and mature zymogen storage granules containing proteases are stored, and then to the ductal surface of the cell, from which they are extruded by exocytosis. During this phase, the proteolytic enzymes are in an inactive form, the maintenance of which is important in preventing pancreatitis.

INVESTIGATIONS

Estimation of pancreatic enzymes in body fluids

When the pancreas is damaged, enzymes such as amylase, lipase, trypsin, elastase and chymotrypsin are released into the serum. Measurement of serum amylase is the most widely used test of pancreatic damage (serum lipase is more sensitive and specific, but is not widely available). The serum amylase rises within a few hours of pancreatic damage and declines over the next 4–8 days. A markedly elevated serum level is highly suspicious but not diagnostic of acute pancreatitis (Summary box 68.2). Urinary amylase and amylase–creatinine clearance ratios add little to diagnostic accuracy. If confirmation of the diagnosis is required, computed tomography (CT) of the pancreas is of greater value (Table 68.2).

Summary box 68.2

Causes of raised serum amylase level other than acute pancreatitis

- Upper gastrointestinal tract perforation
- Mesenteric infarction
- Torsion of an intra-abdominal viscus
- Retroperitoneal haematoma
- Ectopic pregnancy
- Macroamylasaemia
- Renal failure
- Salivary gland inflammation

Table 68.2 Investigation of the pancreas.

Serum enzyme levels		
Pancreatic function tests		
Morphology	Ultrasound scan	
	Computed tomography	
	Magnetic resonance imaging	
	Endoscopic retrograde cholangiopancreatography	
	Endoscopic ultrasound	
	Plain radiography	Chest
		Upper abdomen

Pancreatic function tests

Pancreatic exocrine function can be assessed by directly measuring pancreatic secretion in response to a standardised stimulus. The stimulus to secretion can be physiological, e.g. ingestion of a test meal, as in the Lundh test, or pharmacological, e.g. intravenous injection of a hormone, such as secretin or CCK. Duodenal intubation has to be performed with a triple-lumen tube so that the gastric and duodenal juices can be aspirated, and a non-absorbable marker, such as polyethylene glycol, is used to assess the completeness of the aspiration. The nitroblue tetrazolium–*para*-aminobenzoic acid (NBT–PABA) test provides an indirect measure of pancreatic function. The substance is administered orally and degraded in the gut by a pancreatic enzyme, and the breakdown product (PABA) is absorbed by the intestine and excreted in the urine; its urinary level is measured. The Pancreolauryl test works on a similar principle. These tests are cheap and easy to perform, but are non-specific, especially following gastrectomy and in conditions that may alter gastrointestinal transit and intestinal absorptive capacity. Measurement of the enzyme elastase in stool is simple, specific and now used widely. A low level of faecal elastase indicates exocrine insufficiency.

Imaging investigations

Ultrasonography

Ultrasonography is the initial investigation of choice in patients with jaundice to determine whether or not the bile duct is dilated, the coexistence of gallstones or gross disease within

Camillo Golgi, 1844–1926, Professor of Anatomy and Histology at Pavia, and later at Sienna, Italy. Developed silver staining of neural tissue, and received the Nobel Prize in 1906 (with Ramon y Cajal) for his studies in neuroanatomy.

the liver, such as metastases. It may also define the presence or absence of a mass in the pancreas (Figure 68.6). However, obesity and overlying bowel gas often make interpretation of the pancreas itself unsatisfactory.

Computed tomography

Most significant pathologies within the pancreas can be diagnosed on high-quality CT scans, with three-dimensional reconstruction if necessary. A specific pancreatic protocol should be followed. An initial unenhanced CT scan is essential to determine the presence of calcification within the pancreas and gall bladder (Figure 68.7). Then, following rapid injection of intravenous contrast, scanning is performed in the arterial and venous phases. The stomach and duodenum should be outlined with water and distended to define the duodenal loop. Pancreatic carcinomas of 1–2 cm in size can usually be demonstrated whether in the head, body or tail of the pancreas (Figure 68.8). Endocrine tumours are also well imaged on CT (Figure 68.9). In patients with pancreatitis, necrotic areas within the gland can be identified by the absence of contrast enhancement on CT. Inflammatory collections and pseudocysts can be seen (Figure 68.10). CT-guided drainage is helpful in the treatment of pancreatic collections, cysts and pseudocysts, and facilitates percutaneous fine-needle or Trucut biopsy.

Magnetic resonance imaging

With magnetic resonance imaging (MRI), the pancreas can be clearly identified, and the anatomy of the bile duct and the pancreatic duct, together with fluid collections, can be defined. Magnetic resonance cholangiography and pancreatography (MRCP) may well replace diagnostic endoscopic retrograde cholangiography and pancreatography (ERCP) as it is non-invasive and less expensive (Figure 68.11). Using the technique in conjunction with intravenous injection of secretin, emptying of the pancreatic duct can be demonstrated to show the absence or presence of obstruction.

Endoscopic retrograde cholangiopancreatography

ERCP is performed using a side-viewing fibreoptic duodenoscope. The ampulla of Vater is intubated, and contrast is

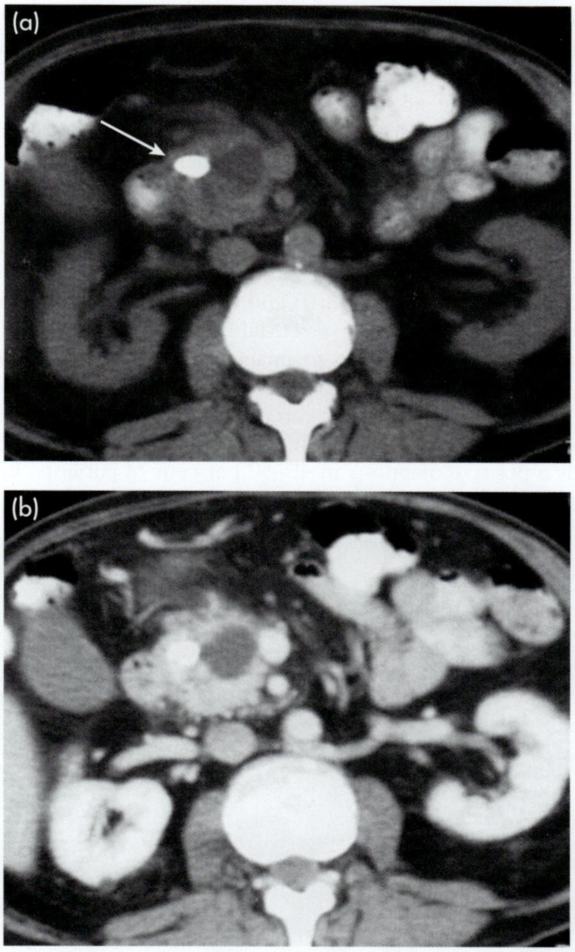

Figure 68.7 (a) Unenhanced computed tomography scan of a man with chronic pancreatitis, showing a focus of calcification (marked by an arrow) in the head of the pancreas and a cyst adjacent to that. Oral contrast has been administered. (b) The same area after injection of intravenous contrast.

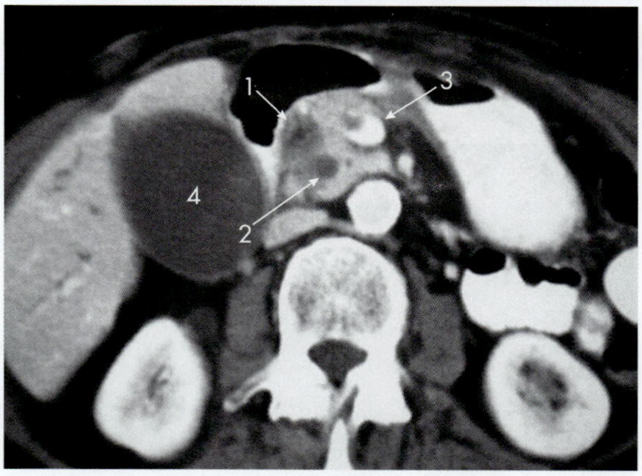

Figure 68.8 Contrast-enhanced computed tomography scan of a patient with a carcinoma of the pancreatic head. The main bulk of the tumour lies inferior to the section shown here. The dilated bile duct (1) and main pancreatic duct (2) can be seen, with tumour infiltration around them. There is a thrombus in the superior mesenteric vein (3). The gall bladder is distended (4).

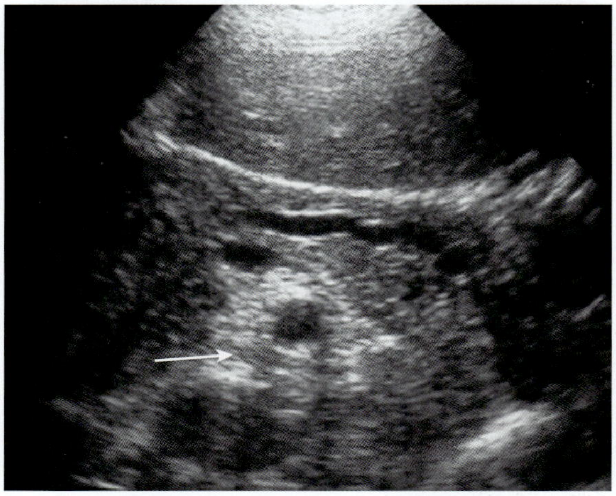

Figure 68.6 Ultrasound scan showing a mass in the head of the pancreas (marked by an arrow) and a dilated pancreatic duct in the body of the gland (courtesy of Dr Alison McLean).

Abraham Vater, 1684–1751, Professor of Anatomy and Botany, and later of Pathology and Therapeutics, Wittenberg, Germany. Apart from the ampulla, he also described what later came to be known as Pacinian corpuscles in the skin.

injected into the biliary and pancreatic ducts to display the anatomy radiologically (Figure 68.12). In pancreatic carcinoma, the main pancreatic duct may be narrowed or completely obstructed at the site of the tumour (Figure 68.13), or the distal bile duct may be narrowed. Concurrent narrowing of both ducts results in the so-called double duct sign (Figure 68.14). Changes seen in chronic pancreatitis include the presence of pancreatic duct strictures, dilatation of the main pancreatic duct with stones, abnormalities of pancreatic duct side branches, communication of the pancreatic duct with cysts, and bile duct strictures (Figures 68.15, 68.16 and 68.17). A plain radiograph before contrast studies is essential to delineate calcification (Figure 68.18). In addition to imaging, bile or pancreatic fluid and brushings from duct strictures can yield cells that confirm the suspected diagnosis of carcinoma (Figure 68.19). Brush cytology taken from malignant strictures at the time of ERCP yields a positive diagnosis in 40–50 per cent of patients. ERCP also allows the placement of biliary and pancreatic stents.

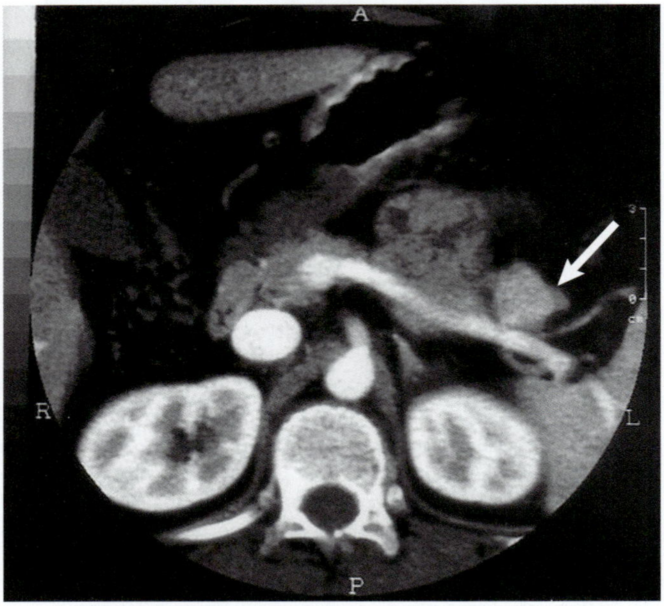

Figure 68.9 Computed tomography scan showing a hypervascular insulinoma adjacent to the splenic vein. Local excision of the tumour resulted in normoglycaemia.

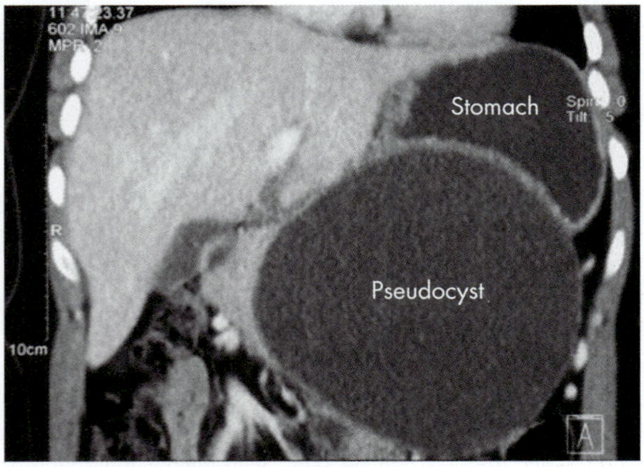

Figure 68.10 Computed tomography scan of a large pseudocyst in relation to the body and tail of the pancreas.

Endoscopic ultrasound

Endoscopic ultrasound (EUS) is performed using a special endoscope that has a high-frequency ultrasonic transducer at its tip. When the endoscope is in the lumen of the stomach or duodenum, the pancreas and its surrounding vasculature and

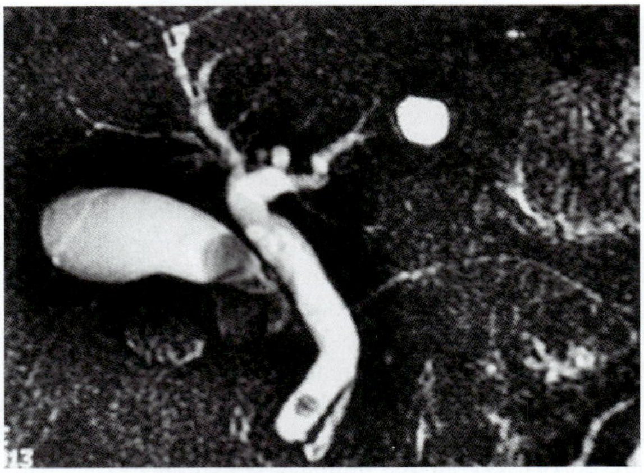

Figure 68.11 Magnetic resonance cholangiopancreatography in a patient with obstructive jaundice. A dilated common bile duct was seen on ultrasound, but no pancreatic mass lesion was visible on computed tomography. The bile duct and the main pancreatic duct are seen very well, with a stone visible in the lower part of the bile duct and another in the neck of the gall bladder.

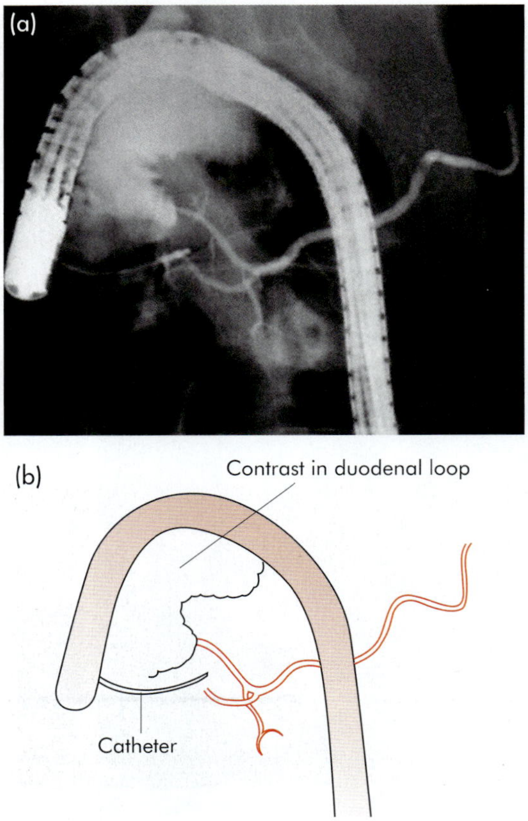

Figure 68.12 (a) Endoscopic retrograde cholangiopancreatography: normal pancreatic duct with filling of the duct of Santorini from the duct of Wirsung. (b) Diagrammatic outline of (a).

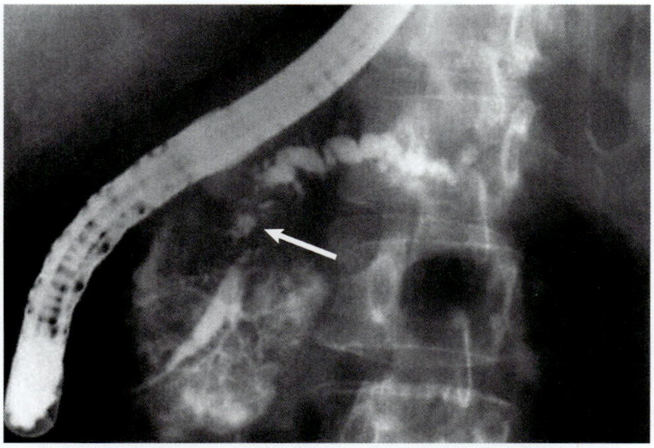

Figure 68.13 Endoscopic retrograde cholangiopancreatography: pancreatic carcinoma. Irregular stricture of the main pancreatic duct (marked by an arrow) with dilatation distal to the obstruction.

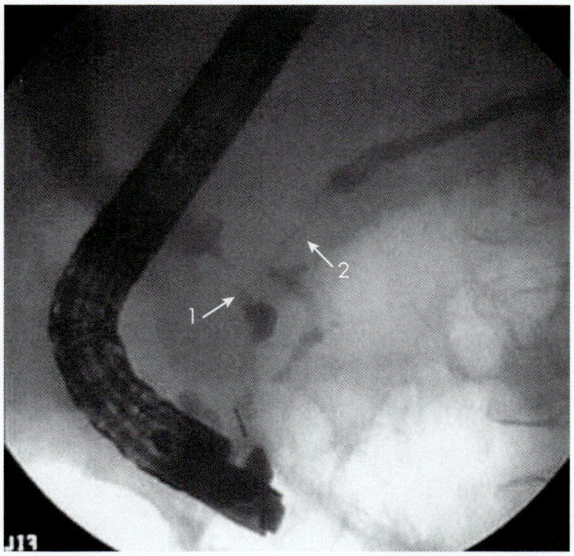

Figure 68.14 Endoscopic retrograde cholangiopancreatography depicting a malignant stricture in the lower part of the common bile duct (1) and in the main pancreatic duct (2), an appearance referred to as the double duct sign (courtesy of Dr George Webster).

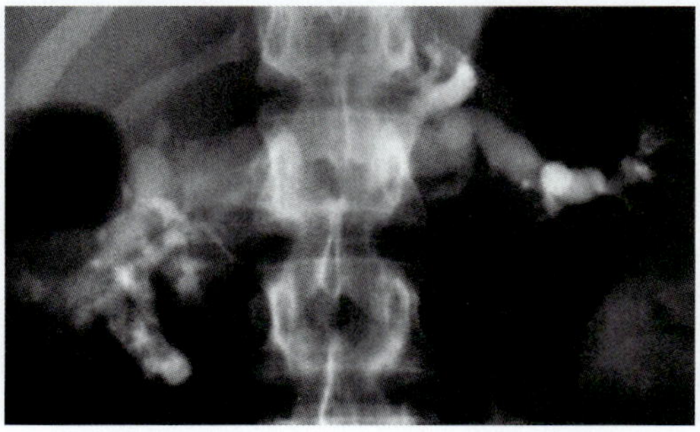

Figure 68.15 Endoscopic retrograde cholangiopancreatography: chronic pancreatitis. Most of the opacities lie within the duct system and are stones. Gross dilatation of ducts in the body and tail are due to obstructions by stones in the head of the pancreas.

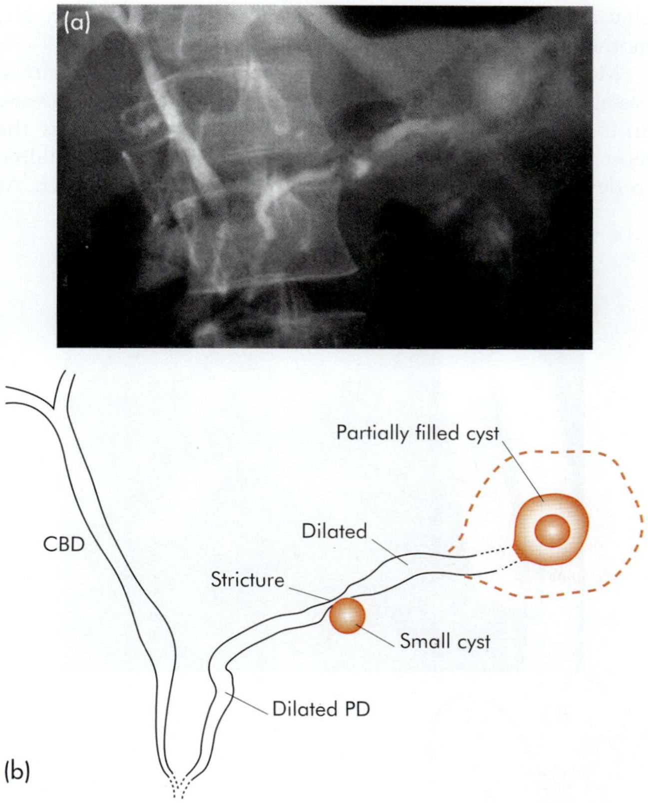

Figure 68.16 (a) Endoscopic retrograde cholangiopancreatography: relapsing acute pancreatitis. Normal biliary tree. Pancreatogram shows stricture of the main duct in the body with distal dilatation and cyst formation. (b) Diagrammatic outline of (a). CBD, common bile duct; PD, pancreatic duct.

lymph nodes can be assessed (Figure 68.20). This is particularly useful in identifying small tumours that may not show up well on CT or MRI, and in demonstrating the relationship of a pancreatic tumour to major vessels nearby. EUS can clarify the relationship of a neuroendocrine tumour to the main pancreatic duct (important if enucleation is being considered). It helps to distinguish cystic tumours from pseudocysts. Transduodenal or transgastric fine needle aspiration (FNA) or Trucut biopsy performed under EUS guidance avoids spillage of tumour cells into the peritoneal cavity.

CONGENITAL ABNORMALITIES

Cystic fibrosis

This is inherited as an autosomal recessive condition. It occurs most frequently among Caucasians, in whom it is the most common inherited disorder (incidence of 1:2500 live births in the UK). Cystic fibrosis (CF) develops when there is a mutation in the *CFTR* (cystic fibrosis transmembrane conductance regulator) gene on chromosome 7. This gene creates a cell membrane protein that helps to control the movement of chloride across the cell membrane.

CF is a multisystem disorder of exocrine glands that affects the lungs, intestines, pancreas and liver, and is characterised by elevated sodium and chloride ion concentrations in sweat. The mother may notice that the child is salty when kissed.

Most of the organ damage is due to blockage of narrow passages by thickened secretions. Chronic pulmonary disease arises from plugging of bronchi and bronchioles. CF is the most common cause of chronic lung disease among children in developed countries. Cor pulmonale may develop later. At birth, the meconium may set in a sticky mass and produce intestinal obstruction (meconium ileus) (see Chapter 8). Secretions precipitate in the lumen of the pancreatic duct causing blockage, which results in duct ectasia and fatty replacement of exocrine acinar tissue. Pancreatic exocrine insufficiency leads to fat malabsorption. Steatorrhoea is usually present from birth, resulting in stools that are bulky, oily and offensive. The islets

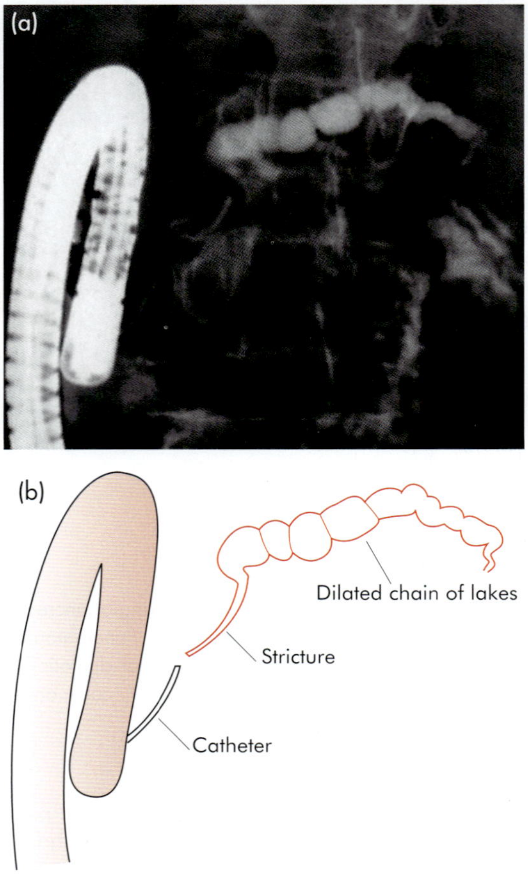

Figure 68.17 (a) Endoscopic retrograde cholangiopancreatography: chronic pancreatitis. Long stricture of the pancreatic duct in the head; distal pancreatic duct shows sacculation with intervening short strictures, 'chain of lakes'. (b) Diagrammatic outline of (a).

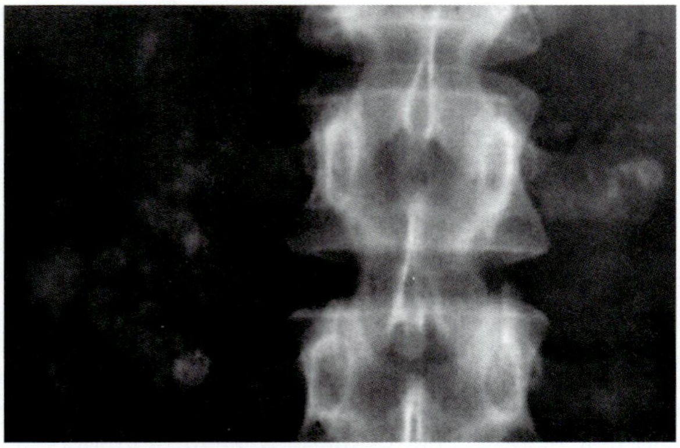

Figure 68.18 Plain abdominal radiograph: chronic pancreatitis. Multiple opacities can be seen in the region of the head and tail of the pancreas.

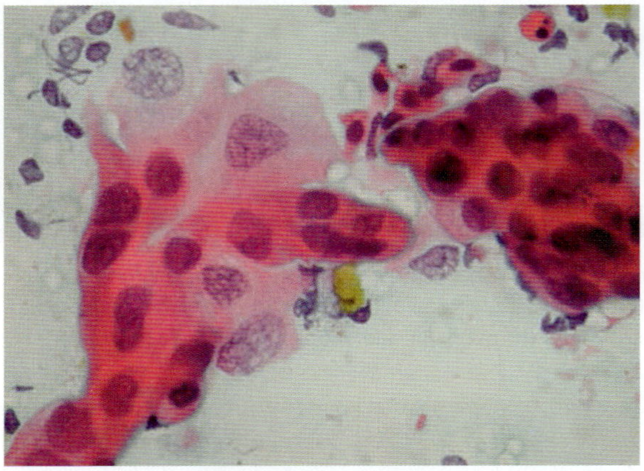

Figure 68.19 A group of adenocarcinoma cells identified in pancreatic juice collected at the time of endoscopic retrograde cholangiopancreatography (courtesy of Professor Roger Feakins).

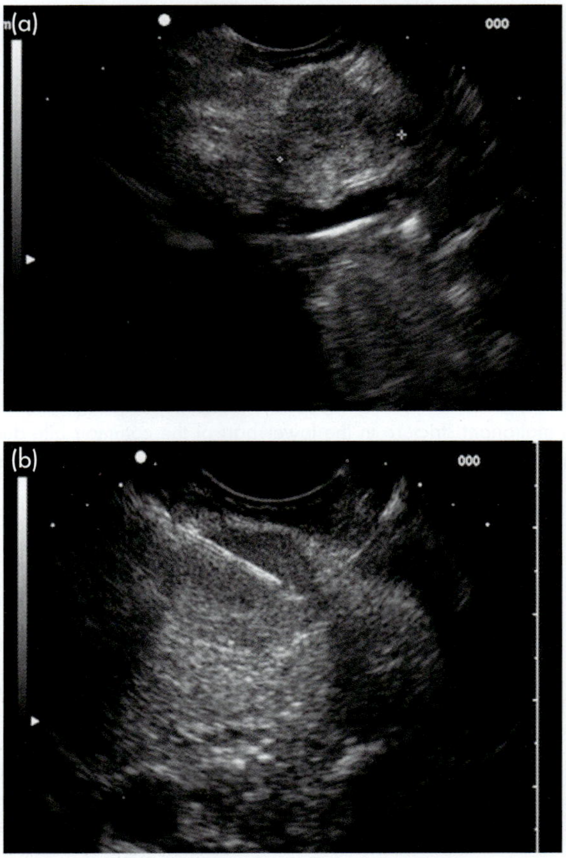

Figure 68.20 (a) Carcinoma of the pancreatic head as seen on endoscopic ultrasound (EUS). (b) Aspiration biopsy carried out under EUS guidance: needle seen entering the tumour (courtesy of Dr Peter Fairclough).

of Langerhans usually appear normal, but diabetes mellitus can occur in older patients. The liver may become cirrhotic as a result of bile duct plugging, and signs of portal hypertension may appear. Infertility is common, due to the absence of the vas deferens in men and thick cervical mucus in women.

Outside the newborn period, the earliest clinical signs of CF are poor growth, poor appetite, rancid greasy stools, abdominal distension, chronic respiratory disease and finger clubbing. The appearance of secondary sexual characteristics may be delayed. The diagnosis can be made by genetic testing (which may be part of prenatal or newborn screening) and by the sweat test. Levels of sodium and chloride ions in the sweat above 90 mmol/L confirm the diagnosis.

Treatment is aimed at control of the secondary consequences of the disease. Pulmonary function is preserved with aggressive physiotherapy and antibiotics. Malabsorption is treated by administration of oral pancreatic enzyme preparations. The diet should be low in fat but contain added salt to replace the high losses in the sweat. With early diagnosis and optimal treatment, patients in the western world can now expect to survive to their mid-thirties. Those with end-stage lung disease may be considered for lung transplantation. Heterozygous carriers of the various gene mutations are asymptomatic, but can be identified by DNA analysis. There is a suggestion that such patients may develop pancreatitis later in life.

Pancreas divisum

Pancreas divisum occurs when the embryological ventral and dorsal parts of the pancreas fail to fuse (Figure 68.3). The dorsal pancreatic duct becomes the main pancreatic duct and drains most of the pancreas through the minor or accessory papilla. The incidence of pancreas divisum ranges from 5 per cent in autopsy series to 10 per cent in some ERCP and MRCP series. Pancreas divisum found incidentally in an asymptomatic person does not warrant any intervention. However, the incidence of pancreas divisum ranges from 25 to 50 per cent in patients with recurrent acute pancreatitis, chronic pancreatitis and pancreatic pain. The minor papilla is substantially smaller than the major papilla (and many of these patients probably have papillary stenosis). A large volume of secretions flowing through a narrow papilla probably leads to incomplete drainage, which may then cause obstructive pain or pancreatitis. Certainly in patients with idiopathic recurrent pancreatitis, pancreas divisum should be excluded. The diagnosis can be arrived at by MRCP, EUS or ERCP, augmented by injection of secretin if necessary. There may be changes indicative of obstruction or chronic inflammation in the dorsal duct system. Endoscopic sphincterotomy and stenting of the minor papilla may relieve the symptoms. Surgical intervention can take the form of sphincteroplasty, pancreatojejunostomy or even resection of the pancreatic head.

Annular pancreas

This is the result of a failure of complete rotation of the ventral pancreatic bud during development, so that a ring of pancreatic tissue surrounds the second or third part of the duodenum. It is most often seen in association with congenital duodenal stenosis or atresia and is therefore more prevalent in children with Down's syndrome. Duodenal obstruction typically causes vomiting in the neonate (see Chapter 8). The usual treatment is bypass (duodenoduodenostomy). The disease may occur in later life as one of the causes of pancreatitis, in which case resection of the head of the pancreas is preferable to lesser procedures.

Ectopic pancreas

Islands of ectopic pancreatic tissue can be found in the submucosa in parts of the stomach, duodenum or small intestine (including Meckel's diverticulum), the gall bladder, adjoining the pancreas, in the hilum of the spleen and within the liver. Ectopic pancreas may also be found in the wall of an alimentary tract duplication cyst (see Chapter 8).

Congenital cystic disease of the pancreas

This sometimes accompanies congenital disease of the kidneys and liver, and occurs as part of the von Hippel–Lindau syndrome.

INJURIES TO THE PANCREAS

External injury

Presentation and management

The pancreas, thanks to its somewhat protected location in the retroperitoneum, is not frequently damaged in blunt abdominal trauma. If there is damage to the pancreas, it is often concomitant with injuries to other viscera, especially the liver, the spleen and the duodenum. Occasionally, a forceful blow to the epigastrium may crush the body of the pancreas against the vertebral column. Penetrating trauma to the upper abdomen or the back carries a higher chance of pancreatic injury. Pancreatic injuries may range from a contusion or laceration of the parenchyma without duct disruption to major parenchymal destruction with duct disruption (sometimes complete transection) and, rarely, massive destruction of the pancreatic head. The most important factor that determines treatment is whether the pancreatic duct has been disrupted.

Blunt pancreatic trauma usually presents with epigastric pain, which may be minor at first, with the progressive development of more severe pain due to the sequelae of leakage of pancreatic fluid into the surrounding tissues. The clinical presentation can be quite deceptive; careful serial assessments and a high index of suspicion are required. A rise in serum amylase occurs in most cases. A CT scan of the pancreas will delineate the damage that has occurred to the pancreas (Figure 68.21). If there is doubt about duct disruption, an urgent ERCP should be sought. MRCP may also provide the answer, but the images can be difficult to interpret. Support with intravenous fluids and a nil by mouth regimen should be instituted while these investigations are performed. There is no need to rush to a laparotomy if the patient is haemodynamically stable, without peritonitis. It is preferable to manage conservatively at first, investigate and, once the extent of the damage has been ascertained, undertake appropriate action. Operation is indicated if there is disruption of the main pancreatic duct; in almost all other cases, the patient will recover with conservative management. In penetrating injuries, especially if other organs are injured and the patient's condition

Eugen von Hippel, 1867–1939, Professor of Ophthalmology, Göttingen, Germany.
Arvid Lindau, 1892–1958, Pathologist, Lund, Sweden, established the link between the retinal angiomatosis described by von Hippel and the cerebellar and visceral components of the syndrome.

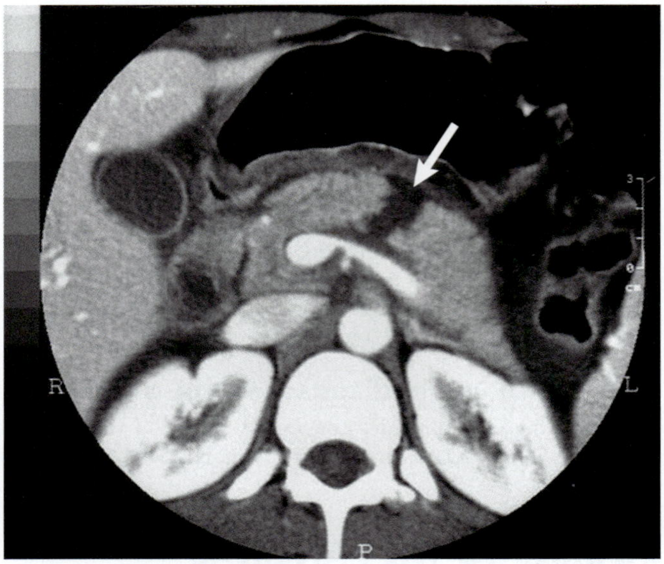

Figure 68.21 Computed tomography scan showing a pancreatic transection due to a bicycle handlebar injury. A distal pancreatectomy was performed.

is unstable, there is a greater need to perform an urgent surgical exploration.

Assessment of pancreatic damage and duct disruption at the time of surgery can be difficult, because the bruising associated with the retroperitoneal damage prevents clear visualisation of the pancreas. A patient and thorough examination of the gland should be carried out. Haemostasis and closed drainage is adequate for minor parenchymal injuries. If the gland is transected in the body or tail, a distal pancreatectomy should be performed, with or without splenectomy. However, if the plane of transection is flat and clean, it may be possible to anastomose the stump of the distal pancreas to a Roux loop of jejenum as an end-to-side pancreatojejunostomy. If damage is purely confined to the head of the pancreas, haemostasis and external drainage is normally effective. In the emergency setting, in an unstable patient with concomitant injuries, a surgeon unaccustomed to pancreatic surgery should refrain from trying to ascertain whether the duct in the pancreatic head is intact or embarking on a major resection. However, if there is severe injury to the pancreatic head and duodenum, then a pancreatoduodenectomy may be necessary (Summary box 68.3).

Summary box 68.3

External injury to the pancreas

- Other organs are likely to be injured
- It is important to ascertain whether the pancreatic duct has been disrupted
- CT and ERCP are the most useful tests
- Surgery is indicated if the main pancreatic duct is disrupted

Prognosis

The most common cause of death in the immediate period is bleeding, usually from associated injuries. Once the acute phase has passed, the mortality and morbidity related to the pancreatic injury itself are treatable, with a complete return to normal activity the usual outcome.

Persistent drain output occurs in up to a third of patients (see below under Pancreatic fistula). Sometimes, in the aftermath of trauma that has been treated conservatively, duct stricturing develops, leading to recurrent episodes of pancreatitis. The appropriate treatment in such cases is resection of the tail of the pancreas distal to the site of duct disruption.

Also, a pancreatic pseudocyst may develop. If the main duct is intact, the cyst can be aspirated percutaneously in the first instance; it may not be necessary to undertake a cystgastrostomy. If the cyst develops in the presence of complete disruption of the pancreas, there is no alternative but to undertake a cystgastrostomy or even a distal resection or, occasionally, a pancreatojejunostomy with a Roux-en-Y loop. In a patient who presents with a peripancreatic cyst and a history of previous blunt abdominal trauma, do not assume that it is a post-traumatic pseudocyst. The possibility of a cystic neoplasm should be considered and excluded.

Iatrogenic injury

This can occur in several ways:

- Injury to the tail of the pancreas during splenectomy, resulting in a pancreatic fistula.
- Injury to the accessory pancreatic duct (Santorini), which is the main duct in 7 per cent of patients, during Billroth II gastrectomy. A pancreatogram performed by cannulating the duct at the time of discovery of such an injury will demonstrate whether it is safe to ligate and divide the duct. If no alternative drainage duct can be demonstrated, then the duct should be reanastomosed to the duodenum.
- Enucleation of islet cell tumours of the pancreas can result in fistulae.
- Duodenal or ampullary bleeding following sphincterotomy. This injury may require duodenotomy to control the bleeding.

Pancreatic fistula

Pancreatic fistula usually follows operative trauma to the gland or occurs as a complication of acute or chronic pancreatitis. It is important to define the site of the fistula and the epithelial structure with which it communicates (e.g. externally to skin or internally to bowel). If there is uncertainty about whether the fluid issuing from a drain site or a wound is pancreatic, measurement of the amylase content will be diagnostic.

Management includes correction of metabolic and electrolyte disturbances and adequate drainage of the fistula into a stoma bag with protection of the skin. Investigation of the cause of the fistula is required as the underlying cause must be treated before the fistula will close. Frequently, the cause is related to obstruction within the pancreatic duct, which can be overcome by the insertion of a stent or catheter endoscopically into the pancreatic duct. While waiting for closure of the fistula, the patient should be given parenteral or nasojejunal nutritional support (as opposed to nasogastric or oral feeding; the rationale is that parenteral or nasojejunal feeding reduces the volume of pancreatic secretion). The use of octreotide will also suppress pancreatic secretion (Summary box 68.4) (see also Chapter 20).

Giovanni Domenico Santorini, 1681–1737, Professor of Anatomy and Medicine, Venice, Italy. His drawings of the accessory pancreatic duct were published after his death.
Christian Albert Theodor Billroth, 1829–1894, Professor of Surgery, Vienna, Austria. A hugely influential surgical teacher and an early proponent of surgical audit, Billroth performed the first oesophagectomy, first laryngectomy and first successful gastrectomy. He was also a talented musician and a friend of the composer Brahms.

Summary box 68.4

Management of pancreatic fistulae

- Tests
  - Measure amylase level in fluid
  - Determine the anatomy of the fistula
  - Check whether the main pancreatic duct is blocked or disrupted
- Measures
  - Correct fluid and electrolyte imbalances
  - Protect the skin
  - Drain adequately
  - Parenteral or nasojejunal feeding
  - Octreotide to suppress secretion
  - Relieve pancreatic duct obstruction if possible (ERCP and stent)
  - Treat underlying cause

PANCREATITIS

Pancreatitis is inflammation of the gland parenchyma of the pancreas. For clinical purposes, it is useful to divide pancreatitis into acute, which presents as an emergency, and chronic, which is a prolonged and frequently lifelong disorder resulting from the development of fibrosis within the pancreas. It is probable that acute pancreatitis is but a phase of chronic pancreatitis.

Acute pancreatitis is defined as an acute condition presenting with abdominal pain and is usually associated with raised pancreatic enzyme levels in the blood or urine as a result of pancreatic inflammation. Acute pancreatitis may recur.

The underlying mechanism of injury in pancreatitis is thought to be premature activation of pancreatic enzymes within the pancreas, leading to a process of autodigestion. Anything that injures the acinar cell and impairs the secretion of zymogen granules, or damages the duct epithelium and thus delays enzymatic secretion, can trigger acute pancreatitis. Once cellular injury has been initiated, the inflammatory process can lead to pancreatic oedema, haemorrhage and, eventually, necrosis. As inflammatory mediators are released into the circulation, systemic complications can arise, such as haemodynamic instability, bacteraemia (due to translocation of gut flora), acute respiratory distress syndrome and pleural effusions, gastrointestinal haemorrhage, renal failure and disseminated intravascular coagulation (DIC).

Acute pancreatitis may be categorised as mild or severe. **Mild acute pancreatitis** is characterised by interstitial oedema of the gland and minimal organ dysfunction. Eighty per cent of patients will have a mild attack of pancreatitis, the mortality from which is around 1 per cent. **Severe acute pancreatitis** is characterised by pancreatic necrosis, a severe systemic inflammatory response and often multi-organ failure. In those who have a severe attack of pancreatitis, the mortality varies from 20 to 50 per cent. About one-third of deaths occur in the early phase of the attack, from multiple organ failure, while deaths occurring after the first week of onset are due to septic complications.

Chronic pancreatitis is defined as a continuing inflammatory disease of the pancreas characterised by irreversible morphological change typically causing pain and/or permanent loss of function. Many patients with chronic pancreatitis have painful exacerbations, but the condition may be completely painless.

Acute pancreatitis

Incidence

Acute pancreatitis accounts for 3 per cent of all cases of abdominal pain among patients admitted to hospital in the UK. The hospital admission rate for acute pancreatitis is 9.8 per year per 100 000 population in the UK, although worldwide, the annual incidence may range from 5 to 50 per 100 000. The disease may occur at any age, with a peak in young men and older women.

Aetiology

The two major causes of acute pancreatitis are biliary calculi, which occur in 50–70 per cent of patients, and alcohol abuse, which accounts for 25 per cent of cases. Gallstone pancreatitis is thought to be triggered by the passage of gallstones down the common bile duct. If the biliary and pancreatic ducts join to share a common channel before ending at the ampulla, then obstruction of this passage may lead to reflux of bile or activated pancreatic enzymes into the pancreatic duct. Patients who have small gallstones and a wide cystic duct may be at a higher risk of passing stones. The proposed mechanisms for alcoholic pancreatitis include the effects of diet, malnutrition, direct toxicity of alcohol, concomitant tobacco smoking, hypersecretion, duct obstruction or reflux, and hyperlipidaemia. The remaining cases may be due to rare causes or be idiopathic (Summary box 68.5).

Summary box 68.5

Possible causes of acute pancreatitis

- Gallstones
- Alcoholism
- Post-ERCP
- Abdominal trauma
- Following biliary, upper gastrointestinal or cardiothoracic surgery
- Ampullary tumour
- Drugs (corticosteroids, azathioprine, asparaginase, valproic acid, thiazides, oestrogens)
- Hyperparathyroidism
- Hypercalcaemia
- Pancreas divisum
- Autoimmune pancreatitis
- Hereditary pancreatitis
- Viral infections (mumps, Coxsackie B)
- Malnutrition
- Scorpion bite
- Idiopathic

Among patients who undergo ERCP, 1–3 per cent develop pancreatitis, probably as a consequence of duct disruption and enzyme extravasation. Patients with sphincter of Oddi dysfunction or a history of recurrent pancreatitis, and those who undergo sphincterotomy or balloon dilatation of the sphincter, carry a higher risk of developing post-ERCP pancreatitis. Patients who have undergone upper abdominal or cardiothoracic surgery may develop acute pancreatitis in the postoperative phase, as may those who have suffered blunt abdominal trauma.

Hereditary pancreatitis is a rare familial condition associated with mutations of the cationic trypsinogen gene. Patients have a tendency to suffer acute pancreatitis while in their teens, progress to chronic pancreatitis in the next two decades and

Ruggero Oddi, 1864–1913, anatomist and physiologist, Perugia, Italy, wrote about the structure and function of the ampullary sphincter in 1887, when still a student. He struggled in later life with drug addiction.

have a high risk (possibly up to 40 per cent) of developing pancreatic cancer by the age of 70 years.

Occasionally, tumours at the ampulla of Vater may cause acute pancreatitis. It is important to check the serum calcium level, a fasting lipid profile, autoimmune markers and viral titres in patients with so-called idiopathic acute pancreatitis. It is equally important to take a detailed drug history and remember the association of corticosteroids, azathioprine, asparaginase and valproic acid with acute pancreatitis. A careful search for the aetiology must be made in all cases, and no more than 20 per cent of cases should fall into the idiopathic category (Summary box 68.6).

Summary box 68.6

Aetiology of acute pancreatitis

- It is essential to establish the aetiology
- Investigate thoroughly before labelling it as 'idiopathic'
- After the acute episode resolves, remember further management of the underlying aetiology
- If the aetiology is gallstones, cholecystectomy is desirable during the same admission

Clinical presentation

Pain is the cardinal symptom. It characteristically develops quickly, reaching maximum intensity within minutes rather than hours and persists for hours or even days. The pain is frequently severe, constant and refractory to the usual doses of analgesics. Pain is usually experienced first in the epigastrium but may be localised to either upper quadrant or felt diffusely throughout the abdomen. There is radiation to the back in about 50 per cent of patients, and some patients may gain relief by sitting or leaning forwards. The suddenness of onset may simulate a perforated peptic ulcer, while biliary colic or acute cholecystitis can be mimicked if the pain is maximal in the right upper quadrant. Radiation to the chest can simulate myocardial infarction, pneumonia or pleuritic pain. In fact, acute pancreatitis can mimic most causes of the acute abdomen and should seldom be discounted in differential diagnosis.

Nausea, repeated vomiting and retching are usually marked accompaniments. The retching may persist despite the stomach being kept empty by nasogastric aspiration. Hiccoughs can be troublesome and may be due to gastric distension or irritation of the diaphragm.

On examination, the appearance may be that of a patient who is well or, at the other extreme, one who is gravely ill with profound shock, toxicity and confusion. Tachypnoea is common, tachycardia is usual, and hypotension may be present. The body temperature is often normal or even subnormal, but frequently rises as inflammation develops. Mild icterus can be caused by biliary obstruction in gallstone pancreatitis, and an acute swinging pyrexia suggests cholangitis. Bleeding into the fascial planes can produce bluish discolouration of the flanks (Grey Turner's sign) or umbilicus (Cullen's sign). Neither sign is pathognomonic of acute pancreatitis; Cullen's sign was first described in association with rupture of an ectopic pregnancy. Subcutaneous fat necrosis may produce small, red, tender nodules on the skin of the legs.

Abdominal examination may reveal distension due to ileus or, more rarely, ascites with shifting dullness. A mass can develop in the epigastrium due to inflammation. There is usually muscle guarding in the upper abdomen, although marked rigidity is unusual. A pleural effusion is present in 10–20 per cent of patients. Pulmonary oedema and pneumonitis are also described and may give rise to the differential diagnosis of pneumonia or myocardial infarction. The patient may be confused and exhibit the signs of metabolic derangement together with hypoxaemia.

George Grey Turner, 1877–1951, Professor of Surgery, The University of Durham, Durham (1927–1934), and at the Postgraduate Medical School, Hammersmith, London, UK (1934–1945). The Grey Turner Travelling Surgical Club was named after him.
Thomas Stephen Cullen, 1868–1953, Professor of Gynecology, The Johns Hopkins University, Baltimore, MD, USA. Described bluish discolouration of the periumbilical skin as a sign of ruptured ectopic pregnancy.

Investigations

Typically, the diagnosis is made on the basis of the clinical presentation and an elevated serum amylase level. A serum amylase level three to four times above normal is indicative of the disease. A normal serum amylase level does not exclude acute pancreatitis, particularly if the patient has presented a few days later. If the serum lipase level can be checked, it provides a slightly more sensitive and specific test than amylase. If there is doubt, and other causes of acute abdomen have to be excluded, contrast-enhanced CT is probably the best single imaging investigation (see below under Imaging) (Summary box 68.7).

Summary box 68.7

Investigations in acute pancreatitis should be aimed at answering three questions:

- Is a diagnosis of acute pancreatitis correct?
- How severe is the attack?
- What is the aetiology?

Assessment of severity

On account of the difference in outcome between patients with mild and severe disease, it is important to define that group of patients who will develop severe pancreatitis. Various scoring systems have been introduced, such as the Ranson and Glasgow scoring systems (Table 68.3). The APACHE II scoring system, used in intensive care units, can also be applied. A severe attack may be heralded by an initial clinical impression of a very ill patient and an APACHE II score above 8. At 48 hours after the onset of symptoms, a Glasgow score of 3 or more, a C-reactive protein level greater than 150 mg/L and a worsening clinical state with sepsis or persisting organ failure indicate a severe attack. Severity stratification should be performed in all patients within 48 hours of diagnosis. Patients with a body mass index over 30 are at higher risk of developing complications.

Imaging

Plain erect chest and abdominal radiographs are not diagnostic of acute pancreatitis, but are useful in the differential diagnosis. Non-specific findings in pancreatitis include a generalised or local ileus (sentinel loop), a colon cut-off sign and a renal halo

John HC Ranson, 1938–1995, Professor of Surgery, The New York University School of Medicine, New York, NY, USA, was born in India, trained at St Bartholomew's Hospital, London, UK. Described his criteria for severity of acute pancreatitis in 1974.

Table 68.3 Scoring systems to predict the severity of acute pancreatitis: in both systems, disease is classified as severe when three or more factors are present.

Ranson score	Glasgow scale
On admission	**On admission**
Age >55 years	Age >55 years
White blood cell count >16 × 10^9/L	White blood cell count >15 × 10^9/L
Blood glucose >10 mmol/L	Blood glucose >10 mmol/L (no history of diabetes)
LDH >700 units/L	Serum urea >16 mmol/L (no response to intravenous fluids)
AST >250 Sigma Frankel units per cent	Arterial oxygen saturation (PaO_2) <8 kPa (60 mmHg)
Within 48 hours	**Within 48 hours**
Blood urea nitrogen rise >5 mg per cent	Serum calcium <2.0 mmol/L
Arterial oxygen saturation (PaO_2) <8 kPa (60 mmHg)	Serum albumin <32 g/L
Serum calcium <2.0 mmol/L	LDH >600 units/L
Base deficit >4 mmol/L	AST/ALT >600 units/L
Fluid sequestration >6 litres	

ALT, alanine aminotransferase; AST, aspartate aminotransferase; LDH, lactate dehydrogenase; PaO_2, arterial oxygen tension.

sign. Occasionally, calcified gallstones or pancreatic calcification may be seen. A chest radiograph may show a pleural effusion and, in severe cases, a diffuse alveolar interstitial shadowing may suggest acute respiratory distress syndrome.

Ultrasound does not establish a diagnosis of acute pancreatitis. The swollen pancreas may be seen, but ultrasonography should be performed within 24 hours in all patients to detect gallstones as a potential cause, rule out acute cholecystitis as a differential diagnosis and determine whether the common bile duct is dilated.

CT is not necessary for all patients, particularly those deemed to have a mild attack on prognostic criteria. However, a contrast-enhanced CT is indicated in the following situations:

- if there is diagnostic uncertainty;
- in patients with severe acute pancreatitis, to distinguish interstitial from necrotising pancreatitis (Figure 68.22). In the first 72 hours, CT may underestimate the extent of necrosis. The severity of pancreatitis detected on CT may be staged according to the Balthazar criteria;
- in patients with organ failure, signs of sepsis or progressive clinical deterioration;
- when a localised complication is suspected, such as fluid collection, pseudocyst or a pseudoaneurysm.

Cross-sectional MRI can yield similar information to that obtained by CT. EUS and MRCP can help in detecting stones in the common bile duct and directly assessing the pancreatic parenchyma, but are not widely available. ERCP allows the identification and removal of stones in the common bile duct in gallstone pancreatitis. In patients with severe acute gallstone pancreatitis and signs of ongoing biliary obstruction and cholangitis, an urgent ERCP should be sought (see below under Management).

Emil J Balthazar, contemporary, Professor Emeritus, The Department of Radiology, The New York University, New York, NY, USA.

The presentation is so variable that sometimes even an experienced clinician can be mistaken. While this is not desirable, occasionally the diagnosis is only made at laparotomy. The appearances at laparotomy are characteristic (Figure 68.23).

Management

If after initial assessment a patient is considered to have a mild attack of pancreatitis, a conservative approach is indicated with intravenous fluid administration and frequent, but non-invasive, observation. A brief period of fasting may be sensible in a

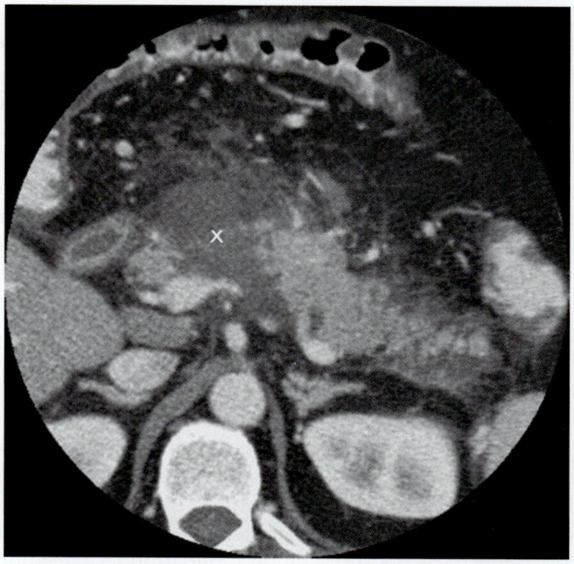

Figure 68.22 Contrast-enhanced computed tomography scan showing acute necrotising pancreatitis. Note the area of reduced enhancement in the pancreas (marked X), the peripancreatic oedema and stranding of the fatty tissues (courtesy of Dr Niall Power).

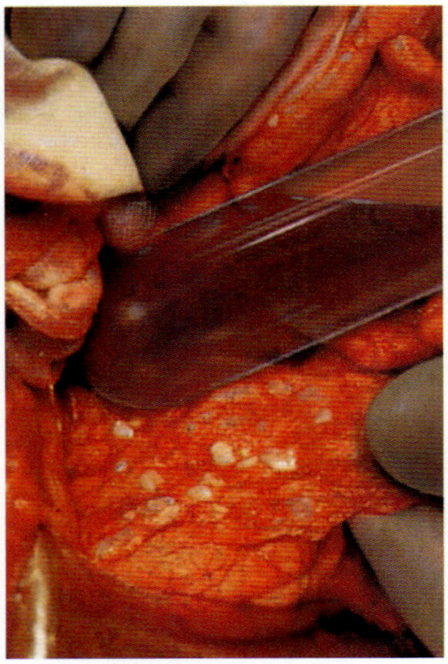

Figure 68.23 Widespread fat necrosis of the omentum. A test tube has been filled with blood-stained peritoneal fluid. This specimen was rich in amylase. Fat necroses are dull, opaque, yellow-white areas suggestive of drops of wax. They are most abundant in the vicinity of the pancreas, but are widespread in the greater omentum and the mesentery. At necropsy, they can sometimes be demonstrated beneath the pleura and pericardium, and even in the subsynovial fat of the knee joint. Fat necroses consist of small islands of saponification caused by the liberation of lipase, which splits into glycerol and fatty acids. Free fatty acids combine with calcium to form soaps (fatty necrosis) (courtesy of Dr GD Adhia, Mumbai, India).

patient who is nauseated and in pain, but there is little physiological justification for keeping patients on a prolonged 'nil by mouth' regimen. Antibiotics are not indicated. Apart from analgesics and anti-emetics, no drugs or interventions are warranted, and CT scanning is unnecessary unless there is evidence of deterioration. However, if a stable patient meets the prognostic criteria for a severe attack of pancreatitis, then a more aggressive approach is required, with the patient being admitted to a high-dependency or an intensive care unit and monitored invasively.

Patients with a severe attack should be admitted to an intensive care or high-dependency unit (Table 68.4). Adequate analgesia should be administered. Aggressive fluid resuscitation is important, guided by frequent measurement of vital signs, urine output and central venous pressure. Supplemental oxygen should be administered and serial arterial blood gas analysis performed. The haematocrit, clotting profile, blood glucose and serum levels of calcium and magnesium should be closely monitored.

A nasogastric tube is not essential but may be of value in patients with vomiting. Specific treatments, such as aprotinin, somatostatin analogues, platelet-activating factor inhibitors and selective gut decontamination, have failed to improve outcome in numerous clinical trials and should not be given. There are no data to support a practice of 'resting' the pancreas and feeding only by the parenteral or nasojejunal routes. If nutritional support is felt to be necessary, enteral nutrition (e.g. feeding via a nasogastric tube) should be used.

There is some evidence to support the use of prophylactic antibiotics in patients with severe acute pancreatitis, but there is no consensus. The rationale is to prevent local and other septic complications. The regimens used include intravenous cefuroxime, or imipenem, or ciprofloxacin plus metronidazole. The duration of antibiotic prophylaxis should not exceed 14 days. Additional antibiotic use should be guided by microbiological cultures.

Table 68.4 Early management of severe acute pancreatitis.

Admission to HDU/ICU
Analgesia
Aggressive fluid rehydration
Oxygenation
Invasive monitoring of vital signs, central venous pressure, urine output, blood gases
Frequent monitoring of haematological and biochemical parameters (including liver and renal function, clotting, serum calcium, blood glucose)
Nasogastric drainage
Antibiotic prophylaxis can be considered (imipenem, cefuroxime)
CT scan essential if organ failure, clinical deterioration or signs of sepsis develop
ERCP within 72 hours for severe gallstone pancreatitis or signs of cholangitis
Supportive therapy for organ failure if it develops (inotropes, ventilatory support, haemofiltration, etc.)
If nutritional support is required, consider enteral (nasogastric) feeding

CT, computed tomography; ERCP, endoscopic retrograde cholangiopancreatography; HDU, high-dependency unit; ICU, intensive care unit.

If gallstones are the cause of an attack of predicted or proven severe pancreatitis, or if the patient has jaundice, cholangitis or a dilated common bile duct, urgent ERCP should be carried out within 72 hours of the onset of symptoms. There is evidence that sphincterotomy and clearance of the bile duct can reduce the incidence of infective complications in these patients. In patients with cholangitis, sphincterotomy should be carried out or a biliary stent placed to drain the duct. ERCP is an invasive procedure and carries a small risk of worsening the pancreatitis.

Systemic complications

Pancreatitis may involve all organ systems (Table 68.5) and place demands on the surgeon beyond his or her skills. Patients with systemic complications should be managed by a multidisciplinary team that includes intensive care specialists. When there is organ failure, appropriate supportive therapies may include inotropic support for haemodynamic instability, haemofiltration in the event of renal failure, ventilatory support for respiratory failure and correction of coagulopathies (including DIC). There is no role for surgery during the initial period of resuscitation and stabilisation; surgical intervention is contemplated only in the patient who deteriorates as a result of local complications following successful stabilisation.

Local complications and their management

Once the acute phase has been survived, usually by the end of

Table 68.5 Complications of acute pancreatitis.

Systemic	Local
(More common in the first week)	*(Usually develop after the first week)*
Cardiovascular	Acute fluid collection
Shock	Sterile pancreatic necrosis
Arrhythmias	Infected pancreatic necrosis
Pulmonary	Pancreatic abscess
ARDS	Pseudocyst
Renal failure	Pancreatic ascites
Haematological	Pleural effusion
DIC	Portal/splenic vein thrombosis
Metabolic	Pseudoaneurysm
Hypocalcaemia	
Hyperglycaemia	
Hyperlipidaemia	
Gastrointestinal	
Ileus	
Neurological	
Visual disturbances	
Confusion, irritability	
Encephalopathy	
Miscellaneous	
Subcutaneous fat necrosis	
Arthralgia	

ARDS, acute respiratory distress syndrome; DIC, disseminated intravascular coagulation.

the first week, and major organ failure is under control, then local complications become pre-eminent in the management of these patients. The course of the patient should be followed carefully and, if clinical resolution does not take place or signs of sepsis develop, a CT scan should be performed. It is important to be clear about the definitions. Certain terms are confusing, such as 'phlegmon', which may refer to an abscess or to an inflammatory mass in the pancreas. Local complications in pancreatic disease are serious and carry a significant mortality. The management approach is conservative on the whole, with surgery restricted to situations in which conservative management has failed.

Acute fluid collection

This occurs early in the course of acute pancreatitis and is located in or near the pancreas. The wall encompassing the collection is ill defined. The fluid is sterile and most such collections resolve. No intervention is necessary unless a large collection causes symptoms or pressure effects, in which case it can be percutaneously aspirated under ultrasound or CT guidance. Transgastric drainage under EUS guidance is another option. An acute fluid collection that does not resolve can evolve into a pseudocyst or an abscess if it becomes infected.

Sterile and infected pancreatic necrosis

The term 'pancreatic necrosis' refers to a diffuse or focal area of non-viable parenchyma that is typically associated with peripancreatic fat necrosis. Necrotic areas can be identified by an absence of contrast enhancement on CT. These are sterile to begin with, but can become subsequently infected, probably due to translocation of gut bacteria. Infected necrosis is

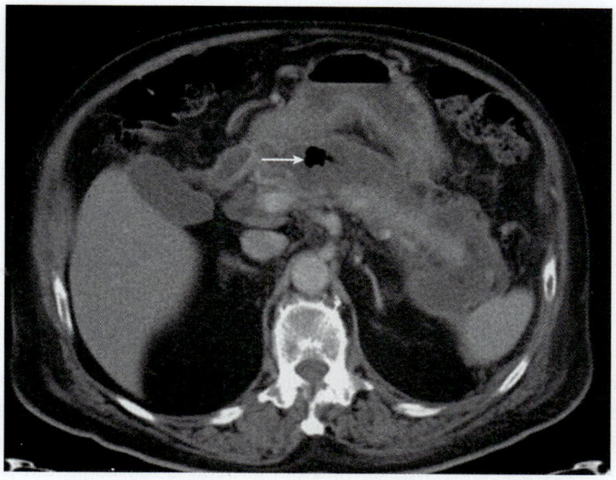

Figure 68.24 Infected pancreatic necrosis in an elderly patient. Note the areas of reduced enhancement in the pancreas and the peripancreatic fluid collection with pockets of gas within it (arrow). This resolved after percutaneous drainage and antibiotic therapy.

associated with a mortality rate of up to 50 per cent. Sterile necrotic material should not be drained or interfered with. However, if the patient shows signs of sepsis, then one should determine whether the necrotic pancreas or the peripancreatic fluid is infected (Figure 68.24). A CT scan should be performed and a needle passed into the area under CT guidance, choosing a path that does not traverse hollow viscera. This may be done under ultrasonographic guidance as well. If the aspirate is purulent, percutaneous drainage of the infected fluid should be carried out. The tube drain inserted should have the widest bore possible. The aspirate should be sent for microbiological assessment, and appropriate antibiotic therapy should be commenced as per the sensitivity report. The fluid can be quite viscous with particulate matter, and the drain may need regular flushing with full aseptic precautions. Often, repeated imaging and repeated insertion of drains is necessary.

If the sepsis worsens despite this, then a pancreatic necrosectomy should be considered. This is a challenging operation that carries a high morbidity and mortality, and is best carried out in a specialist unit. The overwhelming majority of patients with peripancreatic sepsis can be successfully treated by conservative means, and necrosectomy should be necessary in a very small proportion of patients. The surgical approach may be through a mid-line laparotomy, especially if the area involved is around the head of the gland. The duodenocolic and gastrocolic ligaments should be divided and the lesser sac opened. Thorough debridement of the dead tissue around the pancreas should be carried out. If the body and tail of the gland are primarily involved (Figure 68.25), a retroperitoneal approach though a left flank incision may be more appropriate. The tissues are inevitably friable, and one should be careful not to precipitate excessive bleeding or inadvertently breach the bowel wall. Blunt dissection is preferable to sharp dissection. A feeding jejunostomy may be a useful adjunct to the procedure. If gallstones are the precipitating factor of the pancreatitis, a cholecystectomy should be included. Some prefer a minimally invasive approach to a formal laparotomy. A rigid laparoscope is inserted into the peripancreatic area through a retroperitoneal approach, and vigorous

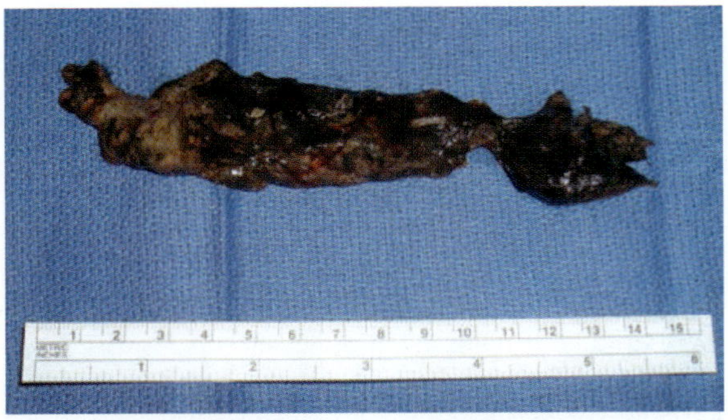

Figure 68.25 Necrotic body and tail of the pancreas removed as an intact specimen rather than piecemeal. The patient had suffered severe necrotising gallstone pancreatitis complicated by persistent pancreatic sepsis. Necrosectomy was carried out through a left flank retroperitoneal approach.

irrigation and suction is combined with a gradual nibbling away of the necrotic debris.

Once a necrosectomy has been completed, further necrotic tissue may form. There are several possible ways of dealing with this (listed below), none of which has been proved to be more effective than the others. The last two approaches make greater logistic demands as one is committed to a re-exploration every 48–72 hours.

- **Closed continuous lavage.** Tube drains are left in and the raw area flushed (Beger) (Figure 68.26).
- **Closed drainage.** The incision is closed, but the cavity is packed with gauze-filled Penrose drains and closed suction drains. The Penrose drains are brought out through the flank and slowly pulled out and removed after 7 days.
- **Open packing.** The incision is left open and the cavity is packed with the intention of returning to the operating theatre at regular intervals and repacking until there is a clean granulating cavity.

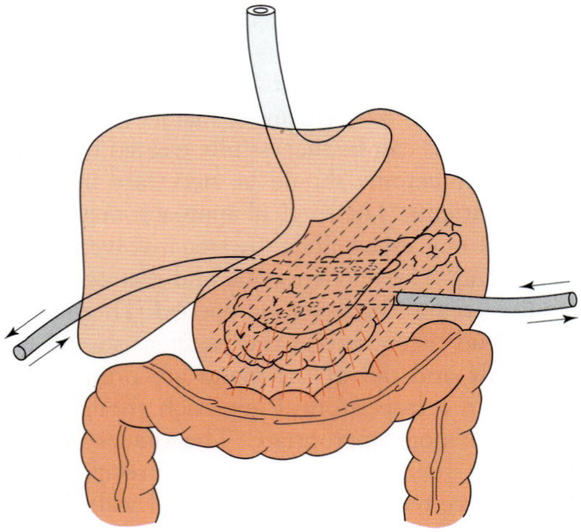

Figure 68.26 Continuous postoperative closed lavage of the lesser sac as advised by Beger. Lavage is carried out through several double-lumen and single-lumen catheters. Each time, 1 litre of saline is infused through and then drained over a period of hours, and the process is repeated.

- **Closure and relaparotomy.** The incision is closed with drains with the intention of performing a series of planned relaparotomies every 48–72 hours until the raw area granulates (Bradley).

There is a subgroup of patients who respond initially to percutaneous treatment but then develop recurrent sepsis that requires repeated insertion of drains, and fail to thrive. Necrosectomy should be considered in these patients, but it can be a difficult judgement call.

Patients with peripancreatic sepsis are ill for long periods of time, and may require management in an intensive care unit. Nutritional support is essential. The parenteral and nasojejunal approaches are more popular (on the assumption that they rest the pancreas), although there is little evidence to show that nasogastric feeding, if tolerated, is harmful in any way.

Pancreatic abscess

This is a circumscribed intra-abdominal collection of pus, usually in proximity to the pancreas. It may be an acute fluid collection or a pseudocyst that has become infected. The principles of diagnosis and management are as outlined above for infected pancreatic necrosis. Percutaneous drainage with the widest possible drains placed under imaging guidance is the treatment, along with appropriate antibiotics and supportive care. Repeated scans may be required depending on the progress of the patient, and drains may need to be flushed, repositioned or reinserted. Very occasionally, open drainage of the abscess may be necessary.

Pancreatic ascites

This is a chronic, generalised, peritoneal, enzyme-rich effusion usually associated with pancreatic duct disruption. Paracentesis will reveal turbid fluid with a high amylase level. Adequate drainage with wide-bore drains placed under imaging guidance is essential. Measures that can be taken to suppress pancreatic secretion include parenteral or nasojejunal feeding and administration of octreotide. An ERCP may allow demonstration of the duct disruption and placement of a pancreatic stent.

Pancreatic effusion

This is an encapsulated collection of fluid in the pleural cavity, arising as a consequence of acute pancreatitis. Concomitant pancreatic ascites may be present, or there may be a communication with an intra-abdominal collection. Percutaneous drainage under imaging guidance is necessary.

Haemorrhage

Bleeding may occur into the gut, into the retroperitoneum or into the peritoneal cavity. Possible causes include bleeding into a pseudocyst cavity, diffuse bleeding from a large raw surface, or a pseudoaneurysm. The last is a false aneurysm of a major peripancreatic vessel confined as a clot by the surrounding tissues and often associated with infection. Recurrent bleeding is common, often culminating in fatal haemorrhage. CT, angiography or magnetic resonance angiography (MRA) helps to make the diagnosis. Treatment involves embolisation or surgery.

Portal or splenic vein thrombosis

This may often develop silently and is identified on a CT scan. A marked rise in the platelet count should raise suspicions. In

Hans Günther Beger, contemporary, Emeritus Professor of Surgery, Ulm, Germany.
Charles Bingham Penrose, 1862–1925, Professor of Gynecology, The University of Pennsylvania, Philadelphia, PA, USA.
Edward Bradley III, contemporary, professor, The Department of Clinical Sciences, Florida State University College of Medicine, FL, USA.

the context of acute pancreatitis, treatment is usually conservative. The patient should be screened for pro-coagulant tendencies. If varices or other manifestations of portal hypertension develop, they will require treatment, such as endoscopic injection or banding, β-blockade, etc. Thrombocytosis may mandate the use of aspirin or other anti-platelet drugs for a period. Systemic anticoagulation, if instituted early in the process, may achieve recanalisation of the vein, but it is not routinely used as it carries considerable risks in a patient with ongoing pancreatitis.

Pseudocyst

A pseudocyst is a collection of amylase-rich fluid enclosed in a wall of fibrous or granulation tissue. Pseudocysts typically arise following an attack of acute pancreatitis, but can develop in chronic pancreatitis or after pancreatic trauma. Formation of a pseudocyst requires 4 weeks or more from the onset of acute pancreatitis (Figure 68.27; see also Figure 68.10). They are often single but, occasionally, patients will develop multiple pseudocysts. If carefully investigated, more than half will be found to have a communication with the main pancreatic duct.

A pseudocyst is usually identified on ultrasound or a CT scan. It is important to differentiate a pseudocyst from an acute fluid collection or an abscess; the clinical scenario and the radiological appearances should allow that distinction to be made. Occasionally, a cystic neoplasm may be confused with a chronic pseudocyst. EUS and aspiration of the cyst fluid is very useful in such a situation. The fluid should be sent for measurement of carcinoembryonic antigen (CEA) levels, amylase levels and cytology. Fluid from a pseudocyst typically has a low CEA level, and levels above 400 ng/mL are suggestive of a mucinous neoplasm. Pseudocyst fluid usually has a high amylase level, but that is not diagnostic, as a tumour that communicates with the duct system may yield similar findings. Cytology typically reveals inflammatory cells in pseudocyst fluid. If there is no access to EUS, then percutaneous FNA is acceptable (just aspiration, not percutaneous insertion of a drain). ERCP and MRCP may demonstrate communication of the cyst with the pancreatic duct system, demonstrate ductal anomalies or diagnose chronic pancreatitis and thus help in planning treatment.

Pseudocysts will resolve spontaneously in most instances, but complications can develop (Table 68.6). Pseudocysts that are thick-walled or large (over 6 cm in diameter), have lasted for a long time (over 12 weeks) or have arisen in the context of chronic pancreatitis are less likely to resolve spontaneously, but these factors are not specific indications for intervention. Therapeutic interventions are advised only if the pseudocyst causes symptoms, if complications develop or a distinction has to be made between a pseudocyst and a tumour.

There are three possible approaches to draining a pseudocyst: percutaneous, endoscopic and surgical. Percutaneous drainage to the exterior under radiological guidance should be avoided. It carries a very high likelihood of recurrence. Moreover, it is not advisable unless one is absolutely certain that the cyst is not neoplastic and that it has no communication with the pancreatic duct (or else a pancreaticocutaneous fistula will develop). A percutaneous transgastric cystgastrostomy can be done under imaging guidance, and a double-pigtail drain placed with one end in the cyst cavity and the other end in the gastric lumen. This requires specialist expertise but, in experienced hands, the recurrence rates are no more than 15 per cent. Endoscopic drainage usually involves puncture of the cyst through the stomach or duodenal wall under EUS guidance, and placement of a tube drain with one end in the cyst cavity and the other end in the gastric lumen. The success rates depend on operator expertise. Occasionally, ERCP and placement of a pancreatic stent across the ampulla may help to drain a pseudocyst that is in communication with the duct. Surgical drainage involves internally draining the cyst into the gastric or jejunal lumen (Figure 68.28). Recurrence rates should be no more than 5 per cent, and this still remains the standard against which the evolving radiological and endoscopic approaches are measured. The approach is conventionally through an open incision, but laparoscopic cystgastrostomy is also feasible. Pseudocysts that have developed complications are best managed surgically (Summary box 68.8).

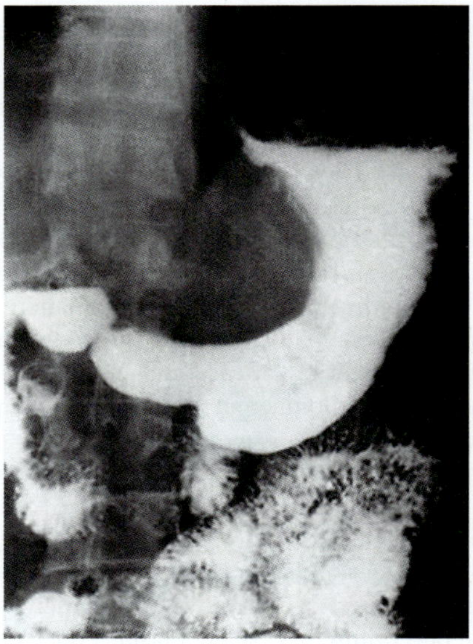

Figure 68.27 Barium meal. Pseudocyst displacing the stomach (courtesy of Professor VK Kapoor, Lucknow, India).

Table 68.6 Possible complications of a pancreatic pseudocyst.

Process	Outcomes
Infection	Abscess Systemic sepsis
Rupture	
Into the gut	Gastrointestinal bleeding Internal fistula
Into the peritoneum	Peritonitis
Enlargement	
Pressure effects	Obstructive jaundice from biliary compression Bowel obstruction
Pain	
Erosion into a vessel	Haemorrhage into the cyst Haemoperitoneum

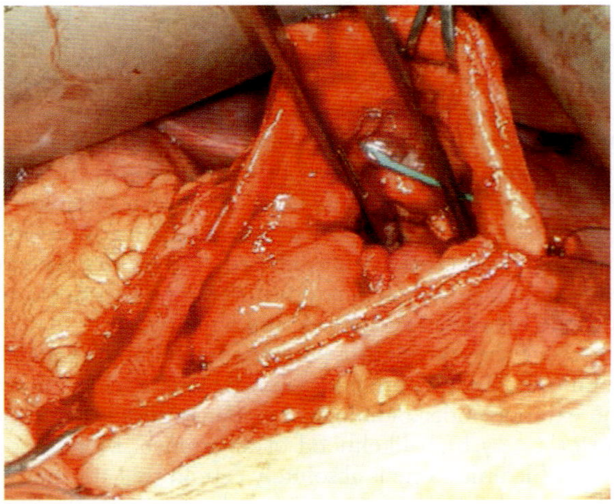

Figure 68.28 Cystgastrostomy for the pancreatic pseudocyst shown in Figure 68.10. The anterior wall of the stomach has been opened and the edges drawn back, held by Babcock's forceps. An opening has been made through the posterior wall of the stomach into the pseudocyst, and the tips of the dissecting forceps are in the cavity of the pseudocyst, which is lined by slough and granulation tissue. The tip of a nasogastric tube is visible. A running stitch will next be placed along the edges of this opening, suturing the full thickness of the posterior gastric wall to the capsule of the pseudocyst.

Summary box 68.8

Distinguishing a pseudocyst from a cystic neoplasm

- History
- Appearance on CT and ultrasound
- FNA of fluid, preferably under EUS guidance
  - CEA (high level in mucinous tumours)
  - Amylase (level usually high in pseudocysts, but occasionally in tumours)
  - Cytology

Outcomes and follow up of acute pancreatitis

The overall mortality from acute pancreatitis has remained at 10–15 per cent over the past 20 years. There is a clear responsibility before the patient is discharged to determine the aetiology of the attack of pancreatitis, and the causes listed in Summary box 68.5 must be looked for and excluded. Failure to remove a predisposing factor could lead to a second attack of pancreatitis, which could be fatal. A proportion of patients in the idiopathic group who suffer repeated attacks may prove to have biliary microlithiasis, which can be identified only by bile sampling at ERCP or by endoscopic ultrasound. In a patient who has gallstone pancreatitis, the gallbladder and gallstones should be removed as soon as the patient is fit to undergo surgery and, preferably, before discharge from hospital.

Chronic pancreatitis

Chronic pancreatitis is a progressive inflammatory disease in which there is irreversible destruction of pancreatic tissue. Its clinical course is characterised by severe pain and, in the later stages, exocrine and endocrine pancreatic insufficiency. In the early stages of its evolution, it is frequently complicated by attacks of acute pancreatitis, which are responsible for the recurrent pain that may be the only clinical symptom. The incidence of chronic pancreatitis in several European, North American and Japanese studies ranges from two to ten new cases per 100 000 population per year, with a prevalence of around 13 cases per 100 000, although there are suspicions that the prevalence is actually higher. In certain parts of the world, such as southern India, the prevalence is much higher (100–200 per 100 000). The disease occurs more frequently in men (male to female ratio of 4:1), and the mean age of onset is about 40 years.

Aetiology and pathology

High alcohol consumption is the most frequent cause of chronic pancreatitis, accounting for 60–70 per cent of cases, but only 5–10 per cent of people with alcoholism develop chronic pancreatitis. The exact mechanism of how alcohol causes chronic inflammation in these patients is unclear; genetic and metabolic factors may be at play.

Other causes include pancreatic duct obstruction resulting from stricture formation after trauma, after acute pancreatitis or even occlusion of the duct by pancreatic cancer. Congenital abnormalities, such as pancreas divisum and annular pancreas, if associated with papillary stenosis, are rare causes of chronic pancreatitis.

Hereditary pancreatitis, CF, infantile malnutrition and a large unexplained idiopathic group make up the remainder. Normally, if trypsinogen does become prematurely activated within the pancreas, it is inhibited by *SPINK1* and then gets destroyed. Hereditary pancreatitis is an autosomal dominant disorder with an 80 per cent penetrance, associated with a gain-of-function mutation in the cationic trypsinogen gene (*PRSS1*) on chromosome 7, which leads to production of a degradation-resistant form of trypsin. A loss-of-function mutation in *SPINK1* also predisposes to idiopathic pancreatitis. Some patients with idiopathic chronic pancreatitis have mutations in the *CFTR* gene. Idiopathic chronic pancreatitis accounts for approximately 30 per cent of cases and has been subdivided into early-onset and late-onset forms.

Tropical pancreatitis is a form of idiopathic pancreatitis that begins at a young age and is associated with a high incidence of diabetes mellitus and stone formation. This has been described in Kerala, in southern India, as well as in other developing countries in Asia, Africa and central America. Malnutrition, ingestion of cyanogenic glycosides in cassava, and exposure to hydrocarbons released by kerosene or paraffin lamps have been proposed as possible mechanisms for tropical pancreatitis. The importance of hereditary pancreatitis and pancreatitis occurring at a young age is that there is a markedly increased risk of developing pancreatic cancer, particularly if the patient smokes tobacco. Hyperlipidaemia and hypercalcaemia can lead to chronic pancreatitis.

Autoimmune pancreatitis has been described relatively recently. Features include diffuse enlargement of the pancreas, diffuse and irregular narrowing of the main pancreatic duct. It may occur in association with other autoimmune diseases, as a multi-system disorder, or may affect the pancreas alone. The changes may be confused with neoplasia. Autoantibodies may be present and levels of the immunoglobulin subtype IgG4 are elevated.

William Wayne Babcock 1872–1963, surgeon, Philadelphia, PA, USA.

At the onset of the disease when symptoms have developed, the pancreas may appear normal. Later, the pancreas enlarges and becomes hard as a result of fibrosis. The ducts become distorted and dilated with areas of both stricture formation and ectasia. Calcified stones weighing from a few milligrams to 200 mg may form within the ducts. The ducts may become occluded with a gelatinous proteinaceous fluid and debris, and inflammatory cysts may form. Histologically, the lesions affect the lobules, producing ductular metaplasia and atrophy of acini, hyperplasia of duct epithelium and interlobular fibrosis.

Clinical features

Pain is the outstanding symptom in the majority of patients. The site of pain depends to some extent on the main focus of the disease. If the disease is mainly in the head of the pancreas, then epigastric and right subcostal pain is common, whereas if it is limited to the left side of the pancreas, left subcostal and back pain are the presenting symptoms. In some patients, the pain is more diffuse. Radiation to the shoulder, usually the left shoulder, occurs. Nausea is common during attacks and vomiting may occur. The pain is often dull and gnawing. Severe flare up of pain may occur superimposed on background discomfort. All the complications of acute pancreatitis can occur with chronic pancreatitis. Weight loss is common, because the patient does not feel like eating. The pain prevents sleep and time off work is frequent. The number of hospital admissions for acute exacerbations is a pointer towards the severity of the disease. Analgesic use and abuse is frequent. This, too, gives an indication of the severity of the disability. The patient's lifestyle is gradually destroyed by pain, analgesic dependence, weight loss and inability to work. Loss of exocrine function leads to steatorrhoea in more than 30 per cent of patients with chronic pancreatitis. Loss of endocrine function and the development of diabetes are not uncommon, and the incidence increases as the disease progresses. Complications frequently bring the patient to the attention of the surgeon. Infection is not infrequent, possibly related to the diabetes mellitus.

Investigations

Only in the early stages of the disease will there be a rise in serum amylase. Tests of pancreatic function merely confirm the presence of pancreatic insufficiency or that more than 70 per cent of the gland has been destroyed.

Pancreatic calcifications may be seen on abdominal x-ray (see Figure 68.18). CT or MRI scan will show the outline of the gland, the main area of damage and the possibilities for surgical correction (Figure 68.29; see also Figure 68.7). Calcification is seen very well on CT, but not on MRI. An MRCP will identify the presence of biliary obstruction and the state of the pancreatic duct (Figure 68.30). The use of intravenous secretin during the study may demonstrate a pancreatic duct stricture that is not apparent on a standard MRCP, but a normal-looking pancreas on CT or MRI does not rule out chronic pancreatitis. ERCP is the most accurate way of elucidating the anatomy of the duct and, in conjunction with the whole organ morphology, can help to determine the type of operation required, if operative intervention is indicated (Figures 68.15 and 68.17). Histologically proven chronic pancreatitis can, however, occur in the setting of normal findings on pancreatography. EUS can also be very useful. Sonographic findings characteristic of chronic pancreatitis include the presence of stones, visible side branches, cysts, lobularity, an irregular main pancreatic duct, hyperechoic foci and strands, dilation of the main pancreatic duct and hyperechoic margins of the main pancreatic duct. The presence of four or more of these features is highly suggestive of chronic pancreatitis.

Treatment

Most patients can be managed with medical measures. There is no single therapeutic agent that has been shown to relieve symptoms (Summary box 68.9).

Endoscopic, radiological or surgical interventions are indicated mainly to relieve obstruction of the pancreatic duct, bile duct or the duodenum, or in dealing with complications (e.g. pseudocyst, abscess, fistula, ascites or variceal haemorrhage). Decompressing an obstructed pancreatic duct can provide pain relief in some patients (the assumption is that ductal hypertension causes the pain).

Endoscopic pancreatic sphincterotomy might be beneficial in patients with papillary stenosis and a high sphincter pressure and pancreatic ductal pressure. Patients with a dominant pancreatic duct stricture and upstream dilatation may benefit by placement of a stent across the stricture. The stent should be left in for no more than 4–6 weeks as it will block. The complication rate is high, and less than two-thirds of patients experience pain relief,

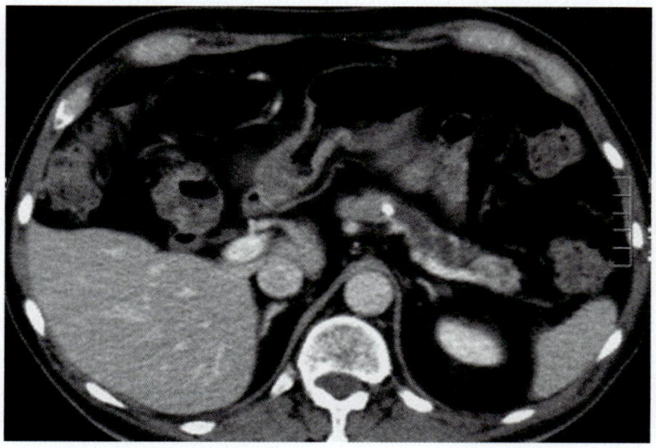

Figure 68.29 Computed tomography scan in a patient with chronic pancreatitis. There is a stone obstructing the main pancreatic duct in the body of the gland with marked dilatation of the duct distal to the stone.

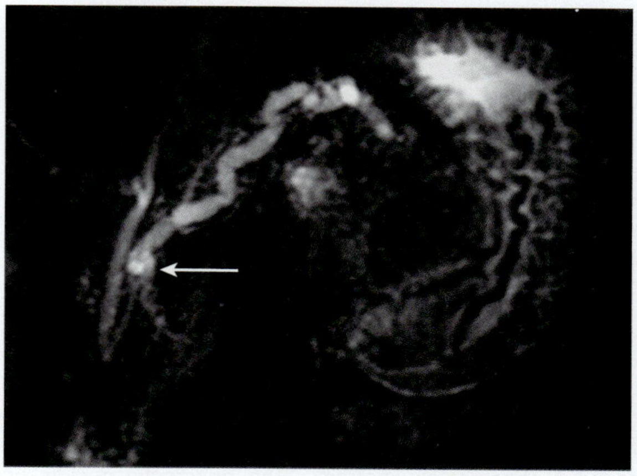

Figure 68.30 Magnetic resonance cholangiopancreatography in a patient with chronic pancreatitis. Stricture of the pancreatic duct in the body of the gland (arrow), with dilatation upstream.

PART 11 | ABDOMINAL

Summary box 68.9

Medical treatment of chronic pancreatitis

- Treat the addiction
  - Help the patient to stop alcohol consumption and tobacco smoking
  - Involve a dependency counsellor or a psychologist
- Alleviate abdominal pain
  - Eliminate obstructive factors (duodenum, bile duct, pancreatic duct)
  - Escalate analgesia in a stepwise fashion
  - Refer to a pain management specialist
  - For intractable pain, consider CT/EUS-guided coeliac axis block
- Nutritional and pharmacological measures
  - Diet: low in fat and high in protein and carbohydrates
  - Pancreatic enzyme supplementation with meals
  - Correct malabsorption of the fat-soluble vitamins and vitamin B12
  - Micronutrient therapy with methionine, vitamins C and E, selenium (may reduce pain and slow disease progression)
  - Steroids (only in autoimmune pancreatitis, for relief of symptoms)
  - Medium-chain triglycerides in patients with severe fat malabsorption (they are directly absorbed by the small intestine without the need for digestion)
  - Reducing gastric secretions may help
- Treat diabetes mellitus

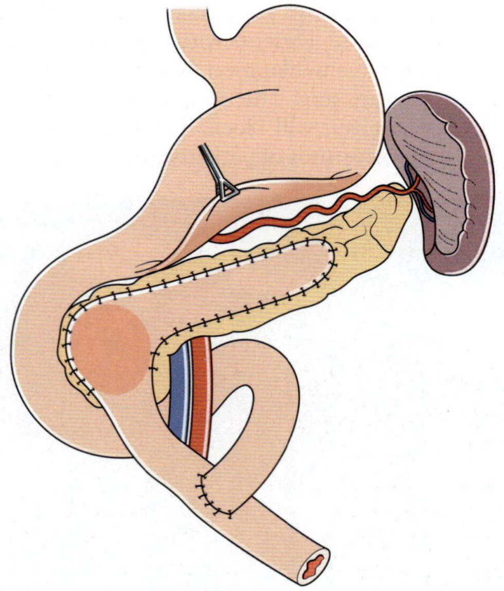

Figure 68.31 Pancreatojejunostomy. The pancreatic duct is opened longitudinally, and a loop of jejunum is sutured to the duct. In the Frey procedure, the superficial part of the head of the pancreas is removed to achieve drainage.

but those who do get relief may benefit from a surgical bypass. Pancreatic duct stones may be extracted at ERCP, and this may sometimes be combined with extracorporeal shock wave lithotripsy. Pseudocysts may be drained internally under EUS guidance. Percutaneous or transgastric drainage of pseudocysts under ultrasound or CT guidance may be performed.

The role of surgery is to overcome obstruction and remove mass lesions. Some patients have a mass in the head of the pancreas, for which either a pancreatoduodenectomy or a Beger procedure (duodenum-preserving resection of the pancreatic head) is appropriate. If the duct is markedly dilated, then a longitudinal pancreatojejunostomy or Frey procedure can be of value (Figure 68.31). The natural evolution of the disease may not be altered significantly, but around half the patients get long-term pain relief. The rare patient with disease limited to the tail will be cured by a distal pancreatectomy. Patients with intractable pain and diffuse disease may plead for a total pancreatectomy in the expectation that removing the offending organ will relieve their pain. However, one should keep in mind that pancreatic function and quality of life are significantly impaired after this procedure, and the operative mortality rate is not trivial. Moreover, there is no guarantee of pain relief (approximately a third of patients get resolution, a third show some benefit, and a third see no benefit at all). Total pancreatectomy and islet autotransplantation has been reported in selected patients, but it is difficult to demonstrate any overall benefit.

Prognosis

Chronic pancreatitis is a difficult condition to manage. Patients often suffer a gradual decline in their professional, social and personal lives. The pain may abate after a surgical or percutaneous intervention, but tends to return over a period of time. In a proportion of patients, the inflammation may gradually burn out over a period of years, with disappearance of the pain, leaving only the exocrine and endocrine insufficiencies. Development of pancreatic cancer is a risk in those who have had the disease for more than 20 years. New symptoms or a change in the pattern of symptoms should be investigated and malignancy excluded.

Sphincter of Oddi dysfunction

Separate mention is warranted of this condition, which should be considered in the differential diagnosis of chronic biliary or pancreatic pain. The sphincter of Oddi is 6–10 mm long and lies within the duodenal wall. A part of it encircles the common channel, and then there are separate biliary and pancreatic components (see Figure 68.5). Scarring or stenosis of the sphincter can result from passage of stones, pancreatitis or prior endoscopic sphincterotomies. Sphincter of Oddi dyskinesia or dysfunction (SOD) is a clinical syndrome in which pain, biochemical abnormalities and dilatation of the bile duct and/or pancreatic duct are attributed to abnormal function of the sphincter of Oddi. The true incidence of SOD is unknown. Females are more commonly affected than males.

There are two types of SOD. Biliary-type SOD is characterised by biliary pain, which may be accompanied by abnormally raised liver enzymes and/or dilation of the bile duct and/or evidence of delayed emptying on biliary scintigraphy. It may be a cause of persistent post-cholecystectomy symptoms. A predominance of pancreatic problems, especially recurrent episodes

Charles Frederick Frey, born 1929, Professor of Surgery, The University of California, Davis, CA, USA.

of acute pancreatitis, is known as pancreatic-type SOD. The biliary and pancreatic sphincters can be evaluated at the time of ERCP with manometry, and high sphincter pressures may be demonstrated. Sphincterotomy and/or stenting of the involved duct system may be performed if deemed appropriate. SOD is, however, associated with a particularly high risk of post-ERCP pancreatitis, and such treatments are best carried out in tertiary units by expert gastroenterologists.

In a small subgroup of patients who have experienced significant but short-lived relief with sphincterotomy or stenting, surgical transduodenal sphincteroplasty may be considered. Although SOD can cause severe symptoms (and the patient may therefore be keen to have something done), it is not fatal. However, post-ERCP pancreatitis and surgery both carry a small but definite risk of mortality.

CARCINOMA OF THE PANCREAS

Pancreatic cancer is the sixth leading cause of cancer death in the UK, and the incidence is ten cases per 100 000 population per year. Worldwide, it constitutes 2–3 per cent of all cancers and, in the United States, is the fourth highest cause of cancer death. The incidence has declined slightly over the last 25 years. There is no simple screening test; however, patients with an increased inherited risk of pancreatic cancer (Table 68.7) should be referred to specialist units for screening and counselling.

Table 68.7 Risk factors for the development of pancreatic cancer.

Demographic factors	Age (peak incidence 65–75 years) Male gender Black ethnicity
Environment/lifestyle	Cigarette smoking
Genetic factors and medical conditions	Family history Two first-degree relatives with pancreas cancer: relative risk increases 18- to 57-fold Germline *BRCA2* mutations in some rare high-risk families Hereditary pancreatitis (50- to 70-fold increased risk) Chronic pancreatitis (5- to 15-fold increased risk) Lynch syndrome Ataxia telangiectasia Peutz–Jeghers syndrome Familial breast–ovarian cancer syndrome Familial atypical multiple mole melanoma Familial adenomatous polyposis – risk of ampullary/duodenal carcinoma Diabetes mellitus

Pathology

More than 85 per cent of pancreatic cancers are ductal adenocarcinomas. The remaining tumours constitute a variety of pathologies with individual characteristics. Endocrine tumours of the pancreas are rare. They are covered in Chapter 52.

Ductal adenocarcinomas arise most commonly in the head of the gland. They are solid, scirrhous tumours, characterised by neoplastic tubular glands within a markedly desmoplastic fibrous stroma. Fibrosis is also a characteristic of chronic pancreatitis, and histological differentiation between tumour and pancreatitis can cause diagnostic difficulties. Ductal adenocarcinomas infiltrate locally, typically along nerve sheaths, along lymphatics and into blood vessels. Liver and peritoneal metastases are common. Proliferative lesions in the pancreatic ducts can precede invasive ductal adenocarcinoma. These are termed 'pancreatic intraepithelial neoplasia' or PanIN, and can demonstrate a range of structural complexity and cellular atypia.

Cystic tumours of the pancreas may be serous or mucinous. Serous cystadenomas are typically found in older women, and are large aggregations of multiple small cysts, almost like bubblewrap. They are benign. Mucinous tumours, on the other hand, have the potential for malignant transformation. They include mucinous cystic neoplasms (MCNs) and intraductal papillary mucinous neoplasms (IPMNs). MCNs are seen in perimenopausal women, show up as multilocular thick-walled cysts in the pancreatic body or tail and, histologically, contain an ovarian-type stroma. IPMNs are more common in the pancreatic head and in older men, but an IPMN arising from a branch duct can be difficult to distinguish from an MCN. IPMNs arising within the main duct are often multifocal and have a greater tendency to prove malignant. Thick mucus seen extruding from the ampulla at ERCP is diagnostic of a main duct IPMN. Mucinous tumours can be confused with pseudocysts (see Summary box 68.8). Occasionally, lymphoepithelial cysts, lymphangiomas, dermoid cysts and intestinal duplication cysts can show up in the pancreas. Solid pseudopapillary tumour is a rare, slowly progressive but malignant tumour, seen in women of childbearing age, and manifests as a large, part-solid, part-cystic tumour.

Tumours arising from the ampulla or from the distal common bile duct can present as a mass in the head of the pancreas, and constitute around a third of all tumours in that area. Adenomas of the ampulla of Vater are diagnosed at endoscopy as polypoid submucosal masses covered by a smooth epithelium. They can harbour foci of invasive carcinoma; the larger the adenoma, the greater the risk. Biopsies taken at endoscopy may not always include the malignant focus. Endoscopic surveillance, endoscopic resection or even surgical transduodenal ampullary excision should be considered (Figure 68.32). Patients with familial adenomatous polyposis (FAP) can present with multiple duodenal polyps. Malignant transformation in a duodenal polyp is a significant cause of mortality in these patients, mandating endoscopic follow up and pancreatoduodenectomy in selected patients with high-grade dysplasia within the polyp.

Ampullary adenocarcinomas often present early with biliary obstruction. Their natural history is distinctly more favourable compared with pancreatic ductal adenocarcinoma. Ampullary carcinomas are relatively small when diagnosed, which may account for their better prognosis. Occasionally, other malignant neoplasms can arise at the ampulla, such as carcinoid tumours and high-grade neuroendocrine carcinomas.

Clinical features

Jaundice secondary to obstruction of the distal bile duct is the most common symptom that draws attention to ampullary and pancreatic head tumours. It is characteristically painless jaundice but may be associated with nausea and epigastric

John Law Augustine Peutz, 1886–1968, Chief Specialist for Internal Medicine, St John's Hospital, The Hague, The Netherlands.
Harold Joseph Jeghers, 1904–1990, Professor of Internal Medicine, The New Jersey College of Medicine and Dentistry, Jersey City, NJ, USA.
Henry Lynch, contemporary, Professor of Medicine, Creighton University, Omaha, Nebraska, USA, described the family cancer syndrome that now bears his name. Formally known as HNPCC (hereditary non-polyposis colon cancer) due to the frequency of colorectal cancers in the absence of polyposis.

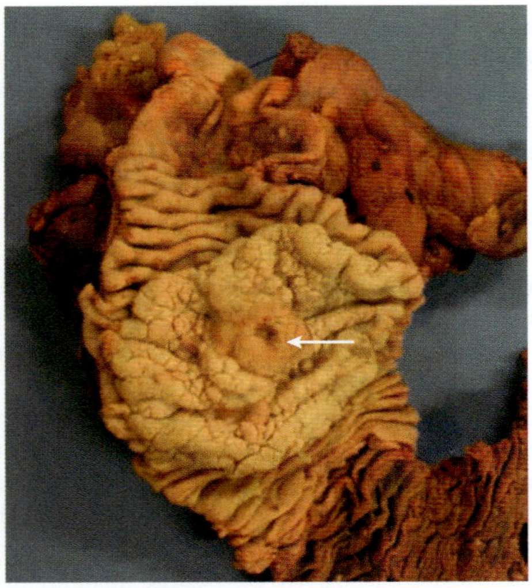

Figure 68.32 A large ampullary adenoma that turned into an adenocarcinoma; the arrow indicates the ampulla. Photograph taken after resection in the form of a pancreatoduodenectomy (courtesy of Dr Joanne Chin-Aleong).

discomfort. Pruritus, dark urine and pale stools with steatorrhoea are common accompaniments of jaundice. In the absence of jaundice, symptoms are often non-specific, namely vague discomfort, anorexia and weight loss, and are frequently dismissed by both patient and doctor. Upper abdominal symptoms in a recently diagnosed diabetic, especially in one above 50 years of age, with no family history or obesity, should raise suspicion. Occasionally, a patient will present with an unexplained attack of pancreatitis; all such patients should have follow-up imaging of the pancreas. Tumours of the body and tail of the gland often grow silently, and present at an advanced unresectable stage. Back pain is a worrying symptom, raising the possibility of retroperitoneal infiltration.

On examination, there may be evidence of jaundice, weight loss, a palpable liver and a palpable gall bladder. Courvoisier first drew attention to the association of an enlarged gall bladder and a pancreatic tumour in 1890, when he noted that, when the common duct is obstructed by a stone, distension of the gall bladder (which is likely to be chronically inflamed) is rare; when the duct is obstructed in some other way, such as a neoplasm, distension of the normal gall bladder is common. Other signs of intra-abdominal malignancy should be looked for with care, such as a palpable mass, ascites, supraclavicular nodes and tumour deposits in the pelvis; when present, they indicate a grim prognosis.

Investigation

In a jaundiced patient, the usual blood tests and ultrasound scan should be performed. Ultrasound will determine whether or not the bile duct is dilated. If it is, and there is a genuine suspicion of a tumour in the head of the pancreas, the preferred test is a contrast-enhanced CT scan (see Figure 68.8). In the majority of instances, this should establish if there is a tumour in the pancreas and if it is resectable. The presence of hepatic or peritoneal metastases, lymph node metastases distant from the pancreatic head, encasement of the superior mesenteric, hepatic or coeliac artery by tumour are clear contraindications to surgical resection. Tumour size, continuous invasion of the duodenum, stomach or colon, and lymph node metastases within the operative field are not contraindications. If the tumour abuts or minimally invades the portal or superior mesenteric vein, this is not a contraindication to surgery (as part of the vein can be resected if necessary), but complete encasement and occlusion of the vein is. MRI and MRA can provide information comparable to CT.

ERCP and biliary stenting should be carried out if there is any suggestion of cholangitis, if there is diagnostic doubt (small ampullary lesions may not be seen on CT, and ERCP is the best way to identify them), if the patient is deeply jaundiced (serum bilirubin >250 μmol/L), or there are distressing symptoms (e.g. pruritus) and there is likely to be a delay between diagnosis and surgery. It relieves the jaundice and can also provide a brush cytology or biopsy specimen to confirm the diagnosis (see Figures 68.13, 68.14 and 68.19). Otherwise, however, preoperative ERCP and biliary stenting is not mandatory in patients with resectable disease; there is evidence to suggest that it is associated with a slightly higher incidence of infective complications after surgery. The prothrombin time should be checked, and clotting abnormalities should be corrected with vitamin K or fresh-frozen plasma prior to ERCP. If a stent is placed in a patient who may undergo resection, it should be a plastic stent or a **covered** metal stent that can be easily removed.

EUS is useful if CT fails to demonstrate a tumour, if tissue diagnosis is required prior to surgery (e.g. a mass has developed on a background of chronic pancreatitis and a distinction needs to be made between inflammation and neoplasia), if vascular invasion needs to be confirmed and in separating cystic tumours from pseudocysts (Figure 68.33; see also Figure 68.20). Transduodenal or transgastric FNA or Trucut biopsy performed under EUS guidance avoids spillage of tumour cells into the peritoneal cavity. Percutaneous transperitoneal biopsy of potentially resectable pancreatic tumours should be avoided as far as possible. Histological confirmation of malignancy is desirable but not essential, particularly if the imaging clearly demonstrates a resectable tumour. The lack of a tissue diagnosis should not delay appropriate surgical therapy. In patients judged to have unresectable disease, tissue diagnosis should be obtained prior to starting palliative therapy.

Diagnostic laparoscopy prior to an attempt at resection can spare a proportion of patients an unnecessary laparotomy by identifying small peritoneal and liver metastases. It can be combined with laparoscopic ultrasonography. The tumour marker CA19-9 is not highly specific or sensitive, but a baseline level should be established; if it is initially raised, it can be useful later in identifying recurrence.

Management

At the time of presentation, more than 85 per cent of patients with ductal adenocarcinoma are unsuitable for resection because the disease is too advanced. If imaging shows that the tumour is potentially resectable, the patient should be considered for surgical resection, as that offers the only (albeit small) chance of a cure. Comorbidities should be carefully taken into account. Biological rather than chronological age should be the consideration. If a cystic tumour is encountered, no matter how large, surgical resection should be considered, as it carries a reasonable chance of cure. Tumours of the ampulla have a good prognosis and should, if at all possible, be resected. Some of the rare

Ludwig Courvoisier, 1843–1918, surgeon, Basle, Switzerland, was one of the first surgeons to remove stones from the common bile duct.

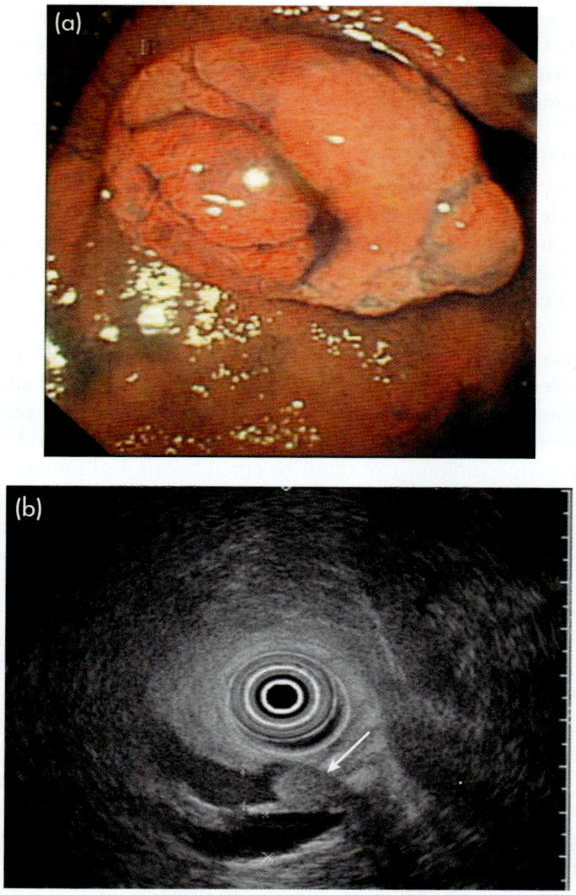

Figure 68.33 (a) Carcinoma of the ampulla as seen at endoscopy. (b) Appearance of the same tumour (arrow) on endoscopic ultrasound (courtesy of Dr Peter Fairclough).

tumours and the neuroendocrine lesions should also be resected if at all possible. For those patients who have inoperable disease, palliative treatment should be offered.

Surgical resection

The standard resection for a tumour of the pancreatic head or the ampulla is a pylorus-preserving pancreatoduodenectomy (PPPD). This involves removal of the duodenum and the pancreatic head, including the distal part of the bile duct. The original pancreatoduodenectomy as proposed by Whipple included resection of the gastric antrum. Preserving the antrum and the pylorus is thought to result in a more physiological outcome with no difference in survival or recurrence rates. The Whipple procedure is now reserved for situations in which the entire duodenum has to be removed (e.g. in FAP) or where the tumour encroaches on the first part of the duodenum or the distal stomach and a PPPD would not achieve a clear resection margin. Total pancreatectomy is warranted only in situations where one is dealing with a multifocal tumour (e.g. a main duct IPMN), or the body and tail of the gland are too inflamed or too friable to achieve a safe anastomosis with the bowel. The PPPD procedure includes a local lymphadenectomy. Extended lymphadenectomy has not been shown to be beneficial in improving survival and is associated with increased morbidity. If the tumour is adherent to the portal or superior mesenteric vein, but can still be removed by including a patch or a short segment of vein in the resection, with an appropriate reconstruction of the vessel, then that should be done. This is not associated with an increase in the morbidity or mortality of the procedure, and the outcomes are similar.

> **Allen Oldfather Whipple**, 1881–1963, Director of Surgical Services, The Presbyterian Hospital, and Professor of Surgery, Columbia University, New York, NY, USA, began to perform two-stage pancreatoduodenectomies in 1934 and shortened the procedure into a one-stage process in 1940.
> **Alessandro Codivilla** (1861–1912) and **Walter Kausch** (1867–1928) had performed the operation before him, but Whipple was the surgeon who established pancreatoduodenectomy as an operation.

For tumours of the body and tail, distal pancreatectomy with splenectomy is the standard. Infiltration of the splenic artery or vein by the tumour is not a contraindication to resection. When resecting the pancreatic tail for a benign lesion, one may attempt to preserve the spleen if possible. When removing the spleen, prior vaccinations against pneumococci, meningococci and *Haemophilus influenzae* B should be administered, and subsequent antibiotic prophylaxis given (see Chapter 66).

Attempts to downstage unresectable disease with chemotherapy or chemoradiation and render it resectable are rarely successful. Neoadjuvant chemotherapy or chemoradiation for resectable disease should only be considered within a clinical trial; it carries the risk that the disease may progress despite the neoadjuvant therapy and become unresectable.

Pancreatoduodenectomy

The patient's coagulation screen should be checked preoperatively and adequate hydration ensured. The patient should be aware of the diagnosis, the gravity of the operation and the risks involved. The operation has three distinct phases:

- exploration and assessment;
- resection;
- reconstruction.

A cholecystectomy is performed. The bile duct and hepatic artery are exposed, removing the lymphatic tissue in this area. Exposure of the hepatic artery enables division of the gastroduodenal artery and visualisation of the portal vein. The distal part of the gastric antrum is mobilised. The duodenum and right colon are mobilised from the retroperitoneal tissues. The superior mesenteric vein is exposed inferior to the pancreatic neck. Careful dissection into the plane between the vein and the pancreatic substance (see Figure 68.2) will reveal whether the tumour is adherent to the vein. At this juncture, a decision has to be made whether to proceed to the next phase of resection or not. If resection is to be performed, the fourth part of the duodenum is dissected and freed from the ligament of Treitz so that the upper jejunum can be brought into the supracolic compartment. The jejunum is divided 20–30 cm downstream from the duodenojejunal flexure, and the mesentery of the proximal jejunum is detached. The first part of the duodenum is divided. The neck of the pancreas is divided, and then the uncinate process is separated from the superior mesenteric artery and vein working up towards the upper bile duct, which is divided, releasing the specimen (Figure 68.34). Retroperitoneal lymph nodes within

> **Wenzel Treitz**, 1819–1872, Professor of Anatomy and Pathology, at Krakow, Poland, and later at Prague, Czech Republic. He was involved in the struggle for Czech nationalism.

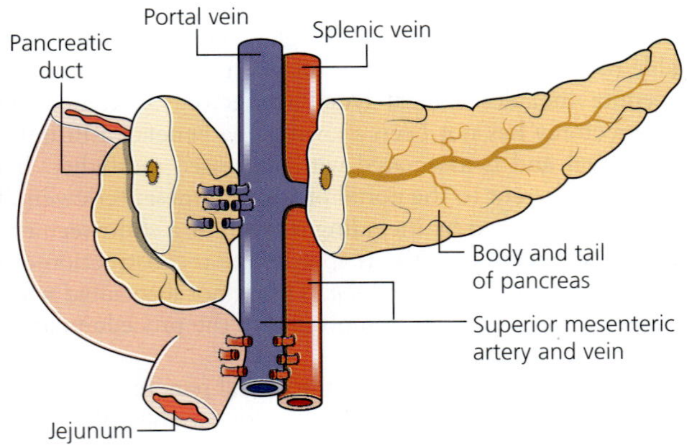

Figure 68.34 Resection of the head of the pancreas in a pylorus-preserving pancreatoduodenectomy.

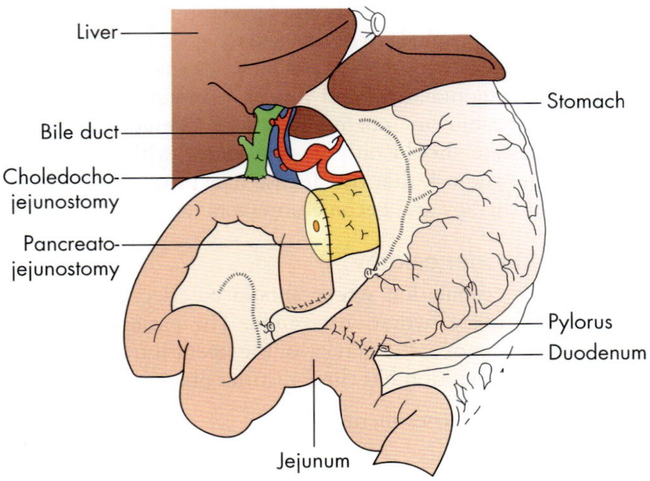

Figure 68.35 Reconstruction after a pylorus-preserving pancreatoduodenectomy.

the operative field are completely removed with the specimen. Reconstruction is carried out as in Figure 68.35. The pancreatic stump, the divided bile duct and the duodenal stump are anastomosed on to jejunum, in that order. Some surgeons prefer to anastomose the pancreas to the posterior wall of the stomach instead; others prefer to create a separate Roux loop of the jejunum and anastomose the pancreas to that. The operation should take between 3 and 6 hours. Blood loss should be low, and transfusion is often not necessary. The patients are usually nursed in a high dependency area for the first 24–48 hours after surgery. Prolonged nasogastric drainage is unnecessary, and early feeding can be commenced.

Resection for pancreatic cancer should be carried out in specialist units. There is a clear correlation between higher caseload volume and lower hospital mortality and morbidity. PPPD should carry a mortality of no more than 3–5 per cent. The morbidity remains high, with some 30–40 per cent of patients developing a complication in the postoperative period. These complications are usually infective, but a leak from the anastomosis between the pancreas and the bowel is known to occur in at least 10 per cent of patients, and this may give rise to major complications. Octreotide may be administered in the perioperative period to suppress secretion and reduce the likelihood of a leak, but the evidence for its efficacy is still debatable. Following surgical resection, the pathological tumour–node–metastasis (TNM) stage should be documented.

Adjuvant therapy

The reported five-year survival following resection of a pancreatic adenocarcinoma ranges from 7 to 25 per cent. The median survival is 11–20 months. Considering that, at best, 15 per cent of patients have resectable disease to begin with, this means only two or three of 100 patients with this disease can expect to survive to five years. Moreover, recurrences can and do show up even beyond the five-year cut off. It should be emphasised, however, that these depressing statistics apply to ductal adenocarcinomas. Patients with resected ampullary tumours have a five-year survival of 40 per cent, and cystic tumours and neuroendocrine tumours can often be cured by surgical resection.

The high recurrence rate following resection has inevitably led to the consideration of adjuvant treatments to improve outcome. In a large multicentre European study (ESPAC-1), adjuvant radiotherapy or chemoradiotherapy was shown to confer no advantage, but chemotherapy with 5-fluorouracil (5-FU) provided an overall benefit; median survival with chemotherapy was 20 months compared with 16 months without. Another trial (ESPAC-3) showed that gemcitabine works equally well. Most patients with resected ductal adenocarcinoma are now offered adjuvant chemotherapy, using gemcitabine or 5-FU. A further trial is in progress of gemcitabine alone versus gemcitabine with capecitabine (a fluorouracil that can be taken orally). Some centres continue to offer chemoradiotherapy, particularly in patients with involved (R1) resection margins, and further trials of adjuvant chemoradiation are also in progress.

Palliation

The median survival of patients with unresectable, locally advanced, non-metastatic pancreatic cancer is between six and ten months and, in patients with metastatic disease, it is two to six months.

If unresectable disease is found in the course of a laparotomy that was commenced with the intent to resect, a choledochoenterostomy and a gastroenterostomy should be carried out to relieve (or pre-empt) jaundice and duodenal obstruction. The bile duct may be anastomosed to the duodenum, or to a loop of jejunum. It is preferable to use the bile duct rather than the gall bladder. Cholecystojejunostomy is easier to perform, but the bile must then drain through the cystic duct, which is narrow and, if the cystic duct is inserted low into the bile duct, it is vulnerable to occlusion by tumour growth. A coeliac plexus block can also be administered. A transduodenal Trucut biopsy of the tumour should be obtained.

In patients found to have unresectable disease on imaging, jaundice is relieved by stenting at ERCP (Figure 68.36b). Stents may be made of plastic or self-expanding metal mesh. Plastic stents are cheaper but tend to occlude faster and, if the patient is likely to have a longer life expectancy, a metal stent can be used. If the patient is not a suitable candidate for endoscopic biliary stenting, a percutaneous transhepatic stent can be placed (Figure 68.36a). Obstruction of the duodenum occurs in approximately 15 per cent of cases. If this occurs early in the course of the disease, surgical bypass by gastrojejunostomy is appropriate but, if it is late in the course of the disease, then the use of expanding

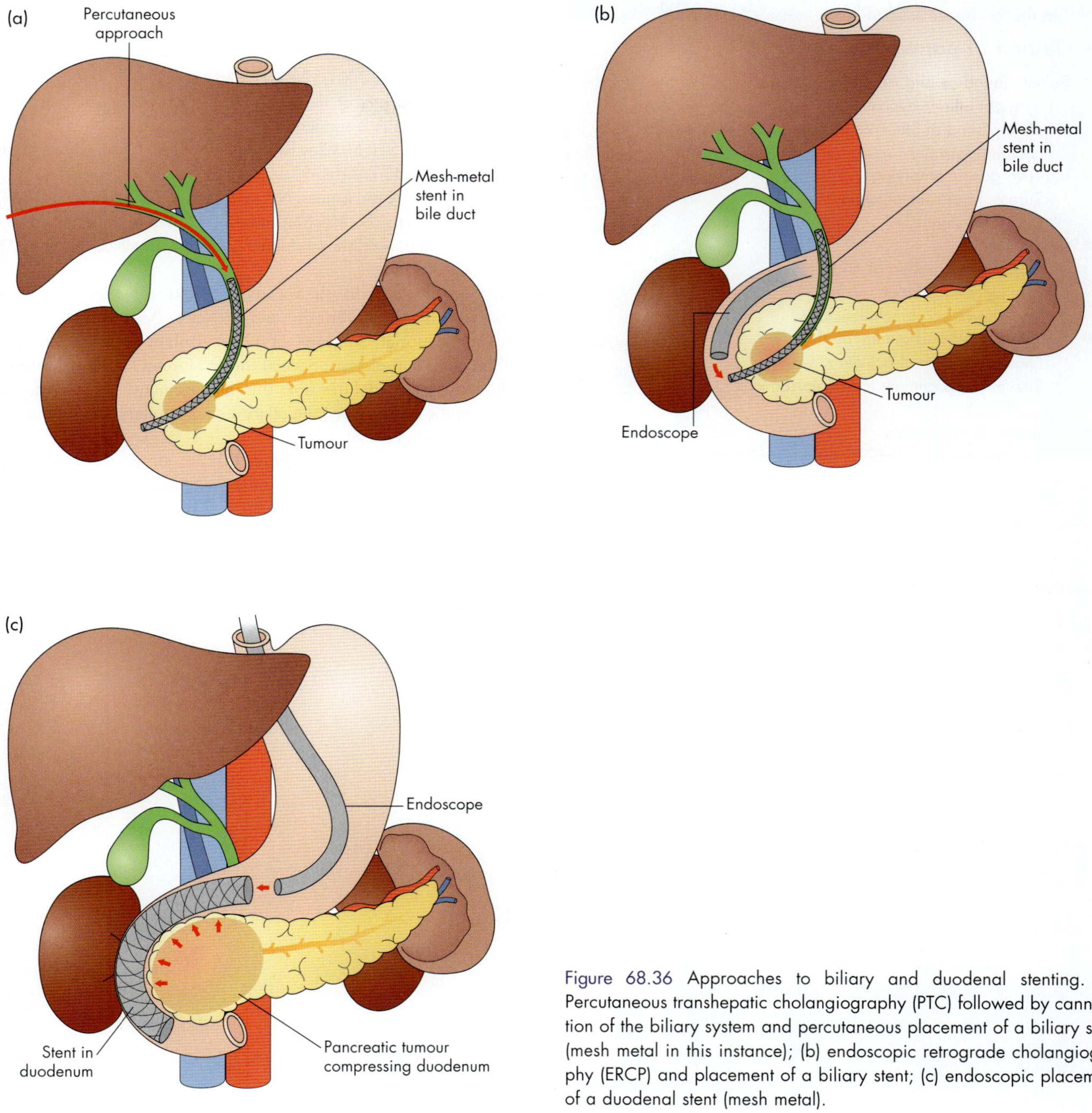

Figure 68.36 Approaches to biliary and duodenal stenting. (a) Percutaneous transhepatic cholangiography (PTC) followed by cannulation of the biliary system and percutaneous placement of a biliary stent (mesh metal in this instance); (b) endoscopic retrograde cholangiography (ERCP) and placement of a biliary stent; (c) endoscopic placement of a duodenal stent (mesh metal).

metal stents inserted endoscopically is preferable, as many of these patients have prolonged delayed gastric emptying following surgery (Figure 68.36c). If both biliary and duodenal metal stents are to be placed endoscopically, the biliary one should be placed first.

If no operative procedure is undertaken, an EUS-guided or percutaneous biopsy of the tumour should be performed before consideration of chemotherapy or chemoradiation. The role of chemotherapy in the management of pancreatic cancer remains ill defined. If the tumour is a lymphoma, then benefit is without doubt. Lymphomas of the pancreas are rare and constitute less than 3 per cent of all pancreatic cancers. For patients with ductal adenocarcinoma, 5-FU or gemcitabine will produce a remission in 15–25 per cent, while the remainder will receive no benefit from the therapy. No long-term cures have been described with chemotherapy or radiotherapy.

Steatorrhoea is treated with enzyme supplementation. Diabetes mellitus, if it develops, is treated with oral hypoglycaemics or insulin as appropriate, and pain with either analgesics or an appropriate nerve block (Summary box 68.10).

Summary box 68.10

Palliation of pancreatic cancer

- Relieve jaundice and treat biliary sepsis
  - Surgical biliary bypass
  - Stent placed at ERCP or percutaneous transhepatic cholangiography
- Improve gastric emptying
  - Surgical gastroenterostomy
  - Duodenal stent
- Pain relief
  - Stepwise escalation of analgesia
  - Coeliac plexus block
  - Transthoracic splanchnicectomy
- Symptom relief and quality of life
  - Encourage normal activities
  - Enzyme replacement for steatorrhoea
  - Treat diabetes
- Consider chemotherapy

FURTHER READING

Ayub K, Imada R, Slavin J. Endoscopic retrograde cholangiopancreatography in gallstone-associated acute pancreatitis. *Cochrane Database Syst Rev* 2004; (**2**): CD003630.

Blumgart LH. *Surgery of the liver, biliary tract and pancreas*, 4th edn. Philadelphia, PA: Saunders, 2006.

Braganza JM, Lee SH, McCloy RF, McMahon MJ. Chronic pancreatitis. *Lancet* 2011; **377**: 1184–97.

Hidalgo M. Pancreatic cancer. *N Engl J Med* 2010; **362**: 1605–17.

Moss AC, Morris E, MacMathuna P. Palliative biliary stents for obstructing pancreatic carcinoma. *Cochrane Database Syst Rev* 2006; (**2**): CD004200.

Pancreatic Section, British Society of Gastroenterology; Pancreatic Society of Great Britain and Ireland; Association of Upper Gastrointestinal Surgeons of Great Britain and Ireland; Royal College of Pathologists; Special Interest Group for Gastro-Intestinal Radiology. Guidelines for the management of patients with pancreatic cancer, periampullary and ampullary carcinomas. *Gut* 2005; **54** (Suppl. V): 1–16.

Sewnath ME, Karsten TM, Prins MH *et al.* A meta-analysis on the efficacy of preoperative biliary drainage for tumors causing obstructive jaundice. *Ann Surg* 2002; **236**: 17–27.

Working Party of the British Society of Gastroenterology; Association of Surgeons of Great Britain and Ireland, Pancreatic Society of Great Britain and Ireland; Association of Upper GI Surgeons of Great Britain and Ireland. UK guidelines for the management of acute pancreatitis. *Gut* 2005; **54** (Suppl. III): 1–9.

CHAPTER 69

The small and large intestines

LEARNING OBJECTIVES

To appreciate:
- The basic anatomy and physiology of the small and large intestines
- The range of conditions that may affect the intestines

To understand:
- The aetiology and pathology of common intestinal conditions
- The principles of investigation of intestinal symptoms
- The importance of non-surgical management of intestinal problems
- The principles of intestinal surgery
- That complex intestinal problems are best managed by a multidisciplinary team
- The management of acute surgical problems of the intestines

ANATOMY OF THE SMALL AND LARGE INTESTINES

Small intestine

Although the duodenum is anatomically indistinguishable from the small intestine, it is subject to some specific pathologies and surgical therapies, so, in purely surgical terms may be regarded as a distinct entity, covered in Chapter 63. The length of the small bowel may vary from 300 to 850 cm between the duodenojejunal (DJ) flexure to the ileocaecal valve. It is notoriously difficult to establish the length of the small intestine, and estimates gathered at surgery, post-mortem and during radiological investigations vary widely, even in the same individual. In addition, there may be considerable interindividual variability and the small intestine is believed to be longer in men.

The proximal 40 per cent of the small intestine is referred to as the jejunum; the remainder is the ileum. There is no clear demarcation between jejunum and ileum, but the small bowel does change gradually in character from proximal to distal. The jejunum tends to have a wider diameter and a thicker wall, with more prominent mucosal folds (**valvulae conniventes**), while the ileum has a thicker, more fatty mesentery with more complex arterial arcades. The ileum also contains larger aggregates of lymph nodes (Peyer's patches), which can occasionally become lead points in intussusception in childhood.

The small intestine has a very rich blood supply, from the superior mesenteric artery, while venous drainage is via the portal venous system, into which the superior mesenteric vein drains blood rich in nutrients after a meal. This arrangement facilitates processing of the nutrients by the liver, into which the portal vein drains in turn. The lymphatic drainage of the small intestine follows the arterial supply. The small intestine has a rich autonomic innervation arising from the splanchnic nerves, which contribute a dense network of sympathetic fibres around the superior mesenteric artery and its branches. Referred pain from the small intestine is usually felt in the periumbilical region (T10). The blood and nerve supply to the small intestine all runs in the attached mesentery which originates on the posterior abdominal wall and runs obliquely downwards to the right between the DJ flexure to the left of the second lumbar vertebra and the right sacroiliac joint. Surgical resection of the small bowel requires careful division not only of the arteries and veins, but also the mesentery (see Summary box 69.1).

Summary box 69.1

Anatomy of the small and large intestine

- Small intestine
  - Comprises jejunum and ileum
  - Has valvulae conniventes
  - Blood supply from superior mesenteric artery
- Large intestine
  - Comprises caecum, ascending, transverse, descending and sigmoid colon
  - Has appendices epiploicae and taenia coli
  - Blood supply from branches of superior and inferior mesenteric arteries
  - Marginal artery runs round the length of the colon

Valvulae conniventes describes a fold of mucus membrane that passes across two-thirds of the bowel circumference.
Johann Conrad Peyer, 1653–1712, Professor of Logis, Rhetoric and Medicine, Schaffausen, Switzerland, described the lymph follicles in the intestine in 1677.
Eric Adolph von Willebrand, 1879–1949, physician, Diakonissanstaltens Hospital, Helsinki (Helsingfors), Finland, described hereditary pseudo-haemophilia in 1926.
Norman Stanley Williams, contemporary, President, Royal College of Surgeons of England and Professor of Surgery, Barts and The London School of Medicine and Dentistry, London, UK.

Large intestine

The large intestine begins at the ileocaecal valve and extends to the anus. It is divided into the caecum, with its attached vermiform appendix (discussed in Chapter 71), the ascending colon, which runs up to the hepatic flexure, the transverse colon with attached greater omentum, running up to the splenic flexure, the descending colon, sigmoid and rectum (discussed separately in Chapter 72). The large intestine is approximately 1.5 m long, although at colonoscopy the bowel can be straightened so the caecum can be reached with as little as 70 cm of colonoscope.

The large intestine is less mobile than the small bowel as the ascending and descending colon are fixed to the retroperitoneum following embryological rotation. The colon is also distinguished by having fat-filled peritoneal tags known as **appendices epiploicae** and the presence of **taeniae**. The **taenia coli** are three flat bands of longitudinal muscle that run the length of the large intestine from the appendix base to the rectosigmoid junction and they act to pull the colon into its typical sacculated state, producing a series of **haustrations**. Distended small and large intestine can be distinguished on an abdominal radiograph as the small bowel has complete transverse markings caused by the valvulae conniventes, while the colon has incomplete lines from the sacculation caused by the taeniae. The important posterior relations of the caecum and ascending colon are the right ureter, right gonadal vessels and duodenum, and these must be carefully protected at surgery. Similarly, the left ureter, left gonadal vessels and tail of the pancreas must be protected when operating on the left colon.

The blood supply of the large intestine is derived from branches of the superior mesenteric artery proximally as far as the distal transverse colon (which is derived embryologically from the primitive midgut) and the inferior mesenteric artery and its branches more distally (derived from the primitive hindgut). Adjacent branches of the superior and inferior mesenteric arteries anastomose so there is usually a complete vascular supply along the colon named the 'marginal artery of Drummond'. This vessel is often the key blood supply to the vascular arcades ensuring adequate perfusion of a colonic anastomosis, but blood flow in the 'watershed' area of the splenic flexure representing the junction between the superior and inferior mesenteric supply may be quite tenuous. The consequences of this might be, for example, that sudden occlusion of the inferior mesenteric artery may leave the area of the splenic flexure (at the most distal point of supply from the superior mesenteric artery) poorly perfused, leading to an ischaemic colitis. Venous and lymphatic drainage of the colon follows the arterial supply and as for the small intestine system, venous drainage is into the portal system. High ligation of the artery supplying a segment of colon will therefore remove the lymph nodes draining the area, a key technical point in cancer surgery. The nerve supply to the large intestine is derived from the splanchnic nerves, via a dense sympathetic plexus surrounding the superior and inferior mesenteric arteries. Visceral pain from the part of the colon supplied by the superior mesenteric artery is thus felt, like that of the small intestine, in the periumbilical region, while pain from the colon distal to that point is felt suprapubically (T12–L1).

Charles Horace Mayo, 1865–1939, surgeon, The Mayo Clinic, Rochester, MN, USA. He and his brother, William James Mayo (1861–1939), joined their father's private practice in Rochester. This practice became The Mayo Clinic. Their father, William Worrall Mayo, was born in Manchester, UK, in 1919.

PHYSIOLOGY OF THE SMALL AND LARGE INTESTINES

Small intestine

The main function of the small intestine is the digestion of food and the absorption of nutrients and fluid. Carbohydrates and proteins are broken down by pancreatic enzymes, but the final hydrolysis takes place at the brush border of the jejunum after which they are absorbed. The products of fat digestion, fatty acids and monoglycerides separate from bile salts in the jejunum and are absorbed for further processing. The jejunum is the principal site for digestion and absorption of fluid, electrolytes, iron, folate, fat, protein and carbohydrate, but the absorption of bile salts and vitamin B12 occurs in the terminal ileum where there are specific transporters. If the jejunum is resected, the ileum can assume all the required absorptive functions, but resection of the terminal ileum will result in a diminished bile salt pool, B12 deficiency and may lead to deficiency of the fat-soluble vitamins A, D and K.

The small intestine plays an important role in the metabolism of plasma lipoproteins, as it is the main site of synthesis of high-density, low-density and very low-density lipoproteins (HDL, LDL, VLDL). The small bowel also synthesises intestinal hormones, which interact with the enteric nervous system to modulate intestinal function, growth and differentiation.

Large intestine

The principal function of the colon is absorption of water; 1000 mL of ileal contents enter the caecum every 24 hours of which only about 150–250 mL is excreted as faeces. Sodium absorption is efficiently accomplished by an active transport system, while chloride and water are absorbed passively following gradients established by the sodium pump. Fermentation of dietary fibre in the colon by the normal colonic microflora (principally anaerobic bacteria, such as bacteroides and bifidobacteria) leads to the generation of short chain fatty acids (SCFAs) such as butyrate, which is an important metabolic fuel for the colonic mucosa and may also contribute to normal daily energy requirements. Thus, diversion of the faecal stream (for example by a temporary 'loop' ileostomy) may lead to inflammatory changes in the colon downstream, a condition referred to as 'diversion colitis'. Some absorption of nutrients including glucose, fatty acids, amino acids and vitamins can also take place in the colon, although under normal circumstances only a tiny amount of this occurs.

Colonic motility is variable. In general, faecal residue reaches the caecum 4 hours after a meal and the rectum after 24 hours. Passage of stool is not orderly, however, because of mixing within the colon. It is thus common for residue from a single meal to still be passed 4 days later.

INFLAMMATORY BOWEL DISEASE

By definition, the term 'inflammatory bowel disease' is reserved for conditions characterised by the presence of **idiopathic** intes-

Sir David Drummond, 1852–1932, English physician.
Gabrielle Fallopio (Fallopius), 1523–1562, Professor of Anatomy, Surgery and Botany, Padua, Italy.

tinal inflammation, i.e. ulcerative colitis (UC) and Crohn's disease (CD). Conditions such as infective or ischaemic colitis or enteritis are thus excluded. Although the availability of population genetics and molecular biology has contributed to our understanding of the pathogenesis of inflammatory bowel disease, the cause of these conditions remains unknown.

ULCERATIVE COLITIS

Ulcerative colitis is a disease of the rectum and colon with extraintestinal manifestations. The incidence is 10 per 100 000 in the UK with a prevalence of 160 per 100 000. The prevalence of UC is stable (unlike Crohn's disease, which is increasing). UC is said to be more common in the Ashkenazi Jewish population and affects men and women equally in early life, although it is said to be more common in males in later life. It is most commonly diagnosed between the ages of 20 and 40. There is a marked geographical distribution of the disease which is far more common in the United States and Western Europe, but relatively rare in the Far East and the Tropics. The incidence in the Asian population of the UK seems to be determined by where childhood was spent. Asians who spent their childhood before the age of 14 in Asia have a much lower incidence of UC than Asians born and raised in the UK, suggesting an important effect of environmental exposure in childhood.

Aetiology

The cause of UC is unknown. There is clearly a genetic contribution as 10–20 per cent of patients with UC have a first-degree relative with inflammatory bowel disease. UC is more common in Caucasians than in the Afro-Caribbean or Asian population. No causative link with any specific organisms has been identified, although studies of patients with severe colitis have suggested a reduction in the number of anaerobic bacteria and a reduction in the variability of bacterial strains in the colon. Whether this is a primary feature of the disease or a secondary consequence of mucosal inflammation is unclear. Animal studies, using models of colitis, have suggested that the presence of a bacterial flora is important in the development of colitis, even if no specific organism is involved. For example, mice with a genetic deficiency predisposing them to colitis (e.g. strains with the genes for IL-10 or PGP knocked out) appear to be protected if reared in a germ-free environment. Although it has been suggested that the mechanism of UC may relate to a primary abnormality of mucosal permeability, resulting in bacterial antigens being able to cross the colonic mucosal barrier and thus triggering an inflammatory response, the data to support this hypothesis are unclear and more recent studies in animal models have shown that genes involved in mucosal inflammation and bacterial recognition are already activated long before evidence of abnormal permeability or overt inflammation appear. This suggests that the demonstration of increased colonic mucosal permeability in colitis may be a consequence, rather than a cause of the disease. Unlike Crohn's disease, smoking seems to have a protective effect in UC and has even been the basis of therapeutic trials of nicotine therapy. Patients often comment that relapses are associated with periods of stress, but personality and psychiatric profiles in patients with UC are the same as those of the normal population.

Pathology

In virtually all cases, the disease starts in the rectum and extends proximally in continuity. The rectum is involved in all circumstances except in those using topical rectal preparations (rectal sparing). Failure of colonic inflammation to adhere to this pattern should lead to strong suspicion that the diagnosis is not one of UC. Colonic inflammation in UC is diffuse, confluent and superficial, primarily affecting the mucosa and superficial submucosa. In very severe cases, the inflammation may extend full thickness through the wall of the colon, making interpretation difficult. Chronic mucosal ulceration is associated with formation of granulation tissue and regeneration, leading to a polyp-like appearance, 'pseudopolyposis', which occurs in almost one-quarter of cases. Stricturing in UC is very unusual and should prompt urgent assessment because of the possibility of coexisting carcinoma. A small proportion of patients with colonic dysplasia may develop irregular mucosal swellings (dysplasia-associated lesions or mass, DALMs), which are highly predictive of the likelihood of coexisting carcinoma.

Histological examination reveals an increase in inflammatory cells in the lamina propria, the walls of the crypts of Lieberkuhn are infiltrated by inflammatory cells and there are crypt abscesses. There is depletion of goblet cell mucin. With time, precancerous changes can develop (dysplasia). The precise incidence of dysplasia in UC is unclear. It seems to increase with time and may range from 2 per cent, up to 18 per cent at 30 years. Dysplasia is classified into low- or high-grade dysplasia. In general, high-grade dysplasia is regarded as an absolute indication for colectomy, as 40 per cent of colectomy specimens in which high-grade dysplasia was detected will have evidence of a colorectal cancer. In contrast, optimum management of low-grade dysplasia is currently controversial. Although the decision to proceed to colectomy must be individualized, 10–30 per cent of patients with low-grade dysplasia will have a cancer at colectomy. The progression rate of low-grade dysplasia to invasive cancer is unclear, and it is likely that many cancers in patients with low-grade dysplasia develop without an intervening period of high-grade dysplasia.

Symptoms

Clinical presentation depends in large part on the extent of disease and the presence or otherwise of complications (see Summary box 69.2). If confined to the rectum (proctitis), there is usually no systemic upset and extra-alimentary manifestations are rare. The main symptoms will be rectal bleeding, tenesmus and mucous discharge. The disease remains confined to the rectum in 90 per cent of cases but proctitis may spread proximally over time. Colitis is almost always associated with bloody diarrhoea and urgency that can be incapacitating. Pain is unusual. Children with poorly controlled colitis may have impaired growth. The more extensive the disease, the more likely extraintestinal manifestations are to occur. Extensive colitis is also associated with systemic illness, characterised by malaise, loss of appetite and fever. Diarrhoea may be profuse and bloody, resulting in anaemia, hypoproteinaemia and electrolyte disturbance. Approximately 30 per cent of patients have inflammation extending to the sigmoid colon and spread proximal to the splenic flexure occurs in 20 per cent.

Summary box 69.2

Complications of ulcerative colitis

- Acute
  - Toxic dilatation
  - Perforation
  - Haemorrhage
- Chronic
  - Cancer
  - Extra-alimentary manifestations: skin lesions, eye problems and liver disease

Classification of colitis severity

The assessment of severity of UC is determined by frequency of bowel action and the presence of systemic signs of illness:

- **Mild disease** is characterised by fewer than four stools daily, with or without bleeding. There are no systemic signs of toxicity, and a normal erythrocyte sedimentation rate (ESR).
- **Moderate disease** corresponds to more than four stools daily, but with few signs of systemic illness. There may be anaemia (but not sufficient to require transfusions). Abdominal pain may occur. Inflammatory markers, including ESR and C-reactive protein (CRP) are often raised.
- **Severe disease** corresponds to more than six bloody stools a day, and evidence of systemic illness with fever, tachycardia, anaemia and raised inflammatory markers. Hypoalbuminaemia is common and an ominous finding.
- **Fulminant disease** is associated with more than ten bowel movements daily, fever, tachycardia, continuous bleeding, anaemia, hypoalbuminaemia, abdominal tenderness and distension, blood transfusion requirement and in the most severe cases, progressive colonic dilation ('toxic megacolon'). This is a very significant finding, suggestive of disintegrative colitis and an indication for immediate surgery if colonic perforation is to be avoided.

Extraintestinal manifestations

Arthritis occurs in around 15 per cent of patients and is of the large joint polyarthropathy type, affecting knees, ankles, elbows and wrists. Sacroiliitis and ankylosing spondylitis are 20 times more common in patients with UC than the general population and are associated with HLA-B27. Sclerosing cholangitis is associated with UC and can progress to cirrhosis and hepatocellular failure. Patients with UC and sclerosing cholangitis are also at a greater risk of development of large bowel cancer. Cholangiocarcinoma is an extremely rare association and its frequency is not influenced by colectomy. The skin lesions erythema nodosum and pyoderma gangrenosum are associated with UC and both normally get better with good colitis control. The eyes can also be affected with uveitis and episcleritis.

Acute colitis

Around 5 per cent of patients present with severe acute (fulminant) colitis characterised by frequent bloody diarrhoea, weight loss and dehydration. Intensive medical treatment and fluid resuscitation leads to remission in 70 per cent, but the rest will require urgent surgery. Toxic dilatation should be suspected in patients with active colitis who develop severe abdominal pain and confirmed by the presence on a plain abdominal radiograph of colon with a diameter of more than 6 cm (megacolon, Figure 69.1). A reduction in stool frequency is not always a sign of improvement in patients with severe UC, and the presence of a falling stool frequency, abdominal distension and abdominal pain (resulting from progression of the inflammatory process through the colonic wall) are strongly suggestive of the development of disintegrative colitis and impending perforation. Severe UC must be differentiated from dysentery, typhoid and amoebic colitis (which can also lead to colonic perforation). Plain abdominal radiographs should be obtained daily in patients with severe colitis, and a progressive increase in diameter in spite of medical therapy is an indication for surgery. Colonic perforation in UC is a grave complication with a mortality rate of 40 per cent. Steroids may mask the physical signs. Severe haemorrhage is uncommon (1–2 per cent), but may occasionally require urgent surgical intervention.

Cancer risk in colitis

The risk of cancer in ulcerative colitis increases with duration of disease. At ten years from diagnosis, it is around 1 per cent. This increases to 10–15 per cent at 20 years and may be as high as 20 per cent at 30 years. There is some evidence to suggest that these figures may be an overestimate of cancer risk and that good control of colonic inflammation may significantly reduce risk. Nevertheless, most patients with pancolitis of more than ten years' duration should be entered into screening programmes in order to detect clinically silent dysplasia, which is predictive of increased cancer risk. The value of screening programmes remains somewhat controversial, however, with most UC patients who develop cancer (approximately 3.5 per cent) presenting with their tumours in between attendances for screening colonoscopy. Carcinoma is more likely to occur if the whole colon is involved (Figure 69.2) or if the disease started early in life. Carcinomatous change, often atypical and high grade, may occur at many sites at once. Colonoscopic

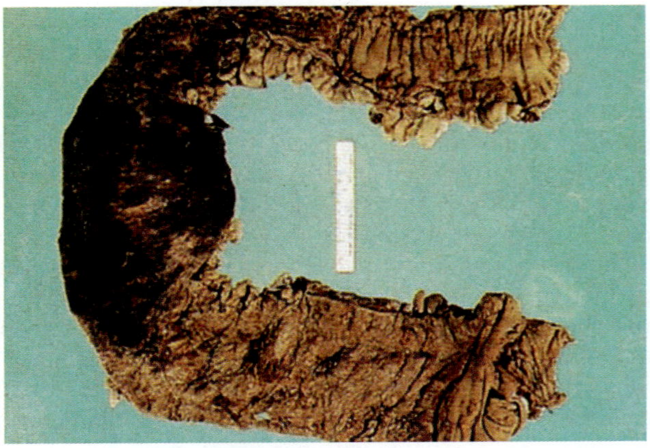

Figure 69.1 Fulminating ulcerative colitis with toxic dilatation of the transverse colon (courtesy of Dr Ian Talbot, St Mark's Hospital, London).

surveillance with multiple biopsies is advised to detect dysplasia, which can occur in a flat mucosa, or a DALM. If on biopsy, there is epithelial dysplasia, surgery should be considered, as cancers may be found in 40 per cent of colectomy specimens for colitis-associated dysplasia.

Investigations

Endoscopy and biopsy

Rigid/flexible sigmoidoscopy can detect proctitis in the clinic: the mucosa is hyperaemic and bleeds on touch, and there may be a purulent exudate. Where there has been remission and relapse, there may be the presence of regenerative mucosal nodules or pseudopolyps. Later, tiny ulcers may be seen that appear to coalesce. This is quite different from the picture of amoebic dysentery, in which there are large, deep ulcers with intervening normal mucosa. Colonoscopy and biopsy has a key role in diagnosis and management:

- to establish the extent of inflammation;
- to distinguish between UC and Crohn's colitis (although this can be exceptionally difficult, Table 69.1);
- to monitor the response to treatment;
- to assess long-standing cases for malignant change.

In the last case, detailed colonoscopic assessment using dye-spray to look for subtle mucosal abnormalities and taking multiple random biopsies every 10 cm is required.

Radiology

A plain abdominal film may indicate the severity of disease in the acute setting and is particularly valuable in demonstrating the development of toxic megacolon (Figure 69.3). Faeces are present only in parts of the colon that are normal or only mildly inflamed. Mucosal islands can sometimes be seen. Small bowel loops in the right lower quadrant may be a sign of severe disease.

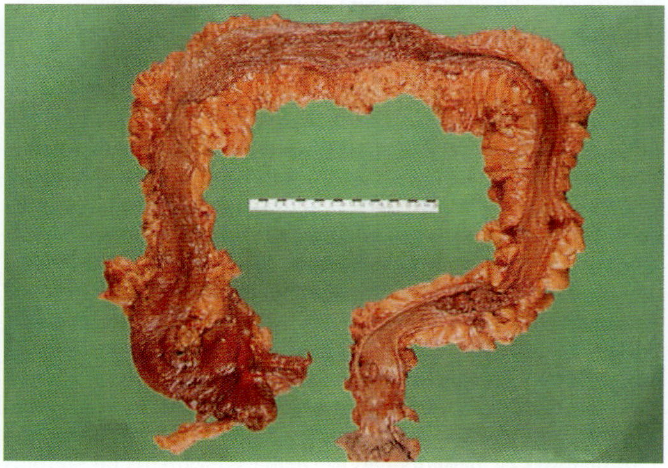

Figure 69.2 Resection specimen from a patient with long-standing ulcerative colitis showing a narrow tubular colon with areas of cancerous change in the rectum and sigmoid (courtesy of Dr B Warren, John Radcliffe Hospital, Oxford, UK).

Table 69.1 Distinguishing ulcerative colitis and Crohn's disease.

	Ulcerative colitis	Crohn's disease
Macroscopic		
Distribution	Colon/rectum	Anywhere in the gastrointestinal tract
Rectum	Always involved	Often spared
Perianal disease	Rare	Common
Fistula formation	Rare	Common
Stricture	Rare	Common
Microscopic		
Layers involved	Mucosa/submucosa	Full thickness
Granulomas	No	Common
Fissuring	No	Common
Crypt abscesses	Common	Rare

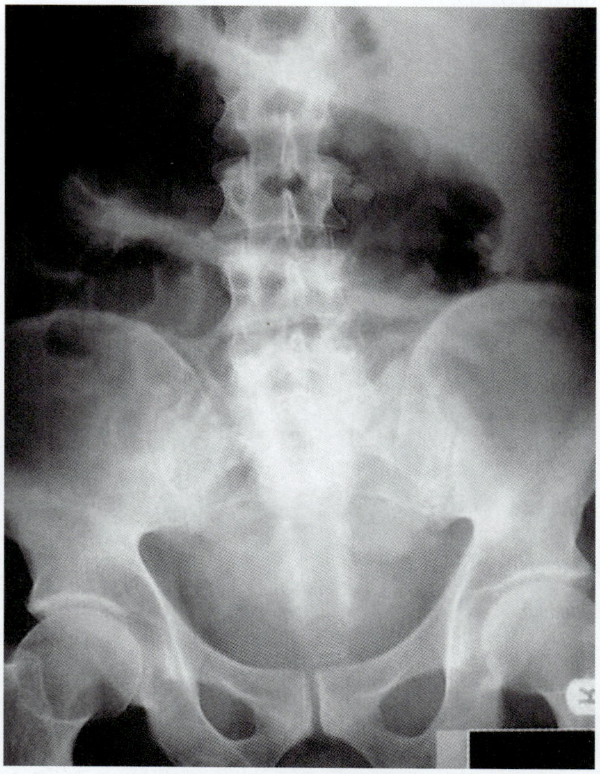

Figure 69.3 Supine abdominal radiograph in toxic megacolon. The transverse colon is dilated (7 cm), there is no formed residue in the colon, and large mucosal islands are present in the ascending colon and hepatic flexure. No haustration is present in the transverse colon, which distinguishes this from ileus of obstruction. Mucosal islands are due to oedematous remnants or mucosa where there has been extensive ulceration (courtesy of Dr C Bartram, St Mark's Hospital, London, UK).

Barium enema has been replaced by computed tomography (CT) in the majority of centres, although a contrast study will give an excellent view of loss of haustra, especially in the distal colon, pseudopolyps and in chronic cases a narrow, featureless, shortened 'hosepipe' colon (Figure 69.4). CT findings in pancolitis may show significant thickening of the colonic wall, as well as inflammatory stranding in the colonic mesentery (Figure 69.5).

Bacteriology

A stool specimen should be sent for microbiology analysis when UC is suspected, in order to exclude infective colitides, notably *Campylobacter*, which may be very difficult to distinguish from acute severe UC. Other infective causes include *Shigella* and *amoebiasis*. Pseudomembranous colitis occurs in hospital patients on antibiotic treatment and, occasionally, those on non-steroidal anti-inflammatory drugs (NSAIDs). The causative organism is *Clostridium difficile*. Immunocompromised patients are at risk of infective proctocolitis from cytomegalovirus and *cryptosporidia*.

Treatment

Effective treatment of UC requires a multidisciplinary approach to management. This involves the gastroenterologist, nurses, nutritionist, enterostomal therapists and occasionally clinical psychologists and social workers, as well as the surgeon (see Summary box 69.3).

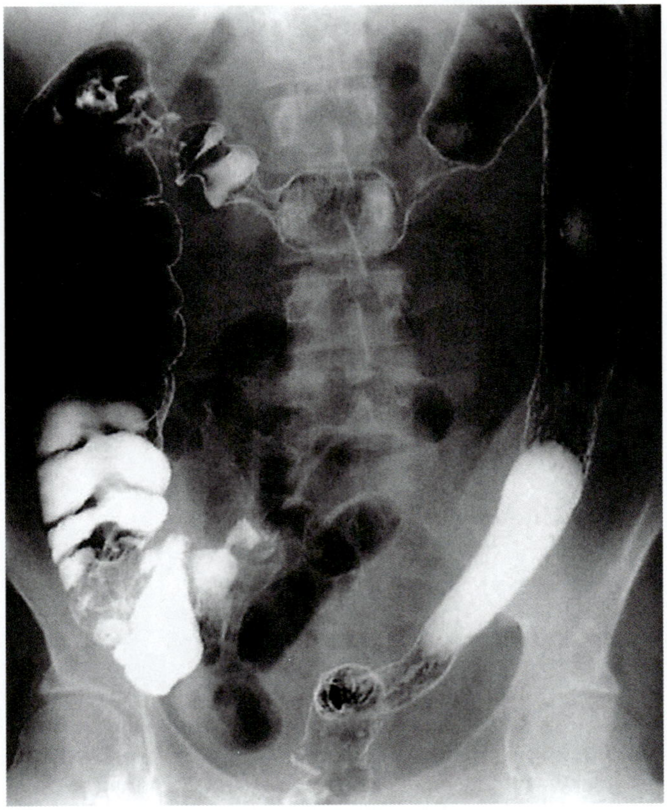

Figure 69.4 Double-contrast barium enema showing left-sided ulcerative colitis with a tubular left colon compared with a normal right colon (courtesy of Dr D Nolan, John Radcliffe Hospital, Oxford, UK).

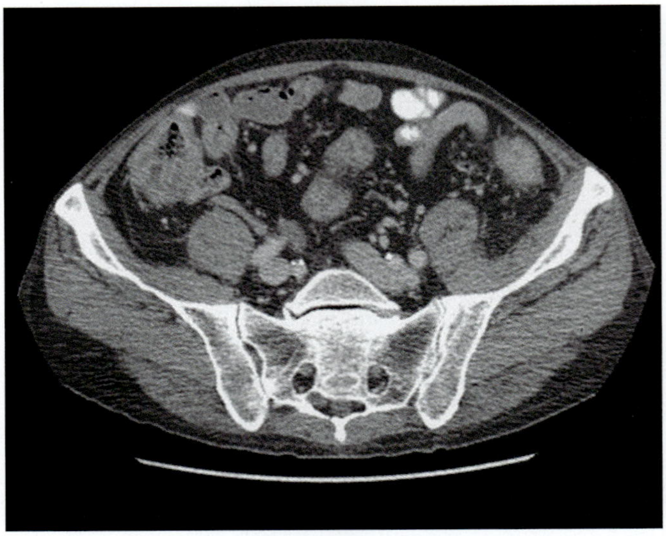

Figure 69.5 Computed tomographic scan demonstrating colitis with thickened colonic wall and inflammatory stranding in the mesentery (courtesy of Dr D Kasir, Hope Hospital, Salford, UK).

Summary box 69.3

Principles of management of ulcerative colitis

- Many patients can be adequately maintained for years on medical therapy
- Toxic dilatation must be suspected in any colitic patient who develops severe abdominal pain; missed colonic perforation is associated with a high mortality
- Colitic patients are at increased risk of developing cancer; those with pancolitis of long duration are most at risk

Medical treatment

Medical therapy is based on anti-inflammatory agents. The 5-aminosalicylic acid (5-ASA) derivatives can be given topically (per rectum) or systemically. They act as inhibitors of the cyclo-oxygenase (COX) enzyme system and are formulated to protect the aspirin-related drug from degradation before reaching the colon. They can be used long term as maintenance therapy. Corticosteroids are the mainstay of treatment for any 'flare up', either topically or systemically and have a widespread anti-inflammatory action. The immunosuppressive drugs azathioprine and cyclosporin can be used to maintain remission and as 'steroid-sparing' agents. More recently, monoclonal antibodies have entered clinical practice; infliximab and adalimumab both act against tumour necrosis factor alpha, which has a central role in inflammatory cascades.

Proctitis

The majority of patients can be managed with rectal steroids for an acute attack and oral 5-ASA compounds to maintain remission. Occasionally, a reducing course of oral steroids is required. It is very unusual for patients with purely rectal disease to require surgery.

Kiyoshi Shiga, 1870–1957, a Japanese bacteriologist reported his discovery of the dysentery bacillus in 1898.

Acute colitis

Patients with a mild attack (up to four motions a day) usually respond to a course of oral prednisolone given over a 3- to 4-week period. One of the 5-ASA compounds can be given concurrently. A moderate attack often responds to oral prednisolone, twice-daily steroid enemas and 5-ASA. Failure to achieve remission as an outpatient is an indication for admission. Severe attacks of UC occur in up to 10 per cent of patients and are emergencies requiring hospital admission. Regular assessment of vital signs, weight and the abdomen is required. A stool chart should be kept and a plain abdominal radiograph is taken daily and inspected for dilatation of the transverse colon. The presence of mucosal islands or intramural gas on plain radiographs (see Figure 69.6), increasing colonic diameter or a sudden increase in pulse and temperature may indicate a colonic perforation. Fluid and electrolyte balance is maintained, anaemia corrected and adequate nutrition is provided, sometimes intravenously in severe cases. If the patient is not having immediate surgery, then oral nutrition is important. It is important to ensure that calorie and nitrogen requirements are met by dietary supplementation or intravenous feeding. The patient is treated with intravenous hydrocortisone four times daily, as well as rectal steroids. There is no evidence that antibiotics modify the course of a severe attack. If there is failure to gain an improvement within 48 hours of commencing high-dose intravenous steroids, then surgery should be seriously considered and it is certainly advisable if there has been no improvement within 3–5 days. Regular and joint review by gastroenterologist and surgeon is essential to identify patients who are failing to make anticipated progress and to ensure that surgery is neither inappropriately delayed nor undertaken. Some gastroenterologists will use azathioprine, cyclosporin A or infliximab in severe attacks to try and induce remission.

Indications for surgery

The greatest likelihood of a patient with UC requiring surgery is during the first year after diagnosis. The overall risk of colectomy is 20 per cent. Indications for surgery in UC are:

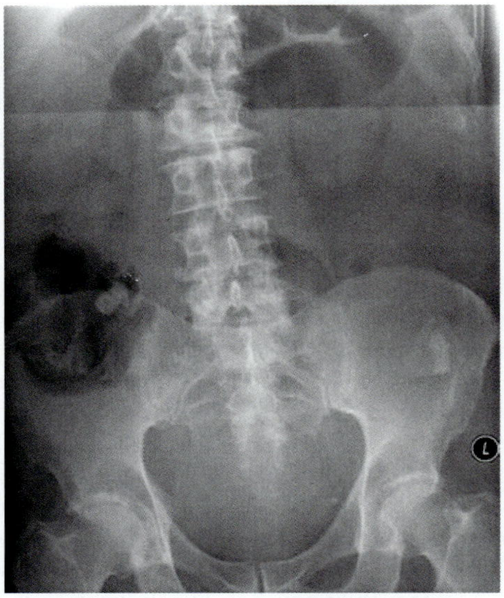

Figure 69.6 Abdominal radiograph demonstrating gas in the wall of the caecum (courtesy of Dr D Kasir, Hope Hospital, Salford, UK).

- severe or fulminating disease failing to respond to medical therapy;
- chronic disease with anaemia, frequent stools, urgency and tenesmus;
- steroid-dependent disease (here, the disease is not severe, but remission cannot be maintained without substantial doses of steroids);
- inability of the patient to tolerate medical therapy required to control the disease (steroid psychosis or other side effects, azathioprine-induced pancreatitis), such that remission cannot be maintained;
- neoplastic change: patients who have severe dysplasia or carcinoma on review colonoscopy;
- extraintestinal manifestations;
- rarely, severe haemorrhage or stenosis causing obstruction.

Operative treatment for UC

Emergency

In the emergency situation (or for a patient who is malnourished or on steroids), the 'first aid procedure' is a subtotal colectomy and end ileostomy. The rectal stump (really rectosigmoid) is left long and can either be brought out as a mucous fistula or closed just beneath the skin. Ideally, the rectal stump is exteriorised as a mucous fistula in the left iliac fossa, and not through the lower end of the wound, which creates significant problems for stoma management. This operation has the advantages that the patient avoids a pelvic operation while unstable, that colonic histology can be assessed and restorative surgery can be contemplated at a later date when the patient is no longer on steroids and has fully recovered from systemic illness and is optimally nourished. The operation is performed in a similar manner to an extended right hemicolectomy – the omentum should be preserved if possible and the dissection of the left colon is continued to divide the sigmoid at a level which will comfortably reach the skin as a mucous fistula. In colitis, it is not necessary to take the mesenteric vessels at their origin. Unless the rectosigmoid is itself disintegrating, the temptation to close the rectal stump and leave it stapled off in the pelvis should be avoided if at all possible. The diseased rectum may disintegrate, causing a pelvic abscess and severe sepsis, with potentially fatal consequences. Allowing the rectal remnant to discharge through the mucus fistula not only minimises the risk of this serious complication, but may also allow the delivery of high-dose topical steroid or 5-ASA compound, via the mucous fistula, into the isolated rectum.

Elective surgery

The indications for elective surgery include:

- failure of medical therapy/steroid dependence;
- growth retardation in the young;
- extraintestinal disease (polyarthropathy and pyoderma gangrenosum respond to colectomy);
- malignant change.

In the elective setting, four operations are available:

1. Subtotal colectomy and ileostomy (as in an emergency)
2. Proctocolectomy and permanent end ileostomy
3. Restorative proctocolectomy with ileoanal pouch
4. Subtotal colectomy and ileorectal anastomosis.

Segmental resections are not recommended as even when the right side is not obviously involved, there is a high recurrence rate in the remaining colon. Subtotal colectomy with ileostomy is performed electively for a frail patient, a patient who cannot be weaned from steroids and when there is doubt as to whether the colitis may represent Crohn's disease. A pouch, a completion proctectomy and even an ileorectal anastomosis can all then be considered at a future date. All of these procedures including formation of a pouch, can be performed laparoscopically in experienced hands.

Proctocolectomy and ileostomy

This operation removes all the colon and rectum, removing any risk of colorectal neoplasia or colitic symptoms, but it leaves a permanent stoma. It has a lower complication rate compared with a pouch procedure, although the perineal wound can be problematic (10 per cent fail to heal) and stoma problems are common. It is indicated for patients who are not candidates for restorative surgery due to sphincter problems or patient preference. The colectomy is performed as above. Provided there is no concern around rectal cancer a close rectal dissection may be performed to minimise damage to the pelvic nerves, avoiding erectile and bladder dysfunction. An intersphincteric excision of the anus is undertaken, which results in a smaller perineal wound and fewer healing problems. A permanent end ileostomy is formed, as described later, with scrupulous attention to detail to ensure a good functional and cosmetic result. It is particularly important to ensure that an adequate spout is created and the stoma is sited adequately to ensure that it is appropriate for the patient's build. The position of the ileostomy should be carefully chosen by the patient with the help of a stoma care nurse specialist. There is an argument for making the trephine incision before entering the abdomen to prevent any problems of distortion of the abdominal wall after opening. If performed laparoscopically, the specimen is removed through the perineal wound and so there is no requirement for any abdominal incision other than the port sites.

Restorative proctocolectomy with an ileoanal pouch (Parks)

In this operation, a pouch is made out of ileum (Figure 69.7) as a substitute for the rectum and sewn or stapled to the anal canal. This avoids a permanent stoma. It is reserved for patients with adequate anal sphincters and should be avoided when Crohn's disease is a possibility. Various pouch designs have been described, but the 'J' is the most popular and the most easily made using staplers (Figure 69.8). The 'S' (three loop) has been associated with evacuation difficulties due to the short efferent spout. The 'W' (four loop) pouch has a larger reservoir, which results in less bowel frequency. There is some controversy over the correct technique for ileoanal anastomosis. In the earliest operations, the mucosa from the dentate line up to midrectum was stripped off the underlying muscle, but it is now known that a long muscle cuff is not needed. Although mucosectomy of the upper anal canal with an anastomosis at the dentate line is claimed to remove all of the at-risk mucosa and any problem of subsequent cancer, it may also increase the risk of incontinence with nocturnal seepage. The alternative is an anastomosis double-stapled to the top of the anal canal, preserving the upper anal canal

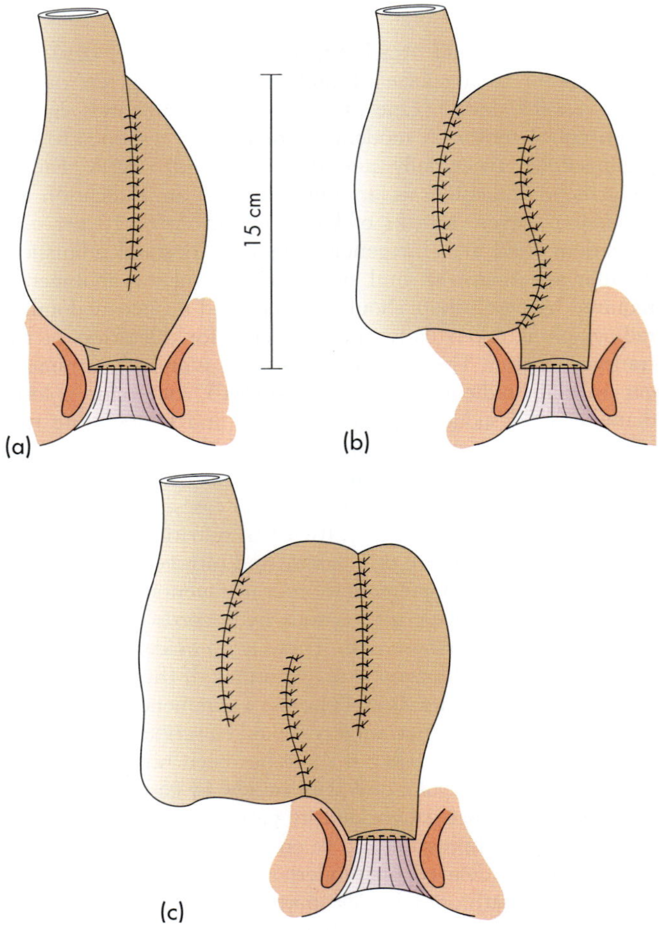

Figure 69.7 Ileoanal anastomosis with pouch. A substitute rectum is made from joined folds of ileum to form an expanded pouch of small intestine. The pouch is then joined directly to the anus at the level of the dentate line, all other rectal mucosa having been removed. Three ways of forming a pouch are illustrated: (a) a simple reversed 'J'; (b) an 'S' pouch; (c) a 'W' pouch.

mucosa. Continence appears to be better, but there is a theoretical risk of leaving inflamed mucosa behind. The procedure can be carried out in stages. In most cases, a covering loop ileostomy is used as described later.

Complications include pelvic sepsis (usually resulting from a leak at the ileoanal anastomosis or, in a J pouch, from the top of the 'J'), postoperative small bowel obstruction (which may occur in as many as 10–15 per cent of patients) and pouch vaginal fistula. Frequency of evacuation is determined by pouch volume, completeness of emptying, reservoir inflammation and intrinsic small bowel motility, but is typically between three and eight evacuations in each 24-hour period. Increased frequency, urgency and faecal incontinence can be seen (20, 5 and 5 per cent, respectively), but these reduce with time. Approximately 50 per cent of patients with ileoanal pouches have a very good quality of life, whereas 35 per cent of patients are less satisfied but choose to retain their pouches. Pouch function is so poor in 15 per cent that the pouch is removed. The main reasons for failure are pelvic sepsis (50 per cent), poor function (30 per cent)

Sir Alan Guyatt Parks, 1920–1982, surgeon, St Mark's Hospital and the London Hospital, London, UK, former President of the Royal College of Surgeons of England.

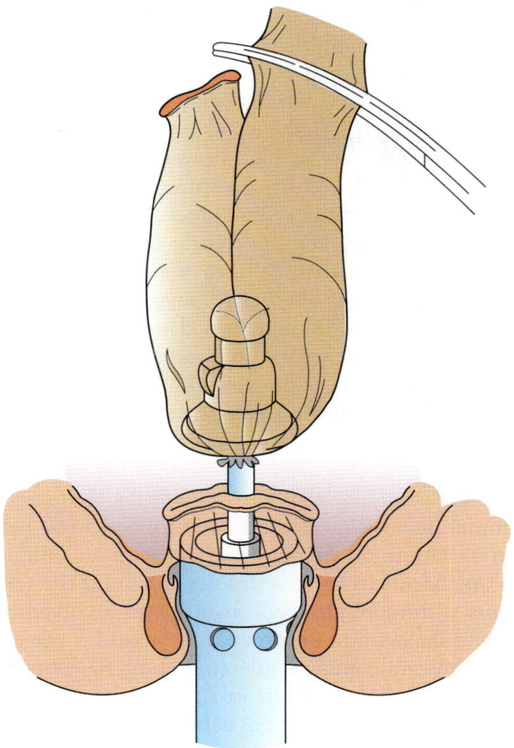

Figure 69.8 Stapled 'J' pouch with stapler creating a pouch–anus anastomosis.

and pouchitis or inflammation of the pouch (10 per cent). It is also important for women of reproductive age to be advised that they may suffer from reduced fertility, as well as vaginal dryness, due to denervation of the secretory glands of the vaginal mucosa. Women who have not completed their families may elect for a colectomy with ileostomy and a pouch later. If it turns out that the patient actually has Crohn's disease, there is a high rate of pouch failure and the operation is not usually recommended in this disease.

In expert hands, a restorative proctocolectomy can be peformed safely laparoscopically. This has a longer operative time but is likely to result in shorter lengths of stay. In young patients, the better cosmetic result with preservation of body image is a consideration. Striking images of well patients with tiny laparoscopic scars and no stoma can act as an advert for the laparoscopic approach. There is also the as yet unproven possibility that laparoscopic pouch surgery will result in a reduction in incisional hernias and small bowel obstruction and less effect on female fertility than open surgery. The key factors still to be determined for the laparoscopic approach are functional outcomes as there is a significant technical challenge to cross-stapling at the pelvic floor and there is the potential to leave a longer rectal cuff, than via an open approach, although this might be circumvented by a new perineal approach dubbed the APPEAR technique.

Pouchitis describes an inflammatory condition, which may affect 30 per cent of patients with an ileoanal pouch. It is characterised not only by the presence of inflammation in the pouch (which is common and frequently asymptomatic), but also by symptoms of pouch dysfunction (increased frequency, tenesmus, bleeding, purulent discharge) and systemic illness (malaise, fever, raised inflammatory markers). The cause of pouchitis is unknown, but it appears to relate to inflammatory bowel disease (pouchitis does not seem to occur in pouches created for patients for other indications). Alterations in bacteria flora in the pouch may be relevant as pouchitis usually responds to a short course of antibiotic therapy, notably with metronidazole or ciprofloxacin.

Colectomy and ileorectal anastomosis

This procedure is occasionally performed in UC if there is minimal rectal inflammation after total colectomy. It is rarely appropriate as a very considerable percentage (at least 50 per cent) of patients with a quiescent rectum after total colectomy will develop significant mucosal inflammation in the rectum, once the faecal stream has been re-established. Although rectal inflammation can be controlled with medical treatment, functional results may be disappointing. If the rectum is preserved, then annual rectal inspection is advocated. Although this procedure has the advantage of avoiding a stoma and the risk to sexual function associated with rectal dissection, it has fallen out of favour due to the ongoing risk of persisting inflammation and malignancy in the retained rectum.

INDETERMINATE COLITIS

Ten per cent of patients with colitis present with histological features that make their disease difficult to characterise. They may, for example, have a patchy colitis, with evidence of fissuring and/or transmural ulceration, or cobblestoning of the colonic mucosa, raising the possibility of Crohn's disease, but without clear pathognomonic features of Crohn's disease, such as epithelioid granulomata (see below); such patients may be said to have an 'indeterminate colitis'. Indeterminate colitis is not, therefore, a specific disease entity so much as an indication by a pathologist that the underlying pattern of colitis (and therefore the course of the illness) is unclear. While the clinical history may suggest the diagnosis in some cases (for example, a history of recurrent perianal sepsis and fistulation would make a diagnosis of Crohn's disease more likely), in others, it may remain, despite colectomy, unclear whether a patient has UC or Crohn's disease. In such cases, it may still be appropriate to offer a pouch, but the risks of pouch failure appear to be significantly higher (up to 25–30 per cent) and patients should be advised accordingly.

CROHN'S DISEASE (REGIONAL ENTERITIS)

The label 'Crohn's disease' became attached to a chronic inflammatory disease of the ileum following a key publication by Burrill Crohn and colleagues in 1932. CD is characterised by a chronic full thickness inflammatory process that can affect any part of the gastrointestinal tract from the lips to the anal margin. It is most common in North America and Northern Europe with an incidence of 5 per 100 000. Prevalence rates of around 50 per 100 000 have been reported in the UK. Over the last four decades, there seems to have been a rise in the incidence, which

Burrill Bernard Crohn, 1884–1983, gastroenterologist, Mount Sinai Hospital, New York, NY, USA, along with Leon Ginzburg and Gordon Oppenheimer described regional ileitis in 1932.

cannot be accounted for by increased diagnosis. It is slightly more common in women than in men, and is most commonly diagnosed in young patients between the ages of 25 and 40 years. There does, however, seem to be a second peak of incidence around the age of 70 years. In those countries with high prevalence of CD, the groups with the highest prevalence seem to be Caucasian, notably American Whites and Northern Europeans, whereas it is less common, even in high prevalence countries, in those originating from Central Europe and less prevalent still in those originating from South America, Asia and Africa. CD seems to be especially prevalent (three- to five-fold higher) in the Ashkenazi Jewish population, although interestingly, the prevalence of CD in the Jewish population in Israel is lower than that in Europe or the United States, suggesting the importance of environmental factors.

Aetiology

The aetiology of Crohn's disease is incompletely understood but is thought to involve a complex interplay of genetic and environmental factors. Although CD shares some features with chronic infection, no causative organism has ever been demonstrated. An intriguing similarity to Johne's disease of cattle, a chronic inflammatory enteropathy resulting from infection with *Mycobacterium paratuberculosis*, suggests that CD in man may share a common aetiology. Some studies in which molecular biological analyses of tissue affected by CD have identified mycobacterial DNA more frequently in patients with CD than in controls, but others have been less conclusive and, in particular, randomised controlled trials have failed to show a significant therapeutic benefit of treating CD with antituberculous drugs. A wide variety of foods have been implicated, and in particular, a diet high in refined foodstuffs, but none conclusively. An association with high levels of sanitation in childhood has been suggested. Smoking increases the relative risk of CD threefold and is certainly an exacerbating factor after diagnosis, contrary to the protective effect seen in UC. Genetic factors are clearly important. Approximately 10 per cent of patients have a first-degree relative with the disease, and concordance has been shown to approach 50 per cent in monozygotic twins. Inheritance is thought to involve multiple genes with low penetrance. The *NOD2/CARD15* gene has excited particular interest as variants of this gene have been shown to have strong associations with CD. Genetic manipulation of these genes in mice seems to induce the development of a disease resembling CD and abnormalities of these genes have been shown to be present in some members of families with a particularly high incidence of CD. It should be noted, however, that abnormalities of these genes have not been found in the vast majority of individuals with CD. Since these genes are involved in intracellular recognition of bacteria, their discovery provides potentially valuable insight into the pathogenesis of CD, as a disease in which the relationship between the gut mucosa and the normal gut bacteria becomes deranged, resulting in uncontrolled intestinal inflammation.

Pathogenesis

As in UC, there is thought to be an increased permeability of the mucous membrane. This may lead to increased passage of luminal antigens, which then induce a cell-mediated inflammatory response. This results in the release of proinflammatory cytokines, such as interleukin-2 and tumour necrosis factor, which coordinate local and systemic inflammatory responses. It has been suggested that CD is associated with a defect in suppressor T cells, which usually act to prevent escalation of the inflammatory process. As in UC, however, it remains unclear whether the proposed increase in intestinal permeability is a cause or consequence of the disease process. Studies of intestinal permeability in healthy and apparently unaffected first degree relatives of patients with CD have also, however, suggested that gut permeability is increased, suggesting that a global, and potentially genetically determined increase in gut permeability, combined perhaps with an abnormal immune-mediated response to colonisation of the gut with subspecies of the normal enteric microflora, may initiate the disease.

Pathology

The terminal ileum is most commonly involved (60 per cent), either in isolation or in combination with colonic disease. Colitis alone occurs in up to a third of cases and the remainder are patients with more proximal small bowel involvement. The stomach and duodenum are affected in around 5 per cent, but perianal lesions are common, affecting up to 50–75 per cent of patients. Perianal disease occurs in 25 per cent of patients with small bowel disease, but in 75 per cent of patients with Crohn's colitis.

Macroscopically, resection specimens show a fibrotic thickening of the intestinal wall with a narrow lumen and fat wrapping (encroachment of mesenteric fat around the bowel, Figure 69.9). There is usually dilated bowel just proximal to the stricture and deep mucosal ulcerations with linear or snake-like patterns in the strictured area itself. Oedema in the mucosa between the ulcers gives rise to a cobblestone appearance. The transmural inflammation (which is a key feature of CD) may lead to segments of bowel becoming adherent to each other and to surrounding structures, inflammatory masses with mesenteric abscesses and fistulae into adjacent organs. The serosa is usually opaque, with thickening of the mesentery and enlarged

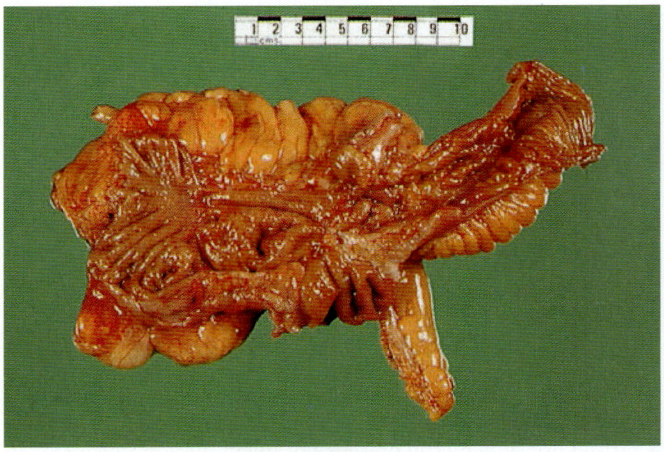

Figure 69.9 Crohn's disease of the ileocaecal region showing typical thickening of the wall of the terminal ileum with narrowing of the lumen (courtesy of Dr B Warren, John Radcliffe Hospital, Oxford, UK).

Eugen (Janö) Alexander Polya, 1876–1944, surgeon, St Stephen's Hospital, Budapest, Hungary.
Sir Walter Fred Bodmer, b. 1936, German-born English geneticist, University of Oxford, Director of Research, Imperial Cancer Research Fund, London, UK.

mesenteric lymph nodes. CD is characteristically discontinuous, with inflamed areas separated from normal intestine, so-called 'skip' lesions.

Microscopically, there are focal areas of chronic inflammation involving all layers of the intestinal wall with lymphoid aggregates. Non-caseating giant cell granulomas are found in 60 per cent of patients and clearly define Crohn's disease. They are most common in anorectal disease. Multifocal arterial occlusions are found in the muscularis propria, which is thickened. There is deep, fissuring ulceration within affected areas. Characteristically, and unlike in UC, there may be completely normal areas immediately next to areas of severe inflammation.

Clinical features

Presentation depends upon the pattern of disease. Very infrequently, CD presents acutely with acute ileal inflammation and symptoms and signs resembling those of acute appendicitis, or even free perforation of the small intestine, resulting in a local or diffuse peritonitis. CD may present with fulminant colitis but this is considerably less common than in UC (see Summary box 69.4).

Summary box 69.4

Differences between ulcerative colitis and Crohn's disease

- Ulcerative colitis affects the colon; Crohn's disease can affect any part of the gastrointestinal tract, but particularly the small and large bowel
- UC is a mucosal disease, whereas CD affects the full thickness of the bowel wall
- UC produces confluent disease in the colon and rectum, whereas CD is characterised by skip lesions
- CD more commonly causes stricturing and fistulation
- Granulomas may be found on histology in CD, but not in UC
- CD is often associated with perianal disease, whereas this is unusual in UC
- CD affecting the terminal ileum may produce symptoms mimicking appendicitis, but this does not occur in UC
- Resection of the colon and rectum cures the patient with UC, whereas recurrence is common after resection in CD

Crohn's disease more commonly presents with features of chronicity. Chronic small bowel CD often manifests as mild diarrhoea extending over many months, occurring in bouts accompanied by intestinal colic. Patients may complain of pain, particularly in the right iliac fossa, and a tender mass may be palpable. Intermittent fevers, secondary anaemia and weight loss are common. After months of repeated attacks with acute inflammation, the affected area of intestine begins to narrow with fibrosis, causing obstructive symptoms. Children developing the illness before puberty may have retarded growth and sexual development. With progression of the disease, adhesions and transmural fissuring, intra-abdominal abscesses and fistula tracts may develop.

Fistulation may occur into adjacent loops of bowel (enteroenteric fistulae), and, most notably the (healthy) sigmoid loop may become adherent to the affected terminal ileum, resulting in ileosigmoid fistulation and profuse diarrhoea. Fistulation may also occur into the bladder (ileovesical) or the female genital tract and, less commonly, the duodenum. Fistulation into the abdominal wall (enterocutaneous fistulation) may also develop spontaneously, but more commonly occurs as a complication of abdominal surgery.

Colonic CD presents with symptoms of colitis and proctitis as described for UC, although toxic megacolon is much less common (Figure 69.10).

Many patients with CD present with perianal problems. In the presence of active disease, the perianal skin appears bluish. Superficial ulcers with undermined edges are relatively painless and can heal with bridging of epithelium. Deep cavitating ulcers are usually found in the upper anal canal; they can be painful and cause perianal abscesses and fistulae, discharging around the anus and sometimes forwards into the genitalia. Fistulation through the posterior wall of the vagina may lead to rectovaginal fistula and continuous leakage of gas and/or faeces per vagina.

The rectal mucosa is often spared and may feel normal on rectal examination. If it is involved however, it will feel thickened, nodular and irregular. Perianal disease is frequently associated with dense, fibrous stricturing at the anorectal junction. Incontinence may develop as a result of destruction of the anal sphincter musculature because of inflammation, abscess formation, fibrotic change and repeated episodes of surgical drainage. In severe cases, the perineum may become densely fibrotic, rigid and covered with multiple discharging openings (watering-can perineum).

Extraintestinal manifestations

The extraintestinal manifestations of Crohn's disease are similar to those that occur in UC and are outlined in Summary box 69.5. Gallstones are common due to an inflamed or excised terminal ileum leading to reduced absorption of bile salts. Amyloidosis is common at post-mortem, but is rarely symptomatic. 'Metastatic' CD can occur in the vagina or skin with nodular ulcers, which demonstrate non-caseating granulomas when biopsied. The appearances can be indistinguishable macroscopically from hidradenitis suppurativa.

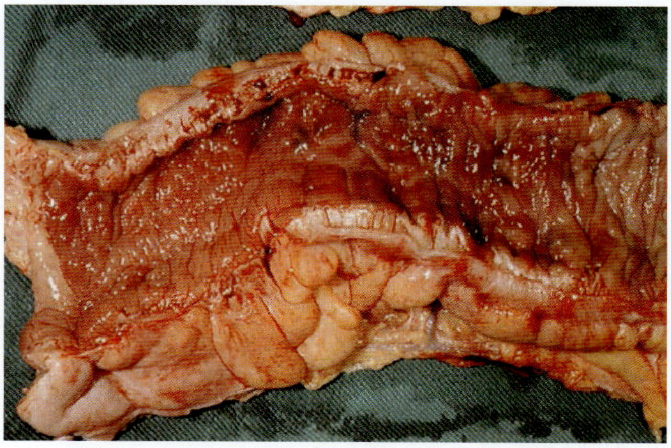

Figure 69.10 Colonic Crohn's disease. Note the normal mucosa on either side of the inflammatory stricture (courtesy of Dr B Warren, John Radcliffe Hospital, Oxford, UK).

Summary box 69.5

Extraintestinal manifestations of Crohn's disease

- Related to disease activity
  - Erythema nodosum
  - Pyoderma gangrenosum
  - Arthropathy
  - Eye complications (iritis/uveitis)
  - Aphthous ulceration
  - Amyloidosis
- Unrelated to disease activity
  - Gallstones
  - Renal calculi
  - Primary sclerosing cholangitis
  - Chronic active hepatitis
  - Sacroiliitis

Investigations

Laboratory

A full blood count should be performed, as anaemia is common and usually multifactorial, it may result from the anaemia of chronic disease, or from iron deficiency as a result of blood loss or malabsorption. Vitamin B12 deficiency may occur as a consequence of terminal ileal disease or resection. Active inflammatory disease is usually associated with a fall in serum albumin, magnesium, zinc and selenium. Acute phase protein measurements (C-reactive protein and orosomucoid) may correlate with disease activity.

Endoscopy

Colonoscopic examination may be normal or show patchy inflammation. There will be areas of normal colon or rectum in between areas of inflamed mucosa that are irregular and ulcerated, with a mucopurulent exudate. The earliest appearances are aphthous ulcers surrounded by a rim of erythematous mucosa. These become larger and deeper with increasing severity of disease. There may be stricturing, and it is important to exclude malignancy in these sites. An irregular Crohn's stricture with polypoid mucosa may be almost indistinguishable from malignancy. The terminal ileum may be ulcerated and strictured. In patients who have had previous ileocaecal resection, recurrent disease usually presents first with aphthous ulceration proximal to the anastomosis.

Upper gastrointestinal symptoms may require upper gastrointestinal endoscopy, which may reveal deep longitudinal ulcers and cobblestone mucosa in the duodenum, stomach or, rarely, in the oesophagus. Enteroscopy may reveal jejunal ulceration and stricturing. Capsule endoscopy should not be undertaken where there is a risk of stricture, because of the possibility of the capsule becoming stuck in the narrow segment. It may, however, have a useful role in those patients with evidence of chronic gastrointestinal blood loss where no evidence of ulceration can be found with more conventional endoscopic assessment.

Imaging

High-resolution ultrasound in expert hands can demonstrate inflamed and thickened bowel loops, as well as fluid collections and abscesses. The small intestine is traditionally imaged by a small bowel enema (Figure 69.11). This will show up areas of stricturing and prestenotic dilatation. The involved areas tend to be narrowed, irregular and, sometimes, when a length of terminal ileum is involved, there may be the string sign of Kantor. CT scans with luminal contrast are widely used in the investigation of abdominal symptoms and can demonstrate fistulae, intra-abdominal abscesses and bowel thickening or dilatation (Figure 69.12). Magnetic resonance imaging (MRI) is useful in assessing complex perianal disease, but more recently has been shown to be an excellent method for investigating the small bowel. MR enteroclysis is particularly effective at demonstrating small bowel stricturing (Figure 69.13) and avoids the need for repeated exposure to large doses of ionising radiation in young patients. In patients with enterocutaneous fistulae, fistulography will be required to demonstrate the anatomy and complexity of fistulae and allow adequate planning for future surgery.

TREATMENT

Medical treatment

Steroids

Steroids are the mainstay of treatment for CD. They induce remission in 70–80 per cent of cases with moderate to severe disease. They should be used in short courses and tapered after response has been achieved. They reduce inflammation and will not therefore be effective against fibrostenotic disease, where the symptoms relate mainly to obstruction. Steroids can also be used as topical agents in the rectum with reduced sys-

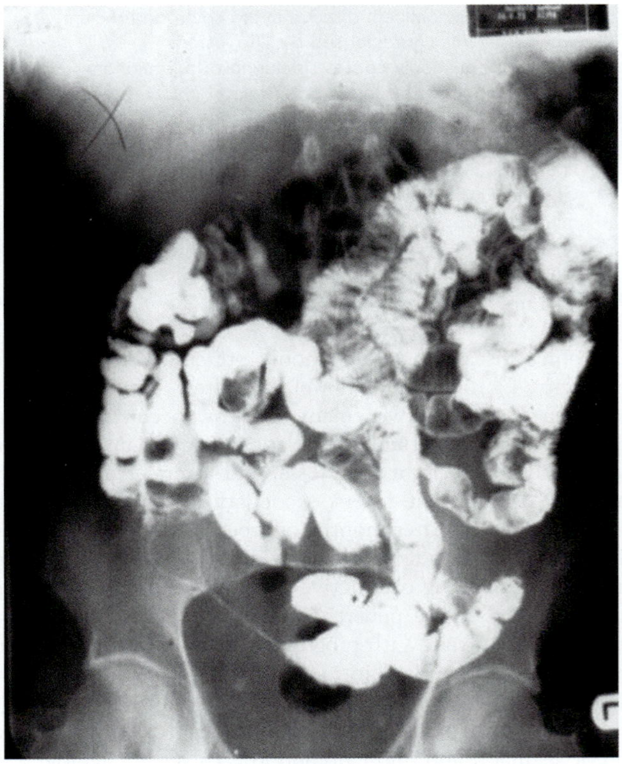

Figure 69.11 Small bowel enema examination showing a narrowed terminal ileum involved with Crohn's disease – the 'string' sign of Kantor.

John Leonard Kantor, 1890–1947, gastroenterologist, the Presbyterian Hospital, New York, NY, USA, described his 'string sign' in 1934.

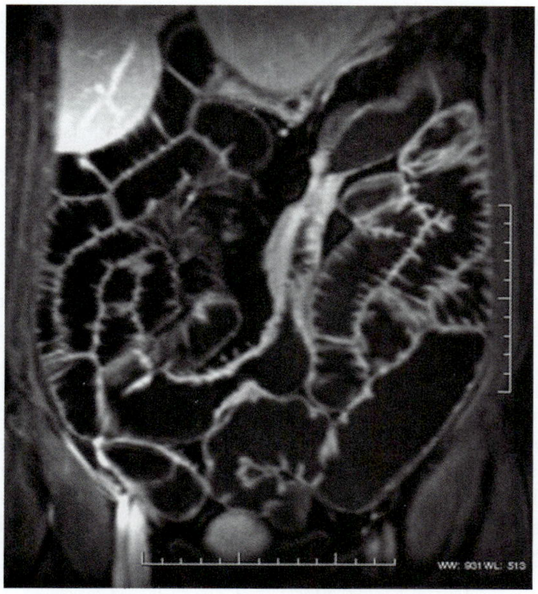

Figure 69.12 Computed tomographic enteroclysis showing small bowel dilatation secondary to strictured terminal ileum involved with Crohn's disease (courtesy of Dr H Bungay, John Radcliffe Hospital, Oxford, UK).

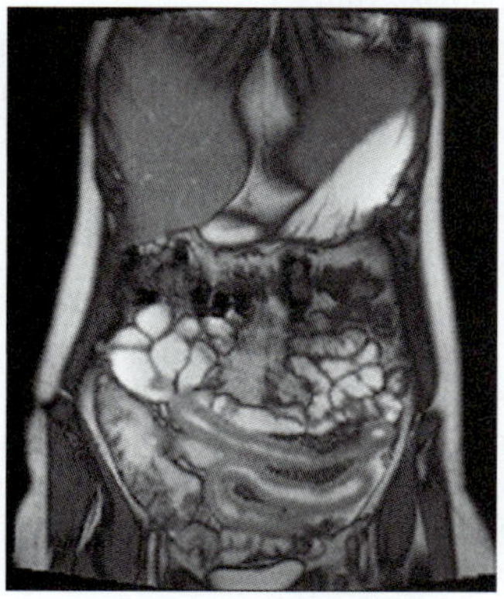

Figure 69.13 Magnetic resonance enteroclysis demonstrating small bowel stricture (courtesy of Dr D Kasir, Hope Hospital, Salford, UK).

temic bioavailability, but long-term use can still cause adrenal suppression. More recent oral steroid formulations have been devised to ensure that the steroid moiety is removed from the portal circulation, reducing systemic side effects. Steroids should not be used for maintenance therapy for CD and are usually replaced with immunomodulatory agents (see below under Immunomodulatory agents) in order to minimise the risk of side effects associated with long-term steroid use.

Aminosalicylates

Colonic symptoms can be treated by 5-ASA agents in a similar manner to that in UC. These agents have been traditionally believed to help with management of small bowel CD, but this has recently been questioned. Some studies of patients who have undergone previous resection have suggested that 5-ASA drugs may reduce the incidence of recrudescent disease.

Antibiotics

Metronidazole and ciprofloxacin may be used, particularly for periods of a few weeks at a time, especially in perianal disease. Long-term use of metronidazole is to be especially avoided, as there is a risk of peripheral neuropathy. Antibiotics may also be used when there is evidence of a mass or an abscess. In general, however, a confirmed abscess should be treated by drainage plus or minus resection as antibiotics alone will not treat a Crohn's mass effectively.

Immunomodulatory agents

Azathioprine is used for its additive and steroid-sparing effect and is now standard maintenance therapy. It is a purine analogue, which is metabolised to 6-mercaptopurine (6-MP) and works by inhibiting cell-mediated immune responses. 6-Mercaptopurine may be given directly for the same reasons. Cyclosporin also acts by inhibiting cell-mediated immunity. Short-course intravenous cyclosporin treatment is associated with 80 per cent remission; however, there is relapse after completion of treatment.

Monoclonal antibody

Several commercially available agents have been developed based upon monoclonal antibodies targeting tumour necrosis factor alpha. Infliximab, the murine chimaeric monoclonal antibody and Adalimumab (human monoclonal) are used for patients with severe, active disease who are refractory to other forms of treatment and who would otherwise be at high risk of requiring surgical intervention. There is some evidence to suggest that early and aggressive use of these agents in patients with evidence of early recrudescent disease after surgery (for example, by colonoscopy showing aphthous ulceration at the anastomosis at one year) may reduce the need for subsequent surgery. These agents also appear to be effective treatments for fistulae, particularly in perianal disease. Recent studies have suggested, however, that they reduce the inflammation associated with the process of fistulation and that the fistula tracks may remain unhealed, even if the skin defects close. Cessation of therapy is associated with a high risk of reactivation of the fistulae. These are very expensive forms of treatment and active infection, tuberculosis and a past history of malignancy are contraindications.

Nutritional support

It is essential that nutritional status is evaluated in all patients with CD. Nutritional support is frequently required. Patients with moderate nutritional impairment will require nutritional supplementation and severely malnourished patients may require nasoenteric or even intravenous feeding. Anaemia, hypoproteinaemia and electrolyte, vitamin and metabolic bone problems must all be addressed. Elemental diet or parenteral nutrition can induce remission in up to 80 per cent of patients, an effect comparable to steroids. Almost all patients relapse rapidly after cessation of therapy (Summary box 69.6).

Non-operative management of Crohn's disease

Although perforating and fistulating disease will require surgical treatment (see below under Surgery), stricturing may be amenable to endoscopic treatment, provided the strictures can be reached with an endoscope and negotiated with a guide

Summary box 69.6

Principles of management of Crohn's disease

- Close liaison between physician and surgeon is crucial
- Medical therapy should always be considered as an alternative to surgery, although surgery should not be delayed when a clear indication for surgery exists
- Patients must be optimised as far as possible prior to surgery, and this may require preoperative total parenteral nutrition
- Crohn's disease is a chronic relapsing disease with a high likelihood of reoperation; the surgeon must take every reasonable effort to preserve bowel length and sphincter function

wire. This may be accomplished by enteroscopy or colonoscopy, depending upon the site of the stricture. Dilatation of an inflamed and ulcerated stricture is contraindicated because of the risks of perforation, but balloon dilatation of fibrostenotic disease may result in substantial symptomatic improvement and obviate the need for surgery in selected cases.

Indications for surgery

Surgical resection will not cure CD. Surgery therefore focuses on the complications of the disease. As many of these indications for surgery may be relative, joint management by an aggressive physician and a conservative surgeon is thought to be ideal (see Figure 69.6). These complications include:

- recurrent intestinal obstruction
- bleeding
- perforation
- failure of medical therapy
- intestinal fistula
- fulminant colitis
- malignant change
- perianal disease.

Surgery

The main surgical principle is to preserve gut length and maintain adequate function. The whole of the gastrointestinal tract should be examined carefully at laparotomy/laparoscopy and intestinal resection kept to the minimum required to treat the local consequences of disease. If, on occasion, CD is diagnosed during the course of an operation for suspected appendicitis, it is reasonable to remove the appendix, although there may be concern about fistulation. If the ileum is thick, rigid and inflamed, an ileocaecal resection can be carried out immediately, although it is equally reasonable to try a period of medical therapy. A senior opinion is important to determine the optimum therapy, taking into account the patient's history, fitness, comorbidity and operative findings.

The course of the disease after surgery is unpredictable, but recrudescence (a better term than 'recurrence' as surgery cannot cure) is common. Symptomatic recrudescence does not seem to be related to the presence of disease at the resection line. The cumulative probability of recrudescence requiring surgery for ileal disease is of the order of 20, 40, 60 and 80 per cent at 5, 10, 15 and 20 years, respectively, after previous resection.

Crohn's surgery is technically demanding as mesenteries are thickened and oedematous, the bowel may be fragile and the patient may be malnourished, immunosuppressed or septic. A key decision has to be made after resection between anastomosis and defunctioning, as leaks and fistulation are a notorious problem. It has been established that anastomotic complications are more common with one or more of the following risk factors:

- steroids
- low albumin
- abscess
- fistula.

If more than two factors are present it is safer (and if all, imperative) to exteriorise the bowel and consider delayed anastomosis when the patient has fully recovered.

Laparoscopic surgery is possible for ileocaecal or colonic resections and has the potential advantage of smaller incisions and potentially shorter recovery time. Reoperative surgery is technically demanding but experienced laparoscopic surgeons have been able to carry out such procedures. A great range of operations is performed for Crohn's disease depending on disease pattern – the most common are outlined below:

- Ileocaecal resection is the usual procedure for terminal ileal Crohn's with a primary anastomosis between the ileum and the ascending or transverse colon, depending on the extent of the disease.
- Segmental resection of short segments of small or large bowel strictures can be performed.
- Colectomy and ileorectal anastomosis is commonly performed for colonic CD with rectal sparing and a normal anus.
- Subtotal colectomy and ileostomy for Crohn's colitis accounts for 8 per cent of such procedures for acute colonic disease. The indications are similar to those for UC.
- Temporary loop ileostomy. This can be used either in patients with acute distal CD, allowing remission and later restoration of continuity, or in patients with severe perianal or rectal disease.
- Proctocolectomy. Patients with colonic and anal disease failing to respond to medical treatment will eventually require a permanent ileostomy.
- Strictureplasty. Multiple strictured areas of CD (Figure 69.14) can be treated by a local widening procedure, strictureplasty, to avoid small bowel resection (Figure 69.15).

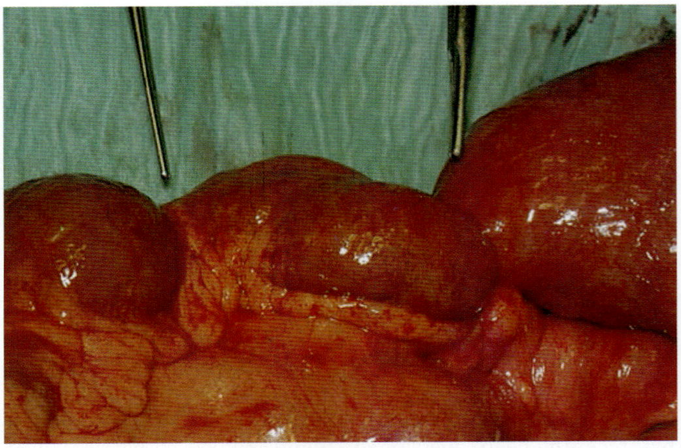

Figure 69.14 Small bowel strictures in Crohn's disease with dilatation between strictures.

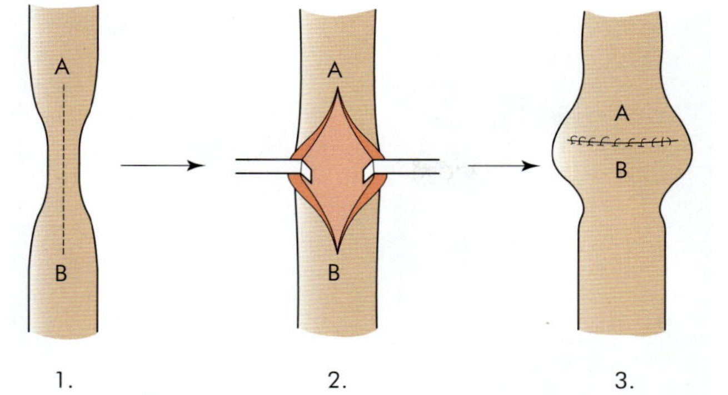

Figure 69.15 Strictureplasty. (1) A strictured length of intestine is incised along its length. (2) The bowel is opened and the walls are retracted as shown. (3) The bowel is resutured transversely to widen the narrowed segment.

- Anal disease should be treated conservatively to avoid sphincter injury by simple drainage of abscesses and the use of setons through fistulae.

INFECTIONS OF THE SMALL AND LARGE INTESTINE

Campylobacter

Infection with *Campylobacter jejuni* (a Gram-negative rod with a distinctive spiral shape) is the most common form of gastroenteritis in the UK, typically acquired from eating infected poultry. It causes diarrhoea and abdominal pain and may mimic an acute abdomen. Severe cases may resemble UC and cause diagnostic difficulty. The organism is very sensitive and may take several days to isolate on stool culture. Treatment is supportive as it usually resolves without antibiotics. It is a notifiable disease.

Yersinia

Yersinia enterocolitica is a Gram-negative rod, which can infect the terminal ileum, appendix, ascending colon and mesenteric lymph nodes, and can cause a granulomatous inflammatory process that mimics Crohn's disease. Yersinia typically causes a fever and gastroenteritis, but may persist and cause a terminal ileitis, which, on occasion, may even perforate. The diagnosis may be made on stool culture, but is more often confirmed serologically. If discovered at laparotomy, the terminal ileum and mesenteric nodes will look thickened and inflamed and a lymph node biopsy can be taken. The disease is normally self-limiting, but also responds to treatment with co-trimoxazole or chloramphenicol.

Intestinal amoebiasis

Amoebiasis is an infestation with *Entamoeba histolytica*. This parasite has a worldwide distribution and is transmitted mainly in contaminated drinking water. It can cause colonic ulcers, which are described as 'bottlenecked' because they have considerably undermined edges. The ulcers typically also have a yellow necrotic floor, from which blood and pus exude. In the majority of cases, they are confined to the distal sigmoid colon and the rectum.

Clinically amoebiasis can mimic UC, most commonly causing bloody diarrhoea but more severe colonic complications can occur, including severe haemorrhage, stricture formation or perforation. A pericolitis is not uncommon and results in adhesions and may cause intestinal obstruction. Amoebiasis may cause liver abscesses or an amoebic mass (amoeboma) of the caecum or sigmoid which is difficult to distinguish from a carcinoma. Surgery is fraught with danger as the bowel is extremely friable.

Endoscopic biopsies or fresh hot stools are examined to look for the presence of amoebae (Figure 69.16). It is important to emphasise, however, that the presence of the parasite does not indicate that it is pathogenic. It is especially important to exclude amoebic infection in patients suspected of having UC.

Treatment is by metronidazole (Flagyl) in the acute setting, three times daily for 7–10 days. Diloxanide furoate is effective against chronic infections associated with the passage of cysts in stools.

Salmonellosis, typhoid and paratyphoid

Salmonella are a family of Gram-negative rods that can cause a range of enteric infections. Salmonella gastroenteritis is typically caused by *S. enteritidis* from poultry, and is most often a self-limiting illness comprising headache, fever and watery diarrhoea. When severe, antibiotics and indeed hospitalisation and intravenous fluids may be needed. The diagnosis is based on stool culture. *Shigella* and enteropathogenic strains of *E. coli* may cause similar diarrhoeal illnesses.

Typhoid fever is caused by *S. typhi* and presents with fever and abdominal pain after an incubation period of 10–20 days. Over the next week, the patient can develop distension, diarrhoea, splenomegaly and characteristic 'rose spots' on the abdomen caused by a vasculitis. A number of surgical complications can result:

- paralytic ileus
- intestinal haemorrhage
- perforation
- cholecystitis.

In addition, invasion of the systemic circulation, which is a characteristic feature of salmonellosis, may cause severe Gram-negative sepsis and septic shock may develop. Some patients develop metastatic sepsis, including septic arthritis and osteomyelitis, meningitis, encephalitis, disseminated intravascular coagulation and pancreatitis.

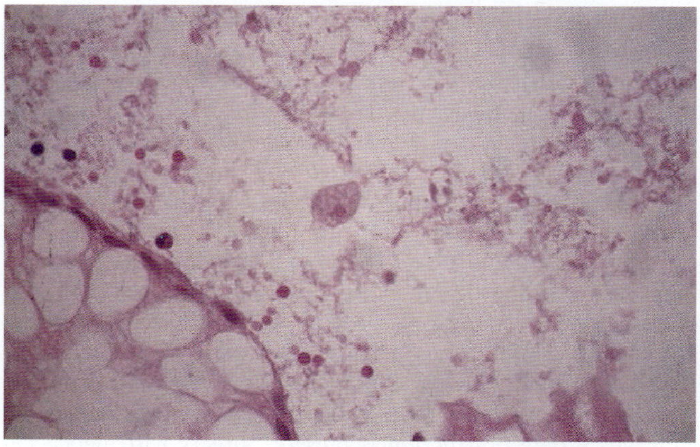

Figure 69.16 An amoeba in a rectal biopsy.

Emanuel Cecil Gruebel Lee, 1933–1986, surgeon, The Radcliffe Infirmary, Oxford, UK, developed strictureplasty for Crohn's disease.
A first-degree relative, defined as the individual's parents, siblings or children.

Perforation of a typhoid ulcer usually occurs during the third week and is sometimes the first sign of the disease. The ulcer is parallel to the long axis of the gut and is usually situated in the distal ileum. Diagnosis is confirmed by culture of blood or stool. Treatment is by antibiotics, usually chloramphenicol. Perforation requires surgery to wash out and close the perforated ulcer – resection is usually avoided. In unstable patients, notably with evidence of septic shock, the bowel should be exteriorised and the perforation closed after recovery. Paratyphoid infection (with *S. paratyphi*) resembles typhoid fever and is treated in a similar manner.

Tuberculosis of the intestine

Tuberculosis, like Crohn's disease, can affect any part of the gastrointestinal tract from the mouth to the anus. The sites affected most often are the ileum, proximal colon and peritoneum. There are two principal presentations.

Ulcerative tuberculosis

Ulcerative tuberculosis is secondary to pulmonary tuberculosis and arises as a result of swallowing tubercle bacilli. Multiple ulcers, lying transversely, develop in the terminal ileum and the overlying serosa is thickened, reddened and covered in tubercles. Patients typically present with diarrhoea and weight loss, although subacute obstruction and even local perforation and fistula formation can occur. A barium follow-through or CT examination show absent filling of the lower ileum, caecum and the ascending colon as a result of narrowing of the ulcerated segment (Figure 69.17).

A course of chemotherapy (antituberculous antibiotics) usually leads to cure, provided the pulmonary tuberculosis is adequately treated. Surgery is usually undertaken only in the rare event of a perforation or complete intestinal obstruction.

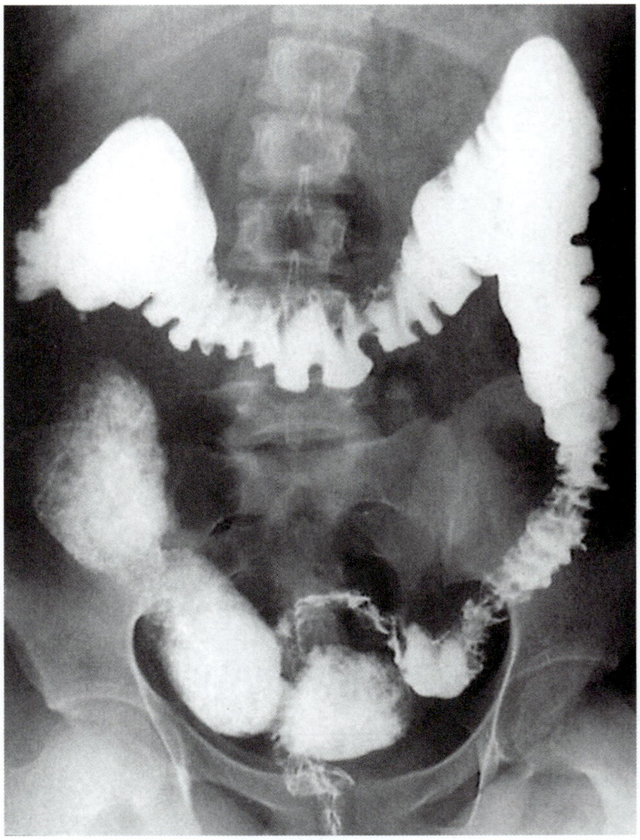

Figure 69.17 Ileocaecal tuberculosis; absent ascending colon and caecum with dilatation of terminal ileum (courtesy of Dr VK Kapoor, Delhi, India).

Hyperplastic tuberculosis

This is caused by the ingestion of *Mycobacterium tuberculosis* by patients with a high resistance to the organism. The infection usually occurs in the ileocaecal region, although solitary and multiple lesions in the lower ileum are also sometimes seen. The infection establishes itself in lymphoid follicles, and the resulting chronic inflammation causes thickening of the intestinal wall and narrowing of the lumen. There is early involvement of the regional lymph nodes, which may caseate. Unlike in Crohn's disease, abscess and fistula formation is rare.

Patients usually present with attacks of abdominal pain and intermittent diarrhoea. There is incomplete ileal obstruction, leading to stasis and bacterial overgrowth. This in turn causes steatorrhoea, anaemia and loss of weight. Patients may present with a mass in the right iliac fossa and vague ill health. The differential diagnosis is that of an appendix mass, lymphoma, carcinoma of the caecum, CD, tuberculosis or actinomycosis.

A barium follow-through or small bowel enema will show a long narrow filling defect in the terminal ileum. CT will also demonstrate the narrowed segment with proximal distension and can also demonstrate the lymphadenopathy. When the diagnosis is certain and the patient has not yet developed obstructive symptoms, treatment with chemotherapy is advised and may be curative. Where obstruction is present, surgery with ileocaecal resection is often required.

Actinomycosis

Abdominal actinomycosis is rare. It is caused by infection with *Actinomyces israelii* and infection usually develops several weeks after an apparently straightforward perforated appendicitis. A local abscess develops and spreads to the retroperitoneal tissues and the adjacent abdominal wall, becoming the seat of multiple indurated discharging sinuses. At first, the discharge from the sinuses is thin, watery and inoffensive, but it may later become thicker and malodorous. Secondary fistulation may occur and the tissues may become extensively indurated and woody. In contrast to tuberculosis, however, mesenteric lymph nodes are not involved and the lumen of the intestine is not narrowed. Haematogenous spread via the portal vein may lead to multiple liver abscesses.

Pus should be sent for bacteriological examination, which will reveal the characteristic sulphur granules. Penicillin or cotrimoxazole treatment should be prolonged and in high dosage.

Human immunodeficiency virus

Human immunodeficiency virus (HIV) infection is associated with a number of proctological problems as discussed in Chapter 73. Intestinal complications are common after the development of AIDS when opportunistic organisms can cause gastroenteritis (see Summary box 69.7). HIV1 may also cause a specific enter-

James Israel, 1848–1926, first found sulphur granules in pus from a discharging sinus in a man's neck. Later, he became a famous Berlin urologist.

opathy. Treatment is directed towards the responsible organism and surgery should be avoided.

Summary box 69.7

Opportunistic intestinal infections in patients with AIDS

- Bacteria
  - Salmonella
  - Shigella
  - Yersinia
  - Campylobacter
  - *Mycobacterium avium intracellulare* (MAI)
- Viral
  - Cytomegalovirus
- Protozoa
  - Cryptosporidium
  - Giardia
- Fungal
  - *Candida albicans*

Clostridium difficile

Clostridium difficile is a toxin producing Gram-positive bacillus that is an increasing worry in many hospitals. Although normally present in around 2 per cent of the population, it seems to proliferate after antibiotic treatment (especially cephalosporins) and can cause antibiotic-associated diarrhoea and pseudomembranous colitis.

Clinically, *C. difficile* infection presents with diarrhoea, abdominal pain and fever. It may progress to pseudomembranous colitis, so called because on visualisation of the bowel, plaques of inflammatory exudate between oedematous mucosa are seen.

Treatment is by metronidazole or vancomycin alongside supportive care. If the colitis does not settle, an emergency subtotal colectomy and ileostomy may be necessary.

TUMOURS OF THE SMALL INTESTINE

Small bowel tumours are rare and in total account for less than 10 per cent of gastrointestinal neoplasia.

Benign

The majority of small bowel neoplasms are benign, comprising adenomas, lipomas, haemangiomas and neurogenic tumours. They are frequently asymptomatic and identified incidentally, but can present with intussusception, small bowel obstruction and bleeding that may cause anaemia or may even be overt. Where these lesions do cause anaemia, the cause can be difficult to diagnose, as CT or small bowel contrast studies do not show them easily. Capsule endoscopy or small bowel endoscopy have been used successfully where the facilities exist. Symptomatic lesions can be treated by small bowel resection and anastomosis.

Peutz–Jeghers syndrome

This is an autosomal dominant disease characterised by melanosis of the mouth and lips and multiple hamartomatous (benign tumour-like malformation resulting from faulty development in an organ) polyps in the small bowel and colon (Figure 69.18).

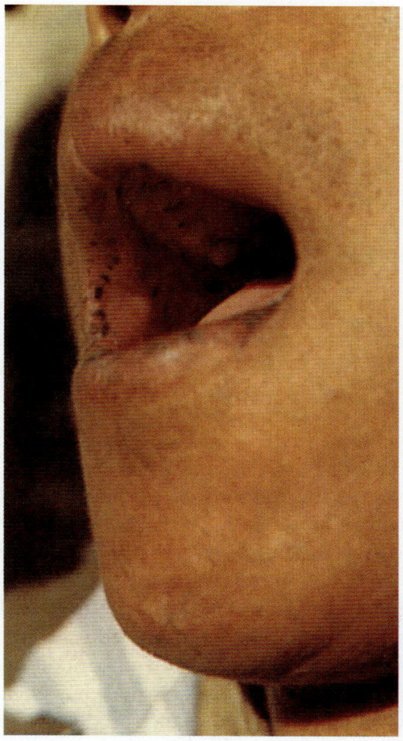

Figure 69.18 Melanin spots on the lips of a patient afflicted with Peutz–Jeghers syndrome (courtesy of Major PCM Manta, Indian Medical Service).

Melanin spots can also occur on the digits and perianal skin. The gene *STK11* on chromosome 19 has been found in a proportion of patients with this condition. Long-term follow up of the original family described by Peutz has shown reduced survival, as a consequence of complications of bowel obstruction and the development of a wide range of cancers. It is logical to perform regular colonic surveillance and encourage female patients to attend breast and cervical screening.

Malignant change in the polyps rarely occurs and, in general the polyps can be left alone. Resection may be indicated for heavy and persistent or recurrent bleeding or intussusception. Polyps may be removed by enterotomy, or, at laparotomy, snared via a colonoscope introduced via an enterotomy. Heavily involved segments of small intestine may occasionally be resected.

Malignant

These are rare and classically present late, most often diagnosed after surgery for small bowel obstruction. Four types will be considered which account for over 99 per cent of small bowel malignancies: adenocarcinoma, carcinoid tumours, lymphomas and mesenchymal tumours (gastrointestinal stromal tumours (GIST)).

Gregor Johann Mendel, 1822–1884, an Austrian monk and naturalist who became Abbot of the Augustinian Monastery at Brunn, Czechoslovakia and discovered the laws of inheritance by studying the edible pea. In 1865, he described 'dominant' and 'recessive' traits in hybrids. His work passed unnoticed for 35 years.

Adenocarcinoma

Small bowel adenocarcinoma is more often found in the jejunum than the ileum and though the aetiology is unknown they are more common in patients with Crohn's disease, coeliac disease, familial adenomatous polyposis (FAP) and Peutz-Jeghers syndrome. They present with anaemia, overt gastrointestinal bleeding, intussusception or obstruction. Prognosis is poor, particularly in patients with Crohn's disease, in whom these tumours often present late because the symptoms may be mistaken for those of Crohn's disease and treated conservatively. When suspected, the advised surgical treatment is a resection of 5 cm of non-involved bowel either side of the lesion and the affected mesentery (Figure 69.19). A right hemicolectomy is likely to be required for tumours of the distal ileum.

Carcinoid tumour

These neuroendocrine tumours occur throughout the gastrointestinal tract, most commonly in the appendix, ileum and rectum in decreasing order of frequency. Appendicular carcinoid tumours are most commonly noted as an incidental finding at appendicectomy. Carcinoid tumours arise from Kulchitsky cells at the base of intestinal crypts (of Lieberkuhn). The primary is usually small, although significant lymph node metastases can occur. In up to one in three cases of small bowel carcinoids, the tumours may be multiple. They may produce dense fibrosis in the surrounding tissues, resulting in distortion and scarring of the bowel and associated mesentery.

The tumours can produce a number of vasoactive peptides, most commonly 5-hydroxytryptamine (serotonin), but also histamine, prostaglandins and kallikrein. When they metastasise to the liver, the carcinoid syndrome can become evident, because the vasoactive substances escape the filtering actions of the liver. The clinical syndrome itself consists of reddish-blue cyanosis, flushing attacks, diarrhoea, borborygmi, asthmatic attacks and, eventually, pulmonary and tricuspid stenosis (Summary box 69.8). Classically, the flushing attacks are induced by alcohol.

Surgical resection is usually sufficient for patients with primary disease, but the incidence of recurrence is significant. The extent of disease can be assessed preoperatively using octreotide scanning, which may detect otherwise clinically apparent primary and secondary tumours. Plasma markers of tumour bulk, such as chromogranin A concentrations, may be useful markers of disease recurrence, as well as of prognostic value.

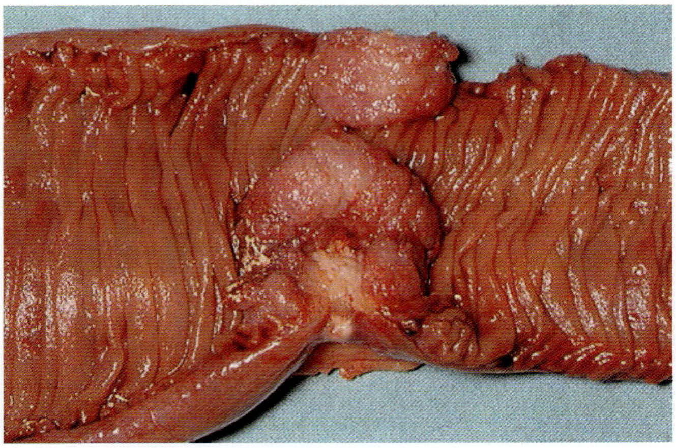

Figure 69.19 Small bowel adenocarcinoma.

Summary box 69.8

Carcinoid syndrome

- Diarrhoea
- Bronchospasm
- Facial/upper chest flushing
- Palpitations
- Tricuspid regurgitation

In patients with metastatic disease, hepatic resection can be carried out. The treatment has been transformed by the use of octreotide (a somatostatin analogue), which reduces both flushing and diarrhoea, and octreotide cover is usually used in patients with a carcinoid syndrome who have surgery to prevent a carcinoid crisis. Carcinoid tumours generally grow more slowly than most metastatic malignancies; the patients may live with the syndrome of metastatic disease for many years. They are not usually sensitive to chemo- or radiotherapy.

Lymphoma

Small bowel lymphoma may be primary, or more commonly secondary to systemic lymphoma. Small bowel lymphoma is also more common in patients with Crohn's disease and immunodeficiency syndromes. The classification of lymphoma is beyond the scope of this chapter, however a number of points are notable for the surgeon. It is rare for Hodgkin's lymphoma to affect the small bowel and most western-type lymphomas are non-Hodgkin's B-cell lymphomas. They present with anaemia, bleeding, perforation, anorexia and weight loss.

T-cell lymphoma develops in patients with coeliac disease. Worsening of the patient's diarrhoea, with pyrexia of unknown origin together with local obstructive symptoms, are the usual features.

Mediterranean lymphoma is found mostly in North Africa and the Middle East and is often widespread at diagnosis. Burkitt's lymphoma can aggressively affect the ileocaecal region, particularly in children. The mainstay of treatment for these conditions is chemotherapy, however surgery may be required for obstruction, perforation or bleeding.

Gastrointestinal stromal tumours

These are mesenchymal tumours and the distinction between benign or malignant types is difficult even on histological examination. Increased size and high levels of c-kit (CD117) staining are associated with malignant potential. GIST tumours are found most commonly in the stomach, but can be found in other parts of the gut. They occur most commonly in the 50- to 70-year age group. Although the cause is unknown, patients with neurofibromatosis have an increased risk of developing these types of tumour.

Patients may be asymptomatic. Symptoms include lethargy, pain, nausea, haematemesis or melaena. Surgery is the most effective way of removing GISTs, as they are radioresistant. Glivec (imatinib) is a tyrosine kinase inhibitor that has been shown to be effective in advanced cases and may also have an adjuvant role.

Thomas Hodgkin, 1798–1866, Lecturer in Morbid Anatomy and Orator of the Museum, Guy's Hospital, London, described lymphadenoma in 1832.

TUMOURS OF THE LARGE INTESTINE

Benign

The term 'polyp' is a clinical description of any protrusion of the mucosa. It encompasses a variety of histologically different tumours shown in Table 69.2. Polyps can occur singly, synchronously in small numbers or as part of a polyposis syndrome. It is important to be sure of the histological diagnosis because colonic adenomas have significant malignant potential.

Adenomatous polyps

Adenomatous polyps vary from a tubular adenoma (Figure 69.20), rather like a berry on a stalk, to the villous adenoma, a flat spreading lesion. Solitary adenomas are usually found during the investigation of colonic symptoms and may be the cause of rectal bleeding. Villous tumours can cause diarrhoea, mucous discharge and, occasionally, hypokalaemia and hypoalbuminaemia. The risk of malignancy developing in an adenoma increases with their size; there is a 10 per cent risk of cancer in a 1-cm diameter tubular adenoma, whereas with villous adenomas over 2 cm in diameter, there may be a 15 per cent chance of carcinoma. Almost one-third of large (>3 cm) colonic adenomas will have an area of invasive malignancy within them at the time of resection. Adenomas larger than 5 mm in diameter are usually excised because of their malignant potential. Colonoscopic snare polypectomy is usually possible for colonic polyps, but larger sessile polyps can require endoscopic mucosal resection (EMR) after saline infiltration. Larger rectal adenomas may require transanal resection or, where the adenoma is too high for safe conventional access, transanal endoscopic microsurgery (TEMS). Massive and extensive villous lesions of the rectum may require proctectomy when the patient is sufficiently fit, or argon beam ablation when the patient is frail but symptomatic.

Table 69.2 Classification of intestinal polyps.

Classification		
Inflammatory	Inflammatory polyps (pseudopolyps in ulcerative colitis)	
Metaplastic	Metaplastic or hyperplastic polyps	
Harmartomatous	Peutz–Jeghers polyp	
	Juvenile polyp	
Neoplastic	Adenoma	Tubular
		Tubulovillous
		Villous
	Adenocarcinoma	
	Carcinoid tumour	

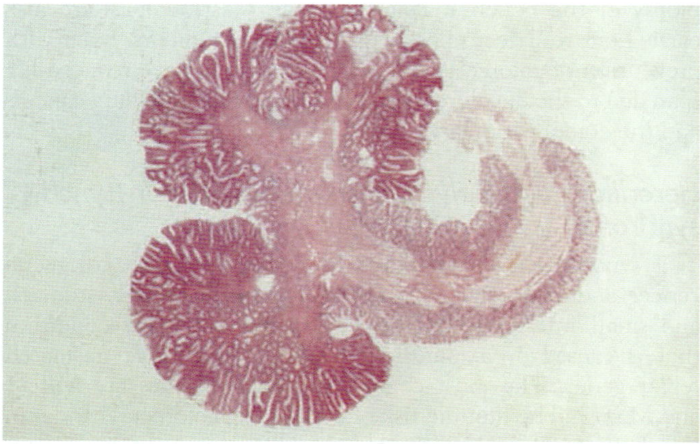

Figure 69.20 Pedunculated adenomatous polyp of the large intestine, longitudinal section (courtesy of Dr P Millard, John Radcliffe Hospital, Oxford, UK).

Familial adenomatous polyposis

FAP is defined clinically by the presence of more than 100 colorectal adenomas, but also characterised by duodenal adenomas and multiple extraintestinal manifestations (Summary box 69.9). Over 80 per cent of cases come from patients with a positive family history. The remainder arise as a result of new mutations in the adenomatous polyposis coli (*APC*) gene. This has been identified on the short arm of chromosome 5. FAP is inherited as an autosomal dominant condition and is consequently equally likely in men and women. Although FAP is less common than hereditary non-polyposis colon cancer (HNPCC), and only accounts for 1 per cent or less of all colon cancer, the risk of colorectal cancer is 100 per cent in patients with FAP. FAP can also be associated with benign mesodermal tumours such as desmoid tumours and osteomas. Epidermoid cysts can also occur (Gardner's syndrome); desmoid tumours in the abdomen spread locally to involve the intestinal mesentery and, although non-metastasising, they can become unresectable. Up to 50 per cent of patients with FAP have congenital hypertrophy of the retinal pigment epithelium (CHRPE), which can be used to screen affected families if genetic testing is unavailable.

Summary box 69.9

Extracolonic manifestations of familial adenomatous polyposis

- Endodermal derivatives
  - Adenomas and carcinomas of the duodenum, stomach, small intestine, thyroid and biliary tree
  - Fundic gland polyps
  - Hepatoblastoma
- Ectodermal derivatives
  - Epidermoid cysts
  - Pilomatrixoma
  - Congenital hypertrophy of the retinal pigment epithelium (CHRPE)
  - Brain tumours
- Mesodermal derivatives
  - Desmoid tumours
  - Osteomas
  - Dental problems

Eldon John Gardner, 1909–1989, geneticist, The University of Utah, Salt Lake City, UT, USA described this syndrome in 1950.

Clinical features

Polyps are usually visible on sigmoidoscopy by the age of 15 years and will almost always be visible by the age of 30 years. Carcinoma of the large bowel occurs 10–20 years after the onset of the polyposis. One or more cancers will already be present in two-thirds of those patients presenting with symptoms at the time of diagnosis (see Summary box 69.10).

> **Summary box 69.10**
>
> **Features of familial adenomatous polyposis**
>
> - Autosomal dominant inherited disease due to mutation of the *APC* gene
> - More than 100 colonic adenomas are diagnostic
> - Prophylactic surgery is indicated to prevent colorectal cancer
> - Polyps and malignant tumours can develop in the duodenum and small bowel

Symptomatic patients

These are either patients in whom a new mutation has occurred or those from an affected family who have not been screened. They may have loose stools, lower abdominal pain, weight loss, diarrhoea and the passage of blood and mucus. Colonoscopy is performed with biopsies to establish the number and histological type of polyps. If over 100 adenomas (Figure 69.21) are present, the diagnosis can be made confidently. If there are no adenomas by the age of 30 years, FAP is unlikely. If the diagnosis is made during adolescence, operation is usually deferred to the age of 17 or 18 years unless symptoms develop.

Screening policy

- At-risk family members are offered genetic testing in their early teens.
- At-risk members of the family should be examined at the age of 10–12 years, repeated every year.
- Most of those who are going to get polyps will have them at 20 years, and these require operation.
- If there are no polyps at 20 years, continue with five-yearly examination until age 50 years; if there are still no polyps, there is probably no inherited gene. Carcinomatous change may exceptionally occur before the age of 20 years. Examination of blood relatives, including cousins, nephews and nieces, is essential, and a family tree should be constructed and a register of affected families maintained. Referral to a medical geneticist is essential.

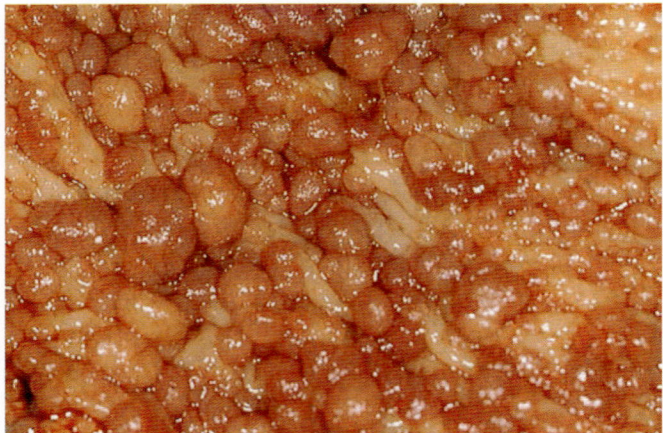

Figure 69.21 Familial adenomatous polyposis.

Treatment

The aim of surgery is to prevent the development of colorectal cancer. The surgical options are:

- colectomy with ileorectal anastomosis (IRA);
- restorative proctocolectomy (RPC) with an ileal pouch-anal anastomosis, the anastomosis may be defunctioned with a loop ileostomy;
- total proctectomy and end ileostomy (normally reserved for patients with a low rectal cancer).

The patient is almost always young and likely to prefer to avoid a permanent stoma and so the choice is normally between the first two options. The advantage of an IRA is that it avoids the temporary stoma frequently required for an RPC and avoids the potential compromise to sexual function that accompanies proctectomy. It also has a lower morbidity and mortality. However, the rectum is left and requires regular surveillance, as there is a risk of adenomas and carcinomas in the residual large bowel. Even with optimal surveillance of the rectal remnant, up to 10 per cent will develop invasive malignancy within a 30-year follow-up period. Restorative proctocolectomy has the advantage of removing the whole colon and rectum (although a small cuff of rectal mucosa may be left behind with a stapled anastomosis). However, there is a pouch failure rate of about 10 per cent. In addition, and particularly where a stapled anastomosis has been created, there remains a very small but definite incidence of cancer developing in the small strip of rectal mucosa between the pouch and the dentate line. This is why some colorectal surgeons advocate complete mucosectomy of the residual rectal cuff and a transanal pouch anal anastomosis, although it is acknowledged that this results in worse function.

Postoperative surveillance

Because of the risk of further tumour formation, follow up is important and takes the form of rectal/pouch surveillance, with biopsy of the pouch-anal anastomosis. Gastroscopies are also carried out to detect upper gastrointestinal tumours. Even with prevention of colorectal cancer, FAP patients have reduced life span due to the development of duodenal and ampullary cancers and the complications of desmoid tumours.

Hereditary non-polyposis colorectal cancer (Lynch syndrome)

This syndrome is characterised by increased risk of colorectal cancer and also cancers of the endometrium, ovary, stomach and small intestines. It is an autosomal dominant condition that is caused by a mutation in one of the DNA mismatch repair genes. The most commonly affected genes are *MLH1* and *MSH2*. The lifetime risk of developing colorectal cancer in Lynch syndrome is 80 per cent, and the mean age of diagnosis is 45 years. Most cancers develop in the proximal colon. Females with HNPCC have a 30–50 per cent lifetime risk of developing endometrial cancer.

Diagnosis

HNPCC can be diagnosed by genetic testing or the Amsterdam II criteria:

- three or more family members with an HNPCC-related cancer (colorectal, endometrial, small bowel, ureter, renal pelvis), one of whom is a first-degree relative of the other two;
- two successive affected generations;
- at least one colorectal cancer diagnosed before the age of 50 years;
- FAP excluded;
- tumours verified by pathological examination.

Patients with HNPCC are subjected to regular (every one to two years) colonoscopic surveillance.

Malignant

Epidemiology

In the UK, colorectal cancer is the second most common cause of cancer death accounting for 16 000 deaths in 2004. About 35 000 patients are diagnosed with colorectal cancer every year in the UK, of which around one-third are in the rectum and two-thirds in the colon. The burden of disease is similar in men and women. Colorectal cancer seems to occur less frequently in the developing world than in industrialised countries.

Aetiology

The accepted model of colorectal cancer development is that it arises from adenomatous polyps after a sequence of genetic mutations influenced by environmental factors. This adenoma–carcinoma sequence is based on strong observational evidence outlined in Summary box 69.11.

Summary box 69.11

Evidence for adenoma–carcinoma sequence

- The prevalence of adenomas and carcinomas is very similar – carcinoma patients are about five years older
- The distribution of adenomas in the colon is the same as that of cancers (70 per cent left sided)
- When small cancers are studied, they almost always have adjacent adenomatous tissue
- Adenomas are found in a third of specimens resected for colorectal cancer
- Sporadic adenomas are identical to the adenomas of familial adenomatous polyposis, which is associated with a 100 per cent chance of colorectal adenocarcinoma unless treated
- Larger adenomas are more likely to be dysplastic and to have higher grades of dysplasia than small adenomas.
- Incidence of colorectal cancer falls within a screening programme that involves colonoscopy and polypectomy

The molecular genetics of sporadic colorectal cancer have been extensively studied. Mutations of the *APC* gene occur in two-thirds of colonic adenomas and carcinomas and are thought to develop early in the carcinogenesis pathway. K-ras mutations result in activation of cell signalling pathways and are more common in larger lesions. This suggests that that they are later events in the mutagenesis pathway. The *p53* gene is frequently mutated in carcinomas, but not in adenomas and is therefore thought to mark the development of invasion. The adenoma–carcinoma sequence is not, however, one of a simple stepwise progression of mutations, but a complicated array of multiple genetic alterations, ultimately resulting in an invasive tumour. While no single mutation is common to all cases of colorectal cancer, knowledge of certain mutations can be used to assess prognosis and, increasingly to direct adjuvant therapy. For example, the K-ras mutation is thought to be associated with an especially poor prognosis.

There has been much interest in the linkage between diet and colon cancer. Worldwide, the prevalence of colorectal cancer is closely associated with intake of red meat. There is ample evidence to suggest effects of red meat components (haem and N-nitroso compounds) on the DNA in the colorectal mucosa. The protective effect of dietary fibre is also suggested by epidemiological studies. The hypothesis is that increased roughage is associated with reduced transit times, and this in turn reduces the exposure of the mucosa to dietary carcinogens. Increased risk for colorectal cancer has also been associated with dietary animal fat, smoking and alcohol. Longstanding ulcerative colitis and Crohn's colitis is associated with increased rates of colorectal cancer as discussed previously. It has been suggested that cholecystectomy may be associated with a slight increase in the risk of right-sided colon cancer, possibly as a consequence of increased bile acid exposure. There is also an increased risk of colorectal cancer after ureterosigmoidostomy, although this procedure is now rarely performed.

Pathology

Macroscopically, the tumour may take one of four forms (Figure 69.22). The annular variety tends to give rise to obstructive symptoms, whereas the others will present more commonly with

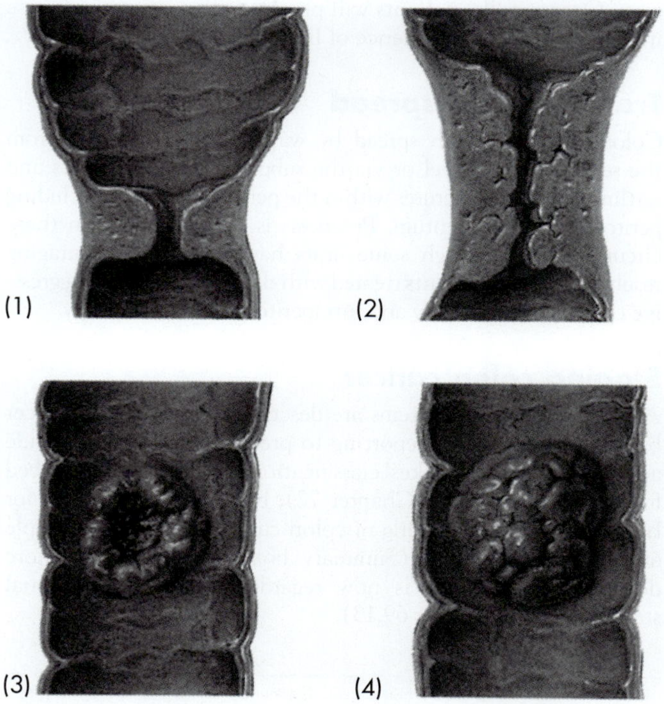

Figure 69.22 The four common macroscopic varieties of carcinoma of the colon. (1) Annular; (2) tubular; (3) ulcer; (4) cauliflower.

bleeding. Microscopically, the neoplasm is an adenocarcinoma originating in the colonic epithelium.

SPREAD OF CARCINOMA OF THE COLON

Direct spread

Colonic cancer can spread locally or via the lymphatics, bloodstream or transcoelomically around the peritoneum. Direct spread can be longitudinal, transverse or radial. Radial spread to adjacent organs has the greatest impact on surgical resectability, as an adequate oncologic resection can still be achieved, despite longitudinal spread, by extension of proximal and distal margins. Radial spread may be retroperitoneal into the ureter, duodenum and posterior abdominal wall muscles, or intraperitoneal into the small intestine, stomach, pelvic organs or the anterior abdominal wall.

Lymphatic spread

In general, involvement of the lymph nodes by the tumour progresses in a gradual manner from those closest to the bowel along the course of the lymphatic vessels to those placed centrally. However, this orderly process does not always occur.

Haematogenous spread

The liver accounts for the majority of distant metastases presumably via the portal vein. Around a third of patients will have liver metastases at the time of diagnosis and 50 per cent will develop liver metastases at some point accounting for the majority of deaths. The lung is the next most common site: metastases to ovary, brain, kidney, brain and bone are less common. Occasionally, patients will present with metastatic disease in the lungs without evidence of liver metastases.

Transcoelomic spread

Colorectal cancer can spread by way of cells dislodging from the serosa of the bowel or via the subperitoneal lymphatics and settling on other structures within the peritoneal cavity, including peritoneum and omentum. Prognosis is typically grave in these circumstances although some units have reported encouraging results in selected patients treated with the combination of aggressive cytoreductive surgery and intraperitoneal chemotherapy.

Staging colon cancer

A variety of staging systems are described for colorectal cancer based on pathological reporting to predict prognosis and guide adjuvant treatment. Dukes' classification was originally described for rectal tumours (see Chapter 72), but has been adopted for histopathological reporting of colon cancer as well. It is simple and widely recognised (Summary box 69.12), but the more detailed TNM system is now regarded as the international standard (Summary box 69.13).

Summary box 69.12

Dukes' staging for colorectal cancer

- A, Invasion of but not breaching the muscularis propria
- B, Breaching the muscularis propria but not involving lymph nodes
- C, Lymph nodes involved

Dukes himself never described a stage D, but this is often used to describe metastatic disease

Summary box 69.13

TNM classification for colonic cancer

- T, Tumour stage
  - T1, Into submucosa
  - T2, Into muscularis propria
  - T3, Into pericolic fat or sub-serosa but not breaching serosa
  - T4, Breaches serosa or directly involving another organ
- N, Nodal stage
  - N0, No nodes involved
  - N1, 1–3 nodes involved
  - N2, Four or more nodes involved
- M, Metastases
  - M0, No metastases
  - M1, Metastases

Clinical features

Carcinoma of the colon typically occurs in patients over 50 years of age and is most common in the eighth decade of life. Colorectal cancer is not rare in early adult life, however. Twenty per cent of cases present as an emergency with intestinal obstruction or peritonitis. An emergency presentation of colorectal cancer is, even when matched for disease stage, associated with a considerably worse prognosis. A careful family history should be taken. Those with first-degree relatives who have developed colorectal cancer at the age of 45 years or below are at higher risk and may be part of one of the colorectal cancer familial syndromes. Tumours of the left side of the colon which are far more common (Figure 69.23) usually present with a change in bowel habit or rectal bleeding, while more proximal lesions typically present later with iron deficiency anaemia or a mass. Patients may present for the first time with metastatic disease. Lesions of the flexures may present with vague upper abdominal symptoms for many months before other, more specific symptoms suggestive of colonic disease appear.

Rupert B Turnbull, 1913–1981, Irish surgeon, Cleveland Clinic, Ohio, reported the presence of cancer cells in the portal vein of patients undergoing resection for colon cancer. He then described in his Moynihan lecture a 'no touch' isolation technique to reduce the manipulation of colonic tumours at surgery.

St Mark's Hospital, Harrow, UK, is recognised as a national and international referral centre for intestinal and colorectal disorders. It was founded in a small room in No 11 Aldersgate Street. Established in 1854 on City Road in Hackney as St Mark's Hospital for Fistula and other Diseases of the Rectum. It was so named as it was opened on St Mark's day, April 25. In 1994, it moved to its present site in Harrow.

Cuthbert Esquire Dukes, 1890–1977, pathologist, St Mark's Hospital, London, UK. The original Dukes' classification in 1932 gave three stages, A–C.

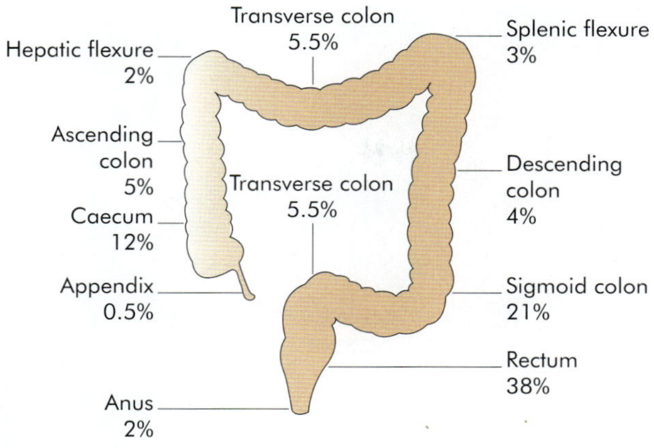

Figure 69.23 Distribution of colorectal cancer by site.

Investigation of colon cancer

Screening

Colon cancer is highly suited to screening as prognosis is better for early stage disease and polypectomy allows the prevention of cancer development. In the UK, a screening programme has been introduced based on faecal occult blood testing of people aged 60–69 years followed by colonoscopy in those who test positive. A guaiac-based test is used which detects the peroxidase-like activity of faecal haematin. Studies have suggested a 15–20 per cent reduction in colorectal cancer mortality in the screened population. Flexible sigmoidoscopy can also be used as the initial screening tool with a similar reduction in colorectal cancer mortality.

Endoscopy

The 60-cm, fibreoptic, flexible sigmoidoscope is increasingly being used in one-stop rectal bleeding clinics. The patient is prepared with an enema and sedation is not usually necessary. It is usually possible to assess the bowel up to the splenic flexure, which will detect up to 70 per cent of cancers and almost all that cause rectal bleeding. Colonoscopy is the investigation of choice if colorectal cancer is suspected, provided the patient is fit enough to undergo the required mechanical bowel preparation (Figure 69.24). It has the advantage of not only picking up a primary cancer, but also having the ability to detect synchronous polyps or even multiple carcinomas, which occur in 3–5 per cent of cases. Ideally, every case should be proven histologically by biopsy before surgery. Full mechanical bowel preparation is necessary, as well as intravenous sedation. There is a small risk of perforation (1:1000) and also even experienced endoscopists may fail to see the caecum in 10 per cent of cases.

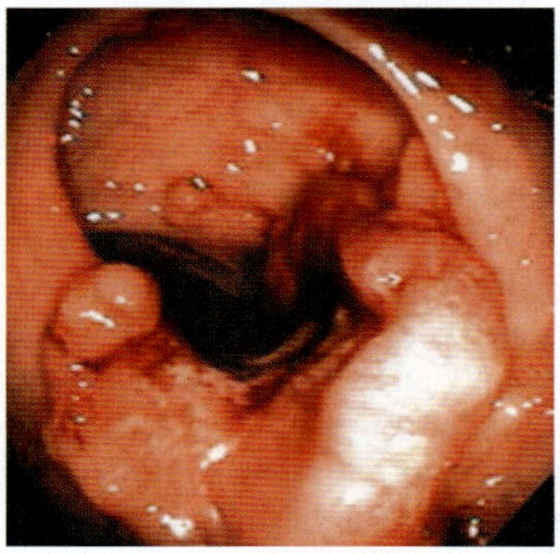

Figure 69.24 A cancer seen at colonoscopy.

Radiology

Double-contrast barium enema shows a cancer of the colon as a constant irregular filling defect often described as looking like an apple core (Figure 69.25). False positives occur in 1–2 per cent of cases and false negatives in 7–9 per cent of cases. CT is used as a diagnostic tool in patients with palpable abdominal masses. Use of spiral CT of the chest and abdomen is now standard to stage colonic cancer by assessing T stage and detecting metastases although chest x-ray and liver ultrasound are an alternative if CT is not readily available. The introduction of CT virtual colonoscopy, which is effective in picking up polyps down to 6 mm (Figure 69.26) provides another diagnostic modality and has largely replaced barium enema in many centres. It has the advantage of being less invasive than colonoscopy, but if a biopsy is required, an endoscopy will still be needed.

Surgical treatment

Preoperative preparation

There is good evidence that there is no benefit for mechanical bowel preparation in colonic cancer surgery and it may in fact be associated with an increased rate of wound infection. Rectal cancer seems to be different and recent trials suggest that mechanical bowel preparation is probably still appropriate. Thromboembolism is common in general surgical patients and the risk is increased by malignant disease, so antiembolic stockings should be fitted and the patient started on prophylactic subcutaneous low molecular weight heparin. If available, manual compression boots can be used perioperatively. Intravenous prophylactic antibiotics are given at the start of surgery, as there is good evidence that these reduce the risk of

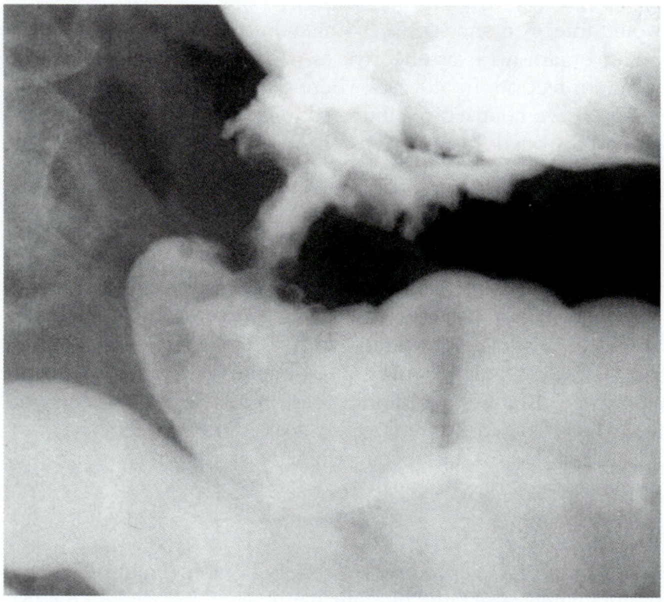

Figure 69.25 Barium enema showing a carcinoma of the sigmoid colon. It may have an 'apple core' appearance, i.e. a short, irregular stenosis with sharp shoulders at each end.

(a)

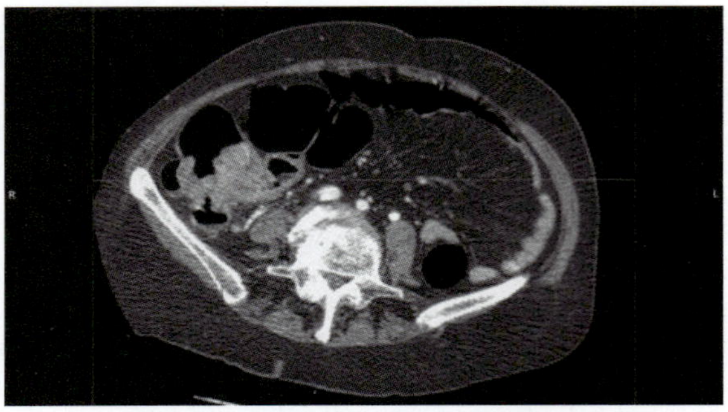

(b)

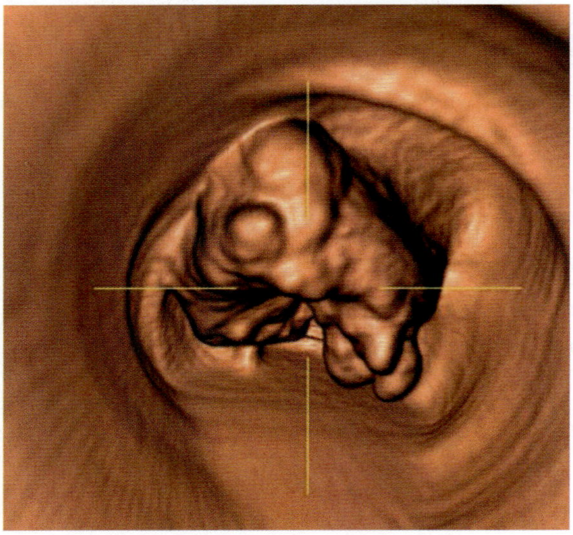

Figure 69.26 Virtual colonoscopy of the right colon. (a) Computed tomography scan of the abdomen showing a caecal tumour. (b) Formatted 'virtual' image of the same lesion as in (a) (courtesy of Dr A Slater, John Radcliffe Hospital, Oxford, UK).

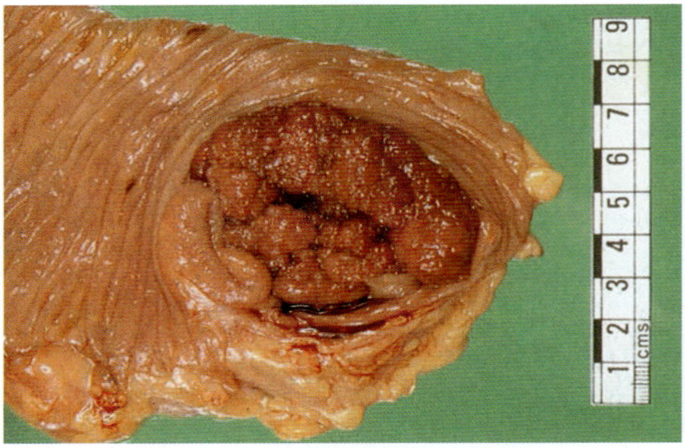

Figure 69.27 Large villous tumour of the caecum with malignant change.

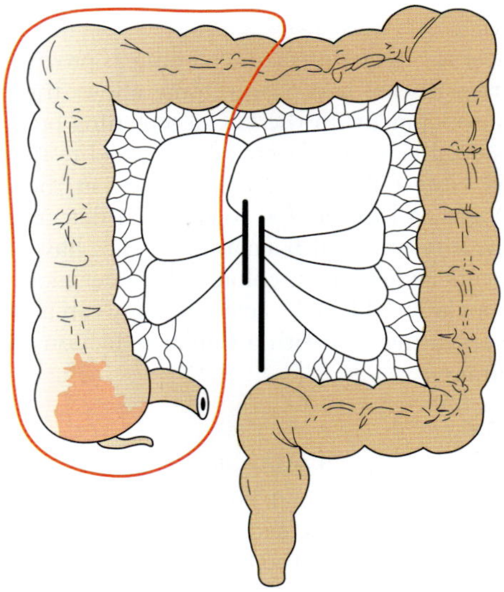

Figure 69.28 Schematic showing right hemicolectomy.

would infection and sepsis. A single dose of antibiotics covering bowel organisms is as effective as multiple doses in preventing wound infection. In all cases where a stoma seems likely, careful preoperative counselling and marking of an appropriate site by an enterostomal therapist is essential.

Operations

The operations described are designed to remove the primary tumour and its draining locoregional lymph nodes. After spiral CT, it is unusual to find unsuspected metastases at laparotomy (or laparoscopy), but the presence of peritoneal metastases may predicate a palliative strategy with a segmental resection and less aggressive lymphadenectomy. The use of stapling and hand-suturing techniques for colonic anastomosis has been compared, and there is little difference in leak rate between the two. Recurrent disease does occur typically at the anastomosis and re-resection can be successful.

Right hemicolectomy

Carcinoma of the caecum or ascending colon (Figure 69.27) is treated when resectable by right hemicolectomy (Figure 69.28). At open surgery, the peritoneum lateral to the ascending colon is incised, and the incision is continued around the hepatic flexure. The right colon is elevated, with the leaf of peritoneum containing its vessels and lymph nodes, from the posterior abdominal wall, taking care not to injure the ureter, gonadal vessels or the duodenum. The ileocolic artery is ligated close to its origin off the superior mesenteric artery ('high-tie') and divided. Where the right colic artery has a separate origin from the superior mesenteric artery (around 10 per cent of patients), this is separately ligated. The leaf of raised peritoneum attached to the caecum, ascending colon and hepatic flexure is divided after ligation of the mesentery of the last 20 cm of ileum and the mesocolon as far as the proximal third of the transverse colon. The greater omentum is divided up to the point of intended division of the transverse colon. When it is clear that there is an adequate blood supply at the resection margins, the right colon is resected, and an anastomosis is fashioned between the ileum and the transverse colon using the surgeon's preferred technique. If the tumour is at the hepatic flexure, the resection must be extended further along the transverse colon and will involve dividing the right branch of the middle colic artery.

Extended right hemicolectomy

Carcinomas of the transverse colon and splenic flexure are most commonly treated by an extended right hemicolectomy. The extent of the resection is from right colon to descending colon. The mobilisation is as for a right hemicolectomy, but dissection continues to take down the splenic flexure and the whole transverse mesocolon is ligated. Some surgeons will perform a left hemicolectomy for a splenic flexure cancer.

Left hemicolectomy

This is the operation of choice for descending colon and sigmoid cancers (Figure 69.29). The left half of the colon is mobilised completely along the 'white line' that marks the lateral attachment of the mesocolon. As the sigmoid mesentery is mobilised, the left ureter and gonadals must be identified and protected. The splenic flexure must be mobilised by extending the dissection from below and from the transverse colon side by entering the lesser sac. The inferior mesenteric artery below its left colic branch, together with the related paracolic lymph nodes, are included in the resection by ligating the inferior mesenteric artery close to its origin – 'high-tie'. For full mobility, the inferior mesenteric vein is also ligated and divided at the lower border of the pancreas. The bowel and mesentery can now be resected to allow a tension-free anastomosis, which can be stapled with an end–end stapling device or hand-sewn. Where there are technical difficulties or concern about the anastomosis, a temporary diverting stoma may be fashioned upstream, usually by formation of a loop ileostomy.

Laparoscopic surgery

Laparoscopic surgery for colonic cancer has now been shown to have equivalent overall and cancer-related outcomes to open surgery. Lymph node harvests are equivalent to open surgery and initial concerns about reports of port site recurrence have been dispelled as the world experience has grown. In the UK, the National Institute for Health and Clinical Excellence (NICE) has endorsed laparoscopic colorectal surgery and has stated it should be offered to suitable patients. Operative times are longer but wound infection rates, blood loss and postoperative pain scores are lower than for open surgery. It is hoped that these factors will lead to shorter hospital stay and faster return to full activity, but this has yet to be firmly demonstrated. The costs of laparoscopic surgery are generally higher and this may be particularly relevant where funds are limited.

It is not possible to palpate lesions, so if laparoscopic surgery is planned, it is ideal to tattoo the lesion. Different surgeons advocate different port positions. The laparoscopic operation has particular advantages if performed in a medial to lateral manner – that is, starting the dissection by controlling and dividing the major vascular pedicles and only taking the lateral peritoneal reflection once the mesocolon is completely free. Specimen retrieval and bowel anastomosis can then be performed via small incisions. Training in laparoscopic surgery is important, as there is a steep learning curve and in the UK is currently part of a national training programme.

Emergency surgery

In the UK, 20 per cent of patients with colonic cancer will present as an emergency, the majority with obstruction, but occasionally with haemorrhage or perforation. If the lesion is right sided, it is usually possible to perform a right hemicolectomy and anastomosis in the usual manner; this can be facilitated by decompressing the bowel at the start of the operation. If there has been perforation with substantial contamination or if the patient is unstable, it may be advisable to bring out an ileo/colostomy rather than anastomosing bowel in these circumstances. For a left-sided lesion, the decision-making process is similar to that in diverticular disease between a Hartmann's procedure and resection and anastomosis. Where facilities are present, an obstructing left-sided lesion can be treated with an expanding metal stent (Figure 69.30). This has the great advantage of converting an emergency operation with a high chance of a stoma to a situation which can be managed semi-electively with a resection and anastomosis. It is currently unclear whether

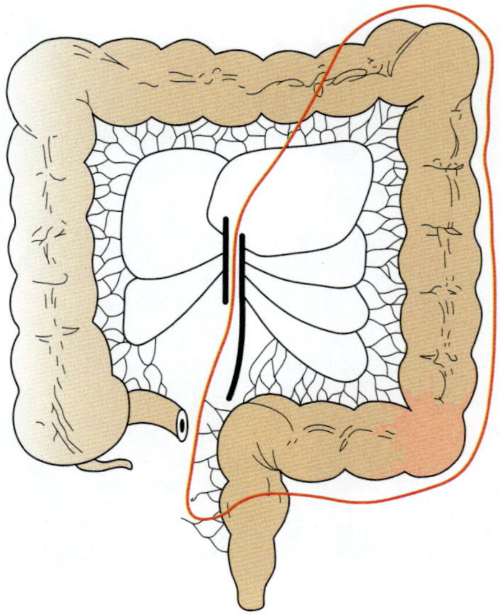

Figure 69.29 Schematic showing left hemicolectomy.

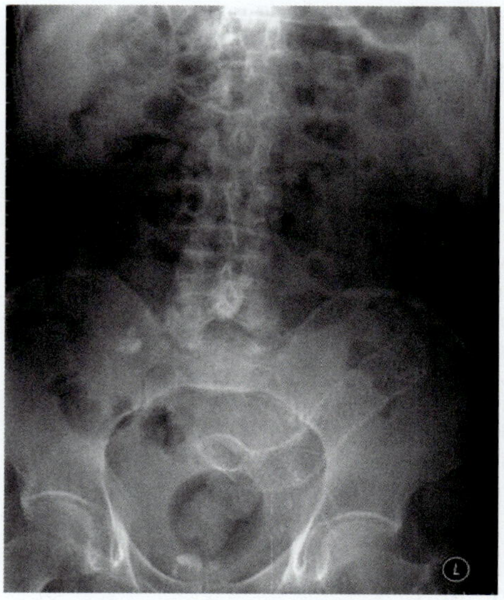

Figure 69.30 Abdominal radiograph demonstrating a colonic stent in position (courtesy of Dr D Kasir, Hope Hospital, Salford, UK).

Henri Albert Antoine Hartmann, 1860–1952, Professor of Clinical Surgery in the Faculty of Medicine, University of Paris, France.

the overall morbidity and mortality of staged management of an obstructing colorectal cancer by initial stenting and later surgery are lower than primary emergency surgery. Results from two European trials have so far failed to demonstrate a benefit and the patients in whom stenting proved impossible seemed to have a higher morbidity and mortality, possibly because of the inherent delay in undertaking definitive surgical treatment. A larger multicentre trial is currently in progress.

Postoperative care

After colonic surgery, patients should be closely monitored, as there is a small incidence of postoperative bleeding. Antithrombosis measures prophylaxis against venous thromboembolism should be continued as discussed above under Preoperative preparation. There is no advantage to placing intra-abdominal drains after colonic surgery. Wound infections are sadly common after colonic surgery and may well be more frequent than the quoted 10 per cent. The most feared postoperative complication of anastomotic breakdown or leak occurs in 4–8 per cent of ileocolic or colocolic anastomoses. It should be kept in mind for any patient not progressing as expected or who is developing temperatures and worsening abdominal pain. Early investigation with contrast-enhanced CT scan is appropriate. In the presence of sepsis or peritonitis, early return to theatre and taking down the leaking anastomosis with the formation of stomas is advised.

Traditional practices after bowel surgery were prolonged nasogastric drainage and very cautious introduction of oral fluid and then diet. There is increasing interest after bowel surgery in enhanced recovery programmes (ERPs) which have been shown to reduce length of hospital stay from the traditional 10–14 days, to as little as 2–3 days by modulating the surgical stress response and reducing postoperative ileus. It is important to appreciate that these programmes require multiple interventions to be instituted and considerable time, effort and education from the surgical, anaesthetic and ward teams (Summary box 69.14).

Summary box 69.14

Key elements of an enhanced recovery programme

- Pre-admission counselling
- Avoidance of mechanical bowel preparation
- Preoperative carbohydrate loading
- Avoidance of preoperative dehydration
- No nasogastric tubes
- Short, transverse incisions (or laparoscopic procedure)
- Short-acting anaesthetic drugs
- Avoidance of perioperative fluid/salt overload
- Thoracic epidurals
- Avoidance of opiate analgesia
- Maintenance of perioperative temperature
- Prevention of postoperative nausea and vomiting
- Early mobilisation
- Early introduction of oral fluids/diets/supplements
- Early removal of urinary catheters
- Continual audit of outcomes

Adjuvant therapy

This is discussed in more detail in Chapter 72 under rectal cancer. In colonic cancer, there is no current role for preoperative chemotherapy although a trial is underway. There is evidence of improved outcome after surgery with 5-fluorouracil (5-FU)-based chemotherapy in node-positive disease (Dukes' C/N1,2).

Metastatic disease

Hepatic metastases can be resected and series have demonstrated five-year survival of over 30 per cent in resectable disease. Liver surgeons are increasingly aggressive in treatment and the only absolute limitation on what can be resected is in terms of leaving enough functional liver behind, although this clearly has to be moderated in terms of patient factors. It is important not to biopsy potentially resectable hepatic metastases as this may cause tumour dissemination. Imaging will usually correctly identify colorectal metastases and assess patients' suitability for liver resection (Figure 69.31). The role of chemotherapy and the timing of colonic and hepatic surgery in synchronous metastases is still a matter of debate and such cases should be carefully discussed by a multidisciplinary team. Isolated lung metastases may also in occasional cases be suitable for resection, but generally they are accompanied by metastases elsewhere. In patients with widespread disease, palliative chemotherapy can be offered alongside symptomatic treatment and support by a palliative care team.

Prognosis

Overall five-year survival for colorectal cancer is approximately 50 per cent. The most important determinant of prognosis is tumour stage and, in particular, lymph node status. Patients with disease confined to the bowel wall (Dukes' stage A) will

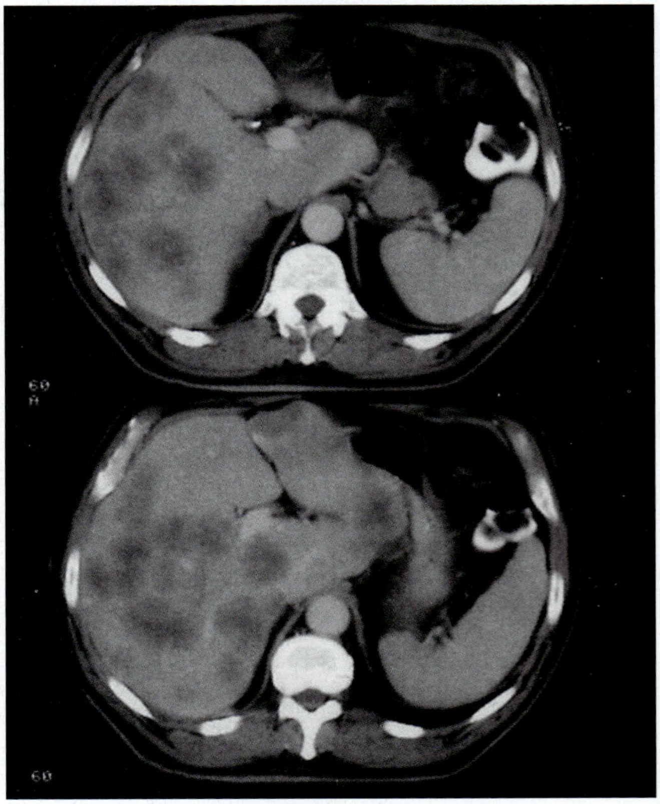

Figure 69.31 Computed tomography scan of the liver showing multiple metastases from carcinoma of the colon.

usually be cured by surgical resection alone and 90 per cent of such patients will have disease-free survival at five years. Spread beyond the bowel wall reduces five-year survival to approximately 60–70 per cent. Patients with lymph node metastases have a five-year survival of 30 per cent, while fewer than 10 per cent of patients presenting with metastatic disease at outset will be alive five years later.

Colorectal cancer follow up

Since the advent of safe liver resection for metastases, the outcome benefit of follow up has become evident and has been demonstrated by meta-analysis. Follow up aims to identify synchronous bowel tumours that were not picked up at original diagnosis due to emergency presentation or incomplete assessment (3 per cent of patients will have a second bowel cancer at diagnosis). Similarly, 3 per cent of patients will develop a metachronous (at a different time) colonic cancer and surveillance colonoscopy is designed to diagnose these. Up to a half of patients with colorectal cancer will have liver metastases at some point and regular imaging of the liver (ultrasound and CT scan) and measurement of carcinoembryonic antigen (CEA) is designed to diagnose this early, in order to allow the possibility of curative metastectomy. Trials of the optimum follow-up pathway are ongoing.

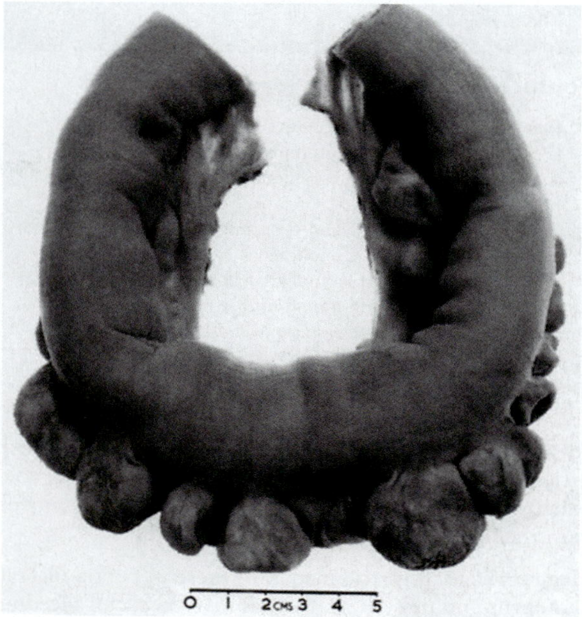

Figure 69.32 Jejunal diverticula.

INTESTINAL DIVERTICULA

Diverticula (hollow out-pouchings) are a common structural abnormality that can occur from the oesophagus to the rectosigmoid junction (but not usually in the rectum). They can be classified as:

- **Congenital**. All three coats of the bowel are present in the wall of the diverticulum, e.g. Meckel's diverticulum.
- **Acquired**. There is no muscularis layer present in the diverticulum, e.g. sigmoid diverticula.

Jejunal diverticula

These arise from the mesenteric side of the bowel as a result of mucosal herniation at the point of entry of the blood vessels. They can vary in size and are often multiple. They are most often asymptomatic and an incidental finding at surgery or on radiological imaging (Figure 69.32); however, they can result in malabsorption, as a result of bacterial stasis, or present as an acute abdominal emergency if they become inflamed or perforate. Bleeding from a jejunal diverticulum is a rare complication. Elective resection of an affected small bowel segment that is causing malabsorption can be effective. If perforated jejunal diverticulitis is found at emergency laparotomy, a small bowel resection should be performed and a decision made between anastomosis and stoma formation. This will depend on degree of contamination, physiological stability and local resource for managing a patient with a high output jejunostomy. Extensive jejunal diverticulosis can be very difficult to treat. In severe cases, much of the proximal small intestine may be involved, effectively precluding resection. In addition, limited resection, while feasible, may fail to deal adequately with recurrent attacks of inflammation or bleeding.

Meckel's diverticulum

A Meckel's diverticulum is a persistent remnant of the vitellointestinal duct and is present in about 2 per cent of the population. It is found on the antimesenteric side of the ileum, commonly at 60 cm from the ileocaecal valve and is classically 5 cm long (Figure 69.33). A Meckel's diverticulum contains all three coats of the bowel wall and has its own blood supply. It is vulnerable to obstruction and inflammation in the same way as the appendix; indeed, when a normal appendix is found at surgery for suspected appendicitis, a Meckel's diverticulum should be looked for by examining the small bowel particularly if free fluid or pus is found (Summary box 69.15).

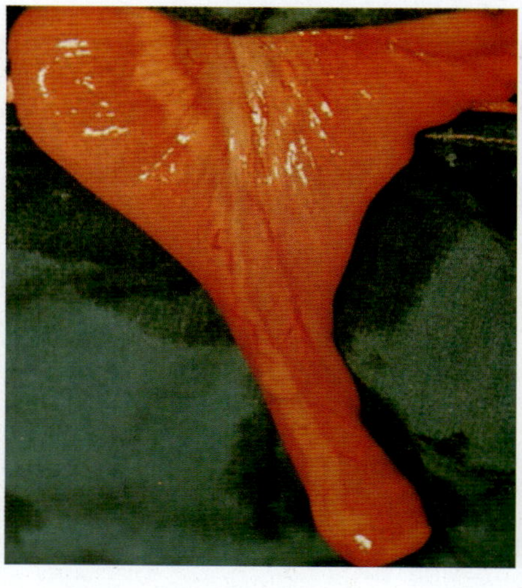

Figure 69.33 Meckel's diverticulum.

Johann Friedrich Meckel (the younger), 1781–1833, Professor of Anatomy and Surgery, Halle, Germany, described the diverticulum in 1809.

Summary box 69.15

Features of Meckel's diverticulum

- Remnant of vitellointestinal duct
- Occurs in 2 per cent of patients, 2 inches (5 cm long), 2 feet (60 cm) from the ileocaecal valve, 20 per cent heterotopic epithelium
- Should be looked for when a normal appendix is found at surgery for suspected appendicitis
- If a Meckel's is found incidentally at surgery, it can be left provided it has a wide mouth and is not thickened
- Can be source of gastrointestinal bleeding if it contains ectopic gastric mucosa

In around 20 per cent of cases, the mucosa of a Meckel's diverticulum contains heterotopic epithelium of gastric, colonic or pancreatic type. A Meckel's diverticulum can present clinically in the following ways:

- **Haemorrhage**. If gastric mucosa is present, peptic ulceration can occur and present as painless maroon rectal bleeding or melaena. If the stomach, duodenum and colon are cleared by endoscopy, radioisotope scanning with technetium-99m may demonstrate a Meckel's. (A Meckel's is notoriously difficult to see with contrast radiology.)
- **Diverticulitis**. Meckel's diverticulitis presents like appendicitis, although if perforation occurs the presentation may resemble a perforated duodenal ulcer.
- **Intussusception**. A Meckel's can be the lead point for ileoileal or ileocolic intussusception.
- **Chronic ulceration**. Pain is felt around the umbilicus, as the site of the diverticulum is midgut in origin.
- **Intestinal obstruction**. A band between the apex of the diverticulum and the umbilicus (also part of the vitellointestinal duct) may cause obstruction directly or by a volvulus around it.
- **Perforation**. (Figure 69.34).

The vast majority of Meckel's are asymptomatic. When found in the course of abdominal surgery, a Meckel's can safely be left alone provided it has a wide mouth and is not thickened. When there is doubt, it can be resected. The finding of a Meckel's diverticulum in an inguinal or femoral hernia has been described as Littre's hernia.

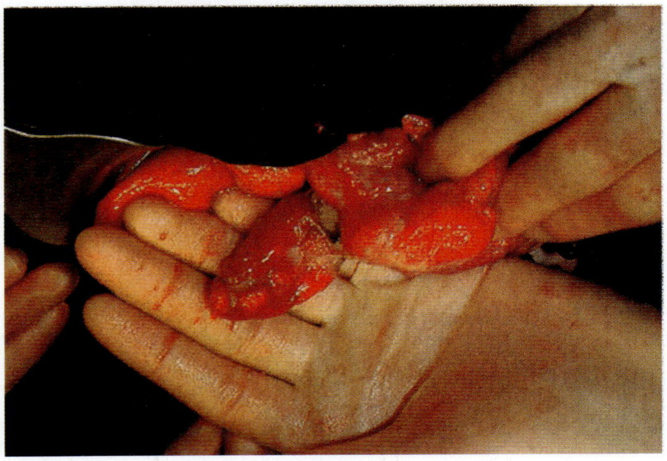

Figure 69.34 Gangrenous Meckel's diverticulitis.

Meckel's diverticulectomy

A broad-based Meckel's diverticulum should not be amputated at its base and invaginated (as for an appendix), as there is the risk of stricture and of leaving heterotopic epithelium behind. It is safer simply to excise the diverticulum, either by resecting it and suturing the defect at its base, or with a linear stapler-cutter. If the base of the diverticulum is indurated, it is on balance more logical to perform a limited small bowel resection of the involved segment followed by an anastomosis.

Diverticular disease of the large intestine

Diverticula are found in the left colon in around 75 per cent of over 70 year olds in the Western world. The condition is overwhelmingly found in the sigmoid, but diverticula are found in the caecum and can affect the whole colon (but not the rectum). Interestingly, in South-East Asia, right-sided diverticular disease is more common. Diverticula are most often asymptomatic (diverticulosis) and found incidentally, but can present clinically with sepsis or haemorrhage.

Aetiology

Epidemiology supports the widely held view that diverticular disease is a consequence of a refined Western diet deficient in dietary fibre. The combination of altered collagen structure with ageing, disordered motility and increased intraluminal pressure most notably in the narrow sigmoid colon results in herniation of mucosa, protruding through the circular muscle at the points where blood vessels penetrate the bowel wall. The rectum has a complete muscular coat and a wider lumen and is thus very rarely affected. Diverticular disease is rare in Africa and Asia where the diet is high in natural fibre.

Complications of diverticular disease

The majority of patients with diverticula are asymptomatic; historical studies suggest somewhere between 10 and 30 per cent will have symptomatic complications (Summary box 69.16). These complications are:

- **Pain and inflammation** (diverticulitis).
- **Perforation**: most often contained leading to pericolic abscess formation, but occasionally free leading to generalised peritonitis.
- **Intestinal obstruction**: progressive fibrosis can cause stenosis of the sigmoid and large bowel obstruction or loops of small intestine can adhere to an inflamed sigmoid resulting in small bowel obstruction.
- **Haemorrhage**: diverticulitis may present with profuse colonic haemorrhage.
- **Fistula formation**: (colovesical, colovaginal, enterocolic, colocutaneous) occurs in 5 per cent of cases, colovesical fistulation is most common.

Alexis Littre, 1658–1726, surgeon and Lecturer in Anatomy, Paris, France. Described Meckel's diverticulum in a hernial sac in 1700, 81 years before Meckel was born.

Summary box 69.16

Complications of diverticular disease

- Diverticulitis
- Abscess
- Peritonitis
- Intestinal obstruction
- Haemorrhage
- Fistula formation

Clinical features

In mild cases, symptoms such as distension, flatulence and a sensation of heaviness in the lower abdomen may be indistinguishable from those of irritable bowel syndrome. These symptoms are thought to result from a combination of increased luminal pressure affecting wall tension and increased visceral hypersensitivity. The difficulty in distinguishing between otherwise uncomplicated diverticular disease and irritable bowel syndrome is such that surgical treatment is rarely, if ever, appropriate for diverticular disease in the absence of complications.

Diverticulitis typically presents as persistent lower abdominal pain, usually in the left iliac fossa accompanied by loose stools or indeed constipation. Fever, malaise and leukocytosis can differentiate diverticulitis from painful diverticulosis. The lower abdomen is tender, especially on the left, but occasionally also in the right iliac fossa, if the sigmoid loop lies across the midline. The sigmoid colon may be tender and thickened on palpation and rectal examination may reveal a tender mass if an abscess has formed. Distinguishing between diverticulitis and abscess formation is difficult on clinical grounds alone and radiological imaging assessment is important. Generalised peritonitis as a result of free perforation presents in the typical manner with systemic upset and generalised tenderness, guarding and rebound. Similarly, large and/or small bowel obstruction due to diverticular disease has the same clinical features as other causes (see Chapter 69) and the aetiology is likely to be discovered only by imaging or at laparotomy.

Haemorrhage from colonic diverticula is typically painless and profuse. When from the sigmoid, it will be bright red with clots, whereas right-sided bleeding will be darker. Torrential bleeding is fortunately rare and in fact more commonly due to angiodysplasia but diverticular bleeding may persist or recur requiring transfusion and indeed resection. The presentation of a fistula resulting from diverticular disease depends on the site. The most common colovesical fistula results in recurrent urinary tract infections and pneumaturia (flatus in the urine) or even faeces in the urine. Colovaginal fistulae are more common in patients who have had a hysterectomy. Colocutaneous fistulation is rare in the absence of prior intervention (e.g. radiological drainage). Rarely, diverticular disease may perforate into the retroperitoneum leading to a psoas abscess, and then presenting in the groin with fistulation.

Classification of contamination

The degree of sepsis has a major impact on outcome in acute diverticulitis. Those with inflammatory masses have a lower mortality than those with perforation (3 versus 33 per cent). Classification systems have been developed for acute diverticulitis to try and rationalise the literature, the most commonly used is the Hinchey classification (Table 69.3).

Table 69.3 Hinchey classification of complicated diverticulitis.

Grade	
I	Mesenteric or pericolic abscess
II	Pelvic abscess
III	Purulent peritonitis
IV	Faecal peritonitis

Radiology

Plain chest and abdominal radiographs can demonstrate a pneumoperitoneum. Where available, spiral CT has excellent sensitivity and specificity for identifying bowel wall thickening, abscess formation and extraluminal disease and has revolutionised the assessment of complicated diverticular disease (Figure 69.35). On identification of abscesses in stable patients, drainage may be carried out percutaneously, avoiding the need for laparotomy/laparoscopy. If access to CT is limited, a water-soluble contrast enema can demonstrate intraluminal inflammation and contrast extravasation. This investigation also has a role in large bowel obstruction to distinguish mechanical blockage from pseudo-obstruction, however distinguishing between a malignant and a diverticular stricture may be difficult.

Barium enemas (and colonoscopy/flexible sigmoidoscopy) are usually avoided in the acute setting for fear of causing perforation or peritonitis. However, they are used after an attack has settled to exclude a coexisting carcinoma and assess

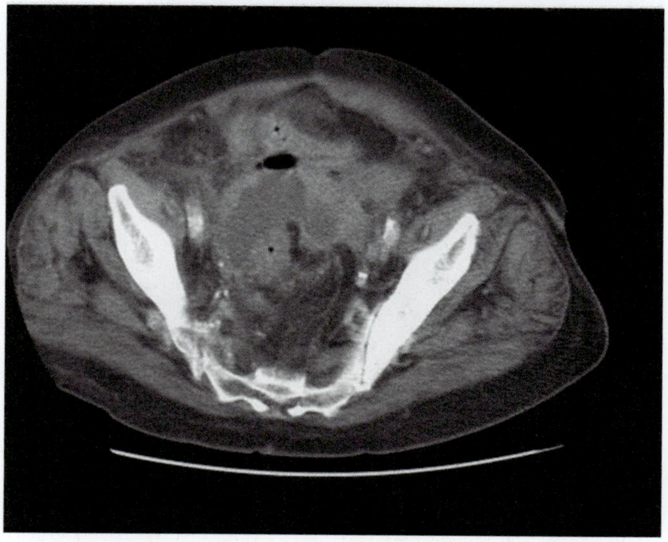

Figure 69.35 Computed tomographic scan demonstrating an abscess associated with diverticulitis (courtesy of Dr D Kasir, Hope Hospital, Salford, UK).

the extent of diverticular disease (Figure 69.36). Colovesical fistulae should be evaluated with cystoscopy and biopsy in addition. Contrast examinations or CT may demonstrate the fistula clearly. The differential diagnosis for colovesical fistula includes cancer, radiation injury, Crohn's disease, tuberculosis and actinomycosis.

Colonoscopy

Colonoscopy is normally deferred until 6 weeks after an acute attack of diverticulitis. It may demonstrate the necks of diverticula within the bowel lumen (Figure 69.37). A narrowed area of diverticular disease may be impassable because of the severity of disease and there is a significant risk of endoscopic perforation. Colonoscopy in these circumstances requires judgement and experience. The differential diagnosis from a carcinoma can be impossible if a tight stenosis prevents colonoscopy. Biopsies may be taken if possible and corroboration with barium enema or CT virtual colonoscopy is required.

Management

Patients are frequently recommended to take a high-fibre diet and bulk-forming laxatives, although the evidence for the effectiveness of these in diverticulosis or after an attack of diverticulitis is limited. Antispasmodics may have a role if recurrent pain is a problem. Acute diverticulitis is treated by intravenous antibiotics (to cover Gram-negative bacilli and anaerobes) alongside appropriate resuscitation and analgesia. Nil by mouth to 'rest the bowel' and catheterisation to reduce the risk of colovesical fistulation are often advocated, but there is little evidence to support these practices. A CT scan can confirm the diagnosis and assess for complications. After the acute attack has subsided and if CT has not already confirmed the diagnosis, the bowel should be investigated by endoscopy, barium enema or CT virtual colonoscopy. An abscess can be drained percutaneously, 5 cm is frequently regarded as a cut off between an abscess likely to settle with antibiotics and one likely to require intervention.

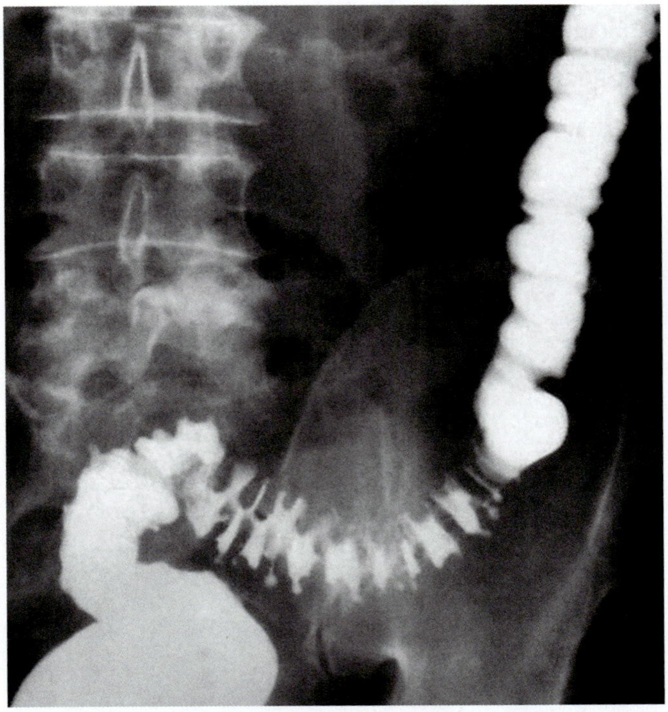

Figure 69.36 Barium enema showing sigmoid diverticular disease 'saw-teeth' and diverticula (courtesy of Dr D Nolan, John Radcliffe Hospital, Oxford, UK).

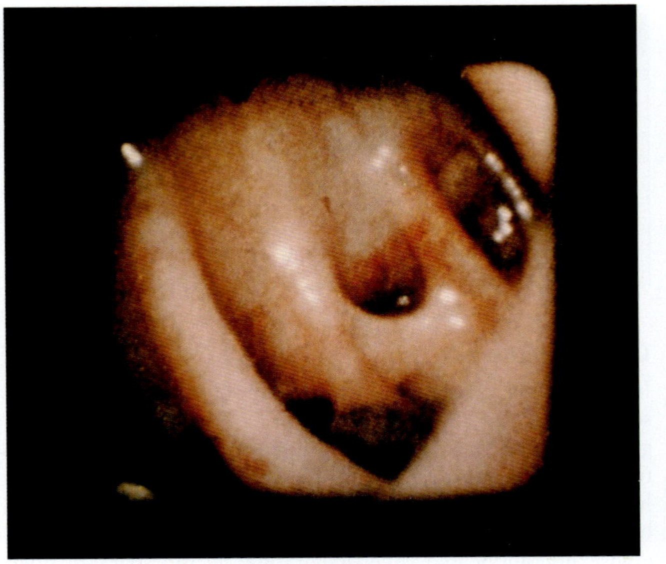

Figure 69.37 Colonoscopic view of sigmoid diverticula. Note the mouths of diverticula between the hypertrophied colonic walls.

Operative procedures for diverticular disease

The aim of emergency surgery is to control peritoneal sepsis; indications are generalised peritonitis and failure to respond to best medical management (Summary box 69.17). Laparotomy for diverticular disease in the acute setting has considerable risk with mortality in most series around 15 per cent and in the case of faecal peritonitis mortality approaches 50 per cent. Alongside operative technique, resuscitation, anaesthesia and postoperative management should be optimised.

Summary box 69.17

Principles of surgical management of diverticular disease

- Hartmann's procedure is the safest option in emergency surgery
- Primary anastomosis can be considered in selected patients
- Elective resection may be offered for recurrent attacks
- Definitive treatment of colovesical fistula will require resection

It is logical to perform a rigid sigmoidoscopy to avoid missing a rectal carcinoma. Laparotomy and thorough washout of contamination are performed and then a choice has to be made between a Hartmann's procedure (sigmoid resection with formation of left iliac fossa colostomy and closure of the rectal stump) and resection with colonic washout and anastomosis (± defunctioning loop ileostomy). Primary anastomosis should be used selectively but is appealing in a young fit patient without gross contamination or overwhelming sepsis. However, this is a relatively rare scenario and the majority of emergency operations for perforated diverticular disease are Hartmann's procedures (Figure 69.38). There is good evidence that simple defunctioning with a proximal stoma is associated with higher mortality than a resection. There may be an emerging role for emergency laparoscopy in diverticular disease with washout if there is no faecal contamination (i.e. Hinchey grade III or less), avoiding sigmoid resection. At present, this remains in the domain of the experienced laparoscopic surgeon.

Indications for surgery in an elective setting are controversial. There are undoubtedly a small number of patients with recurrent attacks who should be offered an elective sigmoid colectomy (with anastomosis). This could be performed laparoscopically in experienced hands with a likely but not clearly proven swifter recovery, as well as improved cosmesis. Cohort series studies suggest that of younger patients (under 50 years old) admitted with diverticulitis, 25 per cent will get a further episode. This is used as an argument for offering elective resection, but equally suggests 75 per cent will not have another severe attack. Many surgeons would discuss the pros and cons of elective surgery after two emergency admissions, although general health must be carefully considered. There has been an increasing tendency, in recent years, to treat even patients with recurrent attacks of diverticulitis conservatively in the absence of complications.

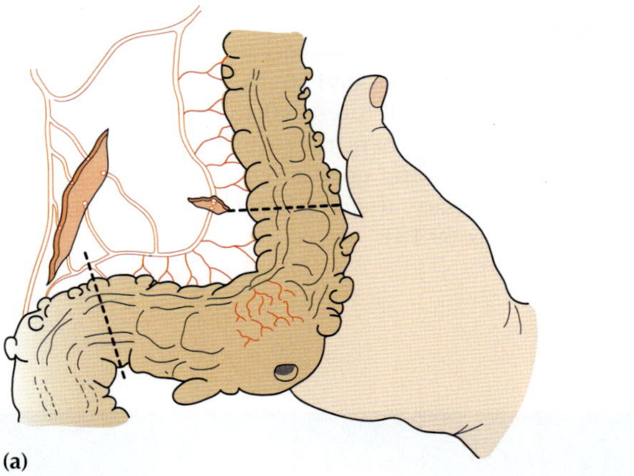

(a)

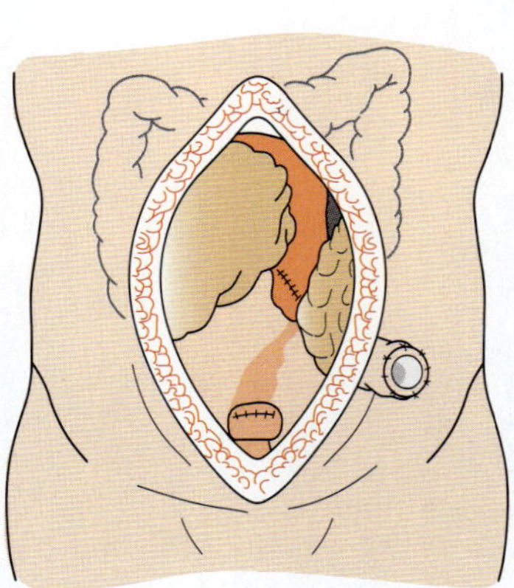

(b)

Figure 69.38 (a) Perforated sigmoid diverticular disease. (b) The Hartmann procedure – oversewn rectal stump and left iliac fossa colostomy.

Diverticular fistulae can only be cured by resection of the affected bowel, although a defunctioning stoma can ameliorate symptoms. In the most common scenario of a colovesical fistula, the sigmoid can often be pinched off the bladder and the sigmoid resected. If an anastomosis is performed, it is wise to place an omental pedicle to prevent recurrent fistulation. There will be occasions when a bladder resection is required and it is ideal to involve a urologist or general surgeon experienced in bladder surgery.

Haemorrhage from diverticular disease should be distinguished from angiodysplasia. It usually responds to conservative management and only occasionally requires resection. Where available angiography is helpful to localise bleeding points. On-table lavage and colonoscopy may be necessary to localise the bleeding site. If the source cannot be located, then subtotal colectomy and ileostomy is the safest option.

VASCULAR ANOMALIES OF THE INTESTINE

Mesenteric ischaemia

Mesenteric vascular disease may be classified as acute intestinal ischaemia – with or without occlusion – venous, chronic arterial, central or peripheral. The superior mesenteric vessels are the visceral vessels most likely to be affected by embolisation or thrombosis, with the former being most common. Occlusion at the origin of the superior mesenteric artery (SMA) is almost invariably the result of thrombosis, whereas emboli lodge at the origin of the middle colic artery. Inferior mesenteric involvement is usually clinically silent because of a better collateral circulation.

Possible sources for the embolisation of the SMA include a left atrium associated with fibrillation, a mural myocardial infarction, an atheromatous plaque from an aortic aneurysm and a mitral valve vegetation associated with endocarditis.

Primary thrombosis is associated with atherosclerosis and thromboangitis obliterans. Primary thrombosis of the superior mesenteric veins may occur in association with factor V Leiden, portal hypertension, portal pyaemia and sickle cell disease and in women taking the contraceptive pill.

Irrespective of whether the occlusion is arterial or venous, haemorrhagic infarction occurs. The mucosa is the only layer of the intestinal wall to have little resistance to ischaemic injury. The intestine and its mesentery become swollen and oedematous. Blood-stained fluid exudes into the peritoneal cavity and bowel lumen. If the main trunk of the SMA is involved, the infarction covers an area from just distal to the duodenojejunal flexure to the splenic flexure. Usually, a branch of the main trunk is implicated and the area of infarction is less.

Clinical features

The most important clue to an early diagnosis of acute mesenteric ischaemia is the sudden onset of severe abdominal pain in a patient with atrial fibrillation or atherosclerosis. The pain is typically central and out of all proportion to physical findings. Persistent vomiting and defaecation occur early, with the subsequent passage of altered blood. Hypovolaemic shock rapidly ensues. Abdominal tenderness may be mild initially with rigidity being a late feature.

Investigation will usually reveal a profound neutrophil leukocytosis with an absence of gas in the thickened small intestine on abdominal radiographs. The presence of gas bubbles in the mesenteric veins is rare but pathognomonic.

Treatment needs to be tailored to the individual. In conjunction with full resuscitation, embolectomy via the ileocolic artery or revascularisation of the SMA may be considered in early embolic cases. The majority of cases, however, are diagnosed late. In the young, all affected bowel should be resected, whereas in the elderly or infirm the situation may be deemed incurable. Anticoagulation should be implemented early in the postoperative period.

After extensive enterectomy, it is usual for patients to require intravenous alimentation. The young, however, may sometimes develop sufficient intestinal digestive and absorptive function to lead relatively normal lives. In selected cases, consideration may be given to small bowel transplantation.

Infarction of the large intestine alone is relatively rare. Involvement of the middle colic artery territory should be treated by transverse colectomy and exteriorisation of both ends, with an extended right hemicolectomy in selected cases.

Ischaemic colitis describes the structural changes that occur in the colon as a result of the deprivation of blood. They are most common in the splenic flexure, whose blood supply is particularly tenuous. They have been classified by Marston into gangrenous, transient and stricturing forms; only stricturing forms cause obstruction and only a few such patients require resection.

Angiodysplasia

Angiodysplasia is a vascular malformation that is a cause of haemorrhage from the colon, typically in patients over 60 years. The lesions are also called angiomas, haemangiomas and arteriovenous malformations. Angiodysplasias occur particularly in the ascending colon and caecum of elderly patients. The malformations consist of dilated tortuous submucosal veins and in severe cases the mucosa is replaced by massive dilated deformed vessels.

Clinical features

In the majority, the symptoms are subtle and patients can present with anaemia. About 10–15 per cent of patients have brisk bleeds, which may present as melaena or significant rectal bleeding. It is likely that in many patients in whom rectal bleeding has been attributed to diverticular disease, bleeding was in fact from angiodysplasia. There is an association with aortic stenosis (Heyde's syndrome).

Investigation

If the bleeding is not too brisk, colonoscopy may show the characteristic lesion in the right colon. The lesions are only a few millimetres in size and appear as reddish, raised areas at endoscopy. Capsule endoscopy is a relatively new technology that may detect small bowel lesions. Selective superior and inferior mesenteric angiography shows the site and extent of the lesion by a 'blush' of contrast provided bleeding is above 1 mL/min. If this fails, a technetium-99m (99mTc)-labelled red cell scan may confirm and localise the source of haemorrhage.

Treatment

The first principle is to stabilise the patient. Following this, the bleeding needs to be localised. Colonoscopy may allow cauterisation to be carried out. In severe uncontrolled bleeding, surgery becomes necessary. On-table colonoscopy is carried out to confirm the site of bleeding. Angiodysplastic lesions are sometimes demonstrated by transillumination through the caecum (Figure 69.39). If it is still not clear exactly which segment of the colon is involved, then a subtotal colectomy may be necessary.

Ischaemic colitis

Ischaemia of the colon typically results from thrombosis or embolism. Sudden embolic events present with severe pain out of proportion to the degree of peritonism, bloody diarrhoea, severe haemodynamic instability and acidosis. Resuscitation and laparotomy are required with resection of gangrenous bowel and exteriorisation of the bowel. Mortality is extremely high. If the disease process is thrombotic in the context of global atherosclerosis, the presentation tends to be less dramatic with intermittent abdominal pain and rectal bleeding. Abdominal radiographs may show 'thumbprinting' and endoscopy may demonstrate haemorrhagic oedema. The left colon and, in particular, the splenic flexure are usually the worst affected. Angioplasty and bypass procedures can be performed in these circumstances, but are rarely required as symptoms usually settle spontaneously. In some cases, ulceration at the splenic flexure associated with ischaemic colitis may heal with stricturing and present with subsequent large bowel obstruction.

STOMAS

A colostomy (or ileostomy) stoma is an artificial opening made in the colon (or small intestine) to divert faeces and flatus outside the abdomen where they can be collected in an external appliance. Depending on the purpose for which the diversion has been necessary, a stoma may be temporary or permanent (Summary box 69.18).

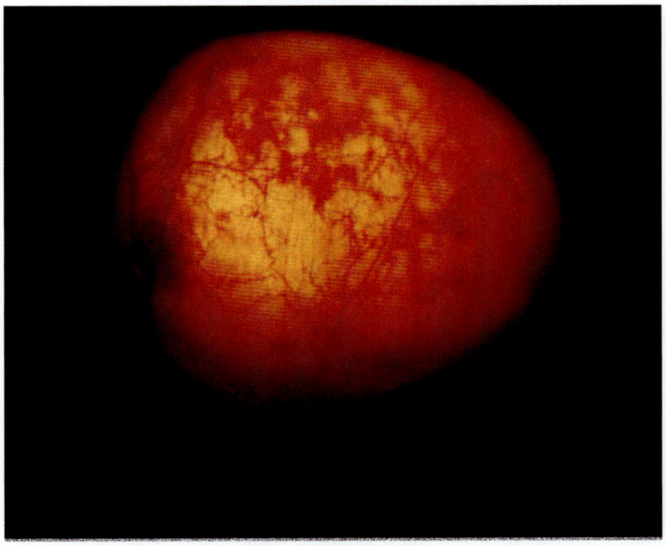

Figure 69.39 Angiodysplasia of the caecum demonstrated by transillumination with a colonoscope intraoperatively.

Jeffery Adrian Priestley Marston, b. 1927, formerly surgeon, The Middlesex Hospital, London, UK.
Edward Heyde, American internist, published his findings on the association between aortic valve stenosis and angiodysplasia in a letter to the *New England Journal of Medicine* in 1958.

Summary box 69.18

Stomas

- May be colostomy or ileostomy
- May be temporary or permanent
- Temporary or defunctioning stomas are usually fashioned as loop stomas
- An ileostomy is spouted; a colostomy is flush
- Ileostomy effluent is usually liquid, whereas colostomy effluent is usually solid
- Ileostomy patients are more likely to develop fluid and electrolyte problems
- An ileostomy is usually sited in the right iliac fossa
- End-colostomy is usually sited in the left iliac fossa
- Whenever possible, patients should be counselled and sited by a stoma care nurse before operation

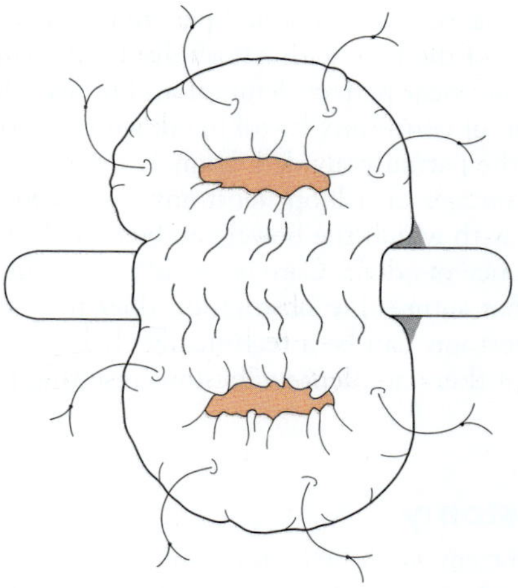

Figure 69.40 Temporary (loop) colostomy opened over a rod, and immediate suture of the colon wall to surrounding skin (alternatively, a skin bridge is used).

Loop colostomy

A transverse loop colostomy has in the past been used to defunction an anastomosis after an anterior resection. It is now less commonly employed, as it is difficult to manage and potentially disrupts the marginal arterial supply to the anastomosis. Loop transverse colostomies are also particularly prone to prolapse. A loop ileostomy is now more commonly used.

A loop left iliac fossa colostomy is still sometimes used to prevent faecal peritonitis developing following traumatic injury to the rectum, to facilitate the operative treatment of a high fistula in ano, for incontinence and to defunction a near obstructing rectal cancer prior to long course chemoradiotherapy (see Chapter 72).

A temporary loop colostomy is made by bringing a mobilised loop of colon to the surface, where it is held in place by a plastic bridge passed through a mesenteric window created just at the junction with the colon. Once the abdomen has been closed, the colostomy is opened, and the edges of the colonic incision are sutured to the adjacent skin margin (Figure 69.40). When firm adhesion of the colostomy to the abdominal wall has taken place, the bridge can be removed.

Following healing of the distal lesion for which the temporary stoma was constructed, the colostomy can be closed. It is usual to perform a contrast examination (proctogram) to check that there is no distal obstruction or continuing problem at the site of previous surgery. Colostomy closure is most easily and safely accomplished if the stoma is mature, typically after the colostomy has been established for two months. Closure is usually possible with a circumstomal incision, which avoids a full laparotomy, but it is important for patient and surgeon to consider the risks of closure carefully as it does involve a bowel anastomosis. In some cases, a full laparotomy may be required for safe closure of the stoma.

End colostomy

This is formed after an abdominoperineal excision of the rectum or as part of a Hartmann's procedure bringing the divided colon through a left iliac fossa trephine in rectus abdominis and skin. The colonic margin is then sutured to the adjoining skin.

The point at which the colon is brought to the surface must be carefully selected to allow a colostomy bag to be applied without impinging on the bony prominence of the anterosuperior iliac spine. The best site is usually through the lateral edge of the rectus sheath, above and medial to the bony prominence (Figure 69.41).

Closure of the lateral space between the intraperitoneal segment of the sigmoid colon and the peritoneum of the pelvic wall, to prevent internal herniation or strangulation of loops of small bowel through the deficiency, has been practised, but there is no good evidence that it is effective.

Loop ileostomy

A loop ileostomy is often used for defunctioning a low rectal anastomosis or an ileal pouch. A knuckle of ileum is pulled out through a skin trephine in the right iliac fossa. An incision is made in the distal part of the knuckle, and this is then pulled

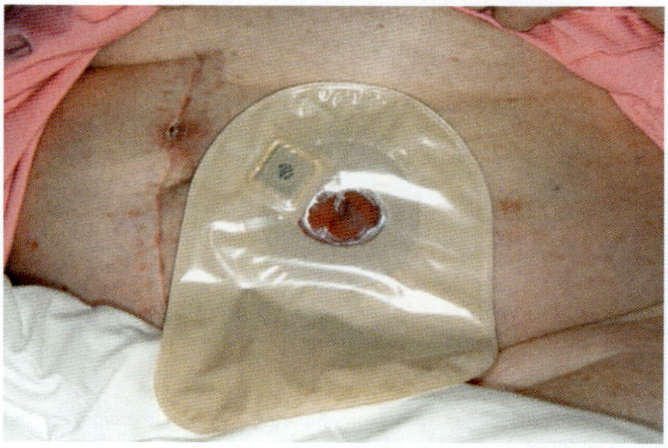

Figure 69.41 A colostomy in the left iliac fossa.

Nils Kock, b. 1924 in Finland, Professor of Surgery, University of Goteborg, Sweden, pioneered the creation of an artificial reservoir within the abdomen from loops of small intestine in 1969.

over the top of the more proximal part to create a spout on the proximal side of the loop with a flush distal side still in continuity. This allows near perfect defunction, but also the possibility of restoration of continuity by taking down the spout and reanastomosing the partially divided ileum.

The advantages of a loop ileostomy over a loop colostomy are the ease with which the bowel can be brought to the surface and the absence of odour. Care is needed when the ileostomy is closed, so that suture line obstruction does not occur. Closure of a loop ileostomy can be a technically challenging procedure, particularly if there are dense adhesions resulting from previous surgery.

End ileostomy

An end ileostomy is formed after a subtotal colectomy without anastomosis when it may later be reversed or may be permanent after a panproctocolectomy. The ileum is normally brought through the rectus abdominis muscle. Careful attention to the terminal ileal mesentery should be taken to ensure that it is not too bulky. The use of a spout was originally described by Bryan Brooke; this should project some 4 cm from the skin surface (Figure 69.42). A disposable appliance is placed over the ileostomy so that it is a snug fit at skin level.

There may be an 'ileostomy flux' while the ileum adapts to the loss of the colon. While ileostomy output can amount to 4 or 5 litres per day, losses of 1–2 litres are more common. A consistent ileostomy output in excess of 1.5 litres is usually associated with dehydration and sodium depletion in the absence of intravenous therapy. The stools thicken in a few weeks and are semisolid in a few months. The help, skill and advice of the stoma care nurse specialist are essential. Modern appliances have transformed stoma care, and skin problems are unusual (Figure 69.43). Complications of an ileostomy include prolapse, retraction, stenosis, bleeding, fistula and parastomal hernia.

Stoma bags and appliances

Stoma output is collected in disposable adhesive bags. Ileostomy appliances tend to be drainable bags, which are left in place for 48 hours, while colostomy appliances are simply changed two or three times each day. A wide range of such bags is currently available. Many now incorporate an adhesive backing, which can be left in place for several days. In most hospitals, a stoma care service is available to offer advice to patients, to acquaint them with the latest appliances and to provide the appropriate psychological and practical help.

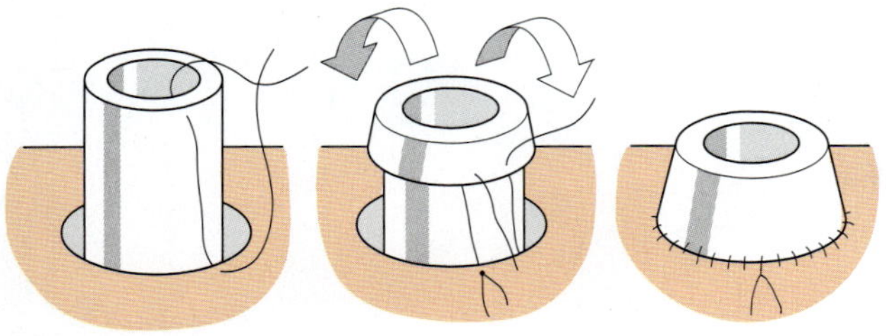

Figure 69.42 Ileostomy formation. Suturing the free extremity of the proximal ileum to the skin edges after eversion to form a spout (after Brooke).

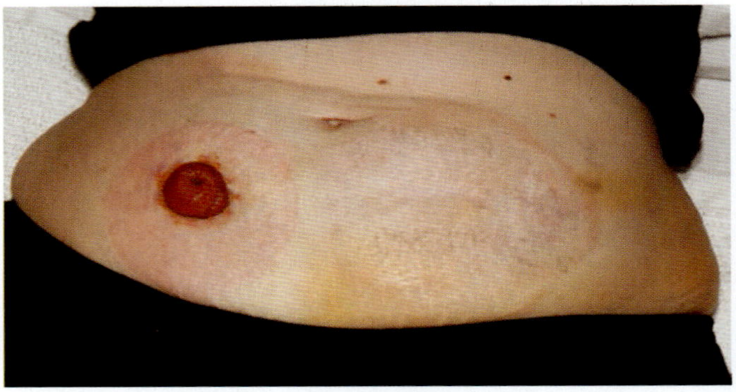

Figure 69.43 Spouted ileostomy in the right iliac fossa.

Caecostomy

In unstable patients with advanced obstruction, a caecostomy may be useful. In late cases of obstruction, the caecum may become so distended and ischaemic that rupture of the caecal wall may be anticipated. This can occur spontaneously, giving rise to faecal peritonitis, or at operation, when an incision in the abdominal wall reduces its supportive role and allows the caecum to expand. In such a situation, it should be decompressed by suction as soon as the abdomen is opened. In thin patients, it may then be possible to carry out direct suture of the incised or perforated caecal wall to the abdominal skin of the right iliac fossa, although resection of this area is really the best treatment preferable. Following on-table lavage, via the appendix stump, the irrigating catheter can be left in place as a tube caecostomy.

Complications of stomas

Stoma complications are underestimated and common (Summary box 69.19). On occasion, these complications require surgical revision. Sometimes, this can be achieved with an incision immediately around the stoma, but on occasion reopening the abdomen and freeing up the stoma may be necessary. Repair of parastomal hernias is particularly technically challenging and the recurrence rate is high. Simple suture of the parastomal hernia is associated with an almost 100 per cent risk of recurrence and transfer to the opposite side of the abdomen, or insertion of a piece of prosthetic material within the abdominal wall around the stoma may be necessary.

Summary box 69.19

Stoma complications

- Skin irritation
- Prolapse
- Retraction
- Ischaemia
- Stenosis
- Parastomal hernia
- Bleeding
- Fistulation

Bryan Nicholas Brooke, 1915–1998, Professor of Surgery, St George's Hospital, London, UK.

CONDITIONS CAUSING MALABSORPTION

Coeliac disease

Coeliac disease is the most common cause of malabsorption in the UK with a stated prevalence of 1:1800, although this may be an underestimate. It is characterised by a hypertrophic small bowel mucosa with atrophic villi and deep crypts. It is thought that loss of surface area and brush border enzymes results in malabsorption.

Coeliac disease is caused by gluten, a cereal protein although the exact mechanism remains unclear. There is a genetic component as the disease is more common in first-degree relatives and has an association with HLA B8. In children, coeliac disease presents with steatorrhoea and growth retardation. In adults, it results in diarrhoea, weight loss and anaemia.

The diagnosis is made after an endoscopic duodenal biopsy allows pathological examination of mucosa. The antiendomysial antibody tests have a very high sensitivity and specificity for coeliac disease, but many gastroenterologists would still want a biopsy to be entirely certain of the diagnosis.

Patients with coeliac disease have an increased risk of small bowel lymphoma and adenocarcinoma. Extraintestinal complications are dermatitis herpetiformis and neurological problems.

The key treatment for coeliac disease is withdrawal of gluten from the diet by avoiding wheat, rye and barley. Surgery is reserved for malignancy.

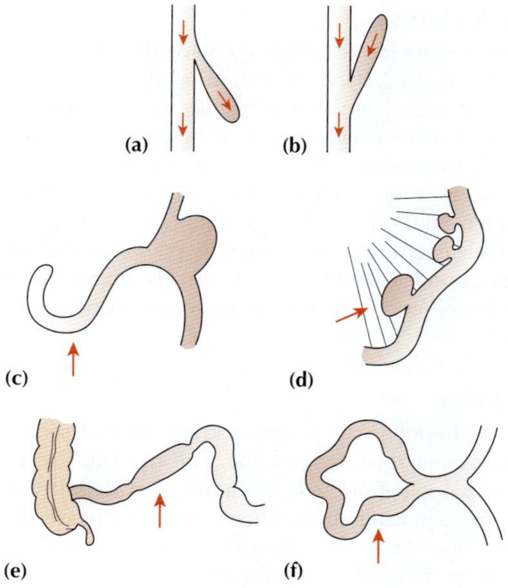

Figure 69.44 Common types of blind loop. (a) Self-filling: deficiency occurs; (b) self-emptying: no deficiency occurs; (c) long afferent loop stasis in Pólya gastrectomy; (d) jejunal diverticula; (e) intestinal stricture causing stasis; (f) 'stenosis–anastomosis loop' syndrome.

Bacterial overgrowth

The small intestine can become colonised with bacteria normally confined to the colon if there is stasis resulting in delayed bacterial clearance (blind loop syndrome, Figure 69.44). If this occurs in the upper intestine, the defect is chiefly of fat absorption; if in the lower intestine, there is vitamin B12 deficiency. There is relatively little effect on carbohydrate or protein metabolism.

Essentially, the stasis produces an abnormal bacterial flora, which prevents proper breakdown of fat and mops up the vitamins that are present. Sometimes, the only manifestation is anaemia, resulting from vitamin B12 deficiency but, if steatorrhoea occurs, other serious malabsorption features may follow including glossitis, osteomalacia, paraesthesia and peripheral neuropathy.

Improvement normally follows after intermittent therapy with oral antibiotics; metronidazole, ciprofloxacin and tetracycline are commonly used. Definitive treatment is surgical to remove the 'blind loop', but this is not always feasible.

FUNCTIONAL ABNORMALITIES

Constipation

There is no single definition of constipation; however, a bowel frequency of less than one every 3 days is commonly considered to be abnormal. Although constipation is often regarded as a trivial symptom, some patients are greatly disabled by abdominal pain, distension, reliance on laxatives and difficulty with defaecation. It is an extremely prevalent complaint in western society. Some reports have put the annual prescription sales for laxatives in the UK at around £50 million. These are usually otherwise healthy individuals who seek help for constipation, but eat a normal diet and have a normal colon on endoscopy and barium enema. Constipation can be divided into:

- megacolon:
  - Hirschsprung's disease;
  - non-Hirschsprung's megacolon and megarectum;
- non-megacolon:
  - secondary to drugs or illness;
  - primary colonic problem.

Hirschsprung's disease

The nature and treatment of Hirchsprung's disease is discussed with other congenital disorders in Chapter 70.

Idiopathic megacolon and megarectum

This is a rare condition and the cause is not known, although in some it may result from poor toilet training during infancy and in others from a congenital abnormality of the intestinal myenteric plexus. In South America, Chagas disease is a common cause of megacolon resulting from infection with *Trypanosoma cruzi*. Volvulus and perforation can occur and treatment may require surgical resection.

Sir Frederick Treves, 1823–1953, surgeon, The London Hospital, attributed Hirschsprung's disease to congenital spasm of the distal segment, thus preceding the rediscovery of this concept by 50 years.

Harald Hirschsprung, 1830–1916, physician, The Queen Louise Hospital for Children, Copenhagen, Denmark described congenital megacolon in 1887.

Clinical features

Idiopathic megacolon usually presents with severe constipation before the age of 20. Patients with idiopathic megarectum often present with faecal incontinence due to rectal faecal loading that requires manual evacuation. Patients with megacolon are more likely to present with abdominal distension and pain. On clinical examination, there may be a hard faecal mass arising out of the pelvis and, on rectal examination, there is a large faecal mass in the lumen. The anus is usually patulous, perianal soiling is common, and sigmoidoscopy is usually impossible but may show melanosis coli if the patient has been taking laxatives over many years.

Investigation

Anorectal physiology tests demonstrate delayed sensation and raised maximum tolerated volume. Full-thickness rectal biopsy shows normal ganglion cells, a finding that definitively distinguishes this condition from Hirschsprung's disease. Radiology studies will show gross faecal loading of the enlarged rectum and colon and an enlarged colon (Figure 69.45).

Medical treatment

This is directed at emptying the rectum and keeping it empty with enemas, washouts and occasionally, manual evacuation under anaesthesia. Thereafter, the patient is encouraged to develop a regular daily bowel habit, with the use of osmotic laxatives to help the passage of semiformed stool. Rectal evacuation with suppositories and biofeedback therapy may be useful in resistant cases.

Surgical treatment

Surgical treatment is sometimes necessary if medical therapy fails. Options that are available include:

- resection of the dilated rectum and colon (Figure 69.46) back to normal-diameter colon followed by reconstruction with a coloanal anastomosis;
- colectomy with the formation of an ileorectal anastomosis if the rectum is spared;
- restorative proctocolectomy;
- vertical reduction rectoplasty, which is a procedure designed to reduce the volume of the rectum by at least 50 per cent;
- stoma formation, which may be used either as a salvage operation for failure of previous surgery or as a primary intervention.

Non-megacolon constipation

Drugs and a range of illnesses can result in constipation (see Summary boxes 69.20 and 69.21). Altering medication or addition of laxatives can be helpful for drug-related constipation, correction of underlying illness is clearly ideal where possible for the conditions in Summary box 69.21.

Summary box 69.20

Drugs that can cause constipation

- Benzodiazepines
- Carbamazepine
- Chlorpromazine
- Cholestyramine
- Iron
- Opiates, particularly codeine and morphine
- Tricyclic antidepressants
- Statins

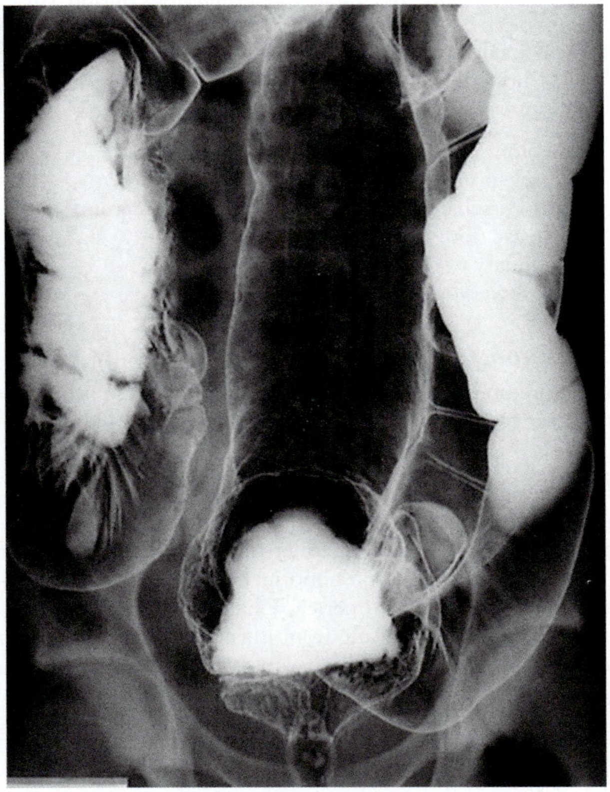

Figure 69.45 Double-contrast barium enema showing megarectum and a huge megasigmoid with normal left colon alongside for comparison (courtesy of Dr D Nolan, John Radcliffe Hospital, Oxford, UK).

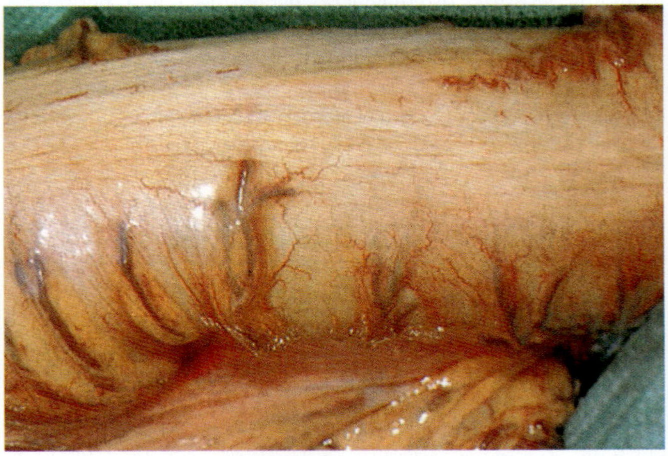

Figure 69.46 Megacolon.

Summary box 69.21

Illnesses associated with constipation

- Neurological conditions
- Parkinson's disease
- Multiple sclerosis
- Diabetic nephropathy
- Spinal cord lesion
- Endocrine conditions
- Hypothyroidism
- Hypercalcaemia

There remain a group of patients with significant constipation who do not have any structural, pharmacological or other pathology to explain their symptoms. Some will have obstructed defaecation and this is discussed in Chapter 72. Others will have slow colonic transit, a disorder usually seen in women, which may have been present since childhood or may suddenly follow abdominal or pelvic surgery. Marker studies will reveal delayed transit, and the patient may or may not be able to empty the rectum normally.

Investigation

Whole-gut transit time can be measured by asking the patient to stop all laxatives and take a capsule containing radio-opaque markers (Figure 69.47). Retention of more than 80 per cent of the shapes, 120 hours after ingestion, is abnormal.

Defaecating proctography will demonstrate intussusception and rectocoele if they are causing obstructed defaecation (Chapter 72).

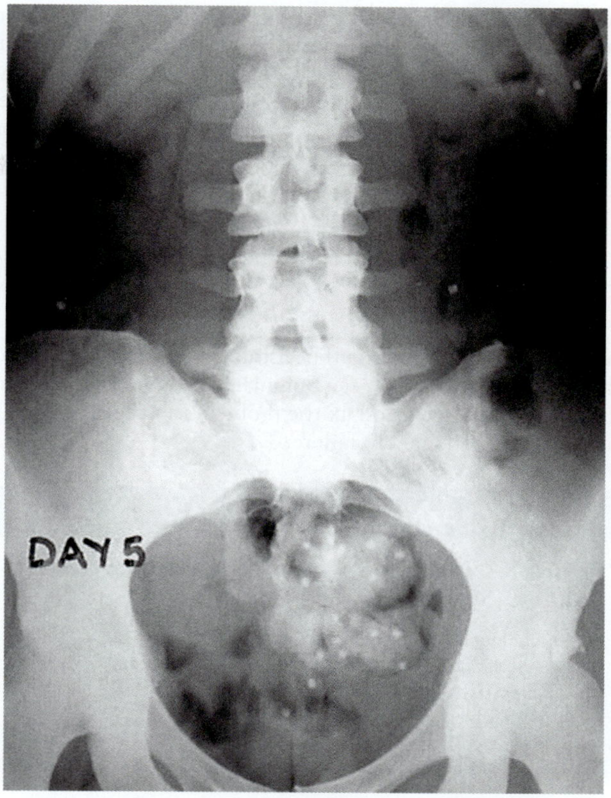

Figure 69.47 Whole-gut transit studied using radio-opaque markers. More than 80 per cent should have passed by day 5, demonstrating delayed transit here (courtesy of Dr D Nolan, John Radcliffe Hospital, Oxford, UK).

Treatment of slow colonic transit

- **Dietary fibre**. This is the first-line treatment for people with mild constipation. Constipation only resolves after several weeks of therapy and usually needs to be continued in the long term.
- **Laxatives**. It is important that patients do not fall into a cycle of laxative abuse. A number of types are available which include bulk, osmotic and stimulant agents.
- **Biofeedback**. This involves conditioning and coordination of the abdominal and pelvic compartments. It has been shown to be effective in those with a rectal evacuation problem and has also been used in slow transit with some benefit.
- **Surgery**. This is a difficult condition to treat medically; dietary measures are usually unsuccessful, and surgical treatment is justified after careful studies and when medical treatment has been exhausted. Total colectomy and ileorectal anastomosis is the preferred procedure, but the results are unpredictable. Studies show complications of intermittent small bowel obstruction (60 per cent), further surgery (30 per cent), constipation (25 per cent), diarrhoea (25 per cent) and incontinence (10 per cent). This may be explained in part by the argument that colectomy does not address the functional problem of the remaining bowel. Patients need to be carefully selected for surgery and psychological evaluation may be of benefit. Other types of surgery performed for slow transit constipation include stoma creation and segmental resection, but results are variable.

Irritable bowel syndrome

The term 'irritable bowel syndrome' (IBS) covers a range of symptom patterns that have a functional basis, i.e. no anatomical abnormality has been found. The clinical features are therefore variable but abdominal pain, bloating, irregularity of bowel habit and passage of mucous are common. Colonic investigations are typically performed to rule out organic disease (colonoscopy, barium enema or CT virtual colonoscopy).

Treatment is difficult by its nature. Many patients benefit from reassurance that there is no sinister pathology and symptomatic treatment; fibre or Fybogel for constipation, loperamide for diarrhoea. Reduction of caffeine intake and nicotine intake may be helpful. Antispasmodic agents are commonly prescribed, but the evidence base for this is poor. There is evidence of benefit for low-dose tricyclic antidepressants, but some patients are reluctant to use them because of a perceived stigma. Psychological treatments have been shown to be beneficial including hypnotherapy and cognitive behavioural therapy.

ENTEROCUTANEOUS FISTULA

An abnormal connection between small bowel and skin can occur in fistulating Crohn's disease or as a result of radiotherapy or abdominal trauma, but most commonly follows a surgical

James Parkinson, 1755–1824, a general practitioner of Shoreditch, London, UK, published 'An Essay on the Shaking Palsey' in 1817.

complication – either a leak from an anastomosis or an inadvertent enterotomy during dissection. This can be very challenging to manage in patients with a high-output fistula (>500 mL/day). Low-output fistulae (<500 mL/day) can be expected to heal spontaneously, provided there is no distal obstruction. Reasons for failure of spontaneous healing also include:

- epithelial continuity between the gut and the skin;
- the presence of active disease where, for example, there is Crohn's disease or carcinoma at the site of the anastomosis or in the fistula track;
- an associated complex abscess.

The management of high output fistulae is based on well-established principles ('SNAP', see Summary box 69.22), as an early return to theatre to try and fix the problem in a septic, malnourished patient is doomed to failure.

Summary box 69.22

Principles of management of enterocutaneous fistulae (SNAP)

- **S**, elimination of Sepsis and skin protection
- **N**, Nutrition – a period of parenteral nutrition may well be required
- **A**, Anatomical assessment
- **P**, definitive Planned surgery

Infected collections are best identified at CT (Figure 69.48) and can be drained percutaneously. Skin protection is important, as small bowel effluent is caustic. Nutritional support must include fluid and electrolytes, which can be lost in high quantities from a proximal fistula as well as carbohydrates, protein, fat and vitamins. Judgements have to be made between enteral and parenteral feeding – enteral feeding has advantages but if the fistula is proximal or high output, total parenteral nutrition (TPN) will be required. Defining anatomy is best done after careful discussion with the radiologist – a sequence of contrast studies (follow-through, fistulogram and enema) may well be required to define bowel length and plan a surgical strategy. The surgery can on occasion be extremely technically demanding, and an anastomosis should not be fashioned in the presence of continuing intra-abdominal sepsis or when the patient is hypoproteinaemic.

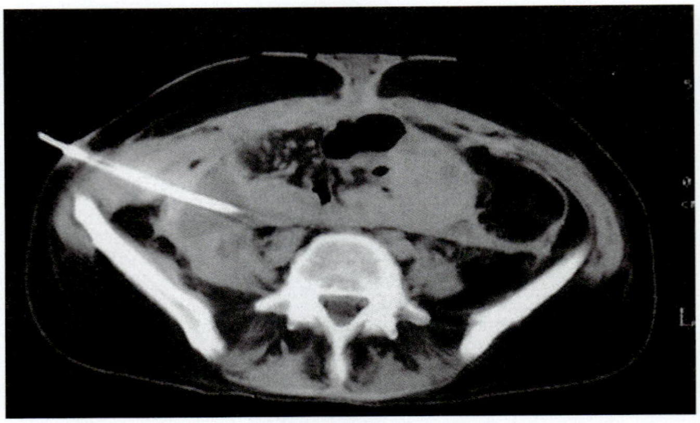

Figure 69.48 Computed tomography scan in a patient with a complex enterocutaneous fistula and an intra-abdominal abscess being drained with a CT-guided catheter.

FURTHER READING

Keighley MRB, Williams NS. *Surgery of the anus, rectum and colon*, 3rd edn. Philadelphia: Elsevier Saunders, 2008.

Phillips RKS. *Colorectal surgery: a companion to specialist surgical practice*, 4th edn. Philadelphia: Elsevier Saunders, 2009.

CHAPTER 70

Intestinal obstruction

LEARNING OBJECTIVES

To understand:

- The pathophysiology of dynamic and adynamic intestinal obstruction
- The cardinal features on history and examination
- The causes of small and large bowel obstruction
- The indications for surgery and other treatment options in bowel obstruction

CLASSIFICATION

Intestinal obstruction may be classified into two types:

- **Dynamic**, in which peristalsis is working against a mechanical obstruction. It may occur in an acute or a chronic form (Figure 70.1 and Summary box 70.1).
- **Adynamic**, in which there is no mechanical obstruction; peristalsis is absent or inadequate (e.g. paralytic ileus or pseudo-obstruction).

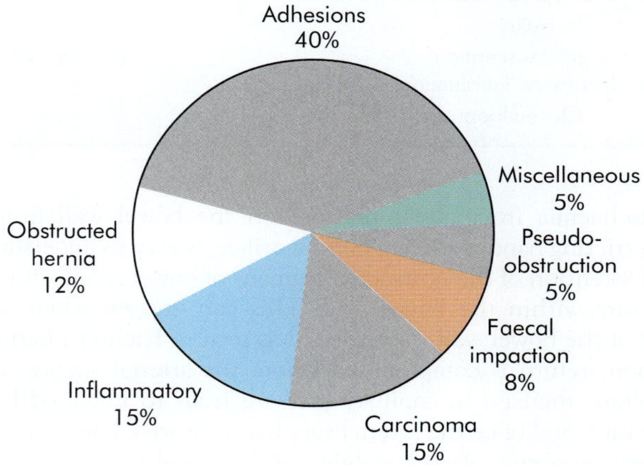

Figure 70.1 Pie chart showing the common causes of dynamic intestinal obstruction and their relative frequencies.

Summary box 70.1

Causes of intestinal obstruction

Dynamic
- Intraluminal
  - Faecal impaction
  - Foreign bodies
  - Bezoars
  - Gallstones
- Intramural
  - Stricture
  - Malignancy
  - Intussusception
  - Volvulus
- Extramural
  - Bands/adhesions
  - Hernia

Adynamic
- Paralytic ileus
- Pseudo-obstruction

PATHOPHYSIOLOGY

Irrespective of aetiology or acuteness of onset, in dynamic (mechanical) obstruction the bowel proximal to the obstruction dilates and the bowel below the obstruction exhibits normal peristalsis and absorption until it becomes empty and collapses. Initially, proximal peristalsis is increased in an attempt to overcome the obstruction. If the obstruction is not relieved, the bowel continues to dilate, ultimately there is a reduction in peristaltic strength, resulting in flaccidity and paralysis.

The distension proximal to an obstruction is caused by two factors:

- **Gas**: there is a significant overgrowth of both aerobic and anaerobic organisms, resulting in considerable gas production. Following the reabsorption of oxygen and carbon dioxide, the majority is made up of nitrogen (90 per cent) and hydrogen sulphide.
- **Fluid**: this is made up of the various digestive juices (saliva 500 mL, bile 500 mL, pancreatic secretions 500 mL, gastric secretions 1 litre – all per 24 hours). This accumulates in the gut lumen as absorption by the obstucted gut is retarded. Dehydration and electrolyte loss are therefore due to:
  – reduced oral intake;

- defective intestinal absorption;
- losses as a result of vomiting;
- sequestration in the bowel lumen;
- transudation of fluid into the peritoneal cavity.

STRANGULATION

It is important to appreciate that the consequences of intestinal obstruction are not immediately life-threatening unless there is superimposed strangulation. When strangulation occurs, the blood supply is compromised and the bowel becomes ischaemic (Summary box 70.2).

Summary box 70.2

Causes of strangulation

- Direct pressure on the bowel wall
  - Hernial orifices
  - Adhesions/bands
- Interrupted mesenteric blood flow
  - Volvulus
  - Intussusception
- Increased intraluminal pressure
  - Closed-loop obstruction

Ischaemia from direct pressure on the bowel wall from a constricting band, such as a hernial orifice, is easy to understand.

Distention of the obstructed segment of bowel results in high pressure within the bowel wall. This can happen when only part of the bowel wall is obstructed as seen in Richter's hernias. Venous return is compromised before the arterial supply. The resultant increase in capillary pressure leads to impaired local perfusion and once the arterial supply is impaired, haemorrhagic infarction occurs. As the viability of the bowel is compromised, translocation and systemic exposure to anaerobic organisms and endotoxin occurs.

The morbidity and mortality associated with strangulation are largely dependent on the duration of the ichaemia and its extent. Elderly patients and those with comorbidities are more vulnerable to its effects. Although in strangulated external hernias the segment involved is often short, any length of ischaemic bowel can cause significant systemic effects secondary to sepsis and obstruction proximal to the obstruction can result in significant dehydration. When bowel involvement is extensive circulatory failure is common.

Closed-loop obstruction

This occurs when the bowel is obstructed at both the proximal and distal points (Figure 70.2). The distention is principally confined to the closed loop, distention proximal to the obstructed segment is not typically marked.

A classic form of closed-loop obstruction is seen in the presence of a malignant stricture of the colon with a competent ileocaecal valve (present in up to one-third of individuals). This can occur with lesions as far distally as the rectum. The inability of the distended colon to decompress itself into the small bowel results in an increase in luminal pressure, which is greatest at the caecum, with subsequent impairment of blood flow in the wall. Unrelieved, this results in necrosis and perforation (Figure 70.3).

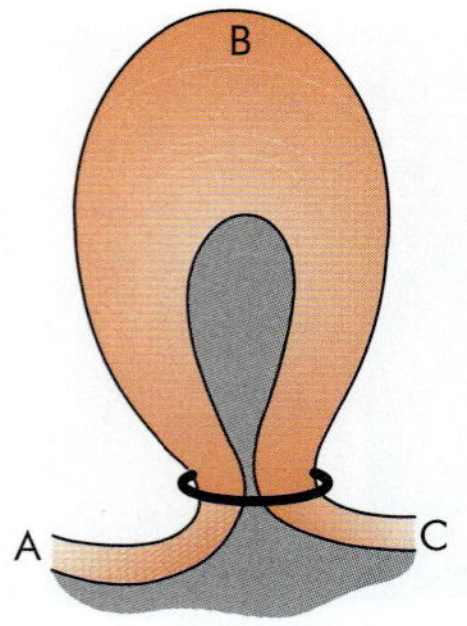

Figure 70.2 Distension. Closed-loop obstruction with no proximal (A) or distal (C) distension and impending strangulation (B).

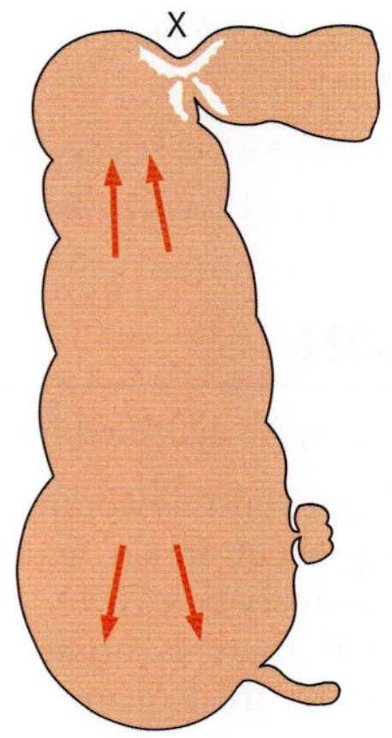

Figure 70.3 Carcinomatous stricture (X) of the hepatic flexure: closed-loop obstruction.

SPECIAL TYPES OF MECHANICAL INTESTINAL OBSTRUCTION

Internal hernia

Internal herniation occurs when a portion of the small intestine becomes entrapped in one of the retroperitoneal fossae or in a congenital mesenteric defect.

The following are potential sites of internal herniation (all are rare):

- the foramen of Winslow;
- a defect in the mesentery;
- a defect in the transverse mesocolon;
- defects in the broad ligament;
- congenital or acquired diaphragmatic hernia;
- duodenal retroperitoneal fossae – left paraduodenal and right duodenojejunal;

Jacob Benignus Winslow, 1669–1760, Professor of Anatomy, Physic and Surgery, Paris, France.

- caecal/appendiceal retroperitoneal fossae – superior, inferior and retrocaecal;
- intersigmoid fossa.

Internal herniation in the absence of adhesions is rare and a preoperative diagnosis is unusual. The standard treatment of an obstructed hernia is to release the constricting agent by division. This should not be undertaken in cases of herniation involving the foramen of Winslow, mesenteric defects and the paraduodenal/duodenojejunal fossae as major blood vessels run in the edge of the constriction ring. The distended loop in such circumstances must first be decompressed (minimising contamination) and then reduced.

Obstruction from enteric strictures

Small bowel strictures usually occur secondary to tuberculosis or Crohn's disease. Malignant strictures associated with lymphoma are uncommon, whereas carcinoma and sarcoma are rare. Presentation is usually subacute or chronic. Standard surgical management consists of resection and anastomosis. Resection is important to establish a histological diagnosis as this can be uncertain clinically. In Crohn's disease, strictureplasty may be considered in the presence of short multiple strictures without active sepsis.

Bolus obstruction

Bolus obstruction in the small bowel may be caused by gallstones, food, trichobezoar, phytobezoar, stercoliths and worms.

Gallstones

This type of obstruction tends to occur in the elderly secondary to erosion of a large gallstone directly through the gall bladder into the duodenum. Classically, there is impaction about 60 cm proximal to the ileocaecal valve. The patient may have recurrent attacks as the obstruction is frequently incomplete or relapsing as a result of a ball-valve effect. The characteristic radiological sign of gallstone ileus is Rigler's triad, comprising: small bowel obstruction, pneumobilia and an atypical mineral shadow on radiographs of the abdomen. The presence of two of these radiological signs has been considered pathognomic of gallstone ileus and is encountered in 40–50 per cent of the cases (note than pneumobilia is common following endoscopic retrograde cholangiopancreatography (ERCP) with sphincterotomy). At laparotomy, the stone is milked proximally away from the site of impaction; it may be possible to crush the stone within the bowel lumen, if not, the intestine is opened at this point and the gallstone removed. If the gallstone is faceted, a careful check for other enteric stones should be made. The region of the gall bladder should not be explored.

Food

Bolus obstruction may occur after partial or total gastrectomy when unchewed articles can pass directly into the small bowel. Fruit and vegetables are particularly liable to cause obstruction. The management is similar to that for gallstone, with intraluminal crushing usually being successful.

Trychobezoars and phytobezoars

These are firm masses of undigested hair ball and fruit/vegetable fibre, respectively. The former is due to persistent hair chewing or sucking, and may be associated with an underlying psychiatric abnormality. Predisposition to phytobezoars results from a high fibre intake, inadequate chewing, previous gastric surgery, hypochlorhydria and loss of the gastric pump mechanism. When possible, the lesion may be kneaded into the caecum, otherwise open removal is required. A peroperative diagnosis is difficult even with high resolution computed tomography (CT) scanning.

Stercoliths

These are usually found in the small bowel in association with a jejunal diverticulum or ileal stricture. Presentation and management are identical to that of gallstones.

Worms

Ascaris lumbricoides may cause low small bowel obstruction, particularly in children, the institutionalised and those near the tropics (Figure 70.4). An attack may follow the initiation of antihelminthic therapy. Debility is frequently out of proportion to that produced by the obstruction. If worms are not seen in the stool or vomitus, the diagnosis may be indicated by eosinophilia or the sight of worms within gas-filled small bowel loops on a plain radiograph (Naik). At laparotomy, it may be possible to knead the tangled mass into the caecum; if not it should be removed. Occasionally, worms may cause a perforation and peritonitis, especially if the enteric wall is weakened by such conditions as ameobiasis.

Obstruction by adhesions and bands

Adhesions

In Western countries where abdominal operations are common, adhesions and bands are the most common cause of intestinal obstruction. The lifetime risk of requiring an admission to hospital for adhesional small bowel obstruction subsequent to abdominal surgery is around 4 per cent and the risk of requiring a laparotomy around 2 per cent. Adhesions start to form within

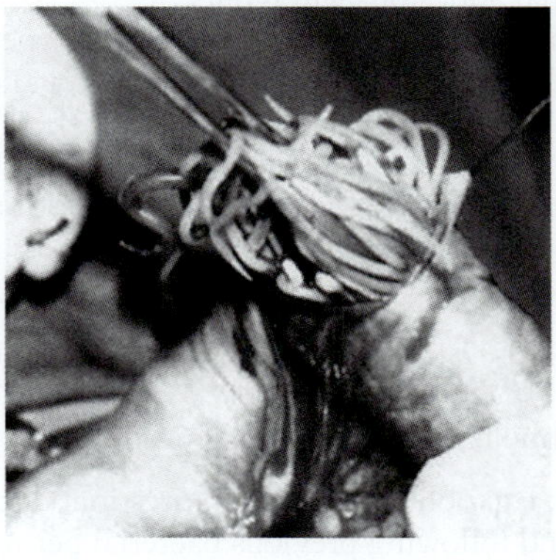

Figure 70.4 Obstruction of the small intestine due to *Ascaris lumbricoides* (courtesy of Asal Y Izzidien, Nenavah, Iraq).

Vinod C Naik, a doctor from Navsari, India.

Table 70.1 The common causes of intra-abdominal adhesions.

Acute inflammation	Sites of anastomoses, reperitonealisation of raw areas, trauma, ischaemia
Foreign material	Talc, starch, gauze, silk
Infection	Peritonitis, tuberculosis
Chronic inflammatory conditions	Crohn's disease
Radiation enteritis	

hours of abdominal surgery. In the early postoperative period, the onset of such a mechanical obstruction may be difficult to differentiate from paralytic ileus.

The causes of intraperitoneal adhesions are shown in Table 70.1. Any source of peritoneal irritation results in local fibrin production, which produces adhesions between apposed surfaces. Early fibrinous adhesions may disappear when the cause is removed or they may become vascularised and be replaced by mature fibrous tissue.

There are several factors that may limit adhesion formation (Summary box 70.3).

Summary box 70.3

Prevention of adhesions

Factors that may limit adhesion formation include:

- Good surgical technique
- Washing of the peritoneal cavity with saline to remove clots
- Minimising contact with gauze
- Covering anastomosis and raw peritoneal surfaces

Numerous substances have been instilled in the peritoneal cavity to prevent adhesion formation, including hyaluronidase, hydrocortisone, silicone, dextran, polyvinylpropylene (PVP), chondroitin and streptomycin, anticoagulants, antihistamines, non-steroidal anti-inflammatory drugs and streptokinase. Currently, no single agent or combination of agents has been convincingly shown to be effective. It is hoped that with the more widespread use of laparoscopic surgery, the incidence of intra-abdominal adhesions will reduce.

Adhesions may be classified into various types by virtue of whether they are early (fibrinous) or late (fibrous) or by underlying aetiology. From a practical perspective, there are only two types – 'easy' flimsy ones and 'difficult' dense ones.

Postoperative adhesions giving rise to intestinal obstruction usually involve the lower small bowel and almost never involve the large bowel.

Bands

Usually only one band is culpable. This may be:

- congenital, e.g. obliterated vitellointestinal duct;
- a string band following previous bacterial peritonitis;
- a portion of greater omentum, usually adherent to the parietes.

Acute intussusception

This occurs when one portion of the gut invaginates into an immediately adjacent segment; almost invariably, it is the proximal into the distal.

The condition is encountered most commonly in children, with a peak incidence between five and ten months of age. About 90 per cent of cases are idiopathic, but an associated upper respiratory tract infection or gastroenteritis may precede the condition. It is believed that hyperplasia of Peyer's patches in the terminal ileum may be the initiating event. Weaning, loss of passively acquired maternal immunity and common viral pathogens have all been implicated in the pathogenesis of intussusception in infancy.

Children with intussusception associated with a pathological lead point such as Meckel's diverticulum, polyp, duplication, Henoch–Schönlein purpura or appendix are usually older than those with idiopathic disease. After the age of two years, a pathological lead point is found in at least one-third of affected children. Adult cases are invariably associated with a lead point, which is usually a polyp (e.g. Peutz–Jeghers syndrome), a submucosal lipoma or other tumour.

Pathology

An intussusception is composed of three parts (Figure 70.5):

- the entering or inner tube (intussusceptum);
- the returning or middle tube;
- the sheath or outer tube (intussuscipiens).

The part that advances is the apex, the mass is the intussusception and the neck is the junction of the entering layer with the mass.

Intussusception may be anatomically defined according to the site and extent of invagination (Table 70.2). In most children, the intussusception is ileocolic (see Chapter 8, Figure 6.16). In adults, colocolic intussusception is more common (Summary box 70.4). The degree of ischaemia is dependent on the tightness of the invagination, which is usually greatest as it passes through the ileocaecal valve. On CT scanning, the target sign may be evident and if present is pathognomonic. It is worth noting that rarely, intussusception has been noted on CT scanning in asymptomatic adults.

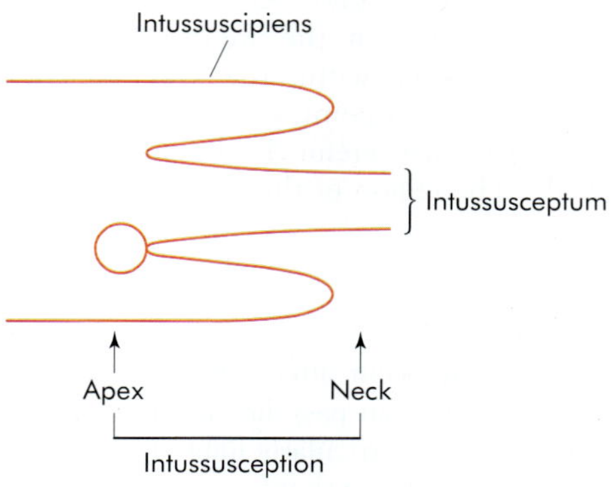

Figure 70.5 Mechanism and nomenclature of intussusception.

Table 70.2 Types of intussusception in children (after RE Gross) (n = 702).

	Percentage of series
Ileoileal	5
Ileocolic	77
Ileoileocolic	12
Colocolic	2
Multiple	1
Retrograde	0.2
Others	2.8

Summary box 70.4

Intussusception

- Most common in children
- Adult cases are secondary to intestinal pathology, e.g. polyp, Meckel's diverticulum
- Ileocolic is the most common variety
- Can lead to an ischaemic segment
- Radiological reduction is indicated in most paediatric cases
- Adults require surgery

Volvulus

A volvulus is a twisting or axial rotation of a portion of bowel about its mesentery. The rotation causes obstruction to the lumen (>180° torsion) and if tight enough also causes vascular occlusion in the mesentery (>360° torsion). Bacterial fermentation adds to the distention and increasing intraluminal pressure impairs capillary perfusion. Mesenteric veins become obstructed as a result of the mechanical twisting and thrombosis results and contributes to the ischaemia.

Volvuli may be primary or secondary. The primary form occurs secondary to congenital malrotation of the gut, abnormal mesenteric attachments or congenital bands. Examples include volvulus neonatorum, caecal volvulus and sigmoid volvulus. A secondary volvulus, which is the more common variety, is due to rotation of a segment of bowel around an acquired adhesion or stoma (Summary box 70.5).

Summary box 70.5

Volvulus

- May involve the small intestine, caecum or sigmoid colon; neonatal midgut volvulus secondary to midgut malrotation is life-threatening
- The most common spontaneous type in adults is sigmoid
- Sigmoid volvulus can be relieved by decompression per anum
- Surgery is required to prevent or relieve ischaemia

Volvulus neonatorum

This occurs secondary to intestinal malrotation (see Chapter 8) and is potentially catastrophic.

Sigmoid volvulus

This is uncommon in Europe and the United States, but more common in Eastern Europe and Africa. Indeed, it is the most common cause of large bowel obstruction in the indigenous Black African population. Rotation nearly always occurs in the anticlockwise direction. The predisposing causes are summarised in Figure 70.6. Other predisposing factors include a high residue diet and constipation. In Western populations, the condition is seen most often in elderly patients with chronic constipation; comorbidities are common and chronic psychotropic drug use is associated with this condition. Younger patients present earlier and the prognosis is inversely related to the duration of symptoms. Presentation can be classified as:

- **Fulminant**: sudden onset, severe pain, early vomiting, rapidly deteriorating clinical course;
- **Indolent**: insidious onset, slow progressive course, less pain, late vomiting.

Compound volvulus

This is a rare condition also known as ileosigmoid knotting. The long pelvic mesocolon allows the ileum to twist around the sigmoid colon, resulting in gangrene of either or both segments of bowel. The patient presents with acute intestinal obstruction, but distension is comparatively mild. Plain radiography reveals distended ileal loops in a distended sigmoid colon. At operation, decompression, resection and anastomosis are required.

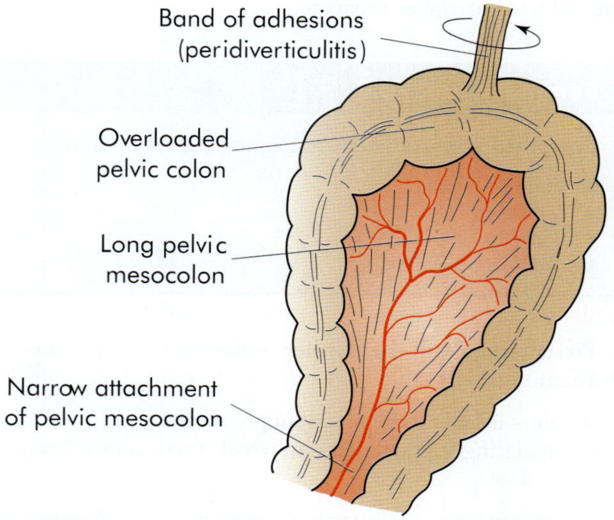

Figure 70.6 Causes predisposing to volvulus of the sigmoid colon. Idiopathic megacolon usually precedes the volvulus in African people.

CLINICAL FEATURES OF INTESTINAL OBSTRUCTION

Dynamic obstruction

The diagnosis of dynamic intestinal obstruction is based on the classic quartet of pain, distension, vomiting and absolute constipation. Obstruction may be classified clinically into two types:

- small bowel obstruction – high or low;
- large bowel obstruction (Summary box 70.6).

Summary box 70.6

Features of obstruction

- In **high small bowel obstruction**, vomiting occurs early, is profuse and causes rapid dehydration. Distension is minimal with little evidence of dilated small bowel loops on abdominal radiography
- In **low small bowel obstruction**, pain is predominant with central distension. Vomiting is delayed. Multiple dilated small bowel loops are seen on radiography
- In **large bowel obstruction**, distension and pronounced. Pain is less severe and vomiting and dehydration are later features. The colon proximal to the obstruction is distended on abdominal radiography. The small bowel will be dilated if the ileocaecal valve is incompetent

The nature of the presentation will also be influenced by whether the obstruction is:

- complete
- incomplete.

A complete small bowel obstruction has all the cardinal features (Summary box 70.7). In cases of complete large bowel obstruction, there is often a surprising lack of preceding symptoms. Both small and large bowel obstruction can present with more chronic symptoms in which the symptoms are intermittent or the obstruction is incomplete. Incomplete obstruction is also referred to as partial or subacute.

Summary box 70.7

Cardinal clinical features of acute obstruction

- Abdominal pain
- Distension
- Vomiting
- Absolute constipation

Presentation will be further influenced by whether the obstruction is:

- simple – in which the blood supply is intact;
- strangulating/strangulated – in which there is interference to blood flow.

The common causes of intestinal obstruction in Western countries and their relative frequencies are shown in Figure 70.1. The underlying mechanisms are shown in Summary box 70.2.

The clinical features vary according to:

- the location of the obstruction;
- the duration of the obstruction;
- the underlying pathology;
- the presence or absence of intestinal ischaemia.

Late manifestations of intestinal obstruction that may be encountered include dehydration, oliguria, hypovolaemic shock, pyrexia, septicaemia, respiratory embarrassment and peritonism. In all cases of suspected intestinal obstruction, the hernial orifices must be examined.

Pain

Pain is the first symptom encountered; it occurs suddenly and is usually severe. It is colicky in nature and usually centred on the umbilicus (small bowel) or lower abdomen (large bowel). The pain coincides with increased peristaltic activity. With increasing distension, the colicky pain is replaced by a mild and more constant diffuse pain. If there is no ischaemia and the obstruction persists over several days, pain reduces and can disappear.

The development of severe pain is suggestive of the presence of strangulation, especially if that severe pain is continuous. Beware the patient whose pain is not controlled with intravenous opiates. Colicky pain may not be a significant feature in postoperative simple mechanical obstruction and pain does not usually occur in paralytic ileus.

Vomiting

The more distal the obstruction, the longer the interval between the onset of symptoms and the appearance of nausea and vomiting. As obstruction progresses, the character of the vomitus alters from digested food to faeculent material, as a result of the presence of enteric bacterial overgrowth.

Distension

In the small bowel, the degree of distension is dependent on the site of the obstruction and is greater the more distal the lesion. Visible peristalsis may be present (Figure 70.7). This can sometimes be provoked by 'flicking' the abdominal wall. Distension is a later feature in colonic obstruction.

Constipation

This may be classified as absolute (i.e. neither faeces nor flatus is passed) or relative (where only flatus is passed). Absolute constipation is a cardinal feature of complete intestinal obstruction. Some patients may pass flatus or faeces after the onset of obstruction as a result of the evacuation of the distal bowel contents. The administration of enemas should be avoided in cases of suspected obstruction. This merely stimulates evacuation of bowel contents distal to the obstruction and confuses the clinical picture.

The rule that absolute constipation is present in intestinal obstruction does not apply in:

- Richter's hernia;
- gallstone ileus;
- mesenteric vascular occlusion;
- functional obstruction associated with pelvic abscess;
- all cases of partial obstruction (in which diarrhoea may occur).

August Gottlieb Richter, 1742–1812, lecturer in surgery, Göttingen, Germany, described this form of hernia in 1777.

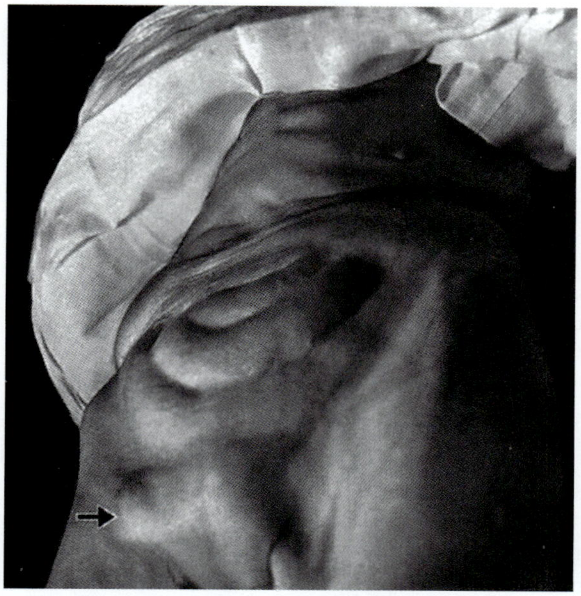

Figure 70.7 Visible peristalsis. Intestinal obstruction due to a strangulated right femoral hernia, to which the arrow points.

Other manifestations

Dehydration

Dehydration is seen most commonly in small bowel obstruction because of repeated vomiting and fluid sequestration. It results in dry skin and tongue, poor venous filling and sunken eyes with oliguria. The blood urea level and haematocrit rise, giving a secondary polycythaemia.

Hypokalaemia

Hypokalaemia is not a common feature in simple mechanical obstruction. An increase in serum potassium, amylase or lactate dehydrogenase may be associated with the presence of strangulation, as may leukocytosis or leukopenia.

Pyrexia

Pyrexia in the presence of obstruction is rare and may indicate:

- the onset of ischaemia;
- intestinal perforation;
- inflammation or abscess associated with the obstructing disease.

Hypothermia indicates septicaemic shock or neglected cases of long duration.

Abdominal tenderness

Localised tenderness indicates impending or established ischaemia. The development of peritonism or peritonitis indicates impending or overt infarction and/or perforation. In cases of large bowel obstruction, it is important to elicit these findings in the right iliac fossa as the caecum is most vulnerable to ischaemia.

Bowel sounds

High-pitched bowel sounds are present in the vast majority of patients with intestinal obstruction. Normal bowel sounds are of negative predictive value. Bowel sounds may be scanty or absent if the obstruction is long-standing and the small bowel has become inactive.

Clinical features of strangulation

It is vital to distinguish strangulating from non-strangulating intestinal obstruction because the former is a surgical emergency. The diagnosis is almost entirely clinical; the clinical features are shown in Summary box 70.8.

Summary box 70.8

Clinical features of strangulation

- Constant pain, severe pain
- Tenderness with rigidity and peritonism
- Shock

In addition to the features above, it should be noted that:

- The presence of shock suggests underlying ischaemia especially if the shock is resistant to simple fluid resuscitation.
- In impending or established strangulation, pain is never completely absent.
- The presence and character of any local tenderness are of great significance and, however mild, tenderness requires frequent reassessment.
- Generalised tenderness and the presence of rigidity indicate the need for early laparotomy.
- In cases of intestinal obstruction in which pain persists despite conservative management, even in the absence of the above signs, strangulation should be presumed.
- When strangulation occurs in an external hernia, the lump is tense, tender and irreducible and there is no expansile cough impulse. Skin changes with erythema or purplish discolouration are associated with underlying ischaemia (Figures 70.8 and 70.9).

Clinical features of intussusception

The classical presentation of intussusception is with episodes of screaming and drawing up of the legs in a previously well male infant. The attacks last for a few minutes and recur repeatedly. During attacks the child appears pale; between episodes he may be listless. Vomiting may or may not occur at the outset but becomes conspicuous and bile-stained with time. Initially, the passage of stool may be normal, whereas, later, blood and mucus are evacuated – the 'redcurrant jelly' stool.

Whenever possible, examination should be undertaken between episodes of colic, without disturbing the child. Classically, the abdomen is not initially distended; a lump that hardens on palpation may be discerned but this is present in only 60 per cent of cases (Figure 70.10). There may be an associated feeling of emptiness in the right iliac fossa (the sign of Dance). On rectal examination, blood-stained mucus may be found on the finger. Occasionally, in extensive ileocolic or colocolic

Jean Baptiste Hippolyte Dance, 1797–1832, physician, Hôpital Cochin, Paris, France.

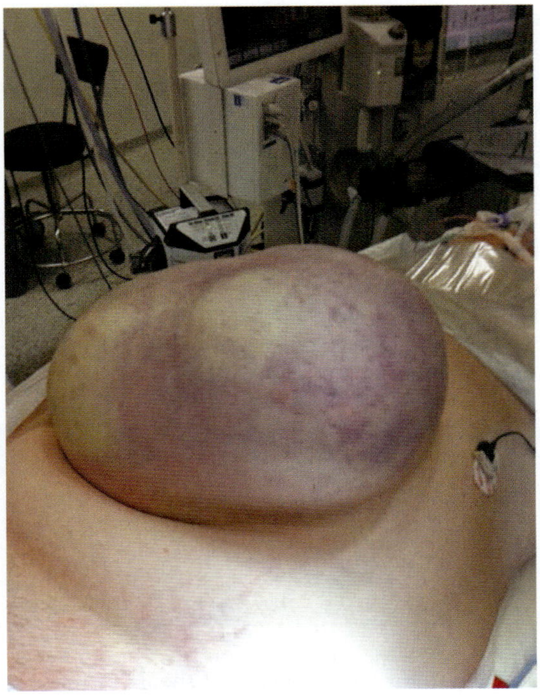

Figure 70.8 Skin discolouration over a strangulated incisional hernia.

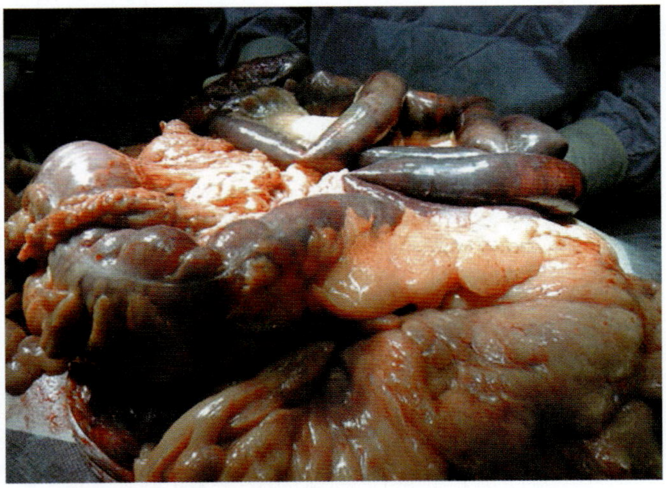

Figure 70.9 Ischaemic small and large bowel in the strangulated incisional hernia.

intussusception, the apex may be palpable or even protrude from the anus.

Unrelieved, progressive dehydration and abdominal distension from small bowel obstruction will occur, followed by peritonitis secondary to gangrene. Rarely, natural cure may occur as a result of sloughing of the intussusception.

Differential diagnosis

Acute gastroenteritis

Although abdominal pain and vomiting are common in acute gastroenteritis, with occasional blood and mucus in the stool,

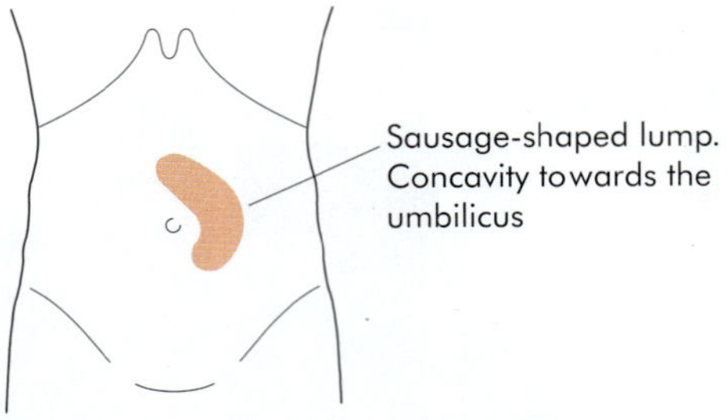

Figure 70.10 The physical signs as recorded by Hamilton Bailey in a typical case of intussusception in an infant.

diarrhoea is a leading symptom and faecal matter or bile is always present in the stool.

Henoch–Schöenlein purpura

Henoch–Schöenlein purpura is associated with a characteristic rash and abdominal pain; intussusception may occur.

Rectal prolapse

This may be easily differentiated by the fact that the projecting mucosa can be felt in continuity with the perianal skin whereas in intussusception the finger may pass indefinitely into the depths of a sulcus.

Clinical features of volvulus

Volvulus of the small intestine

This may be primary or secondary and usually occurs in the lower ileum. It may occur spontaneously in African people, particularly following the consumption of a large volume of vegetable matter, whereas in the West, it is usually secondary to adhesions passing to the parietes or female pelvic organs.

Caecal volvulus

This may occur as part of volvulus neonatorum or *de novo* and is usually a clockwise twist. It is more common in females in the fourth and fifth decades and usually presents acutely with the classic features of obstruction. Ischaemia is common. At first the obstruction may be partial, with the passage of flatus and faeces. In 25 per cent of cases, examination may reveal a palpable tympanic swelling in the midline or left side of the abdomen. The volvulus typically results in the caecum lying in the left upper quadrant. The diagnosis is not usually made preoperatively.

Sigmoid volvulus

The symptoms are of large bowel obstruction. Presentation varies in severity and acuteness, with younger patients appearing to develop the more acute form. Abdominal distension is an early and progressive sign, which may be associated with hiccough and retching. Constipation is absolute. In the elderly, a more chronic form may be seen. In some patients, the grossly distended torted left colon is visible through the abdominal wall.

Henry Hamilton Bailey, 1894–1961, surgeon, The Royal Northern Hospital, London, UK.

IMAGING

Erect abdominal films are no longer routinely obtained and the radiological diagnosis is based on a supine abdominal film (Figure 70.11). An erect film may subsequently be requested when further doubt exists.

When distended with gas, the jejunum, ileum, caecum and remaining colon have a characteristic appearance in adults and older children that allows them to be distinguished radiologically (Summary box 70.9).

In intestinal obstruction, fluid levels appear later than gas shadows as it takes time for gas and fluid to separate (Figure 70.12). These are most prominent on an erect film. In adults, two inconstant fluid levels – one at the duodenal cap and the other in the terminal ileum – may be regarded as normal. In infants (less than one year old), a few fluid levels in the small bowel may be physiological. In this age group, it is difficult to distinguish large from small bowel in the presence of obstruction, because the characteristic features seen in adults are not present or are unreliable.

During the obstructive process, fluid levels become more conspicuous and more numerous when paralysis has occurred. When fluid levels are pronounced, the obstruction is advanced. In the small bowel, the number of fluid levels is directly proportional to the degree of obstruction and to its site, the number increasing the more distal the lesion.

In patients without evidence of strangulation, there is a role for other imaging modalities. A recent systematic review and meta-analysis of the diagnostic and therapeutic role of 50–100 mL water-soluble contrast agent in adhesive small bowel obstruction included 14 prospective studies. The appearance of contrast in the colon 4–24 hours after administration had a sensitivity of 96 per cent and a specificity of 98 per cent in predicting resolution of small bowel obstruction. If contrast does not reach the colon, surgery is required in about 90 per cent of patients. Administration of a water-soluble agent was also effective in reducing the need for surgey (OR 0.62; $p = 0.007$) and shortening hospital stay.

In contrast, low colonic obstruction does not commonly give rise to small bowel fluid levels unless advanced, whereas high colonic obstruction may do so in the presence of an incompetent ileocaecal valve. Colonic obstruction is usually associated with a large amount of gas in the caecum. A limited water-soluble enema should be undertaken to differentiate large bowel obstruction from pseudo-obstruction. A barium follow-through is contraindicated in the presence of acute obstruction and may be life-threatening.

Summary box 70.9

Radiological features of obstruction (on plain x-ray)

- The obstructed small bowel is characterised by straight segments that are generally central and lie transversely. No/minimal gas is seen in the colon
- The jejunum is characterised by its valvulae conniventes, which completely pass across the width of the bowel and are regularly spaced, giving a 'concertina' or ladder effect
- Ileum – the distal ileum has been piquantly described by Wangensteen as featureless
- Caecum – a distended caecum is shown by a rounded gas shadow in the right iliac fossa
- Large bowel, except for the caecum, shows haustral folds, which, unlike valvulae conniventes, are spaced irregularly, do not cross the whole diameter of the bowel and do not have indentations placed opposite one another

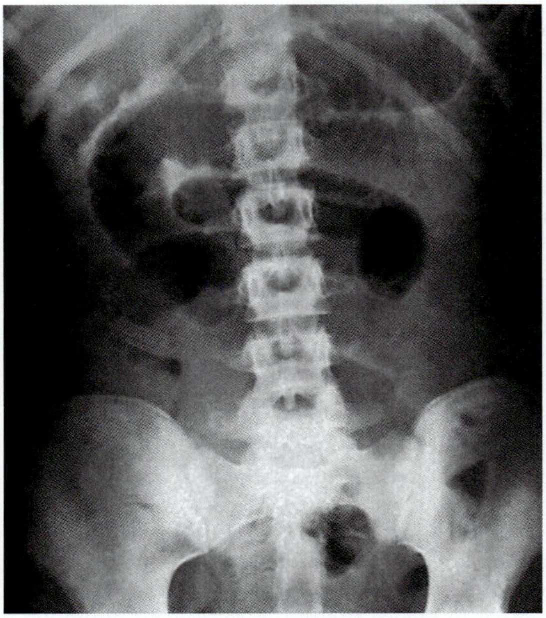

Figure 70.11 Gas-filled small bowel loop; patient supine.

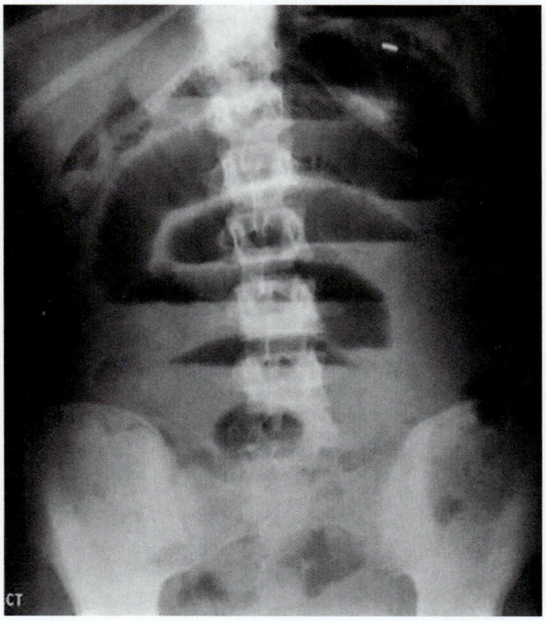

Figure 70.12 Fluid levels with gas above; 'stepladder pattern'. Ileal obstruction by adhesions; patient erect.

Owen Harding Wangensteen, 1898–1981, Professor of Surgery, The University of Minnesota, Minneapolis, MN, USA.

The CT scan is now used very widely to investigate all forms of intestinal obstruction. It is highly accurate and its only limitations are in diagnosing ischaemia. It is important to remember that even with the best imaging techniques, the diagnosis of strangulation remains a clinical one.

Impacted foreign bodies may be seen on abdominal radiographs. It is noteworthy that gas-filled loops and fluid levels in the small and large bowel can also be seen in established paralytic ileus and pseudo-obstruction. The former can, however, normally be distinguished on clinical grounds, whereas the latter can be confirmed radiologically. Fluid levels may also be seen in non-obstructing conditions such as gastroenteritis, acute pancreatitis and intra-abdominal sepsis.

Imaging in intussusception

A plain abdominal field usually reveals evidence of small or large bowel obstruction with an absent caecal gas shadow in ileocolic cases. A soft tissue opacity is often visible in children. A barium enema may be used to diagnose the presence of an ileocolic intussusception (the claw sign) (Figure 70.13), but does not demonstrate small bowel intussusception. An abdominal ultrasound scan has a high diagnostic sensitivity in children, demonstrating the typical doughnut appearance of concentric rings in transverse section. CT scan is currently considered the most sensitive radiologic method to confirm intussusception, with a reported diagnostic accuracy of 58–100 per cent. The characteristic features of CT scan include a 'target' or 'sausage'-shaped soft-tissue mass with a layering effect, mesenteric vessels within the bowel lumen are also typical.

Imaging in volvulus

- In **caecal volvulus**, radiological abnormalities are identifiable in nearly all patients, but are often non-specific, with caecal dilatation (98–100 per cent), single air-fluid level (72–88 per cent), small bowel dilatation (42–55 per cent) and absence of gas in distal colon (82 per cent) reported as the most common abnormalities. A barium enema may be used to confirm the diagnosis if there are no concerns about ischaemia, with an absence of barium in the caecum and a bird beak deformity. CT scanning is replacing barium enema as the imaging of choice in these less urgent cases.
- In **sigmoid volvulus**, a plain radiograph shows massive colonic distension. The classic appearance is of a dilated loop of bowel, the two limbs are seen running diagonally across the abdomen from right to left, with two fluid levels seen, one within each loop of bowel (if an erect film is taken).
- In **volvulus neonatorium**, the abdominal radiograph shows a variable appearance. Initially, it may appear normal or show evidence of duodenal obstruction but, as the intestinal strangulation progresses, the abdomen becomes relatively gasless.

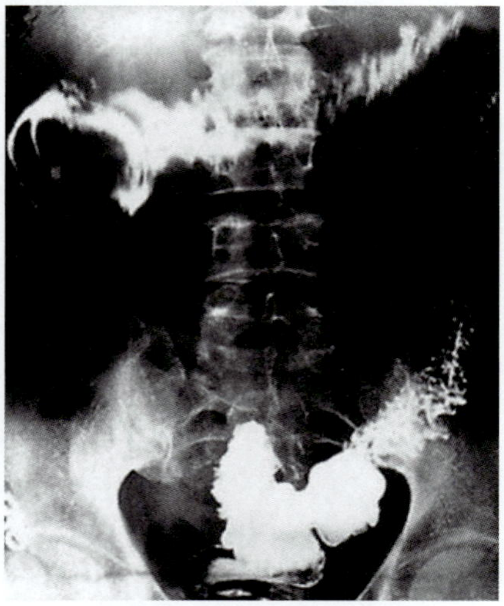

Figure 70.13 'Claw' sign of iliac intussusception. The barium in the intussusception is seen as a claw around a negative shadow of the intussusception (courtesy of RS Naik, Durg, India).

TREATMENT OF ACUTE INTESTINAL OBSTRUCTION

There are three main measures used to treat acute intestinal obstruction (Summary box 70.10).

Summary box 70.10

Treatment of acute intestinal obstruction

- Gastrointestinal drainage via a nasogastric tube
- Fluid and electrolyte replacement
- Relief of obstruction

Surgical treatment is necessary for most cases of intestinal obstruction but should be delayed until resuscitation is complete, provided there is no sign of strangulation or evidence of closed-loop obstruction

The first two steps are always necessary before attempting the surgical relief of obstruction and are the mainstay of postoperative management.

The three principles of surgical intervention are shown in Summary box 70.11.

Summary box 70.11

Principles of surgical intervention for obstruction

Management of:

- The segment at the site of obstruction
- The distended proximal bowel
- The underlying cause of obstruction

Supportive management

Nasogastric decompression is achieved by the passage of a non-vented (Ryle) or vented (Salem) tube. The tubes are normally placed on free drainage with 4-hourly aspiration, but may be placed on continuous or intermittent suction. As well as facilitating decompression proximal to the obstruction, they are essential to reduce the risk of subsequent aspiration during induction of anaesthesia and post-extubation.

John Alfred Ryle, 1889–1950, Regius Professor of Physics, The University of Cambridge, and later Professor of Social Medicine, The University of Oxford, UK, introduced the Ryle's tube in 1921.

The basic biochemical abnormality in intestinal obstruction is sodium and water loss, and therefore the appropriate replacement is Hartmann's solution or normal saline. The volume required varies and should be determined by clinical haematological and biochemical criteria.

Antibiotics are not mandatory but many clinicians initiate broad-spectrum antibiotics early in therapy because of bacterial overgrowth. Antibiotic therapy is mandatory for all patients undergoing surgery for intestinal obstruction.

Surgical treatment

The timing of surgical intervention is dependent on the clinical picture. There are several indications for early surgical intervention (Summary box 70.12).

Summary box 70.12

Indications for early surgical intervention

- Obstructed external hernia
- Clinical features suspicious of intestinal strangulation
- Obstruction in a 'virgin' abdomen

The classic clinical advice that 'the sun should not both rise and set' on a case of unrelieved acute intestinal obstruction was based on the concern that intestinal ischaemia would develop while the patient was waiting for surgery. If there is complete obstruction, but no evidence of intestinal ischaemia, it is reasonable to defer surgery until the patient has been adequately resuscitated. Where obstruction is likely to be secondary to adhesions, conservative management may be continued for up to 72 hours in the hope of spontaneous resolution.

If the site of obstruction is unknown, adequate exposure is best achieved by a midline incision. Assessment is directed to:

- the site of obstruction;
- the nature of the obstruction;
- the viability of the gut.

In cases of small bowel obstruction, the first manoeuvre is to deliver the distended small bowel into the wound. This permits access to the site of obstruction. The small bowel should be covered with moist swabs and the weight of the fluid-filled bowel supported such that the blood supply to the mesentery is not impaired.

Operative decompression should be performed whenever possible. This reduces pressure on the abdominal wound reducing pain and improving diaphragmatic movement. The simplest and safest method is to insert a large bore orogastric tube and to milk the small bowel contents in a retrograde manner to the stomach for aspiration. All volumes of fluid removed should be accurately measured and appropriately replaced. It is important to ensure that the stomach is empty at the end of the procedure to prevent postoperative aspiration.

Rarely, decompression using Savage's decompressor within a seromuscular purse-string suture may be required. Its benefits should be balanced against the potential risk of septic complications from spillage and the risk of leakage from the suture line postoperatively. The type of surgical procedure required will depend upon the cause of obstruction – division of adhesions (enterolysis), excision, bypass or proximal decompression.

Following relief of obstruction, the viability of the involved bowel should be carefully assessed (Table 70.3). Although frankly infarcted bowel is obvious, the viability status in many cases may be difficult to discern. If in doubt, the bowel should be wrapped in hot packs for 10 minutes with increased oxygenation and then reassessed. The state of the mesenteric vessels and pulsation in adjacent arcades should be sought. Viability is also confirmed by colour, sheen and peristalsis. If at the end of this period, there is still uncertainty about gut viability, the gut should be resected if this does not result in short bowel syndrome. If the patient is septic such that they require inotropic therapy or would require postoperative level 3 intensive care treatment following resection, consideration should be given to raising both ends of the bowel as stomas. This is not only safe, but also allows regular assessment of the bowel.

Intestinal ischaemia/reperfusion injury has been described following reperfusion of ischaemic bowel with remote lung injury resulting from the release of inflammatory mediators. This should be borne in mind when dealing with ischaemic bowel. For example, if there is a volvulus with established infarction, detorsion should be avoided until the affected mesentery has been clamped and thus reperfusion injury prevented. When no resection has been undertaken or there are multiple ischaemic areas (mesenteric vascular occlusion), a second-look laparotomy at 24–48 hours may be required.

Special attention should always be paid to the sites of constriction at each end of an obstructed segment. If of doubtful viability they should be infolded by the use of a seromuscular suture and can also be covered with omentum (Figures 70.14 and 70.15).

The surgical management of massive infarction is dependent on the patient's overall prognostic criteria. In the elderly, infarction of the small bowel from the duodenojejunal flexure to the right colon may be considered incurable, whereas in the young, with the potential for long-term intravenous alimentation and small bowel transplantation, a policy of excision may be justified.

Whenever the small bowel is resected, the exact site of resection, the length of the resected segment and that of the residual bowel should be recorded.

Table 70.3 Differentiation between viable and non-viable intestine.

	Viable	Non-viable
Circulation	Dark colour becomes lighter	Dark colour remains
	Visible pulsation in mesenteric arteries	No detectable pulsation
General appearance	Shiny	Dull and lustreless
Intestinal musculature	Firm	Flabby, thin and friable
	Peristalsis may be observed	No peristalsis

Paul Thwaites Savage, formerly surgeon, The Whittington Hospital, London, UK.

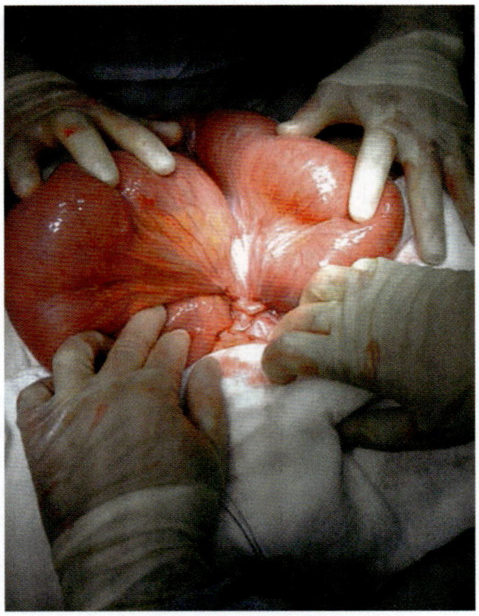

Figure 70.14 Band adhesion causing closed-loop obstruction.

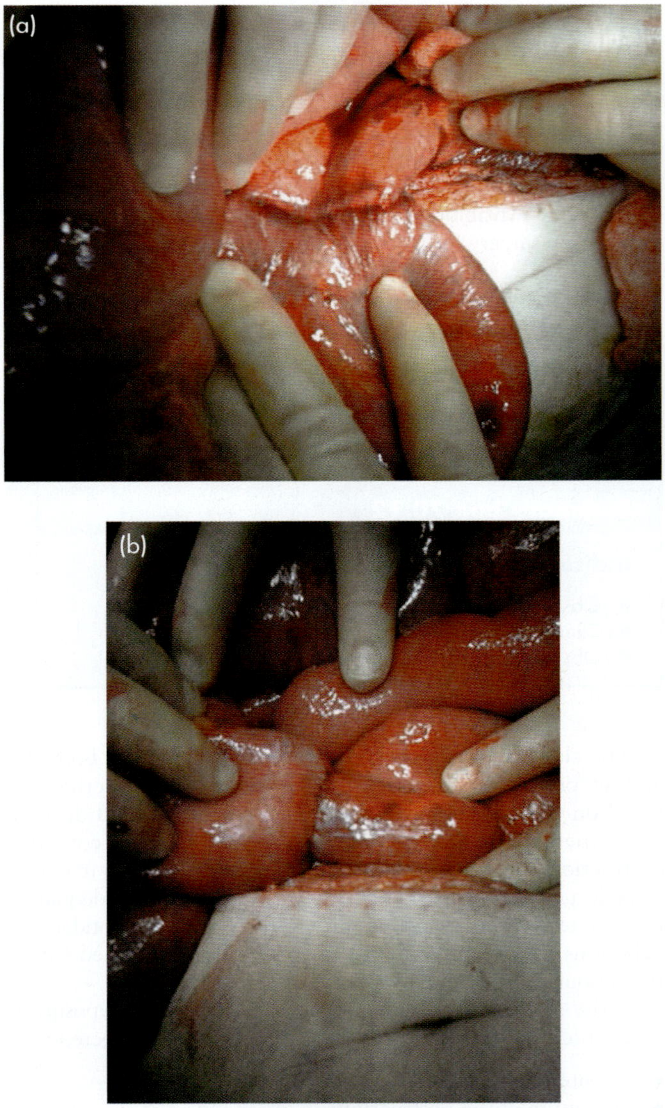

Figure 70.15 (a,b) Wall injury resulting from band compression, oversewn with an absorbable seromuscular suture.

As laparoscopic surgery is now so common, it is important to note that small bowel obstruction and strangulation occur in relation to port site hernias. The risk of port site herniation is related to older age, higher body mass, trocar diameter and extension of the port site for tissue extraction. For laparoscopic cholecystectomy, the hernia rate is reported to be around 2 per cent. Obstruction and strangulation have even been reported through 5-mm port sites. Complications from these hernias may present in the early postoperative period and as a Richter's hernia. They can be easily overlooked and careful examination of port sites in patients with small bowel obstruction is essential.

Treatment of adhesions

Initial management is based on intravenous rehydration and nasogastric decompression; occasionally, this treatment is curative. Although an initial conservative regimen is considered appropriate, regular assessment is mandatory to ensure that strangulation does not occur. Conservative treatment should not usually be prolonged beyond 72 hours.

When laparotomy is required, although multiple adhesions may be found, only one may be causative. If there is absolute certainty that this is the cause of the obstruction, this should be divided and the remaining adhesions can be left *in situ* unless severe angulation is present. Division of these adhesions will only cause further adhesion formation.

When obstruction is caused by an area of multiple adhesions, the adhesions should be freed by sharp dissection from the duodeno-jejunal junction to the caecum. Following the release of band obstruction, the constriction sites that have suffered direct compression should be carefully assessed and, if they show residual colour changes, invaginated with a seromuscular suture (Figure 70.15).

Laparoscopic adhesiolysis may be considered in highly selected cases of small bowel obstruction (Summary box 70.13). This is classed as an advanced laparoscopic procedure and should only be undertaken by surgeons with advanced laparoscopic skills.

Summary box 70.13

Treatment of adhesive obstruction

- Initially treat conservatively provided there are no signs of strangulation; should rarely continue conservative treatment for longer than 72 hours
- At operation, divide only the causative adhesion(s) and limit dissection
- Repair serosal tears; invaginate (or resect) areas of doubtful viability
- Laparoscopic adhesiolysis in the hands of advanced laparoscopic practitioners

Treatment of recurrent intestinal obstruction caused by adhesions

Several procedures may be considered in the presence of recurrent obstruction including:

- repeat adhesiolysis (enterolysis) alone;
- Noble's plication operation;
- Charles–Phillips transmesenteric plication;
- intestinal intubation.

The latter three operations are now very rarely performed and can probably be consigned to the history books (they have never been required by the author).

Postoperative intestinal obstruction

Differentiation between persistent paralytic ileus and early mechanical obstruction may be difficult in the early postoperative period. Mechanical obstruction is more likely if the patient has regained bowel function postoperatively which subsequently stops. Obstruction is usually incomplete and the majority settle with continued conservative management. Postoperative intra-abdominal sepsis is a potent cause of postoperative obstruction; CT scanning with oral contrast is of particular value in the assessment of the postoperative abdomen. A water-soluble contrast agent (50–100 mL) by mouth with a delayed plain abdominal x-ray is also of value (see p. 1189).

Treatment of intussusception

In the infant with ileocolic intussusception, after resuscitation with intravenous fluids, broad-spectrum antibiotics and nasogastric drainage, non-operative reduction can be attempted using an air or barium enema (see Chapter 8, Figure 6.17). Successful reduction can only be accepted if there is free reflux of air or barium into the small bowel, together with resolution of symptoms and signs in the patient. Non-operative reduction is contraindicated if there are signs of peritonitis or perforation, there is a known pathological lead point or in the presence of profound shock. In experienced units, more than 70 per cent of intussusceptions can be reduced non-operatively. Strangulated bowel and pathological lead points are unlikely to reduce. Perforation of the colon during pneumatic or hydrostatic reduction is a recognised hazard, but is rare. Recurrent intussusception occurs in up to 10 per cent of patients after non-operative reduction.

Surgery is required when radiological reduction has failed or is contraindicated. After resuscitation, a transverse right-sided abdominal incision provides good access. Reduction is achieved by gently compressing the most distal part of the intussusception toward its origin (Figure 70.16), making sure not to pull. The last part of the reduction is the most difficult (Figure 70.17). After reduction, the terminal part of the small bowel and the appendix will be seen to be bruised and oedematous. The viability of the whole bowel should be checked carefully. An irreducible intussusception or one complicated by infarction or a pathological lead point requires resection and primary anastomosis.

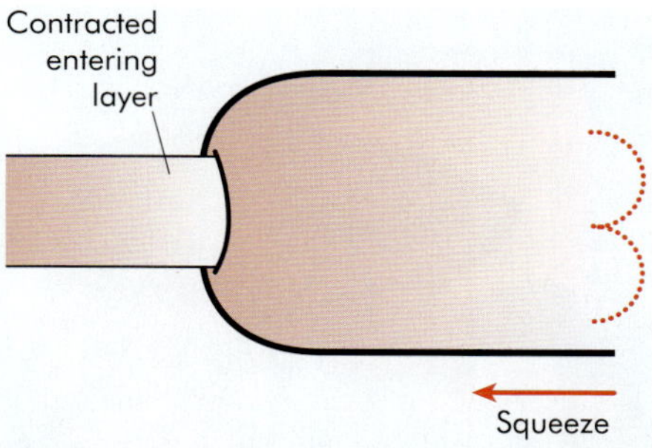

Figure 70.16 Diagram showing the method used to reduce an intussusception.

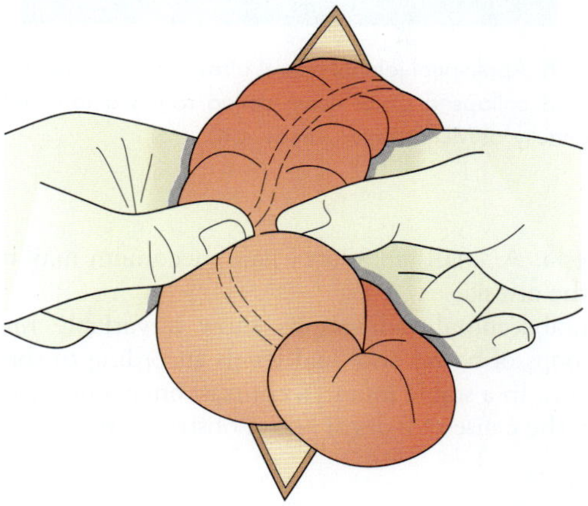

Figure 70.17 Reducing the terminal part of the intussusception (after RE Gross).

Acute intestinal obstruction of the newborn

Neonatal intestinal obstruction has many potential causes. Congenital atresia and stenosis are the most common. Intestinal malrotation with midgut volvulus, meconium ileus, Hirschsprung's disease, imperforate anus, necrotising enterocolitis and an incarcerated inguinal hernia may also be responsible. Many of these conditions are discussed in Chapter 8.

Intestinal atresia

Duodenal atresia and stenosis are the most common forms of intestinal obstruction in the newborn (see Chapter 8). Jejunal or ileal atresias are next in frequency, whereas colonic atresia is rare. The possibility of multiple atresias makes intraoperative assessment of the whole small and large bowel mandatory. As with all congenital anomalies, associated malformations are common and should be excluded.

There are four main types of jejunal/ileal atresia, ranging from an obstructing membrane with continuity of the bowel wall, through blind-ended segments of bowel separated by a fibrous cord or V-shaped mesenteric defect (including the so-called apple-peel atresia) (Figure 70.18), to multiple atresias ('string of sausages'). The obstructed proximal bowel is at risk of perforation, which may happen prenatally causing meconium peritonitis in the fetus.

Small bowel atresias present with intestinal obstruction soon after birth. Bilious vomiting is the dominant feature in jejunal atresia, whereas abdominal distension is more prominent with

Thomas Benjamin Noble, 1895–1965, surgeon, The Community Hospital, Indianapolis, IN, USA.
Richard V Phillips, surgeon, Albuquerque, NM, USA.
Friedrich Oskar Witzel, 1856–1925, a surgeon in Bonn, Germany.

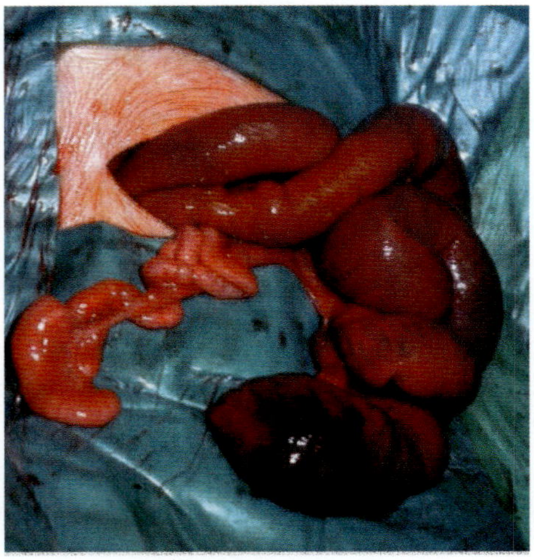

Figure 70.18 Apple-peel jejunal bowel atresia with obstructed proximal jejunum and collapsed distal ileum coiled round a remnant ileocolic artery (courtesy of MD Stringer, Leeds, UK).

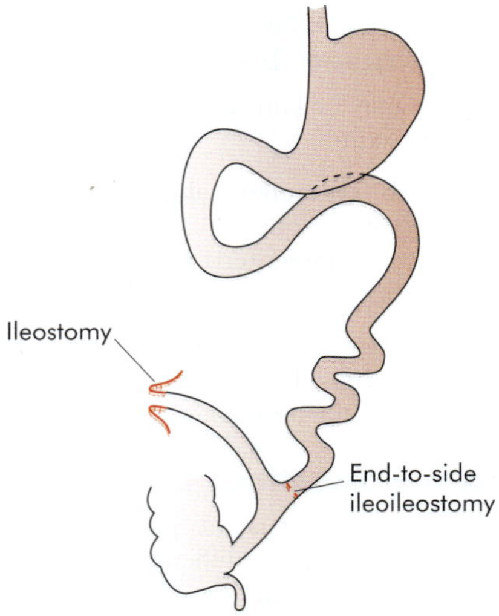

Figure 70.19 Bishop–Koop operation. This shows the completed procedure after grossly distended ileum has been resected. Because intestinal continuity is preserved, early closure of the ileostomy is not essential.

ileal atresia. A small amount of pale meconium may be passed despite the atresia.

Plain abdominal radiographs show a variable number of dilated loops of bowel and fluid levels according to the level of obstruction. In a stable infant, a contrast enema may be required to clarify the cause of a distal bowel obstruction.

Surgery

Duodenal atresia is corrected by a duodenoduodenostomy. In most cases of jejunal/ileal atresia, the distal end of the dilated proximal small bowel is resected and a primary end-to-end anastomosis is possible. If the proximal bowel is extremely dilated it may need to be tapered to the distal bowel before anastomosis. Occasionally, a temporary stoma is required before definitive repair.

Meconium ileus

Cystic fibrosis is almost always the underlying cause of this condition. Meconium is normally kept fluid by the action of pancreatic enzymes. In meconium ileus, the terminal ileum becomes filled with thick viscid meconium, resulting in progressive intestinal obstruction. A sterile meconium peritonitis may have occurred *in utero*.

Visibly dilated loops of bowel are often palpable in the newborn with meconium ileus. An abdominal radiograph may show a dilated small intestine with mottling. Fluid levels are generally not seen. Unlike ileal atresia there is no abrupt termination of the gas-filled intestine. A contrast enema shows an unused microcolon. As the condition is caused by an autosomal recessive genetic defect, a family history may not be present. Further assessment includes gene mutation analysis and, beyond the neonatal period, a sweat test, which shows elevated sodium and chloride levels (>70 mmol/L).

Uncomplicated meconium ileus may respond to treatment with a hyperosmolar gastrografin enema. This draws fluid into the gut lumen and also has detergent properties, which help to liquefy the meconium. Infants treated in this way need extra intravenous fluids to compensate for fluid shifts. Meconium ileus complicated by intestinal perforation, volvulus or atresia, or unresponsive to enemas, demands surgery. Various surgical procedures are used including intestinal resection and temporary stoma formation, resection and primary anastomosis, and, in uncomplicated cases, enterotomy and irrigation of the bowel. The Bishop–Koop operation (Figure 70.19) with its irrigating stoma is now only rarely used.

TREATMENT OF ACUTE LARGE BOWEL OBSTRUCTION

Large bowel obstruction is usually caused by an underlying carcinoma or occasionally diverticular disease, and presents in an acute or chronic form. The condition of pseudo-obstruction should always be considered and excluded by a limited contrast study or CT scan to confirm organic obstruction.

After full resuscitation, the abdomen should be opened through a midline incision. Care should be taken to ensure that the loss of tamponade of the abdominal wall does not lead to increased caecal distension and rupture (this starts with splitting along the line of the taenia coli on the antimesenteric border). Distension of the caecum will confirm large bowel involvement. Identification of a collapsed distal segment of the large bowel and its sequential proximal assessment will readily lead to identification of the cause. As surgery for malignant bowel cancer is technically challenging, wherever possible a suitably trained surgeon should perform the procedure. When a removable lesion is found in the caecum, ascending colon, hepatic flexure or proximal transverse colon, an emergency right hemicolectomy should be performed. A primary anastomosis is safe if the patient's general condition is reasonable. If the lesion is irremovable (this is rarely the case), a proximal stoma (colostomy or ileosotomy if the ileocaecal valve is incompetent) or ileotransverse bypass should be considered. Obstructing lesions at the splenic flexure should be treated by an extended right hemicolectomy with ileo-descending colonic anastomosis.

For obstructing lesions of the left colon or rectosigmoid junction, immediate resection should be considered unless there are clear contraindications (Summary box 70.14).

Summary box 70.14

Management of left-sided large bowel obstruction

Contraindications to immediate resection include:

- Inexperienced surgeon
- Moribund patient
- Advanced disease

In rare instances, or when caecal perforation is imminent, additional time to improve the patient's clinical condition can be bought by performing an emergency caecostomy (or ileosotomy in the presence of an incompetent ileocaecal valve).

In the absence of senior clinical staff, it is safest to bring the proximal colon to the surface as a colostomy. When possible, the distal bowel should be brought out at the same time (Paul–Mikulicz procedure) to facilitate subsequent closure. In the majority of cases, the distal bowel will not reach and is closed and returned to the abdomen (Hartmann's procedure). A second-stage colorectal anastomosis can be planned when the patient is fit.

If an anastomosis is to be considered using the proximal colon, in the presence of obstruction, it must be decompressed and cleaned by an on-table colonic lavage.

Decompression of the obstructed left colon using endoscopically placed stents often as a bridge to surgery has been widely reported. However, as yet randomised trials have not shown improved outcomes compared to standard surgical treatment (Figure 70.20).

Treatment of caecal volvulus

At operation, the volvulus is usually found to be ischaemic and needs resection. If, viable, the volvulus should be reduced. Sometimes, this can only be achieved after decompression of the caecum using a needle. Further management consists of fixation of the caecum to the right iliac fossa (caecopexy) and/or a caecostomy. Recurrence of volvulus after caecopexy has been reported in up to 40 per cent of cases.

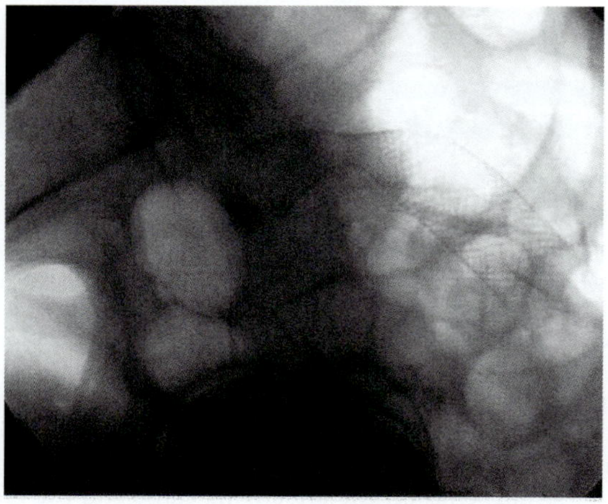

Figure 70.20 X-ray of stent inserted for malignant colonic obstruction.

Treatment of sigmoid volvulus

Flexible sigmoidoscopy or rigid sigmoidoscopy and insertion of a flatus tube should be carried out to allow deflation of the gut. The tube should be secured in place with tape for 24 hours and a repeat x-ray taken to ensure that decompression has occurred. Successful deflation, as long as ischaemic bowel is excluded, will resolve the acute problem.

In young patients, an elective sigmoid colectomy is required. It is reasonable not to offer any further treatment following successful endoscopic decompression in the elderly as there is a high death rate (~80 per cent at two years) from causes other than recurrent volvulus. In elderly patients with comorbidities and recurrent episodes of volvulus, the options are resection or two point fixation with combined endoscopic/percutaneous tube insertion (gastrostomy tubes are frequently used for this purpose). Failure results in an early laparotomy, with untwisting of the loop and per anum decompression (Figure 70.21). When the bowel is viable, fixation of the sigmoid colon to the posterior abdominal wall may be a safer manoeuvre in inexperienced hands. Resection is preferable if it can be achieved

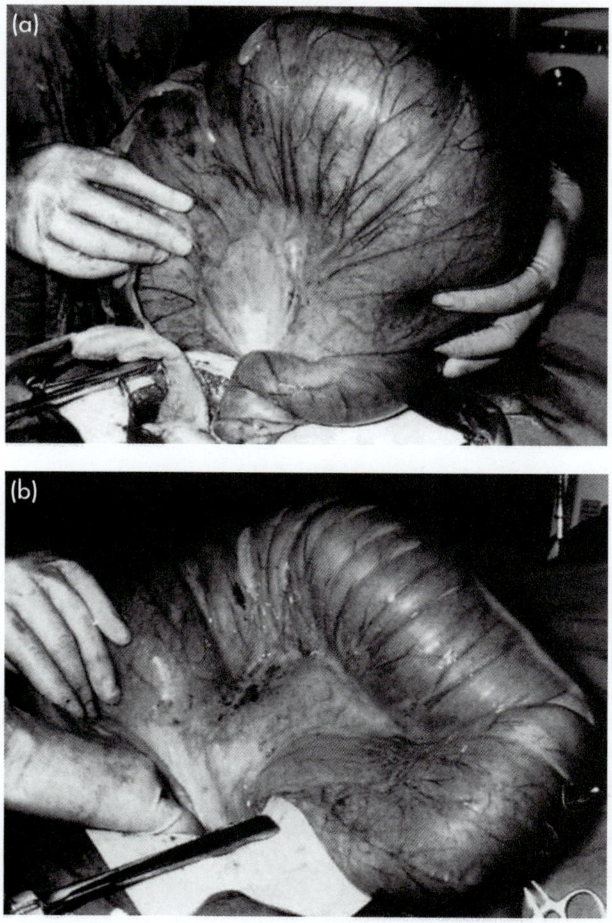

Figure 70.21 Volvulus of the sigmoid colon (a) before and (b) after untwisting (courtesy of SU Rahman, Manchester, UK).

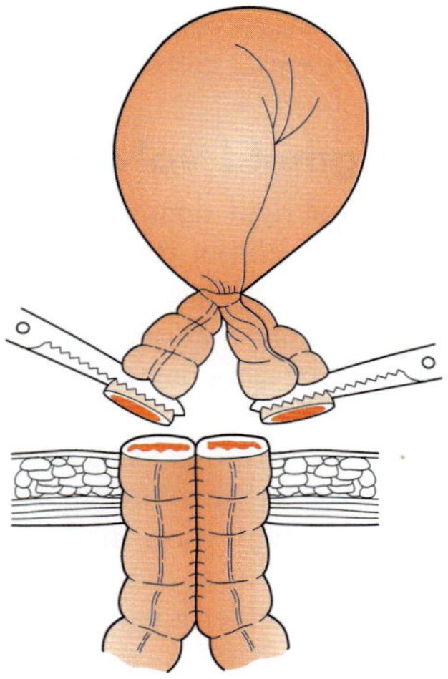

Figure 70.22 The Paul–Mikulicz operation applied to volvulus of the pelvic colon.

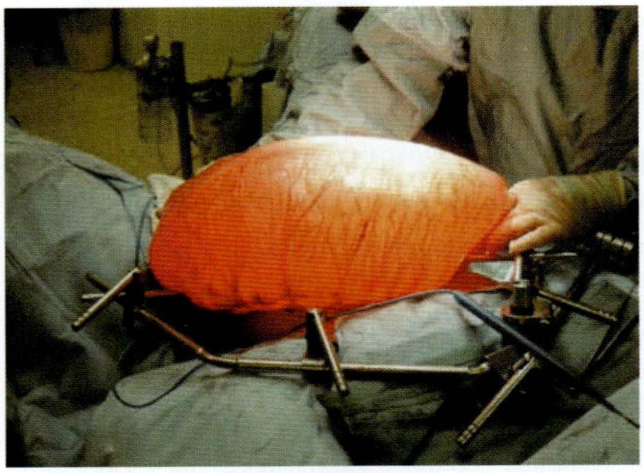

Figure 70.23 Gross functional distension.

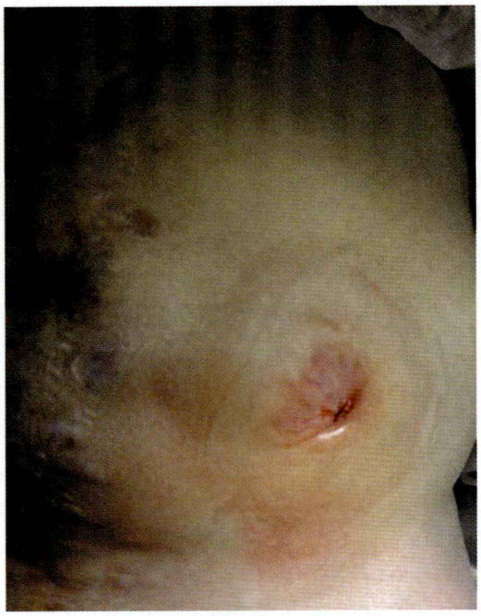

Figure 70.24 Stomal stenosis causing large bowel obstruction.

safely. A Paul–Mikulicz procedure is useful, particularly if there is suspicion of impending gangrene (Figure 70.22); an alternative procedure is a sigmoid colectomy and, when anastomosis is considered unwise, a Hartmann's procedure with subsequent reanastomosis can be carried out.

CHRONIC LARGE BOWEL OBSTRUCTION

The symptoms of chronic intestinal obstruction may arise from two sources – the cause and the subsequent obstruction.

The causes of obstruction may be organic:

- intraluminal (rare) – faecal impaction;
- intrinsic intramural – strictures (Crohn's disease, ischaemia, diverticular), anastomotic stenosis;
- extrinsic intramural (rare) – metastatic deposits (ovarian), endometriosis, stomal stenosis;

or functional:

- Hirschsprung's disease, idiopathic megacolon, pseudo-obstruction.

The symptoms of chronic obstruction differ in their predominance, timing and degree from acute obstruction. In functional cases, the symptoms may have been present for months or years. Constipation appears first. It is initially relative and then absolute, associated with distension. In the presence of large bowel disease, the point of greatest distension is in the caecum, and this is heralded by the onset of pain. Vomiting is a late feature and therefore dehydration is less severe. Examination is unremarkable, save for confirmation of distension (which can be profound) (Figure 70.23) and the onset of peritonism in late cases. Rectal examination may confirm the presence of faecal impaction or a tumour.

Investigation

Plain abdominal radiography confirms the presence of large bowel distension. All such cases should be investigated by a subsequent single-contrast water-soluble enema study, CT scan or endoscopic assessment to rule out functional disease (Summary box 70.15).

Summary box 70.15

Principles of investigation of possible large bowel obstruction

- In the presence of large bowel obstruction, a single contrast water-soluble enema or CT should be undertaken to exclude a functional cause

Organic disease requires decompression with either a laparotomy or stent. Stomal stenosis can usually be managed at the abdominal wall level (Figure 70.24). Surgical management after resuscitation depends on the underlying cause and the relevant chapters in this book should be consulted.

Frank Thomas Paul, 1851–1941, surgeon, The Royal Infirmary, Liverpool, UK.
Johann von Mikulicz-Radecki, 1850–1905, Professor of Surgery, Breslau, Germany (now Wroclaw, Poland).

Functional disease requires colonoscopic decompression in the first instance and conservative management. Intestinal perforation can occur in patients with functional obstruction. Those at risk have such gross distension that the abdomen is rigid on palpation (Figure 70.23).

ADYNAMIC OBSTRUCTION

Paralytic ileus

This may be defined as a state in which there is failure of transmission of peristaltic waves secondary to neuromuscular failure (i.e. in the myenteric (Auerbach's) and submucous (Meissner's) plexuses). The resultant stasis leads to accumulation of fluid and gas within the bowel, with associated distension, vomiting, absence of bowel sounds and absolute constipation.

Varieties

The following varieties are recognised:

- **Postoperative**. A degree of ileus usually occurs after any abdominal procedure and is self-limiting, with a variable duration of 24–72 hours. Postoperative ileus may be prolonged in the presence of hypoproteinaemia or metabolic abnormality (see below).
- **Infection**. Intra-abdominal sepsis may give rise to localised or generalised ileus.
- **Reflex ileus**. This may occur following fractures of the spine or ribs, retroperitoneal haemorrhage or even the application of a plaster jacket.
- **Metabolic**. Uraemia and hypokalaemia are the most common contributory factors.

Clinical features

Paralytic ileus takes on a clinical significance if, 72 hours after laparotomy:

- there has been no return of bowel sounds on auscultation;
- there has been no passage of flatus.

Abdominal distension becomes more marked and tympanitic. Colicky pain is not a feature. Distension increases pain from the abdominal wound. In the absence of gastric aspiration, effortless vomiting may occur. Radiologically, the abdomen shows gas-filled loops of intestine with multiple fluid levels (if an erect film is felt necessary).

Management

Nasogastric tubes are not required routinely after elective intra-abdominal surgery. Paralytic ileus is managed with the use of nasogastric suction and restriction of oral intake until bowel sounds and the passage of flatus return. Electrolyte balance must be maintained. The use of an enhanced recovery programme with early introduction of fluids and solids is, however, becoming increasingly popular.

Specific treatment is directed towards the cause, but the following general principles apply:

- If a primary cause is identified, this must be treated.
- Gastrointestinal distension must be relieved by decompression.
- Close attention to fluid and electrolyte balance is essential.
- There is no place for the routine use of peristaltic stimulants. Rarely, in resistant cases, medical therapy with a gastroprokinetic agent, such as domperidone or erythromycin may be used, provided that an intraperitoneal cause has been excluded.
- If paralytic ileus is prolonged, CT scanning is the most effective investigation; it will demonstrate any intra-abdominal sepsis or mechanical obstruction and therefore guide any requirement for laparotomy. Otherwise the decision to take a patient back to theatre in these circumstances is always difficult. The need for a laparotomy becomes increasingly likely the longer the bowel inactivity persists, particularly if it lasts for more than 7 days or if bowel activity recommences following surgery and then stops again.

Pseudo-obstruction

This condition describes an obstruction, usually of the colon, that occurs in the absence of a mechanical cause or acute intra-abdominal disease. It is associated with a variety of syndromes in which there is an underlying neuropathy and/or myopathy and a range of other factors (Summary box 70.16).

Summary box 70.16

Factors associated with pseudo-obstruction

- Metabolic
  - Diabetes
  - Hypokalaemia
  - Uraemia
  - Myxodoema
  - Intermittent porphyria
- Severe trauma (especially to the lumbar spine and pelvis)
- Shock
  - Burns
  - Myocardial infarction
  - Stroke
  - Idiopathic
  - Septicaemia
  - Postoperative (for example, fractured neck of femur)
- Retroperitoneal irritation
  - Blood
  - Urine
  - Enzymes (pancreatitis)
  - Tumour
- Drugs
  - Tricyclic antidepressants
  - Phenothiazines
  - Laxatives
- Secondary gastrointestinal involvement
  - Scleroderma
  - Chagas' disease

Small intestinal pseudo-obstruction

This condition may be primary (i.e. idiopathic or associated with familial visceral myopathy) or secondary. The clinical picture consists of recurrent subacute obstruction. The diagnosis is made by the exclusion of a mechanical cause. Treatment consists of initial correction of any underlying disorder. Metoclopramide and erythromycin may be of use.

Leopold Auerbach, 1828–1897, Professor of Neuropathology, Breslau, Germany (now Wroclaw, Poland), described the myenteric plexus in 1862.
Georg Meissner, 1829–1905, Professor of Physiology, Gottingen, Germany, described the submucous plexus of the alimentary tract in 1852.
Carlos Justiniano Ribeiro Chagas, 1879–1934, Director of The Oswald Cruz Institute, and Professor of Tropical Medicine, The University of Rio de Janeiro, Brazil.
Sir William Heneage Ogilvie, 1887–1971, surgeon, Guy's Hospital, London, UK, reported his syndrome in 1948.

Colonic pseudo-obstruction

This may occur in an acute or a chronic form. The former, also known as Ogilvie's syndrome, presents as acute large bowel obstruction. Abdominal radiographs show evidence of colonic obstruction, with marked caecal distension being a common feature. Indeed, caecal perforation is a well-recognised complication. The absence of a mechanical cause requires urgent confirmation by colonoscopy or a single-contrast water-soluble barium enema or CT. Once confirmed, pseudo-obstruction requires treatment of any identifiable cause. If this is ineffective, intravenous neostigmine should be given (1 mg intravenously), with a further 1 mg given intravenously within a few minutes if the first dose is ineffective. During this procedure, it is best to sit the patient on a commode. ECG monitoring is required and atropine should be available. If neostigmine is not effective, colonoscopic decompression should be performed. Caecal perforation can occur in pseudo-obstruction. Abdominal examination should pay attention to tenderness and peritonism over the caecum and as with mechanical obstruction, caecal perforation is more likely if the caecal diameter is 14 cm or greater. Surgery is associated with high morbidity and mortality and should be reserved for those with impending perforation when other treatments have failed or perforation has occurred.

Rarely, an endoscopically placed tube colostomy is used as a vent for patients with those with a chronic unremitting condition.

FURTHER READING

Becker JM, Stucchi AF. Intra-abdominal adhesion prevention: are we getting any closer? *Ann Surg* 2004; **240**: 202–4.

Bickell NA, Federman AD, Aufses AH. Influence of time on risk of bowel resection in complete small bowel obstruction. *J Am Coll Surg* 2005; **201**: 847–54.

Branco BC, Barmparas G, Schnuriger B *et al.* Systematic review and meta-analyis of the diagnostic and therapeutic role of water-soluble contrast agent in adhesive small bowel obstruction. *Br J Surg* 2010; **97**: 470–8.

Fazio VW, Cohen Z, Fleshman JW *et al.* Reduction in adhesive small-bowel obstruction by Seprafilm (R) stop adhesion barrier after intestinal resection. *Dis Colon Rectum* 2006; **49**: 1–11.

Fevang BT, Fevang J, Lie SA *et al.* Long-term prognosis after operation for adhesive small bowel obstruction. *Ann Surg* 2004; **240**: 193–201.

Raveenthiran V, Madiba TE, Atamanalp SS. Volvulus of the sigmoid colon. *Colorectal Dis* 2010; **12**: 1–17.

Sajja SB, Schein M. Early postoperative small bowel obstruction. *Br J Surg* 2004; **91**: 683–91.

Williams SB, Greenspon J, Young HA, Orkin BA. Small bowel obstruction: conservative vs. surgical management. *Dis Colon Rectum* 2005; **48**: 1140–6.

CHAPTER 71

The vermiform appendix

LEARNING OBJECTIVES

To understand:

- The aetiology and surgical anatomy of acute appendicitis
- The clinical signs and differential diagnoses of appendicitis
- The investigation of suspected appendicitis
- Evolving concepts in management of acute appendicitis
- Basic surgical techniques, both open and laparoscopic
- The management of postoperative problems
- Less common conditions encountered

INTRODUCTION

The vermiform appendix is considered by most to be a vestigial organ; its importance in surgery results only from its propensity for inflammation, which results in the clinical syndrome known as 'acute appendicitis'. Acute appendicitis is the most common cause of an 'acute abdomen' in young adults and, as such, the associated symptoms and signs have become a paradigm for clinical teaching. Appendicitis is sufficiently common that appendicectomy (termed 'appendectomy' in North America) is the most frequently performed urgent abdominal operation and is often the first major procedure performed by a surgeon in training. Advances in modern radiographic imaging have improved diagnostic accuracy, however the diagnosis of appendicitis remains essentially clinical, requiring a mixture of observation, clinical acumen and surgical science and as such it remains an enigmatic challenge and a reminder of the art of surgical diagnosis.

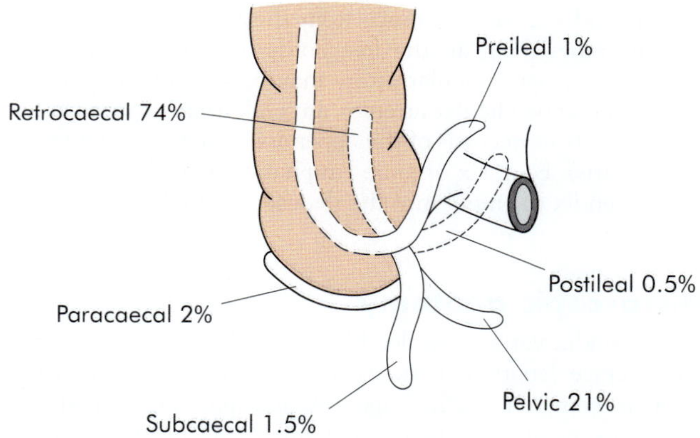

Figure 71.1 The various positions of the appendix (after Sir C Wakeley, London, formerly PRCS).

ANATOMY

The vermiform appendix is present only in humans, certain anthropoid apes and the wombat. It is a blind muscular tube with mucosal, submucosal, muscular and serosal layers. Morphologically, it is the undeveloped distal end of the large caecum found in many lower animals. At birth, the appendix is short and broad at its junction with the caecum, but differential growth of the caecum produces the typical tubular structure by about the age of two years (Condon). During childhood, continued growth of the caecum commonly rotates the appendix into a retrocaecal but intraperitoneal position (Figure 71.1). In approximately one quarter of cases, rotation of the appendix does not occur, resulting in a pelvic, subcaecal or paracaecal position. Occasionally, the tip of the appendix becomes extraperitoneal, lying behind the caecum or ascending colon. Rarely, the caecum does not migrate during development to its normal position in the right lower quadrant of the abdomen. In these circumstances, the appendix can be found near the gall bladder or, in the case of intestinal malrotation, in the left iliac fossa, causing diagnostic difficulty if appendicitis develops (Figure 71.2).

The position of the base of the appendix is constant, being found at the confluence of the three taeniae coli of the caecum, which fuse to form the outer longitudinal muscle coat of the appendix. At operation, use can be made of this to find an elusive appendix, as gentle traction on the taeniae coli, particularly the anterior taenia, will lead the operator to the base of the appendix.

The mesentery of the appendix or mesoappendix arises from the lower surface of the mesentery or the terminal ileum and is itself subject to great variation. Sometimes, as much as the

A **wombat** is a nocturnal burrowing Australian marsupial.
Robert E Condon, contemporary, Emeritus Professor of Surgery, The Medical College of Wisconsin, WI, USA.

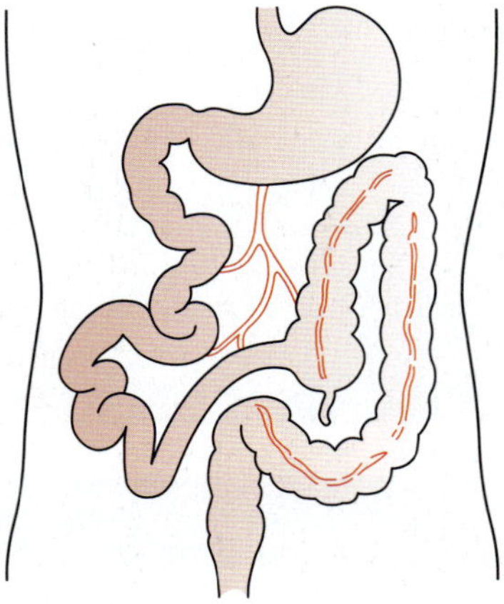

Figure 71.2 Left-sided caecum and appendix due to intestinal malrotation (after Findley and Humphreys).

distal one-third of the appendix is bereft of mesoappendix. Especially in childhood, the mesoappendix is so transparent that the contained blood vessels can be seen (Figure 71.3). In many adults, it becomes laden with fat, which obscures these vessels. The appendicular artery, a branch of the lower division of the ileocolic artery, passes behind the terminal ileum to enter the mesoappendix a short distance from the base of the appendix. It then comes to lie in the free border of the mesoappendix. An accessory appendicular artery may be present but, in most people, the appendicular artery is an 'end-artery', thrombosis of which results in necrosis of the appendix (synonym: gangrenous appendicitis). Four, six or more lymphatic channels traverse the mesoappendix to empty into the ileocaecal lymph nodes.

Microscopic anatomy

The appendix varies considerably in length and circumference. The average length is between 7.5 and 10 cm. The lumen is irregular, being encroached upon by multiple longitudinal folds of mucous membrane lined by columnar cell intestinal mucosa of colonic type (Figure 71.4). Crypts are present, but are not numerous. In the base of the crypts lie argentaffin cells

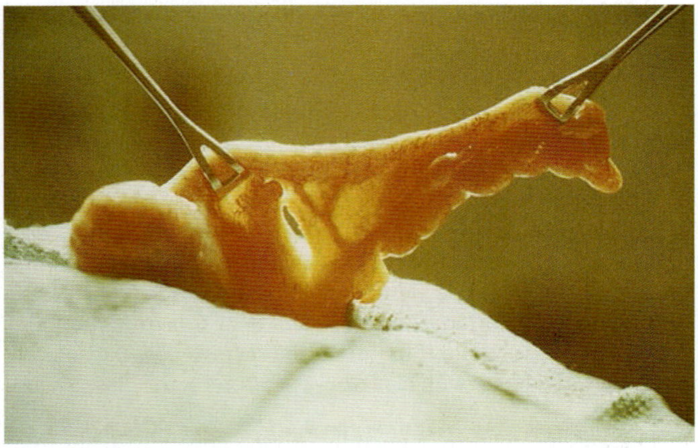

Figure 71.3 Mesoappendix displayed demonstrating the appendicular artery.

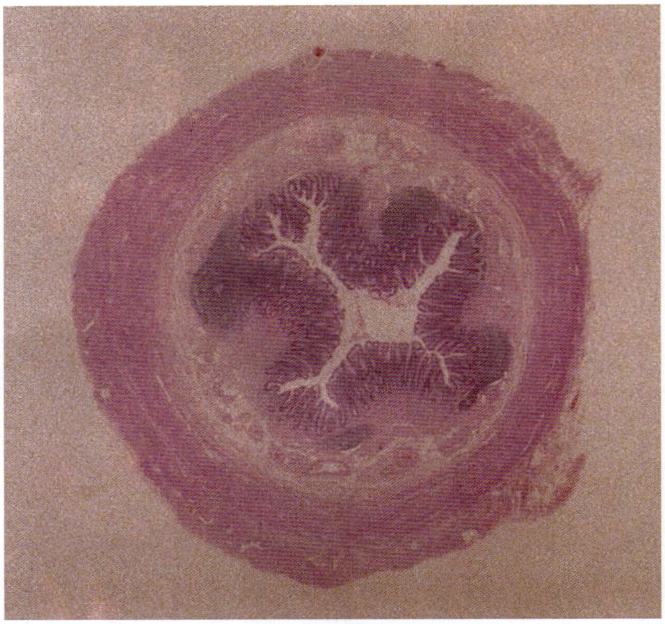

Figure 71.4 Normal vermiform appendix. The narrow lumen is bounded by mucosa which may be arranged in folds. There is usually abundant lymphoid tissue in the mucosa, especially in younger individuals. This may encroach on and further narrow the lumen. The mucosa is bounded by a relatively thin muscularis mucosa (courtesy of Dr P Kelly, FRCPath, Dublin, Ireland).

(Kulchitsky cells), which may give rise to carcinoid tumours (see below under Carcinoid tumours). The appendix is the most frequent site for carcinoid tumours, which may present with appendicitis due to occlusion of the appendiceal lumen. The submucosa contains numerous lymphatic aggregations or follicles. While no discernible change in immune function results from appendicectomy, the prominence of lymphatic tissue in the appendix of young adults seems to be important in the aetiology of appendicitis (see below under Aetiology).

ACUTE APPENDICITIS

While there are isolated reports of perityphlitis (fatal inflammation of the caecal region) from the late 1500s, recognition of acute appendicitis as a clinical entity is attributed to Reginald Fitz, who presented a paper to the first meeting of the Association of American Physicians in 1886 entitled 'Perforating inflammation of the vermiform appendix'. Soon afterwards, Charles McBurney described the clinical manifestations of acute appendicitis including the point of maximum tenderness in the right iliac fossa that now bears his name.

The incidence of appendicitis seems to have risen greatly in the first half of the twentieth century, particularly in Europe, America and Australasia, with up to 16 per cent of the population undergoing appendicectomy. In the past 30 years, the

Nicolai Kulchitsky, 1856–1925, Professor of Histology, Krakov, Ukraine, who left Russia after the revolution of 1917, and later worked at University College, London. He described these cells in 1897.

Reginald Heber Fitz, 1843–1913, Professor of Medicine, Harvard University, Boston, MA, USA.

incidence has fallen dramatically in these countries, such that the individual lifetime risk of appendicectomy is 8.6 and 6.7 per cent among males and females, respectively.

Acute appendicitis is relatively rare in infants, and becomes increasingly common in childhood and early adult life, reaching a peak incidence in the teens and early 20s. After middle age, the risk of developing appendicitis is quite small. The incidence of appendicitis is equal among males and females before puberty. In teenagers and young adults, the male–female ratio increases to 3:2 at age 25; thereafter, the greater incidence in males declines.

Aetiology

There is no unifying hypothesis regarding the aetiology of acute appendicitis. Decreased dietary fibre and increased consumption of refined carbohydrates may be important. As with colonic diverticulitis, the incidence of appendicitis is lowest in societies with a high dietary fibre intake. In developing countries that are adopting a more refined western-type diet, the incidence continues to rise. This is in contrast to the dramatic decrease in the incidence of appendicitis in western countries observed in the past 30 years. No reason has been established for these paradoxical changes; however, improved hygiene and a change in the pattern of childhood gastrointestinal infection related to the increased use of antibiotics may be responsible.

While appendicitis is clearly associated with bacterial proliferation within the appendix, no single organism is responsible. A mixed growth of aerobic and anaerobic organisms is usual. The initiating event causing bacterial proliferation is controversial. Obstruction of the appendix lumen has been widely held to be important, and some form of luminal obstruction, either by a faecolith or a stricture, is found in the majority of cases.

A faecolith (sometimes referred to as an 'appendicolith') is composed of inspissated faecal material, calcium phosphates, bacteria and epithelial debris (Figure 71.5). Rarely, a foreign body is incorporated into the mass. The incidental finding of a faecolith is a relative indication for prophylactic appendicectomy or an interval appendicetomy in a patient treated conservatively (see below) (Figure 71.6). A fibrotic stricture of the appendix usually indicates previous appendicitis that resolved without surgical intervention (Figure 71.7). Obstruction of the appendiceal orifice by tumour, particularly carcinoma of the caecum, is an occasional cause of acute appendicitis in middle-aged and elderly patients. Intestinal parasites, particularly *Oxyuris vermicularis* (pinworm), can proliferate in the appendix and occlude the lumen.

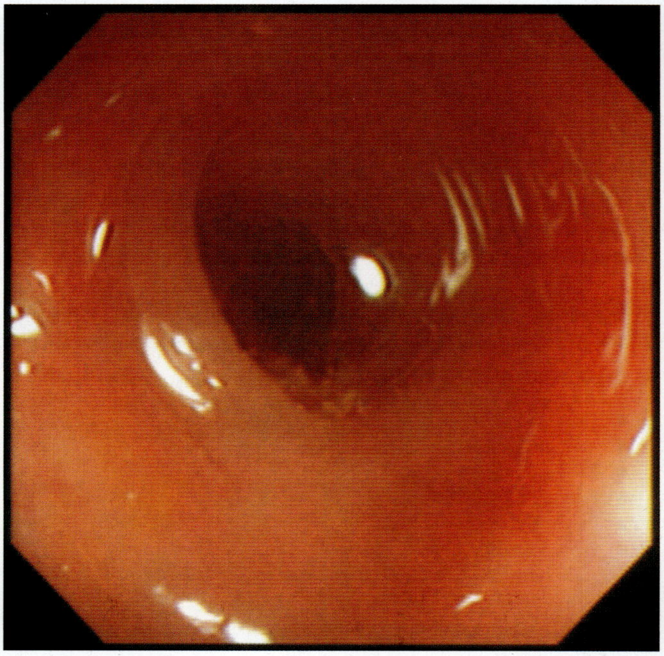

Figure 71.5 Colonoscopic view of the lumen of the appendix showing intraluminal debris (courtesy of Professor D Winter, FRCSI, Dublin, Ireland).

Pathology

Obstruction of the appendiceal lumen seems to be essential for the development of appendiceal gangrene and perforation. Yet, in many cases of early appendicitis, the appendix lumen is patent despite the presence of mucosal inflammation and lymphoid hyperplasia. Occasional clustering of cases among children and young adults suggests an infective agent, possibly viral, which initiates an inflammatory response. Seasonal variation in the incidence is also observed, with more cases occurring between May and August in Northern Europe than at other times of the year.

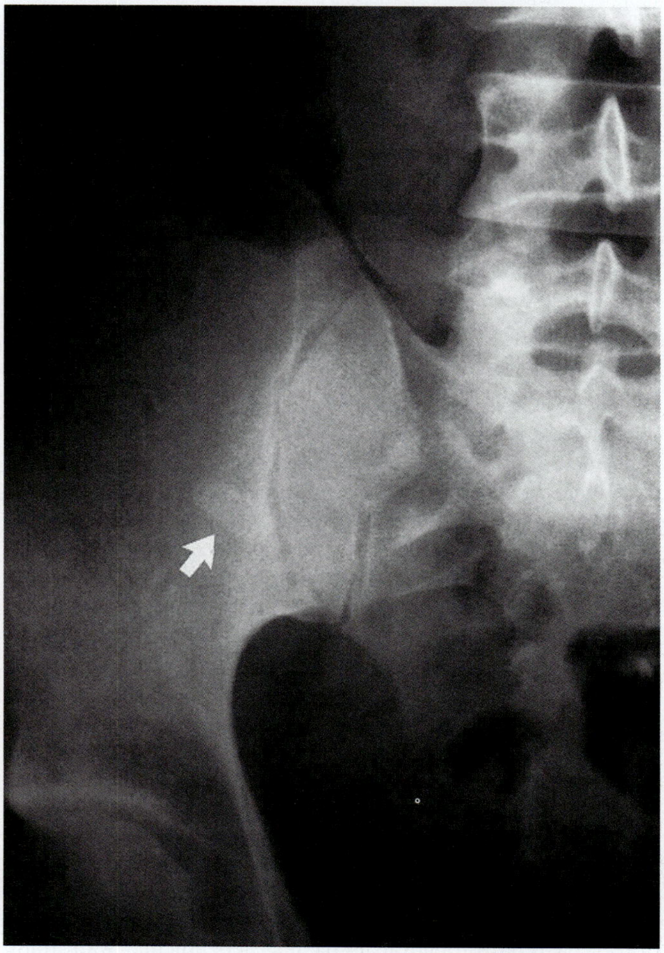

Figure 71.6 Supine abdominal radiograph showing the presence of a large faecolith in the right iliac fossa (arrow).

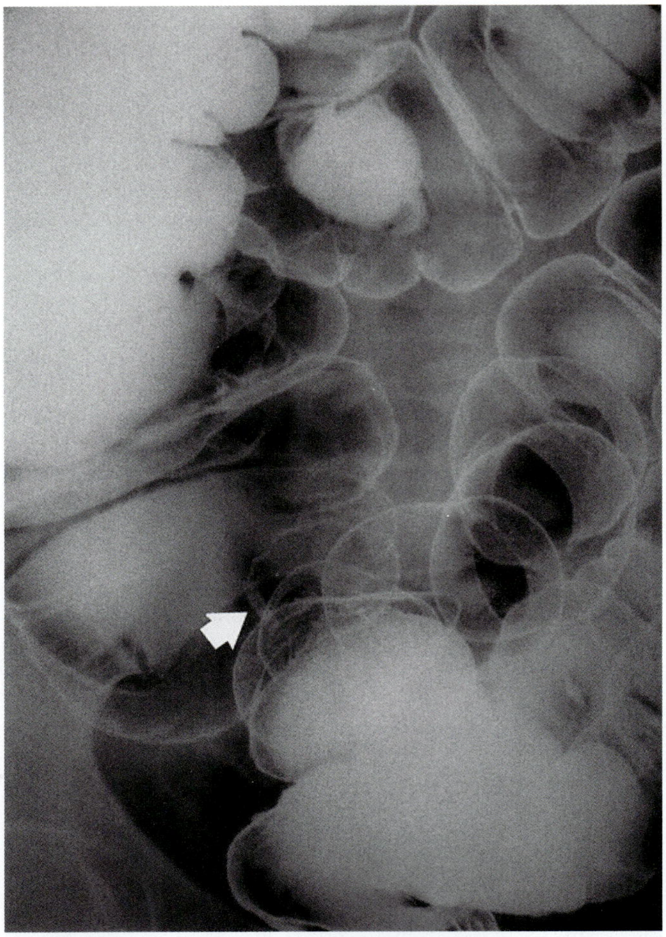

Figure 71.7 Barium enema radiograph demonstrating faecoliths of the appendix (arrow) with distal stricture of the appendix.

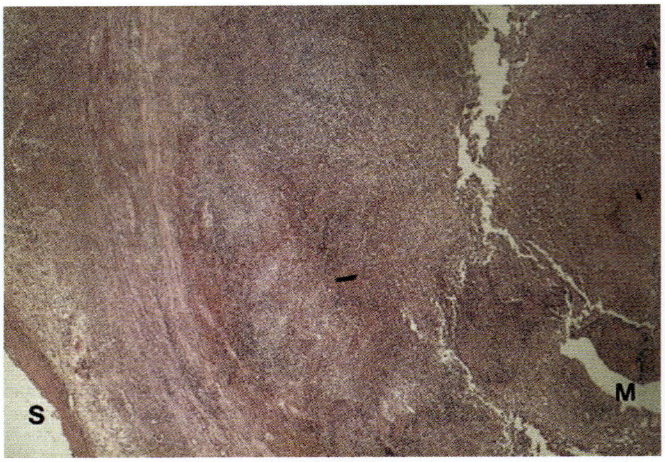

Figure 71.8 Acute appendicitis. A heavy acute inflammatory infiltrate extends through the full thickness of the wall of the appendix, destroying the mucosa, of which only a small island (M) remains, and the smooth muscle. The inflammation extends to involve the serosa (S) (courtesy of Dr P Kelly, FRCPath, Dublin, Ireland).

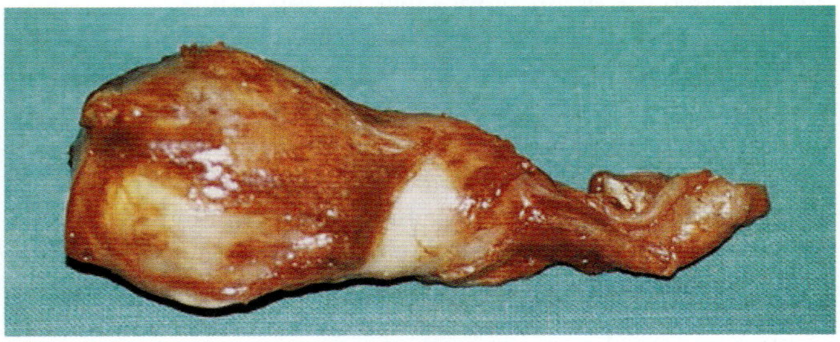

Figure 71.9 Mucocoele of the appendix, following excision.

Lymphoid hyperplasia narrows the lumen of the appendix, leading to luminal obstruction. Once obstruction occurs, continued mucus secretion and inflammatory exudation increase intraluminal pressure, obstructing lymphatic drainage. Oedema and mucosal ulceration develop with bacterial translocation to the submucosa. Resolution may occur at this point either spontaneously or in response to antibiotic therapy. If the condition progresses, further distension of the appendix may cause venous obstruction and ischaemia of the appendix wall. With ischaemia, bacterial invasion occurs through the muscularis propria and submucosa, producing acute appendicitis (Figure 71.8). Finally, ischaemic necrosis of the appendix wall produces gangrenous appendicitis, with free bacterial contamination of the peritoneal cavity. Alternatively, the greater omentum and loops of small bowel become adherent to the inflamed appendix, walling off the spread of peritoneal contamination, and resulting in a phlegmonous mass or paracaecal abscess. Rarely, appendiceal inflammation resolves, leaving a distended mucus-filled organ termed a 'mucocoele' of the appendix (Figure 71.9).

It is the potential for diffuse peritonitis that is the great threat of acute appendicitis. Peritonitis occurs as a result of free migration of bacteria through an ischaemic appendicular wall, frank perforation of a gangrenous appendix or delayed perforation of an appendix abscess. Factors that promote this process include extremes of age, immunosuppression, diabetes mellitus and faecolith obstruction of the appendix lumen, a free-lying pelvic appendix and previous abdominal surgery that limits the ability of the greater omentum to wall off the spread of peritoneal contamination. In these situations, a rapidly deteriorating clinical course is accompanied by signs of diffuse peritonitis and systemic sepsis syndrome (Summary box 71.1).

Summary box 71.1

Risk factors for perforation of the appendix

- Extremes of age
- Immunosuppression
- Diabetes mellitus
- Faecolith obstruction
- Pelvic appendix
- Previous abdominal surgery

Clinical diagnosis

History

The classical features of acute appendicitis begin with poorly localised colicky abdominal pain. This is due to midgut visceral discomfort in response to appendiceal inflammation and obstruction. The pain is frequently first noticed in the periumbilical region and is similar to, but less intense than, the colic of small bowel obstruction. Central abdominal pain is associated with anorexia, nausea and usually one or two episodes of vomiting that follow the onset of pain (Murphy). Anorexia is a useful and constant clinical feature, particularly in children. The patient often gives a history of similar discomfort that settled spontaneously. A family history is also useful as up to one-third of children with appendicitis have a first-degree relative with a similar history (Summary box 71.2).

Summary box 71.2

Symptoms of appendicitis

- Periumbilical colic
- Pain shifting to the right iliac fossa
- Anorexia
- Nausea

With progressive inflammation of the appendix, the parietal peritoneum in the right iliac fossa becomes irritated, producing more intense, constant and localised somatic pain that begins to predominate. Patients often report this as an abdominal pain that has shifted and changed in character. Typically, coughing or sudden movement exacerbates the right iliac fossa pain.

The classic visceral–somatic sequence of pain is present in only about half of those patients subsequently proven to have acute appendicitis. Atypical presentations include pain that is predominantly somatic or visceral and poorly localised. Atypical pain is more common in the elderly, in whom localisation to the right iliac fossa is unusual. An inflamed appendix in the pelvis may never produce somatic pain involving the anterior abdominal wall, but may instead cause suprapubic discomfort and tenesmus. In this circumstance, tenderness may be elicited only on rectal examination and is the basis for the recommendation that a rectal examination should be performed on every patient who presents with acute lower abdominal pain.

During the first 6 hours, there is rarely any alteration in temperature or pulse rate. After that time, slight pyrexia (37.2–37.7°C) with a corresponding increase in the pulse rate to 80 or 90 is usual. However, in 20 per cent of patients, there is no pyrexia or tachycardia in the early stages. In children, a temperature greater than 38.5°C suggests other causes, e.g. mesenteric adenitis (see below under Children).

Typically, two clinical syndromes of acute appendicitis can be discerned, **acute catarrhal (non-obstructive)** appendicitis and **acute obstructive** appendicitis, the latter characterised by a more acute course. The onset of symptoms is abrupt, and there may be generalised abdominal pain from the start. The temperature may be normal and vomiting is common, so that the clinical picture may mimic acute intestinal obstruction.

John Benjamin Murphy, 1857–1916, Professor of Surgery, Northwestern University, Chicago, IL, USA, described his sign in 1903. In 1896, he was the first person to successfully suture a severed femoral artery; in 1898, he was the first person to do thoracoplasty for pulmonary tuberculosis and pioneered bone grafting techniques. William Mayo said of him 'the surgical genius of our generation'.

Signs

The diagnosis of appendicitis rests more on thorough clinical examination of the abdomen than on any aspect of the history or laboratory investigation. The cardinal features are those of an unwell patient with low-grade pyrexia, localised abdominal tenderness, muscle guarding and rebound tenderness. Inspection of the abdomen may show limitation of respiratory movement in the lower abdomen. The patient is then asked to point to where the pain began and where it moved (the pointing sign). Gentle superficial palpation of the abdomen, beginning in the left iliac fossa moving anticlockwise to the right iliac fossa will detect muscle guarding over the point of maximum tenderness, classically McBurney's point. Asking the patient to cough or gentle percussion over the site of maximum tenderness will elicit rebound tenderness (Summary box 71.3).

Summary box 71.3

Clinical signs in appendicitis

- Pyrexia
- Localised tenderness in the right iliac fossa
- Muscle guarding
- Rebound tenderness

Deep palpation of the left iliac fossa may cause pain in the right iliac fossa, Rovsing's sign, which is helpful in supporting a clinical diagnosis of appendicitis. Occasionally, an inflamed appendix lies on the psoas muscle, and the patient, often a young adult, will lie with the right hip flexed for pain relief (the psoas sign). Spasm of the obturator internus is sometimes demonstrable when the hip is flexed and internally rotated. If an inflamed appendix is in contact with the obturator internus, this manoeuvre will cause pain in the hypogastrium (the obturator test; Zachary Cope). Cutaneous hyperaesthesia may be demonstrable in the right iliac fossa, but is rarely of diagnostic value (Summary box 71.4).

Summary box 71.4

Signs to elicit in appendicitis

- Pointing sign
- Rovsing's sign
- Psoas sign
- Obturator sign

Charles McBurney, 1854–1913, Professor of Surgery, Columbia College of Physicians and Surgeons, New York, NY, USA. In 1889, McBurney published a paper on appendicitis in which he stated 'I believe in every case the seat of greatest pain determined by the pressure of one finger has been very exactly between an inch and a half and two inches from the anterior spinous process of the ilium on a straight line drawn from that process to the umbilicus'.

Sir Vincent Zachary Cope, 1881–1975, surgeon, St Mary's Hospital, London, UK. He was a poet who wrote a poetry book under a pseudonym 'Zeta' describing the acute abdomen: 'The Acute Abdomen in Rhyme'. He described the differential diagnosis of acute appendicitis as:

Distension, rigidity, vomiting, pain,
Are actors abdominal which often deign
To act on behalf of the chest, spine or brain,
Or general ills of which typhoid's the main.

Thorkild Rovsing, 1862–1937, Professor of Surgery, Copenhagen, Denmark.

Special features, according to position of the appendix

Retrocaecal

Rigidity is often absent, and even application of deep pressure may fail to elicit tenderness (silent appendix), the reason being that the caecum, distended with gas, prevents the pressure exerted by the hand from reaching the inflamed structure. However, deep tenderness is often present in the loin, and rigidity of the quadratus lumborum may be in evidence. Psoas spasm, due to the inflamed appendix being in contact with that muscle, may be sufficient to cause flexion of the hip joint. Hyperextension of the hip joint may induce abdominal pain when the degree of psoas spasm is insufficient to cause flexion of the hip.

Pelvic

Occasionally, early diarrhoea results from an inflamed appendix being in contact with the rectum. When the appendix lies entirely within the pelvis, there is usually complete absence of abdominal rigidity, and often tenderness over McBurney's point is also lacking. In some instances, deep tenderness can be made out just above and to the right of the symphysis pubis. In either event, a rectal examination reveals tenderness in the rectovesical pouch or the pouch of Douglas, especially on the right side. Spasm of the psoas and obturator internus muscles may be present when the appendix is in this position. An inflamed appendix in contact with the bladder may cause frequency of micturition. This is more common in children.

Postileal

In this case, the inflamed appendix lies behind the terminal ileum. It presents the greatest difficulty in diagnosis because the pain may not shift, diarrhoea is a feature and marked retching may occur. Tenderness, if any, is ill defined, although it may be present immediately to the right of the umbilicus.

Special features, according to age

Infants

Appendicitis is relatively rare in infants under 36 months of age and, for obvious reasons, the patient is unable to give a history. Because of this, diagnosis is often delayed, and thus the incidence of perforation and postoperative morbidity is considerably higher than in older children. Diffuse peritonitis can develop rapidly because of the underdeveloped greater omentum, which is unable to give much assistance in localising the infection.

Children

It is rare to find a child with appendicitis who has not vomited. Children with appendicitis usually have complete aversion to food.

The elderly

Gangrene and perforation occur much more frequently in elderly patients. Elderly patients with lax abdominal walls or obesity may harbour a gangrenous appendix with little evidence of it, and the clinical picture may simulate subacute intestinal obstruction. These features, coupled with coincident medical conditions, produce a much higher mortality for acute appendicitis in the elderly.

The obese

Obesity can obscure and diminish all the local signs of acute appendicitis. Delay in diagnosis, coupled with the technical difficulty of operating in the obese, makes it wiser to consider operating through a midline abdominal incision. Laparoscopy is particularly useful in the obese as it may obviate the need for a large abdominal incision.

Pregnancy

Appendicitis is the most common extrauterine acute abdominal condition in pregnancy, with a frequency of 1:1500–2000 pregnancies. Diagnosis is complicated by delay in presentation as early non-specific symptoms are often attributed to the pregnancy. Obstetric teaching has been that the caecum and appendix are progressively pushed to the right upper quadrant of the abdomen as pregnancy develops during the second and third trimesters. However, pain in the right lower quadrant of the abdomen remains the cardinal feature of appendicitis in pregnancy. Fetal loss occurs in 3–5 per cent of cases, increasing to 20 per cent if perforation is found at operation.

Differential diagnosis

Although acute appendicitis is the most common abdominal surgical emergency, the diagnosis can be extremely difficult at times. There are a number of common conditions that it is wise to consider carefully and, if possible, exclude. The differential diagnosis differs in patients of different ages; in women, additional differential diagnoses are diseases of the female genital tract (Table 71.1).

Children

The diseases most commonly mistaken for acute appendicitis are **acute gastroenteritis** and **mesenteric lymphadenitis**. In mesenteric lymphadenitis, the pain is colicky in nature and cervical lymph nodes may be enlarged. It may be impossible to clinically distinguish **Meckel's diverticulitis** from acute appendicitis. The pain is similar; however, signs may be central or left sided. Occasionally, there is a history of antecedent abdominal pain or intermittent lower gastrointestinal bleeding.

It is important to distinguish between acute appendicitis and **intussusception**. Appendicitis is uncommon before the age of two years, whereas the median age for intussusception is 18 months. A mass may be palpable in the right lower quadrant, and the preferred treatment of intussusception is reduction by careful barium enema.

Henoch–Schönlein purpura is often preceded by a sore throat or respiratory infection. Abdominal pain can be severe and can be confused with intussusception or appendicitis. There is nearly always an ecchymotic rash, typically affecting the extensor surfaces of the limbs and on the buttocks. The face is usually spared. The platelet count and bleeding time are within normal limits. Microscopic haematuria is common.

Lobar pneumonia and pleurisy, especially at the right base, may give rise to right-sided abdominal pain and mimic appendicitis. Abdominal tenderness is minimal, pyrexia is marked,

James Douglas, 1675–1742, anatomist and 'man-midwife' who practised in London, UK, described the Douglas pouch in 1730.

Table 71.1 Differential diagnosis of acute appendicitis.

Children	Adult	Adult female	Elderly
Gastroenteritis	Regional enteritis	Mittelschmerz	Diverticulitis
Mesenteric adenitis	Ureteric colic	Pelvic inflammatory disease	Intestinal obstruction
Meckel's diverticulitis	Perforated peptic ulcer	Pyelonephritis	Colonic carcinoma
Intussusception	Torsion of testis	Ectopic pregnancy	Torsion appendix epiploicae
Henoch–Schönlein purpura	Pancreatitis	Torsion/rupture of ovarian cyst	Mesenteric infarction
Lobar pneumonia	Rectus sheath haematoma	Endometriosis	Leaking aortic aneurysm

and chest examination may reveal a pleural friction rub or altered breath sounds on auscultation. A chest radiograph is diagnostic.

Adults

Terminal ileitis in its acute form may be indistinguishable from acute appendicitis unless a doughy mass of inflamed ileum can be felt. An antecedent history of abdominal cramping, weight loss and diarrhoea suggests regional ileitis rather than appendicitis. The ileitis may be non-specific, due to Crohn's disease or *Yersinia* infection. *Yersinia enterocolitica* causes inflammation of the terminal ileum, appendix and caecum with mesenteric adenopathy. If suspected, serum antibody titres are diagnostic, and treatment with intravenous tetracycline is appropriate. If *Yersinia* infection is suspected at operation, a mesenteric lymph node should be excised and divided, with half submitted for microbiological culture (including tuberculosis) and half for histological examination.

Ureteric colic does not commonly cause diagnostic difficulty, as the character and radiation of pain differs from that of appendicitis. Urinalysis should always be performed, and the presence of red cells should prompt a supine abdominal radiograph. Renal ultrasound or intravenous urogram is diagnostic.

Right-sided acute pyelonephritis is accompanied and often preceded by increased frequency of micturition. It may cause difficulty in diagnosis, especially in women. The leading features are tenderness confined to the loin, fever (temperature 39°C) and possibly rigors and pyuria.

In perforated peptic ulcer, the duodenal contents pass along the paracolic gutter to the right iliac fossa. As a rule, there is a history of dyspepsia and a very sudden onset of pain that starts in the epigastrium and passes down the right paracolic gutter. In appendicitis, the pain starts classically in the umbilical region. Rigidity and tenderness in the right iliac fossa are present in both conditions but, in perforated duodenal ulcer, the rigidity is usually greater in the right hypochondrium. An erect chest radiograph will show gas under the diaphragm in 70 per cent of patients. An abdominal computed tomography (CT) examination is valuable when there is diagnostic difficulty.

Testicular torsion in a teenage or young adult male is easily missed. Pain can be referred to the right iliac fossa, and shyness on the part of the patient may lead the unwary to suspect appendicitis unless the scrotum is examined in all cases.

Acute pancreatitis should be considered in the differential diagnosis of all adults suspected of having acute appendicitis and, when appropriate, should be excluded by serum or urinary amylase measurement.

Rectus sheath haematoma is a relatively rare but easily missed differential diagnosis. It usually presents with acute pain and localised tenderness in the right iliac fossa, often after an episode of strenuous physical exercise. Localised pain without gastrointestinal upset is the rule. Occasionally, in an elderly patient, particularly one taking anticoagulant therapy, a rectus sheath haematoma may present as a mass and tenderness in the right iliac fossa after minor trauma.

Adult female

It is in women of childbearing age that pelvic disease most often mimics acute appendicitis. A careful gynaecological history should be taken in all women with suspected appendicitis, concentrating on menstrual cycle, vaginal discharge and possible pregnancy (see also Chapter 80). The most common diagnostic mimics are pelvic inflammatory disease (PID), Mittelschmerz, torsion or haemorrhage of an ovarian cyst and ectopic pregnancy.

Pelvic inflammatory disease

PID comprises a spectrum of diseases that include salpingitis, endometritis and tubo-ovarian sepsis. The incidence of these conditions is increasing and the diagnosis should be considered in every young adult female. Typically, the pain is lower than in appendicitis and is bilateral. A history of vaginal discharge, dysmenorrhoea and burning pain on micturition is a helpful differential diagnostic point. The physical findings include adnexal and cervical tenderness on vaginal examination. When suspected, a high vaginal swab should be taken for *Chlamydia trachomatis* and *Neisseria gonorrhoeae* culture, and the opinion of a gynaecologist should be obtained. Treatment is usually a combination of ofloxacin and metronidazole for 14 days. Transvaginal ultrasound can be particularly helpful in establishing the diagnosis. When serious diagnostic uncertainty persists, diagnostic laparoscopy should be undertaken.

Mittelschmerz

Midcycle rupture of a follicular cyst with bleeding produces lower abdominal and pelvic pain, typically midcycle. Systemic upset is rare, a pregnancy test is negative, and symptoms usu-

Alexandre Emile Yersin, 1863–1943, bacteriologist, Paris, France.

ally subside within hours. Occasionally, diagnostic laparoscopy is required. Retrograde menstruation may cause similar symptoms.

Torsion/haemorrhage of an ovarian cyst

This can prove a difficult differential diagnosis. When suspected, pelvic ultrasound and a gynaecological opinion should be sought. If encountered at operation in women of childbearing years, untwisting of the involved adnexa and ovarian cystectomy should be performed, if necessary. Documented visualisation of the contralateral ovary is an essential medicolegal precaution prior to oophorectomy for any reason.

Ectopic pregnancy

It is unlikely that a ruptured ectopic pregnancy, with its well-defined signs of haemoperitoneum, will be mistaken for acute appendicitis, but the same cannot be said for a right-sided tubal abortion, or still more for a right-sided unruptured tubal pregnancy. In the latter, the signs are very similar to those of acute appendicitis, except that the pain commences on the right side and stays there. The pain is severe and continues unabated until operation. Usually, there is a history of a missed menstrual period, and a urinary pregnancy test may be positive. Severe pain is felt when the cervix is moved on vaginal examination. Signs of intraperitoneal bleeding usually become apparent, and the patient should be questioned specifically regarding referred pain in the shoulder. Pelvic ultrasonography should be carried out in all cases in which an ectopic pregnancy is a possible diagnosis.

Elderly

Diverticulitis

In some patients with a long sigmoid loop, the colon lies to the right of the midline, and it may be impossible to differentiate between diverticulitis and appendicitis. Abdominal CT scanning is particularly useful in this setting and should be considered in the management of all patients over the age of 60 years. A trial of conservative management with intravenous fluids and antibiotics is often appropriate, with a low threshold for laparoscopy or exploratory laparotomy in the face of deterioration or lack of clinical response. Right-sided diverticulitis is unusual and may be clinically indistinguishable from appendicitis. Abdominal CT scanning is particularly useful in making the distinction. As with left-sided diverticulitis, treatment should be conservative with intravenous antibiotics with recourse to laparoscopy or laparotomy in the face of deterioration.

Intestinal obstruction

The diagnosis of intestinal obstruction is usually clear; the subtlety lies in recognising acute appendicitis as the occasional cause in the elderly. As with diverticulitis, intravenous fluids, antibiotics and nasogastric decompression should be instigated, with early resort to laparotomy.

Carcinoma of the caecum

When obstructed or locally perforated, carcinoma of the caecum may mimic or cause obstructive appendicitis in adults. A history of antecedent discomfort, altered bowel habit or unexplained anaemia should raise suspicion. A mass may be palpable (see below under Carcinoid tumour) and an abdominal CT scan diagnostic.

Rare differential diagnoses

Preherpetic pain of the right 10th and 11th dorsal nerves is localised over the same area as that of appendicitis. It does not shift and is associated with marked hyperaesthesia. There is no intestinal upset or rigidity. The herpetic eruption may be delayed for 3–8 hours.

Tabetic crises are now rare. Severe abdominal pain and vomiting usher in the crisis. Other signs of tabes confirm the diagnosis.

Spinal conditions are sometimes associated with acute abdominal pain especially in children and the elderly. These may include tuberculosis of the spine, metastatic carcinoma, osteoporotic vertebral collapse and multiple myeloma. The pain is due to compression of nerve roots and may be aggravated by movement. There is rigidity of the lumbar spine and intestinal symptoms are absent.

The abdominal crises of **porphyria** and **diabetes mellitus** need to be remembered. A urinalysis should be undertaken in every abdominal emergency. In cyclical vomiting of infants or young children, there is a history of previous similar attacks and abdominal rigidity is absent. Acetone is found in the urine but is not diagnostic as it may accompany starvation.

Typhlitis or leukaemic ileocaecal syndrome is a rare but potentially fatal enterocolitis occurring in immunosuppressed patients. Gram-negative or **clostridial septicaemia** (especially *Clostridium septicum*) can be rapidly progressive. Treatment is with appropriate antibiotics and haematopoietic factors. Surgical intervention is rarely indicated.

Investigation

The diagnosis of acute appendicitis is essentially clinical; however, a decision to operate based on clinical suspicion alone can lead to the removal of a normal appendix in 15–30 per cent of cases. The premise that it is better to remove a normal appendix than to delay diagnosis does not stand up to close scrutiny, particularly in the elderly. A number of clinical and laboratory-based scoring systems have been devised to assist diagnosis. The most widely used is the Alvarado score (Table 71.2). A score of 7 or more is strongly predictive of acute appendicitis.

In patients with an equivocal score (5–6), abdominal ultrasound or contrast-enhanced CT examination further reduces the rate of negative appendicectomy. Abdominal ultrasound examination is more useful in children and thin adults, particularly if gynaecological pathology is suspected, with a diagnostic accuracy in excess of 90 per cent (Figure 71.10). Contrast-enhanced CT scan (Figure 71.11) is most useful in patients in whom there is diagnostic uncertainty, particularly older patients, in whom acute diverticulitis, intestinal obstruction and neoplasm are likely differential diagnoses. Selective use of CT scanning may be cost-effective by reducing both the negative appendicectomy rate and the length of hospital stay (Summary box 71.5).

Treatment

The traditional treatment for acute appendicitis is appendicectomy. While this remains standard teaching, there is an

Alfredo Alvarado, trained in medicine in Bogota, Columbia, contemporary, surgeon, Plantation, FL, USA, described his scoring system in 1986.

Table 71.2 The Alvarado (MANTRELS) score.

		Score
Symptoms	**M**igratory RIF pain	1
	Anorexia	1
	Nausea and vomiting	1
Signs	**T**enderness (RIF)	2
	Rebound tenderness	1
	Elevated temperature	1
Laboratory	**L**eukocytosis	2
	Shift to left	1
Total		10

RIF, right iliac fossa.

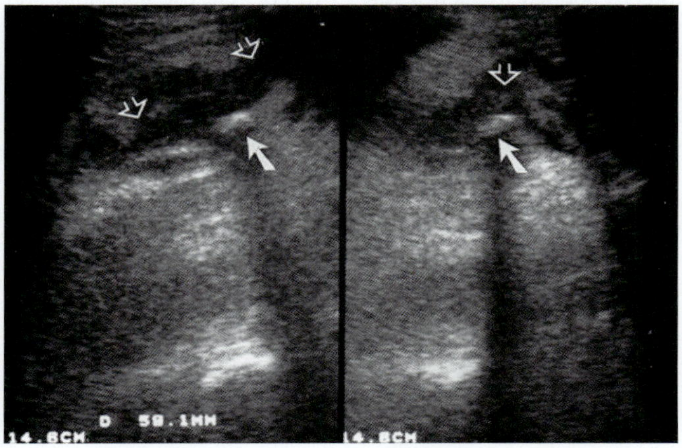

Figure 71.10 Abdominal ultrasound examination showing features of acute appendicitis, distended oedematous appendix (open arrows), longitudinal scan (left) and transverse scan (right). A faecolith is seen (closed arrow) (courtesy of Dr M Behan, FRCR, Dublin, Ireland).

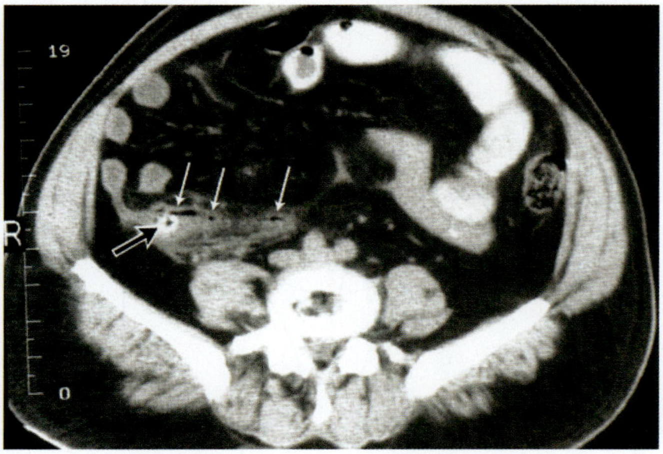

Figure 71.11 Abdominal contrast-enhanced computed tomography scan showing a faecolith (open arrow) at the base of a distended (>0.6 cm) appendix with intramural gas (white arrows) (courtesy of Professor H Fenlon, FRCR, Dublin, Ireland).

Summary box 71.5

Preoperative investigations in appendicitis

- Routine
  - Full blood count
  - Urinalysis
- Selective
  - Pregnancy test
  - Urea and electrolytes
  - Supine abdominal radiograph
  - Ultrasound of the abdomen/pelvis
  - Contrast-enhanced abdomen and pelvic computed tomography scan

emerging body of literature to support a trial of conservative management in those thought not to have obstructive appendicitis. Treatment is bowel rest and intravenous antibiotics, usually metranidazole and third-generation cephalosporin. The available data indicate successful outcomes in 80–90 per cent of patients, however there is an approximately 15 per cent recurrence rate within one year. This approach should be considered in patients with high operative risk (multiple comorbidities). As with conservative treatment of an appendix mass, patients over the age of 40 should be followed up to ensure there is no underlying malignancy (see below under Management of an appendix mass).

With regard to appendicectomy, there is a perception that emergency, often out of hours, operation is essential to prevent the increased morbidity and mortality of peritonitis. While there should be no unnecessary delay, all patients, particularly those most at risk of serious morbidity, benefit by a short period of intensive preoperative preparation. Intravenous fluids, sufficient to establish adequate urine output (catheterisation is needed only in the very ill), and appropriate antibiotics should be given. There is ample evidence that in the absence of purulant peritonitis, a single preoperative dose of antibiotics reduces the incidence of postoperative wound infection. When peritonitis is suspected, therapeutic intravenous antibiotics to cover Gram-negative bacilli, as well as anaerobic cocci, should be given. Hyperpyrexia in children should be treated with salicylates in addition to antibiotics and intravenous fluids. With appropriate use of intravenous fluids and parenteral antibiotics, a policy of deferring appendicectomy after midnight to the first case on the following morning does not increase morbidity. However, when acute obstructive appendicitis is recognised, operation should not be deferred longer than it takes to optimise the patient's condition.

Appendicectomy

Claudius Amyand successfully removed an acutely inflamed appendix from the hernial sac of a boy in 1736. The first surgeon to perform deliberate appendicectomy for acute appendicitis was Lawson Tait in May 1880. The patient recovered; however, the case was not reported until 1890. Meanwhile, Thomas Morton was the first to diagnose appendicitis, drain the abscess and remove the appendix with recovery, publishing his findings in 1887.

Claudius Amyand, 1685–1740, surgeon, St George's Hospital, London, UK.

Appendicectomy should be performed under general anaesthetic with the patient supine on the operating table. When a laparoscopic technique is to be used, the bladder must be empty (ensure that the patient has voided before leaving the ward). Prior to preparing the entire abdomen with an appropriate antiseptic solution, the right iliac fossa should be palpated for a mass. If a mass is felt, it may, on occasion, be preferable to adopt a conservative approach (see below under Management of an appendix mass). Draping of the abdomen is in accordance with the planned operative technique, taking account of any requirement to extend the incision or convert a laparoscopic technique to an open operation.

Conventional appendicectomy

When the preoperative diagnosis is considered reasonably certain, the incision that is widely used for appendicectomy is the so-called gridiron incision (*gridiron*: a frame of cross-beams to support a ship during repairs). The gridiron incision (described first by McArthur) is made at right angles to a line joining the anterior superior iliac spine to the umbilicus, its centre being along the line at McBurney's point (Figure 71.12). If better access is required, it is possible to convert the gridiron to a Rutherford Morison incision (see below) by cutting the internal oblique and transversus muscles in the line of the incision.

In recent years, a transverse skin crease (Lanz) incision has become more popular, as the exposure is better and extension, when needed, is easier. The incision, appropriate in length to the size and obesity of the patient, is made approximately 2 cm below the umbilicus centred on the midclavicular–midinguinal line (Figure 71.13). When necessary, the incision may be extended medially, with retraction or suitable division of the rectus abdominis muscle.

When the diagnosis is in doubt, particularly in the presence of intestinal obstruction, a lower midline abdominal incision is to be preferred over a right lower paramedian incision. The latter, although widely practised in the past, is difficult to extend, more difficult to close and provides poorer access to the pelvis and peritoneal cavity.

Rutherford Morison's incision is useful if the appendix is para- or retrocaecal and fixed. It is essentially an oblique muscle-cutting incision with its lower end over McBurney's point and extending obliquely upwards and laterally as necessary. All layers are divided in the line of the incision.

Removal of the appendix

The caecum is identified by the presence of taeniae coli and, using a finger or a swab, the caecum is withdrawn. A turgid appendix may be felt at the base of the caecum. Inflammatory adhesions must be gently broken with a finger, which is then hooked around the appendix to deliver it into the wound. The appendix is conveniently controlled using a Babcock or Lane's forceps applied in such a way as to encircle the appendix and yet not damage it. The base of the mesoappendix is clamped in artery forceps, divided and ligated (Figure 71.14a). When the mesoappendix is broad, the procedure must be repeated with a second or, rarely, a third artery forceps. The appendix, now completely freed, is crushed near its junction with the caecum in artery forceps, which is removed and reapplied just distal to the crushed portion. An absorbable 2/0 ligature is tied around the crushed portion close to the caecum. The appendix is amputated between the artery forceps and the ligature (Figure 71.14b). An absorbable 2/0 or 3/0 purse-string or 'Z' suture may then be inserted into the caecum about 1.25 cm from the base (Figure 71.14c). The stitch should pass through the muscle

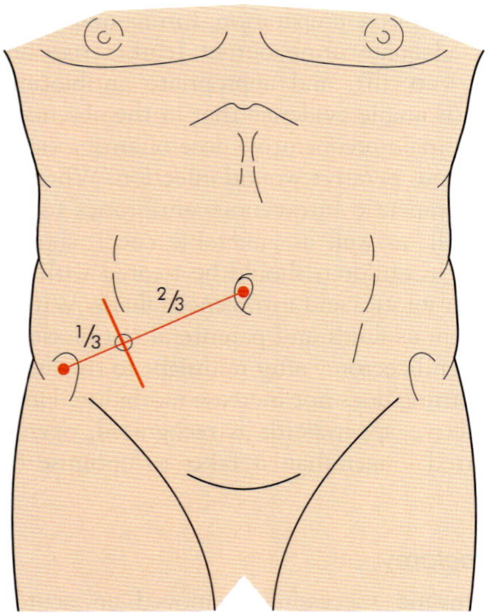

Figure 71.12 Gridiron incision for appendicitis, at right angles to a line joining the anterior superior iliac spine and umbilicus, centred on McBurney's point (courtesy of Professor M Earley, FRSCI, Dublin, Ireland).

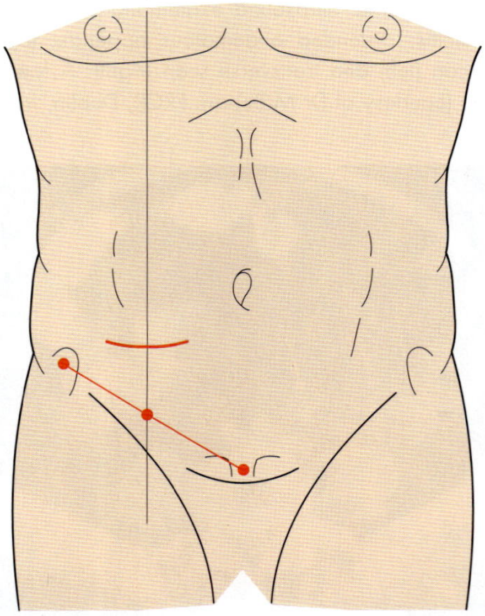

Figure 71.13 Transverse or skin crease (Lanz) incision for appendicitis, 2 cm below the umbilicus, centred on the midclavicular–midinguinal line (courtesy of Professor M Earley, FRSCI, Dublin, Ireland).

Robert Lawson Tait, 1845–1899, surgeon, The Hospital for Diseases of Women, Birmingham, UK.
Thomas George Morton, 1835–1903, surgeon, Philadelphia, PA, USA.
Lewis Linn McArthur, 1858–1934, surgeon, St Luke's Hospital, Chicago, IL, USA.
James Rutherford Morison, 1853–1939, Professor of Surgery, The University of Durham, Durham, UK.
Otto Lanz, 1865–1935, surgeon, Amsterdam, The Netherlands.
William Wayne Babcock, 1872–1963, surgeon, Philadelphia, PA, USA.
Sir William Arbuthnot Lane, 1855–1943, surgeon, Guy's Hospital, London, UK.

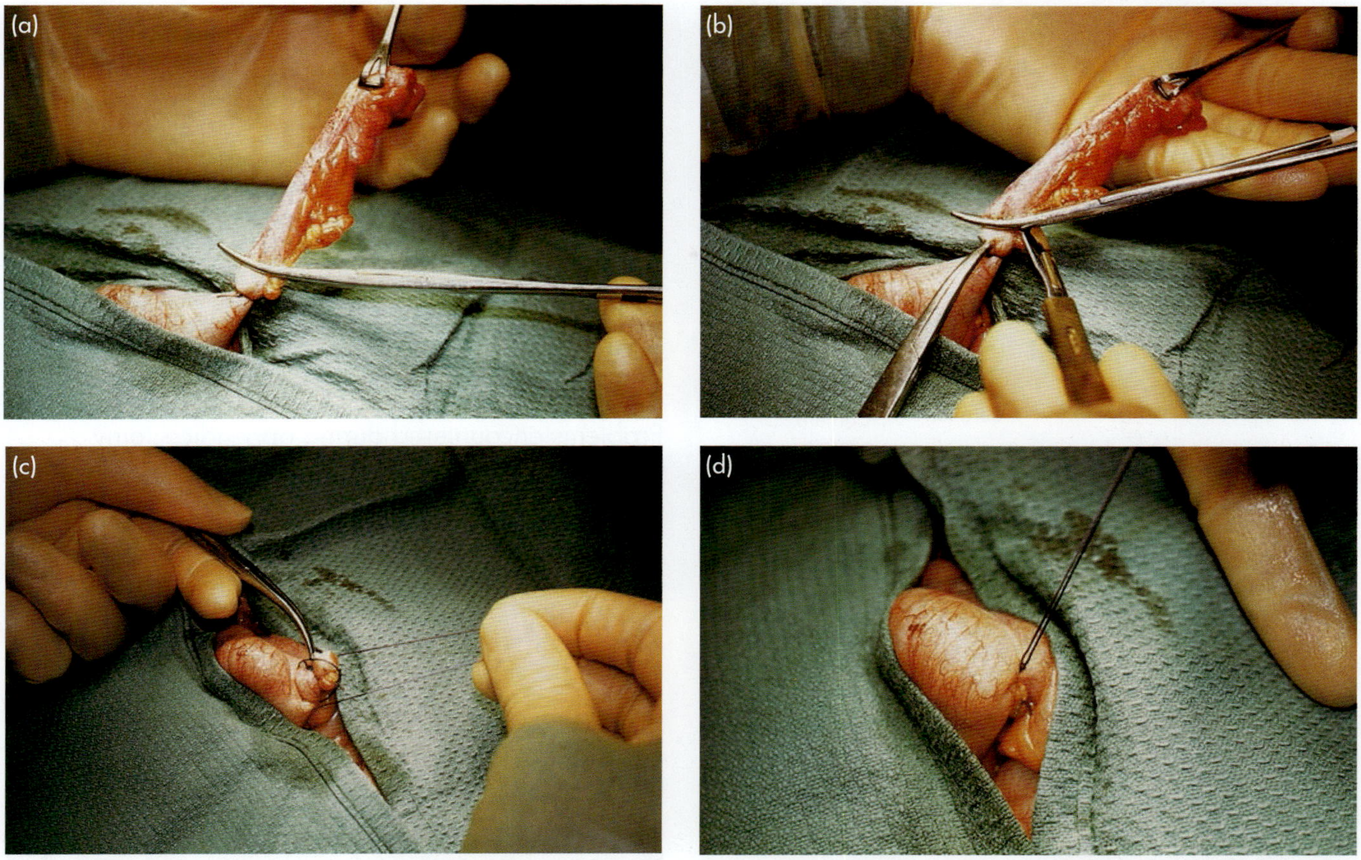

Figure 71.14 (a) Mesoappendix divided between artery forceps and ligated. (b) Appendix crushed and ligated at its base and about to be divided. (c) 'Z' suture inserted prior to inversion of the appendiceal stump. (d) Appendiceal stump inverted, the 'Z' suture having been tied.

coat, picking up the taeniae coli. The stump of the appendix is invaginated (Figure 71.14d) while the purse-string or 'Z' suture is tied, thus burying the appendix stump. Many surgeons believe invagination of the appendiceal stump is unnecessary.

Methods to be adopted in special circumstances

When the caecal wall is oedematous, the purse-string suture is in danger of cutting out. If the oedema is of limited extent, this can be overcome by inserting the purse-string suture into more healthy caecal wall at a greater distance from the base of the appendix. Occasions may arise when, because of the extensive oedema of the caecal wall, it is better not to attempt invagination.

When the base of the appendix is inflamed, it should not be crushed, but ligated close to the caecal wall just tightly enough to occlude the lumen, after which the appendix is amputated and the stump invaginated. Should the base of the appendix be gangrenous, neither crushing nor ligation should be attempted. Two stitches are placed through the caecal wall close to the base of the gangrenous appendix, which is amputated flush with the caecal wall, after which these stitches are tied. Further closure is effected by means of a second layer of interrupted seromuscular sutures.

Retrograde appendicectomy

When the appendix is retrocaecal and adherent, it is an advantage to divide the base between artery forceps. The appendiceal vessels are then ligated, the stump ligated and invaginated, and gentle traction on the caecum will enable the surgeon to deliver the body of the appendix, which is then removed from base to tip. Occasionally, this manoeuvre requires division of the lateral peritoneal attachments of the caecum.

Laparoscopic appendicectomy

The most valuable aspect of laparoscopy in the management of suspected appendicitis is as a diagnostic tool, particularly in women of child-bearing age. The placement of operating ports may vary according to operator preference and previous abdominal scars. The operator stands to the patient's left and faces a video monitor placed at the patient's right foot (Figure 71.15). A moderate Trendelenburg tilt of the operating table assists delivery of loops of small bowel from the pelvis. The appendix is found in the conventional manner by identification of the caecal taeniae and is controlled using a laparoscopic tissue-holding forceps. By elevating the appendix, the mesoappendix is displayed (Figure 71.16a). A dissecting forceps is used to create a window in the mesoappendix to allow the appendicular vessels to be coagulated or ligated using a clip applicator. The appendix, free of its mesentery, can be ligated at its base with an absorbable loop ligature (Figure 71.16b), divided (Figure 71.16c) and removed through one of the operating ports. It is not usual to invert the stump of the appendix (Figure 71.16d). A single absorbable suture is used to close the linea alba at the

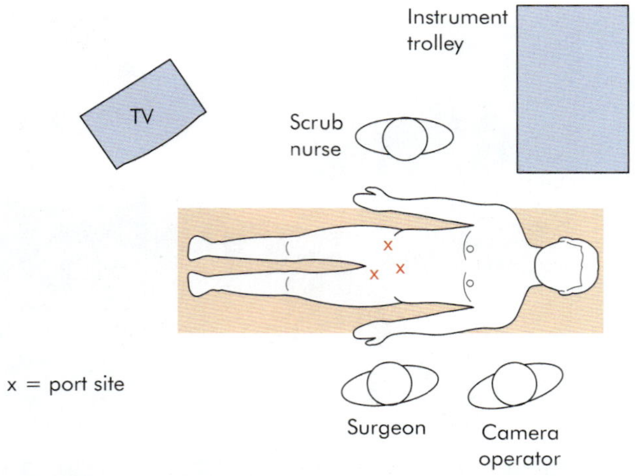

Figure 71.15 Position of surgeon, assistants and equipment for laparoscopic appendicectomy.

umbilicus, and the small skin incisions may be closed with subcuticular sutures.

Patients who undergo laparoscopic appendicectomy are likely to have less postoperative pain and to be discharged from hospital and return to activities of daily living sooner than those who have undergone open appendicectomy. While the incidence of postoperative wound infection is lower after the laparoscopic technique, the incidence of postoperative intra-abdominal sepsis may be higher in patients operated on for gangrenous or perforated appendicitis. There may be an advantage for laparoscopic over open appendicectomy in obese patients and early pregnancy. At present, there seems little, if any, benefit from single incision laparoscopic surgery (SILS) for acute appendicitis.

Problems encountered during appendicectomy

- **A normal appendix is found.** This demands careful exclusion of other possible diagnoses, particularly terminal ileitis, Meckel's diverticulitis and tubal or ovarian causes in women. It is usual to remove the appendix to avoid future diagnostic difficulties, even though the appendix

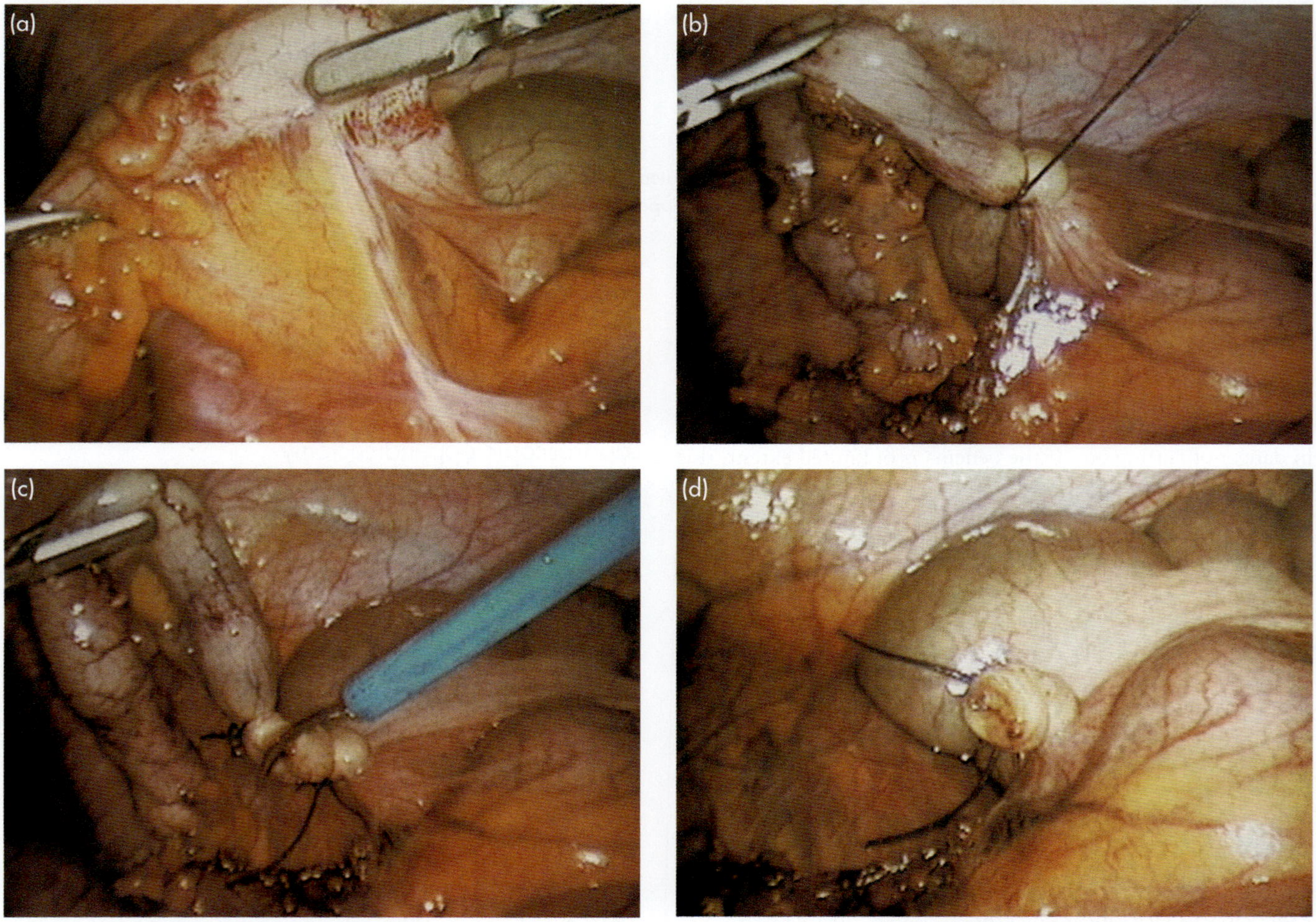

Figure 71.16 Laparoscopic appendicectomy. (a) Mesoappendix displayed; (b) ligation at the base of the appendix; (c) division of base; (d) appendicectomy complete (courtesy of Professor O McAnena, FRCSI, Galway, Ireland).

is macroscopically normal, particularly if a skin crease or gridiron incision has been made. A case can be made for preserving the macroscopically normal appendix seen at diagnostic laparoscopy, although approximately one-quarter of seemingly normal appendices show microscopic evidence of inflammation.

- **The appendix cannot be found.** The caecum should be mobilised, and the taeniae coli should be traced to their confluence on the caecum before the diagnosis of 'absent appendix' is made.
- **An appendicular tumour is found.** Small tumours (under 2.0 cm in diameter) can be removed by appendicectomy; larger tumours should be treated by a right hemicolectomy (see below).
- **An appendix abscess is found and the appendix cannot be removed easily.** This eventuality is rare in the era of modern diagnostic imaging. Percutaneous drainage of the abscess and intravenous antibiotic treatment is to be preferred. If found at operation, the abscess should be drained and intravenous antibiotics administered. Very rarely in the face of a frankly necrotic appendix, a caecectomy or partial right hemicolectomy is required. (The first recorded operation for an appendix abscess was by Henry Hancock of Charing Cross Hospital, London, in 1848.)

Appendicitis complicating Crohn's disease

Occasionally, a patient undergoing surgery for acute appendicitis is found to have concomitant Crohn's disease of the ileocaecal region. Providing that the caecal wall is healthy at the base of the appendix, appendicectomy can be performed without increasing the risk of an enterocutaneous fistula. Rarely, the appendix is involved with the Crohn's disease. In this situation, a conservative approach may be warranted, and a trial of intravenous corticosteroids and systemic antibiotics can be used to resolve the acute inflammatory process.

Appendix abscess

Failure of resolution of an appendix mass or continued spiking pyrexia usually indicates that there is pus within the phlegmonous appendix mass. Ultrasound or abdominal CT scan may identify an area suitable for the insertion of a percutaneous drain. Rarely, this is unsuccessful and laparotomy through a midline incision is indicated.

Pelvic abscess

Pelvic abscess formation is an occasional complication of appendicitis and can occur irrespective of the position of the appendix within the peritoneal cavity. The most common presentation is a spiking pyrexia several days after appendicitis; indeed, the patient may already have been discharged from hospital. Pelvic pressure or discomfort associated with loose stool or tenesmus is common. Rectal examination reveals a boggy mass in the pelvis, anterior to the rectum, at the level of the peritoneal reflection (Figure 71.17). Pelvic ultrasound or CT scan will confirm. Traditionally, treatment has been through transrectal drainage under general anaesthetic, however increasing availability of radiologically guided percutaneous drainage has reduced the need considerably.

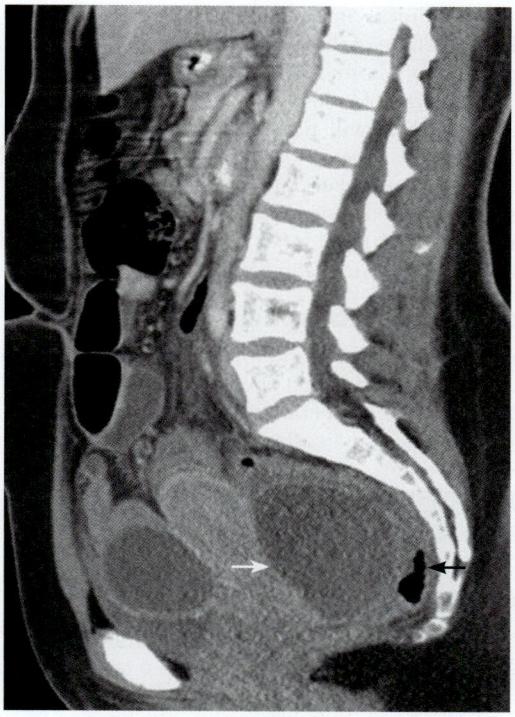

Figure 71.17 Sagittal computed tomography scan of pelvis showing pelvic abscess (white arrow). Note relationship with rectum (black arrow).

Management of an appendix mass

If an appendix mass is present and the condition of the patient is satisfactory, the standard treatment is the conservative Ochsner–Sherren regimen. This strategy is based on the premise that the inflammatory process is already localised and that inadvertent surgery is difficult and may be dangerous. It may be impossible to find the appendix and, occasionally, a faecal fistula may form. For these reasons, it is wise to observe a non-operative programme but to be prepared to operate should clinical deterioration occur (Summary box 71.6).

> **Summary box 71.6**
>
> **Criteria for stopping conservative treatment of an appendix mass**
>
> - A rising pulse rate
> - Increasing or spreading abdominal pain
> - Increasing size of the mass

Careful recording of the patient's condition and the extent of the mass should be made and the abdomen regularly re-examined. It is helpful to mark the limits of the mass on the abdominal wall using a skin pencil. A contrast-enhanced CT examination of the abdomen should be performed and antibiotic therapy instigated. An abscess, if present, should be drained radiologically. Temperature and pulse rate should be recorded 4-hourly and a fluid balance record maintained. Clinical deterioration or evidence of peritonitis is an indication for early

Albert John Ochsner, 1858–1925, Professor of Clinical Surgery, The University of Illinois College of Medicine, Chicago, IL, USA.
James Sherren, 1872–1945, surgeon, The London Hospital, London, UK.

laparotomy. Clinical improvement is usually evident within 24–48 hours. Failure of the mass to resolve should raise suspicion of a carcinoma or Crohn's disease. Using this regimen, approximately 90 per cent of cases resolve without incident. The great majority of patients will not develop recurrence, and it is no longer considered necessary to remove the appendix after an interval of 6–8 weeks. Patients over the age of 40 should have colonoscopy and follow-up imaging to ensure resolution as a small minority (less than 5 per cent) may have an underlying appendicular or colonic malignancy.

Postoperative complications

Postoperative complications following appendicectomy are relatively uncommon and reflect the degree of peritonitis that was present at the time of operation and intercurrent diseases that may predispose to complications (Summary box 71.7).

Summary box 71.7

Checklist for unwell patient following appendicectomy

- Examine the wound and abdomen for an abscess
- Consider a pelvic abscess and perform a rectal examination
- Examine the lungs – pneumonitis or collapse
- Examine the legs – consider venous thrombosis
- Examine the conjunctivae for an icteric tinge and the liver for enlargement, and enquire whether the patient has had rigors (pylephlebitis)
- Examine the urine for organisms (pyelonephritis)
- Suspect subphrenic abscess

Wound infection

Wound infection is the most common postoperative complication, occurring in 5–10 per cent of all patients. This usually presents with pain and erythema of the wound on the 4th or 5th postoperative day, often soon after hospital discharge. Treatment is by wound drainage and antibiotics when required. The organisms responsible are usually a mixture of Gram-negative bacilli and anaerobic bacteria, predominantly Bacteroides species and anaerobic streptococci.

Intra-abdominal abscess

Approximately 8 per cent of patients following appendectomy will develop a postoperative intra-abdominal abscess. In an era of hospital discharge 24 to 48 hours following appendectomy, patients should be advised prior to discharge that a spiking fever, malaise and anorexia developing 5–7 days after operation is suggestive of an intraperitoneal collection and that urgent medical advice should be obtained. Interloop, paracolic, pelvic and subphrenic sites should be considered. Abdominal ultrasonography and CT scanning greatly facilitate diagnosis and allow percutaneous drainage. Laparotomy should be considered in patients suspected of having intra-abdominal sepsis, but in whom imaging fails to show a collection, particularly those with continuing ileus.

Ileus

A period of adynamic ileus is to be expected after appendicectomy, and this may last a number of days following removal of a gangrenous appendix. Ileus persisting for more than 4 or 5 days, particularly in the presence of a fever, is indicative of continuing intra-abdominal sepsis and should prompt further investigation (see above). Rarely, early during postoperative recovery, a Richter's type of hernia may occur at the site of a laparoscopic port insertion and may be confused with a postoperative ileus. A CT scan is usually definitive.

Respiratory

In the absence of concurrent pulmonary disease, respiratory complications are rare following appendicectomy. Adequate postoperative analgesia and physiotherapy, when appropriate, reduce the incidence.

Venous thrombosis and embolism

These conditions are rare after appendicectomy, except in the elderly and in women taking the oral contraceptive pill. Appropriate prophylactic measures should be taken in such cases.

Portal pyaemia (pylephlebitis)

This is a rare but very serious complication of gangrenous appendicitis associated with high fever, rigors and jaundice. It is caused by septicaemia in the portal venous system and leads to the development of intrahepatic abscesses (often multiple). Treatment is with systemic antibiotics and percutaneous drainage of hepatic abscesses as appropriate. A screen for underlying thrombophilia should be considered.

Faecal fistula

Leakage from the appendicular stump occurs rarely, but may follow if the encircling stitch has been put in too deeply or if the caecal wall was involved by oedema or inflammation. Occasionally, a fistula may result following appendicectomy in Crohn's disease. Conservative management with low-residue enteral nutrition will usually result in closure.

Adhesive intestinal obstruction

This is the most common late complication of appendicectomy. At operation, a single band adhesion is often found to be responsible. Occasionally, chronic pain in the right iliac fossa is attributed to adhesion formation after appendicectomy. In such cases, laparoscopy is of value in confirming the presence of adhesions and allowing division.

Recurrent acute appendicitis

Appendicitis is notoriously recurrent. It is not uncommon for patients to attribute such attacks to 'biliousness' or dyspepsia. The attacks vary in intensity and may occur every few months, and the majority of cases ultimately culminate in severe acute appendicitis. If a careful history is taken from patients with acute appendicitis, many remember having had milder but similar attacks of pain. The appendix in these cases shows fibrosis indicative of previous inflammation (Figure 71.18). Chronic appendicitis, per se, does not exist; however, there is evidence of altered neuroimmune function in the myenteric nerves of patients with so-called recurrent appendicitis (Büchler).

Neoplasms of the appendix

Carcinoid tumours

Carcinoid tumours (synonym: argentaffinoma) arise in argentaffin tissue (Kulchitsky cells of the crypts of Lieberkühn) and are most common in the vermiform appendix. Carcinoid tumour is found once in every 300–400 appendices subjected to histological examination and is ten times more common than any other neoplasm of the appendix. In many instances, the appendix had been removed because of symptoms of subacute or recurrent appendicitis. The tumour can occur in any part of the appendix, but it is frequently found in the distal third. The neoplasm feels moderately hard and, on sectioning the appendix, it can be seen as a yellow tumour between the intact mucosa and the peritoneum. Microscopically, the tumour cells are small, arranged in small nests within the muscle and have a characteristic pattern using immunohistochemical stain for chromogranin B (Figure 71.19). Unlike carcinoid tumours arising in other parts of the intestinal tract, carcinoid tumour of the appendix rarely gives rise to metastases. Appendicectomy has been shown to be sufficient treatment, unless the caecal wall is involved, the tumour is 2 cm or more in size or involved lymph nodes are found, when right hemicolectomy is indicated.

Other appendiceal tumours

Goblet cell carcinoid tumour is an unusual variant, which exhibits a combination of endocrine and glandular differentiation. It has a more aggressive natural history and right hemicolectomy is indicated if the tumour is 2 cm or more in size, has greater than two mitoses per high power field, involved margins or lymphovascular invasion.

Primary adenocarcinoma of the appendix is extremely rare. It is usually of the colonic type and should be treated by right hemicolectomy (as a second-stage procedure if the condition is not recognised at the first operation).

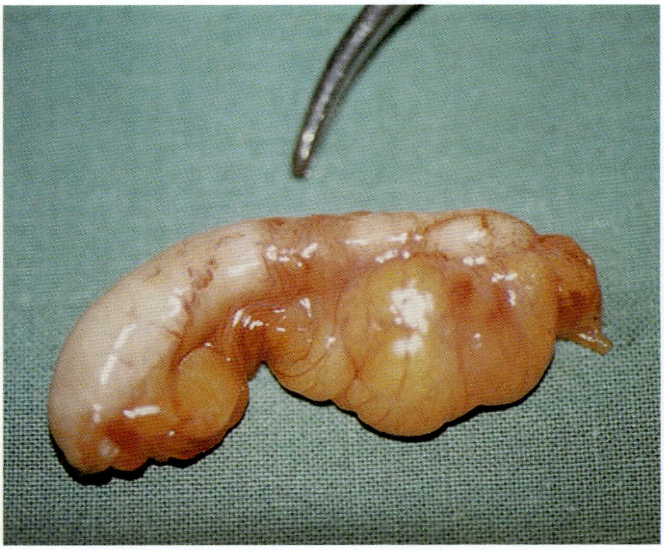

Figure 71.18 Excised appendix showing the point of luminal obstruction with distal fibrosis.

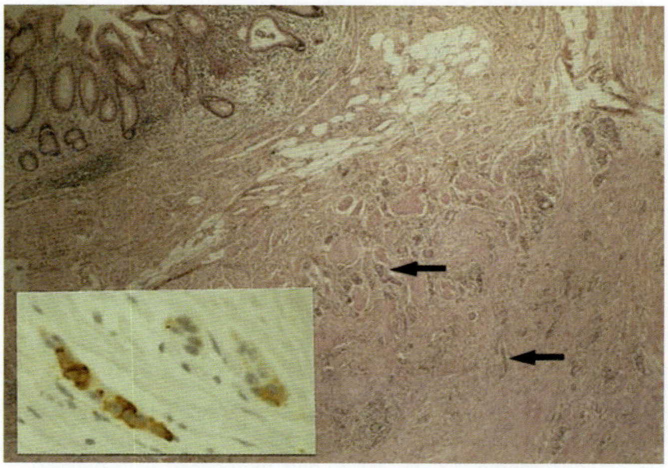

Figure 71.19 Carcinoid tumour. A small incidental carcinoid tumour of the appendix. The tumour cells infiltrate the muscle arranged in small nests and trabeculae (arrows). Tumour cells are small and have inconspicuous nuclei. Inset: higher magnification of an immunohistochemical stain for chromogranin B shows a strong positive reaction (brown) of tumour cells (courtesy of Dr P Kelly, FRCPath, Dublin, Ireland).

Mucinous cystadenoma

A mucin-secreting adenoma of the appendix may rupture into the peritoneal cavity (Figure 71.20), seeding it with mucus-secreting cells. Presentation is often delayed until the patient has gross abdominal distension as a result of pseudomyxoma peritoneii, which may mimic ascites (Figure 71.21). Treatment consists of radical resection of all involved parietal peritoneal surfaces and aggressive intraperitoneal chemotherapy (Sugarbaker). When diagnosed, patients should be referred to specialist centres that have the requisite facilities and experience to undertake the prolonged and complex surgery involved.

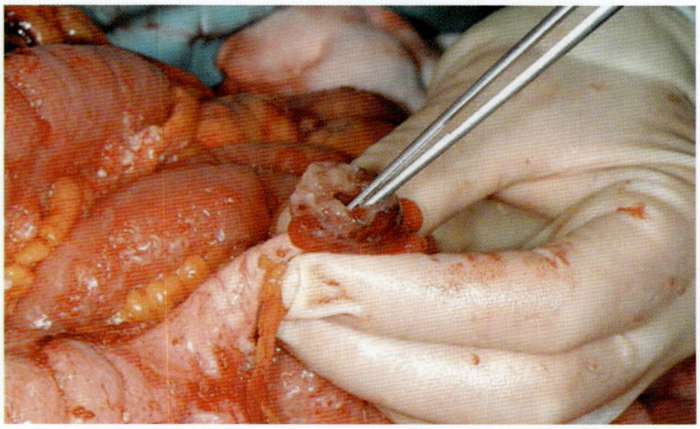

Figure 71.20 Perforated mucin producing tumour of the appendix (courtesy of Mr Brendan Moran, FRCSI, FRCS, and reproduced with permission Basingstoke and North Hampshire NHS Foundation Trust, UK).

Marcus Büchler, contemporary, Professor of Surgery, Heidelberg, Germany.
Johann Nathaniel Lieberkühn, 1711–1756, physician and anatomist, Berlin, Germany, described these glands in 1745, in anatomical preparations in London. He was made a Fellow of the Royal Society in 1740.
Paul H Sugarbaker, contemporary, surgeon, Washington DC, USA.

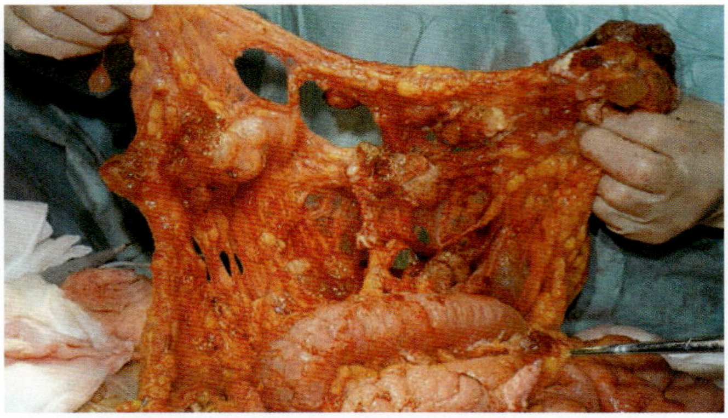

Figure 71.21 Pseudomyxoma peritoneii. Operative photograph illustrating the extensive peritoneal seeding by mucin-producing cells (courtesy Mr Brendan Moran, FRCSI, FRCS, and reproduced with permission Basingstoke and North Hampshire NHS Foundation Trust, UK).

FURTHER READING

Andersen BR, Kallehave FL, Andersen HK. Antibiotics versus placebo for prevention of postoperative infection after appendicectomy. *Cochrane Database Syst Rev* 2005; (**3**): CD001439.

Berry J, Malt RA. Appendicitis near its centenary. *Am J Surg* 1984; **2000**: 567–75.

Ingraham AM, Cohen ME, Bilimoria KY *et al.* Comparison of outcomes after laparoscopic versus open appendectomy for acute appendicitis at 222 ACS NSQIP hospitals. *Surgery* 2010; **148**: 625–35.

Ingraham AM, Cohen ME, Bilimoria KY *et al.* Effect of delay to operation on outcomes in adults with acute appendicitis. *Arch Surg* 2010; **145**: 886–92.

Kaminski A, Liu IL, Applebaum H *et al.* Routine interval appendectomy is not justified after initial non-operative treatment of acute appendicitis. *Arch Surg* 2005; **140**: 897–901.

Murphy EMA, Farquharson SM, Moran BJ. Management of an unexpected appendiceal neoplasm. *Br J Surg* 2006; **93**: 783–92.

Poortman P, Oostvogel HJ, Bosma E *et al.* Improving diagnosis of acute appendicitis: results of a diagnostic pathway with standard use of ultrasonography followed by selective use of CT. *J Am Coll Surg* 2009; **208**: 434–41.

Styrud J, Eriksson S, Nilsson I *et al.* Appendectomy versus antibiotic treatment in acute appendicitis: a prospective multicentre randomized controlled trial. *World J Surg* 2006; **30**: 1033–7.

Vettoretto N, Gobbi S, Corradi A *et al.* Consensus conference on laparoscopic appendectomy: development of guidelines. *Colorectal Dis* 2011; **13**: 748–54.

CHAPTER

72 The rectum

LEARNING OBJECTIVES

To understand:

- The anatomy of the rectum and its relationship to surgical disease and its treatment
- The pathology, clinical presentation, investigation, differential diagnosis and treatment of diseases that affect the rectum

To appreciate that:

- Carcinoma of the rectum is common and its symptoms are similar to those of benign disease and, hence, patients with such symptoms must be carefully evaluated

ANATOMY

Surgical anatomy

The rectum begins where the taenia coli of the sigmoid colon join to form a continuous outer longitudinal muscle layer at the level of the sacral promontory. The rectum follows the curve of the sacrum, and ends at the anorectal junction. The puborectalis muscle encircles the posterior and lateral aspects of the junction, creating the anorectal angle (normally 120°). The rectum has three lateral curvatures: the upper and lower are convex to the right, and the middle is convex to the left. On the luminal aspect, these three curves are marked by semicircular folds (Houston's valves) (Figure 72.1).

The adult rectum is approximately 12–18 cm in length and is conventionally divided into three equal parts: the upper third, which is mobile and has a peritoneal covering anteriorly and laterally; the middle third, where the peritoneum covers only the anterior and part of the lateral surfaces; and the lowest third, which lies deep in the pelvis surrounded by fatty mesorectum and is separated from adjacent structures by fascial layers.

The lower third of the rectum is separated by a fascial condensation (Denonvilliers' fascia) from the prostate/vagina in front, and behind by another fascial layer (Waldeyer's fascia) from the coccyx and lower two sacral vertebrae (Table 72.1). These fascial layers are surgically important as they are a barrier to malignant invasion (Summary box 72.1).

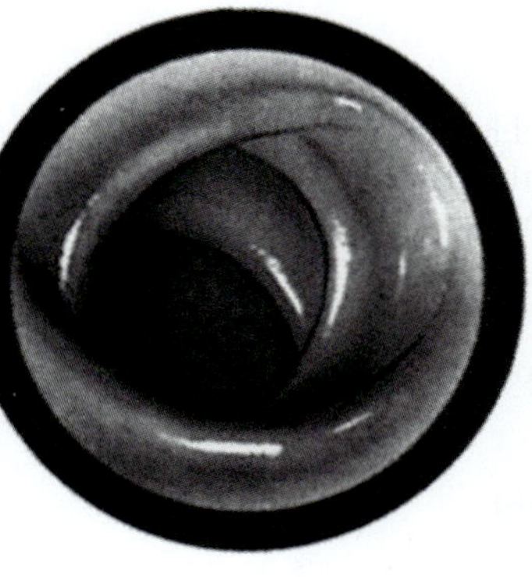

Figure 72.1 Houston's valves as seen through a sigmoidoscope.

Table 72.1 Relations of the rectum.

	Male	Female
Anterior	Bladder Seminal vesicles Ureters Prostate Urethra	Pouch of Douglas Uterus Cervix Posterior vaginal wall
Lateral	Lateral ligaments Middle rectal artery Obturator internus muscle Side wall of pelvis Pelvic autonomic plexus Levator ani muscle	Lateral ligaments Middle rectal artery Obturator internus muscle Side wall of pelvis Pelvic autonomic plexus Levator ani muscle
Posterior	Sacrum and coccyx Loose areolar tissue Fascial condensation Superior rectal artery Hypogastric nerves Lymphatics	Sacrum and coccyx Loose areolar tissue Fascial condensation Superior rectal artery Hypogastric nerves Lymphatics

John Houston, 1802–1845, physician, City of Dublin Hospital and Lecturer in Surgery, Dublin, Ireland.
Charles Pierre Denonvilliers, 1808–1872, Professor of Anatomy and later of Surgery, Paris, France.
Heinrich Wilhelm Gottfried Waldeyer-Hartz, 1836–1921, Professor of Pathological Anatomy, Berlin, Germany.

Summary box 72.1

Anatomy of the rectum

- The rectum measures approximately 15 cm in length
- It is divided into lower, middle and upper thirds
- The blood supply consists of superior, middle and inferior rectal vessels
- Although the lymphatic drainage follows the blood supply, the principal route is upwards along the superior rectal vessels to the para-aortic nodes

Blood supply

The **superior rectal artery** is the direct continuation of the inferior mesenteric artery and is the main arterial supply of the rectum. The arteries and their accompanying lymphatics lie within the loose fatty tissue of the mesorectum, surrounded by a sheath of connective tissue (the mesorectal fascia).

The **middle rectal artery** arises on each side from the internal iliac artery (Figure 72.2) and passes to the rectum in the lateral ligaments. It is usually small (and often only present on one side) and breaks up into several terminal branches.

The **inferior rectal artery** arises on each side from the internal pudendal artery as it enters Alcock's canal. It hugs the inferior surface of the levator ani muscle as it crosses the roof of the ischiorectal fossa to enter the anal muscles (Figure 72.2).

Venous drainage

The superior haemorrhoidal veins draining the upper half of the anal canal above the dentate line pass upwards to become the rectal veins: these unite to form the **superior rectal vein**, which later becomes the **inferior mesenteric vein**. This forms part of the portal venous system and ultimately drains into the splenic vein. Middle rectal veins exist but are small, unimportant channels unless the normal paths are blocked.

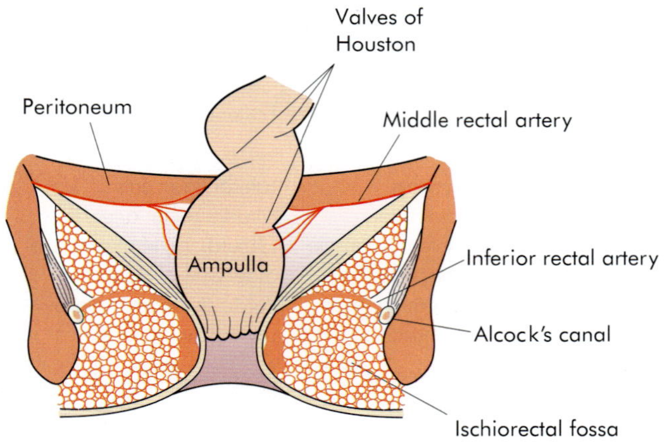

Figure 72.2 The rectum lying in the pelvis (coronal view). Note the curvatures corresponding to Houston's valves.

Lymphatic drainage

The lymphatics of the mucosal lining of the rectum communicate freely with those of the muscular layers. The usual drainage flow is upwards, and only to a limited extent laterally and downwards. For this reason, surgical clearance of malignant disease concentrates mainly on achieving wide resection of proximal lymph nodes. However, if the usual upwards routes are blocked (for example, by carcinoma), flow can reverse, and it is then possible to find metastatic lymph nodes on the side walls of the pelvis (along the middle rectal vessels) or even in the inguinal region (along the inferior rectal artery).

CLINICAL FEATURES OF RECTAL DISEASE

Symptoms

Rectal diseases are common and serious and can occur at any age. The symptoms of many of them overlap. In general, the inflammations affect younger age groups, while the tumours occur in the middle-aged and elderly. The common symptoms of rectal disease are shown in Summary box 72.2.

Summary box 72.2

Main symptoms of rectal disease

- Bleeding per rectum
- Altered bowel habit
- Mucus discharge
- Tenesmus
- Prolapse

Bleeding

This is often bright red in colour but may be darker, and should be carefully investigated at any age.

Altered bowel habit

Early-morning stool frequency ('spurious diarrhoea') is a symptom of rectal carcinoma, while blood-stained frequent loose stools characterise the inflammatory diseases.

Discharge

Mucus and pus are associated with rectal pathology.

Tenesmus

Often described by the patient as 'I feel I want to go, but nothing happens', this is normally an ominous symptom of rectal cancer, but can occur with any rectal pathology.

Prolapse

This usually indicates either mucosal or full-thickness rectal wall descent.

Loss of weight

This usually indicates serious or advanced disease, e.g. hepatic metastases.

Charles Alexander Wells, 1898–1989, Professor of Surgery, University of Liverpool, Liverpool, UK.
Aubrey York Mason, 1910–1993, surgeon, St Helier Hospital, Carshalton, Surrey, UK.

Signs

Because the rectum is accessible via the anus, these can be elicited by systematic examination. The patient is either positioned in the left lateral (Sims) position or examined in the knee–elbow position (Figure 72.3).

Inspection

Visual examination of the anus precedes rectal examination to exclude the presence of anal disease, e.g. fissure or fistula.

Digital examination

The index finger used with gentleness and precision remains a valuable test for rectal disease (Figure 72.4). Tumours in the lower and middle thirds of the rectum can be felt and assessed; by asking the patient to strain, even some tumours in the upper third can be 'tipped' with the finger. After it is removed, the finger should be examined for tell-tale traces of mucus, pus or blood. It is always useful to note the normal, as well as the abnormal findings on digital examination, e.g. the prostate in the male. Digital findings can be recorded as intraluminal (e.g. blood, pus), intramural (e.g. tumours, granular areas, strictures) or extramural (e.g. enlarged prostate, uterine fibroids).

Proctoscopy

This procedure can be used to inspect the anus, anorectal junction and lower rectum (up to 10 cm) (Figure 72.5). Biopsy can be performed of any suspicious areas.

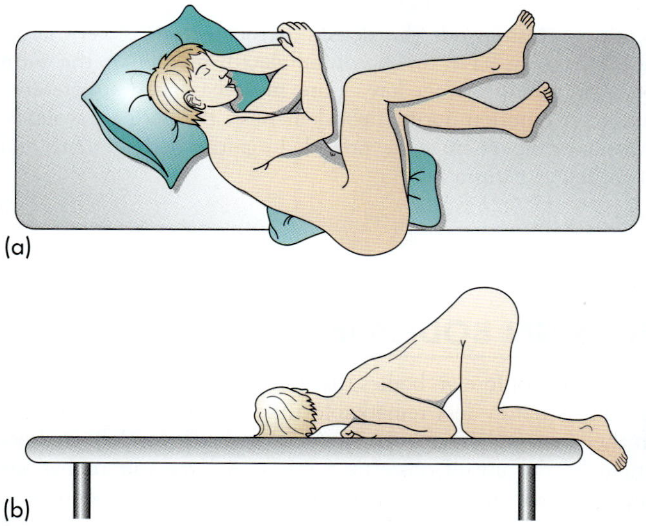

Figure 72.3 Positions for digital rectal examination. (a) Left lateral (Sims). (b) Knee–elbow. Redrawn with permission from Corman ML. *Colon and rectal surgery*, 3rd edn. London: JB Lippincott, 1992.

James Marion Sims, 1813–1883, gynaecological surgeon, the State Hospital for Women, New York, NY, USA, introduced this position to give access to the anterior vaginal wall during operations for the closure of vaginovesical fistulae.

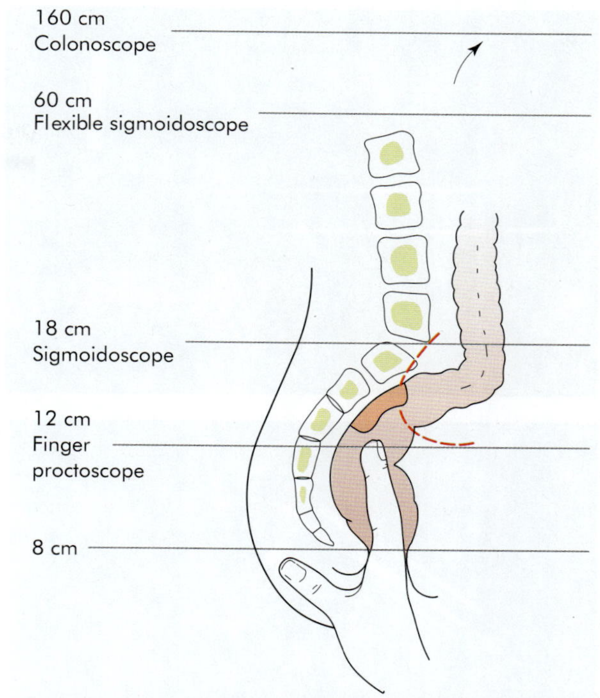

Figure 72.4 Illustration showing how the various methods of examining the rectum reach different levels. Note that even cancers in the upper part of the rectum can be felt with the index finger, especially if the patient is asked to 'strain down' (courtesy of CV Mann).

Sigmoidoscopy

In the past, the sigmoidoscope was a rigid stainless steel instrument of variable diameter and normally 25 cm in length (Figure 72.5). This has in the main been replaced by a disposable plastic instrument. The rectum must be empty for proper inspection with a sigmoidoscope. Gentleness and skill are required for its use, and perforations can occur if care is not taken.

Flexible sigmoidoscope

The 'flexiscope' can be used to supplement or replace rigid sigmoidoscopy (Figure 72.6). It requires skill and experience, and the lower bowel should be cleaned out with preliminary enemas. In addition to the rectum, the whole sigmoid colon is within visual reach of this instrument (Summary box 72.3).

Summary box 72.3

Examination of the rectum

- Visual inspection of the perineum
- Digital examination
- Proctoscopy
- Sigmoidoscopy – rigid or flexible

INJURIES

The rectum or anal canal may be injured in a number of ways, all uncommon:

Charles Victor Mann, formerly surgeon, St Mark's Hospital and Royal London Hospital, London, UK.

(a)

(b)

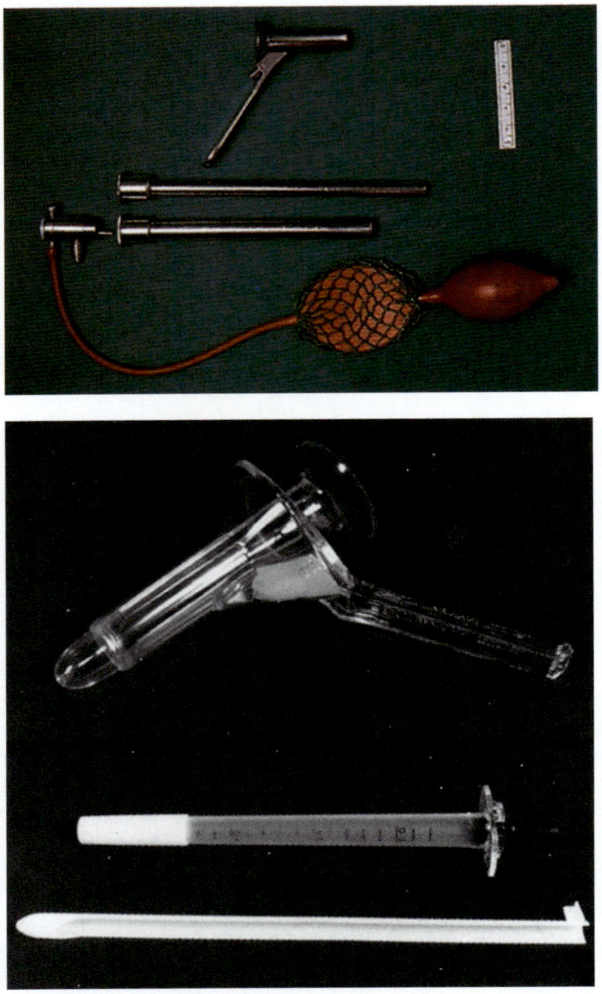

Figure 72.5 (a) A metal proctoscope and two different-sized metal Lloyd-Davies rigid sigmoidoscopes – small (diameter 20 mm). Since the advent of greater awareness of transmitted infection, disposable proctoscopes and sigmoidoscopes (b) have replaced the reusable metal types.

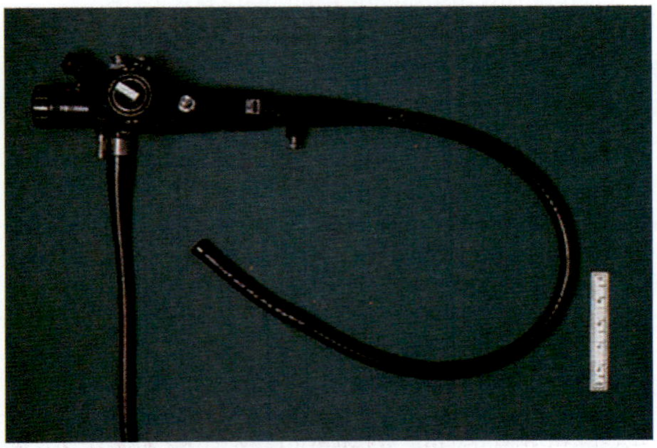

Figure 72.6 The flexible (60 cm) endoscope ('flexiscope').

- by falling in a sitting posture onto a pointed object: the upturned leg of a chair, handle of a broom, floor-mop, pitchfork or a broken shooting stick have all resulted in rectal impalement;
- by penetrating injury (including gunshots) to the buttocks;
- by sexual assault or sexual activity involving anal penetration;
- by the fetal head during childbirth, especially forceps-assisted.

Diagnosis

The anus should be inspected and the abdomen palpated. If rigidity or tenderness is present, early laparotomy or laparoscopy is indicated. A water-soluble contrast enema or computed tomography (CT) scan with rectal contrast is useful to identify perforation. Prior to the operation, a urethral catheter is passed, but if there is any possibility of urethral injury (suggested by difficulty passing urine, haematuria or high prostate on digital examination), a urethrogram should be performed first (see Chapters 76 and 78).

Treatment

If perforation is suspected, the rectum is examined under general anaesthetic with a finger and a sigmoidoscope, particular attention being directed to the anterior wall. If penetrating injury is confirmed, laparotomy or laparoscopy is then performed. If an intraperitoneal rupture of the rectum is found, the perforation is closed with sutures. A defunctioning colostomy is usually required, constructed in the left iliac fossa. If the rectal injury is below the peritoneal reflection, wide drainage from below is indicated, with rectal washout and a defunctioning colostomy. If the defect in the rectum is very large, resection may have to be contemplated, usually in the form of a Hartmann's procedure. Care must be taken to preserve sphincter function during debridement of the perineal wounds. Antibiotic cover must be provided against both aerobic and anaerobic organisms.

FOREIGN BODIES IN THE RECTUM

The variety of foreign bodies that have found their way into the rectum is hardly less remarkable than the ingenuity displayed in their removal (Figure 72.7). A turnip has been delivered per anum by the use of obstetric forceps. A large soft rubber sex toy has been withdrawn by inserting a myomectomy screw into its lower end. A tumbler, mouth open downwards, has been extracted by filling the interior with a wet plaster of Paris bandage, leaving the end of the bandage protruding and allowing the plaster to set.

If insurmountable difficulty is experienced in grasping any foreign body in the rectum, a laparotomy is usually necessary, which allows the object to be pushed from above into the assistant's fingers in the rectum. If there is considerable laceration of the mucosa, a temporary colostomy is advisable (Summary box 72.4).

Charles Bowesman, ?1907–1993, surgical specialist, Colonial Medical Service, Kumasi, Ghana.

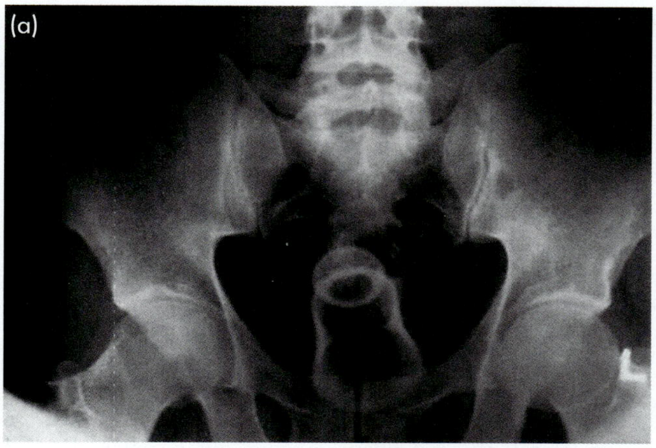

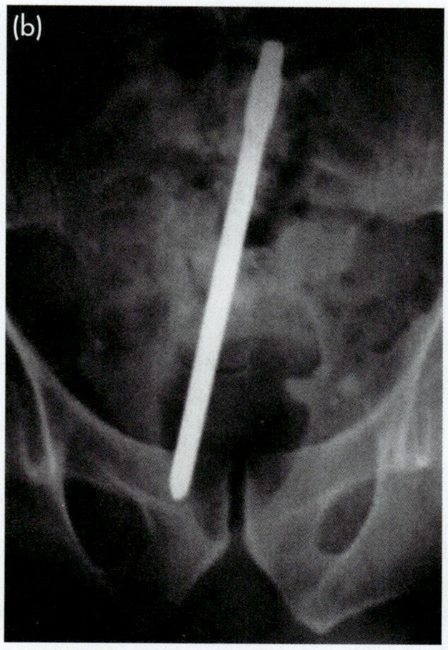

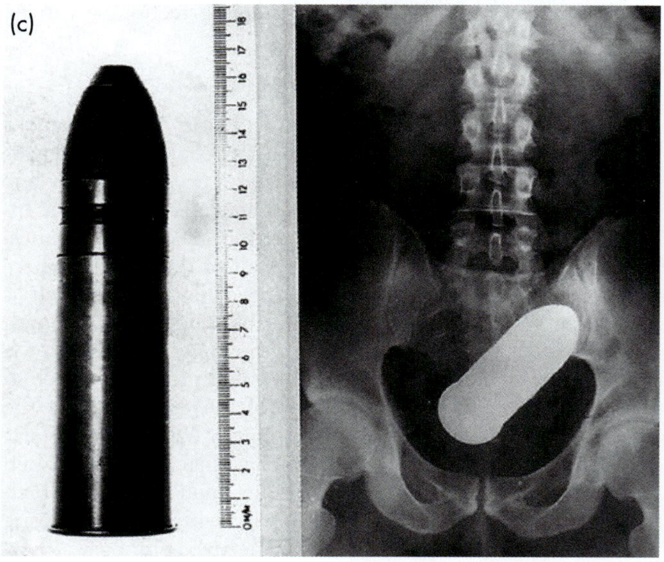

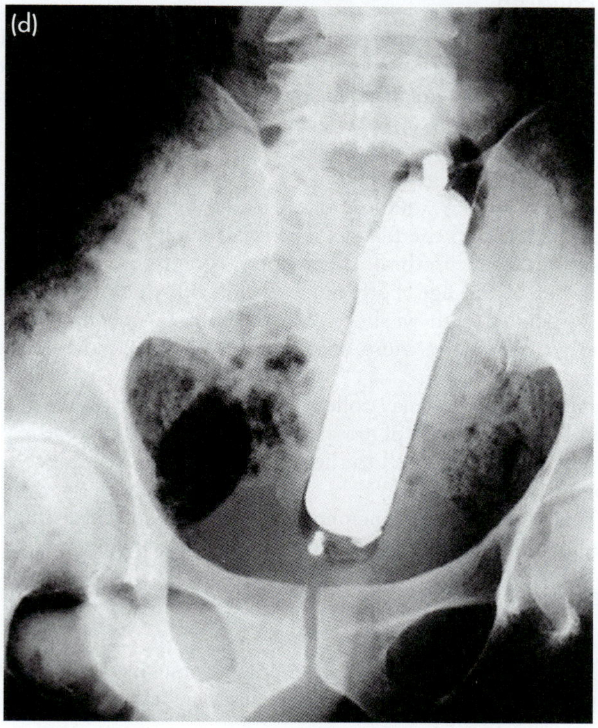

Figure 72.7 (a) Pepper pot in the rectum. On removal, it was found to be inscribed 'A present from Margate' (courtesy of Dr LS Carstairs, Royal Northern Hospital, London). (b) A screwdriver with a plastic handle (courtesy of Dr AK Sharma, Agra, India). (c) A live shell, which needed careful handling. (d) A large vibrator, which had pierced the lateral intraperitoneal rectal wall and caused peritonitis.

Summary box 72.4

Injuries to the rectum are serious and invariably require surgery

- A temporary colostomy is often necessary
- There is a serious risk of associated necrotising fasciitis, and broad-spectrum antibiotics are mandatory
- There may be associated bladder or urethral damage

PROLAPSE

Mucosal prolapse

The mucous membrane and submucosa of the rectum protrude outside the anus for approximately 1–4 cm. When the prolapsed mucosa is palpated between the finger and thumb, it is evident that it is composed of no more than a double layer of mucous membrane (see below under Full-thickness prolapse) (Summary box 72.5).

Summary box 72.5

Rectal prolapse

- It may be mucosal or full thickness
- If full thickness, the whole wall of the rectum is included
- It commences as a rectal intussusception
- In children, the prolapse is usually mucosal and should be treated conservatively
- In the adult, the prolapse is often full thickness and is frequently associated with incontinence
- Surgery is necessary for full-thickness rectal prolapse
- The operation is performed either via the perineum or via the abdomen

In infants

The direct downward course of the rectum, due to the as-yet undeveloped sacral curve (Figure 72.8), predisposes to this condition, as does the reduced resting anal tone, which offers diminished support to the mucosal lining of the anal canal.

In children

Mucosal prolapse often commences after an attack of diarrhoea, or from loss of weight and consequent loss of fat in the ischiorectal fossae. It may also be associated with cystic fibrosis, neurological causes and maldevelopment of the pelvis.

In adults

The condition in adults is often associated with third-degree haemorrhoids. In the female, a torn perineum, and in the male straining from urethral obstruction, predispose to mucosal prolapse. In old age, both mucosal and full-thickness prolapse are associated with weakness of the sphincter mechanism, but whether this is the cause of the problem or secondary to it is unknown.

Partial prolapse may follow an operation for fistula *in ano* where a large portion of muscle has been divided. Here, the prolapse is usually localised to the damaged quadrant and is seldom progressive.

Prolapsed mucous membrane is pink; prolapsed internal haemorrhoids are plum coloured and more pedunculated.

Treatment

In infants and young children

- **Digital repositioning**. The parents are taught to replace the protrusion, and any underlying causes are addressed.
- **Submucosal injections**. If digital repositioning fails after 6 weeks' trial, injections of 5 per cent phenol in almond oil are carried out under general anaesthetic. As a result of the aseptic inflammation following these injections, the mucous membrane becomes tethered to the muscle coat.
- **Surgery**. Occasionally, surgery is required and, in such cases, the child is placed in the prone jack-knife position, the retrorectal space is entered, and the rectum is sutured to the sacrum.

In adults

- **Local treatments**. Submucosal injections of phenol in almond oil or the application of rubber bands are sometimes successful in cases of mucosal prolapse.
- **Excision of the prolapsed mucosa**. When the prolapse is unilateral, the redundant mucosa can be excised or, if circumferential, an endoluminal stapling technique can be used.

Full-thickness prolapse

Full-thickness prolapse (synonym: procidentia) is less common than the mucosal variety. The protrusion consists of all layers of the rectal wall and is usually associated with a weak pelvic floor. The prolapse is thought to commence as an intussusception of the rectum, which descends to protrude outside the anus. The process starts with the anterior wall of the rectum, where the supporting tissues are weakest, especially in women. It is more than 4 cm and commonly as much as 10–15 cm in length (Figure 72.9). On palpation between the finger and thumb, the prolapse feels much thicker than a mucosal prolapse, and obviously consists of a double thickness of the entire wall of the rectum. Any prolapse over 5 cm in length contains anteriorly between its layers a pouch of peritoneum (Figure 72.10). When large, the peritoneal pouch may contain small intestine, which returns to the general peritoneal cavity with a characteristic gurgle when the prolapse is reduced. The anal sphincter is characteristically patulous and gapes widely on straining to allow the rectum to prolapse. Complete prolapse is uncommon in children. In adults, it can occur at any age, but it is more common in the elderly. Women are affected six times more often than

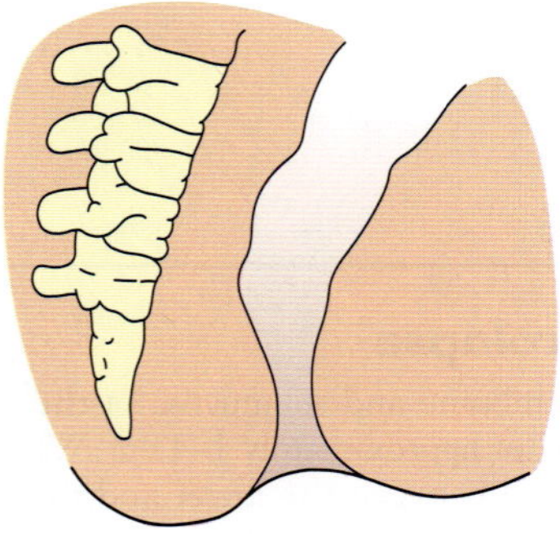

Figure 72.8 The absence of the normal sacral curve predisposes to rectal prolapse in an infant.

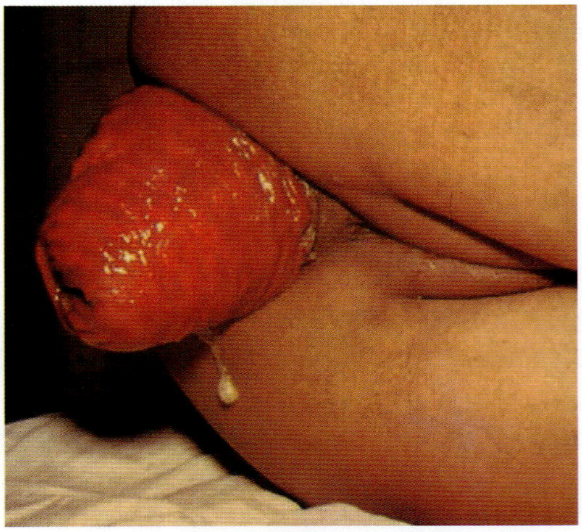

Figure 72.9 Full-thickness rectal prolapse (courtesy of GD Adhia, Bombay, India).

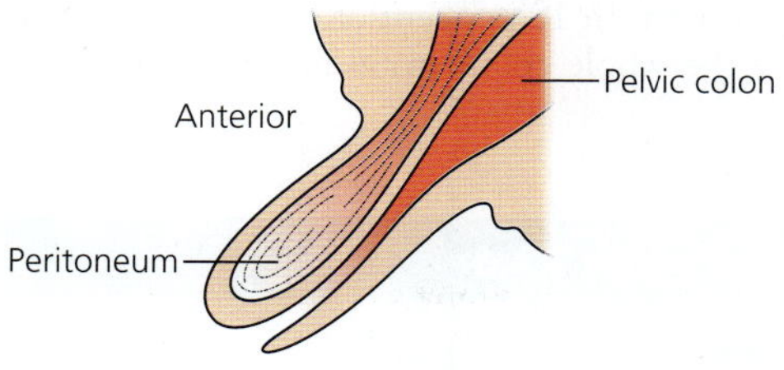

Figure 72.10 Rectal prolapse containing a pouch of peritoneum.

men, and it is commonly associated with prolapse of the uterus. In approximately 50 per cent of adults, faecal incontinence is also a feature.

Differential diagnosis

In the case of a child with abdominal pain, prolapse of the rectum must be distinguished from **ileocaecal intussusception** protruding from the anus. Figures 72.11 and 72.12 make the differential diagnosis clear. In **rectosigmoid intussusception** in the adult, there is a deep groove (5 cm or more) between the emerging protruding mass and the margin of the anus, into which the finger can be placed.

Treatment

Surgery is required, and the operation can be performed via the perineal or the abdominal approaches. An abdominal rectopexy has a lower rate of recurrence but, when the patient is elderly and very frail, a perineal operation, sometimes performed under spinal anaesthetic, is usually safer. As an abdominal procedure risks damage to the pelvic autonomic nerves, resulting in possible sexual dysfunction, a perineal approach is often preferred in young men.

Perineal approach

These procedures have been used most commonly:

- **Thiersch operation**. This procedure, which aimed to place a steel wire or, more commonly, a silastic or nylon suture around the anal canal, has become obsolete. The reasons for its lack of popularity were that the suture would often break or cause chronic perineal sepsis, or both, or the anal stenosis so created would produce severe functional problems.
- **Delorme's operation**. In this procedure, the rectal mucosa is removed circumferentially from the prolapsed rectum over its length (Figure 72.13). The underlying muscle is then plicated with a series of sutures, so that, when these are tied, the rectal muscle is concertinaed towards the anal canal. The anal canal mucosa is then sutured circumferentially to the rectal mucosa remaining at the tip of the prolapse. The prolapse is reduced, and a ring of muscle is created above the anal canal, which prevents recurrence.
- **Altemeier's procedure**. This consists of excision of the prolapsed rectum and associated sigmoid colon from below, and construction of a coloanal anastomosis.

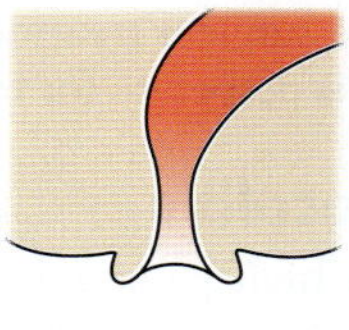

Figure 72.11 Partial prolapse of the rectum.

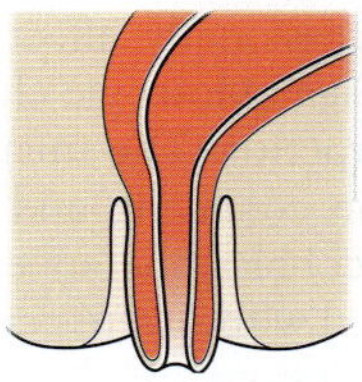

Figure 72.12 Intussusception protruding from the anus.

Abdominal approach

The principle of all abdominal operations for rectal prolapse is to fix the rectum in its proper position. Many variations have been described, including inserting a sheet of polypropylene mesh between the rectum and the sacrum, hitching up the rectosigmoid junction with a Teflon sling to the front of the sacrum (Figure 72.14) or simply suturing the mobilised rectum to the sacrum using four to six interrupted non-absorbable sutures – so-called 'sutured rectopexy'. Recently, the technique has been performed laparoscopically, thus reducing the operative trauma and limiting the time in hospital.

As an abdominal rectopexy may lead to severe constipation, some surgeons recommend combining this procedure with resection of the sigmoid colon, so-called 'resection rectopexy'. Recently, an anterior mesh rectopexy has gained favour. In this procedure, a piece of mesh is fixed to the upper sacrum. The plane between the rectum and vagina is dissected, and the mesh placed into it and sutured to the rectum. This has the advantage of fixing the rectum in place anteriorly, where the prolapse starts, and reinforcing the rectovaginal septum which can bulge forward as a rectocoele.

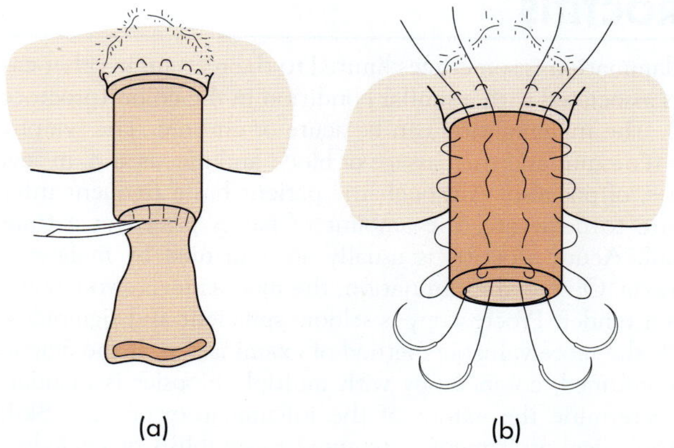

Figure 72.13 Delorme's operation for rectal prolapse. (a) The mucosa has been removed from the prolapse. (b) Interrupted sutures have been placed in the underlying muscle so that, when tied, the muscle is plicated. Redrawn with permission from Keighley MRB, Williams NS. *Surgery of the anus, rectum and colon*. London: WB Saunders, 1999.

Karl Thiersch, 1822–1895, Professor of Surgery, Leipzig, Germany.
Edmond Delorme, 1847–1929, Professor of Surgery, Val-de-Grace Military Hospital, Paris, France.
William Altemeier, 1910–1983, Professor of Surgery, Cincinnati, USA.

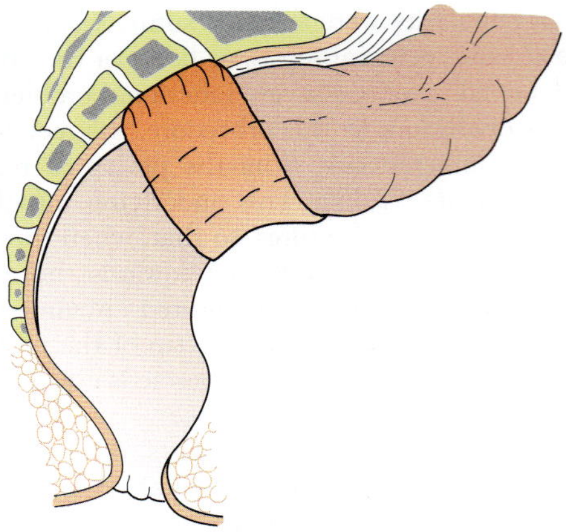

Figure 72.14 Abdominal rectopexy for rectal prolapse. The rectum is mobilised and fixed to the sacrum with a sheet of polypropylene mesh. Redrawn with permission from Corman ML. *Colon and rectal surgery*, 3rd edn. London: JB Lippincott, 1992.

SOLITARY RECTAL ULCER

This is becoming a more commonly diagnosed problem. Classically, it takes the form of an ulcer on the anterior wall of the rectum. In this form, it can be mistaken for a rectal carcinoma or inflammatory bowel disease, particularly Crohn's disease. It may heal, leaving a polypoid appearance. Proctographic studies indicate that it is due to a combination of internal intussusception or anterior rectal wall prolapse and an increase in intrarectal pressure, usually caused by chronic straining as a result of constipation. The histological appearances confirm the diagnosis and are similar to the appearance of biopsies from a full-thickness overt rectal prolapse. The condition, although benign, is difficult to treat. Symptomatic relief from bleeding and discharge may sometimes be achieved by preventing the internal prolapse by biofeedback, an intrarectal stapling procedure or an abdominal rectopexy. In rare cases, rectal excision may be required.

PROCTITIS

Inflammation is sometimes limited to the rectum; in other cases, it is associated with a similar condition in the colon (proctocolitis). The inflammation can be acute or chronic. The symptoms are tenesmus and the passage of blood and mucus and, in severe cases, of pus also. Although the patient has a frequent intense desire to defaecate, the amount of faeces passed at a time is small. Acute proctitis is usually accompanied by malaise and pyrexia. On rectal examination, the mucosa feels swollen and is often tender. Proctoscopy is seldom sufficient and sigmoidoscopy is the more valuable method of examination. If the diagnosis is confirmed, colonoscopy with multiple biopsies is mandatory to determine the extent of the inflammatory process. Skilled pathological assessment is required to establish or exclude the diagnosis of specific infection by bacteriological examination and culture of the stools, examination of scrapings or swabs from ulcers and serological tests.

Non-specific proctitis is an inflammatory condition affecting the mucosa and, to a lesser extent, the submucosa, confined to the distal rectum. In 10 per cent of cases, the condition extends to involve the whole colon (total ulcerative colitis) (Summary box 72.6).

> **Summary box 72.6**
>
> **Proctitis**
>
> - May be non-specific or related to a specific infective agent
> - Non-specific proctitis usually remains confined to the distal bowel, but can spread to the proximal colon
> - Causes bleeding, diarrhoea and tenesmus
> - Treatment is usually conservative

Aetiology

This is unknown. The concept that the condition is a mild and limited form of ulcerative colitis (although actual ulceration is often not present) is the most acceptable hypothesis.

Clinical features

The patient is usually middle-aged and complains of slight loss of blood in the motions. Often, the complaint is one of diarrhoea but, on closer questioning, it transpires that usually one relatively normal action of the bowels occurs each day, although it is accompanied by some blood. During the day, the patient attempts to defaecate, with the passage of flatus and a little blood-stained faecal matter, which is interpreted as diarrhoea. On rectal examination, the mucosa feels warm and smooth. Often, there is some blood on the examining finger. Proctoscopic and sigmoidoscopic examination shows inflamed mucosa of the rectum, but usually no ulceration. The inflammation usually extends for only 5–15 cm from the anus, with the mucosa above this level being normal.

Treatment

The condition is usually self-limiting, but treatment with topical 5-aminosalicylic acid (5-ASA) compounds (Asacol, Pentasa) in the form of suppositories or foam enemas is usually effective. Topical steroids are a less effective alternative. In very severe resistant cases, oral steroids may have to be used to obtain remission. Rarely, surgical treatment is required as a last resort when the patient is desperate for relief of symptoms.

Ulcerative proctocolitis

Proctitis is present in a high percentage of cases of ulcerative colitis, and the degree of severity of the rectal involvement may influence the type of operative procedure (see Chapter 69).

Proctitis due to Crohn's disease

Crohn's disease can occasionally affect the rectum, although classically it is spared. Sigmoidoscopic characteristics differ from those in non-specific proctitis. The inflammatory process tends to be patchy rather than confluent, and there may be fissuring, ulceration and even a cobblestone appearance. Rectal Crohn's disease is often associated with severe perineal disease characterised by fistulation. Skip lesions are also often present in the rest of the colon or small bowel, or both.

Proctitis due to specific infections

Clostridium difficile

An acute form of proctocolitis caused by infection with *Clostridium difficile* can follow broad-spectrum antibiotic administration. A 'membrane' can sometimes be seen on proctoscopy ('pseudomembranous' colitis).

Bacillary dysentery

The appearance is that of an acute purulent proctitis with multiple small, shallow ulcers. The examination of a swab taken from the ulcerated mucous membrane is more certainly diagnostic than stool microscopy.

Amoebic dysentery

The infection is more liable to be chronic, and exacerbations after a long period of freedom from symptoms often occur. Proctoscopy and sigmoidoscopy are not painful. The appearance of an amoebic ulcer is described in Chapter 69. Scrapings from the ulcer should be immersed in warm isotonic saline solution and sent to the laboratory for immediate microscopic examination.

Amoebic granuloma

This presents as a soft mass, usually in the rectosigmoid region. This lesion is frequently mistaken for a carcinoma. Sigmoidoscopy shows an ulcerated surface, but the mass is less friable than a carcinoma. A scraping should be taken, preferably with a small, sharp spoon on a long handle, and the material sent for immediate microscopic examination, as detailed above. A biopsy can also help. Treatment is as described in Chapter 69. Amoebic granuloma of the rectum is encountered from time to time in a patient who has never visited a country in which the disease is endemic.

Tuberculous proctitis

This is nearly always associated with active pulmonary tuberculosis or tuberculous ulceration of the anus. Submucous rectal abscesses burst and leave ulcers with an undermined edge. A hypertrophic type of tuberculous proctitis occurs in association with tuberculous peritonitis, or tuberculous proctitis occurs in association with tuberculous peritonitis or tuberculous salpingitis. This type of tuberculous proctitis requires biopsy for confirmation of the diagnosis.

Gonococcal proctitis

Gonococcal proctitis occurs in both sexes as the result of rectal coitus and, in the female, from direct spread from the vulva. In the acute stage, the mucous membrane is hyperaemic, and thick pus can be expressed as the proctoscope is withdrawn. In the early stages, the diagnosis can be readily established by bacteriological examination but, later, when the infection is mixed, it is more difficult to recognise. Systemic treatment is so effective that local treatment is unnecessary.

Lymphogranuloma venereum

The modes of infection are similar to those of gonococcal proctitis but, in the female, chlamydial infection spreading from the cervix uteri via lymphatics to the pararectal lymph nodes is common. The proctological findings are similar to those of gonococcal proctitis. The diagnosis of lymphogranuloma venereum should be suspected when the inguinal lymph nodes are greatly enlarged, although the enlargement may be subsiding by the time proctitis commences.

Acquired immunodeficiency syndrome

Acquired immunodeficiency syndrome (AIDS) due to human immunodeficiency virus (HIV) may present with a particularly florid type of proctitis. In such patients, unusual organisms such as cytomegalovirus (CMV), herpes simplex virus and organisms such as *Cryptosporidium* are often found.

'Strawberry' lesion of the rectosigmoid

This results from an infection by *Spirochaeta vincenti* and *Bacillus fusiformis*. The leading symptom is diarrhoea, often scantily blood-stained. Occasionally, the diagnosis can be made by the demonstration of the specific organisms in the stools. More often, sigmoidoscopy is required. The characteristic lesion is thickened, somewhat raised mucosa with superficial ulceration in the region of the rectosigmoid. The inflamed mucous membrane oozes blood at numerous pinpoints, giving the appearance of an over-ripe strawberry. A swab should be taken from the lesion and examined for Vincent's and fusiform organisms. Swabs from the gums and the throat are also advisable.

Rectal bilharziasis

Rectal bilharziasis is caused by *Schistosoma mansoni*, which is endemic in many tropical and subtropical countries, and particularly in the delta of the Nile.

In stage 1, a cutaneous lesion develops at the site of entrance of the cercariae (parasites of freshwater snails). Stage 2 is characterised by pyrexia, urticaria and a high eosinophilia. Both these stages are frequently overlooked. Stage 3 results from deposition of the ova in the rectum (much more rarely in the bladder; Chapter 76) and is manifested by bilharzial dysentery. On examination in the later stages, papillomas are frequently present. The papillomas, which are sessile or pedunculated, contain the ova of the trematode, the life cycle of which resembles that of *Schistosoma haematobium*.

Untreated, the rectum becomes festooned, and prolapse of the diseased mucous membrane is usual. Multiple fistulae *in ano* are prone to develop.

Treatment

The primary treatment is systemic and should be undertaken by a specialist in tropical medicine. When the papillomas persist in spite of general treatment, they should be treated by local destruction.

Proctitis due to herbal enemas

This is a well-known clinical entity to those practising in tropical Africa. Following an enema consisting of a concoction of ginger, pepper and bark, administered by a witch doctor, a virulent proctitis sets in. Pelvic peritonitis frequently supervenes. Not infrequently, a complete gelatinous cast of the mucous membrane of the rectum is extruded. Very large doses of morphine, together with antibiotics, often prevent a fatal outcome if commenced early. Temporary colostomy is often advisable.

Jean Hyacinthe Vincent, 1862–1950, Professor of Epidemiology, Val-de-Grace Military Hospital, Paris, France.
Theodor Maximillan Bilharz, 1825–1862, Professor of Zoology, Cairo, Egypt.

Treatment

General treatments should include bed rest in extreme cases. The stools should be kept soft. Suppositories of 5-ASA are often beneficial. Infective causes require specific treatment.

BENIGN TUMOURS

The rectum, along with the sigmoid colon, is the most frequent site of polyps (and cancers) in the gastrointestinal tract. Adenomatous polyps of the colon and rectum have the potential to become malignant. The chance of harbouring invasive cancer is enhanced if the polyp is more than 1 cm in diameter. Removal of all polyps is recommended to give complete histological examination and exclude (or confirm) carcinoma, and also to prevent local recurrence. This is best done using endoscopic hot biopsy or snare polypectomy techniques. If one or more rectal polyps are discovered on sigmoidoscopic examination, a colonoscopy must be performed, as further polyps are frequently found in the colon and treatment may be influenced. No rectal polyp should be removed until the possibility of a proximal carcinoma has been ruled out, otherwise local implantation of cancer cells may occur in the distally situated rectal wound.

The rectum shares substantially the same spectrum of polyps as the colon. Polyps are described chiefly in terms of their tissue organisation. Certain polyps that have features relevant to the rectum are now described.

Polyps relevant to the rectum

Villous adenomas

These have a characteristic frond-like appearance. They may be very large, and occasionally fill the entire rectum. These tumours have an enhanced tendency to become malignant – a change that can sometimes be detected by palpation with the finger; any hard area should be assumed to be malignant and should be biopsied. Rarely, the profuse mucous discharge from these tumours, which is rich in potassium, causes dangerous electrolyte and fluid losses (Figure 72.15).

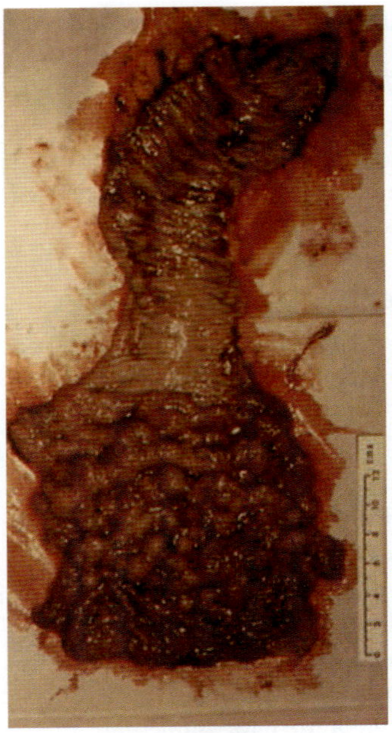

Figure 72.15 Huge villous adenoma which occupied the lower half of the rectum and caused hypokalaemia.

Provided cancerous change has been excluded, these tumours can be removed by submucosal resection endoscopically, surgically *per anum* or by sleeve resection from above. Only very occasionally is rectal excision required. A technique known as transanal endoscopic microsurgery (TEM) has been developed, which has improved the endoanal approach for the local removal of villous adenomas. The method requires the insertion of a large operating sigmoidoscope. The rectum is distended by carbon dioxide insufflation, the operative field is magnified by a camera inserted via the sigmoidoscope, and the image is displayed on a monitor (Figure 72.16). The lesion is excised using specially designed instruments. The technique is highly specialised and takes a considerable amount of time to master.

Familial adenomatous polyposis

This autosomal dominantly inherited condition is characterised by the development of multiple rectal and colonic adenomas around puberty. It is due to mutation of the adenomatous polyposis coli (*APC*) gene, allowing genetic testing in the 75 per cent of families in which a mutation can be identified. A colonoscopy and biopsy will confirm the diagnosis. As this condition is premalignant, a total colectomy must be performed; often, the rectum can be preserved, but regular flexible endoscopy and removal of polyps before they develop carcinoma are required. The operation of restorative proctocolectomy with ileal pouch–anal anastomosis is an alternative if proctectomy is required: the rectum is replaced by a 'pouch' of folded ileum (Chapter 69). A pan-proctocolectomy with permanent ileostomy is necessary in some instances, especially when patient follow up may be impractical.

Hyperplastic polyps

These are small, pinkish, sessile polyps, 2–4 mm in diameter and frequently multiple. They are common and generally harmless.

Inflammatory pseudopolyps

These are oedematous islands of mucosa. They are usually associated with colitis in the UK, but most inflammatory diseases (including tropical diseases) can cause them. They are more likely to cause radiological difficulty as the sigmoidoscopic appearances are usually associated with obvious signs of the inflammatory cause.

Juvenile polyp

This is a bright-red glistening pedunculated sphere ('cherry tumour'), which is found in infants and children. Occasionally, it persists into adult life. It can cause bleeding, or pain if it prolapses during defaecation. It often separates itself, but can be removed easily with forceps or a snare. A solitary juvenile polyp has virtually no tendency to malignant change, but should be treated if it is causing symptoms. It has a unique histological structure of large mucus-filled spaces covered by a smooth surface of thin rectal cuboidal epithelium (Figure 72.17). The rare autosomal dominantly inherited syndrome juvenile polyposis does confer an increased risk of gastrointestinal cancers. It is characterised by multiple juvenile polyps and a positive family history (Summary box 72.7).

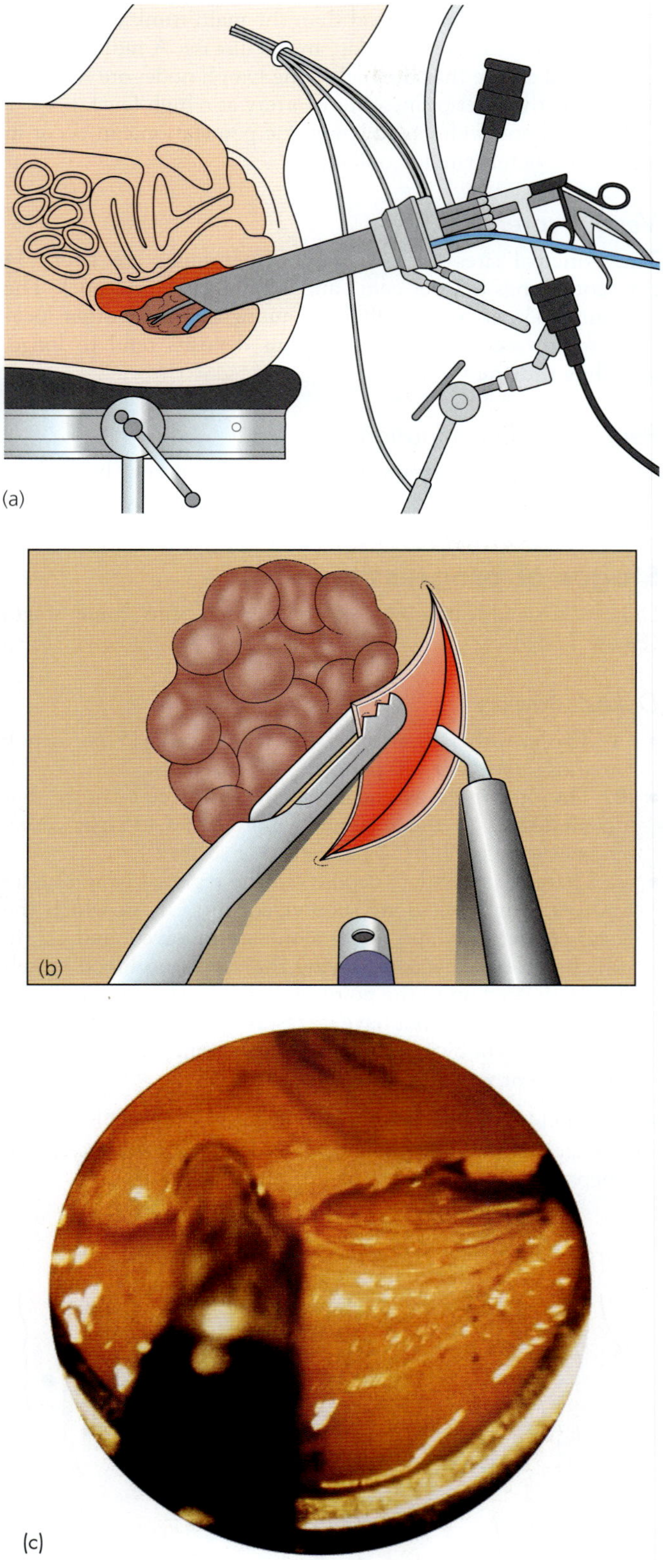

Figure 72.16 (a–c) Transanal endoscopic microsurgery technique (see text).

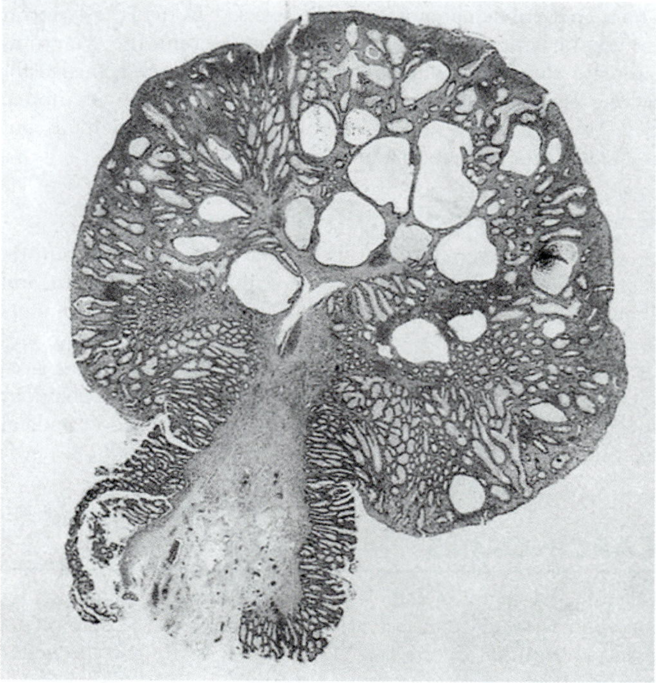

Figure 72.17 Microscopic appearance of a juvenile polyp.

Summary box 72.7

Polyps in the rectum

- Are either single or multiple
- Adenomas are the most frequent histological type
- Villous adenomas may be extensive and undergo malignant change more commonly than tubular adenomas
- All adenomas must be removed to avoid carcinomatous change
- All patients must undergo colonoscopy to determine whether further polyps are present
- Most polyps can be removed by endoscopic techniques, but sometimes major surgery is required

Endometrioma

Endometrioma is rare and may be misdiagnosed as a carcinoma. The focus of ectopic endometrial tissue produces either a constricting lesion of the rectosigmoid or a tumour invading the rectum from the rectovaginal septum. The latter variety gives rise to a very tender submucous elevation of the rectal wall. Endometrioma occurs usually between 20 and 40 years of age. Dysmenorrhoea and rectal bleeding (particularly coinciding with the menses) are the main symptoms. On sigmoidoscopy, endometriosis involving the rectosigmoid junction usually presents as a stricture, with the mucous membrane intact. Hormonal manipulation is the first line of therapy, but sometimes total abdominal hysterectomy and bilateral salpingo-oophorectomy and even bowel resection is required.

Haemangioma

Haemangioma of the rectum is an uncommon cause of serious haemorrhage. When localised in the lower part of the rectum or anal canal, a haemangioma can be excised. When the lesion is diffuse, or lying in the upper part of the rectum, the symptoms simulate ulcerative colitis, and the diagnosis is often missed for a long period, or it is mistakenly thought to be a carcinoma. Selective angiography and embolisation may be helpful, but excision of the rectum is sometimes required.

Gastrointestinal stromal tumour

Smooth muscle tumours of the rectum are rare. If the mitotic rate is high, and if there is variation in nuclear number, size and shape, hyperchromasia and frequent bizarre cells, these tumours are likely to metastasise. In these circumstances, they should be classified as malignant gastrointestinal stromal tumours (formerly leiomyosarcomas). The uncertainty in their behaviour means that treatment should, whenever possible, be by radical excision.

CARCINOMAS

Overall, colorectal cancer is the second most common malignancy in western countries, with approximately 18000 patients dying per annum in the UK. The rectum is the most frequent site involved.

Origin

It is now accepted that colorectal cancer arises from adenomas in a stepwise progression in which increasing dysplasia in the adenoma is due to an accumulation of genetic abnormalities (the adenoma–carcinoma sequence). In approximately 5 per cent of cases, there is more than one carcinoma present. Usually, these carcinomas present as an ulcer, but polypoid and infiltrating types are also common.

Types of carcinoma spread

Local spread

Local spread occurs circumferentially rather than in a longitudinal direction. After the muscular coat has been penetrated, the growth spreads into the surrounding mesorectum, but is initially limited by the mesorectal fascia. If penetration occurs anteriorly, the prostate, seminal vesicles or bladder become involved in the male; in the female, the vagina or the uterus is invaded. In either sex, if the penetration is lateral, a ureter may become involved, while posterior penetration may reach the sacrum and the sacral plexus. Downward spread for more than a few centimetres is rare.

Lymphatic spread

Lymphatic spread from a carcinoma of the rectum above the peritoneal reflection occurs almost exclusively in an upward direction; below that level, the lymphatic spread is still upwards, but when the neoplasm lies within the field of the middle rectal artery, primary lateral spread along the lymphatics that accompany it is not infrequent.

Downward spread is exceptional, with drainage along the subcutaneous lymphatics to the groins being confined, for practical purposes, to the lymph nodes draining the perianal rosette and the epithelium lining the distal 1–2 cm of the anal canal.

Metastasis at a higher level than the main trunk of the superior rectal artery occurs only late in the disease. A radical operation should ensure that the high-lying lymph nodes are removed by ligating the inferior mesenteric artery at a high level.

Atypical and widespread lymphatic permeation can occur in highly undifferentiated neoplasms.

Venous spread

The principal sites for blood-borne metastases are liver (34 per cent), lungs (22 per cent) and adrenals (11 per cent). The remaining 33 per cent are divided among the many other locations where secondary carcinomatous deposits tend to lodge, including the brain.

Peritoneal dissemination

This may follow penetration of the peritoneal coat by a high-lying rectal carcinoma.

Stages of progression

Dukes classified carcinoma of the rectum into three stages (Figure 72.18).

Dukes' staging

- **A**, The growth is limited to the rectal wall (15 per cent): prognosis excellent (90 per cent year survival).
- **B**, The growth is extended to the extrarectal tissues, but no metastasis to the regional lymph nodes (35 per cent): prognosis reasonable (70 per cent year survival).
- **C**, There are secondary deposits in the regional lymph nodes (50 per cent). These are subdivided into C1, in which the local pararectal lymph nodes alone are involved, and C2, in which the nodes accompanying the supplying blood vessels are implicated up to the point of division. This does not take into account cases that have metastasised beyond the regional lymph nodes or by way of the venous system: prognosis is poor (40 per cent year survival).

A stage D is often included, which was not described by Dukes. This stage signifies the presence of widespread metastases, usually hepatic.

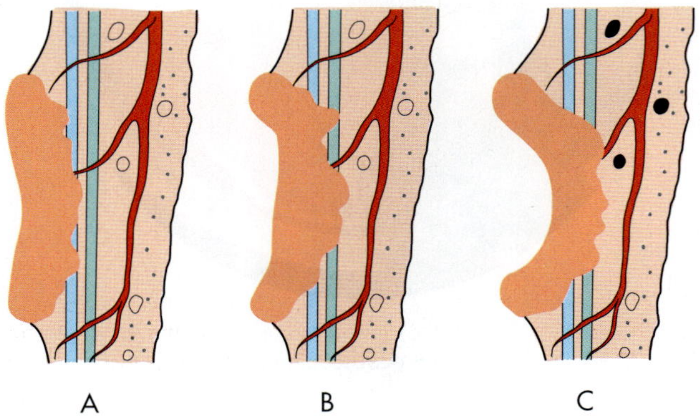

Figure 72.18 The three cardinal stages of progression of the neoplasm (after C Dukes, FRCS).

Sir Walter Fred Bodmer, geneticist, Director of Research, Imperial Cancer Research Fund, London, UK.

Other staging systems have been developed (e.g. Astler–Coller, TNM) to improve prognostic accuracy, but the tumour–node–metastasis (TNM) classification is now recognised internationally as the optimum classification for staging.

TNM staging

T represents the extent of local spread and there are four grades:

- T1 tumour invasion through the muscularis mucosae, but not into the muscularis propria;
- T2 tumour invasion into, but not through the muscularis propria;
- T3 tumour invasion through the muscularis propria, but not through the serosa (on surfaces covered by peritoneum) or mesorectal fascia;
- T4 tumour invasion through the serosa or mesorectal fascia.

N describes nodal involvement:

- N0 no lymph node involvement;
- N1 between one and three involved lymph nodes;
- N2 four or more involved lymph nodes.

M indicates the presence of distant metastases:

- M0 no distant metastases;
- M1 distant metastases.

The prefix 'p' indicates that the staging is based on histopathological analysis, and 'y' that it is the stage after neoadjuvant treatment, which may have resulted in downstaging.

Histological grading

In the great majority of cases, carcinoma of the rectum is a columnar-celled adenocarcinoma. The more nearly the tumour cells approach normal shape and arrangement, the less aggressive the tumour is. Conversely, the greater the percentage of cells of an undifferentiated type, the more aggressive the tumour is:

- Low grade, well-differentiated 11 per cent prognosis good;
- Average grade, 64 per cent prognosis fair;
- High grade, undifferentiated tumours 25 per cent prognosis poor.

Vascular and perineural invasion are poor prognostic features, as is the presence of an infiltrating (rather than pushing) margin and tumour budding. In a small number of cases, the tumour is a primary mucoid carcinoma. The mucus lies within the cells, displacing the nucleus to the periphery, like the seal of a signet ring. Primary mucoid carcinoma gives rise to a rapidly growing bulky growth that metastasises very early and the prognosis of which is very poor (Summary box 72.8).

Summary box 72.8

Pathology and staging of rectal cancer

- Tumours are adenocarcinomas and are well, moderately or poorly differentiated
- They spread by local, lymphatic, venous and transperitoneal routes
- Circumferential local spread is the most important as this profoundly affects surgical treatment
- Although lymphatic spread follows the blood supply of the rectum, most occurs in an upwards direction via the superior rectal vessels to the para-aortic nodes
- The TNM classification is the internationally recognised staging system

Clinical features

Carcinoma of the rectum can occur early in life, but the age of presentation is usually above 55 years, when the incidence rises rapidly. Often, the early symptoms are so insignificant that the patient does not seek advice for six months or more (Summary box 72.9), and the diagnosis is often delayed in younger patients as these symptoms are attributed to benign causes. Initial rectal examination and a low threshold for investigating persistent symptoms are essential to prevent this.

Summary box 72.9

Early symptoms of rectal cancer

- Bleeding per rectum
- Tenesmus
- Early morning diarrhoea

Bleeding

Bleeding is the earliest and most common symptom. There is nothing characteristic about the time at which it occurs, nor is the colour or the amount of blood distinctive; often, the bleeding is slight in amount and occurs at the end of defaecation, or is noticed because it has stained underclothing. Indeed, more often than not, the bleeding in every respect simulates that of internal haemorrhoids (haemorrhoids and carcinoma sometimes coexist).

Sense of incomplete defaecation

The patient's bowels open, but there is the sensation that there are more faeces to be passed (**tenesmus**, a distressing straining to empty the bowels without resultant evacuation). This is a very important early symptom and is almost invariably present in tumours of the lower half of the rectum. The patient may endeavour to empty the rectum several times a day (spurious diarrhoea), often with the passage of flatus and a little blood-stained mucus ('bloody slime').

Alteration in bowel habit

This is the next most frequent symptom. The patient may find it necessary to start taking an aperient or to supplement the usual dose. A patient who has to get up early in order to defaecate, or one who passes blood and mucus in addition to faeces ('early-morning bloody diarrhoea'), is usually found to be suffering from carcinoma of the rectum. Often, it is the patient with an annular carcinoma at the rectosigmoid junction who suffers with increasing constipation, and the one with a growth in the ampulla of the rectum who has early-morning diarrhoea.

Pain

Pain is a late symptom, but pain of a colicky character may accompany advanced tumours of the rectosigmoid, and is caused

Sir John Bruce, 1905–1975, Professor of Surgery, Edinburgh, UK.

by some degree of intestinal obstruction. When a deep carcinomatous ulcer of the rectum erodes the prostate or bladder, there may be severe pain. Pain in the back, or sciatica, occurs when the cancer invades the sacral plexus.

Weight loss is suggestive of hepatic metastases.

Investigation

Abdominal examination

Abdominal examination is normal in early cases. Occasionally, when an advanced annular tumour is situated at the rectosigmoid junction, signs of obstruction of the large intestine are present. By the time the patient seeks advice, metastases in the liver may be palpable. When the peritoneum has become studded with secondary deposits, ascites usually results.

Rectal examination

In many cases, the neoplasm can be felt digitally: in early cases as a nodule with an indurated base. When the centre ulcerates, a shallow depression will be found, the edges of which are raised and everted. On bimanual examination, it may be possible to feel the lower extremity of a carcinoma situated in the rectosigmoid junction. After the finger has been withdrawn, if it has been in direct contact with a carcinoma, it is smeared with blood or mucopurulent material tinged with blood. When a carcinomatous ulcer is situated in the lower third of the rectum, involved lymph nodes can sometimes be felt as one or more hard, oval swellings in the mesorectum posteriorly or posterolaterally above the tumour. In females, a vaginal examination should be performed and, when the neoplasm is situated on the anterior wall of the rectum, with one finger in the vagina and another in the rectum, very accurate palpation can be carried out.

Proctosigmoidoscopy

Proctosigmoidoscopy will always show a carcinoma, if present, provided that the rectum is emptied of faeces beforehand.

Biopsy

Using biopsy forceps (Figure 72.19) via a sigmoidoscope, a portion of the edge of the tumour can be removed. If possible, another specimen from the more central part of the growth should also be obtained.

Colonoscopy

A colonoscopy is required if possible in all patients to exclude a synchronous tumour, be it an adenoma or a carcinoma. If a proximal adenoma is found, it can be conveniently snared and removed via the colonoscope. If a synchronous carcinoma is present, the operative strategy will need changing. If a full colonoscopy is not possible, a CT colonography or barium enema can be performed.

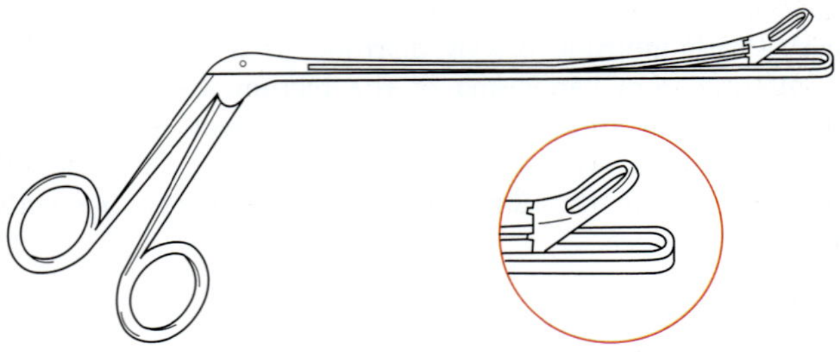

Figure 72.19 Yeoman's biopsy forceps.

When a stenosing carcinoma is present, it may not be possible using these investigations, especially colonoscopy, to visualise the proximal colon. However, in view of the high incidence of synchronous tumours, it is imperative that a colonoscopy is always performed either before or within a few months of surgical resection.

Differential diagnosis

When an adenoma shows evidence of induration or unusual friability, it is almost certain that malignancy has occurred, even in spite of biopsy findings to the contrary. On the other hand, biopsy is invaluable in distinguishing carcinoma from an inflammatory stricture or an amoebic granuloma. The possibility of a neoplasm being an endometrioma should always be considered in patients with dysmenorrhoea. The possibility of a carcinoid tumour in atypical cases must be remembered. In the last four instances, biopsy should establish the correct diagnosis. The solitary ulcer syndrome has already been mentioned above (Summary box 72.10).

Summary box 72.10

Diagnosis and assessment of rectal cancer

All patients with suspected rectal cancer should undergo:

- Digital rectal examination
- Sigmoidoscopy and biopsy
- Colonoscopy if possible (or CT colonography or barium enema)

All patients with proven rectal cancer require staging by:

- Imaging of the liver and chest, preferably by CT
- Local pelvic imaging by magnetic resonance imaging and/or endoluminal ultrasound

Treatment

Some form of excision of the tumour remains the mainstay of treatment, if at all possible, because of the extreme suffering entailed if the neoplasm remains. However, the management of rectal cancer has become increasingly complex, because of the various surgical, neoadjuvant and adjuvant options available, and is best delivered in a multidisciplinary setting. Before treatment can be planned, it is necessary to assess:

- the fitness of the patient;
- the extent of spread of the tumour.

Assessment of spread should include CT of the chest and abdomen to exclude distant metastases (Figure 72.20). Ultrasonography of the liver and a chest radiograph are decreasingly used alternatives. Positron emission tomography (PET) scanning can be helpful in identifying metastases if imaging is otherwise equivocal.

Endoluminal ultrasound, performed using a probe placed in the rectal lumen, can be used to assess the local spread of the tumour (Figure 72.21), and is particularly accurate in staging the degree of penetration through the rectal wall in early tumours. CT is not particularly accurate in local staging, which is usually performed using magnetic resonance imaging (MRI), which allows assessment of the circumferential resection margin and adjacent structures (Figure 72.22).

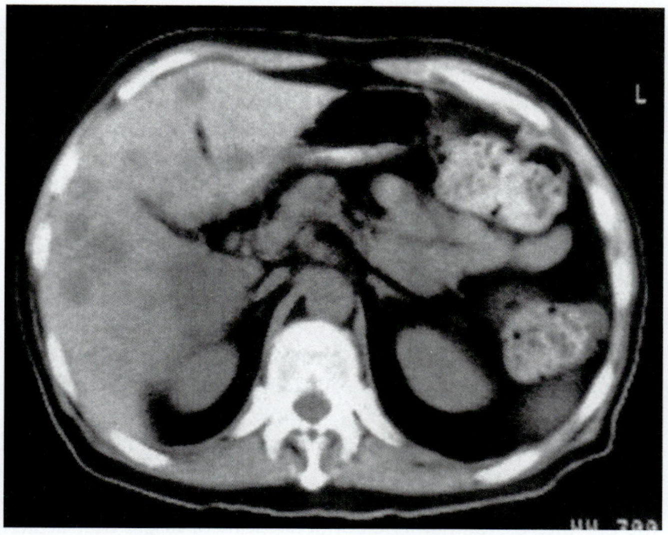

Figure 72.20 Computed tomography scan of the liver in a patient with a rectal cancer showing multiple liver metastases.

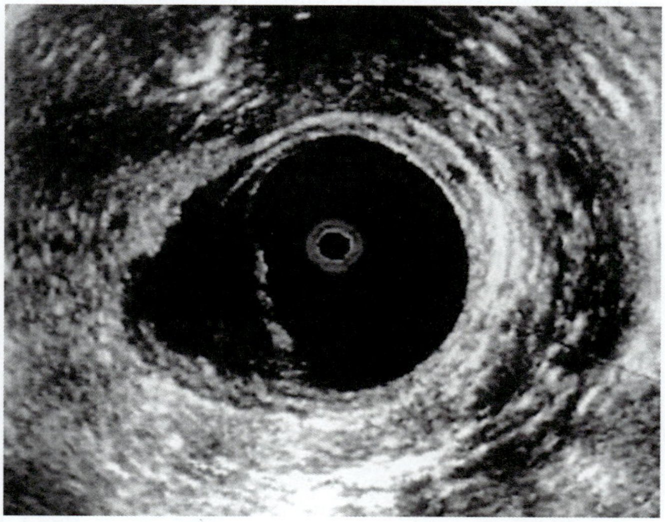

Figure 72.21 Endoluminal ultrasound. The probe is in the rectal lumen and shows a rectal tumour invading through the rectal wall.

Principles of surgical treatment

Radical excision of the rectum, together with the mesorectum and associated lymph nodes, should be the aim in most cases. Even in the presence of widespread metastases, a rectal excision should be considered, as this is often the best means of palliation. The presence of liver metastases does not necessarily rule out the feasibility of cure: the results of surgery for liver metastases have greatly improved, with long-term survival being achieved in over a third of patients.

When a tumour appears to be locally advanced (i.e. invading a neighbouring structure or threatening to breach the circumferential resection margin), the administration of a course of neoadjuvant (preoperative) chemoradiotherapy over approximately 6 weeks may reduce its size and make curative surgery

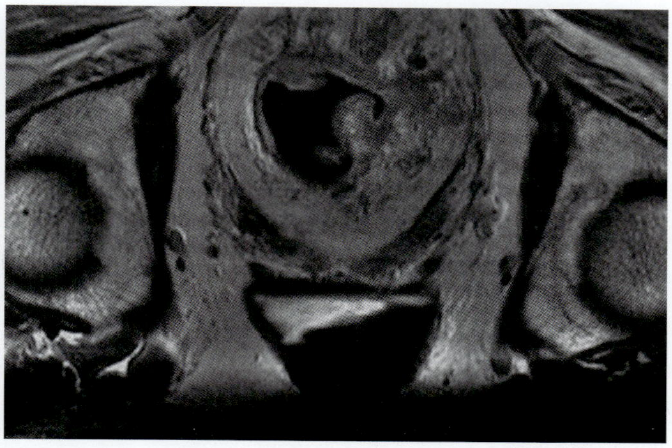

Figure 72.22 Magnetic resonance imaging scan of pelvis showing extensive T3 rectal carcinoma invading the left side of the mesorectum.

possible. The administration of preoperative 'short-course' (5 days) neoadjuvant radiotherapy in resectable rectal cancer cases significantly reduces the incidence of local recurrence, but at the cost of some increase in complication rates.

For patients who are unfit for radical surgery, who have very early tumours or who have widespread metastases, a local procedure such as transanal excision, laser destruction or interstitial radiation should be considered.

When a rectal excision is possible, the aim should be to restore gastrointestinal continuity and continence by preserving the anal sphincter whenever feasible. A sphincter-saving operation (anterior resection) is usually possible for tumours whose lower margin is ≥2 cm above the anal canal. Although removal of the rectum and anus with a permanent colostomy (abdominoperineal excision) was often required for tumours of the lower third of the rectum in the past, the introduction of the stapling gun has enabled many more of these patients to be treated by a sphincter-saving procedure. The principles of the operation involve radical excision of the neoplasm, removal of the mesorectum that surrounds it and high proximal ligation of the inferior mesenteric lymphovascular pedicle. Once the rectum has been adequately mobilised, it is removed, and the rectal stump is washed out. Restoration of continuity by direct end-to-end anastomosis (manually or by stapling) must be carried out by a meticulous technique to reduce the risks of anastomotic breakdown.

Rectosigmoid tumours and those in the upper third of the rectum are removed by 'high anterior resection', in which the rectum and mesorectum are taken to a margin 5 cm distal to the tumour, and a colorectal anastomosis is performed. This does not usually require defunctioning. The retention of at least a part of the rectum results in good postoperative function.

For tumours in the middle and lower thirds of the rectum, complete removal of the rectum and mesorectum is required, i.e. total mesorectal excision (TME). A temporary protecting stoma is usually formed after TME (see below under Anterior resection).

Preoperative preparation

Traditionally, the bowel was prepared by mechanical cleansing using a combination of diet, purgatives and enemas (e.g. senna,

Picolax). This approach is now used more selectively, with many surgeons reserving full bowel preparation for those undergoing a low anterior resection, and clearing only the distal bowel using enemas in the rest. Prophylactic systemic antibiotics are given peroperatively. The antibiotic regimen must be active against both aerobic and anaerobic organisms. At present, a suitable prescription would be cefuroxime 750 mg plus metronidazole 500 mg given on induction of anaesthesia. If a patient comes to surgery with a loaded colon, on-table intraoperative irrigation can be performed.

All patients should see a stoma care nurse preoperatively and be sited for a temporary or permanent ileostomy or colostomy. They must also be counselled as to the complications of the procedure, and particularly about the risks of pelvic autonomic nerve damage causing bladder and sexual disturbance, especially impotence.

Blood and electrolyte deficiencies are corrected. Before commencing the operation, an indwelling catheter is inserted into the bladder (Summary box 72.11).

Summary box 72.11

Preoperative preparation

- Counselling and siting of stomas
- Correction of anaemia and electrolyte disturbance
- Cross-matching of blood
- Bowel preparation
- Deep vein thrombosis prophylaxis
- Prophylactic antibiotics
- Insertion of urinary catheter

Local operations

For small, low-grade T1 tumours, local removal should be curative in the vast majority; only a small percentage of these will have involved lymph nodes which are left undetected and unremoved by this approach. For these tumours, especially in the unfit or in patients who will not accept a colostomy, local removal has been used. This is usually done via the anus and the TEM technique is often used.

There is considerable controversy, however, as to whether such local techniques should be used for potentially curable lesions as they do not allow full histopathological staging or deal with the mesorectal or lymphatic spread of the tumour. Certainly the local recurrence rate (mostly due to lymph node metastases within the mesorectum) after local excision of T2 tumours is in the region of 20 per cent, which is unacceptable in all but those in whom radical surgery is associated with very high risk. Combined local excision with chemotherapy and radiotherapy has been suggested as a curative treatment for T1 and T2 tumours, but is not widely accepted.

Anterior resection

In the last 30 years, there has been a move to extend sphincter-saving operations to treat most tumours of the middle third of the rectum, and indeed many in the lower third. Over the last five years it has become clear that this surgery can be performed laparoscopically with at least equivalent oncological outcomes. This is, however, technically challenging and should only be performed in this way by adequately trained and experienced surgeons.

Following a midline incision, the liver and the peritoneum are examined for metastases. The sigmoid and descending colon are freed by dividing the peritoneal reflection on the left side and mobilised to the midline on their mesentery. The splenic flexure is dissected and the left ureter and testicular or ovarian vessels are identified. The mesocolon is divided at the site of the proposed division of the colon and the trunk of the inferior mesenteric artery (Figure 72.23) is ligated and divided. Most surgeons divide the descending colon at this point.

The rectosigmoid mesentery is separated from the sacrum by sharp dissection with scissors or, more usually, diathermy. Great care is exercised to ensure that the hypogastric nerves are identified and preserved. It is essential that, as the distal dissection proceeds, the surgeon remains outside the mesorectal fascia and stays within the bloodless 'holy' plane outside it. The peritoneal incision is carried anteriorly around the rectum, and the seminal vesicles or the vaginal wall are identified so that Denonvilliers' fascia behind them is cleared by a dissection leading down to the prostate or vagina. The condensations of fascia that attach the rectum to the pelvic side walls and are known as the lateral ligaments are dissected by diathermy. This tissue contains the middle rectal vessels, which sometimes require separate ligation and division.

The rectum is mobilised to the pelvic floor, and a right-angled clamp is placed at least 1 cm below the tumour. The rectum can then be stapled transversely. After the rectum and sigmoid colon have been excised, continuity is re-established by the method depicted in Figure 72.24. Although a single loop of colon is often used for the anastomosis, a short J-shaped colonic pouch may be

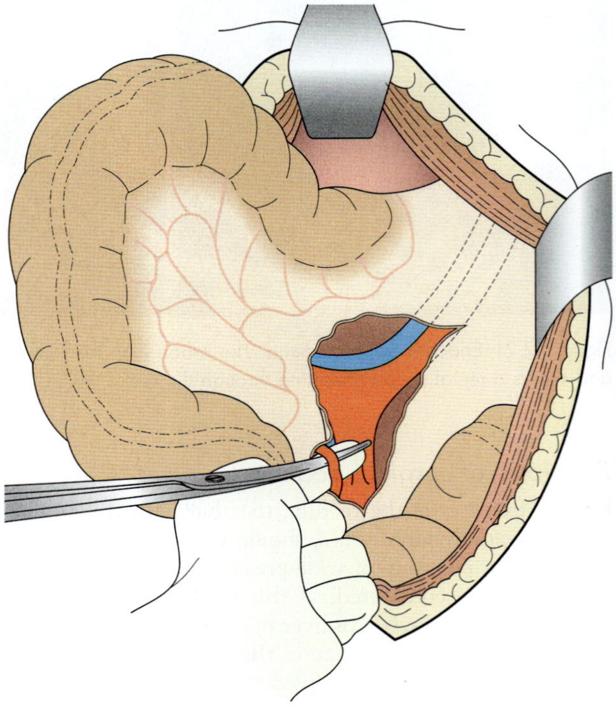

Figure 72.23 Exposure and division of the inferior mesenteric vessels flush with the aorta (high tie) in the course of an abdominoperineal excision of the rectum. Redrawn with permission from Keighley MRB, Williams NS. *Surgery of the anus, rectum and colon*. London: WB Saunders, 1999.

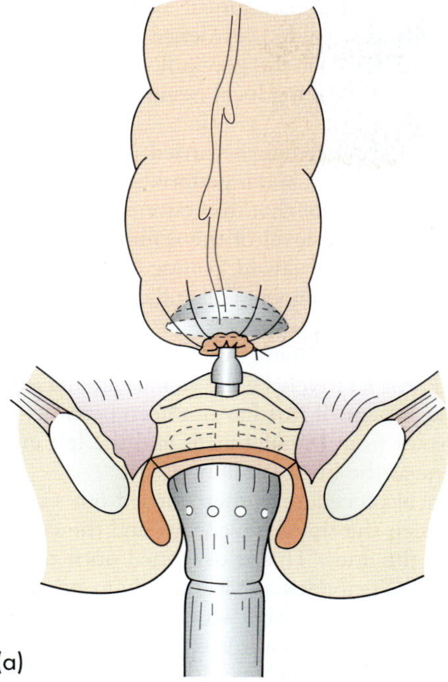

(a)

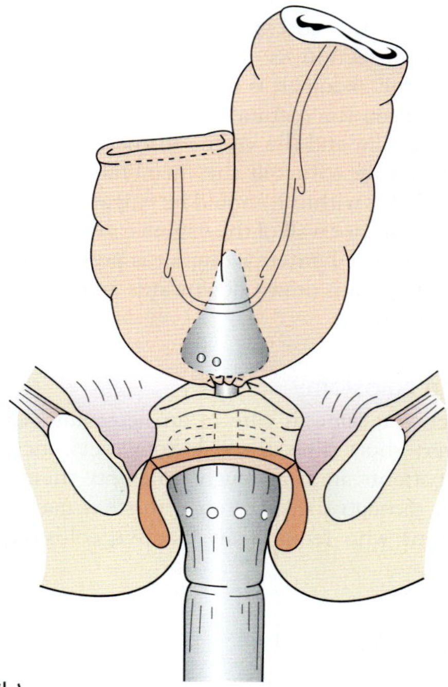

(b)

Figure 72.24 Low anterior resection by the double stapling method. The rectum has been excised, and the distal anorectal stump has been transected with a transverse stapling device. A circular stapling gun is used to construct (a) a straight low coloanal anastomosis or (b) a colonic pouch–anus anastomosis.

constructed with the aim of increasing neorectal capacity and thus reducing postoperative bowel frequency and urgency. Many surgeons believe that such a temporary defunctioning stoma is required for all colorectal and coloanal anastomoses that are constructed below the peritoneal reflection.

Occasionally, although the rectum, together with its tumour, can be removed adequately, continuity cannot be restored by a stapling technique. In such cases, it may still be possible to restore continuity by bringing the colon down to the anal canal and constructing a sutured coloanal anastomosis via the transanal route (Figure 72.25).

It is important to ensure that any free tumour cells released by mobilisation of the rectum are destroyed by irrigation of the rectal lumen with a cancercidal solution such as 1 per cent cetrimide. By so doing, the implantation of such cells and subsequent local recurrence is prevented. However, it should be realised that, although a small percentage of local recurrences are due to implantation of shed cells, the majority result from inadequate removal of the tumour at the time of the initial operation. It is now known that micrometastases are present in the mesorectum, and these are the most likely cause of local recurrence after rectal excision. It is essential to remove all the mesorectum during anterior resection or abdominoperineal

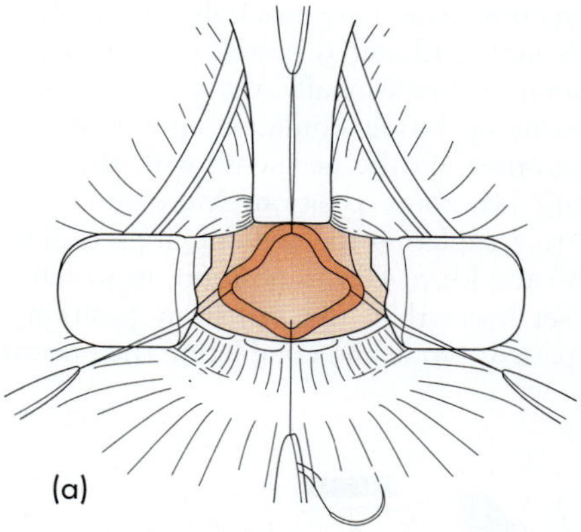

(a)

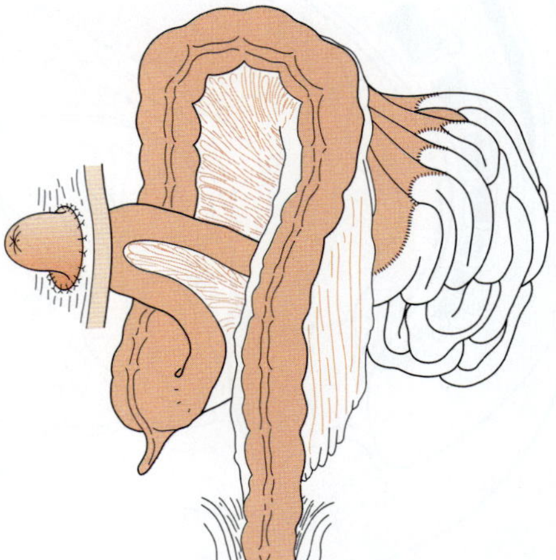

(b)

Figure 72.25 Abdominotransanal–coloanal anastomosis. (a) The rectum has been excised, and the mucosa from the distal anorectal stump has been removed, leaving the rectal muscle intact. The proximal colon has been brought down through the rectal muscular cuff to be anastomosed to the anal mucosa via the transanal route. (b) The completed coloanal anastomosis. A covering ileostomy has been performed to allow the anastomosis to heal.

excision, the procedure known as TME. TME is now being practised worldwide and appears to reduce the risks of local recurrence substantially (Figure 72.26). This has been largely due to the work of Heald, who has shown that training in the technique improves local recurrence rates, and has been central to its widespread adoption. However, it is unlikely that surgery alone will deal adequately with all the micrometastases in the pelvis. Consequently, neoadjuvant radiotherapy may have added benefit (see below under Radiotherapy).

Hartmann's operation

This is an excellent procedure in an old and frail patient in whom there is concern about anal sphincter function or the viability of an anastomosis. Through an abdominal incision, the rectum is excised, the anorectal stump is transected, usually with a stapler and an end colostomy is formed.

Abdominoperineal excision of the rectum

This operation is still required for some tumours of the lower third of the rectum, which are unsuitable for a sphincter-saving procedure. A large catheter is passed to allow easy identification of the urethra. Traditionally, the procedure was performed by two surgeons operating simultaneously, one via the abdomen and the other via the perineum with the patient in the Trendelenburg lithotomy position. More recently, there has been a shift to completing the abdominal procedure first (with the patient in the Lloyd-Davies position, in which the legs are in supports set lower than the lithotomy position), and then placing the patient prone and completing the operation via the perineum from behind (cylindrical or extra-levator abdominoperineal excision). There is evidence that this allows a wider dissection at the level of the pelvic floor, increasing complete resection rates and reducing local recurrence, although increasing morbidity.

The abdominal procedure is carried out laparoscopically or via a midline laparotomy, and is performed in the same way as an anterior resection, except that dissection stops before the pelvic floor is reached (at the level of the seminal vesicles in men or the cervix in women), to avoid 'coning down' onto the tumour at the level of the pelvic floor. The end colostomy is formed and the wounds closed.

The site for the colostomy in the left iliac fossa should have been marked preoperatively by the stoma care nurse in consultation with the patient. If this has not been possible, it should be sited equidistant from the umbilicus and the left anterior superior iliac spine at the linea semilunaris.

The perineal procedure is then carried out via an elliptical incision between the tip of the coccyx and the central perineal point around the anus. This is deepened until the pelvic floor is reached. This is divided as far laterally as possible, to maximise clearance of the tumour, which will be lying at this level (Figure 72.27). The dissection is extended posteriorly by incising Waldeyer's fascia, which is a thick condensation of pelvic fascia lying between the rectum and the sacrum. Some surgeons routinely remove the coccyx to improve access and surgical margins. The dissection is deepened until the mobilisation performed via the abdomen is reached posteriorly and laterally. The plane between the rectum and the prostate in the male or between the rectum and the vagina in the female is developed, with particular care to avoid the membranous urethra in the male. The catheter within it should be palpated so that it can be avoided. The posterior wall of the vagina can be excised with the rectum if an advanced anterior tumour is present. The whole of the anus and rectum is drawn downwards and removed through the perineal wound.

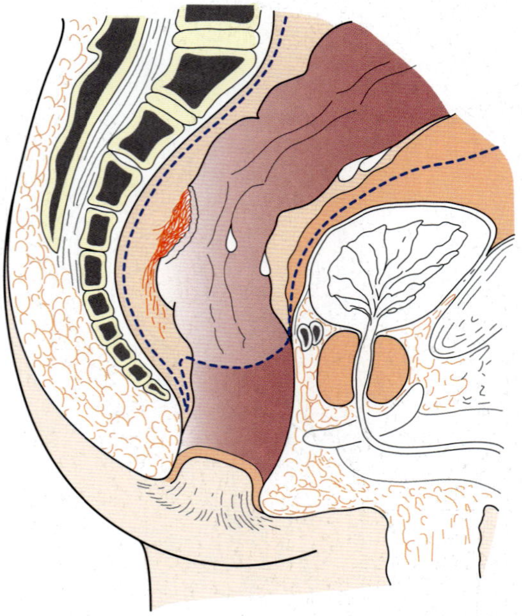

Figure 72.26 Plane of dissection for total mesorectal excision.

Friedrich Trendelenburg, 1844–1924, Professor of Surgery successively at Rostock (1875–1882), Bonn (1882–1895), Leipzig (1895–1911), Germany. The Trendelenburg position was first described in 1885.

Care of the colostomy

This is much the same as care of an ileostomy (Chapter 69). Within a very short time, the colostomy acts once or twice a day. Many patients are now taught to empty their lower colon by irrigation through the colostomy: this has many advantages for the patient who requires an inactive colostomy while at work.

Endoluminal stenting

An increasingly used alternative is placement of an endoluminal stent, which can be done endoscopically, often with fluoroscopic guidance. This can either be used as a palliative procedure, or to relieve obstruction and permit elective rather than emergency surgery to be undertaken. Only colonic and upper rectal tumours are suitable for stenting.

Palliative colostomy

This is indicated only in cases giving rise to intestinal obstruction, or where there is gross infiltration of the neoplasm. It is sometimes possible to resect the tumour later (e.g. after chemoradiotherapy) and, in some cases, cure, rather than palliation, is achieved.

Oswald Vaughan Lloyd-Davies, 1905–1987, St Mark's Hospital and The Middlesex Hospital, London, UK.
Richard John (Bill) Heald, consultant colorectal surgeon, Basingstoke, UK.

Other palliative procedures

Occasionally, a neodymium:yttrium–aluminium–garnet (Nd: YAG) laser can be used to deal with an obstructing or bleeding lesion, and intraluminal debulking has also been described.

More extensive operations

When the carcinoma of the rectum has spread to contiguous organs, the radical operation can often be extended to remove these structures. Thus, in the male, in whom spread is usually to the bladder, a cystectomy and resection of the rectum can be performed. In the female, the uterus acts as a barrier, usually preventing spread from the rectum to the bladder. Accordingly, a hysterectomy should be undertaken in addition to excision of the rectum. Pelvic evisceration for carcinoma of the rectum is justifiable only when the surgeon is confident that the growth can be completely removed.

Pelvic exenteration (Brunschwig's operation)

The aim is to remove all the pelvic organs, together with the internal iliac and the obturator groups of lymph nodes (Figure 72.28). Ligation of both internal iliac arteries diminishes the blood loss. A rectus abdominis flap can be used to fill the empty pelvis. Special care must therefore be taken to suture the perineal skin accurately, and to avoid pressure necrosis of the perineal incision by nursing the patient on alternate sides. Some form of urinary diversion is necessary, usually an ileal conduit.

Liver resection

Single or several well-localised liver metastases can now be resected with relatively low mortality and morbidity. Provided the patients are carefully selected, a reasonable long-term

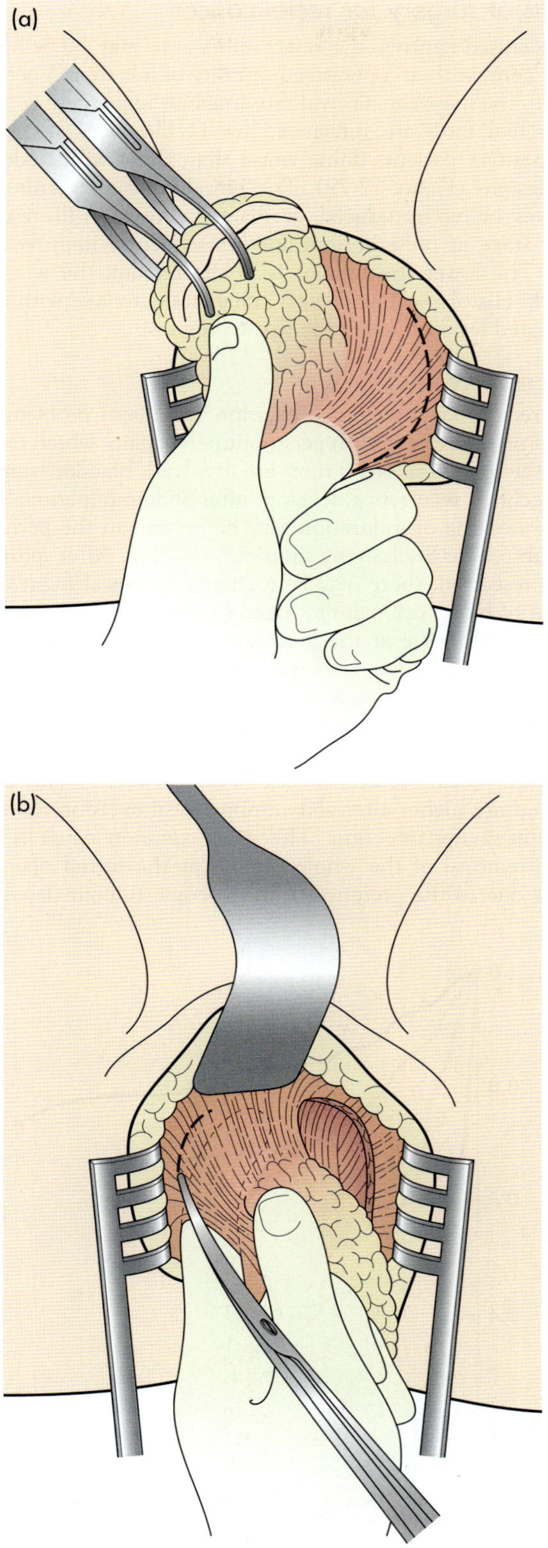

Figure 72.27 (a, b) Separation and division of the pubococcygeus and puborectalis muscles in the course of the perineal phase of an abdominoperineal excision of the rectum. Redrawn with permission from Keighley MRB, Williams NS. *Surgery of the anus, rectum and colon*. London: WB Saunders, 1999.

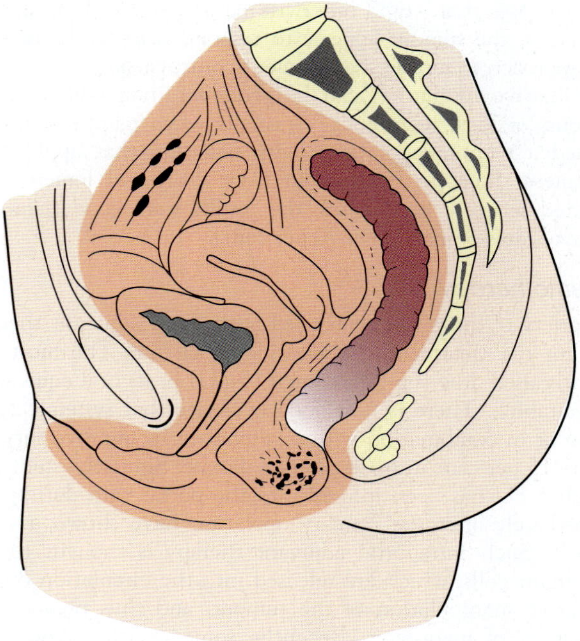

Figure 72.28 Radical pelvic exenteration, indicating the extent of the dissection and the viscera removed. Redrawn with permission from Keighley MRB, Williams NS. *Surgery of the anus, rectum and colon*. London: WB Saunders, 1999.

Alexander Brunschwig, 1901–1969, gynaecologist, the Memorial Hospital for the Treatment of Cancer, New York, NY, USA.

survival rate can be achieved (approximately 40 per cent in some series). Such surgery is usually carried out in a specialised liver unit, and it is generally advised that it takes place after the primary lesion has been dealt with (Summary box 72.12).

Summary box 72.12

Surgery for rectal cancer

- Surgery is the mainstay of curative therapy
- The primary resection consists of rectal excision with total mesorectal excision
- Most cases can be treated by anterior resection with the colorectal anastomosis being achieved with a circular stapling gun
- A smaller group of low, extensive tumours require an abdominoperineal excision with a permanent colostomy
- Preoperative radiotherapy can reduce local recurrence
- Adjuvant chemotherapy can improve survival in node-positive disease
- Liver resection in carefully selected patients offers the best chance of cure for single or well-localised liver metastases

Radiotherapy

Various trials have been performed to investigate the effect of adjuvant radiotherapy given either pre- or postoperatively. The overall results suggest that, provided an adequate dose is given, neoadjuvant radiotherapy can reduce the incidence of local recurrence; however, long-term survival is not affected. Recent studies have combined radiotherapy with chemotherapy in an attempt to shrink an extensive tumour prior to surgical excision. In some cases using this combined therapy, the results can be spectacular, and it has become the standard initial treatment for locally advanced tumours, allowing potentially curative resection in cases that would otherwise be inoperable. Indeed, in a few cases, the tumour appears to respond completely, making the approach to further management controversial.

Palliative irradiation can be given for inoperable primary tumours or local recurrence, especially when painful. Papillon refined a technique of intracavity radiation that applies the treatment direct to the tumour from the rectal lumen. In a selected series of early cases, the results were good (five-year survival rates of more than 70 per cent).

Chemotherapy

A variety of drugs has been tried both as an adjuvant therapy and for the treatment of disseminated disease. The most frequently used drug is 5-fluorouracil (5-FU) or its oral equivalent capecitabine. There is now good evidence that systemic 5-FU alone or in combination with oxaliplatin can improve survival by 10–15 per cent in node-positive disease. Similarly, studies in which 5-FU has been infused into the portal vein during and immediately after the primary operation have shown a small benefit. Such intraportal adjuvant therapy is thought to kill malignant cells, which are released into the circulation during operative manipulation of the tumour, and thus prevent the formation of metastases. Recently, some exciting new drugs have become available, the most notable being irinotecan and cetuximab. Both agents have been shown to have a moderate but beneficial effect in disseminated disease, but it remains to be seen whether they will be effective in an adjuvant setting.

Results of surgery for rectal cancer

In specialised centres, the resectability rate may be as high as 95 per cent, with an operative mortality of less than 5 per cent. Overall, the five-year survival rate is about 50 per cent.

Survival rates are influenced by TNM/Dukes' stage, with node-positive patients doing worse than those with node-negative lesions (Figure 72.29). The bowel cancer screening programmes being introduced in many countries will result in earlier stage at presentation, and consequently improved outcome. The lower the tumour is in the rectum, the worse the outlook. Histological grade also influences outcome, with undifferentiated lesions having the worse prognosis.

Local recurrence

Local recurrence after rectal excision is a major problem. The patient often presents with persistent pelvic pain, which radiates down the legs if the sacral roots are involved. Bladder symptoms may occur. If recurrence develops after abdominoperineal excision, a swelling or induration may be present in the perineum, or an abscess or discharging sinus may develop. After sphincter-saving resection, there may be a change in bowel habit or the passage of blood per rectum. Sigmoidoscopic examination may reveal friable tissue at the anastomosis which, when biopsied, confirms the diagnosis. However, the recurrence is usually situated extrarectally, and is detected either as induration on digital examination or by endoluminal ultrasonography, CT or MRI. These investigations can also detect recurrence before it causes symptoms. Local recurrence rates vary between 2 and 25 per cent and are higher after abdominoperineal excision than after sphincter-saving resection. The most common cause is inadequate removal of the whole tumour at the initial operation. This is due to the presence of microscopic tumour deposits in

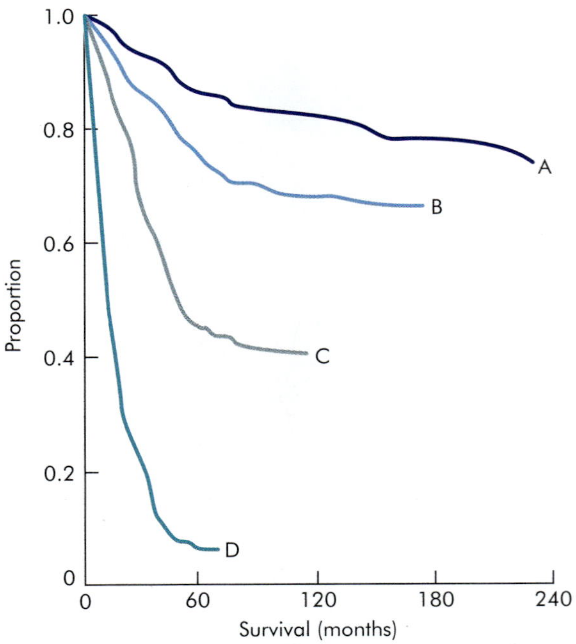

Figure 72.29 Cancer-specific survival rates following surgery for rectal cancer according to Dukes' stages. Redrawn with permission from Keighley MRB, Williams NS. *Surgery of the anus, rectum and colon.* London: WB Saunders, 1999.

the mesorectum. If the mesorectum is removed in its entirety, the local recurrence rate can be reduced to less than 5 per cent.

Less common causes of local recurrence include implantation of viable cells on the suture line and the development of a new primary tumour. Eighty per cent of all local recurrences develop within two years following surgery, and they are very difficult to treat. The best prospect of salvage is by surgical resection. However, it is possible to achieve apparently complete removal in only a minority of cases, and will usually involve hysterectomy, bladder resection and even partial sacrectomy. Radiotherapy also has an important role, but many patients will have already been exposed to a maximal dose during the treatment of the primary tumour.

Carcinoid tumour

Carcinoid tumour originates in the submucosa, with the mucous membrane over it being intact. Consequently, it seldom produces evidence of its presence in the early stages, when it presents as a small plaque-like elevation. The incidence of clinical malignancy, i.e. the occurrence of metastases, is 10 per cent. This is much less than that for carcinoid tumour of the small intestine, but it is greater than that for carcinoid tumour of the appendix. Multiple primary carcinoid tumours of the rectum are not infrequent. The neoplasm is of slow progression, and usually metastasises late. Large carcinoids (over 2 cm) are almost always malignant.

Treatment

Local excision is sufficient treatment for small carcinoids. Resection of the rectum is advisable if the growth is more than 2.5 cm in diameter, if recurrence follows local excision or if the growth is fixed to the perirectal tissues. Even when metastases are present, resection may prolong life.

FURTHER READING

Keighley MRB, Williams NS (eds). *Surgery of the anus, rectum and colon*, 3rd edn. London: WB Saunders, 2008.

Phillips RKS (ed.). *A companion to specialist surgical practice: colorectal surgery*, 4th edn. London: Elsevier, 2009.

CHAPTER 73 The anus and anal canal

LEARNING OBJECTIVES

To understand:

- The anatomy of the anus and anal canal and their relationship to surgical disease and its treatment
- The pathology, clinical presentation, investigation, differential diagnosis and treatment of diseases that affect the anus and anal canal
- That anal disease is common and its treatment tends to be conservative, although surgery may be required
- That too aggressive or inappropriate surgery may render the patient permanently disabled

ANATOMY AND PHYSIOLOGY

Surgical anatomy

The anal canal commences at the level where the rectum passes through the pelvic diaphragm and ends at the anal verge. The muscular junction between the rectum and anal canal can be felt with the finger as a thickened ridge – the anorectal 'bundle' or 'ring'.

Anal canal anatomy

The anorectal ring

The anorectal ring marks the junction between the rectum and the anal canal (Figure 73.1). It is formed by the joining of the puborectalis muscle (Figure 73.2), the deep external sphincter, conjoined longitudinal muscle and the highest part of the internal sphincter. The anorectal ring can be clearly felt digitally, especially on its posterior and lateral aspects.

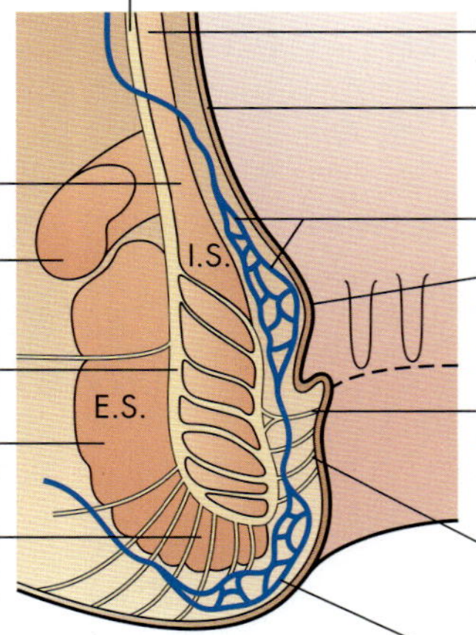

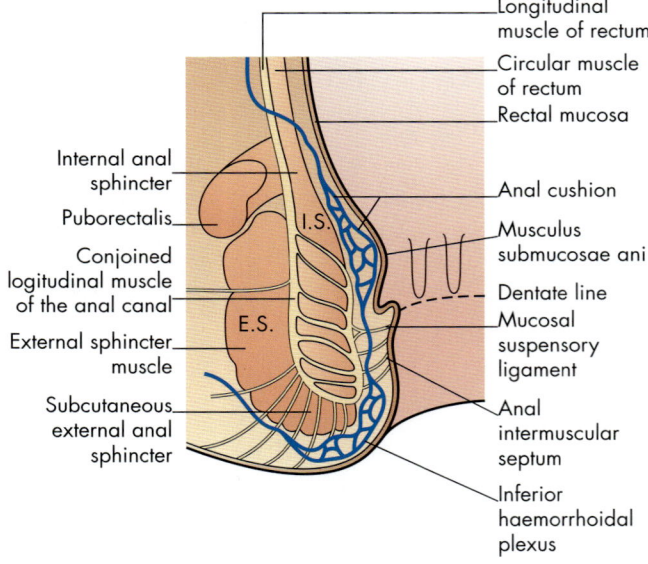

Figure 73.1 Relevant anatomy of the anus. Redrawn with permission from Mann CV. *Surgical treatment of haemorrhoids*. London: Springer, 2002.

The puborectalis muscle

Puborectalis, part of the funnel-shaped muscular pelvic diaphragm, maintains the angle between the anal canal and rectum and hence is an important component in the continence mechanism (Figure 73.2). The muscle derives its nerve supply from the sacral somatic nerves, and is functionally indistinct from the external anal sphincter. The position and length of the anal canal, as well as the angle of the anorectal junction, depend to a major extent on the integrity and strength of the puborectalis muscle sling. It gives off fibres that contribute to the longitudinal muscle layer.

The external sphincter

The external sphincter forms the bulk of the anal sphincter complex and, although traditionally it has been subdivided into deep, superficial and subcutaneous portions, it is a single muscle (Goligher), which is variably divided by lateral extensions from the longitudinal muscle layer. Some of its fibres are attached posteriorly to the coccyx, whereas anteriorly they fuse with the perineal muscles. Being a somatic voluntary muscle, the external sphincter is red in colour and is innervated by the pudendal nerve.

John Cedric Goligher, 1912–1998, Professor of Surgery, University of Leeds, Leeds, UK. Goligher is reputed to have said to his staff: 'It is a simple system here: if you do not agree with the style or requirements of the man above you, leave'.

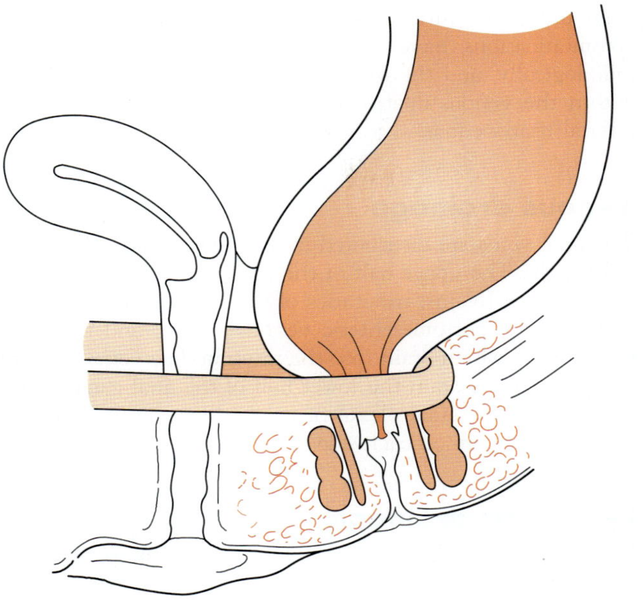

Figure 73.2 The disposition of the puborectalis muscle. Note how it maintains the rectoanal angle.

The intersphincteric plane

Between the external sphincter muscle laterally and the longitudinal muscle medially exists a potential space, the intersphincteric plane. This plane is important as it contains intersphincteric anal glands (see below under The anal glands) and is also a route for the spread of pus, which occurs along the extensions from the longitudinal muscle layer. The plane can be opened up surgically to provide access for operations on the sphincter muscles.

The longitudinal muscle

The longitudinal muscle is a direct continuation of the smooth muscle of the outer muscle coat of the rectum, augmented in its upper part by striated muscle fibres originating from the medial components of the pelvic floor. Most of the muscle continues caudally before splitting into multiple terminal septa that surround the muscle bundles of the subcutaneous portion of the external sphincter to insert into the skin of the lowermost part of the anal canal and adjacent perianal skin. Milligan and Morgan named the most medial of these septa, passing around the inferior border of the internal sphincter, the 'anal intermuscular septum'. As it descends, however, it gives off fibres that pass medially across the internal sphincter to reach the submucosal space, and laterally across the external sphincter and ischiorectal space to reach the fascia of the pelvic side walls. As well as providing a supportive mesh for the anal canal and other muscular components, its ramifications provide potential pathways for the spread of infection. During defaecation, its contraction widens the anal lumen, flattens the anal cushions, shortens the anal canal and everts the anal margin; subsequent relaxation allows the anal cushions to distend and thus contribute to an airtight seal.

The internal sphincter

The internal sphincter is the thickened (2–5 mm) distal continuation of the circular muscle coat of the rectum, which has developed special properties and which is in a tonic state of contraction. This involuntary muscle commences where the rectum passes through the pelvic diaphragm and ends above the anal orifice, its lower border palpable at the intersphincteric groove, below which lie the most medial fibres of the subcutaneous external sphincter, and separated from it by the anal intermuscular septum. When exposed during life, it is pearly-white in colour and its circumferentially placed fibres can be seen clearly. Although innervated by the autonomic nervous system, it receives intrinsic non-adrenergic and non-cholinergic (NANC) fibres, stimulation of which causes release of the neurotransmitter nitric oxide, which induces internal sphincter relaxation.

The epithelium and subepithelial structures

The pink columnar epithelium lining the rectum extends through the anorectal ring into the surgical anal canal. Passing downwards, the mucous membrane becomes cuboidal and redder in colour (Figure 73.3), whereas above the anal valves it is plum coloured. Just below the level of the anal valves there is an abrupt, albeit wavy, transition to stratified squamous epithelium, which is the colour of parchment. This wavy junction constitutes the dentate line. The dentate line is a most important landmark both morphologically and surgically, representing the site of fusion of the proctodaeum and postallantoic gut, and being the site of the crypts of Morgagni (synonym: anal crypts, sinuses). The latter are small pockets between the inferior extremities of the columns of Morgagni through which anal ducts that communicate with deeper placed anal glands open into the anal lumen. The squamous epithelium lining the lower anal canal is thin and shiny and is known as the anoderm; it differs from the true skin in that it has no epidermal appendages, i.e. hair and sweat glands. At the dentate line, the anoderm is attached more firmly to deeper structures. The mucosa and submucosa above the dentate line is uneven and thrown into folds, the so-called anal

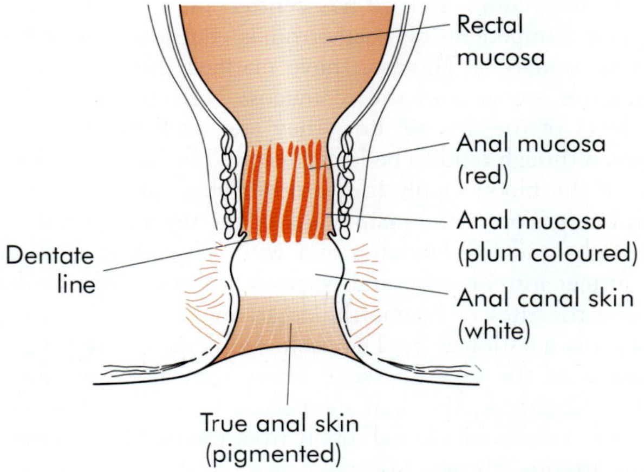

Figure 73.3 The lining membrane of the anal canal (after Sir Clifford Naunton Morgan, London).

Edward Thomas Campbell Milligan, 1886–1972, surgeon, St Mark's Hospital, London, UK.
Sir Clifford Naunton Morgan, 1901–1986, surgeon, St Mark's Hospital and St Bartholomew's Hospital, London, UK.

cushions. There are variations in the numbers and positions of these cushions, but there are usually three, corresponding to those seen in later life. These are described classically as occupying the left lateral, right posterior and right anterior positions, and they continue proximally as the primary rectal foldings. Secondary foldings (the rectal columns of Morgagni) lie both over and between the primary folds. This area is the caudal limit of the so-called epithelial transitional zone, below which the stratified squamous epithelium is richly innervated by sensory nerve endings serving several modalities including touch, pain and temperature. The bulk of the anal cushions themselves, situated in the upper part of the anal canal, receive only visceral afferent innervation and, although there is perception of stretching, sensitivity to noxious stimuli is much more blunted than distally.

Between the epithelial layer and the internal sphincter lies the submucosa, consisting of vascular, muscular and connective tissue supportive elements. From the longitudinal muscle, medial extensions cross the internal anal sphincter and form part of the supporting meshwork of the submucosa, blending with the true submucosal smooth muscle layer and thereby supporting the mucosa itself. Parks described the increased density of fibres that insert into the mucosa of the anal crypts at the level of the dentate line, termed the 'mucosal suspensory ligament'. One feature of this structure is that it separates the superior (portal) and inferior (systemic) haemorrhoidal plexuses, another is that the mucosa is more firmly tethered to underlying tissues at this level than above. It is important to appreciate that the meshwork of supporting tissues (muscle fibres and connective tissue) within the subepithelial space is intimately linked to deeper structures within the anal sphincter complex, including the internal sphincter, longitudinal muscle layer and external anal sphincter, and indeed structures beyond the sphincter complex. With age, the smooth muscle component of this mesh is reduced and muscle fibres are gradually replaced with fibroelastic connective tissue, which in turn becomes fragmented.

Blood supply

In addition to the meshwork support of the lining of the anal canal, the subepithelial space contains venous dilatations supported by the same fibroelastic connective tissue and smooth muscle scaffolding. Debate has centred on the nature of the vascular component of haemorrhoids, but the seminal anatomical studies of Thomson have clarified this issue. Venous dilatations are seen in the submucosa both above and below the level of the dentate line; they are much more numerous above, although tend to be larger below. The historical description of the blood supply to the upper anal canal as constant, with bifurcation of the main trunk of the superior rectal artery into right and left branches and with subsequent division of the former into anterior and posterior divisions thereby determining the sites of haemorrhoids around the anal circumference, was questioned by Thomson. He demonstrated that the divisions of the superior rectal artery were not constant and that, furthermore, the anal submucosa in a proportion of his specimens received a blood supply from the middle and inferior rectal arteries. He was also able to show the presence of free communications between tributaries of the superior, middle and inferior rectal veins, as well as tiny direct arteriovenous communications with the submucosal venous dilatations. These communications have been shown both histologically and radiologically, and the oxygen tension of the blood contained within the venous dilatations (as well as the colour) is more arterial than venous.

Venous drainage

The anal veins are distributed in a similar fashion to the arterial supply. The upper half of the anal canal is drained by the superior rectal veins, tributaries of the inferior mesenteric vein and thus the portomesenteric venous system, and the middle rectal veins, which drain into the internal iliac veins. The inferior rectal veins drain the lower half of the anal canal and the subcutaneous perianal plexus of veins: they eventually join the internal iliac vein on each side.

Lymphatic drainage

Lymph from the upper half of the anal canal flows upwards to drain into the postrectal lymph nodes and from there goes to the para-aortic nodes via the inferior mesenteric chain. Lymph from the lower half of the anal canal drains on each side first into the superficial and then into the deep inguinal group of lymph glands. However, if the normal flow is blocked, e.g. by tumour, the lymph can be diverted into the alternative route (Summary box 73.1).

Summary box 73.1

Anal canal anatomy

- The internal sphincter is composed of circular, non-striated involuntary muscle supplied by autonomic nerves
- The external sphincter is composed of striated voluntary muscle supplied by the pudendal nerve
- Extensions from the longitudinal muscle layer support the sphincter complex
- The space between sphincters is known as the intersphincteric plane
- The superior part of the external sphincter fuses with the puborectalis muscle, which is essential for maintaining the anorectal angle, necessary for continence
- The lower part of the anal canal is lined by sensitive squamous epithelium
- Blood supply to the anal canal is via superior, middle and inferior rectal vessels
- Lymphatic drainage of the lower half of the anal canal goes to inguinal lymph nodes

The anal glands

Anal glands (which are not vestigial remnants of sexual scent glands) may be found in the submucosa and intersphincteric space (Figure 73.4), and normally number between 0 and 10 in an individual. They drain via ducts into the anal sinuses at the level of the dentate line. Not all sinuses have a duct draining into them and, occasionally, more than one gland can discharge into the same sinus. Their function is unknown, although they secrete mucin (distinct from that secreted by the rectal epithe-

Giovani Battista Morgagni, 1682–1771, Professor of Anatomy, Padua, Italy, for 59 years. He is regarded as the founder of morbid anatomy.
William Hamish Fearon Thomson, retired surgeon, The Gloucestershire Royal Infirmary, Gloucester, UK.

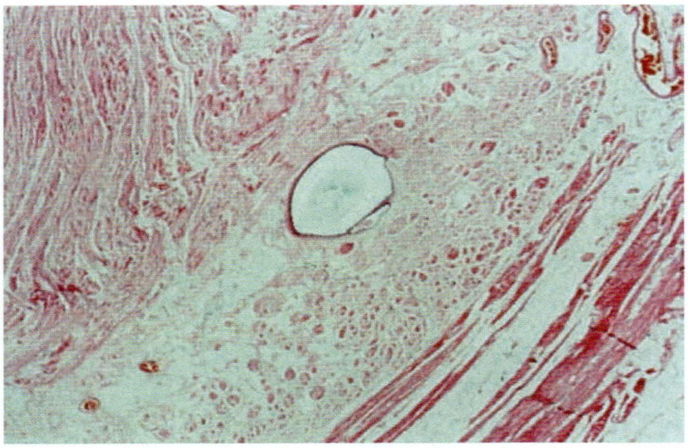

Figure 73.4 Intersphincteric anal gland lying between the voluntary muscle of the external sphincter and the longitudinal muscle. The internal sphincter is also seen. Reproduced with permission from Nicholls RJ, Dozois RR. *Surgery of the colon and rectum*. Edinburgh: Churchill Livingstone, 1997.

lium), which perhaps lubricates the anal canal to ease defaecation. The importance of intersphincteric anal glands is that they are widely considered to be the potential source of anal sepsis, either acute, presenting as perianal, ischiorectal or even pelvic sepsis, or chronic, presenting as a cryptoglandular (non-specific) anal fistula.

EXAMINATION OF THE ANUS

Careful clinical examination will be diagnostic in the vast majority of patients complaining of anal symptoms, but it requires a relaxed patient who is informed of what the examination will entail, a private environment, a chaperone (for the security of both parties) and good light. Most commonly, the patient is examined in the left lateral (Sims) position with the buttocks overlying the edge of the examination couch and with the axis of the torso crossing, rather than parallel with, the edge of the couch. Alternatively, in younger patients, the prone jack-knife or knee–elbow positions may be used (Figure 73.5). The examining couch should be of sufficient height to allow easy inspection and access for any necessary manoeuvres. A protective glove should be worn.

Inspection

The buttocks are gently parted to allow inspection of the anus and perineum: the presence of any skin lesions and whether they are confined to the perineum or evident elsewhere on general examination, e.g. psoriasis, lichen planus, or on genital examination, e.g. warts, candidiasis, lichen sclerosus et atrophicus, the vesicles of herpes simplex virus (HSV); evidence of anal leakage; whether the anus is closed or patulous; and the position of the anus and perineum at rest and on bearing down (the latter may reveal prolapse of haemorrhoids or even the rectum). Pain on parting the buttocks, perhaps together with the presence of a sentinel tag, may indicate the presence of an underlying fissure, but may also prompt the need for examination under anaesthesia to exclude more suspicious pathology, for example squamous cell carcinoma of the anal canal.

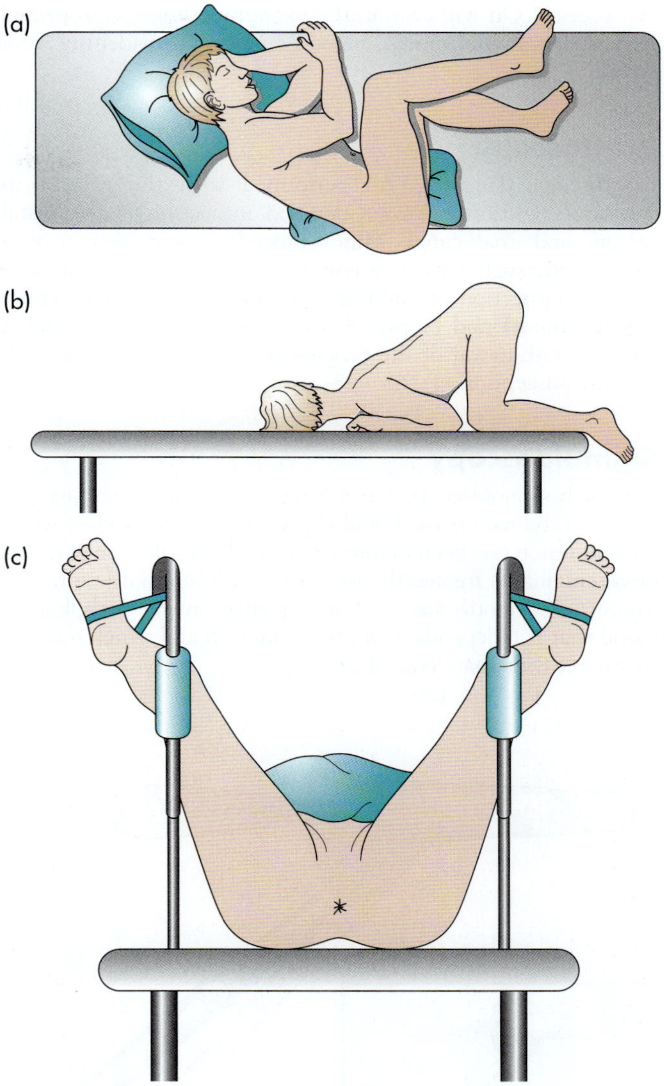

Figure 73.5 The left lateral (a), knee–elbow (b) and lithotomy (c) positions for examination. Redrawn with permission from Mann CV. *Surgical treatment of haemorrhoids*. London: Springer, 2002.

Digital examination with the index finger

With an adequately lubricated index finger, the soft tissues around the anus are palpated for induration, tenderness and subcutaneous lesions. The index finger is then introduced gently into the anal canal along its posterior aspect. At the apex of the canal, the sling of puborectalis is felt posteriorly; supralevator induration feels bony hard and is more easily appreciated if unilateral. The posterior surface of the prostate gland with its median sulcus can be palpated anteriorly in male patients; in female patients, the uterine cervix can be palpated. The presence of any distal intrarectal, intra-anal or extraluminal mass is recorded. Sphincter length, resting tone and voluntary squeeze are assessed. On withdrawal, the examining finger is inspected for the presence of mucus, blood or pus, and to identify stool colour.

Proctoscopy

Proctoscopy (Figure 73.6), performed with the patient in the same position, allows a detailed inspection of the distal rectum and anal canal. Minor procedures can also be carried out through this instrument, e.g. treatment of haemorrhoids by injection or banding (see below Management under Haemorrhoids) and biopsy. Asking the patient to bear down on slow withdrawal of the proctoscope may reveal a descending intussusception.

Sigmoidoscopy

Although sigmoidoscopy (see Chapter 72) is strictly an examination of the rectum, it should always be carried out even when an anal lesion has been confirmed. Rectal pathology, e.g. colitis or carcinoma, is frequently associated with an anal lesion, e.g. fissure or haemorrhoids. Not infrequently, rectal pathology is found that is independent of the anal lesion and which requires treatment (Summary box 73.2).

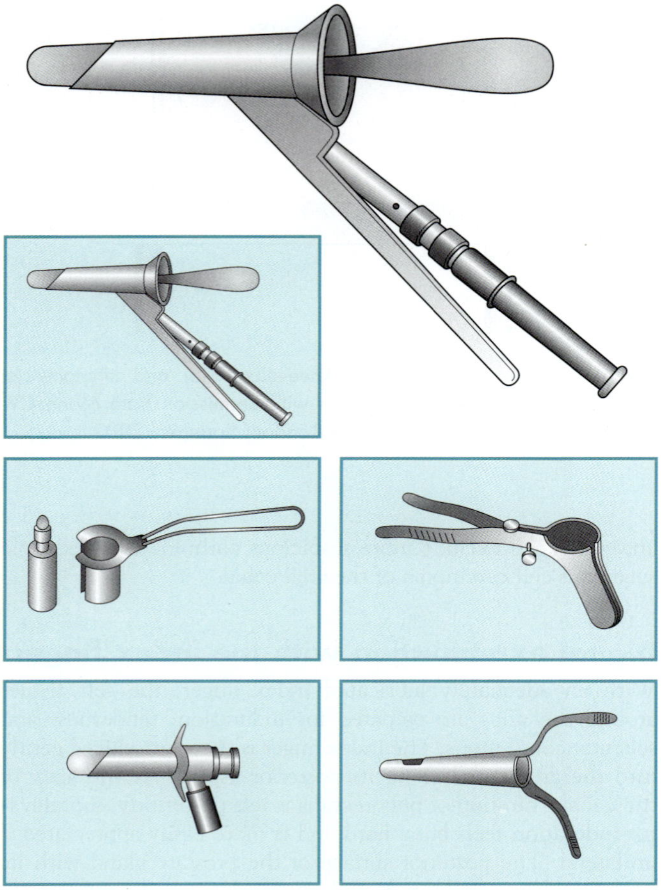

Figure 73.6 Various types of proctoscope. Redrawn with permission from Mann CV. *Surgical treatment of haemorrhoids*. London: Springer, 2002.

Summary box 73.2

Examination of anal canal

- A rectal examination is essential for any patient with anorectal and/or bowel symptoms – 'If you don't put your finger in, you might put your foot in it'
- A proctosigmoidoscopy is essential in any patient with bowel symptoms, and particularly if there is rectal bleeding

PHYSIOLOGICAL ASPECTS OF THE ANAL SPHINCTERS AND PELVIC FLOOR, AND SPECIAL INVESTIGATIONS

Anal continence and defaecation are highly complex processes that necessitate the structural and functional integrity of the cerebral, autonomic and enteric nervous systems, the gastrointestinal tract (especially the rectum) and the pelvic floor and anal sphincter complex, any of which may be compromised and lead to disturbances of function of varying severity. The sphincter mechanism provides the ultimate barrier to leakage and its integrity can be assessed fairly simply and objectively in the physiology laboratory (Swash and Henry). Perineal position and degree of descent on straining (markers of pelvic floor and pudendal nerve function) can be quantified, and functional anal canal length, resting tone (reflective predominantly of internal sphincter activity) and squeeze increment (reflective of external sphincter function) can be measured by a variety of simple manometric techniques (Figure 73.7). The structural integrity of the sphincters can be visualised with endoluminal ultrasound (Figure 73.8), and neuromuscular function can be measured by assessment of conduction velocity along the pudendal nerve on each side, or, more painfully, by needle electromyogram (EMG) studies (Figures 73.9 and 73.10). In the elderly especially, but also in younger patients, disorders relating to rectal sensorimotor dysfunction can lead to 'overflow' of rectal contents through what may be an otherwise normal sphincter. The dynamics of defaecation can also be assessed radiologically by evacuation proctography, in which radio-opaque pseudo-stool is inserted into the rectum and the patient asked to rest, squeeze and then bear down to evacuate the rectal contents under real-time imag-

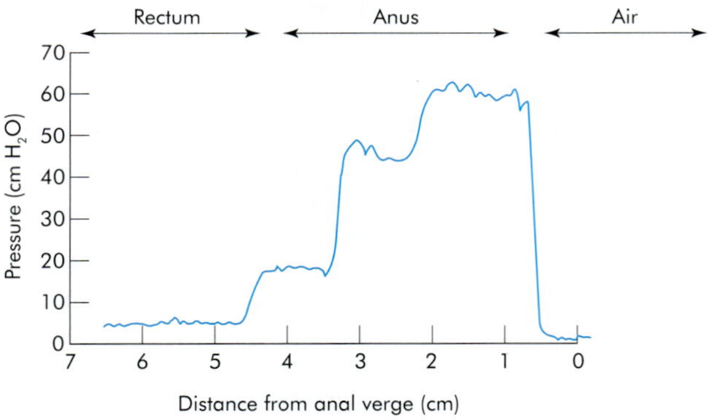

Figure 73.7 A typical, normal 'pull-through' manometric study of the anal canal (3.5 cm long; maximal pressure approximately 60 cmH_2O).

Michael Swash, formerly Professor of Neurology, St Bartholomew's and The Royal London Hospital, London, UK.
Michael Meldrum Henry, formerly Surgeon, The Chelsea and Westminster Hospital, London, UK.

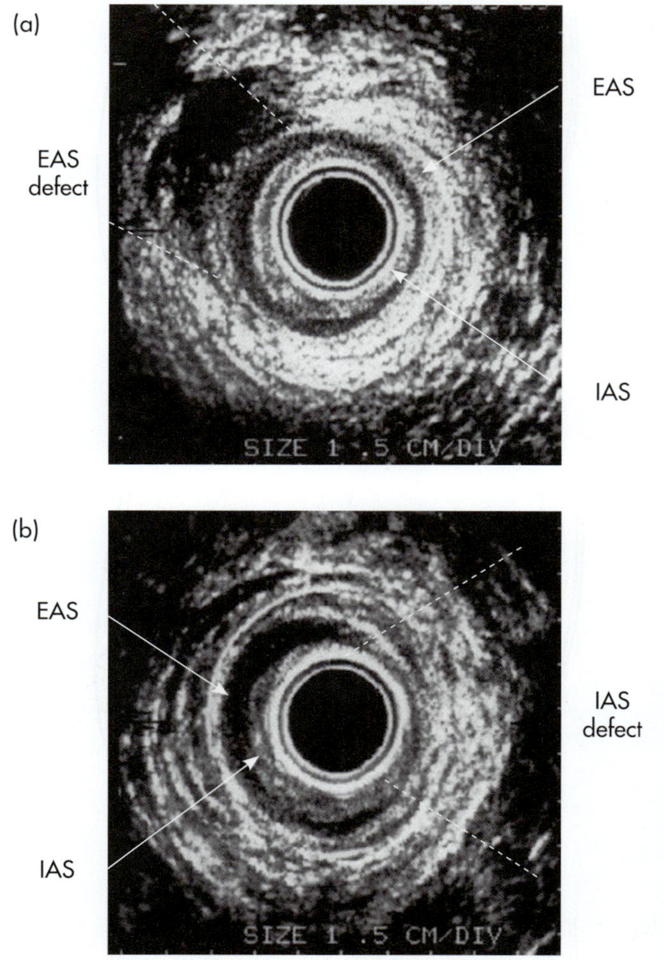

Figure 73.8 Endoanal ultrasonography. (a) External anal sphincter (EAS) defect caused by obstetric injury. (b) Internal anal sphincter (IAS) defect post-sphincterotomy.

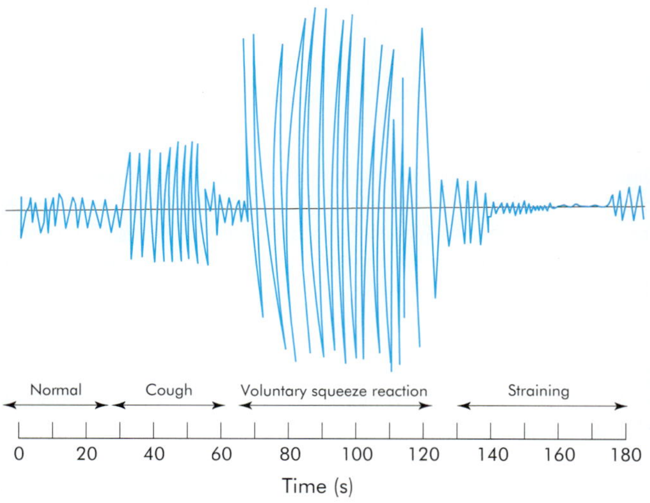

Figure 73.9 A typical, normal electromyographic study of the external sphincter during various activities.

ing. Proctography can be combined with synchronous EMG and pressure studies (Williams) (Figure 73.11) to yield more information about possible reasons (mechanical (rectocoele, intussusception) or functional (anismus, lack of effort)) for disordered defaecation in an individual. More recently, use of the

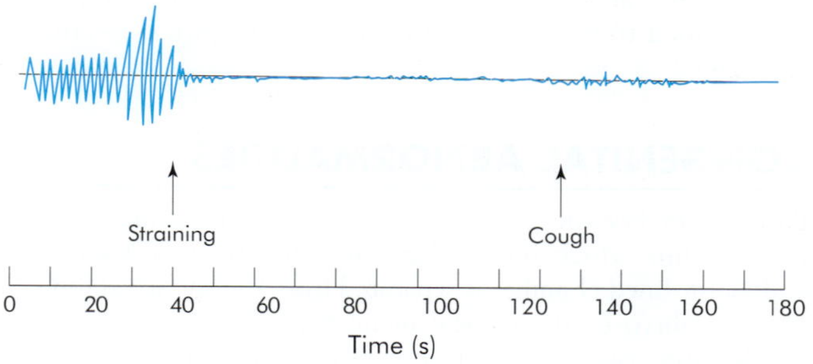

Figure 73.10 An electromyographic study of the external sphincter showing prolonged inhibition on straining and absent cough reflex. This is typical of a denervated patulous sphincter.

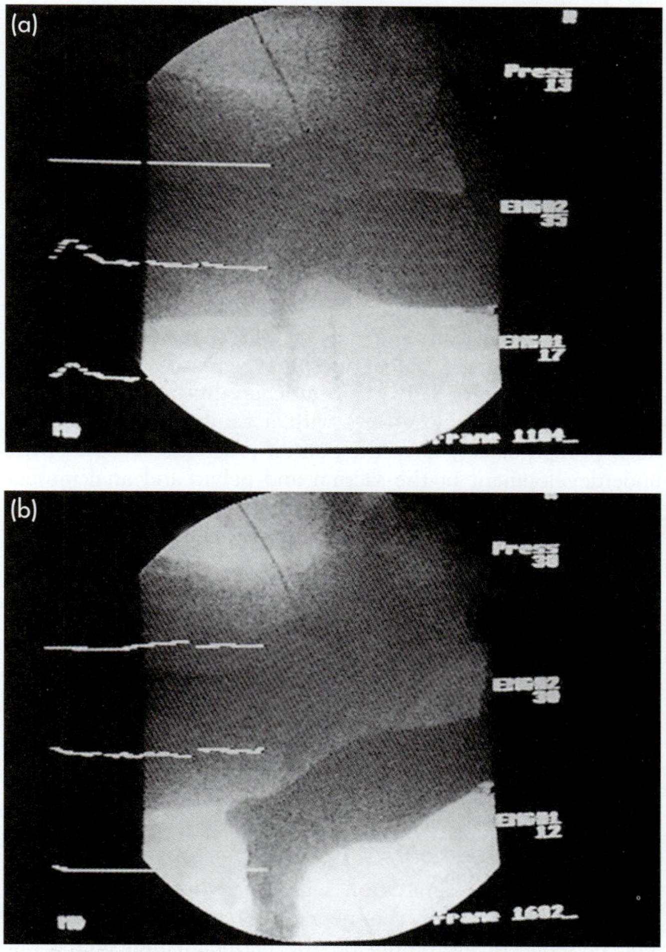

Figure 73.11 Integrated dynamic proctography. (a) At rest; (b) during evacuation. Visualisation of the rectum is achieved using barium-impregnated 'synthetic stool'. The effects of straining and evacuation on the electromyographic activity of the sphincter muscles and intrarectal pressure can be simultaneously recorded (Williams).

much more expensive modality of dynamic magnetic resonance proctography has become more widespread, although studies in which the subject is asked to evacuate in the supine position may be less physiological than those in which the subject adopts a sitting position within an open magnet. Results of all physiological and imaging tests have to be compared with a robust normal range and within the context of the patient's symptoms, and are used to guide rational rather than empirical treatment strategies.

CONGENITAL ABNORMALITIES

Early in embryonic life there is a common chamber – the cloaca – into which the hind gut and the allantois open. This endoderm-lined chamber is separated from the surface ectoderm of the embryo by the cloacal membrane. The cloaca becomes divided into two parts, dorsal (rectum) and ventral (urogenital sinus), by the downgrowth of a septum. The dorsal part of the cloacal membrane, known as the anal membrane, is thus composed of an outer layer of ectoderm and an inner layer of endoderm. Resorption of this anal membrane by the 8th week of embryonic life creates the anal canal.

Imperforate anus

Imperforate anus (see Chapter 8) (strictly, it should be anal 'agenesis' or 'atresia') has historically been divided into two main groups – high and low – depending on the level of termination of the rectum in relation to the pelvic floor. Treatment and prognosis are influenced by any associated abnormalities of the sacrum and genitourinary systems. In both sexes, low defects embrace rectoperineal fistula (Figure 73.12), covered anus and anal membrane. The most frequent defect in boys with imperforate anus is one in which the distal rectum is sited within the puborectalis sling, but terminates as a fistula into the bulbar urethra (Figure 73.13) (see also Chapter 8, Figure 6.32) or prostatic urethra above the main anal sphincter complex. Boys with a fistula into the bladder neck (a high defect) have the poorest prognosis because of the underdevelopment of the sacrum and pelvic and anal musculature. The most common defect in girls is a rectovestibular fistula, in which the fistula opens into the posterior vestibule (not the vagina) (Figure 73.12). The finding of a single perineal orifice indicates a persistent cloaca in which the rectum, vagina and urinary tract form a confluence (Figure 73.13); the longer the common channel, the greater the likelihood of more complex defects, including vaginal and uterine septation, duplication or atresia. An anterior anus, although not imperforate, is not fully located within the sphincter mechanism and is regarded as part of the spectrum of anorectal malformations (Figure 73.12).

(a) (b) (c)

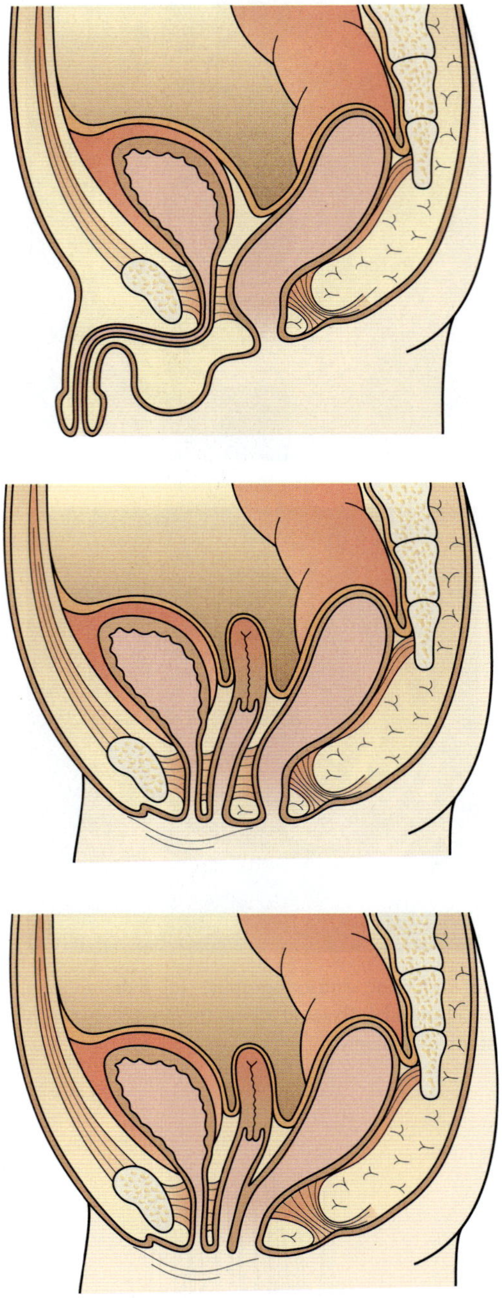

Figure 73.12 Low anorectal malformations. (a) Rectoperineal fistula in a boy; (b) rectoperineal fistula in a girl (anterior anus); (c) rectovestibular fistula. Courtesy of Alberto Pena and Springer-Verlag. From *Atlas of surgical management of anorectal malformations* by Alberto Pena, 1990. Copyright Springer-Verlag.

Clinical management

Careful perineal examination will usually provide the most important clues about the neonate's type of malformation. The presence of meconium on the perineum indicates a low defect and meconium in the urine is evidence of a urinary tract fistula. During the first 24 hours, the baby should receive intravenous fluids and antibiotics, and should be evaluated for associated congenital anomalies. By 24 hours, the distal limit of air within the rectum, seen on a lateral prone radiograph, indicates the distance between the rectal stump and perineum (Figure 73.14).

Treatment

Low anomalies with a perineal fistula can be treated by an anoplasty. More complex malformations require early colostomy, with definitive repair performed several months later. This may

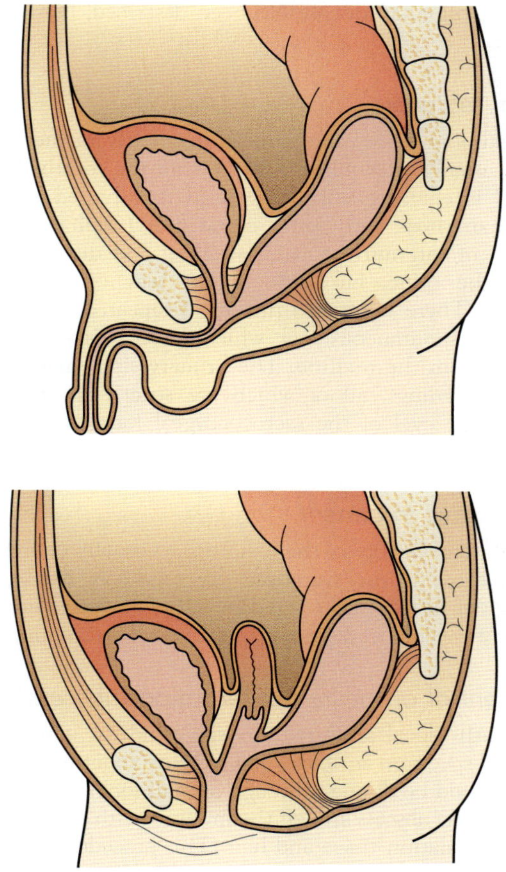

Figure 73.13 More complex anorectal malformations. (a) Rectobulbar fistula; (b) cloacal malformation. Courtesy of Alberto Pena and Springer-Verlag. From *Atlas of surgical management of anorectal malformations* by Alberto Pena, 1990. Copyright Springer-Verlag.

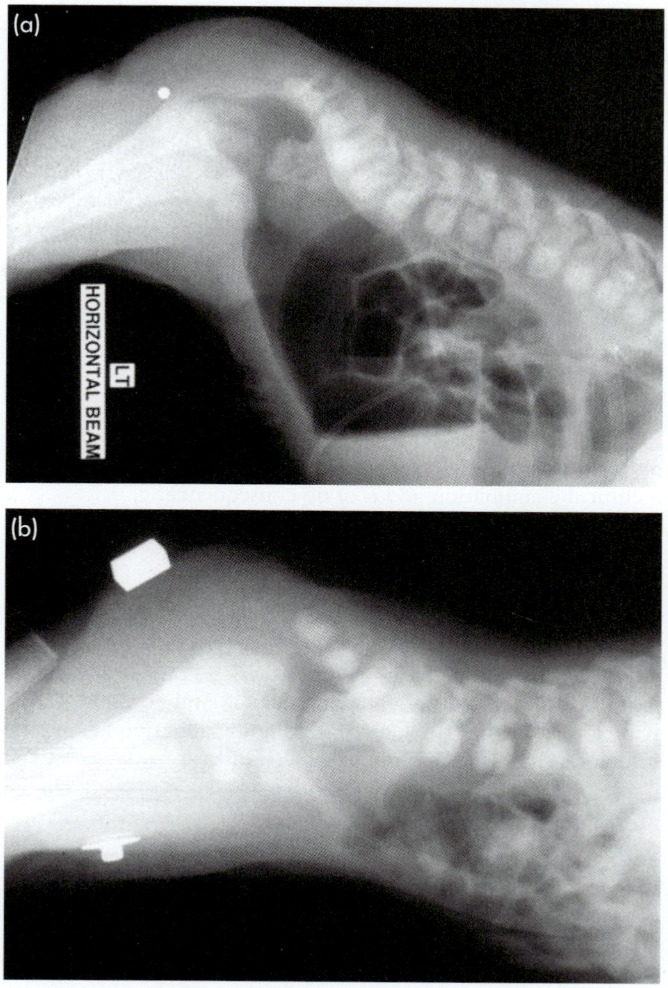

Figure 73.14 Lateral prone shoot-through radiograph of a neonate with (a) low and (b) high anorectal malformation. A radio-opaque marker has been placed on the anal dimple (courtesy of Mark D Stringer, Leeds, UK).

involve posterior sagittal anorectoplasty (PSARP, Pena) with or without transabdominal mobilisation of the left colon and division of any communication with the urinary tract. In girls with a cloaca and long common channel, urinary and vaginal reconstruction is also required. Postoperatively, a programme of anal dilatation is instituted, and any residual colostomy is closed at a later date. Ultimate bowel function (voluntary bowel movements, continence, constipation) is related to the type of anorectal abnormality and the presence of associated defects, especially sacral (Summary box 73.3).

Summary box 73.3

Imperforate anus

- A rare congenital disorder
- Classified as being high or low depending on the site of the rectal termination in relation to the pelvic floor
- Low defects: relatively easy to correct, but prone to constipation
- High defects: more difficult to correct and prone to faecal incontinence

Post-anal dermoid

The space in front of the lower part of the sacrum and coccyx may be occupied by a soft, cystic swelling – a post-anal dermoid cyst. Hidden in the hollow of the sacrum, it is unlikely to be discovered unless a sinus communicating with the exterior is present or it develops as a result of inflammation. Such a cyst usually remains asymptomatic until adult life, when it is prone to becoming infected. Exceptionally, because of its size, it gives rise to difficulty in defaecation. The cyst is easily palpable on rectal examination.

Differential diagnosis

Especially in a child, an anterior sacral meningocoele must be excluded. This enlarges when the child cries and is frequently associated with paralysis of the lower limbs and incontinence. When a discharging sinus is present, a post-anal dermoid will probably be mistaken for a pilonidal sinus or even an anal fistula. Pressure over the sacrococcygeal region with a finger in the

Alberto Pena, contemporary, Professor of Pediatric Surgery, Schneider Children's Hospital, New York, NY, USA.

rectum may cause a flow of sebaceous material, and injection of contrast media followed by radiography reveals a bottle-necked cyst in front of the coccyx.

Treatment

Treatment involves complete excision of the cyst and, if present, the sinus. In the case of large cysts, it is necessary to remove the coccyx to gain access. The coccyx should also be removed *en bloc* in any child with a presacral dermoid because of the risk of sacrococcygeal teratoma.

Post-anal dimple

A post-anal dimple (synonym: fovea coccygea) is a dimple in the skin beneath the tip of the coccyx, sometimes amounting to a short blind pit. It is noticed from time to time in the course of a clinical examination and is of no consequence.

Pilonidal sinus

The term 'pilonidal sinus' describes a condition found in the natal cleft overlying the coccyx, consisting of one or more, usually non-infected, midline openings, which communicate with a fibrous track lined by granulation tissue and containing hair lying loosely within the lumen. A common affliction among the military, it has been referred to as 'jeep disease'.

Aetiology and pathology

Although acquired theories of development are better accepted than the more historical congenital theories, exact mechanisms of development are speculative. Evidence that supports the acquired theory of origin of pilonidal sinuses can be summarised as follows:

- Interdigital pilonidal sinus is an occupational disease of hairdressers, the hair within the interdigital cleft or clefts being from the customers. Pilonidal sinuses of the axilla and umbilicus have also been reported.
- The age incidence of the appearance of pilonidal sinus (82 per cent occur between the ages of 20 and 29 years) is at variance with the age of onset of congenital lesions.
- Hair follicles have almost never been demonstrated in the walls of the sinus.
- The hairs projecting from the sinus are dead hairs, with their pointed ends directed towards the blind end of the sinus.
- The disease mostly affects men, in particular hairy men.
- Recurrence is common, even though adequate excision of the track is carried out.

It is thought that the combination of buttock friction and shearing forces in that area allows shed hair or broken hairs which have collected there to drill through the midline skin, or that infection in relation to a hair follicle allows hair to enter the skin by the suction created by movement of the buttocks, so creating a subcutaneous, chronically infected, midline track. From this primary sinus, secondary tracks may spread laterally, which may emerge at the skin as granulation tissue-lined, discharging openings. Usually, but not invariably (when diagnosis may be confused with anal fistula or hidradenitis suppurativa), the sinus runs cephalad. Carcinoma arising in chronic pilonidal disease has been described, but is exceedingly rare.

Clinical features

The condition is seen much more frequently in men than in women, usually after puberty and before the fourth decade of life, and is characteristically seen in dark-haired individuals rather than those with softer blond hair (Oldham). Patients complain of intermittent pain, swelling and discharge at the base of the spine, but little in the way of constitutional symptoms. There is often a history of repeated abscesses that have burst spontaneously or which have been incised, usually away from the midline. The primary sinus may have one or many openings, all of which are strictly in the midline between the level of the sacrococcygeal joint and the tip of the coccyx.

Conservative treatment

As the natural history of the condition is usually one of regression, in those whose symptoms are relatively minor, simple cleaning out of the tracks and removal of all hair, with regular shaving of the area and strict hygiene, may be recommended.

Treatment of an acute exacerbation (abscess)

If rest, baths, local antiseptic dressings and the administration of a broad-spectrum antibiotic fail to bring about resolution, the abscess should be drained through a small longitudinal incision made over the abscess and off the midline, with thorough curettage of granulation tissue and hair. This procedure may or may not be associated with complete resolution.

Surgical treatment of chronic pilonidal disease

The multitude of surgical procedures advocated to eradicate pilonidal disease, combined with the lack of prospective trials, attests to the lack of overall superiority of one method over the others. Time spent off work and perceived recurrence rates, but more usually surgeon preference, influence the choice of method, which includes the laying open of all tracks with or without marsupialisation, the excision of all tracks with or without primary closure, and the excision of all tracks and then closure by some other means designed to avoid a midline wound (Z-plasty, Karydakis procedure (Figure 73.15)). Bascom's procedure involves an incision lateral to the midline to gain access to the sinus cavity, which is rid of hair and granulation tissue (Figure 73.16), and excision and closure of the midline pits (Figure 73.17). The lateral wound is left open (Figure 73.18). Irrespective of procedure, postoperative wound care is important and centres around elimination of hair (ingrown, local or other) from the wound.

Recurrent pilonidal sinus

Three possibilities account for this disappointment:

- part of the sinus complex has been overlooked at the primary operation;
- new hairs enter the skin or the scar;
- there is persistence of a midline wound caused by shearing forces and scarring; in this situation, revisional surgery may include re-excision followed by wound closure and

A **jeep** is a small military, general purpose, vehicle with hard springing, which gives its occupants a very bouncy ride when driven over rough terrain.
James Bagot Oldham, 1899–1977, surgeon, the United Liverpool Hospitals, Liverpool, UK.
Col Dr Karydakis, surgeon, Athens, Greece.
J Bascom, American surgeon.

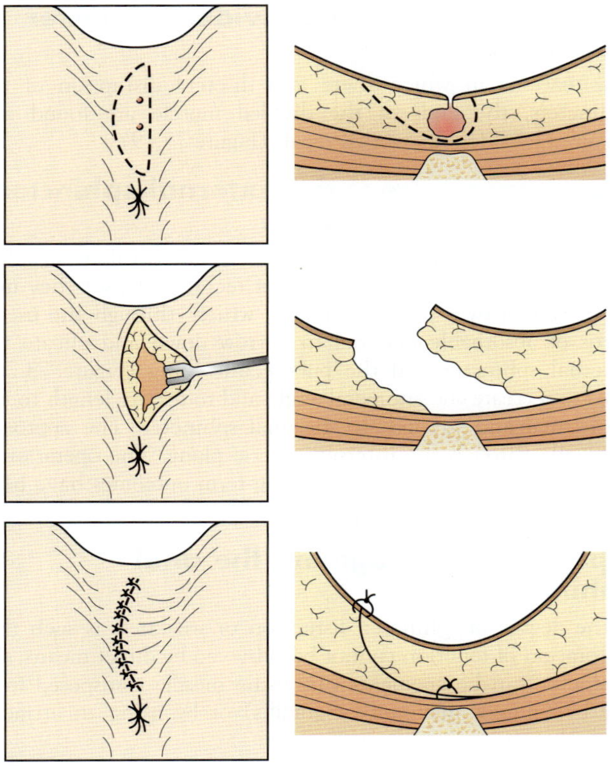

Figure 73.15 Karydakis's operation for pilonidal sinus. A semilateral incision is made around the sinus complex, the diseased component excised and the flap mobilised to allow tension-free closure of the wound off the midline. Reproduced with permission from Nicholls RJ, Dozois RR. *Surgery of the colon and rectum*. Edinburgh: Churchill Livingstone, 1997.

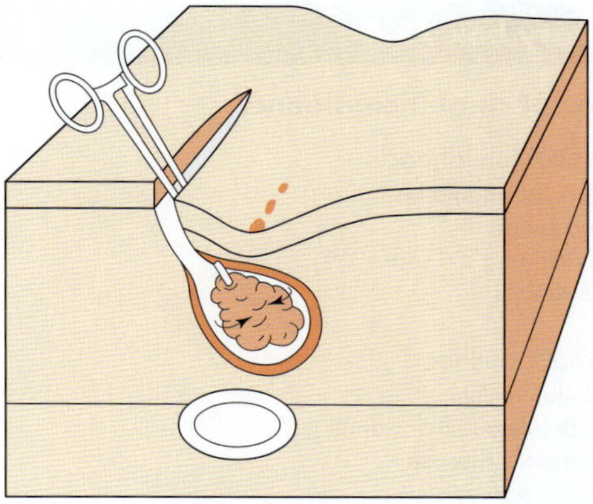

Figure 73.16 Bascom's technique for pilonidal sinus: 1.

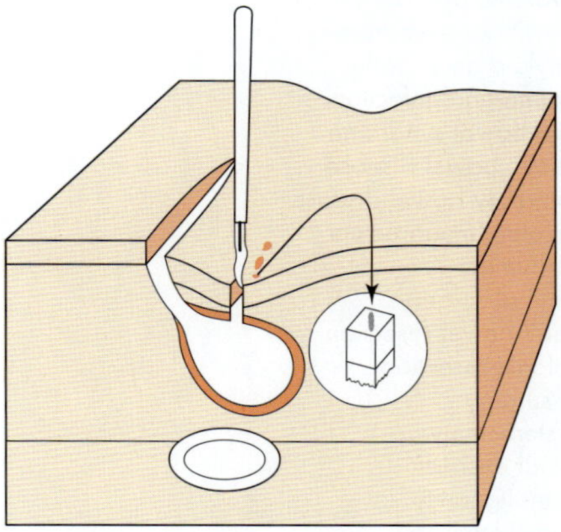

Figure 73.17 Bascom's technique for pilonidal sinus: 2.

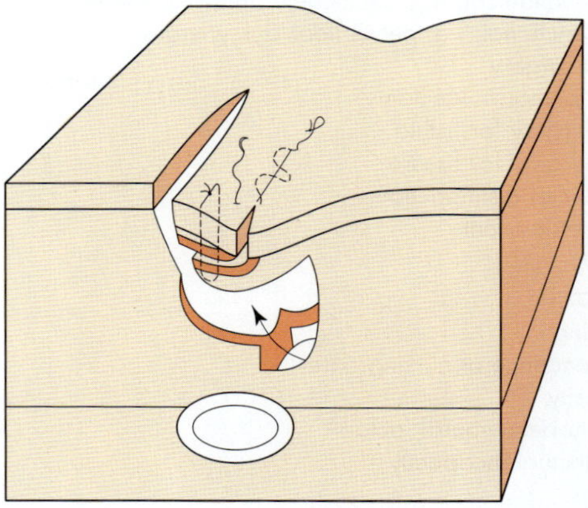

Figure 73.18 Bascom's technique for pilonidal sinus: 3.

obliteration of the natal cleft either by myocutaneous rotational buttock flap or cleft closure (Bascom).

ANAL INCONTINENCE

Aetiology

As continence is dependent upon the structural and functional integrity of both the neurological pathways and the gastrointestinal tract, the risk factors for anal incontinence are many (Summary box 73.4). Patients complaining of the involuntary loss of rectal contents require a comprehensive assessment of the nature and severity of symptoms; past history, especially of gastrointestinal disease, neurological conditions, obstetric events and anal surgery; and careful clinical examination (in the elderly, incontinence is often one of overflow secondary to rectal impaction, and proctitis may lead to such an irritable rectum that even the strongest sphincter is occasionally overwhelmed). A combination of history and examination will usually be diagnostic, but special investigations are then usually required to clarify the exact cause, including exclusion of an underlying malignancy, and to direct management.

Sphincteric causes of incontinence may be classified as structural, in which there is disruption (or atrophy) of part of the sphincter muscles, neuropathic (previously termed idiopathic), in which the nerve supply to the sphincters is damaged, usually by chronic straining or complicated vaginal delivery (prolonged second stage), or a combination of the two. The most common causes of sphincteric disruption are obstetric damage, anal surgery (following haemorrhoidectomy, dilatation or sphincterotomy for anal fissure, and fistulotomy for anal fistula) and trauma (including anal intercourse, forced or otherwise).

Summary box 73.4

Causes of anal incontinence

Congenital/childhood
- Anorectal anomalies
- Spina bifida
- Hirschsprung's disease
- Behavioural

Acquired/adulthood
- Diabetes mellitus
- Cerebrovascular accident
- Parkinson's disease
- Multiple sclerosis
- Spinal cord injury
- Other neurological conditions:
  - Myotonic dystrophy
  - Shy–Drager syndrome
  - Amyloid neuropathy
- Gastrointestinal infection
- Irritable bowel syndrome
- Metabolic bowel disease
- Inflammatory bowel disease
- Megacolon/megarectum
- Anal trauma
- Abdominal surgery:
  - Small bowel resection
  - Colonic resection
- Pelvic surgery:
  - Hysterectomy
  - Rectal excision
- Pelvic malignancy
- Pelvic radiotherapy
- Rectal prolapse
- Rectal evacuatory disorder:
  - Mechanical, e.g. rectocoele, intussusception
  - Functional, i.e. pelvic floor dyssynergia
- Anal surgery:
  - Haemorrhoidectomy
  - Surgery for fistula
  - Surgery for fissure
  - Rectal disimpaction
- Obstetric events

General
- Ageing
- Dependence of nursing care
- Obesity
- Psychobehavioural factors
- Intellectual incapacity
- Drugs:
  - Primary constipating and laxative agents
  - Secondary effects

In general, conservative measures to reduce symptoms are employed initially. These may be in the form of stool bulking or constipating agents, nurse-led bowel retraining including specific biofeedback programmes, or anal plugs, which expand within and thus seal the anal canal. Failure of such measures and severity of symptoms may result in selection for surgery.

Operations to reunite divided sphincter muscles

In situations in which there is a discrete disruption of the sphincters, the ends of the divided muscle are found and reunited by a double overlap repair (Figure 73.19).

Operations to reef the external sphincter and puborectalis muscle

If the sphincter muscles are stretched and patulous (as they often are in old age and in cases of rectal prolapse) they may be tightened by a post-anal repair, which, through the use of darns of absorbable material to narrow down and plicate the external sphincter and the puborectalis sling (Figure 73.20), aims to recreate the anorectal angle and to restore length to the anal canal and strength to the anal sphincter. The approach is usually through the intersphincteric plane. The operation is now much less popular because long-term outcomes have been reported as poor.

Operations to augment the anal sphincters

If the degree of sphincter disruption or weakness is such that restoration of function cannot be achieved by direct means, the sphincter can be augmented by using muscle transposed from nearby (gluteus maximus or gracilis) or by using an artificial

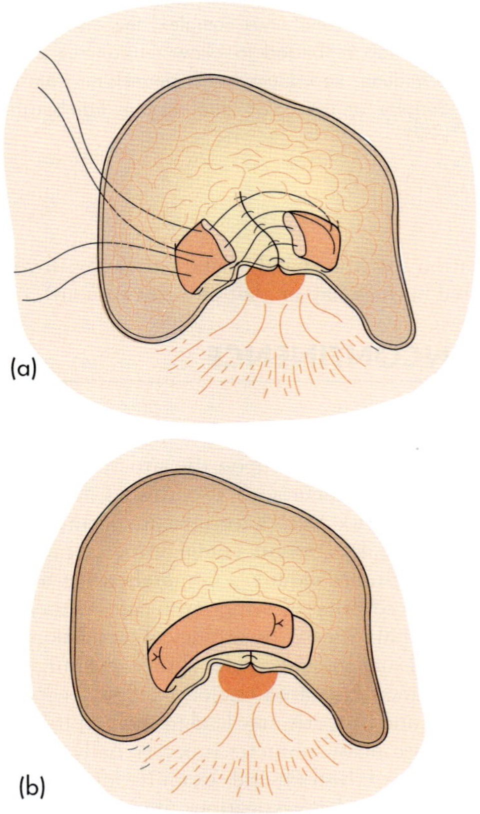

Figure 73.19 Direct sphincter repair in which (a) the sphincter defect is excised and (b) the remaining muscle is overlapped. Redrawn with permission from Mann CV, Glass RE. *Surgical treatment of anal incontinence*. New York: Springer, 1991.

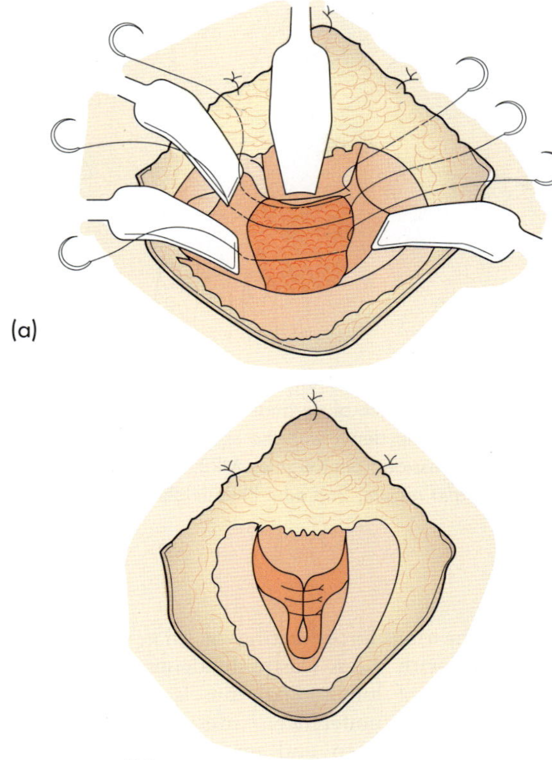

Figure 73.20 Post-anal repair in which (a) the sphincter muscle is plicated posterior to the anal canal, thus restoring the anorectal angle. (b) The completed repair. Redrawn with permission from Mann CV, Glass RE. *Surgical treatment of anal incontinence*. New York: Springer, 1991.

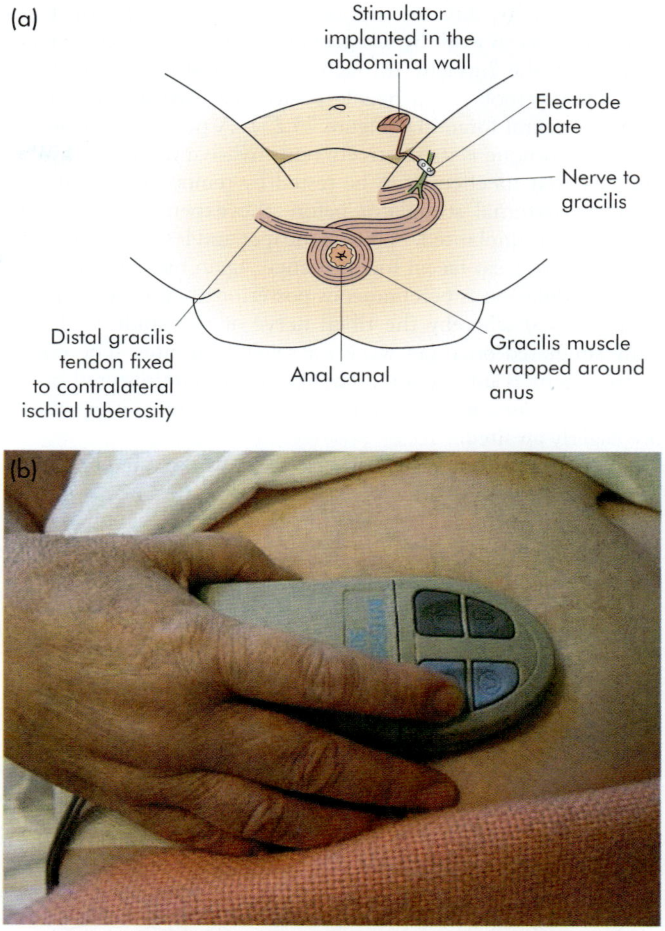

Figure 73.21 (a) The electrically stimulated gracilis neosphincter or dynamic graciloplasty. (b) Hand-held radiotelemetry controller, which allows the patient to turn the stimulator on and off.

sphincter. Transposition of the gracilis muscle around the anal canal is followed by electrical stimulation, with conversion from a fast-twitch to a less fatiguable slow-twitch muscle by an implanted pacemaker (Williams) (Figure 73.21). Because of its magnitude, this technique is performed only in highly selected and motivated patients, most of whom have had more conventional treatment that has failed to cure their incontinence; it is effective in approximately 60 per cent of patients in the long term. A simpler means of augmenting the sphincter, developed initially for urinary incontinence, is the placement of an inflatable silastic cuff around the anal canal. When evacuation is required, the cuff is deflated by squeezing a small balloon positioned in the scrotum or labia, the balloon being attached to a subcutaneous reservoir (Figure 73.22). However, because this device is a foreign body that exerts pressure on the bowel wall, erosion and infection have been found to be common problems. To reduce the risk of septic complications the operation should be covered by antibiotics active against both aerobic and anaerobic organisms. Paradoxically, all of these methods used to treat incontinence may be associated with difficulties in rectal evacuation.

More recently, again as a result of its use in urinary incontinence, sacral nerve stimulation has been used to treat faecal incontinence, with encouraging short- and medium-term results.

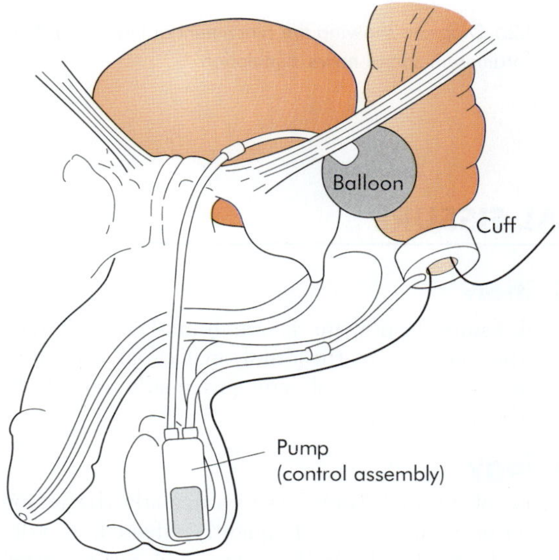

Figure 73.22 Artificial bowel sphincter. A cuff is placed around the anal canal. An inflatable pump control assembly is placed in the scrotum and the balloon reservoir is placed under the symphysis pubis.

Rather than any direct action on sphincter strength, this technique appears to work by sensorimotor neurophysiological modulation of the hindgut through electrical stimulation of the sacral nerve roots via a needle positioned through one of the posterior sacral foramina (Figure 73.23). A potential advantage of this technique is its relatively non-invasive nature, as well as the fact that its effects can be tested by temporary stimulation using an external stimulator before the expensive permanent pacemaker is implanted. A much cheaper and less invasive novel technique to treat faecal incontinence, again mediated through neuromodulation is percutaneous posterior tibial nerve stimulation (PTNS) whereby the tibial nerve at the ankle is electrically simulated once per week for several minutes. The course of treatment is usually for 12 weeks and is administered on an outpatient basis. Results from prospective comparative studies are eagerly awaited.

For some patients, and in those in whom quality of life remains poor despite attempts at restoring continence, a permanent stoma can provide relief from a condition which is both disabling and socially isolating.

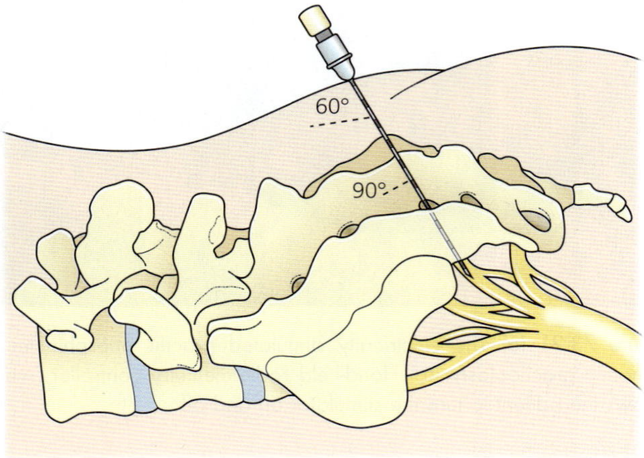

Figure 73.23 Diagram showing the placement of the electrode through a sacral foramen in sacral nerve stimulation.

ANAL FISSURE

Definition

An anal fissure (synonym: fissure-*in-ano*) is a longitudinal split in the anoderm of the distal anal canal (Figure 73.24), which extends from the anal verge proximally towards, but not beyond, the dentate line.

Aetiology

The cause of an anal fissure, and particularly the reason why the posterior midline is so frequently affected, is not completely understood. Classically, acute anal fissures arise from the trauma caused by the strained evacuation of a hard stool or, less commonly, from the repeated passage of diarrhoea. The location in the posterior midline perhaps relates to the

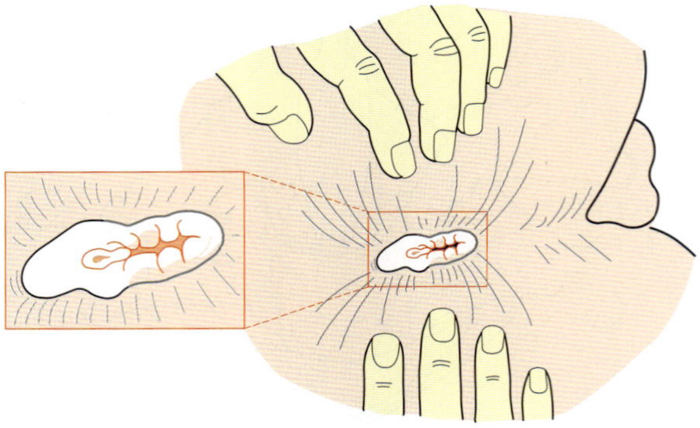

Figure 73.24 The appearance of an anal fissure. If the buttocks are gently parted, the presence of an anal fissure can usually be detected as an ulcer of variable depth with the skin tag and an anal papilla. Redrawn with permission from Keighley MRB, Williams NS. *Surgery of the anus, colon and rectum*, 2nd edn. Philadelphia, PA: WB Saunders, 1999.

exaggerated shearing forces acting at that site at defaecation, combined with a less elastic anoderm endowed with an increased density of longitudinal muscle extensions in that region of the anal circumference. Anterior anal fissure is much more common in women and may arise following vaginal delivery. Perpetuation and chronicity may result from repeated trauma, anal hypertonicity and vascular insufficiency, either secondary to increased sphincter tone or because the posterior commissure is less well perfused than the remainder of the anal circumference.

Clinical features

Simple epithelial splits, because of their location involving the exquisitely sensitive anoderm, acute anal fissures are characterised by severe anal pain associated with defaecation. This usually resolves spontaneously after a variable time only to recur at the next evacuation, as well as the passage of fresh blood, normally noticed on the tissue after wiping. Chronic fissures are characterised by a hypertrophied anal papilla internally and a sentinel tag externally (both consequent upon attempts at healing and breakdown), between which lies the slightly indurated anal ulcer overlying the fibres of the internal sphincter. When chronic, patients may also complain of itching secondary to irritation from the sentinel tag, discharge from the ulcer or discharge from an associated intersphincteric fistula, which has arisen through infection penetrating via the fissure base. Although most sufferers are young adults, the condition can affect any age, from infants to the elderly. Men and women are affected equally. Anterior fissures account for about 10 per cent of those encountered in women, but only 1 per cent in men. A fissure sited elsewhere around the anal circumference or with atypical features should raise the suspicion of a specific aetiology, and failure of adequate examination in the clinic should prompt early examination under anaesthesia, with biopsy and culture to exclude Crohn's disease, tuberculosis, sexually transmitted or human immunodeficiency virus (HIV)-related ulcers (syphilis, *Chlamydia*, chancroid, lymphogranuloma venereum, HSV, cytomegalovirus, Kaposi's sarcoma, B-cell lymphoma) and squamous cell carcinoma (Summary box 73.5).

Summary box 73.5

Anal fissure

- Acute or chronic
- Ischaemic ulcer in the midline of the anal canal
- Ectopic site suggests a more sinister cause
- Symptoms:
  - Pain on defaecation
  - Bright-red bleeding
  - Mucous discharge
  - Constipation

Treatment

After confirmation of the diagnosis in the clinic or under anaesthesia, with exclusion of secondary causes of anal ulceration, conservative management should result in the healing of almost all acute and the majority of chronic fissures. Emphasis must be placed on normalisation of bowel habits such that the passage of stool is less traumatic. The addition of fibre to the diet to bulk up the stool, stool softeners and adequate water intake are simple and helpful measures. Warm baths and topical local anaesthetic agents relieve pain; however, providing patients with anal dilators is usually associated with low compliance and consequently little effect. The mainstay of current conservative management is the topical application of pharmacological agents that relax the internal sphincter, most commonly nitric oxide donors (Scholefield); by reducing spasm, pain is relieved, and increased vascular perfusion promotes healing. Such agents include glyceryl trinitrate (GTN) 0.2 per cent applied four times per day to the anal margin (although this may cause headaches) and diltiazem 2 per cent applied twice daily.

Operative measures

Historically, under regional or general anaesthesia, forceful manual (four- or eight-digit) sphincter dilatation was used to reduce sphincter tone; however, this was achieved in an uncontrolled fashion with potential disruption at multiple sites of the internal (and even external) sphincter. The risk of incontinence following this procedure has now made it unpopular, although more conservative controlled stretching is still practised in young men with very high sphincter tone.

Fissure healing can also be achieved by a posterior division of the exposed fibres of the internal sphincter in the fissure base, but this is associated with prolonged healing, as well as passive anal leakage thought mainly to be due to the resulting keyhole gutter deformity; however, it may be indicated if there is an associated intersphincteric fistula.

Lateral anal sphincterotomy

In this operation, the internal sphincter is divided away from the fissure itself – usually either in the right or the left lateral positions (Notaras). The procedure can be carried out using an open or a closed method, under local, regional or general anaesthesia, and with the patient in the lithotomy or prone jackknife position. The distal internal sphincter is palpated with a bivalved speculum at the intersphincteric groove. In the closed method, a small longitudinal incision is made over this, and the submucosal and intersphincteric planes are carefully developed to allow precise division of the internal sphincter with a knife or scissors to the level of the apex of the fissure; the wound is then closed with absorbable sutures. Alternatively, either plane can be entered using a scalpel (No. 11 blade), with the blade advanced parallel to the sphincter and then rotated such that the sharp edge faces the internal sphincter, which can then be divided along its distal third. Pressure should be applied to the wound for a few minutes to prevent haematoma formation. In the open technique, the anoderm overlying the distal internal sphincter is divided longitudinally to expose the sphincter, which is divided, and the wound is closed with absorbable sutures. Although the fissure needs no specific attention, problematic papillae and external tags can be excised concomitantly.

Early complications of sphincterotomy include haemorrhage, haematoma, bruising, perianal abscess and fistula. Despite low recurrence rates, the most important complication is incontinence of a variable nature and severity, which may affect up to 30 per cent of patients, particularly women, who have weaker, shorter sphincter complexes and in whom there may already have been covert sphincter compromise incurred by childbirth.

Anal advancement flap

The recognition of the risk to continence following internal sphincterotomy has led some to advocate a different approach, especially in women and those with normal or low resting anal pressures, developed from the treatment of anal stenosis. After excision of the edges of the fissure and, if necessary, its base overlying the internal sphincter, an inverted house-shaped flap of perianal skin is carefully mobilised on its blood supply and advanced without tension to cover the fissure, and then sutured with interrupted absorbable sutures (Figure 73.25). The patient is maintained on stool softeners and bulking agents postoperatively, and usually also on topical sphincter relaxants; minor breakdown of one anastomotic edge does not herald ultimate failure (Summary box 73.6). The technique appears to work irrespective of sphincter hypertonicity or patient gender.

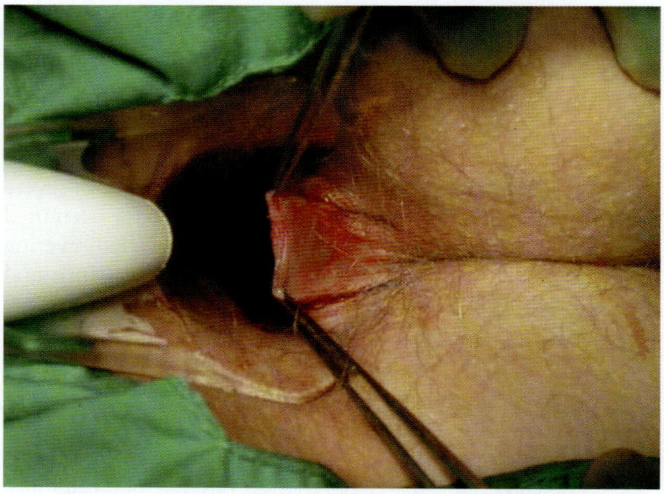

Figure 73.25 Mobilised skin flap prior to suturing intra-anally over the debrided and freshened posterior fissure base.

John Howard Scholefield, contemporary, Professor of Surgery, The University of Nottingham, Nottingham, UK.
Mitchell James Notaras, surgeon, Barnet General Hospital, Barnet, UK.

Summary box 73.6

Treatment of an anal fissure

- Conservative initially, consisting of stool-bulking agents and softeners, and chemical agents in the form of ointments designed to relax the anal sphincter and improve blood flow
- Surgery if above fails, consisting of lateral internal sphincterotomy or anal advancement flap

Hypertrophied anal papilla

Anal papillae occur at the dentate line and are remnants of the ectodermal membrane that separated the hindgut from the proctodaeum. As these papillae are present in 60 per cent of patients examined proctologically, they should be regarded as normal structures. Anal papillae can become elongated, as they frequently do in the presence of an anal fissure. Occasionally, an elongated anal papilla may be the cause of pruritus. An elongated anal papilla associated with pain and/or bleeding at defaecation is sometimes encountered in infancy. Haemorrhage into a hypertrophied anal papilla can cause sudden rectal pain. A prolapsed papilla may become nipped by contraction of the sphincter mechanism after defaecation. Occasionally, a red oedematous papilla is encountered, with local pain and a purulent discharge from the associated crypt. This condition of 'cryptitis' may be cured by laying open the mouth of the infected anal gland and excising the papilla. Troublesome papillae may be simply excised.

Proctalgia fugax

This problem is characterised by attacks of severe pain arising in the rectum, recurring at irregular intervals and apparently unrelated to organic disease. The pain is described as cramp-like, often occurs when the patient is in bed at night, usually lasts only for a few minutes and disappears spontaneously. It may follow straining at stool, sudden explosive bowel action or ejaculation. It seems to occur more commonly in patients suffering from anxiety or undue stress, and it is also said to afflict young doctors. The pain may be unbearable – it is possibly caused by segmental cramp in the pubococcygeus muscle. It is unpleasant and incurable, but is fortunately harmless and gradually subsides. If patients have frequent attacks, they may benefit from amitryptiline. Salbutamol inhalers have been suggested as treatment for acute attacks. A more chronic form of the disease has been termed the 'levator syndrome' and can be associated with severe evacuatory dysfunction. Biofeedback techniques have been used to help such patients; in the past, some surgeons tried severing the puborectalis muscle, but this can cause incontinence and should never be carried out.

HAEMORRHOIDS

The prevalence of haemorrhoids when patients are assessed proctoscopically far outweighs the prevalence of symptoms, and the term should only be used when patients have symptoms referable to them. Occasionally, patients with portal hypertension develop rectal varices, but these should not be confused with haemorrhoids as the consquences may be disastrous. Internal haemorrhoids (Greek: *haima*, blood; *rhoos*, flowing; synonym: piles, Latin: *pila*, a ball) are symptomatic anal cushions and characteristically lie in the 3, 7 and 11 o'clock positions (with the patient in the lithotomy position). In addition, haemorrhoids may be observed between the main pile masses, in which case they are internal haemorrhoids at the secondary position. External haemorrhoids relate to venous channels of the inferior haemorrhoidal plexus deep in the skin surrounding the anal verge and are not true haemorrhoids; they are usually only recognised as a result of a complication, which is most typically a painful solitary acute thrombosis. External haemorrhoids associated with internal haemorrhoids ('interoexternal piles') result from progression of the latter to involve both haemorrhoidal plexuses and are best thought of as being external extensions of internal haemorrhoids. Secondary internal haemorrhoids arise as a result of a specific condition, although the mechanisms involved may be the same as those involved in the formation of primary internal haemorrhoids. The most important cause, albeit relatively uncommon, is carcinoma of the anorectum (Figure 73.26), but there are many other causes, which may be categorised as follows:

- local, e.g. anorectal deformity, hypotonic anal sphincter;
- abdominal, e.g. ascites;
- pelvic, e.g. gravid uterus, uterine neoplasm (fibroid, carcinoma of the uterus or cervix), ovarian neoplasm, bladder carcinoma;
- neurological, e.g. paraplegia, multiple sclerosis.

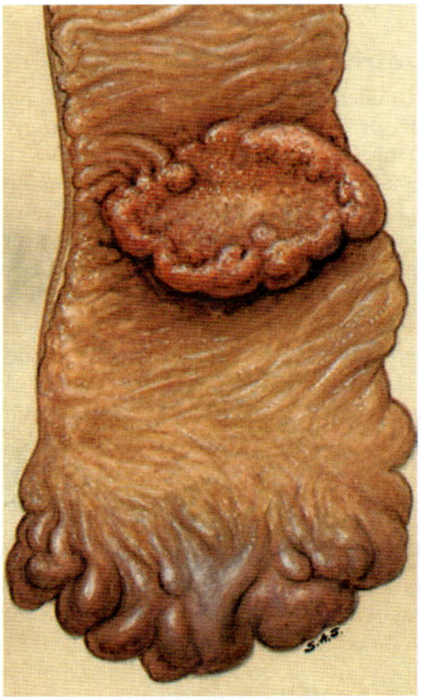

Figure 73.26 Carcinoma of the rectum associated with haemorrhoids, a not infrequent diagnostic pitfall.

Primary internal haemorrhoids

Theories of development

Portal hypertension and varicose veins

Misconceptions concerning the vascular anatomy of the anal canal (specifically the lack of appreciation of communications between portal and systemic systems and the 'normality' of venous dilatations) led to theories of development of primary internal haemorrhoids that lasted for several centuries. Man's upright posture (we know little about haemorrhoidal problems in animals), lack of valves in the portal venous system and raised abdominal pressure were thought to contribute to the development of anal varicosities. If raised portal venous pressure were indeed the cause, one would expect a high incidence in subjects suffering from portal hypertension; however, although such patients have a higher incidence of anorectal varices, these are a separate anatomical and clinical entity from haemorrhoids, which are seen no more frequently than in those without cirrhosis, portal hypertension and oesophageal varices.

Other vascular causes

Historically, some considered haemorrhoids to be haemangiomatous or to result from changes in the erectile tissue that forms part of the continence mechanism, such as hyperplasia of the 'corpus cavernosum recti'.

Infection

Repeated infection of the anal lining, secondary to trauma at defaecation, has been postulated as a cause of weakening and erosion of the walls of the veins of the submucosa. This hypothesis is difficult to accept, as one of the truly incredible properties of the anal canal is its resistance to infection, as well as the ability of its mucosa to heal after surgical intervention despite the torrent of micro-organisms passing over it.

Diet and stool consistency

Much emphasis has been placed on the role of constipation in the development of haemorrhoids and, indeed, much of the management of sufferers involves attempts to 'normalise' bowel habits. A fibre-deficient diet results in a prolonged gut transit time, which is associated with the passage of smaller, harder stools that require more straining to expel. The presence of a hard faecal mass in the rectum could obstruct venous return, resulting in engorgement of the anal veins with the act of straining at stool or sitting for prolonged periods on the lavatory with a relaxed perineum, causing a disturbance of vascular flow. However, the epidemiological pattern of constipation is different from that of haemorrhoidal disease and, indeed, an association has been demonstrated between haemorrhoids and diarrhoeal disorders.

Anal hypertonia

The association between raised anal canal resting pressure and haemorrhoids is well known, but whether anal hypertonia causes symptoms attributable to haemorrhoids or whether anal cushion hypertrophy causes anal hypertonia is a subject of debate. The fact that surgical haemorrhoidectomy restores resting pressures to the normal range is not absolute evidence that the pile masses themselves are the cause of the hypertonia. It should be remembered, however, that there are a significant proportion of patients who suffer haemorrhoidal symptoms in whom the anal canal is relatively patulous, and there is mucosal prolapse, which is associated with perineal descent and pudendal neuropathy.

Ageing

In contrast to the anal cushion of early life, with age, the supporting structures show a higher proportion of collagen than muscle fibres and are fragmented and disorganised. Presumably, these changes arise over time with continued use of the anal canal for defaecation; however, similar changes are noted histologically in surgically excised haemorrhoids in younger patients.

Current view

Shearing forces acting on the anus (for a variety of reasons) lead to caudal displacement of the anal cushions and mucosal trauma. With time, fragmentation of the supporting structures (a normal consequence of ageing, but perhaps accelerated in those with haemorrhoids) leads to loss of elasticity of the cushions such that they no longer retract following defaecation.

Clinical features

Bleeding, as the name haemorrhoid implies, is the principal and earliest symptom. The nature of the bleeding is characteristically separate from the motion and is seen either on the paper on wiping or as a fresh splash in the pan. Very rarely, the bleeding may be sufficient to cause anaemia. Pain is not commonly associated with the bleeding and its presence should make the clinician alert to the possibility of another diagnosis; however, pain may result from congestion of pile masses below a hypertonic sphincter. Piles associated with bleeding alone are called first-degree haemorrhoids (Summary box 73.7).

Summary box 73.7

Haemorrhoids: clinical features

- Haemorrhoids or piles are symptomatic anal cushions
- They are more common when intra-abdominal pressure is raised, e.g. in obesity, constipation and pregnancy
- Classically, they occur in the 3, 7 and 11 o'clock positions with the patient in the lithotomy position
- Symptoms of haemorrhoids:
  - bright-red, painless bleeding
  - mucous discharge
  - prolapse
  - pain only on prolapse

Patients may complain of true 'piles', lumps that appear at the anal orifice during defaecation and which return spontaneously afterwards (second-degree haemorrhoids), piles that have to be replaced manually (third-degree haemorrhoids) (Figure 73.27) or piles that lie permanently outside (fourth-degree haemorrhoids). By this stage, there is often a significant cutaneous component to the pile masses, which arise through repeated congestion and oedema. In addition to the main symptoms of pain and prolapse, patients may complain of anal irritation, which may occur as a result of mucus secretion from the caudally displaced rectal mucosa, minor leakage through a now imperfect anal seal or difficulties in cleaning after defaecation because of the irregularity of the anal verge (Summary box 73.8).

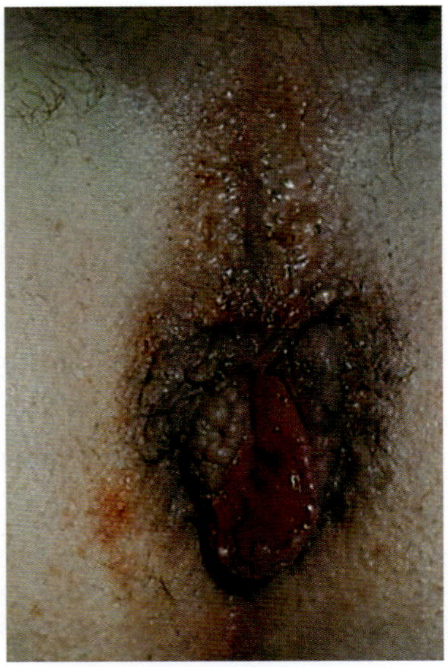

Figure 73.27 Third-degree haemorrhoids (courtesy of CV Mann, The Royal London Hospital, London, UK).

Summary box 73.8

Four degrees of haemorrhoids

- First degree – bleed only, no prolapse
- Second degree – prolapse, but reduce spontaneously
- Third degree – prolapse and have to be manually reduced
- Fourth degree – permanently prolapsed

Complications

Profuse haemorrhage is uncommon. The bleeding mainly occurs externally but it may continue internally after the bleeding haemorrhoid has retracted or has been returned. In these circumstances, the rectum is found to contain blood (Summary box 73.9).

Summary box 73.9

Complications of haemorrhoids

- Strangulation and thrombosis (Figure 73.28)
- Ulceration
- Gangrene
- Portal pyaemia
- Fibrosis

Treatment of complications

- **Strangulation, thrombosis and gangrene.** In these cases, it was formerly believed that surgery would promote portal pyaemia. However, if adequate antibiotic cover is given from the start, this is not found to be so, and immediate surgery can be justified in many patients. The other risk if surgery is performed at this stage, that of postoperative stenosis, results in some surgeons reviewing the situation much later and carrying out haemorrhoidectomy only if necessary. Besides adequate pain relief, bed rest with frequent hot baths and warm or cold saline compresses with firm pressure usually cause the pile mass to shrink considerably in 3–4 days (the authors' preference is shrinkage through external application of small bags of frozen peas). An anal dilatation technique has in the past been used as an alternative treatment to surgery for painful 'strangulated' haemorrhoids (Figure 73.28). However, because of the risk of incontinence this is no longer advised.
- **Severe haemorrhage.** The cause usually lies in a bleeding diathesis or the use of anticoagulants. If such causes are excluded, a local compress containing adrenaline solution, with an injection of morphine and blood transfusion if necessary, will usually suffice. However, after adequate blood replacement, ligation and excision of the piles may be required.

Management

Exclusion of other causes of rectal bleeding, especially colorectal malignancy, is the first priority. In the absence of a specific predisposing cause, important measures include attempts at normalising bowel and defaecatory habits: only evacuating when the natural desire to do so arises, adopting a defaecatory position to minimise straining, and the addition of stool softeners and bulking agents to ease the defaecatory act. Various proprietary creams can be inserted into the rectum from a collapsible tube fitted with a nozzle, at night and before defaecation. Suppositories are also useful.

In those with first- or second-degree piles whose symptoms are not improved by conservative measures, injection sclerotherapy (Mitchell), the submucosal injection of 5 per cent phenol in arachis oil or almond oil, may be advised. Any invasive treatment, however, must be with full agreement of the patient, who should be informed of the potential risks of such interventions. The aim is to create fibrosis, cause obliteration of the vascular channels and hitch up the anorectal mucosa.

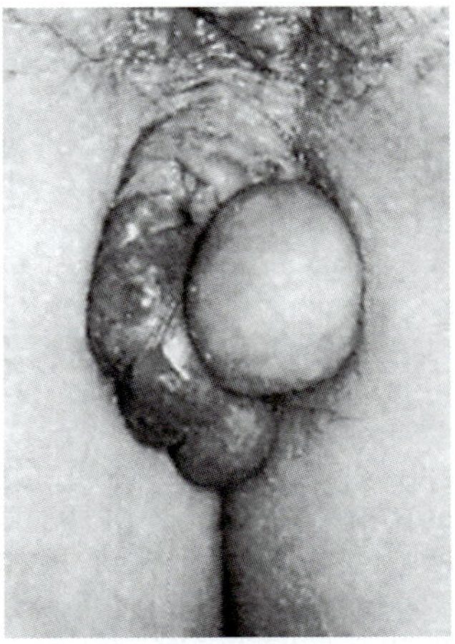

Figure 73.28 An attack of piles. Prolapsed strangulated piles, as commonly seen, on the left. A less common mass on the right with fibrofatty covering.

Clinton Mitchell of Illinois, IL, USA was the first to use carbolic acid for injecting haemorrhoids. Itinerant irregular practitioners exploited the method.

With the awake patient in the left lateral position and under direct vision with a proctoscope, about 5 mL of sclerosant is injected into the apex of the pile pedicle (Figure 73.29) using a (now) disposable needle and syringe (Figure 73.30). The procedure is repeated for each pile and the patient reassessed after 8 weeks; if necessary, the injections are repeated. Pain upon injection means that the needle is in the wrong place and should be withdrawn. Injections that are too superficial are heralded by the rapid bulging of the mucosa, which turns white; this leads to superficial ulceration but rarely serious septic sequelae. However, injections placed too deeply can have disastrous consequences, including pelvic sepsis, prostatitis, impotence and rectovaginal fistula.

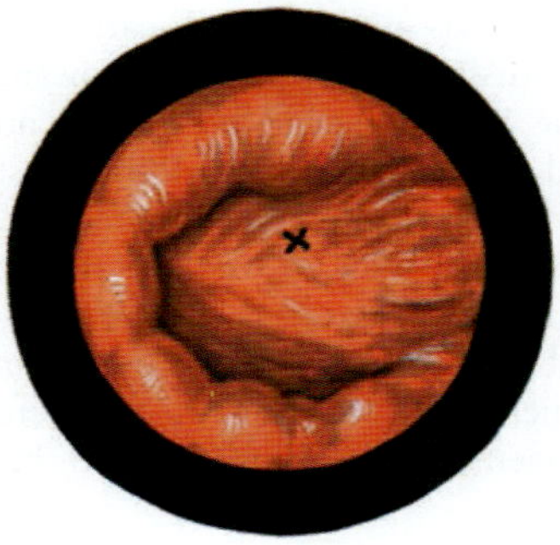

Figure 73.29 Correct site (cross) for injecting a haemorrhoid (after WB Gabriel, London, UK).

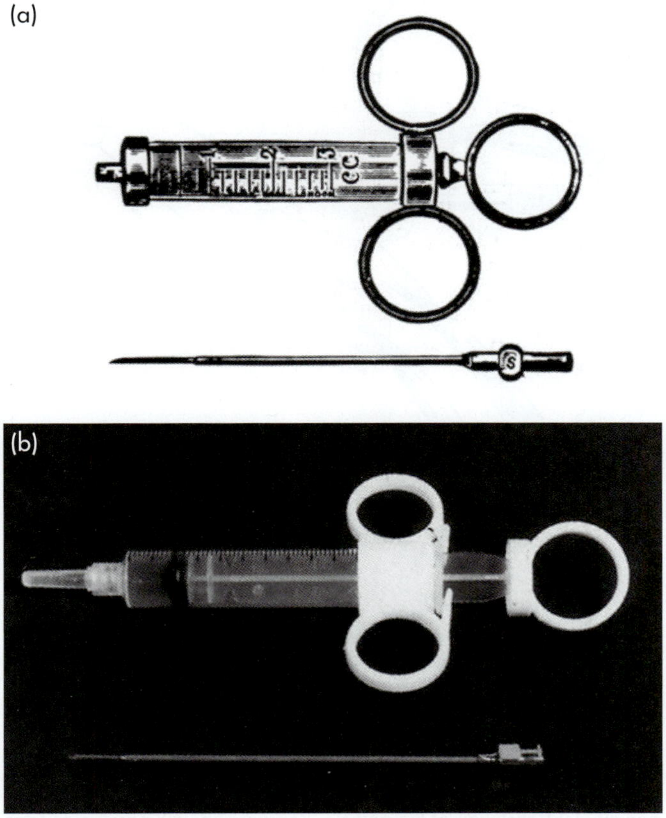

Figure 73.30 Gabriel's syringe (a) has now been replaced by disposable syringes (b).

For more bulky piles, banding has been shown to be efficacious, but it is associated with more discomfort. The Barron's bander is a commonly available device used to slip tight elastic bands onto the base of the pedicle of each haemorrhoid (Figure 73.31). The bands cause ischaemic necrosis of the piles, which slough off within 10 days; this may be associated with bleeding, about which the patient must be warned. As with sclerotherapy, three piles may be treated at one session, and the process may be repeated after several weeks if necessary. The techniques of cryotherapy (Lloyd Williams) and infrared photocoagulation (Leicester) are not often used nowadays.

Operation

Indications

The indications for haemorrhoidectomy include:

- third- and fourth-degree haemorrhoids;
- second-degree haemorrhoids that have not been cured by non-operative treatments;
- fibrosed haemorrhoids;
- interoexternal haemorrhoids when the external haemorrhoid is well defined.

If there is any doubt about the diagnosis of haemorrhoids, examination under anaesthesia and, if indicated, biopsy are necessary. The other strong indication for surgery is haemorrhoidal bleeding sufficient to cause anaemia. Beyond these, the indications summarised above are more relative than absolute, because in these situations surgery aims simply to improve symptoms and, of course, is not without risk. For instance, elderly multiparous women with hypotonic sphincters who are just continent before haemorrhoidectomy may find that the procedure results in frank incontinence, a far worse condition than that for which they originally sought help.

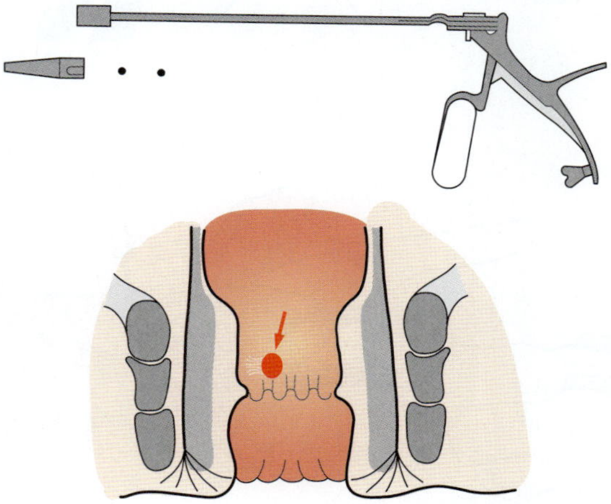

Figure 73.31 Barron's banding apparatus, with the appearance of a typical 'banded' haemorrhoid.

John Barron, surgeon, Chicago, IL, USA.
William Bashall Gabriel, 1893–1975, surgeon, St Mark's Hospital and the Royal Northern Hospital, London, UK.
Kenneth Lloyd Williams, deceased, surgeon, The Royal United Hospitals, Bath, UK.
Roger James Leicester, surgeon, St George's Hospital, London, UK.

Technique

It is usual for the patient to have been taking stool softeners in the days before surgery and a preoperative enema to empty the rectum is administered. The procedure is usually performed under general or regional anaesthesia with the patient in the lithotomy or prone jack-knife position. The perianal skin is shaved and a formal examination performed. Haemorrhoidectomy can be performed using an open or a closed technique. The open technique is most commonly used in the UK and is known as the Milligan–Morgan operation – named after the surgeons who described it. The closed technique is the popular technique in the United States. Both involve ligation and excision of the haemorrhoid, but in the open technique the anal mucosa and skin are left open to heal by secondary intention, and in the closed technique the wound is sutured.

- **Open technique.** The anoderm and subcutaneous tissues between the pile masses may be injected with dilute adrenaline (epinephrine, 1:300 000 dilution) to reduce bleeding and aid preservation of the skin bridges left following excision. Artery forceps are applied to the skin-covered external components of the piles and traction exerted to reveal the internal components, which are also grasped by artery forceps. When held out by the assistant, these pairs of artery forceps form a triangle (Figure 73.32a). The operator takes the left lateral pair of artery forceps in the palm of the hand and places the extended forefinger in the anal canal to support the internal haemorrhoid. In this way, traction is applied to the skin of the anal margin. With scissors or cutting diathermy, a V-shaped cut is made through the skin and those fibres inserting into it around the skin-holding artery forceps. Traction by both operator and assistant, combined with careful dissection, will expose the lower border of the internal sphincter. The dissection proceeds up the anal canal, with the sides of the mucosal dissection converging towards the pile apex and with the internal sphincter visible and separate from the dissected pile (Figure 73.32b). A transfixion ligature of strong Vicryl is applied to the pedicle at this level (Figure 73.32c), the pile is excised well distal to the ligature and, after ensuring haemostasis, the ligature is cut long. Each haemorrhoid is dealt with in this manner, taking care to leave mucocutaneous bridges. If there are significant secondary haemorrhoids under these bridges, they can

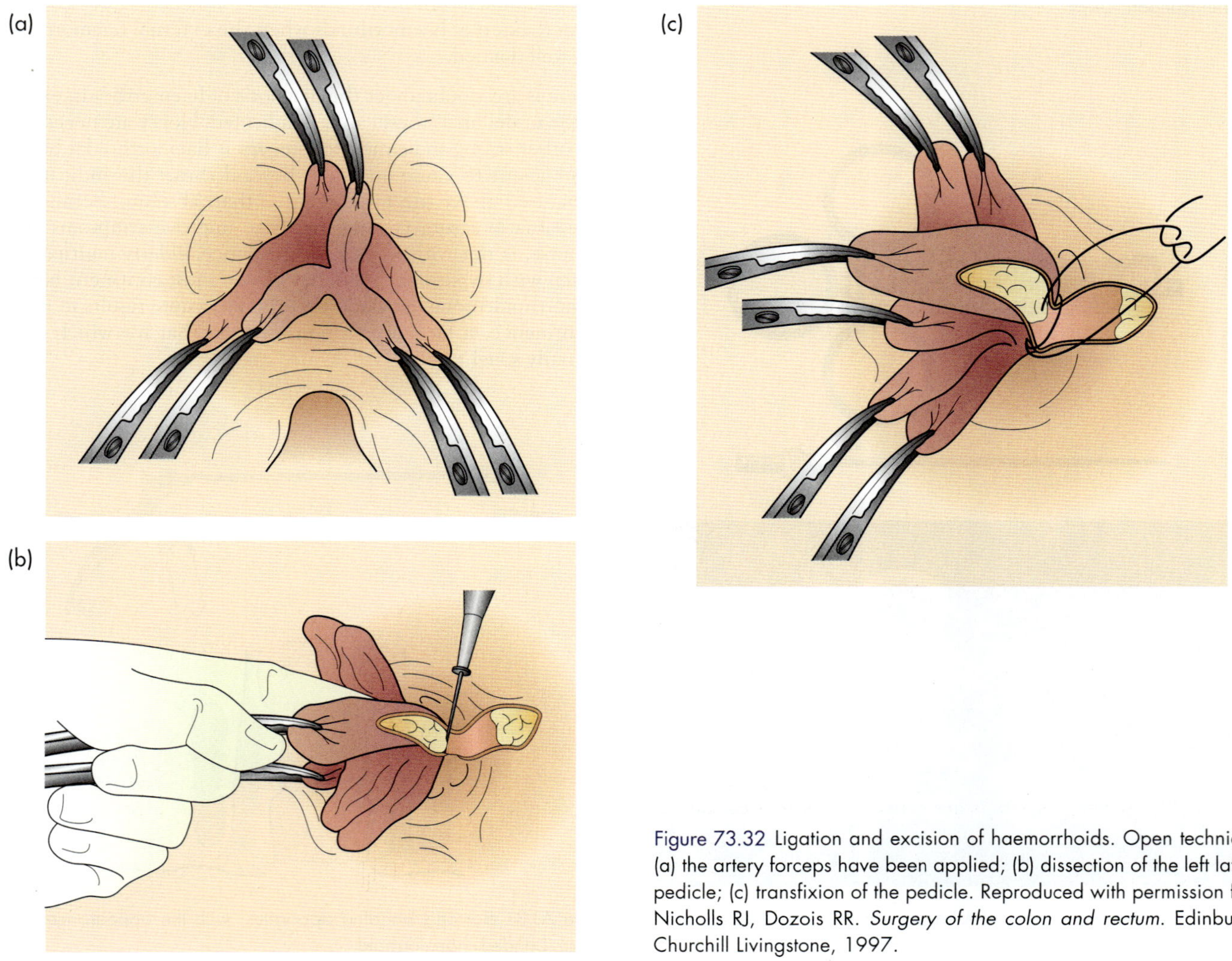

Figure 73.32 Ligation and excision of haemorrhoids. Open technique: (a) the artery forceps have been applied; (b) dissection of the left lateral pedicle; (c) transfixion of the pedicle. Reproduced with permission from Nicholls RJ, Dozois RR. *Surgery of the colon and rectum*. Edinburgh: Churchill Livingstone, 1997.

be filleted out by scissor dissection. Haemostasis must be absolute at the end of the procedure, when a soft absorbable anal dressing is inserted. The margins of the skin wounds are trimmed so as not to leave overhanging edges (Figure 73.33). Bleeding subcutaneous arteries having been secured, the areas denuded of skin are dressed with three pieces of petroleum jelly gauze. A pad of gauze and wool and a firmly applied T-bandage complete the operation.

- **Closed technique.** The haemorrhoid is excised, together with the overlying mucosa, as illustrated in Figure 73.34a. The haemorrhoid is dissected carefully from the underlying sphincter and haemostasis is achieved. The pedicle is transfixed and ligated with 3/0 Vicryl or Dexon. Any residual small haemorrhoids should be removed by filleting them out after undermining the edges of the cut mucosa. The mucosal defect is then closed completely with a continuous suture using the same stitch that was employed to ligate the haemorrhoid pedicle. The remaining haemorrhoids are excised and ligated in a similar fashion, ensuring that there are adequate mucosal and skin bridges between each area of excision to avoid a subsequent stenosis.

With the aim of symptom relief but preservation of the anal cushions, the technique of stapled haemorrhoidopexy (Longo), which utilises a purpose-designed stapling gun (PPH, Ethicon Inc.), has recently been described. This procedure excises a strip of mucosa and submucosa (together with the vessels travelling within them) circumferentially, well above the dentate line. Activation of the gun also simultaneously repairs the cut mucosa and submucosa by stapling the edges together (Figure 73.35). This procedure is quick to perform, and controlled trials suggest that it is less painful and less traumatic than conventional haemorrhoidectomy and, at least in the short term, it seems to be equally efficacious. However, evidence is emerging that the technique is associated with higher recurrence rates than following conventional haemorrhoidectomy, and associated with more additional surgery. The patient, after counselling, may choose to accept a higher recurrence rate to take advantage of the short-term benefits, or not (Summary box 73.10).

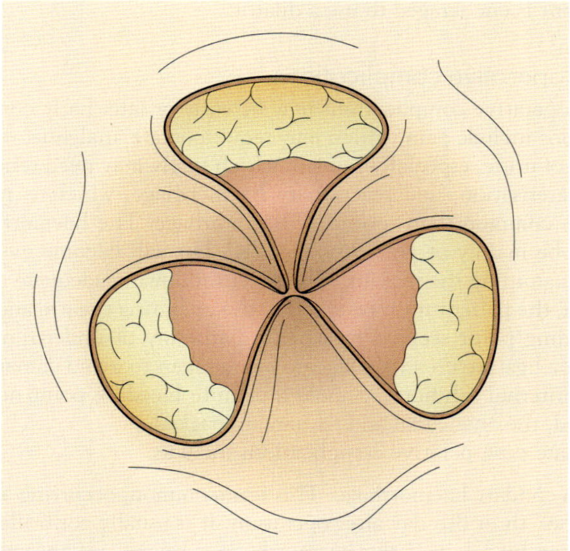

Figure 73.33 The appearance of the anus at the conclusion of the operation. (Note that to avoid stricture formation, it is necessary to ensure that a bridge of skin and mucous membrane remains between each wound.) 'If it looks like a clover the trouble is over, if it looks like a dahlia, it is surely a failure.' Reproduced with permission from Nicholls RJ, Dozois RR. *Surgery of the colon and rectum*. Edinburgh: Churchill Livingstone, 1997.

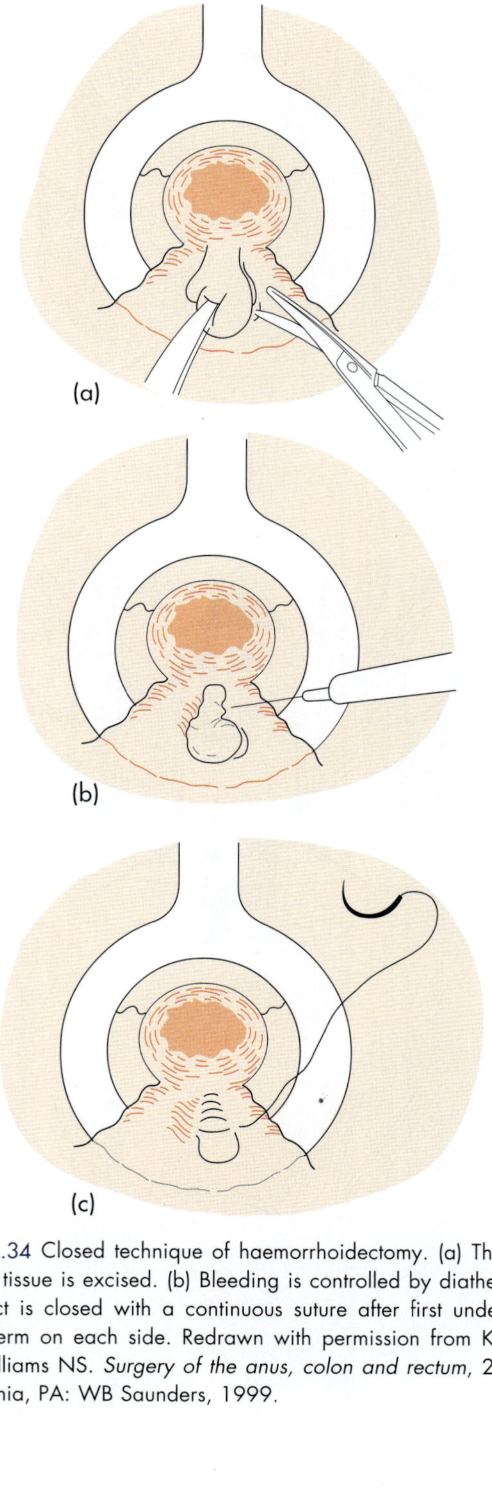

Figure 73.34 Closed technique of haemorrhoidectomy. (a) The haemorrhoidal tissue is excised. (b) Bleeding is controlled by diathermy. (c) The defect is closed with a continuous suture after first undermining the anoderm on each side. Redrawn with permission from Keighley, MRB, Williams NS. *Surgery of the anus, colon and rectum*, 2nd edn. Philadelphia, PA: WB Saunders, 1999.

A Longo, surgeon, Sicily, Italy.

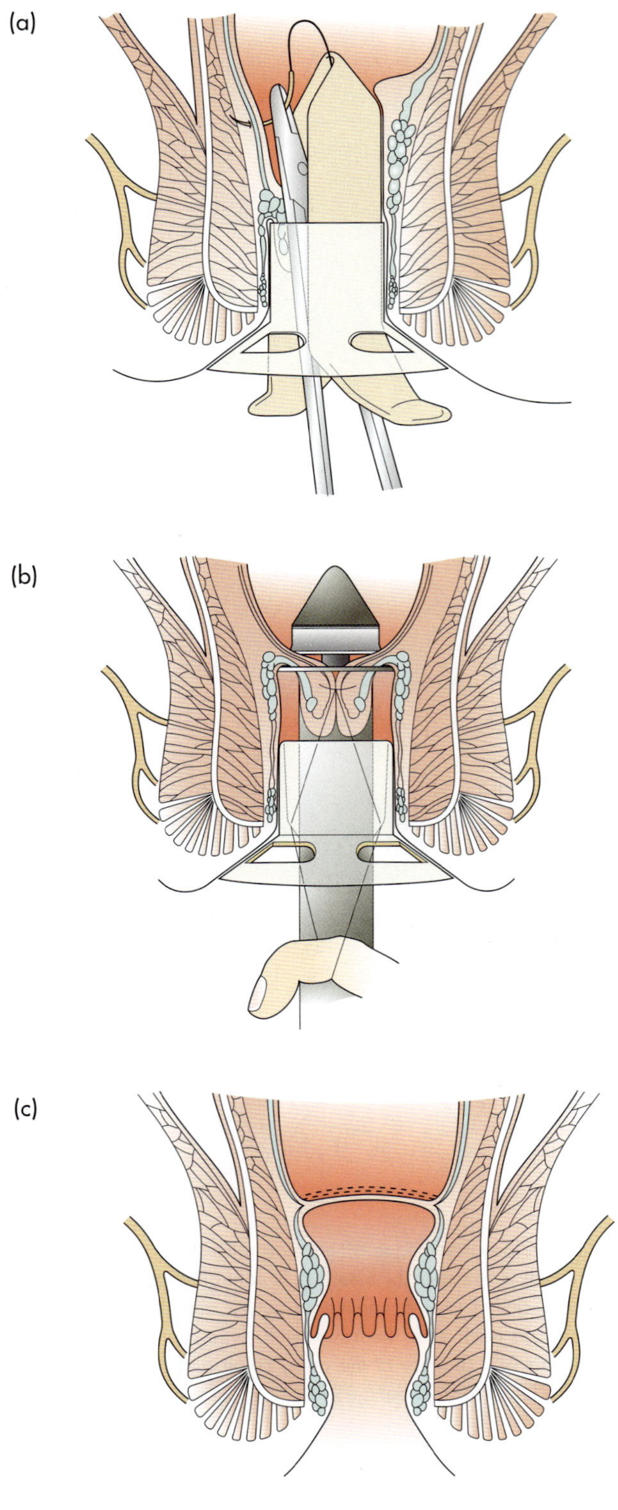

Figure 73.35 Stapled haemorrhoidectomy. (a) The purse-string suture is placed several centimetres above the dentate line. (b) The anvil of the fully opened stapling gun is inserted endoanally so that it is above the purse-string suture, which is then tied around the shaft of the gun. The gun is closed and fired. (c) After firing, a 3–4 cm strip of mucosa and submucosa containing the haemorrhoids is excised and the mucosal edges are simultaneously stapled together.

Summary box 73.10

Treatment of haemorrhoids

- Symptomatic – advice about defaecatory habits, stool softeners and bulking agents
- Injection of sclerosant
- Banding
- Transanal haemorrhoidal dearterialisation/ haemorrhoidopexy
- Haemorrhoidectomy

Transanal haemorrhoidal dearterialisation

Transanal haemorrhoidal dearterialisation (THD) is used for the treatment of second- and third-degree haemorrhoids. Some have recently advocated transanal Doppler-guided ligation of those vessels feeding the haemorrhoidal masses, to which others have added suture 'mucopexy' to deal with any prolapse. Long-term outcomes are unknown, but recurrence rates for fourth-degree haemorrhoids (certainly when additional procedures are not incorporated) are high.

Postoperative care

In these days of economic stringencies, the patient is discharged from hospital within a day or two of the operation. In many countries, the procedure is often performed on a day-care basis. The patient is instructed to take two warm baths each day and is given a bulk laxative to take twice daily together with appropriate analgesia. There is some evidence that a 5-day course of oral metronidazole may reduce pain. Dry dressings are applied as necessary, a sterile sanitary towel usually being ideal. The patient is seen again 3–4 weeks after discharge and a rectal examination is performed. If there is evidence of stenosis, the patient is encouraged to use a dilator.

Postoperative complications

Postoperative complications may be early or late. Early complications include pain, which may require opiate analgesia; retention of urine, especially in men, which rarely may need relief by catheterisation; and reactionary haemorrhage, which is much more common than secondary haemorrhage. The haemorrhage may be mainly or entirely concealed, but will become evident on examining the rectum. If persistent following adequate analgesia, the patient must be taken to the operating theatre and the bleeding point secured by careful diathermy or under-running with a ligature on a needle, care being taken to avoid damage to the internal sphincter. Should a definite bleeding point not be found, the anal canal and rectum are packed.

Late postoperative complications include:

- Secondary haemorrhage. This is uncommon, occurring about the 7th or 8th day after operation. It is usually controlled by morphine but, if the haemorrhage is severe, an anaesthetic should be given and the bleeding controlled.
- Anal stricture, which must be prevented at all costs. A rectal examination at the postoperative review will indicate whether stricturing is to be expected. It may then be necessary to give a general anaesthetic and dilate the anus. After that, daily use of the dilator should give a satisfactory result.
- Anal fissures and submucous abscesses.

- Incontinence, especially if there has been inadvertent damage to the underlying internal sphincter. Although uncommon, this is obviously a very serious problem that is difficult to treat (Summary box 73.11).

Summary box 73.11

Complications of haemorrhoidectomy

- Early
  - Pain
  - Acute retention of urine
  - Reactionary haemorrhage
- Late
  - Secondary haemorrhage
  - Anal stricture
  - Anal fissure
  - Incontinence

External haemorrhoids

A thrombosed external haemorrhoid relates anatomically to the veins of the superficial or external haemorrhoidal plexus and is commonly termed a 'perianal haematoma'. It presents as a sudden onset, olive-shaped, painful blue subcutaneous swelling at the anal margin and is usually consequent upon straining at stool, coughing or lifting a heavy weight (Figure 73.36). The thrombosis is usually situated in a lateral region of the anal margin. If the patient presents within the first 48 hours, the clot may be evacuated under local anaesthesia. Untreated it may resolve, suppurate, fibrose and give rise to a cutaneous tag, burst and the clot extrude, or continue bleeding. In the majority of cases, resolution or fibrosis occurs. Indeed, this condition has been called 'a 5-day, painful, self-curing lesion' (Milligan).

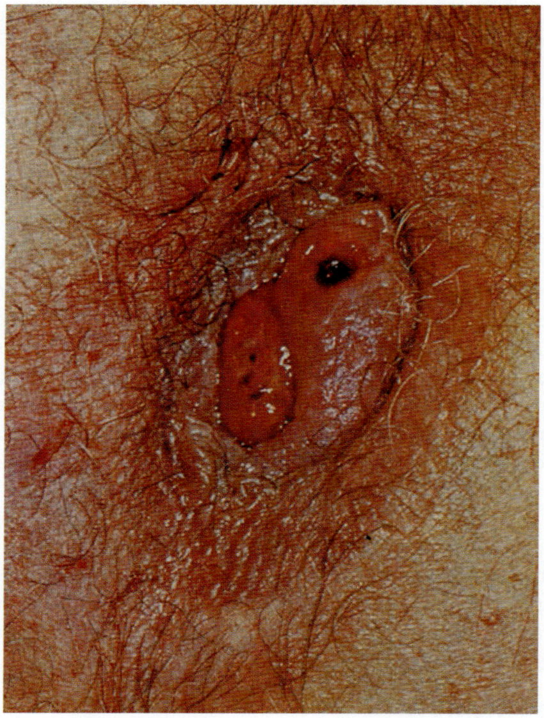

Figure 73.36 A thrombosed external haemorrhoid that has burst. There is also a mucosal prolapse, which is separate from the cutaneous lesion.

PRURITUS ANI

This is intractable itching around the anus, a common and embarrassing condition. Usually, the skin is reddened and hyperkeratotic and it may become cracked and moist.

Causes

The causes are numerous. A useful mnemonic is 'pus, polypus, parasites, piles, psyche':

- **Lack of cleanliness**, excessive sweating and wearing rough or woollen underclothing.
- An **anal or perianal discharge** that renders the anus moist. The causative lesions include an anal fissure, fistula-*in-ano*, prolapsed internal or external haemorrhoids, genital warts and excessive ingestion of liquid paraffin. A mucous discharge is an intense pruritic agent and a polyp can be the cause.
- A **vaginal discharge**, especially caused by *Trichomonas vaginalis* infection.
- **Parasitic causes**. Threadworms should be excluded, especially in young subjects. Children suffering from threadworms should wear gloves at night, lest they scratch the perianal region and are reinfested with ova by nail biting – 'parasites lost, parasites regained'. Scabies and pediculosis pubis may infest the anal region.
- **Epidermophytosis** is a common cause, especially if the skin between the toes is also infected; microscopic and cultural examinations are essential. Half-strength Whitfield's ointment quickly gives relief and is the sheet anchor of treatment.
- **Allergy** is sometimes the cause, in which case there is likely to be a history of other allergic manifestations, such as urticaria, asthma or hay fever. Antibiotic therapy may be the precipitating factor.
- **Skin diseases** localised to the perianal skin: psoriasis, lichen planus and contact dermatitis.
- **Bacterial infection**, such as intertrigo resulting from a mixed bacterial infection. Erythrasma caused by *Corynebacterium minutissimum* is responsible for some cases and its presence is detected by ultraviolet light, which induces a pink fluorescence.
- A **psychoneurosis**. It is alleged that in a few instances neurotic individuals become so immersed in their complaint that a pain–pleasure complex develops, the pleasure being the scratching. Possibly this is true, but such a syndrome should not be assumed without firm grounds for coming to this conclusion.
- **Diabetes** can sometimes present with pruritus ani, and the urine should be tested in all patients.

Treatment

The cause is treated. Symptomatic treatment includes the following:

- **Hygiene measures**. Cotton wool should be substituted for toilet paper. Soap is avoided and replaced by water alone,

Arthur Whitfield, 1867–1967, Professor of Dermatology, King's College Hospital, London, UK. Whitfield's ointment is 'compound ointment of benzoic acid'.

and the area pat-dried rather than rubbed. These measures alone, combined with wearing cotton underwear and the application of calamine lotion or zinc and castor oil, are all that is necessary to cure some cases. If there is much anal hair trapping the moisture and discharge, shaving can be very helpful.

- **Hydrocortisone.** In patients with dermatitis, and only in patients with dermatitis, the topical application of 0.5 or 1 per cent prednisolone cream is often beneficial; sometimes after discontinuation of the therapy, the pruritus is liable to return, in which case 5 per cent lidocaine hydrochloride (Xylocaine) ointment can be substituted for a time.
- **Strapping the buttocks** keeps moist opposing surfaces apart, but is not well tolerated. If the moistness originates from anal discharge, a cotton wool anal plug will seal the anal orifice.

Operative treatment

This may be necessary for a concomitant lesion of the anorectum that is thought to initiate or contribute to the pruritus. Otherwise, surgery is not indicated (Summary box 73.12).

Summary box 73.12

Pruritus ani

- Common
- Numerous causes including skin diseases, parasites (threadworm), anal discharge, allergies, diabetes
- Treat the cause if possible
- Symptomatic treatment is the mainstay

ANORECTAL ABSCESSES

Acute sepsis in the region of the anus is common. A fundamental distinction that has to be made is whether the sepsis is in that area by chance (simple boil, skin appendage infection) or whether it has arisen as a consequence of the presence of the anorectum, specifically the anal glands. Overall, anorectal sepsis is more common in men than women, although infections with skin-type organisms (and thus unrelated to fistula) are evenly distributed. The cryptoglandular theory of intersphincteric anal gland infection (Parks) holds that, upon infection of a gland, pus, which travels along the path of least resistance, may spread caudally to present as a perianal abscess, laterally across the external sphincter to form an ischiorectal abscess or, rarely, superiorly above the anorectal junction to form a supralevator intermuscular or pararectal abscess (depending on its relation to the longitudinal muscle), as well as circumferentially in any of the three planes: intersphincteric/intermuscular, ischiorectal or pararectal supralevator (Figure 73.37). Sepsis unrelated to anal gland infection may occur at the same or at other sites (Figure 73.38), including submucosal abscess (following haemorrhoidal sclerotherapy, which usually resolve spontaneously), mucocutaneous or marginal abscess (infected haematoma), ischiorectal abscess (foreign body, trauma, deep skin-related infection) and pelvirectal supralevator sepsis originating in pelvic disease. Underlying rectal disease, such as neoplasm and particularly Crohn's disease, may be the cause. Similarly,

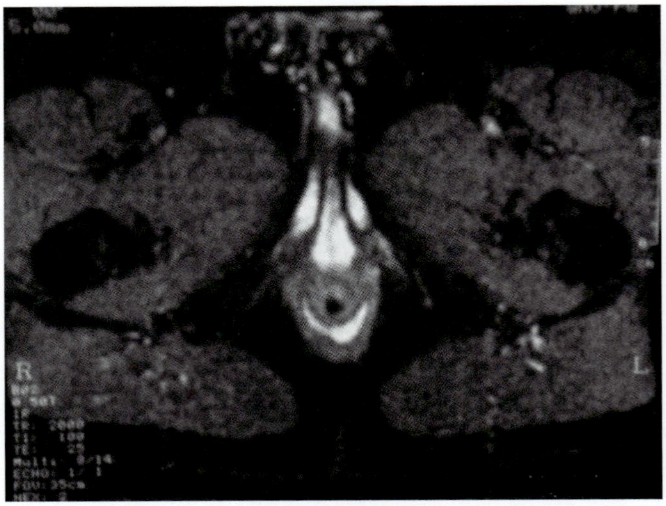

Figure 73.37 Axial magnetic resonance imaging (MRI) scan (STIR sequence) showing posterior horseshoe spread of sepsis within the intersphincteric space.

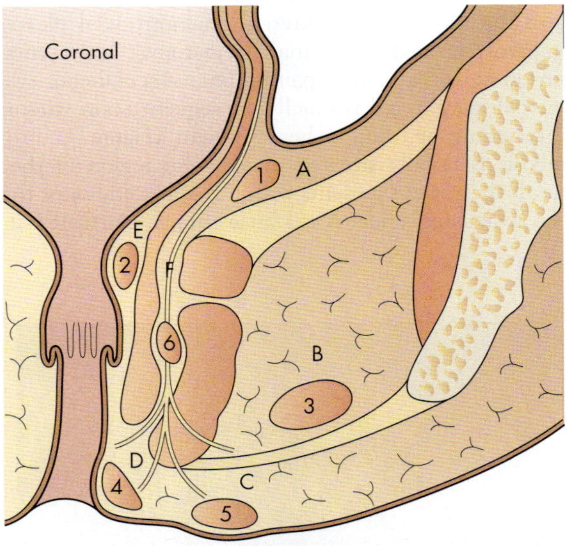

Figure 73.38 Diagram showing the spaces in relation to the anus and types of anorectal abscess in coronal section: A, pelvirectal supralevator space; B, ischiorectal space; C, perianal or superficial ischiorectal space; D, marginal or mucocutaneous space; E, submucous space; F, anorectal intermuscular (intersphincteric) space; 1, pelvirectal supralevator abscess; 2, submucous abscess; 3, ischiorectal abscess; 4, marginal abscess; 5, perianal abscess; 6, intersphincteric abscess. Reproduced with permission from Nicholls RJ, Dozois RR. *Surgery of the colon and rectum*. Edinburgh: Churchill Livingstone, 1997.

patients with generalised disorders, such as diabetes and acquired immunodeficiency syndrome (AIDS), may present with an anorectal abscess; in these patients, abscesses may run an aggressive course.

Presentation

A perianal abscess, confined by the terminal extensions of the longitudinal muscle, is usually associated with a short (2–3 day) history of increasingly severe, well-localised pain and a palpable tender lump at the anal margin. Examination reveals an indurated hot tender perianal swelling. Patients with infection in the larger fatty-filled ischiorectal space, in which tissue tension is much lower, usually present later, with less well-localised symptoms but more constitutional upset and fever. On examination, the affected buttock is diffusely swollen with widespread induration and deep tenderness. If sepsis is higher, deep rectal pain, fever and sometimes disturbed micturition may be the only features, with nothing evident on external examination but tender supralevator induration palpable on digital examination above the anorectal junction.

Differential diagnosis

The only conditions with which an anorectal abscess is likely to be confused are abscesses connected with a pilonidal sinus, Bartholin's gland or Cowper's gland.

Management

Management of acute anorectal sepsis is primarily surgical, including careful examination under anaesthesia, sigmoidoscopy and proctoscopy, and adequate drainage of the pus. For perianal and ischiorectal sepsis (with an incidence of 60 and 30 per cent, respectively), drainage is through the perineal skin, usually through a cruciate incision over the most fluctuant point, with excision of the skin edges to deroof the abscess (Figure 73.39). Pus is sent for microbiological culture (Grace) and tissue from the wall is sent for histological appraisal to exclude specific causes. With a finger in the anorectum to avoid creation of a false opening, the cavity is carefully curetted. A gentle search may be made for an underlying fistula if the surgeon is experienced, and, if obvious, a loose draining seton may be passed; injudicious probing in the acute stage is, however, potentially dangerous and may lead to a much more difficult situation. Unless by highly experienced hands, immediate fistulotomy should not be performed. After irrigation of the cavity, the wound is lightly tucked; antibiotics are prescribed if there is surrounding cellulitis and especially in those less resistant to infection, such as diabetics. If the pus subsequently cultures skin-type organisms, there will be no underlying fistula and the patient can be reassured. If gut flora are cultured, it is likely, but not inevitable, that there is an underlying fistula.

The management of supralevator sepsis is dependent upon its exact anatomy (within or outside the rectal wall) and its origin. Sepsis originating in pelvic disease necessitates appropriate management of the underlying cause (appendiceal, gynaecological, diverticular, Crohn's disease, malignancy), although intrarectal drainage may be apt to avoid creation of an extrasphincteric fistula. Cephalad extension of an intersphincteric fistula can be safely drained into the rectum, whereas supralevator extension of a trans-sphincteric fistula should be drained via the skin of the buttock. Rarely, a colostomy may be necessary to control severe sepsis, especially in the immunocompromised individual (Summary box 73.13).

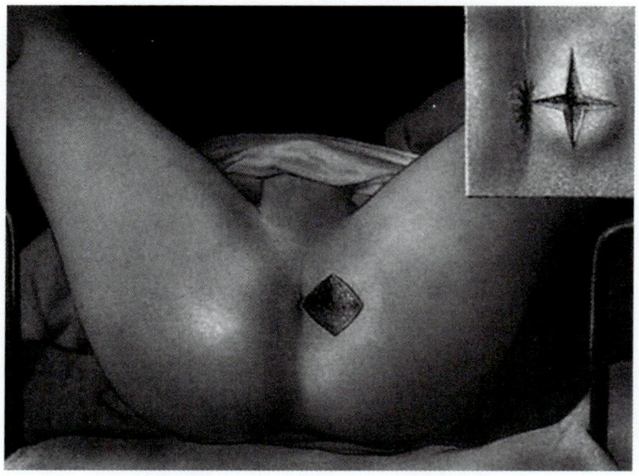

Figure 73.39 Incision of an ischiorectal abscess. The cavity is explored and, if septa exist, they should be broken down gently with a finger and the necrotic tissue lining the walls of the abscess removed by the finger wrapped in gauze. It is wise to biopsy the wall and send the pus for culture. Nothing further is done at this stage.

Summary box 73.13

Anorectal abscess

- Usually produces a painful, throbbing swelling in the anal region. The patient often has swinging pyrexia
- Subdivided according to anatomical site into perianal, ischiorectal, submucous and pelvirectal
- Underlying conditions include fistula-*in-ano* (most common), Crohn's disease, diabetes, immunosuppression
- Treatment is drainage of pus in first instance, together with appropriate antibiotics
- Always look for a potential underlying problem

FISTULA-*IN-ANO*

A fistula-*in-ano*, or anal fistula, is a chronic abnormal communication, usually lined to some degree by granulation tissue, which runs outwards from the anorectal lumen (the internal opening) to an external opening on the skin of the perineum or buttock (or rarely, in women, to the vagina). Anal fistulae may be found in association with specific conditions, such as Crohn's disease, tuberculosis, lymphogranuloma venereum, actinomycosis, rectal duplication, foreign body and malignancy (which may also very rarely arise within a longstanding fistula), and suspicion of these should be aroused if clinical findings are unusual. However, the majority are termed non-specific, idiopathic or cryptoglandular, and intersphincteric anal gland infection is deemed central to them.

Presentation

For reasons that are unknown, non-specific anal fistulae are more common in men than women. The overall incidence is about nine cases per 100000 population per year in Western Europe, and those in their third, fourth and fifth decades of life are most commonly affected. Patients usually complain of intermittent purulent discharge (which may be bloody) and pain (which increases until temporary relief occurs when the pus discharges). There is often, but not invariably, a previous episode of acute anorectal sepsis that settled (incompletely) spontaneously or with antibiotics, or which was surgically drained. The passage of flatus or faeces through the external opening is suggestive of a rectal rather than an anal internal opening.

Caspar Bartholin, Secundus, 1655–1709, Professor of Medicine, Anatomy and Physics, Copenhagen, Denmark, described these glands in 1677.
William Cowper, 1666–1709, London surgeon, described these glands in 1697.
Roger Hew Grace, formerly Professor of Colorectal Surgery, The Royal Wolverhampton Hospital, Wolverhampton, UK.

Classification

The most widespread and useful classification of anal fistulae is that proposed by Parks, based on the centrality of intersphincteric anal gland sepsis (the internal opening is usually at the dentate line), which results in a primary track whose relation to the external sphincter defines the type of fistula and which influences management (Figure 73.40). Classifications based simply on level are less practical because they mean different things to different people, although the description of a fistula as high, indicating a high risk of incontinence if laid open, or low, with a lower but still some risk to function, is often used. Similarly, 'simple' and 'complex' are commonly used adjectives – complexity may be endowed by the level at which the primary track crosses the sphincters, the presence of secondary extensions or the difficulties faced in treatment. The vast majority of fistulae are intersphincteric or trans-sphincteric.

Intersphincteric fistulae (45 per cent) do not cross the external sphincter (bar, for the purist, the most medial subcutaneous fibres running below the distal border of the internal sphincter); most commonly they run directly from the internal to the external openings across the distal internal sphincter, but may extend proximally in the intersphincteric plane to end blindly with or without an abscess, or enter the rectum at a second internal opening.

Trans-sphincteric fistulae (40 per cent) have a primary track that crosses both internal and external sphincters (the latter at a variable level) and which then passes through the ischiorectal fossa to reach the skin of the buttock. The primary track may have secondary tracks arising from it, which often reach the roof of the ischiorectal fossa, which may rarely pass through the levators to reach the pelvis and which may spread circumferentially (horseshoe). Circumferential spread of sepsis may occur in the intersphincteric and pararectal planes, as well as in the ischiorectal plane.

Suprasphincteric fistulae are very rare, are thought by some to be iatrogenic and are difficult to distinguish from high-level trans-sphincteric tracks (for which, fortunately, management strategies are similar). Extrasphincteric fistulae run without specific relation to the sphincters and usually result from pelvic disease or trauma.

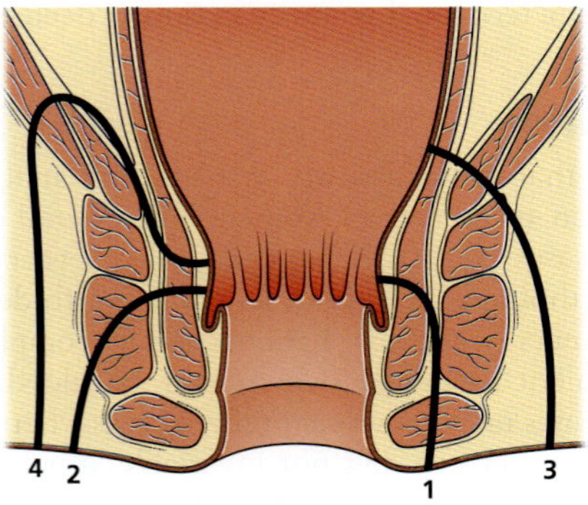

Figure 73.40 Types of anal fistula (Parks' classification): 1, intersphincteric; 2, trans-sphincteric; 3, suprasphincteric; and 4, extrasphincteric primary tracks.

Clinical assessment

A full medical (including obstetric, gastrointestinal, anal surgical and continence) history and proctosigmoidoscopy are necessary to gain information about sphincter strength and to exclude associated conditions. The key points to determine are the site of the internal opening; the site of the external opening(s); the course of the primary track; the presence of secondary extensions; and the presence of other conditions complicating the fistula. Palpable induration between external opening and anal margin suggests a relatively superficial track, whereas supralevator induration suggests a primary track above the levators or high in the roof of the ischiorectal fossa, or a high secondary extension. Intersphincteric fistulae usually have an external opening close to the anal verge. Goodsall's rule (Figure 73.41), used to indicate the likely position of the internal opening according to the position of the external opening(s), is helpful but not infallible. The site of the internal opening may be felt as a point of induration or seen as an enlarged papilla. Probing in an awake patient is painful, unhelpful and can be dangerous. Full examination under anaesthesia should be repeated before surgical intervention. Dilute hydrogen peroxide, instilled via the external opening, is a very useful way of demonstrating the site of the internal opening; gentle use of probes (Figure 73.42) and a finger in the anorectum usually delineates primary and secondary tracks and their relations to the sphincters. Any concerns about fistula topography at clinical examination or examination under anaesthesia (more common after previous unsuccessful surgery) should prompt further investigations before surgical intervention.

Special investigations

A successful outcome after fistula surgery requires an accurate assessment of the fistula itself, the sphincter through which it passes and patient expectations (especially in terms of risk to continence). Clinical examination will give some indication

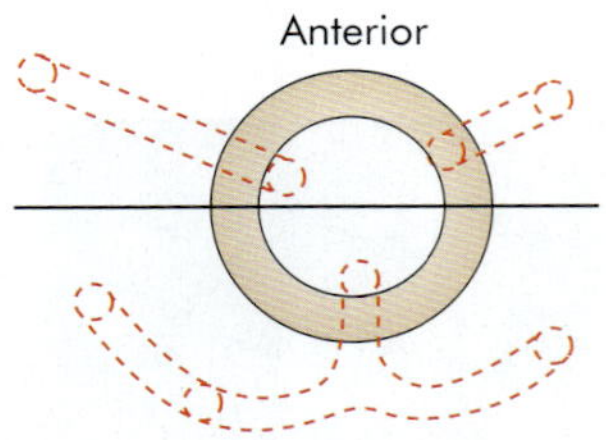

Figure 73.41 Goodsall's rule.

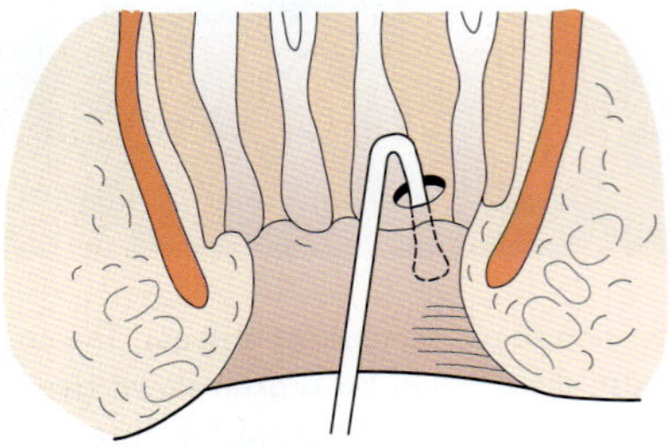

Figure 73.42 Retrograde probing of an anal canal sometimes reveals the internal orifice of the fistula.

David Henry Goodsall, 1843–1906, surgeon, St Mark's Hospital, London, UK.

of functional anal sphincter length, resting tone and voluntary squeeze; these may be more objectively assessed by manometry, whereas endoanal ultrasound gives useful information about sphincter integrity – the knowledge so gained may well influence surgical strategy. Endoanal ultrasound, especially with hydrogen peroxide, can also be used to delineate fistulae, although definition of sepsis outside or above the sphincters is limited by the probe's focal range and scarring makes interpretation difficult. Nonetheless, ultrasound, which is more accurate than clinical examination, is useful to determine whether a fistula is relatively straightforward or not. Magnetic resonance imaging (MRI) is acknowledged to be the 'gold standard' for fistula imaging, but it is limited by availability and cost and is usually reserved for difficult recurrent cases. The great advantage of MRI is its ability to demonstrate secondary extensions, which may be missed at surgery and which are the cause of persistence (Figure 73.43). Fistulography and computed tomography (CT) both have limitations but are useful techniques if an extrasphincteric fistula is suspected.

Surgical management

Patients with minimal symptoms, especially if they have compromised sphincters, may be managed expectantly. Eradication of sepsis requires surgery, the aim of which must be balanced with the preservation of continence. Most fistulae are relatively straightforward to deal with; however, a minority are extremely problematic and are not the realm of the 'occasional proctologist'. The multitude of strategies advocated attests to these difficult situations; comparisons between techniques are difficult to make because of the heterogeneity of patient groups, the variability in classification, the inapplicability of certain techniques in some situations, inadequate reporting of functional outcomes, inadequate follow up and surgeon preference over-riding entry into prospective randomised trials.

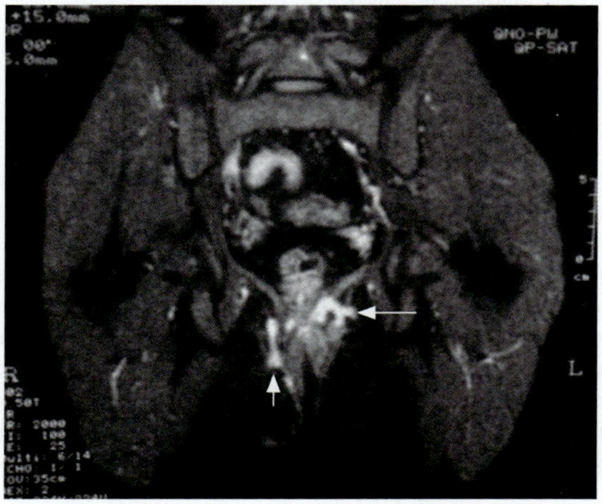

Figure 73.43 Coronal magnetic resonance imaging (MRI) scan (STIR sequence) demonstrating a primary track running up the right ischiorectal space (short white arrow), which then crosses the sphincters to open into the anal canal just below the puborectalis. However, there is a blind secondary extension (long white arrow) passing to the contralateral side in the roof of the left ischiorectal fossa (and involving the levators), which was missed at surgery and which was the cause of fistula persistence.

Fistulotomy

That the fistulous track must be laid open from its termination to its source was a rule promulgated by John of Arderne more than 600 years ago. Fistulotomy, or laying open, is the surest way of getting rid of a fistula, but, by definition, it involves division of all those structures lying between the external and internal openings. It is therefore applied mainly to intersphincteric fistulae and trans-sphincteric fistulae involving less than 30 per cent of the voluntary musculature (but not anteriorly placed fistulae in women); however, even then, it is not immune to postoperative defects in continence. After full examination under anaesthesia in the lithotomy or prone jack-knife position, during which the internal opening should have been identified, a grooved fistula probe is passed from the external to the internal opening (Figure 73.44), the amount of sphincter below and above the probe is noted and, if indicated, the track is laid open over the probe. Granulation tissue is curetted and sent for histological appraisal and the wound edges are trimmed. Secondary tracks, often identified as granulation tissue that persists despite curettage, should be laid open or drained. Marsupialisation reduces wound size and speeds up healing. Primary tracks crossing the external sphincter more deeply have been managed with good outcomes by fistulotomy and immediate reconstitution of the divided muscle – failure to eradicate all sepsis and subsequent breakdown of the repair, however, are very problematic. Alternatively, a staged fistulotomy may be carried out in which secondary tracks are laid open and only part of the sphincter enclosed by the primary track is divided, with the remainder encircled by a loose seton. After sufficient time for healing of the wound and fibrosis, the seton-enclosed track is divided at a second stage.

Fistulectomy

This technique involves coring out of the fistula, usually by diathermy cautery; it allows better definition of fistula anatomy than fistulotomy, especially the level at which the track crosses the sphincters and the presence of secondary extensions. If the sphincteric component of the fistula is deemed low enough to allow safe fistulotomy, then this may proceed (at the expense of longer healing times than conventional fistulotomy). If laying open is not advisable, then the sphincteric component can be managed by another method.

Setons

Setons (Latin: *seta*, bristle) have been used in a variety of ways in fistula surgery and it is important for surgeons to be clear about what they are trying to achieve in a particular situation. Loose setons are tied such that there is no tension upon the encircled tissue; there is no intent to cut the tissue. A variety of materials have been used, but the seton should be non-absorbable, non-degenerative and comfortable. Tight or cutting setons are placed with the intention of cutting through the enclosed muscle.

John of Arderne, 1307–1390, was the first English surgeon of note. He practised at Newark-upon-Trent, Nottinghamshire and, from 1370, in London, UK. He described his operation for the treatment of fistula in about 1376.

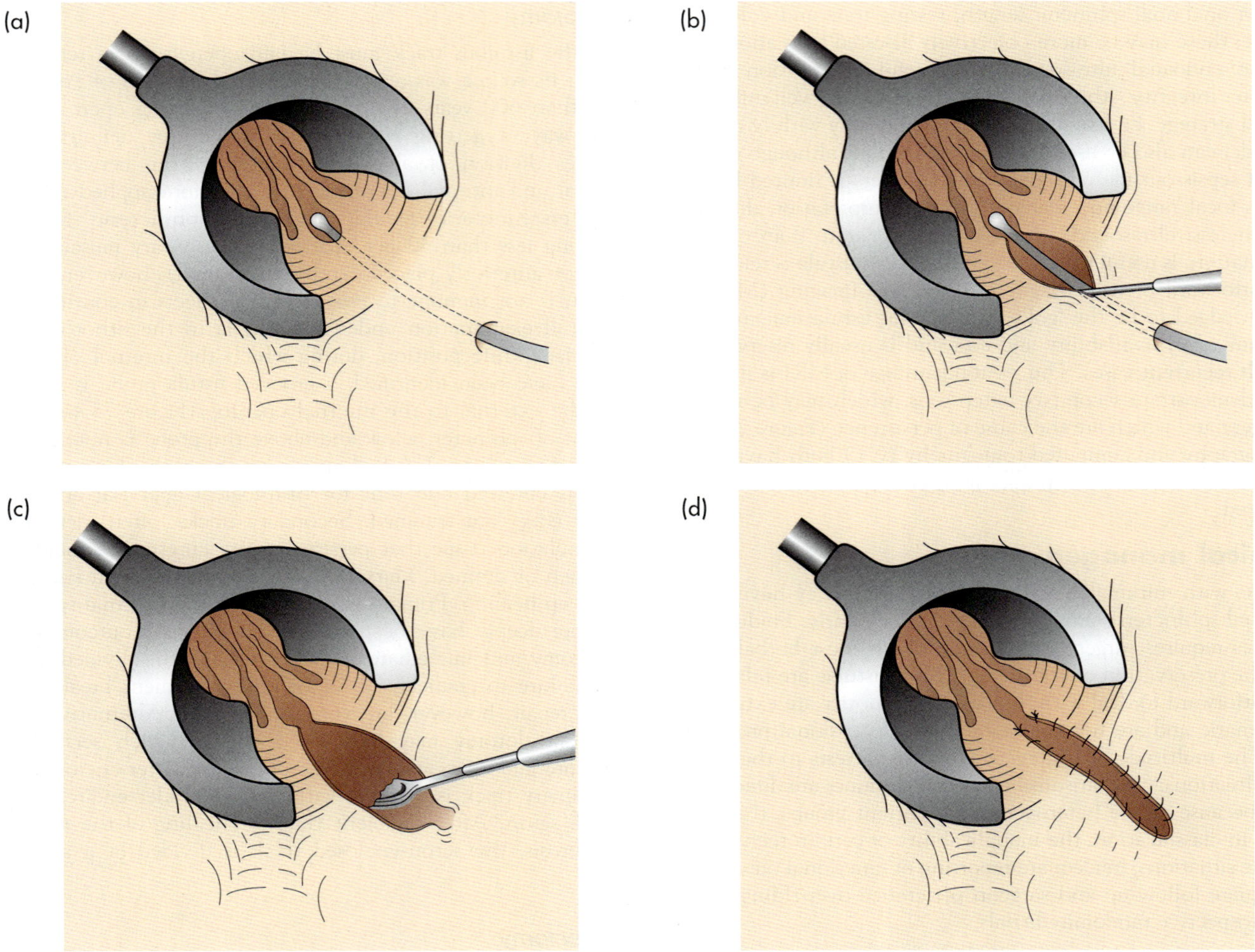

Figure 73.44 Fistulotomy. A grooved probe is passed from the external to internal openings (a) and the track laid open over the probe (b). The track is curetted to remove granulation tissue (c), the edges of the wound are trimmed and the wound may then be marsupialised (d). Reproduced with permission from Nicholls RJ, Dozois RR. *Surgery of the colon and rectum*. Edinburgh: Churchill Livingstone, 1997.

Uses of loose setons

- For long-term palliation to avoid septic and painful exacerbations by establishing effective drainage; most often in Crohn's disease and in those with problematic fistulae not wishing to countenance the possibility of incontinence.
- Used before 'advanced' techniques (fistulectomy, advancement flap, cutting seton); acute sepsis and secondary extensions are eradicated and a loose seton is passed across the sphincteric component of the primary track to simplify the fistula and allow fibrosis.
- As part of a staged fistulotomy.
- As part of a therapeutic strategy to preserve the external sphincter in trans-sphincteric fistulae. Secondary tracks in the ischiorectal fossa are laid open. Access to the site where the primary track crosses the external sphincter may sometimes necessitate division of the anococcygeal ligaments to reach the deep post-anal space. The internal sphincter is laid open to the level of the internal opening (or higher if there is a cephalad intersphincteric extension) to eradicate the presumed source and the sepsis in the intersphincteric space. A seton is then passed along the residual track around the denuded external sphincter and tied loosely, and the wounds are dressed. Initial postoperative management includes daily wound irrigation and light wound redressing. The seton is left in place for three months and, if there is evidence of good healing, simply removed. Such a strategy certainly protects against the consequences of external sphincter division, with an incidence of healing in the short term of 50–60 per cent.

Uses of cutting setons

Cutting setons aim to achieve the high fistula eradication rates associated with fistulotomy, but without the degree of functional impairment endowed by division of the sphincters at a single stage. The enclosed muscle is gradually severed ('cheese wiring through ice') such that the divided muscles do not spring apart, and the site of the fistula track is replaced by a thin line of fibrosis as it is brought down. Some recommend prior internal sphincter division, others incorporation of the internal sphincter within the cutting seton. A variety of seton material has been used, either elastic and 'self-cutting' or non-elastic and tightened at intervals, with the sphincter being divided at varying speeds. In eastern parts of the world, the same aim has been achieved by chemical cautery using an Ayurvedic method, known in India as Kshara sutra, in which a specially prepared seton thread burns through the enclosed tissue. This outpatient method has been shown to be equivalent to one-stage fistulotomy in patients with intersphincteric and distal trans-sphincteric fistulae.

Advancement flaps

When the sphincter complex is not too indurated and adequate intra-anal access can be obtained, the advancement flap technique can be employed, which aims to preserve both anatomy and function. The principles are prior elimination of acute sepsis and secondary tracks, with ideally a direct track from internal to external openings; coring out of the entire track; and closure of the communication with the anal lumen with an adequately vascularised flap consisting of mucosa and internal sphincter, sutured without tension to the anoderm, well distant from the site of the (excised) internal opening. Modifications include flap orientation (proximally or distally based) and thickness (mucosal, partial or full-thickness internal sphincter), and treatment of the external wound.

Biological agents

The functional consequences of fistulotomy and the poorer eradication rates of sphincter-preserving techniques have led to a search for agents that essentially plug and seal the track and allow ingrowth of healthy tissue to replace it (Summary box 73.14). Intuitively, success must depend on the biomaterial itself and the environment into which it is placed. The poor long-term results of fibrin glue probably result from its relatively rapid resorption, and thus inadequate time for host tissue incorporation. The variable short-term results associated with porcine small intestinal submucosa may reflect early extrusion, premature degradation within an infected field, or the protocol advocated for its use which does not include meticulous eradication of secondary extensions, or the lining of the primary track itself, whether epithelial or granulation tissue. Cross-linked porcine dermal collagen has also, more recently, been studied, but only short-term outcomes (albeit optimistic) are known. Research into biological agents must continue.

Summary box 73.14

Anorectal fistulae

- Are common and may be simple or complex
- Are classified according to their relationship to the anal sphincters
- May be associated with underlying disease, such as tuberculosis or Crohn's disease
- Laying open is the surest method of eradication, but sphincter division may result in incontinence

HIDRADENITIS SUPPURATIVA

This is a chronic suppurative condition of apocrine gland-bearing skin, which is found in the axillae, submammary regions, nape of the neck, groin, mons pubis, inner thighs and sides of the scrotum, as well as the perineum and buttocks, and is a source of considerable physical and psychological morbidity. There is no confirmatory test or specific characteristic for diagnosis, which makes definition difficult. Acne, pilonidal sinus and chronic scalp folliculitis may coexist with hidradenitis suppurativa in the condition 'follicular occlusion tetrad'.

Pathology

Occlusion of gland ducts leads to bacterial proliferation, gland rupture and spread of infection and epithelial components into the surrounding soft tissue and to adjacent glands. Secondary infection (with *Staphylococcus aureus*, *Streptococcus milleri* and anaerobes) causes further local extension, skin damage and deformity, with multiple communicating subcutaneous fistulae. There is some evidence that the disease may be related to a relative androgen excess.

Presentation

The condition is not seen before puberty and rarely presents after the fourth decade of life. Overall, it is three times more common in women than men, although anogenital disease is more common in men, and obesity is a common association. When affecting the perineum, lesions begin as multiple raised boils, with recurrent lesions within the same vicinity leading to sinus tract formation, bridged scarring and multiple points of discharge. Rarely, it may involve the anal canal anoderm, but it does not extend above the dentate line or involve the sphincter muscles themselves.

Differential diagnosis

In the early stages, distinction from furunculosis can be difficult. Crohn's disease, cryptoglandular fistula, pilonidal sinus, tuberculosis, actinomycosis, lymphogranuloma venereum and granuloma inguinale must be considered when later stages present.

Treatment

In the early stages, general measures, including weight reduction and antiseptic soaps, may be helpful. Antibiotics may induce remission, but often the disease relapses and progresses, at which point surgery is indicated. Inadequate treatment may lead to prolonged morbidity but any surgery should be less debilitating than the condition. Surgical intervention ranges from simple incision and drainage of acute sepsis to radical excision of all apocrine gland-bearing skin. Careful laying open of all tracts, possibly as a staged procedure according to anatomical location, is an option that appeals to many patients. Radical excision requires closure by skin graft or rotation flap and, occasionally, a defunctioning colostomy to allow healing.

CONDYLOMATA ACCUMINATA (ANAL WARTS)

There is increasing evidence that sexually transmitted infection with human papillomavirus (HPV) forms the aetiological basis of anal and perianal warts, anal intraepithelial neoplasia (AIN) and squamous cell carcinoma of the anus. In those areas of the

The **Ayurvedic method** is derived from the Ayurveda, the most ancient system of Hindu medicine whose origin is ascribed to Brahma and dates from circa 1400 to 1200BC.

world where sexual promiscuity (especially anal intercourse) is more common, and in immunocompromised individuals (HIV-infected individuals and transplant recipients), there have been dramatic increases in the incidence of these conditions over the last 30 years, most importantly of AIN and anal cancers. Similar virally induced changes have been noted in the genital tracts of women (vulval intraepithelial neoplasia (VIN), cervical intraepithelial neoplasia (CIN) and cancers). There are over 80 subtypes of HPV but certain subtypes (16, 18, 31, 33) are associated with a greater risk of progression to dysplasia and malignancy.

Condylomata accuminata is the most common sexually transmitted disease encountered by colorectal surgeons and is most frequently observed in homosexual men. Associated warts on the penis and along the female genital tract are common.

Presentation

Many are asymptomatic but pruritus, discharge, bleeding and pain are usual presenting complaints. In the early stages, examination reveals separate pinkish-white warts close to the anal margin and also often on the anoderm within the distal anal canal. Later, the warts enlarge, coalesce and carpet the skin. Rarely, relentless growth results in giant condylomata (Buschke–Löwenstein tumour), which may obliterate the anal orifice. The diagnosis is aided by aceto-whitening upon application of acetic acid but confirmed by biopsy, which will also indicate the presence or absence of dysplasia.

Treatment

Because of the field effect endowed by viral skin infection, long-term resolution can be problematic. Careful serial application of 25 per cent podophyllin to discrete warts on the perianal skin is often used; however, it cannot be used intra-anally. Surgical excision under local, regional or general anaesthesia involves raising and separating the lesions with local infiltration of dilute adrenaline, which allows more accurate scissor or electrocautery excision to maximise the preservation of normal skin.

ANAL INTRAEPITHELIAL NEOPLASIA

Anal intraepithelial neoplasia (Figure 73.45) is a multifocal virally induced dysplasia of the perianal or intra-anal epidermis which is associated with the human papilloma virus (most frequently subtypes 6, 11, 16 and 18). The prevalence is <1 per cent of the population with a rising incidence especially in those areas where anoreceptive intercourse and HIV are prevalent. At-risk groups include patients with HIV, as well as immunocompromised patients, women with a history of other genital intraepithelial neoplasia (VIN and CIN) and patients with extensive anogenital condylomata. Patients may be asymptomatic and the diagnosis is often a histological surprise, although increasing numbers in high-risk groups are picked up on anal cytology. It is classified according to the degree of dysplasia on biopsy into AIN I, AIN II and AIN III, according to the lack of keratocyte maturation and extension of the proliferative zone from the lower third (AIN I) to the full thickness of the epithelium (AIN III), in the same manner as cervical or vulval dysplasia. The natural history is uncertain, but progression from AIN II to AIN III to invasive carcinoma has been observed, notably in the immunocompromised. The term Bowen's disease should probably be avoided.

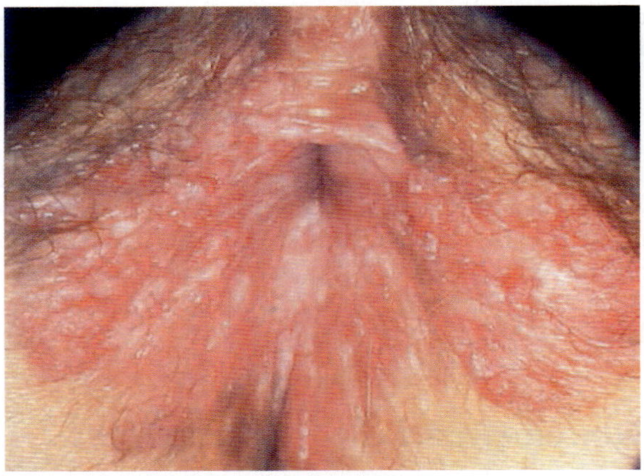

Figure 73.45 Extensive anal intraepithelial neoplasia (AIN), which extends intra-anally.

Presentation

Around 10 per cent of AIN lesions are diagnosed by the pathologist after excision of abnormal skin lesions. Low-grade lesions may be raised and similar to anal condylomata; however, AIN III lesions are more often flat and may be white, grey, purple or brown in colour. Ulceration would suggest progression to invasive anal carcinoma. Patients' symptoms include pruritis, pain, bleeding and discharge. AIN is present in 28–35 per cent of excised anal warts. Approximately 10 per cent of AIN III lesions will progress to anal carcinoma at five years. Regression of AIN III rarely occurs, but AIN I and AIN II may regress. The association between AIN III and carcinoma is strengthened by the findings of AIN III in 80 per cent of anal cancer biopsies.

Diagnosis and management

A high index of suspicion and targeted biopsy yields the diagnosis, whereas multiple (mapping) biopsies give an indication of the extent and overall severity of the disease. AIN II and III should be regularly monitored clinically and, if necessary, by repeat biopsy to exclude invasive disease. Specialised centres may offer colposcopy of the anus (anoscopy) utilising 5 per cent acetic acid with Lugol's iodine to assess *in vivo* the dysplastic areas of the anus. The affected areas show up white and can be biopsied. Focal disease may be excised and local excision is effective for lesions <30 per cent of the circumference of the anus. More widespread disease can be dealt with surgically by wide local excision and closure of the resultant defect by flap or skin graft, with or without covering colostomy (especially if there is intra-anal disease). However, for a condition with uncertain malignant potential, this approach should be used with caution as it carries with it significant morbidity. It is important to remember that female patients are at risk of other anogenital intraepithelial neoplasia; it is recommended that those with AIN III have a yearly cervical smear test.

Topical imiquimod, 5 per cent, or oral retinoids have some effect on the progression of dysplasia and can cause regression by at least two histological grades. Other newer options may include anti-human papilloma virus treatment and vaccination may reduce the incidence long term.

Abraham Buschke, 1868–1943, a German dermatologist.
LW Löwenstein described this condition in 1939.
John Templeton Bowen, 1857–1941, Professor of Dermatology, Harvard University Medical School, Boston, MA, USA, described this intradermal precancerous skin lesion in 1912.

NON-MALIGNANT STRICTURES – ANAL STENOSIS

Spasmodic

An anal fissure causes spasm of the internal sphincter. Rarely, a spasmodic stricture accompanies secondary megacolon, possibly as a result of the chronic use of laxatives.

Organic

Anal stenosis is a rare but serious complication of anorectal surgery, 90 per cent are seen after haemorrhoidectomy. Other causes include trauma, inflammatory bowel disease, radiation treatment, sexually transmitted disease, tuberculosis and some skin conditions, e.g scleroderma.

Postoperative stricture

This sometimes follows a haemorrhoidectomy performed incorrectly. Removal of excess anoderm and mucosa without adequate skin bridges can lead to scarring and structuring. Stenosis can be seen after stapled haemorrhoidopexy (0.8–5 per cent) and low coloanal anastomoses, especially if a stapling gun is used, but these are really low rectal stenoses.

Irradiation stricture

This is an aftermath of irradiation and is particularly seen after chemoradiation for anal carcinoma when a wide area of skin and anoderm are irradiated. It can be seen after irradiation for any pelvic tumours.

Senile anal stenosis

A condition of chronic internal sphincter contraction is sometimes seen in the elderly. Increasing constipation is present, with pronounced straining at stool. Faecal impaction is liable to occur. The muscle is rigid and feels like a tight rubber ring. There is no evidence of a fissure-*in-ano*. The treatment is dilatation at frequent intervals.

Lymphogranuloma inguinale

Lymphogranuloma inguinale (see Chapter 72) is by far the most frequent cause of a tubular inflammatory stricture of the rectum and 80 per cent of the sufferers are women. Frei's reaction is usually positive. This variety of rectal stricture is particularly common in black populations and may be accompanied by elephantiasis of the labia majora. In the early stages, antibiotic treatment may lead to cure. In advanced cases, excision of the rectum is required.

Inflammatory bowel disease

Stricture of the anorectum may complicate Crohn's disease and, in this instance, the stricture is annular and often more than one is present. These stenoses are characterised by transmural scarring and inflammation. Occasionally, an anal stricture may occur in ulcerative colitis. Until a biopsy is obtained, a carcinoma should be suspected if a stricture is found.

> **Wilhelm Sigmund Frei**, 1885–1943, Professor of Dermatology, the State Hospital, Spandau, Berlin, who later settled in New York, NY, USA, described his test for lymphogranuloma inguinale in 1925.
> **George Grey Turner**, 1877–1951, Professor of Surgery, The University of Durham (1927–1934) and at The Royal Postgraduate Medical School, Hammersmith Hospital, London, UK (1935–1946). The surgical club Grey Turner Surgical Club was named after him. It is said that he dressed shabbily so that when his friends met him they used to ask him to 'mend the clock'. He had a habit of keeping his cup of tea warm by covering it with his bowler hat!

Endometriosis

Endometriosis of the rectovaginal septum may present as a stricture. There is usually a history of frequent menstrual periods with severe pain during the first 2 days of the menstrual flow.

Neoplastic

When free bleeding occurs after dilatation of a supposed inflammatory stricture, carcinoma should be suspected (Grey Turner) and a portion of the stricture should be removed for biopsy. Sometimes in these cases, repeated biopsies show inflammatory tissue only. If, however, the symptoms show a marked progression, malignancy should be strongly suspected.

Clinical features

Increasing difficulty in defaecation is the leading symptom. The patient finds that increasingly large doses of aperients are required and, if the stools are formed, they are 'pipe-stem' in shape. In cases of inflammatory stricture, tenesmus, bleeding and the passage of mucus are superadded. Sometimes the patient comes under observation only when subacute or acute intestinal obstruction has supervened.

Rectal examination

The finger encounters a sharply defined shelf-like interruption of the lumen. If the calibre is large enough to admit the finger, it should be noted whether the stricture is annular or tubular. Sometimes this point can be determined only after dilatation. A biopsy of the stricture must be taken. Often the examination will be painful and needs to be performed under general anaesthesia when biopsies and gentle, graduated dilatation may be undertaken.

Treatment

Before starting treatment, it is important to ascertain the cause of the stricture. If associated with Crohn's disease, an anoplasty is contraindicated. Non-operative treatment is recommended for mild stenosis. The use of stool softeners and fibre supplements helps aid the passage of stools.

Prophylactic

The passage of an anal dilator during convalescence after haemorrhoidectomy greatly reduces the incidence of postoperative stricture. Efficient treatment of lymphogranuloma inguinale in its early stages should lessen the frequency of stricture from that cause.

Dilatation

Anal dilatation can be performed under general anaesthesia and then, by the patient, using an anal dilator. For anal and many rectal strictures, dilatation at regular intervals is all that is required.

Anoplasty

For severe anal stenosis, an anoplasty is used to replace loss of anal tissue. The stricture is incised and a rotation or advancement flap of skin and subcutaneous tissue replaces the defect and enlarges the anal orifice (Figure 73.46). This technique is particularly useful for postoperative strictures.

Colostomy

Colostomy must be undertaken when a stricture is causing intestinal obstruction and in advanced cases of stricture complicated by fistulae-*in-ano*. In selected cases, this can be followed by restorative resection of the stricture-bearing area. If this step is anticipated, a loop ileostomy is constructed.

Rectal excision and coloanal anastomosis

When the strictures are at or just above the anorectal junction and are associated with a normal anal canal, but irreversible changes necessitate removal of the area, excision can be followed by a coloanal anastomosis with good functional results (Summary box 73.15).

Summary box 73.15

Benign anal stricture

- May be spasmodic or organic
- May be iatrogenic, e.g. after haemorrhoidectomy or repair of imperforate anus
- Biopsy must be taken to rule out malignancy
- Can usually be managed by regular dilatation
- Severe anal stenosis may require an anoplasty

MALIGNANT TUMOURS

Malignant lesions of the anus and anal canal

Anal malignancy is rare and accounts for less than 2 per cent of all large bowel cancers. The crude incidence rate is 0.65 per 100 000. Those arising below the dentate line are usually squamous, whereas those above are variously termed basaloid, cloacogenic or transitional. Collectively, they are known as epidermoid carcinomas, and management and prognosis is similar for this group, which accounts for >70 per cent of anal malignancies. Adenocarcinomas are the next most common. Other tumours include melanoma, lymphoma and sarcoma.

Squamous cell carcinoma

Although rare, the incidence of anal squamous cell carcinoma (SCC) is rising, with a direct association with HPV infection, AIN and immunosuppression. Anal SCC is associated with HPV (especially subtypes 16, 18, 31 or 33) in 70–90 per cent of cases (Figure 73.47). Patients at increased risk are those with HIV infection, recipients of organ transplants (renal transplant patients have a 100-fold increased risk) and those with a past history of cancers at 'sexually accessible' sites (usually genital). Pain and bleeding are the most common symptoms and the disease is thus often initially misdiagnosed as a benign condition, highlighting the need for a level of suspicion and adequate examination. A mass, pruritus or discharge is less common. Advanced tumours may cause faecal incontinence by invasion of the sphincters and, in women, anterior extension may result in anovaginal fistulation. On examination, anal margin tumours look like malignant ulcers. There may be associated HPV lesions. Anal canal tumours are palpable as irregular indurated tender ulceration. Sphincter involvement may be evident.

Management

Historically, early anal margin tumours were treated by local excision and anal canal tumours by abdominoperineal excision of the rectum. Nowadays, primary treatment is by chemoradiotherapy (combined modality therapy (CMT)) (Nigro), the chemotherapy usually including a combination of 5-fluorouracil (5-FU) with mitomycin C or cisplatin. Metastases are rare at presentation (5 per cent) and treatment is aimed at local control. Initial staging involves a clinical examination and biopsy of the primary tumour, as well as examination of inguinal nodes. Local staging is by MRI scanning and CT is used to assess lungs and abdomen for metastatic spread. Positron emission tomography (PET) CT may help in equivocal inguinal node assessment. The surgeon has an important role in management: initial diagnosis is surgical; small marginal tumours are still best treated by local excision; radical surgery is indicated in those with persistent or recurrent disease following CMT; and a defunctioning stoma may be indicated for those in whom treatment and disease regression is associated with radionecrosis, incontinence or fistula. Despite good results with chemoradiotherapy 20–25 per cent of patients will have local disease relapse. After thorough assessment, these patients may require radical abdominoperineal resection, including excision of the posterior wall of the vagina in 70 per cent of women and reconstruction of the perineum using myocutaneous flaps.

Other anal malignancies

Adenocarcinomata within the anal canal are usually extensions of distal rectal cancers. Rarely, adenocarcinoma may arise from anal glandular epithelium or develop within a longstanding

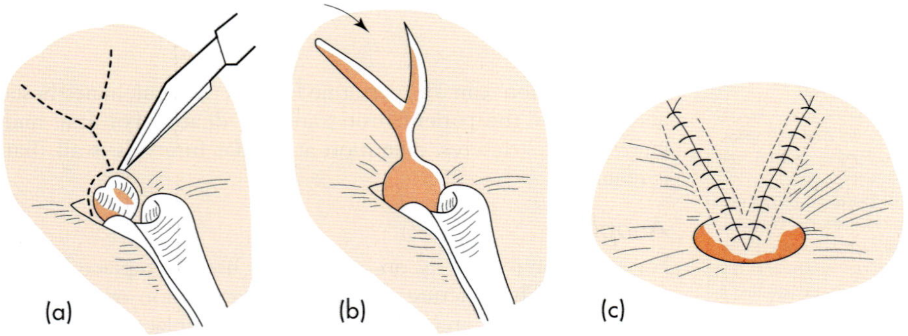

Figure 73.46 (a–c) Y–V advancement flap for anal stenosis.

N Nigro, surgeon, Wayne State University, Detroit, MI, USA.

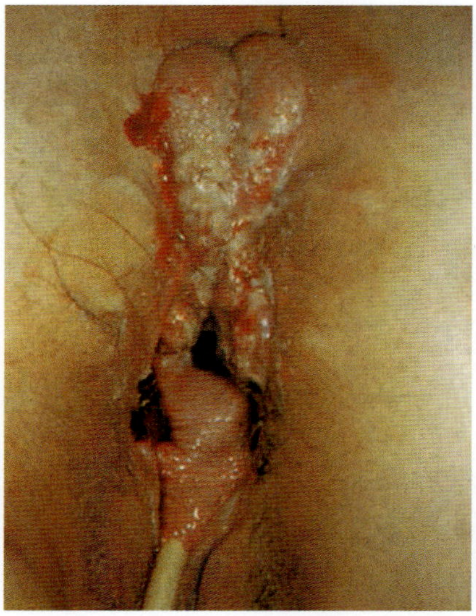

Figure 73.47 Neglected papillomas of the anus that have become malignant.

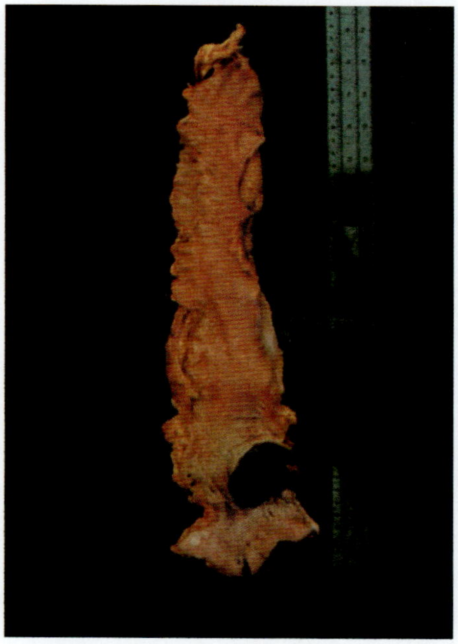

Figure 73.48 Malignant melanoma of the anal canal (courtesy of Mr B Thomas, Kalushi, Zambia).

(usually complex) anal fistula; treatment is as for low rectal cancers (i.e. abdominoperineal excision of the rectum (APER) with or without previous radiotherapy or chemoradiotherapy), but prognosis is less good. Melanocytes can be found in the transitional zone of the anal canal. Malignant melanoma of the anus is very rare and usually presents as a bluish-black soft mass that may mimic a thrombosed external pile, although it may be amelanotic (Figure 73.48). The prognosis, irrespective of treatment, is extremely poor. Perianal Paget's disease is exceedingly rare (Summary box 73.16).

Summary box 73.16

Anal cancer

- Uncommon tumour, which is usually a squamous cell carcinoma
- Associated with human papilloma virus (HPV)
- More prevalent in patients with HIV infection
- May affect the anal verge or anal canal
- Lymphatic spread is to the inguinal lymph nodes
- Treatment is by chemoradiotherapy in the first instance
- Major ablative surgery is required if the above fails

FURTHER READING

Fielding LP, Goldberg S (eds). *Rob and Smith's operative surgery: surgery of the colon, rectum and anus*, 2nd edn. London: Chapman & Hall, 1999.

Keighley MRB, Williams NS. *Surgery of the anus, rectum and colon*, 3rd edn. London: WB Saunders, 2008.

Sir James Paget, 1814–1899, surgeon, St Bartholomew's Hospital, London, UK, described this disease in 1874

PART

12 Genitourinary

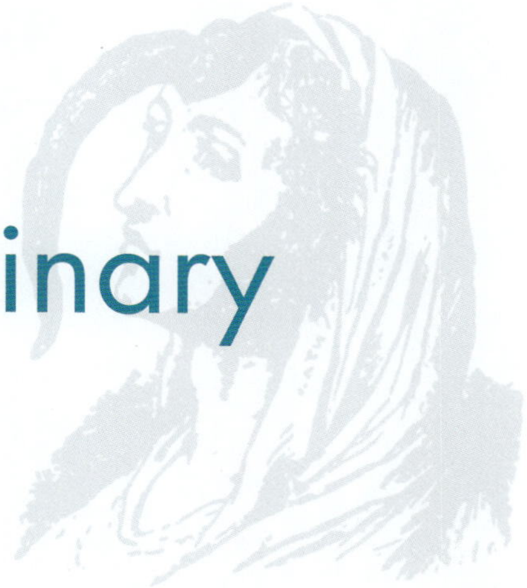

CHAPTER 74

Urinary symptoms and investigations

LEARNING OBJECTIVES

To recognise and understand:

- The major symptoms of urological disease
- The most common urological investigations

URINARY SYMPTOMS

Haematuria

Blood in the urine (haematuria) may be the only indication of cancer and other pathology in the urinary tract (Figure 74.1). Microscopic haematuria may be detected by dipstick testing in a routine health check. A substantial haemorrhage imparts a red or brownish tinge to the urine (macroscopic haematuria) and the patient may pass clots. False-positive stick tests and the discoloured urine caused by beetroot and some drugs (e.g. Dindevan (phenindione), Pyridium (phenazopyridine) and Furadantin (nitrofurantoin)) are distinguishable by the absence of red blood cells on urinary microscopy.

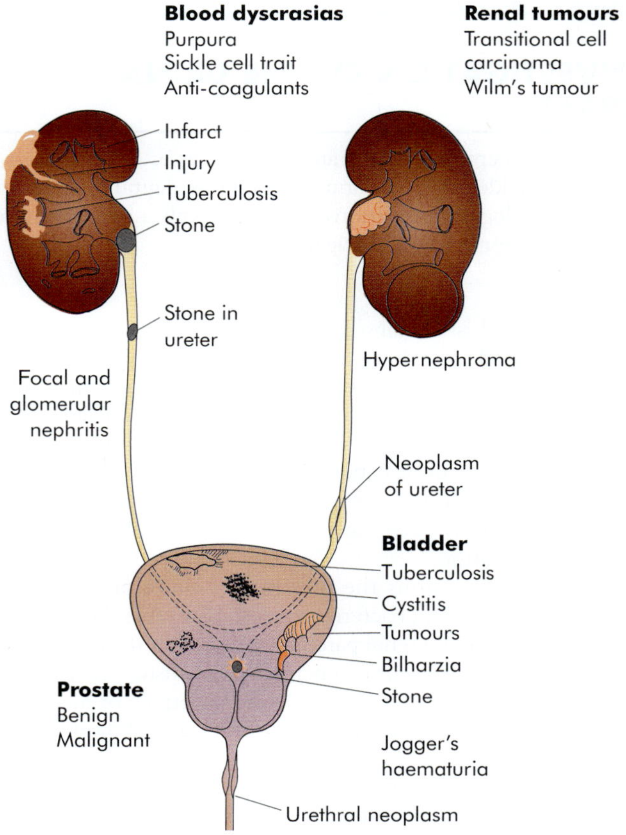

Figure 74.1 The more common causes of haematuria.

Haematuria may be intermittent or persistent. If the patient experiences pain with haematuria, the characteristics of the pain may help to identify the source of the bleeding. If there is a malignant cause for the haematuria, there is usually no pain.

In practice, all patients with haematuria should be investigated even if they are taking anticoagulant drugs. In many, all tests will be negative: the chance of finding a urological cause in patients under 40 years of age with microscopic haematuria is small. However, bleeding into the urinary tract may be caused by an occult nephropathy so it is important to check for significant proteinuria and hypertension in these patients (Summary box 74.1).

Pain

Renal pain

A deep-seated, sickening ache in the loin characterises acute upper urinary tract inflammation or obstruction, probably as the result of stretching of the capsule of the kidney. Even small and peripheral kidney stones may cause pain, even in the absence of infection. Large slow-growing masses such as tumours or cysts

Summary box 74.1

Haematuria

- Is always abnormal whether microscopic or macroscopic
- May be caused by a lesion anywhere in the urinary tract
- Is investigated by:
  - examination of midstream specimen for infection
  - cytological examination of a urine specimen
  - intravenous urogram and/or urinary tract ultrasound scan
  - flexible or rigid cystoscopy
- Is commonly caused by urinary infection, especially in young women

Summary box 74.2

Pain from the upper urinary tract

- Pain of acute obstruction of the renal pelvis is typically deep in the loin and 'bursting' in character
- Ureteric colic (usually due to stone) is characterised by sharp exacerbations against a constant background
- Pain is referred to the groin, scrotum or labium as calculus obstruction moves distally in the ureter

Summary box 74.3

Pain from the lower urinary tract

- Is commonly felt as subrapubic discomfort, worsening as the bladder fills
- Cystitis causes burning or scalding urethral pain (dysuria)
- May be referred to the tip of the penis in men, even when lesion is in the bladder

are commonly painless. When the cause is inflammatory, there may be local deep tenderness and occasionally reflex spasm of the psoas muscle and involuntary flexion of the hip joint.

Ureteric colic

This is an acute pain felt in the loin and radiating to the ipsilateral iliac fossa and genitalia. The patient often rolls around in agony as waves of excruciating pain are imposed upon a continuing background of discomfort. Contrast this with the patient suffering from peritoneal pain, who lies still because movement hurts.

Blood clot or a sloughed renal papilla may give identical pain. The site of the pain is a partial guide to the progress of a stone: the more the pain radiates into the groin, the more distal the stone. Local tenderness is much less than would be expected from the severity of the pain (Summary box 74.2).

Bladder pain

Bladder pain is a suprapubic discomfort worsened by bladder filling. In men, a sharp pain misleadingly referred to the tip of the penis may be the result of irritation of the bladder trigone. Severe inflammation of the bladder can cause strangury, an extreme wrenching discomfort at the end of micturition.

Perineal pain

This is experienced as a penetrating ache in the perineum and rectum, sometimes with associated inguinal discomfort. The patient is characteristically depressed by the relentless pain. Pelvic pain is often blamed on 'chronic prostatitis', 'prostadynia' or 'chronic prostate pain syndrome', but it occurs in both men and women. It is notoriously difficult to treat, a characteristic shared with various chronic scrotal pain syndromes.

Urethral pain

Urethral pain is a scalding or burning felt in the vulva or penis, especially during voiding (Summary box 74.3).

Altered bladder function

The normal bladder has two phases of function. During the filling phase, the bladder acts as a reservoir to collect urine until it is emptied in the voiding phase. Inappropriate contraction of the bladder detrusor muscle during filling (instability) is perceived as a sensation of urgency. There may be frequent micturition with or without urge incontinence. Sleep may be disturbed by nocturia. Instability may be idiopathic in both sexes or part of the bladder response to outflow obstruction, notably in prostatic disease. When detrusor instability has a demonstrable neurological cause, it is known as hyperreflexia.

Symptoms of impaired emptying are most commonly the result of bladder outflow obstruction, but detrusor failure presents a similar picture. The patient has difficulty initiating voiding (hesitancy) and the stream is variable or slow. Abdominal straining improves the weak flow. When micturition is complete, the bladder may still feel full. With time, the bladder becomes chronically overfilled. Urine spills out, typically at night when sleep halts trips to the lavatory (chronic retention with overflow) (Summary box 74.4).

Summary box 74.4

Altered bladder function

- Failure bladder storage function leads to urgency and frequency of micturition, often by day and by night
- Failure of bladder emptying function is most commonly caused by obstruction to the bladder outflow (e.g. by prostatic enlargement) but can also be caused by weakness of the detrusor muscle
- Chronic retention of urine may present as nocturnal bedwetting

INVESTIGATION OF THE URINARY TRACT

With the exception of renal and scrotal masses or tenderness, a palpable bladder or an abnormal prostate on digital rectal examination, urological conditions are most likely to be diagnosed from the history or by investigations.

Urine

Dipsticks (Multistix, Labstix) are a convenient way to screen urine for blood, protein or nitrites. When the urine is macroscopically clear and negative on dipstick testing, microscopy and culture of a midstream clean-catch specimen are usually negative. The presence of protein and nitrites (produced by organisms in the urine) indicates the likelihood of infection. The significance of microscopic haematuria is discussed above. Some dipsticks also give an indication of the pH and specific gravity of the urine.

Microscopy confirms the presence of white and red blood cells in the urine, and bacteria may also be visible. Protein casts suggest disease of the renal parenchyma, as does red cell dysmorphia seen on phase contrast microscopy. Schistosoma ova have a typical appearance (Figure 74.2), and vegetable or meat fibres may be present if there is a fistula connecting the bowel with the urinary tract.

Cytological examination of the urinary sediment is sensitive and specific for poorly differentiated transitional cell tumours anywhere in the urinary tract. However, false negatives are common when the cancer is well differentiated. A chemical test

pis-en-deux is French to urinate twice.

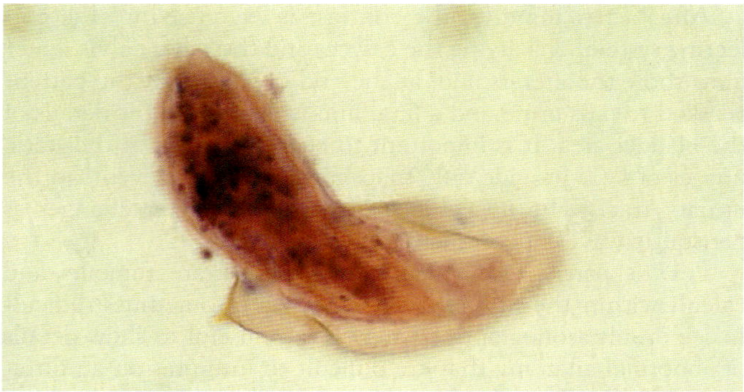

Figure 74.2 Schistosoma ovum (courtesy of Dr Nawal Derius).

(BTA-Bard) for bladder tumour antigen in the urine can complement cytological examination.

Bacteriological culture of a clean-catch midstream specimen of the urine is the standard means of identifying urinary pathogens. Organisms at a level of >10^5/mL is deemed to indicate the presence of infection rather than contamination of the urine by bacteria. If there are pus cells in the urine but there is no growth on the routine culture media (sterile pyuria), it is worth testing for more fastidious organisms. The centrifuged sediment of multiple early-morning urine specimens are cultured on Löwenstein–Jensen medium to detect urinary tract tuberculosis. Chlamydia is another common urinary pathogen that will not be detected on routine culture.

Biochemical examination for electrolytes, glucose, bilirubin, haemoglobin and myoglobin is essential to detect abnormal amounts of these substances in the urine. Analysis of a 24-hour specimen of urine will quantify the rate of loss, and is especially useful in the investigation of calculus disease caused by abnormal excretion of calcium, oxalate, uric acid and other products of metabolism (Summary box 74.5).

Summary box 74.5

Microscopic, cytological, bacteriological and biochemical examination of urine

- Abnormalities found on Multistik testing of the urine should be confirmed by microscopy and culture
- More than 10^5 organisms per mL of urine is deemed to indicate a significant urinary infection
- Cytological examination of the urine will usually detect a poorly differentiated transitional cell tumour

Tests of renal function

More than 70 per cent of kidney function must be lost before renal failure becomes evident: there is a large functional reserve. It follows that renal damage must be extensive before changes occur in blood constituents whose level is controlled by renal excretion. Such damage is of three main types: reduction of renal plasma flow, destruction of glomeruli and impairment of tubular function. In severe hypertension or renal artery stenosis, the plasma flow is impaired. In glomerulonephritis or acute cortical necrosis, there is a loss of glomeruli, whereas in pyelonephritis, tubular function is most severely affected. In obstructive nephropathy, back pressure on the renal parenchyma causes all three types of damage.

Levels of blood urea and serum creatinine can be affected by various factors but, when taken together they serve as a useful clinical guide to overall renal function. A creatinine clearance test will give an approximate value for glomerular filtration rate but is prone to error. A more accurate assessment of glomerular function can be obtained from an estimate of the clearance of chromium-51-labelled ethylenediaminetetraacetic acid. Surgeons will usually call on their nephrological colleagues for more detailed investigations of tubular function and renal blood flow.

The specific gravity of the urine is fixed at a low level when the kidney loses the power to concentrate because of renal tubular dysfunction. Estimation of the urinary loss of sodium, β_2-microglobulin or the tubular enzyme *N*-acetylglucosamine (NAG) will further define the nature of any functional impairment (Summary box 74.6).

Summary box 74.6

Tests of renal function

- Elevated blood urea and serum creatinine levels usually indicate a significant impairment of renal function
- More sophisticated renal assessment is required to quantify the functional deficit

Imaging

A plain abdominal x-ray showing the kidneys, ureters and bladder (the KUB) is a simple and useful test. Abnormalities of the spine and other bony structures including scoliosis, spina bifida, degenerative disease of the spine, metastases, fractures and arthritis may be relevant to the urological diagnosis. The soft-tissue renal shadows, outlined by their more radiolucent fatty coverings, overlie the upper attachments of the psoas muscles. A full bladder often presents a hazy outline arising from the pelvis.

Most urinary calculi absorb x-rays and lie in the region of the renal shadows and along the course of each ureter. These normally follow the tips of the transverse processes of the vertebrae, cross the sacroiliac joints and head for the ischial spine before hooking medially towards the bladder base. Stones with a low calcium content and those overlying bony structures may be difficult to see on the plain film. Pelvic phleboliths are very common and can look like lower ureteric calculi. Uric acid stones are the most common radiolucent calculi (Summary box 74.7).

Summary box 74.7

Straight abdominal radiograph

- Most urinary calculi are radiodense
- Uric acid calculi are typically radiolucent

Ernst Lowenstein, 1878–1949, pathologist, Vienna, Austria.
Carl Oluf Jensen, 1864–1934, veterinary surgeon and pathologist, Copenhagen, Denmark.

Intravenous urography (urography)

Excretion renography has been a mainstay of urological investigation since the introduction of intravenous contrast media in the 1930s. These are organic chemicals to which iodine atoms are attached to absorb x-rays. When such a chemical is injected intravenously, it is filtered from the blood by the glomeruli and does not undergo tubular absorption. As a result, it rapidly passes through the renal parenchyma into the urine, which it renders radio-opaque.

Although intravenous urography (IVU) gives excellent images of the urinary tract (Figure 74.3), its use should be restricted because in a few patients the iodine in the contrast medium may cause an anaphylactic reaction. Patients with a history of allergy, atopy and eczema are particularly vulnerable, but severe reactions may occur without warning. Less invasive and dangerous imaging techniques are clearly to be preferred if they are able to give comparable diagnostic information (Summary box 74.8).

Summary box 74.8

Intravenous urography

- IVU can cause a dangerous hypersensitivity reaction in a small number of patients

Preparation

A laxative will clear faeces that might otherwise obscure details of urinary tract anatomy. Modest fluid restriction is permissible, but dehydration is dangerous because it may precipitate acute renal failure.

Technique

The patient is observed carefully while the first few drops of contrast medium (Urografin or Niopam 370) are injected. The earliest films show the renal parenchyma opacified by contrast medium – the nephrogram phase. A delayed nephrogram on one side indicates unilateral functional impairment. Distortion of the renal outline or failure of part of the kidney to function suggests a space-occupying lesion.

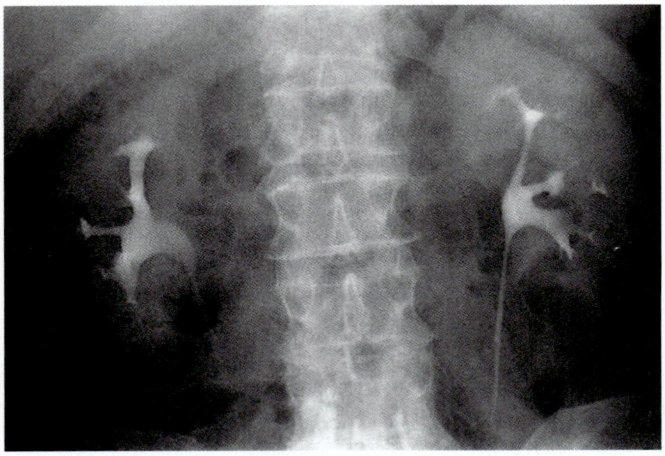

Figure 74.3 Normal intravenous urogram showing the outline of both kidneys with the collecting system and upper ureters highlighted by the contrast medium.

After a few minutes, the contrast is excreted into the collecting system, opacifying the calyces and the renal pelvis. Later films show the ureters and, at the end of the study, the patient is asked to pass urine and a final film is taken to show details of the bladder area. It is important to bear in mind that the static images of IVU provide only snapshots of dynamic events in the urinary tract. The appearance of a normal ureter changes as peristaltic waves of contraction pass along it.

IVU is particularly valuable to demonstrate tumours and calculi within the urinary tract, which are sometimes difficult to see on ultrasonography. It may also be useful to show details of abnormal anatomy that are difficult to interpret on an ultrasonogram.

As ultrasonography and other forms of scanning have become more sophisticated, the indications for the urogram are fewer and it may eventually fall into disuse. Obstruction to the upper urinary tract interferes with transport of contrast medium into the urine, which will show up as a non-functioning kidney on the standard urogram films. In these circumstances, a further x-ray taken many hours after injection of the contrast medium may show hazy opacification of a dilated system. Distortion of the calyces or the renal outline can equally be caused by a tumour or by harmless simple cysts. In each of these cases, more information can be obtained from ultrasonography or computed tomography (CT).

Retrograde ureteropyelography (synonym: retrograde ureterogram)

A ureteric catheter is passed into the ureteric orifice through a cystoscope (Figure 74.4). Contrast medium injected through the catheter will demonstrate the anatomy of the upper urinary tract. This is particularly useful if there is doubt about an intraluminal lesion (Figure 74.5) or if renal function is deficient (before surgery for pelviureteric junction obstruction, for instance). When a transitional tumour is found, it can be sampled by aspiration of urine from the upper tract or by brush biopsy. Retrograde ureteropyelography is possible under topical urethral anaesthesia using a flexible cystoscope. Introducing infection into a poorly draining part of the system carries a serious risk of septicaemia. If there is to be any delay in correcting the blockage surgically, facilities must be available to decompress the kidney by retrograde stenting or percutaneous nephrostomy.

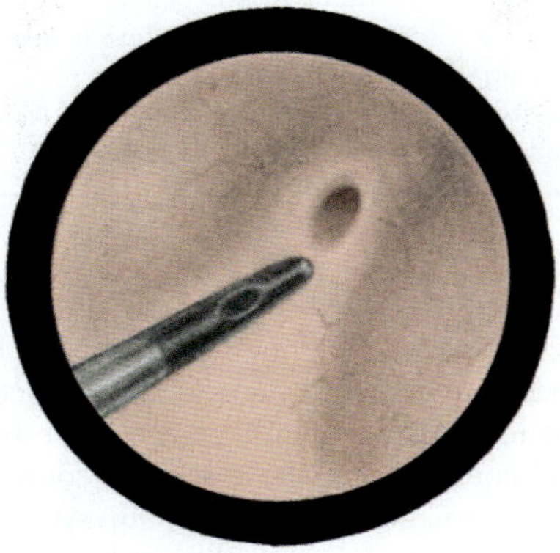

Figure 74.4 A ureteric catheter about to enter the left ureteric orifice. Cystoscopic view.

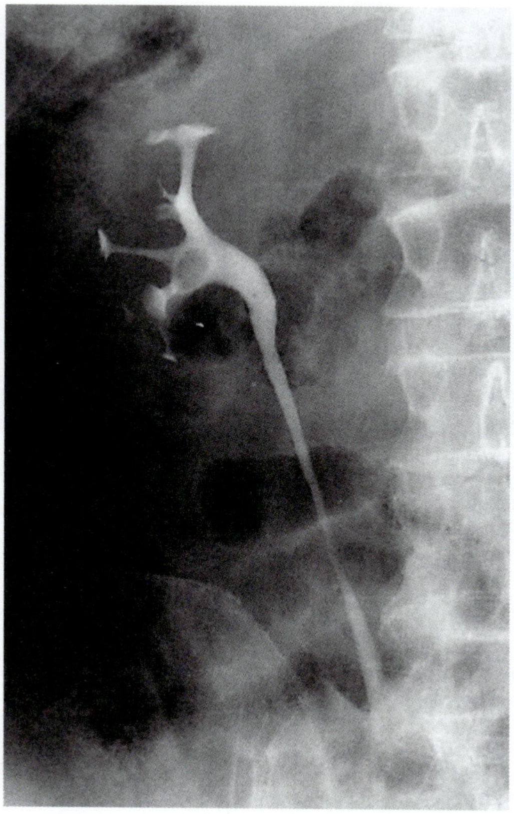

Figure 74.5 Retrograde ureterogram demonstrating the collecting system. The radiolucent filling defect in the renal pelvis is caused by a uric acid calculus.

Antegrade pyelography

Percutaneous puncture of a dilated renal collecting system is reasonably simple. The most common indication is the placement of a nephrostomy tube to drain an obstructed infected kidney or to provide access for percutaneous nephrolithotomy. Antegrade pyelography – in which contrast medium is introduced through the nephrostomy – can be helpful when retrograde studies are prevented by obstruction at the extreme lower end of the ureter.

Digital subtraction arteriography

Refinements in radiological imaging have now almost eliminated the need for translumbar aortography. Satisfactory imaging of the renal vessels can be achieved by digital subtraction angiography after intravenous injection of contrast medium. More precise information can be obtained by intra-arterial injection through a fine catheter inserted into the femoral artery using the Seldinger technique. Arteriography is now rarely used to demonstrate tumour vasculature in a hypernephroma (Figure 74.6), but a flush venogram is useful when CT suggests tumour invasion of the renal vein and vena cava.

Cystography

Cystography is now most commonly a component of videourodynamic assessment (see Chapter 76). Its role in assessing ureteric reflux in children has been largely superseded by radioisotope scanning and dynamic ultrasonography.

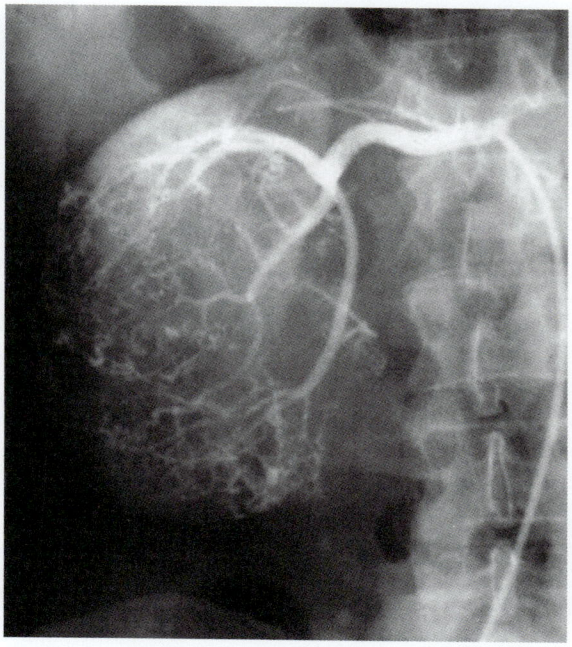

Figure 74.6 A selective renal arteriogram showing abnormal vessels in a renal cell carcinoma.

Urethrography

Ascending urethrography is valuable to demonstrate the extent of a urethral stricture (Figure 74.7) and the presence of false passages and diverticula associated with it. A urethrogram can be used to assess the extent of urethral trauma, but there is a serious danger that contrast medium may pass into the circulation. Lipiodol carries the danger of fat embolus and should never be used, and death has followed the use of barium emulsion. Umbradil viscous V is a radio-opaque water-soluble gel that contains the local anaesthetic lignocaine. It can be injected gently and safely using Knutsson's apparatus even if the urothelium is breached.

Venography

Extension of a renal carcinoma from the renal vein into the vena cava can usually be demonstrated by ultrasound or CT, but venography was used for this purpose.

Ultrasonography

Ultrasonography is perhaps the imaging technique most widely used in urology. Kidney size, the thickness of its cortex and the presence and degree of hydronephrosis can be measured with great accuracy. Intrarenal masses can be diagnosed as smooth walled and fluid filled (simple cysts) or solid and complex (possible tumours). Stones produce a bright ultrasonic reflection and cast an acoustic shadow (Figure 74.8).The volume of urine in the bladder before and after micturition can be calculated, and even tiny filling defects within it detected. Scrotal contents can be displayed in great detail. The prostate is accessible by the transrectal route. Only the lower ureter resists effective investigation by transabdominal ultrasonography because of its small calibre and its proximity to the large bones of the pelvis and spine (Summary box 74.9).

Sven Ivar Seldinger, b. 1921, radiologist, Karolinska Sjukhuset, Stockholm, Sweden.
Folke Knutsson, Director, The Roentgen Department, The University Hospital, Uppsala, Sweden.

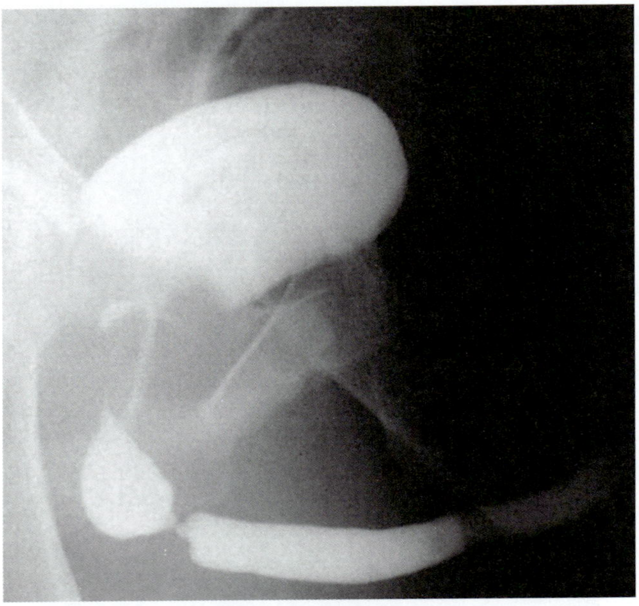

Figure 74.7 Ascending urethrogram demonstrating a tight stricture in the bulbar urethra. Above the stricture the contrast outlines the prostatic urethra and bladder.

Summary box 74.9

Ultrasonography

- Ultrasound scanning provides broadly similar anatomical information to an intravenous urogram but without the risks

Transrectal ultrasonography

This has become a routine component of the investigation of suspected carcinoma of the prostate. Most commonly, suspicion has arisen because the level of prostate-specific antigen is raised or there is an abnormality of the texture or outline of the prostate on digital rectal examination. The features of carcinoma or benign enlargement of the prostate, although not absolutely specific, are sufficiently well recognised to allow an experienced ultrasonographer to identify promising sites for transrectal fineneedle biopsy.

Computed tomography

CT is particularly useful to assess structures in the retroperitoneum (Figure 74.9). In renal carcinoma it will show:

- the size and site of the tumour and the degree of invasion of adjacent tissue;
- the presence of enlarged lymph nodes at the renal hilum;
- invasion of the renal vein and vena cava.

CT is of crucial importance in the initial staging and follow up of men with testicular cancer, in whom the presence of retroperitoneal lymph node masses features in advanced disease. It has also been used to stage bladder and prostate cancer, but its value is less clearcut in these diseases. Non-contrast CT is also

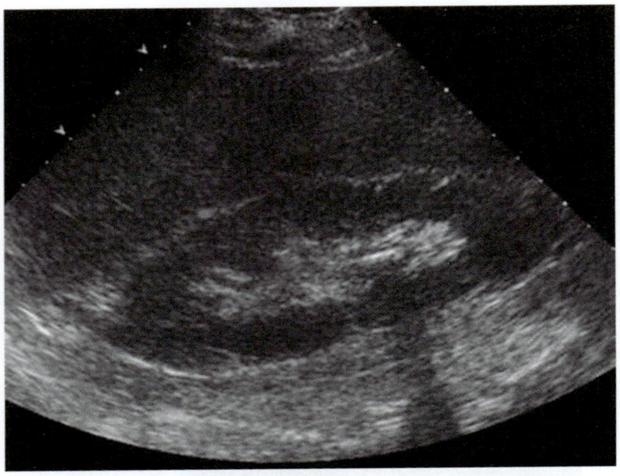

Figure 74.8 A calculus in the kidney casts an acoustic shadow (courtesy of Dr Matthew Matson).

used routinely in the diagnosis of urinary calculi (Figures 74.10 and 74.11).

Magnetic resonance imaging and positron emission tomography

These technologies give information about the function of organs as well as detailed structural images. As they become more widely available, they are replacing many of the routine imaging techniques.

Radioisotope scanning

Radioisotope scanning is used to obtain information about function in individual renal units. Diethyltriaminepentaacetic acid (DTPA) behaves in the kidney like inulin: it is filtered by the glomeruli and not absorbed by the tubules. Using a gamma camera, DTPA labelled with technetium-99m can be followed during its transit through individual kidneys to give a dynamic representation of renal function. A 99mTc-DTPA scan is particularly useful to prove that collecting system dilatation is caused by obstruction. In obstruction, radioactivity will remain in the kidney even if urine flow is stimulated by administra-

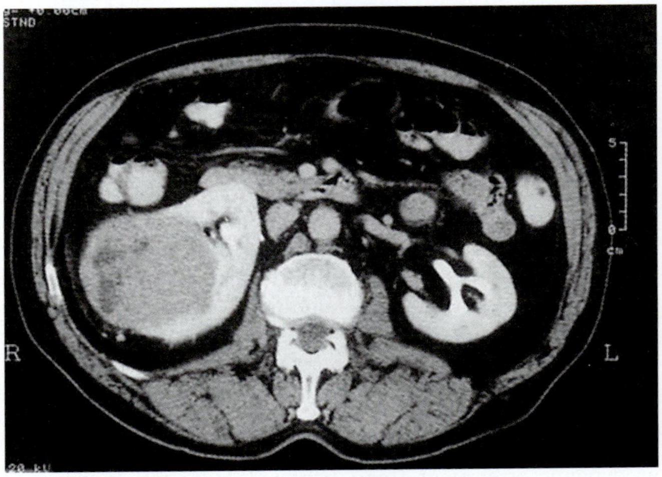

Figure 74.9 Computed tomography showing renal cell carcinoma of the right kidney.

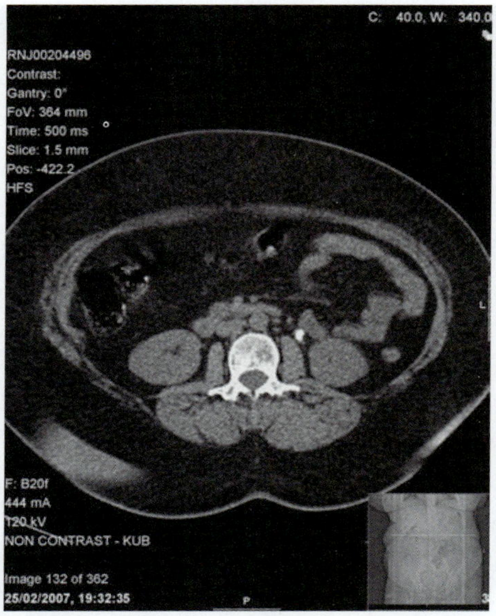

Figure 74.10 A non-contrast computed tomography scan clearly shows a calculus in the left upper ureter (courtesy of Dr Matthew Matson).

tion of a diuretic like frusemide (furosemide). Other substances (dimercaptosuccinic acid (DMSA), mercaptoacetylglycine (MAG-3) and sodium orthoiodohippurate (Hippuran)) labelled with suitable radioactive isotopes have similarly been used to investigate renal function (Figure 74.12).

Isotope bone scanning is fundamental to the staging of kidney and prostate cancers, which typically metastasise to the skeleton.

Endoscopy

Visual inspection of the lower urinary tract has been possible since 1877, when Nitze invented his cystoscope. A leap forward in urological endoscopy came with the introduction by Hopkins of the rod lens telescope and fibreoptic illumination. This allowed development of a family of endoscopes, which allow the urologist to visualise the upper and lower urinary tracts for diagnosis and therapy. Finally, in the early 1980s, the small calibre flexible fibrescopic cystoscope was introduced. This allows simple diagnostic cystourethroscopy, bladder biopsy and retrograde ureterography to be performed under topical urethral anaesthesia with minimal discomfort to the patient (Summary box 74.10).

Summary box 74.10

Diagnostic examination

- Diagnostic examination of the bladder is performed painlessly under local anaesthesia using a flexible cystoscope

ANURIA

Anuria is defined as the complete absence of urine production. Oliguria is present when less than 300 mL of urine is excreted in a day (Summary box 74.11).

Summary box 74.11

Diagnosing anuria

- Check that the bladder is empty before diagnosing anuria
- Ultrasound the bladder

The maintenance of renal function and urine production depends upon perfusion of the kidneys with oxygenated blood. Reduced renal blood flow or hypoxia impairs renal function. When both are present, the danger of acute renal failure is even greater.

Renal failure is traditionally divided into:

- prerenal;
- renal;
- postrenal (obstructive).

Prerenal

Prerenal causes of acute renal failure include:

- hypovolaemia;
- blood loss;
- sepsis;
- cardiogenic shock;
- anaesthesia;
- hypoxia.

Hypovolaemia

This may result from inadequate fluid intake or from excessive loss of body water. Dehydration, prolonged vomiting, diarrhoea and other abnormal gastrointestinal fluid losses, burns and excessive sweating are all common causes of hypovolaemia.

Blood loss

This is usually caused by trauma or surgery, but acute blood loss from the gastrointestinal tract or haemorrhage associated with childbirth may be sufficient to cause hypovolaemic renal impairment.

Sepsis

Gram-negative septicaemia from a urinary tract source is a particularly potent cause of bacteraemic shock. Sepsis from the biliary tract and overwhelming infection from other sites, especially in the immunocompromised individual, are also associated with acute renal failure.

Cardiogenic shock

Acute dysrhythmia secondary to myocardial infarction, cardiac tamponade and pulmonary embolus may all result in reduced cardiac output of often poorly oxygenated blood.

Anaesthesia

Hypotension is a hazard of epidural and spinal anaesthesia.

Hypoxia

Prolonged hypoxia from any cause may occasionally be responsible.

Bozzini, at Frankfurt in 1806, devised the first cystoscope. However, Nitze, a urologist from Berlin, in 1877 is credited to have been the first to demonstrate the use of the cystoscope helped in some way by Beneche, a Viennese optician.

Max Nitze, 1848–1906, urological surgeon, Vienna, Austria.
Harold Horace Hopkins, 1918–1994, Professor of Applied Optics, The University of Reading, Reading, UK.

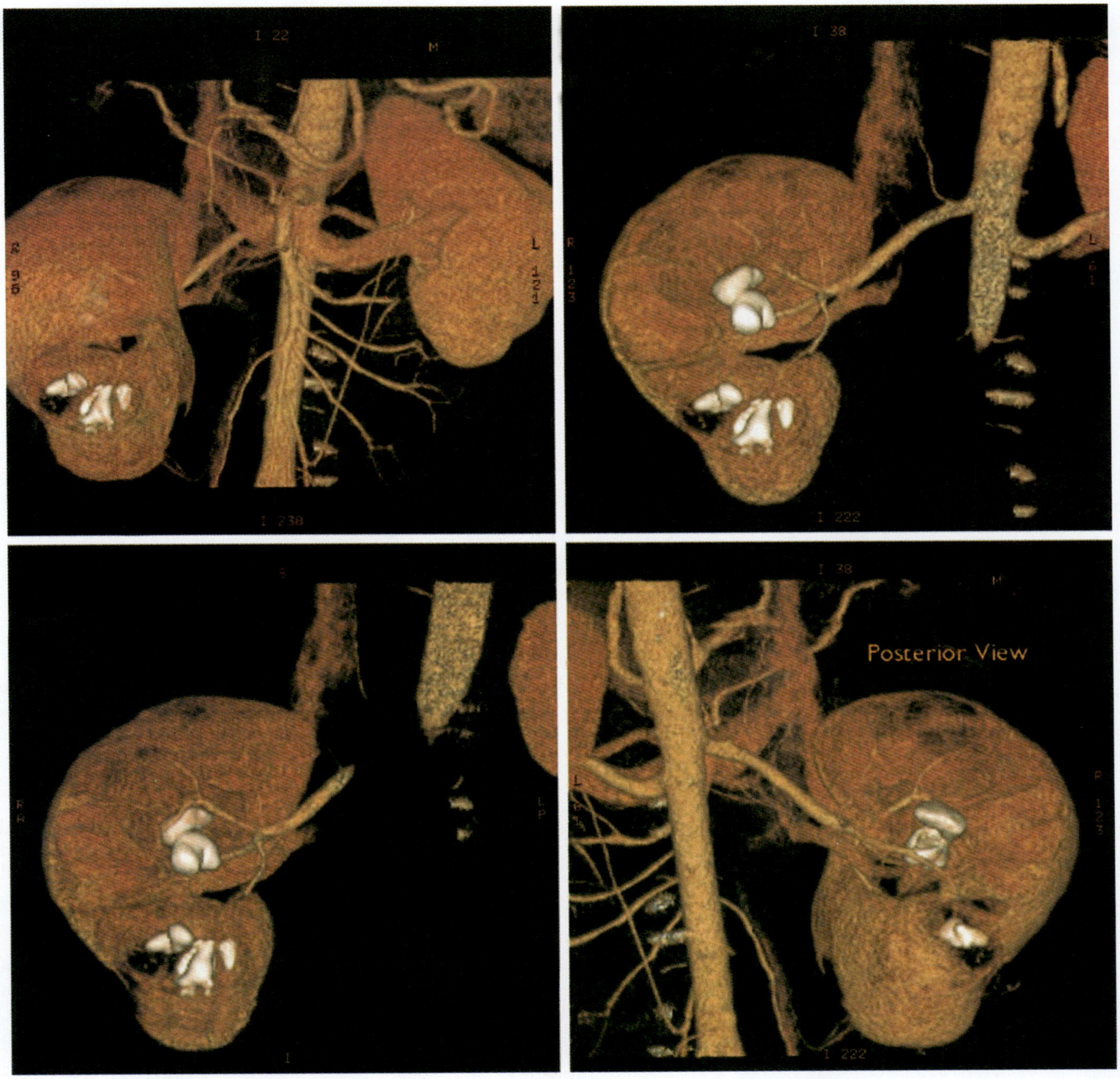

Figure 74.11 Reconstructed spiral computed tomography scan showing calculi in the right kidney (courtesy of Professor R Resnek).

Renal

Renal causes of acute renal failure include:

- drugs;
- poisons;
- contrast media;
- eclampsia;
- myoglobinuria;
- incompatible blood transfusion;
- disseminated intravascular coagulation.

Drugs

Aminoglycosides, cephalosporins and diuretics can be nephrotoxic, particularly if used in combination. They are quite commonly used in patients whose renal function is already compromised by sepsis or circulatory abnormalities. Prolonged use of non-steroidal anti-inflammatory drugs (NSAIDs) can cause a chronic interstitial nephritis and papillary necrosis; they also reduce renal plasma flow and therefore have nephrotoxic properties. Angiotensin-converting enzyme inhibitors used for the control of hypertension can cause a rapid reduction in the

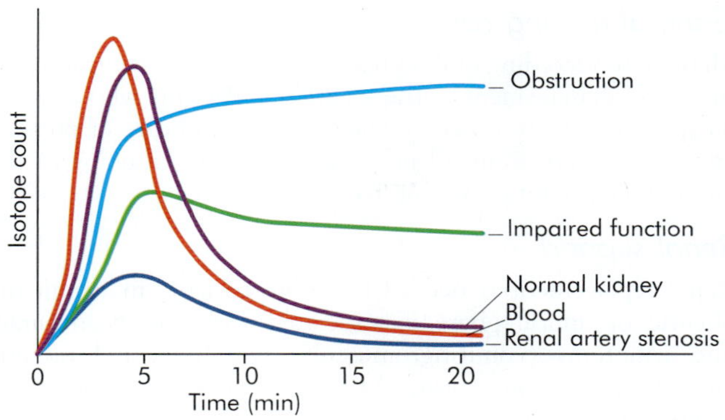

Figure 74.12 Radioisotope renogram.

glomerular filtration rate; this is particularly liable to occur in patients who have a reduced renal blood flow.

Poisons

Some of these are nephrotoxic.

Contrast media

Even modern contrast media may cause renal failure when injected into a dehydrated patient with compromised renal function.

Eclampsia

The early recognition of pre-eclampsia is vital to avoid the nephrotoxic consequences of toxaemia and uncontrolled hypertension.

Myoglobinuria

The presence of myoglobin in the urine is associated with the 'crush' syndrome after major trauma. Less severe injuries can also cause the syndrome, especially if a compartment syndrome is unrecognised or pressure areas break down.

Incompatible blood transfusion

This may lead to renal failure with myoglobinuria.

Disseminated intravascular coagulation

Disseminated intravascular coagulation usually follows major sepsis or massive blood transfusion and may occur post-partum.

Obstructive

Obstructive causes of acute renal failure include:

- calculi;
- pelvic malignancy;
- surgery;
- retroperitoneal fibrosis;
- bilharzia;
- crystalluria.

Calculi

Renal calculus disease is probably the most common cause of acute obstruction leading to anuria. The patient is likely to have unilateral renal colic against a background of non-function of the contralateral kidney, often due to previous surgery or pre-existing obstruction by calculus.

Pelvic malignancy

Carcinomas arising from the bladder, prostate, cervix, ovary or rectum can all lead to obstruction of one or both ureters. A history of haematuria and vaginal or rectal bleeding signpost the diagnosis. A large pelvic mass is commonly palpable on bimanual examination.

Surgery

The ureters are vulnerable to damage during pelvic and retroperitoneal surgery, but injury should be avoided if proper care is taken. It is unusual, but not impossible, to damage both ureters.

Retroperitoneal fibrosis

For details of retroperitoneal fibrosis, see Chapter 75.

Bilharzia

Schistosomiasis may lead to ureteric fibrosis and stenosis, and may be responsible for the development of squamous cell carcinoma of the bladder.

Crystalluria

Uric acid crystalluria can develop in patients receiving chemotherapy for leukaemia or lymphoma unless they are given prophylactic treatment with allopurinol.

Clinical aspects

Answers to the following questions should indicate the probable cause of reduced urine output.

- **Is urine being produced?** Bladder catheterisation is essential if a voided sample cannot be obtained. If urine is available, check the specific gravity, look for the presence of casts (implying a renal cause), test for myoglobinuria and send a sample for culture and microscopy.
- **Is there an obvious prerenal cause?** This can usually be answered by clinical examination, assessment of the patient's vital signs, examination of the fluid balance chart and measurement of the arterial oxygen concentration.
- **Is there ureteric obstruction?** Hydronephrosis may not be marked in acute obstruction, but ultrasonography will usually show some degree of ureteric dilatation. A plain abdominal x-ray should be checked for calculi.
- **What drugs have been given recently?** If a drug is thought to be responsible for renal impairment, it should obviously be withdrawn unless its use is vital.
- **Is this a progression to chronic renal failure?** The presence of shrunken kidneys on ultrasound, normochromic anaemia and hypertension suggest progression to a chronic state even if a previous history of renal failure is not available.

Management and treatment

Renal failure caused by acute tubular necrosis may progress through three recognisable phases:

1. oliguria;
2. the diuretic phase;
3. recovery.

The initial management is aimed at prompt restoration of the circulating volume deficit and correction of tissue hypoxia. Most patients will require a level of care that is available only in a specialised unit. As a minimum, monitoring with a pulse oximeter and central venous pressure measurements will supplement basic observations. For patients with hypovolaemia or sepsis, inotropic support with dopamine may improve cardiac efficiency and increase renal blood flow. If urine production is not promptly restored, frusemide (furosemide) can be given, but this is not always successful and the drug itself may be nephrotoxic. Mannitol may be used as a plasma expander and osmotic diuretic, but care must be taken not to overload the circulation. The aim is to achieve the best possible blood pressure, with a central venous pressure of 7–9 cmH_2O. It may be that 100 per cent oxygen is needed to maintain the oxygen tension (PO_2).

If these measures fail, acute tubular necrosis has supervened. Excess fluid loads must be avoided and fluid input restricted to match the reduced output plus insensible losses (500–800 mL per 24 hours depending on ambient conditions). Abnormal losses due to vomiting, nasogastric aspiration, diarrhoea or fistulae should be monitored and replaced.

A hyperkalaemic acidosis is the characteristic metabolic abnormality of the oliguric phase of renal failure. Correction of the metabolic acidosis with intravenous bicarbonate is tempting but not always advisable. Rising serum potassium is life-threatening and requires effective intervention. A calcium resonium enema is the simplest remedy. The ion-exchange resin can also be administered orally but is unpalatable. Cautious use of intravenous dextrose and insulin should be considered if ion exchange fails. The help of a renal physician is highly desirable because urgent dialysis may become necessary to save life (Summary box 74.12).

Summary box 74.12

Shared management with nephrologist

- Enlist the help of a nephrologist at an early stage in the management of renal failure

The diuretic phase traditionally occurs between the eighth and tenth day but may be delayed as long as 6 weeks. Glomerular filtration recommences but tubular function takes longer to recover. A heavy loss of sodium and potassium can be expected, and fluid and electrolyte requirements must be carefully judged. In most patients the diuretic phase is followed by the recovery phase, but some never recover and will need renal replacement therapy if they are to survive.

Factors that influence the outcome of acute renal failure include the need for artificial ventilation, the need for inotropic support and the presence of jaundice. There is a significant mortality rate.

Nutritional support

Many patients are unable to eat. If enteral feeding is impossible, parenteral nutrition must be administered, with extreme care to avoid circulatory overload.

Infection

These patients are at increased risk of generalised infection. Swabs taken from the nose and throat, sputum specimens and urine, if available, should be sent for culture. If antibiotics are required, they should be non-nephrotoxic.

General nursing care

Meticulous recording of fluid balance is obviously central to the successful management of these patients. Patients who are seriously ill or comatose need regular turning and care of pressure areas if they are to avoid pressure sores. Physiotherapy to the chest and extremities will aid recovery.

Renal support

Renal replacement is needed for those patients in whom the oliguric or anuric phase is associated with significant uraemic symptoms (vomiting, muscular twitching, itching and altered states of consciousness) or uncontrollable hyperkalaemia (Summary box 74.13).

Summary box 74.13

Life-threatening hyperkalaemia

- In acute renal failure, significant hyperkalaemia is life-threatening and should be corrected at an early stage

Peritoneal dialysis

Provided that the patient has not had recent abdominal surgery, peritoneal dialysis can be performed by insertion of a fenestrated catheter under local anaesthetic. This is placed just inferior to the umbilicus in the midline. Sterile dialysis fluid is then run into the peritoneal cavity, where it equilibrates with the extracellular fluid using the peritoneum as a dialysis membrane. After a variable time, the fluid is drained into a closed drainage system. The process is repeated in cycles. Occasionally, when anuria is prolonged, a cuffed catheter needs to be inserted, as used in chronic ambulatory peritoneal dialysis. The disadvantages of acute peritoneal dialysis are the potential for introducing infection into the peritoneum and the rather slow rate of correcting metabolic imbalance, particularly hyperkalaemia.

Haemodialysis

A few sessions of haemodialysis may be life-saving. A double lumen catheter is placed over a guidewire into one of the great veins (jugular, subclavian or femoral). Between sessions of dialysis the lines are kept patent by filling them with heparin solution. Haemodialysis can result in a rapid correction of metabolic abnormalities, but also tends to result in considerable fluctuations of the overall fluid balance. The other disadvantage is that heparinisation is necessary, and this may be undesirable after a recent surgical procedure.

Haemofiltration

This, like haemodialysis, requires the use of an extracorporeal machine but causes much less haemodynamic upset. This may be of critical importance for the acutely ill patient.

Obstructive renal failure

When the patient is too ill for surgery to remove the cause of obstruction to the upper urinary tract, the treatment of obstructive renal impairment is drainage, either externally using a nephrostomy or internally using an indwelling stent (Summary box 74.14).

Summary box 74.14

Catheterisation and stents

- Urethral or suprapubic catheterisation will relieve obstruction distal to the bladder
- Indwelling stents to relieve ureteric obstruction can be inserted cystoscopically or percutaneously

Percutaneous nephrostomy

Under ultrasonographic guidance and local anaesthetic, a fine bore hollow needle is introduced via the flank through the parenchyma and into the expanded collecting system of the obstructed kidney. Once it penetrates the system, contrast medium can be injected through the needle to define its exact position. A wire passed through the lumen of the needle is used to guide the insertion of a series of dilators, which enlarge the track until it will accept a suitably sized nephrostomy tube (Figure 74.13). This will drain urine and pus, provided that the latter is not too viscous. The tube is anchored firmly in place to allow continued drainage as renal function recovers.

Insertion of a J-stent

The ureter can be drained into the bladder by the insertion of a pigtail- or J-stent (see Figure 74.13). The procedure begins with a retrograde ureterogram under fluoroscopic control to provide an image of the ureter. This will often give an indication of the cause of the obstruction. A guidewire is introduced through the ureteric orifice and guided up the ureter into the renal pelvis. The stent is rail-roaded over the guidewire until its distal end also lies within the renal pelvis above the obstruction. When the guidewire is removed, the ends of the stent curl to form a J-shape or a pigtail to secure the device against migration. Stents can be placed under topical urethral anaesthesia using the flexible cystoscope and may be safely left in position for several months. As a foreign body in the urinary tract, stents are prone to infection and encrustation if neglected. It is vital to keep careful records to account for all stents inserted.

If the J-stent cannot be inserted cystoscopically, it may be placed from above through a nephrostomy.

Open surgery

This is a rarity when the minimally invasive methods described above are available. Retrograde insertion of a nephrostomy through an incision in the renal pelvis is the preferred method because it can be surprisingly difficult to locate even dilated calyces by blind puncture of the renal parenchyma.

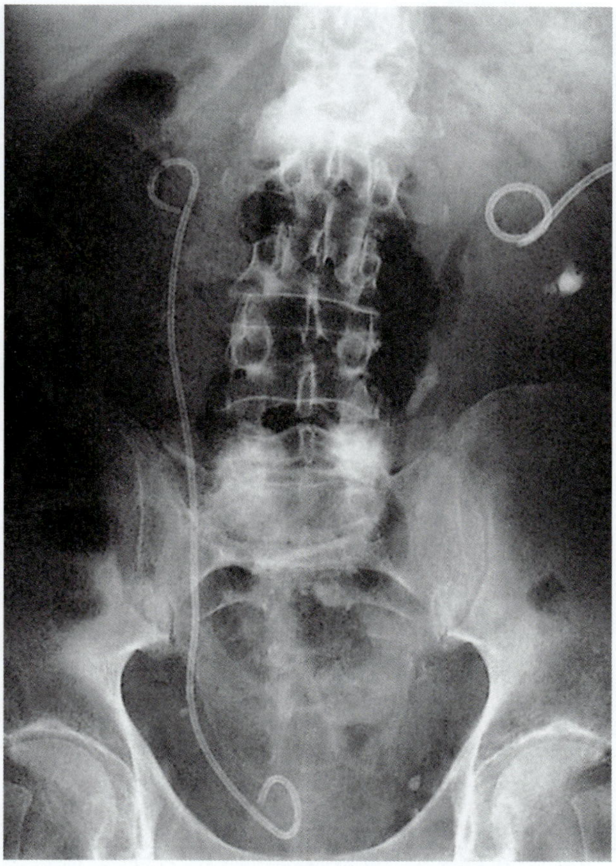

Figure 74.13 X-ray showing a left-sided, pigtail nephrostomy tube draining a kidney obstruction by a ureteric calculus, seen at the level of L3–4. A J-stent is in the right ureter, which has been cleared of stones.

FURTHER READING

Blandy JP, Kaisary AV. *Lecture notes: urology*, 6th edn. Oxford: Blackwell, 2007.

Tanagho EA, McAnich JW (eds). *Smith's general urology*, 15th edn. New York: McGraw-Hill/Appleton & Lange, 2000.

Wein AJ, Kavoussi LR, Novick AC *et al. Campbell–Walsh urology*, 9th edn. Philadelphia, PA: WB Saunders, 2007.

Weiss G, Weiss RM, O'Reilly PH (eds). *Comprehensive urology*. Amsterdam: Elsevier Science, 2001.

CHAPTER 75

The kidneys and ureters

LEARNING OBJECTIVES

To recognise and understand:

- Important congenital abnormalities of the upper urinary tract
- Important cystic diseases of the kidney
- The management of open and closed trauma to the kidney and ureter
- The aetiology, presentation and surgical management of obstruction to the upper urinary tract
- The pathophysiology of renal stone formation
- The management of urinary tract calculi
- The management of sepsis in the upper urinary tract
- Important renal neoplasms and their presentation
- The surgery of upper urinary tract tumours

SURGICAL ANATOMY

The parenchyma of each kidney usually drains into seven calyces, three upper, two middle and two lower calyces (Figure 75.1). Each of the three segments represents an anatomically distinct unit with its own blood supply. One or more renal arteries are present as physiological end arteries that provide the sole blood supply to the tissue they serve. The renal veins are commonly multiple, variable and richly anastomotic. When approached anteriorly, the main artery is typically hidden behind the renal vein.

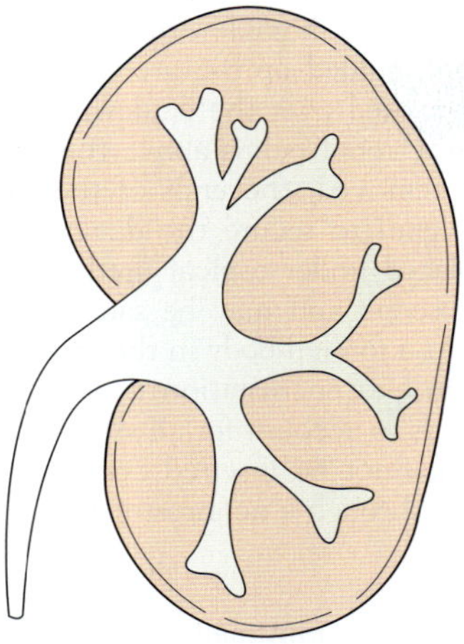

Figure 75.1 The arrangement of renal calyces.

CONGENITAL ABNORMALITIES OF THE KIDNEY

Absence of one kidney

About one in 1400 people have a single kidney (Table 75.1). Sometimes a ureter and renal pelvis are present with no kidney. The contralateral kidney is typically hypertrophied. The possible absence of the contralateral kidney must be considered when planning nephrectomy.

Renal ectopia

Ectopic kidneys are found in one in 1000 people, usually on the left near the pelvic brim. The other kidney is generally normal. A diseased ectopic kidney may present diagnostic problems and may be mistakenly excised as an unexplained pelvic mass.

Horseshoe kidney

A horseshoe kidney is a pair of ectopic kidneys fused usually at their lower poles and lying in front of the fourth lumbar vertebra and great vessels. It is found in one in 1000 necropsies and is more common in men. Upper pole fusion is rare.

Clinical features

Horseshoe kidneys are vulnerable to disease, possibly because the ureters are angulated (Figure 75.2) causing urinary stasis, infection and nephrolithiasis. A pelviureteric junction obstruction (see below) has the same consequences. Horseshoe kidney is usually a radiological diagnosis. Usually the urogram shows the lower pole calyces bilaterally point towards the midline. Rarely, all or most of the calyces are reversed (Figure 75.3). Horseshoe kidney is not a contraindication to pregnancy but may predispose to urinary complications.

Kaspar Friedrich Wolff, 1733–1794, Professor of Anatomy and Physiology, St Petersburg, Russia, described the mesonephric duct and body in 1759.

Division of the relatively avascular isthmus between the kidneys is usually only indicated in the course of surgery for abdominal aortic aneurysm. The blood supply of the horseshoe comes unpredictably from nearby major vessels (Summary box 75.1).

Table 75.1 Congenital abnormalities of the kidney and ureter.

Renal agenesis	
Renal ectopia	Pelvic kidney
	Horseshoe kidney
	Crossed dystopia
	Infantile polycystic disease
	Unilateral multicystic dysplastic kidney
Aberrant renal vessels	Multiple renal arteries and veins
Duplication	Duplex kidney
	Duplex renal pelvis
	Duplex kidney and ureter
Others	Congenital hydronephrosis
	Retrocaval ureter
	Congenital megaureter

Summary box 75.1

Horseshoe kidneys

- Horseshoe kidneys are liable to pelviureteric obstruction, infection and stone
- An unrecognised pelvic kidney may cause diagnostic confusion during surgery

Unilateral fusion

Unilateral fusion (synonyms: crossed dystopia, cross fused renal ectopia) is rare but the urogram is striking. Both kidneys are in one loin and usually fused. The ureter of the lower kidney crosses the midline to enter the bladder on the contralateral side. Both renal pelves can lie one above each other medial to the renal parenchyma (unilateral long kidney) or the pelvis of the crossed kidney faces laterally (unilateral S-shaped kidney; Figure 75.4).

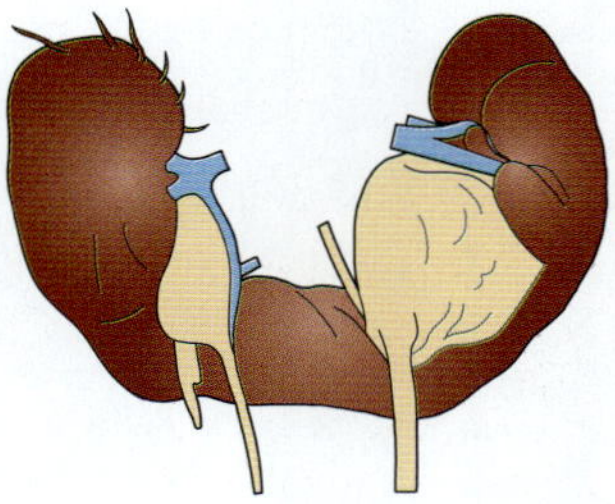

Figure 75.2 Horseshoe kidney. Note the ureters passing in front of the fused lower poles.

Congenital cystic kidneys

Congenital cystic kidneys (synonym: polycystic kidneys) are hereditary, potentially lethal and transmitted by either parent as an autosomal dominant trait. Thus, the risk of inheriting the condition is high. The disease does not usually manifest clinically before the age of 30 years.

Pathology

The kidneys are huge: the cysts distort the renal capsule. Cysts of various sizes contain clear fluid, thick brown material or coagulated blood. There may be a congenital cystic disease of the liver. The aetiology is uncertain.

Clinical features in the adult

The condition is slightly more common in women than men. There are six clinical features:

1 an irregular upper quadrant abdominal mass;
2 loin pain;
3 haematuria;
4 infection;
5 hypertension;
6 uraemia.

Renal enlargement

Less florid examples are revealed unexpectedly at laparotomy or on abdominal imaging. Unilateral renal swelling, in which one kidney contains larger cysts than the other, may be confused with a cystic renal tumour.

Pain

Pain is commonly a dull loin ache. Haemorrhage into a cyst causes more severe pain, as does a calculus passing from the diseased kidney.

Haematuria

Cyst rupture into the renal pelvis may cause recurrent haematuria. Profuse haematuria is uncommon.

Infection

Pyelonephritis is common in patients with congenital cystic kidney, presumably because of urinary stasis.

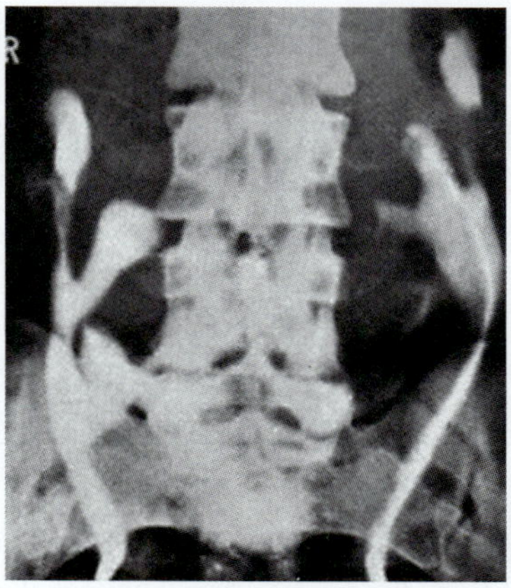

Figure 75.3 Urogram of a horseshoe kidney. Only rarely are all the calyces directed towards the spinal column.

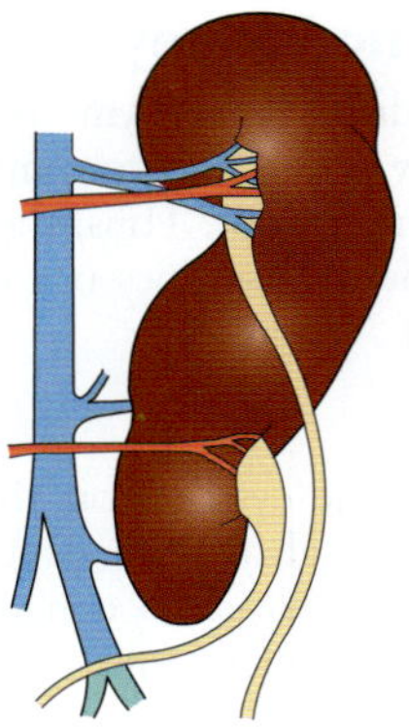

Figure 75.4 Unilateral S-fusion of the kidneys.

Hypertension

After the age of 20 years, most patients are hypertensive.

Uraemia

Congenital cystic kidneys produce large volumes of poor quality urine with a trace of albumin but no casts or cells. Non-specific symptoms of chronic renal failure develop as functioning renal tissue is replaced by cysts. Severe anaemia is common. Signs of renal failure often begin in middle life and the patient soon needs renal replacement therapy.

Imaging

There are multiple cysts in both kidneys and sometimes cysts in the liver and other organs. Blood and debris in the cysts may mimic the heterogeneity of a cystic adenocarcinoma. Simple cysts are usually solitary and have smooth thin walls and homogeneous contents (Figure 75.5). Cytologic examination of cyst fluid obtained by fine-needle aspiration will rule out cancer.

The urogram is typical: the renal shadows are enlarged in all directions; the renal pelvis is compressed and elongated; and the calyces are stretched over the cysts (Figure 75.6).

Treatment

As kidney failure develops, a low-protein diet postpones the inevitability of renal replacement therapy. Infection, anaemia, hypertension and disturbances of calcium metabolism also need treatment by a nephrologist.

Surgery to uncap the cysts (Rovsing's operation) is rarely indicated (Summary box 75.2).

Summary box 75.2

Polycystic kidney disease

- Inherited as an autosomal dominant trait
- An important cause of end-stage renal failure
- Pain, haematuria, infection and hypertension are common
- Often fatal in early middle age

Infantile polycystic disease

Infantile polycystic disease is a rare autosomal recessive condition. The kidneys are large and may obstruct birth. Many patients are stillborn or die from renal failure early in life. In some children, associated congenital hepatic fibrosis is a major problem.

Unilateral multicystic disease

Multicystic dysplastic kidney is more common. It presents as a mass in the flank. Excision is the treatment of choice. Wilms' tumour (see below), neuroblastoma and congenital hydronephrosis are all rarer childhood causes of flank masses.

Simple cyst of the kidney

Simple renal cysts are often discovered incidentally on imaging: they rarely give symptoms and are often multiple (Figure 75.5). A palpable mass, pain from haemorrhage into the cyst and infection are uncommon presentations. Occasionally, a cyst in the hilum of the kidney (a parapelvic cyst) presses on the pelviureteric junction and causes obstruction.

The true nature of a cyst will be apparent by its appearance on ultrasound or computed tomography (CT). Percutaneous cyst puncture for cytology is rarely necessary (Summary box 75.3).

Summary box 75.3

Simple renal cysts

- Common
- Often multiple
- Diagnosed on ultrasound
- Rarely require treatment
- Treat only if causing obstruction

Differential diagnosis

In sheep-rearing districts, hydatid cysts of the kidney are common. On the right side, they can be mistaken for a hydatid cyst of the liver. Occasionally, the patient complains of passing 'grape skins' (ruptured daughter cysts) in the urine. Removal of the cyst must follow the principles used in excision of hydatid cyst of the liver. For a large cyst, nephrectomy may be safer.

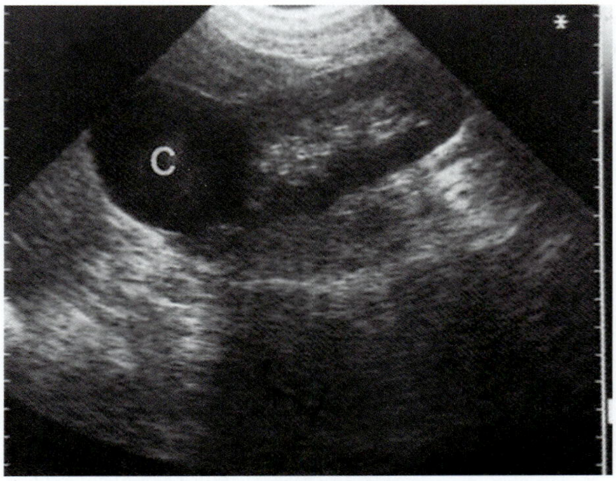

Figure 75.5 Simple cyst (C) of the lower pole shown on a longitudinal ultrasound scan of the kidney.

Nils Thorkild Rovsing, 1862–1927, Professor of Surgery, Copenhagen, Denmark.

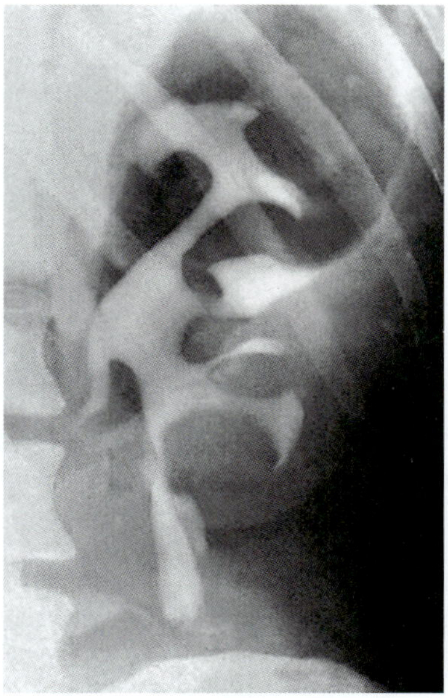

Figure 75.6 Polycystic kidney: urographic appearance. Note the length of the kidney and the bell-like calyces stretched over the cysts.

Aberrant renal vessels

Multiple renal arteries are most common on the left. The renal arteries are functional end-arteries, so division of an aberrant renal artery leads to infarction of a section of parenchyma. Aberrant renal veins are common and can be divided with impunity. Aberrant arteries probably do not cause hydronephrosis, although a hydronephrotic renal pelvis may bulge between renal vessels, making them noticeable (Figure 75.7).

CONGENITAL ABNORMALITIES OF THE RENAL PELVIS AND URETER

Duplication of a renal pelvis

Duplication of a renal pelvis, usually unilateral and left-sided (Figure 75.8), is found in about 4 per cent of patients. The small upper renal pelvis drains the upper calyces; the larger lower renal pelvis drains the middle and lower groups of calyces.

Duplication of a ureter

Duplicated ureter is found in about 3 per cent of urograms often joining in the lower third of their course (Figure 75.9) with a common ureteric orifice. When the ureters open independently into the bladder, the ureter from the upper pelvis opens distally and medially (Figure 75.10).

Clinical features

Infection, calculus formation and pelviureteric junction obstruction are more common than in normal kidneys but most are discovered by chance. One moiety may be dysplastic and non-functioning. Two ureters opening separately may both be abnormal in function, position or both. In children, this may result in a refluxing lower pole ureter and an upper pole ureter terminating in a ureterocele with a risk of infection and/or obstruction.

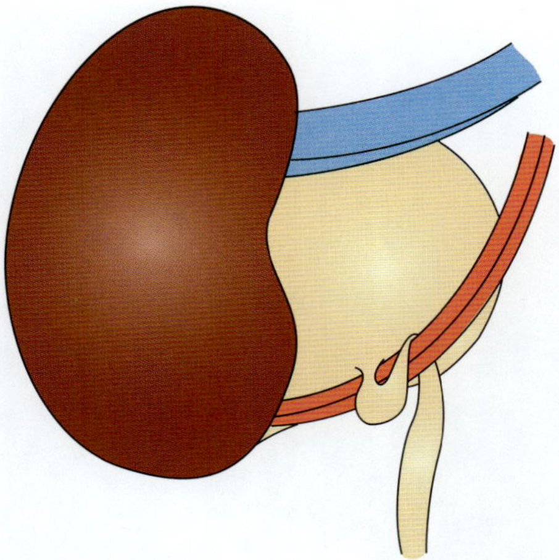

Figure 75.7 Aberrant accessory renal artery with hydronephrosis. The dilated renal pelvis bulges over the vessel.

An ectopic second ureteric opening is a rare cause of puzzling symptoms. In females, an ectopic ureter opens either into the urethra below the sphincter (Figure 75.11) or into the vagina. The history suggests the diagnosis which is confirmed by urography. A girl or woman who voids normally but who has dribbled urine for as long as she can remember probably has an ectopic ureteric orifice. The orifice is difficult to see because it is guarded by a valve.

In the male, the aberrant opening is above the external urethral sphincter so the patient is continent. The ureteric orifice at the apex of the trigone, the posterior urethra, in a seminal vesicle or in an ejaculatory duct is likely to be functionally abnormal, and infection is common.

Treatment

Asymptomatic duplication of the kidney is harmless. A severely diseased or atropic moiety is effectively treated by partial nephrectomy. A refluxing ureter may need reimplanting. An ectopic ureter in the female frequently drains hydronephrotic and chronically infected renal tissue, which is best excised. Rarely, the incontinence can be cured and renal function preserved by implanting the ectopic ureter into the bladder or contralateral ureter (Summary box 75.4).

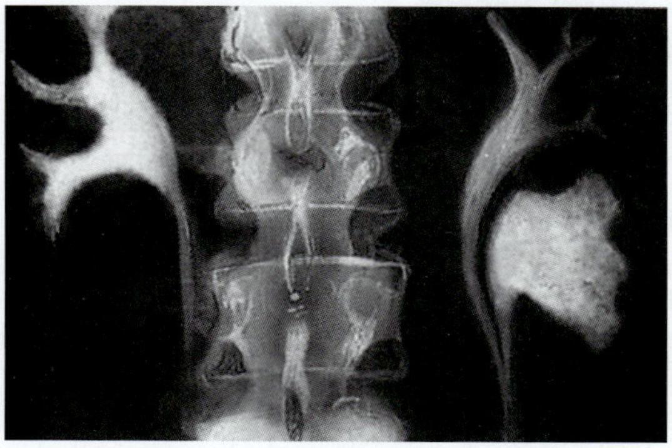

Figure 75.8 Urogram showing a left kidney with double pelvis.

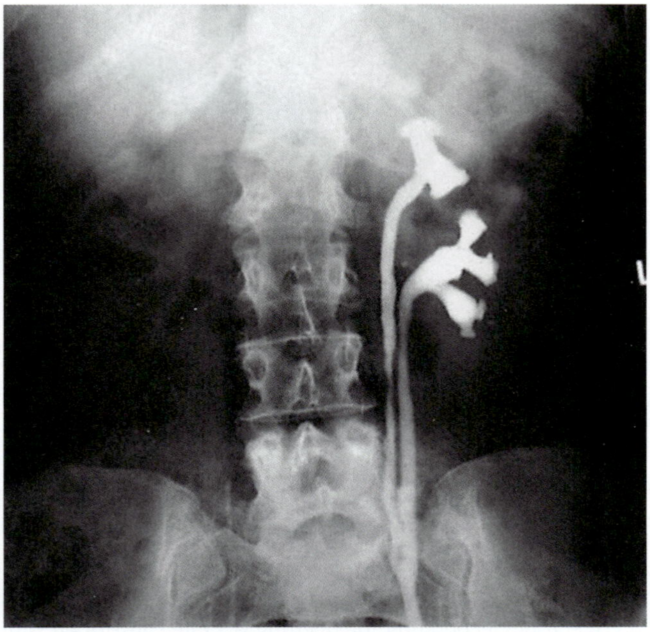

Figure 75.9 Retrograde ureterogram showing a double ureter on the left.

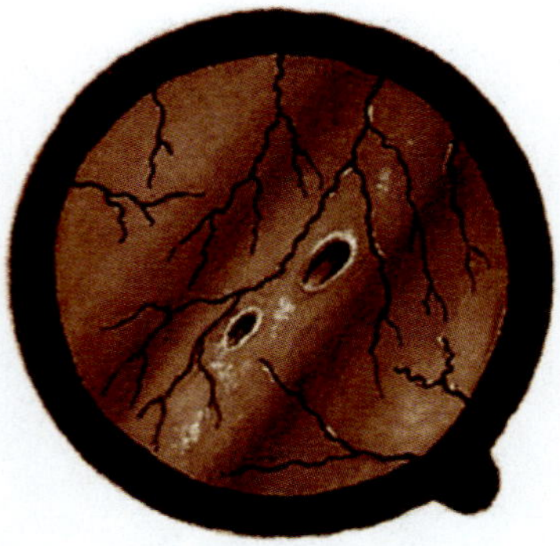

Figure 75.10 Complete ureteric duplication. Two ureteric orifices are seen on cystoscopy: the lower and more medial drains the upper renal pelvis.

Summary box 75.4

Duplication of the kidneys and ureters

- Is commonly asymptomatic and harmless
- One or both moieties may be dysplastic
- There may be urinary reflux, incontinence or obstruction

Congenital megaureter

Congenital megaureter is a rare oddity that may be bilateral and associated with other congenital anomalies. Functional obstruction at the lower end of the ureter ends in progressive dilatation and infection. The ureteric orifice appears normal and a ureteric catheter passes easily. Reflux is not a feature of the untreated condition but occurs if the ureteric orifice is opened endoscopically. Spontaneous improvement occurs but infection or deteriorating function will require refashioning and reimplantion of the affected ureter.

Post-caval ureter

The right ureter passes behind the vena cava instead of lying to the right. If this causes obstructive symptoms, the ureter can be divided and rejoined in front of the cava. Unusually, the retrocaval portion of the ureter is fibrotic and must be excised.

Ureterocele

Ureterocele is a cystic enlargement of the intramural ureter, probably due to congenital atresia of the ureteric orifice. Present from childhood, the condition is often unrecognised until adult life. The 'adder head' on excretory urography (Figure 75.12) is typical. Ureterocele is confirmed by the cystoscopic appearance of a translucent cyst enlarging and collapsing as urine flows in to it (Figure 75.13). Treatment should be avoided unless there are symptoms arising from infection and/or stone formation. Ureterocele is most common in women; occasionally, the cyst may cause obstruction to the bladder outflow by prolapsing into the internal urethral opening.

Endoscopic diathermy incision is effective treatment for a symptomatic ureterocele, although a micturating cystogram is advisable to detect postoperative urinary reflux. In advanced unilateral cases with hydronephrosis or pyonephrosis, consider nephrectomy.

Adder head. An adder is a venomous snake of the family Viperidae which is found in the UK and other parts of the world. It has a triangular shaped head.

INJURIES TO THE KIDNEY

In civilian life, injuries to the kidney result most often from either blows or falls on the loin or crushing injury to the abdomen, typically in a road traffic accident. Haematuria after trivial injury to the kidney should suggest the possibility of a pre-existing disease, e.g. calculus, hydronephrosis or tuberculosis.

The range of injury extends from a small sub-capsular haematoma to a complete tear through the kidney (Figure 75.14).

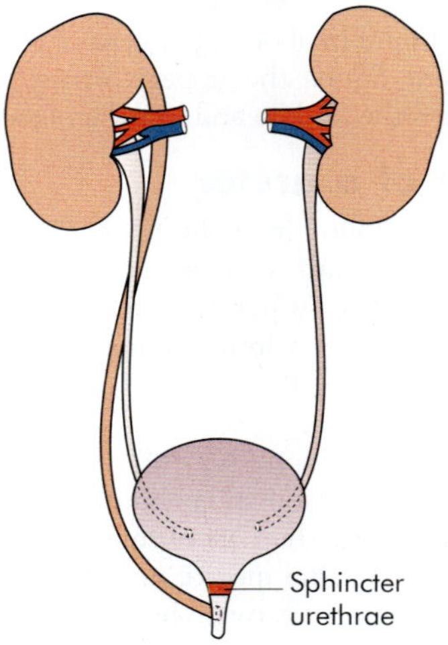

Figure 75.11 In women, one ureteric orifice may open below the sphincter, causing intractable incontinence of urine.

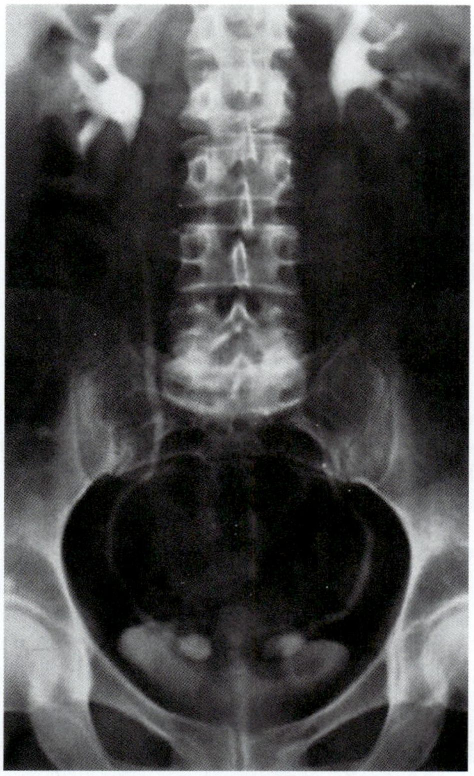

Figure 75.12 Adder-head appearance of a ureterocele.

The kidney may be partially or wholly torn from its vascular pedicle; one pole may be completely detached.

Closed renal injury is usually extraperitoneal. In young children with little extraperitoneal fat, the peritoneum, which is closely applied to the kidney, can tear with the renal capsule, leaking blood and urine into the peritoneum (Summary box 75.5).

> **Summary box 75.5**
>
> **Haemorrhage**
>
> - Lethal haemorrhage is a serious risk in kidney trauma

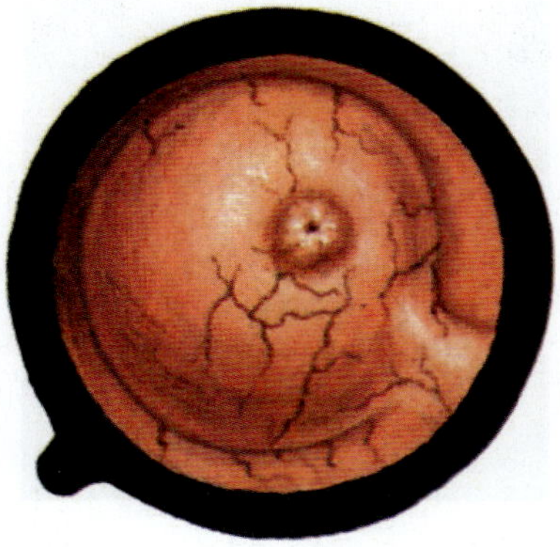

Figure 75.13 Ureterocele on cystoscopy.

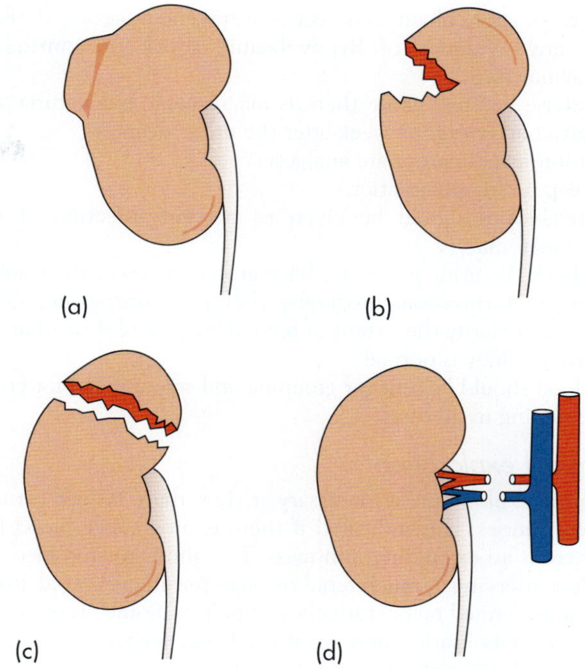

Figure 75.14 Types of closed renal trauma: (a) subscapular haematoma; (b) laceration; (c) avulsion of one pole; (d) avulsion of the renal pedicle.

Clinical features of closed renal trauma

There is local pain and tenderness, sometimes with superficial soft-tissue bruising.

Haematuria

Haematuria may not appear until days after the injury. Profuse bleeding may cause clot colic.

Severe delayed haematuria

Sudden haematuria between the third day and third week after trauma in a recovering patient is caused by a clot becoming dislodged.

Meteorism

Abdominal distension 24–48 hours after renal injury is probably a result of retroperitoneal haematoma implicating splanchnic nerves (Summary box 75.6).

> **Summary box 75.6**
>
> **Clinical features of closed renal trauma**
>
> - There may be no external bruising
> - Haematuria indicates kidney damage and should prompt careful monitoring and urgent investigation
> - Delayed haemorrhage may occur

Management and treatment

Watchful treatment of closed renal trauma is often successful. Consider the possibility of injury to other organs at an early stage.

- Cross-match blood and secure intravenous access if there is any evidence of hypovolaemic shock or continuing haemorrhage.
- Advise bed-rest while there is macroscopic haematuria and retrict activity for a week after the urine clears.
- Administer appropriate analgesia.
- Keep hourly observations.
- Antibiotics should be given to prevent infection of the haematoma.
- Check the urine passed for haematuria and chart the result.
- Urgent intravenous urography (IVU) or contrast-enhanced CT will clarify the extent of renal damage and show that the other kidney is normal.
- Blood should be sent for grouping and serum saved for cross-matching in all cases.

Surgical exploration

Surgical exploration is necessary in less than 10 per cent of closed injuries; it is indicated if there is progressive blood loss or there is an expanding loin mass. The aim is to stop bleeding while conserving as much renal tissue as possible. A renal arteriogram performed preoperatively will help to frame an operative strategy. Embolisation may arrest the haemorrhage if a bleeding vessel can be identified.

Damage to other abdominal organs is checked during a transperitoneal approach. Release of the tamponading effect of the perirenal haematoma can result in massive haemorrhage and the surgeon must be prepared for this. When the kidney is irretrievably ruptured or avulsed from its pedicle, nephrectomy is the only course. Small tears can be sutured over a haemostatic sponge or a piece of detached muscle. Large single rents in the kidney are best dealt with by passing a tube nephrostomy through the defect and suturing the renal tissue around it. Partial nephrectomy may be practicable for localised injury.

When a solitary kidney is sufficiently damaged to need exploration, it must be repaired. Failing this, the wound is packed firmly with gauze to stop the bleeding in the hope that some renal function may be retained when the ruptured kidney heals (Summary box 75.7).

Summary box 75.7

Surgical treatment in closed renal trauma

- Exploration of the kidney may be associated with massive blood loss as the haematoma is opened
- Check that the contralateral kidney is functioning because nephrectomy is a possibility

Complications

Heavy haematuria may lead to clot retention requiring bladder washout.

Pararenal pseudohydronephrosis may occur weeks later from a combination of complete cortical tear and ureteric obstruction caused by scarring.

Hypertension, resistant to drugs, resulting from renal fibrosis, may occur long after injury. Nephrectomy may be necessary.

Post-traumatic aneurysm of the renal artery (Figure 75.15) is rare. There is loin pain and a non-tender swelling may be felt if the aneurysm is large. Congestion of the parenchyma leads to intermittent haematuria. Aortography is diagnostic. Excision or nephrectomy is indicated to prevent fatal rupture of the aneurysm.

INJURIES TO THE URETER

Rupture of the ureter

This is an uncommon result of a hyperextension injury of the spine. The diagnosis is rarely made until there is swelling in the loin or iliac fossa associated with a reduced urine output. An IVU or contrast-enhanced CT shows extravasation of contrast.

Injury to one or both ureters during pelvic surgery

This occurs most often during vaginal or abdominal hysterectomy when the ureter is mistakenly divided, ligated, crushed or excised. Pre-emptive ureteric catheterisation makes it easier to identify the ureters.

Injury recognised at the time of operation

Ureterovesical continuity should be restored by one of the methods described below unless the patient's condition is poor. Deliberate ligation of the proximal ureter and temporary percutaneous nephrostomy is then the best course until the patient is well enough for a repair (Summary box 75.8).

Summary box 75.8

Ureteric injury during operation

- Surgical trauma during pelvic surgery is the most common cause of ureteric trauma
- Preoperative catheterisation of the ureters makes them easier to protect
- Injuries discovered during surgery should be repaired immediately

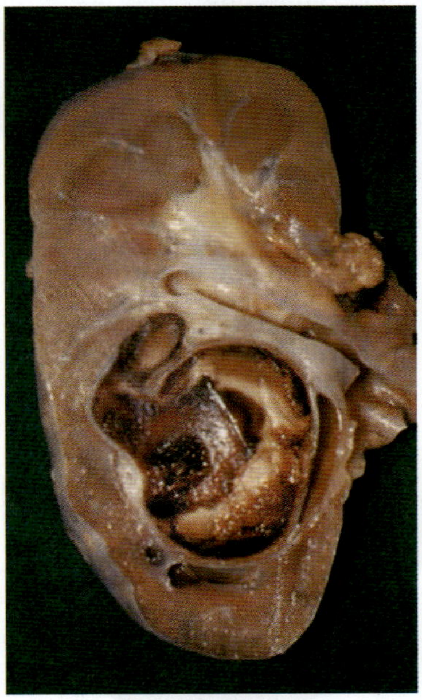

Figure 75.15 Aneurysm of the renal artery containing lamellated thrombus.

Injury not recognised at the time of operation

Unilateral injuries

There are three possibilities:

1 **No symptoms**. Ligation of a ureter may lead to silent atrophy of the kidney. The injury may be unsuspected until the patient undergoes urological imaging.
2 **Loin pain and fever**, possibly with pyonephrosis, occur with infection of the obstructed system. Loss of function will be permanent unless obstruction is relieved by promptly inserting a percutaneous nephrostomy.
3 **A urinary fistula** develops through the abdominal or vaginal wound. The IVU or contrast-enhanced CT shows extravasation with or without obstruction of one or both ureters. Nephrostomies may be inserted and repair postponed until oedema and inflammation have subsided, but delayed repair often leaves the patient incontinent. Early repair is safe if the patient is fit for surgery.

Bilateral injury

Ligation of both ureters leads to anuria. Ureteric catheters will not pass and urgent nephrostomy or immediate surgery is essential.

Repair of the injured ureter

An open repair may be avoidable if a stent will pass the obstruction (Table 75.2). If the cut ends of the ureter can be apposed without tension, they should be joined by a spatulated anastomosis over a double pigtail catheter.

If the division is low, the bladder may be hitched and the ureter can be reimplanted. Extra length may be obtained by mobilising the kidney.

In the Boari operation (Figure 75.16), a flap of bladder wall is fashioned into a tube to replace the lower ureter. The disadvantage of implanting the ureter end to side into the contralateral ureter (a transureteroureterostomy) is that it risks converting a unilateral injury into a bilateral one.

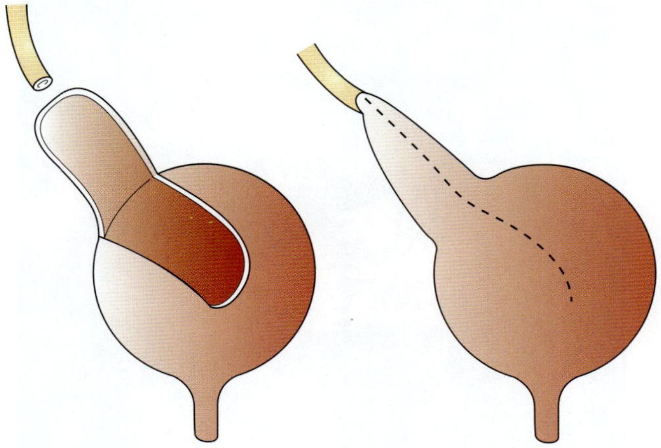

Figure 75.16 Boari operation: a strip of bladder wall is fashioned into a tube to bridge the gap between the cut ureter and the bladder.

Achille Boari, 19th century Italian, urological surgeon from Ferrara; he described the technique of a bladder flap in dogs in 1894; it was first performed in a patient in 1936.

Table 75.2 Methods for repairing a damaged ureter.

If there is no loss of length	Spatulation and end-to-end anastomosis without tension
If there is little loss of length	Mobilise kidney
	Psoas hitch of bladder
	Boari operation
If there is marked loss of length	Transureteroureterostomy
	Interposition of isolated bowel loop or mobilised appendix
	Nephrectomy

Nephrectomy may be best when the patient's outlook is poor and the other kidney is normal. When conservation of all renal tissue is vital, replacement of the damaged ureter by a segment of ileum is necessary (Summary box 75.9).

Summary box 75.9

Repair of ureteric injury

When surgical damage to a ureter is discovered postoperatively:

- Repair need not be delayed
- Ideally surgical repair should be performed by a urologist

HYDRONEPHROSIS

Hydronephrosis is an aseptic dilatation of the kidney caused by obstruction.

Unilateral hydronephrosis

See Summary box 75.10.

Summary box 75.10

Causes of unilateral ureteric obstruction

Extramural obstruction

- Tumour from adjacent structures, e.g. cervix, prostate, rectum, colon or caecum
- Idiopathic retroperitoneal fibrosis
- Retrocaval ureter

Intramural obstruction

- Congenital stenosis, physiological narrowing of the pelviureteric junction leading to pelviureteric junction obstruction
- Ureterocele and congenital small ureteric orifice
- Inflammatory stricture following removal of ureteric calculus, repair of a damaged ureter or tuberculous infection
- Neoplasm of the ureter or bladder cancer involving the ureteric orifice

Intraluminal obstruction

- Calculus in the pelvis or ureter
- Sloughed papilla in papillary necrosis (especially in diabetics, analgesic abusers and sickle cell disease)

Bilateral hydronephrosis

Bilateral hydronephrosis is usually the result of urethral obstruction, but the lesions described above may occur bilaterally.

When due to lower urinary obstruction, the cause may be:

- congenital:
  - posterior urethral valves;
  - urethral atresia;
- acquired:
  - benign prostatic enlargement or carcinoma of the prostate;
  - postoperative bladder neck scarring;
  - urethral stricture;
  - phimosis.

The ureters can be obstructed in their intramural course by detrusor hypertrophy caused by urethral obstruction.

Pathology

There is calyceal dilatation and pressure atrophy of the kidney. A kidney destroyed by longstanding hydronephrosis is a thin-walled, lobulated, fluid-filled sac.

Clinical features

Unilateral hydronephrosis

Unilateral hydronephrosis (commonly caused by idiopathic pelviureteric junction obstruction or calculus) is more common in women and on the right.

Presenting features include the following:

- Mild pain or dull aching in the loin, often a dragging heaviness worstened by excessive fluid intake. The kidney may be palpable.
- Intermittent hydronephrosis (Dietl's crisis). Loin swelling is associated with acute renal pain. The pain goes and the swelling disappears when a large volume of urine is passed.
- Antenatal detection in the fetus by ultrasound scan. Many of these cases are benign, but postnatal investigation is required to detect those with significant pelviureteric junction obstruction (Summary box 75.11).

Summary box 75.11

Idiopathic pelviureteric obstruction

- May be asymptomatic
- Can present as intermittent loin pain often exacerbated by a fluid load

Bilateral hydronephrosis

From lower urinary obstruction

Symptoms of bladder outflow obstruction predominate. The kidneys are usually impalpable because renal failure intervenes before they enlarge.

From bilateral upper urinary tract obstruction

Idiopathic retroperitoneal fibrosis affects both ureters and idiopathic pelviureteric junction obstruction can be bilateral. Symptoms may be referred to one side.

From pregnancy

Dilatation of the ureters and renal pelves occurs early in pregnancy up to the 20th week. It results from the effects on the ureteric smooth muscle of high levels of circulating progesterone and is part of normal pregnancy. The ureters return to their normal size within 12 weeks of delivery. This physiological condition is associated with an increased liability to infection and there is a possibility that abdominal pain during pregnancy may be erroneously ascribed to ureteric obstruction (Summary box 75.12).

Summary box 75.12

Ureteric dilatation in pregnancy

- Physiological dilatation of the ureter is common in pregnancy

Imaging

Ultrasound scanning (Figure 75.17) is the least invasive means of detecting hydronephrosis and is regularly used to diagnose pelviureteric junction obstruction *in utero*.

IVU helps only if there is significant function in the obstructed kidney. The extrarenal pelvis is dilated and the minor calyces lose their normal cupping and become 'clubbed'. If the level of obstruction is in doubt, it can help to take follow-up films 36 hours after the contrast has been injected. Contrast slowly diffuses to fill the obstructed system down to the blockage.

Isotope renography is the best test to confirm obstructive dilatation of the collecting system. A substance (usually diethylenetriaminepenta-acetic acid (DTPA) or MAG-3) is injected intravenously. The DTPA is labelled with technetium-99m, a gamma-ray emitter, so that the passage of 99mTc-labelled DTPA through the kidneys can be tracked using a gamma camera. 99mTc-DTPA is cleared from a normal kidney but stays

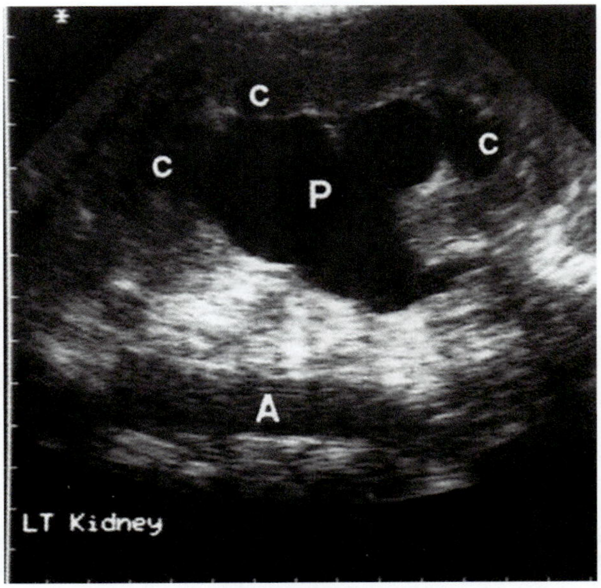

Figure 75.17 Ultrasound of a hydronephrotic kidney. A, artery; C, calyces; P, pelvis.

Joseph Dietl, 1804–1878, Professor of Pathology and Therapeutics, Krakau, Poland.

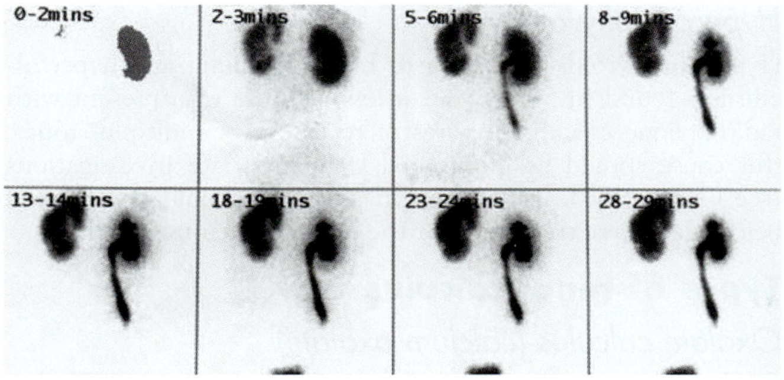

Figure 75.18 Isotope renogram series shows a late accumulation and persistence of radioactivity in the left kidney (the image is a posterior view).

in the renal pelvis on the obstructed side and is retained even if urine flow is increased by administering frusemide (Figure 75.18).

Very occasionally, a Whitaker test is indicated. A percutaneous puncture of the kidney is made and fluid is infused at a constant rate with monitoring of intrapelvic pressure. An abnormal rise in pressure confirms obstruction. Retrograde pyelography (Figure 75.19) is rarely indicated but will confirm the site of obstruction immediately before corrective surgery (Summary box 75.13).

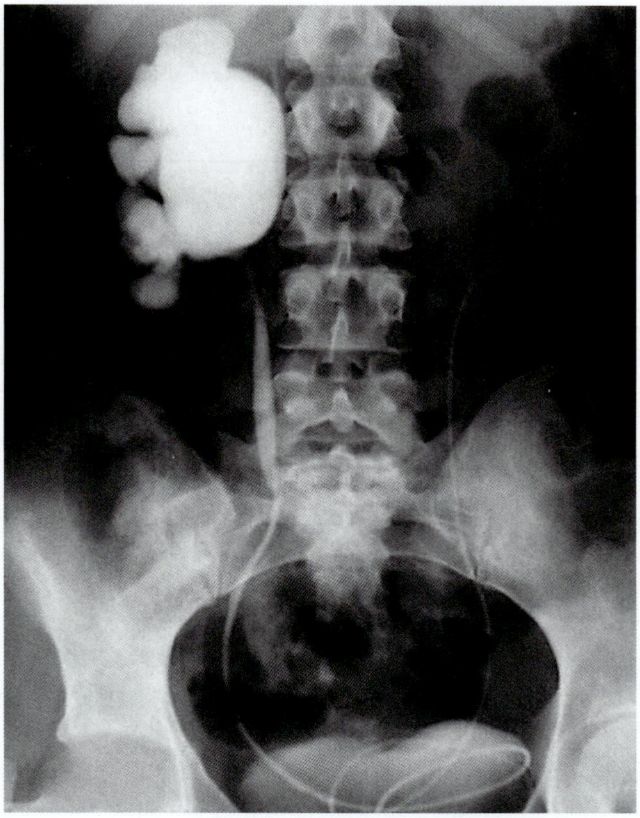

Figure 75.19 Retrograde ureteropyelogram showing hydronephrosis with greatly enlarged pelvis and dilated 'clubbed' calyces.

Summary box 75.13

Imaging

- Obstruction of the ureter is diagnosed by a combination of ultrasound scanning and isotope renography
- An obstructed kidney is worth preserving if it is contributing more than 20 per cent of total renal function

Treatment

The indications for operation are bouts of renal pain, increasing hydronephrosis, evidence of parenchymal damage and infection. Nephrectomy should be considered only when the kidney has been largely destroyed. Mild cases should be followed by serial ultrasound scans and operated upon if dilatation is increasing.

Pyeloplasty

In the Anderson–Hynes operation (Figure 75.20), the upper third of the ureter and the renal pelvis are mobilised. A renal vein overlying the distended pelvis can be divided, but an artery in this situation should be preserved to avoid infarction of the territory that it supplies. The anastomosis is made in front of such an artery. A nephrostomy tube or a ureteric stent protects the anastomosis. Laparoscopic pyeloplasty is becoming increasingly popular.

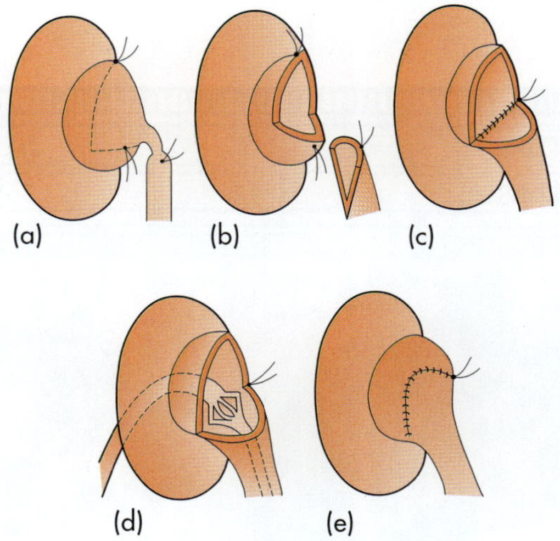

Figure 75.20 (a–e) Anderson–Hynes disjunction pyeloplasty.

Endoscopic pyelolysis

Disruption of the pelviureteric junction by a balloon passed up the ureter and distended under radiographic control has been used to treat idiopathic pelviureteric junction obstruction.

Robert Whitaker, urologist, Addenbrooke's Hospital, Cambridge, UK.

James Christie Anderson, 1899–1984, urologist, The Royal Hallamshire Hospital, Sheffield, UK.

Wilfred Hynes, 1903–1991, plastic surgeon, The Plastic and Jaw Department, The Royal Sheffield Hospital, Sheffield, UK. Anderson and Hynes devised the operation in 1949. It is nowadays done laparoscopically, particularly in children. Robotically assisted laparoscopic dismembered pyeloplasty has also been carried out.

The long-term efficacy of this and various forms of endoscopic pyelotomy has still to be proved. The alternative minimal access procedure, laparoscopic pyeloplasty, is increasingly popular.

RENAL CALCULI

Aetiology

This subject is complex and the following represents a brief summary of current opinion.

Dietetic

Deficiency of vitamin A causes desquamation of epithelium forming a nidus on which a stone is deposited. This mechanism is probably active in the formation of bladder calculi.

Altered urinary solutes and colloids

Dehydration concentrates urinary solutes until they precipitate. Reduction of urinary colloids, which adsorb solutes, or mucoproteins, which chelate calcium, might tend to crystal and stone formation.

Decreased urinary citrate

The presence of citrate in urine, 300–900 mg per 24 hours (1.6–4.7 mmol per 24 hours) as citric acid, keeps relatively insoluble calcium phosphate and citrate in solution.

Renal infection

Infection favours the formation of urinary calculi. Clinical and experimental stone formation are common when urine is infected with urea-splitting streptococci, staphylococci and especially *Proteus* spp.

Inadequate urinary drainage and urinary stasis

Stones are liable to form when urine is static.

Prolonged immobilisation

Immobilisation is liable to result in skeletal decalcification and an increase in urinary calcium favouring the formation of calcium phosphate calculi.

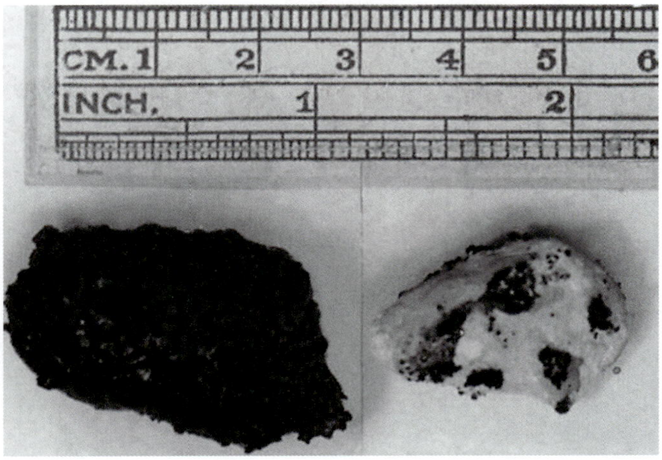

Figure 75.21 Oxalate calculi. The larger one removed from the right kidney is blackened by the deposition of altered blood.

Hyperparathyroidism

Hyperparathyroidism leading to hypercalcaemia and hypercalciuria is found in 5 per cent or less of those who present with radio-opaque calculi. In cases of recurrent or multiple stones, this cause should be eliminated by appropriate investigations (see Chapter 51). A parathyroid adenoma should be removed before definitive treatment for the urinary calculi.

Types of renal calculus

Oxalate calculus (calcium oxalate)

Oxalate stones are irregular with sharp projections (Figure 75.21). A calcium oxalate monohydrate stone is hard and radiodense.

Phosphate calculus

A phosphate calculus (calcium phosphate often with ammonium magnesium phosphate (struvite)) is smooth and dirty white. It grows in alkaline urine, especially when urea-splitting *Proteus* organisms are present. The calculus may enlarge to fill most of the collecting system, forming a stag-horn calculus (Figure 75.22). Even a large stag-horn calculus may be asymptomatic for years until it presents with haematuria, urinary infection or renal failure.

Uric acid and urate calculi

These are hard, smooth and often multiple and multifaceted. Pure uric acid stones are radiolucent. CT will distinguish them from other causes of filling defects including tumours of the ureter. Most uric acid stones contain some calcium, so they cast a faint radiological shadow.

Cystine calculus

An uncommon congenital error of metabolism leads to cystinuria. Cystine stones are often multiple and may grow to form a cast of the collecting system. Cystine stones are radio-opaque and very hard.

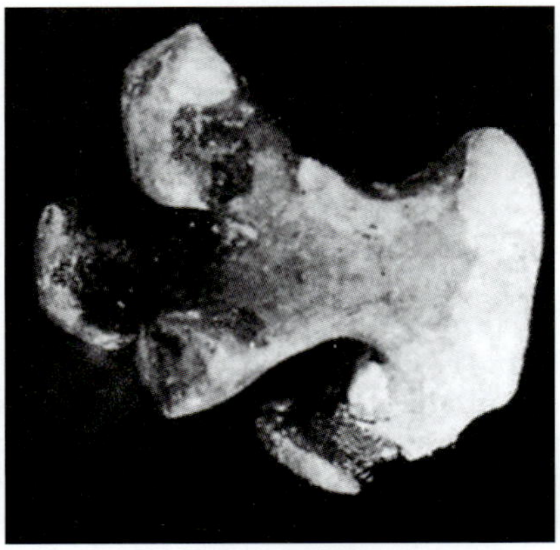

Figure 75.22 Stag-horn calculus.

The first nephrolithotomy was performed by Ambrose Paré (1509–1590) on a prisoner condemned to death by hanging. Paré cut out two stones from his kidney following which he was cured. As he recovered from this procedure, he secured remission from his death penalty and was given a grant of money.' Paré said: 'I dressed his wounds, but God healed them'.

Theodor Escherich, 1857–1911, Professor of Paediatrics, Vienna, Austria, discovered the bacterium coli commune in 1886.

Clinical features

Renal calculi are common. Approximately 50 per cent of patients present between the ages of 30 and 50 years. The male–female ratio is 4:3 (Summary box 75.14).

> **Summary box 75.14**
>
> **Renal stones**
>
> - Are common
> - May be clinically silent even when large
> - Are usually visible on a plain abdominal radiograph
> - May be radiolucent when composed of uric acid

Silent calculus

Renal failure may be the first indication of bilateral silent calculi, although secondary infection usually produces symptoms first.

Pain

Pain occurs in 75 per cent of people with urinary stones. Fixed renal pain occurs in the renal angle (Figure 75.23), the hypochondrium, or in both. It may be worse on movement.

Ureteric colic is an agonising pain passing from the loin to the groin. Pain resulting from renal stones rarely lasts more than 8 hours in the absence of infection. There is no pyrexia, although the pulse rate rises because of the severe pain. Ureteric colic is often caused by a stone entering the ureter but it may also occur when a stone becomes lodged in the pelviureteric junction. The severity of the colic is not related to the size of the stone (Summary box 75.15).

> **Summary box 75.15**
>
> **Ureteric colic**
>
> - Severe exacerbations on a background of continuing pain
> - Radiates to the groin, penis, scrotum or labium as the stone progresses down the ureter
> - Severity of pain is not related to stone size
> - Haematuria is very common
> - There may be few physical signs

Abdominal examination

During an attack of ureteric colic, rigidity may be present but not prominent. Percussion over the kidney produces a stab of pain and there may be tenderness on gentle deep palpation. Hydronephrosis or pyonephrosis leading to a palpable loin swelling is rare.

Haematuria

Haematuria, usually small in amount, is common and sometimes is the only symptom of stone disease.

Pyuria

Infection is particularly dangerous when the kidney is obstructed. Pressure builds in the system, organisms are forced into the circulation and a septicaemia can quickly develop.

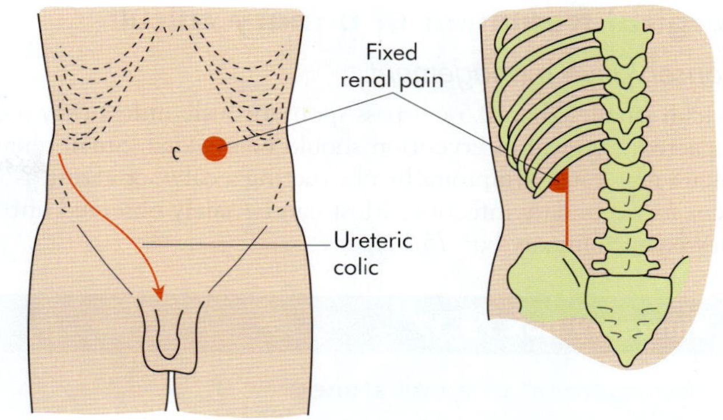

Figure 75.23 The usual distribution of renal pain.

Stones may cause pyuria by irritating the urothelium even in the absence of infection.

Investigation of suspected urinary stone disease

X-ray

The 'KUB' film shows the kidney, ureters and bladder. A branched stone is unmistakable. (Figure 71.24). An opacity maintaining its position relative to the urinary tract during respiration is likely to be a calculus.

Calcified mesenteric nodes and opacities within the gut will be anterior to the vertebral bodies on a lateral x-ray and thus outside the urinary tract (Summary box 75.16).

> **Summary box 75.16**
>
> **Opacities on a plain abdominal radiograph that may be confused with renal calculus**
>
> - Calcified mesenteric lymph node
> - Gallstones or concretion in the appendix
> - Tablets or foreign bodies in the alimentary canal (e.g. cyclopenthiazide (Navidrex-K))
> - Phleboliths – calcification in the walls of veins, especially in the pelvis
> - Ossified tip of the 12th rib
> - Calcified tuberculous lesion in the kidney
> - Calcified adrenal gland

Contrast-enhanced CT

CT, preferably spiral, has become the mainstay of investigation of acute ureteric colic.

Excretion urography

IVU will establish the presence and position of a calculus and the function of the other kidney.

Ultrasound scanning

Ultrasound scanning is of most value in locating stones for treatment by extracorporeal shock wave lithotripsy (ESWL) (see below).

Surgical treatment of urinary calculi

Conservative management

Calculi smaller than 0.5 cm pass spontaneously unless they are impacted. Surgical intervention should be avoided. Small renal calculi may cause symptoms by obstructing a calyx or acting as a focus for secondary infection. Most can be safely observed until they pass (Summary box 75.17).

Summary box 75.17

Management of small stones

- Most small urinary calculi will pass
- Infection in an upper urinary tract obstructed by stone is dangerous and needs urgent surgical intervention

Preoperative treatment

Antibiotic treatment starts before surgery and continues afterwards.

Operation for stone

Most stones should be treated by minimal access and minimally invasive techniques. Open operations are still needed when appropriate expertise is not available or newer techniques have failed (Summary box 75.18).

Summary box 75.18

Kidney stone removal

- Most urinary calculi can be treated by minimal access techniques

Modern methods of stone removal

Kidney stones

Percutaneous nephrolithotomy

Endoscopic instruments are passed into the kidney by a percutaneous technique (Figure 75.25). Small stones may be grasped under vision and extracted whole. Larger stones are fragmented by an ultrasound, laser or electrohydraulic probe and removed in pieces.

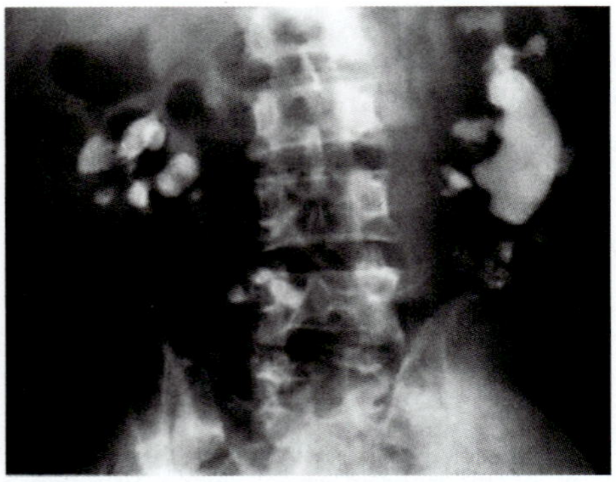

Figure 75.24 Plain abdominal x-ray showing complete stag-horn calculi.

The aim is to remove all fragments. A nephrostomy drain is left in the system when the procedure is complete. This decompresses the kidney and allows repeated access if necessary. Percutaneous nephrolithotomy is sometimes combined with ESWL in the treatment of complex (stag-horn) calculi.

Complications of percutaneous nephrolithotomy include: (1) haemorrhage from the punctured renal parenchyma; (2) perforation of the collecting system with extravasation of saline irrigant; (3) perforation of the colon or pleural cavity during placement of the percutaneous track.

Extracorporeal shock wave lithotripsy

Crystalline stones disintegrate under the impact of shock waves produced by the ESWL machine.

The shocks may be aimed by ultrasound or x-ray imaging (Figure 75.26). The devices also differ in the disruptive force that they can develop. Less powerful machines break stones less effectively and several treatments may be necessary. Weaker shocks hurt less and treatment can be given without general anaesthesia.

Ureteric colic is common after ESWL, and the patient needs analgesia, usually in the form of a non-steroidal anti-inflammatory drug. Bulky stone fragments may impact in the ureter, causing obstruction. To avoid this, a stent should be placed in the ureter to drain the kidney while stone fragments pass. Occasionally, impacted fragments have to be removed ureteroscopically (see below).

The principal complication of ESWL is infection. Many calculi contain bacteria, which are released from the broken stone. It is wise to give prophylactic antibiotics before ESWL, and an obstructed system should be decompressed by a ureteric stent or percutaneous nephrostomy before treatment.

The clearance of stone from the kidney will depend upon the consistency of the stone and its site. Most oxalate and phosphate stones fragment well and, if lying in the renal pelvis, will clear within days. The results with harder stones, especially cystine stones, are less satisfactory. When treating calyceal stones, the patients should be warned that the clearance may take months.

Open surgery for renal calculi

Operations for kidney stone are usually performed via a loin or lumbar approach (Figure 75.27). All of the procedures are difficult unless the kidney is fully mobilised and its vascular pedicle controlled. A sling should be placed around the upper ureter to stop stones migrating downwards.

Pyelolithotomy

Pyelolithotomy is indicated for stones in the renal pelvis. When the wall of the renal pelvis has been dissected from its surrounding fat, an incision is made in its long axis directly on to the stone. The stone is removed with gallstone forceps. Stone fragments in peripheral calyces may be detected by direct palpation or by intraoperative x-ray or nephroscopy. If there is sepsis, a nephrostomy is essential to drain the system.

Extended pyelolithotomy

The plane between the renal sinus and the wall of the collecting system is developed on the posterior surface of the kidney. This avoids major vessels and allows incisions into the calyces so that even large stag-horn stones can be removed intact.

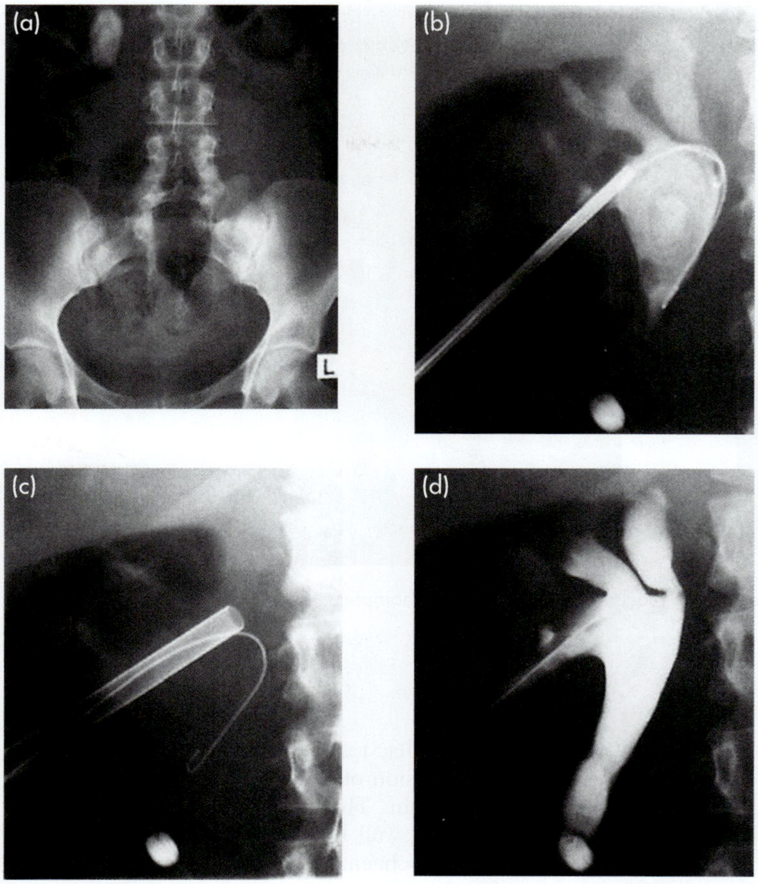

Figure 75.25 Percutaneous renal stone removal. (a) The stone is in the right renal pelvis. (b) Placement of a cannula under radiological control into the renal pelvis and through it a balloon catheter to stop fragments migrating into the upper ureter. (c) The stone is disrupted by contact lithotripsy and the fragments have been successfully removed by irrigation. (d) A nephrostogram confirms that the renal pelvis is intact.

Nephrolithotomy

If there is a complex calculus branching into the most peripheral calyces, it may be necessary to make incisions into the renal parenchyma to clear the kidney. Nephrolithotomy may also be necessary when the adhesions from previous surgery complicate access to the renal pelvis. The renal pedicle is temporarily cross-clamped to reduce bleeding from the vascular renal tissue. Incisions are made posterior and parallel to the most prominent part of the convex renal border, where the territories of the anterior and posterior branches of the renal artery meet (Brödel's line). Cooling the kidney extends the ischaemia. Nephrolithotomy incisions must be closed with haemostatic sutures and the patient observed for signs of reactionary haemorrhage.

Partial nephrectomy is sometimes preferable for a stone in the lowermost calyx with infective damage to the adjacent parenchyma.

A functionless kidney destroyed by stone disease should be removed, particularly when there is xanthogranulomatous pyelonephritis. This stone-related inflammatory mass must be removed with care because it is liable to be attached to adjacent structures such as the colon.

Treatment of bilateral renal stones

Usually the kidney with better function is treated first, unless the other kidney is more painful or there is pyonephrosis which needs urgent decompression.

Prevention of recurrence

Ideally, stone formers should be investigated to exclude metabolic factors, although the diagnostic yield is low in patients with a single small stone. The urine should be screened for infection. The following investigations are appropriate in bilateral and recurrent stone formers:

- serum calcium, measured fasting on three occasions to exclude hyperparathyroidism;
- serum uric acid;
- urinary urate, calcium and phosphate in a 24-hour collection; the urine should also be screened for cystine;
- analysis of any stone passed.

Dietary advice is not usually helpful in avoiding stone recurrence in people who have a balanced diet. Those who consume excessive amounts of milk products (calcium stones), rhubarb, strawberries, plums, spinach and asparagus (calcium oxalate stones) should be advised to be more moderate.

Patients with hyperuricaemia should avoid red meats, offal and fish, which are rich in purines, and should be treated with allopurinol. Eggs, meat and fish are high in sulphur-containing proteins and should be restricted in cystinuria.

Max Brödel, 1870–1941, medical artist who founded 'The Department of Art as Applied to Medicine' at the Johns Hopkins Hospital, Baltimore, MD, USA.

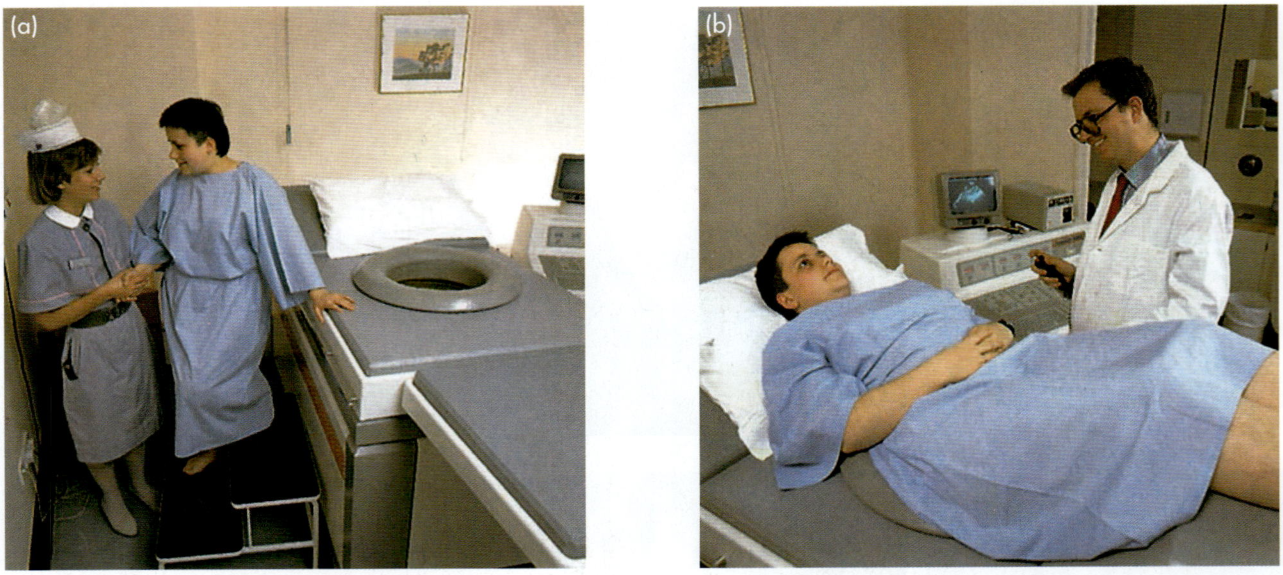

Figure 75.26 Extracorporeal shock wave lithotripsy. (a) The patient being placed on the ultrasound lithotripter. (b) Positioning of the patient being checked by ultrasound.

Stone sufferers should drink plenty to keep their urine dilute.

Drug treatment is largely ineffective except in those few patients who are shown to have idiopathic hypercalciuria. Bendroflumethiazide (5 mg) and a calcium-restricted diet reduce urinary calcium (Summary box 75.19).

Summary box 75.19

Recurrent stone formation

- Stones are more common in those who have had a previous stone
- Unless there is a specific biochemical abnormality, high fluid intake is the best prophylactic measure

URETERIC CALCULUS

A stone in the ureter usually comes from the kidney. Most pass spontaneously.

Clinical features

A stone passing down the ureter often causes intermittent attacks of ureteric colic.

Ureteric colic

The waves of agonising loin pain are typically referred to the groin, external genitalia and the anterior surface of the thigh. As the stone enters the bladder, the pain can be referred to the tip of the penis.

Impaction

There are five sites of narrowing where the stone may be arrested (Figure 75.28). An impacted stone causes a more consistent dull pain, often in the iliac fossa and increased by exercise and lessened by rest. Distension of the renal pelvis due to obstruction may cause loin pain. The stone may become embedded as the adjacent ureteric wall becomes eroded and oedematous as a result of pressure ischaemia. Perforation of the ureter and extravasation of urine is a rare complication.

Severe renal pain subsiding after a day or so suggests complete ureteric obstruction. If obstruction persists after 1–2 weeks, the calculus should be removed to avoid pressure atrophy of the renal parenchyma.

Haematuria

Almost all ureteric colic is associated with transient microscopic haematuria. Serious bleeding is uncommon and should suggest clot colic.

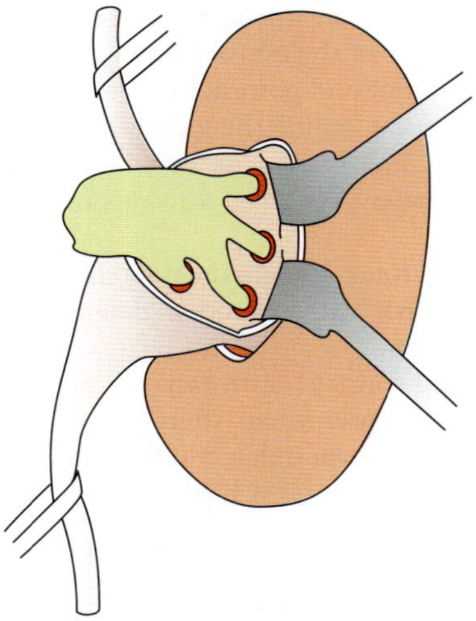

Figure 75.27 Open operations for renal calculus.

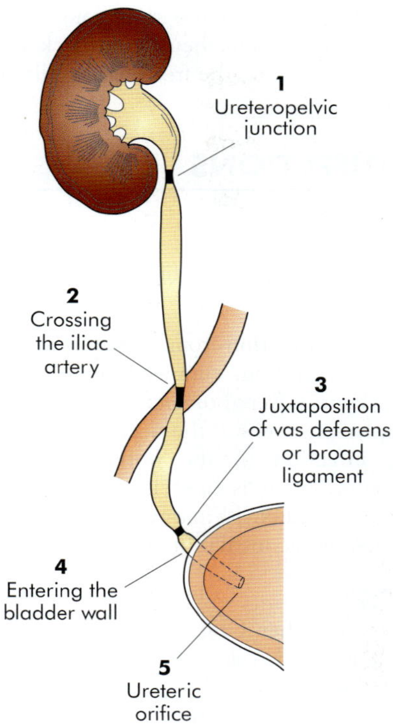

Figure 75.28 Normal anatomical narrowings (1–5) of the ureter.

Abdominal examination

There is tenderness and some rigidity over some part of the course of the ureter. The presence of haematuria does not rule out appendicitis because an inflamed appendix can give rise to a local ureteritis leaking some red cells into the urine. The patient with acute ureteric colic is usually in greater pain and less ill than one with appendicitis or acute cholecystitis.

Imaging

Most urinary calculi are radio-opaque. Stones are difficult to see if small or obscured by bowel contents or nearby bones. IVU while the patient has pain can confirm the diagnosis, although spiral CT is preferable. In ureteric colic, there will probably be little or no excretion on the affected side. Occasionally, there is an extravasation of contrast from the dilated system. Late x-rays, taken up to 36 hours after the injection of contrast, may show dilatation of the ureter down to an obstructing calculus. A radiolucent uric acid stone may be demonstrated as a filling defect in the contrast-filled system.

Analgesic abusers occasionally fake symptoms to obtain drugs, and emergency imaging is useful in excluding renal colic. If the CT or urogram is normal during an attack, the patient does not have renal colic. The absence of blood in the urine makes colic less likely but its presence can be simulated.

Cystoscopy is not indicated routinely but may reveal oedema around the ureteric orifice when the stone is nearby.

Retrograde ureterography is performed as an immediate preliminary to an endoscopic operation to remove a calculus.

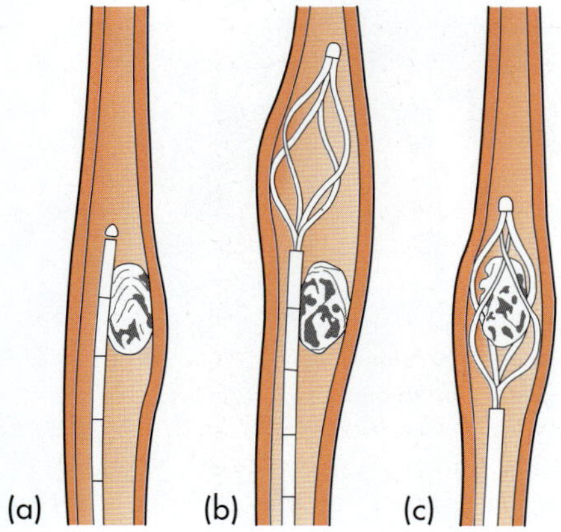

Figure 75.29 Dormia stone-catching basket in use: (a) basket introduced past stone; (b) opened; and (c) enclosing stone, ready for withdrawal.

Treatment

Pain

Non-steroidal anti-inflammatory drugs, such as diclofenac and indomethacin, have replaced opiates as the first line of treatment for renal colic. The value of smooth muscle relaxants, such as propantheline (Pro-Banthine), is debatable.

Removal of the stone

Expectant treatment is appropriate for small stones likely to pass naturally (Summary box 75.20). If the patient is not disabled by recurrent attacks of colic, progress can be followed by x-rays every 6–8 weeks.

Summary box 75.20

Indications for surgical removal of a ureteric calculus

- Repeated attacks of pain and the stone is not moving
- Stone is enlarging
- Complete obstruction of the kidney
- Urine is infected
- Stone is too large to pass
- Stone is obstructing solitary kidney or there is bilateral obstruction

Endoscopic stone removal

Dormia basket

The use of wire baskets under image intensifier control has been replaced by ureteroscopic techniques but they may be useful when the instruments and expertise are not available (Figure 75.29). There is a danger of ureteric injury even with small stones.

Ureteric meatotomy

Endoscopic incision with a diathermy knife will enlarge the opening and free a stone lodged in the intramural ureter. The consequent urinary reflux rarely causes problems.

Ureteroscopic stone removal

A ureteroscope is introduced transurethrally across the bladder into the ureter (Figure 75.30) to remove stones impacted in the

Enrico Dormia, 1928–2009, Professor of Urology, University of Milan and Chief of the Department of Urology, S Carlo Hospital, Milan.

ureter. Stones that cannot be caught in baskets or endoscopic forceps under direct vision are fragmented using an electrohydraulic, percussive or laser lithotripter.

Push bang

A stone in the middle or upper part of the ureter can often be flushed back into the kidney using a ureteric catheter. A J-stent secures the calculus in the kidney for subsequent treatment with ESWL.

A flexible fibreoptic ureteroscope can be used for laser destruction of calculi in the renal collecting system or ureter and to retrieve small stones from the kidney.

Lithotripsy *in situ*

A stone in a part of the ureter that can be identified by the imaging system of the lithotripter can be fragmented *in situ*. This form of treatment is not appropriate if there is complete obstruction or if the stone has been impacted for a long time.

Open surgery

Ureterolithotomy

An x-ray confirms the position of the stone immediately before surgery.

The skin incision must be appropriate for the position of the stone. Calculi in the upper third of the ureter are approached through a loin or upper quadrant transverse incision as used for a stone in the renal pelvis. Access to midureteric stones is through a muscle-cutting iliac fossa incision; lower ureteric stones are best reached through a Pfannenstiel incision. For stones close to the bladder, exposure is improved by ligating and dividing the superior vesical vascular pedicle. The ureter is exposed in the retroperitoneum and slings are applied above and below the calculus to stop it from escaping. The ureter is incised longitudinally, directly on to the stone, which is freed by blunt dissection and removed with stone forceps. Soft catheters are passed upwards and downwards to ensure that the ureter is clear. The ureterotomy is closed with interrupted absorbable sutures and a drain left to drain urine leakage. The operation can be performed laparoscopically, but alternative minimal access techniques described above are usually preferable.

IDIOPATHIC RETROPERITONEAL FIBROSIS

In this rare condition, one or both ureters are bound in progressive fibrosis of the retroperitoneal tissues. Most cases are idiopathic but some may be drug related. A similar clinical picture occurs in patients with leaking aortic aneurysm and infiltrating retroperitoneal malignancy.

The patient complains of persistent backache. The onset of anuria and renal failure prompts investigation of the renal tract, which reveals hydronephrosis. The IVU typically shows medial displacement of the ureters and the CT appearances are diagnostic. The sedimentation rate is markedly raised.

Treatment

It may be possible to insert temporary ureteric stents while renal function recovers. If not, percutaneous nephrostomies will drain the obstructed kidneys. Some patients need dialysis. Some advocate conservative treatment with steroids. Surgery involves dissection of the ureters from their fibrous jacket (ureterolysis). Wrapping omentum around the freed ureters discourages recurrent obstruction.

KIDNEY INFECTIONS

Aetiology

Renal infections arise in the following ways (Summary box 75.21):

- **Haematogenous infection** from a primary site in the tonsils or carious teeth or from cutaneous infections, particularly boils or a carbuncle. Renal tuberculosis occurs by bloodborne spread from lymph nodes in the neck, chest or abdomen.
- **Ascending infection** in the urinary tract is the most common route, and it is most likely to occur when there is vesicoureteric reflux. Urinary stasis and the presence of calculi are common contributory factors.

Bacteriology

Escherichia coli and other Gram-negative organisms are commonly responsible. In *E. coli* and streptococcal infections, the urine is acidic. *Proteus* spp. and staphylococci split urea to form ammonia, which makes the urine alkaline and promotes the formation of calculi.

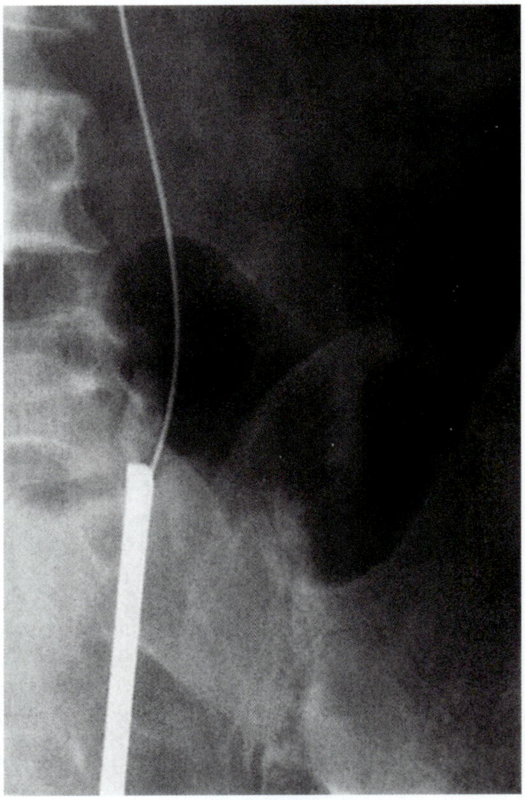

Figure 75.30 Ureteroscopy. X-ray showing a ureteroscope and guidewire in the lower ureter.

Herman Johann Pfannenstiel, 1862–1909, gynaecologist, Breslau, Germany, (now Wroclaw, Poland) described this incision in 1900.

Summary box 75.21

Kidney infection

- Acute pyelonephritis:
  - In childhood
  - In pregnancy
  - With urinary obstruction
- Chronic pyelonephritis:
  - Reflux nephropathy
- Pyonephrosis
- Renal abscess
- Perinephric abscess

Acute pyelonephritis

Acute pyelonephritis is more common in females, especially during childhood, at puberty, after intercourse, during pregnancy and during menopause. It occurs more on the right and is frequently bilateral.

Clinical features

There may be prodromal headache, lassitude and nausea, but the onset of pain is usually sudden, often with a rigor and vomiting. There is acute pain in the flank and hypochondrium. The remitting temperature rises to 39°C or more. The symptoms of cystitis commonly set in, with urgency, frequency and scalding dysuria. There is tenderness in the hypochondrium and in the loin. Rarely, in cases of severe bilateral pyelonephritis, especially when there is an associated obstruction, renal dysfunction may be sufficient to cause uraemia. The risk of life-threatening septicaemia is ever present (Summary box 75.22).

Summary box 75.22

Clinical features of kidney infections

- More common in women
- Often associated with septicaemia leading to pyrexia and rigors
- Associated with pyuria and occasionally haematuria
- Should be initially treated with broad-spectrum parenteral antibiotics
- Extremely dangerous if the kidney is obstructed

Bacteriological examination of the urine

A midstream urine specimen should be collected into a sterile container; the urine is centrifuged and the sediment examined microscopically. In early acute pyelonephritis, there are usually pus cells and many bacteria. The urine may be misleadingly clear to the eye until the infection becomes established. Culture and sensitivity testing of the causative organisms allows a rational choice of antibiotic, but parenteral treatment with a broad-spectrum antibiotic should be started before the results are available.

Severe cases

There are rigors and a temperature of 40°C or more, often without a corresponding tachycardia. There is vomiting, sweating and thirst; the patient feels awful. Blood culture is usually positive, especially if the specimen has been taken during a rigor.

Differential diagnosis

It may be difficult to be sure that the patient does not have pneumonia, acute appendicitis or acute cholecystitis. The urgent need is to distinguish acute pyelonephritis from appendicitis, and the site of pain and the presence of marked peritonism are usually helpful. A plain abdominal x-ray may show the outline of a swollen kidney and, if the infection is severe, a ultrasonographer may confirm the appearance of pyelonephritis.

Special cases

Pyelonephritis of pregnancy

Pyelonephritis of pregnancy usually occurs between the fourth and sixth months of gestation in women with a past history of recurrent urinary infection. In about 10 per cent of cases, the disease runs a severe and protracted course and occasionally leads to abortion or premature birth.

Urinary infection in childhood

Urinary infection in childhood may damage the growing kidney. In young children, symptoms are often non-specific but the child may pass cloudy or offensive urine. The possibility of urinary sepsis should be considered if a child fails to thrive or suffers unexplained pyrexia. Pain or screaming on micturition may occur. The older child may complain of loin pain and may develop urinary frequency and secondary enuresis.

Up to 50 per cent of children with urinary infection have an underlying anatomical abnormality (e.g. reflux or obstruction). The diagnosis of infection is confirmed by examination of a clean-catch specimen or a specimen obtained by suprapubic needle puncture. On culture, a pure growth of more than 10^5 organisms/mL with a significant pyuria is evidence of infection. Such children should be investigated for underlying urinary tract abnormalities and to assess renal function and scarring.

Vesicoureteric reflux of urine is detectable in about 35 per cent of children with recurrent urinary infection. Renal damage results from the combination of reflux and urinary infection early in life, and reflux nephropathy is a common cause of end-stage renal failure in the UK. Long-term prophylactic antibiotic treatment has become the favoured treatment for recurrent urinary infections resulting from reflux. Surgical reimplantation of the ureters is reserved for those in whom conservative measures fail. However, reimplantation in these patients may fail to cure reflux (Summary box 75.23).

Summary box 75.23

Urinary infection in childhood

- A single proven urinary infection in a child should prompt referral to a paediatric urologist

Acute pyelonephritis associated with urinary retention

Acute pyelonephritis is a relatively uncommon complication of chronic urinary retention. Often the organisms are introduced during instrumentation. Patients with a significant postmicturition urinary residue need prophylactic antibiotics to cover transurethral procedures.

Treatment

The treatment of acute pyelonephritis should be prompt, appropriate and prolonged. Investigation to exclude underlying abnormalities in the urinary tract should be undertaken when the acute illness subsides.

While awaiting the bacteriological report and the results of sensitivity tests, a broad-spectrum antibiotic, such as amoxicillin or gentamicin, should be administered, parenterally if necessary. When pain is severe, a morphine-like analgesic drug may be necessary if non-steroidal anti-inflammatory agents are ineffective. The patient should drink copiously; if this is not possible because of nausea and vomiting, an intravenous infusion should be set up.

Most urinary infections acquired outside hospital are sensitive to agents such as trimethoprim and amoxicillin. Hospital-acquired infections are much more likely to be resistant and second-line antibiotics may be needed. Gentamicin and carbenicillin are suitable for infections with more resistant strains of *Pseudomonas pyocyanea*, *Proteus* spp. and *Klebsiella* spp. Ciprofloxacin is particularly useful against *Pseudomonas* spp. in patients who do not have septicaemia. Despite the efficacy of modern antibacterial drugs, recurrent infection is likely if there is an untreated underlying abnormality of the urinary tract such as a stone, vesicoureteric reflux, fistula to the gastrointestinal tract or retention of urine.

Chronic pyelonephritis

Chronic pyelonephritis is often associated with vesicoureteric reflux, sometimes called 'reflux nephropathy', is an important cause of renal damage and end-stage renal failure.

Pathology

There is interstitial inflammation and scarring of the renal parenchyma with a patchy distribution.

Clinical features

The condition is almost three times as common in women as it is in men. Two-thirds of female patients are under 40 years of age, whereas 60 per cent of male patients are over 40.

It is possible, but unusual, for chronic pyelonephritis to remain clinically silent until the symptoms of advanced renal insufficiency appear.

Lumbar pain, dull and non-specific in character, is present in 60 per cent of cases. Increased urinary frequency and dysuria are common. Hypertension, present in 40 per cent of cases, may be of the accelerated ('malignant') type. Tiredness, malaise, anorexia, nausea and headache constitute the main complaint in 30 per cent of cases. The true cause of these nonspecific symptoms may elude diagnosis for years.

Normochromic anaemia due to unsuspected renal impairment is an occasional presenting feature (Summary box 75.24).

Investigations

The glomeruli are relatively preserved so proteinuria is less marked than in glomerulonephritis (<3 g daily). Casts are not usually present but white cells are plentiful.

Summary box 75.24

Chronic pyelonephritis

- A common cause of end-stage renal failure
- Often associated with ureteric reflux
- May be symptomatically silent
- Leads to progressive renal scarring

Escherichia coli, *Streptococcus faecalis*, *Proteus* spp. or *Pseudomonas* spp. are found in the urine.

Treatment

Treatment aims at eradicating predisposing factors such as obstruction or stones and treating the infection, often with repeated courses of antibiotic. Scarred parenchyma is vulnerable to blood-borne organisms and reinfection is likely. Consequently, antibiotics confer only temporary benefit and progressive renal damage is common.

Surgery is indicated only when the disease is confined to one kidney. This is unusual but in such cases nephrectomy or partial nephrectomy may stop the symptoms of infection and make hypertension easier to control. Patients with end-stage renal failure require renal replacement therapy.

Pyonephrosis

Pyonephrosis results from infection of a hydronephrosis, follows acute pyelonephritis or, most commonly, arises as a complication of renal calculus disease. The kidney becomes a multilocular sac containing pus or purulent urine.

Clinical features

The classical triad of symptoms is anaemia, fever and a swelling in the loin. When the condition arises as an infected hydronephrosis, the swelling may be very large and the pyrexia very high and associated with rigors. Symptoms of cystitis may be prominent.

Investigations

Imaging may show a calculus and will demonstrate dilatation of the pus-filled collecting system.

Treatment

Pyonephrosis is a surgical emergency because permanent renal damage and lethal septicaemia threaten. Parenteral antibiotics should be given and the kidney drained. If the pus is too thick to be aspirated through a large percutaneous nephrostomy, consider open nephrostomy. When there is a stone, it should be removed. Nephrectomy may be appropriate when the kidney is destroyed and function on the other side is good.

Renal carbuncle

An abscess may form in the renal parenchyma as the result of blood-borne spread of organisms, especially coliforms or *Staphylococcus aureus*. Renal carbuncle is most commonly seen in diabetics, intravenous drug abusers, those debilitated by chronic disease and patients with acquired immunodeficiency.

Pathology

The renal parenchyma contains an encapsulated necrotic mass.

Clinical features

There is an ill-defined tender swelling in the loin, persistent pyrexia and leukocytosis, simulating a perinephric abscess. Initially there is no pus or bacteria in the urine, but these appear later. The mass in the kidney may be confused with a renal adenocarcinoma (Figure 75.31).

Treatment

Resolution by antibiotic treatment alone is unusual. Formal open incision of the abscess may be necessary if the pus is too thick to be drained by percutaneous aspiration.

Perinephric abscess

The common causes of perinephric abscess are shown in Figure 75.32. Other causes are infection of a perirenal haematoma and perinephric discharge of an untreated pyonephrosis or renal carbuncle. A mycobacterial perinephric abscess may arise by extension from a nearby tuberculous vertebra.

Clinical features

There is swinging pyrexia, abdominal tenderness and fullness in the loin (Figure 75.33). Local signs present early if the infection starts in the lower part of the perinephric fat. Infection at the upper pole is masked by the lower ribs and signs in the loin are less. The white cell count is always markedly raised but there are characteristically no pus cells or organisms in the urine.

Imaging

Ultrasonography and CT are diagnostic.

Treatment

Open drainage may be necessary if the abscess cannot be aspirated through a percutaneous needle. A lumbar incision is made under antibiotic cover large enough to allow the surgeon to open pockets of pus and to explore for an unruptured cortical abscess. Pus is sent for culture and the wound is closed over a tube drain (Summary box 75.25).

> **Summary box 75.25**
>
> **Management of perinephric abscess**
>
> - Collections of pus in or around the kidney should be drained

Renal tuberculosis

Aetiology and pathology

Tuberculosis of the urinary tract arises from haematogenous infection from a distant focus. The lesions are usually unilateral. Tuberculous granulomas in a renal pyramid coalesce to form an ulcer. Mycobacteria and pus cells discharge into the urine. Untreated lesions enlarge and a tuberculous abscess may form in the parenchyma. The necks of the calyces and the renal pelvis stenosed by fibrosis confine the infection so that there is tuberculous pyonephrosis, sometimes localised to one pole of the kidney. Extension of pyonephrosis or tuberculous renal abscess leads to perinephric abscess and the kidney is progressively replaced by caseous material (putty kidney), which may

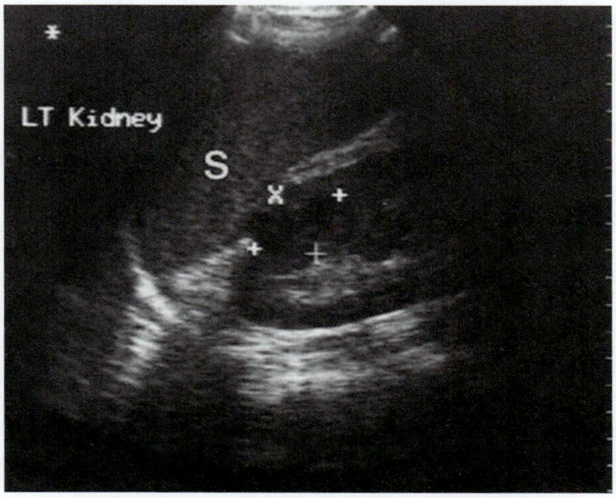

Figure 75.31 Longitudinal ultrasound scan through the upper pole of the left kidney demonstrates a renal carbuncle, outlined by crosses. S, spleen.

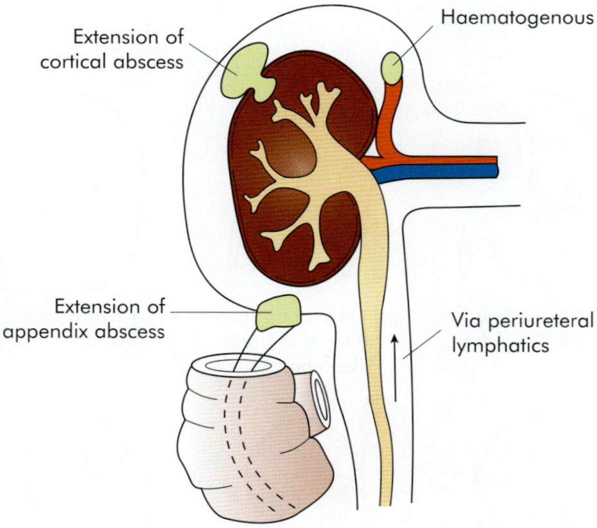

Figure 75.32 Sources of perinephric abscess.

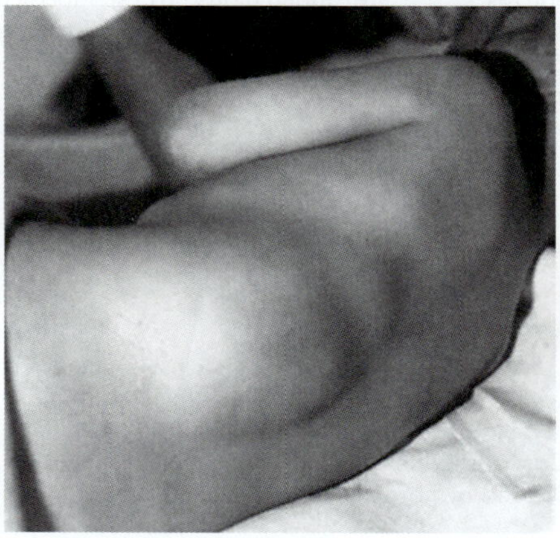

Figure 75.33 A large perinephric abscess.

be calcified (cement kidney). At any stage, the plain x-ray may show areas of calcification (pseudocalculi). Less commonly, the kidneys may be bilaterally affected as part of the generalised process of miliary tuberculosis (Figure 75.34).

Renal tuberculosis is often associated with tuberculosis of the bladder and typical tuberculous granulomas may be visible in the bladder wall. In men, tuberculous epididymo-orchitis may occur without apparent infection of the bladder.

Clinical features

Renal tuberculosis usually occurs between 20 and 40 years of age, and is more common in men than women.

Urinary frequency is often the earliest symptom and may be the only one. The patient complains of a progressive increase in both daytime and night-time frequency.

'Sterile' pyuria

Routine urine culture is negative but there are white cells in the urine.

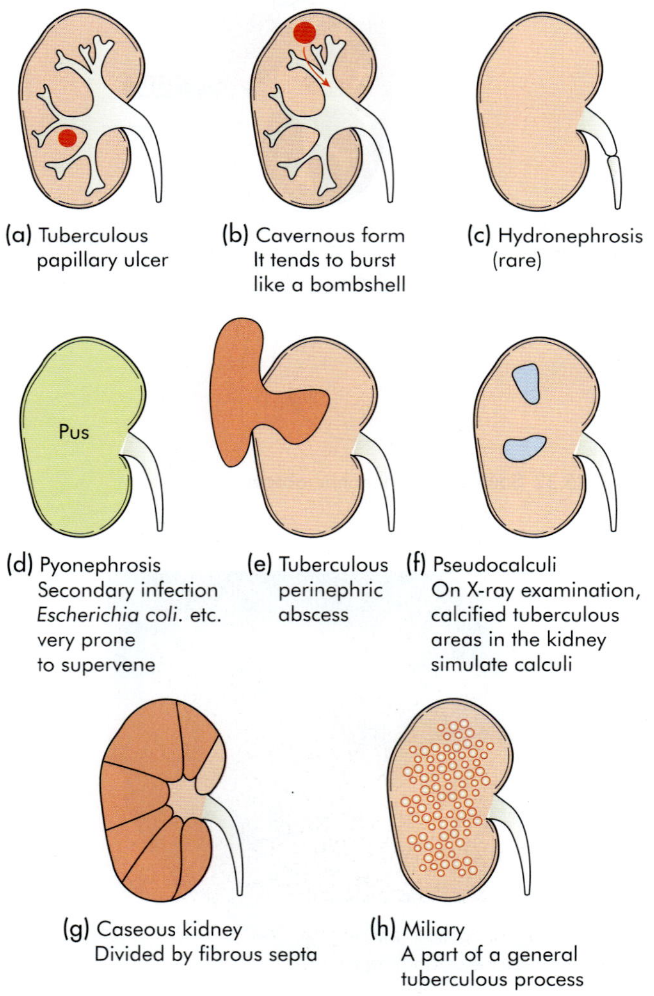

Figure 75.34 Types of lesion in renal tuberculosis.

Pain

Painful micturition is a feature of tuberculous cystitis. First, there is a suprapubic pain if voiding is delayed; later, a burning pain accompanies micturition. When there is secondary infection, a superadded agonising pain referred to the tip of the penis or to the vulva is often associated with haematuria and strangury.

Renal pain is often minimal but there may be a dull ache in the loin.

Haematuria

In 5 per cent of cases, the first symptom is haematuria occurring from an ulcer on a renal papilla. The tuberculous lesion may be difficult to detect radiologically and mycobacteria may not be cultured from the urine until months later.

A tuberculous kidney is oedematous and friable and is more liable to damage than a normal kidney.

Malaise and weight loss are usual and a low-level evening pyrexia is typical. A high temperature suggests secondary infection or dissemination, i.e. miliary tuberculosis.

On examination

It is unusual for a tuberculous kidney to be palpable. The prostate, seminal vesicles, vasa and scrotal contents should be examined for nodules or thickening (Summary box 75.26).

Summary box 75.26

Renal tuberculosis

- Consider when symptoms of cystitis continue despite treatment with antibiotics
- Is a cause of 'sterile pyuria'
- Causes chronic inflammation and scarring throughout the urinary tract, which may continue after antituberculous treatment has been instituted
- May cause obstructive lesions throughout the urinary tract

Investigation

Bacteriological

Three complete specimens of early-morning urine should be sent for microscopy and culture before specific chemotherapy is started. Staining of the urine sediment with the Ziehl–Neelsen stain occasionally shows the presence of acid-fast bacilli, but proof that these are pathological mycobacteria must await culture on Löwenstein–Jensen medium. When the clinical picture is convincing, it is permissible to start anti-tuberculous therapy in anticipation of the culture results some 6 weeks later.

X-ray

An abdominal x-ray may show calcified lesions.

Intravenous urography

Early in the disease, the clear-cut outline of a renal papilla may be rendered indistinct by the presence of ulceration. Later, there may be calyceal stenosis (Figure 75.35) and/or hydronephrosis caused by stricture of the renal pelvis or the ureter draining the affected kidney (Figure 75.36). A tuberculous abscess appears as a space-occupying renal lesion. The bladder may appear shrunken, with its wall irregular or thickened.

Cystoscopy

Cystoscopy is not routine in the investigation of urinary tuberculosis but is often performed because there has been haematuria or unexplained bladder symptoms. The tuberculous urothelium is studded with granulomas that cluster particularly around the ureteric orifices, sometimes with ulceration. As the bladder wall fibroses, the bladder capacity decreases. Contraction of the fibrosed ureter tugs at the ureteric orifice, which is displaced upwards, its mouth wide open (the so-called 'golf-hole' orifice).

Chest x-ray

A chest x-ray will exclude an active lung lesion.

Treatment

Anti-tuberculous chemotherapy is best managed by a specialist. The surgeon must ensure that the state of the urinary tract is reviewed during the first few weeks of therapy because scarring and stricture continue after treatment has started.

Prognosis in renal tuberculosis is good if the patient completes the course of chemotherapy.

Operative treatment

Operative treatment should be conservative, aiming to remove large foci of infection, which are difficult to treat with drugs, and correct the obstruction caused by fibrosis. The optimum time for surgery is between 6 and 12 weeks after the start of anti-tuberculous chemotherapy.

A repertoire of procedures is needed to deal with various potential effects of urinary tuberculosis. An obstructed lower pole calyx may be drained into the upper ureter. A strictured renal pelvis needs a pyeloplasty. Ureteric stenosis and shortening may require a Boari operation or a bowel interposition, depending on the level and extent of the fibrosis. If the kidney has no function it is best to perform a nephroureterectomy (Figure 75.37). A badly contracted bladder may be replaced with a neobladder fashioned from a loop of bowel in a substitution cystoplasty.

NEOPLASMS OF THE KIDNEY

Neoplasms of the kidney are summarised in Summary box 75.27.

Summary box 75.27

Renal neoplasms

Benign neoplasms
- Adenoma
- Angioma
- Angiomyolipoma

Malignant neoplasms
- Wilms' tumour (nephroblastoma in children)
- Grawitz's tumour (adenocarcinoma, hypernephroma)
- Transitional cell carcinoma of the renal pelvis and collecting system
- Squamous cell carcinoma of the renal pelvis

Benign neoplasms

Adenoma

Pea-like cortical adenomas are occasionally discovered. They are asymptomatic and are benign.

Angioma

Angioma may cause profuse haematuria, often in young adults. The bleeding source may be difficult to diagnose without renal angiography.

Angiomyolipoma

Angiomyolipoma is an unusual tumour of the kidney often but not always associated with tuberous sclerosis. Its high fat

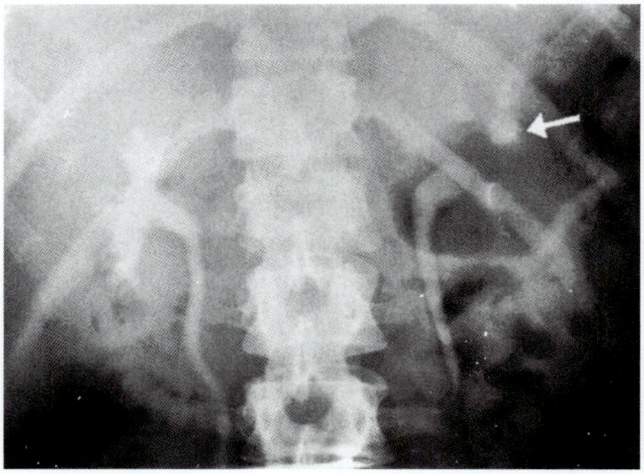

Figure 75.35 Intravenous urogram showing a small localised tuberculous lesion with hydrocalyx (arrow). Healing took place with conservative treatment.

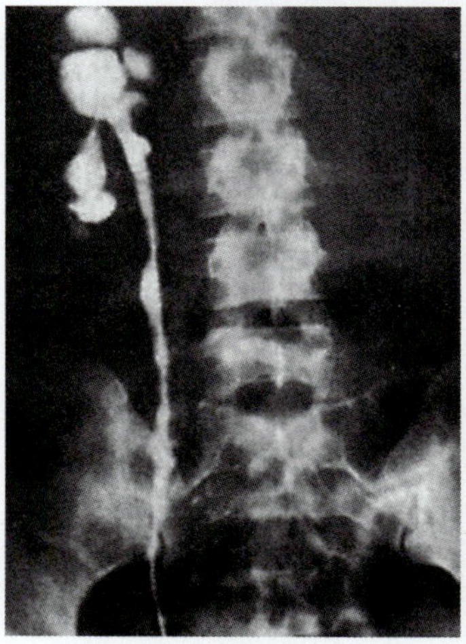

Figure 75.36 Retrograde ureterogram showing advanced tuberculosis of the right kidney. Right retrograde study shows multiple ureteric strictures and gross distortion of the internal architecture of the affected kidney.

content has a typical appearance on CT. Malignant elements are present in about one-quarter and may metastasise.

Malignant neoplasms

Renal neoplasm in children

Wilms' tumour (synonym: nephroblastoma)

This mixed tumour contains elements from embryonic nephrogenic tissue (Figure 75.38). Nephroblastoma is usually discovered during the first five years of life, usually in one pole of one kidney. Bilateral tumours pose a difficult problem.

Pathology

A rapidly growing tumour is likely to be friable in consistency.

Clinical features

An abdominal tumour grows rapidly in a poorly child. The mass may be very large. Some patients are hypertensive.

Haematuria is an unfavourable symptom denoting extension of the tumour into the renal pelvis.

Imaging confirms a solid space-occupying lesion in the kidney, with or without venous invasion, contralateral disease and distant spread.

Metastasis to the lungs occurs early. Liver, bone and brain metastases are rare. Lymphatic spread is uncommon.

Treatment

These children are best treated in specialist paediatric oncology units. Most unilateral tumours are treated by chemotherapy followed by nephrectomy. Partial nephrectomy may be possible in patients with bilateral disease.

Prognosis

Eighty per cent survive long term with modern chemotherapy and surgery. The prognosis is worse in those with metastases and in older children (Summary box 75.28).

Summary box 75.28

Nephroblastoma (Wilms' tumour)

- Usually presents in the first five years of life
- Typically presents with an abdominal mass
- May cause haematuria, abdominal pain or fever
- Metastasises to the lung
- Is best treated in a specialist paediatric oncology unit

Renal neoplasm in adults

Hypernephroma (synonym: Grawitz's tumour)

This adenocarcinoma, the most common neoplasm of the kidney (75 per cent incidence), arises from renal tubular cells.

Pathology

The cut surface is usually yellowish or dull white, semi-transparent, with areas of haemorrhage (Figure 75.39). The tumour is often divided into lobules, some of which are cystic. Larger tumours are irregular in shape with central haemorrhage and necrosis.

Microscopic structure

The most common pattern is of solid areas of polyhedral or cubical clear cells with deeply stained, small, rounded nuclei and abundant cytoplasm containing lipids, cholesterol and glycogen. The cells are occasionally arranged as papillary cysts or tubules. Less commonly, the cells are granular (dark), and both clear and dark cells may be represented in the same tumour. The scanty stroma is richly vascular.

Spread

The tumour is prone to grow into the renal vein. Cells enter the circulation and reach the lungs, where they grow to form can-

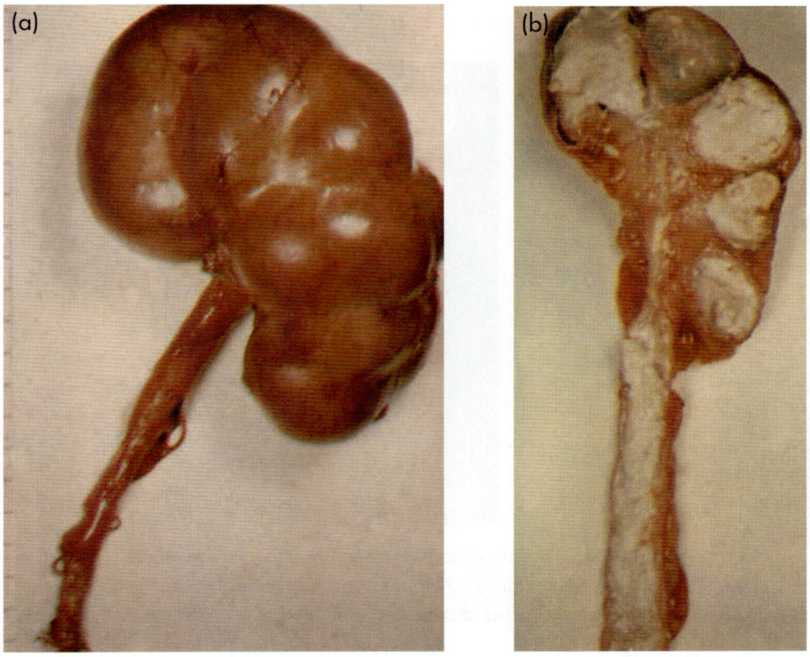

Figure 75.37 (a and b) Nephroureterectomy specimen from a patient with a kidney destroyed by tuberculous pyonephrosis.

Paul Albert Grawitz, 1850–1932, Professor of Pathology, Greifswald, Germany, described adeno-carcinoma of the kidney in 1884.

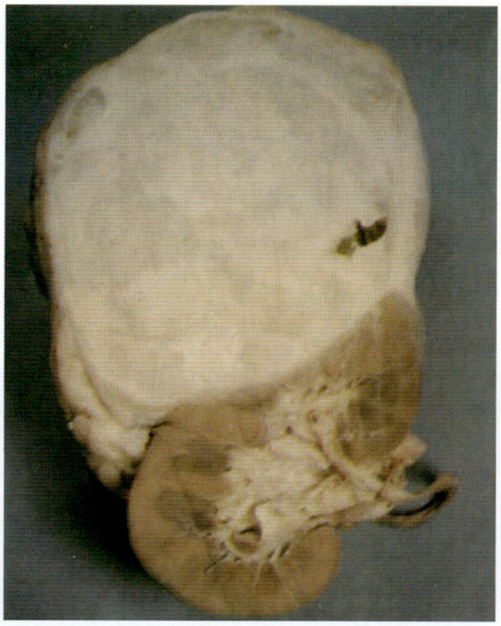

Figure 75.38 Wilms' tumour.

nonball secondary deposits (Figure 75.40). Metastasis to bone also occurs and a secondary deposit in a long bone may be the only sign of distant spread for a year or more. Highly vascular metastases may pulsate. Tumour extending beyond the renal capsule is liable to metastasise via the lymph nodes in the hilum of the kidney to the para-aortic nodes and beyond.

Clinical features

Adenocarcinoma of the kidney is more common in men. Haematuria is usually the presenting symptom, sometimes with clot colic. There may be a dragging discomfort in the loin or the patient may detect a mass. In men, a rapidly developing varicocele is a rare but impressive sign, most often on the left side because the left gonadal vein is obstructed where it joins the left renal vein.

Atypical presentations

In 25 per cent of cases there are no local symptoms. The patient presents with symptomatic secondary deposits in bone (Figure 75.41) or the lung (persistent cough or haemoptysis).

Occasionally, persistent pyrexia (37.8–38.9°C) with no evidence of infection is the only symptom. Pyrexia after nephrectomy suggests metastases.

A few patients present with constitutional symptoms and anaemia.

Polycythaemia occurs in 4 per cent of cases as a result of the production of erythropoietin by tumour cells. The erythrocyte sedimentation rate is always raised above the 1–2 mm found in idiopathic polycythaemia vera. The blood count returns to normal after nephrectomy unless there are metastases. Other hormones, such as renin and calcitonin, may be produced by the tumour. Hypercalcaemia is common.

Nephrotic syndrome has been reported as a rare presentation of hypernephroma.

Investigation

IVU is being supplanted by CT in the investigation of haematuria. There is typically abnormal calcification and distortion of the renal outline. The calyces may be stretched and distorted. It is important to know whether the contralateral kidney is working (Figure 75.42). CT with enhancement will demonstrate the extent of the lesion and will show whether the hilar lymph nodes or renal vein are involved (Figure 75.43).

Enthusiasm for renal angiography and preoperative embolisation has waned. Occasionally, a flush inferior cava shows the extent of caval involvement by tumour growing in from the renal vein.

A chest x-ray is essential to detect lung secondaries. An isotope bone scan will reveal deposits in bone.

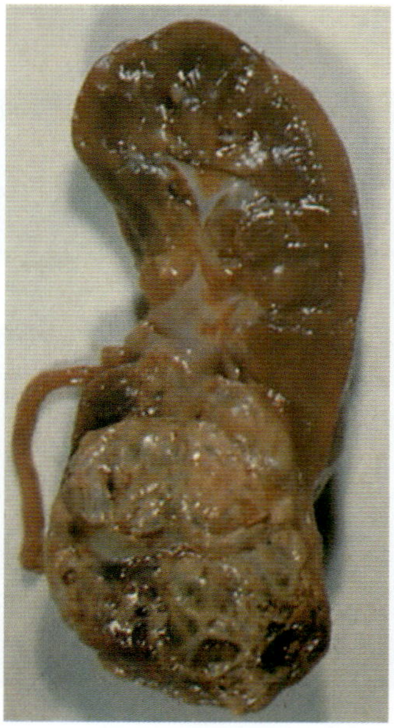

Figure 75.39 Adenocarcinoma of the kidney (Grawitz's tumour).

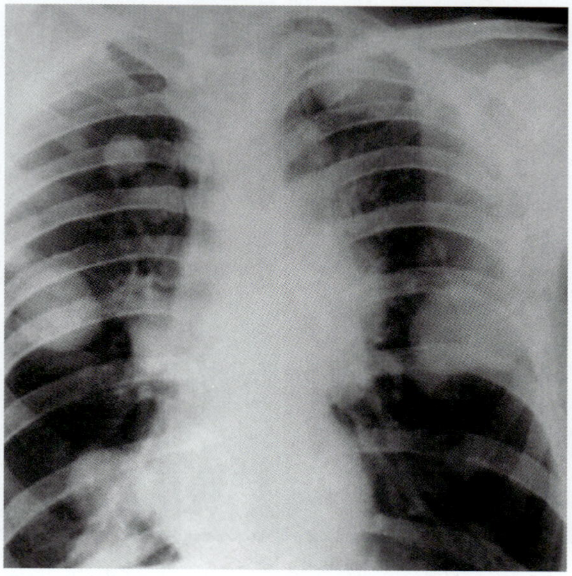

Figure 75.40 Cannonball secondaries from a hypernephroma.

Treatment

Nephrectomy can be performed through a loin or a transverse or oblique upper abdominal incision. The transabdominal approach has the advantage that the renal pedicle and the inferior vena cava can be widely exposed.

The vascular pedicle should be ligated before the kidney is mobilised because handling the tumour may cause malignant cells to be released into the circulation. The first step in the procedure is to ligate the renal artery in continuity. Once the artery is occluded, the tumour loses most of its profuse blood supply and massive bleeding during mobilisation becomes less likely. Gentle palpation of the renal vein ensures that there is no tumour in its lumen. An empty vein can be divided between ligatures. The renal artery is then divided and the kidney mobilised within its coverings. Aberrant vessels feeding the tumour must be ligated or coagulated to avoid troublesome bleeding. The ureter is then traced downwards as far as is safe, tied and divided.

If the renal vein or the inferior vena cava is invaded, the surgeon must obtain early control of the cava above and below the tumour extension. If there is extension into the thorax, the cardiac team may be needed to put the patient on cardiac bypass so that tumour can, if necessary, be removed from the right side of the heart.

Renal adenocarcinoma responds poorly to radiotherapy or conventional chemotherapy. There have been early promising results from clinical trials of the cytokine interleukin-2 in this condition.

Prognosis

Removal of even a large neoplasm may be curative. In operable cases, 70 per cent of patients are well after three years and 60 per cent after five years. Macroscopic involvement of the renal vein or its tributaries, invasion beyond the capsule and lymphatic involvement all worsen the prognosis (Summary box 75.29).

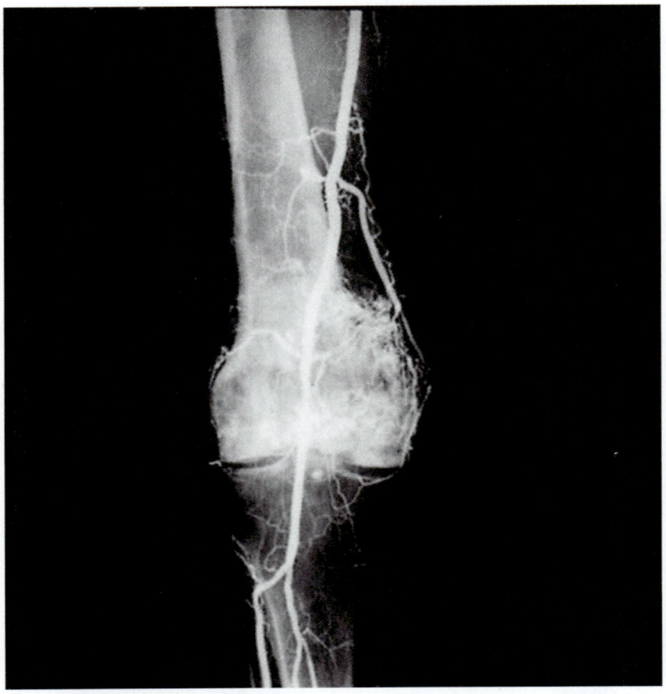

Figure 75.41 Arteriogram showing a vascular 'blush' due to metastasis in the femur from a Grawitz's tumour.

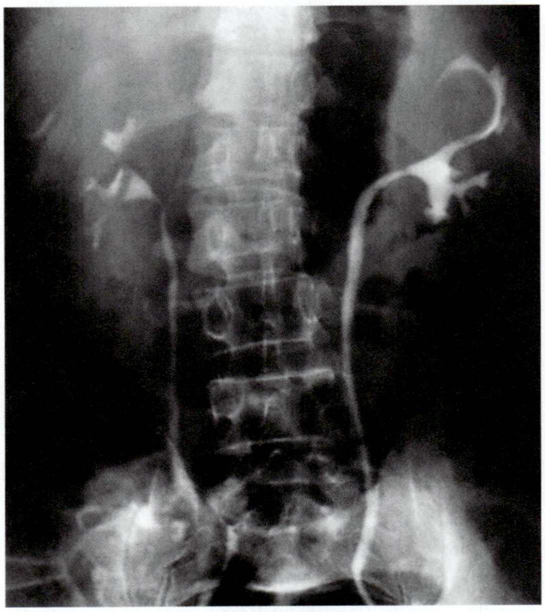

Figure 75.42 Intravenous urogram in a case of hypernephroma of the left kidney. The only symptom was one attack of painless haematuria. Note the displacement of the upper pole calyces by the mass.

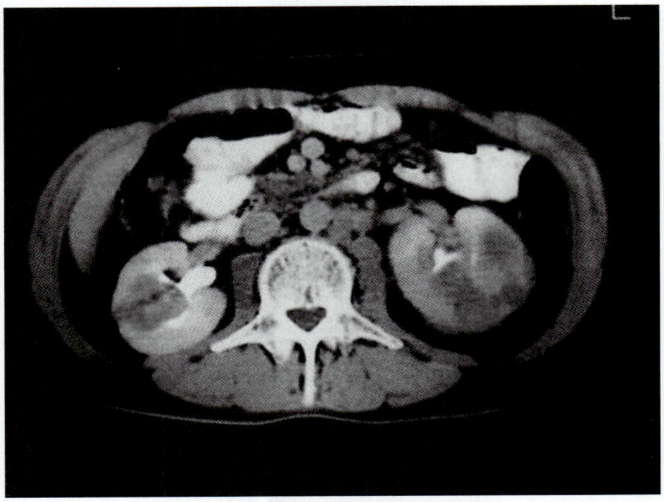

Figure 75.43 Computed tomography scan showing large bilateral renal adenocarcinomas.

Summary box 75.29

Adenocarcinoma of the kidney

- Often presents with haematuria
- May be associated with pyrexia of unknown origin, polycythaemia, hypercalcaemia, anaemia and other paraneoplastic symptoms
- Metastasises via the bloodstream to bone, liver and lung (cannonball secondaries)
- Renal vein extension may embolise to the pulmonary circulation during nephrectomy

Papillary transitional cell tumours of the renal pelvis

These resemble those of the bladder but are much less common (Figure 75.44). They may invade the renal parenchyma, be multifocal and metastasise. Multiple ureteric tumours are thought to arise from a field change that predisposes the whole urothelium to metaplasia rather than seeding down the ureter. Whether the carcinogen is chemical or viral is uncertain.

Clinical features

Haematuria is the most common clinical symptom.

The presence of malignant cells in the urine may indicate whether the tumour is well or poorly differentiated. There is some evidence that those with poorly differentiated tumours do better if they have preoperative radiotherapy. It is therefore useful to obtain cells from the tumour by sampling using a brush or catheter passed up the ureter under radiological control.

Intravenous urography usually demonstrates the tumour (Figure 75.45). Retrograde pyelography may be helpful if the urogram is indistinct.

Treatment

Conventional surgical treatment is by nephroureterectomy. The ureter must be disconnected with a cuff of bladder wall. If this is done by open surgery a second incision is needed to remove the kidney. Alternatively, the ureteric orifice can be widely resected with a resectoscope and the ureter delivered by blunt dissection from the upper abdominal wound used to remove the kidney. Some urologists argue that well-differentiated upper urinary tract transitional tumours should be treated conservatively by resection with appropriate steps taken to avoid the growth of tumour seeded in the percutaneous track.

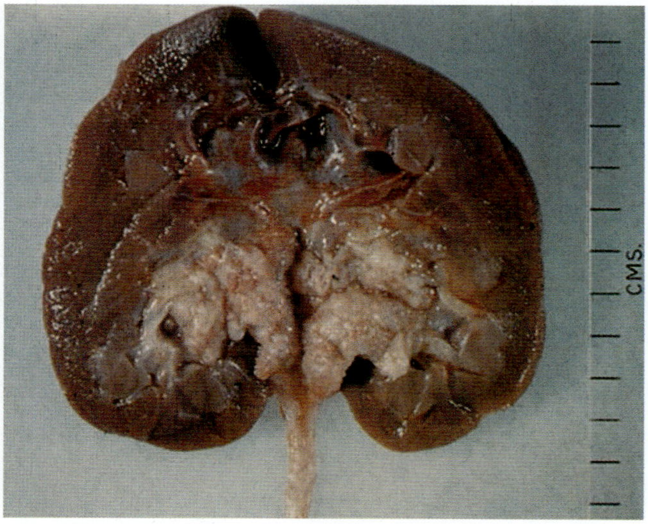

Figure 75.44 Papillary transitional cell tumour of the renal pelvis.

Squamous cell carcinoma of the renal pelvis

This is rare and often associated with chronic inflammation and leucoplakia resulting from stone. The tumours are radiosensitive but metastasise early and the prognosis is poor.

Transitional cell tumours of the ureter

These are rare and behave like tumours of the renal pelvis. Treatment is by nephroureterectomy.

About half of patients with tumours of the upper urinary tract will have tumours in the bladder at some stage. Follow up by cystoscopy with regular urography is therefore necessary to detect recurrent tumours.

Balkan nephropathy

Transitional cell tumours of the upper urinary tract have a very high incidence in certain areas of the Balkans. The same population has a high incidence of a form of primary nephropathy. The causative agent has not been identified with certainty but there seems to be an association with the consumption of grain products stored in a damp environment. Tumours that develop against a background of Balkan nephropathy should be treated by nephron-sparing surgery in view of the impaired overall renal function.

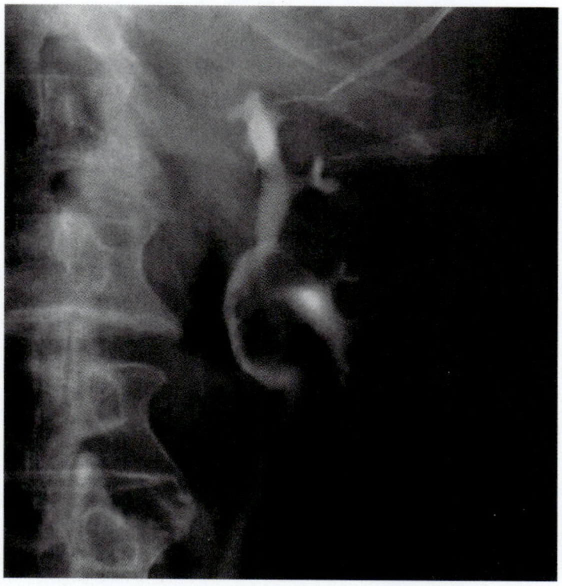

Figure 75.45 Intravenous urogram showing a filling defect in the left renal pelvis due to transitional cell carcinoma.

The Balkans are the countries of the south-east of Europe. They lie south of the Danube and Sava rivers, and form a peninsula bounded on the east by the Aegean and Black Seas, on the west by the Adriatic and Ionian Seas, and on the south by the Mediterranean.

Nephrectomy for benign disease

Nephrectomy is now rarely performed for benign disease except when the kidney is atrophic or dysplastic or the cause of accelerated hypertension. Non-functioning kidneys resulting from longstanding obstruction or stone disease are a potential site for infection and even malignancy. In a simple nephrectomy, the kidney is dissected free through the convenient plane between the capsule and its fatty coverings. If this plane is obscured by the scarring of previous surgery, a subcapsular nephrectomy may be safer.

Laparoscopic renal surgery

The benefits of laparoscopy are being progressively applied to the whole range of renal surgery. Laparoscopic nephrectomy is certainly possible for small kidneys destroyed by benign disease. The technique requires special skills and the full costs and benefits are under evaluation. More complex techniques are necessary when there is bulky excised tissue to be extracted. Laparoscopic surgery for pyelopasty, ureterolysis and nephrectomy for renal malignancy have all been described.

Hypertension and a unilateral renal lesion

Ischaemia of the renal parenchyma leads to the release of pressor agents that cause arterial hypertension. When a renal lesion is discovered during the investigation of hypertension, nephrectomy may make the hypertension more amenable to drug treatment.

FURTHER READING

Blandy JP, Kaisary AV. *Lecture Notes: urology*, 6th edn. Oxford: Blackwell, 2007.

Reynard J, Brewster S, Biers S. *Oxford handbook of urology*. Oxford: Oxford University Press, 2009.

Tanagho EA, McAnich JW (eds). *Smith's general urology*, 17th edn. New Europe: McGraw-Hill Education, New 2008.

Wein AJ, Kavoussi LR, Novick AC *et al. Campbell–Walsh urology*, 10th edn. Philadelphia, PA: Elsevier – Health Sciences Division Saunders, 2011.

CHAPTER 76

The urinary bladder

LEARNING OBJECTIVES

To understand:

- The anatomy, vascular supply and innervation of the bladder in relation to function and disease
- The principles of management of bladder trauma, incontinence and fistulae
- The common causes of acute and chronic urinary retention and management
- The different types of bladder cancer and the principles of management

SURGICAL ANATOMY OF THE BLADDER

- It is lined by transitional epithelium covering the connective tissue lamina propria, which contains a rich plexus of vessels and lymphatics.
- When the detrusor muscle hypertrophies, the inner layer, covered by urothelium, stands out, resulting in the appearance of trabeculation.
- Over the trigone is a thin layer of smooth muscle to which the epithelium is closely adherent and which extends as a sheath around the lower ureters and into the proximal urethra.
- Around the male bladder neck is the smooth muscle internal sphincter innervated by adrenergic fibres, which prevents retrograde ejaculation.
- The distal urethral sphincter is a horseshoe-shaped mass of striated muscle that lies anterior and distal to the prostate, or in the proximal two-thirds of the female urethra. It is distinct from the pelvic floor and is supplied by S2–S4 fibres via the pudendal nerve and by somatic fibres passing through the inferior hypogastric plexus.

Fascial and ligamentous supports of the bladder

At the posterolateral bladder neck, condensations of fascia pass forward medially and laterally to the ureter to join with the prostatic fascia; this fascia needs to be divided during cystectomy. The puboprostatic ligaments are well-defined condensations of the anterior endopelvic fascia; they stretch from the front of the prostate to the periosteum of the pubis and lie lateral to the dorsal vein complex. The urachus and obliterated hypogastric arteries, together with the folds of peritoneum overlying them, are called the median and lateral umbilical ligaments. Condensations of fascia also occur around the superior and inferior vascular pedicles.

Arteries

The superior and inferior vesical arteries are derived from the anterior trunk of the internal iliac artery. Branches from the obturator and inferior gluteal arteries (and from the uterine and vaginal arteries in females) also help to supply the bladder.

Veins

The veins form a plexus on the lateral and inferior surfaces of the bladder. In the male, the prostatic plexus is continuous with the vesical plexus, which drains into the internal iliac vein. In the female, similar large veins are continuous with the vaginal plexus.

Lymphatics

These accompany the veins and drain to nodes along the internal iliac vessels and then to the obturator and external iliac chains. Some lymphatics pass to nodes that are situated posteriorly to the internal iliac artery (hypogastric nodes).

INNERVATION

The parasympathetic input

This is derived from the anterior primary divisions of the second, third and fourth sacral segments (mainly S2 and S3). Fibres pass through the pelvic splanchnic nerves to the inferior hypogastric plexus, from where they are distributed to the bladder (Figure 76.1). The pelvic plexus can be damaged during deep pelvic operations.

The sympathetic input

This arises in the 11th thoracic to the second lumbar segments; fibres pass via the presacral hypogastric nerve (rather than via the sympathetic chains) to the inferior hypogastric plexus.

Somatic innervation

A somatic innervation passes to the distal sphincter mechanism via the pudendal nerves and also via fibres that pass through the inferior hypogastric plexus.

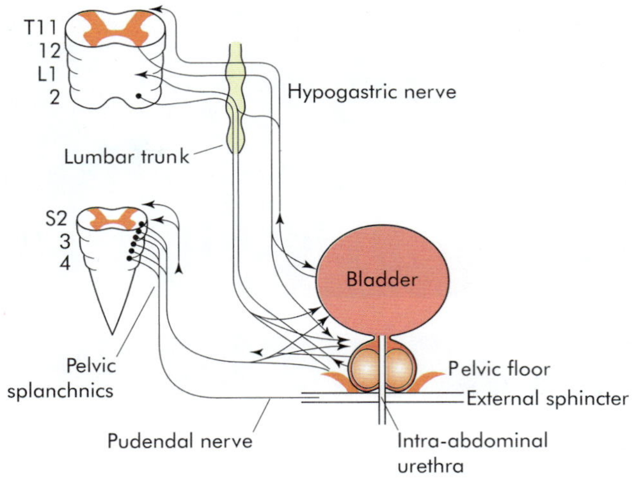

Figure 76.1 The nervous control of the bladder. Micturition is partly a reflex and partly a voluntary act.

Functional aspects

Sympathetic nerves convey afferents from the fundus. Afferents arise from the mucosa, where they respond to touch, temperature and pain, and from the detrusor and lamina propria, where they convey stretch information. Afferents pass via the inferior hypogastric plexus to the posterior roots of S2–S4. Some aspects of micturition are centred in the pons, where detrusor contraction is coordinated with inhibition of the distal sphincter. Interruption of this pathway below the pons with preservation of the sacral cord is likely to result in a contractile detrusor and tonically active distal sphincter that will not relax during voiding (detrusor–sphincter dyssynergia).

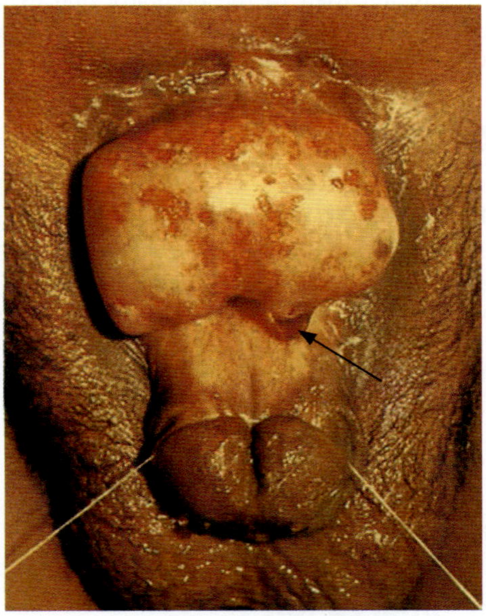

Figure 76.2 Ectopia vesicae in a male. A drop of urine (arrow) is seen at the left ureteric orifice, the corona glandis being retracted by threads (courtesy of GD Adhia, Bombay, India).

CONGENITAL DEFECTS OF THE BLADDER

Bladder exstrophy

Clinical features

Bladder exstrophy occurs in 1:50000 births (male–female ratio 4:1) (Figure 76.2). In the male, the penis is broad and short, and bilateral inguinal herniae may be present. There is separation of the pubic bones (Figure 76.3). In epispadias alone, the pubes are united and external genitalia are almost normal, although in the female the clitoris is bifid (Figure 76.4).

Treatment

The bladder is closed in the first year of life, usually following osteotomy of both iliac bones just lateral to the sacroiliac joints. Later, reconstruction of the bladder neck and sphincters is required. In some patients the reconstructed bladder remains small and requires augmentation. One-stage reconstruction is being practised in some major centres.

Less satisfactorily, urinary diversion can be carried out by means of ureterosigmoid anastomosis, an ileal or colonic conduit, or continent urinary diversion. Long-term complications include: (1) stricture at the site of anastomosis with bilateral hydronephrosis and infection; (2) hyperchloraemic acidosis; and (3) an increased (20-fold) risk of tumour formation (adenoma and adenocarcinoma) at the site of a ureterocolic anastomosis.

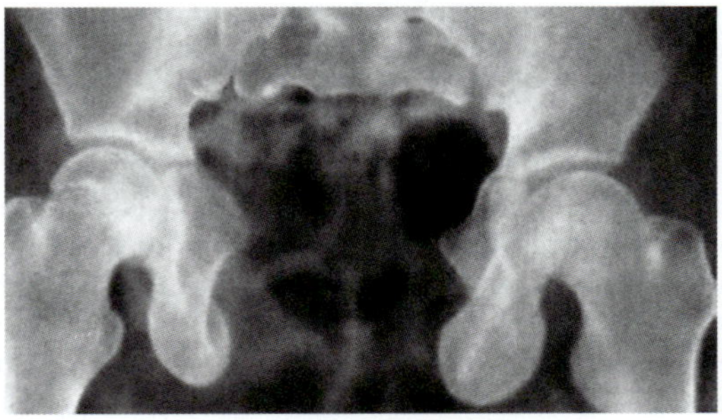

Figure 76.3 Separation of the pubes in a case of ectopia vesicae (courtesy of the late Professor Grey Turner, London, England).

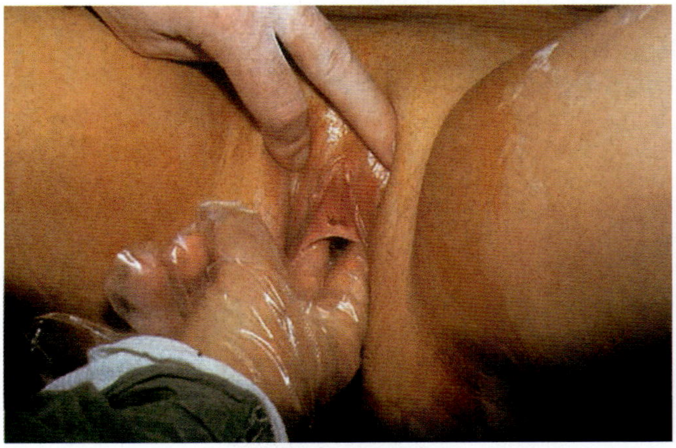

Figure 76.4 Female epispadias showing deficient sphincter and bifid clitoris.

BLADDER TRAUMA

Bladder rupture

This can be intraperitoneal (20 per cent) or extraperitoneal (80 per cent) (Figures 76.5 and 76.6). Intraperitoneal rupture is usually secondary to a blow or fall on a distended bladder, more rarely to surgical damage. Extraperitoneal rupture is caused by blunt trauma or surgical damage. Gross haematuria can be absent. It may be difficult to distinguish extraperitoneal rupture from rupture of the membranous urethra (see Chapter 78). Intraperitoneal rupture is associated with sudden severe pain in the hypogastrium, often accompanied by syncope. The shock subsides and the abdomen distends and there is no desire to micturate. Peritonitis does not follow immediately if the urine is sterile; varying degrees of rigidity are present on examination.

Investigation

Computed tomography (CT) is ideal. Plain erect x-rays may show a ground-glass appearance (fluid). Intravenous urography (IVU) may confirm a leak. Retrograde cystography will confirm the diagnosis (Figure 76.7). It is important to image the patient after drainage of contrast as the full bladder may mask extravasation (Summary box 76.1).

Summary box 76.1

Bladder trauma

- Intraperitoneal or extraperitoneal
- Suspected if there is trauma and damage to the pelvis
- May be diagnosed by retrograde cystography

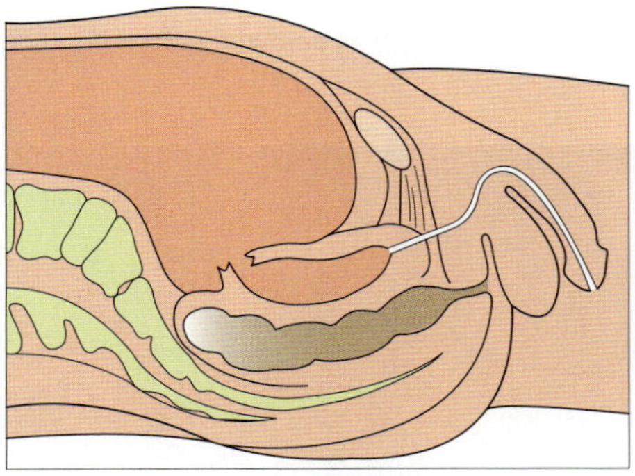

Figure 76.5 Intraperitoneal extravasation of urine.

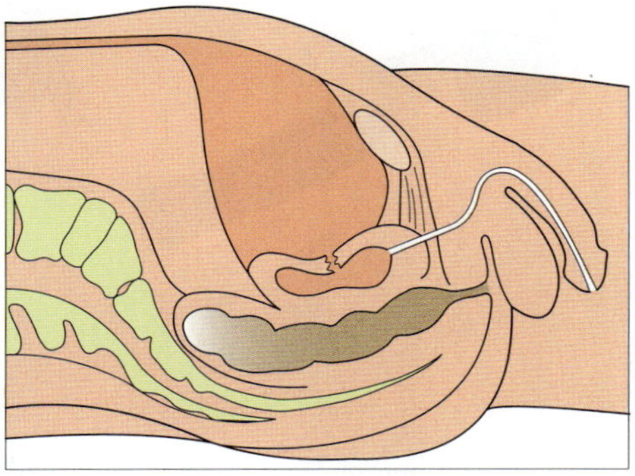

Figure 76.6 Extraperitoneal extravasation of urine.

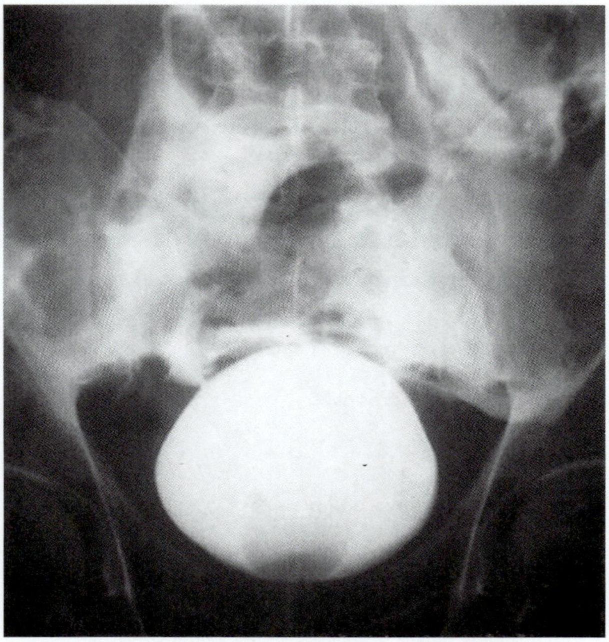

Figure 76.7 Cystogram of a patient who has fallen over and developed severe abdominal pain. Leakage of contrast into the peritoneal cavity is seen.

Treatment of intraperitoneal rupture

A lower midline laparotomy should be performed; the edges of the rent are trimmed and sutured with a single-layer 2/0 absorbable suture. A suprapubic and a urethral catheter are placed. Very rarely, the rupture will be through an unsuspected tumour; a biopsy can be taken before suturing the defect. Laparoscopic approaches are also now being used.

Injury to the bladder during operation

The bladder may be injured in: (1) inguinal or femoral herniotomy; (2) hysterectomy; and (3) excision of the rectum. If the injury is recognised, the bladder must be repaired and catheter drainage maintained for 7 days. If it is not recognised, the treatment is similar to that of rupture of the bladder.

When accidental extraperitoneal perforation of the bladder occurs during endoscopic resection, drainage of the bladder with a urethral catheter and the administration of antibiotics usually suffice. If a mass of extravasated fluid is present it is best to place a small drain through a stab incision. A laparotomy will usually be required if an intraperitoneal perforation is caused by transurethral resection (Summary box 76.2).

Summary box 76.2

Management of bladder trauma

- Extravesical injury – catheter drainage for 10 days
- Intraperitoneal injury – laparotomy, repair and bladder drainage

RETENTION OF URINE

Acute retention

There are many possible causes of acute retention of urine (see also Chapter 77) (Summary box 76.3).

Summary box 76.3

The most frequent causes of acute retention

Male
- Bladder outlet obstruction (the commonest cause)
- Urethral stricture
- Acute urethritis or prostatitis
- Phimosis

Female
- Retroverted gravid uterus
- Bladder neck obstruction (rare)

Both
- Blood clot
- Urethral calculus
- Rupture of the urethra
- Neurogenic (injury or disease of the spinal cord)
- Smooth muscle cell dysfunction associated with ageing
- Faecal impaction
- Anal pain (haemorrhoidectomy)
- Intensive postoperative analgesic treatment
- Some drugs
- Spinal anaesthesia

Clinical features

- No urine is passed for several hours.
- Pain is present.
- The bladder is visible, palpable, tender (Figure 76.8) and dull to percussion.
- Potential neurological causes should be excluded by checking reflexes in the lower limbs and perianal sensation.

Treatment

Treatment is to pass a fine urethral catheter (14F – French gauge is defined as the circumference in millimetres) and arrange urological management. Occasionally, in postoperative retention a warm bath can help (Figures 76.9, 76.10, 76.11 and 76.12).

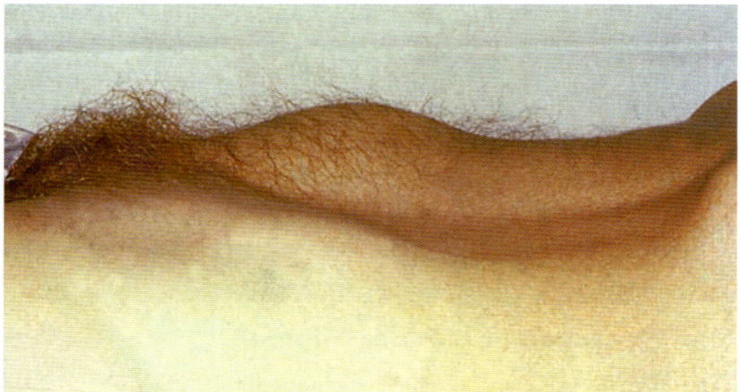

Figure 76.8 Distended bladder in a man who presented with retention of urine.

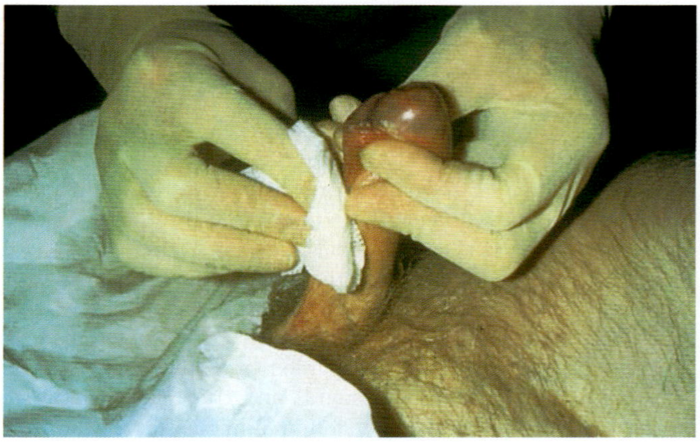

Figure 76.9 Cleaning of the penis before catheterisation.

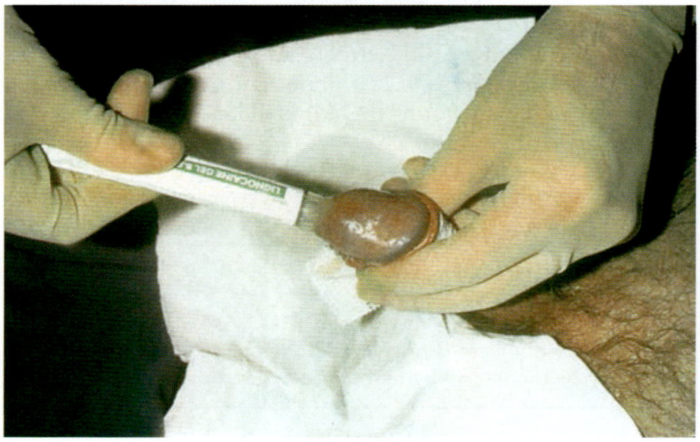

Figure 76.10 Insertion of local anaesthetic before insertion of a catheter.

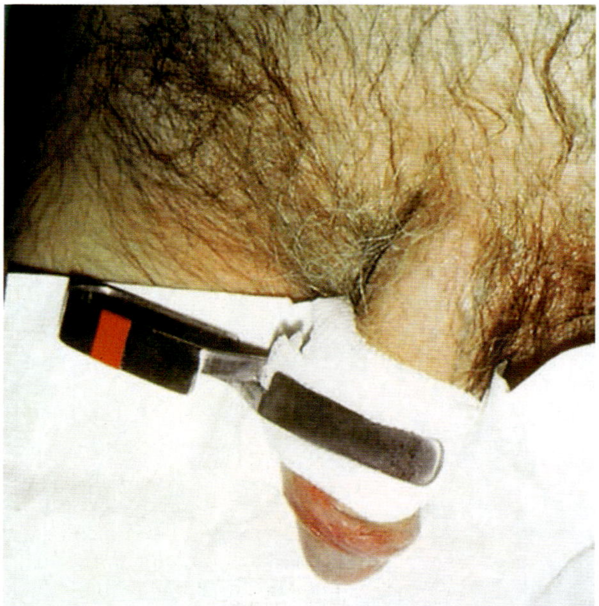

Figure 76.11 The use of a penile clamp to ensure that sufficient time is given to allow the anaesthetic to work before the catheter is inserted.

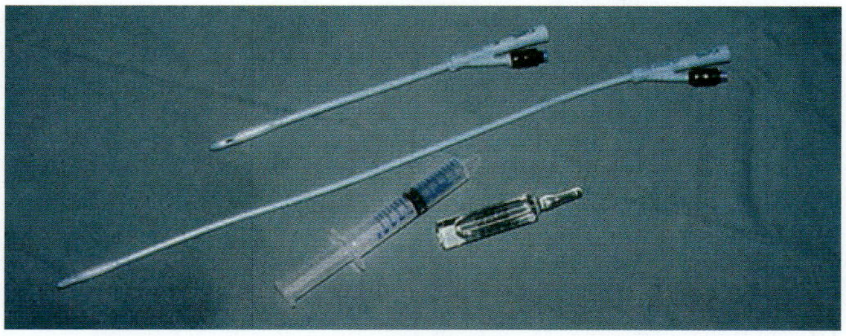

Figure 76.12 A selection of silicone catheters.

Urethral catheterisation

Following a thorough hand wash, sterile gloves are donned. The genitalia are cleaned using soapy antiseptic. Lignocaine gel is inserted into the urethra, warning the patient that this may create stinging. The jelly should be massaged posteriorly in an attempt to anaesthetise the sphincter region, and it is of advantage to place a penile clamp for several minutes. A small Foley catheter should be passed while the penis is held taut. In a female patient, the labia should be parted using the middle and index fingers of the left hand, which should not be moved once cleaning has been performed. Providing a stricture is not the cause, the catheter should pass freely. Once urine begins to drain, it is wise to pass a few more centimetres of catheter into the bladder before the balloon is inflated to avoid inflation in the prostate. Force must not be used (Summary box 76.4).

Summary box 76.4

Catheterisation for acute retention of urine

Following catheterisation:

- Record the volume of urine drained
- Examine the abdomen to exclude other pathology (rupture of an aortic aneurysm, ureteric colic or diverticulitis can cause confusion)

If the catheter will not pass, it is usually due to poor technique, lack of anaesthesia, traumatisation of the urethra or a urethral stricture. Occasionally, a large prostatic middle lobe may prevent the catheter entering the bladder; sometimes a coudé catheter will pass. If a catheter cannot be passed the following plan should be pursued.

Suprapubic puncture

Suprapubic puncture with commercially available catheters such as Cystofix or Lawrence Add-a-Cath catheters is straightforward provided that the bladder is palpable. The skin, fascia and retropubicspace are anaesthetised with 0.5 per cent lignocaine. Correct placement is confirmed by aspiration. A large-bore needle is then placed into the bladder, down which a fine catheter is passed (Cystofix) and then secured in position. The other option is to place a plastic suprapubic trocar and cannula, which has a removable plastic strip on the side. A standard 12F Foley catheter can be passed down the cannula, the balloon is inflated, the cannula is extracted and the strip is pulled away from the catheter (Add-a-Cath). If urine cannot be aspirated through the fine-bore needle, passing a suprapubic trocar should not be attempted.

If these devices are not available, a catheter can be placed in the bladder under direct vision through a small incision under local anaesthetic.

Urethral instrumentation

In a patient with a known stricture, an experienced urologist may elect to dilate the stricture or to take the patient to theatre to carry out an optical urethrotomy (see Chapter 78).

Chronic retention

In chronic retention there is no pain. These patients are at risk of upper tract dilatation because of high intravesical tension – they require urgent urological referral. Men with impaired renal function may develop post-obstructive diuresis following catheterisation. Such men need careful monitoring, with replacement of inappropriate urinary losses by intravenous saline; they are also at risk of haematuria as the distended urinary tract empties. Often it is several days before full renal recovery occurs.

Retention with overflow

The patient is incontinent with small amounts of urine passing involuntarily from the distended bladder. It usually follows a neglected retention.

Indwelling catheters and closed systems of catheter drainage

The risk of ascending infection is decreased by connecting the catheter to sterile tubing connected to a collecting bag. Irrigations should be avoided unless clot retention occurs. When a catheter has been *in situ* for a few days, some degree of urethritis and bacteriuria is likely; changing a catheter then entails risks of severe infection if prophylactic antibiotics are not used (Figure 76.13).

Acute retention due to drugs

A number of drugs can induce retention, including antihistamines, anti-hypertensives, anti-cholinergics and tricyclic antidepressants.

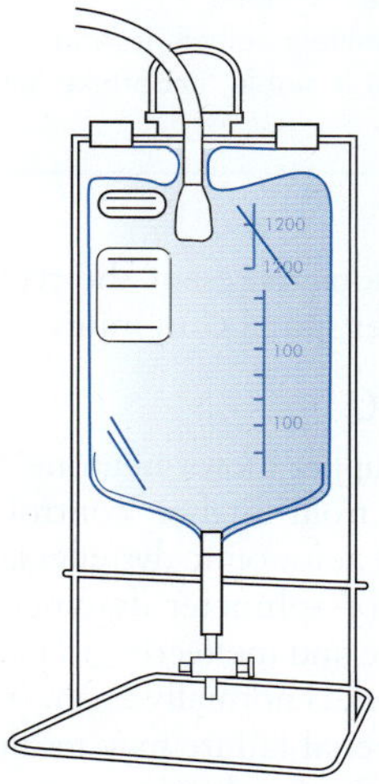

Figure 76.13 Modern Simpla bag used for continuous bladder drainage. (The nurse who is emptying the bag should be wearing disposable gloves to avoid contaminating the hands with organisms.)

Frederic Eugene Basil Foley, 1891–1966, Urologist, Anker Hospital, St Paul, MN, USA.

The acute neuropathic bladder

1 Immediately after spinal cord injury, 'spinal shock' occurs (see Chapter 35), which may last for days or months. The detrusor is not able to contract, the bladder distends and overflow incontinence occurs. Neglected bladder distension will lead to damage to the detrusor, infection and ultimately renal failure. Management is as follows:
2 The bladder must be emptied by aseptic intermittent catheterisation performed two or three times daily or the use of an indwelling urethral catheter on continuous drainage, making sure that the patient has a high urinary output (3 litres per day) to combat infection. Currently, intermittent catheterisation is preferred as soon as the patient's spinal injury is stable.
3 Neurological examination must be performed to assess the level of sensory and motor loss. Ischaemic necrosis of the cord may extend below the upper level of cord injury. When sensory loss below the upper level is total, recovery is unlikely. Incomplete lesions may recover somatic and bladder function.
4 Demonstration of intact bulbocavernosus and anal reflexes indicates that the sacral cord and nerves are intact and that reflex bladder contractions are likely to develop, though they may be insufficient to empty the bladder. If there is persistent total loss of reflexes and perineal sensation then either the sacral cord or cauda equina is damaged. In such circumstances, an acontractile bladder is likely. In cauda equina lesions, there may be sensory, motor or mixed loss.
5 Full urodynamic assessment of bladder function should be undertaken when the injury is stable. This allows an accurate assessment of bladder and sphincter activity and will enable decisions to be made about further management; the prime aim is to prevent upper tract damage by promoting good bladder emptying (Summary box 76.5).

Summary box 76.5

Clinical management of spinal injury

- The bladder should be emptied during spinal shock by catheterisation
- Encourage high fluid intake
- Commence intermittent catheterisation
- When the patient is stable, undertake full urodynamic evaluation

The following situations represent the typical patterns of bladder function seen after spinal cord injury.

Lesions above T10

Usually leads to an 'upper motor neurone' bladder with reflexes intact but isolated from higher control mechanisms. Such patients are at risk of autonomic dysreflexia.

Because of detrusor–sphincter dyssynergia, bladder contractions are high pressure and ineffective in producing bladder emptying; the bladder neck is normally open. If left untreated, upper tract dilatation and renal failure may result. Bladder capacity is usually decreased with the development of trabeculation and a typical 'fir-tree' appearance. Patients are incontinent during high-pressure phasic contractions because the sphincter resistance suddenly diminishes.

Some patients with low-pressure bladders that empty may be managed by means of condom drainage. Others will require clean intermittent self-catheterisation (CISC), popularised by Lapides. Patients with poor emptying, low bladder capacity and upper tract dilatation require treatment with endoscopic sphincterotomy and condom drainage. Some carefully selected patients may require bladder reconstruction.

Lesions involving the sympathetic outflow (T11, T12, L1, L2)

These patients are usually similar to the group with lesions above T10.

Damage to the sacral centre S2, S3, S4 and cauda equina lesions

Usually leads to a 'lower motor neurone' bladder, also found in spina bifida (myelodysplasia); the detrusor is acontractile. Abdominal straining can produce reasonable emptying but the mainstay is CISC. Some patients may have sensation of filling through the hypogastric nerves, if T11 and T12 are intact. The bladder capacity may be good, but some patients have high resting pressures and high increases during bladder filling, which means that there is a risk to the upper urinary tract. The bladder neck is usually open and the distal sphincter mechanisms may be paralysed but of fixed resistance. Vesicoureteric reflux is common and upper tract damage is frequent in neglected cases. Patients who can achieve satisfactory bladder emptying by means of CISC usually have reasonable continence.

Bladder dysfunction after excision of the rectum or radical hysterectomy

Between 10 and 15 per cent of patients undergoing radical rectal excision for cancer sustain damage to the inferior hypogastric plexus, leading to impotence in the male and neurogenic bladder dysfunction. This type of bladder dysfunction is similar to the cauda equina lesion. Postoperative retention in other patients may also be caused by simple bladder outlet obstruction. The best plan is to catheterise the patient to allow postoperative recovery and then carry out urodynamic investigation to determine the appropriate treatment.

INCONTINENCE OF URINE

Overall, urinary incontinence occurs in 5 per cent of men and 20 per cent of women. Up to 40 per cent of women over the age of 60 years and 50 per cent of institutionalised elderly patients experience regular episodes of urinary incontinence. Health problems include skin breakdown and depression, and loss of esteem and sexual activity. Continence is dependent on normal mobility and brain function allowing a perception of when it is socially acceptable to void, normal bladder sensation, normal voluntary detrusor contraction producing good bladder emptying, a normally competent sphincter mechanism, which relaxes appropriately during a voluntary detrusor contraction allowing good bladder emptying, and good bladder capacity with normally low pressures during filling. This is clearly a fine balance and several factors can cause incontinence. In children, non-neurogenic incontinence is often associated with other dysfunctional conditions such as infections, constipation, psychological factors, increased fluid intake, intentional misconduct or an overactive bladder. Several investigations are required for diagnosis of urinary incontinence (Summary box 76.6).

Summary box 76.6

Diagnosis of urinary incontinence

The following investigations are required:

- A careful history and physical examination and completion of frequency voiding charts
- Urodynamic testing in most patients and in all patients in whom surgical intervention is proposed
- Urine culture to exclude infection and measurement of serum creatinine

In selected cases, IVU is carried out if a ureteric fistula is suspected, although ultrasound examination will often provide adequate details.

Urodynamic testing

The key to the practical management of lower urinary tract dysfunction, and particularly incontinence, lies with urodynamic investigation. The principle is to artificially simulate bladder filling and emptying while obtaining pressure measurements (Figure 76.14).

The patient attends with a full bladder and is allowed to void in private to measure the maximum urinary flow rate. After voiding, the residual urine is measured by ultrasound. A pair of catheters or a twin-lumen catheter is passed into the bladder, which allows the bladder to be filled at a rate of 50 mL/min while a continuous recording of intravesical pressure is made. To obtain 'true' detrusor pressure, a second channel is required to assess intra-abdominal pressure, measured by means of a small intrarectal or intravaginal balloon. The bladder is filled until the patient states that the bladder is full. X-ray screening may be carried out to assess bladder neck closure and urinary leakage during movement or coughing (stress incontinence) or during bouts of phasic detrusor pressure (detrusor instability). The patient is then asked to void at the end of bladder filling after the filling catheter has been removed (Figure 76.15).

The normal bladder will accept approximately 400–550 mL when filled at room temperature at a rate of <50 mL/min. The pressure increase in the bladder should be less than 15 cmH_2O. In addition, phasic pressure increases should not be seen. The normal voiding pressure should not exceed 60 cmH_2O in men and about 40 cmH_2O in women, with a flow rate of between 20 and 25 mL/s.

Common abnormalities identified during urodynamic testing in incontinence

The overactive bladder

Phasic increases in pressure give rise to urgency and urge incontinence (detrusor overactivity; Figure 76.16). This abnormality is found in patients with neurogenic bladder dysfunction, such as in multiple sclerosis (MS) or Parkinson's disease or following a stroke or spinal injury, when it is known as detrusor hyperreflexia. About 50 per cent of men with bladder outflow obstruction have detrusor instability, and in about half of them the instability resolves after prostatectomy. Idiopathic detrusor overactivity is common and must be distinguished from genuine stress incontinence (GSI) in women before performing bladder neck suspension procedures. In children, overactive bladder symptoms must be carefully investigated and treated with conservative measures before initiating antimuscarinic therapy.

Genuine stress incontinence

This is defined as urinary leakage occurring during increased bladder pressure when this is solely due to increased abdominal pressure and not to increased true detrusor pressure (see Figure 76.15). It is caused by sphincter weakness.

Chronic urinary retention

Chronic urinary retention with overflow incontinence is recognised by a large residual volume of urine (Figure 76.17) and is usually associated with high pressures during bladder filling.

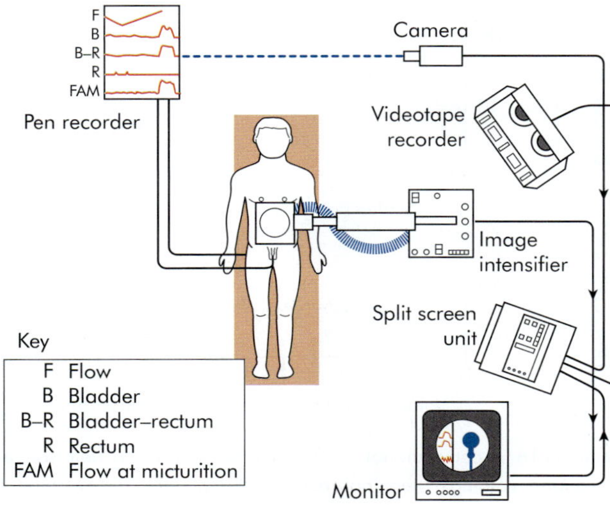

Figure 76.14 Urodynamic study.

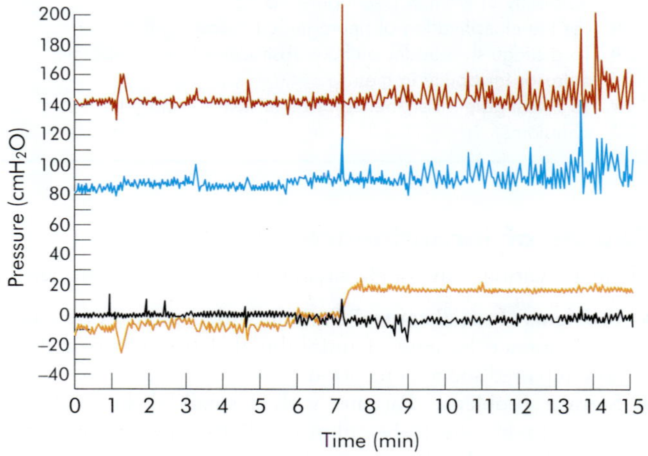

Figure 76.15 A section of an ambulatory, natural-fill urodynamic trace. The rectal pressure is in red, the bladder pressure in blue and the subtracted detrusor trace in black. The orange trace is the output of an electronic nappy, which records urinary leakage. A cough is shown, which results in genuine stress incontinence.

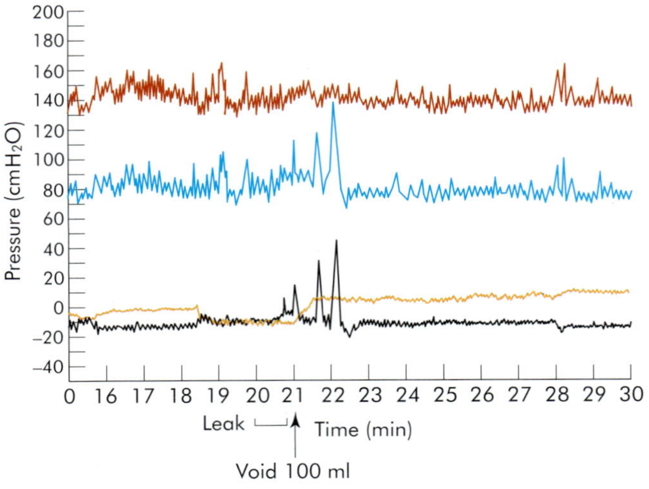

Figure 76.16 A section of an ambulatory, natural-fill urodynamic trace. The rectal pressure is in red, the bladder pressure in blue and the subtracted detrusor trace in black. The orange trace is the output of an electronic nappy which records urinary leakage. Phasic activity is shown, which is detrusor instability resulting in urge incontinence.

Bladder outflow obstruction

Bladder outflow obstruction is associated with increased voiding pressures, often in excess of 90 cmH_2O (Figure 76.18), coupled with low urinary flow rates.

Neurogenic dysfunction

Neurogenic bladder dysfunction may also be identified (Summary box 76.7).

Summary box 76.7

Uses of urodynamic testing

- To distinguish GSI (due to sphincter weakness) from detrusor instability in women (see Figure 76.15)
- For the classification of neurogenic bladder dysfunction
- To distinguish bladder outflow obstruction from idiopathic detrusor instability in men
- To investigate incontinence or other lower urinary tract symptoms

Causes of incontinence

There are various ways of classifying the causes of incontinence.

- **Problems of social control**. Patients with dementia often have incontinence because of uninhibited detrusor hyperreflexia and impaired social perception.
- **Storage problems**. Patients with a small bladder capacity owing to fibrosis (tuberculosis, radiotherapy or interstitial cystitis) can develop incontinence. Patients with a small functional capacity owing to severe detrusor instability, neurogenic dysfunction or infection can develop incontinence.
- **Impairment of emptying**. Patients with chronic retention or neurogenic bladder dysfunction have small functional bladder capacities with detrusor overactivity causing incontinence, despite having large residual volumes of urine.
- **Weak sphincter**. This leads to GSI and can follow surgical procedures such as radical prostatectomy in men.
- **Fistulae**. Leakage from fistulae or upper tract duplication with an ectopic ureter.
- **In children**, the causes must be carefully investigated and treated with conservative measures before initiating antimuscarinic therapy.

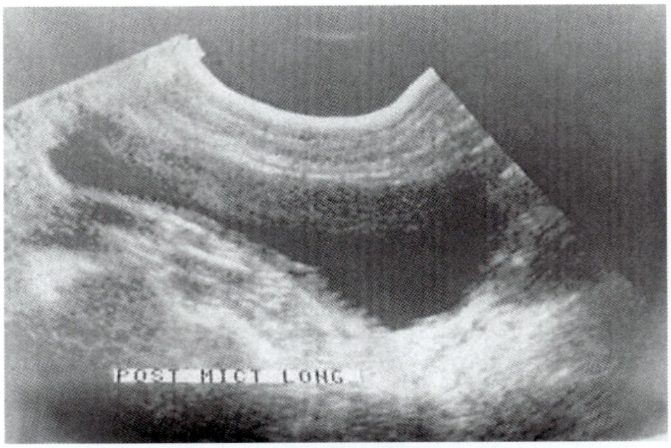

Figure 76.17 An ultrasound scan showing a large post-void residual urine.

The common causes may be classified into male, female or mixed-sex groups.

Male incontinence

Chronic urinary retention with overflow

This may be due to benign prostatic hypertrophy, carcinoma

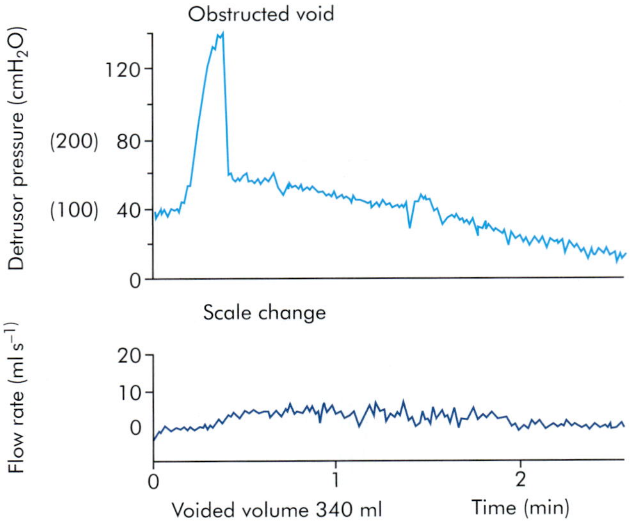

Figure 76.18 A conventional urodynamic trace showing detrusor pressure during voiding. There has been a change of scale because the pressure was so high; voiding pressures are increased with a low flow rate, which is diagnostic of bladder outflow obstruction.

of the prostate, urethral stricture and, in younger men, hypertrophy of the bladder neck. Examination may reveal that the bladder is distended, and it can be confirmed by ultrasound scanning. The treatment is discussed in Chapter 77.

Post-prostatectomy

Post-prostatectomy incontinence may result from injury to the external sphincter mechanism. Treatment should be conservative initially with pelvic floor exercises, and an anstomotic stricture must be excluded. The condition may necessitate insertion of an artificial urethral sphincter (Figure 76.19).

Female incontinence

Stress incontinence

The most common cause is GSI, although in some parts of the world, vesicourethral fistulae as a result of neglected labour are common. It is usually found in multiparous women with a history of difficult labour. It can be found in normal young women who indulge in competitive trampolining and in patients with epispadias. The classical symptom is urine loss during coughing, laughing, sneezing or a sudden change of posture. The symptoms may change with the menstrual cycle. The volume of urine loss can be measured during an exercise test, which is performed by putting the patient through a standard set of tests with 300 mL of fluid in the bladder; in GSI the fluid losses usually range from 10 to 50 mL. Urinary frequency and urgency are often found in such patients as they try to avoid incontinence by frequent voiding.

Idiopathic detrusor instability can mimic GSI and coexist with it. It is important to make a correct preoperative diagnosis by urodynamic measurements, as the outcome of surgery is suboptimal in women with idiopathic detrusor instability.

Minor to moderate stress urinary incontinence can be controlled by pelvic floor exercises. However, if this fails, surgery is indicated. Standard operations include open colposuspension or the use of a minimally invasive approach involving the insertion of a transvaginal tape (TVT procedure).

Open colposuspension

This operation is carried out through a Pfannenstiel incision with the patient in the Lloyd-Davies position. The vaginal fascia is identified by sweeping the bladder off the vagina and three sutures are placed on each side between the vaginal fascia and the iliopubic ligament. A suprapubic catheter is placed. Voiding difficulties are frequent but usually temporary. It is best to warn women with large bladder capacities and low voiding pressures that this complication may occur and that they may be required to carry out CISC for a period. The operation is very successful for the treatment of GSI, with good results at one year in 90 per cent of patients, which are maintained in about 80 per cent of patients at five years.

Modifications of bladder neck suspension can also be achieved by minimally invasive approaches such as the transvaginal sling. This technique does reduce both hospital stay and postoperative morbidity.

Incontinence common to both sexes

Idiopathic detrusor overactivity

Phasic increases in bladder pressure may occur during filling in otherwise normal patients (idiopathic) or it may be found in neurogenic bladder dysfunction (when it is known as detrusor hyperreflexia) and bladder outflow obstruction. Idiopathic detrusor overactivity may be symptomless but usually results in symptoms of frequency, urgency, urge incontinence, nocturia or nocturnal incontinence (enuresis) depending on the severity of the instability. It must be distinguished from GSI and from bladder outflow obstruction before surgical treatment. Infection, tuberculosis or carcinoma *in situ* (CIS) should be excluded. The mainstay of treatment is the use of various anti-cholinergic medications (oxybutynin and tolterodine). Severe symptoms resistant to conventional conservative treatment resulting in major impairment of quality of life may need more aggressive treatment, such as enterocystoplasty or the injection of small doses of botulinum toxin (the toxin from *Clostridium botulinum*), known as BoTox, which blocks cholinergic neuromuscular transmission, at least for a time.

Ageing

Ageing can result in smooth muscle cell dysfunction, which can cause combinations of small functional capacity, detrusor overactivity, impaired bladder emptying and symptoms of lower urinary tract dysfunction.

Congenital

Congenital causes include ectopic vesicae and severe epispadias. The abnormal entry of an ectopic ureter distal to the sphincter complex or into the vagina in a female patient should theoretically result in total urinary incontinence. This is discussed in Chapters 6 and 75.

Trauma

Trauma, whether from pelvic surgery or associated with pelvic fracture, may result in disruption of the nerve supply to the bladder or urethra, or in fistula formation.

Infection

Lower urinary tract infection (UTI) may be sufficient to induce urinary incontinence. A history of frequency, burning and a fever should prompt the diagnosis. Symptoms will usually settle with a course of antibiotics, but in the case of recurrent infection further investigation of the urinary tract will clearly be indicated.

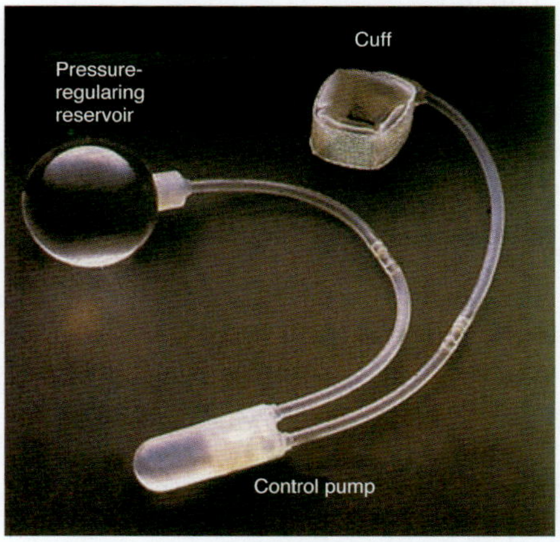

Figure 76.19 The artificial urinary sphincter made by American Medical Systems.

Neoplasia

Locally advanced cancers in the pelvis, particularly carcinoma of the cervix in a woman and carcinoma of the prostate in a man, may result in direct invasion of the sphincter mechanism causing incontinence; occasionally, fistula formation may occur in women.

Other causes

Constant dribbling of urine coupled with normal micturition

This occurs when there is a ureteric fistula or an ectopic ureter associated with a duplex system opening into the urethra beyond the urethral sphincter in females or into the vagina. The history is diagnostic, and intravenous pyelography or ultrasound scanning may reveal the upper pole segment, which is often poorly functioning. Treatment is by excision of the aberrant ureter and portion of kidney. A ureteric fistula can be difficult to diagnose and its demonstration may require retrograde ureterography and a high degree of suspicion.

Nocturnal enuresis

This is a condition of young children and young adults. Of course, the time at which children become dry at night varies and, in some, nocturnal enuresis is merely a delayed onset of continence. In others, it persists until late adolescence and is classified into primary and secondary nocturnal enuresis. In children, once neurogenic dysfunction has been excluded, the condition can be associated with other symptoms such as intentional misconduct, infections, constipation and increased fluid intake. These causes must be ruled out before medication is considered.

Primary nocturnal enuresis occurs in patients with nocturnal symptoms alone, which are absent during the day. Often, they have been dry for a period, and the vast majority of patients will eventually become dry. In the meantime, a sympathetic approach to these children is essential. They often respond to a system of rewards using a 'star' chart. In addition, the use of DDAVP (a vasopressin analogue) can produce increased urinary concentration at night with a decrease in nocturnal incontinence. Other treatments include the use of an alarm that wakes the child (or at least the child's parents) when incontinence occurs and medication in the form of an anticholinergic drug such as oxybutynin.

Treatments for incontinence

Treatments are listed below. Management is dependent on making a correct diagnosis.

Management and treatment

Following careful assessment and investigation, many cases of incontinence can improve with simple measures such as lifestyle interventions, pelvic floor exercises with biofeedback, bladder training and incontinence devices where necessary. In mixed urge and stress incontinence, the major component has to be treated first.

Problems of social functioning

Patients with dementia may respond to regular toileting. Anticholinergic agents can cause increased confusion in these patients and often, in severe cases, an indwelling catheter is needed.

Storage problems

Patients with a small bladder capacity because of fibrosis may require augmentation cystoplasty. Detrusor overactivity will require treatment with anti-cholinergic medication but, in severe cases, particularly in neuropathic patients at high risk of upper tract dilatation, bladder substitution (near-total supratrigonal cystectomy followed by the need for detubularised ileocaecal segment bladder substitution) or augmentation (enterocystoplasty) may be needed. These procedures should be carried out only after careful assessment in units used to dealing with such problems. Patients with very impaired mobility and MS may require ileal conduit diversion. The use of intravesical injections of BoTox has provided good improvements, and it may avoid or delay the need for major surgery.

Impaired bladder emptying

Patients with overflow incontinence because of bladder outflow obstruction will usually respond well to prostatectomy. Patients with impaired bladder emptying because of neurogenic bladder dysfunction should be treated in the first place by means of CISC.

Weak sphincter

Patients with GSI should be treated by means of pelvic floor exercises initially. Duloxetine can be used as medical treatment for GSI. Bulking agents, such as macroplastique, can be used and can provide good temporary solutions. Surgical treatment by means of colposuspension or TVT may be needed. Those with post-prostatectomy incontinence or neurogenic bladder dysfunction may need to be fitted with an artificial urinary sphincter (Figure 76.19), if they are well motivated and mobile, but careful assessment is required.

Use of appliances

An indwelling catheter drained constantly into a leg urinal may be a satisfactory solution although, in some instances, diversion via an ileal conduit is necessary. In men, a condom urinary appliance may be satisfactory and can avoid an indwelling catheter.

More major surgical treatments

Various types of urinary diversion

Urinary diversion may be required for the treatment of end-stage incontinence that is not otherwise treatable (see later in this chapter).

Bladder substitution procedures

The principle behind these operations is the creation of a low pressure, large-capacity reservoir, which can be made using any segment of bowel isolated on its vascular pedicle (Figures 76.20, 76.21 and 76.22). This is then detubularised by dividing its anti-mesenteric border and suturing this into a plate, which is then reconfigured into a spherical structure. This reservoir can then be anastomosed to the bladder remnant after excision of the fundus above the trigone. If necessary, the ureters can be reimplanted into the bowel segment. This new bladder will need to be emptied by means of CISC in up to 30 per cent of cases.

'Clam' enterocystoplasty

This procedure was originally described by Bramble for the treatment of nocturnal enuresis. It has been used in the treatment of idiopathic detrusor instability (Figure 76.23). This procedure can also be used as an augmentation procedure in patients with neurogenic bladder dysfunction and a reasonable bladder capacity (approximately 300 mL).

Fitment of artificial urinary sphincter

See Figure 76.19.

Summary

Treatments for incontinence can be summarised as follows:

1 Conservative measures such as lifestyle interventions, pelvic floor muscle and bladder training.
2 Devices for collection: external penile condom, or an indwelling urethral or suprapubic catheter.
3 Drugs: to decrease the strength of the bladder neck (e.g. adrenergic blockers); with mixed action on the bladder neck and central nervous system (e.g. tricyclic drugs); to inhibit bladder activity (e.g. anti-cholinergic drugs). Botulinum toxin A is used in selected patients. Duloxetine can be used as medical treatment for GSI – it is a serotonin–noradrenaline (norepinephrine) reuptake inhibitor.
4 Intermittent self-catheterisation: to improve emptying.
5 Increasing outlet: pelvic floor physiotherapy; resistance colposuspension or TVT tapes or slings; periurethral injections of 'bulking agents' such as cross-linked collagen or other particles; use of the artificial urinary sphincter.
6 Denervation of bladder: S3 sacral nerve blockade, neurectomy or surgical transection of the bladder to inhibit bladder activity and improve functional capacity. These are rarely used nowadays because of the use of botulinum toxin and the clam cystoplasty or S3 nerve stimulation (see point 7).
7 Sacral nerve stimulation devices can improve incontinence. They involve percutaneous insertion of electrodes through the sacral foramina under radiological control and implantation of an electronic stimulator.
8 Augmentation of bladder: 'clam' enterocystoplasty, bladder capacity substitution with detubularised bowel segment.
9 Urinary diversion: ileal conduit, continent urinary diversion.

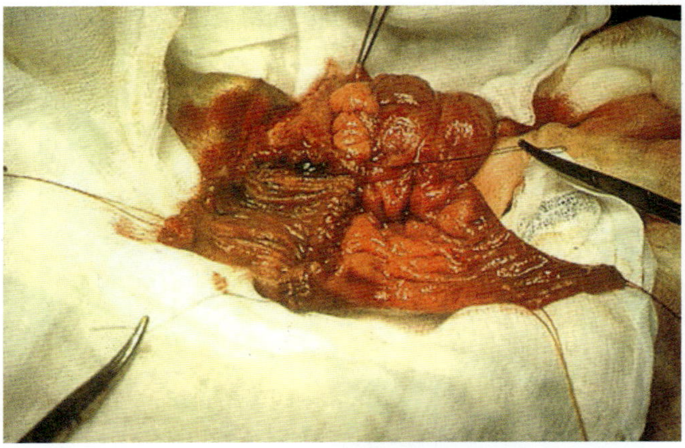

Figure 76.20 A vascularised ileocaecal segment being detubularised.

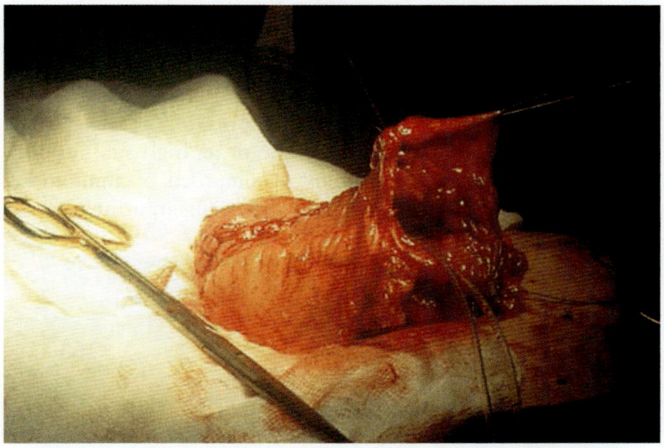

Figure 76.22 A capacious ileocaecal reservoir to be used in a patient requiring bladder substitution. These segments may be used for total bladder replacement, bladder substitution and the construction of continent diversion with a Mitrofanoff-type anti-incontinence mechanism (see later in the chapter).

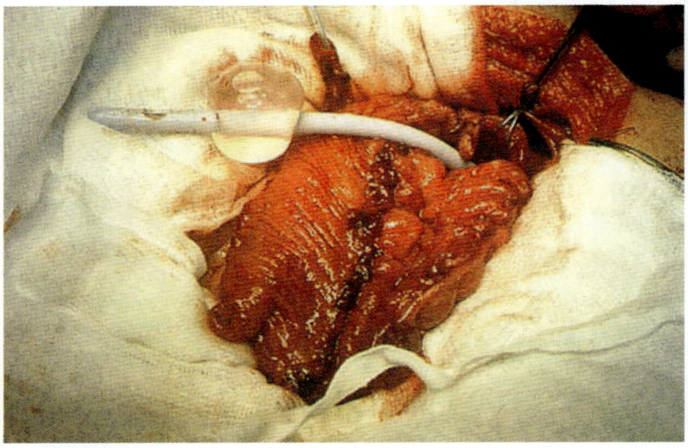

Figure 76.21 An ileocaecal segment being anastomosed to the trigone after near-total cystectomy; the left ureter is about to be implanted by means of a Camay–Le Duc anastomosis.

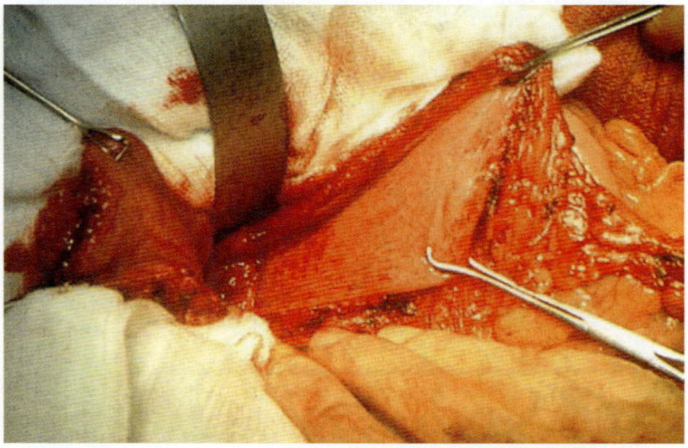

Figure 76.23 A 'clam' cystoplasty being performed. The ureteric orifices can be seen with the interureteric bar; the defect will be filled by a segment of detubularised ileum, performing a bladder augmentation.

Frank James Bramble, formerly urologist, The Royal Victoria Hospital, Bournemouth, UK.

BLADDER STONES

Definition

A primary bladder stone is one that develops in sterile urine; it often originates in the kidney. A secondary stone occurs in the presence of infection, outflow obstruction, impaired bladder emptying or a foreign body.

Incidence

Until the twentieth century, bladder stone was a prevalent disorder among poor children and adolescents. Because of improved diet, especially an increased protein–carbohydrate ratio, primary vesical calculus is rare.

Composition and cystoscopic appearance

Most vesical calculi are mixed. An oxalate calculus is a primary calculus that grows slowly; usually, it is of moderate size and solitary, and its surface is uneven (Figure 76.24). Although calcium oxalate is white, the stone is usually dark brown or black because of the incorporation of blood pigment. Uric acid calculi are round or oval, smooth and vary in colour from yellow to brown (Figure 76.25). They occur in patients with gout but are also found in patients with ileostomies or with bladder outflow obstruction. A cystine calculus occurs only in the presence of cystinuria and is radio-opaque because of its high sulphur content. A triple phosphate calculus is composed of ammonium, magnesium and calcium phosphates and occurs in urine infected with urea-splitting organisms. It tends to grow rapidly. In some instances it occurs on a nucleus of one of the other types of calculus; more rarely it occurs on a foreign body (Figures 76.26 and 76.27). It is dirty white in colour and of chalky consistency.

A bladder stone is usually free to move in the bladder and it gravitates to the lowest part of the bladder. Less commonly, the stone is wholly or partially in a diverticulum, where it may be hidden from view.

Clinical features

Men are affected eight times more frequently than women. Stones may be asymptomatic and found incidentally.

Symptoms

Frequency is the earliest symptom and there may be a sensation of incomplete bladder emptying. Pain (strangury) is most often found in patients with a spiculated oxalate calculus. It occurs at the end of micturition and is referred to the tip of the penis or to the labia majora; more rarely, it is referred to the perineum or suprapubic region. The pain is worsened by movement. In young boys, screaming and pulling at the penis with the hand at the end of micturition are indicative of bladder stone. Haematuria is characterised by the passage of a few drops of bright-red blood at the end of micturition, and is due to the stone abrading the vascular trigone. Interruption of the urinary stream is due to the stone blocking the internal meatus. Urinary infection is a common presenting symptom.

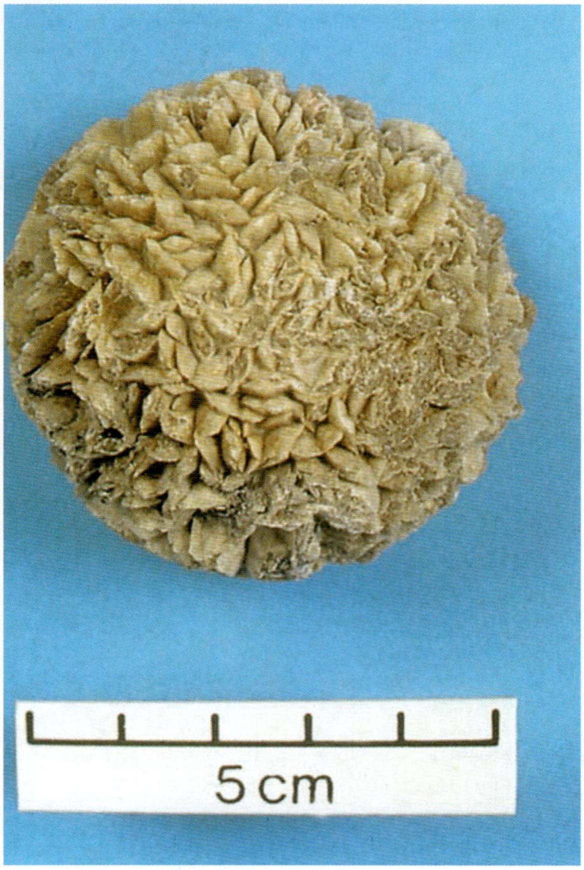

Figure 76.24 A rough bladder stone.

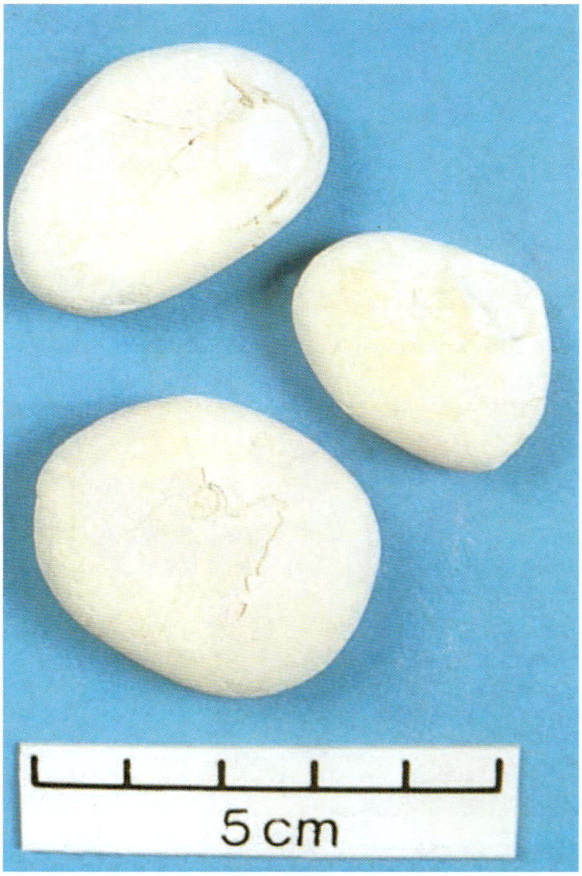

Figure 76.25 Smooth uric acid-type stones.

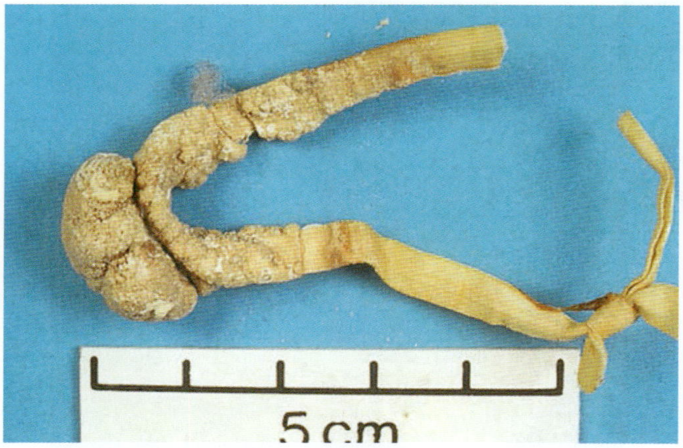

Figure 76.26 Stone on a vaginal sling that had eroded into the bladder.

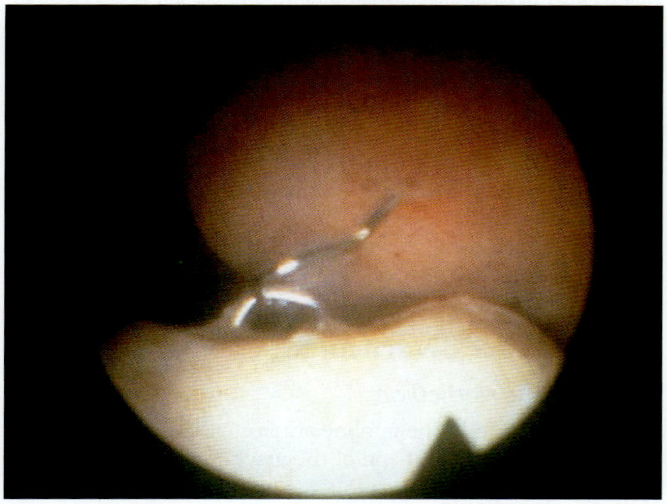

Figure 76.27 Uric acid stones that had formed on metal staples used to construct a colonic bladder augmentation.

Examination

Rectal or vaginal examination is normal; occasionally, a large calculus is palpable in the female. Examination of the urine reveals microscopic haematuria, pus or crystals that are typical of the calculus, for example envelope-like in the case of an oxalate stone or hexagonal plates in the case of cystine calculi. In most patients, the stone is visible on ultrasound or on a plain x-ray (Figure 76.28). Imaging of the whole of the urinary tract should be undertaken to exclude an upper tract stone. Nearly all stones can be dealt with endoscopically. In men with bladder outflow obstruction, endoscopic resection of the prostate should be performed at the same time as the stone is dealt with.

Treatment

The cause of the stone should be sought and treated; this may include bladder outflow obstruction or incomplete bladder emptying in patients with neurogenic bladder dysfunction.

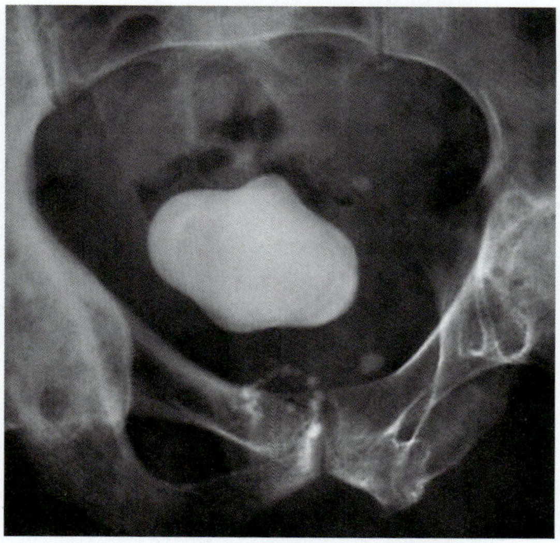

Figure 76.28 Radiograph showing a vesical calculus (no contrast has been used).

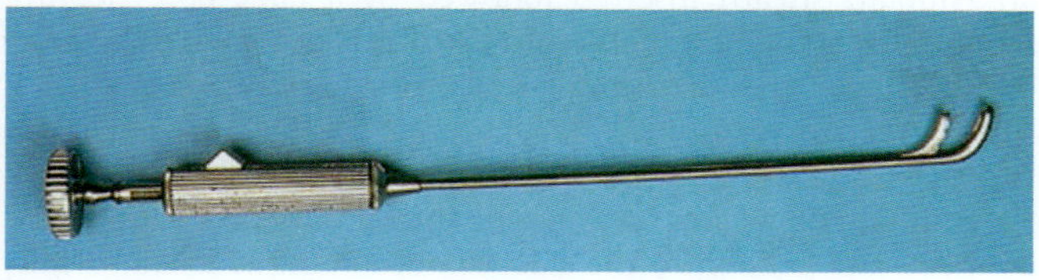

Figure 76.29 'Blind' lithotrite used to crush bladder stones.

Litholapaxy

The blind lithotrite (Figure 76.29) was an early type of minimally invasive technique. Standard management now includes the optical lithotrite, electrohydraulic lithotrite, Holmium laser or ultrasound probe (Figure 76.30). Other devices include the stone punch, which is useful to crush small fragments further so that they can be evacuated with an Ellik evacuator. Contraindications to perurethral litholapaxy are extremely rare:

- urethral: a urethral stricture that cannot be dilated sufficiently; when a patient is aged below ten years;
- bladder: a contracted bladder;
- stone characteristics: a very large stone.

Ultrasound lithotripsy is extremely safe but appropriate only for small stones. Laser lithotripsy with the holmium laser can deal with most large stones. Once small fragments are produced, the optical lithotrite can be used to finish the job. For evacuation of the fragments, fluid (200 mL) is introduced into the bladder. The evacuator, filled with solution, is fitted on to the sheath. The bulb is compressed slowly and then permitted to expand; the returning solution carries with it fragments of stone.

Milo Ellik, b. 1905, American urologist. One of the original members of the Los Angeles Urological Society. In 1932 Dr Alcock, a pioneer of transurethral resection of prostate, persuaded one of his residents, Milo Ellik, to go to the Chemistry Department glass blowing shop where he devised his evacuator. Unfortunately he never had a patent on his device which was patented by Bard, the surgical company, in the 1940s.

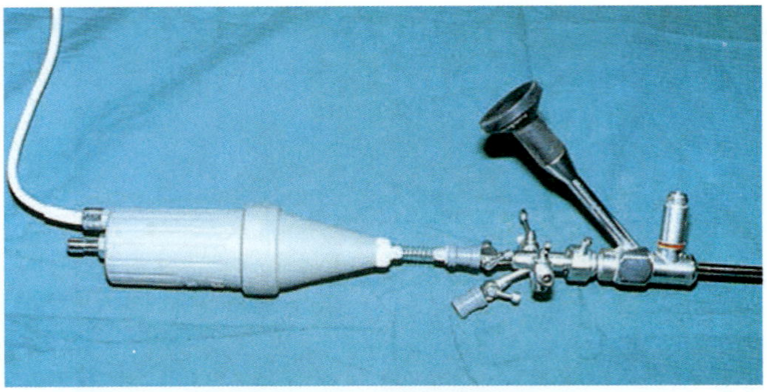

Figure 76.30 An endoscopic ultrasound probe, which is used to fragment bladder or kidney stones.

Percutaneous suprapubic litholapaxy

It is possible to insert a needle into the bladder and then pass a guidewire. As in percutaneous nephrolithotomy, Alken metal dilators can be passed over the guidewire to dilate the track and an Amplatz sheath inserted followed by a large-bore nephroscope. This is the best method to use if it is not possible to carry out litholapaxy per urethram because of a narrow urethra.

Removal of a retained Foley catheter

A retained Foley catheter is usually caused by the channel that connects the balloon to the side arm becoming blocked, usually at the end near the balloon. The best way of dealing with this problem is to further inflate the balloon with 20 mL of water and then burst the balloon percutaneously using a needle under ultrasound screening. If the balloon bursts, it is important to subsequently cystoscope the patient to ensure that any fragments are removed before they can form a foreign body calculus. Cutting off the side arm and attempting to clear the channel with a wire is only occasionally successful.

FOREIGN BODIES IN THE BLADDER

The most common foreign body in the bladder is a fragment of catheter balloon (see above). Occasionally, a foreign body enters through the wall of the bladder, for example nonabsorbable sutures used in an extravesical pelvic operation. Complications include:

- lower UTI;
- perforation of the bladder wall;
- bladder stone.

Treatment

A small foreign body can usually be removed per urethram by means of an operating cystoscope. Occasionally, a suprapubic approach using the percutaneous insertion of a cystoscope is needed.

DIVERTICULAE OF THE BLADDER

Definition

The normal intravesical pressure during voiding is about 35–50 cmH_2O; however, pressures as great as 150 cmH_2O may be reached by a hypertrophied bladder endeavouring to force urine past an obstruction. This pressure causes the lining between the inner layer of hypertrophied muscle to protrude, forming multiple saccules. If one or more, but usually one, saccule is forced through the bladder wall, it becomes a diverticulum (Figure 76.31). Congenital diverticula are the result of a developmental defect.

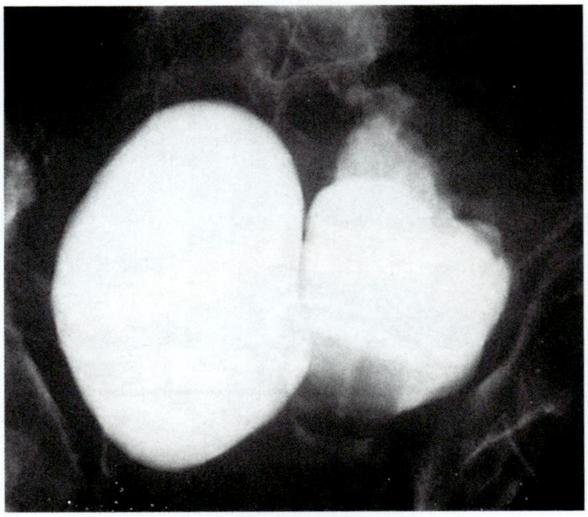

Figure 76.31 Cystogram showing a large diverticulum of the bladder.

Aetiology of diverticulae

Congenital diverticulae

These are situated in the midline anterosuperiorly and represent the unobliterated vesical end of the urachus.

Pulsion diverticula

The usual cause is bladder outflow obstruction.

Pathology

The mouth of the diverticulum is situated above and to the outer side of one ureteric orifice. Exceptionally, it is near the midline behind the interureteric ridge. The size varies from 2 to 5 cm, but they may be larger. Diverticula are lined by bladder mucosa and the wall is composed of fibrous tissue only (compare with a traction diverticulum). A large diverticulum enlarges in a downward direction and sometimes may obstruct a ureter – probably because of peridiverticular inflammation.

Complications

Recurrent urinary infection

As the pouch cannot empty itself efficiently, there remains a stagnant pool of urine within it. Peridiverticulitis can cause dense adhesions between the diverticulum and surrounding structures. Squamous cell metaplasia and leukoplakia are infrequent complications.

Bladder stone

This develops as a result of stagnation and infection. The stone often protrudes into the bladder.

P Alken, urologist, The University of Heidelberg, Germany.

Hydronephrosis and hydroureter

This is extremely rare and is a consequence of peridiverticular inflammation and fibrosis.

Neoplasm

Neoplasm arising in a diverticulum is an uncommon complication (<5 per cent). The prognosis is dependent on the stage of the tumour (see below).

Clinical features

An uninfected diverticulum of the bladder usually causes no symptoms. The patient is nearly always male (95 per cent) and over 50 years of age. Symptoms are those of associated urinary tract obstruction, recurrent infection and pyelonephritis. Haematuria (due to infection, stone or tumour) is a symptom in about 30 per cent. In a few patients micturition occurs twice in rapid succession (the second act may follow a change of posture).

Diagnosis

Diverticula are usually discovered incidentally on cystoscopy or ultrasound (Figures 76.32, 76.33 and 76.34).

Indications for operation

Operation is necessary only for the treatment of complications. Provided the diverticulum is small and associated outflow obstruction has been dealt with by prostate resection, there is no reason to resect the diverticulum. Even a large diverticulum may not require treatment in the absence of infection or other complications.

Combined intravesical and extravesical diverticulectomy

A ureteric stent is passed up the ureter on the affected side and the anterior bladder wall is exposed through a suprapubic incision. The bladder is incised in the midline and the diverticulum is packed with a strip of gauze. The neck of the diverticulum is separated from the ureter and, when the pouch is free, it is severed from the bladder. The resulting defect is closed in a single layer with 2/0 absorbable sutures. A suprapubic catheter is left in place and an extravesical drain is inserted. An alternative method, if the sac is densely adherent, is to carry the incision in the bladder down to the rim of the diverticular orifice, then to detach the diverticulum together with its fibrous rim. The incision in the bladder is closed and the diverticulum left in position with a corrugated drain placed into it for 2–3 days. The track fibroses rapidly after removal of the drain. If bladder outlet obstruction is present, prostatectomy should be carried out at the same time as the diverticulectomy, using any appropriate method (transurethral resection of the prostate (TURP), laser or open) (Summary box 76.8).

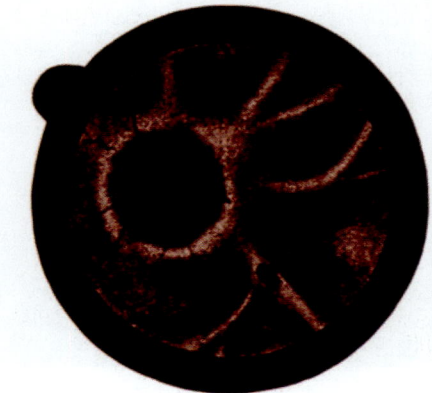

Figure 76.32 Cystoscopic appearance of the orifice of a diverticulum and trabeculation of the bladder.

Summary box 76.8

Bladder diverticula

- Bladder diverticula are most frequently diagnosed incidentally by cystoscopy or urinary tract imaging
- The presence of a diverticulum – even quite a large one – is not an indication for diverticulectomy unless symptoms or cancer are present

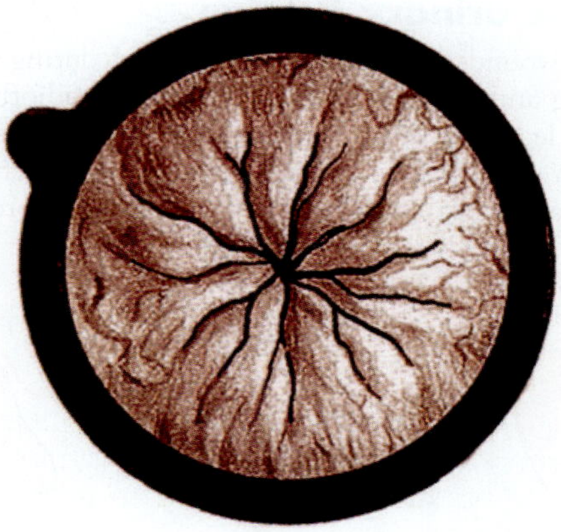

Figure 76.33 Occasional appearance of a diverticulum with inadequate distension of the bladder.

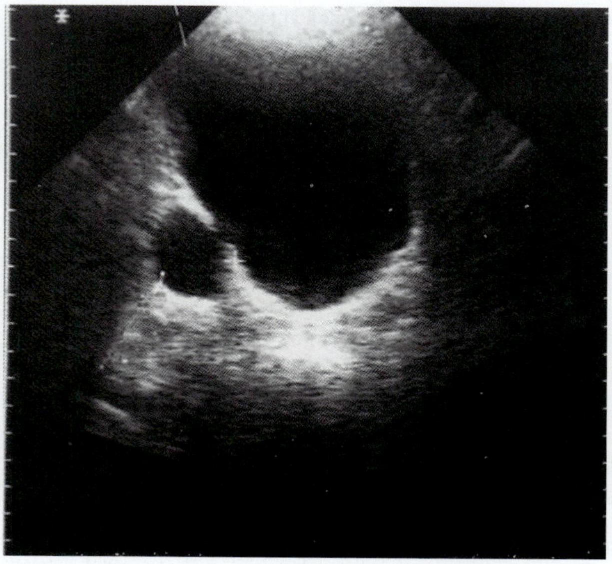

Figure 76.34 Bladder diverticulum demonstrated by ultrasound.

Traction diverticulum (synonym: hernia of the bladder)

A portion of the bladder protruding through the inguinal or femoral hernial orifice occurs in 1.5 per cent of such herniae treated by operation (Figure 76.35).

URINARY FISTULAE

Congenital urinary fistulae

The causes of congenital urinary fistulae include:

- ectopia vesicae;
- a patent urachus – the presence of a urinary leak from the umbilicus, present at birth or commencing soon after, suggests this diagnosis. In adult life, infection in a urachal cyst may produce a fistula and adenocarcinoma may occur (Figures 76.36 and 76.37). Treatment is by means of excision of the urachal tract and closure of the bladder once distal obstruction has been excluded;
- in association with imperforate anus (see Chapters 8 and 73).

Traumatic urinary fistulae

Perforating wounds, damage not recognised during surgery or poor healing and avascular necrosis following radiotherapy and surgery may lead to fistula formation. Also, clot retention occurring after an open bladder operation may lead to dehiscence of the wound and a fistula, which will heal quickly provided the bladder is kept empty with an indwelling catheter.

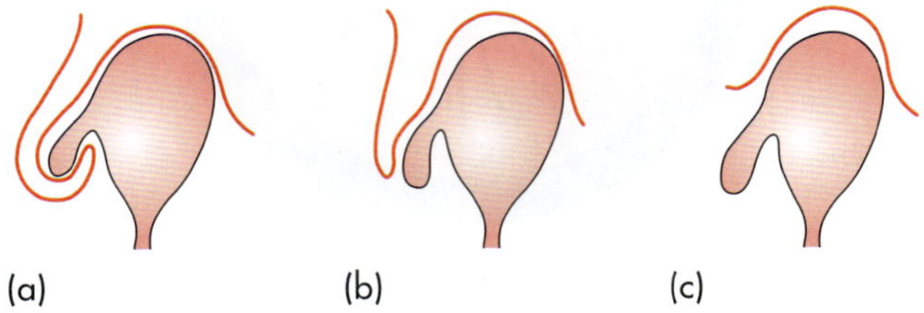

Figure 76.35 (a) Intraperitoneal, (b) paraperitoneal and (c) extraperitoneal hernia of the bladder, in relation to a hernial sac.

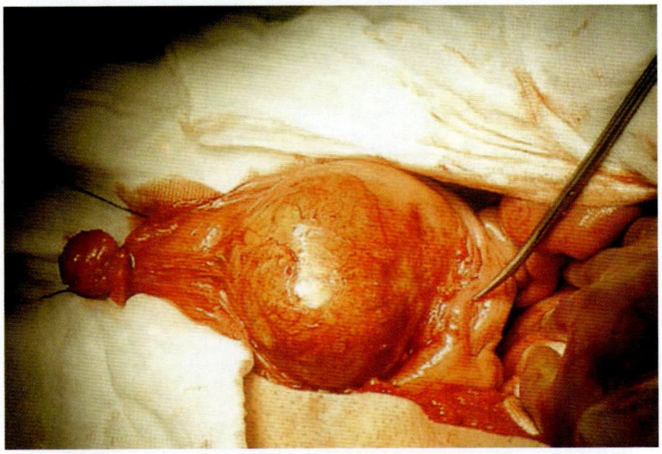

Figure 76.36 An operative photograph showing a large urachal cyst in which adenocarcinoma formation has occurred. A partial cystectomy with total removal of the urachal remnant is about to be carried out.

Vesicovaginal fistulae

Aetiology

- **Obstetric**. The usual cause is protracted or neglected labour.
- **Gynaecological**. The operations chiefly causing this complication are total hysterectomy and anterior colporrhaphy.
- **Radiotherapy**.
- **Direct neoplastic infiltration**. Exceptionally, carcinoma of the cervix ulcerates through the anterior fornix to implicate the bladder.

When an injury to the bladder is recognised and repaired, leakage is uncommon, but escape of urine will quickly follow if such damage passes unnoticed. However, most vesicovaginal fistulae are the result of ischaemic necrosis of the bladder because of prolonged pressure of the fetal head in obstetric cases. In gynaecological cases, the ischaemia is brought about by grasping the bladder wall in an artery forceps, including the bladder wall in a suture or perhaps even by local oedema or haematoma. Leakage because of necrosis of tissue seldom manifests itself before 7 days after the operation. An intractable fistula following radiotherapy for carcinoma of the cervix uteri may arise from avascular necrosis years after the apparent cure of the original lesion.

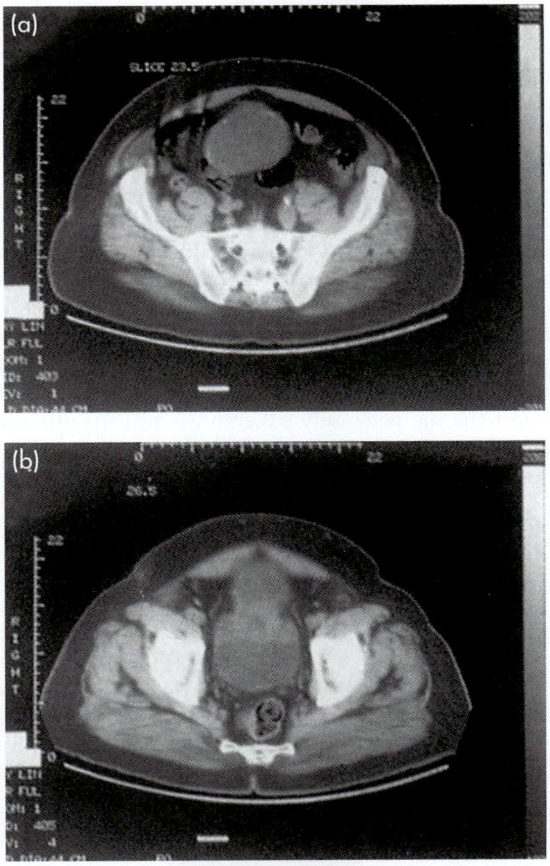

Figure 76.37 A computed tomography scan of the same patient as in Figure 76.36, showing a large urachal cyst closely approximated to the dome of the bladder.

Clinical features

There is leakage of urine from the vagina and excoriation of the vulva. Vaginal examination may reveal a localised thickening on its anterior wall or in the vault. On inserting a vaginal speculum, urine will be seen escaping from an opening in the anterior vaginal wall.

The 'three-swab test'

The differential diagnosis between a ureterovaginal and vesicovaginal fistula can be made by placing a swab in the vagina and injecting a solution of methylene blue through the urethra; the vaginal swab becomes coloured blue if a vesicovaginal fistula is present. Cystoscopy and bilateral retrograde ureterography provide a more reliable demonstration. An IVU should be performed to exclude a coincidental ureterovaginal fistula (ureterovaginal fistula occurs with vesicovaginal fistula in about 10 per cent of cases). Usually, the IVU shows some upper tract dilatation resulting from partial obstruction.

Treatment

Just occasionally, conservative management of a vesicovaginal fistula following hysterectomy, by urethral bladder drainage, is successful; however, the majority of fistulae will require definitive surgical repair. A low fistula (subtrigonal) is best repaired per vaginam. The fistula is exposed, the bladder is closed using absorbable sutures and the vagina subsequently closed with a separate layer. A urethral catheter should be left *in situ* for at least 10 days. For higher (supratrigonal) fistulae, a transvaginal approach can be difficult. These patients should always be cystoscoped before the repair procedure and bilateral ureterograms performed. For high fistulae, a suprapubic approach is the best method in most hands; however, some experts will aim to carry out vaginal closure in most cases that have not involved complex surgery or radiotherapy.

To repair a ureterovaginal fistula, an extraperitoneal approach to the ureter via the previous Pfannenstiel incision is made. Considerable adhesions will be encountered, but the ureter can usually be found above the level of the injury and followed down. Reimplantation into the bladder is often required. Depending on the amount of ureter lost, it may be possible to achieve reimplantation with a psoas hitch procedure. If the gap is too large, a Boari flap of anterior bladder wall should be cut and brought over to meet the ureter and a reimplant performed. The most important principle of ureteric reimplantation is that there should be no tension on the repair.

Fistulae from renal pelvis to skin or gut

Tuberculosis of a kidney may result in a fistula to the duodenum, colon or skin. Similarly, a pyonephrosis may discharge into the gut or onto the skin. Duodenal ulcer involving the pelvis of the right kidney, Crohn's disease involving the renal pelvis or ureter, or cases of xanthogranulomatous pyelonephritis may cause fistulae. A longstanding urinoma will occasionally fistulate into the gut.

Fistulae arising from infection

The most common cause is diverticulitis of the colon. Fistulae may also follow Crohn's disease, appendix abscess or pelvis sepsis after acute salpingitis, or pelvic surgery.

The onset of a fistula from diverticular disease may well be treated as a simple urinary infection. The diagnosis can be difficult to make, but on cystoscopy a patch of oedema on the left side of the vault is suggestive and bubbles of gas may be seen (Figure 76.38). A cystogram may reveal the fistula. The passage of gas per urethram in a patient is most suggestive (provided that diabetes resulting in urinary infection with a gas-forming organism is excluded).

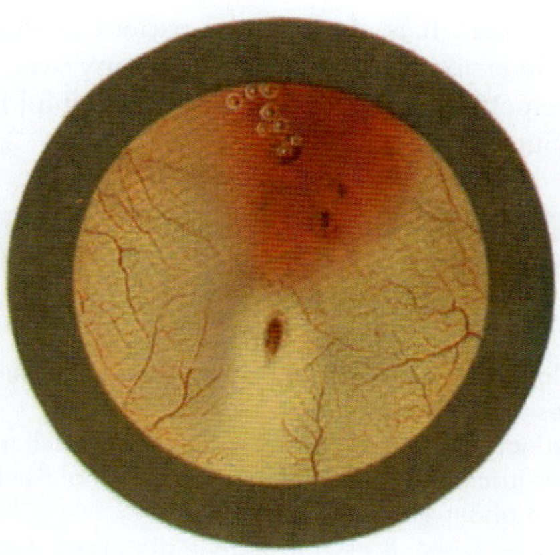

Figure 76.38 Cystoscopic view of a vesicointestinal fistula. Bubbles of gas can be seen issuing from the orifice of the fistula.

Treatment of fistulae caused by diverticular disease

In most patients a single-stage operation is indicated provided that the surgeon is experienced in colonic surgery. At laparotomy, the communication is separated, the hole in the bladder being closed and patched with omentum, and the segment of diseased bowel resected; it is most important to ensure that the left colon and, if necessary, the splenic flexure are fully mobilised to facilitate a tension-free, well-vascularised anastomosis. The bladder is drained by a urethral catheter.

Fistulae caused by carcinoma

By the time that a fistula between the bowel and the bladder has developed, the tumour is usually locally advanced but may be operable.

Urethral fistulae in the male

These occur as the result of infection above a stricture producing a paraurethral abscess that ruptures into the urethra, allowing extravasation to occur suddenly into the scrotum and perineum. Urine and infection extend into the upper 2.5 cm of the thigh and lower abdominal wall. Widespread cellulitis and tissue necrosis (which may lead to Fournier's gangrene) may occur unless drainage of urine is achieved by suprapubic cystotomy and the tissue planes are freely drained by inguinal and scrotal incisions.

Neoplastic fistulae

Primary bladder tumours very rarely produce fistulae. Involvement of the bladder by tumours of the cervix, uterus, colon and rectum can produce fistulae, as may sarcoma of the small gut. Carcinoma of the prostate rarely produces a rectal fistula. Treatment is difficult and in most cases only palliative relief can be given. It is rarely in the patient's interest to carry out urinary diversion, although minimally invasive techniques, such as placement of ureteric stents, can be helpful in palliating symptoms (Summary box 76.9).

Summary box 76.9

Fistulae

- A fistula is a communication between two epithelium-lined surfaces
- Most urinary fistulae are vesicovaginal and result from obstetric trauma; an associated ureterovaginal fistulae occurs in about 10 per cent of cases
- A 'three-swab test' is used to aid the diagnosis. An examination under anaesthesia, vaginoscopy, and cystoscopy and IVU should be performed and, if necessary, retrograde ureterography
- Conservative management is rarely successful
- The principles of repair include good exposure, excision of diseased tissue and tension-free vascularised repair in anatomic layers
- Fistulae caused by radiation, cancer and sepsis can be complex with multiple tracts
- The persistence of a fistula on the skin implies the presence of distal obstruction, chronic infection, such as tuberculosis, or a foreign body, such as a stone or non-absorbable ligature

LOWER URINARY TRACT INFECTION AND CYSTITIS

Infection of the bladder gives rise to symptoms of frequency, urgency, suprapubic discomfort, dysuria and cloudy offensive urine. These symptoms are often known as 'cystitis'. Lower UTIs are much more common in women than in men, particularly in the under 50s. It should be remembered that a lower UTI is often associated with upper tract colonisation and the presence of associated loin pain, pyrexia, rigors and malaise (these symptoms represent complicated infection and should be taken seriously as serious sepsis can ensue).

Isolated infection

A single episode of lower tract infection occurs frequently in females and is rarely complicated.

Recurrent infection

Recurrent infection may be associated with an underlying predisposing cause or may be a result of bacterial resistance. In healthy women, infection after intercourse can occur without any demonstrable abnormality of the urinary tract. Repeated attacks of UTI in women, or a single attack in a man or a child of either sex, should always be followed by investigation to discover and treat the cause; sometimes, however, no cause can be found. Asymptomatic bacteriuria is common and investigation may fail to demonstrate any underlying cause.

Infection in males

Although more common in female adults, the incidence of infection is higher in male infants as underlying urinary tract abnormalities are more frequent. Complicated or recurrent infection in adult males warrants prompt antibiotic therapy and investigation to exclude an underlying cause.

Infection in pregnancy

The incidence of asymptomatic bacteriuria in pregnant women is twice as high as in non-pregnant women. Simple uncomplicated infection can be treated following urine culture with an appropriate antibiotic that is not contraindicated in pregnancy, such as cephalosporin or ampicillin. Non-responsive infection may require intravenous therapy and an ultrasound scan.

Predisposing causes of urinary tract infection

- Incomplete emptying of the bladder, secondary to bladder outflow obstruction, a bladder diverticulum, neurogenic bladder dysfunction or decompensation of the detrusor muscle.
- A calculus, foreign body or neoplasm.
- Incomplete emptying of the upper tract, dilatation of the ureters associated with pregnancy, or vesicoureteric reflux. In childhood, the mainstay of treatment of vesicoureteric reflux is antibiotic therapy; operation is reserved for those with recurrent infection despite antibiotics or with severe upper tract dilatation.
- Oestrogen deficiency, which may give rise to lowered local resistance.
- Colonisation of the perineal skin by strains of *Escherichia coli* expressing molecules that facilitate adherence to mucosa.
- Diabetes.
- Immunosuppression.

Avenues of infection

Ascending infection from the urethra is the most common route (see Chapter 74). The organisms originate in the bowel, contaminate the vulva and reach the bladder. The passage of urethral instruments may cause infection in either sex, especially when the bladder contains residual urine (Figure 76.39). Other routes are less common and include descending infection from the kidney (tuberculosis), haematogenous spread, lymphogenous spread and spread from adjoining structures (Fallopian tube, vagina or gut).

Bacteriology

Bacterial virulence factors affect the ability of a pathogen to infect the host. The possession of pili (rod-shaped structures) that project from the outer membrane increases adhesiveness. The type of pilus can be used to classify the pathogen involved. *Escherichia coli* is the most common organism followed by *Proteus mirabilis*, *Staphylococcus epidermidis* and *Streptococcus faecalis*. Infection with other organisms or infection with mixed organisms is found in patients with neurogenic bladder dysfunction or those with a longstanding indwelling urethral catheter. These organisms include *Pseudomonas*, *Klebsiella*, *Staphylococcus aureus* and various streptococci. Tuberculous infection is considered below. The presence of pus cells without organisms calls for examination for *Mycobacterium tuberculosis* and *Neisseria gonorrhoeae*. Having eliminated these possibilities, the underlying condition may be abacterial cystitis, carcinoma *in situ*, renal papillary necrosis, stones or incomplete treatment of a urinary infection.

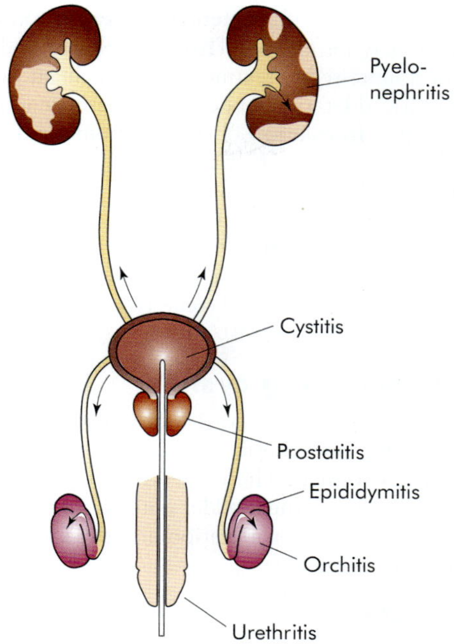

Figure 76.39 Complications liable to follow the changing of a urethral catheter in the presence of urethritis (courtesy of CG Scorer, FRCS, London, UK).

Clinical features

These include frequency, pain, haematuria and pyuria. Pyrexia and rigors are not associated with a simple UTI, but are a sign of upper tract infection or septicaemia.

Examination

On examination, there is tenderness over the bladder. Initial and midstream urine specimens should be collected in a male as acute prostatitis may be present (see below), which will lead to threads in the initial specimen. The midstream specimen must be subjected to microscopy and culture, and the sensitivity of any organisms assessed.

Treatment

Treatment should be commenced immediately and modified if necessary when the bacteriological report is to hand. The patient is urged to drink. Appropriate first-line antibiotics depend on local likely sensitivities, but would include trimethoprim or one of the quinolones. Failure to respond indicates the need for further investigation to exclude predisposing factors. It is important to check for associated allergies or other drugs or conditions that might preclude the use of some antibiotics (e.g. concomitant administration of methotrexate and trimethoprim (both inhibit tetrahydrofolate reductase)).

Investigation

Investigation may be needed in the male or when recurrent infection occurs. This includes measurement of urinary flow rates and post-void residual urine. IVU, ultrasound scan or CT scanning will usually be carried out together with cystoscopy.

Summary box 76.10

UTI in adults

- Isolated UTI in adults is not infrequent and is more common in women
- Recurrent or complicated infection (haematuria, rigors) warrants appropriate antimicrobial therapy and investigation
- Investigation to exclude a predisposing cause includes urinalysis, microscopy and culture, upper tract imaging and cystoscopy
- *Mycobacterium tuberculosis, Neisseria gonorrhoeae* or *Mycoplasma genitalium* should be suspected if pus cells are present but urine culture is negative
- Cancer, especially CIS, masquerading as infection may be diagnosed as abacterial cystitis

Difficult cases may require urodynamic investigation (Summary box 76.10).

SPECIAL FORMS OF LOWER URINARY TRACT INFECTION

Acute abacterial cystitis (acute haemorrhagic cystitis)

The patient presents with severe UTI. Pus is present in the urine but no organism can be cultured. It is commonly sexually acquired, but tuberculous infection and CIS must be ruled out. The underlying causative organism may be *Mycoplasma* or herpes simplex virus. Cyclophosphamide can also cause this problem.

Frequency–dysuria syndrome (urethral syndrome)

This consists of symptoms of lower tract infection but with negative urine cultures. CIS, tuberculosis and interstitial cystitis should be excluded. Most urologists advise patients to adopt general measures such as wearing cotton underwear, using simple soaps, adopting general perineal hygiene measures and voiding after intercourse. Other treatments include cystoscopy and urethral dilatation, although the benefits remain doubtful.

Tuberculous urinary infection

Tuberculous urinary infection is secondary to renal tuberculosis. Early tuberculosis of the bladder commences around the ureteric orifice or trigone, the earliest evidence being pallor of the mucosa due to submucous oedema. Subsequently, tubercles may be seen and, in longstanding cases, there is marked fibrosis and the capacity of the bladder is greatly reduced (Figure 76.40).

Treatment

Tuberculous infection usually responds rapidly to anti-tuberculous drugs but occasionally the involved kidney and ureter have to be removed. If the bladder remains of low capacity, patients will have severe symptoms and the upper tracts are at risk because of high filling pressures and vesicoureteric reflux. Such

Albert Ludwig Siegmund Neisser, 1855–1916, Director of the Dermatological Institute, Breslau, Germany (now Wroclaw, Poland).

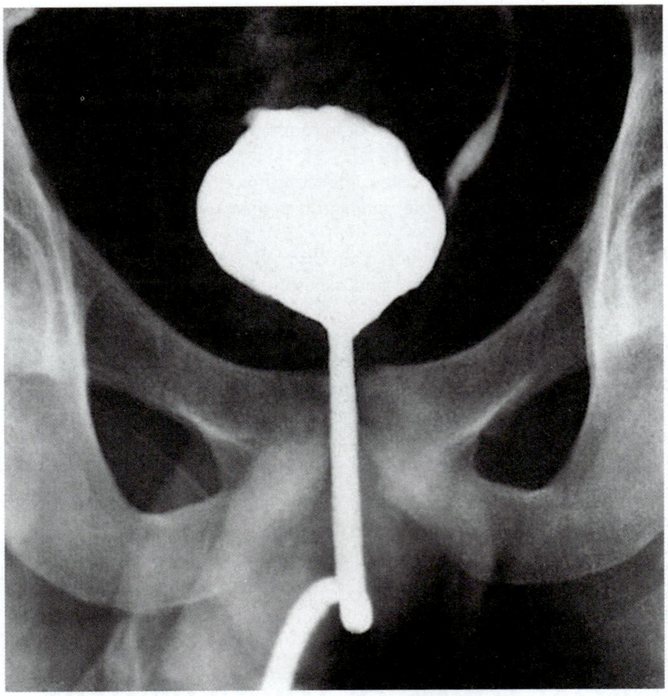

Figure 76.40 Retrograde cystograph showing an exceedingly contracted ('thimble') bladder in a case of tuberculous cystitis.

patients, after appropriate chemotherapy, respond well to bladder augmentation. The ureters may need reimplantation.

Bladder augmentation by ileocystoplasty or caecocystoplasty

The fibrosed supratrigonal bladder is removed and the bladder augmented with a segment of bowel. This may consist of intact caecum, a detubularised segment of ileum or a detubularised ileocaecal segment (see Figures 76.20, 76.21 and 76.22).

Interstitial cystitis (Hunner's ulcer)

For practical purposes, this is confined to women. The first symptom is increased frequency; pain, relieved by micturition and aggravated by jarring and overdistension of the bladder, is another characteristic symptom. In most patients, pyuria and urinary infection are absent. Haematuria also occurs. The aetiology remains as obscure as it was when Guy Hunner described the condition in 1914. It consists of a chronic pancystitis, often with marked infiltration with lymphocytes and macrophages. Fibrosis of the vesical musculature and areas of avascular atrophy of the epithelium occur. Ulceration of the mucosa occurs in the fundus of the bladder. In severe cases, the bladder capacity is reduced to 30–60 mL. The characteristic linear bleeding ulcer is caused by splitting of the mucosa when the bladder is distended under anaesthesia. Inflammation of all coats of the bladder is present with granulation tissue in the submucosa underlying the ulcer. The muscularis is hypertrophied and the peritoneum in proximity to the area of maximum disease is thickened. The inflammation may involve the trigone, the urethra and, in severe cases, the peritoneum. Pronounced mast cell infiltration is seen but is not specific. It is important to check urinary cytology and to biopsy the mucosa to exclude underlying neoplastic disease.

On cystoscopy, the characteristic ulcer is found in the fundus, but it may be absent. This area bleeds readily as the bladder is decompressed. Treatment is difficult and unsatisfactory. Hydrostatic dilatation under anaesthesia may give relief for some months. Instillation of dimethylsulphoxide results in improvement in some patients. Other drugs that have been tried include intravesical heparin, oral ranitidine and steroid therapy. Patients with severe symptoms may well require cystectomy and orthotopic bladder substitution. In patients with severe inflammation involving the trigone and urethra, this operation may not result in complete relief and some type of urinary diversion may be needed.

Alkaline encrusting cystitis

Alkaline encrusting cystitis is rare and is due to urea-splitting organisms causing phosphatic encrustations on the bladder mucosa of elderly women. There are symptoms of chronic UTI and a plain x-ray shows the bladder outline. The encrustations may be removed by bladder irrigation and the infection treated with appropriate antibiotics.

Cystitis cystica

Under the influence of chronic inflammation, the surface epithelium sends down buds, resulting in minute cysts filled with clear fluid, most abundant on the trigone. This is frequently found in patients with recurrent frequency and dysuria.

SCHISTOSOMIASIS OF THE BLADDER

Geographical distribution

The disease is endemic in Egypt, parts of Africa, Israel, Syria, Saudi Arabia, Iran, Iraq and the shores of China's great lakes. Dwellers of the Nile valley have suffered for centuries. Marshes or slow-running fresh water provide the habitat for the freshwater snail (*Bulinus truncatus*) that is the intermediate host (see Chapter 6).

Mode of infestation

The disease is acquired through exposure of the skin to infected water, which usually occurs while bathing. The free-swimming, bifid-tailed embryos (cercariae) of the trematode *Schistosoma haematobium* penetrate the skin. Shedding their tails, they enter blood vessels and are swept to all parts of the body but they flourish in the liver where they live on erythrocytes and develop into male and female worms. Sexual maturity having been attained, the nematodes leave the liver and enter the portal vein. The male worm bends into the shape of a gutter (the gynaecophoric canal) into which a female worm nestles, and the pair makes its way towards the inferior mesenteric vein. *Schistosoma haematobium* has an affinity for the vesical venous plexus, which it reaches through the portosystemic anastomotic channels.

Having reached the bladder, the female worm eventually enters a submucous venule which is so small that it completely blocks it. It now proceeds to lay about 20 ova in a chain; each ovum is provided with a terminal spine that penetrates the vessel wall. A heavily infected subject passes hundreds of ova a day. If the ova reach fresh water, the low osmotic pressure causes rupture and the ciliated miracidium emerges. To survive, it must reach and penetrate the intermediate snail host within 36 hours. Within the snail's liver, the miracidium enlarges and gives rise

Guy Leroy Hunner, 1868–1951, gynaecologist, The Johns Hopkins Hospital, Baltimore, MD, USA.

to myriads of daughter cysts, which are set free on the death of the snail. A single miracidium begets thousands of cercariae to complete the life cycle.

Clinical features

After penetration of the skin, urticaria lasting about 5 days can occur (swimmer's itch). Following an incubation period of 4–12 weeks, a high evening temperature, sweating and asthma, together with leukocytosis and eosinophilia, occur. Usually, an asymptomatic period of several months supervenes before the ova are released, causing the typical early sign and symptom of intermittent, painless, terminal haematuria. Men are affected three times more frequently than women.

Examination of the urine

The last few millilitres of an early-morning urine specimen are collected and centrifuged. Examination on several consecutive days may be required, but a negative result does not exclude bilharziasis, especially in patients no longer resident in bilharzial districts. Antibody detection by enzyme-linked immunoabsorbent assay (ELISA) using *Schistosoma mansoni* adult microsomal antigen (MAMA) can be performed. The test is positive one month after infection and is specific for *Schistosoma mansoni* and *Schistosoma haematobium*.

Cystoscopy

Depending on the length of time for which the disease has remained untreated, cystoscopy will reveal one or more of the following:

1. **Bilharzial pseudotubercles** are the earliest specific appearance of the disease (Figure 76.41);
2. **Bilharzial nodules** (Figure 72.42) are caused by the fusion of tubercles;
3. **'Sandy patches'** are the result of calcified dead ova with degeneration of the overlying epithelium (Figure 76.43);
4. **Ulceration** is the result of sloughing of the mucous membrane containing dead ova (Figure 76.44);
5. **Fibrosis** is mainly the result of secondary infection;
6. **Granulomas**. Bilharzial masses are caused by the aggregation of nodules;
7. **Papillomas** are more pedunculated (Figure 76.45);
8. **Carcinoma** is a common end result in grossly infected bilharziasis of the bladder that has been neglected for years.

Treatment

Safe and effective drugs are available for the treatment of schistosomiasis, including praziquantel taken in three doses of 20 mg/kg (total 60 mg/kg) 4 hours apart. It takes many months for dead ova to be expelled and, even after repeated courses and healing of the bladder lesion, living bilharzial worms have been found at necropsy in the portal system.

Other complications, requiring specific treatment, include the following:

- burinary calculi;
- stricture of the ureters;
- prostatoseminal vesiculitis;
- fibrosis of the bladder and bladder neck (Figure 76.46);
- bilharzial urethral strictures;
- squamous bladder cancer.

Sir Patrick Manson, 1844–1922, practised in Formosa (now Taiwan), and Hong Kong before becoming Physician to the Dreadnought Hospital, Greenwich, London, UK. He is regarded as The Founder of Tropical Medicine.

NEOPLASMS OF THE BLADDER

In total, 95 per cent of primary bladder tumours originate in transitional epithelium; the remainder arise from connective tissue (angioma, myoma, fibroma and sarcoma) or are extra-adrenal phaeochromocytomas.

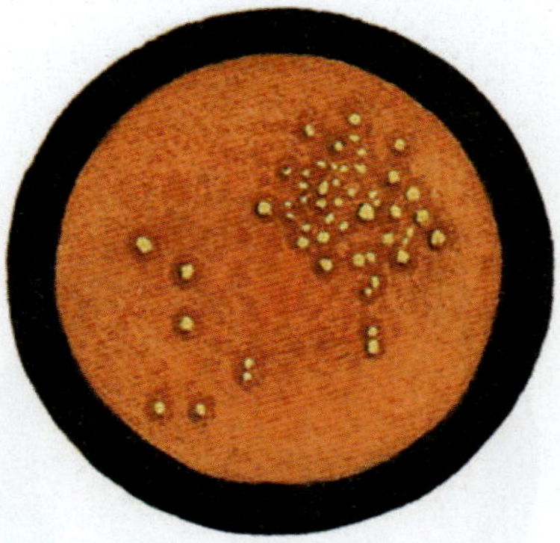

Figure 76.41 Bilharzial tubercles (courtesy of N Makar).

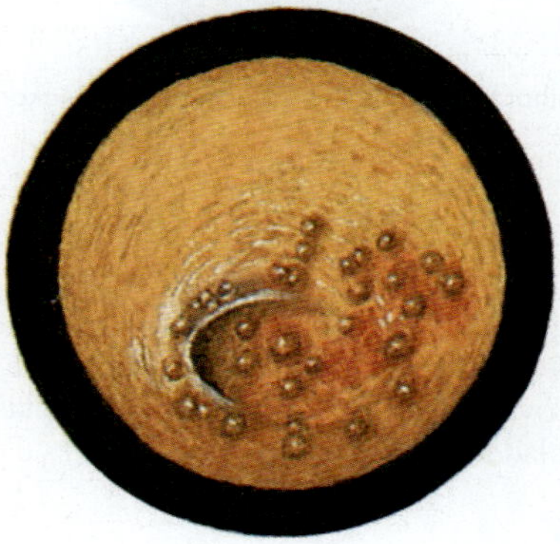

Figure 76.42 Bilharzial nodules (courtesy of N Makar).

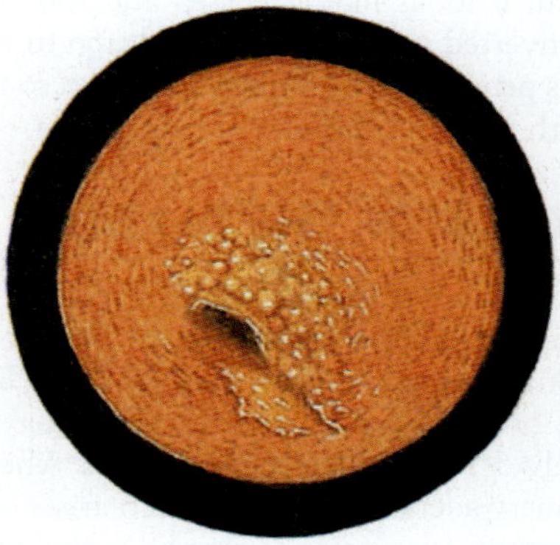

Figure 76.43 'Sandy patches' (courtesy of N Makar).

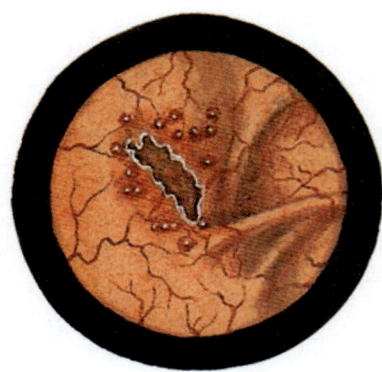

Figure 76.44 Bilharzial ulcer (courtesy of N Makar).

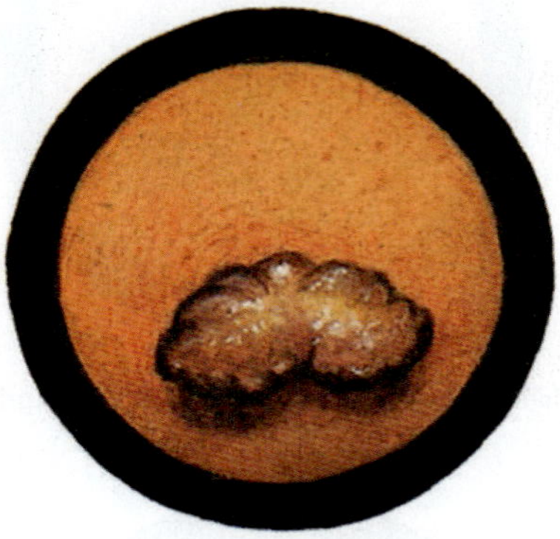

Figure 76.45 Bilharzial papilloma (courtesy of N Makar).

Secondary tumours of the bladder are common and most frequently arise from the sigmoid and rectum, the prostate, the uterus or the ovaries, although bronchial neoplasms may also spread to the bladder.

Pathology

Benign papillary tumours

The papilloma consists of a single frond with a central vascular core with villi; it looks like a red sea anemone (Figures 76.47 and 76.48). Inverted papilloma is a condition in which the proliferative cells penetrate under normal mucosa so that the lesion is covered with smooth urothelium. It is benign.

CARCINOMA OF THE BLADDER

Histological types of bladder cancer include urothelial, squamous and adenocarcinoma (or mixed, as a result of metaplasia in a transitional cell carcinoma (TCC)). Over 90 per cent are urothelial in origin. Pure squamous carcinoma is uncommon (approximately 5 per cent), except in areas where bilharzia is endemic. Primary adenocarcinoma, which arises either from the urachal remnant or from areas of glandular metaplasia, accounts for 1–2 per cent of cases.

Urothelial cell carcinoma

Aetiology

Cigarette smoking is the main aetiological factor (40 per cent of cancers). Occupational exposure to urothelial carcinogens remains common. The first suspicion of a chemical cause for bladder cancer was raised by Rehn in 1895 when he recorded a series of tumours in workers in aniline dye factories. Hueper showed that 2-naphthylamine was carcinogenic in dogs. Subsequent investigation demonstrated that the following compounds may be carcinogenic:

- 2-naphthylamine;
- 4-aminobiphenyl;
- benzidine;
- chlornaphazine;
- 4-chloro-*o*-toluidine;
- *o*-toluidine;
- 4,4′-methylene bis(2-choloroaniline);
- methylene dianiline;
- benzidine-derived azo dyes.

Occupations associated with an increased risk of bladder cancer are:

- textile workers;
- dye workers;
- tyre rubber and cable workers;
- petrol workers;
- leather workers;
- shoe manufacturers and cleaners;
- painters;
- hairdressers;
- lorry drivers;
- drill press operators;
- chemical workers;
- rodent exterminators and sewage workers.

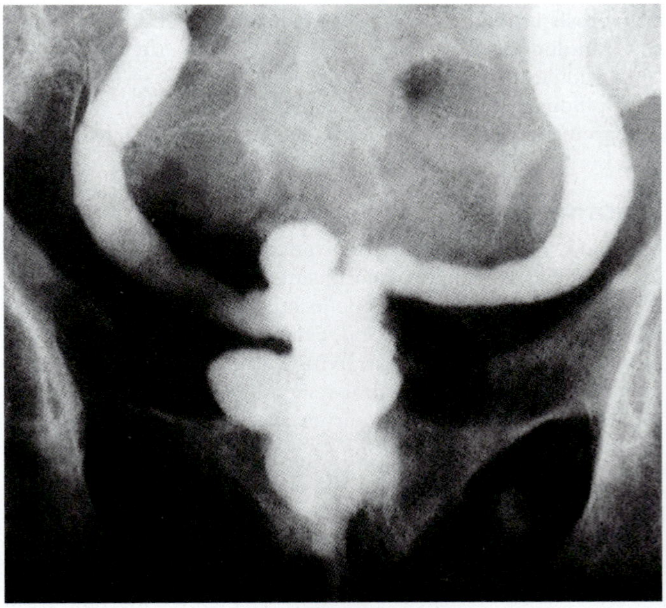

Figure 76.46 Bilharzial contracture of the bladder, with ureteric reflux (courtesy of H Talib, Baghdad, Iraq).

Ludwig Rehn, 1849–1930, surgeon, Frankfurt am Main, Germany.

Bladder cancer became a prescribed industrial disease (No. 39) in 1953, and previously exposed workers may be entitled to compensation. Balkan nephropathy is associated with an increased incidence of upper tract urothelial tumours (see Chapter 75).

A series of genetic events has been clearly implicated in cancer formation but is outside the remit of this chapter. Activation of dominantly acting oncogenes such as *ras* and c-*erbB*-1 and -2, and transcription factors such as E2F3, have been reported in bladder cancer, as has the inactivation of tumour-suppressor genes such as *p53*, *p21*, *p16* and the retinoblastoma gene. Activation of many other genes occurs including those coding for enzymes that dissolve the basement membrane, such as the metalloproteinases (stromelysin, collagenases and elastase), lysosomal enzymes such as the cathepsins and others including urinary plasminogen activators; angiogenic factors (e.g. vascular endothelial growth factor (VEGF)) and other peptide growth factors such as the epidermal growth factor and its receptor (EGFR) also have a role to play, as well as the fibroblast growth factor and its receptor-3 (FGFR-3) which was found to be altered mostly in non-muscle invasive disease. These changes are common to several tumour types, including prostate cancer (Summary box 76.11). More recently, new approaches through genome-wide association studies allowed the investigation of genetic susceptibility for urothelial cancer. Several new loci were identified, but to date, only two, NAT2 (N-acetyltransferase 2) and GSTM1 (glutathione S-transferase Mu 1) have been demonstrated to be consistent germline susceptibility markers. These genetic markers do not yet have sufficient discriminatory ability to be used for clinical decision making.

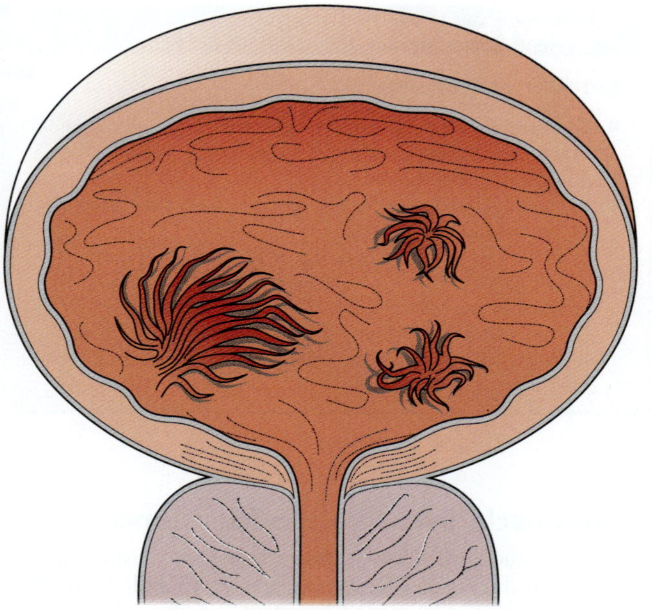

Figure 76.47 Papillary tumour with daughter implantation ('kiss' cancer).

Tumour staging and grading

Study of the biological behaviour of transitional cell cancer of the bladder shows that cancers fall into the three following groups. Depth of invasion (T) from the tumour–node–metastasis (TNM) classification and grade (World Health Organization I, II or III) are important factors in planning treatment and determining prognosis in bladder cancer.

- Non-muscle-invasive pTa (Figure 76.48) and pT1 tumours account for 70 per cent of all new cases; the previous terminology of 'superficial' bladder cancer in this category has now been abandoned; it is important to distinguish however 'low-risk' uothelial cancers which are unlikely to progress, such as well differentiated (G1) pTa tumours (not invading lamina propria), from 'high-risk' cancers such as poorly differentiated (G3) pT1 cancers (invading lamina propria), which should be followed up carefully and treated aggressively as necessary. This can be determined by careful histological examination. Single papillary pTa tumours account for a significant proportion of bladder cancers and carry an excellent prognosis.
- Muscle-invasive disease (pT2) accounts for 25 per cent of new cases. Such tumours carry a much worse prognosis as they are subject to local invasion and distant metastasis.
- Flat, non-invasive CIS (primary CIS) accounts for 5 per cent of new cases. Unless diagnosed and treated promptly, it carries a poor prognosis (Summary box 76.12). The highest risk non-muscle invasive cancer is found with multifocal poorly differentiated tumours invading lamina propria (pT1G3) in the presence of CIS.

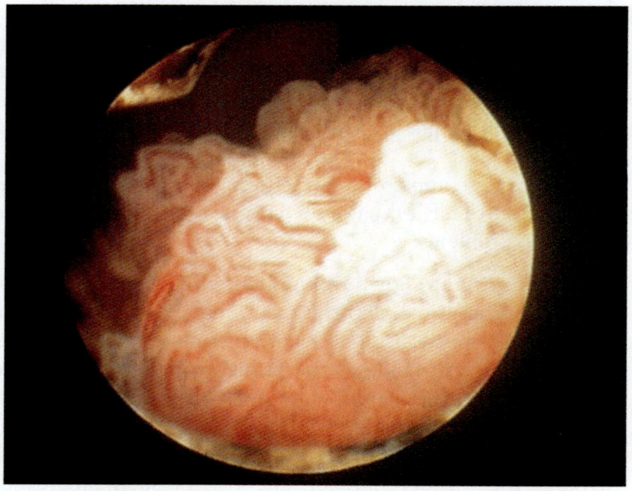

Figure 76.48 Endoscopic photograph of a pTa bladder tumour about to be resected.

Summary box 76.11

Urothelial cell carcinoma of the bladder

- The fourth most common non-dermatological malignancy in men (male–female ratio 3:1)
- Strongly associated with smoking and chemical exposure in western societies
- Strongly associated with *Schistosoma haematobium* infection (bilharzial bladder cancer) in regions where the parasite is endemic
- Reducing in incidence in countries where smoking is decreasing

Summary box 76.12

Bladder cancer staging

- Cystoscopy and resection of tumour with separate resection of the tumour base is essential for accurate analysis of invasion into detrusor muscle
- Bimanual examination should be performed after resection of the tumour
- Complete urinary tract imaging is required using contrast CT urography, MR or intravenous urography where other techniques are not available. Cross-sectional imaging by CT or MR is essential in high-risk and muscle invasive disease to stage the tumour further including lymph node status for metastasis.

Non-muscle invasive bladder cancer

These are usually papillary tumours that grow in an exophytic fashion into the bladder lumen (Figures 76.47 and 76.48). They may be single or multiple and may appear pedunculated, arising on a stalk with a narrow base, but if the tumours are less well differentiated they are more solid with a wider base. The mucosa around the tumour is often rather oedematous, with angry-looking, dilated blood vessels. These areas may contain *in situ* changes (concomitant CIS).

The urothelium elsewhere in the bladder may appear rather oedematous and velvety; this suggests a generalised 'field change' with the presence of widespread CIS. The most common sites for superficial tumours are the trigone and lateral walls of the bladder.

After initial complete treatment by endoscopic transurethral resection (TURT), patients with pTa or pT1 disease may develop two problems:

1 About 50–70 per cent develop recurrent tumours that may be single or multiple, and the recurrences may occur on one or on many occasions. The recurrent tumours are usually of the same stage or grade as the primary tumour. High-grade, multiple tumours with concomitant CIS are most likely to develop recurrent disease.
2 About 15 per cent will develop a recurrent tumour that invades the bladder muscle. The risk of such progression increases with high-grade disease, pT1 disease, multiple primary disease and concomitant CIS. Many urologists now regard the presence of pT1 grade 3 tumours as an indication for offering the patient immediate cystectomy because of the excellent outcome.

This behaviour provides the rationale for performing check cystoscopies. The factors that result in an increased recurrence and progression rate are:

- high grade;
- pT1 disease;
- concomitant CIS;
- multiple primary tumours;
- recurrent disease at the first check cystoscopy three months after diagnosis.

Patients presenting with a solitary grade 1 or grade 2 pTa tumour without concomitant CIS, which does not recur within the first six months, have an excellent outcome. Patients with recurrent low-grade disease can be treated with intravesical instillations of a chemotherapeutic agent such as mitomycin-C or epirubicin with regular cystocopic checkups and repeat biopsies, or immunotherapy using regular intravesical instillations of Bacille Calmette–Guérin (BCG), an attenuated form of the anti-tuberculosis vaccine. Patients with high-grade pTa or pT1 disease are at high risk and should be counselled very carefully. The options include immediate cystectomy or a more conservative approach with a course of BCG) followed by careful cystosopic assessment and maintenance instillations. assessment. The presence of persistent disease after BCG therapy is reason to offer cystectomy (Summary box 76.13).

Summary box 76.13

Non-muscle-invasive bladder cancer (NMIBC)

- Does not invade the detrusor muscle but can extend to the lamina propria
- Extension to the lamina propria (pT1) is a significant risk factor for progression to invasive disease, especially if associated with high-grade disease and CIS
- The incidence of recurrence of this disease can be reduced by intravesical chemotherapy and immunotherapy
- High-risk superficial disease (any grade 3 disease) is best managed by BCG immunotherapy followed by radical treatment if disease persists

Muscle-invasive bladder cancer

Muscle-invasive tumours are nearly always solid (Figure 76.49), although there may be a low tufted surface. These tumours are often large and broad based, having an irregular, ulcerated, appearance within the bladder. The incidence of metastases, whether from lymphatic invasion in the pelvis or blood-borne to the lung, liver or bones, is much more common and will cause the death of 30–50 per cent of patients (Summary box 76.14).

Summary box 76.14

Muscle-invasive bladder cancer

- Muscle-invasive bladder cancer should be staged by an accurate bimanual examination performed under anaesthesia before and after resection of the tumour
- Complete urinary tract assessment should be performed, including CT, MR or IV urography, as well as cross-sectional imaging identify lymph node involvement and distant spread
- Radical primary treatment options include radical cystectomy, urinary diversion and thorough lymph node dissection which tends to be offered as first line, or radical external beam radiotherapy
- Neoadjuvant chemotherapy improves survival rates as well as adjuvant chemotherapy in some cases particularly in the presence of nodal and distant disease
- Locally advanced disease may be downstaged by radiotherapy or chemotherapy to enable salvage cystectomy

Albert Leon Charles Calmette, 1863–1933, and Jean-Marie Camille Guérin, 1872–1961, microbiologists at the Institute Pasteur, at Lille in France, introduced the Bacille Calmette–Guérin in 1908.

In situ carcinoma

The histological appearance of irregularly arranged cells with large nuclei and a high mitotic index replacing the normally well-ordered urothelium is known as CIS. It may occur alone (primary CIS) or in association with a new tumour (concomitant CIS) or it may occur later in a patient who has previously had a tumour (secondary CIS). It can only be diagnosed when a biopsy is examined under the microscope. It may cause severe symptoms of dysuria, suprapubic pain and frequency (hence its old name of malignant cystitis). It carries a risk for the patient of developing a malignant muscle-invasive cancer. Without treatment, 50 per cent will die of invasive bladder cancer. It can be treated initially with intravesical BCG, but failure of response is an indication for cystectomy. CIS cannot be treated with external beam radiotherapy

Pure squamous cell carcinoma of the bladder

Squamous cell tumours tend to be solid and are nearly always associated with muscle invasion. This is the most prevalent form of bladder cancer in areas where bilharzia is endemic. Squamous cell tumours may be associated with chronic irritation caused by stone disease in the bladder as a result of metaplasia.

Pure adenocarcinoma

Adenocarcinoma accounts for approximately 1–2 per cent of all bladder cancers. It usually arises in the fundus of the bladder at the site of the urachal remnant. Occasionally, primary adenocarcinomas arise at other sites and probably originate from areas of glandular metaplasia. Such tumours need to be distinguished from secondary cancer, and can be treated with partical cystectomy

CLINICAL FEATURES OF BLADDER CARCINOMA

Painless gross haematuria is the most common symptom and is indicative of a bladder carcinoma until proven otherwise. Often, however, the patient fails to declare the symptom to their GP. The bleeding may give rise to clot formation and clot urinary retention.

Constant pain in the pelvis usually heralds extravesical spread. There is often frequency and discomfort associated with urination. Pain in the loin or pyelonephritis may indicate ureteric obstruction and hydronephrosis. A late manifestation is nerve involvement causing pain that is referred to the suprapubic region, groins, perineum, anus and into the thighs.

It is also important to assess the patient as a whole. Many are elderly men who have been lifelong smokers and who suffer from chronic obstructive airway disease or cardiovascular disease. Their suitability for major surgery must be borne in mind.

INVESTIGATION OF BLADDER CARCINOMA

Urine

Urine should be cultured and examined cytologically for malignant cells. This is not a good screening test but a positive result is highly specific, and it is mostly helpful with high grade disease

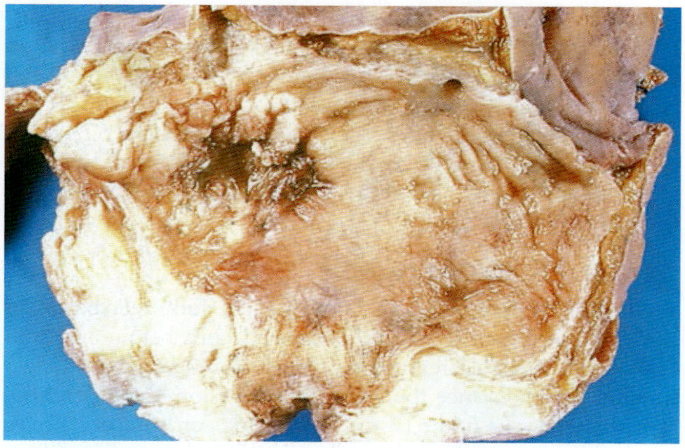

Figure 76.49 Radical cystectomy specimen showing a large solid bladder cancer with total removal of the bladder and prostate.

and CIS. New tests are being developed based on the presence of antigens such as nuclear matrix proteins (NMP22) or minichromosome maintenance (MCM) proteins, which may be able to detect new or recurrent tumours; and epigenetic events such as methylated panels of markers or microRNA fragments. These tests continue to be under evaluation and are not used routinely.

Blood

Estimation of haemoglobin and the level of serum electrolytes and urea should be carried out.

CT, magnetic resonance, IVU or ultrasound scanning

This should be performed on all patients with painless haematuria. Occasionally, the preliminary film shows a faint shadow of an encrusted neoplasm of the bladder. The most common radiological sign is a filling defect (Figure 76.50). Occasionally, irregularity of the bladder wall may herald the presence of an invasive tumour. Hydronephrosis may occur if a superficial tumour grows up the intramural ureter or if direct invasion of the ureteric wall occurs. Ultrasound scanning should be carried out if the kidney is non-functioning to determine its presence and the possibility of an obstructed system.

Cross-sectional imaging

Non-contrast CT or magnetic resonance (MR) imaging is being used in some centres instead of IVU or ultrasound scanning for the immediate management of patients with gross painless haematuria. For staging when a muscle-invasive bladder cancer is suspected, contrast-enhanced CT is used, ideally before TURT. False-positive pT3 disease can be diagnosed if cross-sectional imaging is carried out soon after TURT. Magnetic resonance imaging is being used more frequently (Figure 76.51) and can demonstrate lymph node metastasis or muscle invasion.

Cystourethroscopy

Cystourethroscopy is the mainstay of diagnosis and should always be performed on patients with haematuria. It can be carried out with a rigid instrument under general anaesthesia or with a flexible instrument under local anaesthesia. The urethra is inspected at the initial insertion of the instrument (urethroscopy) and the bladder is then examined in a systematic fashion (cystoscopy). Conventional 'white' light cystoscopy has been improved recently by the introduction of photodynamic 'blue' light cystoscopy which relies on the photosensitiser hexaminolevulinate. It is now recommended in patients with high suspicion of the disease and negative initial findings and in follow up of patients with CIS.

Bimanual examination

A bimanual examination with the patient fully relaxed under general anaesthesia should be performed both before and after endoscopic surgical treatment of these tumours. The bladder should be empty. Once there is muscle invasion, the differentiation between pT2 and pT3 disease depends on whether a mass is palpable bimanually at the end of the procedure (pT3). When invasion has spread into the prostate in a man or the vagina in a woman, it is classified as pT4a. If the tumour is fixed to the lateral pelvic side wall, it is staged as pT4b.

TREATMENT FOR CARCINOMA OF THE BLADDER

Non-muscle invasive tumours

Endoscopic surgery

The tumour should be carefully resected in layers using a resectoscope. The base of the tumour is sent separately for histological examination. Small pinch biopsies are taken near to and distant from the primary lesion when CIS is suspected (inflamed or velvety appearance). After removal of the tumour, two or three further loops of tissue from the base should be sent separately so that the pathologist can accurately determine whether there is lamina propria or muscle invasion. The base of the tumour is then coagulated, so achieving haemostasis. The appearance of pale-yellow glistening fat will indicate a perforation of the bladder. Should this occur before the resection is complete, it may be prudent to stop the resection and leave a catheter in the bladder for a few days. In this instance, the procedure could be completed some 2 weeks later. The bimanual examination is repeated at the end of the endoscopic procedure. Following these procedures, an irrigating catheter is left *in situ* for 48 hours to prevent clot retention of urine. There is good evidence that a single dose of mitomycin (mitomycin C; 40 mg in 60 mL of fluid) instilled into the bladder before catheter removal decreases the risks of recurrence in patients with pTa and pT1 grade 1 and 2 disease.

Patients with larger solid tumours should have adequate material resected for histological staging and grading. If possible and straightforward, the mass of the tumour should be resected as completely as possible – even when pT2 or pT3 disease is suspected.

Follow up

Most urologists agree that patients with a single low- or medium-grade pTa tumour can safely be treated by resection alone plus a single instillation of mitomycin, followed up with regular cystoscopies.

The treatment of patients with multiple low- or medium-grade pTa tumours can be by either resection alone or resection

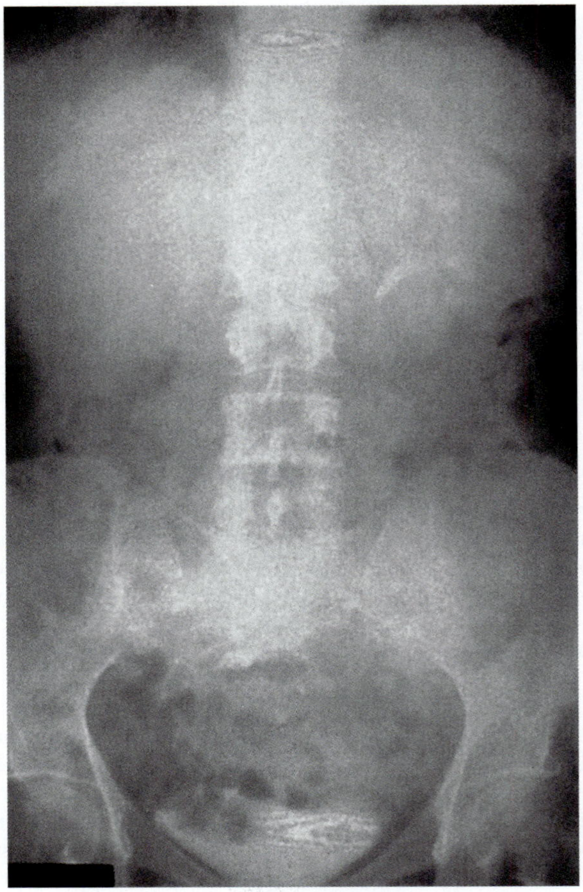

Figure 76.50 Intravenous urography showing a filling defect in the region of the right ureteric orifice.

followed by a 6-week course of intravesical chemotherapy with mitomycin, doxorubicin or epirubicin.

The treatment of pT1 disease is difficult. Approximately 30 per cent of tumours are understaged at first resection. For this reason, a repeat cystoscopy and resection of the tumour base is advocated within 6 weeks. Some urologists would offer immediate cystectomy to a patient with a high-grade pT1 tumour, particularly if it were multiple or accompanied by CIS, because of the 30–50 per cent risk of progression to muscle invasion. Others will treat such patients by endoscopy followed by immunotherapy with intravesical BCG. The most effective treatment of solitary medium-grade pT1 disease remains uncertain, but a reasonable approach would be endoscopic resection followed by reresection of the area after 6 weeks, followed by intravesical BCG.

Follow-up cystoscopies are essential; they may be carried out under local anaesthesia with a flexible cystoscope or under general anaesthesia if the urologist feels that the patient is at high risk of recurrence. They should be performed at three-monthly intervals over the first year; following this the time interval between cystoscopies can be determined according to the presence or absence of further disease. In total, 30 per cent of patients will never develop another tumour so that, if the bladder has remained clear after two years, annual inspection

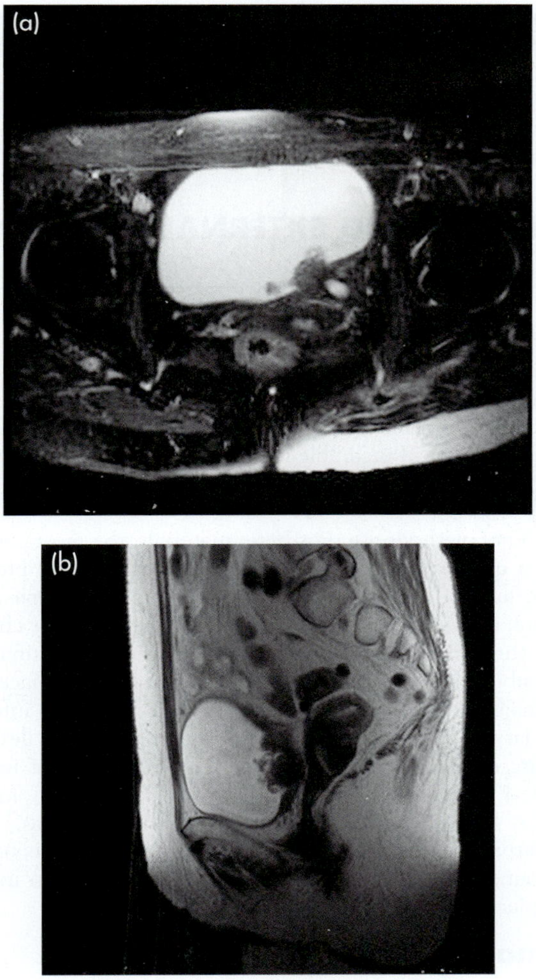

Figure 76.51 (a) Cross-sectional magnetic resonance imaging showing a 'cystogram' and a bladder cancer. (b) Cross-sectional magnetic resonance imaging showing invasive bladder cancer.

may be adequate. For patients who go on to develop multiple recurrences within the bladder at each examination, the cystoscopies need to be maintained at frequent intervals so that the growths can be resected. These patients are at a greater risk of their disease progressing; although intravesical chemotherapy can decrease the recurrence rate, no reduction in progression rates has been found.

Open surgical excision

This should be totally avoided. If by some error a bladder containing a tumour is entered, then the tumour may be removed with a diathermy needle and the base coagulated and the bladder closed. Postoperative radiotherapy to the wound will diminish the chance of tumour implantation.

Muscle-invasive tumours

The treatment of cancer with proven muscle invasion remains a subject for debate. Whatever the modality of treatment employed, few centres have five-year survival figures of more than 50 per cent. There is a move towards primary surgical treatment in most centres. The use of systemic chemotherapy with a combination of agents – cisplatin, methotrexate, doxorubicin and vinblastine (M-VAC) or cisplatin plus gemcitabine given before (neoadjuvant) radical cystectomy – has been shown to be of benefit. The current evidence is that neoadjuvant chemotherapy improves survival by about 5–7 per cent.

Radiotherapy

External beam radiotherapy

External beam radiotherapy is usually given at 60 Gy over a 4- to 6-week period. There is a complete response rate of 40–50 per cent. Unfortunately, some patients do not respond and others exhibit only a partial response, with pTa or pT1 tumour remaining in the bladder giving rise to a risk of recurrence. Patients with residual disease after radiotherapy should be offered 'salvage cystectomy' if they are fit. Proponents of radiotherapy claim that it avoids the need to remove the bladder in some patients and allows men to retain potency. Radiotherapy is not without complications, and during the course of treatment will cause urinary frequency and also diarrhoea. Late complications can leave the bladder contracted and fibrosed, in which case it may need to be removed for palliative reasons. Late complications affecting the rectum should be uncommon, especially if lateral fields of irradiation are employed.

Surgery

Partial cystectomy

This should be limited to the treatment of small adenocarcinomas of the bladder.

Radical cystectomy and pelvic lymphadenectomy

This is now standard treatment for localised pT2–pT3 disease without evidence of secondary spread or of CIS that has not responded to BCG. Before contemplating radical surgery to remove the bladder, it is important to have evidence that surgical cure is attainable. Cross-sectional imaging of the pelvis may locally overstage the bladder if a recent resection has been carried out, although the finding of grossly enlarged pelvic, iliac or para-aortic nodes or liver metastases will alter the decision for cystectomy. A bone scan (using technetium-99m (99mTc)) will help to show whether there is spread to bone, and a chest plain x-ray should be performed to exclude pulmonary metastases, although many centres now perform routine CT imaging of the chest preoperatively and it tends to be more sensitive than plain x-ray in detecting small lung lesions.

Operation

Alternative drainage for urine is necessary following removal of the bladder. The standard procedure is to perform an ileal conduit diversion. Male patients should be counselled about the onset of erectile impotence and absent ejaculation following the operation, although in some cases the nerve supply for erectile function can be preserved through careful dissection; they should also be told about alternative forms of urinary diversion, which include continent urinary diversions and orthotopic bladder replacement.

Patients should be seen by a stoma care therapist, who will help to advise the patient and will try different ileostomy bags to ensure that the correct site is chosen, avoiding skin creases so that one does not end up with the disaster of a leaking urinary ileostomy. A decision is made about whether the male urethra is to be removed (depending on the estimated risk of recurrence within the urethra); a urethrectomy is usually indicated in patients with primary CIS or those with tumour invading the prostate stroma. Many surgeons are now offering total replacement of the bladder after cystectomy.

The patient should receive prophylactic antibiotics including metronidazole, cefuroxime and amoxicillin, and low-dose heparin or equivalent thrombo-embolic prophylaxis including physical means such as stockings and inflatable devices applied to the legs peroperatively to promote venous circulation.

The abdomen is opened through a midline incision extending down to the symphysis pubis. The liver and the retroperitoneum are checked for evidence of metastases, and the operability of the bladder is assessed. A bilateral pelvic lymphadenectomy is performed, removing external iliac nodes, internal iliac nodes and the nodes in the obturator fossae. Some surgeons will remove lymph nodes up to the aortic bifurcation or higher with some evidence of improved long-term oncological outcomes. The vessels passing to the bladder from the side wall of the pelvis are ligated and divided; these include the obliterated hypogastric vessels, the superior vesical artery, the middle vesical veins, and the inferior vesical arteries and veins. The ureters are then divided. The posterior ligaments extending from the pararectal area to the back of the bladder are ligated and divided, and the layer posterior to Denonvilliers's fascia is opened up. The endopelvic fascia is then divided on each side and the puboprostatic ligaments are divided. A ligature is passed between the dorsal vein complex and the urethra, and the former is ligated and divided. The urethra is then mobilised and divided. The ligaments lateral to the prostate are divided and the bladder is removed. In women, the uterus and anterior vaginal wall need to be included. Women must be counselled about the loss of ovarian and uterine function.

An isolated loop of ileum is then prepared on its own mesentery, and continuity of the small bowel restored. The ureters are then implanted into the bowel segment and the ileostomy is created. Meticulous care must be taken to close all mesenteric windows, thus avoiding internal hernias. If the bladder is to be replaced orthotopically, a reservoir made from detubularised bowel (usually a segment of well vascularised ileum) is created and anastomosed to the urethra after implantation of the ureters.

The operative mortality rate associated with cystectomy used to be considerable but is now <2 per cent. Late complications include urethral recurrence (about 5–8 per cent), which is increased in the presence of multifocal tumours, CIS and, particularly, invasion of prostatic stroma (Figure 76.52).

Leukoplakia

This condition is simply squamous metaplasia of the bladder. Profuse production of keratin may result in the passing of white particles in the urine. It cannot be treated easily. Localised areas may be resected endoscopically. Diffuse leukoplakia of the bladder is pre-malignant and results in squamous cancer of the bladder. Careful cystoscopic assessment is required and the condition may require cystectomy.

Endometriosis

Endometriosis within the bladder wall is rare but can have the appearance of a vascular bladder tumour or a tumour that contains chocolate-coloured or bluish cysts. The swelling enlarges and bleeds during menstruation. If medical management fails, by means of danazol or luteinising hormone-releasing hormone (LHRH) agonists, further treatment is usually by means of partial cystectomy or full-thickness endoscopic resection, depending on its site. The condition may be part of more widespread disease. Endometriosis is also a cause of ureteric stricture.

INTERNAL AND EXTERNAL URINARY DIVERSION

Indications

Diversion of the urine may be either a temporary expedient to relieve distal obstruction or a permanent procedure when the bladder has been removed or has lost normal neurological control and in cases of incurable fistula or irremovable obstruction.

Methods of urinary diversion

Temporary methods use prosthetic materials, the most common being a urinary catheter. In elderly patients unfit for prostatectomy, and in some patients with terminal carcinoma of the prostate, an indwelling silicone urethral Foley catheter changed every three months is a satisfactory method of drainage. A suprapubic placement is an alternative to urethral placement. The major drawback of long-term catheterisation is infection secondary to the associated bacteriuria that invariably develops. Ureteric obstruction can be relieved by placement of internal 'double-J' pigtail ureteric stents, which can remain for 4–5 months, but are usually changed every three months. As an alternative, a nephrostomy tube, inserted percutaneously by ultrasound and fluoroscopic imaging, is effective when internal stent placement is not feasible.

Permanent urinary diversion

External diversion

Ileal conduit

Permanent urinary tract diversion is most commonly performed by conduit diversion. The ureters are implanted into a short, isolated segment of ileum (Figure 76.53a) or, less commonly, colon. The conduit diverts the urine onwards to a cutaneous stoma for collection in an ileostomy bag. This form of diversion is well established and associated with a low complication rate of less than 10 per cent. The main complication is ureteroileal stricture, which can be limited by spatulation of the distal ureters and an end-to-end anastomosis as described by Wallace (Figure 76.53a). Stenosis at the ileocutaneous site is

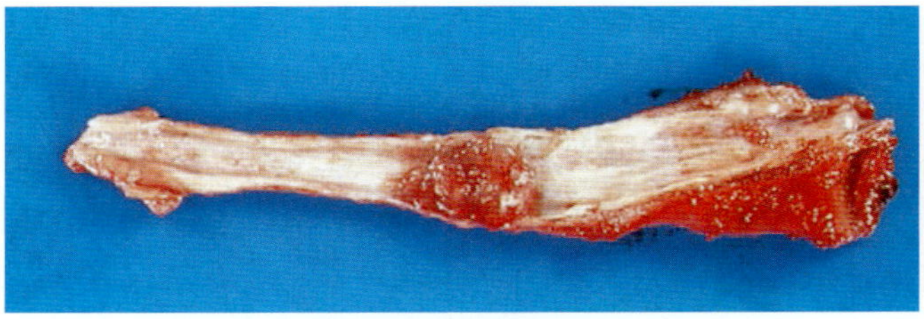

Figure 76.52 Urethrectomy specimen from a patient who has previously undergone a radical cystectomy showing new transitional cell tumour formation in the urethra.

Charles Pierre Denonvilliers, 1808–1872, Professor of Anatomy, and later of Surgery, Paris, France.

less frequent, and a short isoperistaltic conduit limits the formation of a residual urine volume, reducing infection and avoiding the problems of reabsorption of urine. In some cases, when the pelvic area has been subjected to radiation, the lower ureters may be unhealthy; a high division with insertion of the ureters into an ileal loop above the root of the mesentery may then be wiser (Figure 76.54).

The site for the stoma must be chosen before operation, in consultation with a stoma care therapist; the site is marked indelibly on the skin.

Operative details

A coil of ileum, approximately 15–20 cm long and 30 cm from the ileocaecal valve, with its blood supply intact, is isolated. The left ureter is brought behind the mesorectum. The ureters may be joined to the ileum either end-to-side or end-to-end after anastomosing of the distal spatulated ureters to form a plate (Wallace). The distal end of the coil is brought out through an incision made at the site identified before operation; a disc of skin and fat is removed, a cruciate incision is made in the fascia and the muscle is split. The stoma is made about 2–3 cm long. It is evaginated initially by means of four sutures passing through the skin, the ileal loop as it passes through the opening and the cut edge of the ileum.

Internal urinary diversion

Colon and rectum

The advantage of diverting urine into the colon is that no collecting apparatus is necessary. Clearly, however, the anal sphincter must be competent. Before ureterosigmoidostomy is undertaken, the patient must prove that he or she can control at least 200 mL of fluid in the rectum. The disadvantage of the operation is that the renal tract is exposed continuously to infection from the faeces; this can be minimised by constructing an anti-reflux procedure. Various diversions are described; the Mainz II ureterosigmoidostomy creates a cul-de-sac type low-pressure reservoir in the sigmoid into which the ureters are placed (see Figure 76.53b). This reduces reflux, and bowel content, although in contact with urine, takes a direct route to the rectum. In the long term, cancer can develop at long-standing ureterocolic junctions (Figure 76.55).

Bladder reconstruction

Over the past decade, several techniques have been developed to allow a near-spherical urinary reservoir to be formed out of various lengths of bowel that are detubularised. These may consist of ileum, ileum and caecum or sigmoid colon (see Figure 76.53c). The ureters can then be reimplanted in these reservoirs in an anti-reflux manner and the reservoir anastomosed to the membranous urethra in the male (see Figures 76.20, 76.21 and 76.22). This is only indicated when the urethra can be preserved, with no evidence of tumour at the junction between the urethra and the prostate in the male, and bladder neck in the female. About 15–30 per cent of patients cannot empty the neobladder completely and will need to perform intermittent self-catheterisation. The results are good after radical cystectomy, particularly in younger well motivated patients.

Continent urinary diversion

A similar concept is used in the construction of continent diversions. A urinary reservoir is made as described above and the

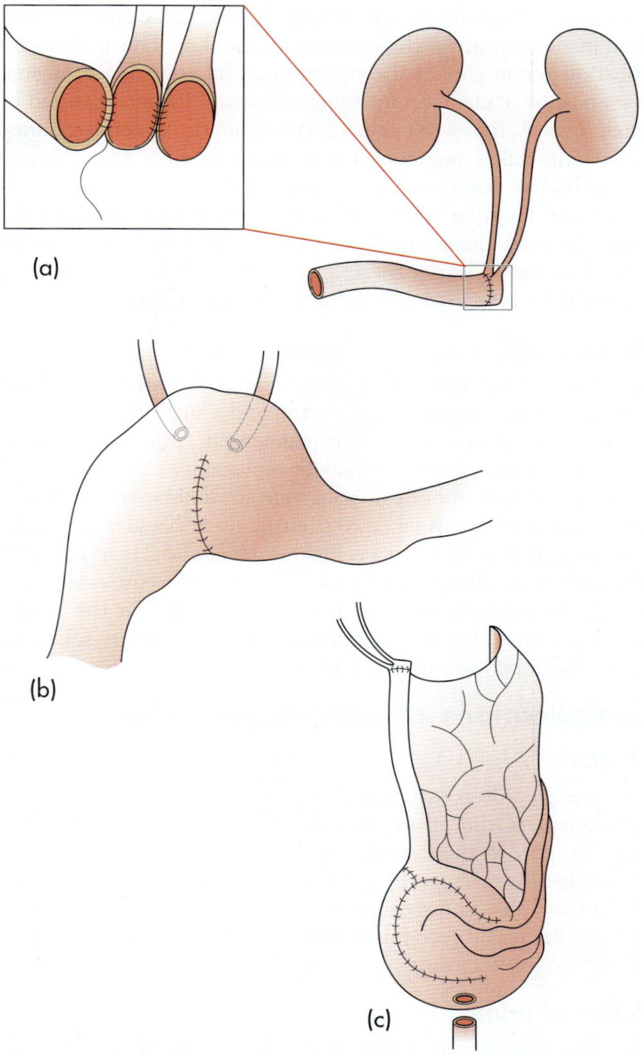

Figure 76.53 Diversion of urine. Favoured methods: (a) ileal conduit; the ureters are spatulated and anastomosed to ileum end-to-side (insert); (b) ureterosigmoidostomy; (c) ileal neobladder with anti-reflux long afferent limb.

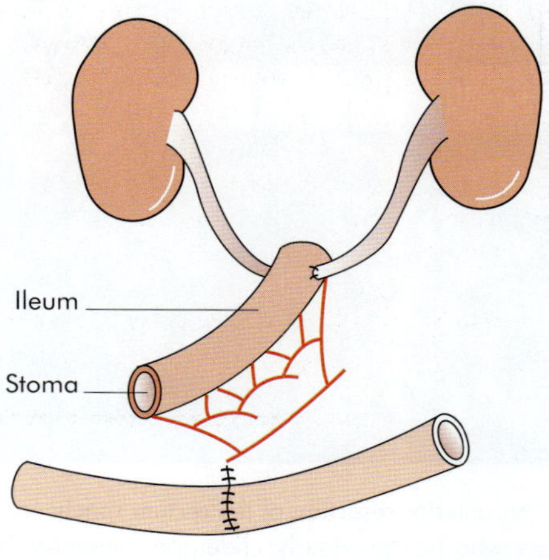

Figure 76.54 Ureteroileostomy (after DM Wallace, FRCS).

David Mitchell Wallace, 1913–1992, urologist, St Peter's Hospital, London, UK.

ureters are attached to the reservoir. A continence mechanism is then made to connect the reservoir to the skin. This is the complication-prone part of the operation. The continence mechanism may be made of an invaginated loop of ileum supported by three rows of staples (Kock pouch) or from the appendix, buried in an anti-reflux manner in a submucosal tube (Mitrofanoff; Figure 76.56). Alternatively, a length of ileum can be made into a tube (of a similar size to the appendix) after excision of the antimesenteric ileum and buried in a submucosal tunnel in an antireflux way. Clearly, these operations are complex, with the potential for increased postoperative complications.

Bladder substitution and augmentation

In patients with contraction of the bladder because of tuberculosis or with neuropathic dysfunction and a small bladder capacity, the bladder may need to be augmented. Similar techniques to those used to perform a bladder replacement can be utilised to make a near-spherical pouch from detubularised bowel, which can then be attached to the trigone or bladder neck after a near-total cystectomy (see Figures 76.20, 76.21 and 76.22). The ureters are then reimplanted. The facility to provide a continence mechanism must be available if needed in the neuropathic patient. This may comprise an artificial urinary sphincter or a colposuspension in the female.

Complications of internal diversion

Stricture

Ureterosigmoidostomy was first used by Chaput in 1894. Subsequent modifications included those made by Coffey and Grey Turner. In these methods, the ureters were cut obliquely and pulled into the gut by a stitch – the ends were not stitched to the gut wall – and stenosis was common. Nesbit, Cordonnier and Leadbetter all recognised that these strictures could be prevented by anastomosing mucosa to mucosa.

Reflux of urine

High-pressure activity within a segment of gut can cause reflux of potentially infected urine at high pressure to the kidneys. In the long term, this can cause renal impairment. The principle of a low-pressure reservoir for both neobladder and ureterosigmoidostomy (Mainz II) reduces this. In addition, an anti-reflux mechanism, used in neobladder construction, is created by anastomosing the ureters to a non-detubularised 20-cm segment of small bowel, which is in continuity with the neobladder (see Figure 76.53c).

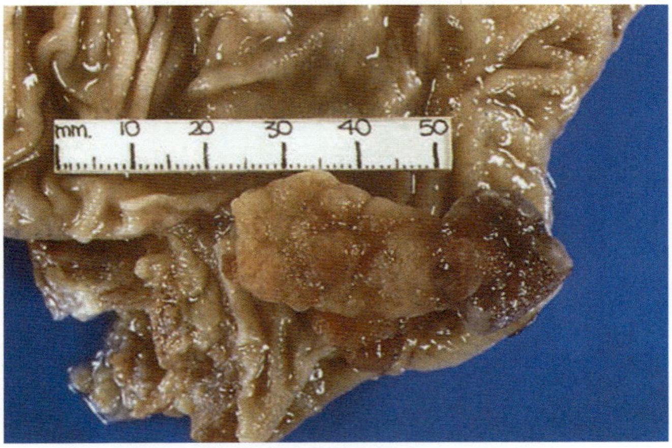

Figure 76.55 An anterior resection of the rectum specimen in a patient aged 18 years who has previously undergone ureterosigmoidostomy for the treatment of bladder exstrophy.

Metabolic consequences of internal diversion

Resorption of solutes

This depends upon the following factors: (1) the area of bowel that is exposed to urine; and (2) the length of time that the urine is in contact with the bowel epithelium.

The biochemical changes associated with urinary diversion are due to a combination of reabsorption of chloride and urea and progressively diminishing tubular function as a result of pyelonephritis. Diarrhoea with loss of potassium-containing mucus may exacerbate the loss of potassium. The typical changes of a hyperchloraemic acidosis with potassium depletion occur more frequently with ureterosigmoid diversion than with a colonic and ileal neobladder. When severe, the patient develops loss of appetite, weakness, thirst and diarrhoea. Coma may ensue. Mild acidosis, unrecognised over a long period, produces osteomalacia. Bone pain and even pathological fracture can occur. Renal impairment from pyelonephritis and reabsorption from the mucosa are seen less frequently after ileal or colonic conduit formation, continent urinary diversion or orthotopic bladder substitution. In fact, they are seen very infrequently except in patients with pre-existing renal impairment and unsatisfactory emptying of the urinary reservoir. Malabsorption can occur with the loss of terminal ileum and small bowel. The loss of terminal ileum can result in vitamin B12 deficiency and so monitoring of vitamin B12 and folate is recommended after the first year.

Treatment

Patients should be instructed to empty the rectum or conti-

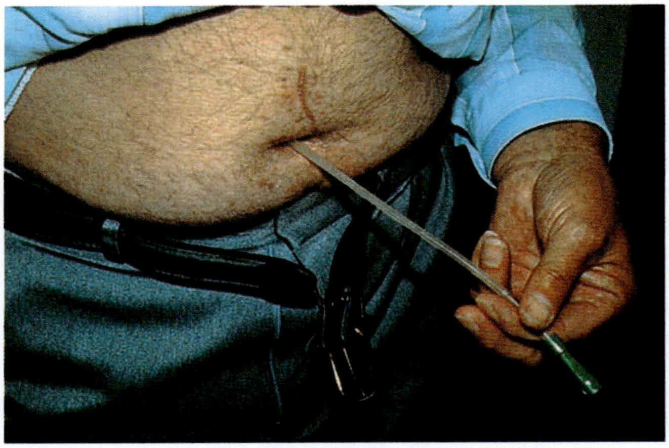

Figure 76.56 A patient with a pT3a bladder cancer who has previously undergone cystoprostatectomy and urethrectomy. A detubularised ileocaecal reservoir has been made with the ureters implanted in submucosal tunnels. The appendix has been implanted within the reservoir in a submucosal tunnel to provide the continence mechanism. The appendix has been brought to the umbilicus and is catheterised 4- to 6-hourly to empty the reservoir.

Paul Mitrofanoff, b. 1934, Professor of Paediatric Surgery, Rouen, France.
Henri Victor Chaput, 1857–1919, surgeon, La Salpêtrière, Paris, France.
Robert Calvin Coffey, 1869–1933, surgeon, Nashville, TN, USA.

nent reservoir or neobladder 3-hourly by day. In patients who have undergone ureterosigmoidostomy and in whom acidosis is present, a rectal tube should be inserted at night to drain the urine continuously. The patient should take a mixture of potassium citrate and sodium bicarbonate three times a day (2 g of each, either as crystals or as tablets). Regular serum biochemical analyses, including calcium, are required.

Established hyperchloraemic acidosis is usually associated with marked dehydration and the mainstay of treatment is administration of intravenous saline. The patient may be given small doses of sodium bicarbonate to half-correct the pH deficit if it is severe and additional intravenous potassium. This should be coupled with appropriate systemic antibiotic treatment.

Risk of malignancy

There is a risk of cancer developing in bowel used to reconstruct the urinary tract. When the urine is not mixed with faeces, the incidence is small, becoming significant after 15–18 years. The major risk of malignancy was discovered when ureterosigmoidostomy construction enabled free mixing of urine and faeces. The development of sigmoid reservoirs into which the ureters are inserted has reduced this risk.

FURTHER READING

Cardozo L, Staskin DR. *Textbook of female urology and urogynecology*, 3rd edn. London: Informa Healthcare, 2010.

Mundy AR, Fitzpatrick J, Neal DE, George NJ. *The scientific basis of urology*, 3rd edn. London: Informa Healthcare, 2010.

Scardino PT, Marston Linehan W, Zelefski MJ *et al. Comprehensive textbook of genitourinary oncology*, 4th edn. Philadelphia, PA: Lippincott Williams and Wilkins, 2011.

Wein AJ, Kavoussi LR, Novick AC *et al. Campbell-Walsh urology*, 10th edn. Philadelphia, PA: Saunders, 2011.

CHAPTER 77

The prostate and seminal vesicles

LEARNING OBJECTIVES

To understand:

- The relationship of anatomical structure and biochemical function to the development and treatment of benign and malignant disease of the prostate
- The terminology used to describe lower urinary tract symptoms and to know their causes as well as the treatment options available
- Which investigations are appropriate for carcinoma of the prostate
- Clinical staging of carcinoma of the prostate and how staging contributes to the complex decision-making process for the best treatment option

EMBRYOLOGY

From the primitive urethra, a series of solid epithelial buds develop and become canalised in a matter of weeks. The surrounding mesenchyme forms the muscular and connective tissue of the gland and has a major role in differentiation (stromal epithelium interactions). Skene's tubules, which open on either side of the female urethra, are the homologue of the prostate.

SURGICAL ANATOMY

The contemporary classification of the prostate into different zones was based on the work of McNeal (Figure 77.1). He showed that it is divided into the peripheral zone (PZ), which lies mainly posteriorly and from which most carcinomas arise, and a central zone (CZ), which lies posterior to the urethral lumen and above the ejaculatory ducts as they pass through the prostate; the two zones are rather like an egg in an egg-cup. There is also a periurethral transitional zone (TZ), from which most benign prostatic hyperplasia (BPH) arises. Smooth muscle cells are found throughout the prostate but, in the upper part of the prostate and bladder neck, there is a separate sphincter muscle that subserves a sexual function, closing during ejaculation. Resection of this tissue during prostatectomy is responsible for retrograde ejaculation. The distal striated urethral sphincter muscle is found at the junction of the prostate and the membranous urethra; it is horseshoe shaped with the bulk lying anteriorly and is quite distinct from the muscle of the pelvic floor (Figure 77.1).

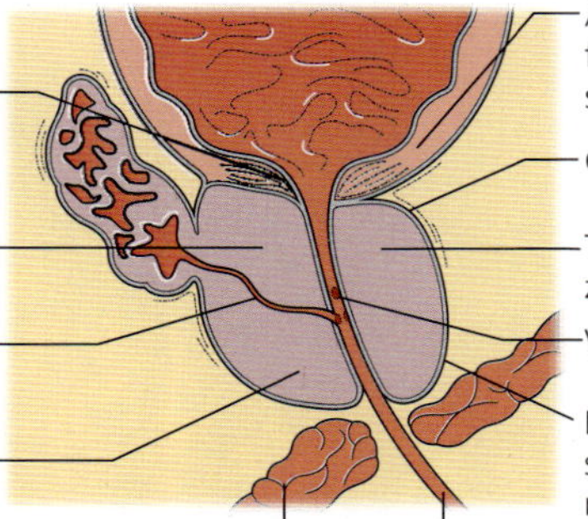

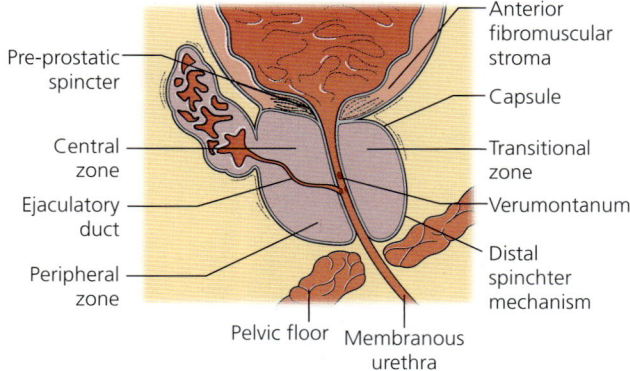

Figure 77.1 Sagittal diagram of the prostate just lateral to the urethra showing the division into the different zones described by McNeal. The transitional zone is the area from which most benign prostatic hyperplasia (BPH) arises.

The glands of the peripheral zone (Figure 77.2), lined by columnar epithelium, lie in the fibromuscular stroma, and their ducts, which are long and branched, open into posterolateral grooves on either side of the verumontanum. The glands of the CZ and TZ are shorter and unbranched. All these ducts, the common ejaculatory ducts and the prostatic utricle open into the prostatic urethra.

Benign prostate hypertrophy starts in the periurethral transitional zone and, as it increases in size, it compresses the outer PZ of the prostate, which becomes the false capsule. There is also the outer true fibrous anatomical capsule, and external to this lie condensations of endopelvic fascia known as the periprostatic sheath of endopelvic fascia. Between the anatomical capsule and the prostatic sheath lies the abundant prostatic venous plexus. The prostatic sheath is contiguous with the fascia of Denonvilliers, which separates the prostate and its coverings from the rectum. The neurovascular bundles supplying autonomic innervation to the corpora of the penis are in very close

Alexander Johnston Chalmers Skene, 1828–1900, Professor of Gynecology, Long Island Hospital, Brooklyn, New York, NY, USA.

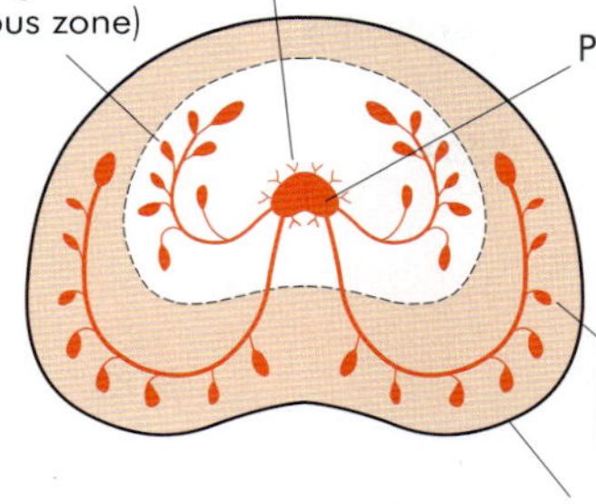

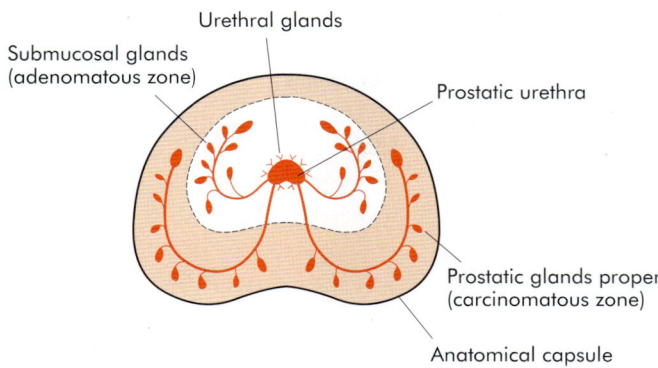

Figure 77.2 A transverse section of the prostate. The peripheral zone is the area from which most prostate cancers arise. The 'adenomatous' zone comprises the central and transitional zones.

relationship to the posterolateral aspect of the prostatic capsule and are at risk of damage during radical cystoprostatectomy or radical prostatectomy; inadvertent diathermy in the region of these nerves may be the cause of uncommon erectile impotence after transurethral prostatectomy.

PHYSIOLOGY

The prostate has a sexual function, but it is unclear how important its secretions are to human fertility. That the normal adult prostate undergoes atrophy after castration was known to John Hunter.

Systemic hormonal influences (endocrine) and local growth factors (paracrine and autocrine)

The growth of the prostate is governed by many local and systemic hormones whose exact functions are not yet known. The main hormone acting on the prostate is testosterone, which is secreted by the Leydig cells of the testes under the control of luteinising hormone (LH), itself secreted from the anterior pituitary under the control of hypothalamic luteinising hormone-releasing hormone (LHRH). LHRH has a short half-life and is released in a pulsatile manner. This pulsatile release is important, as receptors for LHRH will become desensitised if permanently occupied. The administration of LHRH analogues in a continuous, non-pulsatile manner exploits the concept of receptor desensitisation and forms the basis for androgen deprivation therapy in prostate cancer. Testosterone is converted to 1,5-dihydrotestosterone (DHT) by the enzyme 5α-reductase, which is found in high concentration in the prostate and the perigenital skin (type II). Other androgens are secreted by the adrenal cortex, but their effects are minimal in the normal male. Oestrogenic steroids are also secreted by the adrenal cortex and, in the ageing male, may play a part in disrupting the delicate balance between DHT and local peptide growth factors, and hence increase the risk of BPH. Increased levels of serum oestrogens, by acting on the hypothalamus, decrease the secretion of LHRH (and hence LH) and thereby decrease serum testosterone levels. Thus, pharmacological levels of oestrogens cause atrophy of the testes and prostate by means of reductions in testosterone.

Other locally acting peptides are secreted by the prostatic epithelium and mesenchymal stromal cells in response to steroid hormones. These include epidermal growth factor, insulin-like growth factors, basic fibroblast growth factor and transforming growth factors alpha and beta. These undoubtedly play a part in normal and abnormal prostatic growth, but as yet their functions are unclear (Summary box 77.1).

Summary box 77.1

Androgenic hormones

- Androgenic hormones, which drive prostate growth, are derived from several sources
- The majority of testosterone (90 per cent) is secreted by the Leydig cells of the testes under the control of LH, secreted from the anterior pituitary
- Metabolised adrenal androgen accounts for the remaining 5–10 per cent of testosterone
- Testosterone is converted to DHT by the enzyme 5α-reductase type II, which is found in high concentration in the prostate and the perigenital skin
- DHT has five times the potency of testosterone

Elaboration and secretion of prostate-specific antigen and acid phosphatases

Prostate-specific antigen (PSA) is a glycoprotein that is a serine protease. Its function may be to facilitate liquefaction of semen, but it is a marker for prostatic disease. It is measured by an immunoassay, and the normal range can differ a little from laboratory to laboratory. There is no real normal upper limit. The levels increase with age, with prostate cancer and with BPH. There are age-related values but, in general, in men aged 50–69 years, a level of about 3–4 ng/mL would prompt a discussion about the need for prostate biopsy. Its level in men with metastatic prostate cancer is usually increased to >30 ng/mL and falls to low levels after successful androgen ablation. Men with locally confined prostate cancer usually have serum PSA levels <10–15 ng/mL. Although PSA is a reliable marker for the progression of advanced disease, it is neither specific nor sensitive in the differential diagnosis of early prostate cancer and BPH, as both diseases are compatible with PSA in the range of 3–15 ng/mL. PSA measurement has superseded measurement of serum acid phosphatase. In summary, about 25 per cent of men with a PSA of 4–10 ng/mL have prostate cancer (i.e. it is not very specific), and about 15–20 per cent of men with a PSA of 1–4 ng/mL have prostate cancer. In general, one would advise men aged 50–69 years to undergo prostate biopsy if the PSA was more than ~3 ng/mL. The threshold would be lower in younger men with a strong family history.

BENIGN PROSTATIC HYPERPLASIA

Aetiology of benign prostatic hyperplasia

Hormones

Serum testosterone levels slowly but significantly decrease with advancing age; however, levels of oestrogenic steroids are not decreased equally. According to this theory, the prostate enlarges because of increased oestrogenic effects. It is likely that the secretion of intermediate peptide growth factors plays a part in the development of BPH (Summary box 77.2).

Franz von Leydig, 1821–1908, Professor of Histology successively at Wurzburg, Tubingen and Bonn, Germany.

Summary box 77.2

Benign prostatic hyperplasia (BPH)

- Occurs in men over 50 years of age; by the age of 60 years, 50 per cent of men have histological evidence of BPH
- Is a common cause of significant lower urinary tract symptoms in men and is the most common cause of bladder outflow obstruction in men >70 years of age

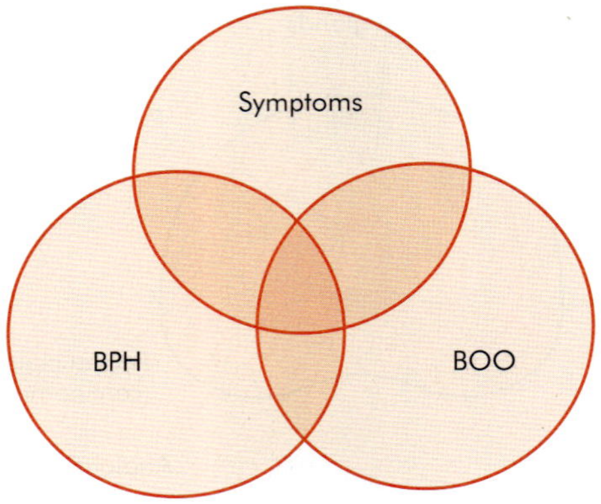

Figure 77.4 Diagrammatic representation of the relation between symptoms of prostatism, benign prostate hyperplasia (BPH) and urodynamically proven bladder outflow obstruction (BOO).

Pathology

BPH affects both glandular epithelium and connective tissue stroma to variable degrees. These changes are similar to those occurring in breast dysplasia (see Chapter 53), in which adenosis, epitheliosis and stromal proliferation are seen in differing proportions. BPH typically affects the submucous group of glands in the transitional zone, forming a nodular enlargement. Eventually, this overgrowth compresses the PZ glands into a false capsule and causes the appearance of the typical 'lateral' lobes.

When BPH affects the subcervical CZ glands, a 'middle' lobe develops that projects up into the bladder within the internal sphincter (Figure 77.3). Sometimes, both lateral lobes also project into the bladder, so that, when viewed from within, the sides and back of the internal urinary meatus are surrounded by an intravesical prostatic collar.

Effects of benign prostatic hyperplasia

It is important to realise that the relationship between anatomical prostatic enlargement, lower urinary tract symptoms (LUTS) and urodynamic evidence of bladder outflow obstruction (BOO) is complex (Figure 77.4). Pathophysiologically, BOO may be caused in part by increased smooth muscle tone, which is under the control of α-adrenergic agonists (Summary box 77.3).

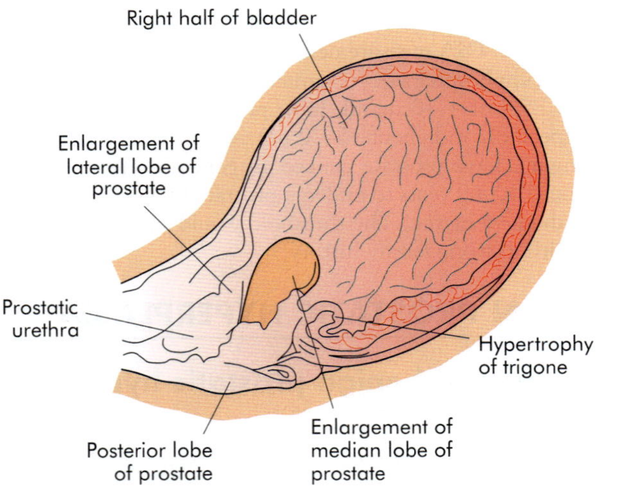

Figure 77.3 Diagram of late-stage bladder outflow obstruction (BOO) showing enlargement of the prostate from benign prostatic hyperplasia (BPH), trabeculation of the bladder with smooth muscle hypertrophy and fibrosis.

Summary box 77.3

Consequences of BPH

- No symptoms, no BOO
- No symptoms, but urodynamic evidence of BOO
- Lower urinary tract symptoms, no evidence of BOO
- Lower urinary tract symptoms and BOO
- Others (acute/chronic retention, haematuria, urinary infection and stone formation)

Anatomically, the effects are as follows:

- **Urethra**. The prostatic urethra is lengthened, sometimes to twice its normal length, but it is not narrowed anatomically. The normal posterior curve may be so exaggerated that it requires a curved catheter to negotiate it. When only one lateral lobe is enlarged, distortion of the prostatic urethra occurs.
- **Bladder**. If BPH causes BOO, the musculature of the bladder hypertrophies to overcome the obstruction and appears trabeculated (Figure 77.5). Significant BPH is associated with increased blood flow, and the resultant veins at the base of the bladder are apt to cause haematuria.

Lower urinary tract symptoms

In both sexes, non-specific symptoms of bladder dysfunction become more common with age, probably owing to impairment of smooth muscle function and neurovesical coordination. Not all symptoms of disturbed voiding in ageing men should therefore be attributed to BPH causing BOO. Urologists prefer the term LUTS and discourage the use of the descriptive term 'prostatism'.

The following conditions can coexist with BOO, leading to difficulty in diagnosis and in predicting the outcome of treatment:

- idiopathic detrusor overactivity (see Chapter 76);
- neuropathic bladder dysfunction as a result of diabetes, strokes, Alzheimer's disease or Parkinson's disease (see Chapter 76);

Alois Alzheimer, 1864–1915, a neurologist who worked at Heidelberg and Munich, before being appointed Professor of Psychiatry at Breslau, Germany (now Wroclaw, Poland).

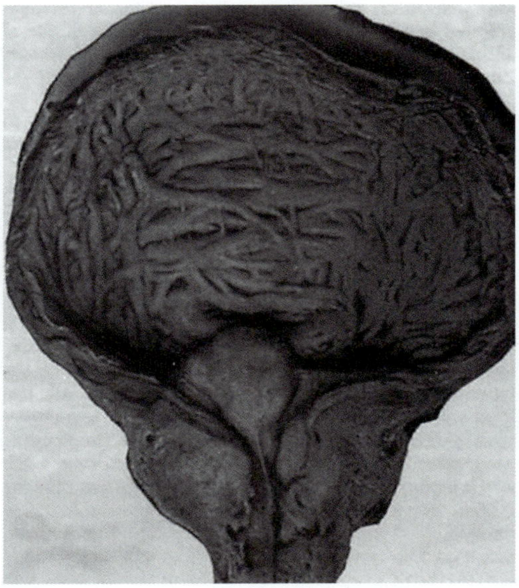

Figure 77.5 Trabeculation of the bladder from prostatic obstruction. When viewed from within, bands of muscle fibres can be seen – trabeculation. Between these hypertrophied bundles, there are shallow depressions, i.e. sacculations. Sometimes, one of the saccules (rarely two or more) continues to enlarge and forms a diverticulum (courtesy of the late Professor KAL Aschoff, Freiburg, Germany).

- degeneration of bladder smooth muscle giving rise to impaired voiding and detrusor instability;
- BOO due to BPH.

LUTS can be described as:

- voiding
  - hesitancy (worsened if the bladder is very full);
  - poor flow (unimproved by straining);
  - intermittent stream – stops and starts;
  - dribbling (including after micturition);
  - sensation of poor bladder emptying;
  - episodes of near retention;
- storage
  - frequency;
  - nocturia;
  - urgency;
  - urge incontinence;
  - nocturnal incontinence (enuresis).

LUTS are usually assessed by means of scoring systems, which give a semi-objective measure of severity. However, some symptoms do not give an accurate picture of the underlying pathophysiological problem. For instance, a man with severe detrusor instability may void only small volumes and hence he will have a sensation of poor flow because low voided volumes (<100 mL) are associated with low flow rates.

Severe irritative symptoms are usually associated with detrusor instability. Post-micturition dribbling is now known not to be a consequence of BOO and is not usually improved by prostatectomy.

Bladder outflow obstruction

This is a urodynamic concept based on the combination of low flow rates in the presence of high voiding pressures. It can be diagnosed definitively only by pressure-flow studies. This is because symptoms are relatively non-specific and can result from detrusor instability, neurological dysfunction and weak bladder contraction. Even low measured peak flow rates (<10–12 mL/s) are not absolutely diagnostic because, in addition to BOO, weak detrusor contractions or low voided volumes (owing to instability) can be the cause. Nonetheless, flow rates provide a useful guide for everyday clinical management.

Urodynamically proven BOO may result from:

- BPH;
- bladder neck stenosis;
- bladder neck hypertrophy;
- prostate cancer;
- urethral strictures;
- functional obstruction due to neuropathic conditions.

The primary effects of BOO on the bladder are as follows:

- **Urinary flow rates decrease** (for a voided volume >200 mL, a peak flow rate of >15 mL/s is normal (Figure 77.6), one of 10–15 mL/s is equivocal and one <10 mL/s is low (Figure 77.7).
- **Voiding pressures increase** (pressures >80 cmH_2O are high (Figure 77.8), pressures between 60 and 80 cmH_2O are equivocal and pressures <60 cmH_2O are normal).

The long-term effects of bladder outflow obstruction are as follows:

- The bladder may decompensate so that detrusor contraction becomes progressively less efficient and a residual urine develops.
- The bladder may become more irritable during filling with a decrease in functional capacity partly caused by detrusor overactivity (see Chapter 76), which may also be caused by neurological dysfunction or ageing, or may be idiopathic.

Aside from symptoms, the complications of BOO are as follows:

- Acute retention of urine is sometimes the first symptom of BOO. Postponement of micturition is a common precipitating cause; overindulgence in beer and confinement to bed on account of intercurrent illness or operation are other causes.
- Chronic retention. In patients in whom the residual volume is >250 mL or so (Figure 77.9), the tension in the bladder wall increases owing to the combination of a large volume of residual urine and increased resting and

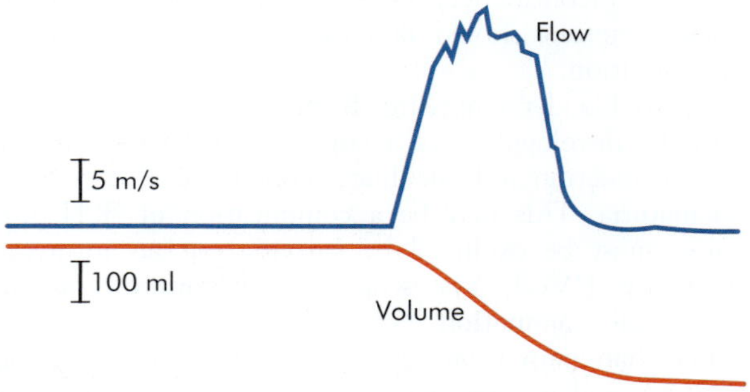

Figure 77.6 Normal flow rate. The voided volume is well in excess of 350 mL, and the maximum flow rate is in excess of 25 mL/s.

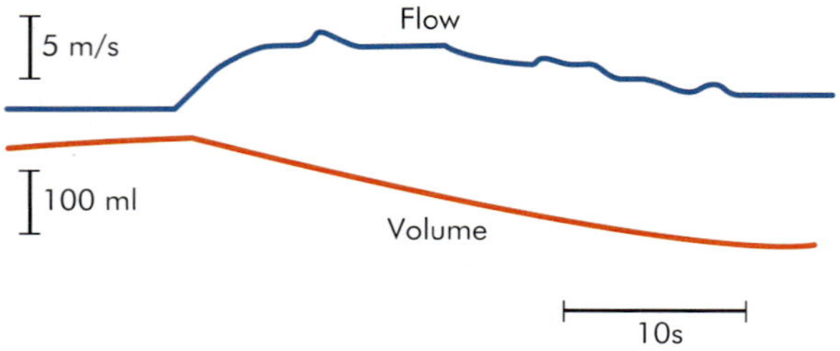

Figure 77.7 Diagram of a low flow rate showing a rather low voided volume of about 200 mL, but with markedly decreased flow rate. Such a flow rate could be caused by a urethral stricture, bladder outflow obstruction or a weak detrusor.

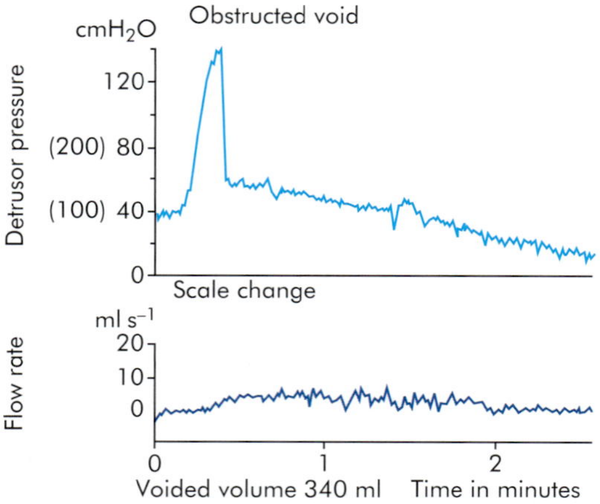

Figure 77.8 Conventional urodynamic trace showing detrusor pressure during voiding. There has been a change in scale because the pressure was so high; voiding pressures are increased with a low flow rate. This is diagnostic of bladder outflow obstruction.

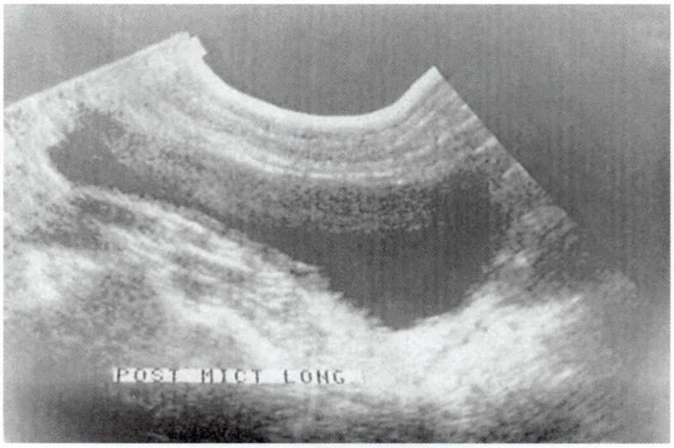

Figure 77.9 An ultrasonogram showing a large post-void residual urine.

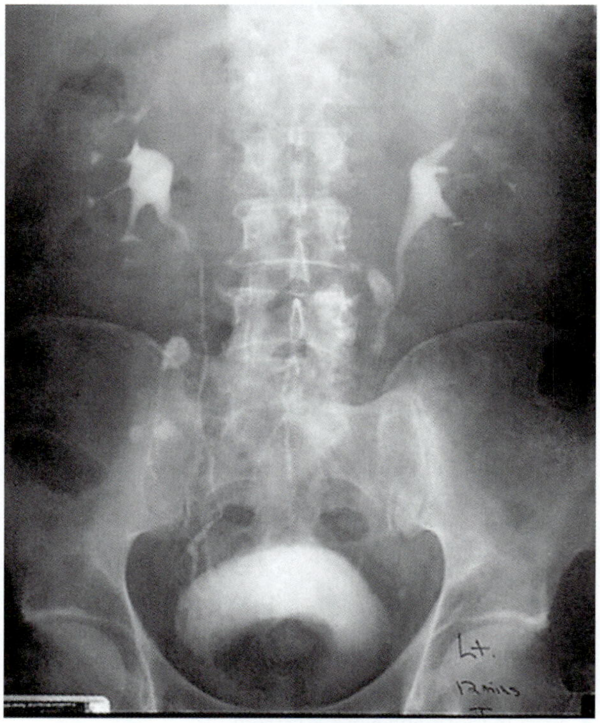

Figure 77.10 Intravenous urogram from a patient with symptoms of outflow obstruction and a moderate post-micturition residual urine. The patient did not undergo treatment.

filling bladder pressures (a condition known as high-pressure chronic retention). The increased intramural tension results in functional obstruction of the upper urinary tract with the development of bilateral hydronephrosis (Figures 77.10 and 77.11). As a result, upper tract infection and renal impairment may develop. Such men may present with overflow incontinence, enuresis and renal insufficiency. These symptoms should alert the doctor to the presence of this condition.

- Impaired bladder emptying. If the bladder decompensates with the development of a large volume of residual urine, urinary infection and calculi are prone to develop.
- Haematuria. This may be a complication of BPH. Other causes must be excluded by carrying out an intravenous urography (IVU), cystoscopy, urine culture and urine cytological examination.
- Other than pain from retention, pain is not a symptom of BOO, and its presence should prompt the exclusion of acute retention, urinary infection, stones, carcinoma of the prostate and carcinoma *in situ* of the bladder.

ASSESSMENT OF THE PATIENT WITH LOWER URINARY TRACT SYMPTOMS

History

Symptom score sheets such as the International Prostate Symptom Score (IPSS) assign a score which gives information regarding the severity of symptoms at the outset and changes over time and following intervention. The IPSS assessment should include an assessment of quality of life, which is a reflec-

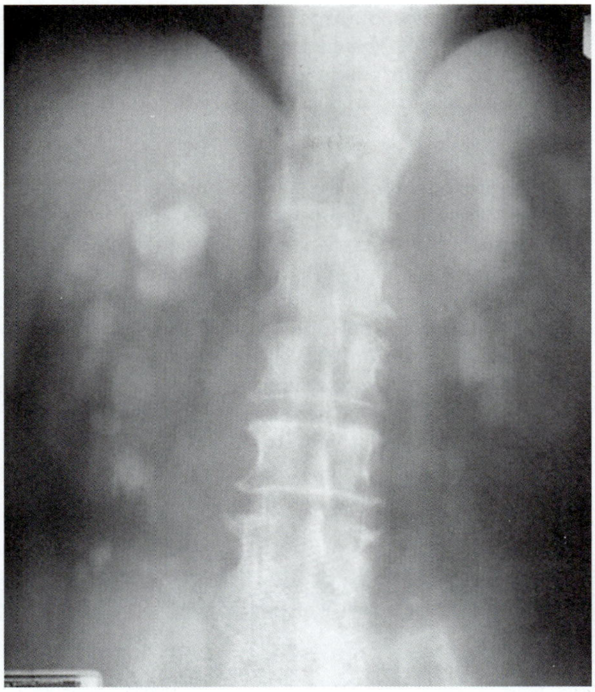

Figure 77.11 Intravenous urogram from the same patient as in Figure 77.10 but carried out some years later. The patient had developed chronic urinary retention and renal impairment owing to upper urinary dilatation.

tion of the degree of 'bother' caused by a patient's symptoms. In addition to the IPSS, a frequency-volume diary completed by the patient before attending the clinic is invaluable in revealing fluid intake habits, diurnal variation in outputs and low-volume, frequent voiding. These assessments are routinely performed at lower urinary tract clinics but can be elicited by a thorough clinical history (Summary box 77.4).

Summary box 77.4

Investigations of men with LUTS

Essential investigations

- Urine analysis by dipstick for blood, glucose and protein
- Urine culture for infection
- Serum creatinine
- Urinary flow rate and residual volume measurement

Additional investigations

- PSA if indicated
- Pressure-flow studies

Abdominal examination

Abdominal extension is usually normal. In patients with chronic retention, a distended bladder will be found on palpation, on percussion and sometimes on inspection with loss of the transverse suprapubic skin crease. General physical examination may demonstrate signs of chronic renal impairment with anaemia and dehydration. The external urinary meatus should be examined to exclude stenosis, and the epididymides are palpated for signs of inflammation.

Rectal examination

In benign enlargement, the posterior surface of the prostate is smooth, convex and typically elastic, but the fibrous element may give the prostate a firm consistency. The rectal mucosa can be made to move over the prostate. Residual urine may be felt as a fluctuating swelling above the prostate. It should be noted that, if there is a considerable amount of residual urine present, it pushes the prostate downwards, making it appear larger than it is.

The nervous system

The nervous system is examined to eliminate a neurological lesion. Diabetes mellitus, tabes dorsalis, disseminated sclerosis, cervical spondylosis, Parkinson's disease and other neurological states may mimic prostatic obstruction. If these are suspected then a pressure-flow urodynamic study should be carried out to diagnose BOO. Examination of perianal sensation and anal tone is useful in detection of an S2 to S4 cauda equina lesion.

Serum prostate-specific antigen

The difficulty here is the uncertain benefit of early detection and radical treatment of prostate cancer – this is dealt with in the section on prostate cancer. Certainly, men should be informed about the test, the risks of the prostate biopsy that might be required and the risks of the detection of a cancer that we are not certain how best to treat, as well as the positive aspects of the early discovery of a small prostate cancer. After suitable counselling, measurement of serum PSA may be helpful. Men in whom a diagnosis of early prostate cancer might influence treatment option (such as those under 70 years or those with a positive family history who might be offered radical treatment) should be offered a PSA measurement. If this is in excess of 2.5–4 nmol/L, then transrectal ultrasound scanning (TRUS) plus multiple transrectal biopsies (10 biopsies) should be considered.

If rectal examination is quite normal with no suspicion of cancer, and if no change in treatment policy would in any case result from the diagnosis of early prostate cancer, then there is little point in the routine measurement of PSA in men with uncomplicated BOO. However, because of the fear of future litigation, many find it easier to offer a PSA test.

Flow rate measurement

For this to be meaningful, two or three voids should be recorded, and the voided volume should be in excess of 150–200 mL. This usually means the patient attending a special flow rate clinic. A typical history and a flow rate <10 mL/s (for a voided volume of >200 mL; Figure 77.7) will be sufficient for most urologists to recommend treatment. Usually, a flow rate measurement will be coupled with ultrasound measurement of post-void residual urine.

There are pitfalls in the measurement of flow rates. The machine must be accurately calibrated. The patient must void volumes in excess of 150 mL, and two or three recordings are needed to obtain a representative measurement. Decreased flow rates and symptoms of prostatism may be seen in:

- BOO;
- low voided volumes (characteristically in men with detrusor instability);

- men with weak bladder contractions (low pressure-flow voiding).

Pressure-flow urodynamic studies

Details of these studies are outlined in Chapter 76 (see Figure 77.8). They should be performed on the following patients:

- men with suspected neuropathy (Parkinson's disease, dementia, longstanding diabetes, previous strokes, multiple sclerosis);
- men with a dominant history of irritative symptoms and men with lifelong urgency and frequency;
- men with a doubtful history and those with flow rates in the near normal range (~ or >15 mL/s);
- men with invalid flow rate measurements (because of low voided volumes).

Blood tests

Serum creatinine, electrolytes and haemoglobin should be measured.

Examination of urine

The urine is examined for glucose and blood; a midstream specimen should be sent for bacteriological examination, and cytological examination may be carried out if carcinoma *in situ* is thought possible.

Upper tract imaging

Most urologists no longer carry out imaging of the upper tract in men with straightforward symptoms. Obviously, if infection or haematuria is present, then the upper tract should be imaged by means of intravenous urogram or ultrasound scan.

Cystourethroscopy

Inspection of the urethra, the prostate and the urothelium of the bladder should always be done immediately prior to prostatectomy, whether it is being done transurethrally or by the open route to exclude a urethral stricture, a bladder carcinoma and the occasional non-opaque vesical calculus. The decision of whether to perform prostatectomy must be made before cystoscopy. This should be based on the patient's symptoms, signs and investigations. Direct inspection of the prostate is a poor indicator of BOO and the need for surgery.

Transrectal ultrasound scanning

There is no need to carry this out routinely. Accurate estimation of prostatic size is also possible by means of transrectal or transabdominal ultrasound scanning.

MANAGEMENT OF MEN WITH BENIGN PROSTATIC HYPERPLASIA OR BLADDER OUTFLOW OBSTRUCTION

Strong indications for treatment (usually prostatectomy) include:

- **Acute retention** (see Chapter 76) in fit men with no other cause for retention (drugs, constipation, recent operation, etc.) (accounts for 25 per cent of prostatectomies).
- **Chronic retention and renal impairment**: a residual urine of 200 mL or more, a raised blood urea, hydroureter or hydronephrosis demonstrated on urography and uraemic manifestations (accounts for 15 per cent of prostatectomies).
- **Complications of bladder outflow obstruction**: stone, infection and diverticulum formation.
- **Haemorrhage**: occasionally, venous bleeding from a ruptured vein overlying the prostate will require prostatectomy to be performed.
- **Elective prostatectomy for severe symptoms**: this accounts for about 60 per cent of prostatectomies. Increasing difficulty in micturition, with considerable frequency day and night, delay in starting and a poor stream are the usual symptoms for which prostatectomy is advised. Frequency alone is not a strong indication for prostatectomy. The natural progression of outflow obstruction is variable and rarely gets worse after ten years. Severe symptoms, a low maximum flow rate (<10 mL/s) and an increased residual volume of urine (100–250 mL) are relatively strong indications for operative treatment. The exact cut-off for operative or non-operative treatment will depend on careful discussion between the patient and the urologist (Summary box 77.5).

Summary box 77.5

Options for treatment of LUTS secondary to BPH

- Conservative measures include watchful waiting in conjunction with fluid restriction and reduction in caffeine intake
- Drug therapy is with α-blockers or, in men with a large prostate, a 5α-reductase inhibitor, or both
- Interventional measures include transurethral resection of the prostate (TURP), which remains the 'gold standard'; consider open prostatectomy for large glands

Acute retention

The management of retention is discussed in detail in Chapter 76. Once the bladder has been drained by means of a catheter, the patient's fitness for treatment is determined. If retention was not caused by drugs or constipation, then prostatectomy would usually be the correct management. Unfit men or those with dementia may be treated by means of indwelling prostatic stents or a catheter. Similar comments apply to men with chronic retention once renal function has been stabilised by catheterisation. The role of α-adrenergic drugs followed by a trial of catheter has been tested and found to be successful in certain groups with a short history and a low residual volume of urine, but the recurrence rate becomes cumulatively high.

Special problems in the management of chronic retention

Men with chronic retention who have relatively low volumes of residual urine and who do not have symptoms suggestive of coexistent infection and with good renal function do not necessarily require catheterisation before proceeding to prostatectomy on the next available list. For those who are uraemic, urgent catheterisation is mandatory to allow renal function to recover and stabilise. Haematuria often occurs following catheterisation owing to collapse of the distended bladder and upper tract, but settles within a couple of days (see Chapter 76 for general management of retention).

Uraemic patients with chronic retention are often dehydrated at the time of admission. Owing to the chronic back pressure on the distal tubules within the kidney, there is loss of the ability to reabsorb salts and water. The result, following release of this pressure, may be an enormous outflow of salts and water, which is known as post-obstructive diuresis. It is for this reason that a careful fluid chart, daily measurements of the patient's weight and serial estimations of creatinine and electrolytes are essential. Intravenous fluid replacement is required if the patient is unable to keep up with this fluid loss. These patients are often anaemic and may require a blood transfusion once fluid balance is stabilised (if haemoglobin is <9 g/L).

Indications for elective treatment in men with LUTS secondary to BPH

Following careful assessment (see above under Assessment of the patient with lower urinary tract symptoms), the following questions should be answered:

1. Have they failed a preliminary trial of medical therapy? Commonly, men will have been treated with α-blockers or 5α-reductase inhibitors and will have failed treatment. They are then referred by their general practitioner to the urologist.
2. Is BOO present? In many cases, the findings of significant symptoms (assessed by symptom scoring), a benign prostate supplemented by the finding of a low maximum flow rate (<10–12 mL/s for a good voided volume (>200 mL)) will suffice to make a reasonable working diagnosis of BOO. In some men, particularly those with irritative symptoms, suspected neurological disease or those with technically imperfect flow rate measurements, pressure–flow studies will need to be performed.
3. How severe are the symptoms and what are the risks of doing nothing? Severe symptoms and a large residual volume of urine will usually require treatment. Men with mild symptoms, good flow rates (>15 mL/s) and good bladder emptying (residual urine <100 mL) may be safely managed by reassurance and review: such patients rarely develop severe complications such as retention in the long term.
4. Is the man fit for operative treatment?
5. What treatments are available, what are the outcomes and do the side-effects justify treatment?

Treatment

Men with symptoms attending for elective treatment (excluding acute and chronic retention)

Conservative treatment

It is in men with relatively mild symptoms, reasonable flow rates (>10 mL/s) and good bladder emptying (residual urine <100 mL) that careful discussion over the merits and side effects of operative treatment is warranted. Waiting for a period of six months after careful discussion of the diagnosis is indicated. After this, a repeat assessment of symptoms, flow rates and ultrasound scan is helpful; many men with stable symptoms will elect to leave matters be. Advice over limiting fluid intake in the evening and careful use of anti-muscarinics to help with irritative symptoms is also useful.

Drugs

In men who are very concerned about the development of sexual dysfunction after transurethral resection of the prostate (TURP), the use of drugs may be helpful. Two classes of drug have been used in the treatment of men with BOO. α-Adrenergic blocking agents inhibit the contraction of smooth muscle that is found in the prostate. The other class of drug is the 5α-reductase inhibitors, which inhibit the conversion of testosterone to DHT, the most active form of androgen. These drugs, when taken for a year, result in a 25 per cent shrinkage of the prostate gland. Both groups of drugs are effective; however, α-blockers work more quickly and, although the 5α-reductase inhibitors have fewer side effects, they need to be taken for at least six months, and their effect is greatest in patients with large (>50 g) glands. Drug therapy results in improvements in maximum flow rates by about 2 mL/s more than placebo and results in mild (20 per cent) improvement in symptom scores. TURP, however, results in improvements in maximum flow rates from 9 to 18 mL/s and a 75 per cent improvement in symptom scores. These drugs are expensive in comparison with their effectiveness, and a significant proportion of men who try these drugs will subsequently undergo TURP. They may be best targeted at men who have failed an initial trial of watchful waiting and who wish to avoid surgery for a period.

Operative treatment

Apart from the strong indications for operative treatment mentioned above, the most common reason for TURP is a combination of severe symptoms and a low flow rate <12 mL/s. The key is to assess symptoms carefully and to counsel men about side effects and likely outcome before advising operative treatment.

Counselling men undergoing prostatectomy

Men undergoing prostatectomy need to be advised about the following:

- **Retrograde ejaculation**. This occurs in about 65 per cent of men after prostatectomy.
- **Erectile impotence**. This occurs in about 5 per cent of men, usually those whose potency is waning.
- **The success rate**. On the whole, men with acute and chronic retention do well from the symptomatic point of view. Ninety per cent of men undergoing elective operation for severe symptoms and urodynamically proven BOO do well in terms of symptoms and flow rates. Only about 65 per cent of those with mild symptoms or those with weak bladder contraction as the cause of their symptoms do well. Men with unobstructed detrusor instability do not respond well to TURP. This is the reason for carefully documenting the severity of symptoms and flow rates (supplemented when necessary by pressure–flow studies) before deciding on treatment.
- **The risk of reoperation**. After TURP, this is about 15 per cent after 8–10 years.
- **The morbidity rate**. Death after TURP is infrequent (<0.5 per cent), severe sepsis is found in about 6 per cent and severe haematuria requiring transfusion of more than two units of blood occurs in about 3 per cent. After discharge, about 15–20 per cent of men subsequently require antibiotic treatment for symptoms of urinary infection. Risk factors for complications include admission with retention, prostate cancer, renal impairment and advanced age.

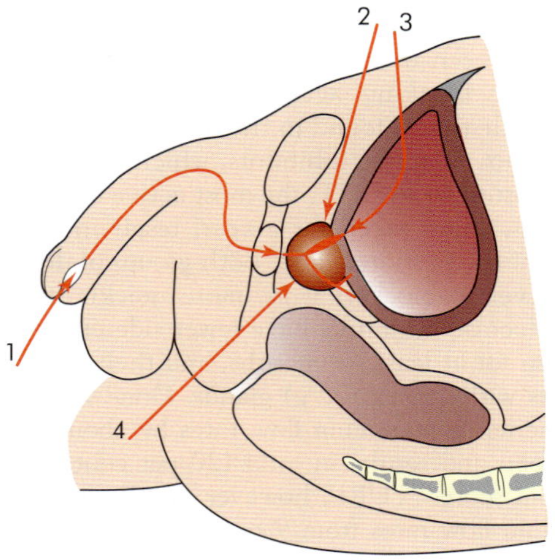

Figure 77.12 The surgical approaches to the prostate.

Methods of performing prostatectomy

The prostate can be approached (1) transurethrally (TURP), (2) retropubically (RPP), (3) through the bladder (transvesical; TVP) or (4) from the perineum (Figure 77.12).

Transurethral resection of the prostate

TURP has largely replaced other methods unless diverticulectomy or the removal of large stones necessitates open operation; over 95 per cent of men being treated by urologists can be dealt with by TURP. Perhaps the greatest advance in the history of transurethral surgery was marked by the development of the rigid lens system of Professor Harold Hopkins. His lenses, illuminated by a fibreoptic light source, permit unparalleled visualisation of the working field. Men with indwelling catheters, those with recent urinary infection, those with chronic retention or those with prosthetic material or heart valves should receive broad spectrum prophylactic antibiotics with amoxicillin plus cefuroxime or gentamicin intravenously at induction of anaesthesia.

Strips of tissue are cut from the bladder neck down to the level of the verumontanum (Figure 77.13). Cutting is performed by a high-frequency diathermy current, which is applied across a loop mounted on the hand-held trigger of the resectoscope. Coagulation of bleeding points can be accurately achieved, and damage to the external sphincter is avoided provided one uses the verumontanum as a guide to the most distal point of the resection. The 'chips' of prostate are then removed from the bladder using an Ellik evacuator. The risks of hyponatraemia are reduced by using 1.5 per cent isotonic glycine for irrigation, and the recent introduction of continuous-flow resectoscopes makes the procedure swift and safe in experienced hands. At the end of the procedure, careful haemostasis is performed, and a three-way, self-retaining catheter irrigated with isotonic saline is introduced into the bladder to prevent any further bleeding from forming blood clots. Irrigation is continued until the outflow is pale pink, and the catheter is usually removed on the second or third postoperative day. In men with small prostates or bladder neck dyssynergia or stenosis, it is better to divide the bladder neck and prostatic urethra with a diathermy 'bee-sting' electrode.

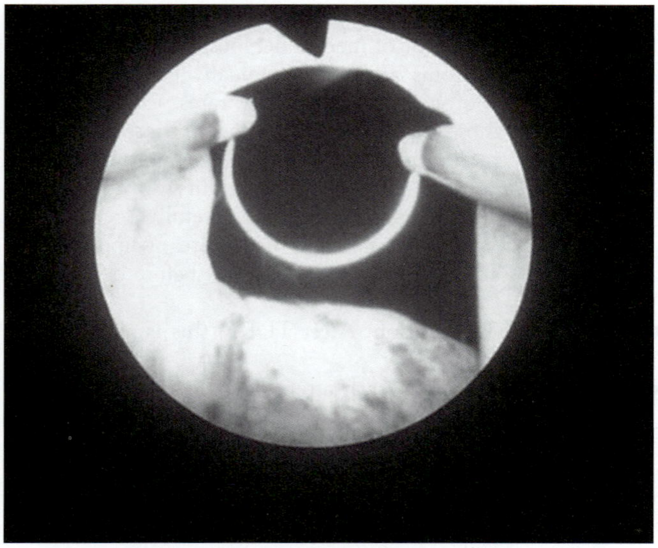

Figure 77.13 Endoscopic photograph of transurethral prostatectomy.

Retropubic prostatectomy (Millin)

Using a low, curved transverse suprapubic Pfannenstiel incision, which includes the rectus sheath, the recti are split in the midline and retracted to expose the bladder. With the patient in the Trendelenburg position, the surgeon separates the bladder and the prostate from the posterior aspect of the pubis. In the space thus obtained, the anterior capsule of the prostate is incised with diathermy below the bladder neck, care being taken to obtain complete control of bleeding from divided prostatic veins by suture ligation. The prostatic adenoma is exposed and enucleated with a finger. A wedge is taken out of the posterior lip of the bladder neck to prevent secondary stricture in this region. The exposure of the inside of the prostatic cavity is good, and control of haemorrhage is achieved with diathermy and suture ligation of bleeding points before closure of the capsule over a Foley catheter (inserted per urethram) draining the bladder.

Transvesical prostatectomy

The bladder is opened, and the prostate enucleated by putting a finger into the urethra, pushing forwards towards the pubes to separate the lateral lobes, and then working the finger between the adenoma and the false capsule. In Freyer's operation (1901), the bladder was left open widely and drained by

Terence John Millin, 1903–1980, surgeon, The Westminster Hospital, London, UK, described the operation of retropubic prostatectomy in 1945. Honorary surgeon, All Saints' Hospital for Genitourinary Diseases, London, UK; he was regarded as 'the greatest of Irish urologists' and 'the pioneer of the retropubic space'. To facilitate his operation, he devised a self-retaining retractor that goes by his name and the 'boomerang' needle to close the prostatic capsule. He used to be invited all over the world to operate on VIPs. He was a former President of the Royal College of Surgeons in Ireland. He gave up operating at the age of 57 to enjoy his farm in County Wicklow where he died of laryngeal carcinoma. He played international rugby for Ireland.

Sir Peter Johnston Freyer, 1852–1921, an Irish born surgeon who performed the first successful prostatectomy in 1900 at St Peter's Hospital, London. He used to give a running commentary to his visiting surgeons in French and Hidustani. Surgeon, St Peter's Hospital for Stone, London, UK.

a suprapubic tube with a 16-mm lumen in order to allow free drainage of blood and urine. Harris (1934) advocated control of the prostatic arteries by lateral stitches inserted with his boomerang needle, the bladder wall was closed and the wound drained.

Perineal prostatectomy (Young)

This has now been abandoned for the treatment of BPH.

After treatment

Most urologists irrigate the bladder with sterile saline by means of a three-way Foley catheter for 24 hours or so.

Complications

Local

Haemorrhage is a major risk following prostatectomy whatever the surgical approach. Care should be taken in diathermising arterial bleeding points after TURP; they are often better seen when the rate of inflow of fluid is decreased. In the recovery room, one should check that the bladder is draining adequately; if it is not, this may indicate that a clot is blocking the eye of the catheter. The bladder should be promptly washed out using strict aseptic technique. The catheter should be changed by the surgeon. Only rarely is it necessary to return the patient to the operating room.

Secondary haemorrhage tends to occur after the patient has been discharged. All men should be warned about this possibility and given appropriate advice to rest and to have a high fluid intake. It is usually minor in degree but if clot retention occurs, the patient will need to be readmitted, a catheter will have to be passed and the bladder washed out.

Perforation of the bladder or the prostatic capsule can occur at the time of transurethral surgery. This usually occurs from a combination of inexperience in association with a large prostate or heavy blood loss. If the field of vision becomes obscured by heavy blood loss, it is often prudent to achieve adequate haemostasis and abandon the operation, swallowing one's pride on the understanding that a second attempt may be necessary. A large perforation with marked extravasation may require the insertion of a small suprapubic drain. Rectal perforation should be extremely rare.

Sepsis

Bacteraemia is common even in men with sterile urine and occurs in over 50 per cent of men with infected urine, prolonged catheterisation or chronic retention. Septicaemia can occur in these patients shortly after operation or when the catheter is removed. In men at high risk, the use of prophylactic antibiotics is recommended. Wound infection following open prostatectomy is common if a urethral catheter has been *in situ* for a number of days before the operation. The most worrying aspect of infection is the early rigor following surgery. If left undetected and untreated, this may progress to frank septicaemia with profound hypotension. A blood culture should be taken and broad spectrum antibiotics with Gram-negative activity given parenterally, e.g. augmentin and gentamicin.

Incontinence

Incontinence is inevitable if the external sphincter mechanism is damaged. The bladder neck is rendered incompetent by any prostatectomy and, therefore, an intact distal sphincter mechanism is essential for continence. Damage to the sphincter may occur at open prostatectomy and following transurethral surgery if the resection extends beyond the verumontanum. If pelvic floor physiotherapy is ineffective, then the only satisfactory treatment is the fitting of an artificial urinary sphincter. In some patients, detrusor instability contributes to the incontinence. The use of anti-cholinergic agents or imipramine or duloxetine may help.

Retrograde ejaculation and impotence

Impotence in men with good sexual function before surgery is uncommon, but retrograde ejaculation occurs commonly (>50 per cent) because of disruption to the bladder neck mechanism.

Urethral stricture

This may be secondary to prolonged catheterisation, the use of an unnecessarily large catheter, clumsy instrumentation or the presence of the resectoscope in the urethra for too long a period. These strictures arise either just inside the meatus or in the bulbar urethra. An early stricture can usually be managed by simple bouginage but, later on, it may be necessary to cut the densely fibrotic stricture with the optical urethrotome. The routine use of an Otis urethrotomy prior to TURP reduces the incidence of postoperative stricture.

Bladder neck contracture

Occasionally, a dense fibrotic stenosis of the bladder neck occurs following overaggressive resection of a small prostate. It may be due to the overuse of coagulating diathermy. Transurethral incision of the scar tissue is necessary.

Reoperation

It is now well known that, after eight years, 15–18 per cent of men with BPH will undergo repeat TURP (the rate after open prostatectomy is about 5 per cent). The reasons include a technically imperfect primary procedure and a speculative repeat operation in men with symptoms who are cystoscoped after operation.

General complications

Death occurs in about 0.2–0.3 per cent of men undergoing elective prostatectomy. In very elderly men, in men with prostate cancer admitted as an emergency with acute or chronic retention or in those with very large prostates, the 30-day death rate may be in the order of 1 per cent.

Cardiovascular

Pulmonary atelectasis, pneumonia, myocardial infarction, congestive cardiac failure and deep venous thrombosis are all potentially life-threatening conditions that can affect this elderly and often frail group of men.

Water intoxication (also known as TUR syndrome)

The absorption of water into the circulation at the time of transurethral resection can give rise to congestive cardiac failure, hyponatraemia and haemolysis. Accompanying this, there is frequently confusion and other cerebral events often mimicking a stroke. The incidence of this condition has been reduced since the introduction of isotonic glycine for performing the

Samuel Harry Harris, 1881–1937, urologist, Lewisham Hospital, Sydney, NSW, Australia.
Hugh Hampton Young, 1870–1945, Director, The James Buchanan Brady Urological Institute, Baltimore, MD, USA.
Fessenden Nott Otis, 1825–1900, a nineteenth century American urologist.

resections and the use of isotonic saline for postoperative irrigation. The treatment consists of fluid restriction.

Osteitis pubis

This is rare.

Newer treatments

In general, newer, minimally invasive treatments occupy a position intermediate between TURP and drug treatment. In the last decade, technological innovations led to the introduction of novel minimally invasive treatments for prostatectomy. Tissue ablative techniques using hyperthermia and laser energy were associated with minimal morbidity and could often be performed as outpatient procedures. Many of the initial studies reporting treatment success were poorly designed and over a short duration. Longer-term follow up and randomised controlled trials have failed to confirm significant benefit from these techniques. More recently, the holmium laser, a pulsed solid-state laser, has been used to enucleate the prostate adenoma. This approach involves excision of parts of the prostate using a cutting laser and then morcellating the excised prostate fragments, which fall back into the bladder so that they can be removed. Morbidity with this procedure is low and short-term results favourable; long-term follow up will be necessary to determine whether this treatment will have a role to play in the management of BOO. The green light laser is now being used to vaporise the prostate tissue, but has not yet been shown to be as durable as holmium laser treatment or TURP, because the amount of tissue removed is usually less. Recently, the development of bipolar resectoscopes, which allow irrigation with normal saline, has allowed the resection of larger prostates without the risk of causing water intoxication.

Intraurethral stents

These devices are possibly helpful in the management of men with retention who are grossly unfit (classified by the American Society of Anesthesiologists as ASA grade IV) (Figure 73.14). These men are rare cases.

BLADDER OUTFLOW OBSTRUCTION CAUSED BY THE BLADDER NECK

Aetiology

This condition usually occurs in men, but can rarely affect children of both sexes and women. It may be due to muscular hypertrophy or fibrosis of the tissues at the bladder neck following TURP.

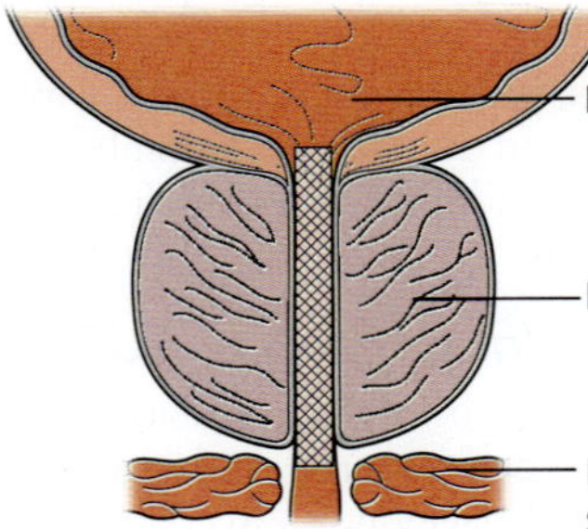

Figure 77.14 Diagram showing one type of prostatic stent *in situ*.

Clinical syndromes

Owing to muscle hypertrophy or dyssynergia

Marion described a series of cases in which muscular hypertrophy of the internal sphincter in a young person had resulted in the development of a vesical diverticulum or hydronephrosis (Marion's disease or 'prostatism sans prostate'). It is thought that dyssynergic contraction of the smooth muscle of the bladder neck (bladder neck dyssynergia) may account for some cases of BOO.

Owing to fibrosis

The symptoms are similar to those of prostatic enlargement but are a consequence of scarring after TURP.

Treatment

The management of these patients depends on achieving an accurate diagnosis. For this, urodynamic investigation is often necessary, which should demonstrate raised voiding pressures and diminished flow rate.

Drugs

The presence of α-adrenergic receptors in the region of the bladder neck and prostatic urethra allows pharmacological manipulation of the outflow to the bladder.

α-Blocking drugs

Alfuzosin, 2.5 mg bd to tds (to a total maximum of 10 mg/day), doxazosin, 1 mg nocte (up to a maximum of 8 mg/day), indoramin, 20 mg bd (increased to a total maximum of 100 mg/day in divided doses), prazosin 500 mg bd (maintenance up to 2 mg/day) and terazosin, 1 mg nocte (to a total maximum of 10 mg/day), can be very useful, causing relaxation of the bladder neck. Modified release tamsulosin 400 mg can be taken once daily. These drugs are not target specific, and patients must be warned of the possibility of postural hypotension.

Transurethral incision

Transurethral incision of the bladder neck is the operation of choice. Sometimes symptoms recur, but this is usually due to inadequate division of the fibres of the bladder neck.

Congenital valves of the prostatic urethra

See Chapter 78.

PROSTATIC CALCULI

Prostatic calculi are of two varieties: endogenous, which are common, and exogenous, which are comparatively rare.

An exogenous prostatic calculus is a urinary (commonly ureteric) calculus that becomes arrested in the prostatic urethra. This is considered in Chapter 75.

Endogenous prostatic calculi are usually composed of calcium phosphate combined with about 20 per cent organic material.

Clinical features

Prostatic calculi are usually symptomless, being discovered on

Jean Baptiste Camile Marion, 1869–1932, Professor of Urology, The Faculty of Medicine, Paris, France.

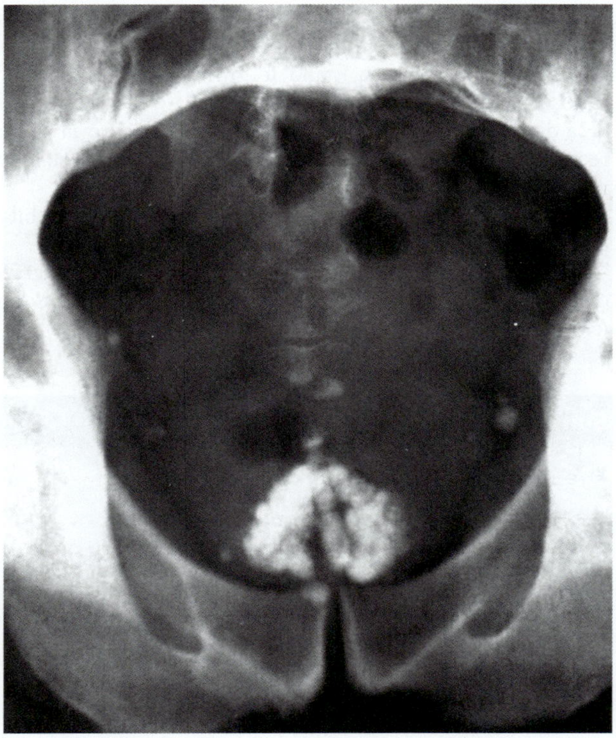

Figure 77.15 Endogenous prostatic calculi.

TRUS, on radiography of the pelvis, during prostatectomy or associated with carcinoma of the prostate or chronic prostatitis. In cases associated with severe chronic prostatic infection, the associated fibrosis and nodularity are difficult to differentiate from carcinoma. On radiographs or ultrasound scans, these stones are often seen to form a horseshoe (Figure 77.15) or a circle.

Treatment of prostatic calculi

They usually require no treatment.

Conservative measures

Associated chronic prostatic infection may be treated by means of ciprofloxacin or trimethoprim.

Transurethral resection

Transurethral resection will often release small calculi as the strips of prostatic tissue are excised. Others are passed per urethram at a later date.

Corpora amylaceae

Corpora amylaceae are tiny calcified lamellated bodies found in the glandular alveoli of the prostates of elderly men and apes, but not in the prostates of animals lower in the phylogenetic scale than anthropoids. Corpora amylaceae are probably the forerunners of endogenous prostatic calculi.

CARCINOMA OF THE PROSTATE

Carcinoma of the prostate is the most common malignant tumour in men over the age of 65 years. In England and Wales in 2008, 37000 men were registered and 10000 died from it; the corresponding figures in the USA were 186000 and 28000, respectively. If histological section of prostates at autopsy is performed, increasingly frequent foci of microscopic prostate cancers are found with increasing age. These foci of prostate cancer have variable potential for progressing clinically to metastatic disease. About 10–15 per cent of younger men who develop prostate cancer have a positive family history of the disease, but the aetiology is unclear. Throughout the world, rates of microscopic foci of prostate cancer are constant, but rates of clinically evident disease are low in men in Japan and China. Carcinoma of the prostate usually originates in the PZ of the prostate (Figure 77.2), so 'prostatectomy' for benign enlargement of the gland confers no protection from subsequent carcinoma.

Pathology

Serial sections of prostates obtained at routine necropsy demonstrate prostate carcinoma in 25 per cent of men between 50 and 65 years of age. The incidence in men over 80 years is in the region of 70 per cent (Franks). Most of these neoplasms are tiny and (if life had continued) might have remained latent for years.

The following types of prostate cancer occur:

- microscopic latent cancer found on autopsy or at cystoprostatectomy;
- impalpable tumours found incidentally during TURP (T1a and T1b) or following screening by PSA measurement (T1c);
- early, palpable, localised prostate cancer (T2);
- advanced local prostate cancer (T3 and T4);
- metastatic disease, which may arise from a clinically evident tumour (T2, T3 or T4) or from an apparently benign gland (T0, T1), i.e. occult prostate cancer.

It should be noted that only the last two groups cause symptoms, and such tumours are not curable. Only screening or the treatment of incidentally found tumours can result in cure of the disease. The problem is that many such tumours would never progress during the patient's lifetime; herein lies the problem with prostate cancer (Summary box 77.6).

Summary box 77.6

Prostate cancer detection

- The incidence has increased, and opportunistic PSA testing has enabled the detection of early-stage disease
- It is not yet clear whether national screening programmes for prostate cancer should be instigated
- Patients should be counselled about the investigations and treatment options available before a PSA test is performed

Screening for prostate cancer

The cancer detection rate using measurement of PSA is between 2 and 4 per cent, and approximately 30 per cent of men with an elevated PSA will have prostate cancer confirmed by biopsy. Unfortunately, 20 per cent of men with clinically significant prostate cancer will have PSA values within the normal range. There is therefore controversy over the usefulness of PSA alone as a screening procedure. One of the two recent prospective screening trials (the other was inconclusive due to contamination) suggests that screening with PSA does prevent death due to prostate cancer, but that a lot of men must be screened and treated to prevent one death. At present, in Europe, population-based screening is performed only within the confines of clinical trials.

Histological appearances

The prostate is a glandular structure consisting of ducts and acini; thus, the histological pattern is one of an adenocarcinoma. The prostatic glands are surrounded by a layer of myoepithelial cells. The first change associated with carcinoma is the loss of the basement membrane, with glands appearing to be in confluence. As the cell type becomes less differentiated, more solid sheets of carcinoma cells are seen. A classification of the histological pattern based on the degree of glandular de-differentiation and its relation to stroma has been devised by Gleason. Prostate cancers exhibit heterogeneity within tissue, and so two histological areas of prostate are each scored between 1 and 5. The scores are added to give an overall Gleason score of between 2 and 10; this (and the volume of the cancer) appears to correlate well with the likelihood of spread and the prognosis.

Local spread

Locally advanced tumours tend to grow upwards to involve the seminal vesicles, the bladder neck and trigone and, later, the tumours tend to spread distally to involve the distal sphincter mechanism. Further upward extension obstructs the lower end of one or both ureters, obstruction of both resulting in anuria. The rectum may become stenosed by tumour infiltrating around it, but direct involvement is rare.

Spread by the bloodstream

Spread by the bloodstream occurs particularly to bone; indeed, the prostate is the most common site of origin for skeletal metastases, followed in turn by the breast, the kidney, the bronchus and the thyroid gland. The bones involved most frequently by carcinoma of the prostate are the pelvic bones and the lower lumbar vertebrae. The femoral head, rib cage and skull are other common sites.

Lymphatic spread

Lymphatic spread may occur (1) via lymphatic vessels passing to the obturator fossa or along the sides of the rectum to the lymph nodes beside the internal iliac vein and in the hollow of the sacrum and (2) via lymphatics that pass over the seminal vesicles and follow the vas deferens for a short distance to drain into the external iliac lymph nodes. From retroperitoneal lymph nodes, the mediastinal nodes and occasionally the supraclavicular nodes may become implicated.

Staging using the tumour, node, metastasis (TNM) system (Figure 77.16)

1 **T1a, T1b and T1c**. These are incidentally found tumours in a clinically benign gland after histological examination of a prostatectomy specimen. T1a is a tumour involving less than 5 per cent of the resected specimen; these tumours are usually well or moderately well differentiated. T1b is a tumour involving >5 per cent of the resected specimen. T1c tumours are impalpable tumours found following investigation of a raised PSA.
2 **T2a** disease presents as a suspicious nodule (Figure 77.17) on rectal examination confined within the prostate capsule and involving one lobe. T2b disease involves both lobes.
3 **T3** tumour extends through the capsule (T3a, uni- or bilateral extension. T3b, seminal vesical extension).
4 **T4** is a tumour that is fixed or invading adjacent structures other than seminal vesicles – rectum or pelvic side wall (Summary box 77.7).

Donald F Gleason, 1920–2008, pathologist, University of Minnesota, Minneapolis, MN, USA. He published The Gleason System in 1966. He spent his last 20 years sailing, baking bread and playing bridge.

Summary box 77.7

The natural history of prostate cancer

This depends on the stage and grade of disease:

- T1 and T2
  The progression rate of well-differentiated T1a prostate cancer is very low: 10–14 per cent after eight years. For moderately differentiated tumours, the rate is about 20 per cent
  For T1b and T2 tumours, the rate is in excess of 35 per cent
- T3 and T4 (MO)
  About 50 per cent progress to bony metastases after 3–5 years
- M1
  The median survival of men with metastatic disease is about three years

Clinical features

Only advanced disease gives rise to symptoms, but even advanced disease may be asymptomatic. Symptoms of advanced disease include:

- BOO;
- pelvic pain and haematuria;
- bone pain, malaise, 'arthritis', anaemia or pancytopenia;
- renal failure;
- locally advanced disease or even asymptomatic metastases, which may be found incidentally on investigation of other symptoms.

Early prostate cancer is asymptomatic and may be found:

- incidentally following TURP for clinically benign disease (T1);
- as a nodule (T2) on rectal examination (Summary box 77.8).

Rectal examination

Rectal examination can detect nodules within the prostate and advanced disease. TRUS may be used to access the local stage and can be combined with a needle core biopsy (Figure 77.18). Irregular induration, characteristically stony hard in part or in the whole of the gland (with obliteration of the median sulcus), suggests carcinoma. Extension beyond the capsule up into the

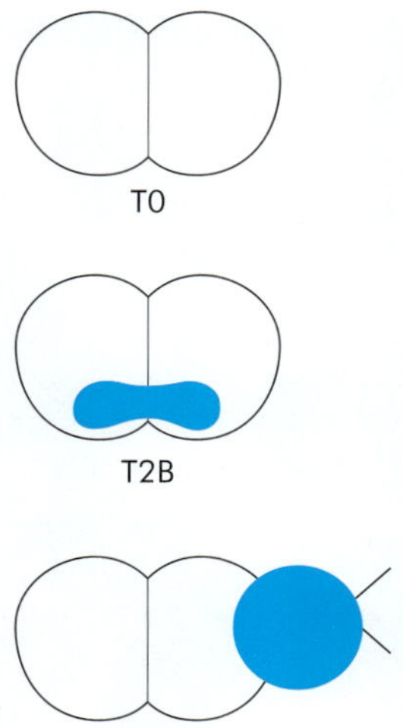

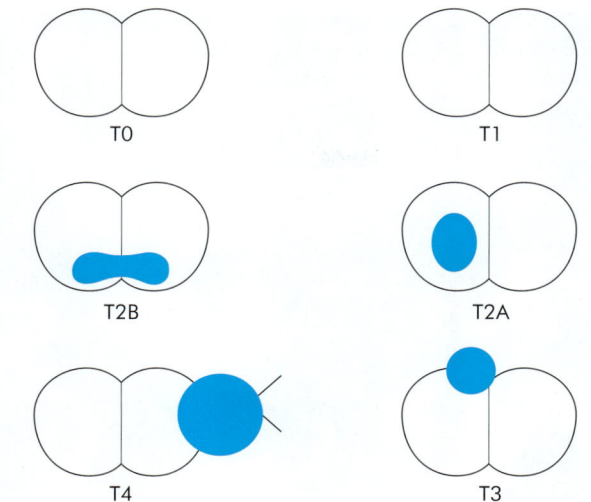

Figure 77.16 Tumour, node, metastasis (TNM) staging system for prostate cancer.

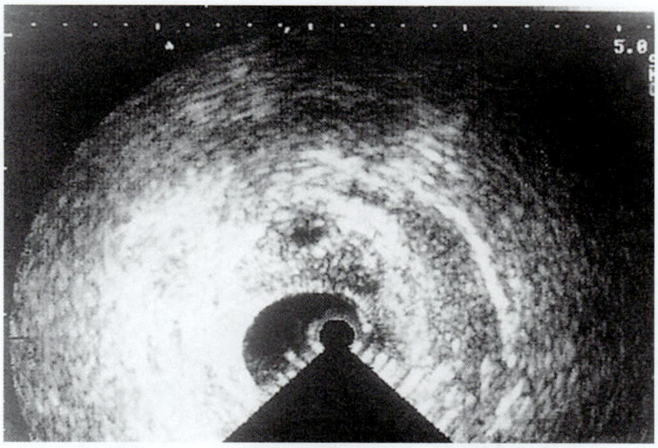

Figure 77.17 Transrectal ultrasound scan of a T2 nodule in the prostate.

Summary box 77.8

The presentation of men with prostate cancer

- Often men are asymptomatic, and detection is by opportunistic PSA testing
- Cancer is detected in men describing LUTS or may present with symptoms from metastatic disease

bladder base and vesicles (Figure 77.19 demonstrates normal vesicles) is diagnostic, as is local extension through the capsule (Figure 77.20).

Prostatic biopsy

If there is suspicion of prostate cancer, because of local findings, a raised PSA or metastatic disease, then a transrectal biopsy using an automated gun is recommended. Routine local anaesthetic is used to decrease pain. About ten systematic biopsy cores are obtained, as well as biopsy of any suspicious areas. Broad spectrum antibiotic cover is given to all patients to reduce the incidence of sepsis.

If there are associated symptoms of BOO, then either:

- a TURP can be performed, which will provide diagnostic material and symptomatic relief;
- a transrectal biopsy can be carried out. If the diagnosis is positive and there is locally advanced disease, then hormone ablation can provide good symptomatic relief without the need for operation.

General blood tests

These are normal in early disease but, in metastatic disease, there may be leuko-erythroblastic anaemia secondary to extensive marrow invasion, or anaemia may be secondary to renal failure. There may be thrombocytopenia and evidence of disseminated intravascular coagulopathy with increased fibrinogen degradation products (FDPs).

Liver function tests

These will be abnormal if there is extensive metastatic invasion of the liver. The alkaline phosphatase may be raised from either hepatic involvement or secondaries in the bone. These can be distinguished by measurement of isoenzymes or gamma-glutamyltransferase.

Prostate-specific antigen

This is discussed earlier in this chapter. It is good at following the course of advanced disease. It is lacking in sensitivity and specificity in the diagnosis of early localised prostate cancer. Nevertheless, the finding of a PSA >10 nmol/mL is suggestive of cancer and >35 ng/mL is almost diagnostic of advanced prostate cancer. A decrease in PSA to the normal range following hormonal ablation is a good prognostic sign.

Acid phosphatase

Acid phosphatase has been superseded by measurement of PSA.

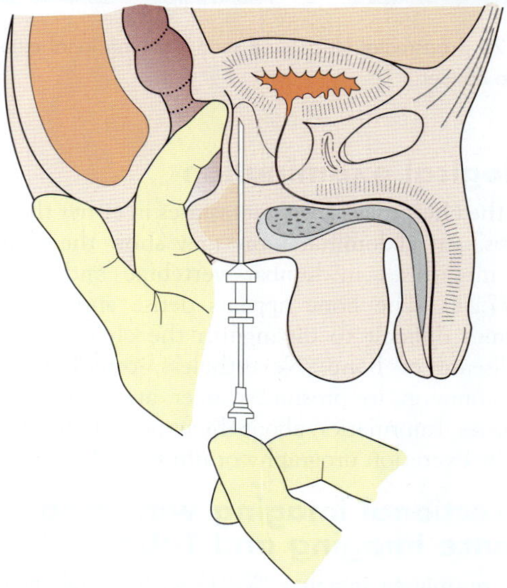

Figure 77.18 Obtaining a specimen of prostatic tissue by means of a TruCut biopsy needle.

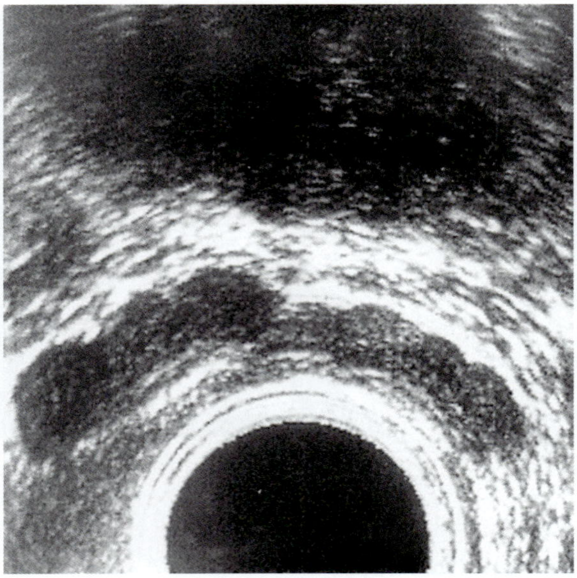

Figure 77.19 Transrectal ultrasound scan showing normal seminal vesicles.

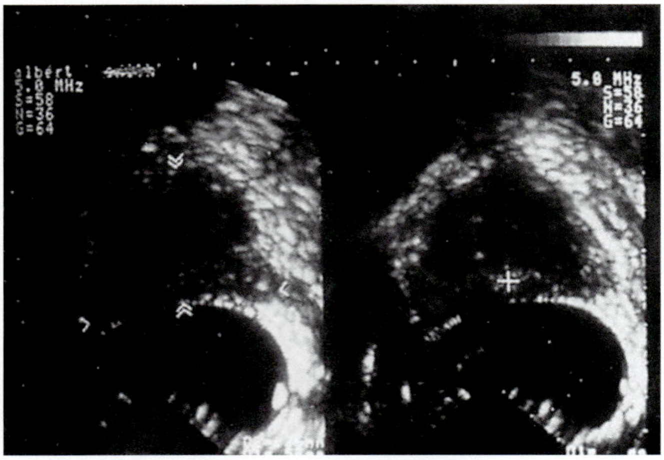

Figure 77.20 Transrectal ultrasound scan showing local extension of a T3 prostate cancer.

Radiological examination

X-rays of the chest may reveal metastases in either the lung fields or the ribs. An abdominal x-ray may show the characteristic sclerotic metastases in lumbar vertebrae and pelvic bones (Figure 77.21). The bone appears dense and coarse, and it is sometimes difficult to distinguish the change from that in Paget's disease of bone. Nevertheless, osteolytic metastases are very common in prostate cancer and may coexist with sclerotic ones. Information about the upper urinary tracts can be obtained by excretion urography or ultrasound.

Cross-sectional imaging with magnetic resonance imaging and TRUS

Magnetic resonance imaging (MRI) with a high tesla magnet (1.5–3 T) is the most accurate method of staging local disease.

Transrectal ultrasound scanning can also be used. Locally extensive disease (T2) can be diagnosed with increased sensitivity by TRUS (Figure 77.17) compared with rectal examination, but many tumours will still be missed. This problem remains a real one in screening for early prostate cancer; in comparison with breast cancer, with mammography detecting 70–80 per cent of tumours, TRUS plus rectal examination and measurement of PSA will detect only 30–50 per cent of cancers that are known to be present on autopsy studies (although it may detect the larger, more significant cancers).

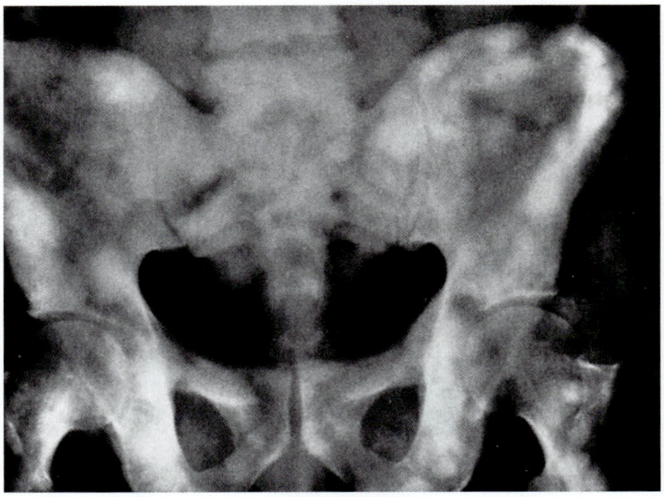

Figure 77.21 Osseous metastases of the pelvic bones in carcinoma of the prostate (courtesy of LN Pyrah, Leeds, UK).

Bone scan

Once the diagnosis has been established, it would be normal to perform a bone scan as part of the staging procedure if the PSA were >10 nmol/mL or if the biopsy showed high-grade cancer. If the PSA is <10 nmol/mL, then a bone scan would be performed only on clinical indications. The bone scan is performed by the injection of technetium-99m, which is then monitored using a gamma camera. It is more sensitive in the diagnosis of metastases (Figure 77.22) than a skeletal survey, but false positives occur in areas of arthritis, osteomyelitis or a healing fracture.

Lymphangiography

This is no longer carried out. If accurate information is required, then pelvic lymphadenectomy can be performed by means of laparoscopic surgery.

Bone marrow aspiration

Sometimes, examination of the bone marrow will reveal the presence of metastatic carcinoma cells.

Treatment of carcinoma of the prostate

Early disease

Curative treatment can only be offered to patients with early disease (T1a, T1b, T1c and T2). T1a disease found incidentally at TURP is by definition low volume and usually well differentiated. This stage can often be managed by active surveillance, with three- to six-monthly digital rectal examination (DRE)

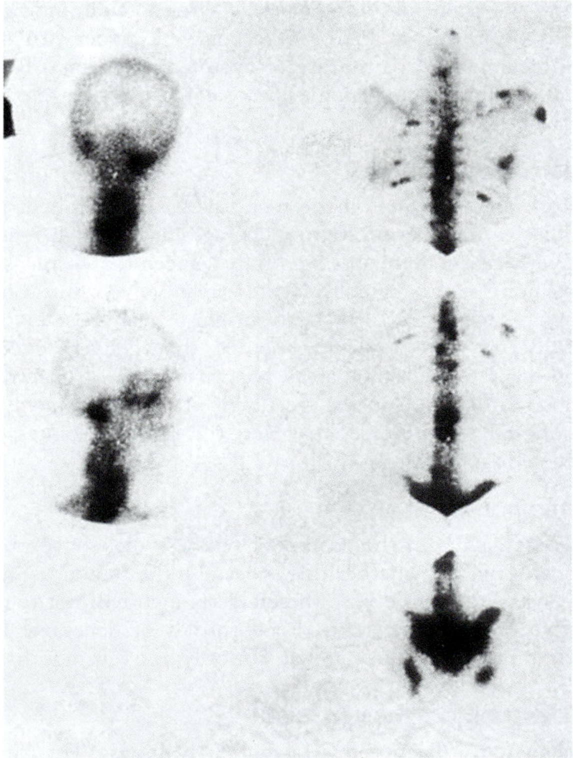

Figure 77.22 Bone scan showing multiple hot-spots suggestive of metastatic disease in a man with prostate cancer.

and PSA measurement, considering treatment if there is evidence of disease progression. The options available for T1b, T1c and T2 disease need to take into account patient age, performance status and lifestyle preferences. The treatment of patients with advanced disease (T3, T4 or any M0) is only palliative (Summary box 77.9).

Summary box 77.9

Treatment and stage

- Treatment options for prostate cancer depend on stage of disease, life expectancy of the patient and patient preference
- PSA, DRE and biopsy Gleason grade are used to predict pathological stage
- Localised cancer can be treated by radical prostatectomy, radiation therapy and active monitoring
- Treatment of advanced disease is palliative, and hormone ablation remains the first-line therapy

Radical prostatectomy

Radical prostatectomy is only suitable for localised disease (T1 and T2) and should be carried out only in men with a life expectancy of >10 years. Exclusion of metastases would require a negative bone scan, chest x-ray and a serum PSA <20 nmol/mL. It is a procedure that should be performed only by experienced surgeons when there is a high chance of cure. It results in a high incidence of impotence, but a low incidence of severe stress incontinence (<2 per cent), which may require the fitting of an artificial urinary sphincter. It involves removal of the prostate down to the distal sphincter mechanism in addition to the seminal vesicles (Figure 77.23). The bladder neck is reconstituted and anastomosed to the urethra. Recent modifications to this operation by Professor Patrick Walsh of the Johns Hopkins Hospital in Baltimore have led to the realisation that careful dissection in early-stage disease can lead to preservation of the neurovascular bundles that lie behind the prostate. This modification has led to the preservation of erectile function in about 60–70 per cent of cases. Recently, laparoscopic approaches to radical prostatectomy, sometimes supported by robotic techniques, have been introduced.

Radical radiotherapy for early prostate cancer

External beam radiotherapy (EBRT) can be administered in fields that conform to the contours of the prostate, thereby limiting exposure of adjacent tissues. Survival rates following the treatment of T1 and low-volume T2 disease are not greatly different from those following radical prostatectomy, although histological evidence of persistent tumour is found within the prostate in about 30 per cent of treated patients. The treatment of T3 disease which has spread through the capsule of the gland is controversial. Surgery, radiotherapy, androgen ablation or combinations of the above are used. The treatment requires the patient to attend hospital on a daily basis for between 4 and 6 weeks. Some local complications are inevitable, namely irritation of the bladder with urinary frequency, urgency and sometimes urge incontinence and similar problems affecting the rectum with diarrhoea and, occasionally, late radiation proctitis. Development of erectile dysfunction occurs less frequently than following radical prostatectomy, but is present in up to 30 per cent of cases.

Brachytherapy

Under transrectal ultrasound guidance, radioactive seeds are permanently implanted into the prostate. A computer program converts accurate ultrasound measurements of the prostate gland to construct a plan of the gland. Under anaesthesia, the patient is placed in the lithotomy position and, according to the template plan, seeds are placed through transperineal needles.

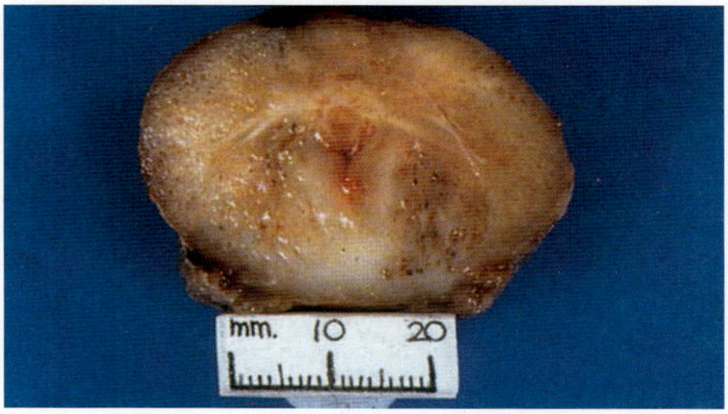

Figure 77.23 Radical prostatectomy specimen for a T2a prostate cancer. Preoperative PSA was 6 ng/L; postoperative levels remained undetectable at eight years. The patient is fully continent.

Patrick C Walsh, Professor of Urology, Johns Hopkins Hospital, Baltimore, MD, USA. Recipient of 2007 National Physician of the Year Clinical Excellence Award.

The radioisotopes commonly used are iodine-125 and palladium-103. These isotopes deliver an intense, confined radiation dose, which falls off rapidly to spare the surrounding structures. Brachytherapy is gaining widespread acceptance for the treatment of lower grade low-volume T1 disease. A major factor is the reduced peroperative complications and generally low morbidity. Long-term cancer survival results from institutions specialising in the procedure are encouraging.

Advanced disease

There is still debate about the timing of androgen ablation treatment in patients with locally advanced or metastatic disease without symptoms. The options are androgen deprivation at diagnosis or careful review, reserving active treatment for the later development of symptoms. Patients with poorly differentiated disease are at risk of a catastrophic event such as spinal cord compression; in these patients, early androgen ablation can prolong the time to complications. Also, patients with local or general symptoms should be offered androgen deprivation.

Orchidectomy

Orchidectomy is performed to carry out androgen ablation in the treatment of locally advanced (T3 or T4) disease or of metastatic disease. In 1941, prostate cancer was shown to be responsive to such treatment by Charles Huggins, the only urologist to win a Nobel Prize. Bilateral orchidectomy, whether total or subcapsular, will eliminate the major source of testosterone production.

Medical castration

Medical forms of androgen ablation have been available since the discovery of stilbestrol. The other commonly available treatment to reduce testosterone levels to the castrate range is LHRH agonists. These agents initially stimulate hypothalamic LHRH receptors but, because of their constant presence (rather than the normal diurnal rhythm), they then downregulate them, resulting in cessation of pituitary LH production and, hence, a decrease in testosterone production. In the first 10 days or so, serum testosterone levels may increase, and it is wise to give flutamide, bicalutamide or cyproterone acetate for this period. LHRH agonists may be given by monthly or three-monthly depot injection.

Other treatments that block the androgen receptor have become available recently. Cyproterone acetate also has some progestogenic effect, while flutamide and bicalutamide are pure anti-androgen. In general, oral anti-androgen monotherapy has not been shown to be as good as LHRH agonists or orchidectomy. New types of drugs affecting the LHRH–androgen axis, such as LHRH antagonists, superpotent androgen receptor antagonists and drugs inhibiting androgen biosynthesis, are in clinical trials. The role of these drugs is yet to be established.

Complete androgen blockade

Complete androgen blockade has been advocated as being likely to result in increased life expectancy and an increased time to progression in a fitter subgroup of men with advanced prostate cancer. The concept is that of abolishing the testicular secretion of testosterone by means of orchidectomy or the use of LHRH therapy and then inhibiting the effects of adrenal androgenic steroids by means of androgen receptor blockade with flutamide, bicalutamide or the use of cyproterone acetate. Recent overviews of randomised trials do not confirm earlier reports of effectiveness.

Charles Brenton Huggins, 1901–1997, (Canadian born), Professor of Surgery, The University of Chicago, IL, USA, shared the 1966 Nobel Prize for Physiology or Medicine for his discoveries concerning hormonal treatment of prostate cancer.

General radiotherapy

Radiotherapy for symptomatic metastases is an excellent form of palliative treatment, often producing dramatic pain relief in men with hormone-relapsed prostate cancer that can last up to six months. When multiple sites are involved, intravenous radiopharmaceuticals such as strontium-89 can be employed. Strontium is a bone-seeking isotope that delivers effective radiotherapy to metastatic areas. It appears to be as effective as hemibody irradiation in the treatment of men with metastatic hormone-relapsed disease; however, the duration of response has been disappointing.

Chemotherapy

Cytotoxic agents in the treatment of these men have proved disappointing, but whether this is because the tumour is inherently insensitive or because these elderly men will not tolerate effective doses is uncertain. Recent trials of docetaxel have shown improvements in survival, but only by a few months.

Summary of treatment

1. **Incidentally diagnosed T1a and T1b disease**. For men in their 70s, conservative treatment would usually be the correct approach. Radical surgical treatment might be considered in the younger (<70 years) man with this form of the disease, although even in this group, some men will elect to pursue a conservative course when counselled about risks versus benefits.
2. **Localised T1c and T2 disease**. In younger, fitter men (<70 years), this may be treated by radical prostatectomy or radical radiotherapy. Active monitoring remains an option, particularly for more elderly patients with low-grade disease. In the elderly patient with outflow obstruction, transurethral resection with or without hormone therapy is indicated. The benefit of radical treatment over a conservative approach is likely to be about 25 per cent, given that progression to metastatic disease is of this order of magnitude after 10 years.
3. **Locally advanced T3 and T4 disease**. These patients are at significant risk of disease progression. Early androgen ablation is favoured if close follow up is not possible. For the sexually active, a careful conservative approach with the adoption of androgen ablation when symptoms arise is reasonable. Androgen ablation coupled with radiotherapy is standard treatment for younger men with T3 disease.
4. **Metastatic disease**. Once metastases have developed, the outlook is poor. For patients with symptoms, there is no dilemma; androgen ablation will provide symptomatic relief in over two-thirds of patients. For patients with asymptomatic metastases, the timing of treatment is less clear. Systemic chemotherapy with docetaxel should be considered in younger, fitter men.

PROSTATITIS

In both acute and chronic prostatitis, the seminal vesicles and posterior urethra are usually also involved.

Acute prostatitis

Aetiology

Acute prostatitis is common, but underdiagnosed. The usual organism responsible is *Escherichia coli*, but *Staphylococcus aureus*, *Staphylococcus albus*, *Streptococcus faecalis*, *Neisseria gonorrhoeae* or *Chlamydia* may be responsible. The infection may be haematogenous from a distant focus, or it may be secondary to acute urinary infection.

Clinical features

General manifestations overshadow the local: the patient feels ill, shivers, may have a rigor, has 'aches' all over, especially in the back, and may easily be diagnosed as having influenza. The temperature may be up to 39°C. Pain on micturition is usual, but not invariable. The urine contains threads in the initial voided sample, which should be cultured. Perineal heaviness, rectal irritation and pain on defaecation can occur; a urethral discharge is rare. Frequency occurs when the infection involves the bladder. Rectal examination reveals a tender prostate; one lobe may be swollen more than the other, and the seminal vesicles may be involved. A frankly fluctuant abscess is uncommon.

Treatment

Treatment must be rigorous and prolonged or the infection will not be eradicated and recurrent attacks may ensue. Spread of infection to the epididymides and testes may occur. Prolonged treatment with an antibiotic that penetrates the prostate well is indicated (trimethoprim or ciprofloxacin).

Prostatic abscess

In addition to the foregoing symptoms and signs, the advent of a prostatic abscess is heralded by the temperature rising steeply with rigors. Antibiotics disguise these features. Severe, unremitting perineal and rectal pain with occasional tenesmus often cause the condition to be confused with an anorectal abscess. Nevertheless, if a rectal examination is performed, the prostate will be felt to be enlarged, hot, extremely tender and perhaps fluctuant. Retention of urine is likely to occur and, in such men, suprapubic catheterisation is best.

Treatment

The abscess should be drained without delay:

- The abscess can be drained by perurethral resection – unroofing the whole cavity.
- The perineal route is rarely indicated unless there is marked periprostatic spread.

Chronic prostatitis

Many urologists find the diagnosis of chronic prostatitis and 'prostatodynia' very difficult, for many men present with perigenital pain, testicular pain, prostatic pain exacerbated by sexual intercourse or pain that apparently renders sexual intercourse out of the question. Psychosexual dysfunction in such patients may be the underlying problem. The diagnosis of chronic prostatitis has to be based on:

- persistent threads in voided urine;
- prostatic massage showing pus cells with or without bacteria in the absence of urinary infection.

Aetiology

This is thought to be the sequel of inadequately treated acute prostatitis. While pus is present in the prostatic secretion, the responsible organism is often difficult to find. Other organisms such as *Chlamydia* species may be responsible for chronic abacterial prostatitis.

Clinical features

The clinical features are extremely varied. Only men with symptoms of posterior urethritis, prostatic pain and perigenital pain accompanied by intermittent fever and pus cells or bacteria in the post-prostatic massage specimen should be diagnosed as having chronic prostatitis.

Diagnosis

The three-glass urine test is valuable. If the first glass with the initial voided sample shows urine containing prostatic threads, prostatitis is present.

Rectal examination of the prostate may be normal or may show a soft, boggy and tender prostate.

Examination of the prostatic fluid obtained by prostatic massage should show pus cells and bacteria.

Urethroscopy may reveal inflammation of the prostatic urethra, and pus may be seen exuding from the prostatic ducts. The verumontanum is likely to be enlarged and oedematous. In many men with the symptoms described above, all investigations are normal.

Treatment

Antibiotic therapy should be administered only in accordance with bacteriological sensitivity tests. Trimethoprim penetrates well into the prostate. If *Trichomonas* or anaerobes are the responsible agent, a rapid response is obtained from administration of flagyl (metronidazole, 200 mg tds for 7 days to both partners). If *Chlamydia* is suspected, doxycycline is the antibiotic treatment of choice. It is uncertain whether prostatic massage helps in eradicating the infection.

Prostatodynia

This diagnosis is made by the presence of perigenital pain in the absence of any objective evidence of prostatic inflammation. Whether the syndrome has any relationship with the prostate is unclear.

TUBERCULOSIS OF THE PROSTATE AND SEMINAL VESICLES

Tuberculosis of the prostate and seminal vesicles is rare and associated with renal tuberculosis. In 30 per cent of cases, there is a history of pulmonary tuberculosis within five years of the onset of genital tuberculosis.

Tuberculosis of one or both seminal vesicles may be found when examining a patient with chronic tuberculous epididymitis, no symptoms being referable to the internal genitalia. On rectal examination, the affected vesicle is found to be nodular.

When the prostate is involved, rectal examination reveals nodules in one or both lateral lobes. Patients with tuberculous prostatitis usually present with the following:

- urethral discharge;

- painful, sometimes blood-stained, ejaculation;
- mild ache in the perineum;
- infertility;
- dysuria;
- abscess formation.

Special forms of investigation

X-ray sometimes displays areas of calcification in the prostate and/or the seminal vesicles.

Bacteriological examination of the seminal fluid yields positive cultures for tubercle bacilli.

Treatment

The general treatment is that for tuberculosis. If a prostatic abscess forms, it should be drained transurethrally.

SEMINAL VESICLES

Acute seminal vesiculitis

Acute seminal vesiculitis occurs in association with prostatitis. Prior to the antibiotic treatment of gonorrhoea, gonococcal vesiculitis was common.

Chronic seminal vesiculitis

Chronic seminal vesiculitis usually presents with haematospermia and pain on intercourse. TRUS demonstrates the features of distension and thickening and the presence of turbid fluid. The treatment is the same as for chronic prostatitis.

Tuberculous seminal vesiculitis

The clinical features and treatment have been discussed above.

Diverticulum of the seminal vesicle

Diverticulum of the seminal vesicle occurs occasionally. In such cases, the kidney of that side is absent, and the diverticulum represents an abortive ureteric bud. It is a cause of persistent infection.

Cyst of the seminal vesicle

A cyst of the seminal vesicle is uncommon and rarely requires treatment. It may be removed by dissection through an incision similar to that for perineal prostatectomy, if it is large or giving rise to symptoms.

FURTHER READING

Mundy AR, Fitzpatrick J, Neal DE, George NJR. *The scientific basis of urology*, 3rd edn. London: Informa Healthcare, 2010.

Vogelzan NJ, Scardino PT, Shipley WU *et al. Comprehensive textbook of genitourinary oncology*, 3rd edn. Philadelphia, PA: Lippincott Williams & Wilkins, 2006.

Wein AJ, Kavoussi LR, Novick AC *et al. Campbell's urology*, 9th edn. Philadelphia, PA, Saunders, 2007.

CHAPTER 78

Urethra and penis

LEARNING OBJECTIVES

To recognise and understand:

- The common congenital abnormalities of the urethra
- The diagnosis and management of urethral trauma
- The diagnosis and management of urethral stricture
- The diagnosis and management of phimosis
- The principles of management of a man with erectile dysfunction
- The common diseases of the penis and the principles of their surgical management

THE MALE URETHRA

Anatomy

The male urethra is a tubular structure extending from the bladder neck to the external urinary meatus at the tip of the glans penis. It has four components which are named (from proximal to distal), the prostatic, membranous, bulbar and penile urethra. The prostatic urethra extends from the bladder neck to the verumontanum and is compressed on either side by the lateral lobes of the prostate, giving it a slit-like configuration. The verumontanum is a small hillock of tissue indented at its crown by a pit called the utriculus masculinus which marks the proximal extent of the external urethral sphincter and is an important landmark for urologists performing transurethral resection of the prostate. The membranous urethra lies just distal to the verumontanum and is located where the urethra penetrates the pelvic floor and it is the usual site of urethral rupture at the time of a pelvic fracture. It is the primary location of continence as a consequence of the surrounding pelvic floor musculature and external urethral sphincter. The bulbar urethra extends from the membranous urethra to the penoscrotal junction and is anteriorly located within the corpus spongiosum. The penile urethra is normally flattened anteroposteriorly, but distends when filled with fluid. The penile urethra becomes dilated within the glans penis where it is named the 'navicular fossa'.

The external urethral sphincter is composed of circular striated muscle within the urethral wall. The bladder neck contributes to maintenance of continence in the man, although its main role is as a genital sphincter that closes at the time of ejaculation.

Congenital abnormalities

Posterior urethral valves

Posterior urethral valves occur in around one in 5000–8000 live male births. The valves are membranes which typically lie just distal to the verumontanum and cause obstruction to the urethra of boys. They are flap valves and so although they are obstructive to antegrade urinary flow, a urethral catheter can be passed retrogradely without any difficulty. The diagnosis is commonly made antenatally with ultrasound which demonstrates bilateral hydronephrosis above a distended bladder. If the diagnosis is not made antenatally, then patients typically present with urinary infection in the neonatal period or with uraemia and renal failure. Rarely the valves are incomplete and the patient is symptom free until adolescence or adulthood when again urinary infection or renal impairment can supervene.

Diagnosis

Posterior urethral valves need to be detected and treated as early as possible to minimise the degree of renal failure. The valves can be difficult to see on urethroscopy because the flow of irrigant sweeps them into the open position. If the bladder is filled with contrast medium, the dilatation of the urethra above the valves can be demonstrated on a voiding cystogram (Figure 78.1). The bladder is hypertrophied and often shows diverticula. Typically, there is vesicoureteric reflux into dilated upper tracts (Summary box 78.1).

Summary box 78.1

Posterior urethral valves

- Posterior urethral valves are congenital membranes that cause obstruction to the urinary tract in baby boys
- Antenatal ultrasound typically shows urinary tract dilatation
- If not recognised antenatally, they may cause recurrent urinary infection, urinary retention and uraemia
- Treatment is valve destruction accompanied by treatment of urinary infection and renal impairment

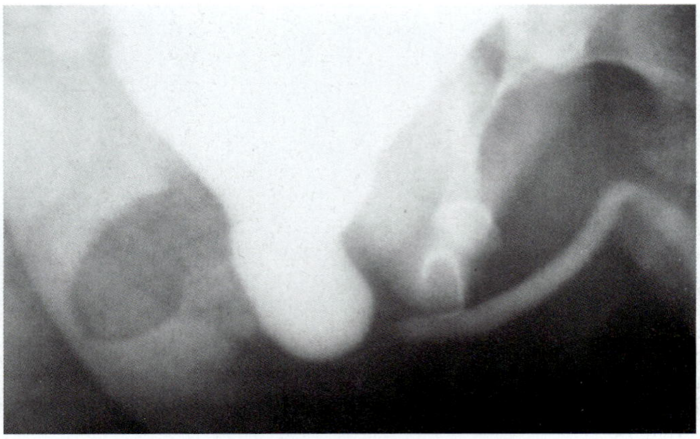

Figure 78.1 A voiding cystogram showing a dilated bladder with a dilated prostatic urethra above an obstruction at the level of the posterior urethral valve.

Treatment

Initial treatment is by catheterisation to relieve the back pressure and to allow the effects of renal failure to improve. Definitive treatment is by endoscopic destruction of the valves with continuing supportive treatment of the dilated urinary tract, the recurrent urinary infections and the uraemia (Summary box 78.1).

Hypospadias

Hypospadias occurs in around one in 200–300 male live births and is the most common congenital abnormality of the urethra (see also Chapter 8). There are three characteristic features. Firstly the external meatus opens on the underside of the penis or the perineum, secondly the ventral aspect of the prepuce is poorly developed ('hooded prepuce') and thirdly there is a ventral deformity of the erect penis (chordee).

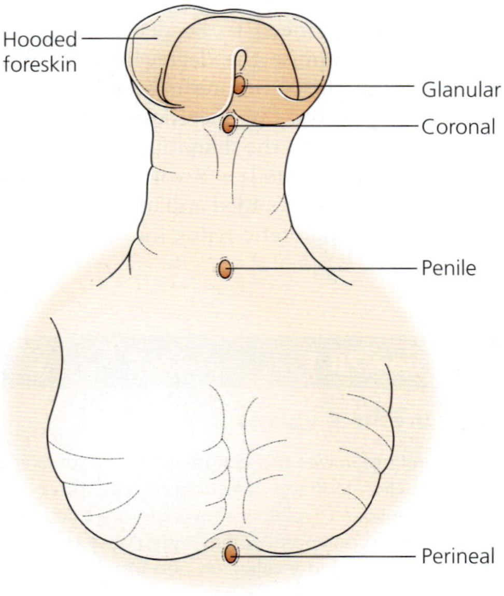

Figure 78.2 Hypospadias classification.

Hypospadias is classified according to the position of the meatus (Figure 78.2).

- **Glanular hypospadias.** The ectopic meatus is placed on the glans penis, but proximal to the normal site of the external meatus which is marked by a blind pit. Occasionally the two are connected by a channel.
- **Coronal hypospadias.** The meatus is placed at the junction of the underside of the glans and the body of the penis.
- **Penile and penoscrotal hypospadias.** The meatus is on the underside of the penile shaft.
- **Perineal hypospadias.** This is the rarest and most severe abnormality. The scrotum is bifid and the urethra opens between its two halves. There may be testicular maldescent, which may make it difficult to determine the sex of the child.

The more severe varieties of hypospadias represent an absence of the urethra and corpus spongiosum distal to the ectopic opening. The absent structures are represented by a fibrous cord, which deforms the penis in a downward direction (chordee).

Treatment

Hypospadias does not cause either obstruction or urinary tract infection. Surgery is indicated to improve sexual function, to correct problems with the urinary stream and for cosmetic reasons. A variety of plastic surgical procedures have been described to correct the chordee and to re-site the urethral opening. Some techniques utilise the foreskin and therefore circumcision should be avoided before the hypospadias has been repaired. Operations for hypospadias are best performed by a paediatric urologist and are typically undertaken before the age of one year (Summary box 78.2).

Summary box 78.2

Hypospadias

- Hypospadias is characterised by the combination of a ventrally placed urethral meatus, a hooded foreskin and chordee
- Avoid circumcision as the prepuce may be used in procedures to correct the abnormality
- Surgical treatment should be undertaken by a paediatric urologist

Epispadias

Epispadias is very rare. In penile epispadias, the urethral opening is on the dorsum of the penis and is associated with an upward curvature of the penis (Figure 78.3). Epispadias often coexists with bladder exstrophy and other severe developmental defects.

Urethral diverticulum

This is usually congenital and represents a partial duplication of the urethra. Acquired cases are uncommon but are sometimes seen as a result of increased intraurethral pressure behind a stricture. Others are caused by the longstanding presence of a foreign body such as a stone or calculus in the urethra.

Typically, patients present in adult life with a history of postmicturition dribbling and diagnosis is made at cystoscopy (Figure 78.4) or via a urethrogram. Treatment is often unnecessary, but they can be treated endoscopically by incising the flap of urethral

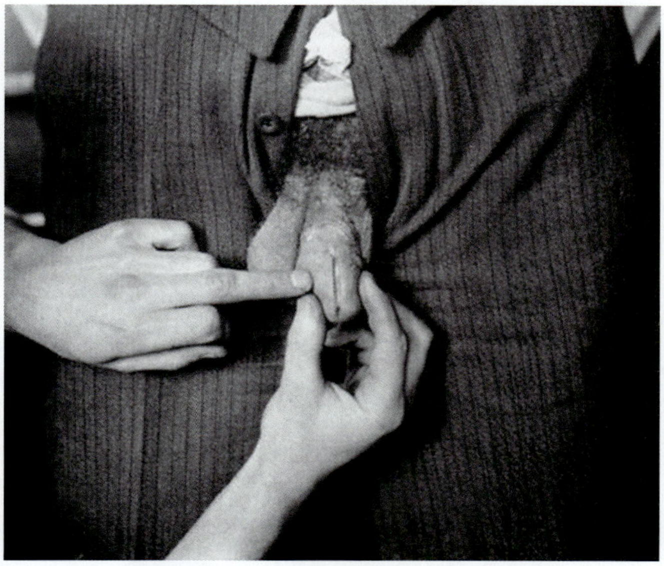

Figure 78.3 Glandular epispadias.

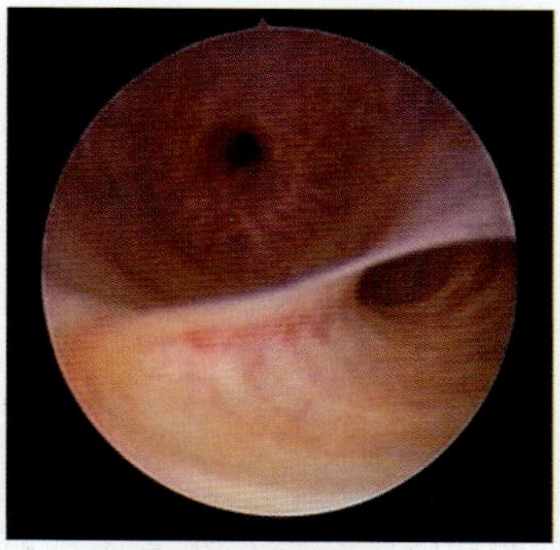

Figure 78.4 Cystoscopic appearance of a urethral diverticulum. The normal urethra can be seen to extend superiorly to the urethral sphincter, while the blind ending diverticulum is seen inferiorly.

mucosa between the two lumens, or in severe cases by excision of the diverticulum.

Injuries to the male urethra

Rupture of the bulbar urethra

There is a history of a blow to the perineum, usually due to a fall astride injury. The bulbar urethra is crushed upwards onto the pubic bone, typically with significant bruising. In the days of sailing ships, the common cause was falling astride a spar and the modern equivalent is seen among workers losing their footing on scaffolding. Cycling accidents, loose manhole covers and gymnasium accidents astride the beam account for a number of cases. Almost certainly King William I of England died in 1087 following a ruptured bulbar urethra that he sustained when falling off his horse. It is thought that he ruptured the urethra on the saddle's pommel and he subsequently developed urinary retention and sepsis secondary to infection of the haematoma and he died some days after the accident.

Extravasation of urine is common and the extravasated urine is confined in front of the midperineal point by the attachment of Colles' fascia to the triangular ligament and by the attachment of Scarpa's fascia just below the inguinal ligament. The external spermatic fascia stops it getting into the inguinal canals. Extravasated urine collects in the scrotum and penis and beneath the deep layer of superficial fascia in the abdominal wall.

Clinical features

The signs of a ruptured bulbar urethra are perineal bruising and haematoma, typically with a butterfly distribution. There is usually bleeding from the urethral meatus and retention of urine is also typically present.

Management

If the diagnosis is suspected, the patient should be treated with appropriate analgesia and antibiotics should be administered. He should be discouraged from passing urine. A full bladder should be drained with a catheter placed by percutaneous suprapubic puncture (Figure 78.5). This reduces urinary extravasation and allows investigations to establish the extent of the urethral injury. If the patient has passed urine when first seen and there is no extravasation, the rupture, if any, is partial and a suprapubic catheter is not usually needed. Diagnosis is made by urethrography using water soluble contrast.

If there is significant extravasation, then the perineal collection should be drained.

If the urethral tear is complete, the suprapubic catheter should remain *in situ* while the bruising and extravasation settle down. A stricture will typically develop at the site of the injury. The optimal treatment is delayed anastomotic urethroplasty after the swelling and bruising have settled down (typically 8–12 weeks later), with excision of the traumatised section and spatulated end-to-end reanastomosis of the urethra (Summary box 78.3).

Summary box 78.3

Bulbar urethral injury

- Suspect urethral injury after blunt perineal trauma when the man cannot void, when there is perineal bruising and when there is blood at the urethral meatus
- The safest initial management is to insert a suprapubic catheter
- Beware of urinary extravasation and sepsis in the perineal haematoma
- Delayed urethroplasty is the preferred definitive management of complete disruptions

Rupture of the membranous urethra

Rupture of the membranous urethra typically occurs in association with a fractured pelvis and may be associated with an extraperitoneal rupture of the bladder. When the pelvis fractures, the membranous urethra is ruptured as it passes through the bony ring of the pelvis. The urethra is elastic at this point, and if the fracture results in only a minor displacement, then the tear may only be partial, but more typically the rupture is complete, such that the two ends are completely displaced, with the develop-

Antonio Scarpa, 1747–1832, Professor of Anatomy, Pavia, Italy.

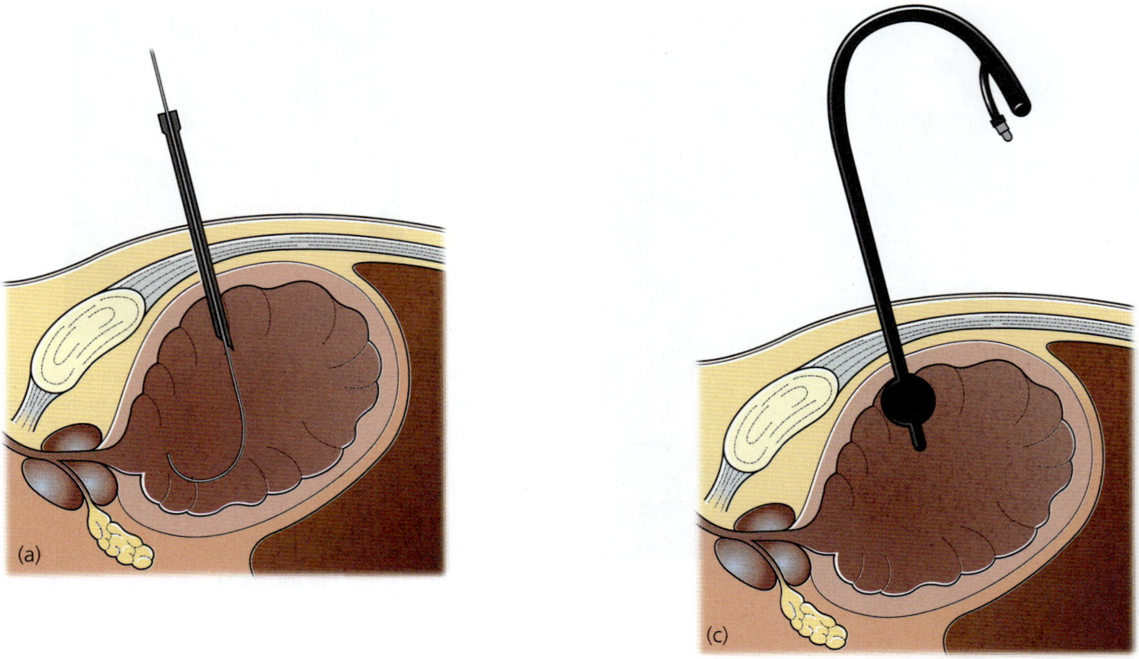

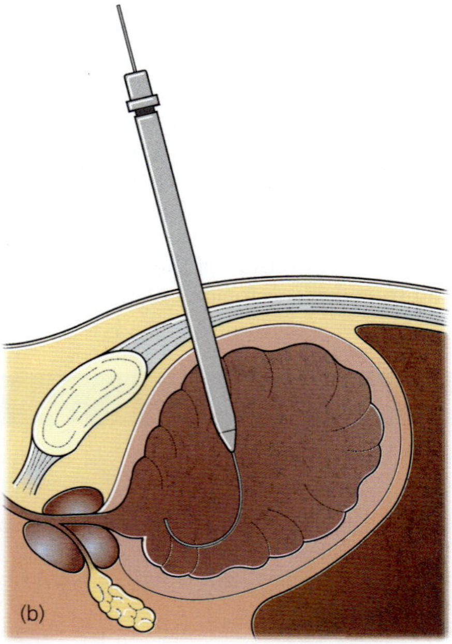

Figure 78.5 (a) Percutaneous puncture of bladder with passage of a guidewire into the bladder followed by dilatation of track over the guidewire (b), thereby allowing placement of catheter into the bladder (c).

ment of a significant interposing haematoma. About 5 per cent of cases of fractured pelvis have an associated urethral injury and such injuries are almost universally seen in men.

Clinical features

The most common causes of pelvic fracture are road traffic accidents, severe crush injuries and falls. Typically there are multiple associated injuries that may be immediately life threatening and the overriding priority is to keep the patient alive by appropriate resuscitation. Under these circumstances, the management of the other injuries takes precedence.

The clinical features include urinary retention, blood at the urethral meatus and a high riding prostate on digital rectal examination. If the diagnosis is suspected, a urethrogram performed with water soluble contrast media is confirmatory (Figure 78.6).

A suprapubic catheter should be inserted as soon as practicable. The distended bladder may be palpable making suprapubic catheterisation straightforward, but often the bruising and swelling associated with the fracture makes this difficult and ultrasound guidance is required. In the presence of a coexistent extraperitoneal bladder injury, no bladder will be apparent on ultrasound examination, and surgical exploration, bladder repair, suprapubic catheter placement and drainage of the retropubic space are needed.

Complications

Urethral disruption injury

The two ends of the urethra, having been torn apart, become separated by a haematoma. With time, this haematoma resolves and is replaced by fibrosis. This pelvic fracture urethral disruption injury is technically not a stricture of the urethra but is often erroneously described as being one. The conventional management of such an injury is delayed surgical reconstruction with excision of the scar tissue and end to end anastomosis. This surgery should be delayed until the patient has recovered from any other injuries and is usually undertaken 3–6 months later. It is a highly challenging technical procedure and should be undertaken only in specialist centres. Some surgeons continue to undertake early attempts to realign the urethral ends endo-

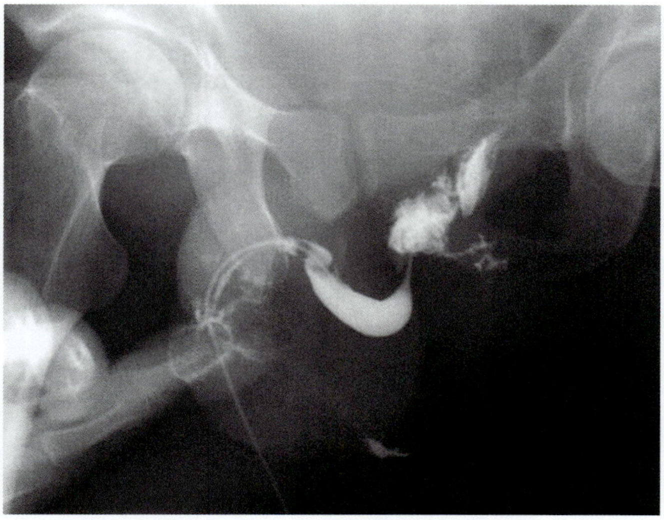

Figure 78.6 An ascending urethrogram demonstrating extravasation of contrast from the membranous urethra at the site of a urethral injury. Note the associated pelvic fracture with disruption of the inferior pubic rami.

scopically, and while there are some successful reports, most experts feel that there is an increased risk of sepsis, (true) stricture, incontinence and erectile dyfsunction.

Urinary incontinence

The site of the urethral rupture is at or close to the striated urethral sphincter. If the external urethral sphincter is damaged or destroyed, continence of urine will depend upon the bladder neck mechanism. While this is usually adequate to maintain complete continence (only 5–10 per cent of men suffer stress urinary incontinence after urethroplasty), subsequent surgical manoeuvres, which destroy the bladder neck (such as transurethral prostatectomy), may cause incontinence.

Erectile dysfunction

Erectile dysfunction is common after pelvic fracture with urethral injury and is due to damage of either the cavernosal nerves which innervate the penis or the penile arteries, which also lie close to the site of the urethral disruption. Indeed, surgical treatment of the urethral disruption can itself cause erectile dysfunction by similar mechanisms. If this does occur, treatment is with an orally active agent such as sildenafil, or if that fails with intracavernosal prostaglandin injections, a vacuum device or a penile implant.

Extravasation of urine

This can occur with extraperitoneal rupture of the bladder, pelvic fracture urethral disruption or in the rare cases where the level of the disruption is the prostatic urethra. Urine extravasates in the layers of the pelvic fascia and the retroperitoneal tissues. Treatment is by suprapubic cystostomy. In rare cases where the extravasation persists despite the suprapubic tube, then drainage of the retropubic space and the definitive repair of the urethral, prostatic or bladder rupture is required (Summary box 78.4).

Summary box 78.4

Pelvic fracture urethral disruption injury

- Suspect the diagnosis in cases of pelvic fracture, when the patient has not voided and when there is blood at the urethral meatus
- A water soluble urethrogram confirms the diagnosis
- Initial management is insertion of a suprapubic catheter
- Surgical exploration is needed if there is coexistent rupture of the bladder
- Delayed anastomotic urethroplasty is the preferred definitive management

Inflammation of the urethra

Inflammatory conditions of the urethra include:

- meatal ulcer
- urethritis
- gonococcal urethritis
- non-specific urethritis
- Reiter's disease
- peri-urethral abscess.

Ulceration of the urethral meatus

Meatal ulcer is an uncommon complication of neonatal circumcision and may develop up to two years after the circumcision. Lack of protection by the prepuce seems to be the primary cause, with friction from clothing and ammoniacal dermatitis also being contributory factors. Devascularisation caused by ligation of the frenular artery may also possibly play a part. The ulcer forms a scab that blocks the meatus and the child can pass urine only by bursting the scab. This hurts, so the boy screams; a tiny amount of blood may be passed as well. The process causes fibrosis, which can result in an acquired pinhole meatus. Local measures to soften the scab and alkalinise the urine are often curative although a few do need meatotomy.

Gonorrhoeal urethritis

Gonorrhoea is a sexually transmitted disease caused by *Neisseria gonorrhoeae* (gonococcus), a Gram-negative kidney-shaped diplococcus that infects the anterior urethra in men, the urethra and cervix in women and the oropharynx, rectum and anal canal in both sexes, but especially men. It is transmitted by unprotected sexual intercourse.

Most men have symptoms typical of urethral discomfort and urethral discharge. There is often scalding dysuria. In women it is often asymptomatic. Symptoms, which are present in 50 per cent or less, usually consist of a mild dysuria or slight urethral discharge, which can go unnoticed by the patient. Cervicitis can occur with about 10 per cent suffering from pelvic inflammatory disease (salpingitis), which, if bilateral, may lead to infertility. A mother may transmit gonorrhea to her newborn during childbirth with the risk that blindness of the child can result. In addition, in both men and women exposed orally or anally, gonococcal infections can cause a predominantly asymptomatic pharyngitis or proctitis.

Investigations

Traditionally the diagnosis was made by identification of pus and gonococci in a Gram-stained urethral smear with subsequent culture. However, more recently PCR-based techniques, which are more sensitive, are the norm.

Complications

Complications are prevented by effective early treatment. In men, complications include posterior urethritis, prostatitis (acute or chronic), acute epididymo-orchitis, periurethral abscess and urethral stricture. Gonococcal arthritis, iridocyclitis, septicaemia and endocarditis are unusual.

Treatment

Treatment is with antibiotics, with ceftriaxone currently the treatment of choice as a consequence of the increasing prevalence of antibiotic resistance to more traditional antibiotics such as ciprofloxacin or penicillin. Contact tracing is important in controlling the spread of the disease and management is usually by a genitourinary physician.

Non-specific urethritis (synonym: non-gonococcal urethritis)

Non-specific urethritis (NSU) is a sexually transmitted infection that in around 40 per cent of cases is due to *Chlamydia trachomatis* with other cases being caused by *Ureaplasma urealytica* or *Mycoplasma genitalium*. The causative agent in up to 50 per cent of cases is unknown.

Clinical features

In men, dysuria and a white mucopurulent urethral discharge appear up to 6 weeks after sexual intercourse. The urine appears to be clear but may contain 'threads' or pus cells. Epididymitis is common and urethral stricture can result. In women, the condition is usually asymptomatic although it can present as vaginal discharge or as a form of urethrotrigonitis. It may result in cervicitis or pelvic inflammatory disease.

Treatment

Exclusion of gonorrheal infection is important. Chlamydial infection is diagnosed by PCR techniques on a urethral swab or a urine sample. Treatment with oxytetracycline or doxycycline is usually effective although relapse is common, especially in men, in whom the prostate may act as a reservoir of infection. Azithromycin is an alternative treatment taken as a single oral dose. It is important to treat both partners as reinfection is probable if this is not done.

Reiter's disease (synonym: sexually acquired reactive arthritis)

Reiter's disease is an autoimmune disease characterised by the triad of urethritis or diarrhoea, conjunctivitis and polyarthritis. Common triggers include *Chlamydial urethritis*, less commonly gonococcal urethritis and diarrhoea secondary to *Salmonella*, *Shigella* or *Campylobacter*. It is an HLA-B27 associated condition. The conjunctivitis (present in around 50 per cent) and arthritis typically occur 1–3 weeks after the primary infection. Diagnosis is made on clinical grounds and treatment is largely symptomatic, although antibiotic treatment of the precipitating infection is important. The urethritis and conjunctivitis frequently subside after a few weeks but the arthritis may persist for months. Severe anterior uveitis and frequently recurrent attacks suggest a poor outlook.

Hans Conrad Julius Reiter, 1881–1969, President of the Health Service and Honorary Professor of Hygiene, Berlin, Germany, described this condition in 1916. He was subsequently convicted of war crimes as a consequence of his involvement in the death of hundreds of inmates in Buchenwald.

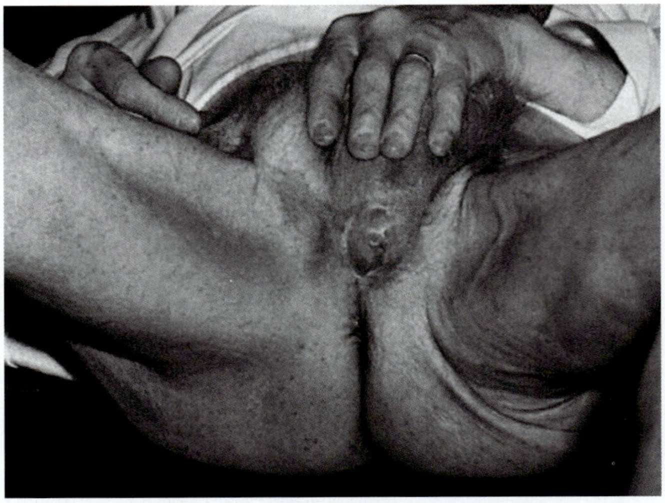

Figure 78.7 Chronic periurethral abscess.

Periurethral abscess

Periurethral abscesses can be penile, bulbar or chronic.

Penile periurethral abscess

A penile periurethral abscess arises as an acute gonococcal infection of one of the glands of Littre. The tender induration felt on the underside of the penis points and discharges externally, often leaving a fistula. An anterior urethrotomy will encourage the abscess to burst into the urethra. When the abscess lies behind a stricture, it should be opened externally.

Bulbar periurethral abscess

A bulbar periurethral abscess is a spreading cellulitis caused by infection with streptococci and anaerobic organisms, possibly associated with a stricture. Extravasation of urine is not unusual. There is perineal pain with pyrexia, rigors and tachycardia. Tenderness and swelling rapidly spread from the perineum to the penis and the anterior abdominal wall. Antibiotics are essential. Collections of pus should be drained and the urethra should be defunctioned by a suprapubic urinary catheter.

Chronic periurethral abscess

A chronic periurethral abscess sometimes results from a long-standing urethral stricture (Figure 78.7). The multiple loculi of pus should be drained and the stricture treated. Urethral fistula occurs either spontaneously or as a result of incision of the abscess.

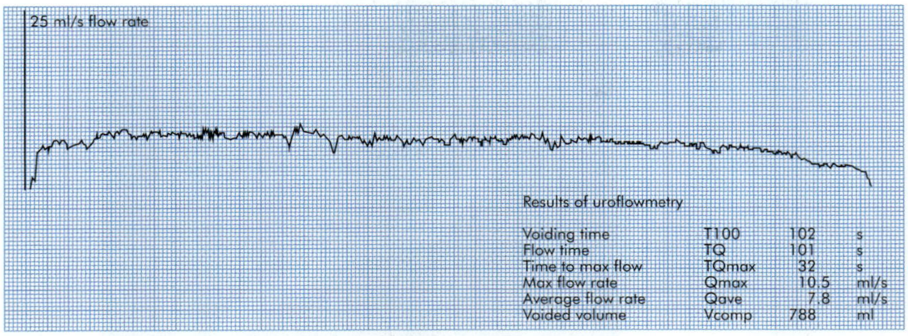
25 ml/s flow rate
Results of uroflowmetry
Voiding time T100 102 s
Flow time TQ 101 s
Time to max flow TQmax 32 s
Max flow rate Qmax 10.5 ml/s
Average flow rate Qave 7.8 ml/s
Voided volume Vcomp 788 ml

Figure 78.8 Urinary flow rate trace from a patient with a urethral stricture. Note the prolonged flow with the typical plateau shape of the curve.

Urethral stricture

Causes

The common causes of urethral stricture are:

- Inflammatory
  - Secondary to urethritis
  - Secondary to balanitis xerotica obliterans
- Traumatic
  - Bulbar urethral injury
  - Pelvic fracture urethral disruption injury
- Iatrogenic
  - Secondary to urethral instrumentation
  - Secondary to urethral catheterisation
  - Secondary to transurethral prostatectomy
  - Secondary to radical prostatectomy
- Idiopathic.

Pathophysiology

Post-inflammatory strictures are less common since the introduction of effective antibiotic treatment of gonorrhoea. The stricture is most commonly seen in the bulbar urethra but submeatal strictures also occur. There is infection in the periurethral glands which persists after inadequately treated gonorrhoea. The infection spreads to cause a periurethritis, which heals by fibrosis. Most strictures appear within one year of infection but may not cause difficulty in micturition for some time later.

Balanitis xerotica obliterans is a rare condition characterised by fibrosis of the foreskin resulting in phimosis. In around 10 per cent of cases, the glans penis is also affected causing meatal stenosis and, in a proportion of these cases, there is also fibrosis and stricturing of the penile urethra. The cause of the condition is unknown, but the strictures produced are typically long and difficult to treat.

Post-traumatic strictures have been discussed previously.

Post-instrumentation strictures follow endoscopy or catheterisation and may affect any part of the urethra. Some surgeons recommend prophylactic dilatation or urethrotomy before transurethral prostatectomy in order to try to avoid this complication. Some cases of stricture seem to be due to sensitivity to chemicals from a catheter, but most are the result of a combination of trauma, infection and pressure necrosis.

Bladder neck stenosis can occur following transurethral resection of the prostate (TURP) and following radical prostatectomy for the treatment of prostate cancer. If it cannot be managed by dilatation, bladder neck stenosis should be treated by transurethral incision and resection of the stricture, although in the man who has undergone radical prostatectomy, this will result in urinary incontinence.

Clinical features

Symptoms are usually hesitancy of micturition, straining to void and a poor urinary stream. The relative youthfulness of the patient often rules out prostatic enlargement, which characteristically occurs after the age of 50. As the stream becomes narrower, micturition is prolonged and is followed by post-micturition dribbling as a result of urine trickling from the dilated urethra proximal to the stricture. Urinary frequency by day and night is common and is due to incomplete bladder emptying, coexistent detrusor overactivity or urinary infection. The urinary flow rate is typically prolonged and plateau shaped (Figure 78.8).

A well-established stricture may be palpable as scarring along the line of the urethra. If the stricture is tight enough, the patient will go into acute retention, although this is rare. If this happens there is a danger that clumsy attempts to pass a urethral catheter will result in a false passage. If a patient has gone into retention because of a urethral stricture, its lumen will be too narrow to pass even a tiny catheter and suprapubic catheterisation is required.

Urethroscopy allows the stricture to be viewed as a circumferential scar (Figure 78.9). Openings of false passages commemorate previous misguided attempts to pass a urethral catheter.

Urethrography using a water-soluble contrast medium will show the extent and severity of the stricture (Figures 78.10 and 78.11).

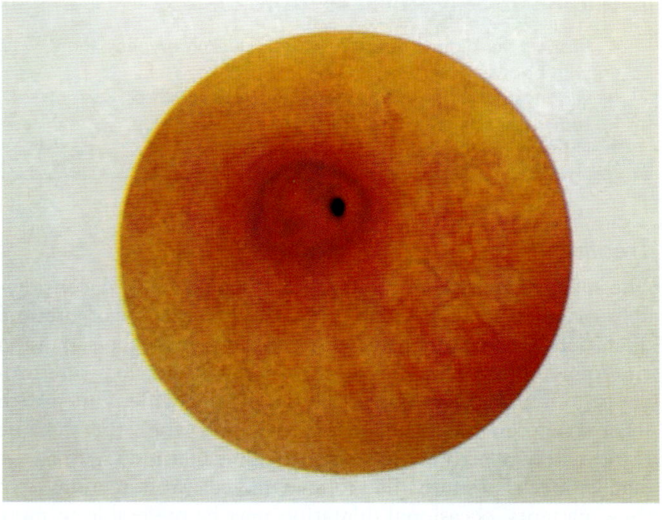

Figure 78.9 Urethroscopic appearance of a urethral stricture.

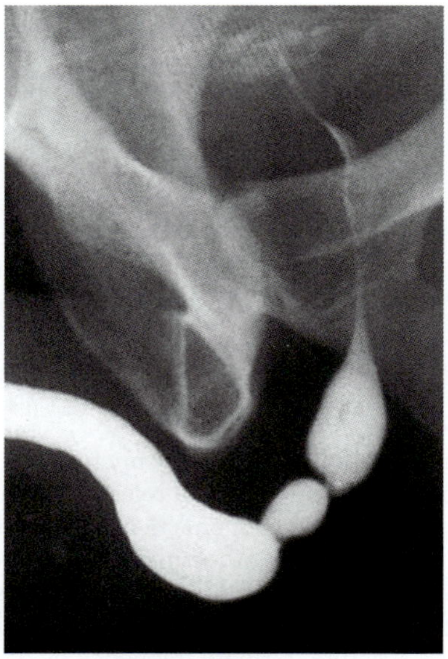

Figure 78.10 Ascending urethrogram showing urethral stricture of the bulbar urethra.

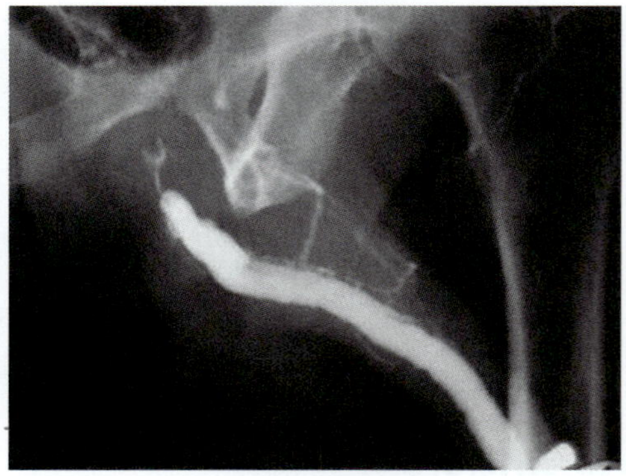

Figure 78.11 Gonorrhoeal stricture of the bulbar urethra. Note that some of the contrast has entered the penile veins.

Complications

The most common complication of a urethral stricture is urinary tract infection, which usually responds to antibiotic treatment although there is a tendency for them to recur as a consequence of the increased residual urines within the bladder. Any of the complications of bladder outflow obstruction can occur, including bladder calculi and upper tract dilatation with renal impairment, although the latter is rare. Similarly, retention of urine is also rare, and should be treated by suprapubic catheterisation. Rare complications include urethral diverticulum and paraurethral abscess (Summary box 78.5).

Summary box 78.5

Diagnosis of urethral stricture

- Suspect the diagnosis of urethral stricture in a young man with poor urinary stream
- Diagnosis is made either by visualisation (urethroscopy) or radiologically (by urethrography)
- Urinary infection should be excluded

Treatment

The management of urethral strictures has changed considerably over the past 20 years. The old treatments of urethral dilatation have largely been superceded by endoscopic incision (internal urethrotomy) or by formal reconstruction (urethroplasty). Urethral dilatation still has a place in elderly men with short strictures that recur infrequently and when the stricture is intimately related to the continence mechanism (such as the bladder neck stricture that follows radical prostatectomy). In these patients, occasional dilatation may be preferable to more complex procedures.

Internal urethrotomy cures around 50 per cent of short strictures. Success rates are highest when the stricture is short and when it is present within the bulbar urethra. In contrast, failure rates are highest in long strictures, strictures within the penile urethra and in recurrent strictures. In patients with recurrent strictures who are unable or unwilling to undergo urethroplasty, then intermittent self-dilatation with soft hydrophilic catheters on a regular (daily) basis can prevent stricture recurrence, although such self-dilatation is needed lifelong.

Short strictures with a clear traumatic history should be treated by urethroplasty since cure rates in excess of 90 per cent can be achieved by excision of the stricture with end to end anastamosis. Therefore, a conventional therapeutic algorithm is to offer an internal urethrotomy to all newly diagnosed strictures (excluding post-traumatic strictures), and to reserve the more major urethroplasty procedures for recurrent strictures.

Urethral dilatation

This is the old treatment for stricture. Under aseptic conditions, the urethra is stretched using graduated dilators. With care and gentleness, the procedure can be performed under local urethral anaesthesia with lignocaine gel. The drawback of dilatation is that it is performed 'blind', so there is always a danger of causing a false passage. This is most likely with an inexperienced operator unfamiliar with the complexities of an individual patient's urethra.

Strictures have been treated by surgeons for centuries and there are many different dilating instruments. A simple stricture may be dilated using metal sounds (Figure 78.12), so called because they were originally used to 'sound' for stones in the bladder. These must be wielded with great care as it is easy to make a false passage.

Endoscopic (internal) urethrotomy

Internal urethrotomy is performed using the optical urethrotome. The stricture is cut under visual control using a knife passed through the sheath of a rigid urethroscope. The stricture is usually cut at the 12 o'clock position, taking care not to cut too deeply into the vascular spaces of the corpus spongiosum that surrounds the urethra. Other cuts can be made

Auguste Nélaton, 1807–1873, Professor of Surgery, Paris, France.

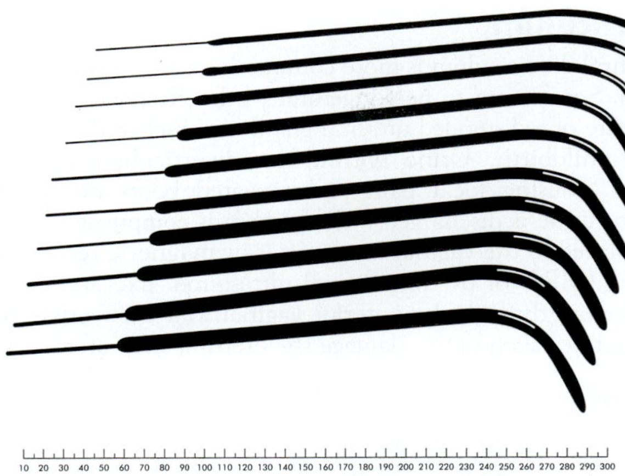

Figure 78.12 Metal dilators ('sounds').

until there is a wide passage through the strictured segment of urethra. Many surgeons leave a catheter for 1–2 days afterwards. A single urethrotomy seems to give a permanent cure of an uncomplicated stricture in about 50 per cent of patients. The main complications are infection and bleeding. It is possible to get lost when trying to cut a way through a very tight stricture and this is especially true when there are false passages because of previous dilatation attempts. Accordingly, a guidewire should be passed through to the bladder prior to incision of the stricture in order to establish the true lumen of the urethra.

Urethroplasty

The simplest urethroplasty involves excision of the stenosed length of urethra and reanastomosis of the spatulated cut ends. This operation is possible only if the stricture is relatively short because there must be no tension at the suture line. If an end-to-end anastomosis is not feasible, a large number of different surgical procedures can be used to reconstruct the fibrosed urethra. The operations using myocutaneous flaps of penile and scrotal skin that dominated the field 20 years ago have largely been replaced by operations that utilise free grafts, usually of buccal mucosa, but also occasionally of penile skin, lingual mucosa and bladder mucosa. The advantage of buccal mucosa is that there is a plentiful supply (approximately 6–7 cm can be obtained from each cheek), it is tough with an excellent vascular plexus, it is used to being wet and the donor site cannot be seen. Indeed, the morbidity associated with the donor site is minimal.

Urethroplasty should be considered when the stricture has arisen following trauma, and when a stricture has recurred following endoscopic treatment. The actual technique used should depend upon the site of the stricture, the length of the stricture and the cause of the stricture. Careful preoperative assessment with ascending and descending urethrography is vital.

Anastomotic urethroplasty has a success rate of around 90 per cent while substitution urethroplasty has success rates at ten years of around 80 per cent (Summary box 78.6).

Ahmad Orandi, urological surgeon, Fergus Falls, MN, USA. Born in Iran, he retired in 1991 at the age of 59 and went into the stock market, real estate and pistachio farming in California – a family tradition from Iran, that he restarted as a business called A & R Pistachios, the initials representing his and his wife's names.

Summary box 78.6

Treatment of urethral strictures

- Newly diagnosed strictures are best treated initially by internal urethrotomy with a 50 per cent success rate
- Intermittent self-dilatation increases the success rate of internal urethrotomy alone
- Urethroplasty should be considered in traumatic strictures and in recurrent strictures
- Treatment by intermittent self-dilatation should be considered in strictures closely related to the external sphincter mechanism

OTHER CONDITIONS OF THE URETHRA

Urethral fistula

The most frequent cause of urethral fistula is bursting or incision of a periurethral abscess. If the fistula arises behind a tight stricture, there may be multiple openings (watering-can perineum). A fistula can also follow urethroplasty if there is necrosis of part of the graft or flap. The stricture should be treated, in which case some fistulae heal themselves. Occasionally, formal urethroplasty is indicated.

Urethral calculi

Urethral calculi can arise primarily behind a stricture or in an infected urethral diverticulum. More commonly, the stone is a renal calculus that has migrated to the urethra via the bladder.

Clinical features

Migratory calculi cause sudden pain in the urethra soon after an attack of ureteric colic. There is blockage to the flow of urine and, if the stone is small, the force of the jet will usually expel it from the urethral meatus. Larger stones get stuck and must be removed endoscopically. It is sometimes possible to feel the calculus as a hard lump in the urethra, but if there is doubt the diagnosis is confirmed by urethroscopy.

A stone formed within the urethra is less likely to cause recognisable symptoms and is usually detected during urethroscopy or bouginage.

Treatment

A stone lodged within the prostatic urethra should be displaced back into the bladder and treated by lithopaxy or suprapubic cystotomy as if it were a bladder stone. Calculi in more distal parts of the urethra are removed by basketing under vision or fragmented *in situ* using the electrohydraulic or ultrasonic lithotripter. It may be necessary to perform a meatotomy to deliver the stone. Open removal by external urethrotomy is rarely necessary.

Neoplasms

Polyps are a relatively common finding in the prostatic urethra, where they may result from chronic infection. Genital warts acquired by sexually transmitted infection are sometimes found in the anterior urethra as an extension of warts on the skin of the glans penis. Angioma of the urethra is a very rare cause of urethral bleeding.

John Peter Blandy, 1927–2011, formerly Professor of Urology, The London Hospital Medical College, London, UK.
Richard Trevor Turner-Warwick, b. 1925, contemporary, formerly urologist, The Middlesex Hospital, London, UK.

Carcinoma of the urethra is relatively rare. Multifocal transitional cell cancers of the bladder are sometimes associated with tumours in the prostatic urethra and occasionally more distally. Though superficial and susceptible to local ablation by diathermy or laser, they are associated with a tendency to distant spread. Squamous carcinoma can develop in an area of squamous metaplasia sometimes seen with a urethral stricture. It carries a poor prognosis even if the patient is treated by radical surgery. Bloody urethral discharge without infection should raise the suspicion that the patient has a urethral tumour.

THE FEMALE URETHRA

Anatomy

The female urethra is around 2–3 cm long, extending from the bladder neck to the external urethral meatus. Continence is maintained by the external striated urethral sphincter, which in women extends for almost the whole length of the urethra. There is extra support from the surrounding pelvic floor musculature. In contrast to men, the female bladder neck has little role in the maintenance of continence.

Abnormalities of the female urethra include:

- prolapse
- stricture
- Fowler's syndrome (dysfunction of the striated urethral sphincter)
- diverticulum
- caruncle
- papillomata acuminata
- carcinoma.

Prolapse (synonym: urethrocele)

Weakening of the tissues that hold the urethra in place can cause it to move and to put pressure on the vagina, leading to the prolapse of the anterior distal wall of the vagina. Urethroceles often occur with cystoceles. Prolapse occurs in later life and is usually, in part, due to the trauma of childbirth. Prolapse of the urethral lining also occurs as a congenital abnormality, when it causes discomfort proportional to the degree of prolapse.

Stricture

Urethral strictures are uncommon in women but may follow urethritis or more commonly the trauma of a difficult labour. Urinary retention is an occasional consequence and is usually chronic. True urethral strictures in women respond well to dilatation.

Fowler's syndrome

This condition, which was described by Fowler and Kirby, is associated with an abnormal myotonic discharge in the striated urethral sphincter, which can be detected by electromyography. It causes urinary retention in women and should not be confused with a urethral stricture. Urethral dilatation is ineffective and the retention is best treated by intermittent self-catheterisation. There is some evidence that sacral neuromodulation can be effective.

Diverticulum

A urethral diverticulum is more commonly seen in women than in men. Some seem to be congenital while others are acquired by rupture of a distended urethral gland or injury of the urethra during childbirth. Urine within the diverticulum becomes infected, causing local pain and repeated bouts of cystitis. Purulent urine is discharged if the urethra is compressed with a finger placed in the vagina. Diagnosis is by magnetic resonance imaging (MRI) or by transvaginal ultrasound. Excision of the diverticulum through the anterior vaginal wall is effective, but care must be taken not to damage the urethral sphincter.

Caruncle

This is common in elderly women. It presents as a soft, raspberry-like, pedunculated granulomatous mass about the size of a pea, attached to the posterior urethral wall near the external meatus. It is composed of highly vascular connective tissue stroma infiltrated with pus cells. There may be frequency of micturition and urethral pain afterwards. Occasionally, there is bleeding. A urethral prolapse is less tender and is not pedunculated. Treatment is by excision and diathermy coagulation of the base of the stalk. The patient should be given antibiotics to treat the underlying chronic urethritis.

Papillomata acuminata

Papillomata acuminata are the same as the sexually transmitted warts that occur on the penis. They are treated in the same way. In African women, papillomata acuminata are common and may grow to such a large size during pregnancy that they obstruct labour and necessitate a caesarean section.

Carcinoma of the urethra

This occurs twice as often in women as in men. Whether a caruncle can become malignant is disputed, but caruncles and tumours often occur close together. Malignant swellings of the urethra feel harder than benign ones. Treatment by radiotherapy or radical surgery is often ineffective. The overall prognosis is poor.

THE PENIS

Anatomy

The penis is composed of three tubular structures. The upper two structures, which are apposed to each other, are called the corpora cavernosa and are anchored posteriorly onto the pubic rami. They provide the erectile function. The third tubular structure is the corpus spongiosum, which contains the urethra and it expands distally to form the glans penis. The corpora cavernosa have an outer covering of tunica albuginea which is relatively inelastic and which also forms the septum between them. The tunica albuginea encloses the erectile tissue itself which has

A **caesarean section** is the operation of delivering the fetus by an incision into the uterus, usually through the abdominal wall. More than one explanation has been given as the origin of the term. The word 'caesarean' could be a derivative of the Latin term 'caedo', which means to cut. The thought that it derives from the name of the Roman Emperor Julius Caesar is untrue as his mother Aurelia successfully gave birth to her son by natural means and later was an advisor to him. The most plausible explanation is that the Roman or Caesarean Law (law during Caesar's time) demanded that when a pregnant woman died, her body could not be buried until the fetus had been removed.)

Clare Juliet Fowler, contemporary, Professor of Uro-neurology, The National Hospital for Nervous Diseases, Queen Square, London, UK.
Roger Sinclair Kirby, contemporary, Professor of Urology, St George's Hospital, London, UK.
Charles Bowesman, 1907–1993, Professor of Surgery, Kumasi, Ghana.

a trabecular structure with a network of sinusoidal spaces lined by endothelium within which the blood pools during erection. The central arterial blood supply (the central penile artery) is a branch of the internal pudendal artery. Erection occurs when the parasympathetic nerves that innervate the penis cause smooth muscle relaxation with increased arterial inflow and dilatation of the sinusoids, such that blood accumulates within the trabecular spaces.

DISEASES OF THE FORESKIN

Phimosis

Phimosis is overdiagnosed in children (see also Chapter 8). At birth, the foreskin is normally adherent to the glans penis. These physiological adhesions between the foreskin and the glans penis may persist until six years of age or more, giving the false impression that the prepuce will not retract. This condition (sometimes known as physiological phimosis) should not be confused with true phimosis in boys, with scarring of the prepuce such that it will not retract without fissuring of the foreskin (Figure 78.13). In these cases, the aperture in the prepuce may be so tight as to cause urinary obstruction. Urinary difficulty with residual urine and back pressure effects on the ureters and kidney is far more commonly caused by meatal stenosis, which may be masked by the prepuce.

In adults, phimosis is due to scarring of the foreskin as a consequence of balanitis (inflammation of the glans penis), posthitis (inflammation of the foreskin), forcible retraction of the foreskin or lichen sclerosus et atrophicus (synonym: balanitis xerotica obliterans or BXO).

BXO is an uncommon condition in which the normally pliant foreskin becomes thickened. It typically becomes whitish in appearance and forms a constricting band (cicatrix) which prevents retraction (Figure 78.14a,b). BXO may also affect the glans penis (causing meatal stenosis) (Figure 78.15) and the penile urethra (causing urethral stricture). As a consequence it is difficult to keep the penis clean, there may be recurrent attacks of balanitis and there is both a problem with hygiene and, in later life, an increased susceptibility to carcinoma.

Treatment.

In a young child with a non-retractile foreskin, no treatment is necessary or appropriate. When the foreskin is mildly scarred, then preputioplasty is possible. For all other cases, circumcision is the appropriate treatment. In cases of BXO, circumcision is often curative, although when the condition affects the glans penis, topical steroid cream may be helpful. In resistant cases, formal meatotomy is necessary. In emergency situations, such as when catheterisation is required, but is impossible, then it is possible to divide the foreskin dorsally under local anaesthetic (a so-called dorsal slit).

Preputioplasty

This is an application of the Heineke Mikulicz principle whereby the tight ring of the foreskin is divided longitudinally and sewn transversely, thereby allowing retraction of the preserved foreskin. There is a recurrence rate and it is only indicated in mild cases with minimal scarring. If it fails, then circumcision is indicated.

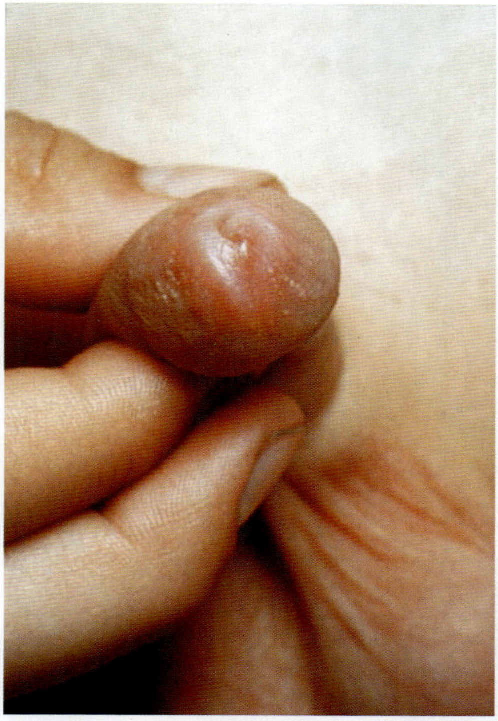

Figure 78.13 Non retractile foreskin. Recent history of symptoms. Examination reveals thickening and scarring with a true phimosis (picture courtesy of Kim Hutton).

Circumcision

Apparently, circumcision did not originate among the Jewish people: they took the practice either from the Babylonians or from African tribes, probably the latter. It had been practised in West Africa for over 5000 years.

Indications

In infants and young boys, circumcision is most usually performed at the request of the parents for social or religious reasons. Medical indications for circumcision in boys include true phimosis, BXO (rare under the age of five years), recurrent attacks of balanoposthitis and recurrent urinary tract infections with an abnormal upper urinary tract. Phimosis may result from misguided attempts by parents to expose the glans forcibly.

In adults, circumcision is indicated because of an inability to retract the foreskin for intercourse, for splitting of an abnormally tight frenulum or for recurrent balanitis.

Recently evidence has emerged that circumcision protects against the spread of human immunodeficiency virus (HIV), and a large scale programme of adult circumcision under the auspices of the World Health Organisation is planned for some African countries where HIV is a major health problem.

Technique in an infant

Applying a clamp or bone forceps across the prepuce distal to the glans with blind division of the foreskin is to be condemned. To see one boy with partial or total amputation of the glans is enough to realise the folly of this technique. It is far better to perform a proper circumcision under direct vision as in an adult.

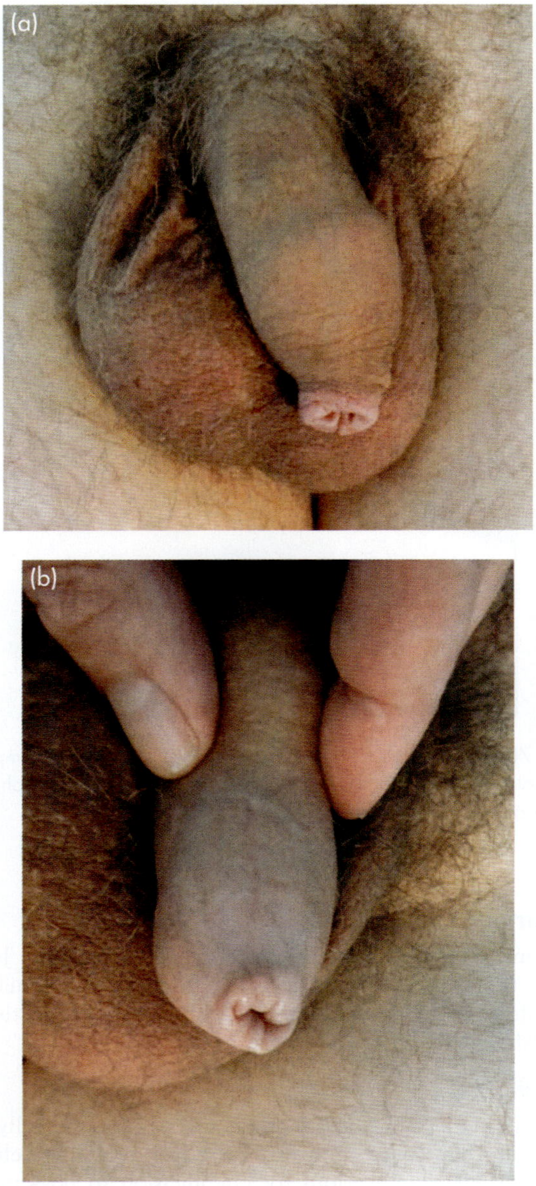

Figure 78.14 Phimosis secondary to balanitis xerotica obliterans. Note the white and thickened appearance of the preputial skin (a) with a constriction such that the foreskin cannot be retracted (b).

The Plastibel device can be used in infants (Hollister) and its use is shown in Figure 78.16a–c: the ring separates between 5 and 8 days postoperatively.

Technique in adolescents and adults

In adolescents and adults, the following method is preferable. The prepuce is held in artery forceps and put on a gentle stretch. A circumferential incision in the penile skin is made at the level of the corona using a knife. Marking the skin with a pen is often helpful prior to the incision to ensure that excess skin is not removed. The prepuce is then slit dorsally in the midline to within 1 cm of the corona. This converts the foreskin into two flaps connected at the midline anteriorly. When the undersurface of the prepuce has been separated from the glans, the inner layer of each flap is incised with a second circumferential incision, leaving about 0.5 cm of the inner layer of the preputial skin. Cutting the remaining connective tissue completes the excision (Figure 78.17a–e). Monopolar diathermy must be avoided in operations on the penis in small boys because there is a danger that the current path will cause coagulation at the base of the penis. Haemostasis is important in circumcision however, and vessels should be secured with bipolar diathermy or with absorbable ligatures. The cut edges of the skin are approximated using interrupted sutures being certain that the frenular vessels are ligated (Summary box 78.7).

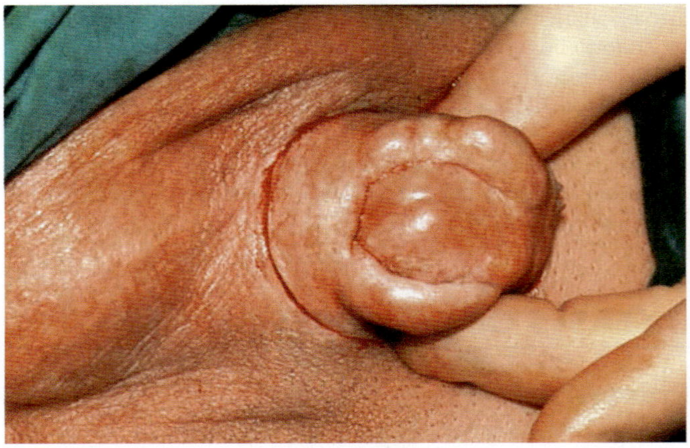

Figure 78.15 Severe balanitis xerotica obliterans causing meatal stenosis, thickened and scarred preputial and penile skin. There was also a severe penile urethral stricture.

Summary box 78.7

Circumcision

- Is most commonly performed for cultural reasons
- Is not indicated for failure of retraction caused by congenital adhesions between the glans penis and the prepuce
- Is indicated when there is true phimosis with balanoposthitis or obstruction to urinary flow
- Never use monopolar diathermy when performing circumcision

Frenulum breve

Phimosis should not be confused with this condition, where the frenulum is short, such that it causes pain when the foreskin is retracted. Another possible presentation is tearing of the frenulum during sexual activity. Treatment is by frenuloplasty, which utilises the Heineke Mikulicz principle to 'lengthen' the frenulum.

Paraphimosis

A tight foreskin once retracted may be difficult to return and a paraphimosis results. In this condition, the venous and lymphatic return from the glans and distal foreskin is obstructed and these structures swell, causing even more pressure within

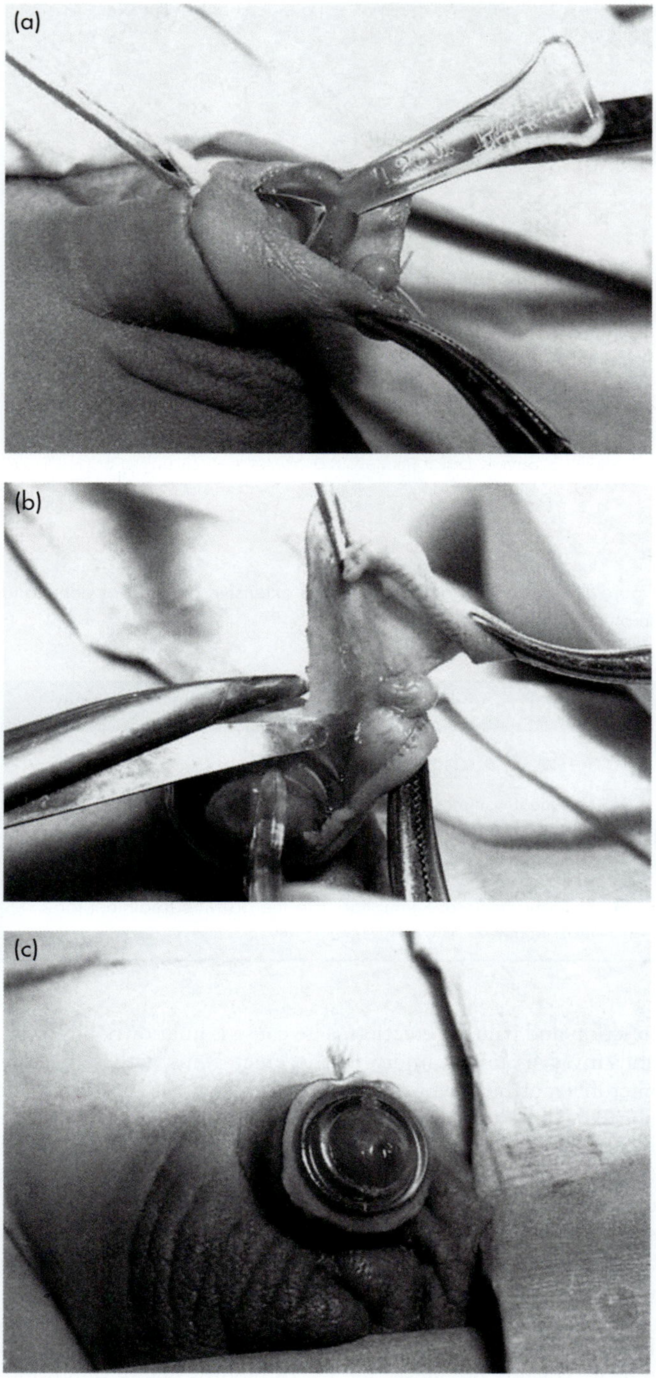

Figure 78.16 The Plastibel (Hollister) device for circumcision in infants. (a) The foreskin is freed and retracted. (b) After the Plastibel device has been slipped into place over the glans penis, the foreskin is ligated over the groove of the bell and redundant foreskin is cut away. (c) This shows the completed operation (courtesy of Professor Asal Y Izzidien Al-Samarrai, King Saud University, Riyadh, Saudi Arabia).

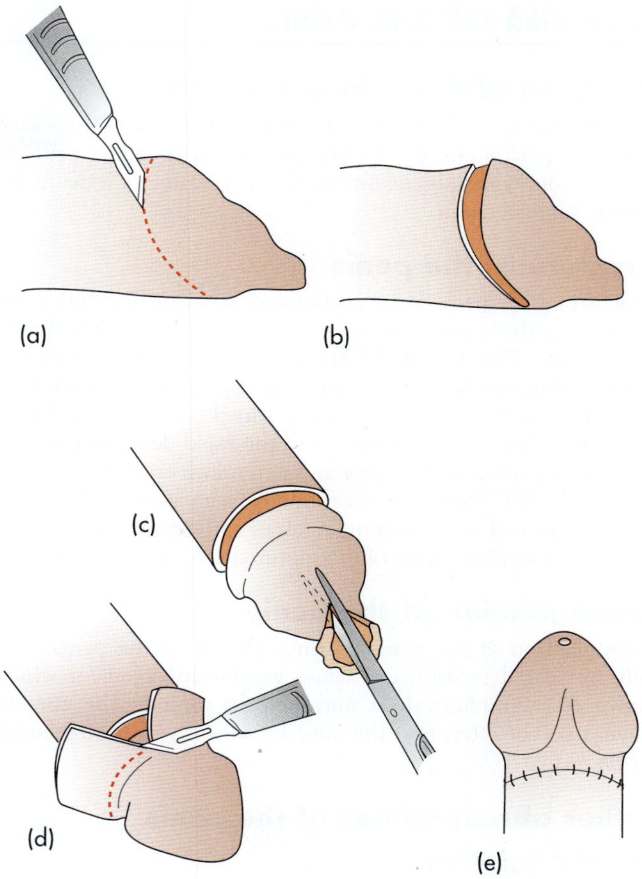

Figure 78.17 (a–e) Stages in circumcision.

the obstructing ring of prepuce. Icebags, gentle manual compression and injection of a solution of hyaluronidase in normal saline may help to reduce the swelling. Such patients can be treated by circumcision if careful manipulation fails. A dorsal slit of the prepuce under local anaesthetic may be enough in an emergency.

Balanoposthitis

Inflammation of the prepuce is known as posthitis; inflammation of the glans is balanitis. The opposing surfaces of the two structures are often involved, hence the term 'balanoposthitis'. Skin conditions such as lichen planus and psoriasis affect the penis and, indeed, may be localised there. Drug hypersensitivity reactions can affect the skin of the penis. In mild cases, the only symptoms are itching and some discharge. In more severe inflammation, the glans and foreskin are red-raw and pus exudes. Balanoposthitis is associated with penile cancer, diabetes and phimosis. Monilial infections are quite common under the prepuce. Treatment is by broad-spectrum antibiotics and local hygiene measures. If there is associated phimosis, then a circumcision is required.

Preputial calculi

Later in life, chronic posthitis may lead to adhesions between the prepuce and the glans and closure of the orifice of the preputial sac. Preputial calculi result from the accumulation beneath a non-retractable foreskin of inspissated smegma, urinary salts or both.

INJURIES OF THE PENIS

Avulsion of the skin of the penis

Entanglement of clothing in rotating machinery is the usual cause. Repair is effected by burying the shaft of the penis in the scrotum with subsequent release at the time of a definitive plastic surgical repair.

Fracture of the penis

Fracture of the penis is an uncommon accident, usually occurring when the erect penis is bent violently downwards during intercourse. The forced deformity results in a rupture of the tunica albuginea with immediate extravasation of blood from within the penis. There is typically a loud cracking sound with immediate loss of the erection, and the rapid development of a large bruise around the penis and extending onto the scrotum (Figure 78.18). There may occasionally be an associated urethral injury. Optimal management involves early exploration of the penis with surgical repair of the ruptured tunica albuginea.

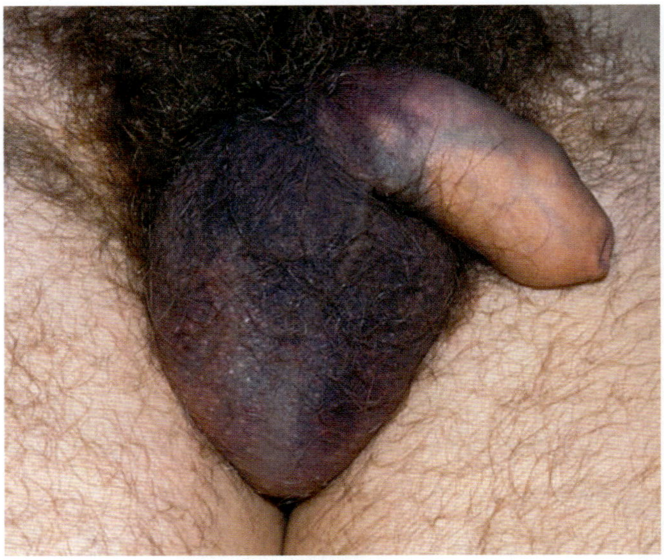

Figure 78.18 Penile fracture. Note the extensive bruising of penis and scrotum.

Strangulation of the penis

Strangulation of the penis by rings placed on the penis, usually for sexual reasons, can cause venous engorgement which prevents their removal. It may help to aspirate the corpora cavernosa but often the ring must be cut off with a ring cutter or hacksaw.

Other abnormalities of the penis

Erectile dysfunction

Failure to attain or maintain an erection is called erectile dysfunction (ED). It is a symptom, rather than a condition in itself. It can arise as a consequence of psychological issues, but the most common cause is vascular disease, and as such ED is associated with diabetes, hypertension, dyslipidaemia and smoking. Other rarer causes include endocrine disease (hypogonadism and prolactin secreting pituitary tumours), neurological disease (multiple sclerosis, spinal cord injury and prolapsed intervertebral disc), iatrogenic damage to the cavernosal nerves due to radical pelvic surgery (e.g. radical prostatectomy, abdominoperineal excision of the rectum and radical cystectomy), neuropathy secondary to pelvic radiotherapy and drug-induced cases (including anti-hypertensive agents, antidepressants and antipsychotics).

Assessment involves confirmation of the diagnosis by taking a careful history, assessing the patient for underlying risk factors, and trying to identify the rare case that can be cured as opposed to being treated. Physical examination of the genitalia, the blood pressure and assessment of the secondary sexual characteristics is required and biochemical assessment of the blood sugar, the serum lipid profile and the serum testosterone is necessary in all cases.

Treatment for most patients involves the use of the phosphodiesterase type 5 inhibitors (such as sildenafil) with intracavernosal injection of prostaglandin, vacuum pumps and penile implants reserved for resistant cases (Summary box 78.8).

Summary box 78.8

Erectile dysfunction

- The most common cause of erectile dysfunction is atherosclerosis
- Appropriate investigation involves identification of vascular risk factors
- Phosphodiesterase inhibitors are the first line treatment for most men

Peyronie's disease

Peyronie's disease is characterised by penile deformity (Figure 78.19), palpable penile plaques within the penis, erectile dysfunction and pain on erection. The cause is unknown, but probably involves minor injury to the erect penis with secondary microhaemorrhage beneath the tunica albuginea and secondary fibrosis. The latter results in the palpable plaques that can be identified on examination. The plaques may rarely be calcified (Figure 78.20). The presence of these relatively inelastic plaques causes the erect penis to bend, often dramatically, towards the side of the plaque. The most common direction of deformity is dorsally (towards the abdomen) and the deformity may be so great as to prevent penetrative sexual intercourse.

While the aetiology is uncertain, there is an association with Dupuytren's contracture. The natural history of the condition is that it typically progresses for 18–24 months before stabilising. During this active phase of the disease, surgery is not indicated, and a variety of medical treatments have been tried, although none with any good evidence of benefit.

When the disease has stabilised, the crucial issue is whether the patient is still able to have sexual intercourse. If he can then no treatment is indicated, while if the deformity prevents penetration, or makes it difficult, then corrective surgery is indicated. Using this criterion, only around a quarter of men come to surgery. The most common procedure is the Nesbitt procedure which corrects the deformity by plicating the convex side of the deformity, thereby straightening the penis, with some accompanying loss of length (Summary box 78.9).

Francois de la Peyronie, 1678–1747, surgeon to King Louis XIV of France, and founder of the Royal Academy of Surgery, Paris, France.
Reed Nesbitt, urological surgeon, Nashville, TN, USA.

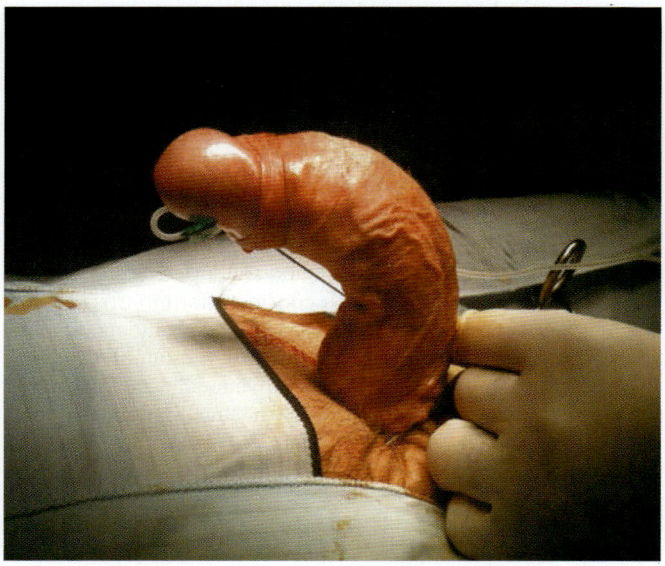

Figure 78.19 An artificial erection obtained peri-operatively demonstrating the dorsal deformity of the erect penis that is typical of Peyronie's disease.

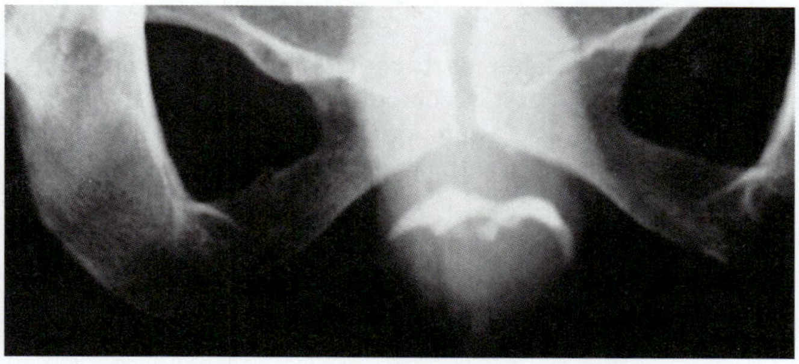

Figure 78.20 Penile calcification in Peyronie's disease (courtesy of Dr SS Rawat, Riyadh, Saudi Arabia).

Summary box 78.9

Peyronie's disease

- Medical treatments during the active phase have little evidence of efficacy
- The disease has a natural history of 18–24 months active disease before it stabilises
- Surgery may be indicated to correct deformity that interferes with sexual activity
- Surgical treatment will shorten the erect penile length

Chordee

Chordee (French = corded) is a fixed bowing of the penis caused by hypospadias or, more rarely, chronic urethritis. Erection is deformed and sexual intercourse may be impossible. Treatment is usually surgical.

Priapism

Priapism means persistent erection lasting longer than 4 hours and it is a surgical emergency. There are two main types of priapism, ischaemic and non-ischaemic.

Ischaemic priapism

Ischaemic or venogenic priapism is the more common and is due to venous congestion, with consequent thrombosis and ischaemia. The penis remains erect and becomes painful. This is a pathological erection and the glans penis and corpus spongiosum are not involved. The condition is most commonly seen as a side effect of medication, most notably anti-psychotic medication and intracavernosal injections, but it can also arise as a complication of a hypercoagulable blood disorder such as sickle cell disease or leukaemia. A tiny proportion of cases are caused by malignant disease in the corpora cavernosa or the pelvis.

The clinical features are of a painful erection not involving the glans penis. Blood taken from the penis shows hypoxia, hyerpcapnoea and acidosis, while Doppler scanning shows an absence of blood flow within the penis.

An underlying cause should be excluded. The patient should be referred for specialist urological care. Treatment is an emergency, since a delay of 6–12 hours results in irreversible damage to the corpus cavernosal tissue with subsequent fibrosis and erectile dysfunction. Aspiration of the sludged blood in the corpora cavernosa is the first-line therapy, but if this fails then intracavernosal injection of phenylephrine (an alpha adrenoceptor agonist) is the next line of therapy. If that proves ineffective, it may be necessary to decompress the penis by creating a shunt between the corpus cavernosum and either the glans penis or the corpus spongiosum. The outlook for normal erectile function is poor if treatment is delayed (Summary box 78.10).

Summary box 78.10

Ischaemic priapism

- The characteristic clinical features are a painful erection not involving the glans penis
- Blood gas analysis from the penis shows hypoxia, hypercapnoea and acidosis
- Detumescence should be ideally achieved within 6–12 hours to avoid long-term erectile dysfunction

Non-ischaemic priapism

The rarer form of priapism arises as a consequence of traumatic damage to the central penile artery, usually as a consequence of blunt perineal trauma. A fistula develops between the artery and the sinusoidal space which results in a persistent erection, which in contrast to the ischaemic priapism is painless. Blood gas analysis shows arterial blood and Doppler scanning demonstrates the fistula (Figure 78.21a,b). Treatment is not an emergency, since there is no ischaemia, and is most appropriately achieved by selective arterial embolisation.

CARCINOMA OF THE PENIS

Penile cancer is rare in the UK, with only around 600 cases being recorded annually. It is much more common in other parts of the world, most notably South America, where it is one of the most common cancers.

Aetiology

Circumcision soon after birth confers immunity against carcinoma of the penis. Later circumcision does not seem to have the same benefit, with the assumption that smegma is in some way carcinogenic. Human papillomavirus infection with penile warts is a risk factor, as is BXO and smoking. Phimosis and chronic balanoposthitis are known to be contributory factors, and there are definite precarcinomatous states including leukoplakia of the glans, which is similar to the condition seen on the tongue, and carcinoma *in situ* of the penis.

Carcinoma *in situ* of the penis (synonym Bowen's disease, erythroplasia of Queryat)

Carcinoma *in situ* of the penis is typically seen as a red cutaneous patch on the penis. When it occurs on the glans penis, it is known as erythroplasia of Queryat and when it occurs on the shaft of the penis it is called Bowen's disease. There are several other benign causes of red patches on the penis, and when in doubt a biopsy is indicated. When the diagnosis of carcinoma *in situ* is confirmed, treatment is by means of topical 5-FU cream, CO_2 laser ablation or surgical excision.

Pathology

Carcinoma of the penis is most typically a squamous cell carcinoma arising in the skin of the glans or the prepuce. It may be flat and infiltrating or warty in appearance (Figure 78.22). The former often starts as leukoplakia and the latter results from an existing papilloma. Local growth continues for months or years. T1 tumours are confined to the skin, with T2 tumours invading the corpus spongiosum or the corpus cavernosum. T3 tumours invade the urethra and T4 tumours invade adjacent structures. The earliest lymphatic spread is to the inguinal (N1 and N2 disease) and then to the iliac nodes (N3 disease) (Figure 78.23). Distant metastatic deposits are infrequent.

Clinical features

Many patients present late (Figure 78.24), either because of embarrassment or because of misdiagnosis. About 10 per cent of patients are under 40 years of age. By the time the patient presents, the growth is often large and secondary infection causes a foul bloody discharge. There is typically little or no pain.

Around 50 per cent have inguinal lymph node enlargement at presentation, but the nodal enlargement often reflects infection. In many, the prepuce is non-retractile and must be split to view the lesion. A biopsy should be performed to make the diagnosis. Untreated, the whole glans may be replaced by a fungating offensive mass. Later, the inguinal nodes can erode the skin (Figure 78.23) of the groin and in rare cases death of the patient can result from erosion of the femoral or external iliac vessels.

Treatment

Management is divided into treatment of the primary tumour and treatment of the inguinal nodes. For the primary tumour surgical excision is the mainstay of treatment, with the tradi-

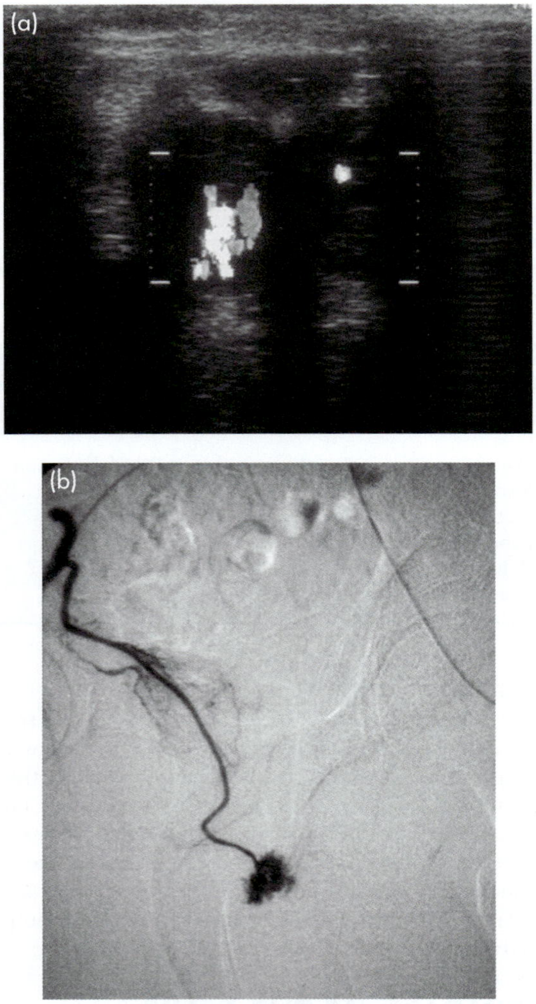

Figure 78.21 (a) Colour Doppler scan of a high flow (non-ischaemic) priapism showing turbulence at the site of the arterial injury. Compare the high unilateral signal (turbulence) with normal contralateral flow. (b) Selective pudendal arteriogram showing the site of the fistula (the arterial blush) between the central penile artery and the corpus cavernosum.

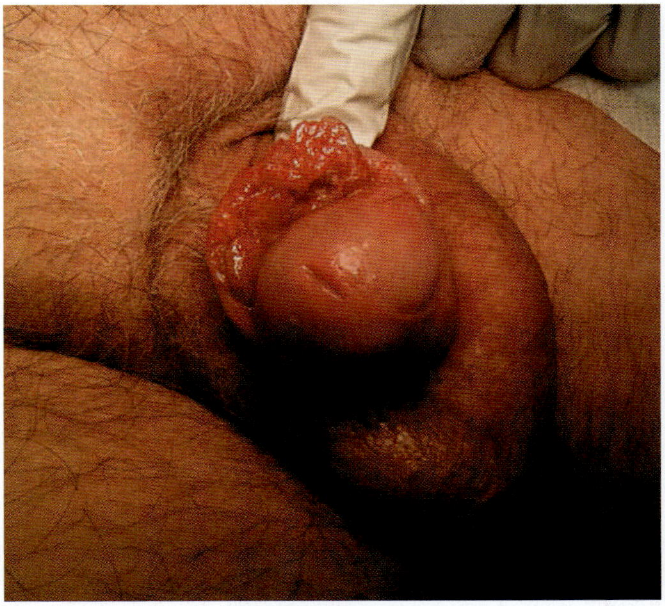

Figure 78.22 A squamous cell cancer arising from the inner aspect of the prepuce.

Auguste Queyrat, 1872–1933, Dermatologist, Paris, France, described this condition in 1911.

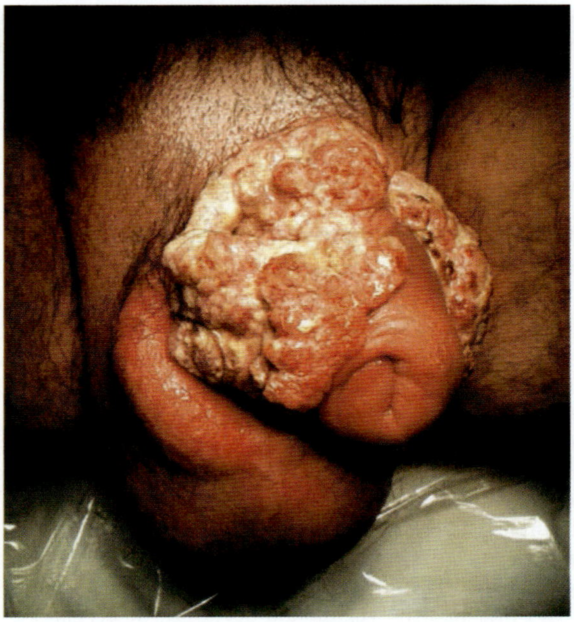

Figure 78.23 A late presenting squamous cell cancer of the penis.

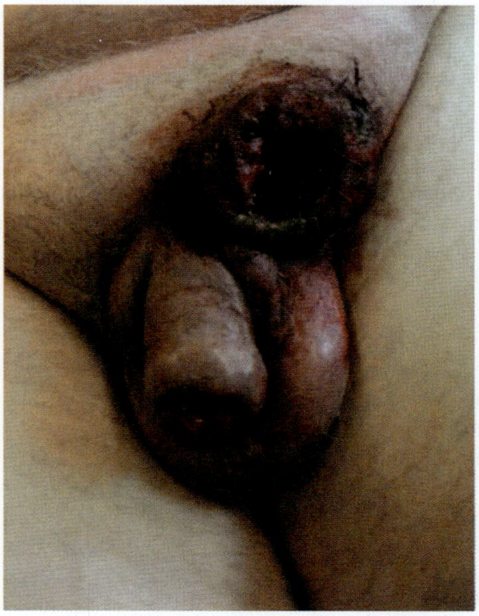

Figure 78.24 A squamous cell cancer of the penis with an ulcerating groin node.

tional view that a 2 cm margin of normal tissue be removed being superceded by a more recent, more conservative view, such that penile preserving surgery with excision of much lower margins of normal tissue are now accepted. Tumours affecting the glans penis require glansectomy, with more advanced tumours requiring partial penectomy. In advanced cases, total penectomy is required with formation of a perineal urethrostomy. Such surgery is indicated even in advanced metastatic disease for reasons of local control.

Treatment of any associated enlarged inguinal lymph nodes should be delayed until at least 3 weeks after local treatment of the primary lesion. Enlargement caused by infection will usually show signs of subsiding with antibiotic treatment. For palpable nodes, ultrasound-guided fine needle aspiration will confirm the diagnosis and a block dissection of both groins should be undertaken. The management of the nodes when there is no palpable disease is more controversial with most protocols dictating prophylactic lymph node dissection for tumours that are T2 or greater and for those that are poorly differentiated because of the risk of microscopic disease. A recent development is the use of sentinel node biopsy for impalpable nodes in high risk cases.

Management of the pelvic nodes is even more controversial. When they are involved on computed tomography (CT) scanning, surgery probably has little role, but when the iliac nodes are not enlarged in the presence of N2 disease, the options are observation, pelvic lympadenectomy or radiotherapy. The prognosis for tumours confined to the penis is good with five-year survival rates in excess of 80 per cent. With nodal involvement, the five-year survival rate falls to around 40 per cent (Summary box 78.11).

Buschke–Löwenstein tumour

Buschke–Löwenstein tumour is uncommon. It has the histological pattern of a verrucous carcinoma. It is locally destructive and invasive but appears not to spread to lymph nodes or to metastasise. Treatment is by surgical excision.

Summary box 78.11

Carcinoma of the penis

- A relatively uncommon tumour in the UK
- Enlargement of superficial inguinal lymph nodes may be caused by infection or metastatic spread
- Surgery is the mainstay of treatment
- Nodal involvement indicates a poor prognosis

Malignant melanoma of the penis

This is an uncommon tumour, with the principles of management being the same as for squamous cell carcinoma. Bloodborne metastatic disease is, however, more common.

SEXUALLY TRANSMITTED GENITAL INFECTIONS

Genital ulcers

The most common cause of a genital ulcer is genital herpes. Other less common causes include syphilis and chancroid.

Genital herpes

Genital herpes is caused by sexual transmission of the herpes simplex virus (usually type 2, occasionally type 1). Recurrent attacks occur in 50 per cent or more of cases. Pain along the distribution of the sensory nerve, usually the genitofemoral nerve, precedes the eruption by 2 days and may be particularly severe around the anus. A group of tiny vesicles rapidly erodes to form shallow ulcers which are painful. The first attack is typically accompanied by fever and myalgia. In female patients, the ulcers often spread on to the thighs during the attack. Involvement of the urethra may cause retention of urine, which may persist for

Abraham Buschke, 1868–1943, dermatologist, Berlin, Germany.
Ludwig Loewenstein, 1885–1959, dermatologist, Berlin, Germany.

up to 14 days if there is radiculitis of the S2 and S3 nerve roots. The diagnosis is made clinically, or when there is doubt by either cell culture or by PCR-based techniques. Acyclovir and valacyclovir have been shown to be effective in treating genital herpes but they do not prevent recurrences.

A child born to a mother with active infection is susceptible to a fatal generalised herpes infection in the neonatal period. Caesarean section should be considered in these circumstances. There is an increased risk of carcinoma of the cervix and annual cytology for life is recommended.

Syphilis

Syphilitic ulcers are typically painless, rubbery and indurated. Due to the spirochaete *Treponema pallidum*, diagnosis was traditionally achieved by dark field microscopy, but modern serological techniques are nowadays more appropriate. The incidence of syphilis is increasing since the advent of the retrovirals used to treat HIV in mid-1990s. Treatment is by use of a long-acting penicillin.

Lymphogranuloma venereum

Lymphogranuloma venereum is a sexually transmitted disease caused by *Chlamydia trachomatis* (Chlamydia A) types L1–L3 and is primarily an infection of the lymphatics and lymph nodes. The primary lesion is a fleeting, painless, genital papule or ulcer which is often unnoticed by the patient. It can affect both sexes. While it was considered rare in developed countries, some recent outbreaks in Europe have occurred, usually in conjunction with HIV.

The inguinal glands become enlarged and painful between two and four months after infection. The masses of nodes mat together above and below the inguinal ligament to give the 'sign of the groove'. The overlying skin reddens and there may be fluctuance. There may be a proctitis, which can go on to produce a rectal stricture if untreated. Lymphatic obstruction leads to lymphoedema in the perineum and occasionally the lower limbs. Urethritis and urethral stricture occur in men.

The diagnosis is confirmed clinically and by the detection of antibodies against the organism. Treatment is by a combination of antibiotics, which may include sulphonamides, oxytetracycline and erythromycin. The multilocular lymphatic masses should not be incised; aspiration is permissible to reduce discomfort.

Granuloma inguinale

This is a chronic and slowly progressive ulcerative tropical disease affecting the genitals and surrounding tissue but occasionally occurring elsewhere in the body. It is usually sexually transmitted and is caused by *Klebsiella granulomatis* and is most commonly seen among socially deprived people. The incubation period varies greatly but is typically between 7 and 30 days.

A painless vesicle or indurated papule, usually on the external genitals but occasionally elsewhere on the skin, gradually erodes into a slowly extending ulcer with a beefy-red, granulomatous base. More chronic lesions may become greyish, especially at the edges, where, after months or years, malignant change may develop. The ulcerated area may bleed if touched but is usually surprisingly painless. Without treatment, healing is only partial and keloid is common.

Diagnosis is by microscopy of material from the edges of the ulcer, which shows the presence of short Gram-negative rods within the cytoplasm of the large mononuclear cells. Treatment is by erythromycin, oxytetracycline or streptomycin.

> Syphilis derives its name from a poem by a physician, Girolamo Fracastoro, published in Venice in 1530. The poem tells of the shepherd Syphilus, who was struck down by the disease as a punishment for neglecting the worship of Apollo. On his return from Haiti to Barcelona in 1493, Columbus 'brought back syphilis, parrots and rare plants'. The King and Queen of Spain received him with the highest honours.

Condylomata acuminata (synonym: genital warts)

Genital warts are caused by infection with human papillomavirus (HPV) and are sexually transmitted. Infection is very common with only a small proportion of infected patients actually having visible warts. Most commonly due to HPV types 6 and 11, these viruses do not cause cervical cancer. Ordinary skin warts can occur on the genitals by direct contact with a finger lesion, but they are less moist and soft and less often pedunculated than the genital variety. The lesions most commonly occur under the prepuce in the coronal sulcus but may be found elsewhere, including inside the urinary meatus (Figure 78.25). In women, genital warts are most commonly found on the vulva but they may line the vagina and occur on the cervix. Perianal warts are common.

Other associated sexually transmitted diseases should be excluded: in women mainly candidiasis and Trichomonas infection and in men syphilis or gonorrhoea. Genital warts may complicate HIV infection.

Treatment is by chemical or physical means. Podophyllin is often effective as a topical application. It is applied to the wart, taking great care to avoid the surrounding skin, and washed off after 6 hours or so. An alternative agent is Imidaquod. If chemical methods fail, the warts can be excised or they can be ablated with cryosurgery, electrosurgery or laser. Circumcision is sometimes advised if there are florid lesions under the foreskin.

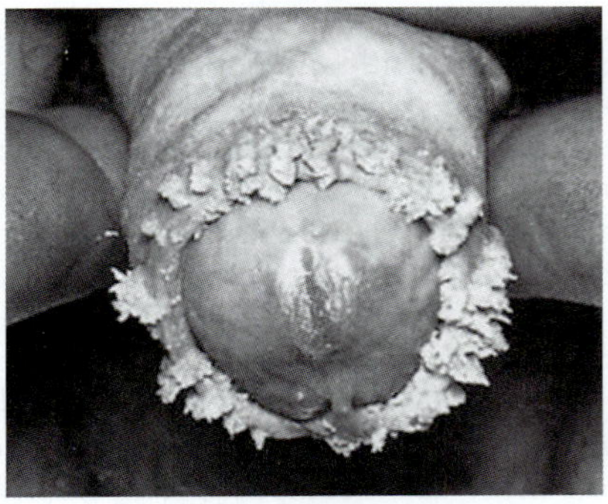

Figure 78.25 Penile warts.

FURTHER READING

Blandy JP, Kaisary AV. *Lecture notes: urology*, 6th edn. Oxford: Blackwell, 2007.

Wein AJ, Kavoussi LR, Novick AC, Partin AW. *Campbell-Walsh urology*, 10th edn. Philadelphia: Elsevier, 2010.

CHAPTER

79 Testis and scrotum

LEARNING OBJECTIVES

To recognise and understand:

- Testicular maldescent and to appreciate the reasons for intervention
- Testicular torsion as a urological emergency
- The management of the common scrotal swellings (varicocele, hydrocele and epididymal cysts)
- The management of testicular tumours
- The treatment options for infertile men

EMBRYOLOGY AND ANATOMY OF THE TESTIS

The testes develop in the retroperitoneum below the kidneys at around the 10th thoracic level. During the 7th week of fetal development, the gubernaculum forms within the folds of the peritoneum. The upper end is attached to the developing testis and the lower end is attached to the fascia between the developing abdominal wall muscles. At the same time an evagination of the peritoneum itself, the processus vaginalis, develops adjacent to the gubernaculum and over the subsequent weeks evaginates through the abdominal wall to create the inguinal canal. The processus vaginalis initially picks up fibres of the internal oblique (which become the cremasteric muscle) and then fibres of the external oblique (which become the external spermatic fascia). As it elongates, the processus carries with it the gubernaculum, which contains muscle fibres, although it is not fully clear what part it plays in testicular descent. What is clear is that the testes lie at the internal inguinal ring at three months' gestation and descend to the scrotum between seven and nine months. This latter descent into the scrotum is accompanied by shortening of the gubernaculum. Final descent from the external ring to the base of the scrotum takes 4–6 weeks and is usually complete by birth.

The mechanisms that result in testicular descent are poorly understood but probably involve Müllerian inhibiting substance. Maternal chorionic gonadotrophin stimulates growth of the testis and may stimulate its migration. Imperfectly developed testes tend to descend incompletely.

The anatomy of the adult testis reflects its embryonic development. The testicular arteries originate high up in the retroperitoneum from the abdominal aorta, just below the renal arteries. The testicular veins drain into the renal vein on the left and the inferior vena cava on the right. For much of their course, the testicular artery and vein run parallel to the ipsilateral ureter, for which they may be mistaken during retroperitoneal surgery.

The epididymis lies on the posterior aspect of the testis and is palpable as a separate structure, with a head, a body and a tail. The seminiferous tubules enter the epididymis at the upper end of the epididymis (the head). From the head, sperm travel through the body and tail of the epididymis to enter the vas deferens at the lower pole of the testis. The vas curves up behind the testis and can be felt above the testis as a firm tubular structure entering the external inguinal ring. In the inguinal canal, the vas deferens is invested by the cremasteric muscle along with the other components of the spermatic cord.

INCOMPLETELY DESCENDED TESTIS

Definitions

Incomplete descent of the testis occurs when the testis is arrested in some part of its normal path to the scrotum. An ectopic testis is a testis that is abnormally placed outside this path (see also Chapter 8).

Incidence

About 4 per cent of boys are born with one or both testes incompletely descended. About two thirds of these reach the scrotum during the first three months of life, but full descent after that is uncommon. The incidence of testicular maldescent at the age of one year is around 1 per cent. The condition is sometimes missed in the neonatal period and only discovered later in life. In a few cases, the presence of a hernia, testicular pain or acute torsion directs attention to the abnormality. In 10 per cent of unilateral cases, there is a family history.

True testicular pain can be situated in the lower abdomen at the level of the internal inguinal ring in accordance with Brown's Law. **Francis Robert Brown**, former Reader in Surgery, St Andrew's University, UK. Brown's law: Pain, produced in an organ which has migrated from its primary position, and which has not acquired an additional nerve supply in its secondary or permanent position, is invariably localised in the primary relative of that organ.

Sir Astley Cooper, 1768–1841, surgeon, Guy's Hospital, London and First President of the Royal College of Surgeons of England, taught that patients with bilateral retained testes were usually sterile, whereupon one of his pupils, a cryptorchid, left the room and committed suicide. At the post-mortem motile spermatozoa were demonstrated.

Kaspar Friedrich Wolff, 1733–1794, Professor of Anatomy and Physiology, St Petersburg, Russia.

Pathology

The condition is more common on the right and is bilateral in 20 per cent of cases. In adults, secondary sexual characteristics are typically normal.

The testis may be:

- intra-abdominal; usually lying extraperitoneally just inside the internal inguinal ring;
- intra-canalicular; it may or may not be palpable (Figure 79.1);
- extra-canalicular; usually at the scrotal neck;
- ectopic; the most common site is within the superficial inguinal pouch which lies just inferior and medial to the superficial inguinal ring. Other rarer ectopic sites include the femoral triangle, the root of the penis and perineum.

Incompletely descended testes are often macroscopically normal in early childhood, but by puberty the testis is typically smaller compared with its intrascrotal counterpart. Microscopic changes are apparent from 1–2 years, including loss of Leydig cells, degeneration of Sertoli cells and decreased spermatogenesis. The higher the testis, the greater the degree of histological change.

Consequences

Infertility

Impaired fertility is a well-recognised consequence of testicular maldescent with paternity rates around two-thirds of normal for unilateral undescended testes and one-third of normal for bilateral undescended testes. Although there has been a recent tendency to undertake surgical orchidopexy earlier in life, evidence to show that this might benefit fertility is currently lacking.

Malignancy

The cancer risk for adults after cryptorchidism in childhood is 5–10 times greater than normal. The most common cancer is a seminoma and, as with fertility, it is unclear whether early orchidopexy reduces the risk of malignancy. However, if a testicular tumour does develop, it is undoubtedly easier to identify in a testis that is within the scrotum.

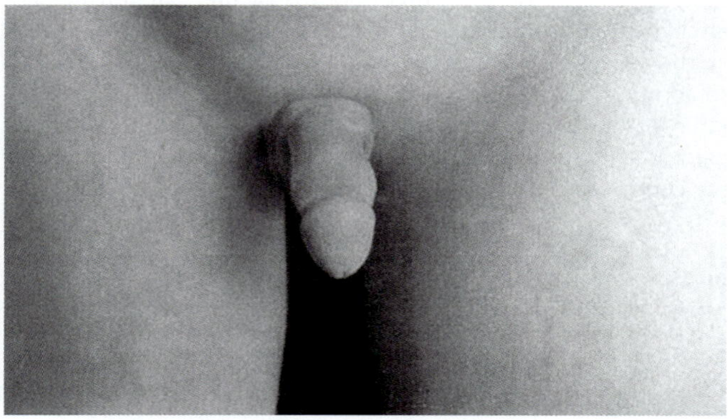

Figure 79.1 Undescended testes in a boy aged 12 years. Note the bilateral undescended testes with the underdeveloped scrotum. In cases of retractile testis, the scrotum is relatively well developed.

Hernia

Around 90 per cent of boys with an undescended testis have a patent processus vaginalis, although the incidence of a clinically apparent hernia is much lower.

Testicular torsion

The undescended testis is more prone to testicular torsion, largely as a consequence of a developmental abnormality between the testis and its mesentery (Summary box 79.1).

Summary box 79.1

Undescended testis

- Testes that are absent from the scrotum after three months of age are unlikely to descend
- Histological changes in the testis can be seen from one year of age
- An incompletely descended testis tends to atrophy as puberty approaches
- Boys with undescended testes are at greater risk of infertility, testicular malignancy, hernia and testicular torsion

Clinical features

During childhood, the testes are mobile and the cremasteric reflex is active. In some boys, any stimulation of the skin of the scrotum or thigh causes the testis to ascend and to temporarily disappear into the inguinal canal. This is called a retractile testis. In comparison to a true undescended testis, the scrotum of a boy with a retractile testis is normal as opposed to underdeveloped. When the cremaster relaxes, the testis reappears only to vanish when the scrotal skin is touched again. A retractile testis can be gently milked from its position in the inguinal region to the bottom of the scrotum. A diagnosis of true incomplete descent should be made only if this is not possible. It is helpful to have the boy as relaxed as possible and for him to be examined in a warm room, usually in a supine position.

When the testis is impalpable, ultrasound may be helpful in identifying the intracanalicular testis, while laparoscopy may be needed to differentiate between the abdominal testis and a truly absent testis (Summary box 79.2).

Summary box 79.2

Retractile testis

- Retractile testes should be differentiated from true undescended testes
- This is most easily done with the child relaxed in a warm room
- Retractile testes are more common than true undescended testes
- Retractile testes require no treatment

Surgical treatment

Orchidopexy

Orchidopexy is usually performed before the boy reaches 12 months of age in an attempt to prevent the consequences described earlier. The testis and spermatic cord are mobilised

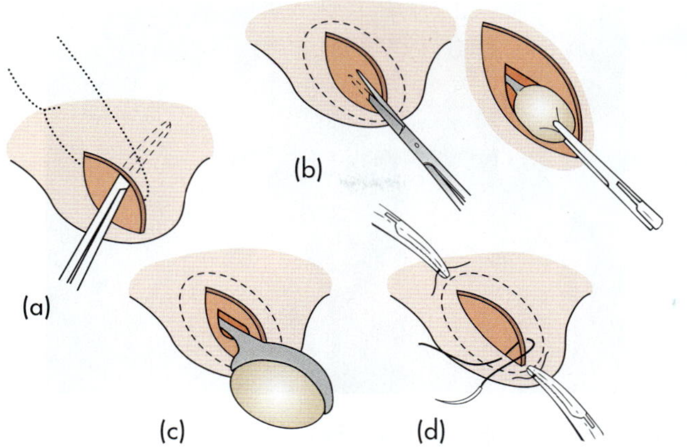

Figure 79.2 The testis is mobilised and retained in a pouch constructed between the dartos muscle and skin.

and the testis is repositioned in the scrotum. The operation is performed through a short incision over the deep inguinal ring. The inguinal canal is exposed by division of the external oblique aponeurosis in the direction of its fibres.

Three manoeuvres help to gain the length required to bring the testis down into the bottom of the scrotum. First the patent processus vaginalis should be identified, separated and ligated. Second the coverings of the spermatic cord (including the cremasteric muscle) should be divided and third, lateral fibrous bands just inside the internal inguinal ring should be divided. Although these techniques are usually effective, the tiny vas and testicular vessels are vulnerable to injury. The empty hemiscrotum is stretched with a finger passed into it through the inguinal incision to give enough room for the testis which is placed in a pouch constructed between the dartos muscle and the skin (Figure 79.2).

Failure to bring the testis down

Sometimes for a high undescended testis a two-stage surgical procedure is necessary. The testis is mobilised as far as possible and anchored with a suture and the mobilisation is completed six months later. An alternative approach involves initial division of the gonadal artery (which is usually 'tighter' than the vas deferens), such that the testis becomes dependent for its blood supply upon the vasal artery. The second stage procedure involves conventional orchidopexy. Orchidectomy should be considered if the incompletely descended testis is atrophic, particularly in the post-pubertal boy if the other testis is normal.

INJURIES TO THE TESTIS

The testis can be damaged either by blunt or by penetrating trauma. Injuries can range from simple bruising, through significant intra-testicular haematomas to rupture of the tunica albuginea with very significant collections of blood within the tunica vaginalis (haematocele) (Figure 79.3). If the tunica ruptures, the blood can track into the groin and perineum. Ultrasound examination is a useful adjunct to clinical examination and surgical exploration is indicated for significant injuries including testicular rupture. The objective is to repair the tunica albuginea and preserve the testis, but on occasions orchidectomy is necessary (Summary box 79.3).

Summary box 79.3

Scrotal trauma

- Scrotal exploration should be considered when there is massive swelling and pain after scrotal trauma
- Ultrasound is valuable in the assessment of the injury

ABSENT TESTIS

'Vanishing' testis describes a condition in which a testis develops but disappears before birth. The most likely cause for this is prenatal torsion. True agenesis of the testis is rarer. Laparoscopy is useful in distinguishing these causes of clinically absent testis from intra-abdominal maldescent.

TORSION OF THE TESTIS

Pathophysiology

Testicular torsion is a condition whereby the testicle twists in such a way that its blood supply becomes compromised. If left untreated, the blood flow to the testicle ceases and the testicle dies. The earlier the surgery to untwist the testis can be undertaken the better the results, with a testicular salvage rate of 100 per cent if the testicle can be untwisted within 6 hours of the torsion taking place compared with an approximate 20 per cent salvage rate if the surgery is delayed for 24 hours.

Torsion of the testis is uncommon because the normal testis is anchored and cannot rotate. For torsion to occur, one of several abnormalities must be present:

- Inversion of the testis is the most common predisposing cause. The testis is rotated so that it lies transversely or upside down.
- High investment of the tunica vaginalis causes the testis to hang within the tunica like a clapper in a bell (Figure 79.4).
- Separation of the epididymis from the body of the testis permits torsion of the testis on the pedicle that connects the testis with the epididymis (Figure 79.5).

Normally, when there is a contraction of the abdominal muscles, the cremaster contracts as well. In the presence of one of the abnormalities described above, the spiral attachment of

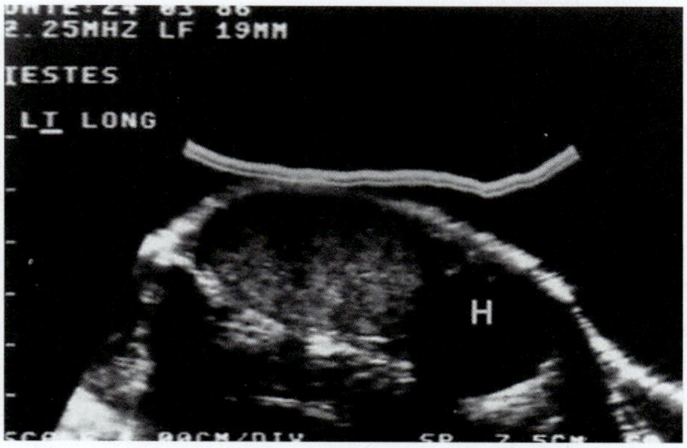

Figure 79.3 Longitudinal scan of testicle with haematocele (H) at lower pole.

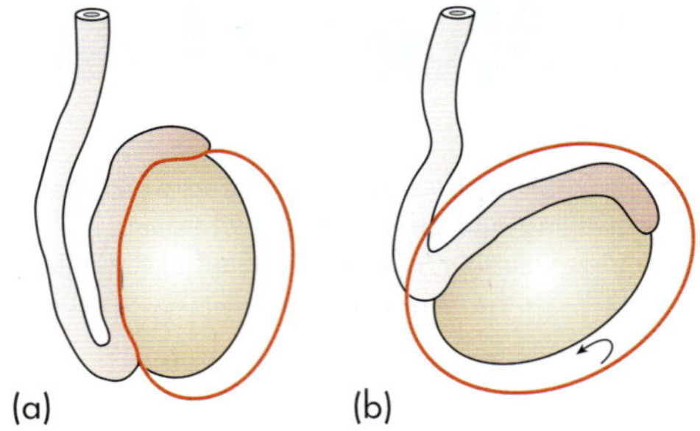

Figure 79.4 Testicular torsion. (a) Normal attachment. (b) An abnormally high attachment of the tunica vaginalis predisposes to torsion – the 'bell-clapper'.

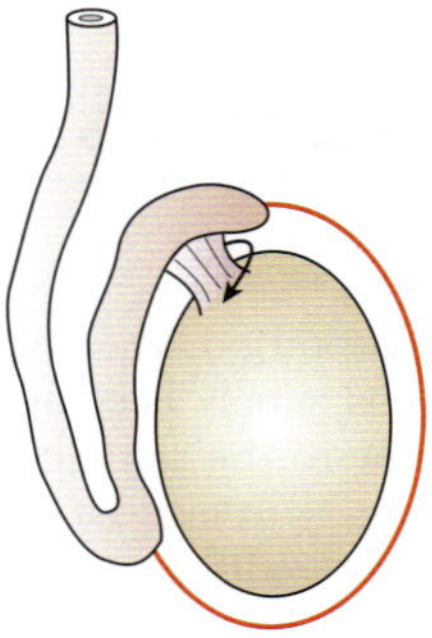

Figure 79.5 Testicular torsion. Separation of the testis from the epididymis – torsion about the pedicle between them.

the cremaster favours rotation of the testis around the vertical axis. Straining on stool, lifting of a heavy weight and coitus are all possible precipitating factors. Alternatively, torsion may develop spontaneously during sleep.

Clinical features

Testicular torsion is most common between 10 and 25 years of age, although a few cases occur in infancy. Typically, there is sudden agonising pain in the groin and the lower abdomen. The patient feels nauseated and may vomit. Torsion of a fully descended testis is usually easily recognised. The testis seems high and the tender twisted cord can be palpated above it. The cremasteric reflex is lost.

Differential diagnosis

Redness of the skin and a mild pyrexia may result in the condition being confused with epididymo-orchitis in the older patient; however, in epididymo-orchitis there will usually be dysuria associated with the accompanying urinary infection. Elevation of the testis reduces the pain in epididymo-orchitis and makes it worse in torsion.

Torsion of a testicular appendage cannot always be distinguished with certainty from testicular torsion. The most common structure to twist is the appendix of the testis (the pedunculated hydatid of Morgagni). The twisted testicular appendages can sometimes be visible through the scrotal wall. If the diagnosis is made clinically, then conservative management is possible, but if in doubt then surgical exploration should be undertaken with ligation and amputation of the twisted appendage.

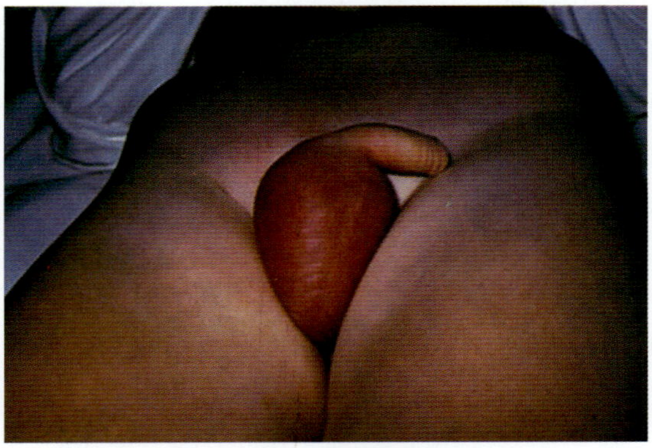

Figure 79.6 Idiopathoc oedema of the scrotum.

In mumps orchitis the cord is not particularly thickened and the condition is often bilateral.

Idiopathic scrotal oedema is an oddity that occurs between the age of four and 12 years and must be differentiated from torsion. The scrotum is very swollen but there is little pain or tenderness. The swelling is usually bilateral and may extend into the perineum, groin and penis. It is thought to be an allergic phenomenon; occasionally there is eosinophilia. The swelling subsides after a day or so but may recur (Figure 79.6).

Very occasionally, torsion can be convincingly mimicked by a small tense strangulated inguinal hernia compressing the cord and causing compression of the pampiniform plexus.

Management

The management of the case should be determined primarily on clinical grounds. If there is any doubt as to the diagnosis, then urgent scrotal exploration is indicated. While Doppler ultrasound scanning can confirm the absence of the blood supply to the affected testis, false positive results can be seen, so it is not routinely recommended.

Exploration for torsion should be performed through a scrotal incision. If the testis is viable when the cord is untwisted it should be prevented from twisting again by fixation with non-absorbable sutures between the tunica vaginalis and the tunica albuginea. The other testis should also be fixed because the anatomical predisposition is likely to be bilateral. An infarcted testis should be removed – the patient can be counselled later about a prosthetic replacement.

In cases where there is a history of pain for several days, the affected testis will be dead. It is not possible to recover such a testis and although little is gained (other than pain relief) by immediate exploration it is necessary to fix the contralateral testis (Summary box 79.4).

VARICOCELE

A varicocele is a varicose dilatation of the veins draining the testis.

Surgical anatomy

The veins draining the testis and the epididymis form the pampiniform plexus. The veins gradually join each other as they traverse the inguinal canal and, at or near the inguinal ring, there are only one or two testicular veins, which pass upwards

Summary box 79.4

Testicular torsion

- If the diagnosis of testicular torsion is possible, then surgical exploration is indicated
- Prompt exploration, untwisting and fixation is the only way to save the torted testis
- The patient should be counselled and consented for orchidectomy before exploration
- The anatomical abnormality is bilateral and the contralateral testis should also be fixed

within the retroperitoneum. The left testicular vein empties into the left renal vein, the right into the inferior vena cava below the right renal vein. The testicular veins usually have valves near their terminations, but these are sometimes absent. There is an alternative (collateral) venous return from the testes through the cremasteric veins, which drain mainly into the inferior epigastrics.

Aetiology

Varicoceles are common, affecting perhaps 15–20 per cent of males. Ninety per cent are left-sided, reflecting the proximal venous anatomy. In some cases, the dilated vessels are cremasteric veins and not part of the pampiniform plexus. The usual cause is absence or incompetence of valves in the proximal testicular vein. While most varicoceles are idiopathic, obstruction of the left testicular vein by a renal tumour or nephrectomy is a cause of varicocele in later life; characteristically, in such cases the varicocele does not decompress in the supine position.

Clinical features

While most varicoceles are asymptomatic, those that are symptomatic tend to present in adolescence or early adulthood when there may be an annoying dragging discomfort that is worse on standing at the end of the day. This presumably reflects distension of the testicular veins. When examined in the erect position, the scrotum on the affected side hangs lower than normal (Figure 79.7), and on palpation, with the patient standing, the varicose plexus feels like a bag of worms. There may be a cough impulse. If the patient lies down the veins empty by gravity and this provides an opportunity to ensure that the underlying testis is normal to palpation. In longstanding cases, the affected testis is smaller and softer than its fellow owing to a minor degree of atrophy.

Ultrasonography can be helpful in the diagnosis of small varicoceles (Figure 79.8) and in older men with an apparently recent onset of varicocele, ultrasonography of the kidneys is important in excluding a left renal tumour.

Varicocele and spermatogenesis

Of all the possible causes of primary infertility, oligozoospermia (reduced numbers of sperm in the ejaculate) is one of the most difficult to treat. Because varicoceles are relatively common, some men with oligozoospermia will have a varicocele, and it is tempting to blame this for the infertility. Certainly the varicocele will tend to 'warm' the testis, which is usually around 2.5°C below rectal temperature, and there is conflicting evidence regarding the effect of this temperature difference upon spermatogenesis. Unfortunately, there is little evidence that varicocelectomy improves semen quality or the rate of conception.

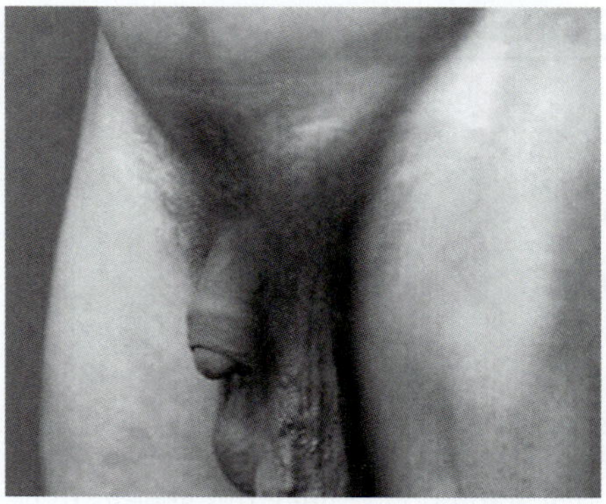

Figure 79.7 Large varicocele in a pendulous scrotum. Note the left inguinal hernia.

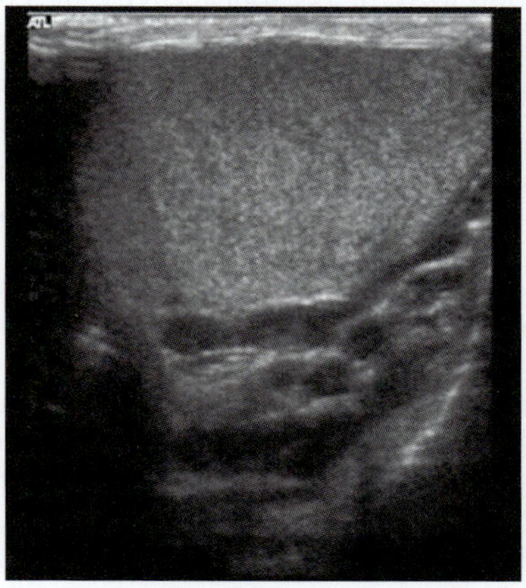

Figure 79.8 Ultrasound of a varicocele. Note the dilated veins at the lower pole of the testis.

Treatment

Operation is not indicated for an asymptomatic varicocele. When the discomfort is significant, then embolisation of the gonadal veins is the usual first line intervention. If this is not possible, or if the varicocele recurs (as it does in around 20 per cent after embolisation), then surgical ligation of the testicular veins is the appropriate treatment, although recurrence can occur even after such surgery (Summary box 79.5).

Summary box 79.5

Varicocele

- Varicocele is a common condition and 90% are left sided
- Development of a left-sided varicocele in later life may indicate the presence of a renal tumour
- They are usually asymptomatic and as such rarely need treatment
- First-line treatment is embolisation in symptomatic cases
- Varicoceles often recur, even after surgical treatment
- The association of varicoceles with subfertility is controversial

HYDROCELE

A hydrocele is an abnormal collection of serous fluid in a part of the processus vaginalis, usually the tunica vaginalis. Acquired hydroceles are primary or idiopathic, or secondary to epididymal or testicular disease.

Aetiology

A hydrocele can be produced in four different ways (Figure 79.9):

1 By excessive production of fluid within the sac, e.g. a secondary hydrocele
2 By defective absorption of fluid; this appears to be the explanation for most primary hydroceles, although the reason why the fluid is not absorbed is obscure
3 By interference with lymphatic drainage of scrotal structures
4 By connection with the peritoneal cavity via a patent processus vaginalis (congenital).

Hydrocele fluid contains albumin and fibrinogen. If the contents of a hydrocele are allowed to drain into a collecting vessel, the liquid does not clot; however, the fluid coagulates if mixed with even a trace of blood that has been in contact with damaged tissue.

A secondary hydrocele is most frequently associated with acute or chronic epididymo-orchitis. It is also seen with torsion of the testis and with some testicular tumours. A secondary hydrocele is usually lax and of moderate size: the underlying testis is palpable. If a tumour is suspected, the hydrocele should not be punctured for fear of needle-track implantation of malignant cells. A secondary hydrocele subsides when the primary lesion resolves.

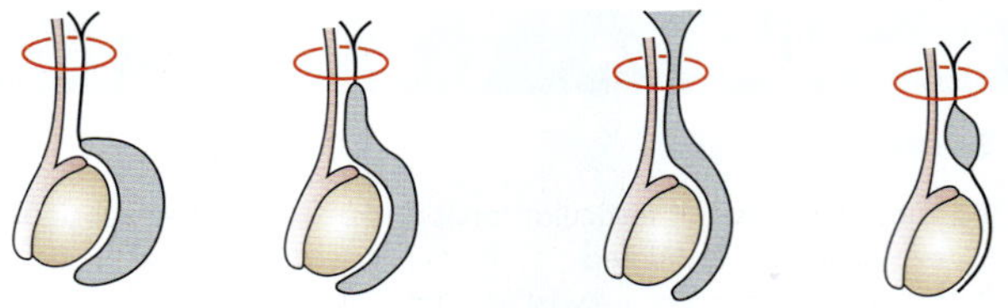

Figure 79.9 (a) Vaginal hydrocele (very common); (b) 'infantile' hydrocele; (c) congenital hydrocele; (d) hydrocele of the cord.

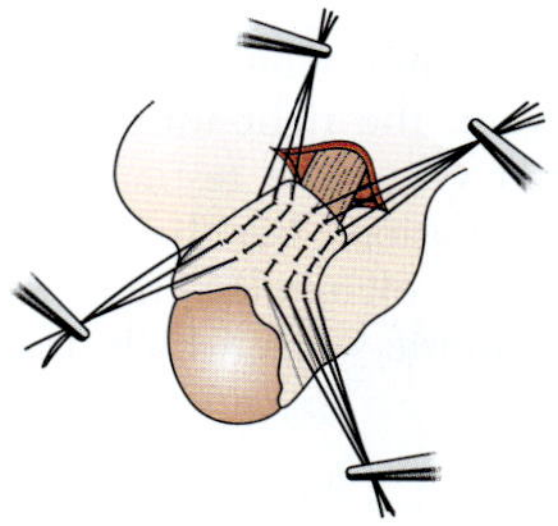

Figure 79.10 Lord's operation. A series of interrupted absorbable sutures is used to plicate the redundant tunica vaginalis. When these are tied, the tunica bunches at its attachment to the testis.

Clinical features

Hydroceles are typically translucent and it is possible to 'get above the swelling' on examination of the scrotum. The swelling usually surrounds the testis and epididymis such that they may become impossible to palpate separately.

A primary vaginal hydrocele is seen most commonly in middle and later life but can also occur in older children. The condition is particularly common in hot countries. Because the swelling is usually painless it may reach a prodigious size before the patient presents for treatment. The testis may be palpable within a lax hydrocele, but an ultrasound scan is necessary to visualise the testis if the hydrocele sac is tense. Be wary of an acute hydrocele in a young man since there may be a testicular tumour.

In congenital hydrocele, the processus vaginalis is patent and connects with the peritoneal cavity. The communication is usually too small to allow herniation of intra-abdominal contents. Pressure on the hydrocele does not always empty it but the hydrocele fluid may drain into the peritoneal cavity when the child is lying down; thus, the hydrocele may be intermittent. Ascites should be considered if the swellings are bilateral.

Encysted hydrocele of the cord is a smooth oval swelling near the spermatic cord, which is liable to be mistaken for an inguinal hernia. The swelling moves downwards and becomes less mobile if the testis is pulled gently downwards.

Hydrocele of the canal of Nuck is a similar condition in females. The cyst lies in relation to the round ligament and is always at least partially within the inguinal canal.

Edward Gibbon, 1737–1794, the author of 'The Decline and Fall of the Roman Empire', was greatly embarrassed by a large hydrocele. The second time that it was tapped it became infected, and Gibbon died a few days later. The hydrocele was associated with a large scrotal hernia which had probably been punctured.

Treatment

Congenital hydroceles are treated by herniotomy if they do not resolve spontaneously (see Chapter 8).

Small acquired hydroceles do not need treatment. If they are sizeable and bothersome for the patient, then surgical treatment is indicated. Established acquired hydroceles often have thick walls. Unless great care is taken to stop bleeding after excision of the wall, haemorrhage from the cut edge is liable to cause a large scrotal haematoma. Lord's operation is suitable when the sac is reasonably thin-walled (Figure 79.10). There is minimal dissection and the risk of haematoma is reduced. Eversion of the sac with placement of the testis in a pouch prepared by dissection in the fascial planes of the scrotum is an alternative (Jaboulay's procedure) (Figure 79.11).

Aspiration of the hydrocele fluid is simple, but the fluid always reaccumulates within a week or so. It may be suitable for men who are unfit for scrotal surgery, although hydrocele surgery can be undertaken under local anaesthetic. Aspiration can result in bleeding into the hydrocele sac and haematocele formation. Injection of sclerosants such as tetracycline is effective but painful (Summary box 79.6).

Filarial hydroceles and chyloceles

Filarial hydroceles and chyloceles account for up to 80 per cent of hydroceles in tropical countries where the parasite *Wucheria bancrofti* is endemic. Filarial hydroceles follow repeated attacks

Anton Nuck, 1650–1692, Professor of Anatomy and Medicine, Leiden, The Netherlands.
Peter Herent Lord, contemporary, formerly surgeon, Wycombe General Hospital, High Wycombe, UK, described his operation for hydrocele in 1964 and his procedure for haemorrhoids in 1968.

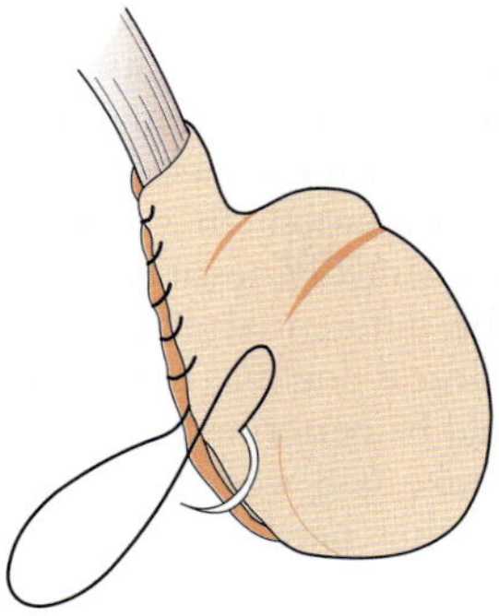

Figure 79.11 Jaboulay's procedure. The hydrocele sac is everted and anchored with sutures.

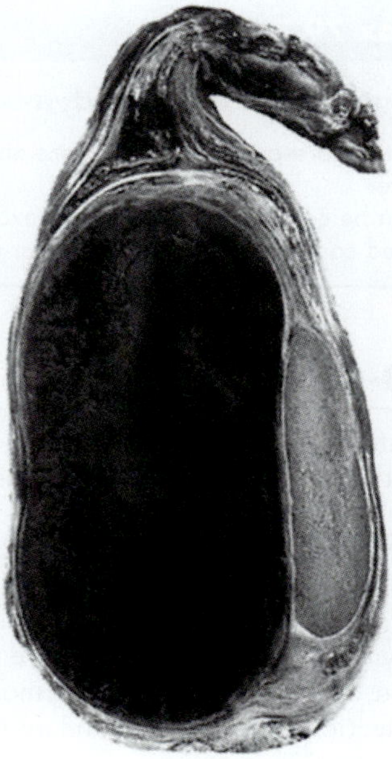

Figure 79.12 A longstanding haematocele. The testis has been flattened by prolonged pressure.

Summary box 79.6

Hydrocele

- A hydrocele is a collection of fluid within the tunica vaginalis
- Primary hydroceles surround the testis and transilluminate brightly
- Ultrasound examination is valuable when the testis and epididymis are impalpable
- Hydroceles can be treated conservatively unless they are large and symptomatic
- Surgery is the mainstay of treatment
- Testicular malignancy is an uncommon cause of hydrocele that can be excluded by ultrasound examination

of filarial epididymo-orchitis. They vary in size and may develop slowly or very rapidly. Occasionally, the fluid contains liquid fat, which is rich in cholesterol. This is caused by rupture of a lymphatic varix with discharge of chyle into the hydrocele. In longstanding chyloceles, there are dense adhesions between the scrotum and its contents. Filarial elephantiasis supervenes in a small number of cases. Treatment is by rest and aspiration. The more usual chronic cases are treated by excision of the sac.

Haematocele

The most common cause of a haematocele is vessel damage during needle drainage of a hydrocele. Prompt refilling of the sac associated with pain, tenderness and reduced transillumination will confirm the diagnosis. Acute haemorrhage into the tunica vaginalis sometimes results from testicular trauma with or without testicular rupture. If the haematocele is not drained, the blood within it clots (Figure 79.12). It becomes painless and may be mistaken for a testicular tumour. Indeed, a tumour may present as a haematocele. Ultrasound scanning usually helps with the differential diagnosis.

CYSTS ASSOCIATED WITH THE EPIDIDYMIS

There are several types of cyst associated with the epididymis including epididymal cysts and spermatoceles.

Epididymal cysts

These are filled with a crystal-clear fluid. They are very common, usually multiple and vary in size at presentation. They represent cystic degeneration of the epididymis. Cysts of the epididymis are usually found in middle age and are often bilateral. The clusters of tense cysts feel like tiny bunches of grapes that lie posterior to and quite separate from the testis. They should transilluminate brilliantly. The diagnosis can be confirmed by ultrasound (Figure 79.13).

Aspiration is useless because the cysts are usually multilocular. If they are causing discomfort, they should be excised. While single large cysts can be excised separately, recurrent or multilocular cysts usually require partial or total epididymectomy. Excision should be expected to interfere with the transportation of sperm from the testis on that side and young men should be counselled regarding this.

Cysts of a testicular appendage

Cysts of a testicular appendage are usually unilateral and are felt as small globular upper pole swellings. Such cysts are liable to torsion and should be removed if they cause symptoms. They are usually very small.

Spermatocele

This is a unilocular retention cyst derived from some portion of the sperm-conducting mechanism of the epididymis. A spermatocele typically lies in the epididymal head above and behind the upper pole of the testis. It is usually softer and laxer than other cystic lesions in the scrotum but, like them, it transilluminates. The fluid contains spermatozoa and resembles barley water in appearance. Spermatoceles are usually small and unobtrusive. Small spermatoceles can be ignored. Larger ones should be aspirated or excised through a scrotal incision (Summary box 79.7).

Mathieu Jaboulay, 1860–1913, Professor of Surgery, Lyons, France.

A patient with a spermatocele often complains that he has a 'third testicle'. He feels lucky that he is unduly provided! The story goes that, in the 14th century, on petition from a patient with a spermatocele, the Pope granted a gentleman to marry two wives because he had 'three testicles'.

Summary box 79.7

Cysts associated with the epididymis

- Lie posterior to and separate from the testis and they transilluminate
- Diagnosis can be confirmed by ultrasound examination
- Can be treated conservatively unless large or uncomfortable

EPIDIDYMO-ORCHITIS

Inflammation confined to the epididymis is epididymitis; infection spreading to the testis is epididymo-orchitis.

Pathophysiology

Infection reaches the epididymis via the vas from a primary infection of the urethra, prostate or seminal vesicles. A general rule is that epididymitis arises in sexually active young men from a genital infection, while in older men it more usually arises from a urinary infection or may be secondary to an indwelling urethral catheter.

In young sexually active men, the most common cause of epididymitis is now *Chlamydia trachomatis*, but gonococcal epididymitis is still occasionally seen. In older men with bladder outflow obstruction, epididymitis may result from a urinary infection – it is proposed that a high pressure in the prostatic urethra might cause reflux of infected urine up the vasa. Blood-borne infections of the epididymis are less common but may be suspected when there is *Escherichia coli*, streptococcal, staphylococcal or *Proteus* infection without evidence of urinary infection and are presumably the only possible mechanism in men who have previously undergone a vasectomy. Acute epididymo-orchitis can follow any form of urethral instrumentation. It is particularly common when an indwelling catheter is associated with infection of the prostate

Clinical features

While there may be initial symptoms of a urinary or a genital infection, such symptoms are not always seen. The development of an ache in the groin and a fever can herald the onset of epididymitis. The epididymis and testis swell and become painful. The scrotal wall, at first red, oedematous and shiny, may become adherent to the epididymis. Urinalysis will usually show leukocytes and may show a formal urinary tract infection. Ultrasound is useful in the initial assessment of epididymitis and will identify abscess formation. In young men, urethral swabs should be taken for chlamydial testing.

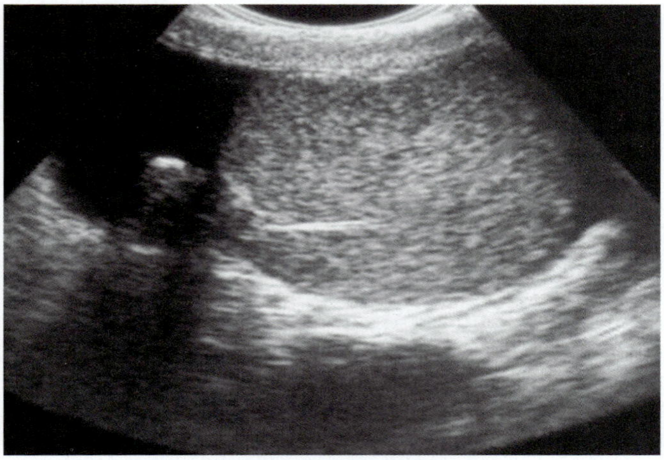

Figure 79.13 Ultrasound of an epididymal cyst.

In adolescents the differential diagnosis is testicular torsion and if there is any clinical doubt as to the diagnosis then testicular exploration should be performed.

Resolution may take 6–8 weeks to complete. Occasionally, an abscess can form that needs surgical drainage. Other complications include testicular atrophy, development of a chronic epididymitis and infertility.

Treatment

Either doxycycline (100–200 mg daily) or a quinolone should be the initial treatment in young men. There should be contact tracing of the partner and treatment if necessary.

In older men, quinolones are the usual initial treatment but if there is evidence of systemic sepsis, then intravenous antibiotics directed at urinary pathogens may be valuable. If an organism is isolated from the urine, this simplifies the choice of antibiotic.

All patients should drink plenty of fluid. Local measures including scrotal support and analgesia are helpful. Antibiotic treatment should continue for at least 2 weeks or until the inflammation has subsided. If suppuration occurs, drainage is necessary.

Chronic disease

Chronic non-tuberculous epididymitis usually follows the failure of resolution of an acute episode of epididymitis. Patients typically complain of intermittent episodes of discomfort and the epididymis feels thickened and tender. Treatment involves use of antibiotics (usually quinolones or doxycycline) and anti-inflammatory agents for 4–6 weeks. Epididymectomy or orchidectomy can be considered if there is no resolution although some patients continue to suffer from pain despite such surgery (Summary box 79.8).

Summary box 79.8

Acute epididymo-orchitis

- In young men usually arises secondary to a sexually transmitted genital infection
- In older men usually arises secondary to urinary infection
- May be a complication of catheterisation or instrumentation of the urinary tract
- May need aggressive treatment with parenteral antibiotics

TUBERCULOUS EPIDIDYMO-ORCHITIS

Chronic tuberculous epididymo-orchitis usually begins insidiously. The frequency with which the lower pole of the epididymis is involved first indicates that the infection is retrograde from a tuberculous focus in the seminal vesicles.

Clinical features

Typically, there is a firm, uncomfortable discrete swelling of the lower pole of the epididymis. The disease progresses until the whole epididymis is firm and craggy behind a normal-feeling testis. There is a lax secondary hydrocele in 30 per cent of cases, and a characteristic beading of the vas may be apparent as a result of subepithelial tubercles. The seminal vesicles feel indurated and swollen. In neglected cases, a tuberculous 'cold' abscess forms, which may discharge. The body of the testis may be uninvolved for years, but the contralateral epididymis often becomes diseased. In two-thirds of cases, there is evidence of renal tuberculosis or previous disease. Otherwise, patients typically appear healthy.

The urine and semen should be examined repeatedly for tubercle bacilli in all patients with chronic epididymo-orchitis. A chest x-ray should be performed as should imaging of the upper urinary tract. Ultrasound will demonstrate a thickened epididymis.

Treatment

Secondary tuberculous epididymitis may resolve when the primary focus is treated.

Treatment with anti-tuberculous drugs is less effective in genital tuberculosis than in urinary tuberculosis. If resolution does not occur within two months, epididymectomy or orchidectomy is advisable. A course of anti-tuberculous chemotherapy should be completed even if there is no evidence of disease elsewhere.

ORCHITIS

Mumps orchitis, which is the most common form of orchitis, develops in 20–30 per cent of post-pubertal patients with a mumps virus infection and it usually develops as the parotid swelling is waning. Evidence of IgM antibodies in the serum supports the diagnosis. The main complication is testicular atrophy, which may cause infertility if the condition is bilateral. Partial testicular atrophy is associated with persistent testicular pain.

Syphilitic orchitis is now uncommon. It can cause bilateral orchitis (which is a feature of congenital syphilis), interstitial fibrosis, which causes painless destruction of the testis or rarely it may lead to a gumma of the testis, which presents as a unilateral slowly growing painless swelling. The latter presentation may be difficult to distinguish from a neoplasm without surgical exploration. Diagnosis is confirmed by serology.

TUMOURS OF THE TESTES

Testicular cancer represents around 1–1.5 per cent of male neoplasms and there is clear evidence of an increased incidence of these tumours in the past 30 years. The vast majority are germ cell tumours and the peak incidence of seminomas is in the fourth decade of life with the non-seminomatous germ cell tumours being more common in the third decade of life. They are the most common form of tumour in young men. Risk factors include a history of testicular maldescent, a history of a contralateral testicular tumour and Klinefelter's syndrome.

Classification and pathology

Tumours of the testis are classified according to their predominant cellular type:

- germ cell tumours (90–95% per cent) (these include seminoma, embryonal cell carcinoma, yolk sac tumor, teratoma, and choriocarcinoma);
- interstitial tumours (1–2 per cent) (these include Leydig cell tumours);
- lymphoma (3–7 per cent);
- other tumours (1–2 per cent).

Seminoma

A seminoma typically has a cut surface which is homogeneous and pinkish cream in colour. It appears to compress neighbouring testicular tissue (Figure 79.14). It consists of oval cells with clear cytoplasm and large, rounded nuclei with prominent acidophilic nucleoli. Sheets of cells resembling spermatocytes are separated by a fine fibrous stroma. Active lymphocytic infiltration of the tumour suggests a good host response and a better prognosis. There are two histological variants, one with a more anaplastic appearance and another that is characterised by cells which closely resemble different phases of maturing spermatogonia (spermatocytic seminoma).

Seminomas metastasise mainly via the lymphatics (Figure 79.15) and haematogenous spread is uncommon. The lymphatic drainage of the testes is to the para-aortic lymph nodes near the origin of the gonadal vessels. The contralateral para-aortic lymph nodes are sometimes involved by tumour spread, but the inguinal lymph nodes are affected only if the scrotal skin is involved.

Non-seminomatous germ cell tumours (NSGCT)

These tumours may be tiny but can reach the size of a coconut. The smaller tumours may not even distort the tunica albuginea (Figure 79.16). The usual type of teratoma is yellowish in colour with cystic spaces containing gelatinous fluid (Figure 79.17). There are a number of histological types of non-seminomatous germ cell tumours (NSGCT), which may coexist within a single tumour:

- **Embryonal carcinoma**. Highly malignant tumours that occasionally invade cord structures.
- **Yolk sac tumour**. Tumours with this component secrete alpha fetoprotein (AFP).
- **Choriocarcinoma**. Often produces human chorionic gonadotrophin (HCG). This is a highly malignant tumour that metastasizes early via both the lymphatics and the bloodstream.
- **Teratoma**. These tumours contain more than one cell type with components derived from ectoderm, endoderm, and mesoderm. Tumours may range from 'mature' with

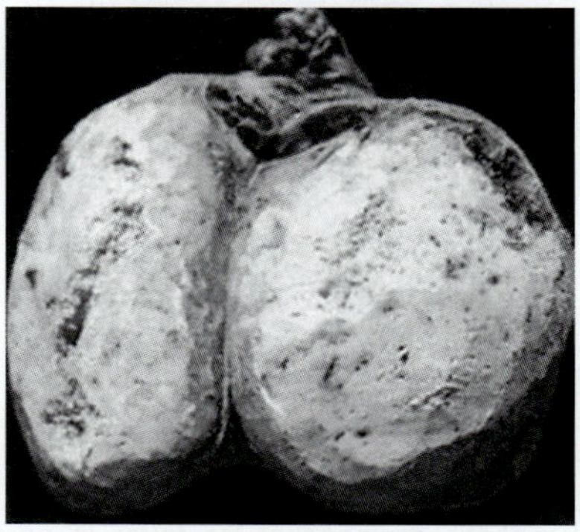

Figure 79.14 Seminoma of the testis.

well-differentiated tissue elements to 'immature' with undifferentiated primitive tissues. All can metastasise.

Interstitial cell tumours

Interstitial cell tumours arise from Leydig or Sertoli cells. A Leydig cell tumour masculinises; a Sertoli cell tumour feminises. They are typically small well circumscribed tumours with a yellow cut surface. Microscopically, the cells are usually uniform and closely packed. Approximately 10 per cent are malignant.

Most prepubertal tumours (which account for around 25 per cent of cases) produce androgens, which cause sexual precocity including prominent external genitalia, suprapubic hair growth and a deep masculinised voice. Regression of the symptoms after orchidectomy may be incomplete. Most post-pubertal interstitial cell tumours produce feminising hormones leading to gynaecomastia, erectile dysfunction, loss of libido and azoospermia.

Clinical features

Usually the patient presents with a painless testicular lump. A sensation of heaviness can occur if the testis is two or three times its normal size, but only a minority of patients experience pain. In a few cases, an episode of trauma calls attention to the swelling. Some cases may simulate epididymo-orchitis and rarely some patients present with severe pain and acute enlargement of the testis because of haemorrhage into the tumour. Such cases can occasionally mimic testicular torsion.

Rarely, the predominant symptoms are those of metastatic disease. Intra-abdominal disease may cause abdominal or lumbar pain and the mass may be discovered in the epigastrium. Lung metastases are usually silent but they can cause chest pain, dyspnoea and haemoptysis in the later stages of the disease. The primary tumour may not have been noticed by the patient, and indeed may be so tiny that it can be detected only by ultrasonography (Figure 79.16).

On examination, there is an intratesticular solid mass. If present, a lax secondary hydrocele does not usually obscure the underlying tumour. The epididymis becomes more difficult to feel when it is flattened or incorporated in the growth. The vas is never thickened and rectal examination is normal. Around 5 per cent of cases have gynaecomastia (mainly the NSGCT). Metastatic disease is rarely apparent clinically and is more usually identified by formal staging investigations. In 1–2 per cent of cases, the tumour is bilateral at the time of diagnosis.

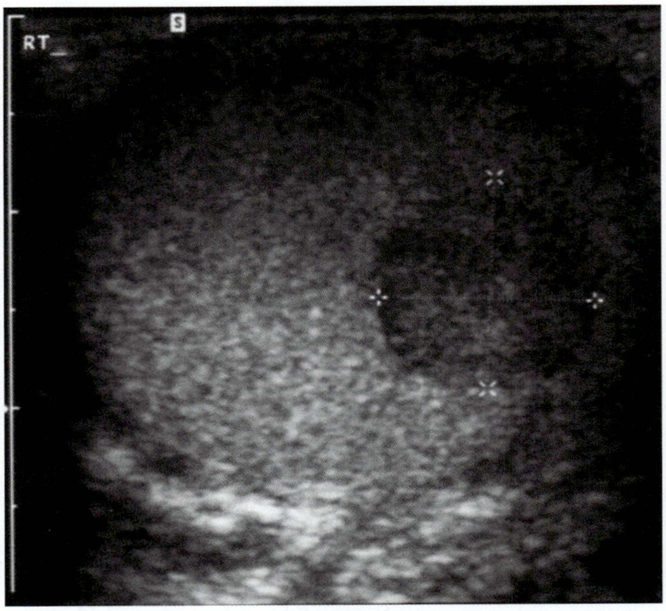

Figure 79.16 Ultrasound of a small intratesticular tumour with minimal distortion of the tunica albuginea.

Investigation and staging

The diagnosis is confirmed by ultrasound scanning of the testis (Figure 79.18) which is also able to assess the contralateral testis. It is a mandatory test in all suspected cases of testicular tumour.

In confirmed cases, staging is an essential step in planning treatment. Blood is taken prior to orchidectomy to measure the levels of tumour markers which are raised in around 50 per cent of cases. A rise in AFP is seen in around 50–70 per cent

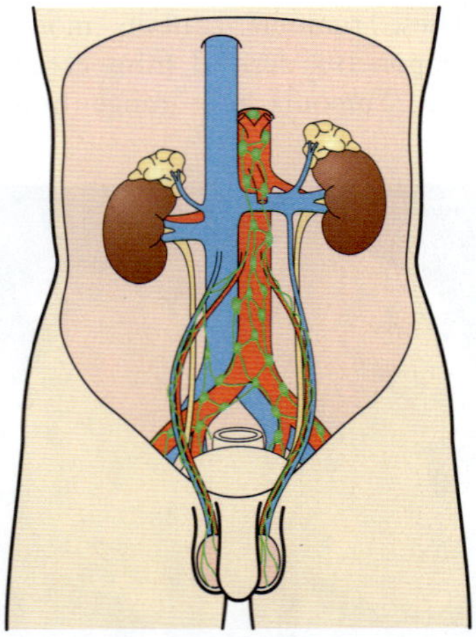

Figure 79.15 Lymphatic drainage of the testes to para-aortic lymph nodes.

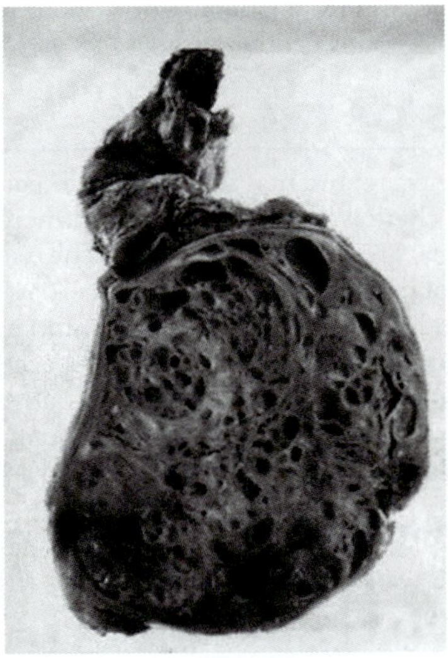

Figure 79.17 Teratoma of the testis – note the solid and cystic areas (courtesy of Dr Keith Simpson, London).

Franz von Leydig, 1821–1908, Professor of Histology successively at Würzburg, Tübingen, and Bonn, Germany.
Enrico Sertoli, 1842–1910, Professor of Experimental Physiology, Milan, Italy.

of NSGCTs and a rise in HCG is seen in 40–60 per cent of NSGCTs and around 30 per cent of seminomas. When raised, these markers are used to monitor the response to treatment. The mean serum half-lives of AFP and HCG are 5–7 days and 2–3 days, respectively, and reassessment of the markers following orchidectomy can indicate whether all the tumour tissue has been removed.

While a chest x-ray will occasionally demonstrate the 'classical' cannon ball metastases (Figure 79.19), computed tomography (CT) of chest and abdomen has taken over as the most useful means of detecting metastatic disease and for monitoring the response to therapy. Such imaging is usually undertaken after the affected testis has been removed.

Staging of testicular tumours

While TNM staging is the most widely used system for the staging of testicular cancer, the older staging system of stages 1–IV is still considered valuable in determining the treatment options:

The stages are:

- Stage I: the tumour is confined to the testis;
- Stage II: nodal disease is present but is confined to nodes below the diaphragm;
- Stage III: nodal disease is present above the diaphragm;
- Stage IV: nonlymphatic metastatic disease (most typically within the lungs) (Summary box 79.9).

Summary box 79.9

Testicular tumours

- A solid testicular lump that cannot be felt separately from the testis may be a malignant tumour
- Lymphatic spread is to the para-aortic lymph nodes
- Ultrasound is a mandatory investigation in all cases of suspected testicular tumour
- Tumour markers (AFP and HCG) should be measured prior to orchidectomy

Treatment

Scrotal exploration and orchidectomy for suspected testicular tumour

The orchidectomy is undertaken via an inguinal incision. The spermatic cord is displayed by dividing the external oblique aponeurosis and a soft clamp is placed across the cord to stop dissemination of malignant cells as the testis is mobilised into the wound. If necessary, the testis should be bisected along its anterior convexity to examine its internal structure. If there is a tumour, the cord should be double transfixed and divided at the level of the internal inguinal ring and the testis removed.

Management by staging and histological diagnosis (after orchidectomy)

The treatment of patients with testicular tumours is usually successful, even in cases that are advanced at presentation. This largely reflects the excellent response of these tumours to platinum-based chemotherapy and (for seminomatous tumours) to radiotherapy. Indeed in recent years the emphasis of clinical trials has been focused upon the identification of those patients who do not need chemotherapy, and who therefore will escape the side effects of treatment.

Stage I tumours

Seminomas are radiosensitive and for many years adjuvant radiotherapy to the para-aortic nodes was the mainstay of treatment for stage I disease. Some years ago, the excellent response to platinum-based chemotherapy led to chemotherapy being introduced for most men with stage 1 seminoma. However, current practice uses CT and tumour marker-based surveillance protocols with chemotherapy being reserved for men who demonstrate relapse.

NSGCTs are not radiosensitive, but they are highly sensitive to combination chemotherapy with bleomycin, etoposide and cis-platinum (so called BEP chemotherapy). Some good prognosis NSGCTs can be managed by surveillance protocols (using regular CT scanning and tumour marker measurement) with the more high risk cases receiving chemotherapy.

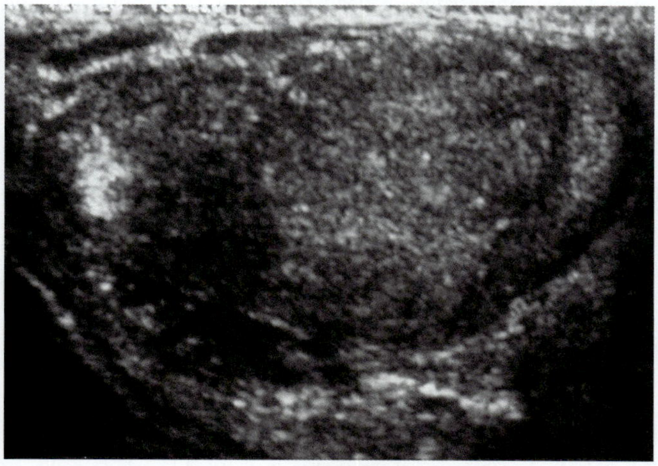

Figure 79.18 Testicular ultrasound: the homogeneous tissue of the testicular teratoma on the left of the image produces multiple ultrasound reflections.

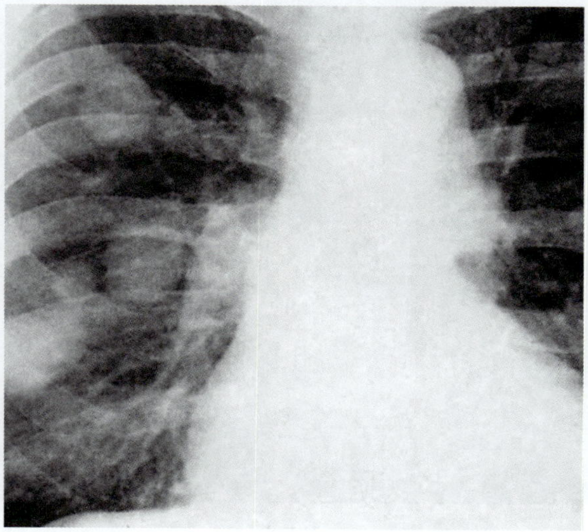

Figure 79.19 Cannon ball metastases from carcinoma of the testis.

Stage II–IV tumours

Combination BEP chemotherapy is the mainstay of treatment for stages II–IV seminoma and NSGCT. Retroperitoneal lymph node dissection is sometimes needed in some cases of NSGCT when retroperitoneal masses remain after chemotherapy (Figure 79.20). The tissue removed may contain only necrotic tissue, but some patients have foci of mature teratoma or active malignancy. The operation can be formidable if the tumour mass is large, and retrograde ejaculation is likely unless steps are taken to preserve the sympathetic outflow to the bladder neck.

Prognosis

The prognosis of testicular tumours depends on several factors including the histological type and the stage at presentation. For seminoma, if there are no metastases, 90–95 per cent of patients will be alive five years after diagnosis. If there are poor prognostic features, the survival rate drops to around 70 per cent. For NSGCTs, a five-year survival rate of more than 90 per cent is achievable in patients with good prognosis tumours while for more advanced tumours the five-year survival rate is about 60 per cent (Summary box 79.10).

Summary box 79.10

Testis tumour staging and treatment

- Tumour markers help to make the diagnosis and to follow the response to treatment
- CT scanning of chest and abdomen is central to the staging of testicular tumours
- Testicular tumours are extremely sensitive to platinum-based chemotherapy
- Prognosis is excellent when the patient is treated with combination chemotherapy in a cancer centre

TESTICULAR TUMOURS IN CHILDREN

These are usually anaplastic teratomas. They occur before the age of three years and are often rapidly fatal.

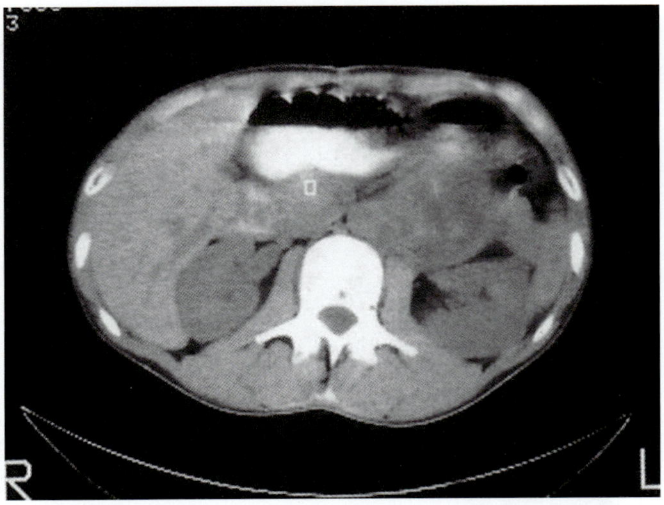

Figure 79.20 Computed tomography scan showing a large residual retroperitoneal mass after chemotherapy.

TUMOURS OF THE EPIDIDYMIS

These may be benign mesothelioma or malignant sarcoma or secondary carcinoma. They are extremely rare but should not be forgotten when the patient presents with a non-cystic lump in the epididymis.

THE SCROTUM

Fournier's gangrene

Fournier's gangrene is an uncommon and nasty condition (Figure 79.21) of infective origin that is characterised by sudden scrotal inflammation, with rapid onset of gangrene leading to exposure of the scrotal contents. Although it can occur in conjunction with sepsis of the testis, epididymis or perianal region, an obvious cause is absent in over half the cases. It can arise following minor injuries or procedures in the perineal area, such as a bruise, scratch, urethral dilatation, injection of haemorrhoids or opening of a periurethral abscess. Many patients have concurrent illnesses that diminish their defences, most notably diabetes mellitus and alcoholism.

There is a mixed infection of aerobic and anaerobic bacteria in a fulminating inflammation of the subcutaneous tissues, which results in an obliterative arteritis of the arterioles to the scrotal skin which in turn results in gangrene. The condition can spread rapidly to involve the fascia and skin of the penis, perineum and abdominal wall.

Clinical features

There is sudden pain in the scrotum associated with prostration, pallor and pyrexia. Cellulitis spreads rapidly (within hours) and progresses to necrosis until the entire scrotal and penile coverings slough, leaving the testes exposed but healthy.

Treatment

Treatment of a case of Fournier's gangrene is a surgical emergency. Urgent wide surgical excision of the dead and infected tissue is essential. This should be accompanied by intravenous antibiotics. Supportive care is essential, because the patients often become severely septic. Early review of the wounds is helpful to confirm that all dead tissue has been removed, and if the patient survives the acute episode, skin grafting is often necessary. Despite best therapy, mortality rates as high as 50 per cent are often reported (Summary box 79.11).

Summary box 79.11

Fournier's gangrene

- Fournier's gangrene requires early and aggressive treatment if the patient is to survive
- Treatment involves urgent surgical debridement of necrotic tissue in combination with intravenous antibiotics

Filarial elephantiasis of the scrotum

Filarial elephantiasis of the scrotum is caused by obstruction of the pelvic lymphatics by worms of which *Wuchereria bancrofti* accounts for 90 per cent of cases. The condition is common in the tropics and is transmitted by mosquitoes. It is often

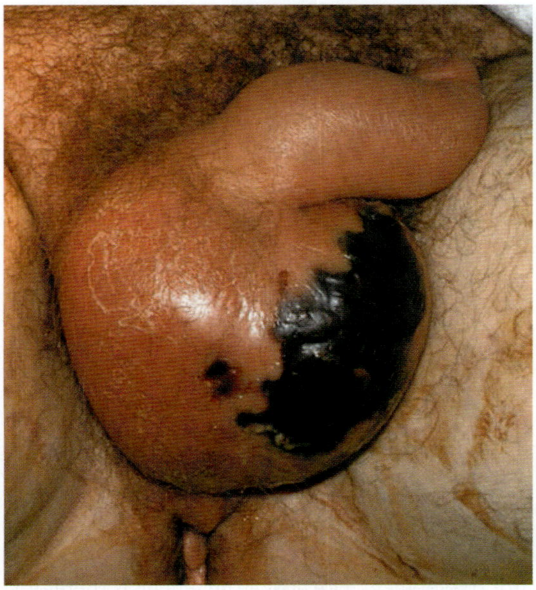

Figure 79.21 Fournier's gangrene with an area of necrotic skin overlying an area of scrotal inflammation.

accompanied by superadded infection and lymphangitis, resulting in swelling of the genital skin and skin of the lower limbs. In longstanding cases, the enormously swollen scrotum may bury the penis (Figure 79.22). Associated symptoms and signs include fever, epididymitis, hydrocele and chyluria. The diagnosis is usually made clinically, although immunological testing can be helpful.

Medical treatment involves the use of diethylcarbamazine (DEC), ivermectin and albendazole, with the exact regime depending upon geographical location. Surgical treatment is rarely helpful, although a range of procedures has been devised to remove redundant skin and to reconstruct the enlarged scrotum.

Non-filarial elephantiasis

Elephantiasis can occur in the absence of filariasis, most notably in sub-Saharan Africa. Non-filarial elephantiasis can result from fibrosis of the lymphatics caused by lymphogranuloma venereum, but in many cases it is thought to arise as a consequence of persistent contact with irritant soils.

Sebaceous cysts

Sebaceous cysts are common in the scrotal skin. They are usually small and multiple (Figure 79.23).

Carcinoma of the scrotum

Chimney sweeps cancer was the first reported occupational cancer (described by Percival Pott in 1775). It is a rare cancer that has also been seen in other workers who come into contact with oil and coal products. Animal studies suggest that aromatic cyclic hydrocarbons are the aetiological factor. Nowadays, this tumour is rarely associated with any obvious aetiological factor. Unlike carcinoma of the penis, carcinoma of the scrotum is almost unknown in India and Asiatic countries.

The growth starts as a wart or ulcer (Figure 79.24) and as it grows it may involve the testis. The tumour should be excised

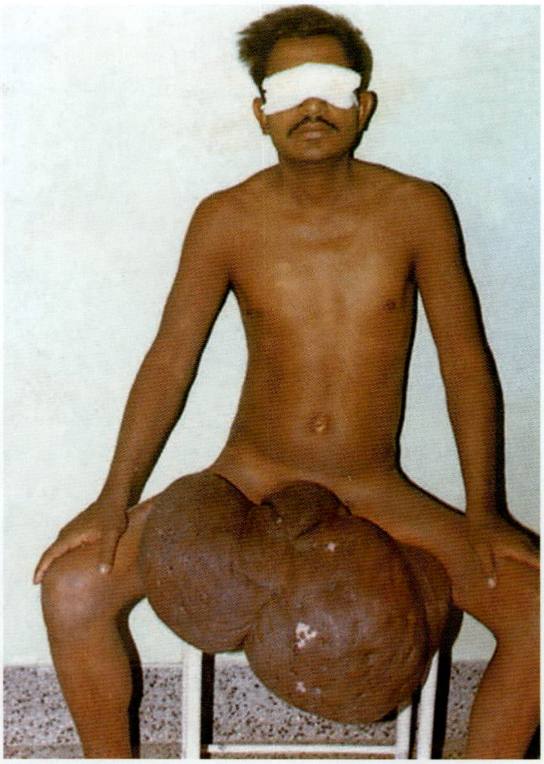

Figure 79.22 Elephantiasis of the scrotum burying the penis (courtesy of Mr S Bhattacharjee, Lucknow, India).

with a margin of healthy skin. The management of the inguinal nodes parallels the management of penile cancer and if nodal enlargement does not settle with antibiotics following treatment of the primary, then a bilateral groin dissection is indicated.

MALE FACTOR INFERTILITY

For couples of unknown fertility status, approximately 15 per cent are unable to achieve a pregnancy within one year. The inability to conceive may be due to female factor infertility, male factor infertility or a combination of these two factors and approximately 20 per cent of cases of infertility are caused entirely by the male factor.

Aetiology

The two main causes of male factor infertility are testicular causes and vasal or epididymal obstruction. A few cases reflect endocrinological abnormalities, such as hypogonadism or hyperprolactinaemia.

Percival Pott, 1714–1788, surgeon, St Bartholomew's Hospital, London, UK, described the 'Puffy tumour' in 1760. In 1756 he sustained a broken leg after a fall from his horse. As he lay on the ground, he sent a servant to buy a door which acted as a stretcher. While his surgeons were contemplating amputating his leg, he persuaded them to splint the leg instead as a result of which he recovered completely. Although some think that Pott's fracture of the ankle was described after this injury of his, it is not so. He sustained a compound fracture of the femur. Nevertheless, history can be controversial. Other authorities feel that Pott actually suffered a fracture-dislocation of the ankle from whence the fracture gets its name. Pott was the first to link an environmental factor to the aetiology of cancer when he demonstrated that chimney sweeps developed squamous cell scrotal cancer. In those days, the chimney sweep's apprentice climbed up inside the chimney.

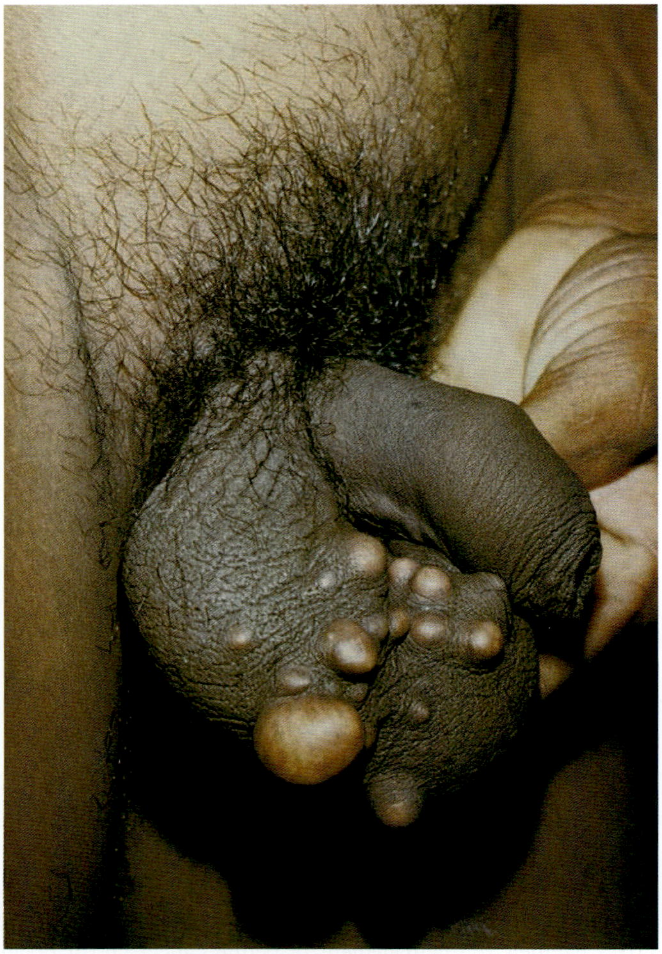

Figure 79.23 Sebaceous cysts of the scrotum (courtesy of Dr R Kaje MS, Jipmer, India).

Testicular causes include chromosomal problems (e.g. Klinefelter's syndrome), microdeletions of the Y chromosome, cryptorchidism, mumps orchitis, drugs and radiation damage. In most cases, however, the cause is unclear. In these cases, there may be reduced numbers of sperm in the ejaculate (oligozoospermia) or a complete absence of sperm in the ejaculate (azoospermia). Obstructive causes include congenital absence of the vasa (often in association with cystic fibrosis), surgical damage to the vasa, epididymitis and azoospermia is inevitable in these cases.

Assessment and investigation

Given the interplay between male and female factors, the man should not be investigated in isolation from his female partner. A careful history is the mainstay of the assessment with a careful search for aetiological factors. Physical examination is usually normal, but occasionally the testes may feel small (suggestive of a testicular cause), the vasa may be absent, there may be evidence of endocrine abnormalities (gynaecomastia or abnormal hair distribution) or there may be a varicocele. The relation of any varicocele to the infertility is controversial and treatment is not usually indicated.

The female should also be assessed. It is important to remember that female fertility declines from the age of 35 years in a way

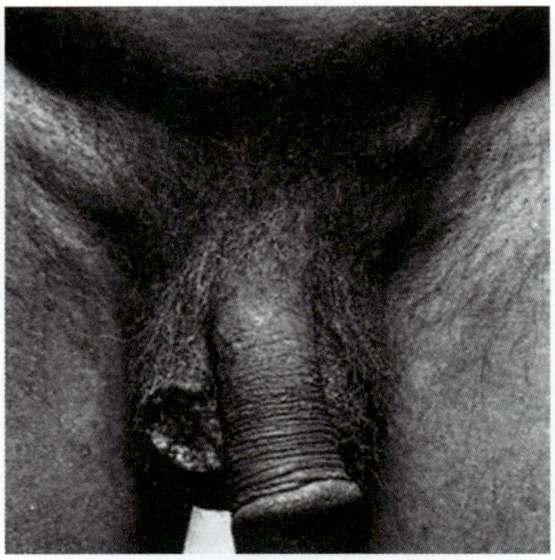

Figure 79.24 Carcinoma of the scrotum with bilateral enlargement of the inguinal lymph nodes (courtesy of Department of Medical Photography, Cardiff Royal Infirmary, Cardiff, UK).

that is not true of men. The age of the female is therefore important and the regularity of menstruation should be confirmed either by temperature testing or by endocrinological testing.

The assessment of the male includes semen analysis, which should be tested within 2 hours of the semen being produced. Two or three samples should be tested. The volume of the ejaculate, the numbers of sperm, their motility and the percentage of abnormal or damaged sperm are all predictive of the male fertility. An endocrine screen should be performed including serum testosterone, prolactin, FSH and LH.

Treatment

Sperm counts of less than 20 million sperm per mL are defined as oligozoospermia. If there is a reversible cause, it should be treated. However, in many cases, some form of assisted conception is required.

Azoospermia (the complete absence of sperm from the ejaculate) is either due to obstruction of the pathway of spermatozoa from the testis to the ejaculatory ducts or due to severe testicular failure. In the latter, the serum FSH is typically raised, while in obstructive cases, the FSH is typically normal. If there is doubt as to the cause, then testicular biopsy is mandated to check for the presence of spermatogenesis combined with vasography to assess the presence and location of any obstructive lesion. If the site of the obstruction can be identified, it may be possible to perform a bypass operation. Unfortunately, even in the best hands, the results of epididymovasostomy are poor.

Assisted conception including *in vitro* fertilisation (IVF) and intracytoplasmic sperm injection (ICSI) has revolutionised the management of male factor infertility regardless of the cause of the problem. In ICSI, spermatozoa harvested from the ejaculate, by aspiration of the epididymis or even from testicular biopsy, can be injected *in vitro* into ova obtained from the mother. Embryos are then transferred into the mother's uterus at the four- to six-cell stage (Summary box 79.12).

Vasectomy for sterilisation

Vasectomy for sterilisation is a common and effective contraceptive procedure. It should be undertaken only after the couple has been carefully counselled. Both partners need to know that the operation is performed to make the man permanently

> **Summary box 79.12**
>
> **Male infertility**
>
> - Atrophy of the testis is associated with raised levels of FSH in the blood
> - Testicular biopsy will show whether azoospermia is a result of obstruction or failure of sperm production
> - If spermatozoa can be harvested they can be used in ICSI with a fertility rate of around 30 per cent

sterile. They should be warned that normal contraceptive precautions should continue until the success of the operation is confirmed by semen analysis performed 12–16 weeks after surgery. They should also be warned of the possibility of spontaneous recanalisation, which may restore fertility unexpectedly and of the possibility of chronic testicular pain which may occur in up to 5 per cent of men.

Vasectomy is easily and painlessly performed under local anaesthetic. The vasa are delivered through tiny bilateral scrotal incisions or through a single midline scrotal incision. For medico-legal reasons, it is wise to remove a segment of each vas to prove that it has been successfully divided. Burying the cut ends or turning them back on themselves helps to prevent them rejoining.

Reversal of vasectomy may not restore fertility even if technically successful because of damage to the testis secondary to the vasectomy. Although patency rates of 80 per cent or more are commonly reported, successful fertility rates are much lower and diminish with increasing delay from the time of vasectomy (Summary box 79.13).

> **Summary box 79.13**
>
> **Vasectomy**
>
> Counselling before vasectomy should include mention that:
>
> - The operation is not immediately effective and that contraceptive precautions should be continued until there have been two negative semen analyses
> - The procedure should be considered irreversible
> - Spontaneous recanalisation is rare, but can occur
> - There is a risk of chronic scrotal pain postoperatively

FURTHER READING

Blandy JP, Kaisary AV. *Lecture notes: urology*, 6th edn. Oxford: Blackwell, 2007.

Wein AJ, Kavoussi LR, Novick AC, Partin AW. *Campbell–Walsh urology*, 10th edn. Oxford: Elsevier, 2010.

CHAPTER

80

Gynaecology

LEARNING OBJECTIVES

To understand:

- Pelvic anatomy and reproductive physiology
- The common causes of vaginal bleeding and acute pain in early pregnancy
- The surgical management of acute pelvic inflammatory disease, endometriosis, uterine fibroids and ovarian tumours

ANATOMY

The female external genitalia are described as the vulva, which is bordered by the mons veneris anteriorly and the labiocrural folds posterolaterally. The introitus tends to be open in parous women, but otherwise appears closed by the apposing labia majora. The labia minora are folds of skin that fuse anteriorly to form the clitoris, which contains erectile tissue similar to the penis. The fourchette is the posterior part of the introitus, which must stretch considerably to allow the delivery of a baby.

The vagina is an elastic, distensible tube, approximately 10 cm long, passing upwards and backwards from the introitus. The cervix protrudes into the vault of the vagina, dividing it into anterior, posterior and lateral fornices. Pelvic structures can be felt in the posterior and lateral fornices on bimanual examination, as the vaginal vault sits just below the pouch of Douglas (the area at the bottom of the pelvic cavity bordered by the uterus anteriorly and rectum posteriorly). The urethra and bladder neck sit above the anterior wall of the vagina; the perineal body and rectum behind the posterior wall (Figure 80.1).

The uterus, consisting of a body and a cervix, is a pear-shaped structure that is flattened anteroposteriorly giving its cavity a flat, triangular shape. The uterus is supported partly by ligaments attached to the cervix (transverse cervical, pubocervical and uterosacral) consisting of condensed connective tissue. The cervix is a canal, approximately 2 cm long, connecting the external os, which can be seen on speculum examination, to the internal os, where the cervix enters the uterine cavity. The length of the uterine cavity, including the cervical canal, is approximately 6 cm in nulliparous women and approximately 8 cm in parous women. The walls of the uterus are 1–2 cm thick and composed of muscular tissue (myometrium). The uterine cavity is lined with endometrium, a tissue that undergoes cyclical changes in response to ovarian hormones (see below under Reproductive physiology).

At the uterine fundus, on either side, are the cornua by which the uterus is connected to each Fallopian tube. These are thin, muscular tubes, approximately 10 cm long, which connect the peritoneal and uterine cavities. They are divided into four parts: intramural, isthmus, ampulla and fimbriated opening, which pick up the oocyte following its release at the time of ovulation. The tubes are very narrow in the isthmic and intramural parts but they widen in the ampullary region. Each tube is contained within the upper part of the broad ligament, a fold of peritoneum on either side of the uterus, which also contains blood vessels and the round and ovarian ligaments. The fimbriated opening and part of the ampulla, however, are free and closely associated with the ovary on either side. The ovaries are flattened, ovoid structures, approximately 3–4 cm long, suspended from the back of the broad ligament on either side of the pelvis. The ovarian blood vessels are contained within the infundibulopelvic ligaments, which are continuations of the broad ligaments to the pelvic brim on either side.

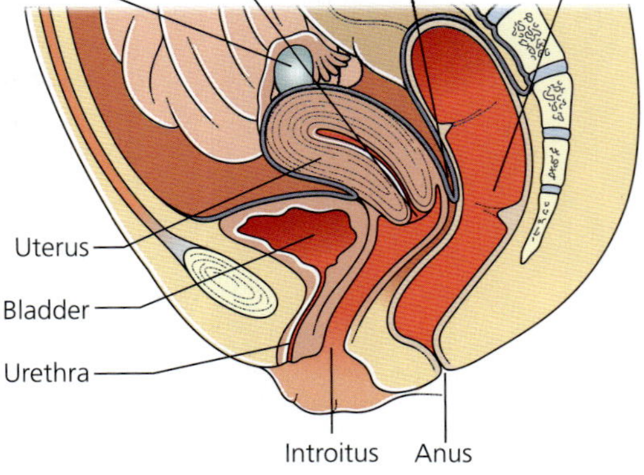

Figure 80.1 Female anatomy.

James Douglas, 1675–1742, anatomist and male midwife, London, UK.
Gabriele Falloppio, (Falloppius), 1523–1563, Professor of Anatomy, Surgery and Botany, Padua, Italy.

The cervix is located in the centre of the bony cavity of the pelvis and the uterus can be pivoted around this point. It is usually angled forwards (anteverted) at approximately 90° relative to the vagina. It is usually freely mobile but filling of the bladder or changes in position may rotate it backwards. In some women, the uterus is retroverted, either because of weak ligaments or because the uterus becomes adherent as the result of a disease process such as endometriosis. The uterus may also be angled forward (anteflexed) relative to the cervix when anteverted or backwards (retroflexed) when retroverted, in which case it can usually be felt in the pouch of Douglas on vaginal examination. The most common cause of an enlarged uterus, aside from pregnancy, is the presence of fibroids (benign tumours of the myometrium) growing inside or outside the uterus. When fibroids are present, the overall size of the uterus is described in terms of weeks of pregnancy as it expands forwards and upwards into the abdominal cavity with increasing gestational age.

REPRODUCTIVE PHYSIOLOGY

The menstrual cycle is under the control of circulating hormones produced within the hypothalamic–pituitary–ovarian axis. Thus, gonadotrophin-releasing hormone (GnRH) produced in the hypothalamus stimulates the pituitary to produce follicle stimulating hormone (FSH) and luteinising hormone (LH), which in turn control how the ovary produces an oocyte on a monthly basis and also the hormones oestrogen and progesterone. These hormones have an effect on many structures in the body, but principally on the endometrium, which prepares itself to receive a fertilised egg during the course of the menstrual cycle. In the first half (proliferative or follicular phase) of the cycle, following menstruation, the endometrium starts to regrow or proliferate in response to oestrogen produced by the growing ovarian follicle. The endometrium becomes thick and spongy during this phase of the cycle, associated with considerable angiogenesis.

Ovulation occurs at mid-cycle, on approximately day 14 (day 1 of the cycle is defined as the first day of menstruation), following which the follicle is transformed into the corpus luteum. In the second half (secretory or luteal phase) of the cycle, the endometrium thickens even more in response to the hormone progesterone, produced by the corpus luteum (Figure 80.2).

If fertilisation occurs, the fertilised egg is transported along a Fallopian tube into the uterine cavity and then implants in the endometrium. If fertilisation does not occur or if the fertilised egg fails to implant, the endometrium is shed and menstruation occurs. Bleeding (a 'period') tends to last for 4 days, but can range from 2–6 days. Typically, about 40 mL of blood is lost during each period; if the bleeding is heavy (i.e. greater than 80 mL), blood clots may form. The whole process then starts again in the next menstrual cycle.

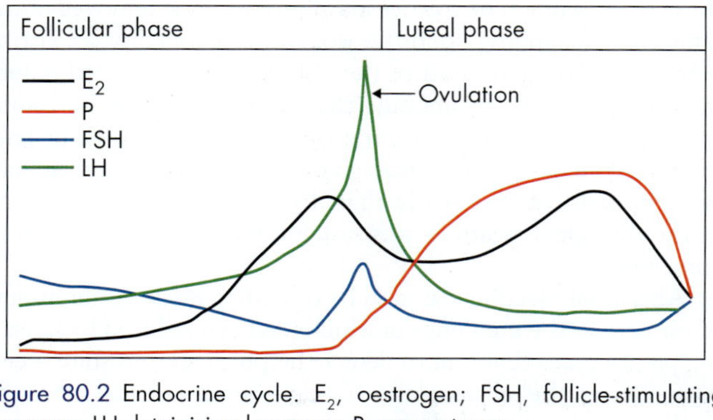

Figure 80.2 Endocrine cycle. E_2, oestrogen; FSH, follicle-stimulating hormone; LH, luteinising hormone; P, progesterone.

If fertilisation does occur, the duration of the pregnancy (gestational age) is traditionally calculated from the first day of the last menstrual period (LMP); however, ovulation may occur earlier or considerably later than day 14 or the woman's recollection of the date of the LMP may be incorrect, which means that calculating gestational age on the basis of the LMP alone may be inaccurate. This explains the alternative practice of calculating gestational age using ultrasound measurements of fetal size.

VAGINAL BLEEDING IN EARLY PREGNANCY

A miscarriage is defined as the spontaneous loss of an intrauterine pregnancy at less than 24 weeks' gestation. A miscarriage usually starts with painless vaginal bleeding, at which point it is defined as a threatened miscarriage. The bleeding may then become heavier with associated uterine cramps, at which point it becomes an inevitable miscarriage. Blood clots and products of conception (i.e. fetal and placental tissue) are passed through the cervical os until the uterus is emptied (defined as a complete miscarriage). Sometimes, not all the products of conception are passed spontaneously (defined as an incomplete miscarriage) and the woman may require an evacuation of retained products of conception (ERPC) to remove what is left of the pregnancy. The operation involves passing a plastic suction curette through the cervix into the uterine cavity. The current (2006) Royal College of Obstetricians and Gynaecologists (RCOG) recommendations are for ERPC to be considered if there is persistent excessive bleeding, haemodynamic instability, evidence of infected retained tissue or suspected gestational trophoblastic disease. Serious operative complications, which are fortunately rare, include uterine perforation with, possibly, intra-abdominal trauma (e.g. bowel damage), cervical tears and haemorrhage.

In the case of a miscarriage, on vaginal examination there is typically no cervical excitation (pain on moving the cervix) or tenderness in the vaginal fornices, which are signs associated with an ectopic pregnancy. The uterus feels the right size or smaller for the gestational age. The internal cervical os, by definition, is closed if the miscarriage is threatened or complete and open if the miscarriage is inevitable or incomplete. If the fetus has not developed (defined as a missed abortion) the uterus will feel small for the gestational age and there may have been no bleeding, in which case the os will be closed. In such circumstances, the os will need to be dilated before performing the ERPC.

An ultrasound scan is usually performed to determine whether there is a viable intrauterine pregnancy present. It may not be possible to determine the precise location of the pregnancy because the woman has had a complete miscarriage, the pregnancy is not sufficiently advanced or she has an ectopic pregnancy that is not visible on ultrasound. For these reasons, it is important to establish the gestational age as accurately as possible, on the basis of the LMP and the length/regularity of the menstrual cycle, as well as with any other relevant information, e.g. fertility treatment. It is still not uncommon, especially in early pregnancy, to make the diagnosis of a miscarriage on clinical grounds alone, for example in the case of:

- heavy vaginal bleeding with clots and associated uterine cramps;
- no history of abdominal pain;
- no cervical excitation or tenderness in the vaginal fornices;
- no risk factors for an ectopic pregnancy, e.g. a past history of pelvic inflammatory disease (PID) or previous tubal surgery.

Vaginal bleeding in early pregnancy may also result from a local cause such as a cervical lesion (which may first manifest as bleeding after intercourse) or, rarely, trauma.

VAGINAL BLEEDING IN THE NON-PREGNANT STATE

Bleeding in the non-pregnant state may occur at the time of an expected menstrual period, between periods (intermenstrual bleeding) or after intercourse (post-coital bleeding). It may also occur after surgical instrumentation of the uterus and/or cervix, including insertion of an intrauterine contraceptive device (IUCD). The principal causes of these types of bleeding are shown in Table 80.1.

The mainstay of management is to identify and treat pathology (except in women <40 years old with heavy, menstrual periods in whom pathology is very rarely found; these women tend to be treated symptomatically). This usually involves ultrasound examination and an endometrial biopsy, either under direct vision at hysteroscopy or blindly with a Pipelle. The indications for endometrial biopsy are shown in Summary box 80.1.

Summary box 80.1

Indications for endometrial biopsy

Endometrial biopsy should be considered in the following women:

- All women >40 years old with excessively heavy, irregular or frequent bleeding
- Younger women with major risk factors for endometrial hyperplasia/cancer:
  - Polycystic ovarian syndrome
  - Obesity
  - Tamoxifen treatment
- Unopposed oestrogen therapy
- Family history of endometrial/colon cancer, especially hereditary non-polyposis colorectal cancer (Lynch syndrome)
- Younger women who fail to respond to conventional treatment

Women taking tamoxifen – the selective oestrogen receptor modulator used in breast cancer treatment – represent a special group because the drug can induce endometrial polyps, hyperplasia, cancer and, rarely, uterine sarcomas, which are much more aggressive. Tamoxifen treatment results in a doubling of the risk of endometrial cancer after one to two years of treatment and a quadrupling after five years. The relationship is time-dependent and dose-independent and the risk does not decrease after stopping treatment. There is no clear consensus regarding the need for screening and which method to use; the alternative, more common, approach is to investigate only those women who develop post-menopausal bleeding with tamoxifen use. Aromatase inhibitors such as anastrozole, letrozole and exemestane, which are also used in the treatment of breast cancer but whose effects are not mediated via the oestrogen receptor, are associated with less endometrial pathology than tamoxifen and it has even been suggested that aromatase inhibitors may reverse abnormalities induced by tamoxifen.

Table 80.1 Causes of vaginal bleeding in the non-pregnant state.

Menstrual	Endometrial polyp/malignancy[a] Fibroids
Intermenstrual	Vaginal trauma/malignancy Cervical polyp/malignancy Endometrial polyp/malignancy
Post-coital	Vaginal malignancy[a] Cervical ectropion/polyp/malignancy

[a]These cancers occur principally in post-menopausal women.

Women with hereditary non-polyposis colorectal cancer (HNPCC) (Lynch syndrome) and those who are at high risk of developing HNPCC are another special group, as the lifetime risk of developing endometrial cancer is as high as 60 per cent. Unlike sporadic cases of endometrial cancer, which are usually diagnosed during the sixth and seventh decades, the mean age at diagnosis in HNPCC patients is the fifth decade. However, it appears that five-year survival rates in HNPCC patients with endometrial cancer are similar to those in women with sporadic disease. International guidelines suggest that these women should be screened annually from the age of 35 years with transvaginal ultrasound, to measure endometrial thickness and look for polyps, and with endometrial biopsy.

Menstrual bleeding may be excessively heavy, irregular or frequent in the absence of pathology; this is known as dysfunctional uterine bleeding. Medical treatments used to reduce the amount of menstrual loss include tranexamic acid, mefenamic acid and the combined oral contraceptive (COC). It may be necessary to stop the bleeding completely using high-dose progestagens, the COC taken continuously or a GnRH agonist, which induces a menopause-like state. Increasingly, an intrauterine system (IUS) similar to a conventional coil, which releases levonorgestrel, is offered to patients as an alternative; it has the added advantage of being a reliable contraceptive.

The surgical treatments for excessive bleeding and their principal operative complications are described in Table 80.2; they are divided into those procedures that retain the uterus and those that do not. The ovaries may or may not be removed at the same time depending upon the woman's age and any coexisting pathology. The aim of all of the ablation methods is to reduce menstrual bleeding by ablating the endometrial layer and some of the underlying myometrium using electrical, thermal or laser energy. Amenorrhoea is not guaranteed, but the procedures are less invasive and costly than hysterectomy. Clearly, none of these surgical treatments is suitable for women who wish to conceive.

Abnormal bleeding can also be caused by invasive carcinoma of the cervix, the incidence of which has been reduced by screening programmes that aim to detect the precancerous state – cervical intraepithelial neoplasia (CIN) – using cervical cytology. In the UK, this is carried out every three to five years in women aged between 25 and 65 years. Infection with certain human papillomavirus (HPV) serotypes (16, 18, 31 and 33) is associated with an increased risk of invasive disease. Abnormalities in cervical cytology are followed up by microscopic examination of the cervix (colposcopy). CIN may be treated with local ablation (cryocautery, cold coagulation, electrodiathermy or laser) or excision (large loop excision of the transformation zone (LLETZ)). However, it is very likely that the incidence of CIN will decrease steadily in the future as a result of vaccination against HPV in young girls and HPV testing.

ACUTE PELVIC PAIN IN EARLY PREGNANCY

Ectopic pregnancy

An ectopic pregnancy is one that grows outside the uterine cavity, almost always in a Fallopian tube (rare sites include the ovary, cervix and broad ligament). As the ectopic grows, the placenta infiltrates blood vessels within the Fallopian tube, which can cause bleeding within the tube and bleeding into the peritoneal cavity. Further growth of the ectopic pregnancy can rupture the Fallopian tube causing substantial intraperitoneal blood loss. It is the most common cause of maternal death in the first trimester and accounts for 9 per cent of maternal deaths in the UK. The major risk factors for ectopic pregnancy are shown in Summary box 80.2.

Summary box 80.2

Risk factors for ectopic pregnancy

- Previous pelvic inflammatory disease
- Smoking
- Older age
- Previous spontaneous miscarriage
- Previous medical termination
- History of infertility
- Previous use of an intrauterine contraceptive device

An ectopic pregnancy may be suspected on clinical grounds, but making the diagnosis can be difficult because the presentation is so variable and can mimic that of a miscarriage (Summary box 80.3).

Summary box 80.3

Differential diagnoses for acute pain in early pregnancy

- Ectopic pregnancy
- Miscarriage
- Urinary tract infection
- Ovarian accident
- Pain unrelated to pregnancy, e.g. acute appendicitis

There may be a history of lower abdominal pain with a small amount of vaginal bleeding at 4–6 weeks' gestation. On vaginal examination, there may be cervical excitation and tenderness in the vaginal fornices; the cervical os is closed. Alternatively, the woman may not have any symptoms or physical findings. The urinary pregnancy test is usually positive. Modern monoclonal antibody-based urine tests can detect the beta subunit of human chorionic gonadotropin (β-hCG) at levels of 25 IU/L, which are reached 9 days post-conception, i.e. on day 23 of the menstrual cycle assuming ovulation occurred on day 14.

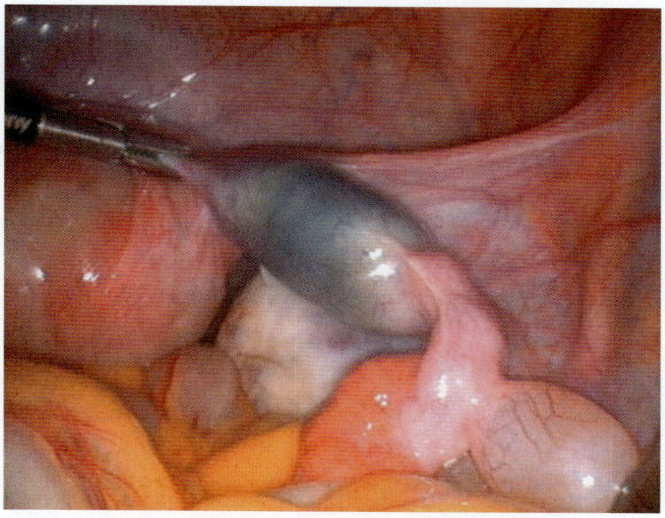

Figure 80.3 Laparoscopy showing an ectopic pregnancy.

A transvaginal ultrasound scan should be performed if the diagnosis is suspected. The complete absence of an intrauterine gestational sac with a positive pregnancy test increases the probability of an ectopic pregnancy unless the pregnancy is not sufficiently advanced for the sac to be seen on ultrasound in the uterus. An ectopic pregnancy is more likely if fluid is seen in the pelvis or an adnexal mass is seen on ultrasound.

In equivocal cases, measuring serum levels of β-hCG can help to establish the diagnosis. β-hCG levels double every 48 hours if the pregnancy is viable and intrauterine. Levels tend to be static or the rise is less than double over a 48-hour period if the pregnancy is ectopic. A single level above approximately 1500 IU/L in association with an empty uterus on ultrasound is highly suggestive of an ectopic pregnancy. The best diagnostic test is laparoscopy (Figure 80.3); occasionally, however, if the pregnancy is not sufficiently advanced, the ectopic pregnancy is too small to be seen in the Fallopian tube. There is also a view that a laparoscopy should only be performed once a miscarriage has been excluded because of the surgical and anaesthetic risks associated with the procedure.

Once an ectopic pregnancy has been diagnosed at laparoscopy, a salpingectomy is usually performed. A salpingostomy may be performed instead as some gynaecologists maintain that subsequent intrauterine pregnancy rates are higher and recurrent ectopic rates lower following conservative surgery. Laparoscopy is the preferred approach because it is associated with shorter operation times, less intraoperative blood loss, shorter hospital stays and similar subsequent intrauterine pregnancy rates.

In practice, the type of operation chosen depends on factors such as the following:

- **The amount of bleeding.** An immediate laparotomy may be required if the woman has lost a great deal of blood.

Table 80.2 Surgical treatments for excessive vaginal bleeding.

Treatment	Route	Major operative risks
Removal of uterus: hysterectomy		
Subtotal (cervix retained)	Abdominal; laparoscopic	Damage to ureter, bladder or bowel; may result in fistula; risks of laparoscopy
Total (cervix removed)	Abdominal; vaginal; laparoscopic; laparoscopic-vaginal	
Retention of uterus: endometrial ablation		
Thermal balloon	Device inserted into uterine cavity	Uterine perforation
Cryotherapy	Device inserted into uterine cavity	Uterine perforation
Microwave	Device inserted into uterine cavity	Uterine perforation; thermal damage to pelvic organs (especially bowel)
Transcervical resection of endometrium	Hysteroscopic	Bleeding; fluid overload; uterine perforation; thermal damage to pelvic organs (especially bowel)

- **The state of the tube**, i.e. the size of the ectopic pregnancy and whether or not it has ruptured (in general, if the ectopic pregnancy is too large the chances of conservative surgery being successful are small; if it has ruptured, there is little point in trying to be conservative).
- **The state of the other tube**. One usually tries to be as conservative as possible if the other tube has been affected by PID (i.e. it is closed or densely adherent to other pelvic organs).
- **Previous ectopic pregnancy or tubal surgery**. One usually performs a salpingectomy if a woman has had a previous ectopic pregnancy or tubal surgery in the same tube.
- **The woman's fertility intentions**. One usually performs a salpingectomy if a woman does not want more children.

Sometimes, the ectopic pregnancy is located at the very end of the tube, in which case it may be possible simply to 'milk' it out, thereby conserving the tube. The principal disadvantage of this method (and salpingostomy) is that some residual trophoblastic tissue can be left inside the tube. The tissue often survives and continues to grow, which can cause intra-abdominal bleeding. The best method for determining whether all of the tissue has been removed at surgery is to measure serial serum β-hCG levels, which should fall to zero over time if all the tissue has been removed; β-hCG levels remain constant or rise if there is residual trophoblastic tissue, which may necessitate another laparoscopy to remove the tube.

In the United States, many women avoid surgery altogether by being treated with intramuscular injections of methotrexate, which is toxic to trophoblastic tissue. The drug has some side effects and the treatment carries the risks associated with residual trophoblastic tissue, namely internal bleeding and the eventual need for a laparoscopy. In the UK, methotrexate seems to be used only in those patients who are at increased surgical risk (e.g. the morbidly obese or those with extensive pelvic adhesions).

After treatment, the patient who still has one or both tubes should be warned that she is at increased risk of another ectopic pregnancy. She should therefore be encouraged to present as early as possible in a subsequent pregnancy to rule out this diagnosis.

INFECTION

The overwhelming majority of cases of acute PID are caused by ascending infection, which is usually sexually transmitted. Rarer causes include spread from other pelvic organs, e.g. the appendix. *Chlamydia trachomatis* is the most common organism responsible for PID; the prevalence of *Neisseria gonorrhoeae* varies depending upon the locality. Infection involves the upper genital tract, particularly the endometrium and Fallopian tubes. Risk factors include young age at first sexual activity, a high number of sexual partners and current use of an IUCD; infection may also follow a surgical procedure, e.g. termination of pregnancy.

There are no definitive criteria for the diagnosis of acute PID. Most clinicians rely instead upon the presence of one or more of the following features, which are suggestive of the diagnosis:

- lower abdominal pain and tenderness;
- deep dyspareunia (pain on intercourse);
- abnormal vaginal or cervical discharge;
- cervical excitation and adnexal tenderness;
- fever >38°C.

The differential diagnoses include endometriosis, urinary tract infection, appendicitis and gastrointestinal dysfunction. A raised neutrophil count and an elevated erythrocyte sedimentation rate (ESR) or C-reactive protein (CRP) level support the diagnosis. Ultrasound may be useful if there appear to be hydrosalpinges present and/or tubo-ovarian abscesses. All women with suspected PID should be screened for *N. gonorrhoeae* and *C. trachomatis* by taking endocervical with or without urethral swabs. *C. trachomatis* is an intracellular organism; therefore, samples obtained for diagnostic purposes should contain cellular material. It is important to wipe off any discharge before inserting the swab inside the cervical os and firmly rotating it against the endocervix.

The current RCOG (2008) guidelines recommend a low threshold for empirical treatment because the consequences of failing to treat acute PID effectively are so significant. Treatment should commence as soon as samples have been obtained for culture even though the results are unavailable; it should include a broad-spectrum antibiotic against coliforms and anaerobic

Albert Ludwig Siegmund Neisser, 1855–1916, Director of the Dermatological Institute, Breslau, Germany (now Wroclaw, Poland).

species, which are responsible for secondary infection. Contact tracing and treatment, if possible, are essential (Summary box 80.4).

Inadequate or inappropriate treatment is associated with a significant risk of developing infertility, ectopic pregnancy, Fitz-Hugh–Curtis syndrome (an extrapelvic manifestation of PID associated with right upper quadrant pain, which probably results from inflammation of the liver capsule and diaphragm) and chronic pelvic pain in the future. The risk of infertility is obviously of great concern. Approximately 20 per cent of women treated for PID will become infertile because of tubal damage; >50 per cent of tubal infertility cases are due to *C. trachomatis* although, interestingly, many of these women do not report a history of PID (Summary box 80.5). In total, 6 per cent of women will have an ectopic in the first pregnancy following an episode of acute PID, a figure that is approximately ten times greater than the rate in the general population.

Summary box 80.4

Treatment of pelvic inflammatory disease

- Because of the lack of definitive clinical diagnostic criteria, a low threshold for the empirical treatment of pelvic inflammatory disease (PID) is recommended
- Women with suspected PID should be screened for gonorrhoea and *Chlamydia*. Testing for gonorrhoea should be with an endocervical specimen, tested via culture (direct inoculation on to a culture plate or transport of the swab to the laboratory within 24 hours) or using a nucleic acid amplification test (NAAT). Screening for *Chlamydia* should also be from the endocervix, preferably using a NAAT. Taking an additional sample from the urethra increases the diagnostic yield for gonorrhoea and *Chlamydia*. A first-catch urine sample provides an alternative sample
- Outpatient antibiotic treatment should be commenced as soon as the diagnosis is suspected. Treatment should be based on one of the following regimens:
  400 mg oral ofloxacin twice a day plus 400 mg oral metronidazole twice a day for 14 days; or
  250 mg intramuscular ceftriaxone immediately or 2 g intramuscular cefoxitin immediately with 1 g oral probenecid, followed by 100 mg oral doxycycline twice a day plus 400 mg metronidazole twice a day for 14 days
- Admission to hospital is appropriate in the following circumstances:
  surgical emergency cannot be excluded
  clinically severe disease
  tubo-ovarian abscess
  PID in pregnancy
  lack of response to oral therapy
  intolerance to oral therapy
- In more severe cases, inpatient antibiotic treatment should be based on intravenous therapy, which should be continued until 24 hours after clinical improvement and followed by oral therapy. Recommended regimens are:
  2 g intravenous ceftriaxone three times a day plus 100 mg intravenous doxycycline twice a day (oral doxycycline may be used if tolerated), followed by 100 mg oral doxycycline twice a day plus 400 mg oral metronidazole twice a day for a total of 14 days; or
  900 mg intravenous clindamycin three times a day, plus intravenous gentamicin: 2 mg/kg loading dose followed by 1.5 mg/kg three times a day (a single daily dose of 7 mg/kg may be substituted), followed by 450 mg oral clindamycin four times a day to complete 14 days or 100 mg oral doxycycline twice a day plus 400 mg oral metronidazole twice a day to complete 14 days or 400 mg intravenous ofloxacin twice a day plus 500 mg intravenous metronidazole three times a day for 14 days

Summary box 80.5

Chlamydia and gonorrhoea testing

There is a need to test women (especially those sexually active under the age of 25 years) who present with:

- Purulent vaginal discharge
- Post-coital/intermenstrual bleeding
- Mucopurulent cervicitis
- Inflamed/friable cervix (which may bleed on contact)
- Urethritis
- Suspected pelvic inflammatory disease
- Reactive arthritis

The majority of suspected cases are treated in the community, but hospital admission is advisable if there is doubt about the diagnosis or symptoms/signs are severe. In hospital, antibiotics should be given intravenously until 24 hours after clinical improvement. If there is an IUCD *in situ*, it should be removed with adequate counselling regarding pregnancy risk (if intercourse has occurred recently) and future contraception.

Severe PID manifests as a tubo-ovarian abscess, so named because the Fallopian tube and ovary become blended into a single, pus-filled, inflammatory mass, which is usually adherent to the uterus and surrounding bowel. The infection may have

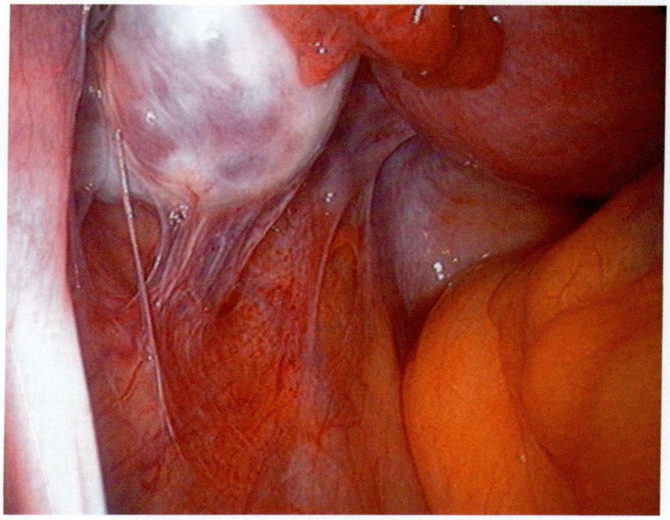

Figure 80.4 Pelvic inflammatory disease.

Thomas Fitz-Hugh Jr, 1894–1963, physician, Chief of the Hematological Section, The University Hospital, The University of Pennsylvania, Philadelphia, PA, USA.
Arthur H Curtis, 1881–1955, Professor of Obstetrics and Gynecology, The Northwestern Medical School, Chicago, IL, USA.

progressed from a milder form of PID or, increasingly, it may result from the introduction of infection or bowel damage at transvaginal oocyte aspiration in a patient undergoing *in vitro* fertilisation (IVF). Modern medical practice is to manage tubo-ovarian abscesses (Figure 80.4) conservatively unless the patient fails to respond to intravenous antibiotics and systemic support. The response is judged to be inadequate if the woman remains systemically unwell, her symptoms do not improve, fever is not reduced, the white blood cell count does not fall and there is no evidence on ultrasound of the abscess becoming smaller. In such circumstances, surgical treatment is necessary, i.e. adhesiolysis and drainage of the abscess, at laparotomy or laparoscopy. As most women with a tubo-ovarian abscess are in the reproductive years, the intention is always to be as conservative as possible at surgery. Rarely, however, if the abscess has ruptured (Figure 80.5) and the patient is extremely ill, then hysterectomy and bilateral salpingo-oophorectomy may be necessary.

Abscess drainage under radiological guidance, e.g. a transgluteal approach via the greater sciatic foramen under computed tomography (CT) guidance, is sometimes performed. Transvaginal ultrasound-guided aspiration has also been advocated. It is clearly less invasive and there are claims that the method is as effective as surgery; however, it carries additional risks such as bowel damage.

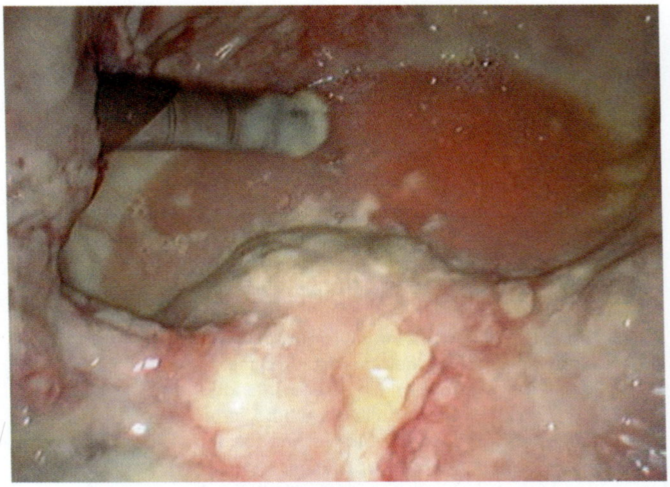

Figure 80.5 Pelvic inflammatory disease with rupture of a pelvic abscess.

UTEROVAGINAL PROLAPSE

Congenital weakness of the pelvic floor ligaments and fascia may be found in conditions such as spina bifida and bladder exstrophy. Far more common, however, are the acquired forms of pelvic floor damage caused by prolonged or difficult labour and multiparity. A gradual increase in denervation of the striated muscle of the pelvic floor with age and oestrogen deficiency at the menopause can also occur in nulliparous women (Figure 80.6).

A minor degree of prolapse may be asymptomatic but with more significant degrees the patient complains of 'something coming down'. A cystocoele (bladder prolapse) and a cystourethrocoele lead to the sensation of a lump in the vagina and may also be associated with incontinence and recurrent urinary infections. Uterine descent can lead to backache; with complete prolapse of the uterus (procidentia) there may be vaginal discharge, ulceration of the vaginal skin and bleeding. A rectocoele (prolapse of the rectum into the vagina) may cause difficulties with defaecation or a sensation of incomplete defaecation, which is relieved by digital reduction of the prolapse.

Non-surgical management of uterovaginal prolapse is with physiotherapy, hormone replacement therapy (HRT) and the use of vaginal rings and pessaries. The vinyl ring is inserted between the posterior fornix and the pubic bone. The main complication is vaginal ulceration and infection leading to discharge and bleeding; it is advisable, therefore, to replace the ring frequently. The aims of surgical management are usually to correct the prolapse, treat any associated incontinence and preserve coital function if appropriate. The surgical procedures are intended to restore the uterovaginal anatomy and position. They may be carried out using a vaginal or abdominal approach or increasingly by a laparoscopic or minimal access approach with the use of vaginal slings and tapes (Table 80.3).

Milton Lawrence McCall, 1911–1963, Founding Chairman, Department of Obstetrics and Gynecology, Magee-Women's Hospital, Pittsburgh, PA, USA described his suture in 1957. Following his untimely death in 1963, the 'Milton Lawrence Professorship and Chair, Department of Obstetrics and Gynecology and Reproductive Sciences' was established in the University of Pittsburgh, PA, USA.

Table 80.3 Surgical treatments for uterovaginal prolapse.

Condition	Treatment
Urethrocele/cystocele (Figure 80.6a)	Traditionally, an anterior vaginal wall repair (anterior colporrhaphy) was performed vaginally; now replaced by vaginally inserted tape (transvaginal tape (TVT) or transobturator tape (TOT)) or mesh slings
Uterine prolapse (Figure 80.6b)	If family complete, a vaginal hysterectomy with an anterior vaginal wall repair if necessary. If the uterus is to be preserved use either amputation of the cervix with suturing of the transverse cervical ligaments vaginally (Manchester repair) or laparoscopic plication of the uterosacral ligaments (McCall suture)
Enterocoele (Figure 80.6c)	Similar technique to repair of a hernia. The vaginal skin is opened and the hernial sac repaired
Vault prolapse (Figure 80.6d)	Sacrospinous fixation or sacrocolpopexy; the vault is attached to the sacrum using a non-absorbable suture
Rectocoele (Figure 80.6e)	Posterior colporrhaphy: the posterior vaginal wall is opened, the rectum returned to its normal position and redundant vaginal skin is excised. A laparoscopic approach to repairing the defect in the pelvic floor with or without the use of a mesh is now more popular and, as there is no resulting scarring in the vaginal skin, the incidence of post-surgery dyspareunia is less

The **Manchester repair** was introduced at St Mary's Hospital for Women and Children, Manchester, UK.

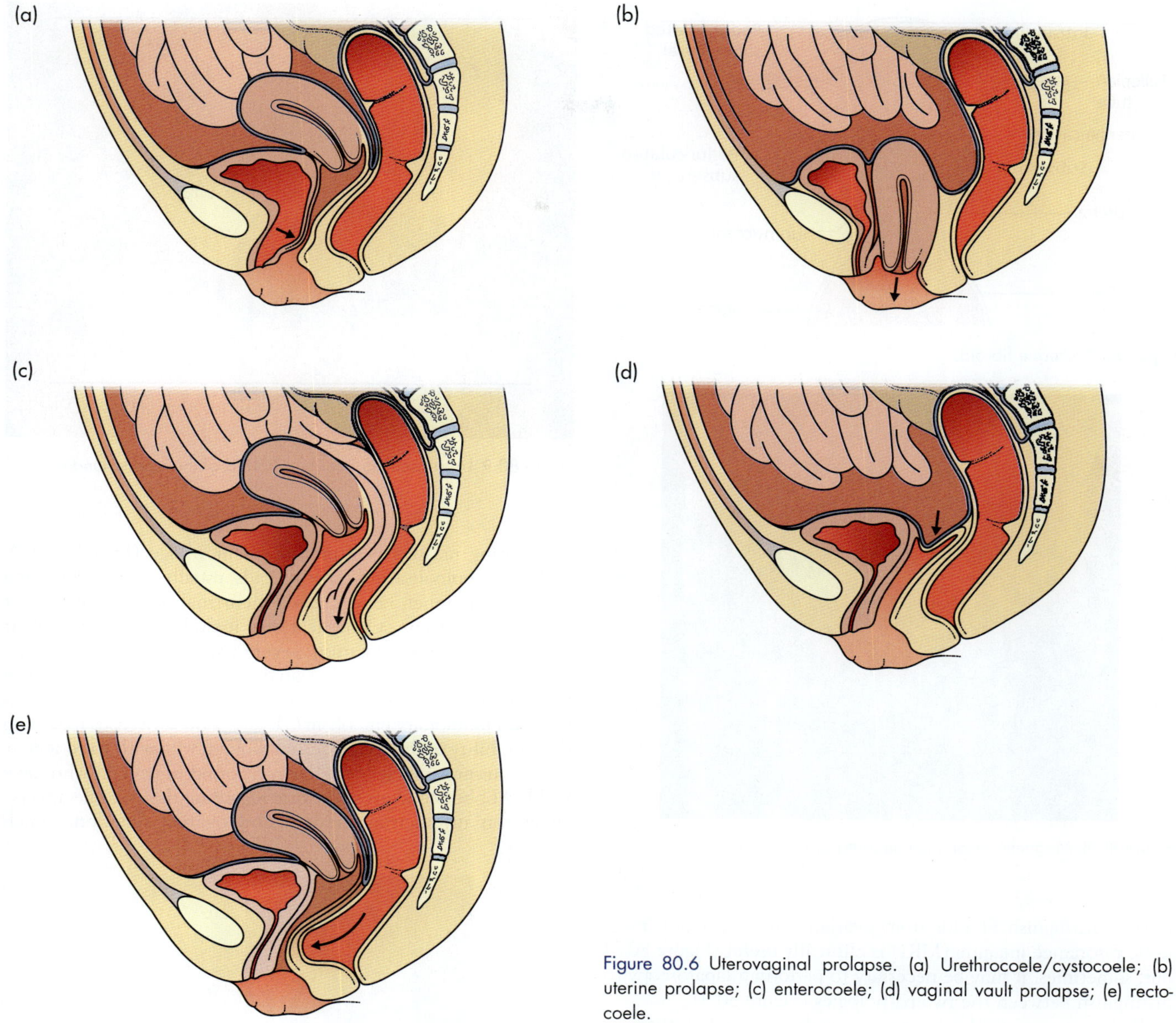

Figure 80.6 Uterovaginal prolapse. (a) Urethrocoele/cystocoele; (b) uterine prolapse; (c) enterocoele; (d) vaginal vault prolapse; (e) rectocoele.

TUMOURS

Uterine fibroids (leiomyomas)

Fibroids are benign, well-circumscribed, smooth muscle tumours of the uterus. Most women will have more than one fibroid, varying in diameter from 1–10 cm, which are typically found in the following locations (Figure 80.7):

- **Subserosal** may cause pressure symptoms (see below); if pedunculated, they can be difficult to distinguish from an ovarian tumour.
- **Intramural** may similarly cause pressure symptoms; associated with infertility and heavy periods.
- **Submucosal** associated with infertility, recurrent pregnancy loss and heavy periods; if pedunculated, may occasionally extrude through the cervical os.
- **Rare** sites include the broad ligament and cervix.

Women with uterine fibroids will present with heavy and/or irregular menstrual bleeding, pressure symptoms or problems conceiving, especially if there is a fibroid in the uterine cavity. The pressure symptoms include pelvic discomfort, urinary incontinence, frequency and retention, constipation and backache. When large fibroids are present, back pressure may cause or exacerbate varicosities. Although these symptoms are common, it is important to note that some women with fibroids are asymptomatic. Rarely, women may present acutely with pain arising from torsion of a pedunculated fibroid or red degeneration, especially in pregnancy.

The diagnosis is usually apparent on bimanual and/or abdominal examination, on the basis of finding an enlarged uterus with attached swellings. The principal differential diagnosis is an ovarian tumour; as a general rule, the uterus is felt separately on vaginal examination if an ovarian tumour is present, although not if the structures are adherent to each other. Ultrasound can

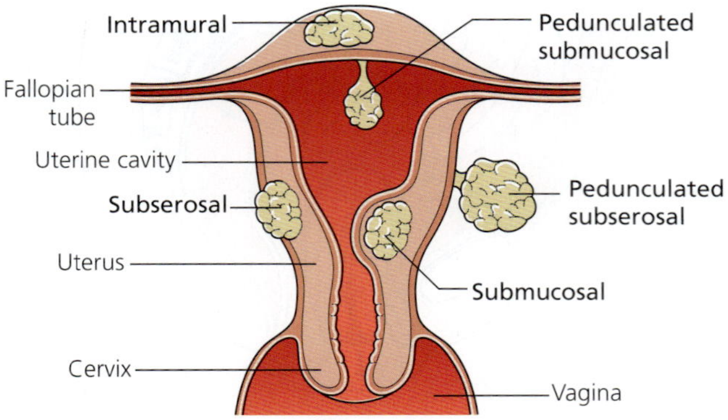

Figure 80.7 Uterine fibroids.

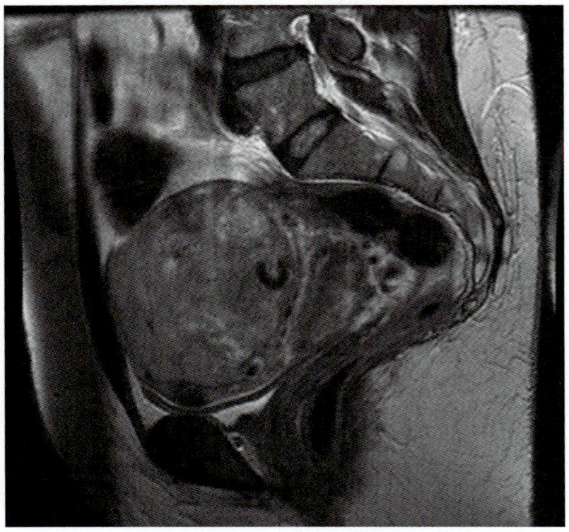

Figure 80.8 Magnetic resonance imaging of uterine fibroids.

usually distinguish fibroids from ovarian tumours; if not, magnetic resonance imaging (MRI) is clinically useful (Figure 80.8) but, sometimes, it may be necessary to perform a laparoscopy to distinguish between the two pathologies (Figure 80.9).

Emergency surgical treatment is only required if there is substantial menstrual bleeding or uncontrollable pain; these are rare events. Otherwise, the woman has time to consider her treatment options, which include shrinkage of the fibroids by inducing a hypo-oestrogenic state with a GnRH agonist, uterine artery embolisation (UAE), myomectomy (removal of the individual fibroids) and hysterectomy. The choice depends upon the woman's age and fertility intentions, the size and number of fibroids and their location. It is also important to know whether there are fibroids in the uterine cavity, especially if the woman is trying to conceive.

A GnRH agonist will usually shrink fibroids, but this class of drug has the disadvantage that treatment cannot be continued indefinitely because of the associated loss in bone mineral density; in addition, the fibroids tend to regrow to their original size when treatment is discontinued. UAE is becoming increasingly popular as an alternative to surgery. It involves blocking the blood supply to the fibroids using a technique in which particles are embolised into each uterine artery via an angiographic catheter in a similar manner to the well-established technique

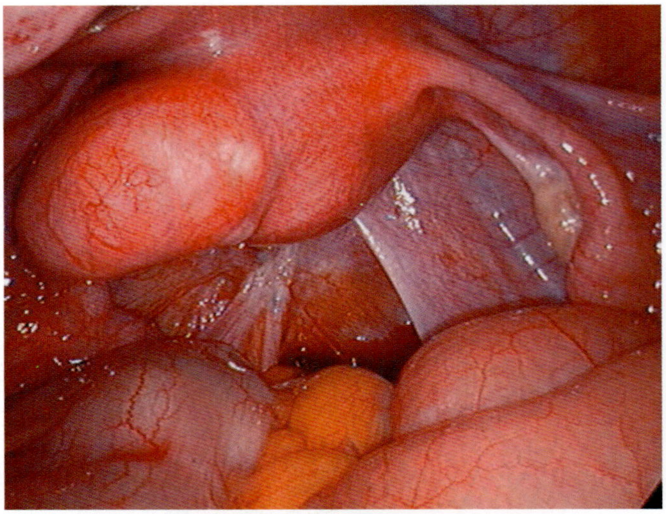

Figure 80.9 Laparoscopic view of a fibroid of the uterine fundus.

for treating massive post-partum haemorrhage (Figure 80.10). Following embolisation, the fibroids usually shrink, bringing symptomatic relief, i.e. decreased menstrual bleeding and fewer pressure symptoms. Complications include arterial injury at the site of catheter insertion, severe pain as a result of uterine ischaemia, infection, and ovarian damage and thromboembolism (a small number of deaths have been reported from uterine infection and pulmonary embolism). There is no consensus regarding the suitability of the technique for women who wish to conceive. Numerous pregnancies have been reported in women who have had UAE, but concern still exists regarding the possible adverse effects on myometrial strength and ovarian function, which

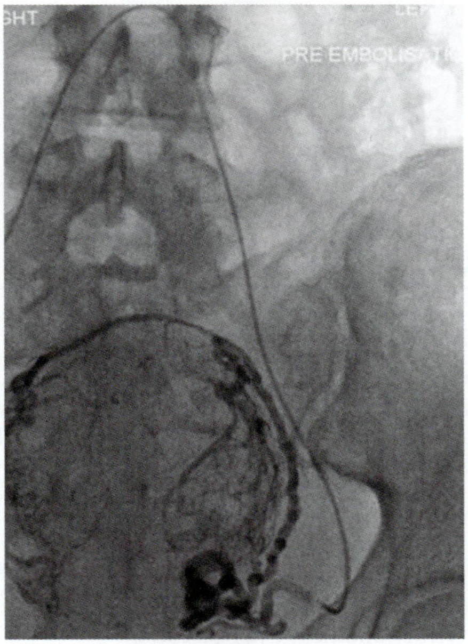

Figure 80.10 Pre-embolisation angiogram showing catheterisation of left uterine artery and blood supply to large fundal fibroid. Image courtesy of Dr Mark Bratby, Consultant Vascular and Interventional Radiologist, John Radcliffe Hospital, Oxford, UK.

might affect a woman's chances of conceiving, carrying the pregnancy and delivering normally.

Myomectomy (performed at laparotomy or increasingly at laparoscopy) involves the removal of pedunculated, subserosal and/or intramural fibroids and closure of any defects left in the uterine wall. Surgical complications are unusual; in exceptional circumstances, however, a hysterectomy may be necessary because of uncontrollable blood loss. Fibroids in the uterine cavity should be removed hysteroscopically; the risks of the procedure are similar to those for transcervical resection of the endometrium (TCRE) (see Table 80.2).

Endometriosis

Endometriosis – defined as the presence of endometrial-like tissue in extrauterine sites – is a complex genetic trait that affects up to 10 per cent of women in the reproductive years. The symptoms associated with the disease include severe dysmenorrhoea, chronic pelvic pain, ovulation pain, deep dyspareunia, cyclical symptoms related to the involvement of other organs (e.g. bowel or bladder) with or without abnormal bleeding, infertility and chronic fatigue. However, the predictive value of any one symptom or set of symptoms remains uncertain as each can have other causes (e.g. irritable bowel syndrome or interstitial cystitis) and a significant proportion of affected women are asymptomatic.

The most commonly affected sites are the pelvic organs and peritoneum, although distant sites such as the lungs are occasionally affected (resulting in symptoms such as recurrent haemoptysis at the time of menstruation). The extent of the disease varies from a few, small lesions on otherwise normal pelvic organs to large, ovarian, endometriotic cysts (endometriomas). There can be extensive fibrosis in structures such as the uterosacral ligaments (Figure 80.11) and adhesion formation causing marked distortion of pelvic anatomy (Figure 80.12). Disease severity can be assessed simply by describing the operative findings or, quantitatively, using various classification systems, but there is little correlation between such systems and the type or severity of pain symptoms.

Endometriosis typically appears as superficial 'powder-burn' or 'gunshot' lesions on the ovaries, serosal surfaces and peritoneum – black, dark-brown or bluish puckered lesions, nodules or small cysts containing old haemorrhage surrounded by a variable extent of fibrosis (Figure 80.13). Atypical or 'subtle' lesions are also common, including red implants (petechial, vesicular, polypoid, haemorrhagic, red flame-like) and serous or clear vesicles. Other appearances include white plaques or scarring and yellow-brown peritoneal discolouration of the peritoneum. Ovarian endometriomas usually contain thick fluid like tar. They are distinguishable from simple haemorrhagic ovarian cysts because, typically, they are densely adherent to the peritoneum of the ovarian fossa. The surrounding fibrosis may involve the bowel. Deeply infiltrating endometriotic nodules represent another disease type. They extend more than 5 mm beneath the peritoneum and may grow into the uterosacral ligaments, vagina, bowel, bladder or ureters; when such lesions grow into the vagina, they may be visible on speculum examination as 'blue-domed' cystic lesions in the posterior fornix. Lesions infiltrating the bowel may mimic cancer in their presentation.

The diagnosis of endometriosis is usually made on visual inspection of the pelvis at laparoscopy; non-invasive diagnostic tools, such as ultrasound scanning, can reliably detect only severe forms of the disease, i.e. endometriomas. The treatment options are limited because the cause is uncertain; these include hormonal drugs to suppress ovarian function, the levonorgestrel-IUS and surgical ablation of endometriotic lesions. Women may require multiple admissions for surgery and/or prolonged treatment with costly drugs that have problematic side effects. Lastly, patients with endometriosis may be at increased risk of ovarian cancer (especially endometrioid and clear-cell types) and non-Hodgkin's lymphoma, which adds to the burden of the disease.

Finding pelvic tenderness, a fixed retroverted uterus, tender uterosacral ligaments or enlarged ovaries on examination is suggestive of endometriosis. The diagnosis is more certain if deeply infiltrating nodules are found on the uterosacral ligaments or in the pouch of Douglas and/or visible lesions are seen in the vagina or on the cervix. The findings may, however, be normal.

For a woman who has completed her family, hysterectomy plus bilateral salpingo-oophorectomy and removal of all the

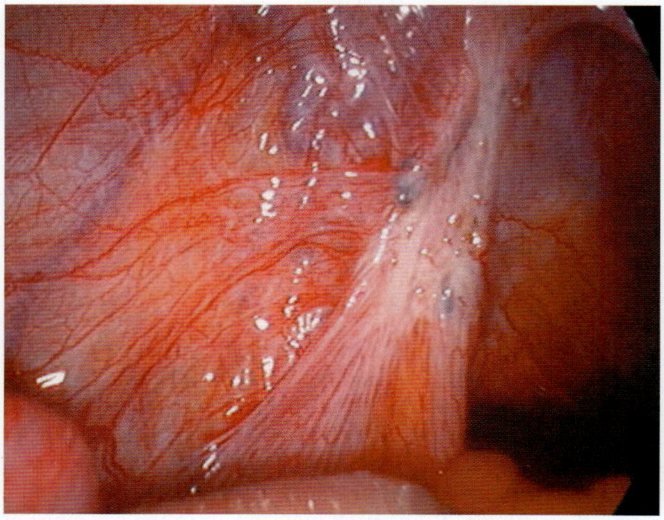

Figure 80.11 Endometriosis seen on the uterosacral ligament.

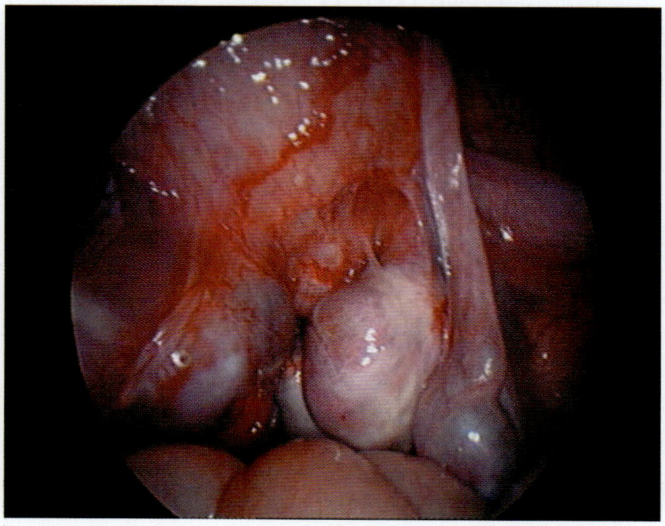

Figure 80.12 Bilateral ovarian endometriosis with pelvic adhesions.

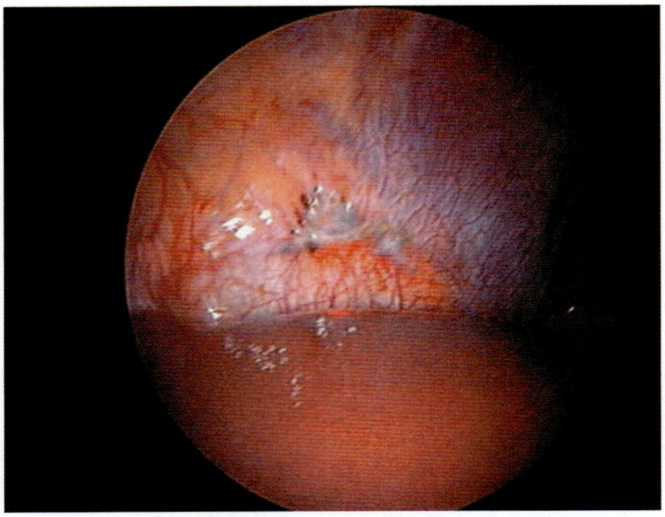

Figure 80.13 Endometriosis seen on the peritoneal surface of the diaphragm.

endometriosis present offers a good chance of cure. However, surgical treatment in a woman who wishes to conceive in the future aims to be as conservative as possible, ensuring in particular that ovarian function is preserved. The aim is to remove all of the endometriotic tissue and restore anatomy to normal by lysing adhesions. The standard (preferably laparoscopic) methods used are ovarian cystectomy and tissue excision or ablation with electrodiathermy, thermal coagulation or laser. The surgical risks include those for any laparoscopic procedure, as well as damage to the ureters and bowel; the risks are increased if deeply infiltrating disease is present, particularly if there is bowel wall involvement. Rarely, infection in an endometrioma will result in the formation of a tubo-ovarian abscess.

Benign ovarian tumour and cysts

Overall, 90 per cent of ovarian tumours are benign, although there is an increased risk of malignancy in older women. Ovarian tumours are subdivided into five main categories according to the World Health Organization's classification system (Table 80.4).

Table 80.4 Classification of ovarian tumours.

Epithelial tumours	Represent about 75% of all ovarian tumours and 90–95% of ovarian malignancies
Sex cord–stromal tumours	Represent about 5–10% of all ovarian neoplasms
Germ cell tumours	Represent about 15–20% of all ovarian neoplasms
Metastatic tumours	Represent about 5% of ovarian malignancies; usually arise from breast, colon, endometrium, stomach and cervical cancers
Other	A small number of other types of neoplasms, which develop from ovarian soft tissue or non-neoplastic processes

The most common solid tumours in young women are cystic teratomas (known more commonly as dermoid cysts), which typically contain a variety of tissues including hair, teeth and bone. Benign ovarian tumours are often asymptomatic and may present coincidentally, for example when an abdominal radiograph reveals the appearance of a tooth in the abdomen or pelvis. Conversely, they may present with pain, abdominal swelling and pressure effects. The pain may be the result of torsion or bleeding inside the cysts. Management will depend, to some extent, on the age of the woman and the characteristics of the cyst. In older women, a conservative approach is reasonable only if the risks of malignancy are low (see Ovarian cancer). In younger women (<35 years), the cyst can be followed by serial ultrasound scanning as many will regress – haemorrhagic corpus luteal cysts, for example, will often shrink after three to four months' treatment with a COC. If there is uncontrollable pain, haemodynamic collapse or a suspicion of torsion, or the cyst does not regress, then laparoscopic ovarian cystectomy with conservation of ovarian tissue is the treatment of choice. As the vast majority of oocytes lie within 5 mm of the surface of the ovary, a carefully carried out cystectomy can leave a normally functioning ovary (Figure 80.14) (Summary box 80.6).

Summary box 80.6

Management of benign ovarian cysts

- Masses are usually detected incidentally but may be suggested by symptoms and signs
- A pregnancy test is done to exclude ectopic pregnancy
- Transvaginal ultrasonography can usually confirm the diagnosis. If results are indeterminate, magnetic resonance imaging or computed tomography scanning may help. Masses with radiographic characteristics of cancer (e.g. cystic and solid components, surface excrescences, multilocular appearance, irregular shape) require removal
- Tumour markers may help in the diagnosis of specific tumours
- In women of reproductive age, simple, thin-walled cystic adnexal masses of 5–8 cm (usually follicular) without characteristics of cancer do not require further investigation unless they persist for more than three menstrual cycles
- Many ovarian cysts resolve without treatment; serial ultrasonography is carried out to document resolution. Cyst removal (ovarian cystectomy) via laparoscopy or laparotomy may be necessary for cysts ≥8 cm, cysts that persist for more than three menstrual cycles and haemorrhagic corpus luteum cysts with signs of peritonitis
- Cystic teratomas require removal via cystectomy if possible. Oophorectomy is carried out for fibromas, cystadenomas, cystic teratomas >10 cm and cysts that cannot be surgically removed from the ovary

Ovarian cancer

Ovarian cancer is the sixth most common malignancy among women worldwide and the leading gynaecological cause of death in the developing world. In the UK, over 6000 women die annually from ovarian cancer. Over 90 per cent of cancers arise from the surface epithelium of the ovary (which has the same embryological origins as the peritoneum); the majority are sporadic rather than inherited. The peak incidence is in the age range of 60–70 years. The overall five-year survival rate is less than 50 per

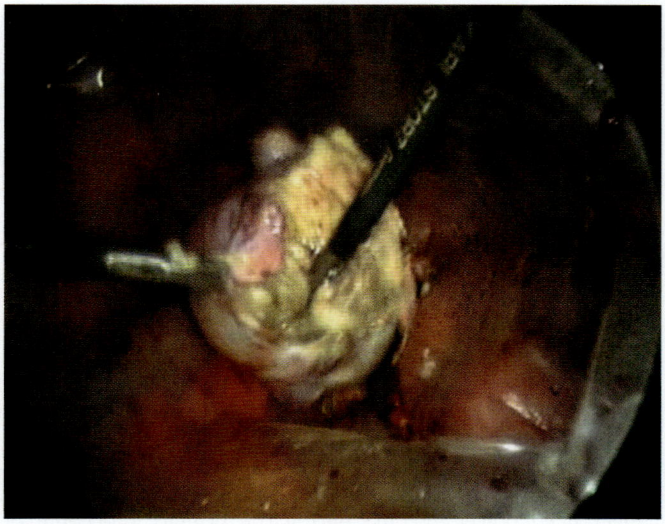

Figure 80.14 Ovarian cystectomy.

cent because approximately two-thirds of women present with advanced disease. The usual presenting symptoms are:

- abdominal distension and/or pain;
- weight gain and increased girth (ascites);
- urinary obstruction.

However, over half of all women present initially to a speciality other than gynaecology, with often vague symptoms caused by metastatic disease, e.g. shortness of breath, gastrointestinal disturbance or a change in bowel habit. Consequently, it is important to include ovarian cancer in the differential diagnosis of any woman presenting with recent onset of persistent, non-specific, abdominal symptoms (including those whose abdomen and pelvis appears normal on clinical examination).

Ultrasound is the first-line investigation if an ovarian mass is suspected on clinical grounds. The features suggestive of malignancy on ultrasound include the presence of:

- cyst complexity (number of locules, wall structure, thickness of septae, fluid echogenicity);
- solid papillary projections into the cyst;
- bilateral lesions;
- ascites;
- intra-abdominal metastases.

The level of cancer antigen 125 (CA-125; a glycoprotein expressed on tissue derived from coelomic and Müllerian epithelia) in serum is measured; the normal cut-off value is 35 U/mL. Elevated levels are found in 50 per cent of patients with stage I disease and >90 per cent of those with advanced disease. However, CA-125 levels are also elevated in other cancers, e.g. pancreas, breast, lung and colon. Levels may even be raised during menstruation; in benign conditions such as endometriosis, PID and liver disease; if ascites or other effusions are present; and after a recent laparotomy. The value of combining the ultrasound and CA-125 measurements is such that a postmenopausal woman with a simple, unilateral, unilocular cyst of <5 cm in diameter and a normal serum CA-125 level should be managed conservatively (Summary box 80.7).

Summary box 80.7

Basic tests on suspicion of ovarian malignancy

- Ultrasonography: findings that suggest cancer include a solid component, surface excrescences, size >6 cm, irregular shape and low vascular resistance on transvaginal Doppler flow studies
- A pelvic mass plus ascites usually indicates ovarian cancer but sometimes indicates Meigs' syndrome (a benign fibroma with ascites and right hydrothorax)
- Computed tomography scan or magnetic resonance imaging is usually carried out before surgery to determine the extent of the cancer
- Tumour markers, including the β-subunit of human chorionic gonadotropin (β-hCG), lactate dehydrogenase, α-fetoprotein, inhibin and CA-125, are also measured
- CA-125 is elevated in 80 per cent of advanced epithelial ovarian cancers, but may be mildly elevated in endometriosis, pelvic inflammatory disease, pregnancy, fibroids, peritoneal inflammation and non-ovarian peritoneal cancer.

Unfortunately, there are still no effective screening methods for ovarian cancer for the general population. Hence, the preliminary results of the UK Collaborative Trial of Ovarian Cancer Screening are of great interest. The study has recruited over 200 000 women, aged 50–74 years, who have been randomised to a control arm or one of two screening strategies: primary screening using measurement of serum CA-125 levels followed by transvaginal ultrasound as a second-line test or transvaginal ultrasound alone. The two screening procedures were similar in terms of sensitivity for all primary ovarian and Fallopian tube cancers, but specificity was higher with combined screening (99.8 versus 98.2 per cent; $p < 0.001$).

There is also no consensus regarding how women who are at high risk because of a family history should be screened, i.e. those with a first-degree relative affected by cancer within a family that meet one of the following criteria:

- Two or more individuals with ovarian cancer, who are first-degree relatives of each other.
- One individual with ovarian cancer at any age and one with breast cancer diagnosed at <50 years, who are first-degree relatives of each other (or second-degree relatives if the transmission is paternal).
- One relative with ovarian cancer at any age and two with breast cancer diagnosed at <60 years, who are connected by first-degree relationships (or second-degree relationships if the transmission is paternal).
- Known carrier of relevant cancer gene mutations (e.g. *BRCA1* or *BRCA2*).
- Untested first-degree relative of a predisposing gene carrier.
- Three or more family members with colon cancer or two with colon cancer and one with stomach, ovarian, endometrial, urinary tract or small bowel cancer in two generations. One of these cancers must be diagnosed at <50 years of age (Lynch syndrome).
- An individual with both breast and ovarian cancer.

Johannes Peter Müller, 1801–1858, Professor of Anatomy and Physiology, Berlin, Germany, described the paramesonephric duct in 1825.
Joe Vincent Meigs, 1892–1964, gynaecological surgeon, Massachusetts General Hospital, Boston, MA, USA.
A first-degree relationship is that between parent and child.
A second-degree relationship is that between siblings (i.e. via the parent), and between a grandparent and a grandchild.

Table 80.5 Staging of ovarian cancer.

Stage I	Growth limited to the ovaries
Stage II	Growth involving one or both ovaries with pelvic extension
Stage III	Tumour involving one or both ovaries with histologically confirmed peritoneal implants outside the pelvis and/or positive retroperitoneal or inguinal nodes. Superficial liver metastasis equals stage III. Tumour is limited to the true pelvis, but with histologically proven extension to the small bowel or omentum
Stage IV	Growth involving one or both ovaries with distant metastases. If pleural effusion is present, there must be positive cytology to classify a case as stage IV. Parenchymal liver metastasis equals stage IV

Some genetic mutations are known to predispose women to ovarian cancer, e.g. *BRCA1* and *BRCA2* and the mismatch repair genes associated with HNPCC (Lynch syndrome) families. *BRCA1* mutations confer a 30 per cent lifetime risk of ovarian cancer up to the age of 60 years; the figure for *BRCA2* mutations is 27 per cent up to the age of 70 years. The mismatch repair genes confer an increased lifetime risk of ovarian cancer of 9–12 per cent, in addition to the increased risk of endometrial cancer (see above under Vaginal bleeding in the non-pregnant state). Referral to a specialist cancer genetics service is advisable. Women at high risk of ovarian cancer may be offered prophylactic oophorectomy, especially as they may also be at increased risk of breast cancer and there is some evidence to suggest that oophorectomy reduces breast cancer risk in these women. Unfortunately, there is no proven role for screening in women at high risk.

Staging (Table 80.5) is performed at laparotomy via a midline incision if disease is suspected preoperatively by:

- Careful evaluation of all peritoneal surfaces.
- Four washings of the peritoneal cavity: diaphragm, right and left abdomen, pelvis.
- Infracolic omentectomy.
- Selected lymphadenectomy of the pelvic and para-aortic lymph nodes.
- Biopsy and/or resection of any suspicious lesions, masses and any adhesions.
- Random blind biopsies of normal peritoneal surfaces, including that from the undersurface of the right hemidiaphragm, bladder reflection, cul-de-sac, right and left paracolic recesses and both pelvic side walls.
- Total abdominal hysterectomy and bilateral salpingo-oophorectomy.
- Appendicectomy for mucinous tumours; if a routine appendicectomy results in an intraoperative suspicion of a mucinous tumour, the surgeon should take washings and a biopsy from any suspicious area.

Surgery is the mainstay of treatment for ovarian cancer. The staging laparotomy and histological findings provide accurate information about prognosis and postoperative therapy. The general principle is cytoreductive surgery followed by combination chemotherapy; only a minority of patients with ovarian cancer need bowel resected during the primary procedure or surgery for recurrent disease. The only exception to this rule is a young woman with stage I disease or a borderline tumour who requests unilateral oophorectomy to conserve her fertility.

Stage I/grade 1 epithelial adenocarcinoma requires no postoperative therapy. Stage I/grade 2 or 3 cancers and stage II cancers require six courses of chemotherapy (typically, paclitaxel and carboplatin). Stage III or IV cancer requires six courses of similar chemotherapy. Intraperitoneal chemotherapy or high-dose chemotherapy with bone marrow transplantation is under study. Radiation therapy is used infrequently. Even if chemotherapy results in a complete clinical response (i.e. normal physical examination, normal serum CA-125 and negative CT scan of the abdomen and pelvis), about 50 per cent of such patients with stage III or IV cancer will have residual tumour. Of patients with persistent elevation of CA-125, 90–95 per cent have residual tumour.

Ovarian stimulation with ooctye or embryo freezing has been reported in patients with low-grade tumours who wish to preserve fertility, but the effect of this on the underlying disease is as yet unknown and it must therefore be carried out with caution.

FURTHER READING

Epithelial ovarian cancer. Available from www.sign.ac.uk.

Pecorelli S. Revised FIGO staging for carcinoma of the vulva, cervix, and endometrium. *Int J Gynaecol Obstet* 2009; **105**: 103–4.

RCOG Green-top guidelines on acute pelvic inflammatory disease, early pregnancy loss, endometriosis, ovarian cysts in postmenopausal women, pregnancy and breast cancer, and ectopic pregnancy. Available from www.rcog.org.uk/womens-health.

PART 13

Transplantation

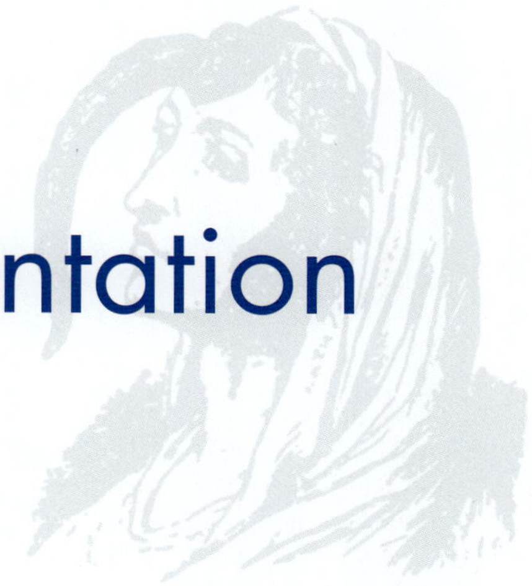

CHAPTER

81 Transplantation

LEARNING OBJECTIVES

- To appreciate the immunological basis of allograft rejection
- To know the principles of immunosuppressive therapy
- To be aware of the side effects of non-specific immunosuppression
- To be familiar with the major issues concerning organ donation
- To appreciate the main indications for organ transplantation
- To know the surgical principles of organ implantation
- To be able to give an account of the causes of graft dysfunction
- To know the likely outcomes after transplantation
- To be aware of potential future developments in transplantation

HISTORICAL PERSPECTIVE

Since early times, the idea of tissue and organ transplantation has captured the imagination of successive generations and, over the centuries, numerous fanciful descriptions of successful transplants have been recorded. One of the most widely cited early examples is that of the Christian Arab Saints Cosmas and Damian. Around ad 300, they were reputed to have successfully replaced the diseased leg of a patient with that from another man who had died several days earlier (Figure 81.1).

The modern era of transplantation began in the 1950s (Table 81.1) and relied on surgical techniques for anastomosing blood vessels that had been developed at the beginning of the twentieth century by Mathieu Jaboulay and Alexis Carrel. The first successful kidney transplant was a living-donor transplant performed between identical twins in 1954 at the Brigham Hospital in Boston by Joseph Murray and colleagues. This, and other kidney transplants between identical twins, demonstrated the technical feasibility of kidney transplantation, but attempts to perform renal transplantation when the donor and recipient were not genetically identical failed because no effective immunosuppressive therapy was available (Figure 81.2). Then, in 1959, Schwartz and Dameshek discovered that 6-mercaptopurine had immunosuppressive properties, and Calne showed that azathioprine, a derivative of 6-mercaptopurine, prevented rejection of canine kidney transplants. From the early 1960s, a combination of azathioprine and corticosteroids was used with moderate success in the clinic to prevent graft rejection after

> **Alexis Carrel**, 1873–1944, was a surgeon from Lyons in France, who worked at the Rockefellar Institute for Medical Research in New York, NY, USA. He received the Nobel Prize for Physiology or Medicine in 1912 'In recognition of his works on vascular suture and the transplantation of blood vessels and organs'.
> **Joseph E Murray**, born 1919, Professor Emeritus of Plastic Surgery, The Harvard University Medical School, Boston, MA, USA. He shared the 1990 Nobel Prize for Physiology or Medicine with E Donnall Thomas for his work on organ and cell transplantation

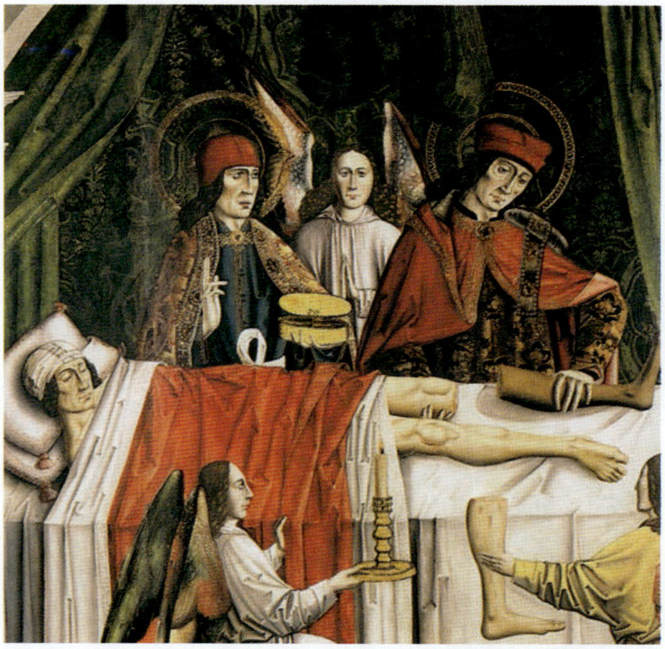

Figure 81.1 Depiction of Saints Cosmas and Damian performing a miraculous transplantation of the leg. Oil painting attributed to the Master of Los Balbases (Wellcome Institute Library, London).

Mathieu Jaboulay, 1860–1913, Professor of Surgery, Lyons, France.
Robert S Schwartz, Professor of Medicine, The Tufts University School of Medicine, Boston, MA, USA.
William Dameshek, 1900–1969, an American physician and haematologist.

Table 81.1 Milestones in organ transplantation.

1954	Joe Murray performed successful kidney transplants between identical twins (Boston, MA, USA)
1962	Roy Calne demonstrated the efficacy of azathioprine in preventing rejection of kidney allografts (Boston, MA, USA)
1963	Tom Starzl performed the first human liver transplant (Denver, CO, USA)
1966	Tom Starzl and colleagues used antilymphocyte globulin immunosuppression (Denver, CO, USA)
1966	Richard Lillehei and William Kelly performed first human whole organ pancreas transplant (along with a kidney transplant) (Minneapolis, MN, USA)
1967	Christiaan Barnard performed the first human heart transplant (Cape Town, South Africa)
1968	Fritz Derom performed the first human lung transplant (Ghent, Belgium)
1969	Geoff Collins developed Collins solution – a new kidney preservation solution
1974	David Sutherland and John Najarin performed the first human pancreatic islet transplant (Minneapolis, MN, USA)
1978	Roy Calne introduced ciclosporin into clinical practice (Cambridge, UK)
1981	Bruce Reitz and Norman Shumway performed the first successful human heart-lung transplant (Stanford, CA, USA)
1987	Fokert Belzer and colleagues developed University of Wisconsin (UW) solution – a new liver and pancreas preservation solution (Wisconsin, USA)
1989	Tom Starzl demonstrated clinical efficacy of FK506 (tacrolimus) (Pittsburgh, PA, USA)
1995	Lloyd Ratner and colleagues first described laparoscopic living-donor nephrectomy (Johns Hopkins University, Baltimore, MD, USA)

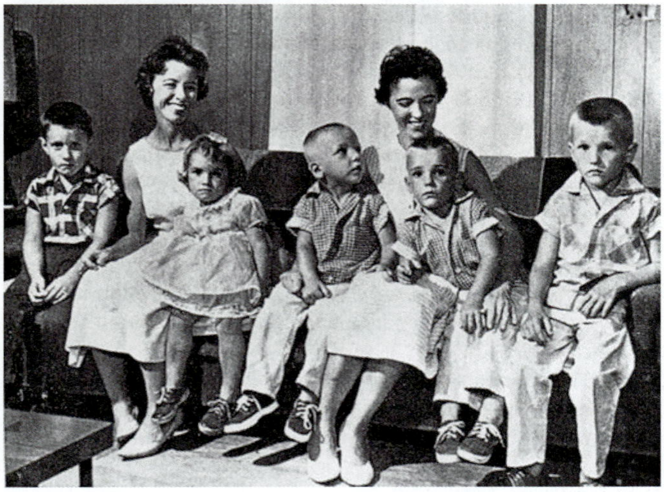

Figure 81.2 One of the early Boston recipients of a kidney transplant from an identical twin, shown here with her twin sister and their children.

kidney transplantation. These chemical agents were sometimes supplemented with a polyclonal antilymphocyte antibody.

The ciclosporin era began in the late 1970s following its discovery by Borel at the Sandoz laboratories in Basle and the demonstration, by Calne in Cambridge, UK, of its potent immunosuppressive properties in clinical transplantation. The introduction of ciclosporin was a major advance and ciclosporin (usually given together with azathioprine and steroids) not only improved the results of renal transplantation, but also allowed transplantation of the heart and liver to be undertaken with acceptable results. Organ transplantation is now well established as an effective treatment for selected patients with end-stage organ failure. Kidney, liver, pancreas, heart and lung transplantation are all routine procedures with good outcome, and transplantation of the small intestine is becoming more widely practised. Transplant activity is limited only by the shortage of donor organs.

Definitions of common terms in the area of organ transplantation are given in Summary box 81.1.

Summary box 81.1

Definitions

- Allograft: an organ or tissue transplanted from one individual to another
- Alloantigen: transplant antigen
- Alloantibody: transplant antibodies
- HLA: human leukocyte antigen, the main trigger to graft rejection
- Xenograft: a graft performed between different species
- Orthotopic graft: a graft placed in its normal anatomical site
- Heterotopic graft: a graft placed in a site different from that where the organ is normally located

GRAFT REJECTION

Allografts provoke a powerful immune response that results in rapid graft rejection unless immunosuppressive therapy is given. The pioneering studies of Medawar in the 1940s and 1950s firmly established that allograft rejection was due to an immune response and not a non-specific inflammatory response and subsequent studies demonstrated that T lymphocytes play an essential role in mediating rejection.

Allografts trigger a graft rejection response because of allelic differences at polymorphic genes that give rise to histocompatibility antigens (transplant antigens) of which ABO blood group antigens and human leukocyte antigens (HLA) are the most important.

ABO blood group antigens

The ABO blood group antigens are expressed not only by red blood cells, but by most other cell types as well. It is vitally

Sir Roy York Calne, Emeritus Professor of Surgery, The University of Cambridge, Cambridge, UK. In 1968 he performed Europe's first liver transplant. He was associated with the world's first liver, heart and lung transplant in 1987. He was elected Fellow of the Royal Society in 1974. He is an accomplished painter who has painted many of his transplant patients and has had exhibitions worldwide.

Sir Peter Brian Medawar, 1915–1987, a zoologist and immunologist and who was Director of the National Institute of Medical Research, London, UK. He shared the 1968 Nobel Prize for Physiology or Medicine with Sir Frank Macfarlane Burnet, for his research into immunological tolerance.

Jean-Francois Borel, a research scientist working in Switzerland.

important, for all types of organ allograft, to ensure that recipients do not unintentionally receive a graft that is ABO blood group compatible otherwise naturally occurring anti-A or anti-B antibodies will likely cause hyperacute graft rejection.

Permissible transplants are:

- group O donor to group O, A, B or AB recipient;
- group A donor to group A or AB recipient;
- group B donor to group B or AB recipient;
- group AB donor to group AB recipient.

There is no need to take account of rhesus antigen compatibility in organ transplantation.

HLA antigens

Allograft rejection (in blood group-compatible grafts) is directed predominantly against HLA – a group of highly polymorphic cell-surface molecules. HLA are strong transplant antigens by virtue of their special physiological role as antigen recognition units for display of antigens from foreign pathogens for recognition by T lymphocytes. It was through their role in stimulating graft rejection responses that their existence was first demonstrated by Dausset in 1958, hence their description as major histocompatibility antigens (Summary box 81.2).

Summary box 81.2

HLA antigens

- Are the most common cause of graft rejection
- Their physiological function is to act as antigen recognition units
- Are highly polymorphic (amino acid sequence differs widely between individuals)
- HLA-A, -B (class I) and -DR (class II) are most important in organ transplantation

Jean Dausset, born 1916, a French immunologist who was Professor of Experimental Medicine at The College of France, Paris, France. He shared the 1980 Nobel Prize for Physiology or Medicine with George Snell and Baruj Benacerraf for his discovery of the HLA antigens.

Table 81.2 HLA class I and HLA class II molecules.

	Class I	Class II
HLA loci	HLA-A, -B and -C	HLA-DR, -DP and -DQ
Structure	Heavy chain and β_2-microglobulin	α- and β-chain
Distribution	All nucleated cells	B cells, dendritic cells, macrophages

There are two types of HLA molecule: HLA class I and HLA class II (Table 81.2). They are broadly similar in structure (Figure 81.3) but have different cell expression profiles. HLA class I antigens are present on all nucleated cells, whereas HLA class II antigens have a more restricted distribution and are expressed most strongly on antigen-presenting cells, such as dendritic cells, macrophages and B lymphocytes. T cells recognize HLA molecules via their T-cell receptor but full T-cell activation also requires the delivery of an additional or second signal delivered by the interaction of costimulatory molecules on the surface of the antigen-presenting cell and T cell (Figure 81.4).

Effector mechanisms of rejection

HLA antigens expressed by graft cells activate T cells and stimulate them to proliferate in response to interleukin-2 (IL-2) and other T-cell growth factors. Activated CD4 T cells, through release of cytokines, play a central role in orchestrating the various effector mechanisms responsible for graft rejection (Figure 81.5). The cellular effectors of graft rejection include cytotoxic CD8 T cells, that recognise donor HLA class I antigens expressed by the graft and cause target cell death by releasing lytic molecules such as perforin and granzyme. Graft-infiltrating CD4 T cells, which recognise donor HLA class II antigens, mediate direct target cell damage and are also able, by releasing proinflammatory cytokines such as interferon-γ, to recruit and activate macrophages that act as non-specific effector cells. Finally, CD4 T cells provide essential T-cell help for B lymphocytes that differentiate into plasma cells and produce

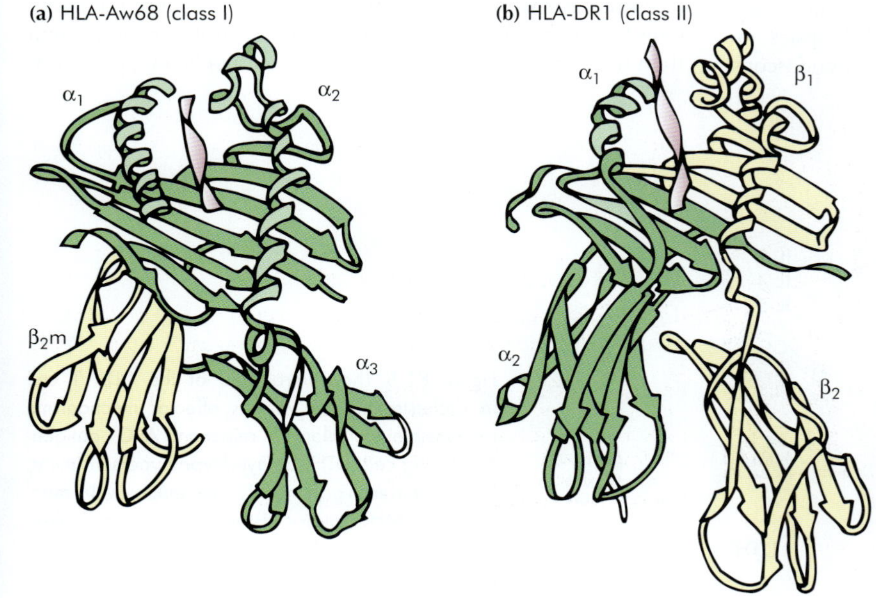

Figure 81.3 The three-dimensional structure of the extracellular domains of human leukocyte antigen (HLA) class I and class II. The α1 and α2 domains of class I and the α1 and β1 domains of class II form a cleft that is floored by a β-pleated sheet and walled by two α-helices. The cleft binds an antigenic peptide and displays it on the cell surface for recognition by a T lymphocyte. (Redrawn with permission from Stern and Wiley (1994) Structure 2: 245–52.)

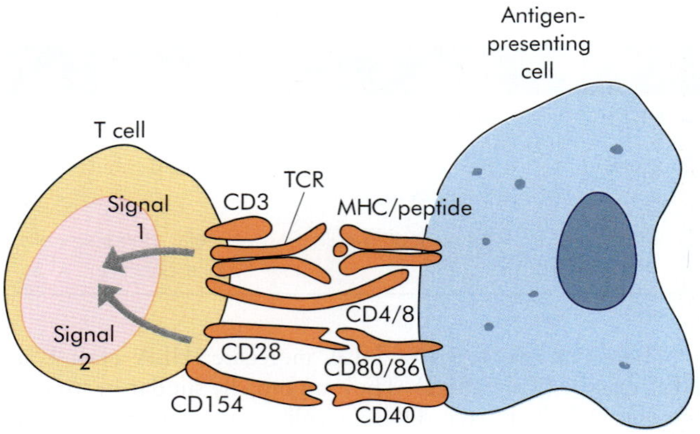

Figure 81.4 Molecular events involved in T-cell activation by an antigen-presenting cell. T-cell activation requires the delivery of two distinct signals to the T cell. The first signal is delivered by ligation of the TCR/CD3 complex with human leukocyte antigen (HLA)/peptide complex. The second signal is delivered following the interaction between pairs of costimulatory molecules such as CD28 with CD80/86 and CD154 with CD40.

Summary box 81.3

Types of graft rejection

- Hyperacute rejection
  - Immediate graft destruction due to ABO or preformed anti-HLA antibodies
  - Characterised by intravascular thrombosis and interstitial haemorrhage
- Acute rejection
  - Usually occurs during first six months
  - T cell dependent
  - May be cell-mediated, antibody-mediated or both
  - Usually reversible
- Chronic rejection
  - Occurs after first six months
  - Most common cause of graft failure
  - Antibodies play an important role
  - Non-immune factors contribute to pathogenesis
  - Characterised by myointimal proliferation in graft arteries leading to ischaemia and fibrosis

alloantibodies that bind to graft antigen and induce target cell injury directly or through antibody-dependent, cell-mediated cytotoxicity.

Types of allograft rejection

Allograft rejection can be divided into three distinct types (Summary box 81.3):

1. hyperacute rejection (occurs immediately);
2. acute rejection (usually occurs in the first six months);
3. chronic rejection (occurs months and years after transplantation).

Allograft rejection manifests itself as functional failure of the transplant and is confirmed by histological examination. Biopsy material is obtained from renal and pancreas grafts by needle biopsy, and from hepatic grafts by percutaneous or transjugular liver biopsy. Cardiac grafts are biopsied by transjugular endomyocardial biopsy and lung grafts by transbronchial biopsy. After small intestinal transplantation, mucosal biopsies are obtained from the graft stoma or more proximally by endoscopy.

A standardised histological grading system, termed the Banff classification (named after the Canadian town where the initial scientific workshop was held), defines the presence and severity of allograft rejection after organ transplantation.

Hyperacute rejection

This is due to the presence in the recipient of preformed antibodies against HLA class I antigens expressed by the donor. These arise from a previous blood transfusion, a failed transplant and pregnancy. This type of rejection also occurs if an ABO blood group-incompatible organ graft is performed inadvertantly. After revascularisation of the graft, antibodies bind immediately to the vasculature, activate the complement system and cause extensive intravascular thrombosis, interstitial haemorrhage and graft destruction within minutes and hours. Kidney transplants are particularly vulnerable to hyperacute graft rejection, whereas heart and liver transplants are relatively resistant. It is not clear why the liver is resistant to hyperacute rejection. One factor may be that that it is less susceptible to ischaemia than the kidney by virtue of its dual blood supply: 60 per cent of

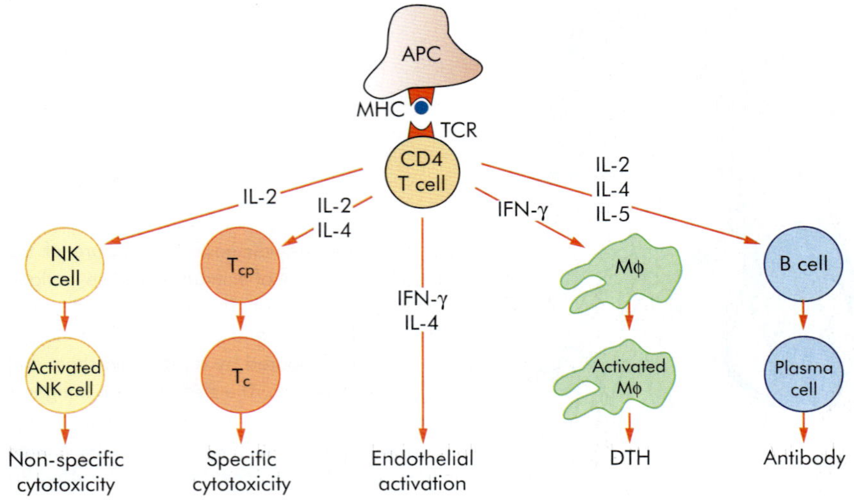

Figure 81.5 The central role of the CD4 T cell in orchestrating the various effector mechanisms responsible for allograft rejection. APC, antigen-presenting cell; DTH, delayed-type hypersensitivity; IFN-γ, interferon-gamma; IL, interleukin; MΦ, macrophage; MHC, major histocompatibility complex; NK, natural killer; Tc, T cytotoxic cell; Tcp, T cytotoxic precursor cell; TCR, T-cell receptor.

the hepatic blood supply is derived from the portal vein and 40 per cent from the hepatic artery.

Hyperacute rejection can be avoided by ensuring ABO blood group compatibility and by performing a cross-match test on recipient serum to ensure that there are no clinically relevant antibodies directed against HLA antigens expressed by a prospective kidney donor.

Acute rejection

This usually occurs during the first six months of transplantation but may occur later. It is mediated predominantly by T lymphocytes, but alloantibodies may also play an important role. Acute rejection is characterised by mononuclear cell infiltration of the graft (Figure 81.6). The mononuclear cell infiltrate is heterogeneous and includes cytotoxic T cells, B cells, NK cells and activated macrophages. Antibody-mediated damage may also be present as evidenced by the deposition of the complement component C4d within the graft microvasculature (Figure 81.7). All types of organ allograft are susceptible to acute rejection, and although relatively common (typically occurring in around 20–30 per cent of grafts), most episodes of acute rejection can be reversed by additional immunosuppressive therapy.

Chronic rejection

This usually occurs after the first six months. All types of transplant are susceptible to chronic rejection, and it is the major cause of allograft failure. Interestingly, the liver is more resistant than other organs to the destructive effects of chronic rejection. The pathophysiology of chronic rejection is not well understood. The underlying mechanisms are immunological, and alloantibodies are thought to be a major cause although cellular effector mechanisms may also contribute. Alloantigen-independent factors also contribute. The risk factors for chronic rejection of a kidney transplant are:

- previous episodes of acute rejection;
- poor HLA match;
- long cold ischaemia time;
- cytomegalovirus (CMV) infection;
- raised blood lipids;
- inadequate immunosuppression (including poor compliance).

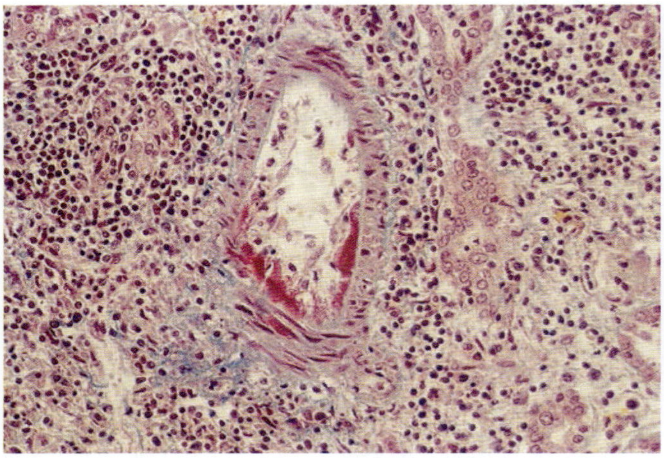

Figure 81.6 Severe acute renal allograft rejection with a heavy mononuclear cell infiltrate and intimal arteritis.

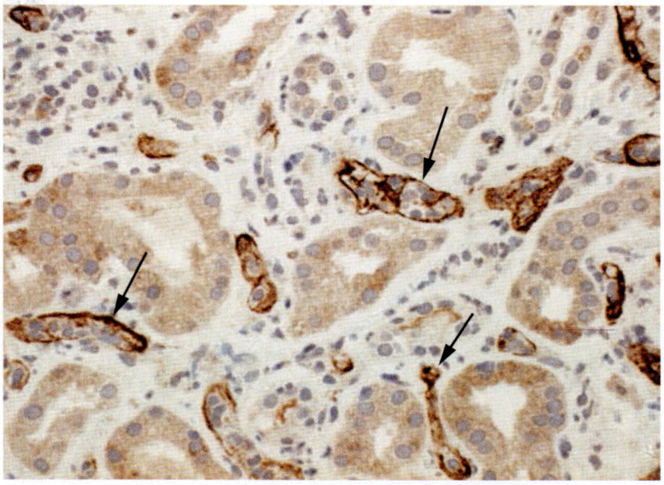

Figure 81.7 Acute antibody-mediated renal allograft rejection. There is widespread staining for the complement component C4d within the peritubular capillaries (arrows) that indicates alloantibody binding to the graft vasculature.

The single most important risk factor for chronic rejection after kidney transplantation is acute rejection (with vascular inflammation) and recurrent episodes of acute rejection. Because non-immune factors often contribute significantly to the long-term failure of a kidney transplant, the term 'chronic allograft nephropathy' is sometimes used.

The histological picture of chronic rejection after organ transplantation is dominated by vascular changes, with the development of myointimal proliferation in arteries, which results in ischaemia and fibrosis (Figure 81.8). In addition to vasculopathy, there are organ-specific features of chronic graft rejection. These are:

- kidney: glomerular sclerosis and tubular atrophy;
- pancreas: acinar loss and islet destruction;
- heart: accelerated coronary artery disease (cardiac allograft vasculopathy);
- liver: vanishing bile duct syndrome;
- lungs: obliterative bronchiolitis.

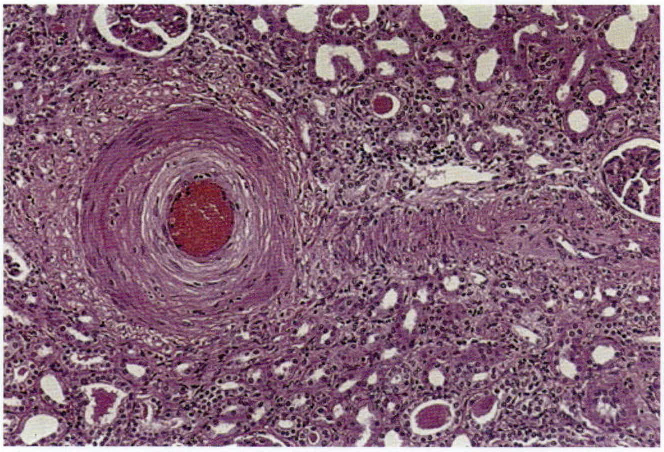

Figure 81.8 Chronic renal allograft rejection. The arteriole shows severe myointimal proliferation and luminal narrowing, resulting in ischaemic fibrosis.

Chronic rejection causes functional deterioration in the graft, resulting after months or years in complete graft failure. Unfortunately, currently available immunosuppressive therapy has had little effect in preventing chronic rejection.

Graft-versus-host disease

Although the main immunological problem after transplantation is graft rejection, the reciprocal problem of graft-versus-host reaction is occasionally seen following certain types of organ transplantation. Some donor organs (particularly liver and small bowel) contain large numbers of lymphocytes, and these may react against HLA antigens expressed by recipient tissues, leading to graft-versus-host disease (GVHD). GVHD frequently involves the skin, causing a characteristic rash on the palms and soles. It may also involve the liver (after small bowel transplantation) and the gastrointestinal tract (after liver transplantation). GVHD is a serious and sometimes fatal complication.

HLA MATCHING

HLA molecules are encoded by the major histocompatibility complex (MHC), a cluster of genes situated on the short arm of chromosome 6 (Figure 81.9). The HLA class I antigens comprise HLA-A, -B and -C, and the HLA class II antigens comprise HLA-DR, -DP and -DQ. Expression of MHC genes is co-dominant, i.e. the genes on both the maternally derived and the paternally derived chromosomes are expressed. Consequently, an individual may express between 6 and 12 different HLA antigens, depending on the degree of homozygosity (shared genes) at individual loci.

The HLA haplotype inherited from each parent is usually inherited as a complete haplotype, according to simple Mendelian genetics (Figure 81.10). In deceased donor renal transplantation (but not other types of organ transplantation), attempts are usually made to match the donor and recipient for as many of the relevant HLA antigens as possible. In addition to reducing the risk of graft loss from rejection, a well-matched kidney allograft that subsequently fails is less likely to cause sensitisation to the HLA antigens that it expresses. It is particularly important in children and young adults to avoid, where possible, grafts that are mismatched for common HLA antigens because, if retransplantation is required subsequently, it may be difficult to find an organ donor who does not express the antigens to which the recipient has become sensitised. In terms of organ transplantation, HLA-A, -B and -DR are the most important antigens to take into account when matching donor and recipient in an attempt to reduce the risk of graft rejection (Figure 81.11).

HLA matching has a relatively small but definite beneficial effect on renal allograft survival (HLA-DR > HLA-B > HLA-A). Recipients who receive well-matched renal allografts may require less intensive immunosuppression and also are troubled less by rejection episodes. It is common practice to express the degree of HLA matching between the donor and recipient in terms of whether or not there are mismatches at each locus for HLA-A, -B and -DR. A '000 mismatch' is a 'full-house' or complete match, whereas a '012 mismatch' is matched at

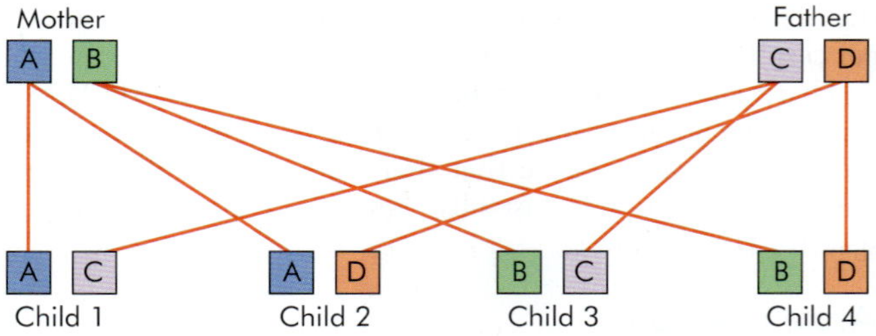

Figure 81.10 Human leukocyte antigen (HLA) inheritance. Children acquire one HLA haplotype (depicted as A–D) from each parent. As shown, child 1 shares one HLA haplotype (haploidentical) with child 2 and child 3, but does not share either haplotype with child 4. The chances that two siblings will share the same parental haplotypes, or that they will share neither HLA haplotype, is one in four. The chance that they will share one HLA haplotype is one in two.

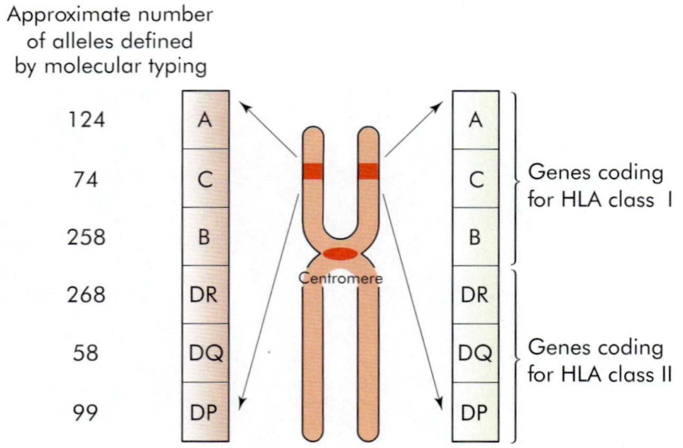

Figure 81.9 The human leukocyte antigen (HLA) system on the short arm of chromosome 6.

Gregor Johann Mendel, 1822–1884, an Austrian monk and naturalist who became Abbot of the Augustinian Monastery at Brunn, the Czech Republic and discovered the laws of inheritance by studying the edible pea. In 1865 he described 'dominant' and 'recessive' traits in hybrids. His work passed unnoticed for 35 years.

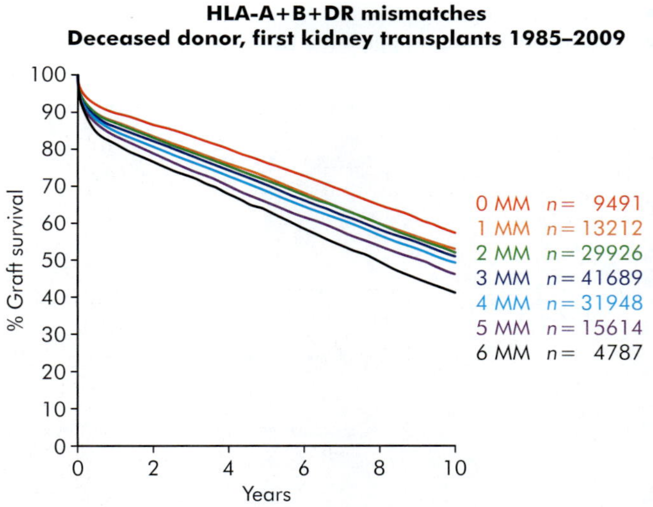

Figure 81.11 Beneficial effect of human leukocyte antigen (HLA) matching (HLA-A, -B and -DR) on first deceased donor renal allograft survival (courtesy of Gerhard Opelz, Collaborative Transplant Study, CTC-K21101-0211). MM, antigen mismatch.

HLA-A loci, has one mismatched HLA-B antigen and is mismatched for both DR antigens. Deceased donor kidneys are allocated in some countries, including the UK, by a points system that optimises HLA matching but also takes into account other factors, such as time on the waiting list, sensitisation to HLA antigens and the age relationship between the donor and recipient. Allocation of organs for transplantation must also take into account the relative size of donor and recipient. This is not an issue in renal transplantation, and adult kidneys can be readily used for paediatric recipients (and vice versa). However, in the case of heart, lung, liver and small bowel transplantation, it is important to consider size compatibility between the donor and recipient. In the case of liver transplants, HLA matching does not confer an advantage and, although it is beneficial in cardiac transplantation, it is not practicable because of the relatively small size of the recipient pool and the short permissible cold ischaemic time.

THE TISSUE-TYPING LABORATORY

Successful organ transplantation requires a close-working relationship between the tissue-typing laboratory and the clinical transplant team. The tissue-typing laboratory carries out three key tasks. First, they determine the HLA type ('tissue type') of all potential organ transplant recipients and organ donors. This is achieved by applying polymerase chain reaction-based DNA-typing techniques to samples of peripheral blood. Second, they perform a cross-match test to exclude the presence in a recipient of clinically significant circulating antibodies to HLA antigens expressed by a potential organ donor that would result in rapid or hyperacute graft rejection. This involves incubating recipient sera with donor lymphocytes prepared from either blood or lymphoid tissue. The presence of antidonor antibodies is detected in a conventional cytotoxic cross-match assay by adding rabbit complement along with indicator dyes and visualising target cell death. More often now a flow cytometric cross-match is performed as well as, or instead of, a cytotoxic cross-match. Third, the tissue-typing laboratory determines the HLA specificity of circulating anti-HLA antibodies in recipients before and after organ transplantation to guide organ allocation and immunosuppressive therapy. This task has been revolutionised by the availability of solid phase assays, particularly Luminex technology, where patient sera are incubated with a panel of latex beads coated with purified HLA molecules and antibody binding detected by flow cytometric analysis.

Patients on the renal transplant waiting list should be screened for the development of HLA antibodies on a regular basis and especially after potential priming to HLA antigens by blood transfusion.

If, when considering renal transplantation the cross-match test is strongly positive, transplantation should not proceed, otherwise hyperacute rejection is likely. Antibodies directed against HLA class II antigens, unlike those to HLA class I, do not usually cause hyperacute rejection but are associated with acute rejection and a poor clinical outcome. Patients awaiting heart transplantation are also screened for the presence of HLA antibodies and those with preformed antibodies are subjected to a prospective cross-match test. Although heart allografts rarely undergo hyperacute rejection, transplantation in the presence of a positive cross-match is associated with graft loss from accelerated acute rejection. Even in the presence of a strongly positive cross-match test, liver transplants rarely undergo hyperacute rejection, although long-term survival is reduced.

IMMUNOSUPPRESSIVE THERAPY

A range of different agents are available that act at different sites during T-cell activation to prevent rejection (Table 81.3 and Figure 81.12). They can be classified according to their principal mode of action.

Table 81.3 Immunosuppressive agents.

Agent	Principal mode of action
Corticosteroids	Widespread anti-inflammatory effects
Azathioprine	Prevents lymphocyte proliferation
Mycophenolic acid preperations	Prevents lymphocyte proliferation
Calcineurin inhibitors (ciclosporin/tacrolimus)	Blocks IL-2 gene transcription
mTOR inhibitors	Blocks IL-2 receptor signal transduction
ALG	Depletion and blockade of lymphocytes
Anti-CD25 mAb	Targets activated T cells
Anti-CD52 mAb	Depletion of lymphocytes
Anti-CD20	Depletion of B lymphocytes
CTLA-4Ig	Blocks T-cell costimulation

IL-2, interleukin-2.

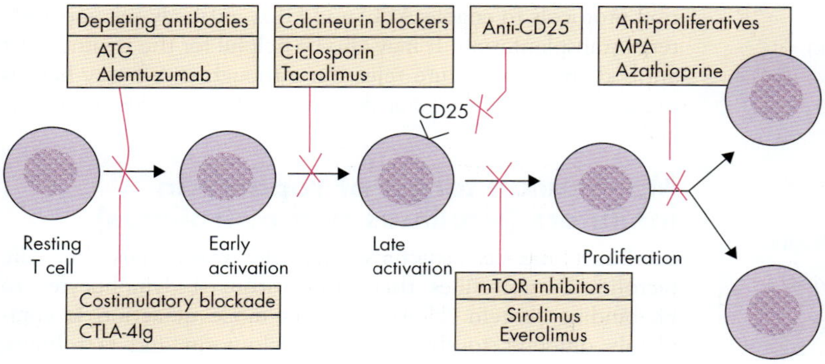

Figure 81.12 Site of action of immunosuppressive agents on T cell. ATG, antithymocyte globulin; MPA, mycophenolic acid derivatives; mTOR, mammalian target of rapamycin.

Calcineurin inhibitors (ciclosporin and tacrolimus)

Ciclosporin and tacrolimus are the mainstay of most modern immunosuppressive protocols for organ transplantation. Although structurally distinct, they exert their principal immunosuppressive effect through the same intracellular pathway. Each of the two agents binds within the T cell to a cytoplasmic protein or immunophilin (ciclosporin binds to cyclophilin and tacrolimus to FK-binding protein). The resulting immunophilin–drug complex then blocks the activity of calcineurin (a phosphatase) within the cytoplasm of the T cell. Calcineurin plays a critical role in facilitating the transcription of IL-2, the main T-cell growth factor, and other cytokines after T-cell activation. By blocking cytokine synthesis, ciclosporin and tacrolimus exert a potent immunosuppressive effect. The two agents share a number of side effects, the most notable of which is nephrotoxicity (Table 81.4). Ciclosporin sometimes causes cosmetic side effects (hirsutism and gingival hypertrophy) that may be distressing, particularly in younger female recipients. The calcineurin inhibitors (CNIs) have a relatively small therapeutic window. Their immunosuppressive action, as well as their side effects, is dependent on their blood concentration, and monitoring of whole-blood drug levels is an important guide to optimal therapy. Ciclosporin and tacrolimus are broadly equivalent in terms of long-term graft survival but increasing evidence suggests tacrolimus is more effective in reducing acute rejection. The choice between the two agents depends on the preference of the transplant unit and on individual patient tolerance to the different side effects of the two agents.

Table 81.4 Agent-specific side effects of immunosuppressive agents used in organ transplantation (all immunosuppressive agents increase the risk of infection).

Agent	Side effects (not comprehensive)
Corticosteroids	Hypertension, dyslipidaemia, diabetes, osteoporosis, avascular necrosis, Cushingoid appearance
Azathioprine	Leukopenia, thrombocytopenia, hepatotoxicity, gastrointestinal symptoms
Mycophenolic acid derivatives	Leukopenia, thrombocytopenia, gastrointestinal symptoms
Ciclosporin	Nephrotoxicity, hypertension, dyslipidaemia, hirsutism, gingival hyperplasia
Tacrolimus	Nephrotoxicity, hypertension, dyslipidaemia, neurotoxicity, diabetes
mTOR inhibitors	Thrombocytopenia, dyslipidaemia, pneumonitis, impaired wound healing
ALG	Infusion reactions, leukopenia and thrombocytopenia
Anti-CD25	Uncommon
CTLA-4Ig	? Increased risk of PTLD
Anti-CD52	Infusion reaction and autoimmune disease
Anti-CD20	Infusion reactions and pulmonary toxicity

ALG, antilymphocyte globulin; mTOR, mammalian target of rapamycin; PTLD, post-transplant lymphoproliferative disease.

Antiproliferative agents (azathioprine and mycophenolate)

Lymphocytes are among the most rapidly proliferating cells in the body, and lymphocyte proliferation and clonal expansion is an integral part of the immune response to an allograft. The antiproliferative agents available for immunoprophylaxis are azathioprine and mycophenolic acid preparations (mycophenolate mofetil (MMF) and mycophenolic acid sodium (MPAS)). Azathioprine is converted in the liver to its active metabolite, 6-mercaptopurine, which blocks purine metabolism and thereby inhibits cellular proliferation. Mycophenolic acid (MPA) preparations are more expensive than azathioprine but have largely replaced it as the agents of choice. After ingestion, MMF is converted to its active metabolite MPA. It inhibits the enzyme inosine monophosphate dehydrogenase, which is the rate-limiting enzyme in the *de novo* pathway of purine nucleotide synthesis. Because lymphocytes do not have a salvage pathway for purine synthesis, their ability to proliferate is selectively impaired. The main side effects of azathioprine and MPA are bone marrow suppression and gastrointestinal symptoms.

Steroids

Steroids are an important component of many immunosuppressive regimens. Glucocorticoids are potent anti-inflammatory agents and have wide-ranging effects on the immune response. Because of their numerous and well-known side effects, some centres attempt to gradually withdraw steroids from patients who have stable graft function after transplantation, but this sometimes precipitates a rejection episode and necessitates recommencement of steroids.

Antibody therapies

Monoclonal antibodies directed against the IL-2 receptor on T lymphocytes (CD25) are commonly given at the time of transplantation to temporarily augment the effects of calcineurin blockade during the early post-transplant period. Their effect lasts for a few weeks only and they lack any significant agent-specific side effects. Polyclonal antibody (antithymocyte globulin (ATG)) and monoclonal antibody preparations (alemtuzumab (anti-CD52 expressed on T cells and dendritic cells) are also quite widely used as more potent and alternative induction agents. They cause a temporary depletion of circulating lymphocytes that reduces rejection but may lead to an increase in infection and malignancy. In addition to their use as induction agents, antibody preparations may be used to treat acute rejection episodes that fail to respond to steroid therapy.

The monoclonal anti-CD20 antibody (rituximab) depletes B lymphocytes and is widely used as a component of desensitisation protocols to enable ABO and HLA antibody-incompatible renal transplantation. It may also be helpful for the treatment of antibody-mediated acute rejection although its efficacy here is limited because it does not deplete antibody-producing plasma cells.

Mammalian target of rapamycin inhibitors (sirolimus and everolimus)

Sirolimus and its structural analogue everolimus are, like tacrolimus, macrolides that bind within T lymphocytes to FK-binding protein. However, their mode of action is completely different to that of both ciclosporin and tacrolimus.

They act by inhibiting an intracellular kinase called mammalian target of rapamycin (mTOR) and interfere with intracellular signalling from the IL-2 receptor, arresting T-cell division in the G1 phase. In contrast to CNIs they are not nephrotoxic. However, their side effect profile includes lymphocoele formation, impaired wound healing, an adverse effect on the blood lipid profile, thrombocytopenia and very occasionally pneumonitis. mTOR inhibitors may have antitumour activity and the potential value of this effect in transplant patients is under investigation. Although the negative effect on wound healing and lymphocoele formation limits the immediate use of mTOR inhibitors after transplantation, switching from CNIs to mTOR inhibitors is being used increasingly as a strategy to minimise CNI-induced nephrotoxicity.

T-cell costimulatory blockers

CTLA-4Ig (belatocept, LEA29Y) is a fusion protein comprising the extracellular domain of CTLA-4 fused to human IgFc. It binds to the costimulatory ligands CD80 and CD86 expressed on antigen-presenting cells and as a result prevents them from delivering the costimulatory signals to the T cells that are required for full T-cell activation. It has recently been shown in renal transplantation to provide an effective alternative to CNIs when given by regular i.v. injection, thereby avoiding the metabolic, cardiovascular and nephrotoxic effects of CNIs. Although its future looks very promising, a potential concern is that it may be associated with an increased risk of post-transplant lymphoproliferative disease (PTLD).

Immunosuppressive regimens

When selecting an immunosuppressive regimen, the challenge is to provide levels of immunosuppression that are sufficient to protect the graft from rejection without exposing the recipient to excessive risk from infection and malignancy as a result of non-specific immunosuppression (Summary box 81.4). Immunosuppressive therapy is started at the time of transplantation and is continued indefinitely (as maintenance therapy), although the requirement for immunosuppression is highest in the first few weeks after transplantation when the risk of acute rejection is greatest. Immunosuppressive protocols vary, but all use a combination of immunosuppressive agents acting at different points in the pathway of lymphocyte activation. Most currently include a CNI (ciclosporin or tacrolimus) as the main agent and often this is supplemented with anti-CD25 monoclonal antibody induction therapy. CNIs are usually combined with an antiproliferative agent (most often MMF) and steroids, so-called triple therapy. Less often, a CNI is used with an antiproliferative agent alone or with steroids alone (dual therapy). When there is particular concern about acute rejection, polyclonal or monoclonal antibody preparations are administered followed by a CNI, an antiproliferative agent and steroids.

The principles of immunoprophylaxis are similar for all types of organ transplantation. Interestingly, liver grafts seem to be less susceptible to rejection for reasons that are still unclear. The mTOR inhibitors have been shown to be effective immunosuppressive agents for preventing acute rejection following kidney transplantation and they provide a non-nephrotoxic alternative to CNIs for maintenance therapy. They have a similar safety profile to CNIs in terms of post-transplant infection but some of their agent-specific side effects are of potential concern and their clinical niche is still to be fully determined. Similarly, the potential role that CTLA-4Ig will find as an alternative to CNIs remains to be seen.

Acute rejection occurs in up to around 30 per cent of transplant recipients but usually responds to a short course of high-dose steroid therapy. If the response to steroids is inadequate or if acute rejection recurs, acute rejection can often be treated successfully by recourse to antilymphocyte globulin (ALG) therapy.

Summary box 81.4

Principles of immunosuppression

- Principles are the same for all types of organ transplantation
- Aim is to maximise graft protection with minimum of side effects
- Most regimens are based on calcineurin blockade and include steroids and an antiproliferative agent
- Need for immunosuppression is highest in the first three months but indefinite treatment is needed
- Immunosuppression increases the risk of infection and malignancy

COMPLICATIONS OF IMMUNOSUPPRESSION

As well as the agent-specific side effects already mentioned, the immunosuppressive agents used in organ transplantation cause non-specific immunosuppression and increase the risk of both infection and malignancy (Summary box 81.5).

Summary box 81.5

Side effects of non-specific immunosuppression

- Infection
  - Transplant recipients are at high risk of opportunistic infection, especially by viruses
  - Bacterial and fungal infections are also common
  - Risk of infection is greatest during first six months
  - Chemoprophylaxis is important for high-risk patients
  - Viral infection may result from reactivation of latent virus or from primary infection
  - Cytomegalovirus is a major problem
  - Pretransplant vaccination against community-acquired infection should be considered
- Malignancy
  - Most types of cancer are more common after transplantation
  - Recipients, especially children, are at risk of post-transplant lymphoproliferative disease (PTLD)
  - There is a very high risk of squamous cancer of the skin and recipients should have regular skin review

Infection

Transplant recipients receiving immunosuppressive therapy are at high risk from opportunistic infection, especially by viruses. Opportunistic infection is a potential problem in all transplant recipients, but those receiving aggressive immunosuppressive therapy are most at risk. Chemoprophylaxis is important in high-risk recipients, and early recognition followed by prompt and aggressive treatment of infection is essential in all transplant recipients. Pretransplant vaccination against community-acquired infections should be considered.

Bacterial infection

The risk of bacterial infection is highest during the first month after transplantation. Transplant recipients are, like any patient undergoing major surgery, at risk of bacterial infections in the wound, respiratory tract and urinary tract. It is standard practice to give a broad-spectrum antibiotic to cover the perioperative period as prophylaxis against wound infection and possible bacterial contamination of the donor organ. The risk of bacterial infection is greatest in transplant recipients who are critically ill before or after surgery and are in the intensive care unit with indwelling catheters and lines. After recovery from surgery, the risk of bacterial infection is much reduced. Tuberculosis is a concern in patients who have previously had mycobacterial infection and in patients from the Indian subcontinent, and it is usual to give them chemoprophylaxis for a period of 6–12 months after transplantation.

Viral infection

The risk of viral infection is highest during the first six months after transplantation and the most common problem is CMV infection. CMV disease may arise because of reactivation of latent infection or because of primary infection that can be transmitted by an organ from a CMV-positive donor. Recipients at most risk from CMV infection are those who are CMV seronegative (i.e. those who have not been infected previously with CMV) and receive an organ from a CMV-seropositive donor (about half of all UK donors are CMV seropositive). Unfortunately, matching seronegative donors with seronegative recipients is not practicable. Without prophylaxis, CMV disease typically presents at 4–8 weeks with a high swinging fever, lethargy and leukopenia. The severity of the disease is variable and the clinical picture depends on the organ system most affected. It may present as:

- pneumonia
- gastrointestinal disease
- hepatatitis
- retinitis
- encephalitis.

Severe CMV disease is potentially fatal. Prophylaxis for CMV consists of administration of antiviral agents, most commonly valganciclovir; aciclovir and valaciclovir are cheaper but less effective alternatives. A diagnosis of active CMV infection is confirmed by polymerase chain reaction (PCR) to detect viral DNA in whole blood, and by histological examination of biopsy material. Treatment is with antiviral agents (either oral valganciclovir or i.v. ganciclovir) and is more effective when given pre-emptively on the basis of increased viral load detected by quantitative PCR analysis of peripheral blood.

Herpes simplex virus (HSV) infection is common after transplantation and is usually due to reactivation of latent infection. It causes mucocutaneous lesions around the mouth and sometimes the genitalia. These usually respond to topical treatment with acyclovir, but in severe cases systemic antiviral therapy is needed. Disseminated HSV infection is rare.

BK virus is emerging as an important cause of graft dysfunction after renal transplantation. Infection with BK virus is almost universal during childhood, with latent infection in the epithelium of the urinary tract. Immunosuppression causes lytic BK virus replication with graft involvement in 1–5 per cent of renal transplants. The only effective treatment is to reduce the level of immunosuppression to allow natural immune mechanisms to regain control of the virus.

Herpes zoster infection, as a result of reactivation of latent varicella zoster virus, occurs more frequently in transplant patients and should be treated with systemic antiviral therapy. Primary varicella zoster virus infection (chickenpox) is potentially very serious in immunosuppressed patients but is relatively uncommon as most adults have acquired immunity.

Fungal infection

Pneumocystis jiroveci (previously designated *Pneumocystis carinii* and wrongly classified as a protozoa) is one of the more important fungal infections after transplantation. It occurs during the first few months and presents with respiratory symptoms. The diagnosis is made by examination of bronchoalveolar lavage fluid or lung biopsy material for evidence of fungal infection (Figure 81.13). Chemoprophylaxis is highly effective and usually continued for up to six months after transplantation.

Other types of invasive fungal infections are uncommon in renal transplant recipients but infection with *Candida* or *Aspergillus* is more common after other types of organ transplantation. Fungal infection usually occurs in the first three months after transplantation, and early diagnosis and aggressive treatment are essential to avoid fatal infection.

Malignancy

After transplantation, there is an increased risk of developing most types of malignant disease but the risk is particularly high for those types of tumour in which viral infection plays an aetiological role. The increased risk of malignancy is particularly high for skin cancer and post-transplant lymphoproliferative disorder. Most of the skin cancers seen are squamous cell car-

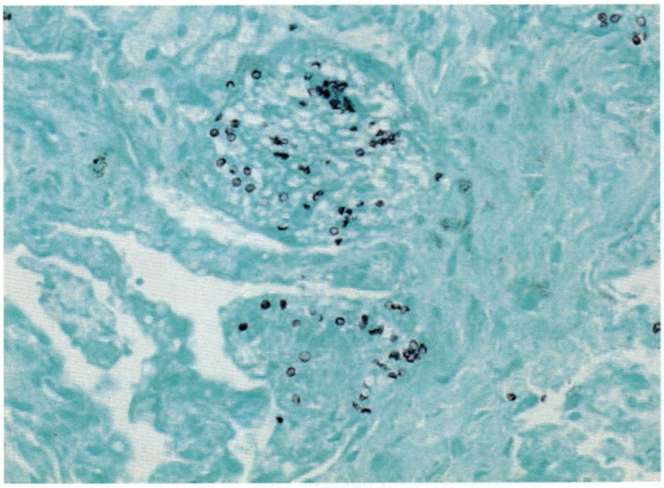

Figure 81.13 Transbronchial lung biopsy from a renal allograft recipient with *Pneumocystis jiroveci* pneumonia. The silver stain used reveals fungal cysts, each containing several intracystic bodies or spores, distributed widely within the biopsy material.

cinomas, but basal cell carcinoma and malignant melanoma are also more common than in the general population. The risk of skin cancer after transplantation rises with age and with exposure to sunlight, and it has been predicted that 50 per cent of transplant patients will develop a skin malignancy within 20 years of transplantation. Patients must be warned of this risk before they undergo transplantation and advised to take precautions to protect their skin from excessive sunlight. They should undergo regular review of their skin to detect early malignancy, and when malignant lesions occur they must be treated promptly and aggressively.

Post-transplant lymphoproliferative disorder is an abnormal proliferation of B lymphocytes, usually in response to Epstein–Barr virus infection. The condition presents in a variety of ways including as an infectious mononucleosis-type illness, as lymphadenopathy or with involvement of extranodal sites such as the tonsils, gastrointestinal tract, lung, liver or the transplanted organ (Figure 81.14). PTLD occurs in around 1–3 per cent of kidney and liver transplant recipients and the incidence is considerably higher in children. Those patients at most risk are those who have received aggressive immunosuppression. PTLD is a serious condition with an overall mortality of up to 50 per cent. If it is identified at an early stage, reduction or cessation of immunosuppressive therapy may cause disease regression and result in a cure. Chemotherapy is often given and antiviral therapy, surgery and radiotherapy may also have a role in treating established disease. Disseminated PTLD and central nervous system (CNS) involvement have a very poor prognosis.

Transplant patients also have a 300-fold increased risk of developing Kaposi's sarcoma, although this malignancy is still very uncommon after transplantation.

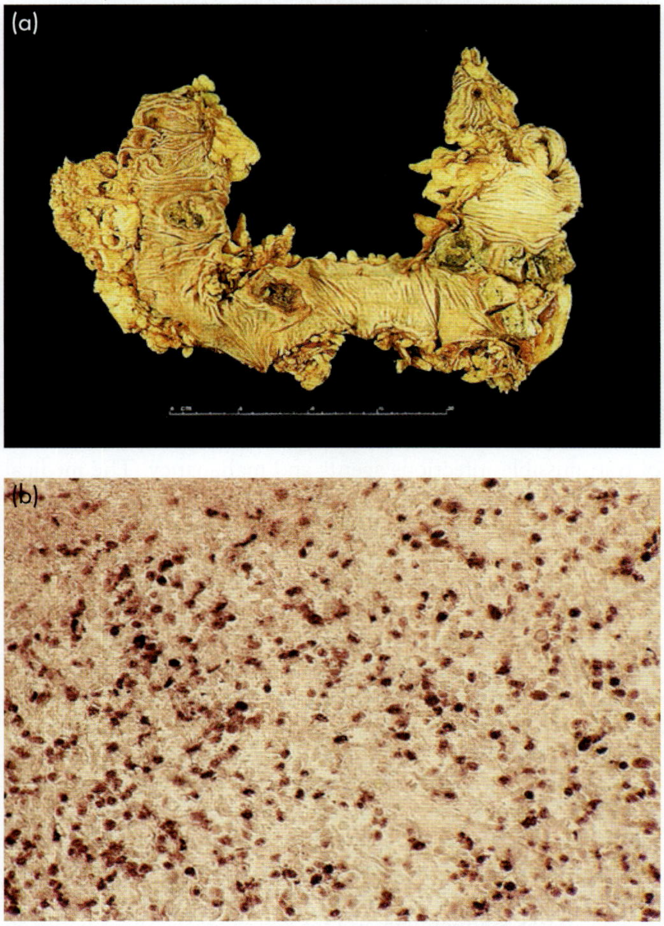

Figure 81.14 (a) Intestinal post-transplant lymphoproliferative disease (PTLD). Note multiple lesions in terminal ileum and colon. (b) Atypical B lymphocytes stained positive with a probe for Epstein–Barr virus (EBV) DNA (courtesy of C Watson, R Chavez-Cartaya and D Wight).

ORGAN DONATION

The number of organs required to satisfy the needs of transplantation far exceeds the number of donor organs available. In the case of renal transplantation in the UK there are approximately 7000 patients waiting for transplantation, but only around 3500 transplants performed annually, which has led to a median waiting time for transplantation of three years. Similar shortages exist for liver and pancreas transplantation. For cardiothoracic organs the shortage is even worse and not all patients who might benefit from transplantation are listed.

Organs may be obtained from living donors or from deceased donors (DD) and DD may be either brainstem-dead heart-beating donors (donation after brain death or DBD donors) or donation after circulatory death (DCD) donors. Living donation is limited to donation of the kidney and, to a much lesser extent, liver or lung lobe. DBD donors provide a majority of organs for transplantation for all organ types although DCD donors provide an increasing number of kidneys, livers, pancreas glands and lungs for transplantation (see Summary box 81.6). The approach to referral and consent for organ donation varies between countries. Some have 'required request' or 'required referral' systems in place where all patients dying in intensive care settings have to be referred for their potential suitability to be organ donors assessed. Some countries (e.g. Austria and Spain) have an 'opt out' or 'presumed consent' system, where the assumption is made that an individual wished to donate their organs for transplantation unless they specifically registered their objection before death. There is debate about whether such a policy alone increases organ donation and a concern expressed by some that individuals who may not have wanted to become organ donors may fail to opt out before death, and that conflict may occur with relatives and next of kin who may oppose organ donation.

Summary box 81.6

Overcoming the shortage of organs for transplantation

- Maximising donation after brain-death (DBD) donation
- Use of marginal DBD deceased donors
- Use of donation after circulatory death (DCD) donors
- Increased use of split liver transplantation
- Increased living donor kidney (and liver) transplantation

Donation after brain death donors

The majority of DD organs are obtained from patients in whom brainstem death has been diagnosed. Such donors were previously called 'heart-beating deceased donors' and in most brain death results from stroke or traumatic head injury. Brain death occurs when severe brain injury causes irreversible loss of the capacity for consciousness combined with the irreversible loss of the capacity for breathing. In most countries, it is accepted that the condition of brain death equates in medical, legal and religious terms with death of the patient. The concept of brain death arose through necessity in the management of patients with irreversible brain damage on life support when there was no prospect for recovery. It was not in the interest of such patients, their relatives or the hospital in which they were being treated to delay their inevitable demise by continuing with futile life support. Acceptance of the concept of brain death had major implications for organ transplantation as it allowed the possibility for removal of viable organs from brain-dead patients before their circulation failed.

In the UK and many other countries, brain death is defined in terms of permanent functional death of the brainstem as neither consciousness nor spontaneous respiration is possible in the absence of a functional brainstem. A diagnosis of brainstem death should be considered only when certain preconditions have been met. The patient must have suffered major brain damage of known aetiology, be deeply unconscious and require ventilatory support. Particular care must be taken to ensure that muscle relaxant agents and drugs with known CNS depressant effects are not contributing to the clinical picture. Hypothermia, profound hypotension and metabolic or hormonal conditions that may contribute to CNS depression and confound the diagnosis of brainstem death must also be excluded. When the necessary preconditions have been satisfied, formal clinical assessment of the brainstem reflexes can be undertaken (Table 81.5). The UK guidelines state that the tests should be performed on two separate occasions by two clinicians experienced in this area. At least one of the two clinicians should be a consultant and neither should be connected with the transplant team. The time that must elapse between the two sets of brainstem tests is not specified in the guidelines and is determined on the basis of clinical judgement. In the UK, there is no requirement to perform electrophysiological or brain perfusion studies to aid the diagnosis of brainstem death. Particular care is required in the diagnosis of brainstem death in neonates and infants.

Donation after circulatory death donors

The number of potential DBD donors has remained relatively static or even declined as a result of changes in neurosurgical practice and improved road safety. To address the rising demand for organ transplantation there has been a major trend towards increasing use of organs from DCD donors.

DCD donors can be grouped according to the Maastricht classification as follows:

- category 1: dead on arrival at hospital;
- category 2: resuscitation attempted without success;
- category 3: 'awaiting cardiac arrest' after withdrawal of support;
- category 4: cardiac arrest while brain dead;
- category 5: cardiac arrest and unsuccessful resuscitation in hospital.

Maastricht categories 1, 2 and 5 donors are sometimes referred to as uncontrolled DCD donors. The warm ischaemic time of organs from these three categories of donor is usually longer and less predictable than in the case of categories 3 and 4 (controlled) donors. The majority of DCD donor organs used for transplantation in the UK, US and several other European countries are from controlled (category 3) donors who have died in intensive care after planned withdrawal of futile cardiorespiratory support.

Kidneys may be also be recovered from carefully selected patients who are dead on arrival at the hospital or who have died following unsuccessful resuscitation. In Spain and France most DCD kidneys are obtained from uncontrolled donors.

Table 81.5 Clinical testing for brainstem death.

Absence of cranial nerve reflexes	Pupillary reflex Corneal reflex
	Pharyngeal (gag) and tracheal (cough) reflex
	Oculovestibular (caloric) reflex
Absence of motor response	The absence of a motor response to painful stimuli applied to the head/face and the absence of a motor response within the cranial nerve distribution to adequate stimulation of any somatic area is an indicator of brainstem death. The presence of spinal reflexes does not preclude brainstem death
Absence of spontaneous respiration	After preventilation with 100% O_2 for at least 5 minutes, the patient is disconnected from the ventilator for 10 minutes to confirm absence of respiratory effort, during which time the arterial P_{CO_2} level should be >8 kPa (60 mmHg) to ensure adequate respiratory stimulation. To prevent hypoxia during the apnoeic period, O_2 (6 L/min) is delivered via an endotracheal catheter

Evaluation of the deceased donor

After a deceased donor has been referred to the transplant team with a view to organ donation, the general suitability of the potential organ donor must be carefully assessed. Particular care must be taken to assess the donor from the point of view of transmissible infectious agents and malignancy. The medical history should be carefully scrutinised and evidence sought of risk factors for human immunodeficiency virus (HIV), such as intravenous drug abuse. The presence of Creutzfeldt–Jakob disease is an absolute contraindication to organ donation. Organs from HIV-infected donors should not be used for transplantation, except sometimes in recipients who are already infected by the HIV virus. Hepatitis B infection (in most countries) and active systemic sepsis, e.g. major abdominal infection, are contraindications to donation. The presence of malignancy within the past five years is usually an absolute contraindication to organ donation with the exceptions of primary tumours of the CNS, non-melanotic tumours of the skin and carcinoma *in situ* of the uterine cervix. If there are no general contradictions to organ donation, consideration is then given to organ-specific selection criteria.

Because of the high demand for donor organs there has been a progressive relaxation in the organ-specific selection criteria. The chronological age of the donor is less important than the physiological function of the organs under consideration for transplantation.

Maastricht is a city in the province of Limburg, in The Netherlands.
In situ is Latin for 'in the place'.

The organs to be donated should generally be free from primary disease. Potential kidney donors should have a reasonable urine output and relatively normal serum urea and creatinine, although acute terminal elevations are acceptable. Liver donors should not have hepatic disease, although impaired liver function tests are common in deceased donors and do not necessarily preclude donation. Heart donors should have a normal electrocardiogram and, in doubtful cases, echocardiography may be necessary. For lung donors the chest radiograph and gas exchange should be satisfactory, and bronchial aspirates should be free from fungal and bacterial infection. Elevations of blood glucose and serum amylase are not uncommon in deceased donors and do not preclude pancreas donation. The use of organs from suboptimal or 'marginal' deceased donors has increased markedly in an attempt to address the demand for transplantation. The definition of a marginal donor depends on the organs being considered for transplantation and varies between countries. In the case of kidney transplantation a marginal donor is defined in the United States as a donor age >60 years or one between the ages of 50 and 60 years with two of the following: hypertension, death from stroke and a terminal creatinine of >132 mmol/L. Organs from 'marginal donors' generally lead to less satisfactory transplant outcomes than those from standard donors.

Organ recovery from deceased donors

In DBD donors, once brainstem death has been confirmed, management of the donor is aimed at preserving the functional integrity of the organs to be recovered. Brainstem death produces profound metabolic and neuroendocrine disturbances leading to cardiovascular instability. Careful monitoring and management of fluid balance is essential. Inotropic support is given and there may be a role for the use of tri-iodothyronine (T3) and argipressin.

Recovery of multiple organs from a DBD donor requires cooperation between the thoracic and abdominal surgical teams. A midline abdominal incision and median sternotomy is used to obtain access. After dissection of the organs to be recovered, they are perfused *in situ*. The heart is perfused with cold cardioplegia solution via a cannula in the ascending aorta and the lungs are perfused via a cannula in the pulmonary artery. The abdominal organs are perfused with chilled organ preservation solution via an aortic and portal cannula. Blood and perfusate are vented from the left atrial appendage and the inferior vena cavae. This produces rapid cooling of the organs, reduces their metabolic activity and preserves their viability. Additional surface cooling of the abdominal organs may be achieved by application of saline ice slush. The heart and lungs are excised followed by the liver and pancreas and then the kidneys, either en bloc or separately. The extent to which the abdominal organs are dissected prior to cold flush depends on the preference of the surgical team. Some surgeons perform minimal dissection prior to cold perfusion and complete the dissection of the abdominal organs *in situ* or on the back table after the organs have been removed en bloc. During recovery of the liver, care is taken to ensure that if there is an aberrant hepatic artery arising from the superior mesenteric artery it is included in the aortic patch. An adult donor liver cannot be transplanted into a child because of the size mismatch, and there are insufficient deceased paediatric donor livers available for transplantation. One solution is to undertake split liver transplantation, which was first performed by Pichlmayr in 1988. The liver from a deceased donor is split and the left lobe or left

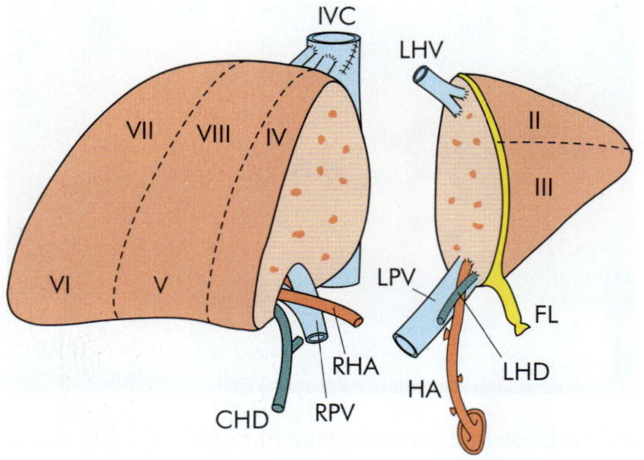

Figure 81.15 An adult liver may be split (according to Couinard's segments) so that the left lateral segment (segments II and III) can be transplanted into a child and the right lobe (together with segment IV) can be transplanted into an adult. CHD, common hepatic duct; FL, falciform ligament; HA, hepatic artery (on aortic patch); IVC, inferior vena cava; LHD, left hepatic duct; LHV, left hepatic vein; LPV, left portal vein; RHA, right hepatic artery; RPV, right portal vein.

lateral segments are used for a paediatric recipient and the right lobe is used for an adult recipient (Figure 81.15).

When removing the donor kidneys care is taken to ensure that any polar renal arteries are included on an aortic patch with the renal artery (Figure 81.16). In older kidney donors with atherosclerosis the aortic segment may be too diseased to use as an arterial patch and the donor renal artery and any polar arteries are divided shortly after their origin and if necessary reconstructed prior to implantation (Figure 81.17). In the case of the pancreas, a Y graft of donor iliac artery is excised and used to reconstruct the divided splenic and superior mesenteric arteries of the graft prior to implantation (Figure 81.18).

In DCD donors there is an inevitable period of warm ischaemia (up to 45 minutes is acceptable) between the diagnosis of death (cardiorespiratory arrest) and cold perfusion of the organs. The aim during organ recovery is to minimise the period of

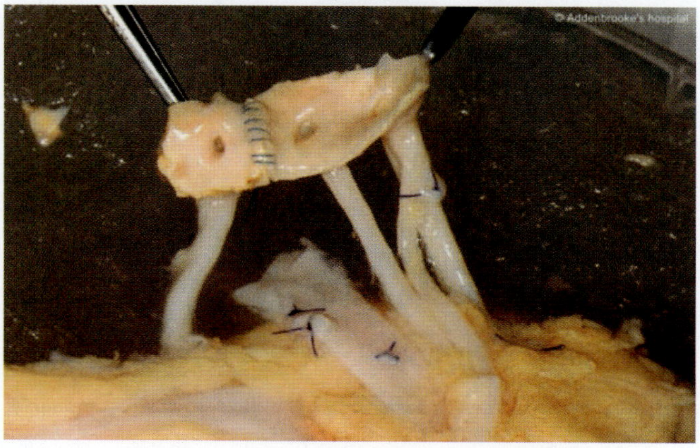

Figure 81.16 Deceased donor kidney with multiple renal arteries on an aortic patch. The aortic patch has been shortened to limit the length of the anastomosis needed when joining the donor patch to the side of the recipient external iliac artery (Medical Photography, Addenbrooke's Hospital).

Rudolph Pichlmayr, 1932–1997, surgeon of Hannover, Germany.

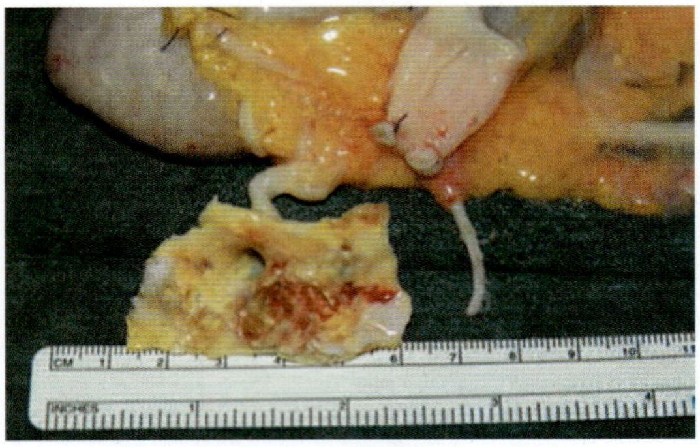

Figure 81.17 Deceased donor kidney from elderly (>70 years) donor illustrating the technical challenges of using kidneys from marginal donors. The aorta shows severe atherosclerosis with extensive plaque formation and ulceration and is not suitable for use as an aortic patch. A lower polar artery has already been divided. The two arteries can be joined together prior to implantation or implanted separately.

warm ischaemia although the approach used differs according to whether the donor is a controlled or uncontrolled DCD donor. It is important to note that only around 50 per cent of all patients considered as potential controlled DCD donors have a cardiorespiratory arrest within the period of time (usually 2 hours) considered practicable for the surgical team to stand by for organ recovery. After cardiorespiratory arrest there is an obligatory 'hands off' period before certification of death of at least 5 minutes before the surgical procedure for organ recovery can begin. If not already in the operating theatre, the DCD donor is transferred immediately to the operating room and the abdomen opened to allow rapid cannulation of the aorta and cold perfusion of the organs to be recovered. In the case of uncontrolled DCD donors the warm ischaemic time can be minimised by rapid insertion of a double balloon catheter introduced into the aorta via a femoral cut-down and used to cool the kidneys *in situ* by chilled perfusate preferably within 30 minutes of circulatory arrest (Figure 81.19). This allows time to gain consent from relatives for organ donation to proceed if it is not already available and to assemble the surgical team for organ recovery.

After removal from the donor, the organs may undergo a further flush with chilled preservation solution before they are placed in double or triple sterile bags and stored at 4°C by immersion in ice while they are transported to the recipient centre and await implantation. Once the donor organs have been excised, samples of donor spleen and mesenteric lymph nodes are obtained for confirmation of tissue type and use in the cross-match test.

Various organ preservation solutions are available for flushing organs before cold storage. They all contain impermeants to limit cell swelling, buffers to counter acidosis and electrolytes, the composition of which reflects that of intracellular rather than extracellular fluid. Commonly used preservation solutions include University of Wisconsin (UW) solution and Euro-Collins solution, but there are many others. The use of UW solution (Table 81.6) (developed by Belzer and colleagues in Wisconsin, USA) is particularly effective for liver grafts, and after perfusion with UW the liver can be stored safely for up to 24 hours. The length of time for which an organ can be stored before transplantation varies depending on the type of organ (Table 81.7). Although minimising the duration of organ storage is important for all organs, it is essential that organs from DCD donors are transplanted with the minimum possible cold storage time. Most organs for transplantation are stored by static cold storage in an ice box. However, there is a recent trend towards storing deceased donor kidneys by pulsatile machine perfusion where the kidneys are placed inside a purpose-designed perfusion machine that pumps cold preservation solution through the renal artery in an attempt to reduce ischaemic injury. Machine perfusion can be started immediately

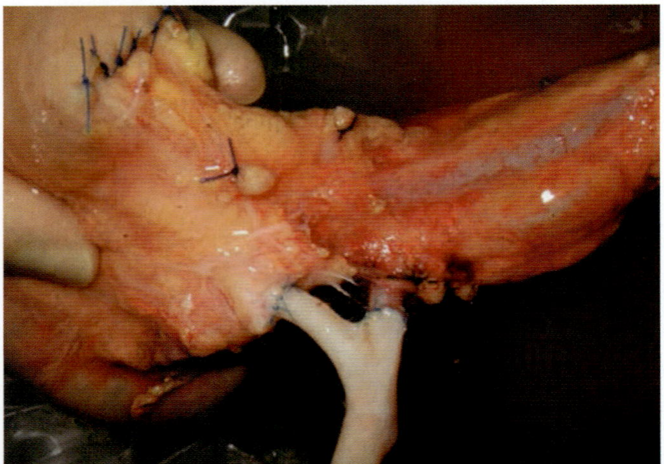

Figure 81.18 Donor pancreas viewed from the posterior aspect after preparatory bench surgery. The duodenal component of the graft has been sutured closed proximally and distally and a Y graft of donor iliac artery used to reconstruct the divided splenic and superior mesenteric arteries. The bile duct (ligated) and portal vein are anterior and not seen in this view.

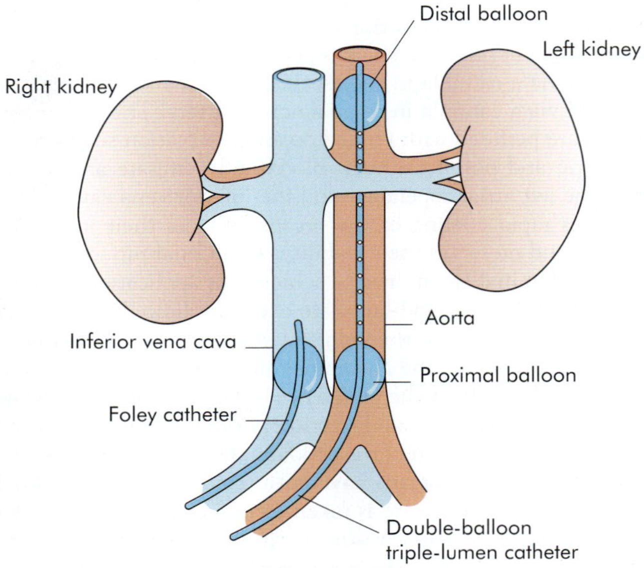

Figure 81.19 *In situ* perfusion of kidneys in a non-heart-beating donor (donation after cardiac death (DCD). A double-balloon aortic catheter is introduced through a groin incision and 10–15 litres of chilled preservation solution is administered. The perfusate is vented through a Foley catheter introduced into the femoral vein.

Table 81.6 Composition of University of Wisconsin (UW) solution.

Potassium lactobionate (mmol/L)	100
Sodium phosphate (mmol)	25
Magnesium sulphate (mmol)	5
Adenosine (mmol/L)	5
Allopurinol (mmol/L)	1
Gluthione (mmol/L)	3
Raffinose (mmol/L)	30
Hydroxethyl starch (g/L)	50
Insulin (U/L)	100
Dexamethasone (mg/L)	8
Potassium (mmol/L)	135
Sodium (mmol/L)	35
Osmolality (mosmol/L)	320
pH	7.4

Table 81.7 Maximum and optimal cold storage times (approximate).

Organ	Optimum (hours)	Safe maximum (hours)
Kidney	<18	36
Liver	<12	18
Pancreas	<10	18
Small intestine	<4	6
Heart	<3	6
Lung	<3	8

(Assuming zero warm ischaemic time and organs obtained from a non-marginal donor.)

after kidney recovery or as soon as practicable thereafter and is usually continued until the time of implantation. The benefit of machine perfusion over simple cold storage is currently the subject of considerable debate.

Living kidney donors

Living-donor renal transplants account for around 30 per cent of the total renal transplant activity in the UK, but in some countries (notably the Scandinavian countries and the US) this figure is much higher (>50 per cent). The justification for living-donor renal transplantation is based on the shortage of deceased donor transplants and the superior results obtained. Traditionally most living-donor transplants were between genetically related individuals. However, living donor kidney transplants performed between genetically unrelated individuals also fare better than even well-matched deceased donor grafts, and this observation gave rise to a steady increase in living unrelated kidney transplantation activity, usually between spouses or partners. It is essential to ensure that in all cases of living donation the prospective donor is fully informed and is free from coercion to donate and that the risk to the donor is small. In the UK, all living donor transplants (irrespective of whether they are genetically related or not) require prior approval by the Human Tissue Authority (HTA). An independent person (one not associated with the transplant team) approved by the HTA must provide confirmation to the HTA that the donor and recipient understand the implications of the proposed operation and that there is no evidence of coercion or financial inducement.

Live donation should proceed only after the prospective donor has undergone rigorous assessment to ensure that they are suitable. Before the donation, it is essential to perform imaging (usually magnetic resonance angiography or computed tomography-guided angiography), to delineate the anatomy of the arterial supply to the kidneys. If the left kidney has a single renal artery (10 per cent of kidneys have two or more renal arteries), it is usually chosen for transplantation because the longer left renal vein simplifies the transplant operation. The presence of multiple renal arteries does not necessarily preclude donation although implantation of living donor kidneys with multiple renal arteries may increase the chances of vascular complications developing after implantation.

Live donor nephrectomy was historically undertaken either through a loin incision and retroperitoneal approach or through a midline abdominal incision and transperitoneal approach. In most transplant units, nephrectomy is now undertaken laparoscopically (totally laparoscopic or hand-assisted). Laparoscopic nephrectomy is associated with less wound pain in the donor, allows more rapid mobilisation after surgery and reduces hospital stay. Initial concerns that kidneys removed by the laparoscopic technique may have more ureteric complications after implantation have proven unfounded. After removal from the donor the kidney is flushed immediately with chilled organ preservation solution (Figure 81.20). The mortality rate for live donation is less than 0.05 per cent, and around one-half of reported deaths are due to pulmonary embolic disease so it is essential to ensure prophylaxis to reduce deep-vein thrombosis (DVT). The major complication rate after live donor nephrectomy is <5 per cent: potential complications include haemorrhage requiring blood transfusion or surgery, infection (chest, abdomen, renal tract and wound), damage to an intra-adominal viscus, adverse reaction to drugs and anaesthetic agents, and DVT and pulmonary embolus.

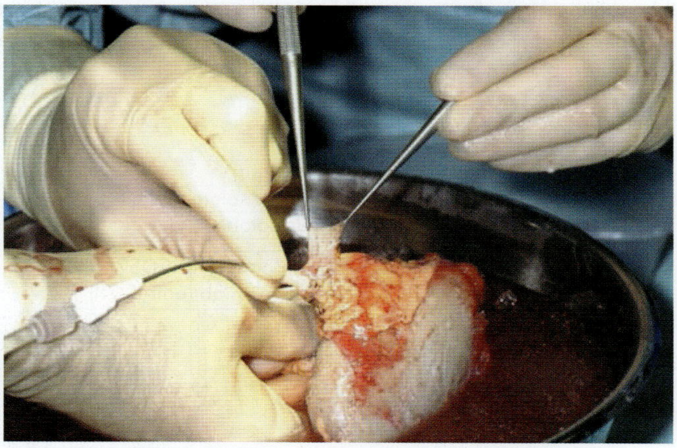

Figure 81.20 After removal from the donor kidney is flushed with chilled organ preservation solution and, if necessary, stored briefly on ice until transplanted into the recipient.

The University of Wisconsin is at Madison, WI, USA.
Fokert O Belzer, 1931–1995, a surgeon of Madison, WI, USA.

In the long term, kidney donors may be at increased risk from hypertension and donors should have their blood pressure and urine checked annually.

Around 35 per cent of potential living donor transplant recipients will be ABO blood group incompatible with their intended donor and until recently this precluded transplantation. However, there are now two potential solutions to this problem. The first is 'paired donation' where incompatible donor/recipient pairs exchange kidneys between pairs to allow ABO-compatible transplantation (Figure 81.21). Recruitment of more than two pairs to facilitate 'pooled donation' increases the likelihood of matching donors with compatible recipients and while such schemes pose considerable logistic challenges they are now operating successfully in several countries. An alternative approach is to transiently deplete ABO antibodies from potential recipients by passing their blood through special absorption columns or by performing plasmaphoresis along with administration of pretransplant immunosuppressive agents (Figure 81.22). Perhaps surprisingly, graft outcome following desensitisation is similar to that after paired donation. Both paired donation and antibody depletion strategies are also potentially applicable to recipients in whom HLA antibodies preclude transplantation from an intended living donor, but graft survival after depletion of HLA antibodies is lower than when the recipient receives a kidney from an HLA antibody-compatible donor.

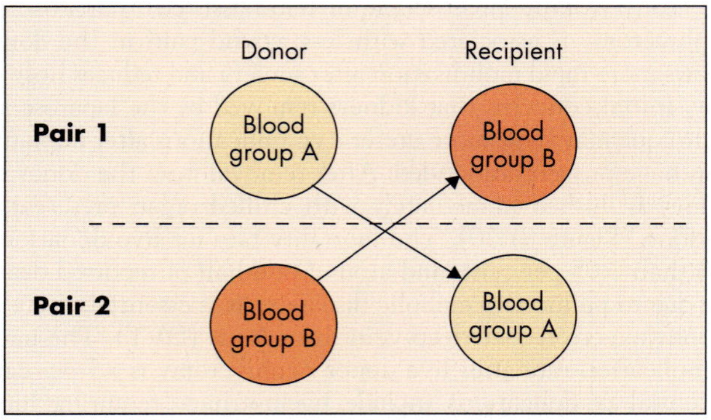

Figure 81.21 Paired living donor kidney transplantation. Paired donation allows patients with willing but blood group-incompatible donors to be transplanted by pairing them with other incompatible donor–recipient pairs. In the example shown, the two willing donors are incompatible with their intended recipient (blood groups A to B and B to A) but by paired donation each recipient can receive an ABO-compatible kidney transplant (blood groups A to A and B to B).

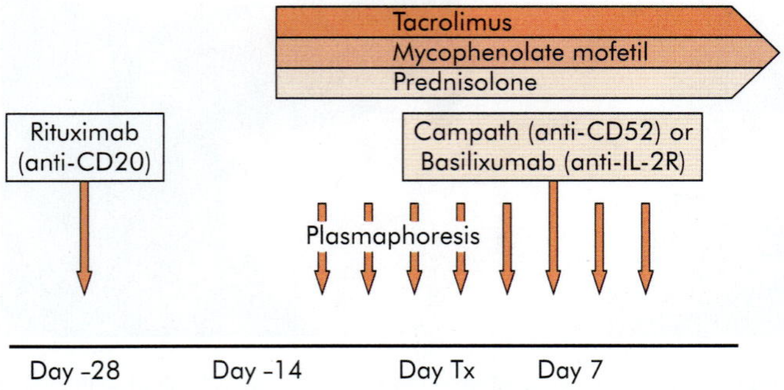

Figure 81.22 Typical desensitisation protocol for ABO or human leukocyte antigen (HLA) antibody incompatible live donor kidney transplant.

Living liver donors

Living donor liver transplantation is now undertaken in a number of transplant centres worldwide and is relatively common practice in some countries where deceased donation is not practised for cultural or religious reasons, notably Japan and Korea. The concept was first pioneered to allow children to receive the left lobe or left lateral segment from an adult donor and has been very successful. It has now been extended to adult-to-adult live liver transplantation (Figure 81.23). The majority of such transplants require a right liver lobe to provide adequate hepatic function. For adult-to-adult live liver donation, the donor procedure has a reported mortality rate of around 0.5 per cent and a major complication rate of up to 15 per cent. One of the more common donor complications is bile leak.

Living donors: other organs

Occasionally, living donors have provided segments of pancreas, small bowel and lung for transplantation, but this is more controversial. In the United States, living donor combined kidney and segmental pancreas transplantation has been undertaken to treat insulin-dependent diabetics with end-stage renal disease. In occasional patients, living-donor small bowel transplantation has been performed using a small bowel graft, which comprises a length of around 1.5 m of ileum. Finally, a small number of living-donor segmental lung transplants have been performed. To provide sufficient pulmonary tissue without compromising the donor, it is necessary to use segments from two different donors for each recipient. The ethical issues raised by living donation for extrarenal organs are understandably complex.

Resumption of function following organ transplantation

It is crucial that following heart, lung or liver transplantation the transplanted organ resumes satisfactory function immediately. If primary non-function occurs, the only option is rapid retransplantation. After kidney, pancreas or small bowel transplantation, immediate graft function is desirable but not vital. The factors that determine the functional integrity of a transplanted organ are shown in Summary box 81.7. Kidneys

Summary box 81.7

Factors determining organ function after transplantation

- Donor characteristics
  - Extremes of age
  - Presence of pre-existing damage in transplanted organ
  - Haemodynamic and metabolic instability
- Procurement-related factors
  - Warm ischaemic time
  - Type of preservation solution
  - Cold ischaemic time
- Recipient-related factors
  - Technical factors relating to implantation
  - Haemodynamic and metabolic stability
  - Immunological factors
  - Presence of drugs that impair transplant function

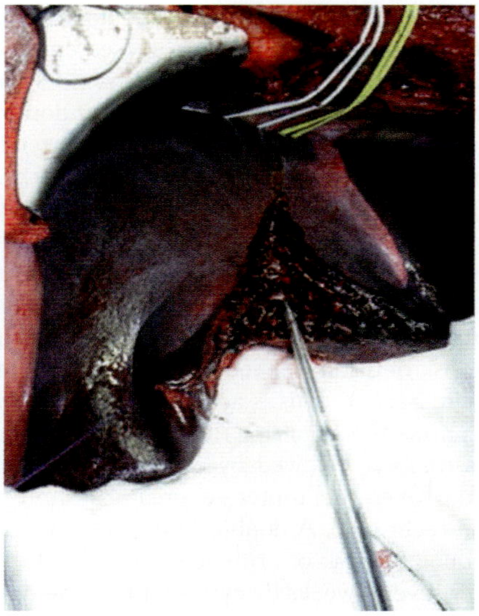

Figure 81.23 Living donor hepatectomy. A CUSA (cavitron ultrasonic aspirator) is being used to divide the right and left lobes of the liver so that the right lobe can be transplanted into an adult recipient.

obtained from DCD donors invariably suffer a variable degree of ischaemic damage, and delayed graft function is more common (typically 50 per cent for category 3 DCD donors) than for kidneys obtained from DBD deceased donors (typically 25 per cent). Irreversible ischaemic necrosis occasionally occurs and the graft never functions adequately (primary non-function). However, graft survival results for kidneys from controlled DCD kidneys are similar to those obtained from DBD deceased donors. Livers obtained from DCD donors have an increased incidence of primary non-function and of biliary complications, including biliary anastomotic strictures, bile leak and ischaemic cholangiopathy.

KIDNEY TRANSPLANTATION

Patient selection

Renal transplantation is the preferred treatment for many patients with end-stage renal disease because it provides a better quality of life for them than dialysis. Transplantation releases patients from the dietary and fluid restrictions of dialysis and the physical constraints imposed by the need to dialyse. Transplantation is also more cost-effective than dialysis and improves patient survival.

In the UK, around 100 people per million of the population develop end-stage renal disease, and the incidence increases with age. The causes of end-stage renal disease are numerous and include the following:

- glomerulonephritis;
- diabetic nephropathy;
- hypertensive nephrosclerosis;
- renal vascular disease;
- polycystic kidney disease;
- pyelonephritis;
- obstructive uropathy;
- systemic lupus erythematosus;
- analgesic nephropathy;
- metabolic disease (oxalosis, amyloid).

Frequently, the primary cause of end-stage renal disease is uncertain. For renal transplantation, as for other types of organ transplantation, careful patient selection is essential. Before acceptance as suitable candidates on the transplant waiting list, a transplant surgeon and nephrologist should formally assess all patients. A significant number of patients are likely to be considered unsuitable for renal transplantation because of major comorbid disease, especially cardiovascular disease. In the UK, around 30–40 per cent of the dialysis population are on the waiting list for renal transplantation.

The nature of the primary renal disease does not generally affect the decision to proceed to transplantation. Many of the glomerulonephritides (especially IgA, focal segmental glomerulosclerosis, and mesangiocapillary glomerulonephritis types I and II) may recur in a kidney transplant, and sometimes can lead to early graft failure (especially focal segmental glomerulosclerosis). In the case of primary oxalosis, combined kidney and hepatic transplantation is usually undertaken to eliminate the metabolic defect and thereby prevent early graft failure from the formation of further oxalate stones.

The age of patients with end-stage renal failure accepted for dialysis has gradually risen over the last two decades, and in the UK the mean age of patients starting dialysis is around 70 years. There is no absolute upper age limit to renal transplantation, but inevitably older patients (over the age of 65 years) are less likely to be considered suitable candidates because of major cardiovascular and other comorbid disease.

A careful assessment of comorbid disease that might significantly reduce the chances of successful outcome after transplantation is essential (Summary box 81.8). Rigorous evaluation of the cardiovascular system is particularly important. Cardiovascular disease is very common in the dialysis population, especially those with diabetes, and is the major cause of death after transplantation. Before listing patients for transplantation, it is important to ensure that their urinary tract is functional and that there is no need for corrective urological surgery. Only when there is intractable renal sepsis or very large polycystic kidneys that intrude into both iliac fossae is native nephrectomy required before transplantation (Figure 81.24). Finally, the prospective transplant recipient must be deemed able to cope with the psychological consequences of transplantation and likely to comply with immunosuppressive therapy.

Summary box 81.8

Evaluation of potential recipients for organ transplantation

- Evaluation undertaken by appropriate multidisciplinary team including surgeon and physician
- Determine presence of comorbid disease
- Exclude malignancy and systemic sepsis
- Evaluate against organ-specific criteria for transplantation
- Determine probable ability to cope psychologically with transplant and comply with immunosuppression
- Evaluate need for any preparative surgery needed to facilitate transplantation
- Optimise recipient condition prior to transplantation

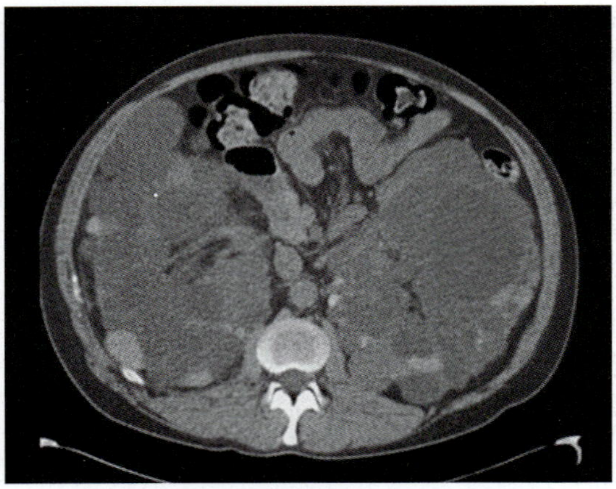

Figure 81.24 Computed tomography scan of a patient with very large polycystic kidneys that extend well into both iliac fossa. The patient requires removal of one of the polycystic kidneys to make room for a subsequent renal transplant. Nephrectomy should be performed several weeks before transplantation.

Immunosuppressive therapy impairs the protective response to both malignancy and infection. Consequently, pre-existing malignancy is an absolute contraindication and, even after curative treatment, transplantation should not usually be considered for at least three years. Similarly, the presence of active infection is a contraindication to transplantation.

Technique of renal transplantation

The transplant kidney is placed in the iliac fossa, in the retroperitoneal position, leaving the native kidneys *in situ*. After induction of general anaesthesia, a central venous line and a urinary catheter are inserted. It is helpful to distend the bladder with saline containing methylene blue to allow it to be identified with certainty prior to ureteric implantation. A curved incision is made in the lower abdomen and, after dividing the muscles of the abdominal wall, the peritoneum is swept upwards and medially to expose the iliac vessels. These are dissected free so that they can be controlled with vascular clamps. The kidney is then removed from ice and the donor renal vein is anastomosed end-to-side to the external iliac vein. The donor renal artery on a Carrel patch of donor aorta is anastomosed end-to-side to the external iliac artery (Figure 81.25a). If the donor renal artery lacks an aortic patch, as in the case of a living-donor transplant, it may be preferable to anastomose the donor artery end-to-end to the recipient internal iliac artery (Figure 81.25b). While the vascular anastomoses are being undertaken, the kidney is kept cold by application of topical ice.

Following completion of the venous and arterial anastomoses, the vascular clamps are removed and the kidney is allowed to reperfuse with blood. The ureter, which is kept reasonably short to avoid the risk of distal ischaemia, is then anastomosed to the bladder (Figure 81.26). This is achieved by direct implantation of the ureter into the dome of the bladder with a mucosa-to-mucosal anastomosis followed by closure of the muscular wall of the bladder over the ureter to create a short tunnel, the Lich–Gregoir technique. A double-J ureteric stent should be left *in situ*, to reduce the risk of urine leak or early obstruction, and removed after several weeks by cystoscopy. If the donor ureter is too short to reach the bladder, the native ureter can be divided

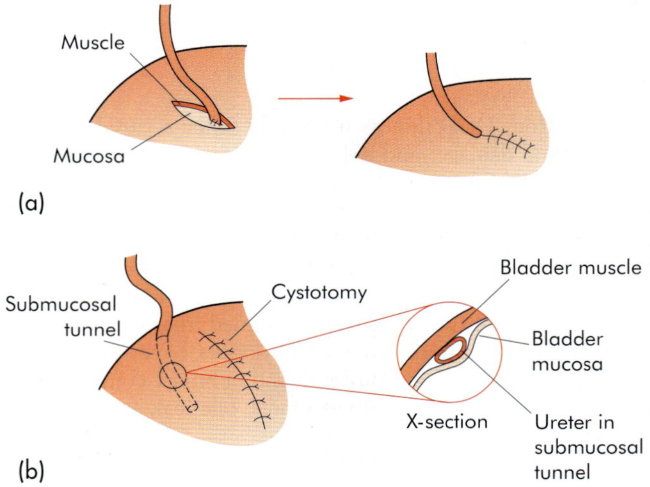

Figure 81.26 Ureteric implantation by direct anastomosis to a small cystomy. (a) Lich–Gregoir technique; (b) Leadbetter–Politano technique.

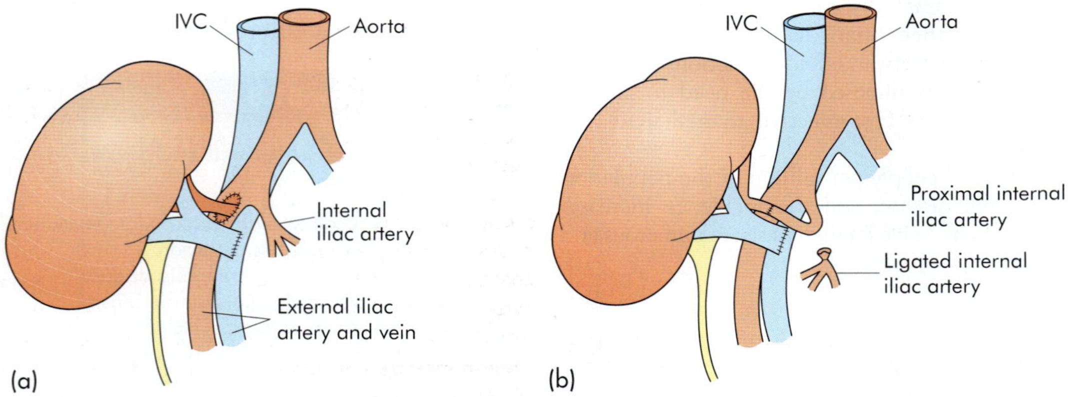

Figure 81.25 Implantation of renal allograft. (a) The renal artery on a Carrel patch is anastomosed to the external ilac artery. (b) The renal artery is anastomosed end-to-end to the internal iliac artery. IVC, inferior vena cava.

Robert Lich Jr, a urologist of Louisville, KY, USA.
Willy Gregoir, Chef de Clinique Urologique, Brussels, Belgium, from 1962 to 1987.
Guy W Leadbetter, a urologist of Cambridge, VT, USA.
Victor A Politano, a urologist who was at the Massachusetts General Hospital, Boston, MA, and now at the University of Florida, FL, USA.

and the distal segment anastomosed to the ureter or renal pelvis of the donor kidney. The proximal segment of the native ureter can usually be ligated and the native kidney left *in situ* without causing a problem. Before closing the transplant wound, it is very important to ensure that the kidney is lying in a satisfactory position without kinking or torsion of the renal vessels. In small children receiving an adult donor kidney, the abdomen is opened through a midline incision and the graft is placed intra-abdominally with anastomosis of the renal vessels to the aorta and vena cava.

Technical complications

Vascular complications

The incidence of vascular complications after renal transplantation is quite low. Renal artery thrombosis occurs in approximately 1 per cent of cases. Renal vein thrombosis is more common (up to 5 per cent of cases) and, although sometimes due to technical error, the aetiology is often uncertain. It presents during the first week after transplantation with sudden pain and swelling at the site of the graft. The diagnosis is confirmed by Doppler ultrasonography. Urgent surgical exploration is indicated, and in most cases transplant nephrectomy is required. The incidence of renal vein thrombosis can be minimised by giving low-dose heparin or aspirin prophylaxis. Renal artery stenosis usually presents late (often years) after transplantation with increasing hypertension and decreasing renal function. It may occur in up to 10 per cent of grafts and is diagnosed by angiography. Renal artery stenosis is best treated by angioplasty, but if angioplasty fails or is not technically possible then the condition can be treated successfully by open surgery and vascular reconstruction.

Urological complications

Urological complications occur in around 5 per cent of patients in the early post-transplant period, but their incidence can be reduced markedly by leaving a temporary ureteric stent *in situ*. Urinary leaks result from technical errors at the ureteric anastomosis or because of ureteric ischaemia. They present with discomfort and leakage of urine from the wound and usually require surgical intervention and reimplantation of the ureter into the bladder or anastomosis of the transplant ureter to the ipsilasteral native ureter. Obstruction of the transplant ureter may occur early or late. Causes of obstruction include technical error, external pressure from a haematoma or lymphocoele and ischaemic stricture. Ureteric obstruction presents with painless deterioration in graft function and is confirmed by demonstrating hydronephrosis and ureteric dilatation on ultrasound examination. Initial treatment is by percutaneous antegrade nephrostomy and insertion of a stent. Some ureteric strictures may be amenable to treatment by balloon dilatation but most are best treated by surgical intervention, reimplanting the donor ureter into the bladder or anastomosing it to the native ureter.

Lymphocoele

Peritransplant lymphocoeles are usually asymptomatic, but occasionally they become large enough to cause ureteric obstruction or oedema of the ipsilateral leg. Initial treatment is usually by ultrasound-guided percutaneous drainage. In the case of large or recurrent lymphocoeles, surgical intervention may be needed to drain a persistent lymphocoele into the peritoneal cavity, and this can often be achieved by an ultrasound-guided laparoscopic approach.

Investigation of graft dysfunction

Graft dysfunction (Summary box 81.9) during the early postoperative period is a common problem. Possible causes are:

- acute tubular necrosis;
- arterial/venous thrombosis;
- urinary leak/obstruction;
- CNI toxicity;
- hyperacute/accelerated acute rejection.

Summary box 81.9

Causes of allograft dysfunction

- Early
  - Primary non-function (irreversible ischaemic damage)
  - Delayed function (reversible ischaemic injury)
  - Hyperacute and acute rejection
  - Arterial or venous thrombosis of the graft vessels
  - Drug toxicity (e.g. CNI toxicity)
  - Infection (e.g. CMV disease in graft
  - Mechanical obstruction (ureter/common bile duct)
- Late
  - Chronic rejection
  - Arterial stenosis
  - Recurrence of original disease in graft (glomerulonephritis, hepatitis C)
  - Mechanical obstruction (ureter, common bile duct)

Delayed graft function (defined as the need for dialysis post-transplantation) as a result of acute tubular necrosis occurs in around 25 per cent of kidneys from DBD and up to 50 per cent of kidneys from DCD donors, but is uncommon (<5 per cent) following living-donor transplantation. Often, recipients produce significant volumes of urine from their native kidneys, making the diagnosis of delayed graft function more difficult. The incidence of delayed function can be minimised by optimising donor management before kidney procurement and reducing the cold ischaemia time by avoiding unnecessary delay before implantation. As a first step in the management of early graft dysfunction, the urinary catheter should be irrigated in case it is occluded by a blood clot. Hypovolaemia, if present, should be corrected with the aid of central venous pressure (CVP) monitoring. A Doppler ultrasound examination of the graft is the single most important investigation as it allows exclusion of vascular thrombosis and urinary obstruction as causes of graft dysfunction. Renal radionucleotide scanning provides information on renal perfusion and excretion and may be helpful but is used infrequently. If graft dysfunction is still present after several days, it is usual to perform an ultrasound-guided needle biopsy of the kidney to ensure that graft rejection is not present and then to repeat the investigation every week or so until graft function occurs. CNI toxicity may cause graft dysfunction and it is important to monitor CNI blood levels to avoid nephrotoxicity. Acute tubular necrosis usually resolves within the first 4 weeks of transplantation, but a small number of grafts (<5 per cent) suffer primary non-function (i.e. never function).

Allograft dysfunction developing late (>1 month after transplant) may be due to:

- acute/chronic rejection;
- drug toxicity;
- ureteric obstruction (lymphocoele/ureteric stricture);
- recurrent disease;
- urinary tract infection.

Blood levels of cyclosporine or tacrolimus are assessed to ensure that they are not unduly elevated, and ultrasound examination of the graft is performed to determine whether ureteric obstruction is present. If obstruction is detected, it is further investigated by percutaneous antegrade pyelography and treated as outlined above. If there is uncertainty about the cause of graft dysfunction, transplant biopsy should be performed to establish whether allograft rejection is present.

Outcome after transplantation

The results of organ transplantation (Summary box 81.10) are generally defined in terms of patient and graft survival. Patient survival after deceased donor renal transplantation is >95 per cent at one year and >85 per cent at five years. Graft survival is around 90 per cent at one year and 80 per cent at five years. Graft survival after a second transplant is only marginally worse than after a first graft. After living-related kidney transplantation, overall graft survival is around 95 per cent at one year and 85 per cent at five years. Graft survival after transplantation can also be expressed in terms of the half-life of the graft. The half-life of grafts obtained from living donors is substantially longer than that of DD grafts:

- deceased donor grafts, 13 years;
- living-unrelated grafts, 15 years;
- living-haploidentical grafts, 16 years;
- living-identical sibling grafts, 27 years.

Summary box 81.10

Outcome after transplantation

- Transplantation improves the quality and duration of life in most recipients
- Transplant outcome has improved progressively over the last two decades and continues to improve
- Improved outcome is due to better immunosuppression, organ preservation, chemoprophylaxis and technical advances
- Graft survival after kidney, liver and heart transplantation is >90 per cent at one year and >80 per cent at five years
- The results of lung and small bowel transplantation are less good
- Chronic rejection is the most common cause of graft failure after all types of solid-organ transplant
- Recurrence of the original disease necessitating transplantation may also lead to graft failure
- Death with a functioning transplant from cardiovascular disease is relatively common
- Up-to-date transplant outcomes for the different organs can be found at the online national and international transplant databases (see end of chapter for website addresses)

If a kidney transplant fails late after transplantation, the graft can often be left *in situ* and immunosuppression stopped, but transplant nephrectomy may be indicated if the graft is causing symptoms. The operation is undertaken via the original wound, but the kidney is dissected free from the renal capsule and delivered into the wound. The renal vessels are then ligated and divided, leaving behind the original vascular anastomosis.

In addition to graft survival, it is important to consider the extent to which transplantation improves the physical and mental well-being of the patient and allows them to lead a satisfactory social life. In the case of kidney, as in other types of solid organ transplant, successful transplantation undoubtedly leads to a substantial improvement in quality of life. However, although some recipients return to a normal or near-normal life, others fare much less well and, for the group overall, the quality of life after transplantation falls short of that seen in normal healthy individuals. Renal transplantation is best regarded, therefore, as an effective form of therapy rather than a complete cure.

PANCREAS TRANSPLANTATION

Successful pancreas transplantation restores normal control of glucose metabolism and obviates the need for insulin therapy in patients with diabetes mellitus. Improved control of blood glucose levels in diabetes reduces the progression of secondary complications such as retinopathy, peripheral vascular disease and nephropathy. However, in considering the indications for pancreas transplantation, these advantages have to be weighed carefully against the risks posed by both the transplant procedure itself and the immunosuppressive therapy required to prevent graft rejection. For most patients with diabetes, the additional risks associated with pancreas transplantation and immunosuppression are such that the operation can be justified only when kidney transplantation for diabetic nephropathy is also being undertaken. The only additional risks of pancreas transplantation in such patients relate to the transplant operation itself. In the United States, around one-half of all diabetic patients undergoing kidney transplantation also receive a pancreas transplant. In most cases, the kidney and pancreas are obtained from the same donor, so-called simultaneous pancreas and kidney (SPK) transplantation. Pancreas transplantation is sometimes performed in patients who have already undergone successful kidney transplantation, pancreas after kidney (PAK) transplantation. Occasionally, pancreas transplantation alone (PTA) can be justified to treat life-threatening diabetic complications such as hypoglycaemic unawareness.

Careful patient selection is essential to avoid excessive mortality and morbidity. The procedure is usually reserved for those patients with type I diabetes who are relatively young (under the age of 55 years) and do not have advanced coronary artery disease or peripheral vascular disease. Investigation of the heart's response to stress, either using echocardiography or nuclear medicine imaging is mandatory.

Surgical technique

The whole pancreas gland together with a segment of duodenum is transplanted, essentially as pioneered by Lillehei in 1966. Segmental pancreas transplantation is performed only occasionally. SPK transplantation is usually performed through a midline incision (Figure 81.27). The pancreas graft is placed intraperitoneally in the pelvis, usually on the right, and the

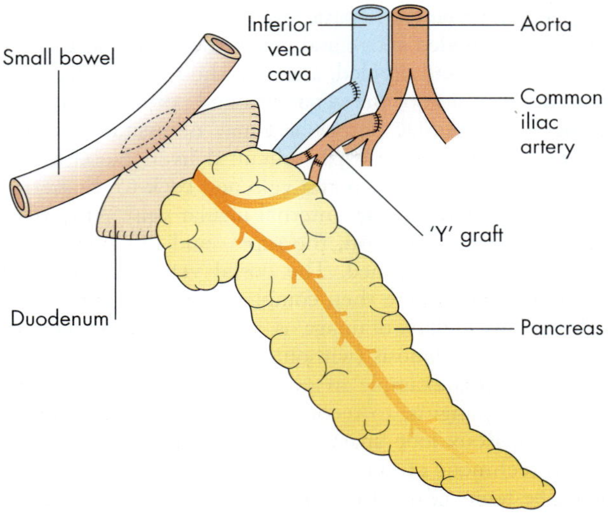

Figure 81.27 Pancreas transplant operation with enteric drainage of the exocrine secretion via a duodenoenterostomy. A 'Y' graft using donor iliac artery is usually used to reconstruct the divided splenic and superior mesenteric arteries of the graft prior to implantation.

kidney graft is placed on the left side. The donor vessels of the pancreas graft are anastomosed to the recipient iliac vessels and the exocrine secretions are most commonly dealt with by anastomosing the graft duodenum to the small bowel (enteric drainage) often via a roux-en-Y loop although the duodenum may sometimes be anastomosed to the bladder (urinary drainage). The pancreas graft functions immediately after revascularisation, although supplementary insulin may be required for a few days. Technical complications usually occur early and include vascular thrombosis of the graft (5 per cent) and duodenal anastomotic leaks. Wound infection occurs in up to 10 per cent of patients, and intra-abdominal infection is relatively common. The specific complications of enteric drainage include intra-abdominal sepsis and adhesive small intestinal obstruction. Bladder drainage of the exocrine pancreas may result in the following complications:

- bladder/duodenal anastomotic leaks;
- cystitis (owing to effect of pancreatic enzymes);
- urethritis/urethral stricture;
- reflux pancreatitis;
- urinary tract infection;
- haematuria;
- metabolic acidosis (due to loss of bicarbonate in the urine).

Urinary drainage of the pancreas has the advantage that urinary amylase levels can be used to monitor for graft rejection. However, after bladder drainage, urinary complications are common, and in around 20 per cent of cases their severity necessitates conversion to enteric drainage. Most centres now prefer primary enteric drainage after SPK transplantation. Acute rejection after SPK transplantation is relatively common (10–20 per cent) and if detected early responds to treatment with steroids. Since it usually involves both the kidney and pancreas graft, serum creatinine can be used as a surrogate marker for pancreas graft rejection. Serum lipase and amylase levels are useful indications of pancreas graft inflammation of which acute rejection is one cause. Urinary drainage has the advantage, after PTA and PAK transplantation, of allowing pancreas graft rejection to be monitored by serial measurement of urinary amylase. A fall in urinary amylase is indicative of acute rejection. Elevation of blood glucose level is a late feature of acute rejection and often indicates the process is beyond reversal.

Results of pancreas transplantation

The principal aim of pancreas transplantation is to prolong life in diabetic patients who otherwise have a high mortality at ten years after receiving a kidney transplant alone. It also provides freedom from insulin treatment and improves quality of life.

The results of pancreas transplantation have improved significantly over the last decade. After SPK transplantation, the one-year patient survival rate is greater than 95 per cent and the one-year graft survival rates for pancreas and kidney grafts are 85 and 95 per cent, respectively. Most deaths are due to cardiovascular complications or overwhelming infection. Patient and kidney graft survival after SPK transplantation in patients with diabetic nephropathy is at least as good as after kidney transplant alone in this group. The results of PTA are not as good as after SPK transplantation (one-year pancreas graft survival 75 per cent) because acute rejection is more difficult to monitor in the absence of a kidney allograft.

Transplantation of isolated pancreatic islets

Treatment of diabetes by transplantation of isolated islets of Langerhans is a more attractive concept than vascularised pancreas transplantation because major surgery and the potential complications of transplanting exocrine pancreas are avoided. Pancreatic islets for transplantation are obtained by mechanically disrupting the pancreas after injection of collagenase into the pancreatic duct. The islets are then purified from the dispersed tissue by density-gradient centrifugation and can be delivered into the recipient liver (the preferred site for transplantation) by injection into the portal vein. Until recently, human islet transplantation had been performed intermittently and with very disappointing results. However, in 2000, Shapiro and colleagues in Edmonton, Canada, reported success with islet transplantation in seven patients with type I diabetes. Sequential islet transplantation from two or three donor pancreas glands was required to produce insulin independence, and although the long-term success is less than initially hoped for, some patients remained free from exogenous insulin and other units are now undertaking islet transplantation with variable results.

As an alternative to preventing islet rejection through immunosuppressive therapy, attempts have been made to protect isolated islet cells from rejection by encapsulating them inside semipermeable membranes. The protective membranes are designed with a pore size that allows insulin to pass through but prevents antibodies and leukocytes from reaching the islets, thereby avoiding the need for immunosuppressive therapy. A major attraction of this approach is that islets isolated from animals can be used and bioartificial pancreas grafts containing xenogeneic islets are currently under evaluation.

LIVER TRANSPLANTATION

Starzl first attempted liver transplantation in 1963 and, by 1967, had achieved prolonged survival. The first liver transplant

Richard Lillehei, surgeon, the University of Minnesota, Minneapolis, MI, USA.
Paul Langerhans, 1847–1888, Professor of Pathological Anatomy, Freiberg, Germany, described the islets in 1869.
Andrew Mark James Shapiro, Chairman of Clinical Research in Transplantation, CHRI/Wyeth Canad, Edmonton, Alberta, Canada.

performed outside the US was performed in Cambridge, UK by Calne in 1968. Throughout the 1970s, liver transplantation remained a hazardous procedure that frequently failed. However, since then, the results have progressively improved as a result of better patient selection, improved immunosuppression and chemoprophylaxis, better organ preservation, refinements in the operative technique, and advances in per- and postoperative management.

Indications and patient selection

The indications for liver transplantation fall into four groups:

1 cirrhosis;
2 acute fulminant liver failure;
3 metabolic liver disease;
4 primary hepatic malignancy.

The most common indication for transplantation is chronic liver failure. In adults the most common causes are alcoholic liver disease, viral liver disease (hepatitis C in Europe and the US and hepatitis B in some other countries), non-alcoholic steatohepatitis, primary biliary cirrhosis and sclerosing cholangitis. In children, who account for around 10–15 per cent of all liver transplants, biliary atresia is the most common indication for transplantation. Acute fulminant liver failure requiring transplantation on an urgent basis accounts for approximately 10 per cent of liver transplant activity and is usually viral or drug induced (e.g. paracetamol overdose in the UK). There are a variety of metabolic diseases for which transplantation offers the prospect of cure. These include Wilson's disease, oxalosis and familial amyloid polyneuropathy. Primary hepatic malignancy is more common in patients with cirrhosis, especially virally induced disease, and may be best treated by transplantation because the field changes in the cirrhotic liver predispose to further primary malignancies. Cholangiocarcinoma has a high recurrence rate and is seldom an indication for liver transplantation.

Technique of liver transplantation

A transverse abdominal incision with a midline extension is usually made and the diseased liver is mobilised (Figure 81.28). Because of portal hypertension, the recipient hepatectomy is often the most difficult part of the operation, especially if there has been previous upper abdominal surgery. The common bile duct is divided, as is the hepatic artery. The inferior vena cava is clamped and divided above and below the liver, and the portal vein is clamped and divided, allowing the recipient liver to be removed. Occlusion of the vena cava and portal vein results in a reduction in cardiac output and may necessitate the use of venovenous bypass. The bypass circuit delivers blood from the inferior vena cava and/or portal vein and back to the heart via a cannula inserted into the internal jugular vein. After placing the donor liver in position, the supra- and infrahepatic caval anastomoses are performed. The portal vein and the hepatic arterial anastomoses are then completed and the graft is reperfused. Finally, biliary drainage is re-established usually by a duct-to-duct anastomosis (without the use of a T-tube). It may be necessary, for example in recipients with biliary atresia or sclerosing cholangitis, to reconstruct the biliary drainage by a bile duct to Roux loop anastomosis. An alternative caval preservation technique of liver transplantation allows the recipient liver to be removed without cross-clamping the vena cava and the donor liver to be implanted using a 'piggyback' technique onto the recipient hepatic veins or using a side-to-side cavo-cavoplasty.

Many patients undergoing liver transplantation are extremely ill, and the surgery involved can be very technically demanding. Optimal perioperative management is crucial to a successful outcome and presents a major challenge. Blood loss during and after the transplant procedure can be very considerable, and management of coagulopathy is particularly important. Coagulation is assessed repeatedly throughout the transplant period and corrected with appropriate clotting factors. Many centres routinely use a thromboelastography to perform dynamic assessment of coagulation (Figure 81.29). In the most widely used system (rotational thromboelastography) this involves placing a blood sample in a small cuvette and then inserting a sensor pin that is subjected to rotational torsion and as clot between the cuvette and the pin forms, the resulting signal is displayed graphically and indicates the speed and strength of clot. Various modifications can be made to the test conditions to maximise the information provided.

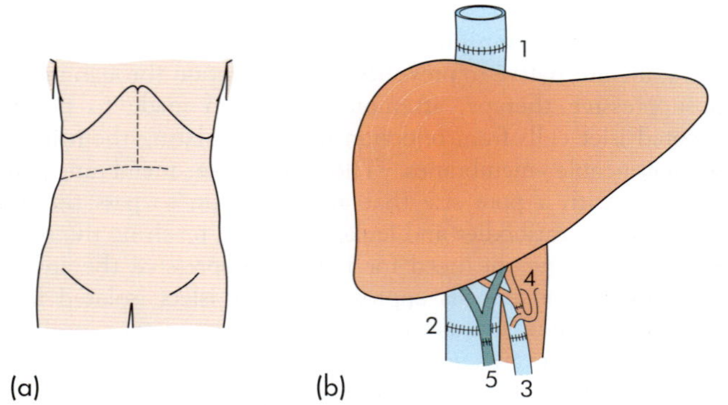

Figure 81.28 (a) Incision used for liver transplantation. (b) Completed implantation. The anastomoses, in order of performance, are: (1) suprahepatic cava; (2) infrahepatic cava; (3) portal vein; (4) hepatic artery; (5) bile duct.

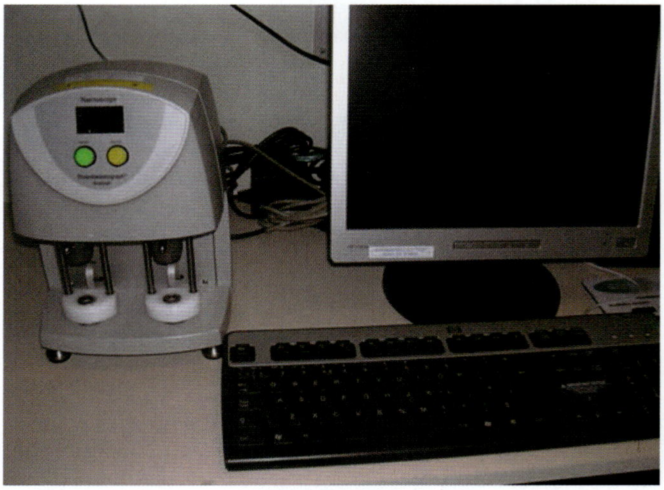

Figure 81.29 Thromboelastogram situated in the operating theatre and used to measure coagulation serially throughout the liver transplant procedure and guide administration of blood products.

Thomas Earl Starzl, Professor of Surgery, Pittsburgh, PA, USA.
Samuel Alexander Kinnier Wilson, 1878–1936, Professor of Neurology, King's College Hospital, London, UK, described this condition in 1912.

Technical complications

Haemorrhage

Meticulous haemeostasis during the transplant operation is important in order to minimise the risk of early haemorrhage. It may be necessary, occasionally, to pack the peritransplant area for 2–3 days to achieve adequate haemostasis when there is diffuse oozing despite correction of coagulopathy. Evacuation of extensive perihepatic haematoma may be required to avoid secondary infection.

Vascular complications

Hepatic artery thrombosis may occur spontaneously or as a result of acute rejection and is more common in paediatric recipients and in adults with primary sclerosing cholangitis. It may present as a rise in serum transaminase levels, unexplained fever or bile leak. Doppler ultrasonography or angiography is used to confirm the diagnosis, and urgent retransplantation is usually required. Portal vein thrombosis is rare and presents with the features of portal hypertension.

Biliary complications

Biliary leaks are now relatively uncommon and biliary stenosis is the more common problem. It usually occurs within the first few months of transplantation and is managed by endoscopic dilatation and stenting or by surgical correction.

Outcome after liver transplantation

The outcome after liver transplantation depends on the underlying liver disease and the best results are seen in patients with chronic liver disease (Figure 81.30). Patients undergoing transplantation as a result of acute liver failure have a higher mortality in the early post-transplant period because of multi-organ failure, but those who make a satisfactory recovery have very good long-term liver allograft survival. Conversely, patients transplanted for tumour have a very good early outcome but ultimately fare much less well because of recurrent malignancy. Patients receiving a liver transplantation following hepatitis B or hepatitis C infection may develop graft failure as a result of recurrent viral disease. However, the availability of improved antiviral therapy has largely eliminated this problem in recipients with hepatitis B infection.

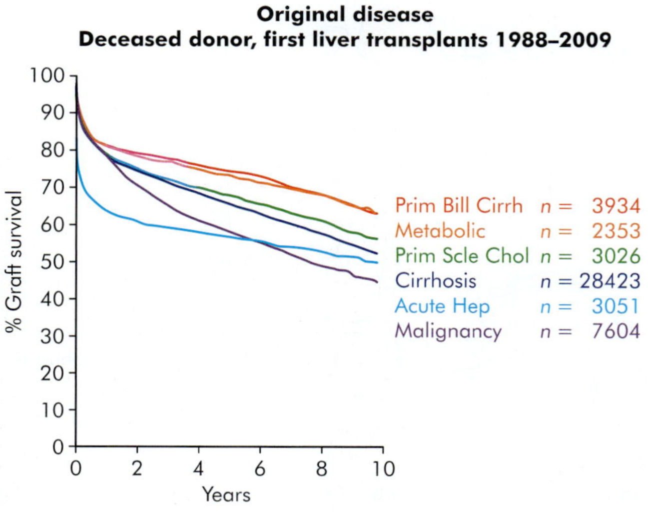

Figure 81.30 Outcome after liver transplantation according to the initial liver disease. Patients transplanted for acute liver disease have a higher early mortality but good long-term outcome. Patients transplanted because of liver tumour have a good initial outcome but survival continues to decline progressively (courtesy of Gerhard Opelz, Collaborative Transplant Study, L-75101-0211).

SMALL BOWEL TRANSPLANTATION

Progress in small bowel transplantation has lagged behind that of other types of organ transplantation but it is now a well-established therapy for highly selected recipients. Intestinal transplants stimulate a particularly strong graft rejection response, probably because the small intestine contains very large amounts of lymphoid tissue. Moreover, ischaemia and rejection increase intestinal permeability and allow translocation of bacteria from the lumen of the bowel. Added to this, the operation is often complex and is made technically difficult because of repeated previous abdominal surgery. Consequently, graft rejection and infection remain major problems after small bowel transplantation and the results obtained are inferior to those seen after other types of organ transplantation. Small bowel transplantation is a treatment option for patients with intestinal failure to an extent that long-term parenteral nutrition is required. Intestinal failure may result from short bowel syndrome after resection of the intestine or from intestinal dysfunction. Conditions that may give rise to intestinal failure include the following:

- intestinal atresia;
- necrotising enterocolitis;
- volvulus;
- disorders of motility;
- mesenteric infarction;
- Crohn's disease;
- trauma;
- desmoids tumours.

Because of the substantial risks associated with small bowel transplantation, the procedure is only considered for those patients in whom long-term total parenteral nutrition (TPN) has failed, usually because venous access has become impracticable or because of frequent life-threatening line sepsis. The need for small bowel transplantation is estimated at around 0.5–1.0 patients per million of the population, and around 50 per cent of cases are children.

Small bowel transplantation may be carried out as an isolated procedure, performed together with a liver transplant or undertaken as a component of a multivisceral transplant. When possible, isolated small bowel transplantation is undertaken because patient survival is higher.

A small bowel transplant from a deceased donor comprises the entire small bowel, and may include the ascending colon in the graft. The superior mesenteric artery of the graft (with an aortic patch) is anastomosed to the recipient aorta, and the superior mesenteric vein is anastomosed to the inferior vena cava or to the side of the portal vein. The proximal end of the small bowel graft is anastomosed to the recipient jejunum or duodenum. The distal end of the graft is anastomosed to the side of the colon (with a loop ileostomy) or is fashioned as an end ileostomy. A gastrostomy tube (to overcome delayed gastric emptying) and a feeding jejunostomy tube are inserted.

About one-half of all patients who require small bowel transplantation have cholestatic liver disease secondary to TPN and require combined liver and small bowel transplantation. Cholestatic liver disease due to TPN is especially common in children. When combined liver and small bowel transplantation is carried out, the two grafts are transplanted en bloc. The donor aorta is fashioned into a conduit including the superior mesenteric and coeliac arteries and anastomosed to the recipient aorta. The portal vein anastomosis is as for isolated liver transplantation (Figure 81.31).

Multivisceral or 'cluster' transplants may be necessary in the case of large desmoid tumours when excision of both the small bowel and adjacent organs is required, when there has been extensive thrombosis of the splanchnic vessels and for generalised disorders of gastrointestinal motility.

The one-year graft survival rate after small bowel transplantation is about 70 per cent for both isolated small bowel transplantation and for combined liver and small bowel transplantation. After three years, the graft survival rate is around 50 per cent. As already noted, however, patient survival is better after isolated small bowel transplantation than after combined liver and small bowel transplantation, when loss of the graft usually equates with death of the recipient. Most of the mortality after small bowel transplantation is due to sepsis and multiorgan failure. The risk of infection after small bowel transplantation is heightened by the additional requirements for immunosuppression in order to control graft rejection. This accounts for the relatively high incidence of lymphoproliferative disease (around 10 per cent) observed in patients who have undergone small bowel transplantation. Because of the large amount of donor lymphoid tissue transplanted, GVHD may be an added complication. Despite the hazards, small bowel transplantation offers patients with intestinal failure a chance to lead an active life free from the constraints of long-term nutritional support.

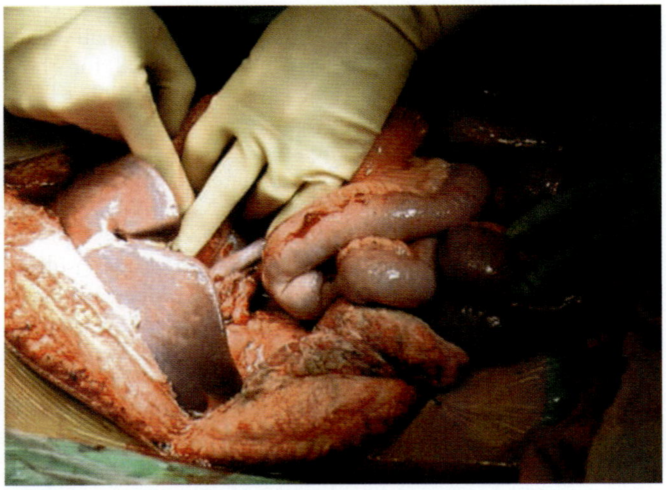

Figure 81.31 Combined liver and small bowel transplant in an adult shortly after reperfusion of the grafts. The small bowel is well perfused via the superior mesenteric artery anastomosed to the aorta on a patch along with the coeliac axis, and the venous blood drains into the portal vein via the superior mesenteric vein.

THORACIC ORGAN TRANSPLANTATION

Heart transplantation

Dr Christiaan Barnard performed the first human heart transplant in Cape Town, South Africa, in 1967. The operation was based on the experimental work of Lower and Shumway in Stanford, and Shumway subsequently went on to pioneer successful cardiac transplantation in the clinic. Heart transplantation is now considered an effective treatment for selected patients with end-stage cardiac failure. The most common indications for heart transplantation are ischaemic heart disease and idiopathic cardiomyopathy, but other indications include valvular heart disease, myocarditis and congenital heart disease.

Transplantation is considered only in patients with end-stage heart disease that has failed to respond to all other conventional therapy and when predicted survival without transplantation is only 6–12 months. Transplantation is usually limited to patients under the age of 65 years who do not have irreversible damage to other organ systems. The preoperative assessment is rigorous, and measurement of pulmonary vascular resistance is mandatory because when it is raised the perioperative mortality is high.

Technique of heart transplantation

A median sternotomy is performed and the patient is given systemic heparin, placed on cardiopulmonary bypass and cooled to 29°C. After cross-clamping the aorta, the recipient heart is excised at the mid-atrial level. The donor heart is then prepared and the left atrium is opened by making incisions (Figure 81.32) in the posterior wall, between the orifices of the pulmonary veins, to create an atrial cuff. The left and then right atrial

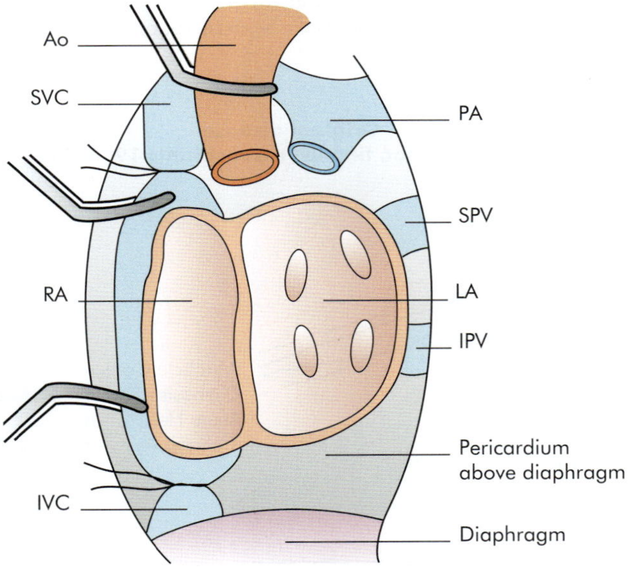

Figure 81.32 Recipient cardiectomy. After median sternotomy, the recipient is placed on cardiopulmonary bypass. Venous cannulae for bypass are sited in the superior vena cava (SVC) and inferior vena cava (IVC) via punctures in the right atrium (RA), and oxygenated blood is returned via a cannula in the ascending aorta (Ao). The diseased recipient heart is excised, leaving behind cuffs of right and left atria. PA, pulmonary artery; IPV/SPV, inferior/superior pulmonary veins; LA, left atrium (courtesy of J Dunning).

Christian Neethling Barnard, 1922–2001, Professor of Cardiac Surgery, the University of Cape Town, Cape Town, the Republic of South Africa.
Richard Rowland Lower, contemporary, thoracic surgeon, Richmond, VA, USA.

anastomoses are performed and the pulmonary and aortic arterial anastomoses are then completed (Figure 81.33). The patient is then rewarmed and weaned from cardiopulmonary bypass. Occasionally, heterotopic cardiac transplantation is undertaken, when the donor heart is placed adjacent to and augments the recipient's own heart.

Heart–lung, single-lung and double-lung transplantations

Pulmonary transplantation became a clinical reality when Dr Bruce Reitz performed the first successful combined heart–lung transplant in 1981. Combined heart–lung transplantation is still sometimes performed, usually in patients with pulmonary vascular disease in whom there is cardiac dysfunction due to congenital (e.g. Eisenmenger syndrome, in which the left-to-right shunt is reversed owing to pulmonary hypertension) or acquired cardiac dysfunction. For most patients with end-stage pulmonary disease, however, single- or double-lung transplantation has now replaced heart–lung transplantation. Lung transplantation is more economical in terms of organ use, although if heart–lung transplantation is undertaken for isolated respiratory disease, the healthy native heart can be used for transplantation, the so-called 'domino procedure'. Heart–lung transplantation is performed through a median sternotomy, taking particular care to avoid injury to the phrenic, vagus and recurrent laryngeal nerves during excision of the recipient heart and lungs. The recipient right atrium and aorta are divided as for orthotopic cardiac transplantation and the donor heart–lung block readied for implantation, incising the right atrium from the divided inferior vena cava. An end-to-end tracheal anastomosis is performed and the right atrial and aortic anastomoses are performed as for cardiac transplantation.

Single- and double-lung transplantation are effective therapies for selected patients with end-stage chronic lung disease, in whom declining lung function limits life expectancy despite optimal medical therapy. Common indications are pulmonary fibrosis, pulmonary hypertension, emphysema and cystic fibrosis. Single-lung transplantation can be performed for pulmonary fibrosis. Single-lung transplantation is performed through a posterolateral thoracotomy and double-lung transplantation through a bilateral thoracotomy or median sternotomy. During lung transplantation, the donor pulmonary veins on a left atrial cuff are anastomosed to the recipient left atrium. Next, the bronchial anastomosis and the pulmonary arterial anastomosis are completed. Cardiopulmonary bypass is usually required if pulmonary hypertension is present. Dehiscence of the airway anastomosis used to be common after heart–lung and lung transplantation, but improvements in organ preservation and surgical technique have dramatically reduced the incidence of this often fatal complication to <5 per cent. Late airway stenosis at the bronchial anastomosis due to ischaemia occurs in around 10 per cent of bronchial anastomoses and is treated by dilatation.

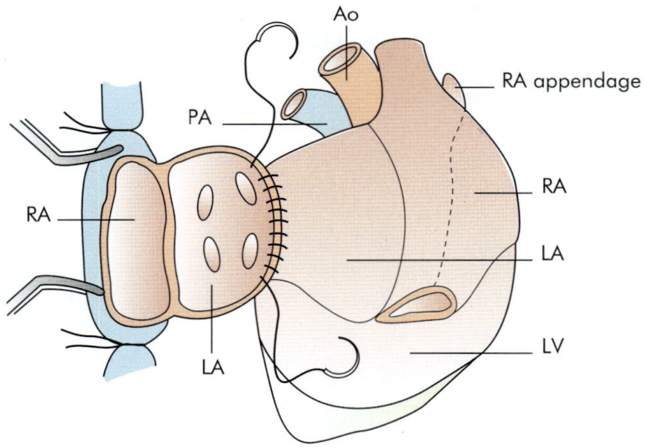

Figure 81.33 Implantation of the donor heart. The donor left atrium is opened by an incision connecting the four pulmonary veins, excising the central portion. The left atrial anastomosis is performed, starting at the lateral wall of the donor and continuing inferiorly and superiorly, concluding with the interatrial septum. The right atrial anastomosis is performed matching the recipient atrium by an incision towards the donor right atrial appendage (dotted line), which avoids the sinus node at the cavoatrial junction. Finally, the pulmonary artery and aortic anastomosis are completed. Abbreviations as for Figure 81.32.

Outcome after thoracic organ transplantation

The one- and five-year graft survival rates after heart transplantation are around 85 and 70 per cent, respectively. The results after heart–lung and lung transplantation are less good, with one-year graft survival rates of around 75 per cent and five-year survival rates of around 50 per cent.

FUTURE PROSPECTS

The two major problems in organ transplantation are:

1 chronic graft rejection and the side effects of non-specific immunosuppression;
2 the shortage of organs for transplantation.

New immunosuppressive agents that have fewer or different agent-specific side effects than existing therapy are likely to enter clinical practice and there is continuing research into the development of non-invasive biomarkers (in urine or blood) that will allow early diagnosis of graft rejection. A long-standing goal in organ transplantation has been the development of strategies for inducing specific immunological tolerance (Summary box 81.11). Transplantation tolerance would eliminate the need for long-term non-specific immunosuppressive agents, leaving the immune system intact for defence against infection. It has long been possible to induce transplant tolerance in experimental animals with a variety of preconditioning regimens that often involve pretreatment schedules using donor bone marrow cells or donor antigen. So far, however, there is no clinically applicable strategy for inducing transplant tolerance.

Summary box 81.11

Future developments in transplantation

- Novel immunosuppressive agents
- Non-invasive biomarkers for early diagnosis of graft rejection
- Donor-specific immunological tolerance
- Xenotransplantation
- Stem cell medicine and tissue engineering

Bruce Arnold Reitz, thoracic surgeon, Stanford University School of Medicine, Palo Alto, CA, USA.
Norman Edward Shumway, 1923–2006, cardiothoracic surgeon, Stanford University School of Medicine, Plao Alto, CA, USA.
Victor Eisenmenger, 1864–1932, German physician.

The demand for human organs for transplantation is so great that deceased donors cannot ever satisfy it. Many consider that the solution is to perfect xenotransplantation, and there is general agreement that the pig is the most suitable source of xenogeneic organs. However, all humans have preformed antibodies directed against carbohydrate antigens expressed by pig organs, and these cause hyperacute rejection. The dominant carbohydrate antigen responsible is gal-1, 3-αgal. Progress has been made towards circumventing hyperacute xenograft rejection and pigs that have been genetically engineered not to express the gal-1, 3-αgal antigen have been produced. However, organs from genetically modified pigs are still rejected within a few weeks by primates, despite the use of potent immunosuppressive agents. In addition to the complex immunological problems posed by xenotransplantation, there is a risk that pig organs may transmit infectious agents, and there is particular concern about the risks posed by porcine endogenous retrovirus (PERV). Lastly, there are unanswered questions regarding the extent to which pig organs are able to fulfil the physiological demands required of them after transplantation into a human.

Finally, looking to the future, there is optimism that human pluripotent stem cells may ultimately provide a source of tissue transplants for treating a wide range of diseases. Attempts are now under way to define the cell signals needed to guide human embryonic and adult-induced pluripotent stem cells to differentiate *in vitro* into functional tissue of the desired cell type. These include insulin-producing cells, cardiac myocytes and neuronal tissue. Although cell transplantation is the initial goal, by combining the developments in stem cell medicine with those taking place in tissue engineering and biomaterials it may one day be possible to engineer more complex vascularised grafts for transplantation.

FURTHER READING

Danovitch GM (ed.). *Handbook of kidney transplantation*, 5th edn. Philadelphia, PA: Lippincott Williams & Wilkins, 2009.

Forsythe JLR (ed.). *Transplantation: a companion to specialist surgical practice*, 4th edn. Philadelphia, PA: WB Saunders, 2009.

Gruessner WG, Sutherland DER (eds). *Transplantation of the pancreas*. New York: Springer, 2004.

Gruessner WG, Benedetti E (eds). *Living donor organ transplantation*. New York: McGraw Hill, 2008.

Hricik D (ed.). *Primer on transplantation*, 3rd edn. Oxford: Wiley-Blackwell, 2011.

Killenberg PG, Clavien PA (eds). *Medical care of the liver transplant patient*, 3rd edn. Oxford: Wiley-Blackwell, 2006.

Morris PJ, Knechtle SJ (eds). *Kidney transplantation: principles and practice*, 6th edn. Philadelphia: WB Saunders, 2008.

Schofield PM, Corris PA. *Management of heart and lung transplantation patients*. Philadelphia, PA: WB Saunders, 1998.

WEBSITE ADDRESSES FOR SELECTED NATIONAL AND INTERNATIONAL TRANSPLANT DATABASES

European Liver Transplant Registry: www.eltr.org
NHS Blood and Transplant: www.nhsbt.nhs.uk
United Network for Organ Sharing (USA): www.unos.org
Collaborative Transplant Study (Europe): www.ctstransplant.org
Scandiatransplant: www.scandiatransplant.org

REFERENCES/WEBSITES FOR USEFUL CLINICAL GUIDELINES IN ORGAN TRANSPLANTATION

UK guidelines for living-donor kidney transplantation: www.bts.org.uk
UK guidelines on CMV in transplantation: www.bts.org.uk
UK guidelines on solid organ transplantation from DCD donors: www.bts.org.uk
Antibody incompatible transplantation: www.bts.org.uk
Surveillance, diagnosis and management of PTLD: www.bcshguidelines.com
Kidney Disease: Improving global outcomes (KDIGO): www.kdigo.org
International Society for Heart and Lung Transplantation: http://www.ishlt.org

In vitro is Latin for 'in the glass'.

APPENDIX 1

Common instruments used in general surgery

This is a list of some of the instruments used in open (as opposed to minimal access surgery) 'general surgery' with information on how they are used and about the people associated with them. It is hoped that this information will help the general surgical trainee answer questions on operative surgery in postgraduate examinations.

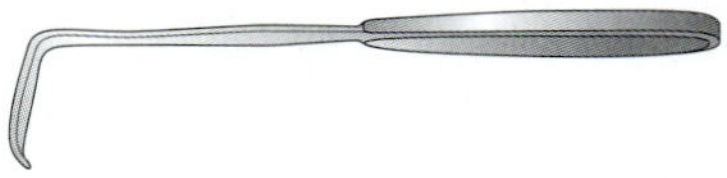

Langenbeck retractor. This small general purpose retractor is useful for holding open wounds, as in an open appendicectomy. They are often used in pairs (one in each of the assistant's hands). They stay in position best if the handles are lifted slightly so that the tips lock in under the fascia. The width of the lip of the retractors varies. Bernhard Rudolf Konrad von Langenbeck (1810–1887) was Professor of Surgery successively at Kiel and Berlin, Germany. He performed the first internal fixation of a femoral neck fracture in 1850.

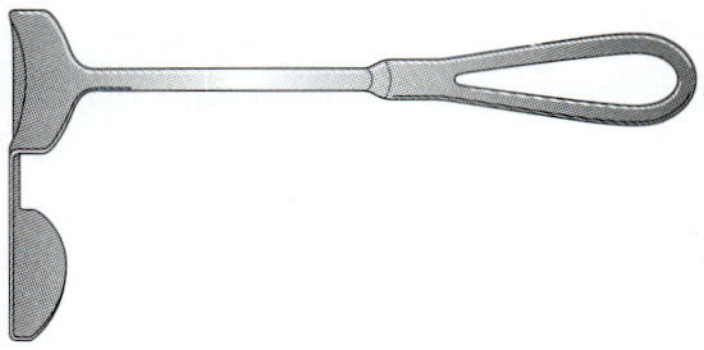

Morris retractor. This is a big retractor which is useful for giving maximum exposure in large incisions such as those used in the abdomen. It can be used to improve visibility on one side of an incision (by pulling firmly in that direction); so is valuable during the initial phase of a laparotomy. Sir Henry Morris (1844–1926) was a surgeon at the Middlesex Hospital, London, UK.

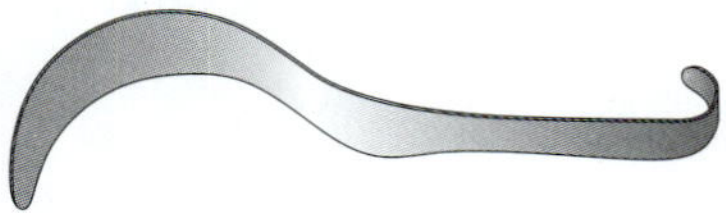

Deaver retractor. This retractor is specifically designed for holding the liver up out of the way during a cholecystectomy. It needs to be used carefully to avoid damaging the liver. Some surgeons protect the liver with an abdominal pack before placing the blade on top. John Blair Deaver (1855–1931) was Professor of Surgery at the University of Pennsylvania Medical School, Philadelphia, PA, USA. He also described a paramedian incision for appendicectomy.

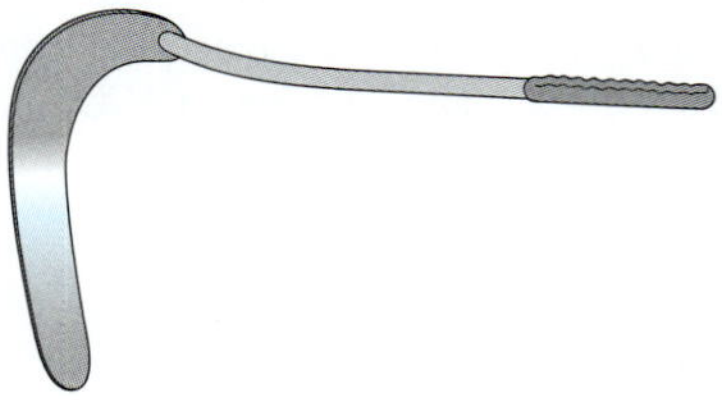

Dyball retractor. Used in major abdominal surgery to retract deeper parts of the abdominal wall or the bladder or the uterus while operating on the rectum and entering the rectovesical or rectouterine pouch. It has a lip at the bottom of the blade to prevent slippage. Care should be taken if it is used to retract the liver in operations in the region of the right upper quadrant as it may damage the liver parenchyma. Brennan Dyball was a distinguished West Country surgeon from Exeter. He also excelled as a carpenter and motor mechanic. He died in 1934 at the age of 62 leaving a great professional legacy to the Royal Devon and Exeter Hospital.

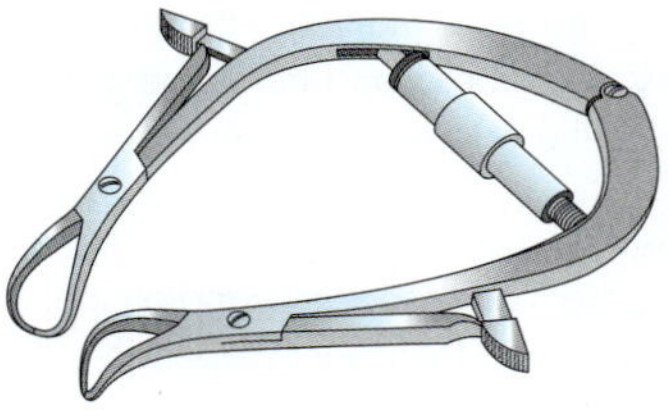

Joll retractor. This is a self-retaining retractor used in thyroid surgery. After making the collar incision and raising the lower and upper flaps fully, this retractor is then inserted. The two clips on the upper and lower edges are attached to the skin preferably with a swab over the skin edge. The central segment is then unscrewed to separate the two edges to obtain full exposure. Cecil Augustus Joll was a surgeon in London who first qualified as a dentist. He was regarded as 'a brilliant technician and an extraordinarily versatile surgeon' who operated on conditions 'from knees to necks and stomach to perineum'. A keen ornithologist, he was a connoisseur of all things good – furniture, pottery, food, wines and cigars. He died in 1945 at the age of 59.

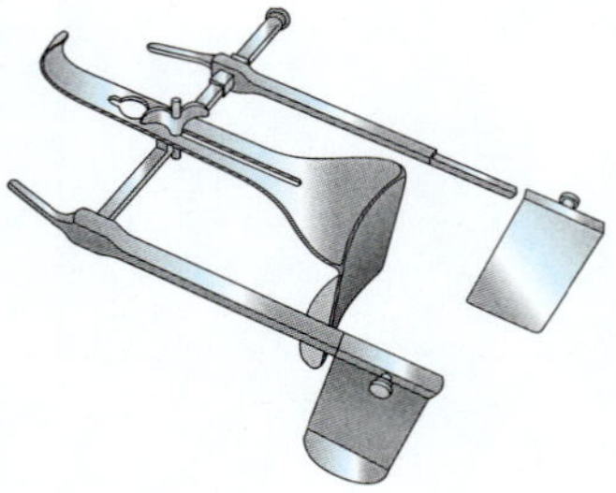

Goligher retractor. This is a self-retaining retractor used in operations on the sigmoid colon and rectum, such as anterior resection and upper end of abdominoperineal resection. Once the abdomen has been opened and laparotomy performed, the patient is placed head down and all the small bowel is packed to the upper end of the abdomen. The retractor is then inserted with the side blades to separate the edges of the abdominal wall. The central blade is then inserted to keep the small bowel well tucked away from the operation site. All three blades come in different widths to fit in with the patient's build. John Cedric Goligher (1912–1998), Ulsterman by birth, Professor of Surgery at Leeds, his contributions to colorectal surgery in the world have been legendary. His operating theatres at Leeds General Infirmary 'have been the Mecca for surgeons from all over the world'. His book, *Surgery of the Anus, Rectum and Colon*, was regarded as the ultimate authority on the subject and had five editions.

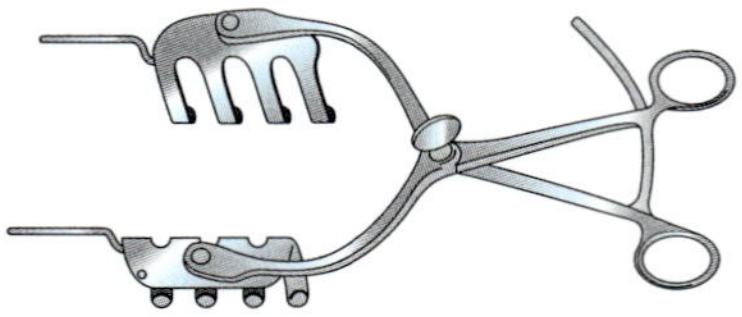

St Mark's perineal retractor. This is used for the perineal part of an abdominoperineal resection. After making the perineal incision and adequate dissection of the perineal wound, the retractor is inserted. As the dissection proceeds, the retractor has to be repositioned. The pointed ends are directed towards the front. St Mark's Hospital, Harrow, UK, is recognised as a national and international referral centre for intestinal and colorectal disorders. It was founded in a small room in No. 11 Aldersgate Street. Established in 1854 on City Road in Hackney as St Mark's Hospital for Fistula and other Diseases of the Rectum. It was so named as it was opened on St Mark's Day, 25 April. In 1994, it moved to its present site in Harrow.

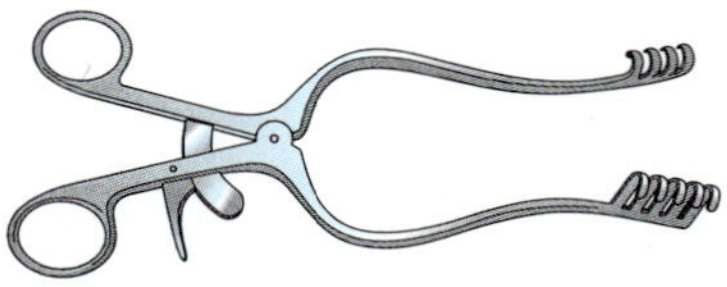

Travers retractor. This is a self-retaining retractor used for intermediate-type operations, such as heriorrhaphy, groin dissection for varicose veins and femoral embolectomy. It retracts skin and subcutaneous tissues; as the incision is deepened, the retractor has to be repositioned. If used incorrectly, it can traumatise the skin. For longer incisions, two such retractors may be used, one at each end of the incision for good exposure. Benjamin Travers (1783–1858) was a surgeon to the London Infirmary for Disease of the Eye (now Moorfields Ophthalmic Hospital). He is regarded as the first general hospital surgeon in England to devote himself specially to disease of the eye. He later became surgeon to St Thomas's Hospital and Vice-President and President of Royal College of Surgeons of England and a Fellow of the Royal Society. As an operator, he was regarded as clumsy and nervous. He had 'exquisite polish of manners, took off his hat and acknowledged salutes more elegantly than any contemporary dandy'.

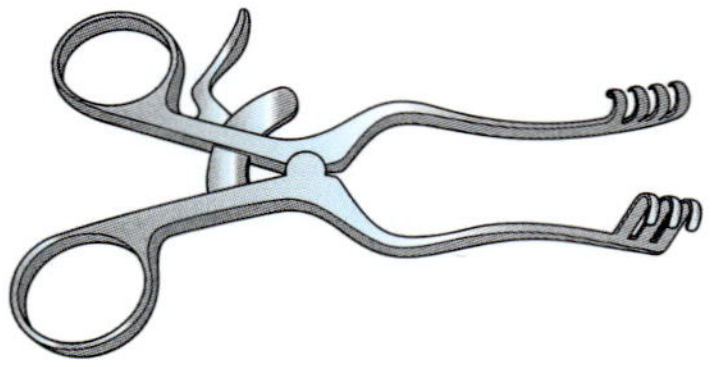

West retractor. Used in a similar manner to the Travers retractor, this is ideal for minor procedures under local anaesthetic where the surgeon is operating without an assistant, e.g. lymph node biopsy, temporal artery biopsy. After making the incision and undermining the edges, the retractor is then inserted and the jaws are prised open gently. Charles Ernest West (1873–1951) 'aural surgeon' of St Bartholomew's Hospital is credited with devising this retractor. It is possible that he got the idea from Franz Weitlaner, an Austrian physician who published the first description of his retractor in the *Vienna Clinical Review* in 1905. He became known as 'the great spreader of surgery'. It would be safe to presume that the present retractor is West's modification of Weitlaner's spreader.

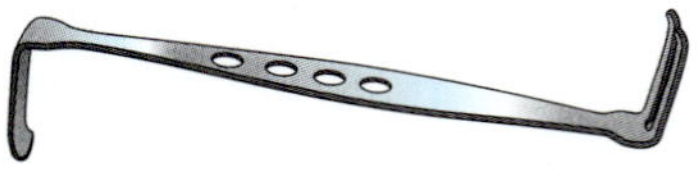

Czerny retractor. This is a double-ended retractor used to retract wound edges for intermediate-type procedures. One end has a blade with a lip which helps to retract without the edge slipping. The other end has two prongs and helps to retract the ends of an incision. When using it, a slight upward tilt gives a better exposure. It is used where a Langenbeck retractor can also be used, but the lip here is broader making it more versatile. Vincenz Czerny (1842–1915) was Professor of Surgery at Freiberg and Heidelberg in Germany. He was a disciple of Theodor Billroth. He was the originator of the concept of multidisciplinary management in cancer.

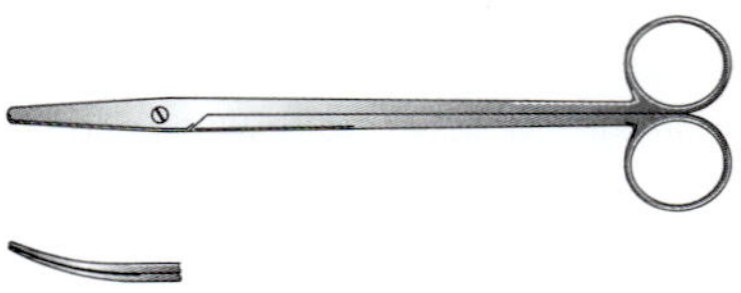

McIndoe scissors are used by surgeons to perform dissection respecting anatomical planes. The closed blades are inserted into a fascial plane, and then gently opened. The tissue to be divided can then be seen clearly and divided without risk of damage to vital structures. Sir Archibald Hector McIndoe (1900–1960) was a plastic surgeon at St Bartholomew's Hospital, London, and the Queen Victoria Hospital, East Grinstead, UK. He was born in New Zealand (cousin of Harold Gillies) and became a consultant plastic surgeon to the RAF during the Second World War. He supervised the rehabilitation of badly disfigured airmen who later formed the Guinea Pig Club.

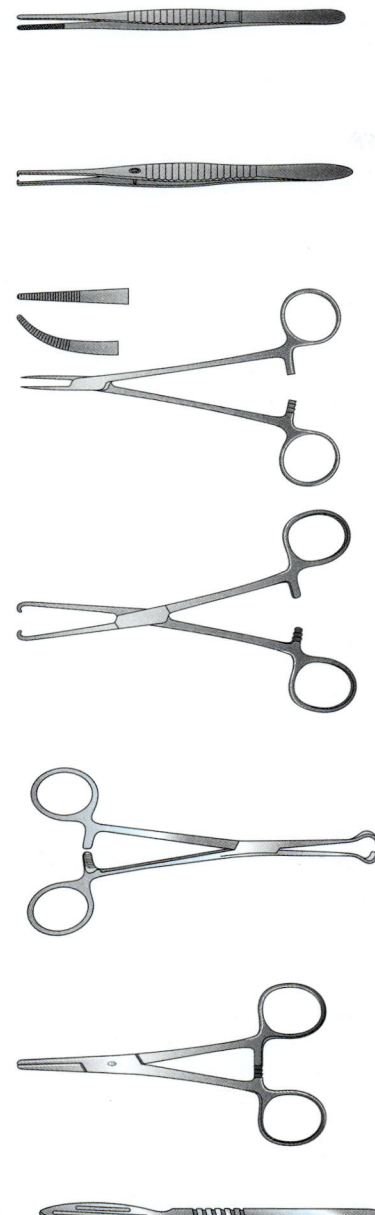

DeBakey forceps allow the surgeon to grasp tissues firmly while minimising damage to the tissue held in the jaws of the forceps. They are useful for holding vessel walls in vascular surgery. Michael Ellis DeBakey (1908–2008) was Professor of Surgery at Baylor University College of Medicine, Houston, TX, USA. He was the first to successfully implant an artificial heart; he also performed the first successful carotid endarterectomy.

Gillies forceps have teeth and are ideal for holding tough tissues, such as skin. Sir Harold Gillies (1882–1960) was a plastic surgeon at St Bartholomew's Hospital, London, UK. He was born in New Zealand (cousin of Archibald McIndoe) and became one of the founders of British plastic surgery. He originated the tubed pedicle flap.

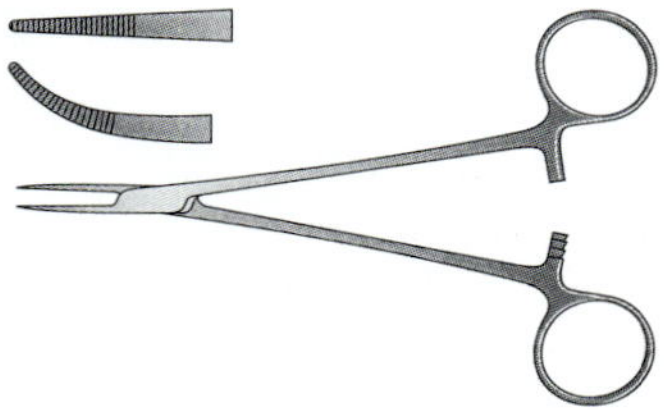

Adson forceps are non-toothed, and so are ideal for holding delicate tissues, such as bowel. Alfred Washington Adson (1887–1951) was Professor of Neurosurgery at the Mayo Clinic, Rochester, MN, USA. He was one of the first to use sympathectomy for the treatment of hypertension, and cervical sympathectomy for Raynaud's syndrome.

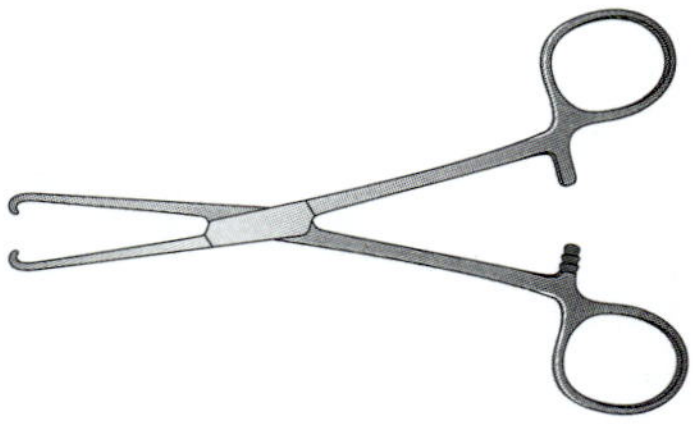

Allis forceps are used to hold soft tissues for a long period while minimising tissue damage. Using the ratchet they can be locked on to tissue, such as bowel, and can be used to provide gentle traction. Oscar Huntington Allis (1836–1921) was a surgeon at the Presbyterian Hospital, Philadelphia, PA, USA.

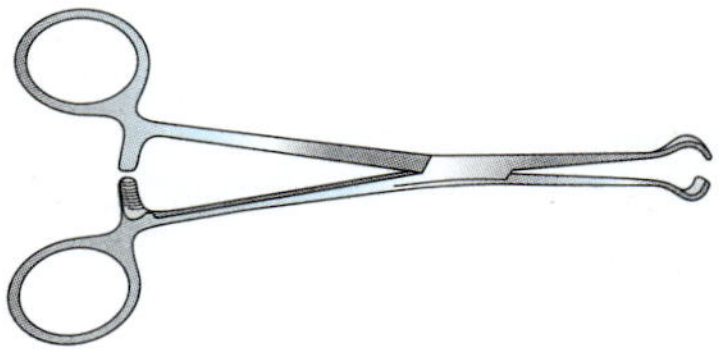

Babcock forceps. This is used to grasp any part of the bowel. The jaws are atraumatic and cause minimal tissue damage. Used commonly in appendicectomy to grasp the appendix and deliver it out of the wound. Care is taken when using it not to perforate the inflamed appendix. William Wayne Babcock (1872–1963), Professor and Head of the Department of Surgery at the Temple University School of Medicine, Philadelphia for 40 years. 'He was the inventor of the acorn-shaped vein stripper, introduced the alloy steel wire sutures, wire mesh in hernia repairs, and zinc chloride in the treatment of osteomyelitic sinus'.

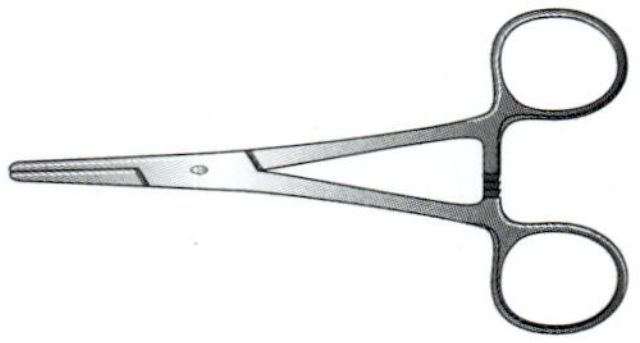

Spencer Wells forceps. These were one of the first ratchet forceps ever designed and are still very useful. They are often used in pairs for clamping an artery before dividing it. The cut ends of the artery are then tied off, and the forceps removed (carefully!). Sir Thomas Spencer Wells (1818–1897) was a surgeon at the Samaritan Free Hospital for Women and Children, London, UK. He was one of the earliest surgeons to make use of anaesthetics in operation.

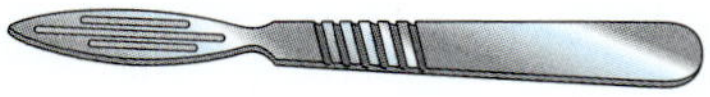

Kocher dissector. This is used during a thyroidectomy to dissect the upper pole of the thyroid. The instrument is blunt and therefore the surgeon is highly unlikely to inadvertently damage the superior thyroid artery or the external laryngeal nerve. It is used to dissect the superior pedicle, the superior thyroid artery. Once it has been isolated, the dissector is pushed under the pedicle. A tie is then put through the eye of the dissector which at this stage doubles up as an aneurysm needle. The pedicle is thus tied three times as close to the gland as possible. With the dissector under the tied pedicle, a fine knife is now used to cut leaving two ties in the patient. The presence of the dissector under the pedicle prevents any damage to the underlying structures. Emil Theodor Kocher (1841–1917), Professor of Surgery at Berne, Switzerland, was awarded the Nobel Prize for Physiology or Medicine in 1909 for his work on the thyroid. The first surgeon to be a Nobel Laureate.

ACKNOWLEDGEMENTS

With thanks to Steven Kerr, Assistant Librarian, Royal College of Surgeons of Edinburgh.

Index

Notes

Page number in **bold** indicate information in figures, tables or boxed material

vs. indicates a comparison or differential diagnosis

To save space in the index, the following abbreviations have been used:

CT - computed tomography

ERCP - endoscopic retrograde cholangiopancreatoduodenography

MRCP - magnetic resonance cholangiopancreatography

MRI - magnetic resonance imaging

PET - positron emission tomography